Manson's Tropical Diseases

Twenty-Third Edition

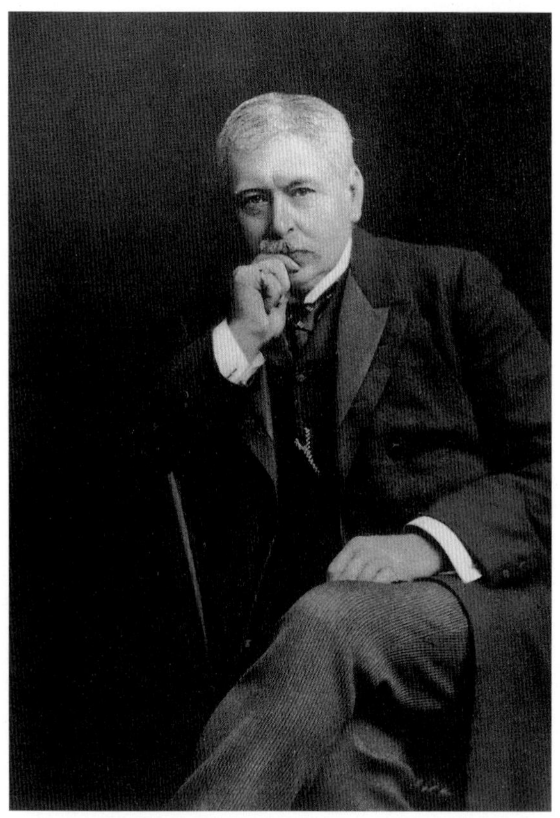

Sir Patrick Manson (1844–1922), GCMG, FRS

Content Strategist: Belinda Kuhn
Content Development Specialist: Poppy Garraway
Content Coordinator: Trinity Hutton, Emma Cole
Project Manager: Sruthi Viswam
Design: Miles Hitchen
Illustration Manager: Jennifer Rose
Illustrator: Richard Tibbitts
Marketing Manager(s) (UK/USA): Katie Alexo

Manson's Tropical Diseases

Twenty-Third Edition

Jeremy Farrar, FRCP, FMedAcSci, DPhil, OBE
Professor of Tropical Medicine
University of Oxford
Oxford, UK
Director
Oxford University Clinical Research Unit
Wellcome Trust Major Overseas Programme
South East Asia Infectious Disease Clinical Research Network
Hospital for Tropical Diseases
Ho Chi Minh City, Vietnam

Peter J. Hotez, MD, PhD, FAAP, FASTMH
Dean, National School of Tropical Medicine
Professor of Pediatrics and Molecular Virology & Microbiology
Baylor College of Medicine
Texas Children's Hospital Endowed Chair of Tropical Pediatrics
President and Director
Sabin Vaccine Institute and Texas Children's Hospital Center for Vaccine Development
Houston, TX, USA

Thomas Junghanss, MD
(Internal Medicine, subspecialties Tropical Medicine and Infectious Diseases), MSc PHDC (Lon)
apl Professor and Head
Section Clinical Tropical Medicine
Department of Infectious Diseases
University Hospital Heidelberg
Heidelberg, Germany

Gagandeep Kang, MD, PhD, FRCPath, FASc, FAAM
Professor and Head
The Wellcome Trust Research Laboratory
Division of Gastrointestinal Sciences
Christian Medical College
Vellore, India

David Lalloo, MB BS, MD, FRCP, FFTM RCPS(Glasg)
Professor of Tropical Medicine
Dean of Clinical Sciences and International Public Health
Liverpool School of Tropical Medicine
Liverpool, UK

Nicholas J. White, OBE, MD, DSc, FRCP, FMedSci, FRS
Professor of Tropical Medicine
Faculty of Tropical Medicine
Mahidol University
Bangkok, Thailand
Nuffield Department of Medicine
University of Oxford
Oxford, UK

ELSEVIER
SAUNDERS

ELSEVIER
SAUNDERS

SAUNDERS is an imprint of Elsevier.

First edition published 1898
Twenty-second edition published 2009

Notices

Knowledge and best practice in this field are constantly changing. As new research and experience broaden our understanding, changes in research methods, professional practices, or medical treatment may become necessary.

Practitioners and researchers must always rely on their own experience and knowledge in evaluating and using any information, methods, compounds, or experiments described herein. In using such information or methods they should be mindful of their own safety and the safety of others, including parties for whom they have a professional responsibility.

With respect to any drug or pharmaceutical products identified, readers are advised to check the most current information provided (i) on procedures featured or (ii) by the manufacturer of each product to be administered, to verify the recommended dose or formula, the method and duration of administration, and contraindications. It is the responsibility of practitioners, relying on their own experience and knowledge of their patients, to make diagnoses, to determine dosages and the best treatment for each individual patient, and to take all appropriate safety precautions.

To the fullest extent of the law, neither the Publisher nor the authors, contributors, or editors, assume any liability for any injury and/or damage to persons or property as a matter of products liability, negligence or otherwise, or from any use or operation of any methods, products, instructions, or ideas contained in the material herein.

ISBN: 9780702051012

Ebook ISBN: 9780702053061

International edition ISBN: 9780702051029

Front cover images (from left to right):
Image 1: Typical place of transmission of T.b. rhodesiense; habitat of G. morsitans. Courtesy of Irene Küpfer (Swiss Tropical and Public Health Institute): Urambo District, Tanzania. From Chapter 45, Human African trypanosomiasis.
Image 2: A villager carrying a heavy load in rural Sri Lanka. Courtesy of Mr Priyanjan De Silva. From chapter 69, Musculoskeletal Disorders.
Image 3: Chest radiography of primary tuberculosis causing right middle lobe pulmonary collapse. Courtesy of Guy Thwaites. From Chapter 40, Tuberculosis.
Image 4: Preparation of eflornithine. Courtesy of François Chappuis (Médecins sans Frontières Switzerland; Banda, Democratic Republic of the Congo. From Chapter 45, Human African trypanosomiasis.
Image 5: Figure 40.4 Granulomatous lymphadenopathy caused by M. tuberculosis. Magnification ×400 (H&E stain) showing a Langhans' multinucleated giant cell with its horseshoe-shaped arrangement of nuclei adjacent to some caseous necrosis. By kind permission of Mr Roger Webb, Consultant Maxillofacial Surgeon and Dr Jon Salisbury, Consultant Histopathologist, King's College Hospital, London, United Kingdom. From Chapter 40, Tuberculosis.
Image 6: Pigs scavenging for food in an African village. Courtesy of Dr. Seth O'Neal. Chapter 57 Other Cestode Infections: Intestinal Cestodes, Cysticercosis, Other Larval Cestode Infections
Image 7: Typical place of transmission of T.b. gambiense where human–fly contact is high; habitat of G. palpalis. Courtesy of Christian Burri (Swiss Tropical and Public Health Institute): Kikongotanga, Democratic Republic of the Congo. From Chapter 45, Human African trypanosomiasis.
Image 8: Diffuse cutaneous leishmaniasis caused by L. aethiopica. Patient from Ethiopia; disease duration: three years. Courtesy of C. Yansouni. From Chapter 47 Leishmaniasis

Printed in China

Last digit is the print number: 9 8 7 6 5 4 3 2

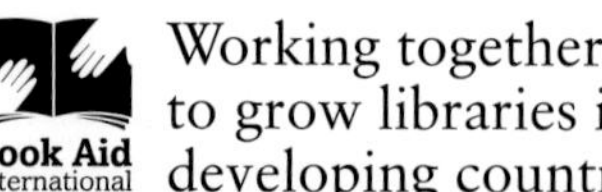

CONTENTS

PREFACE TO THE FIRST EDITION

A manual on the diseases of warm climates, of handy size, and yet giving adequate information, has long been a want; for the exigencies of travel and tropical life are, as a rule, incompatible with big volumes and large libraries. This is the reason for the present work.

While it is hoped that the book may prove of practical service, it makes no pretension to being anything more than an introduction to the important department of medicine of which it treats; in no sense is it put forward as a complete treatise, or as being in this respect comparable to the more elaborate works by Davidson, Schebe, Rho, Laveran, Corre, Roux, and other systematic writers in the same field. The author avails himself of this opportunity to acknowledge the valuable assistance he has received, in revising the text, from Dr. L. Westerna Sambon and Mr David Rees, MRCP LRCP lately Senior House Surgeon, Seamen's Hospital, Albert Docks, London.

He would also acknowledge his great obligation to Mr Richard Muir, Pathological Laboratory, Edinburgh University, for his care and skill in preparing the illustrations.

Patrick Manson
April 1898

PREFACE TO THE TWENTY-THIRD EDITION

In 1898 Sir Patrick Manson (1844–1922), often dubbed the father of tropical medicine, wrote "A Manual of the Diseases of Warm Climates". This preface introduces the 23rd edition. Few textbooks have survived as long as this reference. Manson would have been fascinated by its evolution, as modern medicine has transformed all our lives (although sadly he would still recognize many of the treatments recommended for parasitic diseases). Although much has changed, the improvements in living standards that have greatly lengthened life expectancy have been less in the tropics than in temperate countries, and infectious diseases and nutritional deficiencies continue to exert a substantial toll in these regions. Today, tropical diseases remain leading causes of death and disability in developing countries and there is still an important place for a textbook about these conditions and the challenges of old and new diseases in a changing world. Manson's textbook has always been slightly unusual (some would say eccentric), perhaps a reflection on its originator, and his pioneering colleagues. This edition has been thoroughly revised and reformatted but not at the expense of its character. We hope you will find it refreshing, interesting and useful.

Jeremy Farrar
Peter J. Hotez
Thomas Junghanss
Gagandeep Kang
David Lalloo
Nicholas J. White

CONTRIBUTORS

Steven Abrams, MD
Professor of Pediatrics
Baylor College of Medicine
Attending Physician, Section of Neonatology
Texas Children's Hospital
Houston, TX, USA

Adekunle M. Adesina, MD, PhD, FCAP, FMCPath
Professor of Pathology, Immunology and Pediatrics-Hematology/Oncology
Medical Director
Neuropathology and Molecular Neuropathology
Texas Children's Hospital
Baylor College of Medicine
Houston, TX, USA

Dwomoa Adu, MD, FRCP
Consultant Physician and Nephrologist
Department of Medicine and Therapeutics
University of Ghana Medical School
Accra, Ghana

Sitara S. R. Ajjampur, MB BS, MD, PhD
Associate Professor of Microbiology
Department of Gastrointestinal Sciences
Christian Medical College
Vellore, India

Voahangy Andrianaivoarimanana, PhD
Researcher in Plague Immunology
Plague Unit
Institut Pasteur de Madagascar,
Ambatofotsikely,
Antananarivo, Madagascar

Angelakis Emmanouil, MD, PHD
Faculte de Medecine
Unite de Recherche sur les Maladies Infectieuses et Tropicales Emergentes (URMITE)
Marseille, France

Jeffrey K. Aronson, MA, DPhil, MB ChB, FRCP, FBPharmacolS, FFPM(Hon)
Reader in Clinical Pharmacology
Department of Primary Care Health Sciences
University of Oxford
Oxford, UK

Inoshi Atukorala, MB BS, MD, MRCP(UK)
Lecturer in Clinical Medicine and Consultant Rheumatologist
Department of Clinical Medicine
University of Colombo
Colombo, Sri Lanka

Guy Baily, MD FRCP
Consultant Physician
Infection and Immunity Specialty Group
The Royal London Hospital
Barts Health NHS Trust
London, UK

Till Bärnighausen, MD, ScD, MSc
Associate Professor
Department of Global Health and Population
Harvard School of Public Health
Boston, MA, USA
Senior Epidemiologist
Africa Centre for Health and Population Studies
University of KwaZulu-Natal
Mtubatuba, South Africa

Buddha Basnyat, MD, MSc, FACP, FRCP(Edinburgh)
Director, Oxford University Clinical Research Unit
Medical Director, Nepal International Clinic and Himalayan Rescue Association
Kathmandu, Nepal

Andrew Bastawrous, BSc (Hons), MB ChB, FHEA, MRCOphth
Ophthalmologist & Clinical Research Fellow in International Eye Health
International Centre for Eye Health, Clinical Research Department, Faculty of Infectious & Tropical Diseases
London School of Hygiene & Tropical Medicine
London, UK & Nakuru, Kenya

Imelda Bates, MB BS, MA, MD, FRCP, FRCPath
Professor of Tropical Haematology
Department of International Public Health
Liverpool School of Tropical Medicine
Liverpool, UK

Daniel G. Bausch, MD, MPH&TM
Associate Professor
Department of Tropical Medicine
Tulane School of Public Health and Tropical Medicine
Clinical Associate Professor
Department of Medicine
Section of Adult Infectious Diseases
Tulane Medical Center
New Orleans, LA, USA

Nicholas A. V. Beare, MA, MB ChB, FRCOphth, MD
Consultant Ophthalmologist
St Paul's Eye Unit
Royal Liverpool University Hospital
Honorary Senior Lecturer
Department of Eye and Vision Science
University of Liverpool
Liverpool, UK

Raman Bedi, BDS, MSc, DDS, FDSRCS(Ed), FDSRCS(Eng), FDSRCS (Glas), FGDP, FFPH
Professor
Head, International Centre for Child Oral Health
Director, Global Child Dental Health Taskforce
King's College London
London, UK

Nick J. Beeching, MA, BM BCh, FRCP(L), FRACP, FFTM RCPSGlasg, DCH, DTM&H, Hon FCCP(SL)
Senior Lecturer (Clinical) in Infectious Diseases
Liverpool School of Tropical Medicine
Clinical Director
Tropical and Infectious Disease Unit
Royal Liverpool University Hospital
Liverpool, UK

Nicholas J. Bennett, MA(Cantab), MBBChir, PhD
Assistant Professor in Pediatrics
Division of Pediatric Infectious Diseases and Immunology
Connecticut Children's Medical Center
Hartford, CT, USA

Anita Berlin, MB BS, MA, FRCGP
Senior Lecturer & Sub Dean
Faculty of Population Health and Medical School
University College London
London, UK

Ahmed I. Bhigjee, MB ChB, FRCP, MMed, FCP, PhD, FCN
Professor
Department of Neurology
The Nelson R Mandela School of Medicine
University of KwaZulu-Natal
Durban, South Africa

Zulfiqar A. Bhutta, MB BS, PhD
Richard Harding Chair in Global Child & Policy
Co-Director
SickKids Center in Global Child Health
Toronto, Canada
Professor and Founding Director
Center of Excellence in Women and Child Health
The Aga Khan University
Karachi, Pakistan

David E. Bloom, PhD, MA
Clarence James Gamble Professor of Economics and Demography
Department of Global Health and Population
Harvard School of Public Health
Boston, MA, USA

Lucille Hellen Blumberg, MB BCH, MMED, ID (SA), FFTM (RCP, Glasgow), DTMH, DOH, DCH
Professor and deputy director
National Institute for Communicable Diseases
National Health Laboratory Service
Johannesburg Gauteng, South Africa

Marleen Boelaert, MD, PhD
Professor
Department of Public Health
Institute of Tropical Medicine
Antwerp, Belgium

Francis J. Bowden, MB BS, FRACP, MD, FACSHM
Professor of Medicine
Academic Unit of Internal Medicine
Australian National University Medical School
Canberra, Australia

Bernard J. Brabin, MB ChB, MSc, PhD, FRCPCH
Emeritus Professor of Tropical Paediatrics
Clinical Sciences Division
Liverpool School of Tropical Medicine
Liverpool, UK
Emeritus Professor of International Child Health
Global Child Health Group
Academic Medical Centre
University of Amsterdam, Netherlands

Freddie Bray, BSc, MSc, PhD
Deputy Section Head
Section of Cancer Information
International Agency for Research on Cancer
Lyon, France

Rodney A. Bray, BA, PhD, CBiol, MBS FLS
Scientific Associate
Department of Life Sciences
Natural History Museum
London, UK

Simon J. Brooker, DPhil
Professor of Epidemiology
Faculty of Infectious and Tropical Diseases
London School of Hygiene and Tropical Medicine
London, UK

Matthijs C. Brouwer, MD, PhD
Neurologist
Department of Neurology
Academic Medical Center
University of Amsterdam
Amsterdam, The Netherlands

Reto Brun, PhD
Titulary Professor of Biology
Department of Medical Parasitology and Infection Biology
Swiss Tropical and Public Health Institute
University of Basel
Basel, Switzerland

Enrico Brunetti, MD
Assistant Professor of Infectious Diseases
University of Pavia Staff Physician
Division of Infectious and Tropical Diseases
San Matteo Hospital Foundation
Pavia, Italy

Susan Bull BSc, LLB, MA, PhD
Senior Researcher in Ethics
The Ethox Centre
Nuffield Department of Population Health
University of Oxford
Oxford, UK

Donald A. P. Bundy, PhD
Lead Health and Education Specialist
Human Development Network
The World Bank
Washington, DC, USA

Christian Burri, PhD, MPharm
Professor of Pharmacy and Clinical Pharmacology
Head, Department of Medicines Research
Swiss Tropical and Public Health Institute
Department of Pharmaceutical Sciences
University of Basel
Basel, Switzerland

Amaya Bustinduy, MD, MPH
Paediatric Infectious Diseases Specialist
Department of Parasitology
Liverpool School of Tropical Medicine
Liverpool, UK

Thashi Chang, MB BS MD, MRCP(UK), DPhil(Oxon), FRCP(Lon)
Consultant Neurologist and Senior Lecturer
Department of Clinical Medicine
University of Colombo
Colombo, Sri Lanka

François Chappuis, MD, MCTM, PhD
Associate Professor
Division of Tropical and Humanitarian Medicine
Geneva University Hospitals and Medecins sans Frontières
Operational Center
Geneva, Switzerland

Wirongrong Chierakul, MD, Thai Board of Int Med, PhD
Lecturer
Department of Clinical Tropical Medicine
Mahidol-Oxford Tropical Medicine Research Unit
Faculty of Tropical Medicine
Mahidol University
Bangkok, Thailand

Peter L. Chiodini, BSc, MB BS, PhD, MRCS, FRCP, FRCPath, FFTM RCPS(Glasg)
Consultant Parasitologist
Hospital for Tropical Diseases,
Honorary Professor
London School of Hygiene and Tropical Medicine,
London, UK

John D. Clemens, MD
Executive Director
ICDDR-B
Dhaka, Bangladesh

Gordon C. Cook, MD, DSc, FRCP(Lond), FRCP(Edin), FRACP, FLS
Visiting Professor
Department of Medical Microbiology and Centre for Infectious Diseases
Royal Free and University College London Medical School
London, UK
President
The Royal Society of Tropical Medicine and Hygiene (1993–1995)
Formerly Professor of Medicine
The Universities of Zambia, Riyadh (Saudi Arabia) and Papua New Guinea
Consultant Physician
University College Hospitals Trust
Hospital for Tropical Diseases, London
St Luke's Hospital for the Clergy
Senior Lecturer
London School of Hygiene and Tropical Medicine
London, UK
President
The Fellowship of Postgraduate Medicine
London, UK 2000–2007
President
History of Medicine Section
Royal Society of Medicine, UK

Mark F. Cotton, FCPaed (SA), MMed, PhD, DCH (SA), DTM&H
Professor of Paediatrics and Child Health
Head, Division of Paediatric Infectious Diseases
Faculty of Medicine and Health Sciences
Tygerberg Children's Hospital
Stellenbosch University
Tygerberg, South Africa

John B. S. Coulter, MD, FRCP(I), FRCPCH
Honorary Clinical Lecturer
Liverpool School of Tropical Medicine
Liverpool, UK

Nigel A. Cunliffe, BSc (Hons), MB ChB, PhD, MRCP, FRCPath, DTM&H
Professor
Department of Clinical Infection, Microbiology & Immunology
Institute of Infection and Global Health
University of Liverpool
Liverpool, UK

Bart J. Currie, MB BS, FRACP, FAFPHM, DTM&H
Professor in Medicine and Head of Infectious Diseases
Department of Infectious Diseases
Royal Darwin Hospital and Menzies School of Health Research
Darwin, Northern Territory, Australia

Marian J. Currie, PhD
Academic Unit of Internal Medicine
Australian National University Medical School
Canberra, Australia

David A. B. Dance, MB ChB, MSc, FRCPath
Clinical Research Microbiologist
Lao Oxford Mahosot Hospital Wellcome Trust Research Unit
Microbiology Laboratory, Mahosot Hospital
Vientiane, Lao
Centre for Tropical Medicine
University of Oxford
Honorary Consultant Microbiologist
Public Health England and Oxford University Hospitals NHS Trust
Oxford, UK

Nicholas P. J. Day, MA, BM BCh, DM, FRCP, FMedSci
Professor of Tropical Medicine
University of Oxford
Oxford, UK
Director, Mahidol-Oxford Tropical Medicine Research Unit
Faculty of Tropical Medicine
Mahidol University
Bangkok, Thailand

Kevin DeCock, MD
Director
Center for Global Health
Centers for Disease Control and Prevention
Atlanta, GA, USA

Jacqueline Deen, MD, MSc
Researcher
Global Health Division
Menzies School of Health Research
Casuarina, Northern Territory, Australia

Sarah R Doffman, MB ChB, FRCP
Consultant in Respiratory and General (Internal) Medicine
Brighton and Sussex University Hospitals NHS Trust
Brighton, UK

Arjen Dondorp, MD, PhD
Infectious Diseases and Intensive Care Physician
Professor of Tropical Medicine University of Oxford
Visiting Professor of Clinical Tropical Medicine
Deputy Director, Mahidol-Oxford Tropical Medicine Research Unit
Faculty of Tropical Medicine
Mahidol University
Bangkok, Thailand

H. Rogier van Doorn, MD, PhD
Clinical Virologist
Centre for Tropical Medicine
Oxford University Clinical Research Unit
Ho Chi Minh City, Vietnam

Martin W. Dünser, MD, PD, DESA, EDIC
Head Intensivist
Department of Anesthesiology, Perioperative Medicine and General Intensive Care
Salzburg General Hospital and Paracelsus Private Medical University
Salzburg, Austria

Edward M. Eitzen, Jr., MD, MPH
Adjunct Associate Professor
Department of Military and Emergency Medicine
Uniformed Services University of the Health Sciences
Bethesda, MD
Senior Partner
Biodefense and Public Health Programs
Martin, Blanck and Associates,
Alexandria, VA, USA

Delia A. Enria, MD, MPH
Instituto Nacional de Enfermedades Virales Humanas
Pergamino; Argentina

Jeremy Farrar, FRCP, FMedAcSci, DPhil, OBE
Professor of Tropical Medicine
University of Oxford
Oxford, UK
Director
Oxford University Clinical Research Unit
Wellcome Trust Major Overseas Programme
South East Asia Infectious Disease Clinical Research Network
Hospital for Tropical Diseases
Ho Chi Minh City, Vietnam

Christina Faust, MS, MSc
PhD Candidate
Ecology and Evolutionary Biology
Princeton University
Princeton, NJ, USA

Nicholas A. Feasey, BSc, MSc, MB BS, MRCP, FRCPath, DTM&H
Clinical Research Fellow
Department of Gastroenterology
Institute of Translational Medicine
University of Liverpool
Liverpool, UK

Abebaw Fekadu, MD, PhD, MRCPsych
Doctor
Department of Psychiatry
School of Medicine
Addis Ababa University
Addis Ababa, Ethiopia

Günther Fink, PhD
Assistant Professor of International Health Economics
Harvard School of Public Health, Department of Global Health and Population
Boston, MA, USA

Peter U. Fischer, PhD
Research Associate Professor of Medicine
Infectious Diseases Division
Department of Internal Medicine
Washington University School of Medicine
St. Louis, MO, USA

Carlos Franco-Paredes, MD, MPH
Staff Physician
Infectious Diseases
Phoebe Putney Memorial Hospital
Albany, GA, USA
Clinical Assistant Professor
Hospital Infantil de Mexico Federico Gomez
Mexico City, Mexico

Neil French, MB ChB, PhD, FRCP
Professor of Infectious Diseases & Global Health
Institute of Infection & Global Health
University of Liverpool
Honorary Consultant Physician Tropical & Infectious Disease Unit
Royal Liverpool University Hospital
Liverpool, UK

Hector H. Garcia, MD, PhD
Director, Center for Global Health – Tumbes
Universidad Peruana Cayetano Heredia
Head, Cysticercosis Unit
Instituto Nacional de Ciencias Neurologicas
Lima, Peru

Roger I. Glass, MD, PhD
Director
Fogarty International Center
National Institutes of Health
Bethesda, MD, USA

Melita A. Gordon, BM MCh, MA, MRCP, DTM&H, MD
Reader in Gastroenterology
Department of Gastroenterology
Institute of Translational Medicine
University of Liverpool
Honorary Consultant Gastroenterologist
Royal Liverpool University Hospital
Liverpool, UK

Stephen B. Gordon, MA, MD, FRCP, FRCPE DTM&H
Head, Department of Clinical Sciences
Professor of Respiratory Medicine
Liverpool School of Tropical Medicine
Pembroke Place
Liverpool, UK

Bruno Gottstein, PhD
Professor of Medical and Veterinary Parasitology
Institute of Parasitology
University of Bern
Bern, Switzerland

Stephen M. Graham, MB BS, FRACP, DTCH, PhD
Professor of International Child Health
Department of Paediatrics
University of Melbourne
Melbourne, Victoria, Australia

Andy Haines, MD, FRCP, FRCGP, FFPH, FMedSci
Professor of Public Health and Primary Care
London School of Hygiene and Tropical Medicine
London, UK

Roy A. Hall, BSc, PhD
Professor of Virology
Australian Infectious Diseases Research Centre
School of Chemistry & Molecular Biosciences
University of Queensland
Brisbane, Queensland, Australia

Charlotte Hanlon, BM BChir, MA, MRCPsych, PhD
Associate Professor
Department of Psychiatry
School of Medicine
College of Health Sciences
Addis Ababa University
Addis Ababa, Ethiopia

The late C. Anthony Hart, MB BS, BSc, PhD, FRCPCH, PRCPath
Formerly Professor of Medical Microbiology
Department of Medical Microbiology
University of Liverpool Medical School
Liverpool, UK

Melissa R. Haswell, MSc, PhD
Associate Professor
Muru Marri Indigenous Health Unit
School of Public Health and Community Medicine
University of New South Wales
Sydney, New South Wales, Australia

Sophie Hawkesworth, BSc, MSc, PhD
Research Fellow
MRC International Nutrition Group
London School of Hygiene and Tropical Medicine
London, UK

Roderick J. Hay, DM, FRCP, FMedSci
Professor of Cutaneous Infection
Dermatology
Kings College Hospital
London, UK

Jeannine M. Heckmann, MB ChB, MMed, FCP(Neurol), PhD
Associate Professor of Neurology
Department of Medicine
University of Cape Town
Cape Town, South Africa

Markus M. Heimesaat, MD
Senior Research Associate
Department of Microbiology and Hygiene
Charité – University Medicine Berlin
Berlin, Germany

Anselm J. M. Hennis, MB BS, MSc, PhD, FRCP, FACP
Professor of Medicine and Epidemiology
Chronic Disease Research Centre
Tropical Medicine Research Institute
The University of the West Indies
Cave Hill Campus, Bridgetown, Barbados

Tran Tinh Hien, MD, PhD
Professor of Tropical Medicine
Centre of Tropical Medicine
Oxford University
Oxford University Clinical Research Unit
Ho Chi Minh, Vietnam

Achim Hoerauf, MD
Professor of Microbiology and Parasitology
Chair, Institute of Medical Microbiology, Immunology and Parasitology
University Hospital Bonn
Bonn, Germany

Peter J. Hotez, MD, PhD, FAAP, FASTMH
Dean, National School of Tropical Medicine
Professor of Pediatrics and Molecular Virology & Microbiology
Baylor College of Medicine
Texas Children's Hospital Endowed Chair of Tropical Pediatrics
President and Director
Sabin Vaccine Institute and Texas Children's Hospital Center for Vaccine Development
Houston, TX, USA

Salal Humair, PhD
Research Scientist
Department of Global Health and Population
Harvard School of Public Health
Boston, MA, USA
Associate Professor
School of Science and Engineering
Lahore University of Management Sciences
Lahore, Pakistan

Cheryl A. Johansen, BSc, MSc, W.Aust. PhD Qld
Associate Professor
Arbovirus Surveillance and Research Laboratory
School of Pathology and Laboratory Medicine
The University of Western Australia
Crawley, Australia

Roch Christian Johnson, MD, PhD
Lecturer
Departement of Environment and health sciences (CIFRED)
University of Abomey-Calavi
Cotonou, Bénin

Malcolm K. Jones, BSc, PhD, FASP
Associate Professor
School of Veterinary Sciences
The University of Queensland
Associate Professor
Infectious Diseases
Queensland Institute of Medical Research
Brisbane, Queensland, Australia

Thomas Junghanss, MD
(Internal Medicine, subspecialties Tropical Medicine and Infectious Diseases), **MSc PHDC (Lon)**
apl Professor and Head
Section Clinical Tropical Medicine
Department of Infectious Diseases
University Hospital Heidelberg
Heidelberg, Germany

Sasithorn Kaewkes, PhD
Associate Professor
Department of Parasitology
Faculty of Medicine
Khon Kaen University
Khon Kaen, Thailand

Gagandeep Kang, MD, PhD, FRCPath, FASc, FAAM
Professor and Head
The Wellcome Trust Research Laboratory
Division of Gastrointestinal Sciences
Christian Medical College
Vellore, India

Paul Kelly, MA, MD, FRCP
Reader in Tropical Gastroenterology
Blizard Institute
Barts and The London School of Medicine
Queen Mary, University of London
London, UK
Honorary Lecturer
University of Zambia School of Medicine
Lusaka, Zambia

Charles H. King, MD, MS
Professor of International Health
Center for Global Health and Diseases
Case Western Reserve University
Cleveland, OH, USA

Sandeep P. Kishore, PhD
Chair, Advisory Council
Young Professionals Chronic Disease Network
Tri-Institutional MD/PhD Program
Weill Cornell/Rockefeller/Sloan-Kettering
New York, NY, USA

Patricia Kissinger, PhD
Professor
Department of Epidemiology
Tulane University School of Public Health and Tropical Medicine
New Orleans, LA, USA

David Lalloo, MB BS, MD, FRCP, FFTM RCPS(Glasg)
Professor of Tropical Medicine
Dean of Clinical Sciences and International Public Health
Liverpool School of Tropical Medicine
Liverpool, UK

Trudie Lang, PhD
Research Fellow, Green Templeton College
Centre for Tropical Medicine
Nuffield Department of Medicine
University of Oxford
Oxford, UK

Oliver Liesenfeld, MD
Professor für Medizinische Mikrobiologie und Infektionsimmunologie
Institut für Mikrobiologie und Hygiene
Charité Universitätsmedizin Berlin
Berlin, Germany

Diana N. J. Lockwood, BSc, MD, FRCP
Professor of Tropical Medicine
London School of Hygiene and Tropical Medicine
Consultant Physician and Leprologist
Hospital for Tropical Diseases
London, UK

David C. W. Mabey, DM, FRCP
Professor of Communicable Diseases
Infectious and Tropical Diseases
London School of Hygiene and Tropical Medicine
London, UK

The late M. Monir Madkour, MD, DM, FRCP(L)
Formerly Consultant Physician
Riyadh Military Hospital
Riyadh, Saudi Arabia

Barbara J. Marston, MD
Medical Officer
Center for Global Health
Centers for Disease Control and Prevention,
Atlanta, GA, USA

Refiloe Masekela, MB BCh, MMed(Paeds), Dip Allerg(SA), Cert Paeds Pulm(SA), FCCP, PhD
Professor
Paediatrics and Child Health
University of Pretoria
Pretoria, Gauteng, South Africa

Philippe Mayaud, MD, MSc
Professor of Infectious Diseases and Reproductive Health
Department of Clinical Research
Faculty of Infectious and Tropical Diseases
London School of Hygiene and Tropical Medicine
London, UK

James S. McCarthy, MD, FRACP
Professor of Tropical Medicine and Infectious Diseases
Queensland Institute of Medical Research
University of Queensland
Senior Consultant Infectious Diseases Physician
Royal Brisbane and Womens Hospital
Brisbane, Australia

Rose McGready, MB BS, PhD, Dip, RANZCOG, Dip, LATHE, DTM&H
Centre for Tropical Medicine
Nuffield Department of Medicine
University of Oxford
Oxford, UK
Shoklo Malaria Research Unit
Mahidol-Oxford Tropical Medicine Research Unit
Faculty of Tropical Medicine
Mahidol University
Bangkok, Thailand

Paul S. McNamara, MB BS, MRCPCH, PhD
Reader in Child Health Department of Women's and Children's Health
University of Liverpool
Alder Hey Children's NHS Foundation Trust Hospital
Liverpool, UK

Laura Merson, BSc
Head of Clinical Trials Unit
Centre for Tropical Medicine
University of Oxford
Oxford University Clinical Research Unit
Ho Chi Minh, Vietnam

Robert F. Miller, MB BS, FRCP, FSB
Reader in Clinical Infection and Honorary Consultant Physician
Research Department of Infection and Population Health
Institute of Epidemiology and Health Care
University College London Medical School
London, UK

Glen D. Liddell Mola, MB BS (Melb), DPH(Syd), MRACGP, FRANZCOG, FRCOG, OL
Professor and Head of Reproductive Health, Obstetrics and Gynecology
School of Medicine and Health Sciences
University of Papua New Guinea
Honorary Senior Clinical Consultant
Port Moresby General Hospital
Port Moresby, Papua New Guinea

Kevin Mortimer, MB, BChir, MRCP, MSc, PhD
Senior Clinical Lecturer in Respiratory Medicine
Department of Clinical Sciences
Liverpool School of Tropical Medicine
Honorary Consultant in Respiratory Medicine
Department of Respiratory Medicine
Aintree University Hospital NHS Foundation Trust
Liverpool, UK

Ayesha A. Motala, MB ChB, MD, FRCP, FCP
Professor
Department of Diabetes and Endocrinology
Nelson R Mandela School of Medicine
University of KwaZulu-Natal
Durban, South Africa

Kosta Y. Mumcuoglu, PhD
Research Fellow
Department of Microbiology and Molecular Genetics
The Kuvin Centre for the Study of Infectious and Tropical Diseases
Hebrew University-Hadassah Medical School
Jerusalem, Israel

Flor M. Munoz, MD
Associate Professor
Pediatrics, Section on Infectious Diseases
Molecular Virology and Microbiology
Baylor College of Medicine
Texas Children's Hospital
Houston, TX, USA

Melba Munoz Roldan, MD, PhD
Deutsches Rheuma-Forschungszentrum, Institut der Leibniz-Gemeinschaft
Experimental Immunology, Department of Rheumatology and Clinical Immunology
Charité-University Medicine
Berlin, Germany

Theonest Mutabingwa, MD, MSc, PhD
Professor in Community Medicine
Department of Community Medicine
Hubert Kairuki Memorial University
Dar-es-Salaam, Tanzania

Osamu Nakagomi, MD, PhD
Professor of Molecular Epidemiology
Department of Molecular Microbiology and Immunology
Graduate School of Biomedical Sciences, and Global Centre of Excellence
Nagasaki University
Nagasaki, Japan

Yukifumi Nawa, BM, MD, PhD
Invited Professor/Consultant
Faculty of Tropical Medicine
Mahidol University
Bangkok, Thailand

Robert Newton, MB BS, DPhil, FFPH
Senior Clinical Epidemiologist at Medical Research Council / Uganda Virus Research Institute Research Unit on AIDS
Entebbe, Uganda
Reader in Clinical Epidemiology
University of York
York, UK
Senior Visiting Scientist
World Health Organisation's International Agency for Research on Cancer
Lyon, France

Lisa F. P. Ng, PhD
Principle Investigator/Associate Professor
Singapore Immunology Network (SIgN)
Agency for Science, Technology and Research (A*STAR)
Singapore

François H. Nosten, MD, PhD
Professor of Tropical Medicine
Centre for Tropical Medicine
Nuffield Department of Medicine
University of Oxford
Oxford, UK
Shoklo Malaria Research Unit
Mahidol-Oxford Tropical Medicine Research Unit
Faculty of Tropical Medicine
Mahidol University
Bangkok Thailand

Jennifer O'Hea, MD, FCCP
Intensivist
Department of Critical Care
Banner Good Samaritan Medical Center
Clinical Assistant Professor of Medicine
University of Arizona College of Medicine
Phoenix, AZ, USA

Shirley Owusu-Ofori, BSc, MB ChB, CTM, FGCP
Senior Specialist
Transfusion Medicine
Head
Transfusion Medicine Unit
Komfo Anokye Teaching Hospital
Kumasi, Ghana

Daniel H. Paris, MD, PhD, DTM&H
Research Lecturer, University of Oxford, Oxford, UK
Head of Rickettsiology, Mahidol-Oxford Tropical Medicine Research Unit
Faculty of Tropical Medicine
Mahidol University
Bangkok, Thailand

Michael Parker B Ed, MA, PhD
Professor of Bioethics and Centre Director
The Ethox Centre
Nuffield Department of Population Health
University of Oxford
Oxford, UK

Philip J. Peters, MD, DTM&H
Consultant Parasitologist
Hospital for Tropical Diseases
Honorary Professor
The London School of Hygiene and Tropical Medicine
Director
Public Health England Malaria Reference Laboratory
London, UK

Fraser J. Pirie, MB ChB, MD, FCP
Senior Lecturer
Department of Diabetes and Endocrinology
Nelson R Mandela School of Medicine
University of KwaZulu-Natal
Durban, South Africa

Gerd Pluschke, PhD
Professor, Head of Department
Department of Medical Parasitology and Infection Biology
Swiss Tropical and Public Health Institute
University of Basel
Basel, Switzerland

Andrew M. Prentice, BSc, PhD,
Director
MRC International Nutrition Group
London School of Hygiene and Tropical Medicine
London, UK

Thomas C. Quinn, MD, MSc
Associate Director of International Research
Division of Intramural Research
National Institute of Allergy and Infectious Diseases
National Institutes of Health
Director of Global Health
Professor
Departments of Medicine, Pathology, International Health, Molecular Microbiology and Immunology, and Epidemiology
Johns Hopkins University
Baltimore, MD, USA

Minoarisoa Esther Rajerison, PhD
Head of Plague Unit
Institut Pasteur de Madagascar
Ambatofotsikely
Antananarivo, Madagascar

Didier Raoult, Pr (MD, PhD)
Professor of Microbiology
Unité de Recherche sur les Maladies Infectieuses et Tropicales Emergentes
Aix Marseille UniversitéFaculté de Médecine
Marseille, France

Maherisoa Ratsitorahina, MD
Doctor
Epidemiology Unit
Institut Pasteur de Madagascar
Ambatofotsikely, Antananarivo, Madagascar

K. Srinath Reddy, MD, DM, MB BS
President
Public Health Foundation of India & World Heart Federation
Delhi, India

Steven J. Reynolds, MD, MPH FRCP(C), DTM&H
Senior Clinician
Division of Intramural Research
National Institute of Allergy and Infectious Diseases
National Institutes of Health
Associate Professor
Department of Medicine and Epidemiology
Johns Hopkins University
Baltimore, MD, USA

John Richens, MA, MB BS, MSc, FRCPE
Clinical Lecturer
Department of Sexually Transmitted Diseases
Division of Pathology and Infectious Diseases
Royal Free and University College Medical School
London, UK

Marcus J. Rijken, MD, PhD
Obstetric Department
Shoklo Malaria Research Unit
Mahidol-Oxford Tropical Medicine Research Unit
Faculty of Tropical Medicine
Mahidol University
Bangkok, Thailand

Sara Ritchie, MB ChB, MRCGP, DFFP, MPH, DTM&H, Dip Derm
Honorary Clinical Fellow in Tropical Dermatology
University College London Hospitals NHS Foundation Trust
London, UK

Janet Robinson, FIBS
Global Director, Laboratory Sciences
Laboratory Sciences Division
Asia Pacific Regional Research Director
Bangkok, Thailand

Angela M. C. Rose, BA, MSc
Lecturer in Epidemiology
The University of the West Indies
Director
Barbados National Registry for Chronic NCDs
Chronic Disease Research Centre
The University of the West Indies
St Michael, Barbados

Juan C. Salazar, MD, MPH
Professor of Pediatrics and Immunology
University of Connecticut School of Medicine
Farmington
Director, Division of Pediatric Infectious Diseases and Immunology
Connecticut Children's Medical Center,
Hartford, CT, USA

T. Alafia Samuels, MB BS, MPH, PhD
Senior Lecturer, Public Health & Epidemiology
Faculty of Medical Sciences
The University of the West Indies
Cave Hill, Barbados

Marcus J. Schultz, MD, PhD
Professor of Intensive Care Medicine
Department of Intensive Care Medicine
Academic Medical Center at the University of Amsterdam
Amsterdam, The Netherlands

Crispian Scully, MD, PhD, FDS, FRCPath, FMedSci, DSc
Professor Emeritus
University College London
London, UK

Paul Shears, MD, FRCPath
Consultant Medical Microbiologist
Royal Hallamshire Hospital Sheffield
Teaching Hospitals NHS Foundation Trust
Sheffield, UK

Paul E. Simonsen, PhD
Research Associate Professor
Faculty of Health and Medical Sciences
University of Copenhagen
Copenhagen, Denmark

Paiboon Sithithaworn, PhD
Head, Associate Professor
Department of Parasitology
Liver Fluke and Cholangiocarcinoma Research Center
Faculty of Medicine
Khon Kaen University
Khon Kaen, Thailand

David W. Smith, BMedSc, MB BS, FRCPA, FACTM, FASM, FFSc(RCPA)
Clinical Professor
School of Pathology and Laboratory Medicine
Co-Director
Arbovirus Research and Surveillance Group
The University of Western Australia
Medical Microbiologist/Virologist
Division of Microbiology and Infectious Diseases
PathWest Laboratory Medicine WA
Perth, Western Australia

Tom Solomon, BA, BM BCh, DCH, DTMH, FRCP, PhD
Professor of Neurological Science
Walton Centre NHS Foundation Trust
Director
Institute of Infection and Global Health
University of Liverpool
Liverpool, UK

Vaughan R. Southgate, BSc, PhD, CBiol, FIBiol, FLS
Scientific Associate
Department of Zoology
The Natural History Museum
London, UK

Banchob Sripa, PhD
Professor
Tropical Disease Research Laboratory
Faculty of Medicine
Khon Kaen University
Khon Kaen, Thailand

M. Leila Srour, MD, MPH, DTM&H
Pediatric Development Coordinator
Health Frontiers
Muang Sing
Luang Namtha, Laos

Marija Stojkovic, MD, DTM&H
Section Clinical Tropical Medicine
Department of Infectious Diseases
University Hospital Heidelberg
Heidelberg, Germany

Shyam Sundar, MD, FRCP, FNA
Professor of Medicine
Department of Medicine
Institute of Medical Sciences,
Varanasi, India

Jecko Thachil, MRCP, FRCPath
Consultant Haematologist, Department of Haematology
Central Manchester University Hospitals NHS Foundation Trust
Manchester, UK

Raj Thuraisingham, MD, FRCP
Honorary Senior Lecturer and Consultant Nephrologist
Department of Renal Medicine and Transplantation
Barts Health NHS Trust
London, UK

C. Louise Thwaites, BSc, MB BS, MRCP, MD
Oxford University Clinical Research Unit
Hospital for Tropical Diseases
Ho Chi Minh City, Vietnam

Guy Thwaites, MA, MB BS, MRCP, FRCPath, PhD
Oxford University Clinical Research Unit,
Hospital for Tropical Diseases
Ho Chi Minh City, Vietnam

M. Estée Török, MA, MB BS, PhD, FRCP, FRCPath
Senior Research Associate and Honorary Consultant Physician
Department of Medicine
University of Cambridge
Cambridge, UK

Nigel Unwin, BA, BM BCh, MSc, DM, FRCP, FFPH
Professor of Public Health and Epidemiology
Faculty of Medical Sciences
The University of the West Indies
Cave Hill, Barbados

Diederik van de Beek, MD, PhD
Professor in Neurology
Department of Neurology
Academic Medical Center
Amsterdam, The Netherlands

Francisco Vega-Lopez, MD, MSc, PhD, FRCP, FFTM RCPSG
Consultant
Department of Dermatology
University College London Hospitals – NHS Trust
London, UK
Professor
Department of Dermatology and Medical Mycology
National Medical Centre IMSS, and National University UNAM
Mexico City, Mexico
Former Honorary Professor
Faculty of Infectious and Tropical Diseases
London School of Hygiene & Tropical Medicine
University of London
London, UK

Govinda S. Visvesvara, PhD
Microbiologist
Centers for Disease Control and Prevention
National Center for Emerging and Zoonotic Infectious Diseases
Division of Foodborne, Waterborne & Environmental Diseases
Atlanta, GA, USA

Lorenz von Seidlein, MD, PhD
Clinical Coordinator
Global Health Division
Menzies School of Health Research
Casuarina, Northern Territory, Australia

Katie Wakeham, BSc, MB BS
Wellcome Trust Clinical Training Fellow
MRC/UVRI Research Unit on AIDS
Entebbe, Uganda
University of York
York, UK

Stephen L. Walker, PhD, MRCP(UK), DTM&H
Clinical Research Fellow
Department of Clinical Research
Faculty of Infectious and Tropical Diseases
London School of Hygiene and Tropical Medicine
London, UK

Honorine Ward, MB BS
Professor of Medicine
Tufts University School of Medicine
Division of Geographic Medicine and Infectious Diseases
Tufts Medical Center
Boston, MA, USA

Mary J. Warrell, MB BS, FRCP, FRCPE, FRCPath
Honorary Senior Researcher
Oxford Vaccine Group
University of Oxford
Centre for Clinical Vaccinology & Tropical Medicine
Oxford, UK

David A. Warrell, DM, DSc, FRCP, FRCPE, FMedSci
Emeritus Professor of Tropical Medicine
Nuffield Department of Clinical Medicine
University of Oxford
Oxford, UK

Gary J. Weil, MD
Professor
Internal Medicine and Molecular Microbiology
Washington University School of Medicine
St Louis, MO, USA

Graham B. White, MB ChB
Richmond Surrey, UK

Nicholas J. White, OBE, MD, DSc, FRCP, FMedSci, FRS
Professor of Tropical Medicine
Faculty of Tropical Medicine
Mahidol University
Bangkok, Thailand
Nuffield Department of Medicine
University of Oxford
Oxford, UK

Stephen G. Withington, MB ChB, FRACP, FDRHMNZ
Executive Director
LAMB Hospital & Community Health and Development Programme
Parbatipur, Bangladesh

Vanessa Wong, BM BCh, MA, MRCP, Msc
Wellcome Trust Clinical PhD Fellow
Microbial Pathogenesis
Sanger Institute
University of Cambridge
Specialist Registrar in Medical Microbiology Clinical Microbiology and Public Health Laboratory Addenbrooke's Hospital
Cambridge, UK

Robin Wood, FCP (SA) DSc (Med)
Professor
Desmond Tutu HIV Centre, IIDMM
University of Cape Town
Cape Town, South Africa

Sarah Wyllie, MB ChB, MA, MSc, MRCP, MRCPath
Consultant Microbiologist
Portsmouth Hospitals NHS Trust
Portsmouth, UK

Lam Minh Yen, MD
Director
Tetanus Unit
Hospital for Tropical Diseases
Ho Chi Minh City, Vietnam

Paul R. Young, BSc, PhD, FASM
Professor of Virology
Australian Infectious Diseases Research Centre
School of Chemistry & Molecular Biosciences
Institute for Molecular Bioscience
University of Queensland
Brisbane, Queensland, Australia

Sophie Yacoub, MRCP, MSc, DTM&H
Specialist Registrar in Infectious Diseases
Department of Medicine
Imperial College London
London, UK
Clinical Research Fellow
Infectious Diseases
Oxford University Clinical Research Unit
Hanoi, Vietnam

Ken Zafren, MD, FAAEM, FACEP, FAWM
Associate Medical Director
Himalayan Rescue Association
Kathmandu, Nepal
Nepal Clinical Associate Professor, Division of Emergency Medicine
Stanford University Medical Center
Stanford, CA, USA
USA Staff Emergency Physician – Alaska Native Medical Center
Anchorage, AK, USA

1

History of Tropical Medicine, and Medicine in the Tropics

GORDON C. COOK

European doctors practised in *tropical* countries as early as the seventeenth and eighteenth centuries in the English West Indies (the 'Sugar Islands'), India, the East Indies and later Africa, the western coast of which was widely termed the 'white man's grave'.[1–3] Many also produced monographs describing their experiences, with an outline of the disease pattern at these various locations. Many infections which now fall under the 'tropical' umbrella were widely distributed in northern Europe and northern America during the seventeenth to nineteenth centuries. For example, William Shakespeare (1564–1616) was well aware of malaria in England: 'he is so shak'd by the burning quotidian tertian that it is most lamentable to behold' (*Henry V*, II. i. 123). Thomas Sydenham (1624–1689) successfully used fever-tree bark (containing quinine) in the management of the 'intermittent fevers' during the seventeenth century.[4] Indigenous *Plasmodium vivax* infection remained a clinical problem in south-east England well into the twentieth century. Plague, typhoid, cholera, typhus and smallpox were major health hazards in Britain, London included, during the Victorian era.[5] John Bunyan (1628–1688) was well aware of the consumption (tuberculosis) – now such an important disease in 'tropical' countries – which so often 'took him down to the grave' (*The Life and Death of Mr Badman*).

What then is tropical medicine? Andrew Balfour (1873–1931)[2] summarized the position as he saw it, in his Presidential Address to the Royal Society of Tropical Medicine and Hygiene in 1925: 'there is in one sense no such thing as tropical medicine, and in any case many of the most erudite writings of Hippocrates are concerned with maladies which nowadays are chiefly encountered under tropical or subtropical conditions'. Some, including many historians, consider that 'tropical medicine' originated as a by-product of the British Empire and Raj.[6] The truth of the matter is that 'medicine in the tropics' was exploited by the Colonialists in order that the health of British personnel, both overseas and following return to the UK, could be improved (see below).[3] The specialty, in fact, as a formal discipline, had its origin(s) in a multidisciplinary background: major areas of progress during the nineteenth century were public health (and hygiene), travel and exploration, natural history, evolutionary theory, and a precise knowledge of the causation of disease (the 'germ theory').[3,7–9] The miasmatists and contagionists were previously at loggerheads. The development of clinical parasitology following the work of Manson, Ross and others (see below), and superimposed on this complex backcloth, led to the inevitable genesis of 'tropical medicine' as a formal discipline.[3,9,10]

Development of Tropical Medicine as a Formal Discipline

THE SEAMEN'S HOSPITAL SOCIETY

In London, the Seamen's Hospital Society (SHS) (the 'foster mother of clinical tropical medicine') was formed in 1821, its predecessor being the Committee for Distressed (or destitute) Seamen, which was set up in the winter of 1817–1818; its raison d'être was to provide temporary relief to sick members of the mercantile marine then roaming in large number on the streets of London's docklands.[1,3,11,12] The major objective was thus largely targeted at the management of illnesses (especially fevers and sexually transmitted diseases), many of which had been introduced into London from tropical and subtropical countries.[5] At a meeting held at the City of London Tavern on 8 March 1821 (William Wilberforce MP (1759–1833) was among those present), the committee resolved to establish a *permanent* floating hospital on the Thames for the exclusive use of sick and distressed seamen; the venture was to be supported by voluntary contributions. A series of hulks, HMS *Grampus* (lent by the Admiralty in 1821) (Figure 1.1), HMS *Dreadnought* (1831–1857) and HMS *Caledonia* (renamed *Dreadnought*) (1857–1870) were all anchored in Greenwich Reach and used successively; they had been 48, 98, and 120-gun vessels, respectively.[1,11,12] Although they served a valuable function, major practical problems arose: ventilation was poor, and nosocomial spread of disease occurred; lack of light was a major drawback during the winter months; and other problems (not least noise) associated with the situation in the midst of an extremely busy part of the River Thames proved tiresome.[12,13] In 1870, after protracted negotiations, the Commissioners of the Admiralty granted the SHS a 99-year lease of the Infirmary (and adjoining Somerset Ward) of the Royal Hospital, Greenwich, in lieu of the loan of the ship(s).[1,11,12] This move was made possible by a sharp decline in the number of pensioners residing in the hospital during the peaceful years following the battle of Waterloo (in 1815); the infirmary was therefore no longer required for them. In 1873, the hospital ceased being a permanent home for naval pensioners and became the Royal Naval College (previously based at Portsmouth). The Royal Hospital[14] had been founded in 1694 by William III (1650–1702) and Mary as the naval equivalent of the Royal Hospital, Chelsea, founded by King Charles II, and is still in use for army pensioners today.

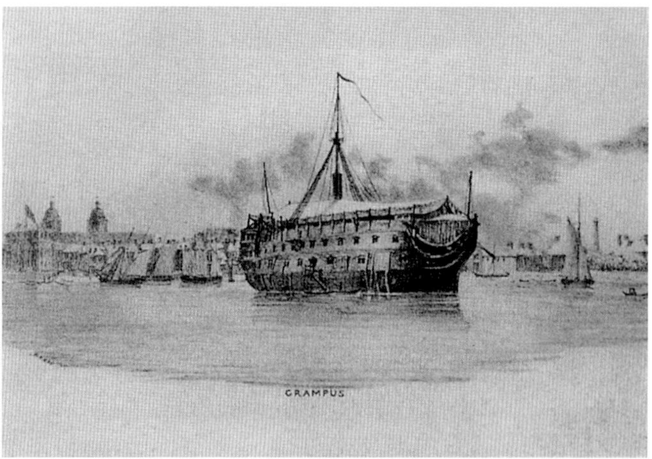

Figure 1-1 HMS *Grampus*. The first of three hospital-ships lent by the Admiralty to the Seamen's Hospital Society, anchored on Greenwich Reach. This disused 48-gun warship served in this capacity from October 1821 to October 1831.

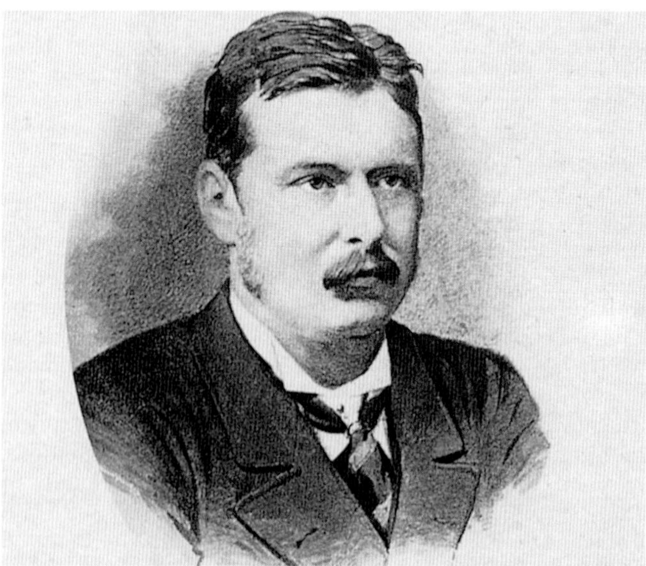

Figure 1-2 Dr (later Sir) Patrick Manson (1844–1922) aged 31 years. This photograph was probably taken while he was on leave in Britain from Amoy in 1875.

EMERGENCE OF THE FORMAL DISCIPLINE IN LONDON

Following his return to London from Formosa and Amoy (where he had made his seminal discovery of man–mosquito transmission of the nematode *Filaria sanguinis hominis* (*Wuchereria bancrofti*), a causative agent of lymphatic filariasis) and Hong Kong, Patrick Manson (1844–1922)[3,8,15] (Figure 1.2) embarked on a series of lectures devoted to 'tropical medicine' at several London medical schools.[1,3,16] The Rt Hon Joseph Chamberlain (1836–1914), Secretary of State for the Colonies, was immediately impressed at the possibility of sending colonial medical staff on leave in Britain to these lectures, to give an update on the prevention and management of those diseases which seriously affected the 'servants of Empire'.[1,3] Regular trade, efficient administration and agricultural production were all seriously hampered by disease; Chamberlain's concept of 'constructive imperialism' could not be adequately developed in the presence of such a great deal of morbidity and mortality. Despite a great deal of opposition,[17] *clinical* tropical medicine emerged as both an important medical specialty and scientific discipline (the importance of parasites and their vectors in transmission of disease had only recently become clear – see above), Chamberlain considered that 'tropical medicine' was an essential component in the future development of British economic and social imperialism. It was, in fact, to become a 'colonial science'.[1,13] At the 1898 meeting of the British Medical Association held in Edinburgh, at which Ronald Ross's (1857–1932) work in Calcutta, India, on the role of the mosquito in *avian* malaria was announced (his initial demonstration at Secundarabad, India, of *Plasmodium* spp. development in the mosquito had been published in the *British Medical Journal* the previous year), a new section devoted to 'Tropical Medicine' was inaugurated.[10] There were several reasons why the discipline had not previously emerged. Many 'tropical diseases' had formerly existed in northern Europe (including England) and northern America. There was also widespread feeling that the high mortality rate affecting the white man in the tropics was inevitable, and that climate would prevent his living and working there successfully. The 'miasmatic theory' still held sway. Furthermore, there was an understandable pessimism regarding the possibility of significant environmental improvement in the foreseeable future, most British colonies being situated on unhealthy coastlines. Also, research had until then taken a very low priority for medical staff working in the tropics; their perceived task was solely to provide medical advice and care to the local British community.

THE MANSON–CHAMBERLAIN COLLABORATION

In order to implement effective development of the 'new' discipline Manson was appointed Medical Officer to the Colonial Office in 1897. Here, with Chamberlain's wholehearted support, he set about establishing a School of Tropical Medicine in London (LSTM).[1,3] A major problem relating to the venue of the proposed institution arose. Manson favoured the branch hospital of the Seamen's Hospital Society, situated near the Royal Albert Dock.[1,3,18] However, hostility to this suggestion arose from several quarters. The War Office favoured the Royal Victoria Hospital, Netley, which, situated on Southampton Water, had been founded in 1863;[1,3,19] it had been established principally for soldiers invalided from the Crimea and was then staffed by officers of the Royal Army Medical Corps. Manson considered this option unacceptable (he was already on the staff of the Albert Dock Hospital): the atmosphere and remote situation from London were, in his opinion, incompatible with the teaching of tropical medicine. The Royal College of Physicians was of the opinion that a new school was unnecessary. The senior medical staff of the Greenwich Hospital felt that removal of the 'tropical' cases to the Albert Dock Hospital (ADH) was a slight on their professional ability and was in any case undesirable because medical students from London's teaching hospitals were accustomed to visiting Greenwich for tuition in the diagnosis and management of these illnesses.[17] The end result was an outburst of acrimonious correspondence in the columns of the *Lancet*, the *British Medical Journal* and *The Times*, which later involved, among others, Sir William Broadbent, Sir William Church, Sir Jonathan Hutchinson and Sir Joseph Fayrer, the doyen of the Indian Medical Service.

However, staunch determination from Manson and Herbert Read (Assistant Private Secretary to Chamberlain) to proceed with the project, strongly supported by Chamberlain himself, led to the rapid establishment of the proposed school at the ADH;[1,16,20] financial assistance to the tune of £3550 came from the Colonial Office. A subcommittee was set up to 'formulate a scheme for organisation and management of the LSTM in connection with the SHS'; the committee of management was to be composed of equal numbers of personnel from the SHS, the medical and surgical staff of the ADH, and teachers from the LSTM.

SCHOOL AND HOSPITAL IN CLOSE PROXIMITY

The LSTM was officially opened on 2 October 1899.[1,3] The hospital (under SHS supervision) and teaching and research facilities at the LSTM were on the same site (Figure 1.3). With (Sir) Perceval Nairne (1841–1921) (Chairman of the SHS) presiding, the inaugural address – written by Manson – was read in his absence. He later declared: 'the school strikes, and strikes effectively, at the root of the principal difficulty of most of our Colonies-disease. It will cheapen government and make it more efficient. It will encourage and cheapen commercial enterprise. It will conciliate and foster the native'.[1,21] Meanwhile, a continuity funding was necessary, and several sources of income were exploited; two charity dinners, at which Chamberlain presided, were held at the Hotel Cecil in 1899 and 1905; they raised £12 000 and £11 000 respectively. At the former, Chamberlain declared:[1] 'The man who shall successfully grapple with this foe of humanity and find the cure for malaria, for the fever desolating our colonies . . . and shall make the tropics livable for white men . . . will do more for the world, more for the British Empire, than the man who adds a new province to the wide Dominions of the Queen'. A 'Tropical Diseases Research Fund' was set up, and the Dean – (Sir) Francis Lovell (1844–1916) – raised funds on several overseas trips. In 1912, the school was enlarged and a new wing opened by Their Majesties King George V and Queen Mary. 'Tropical' cases were relatively few in the early days of the LSTM;[3,22] in fact, the ADH had been founded to care for seafarers and 'landsmen' in the London Docks – most of whom suffered from injuries.

In 1919, a decision was taken to relocate the school and hospital to central London; Endsleigh Palace Hotel, 25 Gordon Street, London WC1, was purchased (by the SHS with funding from the Red Cross) for £70 000 and on 11 November, 1920 the Duke of York (later King George VI) (1895–1952) opened the joint LSTM and Hospital for Tropical Diseases (HTD) in this building.[1,13] The structure, which remains extant (and constitutes the student union of University College), provided five floors (at the top) for clinical tropical medicine, and four for the basic sciences; a radiology department was situated in the basement. Sir Philip Manson-Bahr (1881–1966)[12] considered the building 'dark, awkward and inconvenient, with multitudes of doors and narrow passages', but never before had there been 'more unanimity or good fellowship among the staff of the school and the hospital'. The Wellcome Tropical Museum was nearby and provided invaluable teaching resources.[1,13]

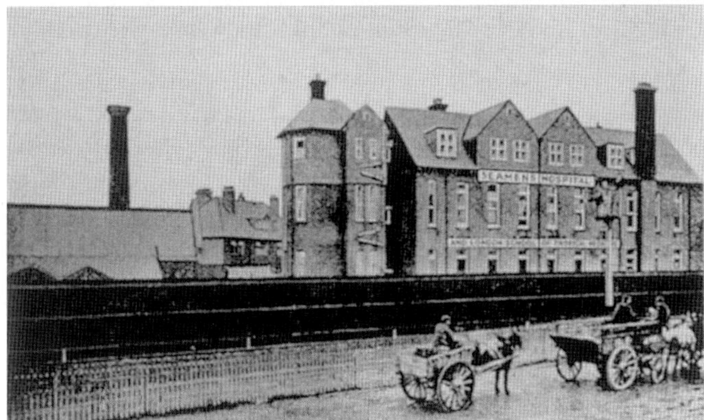

Figure 1-3 Newly opened London School of Tropical Medicine – situated on an adjoining site to the Seamen's Hospital Society's Branch (Albert Dock) Hospital – in October 1899.

Between 1899 and 1929 the clinical specialty and the basic sciences were thus on the same site – first at the ADH[18] and later London WC1;[20] the close proximity was both valuable and productive, a great deal of teaching and clinical research being accomplished. For example, two research projects carried out by the clinical staff clinched the mosquito transmission of malaria saga in *Homo sapiens*. G. C. Low (1872–1952) (later in large part responsible for establishing the Royal Society of Tropical Medicine and Hygiene at Manson's House)[23,24] and three other investigators slept between dusk and dawn, for 3 months, in a mosquito-proof hut about 7 km from Rome, Italy (where *Plasmodium vivax* malaria was prevalent); by so doing they avoided a *P. vivax* infection.[1,3,8] Also, in 1900, three batches of mosquitoes infected with *P. vivax* were sent from Rome to London; Manson's elder surviving son – then a medical student at Guy's Hospital, and captain of rugby football – was exposed to them, and together with a technician, duly acquired a clinical attack of *P. vivax* infection, which responded to quinine.[1,3,7]

FOUNDATION OF THE LONDON SCHOOL OF HYGIENE AND TROPICAL MEDICINE: THE CLOSE RELATIONSHIP BETWEEN TROPICAL PHYSICIANS AND BASIC SCIENTIFIC STAFF ENDS

In 1921, the Postgraduate Medical Committee recommended that an Institute of State Medicine Public Health be created in Bloomsbury, near the University of London; the Rockefeller Foundation was persuaded by Professor R. T. Leiper (1881–1969) to donate US$2 million to the Ministry of Health for the development of this facility.[1,13,20] On 18 July, 1929, the London School of Hygiene and Tropical Medicine (LSHTM) was officially opened at Keppel Street (Gower Street) by the Prince of Wales (later King Edward VIII) (1894–1972). Some years after this, the SHS ceased managing the School, and *clinical* tropical medicine became detached from the basic sciences.

Clinical tropical medicine in London suffered a further temporary setback when the Ross Institute and Hospital for Tropical Diseases (Director: Sir Ronald Ross) was opened at Putney West Hill on 15 July, 1926.[1,13,25,26] It was, however, clear from the outset that there was insufficient clinical material in London to justify two hospitals devoted to the management of tropical disease; the project therefore had no chance of becoming viable from a clinical viewpoint. The institution ultimately became incorporated into the LSHTM, as the Ross Institute for Tropical Hygiene, with four beds at the HTD, in 1934; the Director had died 2 years previously.[3,26]

The itinerant saga of *clinical* tropical medicine in London continued unabated and the survival of Manson's original concept seemed at times in serious jeopardy – not least during World War II (1939–1945), when the specialty had to make do with a mere 10 beds – with no teaching facilities, at the *Dreadnought* (the SHS's land-based flagship) Hospital, Greenwich. For a brief period after the war, a nursing home in Devonshire Street, London W1, housed the discipline. In 1951, the HTD was transferred to St Pancras, NW1 and officially opened on 24 May (Empire Day) by the Duchess of Kent.[1,20] In late 1999, the latest (and possibly the final) move of the clinical discipline, to University College Hospital, took place;[20] regrettably, the facilities in that overcrowded setting were extremely limited.

Regarding the clinical discipline in London, Manson-Bahr[13] later concluded:

> *In recounting the chequered history of this institution, the Hospital for Tropical Diseases, a venture one would have thought essential to the greatest of all Empires, there runs the thread of insecurity . . . the hospital became the whipping boy of medical politics . . . The Board of the SHS was always a representative body of admirals whose interest lay in the sailor, but not in (clinical) tropical medicine.*
>
> *The future of the clinical discipline in London remains anyone's guess!*[1,3,27]

Development of Tropical Medicine in Liverpool

This chapter has concentrated on the LSHTM because the principal catalyst for the 'formal discipline' – Manson (the 'Father of Tropical Medicine') established his school there. However, the Liverpool School of Tropical Medicine had opened about 6 months earlier.[1,3,28,29] Although the concept of a School of Tropical Medicine in Liverpool developed after that in London, the plan of action proceeded more rapidly, and the School was opened to students on 21 April, 1899. In many senses therefore, that one should be designated *the* Pioneer School of Tropical Medicine. The initial momentum had originated in a circular from Chamberlain to the General Medical Council and leading British medical schools (11 March, 1898), and a letter to the Governors of the Colonies (14 June, 1898). The timescale of the first appointments was impressive:[28,30] 20 January, 1899 – Dean appointed; 7 February – Demonstrator in tropical pathology (Dr H. E. Annett); 10 April – Lecturer in tropical medicine (Major Ronald Ross, IMS); 22 April – School officially opened by Lord Lister (1827–1912); May 1899 – teaching started. The Liverpool School was not a 'brainchild' of Manson/Chamberlain (unlike the LSTM), and it did not therefore receive government support – a source of irritation (and perhaps even anger) at the time. It owed its inception to the initiative(s) of Mr (later Sir) Alfred Jones KCMG (1845–1909), a prominent Liverpool (an important seaport) figure, and an energetic leader in the development of Liverpool's overseas trade with the West African Colonies. He controlled the Elder Dempster shipping line, which traded with the Canary Islands and West Africa (and had a thriving business in bananas, groundnuts and oil nuts); local commerce had previously involved the 'triangular trade'. Together with several wealthy and generous Liverpool merchants, he also provided the financial backing for the School's foundation. The other major personality in the project was Dr (later Sir) Rubert Boyce, FRS (1863–1911) – the first Dean.

The project was encouraged by the Royal Society, whose Secretary wrote to the Principal of University College, Liverpool (18 November, 1898):[28,29]

> *I think the idea of starting something at Liverpool about Tropical Diseases in connection with the College, most admirable. The opportunities of studying Tropical Diseases are greater at Liverpool than anywhere else in England, excepting perhaps London. You have to arrange: 1. For teaching. 2. For investigation. No. 2 wants, I think, more support than No. 1. If you had a ward, say at the Southern Hospital, one of the physicians might take charge of it, and give lectures, clinical at the Hospital, and general say at the College – I suppose you might give him a title. For investigation you do not, I think, need a separate Laboratory at College, but a small Clinical Laboratory and the Hospital itself . . . The next point, I am in doubt about. I am inclined to think that the Pathology of Tropical Diseases should belong to the Professor of Pathology, who should, by virtue of this have some connection with the Tropical Diseases Ward in the Hospital, have access to the cases, . . . This system of a Pathologist working with the Physician or Surgeon in Clinical charge of the sick is being very largely worked with great success in America, and in this Tropical Disease seems to offer an opportunity for it. I have talked with Lord Lister (1827–1912) [President of the Royal Society], and he generally approves of what I have proposed, at least, thinks it most desirable that the Hospital and College should lay hold of Tropical Diseases. I myself feel very strong that it is an opportunity of study of these diseases. When the experts on Malaria sent out to Africa get to work on the West Coast, as they will in time do, it will be a great advantage to have an Institution for Tropical Diseases already in work at Liverpool. The experts abroad can work with the men at home.*

At a meeting convened at the offices of Messrs Elder, Dempster and Co. on 23 November, 1898, the following were present:[28,29] Alfred L. Jones; William Adamson, President of the Royal Southern Hospital; R. T. Glazebrook, Principal of University College; William Alexander, Senior Surgeon of the Royal Southern Hospital; William Carter, Physician to the Royal Southern Hospital, Professor of Therapeutics, University College; and Boyce. The resulting minutes were as follows:

> *The following resolutions were unanimously passed: 1. That the gentlemen present form themselves into a Committee, with the approval of their various boards, for promoting the study of Tropical Diseases and to consider the best means of carrying out . . . Jones' intentions in the munificent offer he has made to further the above object. 2. That Mr Charles W. Jones (of Messrs Lamport and Holt) be asked to serve on this Committee. It was decided that the above resolutions should be printed, and that Jones would hand a copy to . . . Chamberlain . . . The Committee recommended that before the next meeting, the Professional Members should meet together to consider and suggest the best means for . . . carrying out these objects.*

At a second meeting (12 December, 1898) a letter from Lord Ampthill (Colonial Office) to the Chairman (1 December) was read:[28]

I have shown your letter of the 28th ult. with regard to the School of Tropical Medicine [to] Chamberlain. He was much interested and very glad to hear of the important work you have thus commenced. You are no doubt aware of what . . . Chamberlain has been doing himself with regard to the establishment of a School of Tropical Medicine [in London] and he considers it a great advantage that Liverpool should be co-operating on similar lines. If it would interest you, I should be very glad to send you particulars of the Colonial Office scheme and information as to what has already been done, but I dare say you have learnt all that is essential from the newspapers.

In December 1898, the *Lancet*[30] reported:

. . . Chamberlain's scheme for the teaching of tropical diseases to colonial surgeons . . . has already borne practical fruit. Mr Alfred Jones [1845–1909] of Liverpool has offered £350 annually to establish and maintain a laboratory in Liverpool for the study of tropical diseases and the scheme will be carried out by a joint committee of the Royal Southern Hospital and of University College. A laboratory for immediate investigation will be built opposite the hospital, whilst prolonged research will be carried out in the pathological laboratory of University College, under the direction of Professor Boyce [1863–1911]. A large number of cases from the West Coast of Africa are taken into the wards of the Royal Southern Hospital, as Liverpool, being the centre of the African trade, is in constant communication with West Africa. We again have to congratulate Liverpool on the munificence of her citizens and would direct the attention of medical men about to practice in any capacity on the West Coast of Africa to the opportunity that is being afforded them for obtaining invaluable information.

In a letter (1 February 1899) from the Colonial Office,[28] read to a Committee meeting, it was stated that 'Chamberlain was very glad to learn that it had been decided to establish this School, but regretting that the Government could not grant any financial aid; however, in the selection of candidates for medical appointments in the Colonies, preference would be given to those who had received instruction in tropical medicine, such as that provided in the Liverpool School'. A further letter from Chamberlain (23 February) stated, however, that 'all doctors appointed to the Colonial Service must be attached to the ADH[3,18] for at least 2 months'. The Committee resolved to: (1) write to the Colonial Office and express regret that Chamberlain did not see his way to dispense with the latter condition in the case of students from the Liverpool School; and (2) approach the Colonial Office on the subject. On 20 March, Professor Boyce announced that Lord Lister (see above) had written stating that he intended to approach Chamberlain on behalf of the School, and it was therefore resolved to postpone further action in the matter pending receipt of information concerning the result of this interview. However, government funding was never forthcoming and there can be no doubt that this led to a significant souring of relationships (some friendly rivalry still exists) between Liverpool and London.

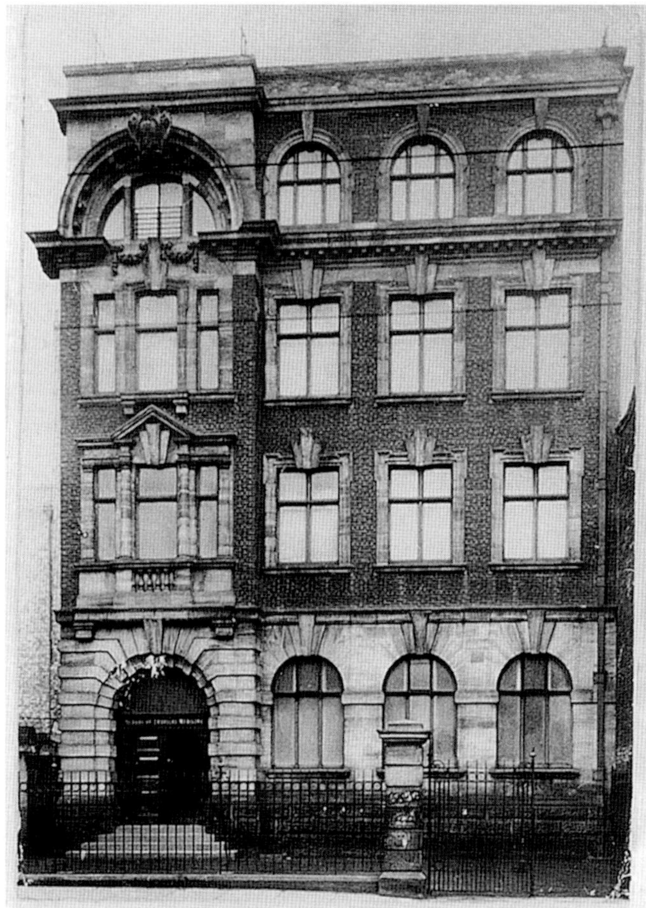

Figure 1-4 Liverpool School of Tropical Medicine; this building opened in 1920.

OPENING OF THE LIVERPOOL SCHOOL

In 1899, *The Lancet*[31] summarized the opening of the Liverpool School (Figure 1.4):

This School was inaugurated under fortunate auspices on April 22nd of this year by Lord Lister. At the annual dinner of the Royal Southern Hospital on Nov. 12th, 1898, Mr. Alfred L. Jones, a prominent Liverpool citizen and West Africa merchant, made an offer of £350 a year to start a school in Liverpool for the study of tropical diseases. The offer was made in the presence of Professor Rubert Boyce of University College, Liverpool, and Dr. William Alexander of the Royal Southern Hospital . . . The great interest subsequently taken in the project by Mr. Alfred L. Jones, aided by the indomitable energy of Professor Boyce, resulted in subscription and donations coming in from all quarters towards the expenses of the proposed school. To those two gentlemen, warmly supported by the committee and medical staff of the Royal Southern Hospital, is due the establishment of the Liverpool School of Tropical Diseases. The management of the school is in the hands of a strong committee, of which Mr. Alfred L. Jones is the chairman and Mr. William Adamson . . . the vice-chairman. The committee also consists of duly appointed representatives of University College, Liverpool, the Royal Southern Hospital, the Liverpool

Chamber of Commerce, the Steamship Owners' Association, and the Shipowners' Association. A sum of over £1700 has already been promised, partly in annual subscriptions and partly in donations, in support of the school, but more pecuniary support is urgently needed if the practical work already begun is to be maintained at its excellent level. A large floor in the Royal Southern Hospital has been set apart for tropical cases. This floor includes a cheerful ward containing 12 beds, now fully occupied, also an extensive laboratory for the examination of blood, urine, faeces, etc., and furnished with the apparatus applicable to modern research. Professor Boyce superintends the pathological department of the school, with Dr. Annett as pathological demonstrator. The committee have been fortunate in securing the services of Major Ronald Ross, IMS [see above], as special lecturer [later professor] on tropical diseases . . . The number of malarial cases treated in Liverpool in 1898 amounted to 294. In the previous year . . . there were 242 cases of malaria, 14 of beri-beri, 30 of dysentery, and 39 of tropical anaemia. With the means of instruction in the varied forms of tropical diseases thus afforded there will be no need for Liverpool students to proceed to London [where there were fewer cases[22]] to obtain that which is ready to hand at their own doors. The authorities of the Liverpool School of Tropical Medicine have lost no time in getting to real work.

In June 1899, Ross (Figure 1.5) gave an inaugural lecture: he committed himself to the practical application of his malaria researches; extirpation of the mosquito, he envisaged, was the answer to the 'great malaria problem'. Ross had thus embarked on the 'sanitation' (or hygiene) tack, which was to dominate much of the Liverpool School's work for the forthcoming century.[3,29]

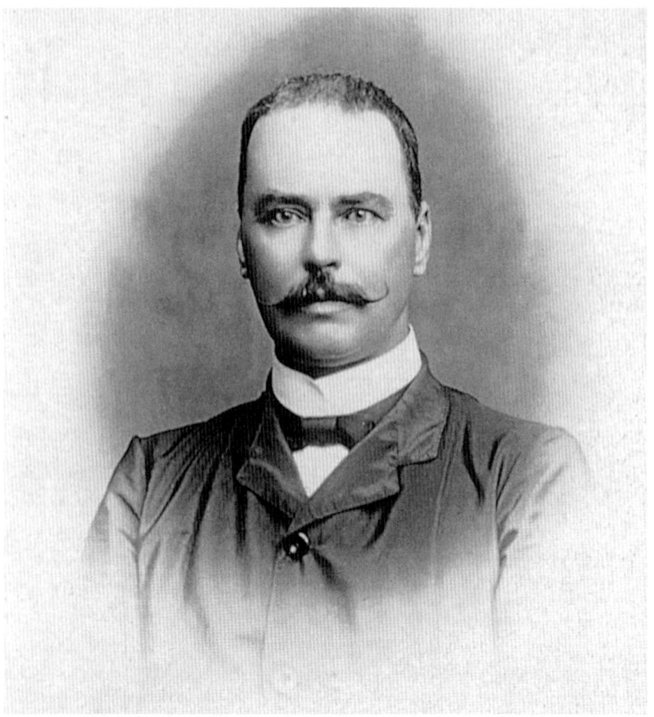

Figure 1-5 Major (later Sir) Ronald Ross (1857–1932).[35] The photograph was probably taken in the early twentieth century.

SUBSEQUENT DEVELOPMENTS IN LIVERPOOL

Shortly after its opening (in April 1899), the Liverpool School started on a series of 'expeditions': the first embarked for Sierra Leone in July, and 11 more had been carried out by the end of 1903. Between its foundation and 1914, a total of 32 scientific expeditions to the tropics had taken place.[28,32] The *Annals of Tropical Medicine and Parasitology* was founded by the School's staff in 1907. The School was compelled, however, to survive by subscription; there was therefore no year-to-year stability.

At the outbreak of the Great War (1914–1918), teaching had been in full swing for 15 years;[33] two full courses were being given annually. An advanced practical course (of 1 month duration) was designed to meet the convenience of practitioners when at home on leave; those who attended this were excused the first month of the other course. Special courses on entomology designed for officers in the West African Medical Service and others were also given three times annually. Special research work was carried out at the School and the Runcorn Research Laboratories (about 16 miles from Liverpool).

Excellent historical accounts of the Liverpool School of Tropical Medicine are due to Miller[29] and Maegraith.[34] The School (unlike LSHTM) has established close collaborative links with some of the recently created Universities and Medical Schools of Africa, and other newly 'emergent' developing countries.

Medicine in the Tropics and Tropical Medicine

The practice of medicine in a tropical country differs in many ways from that in a temperate one – where the classical specialty (exemplified by the London and Liverpool Schools) has dominated the scenario. A major problem arises in the definition of 'tropical medicine'; this was accepted by Manson himself[3] in the preface to the first edition of this textbook in 1898:

The title I have elected to give to this work, TROPICAL DISEASES, is more convenient than accurate. If by 'tropical diseases' be meant diseases peculiar to, and confined to, the tropics, then half a dozen pages might have sufficed for their description . . . If . . . the expression 'tropical diseases' be held to include all diseases occurring in the tropics, then the work would require to cover almost the entire range of medicine. The tropical practitioner [he continued] enjoys opportunities for original research and discovery far superior in novelty and interest to those at the command of his fellow inquirer in the well-worked field of European and American research.

Figures 1.6 and 1.7 summarize some of the highlights in the development of these separate disciplines.[7]

In Britain (and other European countries) and northern America, infectious diseases dominated the medical scene until well into the twentieth century (Figure 1.6); however, following the introduction of improved sanitation/hygiene in Victorian England, their prevalence slowly declined,[1,3,35,36] the downward trend continued with the introduction of antibiotics in the 1940s and 1950s. Only recently has prevalence tended to increase – largely as a result of the HIV/AIDS pandemic. Tropical medicine, as an organized discipline, took off in the 1890s

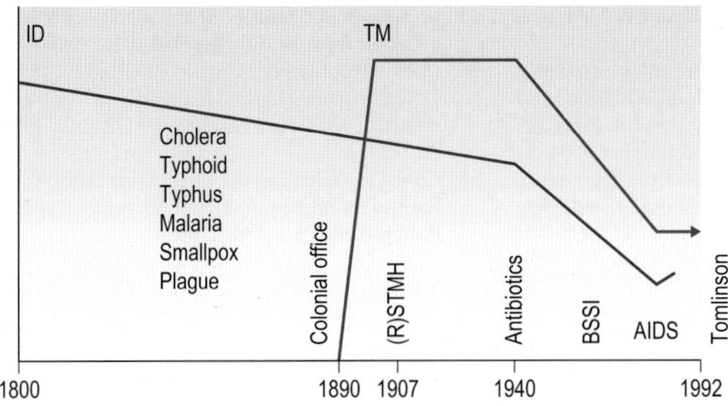

Figure 1-6 Approximate sequence of events in the foundation and development of the formal discipline of Tropical Medicine (TM). ID, infectious diseases; (R)STMH, (Royal) Society of Tropical Medicine and Hygiene; BSSI, British Society for the Study of Infection; AIDS, acquired immune deficiency syndrome; Tomlinson Report, published in 1992, which gave rise to sweeping changes in the British National Health Service.

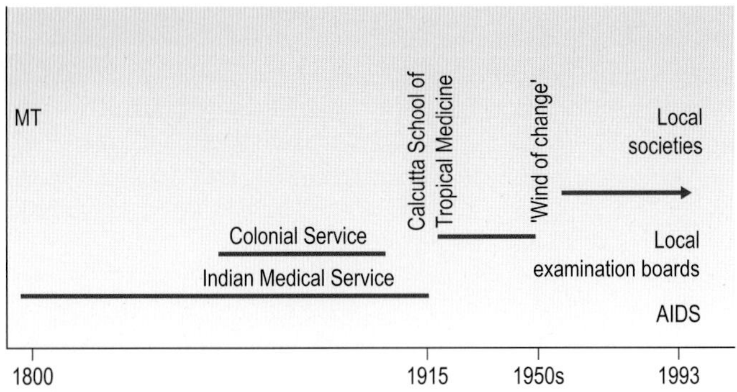

Figure 1-7 Approximate sequence of events in the progress of teaching/research in tropical (developing) countries. Medicine in the tropics (MT). AIDS, acquired immune deficiency syndrome.

(see above) and reached a peak during the first half of the last century. Following World War II (1939–1945), or possibly before, a downward trend set in and as a result, this specialty continues to decline as a specific entity. The introduction of National Health Service 'reforms', following the Tomlinson report (published in 1992) and strategies of recent British governments, have rendered the future of this relatively small discipline extremely vulnerable. The major priority in Britain at present is to maintain a cadre of physicians well versed in the more 'exotic' infections encountered in the UK (e.g. trypanosomiasis, leishmaniasis and schistosomiasis), a requirement which also applies to other 'temperate' countries. More emphasis should also be given to 'travel medicine'.

In countries situated in the tropics (Figure 1.7) the scenario is different.[7] Organized medical services began with the Indian Medical Service; this was followed by the Colonial Medical Service – with a far wider influence. Although Manson had started a Medical School in Hong Kong in 1887, the first School of Tropical Medicine in a tropical country was established by Sir Leonard Rogers (1868–1962) at Calcutta (now Kolkata) in 1920; this was a pioneering achievement.[3] When the former British Colonies acquired 'independence' in the 1950s and later, the 'wind of change' brought in its wake many newly created (indigenous) universities and medical schools, e.g. Makerere University College, Kampala; Ibadan University, Nigeria; and the University (and University Teaching Hospital), Lusaka; this led to much local teaching and research, and also simultaneously the introduction of local medical societies and examining boards.

These are changing times, and the future of the formal discipline specialty Tropical Medicine is at present uncertain. But that must on no account be confused with 'medicine in the tropics'.[3,37]

REFERENCES

1. Cook GC. From the Greenwich Hulks to Old St Pancras: A History of Tropical Disease in London. London: Athlone Press; 1992. p. 338.
2. Balfour A. Some British and American pioneers in tropical medicine and hygiene. Trans R Soc Trop Med Hyg 1925;19:189–231.
3. Cook GC. Tropical Medicine: An Illustrated History of the Pioneers. London: Academic Press; 2007. p. 278.
4. Dewhurst K. Dr Thomas Sydenham (1624–1689): His Life and Original Writings. London: Wellcome Historical Medical Library; 1966. p. 131–9.
5. Singer C, Underwood EA. A Short History of Medicine. 2nd ed. Oxford: Oxford University Press; 1962. p. 221–3.
6. Arnold D. Introduction: diseases, medicine and empire. In: Arnold D, editor. Imperial Medicine and Indigenous Societies. Manchester: Manchester University Press; 1988. p. 1–26.
7. Cook GC. Presidential Address. Evolution: the art of survival. Trans R Soc Trop Med Hyg 1994;89:4–18.
8. Cook GC. Some early British contributions to tropical disease. J Infect 1993;27:325–33.
9. Manson P. Tropical diseases: A Manual of the Diseases of Warm Climates. London: Cassell; 1898. p. 624.
10. Ross R. Memoirs: With a Full Account of the Great Malaria Problem and its Solution. London: John Murray; 1923. p. 547.
11. Cook GC. The Seamen's Hospital Society: a progenitor of the tropical institutions. Postgrad Med J 1999;75:715–17.
12. Cook GC. Disease in the Merchant Navy: A History of the Seamen's Hospital Society. Oxford: Radcliffe; 2007. p. 630.
13. Manson-Bahr P. History of the School of Tropical Medicine in London: 1899–1949. London: HK Lewis; 1956. p. 328.
14. Cook GC. Changing role(s) for the Royal Hospital, Greenwich. Hist Hosp 2001;22:35–46.
15. Manson-Bahr PH, Alcock A. The Life and Work of Sir Patrick Manson. London: Cassell; 1927. p. 273.
16. Manson P. The necessity for special education in tropical medicine. Lancet 1897;ii:842–5.
17. Cook GC. Doctor Patrick Manson's leading opposition in the establishment of the London School of Tropical Medicine: Curnow, Anderson, and Turner. J Med Biog 1995;3:170–7.
18. Cook GC, Webb AJ. The Albert Dock Hospital, London: the original site (in 1899) of Tropical Medicine as a new discipline. Acta Tropica 2001;79:249–55.
19. Hoare P. Spike Island: the Memory of a Military Hospital. London: Fourth Estate; 2001. p. 417.
20. May A. London School of Hygiene and Tropical Medicine 1899–1999. London: LSHTM; 1999. p. 40.
21. Manson P. London School of Tropical Medicine: the need for special training in tropical disease. J Trop Med 1899;2:57–62.
22. Cook GC. 'Tropical' cases admitted to the Albert Dock Hospital in the early years of the London School of Tropical Medicine. Trans R Soc Trop Med Hyg 1999;93:675–7.
23. Low GC. The history of the foundation of the Society of Tropical Medicine and Hygiene. Trans R Soc Trop Med Hyg 1928;22:197–202.
24. Cook GC. George Carmichael Low FRCP: Twelfth President of the Society and underrated pioneer of tropical medicine. Trans R Soc Trop Med Hyg 1993;87:355–60.
25. Cook GC. Aldo Castellani FRCP (1877–1971) and the founding of the Ross Institute and Hospital for Tropical Diseases at Putney. J Med Biog 2000;8:198–205.
26. Cook GC. A difficult metamorphosis: the incorporation of the Ross Institute and Hospital for Tropical Diseases into the London School of Hygiene and Tropical Medicine. Med Hist 2001;45:483–506.

27. Cook GC. Future structure of clinical tropical medicine in the United Kingdom. BMJ 1982; 284:1460–1.
28. Liverpool School of Tropical Medicine. Historical Record 1898–1920. Liverpool: University Press, 1920. p. 103.
29. Miller PJ. 'Malaria, Liverpool': An Illustrated History of the Liverpool School of Tropical Medicine 1898–1998. Liverpool: Liverpool School of Tropical Medicine; 1898. p. 78.
30. The study of tropical diseases in Liverpool. Lancet 1898;ii:1495.
31. The Liverpool School of Tropical Medicine. Lancet 1899;i:1174–6.
32. Worboys M. Manson, Ross and colonial medical policy: tropical medicine in London and Liverpool, 1899–1914. In: Macleod R, Lewis M, editors. Disease, Medicine and Empire: Perspectives on Western Medicine and the Experience of European Expansion. London: Routledge; 1988. p. 21–37.
33. Liverpool School of Tropical Medicine. BMJ 1914;i:324.
34. Maegraith BG. History of the Liverpool School of Tropical Medicine. Med Hist 1972;16:354–68.
35. Cook GC. Joseph William Bazalgette (1819–1891): a major figure in the health improvements of Victorian London. J Med Biog 1999; 7:17–24.
36. Cook GC. What can the Third World learn from the health improvements of Victorian Britain? Postgrad Med J 2005;81:763–4.
37. Cook GC. Tropical medicine. Lancet 1997; 350:813.

2 Global Health

ANDY HAINES | ANITA BERLIN

KEY POINTS

- Unprecedented growth in international travel and global trade, together with an increased flow of information and advances in the technology available to healthcare professionals are having a range of impacts on the determinants of health, the spread of disease and the functioning of health systems.
- Trade in pharmaceuticals is of obvious importance to health. In many other sectors trade liberalisation is having a significant impact on health and health services.
- Evidence suggests that the impacts of climate change will be concentrated on low-income countries where vulnerability is high and the capacity to adapt is limited. There is now growing evidence about the potential of policies which both address climate change goals and improve health.
- Following the financial crisis the growth in development assistance for health (DAH) has slowed. Some EU and G7 nations have reneged on DAH commitments made at the Gleneagles summit in 2005.
- A growing 'health industry' provided by for-profit healthcare organisations, particularly in the emerging economies of the BRIC countries, operates largely outside existing regulation. Deregulation and industrialisation is reflected in education systems with private medical schools leading to overproduction of professionals and a distortion of provision in some areas while others struggle to train and retain sufficient personnel.

Unprecedented growth in international travel, global trade and investment, and an increased flow of information and technology are having a pervasive impact on the determinants of health, the spread of disease and the functioning of health systems. As a consequence it is increasingly recognised that many determinants of health transcend national boundaries and the term 'global health 'is increasingly used to describe this phenomenon. A commonly used definition suggests that the transition from public health to global health occurs 'where the determinants of health or health outcomes circumvent, undermine or are oblivious to the territorial boundaries of states and thus beyond the capacity of individual countries alone to address through domestic institutions'.[1] In contrast international health has been defined as 'the application of the principles of public health to problems and challenges that affect low and middle-income countries and to the complex array of global and local forces that influence them'. International health may therefore imply a focus on improving health in countries other than one's own and, according to some, emphasizes differences rather than similarities between nations and the challenges facing them.[2]

Koplan and colleagues sought to define global health and clarify the differences between global, international and public health.[3] They distinguish between global health on the one hand and public and international health on the other on the grounds that for the former the development and implementation of solutions often requires global cooperation and highly interdisciplinary engagement beyond the health sciences as well as commitment to equitable access to health among nations and for all people. Unsurprisingly the term 'global health' has been contested, with some observers asserting that global health and public health are interchangeable concepts.[4] However, although the focus of both global and public health is on improving population health, some public health issues may be of largely national scope and relevance, for example the introduction of national legislation or taxation on tobacco products or unhealthy foods. Some authorities use the term 'global health' to refer principally to 'the goal of improving health for all people in all nations by promoting wellness and eliminating avoidable disease, disability, and death'.[5] The Institute of Medicine report for example suggests five priority topic areas in which the US Government and non-governmental sector could make contributions to improving health around the world. These comprise: scaling up existing interventions to achieve significant health gains; generating and sharing knowledge to address health problems endemic to the global poor; investing in people, institutions, and capacity building with global partners; increasing US financial commitments to global health; setting the example of engaging in respectful partnerships. Using 'global health' in this sense covers some of the terrain which has traditionally been the focus of 'international health'. In practice many initiatives blur the distinction between the two concepts.

Global health has also been used in the context of the study of the governance and impacts of global institutions that influence health such as the Global Fund to Fight AIDS, Tuberculosis and Malaria, the GAVI Alliance, the World Bank, WHO, the International Monetary Fund, etc.[6] There is also growing activity in the field of global health diplomacy which 'brings together the disciplines of public health, international affairs, management, law and economics and focuses on negotiations that shape and manage the global policy environment for health'. It encompasses interdisciplinary study of the two-way relationship between diplomacy and foreign policy on the one hand and health on the other and promotes education of diplomats in global health together with educational initiatives to improve mutual understanding with a special focus on the negotiation process – particularly the interface between technical and political issues that arise in global health agreements.[7–9]

There are a number of links between tropical medicine and global health, for example where global travel patterns result in significant numbers of imported infections with impacts on national health services and public health. In the case of the UK the Heath Protection Agency runs a 24-hour specialist service for medical professionals for the diagnosis of acute fevers due to travel-related infections, providing: '...expert clinical and microbiological advice to support patient management, infection control and public health interventions, from referral to delivery and interpretation of final results.'[10] Around 1700 imported cases of malaria were reported in the UK in 2011 with eight deaths.[11] Another example is the development in 2006 of The Global Network for Neglected Tropical Diseases (http://www.globalnetwork.org/neglected-tropical-diseases) which advocates for more international funding to address seven diseases which together afflict about one in six people around the world. Global trade patterns can influence vector-borne diseases, for example the spread of dengue has been linked to trade in used car tyres which contributes to the worldwide dispersal of important vector mosquitoes such as *Aedes albopictus* and *Ae. aegypti*.[12]

This chapter focuses on topics that can be encompassed by the definition of Lee and Collin[1], issues that cannot be effectively addressed by national governments working alone. It does not aim to be comprehensive but provides examples of key challenges in global health. It focuses particularly on the relationships between health on the one hand and trade and global environmental change on the other, as well as the effects of global institutions on national health policies and global influences on health professional education and training.

Trade and Health

The wide-ranging impacts of trade on health include the effects of the World Trade Organization's (WTO) Agreement on Trade-Related Aspects of Intellectual Property Rights (TRIPS) which sets global minimum standards for the protection of intellectual property.[13] Its consequence was to extend intellectual property rights, and generate substantial gains for the pharmaceutical industry in high-income country economies. Whilst patents have been the main mechanism by which pharmaceutical companies have assured a healthy return on investment, they have also proved to be barriers to access to affordable medications by poor populations. As a result, low- and middle-income country (LMIC) governments pressed for adoption of the WTO ministerial declaration on the TRIPS agreement and public health (the Doha Declaration) which was agreed in 2001.The Doha Declaration granted rights under article 8 to 'adopt measures necessary to protect public health and nutrition' through a number of provisions in the TRIPS agreement. These flexibilities include: identification of patentability standards that could prevent the patenting of minor modifications to existing drugs; the ability to grant compulsory licences to permit the production or sale of a drug by an independent party, with payment of a royalty to the patent owner, when drugs are not made available to meet public health needs or are not affordable and allowance of parallel imports of patented drugs legitimately sold in another country at lower prices without the consent of the patent holder. In response, the pharmaceutical industry with the support of the US Government and European Commission, has continued to seek increased patent protection, resorting to unilateral or bilateral negotiations to obtain TRIPS-plus conditions. In these cases protection of intellectual-property rights in excess of TRIPS are negotiated in exchange for trade concessions, particularly the promise of free access to markets for agricultural goods. These additional requirements may include: extension of patent rights beyond the usual 20-year term; prohibition of use of an already licensed and off-patent drug for a second indication and; imposing constraints on opposing or reviewing a patent.

Despite these manoeuvres, the pharmaceutical industry is facing unprecedented challenges worldwide with declining numbers of new medicines being licensed, although, at least until recently, expenditure on research and development (R&D) was increasing. Productivity as indicated by sales generated per $ of R&D expenditure has declined 70% between 1996–2004 and 2005–2010.[14] This has been accompanied by seismic changes in the industry resulting in extensive mergers and acquisitions. Generic medications are now becoming dominant even in high-income countries such as the USA, as a result of budgetary pressures which are likely to intensify even further in years to come.

Current mechanisms for financing and undertaking research in the sector are undergoing dramatic changes and are resulting in new relationships between universities, government-funded research institutions and smaller biotech and start-up companies which involves active scanning of the wider research environment for promising new compounds and technologies. This is also resulting in new approaches to intellectual property that promote collaboration whilst preserving the key rights of value to the licensor. In response to longstanding concerns about the failure of current market and publicly funded mechanisms to develop medicines that meet the needs of the poor and are affordable, discussions have taken place over several years under the auspices of WHO resulting in a series of reports and strategy documents including most recently the Consultative Expert Group on Research and Development: Financing and Coordination.[14] This Group has considered a number of financing mechanisms to support R&D against a range of pre-set criteria and highlighted two taxes for consideration, a Financial Transactions Tax and a Tobacco Solidarity Contribution. These, in addition to airline taxes already levied in some countries, could, they proposed, be channelled through international mechanisms to supplement national sources of funding. Whichever proposals are eventually adopted, it is abundantly clear that fundamental changes will be needed to the ways in which drug development is financed and undertaken, particularly to address the needs of the poor but even to meet the requirements of high-income countries.

Although trade in pharmaceuticals is of obvious importance to health, trade in many other sectors is also highly relevant, for example through the impact of trade liberalisation on health.[15] Trade liberalisation has been at the centre of a vigorous debate for many years, both because of its supposed central role in economic development and because of its contested role in contributing to improved health. It now seems likely that uncritical support of trade liberalisation as an engine of economic growth may have been misplaced. It is generally agreed that trade liberalisation by itself is insufficient to stimulate the economy. It appears that trade liberalisation has led to widening of income inequalities particularly as a result of growing rewards for skilled labour but stagnating incomes for many unskilled workers. These have obvious implications for health. In addition there are asymmetries between high- and low-income countries in their trade liberalisation policies. Although many low-income countries in Africa liberalised trade, OECD countries did not reduce their subsidies sufficiently quickly to create fair trading systems such that these still amount to around 376 bn euros annually on the part of the US, EU and Japan, vastly dwarfing their expenditure on development assistance.[16] Although duty and quota-free access for low-income countries is improving there are concerns that many of the benefits are concentrated in a relatively few countries.

Trade liberalisation contributes to profound changes in diet and nutrition for example by increasing the availability and marketing of calorie-rich and nutrient-poor processed food in low- and middle-income countries.[15] Some of the clearest evidence of the effects of such policies on health has been collected through studies of some Pacific Island populations where an increasing prevalence of obesity, diabetes and other non-communicable diseases has resulted.[17]

In response to declining sales in many high-income countries, multinational tobacco companies expanded their markets into Latin America in the 1960s, the emerging economies of Asia in the 1980s and into China, Africa and eastern Europe in the 1990s with a particular emphasis on marketing to young people, notably women.[18] Penetration of tobacco companies into world tobacco markets facilitated by the Uruguay round of trade negotiations, which included for the first time unmanufactured tobacco and regional trade agreements, also contributed to accelerating access by mandating further liberalisation of trade and services including tobacco.

From the perspective of global health a nuanced view of trade liberalisation is needed which seeks to maximise potential benefits from more equitable trade relationships and avoids harmful subsidies which can distort trade and disadvantage poor nations as well as having adverse effects on public health in developed nations. One example of the latter is the EU Common Agricultural Policy which encourages the consumption of high levels of saturated fats through subsidies to beef and dairy production and relatively disadvantages the production of mono- and polyunsaturated vegetable oils (such as olive, rape and sunflower oils) with adverse effects on cardiovascular risk.[19]

Even more fundamentally, the focus on market production (as measured by GDP) as an end in itself has been questioned and a growing number of voices are proposing that it is more appropriate to focus on human wellbeing as an indicator of societal success together with income and consumption at the household level.[20] Health is of course one of the key components of wellbeing but objective data should be complemented by the collection of more subjective measures of quality of life. Furthermore, inequalities in the distribution of economic and wellbeing indicators should be assessed together with the sustainability of policies in the light of threats such as climate change and biodiversity loss.

Global Environmental Change

It has been suggested that nine of the Earth's biophysical boundaries have been or will be exceeded in the foreseeable future, three are likely to have been exceeded already – climate change, the rate of biodiversity loss and nitrogen loading of the biosphere.[21] These boundaries indicate the limits within which there is reasonable assurance that systems can self-regulate and when they are exceeded non-linear, potentially irreversible changes may occur with serious but as yet uncertain consequences. The authors conclude that 'The human pressure on the Earth System has reached a scale where abrupt global environmental change can no longer be excluded'. Examples include melting of much of the polar ice caps or the loss of many coral reefs. Interactions between the boundaries may mean that crossing one may make it more likely that others could be exceeded. Four other boundaries are close to being exceeded – stratospheric ozone depletion, ocean acidification, global freshwater use and changes in land use – and in the cases of aerosol loading of the atmosphere and chemical pollution, the boundaries are highly uncertain.

Climate change, caused by the accumulation of greenhouse gases in the atmosphere largely as a result of fossil fuel combustion and land use change, poses serious challenges for human societies around the world.[22,23] The major greenhouse gas, carbon dioxide, is at its highest concentration in the atmosphere for at least 650 000 years. The first decade of this century has been, by far, the warmest decade on the instrumental record and all three major global surface temperature reconstructions show that Earth has warmed since 1880.[24] Average global temperatures are now some 0.75C° warmer than they were 100 years ago.

Of particular concern is that there may be 'tipping points' within the climate system which if exceeded will result in rapid change with incalculable consequences. The Greenland and Antarctic ice sheets, which between them store the majority of the world's fresh water, have both started to shrink. This melting reveals darker land and water surfaces that were beneath the snow and ice, which absorb more of the sun's heat, causing more warming, in a self-reinforcing cycle. The Greenland ice sheet contains sufficient water to cause a rise of 5–6 metres in sea level if it were to melt completely. Another example is the release of methane, a potent greenhouse gas from the tundra as the world warms.

Climate change is likely to have a range of effects on health, mostly adverse, through a range of mechanisms.[25–27] These include changes in the distribution of vector-borne diseases, increases in diarrhoeal disease, reductions in agricultural productivity particularly in low-income countries, the health consequences of extreme events – floods, droughts, heatwaves and intense tropical cyclones.

It has been known for many years that death rates increase during hot weather and the risk factors for death include being bed bound, inability to care for oneself and pre-existing psychiatric illness.[28] Temperatures are higher in urban areas because of the urban heat island effect. Elderly people are at particular risk and access to home air conditioning confers protection. However, air conditioning may interfere with acclimatization to heat and depends on access to reliable electricity supply which may be subject to grid failure during prolonged heatwaves. In some studies between 20% and 40% of deaths during heatwaves have been attributed to bringing forward the deaths of frail individuals by a few days or weeks. In prolonged heatwaves a higher proportion of deaths might arise in otherwise healthy individuals, or in low-income countries heat-related deaths from infectious diseases might be common.[29] Increased temperatures will also reduce the capacity for heavy physical labour which is common in many occupations, particularly in low-income countries and will therefore reduce economic productivity and increase poverty.[30]

Sub-Saharan Africa (SSA) has contributed the least to the global accumulation of greenhouse gas emissions; however, this region will be more vulnerable to the impacts of climate change than any other. WHO estimates suggest that the highest regional burden of climate change per million population is likely to be borne by SSA, with over one-third of the global disability adjusted life years (DALYs) attributable to climate change occurring there.[31] This conclusion is also shared by the Stern Review which suggests that 'the human consequences of climate change will be most serious and widespread in SSA, where millions more will die from malnutrition, diarrhoea, malaria and dengue fever, unless effective control measures are in place'.[32] Indeed, current evidence suggests that the impacts of climate change will be concentrated in low-income countries where poor populations already have a high burden of disease, health systems are weak, and where vulnerability is high and the capacity to adapt is limited.

Despite the growing awareness of Africa's vulnerability to climate change, there is surprisingly very little empirical evidence published about the effects of climate change on population health in Africa and few African scientists appear to be working on the topic.[33] Much of the work on climate change in SSA makes generalized predictions about the potential continent-wide effects of climate change with very few locally documented population studies. There is particular concern about impacts on agriculture and food security, droughts, floods, malaria and population displacement. The impacts are likely to be compounded by simultaneous exposure to multiple stressors both related to climate change, e.g. floods and malaria and other non-climate stressors (such as HIV/AIDS and poverty).[34] These multiple sources of vulnerability must be considered when designing climate change adaptation strategies.

At global mean temperature increases of above 2°C more than pre-industrial levels the likelihood of a range of serious impacts is high.[35] In the absence of policies to greatly reduce greenhouse gas (GHG) emissions it seems likely that the 2°C threshold will be exceeded, with one estimate suggesting a 5% probability that the upper limit of warming from a doubling of carbon dioxide could exceed 7.1°C. At this point parts of the earth's surface become effectively uninhabitable because they exceed the adaptability limit to thermal stress for human populations.[36] Global emissions will need to be cut by at least 50% of their 1990 levels by 2050 for the world to have a reasonable probability of staying below 2°C. However, that will be difficult to attain as emerging economies such as China and India are rapidly increasing their GHG emissions albeit from a lower base than developed countries. To stabilize atmospheric CO_2 at the current concentration, carbon emissions would need to be reduced to about 5.5 billion tonnes, the amount that is taken up by the oceans and land, this would constitute an immediate 45% reduction in global emissions of CO_2.[37]

The perceived cost of 'low-carbon' technologies and policies often constitute barriers to the deep cuts in emissions that are required but there are also a range of benefits to society that will result from their implementation. For example there is a growing body of evidence about the potential range of policies which could both address climate change goals and improve health. The term 'health co-benefits' is becoming widely used to describe the ancillary or collateral benefits to health arising from low-carbon technologies, policies and lifestyles in a number of sectors. These benefits are additional to those which would result from a reduction in projected climate change. They could offset part, and in some cases all, of the increased costs of action by for example reducing health care costs and increasing labour productivity. The main health co-benefits of policies to reduce greenhouse gas accumulation arise from technologies and policies in the following sectors: transport, food and agriculture, housing and electricity generation, each responsible for large emissions of GHGs and with major influences on health.[38]

In the case of urban transport, increasing active travel (walking and cycling) together with reduced car use and more efficient vehicles with lower emissions of GHGs and fine particulates could have substantial benefits for health, particularly due to increased physical activity. Seven conditions – ischaemic heart disease, cerebrovascular disease, diabetes, depression, breast cancer, colorectal cancer and dementia have been shown by robust epidemiological evidence to be related to sedentary lifestyle and the disease burden arising from them could be reduced by increasing active travel.[39]

Substantial reductions in ischaemic heart disease could result from reducing the consumption of animal products (particularly beef and other red meat) in high consuming populations as a consequence of decreased saturated fat consumption accompanied by increased intake of polyunsaturated fats of plant origin.[40] Agriculture is responsible for around 10–12% of global GHG emissions with additional contributions arising from deforestation to clear land for crops or livestock. Around 80% of GHG emissions in the food and agriculture sector are thought to come from livestock, both nitrous oxide from land used to grow feed crops and methane from ruminants such as cows and sheep.

In the UK the housing sector is currently responsible for around 26% of the total carbon dioxide emissions and many houses use energy inefficiently. A programme of improved insulation and ventilation control for the most tightly sealed houses could reduce deaths, particularly those due to fine particulate pollution, provide warmer indoor environments and cut GHG emissions by over one-third. Switching to renewable or other low-carbon sources of electricity would yield further reductions.[41] In poor countries introducing high-efficiency cookstoves can reduce household air pollution which causes over 3 million deaths per annum, as well as reducing emissions of black carbon and other greenhouse pollutants.[41a]

Reducing coal combustion for electricity generation could lower fine particulate matter ($PM_{2.5}$) air pollution and GHG emissions. Major reductions in deaths due to air pollution could be achieved in countries such as India and China, where background levels of air pollution are high, but even in regions such as the EU where air pollution levels are lower, reducing coal combustion could still result in worthwhile improvements in health.[42]

Recognition of these health co-benefits and their attendant economic benefits can make political decisions in favour of low-carbon policies more palatable, particularly in a time of economic difficulty and should achieve more prominence in international negotiations to reduce GHGs.

Global Health Institutions and Development Aid for Health

Over the past decade or so there has been a dramatic transformation in the institutional landscape of global health with the ascendance of global health initiatives such as the Global Fund to Fight AIDS, TB and Malaria and the GAVI Alliance which have raised large sums of money for essential health care and immunisation programmes respectively. At the same time multiple donors and disease-specific initiatives are operating at global and national levels with their own priorities, contributing to high transaction costs and sometimes distorting national priorities. This can lead to inefficiencies at the country level for example because of the need to prepare different reports for a range of donors.[6] Despite their role in sustaining vital treatment and immunisation programmes there is as yet little evidence that global health initiatives have had a decisive role in strengthening national health systems.[43] A systematic approach to health systems strengthening would require actions to support the ability of the entire health system to collect, pool and spend the necessary finances to become sustainable; to deliver effective, appropriate, efficient and equitable health care; to develop the human and other resources to make this happen and to provide the stewardship for effective governance. This should be distinguished from selective attempts to support specific parts of the health system to enhance the delivery of care for specific diseases.

Following the financial crisis development assistance for health (DAH) is growing at a slower rate than previously, for example having grown strongly over the past decade US DAH grew at only 2% between 2010 and 2011.[44] Growth of DAH for HIV, TB and health systems slowed but DAH for malaria grew rapidly by 50% 2 years in a row and the growth in DAH for maternal, newborn and child health and for non-communicable diseases also accelerated. So far the global financial crisis does not appear to have slowed total public domestic spending on health which amounted to around 16 times the resources contributed by donors.

However, the commitments of some of the EU and G7 countries made at the Gleneagles summit in 2005 have not been kept.[45] The G7 increased their annual development assistance to sub-Saharan Africa by $11.197 billion between 2004 and 2010, delivering 61% of the $18.227 billion increases they promised in 2005. The increases were largely due to the US, Japan and Canada surpassing their (relatively modest) targets and the UK nearly meeting its ambitious commitment. Three countries – Italy, Germany and France – were responsible for most of the G7's shortfall. Germany and Italy fell short of their committed funding goals by a combined $7.11 billion, and France by $1.34 billion. Overall the EU delivered only 35% of its committed increases to the region. However, several members of the EU15 are consistently high donors. Four of these – Denmark, Luxembourg, the Netherlands and Sweden – maintained their target ODA/GNI ratios of 0.7% or above. Only Denmark and Luxembourg have met the official EU target for sub-Saharan Africa. Over the past decade or so, the role of BRICs (Brazil, Russia, India and China) and other emerging economies and the private sector in Sub-Saharan Africa have grown substantially. Though the main impact on Africa will be through increased trade and investment, the role of emerging economies as donors is becoming increasingly salient.[46]

The Task Force on Innovative International Financing for Health Systems (2009)[47] called for an additional $10 bn of international donor funding to support attainment of the UN Millennium Development Goals as well as increased domestic financing of health. This is essential to address the severe lack of funds in low-income countries which spend on average $24 per capita annually on health compared with a typical sum of $4000 in rich countries. The Task Force suggested a number of innovative approaches to raising resources internationally that should be explored. Their recommendations included: expanding the mandatory solidarity levy on airline tickets; assessing the technical viability of other solidarity levies on tobacco and currency transactions; expanding the use of the International Financing Facility for Immunization and other approaches to ensure predictability and providing public catalytic funding for large-scale private giving.

In order to enhance the impact of DAH through global health initiatives and bilateral donors, there needs to be convergence of thinking on what constitutes health systems strengthening and the role of different agencies to make universal coverage with affordable health care a reality. More progress is needed to harmonise the assessment of aid effectiveness, build the evidence base for health systems strengthening and support the development of national mechanisms which enable countries to address their own priorities where governments are committed and able to do so. Investments in disease-specific programmes should aim to support the broader health system, for example by ensuring that the payment of higher salaries to health workers in priority programmes does not result in 'poaching' of staff from elsewhere in the health system or that improved supply chains for one disease also contribute to improving delivery of essential medications for other diseases. In a time of economic difficulty it will be particularly vital to ensure that resources are used efficiently and that expenditure on health by both donors and national governments can be justified to their taxpayers.

Global Influences on Health Professional Education and the Health Professional Marketplace

Globalising phenomena have a significant impact on the healthcare workforce – in terms of their preparation and distribution. Strong health systems require investment in capacity building including human resource development through training and education. A key challenge is ensuring relevance of education focussed primarily on local health needs but also alert to transnational influences, threats and responsibilities. The makeup of the health workforce needs to adapt to demographic, socioeconomic and epidemiological changes but is also a clear reflection of these: the emptying of a bedpan in New York or Stockholm pays a child's school fee or healthcare bill in Sri Lanka or the Philippines.

Globally around a million healthcare professionals are trained each year in nearly 2500 medical schools, 500 schools of public health and an indeterminate number of nursing institutions.[48] Between them China, India, Brazil and the USA now account for more than 600 medical schools whereas 36 countries in SSA have no or one medical school. Reliable data on nursing schools are almost impossible to obtain. However, there are severe shortages with mal-distribution of institutions and trained professionals within and between countries resulting in pronounced gaps worldwide between high- and low-income countries and national urban–rural imbalances. There is little alignment between training provision and burden of disease compounded by the huge mobility of healthcare professionals.[49]

Although there are increasing demands on health care most economies offer relatively unattractive working conditions for health professionals. This combination of increasing demand and relatively poor local rewards stimulates a global market in trained health professionals – with, for instance, British midwives working in Australia, Senegalese nurses in France, and South African doctors in the UK.[50]

The Philippine economy, for example, depends on this market. The health system is weak and health professional training does not always match local need. It is even orientated towards working aboard with the remittances of migrant healthcare workers forming a major stream of income to the national economy.[51] Many European health systems have depended on this human flow for decades.[49] In 2005 at least 10% of all nurses in Europe qualified in another country.[50] In the UK 30% of doctors are not home trained – which represents a considerable saving on training costs for the host health system and a tragic brain drain for many countries.[52] Figures are not available for the proportion of migrant ancillary staff from the global south that mop and scrub European and North American healthcare facilities. Overall around 80% of the global healthcare workforce is female[53] – millions of women are displaced so that it is not just the 'brains' that are drained by economic migration but whole, often educated, women – daughters and mothers – separated from their communities, families and children, in a vicious cycle.

A growing 'health industry' provided by local and multinational for-profit healthcare organisations, particularly in the emerging economies of the BRIC countries, operates largely outside existing regulation. The deregulation and industrialisation of health care is reflected in education systems. For-profit medical schools have led to overproduction of professionals and a distortion of provision. Since the 1980s the number of private medical schools in India has increased eightfold while the public schools have trebled. There have been suggestions of illegal payments[54] to regulatory bodies in India facilitating this growth. In Brazil, although the health system has expanded successfully[55] requiring more doctors and nurses, many new schools are private, for-profit and poorly regulated.[48]

Where training institutions create an oversupply, professionals who do not migrate inevitably compete for income. Coupled with weak health systems and poor regulation this leads to gross distortions of health care provided. In parts of Latin American the most common surgical procedure is breast augmentation, often a birthday present to a teenager, and many countries of the south and east (and increasingly the economically precarious north) actively promote health tourism largely for cosmetic interventions.[56]

Looking back a century the Flexner report on medical education[57] can be seen as a foundation stone in the globalisation of healthcare by establishing a model for science-based university-led medical education with a sustained worldwide reach. Subsequent reports on nursing[58] and public health[59] had similar effects. While raising standards they also ensured a colonial approach to content, assessment and regulation with no regard to local educational and health need or relevance. The interconnected world and the shared impacts of global mobilities and environmental change, coupled with requirements to ensure synergy with appropriate health systems, demand new approaches to the health professional curriculum in the broadest sense. New knowledge grows and spreads fast, and solutions to complex health needs and environmental threats require interdisciplinary thinking and action.

Calls for reforms often focus on the need for relevance and competency in patient- and population-centred care. Many commentators recognise the need for greater teamwork but many are concerned about single professions (see for example, Irby et al , 2010) .[60] The Lancet commission 'Health professionals for a new century'[48] and recent joint WHO/PEPFAR initiatives,[61] explicitly consider the importance of taking a cross-disciplinary perspective.

A focus on explicit competences allows for clarity of training objectives and hugely assists robust assessments. The competences serve to demarcate the core skills of each professional and facilitate accreditation of programmes. However, they emphasise credentialisation with the risk of inflexibility of individual practice and increased tension between professionals rather than promoting greater collaboration.

Despite research evidence of the important role of primary care in effective and efficient health systems[62] and the essential contribution of community health workers particularly in low- and middle-income settings, these tend to be underdeveloped in curricula which are often dominated by specialised hospital clinical care. The potential of a step-ladder approach to 'transprofessional' education – through which health workers can progress if they show ability from a basic health worker to nursing, medical or other healthcare qualifications. The step ladder may serve to attract disadvantaged young people into health care and offers prospects for their future.

Entirely competency-based approaches to curricula tend to constrain practice to a defined list of acceptable behaviours and there is increasing evidence for the use of multiple approaches to training to encourage agency, advocacy and critical thinking in the learner.[63] Without these so-called transformative capabilities future professionals will be unable to adapt their own practice to address the changing and globally interconnected demands on them and their patient populations nor ensure the sustainability of their health systems.

While many nations struggle to establish their own training programmes, universities in the resource-rich countries are internationalising and globalising their enterprises often with the objective of attracting fee-paying overseas students, setting up prestigious off-shore campuses or establishing international educational networks and partnerships.

The worldwide web and mobile technologies are increasingly supporting learning in a myriad of contexts and can reduce educational disparities between rural–urban settings and high- and lower-income nations. Students and staff can collaborate directly across national settings and international publications and course materials can be freely shared. Within countries mobile technologies increasingly supply immediate support in remote locations.[64] This combination of closer institutional links and rapid knowledge exchange draws healthcare workers, current and future, together in an instant but raises questions of relevance, moral authority and power gradients.

Concerns regarding commercial expansion of universities, mal-distribution of health professional institutions and workforce mobility have led to transnational interventions from formal international agencies, aid organisations and unaligned NGOs with a combination of monitoring, funding and campaigning. In an effort to move away from direct aid funders are supporting university partnerships. The largest projects are the Nursing and the Medical Education Partnership Initiatives (NEPI and MEPI) the latter with 30 African partners linked to 20 north American collaborators to the tune of $130 million from the US government as part of America's response to the MDGs.[65] Such programmes have huge potential for good but are fraught with concerns regarding lack of mutuality, paternalism and neo-colonialism.[66,67] Exchange for staff and elective placements for students can be transformative experiences but lead to legitimate accusations of one-way 'edu-tourism' without sustainable investment in the host university infrastructure.

Ostensibly intended to reverse some of the colonial effects of the extensive uptake of the Flexner model, programmes such as MEPI and NEPI designed to support and strengthen local educational development may be at risk of implementing, as with the Flexner model a century ago, curricula that lack relevance to local needs. There is a danger that donor-driven educational and broader capacity building initiatives may promote approaches to the organisation and delivery of health care that reflect the prevailing system in the donor country and do not reflect the needs of the 'recipient' country, particularly with regard to the importance of scaling up primary healthcare programmes. It has been observed that such north–south partnerships need to be more inclusive of local expertise, less reliant on exogenous ideas and may be less effective than south–south collaborations.[68] Clearly thorough evaluation is required.

One response to the challenges posed by health professional migration and partnerships between educational institutions is stewardship through transnational monitoring, governance and regulation. International agencies assume or are given responsibilities previously located in nation-states. Here the sustainability of local health systems and influences on healthcare worldwide coincide and attempt to bridge the divide between global solutions and the need for local adaptability and self-determination. Concerned about the cost and ethics of the healthcare professional market, the WHO produced a Global Code of Practice on the International Recruitment of Health Personnel in 2006, advocating reciprocal support for health system development from recipient to home countries and a commitment to facilitating 'circular migration'.[53] This Code recognises the problem and solution but needless to say is voluntary. Further evidence of genuine concern for achieving a better, more responsible governance of training organisations includes the Global Consensus for Social Accountability of Medical Schools,[69] also voluntary. These documents highlight consensus on complex scientific, practical and ethical challenges. The documents also have implications for the growing number of students studying at off-shore campuses of universities based in high income countries such as the USA and the UK. These students want a US or UK medical degree and the regulatory bodies accrediting them should ask themselves: how is this institution strengthening. The students studying at off-shore campuses want a US or UK medical degree and regulators ask themselves: How is this institution strengthening local healthcare provision? Or how do we licence a medical school when students visit mental hospitals where homosexuals receive compulsory treatment? Healthcare and the training of health professionals in one continent impact on the health system of another and then ricochet back home again across vast distances.

The role of the health professional school goes beyond educating students about biomedical sciences to support interdisciplinary practice cognisant of relevance and context in the broadest sense to protect the health of and provide care for individuals and populations in our ever more vulnerable planet. Increasingly this is likely to involve integrating the emerging knowledge of global health into health professional curricula and ensuring that the many other professions whose actions influence health across national borders are aware of the impacts of their professional activities.

The emerging challenges of global health will undoubtedly feature more prominently in research, policy and education agendas over coming decades. Current institutions are often poorly configured to address these challenges and in order to do so fundamental re-orientation is needed to promote greater transnational and inter-disciplinary collaboration to tackle rapidly evolving threats to health as well as capitalising on new opportunities.

REFERENCES

6. Balabanova D, McKee M, Mills A, et al. What can global health institutions do to help strengthen health systems in low income countries? Health Res Policy Syst 2010;8:22, doi:10.1186/1478-4505-8-22.
9. Drager N, Fidler D. Foreign policy, trade and health: at the cutting edge of global health diplomacy. Bull World Health Organ 2007; 85:162.
15. Consultative Expert Group on Research and Development: Financing and Coordination. Research and Development to Meet Health Needs in Developing Countries; Strengthening Global Financing and Coordination. Geneva: WHO; 2011.
39. Haines A, McMichael AJ, Smith KR, et al. Public health benefits of strategies to reduce greenhouse-gas emissions: overview and implications for policy makers. Lancet 2009;374: 2104–14.
54. World Health Organization. The World Health Report 2006 – Working together for health. Geneva: WHO; 2002. Available at: http://www.who.int/whr/2006/en/ Accessed 20/9/2012.

Access the complete references online at www.expertconsult.com

3

Global Health Governance and Tropical Diseases

TILL BÄRNIGHAUSEN | DAVID E. BLOOM | SALAL HUMAIR

KEY POINTS

- 'Global health governance comprises the means adopted to promote global health decision-making and the actions undertaken to pursue common global health goals,along with the underlying architecture of global health institutions, initiatives and actors that facilitate these means and actions
- GHG is a key factor influencing health outcomes at the global scale.
- Over the past decade, the GHG system has increased dramatically in size and complexity.
- GHG has achieved remarkable successes against some tropical diseases in the past half centurybut, going forward, it faces several challenges.
- The current GHG system has several weaknesses, such as lack of participation, lack of transparency, political unaccountability and operational inefficiency.
- The system also has several strengths such as its capacity for innovation, flexibility, and the ability to attract a motivated workforce and to encourage entrepreneurship.
- To adequately address tropical diseases in the future, the GHG system will need to address some of its weaknesses, while preserving its strengths.

Background

In 2000, in the hopes of dramatically reducing poverty and boosting living standards worldwide, the global community adopted eight Millennium Development Goals (MDGs) to be met by 2015. The level to which the world has been successful in achieving these goals is instructive for combating tropical diseases at the global level.[1] Three of the MDGs are specific to health, and others indirectly involve health as a stepping stone to a better standard of living. However, recent reports suggest that MDG 4 (aiming to reduce child mortality by two-thirds) and MDG 5 (aiming to reduce maternal mortality by three-quarters) are unlikely to be reached by 2015. As for MDG 6, one part of it may be achieved (aiming to halt and reverse the spread of malaria and tuberculosis), but the part that has to do with controlling HIV looks out of reach, as the incidence of new infections continues to outpace the number of people being added to those receiving HIV treatment. It is becoming increasingly clear that reaching these goals hinges on substantially improved and accelerated action by the global community.

What determines these and other critical public health outcomes at the global scale? A key factor is the manner in which the world makes and implements decisions about global health. Broadly, such decisions involve choosing areas of global health the world should focus on (such as health workers, drugs, primary health, specific diseases), raising funds for addressing issues in these areas, creating organizational structures for managing these funds, creating processes for directing these funds to implementing agencies (such as processes for grant or loan solicitation and grant-making), monitoring implementing agencies and evaluating implementation outcomes.

Global health governance comprises the means adopted to promote such decision-making and the actions undertaken to pursue common global health goals,[2] along with the underlying architecture of global health institutions, initiatives and actors[3] that facilitate these means and actions. This architecture plays a vital role in determining health outcomes within countries, and for specific diseases, as evidenced by the advances against HIV in the past decade.

In this chapter, we briefly review the overall system of global health governance and its evolution over the last decade, the emerging challenges it faces, its strengths and weaknesses, and how these strengths and weaknesses affect the system's ability to address tropical diseases in the future.

GLOBAL HEALTH GOVERNANCE TODAY

The system of global health governance has changed dramatically since the World Health Organization (WHO) was founded in 1948.[4] The WHO still remains at the centre of this system, but it increasingly shares responsibility and agenda-setting with other organizations. In fact, the current system is highly fragmented, involving a large array of multinational, national and private organizations with overlapping missions and responsibilities, a diverse set of fundraising and fund disbursement mechanisms, and a range of monitoring and evaluation standards.[5] Table 3.1 lists a limited selection of the key bilateral, multilateral and private actors in global health. To this list other actors could be added, such as multi-country networks (e.g. the 'Group of Eight' and the 'Group of Twenty') and civil society.

One indicator of the influence of these organizations, is the level of funding they provide for global health, for instance, consider Table 3.2 on bilateral official development assistance (ODA), Table 3.3 on multilateral ODA and Table 3.4 on international health grants given by a few US-based foundations in 2010. Even though the numbers in these tables are only a limited snapshot of total giving by some institutions (not including, e.g. the cumulative overseas health expenditures by large non-governmental organizations, such as Food for the Poor, Population Services International, etc.), they do show that the emergence of new multilateral institutions like the GAVI Alliance and the Global Fund to Fight HIV, Tuberculosis and Malaria (GFATM) has reduced the dominance of WHO, other traditional UN agencies and some donor countries. Together with the emergence of global private philanthropy – once relatively insignificant but now a significant fraction of all

TABLE 3.1 A Large Range of Institutions Play An Important Role in Global Health Governance

Multilateral Institutions	Bilateral Institutions	Philanthropic Institutions	Humanitarian Institutions
UN System	AusAID (Australia)	Abbott Fund	(MSF) Médicins Sans Frontières
UNAIDS	ADA (Austria)	Bill & Melinda Gates Foundation	Oxfam
UNFPA	CIDA (Canada)	Ford Foundation	(IRC) International Rescue Committee
UNICEF	DANIDA (Denmark)	The Bloomberg Family Foundation, Inc.	Save the Children
World Health Organization	FINIDA (Finland)	The David and Lucile Packard Foundation	Merlin
World Bank	AFD (France)	The John D. and Catherine T. MacArthur Foundation	
Regional Multi-Laterals	GIZ (Germany)	The Merck Company Foundation	
African Development Bank	Irish Aid (Ireland)	The Rockefeller Foundation	
Asian Development Bank	JICA (Japan)	The Susan Thompson Buffett Foundation	
European Bank for Reconstruction and Development	NZAID (New Zealand)	The William and Flora Hewlett Foundation	
Inter-American Development Bank	NORAD (Norway)	The William and Sue Gross Family Foundation	
Specialized Multi-Laterals	KOICA (Korea)	Wellcome Trust	
Global Fund for AIDS, Tuberculosis, and Malaria	AECID (Spain)		
GAVI Alliance	SIDA (Sweden)		
UNITAID	SDC (Switzerland)		
	DFID (UK)		
	USAID (USA)		

TABLE 3.2 A Few Countries Account for Most Public Health Aid (Overseas Development Assistance for Public Health in 2010 by Development Assistance Committee (DAC) Countries)

	ODA for Public Health	
	US$ Million	% of Total ODA to Public Health
Total DAC countries	15315	13
USA	7809	23
Japan	2226	13
Germany	1016	9
France	859	8
Spain	501	11
Australia	405	11
Canada	347	9
Korea	339	19
UK	282	6
Netherlands	275	4
Denmark	208	12
Sweden	195	6
Norway	194	5
Belgium	138	7
Finland	117	11
Switzerland	114	6
Italy	109	11
Ireland	72	12
Luxembourg	64	21
Austria	24	4
New Zealand	14	5
Portugal	4	1
Greece	2	1

Source: OECD Statistics 2012. Current prices (data extracted on 18 May 2012).
Includes Overseas Development Assistance (ODA) for basic health, population and reproductive health, and water and sanitation.

TABLE 3.3 Numerous Multilateral Institutions Are Active in Public Health (Overseas Development Assistance for Public Health in 2010 by Multilateral Institutions)

	ODA	
	US$ Million	% of ODA to Public Health
Total multilateral funding	8963	19
Global Fund	3128	100
IDA	1827	13
EU Institutions	1383	10
GAVI	697	89
AsDB Special Funds	356	14
UNFPA	316	100
UNICEF	229	22
AfDF	205	9
UNAIDS	164	67
WHO	134	37
OFID	132	21
AFESD	109	9
UNRWA	98	18
Islamic Dev Bank	76	20
IDB Special Fund	59	8
UNDP	25	4

Source: OECD Statistics 2012. Current prices (data extracted on 18 May 2012).
Includes Overseas Development Assistance (ODA) for basic health, population and reproductive health, and water and sanitation.

development aid for health[6] – and the emergence of dominant players like the Bill & Melinda Gates Foundation, the landscape of global health has undergone a major transformation in the past decade.

To understand global health governance, we therefore need to understand how these institutions interact with each other, with the private sector and with civil society to exchange information and technical skills, and establish rules for health programmes that promote health worldwide. Moreover, global health governance matters greatly for tropical diseases, which still are rampant in many developing countries (Box 3.1). The governance system generates funding for these diseases, decides on disease priorities and funding levels, selects the interventions for priority diseases that should receive funding, monitors performance and gives account of its activities.

Challenges Facing the System of Global Health Governance for Tropical Diseases

Several issues shape the ability of the global health governance system to successfully prevent, treat or eliminate tropical diseases. They include the following.

TABLE 3.4 Gates Leads by Far Private Philanthropy for Global Health (Top 20 US Foundations Awarding International Grants for Health in 2010)

Foundation	US$ Million
Bill & Melinda Gates Foundation	1311
The Susan Thompson Buffett Foundation	82
The Bloomberg Family Foundation, Inc.	56
The David and Lucile Packard Foundation	25
Ford Foundation	22
The Rockefeller Foundation	22
The William and Flora Hewlett Foundation	19
The John D. and Catherine T. MacArthur Foundation	15
The Merck Company Foundation	12
The William and Sue Gross Family Foundation	12
Abbott Fund	10
Howard G. Buffett Foundation	10
The Bristol-Myers Squibb Foundation, Inc.	10
The PepsiCo Foundation, Inc.	8
China Medical Board, Inc.	7
Ann and Robert H. Lurie Foundation	6
ExxonMobil Foundation	6
Conrad N. Hilton Foundation	6
The Medtronic Foundation	5
Eli Lilly and Company Foundation	4

Source: Foundation Center 2012. Current prices (data extracted on 18 May 2012).

FUNDING FOR GLOBAL HEALTH IS EITHER STAGNANT OR DECLINING

Although global health has attracted considerable attention and funding over the past decade, enthusiasm for increased or even stable funding by multilaterals and bilaterals is declining. One reason is the economic contraction brought about by the global financial crisis of 2008.[10] In its wake, the global community has been coping with a slow recovery in the USA, natural disasters in Japan, continuing and perhaps worsening perils in the European Union, and a slowdown in China. In the USA, for example, the President's proposed budget for fiscal year 2013 calls for a net reduction in funding for AIDS, counterbalanced only in part by increased funding for TB and malaria. At the global level, bilateral funding for public health continued to rise in 2009 but then fell off in 2010 to below 2008 levels (Table 3.5). Multilateral funding followed a similar path but stayed about the same from 2009 to 2010. Bilateral funding for malaria, TB and STDs suffered only a small decline, but the corresponding multilateral funding declined notably. In addition, some funding commitments for 2009 were not even realized, as shown by higher commitment-to-disbursement ratios in recent years.[11]

Rapid population ageing is perhaps the most salient and dynamic aspect of modern demography. To an ever greater extent, people all over the world are living longer and then dying predominantly of non-communicable diseases (NCDs) – primarily cardiovascular diseases, cancers, chronic obstructive pulmonary diseases and diabetes – rather than from the infectious diseases that were historically the primary cause of death. This trend is particularly prominent in the developed world, where infectious diseases have become much less of a concern, but population ageing is also accelerating in the developing world. As a result, tropical countries are beginning to shoulder a double burden. They still have high rates of infectious diseases (many of which lack a cure) but they are now experiencing

TABLE 3.5 Development Aid for Public Health Is Slipping (Funding Commitment for Public Health and Specific Tropical Diseases)

	2006	2007	2008	2009	2010
Total Public Health Funding					
Total DAC countries	11731	13980	17040	17792	15315
Total multilaterals	5969	7198	6658	8457	8963
Total Funding Malaria, TB, STDs Including HIV/AIDS					
Total DAC countries	3335	5321	6370	6436	6203
Total multilaterals	2371	3206	2651	4737	3559

DAC, Development Assistance Committee; TB, tuberculosis; STD, sexually transmitted diseases. Non-communicable diseases are attracting more attention.
Source: OECD Statistics 2012. Current prices (data extracted on 18 May 2012).

BOX 3.1 A SNAPSHOT OF TROPICAL DISEASES AND GLOBAL HEALTH GOVERNANCE

What exactly are 'tropical diseases'? We use the term in its traditional definition – that is, diseases that are unique to or are more prevalent in tropical and sub-tropical areas and that typically are infectious. Examples include vaccine-preventable diseases such as smallpox and polio; diseases responsible for major epidemics that have received considerable attention over the past decade, such as HIV, tuberculosis (TB) and malaria; and relatively neglected diseases, such as schistosomiasis and dengue. The 'tropics' covers the zone between the Tropic of Cancer and the Tropic of Capricorn; the 'sub-tropics' refers to areas just outside that zone (latitudinally). In this chapter, 'tropical' refers to both areas, in effect encompassing all developing countries and parts of a few developed ones where the disease ecology (e.g. hot climate, abundant rainfall, large number of potential insect vectors, potential vector breeding grounds, large number of potential pathogens) facilitates the transmission of tropical diseases.

Over the past half century, the global health system has had some major successes in the fight against tropical diseases – such as eliminating smallpox, nearly eradicating polio and developing oral rehydration therapy (ORT) for diarrhoea. Smallpox and polio, although not exclusive to the tropics, were major scourges in those regions. In addition to these diseases, the incidence of other infections that are often fatal and extremely common in the tropics has been significantly reduced by the provision of clean water and sanitation, along with ORT.

Because of these successes, people in specific populations live longer, commonly into old age, when they become vulnerable to old-age diseases. For instance, in countries with high HIV prevalence, high antiretroviral treatment (ART) coverage brings into existence a 'new' population group – ageing HIV-infected people receiving ART, who have a bigger risk of cardiovascular disease owing to ageing and the interdependent effects of HIV and ART.[7–9]

Thus, the past successes in combating tropical diseases are creating new challenges for the future, creating a need to modify the governance system appropriately. Moreover, the continued high incidence and prevalence of other tropical diseases (increasingly concentrated in certain regions) and the greater burden of morbidity (rather than mortality) from these diseases, means an outdated global health governance system could lead to poorer health in tropical countries in the future.

increased rates of NCDs as people live longer. Moreover, for several important diseases, successful treatment comes at the price of higher NCD morbidity and mortality.

In recent years, NCDs have registered prominently on the global health agenda. They were the subject of a high-level meeting of the General Assembly of the United Nations, in September 2011, which led to a political commitment from the heads of states to combat them.[12] This was only the second time that a high-level UN meeting has been dedicated to a health topic (the first time being on HIV/AIDS in 2001). Given that developed countries, which control most of the funding on any issue, are highly concerned about NCDs, it is a distinct possibility that funding for the prevention and treatment of tropical diseases may suffer, as scarce resources are directed towards NCDs.

TROPICAL DISEASES, WHERE THEY ARE STILL PREVALENT, IMPOSE A HUGE BURDEN

Where tropical diseases are still prevalent, they not only account for a large share of morbidity and mortality[13,14] but they also disproportionately affect certain subsets of the population and impose a significant economic burden.

Setting aside the big three: HIV, TB and malaria – the group of 17 neglected tropical diseases are endemic in 149 countries and affect over 1 billion people – mostly the poor, and among them, infants and children.[15,16] Children are particularly badly affected, with such diseases having led to the persistence of high infant mortality rates (IMR) in most developing countries. In the world's least developed countries, the IMR fell from 125 infant deaths per thousand live births in 1980–1985 to 73 today (mid-2012), whereas in the more developed regions, it had already declined to 60 by the early 1950s.

A high IMR has also impeded economic growth by limiting progress on reducing the total fertility rate (TFR). For the poorest countries, the TFR declined from 6.5 children per woman in the early 1980s to 4.1 today, whereas in the more developed regions, the TFR had already declined to 2.8 by the early 1950s. The combination of a high IMR and low fertility decline has slowed growth of the working-age share of the population, imposing a constant demographic disadvantage on economies. Further, tropical diseases often impede long-run planning, as periodic outbreaks sap local budgets and, at times, cause political chaos.[17]

Defining 'Good Governance'

Given the challenges that the system of global health governance needs to address to combat tropical diseases over the coming decades, it is important to ask how well-prepared the current system is for this task and how far it needs reform to meet the challenge.

'Good governance' is notoriously difficult to define. Several different definitions have been proposed[18–22] and many have been challenged, because they consist of a set of concepts that are too abstract.[23] Rather than debate what constitutes 'good governance', we simply use some of the commonly identified attributes of 'good governance' to provide an overview of the current thinking on global health governance,[24] and discuss its good and bad aspects. However, our use of these attributes does not imply that we think that they are individually necessary or jointly sufficient for governance to be 'good'. In fact, in the following discussion of the *strengths* of the current system of global health governance for tropical diseases, we discuss how some of the factors that are identified as reasons for weaknesses can also give rise to beneficial effects.

Weaknesses of the Current System of Global Health Governance

PARTICIPATION

The current system of global health governance has been criticized as lacking in participation[25] – which the UN defines as involvement of those who are directly or indirectly affected by a health policy through representation in the system of governance that decides the policy.[16] In a narrow sense, the problem arises because some of the key global health institutions are set up by individual donors or private firms who are not required to invite any particular group of people to participate in their decision-making – whether or not a group is affected by the decisions.

Prominently, this criticism has been levelled at the Bill & Melinda Gates Foundation. For instance, Devi Sridhar asserts that one result of the Gates Foundation's generosity towards global health is that almost every university department, think-tank, civil society group or partnership working on global health issues is directly or indirectly receiving funding from it. She goes on to argue that the new money available for global health, in particular for HIV interventions, 'is radically skewing public health and medical programmes towards the issues of greatest concern to the donors, *but not necessarily of top priority for people in recipient states*' [our emphasis].[4]

For tropical diseases, one hope for increased participation[26] was the formation of new partnerships, widening the involvement of different public and private groups working across different sectors.[25] Such partnerships included: the Global Fund to Fight AIDS, Tuberculosis and Malaria; the GAVI Alliance; Roll Back Malaria; the Stop TB Partnership; and the Global Alliance for Improved Nutrition. However, an analysis of the performance of these partnerships[27] shows that many of the difficulties that motivated their formation persisted. The partnerships encountered the same difficulties (unrealistic goals, lack of concrete plans to implement goals, and unclear distribution of responsibilities across partners) because of lack of participation in decision-making by policy-makers from recipient countries.

TRANSPARENCY

Another criticism of current global health governance is lack of transparency in making political decisions – which the UN defines as freely available and directly accessible information about decisions, to those who are affected by such decisions.[16] One example of lack of transparency is information on financial flows for treatment of tropical diseases.[28] Information on the disbursements of funds for tropical disease programmes to recipient nations is often not publicly available and, when it is, is incomplete and not standardized across different funders, making it difficult to examine and challenge funding decisions.[29] One reason this problem occurs is that the policy actors and their respective roles have changed dramatically over the past years and continue to undergo rapid changes, so it is unclear to most observers who is responsible for which decisions.[25] Another example of lack of transparency is that most routine monitoring and evaluation data and results, which are collected in tropical disease programmes worldwide, are normally not publicly available. Civil society, patients and researchers outside particular programmes are thus unable to independently check claims made by the institutions responsible for the programmes.

ACCOUNTABILITY

A third criticism is a lack of accountability – that is, the need for institutions or individuals to account for their decisions and be held responsible for the consequences of the decisions by those who are affected by them. Transparency is a necessary but insufficient condition for accountability. In addition, political actors need to explain the reasons for their decisions to those affected by the decisions, and the affected need to be able to reward or punish the responsible actors.[30]

The preamble to the 1946 constitution of WHO assigns responsibility for health to governments.[31] Democratically elected policy-makers can be held accountable by the public (through elections) and by legislative bodies (through inquiries, impeachment or votes of no confidence). However, it is far more difficult to hold accountable the non-state actors that have proliferated in recent years in global health – especially the many multilateral, bilateral, philanthropic and humanitarian donor institutions.

Two recent declarations by donors have called for greater accountability in global health governance:

- The Paris *Declaration on Aid Effectiveness* calls for 'enhancing donors' and partner countries' respective accountability to their citizens and parliaments for their development policies, strategies and performance'.[32]
- The *Accra Agenda for Action* supports mutual assessment reviews as an instrument for governments, donors, and the broader public to hold each other accountable for the results of global health investments. 'These reviews will be based on country results reporting and information systems complemented with available donor data and credible independent evidence. They will draw on emerging good practice with stronger parliamentary scrutiny and citizen engagement. With them we will hold each other accountable for mutually agreed results in keeping with country development and aid policies'.[32]

While these declarations are a sign that lack of accountability in global health governance has been identified as a substantial problem, they have yet to be followed by concrete actions to build a system of accountability that encompasses all of the key actors in global health.

EFFECTIVENESS AND EFFICIENCY

A fourth criticism is a lack of effectiveness and efficiency. The reason given for this hypothesized state of the global health governance system is usually a lack of coordination among the different political actors in global health.[33,34] Some have characterized the result of unprecedented funding increases and the proliferation of organizations in global health, as anarchic.[35] While this may be an extreme characterization, the calls for more coordination and control have come from many quarters.

One consequence of poor coordination is duplication of efforts in tropical disease interventions, leading to inefficiencies. For instance, each donor agency usually requires its own funding application and performance reports, even if the different agencies are contributing to funding the same tropical disease programme.[36] Other consequences include a breakdown of political and technical support of particular tropical disease programmes,[27] along with lost opportunities to learn from each other,[36] and to ensure that all necessary components of programmes and interventions are funded, appropriately managed, and monitored and evaluated.

Over the past decade, several initiatives have been started to improve coordination among the many initiatives working in global health. At the global level: the Global Task Team on Improving AIDS Coordination among Multilateral Institutions and International Donors;[37] the Global Implementation Support Team (GIST);[38] the Global Campaign for the Health Millennium Development Goals;[39] and the International Health Partnership (IHP+)[40] have tried to improve coordination among international donors providing aid for tropical disease programmes. However, the extent of their success remains unclear. For instance, GIST has been hampered in fulfilling its mission, because of confusion about its role among the participating institutions, such as World Bank, Global Fund and UNAIDS.[41]

At national levels, institutions such as the National AIDS Commissions (NAC),[42] the Global Fund Country Coordination Mechanisms (CCM) and the United Nations Delivering as One initiative[43] have tried to ensure that various donors' efforts are integrated with countries' health systems and programmes. For instance, the Global Fund CCM has brought together representatives of national governments, civil society, the private sector and multilateral and bilateral donor institutions to help coordinate the development of national proposals, and to help better coordinate Global Fund grants with other national health and broader development programmes.[44] Initial evidence shows that the country-level programmes have improved coordination and transparency, but that they have not yet succeeded in comprehensively coordinating the efforts of all donors.[45] Moreover, in some cases, the different coordinating initiatives have themselves contributed to coordination problems. For instance, in many countries the Global Fund CCMs became 'a new and separate channel which competes with and confuses the role of other bodies'.[46]

Strengths of the Current System of Global Health Governance

While several weaknesses plague the current system of global health for tropical diseases, it is important to emphasize that some of the underlying structural reasons for these faults have also led to strengths. In particular, it is likely that the simultaneous existence of many institutions working in global health – at different levels, with different but overlapping mandates, and with different organizational histories – has been a source of innovation, flexibility, motivation and entrepreneurship.

INNOVATION

One of the greatest achievements in global health in the past decades has been the provision of ART to millions of

HIV-infected patients in developing countries. While a few large initiatives and organizations have played prominent roles in ART scale-up – the US President's Emergency Plan for AIDS Relief, the Global Fund, WHO and UNAIDS – many other institutions have contributed, leading to experimentation with a range of ART delivery models. While the efficiency of exchange of best practices, experiences and scientific results can be improved, meetings, conferences and publications have ensured the exchange of knowledge about the performance of the various ART delivery models.

For instance, in South Africa, ART has been funded and provided by Médecins Sans Frontières (MSF), the Elizabeth Glaser Pediatric AIDS Foundation (EGPAF), and the South African Catholic Bishops' Conference, in addition to PEPFAR. Each of these organizations initially set up their own separate programmes – some of them, such as the Catholic Bishops, many years before PEPFAR started providing ART in the country. The lack of coordination across these different organizations allowed for experimentation and testing of alternative models of ART delivery, leading to innovations that are unlikely to have occurred in a single HIV treatment programme. For instance, MSF piloted so-called adherence clubs in 2007 to improve ART retention and adherence and give ART patients a forum to share experience and support each other. The experience from this innovation – club members are two-thirds less likely to experience ART failure – led the joint government and PEPFAR HIV treatment and care programmes in the South African province of the Western Cape to adopt adherence clubs, and it seems likely that similar clubs will be started in other provinces.[47]

At the global level, the Clinton Health Access Initiative (CHAI) has successfully negotiated substantial price reductions for ART medicines in low-income countries[48] – an innovative approach to improve access to these medicines that is unlikely to have succeeded had CHAI not been added to the institutions that form the global health governance system. It also seems unlikely that the Medicines Patent Pool – which is expected to lower ART prices by facilitating the transfer of licenses for the production of particular drugs from patent holders to companies producing generic drugs[49] – would have come into existence without the emergence of UNITAID as an organization committed to improving access to treatments and diagnostics for tropical diseases through market interventions.

FLEXIBILITY

The fragmented nature of the global health governance system is likely to have yet another advantage. The simultaneous existence of many institutions of different sizes and with different organizational histories and visions may imply that the system as a whole can react quickly to new needs and demands. For instance, procurement processes (such as for new point-of-care machines) or the hiring of short-term consultants (such as for change management) may be substantially faster in small institutions than in larger ones. Changing the current system to a more centrally organized one will likely lead to increased inertia as large organizations usually need more bureaucratic managerial processes and tend to require more intensive internal coordination.

Smaller organizations – as opposed to larger ones – are also usually better able to meet local demands and needs through their organizational culture, intervention delivery, and interactions with people affected by their actions. For instance, community-based organizations (CBOs) have been successful, even if uncoordinated,[50] as providers of HIV interventions to particular geographically or culturally defined communities.[51] A 2005 UNAIDS report attributes the success of CBOs to their fragmented nature and diversity:[50]

> These community-based efforts are diverse and involve different skills, vocations and resource bases. But this diversity is one of the great strengths of the community-based response. The varied responses offer many different ways to introduce, sustain and follow up clients as they receive care and treatment. The diversity and complementary services of community organizations help clients gain access to health care that is adapted to their particular needs at the lowest cost, and is often more comprehensive than services offered in the public sector.

MOTIVATION AND ENTREPRENEURSHIP

Another strength of the global health governance system is that it is likely to lead to a large and motivated workforce. The fragmented architecture of the institutions in global health means that more leadership positions need to be filled than in a less fragmented, more centrally controlled system, and that career progression is likely to be accelerated. The good job market and career prospects, in turn, are likely to attract more – and more qualified – nurses, doctors, managers and researchers. In addition, the existence of institutions with different provenances and commitments is likely to attract a larger variety of people than a system with fewer institutions would.

Currently, people motivated by humanitarian or religious life goals may find an institution involved in tropical disease intervention funding or implementation just as easily as those motivated by opportunities for entrepreneurship or attainment of positional power. In a less fragmented system – such as one in which WHO would be the main supranational actor – a narrower spectrum of people would find an organization that fits their life goals. Supporting evidence comes from medical schools in developed countries, where in recent years the number of students participating in global health experiences and internships[52] and the number of elective courses, academic tracks, and departments to train and conduct research in global health and tropical diseases has increased dramatically.[53–55]

The Way Forward

A range of proposals are being debated to improve the current system of global health governance:

- Partnerships and coordinating mechanisms could improve participation, transparency, and efficiency[45]
- Frequent, routine publication by all donor institutions of all their committed and disbursed contributions to global health would increase transparency, accountability and coordination
- Mutual performance assessment and evaluations among different organizations could increase accountability
- A strengthening of a central organization, such as WHO or a global health monitoring institute, could improve effectiveness and efficiency[4]

- A global health constitution outlining the duties and obligations of actors in global health could improve transparency and effectiveness.[35]

However, none of these proposals has been tested, and it seems plausible that some of them could decrease the level of innovation, flexibility, and motivation and entrepreneurship present in the current system. For instance, organizational centralization through a strengthened WHO may not necessarily improve coordination, because 'WHO itself is a fragmented organization with a cumbersome governance'[56] and has been criticized for being 'ineffective, bureaucratic and political'.[57] Other proposals, such as further coordinating mechanisms, may themselves duplicate existing efforts and require financial investment and technical capacity, which could be employed for alternative uses in the global health sector. It will thus be important that reforms of the current system of global health governance for tropical diseases are carefully selected and that their progress is monitored.

Conclusion

Over the past decade, the system of global health governance has increased dramatically in size and complexity. This has major implications for combating tropical diseases in the future. The system's past successes against tropical diseases may not be replicated in the future because of the challenges in addressing the continued high, and in some areas increasing, morbidity and mortality burdens of tropical diseases; and because of simultaneously increasing disease burdens of NCDs. Funding for tropical disease interventions and global public health in general may be stagnating or declining in the coming decade owing to both economic crises in developed countries and the emergence of new funding priorities, such as NCDs or climate change.

The current global health governance system certainly suffers from a number of weaknesses, such as a lack of participation, low transparency and accountability, and ineffectiveness and inefficiencies stemming from duplication and a lack of coordination among the various institutions that influence global health. However, in thinking of approaches to address these weaknesses, it will be important to preserve the system's strengths – which have provided a fertile ground for innovation, fostered a flexibility that enables actors to react quickly to changes and adapt easily to local conditions, and helped attract and create a highly motivated and entrepreneurial workforce.

Acknowledgement

The authors gratefully acknowledge Larry Rosenberg at the Harvard School of Public Health for his careful and insightful review of this chapter.

REFERENCES

2. Dodgson R, Lee K, Drager N. Global health governance. London: Centre on Global Change and Health. London School of Hygiene & Tropical Medicine; 2002.
4. Sridhar D. Global health – who can lead? The World Today 2009:25–6.
13. Hotez PJ, Molyneux DH, Fenwick A, et al. Control of neglected tropical diseases. N Engl J Med 2007;357:1018–27.
15. Lancet [No authors listed] Progress and challenges in neglected tropical diseases. Lancet 2010;376:1363.
26. Kaul I, Grunberg I, Stern M. Global Public Goods: International Co-operation in the 21st Century. Oxford: Oxford University Press; 1999.
27. Conway MD, Gupta S, Prakash S. Building better partnerships for global health. McKinsey Quarterly 2006;1–8.
33. Garrett L. The challenge of global health. Foreign Affairs 2007;86:14–38.
36. Bloom DE. Governing global health. Finance & Development 2007;31–5.
41. Hellevik SB. 'Making The Money Work': Challenges Towards Coordination of HIV/AIDS Programs in Africa. Houndsmill: Palgrave Macmillan; 2009.
56. Bloom BR. WHO needs change. Nature 2011; 473:143–5.

Access the complete references online at www.expertconsult.com

4

The Economic Case for Devoting Public Resources to Health

DAVID E. BLOOM | GÜNTHER FINK

KEY POINTS

- The world has enjoyed remarkable improvements in population health during the last half century, but major health problems persist, particularly in tropical countries.
- Economic research suggests that better population health can promote economic wellbeing through beneficial changes in age structure, labour productivity, education and investment.
- The economic benefits of improved health can be large, but realizing them depends on a supportive policy environment.

Introduction

Global population health has improved significantly in recent decades. Life expectancy has increased in every single country since 1950, with an average increase of 22 years in the period from 1950 to 2010, and a contemporaneous two-thirds decline in the global under-5 mortality rate. Epidemic polio has ended, the global coverage rate for DTP3 (diphtheria, tetanus and pertussis) vaccination more than quadrupled between 1980 and 2010, and smallpox, which killed 2 million people a year until the late 1960s, has been eradicated.

Although the overall health improvements are remarkable, substantial health deficits persist in a large number of countries, and the gap between developed and developing countries remains large. The gap is particularly large between tropical and non-tropical countries.* As Table 4.1 shows, on average, people in the tropical countries live less long, bear more children, and suffer from lower vaccination rates than those in non-tropical countries. They also experience much higher levels of maternal mortality, infant mortality and under-5 mortality. Although the absolute differences between tropical and non-tropical countries have declined for most indicators since 1980, convergence has been slow, and full catch-up appears unlikely within the next few decades.

One of the primary reasons tropical countries have worse health outcomes than non-tropical countries is their vulnerability to infectious diseases. Table 4.2 shows the 10 principal causes of death for low- and high-income countries as reported by the World Health Organization (2011). Most of the low-income countries in the WHO sample are tropical, while very few of the high-income countries are tropical. As Table 4.2 shows, six of the top 10 causes of death in low-income countries are infectious diseases, while in high-income countries, only one of the top 10 causes (lower respiratory infections) is an infectious disease.

The strong correlation between tropical location and the burden of communicable diseases is also apparent at the regional level. In WHO's 'Africa' region (which closely matches what is generally considered to be 'sub-Saharan Africa'), the share of deaths owing to 'Communicable diseases, maternal and perinatal conditions and nutritional deficiencies' out of deaths other than injuries, is 70%. By contrast, the corresponding share in Europe (i.e. WHO's European region, which includes Central Asia) is 6%.

The simple comparison of disease patterns in tropical versus non-tropical regions is clearly confounded by a large number of country- and region-specific factors, such as income, education and other determinants of health that are partially or entirely unrelated to tropical location.

While the true causal mechanisms underlying the poor health outcomes in tropical countries are complex and hard to disentangle empirically, it is unquestionable that tropical countries striving for improvements in population health will face major challenges in the coming years. For example, communicable diseases remain the primary concern in most tropical countries, but the rapid global increase in the burden of

TABLE 4.1 Big Health Gaps Between Tropical and Non-Tropical Countries (Average Values for Various Health Indicators)

	Year	Tropical	Non-Tropical
Life expectancy at birth (years)	1980	57	69
	2010	64	74
Total fertility rate (births per woman)	1980	5.6	3.5
	2010	3.6	2.1
Immunization, DPT (% of children ages 12–23 months)	1980	39	57
	2010	85	93
Maternal mortality ratio (modelled estimate, per 100 000 live births)	1980	n.a.	n.a.
	2010	287	55
Infant mortality rate (per 1000 live births)	1980	84	43
	2010	45	16
Under-5 mortality rate (per 1000 live births)	1980	133	58
	2010	67	19

Note: Averages are unweighted. n.a., not available.
Source: World Bank, World Development Indicators. Online data, 2012.

*Tropical countries are defined as those with more than half of their land area lying between the Tropic of Cancer and the Tropic of Capricorn. Data are from International Union for Conservation of Nature (1986), http://www.nhm.ac.uk/hosted_sites/bbstbg/tropctry.htm, as updated by the authors.

TABLE 4.2 **Infectious Diseases Still Heavily Burden Tropical Countries (The 10 Leading Causes of Death by Broad Income Group (2008)**

	Deaths in Millions	% of Deaths
Low-Income Countries (40, Including 34 Tropical)		
Lower respiratory infections	1.05	11.3
Diarrhoeal diseases	0.76	8.2
HIV/AIDS	0.72	7.8
Ischaemic heart disease	0.57	6.1
Malaria	0.48	5.2
Stroke and other cerebrovascular disease	0.45	4.9
Tuberculosis	0.40	4.3
Prematurity and low birth weight	0.30	3.2
Birth asphyxia and birth trauma	0.27	2.9
Neonatal infections	0.24	2.6
High-Income Countries (50, Including 6 Tropical)		
Ischaemic heart disease	1.42	15.6
Stroke and other cerebrovascular disease	0.79	8.7
Trachea, bronchus, lung cancers	0.54	5.9
Alzheimer and other dementias	0.37	4.1
Lower respiratory infections	0.35	3.8
Chronic obstructive pulmonary disease	0.32	3.5
Colon and rectum cancers	0.30	3.3
Diabetes mellitus	0.24	2.6
Hypertensive heart disease	0.21	2.3
Breast cancer	0.17	1.9

Note shaded areas are infectious diseases.
Source: World Health Organization. Fact sheet No. 310, updated June 2011; http://www.who.int/mediacentre/factsheets/fs310/en/index.html.

non-communicable diseases (NCDs) means that governments and health policy-makers in tropical countries also get increasingly exposed to new challenges such as diabetes and obesity. This 'double burden of disease' poses a major challenge to health systems, since communicable and non-communicable diseases need to be addressed at the same time with limited resources.

A major global shift of attention towards NCDs, as evidenced in part by the September 2011 United Nations high-level meeting on NCDs, may also mean that global funding toward communicable diseases may decline and thus put populations in tropical countries at risk.

What can be done to ameliorate the situation? One answer lies in a better understanding of the complex links among health, income and poverty. This chapter reviews the classic motives for investing in public health and discusses a new argument for doing so: that such investment can yield significant economic benefits. It then reviews the most recent microeconomic and macroeconomic evidence on causal links from health to income. It concludes with thoughts on how policy-makers and other stakeholders can use these findings to enable governments to invest in health in a timely, cost-effective, efficient manner – and one that is appropriate for the special needs of tropical countries.

Classic Arguments for Spending on Public Health

There are four traditional lines of arguments in favour of devoting public resources to promoting and protecting health:

1. *Ethical arguments*: Moral, ethical and humanitarian considerations dictate that allocating resources to the improvement of population health is ethical, just, and a fair course of action.
2. *Health as a human right*: Health is a fundamental human right, which means that the opportunity to enjoy good health is a legally just claim to which all human beings are entitled.
3. *Health to promote social cohesion and global security*: Health is a key ingredient in forming social capital, and better health will help lead to societies that are cohesive, peaceful, equitable and secure. A nascent political argument that highlights population health as a key determinant of political stability and international security has also been proffered. For example, in a 2000 study commissioned by the CIA,[1] the global model for predicting state failure finds that 'low levels of material well-being, measured by infant mortality rates', 'roughly *doubled* the odds of state failure'. This result is consistent with the view that the inability of a government to satisfy the basic needs of its electorate – including and especially its health – erodes trust and may contribute to repeated cycles of instability and collapse. This appears to be one reason why Richard Holbrooke, then-US Ambassador to the United Nations, masterminded the first-ever UN Security Council meeting on health. At that 2000 meeting, US Vice President Gore said that AIDS was a security issue that the world had to address. In addition, in 2010, the UN General Assembly held a meeting on global health and adopted consensus text on 'Global Health and Foreign Policy'.[2] The text 'encourages Member States to consider the close relationship between foreign policy and global health', acknowledges 'the need to improve research and development in neglected tropical diseases', and [welcomes] in this regard the first World Health Organization report on neglected tropical diseases acknowledges 'that progress in global health is dependent primarily on national policies and actions and on international cooperation and partnerships, which could help to respond to major global challenges and crises' and urges 'Member States to continue to consider health issues in the formulation of foreign policy'.
4. *Health investment to address behavioural externalities*: Since individuals may infect others and not fully take into account the health and financial consequences of their actions, private health behaviour is likely to be suboptimal from a societal perspective. Therefore, welfare improvements can be achieved through government intervention. Public health expenditure, particularly in the realm of disease prevention, can lead to substantial reductions in the costs of treatment and care, and thus have high financial returns.

All four arguments have been important historically, but none have been decisive in their ability to mobilize resources. While the ethical and moral justifications are undoubtedly powerful in theory, they have not proven to be good arguments to substantially increase government expenditure. Arguments built on the spread of infectious diseases have also not carried the day, as evidenced by the fact that although immunization rates have risen greatly, 15% of the world's children are still not being vaccinated for DTP. More broadly, roughly 17% of all deaths under age 5 (and 29% of deaths between 1 month and 5 years) are from vaccine-preventable diseases.

One of the more recent arguments that has generated considerable additional momentum in support of public funding for health in general, and infectious diseases in particular, is the notion that poor health leads to less productive and economically less successful countries. Although the argument has gained considerable traction in recent years, it has a curious history.

Health in Traditional Macroeconomics

One of the oldest, most basic, and yet most difficult questions in the field of economics is why some countries are so much richer than others. While many tropical countries have per capita incomes of less than US$5000 today, most Western countries have per capita incomes well in excess of US$30 000. The fundamental question of why income differentials across countries are so large, was first posed by the father of modern economics, Adam Smith. In his seminal 1776 treatise, *The Wealth of Nations*, Smith first highlighted the importance of the division of labour for labour productivity. Following his original argument, the view that long dominated the field of economics was that income disparities between countries arise from cross-country differences in their stocks of physical capital (tools, plants, equipment, infrastructures like harbours, irrigation systems, communication networks and natural resources) and their technology. According to this view, national income increases via capital accumulation and technological progress. As countries become more productive, the marginal product of workers increases, causing firms that operate in competitive labour markets to offer higher wages.

With increasing data availability in the second half of the twentieth century, this first generation of economic models was challenged by the fact that the cross-country income differences were rather large relative to cross-country differences in capital stock and technology. To address the lack of predictive power of the original model, the notion of capital was augmented to include human capital (in particular, education and skill), in addition to physical or financial resources.[3] However, even the collective differences in physical capital, technology and education were insufficient to account for the observed differences in per capita income, and remained so when positive feedback mechanisms from increased income to capital stock, levels of education and investment in research and development were taken into account.[4]

What role does health have in this literature? Despite the difficulty of accounting for the sources of economic differentials and a large number of attempts to expand existing frameworks, relatively few studies have attempted to directly account for health as a determinant of income in the economic growth literature, although there are some notable exceptions.[5–7]

This one-directional view is well illustrated by Samuel Preston's representation of the changing relationship between income and health. Figure 4.1 shows an updated version of Preston's formulation for both tropical and non-tropical

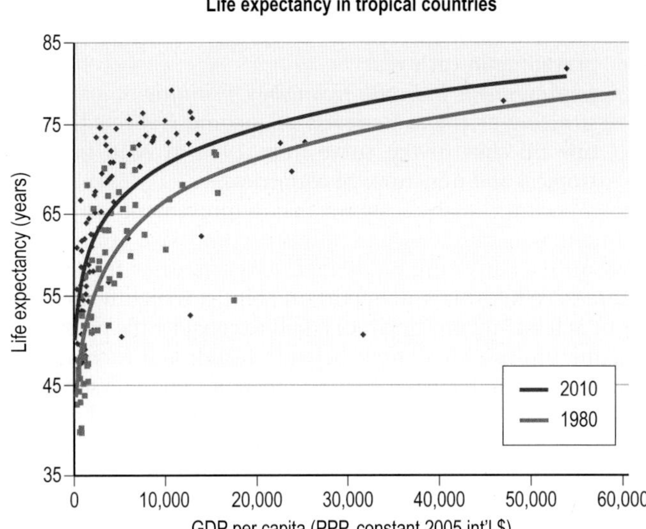

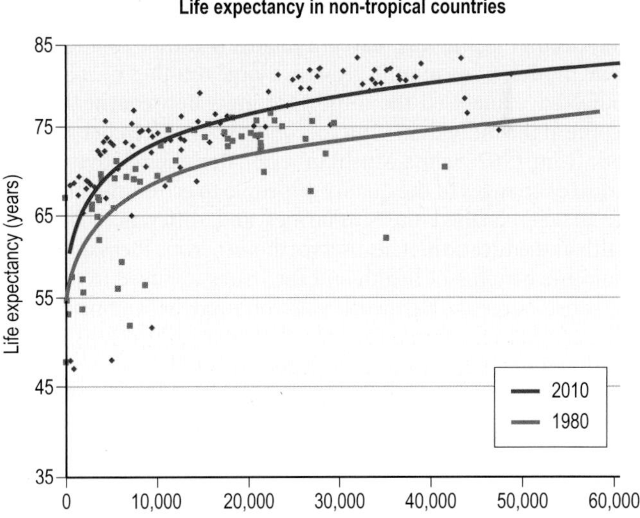

Note: Data points >$60,00 not shown

Figure 4.1 Life expectancy is highly correlated with per capita income. (A) In tropical countries. (B) In non-tropical countries. (Source: *World Bank, World Development Indicators. Online data, 2012.)*

countries.[8] Each panel shows the relationship between income per capita and life expectancy in 1980 and 2010. The basic tendency in both panels is for countries with higher per capita incomes to have healthier populations – a pattern that holds for different income and health measures and at different points in time. The scatterplots also reveal that for a given level of income, the life expectancy that a country can achieve increases substantially over time.

These patterns, displayed in Figure 4.1, are suggestive of a causal link that runs from income to health, since health improvements can either be observed through:

- *Increases in income per capita* (reflected by the tendency of points plotted for 2010 to represent higher income than in 1980, which would indicate higher life expectancy under the positive relationship between health and income prevailing in each year).

- *Improvements in health technology, institutions, and infrastructure* at the same levels of income (reflected in the upward shift of the curve from 1980 to 2010 for both tropical and non-tropical countries).

Decomposition analysis shows that improvements in health technology, institutions and infrastructure have contributed more to overall health gains than have increases in national incomes.[8] While this is an important point, it is slightly misleading or at least incomplete, since it fails to consider the possibility that the positive association between health and income also reflects a causal link from health to income. Some reasons why this might be so – related to labour productivity, education, investment (including foreign direct investment), and demographic change – are discussed below.

Microeconomic Evidence on How Better Health Benefits the Economy

Even though health has played a relatively minor role in traditional models of economic growth, a large number of economic studies have analysed the important links between health and income at the individual ('microeconomic') level. In her seminal work from 1962, Selma Mushkin[9] evaluated the relative contribution of changes in the quality of people to economic progress. Her article clarified the similarities and differences between health and education. It also set forth numerous ideas about the economic benefits of health and the issues involved in estimating those benefits. Her work was followed by a considerable body of microeconomic research that treated health as a form of human capital, akin to knowledge and skill.

Microeconomic studies have considerable potential to inform both researchers and policymakers about the relationships between health and income. By focusing on individuals rather than countries, microeconomic studies have several methodological advantages: more detailed measures of health and income and their determinants, larger sample size, and the ability to analyse natural or true randomized experiments. Randomized controlled trials involve three basic steps: (1) randomly divide the experimental population into a treatment group that participates in a potentially beneficial programme, and a control group that does not; (2) assess outcomes of both groups; and (3) determine whether a significant difference in outcomes exists between the two groups. By contrast, natural experiments occur when a phenomenon (such as an earthquake, a new disease outbreak, or a new policy) induces external variations in individual characteristics that can be explored to investigate the causal impact of the respective characteristic on an outcome of interest. As highlighted in a 2002 review of studies on the links among health, nutrition and prosperity by Duncan Thomas and Elizabeth Frankenberg,[10] such experimental studies are crucial since they allow a careful identification of key biological and behavioural mechanisms of interest.

In their 1998 review of the existing microeconomic literature in this area, John Strauss and Duncan Thomas[11] show that the weight of the evidence points strongly towards the existence of a causal impact of health on productivity, employment and earnings. The review also highlights the contribution of nutrition in childhood to determining adult health and wages. Since then, there have been many compelling microstudies, including a number focused on tropical health. The following section summarizes the main body of work in this area.

RANDOMIZED CONTROLLED STUDIES

De-worming. Intestinal worms (helminths) are a major problem in poorer countries because they can significantly diminish a child's cognitive ability and general health. Ted Miguel and Michael Kremer examined the effects of school-based deworming on educational outcomes in school-age children in Kenya. In a randomized controlled study, the authors found that de-worming led to higher school attendance and provided community-wide benefits.[12] In a follow-up study, they also found large increases in wages among children growing up in treated areas.[13]

Iron Supplements. Along similar lines, but not pertaining to childhood intervention, is the research of Duncan Thomas, Elizabeth Frankenberg, and colleagues that shows the beneficial effect of iron supplementation on productivity and earnings.[14] Their study is based on a randomized, controlled intervention involving over 17 000 30–70-year-olds in Indonesia. Males who were iron-deficient prior to the intervention, and who received the iron supplements, were 'more likely to be working, sleep less, lose less work-time to illness, are more energetic, more able to conduct physically arduous activities, and their psycho-social health is better', and they were earning more on both an hourly and monthly basis. There were lower benefits for women, but in the same positive direction as for males.

Iron and De-worming. Bobonis and colleagues examined the effect of a randomized health intervention that delivered iron supplements and deworming drugs to pre-school children in India.[15] They found significant evidence of weight gain and increased participation in pre-school programmes.

Iodine. Several studies have investigated the impact of iodine supplementation on income. Iodine deficiency can impair the formation of the fetal brain and thus reduce cognitive functioning. In one study, Erica Field and colleagues found evidence of a significant positive effect on educational attainment of an iodine distribution programme in Tanzania.[16] They found larger effects for girls than for boys, which is consistent with the results of laboratory research showing that female fetuses are more sensitive than male fetuses to maternal iodine deprivation. These results confirm the quasi-experimental data collected by Politi and co-authors.[17]

Malaria. Siân Clarke and colleagues used a randomized controlled trial to study the effects on educational outcomes of intermittent treatment for the prevention of malaria in Kenyan schoolchildren.[18] They found that malaria prevention leads to increased attention scores (which measure children's ability to sit still and pay attention to instruction) and lower child parasitaemia at follow-up.

NATURAL OR QUASI-EXPERIMENTAL STUDIES

Malnutrition. Alderman and colleagues studied the effect of malnutrition in pre-school children and found a positive association between early nutrition and both later height (which has widely been found to correlate with earnings) and the amount of schooling completed.[19] They calculated that the 'loss of stature, schooling and potential work experience results in a loss of lifetime earnings of around 14%'.

Hookworm. Hoyt Bleakley conducted a study of hookworm disease in the American South in the early 1900s to evaluate the effect on income and education of the sudden and successful eradication of this disease.[20] At the time, hookworm infected 40% of school-age children and caused listlessness, stunting and anaemia – but not mortality. He shows that areas with higher levels of hookworm infection prior to the Rockefeller Sanitary Commission's intervention experienced: (1) greater increases in school attendance after the intervention (a 23% boost in the likelihood of attendance); (2) subsequent increases in labour earnings; and (3) higher rates of return on investments in education, which imply more human capital accumulation per year of schooling.

Iodine. Politi and colleagues explored historical variations in salt iodization in the USA and found a significant positive effect on cognitive function and a significant negative effect on the prevalence of goiter.[17]

Malaria. Bleakley also studied malaria eradication in the American South and parts of Central and South America.[21] He found evidence that the elimination of malaria led to faster increases in both literacy and wages in regions that were malaria-endemic before the intervention.

How Better Health Benefits the Economy Overall

Several recent studies suggest that the effects of health at the country level may be larger than the effects observed at the individual level,[5,6,22] a conclusion that reached a wide audience through the 2001 report of WHO's Commission on Macroeconomics and Health.[23] On average, each 10-year gain in life expectancy is associated with as much as an additional percentage point of annual growth of income per capita.[24] In a world economy in which per capita income typically grows at 2–3% per year, an additional percentage point is a substantial increase. Even though a 10-year gain in life expectancy may appear large, similar improvements have been frequently reached by several countries in relatively short spans of time.

Another key message is that *improved health is central to alleviating poverty*.[25] The main asset poor people possess is their labour, and the value of that asset is crucially determined by their health. This explains why health figures so prominently in plans to halve the global poverty rate between 1990 and 2015 – the first UN Millennium Development Goal. There is a notable dissent from the general conclusion linking health improvements to economic growth: a prominent paper by Daron Acemoglu and Simon Johnson.[5,6,26] Acemoglu and Johnson address some of the difficulties associated with interpreting the results obtained from studying cross-country data by taking note of the huge innovations in health technology that occurred in the 1940s and 1950s with the advent and diffusion of penicillin and other antibiotics, sulfa drugs, and the use of DDT for malaria control. They show that these sudden and unanticipated breakthroughs led to larger health gains in some countries than others, for example, in Africa as compared with Europe. If the 'healthier means wealthier' hypothesis is true, they reason, the countries with the largest gains from these medical innovations should have grown faster, other things equal, than countries not particularly exposed to the relevant diseases. They found no evidence of this differential effect on the rate of economic growth and strongly challenge the existence of a health-to-wealth link. But the Acemoglu–Johnson analysis has a problem in that the 'potential to benefit' from medical innovation is not independent of health, but rather a reflection of the strength of the country's health systems themselves. Countries with excellent health systems in 1940 had less to gain from the studied health innovations, but were still growing fast. After taking account of initial life expectancy, the health-to-wealth link is statistically restored. In other words, Acemoglu and Johnson's conclusion is fragile and not well supported by their own data.[27–29]

The powerful associations between health and economic development have spurred research to understand the causal links underlying these connections. Four principal channels have emerged through which health is likely to affect output at the country level: productivity, education, investment and demographics.

Labour Productivity Channel. A healthier workforce is characterized by more energy, better mental health and less absenteeism, and is thus more productive.

Education Channel. Education is virtually undisputed among economists, as being one of the most powerful instruments of income growth.[30] Health affects education through three fundamental channels: first, by enhancing children's physical ability to attend school; second, by increasing children's cognitive ability to absorb knowledge presented in school,[31] and third, by providing additional incentives for parents to invest in their children's education, since the returns on such investment can be expected to be earned over a longer period.[32] A recent study[33] finds that in '21 OECD countries over the past two centuries, health has been highly influential for the quantity and quality of schooling, innovations and growth'.

Investment Channel. Healthy populations have longer life expectancies, and thus increased incentives to save for future consumption needs. In response to greater expected longevity, many people might choose to work until a later age, even if public and private pension systems offer disincentives for doing so. A larger domestic savings stock leads to a larger supply of capital, which is presumed to result in further investment, additional physical and human capital, and technological progress – all of which are classic drivers of economic growth. In addition, healthy populations attract foreign direct investment, which often carries with it new technology, job creation and increased trade.[34,35]

Demographic Channel. Better health triggers a set of demographic changes, known as the 'demographic transition', that can ultimately boost economic growth. In fact, there is a growing body of evidence that attributes the 'economic miracles' experienced in the Asian Tigers and the Celtic Tiger (Ireland) largely to high rates of growth of factor inputs – labour, physical capital and human capital – rather than increases in total factor productivity.

The demographic transition typically begins when improvements in health – often spurred by better access to sanitation and safe water and increased use of vaccines and antibiotics – trigger a decline in infant and child mortality rates. In high-mortality populations, such declines cause rapid population growth. The initial boom in population strains capital resources and tends to slow the rate of economic growth (as conventionally measured). As couples realize that the mortality environment has changed, fertility declines and population growth gradually slows down.

As the initial baby boom cohort reaches working age and fertility rates decline, the number of dependent individuals (children and old age) per worker declines. On a per capita basis, productive capacity increases. This effect is further reinforced if mothers who spend less time in child-bearing and child-care participate more in the labour market. Since the working-age group is also the primary contributor to savings, potential output also benefits from increased capital accumulation and subsequent technological innovation. Eventually, the working-age share decreases as the baby boom generation ages and fertility rates converge to a low (replacement) level.

Importantly, during the middle stage of the demographic transition – when the working-age share is high – countries have the opportunity to benefit from what has come to be known as the 'demographic dividend' – that is, they can experience a demographically driven, time-limited economic boom if working-age people are productively employed.[36–39] One of the best examples of such a boom took place in East Asia, where roughly one-third of that region's economic boom between 1965 and 1990 can be attributed to realization of this demographic dividend.

Where are countries now in this demographic transition? The non-tropical countries, as a whole, have already had the opportunity to benefit economically from the rapidly rising ratio of working-age (aged 15–64) to non-working-age individuals (those under 15 or older than 64). Some countries have experienced a demographic dividend, and some not. Non-tropical countries, as a whole, are about to experience a decline in the ratio of their working-age population to their non-working-age population. Tropical countries, as Figure 4.2 shows, have been following a similar demographic trajectory, but with a delay of about 20–25 years. This means they have not yet reached the 'optimal' age structure and are likely to have the opportunity to benefit from demographic change over the next few decades. According to UN demographic projections, fertility rates will decline; however, they will not fall as much as they have in non-tropical countries, so the peak levels of working-age share experienced in non-tropical countries over the past decade are unlikely to be realized in tropical countries.

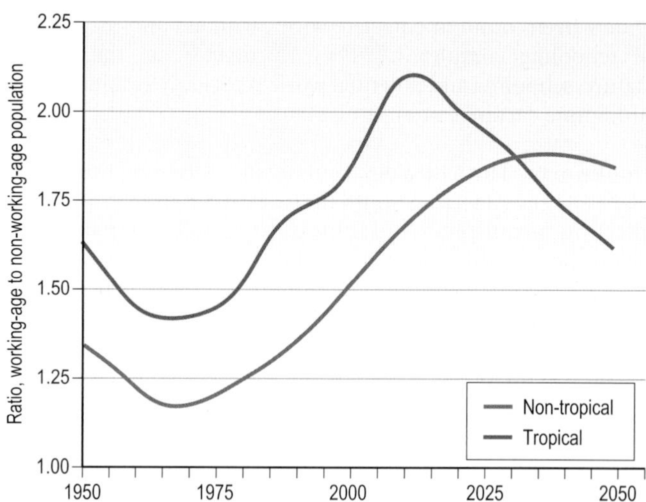

Figure 4.2 Tropical countries have begun to replicate the pattern of non-tropical countries. (Ratio of working-age to non-working age population.) (*Source: United Nations, World Population Prospects. Online data, 2012, and authors' calculations based on list of tropical countries cited above.*)

Economic Effects of Specific Diseases

Malaria is the disease most commonly cited in the context of economic growth. Worldwide, there are 500 million episodes of malaria each year, resulting in about 1 million deaths per year.[40] Malaria has been shown to have an effect on economic growth over and above that created through higher mortality, suggesting that its effects on productivity with a given mortality burden, are greater than other diseases. According to a frequently cited paper by Gallup and Sachs, economies with high malaria prevalence in 1965 grew 1.3 percentage points less per year than others between 1965 and 1990, '*even after other factors such as initial income level, overall health, and tropical location are taken into account*'. In terms of the effect on savings and investment, the eradication of malaria in southern Europe in the 1940s and 1950s spurred economic growth in countries like Greece and Spain, via a large increase in tourism to them.[41]

As for *HIV/AIDS*, the disease has increased mortality rates dramatically, but most researchers do not see a direct impact on income per capita.

- Bloom and Mahal[42] find that HIV/AIDS does not seem to lower income per capita. Mahal[43] corroborates this result, as do Werker and colleagues.[44] One possible reason is that lower output may be matched by lower population numbers owing to high death rates. Also, during the time-frame of these studies, HIV/AIDS had high mortality but the period of sickness before death was relatively short. This mutes the worker productivity effects of the disease; the main effects stem from its impact on demography (that is, a decreased share of working-age people) and the impact of a shortened expected lifespan on life cycle behaviour.
- Bonnel[45] raises the possibility of a negative impact on growth. He reviews the reasons that HIV/AIDS would be likely to *reduce* economic growth and, in conclusions that he says should be viewed as preliminary, he argues that the empirical results match these expectations: '*In the case of a typical sub-Saharan country with a prevalence rate of 20 per cent, the rate of growth of GDP would be some 2.6 percentage points less each year. At the end of a twenty year period GDP would be 67 per cent less than otherwise. One reason for the large impact of HIV/AIDS is that it includes the effect of AIDS-related opportunistic infections and other communicable diseases*'.
- Young[46] argues that AIDS in South Africa is likely to *increase* income per capita, primarily because the reduced

human capital available to nurture orphans is offset by lower fertility.

Important indirect mechanisms also exist. Deaths from HIV/AIDS are concentrated among young adult men and women and depend on socioeconomic factors. These selectivity effects could eventually reduce GDP per capita. Bell and co-authors[47] argue that the creation of a generation of AIDS orphans may lead to lack of care and education for children and to low productivity in the future. The high level of stigma associated with HIV/AIDS can reduce trust in the community, while high mortality and the strains imposed by extreme ill health before death can weaken families, community groups, firms, and government agencies, with long-term consequences for social capital.[48] Resources devoted to preventing and treating HIV/AIDS can reduce consumption of other goods, so consumption and welfare decline even as measured GDP per capita remains steady.

Policy Implications

What policy-relevant implications can we draw from the ideas discussed?

First, *health spending is appropriately regarded as an investment in development.* Health is both an indicator and an instrument of development. As such, health spending is comparable with spending on education, infrastructure, and good governance as a determinant of economic wellbeing.

Second, *health-income spirals can be virtuous or vicious.* The framework described above suggests strong feedback mechanisms between health and income. In an ideal scenario, improvements in health lead to income growth, which can lead to further improvements in health and incomes. The East Asian experience is a good example of this, with simultaneous and rapid increases in economic growth and health. By the same token, this framework also raises the possibility of vicious spirals, in which shocks, such as an infectious disease outbreak, can depress income, which in turn can depress health status and further deteriorate income.

Third, *the overall economic returns on investment in health appear large.* Immunization against infectious disease is a prime example. Vaccinated children tend to avoid the long-term sequelae associated with certain childhood diseases, such as neurological impairments, hearing loss and a variety of other physical disabilities, and they therefore tend to be more productive workers when they grow up. Parents and grandparents of vaccinated children tend to be healthier themselves and can thus work more productively, bringing broader economic benefits to society as a whole. Rough calculations indicate that, taking into account all of the benefits of vaccination, the rate of return on investments in vaccination programmes is at least as large as estimated rates of return on investments in primary school (an investment widely acknowledged to be one of the most fruitful possible). This logic and these kinds of calculations will be more important than ever in the future, because policymakers now have to make spending decisions about a new generation of much more expensive vaccinations – including those against rotavirus, pneumococcal disease and human papilloma virus. More broadly: improved health is not only associated with faster economic growth at the country level, but has also been shown to increase a society's productive capacity by increasing child development, education and savings.

Fourth, *better health improves wellbeing through lower fertility rates.* In societies benefiting from good population health, the expectation that children will grow up healthy naturally leads to families having fewer children. Fewer children means a lower burden of youth dependency, a more educated young generation, and a larger female workforce, which fuels the demographic dividend referred to earlier – an outcome that has been instrumental to many economies in spurring economic growth and reducing poverty. These demographic change processes can be powerfully enabled and further accelerated through sustained family planning programmes.

Fifth, *good population health is not automatically translated into economic wellbeing.* Cuba and Sri Lanka, as well as the Indian state of Kerala, are examples of countries or areas in which populations are healthy but poor. The Soviet Union, too, raised the level of its population's health, but its economic achievements were more mixed. In all situations, a consistent and enabling policy environment is key to realizing the economic benefits that better health can bring. This means sound macroeconomic policies and practices, carefully constructed trade policy, good governance, high-quality education that reaches a high proportion of school-age individuals, and effective labour market practices. A combination of these can lead to economically productive employment, in which people's efforts benefit not only themselves but also the country as a whole. These elements of the policy environment are, of course, important regardless of demographics. But the incentive to adopt and implement them is particularly high in tropical countries that have yet to complete their demographic and health transitions, because the potential benefits are particularly large at this stage of development. Correspondingly, failure to provide an efficient enabling environment can lead to a demographically driven disaster, in which large working-age cohorts are unemployed, with concomitant risks of social and political instability.

Finally, *a large number of diverse interventions can induce and support improvements in population health.* A large medical literature focuses on ways to improve health by improving the availability and quality of health services, including the delivery of specific treatments and vaccines. However, in many other cases, the most effective ways to improve population health may be to reduce exposure to specific diseases. This may in some cases be achieved through simple behavioural change campaigns, and in other cases, through larger infrastructure projects, such as water and sanitation networks. Many other interventions and policies, such as improved schooling, will also have important positive effects, even though they may not directly be considered part of larger health efforts.

Conclusion

Population health matters – not only for the evident humanitarian, legal, and society-building reasons, but also from an economic and welfare perspective. While the links between improvements in health and economic outcomes are complex, the long-run economic returns on investment in health appear large.

REFERENCES

1. Goldstone JA, Gurr TR, Harff B, et al. State Failure Task Force Report: Phase III Findings. Online. Available: http://www.cidcm.umd.edu/publications/papers/SFTF%20Phase%20III%20Report%20Final.pdf.
2. UN General Assembly Document A/65/95. Online. Available: http://www.who.int/mental_health/policy/resolution_global_health_and_foreign_policy.pdf.
5. Bloom DE, Canning D. The health and wealth of nations. Science 2000;287:1207–9.
6. Bloom DE, Canning D, Jamison D. Health, wealth, and welfare. Finance Dev 2004;41(1):10–5.
10. Thomas D, Frankenberg E. Health, nutrition, and prosperity: a microeconomic perspective. Bull World Health Organ 2002;80(2):106–13.
11. Strauss J, Thomas D. Health, nutrition, and economic development. J Econ Lit 1998;36(2):766–817.
23. WHO. Macroeconomics and health: investing in health for economic development. Geneva: Commission on Macroeconomics and Health, WHO; 2001.

Access the complete references online at www.expertconsult.com

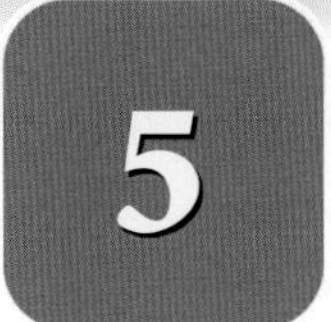

Ethics and Tropical Diseases: Some Global Considerations

SUSAN BULL | MICHAEL PARKER

KEY POINTS

- There are great disparities in health globally. There are strong correlations between the health of populations and national levels of wealth and spending on health.
- Socioeconomic determinants of health in populations include individual levels of income and wealth, as well as access to education and opportunities.
- Neglected tropical diseases primarily affect the poorest 1 billion members of the world's population and their economic costs are very substantial.
- There is debate about the extent of high-income countries' responsibilities to contribute to alleviating global disparities in health.
- Historically only a very small proportion of medical research has been focussed on the problems primarily affecting the world's poorest people.
- Over the last decade, many more actors have become engaged in funding or conducting health research relevant to the needs of developing countries.
- There has also been an increase in large-scale collaborative global health research accompanied by the emergence of complex ethical issues arising out of the interplay between globalized research collaborations and the ways in which such research is manifested locally.
- Approaches to research ethics include those based on considerations of autonomy, those based on considerations of the duties of the parties involved in research and those based on the assessment of the foreseeable consequences of actions.
- While there are many areas of consensus in international research ethics, there are some issues which remain controversial; including the minimal standards of care that it is acceptable to provide to control groups in research and the nature and extent of post-study responsibilities to research participants.
- Where research is necessary to inform strategies for the management and control of disease, care will be needed to ensure research is designed and conducted in a way that conforms to high ethical standards.

Introduction

Enormous global inequalities exist in health measures such as mortality, quality of life and disease. These persist despite increasing levels of overall wealth.[1–3] Low-income countries typically carry substantial and disproportionate burdens of disease and ill-health. Against this background, this chapter considers a range of factors that affect the likelihood of living a long and healthy life, and discusses a number of important ethical questions, including: What responsibilities do rich countries have to contribute to alleviating the burden of ill-health from tropical diseases and to reducing inequitable levels of health? What might such responsibilities encompass and what might be their limits? What are the ethical issues presented by medical research carried out in low-income contexts?

For those children born in 2011, estimated life expectancies (ELE) vary dramatically (Table 5.1). For example, children born in Angola have an ELE of just 38, and another 35 countries have ELEs of less than 60 years.[4] In contrast, 30 countries currently have life expectancies of 80 or above. Infant mortality rates, which inevitably contribute to ELE, also vary dramatically – ranging from 176 to just 1.79 per 1000 live births. Over 70 countries, including Sri Lanka, Chile, Puerto Rico and Cuba, have infant mortality (IM) rates of less than 1%, while five have infant mortality rates of over 10%.[4] Maternal mortality rates vary from 0.02% to over 1% of deliveries, a 50-fold difference. Similar levels of variation in numbers of physicians and hospital beds available are evident. Globally, per 100 000 members of the population, the number of physicians ranges from less than 5 to over 600, and of hospital beds from 10 to more than 800.[4]

Levels of disease, particularly those diseases requiring medical care and facilities for treatment, are often linked to countries' wealth and health spending. The validity of this comparison is reflected to an extent when comparing the ELE and IM figures above to the percentage of Gross Domestic Product (GDP) spent on health by countries, and the amount this equates to in US$ per person, per year. Almost all countries spending more than US$1000/year per person on health, have average ELEs of over 70. Past a certain point, however, higher spending does not necessarily mean a greater ELE – the USA, for example, spends significantly more than any other country at nearly US$7500/person per year – no other country spends more than US$4500 per year. However, approximately 40 countries achieve greater ELEs and lower infant mortality rates than the USA, despite spending between 1100 and 4500 US$/person. There are limits to efficiency – in states that spend less than US$100/person, ELEs are reduced and infant mortality is increased.

These figures are striking, but it is important to remember that levels of health service funding provide a partial, but not complete, indicator about the state of a nation's health. Even within national borders, there may be dramatic variations in health statistics between different populations. When considering where responsibilities might be held to lie for the improvement of health in nations with lower ELEs, it is important to

TABLE 5.1 Estimated Life Expectancies, Infant and Maternal Mortality Rates, Availability of Doctors and Hospital Beds, and Health Expenditure for Selected Countries

Country	Life Expectancy at Birth (2011 Est)	Infant Mortality per 1000 Live Births (2011 Est)	Maternal Mortality per 100 000 Live Births(2008)	Doctors per 1000 (2009)	Hospital Beds per 1000	Health Exp % GDP (2009)	Health Expenditure per Person (US$)[a]
Angola	38.76	175.9	610	0.08	0.8 (2005)	4.6%	377.2
Afghanistan	45.02	149.2	1400	0.21	0.4 (2009)	7.4%	66.6
Chad	48.33	95.31	1200	0.04	0.43 (2005)	7.0%	112
Gabon	52.49	49.95	260	0.29	1.25 (2008)	6.0%	870
Ethiopia	56.19	77.12	470	0.022	0.18 (2008)	3.6%	36
Cote d'Ivoire	56.78	64.78	470	0.144	0.4 (2006)	5.1%	91.8
Botswana	58.05	11.14	190	0.336	1.81 (2008)	10.3%	1442
Burundi	58.78	61.82	970	0.03	0.73 (2006)	13.1%	39.3
Benin	59.84	61.56	410	0.059	0.5 (2005)	4.2%	63
Cambodia	62.67	55.49	290	0.227	0.1 (2004)	5.8%	121.8
Burma	64.88	49.23	240	0.457	0.6 (2006)	2.0%	28
India	66.8	47.57	230	0.599	0.9 (2005)	2.4%	84
Bhutan	67.3	44.48	200	0.023	1.7 (2006)	5.5%	302.5
Azerbaijan	67.36	51.08	38	3.794	7.93 (2007)	5.8%	632.2
Bolivia	67.57	42.16	180	1.22	1.1 (2009)	4.8%	230.4
Belize	68.23	21.95	94	0.828	1.1 (2009)	3.3%	277.2
Bangladesh	69.75	50.73	340	0.295	0.4 (2005)	3.4%	57.8
Bahamas, The	71.18	13.49	49	1.05	3.1 (2008)	7.2%	2066.4
Belarus	71.2	6.25	15	4.869	11.23 (2007)	5.8%	788.8
Fiji	71.31	11	26	0.4529	2.08 (2008)	9.7%	426.8
Vietnam	72.18	20.9	56	1.224	2.87 (2008)	7.2%	223.2
Brazil	72.53	21.17	58	1.72	2.4 (2009)	9.0%	972
Egypt	72.66	25.2	82	2.83	1.7 (2009)	6.4%	396.8
Grenada	73.04	11.43		0.9756	2.4 (2009)	7.1%	724.2
Armenia	73.23	18.85	29	3.697	4.07 (2007)	4.7%	267.9
Estonia	73.33	7.06	12	3.409	5.71 (2008)	4.3%	821.3
El Salvador	73.44	20.3	110	1.596	1.1 (2009)	3.9%	280.8
Bulgaria	73.59	16.68	13	3.635	6.49 (2008)	7.4%	999
Thailand	73.6	16.39	48	0.298	2.2 (2002)	4.3%	374.1
Barbados	74.34	11.86	64	1.811	7.6 (2008)	6.8%	1482.4
Algeria	74.5	25.81	120	1.207	1.7 (2004)	5.8%	423.4
Colombia	74.55	16.39	85	1.35	1 (2007)	6.4%	627.2
China	74.68	16.06	38	1.415	4.06 (2009)	4.6%	349.6
Ecuador	75.73	19.65	140	1.48	1.5 (2008)	5.0%	390
Croatia	75.79	6.16	14	2.59	5.49 (2007)	7.8%	1357.2
Dominica	75.98	12.78		0.5	3.8 (2009)	5.9%	613.6
Brunei	76.17	11.51	21	1.417	2.71 (2008)	3.0%	1548
Argentina	76.95	10.81	70	3.155	4 (2005)	9.5%	1396.5
Georgia	77.12	15.17	48	4.538	3.32 (2007)	11.3%	553.7
Czech Republic	77.19	3.73	8	3.625	7.18 (2008)	7.6%	1945.6
Chile	77.7	7.34	26	1.09	2.1 (2009)	8.2%	1262.8
Cuba	77.7	4.9	53	6.399	5.9 (2009)	11.8%	1168.2
Costa Rica	77.72	9.45	44	1.32	1.2 (2008)	10.5%	1186.5
Cyprus	77.82	9.38	10	2.3	3.72 (2006)	6.0%	1260
Bahrain	78.15	10.43	19	1.442	1.9 (2008)	4.5%	1813.5
USA	78.37	6.06	24	2.672	3.1 (2008)	16.2%	7646.4
Denmark	78.63	4.24	5	3.419	3.57 (2008)	7.0%	2562
Finland	79.27	3.43	8	2.735	6.52 (2008)	11.7%	4141.8
Austria	79.78	4.32	5	4.749	7.71 (2008)	11.0%	4444
Greece	79.92	5	2	6.043	4.77 (2008)	7.4%	2190.4
UK	80.05	4.62	12	2.739	3.38 (2008)	9.3%	3236.4
Germany	80.07	3.54	7	3.531	8.17 (2008)	8.1%	2891.7
France	81.19	3.29	8	3.497	7.11 (2008)	3.5%	1158.5
Canada	81.38	4.92	12	1.9132	3.4 (2008)	10.9%	4294.6
Australia	81.81	4.61	8	2.991	3.82 (2009)	8.5%	3485

[a]Estimated from % of GDP spent on health and most recent figures available for GDP per person in each country.

consider the full range of factors that influence levels of health at a national level. National governments and their healthcare staff have a responsibility to determine how best to deliver equitable and effective healthcare to populations with the resources available.[5] There are a number of examples of very successful initiatives being implemented in resource-poor settings such as the immunization programmes in Bangladesh.

Socioeconomic determinants of health in populations include levels of income and wealth, access to education and opportunities. Furthermore, distributions of rights and powers, including rights to political participation, can have a significant impact on health inequalities. In the relatively impoverished Indian state of Kerala for example, significant investment in education (for women as well as men) in addition to healthcare, and relatively high levels of autonomy and power for women – leading to their control over factors such as reproduction – has led to positive health outcomes, despite slow economic growth overall.[6] Many of the factors influencing levels of health within a population, particularly the broader socioeconomic ones, may fall only partially within the remit of national governments. Some social and cultural traditions, particularly those concerning authority and decision-making powers in the domestic as well as the political arena, will require local support for change and that change may be relatively rapid or take place over a significant period of time.

The following section of this chapter focuses on ethics and appropriate responses to tropical diseases. However, it is also important to remember that the burden of ill-health in tropical regions is not due solely to tropical infectious diseases, but also to inadequate access to hygienic facilities and to shelter, food and safe water – and increasingly – to non-communicable diseases such as diabetes, cardiovascular disease and so on. It is worth remembering that, without health facilities approaching anything available today, basic improvements in hygiene, food, water and shelter produced very dramatic improvements in the life expectancy of populations in European countries during the early 1900s.

Neglected Tropical Diseases

In its 2010 report, 'Working to Overcome the Global Impact of Neglected Tropical Diseases', the World Health Organization (WHO) identifies 17 neglected tropical diseases (NTDs): dengue and other arboviral diseases; rabies; trachoma; Buruli ulcer; yaws; leprosy; Chagas disease; human African trypanosomiasis; leishmaniasis; cysticercosis; dracunculiasis; cystic echinococcosis; food-borne trematodiasis; lymphatic filariasis; onchocerciasis; schistosomiasis; and soil-transmitted helminthiases.[7] It suggests that such diseases share a number of characteristics: they primarily affect hidden (relatively poor and powerless) populations; they tend not to be transmissible beyond such populations; and they are often disfiguring and stigmatizing, as well as causing considerable morbidity, and in some cases, mortality. Such diseases primarily affect the poorest 1 billion members of the world's population and their economic costs are very substantial.

Significant advances have been made in the treatment of some of these diseases (new cases of dracunculiasis reported have, for example, decreased by over 99%, between 1989 and 2009), and relatively safe and simple treatments are available for others, such as trachoma and lymphatic filariasis.[7] However in 2008, only 8% of people with schistosomiasis had access to high-quality medicines because donations of praziquantel from the private sector were insufficient to meet demand and there were not enough other funds available for its production.[7] For other conditions, such as leishmaniasis, affordable effective and non-toxic treatments are needed, or for example in the case of dengue, vaccines are required. Further research is also needed into vector control and veterinary aspects of public health if appropriate environmental responses to such diseases are to be developed. National commitment to implementing comprehensive responses to diseases is also necessary, otherwise successes, such as reduction of endemic treponematoses from 50 million to 2.5 million cases in the 1970s, will not be maintained.[7]

Some medications for tropical diseases have been provided by the private sector, and others are provided via public–private partnerships. However, despite the large numbers of patients with some NTDs, the poverty of the populations affected means that there is not a sufficient economic demand for the development of new and effective treatments. Additionally, given the need for careful monitoring and treatment of cases, as well as public health education and limiting disease transmission, additional resources are required to build capacity in health systems for management and treatment of those conditions for which interventions are available. Consequently, it is unlikely that NTDs will be able to be managed effectively without international support to develop effective treatments, subsidies to make such treatments available for poorer countries and support to develop environmental vector management, public health education, and case monitoring and treatment. Considerable international funding and commitments have already been provided to address many NTDs, but more needs to be done. The following section of this chapter considers what responsibilities those countries without NTDs may have to assist those countries in which they cause a significant burden of disease.

Addressing Inequalities in Health

Notwithstanding the responsibilities of governments in low-income countries themselves, a fundamental ethical issue arising out of the existence of persistent inequalities in health and burdens of disease, concerns the responsibilities of those in high-income countries – including governments, pharmaceutical companies and NGOs.[5] Should governments from wealthier countries divert funds from healthcare for their own citizens to addressing NTDs, for example? If so, on what grounds might they justify this decision? What responsibilities do pharmaceutical companies have to develop and donate treatments to those in greatest need, rather than maximize profit for their shareholders? How should charitable organizations prioritize which diseases and countries should receive their aid, and what kinds of aid should be offered?

A number of different – and sometimes competing – theories have been proposed as an aid to thinking through how to analyse responsibilities to minimize burdens of disease, including tropical disease.

One argument sometimes made in favour of a global responsibility to promote health in low-income countries is grounded in a claim that we have a basic humanitarian obligation to alleviate suffering where it exists and we have the power to do something about it.[8,9] It has sometimes been argued against this position that these obligations are outweighed by the responsibilities we have to alleviate suffering in those nearest to us, such as family and community members and others with whom we have special relationships. However, two strong counterarguments to this are that: (1) it is the existence of preventable harm which is of moral significance, not geographic location and (2) that we do in fact have morally significant and obligation-generating relationships with people in low-income countries.[10] Both these counterarguments re-emphasize the claim that the key morally relevant consideration here is the existence of suffering and that our shared global humanity obliges us to recognize that we have responsibilities to alleviate suffering wherever it exists. From this perspective, everyone has an obligation to do what they can reasonably be expected to do to assist those suffering ill-health, wherever in the world they are based. Clearly, as the use of the term 'reasonably' in the previous sentence recognizes, such obligations are not going to be overriding of all other considerations and may be subject to other competing claims on our time and resources. But they are, nonetheless, important obligations.

An alternative, contrasting approach would be to argue, not that suffering generates obligations to assist but that inequalities in health are fundamentally unjust, and justice – not charity or obligations generated by particular kinds of relationships – requires that they be addressed.[6] We may argue that health has a special moral importance because without health, humans are denied the ability to flourish, thus addressing injustices in health may be prioritized over addressing many other injustices. Issues remain about whether addressing inequalities in health within a nation, or on a global scale should take priority. A related question concerns how competing health needs on a national or international scale can be met fairly when we cannot meet all of them. Considerable literature has been devoted to consider fair means of prioritizing healthcare resources, as even countries with expenditures on health of more than US$1000 per person per year, are unable to meet all the health needs of their populations. Difficult decisions inevitably have to be made. A related consideration is that as wealthier nation states' commitment to their own interests and disproportionate resource use perpetuates global injustices they have an obligation – grounded in justice – to address these. In particular, there is a duty not to exploit vulnerable nations and further limit their abilities to meet the health needs in their own interests. This issue is discussed further below, in relation to migration of health personnel from countries with significant levels of NTDs.

A third argument might be one which appeals not to putative duties to alleviate suffering or the existence of injustices, but to the value of maximizing overall beneficial outcomes. Such a consequentialist approach might be one that argues that reducing the global burden of disease should be prioritized because it will contribute to breaking cycles of poverty and allow people to better themselves, which maximizes productivity. The claim is at least partly that overall everyone is better off if poverty and inequality are reduced. It might also be argued that reducing discrepancies between the richest and poorest populations may reduce the potential for conflicts based on such discrepancies and contribute to global security and prosperity. This would allow further resources to be diverted from national defensive measures and used to promote wellbeing.

A common theme among these three arguments for the addressing of global health disparities is that improving health on a global scale needs to be ranked among other competing claims on resources. This generates a number of additional important questions. How, for example, should health be ranked against education as a priority? Even where a compelling argument is made for prioritizing reduction of burden of ill-health over other considerations or priorities, issues remain about how we should prioritize which diseases to address and how. For example, should resources be focussed on those with the greatest burden of ill-health, on addressing conditions affecting the largest number of people, or on those which are easiest to address quickly – wherever in the world they are based?

TABLE 5.2 Examples of International Responses to Neglected Tropical Diseases

Year	Response
1952	UNICEF and WHO launch Global Yaws Programme
1974	Onchocerciasis Control Programme for West Africa begins
1987	Mectizan Donation Programme created
1997	Programme against African Trypanosomiasis established
	WHO-GET 2020 (Global Elimination of Trachoma by 2020) created
2003	Drugs for Neglected Diseases Initiative established
2005	WHO Department of Control of Neglected Tropical Diseases established
	Bangladesh, India and Nepal sign an agreement to eliminate visceral leishmaniasis by 2015
2006	Collaboration begins between WHO and the Foundation for Innovative New Diagnostics to develop and evaluate new diagnostic tests for human African trypanosomiasis
2008	Launch of the Neglected Tropical Disease Initiative by the US government and
	UK Government Department for International Development commits £50 million to targeting neglected tropical diseases

PRACTICAL RESPONSES TO ADDRESSING INEQUALITIES IN HEALTH

Just as theories about appropriate ways of prioritizing responses to disease on a global scale are still being developed, so are global responses to addressing such needs.[5] Table 5.2 outlines a number of measures to address NTDs being implemented by the WHO, national governments, non-governmental organizations (NGOs) and charities.[7]

The responses captured in Table 5.2 suggest that there is at least some level of commitment among some powerful national and international organizations to reducing burdens of ill-health among poorer populations, even in areas such as NTDs, which are less likely to benefit wealthier populations directly. A greater commitment again is shown to infectious diseases with a broader global reach, including tuberculosis, AIDS and malaria. Many commentators would argue that these measures are insufficient, and that a greater commitment must be demonstrated to reducing inequalities in health around the world.[11]

One argument that commands a great deal of agreement, is that wealthier countries should, at the very least, do all they can to avoid exploiting or exacerbating the burden of ill-health in developing countries. One significant way in which wealthier countries have for many years contributed to increasing the burden of ill-health in developing countries is by allowing the recruitment of healthcare staff from those countries to fulfil their own staff shortages. Entire nursing classes graduating in African and South Asian countries have migrated overseas following recruitment campaigns. From 2000 to 2002 alone, the UK added 13 000 foreign nurses to its NHS staff to contribute to addressing a staff shortage of 20 000 nurses.[6] In 2001, 27% of physicians in the USA were immigrants, 38% of whom were from India, Pakistan or the Philippines.[12,13] In 2002, 30% of doctors trained in Ghana and 20% of doctors trained in Uganda were employed in the USA and Canada.[14]

Migration of skilled health workers is a complex phenomenon, and the means of redressing such brain drain are also complex. Where there are limited or unattractive employment opportunities in countries with greater burdens of disease, migration becomes an increasingly attractive option even for people who are committed to making a difference in their home country. Such problems can be exacerbated by global economic forces. In the 1980s, to take one example, lenders such as the World Bank and International Monetary Fund responded to deteriorating economic conditions in developing countries by requiring them to reduce public funding of healthcare systems among other things. Where such measures lead to under-employment or unemployment of health workers, it is an inevitable consequence that qualified people will seek employment in wealthier nations. While such migration is protected in codes of human rights, wealthier countries can choose to limit recruitment of health staff from countries with unfilled vacancies and to support the development of attractive working conditions in such settings.

The above discussion of staffing has focussed on clinical and medical staff. It is important to remember that WHO recommends that in addition to preventive chemotherapy, the control of NTDs requires appropriate case management, vector control, sanitation and hygiene and veterinary public health.[7] It notes that there are rapidly reducing reserves of expertise in some of these fields in many countries with a high burden of such diseases, so support for improved working conditions for staff working in these fields may also be valuable.

Research

While it is clear from the scope of the discussion above that medical research cannot in itself offer a solution to the persistence of health inequalities, such research is necessary to develop effective responses to some tropical diseases. It is striking that historically, only a very small proportion of medical research has been focussed on the problems primarily affecting the world's poorest people. In 1990, the Commission on Research for Development estimated that about 5% of the world's medical research resources were being applied to health problems arising in developing countries where more than 90% of the global burden of preventable mortality was located.[15] In subsequent years, this disparity has come to be known as the 10/90 gap.

The Council on Health Research for Development (COHRED 1990)[15] and the subsequent reports of the Ad Hoc Committee on Health Research[16] and International Conference on Health Research for Development[17] together established something of a consensus on five core recommendations for the action needed to move towards a more equitable distribution of medical research resources. The five recommendations comprised the need to: (1) correct the 10/90 gap and set priorities; (2) build up the capacity of health research systems in developing countries; (3) create international research networks and public–private partnerships; (4) increase funding for health research by developing countries; and (5) create health research forums to monitor progress in health research.[18]

These recommendations, together with the United Nations' Millennium Development Goals, which included a commitment to work to eradicate infectious diseases such as malaria, have led to a number of important developments. The Global Forum for Health Research 10/90 Report on Health Research 2003–2004 found that the landscape of medical research funding had changed significantly between 1990 and 2003. It reported that there were now 'many more actors engaged in funding or conducting health research relevant to the needs of developing countries' than previously and estimated that global expenditure on research had 'more than quadrupled' by 2003. The Report noted that much of this new research takes the form of emerging international research networks. Among others, the Report identified: The Roll Back Malaria Partnership; the Global Alliance for TB Drug Development.

The developments identified by the Global Forum in 2004 continue.[19] Both the scale of the research being carried out on global health, and the shift towards more collaborative, networked approaches to global health research, have been further encouraged by initiatives such as the Grand Challenges in Global Health Scheme launched in 2003.

The growth in collaborative global health science has also been driven by developments in science and technology. The rapid pace of development in technologies and statistical methods for analysing DNA sequence variation at the level of the whole genome has, for example, made it possible for the first time to contemplate genome-wide analysis of phenotypes such as human resistance to malaria. Such research requires very large sample sets of cases and controls because of the involvement of multiple environmental and genetic factors. The requirement for such large sample sets combined with the importance of cutting-edge sequencing facilities and statistical expertise – to be found largely in developed country sites – means that such research networks are increasingly bringing together research groups in many countries across both the developed and developing worlds. An example is MalariaGEN, which is a genomic epidemiology of malaria consortium funded by the Gates Grand Challenges Scheme and the Wellcome Trust. MalariaGEN involves 24 partners in 21 countries, 15 of which are malaria-endemic.[20]

These forms of collaborative global health research are leading to the parallel emergence of complex ethical issues arising out of the interplay between globalized research collaborations and the ways in which such research is manifested locally. These issues are complementary to and interwoven with the well-described ethical issues arising out of global health inequalities,[6,8,10,21,22] but present qualitatively new challenges. While some issues, such as the standards of care to be provided to control groups, and post-trial responsibilities to participants, have been the subject of debate for over a decade[23–25] and remain the subject of conflicting guidance to date,[26–28] others arising in the building and maintenance of global research collaborations have received less attention. These include issues relating to the importance of achieving shared good practice across a network while remaining sensitive to local variation[29] and reaching agreement about data-sharing and the sharing of biological materials between partners with different values, practices and priorities.[30]

Collaborative global research also has implications for the development of appropriate and effective community engagement;[31,32] for the question of what are to count as appropriate and culturally sensitive modes of obtaining valid consent in the context of complex global collaborations;[33,34] and for the collection, storage and distribution of biological samples. An ethical perspective capable of making sense of these emerging and interdependent phenomena will itself need to be collaborative and multi-sited if it is to be capable of grasping the implications of both global collaboration and the manifestation of the global in the local, where the 'local' is to be found both in developed and developing country sites.[35] Such research will necessarily have a strong empirical component and the issues arising also present new theoretical challenges.[36–38]

APPROACHES TO RESEARCH ETHICS

Against this background of broadly welcome increasing amounts of research – often, but not always involving international collaborations between partners in developed and developing countries – it is nevertheless important to pay attention to the potential ways in which such research, even if well-intentioned, may raise ethical concerns. Before going on to explore some of these issues in depth, it is perhaps worth comparing some of the main theoretical approaches to research ethics. This is important because these different approaches will not only, in some cases, identify different problems as important, they will also have implications for why these problems are problems at all and about what might count as acceptable solutions.

Broadly speaking, there are three main ways of thinking about the ethics of research: *autonomy-based* approaches, *duty-based* approaches, and *consequentialist* approaches.

For *autonomy-based approaches*, as these tend to be conceptualized in the research ethics literature, the question of whether a piece of research is ethical comes down primarily to a question of whether and to what extent the participants' consent to participate in the research was 'valid'. What is important – ethically – for this approach is that people's (research participants') right to live their lives in their own way is respected. And for the autonomy-based approach there are broadly three main ways in which this might fail to be the case. First, it might be that the person has not been provided with all of the information necessary to make an informed choice – or has been provided with information in a form that they are not able to understand. Second, it might be that the person's choice was not voluntary – for example if they were forced to participate or would lose important health benefits if they refused. Third, it might be that the person was not competent to make the decision at the time they were asked. For these reasons, the autonomy-based approach places a great deal of emphasis on the consent processes and the quality of the information provided to participants. However, once *valid* consent has been obtained, the research, even very dangerous research, is ethical – as long as the person understands the risks.

By contrast, the *duty-based approach* to research ethics takes the view that research is ethical to the extent that researchers (who may sometimes also be health professionals) have met their obligations – their 'duties of care' – to research participants. Generally speaking, while this approach would also be likely to emphasize the importance of respecting patients' values and choices and hence also consent, a key difference between this approach and the autonomy approach is that researchers are likely to be seen as having a duty to protect research participants from serious harm. This approach, then, would judge the ethics of a research project not only on the extent to which choices were respected but also on the extent to which participants were going to be subjected to more than minimal risk of harm – even if they were fully aware and willing to take those risks. So, the duty-based approach would place limits upon the kinds of research which participants were allowed to be offered.

The third approach to the ethics of research is the *consequentialist approach*. This approach is one which sees an ethical research project as one in which the foreseeable benefits of the research outweigh the foreseeable harms. This approach differs from the others in that where the benefits of the research outweighed the foreseeable harms the research would be ethical – even, in principle at least, if valid consent was not obtained and/or the harms to participants were significant. The consequentialist would place a great deal of value on the foreseeable benefits of research, e.g. those that might accrue to people in developing countries, but would also, in his or her assessment of the benefits and harms of the research, want to take into account the full range of potential harms including, for example, those which might follow from declining research participation if this was affected by the absence of consent.

These approaches would be in agreement about whether or not a research project was ethical in the majority of straightforward cases, e.g. research with the potential for significant benefits in which competent participants were going to be giving informed and voluntary consent and where the research presents only minimal risks. The approaches will differ in situations where, e.g. research is low risk and has the potential for large benefits but where valid consent is not possible, e.g. research on large numbers of patient records or research in the context of emergencies; or, where research offers the potential for very large benefits to many people but at a cost of significant risk of harm to individual research participants who are – perhaps because of their commitment to medical research – nonetheless willing to provide valid consent.

In the following sections of this chapter, we describe some of the key practical ethical issues arising in the context of research in low-income settings. It will become clear that many of these issues are informed by these different approaches to ethics and research.

ETHICAL ISSUES IN INTERNATIONAL RESEARCH

International research ethics is an expanding area of the field of research ethics, and is, at times, a very controversial topic in the academic literature.[8,39] Overarching themes include appropriate governance and management of large-scale international research efforts, guidance and regulation of global studies, the rights and responsibilities of research actors and issues relating to engaging with research communities and participants. Specific topics include prioritizing research to address local needs, building capacity for ethical review to protect research participants, standards of care it is appropriate to provide to participants in research, how best to seek valid consent to research, benefit sharing and what should happen after research is over. These issues are addressed in turn below.

There are over 1000 national and international guidelines or regulations on research ethics currently in force,[40] which can provide guidance for researchers seeking to determine how to address ethical issues arising in their research. Much of the international guidance is at the level of broad principles and requires careful consideration as to how it should best be given effect on a case-by-case basis in individual research protocols. In such circumstances the role of national governments in supporting the development of national guidelines can be very valuable. National guidelines can provide insights to both local and international research consortia about how general principles of research ethics may be given effect within particular national contexts by highlighting issues of particular importance within local research contexts.

Priority Setting and Research

For research to be of substantive benefit to the population in which it is conducted, it is important that it addresses locally relevant research priorities, rather than just providing information primarily of value to funders seeking to develop interventions for other markets. In relation to tropical diseases potential research areas include, but are not limited to:

- Epidemiological research to map disease aetiology and healthcare priorities in tropical settings
- Operational research to inform appropriate delivery of current treatments and other interventions
- Primary research and upstream research such as genomic studies into mechanisms of disease causation and resistance
- Animal studies
- Phase I–IV studies of novel treatments and prophylactic agents
- Trials of treatments that have proved valuable in other contexts and have the potential to treat or alleviate tropical diseases
- Zoological and environmental research into potential means of reducing transmission of infectious disease
- Social science research into community responses to tropical diseases and the implications of these for research or treatment.

Identifying local research priorities may not necessarily be straightforward however, and may require additional research, and in some cases, the development of new diagnostics to assist in providing a cost-effective and accurate picture of the incidence and effects of a specific disease. For example, at present the characterization and incidence of dengue is uncertain in many regions, although it remains a leading cause of hospitalization and death in children in some countries.[7]

Some research protocols may bring valuable financial and human resources into poorer areas, even if the specific topic being studied is not a direct research priority for the local area. In such cases, centres may wish to permit such research, but should also be able to decline to take part if the opportunity cost of doing so is too great. In particular, it is important that research does not recruit healthcare staff needed to provide services elsewhere in the healthcare system, and thus undermine the current standard of health care provided in the region.

Ethical Review

The requirement of local ethical review is a relatively new but important means of protecting the interests of research participants. The process of establishing and training effective ethics committees around the world is ongoing. It is important that appropriate resources are made available to support ethics review committees, to enable them to have the appropriate training and support to conduct independent and effective ethical review. In some circumstances, it may be appropriate for organizations to build in part of the basic costs of running an ethics committee into proposals being funded, so that those applying for approval meet some of the costs of the approval process.[8]

There are a number of free and subsidised initiatives to support the development of capacity in ethical review in tropical regions. These include the Strategic Initiative for Developing Capacity in Ethical Review (SIDCER); COHRED's MARC project (Mapping African Research Ethics Committees onto capacity needs); the Middle East Research Ethics Training Initiative (MERETI); Training and Resources in Research Ethics Evaluation for Africa (TRREE); and the GlobalHealthReviewers.org website funded by the Bill and Melinda Gates Foundation.

For ethical review to be effective, committees must be able to decline unethical or inappropriate research, or require amendments to protocols where they consider it necessary. For example, institutional research ethics committees should not be pressured to approve problematic research because of the resources that it will bring to their centre. Likewise, in multi-centre trials, it is important that funders and ethics committees from multiple sites interact respectfully with each other. There may be more than one layer of dialogue as committees seek to ensure that protocols are appropriate for their communities while researchers and funders seek a certain measure of consistency across a multi-centre study as a whole.

Consent and Community Engagement in Research

For consent to research to be ethically valid, it must be appropriately informed, and given voluntarily by someone with the capacity to weigh information received about a study and decide whether or not it would be appropriate to take part. Issues relating to information and voluntariness are discussed in more detail below. While there is consensus on fundamental requirements for valid consent in the international guidance and regulation, many issues can arise in practice when seeking consent to studies with impoverished populations.

The provision of information to research participants is one of the most prescriptive and controversial areas in guidance on research ethics. More than one guideline or regulation will often be relevant to an individual research protocol and they may provide conflicting advice about the specific topics that must be covered in a consent form. The eight topics most commonly cited in guidance and regulation as necessary to inform participants of include the aim of the study, what is involved for those taking part (e.g. types of research procedures, duration of participation, etc.), potential risks and benefits of research, the right to decline to take part in a study or to withdraw – without losing access to healthcare to which you would otherwise be entitled, procedures to protect privacy and confidentiality, and the compensation that is available for research-related harms.[26–28] Experienced research teams may also identify additional issues that should be addressed to support participants' understanding and decision-making, such as providing background information about mechanisms of disease causation for the condition being studied. Great care is needed to provide this information about a research protocol in a comprehensible way, and to provide sufficient time and support for prospective participants to ask questions if they wish.

There are a number of factors that may make it difficult for a potential research participant to decline to take part in research. Sociocultural factors include imbalances in power between researchers and prospective participants, and an expectation that medical staff lead decision-making, which may make it difficult to decline what is being offered. In contexts where communitarian decision-making, or hierarchical social structures are in place, it may be difficult for a competent but relatively junior adult to decline to take part in research that appears to be approved of by others with more seniority. Potential economic constraints on free decision-making include a perceived or actual lack of alternatives to research participation, particularly in very impoverished resource contexts. The effects of such constraints are not necessarily overcome by advising participants that research is voluntary and that declining to take part will not mean that they will lose access to treatment to which they would otherwise be entitled.

Engagement with communities in research can have many aims and take many forms.[31,32,41] Engagement with communities may be seen as an end in itself, a way of demonstrating respect for those taking part in research. It can also aim to serve many functions, such as improving communication, information provision and understanding between research populations and researchers, through to soliciting advice on topics such as research priorities or appropriate ways to conduct research. It can also be used as a way of promoting partnership between research organizations and community members, and reducing imbalances of power between these groups. Community engagement can take place at various or all stages of research, from study conception and design, through pre-implementation information-giving and implementation, to feedback and communication of results. Moreover, insights gained from community engagement can improve both the design and conduct of consent processes for research, illustrate the potential overlap and mutual support between community sensitization, community consultation and consent activities.

Standards of Care in Research

During the 1990s, perhaps the most controversial issue in international research ethics related to appropriate standards of care to be provided in clinical trials. Initial debates focussed on whether it was acceptable to provide a placebo to control groups in trials of short-course antiretrovirals to prevent perinatal HIV transmission in resource-poor settings. A fundamental question raised was whether there is a universal best standard of care which should be provided to control groups irrespective of where in the world a study is conducted.[23–25]

One argument concluded that to offer participants in resource-poor settings a lower standard of care than they would receive if the trial was conducted in the wealthier country sponsoring the research was exploitative and unacceptable. Responses to this suggested that if all trials were required to use a universal standard of care as a comparator, it may not be possible to conduct research of specific relevance to resource-poor settings. In particular, if seeking evidence to inform improvements in national healthcare provision, it may be necessary to compare the new proposed treatment to that which would otherwise be available, to determine the value of adopting the new regimen. In such cases it was suggested that control groups may not need to be provided with a universal best standard of care, but instead the best standard of care nationally available within a country.[8]

Appropriate standards of care to be provided to control and intervention groups in research, as well as responsibilities to provide ancillary care to participants for other conditions, or participants' family and community members remain important and controversial issues, which continue to get revised in the international guidance.[27] A related topic concerns the extent of researchers' responsibilities to maximize benefit and minimize harm to participants in non-interventional research, such as epidemiological studies.[42]

What Should Happen after Research?

A second issue which has received extensive attention and debate is what is owed to research participants upon completion of a study.[8,39] In particular, if research has demonstrated the benefit of a new intervention, a question remains whether those who did not receive it during the study should be offered it, and whether others in the community or region should be entitled to preferential access to such a treatment. Additionally, if ongoing treatment is required for a chronic condition, an issue arises about whether it is acceptable to withdraw treatment on completion of research from those who received it during the study.

Issues of post-trial access to research interventions are complicated and have also been the subject of frequent revision in international guidance during the last decade.[27,43,44] Concerns have been raised that making it a requirement of research that effective treatments continue to be provided indefinitely following completion of a study may limit the conduct of relevant research. The extent to which researchers and research funders alone can be appropriately considered responsible for ongoing provision of research interventions beyond the life of the trial has also been debated. Introducing a new treatment into a national healthcare system involves a complicated decision-making process and is fundamentally the responsibility of national governments. Researchers may be considered to have a responsibility to promote their research findings to relevant health authorities, and funders may have a responsibility to enter into agreements with national healthcare providers to provide interventions at preferential rates, or free of charge. However, because ongoing provision of a novel intervention is a complicated process requiring consultation between multiple stakeholders, it may not be possible to guarantee how it will be provided after research before a study has even commenced. Additionally, when trialling a novel treatment, pharmaceutical manufacturers note that they may not be able to make a decision about whether commercial manufacture of a product will be undertaken, or whether to seek approval to market an intervention from the relevant licensing authority, until data from multiple trials is received.

Because of the complexity of managing the responsibilities of multiple stakeholders when rolling out a novel intervention post research, and the variation in responsibilities depending on the mode of research and its findings, some commentators have suggested that what needs to be assured before research begins, is not that a certain type of access will be offered, but that the stakeholders will discuss appropriate measures once research results are available. This is not intended to diminish post-trial responsibilities of stakeholders such as researchers, funders, public–private partnerships, national governments, and others, but rather to ensure that the aspects of the individual study can be taken into account when determining how to maximize post-trial access to beneficial interventions.

Conclusions

We began this chapter by highlighting the fact that enormous global inequalities continue to exist in health measures such as mortality, quality of life and disease and that, as a consequence, low-income countries typically carry substantial and disproportionate burdens of disease and ill-health. Against this background, we have considered a range of factors that affect the likelihood of living a long and healthy life, and discussed a number of important ethical questions relating both to the responsibilities of governments and arising in the practice of health care and research. International collaboration is necessary for the control and eradication of tropical diseases, and a number of such international initiatives are currently successfully reducing burdens of disease. Opinions vary on the extent to which such initiatives are likely in themselves to lead to effective solutions to global health inequalities, and some groups have argued that these need to be complemented by emphasis on reaching international agreement about the nature and scope of responsibilities of various bodies, including governments in both low- and high-income countries.[5] Appeals to global responsibilities to alleviate suffering, to address injustices and to promote prosperity in countries with high burdens of tropical disease support increasing global activity in this area. If such activities are to be successful national governments will need to commit to leading and managing complex initiatives within their borders to address burdens of ill-health. Where research is necessary to inform strategies for the management and control of disease, care will be needed to ensure research is designed and conducted in a way that conforms to high ethical standards.

REFERENCES

6. Daniels N. Just Health: Meeting Health Needs Fairly. Cambridge: Cambridge University Press; 2008.
7. WHO. Working to overcome the impact of neglected tropical diseases. Geneva: World Health Organization; 2010.
8. Nuffield Council on Bioethics. The ethics of research related to healthcare in developing countries. London: Nuffield Council on Bioethics; 2002.
11. Benatar S, Daar A, Singer P. Global health ethics: the rationale for mutual caring. In: Benatar S, Brock G, editors. Global Health and Global Health Ethics. Cambridge: Cambridge University Press; 2011.
15. Council on Health Research for Development (COHRED). Commission's Report – Health Research: Essential Link to Equity in Development. New York: Oxford University Press; 1990.
26. Council for International Organizations of Medical Sciences (CIOMS) International Ethical Guidelines for Biomedical Research Involving Human Subjects. Geneva: CIOMS; 2002.
27. World Medical Association. Declaration of Helsinki. 59th World Medical Assembly, Seoul. 7th ed. World Medical Association; 2008.
33. Chokshi D, Thera M, Parker M, et al. Valid consent for genomic epidemiology in developing countries. PLOS Medicine 2007;4(4): 636–41.

Access the complete references online at www.expertconsult.com

Issues and Challenges of Public-Health Research in Developing Countries

JACQUELINE DEEN | LORENZ VON SEIDLEIN | JOHN D. CLEMENS

KEY POINTS

- There are several aspects of public health research in developing countries that differentiate it from that conducted in more affluent settings, including the need to focus on infectious, perinatal and nutritional disorders especially in children.
- Several methods to assess the burden of and evaluate interventions against infectious diseases are discussed and illustrated with examples.
- Health research in developing countries should comply with current international research standards, so as to assure that the rights, safety and wellbeing of participants are protected and that the study data are credible.
- Public health resources in developing countries are limited. An understanding of the burden of health conditions and the potential impact of interventions and control measures is crucial for rational priority-setting.

Background

Public health is the combination of sciences and skills that aims to protect, promote and restore the wellbeing of a population.[1] Public health research in developing countries is important to quantify health conditions, assess interventions and control measures, as well as inform health policy decisions. There are several aspects of public health research in developing countries that differentiate it from that conducted in more affluent settings.

First, the major health problems in poor populations are infectious, perinatal and nutritional disorders and the highest burden of these problems is found in children. In poor countries, not only are children more vulnerable to disease and death than adults, compared with industrialized nations, they constitute a much larger proportion of the population. Most developing countries have pyramidal populations reflecting high birth rates and short-life spans. By contrast, the age structure of industrialized countries tends to be onion shaped due to decreasing birth rates and longer life expectancy. Recent socioeconomic changes in many poor countries have resulted in a shift in the patterns of disease. As a consequence of lifestyle and behaviour changes, as well as a shift from rural to urban living, developing countries have to cope with chronic noncommunicable illnesses such as adult cardiovascular disease, diabetes and depression, while continuing to struggle with childhood infectious, perinatal and nutritional disorders.[2] Despite these recent developments, the public health sector still tends to focus on children. This is not only because the greatest disease burden still occurs in the youngest age groups, but also because childhood interventions tend to be the most cost-effective and sustainable, and the development of children determines the quality of future populations.

Second, in many parts of sub-Saharan Africa, tropical Asia and Latin America, there is a profound lack of health infrastructure and reliable routinely collected data. Large proportions of births and deaths occur at home and remain unregistered. Many ill patients do not or are unable to seek health care. Treatment facilities are often understaffed and have limited capacity for laboratory-confirmed diagnoses. These factors pose significant challenges for recording accurate morbidity and mortality data. Thus a large fraction of public health research in these settings focuses on health burden assessments to generate the most urgently needed data for public health delivery.

Third, populations in developing countries should be considered as vulnerable in the sense that they have limited financial and political power. It is important that they not be left out of health-related research from which they would benefit, but this research has to be done in accordance with ethical guidelines and principles.

Finally, the bulk of the worldwide disease burden is in developing regions, where only a small fraction of global healthcare funds is available. Epidemiological data are crucial for the rational allocation of these limited resources and to inform decisions about strategies to be implemented. Public health research in developing countries emphasizes the search for cost-effective control and preventive strategies that could potentially benefit large segments of the community rather than expensive treatments for individual patients.

In this chapter, we discuss some important issues and challenges of public-health research in resource-poor settings. This chapter does not cover all aspects of health research in developing countries but will discuss the following: disease burden assessment, outbreak investigation, measuring protection and cost-effectiveness of interventions, good clinical practice in research and using research findings to guide health policy decisions. The focus of all sections will be on infectious diseases.

Methods to Assess the Burden of Infectious Diseases

Improvement of health conditions in a country requires recognition of the main problems, selecting the most appropriate and cost-effective interventions, implementing services efficiently and a continuous assessment of results. On-going analysis of disease burden is essential to the formulation of responsive health policies. There are several epidemiological methods to assess disease burden, the most relevant of which are discussed below.

RETROSPECTIVE REVIEWS OF EXISTING DATA

An assessment of available data provides a general idea about health and disease statistics in a country or region. Collating and analysing existing information is relatively cheap and quick, may be useful to assess trends and may provide a nation- or region-wide picture but its limitations need to be kept in mind. The quality of the assessment depends on the data used to reach it. For example, reliance on public agencies' estimates of a disease, which may be inflated to increase public attention and consequently increase funding, will distort global calculations. The World Health Organization (WHO) compiles more comprehensive health data annually but the accuracy of reporting varies between diseases and across countries.[3] These estimates rely on routine notification, which may be weakened by over- and under-diagnosis, incomplete reporting and delays. Reporting of some diseases may be suppressed due to social taboos (e.g. HIV/AIDS) or the fear of trade sanctions (e.g. cholera).

Systematic reviews and analyses of published and unpublished data on specific diseases may provide more accurate information. For example, Reddy and co-workers conducted a systematic review and meta-analysis of the published literature to assess the burden and the most common aetiologies of community-acquired, non-malaria bloodstream infections in Africa.[4] They found that 13% of adults and 8% of children admitted to hospital with a blood culture taken had a bloodstream infection. The most common isolate was *Salmonella enterica* subspecies (of these, 34% were *S. typhi* and 58% non-typhoidal *Salmonella*) overall in adults and *Streptococcus pneumoniae* in children. Retrospective studies of this nature provide valuable insights for public health planning and research but do not yield detailed and area-specific information. Other limitations include sparse data sources (depending on the health condition of interest) and highly variable or poorly defined methodologies of the original studies. Aside from published findings, there are large amounts of routinely collected and frequently unprocessed disease surveillance reports in health ministries and other institutions. This so-called 'grey literature' may also be included in systematic reviews.

Due to the many weaknesses of using existing data, triangulation of information is recommended, that is comparing and contrasting data from various sources to validate accuracy. Other than WHO publications, peer-reviewed articles and government surveillance reports, innovative sources such as outbreak information from the Program for Monitoring Emerging Diseases (ProMED), which operates as an online forum for infectious disease specialists, microbiologists and public health officials, have also been included in burden of disease assessments.[5]

Traditionally, burden of disease assessments include mortality and morbidity rates, which are useful but do not reflect the total picture. An illness may be uncommon or have low death rates but can still cause considerable burden through chronic disability. In the 1990s, researchers at the Harvard School of Public Health, together with the WHO and the World Bank, estimated the global burden of disease by region and age group, in terms of disability-adjusted life years lost (DALYs). DALYs are the sum of years of life lost due to premature death and years living with disability of specified severity and duration. Using available data from around the world, disease estimates were made for 1990 and mathematical modelling was used to create 5-year projections until 2020.[6] Several parameters are required to calculate DALYs, including age- and gender-specific mortality estimates; incidence of disease estimates; proportion of time individuals are disabled; and severity and duration of disability. Two further adjustments are made: discounting and age-weighing. Future years of healthy life lost are often discounted by 3% per year, i.e. years in the future count for less compared to those in the present. Discounting future health reduces the relative impact of a child death compared with an adult death. The value that is accorded for a year of life lost is also age-weighed, based on the assumption that the relative value of a year of life rises rapidly from zero at birth to a peak in the early 20s, after which it steadily declines. The strengths of this approach are that it incorporates disability and it allows comparison between diseases, populations and time periods. DALYs are now being used in other types of studies, notably economic analyses (see below). In addition, the WHO is also using a new metric, healthy-adjusted life expectancy (HALE) at birth, which adds up expectation of life for different health states, adjusted for severity distribution, making it sensitive to changes over time or differences between countries in the severity distribution of health states. HALE is defined as the average number of years that a person can expect to live in 'full health' by taking into account years lived in less than full health due to disease and/or injury.

To continue the important work on global health statistics, the Institute for Health Metrics and Evaluation (IHME) was launched at the University of Washington in June 2007 (see: http://www.healthmetricsandevaluation.org). The IHME measures population health status and disease burden, identifies the factors that determine health outcomes and evaluates health policies and interventions. Among their earliest projects were new estimates of mortality rates.

In a separate effort, the Child Health Epidemiology Reference Group of WHO and UNICEF estimated global, regional and national causes of child mortality in 2008.[7] They used multi-cause proportionate mortality models to estimate deaths in neonates and under-5-year-old children and selected single-cause disease models and analysis of available vital registration data to estimate causes of child deaths. They found that of the calculated 8.795 million deaths in children younger than 5 years of age worldwide in 2008, infectious diseases caused 68%, with the largest percentages due to pneumonia, diarrhoea and malaria.

These estimates of global disease burden are useful to guide global programmes and donor assistance, but there are uncertainties about the accuracy of these calculations and the estimates may not be applicable to specific locations. Thus, there remains the continuing need for special field research studies to validate these approximations.

SPECIAL PROSPECTIVE SURVEILLANCE STUDIES

Prospective surveillance studies detect a disease of interest in a cohort to calculate incidence, case fraction, case fatality rate or other measures of frequency. These studies provide data on the risk for illnesses or death in a population but may also be implemented in preparation for intervention trials (see below). Prospective surveillance studies are expensive due to the large costs for case-capture, diagnostic verification, treatment and data management. Frequently, it is necessary to conduct a census to have an accurate and up-to-date denominator. The conduct of a census requires technical know-how, a large workforce and hence considerable resources.

For some populations without access to treatment facilities or for rural areas with no laboratories, clinical and diagnostic infrastructure may need to be put in place to carry out surveillance studies. This raises questions of feasibility and increases costs substantially. There is also the problem of long-term sustainability after the surveillance project is completed. However, in an impoverished setting without accurate routine reporting of disease, prospective surveillance studies remain the gold standard for providing as complete and accurate a picture of disease burden as possible.

Geographic sites for prospective surveillance studies should be carefully selected to ensure that they are representative of the population of interest. Generalizing findings from one site to other populations, even within the same country, may be problematic. Multi-site studies may be done to assess the burden of disease in a wider regional area. For example, a prospective surveillance study of *Shigella* diarrhoea was undertaken in study sites in six Asian countries (Bangladesh, China, Pakistan, Indonesia, Vietnam and Thailand), to determine disease burden and prevailing species and serotypes.[8] The overall incidence of shigellosis cases presenting for treatment was two episodes per 1000 residents per year in all ages and was highest among children under 5 years old, at 13/1000 per year. The most frequently isolated *Shigella* species was *S. flexneri* in all sites, except in Thailand, where *S. sonnei* was most frequently detected. Findings such as these may be used to guide potential vaccine development or other interventions.

Detection of Cases (Numerator)

A major decision when conducting prospective studies of disease burden is the choice of how and where to detect cases. Active surveillance detects the disease of interest by regularly visiting or contacting residents of a community. Active surveillance is especially appropriate when the disease of interest is characterized by mild symptoms not likely to cause the patient to present for treatment. Active surveillance, particularly if diagnosis requires laboratory testing and confirmation, is labour-intensive and expensive. In addition, field workers require rigorous training and close supervision to ensure adherence to standardized methods. These logistic complexities limit the population size that can be included in such studies. There is also the danger of fatigue or refusal by the community if the purpose of the study is incompletely understood or if the visits are not conducted in a culturally acceptable fashion.

Passive surveillance captures cases presenting for care at treatment facilities. Passive surveillance may be done through treatment facilities established by the researchers or through existing primary healthcare units. When the burden of disease in a very large population is to be measured, then sentinel surveillance in several selected secondary or tertiary hospitals dispersed over a large geographic area may be conducted. This method is much more cost-efficient but unlike active surveillance, is subject to potential bias, since case detection is influenced by the study population's utilization of treatment. Although passive surveillance may be enhanced by regular community dialogue and household visits to encourage consultation for the disease of interest, it may still underestimate the burden of a disease for which the population usually self-medicates or seeks care with alternative or traditional healers who do not participate in the study. To avoid this bias, the researchers need to understand the community's utilization of healthcare facilities for the disease of interest and design the surveillance method accordingly.

Information from healthcare utilization surveys may be used to adjust disease estimates obtained through surveillance. For example, in a typhoid fever surveillance study in an urban and rural area in Kenya, Breiman and co-workers used health utilization data to adjust crude incidence rates.[9] The crude and adjusted incidence of blood culture-confirmed typhoid fever in the urban area was 247 and 822 cases per 100 000 person-years of observation (pyo), respectively, compared with 29 and 445 cases per 100 000 pyo in the rural area. The results showed dramatic differences in crude and adjusted, urban and rural typhoid incidence and showed rates similar to those in Asian urban settings, which had not been previously available from Africa.

Many diseases have a wide spectrum of presentations, which can range from sub-clinical to life-threatening. Different surveillance methods may capture different entities of the same disease. Active surveillance tends to detect mild illness; passive clinic-based community studies capture conditions that require a patient to present for care; whereas sentinel surveillance in secondary or tertiary hospitals detects the most severe forms of the disease. For example, dengue, a vector-borne viral illness, has a broad range of presentations. The majority of patients recover following a self-limiting febrile illness but a small proportion progress to severe disease, mostly characterized by plasma leakage leading to circulatory failure.[10] Home visits and clinic-based studies are likely to detect dengue fever, whereas hospital-based studies mainly capture the severe forms of the disease (Figure 6.1). If only a small fraction of cases in the population become severe, several sentinel hospitals in a large surveillance area may be needed in order to detect a sufficient number of patients to reach useful research conclusions about the disease.

Estimation of the Population (Denominator)

To calculate incidence rates (usually in terms of cases per 1000 to 100 000 population per year), the researchers need an accurate estimate of the numerator (the number of cases) as well as the source population from which the cases are captured. The study population may be enumerated through a baseline study census; demographic and healthcare utilization data may also be collected at the same time. If the study aims to determine very precise incidence rates (e.g. in preparation for or during intervention studies), baseline and follow-up censuses to monitor deaths, births and migration during the study period are required. When approximate incidence rates are to be measured, projected population size from the last government census may be sufficient. If the referral base of hospitals included in a sentinel surveillance is unclear, incidence cannot be calculated. Instead, the proportion of the disease of interest among all presentations or admissions (i.e. case fraction) may be reported. This is useful as an indicator of the burden of disease among patients who seek hospital care.

Quantification of Sequelae and Deaths

Quantification of sequelae and deaths may be done through follow-up of cases detected during surveillance or through general mortality surveys. In population-based studies, these are usually reported in terms of sequelae and deaths per 1000 to 100 000 population per year. In hospital-based studies, the

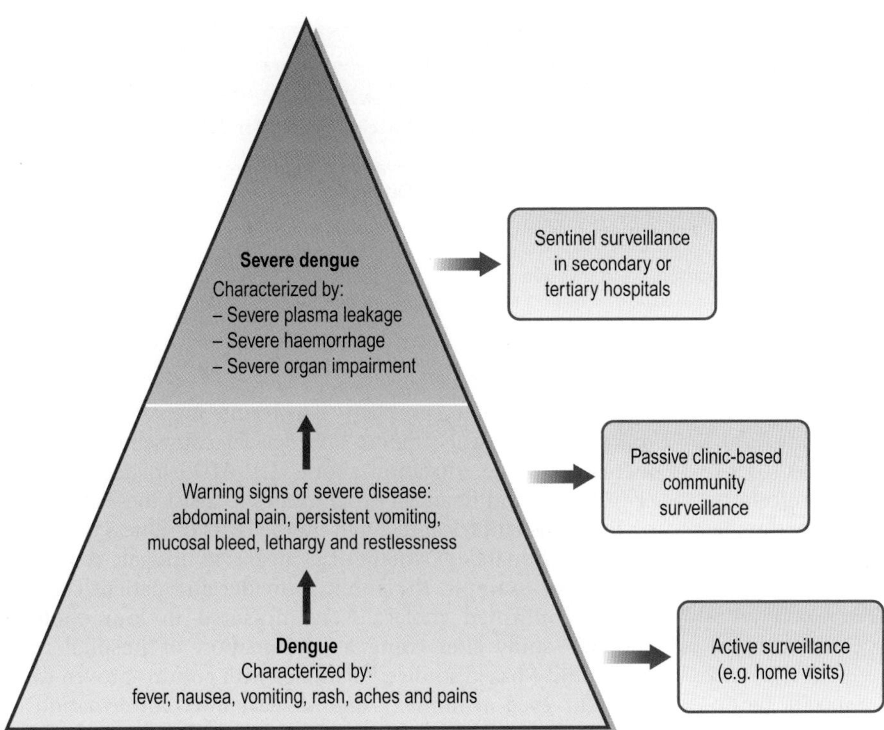

Figure 6.1 The clinical spectrum of dengue related to the surveillance case-capture method. *(Adapted from: WHO. Dengue Guidelines for Diagnosis, Treatment, Prevention and Control. Geneva: World Health Organization; 2009.)*

fraction of presenting or admitted patients who die (case fatality rate) or who develop complications and disability is reported. In prospective surveillance studies, cases have to be immediately and appropriately treated, thus the rates of complications, disability and death are often lower than would be noted outside a research setting. This inherent bias has to be kept in mind when drawing conclusions about sequelae and deaths from prospective research studies.

CROSS-SECTIONAL STUDIES AND CLUSTER SAMPLES

Cross-sectional studies survey a sample of the population at one point in time and estimate the prevalence of a condition, an infection or a disease. The survey tool may be a questionnaire; a physical assessment (e.g. of weight, height or blood pressure); a blood test (e.g. for malaria parasites or HIV infection); or a diagnostic procedure (e.g. chest X-ray). Unlike prospective surveillance studies, cross-sectional surveys do not provide information on incidence, i.e. the number of new cases per population during a specific time period. However, they may provide other important public health information. For example, for diseases that induce life-long antibodies (e.g. HIV, hepatitis A and B), sero-epidemiological studies may show the age groups most affected and when done at different time periods and geographic locations, may indicate the effectiveness of prevention and control strategies. HIV seroprevalence in pregnant women is often used as an indicator of the burden of HIV/AIDS in a community. A major challenge of cross-sectional studies is ensuring that the sample selected and included in the survey is representative of the population of interest.

VERBAL AUTOPSIES

Fatalities in developing countries often go unregistered. Even when death certificates are available and accessible, they may be incomplete or the reported cause of death may be unreliable. Many deaths in developing countries do not occur in hospitals, and officials who had neither treated nor seen the deceased person, may be requested to sign death certificates. Verbal autopsy or verbal postmortem is an alternative method to collect mortality data. It enables investigators to ascribe a probable cause of death, retrospectively. Verbal autopsy consists of a detailed interview of the deceased's next of kin or caregiver and a review of relevant records (e.g. clinic visit records) to determine symptoms and signs of illness before death, so as to establish the most likely cause of death.

There are specific recommendations about the design of verbal autopsies for mortality surveillance.[11] The data collection tool should include structured and unstructured questions; forms for adults and children exist and can be adapted, piloted and validated on-site. The interviewers should be specially trained. The interval between death and interview should be culturally appropriate but not overly long as to affect recall. Algorithms for decoding the completed interviews into causes of death must be clearly pre-defined. For example, two medically trained individuals may independently assess the completed verbal autopsy forms to identify the likely cause of each death. If there is disagreement between the two diagnoses, a third physician may adjudicate the decision. If the physicians cannot determine the cause of death, the death may be recorded as unspecified. Computer-automated methods for assigning cause of death have also been proposed and used. In most studies, the cause of death is assigned according to the International Classification of Diseases, Injuries and Causes of Death codes as recommended by the WHO.[12] Metrics for assessing the performance of different verbal autopsy cause assignment methods have been developed.[13]

Verbal autopsy studies are becoming increasingly common, with the largest to date conducted in India.[14] In this 'One million deaths study', all deaths occurring in 2001–2003 in 1.1 million nationally representative Indian households, were surveyed.

TABLE 6.1 Vaccine Trials Demonstrating Protection against Culture-Proven Invasive Disease, as well as Radiographic Pneumonia

	Vaccine Protection (95% CI) Against	
	Invasive, Culture-Proven Disease	Radiographic Pneumonia
Randomized trial of *Haemophilus influenzae* type-b tetanus protein conjugate for prevention of pneumonia and meningitis in Gambian infants[16]	95% (67–100)	22% (5–35)
Efficacy of nine-valent pneumococcal conjugate vaccine against pneumonia and invasive pneumococcal disease in The Gambia: randomized, double-blind, placebo-controlled trial[18]	77% (51–90)	37% (27–45)

Field staff completed verbal autopsies and two of 130 physicians independently assigned a cause to each death. The estimated 1.5 million child deaths in India in 2005 were attributed to five conditions: prematurity/low birth weight, neonatal infections, birth asphyxia/neonatal trauma, diarrhoeal diseases and pneumonia.[15] Each of these can be addressed with known, highly effective and widely practicable interventions.

VACCINE PROBE ASSESSMENTS

In estimating disease burden, the detection of a specific pathogen through diagnostic tests may be a major problem. The best available tests may fail to confirm many cases of illness caused by some pathogens. If a vaccine is highly effective in preventing disease in such undiagnosed syndromes, vaccine trials may be used to 'probe' the burden of disease that has been missed using the available diagnostic tests. For example, only a proportion of invasive *Haemophilus influenzae* type B (Hib)-associated illness is detectable through blood cultures or even more sensitive diagnostic testing, such as polymerase chain reaction. In a large, randomized trial of the Hib-tetanus protein conjugate vaccine in Gambian infants, protection was shown not only against culture-positive invasive disease, but also against culture-negative pneumonia, presumably because of the insensitivity of cultures in confirming Hib-pneumonia.[16,17] This has also been shown in a pneumococcal vaccine trial.[18] Vaccine probe assessments such as these, demonstrate that the burden of some diseases may be much greater than can be proven with the available diagnostic tools (Table 6.1).

Particularly in less-developed countries, where laboratory confirmation of diagnoses may be difficult and where widespread over-the-counter use of antibiotics may result in false-negative diagnoses, highly protective vaccines may be used to probe the total burden of difficult-to-confirm infectious diseases.

SOCIOECONOMIC RESEARCH

The burden of disease in a population may not only be characterized by rates of disease, death and disability; there are also the social impacts and financial costs of illness. The psychosocial consequences of an illness may be evaluated through socio-behavioural studies including rapid and in-depth qualitative surveys, focus group discussions and interviews on knowledge, attitudes and perceptions. For example, in-depth interviews were conducted with 47 children (ages 8–17 years) experiencing the loss of one or both parents due to HIV/AIDS in two rural counties of central China.[19] The majority of the participants reported some level of stigmatization and described feelings of sadness, fear, anxiety, anger, loneliness, low self-esteem, social withdrawal and sleep problems. The results suggested a need for more psychological support and special counselling services, increased public education about HIV/AIDS to decrease discrimination and financial programmes to assist these children.

Rigorous empirical research on the costs of illness is important for rational deployment of strategies to mitigate economic effects. For example, the public, provider and patient costs of culture-confirmed cholera were measured in four cholera-endemic study sites using a combination of hospital- and community-based studies.[20] Families with culture-proven cases were surveyed at home, 7 and 14 days after confirmation of illness. Hospital-based studies found that the costs of severe cholera were US$32 and US$47 in Matlab (Bangladesh) and Beira (Mozambique), respectively. Community-based studies in North Jakarta (Indonesia) and Kolkata (India) found that cholera cases cost between US$28 and US$206, depending on hospitalization. Patients' cost of illness, as a percentage of average monthly income, was 21% and 65% for hospitalized cases in Kolkata and North Jakarta, respectively. This analysis highlighted the financial burden of an acute diarrhoeal disease on households, often contributing to further poverty. The impact of chronic conditions such as HIV/AIDS on individuals, households and countries is more difficult to quantify. Presumably, HIV/AIDS is an important cause of poverty in many parts of sub-Saharan Africa. And yet, the impoverishing effects of AIDS have been inadequately assessed by existing studies, likely because of methodological challenges.[21]

Policy-maker surveys may be conducted to elicit government opinions about diseases. For example, DeRoeck and co-workers interviewed policy-makers and other influential professionals in four South-east Asian countries (Cambodia, Indonesia, Philippines and Vietnam) to determine their views on the public health importance of dengue, the need for a vaccine and the determinants influencing its potential introduction.[22]

OUTBREAK INVESTIGATIONS

An outbreak is the occurrence of disease episodes in greater numbers than would be expected at a particular time and place. The population at risk may range from a small, localized group to large populations. Infectious disease pathogens may cause epidemics that affect regional areas or pandemics that spread around the world. Recently, outbreak investigation and response have received unprecedented prominence with the severe acute respiratory syndrome (SARS) epidemic and the influenza A (H1N1) pandemic.

Once a report of an outbreak is received, there are several steps in its investigation.[23] Specimens are collected for laboratory verification of the diagnosis. Researchers develop a clinical case definition. Using this definition, cases and deaths are identified and the outbreak is analysed by time, place and person. Starting with the first case identified (index case), the number of cases by day or week is plotted to create an outbreak curve. Cases may be mapped and affected persons described in terms of age, sex and other relevant characteristics. Prevention and control procedures are implemented as soon as possible. Treatment centres may be set-up, guidelines for management disseminated and supplies and other logistics provided.

There are several outbreak patterns, each associated with a distinctive epidemic curve. In a common source outbreak, cases acquire the infection from the same source (e.g. a contaminated water supply). This may be a point source outbreak when the exposure occurs in less than one incubation period or a continuous source outbreak when the exposure occurs over multiple incubation periods. In a propagated outbreak, the pathogen is transmitted from person to person.

It is important to determine how the disease is transmitted in an outbreak, so that interventions can be taken to stop the current epidemic and to prevent future epidemics. A cohort study or a case–control study may be conducted to identify the risk factors that would cause an individual to become ill with the disease causing the outbreak. Cohort studies work best for well-defined populations (e.g. an outbreak that occurs among people who attended a gathering such as a funeral), while case–control studies work best for outbreaks where the population is not well-defined. The decision regarding the type of study that would be appropriate to investigate an outbreak also rests on the magnitude of risk, the latency of exposure to disease, the prevalence of exposure and timing (i.e. in some instances, it may be too late to conduct a cohort study).

Evaluation of Interventions against Infectious Disease

An intervention refers to an intentional change in some aspect of the individual.[1] Public health interventions against infectious diseases are varied and may range from behavioural (e.g. the promotion of hand-washing and breast-feeding; distribution of condoms to control the spread of sexually transmitted diseases; deployment of insecticide-treated bed nets to prevent malaria); structural (e.g. improvement of water supply and sanitation); to pharmacological (vaccine or drug administration). Rational policy-making in developing countries includes the evaluation of potential interventions in terms of safety, efficacy, effectiveness and financial impact.

The protection afforded by many traditional interventions may be widely known and accepted, while that from newer strategies may need to be evaluated. In the assessment of both pharmacological and non-pharmacological interventions, these need to be carried out under ethical conditions and using robust study designs so as to reach valid conclusions. The evaluation of pharmacological compared to non-pharmacological interventions is more stringent; candidate drugs and vaccines require a very careful, phased approach to minimize the potential risks to participants in trials.[24] If there is an intention to license these drugs or vaccines, regulatory agencies (e.g. the US Food and Drug Administration or the equivalent National Regulatory Agency in a developing country) scrutinize the findings of each step in this process.

RANDOMIZED CONTROLLED TRIALS

The randomized controlled trial (RCT) is the gold standard method for evaluating the efficacy of an intervention. The method involves randomly allocating participants into study and control groups, to receive or not receive the intervention being evaluated.[1] The results are assessed by a comparison of rates of disease or other appropriate outcome in the study and control group.

There are practical challenges to doing RCTs in less developed countries, where infrastructure and expertise may not be available. But many infections are geographically limited to developing countries and data on protection against naturally occurring disease can only be obtained in these sites. Even for diseases occurring in both industrialized and developing countries, study results may not necessarily be generalizable because of differences in population characteristics. For example, it has been shown that the immunogenicity of vaccines can be much lower in populations in developing compared with industrialized countries. Poorer performance has been especially problematic for orally administered live vaccines. The efficacy of the Rotarix™ and RotaTeq™ vaccines against severe rotavirus related disease in developing countries of Asia, Africa, and Central America does not appear to be as high as that seen in developed countries.[25–27] Another frequently cited example is the finding that three doses of oral polio vaccine, as formerly used in the USA, resulted in sustained, probably lifelong immunity, whereas many children in developing countries may require >3 doses for adequate seroconversion.[28] The poor performance of these vaccines in developing country populations is not well understood, but could be due to several factors, including high levels of pre-existing natural immunity (either maternal or infection-derived), poor nutritional status, tropical enteropathy and co-existing infections.[29]

Even within the developing world, findings from a randomized, controlled trial done in one region may not be generalizable to another region because of differences in the epidemiology of disease. For example, to seek new and improved treatments for severe falciparum malaria, a large multinational randomized comparison of parenteral artesunate versus the standard therapy of parenteral quinine was conducted in South-east Asia.[30] The trial proved that severe falciparum malaria mortality could be reduced by 30% in Asian adults when artesunate is used, but key decision-makers in Africa felt the results of this study were not generalizable to their populations where severe *falciparum* malaria tends to occur in children, rather than in adults. Over a 5 year period 5000 children with severe malaria in nine African countries participated in a large, multicentre, open-label randomized trial that established the superior efficacy of parenteral artesunate over quinine and led to a change in treatment guidelines.[31,32]

EFFICACY VERSUS EFFECTIVENESS

Conventional efficacy studies focus on the performance of interventions under ideal conditions whereas effectiveness trials address the protection afforded by interventions under real public health conditions.[33] Evidence from efficacy trials may not suffice to convince policymakers to allocate limited resources for new interventions. Effectiveness studies of licensed drugs and vaccines may be conducted in developing countries to collect evidence on feasibility, acceptability, and practical impact or effectiveness. For example, an effectiveness trial of the typhoid Vi vaccine was conducted to provide evidence for wider-scale implementation.[34] Slum-dwelling residents of Kolkata, India, who were 2 years of age or older were randomly assigned to receive a single dose of either Vi vaccine or inactivated hepatitis A vaccine, according to geographic clusters, and were followed for 2 years. The level of protective effectiveness was 61%. Interestingly, the design of the trial also allowed assessment of the protection of unvaccinated neighbours of vaccinated persons. This indirect protection was estimated at 44%. Not only the direct but also the indirect protection by Vi vaccine should be considered in future deliberations about introducing this vaccine in typhoid fever endemic areas.

OTHER DESIGNS

Other than randomized controlled trials, observational studies such as cohort, household contact, case–control, screening and case-cohort studies may be used to assess the effectiveness of an intervention.[35] Since the intervention is not randomly allocated in observational studies, bias is unavoidable. But it may still be possible to obtain sufficiently good estimates of protection from observational studies for public health purposes. Potential biases should be considered in the design phase and steps taken to minimize them if possible. As many more new and innovative interventions become available and the costs of randomized controlled trials escalate, the role of observational methods will become even more important.

ANALYSES OF ECONOMIC IMPACT

The economic impact of an intervention may be assessed using various methods; all of which weigh the costs of an illness with the expenditure for and benefits from an intervention (Figure 6.2). A cost–benefit analysis expresses costs and benefits in terms of money,[36] but monetary value may not be appropriate nor completely capture the benefits from health interventions.

In cost-effectiveness analysis, the cost of the intervention is also measured in monetary units but the benefit gained is expressed in terms of cases, deaths and DALYs averted. For example, in conjunction with the typhoid Vi vaccine effectiveness trial cited above, the cost-effectiveness of vaccination programmes in endemic sites in Asia was calculated.[37] It was estimated that a programme targeting all children ages 2–15 years old would prevent 456, 158 and 258 typhoid cases (and 4.6, 1.6 and 2.6 deaths), and avert 126, 44 and 72 DALYs over 3 years in Kolkata, North Jakarta and Karachi, respectively. The cost was calculated at US$160 and US$549, per DALY averted in Kolkata (India) and North Jakarta (Indonesia), respectively, and considered very cost-effective.

Cost-effective analyses may also compare two or more intervention options. For example, in association with the clinical trial of children with severe malaria in sub-Saharan Africa discussed above,[31] the cost-effectiveness of parenteral artesunate and quinine was compared. The mean cost of treating severe malaria patients was similar in the two study groups: US$63.5 in the quinine and US$66.5 in the artesunate arm. Compared with quinine as a baseline, artesunate showed an incremental cost of US$3.8 per DALY averted and an incremental cost per death averted of US$123. Artesunate was determined to be a highly cost-effective and affordable alternative to quinine for treating children with severe malaria.[38]

Cost-utility analysis estimate the ratio between the cost of a health-related intervention and the benefit it produces in terms of quality-adjusted number of years lived by the beneficiaries. A common metric in the denominator allows comparisons of diverse interventions against diverse diseases. An example is the use of DALYs.

Cost-benefit, cost-effective and cost-utility analyses do not incorporate the populations' stated preferences in decisions to finance new interventions. During the past 20 years, several stated preference studies have been conducted in less-developed countries, some of which have assessed willingness-to-pay for various public health interventions.[39] In general, the studies have shown low willingness to pay for these interventions, which is not surprising considering the competing priorities for food, shelter and other basic necessities. Thus, in the poor regions of the world, local governments and international donors have the obligation to continue to provide and implement much needed interventions.

Good Clinical Practice and Ethical Issues

Health research in developing countries should comply with current international research standards, so as to assure that the rights, safety and wellbeing of participants are protected

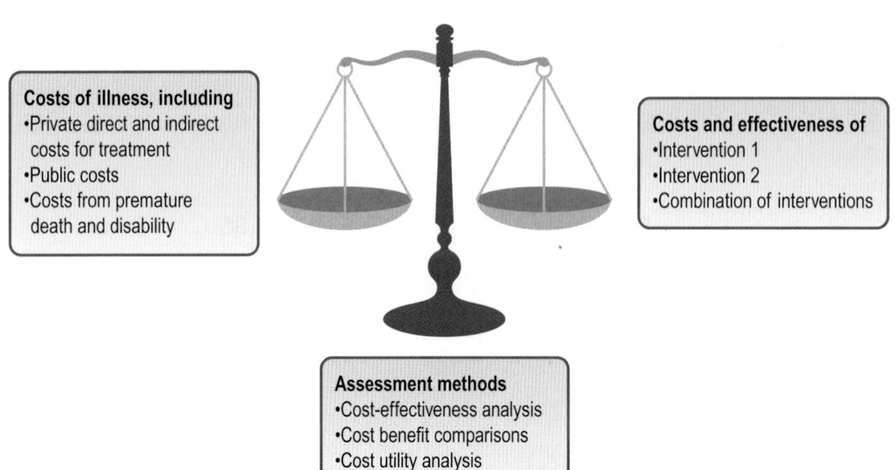

Figure 6.2 Evaluating the economic impact of an intervention.

and that the study data are credible. The ethics of research in developing countries has been the subject of intense discussion.[40] Issues being deliberated include: choosing the appropriate research question and design; use of placebo control groups in randomised controlled trials; capacity-building of local ethics committees to ensure sound and appropriate local review of the study protocol; ensuring that informed consent and assent is obtained which may be especially challenging in impoverished and less educated populations; the potential coerciveness of the offer to participate in research in locations where this may be the only means of obtaining health care; providing equal consideration to participants (including children and pregnant women) in research that would yield results beneficial to them while ensuring the protection of vulnerable participants; ensuring equal distribution of the burden and benefits of the research and minimizing the risk to participants.[41] These concerns are consistent with principles embraced in the World Medical Association's 'Helsinki Declaration' from 1964 and most recently amended in 2008. Special and continuing vigilance is necessary to safeguard the rights of populations in developing countries.

Although general ethical principles apply to all types of research, Good Clinical Practice (GCP) guidelines developed by the International Conference on Harmonization[42] are the standard for conduct of clinical research for licensure of pharmacologic interventions (e.g. vaccine and drugs). The GCP guidelines aim to ensure not only ethical conduct of studies, but generation of credible data. The guidelines' objectives of documenting informed consent, participant safety and data integrity are worthy. However, it has been argued that these GCP guidelines are based on consensus of expert opinions and not on evidence.[43] Not surprisingly, the individual standards as well as the concept of standardization of clinical trials of pharmacological interventions are not free of controversy. There have been increasing calls for the guidelines to be made more scientific, up-to-date, flexible and simple through collaborative and evidence-based efforts.[43,44] For trials in developing countries, rigid adherence to GCP standards as they are now formulated, have both positive and unfavorable consequences.[45] The complexity and expense of clinical trials has risen rapidly in recent years. A portion of this increased expense arises from the extensive documentation and auditing requirements demanded by GCP guidelines. This constitutes a disincentive to the clinical testing of drugs and vaccines for diseases mainly affecting developing countries and for which profitable markets are not foreseen. Furthermore, compliance with the stringent GCP requirements often requires the engagement of expensive contract research organizations, which are, in some cases, highly lucrative publicly traded enterprises. On the other hand, funders are increasingly demanding adherence to GCP and it is unlikely that regulatory agencies will license a new product without the diligence assured by a contract research organization.

Use of Health Research Findings to Guide Health Policy Decisions

We live in an era in which only a fraction of useful health interventions for populations in developing countries are delivered to these populations. This is true both for interventions that are well established as well as for new interventions. There are many reasons. Perhaps the most obvious obstacle is financial, with highly constrained healthcare budgets in developing countries and limited pools of donor resources being inadequate to fund all potentially useful interventions. Because of financial constraints, policy-makers at the global, regional and national levels increasingly demand hard evidence to compare the potential value of alternative interventions and to justify the expenditure of resources to fund the introduction of interventions.

Provision of data on the burden of the disease(s) targeted by the intervention is the most common kind of evidence requested by policy-makers. Evidence about the efficacy of an intervention, often obtained from rigorous clinical trials, is usually also needed. Even for interventions that appear attractive in evaluations of efficacy, there may be uncertainties about the logistic and programmatic feasibility of implementation in public health programmes, as well as about the impact upon desired health outcomes under real-life, public health conditions. Thus, evidence about intervention effectiveness is also relevant to policy deliberations. And, as alluded to above, policy-makers typically require evidence of cost-effectiveness of interventions, ideally expressed as the net cost per DALY averted in order to compare interventions for different diseases, as well as prophylactic versus therapeutic interventions.

Finally, it may be helpful to have an indication of the population demand for the intervention, even including assessment of willingness to pay for the intervention. Table 6.2 provides an outline of a programme of translational research (sometimes called 'implementation research') of this sort used in the Diseases of the Most Impoverished (DOMI) Program – a programme funded by the Bill & Melinda Gates Foundation to accelerate the introduction of new-generation vaccines against cholera, typhoid and shigellosis – for the introduction of killed oral cholera vaccines in several countries of Asia and Africa.[46]

TABLE 6.2 Multidisciplinary, Multi-Country Studies of The 'DOMI Program' to Provide Evidence to Inform Policy on the Introduction of Killed, Oral Cholera Vaccines

	Country						
Type of Activity	Bangladesh	China	India	Indonesia	Mozambique	Pakistan	Vietnam
Prospective disease burden studies	+		+	+	+	+	+
Meta-analysis of disease burden	+	+	+	+		+	+
Cost of illness studies	+		+	+	+		+
Assessment of feasibility, acceptability and impact	+		+		+		+
Cost of delivery studies	+		+		+		+
Cost-effectiveness analyses	+		+	+	+		+
Assessment of demand/willingness to pay studies	+	+	+	+	+	+	+
Policy analyses	+	+	+	+	+	+	+

While the ensemble of evidence generated by the DOMI Program has now become relatively standard in programmes to generate policy-relevant evidence on interventions for developing countries, it is important to note that several additional strategies are helpful if such evidence is to influence or support policy. Programmes to generate evidence should be formulated and conducted in partnership with policy-makers and health-care professionals in the countries where the intervention is being contemplated for introduction. For example, the DOMI Program was based on an initial systematic survey of policy-makers about evidence needs in targeted countries, and the DOMI field research programme was formulated on the basis of these findings.[47] Also, DOMI's multifaceted research programme to generate evidence was implemented in partnership with Ministries of Health in order to ensure that the decision-makers would have a sense of ownership of the findings. Moreover, if the evidence is to have an impact at the regional and global levels, as well as the national level, it may be helpful to construct multi-country programmes of research, with study designs and procedures standardized across countries. As shown in Table 6.2, the DOMI Program employed a standardized, multi-country approach to its studies, to generate evidence to inform policy on the introduction of killed oral cholera vaccines. This led to an evidence base that provided interpretable comparative data across countries.

Beyond generating the data, packaging and presentation of the evidence in a way that is convincing for policy-makers is of critical importance if the evidence is to have an impact on policy. This may require development of both detailed 'investment cases', as well as much shorter policy briefs. Presentation of the information in scientific journals is important, but it is also important to arrange presentations of study findings in both small and large meetings attended by policy-makers. The onus of assuring the attendance of policy-makers at such meetings is on the investigators. Finally, because the WHO has the ear of policy-makers, presentation of the findings at relevant WHO meetings, at both the regional and global levels is critical. An illustration of this approach was provided by efforts to synthesize and communicate the evidence on cholera and oral cholera vaccines. Synthesis of these findings into a white paper, and subsequently an investment case, for WHO's Scientific Advisory Group of Experts led to a greatly strengthened recommendation on oral cholera vaccines by WHO,[48] and provided the background for a recent World Health Assembly resolution, recommending the use of vaccines in the public health armamentarium against cholera.[49]

Summary

Public health research in developing country populations is complicated and challenging, but necessary. When conducted in a well-planned and focused manner, it can yield many important gains including understanding health problems better, informing policy decisions and rational deployment of interventions resulting in large health benefits.

REFERENCES

1. Last JM. A Dictionary of Epidemiology. New York: Oxford University Press; 1995.
2. Heuveline P, Guillot M, Gwatkin DR. The uneven tides of the health transition. Soc Sci Med 2002;55:313–22.
33. Clemens J, Brenner R, Rao M, et al. Evaluating new vaccines for developing countries: Efficacy or effectiveness? JAMA 1996;275:390–7.
36. Boardman NE. Cost-benefit analysis, concepts and practice. 3rd ed. Upper Saddle River: Prentice Hall; 2006.
42. International Conference on Harmonization (ICH) Expert Working Group. ICH Harmonised Tripartite Guideline: Guideline for Good Clinical Practice; 1996. Online. Available: ICHGCP.net
46. Deen JL, von Seidlein L, Clemens JD. Multidisciplinary studies of disease burden in the Diseases of the Most Impoverished Program. J Health Popul Nutr 2004;22:232–9.

Access the complete references online at www.expertconsult.com

Emergency and Intensive Care Medicine in Resource-Poor Settings

ARJEN M. DONDORP | MARTIN W. DÜNSER | MARCUS J. SCHULTZ

KEY POINTS

- Basic principles for the care of critically ill patients are applicable in both resource-rich and resource-poor settings.
- Close monitoring with proper alarm limits prompting appropriate action, use of both short- and long-term treatment plans, good organization of the intensive care unit with accurate patient documentation, and enforcement of strict hygiene rules, are essential ingredients for good critical care management.
- Mechanical ventilation in critically ill patients should make use of lung-protective ventilation strategies, including the use of lower tidal volumes (6 mL/kg predicted body weight).
- Early diagnosis and treatment of sepsis, including control of the infectious focus and a prompt start of antibiotics, reduces morbidity and mortality both in children and adults with severe sepsis independent of the hospital setting.
- Setting-adjusted recommendations derived from the 'surviving sepsis' guidelines can direct the treatment of severe sepsis in resource-poor settings.

Introduction

Care of critically ill patients in resource-poor settings is a challenge. There is often a shortage of nursing and doctor staff, basic supplies like drugs and oxygen are frequently lacking, availability of monitoring and mechanical ventilation is usually sparse, and the supporting infrastructure is frequently not directed to the needs of the critically ill patient. In addition, improvement of emergency and critical care, that is care for acutely and severely ill patients, is often given lower priority than primary care and public health interventions in resource-limited settings.

Without questioning the importance of preventive medicine and primary care, neglecting care for critically ill patients is not justified. As in industrialized countries, primary care and public health systems in resource-poor settings have not eliminated the need for good hospital care. In addition, 'all hospitals have critically ill patients'.[1] One other factor that typically hampers implementation of care for critically ill patients is the misconception of the definition of critical care medicine. Critical care is not necessarily only defined by expensive technology, but may include simple interventions such as oxygen therapy and intensive nursing. The debate about critical care in resource-poor settings should, therefore, not centre around whether it is appropriate, but what aspects are appropriate.[2]

Critical care in resource-poor settings is adaptable to the resource-poor setting and is not by definition unaffordable, but can in fact be highly cost-effective and contribute significantly to reductions in morbidity and mortality.[2,3] This chapter gives a brief outline of the principles of critical care adapted for resource-poor settings. This neglected field is currently attracting more attention, and scientific evidence for setting specific recommendations will grow over time.

Initial Emergency Care

It is recommended that there be a dedicated emergency room (ER) or 'shock room' available for the initial assessment, triage and treatment of medical, neurological and surgical emergencies, as well as trauma patients. This has been shown to contribute to a reduction in mortality in resource-poor settings.[4] A WHO working group has composed a minimum list of equipment for an emergency room at a first referral level health facility (see: http://www.who.int/surgery/publications/EEEGenericList). The list includes: an oxygen source – adult/paediatric resuscitator bag valves, oxygen masks and oropharyngeal airways equipment for endotracheal intubation; a portable suction apparatus; blood pressure cuffs and monitor; an introduction set for emergency chest tubes; equipment for venous access (peripheral and central venous access) and infusion fluids. Other basic requirements include a portable monitor/defibrillator unit with charged batteries, a pulse oximeter with a SpO_2 probe and X-ray facilities. A comprehensive list of essential medication in the emergency unit is beyond the scope of this chapter, however, a collaboration of organizations have generated an Interagency Emergency Health Kit (see: http://whqlibdoc.who.int/publications/2011/9789241502115_eng.pdf). Essential medication includes adrenaline (epinephrine); atropine; lidocaine (lignocaine); dextrose 20%; hydrocortisone; diphenhydramine; aspirin; sublingual nitroglycerin; naloxone (Narcan™); parenteral antibiotics and antimalarials. An ER or 'shock room' is preferably staffed on a 24/7 basis. With limited human resources, however, it will often not be feasible to establish full-time coverage by trained doctors, in which case nurses trained in 'advanced trauma life support' (ATLS) or 'advanced life support' (ALS) may serve as an alternative. Initial assessment and treatment should be aimed at securing vital functions, summarized as 'ABCDE' (Table 7.1): securing the *A*irway; check if the patient is *B*reathing; assessing the *C*irculation by checking the carotid pulse and check for significant

TABLE 7.1 **Summary of a General Approach to Medical Emergencies**

	Assessment	Action
A – Airway	Airway patency Patient's ability to maintain airway Colour of the patient Visible respiratory distress or exhaustion Added noises (e.g. stridor)	Simple airway manoeuvres (with cervical protection in trauma patients) Use of airway suction Guedel and/or nasal airway Upright position Administer oxygen Consider endotracheal intubation
B – Breathing	Inspection, palpation, percussion and auscultation for: Respiratory rate and rhythm Depth/symmetry of respiration Use of accessory muscles Colour of patient (blue, flushed, grey or pale) Assess distress or exhaustion Is there subcutaneous emphysema, tracheal deviation or asymmetry of chest movements? O_2-saturation (pulse oximetry) Additional secondary investigations: Arterial blood gas analysis Chest X-ray (if available)	Administer high-flow O_2 therapy Consider bag-ventilating patient and/or endotracheal intubation Consider bronchodilator therapy Act according to specifics of findings (e.g. emergency chest tube in case of tension pneumothorax)
C – Circulation	Pulse (carotid artery) Blood pressure Capillary refill (after nail pressure) Skin: colour, temperature, perspiration ECG monitor for assessment of cardiac rhythm Check for significant haemorrhage Additional secondary investigations include: – 12 lead ECG – Blood investigations such as blood glucose, electrolytes, full blood counts, others as indicated – If sepsis is suspected, search for infectious focus, and if available obtain blood cultures and other microbiological investigations. – Assess urine output – Other investigation depending on presentation and availability	Establish adequate and reliable IV access: large-bore peripheral vein or central vein Treat rhythm abnormalities: cardioversion or pharmacological rate control as appropriate In case of shock, start fluid therapy and if not quickly responsive, consider vasopressive drugs and inotropes In case of haemorrhage, perform initial haemostasis, start crystalloids solutions and arrange blood transfusion Treat myocardial infarction Treat hypoglycaemia Treat electrolyte disorders If sepsis is suspected, start antibiotics and follow sepsis treatment guidelines (see text)
D – Disability	Check the patient's ability to maintain airway and/or conscious level if cardiovascular parameters such as respiratory rate, oxygen saturation, blood pressure, pulse, blood glucose, temperature are deranged Assess level of consciousness using Glasgow Coma Scale (or Blantyre Coma Score for pre-verbal children; see Table 7.3). An alternative quick neurological assessment is 'APVU' (alert, verbal stimuli response, painful stimuli response, or unresponsive) Check pupil responses (pupil size, pupil reaction, consensual reflex) Check blood glucose level Observe for seizures Pain assessment For *conscious* patients: Check mental state, presence of headaches, speech impairment, lateralizing signs In trauma patients check for spinal cord injury level	If unresponsive consider airway management ('A') and recovery position if the airway is not satisfactorily secured Consider causes; if deranged physiological parameters are associated with a decreased level of consciousness, action must be immediate Correct blood glucose Control seizures and secure airway After initial stabilization, ensure appropriate levels of analgesia
E – Exposure	Undress patient for proper head to toe full assessment: Look for lumps, bumps, swelling, bruises or contusions, rashes, redness or discolouration (e.g. mottling)	Avoid hypothermia Act according to specifics of findings, (severe malnutrition, dehydration, etc.)

A formal course in 'advanced life support' (ALS) or 'advanced trauma life support' (ATLS) is recommended for all doctors and nurses involved in emergency and critical care. Initial assessment and initial actions based on the 'ABCDE' scheme.

haemorrhage; perform a quick neurological assessment ('*D*isability'), including the level of consciousness and pupil size and in the trauma patient also spinal cord injury level; the patient should be undressed for proper assessment whereas hypothermia should be prevented (*E*xposure/environmental control). If the patient has no palpable central pulse, cardiopulmonary resuscitation (CPR) should be started immediately and be followed by advanced life support following a 'shock' (including defibrillation) or a 'non-shock' (not including defibrillation) scenario, depending on whether the observed cardiac rhythm

TABLE 7.2 **Common Reversible Causes of Medical Emergencies in Non-Trauma Patients, Summarized as the 4 Hs and 4 Ts.**

Hs	Ts
Hypotension	Cardiac tamponade
Hypoxia	Tension pneumothorax
Hypokalaemia/hyperkalaemia	Intoxications (including therapeutics/medication)
Hypoglycaemia	
In selected cases also look for: *Hypothermia or hyperthermia, hypocalcaemia/hypercalcaemia/ hypomagnesaemia*	Thromboembolism

on the electrocardiogram is shockable (ventricular fibrillation, ventricular tachycardia or sometimes supraventricular tachycardias) or not shockable (asystole or severe bradycardia, electro-mechanical dissociation). A defibrillator, which can also be used for monitoring the cardiac rhythm, is a prerequisite for ALS. The main drugs which should be available for these emergency situations include adrenaline (epinephrine), used independent of the underlying cardiac rhythm, intravenous amiodarone, used to treat persistent ventricular fibrillation or tachycardia, and atropine, used to treat severe bradycardia.

In non-trauma patients reversible causes of the emergency situation can be summarized as the '4 Hs' and '4 Ts' and should be assessed quickly: *H*ypotension, *H*ypoxia, *H*ypokalaemia/hyperkalaemia (but sometimes also hypocalcaemia/hypercalcaemia/hypomagnesaemia), *H*ypoglycaemia, hypo- or hyperthermia, as well as cardiac *T*amponade, *T*ension pneumothorax, in*T*oxications (including therapeutics/medication) and *T*hromboembolism (Table 7.2). In trauma patients, when the primary survey is completed and vital signs are improving, a secondary survey should start, including a head-to-toe evaluation of the patient.

It is important that the individual roles of all the members of the resuscitation team are well-defined, and practice drills using a variety of possible scenarios can improve team performance. A resuscitation protocol is beyond the scope of this book, but is available on the Worldwide Web (e.g. www.facs.org/trauma/atls/program.html; and outlines on www.en.wikipedia.org). Courses in ATLS and ALS are available in many countries.

Following immediate stabilization, initial surgical or other treatment, the critically ill patient should be admitted to the intensive care unit (ICU) or another appropriate ward. Short communication lines between the emergency department and the ICU or ward are essential, and should occur wherever possible, through dedicated mobile phone numbers.

THE ICU SETTING

Since in most hospitals, ICU beds are in short supply, it is important to implement clear admission criteria in order to identify patients who are likely to benefit most from ICU treatment. This, however, also implies that patients with a grave short-term prognosis are discouraged from ICU admission. In addition to the emergency room, transfers of critically ill patients from other non-ICU hospital wards are an important source of ICU admissions. Guiding of ICU admissions can be optimized by an outreach service, where an ICU nurse and/or physician confirm the indication for ICU treatment prior to ICU admission. Such an outreach service can also prevent ICU admissions by advising ward physicians on, e.g., the management of hypoxia or hypotension.[5]

In resource-poor settings, it is unfortunately common that many patients with a clear indication for ICU care cannot be admitted to an ICU because of a lack of ICU beds or because the patient does not have the financial means to pay for (continuation of) critical care.[6] This can obviously cause important ethical dilemmas. The additional benefit of a prolonged stay in the ICU regarding patient outcome, and the accompanying additional costs, have not been assessed for most conditions in the developing world setting. This is essential knowledge, both for the patient's relatives who might spend an important proportion of their savings on the patient's care, as well as for policy-makers considering more investment in ICU care.

In hospitals without an ICU, a part of the general ward can be used as a high dependency ward dedicated to the care of the most ill patients. This allows implementation of intensified patient monitoring and treatment.

The ICU should be well organized and clean. Appropriate space between beds facilitates patient care and is important in the prevention of hospital-acquired infections, which are a major problem in ICUs around the world.

The rate of hospital-acquired infections in middle- and low-income countries is 3–5 times higher than reported from resource-rich settings.[7] Hospital-acquired infections have been proven to increase length of stay, costs of care, morbidity and mortality.[8] Two important pillars in preventing hospital infections are good hand hygiene and aseptic measures during invasive procedures. The hands of medical personnel are the main culprits in transmitting bacteria from one patient to another.[9] Washing hands before and after each patient contact or whenever hands become contaminated is a crucial step in reducing cross-infections in the hospital. Hospital-wide educational programmes and widespread availability of hand-washing facilities are essential, as these have been shown to improve hand hygiene and reduce the rate of hospital-acquired infections.[10,11] When available, alcohol-based rubs should be used. The use of refillable, pocket-sized containers of hand disinfectant can further improve hand hygiene. When alcohol rub is not available, clean water and soap can be used instead. In all cases, the correct technique of hand-washing must be followed.[12]

Adequate vital organ function monitoring is essential when caring for critically ill patients. The level of sophistication of monitoring will depend on the available resources. Basic low-cost multifunction monitors include 3-lead ECG, non-invasive blood pressure, respiratory rate (electrical impedance) and pulse oximetry. These modalities are recommended as a baseline investment. Ventilation can be assessed non-invasively with end tidal carbon dioxide monitoring. Since power cuts are common in resource-poor settings, equipment should have back-up battery power available, and a stethoscope as well as a sphygmomanometer should be at hand.

A reliable source of oxygen is a first priority for critical care. The choice of oxygen supply depends on the setting. Oxygen cylinders require a constant supply to maintain full tanks. This is expensive and logistically cumbersome. An advantage however, is that they do not require electricity. Oxygen concentrators are cheaper, but require good maintenance and an uninterrupted electricity supply. Piped oxygen from a central oxygen source is the reference standard, but necessitates substantial investment.

Availability of mechanical ventilation is also important. Mechanical ventilators generally require an uninterrupted power supply, making a back-up generator or batteries essential. When choosing a mechanical ventilator, adequate maintenance is pivotal and often complicated in modern lung ventilators. Maintenance contracts by the manufacturer often only apply to the first 3–5 years after purchase, and local availability of skilled bio-technicians can thus be an important asset. Considering the importance of maintenance, it is important to focus on the technical simplicity of mechanical ventilators. Furthermore, it is recommended that one single type of ventilator is used in the ICU, in order to avoid mistakes during handling. In settings without a supply of compressed gasses, mechanical ventilators should contain an internal or external air compressor device. Easy maintenance is important.[13]

Independent of the type of lung ventilator in use, the humidification and warming of inspired gases requires the addition to the ventilator circuit of a heated humidifier. A heat-moisture exchanger (HME) may serve as a good alternative. Apart from the lower costs associated with the use of an HME, compared with a heated humidifier, an HME may also protect against ventilator-associated pneumonia, as water used in heated humidifiers may become colonized with bacteria. A potential hazard of HME is that the inspiratory and expiratory resistance may increase as a result of filter plugging, and can get blocked in cases of excessive sputum production.

For the treatment of unexpected emergencies, certain life-saving drugs and equipment should instantly be available. An emergency tray could contain an emergency supply of these essential drugs and functional equipment. It must be kept on each ward where critically ill patients are cared for. The contents of the emergency tray should be checked daily to ensure completeness.

Essential support for critically ill patients also includes laboratory facilities to assess complete blood counts and basic biochemistry, such as electrolytes, renal function, liver enzymes and cardiac enzymes. Arterial blood gas measurement provides important advantages for assessing gas exchange and acid base disorders, but blood gas analysers are expensive and dependent on appropriate maintenance and regular calibration. Bedside battery-operated devices for point of care assessment of basic haematology, biochemistry and blood gas parameters not requiring additional calibration, are available and an important asset for the ICU. The price of cartridges used in these 'point of care' devices can usually compete with the charges for private laboratories, but a drawback is the limited shelf-life of the cartridges.

A blood bank for storage of blood products and a system of voluntary blood donors is also an essential asset for providing care for critically ill patients. A blood bank should include facilities for cross-matching of blood and tests for blood-borne pathogens.

Availability of bedside imaging techniques including X-ray and ultrasonography can be of great value. Their use for the individual patient should be weighed against the costs of the device and procedure.

PATIENT MONITORING ON THE ICU

Close monitoring of critically ill patients is essential since the condition of the patient can worsen unexpectedly. Monitoring should include at least: blood pressure and peripheral circulation; cardiac rhythm; oxygenation and respiratory rate/work of breathing as well as level of consciousness.

Invasive blood pressure monitoring will generally not be available in resource-poor settings since it is expensive and carries potential dangers if nursing care is inadequate. In most resource-limited settings, non-invasive automated assessment of arterial blood pressure is the modality of choice. If automated non-invasive blood pressure devices are not available, repeated manual measurements should be taken. It is important to realize that a normal arterial blood pressure is not necessarily synonymous with adequate tissue perfusion, since an increase in the peripheral vascular resistance can result in normal blood pressure, whereas blood flow to vital organs can still be compromised. Compensated shock, defined as reduced perfusion without arterial hypotension, is especially common in children. In children, heart rates can be inappropriately high or low for age (infants: <90 or >160/min; children <70 or >150/min). There is no simple test to assess reduced tissue perfusion, but capillary refill time, temperature gradient across the legs and temperature of the acra (toes, fingers, ears, tip of the nose) may serve as useful surrogates.[14] Assessment of the cardiac rhythm requires an ECG. If this is not available, pulse oximetry can be used to measure pulse rate continuously. A central venous catheter for monitoring central venous pressure (CVP) is recommended in case of continuous vasopressor use to assure adequate filling. In other circumstances the usefulness of CVP monitoring is questionable as a measure of end diastolic volume or as a predictor for fluid responsiveness.[15]

Pulse oximetry is a highly valuable tool to measure arterial oxygen saturation, especially if blood gas monitoring is not available. Capnography can be a useful additional tool to monitor ventilation in critically ill patients, typically in those requiring mechanical ventilation. This gives a continuous measurement of carbon dioxide in exhaled air and is more sensitive than pulse oximetry for the detection of alveolar hypoventilation or airway obstruction. In the non-intubated patient, it is important to monitor respiratory rate as well as the 'work of breathing'. Especially in patients with airway obstruction, respiratory insufficiency will often not be revealed by an increase in respiratory rate, whereas the increase in the work of breathing is evident for the closely observing nurse or physician.

The level of consciousness is assessed most easily with the use of the Glasgow Coma Scale (GCS or EMV score) or Blantyre Coma Score (Table 7.3) in pre-verbal children.

Development of acute renal failure is an important threat during the first days of ICU admission, for instance in patients with malaria, bacterial sepsis, certain intoxications or severe trauma. Monitoring of urine output is important. If oliguria is recognized late without appropriate steps being taken, infection, organ failure and death may ensue. However, renal failure can also be 'non-oliguric', and its detection will need assessment of plasma creatinin or blood urea nitrogen (BUN).

If a continuous patient monitor is used, proper alarm limits should be set. Patient monitors allow for continuous surveillance of vital parameters and reduce staff workload. However, it is crucial to remember that monitors can never replace continuous attendance of experienced healthcare staff or repeated clinical examinations. The ICU staff needs to be familiar with the monitor and its technology. It is reasonable to focus on a basic set of parameters such as heart rate, arterial blood pressure, respiratory rate and peripheral oxygen saturation. While

TABLE 7.3 **Quick Assessment of Consciousness Level in Adults (Glasgow Coma Scale) and Pre-Verbal Children (Blantyre Coma Score).**

Adults		Preverbal Children	
Glasgow Coma Scale		Blantyre Coma Scale	
Eye Opening		**Eye Response**	
Spontaneous	4	Follows or watches	1
To loud voice	3	Fails to watch or follow	0
To pain	2		
Nil	1		
Motor[a]		**Motor**[a]	
Obeys verbal commands	6	Localizes painful stimulus	2
Localizes noxious stimuli	5	Withdraws from pain	1
Withdraws (normal flexion)	4	No or inappropriate response	0
Abnormal flexion posturing	3		
Extension posturing	2		
Nil	1		
Verbal		**Verbal**[a]	
Oriented	5	Appropriate cry	2
Confused, disoriented	4	Abnormal cry or moan	1
Inappropriate words	3	No cry	0
Incomprehensible sounds	2		
Nil	1		

[a]This implies the best response to painful stimuli, e.g. pressure on a nail bed, on the sternum or on a supraorbital ridge.

alarm limits set too liberally put the patient at risk by delaying recognition of changes, limits set too tightly bear the risk of over-reporting measurement deviations and 'de-sensitizing' medical staff for truly important alarms.

If continuous monitoring is not feasible, manual assessments of vital signs should be performed frequently. The frequency will depend on the severity of the patient's condition and should be increased in case of cardiopulmonary instability or whenever a change in the patient's condition arises. Concerns expressed about a patient by the nurse or a family member must be taken seriously and lead to careful re-assessment of the patient.

Figure 7.1 shows an example of an early warning system, which can be used to alert both nurses and doctors that the condition of the patient requires additional attention and action.

INVASIVE PROCEDURES

Invasive procedures, such as the insertion of a central venous line, carry the risk of iatrogenic infections. For this reason, full sterile barrier precautions should be applied including sterile draping, caps, gloves, surgical masks and gowns, as well as skin disinfection with chlorhexidine or alcohol- rather than iodine-based disinfectants.[16] Urinary (Foley) catheters should be removed when no longer needed. A prospective study from Thailand revealed that a multifaceted intervention to remind physicians to remove unnecessary urinary catheters could reduce the rate of catheter-associated urinary infections.[17]

DATA DOCUMENTATION ON THE ICU

A medical record including relevant information about demographic data, allergies, medical history and the current disease process should be kept for every patient. Vital signs should be documented regularly on a dedicated patient record form to allow rapid assessment of the disease course and interpret changes in the patient's condition. Depending on the phase of the disease, vital signs should be documented at intervals from at least hourly in unstable patients to 6-hourly in stabilized patients. In addition, body temperature, peripheral perfusion and daily fluid balance should be recorded at least once per shift or when abnormal. Whenever deterioration occurs, it is crucial to not only treat symptomatically (e.g. treat seizures, stabilize haemodynamic and/or respiratory function) but also to identify the underlying causes. Good collaboration between physicians and nurses, with an adequate hand-over between shifts conveying essential information is crucial.[18] Systematic adherence to a standardized protocol, adapted to the local setting, can improve the quality and completeness of information flow. Furthermore, clear definition of daily goals for each patient using a 'daily goal form' increases the proportion of team members understanding

EWS Score:	3	2	1	0	1	2	3
HR		<40	40–50	51–100	101–110	111–130	>130
SBP	<70	70–80	81–100	101–200		>200	
RR		<9		9–14	15–20	21–30	>30
Temperature (°C)		<35	35–36.5	36.6–37.5	>37.5		
Level of consciousness				Alert	Verbal	Pain	Unres-ponsive

Feeling bad:	Add 1 point
Urine output <75ml in the last 4 hours:	Add 1 point
SpO_2 <90%:	Add 3 points

TOTAL SCORE

[If score ≥3, call doctor to evaluate patient]

Figure 7.1 Example of an early warning system.

the goal of care for the day and shortens the intensive care unit length of stay.[19]

DAILY ROUNDS

Daily (or more frequent) rounds by the complete treatment team should be made to formulate a treatment plan for all patients in the ICU or high dependency wards. Round-the-clock care is mandatory, and a detailed written handover should be provided by both doctors and nursing staff to the next shift.

It may be advisable to adopt a standardized approach to evaluation and treatment of critically ill patients, including organ system-based surveys (focused on avoiding diagnostic error and therapeutic delay) and an ICU rounds checklist (e.g. restrictive fluid and transfusion; medication reconciliation; lung protective ventilation; spontaneous awakening and breathing trials with early physical therapy; aspiration precautions; thromboembolism prophylaxis; removal of devices that are no longer needed).

Every critically ill patient should have a dedicated physician and nurse responsible for their care. This implies that nursing care should be patient- rather than task-centred. Task-centred care where several nurses are responsible for different aspects of nursing care concerning the same patient carries the danger of diluting responsibility. A better model is that one nurse has complete nursing responsibility for a small number of critically ill patients, and plays a crucial role in early identification of medical problems, such as arterial hypotension or hypoxia. This requires responsibility empowerment of the nursing staff and appropriate training is a prerequisite for this. Relatively simple tools can be used to identify relevant changes in the patient's condition, such as the use of an 'early warning score' (Figure 7.1), where the number of the score is linked to taking appropriate action by the nursing staff.

ENTERAL FEEDING

Early start of enteral feeding is an established treatment strategy in critically ill patients. Starving deprives the patient from nutritional supplies, vital cell substrates, antioxidants, vitamins and minerals, essential for normal cell function. Furthermore, enteral feeding increases splanchnic blood flow, which protects against development of stress ulcers. In addition, enteral feeding preserves gut integrity and function, preventing translocation of pathogenic gut flora. A meta-analysis of 15 studies in 753 critically ill surgical patients concluded that start of enteral feeding within 36 hours of ICU admission reduced the incidence of invasive infections, the length of hospital stay and costs.[20] In intubated patients, enteral feeding can be administered through a nasogastric tube ideally using a pump for continuous feeding. However, this will not be available in most resource-poor settings where bolus feeding is a good alternative. Before feeding is started, the patient should be positioned with a head tilt of 15–30° above horizontal and the position of the nasogastric tube should be checked. This can be done by X-ray, aspiration of gastric fluids or by auscultation over the gastric region at the moment of inflating air through the nasogastric tube. Feeding should start with small volumes, e.g. 100 mL pureed feeding every 4 hours in order to assess tolerability and gastric retention. Gastric retention should be measured just before the next feed is administered and if cumulative gastric retention per day exceeds 500–1000 mL (~200 mL/4–6 hours), feeding should be discontinued. In these cases, a prokinetic drug can be started, e.g. metoclopramide suppositories in a dose of 20 mg three times a day. Cisapride is no longer used because it affects cardiac repolarisation (QTc prolongation). If the feeding is well tolerated, it can be increased to 300 mL every 4 hours, aiming at delivering around 2000 Kcal/day. However, enteral feeding should not be started in unconscious patients whose airway is not secured (e.g. by an endotracheal tube), since this carries significant risk (33%) of regurgitation, pulmonary aspiration and pneumonia.[21]

BLOOD TRANSFUSION

Availability of pathogen-free blood products, including packed red cells is an important asset for the management of critically ill patients. Full cross-matching of donor and recipient's blood should be a routine assessment before transfusion. When available, packed red cells are preferred over whole blood, because of the latter's greater immunogenicity. If cell separation is not possible, whole blood should be given. Standard tests to exclude the most common blood-borne pathogens, including HIV-1 and HIV-2, hepatitis B and C, syphilis, and where appropriate malaria, Chagas' disease and human T-lymphotropic virus-I/II and/or West Nile virus, should be mandatory before transfusion. Concern about inadvertent transfusion of HIV-positive blood should restrict the use of transfusion, especially in areas where HIV is highly prevalent and facilities for screening are inadequate. In these situations, blood transfusion is indicated only when severe anaemia is accompanied by clinical signs of impaired tissue oxygenation such as shock, cardiac failure, extreme lethargy or severe ongoing blood loss. In patients with chronic anaemia or children, a low haematocrit is often well tolerated. Because the ultimate risk–benefit ratio of transfusion will depend on the setting and condition of the patient, there is no absolute threshold for the administration of packed cell transfusion. WHO guidelines for the management of severe malaria recommended immediate blood transfusion for all children with a haematocrit of ≤12% or Hb ≤4 g/dL. In less severely anaemic children (haematocrit 13–18%; Hb 4–6 g/dL) transfusion is recommended if severe symptoms are present, including shock, impaired consciousness, deep and laboured breathing, and also in case of severe dehydration or very high malaria parastaemia (>10% of red cells with parasites). In areas of high malaria transmission, children often have chronic anaemia and can tolerate low haemoglobin levels surprisingly well. The recommendation for adults is to transfuse all patients with Hb <5 g/dL, and less severely anaemic adults (haematocrit 15–18%; Hb 5–6 g/dL) in cases with severity signs (as in children) or in the presence of cardiac ischaemia or heart failure. In severe sepsis, a threshold of 7 g/dL is often recommended. During transfusion the patient must be closely and repeatedly monitored for adverse events such as hypervolaemic pulmonary oedema. Many patients improve after transfusion but repeated transfusions may be required suggesting ongoing blood loss or abnormally rapid haemolysis of donor erythrocytes. Iron and folic acid supplementation may be necessary when oral medication can be taken, particularly in pregnant patients and in those at risk of a recurrent or chronic hookworm status.

STRESS ULCER PROPHYLAXIS

ICU population's stress ulcer prophylaxis has been shown to be effective in reducing upper gastrointestinal bleeds. Although formally only tested in resource-rich settings, this is also likely to be applicable to resource-poor settings. Stress ulcer prophylaxis can be provided using an H2 blocker such as ranitidine or a proton pump inhibitor such as omeprazole.[22]

DEEP VEIN THROMBOSIS PROPHYLAXIS

It has long been assumed that the prevalence of deep venous thrombosis in many resource-poor settings is too low to warrant widespread antithrombotic prophylaxis, but more recent evidence shows important morbidity and mortality associated with deep venous thrombosis also in middle- and low-income countries.[23,24] Where possible, routine deep vein thrombosis prophylaxis with subcutaneous unfractionated heparin or, whenever available, low-molecular-weight heparins (LMWH) should be administered to all ICU patients, with the exception of patients with increased bleeding risk or ongoing haemorrhage.[25] In settings where no heparin is available, antithrombotic stockings or elastic bandages can be applied on both legs.[26] There are no evidence-based guidelines for use of venous thromboembolism (VTE) prophylaxis in children. However, paediatric ICUs in resource-rich settings often do recommend VTE prophylaxis with LMWH in immobilized children with severe illness. Studies addressing this issue are ongoing.

MOBILIZATION

Prolonged bed-rest and immobilization contributes to important morbidity, e.g., muscular atrophy; prolonged weakness; respiratory compromise; autonomic dysfunction; gastrointestinal paralysis; deep vein thrombosis and delirium.[27] Early mobilization may prevent or counteract these effects and hasten recovery.[28] As soon as the patient is stable, mobilization in- and outside of the bed should actively be encouraged.

Sepsis Treatment Guidelines for Resource-poor Settings

The 'Surviving Sepsis Campaign' document summarizes current best practice for the treatment of severe sepsis and septic shock.[29] The document was written for the ICU setting in resource-rich countries, but has been adapted for the resource-poor setting.[30]

Early diagnosis and treatment, including control of the infectious focus ('drain the pus') and a quick start of broad-spectrum antibiotics, reduces morbidity and mortality both in children and adults with severe sepsis, independent of the hospital setting.[31,32] Initial empirical anti-infective therapy should include one or more drugs that have activity against all likely pathogens (bacterial and/or fungal) and that penetrate, in adequate concentrations, into the presumed source of the infection.[29] The choice of empirical antibiotics will depend on a multitude of factors, including the source of the infection, local antimicrobial resistance patterns, drug intolerance, etc. Recently used antibiotics should generally be avoided. Meticillin-resistant *Staphylococcus aureus* is widely prevalent in developing world settings, so empiric therapy should usually cover this resistant pathogen. Initial broad coverage is essential, and therapy can be narrowed down if the causative organism and antibiotic susceptibilities are defined. Figure 7.2 shows a decision tree for antibiotic choice in a hospital in Orissa, India. It should be emphasized that this flow diagram is for illustration only, and should be adapted to the local setting.

Whenever facilities for microbiology are available, blood and other relevant cultures should be obtained before antibiotic treatment is started, but this should not delay antimicrobial treatment. It is important to recognize the septic patient at an early stage. Febrile patients suspected of having an infection and who show signs of a systemic inflammatory response syndrome (SIRS, summarized in Table 7.4) have sepsis.[33] The listed parameters denoting SIRS are a useful screening tool, although some, such as those requiring blood gas analysis and white blood cell count, will not be generally available in the resource-poor setting. Additional indicators of sepsis in the febrile patient, albeit nonspecific, include a weakened general condition and altered mental status, including obtundation or agitation, which is in particular an early sign in children and the elderly. Hyperglycaemia can be another early manifestation of sepsis in adults, while hypoglycaemia is more common in children. Tissue hypoperfusion characterizes severe sepsis, and is often reflected by peripheral hypoperfusion which can be assessed clinically as prolonged capillary refill time, temperature gradient over the leg, cold extremities, diffuse sweating and skin mottling.[14] Oliguria and altered mental status can be signs of hypoperfusion of kidneys or brain, respectively. Plasma lactate is a frequently used proxy measure of tissue hypoxia, and has a strong prognostic significance in both sepsis and other critical conditions, but assessment of plasma lactate will often not be available in resource-poor settings.[34] Septic shock is characterized by the presence of arterial hypotension, despite adequate fluid loading in combination with signs of tissue hypoperfusion. There is a stepwise increase in mortality in both adults and children from sepsis without organ dysfunction to severe sepsis up to a mortality of 50% or more in septic shock.[35,36]

After rapid initiation of broad-spectrum antibiotics, it is important to prioritize elimination of the source of infection whenever possible. This includes drainage of abscesses, obstructed urinary tracts or deep space infection such as pleural empyema or septic arthritis, as well as surgical treatment of necrotizing soft tissue and wound infections, gastrointestinal perforation and cholangitis. Iatrogenic sources, such as intravascular catheters or urinary (Foley) catheters are frequent sources of infections, especially in intensive care units of middle- and low-income countries.[37] Evidently, infectious sources like pneumonia or meningitis cannot be treated by removing the source and therefore rely on adequate antimicrobial therapy. Antimicrobial therapy needs to be reassessed daily. Worsening or ongoing organ dysfunction and persistence of infectious signs like fever for more than 48–72 hours following initiation of treatment should prompt considering a change of antibiotic therapy. It should be noted that in some infectious diseases such as melioidosis, defervescence usually takes longer, even with adequate antimicrobial therapy. In cases where microbial cultures were obtained at the time of admission (before start of antibiotics), 48–72 hours is the usual time when culture results and pathogen susceptibility become available. This will usually mean reducing the number or narrowing the spectrum of antibiotics (de-escalation), which is important for

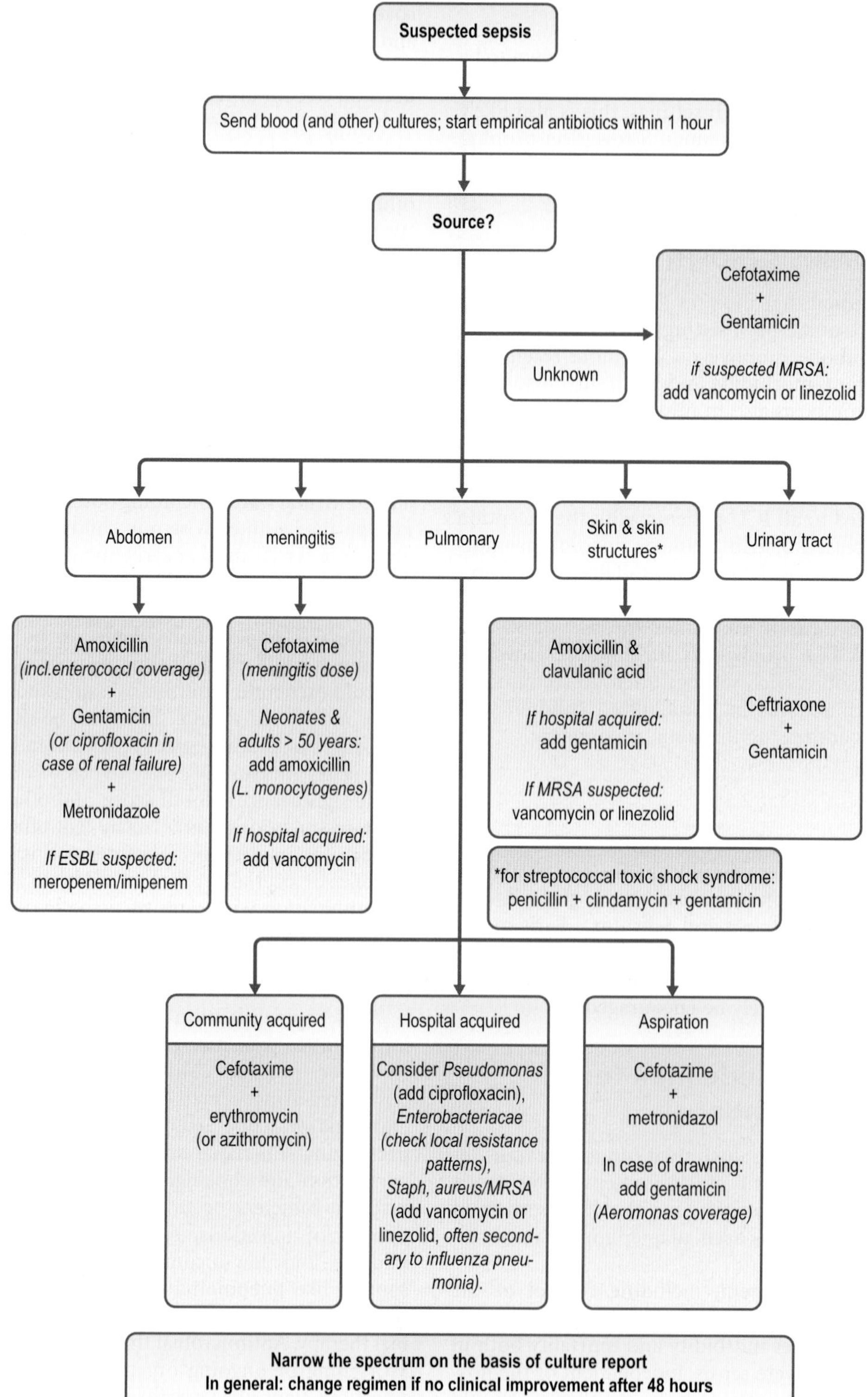

Figure 7.2 Example of a decision tree for choice of antibiotic therapy in patients with severe sepsis. This guideline was developed for an ICU in Orissa, India, based on prevalence and resistance patterns of local pathogens and availability and price of antibiotics. The diagram does not cover the possibility of invasive *Candida* infections, and clinicians should consider whether this is a likely pathogen. Severe malaria is also not included in the diagram; this disease can also present as severe sepsis. The guideline cannot be translated without adaptation to different locations and settings. ESBL = extended-spectrum beta-lactamase-producing Gram-negative bacteria.

TABLE 7.4 **Definition of Infection and Sepsis Syndromes**

	Suggested Sepsis Diagnosis with Limited Resources	Sepsis Diagnosis according to International Consensus[22,23,33]
Sepsis	*Proven or highly suspected infection plus presence of ≥2 of the following conditions:* Heart rate >90 bpm Respiratory rate >20 bpm Temperature <36 or >38°C Malaise and/or apathy	*Proven or highly suspected infection plus presence of ≥2 of the following conditions:* Heart rate >90 bpm Respiratory rate >20 bpm or $PaCO_2$ <32 mmHg Temperature <36 or >38°C WBC <4 or 12 × 10^3/µL or >10% immature forms
Severe sepsis	*Sepsis-induced tissue hypoperfusion or organ dysfunction* *Tissue hypoperfusion* Decreased capillary refill or skin mottling Peripheral cyanosis Arterial hypotension Systolic arterial blood pressure <90 mmHg or a systolic arterial blood pressure decrease >40 mmHg *Pulmonary dysfunction* SpO_2 <90% with or without oxygen Central cyanosis Signs of respiratory distress (e.g. dyspnoea, wheezing, crepitations, unability to talk sentences) *Renal dysfunction* Acute oliguria (urine output <0.5 mL/kg per h or 45 mL/h for at least 2 hours despite adequate fluid resuscitation) Hepatic dysfunction Jaundice *Coagulation dysfunction* Petechiae or ecchymoses Bleeding/oozing from puncture sites *Gastrointestinal dysfunction* Ileus (absent bowel sounds)	*Sepsis-induced tissue hypoperfusion or organ dysfunction* *Tissue hypoperfusion* Decreased capillary refill or skin mottling Hyperlactataemia (>1 mmol/L) Arterial hypotension Systolic arterial blood pressure <90 mmHg; mean arterial blood pressure <70 mmHg; or a systolic arterial blood pressure decrease >40 mmHg *Pulmonary dysfunction* PaO_2/FiO_2 <300 *Renal dysfunction* Acute oliguria (urine output <0.5 mL/kg per hour or 45 mL/h for at least 2 hours despite adequate fluid resuscitation) Creatinine increase >0.5 mg/dL or 44.2 µmol/L Hepatic dysfunction Hyperbilirubinaemia (plasma total bilirubin >4 mg/dL or 70 µmol/L *Coagulation dysfunction* Thrombocytopenia (platelet count, <100 000/µL) Coagulation abnormalities (INR >1.5 or a PTT >60 s) *Gastrointestinal dysfunction* Ileus (absent bowel sounds)
Septic shock	*Sepsis-induced arterial hypotension despite adequate fluid resuscitation (note that patients on inotropics or vasopressors may not be hypotensive despite of presence of shock) and signs of tissue hypoperfusion*	*Sepsis-induced arterial hypotension despite adequate fluid resuscitation (note that patients on inotropics or vasopressors may not be hypotensive despite of presence of shock) and signs of tissue hypoperfusion*

$PaCO_2$, partial arterial carbon dioxide tension; WBC, white blood cell count; SpO_2, plethysmographic oxygen saturation; PaO_2/FiO_2, partial arterial oxygen tension/fractional inspiratory oxygen concentration quotient; INR, international normalized ratio; PTT, partial thromboplastin time.

reducing the likelihood of bacterial selection and induction of resistance. Duration of antibiotic therapy will depend on the source and cause of infections.

In the shocked adult patient, prompt fluid resuscitation should be initiated immediately. In septic shock patients *with* access to mechanical ventilation, liberal initial fluid resuscitation with normal saline should be initiated, which typically improves haemodynamic function and tissue perfusion, thus reducing mortality.[38] In the dehydrated patient, resuscitation with at least 1 L normal saline is often required. If a central venous line is in place, filling up to a CVP of 12 cm H_2O in mechanically ventilated adult patients could be used as a guideline.[29] Alternative more expensive resuscitation fluids have not shown additional benefit, and resuscitation of severe septic patients with colloid hydroxyethyl starch has been associated with increased rates of acute kidney injury.[39] Evidence on the benefit of fluid resuscitation in septic shock is assessed primarily in settings where a mechanical ventilator and staff familiar with its use are readily available. In case fluid therapy results in pulmonary oedema, positive pressure ventilation can counteract this and restore adequate oxygenation. However, in severe sepsis with presence of pulmonary capillary leakage and acute respiratory distress syndrome, adequate oxygenation even with mechanical ventilation can be very difficult. After initial aggressive fluid resuscitation and haemodynamic stabilization in septic patients with acute lung injury, a conservative fluid policy in the following days striving at a negative fluid balance is indicated, since this strategy has been shown to reduce the time on mechanical ventilation[40] and might reduce mortality.[41] It is important to monitor the fluid balance in critically ill patients, who often receive large amount of fluids during the early phase, which has later to be mobilized and removed through diuresis, often with the help of loop diuretics, following stabilization. Electrolyte disturbances can occur in this phase. Hypernatraemia is common, and is most easily treated with drinking water via the oral route or through a nasogastric catheter.

In severely septic patients *without* access to mechanical ventilation, it is often impossible to achieve optimal intravascular filling without causing pulmonary oedema. Nevertheless, patients in septic shock not on ventilatory support, do require fluid resuscitation. There is evidence that withholding fluid resuscitation in adult patients with septic shock increases mortality in resource-poor settings.[42] In the absence of mechanical ventilation, a possible approach for the adult patient with arterial hypotension and suspected hypovolaemia is to give a fluid challenge of 500 mL of crystalloids over 30 min, which can be repeated based on macro- and microcirculatory responses (increase in arterial blood pressure, increase in urine output, improved peripheral perfusion) and tolerance (evidence of intravascular volume overload, especially signs of pulmonary oedema).[42] A benefit of colloids (starches, gelofusine, albumin) above crystalloid fluids (normal saline, Ringer's lactate) has never been shown. Because of associated risks (allergy, acute kidney injury, coagulopathy) and the higher costs of colloids, it may be best to only use crystalloid fluids (i.e. Ringer's lactate or NaCl 0.9%) in resource-poor settings. In African children without ventilator support, a fluid bolus cannot be recommended as an intervention for patients with sepsis and compensated shock (shock without severe hypotension), since this is associated with increased mortality.[43] It is currently unclear as to why fluid bolus therapy is harmful in this group of children.

In patients with septic shock, fluid resuscitation alone will often be insufficient to restore blood pressure and tissue perfusion. This is frequently due to an overwhelming loss of vascular tone ('warm shock'), although cardiac arrhythmias and vascular obstruction caused by tension pneumothorax, cardiac tamponade, massive thromboembolism or abdominal compartment syndrome should be excluded as a cause of fluid-resistant shock. In septic shock which does not respond quickly to fluid-resuscitation, for instance if no improvement is observed after a fluid bolus of 20 mL/kg, vasopressive drugs should be started. Noradrenaline or dopamine are preferred above adrenaline, since adrenaline aggravates lactic acidosis.[44] If vasopressor drugs are used, adequate filling has to be guaranteed. Increasing the blood pressure with vasopressor drugs without adequate circulating volume will be deleterious for tissue perfusion. Because of their strong and potentially harmful vasoconstrictive effects, vasopressive drugs should preferably be infused through a central venous catheter. If central venous catheters are unavailable or the medical staff has insufficient experience of handling them, a peripheral venous large-bore cannula (16G or 18G) may be used instead. It is important to regularly check the site of infusion for signs of drug extravasation, since this may cause substantial skin necrosis. Norepinephrine (noradrenaline) or dopamine should be administered continuously using a syringe or infusion pump. When pumps are unavailable or power cuts frequently occur, vasopressor drugs can be diluted in crystalloid solution (e.g. dopamine 250 mg in 500 mL) and infused using a drop regulator or microinfusion set. Dosing should strictly occur based on the clinical response. In patients requiring vasopressive drugs, arterial blood pressure and heart rate should be measured frequently. Dopamine-refractory shock may be reversed with epinephrine (adrenaline) or norepinephrine (noradrenaline) in children.[45]

Simple oxygen administration through a nasal canula or facemask is crucial in patients developing respiratory insufficiency, but will in most cases not be sufficient for the treatment of septic patients with acute lung injury or respiratory insufficiency. Tracheal intubation and mechanical ventilation can be life-saving in these situations. However, even during mechanical ventilation with high inspiratory oxygen concentrations and appropriate positive end-expiratory pressure, adequate oxygenation may be difficult to achieve in the severely diseased lung. In patients with acute lung injury or the acute respiratory distress syndrome, lung compliance is markedly reduced and unevenly distributed with mismatched ventilation/perfusion and compromised gas diffusion. Guidelines recommend application of positive pressure ventilation with positive end-expiratory pressure (PEEP), avoidance of high tidal volumes (6 mg/kg predicted body weight) and avoidance of prolonged periods of high inspiratory oxygen concentrations in all ICU patients, including those without the acute respiratory distress syndrome. Putting the patient in the prone position can dramatically improve oxygenation and can be recommended as a strategy when adequate tissue oxygenation is at risk despite appropriate ventilator settings and high inspiratory oxygen concentrations.[46] The systematic use of prone positioning, however, failed to improve mortality in a randomized trial in patients with non-malaria- related acute lung injury.[47] Permissive hypercapnia can be a lung-protective strategy in patients with bacterial sepsis, but is not recommended in patients with cerebral malaria, because it may further increase intracranial pressure and exacerbate brain swelling. Good respiratory care is also important, with intermediate bagging and suctioning of secretions, as well as appropriate recruitment procedures. Using an appropriate technique when bagging the patient is important in order to avoid airway pressures being too high. In refractory hypoxaemia, reversal of the inspiratory:expiratory ratio

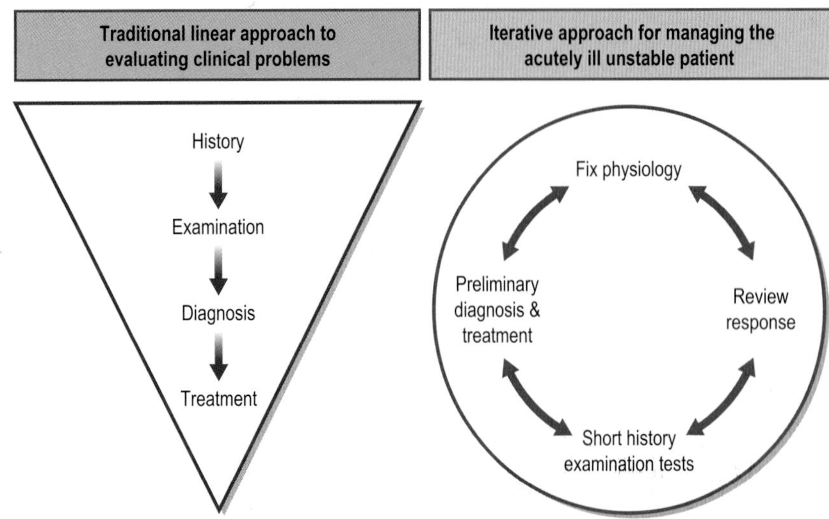

Figure 7.3 Basic differences in clinical management in critically ill patients. *(Adapted from the Patient-centred Acute Care Training (PACT) course, a product of the European Society of Intensive Care Medicine.)*

can be attempted. Some studies report successful management of patients with acute lung injury with non-invasive ventilation, particularly in patients with milder respiratory compromise or quickly reversible causes.

The use of corticosteroids as an adjunctive therapy in sepsis has been the cause of much controversy.[29,48] The current recommendation is that steroids, given as intravenous hydrocortisone in a dose of 100 mg twice a day are only used in adult patients requiring escalating catecholamine doses. An important mechanism is that corticosteroids upregulate adrenergic receptors thus augmenting the catecholamine effects. When vasopressors can be withdrawn in patients receiving corticosteroids, these should be tapered over a couple of days and not be stopped abruptly, in order to avoid rebound hypotension. Corticosteroids are not recommended in patients without shock or who achieve haemodynamic stability with fluid resuscitation and vasopressor therapy, unless there is (suspicion of) adrenal insufficiensy (like with chronic corticosteroid therapy). In children, an Indian pilot randomized study suggested a trend towards earlier shock reversal and less inotrope use when hydrocortisone (5 mg/kg per day in four divided doses followed by half the dose for a total of 7 days) was administered in paediatric patients with septic shock.[49] Until more data are available, use of hydrocortisone can only be recommended as a rescue therapy in paediatric septic shock.

Severe sepsis may be associated with both hypo- and hyperglycaemia. Children and malnourished patients are particular prone to hypoglycaemia. Any change in the level of consciousness should alert the clinician or nurse to check for hypoglycaemia. Since even short episodes of hypoglycaemia carry a risk of permanent neurological damage and increase short-term mortality, blood sugar levels should be measured as early as possible, especially in patients with an impaired mental state. If blood glucose cannot be measured instantly in the unconscious patient, an infusion of glucose should be administered since hypoglycaemia cannot be excluded. If this results in an improvement in the coma score, hypoglycaemia is highly likely to have been present. The benefit of tight glucose control to prevent hyperglycaemia has been trialled in resource-rich settings and might improve outcome, although results are not uniform.[50,51] However, intensive insulin therapy is not recommended in resource-poor settings, since it is difficult to control and carries a high risk of inducing hypoglycaemia.

Conclusion

Care for the critically ill patient requires an iterative process with frequent reassessment of the patient's condition and related treatments, and repeated concomitant appreciation of the overall condition and treatment goals is crucial (Figure 7.3). Although components of critical care medicine can be difficult to implement in resource-poor settings, there are important universal principles applicable to all settings.

REFERENCES

2. Riviello ED, Letchford S, Achieng L, et al. Critical care in resource-poor settings: lessons learned and future directions. Crit Care Med 2011;39(4):860–7.
28. Schweickert WD, Pohlman MC, Pohlman AS, et al. Early physical and occupational therapy in mechanically ventilated, critically ill patients: a randomised controlled trial. Lancet 2009;373 (9678):1874–82.
29. Dellinger RP, Levy MM, Rhodes A, et al. Surviving Sepsis Campaign: international guidelines for management of severe sepsis and septic shock: 2012. Crit Care Med 2013;41(2): 580–637.
30. Dunser MW, Festic E, Dondorp A, et al. Recommendations for sepsis management in resource-limited settings. Intensive Care Med 2012;38 (4):557–74.
41. Murphy CV, Schramm GE, Doherty JA, et al. The importance of fluid management in acute lung injury secondary to septic shock. Chest 2009;136(1):102–9.

Access the complete references online at www.expertconsult.com

8 Ultrasound in Tropical Medicine

ENRICO BRUNETTI

KEY POINTS

- Ultrasound (US) is a radiation-free imaging technique and as such, it is repeatable as often as needed. In addition, it is versatile as all organs can be explored, including lung and, to a limited extent, bone.
- Ultrasound is cost-effective, safe and according to the WHO, should be available worldwide to assist the clinician in the diagnostic process.
- Ultrasound is particularly helpful in a number of 'tropical', poverty-related settings, as it is the first tool to screen, diagnose, treat and follow-up cases even in remote areas. This technique is key in the clinical management of cystic and alveolar echinococcosis, filariasis, schistosomiasis, fascioliasis, amoebic liver abscesses, bacterial abscesses and in a range of other conditions that are widespread in both rural and urban communities.
- Despite all of the above, 60% of the world has still no access to imaging services and the literature on the use of US in tropical medicine is strikingly scarce.
- Large populations in rural areas lack access to basic ultrasound and X-ray, the two key imaging modalities in rural areas. It has been estimated that the two techniques together can meet over 90% of the imaging needs in these settings.
- Ultrasound is operator-dependent, and availability and quality of training remain important issues that need to be addressed to solve the paradox of ultrasound being used least where it is most needed.

Introduction

Ultrasound is a radiation-free imaging technique and as such it is repeatable as often as needed. In addition, it is versatile as all organs can be explored, although the extent to which lungs and bone can be explored with ultrasound is still less than what is possible with other organs.

The wide availability of ultrasound scanners has produced an enormous diffusion of the technique. Thanks to continuous technological advances, portability has increased dramatically, so much so that pocket-sized, hand-held scanners are currently commercially available for relatively modest sums. This has prompted claims that the 'ultrasound stethoscope' has finally arrived.[1,2] This enthusiasm should be tempered, as wide availability has downsides and risks – mainly in the areas of training and certification. Nonetheless, it is a reminder of the opportunities currently available.

Ultrasound in Tropical Medicine

Ultrasound is particularly helpful in a number of 'tropical', poverty-related settings, as it is the first tool to screen, diagnose, treat and follow-up cases even in remote areas. This wide approach applies to helminthic diseases such as echinococcosis, filariasis, schistosomiasis, fascioliasis, but also extends to amoebic liver abscesses, bacterial abscesses and to a range of other conditions that are widespread in both rural and urban communities.[3] While the usefulness varies according to the clinical manifestations (see Tables 8.1–8.3), the diagnosis of many tropical illnesses benefits from ultrasound.

Ultrasound (US) is cost-effective, safe and according to the WHO, should be available worldwide to assist the clinician in the diagnostic process.[4,5] Some articles have documented the impact or change of clinical management due to the use of US in low-resource settings.[6] A comprehensive list of conditions benefiting from ultrasound in such settings has been drawn up by Maru et al.[7]

Despite all of the above, 60% of the world still has no access to radiological services[5] and the literature on the use of US in tropical medicine is strikingly scarce.[6] For instance, large populations in rural areas lack access to basic US and X-ray, the two key imaging modalities in rural areas. It has been estimated that the two techniques together can meet over 90% of the imaging needs in these settings.[7]

This chapter will discuss the most important applications of ultrasound in tropical medicine and the paradox of ultrasound being used least where it is most needed.

CYSTIC ECHINOCOCCOSIS

Cystic echinococcosis (CE) is the parasitic condition that has most benefited from the introduction of US in clinical practice and in epidemiological studies. Together with computed tomography (CT), US has allowed for the first time direct visualization of cystic lesions in the body in a non-invasive way. US has been shown to have a higher sensitivity and specificity than serology and has allowed for population screenings that have demonstrated the true prevalence of disease in the communities studied.[8,9]

The use of ultrasound revolutionized the diagnosis of CE and subsequently the treatment of CE with the introduction of US-guided percutaneous procedures and follow-up. In 1995, the WHO-IWGE (Informal Working Group on Echinococcosis) developed a standardized classification that divided the cysts into three relevant groups according to their biological activity: active (CE1, uniloculated and CE2, with daughter cysts); transitional (CE3) and inactive (CE4 and CE5, solid content with calcifications).[10] CE3 transitional cysts should be differentiated into CE3a (with detached endocyst) and CE3b

TABLE 8.1 Accepted or Established Utility in Diagnosis, Treatment and Screening

Condition	Organ/findings
Cystic echinococcosis	Abdominal, pleural, muscular cysts
Schistosomiasis	Diagnosis and grading in the liver/spleen and bladder
Filariasis	Filaricele
Ascariasis	Hepatobiliary and intestinal helminths
Fascioliasis	Hepatobiliary and extrahepatic helminths and lesions
Toxocariasis	Hepatic and ocular abnormalities
HBV/HCV (with or without HIV) infection	Screening for cirrhosis, ascites, portal hypertension, hepatocellular carcinoma
Tropical pyomyositis	Abscess in muscles
Myiasis	Subcutaneous cavity with moving larvae

Modified from: Walter 'Ted' Kuhn, MD, unpublished.

(active, predominantly solid with daughter cysts), as they respond differently to non-surgical approaches.[11] CE1 and CE3a are early stages, and CE4 and CE5 are late stages. This classification is basically a rearrangement of a previous classification proposed by Hassen Gharbi in 1981.[12]

Sonographic features along with serological results are important for the differential diagnosis of CE. When they are not sufficient, ultrasound-guided aspiration of the cyst and the search for protoscolices in the aspirate can be diagnostic (Figure 8.1).

TABLE 8.2 Demonstrated or Accepted Use as an Adjunct to Diagnosis and Treatment

Condition	Findings
HIV/AIDS	Screening and continuity of care of patients with HIV: mycobacterial, bacterial, fungal and viral infections, lymphomas, Kaposi's sarcoma
Extrapulmonary tuberculosis	Lymphadenopathy, mostly with caseating necrosis, posterior enhancement, hyperechogenic spots due to calcification. Pleural effusions with fibrinous strands Involvement of mesenteric and peripancreatic lymph nodes without involvement of the iliac ones. Hypoechoic lesions in liver and spleen. Mesenteric masses, ascites with fibrinous stranding
Onchocerciasis	Subcutaneous nodules
Opisthorchiasis, clonorchiasis	Hyperechogenic biliary vessels, sludge in gallbladder, cholangiocarcinoma
Haemoglobinopathies common in the tropics	Splenic infarction
Haemorrhagic fevers	Gallbladder wall thickness, haemoperitoneum
Oesophagostomum bifurcum	Abdominal masses

Modified from: Walter 'Ted' Kuhn, MD, unpublished.

TABLE 8.3 May be Useful in Diagnosis, Treatment and Screening (Utility Suggested but to be Ascertained)

Condition	Findings
Cholangiocarcinoma	Screening in patients with clonorchiasis and opisthorchiasis
Cysticercosis	Subcutaneous nodules, demonstration of cysticerci in the eye

Modified from: Walter 'Ted' Kuhn, MD, unpublished.

The WHO-IWGE US classification is important for guiding the choice of treatment and follow-up (see Chapter 56).[11]

SCHISTOSOMIASIS

In acute schistosomiasis, nonspecific hepatosplenomegaly with swelling of perihilar and abdominal lymph nodes may be observed on US.[13] Chronic schistosomiasis has different features depending on the species involved.

Infection with *S. haematobium* is characterized by the presence of granulomas in the bladder wall, followed by wall thickening and calcifications, that are easily detectable with US. Ureters and kidneys can also eventually be involved, with similar aspects (thickening, calcifications), which can cause hydroureteronephrosis and renal failure.[14]

In late stages, bladder shape is distorted, with polypoid masses and calcifications. In addition, a higher incidence of bladder cancer has been observed in individuals with *S. haematobium* infection.

In community-based surveys, US detectable pathology was found to be more common in children than adults and was correlated with intensity and prevalence of infection.[15] In a number of longitudinal studies, US has been used to examine the resolution of uropathy following chemotherapy. Most patients investigated showed a high rate of improvement.[16–18]

US plays an increasingly important role in determining re-treatment intervals, based on the recurrence of morbidity.[19–21]

Liver alterations detectable by US in chronic infection by *S. mansoni* are due to fibrosis, secondary to granulomatous reaction evocated by schistosomal eggs. Ultrasound shows

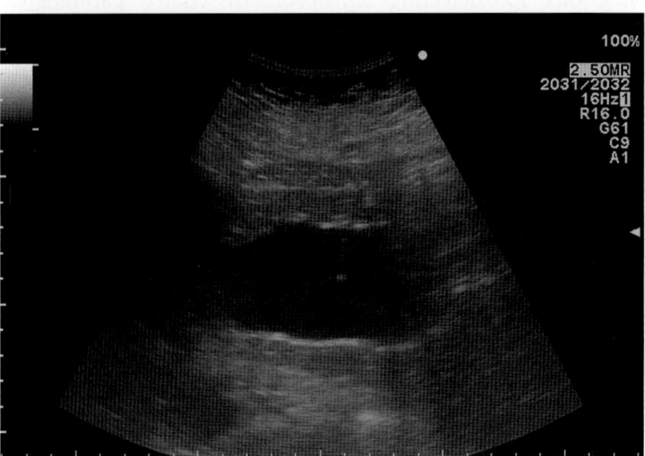

Figure 8.1 CE1 cyst of the left hepatic lobe during the initial phase of PAIR. The echogenic needle tip is visible in the centre of the cavity. *(Copyright © Enrico Brunetti.)*

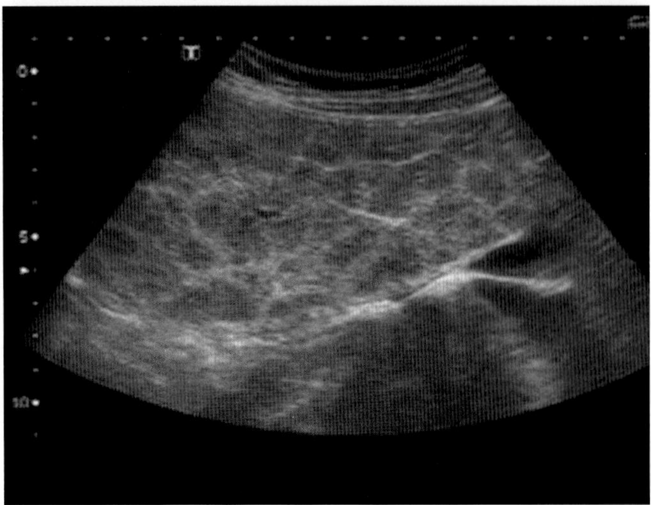

Figure 8.2 Network-like appearance (wide meshes) of *S. japonicum* infection of the liver. *(Copyright © Joachim Richter.)*

periportal fibrosis (Symmers' fibrosis), with the final result of a retracted liver associated with portal hypertension, congestive splenomegaly and gastro-oesophageal varices. US has been used to examine the resolution of hepatic lesions following chemotherapy for *S. mansoni* infection.[22] In a study, reduction in fibrosis was demonstrated 7 months after the administration of praziquantel.[23] In some patients, however, there is a progression of disease. US may be useful in the further study of this phenomenon and in the evaluation of alternative forms of treatment.

Portal fibrosis in Asian schistosomiasis due to *Schistosoma japonicum* and *S. mekongi* is similar to that due to other *Schistosomae*. However, at least in *S. japonicum* infection, a completely distinct pattern, i.e. interseptal fibrosis simultaneously or not to portal fibrosis may occur, which has been called 'network pattern', 'tortoise back' pattern or 'fish scale pattern' (Figure 8.2).[24,25]

US is currently the preferred field and hospital-based method of choice for detecting schistosomiasis-related pathological lesions. Initiatives aiming at the standardization of reporting observations and WHO-funded meetings to provide standardized protocols have been organized.[26,27]

FILARIASIS

The use of ultrasound in human filariasis was introduced between the late 1980s and early 1900s.[28,29] In men with lymphatic filariasis (LF), US of the scrotal area is used to evaluate prevalence and stage of 'filaricele' providing important diagnostic and risk-assessment information, to guide therapeutic options and to monitor responses to antifilarial treatments. Filaricele comprises different conditions such as hydrocele (accumulation of anechoic fluid between the layers of the tunica vaginalis), longstanding hydrocele or chylocele (accumulation of echo-dense fluid with floating particles, at risk of testicular necrosis), lymphocele (dilation of supratesticular lymphatic vessels) and lymphscrotum.[30]

Worm 'nests' in dilated lymphatic vessels can be visualized by US by their typical movement pattern, called 'filarial dance sign (FDS)' using Colour Power Doppler and Pulsed Wave Doppler (Figure 8.3).[31,32] Although primarily used to monitor LF in the scrotal region of men infected with *W. bancrofti*, US has been successfully used also to detect FDS and lymphatic pathology in women[33] and in pathology caused by *B. malayi*, where worm nests are less stable over time.[34]

In onchocerciasis, US complements physical examination, as it is able to detect a proportion of non-palpable nodules[28] and to differentiate onchocercomas from other lesions (e.g. lymph nodes, lipomas). It has also been used to assess the efficacy of antifilarial treatment in clinical trials.[35,36]

Moving worms are only detectable in nodules with cystic areas, where parasites appear as an acoustic enhancement reflected from tissue moving in hypoechoic areas of the nodule, while living worms are not detected in more compact onchocercoma.[36] Moreover, *O. volvulus* movements are rare and slower compared with filariae in the lymphatics. Although not replacing classical diagnostic tools, US has nevertheless been used with success in field trials for the assessment of antifilarial drug efficacy, by virtue of its non-invasiveness and high acceptance by the population.

ASCARIASIS

US is a highly sensitive and specific non-invasive method for the detection of helminths in the biliary tract, although the diagnosis of biliary ascariasis requires a high index of suspicion because the worms move in and out of the biliary tract and can be missed on biliary imaging.[37] In longitudinal sections, adult *A. lumbricoides* have an echogenic non-shadowing tubular structure with a hypo- or anechoic centre, and can be seen moving with a slow-waving pattern. Multiple worms in the bile duct produce a spaghetti-like image, with alternating echogenic and anechoic strips or if densely packed in the bile duct, can appear as a hyperechoic pseudotumor.[38–40] In addition, US can demonstrate worms in the small bowel.[41] In most cases, pathology resolves with pharmacological treatment. The response to treatment can be monitored by ultrasound.[42] Symptoms usually resolve within 3 days in 60–80% of patients, shown by the disappearance of worms on ultrasound.

FASCIOLIASIS

In the liver of patients with fascioliasis, small necrotic lesions form along the migratory paths of juvenile flukes. These can be seen as hypoechoic small lesions, which do not coalesce and are typically arranged along serpiginous tracts, from the surface of the organ to deep within the hepatic parenchyma. They can change in quantity and location over time. This particular lesion arrangement can be helpful in the differential diagnosis of tumours, pyogenic abscesses and visceral larva migrans (Figure 8.4).[43]

In the chronic stage, adult flukes are seen inside the biliary ducts as single or multiple elongated filamentous echoic structures a few centimetres long.[44] Spontaneous movement may be observed. Other ultrasound findings include thickening of the extra-hepatic bile duct and the gallbladder wall, common bile duct dilation, cholelithiasis, small calcifications of the liver parenchyma, liver abscesses, hepatosplenomegaly and ascites.[43,45]

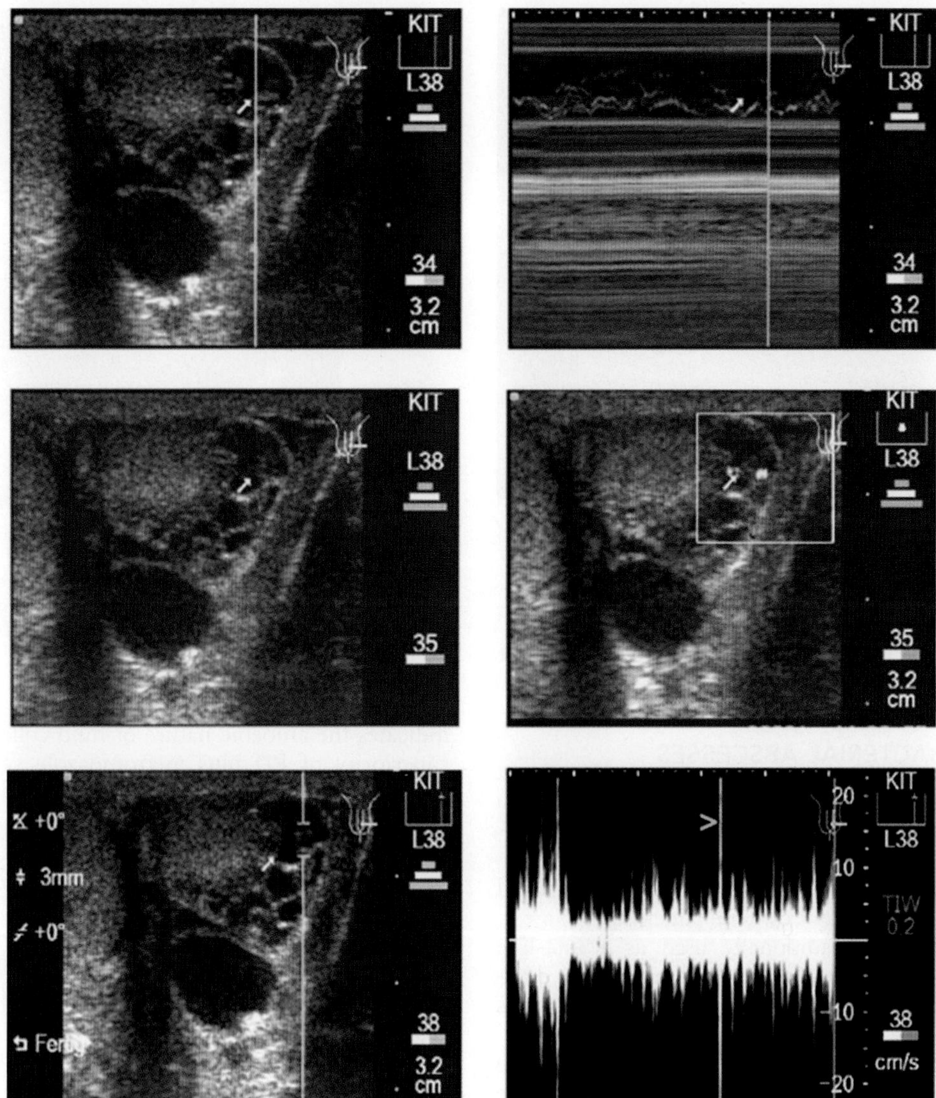

Figure 8.3 Transverse scan of the left testis of a patient with filariasis. Upper left: In para-testicular position an enlarged lymphatic vessel with one or more adult worms can be seen (arrow). The green line depicts the cursor position of the following M-mode (upper right). Middle left: The same worm nest as seen above. Middle right: The use of the colour power Doppler shows that this worm's nest contains much free lymphatic fluid, which induces a red signal due to the worm movements in different parts of the worm nest. Different to vessels, the signal is non-rhythmic and non-pulsating. Lower left: The same worm nests as seen above. Lower right: After switch to the PWD mode the filaria dance sign (FDS) is seen as an undulating band as a function of time, with sharp, irregular peaks (turquoise arrowhead). *(From: Mand S et al. Animated documentation of the filaria dance sign (FDS) in bancroftian filariasis. Filaria J 2003.)*

TOXOCARA

Ultrasonographic abnormalities include non-specific hepatomegaly, lymphadenomegaly and pleuropericardial effusions. Hepatic granulomas appear as multiple small hypoechoic lesions with ill-defined margins, usually oval, angulated or trapezoid in shape and occasionally a central spot or line ('bean sign'). Sometimes lesions conglomerate to form a large area of mixed echogenicity.[46]

The main differential diagnosis of visceral larva migrans (VLM) hepatic lesions is hepatic metastases. Diagnostic clues include: hepatic nodules in toxocariasis have ill-defined margins, they are uniform in size and are usually not spherical in shape.[47]

As toxocariasis is mostly a self-limiting disease, follow-up lesions usually improve and resolve spontaneously unless the patient is re-infected. The position and number of the lesions can change over time due to the migration of the larvae, which supports the diagnosis of VLM. US is also helpful in the diagnosis of ocular complications of toxocariasis (Figure 8.5).[48]

CLONORCHIASIS AND OPISTORCHIASIS

Ultrasound findings reflect the pathology of the bile ducts, namely diffuse intrahepatic bile duct dilatation, truncation and increased periductal echogenicity, and infectious complications, such as pyogenic cholangitis, liver abscesses, stones, pancreatitis and cholangiocarcinoma.[49] Occasionally, flukes or aggregates of eggs are visualized as non-shadowing echogenic foci or casts within the bile ducts (Figure 8.6).[50] Ultrasound is less useful in therapy follow-up and in the differentiation between resolved and active infection, as the pathological

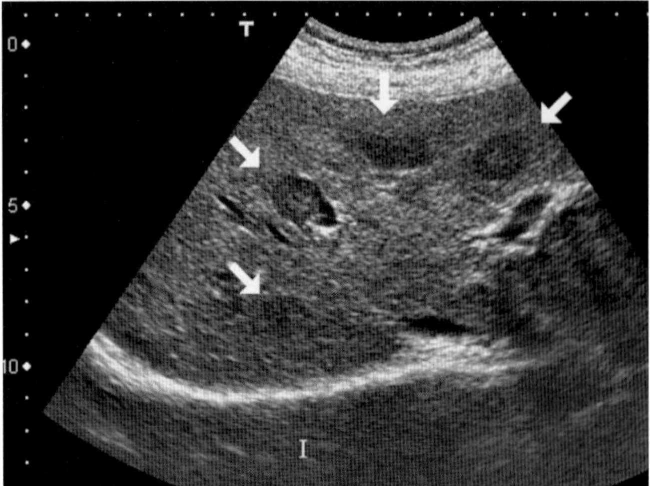

Figure 8.4 Hypoechogenic lesions from *Fasciola* mimicking metastatic disease. *(Copyright © Adnan Kabaalioglu.)*

changes of the bile ducts can persist for years even after the symptoms have resolved.

AMOEBIC AND BACTERIAL ABSCESSES

Over the past three decades, US has gained a central role in the diagnosis and clinical management of abdominal, and particularly hepatic, abscesses. US and US-guided aspiration and percutaneous drainage (PD) of abscesses have dramatically altered both the diagnosis and treatment of these patients.

Ultrasound imaging is traditionally used as a first-line measure to localize a liver abscess, although it may not be diagnostic in some patients as sonographic features of an abscess depend on its stage of evolution.[51] US cannot differentiate pyogenic and amoebic liver abscesses (ALA), (Figure 8.7), but the presence of anchovy-paste material on aspiration or drainage

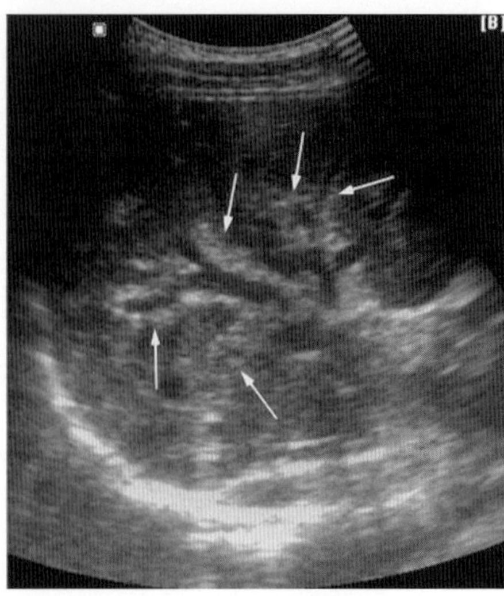

Figure 8.6 Liver scan from a subject with 49 920 *Clonorchis sinensis* eggs per gram of faeces. Transverse images of the central liver show markedly increased periductal echogenicity (arrows) along the dilated bile ducts. *(From: Choi D et al. Sonographic findings of active Clonorchis sinensis infection. J Clin Ultrasound 2004;32(1):17–23.)*

indicates the amoebic nature of fluid collection. For ALA, the superiority of PD plus metronidazole versus metronidazole alone is still debated.[52] However, PD is required when the ALA is at risk of rupture, located in the left lobe of the liver, in pregnant women or when medical treatment has failed.

The mortality in undrained bacterial abdominal abscesses is high, with a rate ranging between 45% and 100%. The outcome in abdominal abscesses, however, has improved thanks to advances in image techniques (especially US as it allows longer procedure) due to guided percutaneous interventional techniques.[53] Although the superiority of percutaneous drainage over surgical drainage remains to be determined,[54] the former

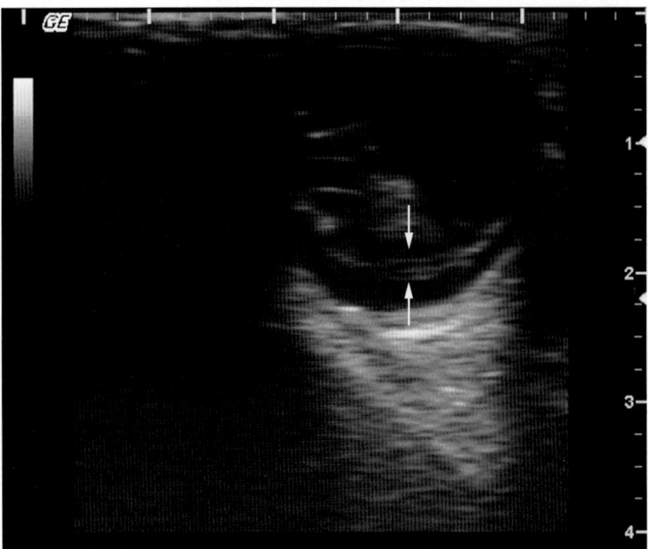

Figure 8.5 Ocular scan (an 8–12 MHz linear transducer was used) of a 5-year-old Peruvian child with *Toxocara*. Retinal detachment is seen in the lower part of the eyeball (arrows). *(Copyright © Walter Kuhn.)*

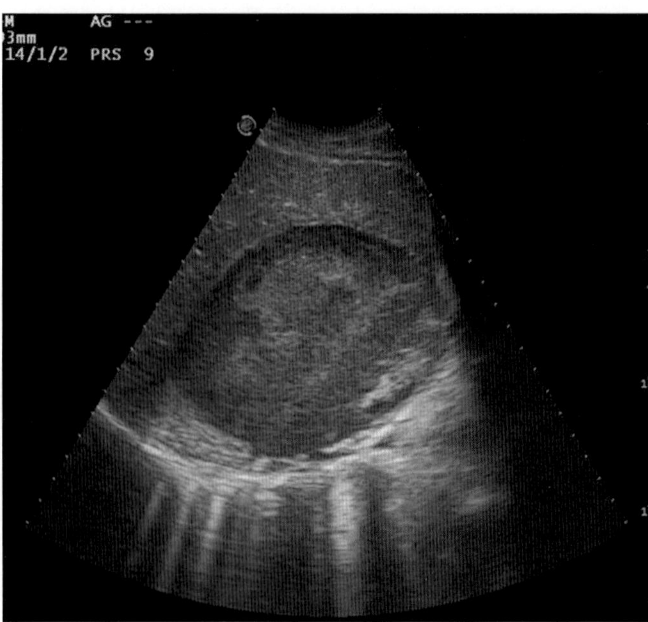

Figure 8.7 Large amoebic abscess in the liver. *(Copyright © Enrico Brunetti.)*

is easier to perform (and less expensive) where surgical facilities are scarce.[55] Despite its usefulness, percutaneous treatment for abscesses is still scarcely used in sub-Saharan Africa[56] where it is most needed.

Finally, US has permitted the determination of the prevalence of subclinical ALA in endemic areas, thus providing important epidemiological information on this condition.[57]

AIDS AND TUBERCULOSIS

Ultrasound has a wide scope of application in AIDS patients[58,59] as it can detect focal lesions in almost all organs and US-guided aspiration biopsy is helpful to differentiate neoplasms from opportunistic infections. US can easily explore liver, biliary system, pancreas, spleen, kidneys and lymph nodes and detect focal lesions, be they neoplastic (Kaposi's sarcoma, AIDS-related lymphomas, hepatocellular carcinoma in HIV-HBV or HIV-HCV coinfected patients) or infectious (fungal abscesses, extrapulmonary *Pneumocystis jiroveci*, mycobacterial lesions, bacillary angiomatosis from *Bartonella henselae*). Lymphadenopathy can also be either neoplastic or infectious (*M. tuberculosis*, MOTT, MAC). Tubercular lymph nodes may have sonographic features such as necrosis and posterior enhancement, and hyperechogenic spots due to calcification, which suggest the diagnosis. In abdominal TB, involvement of peripancreatic and mesenteric lymph nodes, contrasting with rare involvement of those in the lumbar and iliac regions, is noted (Figure 8.8).[60,61] Recent studies have shown that US FNA may be useful in differentiating tubercular from lymphomatous and metastatic nodes,[62] although sensitivity remains low. Many infectious and non-infectious lung conditions due to HIV/TB can be diagnosed and managed by US (e.g. drainage of pleural effusions).

US can be used to diagnose and drain pericardial effusions (Figure 8.9). When they are massive and threaten to be fatal due to cardiac tamponade, US-guided aspiration is a life-saving manoeuvre.[63]

Specific sonographic features such as parenchymal masses, cavities, mucosal thickening of the collecting system and urinary bladder, stenosis of the collecting system, and calcifications have been described in genito-urinary TB.[64]

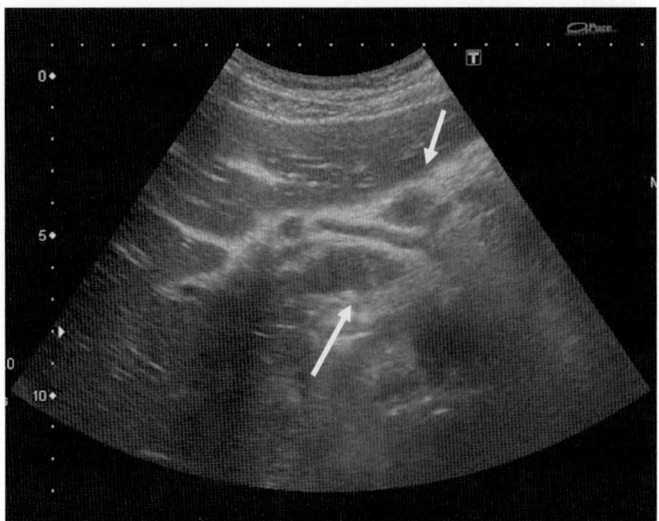

Figure 8.8 Enlarged lymph nodes around the coeliac axis in a patient with HIV and extrapulmonary TB. *(Copyright © Maria Teresa Giordani.)*

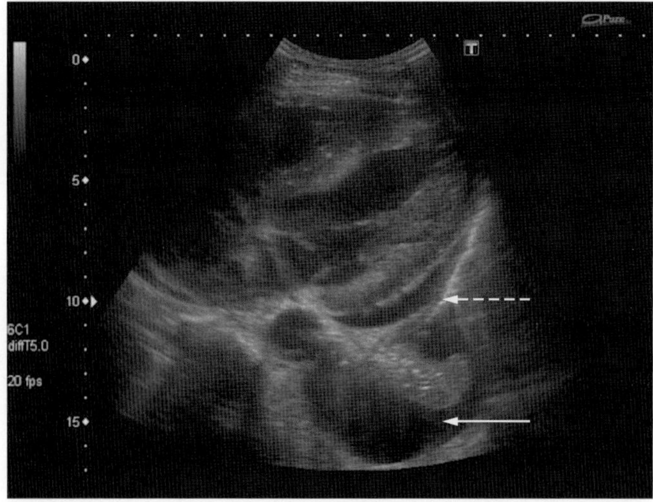

Figure 8.9 Pericardial (dashed arrow) and pleural (solid arrow) effusion in a patient with HIV and TB. *(Copyright © Maria Teresa Giordani.)*

In areas where HIV and TB converge, US presumptive diagnosis of extrapulmonary TB followed by anti-TB treatment is a viable option even in low-resource settings where pathological examination is not affordable.[65]

CHRONIC LIVER DISEASE

Hepatocellular carcinoma (HCC) is one of the most serious complications of chronic liver disease and is the third most lethal cancer worldwide. Symptoms emerge very late in the course of its natural history with an attendant poor outcome. Screening is therefore crucial to treat HCC as early as possible.[66]

Approximately 50% of the underlying aetiologies for the development of HCC worldwide are represented by chronic hepatitis B. Hepatitis C also has a high potential for chronicity. Of the 130–170 million persons worldwide infected with the hepatitis C virus, approximately 350 000 have chronic liver disease. Periodic US surveillance for early detection of HCC is important when curative treatment can still be achieved.[67,68]

US is the method of choice for assessment of the liver, with a high specificity and sensitivity for chronic liver diseases and can even differentiate chronic hepatitis from compensated cirrhosis.[69] Doppler US is also a non-invasive means of assessing haemodynamic changes secondary to chronic liver disease, which are features of portal hypertension.[70]

The accuracy of US in detecting liver abnormalities in patients with chronic viral hepatitis, by assessing liver borders, parenchymal echogenicity, calibre of the portal vein, and largest cross-sectional area of the spleen, correlates well with histopathological results.[71]

LUNG ULTRASOUND

Until recently, the sonographic visualization of pulmonary and pleural diseases was considered impossible, but despite its limitations, lung US is becoming an important diagnostic tool in a growing number of pathological situations such as pneumonia, atelectasis, interstitial-alveolar syndrome, pulmonary embolism, pneumothorax and pleural effusion.[72] The low sensitivity of chest X-ray and the difficulties of performing CT make this technique invaluable for bedside use in the intensive care unit. Further benefits include reduced requirements for computed tomographic scans, therefore decreasing delay, irradiation, cost, and above all, discomfort to the patient.[73–75] The full value of lung US in contexts where CT is not available awaits evaluation.

OBSTETRICS

US is crucial to detect and monitor high-risk pregnancies and to identify the cause of peripartum haemorrhages. Complications during pregnancy are among the most common causes of maternal mortality worldwide and are barriers to achieving the United Nations Maternal Health Millennium Development Goals.[76] Efforts are being made at training non-medical health workers to perform US on specific conditions where physicians are scarce. For example, a pilot project demonstrated that midwives in rural Zambia can be trained to perform basic obstetric ultrasound, a fact that impacts on clinical decision-making.[77]

TRAUMA

Trauma can be rapidly assessed by US and significant thoraco-abdominal trauma manifestations such as pneumothorax, cardiac tamponade, abdominal organ injuries with ensuing hemoperitoneum, etc. can rapidly be diagnosed or ruled out. This is done according to FAST (focused assessment with sonography for trauma) protocols, which were developed in emergency departments in the mid-1990s. With a FAST exam, the physician does not attempt to evaluate the whole abdomen and its organs, but seeks to answer simple and usually relevant binary questions, e.g. 'Is a pericardial effusion present, yes or no?' Findings that are included in the protocol must be: (1) relevant to the immediate treatment of the patient and (2) easy enough to recognize, so that even medical staff without lengthy US training can diagnose them correctly.

Bedside US is also an accurate and convenient method of diagnosing fractures in children.[78]

Training in Resource-Poor Settings

Ultrasound is a highly operator-dependent tool as noted by the World Health Organization (WHO) scientific Group on Clinical Diagnostic Imaging:

> '... *more important than the equipment is the availability of skills. An error in diagnosis because of inadequate education and experience is as dangerous as being without the equipment, and the success of any interventional procedure ... is very dependent on the skills and the experience of the responsible physician*'.[5]

This remains true more than three decades after the introduction of US into clinical practice and is a particularly thorny issue when it comes to training in resource-poor settings and remote environments.[79]

While for most physicians from resource-poor settings training in industrialized countries is costly, sending trainers to tropical countries has its share of problems. Ultrasound training must be planned as a long-time project in order to retain physicians in the health facilities where the training takes place and efforts should be made to train at least a few persons that should in turn become trainers for other local colleagues that are willing to learn the technique.[80] This is a considerable effort in terms of time, money and energy and requires coordination with local health authorities. Only one report apparently exists on the long-term outcome of such training involving three different universities in three continents and the results appear encouraging.[81]

A different approach could be that of teaching a limited number of skills for a short period to untrained physicians or paramedics. This idea extends the concept of FAST protocols (see above), first developed in emergency departments in the mid-1990s. Here the physician seeks to answer simple relevant questions rather than systematically exploring the whole abdomen and the answers must be relevant to the immediate treatment of the patient. This is particularly attractive in resource-poor settings, where the prevalence of certain infectious conditions is high and there is a shortage of physicians trained in ultrasound.[82,77] The idea has recently been applied to infectious conditions such as HIV/TB co-infection[83] and cystic echinococcosis[84] and although these protocols are still in their infancy, they are worth studying.

Where those programmes are not available however, shorter, locally organized courses may be a viable solution.[85]

Training protocols for local healthcare personnel should be developed, standardized and evaluated with the aim of reaching operational independence. Groups such as the World Interactive Network Focused on Critical Ultrasound (WINFOCUS) are already working intensively on critical care sonography training for healthcare providers in underserved areas.[86]

Performance Standards and Quality Assessment

Data monitoring and evaluation programmes are crucial and can be supported via satellite internet connections using the basic 'store and forward' protocol (i.e. attaching scanned or saved in the machine hard disk images to email messages for comments) or electronic databases with low-bandwidth uploading systems to comment on with experts accessed via commercially available software such as Skype. Regular review of images through low-cost telemedicine can help improve clinical work and make continuing medical education possible in remote areas.[87,88]

Acknowledgements

I am grateful to: Sam Goblirsch MD for reviewing the text; Francesca Tamarozzi DVM, MD, MSc, PhD, for editing the section on filaria; Joachim Richter MD, for giving me permission to use Figure 8.2; Adnan Kabaalioglu MD, for Figure 8.4; Walter 'Ted' Kuhn MD, for Figure 8.5; Maria Teresa Giordani MD, for Figures 8.8 and 8.9.

REFERENCES

5. Training in diagnostic ultrasound: essentials, principles and standards. Report of a WHO Study Group. World Health Organ Tech Rep Ser 1998;875(46).
10. International classification of ultrasound images in cystic echinococcosis for application in clinical and field epidemiological settings. Acta Trop 2003;85(2):253–61.
26. Ultrasound in Schistosomiasis: a practical guide to the standardized use of ultrasonography for assessment of schistosomiasis-related morbidity. Geneva: WHO; 2000.
29. Amaral F, Dreyer G, Figueredo-Silva J, et al. Live adult worms detected by ultrasonography in human Bancroftian filariasis. Am J Trop Med Hyg 1994;50(6):753–7.
83. Heller T, Wallrauch C, Lessells RJ, et al. Short course for focused assessment with sonography for human immunodeficiency virus/tuberculosis: preliminary results in a rural setting in South Africa with high prevalence of human immunodeficiency virus and tuberculosis. Am J Trop Med Hyg 2010;82(3):512–15.

Access the complete references online at www.expertconsult.com http://www.isradiology.org/tropical_deseases/tmcr/toc.htm

HIV Epidemiology in the Tropics

PHILIP J. PETERS | BARBARA J. MARSTON | KEVIN M. De COCK

KEY POINTS

- HIV remains a critical public health problem; as of 2010, an estimated 34 million people were living with HIV worldwide.
- International HIV surveillance activities have provided healthcare providers with access to more comprehensive, accurate and timely information on the HIV epidemic than any other infectious disease.
- Globally, most HIV transmission occurs as the result of unprotected sexual contact and prevention of sexual transmission of HIV has proved difficult; young women in sub-Saharan Africa and men who have sex with men worldwide are at particularly high risk.
- As of 2010, half of all persons living with HIV worldwide were unaware of their HIV status, highlighting the need for healthcare providers in settings with a generalized epidemic to offer provider-initiated HIV testing and counselling to all patients.
- The epidemic of HIV has fuelled an increase in tuberculosis disease in countries with a high HIV prevalence and altered the practice of medicine worldwide.
- The epidemiology of HIV varies regionally; there are generalized epidemics throughout sub-Saharan Africa, and epidemics concentrated in high-risk groups in many other regions.
- Expansion of HIV treatment is having a profound effect on the global HIV epidemic by reducing HIV-related deaths and preventing mother-to-child HIV transmission; there is hope that continued expansion will significantly reduce HIV transmission.

Global Snapshot of the HIV Epidemic

As of the end of 2010, the World Health Organization (WHO) and the Joint United Nations Programme on HIV/AIDS (UNAIDS) estimated that 34 million (31.6–35.2 million)*[,1] people were living with human immunodeficiency virus (HIV) infection, globally.[2] HIV infection can be diagnosed with a rapid point-of-care blood test, but only half of all persons living with HIV worldwide are aware of their infection.[2–4] During 2010, an estimated 2.7 million (2.4–2.9 million) new infections occurred worldwide, including an estimated 390 000 among children, and approximately 1.8 million (1.6–1.9 million) people died of AIDS-related causes.[3] Sub-Saharan Africa bears the greatest burden of both prevalent (22.9 million or 68%) and new (1.9 million or 70%) infections. Young people (persons aged 15–24 years), particularly in sub-Saharan Africa, merit specific attention, as approximately 50% of new HIV infections occur in this age group (Figure 9.1), with young women at particular risk.[6–8] There is also increasing awareness that communities of men who have sex with men (MSM) exist in low- and middle-income countries, including Africa, but are often overlooked, despite high rates of HIV infection. Since the late 1990s, significant advances have been made in the prevention and treatment of HIV, resulting in a steady decrease in the annual number of new infections (a 26% decline from 1997 to 2010).[3] The expansion of programmes to treat HIV infection with antiretroviral therapy (ART) between 2004 and 2010 has also resulted in an 18% reduction in acquired immune deficiency syndrome (AIDS)-related deaths.[2] Although ART reduces the risk of HIV transmission, improved survival also contributes to increasing HIV prevalence; thus, despite these prevention successes, the number of new HIV infections still exceeds the number of AIDS-related deaths and the epidemic continues to expand (Figure 9.2).

*Estimates are presented with plausibility bounds in parentheses, based on UNAIDS and WHO methodology.[1] These plausibility bounds reflect the uncertainty surrounding the estimate and are based on a combination of confidence intervals (calculated whenever possible) and expert judgement (if appropriate data for confidence intervals are not available).

Origin and Impact of HIV

The first cases of AIDS were described in the USA in 1981[9] and by 1985, HIV infection had been identified in every region of the world.[10] Analysis of phylogenetic sequences from human and related ape viruses suggests that HIV originated in Central Africa and may have first been transmitted to humans around 1930.[11] In the short time since then, HIV has reduced life expectancy, slowed economic growth and orphaned (loss of one or both parents) over 18 million children.[12] Prior to recent expansions in access to HIV treatment, AIDS was the leading cause of death among people 15–59 years old in low-income countries (especially sub-Saharan Africa);[13] fortunately, recent reports suggest some encouraging reversals of these trends.[14–17]

HIV has had a remarkable impact on the practice of tropical medicine.[18] In many countries in eastern and southern Africa, 50–75% of adult medical in-patients at urban hospitals are HIV-infected.[19–21] The HIV pandemic has also focused attention on health disparities, social justice and human rights and led to an unprecedented mobilization of political, financial and human resources for the expansion of HIV prevention and treatment services.[22–25] This expansion has had positive effects on health systems but we must be vigilant for unintended negative consequences. For example, the expansion of HIV prevention and treatment services in nine countries in eastern and southern Africa has been associated with a greater than 50% reduction in all-cause adult mortality from 2003 to 2008.[26] In

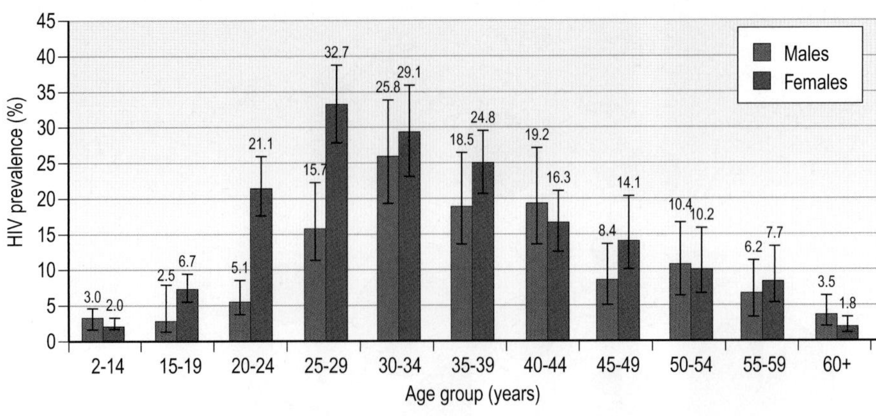

Figure 9.1 HIV prevalence, by sex and age, South Africa 2008. (Shisana O, Rehle T, Simbayi LC, et al. South African national HIV prevalence, incidence, behaviour and communication survey 2008: A turning tide among teenagers? Cape Town: HSRC Press; 2009. (Fig. 3.1).)

addition, improvements in supply chain and laboratory capacity related to HIV may spill over to other health priorities, but implementation of HIV services may also divert resources such as healthcare workers from other priorities.[22]

Molecular Epidemiology

HIV is a retrovirus that uses the viral enzyme reverse transcriptase to transcribe viral RNA into DNA that is incorporated into the host (human) genome. Two main types of HIV cause disease in humans: HIV-1 and HIV-2.

HIV-1

HIV-1 comprises at least three phylogenetically distinct groups, termed group M (main), group O (outlier), and group N (non-M, non-O).[27] A fourth group (group P) has been proposed based on a single infection with a genetically unique HIV strain.[28] Groups M, O, and N likely evolved from independent transmissions of chimpanzee simian immunodeficiency virus (SIVcpz) to humans,[29–31] while group P may have evolved from transmissions of gorilla SIV (SIVgor).[28] Group M viruses cause more than 95% of HIV infections worldwide.[32] Group O infections are less common and occur primarily in Central Africa (especially Cameroon).[33] Group N infections are rare and mainly limited to Cameroon.[34]

Because HIV exhibits rapid replication and very high rates of mutation and recombination, HIV-1 viruses are extremely genetically diverse. There are at least nine distinct subtypes (or clades) of group M and the genetic sequence varies by 17–35% between subtypes. Recombination between subtypes occurs when individuals are infected with more than one subtype, and

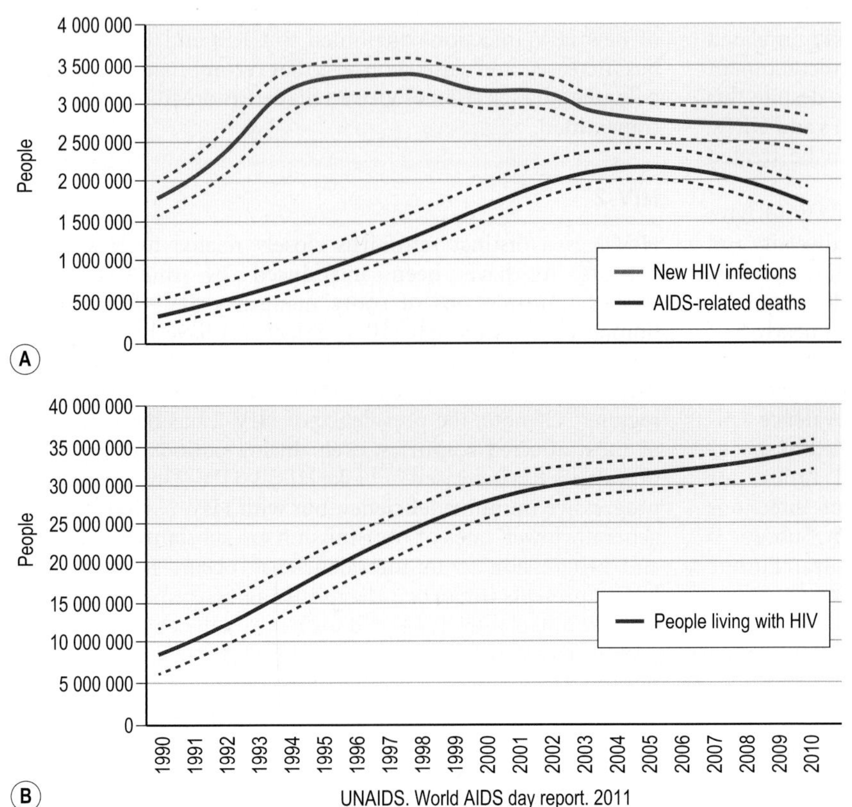

Figure 9.2 New HIV infections and AIDS-related deaths (A) and people living with HIV (B), worldwide 1990–2010.[3] *(UNAIDS. World AIDS Day Report. 2011 (pp 6–7).)*

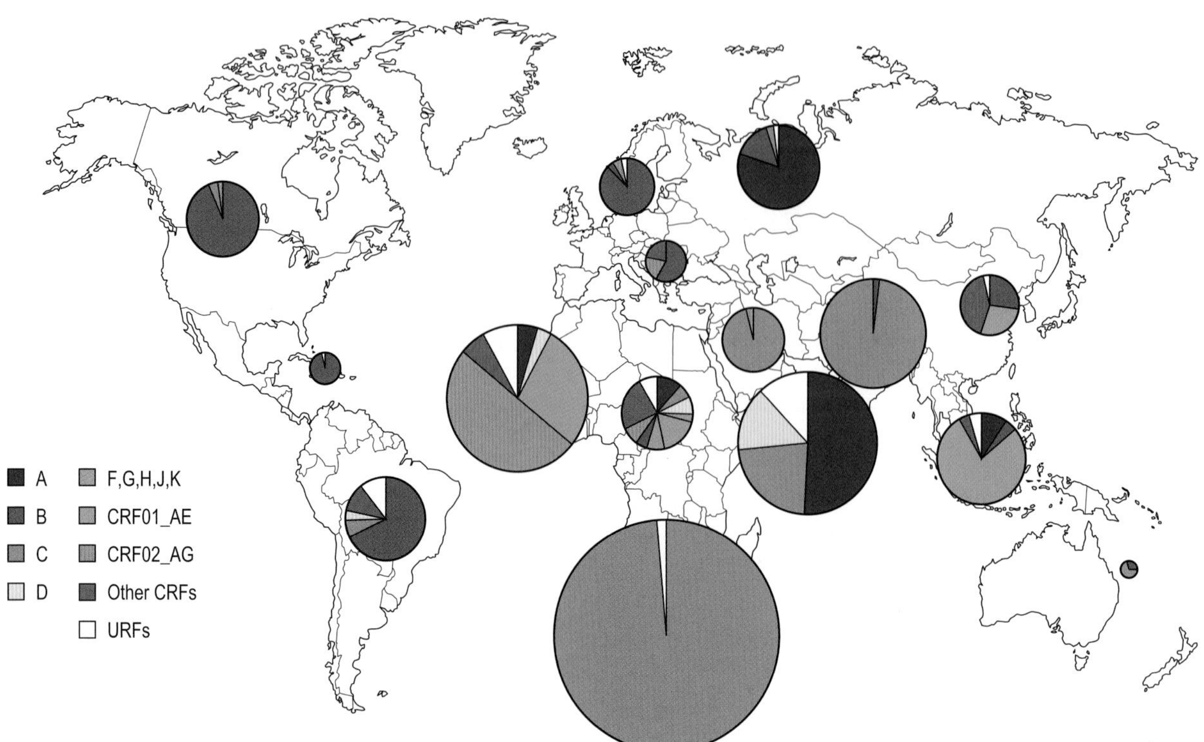

Figure 9.3 Global distribution of HIV-1 subtypes and recombinants, 2004–2007. The pie charts represent the distribution of HIV-1 subtypes and recombinants in each region in 2004–2007. The colors representing the different HIV-1 subtypes are indicated in the legend and the relative size of each pie chart corresponds to the relative numbers of people living with HIV in the region. CRF, circulating recombinant form; URF, unique recombinant form. *(Hemelaar J, Gouws E, Ghys PD, et al., Global trends in molecular epidemiology of HIV-1 during 2000–2007. AIDS 2011;25:679–89.)*

a circulating recombinant form (CRF) is designated when there is evidence that a recombinant virus with a defined mosaic sequence has infected several (>3) epidemiologically unrelated people.[35] Unique recombinant forms (URFs) are recombinant viruses that do not meet CRF criteria. Fortunately, despite this genetic diversity, the vast majority of subtypes, CRFs and URFs, can be detected by HIV diagnostic tests and can be treated effectively with ART.

The initial genetic diversification of HIV is likely to have occurred in Central Africa, where both the greatest diversity and earliest cases of HIV-1 have been identified.[36] Subsequently, HIV-1 subtypes have spread with a geographically heterogeneous distribution (Figure 9.3).[32] Subtype C causes nearly half of HIV infections globally, and is the dominant subtype in southern Africa, Ethiopia and India.[32] The predominance of subtype C, especially in countries with high-prevalence epidemics driven by heterosexual sexual contact, has led to speculation that subtype C may have an increased fitness for transmission.[37,38] Subtype A accounts for 12% of infections worldwide and has a broad geographic distribution. Subtype B predominates in the Americas, western and central Europe and Australia. CRFs are epidemiologically important in South-east Asia, East Asia, West and Central Africa, and the Middle East and North Africa regions.[†,32] URFs are epidemiologically important in Latin America and the East, Central and West Africa regions.[32] In addition, the proportion of new HIV infections attributed to CRFs and URFs globally has increased and raised concern that recombination may contribute to the selection of viruses that are more fit or more easily transmitted.[32,39]

[†]CRFs are estimated to account for the following proportion of HIV infections: South-east Asia (82%), East Asia (69%), West Africa (56%), Central Africa (36%), and the Middle East and North Africa (39%).

HIV-2

HIV-2 is a distinct retrovirus closely related to HIV-1 that appears to have been introduced by multiple cross-species transmissions of sooty mangabey SIV (SIVsmm) to humans.[30,40,41] Although HIV-2 infections have been reported throughout the world, they are most prevalent in western Africa and in countries with economic or cultural ties to the region.[42] Of note, the prevalence of HIV-2 has been declining in most affected countries, even during periods when HIV-1 prevalence has increased.[43,44] Like HIV-1, HIV-2 infection causes progressive immune deficiency, but with HIV-2, viral loads are generally lower, rates of transmission are substantially reduced, and progression to immunodeficiency occurs more slowly.[42] HIV-2 presents important diagnostic and treatment challenges because not all tests developed for HIV-1 will detect HIV-2, and several drugs commonly used to treat HIV-1, particularly the non-nucleoside reverse transcriptase inhibitors nevirapine and efavirenz, may have no or limited benefit for persons with HIV-2.[45] Simultaneous infection with HIV-1 and HIV-2 has been described but the viruses do not appear to recombine with each other.[46]

Interactions between HIV and other Diseases

HIV influences both the epidemiology and the clinical features of many other infectious diseases, malignancies and other illnesses (e.g. renal disease) (see Chapter 10).[47] In HIV-infected patients, immunodeficiency increases the risk that atypical (opportunistic) pathogens will result in clinical illness, and is associated with atypical presentations of some diseases. In addition, HIV-infected patients frequently present with multiple pathologic processes simultaneously, making decisions regarding empiric treatment very challenging. We describe the relationship between HIV and three common infectious diseases that have complex and important interactions.

TUBERCULOSIS

Compared with HIV-negative patients, HIV-infected patients with *Mycobacterium tuberculosis* infection are markedly (21–34 times) more likely to develop active tuberculosis disease.[48] The epidemic of HIV has fuelled an increase in tuberculosis disease in countries with a high HIV prevalence. Many southern and eastern African countries experienced a dramatic increase in the rates of tuberculosis disease and mortality from 1980 to 2004.[48] In 2010, WHO estimated that approximately 12.5% of the 8.8 million incident cases of tuberculosis worldwide were among HIV-infected persons but that 25% of the 1.4 million people who died of tuberculosis had HIV infection.[48] Since 2004, reductions in both the incidence of and mortality from tuberculosis among HIV-infected patients have been attributed to improved tuberculosis diagnosis and treatment, increased HIV testing of patients with tuberculosis, and increased access to ART and cotrimoxazole prophylaxis in HIV/tuberculosis co-infected patients. The epidemiology of these syndemics illustrates the importance of considering and testing for tuberculosis in patients with HIV as well as the importance of HIV testing in all patients with active tuberculosis disease.

MALARIA

Malaria's deleterious effects during pregnancy are substantially magnified by HIV, resulting in increased rates of maternal anemia and low-birth-weight infants.[49] HIV infection is associated with moderately higher malaria parasitemia and greater risk of severe illness, particularly in adults. Additionally, malaria causes an increase in the HIV viral load that is reversed with malaria treatment. Although the clinical consequences of increased malaria parasitemia and HIV viral load may be limited for an individual patient, given the extensive geographic overlap between malaria and HIV, these effects may result in significant consequences at a population level.[50]

HERPES SIMPLEX VIRUS-2 (HSV-2)

HSV-2 has been identified as one of the few factors that distinguish areas of high and low HIV prevalence.[51] HSV-2 seropositivity is associated with a threefold increase in the risk of HIV acquisition, and persons with both HIV and HSV-2 are more likely to transmit HIV. The proportion of HIV that is attributable to HSV-2 infection may increase over time and has been estimated to be as high as 35–48%.[52,53] Efforts to reduce the risk of HIV transmission by treating HSV-2 have been disappointing.[54] Given the strong epidemiologic association between HIV and HSV-2, however, further strategies to prevent HSV-2 transmission (e.g. introduction of an effective HSV-2 vaccine) should be explored.

Modes of Transmission and Risk Factors

HIV is transmitted primarily through sexual contact, contact with infected blood, blood products, or human tissue, and from mother to child.[55,56] Globally, most HIV transmission occurs as the result of unprotected sexual contact. HIV transmission rates per coital act with an HIV-infected partner are estimated to be relatively low (male-to-female: 1.0–3.7 transmissions per 1000 acts; female-to-male: 0.6–1.7 transmissions per 1000 acts; male-to-male anal intercourse: 5 transmissions (receptive) and 0.65 (insertive) transmissions per 1,000 acts)[57] but the risk can be increased substantially if there is disruption of skin or mucous membranes (e.g. by trauma or by sexually transmitted infections that cause genital ulceration) or if the viral load in the source patient is high (e.g. during acute HIV infection).[58] Conversely, ART, which can suppress the viral load to undetectable levels in the plasma, has been demonstrated to reduce the risk of heterosexual transmission of HIV to an HIV-uninfected partner by 96%.[59] Treatment-associated declines in viral load as summarized by mean community viral load[‡] have been associated with decreases in the number of new infections.[60] Rates of HIV transmission in a community are increased when rates of HSV-2 are high and rates of male circumcision are low.[61–63] High numbers of sexual partnerships or concurrent sexual partnerships may increase community transmission[64] although sexual network research indicates that the probability that a sexual partner is HIV-infected is a more important determinant of an individual's HIV risk than the absolute number of partners or concurrent partnerships.[65] Certain genetic factors (e.g. the 32 base-pair deletion in the gene encoding for chemokine receptor 5 (CCR5)) also alter the probability of HIV acquisition.[66,67]

HIV is transmitted by exposure to HIV-infected blood through shared contaminated needles and other injection equipment among persons who inject drugs or as a result of medical procedures that are performed without proper infection control precautions.[68–70] Needle-sharing with an HIV-infected person is a more efficient mode of HIV transmission (6.7 transmissions per 1000 needle sharing events) than sexual contact.[55] There are an estimated 16 million (11–21 million) people who inject drugs worldwide;[71] approximately 80% live in low- and middle-income countries and a majority inject heroin.[72] Outside of sub-Saharan Africa, people who inject drugs account for about 30% of all HIV transmissions and in certain regions this mode of transmission accounts for the majority of HIV transmission (eastern Europe and Central Asia: 60–80%; East Asia and the Pacific: 38–77%).[73]

While unsafe injections in a healthcare setting are currently thought to account for a small proportion of transmissions globally,[74] they may have played a more important role early in the epidemic[75] and outbreaks of HIV infection related to healthcare procedures have been reported.[68,76] The risk of acquiring

[‡]'Mean community viral load' is defined as the average of the most recent viral loads of all persons with known HIV infection in a defined population and during a defined period of time.

HIV from a transfusion with HIV-contaminated blood products is close to 100%.[77] In many parts of the world, increased use of low-risk donors and improved screening practices have reduced the risk of HIV transmission from blood transfusion although further improvements are needed.[2] Although HIV has been isolated from a variety of body fluids, only blood, semen, genital fluids, and breast milk have been proven as sources of infection. HIV is not transmitted through routine household contact or provision of medical care when universal precautions[§] are followed.

TRANSMISSION OF HIV TO CHILDREN

The majority of HIV infections in children occur as the result of mother-to-child transmission. Without interventions, approximately 25–40% of infants born to infected women will acquire HIV about 5% intrapartum, 15% during labour and delivery, and the remainder after birth, primarily through breast-feeding. These risks can be reduced substantially (to <1% in optimal situations) through administration of antiretroviral drugs to the mother, infant or both.[56,78] In 2010, an estimated 64% (57–71%) of pregnant women living with HIV in eastern and southern Africa received an effective antiretroviral regimen to prevent mother-to-child HIV transmission and the percentage of infants born to women living with HIV who received antiretroviral prophylaxis increased from 14% in 2005 to 55% in 2010.[1]

The risk of mother-to-child transmission is increased at all stages of pregnancy if a woman has acquired HIV recently,[79] and transmission during delivery is augmented by certain infections (e.g. HSV-2)[80] and certain obstetric practices (e.g. artificial rupture of membranes, operative vaginal delivery with forceps or a vacuum extractor, and episiotomy).[81] Transmission during breast-feeding appears to occur at a rate of approximately 2% during the first month and 1% per month thereafter – rates of transmission are highest when the infant receives mixed feeding (other infant food in addition to breast milk) in the first 6 months of life rather than being exclusively breast-fed.[56] Acquisition of HIV in utero, compared with acquisition during delivery or from breast-feeding, predicts rapid disease progression in the absence of treatment. Less common modes of HIV transmission to children include pre-chewing or food-mastication[82] and through breast milk from an HIV-infected wet nurse. Sexual abuse of children, which is common in certain settings and often under-reported,[83,84] can be an important contributor to HIV transmission and should be considered when HIV is documented in a child, particularly if the mother does not have HIV.

Methodology for HIV Surveillance and Key Definitions

Internationally, considerable resources have been devoted to HIV surveillance; and healthcare providers have access to more comprehensive, accurate, and timely information on the HIV epidemic than any other infectious disease. The goal of HIV surveillance is to track the epidemic and to generate actionable information that can direct programmes. Surveillance data are used to model key outcomes, which include the estimated number of people living with HIV (prevalence), people newly infected with HIV (incidence), and deaths from HIV-related causes. More recently, programme monitoring systems have supplemented traditional surveillance data by measuring outcomes directly related to HIV prevention interventions (e.g. number of people HIV tested, number of HIV-infected pregnant women who received an intervention to prevent mother-to-child transmission) and HIV treatment and care (e.g. number of people receiving ART).

For the purposes of surveillance, UNAIDS and WHO classify HIV epidemics as generalized, concentrated or low-level.[85] Generalized epidemics are arbitrarily defined by HIV prevalence consistently over 1% in pregnant women, a sentinel population used to assess trends in HIV prevalence and to estimate the adult HIV prevalence among the population 15–49 years old. Such rates indicate that sexual networking in the general population is sufficient to sustain an epidemic independent of high-risk groups. Concentrated epidemics are characterized by HIV prevalence consistently over 5% in at least one defined key population (e.g. MSM, people who inject drugs, commercial sex workers) and an HIV prevalence below 1% in pregnant women in urban areas, indicating that HIV infection is not well established in the general population. Low-level epidemics are defined by an HIV prevalence that has not exceeded 5% in any defined key population.

HIV prevalence can be measured by case reporting or by conducting representative surveys. Few countries currently conduct effective case-based surveillance. Population-based estimates of HIV prevalence are based on results of surveys in key populations in countries with concentrated epidemics and among pregnant women in antenatal care and the general population in countries with generalized epidemics. UNAIDS has developed and validated sophisticated methods to incorporate multiple sources of data, including survey and programmatic data, into estimates of population prevalence.

Full understanding of the HIV epidemic requires accurate data on HIV incidence. However, measuring HIV incidence is complicated because diagnosis of HIV infection often occurs years after the infection is acquired. In the tropics, most estimates of adult HIV incidence have been based on mathematical models that compare trends in observed HIV prevalence data between years and among different age groups.[86,87] Emerging HIV testing technologies have the potential to improve incidence estimates by distinguishing antibody characteristics (e.g. titre or avidity) of recent vs. long-term infections.[88] In addition, as access to HIV testing continues to expand, clinical information on acute and early HIV infections will provide important complementary HIV incidence data.

Substantial capacity has evolved to track implementation of HIV prevention and treatment services. As service delivery becomes more complete, clinical data can replace survey data. For example, when testing rates are consistently high it may be possible to use results of HIV testing in antenatal clinics in place of anonymous surveys of HIV prevalence among pregnant women.[89,90]

Measurement of HIV rates in children presents major challenges. Children have been included in few national surveys, in

[§]'Universal precautions', as defined by CDC, are a set of precautions designed to prevent transmission of bloodborne pathogens, such as HIV, when providing first aid or health care. Information can be found at the UNAIDS website: http://www.unaids.org/en/KnowledgeCentre/Resources/PolicyGuidance/Techpolicies/Univ_pre_technical_policies.asp and the CDC website: http://www.cdc.gov/ncidod/dhqp/bp_universal_precautions.html.

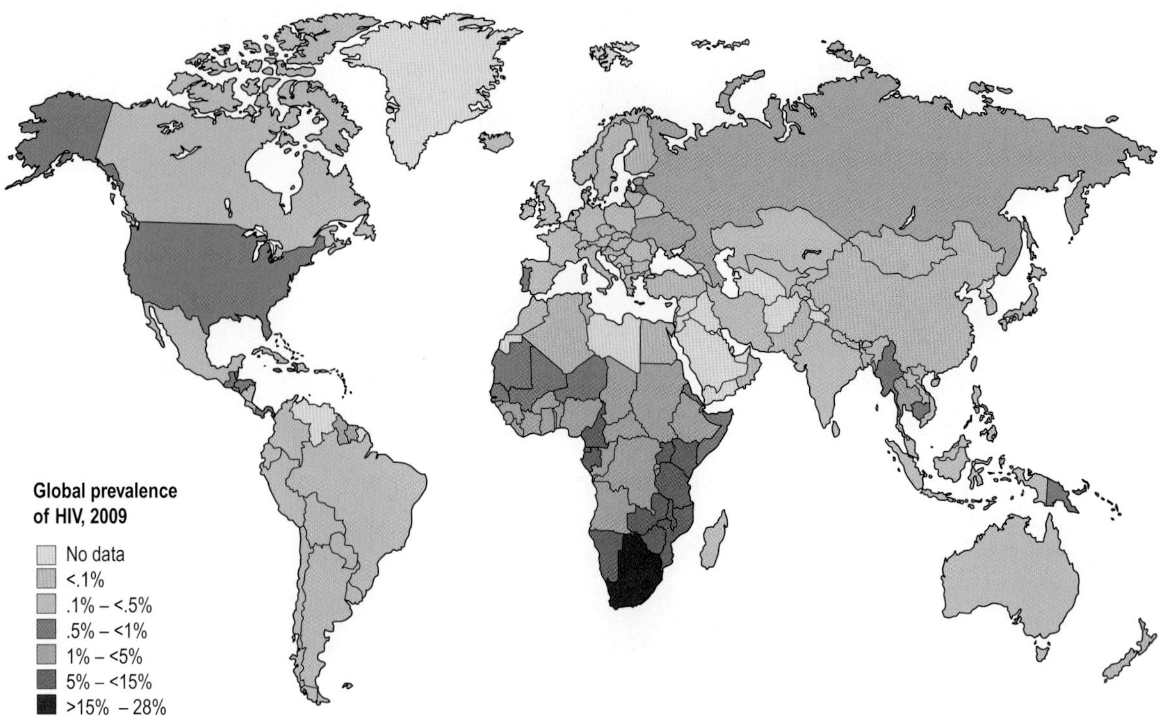

Figure 9.4 Global adult HIV prevalence by country (2009).

part because of ethical issues related to enrolling children in these surveys. More feasible approaches to collection of data on pediatric HIV rates may include conducting HIV testing in the context of immunization, evaluation of school-based cohorts, and surveillance of mortality or specific HIV-related infections.[8]

Geographic Epidemiology (Figure 9.4)

SUB-SAHARAN AFRICA (SOUTH, EAST, CENTRAL, WEST)

HIV has caused a generalized epidemic in many parts of sub-Saharan Africa, which contains 68% of all people living with HIV worldwide but only 12% of the world's total population.[2] An estimated 1.9 million (1.7–2.1 million) people in the region were newly infected with HIV in 2010 (70% of all new HIV infections globally). Overall, the total number of people living with HIV in the region has increased by 12% since 2001. Although considerable efforts have improved access to antiretrovirals, 1.2 million (1.1–1.4 million) Africans still died of AIDS in 2010 (67% of AIDS deaths worldwide).[2]

Southern Africa now has the highest HIV prevalence in the world. Conversely, many West and Central African countries have maintained a relatively low HIV prevalence (<2%). There is also marked geographic variation in HIV prevalence within countries. In Kenya, for example, HIV prevalence estimated in 2007 varied from 0.8% in the northeast part of the country to 14.9% in the western province of Nyanza.[92]

HIV arrived late in southern Africa (South Africa had an HIV prevalence of less than 1% in 1988) but has spread rapidly (Figure 9.5). Southern Africa now has the most intense HIV epidemic in the world with an estimated 34% of all people living with HIV worldwide residing in 10 countries** in the region.[2] Various social and biological factors have played a role in generating and sustaining high prevalence rates; there are data to support the impact of high rates of genital herpes (HSV-2), low rates of male circumcision, intergenerational and age-disparate sex,[††] transactional sex (i.e., the exchange of goods or money for sex), men migrating for work, and gender-based inequalities,[94] although the relative contribution of each of these individual risk factors is neither consistent nor universally relevant in all high-prevalence settings. The importance of concurrent sexual partnerships in generalized, heterosexual HIV epidemics has been debated and is controversial.[95] Rates of male circumcision are high (80–100% prevalence) in many North and West African countries but are low in many southern African and several East African countries with a high HIV prevalence.[‡‡,96] Intergenerational and age-disparate sexual relationships (which often also include transactional sex) are an

**Adult HIV prevalence in 10 southern African countries in 2009: Angola (2%), Botswana (25%), Lesotho (24%), Malawi (11%), Mozambique (12%), Namibia (13%), South Africa (18%), Swaziland (26%), Zambia (14%) and Zimbabwe (14%)

††Intergenerational or cross-generational relationships are often defined as a sexual relationship with a partner who is 10 or more years older. Age-disparate relationships are often defined as a sexual relationship between young people where one partner is 5 or more years older than the other.

‡‡Male circumcision prevalence: Botswana (11%), Nyanza Province of Kenya (47%), Lesotho (52%), Malawi (21%), Mozambique (52%), Namibia (21%), Rwanda (12%), South Africa (42%), Swaziland (8%), Tanzania (67%), Uganda (25%), Zambia (13%), Zimbabwe (10%) (data from surveys conducted between 2005 and 2010).

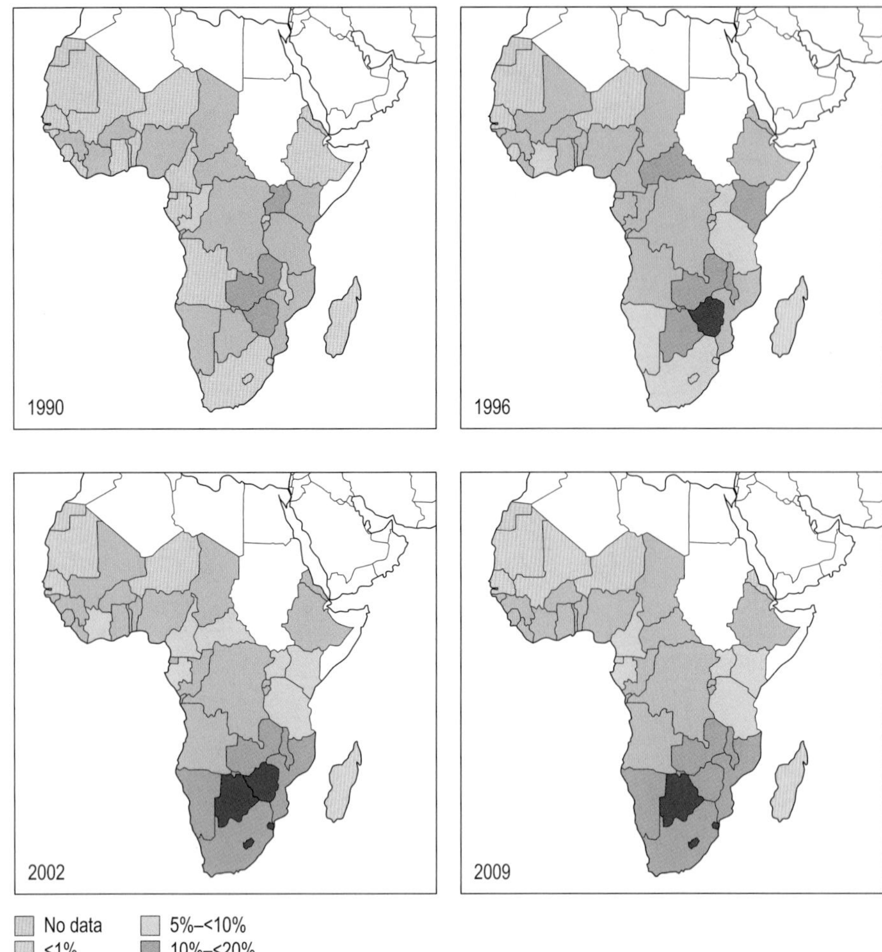

Figure 9.5 HIV prevalence among adults aged 15–49 years in sub-Saharan Africa, 1990 to 2009. *(UNAIDS. Global report: UNAIDS report on the global AIDS epidemic 2010 (Fig. 2.7).)*

important driver of new HIV infections among young women in the region. In a national South African survey in 2008, 28% of sexually active 15-19-year-old females reported having a sexual partner >5 years older compared with only 1% of males. HIV prevalence in 2008 among female and male South Africans aged 20–24 years was 21% vs 5%, respectively.[5]

Before the mid-2000s, AIDS-related deaths led to substantial decreases in life expectancy in many southern African countries.[97] In Botswana, life expectancy fell from 65 years in 1985 to 34 years in 2006; however, with treatment scale-up in which antiretroviral medications became available to approximately 90% of eligible persons in Botswana, AIDS-related deaths have been reduced from an estimated 18 000 in 2002 to 9100 in 2009[91] and life expectancy is rising again. In Malawi, provision of ART has also been linked to a 10% drop in the adult all-cause death rate between 2004 and 2008.[15]

Efforts at preventing new infections are gaining traction. Throughout southern Africa, declining HIV prevalence among young adults, increased testing and counseling services, and provision of perinatal ART for prevention of mother-to-child transmission have reduced new infections among children by 32%.[93] Denial of risk, however, remains a barrier to effective HIV prevention and diagnosis. In a 2005 survey in South Africa, half of people who tested HIV-positive believed they were not at risk of acquiring infection.[98] In a 2007 Kenyan survey of adult men and women who reported not testing for HIV because they were low risk, HIV prevalence was 4.9% and 5.9%, respectively.[92] The epidemiologic importance of HIV infections among MSM[99–103] and among people who inject drugs[104] in sub-Saharan Africa has only recently begun to be appreciated.

ASIA (SOUTH-EAST, SOUTH, EAST, CENTRAL)

Although the adult HIV prevalence is lower in Asia than in sub-Saharan Africa, there were still an estimated 4.8 million (4.3–5.3 million) people living with HIV in 2010.[2] Fortunately in many regions of Asia the HIV transmission rate has declined (from peak rates in the mid-1990s for South and South-east Asia and the mid-2000s for East Asia). With improved access to ART there have also been reductions in HIV-related deaths. As these declines in mortality have exceeded declines in the HIV transmission rate, the total number of people living with HIV in the region has increased by 11% since 2001.[2] The epidemic in Asia is comprised of many concentrated epidemics in specific key populations and the failure of HIV to sustain heterosexual spread in the general population of Asia has provided critical insight into HIV's global epidemiology.[105] There is also significant regional variation in HIV prevalence within and across countries. In China, for example, 5 of 32 provinces account for over 50% of people living with HIV infection.[106]

In many countries in Asia, HIV occurred first among people who inject drugs and among commercial sex workers. More recently (by the mid-2000s), previously undocumented but severe HIV epidemics have been reported among MSM in many Asian countries.[107] For example, in Thailand, HIV spread rapidly among two distinct networks (people who inject drugs and commercial sex workers) beginning in the late 1980s.[108] Surveys indicate that between 0.5–15% adult men in the region buy sex and an HIV prevalence of 1.5–5.6% among male clients of sex workers has been detected. Although commercial sex work has been an important contributor to the epidemic in the region, there is increasing evidence that HIV prevention programmes can prevent HIV transmissions among commercial sex workers and their clients. Thailand's '100% Condom' campaign, for example, which educates sex workers and promotes condom use, has been associated with decreased HIV transmission in female commercial sex workers.[109] Despite Thailand's success in controlling the HIV epidemic among commercial sex workers, however, there is now evidence of a severe HIV epidemic among MSM. In 2003, the HIV prevalence among MSM in Bangkok was 17% and this increased to 25% by 2009, highlighting the urgent need for effective HIV prevention interventions in this population.[110]

The prevalence of HIV has also remained high among people who inject drugs. Harm reduction programmes, which include needle syringe exchange programmes and methadone maintenance treatment programmes, have demonstrated impressive declines in HIV prevalence among people who inject drugs,[111,112] but many countries have been slow to scale-up these programmes as drug dependence is typically viewed as a law enforcement problem instead of a public health issue. Unfortunately, in the absence of harm reduction programmes, the HIV prevalence among people who inject drugs can increase rapidly and achieve dramatically high rates. This has been most recently seen in Cebu, Philippines where the HIV prevalence among people who inject drugs increased from 0.6% in 2009 to 53% in 2011.[113]

LATIN AMERICA AND THE CARIBBEAN

Brazil, the most populous country in Latin America, had an estimated 460 000–810 000 people living with HIV in 2009.[93] In the 1990s, many experts predicted that Brazil's epidemic would rapidly accelerate. However, the country's sustained campaign to promote sex education, condom use, harm reduction, and HIV testing and to provide universal ART has held adult prevalence below 1%.[93] The majority of HIV infections in South America occur among MSM[114] and people who inject drugs.[104] Incarcerated men are at particularly high risk.[115] In addition, in Central America a high proportion of MSM (22%) have reported having sex with at least one female partner in the previous 6 months, underscoring the potential for HIV to bridge to women in this region.[116]

HIV epidemics vary considerably among the countries of the Caribbean from a low HIV prevalence of 0.1% in Cuba to a high prevalence of 3.1% in the Bahamas. Approximately 70% of people living with HIV in the region reside on the island of Hispaniola, which contains the Dominican Republic and Haiti. More women than men are living with HIV in Haiti, the Bahamas, Belize, and the Dominican Republic which illustrates that unprotected sex among men and women, in addition to unprotected sex between men, is a significant driver of new HIV infections in this region.[117]

OCEANIA

Most Pacific island countries and territories are experiencing very small HIV epidemics (fewer than 500 reported HIV cases). Papua New Guinea, however, is experiencing a serious HIV epidemic with an estimated adult prevalence of 0.9% in 2009. Unprotected heterosexual sex is the main mode of HIV transmission in Papua New Guinea. In addition, transactional sex, sex between men, and mother-to-child transmission contribute substantially to the epidemic.[2]

MIDDLE EAST AND NORTH AFRICA

HIV surveillance is limited in this region, but available data indicate that South Sudan and Djibouti are experiencing generalized HIV epidemics. New HIV infections in the region have increased by 34% in 2010 compared with 2001 and new infections among children younger than 15 years have almost doubled during the same time period, indicating that the HIV epidemic is accelerating. In most Middle Eastern and North African countries, except South Sudan[§§] and Djibouti, the national HIV prevalence is low (less than 0.2%), but high rates of HIV have been observed in people who inject drugs (e.g. 14% of people who inject drugs in Iran were living with HIV[2]) and among MSM (e.g. 8% of MSM in Sudan tested HIV-positive[107]).

More detailed global and regional information is published annually by the WHO and UNAIDS: http://www.unaids.org; http://www.who.int/hiv/en/.

Global Response

While the initial response to the HIV pandemic in tropical settings was delayed, global efforts have increased dramatically. Between 1996 and 2010, annual funding for AIDS in low- and middle-income countries increased from US$300 million to US$15 billion.[3] This acceleration of the world's response was facilitated by human rights advocacy from people living with HIV and concerns about the impact of HIV on global economic systems and security.[118] Although funding has been impressive, international assistance contributed by high-income countries declined from US$8.7 billion in 2009 to US$7.6 billion in 2010.[3] An effective global response will depend on sustained funding of effective prevention and treatment programmes until the pandemic can be controlled.

HIV PREVENTION EPIDEMIOLOGY

Comprehensive and sustained prevention programmes have been proven to reduce HIV transmission (see Chapter 12). Unfortunately, HIV prevention interventions have not reached the majority of people at high risk. A major challenge has

[§§]The Republic of South Sudan is included in WHO's Eastern Mediterranean Region and therefore included in this geographic section instead of the sub-Saharan Africa section.

been generating the political will and economic resources to implement proven strategies addressing issues such as sex, sexuality and drug use. Still, there are several encouraging developments in HIV prevention that have impacted global HIV epidemiology.[119]

Safer sexual behaviour is essential to reduce HIV transmission. In Malawi and Zimbabwe, increased condom use, delayed onset of sexual activity, and a reduction in sexual relations with non-regular partners have been associated with declines in HIV prevalence.[120,121] In settings with concentrated epidemics, behavioural interventions focused on people at highest risk of HIV infection have been particularly effective, e.g. the '100% condom' programmes for sex work in Thailand and Cambodia[109] have achieved high levels of condom use in sex work (over 90%) and have been associated with declines in HIV prevalence and sexually transmitted infections among female sex workers. In addition, implementation of these programmes has been associated with declines in HIV prevalence among male army conscripts, pregnant women and blood donors.[122]

Male circumcision reduces a man's risk of acquiring HIV heterosexually by 50–60%.[61–63] In high-prevalence areas where a large fraction of the population is uncircumcised, large-scale implementation of male circumcision has the potential to prevent many new infections. In 2007, WHO and UNAIDS recommended including male circumcision as an HIV prevention intervention for 15–49-year old men in countries with a high HIV and low circumcision prevalence. A total of 13 countries in eastern and southern Africa*** have committed to the goal of achieving 80% coverage among 15–49-year-old men (approx. 20 million men). The number of male circumcisions in 15–49-year-old men increased from 21 000 per year in 2008 to over 400 000 per year in 2010 in these 13 countries but further scale-up is necessary to achieve 80% coverage.[2]

HIV TESTING EPIDEMIOLOGY

Half of all persons living with HIV worldwide are unaware of their status[4] and therefore are not able to access life-saving medical treatment and remain unaware that they need to protect their sex or needle-sharing partners from becoming infected. Many HIV-infected persons will decrease their risk behaviour when they are aware of their positive HIV status.[123,124] Consequently, HIV testing is an important component of primary HIV prevention. Epidemiologic data from population-based surveys in six African countries††† have demonstrated that 31–69% of people living with HIV had never received a prior HIV test.[2] Fortunately, there was a 17% increase in HIV tests performed from 2009 to 2010 in this region.[2] In general, knowledge of HIV status is better among women than men because of the successful expansion of HIV testing among pregnant women in antenatal care. In eastern and southern Africa, the percentage of pregnant women receiving an HIV test increased from 16% in 2005 to 61% in 2010 and similar improvements have also occurred in Latin America and Asia.[2] Conversely, HIV diagnosis among adolescents (aged 10–19 years) has been particularly difficult and it is estimated that the majority of the 2 million adolescents living with HIV have never received an HIV test.[2]

To improve HIV diagnosis in countries with generalized epidemics, WHO now recommends that healthcare providers offer provider-initiated testing and counselling, where the provider offers HIV testing to all patients and the patient has the informed right to accept or refuse. Provider-initiated testing is preferable to relying on client-initiated HIV testing and counselling (also known as voluntary counselling and testing, VCT, where the patient requests an HIV test) in most clinical settings (e.g. antenatal clinics, pediatric and adult general medicine clinics, inpatient settings). In addition, provider-initiated testing can be offered to patients as 'opt-out' HIV testing‡‡‡ to increase the proportion of patients who receive an HIV test. A study from two hospitals in Harare, Zimbabwe demonstrated that 46% of adolescents admitted to the hospital, and 74% of adolescents who died during their hospitalization, were HIV-infected,[125] and highlighted the need for clinicians to initiate opt-out HIV testing as a component of routine clinical care. Couples testing and counselling is another important HIV testing service, particularly in settings with a high HIV prevalence and where transmission is predominately through heterosexual intercourse.[126] A majority of adults in sub-Saharan Africa are in cohabitating unions and among adults living with HIV in a stable relationship, approximately half (49%) have an HIV-negative partner.[127] Couples testing can be linked to ART for the HIV-infected partner, which by suppressing their viral load can reduce transmission to the HIV-negative partner by as much as 96%.[59,128,129] Home-based testing has also been well accepted and can result in early identification of individuals in need of ART.[130]

To achieve the maximum clinical and public health benefits from an HIV diagnosis, linkage to and retention in medical care must be a clinical priority. Limited data indicate that substantial numbers of patients do not successfully transition from HIV testing to a clinical visit to determine ART eligibility (41%); and that a significant percentage of patients deemed eligible do not initiate antiretrovirals (32%).[131]

HIV TREATMENT EPIDEMIOLOGY

Fuelled by individual country efforts and multilateral and bilateral initiatives such as WHO's '3 by 5' campaign, the Global Fund for AIDS, Tuberculosis and Malaria, and the US President's Emergency Plan for AIDS Relief (PEPFAR), the numbers of persons accessing HIV treatment in resource-limited settings rose from barely 40 000 in 2003 to 6.6 million by the end of 2011.[2] By the end of 2010, 10 low- and middle-income countries had achieved treatment coverage levels of at least 80% (Figure 9.6). Scale-up has been facilitated by a public health approach that uses standardized treatment algorithms and

***Countries with a high HIV prevalence and low level of male circumcision are Botswana, Ethiopia (province of Gambella), Kenya, Lesotho, Malawi, Mozambique, Namibia, Rwanda, South Africa, Swaziland, United Republic of Tanzania, Uganda, Zambia and Zimbabwe.

†††Countries that conducted population-based surveys and determined the proportion of adults living with HIV who had never received a prior HIV test (%): Congo (69%), Mozambique (61%), United Republic of Tanzania (61%), Sao Tome and Principe (59%), Lesotho (36%) and Kenya (31%).

‡‡‡'Opt-out HIV testing' is defined as informing patients in defined clinical settings that an HIV test will be included as a part of their clinical care unless they want to specifically decline the test.

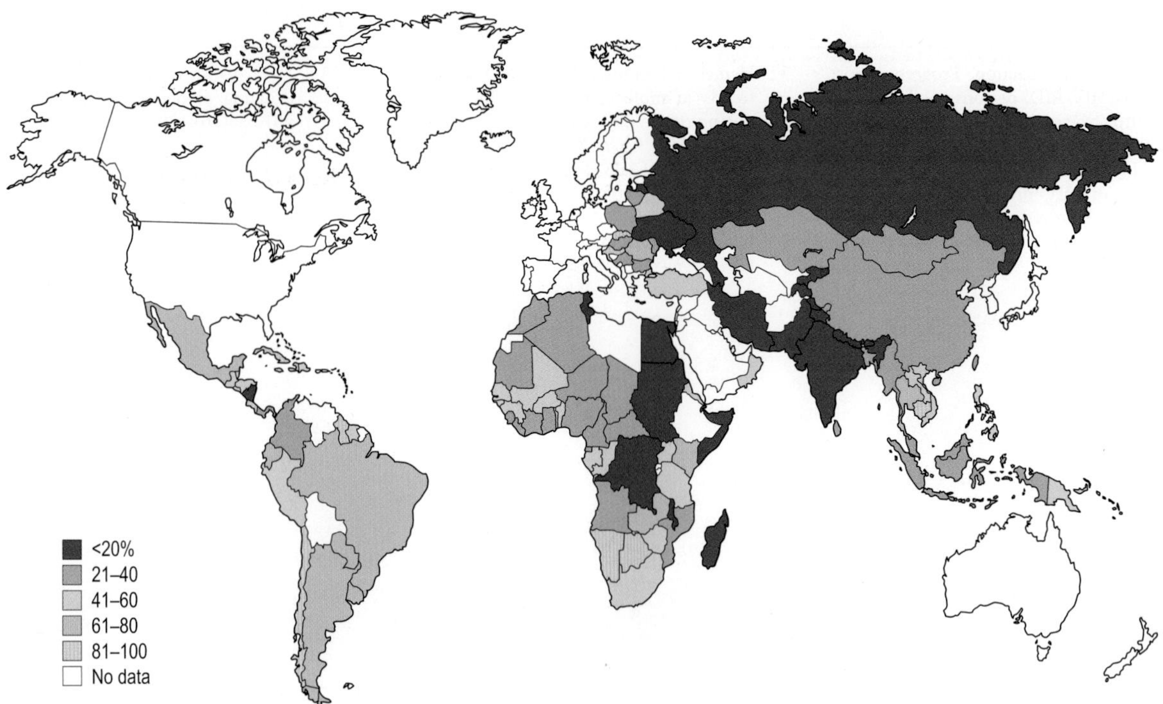

Figure 9.6 Antiretroviral therapy coverage among people with advanced HIV infection in low- and middle-income countries (%). *(Based on WHO 2010 guidelines). WHO. Global Health Observatory. Online. Available:* http://apps.who.int/ghodata *(Accessed 26 March 2012).*

reduced frequency of routine laboratory monitoring compared with high-income settings.[132] Outcomes have generally been good,[133] with adherence rates in low-resourced settings mirroring those in the USA and Europe. A particular challenge, however, has been timely linkage to and initiation of ART as mortality rates have been documented to be extremely high just prior to starting ART in treatment programmes in sub-Saharan Africa.[134,135] High early mortality after ART initiation has also been observed and is attributed to advanced disease at presentation,[136] but the median CD4 cell counts at entry into care and treatment are gradually rising.[137] Finally, in the long-term, achieving sustained retention in care will be a key challenge.

Expansion of HIV treatment is having a profound effect on the global HIV epidemic. Provision of antiretroviral drugs has led to a marked reduction in HIV infections among infants in some settings. Botswana reported the proportion of infants born to HIV-infected mothers who acquired HIV infection declined from 20.7% in 2003 to 3.8% in 2007.[138] In settings like Botswana, as the number of infants with HIV infection declines, clinicians will care for a greater proportion of older children on ART (or with slow disease progression) and children who acquired HIV later in childhood. Population-level implications of the expansion of ART may be less intuitive or predictable. There is mounting evidence that ART reduces HIV transmission both in the setting of stable discordant relationships[59] and at the community level[60] and hope that broad coverage with ART can reduce HIV prevalence. With the expansion of ART in KwaZulu-Natal, South Africa, the risk of HIV acquisition declined significantly among individuals living in communities with relatively high ART coverage (greater than 30% of all HIV-infected adults on ART) compared with individuals living in communities where ART coverage was low (<10% of all HIV-infected adults on ART).[139] This expansion of ART was also associated with an increase in the adult life expectancy from 49.2 years in 2003 to 60.5 years in 2011 (an 11.3 year gain)[140] and an increase in HIV prevalence from 18% in 2003 to 24% in 2011, since reductions in transmission from ART were offset by increased survival on ART. Epidemiological data will be vital to define and monitor the threshold level of antiretroviral coverage required to achieve sustained reductions in HIV transmission.

Summary and Prospects for the Future

HIV has changed the face of global health and the practice of medicine. The response has been heroic, but the remaining challenges are daunting. Even if transmission can be halted, tens of millions of persons will eventually require treatment. The course of the global HIV epidemic will be influenced by the biology of the virus, social and behavioural trends, funding and political priorities, and the continued development of prevention and treatment interventions like simplified antiretroviral regimens. Aspirational interventions such as curative treatment regimens, and therapeutic and preventive vaccines could also have a dramatic impact on the global HIV epidemic if the scientific barriers to their development can be solved. But even with the tools at hand, the epidemic can be turned with broad implementation of evidence-based interventions for prevention, as well as continued support for and expansion of HIV treatment. If declining incidence can be maintained, there is hope that the HIV epidemic can be controlled.

REFERENCES

2. World Health Organization. Progress report 2011: Global HIV/AIDS response. Online. Available: http://www.who.int/hiv/pub/progress_report2011/en/ (Accessed 21 Dec 2011).
15. Jahn A, Floyd S, Crampin AC, et al. Population-level effect of HIV on adult mortality and early evidence of reversal after introduction of antiretroviral therapy in Malawi. Lancet 2008; 371:1603–11.
32. Hemelaar J, Gouws E, Ghys PD, et al. Global trends in molecular epidemiology of HIV-1 during 2000–2007. AIDS 2011;25:679–89.
59. Cohen MS, Chen YQ, McCauley M, et al. Prevention of HIV-1 infection with early antiretroviral therapy. N Engl J Med 2011;365: 493–505.
75. Pepin J. The Origins of AIDS. Cambridge: Cambridge University Press; 2011.
119. De Cock KM, Jaffe HW, Curran JW. The evolving epidemiology of HIV/AIDS. AIDS 2012;26(10):1205–13.

Access the complete references online at www.expertconsult.com

10

Clinical Features and Management of HIV/AIDS

ROBIN WOOD

KEY POINTS

- After 2002, price reductions of branded antiretroviral drugs and increasing competition from cheaper generic formulations decreased the cost of first-line antiretroviral therapy (ART) to less than US$150/year and ART became recognized as a cost-effective medical intervention. Furthermore, there has been an increasing awareness that early initiation of ART may significantly decrease HIV transmission and have a societal prevention benefit additional to individual clinical benefit.
- Knowledge of the natural history of HIV infection in developing countries is incomplete. Nonetheless, there are considerable data to suggest that progression to AIDS and/or death may be faster in developing countries. Many factors may potentially result in shorter survival of HIV-infected patients in resource-poor settings, including more frequent exposure to primary pathogens such as *Mycobacterium tuberculosis* and *Salmonella* spp., limited access to healthcare services, under-resourced medical services, quality of water supply and poor nutritional status.
- Many clinical trials and observational studies have shown that TMP-SMX prophylaxis reduces mortality, morbidity and hospital admissions in HIV-infected adults and children not receiving ART across Africa. In addition to prophylactic activity against *Pneumocystis jirovecii* pneumonia, TMP-SMX is highly effective against *Toxoplasma gondii, Isospora belli, Cyclospora* spp. and has activity against malaria.
- Immunization against infectious agents that commonly affect HIV-infected individuals is an attractive strategy. However, the potential effectiveness of this strategy is undermined by the progressive reduction of vaccine efficacy as the immune deficiency progresses. The impaired immune response to vaccine antigens and the inability to maintain appropriate memory cell populations remains, despite initiation of ART, and may be related to the CD4 count nadir reached prior to ART initiation.
- Tuberculosis is currently the second leading cause of death from infectious disease, responsible for 1.2–1.5 million deaths annually. The clinical presentation of TB is also greatly modified by immune deficiency. Smear-negative pulmonary disease is more frequent in HIV-infected individuals. Early in HIV infection, TB presents with a classic reactivation pattern of pulmonary upper lobe infiltrates with cavitation. With increasing immunodeficiency, the chest radiographic picture often resembles tuberculosis primary infection with adenopathy and mid or lower lobe infiltrates; dissemination to lymph nodes, meninges and pleural, pericardial and peritoneal cavities are also more frequent.

Introduction

Over the last three decades, the world has had to learn to live with an evolving and seemingly unstoppable HIV epidemic. Following the identification of HIV as the cause of AIDS in the early 1980s, the standard of care and treatment changed rapidly in developed countries, resulting in improvements in HIV-associated mortality and morbidity. In contrast, treatment and care in developing countries evolved more slowly. In resource-poor countries, before the full extent of the demographic and social impact of the epidemic became manifest, the emphasis of public health and international agencies focussed on prevention. As the number of patients with AIDS began to overwhelm already over-stressed health systems, care was perceived as an infinite demand, yielding little public health benefit. However, the humanitarian need to alleviate the plight of increasing numbers of people living with HIV/AIDS led to debates pitting care versus prevention. Care was initially limited to cheap chemoprophylaxis and restricted treatment of a few specific opportunistic infections but excluded treatment with antiretroviral drugs, which were considered unaffordable. After 2002, price reductions of branded antiretroviral drugs and increasing competition from cheaper generic formulations decreased the cost of first-line antiretroviral therapy (ART) to less than US$150 per year and ART became recognized as a cost-effective medical intervention.[1,2] Furthermore, there has been increasing awareness that early initiation of ART may significantly decrease HIV transmission and have a societal prevention benefit additional to individual clinical benefit.[3–7]

GLOBAL ACCESS TO HIV TREATMENT

An international consensus has emerged on the need to address HIV/AIDS with a comprehensive response including treatment, care and prevention. In recent years, there has been an unprecedented global effort to address the challenges posed by HIV and AIDS to health in low- and medium-resourced regions of the world.[8] A public health approach to the management of HIV and AIDS including antiretroviral therapy has been developed and continues to evolve in response to increasing scientific knowledge.[9] Access to treatment has improved at a rapid pace and has been accompanied by declining AIDS deaths. The Global Fund to Fight AIDS, Tuberculosis and Malaria was created in 2002. In November 2003, the United Nations General Assembly declared the lack of access to HIV treatment a global emergency. The World Health Organization (WHO) subsequently launched a global effort, in collaboration with other international agencies, to provide antiretroviral therapy to 3 million people living with AIDS by the end of 2005. In 2005, at the World Summit of the United Nations, Heads of State declared that access to HIV treatment was a universal right. The United States Presidents Emergency Plan for AIDS Relief (PEPFAR) to combat global HIV/AIDS, tuberculosis and malaria was implemented in 2004 with a US$15 billion budget and reauthorized in 2008 enabling a US$48 billion expenditure over the next 5 years. These combined funding sources have enabled a continued expansion of antiretroviral treatment and presently 5.2 million of the estimated 15 million people living with HIV in low- and middle-income countries have access to antiretroviral therapy. In 2010 an estimated 10 million people living with HIV were eligible for treatment under the revised WHO treatment guidelines.[10]

RELATIONSHIP BETWEEN HIV AND CO-INFECTION DISEASE

Knowledge of the natural history of HIV infection in developing countries is incomplete. Nonetheless, there are considerable data to suggest that progression to AIDS and/or death may be faster in developing countries. Many factors may potentially result in shorter survival of HIV-infected patients in resource-poor settings, including more frequent exposure to primary pathogens such as *Mycobacterium tuberculosis* and *Salmonella* spp. limited access to healthcare services, under-resourced medical services, quality of water supply and poor nutritional status.

Besides the likely existence of considerable local variation within regions, the cohorts on whom present knowledge is based are subject to selection biases and variable diagnostic criteria.[11–21]

In comparison with reports from developed countries, there are very few reports on early clinical, virological and immunological events after acute infection from developing countries. The subsequent spectrum of clinical presentation of HIV and AIDS varies geographically and is largely determined among indigenous populations by the overlap between prevalent infections and HIV prevalence. The immune compromise associated with HIV infection may change the frequency of disease co-infections and their presentation. The relationship between HIV prevalence in individuals diagnosed with co-infections and the population prevalence of HIV infection is shown in Figure 10.1. The proportion of cases testing HIV-positive in any specific disease is related to the HIV-associated relative risk for that condition and the HIV prevalence of the population at risk. Concomitant HIV infection increases the risk of developing active visceral leishmaniasis by more than 100-fold (Figure 10.1, RR=100). Consequently, in southern Europe, 70% of visceral leishmaniasis cases in adults are associated with HIV infection, although HIV infection is present in only 0.2% of the

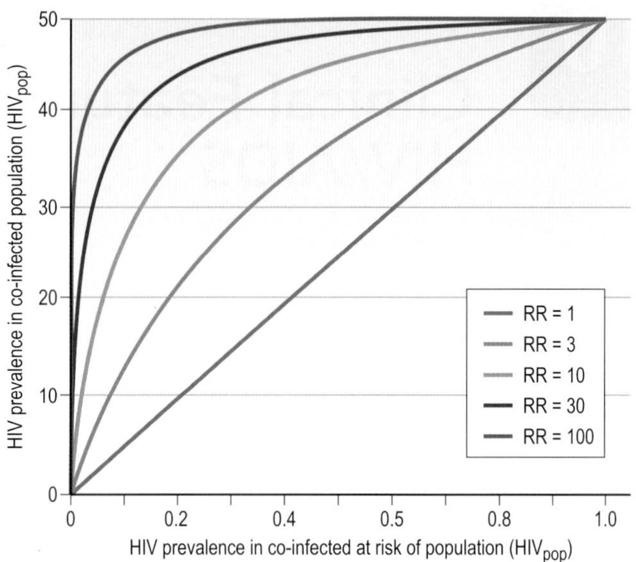

Figure 10.1 The relationship between HIV prevalence in individuals diagnosed with co-infections and the population prevalence of HIV infection.

population. For conditions with slightly lower HIV-associated relative risk such as the endemic mycoses, the proportion of cases that are HIV-positive is still very high even at modest general population HIV prevalences (Figure 10.1, RR=30–100). For conditions with lower relative risks such as bacterial and mycobacterial diseases, HIV prevalence varies markedly with general population HIV prevalence (Figure 10.1, RR=10–30). For diseases where the acquisition of infection is not increased by HIV infection such as some parasitic conditions the prevalence of HIV in diseased and non-diseased populations is similar (Figure 10.1, RR=1).

HIV infection may impact on disease control measures in complex ways by altering disease burden and disease infectivity. The increased parasite load of visceral leishmaniasis in HIV-positive immune-compromised individuals increases both disease burden and transmission probability, thereby transforming leishmaniasis from a sporadic to an endemic threat.[22] HIV infection increases progression to disease following tuberculosis infection resulting in very high TB burdens where there are generalized HIV epidemics. The disease burden of fungal infections such as *Cryptococcus neoformans, Penicillium marneffei*, and *Histoplasma capsulatum* are increased by HIV infection but with no impact on disease transmission. However, even when there is no increase in the burden of disease as a result of HIV infection, the clinical presentation and response to therapy may still be markedly impacted by HIV-associated immune suppression.

PREVENTION OF HIV-RELATED DISEASE

HIV-related morbidity and mortality are due to infections and neoplasms, which tend to occur with increasing frequency as immune suppression progresses. Primary pathogens, such as *Mycobacterium tuberculosis, Streptococcus pneumoniae* and *Plasmodium falciparum*, which can cause disease even in individuals with intact immune systems, occur over a wide range of CD4 counts, whereas less pathogenic organisms, such as *Mycobacterium avium intracellulare* (MAC) and *Penicillium marneffei*, are true opportunistic infections (OIs) and thus occur almost exclusively in individuals in advanced stages of immune deficiency. The best prophylaxis for HIV-related illnesses is the reversal of immune deficiency through the use of ART. However, OIs will still occur, especially if ART is instituted at very low CD4 counts or if the response is suboptimal.

Factors influencing the choice of preventive strategies include the frequency and severity of the OI, the proven efficacy of the intervention in clinical trials and the cost and ease of delivery. Preventive strategies include avoidance of exposure to pathogens, immunization and chemoprophylaxis. Pathogen avoidance measures include access to clean water, sanitation, food hygiene and vector control. HIV services should minimize exposure of HIV-infected persons to *Mycobacterium tuberculosis* by performing sputum collection in the open air or in well-ventilated areas. Those with positive *Mycobacterium tuberculosis* smears or multi-drug resistance should not be in general waiting areas. People living with HIV/AIDS in malaria-endemic areas are particularly vulnerable to malaria and should be provided with insecticide impregnated nets.

Primary Chemoprophylaxis

TMP-SMX CHEMOPROPHYLAXIS

Co-trimoxazole (TMP-SMX) prophylaxis was instituted as an effective and cost-saving intervention in high-income countries prior to availability of combination antiretroviral therapy with the primary aim to prevent *P. jiroveci* pneumonia.[23] It is now routinely used with ART in high-income countries and usually discontinued when CD4 count exceeds 200 cells/µL.[24,25] Many clinical trials and observational studies have shown that TMP-SMX prophylaxis reduces mortality, morbidity and hospital admissions in HIV-infected adults and children not receiving ART across Africa.[26–32] In addition to prophylactic activity against *Pneumocystis jiroveci* pneumonia, TMP-SMX is highly effective against *Toxoplasma gondii*,[33] *Isospora belli*,[34] *Cyclospora* spp.[34] and has activity against malaria.[35] One of the main benefits of TMP-SMX may be a prophylactic effect against malaria; stopping TMP-SMX in patients on ART with a CD4 count >200 cells/µL has been shown to lead to a substantial increase in malaria incidence.[36]

In 2006, the WHO issued guidelines recommending that TMP-SMX prophylaxis be given to all symptomatic adults with CD4 counts lower than 350 cells/µL in resource-limited settings.[37] The dose usually recommended is one double-strength tablet (160 mg of trimethoprin/800 mg of sulphametoxazol) daily, which is generally well tolerated. Nonetheless, cutaneous rashes can occur and may require substitution with dapsone, 50–100 mg daily. While dapsone has some anti-PCP activity, it is not effective against cerebral toxoplasmosis and bacterial infections.[37]

Further analyses have demonstrated that TMP-SMX prophylaxis is highly cost-effective in a variety of low-income settings.[38–40]

The benefits of TMP-SMX alongside ART were demonstrated in a retrospective study of clinics providing ART in Malawi, which reported a 41% reduction in 6-month mortality, compared with those not prescribing TMP-SMX.[41] Observational data from the DART cohort reported that TMP-SMX prophylaxis was associated with a mortality reduction of 59% in the initial 12 weeks of ART and 44% from 12–72 weeks of ART.[42] Use of TMP-SMX prophylaxis in patients with active tuberculosis has been associated with an approximately 40% increase in 2-year survival.[27,28,30]

There has been some fear that widespread implementation of TMP-SMX prophylaxis may engender widespread antimicrobial resistance to TMP-SMX or other antibiotics.[43] However, a systematic review of the published literature concluded that this fear of increased resistance was largely unfounded and that TMP-SMX might protect against resistance against other antibiotics.[44]

MALARIA PROPHYLAXIS

The interaction between HIV and malaria is most marked in areas where malaria transmission is intense and continuous and there is a generalized HIV epidemic. Co-infected pregnant women are particularly vulnerable, since parasitaemia tends to be higher during pregnancy and plasmodia can infect the placenta, resulting in increased risk of anaemia, pre-term birth, intrauterine growth retardation, low-birth-weight infants, and high early mortality. HIV-infected pregnant women also tend to have a poorer response to both prophylaxis and treatment of malaria. Use of insecticide-impregnated mosquito nets should be encouraged to minimize exposure to parasites. HIV-pregnant women at risk of malaria should also receive intermittent preventive therapy, which entails the administration of complete curative doses of an antimalarial at predefined intervals during pregnancy (from the 2nd trimester), regardless of whether or not malaria parasites are identified. Intermittent preventative treatment given in routine antenatal care is a WHO recommended policy adopted in the majority of African malaria-endemic countries. Earlier regimens based on chloroquine and pyrimethamine have been superceded by sulfadoxine-pyrimethamine combination tablets because of increased spread of chloroquine resistance, poor compliance and adverse events especially chloroquine-associated pruritus.

A recent systematic review of the efficacy of various intermittent preventative therapy regimens concluded that three or more treatments with sulfadoxine-pyrimethamine were more effective than two treatments for reduction of placental and blood parasitaemia and increasing birth weight of newborn children.[45] Each treatment course consisted of 3 tablets of sulfadoxine-pyrimethamine at least a month apart. Adverse drug related events included rash, nausea, vomiting, fever, Stevens–Johnson syndrome and neonatal jaundice were generally infrequent (<1%) and not significantly increased in the more frequent regimens.[45]

Concurrent administration of sulfadoxine-pyrimethamine and co-trimoxazole is discouraged because of a possible increase in severe adverse drug reactions. Therefore co-trimoxazole alone is recommended for prevention of malaria in HIV-positive pregnant women with CD4 cell counts below 350 cells/µl. However, the effectiveness of co-trimoxazole alone for malaria prophylaxis is yet to be confirmed and pregnant women may not be adequately protected.

Malarial resistance to chloroquine and sulfadoxine-pyrimethamine is increasingly diminishing the effectiveness of these prophylactic agents. Additionally, widespread use of cotrimoxazole for primary prophylaxis of opportunistic infections may favour development of resistance to sulfadoxine-pyrimethamine in malaria parasites. Therefore, there is a need to develop and investigate alternative drugs and regimens for preventing malaria in HIV-infected pregnant women.

PREVENTION OF TUBERCULOSIS

TB is a major cause of death among people living with HIV/AIDS[46] and may lead to increased HIV disease progression.[47] TB is more common in those with advanced immune suppression but can present across a wide spectrum of CD4 counts.[48] Randomized controlled studies have shown that a 6-month course of isoniazid reduces the risk of active disease in HIV-infected individuals with latent infection with *Mycobacterium tuberculosis*[49] indicated by a positive tuberculin skin test (TST) in the absence of active TB disease. The TST reaction does not distinguish between active and latent infection and also does not have optimal sensitivity and specificity. Although in several trials primary prophylaxis was shown to decrease the incidence of active TB in TST-positive HIV-infected individuals, in only one placebo-controlled trial conducted in Haiti prior to the availability of ART was isoniazid prophylaxis associated with increased survival.[50]

WHO recommends that HIV/AIDS programmes provide isoniazid preventative therapy as part of the package of care for people living with HIV/AIDS.[51] However, exclusion of active tuberculosis is critically important before chemoprophylaxis is started. The recommended regimen is isoniazid 5 mg/kg up to a maximum of 300 mg daily for 6–9 months, during which time patients should be clinically monitored for toxicity and for active tuberculosis.[51]

Programmatic uptake of TB prophylaxis has been low, due to fears of drug resistance emergence, concerns about the short duration of efficacy and the lack of large-scale effectiveness studies. Furthermore, it is programmatically difficult to identify the subset of latently infected patients who would benefit from isoniazid prophylaxis in those accessing ART who have very advanced HIV disease, particularly in high TB-burdened settings. In 2006 in South Africa, a country with an exceptionally high TB burden, 52% of patients presenting to an ART programme had prior or current history of TB, 25% had prevalent TB, 8% were confirmed to have a new TB diagnosis prior to starting ART and a further 3% developed TB soon after starting ART.[52] The concept of short-course TB preventative therapy is also predicated on the assumption that most of the TB disease burden is due to reactivation of latent infection. However, molecular epidemiological evidence suggests that recent infection makes an important contribution to active disease in HIV-infected people living in societies with high TB prevalence.[53,54] Benefits may therefore be less sustained in areas with high force of TB infection resulting in a need for longer treatment periods. Studies of the effectiveness of combined isoniazid with ART are underway and may inform combined therapy approaches.[55]

IMMUNIZATION

Immunization against infectious agents that commonly affect HIV-infected individuals is an attractive strategy. However, the potential effectiveness of this strategy is undermined by the progressive reduction of vaccine efficacy as the immune deficiency progresses. The impaired immune response to vaccine antigens and the inability to maintain appropriate memory cell populations remains despite initiation of ART and may be related to the CD4 count nadir reached prior to ART initiation. Attempts to overcome poor vaccine response in HIV-infected persons include presentation of antigens conjugated with immunogens and increased dose and frequency of administration. Due to the impaired immune response in HIV infection, vaccine research has primarily focused on improving efficacy rather than effectiveness. There are therefore little data on cost-effectiveness of immunization strategies in low-income settings.

Live attenuated vaccines are generally avoided in HIV infection because of concerns of disseminated infection associated with advanced immune suppression. Additionally, viral replication may be temporarily increased following immune stimulation associated with vaccination, an event of uncertain importance. However, any large-scale vaccination campaign, especially if conducted in a country with high HIV prevalence, will inevitably result in inadvertent vaccination of individuals with advanced HIV immune suppression.

Streptococcus Pneumonia Vaccine

Pneumococcal disease has a worldwide distribution and is a major contributor to HIV-related morbidity and mortality. In developed countries, vaccination against pneumococcal infection is widely recommended.[56] Nonetheless, in a randomized controlled trial conducted in Uganda, the use of the 23-valent polysaccharide vaccine (PPV) not only failed to prevent pneumococcal disease or death, but was also associated with an increase in cases of pneumonia in general.[57] Since trial participants had relatively advanced disease, this vaccine was not recommended to be used in similar populations. Protein conjugated vaccines may elicit increased immune responses among those with compromised immune systems including HIV-infected adults.[58] Data indicate effectiveness of the newer conjugated pneumococcal vaccines for prevention of invasive pneumococcal infections in HIV-infected children.[59] A secondary prophylaxis trial of two doses of 7-valent conjugate pneumococcal vaccine (PCV) given to HIV-infected Malawian adults decreased recurrent invasive pneumococcal disease due to the serotypes included in the vaccine but did not impact on mortality.[60] There was additional cross protection against pneumococcal serotype 6A, which was not included in the vaccine. The serotypes included in the vaccine and serotype 6A represent serotypes which are the predominant causes of invasive pneumococcal disease in children but only accounted for approximately 50% of the disease among the adult HIV-positive study population. Furthermore, the protection against invasive disease was CD4 cell dependent and declined rapidly after 12 months. A study of an alternative strategy compared antibody responses to revaccination with a single dose of 7-valent conjugate or 23-valent polysaccharide vaccine in HIV-infected adults who had previously received primary vaccination.[61] Trial subjects had high median CD4 cell counts and most were on antiretroviral therapy but PCV was only transiently more immunogenic than PPV and responses were inferior to HIV-uninfected adults.[61] While results of PCV are encouraging, there is a need for pneumococcal vaccines that produce more robust and sustained immunogenic responses in HIV-infected patients. Furthermore, the serotypes within the vaccines need to be expanded to include the majority of serotypes responsible for adult invasive disease.

Hepatitis B Vaccination

Hepatitis B co-infection is very common in Africa, Asia and South America. Widespread hepatitis vaccination in childhood has been associated with decreased hepatitis B viral prevalence in children but with little change in adult prevalence.[62] To date, no controlled trials of hepatitis B vaccines have been conducted in HIV-infected developing world populations. It is recommended to offer the vaccine to all HIV-infected but hepatitis B seronegative individuals in the USA[63,64] and those with CD4 counts >200/μL in South Africa.[65] However, a long-term follow-up study of an HIV-infected cohort, negative for HBV infection at the time of HIV diagnosis and followed longitudinally after HBV vaccination did not demonstrate a reduced risk of HBV infection.[66] The impaired protection engendered by HBV vaccine in HIV-infected individuals is associated with lower antibody titers and decreased hepatitis B-specific memory cell frequency.[67] Improvements in vaccine delivery and immunogenicity are needed to increase HBV vaccine effectiveness in HIV-infected patients. Post-vaccination testing for HBV surface antibody is recommended and vaccine non-responders should undergo repeat immunization with a full vaccination course. The benefit of repeated dosing, and vaccine response of persons with advanced immunosuppression on antiretroviral therapy remains controversial.[68]

Influenza Vaccines

Influenza has a worldwide distribution. However, the role of influenza vaccine in reducing developing world morbidity and mortality is undefined although annual vaccination is recommended in industrialized countries.[63] A single dose of influenza vaccine in HIV-infected persons resulted in lower levels of protective hemagglutination inhibition or neutralizing antibody than achieved in HIV-uninfected vaccinees.[69] A second dose of vaccine did not significantly increase the frequency or magnitude of antibody responses of either HIV-seropositive or HIV-seronegative subjects over that achieved by a single dose. The two-dose regimen induced a protective level (≥1:64) of hemagglutination-inhibition antibody to influenza A(H1N1) or (H3N2) virus less often in subjects with symptomatic HIV infection than in uninfected control subjects (39% vs 87% or 46% vs 97%, respectively). These results suggest that a substantial proportion of individuals with symptomatic HIV infection might remain unprotected from influenza, even after immunization with a two-dose regimen.[69] However, newer formulations of vaccine may enable boosting.[70] A meta-analysis of clinical efficacy of influenza vaccination studies found only three well-performed studies, all carried out in developed countries, with a pooled relative risk reduction of 66%.[71] A subsequent randomized, double-blind, placebo-controlled trial of trivalent inactivated influenza vaccine performed in South African HIV-infected patients, demonstrated safety and an estimated 75% efficacy, albeit with very wide confidence limits (9.2–95.6%).[72] Although additional information about efficacy among patients with advanced disease and with comorbidities is needed, recommendations to administer influenza vaccine to HIV-infected patients appear justified.[73] It should be noted that a live attenuated influenza vaccine, which is administered by nasal spray, is not recommended for persons with HIV/AIDS.

Yellow Fever Vaccination

Yellow fever vaccine is a live attenuated vaccine recommended for all people over age of 9 months who travel or are resident in areas with yellow fever transmission (Figure 10.2) and mass immunization is the single most important prevention measure. Published studies on the safety and immunogenicity of yellow fever vaccines in HIV-infected persons have been limited to small studies and case reports. Yellow fever vaccine has been demonstrated to evoke protective immune responses[74,75] although less sustained than in HIV-negative individuals.[76] Generally, the vaccine has proven safe although a single case of fatal myeloencephalitis has been reported in an HIV-infected male after receiving yellow fever vaccine.[77] In West and Central Africa, yellow fever vaccine was given to 50 million people between 2007 and 2010 in 10 countries, where an estimated 1–5% of the adult population are HIV-infected. Surveillance from this and other vaccination campaigns in Latin America identified few HIV-positive individuals among those with serious adverse events.[78] There has therefore been no identified problem with mass vaccination in populations with moderate proportions of HIV-prevalence.[78] However, there remains a

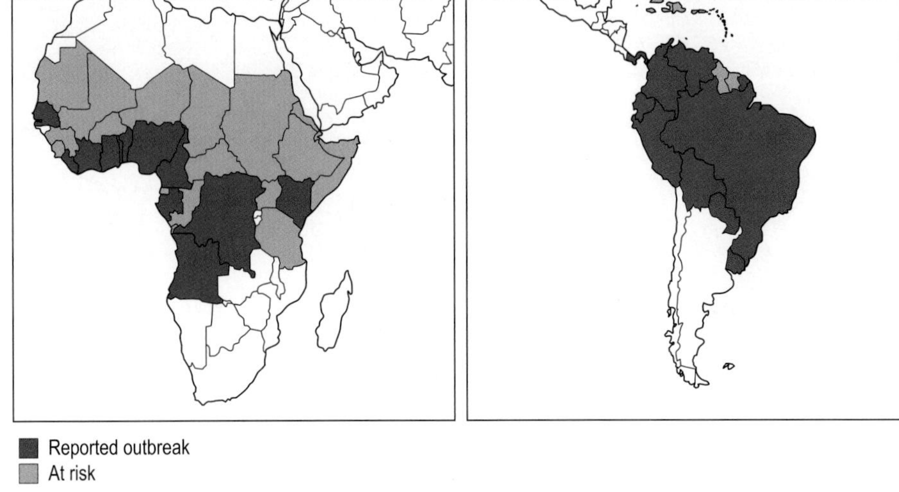

Figure 10.2 Yellow fever 1985–1999.

need for additional safety data but meanwhile the WHO recommendation remains that individuals known to be severely immunocompromised should not receive yellow fever vaccination.[79]

Tuberculosis Vaccines

The existing bacille Calmette–Guérin (BCG) live-attenuated vaccine confers protection against disseminated TB disease when given in the first years of life.[80] However, HIV infection severely impairs BCG specific T-cell responses[81] and together with a significant risk of disseminated BCG infection indicates that BCG should not be given to HIV-infected infants. Several novel TB vaccines are in the development pipeline including: subunit, DNA, rBCG, attenuated *M. tuberculosis* and virally vectored vaccines.[82] Phase 1 studies are planned, targetting specific high-risk populations including HIV-positive adults.[82]

Therapy and Care in Developing Countries

Tuberculosis

There were an estimated 8.8 million incident cases of tuberculosis in 2010, of which 13% were with HIV co-infection. Tuberculosis is currently the second leading cause of death from infectious disease, responsible for 1.2–1.5 million deaths annually. India and China account for 40% of global TB burden and Africa for 24%. HIV is the leading cause of death, resulting in approximately 1.8 million annual deaths.[83] The global distribution of HIV prevalence among TB cases in 2010 is shown in Figure 10.3. There is some uncertainty around these estimates because globally, only 34% of TB patients were tested for HIV infection and in Africa, with a generalized HIV epidemic, the HIV testing proportion was 59%. It is estimated that Africa is responsible for 82% of the global HIV/TB burden.

South Africa is particularly heavily burdened by both HIV and TB epidemics, with 300 000 incident HIV/TB cases in 2010, representing more than 25% of global HIV/TB burden. Of the 53% of TB cases that were tested for HIV co-infection, 60% were HIV-infected. Approximately 10% (5.5 million) of the South African population are living with HIV therefore, with reference to Figure 10.1, the relative risk of TB due to HIV infection in South Africa can be estimated to be approximately 12–14-fold.

HIV co-infection accelerates progression to active disease after exposure to *Mycobacterium tuberculosis* and increases reactivation of latent tuberculous infection. The impact of HIV in sub-Saharan Africa where the annual rate of TB infection and the consequent proportion of the adult population with latent TB infection is high has been devastating. In South Africa, despite a functioning national TB control programme implementing directly observed short course chemotherapy (DOTS), TB incident rates have increased sixfold since 1980. The clinical presentation of TB is also greatly modified by immune deficiency. Smear-negative pulmonary disease is more frequent in HIV-infected individuals. Early in HIV infection, TB presents with a classic reactivation pattern of pulmonary upper lobe infiltrates with cavitation. With increasing immunodeficiency, the chest radiographic picture often resembles tuberculous primary infection with adenopathy and mid or lower lobe infiltrates; dissemination to lymph nodes, meninges and pleural, pericardial and peritoneal cavities is also more frequent.[84,85]

All TB cases should be screened for HIV infection and once an HIV/TB diagnosis is confirmed, subsequent choice of TB chemotherapy and duration of therapy is similar to that recommended for HIV-uninfected TB cases. The latest international recommendations include TB as an indication for ART, which should be instituted as early as possible (see below). As a result of increased HIV-testing among TB suspects, the TB programme has become a major portal to HIV care in high TB

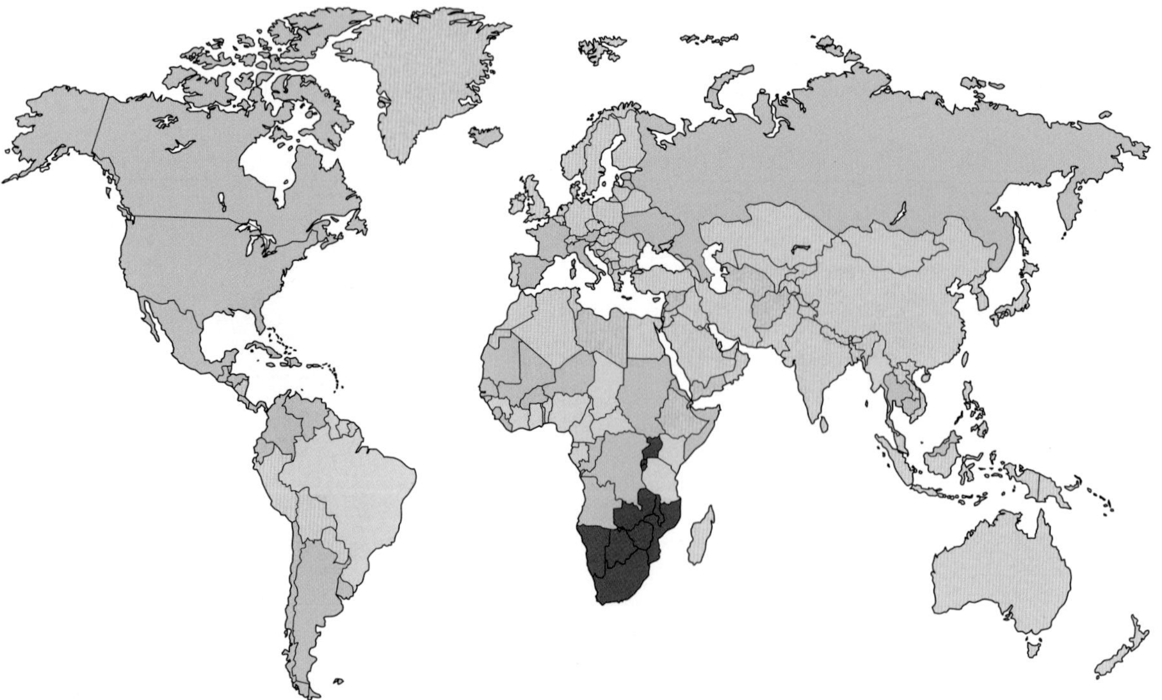

Figure 10.3 Estimated HIV prevalence in new TB cases 2010.

burdened settings. In a Cape Town community ART programme the proportion of patients entering the programme referred from the TB control programme increased from 16.0% of referrals in the period 2002–2005 prior to the introduction of provider-initiated HIV testing, to 34.7% in 2007–2008 (p<0.001).[86]

The frequency of TB co-infection, atypical presentations of TB disease and the urgency to commence ART have posed a diagnostic challenge for ART programmes. Clinical screening lacks specificity and absence of symptoms can therefore be used to 'rule out' TB but is unreliable for disease diagnosis.[87] TB diagnosis in resource-limited settings has remained heavily reliant on smear microscopy using direct Ziehl–Neelsen staining of sputum. Although this method is highly specific, fast, and relatively inexpensive, it is operator-dependent and its use is greatly impaired in the context of HIV infection. A concentration of 10 000 bacilli/mL of sputum is required for a smear result to be positive; the higher the bacillary concentration is above this threshold, the greater the likelihood of positivity. However, lack of pulmonary cavitation and the resulting low bacillary concentrations in sputum means that sputum microscopy results are usually negative in more than half of patients with HIV-associated TB.[88,89] Automated liquid culture is the gold standard for TB diagnosis and of great utility in HIV/TB cases in which most TB is sputum smear-negative. Liquid culture is considerably more rapid and has a greater yield than culture using solid media. The limit of detection of liquid culture is approximately 10–100 organisms/mL. In 2007, these assays were recommended by the WHO to be used in combination with antigen-based species confirmation for TB diagnosis and for drug-susceptibility testing in low- and middle-income countries.[90] However, these culture systems are expensive and prone to contamination. Despite its invaluable role observed in TB diagnosis among patients accessing ART services,[91] culture-based diagnosis is unavailable in most resource-limited settings. As a consequence of inadequate diagnostic capacity, empiric tuberculosis therapy has been frequently initiated after a short course of broad-spectrum antibiotic in patients with very advanced immune suppression. In these situations it is crucial that assessment of response to TB empiric therapy is reviewed after 1 month, by which time an unequivocal clinical response is expected to have occurred. The differential diagnosis of pulmonary infiltrates includes bacterial and fungal pneumonias, and Kaposi's sarcoma.

In December 2010, the WHO endorsed the new rapid molecular GeneXpert® MTB/RIF test as an alternative to direct Ziehl–Neelsen staining of sputum for TB diagnosis.[83] GeneXpert is a close to point-of-care assay, which does not require laboratory isolation facilities and has high specificity and a lower limit of detection of 100–150 bacilli/mL.[92,93] The sensitivity of GeneXpert is therefore close to that achieved by liquid culture systems and much greater than direct sputum smear staining. A further advantage of the molecular assay is the simultaneous read-out of rifampicin resistance. In the 6 months following WHO endorsement, 26 low- and middle-income countries had purchased GeneXpert machines and cartridges.[83]

A urine TB antigen assay for lipoarabinomannan, a cell wall component of *Mycobacterium tuberculosis*, has been developed as a lateral-flow urine dipstick test. This is a truly point-of-care screening test, which has had limited utility because of low sensitivity.[94–96] However, sensitivity is increased in HIV infection, particularly in the subset of patients with extrapulmonary TB disease and CD4 cell counts below 100 cells/μL.[97]

In cohort studies of patients commencing ART from both developed and developing countries, antiretroviral therapy reduced the incidence of TB by 70–90%[98–100] which appears largely related to CD4 cell response to therapy.[91] Widespread ART provision has also been documented to impact on population TB incidence rates in Botswana (Figure 10.4)[83] in South Africa[101] and Malawi.[102]

Mycobacterium Africanum

Mycobacterium africanum, a member of the *Mycobacterium tuberculosis* complex, is endemic to West Africa, where it causes up to half the cases of pulmonary tuberculosis.[103] Sporadic cases of *M. africanum* have been identified outside West Africa. The clinical presentation or disease course is identical to *M. tuberculosis*, although in animal models *M. africanum* appears to be less virulent. Recently it has been suggested that *M. africanum*-infected patients are more likely to be HIV-positive than *M. tuberculosis*-infected patients. The data also suggest that *M. africanum* is more of an opportunist infection than *M. tuberculosis*. It was hypothesized that in areas where rates of HIV are low, *M. africanum* is probably out-competed by *M. tuberculosis*, while increasing HIV prevalence would be associated with an increase in *M. tuberculosis* strain diversity, including lower virulence strains such as *M. africanum*. This, in turn, highlights new complexities associated with the changing pattern of important

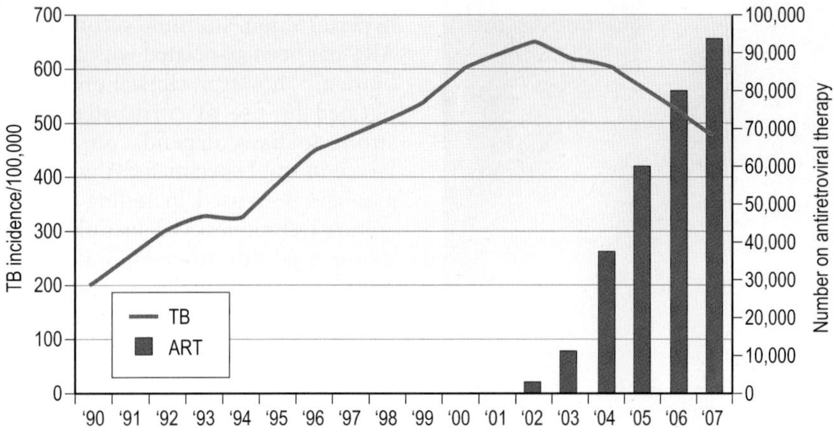

Figure 10.4 Antiretroviral therapy and TB incidence in Botswana.

infectious diseases in the presence of an expanding HIV epidemic.

Salmonella *Septicaemia*

Infection with non-typhoidal *Salmonella*, leading in HIV-infected persons to severe septicaemia, has been reported in Africa[104] and Asia.[105] Bacteraemia is more frequent when the CD4 count falls below 200/μL and is associated with significant mortality (35–60%). Among the survivors, 25–45% have recurrences due to recrudescence of the original infection.[104] Antibiotic resistance patterns vary but fluoroquinolones are particularly useful when there is resistance to other antibiotics. Although secondary chemoprophylaxis is necessary, ART also prevents recurrence.

NEOPLASMS

Kaposi's Sarcoma

Kaposi's sarcoma is the commonest cancer in HIV-infected individuals. In the USA, Europe and Latin America, Kaposi's sarcoma almost exclusively affects male homosexuals. In Africa, it affects males and females equally, often running an aggressive course involving skin, lymph nodes, lungs and the gastrointestinal tract. Skin lesions are variable and can be macular, papular or nodular, with considerable localized oedema when lymph nodes are involved (Figure 10.5). Diagnosis is usually made by clinical appearance although biopsy can be necessary in atypical cases. Although skin lesions frequently resolve after commencement of ART, mucocutaneous and visceral KS may worsen following ART initiation as part of immune restoration disease with increased mortality particularly in patients with visceral KS.[106] Disseminated Kaposi's sarcoma has a significantly higher tumour regression rate when treated with combination chemotherapy with doxorubicin, bleomycin and vincristine in addition to ART.[107] The Kaposi sarcoma risk ratio associated with HIV is lower in areas endemic for HHV-8 compared with non-endemic areas and may be due to the acquisition of infection during childhood rather than by sexual transmission at older ages.[108]

Lymphoma

Although 70% of the global HIV/AIDS epidemic is concentrated in sub-Saharan Africa, the impact of HIV on cancer in this region is incompletely described. The impact of HIV on AIDS-associated cancers in Africa is similar, but less strong, than in the West. Non-Hodgkin's lymphoma is the second most common HIV-related malignancy with an estimated 25 000 cases diagnosed in sub-Saharan Africa in 2002.[109] An increased incidence of NHL has been reported from West,[110] East,[111–113] Central[114] and South Africa[115] associated with increasing HIV-prevalence. Although NHL may be under-reported in resource-poor settings, the risk ratio associated with HIV infection is an estimated 5- to 12.6-fold increase[116] and resultant NHL incidence rates (20–84/100 000 person years) are considerably lower than reported rates in industrialized settings (8000–9000/100 000 person years). Treatment of lymphoma has evolved coincident with improving antiretroviral therapy. Early aggressive dose-intense chemotherapy was associated with poor tolerability and poor response. More conservative dose-modified combination chemotherapy in conjunction with antiretroviral therapy and CNS prophylaxis strategies has resulted in response rates of 20–60% however, median survival remains lower than 1 year, which is considerably worse than expected in high-income countries.[117] There is an urgent need for training and support for pathological diagnosis and treatment of malignancies as part of capacity building in low-resource settings.

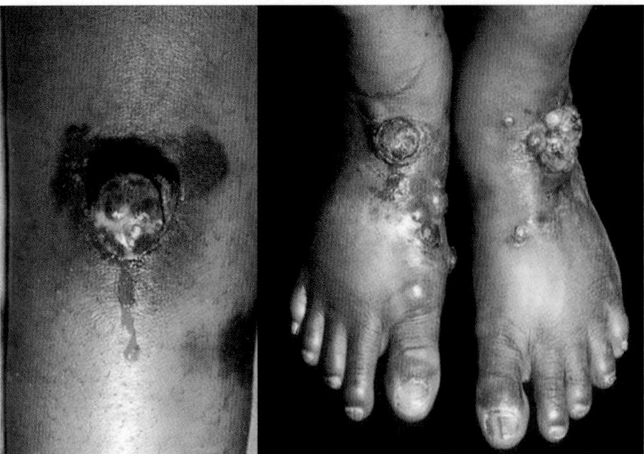

Figure 10.5 Tumoral lesions of Kaposi's sarcoma. *(With permission from www.aids-images.ch.)*

PROTOZOAN INFECTIONS

Strongyloidiasis

Strongyloides stercoralis and *Strongyloidiasis fulleborni* are two intestinal nematodes which infect an estimated 30–100 million people in the warm wet tropical and sub-tropical regions of the world. Both exogenous and endogenous infections occur and adult worms can survive in humans for many years. Clinical presentations include four major clinical syndromes: acute infection; chronic intestinal infection; symptomatic autoinfection and hyperinfection syndrome with dissemination. The prevalence of strongyloides infection has been reported to be increased in HIV-infected populations in Africa and Central and South America.[118–120] Despite occasional reports of HIV-associated hyperinfection syndrome, some complicated by Gram-negative bacteraemia, there has been a surprising dearth of reports of hyperinfection syndrome from strongyloides-endemic regions.[121] It is a conundrum that HIV infection predisposes to strongyloides infection without predisposing to hyperinfection. It has been proposed that an altered immune response may result in a reduced maturation of filiform larvae within the gut and a decreased level of auto-infection and hence hyperinfection. Immune reconstitution following initiation of ART has been associated with a paradoxical increase in parasite burden,[122] however, clinical presentations may have been complicated by use of corticosteroids. A definitive diagnosis of strongyloidiasis depends on microscopic demonstration of larvae in stool specimens. A wide variety of faecal methodologies have been used, including direct smears, concentration and culture techniques. The agar plate culture methodology is commonly used in routine laboratories and has high sensitivity.[123] Treatment with single or repeat doses of ivermectin appears more effective than 7-day courses of albendazole for chronic strongyloidiasis.[124]

Malaria

Malaria and HIV cause more than 4 million deaths per annum, of which 90% occur in tropical Africa where *Plasmodium*

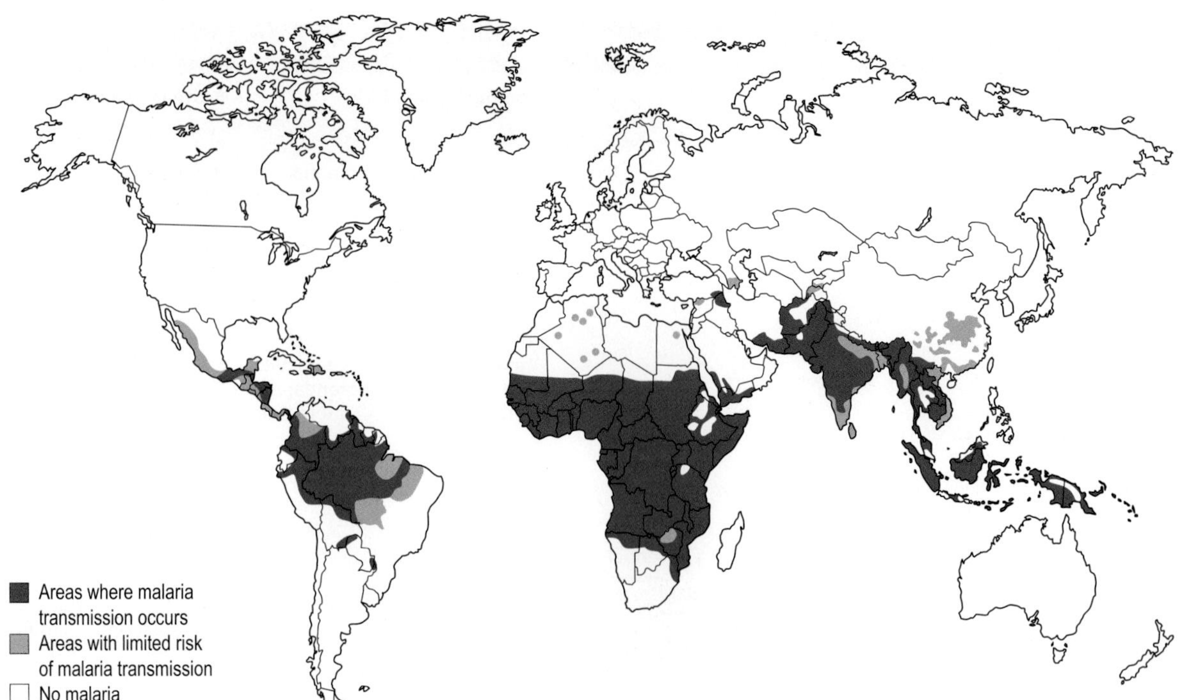

Figure 10.6 Wide overlap between malaria and HIV occurs predominantly in sub-Saharan Africa.

falciparum is the predominant species.[125] Wide overlap between malaria and HIV occurs predominantly in sub-Saharan Africa (Figure 10.6). Cameroon, Central African Republic, Malawi, Mozambique and Zambia are among the most affected countries where 90% of the population are exposed to malaria and HIV prevalence among adults (15–45 years) is more than 10%. Outside Africa, the two diseases overlap in certain at-risk groups in South-east Asia, South America and India. HIV infection is associated with a higher risk of acquiring malarial infection, with higher parasite density, and with increased risk of clinical malaria in adults, especially those with advanced immunosuppression. In regions with unstable malaria, HIV-infected individuals are at increased risk of complicated and severe malaria and death. There are also data to indicate that antimalarial treatment failure may be more common in individuals with low CD4 counts. Although malarial infection, in turn, temporarily increases HIV replication and viral load, there is no evidence that it affects HIV-disease progression, transmission or response to antiretroviral drugs.[126]

Since malaria is associated with anaemia, its presence is a relative contraindication to the use of zidovudine, a nucleoside reverse transcriptase inhibitor frequently associated with anaemia and neutropaenia. Concurrent administration of sulfadoxine-pyrimethamine and co-trimoxazole is also discouraged because of a possible increase in severe adverse drug reactions as both drugs contain sulphonamides. Furthermore, although there have been few specific drug interaction studies there is considerable potential for drug–drug interactions between antiretrovirals and antiprotozoals. Potential drug–drug interactions between commonly used antiretrovirals and antimalarials are shown in Table 10.1. Interactions are more frequent between antimalarials and non-nucleoside reverse transcriptase inhibitors and protease inhibitors. Co-administration of efavirenz (EFV) and amodiaquine results in elevated amodiaquine levels and elevation of liver transaminases and is therefore contraindicated. Halofantrine blocks HERG potassium channels involved in cardiac contractility resulting in a dose-related prolongation of QTc interval on electrocardiogram.[127] Halofantrine is extensively metabolized by the mixed function oxidase enzyme CYP3A4, which is inhibited by atazanavir and lopinavir. Co-administration of atazanavir or lopinavir with halofantrine is therefore contraindicated because resultant elevation of halofantrine levels could result in prolonged QTc interval, torsade de pointes, ventricular arrhythmias or death. A number of studies are currently investigating the clinical significance of potential pharmacokinetic interactions.

Leishmaniasis

Leishmaniasis is a parasitic disease transmitted by the bite of infected sand flies. It is estimated that *Leishmania* spp. infect 12 million people worldwide. Leishmania-endemic regions are expanding and include areas of Central and South America, Southern Europe, Asia, the Middle East, and East Africa. Leishmania/HIV co-infection is emerging as a new serious condition, which is expected to continue to increase in frequency.[128,129]

Three principal clinical forms of leishmaniasis occur: cutaneous, mucocutaneous (espundia) and visceral leishmaniasis (kala azar). HIV infection increases the risk of visceral leishmaniasis by 100–2000 times in endemic areas and leishmaniasis accelerates the progression of HIV disease, thus decreasing life expectancy.[128,130]

It is estimated that 500 000 new cases of visceral leishmaniasis occur annually, 90% of them in five countries, Brazil, Bangladesh, India, Nepal, and Sudan.[128] Visceral leishmaniasis presents in patients with advanced HIV infection with fever, hepatosplenomegaly and pancytopaenia.[128–131] Serological diagnosis in HIV-infected individuals lacks sensitivity and a definitive diagnosis depends on isolation of the parasite, primarily

TABLE 10.1 **Potential Drug–Drug Interactions between Commonly Used Antiretroviral and Antiprotozoal Dugs**

	Nucleoside RTIs				Non-nucleoside RTIs		Protease Inhibitors	
Antiprotozoal	ZDV	TNF	ddI/d4T	3TC/FTC	EFV	NVP	LPV	ATZ
Amodiaquine	√	√	√	√	Contraindicated	Potential interaction	Potential Interaction	Potential interaction
Artemisins	√	√	√	√	Potential interaction	Potential interaction	√	Potential interaction
Atovaquone	√	√	√	√	Potential interaction	Potential interaction	Potential interaction	Potential interaction
Chloroquine	√	√	√	√	√	√	√	√
Halofantrine	√	√	√	√	Potential interaction	Potential interaction	Contra-indicated	Contraindicated
Lumefantrine	√	√	√	√	Potential interaction	Potential interaction	Potential interaction	Potential interaction
Mefloquine	√	√	√	√	√	√	Potential interaction	Potential interaction
Primaquine	√	√	√	√	Unknown	Unknown	Unknown	Unknown
Proguanil	√	√	√	√	Potential interaction	√	Potential interaction	√
Pyrimethamine	None observed	Potential interaction	Potential interaction	Potential interaction	√	√	√	√
Quinine	√	√	√	√	Potential interaction	Potential interaction	Potential interaction	Potential interaction
Sulphadoxine	√	Potential interaction	Potential interaction	Potential interaction	√	√	√	√

from bone marrow aspirates, but also from spleen, liver and peripheral blood. Treatment is based on a number of chemotherapeutic agents that are toxic and/or expensive and are rapidly becoming ineffective. The use of pentavalent antimony is limited by toxicity and resistance, and in some settings the first-line drug is now amphotericin B and liposomal-amphotericin B; the latter is prohibitively expensive. Repeated exposure to single anti-leishmanial drugs predisposes to development of resistance, with relapsed patients potentially acting as reservoirs for drug-resistant strains. There is therefore an urgent public health need for development of combination anti-leishmanial drug regimens to help delay resistance.[132] Alternative therapies include pentamidine, paromomycin, Sitamaquine and miltefosine (an alkylphosphocholine) which was licensed in India in 2002 (see Chapter 47).

There are contradictory data whether highly active antiretroviral therapy prevents visceral leishmaniasis relapses in HIV-infected individuals. A systematic review identified absence of CD4+ cell increase on ART, a previous history of relapse, lack of secondary prophylaxis and a low CD4 cell count at the time of primary diagnosis as predictors of visceral leishmaniasis relapse.[133] Furthermore, antiretroviral therapy may be associated with unmasking of subclinical infection and post-kala-azar dermal leishmaniasis (PKDL), a disfiguring intense cutaneous granulomatous response (Figure 10.7).[122] Secondary prophylaxis should be continued until CD4 count reaches 350 cells/μL.[134]

COCCIDIAL PARASITES

Coccidia is a subclass of microscopic, spore-forming, single-celled intracellular parasites, which must live and reproduce within an animal cell. Coccidian parasites penetrate intestinal cells, feed, grow and go through asexual reproduction (schizogony) followed by sexual reproduction to form an oocyte. Oocytes may be immediately infectious, as in the case of *Cryptosporidium parvum* or may takes days or weeks to become infectious, as in *Toxoplasma gondii* or *Cyclospora cayetanensis*, respectively.[135]

Toxoplasmosis

Toxoplasma gondii is an obligate intracellular parasite with a worldwide distribution and broad host range, which includes most mammals and birds. The sexual cycle of *Toxoplasma* occurs only in the intestine of felines, and human infections usually occur by the ingestion of oocysts shed in cat faeces or more commonly by the ingestion of undercooked meat containing tissue cysts from an intermediate host.[135] In HIV-infected individuals, cerebral toxoplasmosis is the commonest clinical presentation, usually presenting with seizures or a focal neurological deficit in patients with less than 100 CD4 cells/μL.[136] In the Cape Town AIDS cohort, cerebral toxoplasmosis is the third commonest neurological presentation (0.46/100 person years), after cryptococcal meningitis (1.37/100 person years)

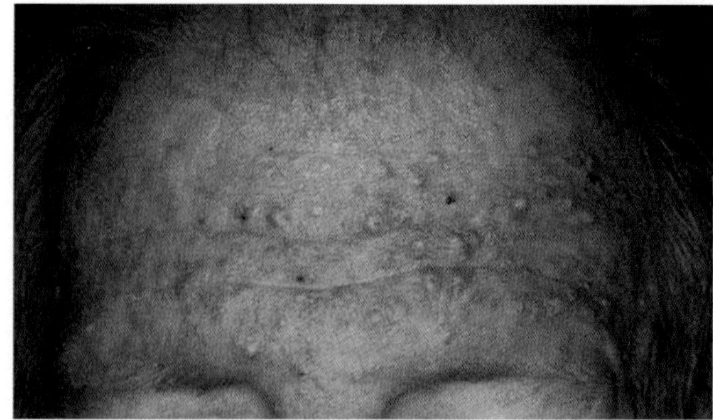

Figure 10.7 Post kala-azar dermal leishmaniasis. Papular non-pruritic rash. *(With permission from www.aids-images.ch.)*

and HIV encephalopathy (0.76/100 person years).[137] An autopsy study from Cote d'Ivoire found that in 10% of the cases, toxoplasmosis was the likely cause of death.[46]

Diagnosis should be entertained in those with focal neurologic signs and ring-enhancing lesions demonstrated through computerized tomography or magnetic resonance imaging. In the absence of radiologic facilities, cerebral toxoplasmosis is strongly suggested by the presence of recently developed focal neurological signs in the absence of meningeal signs in patients with evidence of advanced immune deficiency. In developing countries with a high prevalence of TB, cerebral tuberculomata constitute the primary differential diagnosis and more rarely bacterial abscesses, cryptococcoma, lymphoma and progressive multifocal leukoencephalopathy.

Response to therapy is usually rapid (7–14 days), and a clinical and/or radiological response to a trial of anti-toxoplasma therapy confirms the diagnosis. The recommended standard therapy is with pyrimethamine and sulfadiazine. However, in resource-poor settings there is increasing successful experience with cotrimoxazole 320/1600 mg twice daily for 4 weeks then 180/800 mg twice daily for 3 months.[138–140]

Cryptosporidiosis

Cryptosporidium parvum is a zoonosis infecting a wide spectrum of mammalian and avian hosts and has a worldwide distribution. Recent genetic analyses of *Cryptosporidium* in humans have identified *Cryptosporidium hominis* as a new species specific for humans.[141] Human infection occurs by the faecal–oral route by food or water contaminated with infective oocysts of the parasite which are resistant to routine water chlorination. Sporozoites are released in the small intestine and undergo intracellular asexual and sexual multiplication with subsequent release of oocysts into the intestinal lumen and excretion in faeces. Infection in immune-competent individuals results in a self-limiting diarrhoeal disease lasting 1–2 weeks. The serological prevalence is 30–60% in industrialized countries[142,143] and as high as 95% in tropical and developing countries.[144] In HIV-infected individuals, disease is severe and prolonged with secretory diarrhoea resulting in fluid losses of over 10 L/day. Extraintestinal infections of the liver, biliary tract, pancreas and lungs have been reported. Diagnosis is by identification in the stool of spherical or ovoid refractile oocysts measuring 4–5 µm. Wet mounts are stained by modified acid fast or auramine-rhodamine stains. Passive antibody-based immunotherapy and chemotherapy with macrolides, aminoglycosides and ionophores have shown some activity but results have been mixed. Antiretroviral therapy is the mainstay of management with rapid resolution of symptoms co-incident with CD4 cell increase.[145]

Cyclosporiasis

Cyclospora cayetanensis is acquired via the faecal–oral route and causes a similar spectrum of clinical disease as cryptosporidiosis. The protozoan lives out its life cycle intracellularly within the host's epithelial cells of the gastrointestinal tract. *C. cayetanensis* has previously been confused with other protozoan infections, the most often of which was with *Cryptosporidium parvum*. There are several differences that can be noted between the two including larger oocysts sized 8–10 µm, absence of red staining with modified acid-fast staining and autofluorescence under UV light. Obtaining oocysts from stool specimens is frequently a challenge and amplification by polymerase chain reaction (PCR) of *C. cayetanensis* DNA is an alternative where resources are available.[146] In contrast to *C. parvum* oocysts that are immediately infectious, sporulation within *C. cayetanensis* oocysts takes several weeks before becoming infectious so that person-to-person transmission is unlikely. Treatment and prophylaxis is similar to that described below for cystoisosporiasis infection.

Cystoisosporiasis

Cystoisosporiasis, formerly known as isosporiasis, is an intestinal parasitic disease caused by *Cystoisospora belli* that affects humans. It is found throughout the world but is most common in tropical and sub-tropical areas, where it is typically spread by ingesting oocysts from contaminated food or water. The most common symptom is watery diarrhoea. Diagnosis is by identification of large oocytes which are ovoid and range in size from 23–36 µm by 12–17 µm. The infection is treatable with two double-strength TMP-SMX tablets taken twice a day for 2–4 weeks with pyrimethamine as an alternative therapy.[147] Response to therapy is slower in HIV-infected compared with HIV-uninfected individuals and relapse is more frequent. Relapses are preventable with standard TMP-SMX prophylaxis regimens.

Microsporidiosis

Microsporidia have been classified as protozoans, however, phylogenetic analysis has shown that the microspora phylum is highly divergent and rapidly evolving within the fungi kingdom. Infection is acquired by ingestion, inhalation or inoculation of infective spores. Microsporidiosis can cause infection of the intestine, lung, kidney, brain, sinuses, muscles and eyes. Although there are over 1200 species of microsporidia, the most prevalent pathogens in humans include *Enterocytozoon bieneusi*, *Encephalitozoon cuniculi* and *Encephalitozoon intestinalis*.[148]

Intestinal symptoms that are caused by microsporidia infection include chronic diarrhoea, wasting, malabsorption and gallbladder disease. In patients with AIDS, the chronic diarrhoea may be extremely debilitating and carries a significant mortality risk. Diagnosis is by identification of spores in tissues or body fluids. The gold standard for identification is transmission electron microcopy but this is expensive and not readily available.[146] Light microscopy is hampered by the small size of spores, which are 0.8–1.5 µm. Specific drug therapy with albendazole may be useful for *E. intestinalis* but not for *E. bieneusi*, however eradication usually follows successful ART.

Fungal Infections (Chapter 38)

SUPERFICIAL AND MUCOCUTANEOUS INFECTIONS

Candida spp are the most common fungal infections in HIV-infected individuals. While *C. albicans* is the most common infecting species, *C. tropicalis*, *C. krusei* and *T. glabrata* also cause infection. The degree of skin and mucosal candidal involvement has been used for clinical assessment of HIV prognosis. Candida intertrigo, folliculitis, paronychia and onychomycosis are WHO clinical stage 2 diagnoses. Oral pseudomembranous and atrophic candidosis reflect progression to a WHO stage 3 diagnosis. Candida oesophagitis, which presents with dysphagia, odynophagia and weight loss, is a WHO stage 4 (AIDS) diagnosis. There are many treatment options, however topical clotrimazole or systemic fluconazole are the most widely used. *C. krusei* and *T. glabrata* may be less sensitive to fluconazole and itraconazole is an alternative therapy.

HIV infection is associated with a marked increase in incidence of oral candidiasis and systemic mycoses. However, the prevalence of dermatophyte infections in HIV infection does not appear to be increased when other risk factors are accounted for in data analyses.[149]

CRYPTOCOCCOSIS

Cryptococcosis has a wide global distribution and is the most frequently occurring systemic fungal infection among HIV-infected patients. *Cryptococcus neoformans* meningitis is a major cause of HIV-related deaths in Africa.[150–153] Cryptococcal meningitis (CM) presents as a sub-acute meningoencephalitis. Diagnosis of CM is confirmed by a positive cerebrospinal fluid (CSF) cryptococcal antigen (positive in >95%), CSF culture (positive in >95%) or Indian ink test (positive in 60–90% of cases) and there may be pleocytosis and an elevated CSF pressure.[154] It can also occur as a devastating immune restoration disease (see below) that occurs in the first 2 months after antiretroviral therapy is introduced, at rates of 18.2 (95% CI 8.2–40.6) and 6.2 (95% CI 1.6–25.1) cases/100 persons year in the 1st and 2nd months, respectively.[155]

Cryptococcal antigen screening before initiation of ART in patients with a CD4 cell count <100 cells/mL is highly effective for identifying those at risk of cryptococcal meningitis and death and permits implementation of a targeted preemptive treatment strategy. Development of lateral flow urine test devices for cryptococcal antigen detection allows non-invasive screening of at-risk populations.[156]

Recommended therapy for meningitis is amphotericin B (0.7–1.0 mg/kg per day IV) for 14 days, with or without flucytosine (100 mg/kg per day), followed by 8 weeks of fluconazole (400–800 mg/day), and then fluconazole 200 mg/day as secondary prophylaxis;[157] the higher dose of amphotericin (1 mg/kg per day) may clear the organism from the CSF more rapidly.[158] Mortality during treatment is related to mental status at presentation and a high baseline CSF organism load. Quantitative CSF fungal culture during therapy indicates that a slow rate of clearance of infection is associated with increased mortality at 2 and 10 weeks.

The high rate of cryptococcal immune reconstitution syndrome (see below) in ART programmes in sub-Saharan Africa may be the result of the exclusive use of fluconazole for the treatment of CM. Fluconazole is a fungistatic drug, which is effective as secondary prophylaxis but has less efficacy than amphotericin B in clearing the organism during the initial treatment phase.[158]

PNEUMOCYSTIS PNEUMONIA (CHAPTER 39)

The reported frequency of *Pneumocystis jiroveci* pneumonia (PCP) is highly variable and appears dependent on geography, cohort selection and diagnostic methodology.[159] Studies from Thailand show a prevalence of 27–40% among hospitalized HIV-infected patients.[160,161] Central and South America and the Caribbean also have a large number of PCP cases.[162–165] In contrast, PCP was thought to be rare in African adults,[166] despite high rates of PCP in HIV-infected children. However, PCP has been increasingly recognized among HIV-infected adults in East, Central and Southern African adults.[167–174] PCP might have been under-diagnosed because of the high prevalence of mycobacterial and bacterial respiratory disease together with limited diagnostic resources including few experienced laboratory personnel able to prepare and interpret diagnostic specimens.[159]

Clinical presentation of PCP is a classic triad of dry cough, mild fever and increasing dyspnoea on effort in patients usually, but not exclusively, with less than 200 CD4 cells/μL. Treatment is with co-trimoxazole 15/75/mg/kg per day in divided doses for 21 days; supplemental prednisone (80 mg/day, reducing over 3 weeks) is also recommended for those with hypoxia.[157]

DIMORPHIC MYCOSES

The dimorphic mycoses (see Chapter 38) are a group of pathogenic fungi characterized by an ability to grow as a filamentous form (mycelium) at 25°C and as a yeast at 37°C, a characteristic which appears to be a principal virulence factor. Several yeast-phase-specific genes have been identified which are crucial for host cell adhesion and virulence. The group of dimorphic pathogenic fungi include: *Histoplasma capsulatum*, *Histoplasma capsulatum* var. *duboisii*, *Penicillium marneffei*, *Paracoccidioides brasiliensis*, *Coccidioides immitis*, *Blastomycosis dermatitidis*, *Sporothrix schenckii*.[175,176] These fungi have differing geographic distributions but all have a propensity to cause severe lethal disseminated disease in HIV-infected individuals (Table 10.2).

Histoplasmosis

Histoplasma capsulatum is the most common of the endemic mycoses in patients with AIDS. Although histoplasmosis occurs predominantly in the Americas[175] sporadic cases have been reported in Africa[177] and Asia.[178,179] The most common clinical presentation is a disseminated multiorgan disease, presenting in persons with CD4+ T lymphocyte counts <150 cells/μL with associative systemic symptoms of fever, fatigue and weight loss (Figure 10.8). Respiratory tract symptoms of cough, chest pain and dyspnoea occur in up to 50% of patients.[175] Diagnosis is by identifying the organism in biopsy specimens and *H. capsulatum* can be cultured from blood, bone marrow, respiratory secretions or localized lesions in most cases, but isolation takes 2–4 weeks.[176] Patients with severe disseminated histoplasmosis should be treated initially with intravenous amphotericin B followed by oral therapy itraconazole for 12 weeks, followed by secondary prophylaxis.[180]

African Histoplasmosis

Histoplasma capsulatum var. *duboisii* is an invasive fungal infection, endemic to central, west Africa, Angola and Madagascar that has not been reported outside of Africa. It has been a rarely reported condition with less than 300 case reports up to 1997[181] and remains rare, despite the HIV pandemic in sub-Saharan Africa. In a case series of HIV-infected patients with African histoplasmosis from central and west Africa,[182] systemic symptoms were present in 70%; skin lesions 59%; lymph node 53%; bone lesions in 18% and evidence of dissemination in 85%. Mortality was 24% and a further 12% of patients relapsed after a primary course of therapy. Differentiation from *Histoplasma capsulatum* relies on observation of the large globose yeast phases present in fresh or fixed tissue samples.[183] Treatment is similar to that for *Histoplasma capsulatum*.

TABLE 10.2 **Dimorphic Mycoses in HIV Infection**

Mycosis	Geographic Distribution	Clinical	Treatment
Histoplasma capsulatum	Global: USA: Ohio, Mississippi river valleys, Central and South America, Africa, South-east Asia	Constitutional signs, skin lesions, mucosal ulceration, hepatosplenomegaly, pancytopenia, chorioretinitis, meningo-encephalitis, lung involvement	Severe progressive disseminated disease: Amphotericin B (0.7–1.0 mg/kg/day) 1–2 weeks followed by itraconazole (200 mg twice daily) for 12 months
Histoplasma capsulatum var. *duboisii*	Tropical Africa: Nigeria, Senegal, Congo, Angola, Madagascar	Fever, skin, bone, lymph node and intestinal lesions	As above
Penicillium marneffei	South-east Asia: Thailand, Myanmar, Vietnam, Cambodia, Laos, Southern China, India	Constitutional symptoms, molluscum-contagiosum-like skin lesions reticuloendothelial system, lung and gastrointestinal involvement	Disseminated disease: Amphotericin B (0.6 mg/kg/day) for 2 weeks followed by itraconazole (400 mg/day) for 10 weeks. Secondary prophylaxis itraconazole (200 mg/day)
Paracoccidioides brasiliensis	South America: Brazil, Argentina, Venezuela, Peru, Paraguay	Constitutional symptoms, pulmonary lesions, cervical lymphadenopathy, skin rash, hepatosplenomegaly, oral and CNS involvement	CNS disease: Itraconazole (200 mg/day) or fluconazole (200 mg/day) and trimethoprim-sulfamethoxazole (480/2400 mg/day reducing to 320/1600 mg/day after 2 months). Prolonged treatment necessary (24–84 months)
Coccidioides immitis	South-west USA: Mexico, Guatemala, Honduras, Colombia, Venezuela, Bolivia, Paraguay, Argentina, Brazil	Constitutional symptoms, lungs, kidney, lymph nodes, spleen and brain	Meningitis: Fluconazole (400–1000 mg/day) or itraconazole (400–600 mg/day) for life. Intrathecal amphotericin B may in some cases
Blastomycosis dermatitidis	North and North West USA, Canada, Africa, India, Middle East	Localized pulmonary and disseminated disease. CNS involvement common	Severe pulmonary disease or CNS: amphotericin B (0.7–1.0 mg/kg/day) followed by oral itraconazole (200 mg twice daily) or fluconazole (400–800 mg/day) for at least 12 months
Sporothrix *schenckii* species complex	Global: Tropical and sub-tropical zones. Endemic in Brazil, Mexico, India	Traumatic inoculation, leading to local cutaneous and lymphocutaneous disease. Inhalation and local disease can disseminate to lung, bone and joint, CNS, epididymis and optic tissues	Disseminated disease: amphotericin B (0.7–1.0 mg/kg/day) followed by step-down to oral itraconazole (200 mg twice daily) for at least 12 months

Penicilliosis

Caused by *Penicillium marneffei*, this systemic mycosis occurs exclusively in South-east Asia, Thailand, Vietnam, Laos, Southern China and India. The incidence of this fungal infection has increased in recent years, in parallel with rising HIV-1 seroprevalence. Before the HIV epidemic reached the region, human penicilliosis was uncommon with less than 40 reported cases.[184] Now, the disease is, after tuberculosis and cryptococcosis, the third most frequent opportunistic infection in patients with HIV infection in northern Thailand where approximately 6700 cases of penicilliosis were diagnosed between 1984 and 2004. Marked seasonality of cases suggests that most infections are due to primary infection associated with heavy rains favourable for fungal growth, rather than reactivation of latent infection.[185] The usual presentation is with fever, anaemia, weight loss, skin lesions, generalized lymphadenopathy and hepatomegaly and occurs in patients with advanced immunosuppression (Figure 10.9).[186] Penicilliosis usually presents in severely immune-compromised patients who frequently have other concurrent opportunistic infections. Diagnosis is commonly made by identification of the fungus in clinical specimens by microscopy and culture. Treatment is with amphotericin B (0.6 mg/kg per day), followed by itraconazole 400 mg/day for 10 days.[186] Recurrences occur in approximately 50% of treated cases and secondary prophylaxis with itraconazole 200 mg/day is recommended (Table 10.2). Antiretrovirals should be commenced simultaneously or within 2 weeks of fungal therapy and IRIS has been rarely described.[187] However, drug–drug interactions occur between itraconazole and protease inhibitors and non-nucleoside reverse transcriptase inhibitors.

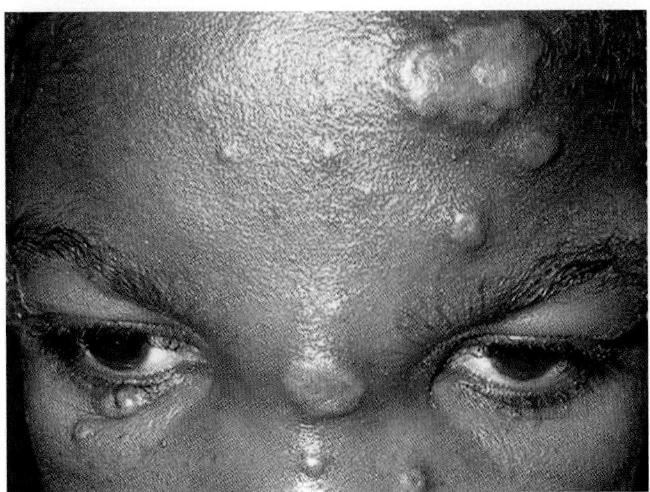

Figure 10.8 Skin lesions of disseminated histoplasmosis. *(With permission from www.aids-images.ch.)*

Paracoccidioidomycosis

This deep systemic fungal infection, caused by *Paracoccidioides brasiliensis*, is common in Brazil and other endemic areas of

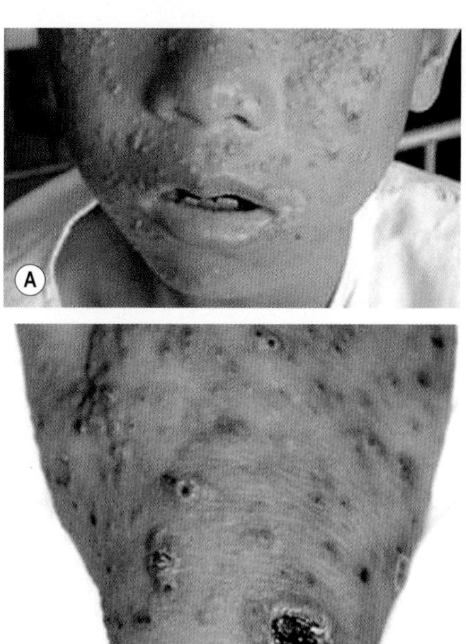

Figure 10.9 Lesions due to *Penicillium marneffei*. Chang Mai, Thailand. *(With permission from www.aids-images.ch.)*

South and Central America, and has also been reported in travellers to these areas.[188] Trimethoprim-sulfamethoxazole prophylaxis against *Pneumocystis jiroveci* pneumonia (PCP) protects against paracoccidioidomycosis. In a series of HIV-infected patients reported from Brazil, clinical presentations were pulmonary in 55%, skin 37%, lymphadenopathy 37%, hepatosplenomegaly 22% and oral mucosa 15%.[188] Central nervous system involvement in this and another large Brazilian case series[189] occurred in approximately 4% of patients with paracoccidioidosis. Neurological presentations were with seizures (57%), hemiplegia (29%), headaches (21%) and ataxia (21%).[189] Diagnosis is confirmed by direct microscopic examination and culture of clinical specimens, such as skin biopsy or lymph node aspirates. Blood and marrow cultures confirm hematogenous dissemination. *P. brasiliensis* is sensitive to a spectrum of antifungals but itraconazole or trimethoprim-sulfamethoxazole are most commonly used (Table 10.2).

Coccidiomycosis

Coccidioides immitis is the causative organism of coccidioidomycosis, a primarily pulmonary disease. Coccidioidomycosis is a common opportunistic infection in HIV-infected individuals living in or who have visited the endemic desert areas of South West USA, Mexico and Central and Southern America. The clinical manifestations of coccidioidomycosis vary with degree of immune suppression. An overwhelming diffuse pulmonary disease with nodules and reticular interstitial infiltrates resembling PCP, occurs at low CD4 cell counts. Dissemination beyond the pleural cavity to meninges, skin and lymph nodes is frequent. At higher CD4 cell counts, presentation with focal pulmonary infiltrates parallels that of immune-competent individuals. Asymptomatic patients may have a positive coccidioidal serologic test and have a high risk of subsequent development of clinically active disease.[190] With wide use of antiretroviral therapy, the incidence of symptomatic coccidioidomycosis has declined and the clinical presentation has become less severe.[191] It has been suggested that patients responding to potent antiretroviral therapy can be treated similarly to immune-competent individuals. Diagnosis is confirmed by serology, histopathology and culture, however, the sensitivity of serology is lower in HIV-infected cases. Treatment is based on azoles with most experience with fluconazole and itraconazole. Meningitis is treated with prolonged high-dose azole therapy with adjunctive intrathecal amphotericin in severe cases.[190]

Blastomycosis

Blastomyces dermatitidis, the cause of North American blastomycosis is a primary pathogen which affects healthy individuals and is a rare opportunistic pathogen in HIV infection.[192] It is the least common of the three endemic mycoses of North America.[175] The highest prevalence of the disease is in the Ohio and Mississippi river basins, where it survives in soil that contains organic debris. The global distribution of *B. dermatitidis* has probably been underestimated as non-imported cases have now been reported from Africa, the Middle East and India. Under-reporting is likely as it clinically mimics tuberculosis and may be under recognized in regions with high tuberculosis burdens.

Immune-suppressed patients typically develop infection following inhalation of spores but reactivation may also occur. While blastomycosis is a chronic granulomatous disease in immune-competent individuals, in HIV infection it is a severe rapidly progressive multisystem disease, which frequently involves the central nervous system. Despite aggressive treatment (Table 10.2), mortality remains high during the first few weeks and subsequent relapse is common. Unlike cryptococcosis and histoplasmosis, there are little data to inform discontinuation of secondary prophylaxis with improved immunological response to antiretroviral therapy and itraconazole chronic suppressive therapy should be continued long term. Serological tests are of limited value in HIV infection and diagnoses in resource-poor settings are usually made by histology or isolation of the organism from biopsy material.[192]

Sporotrichosis

Sporothrix schenckii, the cause of sporotrichoses is a dimorphic fungus found in soil and plant material, with a wide global distribution. Gene sequencing has identified six subspecies within the *S. schenckii* complex; *S. albicans, S. braziliensis, S. globosa, S. luriei, S. mexicana,* and *S. schenckii.* In immune-competent individuals, localized disease follows percutaneous inoculation and disseminated disease is unusual. In contrast, diffuse lesions and systemic dissemination are common in HIV infection. Sporotrichosis is emerging as an increasingly recognized, albeit rare disease in HIV infection. A literature review from 1998 identified only 17 single case reports in the preceding 14 years.[193] However, larger case series have been reported from Brazil[194] and India[195] in recent years. Paradoxical deterioration during antiretroviral therapy of old lesions and unmasking of previous unrecognized sporotrichosis have also been reported.[196] Clinical presentation usually includes diffuse ulcerative skin lesions with dissemination to lymph nodes, lung, bone and joints and central nervous system. The recommended treatment regimen for disseminated sporotrichosis is parenteral amphotericin B followed by prolonged oral itraconazole.[197]

Antiretroviral Therapy

In 2009, more than 5 million people in low- and middle-income countries were receiving ART, representing a 13-fold increase from 2004.[10] Expanded access to ART has contributed to a 19% decline in HIV-related mortality between 2004 and 2009. However, a further 10 million people living with HIV are eligible for therapy under existing guidelines. International funding is currently insufficient to maintain this continued expansion of treatment numbers and domestic expenditure now accounts for 52% of resources available for HIV response in low- and middle-income countries. ART coverage is globally unevenly distributed (Figure 10.10). Approximately 50% of need has been met in Latin America and the Caribbean regions, 30–40% in sub-Saharan Africa and Southern and Eastern Asia but only 10–20% in Eastern Europe, Central Asia, the Middle East and North Africa.

Concerns that expanded access to ART in resource-poor settings would lead to 'antiretroviral anarchy', have proven unjustified.[198] Early reports demonstrated similar virological and immunological responses to those achieved in developed countries.[199–206] However, some have expressed concerns that these results may not necessarily be representative of those currently starting therapy or entering programmes.[207] Early mortality after starting ART is higher in low-income settings,[208] which may reflect more advanced immune suppression, programmatic delays in accessing treatment, paucity of diagnostic and treatment capacity and a higher incidence of severe immune-reconstitution syndromes.[209]

CHALLENGES IN IMPLEMENTING ANTIRETROVIRAL THERAPY IN DEVELOPING COUNTRIES

The global ART scale-up was achieved by widespread implementation of a public health approach, characterized by a limited number of ARV regimens, utilizing a standardized programmatic approach with minimal laboratory monitoring. Drug choices are largely determined by cost. A combination of two nucleoside and one non-nucleoside reverse transcriptase inhibitors allowed construction of an effective regimen costing less than US$150/annum, which enabled the global ARV programme expansion. While high drug costs were the initial major constraint to widespread implementation, lack of infrastructure and adequately trained healthcare workers have become major constraints. As programmes have expanded, human resource shortages have necessitated task-shifting away from conventional doctor-led programmes, including community health workers 'accompagnateurs',[210] 'treatment buddies'[206] and nurses.[211] Similarly, the need to manage programmes within limited national infrastructures has resulted in the exploration of public sector delivery models, including distribution of drugs at district hospitals, community clinics and within tuberculosis services.

Starting Antiretroviral Therapy

ART initiation guidelines used in developing countries have been based on both clinical and laboratory parameters.[212] In the face of high AIDS mortality, initial prioritization was to rapidly expand antiretroviral access to the largest number of patients with advanced clinical disease. Late presentation is costly in terms of morbidity and mortality[213] and utilization of healthcare resources and also limits the potential for restoration of immune function.[214] Treatment of patients with earlier disease is less demanding, results in better outcomes utilizing less health resources and also decreases the proportion of the population progressing to AIDS. In 2010, the WHO changed the recommended CD4 T-cell initiation threshold from 200 to 350 cells/μL in addition to clinical stages 3 and 4.[10] However, implementation of CD4 count criteria only has utility when there is wider access to CD4 counts integrated with voluntary counselling and at all interfaces with the healthcare system.[215] The trend for earlier ART initiation is further supported by recognition of lower HIV transmission from HIV-infected partners of discordant sexual relationships with CD4 cell counts above current treatment thresholds who are receiving effective ART.[5,6] Furthermore, modelling exercises have proposed that universal early initiation of ART has the potential to prevent HIV transmission at a population level.[3,4]

Choice of Antiretroviral Therapy in Resource-poor Settings

Simplified and standardized regimens allow for a limited repertoire of drugs and side-effects with which healthcare workers can become familiar. The maintenance of a secure drug supply is also simpler when a limited number of drugs are used. Many factors impact on regimen selections including cost, tolerability, pill burden, safety, the potential for interaction with other commonly prescribed medications and the need to maintain future treatment options.

Currently recommended first-line therapy is based on a non-nucleoside (NNRTI) in conjunction with two nucleoside reverse

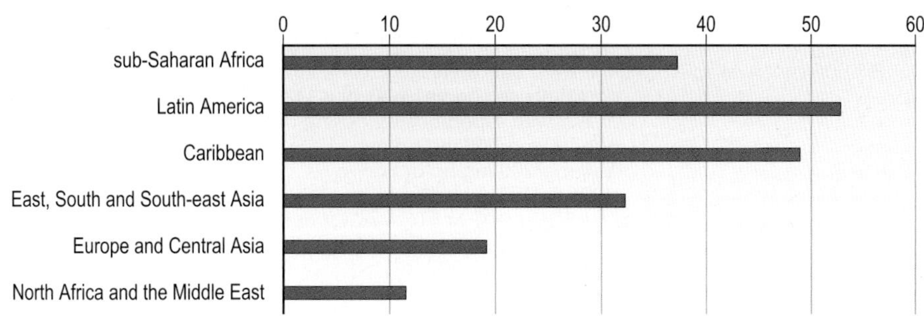

Figure 10.10 Treatment coverage in low- and middle-income countries.

TABLE 10.3 Preferred Adults and Adolescents First-Line ART Treatment Regimens

Target Population		Preferred Options	Comments
HIV+ ARV-naive adults and adolescents		AZT or TDF + 3TC or FTC + EFV or NVP	Select the preferred regimens applicable to the majority of PLHIV. Use fixed-dose combinations
HIV+ pregnant women		AZT + 3TC + EFV or NVP	Do not initiate EFV during first trimester; TDF acceptable option.
HIV+ pregnant women with prior MTCT ARV exposure	Single dose NVP (± antepartum AZT) with no AZT/3TC tail in last 12 months	Initiate a non-NNRTI regimen.	PI preferred over 3 NRTI
	Single dose NVP (± antepartum AZT) with an AZT/3TC tail	Initiate an NNRTI regimen	If possible, check viral load at 3-6 months and if >5000 copies/mL, switch to second-line ART with PI
HIV/TB co-infection		AZT or TDF + 3TC or FTC + EFV	Initiate ART as soon as possible (within the first 8 weeks) after starting TB treatment. NVP or triple NRTIs are acceptable options if EFV cannot be used
HIV/HBV co-infection		TDF + 3TC or FTC + EFV or NVP	Consider HBsAg screening before starting ART, especially when TDF is not the preferred first-line NRTI. Use of two ARVs with anti-HBV activity required

transcriptase inhibitors (NRTI) as outlined in Table 10.3. Stavudine (d4T) because of its low cost has been the most widely used nucleoside in low-income settings, however, the increasing recognition of serious side-effects of dysmorphic changes and life-threatening lactic acidosis has resulted in its removal from the list of preferred regimens.[10] As women of child-bearing potential constitute the majority of patients attending public sector HIV clinics, regimens must be available which are compatible with fertility. Use of single-dose NVP for MTCT has been shown to select for non-nucleoside resistance[216] and appropriate regimens for ARV-exposed women are also shown in Table 10.3. Tenofovir (TDF), lamivudine (3TC) and emtricitabine (FTC) have anti-hepatitis B viral activity[217] and regimens for co-infected patients are also shown in Table 10.3. However, regimens containing AZT or lopinavir/ritonavir are falling out of favour in developed countries and may confer higher risk for emergence of drug resistance than newer regimens.[218]

Recommended second-line therapy regimens based on ritonavir boosted protease inhibitors (PI) are shown in Table 10.4. Second-line PI-based regimens are approximately sixfold more expensive than NNRTI-based first-line regimens[219] and are complicated by drug interactions with TB therapy. Rifampicin is a potent CYP450 enzyme-inducer, which results in lowered plasma levels of protease inhibitors which necessitates increased ritonavir super-boosting. Rifabutin, the rifamycin of choice in the USA for patients on protease inhibitors, is compatible with standard second-line regimens, however, it is rarely available in developing countries due to expense and lack of fixed-dose formulations.

Adherence to ART in Sub-Saharan Africa

Of the 5 million people worldwide taking ART, approximately 80% are in sub-Saharan Africa.[220] The effectiveness of ART is

TABLE 10.4 Preferred Adults and Adolescents Second-Line ART Treatment Regimens

Target Population		Preferred Options	Comments
Adults and adolescents (including pregnant women)	d4T or AZT used in first-line therapy	TDF + 3TC or FTC + ATV/r or LPVr	NRTI sequencing based on availability of FDCs and potential for retained antiviral activity, considering early and late switch scenarios. ATV/r and LPVr are comparable and available as heat-stable FDCs or co-package formulations
	TDF used in first-line therapy	AZT + 3TC + ATV/r or LPVr	
TB/HIV co-infection	Rifabutin available	Same regimens as recommended above for adults and adolescents	No difference in efficacy between rifabutin and rifampicin. Rifabutin has significantly less drug interaction with bPIs, permitting standard bPI dosing
	Rifabutin not available	Same NRTI backbones as recommended for adults and adolescents plus LPVr or SQV/r with superboosted dosing of RTV LPV/r 400 mg/400 mg bd or 800 mg/200 mg bd or SQV/r 400 mg/400 mg bd	Rifampicin significantly reduces the levels of bPIs, limiting the effective options. Use of extra doses of ritonavir with selected bPIs (LPV and SQV) can overcome this effect but with increased rates of toxicity
Hepatitis B co-infection		AZT + TDF + 3TC or FTC + ATV/r or LPVr	In case of ART failure, TDF + 3TC or FTC should be maintained for anti-HBV activity and the second-line regimen should include other drugs with anti-HIV activity

determined by efficacy of the chosen treatment regimen and the ability of patients to be adherent with therapy. Levels of adherence in sub-Saharan African ART programmes are highly variable: from 30% to 98% in a 2006 meta-analysis.[221] A more recent systematic evaluation of adherence strategies in the region from 2003–2010 identified 27 relevant reports from 26 studies of behavioural, cognitive, biological, structural and combination interventions.[222] Despite study diversity and limitations, it was concluded that treatment supporters, directly observed therapy, mobile-phone text messages, diary cards and food rations could effectively increase adherence in sub-Saharan Africa. However, the magnitudes of the benefits were variable, and not demonstrated to be long-lasting. Results from different studies were also frequently discrepant, which may reflect the lack of a 'gold standard' measure of adherence and that interventions may be particularly context-specific.

Choice of Antiretroviral Therapy for HIV-2 Infection

Infection with HIV-2 is common in West Africa, Portugal and countries with close historical links to Portugal. Although HIV-2-infection is associated with similar opportunistic infections as HIV-1, the virus is considered less pathogenic than HIV-1 and the natural history is characterized by a more prolonged asymptomatic phase, resulting in a more favourable prognosis. Additionally, HIV-2 viruses are not susceptible to non-nucleoside reverse transcriptase inhibitors.[223,224] Natural polymorphisms of HIV-2 support PI resistance and unboosted protease inhibitors are also less robust against HIV-2. Experience is limited however, Combivir (AZT/3TC) with or without additional TDF and a boosted PI (LPV/r SQV/r, DRV/r) are recommended regimens.[225]

Immune Restoration Disease

The administration of antiretroviral therapy has greatly ameliorated the interactions between HIV and co-infections. Antiretroviral therapy reverses much of the immune compromise of HIV infection and decreases the individual relative risk of co-infections. However, the rapid restoration of immune responses, particularly during the first 3 months of therapy in those with severe immune compromise, may produce clinical sequelae. A dysregulated immune response can be provoked by many pathogen-specific antigens[122,226,227] but it most frequently occurs with TB,[228] cryptococcal disease[229] and hepatitis B[230] co-infections (Figure 10.11). Three types of clinical manifestation have been described: unmasking of previously latent clinical disease, increased clinical intensity of clinical manifestations and exaggerated dysregulated immunological responses to pathogenic antigens.[231] It has been suggested that the term IRD be restricted to the exaggerated immune response, which when moderate or severe may require adjunct therapy with corticosteroids.[227,231] Mortality is highest in those with exaggerated immune responses or with involvement of the central nervous system.[232,233]

Initiation of ART in Patients with Active Opportunistic Infections

ART may interact with OIs and their specific therapies in a variety of ways. Initiation of ART may be associated with an improved response to specific therapy of an opportunistic infection. However, drugs used for treatment of co-infections may share metabolic pathways or toxicity profiles with antiretrovirals, thereby increasing risk for drug–drug interactions in coinfected patients, or a worsening of the clinical manifestations of the opportunistic infection itself. Concerns about the serious consequences of drug–drug interactions and IRD have led to several trials investigating the timing of initiation of antiretroviral therapy among individuals with co-infections. The collective results were that patients with less than 200 CD4 cells/μL who start ART within the first 2 weeks of treatment for opportunistic infections, including *Pneumocystis jiroveci* pneumonia, serious bacterial infections, cryptococcal meningitis, toxoplasmosis or pulmonary TB have lower mortality compared with patients starting ART at later time-points.[234] In a study conducted in Vietnam, immediate ART in patients with TB meningitis did not confer any survival benefit.[235] Of concern, a study in Zimbabwe of immediate (<72 hours) versus delayed (10 weeks) ART in patients with cryptococcal meningitis treated with fluconazole was discontinued prematurely because of significantly increased mortality in the early treatment arm.[236] Fluconazole is a fungistatic drug which is standard of care for treatment of cryptococcosis in Africa but fungal organisms are cleared less rapidly from the cerebral spinal fluid than amphotericin B fungicidal, which may have predisposed to severe immune reconstitution disease.[237,238] Therefore, early ART is not indicated for African patients receiving fluconazole treatment for cryptococcal meningitis.

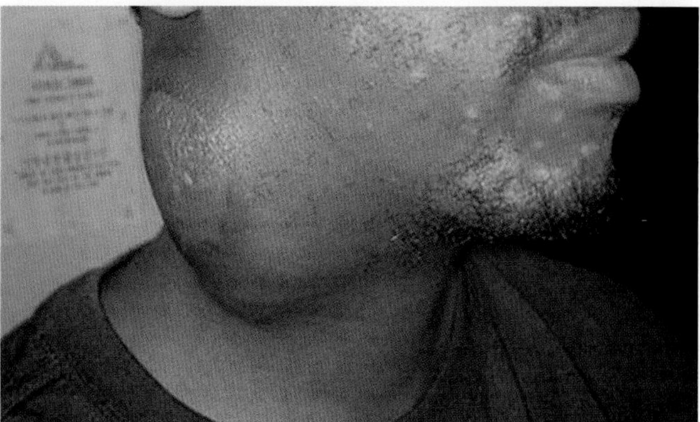

Figure 10.11 Inflammatory Reconstitution Disease, HIV/TB co-infection with cervical lymphadenopathy. *Photograph Rebecca Smith. (With permission from www.aids-images.ch.)*

LABORATORY MONITORING IN RESOURCE-POOR SETTINGS

Screening for HIV and identification of individuals who can benefit by access to care is a prerequisite for treatment programmes and is a very cost-effective activity.[239]

Establishment of individual eligibility for ART is also not controversial, however there is uncertainty and debate about the necessary frequency of CD4 re-testing in those not initially eligible. A recent modeling exercise indicated that frequent CD4 count monitoring of patients with CD4 counts well above the threshold for initiating therapy has a low yield for identification of patients who require therapy. It appeared sufficient to measure CD4 cell count in resource-limited settings 1 year after a count >900 cells/μL when the treatment threshold is 350 cells/μL with increased monitoring reserved for those <900 cells/μL.[240]

Two very different approaches to monitoring patients on antiretroviral therapy (ART) exist. In high-income countries, routine laboratory tests monitor ART efficacy and toxicity, typically 3–4 monthly.[241] In low-income countries, routine monitoring is not widely available due to cost, and infrastructure/personnel constraints result in competing opportunities for improving outcomes for HIV-infected people.[10]

As the numbers on ART have increased, debate about the role of laboratory monitoring have also intensified, in particular, the role of targeted or clinically driven monitoring, rather than routine laboratory monitoring. The focus of the different strategies has been on resulting delays in switching treatment and subsequent harm, and costs of unnecessary switching to expensive second-line ART.

A recent review of 2009–2010 published reports on monitoring of ART[231] in resource-poor settings concluded that CD4 cell counts, HIV RNA viral load and clinical events are frequently discordant; viral load suppression occurs with WHO-defined CD4 failure and, as expected, viral load failure often occurs before CD4 failure. Routine CD4 monitoring provides small but significant mortality and morbidity benefits over clinical monitoring, but, at current prices, is not yet cost-effective in many sub-Saharan African countries. Viral load monitoring is less cost-effective with modelling studies reporting variable results. Most laboratory monitoring for toxicity including hepatic[242] and renal[243] had low yield and was therefore neither effective nor cost-effective.[244]

Additionally, shortages of clinically qualified staff in the rural areas where most needing ART live may make centralized laboratory monitoring less practical. There has therefore been an increasing focus on point-of-care tests,[245] including prescreening for cryptococcal infection,[156] tuberculosis[246] and CD4 cell counts.[247] Dried blood spots may additionally allow batching of samples where storage is limited or absent and enable access to remote laboratory capacity.[248]

Genotyping is both expensive and demanding of laboratory resources and has therefore not played a role in the early roll-out of ART. However, sentinel sites are reporting increasing prevalence of resistance in both treated and naïve patients.[249–251] Continued vigilance will be required to monitor this potential threat to effectiveness of the public health approach to ART.[252]

Conclusions

The last decade has seen an unprecedented global response to the HIV epidemic in resource-poor countries. ART has been able to be delivered in a wide variety of low-resourced settings and has reduced mortality and morbidity. Treatment and management of co-infections have been greatly improved. Consequently, there has been a shift from treatment of only those with pre-morbid disease towards earlier treatment initiation. There remains an increasing tension between the consequent numbers qualifying for ART and the resources available. The recognition that ART has a role in prevention, has further highlighted that resources expended in the short term to put PLWAs on ART, reap long-term epidemiological benefits. However, for many high-burdened countries, the cost of treatment is still unaffordable and has resulted in dependence on international funding sources.

REFERENCES

8. Global report: UNAIDS report on the global AIDS epidemic 2010. Joint United Nations Programme on HIV/AIDS (UNAIDS). Geneva: UNAIDS.
37. WHO Guidelines on co-trimoxazole prophylaxis for HIV-related infections among children, adolescents and adults: recommendations for a public health approach. 2006. Online. Available: http://www.who.int/hiv/pub/guidelines/ctx/en/index.html (Accessed 28 Oct 2011).
56. Kaplan JE, Benson C, Holmes KH, et al. Centers for Disease Control and Prevention (CDC); National Institutes of Health; HIV Medicine Association of the Infectious Diseases Society of America. Guidelines for prevention and treatment of opportunistic infections in HIV-infected adults and adolescents: recommendations from CDC, the National Institutes of Health, and the HIV Medicine Association of the Infectious Diseases Society of America. MMWR Recomm Rep 2009;58(RR-4):1–207.
137. Holmes CB, Wood R, Badri M, et al. CD4 decline and incidence of opportunistic infections in Cape Town, South Africa: implications for prophylaxis and treatment. J Acquir Immune Defic Syndr 2006:42(4):464–9.
231. Lawn SD, Wilkinson RJ, Lipmann MCI, et al. Immune reconstitution and 'unmasking' of tuberculosis during antiretroviral therapy. Am J Respir Crit Care Med 2008;177(7):680–5.

Access the complete references online at www.expertconsult.com

HIV/AIDS in Children

STEPHEN M. GRAHAM | MARK COTTON

KEY POINTS

- HIV infection in children is largely due to mother-to-child transmission and is preventable.
- HIV infection has had a major impact on child mortality in sub-Saharan Africa over the last two decades.
- The major causes of morbidity and mortality in HIV-infected children are the same as for HIV-uninfected children in resource-poor settings, such as pneumonia, malnutrition and invasive sepsis – though with a much higher incidence and case-fatality rate.
- Early initiation of ART before 12 weeks of age significantly reduces mortality and morbidity.
- Pneumocystis pneumonia is common in young HIV-exposed infants not receiving CPT or ART, and is often fatal.
- Tuberculosis is common in HIV-infected children living in tuberculosis-endemic settings.
- Reduction of antenatal HIV prevalence and prevention of mother-to-child transmission are key interventions for HIV prevention in children and are having an impact with a dramatic fall in new paediatric HIV infections an attainable target for the current decade.
- Increasing use of early ART and CPT for HIV-infected infants and children is improving survival and changing the epidemiology of comorbidities.
- The provision of an integrated, community-based continuum of care approach for prevention and management of HIV in children remains a challenge, but is essential.

Introduction

The HIV epidemic has profoundly impacted on child morbidity and mortality over the last three decades, both as a direct consequence of paediatric HIV infection and indirectly through HIV-related morbidity and mortality among parents and carers. Almost all paediatric HIV infection is due to mother-to-child transmission and the majority of children with HIV/AIDS are living in sub-Saharan Africa. Sexual abuse, surrogate breast-feeding, contaminated blood products, feeding of premasticated food and poor injection safety have also been implicated.[1,2] Prior to 2000, the HIV epidemic in children was characterised by a high risk of infection if born to an HIV-infected mother (up to one-third infected), a high prevalence of HIV among infants and young children in HIV-endemic countries, high early mortality (one-third dying as infants and another third before 5 years of age), frequent co-infections and morbidity, and a lack of effective therapeutic or preventive options.

The last decade has seen major improvements in the burden of HIV/AIDS in children. In many settings, the prevalence of maternal HIV has fallen and interventions that prevent mother-to-child transmission (PMTCT) to below 5% are increasingly being implemented.[3,4] The numbers of children infected with HIV globally has fallen to an estimated 370,000 children in 2009 from over 500,000 per year in 2000. Further, interventions that reduce HIV-related morbidity and mortality in children such as co-trimoxazole preventive therapy (CPT) and antiretroviral therapy (ART) are more widely available and are being initiated at an early age, prolonging survival and reducing hospitalizations and the burden of paediatric HIV on the health services. These improvements contribute to the falling global child mortality over the last decade.[5]

This chapter aims to complement Chapter 12 by highlighting common comorbidities in HIV-infected children in the context of a changing epidemic and providing an overview of important preventive and therapeutic strategies to combat HIV/AIDS in children. Consistent with the 'tropical' theme of this textbook, the focus will be on the context of the resource-limited setting where almost all paediatric HIV disease now occurs.

HIV-related Disease in Children

Prior to the ART era, more than 50% of HIV-infected children would die before 2 years of age and the majority died by 5 years of age.[6] Clinical presentations typically related to HIV infection were recognized such as *Pneumocystis* pneumonia (PcP) in infants, severe malnutrition in a breast-fed infant of less than 6 months, or extensive fungal skin disease. However, by far the commonest clinical scenarios in which HIV-infected infants and children presented were those common among all infants and young children in resource-limited settings such as pneumonia, malnutrition, anaemia and invasive bacterial sepsis, and mortality was invariably higher in those with HIV infection.[7–9] Therefore, an HIV test should be routine in the assessment of any sick child in HIV-endemic settings.[10]

Even with the high early mortality that previously characterized the paediatric HIV epidemic, there was still a cohort of HIV-infected children that survived the early years and often did not present with HIV/AIDS until a school-aged child or adolescent, particularly when HIV testing in early childhood illness was not common practice.[11] As this is usually a 'healthy' age even in high child mortality settings, the clinical presentations of malnutrition, anaemia, and acute and chronic lung disease in this age group was a common clinical marker of HIV infection.

COMMON COMORBIDITIES ASSOCIATED WITH HIV INFECTION IN CHILDREN

1. *Pneumonia.* Respiratory disease is the commonest cause of morbidity and mortality in HIV-infected children.[7,12] *Pneumocystis jiroveci* is a common cause of severe pneumonia in HIV-infected infants (especially 2–6 months of age) that is often fatal. Co-infection with cytomegalovirus or bacteria also occurs.[13,14] PcP is a major reason why pneumonia-related mortality is much higher in HIV-infected than HIV-uninfected infants. Overall, the most frequent form of severe pneumonia in HIV-infected infants and children is bacterial pneumonia due to the usual childhood pathogens, especially *Streptococcus pneumoniae*. Gram-negative bacteria may also cause severe pneumonia leading to recommendations of broad-spectrum antibiotics for HIV-infected children with severe pneumonia.[15] *Mycobacterium tuberculosis* causes acute, severe pneumonia especially in HIV-infected infants but the true incidence is uncertain due to difficulties in confirming the diagnosis.[16] The common respiratory viruses of childhood such as RSV and influenza also affect HIV-infected children and compared to HIV-uninfected children are more likely to be associated with co-infections and mortality, and less likely to be associated with wheeze.
2. *Malnutrition.* Severe malnutrition often occurs in HIV-infected children not receiving ART.[8] This may co-exist with acute or chronic diarrhoea. The commonest form is marasmus and HIV infection can present in unusual contexts such as severe malnutrition or failure to thrive in an exclusively breast-fed infant or school-aged child. Response to nutritional rehabilitation alone is often poor and co-infections are common.
3. *Septicaemia.* Bacterial pathogens such as pneumococcus, non-typhoidal *Salmonellae* (NTS) and other Gram-negatives are common causes of septicaemia in HIV-infected children, and have a high case-fatality rate, especially in the young and malnourished.[17] These children present with a nonspecific febrile illness for which malaria may be an alternative diagnosis or co-infection. In contrast to NTS, enteric fever due to *Salmonella typhi* is not an HIV-related condition.
4. *Meningitis.* Common in HIV-infected children due to pneumococcus, NTS or *M. tuberculosis* and is associated with a high mortality.[18] Cryptococcal meningitis occasionally occurs in older children but much less commonly in HIV-infected children than adults.
5. *Tuberculosis.* HIV-infected children living in tuberculosis-endemic countries are at increased risk of infection with *M. tuberculosis* compared to HIV-uninfected children, and are at far greater risk of clinical tuberculosis.[19] The clinical presentation and investigation of tuberculosis in HIV-infected children is similar to that in HIV-uninfected children but outcome is poorer.
6. *Chronic lung disease.* Persistent or recurrent respiratory symptoms are very common in HIV-infected children and pose a particularly difficult diagnostic challenge.[20,21] Tuberculosis should be considered and other common causes include lymphoid interstitial pneumonia, recurrent pneumonia and bronchiectasis. Tuberculosis can be a co-infection of all of these. Older HIV-infected children and adolescents from the pre-ART era may develop severe chronic lung disease such as bronchiolitis obliterans, that is refractory to treatment and extremely debilitating.[11] Digital clubbing is often seen.
7. *Skin disease.* Common manifestations of HIV infection include extensive fungal and bacterial skin infections, molluscum contagiosum or herpes virus infections such as shingles that frequently scars on resolution.
8. *Malignancy.* In tropical HIV-endemic Africa, the commonest HIV-associated malignancy of childhood has been Kaposi's sarcoma (KS). Burkitt's lymphoma, the commonest childhood malignancy in that region, is not HIV-related. HIV-related KS presents differently to endemic non-HIV-related KS with extensive cutaneous lesions or involvement of mucosal surfaces such as palate, conjunctiva and lungs.

These clinical presentations will continue to be common in settings where HIV testing of and/or HIV-related care for mothers and infants is not widespread. In settings where these are available and implemented, the epidemiology and impact of paediatric HIV are changing.

THE IMPACT OF PREVENTIVE AND THERAPEUTIC STRATEGIES ON COMMON COMORBIDITIES

The most important intervention to reduce the burden of HIV-related illness in children is prevention of HIV infection, primarily through implementation of PMTCT for babies born to HIV-infected mothers.[22] Progress has been encouraging with positive impact already evident and with hopes for 'elimination' of new paediatric HIV infections in sight.[3]

For those infants that are still being infected with HIV, improved survival with reduced morbidities is now seen in resource-limited settings. The main strategies of: (1) early commencement of ART in HIV-infected infants, preferably within the first few weeks of life, irrespective of clinical staging or CD4%; (2) Cotrimoxazole prevention therapy (CPT) for all HIV-infected infants and children and for HIV-exposed, uninfected infants, and (3) ART for HIV-infected children and adolescents have dramatically changed the pattern of HIV-related morbidity and mortality in infants and children over the past decade.[23–25] CPT reduces the burden of PcP, bacterial disease and malaria in HIV-infected and -exposed children. Early ART also reduces the incidence and case-fatality associated with these diseases, as well as wasting, skin diseases and typically HIV-related disease such as lymphoid interstitial pneumonitis and KS.

Immunization provides important benefits for HIV-infected children, particularly measles vaccine and bacterial conjugate vaccines against *Haemophilus influenzae* type b and common pneumococcal serotypes.[26,27] Protective efficacy is not as high as for HIV-uninfected children but improves in the setting of early ART and may wane with advanced immunosuppression. However, the protective benefits are still large given the very high incidence of bacterial disease. The routine childhood immunizations are safe in HIV-infected children with the exception of BCG which is not advised for children known to be HIV-infected because of a small risk (around 1%) of developing disseminated BCG disease.[28,29] In practice, BCG is usually given at birth when HIV status is not yet known. This risk is extremely low in the setting of early HIV diagnosis and ART. HIV-infected children without evidence of TB should also receive isoniazid preventive therapy following exposure to a TB case.[30]

Immune reconstitution inflammatory syndrome (IRIS) due to TB and/or BCG immunization is not unusual in infants and children recently commenced on ART. Acute oedematous malnutrition may be precipitated by ART.[31]

The Management of HIV in Children

Recommendations for ART in infants, children and adolescents are often being revised, the most recent versions for resource-limited HIV-endemic settings being published in 2010.[24,25] ART is generally well-tolerated in infants and children – as is also the case for CPT and TB preventive therapy which have a very low risk of serious toxicity. Fixed drug combinations and weight-based dosage guidelines are extremely useful. Adherence is a major challenge and can be influenced by multiple factors including: illness and mortality in caregivers; lack of disclosure of the mother's status in the household; not accepting the need for medication in a 'well' child; the high pill burden; difficulties with access to care; defiance and denial in older children and adolescents; and stigma.

The management of HIV in school-aged children and adolescents can be particularly challenging, dealing with issues such as disclosure and becoming sexually active.[32] The continuing improved survival of HIV-infected children as increasing numbers reach early adulthood provides many challenges for health services to provide a continuum of effective care.

The management of TB/HIV in adults and adolescents is guided by the principles known as the three 'I's: intensified case finding; isoniazid preventive therapy and infection control. These are all relevant to children and a fourth 'I' of 'integration' was recently added to encourage coordination and communication between the health services to provide optimal care.[33]

THE CHALLENGE OF INTEGRATION AND COMMUNITY-BASED CARE

Despite universal acceptance of the need for integrated family-based or community-based care for people living with HIV, the provision of such care is a considerable challenge. The increase in effective interventions reversing the tide of the paediatric HIV epidemic has added to this challenge. It is particularly evident in planning a continuum of care around PMTCT services which is such a critical intervention to reduce the burden of paediatric HIV. Ideally, this might involve some or all of routine antenatal, perinatal and postnatal care; testing, prevention and management of HIV and co-infections such as TB in mother and baby; maternal and child health services; immunization; infant feeding, continued follow-up and integrated management of childhood illness. Training, supervision and task-shifting of community-based health workers are required in addition to coordination and communication in order to achieve the goal of universal access to effective interventions.[34]

REFERENCES

3. UNAIDS. Joint United Nations Programme on HIV/AIDS. Countdown to Zero: Global plan to elimination of new HIV infections among children towards 2015 and keeping their mothers alive, 2011–2015. Geneva: UNAIDS; 2011.
4. WHO. Global health sector strategy on HIV/AID, 2011–2015. Geneva: World Health Organization; 2011.
11. Ferrand RA, Desai SR, Hopkins C, et al. Chronic lung disease in adolescents with delayed diagnosis of vertically acquired HIV infection. Clin Infect Dis 2012;55:145–52.
26. Nunes MC, Madhi SA. Safety, immunogenicity and efficacy of pneumococcal conjugate vaccine in HIV-infected individuals. Hum Vaccin Immunother 2012;8:161–73.
30. WHO. Guidance for National Tuberculosis Programmes on the management of tuberculosis in children. 2nd ed. Geneva: World Health Organization; 2012.
34. Kim MH, Ahmed S, Buck WC, et al. The Tingathe programme: a pilot intervention using community health workers to create a continuum of care in the prevention of mother to child transmission of HIV (PMTCT) cascade services in Malawi. J Int AIDS Soc 2012;15 (Suppl 2):17389.

Access the complete references online at www.expertconsult.com

12 HIV/AIDS Prevention

STEVEN J. REYNOLDS | THOMAS C. QUINN

KEY POINTS

- Approximately 2.7 million people become infected with HIV each year. Despite tremendous improvements in access to care and treatment for infected individuals, effective prevention is urgently needed to reverse the extraordinary toll in human life and public health worldwide due to HIV.
- There is a need for evidence-based, combination prevention including biomedical, behavioural and structural interventions.
- Expanded HIV prevention must be grounded in a systematic analysis of the epidemic's dynamics in local contexts.
- Combination prevention should be based on scientifically derived evidence, with input and engagement from local communities that fosters the successful integration of care and treatment.

Introduction

Curbing the spread of the HIV/AIDS epidemic represents one of the greatest public health challenges of the past quarter-century. Despite considerable knowledge regarding the modes of transmission and spread of the HIV virus, staggering numbers of new infections occur yearly with an estimated 2.7 million new infections occurring in 2011.[1] An effective HIV vaccine is the ultimate solution to reverse the current HIV epidemic, but unfortunately the path to an effective AIDS vaccine may be long and complicated.[2,3] While the modest RV144 or 'Thai' vaccine trial efficacy results in 2009 provided the first hope that a prophylactic HIV vaccine may be possible, there is still a long way to go before an effective vaccine is widely available.[4] With almost 60 million men, women and children having been infected and more than 25 million deaths, 30 years of this epidemic has taken an enormous toll on all populations worldwide.

Results of several new research studies have provided new optimism in the fight against the spread of HIV/AIDS. Medical male circumcision emerged as a major tool after solid scientific evidence provided by three randomized controlled trials proved the efficacy of this strategy. More recent results have shown the potential for antiretroviral treatment to have a dramatic impact on the spread of HIV/AIDS creating both optimism and new challenges for donor funding programmes already struggling to deliver services. The emphasis in prevention research in 2012 has shifted to the design and evaluation of combination prevention packages to demonstrate community effectiveness. HIV prevention programmes need to combine interventions that are feasible, effective, affordable, community- and population-specific and acceptable. This chapter will summarize the available biomedical and behavioural interventions and the evidence of their suitability for inclusion in combination prevention packages.

Due to the complex nature of human behaviours and structural factors driving HIV transmission, prevention packages will not be a 'one size fits all endeavour' and ideal packages will need to be tailored for specific behaviours, regions and risk categories. This requires that policy-makers and public health workers know their local populations and the basis for transmission and thus tailor responses accordingly. The rapidly changing face of the epidemic calls not only for increased epidemiologic HIV transmission and behavioural surveillance but also for nuanced investigation that accounts for preference, social, cultural and gender contexts. UNAIDS has launched a programme entitled 'know your epidemic, know your response', which encourages country-led investigation of the relevant drivers and risk behaviours.[5,6]

Behavioural Strategies

Efforts to modify human behaviours (both sexual and drug-using) to reduce HIV risk have had limited success since the beginning of the HIV epidemic. Behavioural strategies have been defined as interventions to 'motivate behavioural change in individuals and social units by use of a range of educational, motivational, peer-led, skills building approaches as well as community normative approaches'.[7] Some of the first successful examples of behaviour change that led to decreased HIV transmission incidence were reported in men who have sex with men (MSM).[8,9] Subsequently, a number of countries have attributed decreases in HIV incidence to changes in sexual behaviour including Brazil, Cote d'Ivoire, Kenya, Uganda, Malawi, Tanzania, Zimbabwe, Burkino Faso, Namibia and Swaziland.[10,11]

Coates and colleagues have postulated that behavioural strategies were essential, but not sufficient, components of comprehensive HIV prevention and that 'behavioural strategies themselves need to be combinations of approaches at multiple levels of influence'.[7] Although estimates have suggested a decreased incidence of HIV in 33 countries, along with reduced sexual-risk behaviour in young people, weaknesses in the availability of both programme evaluation and behavioural and epidemiological data make causal attribution of these reductions to HIV prevention programming difficult. For example, in Zimbabwe, careful analysis has suggested that incidence declined with behaviour change, but this finding contrasts with a randomized controlled trial of a multipronged prevention intervention in one region of Zimbabwe that failed to show an effect (potentially because of timing or insufficient power).

BEHAVIOURAL INTERVENTION RESEARCH

The HIV literature has several examples of behavioural studies in a variety of settings and target groups, most of which have not objectively altered HIV transmission or acquisition rates. Seven randomized trials of behavioural interventions, described by Padian and colleagues and summarized in Table 12.1, showed neither benefit nor harm.[12] Project EXPLORE is the only interventional study for HIV behaviour with an HIV incidence outcome. Using a counselling intervention to reduce HIV incidence, the average follow-up was 3.25 years and HIV acquisition was reduced by 18.2% in the experimental arm, but this effect was not statistically significant. On more careful examination, there were more dramatic effects on HIV incidence in the first year (39%), but this effect was lost over time. There is also a recurring theme in the literature that behavioural change is hard to maintain.[13,14]

TABLE 12.1 RCTs Assessing Behavioural HIV Prevention Interventions

Author	Citation	Brief Description	Risk-Taking Behaviour Decreased during the Study	
			Intervention	Control
Kamali A, Quigley M, Nakiyingi J, et al.	Syndromic management of sexually transmitted infections and behaviour change interventions on transmission of HIV-1 in rural Uganda: a community randomized trial. Lancet 2003;361:645–52.	Adults in Rural Uganda were randomized to syndromic STI management, behavioural interventions in combination with syndromic STI management and routine care and community development services. The primary outcome was HIV-1 incidence. Secondary outcomes were incidence of STIs and markers of behavioural change.	Yes	Yes
Koblin B, Chesney M, Coates T.	Effects of a behavioural intervention to reduce acquisition of HIV infection among men who have sex with men: the EXPLORE randomized controlled study. Lancet 2004;364:41–50.	Men that have sex with men. The experimental intervention consisted of 10 one-on-one counselling sessions followed by maintenance sessions every 3 months. Outcomes include HIV incidence and assessment of behavioural change including occurrence of unprotected receptive anal intercourse with HIV-positive and unknown-status partners.	Yes	Yes
Ross DA, Changalucha J, Obasi A, et al.	Biological and behavioural impact of an adolescent sexual health intervention in Tanzania: a community-randomized trial. AIDS 2007;21:1943–55	Youth in Tanzania. The intervention had four components: community activities; teacher-led, peer-assisted sexual health education in years 5–7 of primary school; training and supervision of health workers to provide 'youth-friendly' sexual health services; and peer condom social marketing versus standard activities. Impacts on HIV incidence, STI symptoms as well as knowledge, reported attitudes and other sexual health and behavioural outcomes were measured.	NA*	NA*
Corbett EL, Makamure B, Cheung YB, et al.	HIV incidence during a cluster-randomized trial of two strategies providing voluntary counselling and testing at the workplace, Zimbabwe. AIDS 2007;21:483–9.	Business employees in Zimbabwe. Comparison of VCT when counselling and rapid testing were available on-site versus pre-paid vouchers to an external provider (which was the standard VCT).The main outcomes were HIV incidence and VCT uptake.	NR	NR
Jewkes R, Nduna M, Levin J, et al.	Impact of stepping stones on incidence of HIV and HSV-2 and sexual behaviour in rural South Africa: cluster randomized controlled trial. BMJ 2008;337:a506.	Youth (15–26 years) in South Africa. The intervention was Stepping Stones, a 50-hour programme, which aims to improve sexual health by using participatory learning approaches to build knowledge, risk awareness, and communication skills and to stimulate critical reflection versus a three hour intervention on HIV and safer sex. HIV incidence as well as incidence of HSV-2, unwanted pregnancy, reported sexual practices, depression, and substance misuse were measured.	Yes	Yes
Patterson TL, Mausbach B, Lozada R, et al.	Efficacy of a brief behavioral intervention to promote condom use among female sex workers in Tijuana and Ciudad Juarez, Mexico. Am J Public Health 2008;98:2051–57.	Female Sex Workers living in Tijuana, Mexico were provided with a 30-minute behavioural intervention or a didactic control condition. At baseline and 6 months, women underwent interviews and testing for HIV, syphilis, gonorrhea, and chlamydia.	Yes	Yes
Cowan FM, Pascoe SJS, Langhaug LF, et al.	The Regai Dzive Shiri project: results of a cluster randomized trial of a multi-component HIV prevention intervention for rural Zimbabwean adolescents. AIDS 2010;24:2541.	Youth – Community-based HIV prevention intervention for adolescents based in 30 communities in rural Zimbabwe. HIV and STI incidence, pregnancy as well as knowledge, attitude and self- reported sexual behaviour were measured.	NR	NR

Adapted from Padian NS, McCoy SI, Balkus JE, et al. Weighing the gold in the gold standard: challenges in HIV prevention research: Editorial Review. AIDS 2010;24:621–35.
NR: not recorded
NA: not available (changes in behavior are not reported over time for this cohort as many of the participants were not sexually active at study enrollment)

Behavioural prevention for injecting-drug users continues to focus on strategies aimed at mitigating the harmful impacts of drug use, in order to reduce risk behaviour (needle sharing) and HIV incidence. Importantly, most studies have noted that the effect of these programmes is greatly enhanced with combinations of structural (e.g. law reform), biomedical (e.g. ART), and behavioural (e.g. needle and syringe programmes) approaches.

BEHAVIOURAL CHANGE FOR ADHERENCE TO OTHER BIOMEDICAL INTERVENTIONS

Most forms of prevention need continual behaviour modification to be effective. This effect was highlighted in two efficacy trials of pre-exposure prophylaxis (PrEP), one oral.[13,15] Both showed modest efficacy overall but improved efficacy in those participants with highest adherence levels. Future combination prevention packages may contain one or more biomedical interventions depending on the community at risk. The challenge will be to design future prevention studies that embrace this integrated model of combined interventions. In addition, it will be important to monitor at the community level what happens when the combination intervention is scaled up.[16]

Difficulties in measurement of HIV incidence, together with the well-documented problems in self-report of sexual behaviour have presented significant challenges to proving behaviour change interventions in large clinical trial settings. However, large-scale behavioural change is clearly central to reduction of incidence, and behavioural interventions are crucial in amplification and facilitation of other prevention approaches, including driving demand for HIV services such as HIV testing, VMMC, PMTCT, and treatment. Assessment of the effect that these programmes have on service uptake might be useful both alone and as a proxy for effect on HIV incidence. Key questions for implementation of behavioural interventions concern the challenge of bringing community-based programmes to scale while maintaining quality and a better appreciation of the balance between local adaptability and fidelity.

Condoms

Intact latex and polyurethane condoms have been shown in vitro to be impenetrable to particles the size of sexually transmitted pathogens.[17] Consistent condom use has been shown to reduce HIV transmission risk as high as 95%.[18] In most countries with generalized epidemics, condoms are actively promoted for all sexually active individuals as part of a comprehensive prevention approach despite the social, economic and psychological factors that limit their consistent use. Longitudinal cohort studies of serodiscordant couples have estimated the effectiveness of male condoms for prevention of HIV transmission at around 85%.[19] A study in MSM showed 76% efficacy in prevention of HIV if used consistently.[20] The type of lubricant used, rather than strength of condom was reported to be more important in safe usage of condoms in MSM. One of the most cited examples of how campaigns and policy can markedly increase male condom uptake is the much cited '100% condom use policy' in Thailand involving in particular the military and sex workers. Following an increase in condom usage from just over 10% in 1989 to >90% by 1993 in sex workers, the incidence of new sexually transmitted infections (STI) was seven times lower and HIV incidence was 50% lower.[21] Similar success has been described in other female sex worker populations from other parts of the world.[22]

HIV Counselling and Testing

HIV counselling and testing (HCT) services are important entry points for prevention, care and treatment. Studies from different countries have shown that individuals take precautions to protect their partners once they know they are HIV-positive, and modelling studies have found HCT to offer substantial clinical benefits and to be cost-effective even in settings where linkage and access to care is limited.[23–25]

The past decade has seen a rapid global scale-up of HCT to facilitate both access to care and also prevention services.[26,27] Several sociodemographic factors and individual level factors affect uptake of HCT and identification of barriers to access among individuals who have never been tested is important to develop services targeted at first time testers and thus to achieve universal access to HCT.[28,29] Sexually active individuals in high HIV prevalence settings are at continuous risk of infection and should therefore be tested at regular intervals. The World Health Organization (WHO) recommends annual testing in these settings, and a recent study from South Africa found annual screening to be very cost-effective even in the Western Cape, the province with the lowest rates of HIV infection in South Africa.[25]

Studies have demonstrated that many infected persons decrease high-risk sexual or needle-sharing behaviours once they are aware of their positive HIV status. The majority of this research is from high-income countries with the strongest evidence for behaviour change within discordant couples that also received counseling. Most studies that have assessed the effect of HCT on sexual behaviour have focused on the change in behaviour over periods of less than a year.[30]

The challenge is to increase testing coverage and identify those who are positive for care.[26] Strategies to increase testing have included national campaigns, provider-initiated counseling such as has been implemented in Botswana, and couples counseling services and community-level campaigns such as Project Accept (Figure 12.1).[29,31] These alternative strategies not only increase coverage but ensure inaccessible populations such as men, the working population, and asymptomatic HIV-infected individuals are also tested.[32] The role of financial and other positive incentives to increase testing coverage is also being investigated in a number of settings and populations.[33]

This approach, whereby HIV testing is central to the prevention–treatment continuum, moves away from general risk reduction messages for all audiences (e.g. condom use, sexually transmitted infection, treatment) towards specifically tailored approaches for individuals based on their serostatus and prevention needs. Although HIV testing – which has historically been combined with risk-reduction counseling – can prevent inadvertent transmission to sexual and needle-sharing partners in people living with HIV/AIDS, the effect of HIV testing is generally not noted in individuals who are HIV negative (although the community-level benefits of testing on prevention are also being investigated in Project Accept).

Research is focused on streamlining the content of the testing process, particularly in response to the diminishing support for pre-test counseling, by moving assessments of individual risk and plans for risk reduction to post-test sessions. Hence, HIV testing alone is part of a large programme of combination prevention, which is intentionally disaggregated from a broad

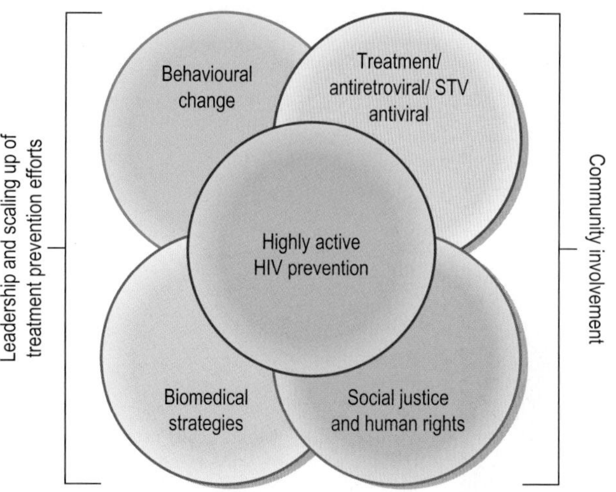

Figure 12.1 Highly active HIV prevention. A term coined by Prof. K. Holmes, University of Washington School of Medicine, Seattle, WA, USA. STI, sexually transmitted infections. *(From Coates, Thomas J, Prof, Richter, Linda, Prof, Caceres, Carlos, Prof – Lancet, Volume 372, Issue 9639, 669–684.)*

approach to HIV testing and counselling. Much of the substantial scale-up in HIV testing has been attributable to worldwide recognition of the value of expanding testing from client-initiated testing (e.g. voluntary counseling and testing) to routine testing, which could normalize and destigmatize HIV testing. Furthermore, such strategies are cost-effective, have individual clinical benefits (via earlier detection), and could potentially greatly reduce new infections when coupled with early start of ART.

However, successful implementation of so-called test-and-treat strategies is challenged by the difficulties of testing of large numbers of healthy people who are not attending healthcare services, incomplete engagement in HIV care, and inadequate technology to detect people with acute HIV infection who are the most infectious. The most crucial question for HIV testing relates to identification of the best strategies to increase demand for, and provide testing services, in both individuals and couples. Currently, overall coverage of testing is low; 17% of women and 14% of men in the general epidemics in sub-Saharan Africa from 2005 to 2009 had ever been tested for HIV infection and knew their results. Demand for HIV testing is a complex function of access to health care, perception of risk, fear, stigma and the threat of violence. Although onsite rapid testing and provider initiated testing can overcome some of these obstacles, approaches to mitigate fear and the threat of violence (particularly for women) are being investigated. Similarly, models of service delivery to optimize uptake of testing and linkage to care and treatment, while protecting patient rights and confidentiality, are an active part of operations research. Home-based, door-to-door testing is a promising model, as are structural interventions, such as economic incentives, which can play an important enabling part. In this way, both supply-side and demand-side barriers as well as inefficiencies can be addressed to improve access to and delivery of this key entry point to HIV prevention services.

Thus, for treatment as prevention to move from a proof of principle in a clinical trial to a public health intervention, lack of testing and linkage to care must be addressed. Furthermore, linkage to care is not enough; we need to determine how best to retain patients in care. This situation is particularly important once individuals have initiated treatment.

Prevention with Positives

Traditional prevention has been thought of as protecting individuals from becoming HIV infected. Positive prevention embraces the concept that individuals who have tested positive may be helped to avoid spreading the infection further. Positive prevention also recognizes that infected individuals may want to remain sexually active and may wish to have children, both of which can be done with minimized harm to others.[34]

RESEARCH IN POSITIVE PREVENTION

ART has dramatically reduced the morbidity and mortality of HIV infection through sustained reduction in HIV viral replication.[35] This reduction in HIV viral load (plasma HIV ribonucleic acid (RNA) levels) reduces infectiousness in the infected individual and as a result, susceptibility for the non-infected partner.[36]

EVIDENCE FOR REDUCED HIV TRANSMISSION

Viral load is the single greatest risk factor for all transmission modes. ART can reduce the plasma and genital HIV viral load in the infected individual to undetectable levels.[37] In a study of 415 HIV serodiscordant couples in Uganda, 21.7% of the initially uninfected partners became infected over 30 months of follow-up, translating to a transmission rate of approximately 12 infections per 100 person years (Figure 12.2).[38] No transmission events occurred in those couples in which the infected partner had a plasma HIV-1 RNA level of less than 1500 copies/mL, and the transmission risk increased as plasma HIV-1 RNA levels increased. For every 10-fold increase in viral load, there was a >twofold risk of transmission. This was similarly shown in HIV serodiscordant couples in Zambia and in the multicountry partner in prevention study.[39,40] Plasma HIV-1 RNA levels generally correlate positively with the concentration of HIV in genital secretions, rectal mucosa, and saliva, although inflammation can stimulate local replication.[41–43] Other studies have shown that transmission events may be observed at a very low plasma HIV-1 RNA level, suggesting that plasma viral load is not the only determinant of transmission.[44,45]

CLINICAL RESEARCH IN DISCORDANT COUPLES

The outcomes of two retrospective clinical studies and two prospective cohort analyses which demonstrated the benefit of ART on HIV transmission have been corroborated by the recent release of early results from a randomized trial, known as HPTN 052.[36,46–48] The deferred treatment study arm was prematurely halted after a scheduled interim review by an independent Data and Safety Monitoring Board, who concluded that initiation of ART by HIV-infected individuals substantially protected their HIV-uninfected sexual partners from acquiring HIV infection, with a 96% reduction in risk of HIV transmission. The study enrolled 1763 mostly heterosexual sero discordant couples in which the infected index case was ART-naive and had a CD4 T cell count of 350–550 cells/mm^3. Treatment was commenced at 250 cells/mm^3 in the control or 'treatment deferment' arm.[49] For each transmission event, genetic analysis was conducted to

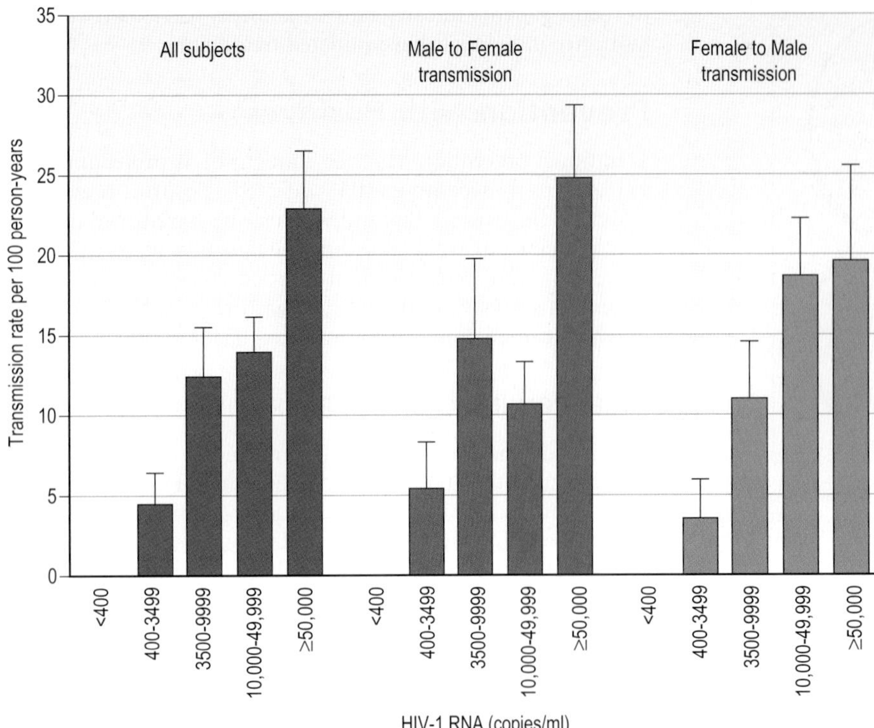

Figure 12.2 Mean (±SE) rate of heterosexual transmission of HIV-1 among 415 couples, according to the sex and the serum HIV-1 RNA level of the HIV-1-positive partner. At baseline, among the 415 couples, 228 male partners and 187 female partners were HIV-1-positive. The limit of detection of the assay was 400 HIV-1 RNA copies/mL. For partners with fewer than 400 HIV-1 RNA copies/mL, there were zero transmissions. *(Taken from Quinn TC, et al. Viral load and heterosexual transmission of human immunodeficiency virus type 1. Rakai Project Study Group. N Engl J Med 2000 March 30;342(13):921–9.)*

determine whether the event was 'linked', meaning that the virus had been transmitted between the members of the enrolled couple, or 'unlinked', meaning that the new infection had been acquired outside of the primary relationship. Among the 877 couples in the delayed ART group, 27 linked HIV transmissions occurred. This finding was in contrast to only one linked transmission that occurred in the immediate ART group. This difference was highly statistically significant. At least 10 unlinked transmission events also occurred, suggesting that the couples counseling provided through the study was not entirely effective. Clinical benefit was also observed in participants receiving early ART. The results of this study have received tremendous attention regarding the potential impact of these findings on the global HIV epidemic and resulted in the journal *Science* choosing the effect of antiretroviral drugs on HIV transmission as the scientific breakthrough of the year for 2011.[50]

MATHEMATICAL MODELS AND POPULATION-LEVEL IMPACT

Extrapolating from this result, reduction of viral load within a population would likely lower the rate of heterosexual transmission within that population. Substantial reduction in the number of anticipated HIV cases in concentrated epidemics of injection drug users and MSM have been reported in at least two population-based studies of HIV incidence before and after the availability of ART.[51–53] Mathematical models have been used to predict the ability of HIV treatment to reduce HIV incidence and prevalence. In a model generated by Gray and colleagues, from the Ugandan transmission study data, ART would be predicted to reduce incident HIV by 80%.[54] Conversely, others have argued that ART could not reduce HIV prevalence in resource-constrained regions.[55] More recently, this has led to the concept of 'Test and Treat', modelled by Granich and co-workers, which espouses universal HIV testing with immediate commencement of ART regardless of clinical or immune status.[56] This controversial model, based on the South African epidemic, with annual testing, heterosexual transmission, and a number of other assumptions, reported that immediate ART initiation could reduce HIV incidence by 95% over a 10-year period. To be considered of course, are the cost and operational challenges (including identification of those infected, the ability to identify early infected individuals and adherence challenges among asymptomatic treated persons) as well as the risk of drug resistance and toxicity.[12] However, this shift from a focus on downstream therapeutic application of ART to more upstream preventive benefits of eliminating HIV transmission has received considerable interest. A number of community-based feasibility studies are underway or planned in the USA and Southern Africa, and it is envisaged that definitive randomized trials will be designed and executed in the next 5–10 years.

HOW TO EXPAND TREATMENT AS PREVENTION: WHOM TO PRIORITIZE?

In prioritizing expansion of treatment, a number of trade-offs will be implicitly or explicitly made and these have consequences for fairness, equity and impact. The choices to be made are only forced on societies and providers of healthcare because of limited resources; without constraints one could choose to provide the best care for everyone. In deciding how to treat, the clinician is too often faced with choices for a limited patient population. The programme manager, policy-maker and international donor must decide more widely between groups of patients. Should resources be used to increase geographical coverage or to increase the range of patients treated in one facility? If some patients are unable to get first-line treatment because of limited resources, is it right that more expensive second-line treatments are available to others? Public health policy requires guidelines on how to use antiretroviral treatment that will maximize their impact on morbidity and mortality. Additional considerations of equity and fairness also need a place in the decision-making process. These considerations will often be in conflict with the ideal clinical management of the individual patient, a conflict that has often been ignored, compromising both equity and coverage.

While focusing on treatment for the benefit of the individual alone, trade-offs in use of resources have been more straightforward than when prevention is included, but both point to those with most advanced disease – as measured by CD4 cell count – as a priority. Addressing the immediate clinical need of those otherwise close to death will save more life years per year of treatment than initiating patients earlier when prognosis is better. Thus, while clinical guidelines call for earlier treatment (<350 cells/μL) with better prognosis, these guidelines have not been implemented in countries, as policy-makers are concerned to ensure good coverage of those with lower CD4 cell counts first. To prevent the most infections it also makes sense to treat those with more advanced disease – not only for their own benefit, but because these individuals are among those with the highest viral load. This does though assume that those in the later stages of infection continue to have unprotected sexual exposures with susceptible partners, which may vary across populations. Despite this caveat it seems probable that treatment of those with low CD4 cell counts is a win–win for both treatment as treatment and treatment as prevention.

Once coverage of those in most immediate need is achieved, that will still leave the incidence of HIV unacceptably high. If antiviral treatment is to be used as prevention then we should consider who among those with higher CD4 cell counts should be prioritized. Since the HPTN trial was done in stable serodiscordant couples, it is tempting to assume this group should be the priority. However, this group was used because it was possible to perform the trial with them. Those HIV positive in a stable relationship with a susceptible partner to whom they have disclosed their status have less risk of transmitting infection than many other HIV-infected persons, particularly sexually active youth who have not disclosed their status to their sexual partners. First, if they have already failed to transmit to that partner, that suggests a lower risk of transmission within the partnership, second if they have only one partner, they will be less likely to transmit to other partners, third, there is good evidence that mutual disclosure in a discordant relationship effectively reduces transmission, suggesting that HIV-positive individuals who are not able to disclose their status are at higher risk of transmitting to their partners. Thus, targeting those with a higher number of partners would be more efficient if it were possible. Should the priority be therefore to treat those in long-term stable discordant partnerships where there is known exposure or those with multiple (unstable) sexual partnerships where treatment could prevent more infections? Is it fair to protect the known susceptible in the clinic while exposing unknown susceptibles to the person with many anonymous partners? Should those in the clinic who are easy to access be the priority or should efforts be increased to seek those HIV infected in the community, increasing demand for treatment among those in greatest need (for their own benefit as well as benefit to others), be the priority? Alternative priorities may be those who are pregnant who are clearly sexually active (or have been recently) and should be treated to prevent mother to child transmission, or those with high viral loads where transmission risk per contact is probably greatest. More work is required: both theoretical work predicting impact, and practical work exploring the feasibility of interventions. These efforts will better inform policy, and will result in the greatest population-level impact.

Community randomized trials of different strategies can help explore directly some of these questions: what is feasible and what impact will they have on AIDS deaths and HIV incidence? Many studies are planned and there is a need for better coordination of the questions they address. Further crucial work is required on optimized testing approaches, linkage and retention in care – and how this can be improved. More research is also needed on how to improve adherence to ARVs in a range of populations and settings.

Pre-exposure Prophylaxis

In addition to the use of antiretroviral drugs to reduce HIV transmission among HIV discordant couples through treatment of the positive partner, additional strategies have been evaluated including ARVs for primary HIV prevention as pre-exposure prophylaxis. The rationale for this approach stems from the demonstration that ARVs prevent transmission of HIV from an infected mother to infant, the cornerstone of mother to child HIV prevention. Several studies have recently been completed in a variety of populations evaluating this approach and are summarized in Table 12.2. Precoital use of 1% tenofovir vaginal gel in the CAPRISA 004 study reduced HIV-1 acquisition by 39%. Daily oral TDF/FTC reduced HIV-1 acquisition by 44% among MSM in the IPrEx study with a greater efficacy observed among individuals in both studies who achieved high levels of adherence. Daily TDF and TDF/FTC reduced HIV acquisition by 66% and 73%, respectively, among HIV-1-uninfected partners in an HIV-1 serodiscordant partnership in the Partners PrEP Study. The efficacy of daily oral TDF/FTC measured among young heterosexuals in Botswana in the TDF2 trial was 66%. Two studies however produced conflicting results with both the FEM-PrEP and VOICE (Vaginal and Oral Interventions to Control the Epidemic) studies in African women finding no efficacy with oral TDF or TDF/FTC. The explanation for these discrepant findings is ongoing but may be due to differences in mucosal penetration of TDF and FTC.[57] This is still an area of active research with policy-makers struggling with implementation issues. The new findings of the IPrEX study among MSM have resulted in policy-makers developing guidelines for using PrEP among MSM as part of a comprehensive prevention package.[58]

Preventing Mother-to-Child Transmission

Prevention of mother-to-child transmission (PMTCT) should include a package including primary prevention services for women of childbearing age, reproductive health services, VCT as part of comprehensive prenatal care, and ART preventive options for both the mother and baby. Safe breast-feeding options have also been a priority in developing countries where alternative feeding options are limited and sometimes associated with increased morbidity. Unfortunately, despite

TABLE 12.2 Ongoing and Planned Pre-Exposure Prophylaxis (PrEP) Trials

Study	Location	Sponsor/ Founder	Population	PrEP Strategies being Tested	Status/Expected Completion
US Extended TDF Safety Trial	USA	CDC	400 MSM	Daily oral TDF	Enrolment started in 2005 Fully enrolled/2010
Bangkok TDF Study	Thailand	CDC	2400 injecting drug users	Daily oral TDF	Enrolment started in 2005 Fully enrolled/2012
TDF-2	Botswana	CDC	1200 heterosexual men and women	Daily oral FTC/TDF (switched from TDF in 2007)	Enrolment started in 2007 Fully enrolled/2011
Partners PrEP	Uganda, Kenya (Partners PrEP study)	BMGF	4700 serodiscordant heterosexual couples	Daily oral TDF vs daily oral FTC/TDF	Enrolment started in 2008 DSMB review in July 2011 showed daily TDF reduced risk of HIV by an average of 62%; daily TDF/FTC reduced risk of HIB by an average of 73%. As a result, placebo arms discontinued but the trial is ongoing with additional data expected in 2013
FEM-PrEP	Kenya, Malawi, South Africa, Tanzania, Zambia (FEMPrEP)	FHI/USAID	3900 high-risk women	Daily oral FTC/TDF	Enrolment started in 2009 Stopped for futility in April 2011, with 29 HIV infections in each arm
IAVI E001, E002 Phase 1/2	Kenya, Uganda	IAVI	150 high-risk women and men	Daily oral FTC/TDF vs intermittent oral FTC/TDF	Enrolment started in 2009 Completed 2010
VOICE, MTN003	South Africa, Uganda, Zambia, Zimbabwe (VOICE study)	NIH/MTN	5000 sexually active women	Daily oral TDF vs daily oral FTC/TDF or daily topical 1% TFV gel	Enrolment started in 2009 Oral TDF and tenofovir gel arms dropped for futility based on data from DSMB reviews. Oral TDF/FTC and oral placebo arms continuing
MTN 001 Phase 2, Adherence	South Africa, Uganda, United States	CONRAD, DAIDS/NIAID, Gilead, MTN	144 heterosexual women	Daily 1% topical TFV gel vs daily oral TDF	Completed/2011
PrEP in YMSM (ATN 082) Phase 2, Safety, Acceptability, Feasibility	USA	ATN, NICHD	99 young men who have sex with men (YMSM)	Daily oral FTC/TDF	Enrolling/2011
PrEP Using TMC278LA Phase 1/2, Safety and Pharmacokinetics	UK	St Stephens AIDS Trust	100 men and women (vaginal and penile/ rectal)	TMC278LA injected intramuscularly	Enrolling/2011
iPrEx Open-label Extension	Brazil, Ecuador, Peru, South Africa, Thailand, USA	NIH	iPrEx trial participants (2499) are offered the opportunity to enroll in this open-label extension	HIV-negative participants offered daily FTC/ TDF; HIV-positive participants offered continued monitoring and risk reduction services	2011 enrolment begins/2013
HPTN 069	USA	NIH	400 MSM	Oral MVC vs MVC/ FTC vs MVC/TDF vs TDF/FTC all once daily	In development
HPTN 067 (ADAPT)	South Africa, Thailand	NIH, Gilead	180 women in Cape Town, 180 men in Bangkok	Intermittent TDF/ FTC	Enrolling 2012

ATN, Adolescent Trial Network; BMGF, Bill & Melinda Gates Foundation; CDC, US Centers for Disease Control and Prevention; FHI, Family Health International; FTC, emtricitabine; IAVI, International AIDS Vaccine Initiative; MSM, men who have sex with men; MTN, Microbicide Trials Network; NIH, US National Institutes of Health; TDF, tenofovir; MVC, Maraviroc; USAID, United States Agency for International Development.
The US Extended TDF Safety Trial and MTN 001 Phase 2 adherence trials have recently been completed but have not been published. These trials are not included in the current AVAC web page.
Adapted from Theodoros Kelesidis & Raphael J. Landovitz. Preexposure Prophylaxis for HIV Prevention. Curr HIV/AIDS Rep 2011;8:94–103.

having tools for effective PMTCT, coverage remained low in many areas due to implementation challenges but recent progress has greatly improved coverage with close to 50% of pregnant women in low- and middle-income countries receiving PMTCT in 2010.[59]

WHO put forth revised guidance in 2009 based on the latest evidence and realities faced in low- and middle-income countries that offers countries some flexibility in how they choose to implement the options. As one option, the guidelines suggest that all HIV-infected pregnant women regardless of CD4 cell count be started on highly active ART as early as 14 weeks gestation and continue through the end of breast-feeding with AZT or NVP given to the baby from birth until 4–6 weeks. Women who needed ART for their own health (CD4 cell count <350 cells/μl or WHO stage III or IV disease) are recommended to continue ART for life. This recommendation has subsequently been extended to include an option where all women are commenced on ART as early as 14 weeks and continue it for life, irrespective of clinical stage or CD4 count. Alternatively, countries may also chose to adopt an alternative strategy which utilizes maternal AZT from 14 weeks and AZT plus 3TC during labour and delivery and for 7 days post-delivery with single-dose NVP given to the infant at birth and NVP or AZT daily until 4–6 weeks of age. Furthermore, for the first time, antiretroviral drug prophylaxis was recommended during breast-feeding in settings where breast-feeding is the safest feeding option for infants. These guidelines are constantly changing to adapt to the increasing amount of evidence aimed at complete elimination of mother-to-child transmission of HIV.

For maximum effect, pregnant women who are HIV positive should receive a series of interventions, including attending antenatal care; being offered, accepting, and receiving the results of an HIV test; and accepting and adhering to antiretroviral-drug prophylaxis for themselves and their exposed infant: the PMTCT cascade. Thus, the success of PMTCT programmes is highly sensitive to the cumulative impact of attrition of mother–infant pairs at each step. Only 15–30% of pairs in high-burden countries complete the cascade.

Worldwide, progress has been made in scaling up PMTCT in resource-poor settings. About 370 000 children born to mothers with HIV infection were newly infected with HIV in 2009 – a decrease of 24% from 2004.[52] Testing coverage of pregnant women also improved from 7% in 2005 to 26% in 2009, and 53% of HIV-positive women in low-income and middle-income countries received antiretroviral drugs to prevent mother-to-child transmission in 2009 – an increase from 45% in 2008 and 15% in 2005. However, a recent demographic model showed that even if new HIV infections in women of reproductive age were halved, the unmet need for contraception was eliminated, the new guidelines had 90% coverage, and the duration of breastfeeding was reduced to 12 months, the reduction in new infections in children and the rate of mother-to-child transmission would still fall short of UNAIDS' objectives by 2015.

Thus, focus on all four prongs of WHO's PMTCT strategy is essential. Understanding women's fertility intentions and the expansion of family planning services to HIV-infected non-pregnant and pregnant women is important to address the second prong of WHO's PMTCT strategy. The provision of contraception to women with HIV who do not want to become pregnant can be more cost-effective than the provision of PMTCT services. In addition, stimulation of demand and strengthening of delivery of services are a major focus of research attention, with particular emphasis on prevention of leakage at every step in the cascade. Low use of antenatal-care services, poor provider knowledge, low coverage of HIV testing, and poor patient documentation and tracking systems have hindered translation of research findings into routine practice. Of the 25 highest-burden countries, only ten had moved from single-dose nevirapine to more effective combination regimens for PMTCT by 2009, although WHO has recommended this approach since 2004. Furthermore, the emphasis on immunological monitoring to establish ART eligibility will need substantial scale-up of CD4 cell testing (in 2008, only 24% of pregnant women with HIV received a CD4 cell count) and complementary implementation research to identify models of service delivery that minimize attrition in view of the added complexity of combination regimens and immunological monitoring.

Male Circumcision

Practiced for cultural and religious reasons over centuries, approximately 30–34% of adult men globally are circumcised.[12] Male circumcision was first proposed in 1986 as an intervention to reduce risk of HIV acquisition.[60] Ecological and observational studies had shown that, in regions where HIV transmission is predominantly heterosexual, the prevalence of HIV and of male circumcision are inversely correlated.[61] The prevalence of HIV has been shown to be significantly higher in uncircumcised than circumcised men in more than 30 cross-sectional studies, and a number of prospective studies have shown a protective effect, ranging from 48% to 88%.[62–67] A meta-analysis of studies from sub-Saharan Africa reported an adjusted relative risk of 0.42 (95% CI 0.34–0.54) in all circumcised men, with a stronger adjusted relative risk of 0.29 (0.20–0.41) in circumcised men who were at higher risk of acquiring HIV.[68]

RANDOMIZED CONTROLLED TRIALS

To definitively document the protective associations of circumcision and eliminate potential confounding due to religious or other factors, three randomized controlled trials were designed and undertaken in three sub-Saharan countries: South Africa, Kenya and Uganda. A total of 11 054 HIV-negative men aged between 15–49 years were randomized and similar to the observational data estimates, there was a protective effect of 58%.[69] Unlike many other biomedical interventions requiring ongoing treatment, support or other, male circumcision is a one-time procedure for which adherence issues are limited to refraining from intercourse during healing. As a result of these three randomized controlled clinical trials, WHO and UNAIDS have now made strong recommendations to roll out male circumcision with all possible urgency.[5] Most recent long-term follow-up from these studies indicate that efficacy does not decrease with time, suggesting that the long-term efficacy of the intervention outweighs any risk compensation should this phenomenon be occurring.[70]

MALE CIRCUMCISION TO PREVENT MALE-TO-MALE HIV TRANSMISSION

Observational studies of male circumcision to reduce HIV transmission between men who have sex with men have shown inconsistent results perhaps because men may adopt both receptive as well as insertive sexual roles. In a cohort study of HIV-negative MSM, no association between circumcision status and HIV acquisition was shown.[71] It is unclear what role male circumcision would have in bisexual men.

MALE CIRCUMCISION TO PREVENT MALE-TO-FEMALE HIV TRANSMISSION

A previous observational study in HIV-discordant couples in Rakai suggested a lower rate of male-to-female HIV transmission from circumcised HIV-infected men, particularly if their viral load was below 50 000 copies per mL.[64] A prospective randomized controlled trial was conducted in discordant couples and examined HIV transmission to female partners of HIV-infected men in Rakai, Uganda. The study was stopped prematurely for futility, however, HIV acquisition was increased in the subgroup of female partners of men who resumed sexual activity early before complete wound healing (relative risk: 2.92, 95% CI 1.02–8.46).

OTHER BENEFITS

The Rakai Male Circumcision study also reported that men circumcised at the beginning of the study had a 50% reduction in rates of genital ulcer disease (GUD) due to herpes, syphilis, or chancroid, a 28% reduction in acquisition of herpes simplex virus type 2, and a 35% reduction in rates of high-risk, cancer-causing, human papillomavirus (HPV). Other studies have shown benefits from circumcision extending to female partners of the circumcised men: a 50% reduction in rates of genital ulcer disease, as well as a dramatic reduction in trichomoniasis, HPV infection, and bacterial vaginosis.[61,72]

CURRENT IMPLEMENTATION PROGRAMMES

While the efficacy of male circumcision on reducing individual risk is clear, the population-level effectiveness of this procedure in reducing HIV transmission will depend heavily on the acceptability of male circumcision programmes in specific populations.[73] Data on its acceptability among adults show this is likely to be highly context-specific and influenced by local cultural norms and practices.[74] A recent modelling study of 13 priority countries with low rates of male circumcision in east and southern Africa suggests that rapid scale-up between 2011 and 2015 to reach 80% coverage of male circumcision could avert 3.36 million new HIV infections by 2025, having a major impact on the current HIV epidemic and potentially saving US$16.51 billion in treatment and care costs.[75]

HIV Vaccines

Unfortunately, the scientific community has faced enormous challenges in the development of an effective HIV vaccine which could form a cornerstone in HIV prevention. To date the only mechanism by which protection from HIV infection can be attained is through the induction of neutralizing antibody responses. These types of antibody responses only emerge in 15–20% of infected individuals and have yet to be elicited through an HIV vaccine. Despite the challenges of HIV vaccine development, recent findings have created optimism in the field. The immune correlates analysis from the RV144 vaccine trial showed a protective effect related to the induction of V1/V2-specific IgG antibodies in the absence of IgA responses against HIV likely mediated through non-neutralizing or weakly neutralizing mechanisms.[76] The second major development has come from a flurry of studies that have recently identified a panel of new broadly neutralizing antibodies, that provide key clues regarding the virus's vulnerabilities. These neutralizing antibodies mark four regions of the viral envelope that represent the virus' 'Achilles heel' that if targeted by a vaccine could provide protection from infection.[77] This new knowledge coupled with novel mechanisms of vaccine development and delivery could provide a fundamental tool in future to achieve an AIDS-free generation.

Sexually Transmitted Infection (STI) Interventions

Longitudinal studies have shown substantial relative risks for HIV infection associated with various STIs with syphilis, chancroid, and genital herpes having larger effects on susceptibility than gonorrhea, chlamydia and trichomonas.[78,79] These ulcerative diseases appear to create an entry point for the virus by disrupting the genital epithelial barrier leading to a greater susceptibility.[80] In addition, studies have shown that HIV viral shedding in the genital tract is substantially increased with a sexually transmitted co-infection, and this replication is reduced after treatment of the STI.[81] As a result, efforts to ensure prompt diagnosis and treatment of STIs along with behavioural risk reduction have been part of HIV prevention programming since the 1980s. In 1989, Pepin and colleagues suggested that the interaction of HIV and STI infections may present an opportunity for intervention.[82] Empirical evidence for this intervention has included uncontrolled intervention studies among sex workers and community-based randomized controlled trials in general populations.[83]

CLINICAL TRIALS OF STI TREATMENT

Eight of the nine randomized controlled trials of STI treatment for HIV prevention showed no effect, although one additional study found a significant reduction on HIV incidence in a subgroup of men who attended programme meetings (Table 12.3).[88] Four community-randomized trials have been conducted to assess the effect on HIV transmission and HIV acquisition through reduction of the incidence of the most common curable STIs. Of all 4 study outcomes, only the Mwanza trial reported significant reduction (38%) in HIV incidence. Many possible reasons for this discrepancy have been cited but most compelling are the differences between the stage of the epidemic in Uganda and Tanzania when the studies were performed. The epidemic in Uganda was more established (HIV prevalence 16% and stable) with lower risk behaviour and lower rates of curable STI. By contrast, the HIV prevalence in Mwanza was 4% and rising with much greater rates of STI.[84] These data would suggest that STI treatment interventions can have an impact where treatable STIs are prevalent and where HIV incidence is very high in the general populations. However, even if the HIV epidemic has matured in the general adult population, adolescents as they sexually debut may initially have low HIV prevalence and constitute a population where STI control may be very important. It is still

TABLE 12.3 The Randomized Trials of Treatment of Sexually Transmitted Infections to Reduce HIV Transmission

Intervention	Country/ Region	Target Population and HIV Incidence (per 100 Person Years or Annual %)	Efficacy/Outcome	Reference
Individual syndromic STI[a] treatment to reduce HIV incidence (CRCT)	Mwanza, Tanzania	General Population; 0.9%	38% reduction in HIV incidence	Grosskurth et al. (2000).[84]
STI therapy[b] to reduce HIV incidence. (everyone treated every 10 months) (CRCT)	Rakai, Uganda	General Population; 1.5 ppy	Nil	Wawer et al. (2009).[85]
Individual RCT of intensive, microscopy-assisted STI[a] screening and treatment to reduce HIV incidence		FSW; 7.6 ppy	Nil	Ghys et al. (2009).[80]
Individual syndromic STI treatment[b] to reduce HIV incidence (CRCT)	Masaka, (rural) Uganda	General population; 0.8 ppy	Nil	Kamali et al. (2003).[86]
Treatable STI[a]; periodic presumptive therapy (Individual RCT)	Kenya	FSW; 3.2 ppy	Nil	Kaul et al. (2004).[87]
Individual syndromic STI treatment[a] to reduce HIV incidence (CRCT)	Manicaland, Zimbabwe	General population; 1.5 ppy	Nil; subgroup of men who attended programme meetings (IRR 0.48; $p = 0.04$)	Gregson et al. 2007.[88]
HSV2 suppression[c]	Tanzania	HSV2 positive women; 4.1 ppy	Nil	Watson-Jones et al. (2008).[89]
HSV2 suppression[c]	Africa; Peru and USA	WSM; MSM HSV2 seropositive; 3.3 ppy	Nil (some benefit in subset of women who took >90% of doses)	Celum et al. (2008).[90]
HSV2 suppression[c]	Africa	HIV/HSV2 positive 2.7 ppy	Nil	Celum et al. (2010).[91]

[a]Treatable Sexually Transmitted Infections: chancroid, syphilis, gonorrhoea, chlamydial infections, trichomonas.
[b]Single dose oral antibiotic.
[c]Acyclovir treatment. CRCT = cluster randomized controlled trial.

recommended that STI treatment should be an essential component of HIV control programmes in communities in which the burden of STIs is substantial.[84,92]

HERPES SIMPLEX VIRUS-2 AND HIV TRANSMISSION

In sub-Saharan Africa, HSV-2 infections have a two- to three-fold increased effect on HIV acquisition in the general population.[93] Initial proof of concept, randomized trials of suppressive treatment with valaciclovir reported reduced HIV shedding in genital secretions of co-infected individuals, suggesting potential for reduced HIV transmission risk.[94,95] Subsequently, in three randomized controlled trials, antivirals for HSV suppression were insufficiently potent to alleviate persistent genital inflammation in HIV-negative HSV2-positive persons, and the reduction in HIV levels in HIV-positive persons was insufficient to reduce HIV transmission.[92] Recent data examining the optimal dose of antiviral therapy to suppress HSV-2 recurrences suggest that even with higher-dose anti-herpes therapy, frequent intermittent shedding of HSV-2 occurs, which could explain why these trials failed to prevent HIV-1 transmission.[96]

HIV Prevention among Injecting Drug Users

HIV prevention for people who inject drugs (commonly referred to as injecting drug users, or IDU) presents a difficult paradox. There is abundant evidence for the efficacy of a number of interventions for this population, and clear and compelling data have emerged on the efficacy of combinations of these interventions in achieving control of HIV spread via this route.[97] Yet IDU remain the least served of any risk group globally for prevention, treatment and care.[98] Epidemics driven by IDU risks, and by risk-enhancing structural and policy environments, continue to expand in 2010.[99] These policy failures include punitive and repressive drug laws, criminalization of drug dependency and possession, and the continued resistance to the provision of evidence-based drug treatment, including methadone maintenance therapy in many states and regions.[100]

HIV spread among IDUs has been driven largely, but not exclusively, by injecting use of heroin. Cocaine, methamphetamine, and combinations are also important substances associated with injecting risks. Heroin predominates in Eastern Europe and Central Asia, North, South and South-east Asia, and Western Europe, encompassing the major populations at risk for HIV through injecting.[101] The most recent global estimate, from the Reference Group to the UN on HIV and Injecting Drug Use was that some 15. 9 million persons (range from 11.0–21.2 million) worldwide were IDU in 2007.[99]

EVIDENCE FOR EFFICACY

The literature on HIV prevention for this population is large and growing.[97] The most compelling recent data suggest, as with prevention of sexual transmission, that no single intervention alone can reduce HIV risks enough to control injecting driven epidemics. Encouragingly, however, recent modeling studies demonstrate that combination approaches to HIV prevention for this population can be synergistic in effect, and have real impact on HIV risks at individual, couple, network, and population levels of spread.[97]

The components of effective prevention services for IDU include individual and higher-level interventions. An essential component is access to safe injecting equipment. Since the primary risk for HIV acquisition and transmission among drug users is the re-use of contaminated injecting equipment, multiple approaches to reducing equipment reuse, termed needle and syringe exchange programmes (NSP), have been developed. The provision of equipment for people who inject has proven politically challenging in many contexts, since this has been seen (based on no empirical evidence) as 'encouraging' injecting. Indeed, the US federal ban on funding for such programmes, lifted in 2010 by the Obama Administration, was based on this unsound premise.[99] A recent global review and modelling exercise of the evidence for efficacy suggests that with high coverage, NSP can reduce HIV incidence at population levels by 20% over 5 years, but the reduction is too modest to control HIV spread.[97]

A second critical component of HIV prevention for IDU is drug treatment. The first agent shown to have efficacy in reduction of HIV transmission among drug users was methadone.[102] Because methadone is an oral-administered liquid, and an opiate agonist, opioid-dependent patients can be maintained on the agent and reduce dramatically their injecting drug use. This simple 'substitution' therapy, as it has come to be known, was shown by Metzger and colleagues to markedly reduce HIV infection rates among IDU in Philadelphia in the 1990s. Newer agents are also now available, but there have been significant obstacles to the widespread use of these agents. Methadone was strongly opposed by the Soviet Union when it was first introduced, and Opioid Substitution Therapy (OST) remains illegal in Russia in 2010.[99]

While NSP and OST in combination can reduce HIV risks, recent modelling work by Hallett and co-workers, reported in the Degenhardt paper,[97] demonstrated that a third element is essential for individuals and for epidemics: access to ARVs. ARV access for IDU alone had roughly the same impact on HIV incidence as the combination of OST and NSP, and was significantly higher when ARVs were available to HIV-infected IDU at higher (<350 CD4 cells/μL) levels. They found a dramatic synergistic impact of provision of NSP, OST, and ARV on reducing HIV incidence over time; with a 39% reduction in population levels of HIV infection over 5 years with the combination approach.[97] This model assumed quite modest levels of efficacy for each component at the individual level (60% for OST, 40% for NSP, and 90% for ARVs when initiated at the higher CD4 level).[97]

CHALLENGES AND OPPORTUNITIES FOR IMPLEMENTATION

While it is tremendously encouraging to demonstrate the synergistic effects of combined preventive interventions on HIV incidence at population levels among IDU, the realities of access to care for this population are sobering. Wolfe and colleagues reviewed access to care for IDU in selected high-burden countries and found that among all populations at risk for HIV infection, IDU remain the least served.[98] An even more telling finding was that in China and Vietnam, the number of drug users in detention is 3 times and 33 times higher, respectively, than those in treatment. Incarceration is not an evidence-based approach to HIV prevention, but rather a well-described risk for HIV infection among drug users.[99]

Strathdee and colleagues used the risk environment framework to investigate another aspect of IDU risks which poses real challenges – the social, policy, and legal environments which can reduce, or drive, HIV risks.[100] They found that structural aspects of risk environments had substantial impacts on HIV risks and disease spread. As IDU risks emerge in new settings, as is happening in East and Southern Africa in 2010, these challenges are likely to continue to undermine our responses.[99]

Combination Preventions

Only the most extremely optimistic scenarios predict that treatment alone can halt the HIV pandemic, and even these assume that treatment enables reductions in sexual risk behaviour. Thus, other primary prevention measures will be required into the future. This argues for combination prevention, but combinations of what? Given the expanded resource needs for treatment, can we cease expenditure on some prevention activities? Here, debate about what is known to work and what creates an environment that enables prevention is intense. Many prevention interventions will be more cost-effective – and some cost-saving – than treatment, for example condom promotion in sex work and medical male circumcision. Sometimes treatment is highly cost-effective, with treatment used to prevent mother-to-child transmission as the most obvious example. Other interventions, such as structural and behavioural interventions could be cost-effective, but have not been amenable to internally valid efficacy studies with an HIV endpoint. Better understanding of combination prevention is also required from community randomized trials and other population-based studies and this should not be neglected in the rush to demonstrate the effectiveness of treatment as prevention. New tools such as oral and topical pre-exposure prophylaxis have been shown efficacious, but only in certain settings. The cost–effectiveness and delivery of such methods as part of a combination prevention approach is the subject of ongoing research.

In summary, evidence suggests that treatment of HIV can be used to directly prevent HIV as well as to improve the environment for other prevention activities. However, there is a need to test how effective it is at a population level; what the optimum programme design would be; and, most importantly, to ensure good treatment coverage of those in immediate clinical need of treatment. In the long run the world needs to stem the flow of new HIV infections if it is to prevent deaths without inexorable increases in the number of people who require treatment. Treatment as prevention adds an important tool in the prevention toolbox that requires careful strategic use to fully maximize the benefits it can generate. The challenges of ensuring widespread testing, linkage to and retention in care and integrating treatment as prevention with other prevention interventions such as circumcision need to be overcome as we move to expand HIV treatment.

Since expanding treatment can potentially absorb all of the currently available resources for treatment and other prevention activities, one of the most pressing policy issues is the definition of what other prevention interventions must be protected as funding is diverted to increase treatment coverage. The UNAIDS-supported HIV investment framework and recent guidance from the President's Emergency Plan for AIDS Relief Scientific Advisory Board both make progress in that direction. The emerging consensus seems to support protecting adult and infant circumcision, PMTCT and condom distribution programmes. Others would argue that sufficient evidence exists to support targeted interventions for most at-risk populations. However, the lack of equally strong evidence in favour of other behavioural and structural interventions does not mean that they are all less cost-effective than treatment as prevention – it just means that we do not have sufficient evidence to be able to make the determination with convincing certainty. This strongly points to the need to generate more robust data on the impact of such interventions where evidence suggests that they may be highly cost-effective.

Conclusion

The aim of the 6th Millennium Development Goal is to halt, and reverse, the spread of HIV by 2015. This chapter has described an impressive array of evidence-based devices (condoms, harm reduction, male circumcision) that can be implemented along with information, skills and services. Concerted HIV prevention efforts from countries as diverse as Thailand, Australia and Senegal have resulted in maintenance of low seroprevalence rates.[8] Other studies conducted in high-risk populations have shown that HIV prevention can work, even in the most challenging settings. Yet, despite this, UNAIDS tells us that only 60% of sex workers, 46% of injection drug users and 40% of MSM were reached with HIV prevention programmes in 2008.[1] The positive results of biomedical interventions in 2010 and those expected over the next several years give promise that a number of other interventions can be added to the menu. The era is one of Highly Active Retroviral Prevention – targeted, strategic and creative combinations of behavioural, biomedical and structural interventions. These programmes will require universal access, wide-scale implementation, careful monitoring and evaluation, financial and technical resources and robust commitment at regional and country levels.[7,103] We may then begin to see a substantial impact on the spread of HIV globally.

REFERENCES

7. Coates TJ, Richter L, Caceres C. Behavioural strategies to reduce HIV transmission: how to make them work better. Lancet 2008;372(9639): 669–84.
12. Padian NS, Buve A, Balkus J, et al. Biomedical interventions to prevent HIV infection: evidence, challenges, and way forward. Lancet 2008;372(9638):585–99.
13. Abdool KQ, Abdool Karim SS, Frohlich JA, et al. Effectiveness and safety of tenofovir gel, an antiretroviral microbicide, for the prevention of HIV infection in women. Science 2010;329(5996):1168–74.
38. Quinn TC, Wawer MJ, Sewankambo N, et al. Viral load and heterosexual transmission of human immunodeficiency virus type 1. Rakai Project Study Group. N Engl J Med 2000;342 (13):921–9.
50. Cohen J. Breakthrough of the year. HIV treatment as prevention. Science 2011;334(6063):1628.
54. Gray RH, Wawer MJ, Brookmeyer R, et al. Probability of HIV-1 transmission per coital act in monogamous, heterosexual, HIV-1-discordant couples in Rakai, Uganda. Lancet 2001;357(9263):1149–53.
56. Granich RM, Gilks CF, Dye C, et al. Universal voluntary HIV testing with immediate antiretroviral therapy as a strategy for elimination of HIV transmission: a mathematical model. Lancet 2009;373(9657):48–57.
64. Gray RH, Kiwanuka N, Quinn TC, et al. Male circumcision and HIV acquisition and transmission: cohort studies in Rakai, Uganda. Rakai Project Team. AIDS 2000;14(15):2371–81.
88. Gregson S, Adamson S, Papaya S, et al. Impact and process evaluation of integrated community and clinic-based HIV-1 control: a cluster-randomised trial in eastern Zimbabwe. PLoS Med 2007;4(3):e102.
97. Degenhardt L, Mathers B, Vickerman P, et al. Prevention of HIV infection for people who inject drugs: why individual, structural, and combination approaches are needed. Lancet 2010;376(9737):285–301.
103. Merson M, Padian N, Coates TJ, et al. Lancet HIV Prevention Series Authors. Combination HIV prevention. Lancet 2008;372(9652):1805–6.

Access the complete references online at www.expertconsult.com

13 Viral Hepatitis

M. ESTÉE TÖRÖK

KEY POINTS

- A number of viruses may present with acute or chronic viral hepatitis – hepatitis A, B, C, D and E are the most frequent causes.
- Hepatitis A is a common cause of acute viral hepatitis with an annual incidence of 1.5 million cases. It is mainly transmitted by the faeco–oral route. Fulminant disease is rare and preventative vaccines are available.
- Hepatitis B is a frequent cause of chronic viral hepatitis, with an estimated 350 million infected cases. It is transmitted sexually, parenterally, vertically or horizontally. Antiviral treatment and vaccines are available.
- Hepatitis C is a common cause of chronic viral hepatitis, with an estimated 130 million chronic cases. It is mainly transmitted parenterally. Antiviral treatment is available and vaccines are under development.
- Hepatitis D is a defective virus that occurs only in patients with hepatitis B, either as co-infection or as super-infection. Antiviral treatment is available.
- Hepatitis E is a frequent cause of acute viral hepatitis transmitted by the faeco–oral route. Fulminant disease is more frequent in pregnancy and chronic disease has been described in solid organ transplant recipients.

Introduction

The first description of hepatitis (epidemic jaundice) is generally attributed to Hippocrates in the fifth century BC. During the seventeenth and eighteenth centuries, outbreaks of infectious hepatitis (hepatitis A) were reported, particularly in the context of military campaigns. The first cases of serum hepatitis (hepatitis B) are thought to have occurred after the administration of smallpox vaccine to German shipyard workers in 1883. In the early twentieth century, serum hepatitis was observed with the use of contaminated needles and syringes and in blood transfusion recipients. In the 1940s, infectious hepatitis (hepatitis A) was epidemiologically differentiated from serum hepatitis (hepatitis B), which had a longer incubation period. The Australia antigen (hepatitis B surface antigen, HBsAg) was described in 1956, followed by the Dane particle (hepatitis B virion) in 1970. In the 1970s, identification of the hepatitis A virus (HAV) and development of serological tests enabled the differentiation of HAV from hepatitis B virus (HBV). After the discovery of HAV and HBV, it became apparent that a large proportion of cases of acute and chronic hepatitis could not be explained by either of these agents. These cases were attributed to another suspected viral agent and called non-A, non-B hepatitis. In 1988, the causative agent was identified and designated hepatitis C virus (HCV). Chronic hepatitis with both hepatitis B and hepatitis C viruses is a significant cause of hepatocellular carcinoma and a serious public health problem in several parts of the developing world. In 1977, Rizetto and colleagues described a new antigen that they had detected in the hepatic nuclei of livers of patients infected with HBV – this was named the delta virus. Hepatitis E was first described in 1978 during an epidemic of acute non-A, non-B hepatitis in India. Collectively, these five agents constitute the major causes of acute and chronic viral hepatitis and affect hundreds of millions of people worldwide. This chapter reviews the epidemiology, virology, pathogenesis, clinical features, diagnosis, management and prevention of these viruses.

Hepatitis A Virus (HAV)

EPIDEMIOLOGY OF HAV INFECTION

HAV infection occurs worldwide (Figure 13.1), with an estimated incidence of 1.5 million cases per year. It remains one of the most commonly reported vaccine-preventable diseases.[1] A recent WHO systematic review reported that in many parts of the world, infection with HAV is decreasing.[2] Several factors contribute to the declining infection rate, including improvements in socioeconomic status, increasing access to clean water and in some areas, the availability of a hepatitis A vaccine that was developed in the 1990s.[3,4] In the USA, vaccination has been recommended for persons considered to be at increased risk of HAV infection and for children living in states with the highest incidence of HAV. Consequently, the incidence of acute HAV infection in the USA has declined substantially from 12 cases/100 000 population per year in 1995, to about one case/100 000 population per year in 2007.

HAV is transmitted by the faeco–oral route and is more prevalent in developing countries or poor socioeconomic areas, where poor hygiene and sanitation facilitate the spread of the infection. In high-income countries, the most commonly reported risk factor is international travel (15%). Other risk factors include: household or sexual contact with another person with HAV infection (10%); male homosexual activity (9%); food- or water-borne outbreaks (7%); attending or working in a child day-care centre (4%); and injection drug use (3%).[5] Nevertheless, HAV infection is sporadic in approximately 40% of cases. Mother-to-child transmission has not been reported. In the childcare setting, most of the children are asymptomatic or have nonspecific symptoms and outbreaks are usually only recognized after staff members develop symptoms.

Community HAV outbreaks caused by contaminated water or food have also been described. In one such report, HAV RNA

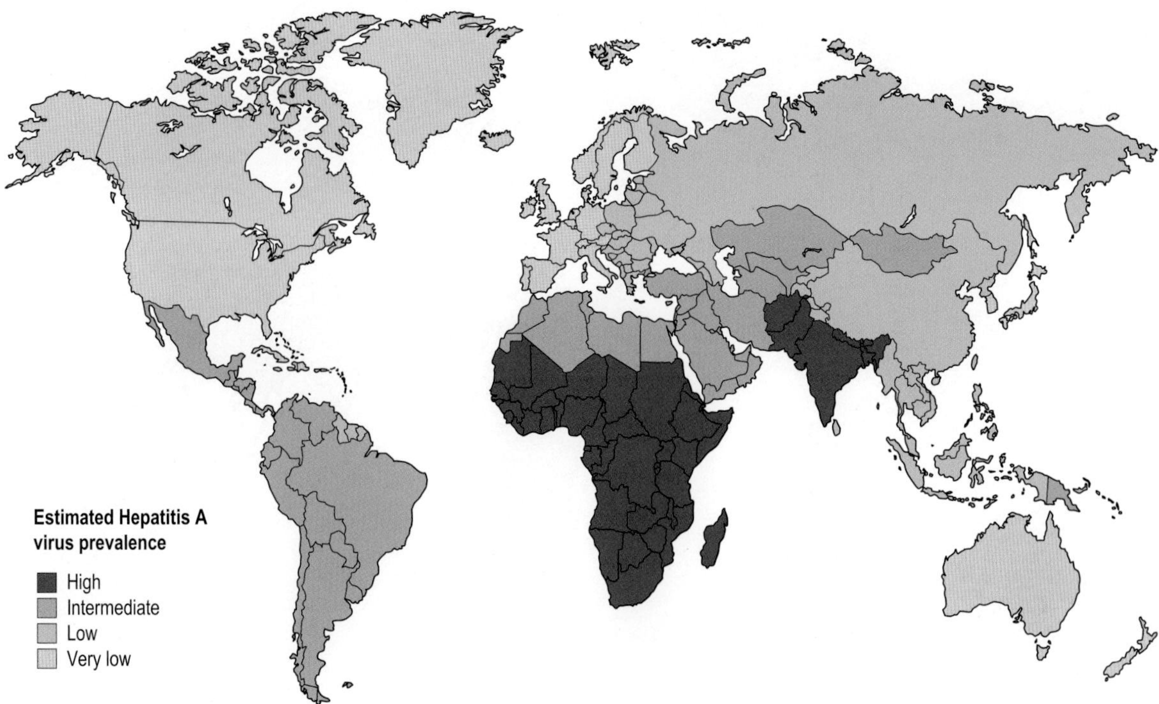

Figure 13.1 Estimated prevalence of hepatitis A virus infection. *(From CDC Health Information for International Travel 2012: The Yellow Book.)*

could be detected in well water 6 months after the initial contamination. HAV can be acquired from contaminated food, often shellfish. In one report, approximately 290 000 people in Shanghai developed acute HAV infection that was traced to clams.[6] Several outbreaks related to consumption of contaminated green onions and frozen strawberries have been described. In the USA, clusters of cases have also been seen in relation to international adoptions; more than half of which occurred in non-travelling contacts of adoptees.[7] Nosocomial spread of HAV is rare, but outbreaks have been reported in neonatal intensive care units, where neonates were infected through blood transfusions and subsequently transmitted the virus to other neonates and staff members.[8]

The global epidemiology of HAV infection is changing, largely as a result of improvements in living conditions in low- to middle-income countries. As a result, fewer children are infected, leading to a larger population of adults, who lack protective antibodies against HAV and are at risk for outbreaks of infection.[1,2]

HAV GENOME

HAV virus is a 27-nm single-stranded, icosahedral, non-enveloped RNA virus that belongs to the Heparnavirus genus of the Picornaviridae. The HAV genome is comprised of 7474 nucleotides divided into three regions: a 5′ untranslated region (742 nucleotides); a single long open reading frame (ORF) that encodes a 2227 amino acid polypeptide (6681 nucleotides); and a 3′ non-coding region (63 nucleotides). The polypeptide encoded by the ORF is processed by a viral protease, resulting in four structural and seven non-structural proteins. Four distinct genotypes of HAV have been identified in humans, although they do not appear to have important biological differences.[9]

PATHOGENESIS OF HAV INFECTION

The degree of hepatic injury during HAV infection depends upon the host's immune response to the virus and is considered a biphasic process.[10] In the first non-cytopathic phase, viral replication occurs exclusively within the cytoplasm of the hepatocyte. This is followed by a second cytopathic phase, characterized by florid portal zone infiltration, necrosis and erosion of the limiting plate. Hepatocellular damage and destruction is not the result of a direct cytopathic effect by HAV but a process mediated by HLA-restricted, HAV-specific, CD8+ T-lymphocytes and natural killer (NK) cells. Interferon-γ appears to have a key role in promoting clearance of infected hepatocytes. An excessive host response, reflected by a marked reduction in HAV RNA during acute infection, is associated with severe hepatitis and a possible fulminant course.

CLINICAL MANIFESTATIONS OF HAV INFECTION

HAV infection is usually silent or subclinical in children. HAV infection in children is typically an acute, self-limited illness associated with general, nonspecific symptoms, such as fever, malaise, anorexia, vomiting, nausea, abdominal pain or discomfort and diarrhoea. During the prodromal period, serum aminotransferases are typically elevated. Jaundice usually occurs 1 week after onset of symptoms, along with dark urine and mild hepatomegaly. Symptomatic hepatitis occurs in approximately 30% of children aged <6 years, some of whom become jaundiced. When it does occur, jaundice usually lasts for less than 2 weeks. Conjugated bilirubin and aminotransferases return to normal within 2–3 months.[11]

In contrast, older children and adults with HAV infection are usually symptomatic for several weeks. Following exposure, there is an incubation period of 15–50 days, after which the

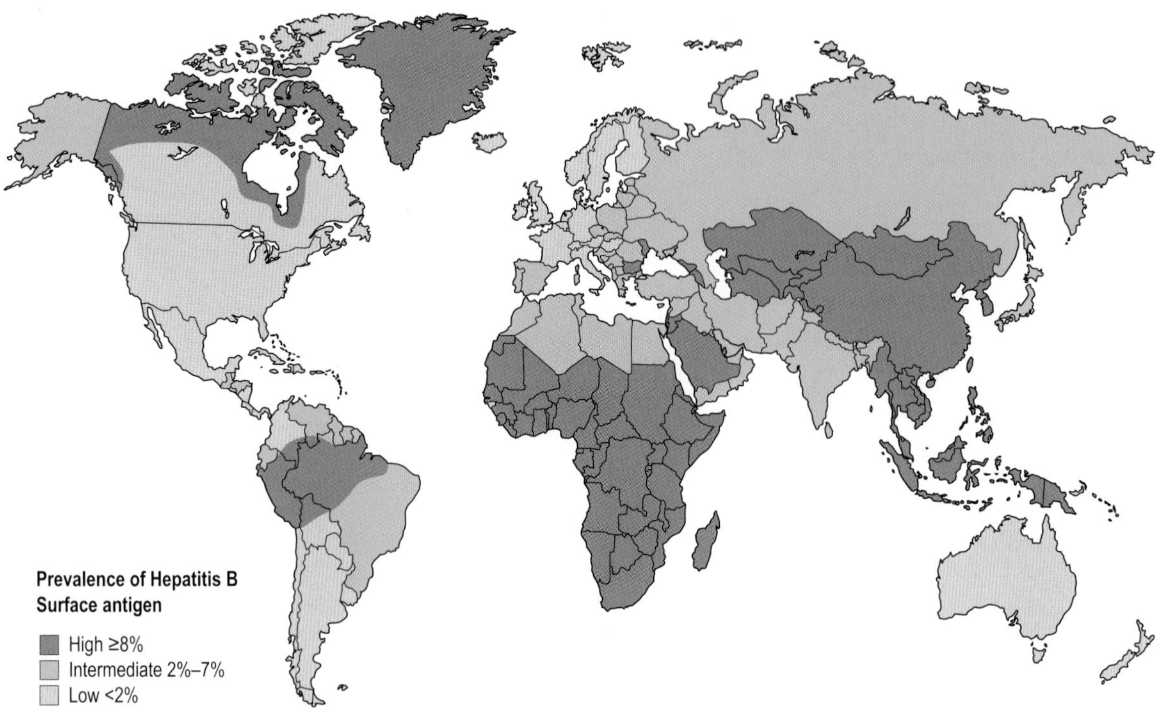

Figure 13.2 Prevalence of chronic infection with hepatitis B, 2006. *(From CDC Health Information for International Travel 2012: The Yellow Book.)*

patient develops prodromal symptoms, including: fatigue, malaise, nausea, vomiting, anorexia, fever and right upper quadrant pain. Within a few days to a week, patients develop dark urine, pale stools, pruritis and jaundice, which typically peaks within 2 weeks. The two most common physical findings are jaundice (Figures 13.2 and 13.3) and hepatomegaly, which occur in 70% and 80% of symptomatic patients, respectively. Less frequent findings include splenomegaly, cervical lymphadenopathy, evanescent rash, arthritis and, rarely, a leucocytoclastic vasculitis. Occasionally, patients may develop prolonged cholestasis or relapsing form of hepatitis.[11] A variety of extrahepatic manifestations have been described in acute HAV infection, including vasculitis, arthritis, optic neuritis, transverse myelitis, thrombocytopenia, aplastic anaemia and red cell aplasia; these conditions are more likely in patients who have protracted illness. HAV is rarely associated with a relapsing or cholestatic clinical illness and may serve as a trigger for autoimmune hepatitis in genetically susceptible individuals.[12]

Acute liver failure is rare in developed countries, occurring in less than 1% of paediatric cases in the USA but is more frequently reported in endemic countries. Hepatitis A-associated fulminant hepatitis is more common in children than adults in developing countries,[13] and also occurs more commonly in patients with underlying liver disease.[14]

Laboratory abnormalities are characterized by marked elevations of serum aminotransferases (>1000 IU/L), bilirubin and alkaline phosphatase. The serum alanine aminotransferase (ALT) is usually higher than the serum aspartate aminotransferase (AST). The serum aminotransferase elevations precede the bilirubin elevation, with the peak bilirubin concentration occurring after the peak aminotransferase elevations. Other laboratory findings include elevations of acute-phase proteins, elevated erythrocyte sedimentation rate and increased immunoglobulin levels.[10,11]

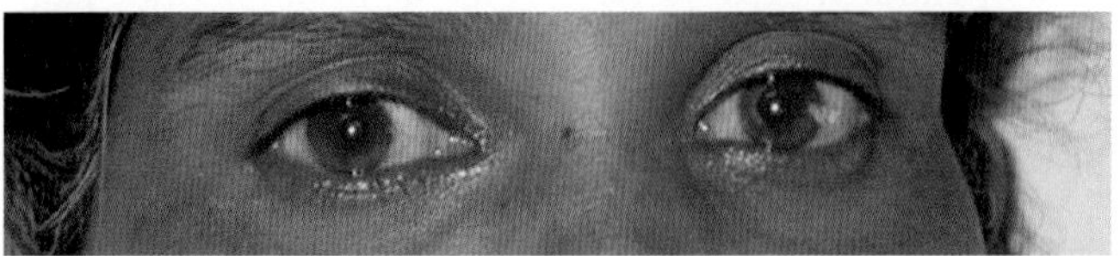

Figure 13.3 Jaundice in viral hepatitis.

LABORATORY DIAGNOSIS OF HAV INFECTION

The diagnosis of acute HAV infection is confirmed by the detection of anti-HAV immunoglobulin M (IgM) antibodies in the serum of a patient with a typical clinical presentation. The presence of anti-HAV IgM antibodies in adults without clinical features of viral hepatitis may indicate asymptomatic infection (which is more common in children), prolonged presence of anti-HAV IgM in a patient with previous acute HAV infection or a false-positive result. Anti-HAV IgM is positive at the onset of symptoms, peaks during the acute or early convalescent phase of the disease and remains positive for approximately 4–6 months. Anti-HAV IgM may persist at a low titre for 12–14 months in patients with a protracted or relapsing course. Anti-HAV IgG antibodies appear early in the convalescent phase of the disease and remain detectable for decades.[15] In adults who are vaccinated against HAV, antibodies become detectable 2 weeks after vaccination, but titres are 10–100-fold lower than levels induced by wild-type infection.

HAV may be detected in the stool and body fluids by electron microscopy. HAV RNA can also be detected by polymerase chain reaction (PCR)-based assays in stool, body fluids, serum and liver tissue. In humans it has been detected for at least 81 days after the onset of disease. In neonates and younger children, HAV RNA can be detected in stools for several months.[16] In practice, these diagnostic methods are infrequently used as they are expensive and not readily available.

TREATMENT OF HAV INFECTION

The disease is usually self-limited and treatment is mainly supportive. Occasionally, patients require hospitalization for severe symptoms. Patients who develop fulminant infection require aggressive supportive therapy and should be transferred to a specialist centre for liver transplantation.

PROGNOSIS OF HAV INFECTION

Approximately 85% of HAV-infected individuals recover within 3 months and nearly all have a complete recovery by 6 months. Serum aminotransferase concentrations decrease more rapidly than the serum bilirubin; the latter normalizes in >85% of individuals by 3 months.[9] The case-fatality of acute HAV infection is low but increased with age and in those co-infected with HCV infection.

PREVENTION OF HAV INFECTION

HAV infection can be prevented by hand washing, heating foods appropriately and avoiding the consumption of contaminated water and food in HAV-endemic areas. Chlorination and certain disinfecting solutions (e.g. household bleach 1:100 dilution) are also effective in inactivating the virus.

Pre-exposure prophylaxis with intramuscular human normal immunoglobulin (HNIG) has been available since the 1950s and can decrease the incidence of HAV infection by more than 90%. Passive immunity lasts for 4–6 months, depending upon the dose of immunoglobulin used, but is only effective if administered within 2 weeks of exposure. There are, however, a number of disadvantages of HNIG prophylaxis including pain at the injection site, the need for repeated administration, interference with development of immunity to live vaccines and the potential risk of transmission of infectious agents such as bloodborne viruses or prions. As a result, HNIG pre-exposure prophylaxis is generally reserved for non-immune individuals exposed to HAV who have contraindications to HAV vaccination.[9]

Several highly effective and safe vaccines are available for HAV; these include formalin-inactivated vaccines, live attenuated vaccines, combined HAV and HBV vaccines and a combination HAV and typhoid vaccine. Monovalent HAV vaccines and combined HAV and typhoid vaccine are given as a single dose; the administration schedule for combined HAV and HBV vaccines is 2 or 3 doses according to the particular product. HAV vaccination is recommended for specific high-risk groups, such as travellers to endemic countries, patients with chronic liver disease or haemophilia, men who have sex with men, injecting drug users, persons at occupational risk of HAV (e.g. laboratory workers, sewage workers) and people living in communities with HAV outbreaks.[5] HAV vaccine is also part of the routine childhood immunization schedule in certain countries such as the USA. A compelling argument for universal vaccination of children is the observation that the disease tends to be more severe when acquired at older ages. Furthermore, as humans are the only known reservoir for HAV, universal vaccination could hypothetically eradicate HAV.[17]

Post-exposure prophylaxis should be considered in non-immune individuals who have been exposed to HAV.[18] Either passive or active immunization, or a combination of the two, may be used.

Hepatitis B Virus (HBV)

EPIDEMIOLOGY OF HBV INFECTION

HBV is a global public health problem with more than 350 million persons estimated to be chronically infected with the virus. HBV can present with a variety of clinical syndromes including acute hepatitis, chronic liver disease, cirrhosis or hepatocellular carcinoma (HCC). HBV-related liver disease accounts for more than half a million deaths per year and 5–10% of cases of liver transplantation.[19] The outcome of HBV infection depends on the age at infection, level of HBV replication, immune status of the host, co-infection with other viruses and comorbidities such as alcohol abuse and obesity.

The prevalence of chronic HBV infection varies from 0.1% to 2% in low-prevalence regions (western Europe, North America and Australia) to 3–5% in intermediate-prevalence areas (the Mediterranean, Central Asia, the Middle East, South America and Japan) to 10–20% in high-prevalence areas (sub-Saharan Africa and South-east Asia) (Figure 13.2).

The predominant mode of transmission of HBV varies in different geographical areas. In high-prevalence areas, perinatal transmission is the most common route of infection. Horizontal transmission, particularly in early childhood, accounts for most cases of chronic HBV infection in intermediate-prevalence areas, whereas unprotected sexual intercourse and injection drug use in adults are the major routes of spread in low-prevalence areas. The rate of progression from acute to chronic HBV infection is inversely related to the age at infection: approximately 90% for perinatal infection; 20–50% for infections acquired between the age of 1 and 5 years; and about 5% for adult-acquired infection.[20]

The high frequency of perinatal transmission in endemic areas is probably related to the high prevalence of HBeAg in women of reproductive age. The risk of maternal–infant transmission is associated with HBeAg status and HBV DNA levels in the mother. Breast-feeding does not appear to increase the risk of transmission. Transmission of HBV from father to infants has been documented. Percutaneous transmission usually happens among intravenous drug users who share syringes and needles. Household contacts can also transmit HBV through the sharing of razors or toothbrushes. Certain practices like acupuncture, tattooing and body piercing have also been associated with transmission of HBV.[21] HBV is the most commonly transmitted blood-borne virus in the healthcare setting. The incidence of transfusion-related HBV infection has decreased significantly since the introduction of HBsAg screening of donors and the exclusion of paid blood donors. Nosocomial transmission generally occurs from patient to patient or from patient to healthcare worker via a sharps injury. Despite the publicity about HBV transmission from healthcare workers to patients, transmission from infected healthcare workers to patients is relatively infrequent compared with transmission from patients to healthcare workers. Transmission of HBV infection has been reported after transplantation of extra-hepatic organs from HBsAg-positive donors.

In Western countries, implementation of vaccination programmes has reduced the prevalence of HBV infection. However, rates of HBV-related hospitalizations, cancers and deaths have increased during the past decade;[22] this may be related to a number of factors including delayed implementation of universal vaccination, immigration from endemic areas and improved diagnosis and reporting of HBV infection.

HBV STRUCTURE AND GENOME

HBV belongs to the family of hepadnaviruses and replicates by reverse transcription via an RNA intermediate, making it prone to mutations. The complete virion (Dane particle) is 42 nm in diameter and consists of an envelope (composed of viral-encoded proteins and host-derived lipid components) and a core (composed of nucleocapsid protein, viral genome and the polymerase protein). HBV also produces non-infectious 22 nm subviral particles composed of envelope proteins. HBV has a circular double-stranded DNA genome of approximately 3200 base pairs in length with four partially overlapping ORFs encoding the envelope (pre-S/S), core (pre-core/core), polymerase and X protein (Figure 13.4).

The pre-S/S ORF consists of the pre-S1, pre-S2 and S regions which encode the large (L), middle (M) and small (S) envelope proteins. The M and S envelope proteins are found in viral and subviral particles whereas the L envelope proteins are only found in complete virions. The precore/core ORF consists of two start codons. Translation from the first start codon produces a precore polypeptide which undergoes post-translational modification to produce the hepatitis B e antigen (HBeAg). Translation from the second codon produces the hepatitis B core antigen (HBcAg). The HBV DNA polymerase gene consists of four regions: a protein primer, a spacer, a reverse transcriptase/DNA polymerase and an RNAase H domain. The X protein is not required for viral replication but acts as a transcriptional activator of many promoters including HBV and cellular oncogenes.[23]

Phylogenetic analyses have resulted in the classification of HBV into eight genotypes (A to H), the clinical significance of which are still under investigation. Genotype A is found mainly in North America, northern Europe, India and Africa, genotypes B and C are prevalent in Asia and genotype D is more common in southern Europe, the Middle East and India. HBV genotypes can be further subdivided into subgroups according to geographic and ethnic origins. For example, two subtypes of genotype B have been described: genotype Ba (which is found in many Asian countries) and genotype Bj (which is predominantly found in Japan).[23] Recombination between different HBV genotypes has been reported and individual patients may also be co-infected with more than one genotype.

HBV was originally classified into four subtypes or serotypes (adr, adw, ayr and ayw) based on the antigenic determinants of the HBsAg. HBV has since been re-classified into nine different serotypes: adrq+; adrq–; adw2; adw4; ayr; ayw1; ayw2; ayw3; and ayw4.[23] Several studies have attempted to investigate the relationships between HBV genotypes and serotypes.

Most of the information on the clinical significance of HBV genotypes has been derived from Asian studies of chronic infection with HBV genotypes B and C. The prevalence of HBeAg appears to be higher in patients with genotype C rather than genotype B, whereas the cumulative rate of HBeAg seroconversion appears to be higher in patients with genotype B than genotype C. Thus HBeAg seroconversion appears to occur earlier and at a higher rate in patients with genotype B infection. There is limited information on the clinical course of patients with HBV genotypes other than B or C.[24] A few studies have suggested that HBV genotype D infection is more likely to be associated with fulminant disease and that HBV genotype A infection is more likely to progress to chronic infection. There are conflicting data on the relationship between HBV genotypes and HCC. Studies conducted in Japan, China, Hong Kong and the USA have shown that patients with HBV genotype C were more likely to develop HCC; in contrast studies from Taiwan have shown that HBV genotype B was more common in younger non-cirrhotic patients with HCC.

Mutations in the precore region of the HBV genome (precore variants) have been described in HBeAg-negative patients with persistent viraemia and active liver disease.[23] The predominant mutation is a change from guanine to adenine at position 1896 (G1896A) which creates a premature stop codon and prevents the production of HBeAg. Selection of the G1896A mutation is

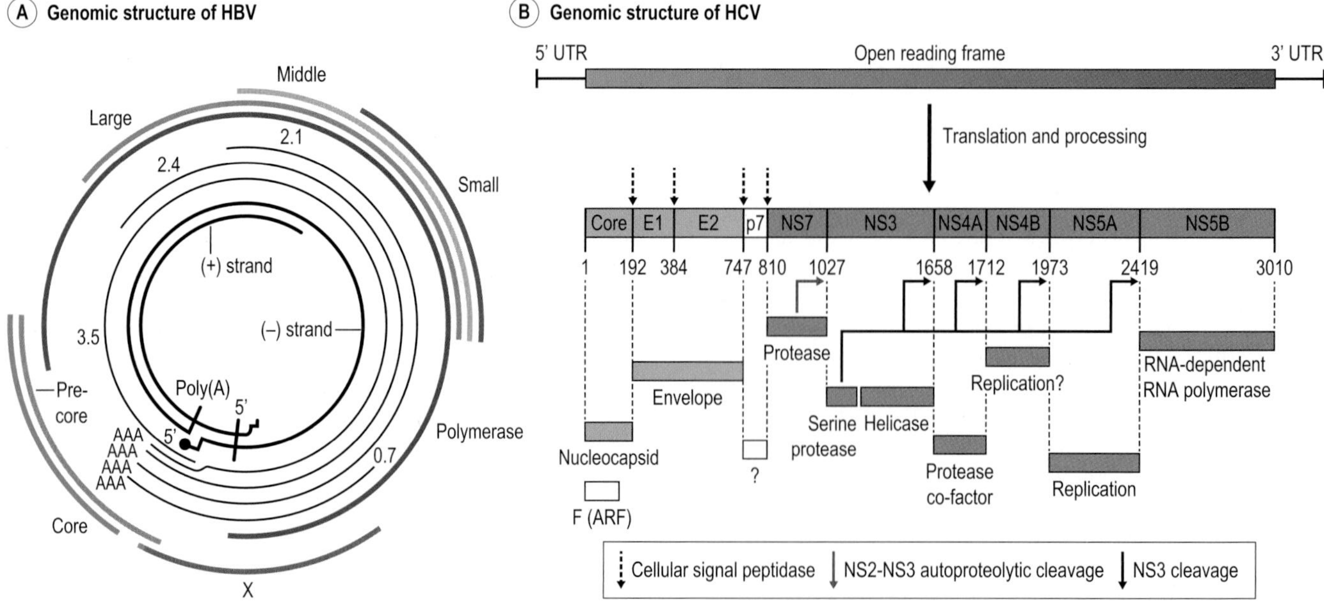

Figure 13.4 Genomic structure of (A) HBV and (B) HCV. *(From Rehermann and Nascimbeni. Nature Reviews Immunology 2005;5:215–29.)*

genotype-dependent and precore variants have been most frequently found in patients with HBV genotype D infections.

Mutations in the core promoter region, located upstream of the precore region, downregulate precore mRNA transcription and HBeAg synthesis.[23] The most common core promoter variants involve a two nucleotide substitution: adenine for thymine at position 1762 (A1762T) and guanine for adenine at position 1764 (G1764A). These mutations were originally described in HBeAg-negative patients but have been seen in some HBeAg-positive patients. Some studies suggest that core promoter variants are associated with increased HBV replication, more severe liver damage and HCC.

PATHOGENESIS OF HBV INFECTION

Chronic HBV infection generally consists of two phases: an early replicative phase with active liver disease and a late/low replicative phase with remission of liver disease. In patients with perinatally acquired HBV infection, there is an additional immune tolerance phase in which virus replication is not accompanied by active liver disease.

In patients with a perinatally acquired HBV infection, the initial phase is characterized by the presence of HBeAg and high levels of HBV DNA in serum, but no evidence of active liver disease as manifested by lack of symptoms, normal serum ALT concentrations and minimal changes on liver biopsy. The lack of liver disease, despite high levels of HBV replication, is believed to be due to immune tolerance to HBV, although the exact mechanisms by which this occurs remain unclear. The immune tolerance phase usually lasts 10–30 years, during which there is a very low rate of spontaneous HBeAg clearance.[25]

The transition from the immune tolerant to the immune clearance phase occurs during the 2nd and 3rd decades in most patients. During this phase, spontaneous HBeAg clearance increases to a rate of 10–20% per year. HBeAg seroconversion is frequently, but not always, accompanied by increases in serum ALT. Exacerbations are often preceded by an increase in serum HBV DNA and a shift of HBcAg from nuclear to cytoplasmic sites within hepatocytes. Most exacerbations are asymptomatic and are discovered during routine follow-up. Some are accompanied by symptoms of acute hepatitis and may lead to the incorrect diagnosis of acute HBV infection in patients who were not previously known to have chronic HBV infection. In a minority of patients, exacerbations result in hepatic decompensation and, rarely, death from hepatic failure. Not all exacerbations lead to HBeAg seroconversion and clearance of HBV DNA from the serum. These patients may develop recurrent exacerbations with intermittent disappearance of serum HBV DNA with or without a transient loss of HBeAg.[22] Such repeated episodes of hepatitis may increase the risk of developing cirrhosis and hepatocellular carcinoma (HCC).[26]

The initial phase in patients with childhood or adult-acquired chronic HBV infection consists of virus replication (with HBeAg positivity and high serum HBV DNA levels) and active liver disease (elevated serum ALT and chronic hepatitis on liver biopsy). The prevalence of HBeAg among non-Asian adults with chronic HBV infection is lower than that seen in Asian adults, but the rate of spontaneous HBeAg clearance appears to be similar at 10–20% per year.

Patients in the low or non-replicating phase/inactive carrier state are HBeAg negative and anti-HBe positive. In some patients, HBV DNA is undetectable in serum and there is no evidence of liver disease, as evidenced by normal serum ALT concentrations and the resolution of hepatic inflammation. Other studies, however, have shown that HBeAg-negative patients with a persistently normal serum ALT may still have significant histologic inflammation and/or fibrosis.

Some patients continue to have moderate levels of HBV replication and active liver disease (elevated serum ALT and chronic inflammation on liver biopsies), but remain HBeAg negative. They have a residual wild-type virus or HBV variants that cannot produce HBeAg as a result of precore or core promoter genetic mutations. Patients with HBeAg-negative chronic hepatitis are older and have more advanced liver disease; they also tend to have fluctuations in HBV DNA and ALT levels.[21]

A few patients with chronic HBV infection become HBsAg negative. The annual rate of delayed clearance of HBsAg has been estimated to be 0.5–2% in Western patients and 0.1–0.8% in Asian countries. In most reports, patients without cirrhosis who cleared HBsAg appeared to have a good prognosis. However, some studies have shown the development of cirrhosis and HCC in patients who had cleared HBsAg.

Many patients who clear HBsAg remained HBV DNA positive, particularly during the first 10 years of HBsAg clearance. A reactivation of HBV replication with reappearance of HBeAg and HBV DNA in serum and recrudescence of liver disease may occur when these patients are immunosuppressed.

CLINICAL MANIFESTATIONS OF HBV INFECTION

The spectrum of clinical manifestations of HBV infection varies in both acute and chronic disease.[27] The incubation period of HBV infection is 1–4 months. A serum sickness-like syndrome may develop during the prodromal period, followed by constitutional symptoms with anorexia, nausea, jaundice and right upper quadrant discomfort. Approximately 70% of patients with acute HBV infection have subclinical/anicteric hepatitis, while 30% develop icteric hepatitis. The disease may be more severe in patients co-infected with other hepatitis viruses or with underlying liver disease. Symptoms and jaundice usually resolve after 1–3 months, but some patients have prolonged fatigue. Fulminant liver failure is rare, occurring in 0.1–0.5% of cases and is believed to be related to immune-mediated lysis of infected hepatocytes.

Laboratory testing during the acute phase reveals elevations in serum aminotransferases (ALT and AST) with values up to 1000–2000 IU/L. The serum bilirubin concentration may be normal in patients with anicteric hepatitis. In patients who recover, normalization of serum aminotransferases usually occurs within one to four months. A persistent elevation of serum ALT for longer than 6 months indicates a progression to chronic hepatitis.

Among patients who recover from acute HBV infection, it was previously thought that the virus was completely cleared by HBV-specific antibodies and cytotoxic T lymphocytes. However, HBV DNA in the blood has been detected by PCR many years after a clinical and serological recovery from acute HAV infection. In one study HBV DNA was detected in the livers of healthy transplant donors who had previously recovered from acute HBV infection. Another study found persistent histological abnormalities up to 10 years after serological recovery from acute infection. These observations suggest that the complete eradication of HBV rarely occurs and that latent infection can maintain the T cell response for decades following clinical recovery, thereby keeping the virus under control. Immunosuppression in such patients may lead to reactivation of the virus.

Many patients with chronic HBV infection are asymptomatic while others have non-specific symptoms such as fatigue. Some patients experience flares of disease which may be asymptomatic or mimic acute hepatitis. Physical examination may be unremarkable or there may be stigmata of chronic liver disease and splenomegaly. Patients with decompensated cirrhosis may present with jaundice, ascites, peripheral oedema and encephalopathy. Laboratory tests may be normal, but most patients have a mild to moderate elevation in serum aminotransferases. During exacerbations, the serum ALT concentration may be as high as 50 times the upper limit of normal. Progression to cirrhosis is suspected if there is evidence of hypersplenism (decreased white blood cell and platelet counts) or impaired hepatic synthetic function (hypoalbuminemia, prolonged prothrombin time, hyperbilirubinemia). HBV is an oncogenic virus and can cause HCC in the absence of cirrhosis. The annual risk of HBV-induced HCC varies according to whether or not cirrhosis is present. In HBV carriers without cirrhosis, the risk is 0.02–03% in Caucasians and 0.4–0.6%/year in Asians. In those with cirrhosis, the risk is 2.2% and 3.7%, respectively, in Caucasians and Asians. HBV likely causes HCC via both indirect (necroinflammation and regeneration injury) and direct (by integration of its DNA in the host genome) pathways. During recent years it has become evident that HBV viral load >2000 IU/mL is associated with a high risk of malignant transformation.[28]

Extra-hepatic manifestations occur in 10–20% of patients with chronic HBV infection and are attributed to circulating immune complexes. Acute HBV infection may be heralded by a serum sickness-like syndrome with fever, skin rashes, arthralgia and arthritis, which usually subsides with the onset of jaundice. Extra-hepatic complications of chronic HBV infection include polyarteritis nodosa, membranous nephropathy, membranoproliferative glomerulonephritis and aplastic anaemia.

HBV infected patients may also be infected with hepatitis C virus (HCV) or hepatitis delta virus (HDV).[29] Acute infection with both HBV and HCV may shorten the duration of HBsAg antigenemia and lower the peak serum aminotransferase concentration compared with acute HBV infection alone. These findings suggest that HCV co-infection may interfere with the replication of HBV, leading to attenuation of liver damage. Acute co-infection with HBV/HCV or acute HCV infection in patients with chronic HBV infection, have also been reported to increase the risk of severe hepatitis and fulminant hepatic failure. Similarly, acute HBV infection in patients with chronic HCV infection can lead to severe hepatitis, but may also lead to clearance of HCV. Coexistent HCV infection has been estimated to be present in 10–15% of patients with HBV-associated chronic hepatitis, cirrhosis or HCC.[29] HCV super-infection in HBsAg carriers appears to reduce HBV DNA levels in serum and liver tissues and to increase the rate of HBsAg seroconversion. Most patients who have dual HCV and HBV infections have detectable serum HCV RNA but undetectable or low HBV DNA levels, indicating that HCV is the predominant cause of liver disease in these patients. Liver disease is usually more severe in dual HBV/HCV infected patients compared with those infected by HBV alone. Patients with dual HBV/HCV infection may also have a higher rate of HCC compared with patients infected by either virus alone, particularly those who are anti-HCV and HBeAg positive.

Acute HBV and HDV co-infection tends to be more severe than acute HBV infection alone and is more likely to result in fulminant hepatitis. HDV super-infection in patients with chronic HBV infection is usually accompanied by a suppression of HBV replication due to interference mechanisms that are not well understood. HDV super-infection in such patients has been associated with more severe liver disease and accelerated progression to cirrhosis in most but not all studies.

LABORATORY DIAGNOSIS OF HBV INFECTION

The diagnosis of HBV infection is based on serological tests for HBV antigens and antibodies as summarized in Figure 13.5 and Table 13.1. Patients with acute HBV infection typically have very high serum aminotransferases compared with patients with chronic HBV infection. HBV DNA detection and quantitation is essential in order to determine the need for treatment and subsequent monitoring.[30] Other causes of chronic liver disease should be systematically excluded: (1) co-infection with HCV, HDV and/or HIV; (2) other causes of chronic liver disease, e.g. alcoholic autoimmune or metabolic liver disease with steatosis or steatohepatitis. A liver biopsy should be performed to determine the degree of necroinflammation and fibrosis in patients with an increased ALT and/or HBV DNA level >2000 IU/mL. A biopsy is also useful to exclude co-existing causes of liver disease.

TREATMENT OF HBV INFECTION

Treatment for acute HBV infection is mainly supportive. In addition, appropriate measures should be taken to prevent infection in exposed contacts. Most patients with acute HBV infection do not require hospitalization. However, patients who are deeply jaundiced, encephalopathic or those who have a coagulopathy should generally be admitted to hospital. Hospitalization may also be considered in patients who have poor oral intake, inadequate social support systems or significant co-morbidities. The benefits of using antiviral therapy in acute HBV infection are not clear – one randomized controlled trial of lamivudine versus placebo failed to demonstrate clinical or biochemical benefit in patients with acute HBV infection. The role of antiviral therapy in patients with severe or protracted acute HBV infection has not been examined but some authors recommend treatment of patients with coagulopathy, jaundice/symptoms lasting longer than 4 weeks, fulminant HBV infection, immunocompromise, co-infection with HCV and HDV, co-existing liver disease or in the elderly. The antiviral agents used include telbivudine, lamivudine, adefovir, entecavir or tenofovir, given as monotherapy. The duration of treatment is usually short and treatment is stopped after confirmation that the patient has cleared HBsAg.

The goal of treatment in chronic HBV infection is to reduce the risk of progressive chronic liver disease, transmission to others and other long-term complications from chronic HBV such as cirrhosis and HCC. This is achieved by suppressing HBV replication and reducing hepatic inflammation, thereby reducing the risk of cirrhosis and HCC. HBV infection cannot be completely eradicated because of the persistence of covalently closed circular DNA in the nucleus of infected hepatocytes.

The indications for treatment of chronic HBV infection are based on a combination of three criteria: (i) HBV DNA level

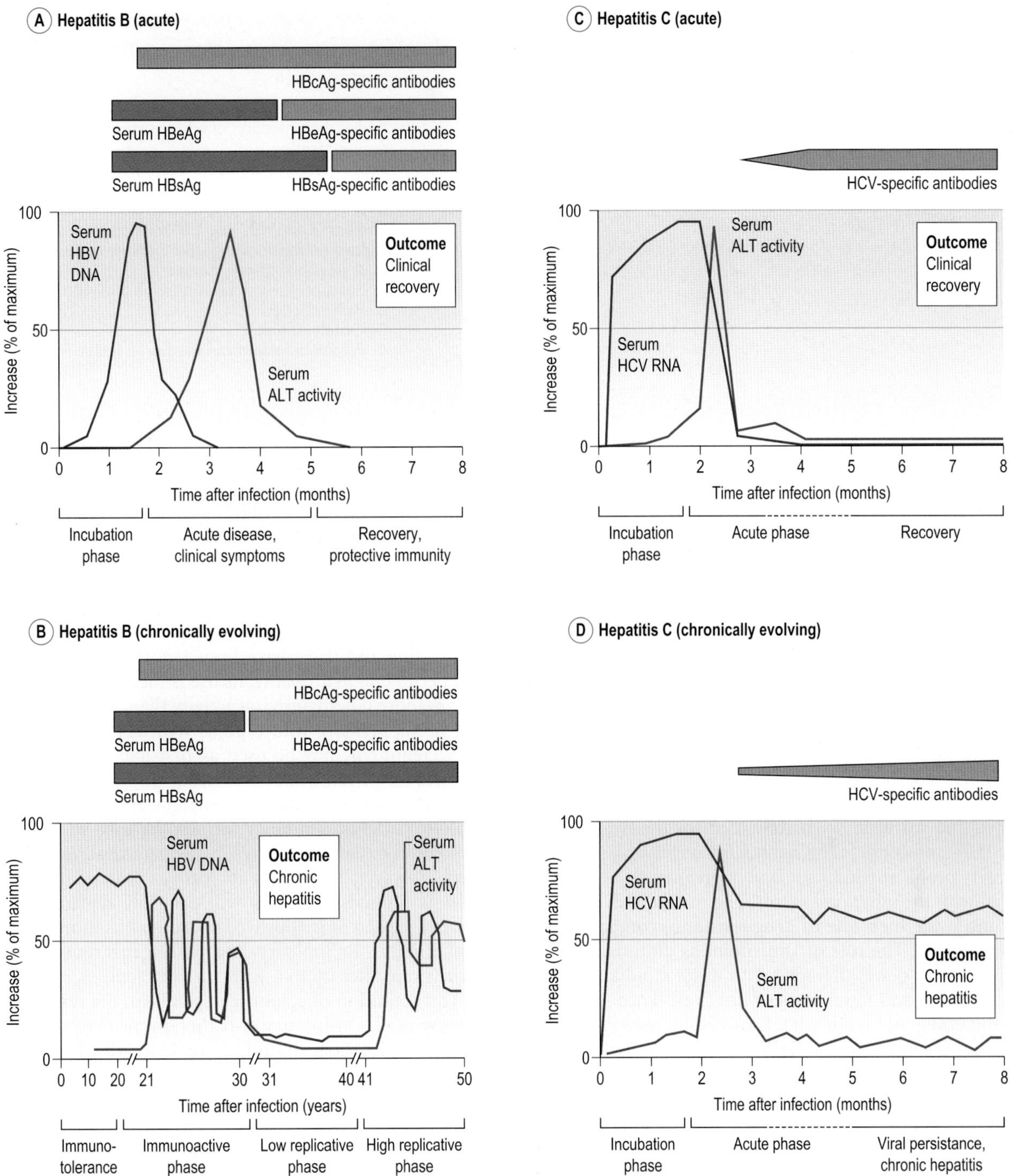

Figure 13.5 Clinical and virological course of (A,B) HBV and (C,D) HCV infection. *(From Rehermann and Nascimbeni. Nature Reviews Immunology 2005;5:215–29.)*

>2000 IU/mL (approx. 10 000 copies/mL); (ii) serum ALT above the upper limit of normal; (iii) liver biopsy showing moderate to severe necroinflammation and/or fibrosis using a standard scoring system (e.g. grade A2 or stage F2 by METAVIR scoring). In addition, patients with compensated cirrhosis and detectable HBV DNA level should be considered for treatment, even if serum ALT is normal and HBV DNA <2000 IU/mL. Patients with decompensated cirrhosis require urgent antiviral treatment but may not respond and should be referred for liver transplantation.

Several drugs are now available for the treatment of chronic HBV infection: interferon-α, pegylated interferon-α and the nucleoside/nucleotide analogues (lamivudine, telbivudine, entecavir, adefovir and tenofovir).[31] The efficacy of these drugs has been assessed in randomized controlled trials; the results may not be directly comparable as they did not compare all agents and used different HBV DNA assays. The aim of therapy is to reduce the level of HBV DNA to as low a level as possible, ideally below the lower limit of detection of a real-time PCR assay (10–15 IU/mL), leading to biochemical

TABLE 13.1 Interpretation of Serological Tests in HBV Infection

HBsAg	Anti-HBc (total)	Anti-HBc (IgM)	Anti-HBs	Interpretation
–	–	–	–	Susceptible
+	–	–	–	Early acute infection or early post-vaccination (<18 days)
+	+	+	–	Acute infection
–	+	+	±	Acute resolving infection
–	+	–	+	Recovered from acute infection and immune
+	+	–	–	Chronic infection
–	–	–	+	Immune if anti-HBs titre ≥10 mIU/mL post-vaccination or passive transfer post-HBV immune globulin
–	+	–	–	Four possible interpretations: 1. Susceptible with false-positive anti-HBc 2. Past infection 3. Occult infection 4. Passive transfer from mother to infant

remission, histological improvement and prevention of complications.

The main role of interferon is for the treatment of young patients with well-compensated liver disease, who do not wish to be on long-term treatment or are planning to be pregnant within the next 2–3 years and in whom drug resistance may limit their treatment options in the future. Interferon is also an attractive option for patients with HBV genotype A infection. The advantages of interferon compared to the other options are its finite duration of treatment, the absence of selection of resistant mutants and a more durable response. On the other hand, side-effects from interferon are troublesome and interferon cannot be used in patients with decompensated disease.

Lamivudine has been extensively used for the treatment of chronic HBV infection.[22] The main advantages of lamivudine are its safety profile (including its use in pregnancy) and its cost compared with the other oral agents. The main disadvantage of lamivudine is the high rate of drug resistance compared with other oral agents. The role of lamivudine is diminishing with the availability of newer therapies with more rapid and potent viral suppression and lower rates of drug resistance (e.g. entecavir, telbivudine and tenofovir). Lamivudine may still have a role in patients coinfected with HIV (in whom lamivudine may be part of the antiretroviral regimen).

Adefovir is active against lamivudine-resistant HBV but has a lower rate of virological suppression and, at the approved dose of 10 mg daily, up to 25% of patients experience minimal or no viral suppression. Adefovir has also been associated with nephrotoxicity, particularly at higher doses. Adefovir resistance was not detected after 1 year of treatment but the rate of drug resistance has been reported to be as high as 29% after 5 years of treatment. In vitro data suggest that adefovir is also effective in suppressing telbivudine- and entecavir-resistant HBV but clinical data are scant. The role of adefovir has diminished since the approval of tenofovir which is both more potent and has low rates of drug resistance than adefovir.

Entecavir has potent antiviral activity and low rates of drug resistance. It has an important role in the primary treatment of HBV infection and may also have an important role in patients with decompensated cirrhosis, although its safety in this patient population has not been well studied. Resistance to entecavir is rare among nucleoside-naïve patients (1% with up to 5 years of treatment) but resistance has been observed in up to 50% of lamivudine-refractory patients after 5 years of treatment. Studies in rodents using high doses have reported increased rates of hepatic tumours, but the clinical relevance of these findings is unclear.

Telbivudine appears to have slightly more potent antiviral effects compared with lamivudine and adefovir but selects the same mutations as lamivudine. It is also more expensive than lamivudine and there have been reported cases of myopathy and peripheral neuropathy. Its use is therefore limited. Tenofovir has more potent antiviral activity than adefovir and is effective in suppressing wild-type as well as lamivudine-resistant HBV. Tenofovir may be used as first-line treatment in treatment-naïve patients and in patients with lamivudine, telbivudine or entecavir resistance, preferably as additional treatment in these patients. Tenofovir can also be used to substitute for adefovir in patients who have inadequate viral response to adefovir. However, its efficacy in patients with adefovir-resistant HBV is limited. Tenofovir will probably replace adefovir in countries where it is approved because of its more potent antiviral activity.[32] Preliminary data indicate that resistance to tenofovir is rare after up to 4 years of treatment.

The definition of response depends on the type of antiviral therapy used. On interferon-α therapy, primary non-response is defined as <1 $\log_{10}$ IU/mL decrease in HBV DNA level from baseline at 3 months. Virological response is defined as an HBV DNA level <2000 IU/mL at 24 weeks of therapy. Serological response is defined by HBeAg seroconversion in those with HBeAg-positive disease. On nucleoside/nucleotide therapy, primary non-response is defined as the same as for interferon-α therapy. However, virological response is defined as an undetectable HBV DNA level within 48 weeks of therapy. A partial virological response is defined as decrease in HBV DNA level to <2000 IU/mL but above the limit of detection. Virological breakthrough is defined as an HBV DNA level of >1 $\log_{10}$ IU/mL compared with nadir HBV DNA level; it usually indicates poor adherence to therapy or development of resistance.

In the case of resistance developing to the first agent, addition of a second agent without cross-resistance is recommended. Discussion of salvage therapy and treatment of complicated cases (e.g. patients with cirrhosis or endstage renal disease, co-infection with HCV, HDV or HIV, infection in children or pregnant women, recurrent HBV after liver transplantation) is beyond the scope of this chapter but further information is available in the references.

PROGNOSIS OF HBV INFECTION

The prognosis of HBV infection appears to vary with the clinical setting. Long-term follow-up studies of HBsAg-positive blood donors have shown that the majority remain asymptomatic, with a very low risk of development of cirrhosis or HCC.[21,25] The prognosis is worse in HBV-infected patients from endemic areas and in patients with chronic HBV infection. The estimated 5-year rates of progression are: chronic hepatitis to cirrhosis 12–20%; compensated cirrhosis to decompensated liver disease 20–30%; compensated cirrhosis to HCC 6–15%. The cumulative survival rate for compensated cirrhosis is 85% at 5 years compared with 14–35% for decompensated cirrhosis.

Among Chinese patients with chronic HBV infection, the life-time risk of a liver-related death has been estimated at 40–50% for men and 15% for women. The risk of progression appears to be greatest in patients who stayed in the immune clearance phase, in patients who have delayed HBeAg seroconversion, in patients who had reactivation of HBV replication after HBeAg seroconversion and who have high viral loads.[33]

A number of studies have evaluated factors influencing survival in patients with chronic HBV infection. Patients with a prolonged replication phase have a worse prognosis, presumably related to prolonged inflammation or recurrent episodes of hepatitis, resulting in the development of cirrhosis and HCC. Other independent factors associated with poor survival were older age, hypoalbuminaemia, thrombocytopenia, splenomegaly and hyperbilirubinaemia. Biochemical remission and clearance of HBeAg or HBV DNA from the serum were significantly associated with a higher rate of survival. The risk of HCC is much higher in patients who are HBeAg positive compared with those who are HBsAg positive but HBeAg negative. Elevated serum HBV DNA levels also appear to be an independent risk factor for HCC.

Among patients who achieve HBeAg seroconversion a subset subsequently experience reactivation. Reactivation can occur in patients who receive immunosuppressive therapy, but can also occur spontaneously. A few studies have identified risk factors for reactivation including HBV genotype C, male gender, serum ALT levels greater than five times the upper limit of normal during the HBeAg-positive phase and age 40 years or older at HBeAg seroconversion.

PREVENTION OF HBV INFECTION

HBV infection may be prevented by immunization, either with a vaccine or with a specific immunoglobulin. Hepatitis B vaccine contains purified recombinant HBsAg adsorbed onto an aluminium hydroxide adjuvant. A combined vaccine containing inactivated HAV and HBsAg is also available. Hepatitis B vaccines are inactivated and cannot cause disease. They are effective in preventing HBV infection if given before or shortly after exposure. However, 10–15% of vaccinees either fail to respond to the vaccine or have a poor response to the vaccine; this is more common in persons aged over 40 years, obesity, alcoholics, advanced liver disease, endstage renal disease and immunosuppressed patients.

Pre-exposure immunization is used for persons who are at increased risk of HBV because of their lifestyle or occupation. In industrialized countries, pre-exposure immunization is recommended for the following groups: injection drug users; individuals who change sexual partners frequently; close family contacts of individuals with chronic HBV infection; families adopting children from countries with high or intermediate HBV prevalence; foster carers; patients with chronic renal failure or chronic liver disease; prison inmates; individuals living or working in residential accommodation for those with learning difficulties; people travelling or going to work in countries with high or intermediate HBV prevalence; and individuals at occupational risk of HBV, e.g. healthcare workers, laboratory workers. In 1992, the World Health Organization recommended that all highly endemic countries include hepatitis B vaccination into their national childhood immunization programmes by 1995 and all other countries by 1997. More than 160 countries have implemented universal hepatitis B vaccination.[34]

Post-exposure immunization is used to prevent infection after accidental inoculation or exposure to HBV-infected blood. Post-exposure prophylaxis is recommended for the following groups: babies born to mothers who have chronic HBV infection or acute HBV infection in pregnancy; sexual partners of cases with acute or chronic HBV infection; and persons who are accidentally inoculated or contaminated with blood from an HBsAg-positive donor.

The standard administration schedule of 0, 1 and 6 months is used where rapid protection is not required and compliance is likely to be good. For pre-exposure prophylaxis of those at high risk and for post-exposure prophylaxis an accelerated schedule of administration at 0, 1 and 2 months is used. For those at increased risk, a fourth dose at 12 months is recommended. One product (Engerix B) has been licenced for very rapid immunization schedule at 0, 7 and 21 days; a fourth dose at 12 months is again recommended. The full duration of protection afforded by HBV vaccine has not been established. Levels of antibody decline over time and vary widely between individuals. It is therefore recommended that a single booster dose of HBV vaccine should be given at 5 years after primary immunization. In those at risk of occupational exposure anti-HBs antibody levels should be checked post-immunization. Responders with an anti-HBs level of ≥100 IU/L do not require further doses but those with an anti-HBs level of 10–100 IU/L should be given another dose. Those with an anti-HBs level of <10 IU/L are considered non-responders and, provided that they are negative for other markers of HBV infection, should be given a second full course of vaccination.

Hepatitis B immunoglobulin (HBIG) provides passive immunity and can give immediate but temporary protection after accidental inoculation or exposure to HBV-infected blood. HBIG is given at the same time as vaccination and does not affect the development of active immunity. HBIG is recommended only in high-risk situations, e.g. babies of highly infectious mothers or vaccine non-responders. It should be given ideally within 48 hours of exposure, although it can be considered for up to 1 week after exposure. If infection has already occurred at the time of immunization, the severity of the illness may be attenuated and chronic infection may be prevented.

Hepatitis C Virus (HCV)

EPIDEMIOLOGY OF HCV INFECTION

HCV is a major global cause of chronic liver disease with an estimated 130 million people infected worldwide.[35] Acute infection is often asymptomatic and liver failure is rare. Acute HCV infection usually leads to chronic infection: 60–80% of cases develop chronic HCV infection and 20–30% of these develop

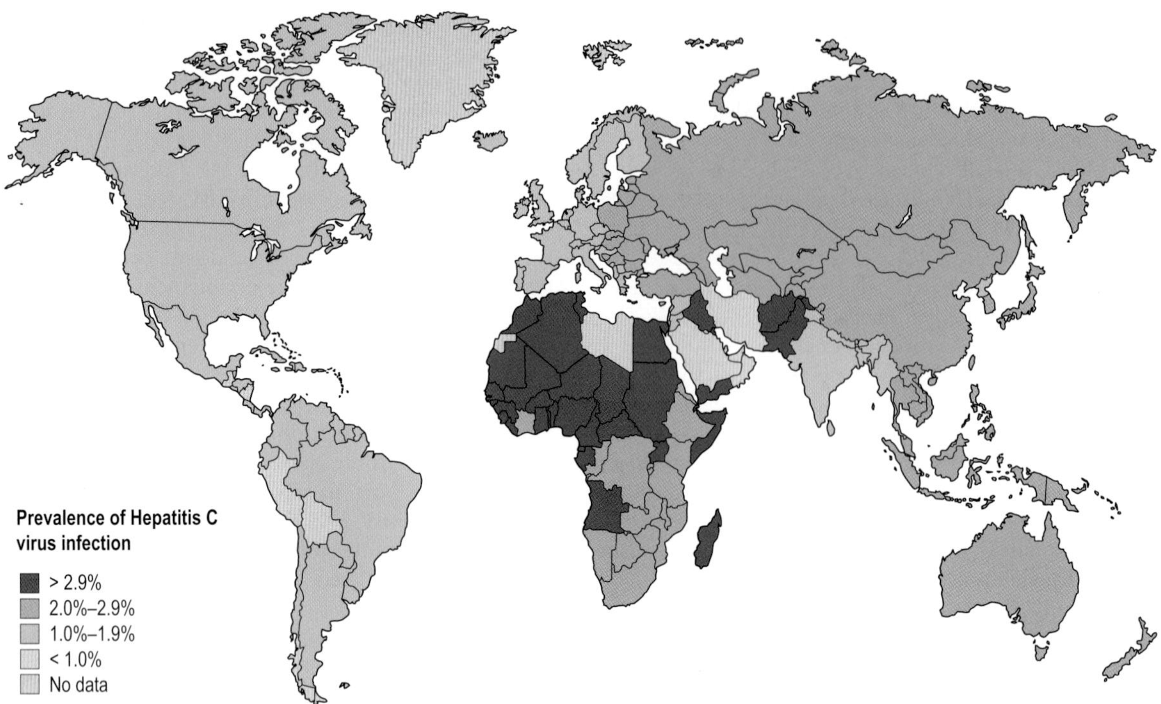

Figure 13.6 Prevalence of chronic hepatitis C virus infection. *(From CDC Health Information for International Travel 2012: The Yellow Book.)*

cirrhosis over a 20–30-year period. Acute HCV infection accounts for 10–20% of cases of acute hepatitis. Chronic HCV infection is the most frequent indication for liver transplantation. Hepatitis C is the cause of 27% of cirrhosis cases and 25% of hepatocellular carcinoma worldwide.

HCV prevalence varies with geographical region and population assessed – in Western Europe HCV prevalence ranges from 0.4–3% whereas in Egypt the overall prevalence is 9%, which rises to 50% in certain rural areas (Figure 13.6). Prior to the 1990s, the main routes of transmission were non-sterile injections, blood transfusion and injection drug use. Multiply transfused patients such as those with haemophilia or thalassaemia have been at particularly high risk of acquiring HCV. With the introduction of routine HCV screening and use of treated or recombinant blood products, the incidence of post-transfusion HCV has declined. Injection drug use remains the most common identifiable source of newly acquired HCV infection. However, up to 10% of patients with HCV infection have no identifiable risk factor. Nosocomial transmission of HCV infection has been reported in the context of medical and surgical procedures. Transplant recipients who receive organs from HCV-positive donors are at high risk of acquiring HCV infection and liver disease. The risk of sexual transmission is low, apart from in men who have sex with men (MSMs) and HIV-infected patients. Haemodialysis is a recognized risk factor for HCV infection with a 0.4–15% incidence of anti-HCV positivity in haemodialysis units. Parenteral transmission related to use of contaminated equipment, traditional medicine practices (e.g. acupuncture, scarification, cupping), tattooing, body piercing and commercial barbering have rarely been reported.

HCV STRUCTURE AND GENOME

HCV is an RNA virus that is classified in the Flaviviridae family. The HCV genome is a positive-sense single-strand RNA molecule of approximately 9500 nucleotides. There are highly conserved 5′ and 3′ untranslated regions flanking a 9000 nucleotide single ORF, which encodes a polyprotein of approximately 3000 amino acids. The polymerase enzyme of HCV lacks proof-reading ability resulting in errors in replication. Many of these nucleotide changes result in a non-functional genome or a lethal mutant. However, others persist and account for the tremendous genetic diversity that is characteristic of HCV.[36] This heterogeneity influences the pathogenesis of infection, response to antiviral therapies and prevents the development of conventional vaccines.

Six major genotypes and more than 50 subtypes have been described. Sequence homology between different genotypes is less than 80%. Genotype 1 is most common in Europe and the USA (60–70% of isolates); genotypes 2 and 3 are less common in these areas and genotypes 4, 5 and 6 are rare. Genotype 3 is most common in India, the Far East and Australia. Genotype 4 is most common in Africa and the Middle East but appears to be emerging in Europe among injection drug users and MSMs. Genotype 5 is most common in South Africa and genotype 6 is most frequent in Hong Kong, Vietnam and Australia.

Quasispecies are families of highly similar strains that develop within an infected host over time; sequence homology is greater than 95%. Differences between quasispecies are usually only apparent in the most rapidly changing parts of the genome (hypervariable regions). The clinical implications of quasispecies are not fully understood although they may be important in the natural history, persistence and response to treatment of the virus.[37] In one study of 59 patients with chronic HCV infection increased quasispecies heterogeneity was associated with longer estimated duration of infection, transmission by transfusion, higher HCV viral load and genotype 1. In another histological study, different quasispecies were compartmentalized in specific regions of the liver and the degree of compartmentalization was greater in histologically advanced disease.

PATHOGENESIS OF HCV INFECTION

HCV usually replicates in hepatocytes. Virus has been observed in other cell types, including lymphocytes and dendritic cells and within the central nervous system, but it is uncertain how this contributes to disease pathogenesis. After natural or experimental infection, virus may be detectable for weeks or months without any apparent clinical, biochemical or immunological disturbance. During this time, virus may replicate to high levels in blood and within the liver, indicating the minimal direct cytopathic effects of the virus in the absence of host immune responses. This silent phase is followed by the onset of acute hepatitis, which is not always clinically apparent. Detailed intrahepatic studies in animal models reveal that the initial responses are production of innate immune mediators (interferons, natural killer cells), followed by an influx of T-lymphocytes (both CD4+ and CD8+). In human studies of acute HCV infection, the emergence of highly activated, virus-specific CD8+ T cells correlates quantitatively and temporally with the peak of the alanine aminotransferase (ALT), suggesting that tissue damage at this stage is a result largely of the host T-cell response.

The subsequent events vary substantially between different patients, but three clinical patterns are observed: clearance of virus below the level of detection in blood; persistence of virus without host control; or an intermediate state, where the virus is transiently controlled, but relapses. The immunological differences determining these outcomes are not clear, but include both innate and adaptive components.[38] Polymorphisms linked to the IL28B gene indicate a major role for interferon-λ in acute outcome. Similarly, the association of specific HLA genes, both class II (such as HLA DR11/DQ3) and class I (such as HLA B27 and HLA B57), with spontaneous resolution point to the importance of T-cell responses. The broader and more sustained in number and function the responses are, the more likely they are to be successful in viral control. B-cell responses are also likely to be involved. However, the rapid emergence of viral escape mutants in the hypervariable envelope regions may limit the efficacy of neutralizing antibody responses in containing viral replication.[37] Viral mutation within T-cell epitopes is also a major cause of persistence despite T-cell responses, although other phenomena such as T-cell exhaustion and the emergence of regulatory T-cell subsets also contribute to T-cell failure.

In the 25% in whom virus is cleared below the level of detection long-term, antibody and T-cell responses may be detected for many years. In most people, virus persists after the acute hepatitis, despite the presence of antibody. T-cell responses in blood at this stage are weak, but infiltrates of T cells may be found within the liver. Viral genotype is not thought to have a major effect on pathogenesis, although genotype 3 has been associated with the development of hepatic steatosis, which might contribute to increased inflammation and fibrosis.

CLINICAL FEATURES OF HCV INFECTION

Acute HCV accounts for approximately 10–20% of cases of acute viral hepatitis. Most acute infections are asymptomatic or have a clinically mild course lasting 2–12 weeks. Symptoms are similar to other forms of acute hepatitis namely malaise, nausea, right upper quadrant pain – jaundice occurs in <25% of cases. Fulminant hepatic failure is very rare but may occur in patients with chronic HBV infection.

Failure to spontaneously eradicate infection occurs in 50–90% of cases. The reasons for persistence of HCV infection remain incompletely understood and may be related to virus or host factors. The high mutation rate and genetic diversity of the virus may allow HCV to escape immune recognition. On the other hand, host factors may influence the ability to clear the virus. For example, polymorphisms of a site close to the interleukin-28B (IL-28B) gene have been associated with higher clearance rates in individuals who had the C/C allele compared with those who had the T/T allele. These alleles also appear to be important predictors of response to antiviral treatment, as discussed below. Other factors that have been implicated in clearance of HCV infection include: the presence of specific HLA-DRB1 and DQB1 alleles; high titres of neutralizing antibodies against HCV structural proteins; persistence of HCV-specific CD4 T-cell responses; Caucasian patients with low levels of HCV viraemia during acute infection; female injection drug users.[39]

In addition to liver damage and hepatocellular carcinoma, HCV-related extrahepatic diseases are also reported. Mixed cryoglobulinaemia, lymphoproliferative disorders, thyroid autoimmune disorders and type 2 diabetes are proposed to be associated with a complex dysregulation of the cytokine/chemokine network, involving proinflammatory and Th1 chemokines.[40]

About 10–30% of chronic infections go on to develop cirrhosis over 30 years. Cirrhosis is more common in those co-infected with hepatitis B or HIV, alcoholics and those of male gender. Those who develop cirrhosis have a 20-fold greater risk of hepatocellular carcinoma at a rate of 1–3% per year and if this is complicated by alcoholism, the risk becomes 100-fold greater.

LABORATORY DIAGNOSIS OF HCV INFECTION

The diagnosis of HCV infection is made by detecting HCV antibody to recombinant HCV proteins in sensitive screening immunoassays. In low-prevalence populations, the probability of a false-positive antibody result is high and supplementary confirmatory tests, e.g. immunoassays using different antigens, should be performed. Alternatively, highly specific line or strip immunoblots (which have individual synthetic or recombinant antigens applied as separate lines to a solid phase) can distinguish different antigens to which the serum is reacting and confirm the presence of anti-HCV antibody.[41] The appearance of anti-HCV antibody after infection can take up to 2 months in immunocompetent people and may be delayed or even absent in immunocompromised patients, such as those with HIV infection or those who are on haemodialysis. By 6 months, 97% of those infected will have developed an antibody response. Recent developments include assays which combine tests for HCV antibody and HCV core antigen. These are useful for the diagnosis of acute infection as the HCV core antigen can be used to detect HCV infection during the window phase of infection. These assays are likely to be particularly useful for screening programmes, e.g. blood donation services and renal dialysis units.

Nucleic acid tests are essential for the diagnosis of acute and chronic HCV infection and should be used as supplementary tests for confirmation of HCV antibody tests. HCV RNA can be detected by polymerase chain reaction (PCR) as early as 2 weeks post-infection, prior to the appearance of HCV antibody.

Several amplification techniques, including reverse transcriptase PCR, transcription-mediated amplification and branched DNA are available.[41] Most commercial assays now produce quantitative results with increasingly sensitive limits of detection. Although quantitative tests may be important to predict the response to interferon (IFN) therapy, they are not useful in predicting disease severity or long-term progression. Some countries have successfully introduced nucleic acid screening of pools of samples for blood donation. Dried blood spot testing for both hepatitis C antibody and RNA is now widely available and can be used to facilitate screening in certain groups, e.g. injection drug users in needle-exchange programmes.

HCV virus genotyping is essential before treatment as it determines the duration of treatment and the response. Most genotyping methods are based on viral sequencing and subsequent phylogenetic analysis or on the detection of nucleic acid mutations specific for individual genotypes.[42]

A pre-treatment liver biopsy is frequently, but not always, performed in order to assess the stage of liver disease. It may also be helpful to exclude other causes of liver disease, guide treatment decisions and surveillance for HCC in those who are found to have cirrhosis. Sampling variability may result in the under-diagnosis of up to 15% of patients with cirrhosis. A number of non-invasive methods of assessing the degree of liver fibrosis using serum markers and assessment of liver stiffness using an ultrasound probe (e.g. Fibroscan, FibroSure/FibroTest) have been developed and are recommended by some centres.

Genotyping of the patient for IL28B polymorphisms can also contribute to pre-treatment evaluation. In genome-wide association studies (GWAS) of interferon/ribavirin therapy for HCV genotype 1 infection, a major impact of those IL28B polymorphisms which favour spontaneous clearance has been shown for treatment response.[43] Together with other clinical markers, this information can now be used to provide an indication of the likelihood of a successful response to therapy.

TREATMENT OF HCV INFECTION

The goal of antiviral therapy is to eradicate HCV RNA and achieve a sustained virological response (SVR), defined as being HCV RNA negative 6 months after completing antiviral therapy. An SVR is associated with a 98–100% chance of being HCV RNA negative in the long-term and is also associated with decreases in liver-related complications and mortality.[44] The decision to treat patients with chronic HCV infection is based on a number of factors including HCV RNA positivity, liver biopsy with chronic hepatitis and fibrosis, compensated liver disease, acceptable haematological and biochemical indices, ability to adhere to treatment and no contraindications to treatment. Additional factors such as alcohol or drug use, chronic kidney disease or prior liver transplantation may also influence treatment decisions.[45]

For many years, the mainstay of treatment for chronic HCV infection has been combination therapy with pegylated interferon and ribavirin, with treatment duration guided by HCV genotype and treatment response. Two formulations of pegylated interferon are available: peginterferon α-2a (given at a dose of 180 μg subcutaneously per week) and peginterferon α-2b (given at a dose of 1.5 mg/kg subcutaneously per week). For HCV genotype 1 and genotype 4 infections, the dose of ribavirin is weight-based and differs with the pegylated interferon preparation used. For HCV genotype 2 and genotype 3 infections the dose of ribavirin is 800 mg daily. Side-effects are frequent in patients treated with peginterferon/ribavirin therapy and the most common ones are anaemia, neutropenia, fatigue, 'flu-like symptoms and neuropsychiatric symptoms, e.g. depression, irritability. Anaemia is usually managed by reducing the dose of ribavirin. The duration therapy is usually 48 weeks for HCV genotype 1 and 4 infections and 24 weeks for HCV genotype 2 and 3 infections.

Once therapy is started the likelihood of achieving a SVR can be predicted by the virological response at 12 weeks of therapy. An early virological response (EVR) is defined as a >2 $\log_{10}$ reduction in HCV RNA or negative HCV RNA at week 12. Patients should also have HCV RNA monitoring at the end of treatment and 24 weeks after completing treatment to determine SVR.

More recently, the NS3/4A protease inhibitors telaprevir and boceprevir have been evaluated in clinical trials and found to markedly improve SVR rates.[46] Telaprevir has been shown to be effective in patients with HCV genotype 1 infections and preliminary data suggest it may have activity against HCV genotype 2, but limited activity against HCV genotypes 3 and 4. It is currently recommended for the treatment of HCV genotype 1 infection and is given orally at a dose of 750 mg three times per day with food. Telaprevir is given from the outset of therapy without a lead-in period of treatment with peginterferon and ribavirin. Boceprevir is a competitive inhibitor of the NS3 protease complex of HCV genotype 1 and does not have significant activity against other HCV genotypes. Boceprevir is given orally at a dose of 800 mg three times per day starting after a 4-week lead-in period of treatment with pegylated interferon and ribavirin. For both drugs the efficacy of treatment is influenced by a patient's prior treatment status and by changes in HCV viral load during therapy, which in turn influences the recommended duration of treatment. Response rates to protease inhibitor-containing regimens vary depending upon the patient's prior treatment: 67–75% in treatment-naïve patients; 69–88% in prior relapsers; 40–59% in prior partial responders; and 23–38% in prior non-responders. Rash is the most frequent side effect with telaprevir and anaemia occurs with both telaprevir and boceprevir.

A number of other directly acting agents are in clinical development. These include other NS3/4A protease inhibitors, NS5A inhibitors and polymerase inhibitors, which inhibit NS5B RNA-dependent RNA polymerase (RdRp) and are either nucleotide/nucleoside analogues or non-nucleoside inhibitors. Another approach to targeting HCV infection is to target host proteins that are required by the virus for its replication. Cyclosporin A is an immunosuppressive agent that inhibits the cellular protein cyclophilin A which in turns affects NS5A function. Alisporivir, a synthetic cyclosporine with potent activity against both HCV and HIV is currently being evaluated in clinical trials. Finally, nitazoxanide, an antiprotozoal agent, has been shown to inhibit HBV and HCV in cell culture systems and is also being evaluated.

PREVENTION OF HCV INFECTION

The development of an HCV vaccine has been hampered by the genetic diversity between HCV genotypes as well as large number of quasispecies within an individual which rapidly generate escape mutants. Furthermore, HCV infection is characterized by the presence of HCV antibodies that are ineffective in clearing the infection. Finally, the lack of a small animal experimental model makes developing a vaccine even more difficult. The strategies of vaccination against HCV may be either preventative (to prevent chronic infection) or therapeutic (to clear chronic infection by boosting the immune response). A number of vaccines are currently in development.[47]

Hepatitis D Virus (HDV)

EPIDEMIOLOGY OF HDV

Hepatitis D virus, also known as hepatitis delta virus, is a defective virus that is closely associated with HBV. Although HDV can replicate autonomously, it requires the presence of HBV for virion assembly and secretion; thus all patients with HDV are coinfected with HBV. Patients may be either simultaneously infected with HBV and HDV or an HBV carrier may be superinfected with HDV.

Approximately 5% of persons infected with HBV are co-infected with HDV. Since the estimated number of persons with HBV infection worldwide is 300 million, approximately 15 million are HDV-infected.[48] Interestingly, the geographical distribution of HDV infection does not completely mirror that of HBV infection, with some HBV-endemic areas having low HDV prevalence. HDV infection is endemic in the Mediterranean basin where infection occurs in children and young adults through mucosal or percutaneous spread, which is usually inapparent. Transmission within families is common and may be associated with poor hygiene and lower socioeconomic status. The prevalence of HDV among HBV carriers in the Far East is variable, ranging from 90% in the Pacific islands to 5% in Japan. HDV transmission has been associated with sexual transmission in Taiwan and injection drug use in Hong Kong. HDV infection is uncommon in industrialized countries and is mainly confined to certain populations, e.g. injection drug users, haemophiliacs and multiply transfused patients. The epidemiology of HDV is changing with in certain countries, e.g. falling rates in Italy as a result of improved socioeconomic conditions and HBV vaccination and prevention programmes. In contrast, other areas of the Mediterranean and Central Europe report rising rates, which may be related to immigration from endemic countries or high-risk behaviours such as injection drug use.[49]

HDV STRUCTURE AND GENOME

The HDV genome is a single-stranded RNA molecule of 1676–1683 nucleotides. There is significant sequence heterogeneity and eight genotypes have been proposed. Hepatitis D antigen (HDAg) is the only antigen of HDV and consists of a phosphoprotein encoded by an ORF on the RNA strand complementary to the genome (antigenomic strand). Approximately 70 molecules of HDAg are complexed with one molecule of HDV RNA to form a core-like structure.[49]

At least eight genotypes of HDV have been described.[50] Genotype 1 predominates in the Western hemisphere and is associated with an increased risk of fulminant infection in acute infection and more rapid progression to cirrhosis in chronic infection. Genotype 2 is the predominant genotype in the Far East and is associated with less severe acute infection and slower disease progression. Genotype 3 is found in South America, particularly in Columbia and Venezuela where severe outbreaks associated with a high incidence of liver failure have been reported. Genotype 2b has been reclassified as genotype 4. Genotypes 5–8 occur in Africa and are less well characterized than genotypes 1–3.

PATHOGENESIS OF HDV

The mechanisms by which HDV causes liver damage are incompletely understood but appear to be related to three factors: HDV-related factors (e.g. HDV genotype and expression of specific HDAg species); HBV-related factors (e.g. HBV genotype and level of replication) and host immune response. Similarly to HBV, HDV appears to cause direct cytopathic damage during acute infection and immune-mediated damage during chronic infection.

CLINICAL FEATURES OF HDV

The clinical manifestations of HDV infection can vary from acute hepatitis to fulminant hepatic failure, from an asymptomatic carrier state to decompensated chronic liver disease. Acute co-infection with HBV and HDV causes an acute hepatitis which is clinically indistinguishable from acute HBV infection. The rate of progression to chronic HDV infection is similar to that of HBV. Super-infection of an HBV carrier with HDV may also present with acute hepatitis; progression to chronic HDV infection occurs in almost all patients. Patients may also present with chronic hepatitis secondary to chronic HDV infection. In most cases of HDV infection HBV replication is suppressed to low levels and liver damage is essentially caused by HDV. Occasionally HBV and HDV may replicate simultaneously resulting in more severe liver disease. As discussed above, the clinical presentation of HDV infection appears to vary with genotype, with genotype 1 being associated with a higher risk of fulminant hepatic failure and chronic disease progression.[51]

LABORATORY DIAGNOSIS OF HDV

The laboratory diagnosis of HBV is dependent on serological tests for both HBV and HDV (Table 13.2). As a result of the dependence of HDV on HBV, all patients with HDV infection are positive for HBsAg. Those with acute HBV/HDV co-infection are also positive for anti-HBc IgM whereas those with HDV super-infection or chronic HDV infection are negative for anti-HBc IgM.

Serum HDAg may be detected early in acute HBV/HDV co-infection or HDV super-infection, but its presence is transient and it frequently missed. HDV antigenaemia is more prolonged in immunosuppressed patients. Serum HDAg is negative in chronic HDV infection. Serum HDV RNA also appears early in the course of acute HBV/HDV co-infection and HDV super-infection; in the former HDV RNA is transient whereas in the latter it is persistent. HDV RNA is also usually detectable in chronic HDV infection.

Serum total anti-HDV antibody is usually detectable 4 weeks after acute HDV infection. In acute HBV/HDV co-infection anti-HDV IgM is transient and may sometimes be the only marker of HDV infection. In HDV super-infection, anti-HDV IgM titres increase rapidly and are persistent. In chronic HDV infection anti-HDV IgM titres are variable and anti-HDV IgG titres are high.

TABLE 13.2 Interpretation of Serological Tests in HDV Infection

Diagnostic Marker	Acute HBV/HDV Co-Infection	Acute HDV Super-Infection	Chronic HDV Infection
HBsAg	+	+	+
Anti-HBc IgM	+	–	–
Serum HDAg	Early, transient	Early, transient	–
Serum HDV RNA	Early, transient	Early, persistent	Usually positive
Anti-HDV total	Late, low titre	Rapidly increasing titre	High titre
Anti-HDV IgM	Transient	Rapidly increasing, persistent	–
Liver HDAg	Not indicated	Positive	Usually positive but may be negative in late stages

Both HDAg and HDV RNA may be detected in liver histopathological specimens. Although the detection of HDAg in liver tissue has been proposed as a gold standard, up to 50% of cases who have been HDV infected for 10 years or more are negative for HDAg.

TREATMENT OF HDV INFECTION

There is no established treatment for acute HDV infection. The aim of treatment of chronic HDV infection is to eradicate or achieve long-term suppression of HDV and HBV replication. For HDV infection the primary aim is suppression of HDV replication (HDV RNA negativity in blood) which is accompanied by normalization of the serum ALT and improvement in hepatic inflammation. A secondary aim is to eradicate HBV infection with conversion of HBsAg to anti-HBs and thus to protect the patient from reinfection with HBV or HDV.[49] There is little evidence that current treatments achieve this goal.

Interferon-α is the only agent that is currently licensed for the treatment of HDV. The mechanism of action of interferon-α against HDV is unclear as it does not appear to have any in vitro activity against HDV; rather its effects may be related to activity against HBV or immunomodulatory effects. A meta-analysis of six trials, including 201 participants in total, concluded that there was a modest benefit in suppressing viral and liver disease activity in some patients, but such benefits were not sustained in the majority of patients.[52] The only factor that was associated with an increased likelihood of response to interferon-α was a short duration of infection.

Pegylated interferon appears to be more effective than standard interferon-α, but again data are limited to a few studies. The largest study included 38 patients who were treated with peginterferon-α2b, with or without ribavirin for 24 weeks. At 48 weeks, 21% of patients had an undetectable HDV RNA, with similar response rates in the monotherapy and combination therapy arms. The response rate was slightly higher in those who had not previously received interferon-α.

The use of nucleoside analogues in combination with pegylated interferon has also been investigated. The largest study of 90 patients compared pegylated interferon alone or in combination with adefovir and adefovir monotherapy. At 48 weeks 25% of patients in the two pegylated interferon arms were HDV RNA negative, compared with 0% in the adefovir monotherapy arm. Furthermore, patients receiving pegylated interferon had a significant decline in HBsAg.[49]

Several other agents (e.g. ribavirin, foscarnet, THF-γ 2, lamivudine and famciclovir) have been investigated for the treatment of HDV infection; overall the results have been disappointing.

PREVENTION OF HDV INFECTION

The mainstay of prevention of HDV infection is vaccination against HBV infection (see Prevention of HBV infection, above). Experimental vaccination studies, using various forms of HDAg in woodchucks, have shown partial protection but human development of these vaccines is unlikely, given the need to screen all potential vaccine recipients for HBsAg prior to vaccination.

Hepatitis E Virus (HEV)

EPIDEMIOLOGY OF HEV INFECTION

Hepatitis E virus, previously known as waterborne or enterically transmitted non-A, non-B hepatitis, was first reported in New Delhi in 1955. Although HEV is found worldwide the highest incidence of infection is in Asia, Africa, the Middle East and Central America (Figure 13.7). In the largest reported outbreak, over 100 000 individuals were infected in China. Large outbreaks have also been reported from Chad, Darfur, Uganda and Sudan.

HEV is transmitted by the faeco-oral route in endemic areas and causes an acute hepatitis. Fulminant infection may occur and is more frequent in pregnancy. High attack rates are seen in adults aged 15–40 years. Person-to-person transmission is uncommon. In endemic areas, HEV can be transmitted by blood transfusion and vertically from mother to child during the third trimester of pregnancy.[53]

Sporadic cases in Western countries have mainly occurred in travellers returning from endemic areas. However, HEV can infect pigs and rodents, suggesting that some human cases may be due to zoonotic transmission. Reports from Japan, Germany and France have documented transmission from consumption of undercooked animal meat and meat products.[54] Zoonotic transmission is also supported by the observation of high anti-HEV seroprevalence among people with occupational contact with animals. Risk factors for exposure remain unclear in some patients and HEV infection appears to be more frequent in industrialized countries than was previously realized. Chronic HEV infection is rare but has been described in solid organ transplant recipients and, rarely, in patients with other forms of immunosuppression.

HEV STRUCTURE AND GENOME

HEV is an icosahedral, non-enveloped single-stranded RNA virus that is approximately 27–34 nm in diameter. It has been classified as the single member of the genus *Hepevirus* in the family Hepeviridae. The genome comprises three large ORFs,

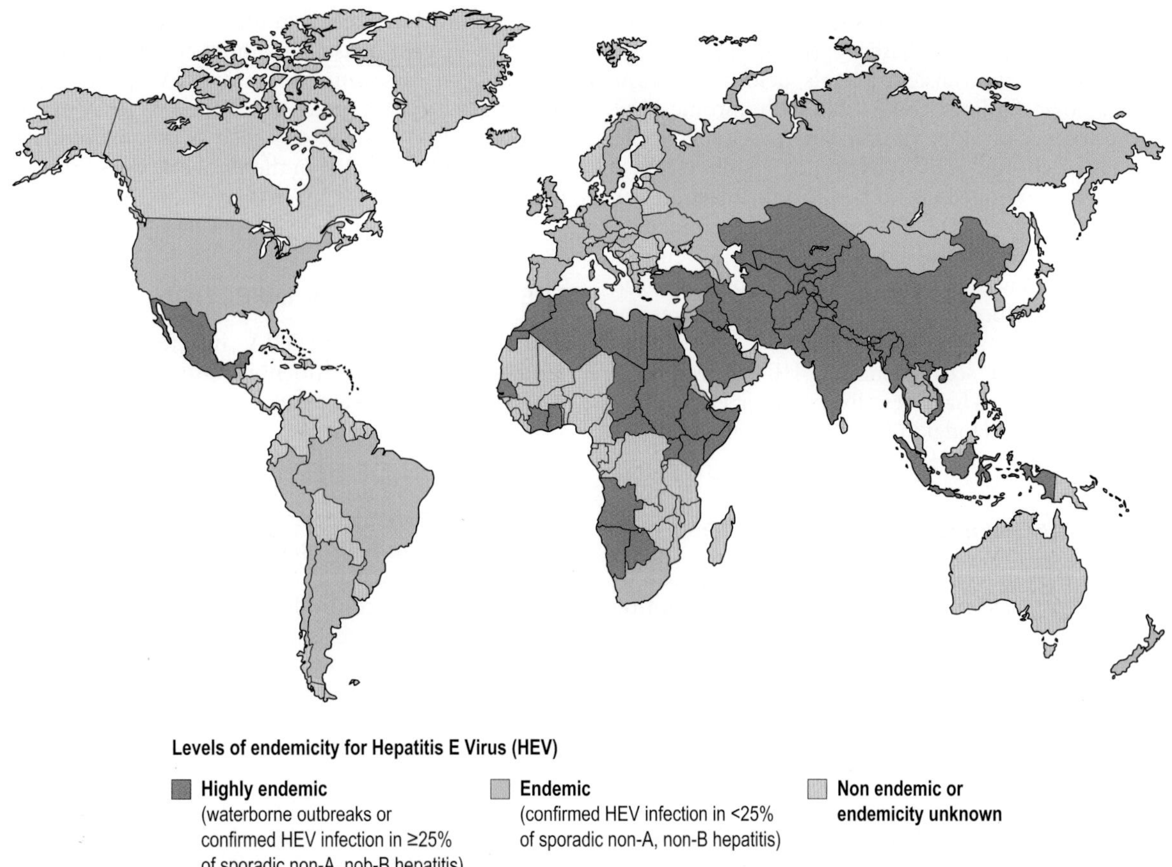

Figure 13.7 Distribution of hepatitis E infection, 2010. *(From CDC Health Information for International Travel 2012: The Yellow Book.)*

the largest of which consists of 1693 codons and codes for the nonstructural proteins that are responsible for the processing and replication of the virus. The second ORF consists of 660 codons and codes for structural proteins, while the third ORF consists of 123 codons and has an undetermined function. The crystal structure of HEV has revealed domains involved in cell-surface binding and cell entry, as well as potential neutralization sites. Phylogenetic analysis suggests that there are four genotypes and up to 24 subtypes. Genotypes 1 and 2 appear to be confined to humans, whereas genotypes 3 and 4 infect both humans and animals. The association between genotype and clinical features is incompletely understood, although genotype 3 has been associated with less severe disease.[55]

PATHOGENESIS OF HEV INFECTION

The histological features of HEV are similar to those seen in other forms of acute viral hepatitis. In the classic presentation, liver biopsy reveals focal necrosis, ballooned hepatocytes and acidophilic degeneration of hepatocytes. In the cholestatic form changes include bile stasis in canaliculi and gland-like transformation of hepatocytes. In fatal cases sub-massive as well as massive hepatic necrosis has been seen.[56]

CLINICAL FEATURES OF HEV INFECTION

HEV generally causes a self-limited acute infection, although fulminant hepatitis can develop, particularly in pregnancy. Chronic hepatitis does not develop after acute HEV infection, except in the transplant setting.

The incubation period of HEV infection ranges from 15 to 60 days. The clinical symptoms and signs are similar to those of other causes of acute viral hepatitis, although some patients have asymptomatic infection. Jaundice is usually accompanied by malaise, anorexia, nausea, vomiting, abdominal pain, fever and hepatomegaly. Laboratory findings include elevated serum concentrations of bilirubin, ALT and AST, which usually resolve 1–6 weeks after the onset of the illness. Prolonged cholestasis has been described in up to 60% of patients. Other less common features include diarrhoea, arthralgia, pruritus and an urticarial rash.[53]

Fulminant hepatitis can occur, resulting in an overall case fatality rate of 0.5–3%. For reasons that are not understood, fulminant hepatic failure occurs more frequently in pregnancy, resulting in a mortality rate of 15–25%, primarily during the 3rd trimester of pregnancy. Pregnant women with acute HEV infection and jaundice appear to have poorer obstetric and fetal outcomes compared with pregnant women with acute viral hepatitis of other causes.

In patients with pre-existing liver disease and those who are malnourished infection with HEV can lead to hepatic decompensation.[57] HEV infection has been reported in solid organ transplant recipients. In a French prospective study of 217 patients, acute HEV infection was diagnosed in 6.5% of patients. In another study, the main risk factor for acute HEV infection was consumption of insufficiently cooked pork or game. A subset of solid organ transplant recipients appear to develop chronic HEV infection based upon the presence of persistently elevated aminotransferase levels, detectable serum HEV RNA, histologic findings compatible with chronic viral hepatitis in the absence of other viral causes. A separate report described a case of chronic HEV infection in a kidney transplant recipient who developed cirrhosis. Chronic infection has been associated with lower CD2, CD3 and CD4 T-lymphocyte counts and the use of tacrolimus immunosuppression. In one report, 30% of patients with chronic HEV infection cleared the infection following reduction of their immunosuppressive therapy.

In the non-transplant setting chronic HEV infection is extremely rare. Case reports have described chronic HEV infection in patients with non-Hodgkin lymphoma receiving rituximab and in one patient with HIV infection.

LABORATORY DIAGNOSIS OF HEV INFECTION

The diagnosis of HEV infection is based on the detection of antibodies to HEV or detection of HEV in serum or stool by PCR.

Anti-HEV IgM appears early in the course of illness and disappears over 4–5 months. Anti-HEV IgG appears shortly after the anti-HEV IgM and increases through the acute phase and convalescent phase, remaining elevated for up to 14 years. Simultaneous assessment of anti-HEV IgA has been recommended to improve specificity as the IgM assay may cross-react with other IgM-based assays such as rheumatoid factor IgM.[53]

HEV can be detected in the stool one week after the onset of illness and persists for up to 2 weeks. HEV viraemia is usually short-lived but can persist up to 4 months.

TREATMENT OF HEV INFECTION

The treatment of acute HEV infection is supportive. Case reports of ribavirin treatment in chronic HEV infection suggest that it may be beneficial but further studies are needed.

PREVENTION OF HEV INFECTION

Travellers to endemic areas should avoid drinking water that is not boiled or purified and consuming uncooked fruits, vegetables, meat and shellfish. HEV vaccines are in development and two randomized controlled trials in endemic settings have shown benefit. There is no evidence to support the use of human normal immune globulin for pre- or post-exposure prophylaxis of HEV infection.[58]

REFERENCES

1. Franco E, Meleleo C, Serino L, et al. Hepatitis A: Epidemiology and prevention in developing countries. World J Hepatol 2012;4(3):68–73.
22. Lok AS, McMahon BJ. Chronic hepatitis B: update 2009. Hepatology 2009;50(3):661–2.
45. Ghany MG, Nelson DR, Strader DB, et al. An update on treatment of genotype 1 chronic hepatitis C virus infection: 2011 practice guideline by the American Association for the Study of Liver Diseases. Hepatology 2011;54(4):1433–44.
49. Hughes SA, Wedemeyer H, Harrison PM. Hepatitis delta virus. Lancet 2011;378(9785):73–85.
53. Aggarwal R, Jameel S. Hepatitis E. Hepatology 2011;54(6):2218–26.

Access the complete references online at www.expertconsult.com

14 Arbovirus Infections

PAUL R. YOUNG | LISA F. P. NG | ROY A. HALL | DAVID W. SMITH | CHERYL A. JOHANSEN

KEY POINTS

- Arbovirus infections are mostly zoonoses; primarily infections of vertebrates other than humans that occasionally spill over into human populations following transmission by an infected insect vector.
- Dengue virus is the most important human arboviral infection causing up to 300 million infections globally each year.
- Ecological and human demographic factors are the driving forces behind changes in arboviral prevalence and spread.
- The impact of climate change on global arbovirus transmission is unknown, but likely to be significant, given the complex interaction these viruses, their hosts and vectors have with their environment.
- Arbovirus evolution plays a major role in the changing patterns of disease and spread, e.g. a single amino acid change in the envelope protein of Chikungunya virus resulted in adaptation to a secondary mosquito vector leading to a dramatic expansion of the geographic range of this virus.
- Despite the large number of arboviruses that cause disease, vaccines for human use are commercially available for only a few, e.g. JEV and TBEV. There are no effective therapeutics available for clinical use, with treatment of patients primarily supportive and symptomatic.
- Arboviruses cause a range of clinical symptoms including systemic febrile disease, haemorrhagic fever, encephalitis and polyarthralgia.

Introduction

Arboviruses (arthropod-borne viruses) are a diverse group of viruses that survive in nature by transmission from infected to susceptible hosts by certain species of mosquitoes, ticks, sandflies or biting midges.[1,2] Following ingestion of a blood meal from an infected host, viruses multiply within tissues of the arthropod during what is referred to as the extrinsic incubation period, often to a high titre, particularly in the salivary glands. They are then passed on to humans or other vertebrates during insect biting. Most diseases caused by arboviruses are zoonoses, that is, they are primarily infections of vertebrates other than humans that can occasionally cause incidental infections in humans. Two major exceptions to this are o'nyong-nyong (ONNV) and dengue (DENV) viruses, as humans are the primary vertebrate host. Indeed passage through humans is essential in maintaining the virus transmission cycle. Monkeys have been implicated as an alternative vertebrate host to humans for dengue in rural settings and it is presumed that there is an unidentified vertebrate host for ONNV. By definition arboviruses are arthropod-borne, however some viruses are classed as arboviruses even though they have not been associated with an arthropod vector, primarily because of their close genetic relationship to those that are.

The names by which these viruses are known are of mixed origin. Some are dialect names for the illnesses they cause (chikungunya, o'nyong-nyong), some are place names (West Nile, Bwamba) and some derive from clinical characteristics (Western equine encephalitis, yellow fever).[1,2]

In this chapter, we will concentrate on the medically important arboviruses. For more detailed information about the viruses and the diseases they cause, a number of major reviews of specific viruses are cited at the beginning of each section.

Aetiology

There are over 500 arboviruses recognized worldwide[2] but only some are implicated in human disease.[3] Some infect humans only occasionally or cause only mild illness, whereas others are of great medical importance and can cause large epidemics with considerable mortality (Table 14.1).

In this chapter viruses are classified according to the ninth report of the International Committee on Taxonomy of Viruses.[4] Most arboviruses causing human disease belong to three major families: Togaviridae (genus *Alphavirus*), Flaviviridae (genus *Flavivirus*) and Bunyaviridae (*Bunyavirus*, *Orthobunyavirus*, *Nairovirus* and *Phlebovirus* genera). The alphaviruses and flaviviruses are enveloped, linear single-stranded, positive-sense RNA viruses. They are spherical in shape, with an underlying capsid and measuring from 40 to 70 nm.[5,6] The *Bunyaviruses* are enveloped, segmented circular negative-strand RNA viruses. They are generally spherical and measure 80–120 nm in diameter.

The flaviviruses are the most important group medically and three infections caused by viruses in this group: yellow fever virus (YFV), dengue virus (DENV) and Japanese encephalitis virus (JEV), are sufficiently prevalent to be of global concern.[7] Others, including tick-borne encephalitis virus (TBEV), Venezuelan equine encephalitis virus (VEEV), St Louis encephalitis virus (SLEV) and West Nile virus (WNV), are usually restricted to specific regions. However, the spread of arboviruses across several regions may cause international health problems.[1] This has occurred most recently with WNV moving from the Middle-East (Israel) into North and South America, Rift Valley fever virus (RVFV) moving from Africa to the Middle East, JEV moving into the Australasian region and chikungunya virus

TABLE 14.1 Arboviruses

Virus[a]	Geographical Distribution	Transmission	Fever	Clinical Form	Rash
Togaviridae					
***ALPHAVIRUS* GENUS**					
Babanki	Africa	Mosquito			
*Barmah Forest virus (BFV)	Australia	Mosquito	+	A	+
*Chikungunya virus (CHIKV)	Africa, India, South-east Asia	Mosquito	+	H/A	+
Getah virus (GETV)	Asia, Australasia	Mosquito	+		
*Mayaro virus (Uruma) (MAYV)	South America	Mosquito	+		+
*O'nyong-nyong virus (ONNV)	Africa	Mosquito	+	A	+
*Ross River virus (RRV)	Australia, South Pacific	Mosquito	+	A	+
*Sindbis virus (SINV)	Africa, Asia, Europe, Australia	Mosquito	+	A	+ (Africa only)
Semliki Forest virus (SFV)	Africa, Russia	Mosquito	+		
*Ockelbo virus (OCKV)	Europe	Mosquito	+	A	+
*Eastern equine encephalitis virus (EEEV)	North and South America	Mosquito	+	E	
*Western equine encephalitis virus (WEEV)	North and South America	Mosquito	+	E	
*Venezuelan equine encephalitis virus (VEEV)	North and South America	Mosquito	+	E	
Flaviviridae					
***FLAVIVIRUS* GENUS**					
Mosquito-Borne					
Banzi virus (BANV)	Southern Africa	Mosquito	+		
Bouboui virus (BOUV)	Central Africa	Mosquito			
Bussuquara virus (BSQV)	Central and South America	Mosquito	+	A	
*Dengue virus-type 1–4	Asia, America, the Caribbean and Pacific Islands, China, Taiwan, Indonesia, Australia	Mosquito	+	H	+
Edge Hill virus (EHV)	Australia	Mosquito	+	A	
Ilhéus virus (ILHV)	South and North America	Mosquito	+	E	
*Japanese encephalitis virus (JEV)	Asia, Australia	Mosquito	+	E	
Karshi virus (KSIV)	Kazakhstan, Uzbekistan	Tick	+		
Kedougou virus (KEDV)	Senegal, Central Africa	Mosquito			
Kokobera virus (KOKV)	Australia, New Guinea	Mosquito	+	A	+
Koutango virus (KOUV)	Senegal	Mosquito	+	A	+
*Kunjin virus (KUNV)	Australia, Indonesia, Malaysia	Mosquito	+	A/E	+
*Murray Valley encephalitis virus (MVEV)	Australia, New Guinea	Mosquito	+	E	
*Rocio virus (ROCV)	Brazil	Mosquito	+	E	
Sepik virus (SEPV)	New Guinea	Mosquito	+		
Spondweni virus (SPOV)	South Africa	Mosquito	+	A	
*St Louis encephalitis virus (SLEV)	Americas	Mosquito	+	E	
Usutu virus (USUV)	Sub-Saharan Africa	Mosquito	+		+
Wesselsbron virus (WESSV)	Africa, Asia	Mosquito	+	E	+
*West Nile virus (WNV)	Africa, India, Europe, North America	Mosquito	+	E	+
*Yellow fever virus (YFV)	Africa, South and Central America	Mosquito	+	H	
Zika virus (ZIKV)	Africa	Mosquito	+		+
Tick-Borne					
*Kyasanur Forest disease virus (KFDV)	India	Ixodid tick	+	H/E	+
Langat virus (LANV)	Malaysia, Asia, Japan	Ixodid tick	+	E	
Louping ill virus (LIV)	Britain, southern Europe	Ixodid tick	+	E	
*Omsk haemorrhagic fever virus (OHFV)	Siberia	Ixodid tick	+	H	+
*Powassan virus (POWV)	Canada, USA, Russia	Ixodid tick	+	E	
*Tick-borne encephalitis virus (TBEV)					
Far-Eastern subtype TBEV (RSSE)	Russia, Siberia, Asia	Ixodid tick	+	E	
European subtype TBEV	Europe	Ixodid tick	+	E	
Siberian subtype TBEV	Russia and Siberia	Ixodid tick	+	E	
Tyuleniy virus (TYUV)	Northern Europe, Russia North America	Tick	+	A	

TABLE 14.1 Arboviruses—cont'd

Virus[a]	Geographical Distribution	Transmission	Fever	Clinical Form	Rash
Other Vectors					
Rio Bravo virus (RBV)	USA, Trinidad	?Bat saliva	+	E, meningitis	
Bunyaviridae					
***BUNYAVIRUS* GENUS**					
Bunyamwera virus (BUNV)	Africa, North and South America	Mosquito	+	E	
Caraparu virus (CARV)	South America, Panama	Mosquito	+		
Itaqui virus (ITQV)	South America	Mosquito	+		
Marituba virus (MTBV)	Trinidad, South/Central America	Mosquito	+		
Oriboca virus (ORIV)	South America	Mosquito	+		
CALIFORNIA GROUP					
*California encephalitis virus (CEV)	USA, Canada	Mosquito	+	E	
Inkoo virus (INKV)	Finland	Mosquito	+	Meningism	
*La Crosse virus (LACV)	USA, Canada	Mosquito	+	E	
*Tahyna virus (Lumbo) (TAHV)	Europe, Africa	Mosquito	+		
Trivittatus virus (TVTV)	USA	Mosquito	+		
Orthobunyavirus Genus					
Bwamba virus (BWAV)	Africa	Mosquito	+		
Guaroa virus (GROV)	South and Central America	Mosquito	+		
*Oropouche virus (OROV)	South America	Mosquito/Culicoides	+	E/A	
Guama virus (GMAV)	South America	Mosquito	+		
Catu virus (CATUV)	South America	Mosquito	+		
***NAIROVIRUS* GENUS**					
CRIMEAN–CONGO GROUP					
*Crimean–Congo haemorrhagic fever virus (CCHFV)	Europe, Africa, Middle East, central Asia, Pakistan	Ixodid tick	+	H	+
Dugbe virus (DUGV)	Africa	Ixodid tick	+		
Nairobi sheep disease virus (NSDV)	Africa, India	Ixodid tick	+	A	
Phlebovirus Genus					
*Sandfly fever virus (Naples, SFNV; Sicily, SFSV)	Africa, Asia, central Europe	Sandflies	+		
Toscana virus (TOSV)	Italy, Portugal, Cyprus	Sandflies		E, meningitis	
*Rift Valley fever virus (RVFV)	Africa, Middle East	Mosquito	+	H/E	
Chandiru virus (CDUV)	Brazil	?	+		
Chagres virus (CHGV)	Panama	?Phlebotomines/ mosquito	+		
OTHER UNASSIGNED *BUNYAVIRIDAE*					
Bhanja virus (BHAV)	India, southern Europe	Tick	+		
Tataguine virus (TATV)	Nigeria	Mosquito	+		
REOVIRIDAE					
***COLTIVIRUS* GENUS**					
*Colorado tick fever virus (CTFV)	North America	Tick	+	H/E (in children)	+
Kemerovo complex	Former USSR and central Europe	Tick	+	E	
Orungo virus (ORUV)	Africa	Mosquito	+		

H, haemorrhagic; E, encephalitis; A, arthralgia. *Of clinical importance. [a]Classification of viruses according to virus taxonomy: 9th Report of the International Committee on Taxonomy of Viruses (2012).[4]

(CHIKV) moving into islands in the South-west Indian Ocean and South-east Asia. The major reasons for virus movement will be discussed later in the chapter.

Epidemiology

For effective arbovirus transmission to occur, three components are necessary: the vector (mosquito, tick, sandfly, biting midge), the vertebrate host(s) and suitable environmental conditions. Transmission cycles range from simple (involving one vector and one host, e.g. DENV) to the highly complex (involving multiple vectors and hosts, e.g. TBEV and JEV). The epidemiology of human arboviral diseases usually involves one of two transmission cycles. In the jungle or sylvatic cycle (where the pathogen is maintained in wild animals), an infected arthropod bites either a human or domestic animal that has strayed into the ecological niche of the virus/vector. This mode of infection results in small clusters of cases initiated at the same site. The second is the urban cycle where a person or domestic animal, infected via the sylvatic mode or moving from another area with urban activity, acts as an amplifier host in the transfer of the virus to other persons or domestic animals in the community. These cases occur as epidemics or epizootics in nature.[2] The vector species involved in the urban cycle may be the same or different to that in the sylvatic cycle. YFV is a good example of an arbovirus that undergoes both modes of transmission.[8] Figure 14.1 shows examples of the types of transmission cycles that can occur in nature. The interactions between vectors, hosts and environmental conditions that are necessary for virus transmission to occur are discussed briefly below.

VERTEBRATE HOSTS

The major hosts for arboviruses are mammals and birds.[1] The potential for virus dispersal is dependent on the type of vertebrate host involved. Migratory birds can facilitate virus movement over large distances whereas most land-based animal hosts result in virus activity tending to be restricted to a particular region. These have been reviewed elsewhere[9] and are summarized below.

Reservoir Hosts

These include hosts that have previously been referred to elsewhere as either maintenance or amplifier hosts. These hosts are responsible for virus transmission and are essential for the continued existence of the virus. The immune status of the host species will affect the rates of transmission of arboviruses. Reservoir hosts become infected by the virus and produce high-titre viraemias enabling virus transmission to occur. However, they are generally not susceptible to disease. Arboviruses may have more than one host species involved in transmission cycles. An example of this is the *flavivirus* JEV, for which birds (particularly herons) are considered to be the major maintenance hosts in natural cycles. However, in Asia pigs are often kept in close proximity to human dwellings and it has been shown that these animals amplify the virus to high titres that are sufficient to infect mosquitoes, which can then transmit the virus to humans. This is thought to have occurred in the Torres Strait (Australia) in 1995, when JEV was detected in the region for the first time.

Disseminating Hosts

These host species may move virus from an area of active transmission to another location. Movement by viraemic waterbirds has been suggested as a mechanism of spread for a number of arboviruses including Murray Valley encephalitis virus (MVEV), JEV, WNV and Eastern equine encephalitis virus (EEEV). Arboviruses can also be introduced into new areas by the movement of humans, particularly as air travel now enables long-distance travel during the few days that they are viraemic. This has been implicated in the spread of DENV between continents. Infected arthropod vectors may also disseminate disease if they are carried on air, marine, rail or road transport. This has been proposed as the most likely mechanism for introduction of WNV into the USA in 1999.

Incidental and Dead-end Hosts

Some hosts become infected but transmission does not occur with sufficient regularity for stable maintenance. For many arbovirus infections humans are usually an incidental host, often, but not always being a dead end in the transmission chain. Incidental hosts may or may not show symptoms and while infected by the virus, do not develop a high enough viraemia to enable transmission to other vectors. Occasionally, one or a few abortive cycles of transmission may occur between these hosts and the vectors, but they cannot be sustained.

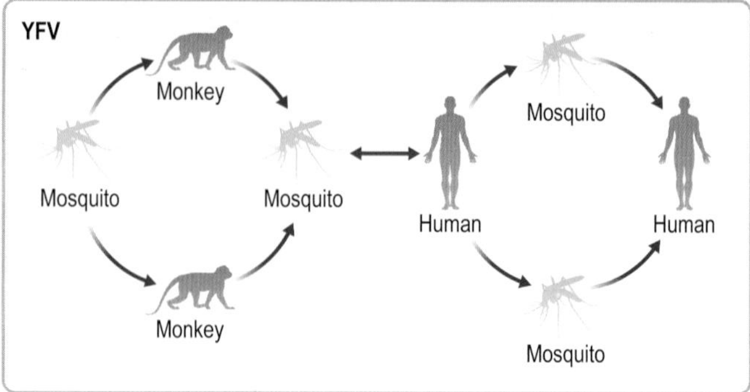

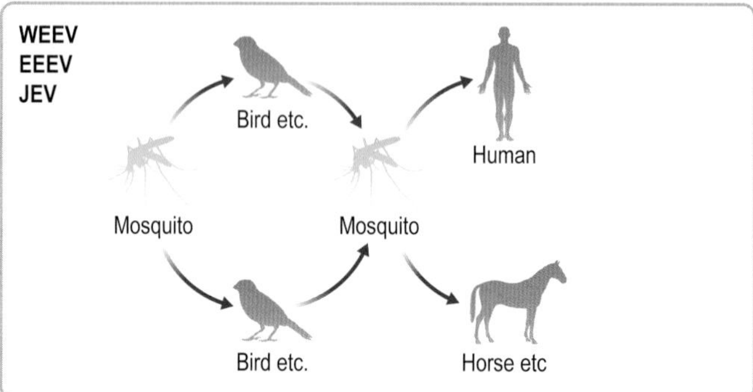

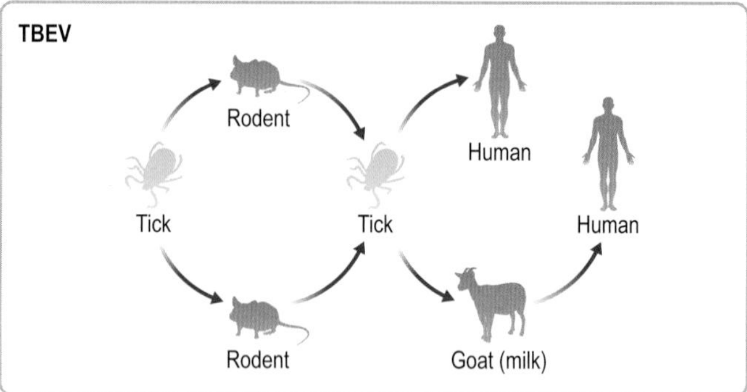

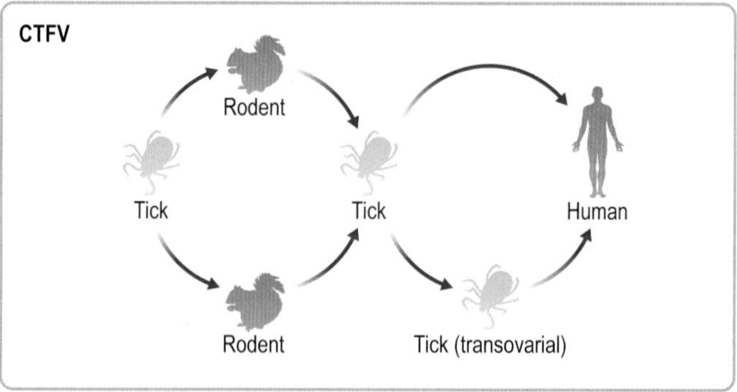

Figure 14.1 Vectors (yellow) and hosts (blue) in the transmission of selected arboviruses. YFV, yellow fever virus; WEEV, Western equine encephalitis virus; EEEV, Eastern equine encephalitis virus; JEV, Japanese encephalitis virus; TBEV, tick-borne encephalitis virus; CTFV, Colorado tick fever virus.

A wide variety of host species have been implicated in arbovirus diseases. As noted above these are commonly birds and mammals (including primates, rodents, marsupials and bats). The host species associated with the major human and animal pathogens described in this chapter are included in the sections on the specific viruses.

VECTORS/INVERTEBRATE HOSTS

Arthropod-borne viruses are distinguished from other animal viruses because of their ability to infect both vertebrate and invertebrate hosts. The virus replicates within the cells of the arthropod vector before being transferred to a susceptible host.[10] Occasionally, arthropods may also transmit viruses by mechanical transmission whereby the vector simply transfers the virus from an infected to a susceptible host without replication in the vector itself. Direct transfer from an infected to an uninfected vector during co-feeding on a naïve host has also been reported (WNV).

Invertebrate hosts include mosquitoes, sandflies, ticks and culicoides (biting midges). Most arboviruses have been recovered from mosquitoes; a list of the vectors is given in Table 14.1. Ixodid ticks are involved in transmission of a closely interrelated subgroup of the flaviviruses and also in some of the other groups. Genera of ticks involved in arbovirus transmission include Haemaphysalis, Ixodes and Dermacentor.

Transmission

Transmission by arthropods involves several processes:

- Ingestion by the arthropods of virus in the blood (usually) or other body fluids of the vertebrate hosts.
- Penetration of the viruses into the tissue of the arthropods, in the gut wall, or elsewhere after passing through the gut wall ('gut barrier').
- Multiplication of the viruses in arthropod cells, including those of the salivary glands.[11]

The time interval between ingestion of a viraemic blood meal and the ability of a vector to transmit the virus is known as the extrinsic incubation period. In mosquitoes, this period is relatively short: approximately 10 days at 30°C (ambient temperature) and longer at lower temperatures. The quantity of blood, and therefore the amount of virus ingested, also affects the length of the extrinsic incubation period. This is extremely important in determining the transmission efficiency of a vector and may also vitally affect the course of an epidemic. Mosquitoes remain infective for life without any apparent ill effects, and their effectiveness as transmitters depends upon longevity and the frequency with which they bite. Different species of female mosquitoes vary in their ability to transmit different arboviruses so that some species are only able to transmit a single virus, while other mosquito species can transmit many arboviruses (e.g. *Culex tarsalis* vectors both Western equine encephalitis virus (WEEV) and SLEV, *Cx. annulirostris* vectors MVEV, JEV, Kunjin virus (KUNV), Ross River virus (RRV) and Barmah Forest virus (BFV)).

Viruses have been reported to persist in overwintering mosquitoes and this could be an important factor in virus survival. This has been shown to occur in *Cx. tritaeniorhynchus* infected with JEV and in *Cx. tarsalis* infected with WEEV (which remain infective by bite for up to 8 months). Transovarial or vertical transmission from one generation to the next via the desiccation-resistant eggs of some *Aedes* species has also been suggested as a possible mechanism of persistence for some arboviruses. However, Turell[12] suggests that other methods, including reintroduction of virus by migratory birds or survival in other vectors, may be more important in the long-term persistence of these viruses. Transmission of virus between the developmental stages (trans-stadial) is normal in ticks and transovarial passage has been observed in some species, and both are of great epidemiological importance. Some arboviruses may also persist for long periods in hibernating mammalian hosts.

IMPORTANT FACTORS IN TRANSMISSION BY ARTHROPODS

- Susceptibility of arthropods to infection and ability to transmit
- Breeding habits of arthropods and preferred habitats, whether near humans and other hosts of the virus
- Biting habits of arthropods – in mosquitoes whether they are anthropophilic (attracted to humans) or zoophilic (attracted to animals), exophilic (feeds outdoors) or endophilic (feeds inside)
- Longevity of arthropods, which depends to a great extent on temperature, humidity and (especially in ticks) the availability of hosts to feed on. Persistence of the virus by overwintering in adult mosquitoes or vertical transmission between generations may carry virus from one year to the next
- Abundance of arthropods. An efficient vector may have a wide range of animals on which to feed, but even if it bites humans only infrequently in the presence of other (and preferred) animals, large vector numbers will still allow significant numbers of human infections. For instance, *Cx. tritaeniorhynchus*, which bites mostly pigs, birds, cattle, dogs, and also humans to a limited extent, can maintain transmission of JEV from pigs to humans by sheer numbers
- Migratory birds can help by spreading virus that is circulating in their blood or by carrying infected ticks
- Interactions in ecological systems are of primary importance in transmission of many mosquito-borne and tick-borne arboviruses. A good example of this is the circulation of YFV in East Africa among forest monkeys and tree-living mosquitoes. Monkeys often leave the forests and raid banana plantations. Hence, YFV can infect mosquitoes in these locations and from there can be transmitted to humans. Similarly, humans become infected with Kyasanur Forest disease virus (KFDV) when they enter the domain of infected monkeys and pick up infected ticks.

Although transmission of arboviruses usually takes place through arthropod bites, it is important to remember that some viruses can, in some instances, be transmitted in other ways. European TBEV can be acquired by drinking the milk of infected goats, VEEV (in cotton rats) apparently via urine or faeces infecting the nasopharynx, WEEV possibly through aerosol from a patient and EEEV (in pheasants) by one bird pecking another. Laboratory infections have been reported with KUNV and DENV and WNV has been transmitted by blood transfusion. DENV, JEV, WNV and CHIKV have all been transmitted from mother to fetus, following infection during pregnancy, but this is rare.

As noted above, humans are usually an incidental host in arbovirus infections. However, it is their behaviour as well as environmental factors that determine the activity and spread of these viruses.[1] Many human activities encourage transmission of these animal viruses to people. The construction of dams and extensive areas of irrigation often promote the breeding of enormous numbers of mosquitoes. For instance, the development of rice fields encourages *Cx. tritaeniorhynchus* in Sarawak, spreading JEV, and *Mansonia uniformis* and *Anopheles gambiae* in Kenya spreading CHIKV, o'nyong-nyong virus (ONNV), possibly WNV and Sindbis virus (SINV). The seasonal cutting of old vegetation in Sarawak produces heavily polluted pools that support massive populations of culicines. The keeping of cattle driven into marginal forest areas in India promotes the growth and transport of ticks, and the intrusion of people into forest areas lays them open to infection with YFV and the tick-borne diseases. In many countries the practice of using large containers for water storage has helped to increase the *Aedes aegypti* populations and hence has increased the transmission of DENV, CHIKV and other viruses vectored by this species.[13] (For further discussion of the effect of human-related behaviour on arbovirus transmission, other reviews should be consulted.[14,15])

Environmental Conditions

Environmental conditions, particularly rainfall, temperature and humidity, have an important role in arbovirus transmission cycles. Arbovirus activity is generally seasonal. For example, the alphaviruses transmitted by mosquitoes in temperate regions cause disease in summer during periods of increased vector activity.[16] In tropical areas, human infections caused by arboviruses usually occur during the wet season, with increased virus activity again coinciding with periods of high vector numbers.

Mosquito larvae and pupae are aquatic and hence require water for breeding.[17] Therefore the abundance of arthropod vectors is directly affected by the amount of rainfall and flooding in a particular region. Rainfall is also required to maintain permanent water bodies, or in some cases create temporary water bodies that provide a sanctuary and breeding grounds for water birds that act both as mechanisms for introducing the virus into that area and for amplifying the virus. A good example of the latter occurred in northern Australia during the 2000 wet season. This resulted in the unprecedented southerly spread of MVEV activity from areas of the tropical north of Western Australia to subtropical and temperate regions. High tides can also lead to increased mosquito breeding and hence increased activity of viruses that are vectored by salt-marsh mosquitoes. Humidity can also play a role, with increased humidity facilitating increased survival of mosquitoes.

High external temperatures may have an adverse effect on vector survival. In addition, some mosquito species are temperature limited in their breeding. For example, *Cx. annulirostris*, the major vector of MVEV, RRV and JEV in Australia, will not breed when the daily temperatures fall below 17.5°C.[18] Temperature can also affect the length of the extrinsic incubation period and most studies have shown that the extrinsic incubation period for mosquitoes is shorter at 30°C than at lower temperatures.[11] Hence, at higher temperatures mosquitoes will become 'infectious' in a shorter time after ingestion of an infected blood meal.

Climate Change

It is predicted that future climate change may affect arbovirus transmission cycles throughout the world[15] by affecting the amount and extent of rainfall, frequency of high tides and actual tide heights, temperature, humidity, movement of vertebrate hosts and movement of human populations. The extent of these environmental changes is unknown but, because of the complex interactions between these viruses, their hosts and vectors and the environment, it seems likely that even minor changes will affect arbovirus activity in different regions. This may result in an increased number of cases or change in the geographical spread of these viruses.[17,19] Human adaptation to climage change is also likely to impact on the distribution and activity of arboviruses, for example the introduction of rainwater tanks to store rainwater. Deterioration of thesse tanks over time will provide new urban breeding grounds for mosquitoes. Climate change impacts on arbovirus transmission are thought to be responsible for the dramatic resurgence of West Nile virus in the USA in 2012. One of the worst outbreaks of WNV infection to hit the USA occurred at the end of the 2012 summer. Despite trends over the last few years suggesting that as WNV has established itself on the American continent, it may be declining as a disease threat, a major outbreak emerged in 2012 that threatened to exceed the peak of infections in 2002. This emergence was linked to a record-breaking drought across the USA, in combination with sporadic end of season rains and local complacency with regards to vector control. Mosquito numbers in metropolitan areas have surged, with consequent increased transmission of WNV.

Ecology of Arboviruses

The last two decades has seen a dramatic increase in the emergence and/or re-emergence of a number of serologically distinct arboviruses.[3,20,21] Ecological factors have played a pivotal role in this expansion with a rich array of demographic, cultural and societal changes impacting arbovirus transmission between vectors and hosts. Understanding some of these mechanisms will provide insight into future predictions of arboviral activity, disease risk assessment and control. South-east Asia in particular has experienced an exponential increase in the number of arbovirus infections. Importantly, it is the dramatic resurgence of a number of well-known arboviruses that were previously thought to be effectively controlled or unimportant that characterizes these renewed threats (DENV, JEV, CHIKV).[3] Their spread has been linked to various complex factors. It is recognized that biodiversity plays an important role for arbovirus maintenance with the South-east Asian tropical regions, particularly rainforests, considered reservoirs for many of these arboviruses. However, it is the demographic and societal changes in the human population during the past 20 years that has had the biggest impact on the revival of arbovirus infections. Unprecedented population growth has been the underlying driver of many of the changes that have affected transmission dynamics. These include rapid urbanization (in Thailand, Malaysia, Indonesia, Vietnam, Philippines, Cambodia, etc.), deforestation (mainly in Indonesia, Malaysia, Thailand and Singapore), new dams (Vietnam, Cambodia, Indonesia, Thailand, etc.), an expansion in irrigation (Malaysia, Thailand), and a lack of closed water storage containers. The resulting increase in mosquito populations and their closer contact with the human population has contributed to increased disease transmission. Moreover, the absence of effective mosquito control strategies has compounded the problem. Perhaps the changing demographics that have resulted from modern transportation have also played a significant role in the distribution and transmission dynamics of arboviruses in several South-east Asian countries.

The most medically significant arboviruses causing human illness in South-east Asia belong mainly to the *Flavivirus* group (e.g. DENV, JEV, and more recently, ZIKV in Cambodia), and to the *Alphavirus* group (CHIKV, SINV and Getah virus). Among them, DENV is the most prevalent in several countries (Indonesia, Thailand, Vietnam, Cambodia, Philippines, Myanmar, Malaysia and Singapore) and constitutes a major public health problem due to high morbidity. JEV is also widespread in the region (Cambodia and Thailand) and infections have been associated with high mortality coupled with severe neurological morbidity. Furthermore, several dengue-like epidemic manifestations that include encephalitis have been reported from Vietnam, Thailand, and on the Cambodia/Lao PDR/Myanmar borders over the past 10 years without any evidence of an aetiological agent. Therefore, significant gaps in our knowledge remain and interdisciplinary approaches are required to further strengthen the fight against rising arboviral infections not only in South-east Asia, but also in many parts of the world.

Arbovirus Evolution and Its Role in Disease and Spread

Globalization and environmental change have heralded the arrival of many new and re-emerging arboviruses creating new challenges for both researchers and policy-makers. While the geographic distribution of some arboviruses and their mosquito vectors has expanded, resulting in recurrent and larger outbreaks (e.g. DENV), others have invaded new geographic regions, having taken advantage susceptible mosquito vectors to become established (e.g. CHIKV).[22–24] Clearly, factors such as the absence of herd immunity and/or ineffective vector control have been instrumental in the re-emergence of several arboviral infections (e.g. CHIKV, JEV, and more recently, ZIKV). The changing epidemiological patterns of arboviruses are complex and unique to each virus, however the realization that virus evolution is an important driver of the emergence of these new disease threats has led to studies attempting to further elucidate the molecular evolution of some of these arboviruses.

One clear example of how virus evolution has re-defined the epidemiology of an arbovirus infection is the re-emergence and spread of CHIKV. Sequence analyses have shown that CHIKV originated from Africa and was later introduced into Asia. Based on partial E1 nucleotide sequences, phylogenetic analysis delineated CHIKV into three distinct clusters: an East-, Central- and South-African cluster (ECSA), an Asian cluster, and a West-African cluster.[25] Phylogenetic analysis of CHIKV strains isolated from the Indian Ocean outbreaks indicated that it was more closely related to the ECSA cluster than the Asian or West African clusters. However, of particular significance, 90% of the CHIKV strains isolated revealed a nucleotide mutation leading to an alanine to valine change at position 226 in the E1 glycoprotein. This single amino acid change was of particular interest as it appeared to be exclusively found in CHIKV isolated from *Ae. albopictus*. This mutation has been shown to be associated with adaptation to *Ae. albopictus* with an increased fitness in this vector attributable to the loss of cholesterol dependence for virus growth. This adaptation has allowed CHIKV to replicate and disseminate more efficiently in *Ae. albopictus*. Interestingly, mutation leading to change in the same amino acid position in SFV (E1 226 Proline → Serine) and SINV also modulated dependence on cholesterol and coincided with rapid growth of SFV in *Ae. albopictus*.[25]

More recently, another arbovirus that has generated significant interest is ZIKV. First isolated in the Zika forest, Uganda, in 1947, it was also isolated in sub-Saharan Africa and South-east Asia.[26] Few human cases were previously noted but in 2007, major human outbreaks were reported in Yap Island, Micronesia. Preliminary phylogenetic data showed two distinct ZIKV lineages circulating in Africa and a third lineage formed by the Micronesia and Malaysia strains.

In a world of rapid travel and transportation, many other arboviruses have the potential to spread geographically and cause serious outbreaks. What is of concern is that most of these new introductions are not detected until an epidemic or some unusual situation signals the alarm, often too late to effect control.

Immune Response to Arbovirus Infection

After inoculation of an arbovirus into the skin of a vertebrate by the arthropod vector, the virus probably multiplies first in local tissues and regional lymph nodes where the earliest immune responses occur.[27,28] As with most viral infections, nonspecific innate responses occur during the first few days. These include the antiviral effects of macrophages, natural killer cells and virus-induced interferon. However, within 4–7 days after infection, the pathogen-specific humoral (antibody) and cell-mediated (T cell) immune responses come into play. IgM antibodies are usually produced within the first few days after onset of illness, while IgG antibodies appear within 7–14 days. One of the characteristics of arbovirus infections is the long-term persistence of IgM, commonly for many months, therefore unlike many other infections, detection of IgM is not, of itself, a completely reliable indicator of recent infection. In general, antibody responses to arbovirus infections appear early and are long-lasting. However, some viruses do not produce high antibody titres in humans while others produce short-lived or late responses.

A person who recovers from an arbovirus infection generally possesses life-long immunity against reinfection with the homologous virus. Neutralizing antibodies can be found as early as a few days after the beginning of the disease and persist for many years. This persistence of immunity does not depend upon re-exposure to the virus. While neutralizing antibodies are a good indication of protective immunity, antibodies that do not neutralize virus in vitro may also provide protection in vivo via other immune mechanisms such as complement-mediated cytolysis (CMC) or antibody-dependent cell-mediated cytotoxicity (ADCC). Non-neutralizing antibodies have also been implicated as a cause of more severe disease due to antibody-dependent enhancement (ADE). The best known example of this is severe dengue, including dengue shock syndrome following secondary dengue infection with a heterologous serotype. This process may also have a role in pathogenesis of arthritis following *alphavirus* infections.[29]

Flaviviruses are known to evoke very broad, cross-reactive antibody responses, particularly IgG responses. Arboviruses are often grouped together according to antigenic similarity. For example, JEV, MVEV and WNV are all members of a single antigenic complex within the *Flavivirus* genus, while the four serotypes of DENV represent another. Infection with any *flavivirus* will usually result in antibody responses that react with antigens from a broad range of other *flaviviruses*, more so within the same antigenic complex. Indeed, recovery from an infection by one member of the group may provide a degree of resistance to a subsequent infection by another member of the same group; for instance, immunity to MVEV may provide subsequent protection against JEV, and vice-versa[30] or may reduce the severity of clinical disease. As mentioned above, cross-reacting non-neutralizing antibody may also increase disease severity due to ADE in dengue. The importance of antibodies in protecting against disease is illustrated by the ability of passively transferred immunoglobulin to protect against a range of *flavivirus* diseases in a mouse model.

The role of the T-cell-mediated immune response is not as clear as that of the antibody response. Broadly cross-reactive $CD8^+$ cytotoxic T cells are induced by infection with flaviviruses and alphaviruses and are likely to have an important role in the clearance of the virus. Paradoxically however, the inflammatory responses and cytolysis caused by these cells contribute to the pathology of some, if not all, arbovirus infections.

Studies on patients infected by arboviruses have revealed that a variety of cytokines and chemokines, such as IL-6, IL-10, IFN-α, MIG and IP-10, are induced during infection.[31–34] Febrile symptoms of CHIKV-infected patients have been found to be associated with high levels of pyrogenic cytokines such as IL-1β and IL-6 produced during the acute phase of infection. In addition, IL-1β, IL-6 and RANTES have been demonstrated to act as biomarkers as they are associated with the severity of CHIKV induced fever. The finding that aberrant type-I interferon signalling in mice led to severe forms of arbovirus disease further highlights the important role cytokines play in pathology. Arthralgia experienced by CHIKV infected patients closely resembles the symptoms induced by other viruses like RRV and Barmah Forest virus (BFV). Such *alphavirus*-induced arthralgia mirrors rheumatoid arthritis, a condition that is characterized by severe joint pains due to inflammation and tissue destruction caused by inflammatory cytokines such as IL-1β, IL-6 and TNF-α. It is thus plausible that CHIKV infection and/or other arthritis-causing alphaviruses induce similar pro-inflammatory cytokines that cause arthralgia, explaining why joint pains are constant ailments of many patients infected with CHIKV even years after recovery from the initial febrile phase.

It is also clear that host factors influence the susceptibility and severity of infections due to arboviruses. Severe manifestations of infection due to flaviviruses and the *alphavirus* CHIKV are more common in young children, the elderly and those with pre-existing illnesses. In contrast, the arthritic manifestations of *alphavirus* infections are less common in children. Genetic factors are also probably important. For example, genetically determined susceptibility to flaviviruses has been shown in mice, and persisting arthritis following RRV infection has been associated with HLA-DR7 positivity in humans.[29]

Clinical Features in General

Arbovirus infections are distributed throughout most of the world, and in areas with endemic or regular epidemic activity infection rates may be quite high within the human population. However, the vast majority of infected individuals will have had either an asymptomatic or nonspecific mild illness and only a handful of those infected will develop one of the recognizable clinical syndromes. For the flaviviruses the case:infection ratio is usually very low (e.g. around 1:300 for encephalitis due to JEV) but varies depending on the virus. It may be higher during epidemic (rather than endemic) disease activity, and will be modified by host susceptibility factors. In particular, the major burden of disease is felt at the extremes of life – the very young and the elderly. For *alphavirus* infections, particularly those causing arthritis, the ratio of symptomatic to asymptomatic infection is much higher, varying from 1:40 to 1:3.

If clinical manifestations arise after infection they do so after an intrinsic incubation period lasting from a few days to a week or more. During that time, the virus replicates at the site of inoculation, then further amplifies within the reticuloendothelial system before it becomes viraemic and spreads to target organs.

The most important clues to a possible arbovirus infection lie in a detailed travel and exposure history, coupled with current knowledge of the viruses circulating in the potential area of exposure. That can be difficult if the patient is a returned traveller, especially if they have travelled through a number of countries during the potential period of infection. Information can be obtained from travel health websites such as those of the World Health Organization (see: http://www.who.int/topics/travel/en/) or the Centers for Disease Control and Prevention in the USA (see: http://www.cdc.gov/travel/). However, it may also be necessary to seek the advice of local experts to get the full picture in difficult cases.

The major clinical syndromes may be grouped as follows:

1. Systemic febrile disease
2. Arboviral haemorrhagic fever
3. Encephalitis
4. Polyarthralgic illness.

SYSTEMIC FEBRILE DISEASE

Arbovirus infection often produces a systemic febrile illness as part of the clinical illness. Fever is very common with *flavivirus* infections, whereas some symptomatic *alphavirus* infections produce fever in 50% or less of those infected. Particularly in the early stages, this illness may be nonspecific or even suggestive of other viral illnesses, including gastrointestinal and respiratory infections. There are some clinical features that are more characteristic of arbovirus infections. Headache is common and may be severe (even with the arboviruses that rarely, if ever, cause encephalitis) and accompanied by meningitis. Muscle and joint aches are also common, especially with *alphavirus* infections where many also develop joint swelling and stiffness. Rash may be present and is usually generalized and maculopapular, although occasionally vesicular. Petechial rashes are less common and may be an early indicator of haemorrhagic fever. In the vast majority of cases febrile illness is followed by recovery. In the remainder, illness progresses to one of the more serious forms of disease, sometimes following a few days of remission. Occasionally, infections have a fulminant course, particularly in young children, where the initial febrile illness is short and advances rapidly to severe illness.

The notable exception to the generally benign nature of the febrile illnesses is YF. This virus produces sufficient liver damage to cause clinical jaundice and a resulting severe febrile illness, even without progressing to haemorrhagic disease.

HAEMORRHAGIC FEVER

Most commonly caused by:

- Flaviviruses: DENV, YFV, KFDV, OHFV
- Alphaviruses: CHIKV
- Phleboviruses: RVFV.

These are the most serious manifestations of arbovirus infection. Haemorrhagic disease most often manifests as bleeding from the gums or gastrointestinal haemorrhage (haematemesis and melaena) and as cutaneous petechiae and purpura. The pathogenesis is complex and poorly understood for most. YF produces sufficient liver dysfunction to cause a reduction of the coagulation factors produced in that organ. However, in severe YF, there is also a consumptive coagulopathy (disseminated intravascular coagulopathy, DIC) due to complement and cytokine activation, resulting in a reduction of most coagulation factors and a rise in the levels of fibrin degradation products. There may also be platelet dysfunction.

Severe dengue is associated with a marked thrombocytopenia and platelet dysfunction, and DIC may develop in severe disease. Complement activation is likely to be important in the induction of the coagulopathy, as is cytokine release from mononuclear cells. However, the major problem in severe dengue relates to endothelial cell dysfunction and increased vascular permeability resulting in loss of fluid from the intravascular into the extravascular spaces. It appears that these processes are triggered by the host immune response, particularly uptake of virus into macrophages, followed by the release of cytokines and other inflammatory mediators from these cells and activated T cells, which in turn leads to complement activation and capillary leakage. There has been considerable interest in the potential role of non-neutralizing antibodies in enhancing uptake of virus into macrophages (i.e. ADE) leading to this excessive immune response. With dengue this may occur when past infection with one serotype results in cross-reactive non-neutralizing antibody if the person gets a subsequent infection with another serotype. This phenomenon has been widely observed in experimental systems with other flaviviruses and with some alphaviruses. Recent studies have pointed to a novel mechanism of ADE in DENV infections involving antibody-facilitated uptake of 'immature' non-infectious virions into macrophages in secondary infections (predominantly by anti-prM antibodies). On uptake, these immature virions are processed to the mature form by host cell furin, rendering them infectious and so substantially enhance the infectious viral burden.[35]

There is little information about KFDV, Omsk haemorrhagic fever virus (OHFV), RVFV and CHIKV, but DIC seems to be an important component of the severe haemorrhagic disease. It is likely that all the arbovirus haemorrhagic diseases will have a similar pathogenesis, but this is complex and not yet fully determined.

Treatment is directed mainly at careful maintenance of intravascular fluid volumes to prevent hypotension, and management of complications such as haemorrhage, pneumonia and renal failure. Replacement of fluid loss in dengue shock syndrome is important and replacement fluids, such as 5% dextrose in saline, plasma, plasma substitutes or colloidal solutions may be used. If the haemoglobin level is falling, blood transfusion is needed.

Fresh frozen plasma may be used to provide coagulation factors, although they need to be used with caution owing to the potential for worsening DIC. In the early stages of YF when there is a selective decline in the hepatic coagulation factors, these can be replaced selectively. Vitamin K has also been suggested, but it is doubtful that the liver will be able to respond to this.

If significant bleeding is occurring as a result of thrombocytopenia, platelet transfusions may be necessary, but they should be used with caution when DIC is established. There is some experimental evidence that ribavirin may be useful for RVFV, but clinical data are lacking.

ENCEPHALITIS

Encephalitis[36] is most commonly caused by:

- Alphaviruses: EEV, WEEV, VEEV
- Flaviviruses: JEV, MVEV, WNV, KUNV, SLEV, TBEV, LIV, KFDV
- Phleboviruses: RVFV.

Many of the arboviruses are capable of infecting the central nervous system. It is assumed that they enter across the blood–brain barrier after the viraemic phase of infection. However, while evidence exists in animal models[37] this has not yet been fully established in human infections. There is also some evidence that entry via the olfactory bulb may be important. In either event, the resulting encephalitis has a fairly characteristic pattern of involvement. The major effects are seen within the central cerebral structures including the midbrain, basal ganglia and brainstem. The cerebellum and upper spinal cord are also often affected, particularly the anterior horn cells of the latter. As a result of the involvement of these essential structures, encephalitis may result in coma, respiratory failure and flaccid paralysis. Milder manifestations include cranial nerve palsies, tremor, cogwheel rigidity, cerebellar ataxia and upper limb weakness. The differential diagnosis in the early stages includes herpes simplex encephalitis, early bacterial cerebritis and tuberculous meningitis. Once signs of involvement of central cerebral structures appear, then it is more characteristic of arboviral encephalitis. Occasionally herpes simplex, postinfectious encephalitis, acute cerebral vasculitis and others may produce a similar picture.

The frequency and nature of sequelae varies with the virus, the severity of the initial illness and the age of the patient. Many survivors are left with mild sequelae and a few unfortunate ones with major intellectual and physical disabilities. Late neuropsychiatric manifestations are also prominent with the arboviral encephalitides, while other patients develop Parkinsonian-type features.

During the acute illness CSF usually shows a mild to moderate lymphocyte pleocytosis (although a neutrophil predominance may be seen in early illness), accompanied by some increase in the levels of protein but a normal glucose concentration. Samples of serum and CSF should be collected for IgM testing as early as possible. If available, virus isolation and/or RNA detection by reverse transcriptase–polymerase chain reaction (RT-PCR) should also be performed on these samples. Computed tomography (CT) may show changes in the affected central structures, but magnetic resonance imaging (MRI) is more sensitive. Late scans in those with chronic disease show destructive changes in the thalamus and other central structures.

Limited data are available on treatment of arboviral encephalitis and no specific antiviral agents are currently available.

Steroids have been shown to be ineffective in JE, but interferon-α may be beneficial. In view of the similarity of the different forms of arbovirus encephalitis, it seems likely that the same will apply to other *flavivirus* infections. Specific immunoglobulin has been used experimentally in mice with *flavivirus* infection, and successful treatment of a patient with WNV encephalitis has also been reported.[38]

However, treatment of these conditions is largely supportive in order to ensure that the patient does not succumb to respiratory failure or haemodynamic instability, or from complications such as pneumonia that may arise with any serious illness.

POLYARTHRALGIC ILLNESS

Most commonly caused by:

- Alphaviruses: CHIKV, RRV, BFV, SINV, ONNV, MAYV
- Flaviviruses: KUNV, KOKV
- Bunyaviruses: OROV
- Phleboviruses: Sandfly fever.

A number of the *Alphavirus* infections have polyarthralgia as a common and prominent component of the presenting illness. This is commonly accompanied by myalgia and fatigue, and may be accompanied by fever and/or rash. Typically, the small joints of the hands and feet, the wrists, elbows, shoulders and knees are involved. Symptoms may consist just of joint pain, but often, there is evidence of true arthritis manifesting as joint swelling and morning stiffness. The tenderness and swelling are largely due to synovitis rather than effusions. Multiple joints are involved, usually in a symmetrical pattern. Back pain is common with some viruses, and neck or jaw pain may occur. Arthralgia is usually accompanied by myalgia and fatigue. Tendonitis and fasciitis may also be clinically evident, and paraesthesiae due to nerve entrapment also occurs in the limbs. Most patients recover within a month, but prolonged arthralgia and myalgia are a feature of *alphavirus* infections, persisting for months or years in up to 50% of patients. There is mounting evidence that *alphavirus* arthritis is due to infection of synovial monocytes/macrophages and synovial cells resulting in release of inflammatory mediators and induction of a cytotoxic T-cell response. The latter is probably important in viral clearance, but also contributes to the inflammatory response. Studies on RRV suggest that the chronic arthritis is due to persistence of the virus in a non-replicating form resulting in an ongoing inflammatory response. The persistence may be due to impaired antiviral cytokines as a result of antibody-dependent enhancement of viral uptake into macrophages.

Flaviviruses less commonly produce polyarthralgia, with the exception of DENV, which causes joint pains but not a true arthritis. KOKV and KUNV are uncommon causes of an *alphavirus*-like polyarthritis.

Acute polyarthritis has a wide differential diagnosis. In some areas more than one arbovirus may be responsible for the illness. In addition there are a number of other causes of polyarthritis with or without rash, including rubella, acute hepatitis B, parvovirus B19 (erythema infectiosum), human immunodeficiency virus (HIV) seroconversion illness, Henoch–Schoenlein purpura, drug-related serum sickness, and the acute onset of other non-infectious arthritides. Subacute or chronic disease following RRV or BFV infection may be confused with rubella or parvovirus B19 arthritis, as well as other chronic arthritides including rheumatoid arthritis, systemic lupus erythematosus and adult Still's disease.

Treatment is symptomatic with rest, gentle exercise, analgesics, and non-steroidal anti-inflammatory drugs. While there are no specific antiviral agents available, inhibitors of macrophage-derived inflammatory mediators, such as monocyte chemotactic protein 1 (MCP1) and macrophage migration inhibition factor (MIF), have been shown to ameliorate *alphavirus*-induced arthralgia in animal models and are promising therapeutic candidates.[39,40] Steroids have also been used to treat some patients with RRV arthritis,[29] but they should be used with caution until further data emerge. Small, uncontrolled trials have found some benefit for arthritis symptoms following CHIKV infection, consistent with its use for treatment of rheumatoid arthritis.

Diagnosis

VIRUS DETECTION

Viraemia lasts for a few days after the onset of illness and virus can be isolated from blood at that time. However, as it is technically demanding, limited in availability and often fails to yield a positive result, virus culture is rarely undertaken as a part of routine diagnosis. They should be reserved for unusual cases or rare pathogens. An unintended consequence of a move away from diagnostic virus culture however, is a drastic reduction in virus isolates available for further study. In cases of meningitis or encephalitis, culture from the CSF may also be undertaken, but with the same constraints as above. Where culture is attempted, blood and/or CSF should be collected as early as possible in the course of illness. Post-mortem tissue may yield virus in the later stages of illness. Many will grow in a variety of cell lines, but maximum sensitivity for the mosquito-borne alphaviruses and flaviviruses is achieved by initially inoculating the sample on to a mosquito cell line (e.g. C6/36, AP-61 or TRA-284) and incubating for 3–4 days at 28°C. In order to obtain a cytopathic effect, this must be blind passaged to Vero, BHK, PS, chick embryo or various other cell lines and incubated at 37°C for a few days. Virus can also be isolated by specimen inoculation into suckling mouse brain or intrathoracic inoculation in appropriate mosquito species. Virus growth in mice manifests as paralysis and death after a few days, and is confirmed by identification of the virus in the brain. For the Bunyaviridae, suckling mouse brain inoculation or culture in mosquito cells (C6/36 or AP-61) are suitable. Coltiviruses grow in suckling mouse brain or in Vero or BHK-21 cell lines.

When an arbovirus is isolated in cell culture, it is most easily identified by monoclonal antibody binding in immunofluorescent antibody (IFA) or enzyme immunoassay (EIA) formats. Neutralization (N) with antisera or complement fixation (CF) assays are used less commonly. Specific reverse transcription PCR (RT-PCR) and/or real-time PCR assays may also be used for identification, and sequencing of the product can provide detailed phylogenetic information.

A variety of antigen detection methods have been described, either by IFA or antigen capture EIA. They have been used for blood, CSF and tissues. Generally they have proved less sensitive than other virus detection methods and many have been replaced by PCR-based diagnosis. An exception is in the detection in patient sera or plasma of the dengue virus protein NS1 which has become a routine diagnostic for early detection of dengue virus infection.[41,42]

Virus may also be detected by amplification of viral RNA by RT-PCR or other nucleic acid amplification tests. Methods have been described for most of the flaviviruses and alphaviruses. They are more sensitive and quicker to perform than virus culture and are now more accessible and, with real-time PCR protocols, results can be available within a few hours. Like culture, they can be performed on blood, CSF or tissues, and should be done as early as possible in the course of illness.

Post-mortem tissues can be used for virus detection if available. The preferred site for sampling is dictated by the major sites of involvement. PCR can be performed on fixed tissues, even if paraffin embedded, but the sensitivity of detection for these samples is lower than fresh material. Amplified nucleic acid can be used for virus identification and characterization directly from patient samples using sequencing, DNA microarrays, or species-specific probes.

SEROLOGICAL DIAGNOSIS

This is the main routine diagnostic method for arboviral infections. Antibody may be detected by enzyme immunoassays, immunofluorescence, haemagglutination inhibition, neutralization or complement fixation (EIA, IFA, HI, N, CF, respectively) assays. Most diagnoses are based on EIA and HI tests, with some use of IFA. The EIA and IFA tests can be formatted to detect either IgG or IgM, or both in the case of competitive EIA formats. HI will detect both IgG and IgM, and differentiation between them requires separation of the antibody classes by sucrose density centrifugation or in chromatography columns. They are now rarely used for IgM detection as they are less sensitive than EIA and IFA, and are more difficult to perform. N assays are regarded as the most specific of the tests, but are confined to specialized laboratories that are able to culture the viruses. Monoclonal antibody epitope-blocking EIAs are used for the identification of specific antibody. These have been applied to a range of flaviviruses, including MVEV, WNV and JEV, and use species-specific epitopes to bind antibodies in patient serum, inhibiting binding of monoclonal antibodies. If inhibition occurs then there is a significant amount of specific antibody in the patient's serum.

Recent infection is best diagnosed by an increase in antibody levels between acute and convalescent samples tested in parallel, but it may take 2–4 weeks before a diagnostic rise is detected. Detection of IgM is helpful in making an earlier diagnosis. IgM usually appears within a few days after onset of illness. A negative IgM using a sensitive test such as EIA or IFA in a sample collected a week or more into the illness makes recent infection very unlikely. For samples collected earlier in the illness or where there is a strong clinical suspicion despite the negative IgM finding, a second sample at least 2 weeks after onset is recommended. As IgM often persists for weeks or months, it does not reliably distinguish between acute infection and recent past infection. Therefore diagnosis of acute infection based on detection of IgM alone requires a clinically consistent illness and a suitable exposure history.

Cross-reactivity between antibodies within the major subgroups of arboviruses is a problem and may result in a misleading diagnosis. *Alphavirus* antibodies show limited cross-reactivity and standard tests are usually sufficient to identify the infecting virus, although it does depend on the particular alphaviruses circulating within that region. However, antibodies to the different flaviviruses generally cross-react widely, so that detection of IgM and/or IgG to one of these viruses in the routine tests is not definitive evidence of infection due to that virus rather than another *flavivirus*. The clinical and epidemiological circumstances may indicate that only one *flavivirus* is possible, for example detection of DENV antibody in a person with clinical dengue during a known epidemic. Otherwise specific serological tests, such as N or epitope-blocking EIA, are needed to identify the antibody.

Diagnosis may be further complicated by the phenomenon of 'original antigenic sin'. This occurs in people who have had previous *flavivirus* infection, and who have a new infection with a different *flavivirus*. Owing to the antigenic similarities, they may mount a vigorous anamnestic antibody response to the original virus before they develop specific antibody to the new virus. As a result, serological tests may initially suggest recent infection with their previous virus. Late convalescent sera may clarify the situation, but sometimes it is not possible to determine the infecting virus. Occasionally a similar phenomenon is seen with closely related alphaviruses such as CHIKV and ONNV.

A detailed travel and exposure history is important for the accurate interpretation of arbovirus serology.

Management

There are no specific antiviral agents currently in use for the treatment of arboviral infections, nor are these likely in the near future. Treatment is supportive and symptomatic. Limited data on steroids, interferon, hydroxychloroquine and ribavirin are discussed under the relevant viruses.

Immunization

Highly effective vaccines have been developed against several arboviruses of public health significance. However, only vaccines against YFV, JEV, KFV and TBEV are licensed for use in the wider community.[27,28,43] A vaccine for RRV is in the final stages of clinical trials and is expected to be available soon.

The YFV 17D vaccine is one of the safest and most successful viral vaccines ever produced. This live vaccine was derived from a highly virulent strain of YFV (Asibi) that has been attenuated by *in vitro* serial passage in mouse embryonic tissue and chick embryo cells. After prolonged propagation in this medium, it was found that neurotropism and viscerotropism were both greatly reduced, but the virus retained its antigenic properties. The 17D vaccine is still widely used and highly effective, giving protection for at least 10 years, and probably longer. Less than 10% of vaccinees experience headache and malaise, while allergic reactions, liver function abnormalities and neurological complications are extremely uncommon. Nevertheless recent reports have indicated that neurological complications may be more common than previously believed and, since 1996, a number of cases of disseminated infection due to vaccine strains have been reported. Estimates of the risk of neurological disease, mainly benign, are 1–16 per million, and of visceral disease is 2.5 per million doses. The vaccine is contraindicated for infants under 6 months of age for whom the frequency of neurological incidents is significantly increased. Depending on the relative risk of natural infection, immunization should also be avoided in pregnant women. Immunization against YFV is required by law before travellers are allowed into certain countries either for their protection or to prevent the importation of the disease to areas where *Ae. aegypti* is present.

An inactivated vaccine derived from infected mouse brain has been in use for several decades, but is gradually being replaced by a more refined version derived from virus grown in cell culture. Immunization is recommended for individuals living in endemic areas, or for travellers visiting regions that are experiencing current outbreaks. This vaccine is also used to immunize military personnel and laboratory workers who may be exposed to the virus. At least three doses of the vaccine at 7–14-day intervals are required to achieve more than 90% seroconversion, with booster doses recommended after 12 months. Minor side-effects such as local tenderness and mild systemic symptoms occur in 10–30% of vaccinees, although more serious neurological complications are rare. Allergic responses, particularly in Western travellers, are not uncommon, with up to 1% of vaccinees experiencing reactions within 7 days of inoculation. A live attenuated vaccine (SA 14–14–2) is also approved for use in China and some Asian countries. A number of other vaccines, including live-attenuated, recombinant, virus-like particles and naked DNA vaccines are at various stages of development.

Inactivated vaccines against TBEV are used widely in several European countries. The highly purified Austrian vaccine induces seroconversion rates of more than 97% in the field with negligible side-effects. Immunization may be warranted for people living in endemic areas or those involved in high-risk activities, such as laboratory workers, military personnel, foresters, farmers or campers. Passive immunization with TBEV immunoglobulin is also used before or after exposure to tick bite in some European countries. As for JEV, a number of other types of vaccines are in development.

An inactivated RVFV vaccine has been shown to be safe and immunogenic in military personnel.[44] It is given as three subcutaneous doses (at 0, 7 and 28 days) and induces a greater than 90% seroconversion rate in recipients. It has been used for the protection of military and laboratory staff, but is not generally available.

There is a clear need for a safe and effective vaccine against DENV and a number of candidate vaccines are in development. However, to avoid vaccine-induced ADE of infection with heterologous serotypes, the vaccine must be delivered as a multivalent preparation so that immunization against each of the four serotypes is concurrent. Obtaining good immune responses to all four serotypes has been problematic. A live recombinant chimeric tetravalent vaccine for DENV was in Phase III clinical trials in 2012. WNV vaccines have been developed for veterinary use, but not yet for humans.

Although no *alphavirus* vaccines have been licensed for widespread human use, several preparations have been used to protect laboratory workers or livestock. Inactivated EEEV and WEEV and VEEV whole-virus vaccines are available for restricted human use and have a veterinary application in horses. Vaccines for CHIKV, RRV and VEEV have had limited testing in volunteers and laboratory workers. There is ongoing commercial interest in *alphavirus* vaccines using new technologies, particularly for the encephalitis viruses, and some may become more widely available over the next few years. An inactivated RRV vaccine is currently in clinical trial and is expected to be available in the next few years.

Control

VECTOR CONTROL

Vector control has been successful in some circumstances, for instance during the construction of the Panama Canal when, by strict discipline, all collections of water capable of breeding *Ae. aegypti* (and vectors of malaria) were eliminated from the area. Similar methods have been applied to cities and towns in South America under the threat of YFV. When DDT was introduced, extensive use in Guyana and elsewhere soon eradicated *Ae. aegypti* and with it the threat of urban YFV. However, in Africa, *Ae. aegypti* became resistant to DDT, and in some areas it is exophilic in habit, so that spraying dwellings with insecticide is ineffective. Forest mosquitoes, of course, are not susceptible to ordinary methods of spraying. Tick control by residual insecticides has, however, achieved some success in the former USSR. However, the problems of vector control, especially in rural areas, are formidable.

Medically Important Arboviruses

The remaining sections describe the distribution, aetiology, transmission cycles, clinical features, diagnosis, treatment, control and epidemiology of individual medically important arboviruses in more detail.

Alphaviruses (Family: Togaviridae, Genus: *Alphavirus*)

BARMAH FOREST VIRUS (BFV)

Geographical Distribution

BFV[45] is confined to the Australian mainland. It was first isolated in south-eastern Australia in 1974. Human infections have been described in all mainland states, but most disease occurs in the tropical north and the temperate coastal region of the south-west and northern and central parts of the east coast.

Aetiology

BFV is an *alphavirus* that occupies its own antigenic group.

Transmission

Transmission is similar to that of RRV (see below).

Clinical Features

Natural History. The incubation period is probably 7–9 days, though it is likely that, like RRV, some patients will have a longer or shorter incubation period. Clinical illness is similar to the more common RRV infection although joint pain is slightly less common (about 85%) and joint swelling or stiffness occurs in only about 30% of cases. Skin rash occurs in 50–100% of patients in different series. It is usually maculopapular, but may be urticarial or vesicular. Chronic illness has been reported in about 10% of patients. BFV disease occurs mainly between the ages of 20 and 60 years of age. Infection of children in endemic or epidemic areas is common, but clinical illness is infrequent.

Diagnosis

The diagnostic methods used are similar to those described for RRV. IgM may persist for many months following acute infection.

Management

In the absence of any controlled data, the infection is usually managed symptomatically, as recommended for RRV disease.

Epidemiology

BFV is found only on the Australian mainland and has an epidemiology similar to that of RRV, although it is less common. It is carried by the same mosquito vectors as RRV, probably uses the

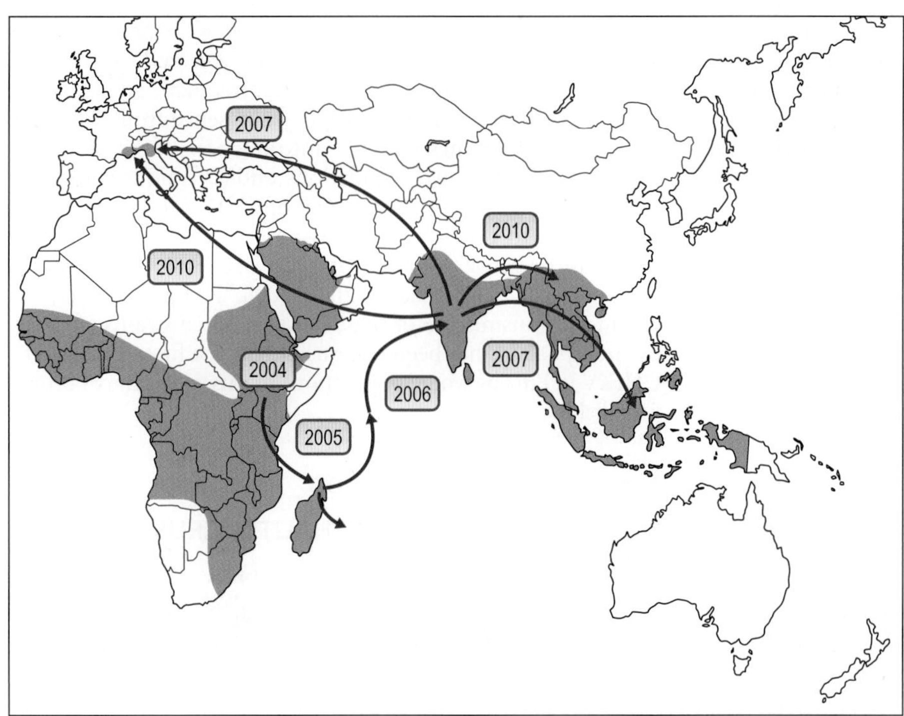

Figure 14.2 Geographical distribution of chikungunya virus. CHIKV was largely restricted to Africa and Asia until successive waves of outbreaks beginning with an epidemic in Kenya in 2004 swept across the globe.

same marsupial vertebrate hosts as RRV and activity requires the same environmental conditions as RRV, but does not necessarily occur at the same time. BFV causes small epidemics as it enters a new area, with low-level seasonal epidemics following that.

CHIKUNGUNYA VIRUS (CHIKV)

Geographical Distribution

CHIKV[16,27,46–50] was first isolated from patients in Tanzania during an epidemic in 1952–1953. Its name is a local word meaning 'that which contorts or bends up'. Infection and human disease are widespread in Africa, and CHIKV is also present in Saudi Arabia, India (Calcutta and southern India), Thailand, Cambodia, Myanmar, Vietnam, Malaysia, Laos, Borneo, Indonesia and the Philippines (Figure 14.2). Large outbreaks have occurred in urban settings in many parts of Africa and Asia, and these may extend over several years. At the beginning of 2005, CHIKV emerged in islands of the southwest Indian Ocean including the Comoros, Mayotte, Seychelles, La Reunion Island, Mauritius and Madagascar, spreading to India and causing imported cases of CHIKV disease in countries in Europe, north and south America, the Caribbean and Australia.[46] It has been estimated that more than 1.25 million cases have occurred in India alone, including several fatalities.[47]

There are two major lineages of the virus, one of which is found worldwide and is further subdivided into Asian and East African sublineages, and the other restricted to West Africa. However, CHIKV continues to evolve and large epidemics are usually due to a unique strain of the virus, as has been seen in the recent Indian Ocean outbreak (see Arbovirus evolution, above).

Aetiology

CHIKV is an *alphavirus* in the Semliki Forest complex, and is most closely related to ONNV.

Transmission

The main vector for humans is *Ae. aegypti*, although a number of other species can transmit infection. *Ae. albopictus* was the most likely vector on La Reunion Island in 2005–2006. In Africa, the virus appears to be maintained in forest and savannahs in a cycle involving non-human primates and a variety of *Aedes* species and *Mansonia africana*. In Asia, *Ae. aegypti* is responsible for urban epidemics (see Table 14.1). During the recent outbreak in the Indian Ocean, there was also evidence for non-vector early maternal–fetal transmission, possibly causing deaths in utero.[48]

Pathology

Although CHIKV fever has often been misdiagnosed as Dengue fever due to similarities of the symptoms, CHIKV patients are plagued by incapacitating arthralgia, a hallmark of the disease, despite recovering from the infection.[51] The arthralgia appears to be commonly bilateral and symmetrical, affecting peripheral small joints such as ankles, toes, fingers, elbows, wrists and knees and chronic arthralgia has also been reported to persist for months and even years. In addition, other symptoms common to CHIKV infection have been reported to occur at variable frequencies and they include lymphopenia, hypocalcaemia, photophobia, lumbar back pain, chills, weakness, nausea and vomiting.

Although CHIKV fever is generally self-limiting and results primarily in considerable morbidity, severe complications of the disease such as myocarditis, meningoencephalitis, and mild haemorrhage have also been reported. Despite being rarely fatal, deaths associated with CHIKV infection were reported during the 2004–2008 outbreaks in various countries. However, these cases have been found to be prevalent in older patients or patients with underlying conditions such as myasthenia, ischaemic cardiopathy and diabetes.

Studies have revealed that CHIKV could be detected in the synovial macrophages of a chronic patient and this has been postulated to mediate arthralgia. Notably, the arthritic condition was associated with the increased infiltration of monocytes, macrophages and natural killer cells, as well as elevated production of pro-inflammatory mediators such as MCP-1, TNF-α and IFN-γ. These findings further support the hypothesis that arthralgia experienced by CHIKF patients could be immune-mediated based on the similarities of symptoms induced by other 'Old World' viruses such as Ross River virus (RRV) and Barmah Forest virus (BFV). Furthermore, arthralgia induced by these viruses resembles rheumatoid arthritis, which is attributed to the dysregulation of pro-inflammatory cytokines such IL-1β, TNF-α, and IL-6, causing inflammation and tissue destruction at the affected joints.[52]

Clinical Features

Natural History. The incubation period is 3–12 days, with an average of 2–7 days. Classical illness begins with the rapid onset of severe arthralgia. Back pain may be prominent. There is associated myalgia, high fever, generalized lymphadenopathy and conjunctivitis. This usually improves after 2–3 days and is followed by the onset of a generalized maculopapular rash in about half. Fever may recur after a break of 1–2 days. Petechiae, bleeding from the gums and a positive tourniquet test have been described in many patients, so that the disease may clinically be mistaken for dengue. More severe haemorrhagic manifestations occur and are more common in children, but overall are rare. Some patients develop a febrile illness without rash or arthralgia. Most patients recover fully over a few weeks, although 5–10% experience chronic joint symptoms including pain, stiffness and swelling that may persist for years. The erythrocyte sedimentation rate is often mildly raised in acute and chronic disease.

In the past, severe and/or fatal illness has been due to haemorrhagic disease in children. However in the recent Indian Ocean outbreak a number of fatalities in the elderly or those with pre-existing illnesses occurred, as well as several cases of encephalitis. Children who are infected are less likely to develop the characteristic clinical illness.

There are no specific treatments, though small, uncontrolled trials of hydroxychloroquine have shown possible beneficial effects on arthritis symptoms.

Diagnosis

The virus can be detected in the serum in the first 3–4 days of illness, with PCR methods being more sensitive than culture. IgM can be detected by IFA or EIA in acute sera and persists for weeks or months. Acute infection can be confirmed by showing rising HI or N antibody titres on paired sera. There are cross-reactions with other alphaviruses, especially Semliki Forest virus (SFV) and ONNV, although they are less frequent with IgM than with IgG. This may pose diagnostic difficulties in Africa where SFV and ONNV are also found, and in travellers who may have been exposed to multiple viruses.

Epidemiology

There is a forest cycle involving monkeys (vervets and baboons) transmitted by *Ae. africanus* and other mosquitoes. Rodents may also be hosts as they show a transient viraemia on being inoculated with virus, whereas monkeys show a high viraemia. This sylvatic cycle results in low-level endemic human infections. Epidemic disease is associated with the wet season and with rises in the number of *Ae. aegypti* and, in Asia, *Ae. albopictus*. These epidemics are large, infrequent, often last 2–3 years and are followed by a prolonged absence from that area. It has been hypothesized that introduction of CHIKV into immunologically naive populations and/or unique molecular changes that have led to adaptation of CHIKV to the *Ae. albopictus* mosquito vector was the reason for the massive outbreak of disease in residents and visitors to islands in the southwest Indian Ocean and India in 2005–2006.[46,49] Furthermore, the enhanced transmission of these newly adapted strains of CHIK by *Ae. alpopictus* has been responsible for the first outbreaks of CHIKV in Europe where populations of this vector have become established.

Equine Encephalitides

WESTERN EQUINE ENCEPHALITIS VIRUS (WEEV)

Geographical Distribution (Figure 14.3)

WEEV[16,27,53] is found in North America in Texas, Colorado and Saskatchewan where it causes disease in horses and humans. It is also found in Argentina, Brazil, Mexico and Guyana, where equine epizootics occur, but human infections have not been described.[53]

Aetiology

WEEV is an *alphavirus* that is in the same group as SINV. It has several antigenic variants, particularly among the South American strains.

Transmission

Transmission is by mosquitoes. *Cx. tarsalis*, which feeds readily on birds, transmits the infection in the western USA, and *Culiseta malanura* in areas where *Cx. tarsalis* does not occur (eastern USA). Transplacental transmission can also occur in humans.

Immunity

Immunity is antibody-mediated and protects against second attacks. Serological surveys show inapparent infections, and children are most affected in epidemics.

Pathology

The CNS shows extensive changes with neuronal necrosis, perivascular inflammatory changes and meningeal inflammation. These are found in the cerebral cortex, striatum, thalamus, pons, cerebellum and spinal cord.

Clinical Features

Natural History. The majority of infections are asymptomatic or nonspecific. Encephalitis occurs in about 1 in 1000 infected adults, but about 1 in 50 infected children, especially infants. The case fatality rate is 3–7% and is highest in the elderly. Severe sequelae are largely confined to infants.

Signs and Symptoms. The incubation period is 5–10 days.

The onset in older children and adults is gradual, with mild fever, malaise, headache, photophobia, nausea, vomiting and sore throat, sometimes with meningism and drowsiness. In the minority who progress to encephalitis, the fever and headache increase, with deterioration of conscious state, possibly with

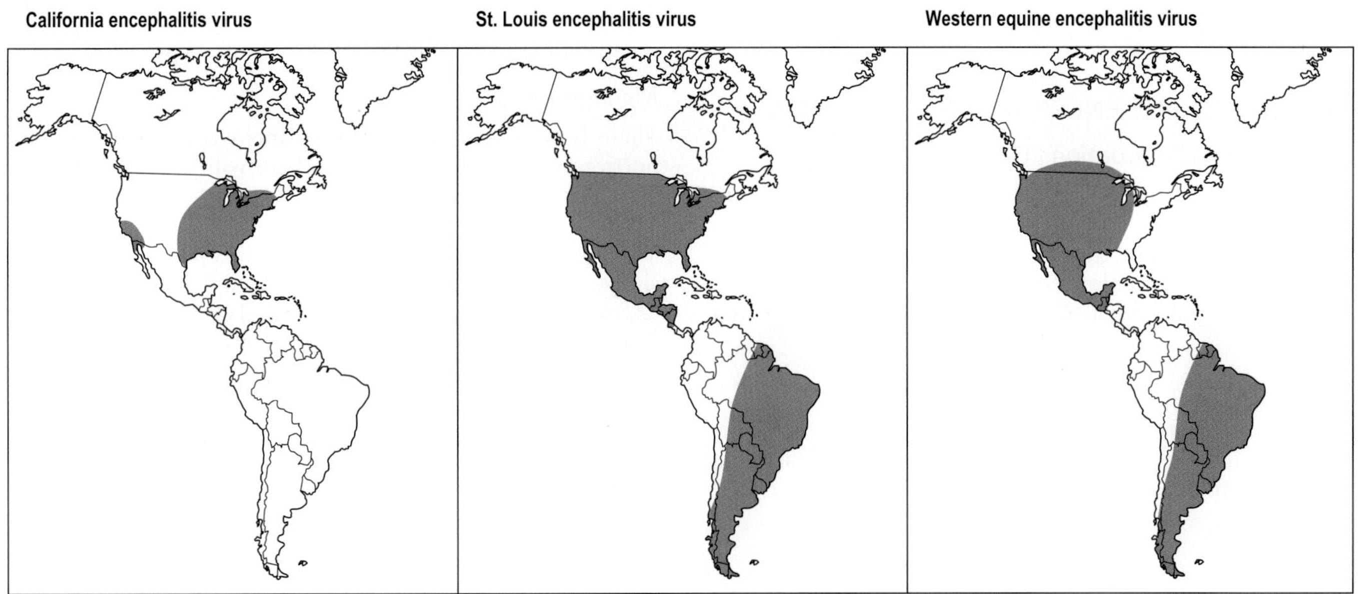

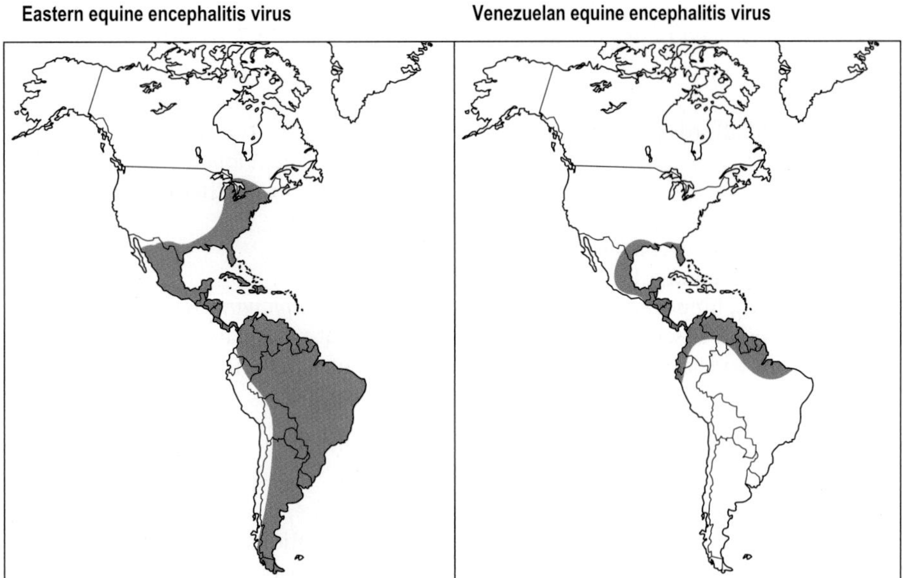

Figure 14.3 Geographical distribution of mosquito-borne encephalitis in the New World.

flaccid or spastic paralysis. Infants have a much more rapid course with fever, convulsions and coma. There is a peripheral leucocytosis in the early stages and the CSF shows a pleocytosis with increased protein levels in those with CNS involvement. Most adults recover fully, although this may take months. Some have residual paralysis, intellectual disability, epilepsy or neuropsychiatric disease. High rates of residual paralysis and severe intellectual impairment are seen in infants, especially those under 3 months.

Diagnosis

The virus may be isolated from serum early in illness, but this is unusual. It can be isolated from post-mortem brain and has been detected in the CSF in some cases. PCR-based tests have also been used successfully. Recent infection can be diagnosed by the detection of rising titres in HI or N tests. IgM detection by EIA is usually positive in the serum at the time of presentation.

Epidemiology

WEEV circulates in more than 75 species of wild birds and some domestic ones. The basic transmission cycle is between *Cx. tarsalis* and birds in the summer. Overwintering of the virus may occur in hibernating mammals but more likely in overwintering mosquitoes. Epizootics in horses acting as amplifying hosts precede human epidemics. In humans, the highest attack rates are in infants and young males in a rural environment.

Control

Anti-mosquito measures are difficult in rural areas, but where small towns are involved, 'fogging' with insecticide may terminate an epidemic. A non-neurotropic strain of virus isolated from birds has been used successfully as a vaccine, but only experimentally.

EASTERN EQUINE ENCEPHALITIS VIRUS (EEEV)

Geographical Distribution (Figure 14.3)

EEEV[16,27,54,55] is found in the eastern USA (where epizootics occur in horses but human cases are rare), Mexico, Panama, Brazil, Argentina and Guyana. Two small human outbreaks have occurred in Dominica and Jamaica, and in 1962 there was a major epidemic of 6762 cases in Venezuela; 0.6% were fatal.

Aetiology

EEEV is an *alphavirus* that occupies its own antigenic group. There are two major variants: North American (including Caribbean strains) and South American.

Transmission

Transmission is by mosquitoes; the *Culiseta* spp. *(Cs. melanura* and *Cs. morsitans)* are the major vectors that maintain the enzootic cycle, while *Aedes* spp. act as sources of transmission to humans and horses. Isolations of virus have been made from other mosquitoes in the field (see Table 14.1).

Immunity

Immunity is antibody-mediated and affords protection against second attacks.

Pathology

The CNS shows extensive changes with neuronal necrosis, perivascular inflammatory changes and meningeal inflammation. These are found in the cerebral cortex, hippocampus and pons, and more severely in the thalamus and basal ganglia. There is little involvement of the cerebellum and spinal cord.

Clinical Features

Natural History. This is the most severe arboviral encephalitis of humans. While most infections are asymptomatic or mild, the rate of encephalitic disease is relatively high, being 5% or more. The mortality rate for encephalitis is 50–75%, with most survivors having severe sequelae. Outcomes are worst in children and the elderly.

Signs and Symptoms. The incubation period is 7–10 days.

The illness begins as a febrile illness lasting up to 2 weeks. In most this resolves, but in about 2% of adults and 6% of children there is sudden onset of encephalitis. Headache, meningism and reduction of conscious state develop. This progresses to coma and convulsions, with most dying in the first few days. There is a peripheral leucocytosis in the early stages, and the CSF usually shows an early polymorph pleocytosis, with a mildly to moderately raised protein level. Those who recover usually have intellectual disability, neuropsychiatric illness and possibly paralysis.

Diagnosis

It is possible to isolate the virus from patients in the prodromal period, but this is rarely achieved in practice. The virus can be isolated from post-mortem brain. Virus has been detected by PCR in horses and humans, but its diagnostic reliability in humans is unknown. Recent infection can be diagnosed by the detection of rising titres in HI or N tests. IgM detection by EIA is usually positive in the serum at the time of presentation.

Management

There is no specific treatment for this virus. High-level supportive therapy is required for patients with encephalitis.

Epidemiology

The virus is maintained in a bird–mosquito cycle across an extensive geographical area. Infection of horses and humans is incidental, and in the centre of the area serological evidence of inapparent human infection can be found. EEEV may cause a high mortality rate in birds, both wild and domestic, though asymptomatic infection with prolonged viraemia is more common. Infection in horses is severe, most dying within a few days.

Control

Vector control is the only approach available. Vaccination is not yet available.

VENEZUELAN EQUINE ENCEPHALITIS VIRUS (VEEV)

Geographical Distribution (Figure 14.3)

Extensive outbreaks with human cases of VEEV[16,27,56,57] have occurred in Venezuela (100 000 equine cases occurred in 1962 – almost wiping out the equine population), Trinidad, Colombia, Brazil and Panama. The virus has also spread through Mexico and the southern USA, with evidence of human infection in Florida.

Aetiology

VEEV is an *alphavirus* with a number of antigenic subtypes. The IABCE subtypes cause epizootic disease, with associated epidemics of human infection. The other subtypes circulate enzootically and cause occasional human infections.

Transmission

The main vectors are *Culex* spp. (particularly the subgenus *Melanoconion*), as well as *Mansonia*, *Psorophora* and *Aedes* species. Isolations have been made from about 40 other species (see Table 14.1). *Simulium* spp. may transmit infections and there is a possibility of person-to-person spread by droplet infection; spread among horses can occur without an insect vector. Aerosol transmission to humans has occurred in laboratory settings.

Immunity

Immunity is antibody-mediated and provides protection against second attacks. It therefore takes about 10 years to build up a susceptible population of humans and equines to sustain a new epidemic.

Clinical Features

Natural History. Most infections are inapparent and the majority of the overt infections are mild and transient, although virulence may vary in epidemics.

Signs and Symptoms. The incubation period is 2–5 days.

The onset is sudden, with fevers, rigors, headache and myalgia. A sore throat and upper respiratory symptoms are common, as are vomiting and conjunctivitis. Some also have diarrhoea. In some cases, and in about 4% of children under 15 years of age, symptoms progress with involvement of the CNS. Neck stiffness, convulsions, coma, and flaccid or spastic paralysis may develop. There is an initial leucopenia and sometimes thrombocytopenia, with pleocytosis and raised protein levels in the CSF. Long-term sequelae seem to be uncommon, but mental depression is common.

Aerosol spread can occur, so appropriate respiratory precautions should be used in hospitals to protect staff, visitors and other patients.

Diagnosis

Virus may be detected by culture or by RT-PCR from the blood in the acute phase, especially within 48 hours of onset, and also from the throat. Recent infection can be diagnosed by the detection of rising titres in HI or N tests. IgM detection by EIA is usually positive in the serum within 1 week of onset.

Aerosol spread can occur and laboratory-acquired infections are well documented. The virus and samples likely to contain virus should be handled with extreme caution, and people working with the virus should be vaccinated.

Management

There is no specific treatment for this virus. High-level supportive therapy is required for encephalitis cases.

Vaccination

A live attenuated vaccine (TC-83) is available for primary immunization against the epidemic strains. It does not elicit good responses in people with previous *alphavirus* infections, nor is it very effective as a booster. An inactivated vaccine (C-84) seems to be better for these applications.

Epidemiology

VEEV circulates silently in small mammals and, with a high rainfall and an increase in the number of mosquitoes and their biting, horses become infected, acting as amplifying hosts. Equine cases precede human cases, most commonly children in whom the disease is more severe. A high proportion of equines develop immunity so that 10 years are necessary to build up another susceptible population.

Control

Mosquito control is difficult in rural conditions.

MAYARO VIRUS (MAYV)

MAYV[58] is an *alphavirus* found initially in Trinidad and has since been recognized in Central America, northern South America and the Amazon basin. Two genotypes have been identified, one of which (Una virus) is restricted to northern Brazil. It is transmitted by *Haemagogus* mosquitoes, and wild vertebrates may serve as the animal hosts. Outbreaks are becoming more common as human populations move into forest areas. Clinically, it resembles CHIKV and some develop persisting arthralgias (see Table 14.1).

O'NYONG-NYONG VIRUS (ONNV)

Geographical Distribution

ONNV[16,27,59,60] is probably endemic in East Africa. A large epidemic beginning in 1959 involved over 2 million people in Uganda, Kenya, Tanzania, Zaire, Malawi, Mozambique, Senegal, Zambia and southern Sudan, and it has also been found in the Central African Republic and Cameroon. The next epidemic occurred in Kenya 35 years later. A variant, Igbo Ora virus is found in West Africa, including Nigeria, the Ivory Coast and the Central African Republic (Figure 14.4).

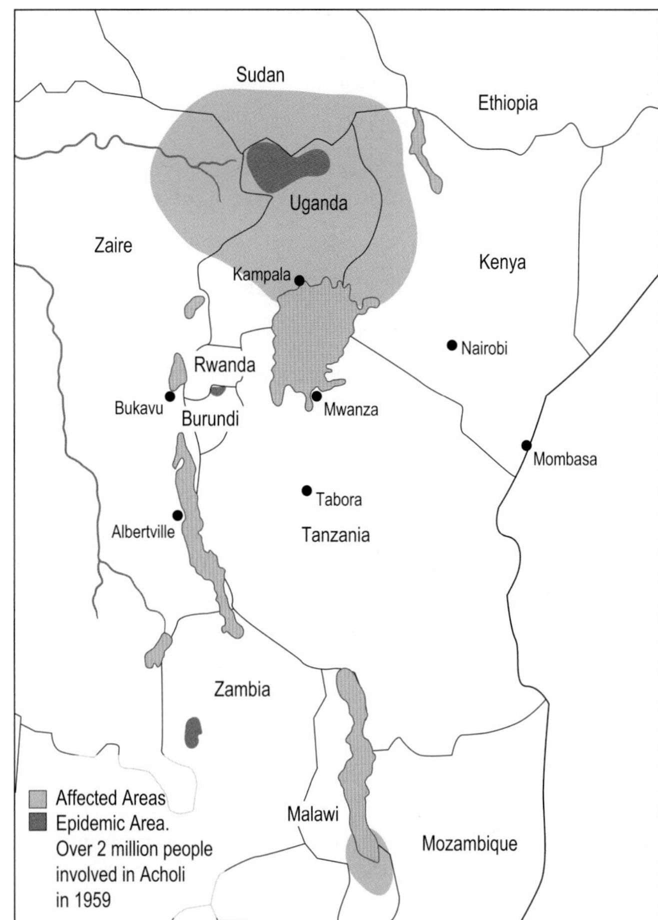

Figure 14.4 Geographical distribution of o'nyong-nyong fever. *(Courtesy of the Department of Entomology, London School of Hygiene and Tropical Medicine.)*

Aetiology

ONNV is an *alphavirus* closely related to CHIKV.

Transmission

Anopheles funestus is the major vector but *An. gambiae* is also involved. A non-human mammalian host has not yet been identified.

Clinical Features

The clinical illness is very similar to CHIKV, with the exception that cervical lymphadenopathy is common, while fever is less prominent. Joint pains may persist for many months.

Epidemiology

There is no animal reservoir identified, though there is likely to be some form of animal–mosquito sylvatic cycle to maintain the virus. Large epidemics occur when the environmental conditions are supportive and there are enough susceptible subjects. Up to 70% of the population may be attacked, with all the age groups affected. Spread of the virus is believed to be by movement of viraemic humans.

Control

Avoidance of mosquito exposure by the use of protective clothing, mosquito nets and mosquito repellents is recommended during epidemic periods.

ROSS RIVER VIRUS (RRV) DISEASE

Geographical Distribution

RRV[16,27,45,61] is named after the area in which it was first isolated from *Aedes vigilax* in 1974. Disease occurs throughout Australia, but most commonly in northern, north-eastern and south-western parts. Epidemics have occurred in Fiji, American Samoa, Cook Islands and New Caledonia. Antibody studies have shown infection to be present in New Guinea, Solomon Islands, the Moluccas and Vietnam.

Transmission

Transmission is by a range of mosquito species including *Ae. vigilax, Ae. camptorhynchus, Cx. annulirostris, Ae. notoscriptus and Ae. sagax* in Australia[62] and *Ae. polynesiensis* in the Cook Islands.[63] *Ae. aegypti* and *Ae. albopictus* are efficient experimental vectors (see Table 14.1).

Pathology

Arthritis is associated with a predominantly mononuclear inflammatory response in the synovium and the synovial fluid. Viral antigen and RNA have been found in joint tissue from patients and RRV is able to replicate in synovial macrophages in vitro. The pathogenesis of *alphavirus* arthritis is discussed earlier.

Clinical Features

Natural History. The incubation period for RRV disease is usually 7–9 days but may vary from 3 to 21 days.

Illness usually begins as joint pains (in a distribution typical of *alphavirus* arthritis) and myalgia, accompanied by lethargy in most patients and fever in about half. A generalized maculopapular rash occurs in 50%, usually after the onset of joint pains but sometimes preceding it. The rash is occasionally vesicular. Headache, photophobia, sore throat and lymphadenopathy may accompany the acute illness. Overall joint pains, swelling and stiffness develop in 80–90% of individuals. The swelling is largely due to synovitis without effusion. The lethargy may be profound and debilitating. The acute illness may resolve over weeks to months, but 10–25% will have joint pains, lethargy and myalgia persisting for over a year, and for several years in some. The chronic illness may follow a relapsing and remitting course.

Diagnosis

Viraemia lasts only a few days and infection is rarely diagnosed by virus isolation. RNA can be detected by PCR in acute serum, but is relatively insensitive. IgG and IgM can be detected by HI, EIA or IFA. There is some cross-reaction with antibody to other *alphavirus* such as BFV, SINV and CHIKV, but IgM reactions are usually limited to the infecting virus. If necessary, specific antibody may be identified by N titres. IgM persists for many months after infection and is therefore only a presumptive indicator of recent infection. Demonstration of seroconversion or a significant rise in IgG levels is required to confirm recent infection.

Management

Treatment is symptomatic, with judicious use of non-steroidal anti-inflammatory agents and simple analgesics for the relief of joint and muscle pains. Physiotherapy and graduated exercise programs help some people. Corticosteroids provide relief of symptoms, but are not currently recommended until there are further data on long-term benefits and risks. A RRV vaccine is currently in clinical trial and promises the opportunity of prophylactic control in the near future.

Epidemiology

Macropods (kangaroos and wallabies) are thought to be the natural vertebrate hosts, but in epidemics the virus can spread from person to person via mosquito vectors. In Australia, cases occur annually between summer and autumn. Explosive epidemics have occurred in Fiji, Samoa and the Cook Islands when the disease encountered a fresh non-immune population. Infection rates were 90%, with 40% of the population showing clinical attacks.

SINDBIS VIRUS (SINV)

Geographical Distribution

SINV[16,27] was first isolated at Sindbis in Egypt, and has since been found to be widely distributed through sub-Saharan Africa, Europe, the Middle East, India, Asia, the Philippines, Australia and New Zealand. However, significant human epidemics occur only in Sweden (where it causes Ockelbo fever), Finland (Pogosta fever), adjacent parts of Russia (Karelian fever) and South Africa. There are two major antigenic lineages: the Oriental/Australian and the Paleoarctic/Ethiopian, with a third lineage being detected in south-western Australia.[64]

Aetiology

SINV is an *alphavirus* in the Western equine encephalitis serogroup. Ockelbo virus is a variant of SINV.

Transmission

A range of bird species, including migratory birds, are susceptible to SINV infection. Transmission to birds is via various *Culex* species, including *Cx. univittatus* and *Cx. pipiens.* Depending on the geographic region, humans may be infected by *Aedes, Culex, Culiseta or Mansonia* species.

Clinical Features

Natural History. Descriptions of clinical illness are most detailed for Ockelbo and Pogosta diseases.[65] The incubation period is up to 1 week. Onset is usually joint pain typical of *alphavirus* infection, usually accompanied by a rash, malaise and fatigue. Fever is mild or absent. The rash is initially widespread and maculopapular. Chronic joint pain is common.

Diagnosis

SINV may be isolated from blood during acute illness and, more often, viral genomic RNA is detected by PCR. HI antibody can be detected but does cross-react with other alphaviruses. IgM can be detected by EIA and IFA, as well as HI.

Management

Treatment is symptomatic, as for other *alphavirus* arthritides.

Epidemiology

SINV is maintained primarily in a mosquito–bird cycle. Birds develop a prolonged viraemia, and infected migratory birds may be responsible for spread of the virus. The patterns of disease vary. Ockelbo outbreaks occur each summer/autumn, Pogosta occurs approximately every seven years, and irregular SINV epidemics occur in South Africa.

Flaviviruses (Family: Flaviviridae, Genus: *Flavivirus*)

DENGUE VIRUS (DENV)

For details on Dengue virus, see Chapter 15.

JAPANESE ENCEPHALITIS VIRUS (JEV)

Geographical Distribution

The geographical range of JEV[66–71] now extends from Japan, maritime Siberia and Korea in the north, through all except two provinces of China to the Philippines in the east, through South-east and southern Asia to Sri Lanka, India, Pakistan and Nepal in the west, and as far south as Indonesia and Papua New Guinea (Figure 14.5). JEV has also been reported to have made an incursion into Cape York, the northern most point of Australia.

Aetiology

JEV is 50 nm in diameter and shares antigens with SLEV, WNV and MVEV.

Transmission

Culex tritaeniorhynchus, a rice-field-breeding mosquito, is the main vector in north Asia and Japan. Other vectors include *Cx. annulirostris* in Guam and northern Australia, *Cx. gelidus* and *Cx. fusocephala* in India, Malaysia and Thailand, and *Cx. vishnui* in India (see Table 14.1). Vertical transmission of JEV in both *Culex* and *Aedes* mosquitoes has been demonstrated.

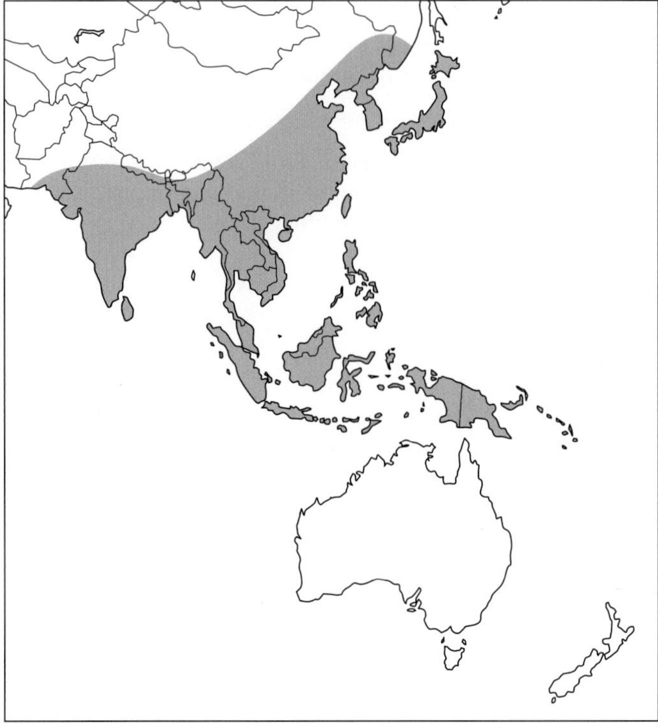

Figure 14.5 Geographical distribution of Japanese encephalitis virus.

Pathology

After inoculation, the virus may replicate in the lymphatic tissues and possibly other organs before invading the CNS. In the brain there are areas of necrosis with small haemorrhages and perivascular cuffing in the grey matter of the cerebral cortex and in the thalamus, midbrain, cerebellum, brainstem and anterior horns of the spinal cord.

Immunity

An antibody-mediated immunity protects against second attacks and builds up resistance in the population.

Clinical Features

Natural History. Many infections are asymptomatic or nonspecific, with encephalitis estimated to occur in only 1 in 300 infections. Encephalitis has a mortality rate of 10–25%, but rises to 40–50% for comatosed patients. Death is more common in children and in the elderly.

The incubation period is 6–16 days.

The onset is sudden, although it may be preceded by gastrointestinal disturbance, especially in children. Fever, headache, altered mental state and, in children, convulsions are the main presenting features. Patients may show generalized weakness or paralysis, cranial nerve palsies and a coarse tremor. A characteristic attitude with head retracted, arms and knees bent, and shoulders pressed to the chest has been described. Some patients make a rapid and complete recovery, but generally severe depression of conscious state and/or evidence of respiratory paralysis are poor prognostic signs. If the acute stage is survived, recovery is slow and 25–50% will have neurological residua. These include paralysis, ataxia, Parkinsonism, mental deterioration, psychiatric disorders and speech difficulties.

The CSF usually shows a pleocytosis, initially due to neutrophils and later lymphocytes, while the protein concentration is normal or moderately raised. Electroencephalography (EEG) and CT findings are usually nonspecific, though the latter may show thalamic and basal ganglia changes in severe cases. MRI has proven more useful in showing these changes.

JEV neurological disease may also present as benign aseptic meningitis, as polio-like acute flaccid paralysis, as an acute psychosis or without overt signs of encephalitis. A variety of psychiatric disturbances occur in many patients several months after recovering from the acute infection.

JEV infection in pregnancy is rare but can result in intrauterine infection and fetal death.

Diagnosis

The virus has occasionally been cultured from human material, mainly CSF in severe cases. The viraemia is short-lived so samples need to be collected early in infection. JEV will grow in mosquito cell lines, a wide range of mammalian cell lines and suckling mouse brain. A number of RT-PCR methods have been described and, if the test is available, it should be performed on early serum samples, CSF and brain tissue where collected. Antigen detection methods have also been used for virus detection in brain. Paired sera taken in the first few days after onset and 2–3 weeks later will show rising antibody levels by HI test, EIA or IFA. IgM is usually detected by EIA or IFA and is present in the serum in the early stages of illness in 80% of cases and virtually all by 10 days after onset. IgM may persist for weeks or months in the serum. It can be detected in CSF in most cases of encephalitis. IgM detection needs to be interpreted with caution in areas where other *flavivirus* infections occur as it may cross-react on tests. IgG antibodies will cross-react broadly with other flaviviruses. The specificity of antibody can be determined by N tests or by monoclonal antibody epitope blocking enzyme immunoassays.

Management

Treatment is supportive, and access to high-level support is important in the survival of severe cases. Neither dexamethasone nor interferon-α has been shown to influence the outcome.

Epidemiology

The main source of infection is rice fields where the vector *Cx. tritaeniorhynchus* breeds, becoming infected from pigs or birds. Three weeks after mosquito breeding begins in the spring, virus can be found in birds and pigs, but humans are not involved until there is a high density of mosquitoes. The virus is amplified by pigs and conveyed to humans. Birds (night herons and egrets) carry the infection from rural to urban areas. There is a seasonal summer incidence, with most activity occurring between June and September in temperate northern regions, with a longer period of transmission further south. In tropical areas transmission is often linked to local monsoonal weather patterns. Most cases are in children and elderly people, although visitors of any age are affected.

Control

Until recently, an inactivated vaccine derived from the attenuated Nakayama strain grown in mouse brain (JE-VAX) was available. The vaccine was given in three injections at 0, 7 and 28 days. Boosters were required every 3 years. Local and systemic reactions to the vaccine were common, and serious hypersensitivity reactions occurred in 1 in 200 people. Several cases of acute encephalomyelitis have also been reported following vaccination, but it is not certain that these were associated with the vaccine. Due to these perceived safety problems with the vaccine, the mouse brain preparation has recently been replaced with a killed vaccine grown in cell culture (JESPECT).[72] Safety profiles of the new vaccine show a slightly improved local tolerability compared to the mouse brain preparation with as yet no serious allergic reactions. A live attenuated vaccine (SA14/14/2) is also used extensively in China. Vector control using chemical larvicides and adulticides has been successful in many areas, although there are increasing problems with insecticide resistance.

KYASANUR FOREST DISEASE VIRUS (KFDV)

Local synonym: 'Monkey disease'.

Geographical Distribution (Figure 14.6)

KFDV[73–75] was first described in 1957 in the Kyasanur Forest of Mysore (now Karnataka) in south-western India, but has been gradually spreading from there. Alkhurma virus is a subtype of KFDV that has been found in Saudi Arabia.

Aetiology

KFDV is a *flavivirus* (see Table 14.1) belonging to the Russian spring summer encephalitis virus group. It is antigenically related to OHFV and POWV, but there is no cross-immunity.

Transmission

KFDV is transmitted by the nymphal stages of ticks that have been infected in the larval stage from a rodent or monkey. The ticks are *Haemaphysalis spinigera*, *H. turturis* and *H. papuana* (kinneari). KFDV is also carried by *Ixodes petauristae* and *I. ceylonensis*, and has been recovered from *Dermacentor* nymphs (see Table 14.1).

Pathology

There are degenerative changes in the large organs. The spleen shows reduction of malpighian corpuscles and erythrophagocytosis. There is focal haemorrhagic bronchopneumonia with focal necrosis of the liver and gastrointestinal tract. The kidneys show acute degeneration of the proximal and collecting tubules. Encephalitis has not been described in human cases.

Immunity

Immunity is antibody-mediated. Little is known about immunity to second attacks, but monkeys that recover are immune. There is no cross-immunity to other flaviviruses.

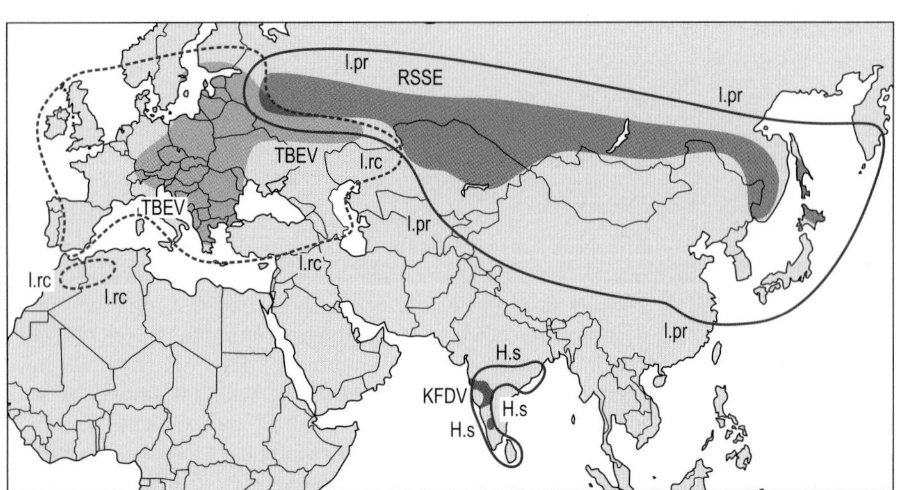

Figure 14.6 Geographical distribution of tick-borne encephalitis virus (TBEV) – RSSE, Russian spring–summer encephalitis (Eastern subtype TBEV); TBEV, European tick-borne encephalitis virus; KFDV, Kyasanur Forest disease virus – and the main vectors. I.pr, *Ixodes persulcatus*; I.rc, *Ixodes ricinus*; H.s, *Haemophysalis spinigera*. *(Courtesy of the Department of Entomology, London School of Hygiene and Tropical Medicine.)*

Clinical Features

Natural History. KFD is mainly a severe febrile illness with complete recovery following a prolonged convalescence. However, meningoencephalitis and/or haemorrhagic disease may develop in a small proportion of cases. The mortality rate is 3–5%, and no sequelae have been reported in survivors.

Signs and Symptoms. The incubation period is 3–8 days after the infective tick bite. In about 20% of cases the disease is biphasic.

The onset is sudden with fever, headache, myalgia, cough, vomiting, diarrhoea, dehydration, hypotension and bradycardia. In the majority of cases there are no haemorrhages, but gastrointestinal bleeding and haemoptysis may occur. After 10 days the illness subsides. In 20% of cases, the fever returns 1–2 weeks after the first phase, lasting 1–7 days. There may then be symptoms of meningoencephalitis, with neck stiffness, mental disturbance, tremors and giddiness, lasting until the fever subsides. After recovery there is a prolonged convalescence, the patient remaining weak for some time. There is a marked leucopenia and a heavy albuminuria with casts in the urine. The CSF is normal in the first phase, but shows increased levels of protein but without cells in the second phase.

Diagnosis

Virus can be isolated from the blood up until the 12th day in suckling mice, hamster, monkey kidney or HeLa cells with cytopathic effect. Serological diagnosis can be made with rising antibody (IFA, HI and N) titres in acute and convalescent sera, as well as by EIA tests.

Management

Treatment is supportive. Care must be taken in the first 12 days to avoid exposure of medical and nursing staff to the patient's blood.

Epidemiology

KFDV circulates in forest rodents, especially the shrew (*Suncus murinus*) but also *Rattus wroughtoni*, *R. blandfordi* and a squirrel (*Funambulus tristriatus*), maintained mainly by larval ticks of *H. spinigera*, *H. turturis* and *H. papuana* (kinneari).

Langur monkeys (*Presbytes entellus*) and bonnet macaques (*Macaca radiata*) acquire larval ticks when foraging on the ground and become infected. Many die, but some recover and are immune for life. When infected, the monkeys show a heavy viraemia. The larvae emerge from the ground as nymphs and come into contact with humans, to whom they transmit the infection as a dead-end infection.

Birds (grey jungle fowl and golden-backed woodpecker) are important in spreading the vector ticks, but are not thought to have a role in maintaining the infection in nature.

The risk of human infection has risen since humans moved into forest environments for rice cultivation, timber felling and cattle ranching. The cattle act as a good food source for the ticks, increasing the infection rates in monkeys thus amplifying the virus and increasing the chance of human exposure.

Control

Control is essentially a breaking of the tick–human contact. Alteration of the environment and keeping cattle out of the forest are important. Personal protection involves regular (daily) de-ticking of the body and the use of repellents and protective clothing. A formalin-inactivated vaccine produced in chick embryo fibroblasts is now used in endemic areas.

KUNJIN VIRUS (KUNV)

KUNV[76,77] is a *flavivirus* in the JE antigenic group and is a subtype of WNV. Human infection and disease have been demonstrated only in Australia. The distribution, reservoirs and transmission seem to be the same as for MVEV. Most infections are asymptomatic, although some produce a febrile illness with headache, with or without arthralgia, myalgia, fatigue and a maculopapular rash. Rare encephalitis cases occur that are clinically identical to MVEV but with a less severe disease and without fatalities. An unusual outbreak of KUNV infection of horses in south-eastern Australia occurred in 2011, resulting in hundreds of cases of severe encephalitis.[78] Although viral isolates from fatal equine cases were shown to be significantly more virulent than reference KUNV strains when tested in mice, there were no recorded cases of human disease due to KUNV infection during the equine outbreak.

LOUPING ILL VIRUS (LIV)

LIV[79,80] is a sheep virus transmitted by *Ixodes ricinus* and found in the UK and parts of southern Europe (Spain, Greece and Turkey). Tick-transmitted cases are rare, with the majority of naturally acquired human infections associated with occupational contact with infected animals. Laboratory-acquired infections are common. It causes an illness very similar to the European subtype TBEV, and the vaccine for that virus will also protect against LIV.

MURRAY VALLEY ENCEPHALITIS VIRUS (MVEV)

Geographical Distribution

MVEV[76,81–84] is found in Australia and New Guinea. Human disease has been identified mainly in the tropical northern areas of Australia, particularly the western and central areas of the north. Epidemic activity occasionally occurs outside these regions, and rarely, it extends to the south-eastern corner of the mainland.

Aetiology

MVEV is a *flavivirus* that lies in the JE antigenic group.

Transmission

Cx. annulirostris is the major mosquito vector. MVEV has also been isolated from a number of *Aedes* species and vertical transmission in these mosquitoes is proposed as a mechanism of persistence in many arid areas.

Pathology

The pathology of MVE is similar to that of JE, with perivascular cuffing in the grey matter, most marked in the thalamus and substantia nigra. These may extend into cerebral white matter, the cerebellum and spinal cord. In more advanced disease there is neuronal loss and areas of focal necrosis in the basal ganglia and thalamus. In severe residual disease these changes are more marked and thalamic necrosis may be seen.

Clinical Features

The majority of infections are asymptomatic or nonspecific. Only about 1 in 500 to 1 in 1000 develop encephalitis.

The incubation period is not well established, but is in the range of 1–3 weeks.

Non-encephalitic illness consists of fever and headache, with or without arthralgia. It settles over 1–2 weeks, although full recovery may take some time. Encephalitic illness in children presents as fever of 1–2 days' duration, almost always with convulsions. Reduction of mental state and respiratory failure may follow. In adults, the encephalitic illness begins with headache, fever and altered mental state. Tremor may be apparent on examination and cranial nerve palsies may develop. The course may then vary from rapid recovery to a prolonged illness with respiratory paralysis or even death. Some patients recover rapidly, whereas others progress to more severe disease characterized by involvement of central brain structures, brain stem and possibly the spinal cord, often with respiratory paralysis. The mortality rate is around 25%, and about 50% of survivors have neurological residua varying from mild cranial nerve palsy to spastic quadriparesis. Death and severe residua are much more likely in the elderly and in infants.

In encephalitis cases the CT findings are usually unremarkable or show nonspecific cerebral oedema, and EEG shows nonspecific changes. MRI in late disease has been reported to show thalamic destruction. Occasionally it mimics herpes simplex encephalitis clinically, and may show temporal lobe changes on CT or MRI scan. The CSF shows a variable leucocyte pleocytosis, usually with lymphocyte predominance, and raised protein levels.

Diagnosis

The virus has rarely been cultured from human material, and the viraemia is likely to be short lived. It will grow in mosquito cell lines and suckling mouse brain. RT-PCR has been used to detect virus in the serum and CSF in the first few days of infection. Paired sera taken shortly after onset and 2–3 weeks later will show rising antibody levels by HI, EIA or IFA, although the HI test is the least sensitive and levels may rise late or not at all. IgM is nearly always present in the serum in the early stages of illness, and can also be detected in about 75% of CSF samples in encephalitis. IgM may persist for weeks or months in the serum. Antibodies will cross-react with other flaviviruses, particularly KUNV and JEV, which may also cause encephalitis in the same geographical area. The specificity of antibody can be determined by N tests or epitope-blocking EIA, although misleading results may occur in patients who have had a previous *flavivirus* infection.

Management

Treatment is supportive, and access to respiratory support is important in the survival of severe cases. Based on the experience with JE, steroids are not recommended, although dexamethasone may be used to reduce intracranial pressure if needed. In contrast, preliminary data on the possible effectiveness of interferon-α for WNV infections suggest that this may be useful.

Epidemiology

The virus is maintained in a cycle involving water birds and mosquitoes. The vector *Cx. annulirostris* becomes infected with MVEV after feeding on birds, which can carry the infection widely by migration. There is also evidence for vertical transmission. A variety of wild and domesticated animals can be infected, but their role in the natural history is unclear (see Table 14.1).

Immunization

There is no specific vaccine for MVEV. Recent data suggest that vaccination with an adjuvanted, inactivated JEV vaccine induces cross protective antibody to MVEV in mice and horses.[21]

OMSK HAEMORRHAGIC FEVER VIRUS (OHFV)

Geographical Distribution

OHFV[73,80] occurs in the Omsk and Novosibirsk regions of western Siberia.

Aetiology

OHFV is a *flavivirus* (see Table 14.1) morphologically similar to but antigenically and genetically distinct from TBEV. The virus can be grown in HeLa cells or chick embryos.

Transmission

The virus is harboured by ticks – *Dermacentor reticulatus* and *D. marginatus* – with trans-stadial and transovarial transmission. The ticks transmit the infection to humans from rodents, mainly muskrats (see Table 14.1). The mechanism of inter-rodent transmission in nature is not known, but mites may transmit the infection between muskrats and other rodents. Infection by direct contact with muskrat carcasses and pelts is common, and inter-human transmission occurs. There is some evidence of infection by the respiratory route.

Pathology

The pathology of fatal cases is that of haemorrhagic fevers with haemorrhage in multiple tissues and necrotic lesions in the liver. Immunity is antibody-mediated; little is known about second attacks.

Clinical Features

OHF is essentially a self-limiting acute infection in the majority of cases, although a small proportion develops haemorrhagic disease. The mortality rate is 1–3%.

The incubation period is 3–7 days.

Signs and Symptoms. The illness is similar to KFD. Complete recovery is usual, although it may take several weeks. Some patients have a biphasic illness with pneumonia, neurological and/or renal disease.

Diagnosis

Virus can be isolated from the blood in the febrile period. Serological diagnosis is made by the CF, HI and N tests, and differentiation needs to be made with TBEV antibody.

Epidemiology and Control

The reservoir of infection is the muskrat and ticks. Human infection depends upon muskrat–human contact, which may be via ticks or the handling of muskrat carcasses and pelts. When there is a great mortality of muskrats then contact is greater and outbreaks occur. TBEV vaccine may offer cross-protection against OHFV.

POWASSAN VIRUS (POWV)

Geographical Distribution

POWV[73,80] is found in Russia, the USA and Canada, and has been isolated from several tick species, including *Ixodes* species, *Dermacentor* species and *Haemaphysalis longicornis*. The natural hosts are mainly wild rodents. Human infections are probably largely asymptomatic. However, some infected individuals develop a nonspecific febrile illness that progresses to meningoencephalitis. The disease may resemble acute herpes simplex encephalitis, while other cases are similar to illness due to the Far-Eastern subtype of TBEV, with upper limb paralysis.

ROCIO VIRUS (ROCV)

ROCV[85,86] emerged as a cause of outbreaks of encephalitis in Brazil in 1975–1976 and since then sporadic cases have continued to be identified but there have not been further epidemics. It is probably carried by wild birds and transmitted by *Psorophora ferox* and *Aedes scapularis* mosquitoes (see Table 14.1). It has an incubation period of 7–14 days, and illness begins with headache, fever, nausea and vomiting, sometimes with pharyngitis and conjunctivitis. Meningitis or encephalitis follows in many, with altered mental state and cerebellar tremor. Convulsions are uncommon. The mortality rate is about 10%. Death occurs in patients of all ages, and neurological sequelae are common. Gait disturbances may appear in survivors. There is no specific therapy or vaccine.

ST LOUIS ENCEPHALITIS VIRUS (SLEV)

Geographical Distribution (Figure 14.3)

SLEV[86–89] was the most important arbovirus in the USA prior to the introduction of WNV. It is widespread throughout North America but has also occurred in Trinidad, Central America, Brazil and Argentina.

Aetiology

SLEV is 30–40 nm in diameter and is antigenically related to JEV and WNV.

Transmission

The basic transmission cycle is between birds and several culicine mosquitoes with most activity in the summer months. This seasonal activity may be due to reintroduction of the virus by migratory waterbirds, or possibly over-wintering in hibernating bats, other mammals or mosquitoes. The main vectors for transmission to humans are *Cx. quinquefasciatus* in urban areas, and *Cx. tarsalis* and *Cx. nigripalpus* in rural areas. Transovarial transmission has been demonstrated in these three species (see Table 14.1).

Pathology

The nervous system shows changes similar to the other *flavivirus* infections, with lymphocytic inflammation and neuronal degeneration in the basal ganglia, brainstem, cerebellum and spinal cord.

Clinical Features

Natural History. The vast majority of infections are asymptomatic or nonspecific. When clinically apparent, infection most often manifests as encephalitis, and less frequently as meningitis or as fever with severe headache. Children are less likely to develop symptomatic disease and it is usually mild. The overall mortality rate is 7%, but is age-dependent with most deaths being in the elderly.

The incubation period is 6–16 days.

Onset is sudden, with fever and severe headache. Neck stiffness and photophobia may occur. Progression to CNS involvement is shown by drowsiness and confusion. Cerebellar ataxia, cranial nerve palsies and cogwheel rigidity may develop, and about 60% have intention tremor. Upper limb paralysis may occur. Convulsions are more common in children and, if severe and prolonged, are a poor prognostic sign. The CSF usually shows a mild to moderate lymphocyte pleocytosis and a raised protein concentration, though a neutrophil predominance may be seen in early infection. Changes in the basal ganglia may be seen on MRI scanning. Following recovery from the acute encephalitis, mild to serious sequelae may be found, particularly in the elderly. Parkinsonism, paralysis, tremor, confusion, gait disturbances and more general declines in cerebral function are seen. Neuropsychiatric disease is a relatively common late effect.

Diagnosis

Virus may be isolated from CSF in the early stages of the illness, but rarely from acute blood. It is best grown in newborn white mice, but also grows in hamster and chicken kidney cell cultures. Antigen may be detected by IFA in brain tissue or CSF mononuclear cells. Nucleic acid detection tests have also been used, but are usually negative by the time patients present. Serological diagnosis is achieved by showing rising antibody levels by HI, CF or N tests, and IgM detection by EIA helps to diagnose early infection. Detection of IgM in the CSF is a reliable indicator of encephalitis. IgM is relatively specific for the infecting virus, though possible cross-reactivity with WNV IgM should be considered. As with other flaviviruses, IgM persists in serum for several months after acute illness. To confirm the specificity of the antibody, N tests are required to differentiate it from antibody to other flaviviruses such as WNV.

Epidemiology

Cx. quinquefasciatus, being an urban mosquito, is responsible for urban outbreaks, while *Cx. tarsalis* and *Cx. nigripalpus* are responsible for rural outbreaks. In urban areas both children and adults are affected equally, but elderly people are most affected. In rural areas people with outdoors occupations are most at risk. Epidemics occur in the late summer and early autumn.

Treatment

Treatment is largely supportive, the level depending on the severity of disease. Interferon-α improves survival in a mouse model and, based on anecdotal experience with WNV encephalitis, it should be considered in severe cases.

Control

Surveillance and vector control are key to managing outbreaks of SLEV. 'Fogging' with insecticides may be necessary during epidemics.

TICK-BORNE ENCEPHALITIS VIRUS (TBEV)

This tick-borne *flavivirus*[73,80,90,91] has three subtypes: the Far-Eastern, the Siberian and the European, although there is considerable overlap. Other names include Russian epidemic encephalitis, Russian Far-East encephalitis, Russian spring–summer, central European encephalitis, Negishi virus and others.

Geographical Distribution (Figure 14.6)

The Far-Eastern subtype is seasonally epidemic in scattered foci in the far eastern part of the former USSR and extending across into China and Japan. The Siberian subtype occurs in the Urals, Siberia and far-eastern Russia, and the European subtype includes most virus isolates from Europe. The Siberian and Far-Eastern subtypes have also been detected in Europe.

Aetiology

TBEV is spherical, 50 nm in diameter, with a dense centre and surface membrane. It shares antigens with LIV, OHFV and KFDV but not JEV.

Transmission

Ixodes ricinus is the major vector of European TBEV, while *Ix. persulcatus* is involved in transmission of the Siberian and Far-Eastern subtypes. *Ix. ovatus, Ix. gibosus, Dermacentor* species and *Haemaphysalis* species have also been implicated. Viral infection is maintained by transovarial and transstadial transmission in ticks, as well as possible horizontal transmission by close proximity. In addition to tick bites, people may also become infected from drinking infected unpasteurized milk and less commonly by entry through injured skin or mucosa, such as crushing an infected tick on the skin. Rare aerosol transmission may occur (see also Table 14.1).

Pathology

The virus enters via a tick bite, ingestion of infected milk or, rarely, through injured skin or mucosa or by inhalation. After multiplying at the site of injection it spreads through the reticuloendothelial system where it is further amplified. In some cases it then invades the CNS. It causes neuronal destruction in the cerebral cortex, basal ganglia, cerebellar cortex, brainstem and anterior horns of the spinal cord.

Clinical Features

Natural History. The infection is often inapparent but when overt, is severe. The Far Eastern subtype (mortality rate 20%) is more severe than the European (mortality rate 1–2%) and Siberian (mortality 1–3%) subtypes.

The incubation period is 3–14 days. Illness due to the Far Eastern subtype usually presents with fever, headache, nausea, and myalgia. Up to 50% develop neurological signs such as meningitis, meningoencephalitis, ataxia, cranial and spinal nerve palsies, and paralysis. Rare haemorrhagic disease has occurred. The European subtype begins as an influenza-like illness that lasts a few days and may lead to a full recovery. In about one-third of cases a second phase begins several days later, with fever and a mild meningoencephalitis. Some have more severe disease resembling the Far Eastern subtype. In rare cases a poliomyelitis-like syndrome with upper limb and respiratory paralysis occurs. The Siberian subtype produces a disease of intermediate severity. Residual neurological disease is common, such as neuropsychiatric disease, progressive weakness and Parkinsonism. The virus has been shown to persist in the brain for over 10 years in some patients.

Diagnosis

Virus can be isolated from the blood in the first week, but this is rarely done in practice. A number of RT-PCR assays have been developed and appear to be highly sensitive for detection of virus in the blood in early infection, prior to the appearance of antibody. Testing of CSF or of blood after the appearance of antibodies has a much lower yield.[92] IgM can be detected in acute serum and possibly the CSF. Serum IgM persists for many months. Paired acute and convalescent sera will show rising IgG levels by HI, CF, IFA, EIA or N tests. Specific antibody can be identified by N tests.

Treatment

Hyperimmune serum may be used in the first week, preferably within the first 3 days of onset of the initial illness, but its effectiveness is not clearly established. Otherwise, treatment is supportive.

Epidemiology

The virus circulates in small wild animals, chiefly rodents, and is transmitted by larval and nymphal ticks which, when they mature, feed on larger mammals, including humans. The incidence of the disease is seasonal – spring and early summer – occurring in small epidemics in the eastern part of the former USSR, where it is a disease of the forest and the taiga. In Europe it is a forest disease and occurs from late spring until early autumn, and outbreaks often follow a period when voles are numerous.

Control

Tick repellents and protective clothing may be of help. Pesticide treatment of large areas or restriction of access has been used.

Immunization

A formalin-inactivated vaccine grown in chick embryo cells is commercially available for the European subtype. The initial vaccine had a high rate of reactions, but that is not a problem with the current purified vaccines. It is 97–98% effective and has been used for mass vaccination in Austria and Germany. It is also recommended for people going to work in or visiting high-risk areas, and for laboratory personnel working with the virus. Hyperimmune globulin can also be used as prophylaxis before and after exposure.

Formalin-inactivated vaccines made from infected mouse brain and later from chick embryo cells have also been produced for the Far Eastern subtype.

WEST NILE VIRUS (WNV)

Geographical Distribution

Serological surveys, virus isolations and reports of disease outbreaks in humans and animals indicate that WNV[28,93] is widely spread throughout Africa, the Middle East, southern Europe, Russia, southern India, parts of South-east Asia, North America and more recently South America (Figure 14.7). In addition, the Australian virus KUNV has now been recognized as a subtype of WNV.[94]

Virus Morphology

WNV is a member of the JE antigenic complex within the *Flavivirus* genus. Similar to other flaviviruses, the virion is roughly

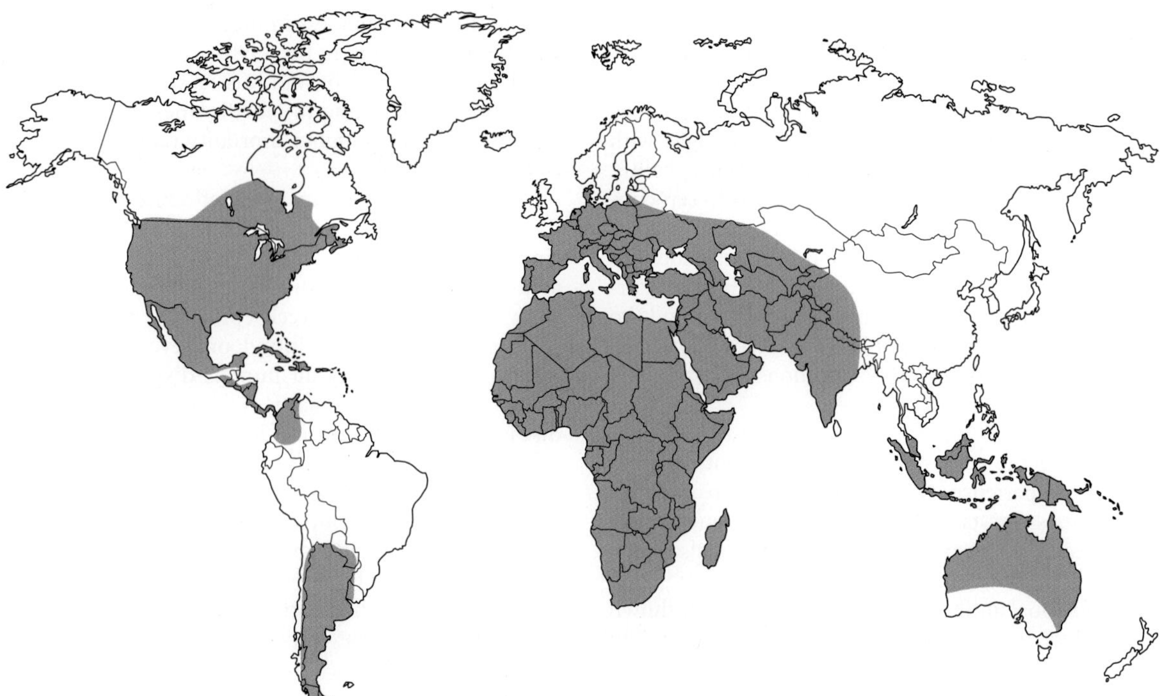

Figure 14.7 Geographical distribution of West Nile and Kunjin viruses.

spherical and approximately 40–50 nm in diameter. A lipid envelope encloses a nucleocapsid that contains the single-stranded, positive-sense RNA genome.

Transmission

Culex mosquitoes, particularly those that feed on birds, have a major role in the transmission of WNV. The virus has also been isolated from mosquitoes of other genera, including *Aedes* and *Mansonia*, which may also serve as natural vectors. WNV has also been isolated from several species of ticks, some of which have been shown to transmit the virus under laboratory conditions. These long-lived vectors may have an important role in the dispersal and overwintering of the virus.

WNV can also be transmitted via blood transfusion. Currently, blood donations in the USA are screened for the presence of WNV, and travel history to WNV-endemic areas is used to screen donors in several countries. This approach has been effective in substantially reducing transfusion-transmission events. Other mechanisms of transmission include organ transplantation, percutaneous exposure, intrauterine infection and possibly via breast milk. Oral transmission occurs among animals by ingestion of infected animals or carcasses. There is some evidence to suggest faecal–oral transmission among confined animals.

Pathology

Following an infected mosquito bite, the virus replicates locally, probably in dendritic cells, then spreads via the reticuloendothelial system and the blood. In those who develop neurological disease, the virus infects neurones of the cerebral cortex, brainstem and spinal cord (especially the anterior horn), resulting in neuronal death. There are infiltrates of microglia and polymorphonuclear leukocytes, perivascular cuffing, neuronal degeneration, and neuronophagia. Immunohistochemical staining has demonstrated viral antigens in neurons, neuronal processes, and areas of necrosis. The histopathologic lesions and immunostaining are more prominent in the brain stem and spinal cord, which may explain the clinical manifestation of muscle weakness in some patients.[95] Virus has been detected in other organs in infected animals and in cancer patients, but this has not been demonstrated in immunocompetent humans.

Clinical Features

Natural History. In the great majority of cases WNV causes an inapparent infection; in others there is an acute dengue-like fever (for which it has often been mistaken) followed by recovery, but a few patients develop meningoencephalitis. Encephalitis has developed in about 1% of infected individuals in the USA, and is much more likely and more severe in adults than in children. The mortality rate from encephalitis is 10–40%.

The incubation period is 2–14 days. Historically the disease has been typically mild, with fever, headache, myalgia, backache and anorexia. Generalized lymphadenopathy, maculopapular rash and nausea are also commonly reported. Other reported manifestations include hepatitis, myocarditis and rhabdomyolysis. Where progression to CNS involvement occurs, the patient develops severe headache, confusion and depression of conscious state, neck stiffness, cranial nerve palsies, tremors and generalized weakness. Presentations with a poliomyelitis-like syndrome and Guillain–Barré syndrome have both been reported. The CSF shows a mild pleocytosis, initially with neutrophil predominance and later lymphocytic, with a raised protein level. CT and MRI scans are usually not helpful in early disease and the EEG shows nonspecific changes. Most survivors have significant neurological residua.

Diagnosis

Virus may be detected in clinical samples by isolation or RNA detection by PCR, especially in the 1st week after onset of illness.[96] A number of test are now available for the detection of WNV-specific IgM in acute-phase serum of patients, and a positive result provides reliable evidence of recent infection. However, it is recommended to also test for IgM to other flaviviruses that may be present in the same area to exclude serological cross-reaction. Indeed, the initial diagnosis of index cases of WN in New York in 1999 was confounded by cross-reactions of WNV IgM with SLEV. Detection of IgM in CSF is a good indicator of encephalitis, but is absent in many cases. Recent infection results in seroconversion or a rise in IgG as measured by HI, IFA or EIA. Specific WNV antibody can be identified using N titres or monoclonal antibody epitope-blocking enzyme immunoassays. It is not currently possible to serologically distinguish between antibody to the different lineages or sublineages of WNV, so KUNV infection is serologically identical to other WNV infections.

Treatment

Supportive therapy is the main component of patient management. Anecdotal experience with interferon-α in a small number of patients suggests that it may be useful, but further experience is needed.[97] Hyperimmune globulin has also been tried and may have some benefits. A potently neutralizing humanized monoclonal antibody to WNV has also been shown to protect hamsters from lethal challenge with WNV when administered up to 5 days post-infection.[98] However the small time window available after the appearance of symptoms will likely limit the efficacy of this treatment.

Epidemiology

WNV is maintained in nature primarily in bird–mosquito cycles. Several species, including crows and pigeons, develop high titres of virus in the blood and provide an infectious blood meal for competent mosquito vectors. Although humans and horses exhibit clinical disease, they are probably dead-end hosts. WNV may be widely dispersed by migration of infected birds.

Following its first isolation from a patient in Uganda in 1937, serological studies in Egypt and the Sudan revealed that human infections with WNV were extremely common, indicating the virus was endemic in parts of Africa. However, the disease had historically manifested as sporadic cases and epidemics of dengue-like febrile illness in that continent, with rare incidents of CNS involvement. In the 1990s, outbreaks of WNV encephalitis occurred in Europe and Russia, with spread to the Western hemisphere, beginning in North America in 1999. These outbreaks had a much higher mortality rate than previously experienced with WNV.

WNV exists as two main genetic lineages (I and II). While the latter appears to be restricted to Africa and parts of Europe (including an outbreak in Greece in 2012) and has been associated primarily with febrile illness (although some fatal cases were reported in the Greek epidemic of 2012), virus strains of lineage I have been found on several continents and are responsible for nearly all human disease, including the outbreaks of WNV encephalitis. Viruses in this lineage also cause disease in horses and death in a range of bird species. Lineage 1 has been subdivided into genetic clades. Clade 1a strains appear to be responsible for the recent outbreaks of severe disease in humans, horses and birds, including those in the West. In contrast clade 1b stains, which are mainly confined to Australia, have rarely caused encephalitis in humans or animals. However, as described earlier, a variant strain that emerged in Australia in 2011 was responsible for an extensive outbreak of encephalitis in horses.[78]

Immunization

Several candidate vaccines are in development or evaluation, including live vaccines, subunit vaccines, recombinant and chimeric vaccines. Immunogenicity, safety and protective efficacy have been shown in animals for some vaccines, but none are yet available for human use. There is also evidence that immunization with the inactivated JE vaccine provides some cross-protection against WNV in mice and horses[30].

YELLOW FEVER VIRUS (YFV)

Geographical Distribution

YFV[3,8,99–101] is found in the tropical forest areas of Africa and South America (Figure 14.8) and until early last century caused

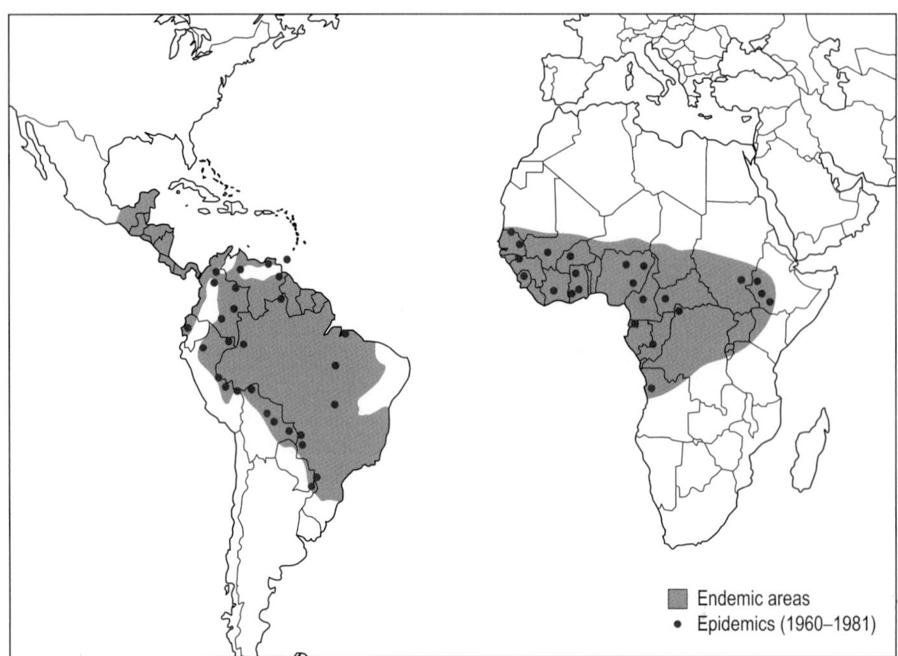

Figure 14.8 Geographical distribution of yellow fever virus.

large epidemics in the Caribbean and the subtropical and temperate regions of North America as far north as Baltimore and Philadelphia. 'Jungle' YF still occurs in Brazil and there was an outbreak in Trinidad in 1978–1979, with 18 cases and eight deaths. Many other epidemics have occurred in South America, and a large epidemic in Ethiopia was responsible for many deaths in 1960–1962, and in Senegal in 1965–1966. YF has caused fatalities in tourists, especially in West Africa, who have not been vaccinated. Over the last decade, there have been several major YFV outbreaks in West and East Africa with fatal cases being imported in Europe, suggesting more intense transmission.

Genetic studies support the hypothesis that YFV probably originated in East and central Africa and was initially introduced into West Africa and then transported to South America, possibly by ships carrying infected mosquitoes in the post-Columbian period. YFV has never been documented in Asia or Australasia although potential vectors (*Ae. aegypti* in South-east Asia) abound. The reasons for this are not clear, but one factor could be that the *Ae. aegypti* mosquitoes in Asia may not be as susceptible to YFV as those in the Americas and Africa.

Aetiology

YFV is a *flavivirus* (see Table 14.1) 25–65 nm in size, which can survive at 4°C for a month and freeze-dried for many years. There are several strains that can infect humans. African strains of YFV possess an antigen absent from American strains. The 17D strain, which is used so successfully as a live vaccine, has acquired an antigen absent from the original 'Asibi' strain from which it was developed. Seven genotypes have been identified, comprising five from Africa and two from South America.

Transmission

Mosquitoes. In nature, mosquitoes of several genera transmit YFV (see Table 14.1). In the Americas the forest cycle is maintained by mosquitoes belonging to the genera *Haemagogus* and *Sabethes*. *Ae. aegypti* is responsible for urban outbreaks. Virus has also been isolated from *Ae. fulvus* in Brazil. In Africa, *Ae. africanus* maintains the monkey–mosquito–monkey cycle in the forest, while *Ae. simpsoni*, which breeds close to humans in the axils of banana plants, becomes infected from monkeys raiding the plantations, and transmits YFV to people. Other *Aedes* involved in the forest cycle include *Ae. luteocephalus*, *Ae. opok*, *Ae. furcifer* and *Ae. taylori*. Vertical transmission of YFV from one generation to another in mosquitoes is thought to be important for virus survival during the dry season. In Africa the urban cycle is maintained by *Ae. aegypti*.

Mosquitoes can become infected from the first to third day of fever in the host. The intrinsic cycle in the mosquito is 4 days at 37°C and 18 days at 18°C. Mosquitoes remain infected for life. The possibility of transovarial transmission has already been mentioned.

Ticks. YFV has been isolated from *Amblyomma variegatum* in Brazil and trans-stadial transmission was demonstrated by infecting nymphs and passing on the infection to uninfected monkeys at the adult stage. The epidemiological significance of this is not clear.

Other methods of transmission have not been identified in nature. However, the high-level viraemia in infected humans and animals raises a potential for transmission though exposure to blood or infected tissues. Caution should be exercised in handling these materials

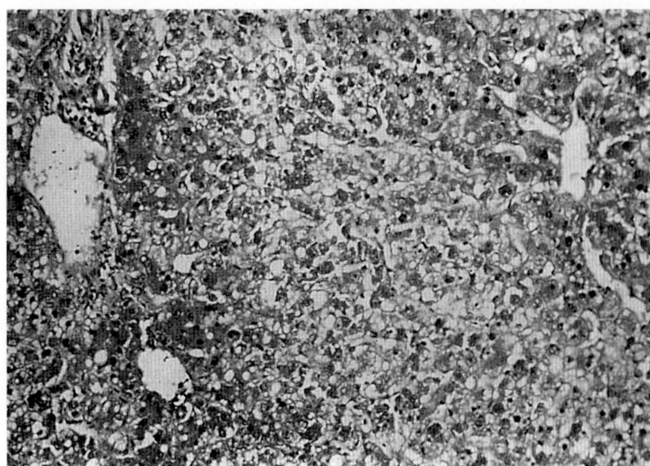

Figure 14.9 Post-mortem appearance of the liver of a rhesus monkey with yellow fever, showing well marked mid-zonal necrosis and minimal inflammatory changes.

Pathology

YFV replicates initially in the reticuloendothelial system before spreading to multiple organs, including liver, spleen, bone marrow, myocardium and skeletal muscle. Pathological changes are seen in all of these organs, characterized by cell damage. The kidneys show acute tubular necrosis, and there is damage of myocardial cells. In the liver of acutely infected patients, YFV produces fatty degeneration of liver cells and central coagulative necrosis of the lobules with sparing of the borders (Figure 14.9). The nuclei of the liver cells are pyknotic and the coagulated contents of the cells stain deeply with eosin, the Councilman bodies resulting from this degeneration taking on a salmon-pink colour (Figure 14.10). These resolve completely in recovered cases. Cerebral changes may occur with oedema and petechial haemorrhages. Haemorrhages may also be seen in other organs such as the lungs, liver and spleen. The bleeding abnormalities are probably a result of a combination of reduced production of coagulation factors by the liver, combined with platelet dysfunction and DIC.

Death usually results from failure of the liver or kidneys or both, although cardiac damage may contribute.

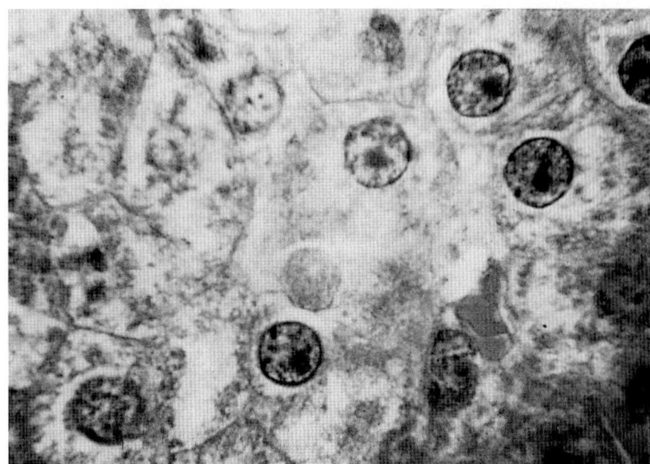

Figure 14.10 Councilman body in the liver cell of a rhesus monkey affected with yellow fever.

Immunity

Immunity is antibody mediated, and lifelong immunity follows infection with YFV. In many endemic areas where contact with virus-carrying mosquitoes is constant (i.e., near the forest), infection in childhood is common, leading to reactivation in later life.

Clinical Features

Natural History. Asymptomatic infections, especially in endemic areas, are common, leading to high levels of immunity within indigenous populations. When disease occurs in endemic areas it is generally mild with a mortality rate of 5–10%. During epidemics the mortality rate is several magnitudes higher, but the exact figure is unclear.

Signs and Symptoms. The incubation period is usually 3–6 days.

Most infections are asymptomatic or mild, with only a small proportion progressing to severe classical YF. The mild form is an acute febrile illness with sudden onset of fever and headache without other symptoms, lasting 48 hours or less. In some other patients, the headache is more severe, accompanied by myalgia, low back pain and slight proteinuria. The characteristic bradycardia in relation to temperature is present and the illness may last several days with recovery.

In severe illness, the onset is abrupt with higher fever, severe headache, nausea, vomiting, abdominal pain and distressing pain in the back, loins and limbs. The patient is dehydrated with a dry tongue and foul breath. Early signs of jaundice may appear in the conjunctivae and skin, and minor bleeding from the gums and nose may be noted. This is called the 'period of infection' corresponding with the viraemia. It lasts about 3 days, and the patient may recover spontaneously after this. If they progress, there may be a 24-hour period of apparent improvement, followed by rapid deterioration. Jaundice worsens and there is frank haemorrhaging from the gastrointestinal tract and other sites. Epigastric pain and vomiting develop and there is a deterioration of renal function and albuminuria. There can be hypotension and heart failure, with a characteristic prolongation of the PR and QT intervals on electrocardiography. The patient may recover rapidly after a period of 3–4 days, or recovery may take over 2 weeks. Death occurs in 20–50%, typically on the seventh to tenth day of illness. Bad prognostic signs are increasing proteinuria, haemorrhages, a rising pulse, hypotension, oliguria and azotaemia.

If the patient recovers from a severe attack, convalescence tends to be long but usually without sequelae. Late deaths after convalescence are very rare and are related to myocardial damage, cardiac arrhythmia or cardiac failure. Disease in children is usually milder and dominated by jaundice.

Diagnosis

Virus can be isolated from the blood in the first few days, or from autopsy samples. Antigen-capture EIA in serum is positive in most cases. RNA detection by RT-PCR appears to be more sensitive and easier than these other techniques.

Serological Diagnosis. IgM can be detected during the acute phase by EIA, IFA or HI, and persists for several months following infection. IFA, HI and N antibodies appear within 1 week of onset and CF antibodies later. Paired acute and convalescent sera showing a rising titre are diagnostic of recent infection, but IgG shows broad cross-reactions with other flaviviruses, though specific IgG can be identified by N titres. Previous YFV vaccination may produce low-level antibodies in serum, and IgM may remain for several months.

Management

There is no specific therapy and treatment is supportive and similar to the management of other haemorrhagic fevers such as DHF. Neither serum nor interferon has been shown to be useful.

Epidemiology

There are two cycles: the forest cycle (jungle yellow fever) and the urban cycle (urban yellow fever).

Forest Cycle (Jungle Yellow Fever). In the Americas, YFV is maintained in rainforests in a cycle involving monkeys and marmosets and *Haemagogus* (tree-hole breeding) mosquitoes. Recurrent epizootics occur in howler (*Alouatta*) monkeys who die in large numbers, starting in Panama and spreading up the east coast of Central America to Guatemala, confirming the belief recorded by Balfour in 1914 that a 'silent forest' where all the howler monkeys had died denoted the presence of YFV. A number of other monkey species also have a role: spider (*Ateles*) monkeys, squirrel (*Saimiris*) monkeys and owl (*Aotus*) monkeys develop fatal infections, while other species such as capuchin (*Cebus*) monkeys are asymptomatic but have viraemia sufficient to be infectious. Humans predominantly contract the disease when clearing forest areas; *Haemagogus* mosquitoes bite in and around houses in forest clearings. *Sabethes* (a drought-resistant mosquito) transmits infection during the dry season.

In the forests of West, Central and East Africa, a jungle cycle exists as an inapparent infection in monkeys, mainly vervet (*Cercopithecus*) monkeys. Other susceptible primates with asymptomatic infections include colobus (important in Ethiopia), mangabeys (*Cercocebus*) and baboons (*Papio*). In East Africa, some species of bushbaby (*Galago*), which are susceptible to the virus, have been shown to have high levels of YFV antibodies and may be involved in transmission cycles. Several different *Aedes* spp. are important vectors of YFV in Africa (see YFV transmission, above). Human infections generally follow the movement of humans into forested areas for agricultural purposes.

An endemic-area population will show a rising percentage of positive antibody tests with age, whereas an epidemic situation will be shown by antibodies in the older age and none in the younger age groups.

Urban Cycle (Urban Yellow Fever). When there is a high population of *Ae. aegypti*, intense transmission among humans occurs, with large epidemics where there are enough non-immunes in the population, which can be brought about by immigration, increased urbanization, poor maintenance of vaccination campaigns or a rising number of people born since the last epidemic. In the early years of the twentieth century huge epidemics of this nature frequently spread throughout the Caribbean and up the east coast of North America. Once *Ae. aegypti* was controlled, these epidemics ceased, and no urban cases of YF were described from the Americas for more than 40 years. However, urban cases continue to occur sporadically and the potential for future epidemics remains.

Regular YF epidemics continue in sub-Saharan Africa. In the Nuba mountains of southern Sudan in 1940 there was an epidemic (17 000 cases; mortality rate 10%) and in south-western Ethiopia along the Omo River in 1960–1962 (15 000–30 000 deaths; mortality rate up to 85%). In 1965–1966 in Senegal, there was an epidemic mainly affecting children under 10 years with a mortality rate of 15%. Since then activity has occurred in a number of countries in sub-Saharan Africa.

Control

Eradication and control of *Ae. aegypti* is the key to the prevention of urban YF in the Americas. This includes an attack on the breeding sites in water containers and tanks, and a monitoring system that gives an *Aedes* index of the numbers of *Aedes* mosquitoes. When this reaches a certain level an epidemic may result. In the presence of an epidemic, adult control by 'fogging' of towns and cities with insecticide will bring the epidemic to a halt. *Ae. aegypti* had been eradicated from the USA but has now returned to Louisiana, once a hotbed of YFV, in its previous numbers.

Vaccination

YF 17D is a safe, live, attenuated vaccine providing a long-lasting immunity. For purposes of certification, 10 years is considered the limit but immunity after 40 years has been documented and it may be lifelong. Vaccination to YFV is imperative for travellers to endemic areas and certificates are demanded for travellers from endemic areas to non-infected tropical areas. Immunity develops within 10 days of vaccination. Serious complications are rare. No consequences for the foetus have been recorded but pregnant women should avoid vaccination unless the risk from YFV is considered great. Vaccination is not recommended for children under 6 months of age, and especially children aged less than 4 months, because of an increased risk of encephalitis. It should also be avoided in immunosuppressed patients. The vaccine is prepared in chick embryos and people sensitive to egg protein may have reactions. Serious side effects are rare with the 17D vaccine. Encephalitis, classical YF and severe multisystem illness have been reported. The risk of neurological disease is 1–16 per million doses, and of visceral disease is 2.5 per million doses.

Bunyaviruses (Family: Bunyaviridae, Genus: *Bunyavirus*)

CALIFORNIA ENCEPHALITIS VIRUS (CEV)

CEV[102] was the first identified member of the California serogroup of bunyaviruses. It was identified as a cause of encephalitis in California in the 1940s, but rarely causes human infection (see Figure 14.3). Human infections occur more commonly with the closely related La Crosse virus and Jamestown Canyon virus. It infects rabbits and rodents, and is transmitted by *Aedes* species.

OROPOUCHE VIRUS (OROV)

OROV[102] is a member of the Simbu group of bunyaviruses (see Table 14.1) and is a major cause of disease in the Amazon region of Brazil and Peru. It is transmitted by the midge *Culicoides paraensis* and some mosquito species. It is maintained in a jungle cycle involving sloths and monkeys. Disease onset is sudden, with fever, chills, headache, myalgia, arthralgia and photophobia being most common. The illness lasts 1–2 weeks and patients make a full recovery. Virus can be detected in blood in the first few days, but diagnosis is usually by serology.

RIFT VALLEY FEVER VIRUS (RVFV)

Geographical Distribution

RVFV[3,103–105] was first recognized in Kenya in 1931 as causing a disease in sheep and humans. Until 1977 it was restricted to humans and domestic animals in sub-Saharan Africa, with epizootics in Kenya, South Africa, Zimbabwe, Sudan, Egypt, Uganda, Tanzania and Zambia. A similar virus (Zinga virus) was found to be present in West Africa (Mali, Nigeria and Zaire) and in Botswana and Mozambique, but without epizootics. In 1977, RVFV spread to Egypt where it caused massive epidemics and epizootics, and showed a capability to spread beyond sub-Saharan Africa (Figure 14.11). The Egyptian episode was centred largely in the Nile Delta where approximately 600 human deaths are thought to have occurred. This was probably preceded by a massive epizootic along the Nile bank from Aswan in the south to Cairo in the north. RVF occurred again in Aswan in 1993 and several cases with ophthalmic complications have been seen in the Nile Delta. The largest ever recorded outbreak of RFV occurred in Kenya and Somalia in 1997–1998 (when up to 89 000 people were affected), and an outbreak was also recorded in the Arabian Peninsula in 2000.

Aetiology

RVFV is a member of the genus *Phlebovirus* in the Bunyaviridae family (see Table 14.1). RVFV is an enveloped virus of up to 120 nm in size, and the RNA genome is divided into three segments.

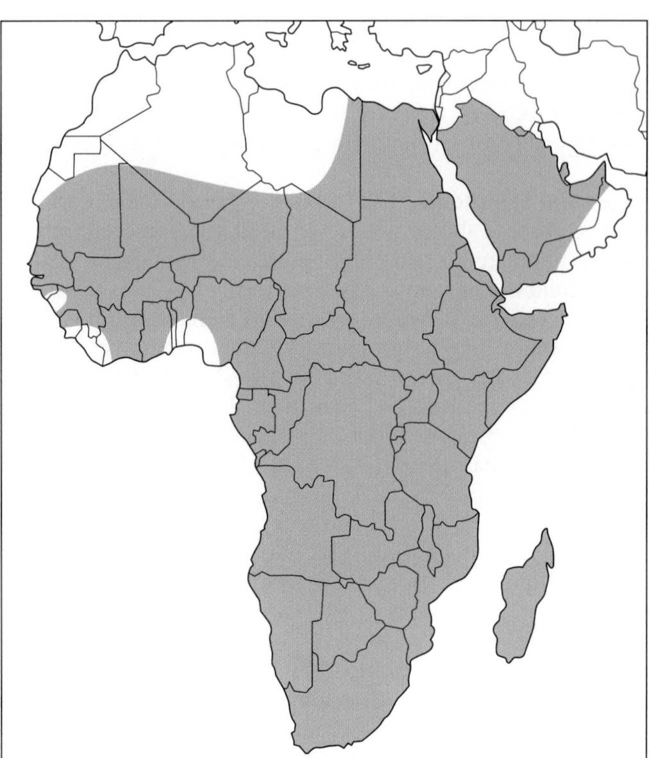

Figure 14.11 Geographical distribution of Rift Valley fever virus.

Pathology

The pathogenesis of RVFV appears to be similar to that of YFV, with initial spread to lymphatic tissue and then to the liver, with necrotic change in the latter. In a small proportion this is followed by haemorrhage which is probably due to a combination of reduced production of coagulation factors and DIC. Cerebral invasion with encephalitis and retinitis may occur 1–4 weeks after recovery.

Transmission

The virus infects a large range of domestic animals. Transmission between the zoonotic hosts is by mosquitoes of the *Eretmapodites, Mansonia, Anopheles, Aedes* and *Culex* groups (see Table 14.1), and possibly to humans by *Ae. caballus* and *Cx. theileri* in South Africa and *Cx. pipiens* in Egypt. Mechanical transmission may also occur by other biting insects including *Culicoides* and *Simulium* species. Direct transmission, especially during epidemics, is by the aerosol route from infected animal tissues. Person-to-person transmission does not occur but acute-phase blood and infected animal tissues are highly infectious, especially in abattoirs. Laboratory-acquired infections have been described and the virus should be handled with extreme caution.

Immunity

Active Immunity. Immunity is antibody-mediated and there is prolonged immunity to reinfection with homologous strains after recovery. Antibodies formed are of the usual viral response (HI, CF and N). HI and CF antibodies are used in diagnosis, and N antibodies give specificity.

Passive Immunity. A passive immunity can be transferred via the placenta to the child and lasts for several months; the possession of antibodies, especially N antibodies, can be used in treatment using convalescent sera.

Clinical Features

Natural History. RVFV is a self-limiting disease in the great majority of infections, with a short, acute, febrile phase and complete recovery. However, in less than 5% of cases, encephalitis, retinal lesions, haemorrhage and hepatic disease develop.

Signs and Symptoms. The incubation period is 2–6 days.

The onset is abrupt with fever, headache, joint and muscle pains, conjunctivitis and photophobia. In the majority of cases this is followed by complete recovery. In a few cases there may be recrudescence of symptoms after the initial short illness and convalescence may be prolonged. Retinal disease develops in 5–10% of cases, between 1 and 3 weeks after the febrile illness, with macular exudates and, in some instances, retinal haemorrhages and vasculitis. About half of the patients are left with permanent impairment of vision. In a further 5%, encephalitis develops, but is rarely fatal. Haemorrhagic disease occurs in approximately 1% of cases and is very similar to YF. Mortality rates are in the region of 10%, but deaths are nearly always found in those with more severe forms of the disease.

Diagnosis

Virus can be detected in blood by culture or PCR in the first week of illness. Antigen detection methods are also available. Detection of IgM by EIA aids diagnosis of early infection.[106] Standard serological diagnosis is by HI test on paired sera, using a standard antigen from the World Health Organization. EIA has also been used for IgG and IgM detection, and the latter can assist early diagnosis. The N tests can be used to show RVF-specific antibody.

Management

High-level supportive care may be needed for the more serious cases. Ribavirin has activity against this virus in animal models and is recommended for treatment of haemorrhagic disease in humans.[107] Immune serum, if available, may also be tried for severe cases.

Epidemiology

RVFV is maintained in the forest in an enzootic fashion between vertebrates and the vector mosquito species. Spectacular epizootics in domestic animals are the result of large numbers of susceptible (European) breeds of cattle and sheep, high arthropod densities (resulting from heavy rainfall or irrigation), and spillover from the forest cycle. The introduction of RVFV into new geographical locations is of particular concern because of its ability to cause catastrophic outbreaks in domestic animals, with severe fatal disease in humans. Originally restricted to domestic animals and humans in sub-Saharan Africa, since 1997 it has spread to Egypt, causing explosive epidemics in humans and domestic animals. The spread was possibly by camels from the Sudan carrying infection or arthropods, establishing new enzootic foci in the changing arthropod and vertebrate population after the construction of the Aswan High Dam. There is evidence in some areas that RVFV maintains endemnicity by transovarial transmission.

Control

Quarantine is not effective, but movements of animals should be controlled and sick animals should be allowed to die or recover, and not be slaughtered, to avoid spreading the infection in abattoirs. Control of abattoirs and vaccination of workers should be enforced. Vector control is also recommended.

Immunization

Vaccination of exposed laboratory workers and veterinary staff using a formalin-inactivated cell culture vaccine (expensive) should be performed.

Veterinary vaccines are the first-line of defence against the spread of RVFV. Both live and inactivated vaccines have been used to control the spread in animals, with some success.

SANDFLY FEVER (NAPLES VIRUS, SFNV; SICILIAN VIRUS, SFSV)

Geographical Distribution

Sandfly fever[108–110] is widespread throughout the Mediterranean and Middle East, Malta, Aegean Islands, Egypt and Iran, North Africa, Red Sea and Arabian Gulf; and in Asia in the Caucasus and Himalayas up to 4000 feet.

Aetiology

The viruses causing sandfly fever are phleboviruses. There are numerous antigenically distinct strains, only two of which, Sicilian and Naples, cause human disease. The others have been isolated from insects and animals.

Transmission

The sandfly responsible for transmission, *Phlebotomus papatsii*, becomes infective 6 days after feeding and remains infective for life. Transovarial transmission occurs so that newly emerged sandflies are capable of transmitting infection. It is possible that a parasitic mite of the sandflies acts as a reservoir.

Clinical Features

Natural History. Sandfly fever is an acute self-limiting disease lasting 2–4 days, with complete recovery and immunity to further attacks, and no mortality.

The incubation period is 3–6 days.

Signs and Symptoms. The onset is abrupt, with high fever, headache, myalgia, arthralgia and neck stiffness. After 3 (range 2–8) days the fever settles. Retro-orbital pain may be prominent and persist after resolution of fever. Mild neck stiffness develops in some patients. Occasionally there is a recrudescence (saddle back fever) lasting for 1–2 days. Rare cases of meningitis have been described.

Diagnosis

The viraemia lasts for only 24–36 hours, so attempts at virus isolation from serum are unlikely to be successful. IgG and IgM enzyme immunoassays have been developed. Paired sera for HI and N antibody tests can show recent infection.

Management

There is no specific treatment.

Epidemiology

There are no animal reservoirs. In endemic areas, transmission lasts from April to October. Epidemics occur among non-immune entrants to the community, especially military forces.

TAHYNA VIRUS (TAHV)

TAHV is a *bunyavirus* transmitted by *Aedes* species and causing occasional outbreaks of an influenza-like illness in central Europe (see Table 14.1).

TOSCANA VIRUS (TOSV)

TOSV[111,112] is a *phlebovirus* currently recognized as a member of the SFNV serological complex. It is found in Italy, Portugal, France and Spain, and possibly occurs in other Mediterranean countries. It is transmitted by *Phlebotomus perniciosus* and *P. perfiliewi* and animal reservoir hosts are not known. TOSV causes a benign meningitis and occasional meningoencephalitis, with full recovery. Serological cross-reactivity occurs between TOSV and other serotypes of SFNV. Diagnosis is usually by serology, but virus can be detected in the CSF by culture and by RT-PCR.

Coltiviruses (Family: Reoviridae, Genus: *Coltivirus*)

COLORADO TICK FEVER VIRUS (CTFV)

CTFV[113] is caused by a *coltivirus*, and is a member of the Reoviridae. It is found in the mountain regions of western USA and Canada, especially in the Rocky Mountain area in Colorado. Clinical illness consists of headache, fever, myalgia, arthralgia, retro-orbital pain, photophobia and neck stiffness, accompanied by a macular, maculopapular or petechial rash in about 10% of cases. It is biphasic in about half the patients, characterized by 2–3 days of illness, then 2 days of remission, followed by 2–3 days' more illness. Children may develop encephalitis. The most important hosts are the chipmunk and the golden-mantled ground squirrel, which infect immature ticks (*Dermacentor andersoni*). Other species of rodents may act as alternative secondary hosts of the virus.

Miscellaneous Arboviruses

There are a large number of other arthropod viruses that only rarely cause human infection or where their role in human disease is uncertain.

ALPHAVIRUSES

Babanki Virus (BBKV). Babanki is related to SINV and has been found in West and Central Africa, and Madagascar. It has been isolated from humans, but its role as a cause of disease is uncertain.

Getah Virus (GETV). This mosquito-borne virus is closely related to RRV. It is distributed widely through Asia, South-east Asia and Australia. Human infection is rare and it is not clearly associated with any disease.

Semliki Forest Virus (SFV). This virus is transmitted by various mosquito species in sub-Saharan Africa. Its role in human disease has not been established, but a laboratory-acquired case of fatal encephalitis has been reported.[114]

FLAVIVIRUSES

Banzi Virus (BANV). BANV is a mosquito-borne rodent virus found in southern and eastern Africa and transmitted by *Culex* species. Febrile illness has been reported.

Bouboui Virus (BOUV). This mosquito-borne virus is found in central Africa and is closely related to BANV. Human infection is asymptomatic.

Bussuquara Virus (BSQV). This is a Central and South American rodent virus transmitted by *Culex* species; it causes fever, headache and arthralgia.

Edge Hill Virus (EHV). EHV has been isolated from *Ae. vigilax* and *Cx. annulirostris* mosquitoes and is widely distributed in Australia. Human infection occurs and a single possible case of polyarthralgic illness has been described.

Ilheus Virus (ILHV). This virus is found in numerous mosquito species. Disease and/or virus has been detected in people in Central and South America and in Trinidad. Rare cases of fever with headache, and a case of encephalitis, have been documented.

Karshi Virus (KSIV). KSV is a tick-borne virus that causes febrile illness. It has been found in Kazakhstan and Uzbekistan.

Kedougou Virus (KEDV). KEDV is a mosquito-borne virus that has been shown to infect children in Senegal and the Central African Republic. No illness has been identified.

Kokobera Virus (KOKV). KOKV is found in Australia and New Guinea and is transmitted by *Ae. vigilax* and *Cx. annulirostris* mosquitoes. Human infections on the east coast of Australia have been documented in serosurveys. Kokobera virus can cause a polyarthralgic illness, sometimes with rash.

Koutango Virus (KOUV). KOUV is a mosquito-borne virus found in Senegal. Natural human infection is not known to occur, but one laboratory-acquired infection caused fever, headache, arthralgia and rash.

Rio Bravo Virus (RBV). This is a *flavivirus*, but does not appear to be arthropod-borne. It is transmitted directly from bats to humans, with one case of febrile illness being reported.

Sepik Virus (SEPV). SEPV has been found in a variety of mosquito species in Papua New Guinea and has caused a case of fever with headache.

Spondweni Virus (SPOV). SPOV is transmitted by several mosquito species in South Africa. It may cause fever, headache and arthralgia. SPOV is closely related to ZIKV.

Tyuleniy Virus (TYUV). TYUV is a tick-borne virus, reported to have caused a single human infection with arthralgia and skin haemorrhages. Meaban virus and Saumarez Reef virus are closely related.

Usutu Virus (USUV). This virus is found in sub-Saharan Africa and Europe. It is primarily an avian virus transmitted by several mosquito species, causing fever and rash.

Wesselsbron Virus (WESSV). WESSV is found in sub-Saharan Africa and Thailand. It is transmitted by several mosquito species. Human illness is characterized by fever, hepatosplenomegaly, rash and sometimes encephalitis, with full recovery.

Zika Virus (ZIKV). This virus is transmitted by *Aedes* species in East, Central and West Africa, and maintained in a cycle similar to that of YFV. It causes fever, headache and rash. ZIKV is closely related to SPOV. Isolated outbreaks outside of Africa have occurred in Indonesia in the 1970s and on Yap Island in the South Pacific in 2007.[115]

BUNYAVIRUSES

There are a large number of bunyaviruses that have been implicated in rare and mild human infection.[116]

NAIROVIRUSES

Congo–Crimean Haemorrhagic Fever Virus (CCHFV)

Geographical Distribution. CCHFV[80,117] is found mainly in Eastern Europe (Kosovo, Bulgaria, Albania, Russia), with first reports in 1944 and 1945 in former Soviet Union troops. It is also distributed throughout the Mediterranean (Turkey, Greece), in north-western China, central Asia (Kazakhstan, Tajikistan, Uzbekistan), southern Europe, Africa (Senegal, Congo, South Africa), the Middle East (Iran), and the Indian subcontinent (Gujarat).

Aetiology. CCHFV is a *Nairovirus* in the family Bunyaviridae. It was first characterized in Crimea in 1944. To date, seven genotypes have been recognized and the virus was hypothesized to have evolved 3100–3500 years ago.

Transmission. CCHFV is transmitted by *Hyalomma* species of ticks, especially *H. marginatum* and *H. anatolicum*, or by crushing those ticks. Nosocomial infection of medical workers after exposure to blood and secretions from patients occurs relatively frequently, and tertiary cases have occurred in family members of medical workers. Infection can also occur through butchering infected animals.

Pathology. Following an incubation period of 2–9 days after exposure to infection, patients present with a sudden onset of disease with fever, nausea, severe headache and myalgia. Gastrointestinal tract symptoms may also be present. Most cases are associated with cutaneous flushing or rash. The haemorrhagic period is short, usually lasting 2–3 days and is characterized by haemorrhage from various sites such as the gastrointestinal, genitourinary, respiratory tracts and the brain. Skin haemorrhagic manifestations, mucous membrane and conjunctival haemorrhage may also present.

Clinical Features. The onset of CCHF is sudden, with initial signs and symptoms including headache, high fever, back pain, joint pain, stomach pain, and vomiting. Red eyes, a flushed face, a red throat, and petechiae (red spots) on the palate are common. Symptoms may also include jaundice, and in severe cases, changes in mood and sensory perception. As the illness progresses, large areas of severe bruising, severe nosebleeds, and uncontrolled bleeding at injection sites can be seen, beginning on about the 4th day of illness and lasting for about 2 weeks.

Diagnosis. Diagnosis of CCHFV infection is determined by serology, evidence of viral antigen in tissue by immunohistochemical staining and microscopic examination, or identification of viral RNA sequence in blood or tissue.

Epidemiology. CCHFV has the widest geographic range of all tick-borne viruses and is endemic in more than 30 countries in Eurasia and Africa. New foci have emerged in several countries in Eastern Europe and Central Asia over the past decade. An essential factor for its resurgence was a rise in the number of *Hyalomma marginatum* ticks.

Dugbe Virus (DUGV). This virus was found to cause a mild febrile illness in Nigeria and Central African Republic, with rare meningitis.

Nairobi Sheep Disease Virus (NSDV). NSDV infects sheep and goats and is transmitted by a number of tick species. Human infection has been reported from East Africa and India, consisting of a fever and arthralgia. The illness is mild and recovery is full.

ORBIVIRUSES

Kemerovo Complex. This is a complex of a large number of viruses found in the former USSR and central Europe. They are tick-borne, and cause illnesses varying from fever to meningoencephalitis.

Orungo Virus (ORUV). Orungo virus is found in West and Central Africa and may be transmitted by a number of mosquito species. It is separated into four serotypes and causes fever and headache, with rare cases of encephalitis.

REFERENCES

2. Bres P. Impact of arboviruses on human and animal health. In: Monath TP, editor. The Arboviruses: Epidemiology and Ecology, vol. I. Florida: CRC Press; 1988. p. 1–18.
19. McMichael AJ, Woodruff RE, et al. Climate change and human health: present and future risks. Lancet 2006;367:859–69.
22. Weaver SC. Evolutionary influences in arboviral disease. Curr Top Microbiol Immunol 2006;299: 285–314.
24. Coffey LL, Vasilakis N, Brault AC, et al. Arbovirus evolution in vivo is constrained by host alteration. PNAS 2008;105:6970–5.
43. Pugachev KV, Guirakhoo F, Monath TP. New developments in flavivirus vaccines with special attention to yellow fever. Curr Opin Infect Dis 2005;18:387–94.

Access the complete references online at www.expertconsult.com

15

Dengue

SOPHIE YACOUB | JEREMY FARRAR

KEY POINTS

- Dengue is the most widely distributed mosquito-borne viral infection of humans, affecting an estimated 100 million people worldwide each year, with 40% (2.5 billion) of the world's population estimated to be at risk for infection. Dengue should be considered in any patient with fever, particularly if there is a recent travel history to endemic regions.
- Dengue severity exists as a continuous spectrum of dengue through to severe dengue.
- Of the many clinical features associated with severe dengue, from the standpoint of threat to life and guiding clinical intervention, the most important is increased vascular permeability leading to the dengue shock syndrome.
- During the critical phase of illness, regular review (every 15–30 min) of vital signs – pulse rate, blood pressure, peripheral temperature and haematocrit – is essential. The mainstay of treatment is prompt, vigorous, but judicious fluid resuscitation. If appropriate volume resuscitation is instituted at an early stage, shock is usually reversible. Careful clinical judgement is required throughout the patient's stay in the hospital to maintain an effective circulation while assiduously avoiding fluid overload. There is increasing interest in developing novel therapeutics for treatment of dengue but currently, no specific drugs exist.
- There is no dengue vaccine available for public health use at present. Many candidate dengue vaccines are in the process of development and the lead candidate is in Phase III trials 2012–2014. Novel technologies showing some promise for future dengue control are biological (*Wolbachia*) and genetic modification of mosquitoes, which are now entering field trials.
- There have been recent advances in our understanding of the clinical management, pathophysiology and identification of therapeutic targets, which should lead to urgently needed treatments. The ability to predict epidemics and to put in place the public health and clinical needs to deal with such massive surges in demand would be a major advance. The development of an effective and safe vaccine to all four dengue serotypes and better control of the vector are needed to address this important and growing global health threat.

Introduction

Dengue infections caused by the four antigenically distinct dengue virus serotypes (DENV1, DENV2, DENV3, DENV4) of the family Flaviviridae are the most important arboviral diseases in humans, in terms of geographical distribution, morbidity and mortality. The global burden of dengue has increased at least fourfold over the last three decades and there are now 2.5 billion people at risk of the disease. An estimated 99 million (95% credible interval 71–137 million) symptomatic dengue infections and 404 million asymptomatic (95% credible interval 304–537 million) infections occur annually in over 100 countries, with 500 000 cases of severe dengue and 20 000 deaths (Figure 15.1). The infection is transmitted from person to person by *Aedes* mosquitoes. Dengue virus infections can cause a wide clinical spectrum of disease, from a mild febrile illness known as 'dengue fever' through to 'severe dengue', previously known as dengue haemorrhagic fever (DHF), which is characterized by capillary leakage leading to hypovolaemic shock, organ impairment and bleeding complications.[1,2] There are currently no antiviral drugs and no available vaccine for dengue and the management relies on judicious fluid replacement of the severe cases.

This chapter will cover epidemiology, transmission and latest developments in pathogenesis and pathophysiology, as well as clinical features and management. It concludes with prevention and future directions.

Epidemiology

Dengue is endemic throughout the tropical and subtropical zones between 30°N and 40°S, where environmental conditions are optimal for dengue virus transmission by *Aedes* mosquitoes. Dengue transmission occurs throughout the year in endemic tropical areas; however, in most countries there is a distinct seasonal pattern, with increased transmission usually associated with the rainy season. Outbreaks occur most frequently in areas where multiple serotypes of dengue virus are simultaneously endemic or sequentially epidemic and infections with heterologous types are frequent. In endemic areas dengue occurs most frequently in children aged between 2 and 15 years. Severe dengue is usually associated with secondary dengue infection and during primary infection in infants less than 1 year, born to dengue-immune mothers.

It is clear that dengue and other arboviruses with similar ecology had a widespread distribution in the tropics as long as 200 years ago.[3] Originating in Africa, it is likely dengue, along with yellow fever, spread to the New World with the African slave trade in the 1600s. One of the first descriptions of a dengue-like illness outbreak occurred in Philadelphia in the USA in 1780, along the Delaware riverfront. Around the same time in Spain, an outbreak of a disease named 'break bone fever' was also being reported.[4] Over the next century, similar reports of dengue-like illness were reported from the Atlantic coast of America, the Caribbean and tropical Australasia.

During and after the Second World War, the global expansion of the vector *Aedes Aegypti* in Asia and later in the Americas

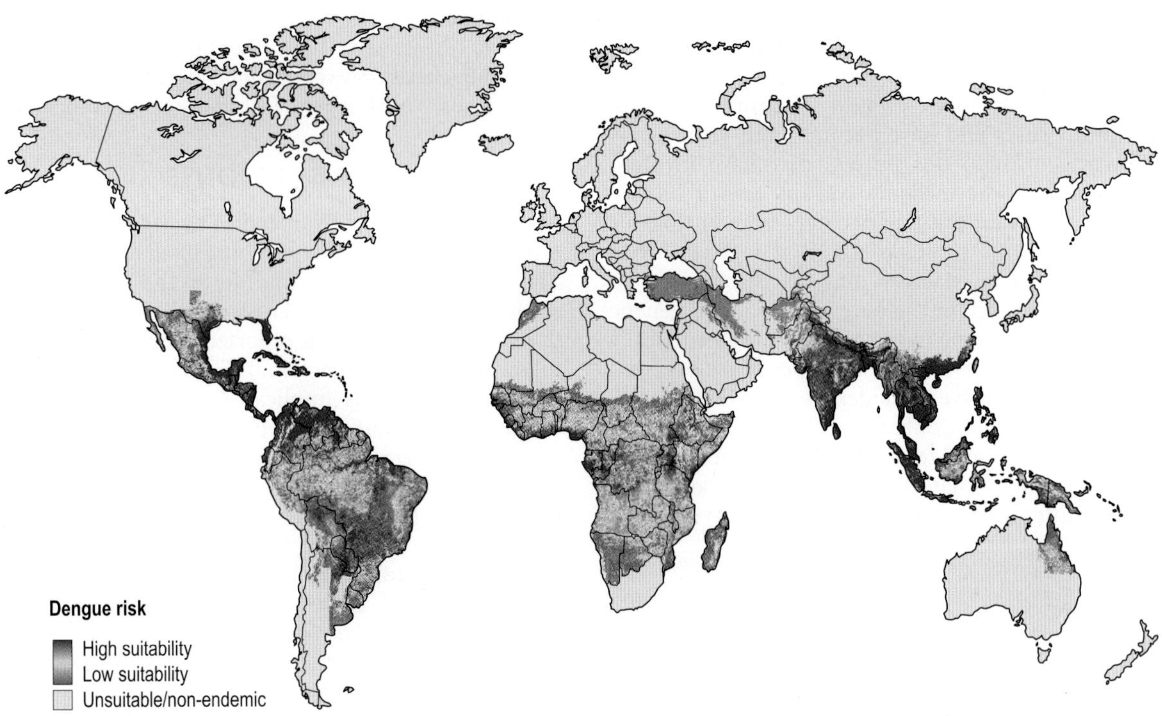

Figure 15.1 Global dengue risk. National level risk status was based on combined reports from the World Health Organization, Centres for Disease Control, Gideon online, ProMED, DengueMap, Eurosurveillance and case reports from returning travellers in addition to the published literature. Additional risk exclusions were made on the basis of a biological model for temperature suitability and areas of hyper-aridity defined by the GlobCover 'bare-areas' land cover classification. Within areas at risk, environmental suitability for dengue transmission was defined using a boosted-regression-trees model drawing on 3700 confirmed point occurrence records and a suite of 40 environmental covariates. *(With permission from Gething PW, Brady O, Hay SI. Dengue. N Engl J Med 2012;366(15):1423–32. Copyright © 2012 Massachusetts Medical Society. All rights reserved.)*

due to increased trade, together with the subsequent urbanization and international travel, saw the incidence of dengue infections increase dramatically. These changes coincided with the emergence of a newly described 'Thai Haemorrhagic Fever' in the 1950s in Thailand and the Philippines. Further outbreaks were then reported from many tropical Asian countries, including Viet nam, Singapore, Malaysia, Myanmar, China and several Pacific Islands. This trend continued and currently over 70% of the global dengue burden occurs in Asia.

Increased epidemic activity was observed in the Pacific Islands and the Caribbean basin in the 1970s and epidemics of all four dengue serotypes were documented in both regions. The first outbreak of DHF to occur outside the South-east Asian and Western Pacific regions was in Cuba in 1981 caused by the Asian genotype DENV 2.[5] This outbreak, which followed a primary DENV1 outbreak in 1997 in Cuba, confirmed the role of secondary infection and particularly the sequence of DENV1–DENV2 infections as risk factors for the occurrence of DHF.

Following this, sporadic cases of DHF have been reported from the Caribbean and small outbreaks occurred in Venezuela in 1989 and Brazil in 1991. An outbreak of secondary DENV 2 in 1995 in Iquitos, Peru, was of interest as there were no documented DHF cases, raising the possibility of lower pathogenicity of the American DENV 2 genotype.

In the last decade, DHF has emerged to become a major public health problem in 28 countries in the Americas with all four serotypes now endemic.[6,7]

In the 1980s, increased dengue activity was observed in Africa, with mild dengue cases being described in Nigeria, Mozambique and East Africa.[8,9] A recent increase in central Africa has been observed, along with Chikungunya cases, possibly due to the expansion of *Aedes Albopictus* in this area.[10] Results of seroprevalence studies show all four dengue serotypes are endemic in most of Africa, although large outbreaks are rare, as are reports of severe dengue. This is likely to be due to a combination of factors including under-reporting, protective genetic host factors, low vector competence and transmission efficiency.[9] A sophisticated systematic assessment of the global burden of disease in Africa suggests 15.6 million symptomatic cases (95% credible interval 10.9–21.6 millions) or approximately 16% of the global total.

The eastern Mediterranean area has also seen an increase in dengue in the last 30 years with recent outbreaks in Yemen, Saudi Arabia and Pakistan.

The World Health Assembly highlighted the importance of dengue as an emerging disease in 2006. Since then, dengue has continued to increase and spread to new areas of the world where the public health systems are not experienced in the prevention of the disease or the surge capacity in clinics and hospitals is not available to deal with an often sudden increase in the number of patients and the clinical experience is limited. In these settings, mortality and morbidity are often higher than in other regions where dengue has been endemic for decades.

The Virus

The dengue virus, a member of genus *Flavivirus* in the family Flaviviridae, is a single-stranded enveloped RNA virus, 30 nm in diameter. There are four distinct but closely related serotypes (DENV1–4). They possess antigens that cross-react with other members in the same genus such as yellow fever, Japanese encephalitis and West Nile viruses.

All four serotypes of DENV evolved independently from ancestral sylvatic viruses and have become both ecologically and evolutionarily distinct; this process may have involved adaptation to peridomestic mosquito vectors and/or human reservoir hosts. Support for this theory comes from phylogenic studies of distinct sylvatic strains of DENV-2 in West Africa and DENV-1, 2 and 4 in Malaysia, but the exact origin of all DENV remains uncertain.[11] There is abundant genetic variation within each serotype in the form of phylogenetically distinct clusters of sequences dubbed subtypes or genotypes.[12] At present, five genotypes have been identified in DENV-1; five in DENV-2 (one of which is only found in non-human primates); four in DENV-3; and four in DENV-4 (with another exclusive to non-human primates). There is some evidence that certain subtypes differ in virulence and their capacity to cause severe disease.[13,14]

Transmission

Dengue virus is transmitted from human to human by different species of *Aedes* mosquitoes. DENV circulation occurs in two cycles: an endemic/epidemic cycle between humans and peridomestic mosquitoes, *Aedes aegypti* and *Ae. albopictus* and a sylvatic enzootic cycle between non-human primates and several arboreal *Aedes* species.

Ae. aegypti is the most efficient of the mosquito vectors because of its domestic habits. The female mosquito bites humans during the day. After feeding on a person whose blood contains the virus, the female *Ae. aegypti* can transmit dengue, either immediately by a change of host when its feeding is interrupted or after an incubation period of 8–10 days, during which time, the virus multiplies in the salivary glands.[15] Once infected, the mosquito host remains infective for life (30–45 days). Other *Aedes* mosquitoes capable of transmitting dengue include *Ae. albopictus*, *Ae. polynesiensis* and several species of the *Ae. scutellaris* complex. Each of these species has its own particular geographical distribution and they are in general less efficient vectors than *Ae. aegypti*. Transovarian transmission of dengue viruses has been documented but its epidemiological importance has not been established.

Pathogenesis

The strong association between the development of severe disease in secondary dengue and the observation that complications occur when the viraemia is in steep decline, has led to the suggestion that the pathogenesis of severe dengue is immune-mediated. Halstead in the 1970s proposed the 'antibody-dependent immune enhancement theory' (ADE) based on in vitro and primate studies.[16] This association of sequential dengue infections being a risk factor for severity has been confirmed repeatedly in epidemiological studies, from different parts of the world.[17,18]

In addition, a particular sequence of infecting serotypes have been linked to severe disease, with several studies suggesting severe dengue is more common in a secondary infection with DENV2.[19,20] During the second infection with a different dengue serotype, pre-existing antibody from the first infection fails to neutralize and may instead enhance viral uptake and replication in mononuclear cells.[21] The resulting higher viral load has been linked to disease severity.[22] Other factors that may contribute to the pathogenesis of severe dengue include more virulent strains of the virus,[14] host genetic factors, age and comorbidities.[23–25]

HUMORAL IMMUNE RESPONSE

After an acute phase of infection by a particular dengue serotype, there is an antibody response to all four dengue serotypes. There is a long-lasting immunity to the homologous serotype of the infecting strain. A cross-reactive heterotypic immunity to all serotypes has been reported for period of 2–12 months following primary infection.[26] The waning cross-reactive heterotypic antibody is implicated in the occurrence of severe dengue through 'antibody dependent enhancement'. This occurs when the heterologous antibody acquired from a previous infection fails to neutralize the current infecting serotype, instead it enhances viral uptake into Fcγ receptor-bearing cells, particularly monocytes and macrophages. ADE, as well as facilitating viral entry into cells, also increases viral replication within the cells, through alterations of innate and adaptive intracellular antiviral mechanisms.[27] Further work identified that cross-reactive antibodies to the structural precursor membrane protein (prM) formed a major component of ADE, even at high titres anti-prM antibodies failed to neutralize the virus.[28]

A different example of ADE is in the setting of severe primary dengue in infants born to dengue-immune mothers.[29,30] Decay of the maternally derived IgG antibody to below neutralization level in infants between age 4–12 months, has been shown epidemiologically and in vitro to cause severe disease through ADE.[31]

CELL-MEDIATED IMMUNITY

The cellular immune response is vital in controlling dengue infections, however recent evidence suggests it also plays an important role in the immunopathogenesis of the severe manifestations of dengue. Studies have shown a greater breadth and magnitude of T-cell responses occurring in severe dengue infection.[32,33] A study of secondary dengue infections showed predominantly expansion of T cells with low avidity for the current infecting viral serotype and high avidity for a presumed previous serotype.[34] This skewing of the immune response to the previous dengue serotype is known as original antigenic sin, which may delay viral control and contribute to a higher peak viraemia and associated severe manifestations.[33] This activation of memory $CD4^+$ and $CD8^+$ T cells, sensitized during a previous infection, leads to rapid proliferation and release of pro-inflammatory cytokines, particularly TNFα and IFNγ.[35] A study investigating T-cell responses to the entire dengue proteome, showed that the response was most marked to the non-structural protein 3 (NS3), with high cytokine and low CD107a (a marker of cell degranulation) predominating.[36] This suggests that in severe dengue the low cytotoxic potential of the T cells fails to obtain early viral control, instead high cytokine-producing cells dominate the response with the excessive pro-inflammatory cytokines causing the tissue damage and plasma leakage. Other studies have linked disease severity to cellular markers of activation in plasma including interleukin-6 and soluble IL-2 receptor.[37]

COMPLEMENT

Complement activation has been suggested to play a role in the pathogenesis of dengue.[38,39] Studies have shown cross-reactive antibodies to the dengue virus can activate complement at the surface of endothelial cells. The release of C3a and C5a anaphylatoxins has been associated temporally with the onset of plasma leakage and shock.[40]

High levels of the major non-structural protein NS1 have been linked to disease severity.[41] A study in Thailand demonstrated NS1 was able to activate complement leading to local and systemic generation of anaphylatoxin C5a and the terminal SC5b-9 complexes. The plasma levels of NS1 and SC5b-9 complexes correlated with disease severity and these complexes were detected in the pleural fluid from patients with severe dengue.[42] In addition, NS1 may have an immune evasion role by modulating the classical and lectin complement pathways through a reduced functional capacity of C4.[43]

These studies suggest a possible role for complement in the pathogenesis of severe dengue, both through excessive local activation at endothelial surfaces contributing to vascular leakage as well as immune modulation leading to a higher viraemia.

Histopathology

From experimental studies in rhesus monkeys, after inoculation the virus reaches the regional lymph nodes and disseminates to the reticuloendothelial system, in which it multiplies and from which it enters the blood.[44] Skin lesions in non-fatal, uncomplicated dengue fever seen in human volunteers were studied by biopsy. The chief abnormality occurred in and around small blood vessels and consisted of endothelial swelling, perivascular oedema and infiltration with mononuclear cells. Extensive extravasation of blood without appreciable inflammatory reaction was observed in the petechial lesions.[45]

Significant changes are found in major organ systems;[46]

- Vascular changes include vasodilatation, congestion, perivascular haemorrhage and oedema of arterial walls
- Proliferation of reticuloendothelial cells with accelerated phagocytic activity is observed frequently
- The lymphoid tissues show increasing activity of the B lymphocyte system with active proliferation of plasma cells and lymphoblastoid cells
- In the liver there is focal necrosis of the hepatic and Kupffer cells, with formation of Councilman-like bodies
- Dengue virus antigen is found predominantly in cells of the spleen, thymus and lymph nodes, in Kupffer cells and in the sinusoidal lining cells of liver and alveolar lining cells of the lung.

Pathophysiology

The pathophysiological hallmarks of severe dengue are plasma leakage and abnormal haemostasis. Clinical evidence supporting plasma leakage includes a rapid rise in haematocrit, hypoproteinaemia, pleural effusions and ascites and reduced plasma volume, leading to haemodynamic compromise and hypovolaemic shock.

Microvascular leakage has been demonstrated using the non-invasive technique of strain gauge plethysmography. A study showed that the filtration capacity was higher in DHF patients than controls, but did not show a difference between the severity grades of DHF.[47] They also showed that age-related changes occur in microvascular permeability, with children having higher filtration capacity than adults, which would explain why dengue shock syndrome is more common in childhood.[48] The transient nature of the leakage implies a functional increase in vascular permeability. The microvascular leak occurs at a time when the viral load is in steep decline and is associated with a more intense immune response.[36] Disruption in the endothelial glycocalyx layer has been implicated, through immune-mediated mechanisms by the virus or the NS1 antigen adhering to the endothelial layer.[49] The NS1 antigen is a glycoprotein secreted from dengue-infected cells and is required for viral replication. Studies have shown that NS1 can selectively bind to heparan sulphate in the glycocalyx layer of microvascular endothelial cells.[50] Thus facilitating immune complex formation and antibody-dependent complement activation causing the endothelial damage and microvascular leakage.[42]

The vascular leakage and hypoproteinaemia seen in the blood at defervescence is also associated with proteinuria. The proteinuria tends to occur more frequently in severe dengue and urinary protein/creatinine ratio has been suggested as a predictor of progression to severe disease.[51,52] A study in Vietnamese children demonstrated a reduction in different size proteins in plasma was associated with increased fractional urinary clearance of the same proteins.[53] The proteinuria resolves in the convalescent period and there is generally no associated renal damage with no increase in creatinine noted. A transient glomerulonephritis has been suggested from renal biopsies, with deposition of dengue immune complexes in the glomerular basement membrane.[54,55]

The abnormalities in haemostasis seen in dengue infections involve all its major components including: (1) vasculopathy; (2) thrombopathy, with impaired platelet function and moderate to severe thrombocytopenia; (3) coagulopathy, with activation of the coagulation system and fibrinolysis, plus in the later stages of severe disease; disseminated intravascular coagulation (DIC); (4) bone marrow changes, including depression of all marrow elements, with maturation arrest of megakaryocytes during the early phase of the illness, which is reversed after defervescence.[56] The most consistent finding in dengue infections is a transient thrombocytopenia. The exact underlying mechanism remains unclear. Studies suggest it is multifactorial, including: suppression of megakaryocytopoiesis,[57] and increased platelet clearance by DENV-induced apoptosis and antiplatelet antibodies.[58,59]

Activation of the coagulation system and fibrinolysis has been demonstrated in different studies and seems to be more pronounced in severe cases. One study showed persistently elevated levels of tissue activator inhibitor levels and an increased thrombin-antithrombin to plasmin-antiplasmin ratio was associated with poor outcomes in dengue patients.[60] Other studies have shown mild prolongation of prothrombin time and partial thromboplastin time and reduced fibrinogen.[61] Fibrinogen degradation products however are rarely raised and not to the levels consistent with a classical DIC picture. Theories to explain these coagulation abnormalities' include; a loss of the various coagulation factors including fibrinogen through the capillary leakage along with other intravascular proteins. The prolongation of the PT and APTT coincides temporally with maximal vascular leakage and is more pronounced in these severe patients. Also, in vitro studies have shown that the virus can bind and activate

BOX 15.1 WARNING SIGNS

- Abdominal pain or tenderness
- Persistent vomiting
- Clinical fluid accumulation
- Mucosal bleed
- Lethargy/restlessness
- Liver enlargement >2 cm
- Laboratory increase in HCT concurrent with rapid decrease in platelet count

Taken from 2009 WHO guidelines.

plasminogen, plus cross-reactive antibodies to plasminogen have been demonstrated in acute and convalescent serum of dengue patients.[62,63]

Clinical Features

Dengue can present with a wide spectrum of clinical features, ranging from a simple febrile illness through to severe features of plasma leakage leading to life-threatening shock. Dengue was previously classified into dengue fever and dengue haemorrhagic fever (DHF) of which there were four grades, with DHF III and IV compiling dengue shock syndrome (DSS). In 2009, the WHO reclassified dengue due to difficulty applying the old classification system in clinical situations and increasing reports of severe cases not fitting the criteria for DHF.[2] The new classification emphasizes levels of severity with patients being classified as dengue with or without warning signs and severe dengue, by encompassing a set of clinical and laboratory parameters (see Box 15.1, for list of warning signs).

Severe dengue is defined as:

- Severe plasma leakage, leading to fluid accumulation with respiratory distress or shock
- Severe organ impairment (including cardiac, liver: ALT>1000 and CNS: altered consciousness)
- Severe bleeding.

Specific organ impairment can occur without shock or any other features of severe dengue, including hepatitis, encephalitis and myocarditis. Although a mild rise in hepatic transaminases is usually present, rarely ALT levels >1000 are seen with associated liver dysfunction.[64] Dengue presenting as an acute encephalitis syndrome without other manifestations of the disease is increasingly recognized in endemic areas.[22] It is more common in children and although rarely fatal a significant proportion are left with neurological sequelae. Different cardiac manifestations have been reported in dengue patients from acute myocarditis, conduction disturbances and myocardial depression.[65,66] These patients need to be identified early in order to tailor their fluid management.

Generally, the clinical course can be divided into febrile, critical and recovery phases (Figure 15.2).

FEBRILE PHASE

Typically, after an incubation period of 5–8 days following an infective mosquito bite, the disease begins with a sudden onset of fever with severe headache and any of the following: chills, pain behind the eyes, particularly on eye movement, backache and pain in the muscles, bones and joints. During the febrile period the temperature can be as high as 40°C; the fever may be sustained for 5–6 days and may occasionally have a biphasic course. Anorexia, vomiting and abdominal pain are common. As the disease progresses the patient becomes anorexic and may show marked weakness and prostration. Other reported symptoms include sore throat, altered taste sensation, constipation and depression.

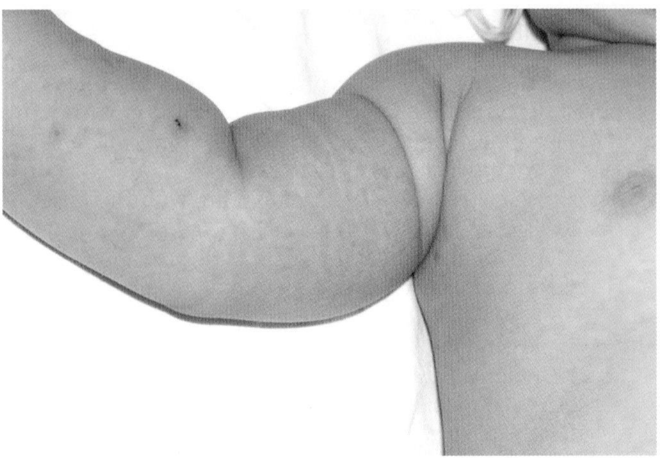

Figure 15.2 Typical skin rash in an infant with dengue.

Several types of skin rash have been described. Initially, diffuse flushing, mottling or fleeting pinpoint eruptions may be observed on the face, neck and chest (Figure 15.2). These are transient in nature. A second type of skin rash is a conspicuous rash that may be maculopapular or scarlatiniform and appears on approximately the 3rd or 4th day. This rash starts on the chest and trunk and spreads to the extremities and face and may be accompanied by itching and dermal hyperaesthesia. Towards the end of the febrile period or immediately after defervescence the generalized rash fades and localized clusters of petechiae may appear over the dorsum of the feet and on the legs, hands and arms. This confluent petechial rash is characterized by a scattered pale round area of normal skin (Figure 15.3).

Mild haemorrhagic complications can occur in the febrile phase, presenting as scattered petechiae on extremities, axillae, trunk and face. A positive tourniquet test and/or tendency to bruise at venepuncture sites are usually present (Figure 15.4). Bleeding into the skin, from the nose, gums and gastrointestinal tract are common but haematuria is rare (Figure 15.5). The liver is often enlarged, but jaundice is generally not observed. A normal white blood count or leucopaenia is common and neutrophils may predominate initially. Towards the end of the febrile phase there is a reduction in the number of total leucocytes and neutrophils shortly before or simultaneously with a relative increase in lymphocytes with the presence of atypical lymphocytes. The leucopaenia usually reaches a nadir shortly before the temperature and platelets drop. This observation is valuable in marking the end of the febrile period and the beginning of the critical phase. Other changes include hypoproteinaemia, hypoalbuminaemia, hyponatraemia and mildly elevated alanine aminotransferase (ALT)/aspartate aminotransferase levels (AST).

CRITICAL PHASE

It is not possible to predict who will have an uneventful defervescence and who will go on to develop severe dengue. However, using the WHO warning signs (Box 15.1) with

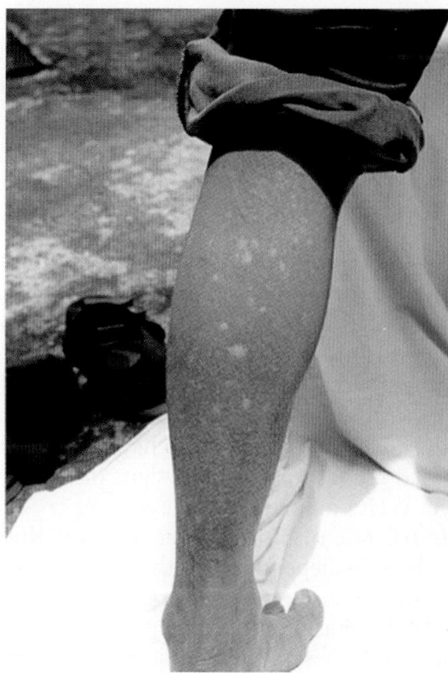

Figure 15.3 Diffuse macular recovery rash in an adult patient with dengue. The rash may appear between 3–6 days after fever onset. Note the 'islands of white' of normal skin surrounded by erythematous rash.

particular vigilance during the critical phase can help identify which patients will require more intensive supportive therapies. The critical phase, which occurs at fever defervescence usually around day 5, is the period where an increase in capillary permeability and plasma leakage can occur. This may present clinically as pleural effusions and/or ascites depending on the degree of plasma leakage and once a critical volume is lost, shock ensues. The skin may be cold and clammy and the pulse pressure becomes narrow (20 mmHg) with elevation of diastolic pressure to meet the systolic pressure. The platelet count drops shortly before or simultaneously with the haematocrit rise (20%) and both changes occur before the subsidence of fever and before onset of shock. Clotting abnormalities are usually present including prolongation of prothrombin and partial thromboplastin time and reduced fibrinogen, which has been shown to correlate to severity of disease but not bleeding.[61,67]

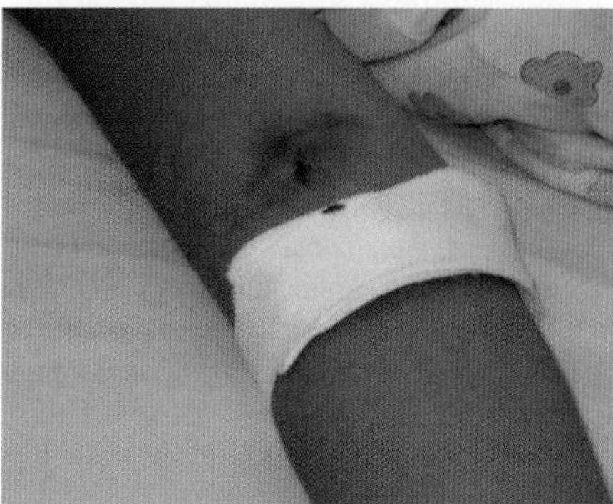

Figure 15.4 Minor bleeding particularly around injection sites is a very common feature in dengue.

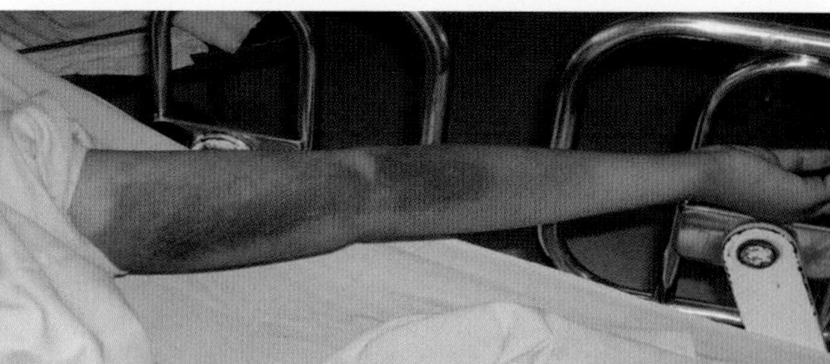

Figure 15.5 Haematoma in a patient with severe dengue. The combination of increased vascular fragility, platelet dysfunction/thrombocytopenia and coagulation disorders are believed to explain the haemorrhagic manifestations in dengue.

Without appropriate fluid resuscitation the patient can deteriorate into profound shock with an imperceptible pulse and blood pressure. Prolonged shock is often complicated by metabolic acidosis, multi-organ impairment and severe bleeding which carries a poor prognosis. The critical phase usually lasts for 24–48 hours, during which time the clinically significant plasma leakage can occur, after which time the recovery period begins.

RECOVERY PHASE

The extravascular fluid begins to be resorbed over the next 48–72 hours. If intravenous fluids are continued into this period there is significant risk of fluid overload, manifesting as respiratory distress from pleural effusions and/or ascites. General symptomatic improvement is seen, with return of appetite, haemodynamic stability and diuresis. During this period, the white cell count begins to rise followed by the platelets, the haematocrit may drop in part due to the dilutional effects of the resorbed extravascular fluid.

Virological Diagnosis

Diagnosis can be confirmed by serological testing and virus detection by molecular techniques or less frequently by virus isolation. No single diagnostic test performed in isolation is sufficiently sensitive to diagnose all the different stages of dengue infection.

In the first 3–5 days of the infection during the febrile phase, RT-PCR techniques to detect DENV RNA in the blood are the most sensitive and specific test, however after defervescence, this method becomes less useful as the viraemia falls.

Serological diagnosis by detection of anti-dengue IgM and IgG by enzyme-linked immunosorbent assay (ELISA) can be used to distinguish primary and secondary infection, but lacks sensitivity in the early stages of the disease. IgG serology lacks sensitivity in early stages of the disease and requires paired serum samples, it also lacks specificity due to cross reactions with other flaviviruses. IgM antibody capture (MAC) – ELISA is specific in distinguishing dengue from other flavivirus infections and has the advantage over the haemagglutination test in that a definite diagnosis can be made from an acute blood specimen alone, with a sensitivity of about 78%; when convalescent sera are tested the sensitivity is 97%.[68]

IgG antibodies to dengue virus antigens increase rapidly in patients with secondary dengue infection. A diagnostic (fourfold) increase in dengue antibody by the haemagglutination inhibition test can be demonstrated from paired sera obtained early in the febrile phase or on admission and 3–5 days later. A third specimen 2–3 weeks after onset is, however, required to confirm diagnosis of primary dengue infection.

More recently an ELISA assay for dengue non-structural protein 1 (NS1) detection has been developed and commercial test kits are now available. They are useful additions to diagnose dengue with excellent sensitivity and specificity in early disease, with limitations later on in the disease and in those with a concurrent humoral immune response.[69]

Management

The initial management (Figure 15.6) of dengue cases involves classification into appropriate severity grades with early recognition of potential complications and warning signs. Early detection of any circulatory compromise and judicious fluid resuscitation is the mainstay of treatment for severe dengue, with delays being associated with worse outcomes.[70] Case fatality rates from severe dengue vary by country but in the hands of experienced nursing and medical staff should be less than 1%, but rates of up to 13% have been reported.[71,72]

It is currently not possible to predict which dengue cases in the early febrile phase will go on to develop severe disease. Therefore, the WHO guidelines focus on the haemodynamic status of the patient plus any of the warning signs (Box 15.1).[2] Initial evaluation of the patient should include careful history and examination, plus a full blood count for a baseline haematocrit and platelets. Further laboratory tests should be performed if indicated and locally available including; electrolytes, urea, creatinine, liver function and cardiac enzymes and lactate. The WHO recommends patients in the early stages of disease with no warning signs can be managed in an outpatient setting with daily follow-up. Parents/guardians are advised to monitor for the following symptoms/signs: persistent vomiting; abdominal pain; lethargy/restlessness; bleeding manifestations; and cold extremities. Antipyretics may be needed to control the high fever. Aspirin and other non-steroidal anti-inflammatory agents should not be used, to avoid gastric irritation and GI bleeding and aspirin, because of the link with Reye syndrome. Oral rehydration solution is recommended to replace losses from vomiting and high fevers. Patients should be seen daily as out-patients until the end of the critical phase.

The following groups of patients should be referred for in-patient management: (1) patients who develop any warning signs; (2) those with any comorbidity (particularly pregnancy, extremes of age, diabetes, chronic renal failure, obesity and any chronic bleeding disorder); (3) any patient that lives alone or far from a health facility.

MANAGEMENT OF PATIENTS WITH WARNING SIGNS

These patients should be monitored in a hospital setting, with emphasis on fluid balance, 4–6-hourly vital signs monitoring, plus peripheral perfusion and urine output. A baseline haematocrit should be obtained and repeated as per WHO protocol.[2] The minimum amount of intravenous fluid should be given to ensure adequate perfusion, clinicians should be guided by vital signs, haematocrit and average urine output of 0.5 mL/kg per hour. An initial rate of 5 mL/kg per hour is suggested, which is decreased gradually over the next 2 hours as per clinical response. Isotonic fluids should be given for the duration of the critical period only (usually 24–48 hours), as there is a significant risk of fluid overload if intravenous fluids are continued into the recovery phase.

MANAGEMENT OF SEVERE DENGUE

Any patient who develops severe plasma leakage with evidence of haemodynamic compromise and/or fluid accumulation with respiratory distress or severe bleeding or organ impairment (hepatitis, myocarditis or encephalitis) needs urgent admission to a hospital with access to an intensive care unit. Immediate resuscitation with intravenous fluids is mandatory for all patients with shock. For patients who have compensated shock (i.e. maintained blood pressure, but signs of circulatory compromise), the WHO guidelines suggest using crystalloid solution at an initial rate of 5 mL/kg per hour for the first hour, with further boluses depending on the clinical response. Particular focus and regular review (every 15 min may be needed during this critical phase) of the patient's blood pressure, pulse, urine output, capillary refill time and pulse pressure and haematocrit will guide the next step. If the patient improves, maintenance fluids should be gradually reduced and maintained on ideal body weight once again for no longer than the critical phase of 24–48 hours. If there is clinical deterioration or no improvement with a falling haematocrit, particularly to levels below the patient's baseline, this indicates significant bleeding, most often gastrointestinal or per vagina in adult women. Blood transfusion should be given as soon as major haemorrhage is suspected, with 5–10 mL/kg packed red cells or 10–20 mL/kg fresh whole blood – and repeated if ongoing signs of bleeding and/or there is no appropriate rise in haematocrit. There is no evidence to support prophylactic platelet transfusions to correct the severe thrombocytopenia seen in severe dengue, but can be considered in cases with massive haemorrhage.[73]

Patients who present with hypotensive shock should be managed with more vigorous protocol of fluid resuscitation, initially receiving 20 mL/kg of crystalloid or colloid solution over 15 minutes, followed by repeated boluses of colloid if the patient remains unstable or has a rising haematocrit. Once the patient's vital signs stabilize, the rate of intravenous fluid can be reduced as per WHO protocol. Oxygen should be given to all cases with shock.

In addition to the laboratory tests mentioned above, severe dengue cases should also have cardiac enzymes, clotting studies and bicarbonate/lactate measurements. Although moderate rises in APTT are common in dengue, DIC is rare, is usually associated with prolonged shock and carries a poor prognosis. Other investigations include ECG to monitor for arrhythmias and an echocardiogram (if available) to detect myocardial dysfunction, and ultrasound to assess gallbladder wall thickening and quantify ascites and pleural effusions.[65,74,75]

Fluid overload is the most common complication of fluid therapy in severe dengue. This may be worsened by a degree of myocardial impairment in addition to the capillary permeability complicating the acute illness. This combination of cardiac dysfunction and plasma loss makes fluid resuscitation a very delicate balance.[65] It is therefore important to adjust the rate of intravenous infusion according to the rate of plasma leakage as guided by regular review of the haematocrit level, vital signs and urine output to avoid excessive fluid

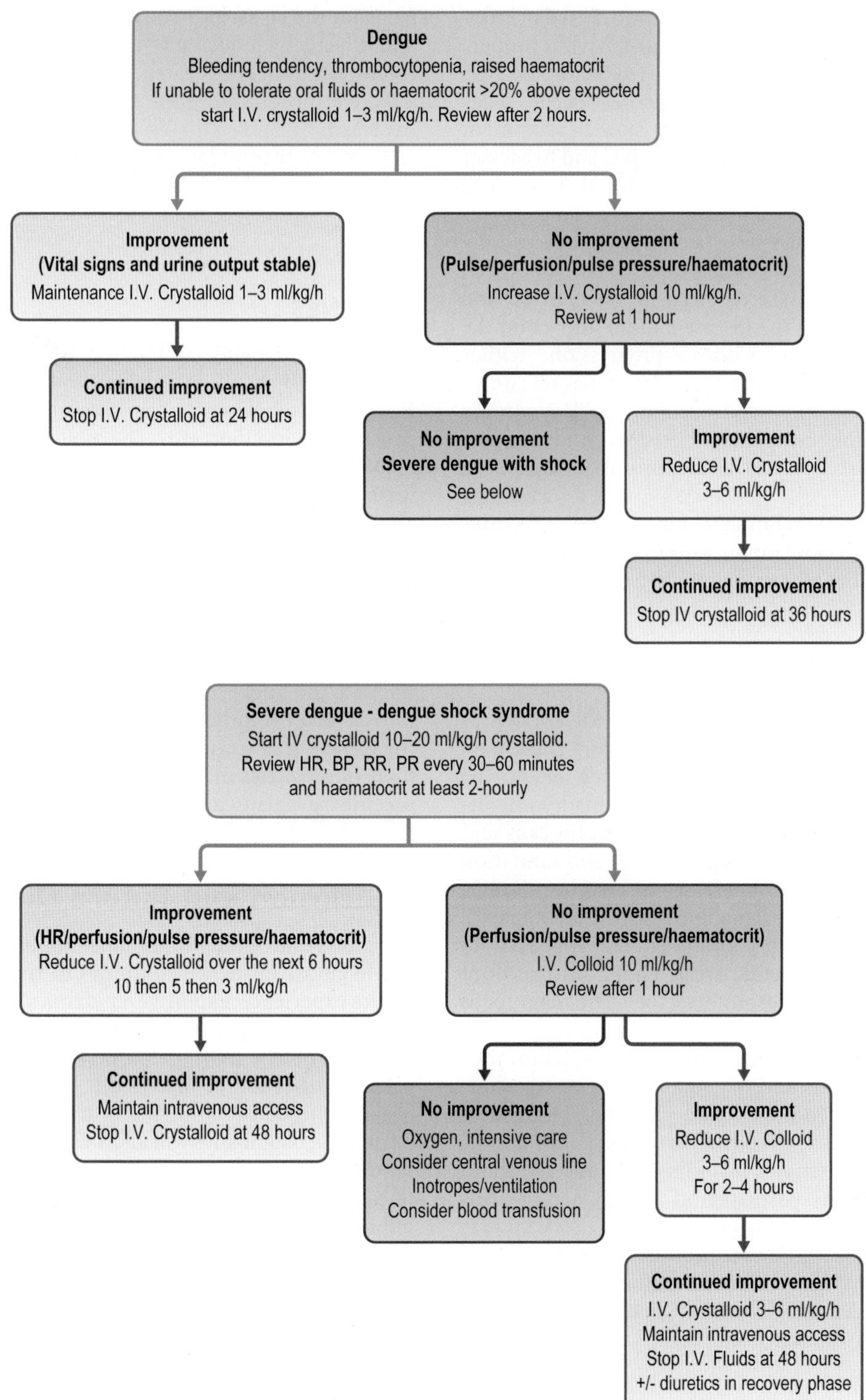

Figure 15.6 Algorithm for treatment of dengue.

replacement. It must be emphasized that the total volume of fluid replacement should be just sufficient to maintain effective circulation during the period of leakage. Fluid replacement must be discontinued when leakage stops after 48 hours. If further fluid replacement is continued after the critical period when extravasated plasma starts to be reabsorbed, it can cause massive pleural effusions, pulmonary oedema and ascites leading to respiratory failure.

ANTIVIRAL AND ADJUNCTIVE THERAPIES

There are currently no licensed antiviral drugs for dengue. Considering the global burden of dengue, the development of potential therapeutics both aimed at the pathogen and immune modulation has been neglected. Research in this area however, has been increasing with recent identification of new compounds with activity against dengue and some promising results in animal models.[76,77] A recent randomized control trial of chloroquine, which had been shown to have anti-flaviviral properties in vitro, did not reduce the duration of viraemia or NS1 antigenaemia in the study group.[78] With earlier specific diagnostics now available and many drugs in late-stage development for other flaviviruses (mostly aimed at hepatitis C and to a lesser extent West Nile Virus), it is to be hoped that this area will develop in the coming years.

Various adjunctive therapies have been tried unsuccessfully to modify disease severity over the last three decades, particularly using corticosteroids. A recent trial in Vietnam of oral corticosteroids given early in the disease had no impact on the development of complications or disease progression.[79] Other trials have also shown no evidence that corticosteroids are of benefit in reducing the fatality rate in dengue shock syndrome or improving the thrombocytopenia.[80,81] A small study showed no benefit of IVIG on recovery of severe thrombocytopenia in dengue.[82]

Therefore, the current treatment for dengue infections remains supportive, with close monitoring of warning signs and judicious fluid replacement for patients with evidence of plasma leakage.

Prevention and Control

The prevention of dengue depends mainly on the control of *Aedes aegypti* mosquitoes, the major global vector. These day-biting, anthropophilic mosquitoes are highly adapted to the urban environment; breeding primarily in man-made containers such as those used for water storage, old jars, tin cans and used tyres. Rapid urbanization with poor water and sanitation planning particularly in South American cities has been implicated in the huge increases in dengue witnessed in the last 2 decades.[83] The WHO advocates an integrated approach to vector control in dengue-endemic areas, taking into account local resources, ecology and mosquito vectors. The main focus is aimed at the elimination of the container breeding sites, through improved access to piped water supplies, removal of rubbish around households and managing water storage containers through frequent drainage and cleaning. The use of larvicides and insecticides is effective, particularly during outbreaks, but has some limitations, including resistance.[84] Health education and community participation are key components for sustained prevention.[85]

Novel technologies showing some promise for future dengue control are biologic and genetic modification of mosquitoes. The intracellular bacterium *Wolbachia*, when introduced into *Aedes* mosquitoes can influence the ability of the insects to transmit the virus, indirectly by reducing the mosquito lifespan and directly by reducing viral replication in the mosquito.[86,87] A recent study demonstrated successful invasion of *Wolbachia*-infected mosquitoes into natural mosquito populations in Australia.[88]

Genetic manipulation of mosquito populations is also now entering field trials, with promising results from a recent trial of engineered male *Aedes* mosquitoes in the Cayman Islands.[89]

VACCINES

There is no dengue vaccine available for public health use at present. Many candidate dengue vaccines, e.g. live-attenuated, inactivated whole virus and recombinant vaccines are in the process of development. The first ever efficacy trial of the recombinant, live-attenuated tetravalent CYD dengue vaccine was reported in September 2012 in Thai children.[90] It showed an overall efficacy of 30.2% (95% CI 13.4–56.6), which varied by serotype. A post hoc analysis suggested vaccine efficacies (VE) varied by serotype: Serotype 1, 55.6 (95% CI −21.6–84); Serotype 2, 9.2 (95% CI −75–51.3); Serotype 3, 75.3 (95% CI −375–99.6); Serotype 4, 100 (95% CI 24.8–100). Although an overall underwhelming result this study was the first to demonstrate the safety of a dengue vaccine in the 1 year follow-up in over 4000 volunteers. There are ongoing phase 3 studies of the same vaccine currently in over 30 000 volunteers in more than 10 countries in Asia and the Americas. A number of other vaccine candidates are in earlier phase development.

Conclusion and Future Directions

Dengue is one of the world's most important emerging diseases, as the global incidence continues to rise and new areas of the world experience explosive epidemics, there are major challenges ahead. There have been recent advances in our understanding of the immunopathogenesis and pathophysiology, plus identification of therapeutic targets, which should lead to urgently needed treatments. In the next few years, a focus on improving diagnostics will allow early disease identification and randomized controlled trials to guide evidence-based practice of cases. The ability to predict epidemics and to put in place the public health and clinical needs to deal with such surges in demand would be a major advance. With ongoing difficulties in the development of an effective and balanced vaccine to all four dengue serotypes, concerted efforts are needed to address this important global health threat.

REFERENCES

1. Simmons CP, Farrar JJ, Nguyen VV, et al. Dengue. N Engl J Med 2012;366:1423–32.
2. WHO. Dengue: Guidelines for Treatment, Prevention and Control. Geneva: World Health Organization; 2009.
21. Halstead SB. Pathogenesis of dengue: challenges to molecular biology. Science 1988;239:476–81.
88. Hoffmann AA, Montgomery BL, Popovici J, et al. Successful establishment of *Wolbachia* in *Aedes* populations to suppress dengue transmission. Nature 2011;476:454–7.
90. Sabchareon A, Wallace D, Sirivichayakul C, et al. Protective efficacy of the recombinant, live-attenuated, CYD tetravalent dengue vaccine in Thai schoolchildren: a randomised, controlled phase 2b trial. Lancet 2012;380(9853):1559–67.

Access the complete references online at www.expertconsult.com

16

Viral Haemorrhagic Fevers

LUCILLE BLUMBERG | DELIA ENRIA | DANIEL G. BAUSCH

KEY POINTS

- Viral HF is an acute systemic febrile syndrome caused by over 30 viruses from four different virus families. Microvascular instability with capillary leak and impaired haemostasis are the pathogenic hallmarks.
- Mortality usually results from an intense inflammatory process akin to septic shock, with insufficient effective circulating intravascular volume leading to hypotension, cellular dysfunction and multi-organ system failure.
- Viral HF is characterized by a short incubation period (usually 1–2 weeks) followed by a rapidly progressive illness usually lasting no longer than 2 weeks. Initial signs and symptoms are usually very nonspecific and include fever, headache and myalgia, followed rapidly by gastrointestinal symptoms and, in some cases, rash and neurologic involvement. Severe cases develop haemodynamic instability, bleeding, shock and multi-organ system failure.
- Mortality rates range from less than 1% to over 80%, depending on the specific viral HF. Survivors generally make a full recovery with few sequelae. There is no chronic carriage of HF viruses. In most cases, infection is thought to confer lifelong immunity in survivors.
- The viruses that cause HF are zoonotic. Consequently, the endemic areas for the various viral HFs are limited to the distribution of their mammalian reservoirs and/or arthropod vectors. Although modern-day ease of travel has made it possible for cases of viral HF to be seen throughout the globe, imported cases remain extremely rare.
- The nonspecific clinical manifestations of viral HF make clinical diagnosis of single cases extremely difficult, especially early in the course of disease. The differential diagnosis is extremely broad. The occurrence of clusters of cases with a compatible clinical syndrome, especially involving healthcare workers, should raise suspicion of viral HF.
- Viral HF should be considered in febrile patients with a compatible clinical syndrome and history of travel and exposure, especially if the patient fails to respond to empiric treatment for the usual infectious diseases prevalent in the area. Despite the name, haemorrhage is not uniformly noted in viral HF and its absence should not be used to exclude the diagnosis.
- Typical laboratory findings in viral HF at presentation include lymphopenia, thrombocytopenia and elevated hepatic transaminases, with AST>ALT. Lymphocytosis and thrombocytosis may be seen in late stages.
- Although many HF viruses may be spread person-to-person, secondary attack rates are generally low as long as routine universal precautions are maintained in patient management. For added safety, specialized viral HF precautions are warranted when there is a confirmed case or high index of suspicion.
- Treatment of viral HF is generally supportive, following guidelines for the management of septic shock. The antiviral drug ribavirin and treatment with convalescent plasma have demonstrated efficacy in a few viral HFs.

Overview

INTRODUCTION

Viral haemorrhagic fever (HF) is a term first coined by Russian physicians in the 1940s to describe a syndrome comprised of fever, a constellation of initially nonspecific signs and symptoms, and a propensity for bleeding and shock. Viral HF may be caused by more than 30 different viruses from four taxonomic families: *Filoviridae*, *Arenaviridae*, *Bunyaviridae* and *Flaviviridae*, although not all members of these families cause viral HF (Table 16.1). Other common elements of viral HF include aspects of their pathogenesis, the fact that they are zoonoses (with the exception of dengue HF) and a tradition of naming HF viruses after the geographic origin of the first recognized case. Nevertheless, there are significant differences in the epidemiology, transmissibility, pathogenesis and clinical picture associated with each specific virus. We first present an overview of the characteristics common to all viral HFs followed by more detailed descriptions of some of the most frequent and important viral HFs. Detailed review of the classic mosquito-borne viral HFs – dengue HF and yellow fever – is provided in Chapters 14 and 15.

EPIDEMIOLOGY

Natural Maintenance and Transmission to Humans

With the exception of dengue virus, for which humans can now be considered to be the reservoir, HF viruses are zoonotic and are maintained in nature in mammals (Table 16.1).[1] The endemic area of any given viral HF is thus restricted by the distribution of its natural reservoir and/or arthropod vector although, for reasons that are often unclear, the distribution of the virus and disease are often less vast than that of the reservoir.

TABLE 16.1 Principal Viruses Causing Haemorrhagic Fever

Virus	Disease	Principal Reservoir/Vector	Geographic Distribution of Disease	Annual Cases	Disease-to-Infection Ratio	Human-to-Human Transmissibility	Case Fatality
Filoviridae							
Ebola[a]	Ebola HF	Fruit bat ('Egyptian fruit bat' or *Rousettus aegyptiacus*, perhaps others)	Sub-Saharan Africa	–[b]	1:1	High	25–85% depending upon species[b]
Marburg	Marburg HF	Fruit bat ('Egyptian fruit bat' or *Rousettus aegyptiacus*, perhaps others)	Sub-Saharan Africa	–[b]	1:1	High	25–85%[c]
Arenaviridae[d]							
OLD WORLD							
Lassa	Lassa fever	Rodent ('multimammate rat' or *Mastomys natalensis*)	West Africa	30 000–50 000	1:5–10	Moderate	25%
Lujo[e]	Lujo HF	Unknown. Presumed rodent	Zambia	Unknown	Unknown	Moderate-to-high	80%
NEW WORLD							
Junin	Argentine HF	Rodent ('corn mouse' or *Calomys musculinus*)	Argentine pampas	<50	1:1.5	Low	15–30%
Machupo	Bolivian HF	Rodent ('large vesper mouse' or *Calomys callosus*)	Beni department, Bolivia	<50	1:1.5	Low	15–30%
Guanarito	Venezuelan HF	Rodent ('cane mouse' or *Zygodontomys brevicauda*)	Portuguesa state, Venezuela	<50	1:1.5	Low	30–40%
Sabiá[f]	Brazilian HF	Unknown. Presumed rodent	Rural area near Sao Paulo, Brazil?	–[f]	1:1.5	Low?	33%
Chapare[g]	Chapare HF	Unknown. Presumed rodent	Cochabamba, Bolivia	Unknown	Unknown	Unknown	Unknown
Bunyaviridae							
OLD WORLD HANTAVIRUSES							
Hantaan, Seoul, Puumala, Dobrava-Belgrade, others	HF with renal syndrome	Rodents (see Table 16.6)	See Table 16.6	50 000–150 000	Hantaan: 1:1.5, Others: 1:20	None	<1–50%, depending on specific virus
NEW WORLD HANTAVIRUSES							
Sin Nombre, Andes, Laguna Negra, others	Hantavirus pulmonary syndrome	Rodents (see Table 16.6)	See Table 16.6	50 000–150 000	Sin nombre: 1:1, Others up to 1:20	None, except for Andes virus	<1–50%, depending on specific virus

TABLE 16.1 Principal Viruses Causing Haemorrhagic Fever—cont'd

Virus	Disease	Principal Reservoir/Vector	Geographic Distribution of Disease	Annual Cases	Disease-to-Infection Ratio	Human-to-Human Transmissibility	Case Fatality
Rift Valley fever	Rift Valley fever	Domestic livestock/ mosquitoes (*Aedes* and others)	Sub-Saharan Africa, Madagascar, Saudi Arabia, Yemen[g]	100–100 000[b,h]	1:100	None	Up to 50% in persons manifesting severe forms
Crimean-Congo HF	Crimean-Congo HF	Wild and domestic vertebrates/tick (primarily *Hyalomma* species)	Africa, Balkans, southern Russia, Middle East, India, Pakistan, Afghanistan, western China	~500	1:1–2	High	15–30%
Flaviviridae							
Yellow fever	Yellow fever	Monkey/mosquito (*Aedes aegypti*, other *Aedes* and *Haemagogus* spp.)	Sub-Saharan Africa, South America up to Panama	5,000–200 000[i]	1:2–20	No	20–50%
Dengue	Dengue HF	Human/mosquito (*Aedes aegypti* and *albopictus*)	Tropics and subtropics worldwide	Dengue HF: 100 000–200 000[h]	1:10–100 depending on age, previous infection, genetic background and infecting serotype	None	Untreated: 10–15% Treated: < 1%
Kyasanur Forest disease	Kyasanur Forest disease	Vertebrate (rodents, bats, birds, monkeys, others)/ tick (*Haemophysalis* species and others)	Karnataka State, India; Yunnan Province, China; Saudi Arabia[j]	~500	Unknown	Not reported, but laboratory infections have occurred	3–5%
Omsk HF	Omsk HF	Rodent/ticks (primarily *Dermacentor* and *Ixodes* species)	Western Siberia	100–200	Unknown	Not reported	1–3%

HF, haemorrhagic fever.

[a]Six species or sub-types of *Ebolavirus* with varying associated case-fatality ratios are recognized: Ebola Zaire, 85%; Ebola Sudan, 55%; Ebola Bundibugyo, 40%; Ebola Cote d'Ivoire, 0 (only one recognized case, who survived); Ebola Reston, 0 (not pathogenic to humans); Lloviu, no human infections recognized. All are endemic to sub-Saharan Africa, with the exceptions of Ebola Reston virus, which is found in the Philippines and Lloviu virus, which was detected in bats in Spain.

[b]Although some endemic transmission of the filoviruses (Ebola>Marburg) and Rift Valley fever virus occurs, these viruses have most often been associated with outbreaks. Filovirus outbreaks are typically less than 100 cases and have never been greater than 500.

[c]The case fatality ratio was 22% in the first recognized outbreak of Marburg HF in Germany and Yugoslavia in 1967 but has been consistently over 80% in outbreaks in central Africa where the virus is endemic. Possible reasons for this discrepancy include differences in quality of care, strain pathogenicity, route and dose of infection, underlying prevalence of immunodeficiency and co-morbid illnesses and genetic susceptibility.

[d]In addition to the arenaviruses listed in the table, Flexal and Tacaribe viruses have caused human disease as a result of laboratory accidents. Another arenavirus, Whitewater Arroyo, has been noted in sick persons in California but its role as a pathogen has not been clearly established.

[e]Discovered in 2008 in an outbreak of five cases (four of them fatal) in South Africa. The index case came to South Africa from Zambia.

[f]Discovered in 1990. Only three cases (one fatal) have been noted; two of them from laboratory accidents.

[g]Discovered in 2003 from a small outbreak in Cochabamba, Bolivia. Blood was obtained from one fatal case and Chapare virus isolated but few other details from the outbreak have been reported.

[h]Although Rift Valley fever virus can be found throughout sub-Saharan Africa, large outbreaks usually occur in East Africa.

[i]Based on estimates from the World Health Organization. Significant underreporting occurs. Incidence may fluctuate widely depending on epidemic activity.

[j]Numerous variants of Kyasanur Forest disease virus have been identified, including Nanjianyin virus in Yunnan Province, China and Alkhumra virus (also spelled 'Alkhurma' in some publications) in Saudi Arabia.

Few data are available on the precise modes of transmission from mammals to humans, but infection is presumed to most often result from inadvertent contact with virus-contaminated excreta of the reservoir, with inoculation into mucus membranes or broken skin. A few HF viruses are arboviruses, spread to humans by mosquitoes or ticks. Aerosol transmission has also been suggested for some viruses, but there are few data to confirm or refute this route of exposure.[2] Empiric observation in the field, including the general absence of clusters of cases in which no direct contact occurred, suggests that aerosol transmission is not a predominant mode of spread, if it occurs at all. Nevertheless, studies in non-human primates show that transmission of many HF viruses is possible when aerosols are artificially produced, with obvious implications for their potential use as bioweapons.[3,4]

Human-to-Human Transmission

Secondary human-to-human transmission occurs with many of the HF viruses, usually through direct contact with contaminated blood or body fluids (Table 16.1). Infection probably occurs most often through oral or mucous membrane exposure in the context of providing care to sick family members in the community or patients in a healthcare institution or during funeral rituals that entail the touching of the corpse prior to burial. Again, there are few data on aerosol spread, although the observation that infection is rare in healthcare workers taking precautions against contact, but not aerosol, transmission suggests that it is rare or non-existent. Large outbreaks are almost always the result of amplification in healthcare settings, in which basic infection control measures have broken down, usually in areas of extreme poverty or civil strife, resulting in the absence of gloves and other personal protective equipment and reuse of unsterilized needles.[5] The risk of transmission during the incubation period or from asymptomatic persons is negligible, although a case of Argentine HF was reported due to blood transfusion from a donor who was asymptomatic. Rarely, sexual transmission of HF viruses (best documented for Ebola, Marburg, Lassa and Junin viruses) during convalescence has been confirmed or strongly suspected.[6]

PATHOGENESIS AND PATHOLOGY

Knowledge of the pathogenesis of viral HF is based on limited data from humans combined with extrapolation from more extensive observations made in animal models.[7–9] Although details of the pathophysiology vary with the specific virus, microvascular instability and impaired haemostasis are the consistent hallmarks. Despite the term 'viral HF', external haemorrhage is not always seen and may even be rare in some viral HFs. Rather, the pathogenesis of viral HF appears to have much in common with septic shock. Mortality usually results not directly from exsanguination, but rather from an intense inflammatory process resulting in insufficient effective circulating intravascular volume leading to hypotension, cellular dysfunction and multi-organ system failure.

The interaction of virus with immune cells, especially macrophages and endothelial cells, results in cell activation and the unleashing of an inflammatory and vasoactive process consistent with the systemic inflammatory response syndrome. Although lymphocytes remain free of infection, they may be destroyed in massive numbers in some viral HFs through apoptosis, as seen in other forms of septic shock.

The synthesis of cell surface tissue factor triggers the extrinsic coagulation pathway. Impaired haemostasis may entail endothelial cell, platelet and/or coagulation factor dysfunction, depending upon the specific infecting virus. Disseminated intravascular coagulopathy (DIC) is frequently noted in some, but not all, viral HFs (Table 16.2).

After inoculation, the virus first replicates in dendritic cells and other local tissues, with subsequent migration to regional lymph nodes followed by dissemination through the lymph and blood monocytes to a broad range of tissues and organs,

TABLE 16.2 Pathobiological and Clinical Aspects of Viral Haemorrhagic Fevers

Disease	Incubation Period (Days)	Onset	Bleeding	Rash	Jaundice	Heart	Lung	Kidney	CNS	Eye
Filoviridae										
Ebola HF	3–21	Abrupt	++	+++	+	++?	+	+	+	+
Marburg HF	3–21	Abrupt	++	+++	+	++?	+	+	+	+
Arenaviridae										
Lassa fever	5–16	Gradual	+	+	0	++	+	0	+	0
Lujo HF	9–13	Abrupt	+	++	0	?	+	+	+	0
South American HFs[a]	4–14	Gradual	+++	+	0	++	+	0	+++	0
Bunyaviridae										
HF with renal syndrome	9–35	Abrupt	+++	0	0	++	+	+++	+	0
Hantavirus pulmonary syndrome	7–35	Gradual	0 (except for Andes virus infection)	0	0	+++	+++	+	+	0
Rift Valley fever[b]	2–5	Abrupt	++	+	++	+?	0	+	++	++
Crimean-Congo HF[c]	3–12	Abrupt	+++	0	++	+?	+	0	+	0
Flaviviridae										
Yellow fever	3–6	Abrupt	+++	0	+++	++	+	++	++	0
Dengue HF	3–15	Abrupt	++	+++	+	++	+	0	+	0
Kyasanur Forest disease	3–8	Abrupt	++	0	0	+	++	0	+++	+
Omsk HF	3–8	Abrupt	++	0	0	+	++	0	+++	+

CNS, central nervous system; HF, haemorrhagic fever; 0, sign not typically noted/organ not typically affected; +, sign occasionally noted/organ occasionally affected; ++, sign commonly noted/organ commonly affected; +++, sign characteristic/organ involvement severe.

[a]Data are insufficient to distinguish between the syndromes produced by the various New World arenaviruses.

[b]HF, encephalitis and retinitis may be seen in Rift Valley fever independently of each other.

[c]The incubation period of Crimean-Congo HF varies with the mode of transmission: typically 1–3 days after tick bite and 5–6 days after contact with infected animal blood or tissues.

including the liver, spleen, lymph nodes, adrenal glands, lungs and endothelium. Migration of tissue macrophages then results in secondary infection of permissive parenchymal cells. The most affected organs vary with the virus (Table 16.2). Tissue damage may be mediated through direct viral infection and necrosis or indirectly through the inflammatory process. Inflammatory cell infiltrates are usually mild.

Cellular immunity is thought to be the primary arm of protection in most viral HFs. With the exception of disease caused by the hantaviruses and some of the flaviviruses, the pathogenesis of viral HF appears to be unchecked viraemia, with most fatal cases failing to mount a significant antibody response. In some viral HFs virus replication and dissemination is facilitated by virus-induced suppression of the host adaptive immune response.

Virus rapidly clears from the blood upon symptom resolution in survivors, but clearance may be delayed (up to 3 months after acute infection) from a few immunologically protected sites, such as the kidney, gonads and chambers of the eye.[6,10] In contrast to the process described above, hantaviruses, yellow fever virus and dengue virus are usually cleared from the blood prior to the most severe phase of the disease. Here, the host immune response is thought to play a detrimental role.

CLINICAL FEATURES

Viral HF is seen in both genders and all age groups, with a spectrum from relatively mild or even asymptomatic infection to severe vascular permeability with shock, multi-organ system failure and death. Although the clinical presentation may differ for each viral HF as it progresses, in most cases it is not possible to distinguish the various syndromes at presentation. Distinct phases of disease and recovery are classically described for HF with renal syndrome and yellow fever, although not seen in all cases. Biphasic illnesses are classically noted for the flavivirus HFs, in which a quiescent period of days (yellow fever and dengue) to weeks (Kyasanur Forest disease and Omsk HF) occurs, after which the most severe manifestations may set in, including haemorrhage, shock, renal failure and meningoencephalitis.

After an incubation period ranging from days to weeks, depending upon the infecting virus (Table 16.2), illness typically begins with fever and constitutional symptoms, including general malaise, anorexia, headache, myalgia, arthralgia, sore throat, chest or retrosternal pain and lumbosacral pain. Neck pain and stiffness, retro-orbital pain and photophobia are common in Rift Valley fever and may be noted in viral HFs, in which meningitis is common, such as Omsk HF and Kyasanur Forest disease. Orthostatic hypotension is common. Gastrointestinal signs and symptoms follow in the first few days of illness, including nausea, vomiting, epigastric and abdominal pain, abdominal tenderness, diarrhoea and constipation. Diarrhoea may become bloody in the later stages of disease. A misdiagnosis of appendicitis or other acute abdominal emergency sometimes occurs, prompting unneeded and dangerous (in terms of risk of nosocomial spread) surgical interventions. Conjunctival injection or haemorrhage is frequent. Various forms of skin rash, including morbilliform, maculopapular, petechial and ecchymotic, may be seen, depending on the specific viral HF (Table 16.2).

In severe cases, towards the end of the first week of illness, patients progress to vascular instability that may be manifested by facial flushing, oedema, bleeding, hypotension, shock and proteinuria. The likelihood of clinically discernible haemorrhage varies with the infecting virus (Table 16.2). Haematemesis, melena, haematochezia, metrorrhagia, petechiae, purpura, epistaxis and bleeding from the gums and venepuncture sites may develop, but haemoptysis and haematuria are infrequent. Significant internal bleeding from the gastrointestinal tract may occur even in the absence of external haemorrhage and misdiagnosis as peptic ulcer disease is common. Central nervous system manifestations, including disorientation, tremor, gait anomalies, convulsions and hiccups, may be noted in end-stage disease in some viral HFs, as is renal insufficiency or failure. Radiographic and electrocardiographic findings are generally nonspecific and correlate with the physical examination.[11] Pregnant women often present with spontaneous abortion and vaginal bleeding, with maternal and fetal mortality approaching 100% in the 3rd trimester.

Convalescence from viral HF may be prolonged, with persistent myalgia, arthralgia, anorexia, weight loss, alopecia orchitis, irritability and memory changes up to a year after infection. Nevertheless, in most cases there are no permanent sequelae. However, the psychological effects of viral HF may also be significant and often overlooked, with some patients experiencing depression or post-traumatic stress, as well as social stigmatization.

DIAGNOSIS

Differential Diagnosis

Many infectious and even non-infectious diseases can mimic viral HF, especially in the early stages, resulting in an extremely broad differential diagnosis that varies by geographic region (Table 16.3 and Figures 16.1–16.4). Initial misdiagnosis of more familiar syndromes is common. Malaria and bacterial septicaemia, including meningococcaemia, are among the most common, although malaria is unlikely to be the cause of severe illness in adults living in malaria-endemic areas. African tick-bite fever and other rickettsial illness should also be considered. Although confirmation of an alternative diagnosis renders viral HF less likely, the possibility of coinfection should be considered, especially taking into account that bacterial septicaemia can occur as a complication of viral HF. Furthermore, a positive test for malaria should not completely exclude viral HF, especially if the patient is not responding to anti-malarial drugs, since pre-existing parasitaemia may be common in holoendemic areas for malaria.

The presence or absence of certain clinical features can help rule out viral HF:

- Haemorrhage is almost never seen in the first few days of illness. Its presence at this early stage should suggest an alternative diagnosis, especially meningococcaemia.
- Although conjunctival injection and sub-conjunctival haemorrhage are frequent in viral HF, they are not accompanied by itching, discharge or rhinitis. The presence of these symptoms should suggest a more common viral upper respiratory tract infection, adenoviral or bacterial conjunctivitis or allergic rhinitis.
- With the exception of yellow fever, jaundice on presentation is not typical of viral HF and should suggest another diagnosis or a complicating factor such as underlying Gilbert's syndrome, drug reaction or co-infection with an

TABLE 16.3 **Differential Diagnosis of Viral Haemorrhagic Fever**

Disease	Distinguishing Characteristics and Comments
Parasites	
Malaria	Classically shows paroxysms of fever and chills; Haemorrhagic manifestations less common; Malaria smears or rapid test usually positive; Co-infection (or baseline asymptomatic parasitaemia) common; Responds to anti-malarials
Amoebiasis	Haemorrhagic manifestations other than bloody diarrhoea generally not seen; Amoebic trophozoites identified in the stool; Responds to anti-parasitics
Giardiasis	Positive stool antigen test and/or identification of trophozoites or cysts in stool; Responds to antiparasitics
African trypanosomiasis (acute stages)	Especially the east African form. Examination of peripheral blood smear/buffy coat may show trypanosomes
Bacteria (including Spirochetes, Rickettsia, Ehrlichia and Coxiella)	
Typhoid fever	Haemorrhagic manifestations other than bloody diarrhoea generally not seen; Responds to antibiotics
Bacillary dysentery (including shigellosis, campylobacteriosis, salmonellosis and enterohaemorrhagic *Escherichia coli* and others)	Haemorrhagic manifestations other than bloody diarrhoea generally not seen; Respond to antibiotics
Capnocytophaga canimorsus	Associated with dog and cat bites, typically in persons with underlying immunodeficiency, notably asplenic patients; Responds to antibiotics
Meningococcaemia	Bacterial-induced DIC may mimic the bleeding diathesis of viral HF; bleeding within the first 24–48 hours after onset of illness and rapidly progressive illness typical; Large ecchymoses typical of meningococcemia are unusual in the viral HFs except for Crimean-Congo HF; Rapid serum latex agglutination tests can be used to detect bacterial antigen in meningococcal septicaemia; May respond to antibiotics (critical to administer early)
Staphylococcaemia	Bacterial-induced DIC may mimic the bleeding diathesis of viral HF; May respond to antibiotics
Septic abortion	History of pregnancy and positive pregnancy test
Septicaemic or pneumonic plague	Bacterial-induced DIC may mimic the bleeding diathesis of viral HF; Large ecchymoses typical of plague are unusual in the viral HFs except for Crimean-Congo HF; Pneumonic plague may mimic HPS; May respond to antibiotics
Streptococcal pharyngitis	May mimic the exudative pharyngitis sometimes seen in Lassa fever
Tuberculosis	Haemoptysis of advanced pulmonary tuberculosis may suggest viral HF, but tuberculosis generally has a much slower disease evolution
Tularaemia	Ulceroglandular and pneumonic forms more common; Responds to antibiotics
Acute abdominal emergencies	Appendicitis, peritonitis and bleeding upper gastrointestinal ulcer
Pyelonephritis and post-streptococcal glomerulonephritis	May mimic HF with renal syndrome
Anthrax (inhalation or gastrointestinal)	Prominent pulmonary manifestations and widened mediastinum on chest X-ray in inhalation form; Responds to antibiotics
Atypical bacterial pneumonia (*Legionella, Mycoplasma, Chlamydophila pneumoniae* and *psittaci*, others)	May mimic hantavirus pulmonary syndrome; Exposure to birds and symptoms often not present until late in the illness in psittacosis; Respond to antibiotics
Relapsing fever	Recurrent fevers and flu-like symptoms, with direct neurologic involvement and splenomegaly; Spirochetes visible in blood while febrile; Responds to antibiotics
Leptospirosis	Jaundice, renal failure and myocarditis in severe cases; Responds to antibiotics
Spotted fever group rickettsia (including African tick bite fever, Boutonneuse fever, Rocky Mountain spotted fever)	Incubation period of 7–10 days after tick bite, compared with 1–3 days in Crimean-Congo HF; Necrotic lesions (eschar) typically seen at site of tick bite in some rickettsial diseases while there may only be slight bruising at the bite site in Crimean-Congo HF; Rash (if present) of Rickettsial infection classically involves palms and soles
Q fever (*Coxiella burnetii*)	Broad spectrum of illness, including hepatitis, pneumonitis, encephalitis and multisystem disease with bleeding; Responds to antibiotics
Ehrlichiosis	Responds to antibiotics
Viruses	
Influenza	Prominent respiratory component to clinical presentation; No haemorrhagic manifestations; Influenza rapid test may be positive; May respond to anti-influenza drugs
Arbovirus infection (including dengue and West Nile fever)	Encephalitis unusual, but when present may mimic the viral HFs with significant neurologic involvement (Kyasanur Forest disease, Omsk HF); Usually less severe than viral HF; Haemorrhage not reported
Viral hepatitis (including hepatitis A, B and E, Epstein-Barr and cytomegalovirus)	Jaundice atypical in HF except yellow fever; Tests for hepatitis antigens positive; Fulminant infection resembling viral HF may be seen in persons with underlying immune deficiencies
Herpes simplex or varicella-zoster	Fulminant infection with hepatitis (with/without vesicular rash); Elevated transaminases and leucopaenia typical; Disseminated disease may be noted in otherwise healthy persons; poor response to acyclovir drugs unless recognized early

TABLE 16.3 Differential Diagnosis of Viral Haemorrhagic Fever—cont'd

Disease	Distinguishing Characteristics and Comments
HIV/AIDS	Seroconversion syndrome or HIV/AIDS with secondary infections, especially septicaemia
Measles	Rash may mimic that seen in early stages of some viral HFs and may sometimes be haemorrhagic; Prominence of coryza and upper respiratory symptoms in measles should help differentiate; Vaccine preventable
Rubella	Rash may mimic that seen in early stages of some viral HFs; Usually a mild disease; Vaccine preventable
Haemorrhagic or flat smallpox	Diffuse haemorrhagic or macular lesions; In contrast to the viral HFs, the rash may involve the oral mucosa, palms and soles; Smallpox in the wild has been eradicated
Alphavirus infection (including chikungunya and o'nyong-nyong)	Joint pain typically a predominant feature
Fungi	
Histoplasmosis	Pulmonary disease may mimic hantavirus pulmonary; Recent entry into mines or caves
Non-infectious Aetiologies	
Heat stroke	History for extreme heat exposure; Absence of sweating; Bleeding not typical but DIC may occur
Idiopathic and thrombotic thrombocytopenic purpura (ITP/TTP)	Presentation usually less acute than viral HF; May have prominent neurologic symptoms in TTP; Coagulation factors normal and DIC absent; Often respond to corticosteroids (ITP) or plasma exchange (TTP)
Acute glaucoma	May mimic the acute ocular manifestations of Rift Valley fever
Haematological malignancies (leukaemia, lymphoma)	May resemble leukemoid reaction occasionally seen in HF with renal syndrome
Drug sensitivity or overdose	Stevens–Johnson's syndrome and anticoagulant (warfarin) overdose
Industrial and agricultural chemical poisoning	Especially anticoagulants, although other symptoms of viral HF absent
Haematoxic snake bite envenomation	History of snake bite

DIC, disseminated intravascular coagulopathy; HF, haemorrhagic fever.

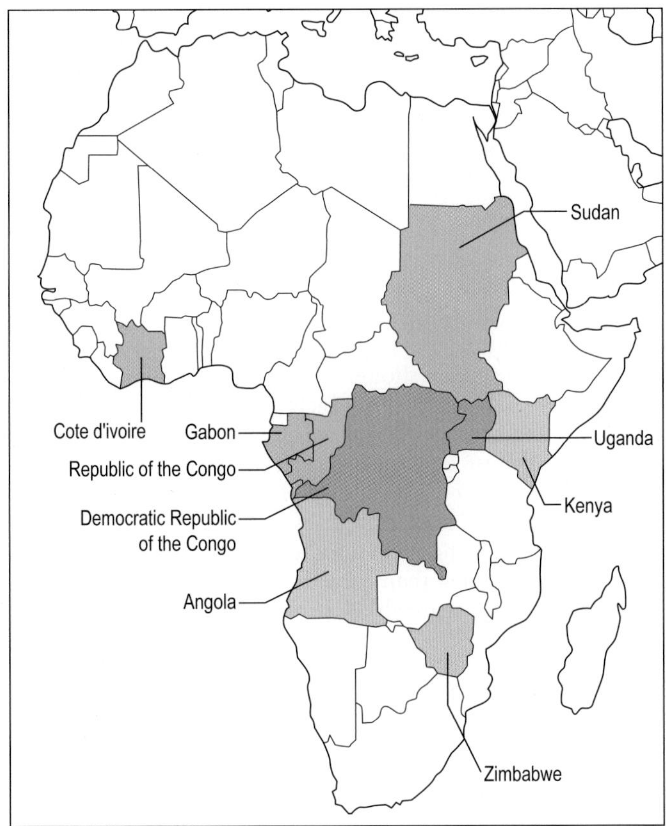

Figure 16.1 Endemic areas for filoviruses. Only filoviruses known to cause haemorrhagic fever are shown. Countries where Ebola and Marburg haemorrhagic fevers have been seen are indicated in green and blue, respectively, with countries in red indicating documentation of both diseases. Incidence and risk of disease may vary significantly within each country.

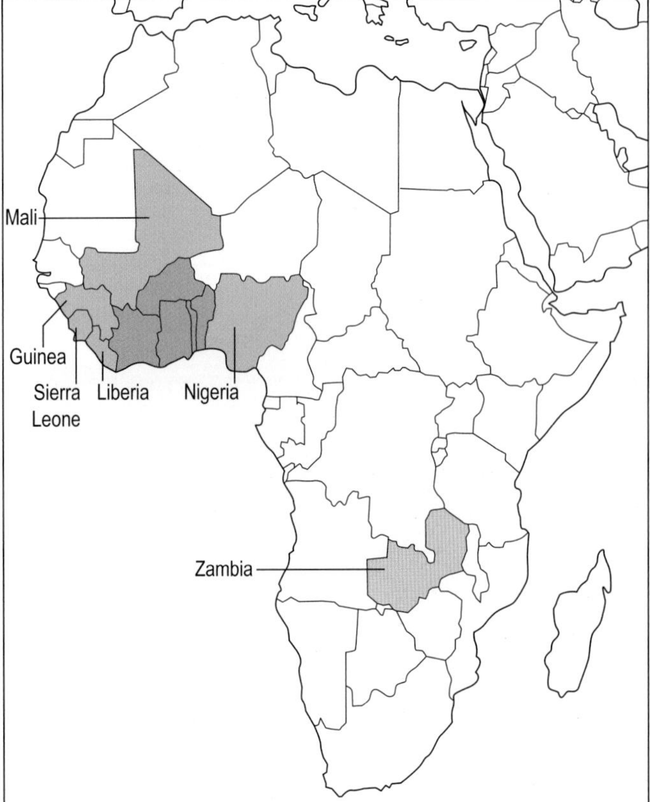

Figure 16.2 Endemic areas for Old World arenaviruses. Only the two arenaviruses, Lassa and Lujo, known to cause haemorrhagic fever are shown. Countries where clinical cases of Lassa fever have been confirmed are depicted in green. Indirect evidence, such as anecdotal reports or seroprevalence data, exists for most of the other countries in West Africa, shown in red. Endemic countries for Lujo virus are depicted by blue. Incidence and risk of disease may vary significantly within each country.

Venezuelan
haemorrhagic fever
(Guanarito virus)
Bolivian
haemorrhagic fever
(Machupo virus)
Chapare
haemorrhagic fever
(Chapare virus)
Argentine
haemorrhagic fever
(Junín virus)
Brazilian
haemorrhagic fever
(Sabiá virus)

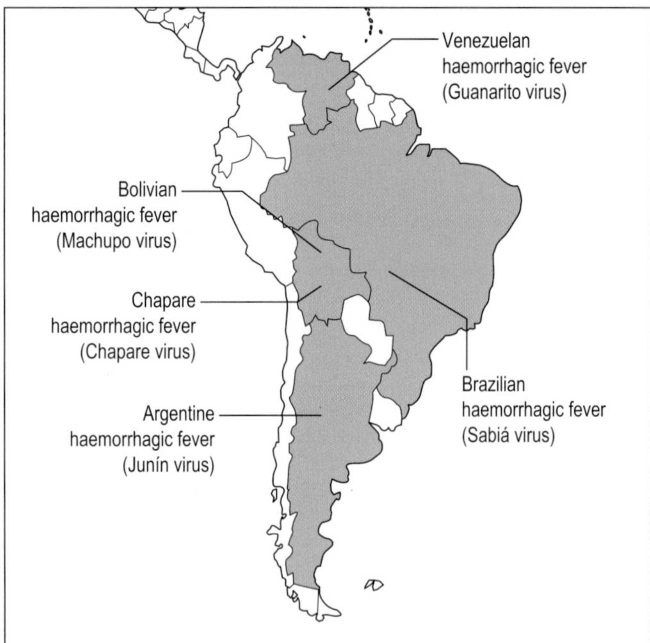

Figure 16.3 Endemic areas for New World arenaviruses. Only the arenaviruses known to cause haemorrhagic fever are shown. Incidence and risk of disease may vary significantly within each country.

organism causing hepatotoxicity or haemolysis, such as malaria.

- Although a dry cough may occasionally be noted in viral HF, sometimes accompanied by a few scattered rales on auscultation, with the exception of hantavirus pulmonary syndrome (HPS), prominent pulmonary symptoms or the presence of productive sputum are not typical of viral HF, although secondary bacterial infection producing these symptoms may occur as disease progresses.

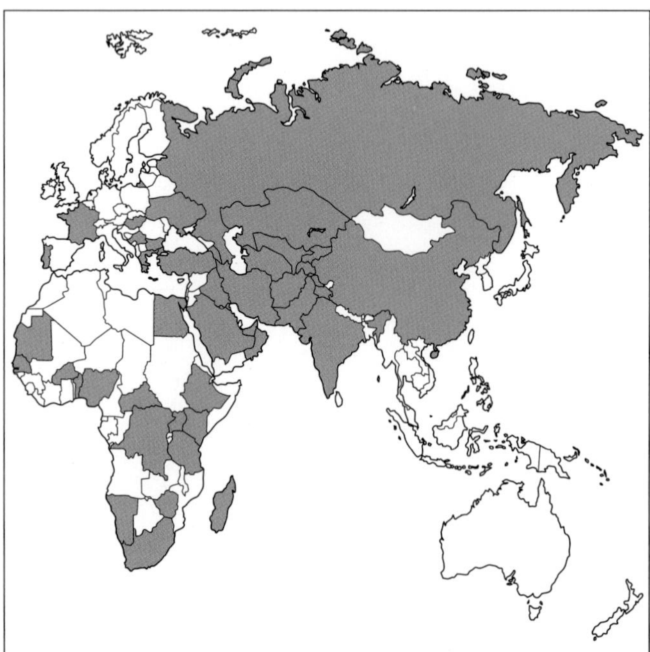

Figure 16.4 Endemic areas for Crimean-Congo haemorrhagic fever virus. Incidence and risk of disease may vary significantly within each country. Variable intensity of surveillance may underlie the absence of confirmed cases in some countries.

Clinical Diagnosis

The nonspecific clinical manifestations of most viral HFs make a clinical diagnosis and detection of single cases extremely difficult, especially early in the course of the disease when haemorrhage and other more identifiable manifestations are usually absent. A detailed epidemiological history and physical examination, along with preliminary basic laboratory results (Table 16.4) are critical in initial consideration of the diagnosis, including details of travel, possible exposures, occupational risks and details of the progression of illness (e.g. timing of haemorrhage relative to onset of illness). A diagnosis of viral HF should be considered in patients with a clinically compatible syndrome who, within the incubation period for the particular viral HF in question (Table 16.2):

- Reside in or travelled to an area where a viral HF is known or suspected to be endemic (Table 16.1 and Figures 16.1–16.4)
- Had potential direct contact with blood or body fluids of someone with a suspected or confirmed viral HF during their acute illness. This group is most often comprised of healthcare workers and laboratory personnel or persons caring for family members at home or preparing bodies for burial
- Had contact with live or recently killed animals in a viral HF-endemic area (although it should be recognized that direct contact with the animal reservoir is not usually reported even in confirmed cases of viral HF). Animals and arthropods in question include non-human primates, rodents, bats, livestock, ticks and mosquitoes, depending upon the viral HF in question. Food potentially recently contaminated by these animals could also be a source of infection
- Worked in a laboratory or animal facility where HF viruses are handled
- Had sex with someone recovering from a viral HF in the last 3 months.

The index of suspicion should be especially high for persons in specific high-risk occupations, including abattoir workers, veterinarians and farm workers, hunters and taxidermists. Acts of bioterrorism must be considered if viral HF is strongly suspected in a patient without any of the aforementioned risk factors, especially if clusters of cases are seen. It should be noted that even persons who meet the above criteria most commonly have a disease other than viral HF, so alternative diagnoses should always be aggressively sought and specific treatment instituted.

Laboratory Diagnosis

If viral HF is still suspected after the initial work-up and laboratory testing, prompt diagnostic laboratory testing is imperative. Rapid access to specialized laboratory testing will vary according to region and is especially a problem in resource-limited areas. Unfortunately, no commercial assays are available for the viral HFs, with the exception of various kits with varying sensitivity and specificity for the serologic diagnosis of dengue fever and HPS. The absence of commercial assays poses a major impediment to both patient diagnosis and research. Recombinant-protein and virus-like particle-based assays for the viral HFs are being developed which may eventually relieve

TABLE 16.4 Indicated Clinical Laboratory Tests and Characteristic Findings in Patients with Viral Haemorrhagic Fever

Test	Characteristic Findings and Comments
Leukocyte count	Early: moderate leukopenia (except for hantavirus infection, in which early leukocytosis with immunoblasts are classically noted); Later: leukocytosis with left shift; Granulocytosis more suggestive of bacterial infection
Haemoglobin and haematocrit	Haemoconcentration (especially noted in haemorrhagic fever with renal syndrome and hantavirus pulmonary syndrome)
Platelet count	Mild-to-moderate thrombocytopenia
Electrolytes	Sodium, potassium and acid–base perturbations, depending upon fluid balance and stage of disease
BUN/creatinine	Renal failure may occur late in disease.
Serum chemistries (AST, ALT, amylase, gamma-glutamyl transferase, alkaline phosphatase, creatinine kinase, lactate dehydrogenase, lactate acid)	Usually increased, especially in severe disease; AST > ALT; A lactate level greater than 4 mmol/L (36 mg/dL) may indicate persistent hypo-perfusion and sepsis. Lactate dehydrogenase is typically markedly increased in hantavirus pulmonary syndrome
Sedimentation rate	Normal or decreased
Blood gas	Metabolic acidosis may be indicative of shock and hypoperfusion
Coagulation studies (PT, PTT, fibrinogen, fibrin split products, platelets, D-dimer)	DIC common in Ebola, Marburg, Lujo virus, Crimean-Congo HF and New World arenavirus infections
Urinalysis	Proteinuria common; Haematuria may be occasionally noted; Sediment may show hyaline-granular casts and round cells with cytoplasmic inclusions
Blood culture	Useful early to exclude viral HF and later to evaluate for secondary bacterial infection; Blood should be drawn before antibiotic therapy is instituted
Stool culture	Useful to exclude viral HF (in favour of haemorrhagic bacillary dysentery)
Thick and thin blood smears	May aid in the diagnosis of blood parasites (malaria and trypanosomes) and bacterial sepsis (meningococcus, capnocytophaga and anthrax); All negative in viral HF unless coinfection
Rapid test, PCR or other assay for malaria	Negative in viral HF unless coinfection with malaria
Febrile agglutinins or other assay for *Salmonella typhi*	Negative in viral HF unless coinfection with *S. Typhi*

ALT, Alanine aminotransferase; AST, aspartate aminotransferase; DIC, disseminated intravascular coagulation; viral HF, viral haemorrhagic fever.

this bottleneck, as well as further improve sensitivity and specificity. Meanwhile, various 'in-house' assays have been developed and are performed in a few specialized laboratories.

The enzyme-linked immunosorbent assay (ELISA), reverse transcriptase polymerase chain reaction (RT-PCR) and cell culture are the mainstays of diagnosis.[12] Although extensive validation of these assays has not been conducted, sensitivities and specificities are generally considered to be over 90%. The immunofluorescent antibody test (IFA) may also be employed but is not as routinely sensitive or specific and is more subjective in its interpretation, varying with the experience of the technician.[13] Post-mortem diagnosis of some viral HFs may be established by immunohistochemical staining of formalin-fixed tissue, especially skin, liver and spleen.[14] All confirmed cases of viral HF should be reported immediately to government health authorities as well as to the World Health Organization in keeping with International Health Regulations. No test can reliably be used to diagnose viral HF before the onset of illness. Consequently, testing of contacts or other asymptomatic persons is not recommended, even if the suspicion of infection is high.

Acute Febrile Stage. In the acute febrile phase of the disease, viral HF is usually diagnosed by identifying virus, virus antigen or nucleic acid in the specimen. These measures also provide prognostic value, since high levels of virus, antigen or nucleic acid in the blood correlate with a poor prognosis in most viral HFs. Serum is the most reliable sample to test, but the virus can be variably isolated from throat washings, urine, CSF, breast milk and various other tissues.[6] ELISAs are high throughput and ELISA antigen tests and RT-PCR can usually be done in a few hours. Multiplex PCR assays have been developed that may allow for simultaneous testing for the HF viruses as well as the many diseases in the differential diagnosis. Furthermore, these assays can be performed with inactivated specimens using standard equipment present in most diagnostic laboratories. In contrast, propagation of most HF viruses in cell culture requires a high containment facility and 2–10 days to detect virus growth, depending on the specific virus and titre in the sample. However, ELISAs may lack sensitivity relative to RT-PCR and cell culture. Nevertheless, cell culture should not be omitted whenever possible because HF viruses have occasionally been isolated from specimens for which ELISA antigen, antibody and RT-PCR tests were all negative – a finding attributable to virus concentrations in the test sample that were below the threshold of detection of these assays or the presence of variant or novel viruses that were not detectable with the antigens and primer sets employed.[15]

Failure to appreciate the intricacies and limitations of the various laboratory assays has occasionally led to false-negative diagnoses and increased risk of nosocomial transmission. Inhibitory substances circulating in the blood have been shown to cause false-negative RT-PCR results in viral HF. Thus, appropriate inhibition controls must be included in all RT-PCR assays.

Although virus is usually present in high titre and relatively easy to detect in the blood of persons with severe disease (with the exception of *Flavivirus* and *Hantavirus* infections), viraemia may be of very short duration or even absent in surviving cases or very early in the course of disease. If clinical suspicion of viral HF remains high, despite a negative result, tests should be repeated in 1–2 days and, if necessary, again in convalescence.

The diagnosis of viral HF can usually be safely discarded if virus, antigen or nucleic acid cannot be detected in blood during the first 7 days of illness and IgM antibody is negative (see below).

False-positive results due to contamination are also a concern with RT-PCR due to its extreme sensitivity, especially when the assay is being performed in more rudimentary facilities in developing countries, where separate spaces for sample preparation and amplification and the routine use of positive and negative controls is not always possible. In the worst case, outbreaks or even bioterrorism could be falsely declared. The use of one-step assays, sequencing of PCR products to distinguish them from reference strains, targeting different portions of the genome and use of multiple supporting diagnostic methods can minimize the risk of false-positives.

Sub-acute and Convalescent Stages. In the sub-acute and convalescent stages of illness, viral HF can be diagnosed through identification of IgM and IgG antibody, respectively, in the blood through ELISA or IFA. Antibody seroconversion (usually interpreted as a fourfold increase in titre) on acute and convalescent serum specimens has also been used to retrospectively diagnose acute disease when assays for detection virus, nucleic acid or antigen are not available. Demonstration of neutralizing antibody can increase the specificity of ELISA antibody results but neutralization assays are not uniformly standardized, are cumbersome to perform and, because they require the use of live virus, must be done in a high containment laboratory for many of the viruses in question. Consequently, they are infrequently performed. The timing of appearance of IgM and IgG antibodies and their duration after infection has not been systematically studied and likely varies with the specific virus. In survivors, IgM generally appears in the first days or weeks of illness and lasts for months after infection, while IgG typically appears during convalescence and is thought to last years, if not decades.

MANAGEMENT AND TREATMENT

Because of their potential severity, risk of secondary spread, high degree of public scrutiny and unfamiliarity on the part of most physicians, consultation with infectious disease specialists or other clinicians with experience in the diagnosis and treatment of viral HFs should be sought when the diagnosis is suspected. The process of performing a work-up for non-viral HF aetiologies, while assuring that proper safety precautions are maintained, nosocomial spread avoided and undue panic is minimized, is a delicate one. The casual inclusion of viral HF in the differential diagnosis has the potential to induce considerable anxiety in patients, hospital staff and the general community. When to 'sound the alarm' of viral HF is a case-by-case decision left to the treating physician in consultation with experts in the field. Knowledge that most viral HFs are rare and that routinely practiced universal precautions are protective in the vast majority of cases (see below) should offer reassurance.

In remote areas of Africa, access to basic laboratory tests and diagnostic tests for the broad range of diseases included in the differential diagnosis of viral HF is very limited and empiric treatment to cover the usual range of infectious agents is the norm. Admission to an isolation ward is based on relatively nonspecific clinical and epidemiological features. Access to accurate on-site specialized diagnostics, typically PCR, may reduce the number of patients potentially exposed to HF viruses in the isolation ward.

Treatment of viral HF can be divided into general supportive measures, antiviral drugs, antibody therapy (including both human convalescent plasma and laboratory-generated mono- and polyclonal antibodies), immune modulators and coagulation modulators.[16–18] However, very few controlled trials in humans have been performed for any treatment strategy for viral HF.

General Supportive Measures

Treatment of viral HF generally follows the guidelines for the management of septic shock.[19] Where possible patients with viral HF should be treated in an intensive care unit since severe microvascular instability, often complicated by vomiting, diarrhoea, decreased fluid intake and third-spacing, may require continuous monitoring and aggressive fluid replacement. Because of the risk of bleeding at insertion sites, intravascular haemodynamic devices are contraindicated. Haemodynamic status should instead be monitored by blood pressure cuff or other non-invasive means. Intramuscular and subcutaneous injections should also be avoided due to the risk of haematoma. Even in resource-limited settings basic supportive care can be safely implemented if contact precautions and sound infection control practices are maintained.

Fluid Management. Fluid management in viral HF poses a particular challenge. Aggressive fluid replacement is warranted and may prevent shock and DIC. However, overaggressive and unmonitored rehydration may lead to significant third-spacing and pulmonary oedema, given the impaired cardiac function present in some viral HFs, especially HPS. Fluid and blood pressure management guidelines for septic shock are recommended for viral HF due to the common elements in the pathogenesis of these two conditions, although there are no efficacy data on their use in viral HF. Crystalloids (Ringers lactate or normal saline) and, if necessary, vasopressors, should be infused to maintain central venous pressure between 8–12 mmHg or mean arterial blood pressure above 65 mmHg in adults. Early use of vasopressors, especially dopamine and norepinephrine, may diminish the risk of fluid overload. Dobutamine should be added if the above measures, and blood transfusion when warranted, fail to maintain the target blood pressure and adequate organ perfusion. Peritoneal and haemodialysis have been used in patients with HF with renal syndrome without major complications, but there is little published experience in other viral HFs. Extreme caution is warranted with this and all procedures that involve potential exposure to blood to avoid virus transmission to healthcare workers.

Clinical Laboratory Findings. A broad range of clinical laboratory parameters should be monitored closely (Table 16.4). Blood samples for clinical laboratory testing can be inactivated by the addition of detergents, such as Triton X-100, although the effect of such inactivation steps on the various possible parameters to be measured has not been firmly established. The anorexia, vomiting and diarrhoea of viral HF frequently result in hypokalaemia, so regular potassium supplementation may be needed, keeping a close eye on renal function, which is often compromised in late disease.

Blood Products and Management of Disseminated Intravascular Coagulopathy. Transfusions, preferably with packed red blood cells, should be used to maintain a haematocrit over 30% while avoiding volume overload, taking into account that chronic anaemia due to malaria and malnutrition may be frequent in patients in certain geographical areas. The possibility of DIC should be assessed through the relevant laboratory parameters (D-dimers are an especially early and sensitive indicator, Table 16.4) if bleeding and thrombocytopenia persist, with transfusion of platelets and/or fresh frozen plasma as required. Transfusion of platelet concentrate (1–2 U/10 kg) should be considered when the platelet count is <50 000/μL in a bleeding patient or <20 000/μL without bleeding. The platelet count should generally rise by at least 2000/μL per unit of platelets transfused, although a lesser response may occur if there is ongoing DIC and platelet consumption. Impaired platelet aggregation may promote haemorrhage in some viral HFs, especially Lassa fever, even when platelet counts are not drastically low. Transfusion of fresh frozen plasma (FFP) (15–20 mL/kg) should be considered when bleeding is present and fibrinogen levels are <100 mg/dL. Fibrinogen concentrates (total dose 2–3 g) or cryoprecipitates (1 U/10 kg) may be administered instead of FFP, although FFP has the theoretical advantage of containing all coagulation factors and inhibitors deficient in DIC but no activated coagulation factors. Vitamin K may be given, especially if underlying malnutrition or liver disease is suspected.

Antibiotics. Patients should be immediately covered with appropriate broad-spectrum antibiotics and/or antiparasitics, with specific consideration of coverage for malaria and tick-borne rickettsial diseases, until a diagnosis of viral HF can be confirmed (Table 16.3). These drugs should be stopped once the diagnosis of viral HF is established unless there is evidence of co-infection. Secondary bacterial infection should be suspected and antibiotics given when patients have persistent or new fever after about 2 weeks of illness, when most viral HFs have either resulted in death or are resolving.

Oxygenation and Ventilation. With the exception of HPS, impaired gas exchange is not typically a prominent feature of viral HF, especially in the absence of iatrogenic pulmonary oedema. Oxygen should be administered by nasal cannula or face mask to patients with unfavourable parameters. Intubation and mechanical ventilation should be avoided because of the risk of barotrauma and pleural-pulmonary haemorrhage except in HPS, in which mechanical ventilation may be life-saving. When required, low tidal volumes (i.e. lung-protective ventilation) are best.

Pain Control and Ulcer Prophylaxis. Acetaminophen, tramadol, opiates or other analgesics should be used for pain control. Salicylates and non-steroidal anti-inflammatory drugs should be avoided due to the risk of bleeding. Prophylactic therapy for stress ulcers with H2 receptor antagonists is appropriate.

Management of Seizures. Seizures sometimes occur in late-stage viral HF and can usually be managed with benzodiazepines or phenytoin, with careful attention to possible respiratory depression. The use of sedatives and neuromuscular blocking agents should be minimized, but haloperidol or a benzodiazepine may be used.

Nutrition. Attention should be given to adequate nutrition, especially if the patient's course is prolonged or the patient is malnourished. Gut feeding is preferable to parenteral alimentation. Nasogastric tubes may be theoretically indicated for patients unable to eat, but there is little practical experience with their use in viral HF. Exacerbation of gastrointestinal bleeding and heightened risk of transmission to healthcare workers during tube placement are concerns.

Management of Pregnant Patients. Uterine evacuation in pregnant patients appears to lower maternal mortality and should be considered given the extremely high maternal and fetal mortality associated with viral HF. However, this procedure must be performed with extreme caution, since it can be considered high-risk with regard to potential nosocomial transmission and may also induce additional maternal haemorrhage.

Antiviral Drugs

Ribavirin. The only currently available antiviral drug for any viral HF is the guanosine analogue ribavirin. Data from the few randomized controlled clinical trials that have been performed combined with empiric observation and anecdotal evidence suggest that ribavirin is efficacious in the treatment of Lassa fever, the South American HFs and HF with renal syndrome.[20] Treatment as early as possible in the course of the diseases is imperative. The mechanism of action is unknown, although lethal mutagenesis is suspected. Although frequently given, more data are needed to make conclusions on ribavirin's efficacy for Crimean-Congo HF. In vitro data show activity against Omsk HF virus as well, but clinical studies have not been performed. Ribavirin is not efficacious and should not be used for Ebola or Marburg HF.

The standard dosing schedule of ribavirin for viral HF is presented in Table 16.5, although pharmacokinetic and pharmacodynamic experiments in relation to each HF virus have not been performed. Although few data are available oral ribavirin may also be effective in some cases, but less so than the intravenous (IV) form, most likely because, with a first-pass metabolism of 50%, the serum concentration achieved through oral administration is on the borderline of the mean inhibitory

TABLE 16.5 Ribavirin Therapy for Viral Haemorrhagic Fever

Indication	Route	Dose	Interval
Treatment	IV[a]	30 mg/kg (max. 2 g)[b]	Loading dose, followed by:
	IV[a]	15 mg/kg (max. 1 g)[b]	Every 6 hours for 4 days, followed by:
	IV[a]	7.5 mg/kg (max. 500 mg)[b]	Every 8 hours for 6 days
Prophylaxis	PO	35 mg/kg (max. 2.5 g)[b]	Loading dose, followed by:
	PO	15 mg/kg (max. 1 g)[b]	Every 8 hours for 10 days

IV, intravenous; PO, oral administration.
[a]The drug should be diluted in 150 mL of 0.9% saline and infused slowly.
[b]Reduce the dose in persons known to have significant renal insufficiency (creatinine clearance of less than 50 mL/min).

concentration of ribavirin for many HF viruses.[21] Furthermore, absorption of oral ribavirin from the gut may also pose a barrier given the vomiting and diarrhoea often present in viral HF. Until more data are available on the efficacy of the oral route, the entire treatment course of ribavirin should be administered IV when possible.

Major adverse effects due to short-term ribavirin therapy are rare.[21,22] The main side-effect is a dose-dependent, mild-to-moderate haemolytic anaemia that infrequently necessitates transfusion and disappears with cessation of treatment. Rigors may occur when ribavirin is infused too rapidly. Relative contraindications include severe anaemia or haemoglobinopathy, coronary artery disease, renal insufficiency, decompensated liver disease, breast-feeding and known hypersensitivity. Jaundice may develop in patients with Gilbert's syndrome. Although findings of teratogenicity and fetal loss in laboratory animals have rendered ribavirin technically contraindicated in pregnancy, its use must still be considered as a life-saving measure given the extremely high maternal and fetal mortality associated with viral HF in pregnancy.

Haemoglobin, haematocrit and bilirubin levels should be checked at initiation of ribavirin therapy and then every few days, with consideration of transfusion of packed red blood cells if significant anaemia develops. Because of the long terminal half-life (~24 hours) and large volume of distribution, ribavirin may still have effect for hours or even days after cessation, particularly in red blood cells where it accumulates.

Patent issues and high cost (up to US$1000/patient from most pharmaceutical sources in Europe and North America) have historically severely limited availability of IV ribavirin. However, the patent is now expired and the World Health Organization has applied to add the drug to the list of essential medicines, which will hopefully significantly lower cost and improve availability. Meanwhile, many countries in Africa import the drug from less-expensive makers in China and Russia.

Other Antiviral Drugs. A number of experimental therapies for viral HFs have shown in vitro activity and, in some cases, therapeutic benefit in animal studies, including nucleoside analogues, inhibitors of S-adenosyl-l-homocysteine hydrolase, small inhibitory RNAs, phosphorodiamidate morpholino oligomers, antisense compounds, tyrosine kinase inhibitors and various other small molecules. None are yet approved or available for clinical use in humans.[16,23]

Antibody Therapy

Although cellular immunity is thought to be the primary arm of protection in most viral HFs, treatment with convalescent immune plasma has often been tried. With the exception of Argentine HF, for which efficacy is clear, there are few controlled trials or objective data on its benefit. Furthermore, there are significant logistical challenges inherent in the use of convalescent immune plasma, including risk of concomitant transmission of other blood-borne pathogens and lack of an existing bank of immune plasma for this purpose. With the exception of treatment of Argentine HF, this therapy should be reserved for severe and refractory cases when ribavirin is not an option, either because it is not available or because the patient has a viral HF for which ribavirin is not efficacious. Numerous mono- and polyclonal antibody preparations for the viral HFs have been tested in animal models over the years, with varying degrees of success.

Immune Modulators

Increasing understanding of the systemic inflammatory response syndrome underlying septic shock and by extension viral HF, has renewed interest in the use of immune modulating drugs for these syndromes. However, trials of various immune modulators in septic shock, including ibuprofen, corticosteroids, anti-TNFα, nitric oxide inhibitors, statins (HMG-CoA reductase inhibitors) and interleukins have not shown conclusive benefit. Ribavirin combined with interferon (IFN)-αcon-1, a consensus IFN, diminished mortality and disease severity in a hamster arenavirus model.[24] Although approved for clinical use in humans, IFN-αcon-1 has not been tested in human viral HF, perhaps in part due to its high cost, systemic toxicity and need for repeated doses. These problems can potentially be overcome through the delivery of a recombinant, replication-deficient type 5 human adenovirus that encodes and elicits the production of IFN-αcon-1 from infected cells. Other immunomodulating approaches being explored include those that enhance immune recognition of infected cells and dampen immune responses through the blockage of toll-like receptors. Corticosteroids should not be administered in viral HF unless adrenal insufficiency is demonstrated, target blood pressure is not maintained despite adequate fluid repletion and vasopressors, or in conjunction with mannitol if cerebral oedema is suspected.

Coagulation Modulators

A growing body of literature suggests that disturbances in the procoagulant–anticoagulant balance play an important role in the mediation of septic shock. Although controversial, recombinant activated protein C, a serine protease that plays a central role in anticoagulation, may be efficacious for some patients with septic shock. Nevertheless, the drug should still be considered experimental for viral HF.[25] At first glance, the major adverse effect of activated protein C – serious bleeding (including intracranial haemorrhage) that has been reported in up to 5% of treated patients – would seem to contraindicate its use in viral HF. However, the mechanism of the drug may not be via direct anticoagulation, but rather through modulation of inflammation. Conceivably, early use could mitigate the pathogenic processes in viral HF that ultimately result in haemorrhage with no additional risk of bleeding due to the drug itself. Other coagulation-modifying drugs that have been explored anecdotally in human cases or in animal models for the viral HFs, with varying degrees of efficacy, include rNAPc2, a potent experimental recombinant inhibitor of the tissue factor/factor VIIa coagulation pathway, recombinant factor VIIa itself (paradoxically, since it would have the opposite effect of rNAPc2), heparin sulphate and antithrombin III. All must presently be considered experimental.

Management of Convalescence

Since the clinical status of patients with viral HF generally correlates with the level of viraemia and infectivity, patients who have recovered from their acute illness can safely be assumed to have cleared their viraemia and can be discharged from the hospital without concern of subsequent transmission at home. However, because of potential delayed virus clearance in the urine and semen, abstinence or condom use is recommended for 3 months after acute illness. Transmission through toilet facilities has not been noted. Nevertheless, simple precautions to avoid contact with excretions in this setting are prudent, including separate toilet facilities and regular hand-washing. Breast-feeding should be avoided during convalescence unless there is no other way to support the baby. Clinical management during convalescence includes the use of warm packs, acetaminophen, non-steroidal anti-inflammatory drugs, cosmetics, hair-growth stimulants, anxiolytics, antidepressants, nutritional supplements and nutritional and psychological counselling as indicated.

PREVENTION

Patient Isolation, Personal Protective Equipment and Nursing Precautions

Infection control of HF viruses relies on classic public health principles of identification and isolation of infected persons. Given the difficulty of clinical diagnosis, all patients with a syndrome clinically compatible with a viral HF should be presumed infectious and isolated until a specific diagnosis is made. It is prudent to place the patient in a negative airflow room when available despite the lack of evidence for natural aerosol transmission between humans. Hermetically sealed isolation chambers are not required and may have profound negative psychological effects on the patient. Although specific viral HF isolation precautions (consisting of surgical mask, double gloves, gown, protective apron, face shield and shoe covers) to prevent contact and droplet exposure to blood and bodily fluids are advised for added security, experience has shown that routine universal precautions are protective in most cases (Figure 16.5).[26] Access to the patient should be limited to a small number of designated staff and family members with specific instructions and training on viral HF infection control guidelines and the use of personal protective equipment. Use of sharps should be minimized and immediate disposal in a sharps box strictly enforced. If the patient is being seen in a facility where mosquito bites are likely, such as the open air wards common in developing countries, insecticide-treated bed nets and/or room screens should be employed to prevent transmission of arthropod-borne HF viruses.

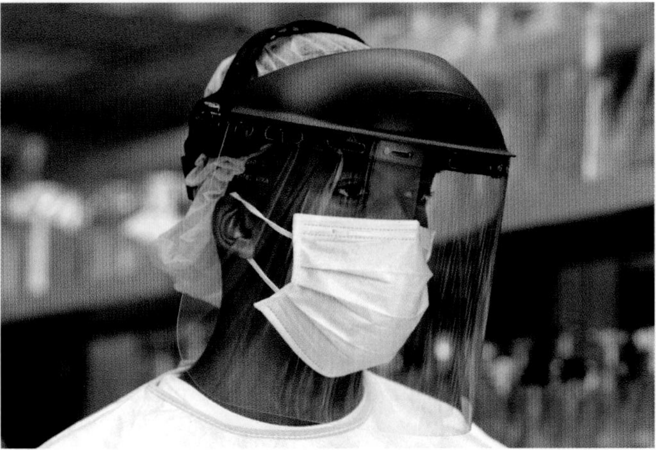

Figure 16.5 Personal protective equipment for the management of viral haemorrhagic fever. Relative to goggles, face shields have the benefits of less fogging, greater protection of the mucus membranes and a better view of the healthcare worker's face, facilitating communication with the patient.

Contact Tracing

Persons with unprotected direct contact with someone during the symptomatic phase of a human-to-human communicable HF virus should be monitored daily for evidence of disease for the duration of the longest possible incubation period starting after their last contact (Table 16.2). Contacts should check their temperature daily and record the results in a log. Despite the lack of evidence for transmission during the incubation period, it is usually recommended that exposed persons remain at home during this time and avoid close contact or activities with household members that might result in exposure to bodily fluids, such as sex, kissing and sharing of utensils. Hospitalization or other confinement of asymptomatic persons is not warranted, but persons who develop fever or other signs and symptoms suggestive of viral HF should be immediately isolated until the diagnosis can be ruled out.

Post-exposure Prophylaxis

Although oral ribavirin has been used as post-exposure prophylaxis for various viral HFs, there are no data on efficacy, dose or duration of administration of the drug for this purpose.[21] Adverse events reported with oral ribavirin, which include nausea, vomiting, dry mouth and metallic taste, myalgia, fatigue, diarrhoea, abdominal pain, headache, jaundice, skin rash, tachycardia, anaemia, thrombocytosis and neurological perturbations (including mood and sleep disturbances), can be mistaken for the early manifestations of viral HF, causing considerable emotional stress and confusion.[22]

Given the lack of efficacy data, generally low secondary attack rates for the HF viruses and the risk of adverse effects, post-exposure ribavirin should be reserved for definitive high-risk exposure to arenaviruses, Crimean-Congo HF virus or Old World hantaviruses, defined as one of the following: (1) Penetration of skin by a contaminated sharp instrument (e.g. needle stick injury); (2) Exposure of mucous membranes or broken skin to blood or bodily secretions (e.g. blood splashing in the eyes or mouth); (3) Participation in emergency procedures without appropriate personal protective equipment (e.g. resuscitation after cardiac arrest, intubation or suctioning) and (4) Prolonged (i.e. hours) and continuous contact in an enclosed space without appropriate personal protective equipment (e.g. a healthcare worker accompanying a patient during medical evacuation in a small airplane).[21] In estimating the risk of infection, clinicians should realize that the most infectious patients are those with severe clinical conditions, usually late in the course of illness. Prophylaxis should not be used when the only exposure was during the incubation period or during convalescence after fever has subsided.

Oral ribavirin should be started immediately after the exposure, but not before counselling between the patient and the physician. Because of the high first-pass metabolism of oral ribavirin, relatively high doses are needed to provide serum levels in the range of the minimum inhibitory concentration of most HF viruses (Table 16.5). The drug should be taken with food. A baseline haemoglobin and haematocrit should be drawn and therapy reconsidered if significant anaemia is present. The patient should be informed that minor adverse effects often occur. If not already performed, the index case should be tested for viral HF, with cessation of ribavirin if the results are negative. Persons taking prophylaxis who develop manifestations of viral HF should also be immediately laboratory tested by the most rapid and sensitive method, usually RT-PCR and converted to IV ribavirin unless the disease can be readily excluded.

Environmental Shedding and Disinfection

The lipid envelope of all HF viruses is relatively easily disrupted, generally limiting virus viability outside a living host.[1] When shed naturally in animal excreta or human body fluids, which would then dry, infectivity appears to be on the order of hours to days, varying with the specific virus and environmental conditions. However, HF viruses have been isolated from samples kept for weeks at ambient temperatures if stored hydrated in a biological buffer, such as blood or serum. Little concern is required regarding HF viruses seeping into ground-water or posing any long-term risk through casual exposures in the general environment, where harsh thermal and pH conditions would likely readily inactivate them.

When contamination may have recently occurred, such as in homes or hospitals treating persons with viral HF, disinfection is warranted. HF viruses can be inactivated by exposure to temperatures above 60°C for 1 hour, gamma irradiation, ultraviolet light (surface disinfection only) and by a wide variety of chemical treatments. Sodium hypochlorite (i.e. household bleach) is the most readily available effective inactivation method, although it is corrosive with repeated use.[26] Bleach solutions should be prepared daily; starting with the usual 5% chlorine concentration, a 1:100 (1%) solution should be used for reusable items such as medical equipment, patient bedding and reusable protective clothing before laundering. A 1:10 (10%) bleach solution should be used to disinfect excreta, corpses and items to be discarded. Workers cleaning areas potentially contaminated by the excreta of small mammals should wear protective materials (gloves and surgical mask) let the area aerate before entering, then spray the area with the 10% bleach solution and let it sit on the surface for at least 15 minutes before mopping or wet sweeping. A site with appropriate security should be dedicated for waste disposal if routine autoclaving is not available. Specific guidelines exist regarding handling and burial of corpses of victims of viral HF.

Vaccines and Reservoir and Vector Control

See individual disease sections for details.

Filovirus Diseases: Ebola and Marburg Haemorrhagic Fevers

The filovirus infections (from the Latin *filo* for 'thread', referring to their filamentous shape), Marburg and Ebola HFs, are perhaps the most severe and feared of all viral HFs. The Filoviridae are comprised of six species of *Ebolavirus* and one *Marburgvirus*, with relatively consistent case fatality ratios associated with each virus (Table 16.1). Although the Marburg genus is limited to a single species, Lake Victoria Marburg virus, numerous strains have been recognized, with possible differences in virulence. All of the known human pathogenic Filoviruses are endemic only in sub-Saharan Africa (Figure 16.1).

EPIDEMIOLOGY

Recent evidence strongly implicates fruit bats as the filovirus reservoir, with human infection likely from inadvertent exposure to infected bat excreta or saliva.[27–30] Miners, spelunkers, forestry workers and others with exposure in environments where bats typically roost are at risk. The association between exposure in caves and mines and *Marburgvirus* infection is particular strong.[31,32] Non-human primates, especially gorillas and chimpanzees and other wild animals may become infected and serve as intermediate hosts that transmit filoviruses to humans through contact with their blood and bodily fluids, usually associated with hunting and butchering.[33,34] These wild animals are presumably also infected by exposure to bats and develop severe and usually fatal disease similar to human viral HF.[35] *Zaire ebolavirus* has caused large die-offs of central chimpanzees and western lowland gorillas in central Africa.[36] Filovirus outbreaks tend to occur at the end of the rainy season.

Filoviruses are probably the most transmissible of all HF viruses, although attack rates are still generally only 15–20% in outbreaks in Africa and much lower if proper universal precautions are maintained.[37] In most outbreaks it appears that there is a single or very few introductions from a zoonotic source into humans followed by nosocomial amplification in a setting of inadequate universal precautions, usually in rural areas of countries where civil unrest has decimated the healthcare infrastructure (Figure 16.1). The largest outbreak of Ebola HF to date was 425 cases in Uganda in 2000–2001 and, of Marburg HF, 252 cases in Angola in 2004–2005. Filovirus outbreaks appear to be occurring more frequently since the mid-1990s, perhaps reflecting societal changes in Africa where healthcare seeking at hospitals, which may sometimes lack appropriate infection control measures, becomes more frequent. Enhanced surveillance for viral HF may also play a role.

PATHOGENESIS AND PATHOLOGY

After initial infection through an as yet unknown receptor, filoviruses disseminate to virtually all organs, causing widespread but focal tissue damage.[8,38] Necrosis is greatest in the liver, spleen, kidney and gonads and is associated with high levels of virus or viral antigen in these organs, suggesting a direct viral-induced effect. Hepatocellular necrosis, Councilman bodies, microvesicular fatty change and Kupffer cell hyperplasia are typically seen in the liver and extensive follicular necrosis and necrotic debris in the spleen and lymph nodes. Diffuse alveolar damage, interstitial oedema and focal haemorrhage may be seen in the lung and myocardial oedema and focal necrosis in the heart. Filovirus antigen can be found in the skin and sweat glands by immunohistochemistry, but the implications of this finding with regard to the potential for virus transmission through skin contact are uncertain.

Pro-inflammatory cytokines, including TNFα and various interleukins, are thought to play a central role in the pathogenesis of filovirus infection, with high levels of IL-10 and IL-1 receptor antagonist correlating with a poor prognosis, as well as neopterin, a marker of cellular immune system activation.[39] This pro-inflammatory state is facilitated by virus-induced suppression of the host adaptive immune response, including the actions of IFN and antiviral RNA interference, by various filovirus proteins, including a secreted glycoprotein. DIC is frequently noted.

CLINICAL FEATURES

Although mild or even asymptomatic cases have been reported, the vast majority of filovirus infections are thought to result in

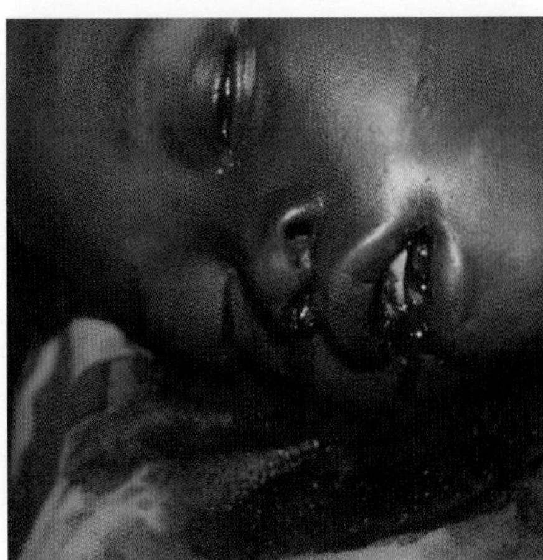

Figure 16.6 Oral bleeding in Ebola haemorrhagic fever. *(From Bausch DG. Viral Hemorrhagic Fevers. In: Schlossberg D, editor. Clinical Infectious Disease. New York, NY: Cambridge University Press; 2008. Used with permission. Photo by D. Bausch.)*

severe disease.[40–42] A fleeting maculopapular rash on the torso or face may be one early and relatively specific, although insensitive, indicator of infection. Abdominal tenderness over the liver is frequently seen and may represent stretching of the liver capsule. External bleeding, especially from the gastrointestinal tract, may be profuse and most fatal cases will manifest oozing from the mucus membranes and skin puncture sites in the late stages (Figures 16.6 and 16.7). Central nervous system manifestations and renal failure are also frequent in end-stage disease. In one unusual case, uveitis with isolation of *Ebolavirus* from the eye was noted 2 months after resolution of acute viral HF.[10]

DIAGNOSIS

Contact with bats or non-human primates and entry into mines, caves or forests in sub-Saharan Africa should enhance suspicion. Advances have been made in recent decades to establish mobile field laboratories that can provide ELISA or PCR-based diagnostics at or near the site of outbreaks.[43,44]

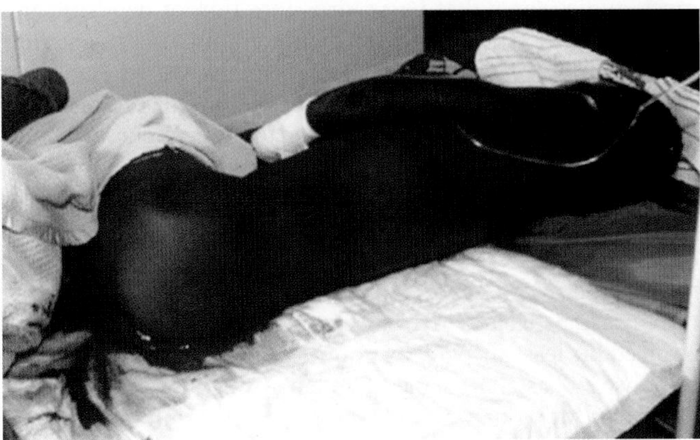

Figure 16.7 Rectal bleeding in Ebola haemorrhagic fever. *(From Bausch DG. Viral Hemorrhagic Fevers. In: Schlossberg D, editor. Clinical Infectious Disease. New York, NY: Cambridge University Press; 2008. Used with permission. Photo by D. Bausch.)*

MANAGEMENT AND TREATMENT

There is presently no specific antiviral therapy for filovirus infection.[45] Nor has the use of convalescent plasma shown convincing efficacy; although 8 of 10 persons treated with convalescent plasma during an Ebola HF outbreak in the Democratic Republic of the Congo survived, in most cases treatment started after the mean time to death for this disease, indicating that the patients were likely to survive anyway.[46] Human-mouse chimeric monoclonal antibodies have recently shown efficacy in animal models of Ebola HF.[47,48] Activated protein C reduces mortality in *Ebolavirus*-infected monkeys but has not been tried in humans with Ebola HF.[49] *Ebolavirus* induces overexpression of the procoagulant tissue factor in nonhuman primate monocytes/macrophages, suggesting that inhibition of the tissue factor pathway could ameliorate filovirus infection. Accordingly, rNAPc2 decreased mortality by 67% in *Ebolavirus*-infected monkeys.[50] A Phase I trial of the drug in humans was recently completed with no safety concerns arising.[51]

PREVENTION

Post-exposure Prophylaxis. Although no post-exposure prophylaxis is available for filovirus infection, a live recombinant vesicular stomatitis virus vector engineered to express the key immunogenic proteins of *Ebolavirus* was administered on a compassionate use basis to a laboratory worker after a needle stick injury, with no apparent detrimental effect.[52] Efficacy could not be assessed because it was not clear that the accident resulted in *Ebolavirus* infection. rNAPc2, small interfering RNAs and monoclonal antibodies have also shown efficacy as post-exposure prophylactics in monkey models.[45,53–55]

Vaccines

A number of experimental approaches for filovirus infection have shown promise;[56] the aforementioned vesicular stomatitis virus vectored vaccine for viral HFs has shown protective immunity in animal models. In addition, a DNA plasmid vaccine for Ebola HF has been shown to be safe and immunogenic in a Phase I trial.[57,58]

Reservoir Control

Avoiding contact with bats, primarily by avoiding entry into caves and mines in endemic areas, is a key prevention measure for the filoviruses. Personal protective equipment may be indicated for miners and other persons who work in these environments. Humans should also avoid exposure to fresh blood, bodily fluids or meat of wild animals, especially non-human primates, in filovirus-endemic areas.

Old World Arenavirus Diseases: Lassa Fever and Lujo Haemorrhagic Fever

Lassa and Lujo viruses are members of the Arenaviridae family, which derives its name from the Latin *arenosus* for 'sandy', referring to the grainy appearance of internal electron-dense particles seen on electron microscopy. Arenaviridae are serologically, phylogenetically and geographically divided into Old World (i.e. Africa) and New World (i.e. the Americas) complexes (Figures 16.2 and 16.3).[59] Although almost 15 Old World arenaviruses have been recognized only two, Lassa and Lujo viruses, have been associated with viral HF.

Lassa virus was first isolated from Nigeria in 1969 and named after the town from which the first case came. Lassa fever is endemic exclusively in West Africa (Figure 16.2).[60] The risk of exposure to Lassa virus varies significantly in a given country and often among regions or even villages within endemic areas. The highest incidence of disease appears to be in areas of eastern Sierra Leone, northern Liberia, south-eastern Guinea and central and southern Nigeria.[61] The reasons for the extreme heterogeneity in incidence across West Africa are not clear, especially considering that the rodent reservoir is often readily found in areas where little or no human Lassa fever has been recognized. Varied intensity of surveillance may contribute to the heterogeneous distribution but cannot completely explain it.

An annual incidence of 300 000–500 000 Lassa virus infections with up to 5000 deaths is often quoted in the scientific literature but these figures are extrapolations from surveillance in the 1970s and 1980s in eastern Sierra Leone where Lassa fever is clearly hyperendemic. Estimating the true incidence and mortality is challenging due to the nonspecific clinical presentation and the civil unrest, unstable governments with underdeveloped surveillance systems, extensive human migration and perturbation of the physical landscape and paucity of laboratories with the capacity to perform the diagnosis in West Africa. The incidence of Lassa fever is consistently highest during the dry season, although cases may be seen throughout the year.

Lujo virus was first identified in 2008 after an outbreak of five cases (four fatal).[15,62] The first case was infected in Zambia and subsequently medically evacuated to Johannesburg, initiating a chain of four nosocomial infections in South Africa (Figure 16.2). The disease has not been seen since.

EPIDEMIOLOGY

Arenaviruses causing viral HF are maintained by chronic infection of rodents with a tight reservoir species-virus pairing, thought to be the result of long-term rodent-virus co-evolution.[1] Rodent populations are usually not uniformly infected across their entire geographic range. There are generally few human cases relative to the frequency of infected rodents. The reservoir for Lassa virus is *Mastomys natalensis*, commonly called the 'multimammate rat', which is almost always found in close association with humans in rural villages and surrounding cultivated fields and, less commonly, in grasslands and at the forest edge.[63] Consumption of rodents and poor-quality housing, which may allow rodents easy entry, have been shown to be risk factors for Lassa fever. Foreign military personnel, peacekeepers and aid workers in rural settings are occasionally infected, sometimes importing Lassa virus back to their countries of origin.[64] Multimammate rats are not typically found in large urban centres, so the risk of rodent transmission of Lassa virus to humans in these environments is negligible. Despite the occurrence of *Mastomys* species throughout sub-Saharan Africa, Lassa virus has not been found outside of West Africa. The reasons for this are unclear, but may relate to evolutionary bottlenecks in dispersal of the virus, reservoir or both. On rare occasions, Lassa virus has been isolated from other rodent species, a finding which is usually considered to be due to spillover infection (i.e. incidental transient infection of a non-reservoir host) or difficulty identifying the rodent species. These animals are not thought to play a role in Lassa virus maintenance.

Transmission of Lassa virus to humans occurs via exposure to rodent excreta, either from direct inoculation to the mucous membranes or from inhalation of aerosols produced when rodents urinate.[1] The relative frequency of these modes of transmission is unknown. Experimental data illustrate that arenavirus infection may also occur by the oral route. Lassa virus may also be contracted when rodents are trapped and prepared for consumption, a common practice in some parts of West Africa. Since HF viruses are easily inactivated by heating, eating cooked rodent meat should pose no danger.[1] It is not known whether Lassa virus can be transmitted through a rodent bite, although the virus has been found in rodent saliva. Transmission of Lassa virus through aerosolized rodent urine or virus-contaminated dust particles is often referred to in the scientific literature, but there are few data to support or refute this mode of transmission. The reservoir for Lujo virus is unknown, but is presumed to be a rodent.

PATHOGENESIS AND PATHOLOGY

The pathogenesis of arenaviral HF is thought to relate more to disruption of cellular function, as opposed to extensive cell death; patients often die without significant bleeding and histopathological lesions (on the few cases in which autopsies have been performed) are usually not severe enough to account for death. Lassa virus can be found in virtually all organs, which is not surprising considering that one of the primary receptors, α-dystroglycan, is expressed on most tissues. The liver is usually the most affected organ, which is consistent with the finding of elevated hepatic transaminases in severe cases. The lowest titres are in the central nervous system, presumably due to protection afforded by the blood–brain barrier. Infection of mesothelial cells can explain the serous effusions sometimes seen in Lassa fever. Lassa virus infection of hormone-secreting cells may relate to the more severe pathophysiology of the disease noted in pregnant women. Gross pathological findings include pulmonary oedema, pleural effusion, ascites and haemorrhage from the gastrointestinal mucosa. Microscopic lesions include hepatocellular and splenic necrosis, renal tubular injury with interstitial nephritis, interstitial pneumonitis and myocarditis.

Although the data are mixed, severe Lassa fever appears to result from an insufficient or suppressed immune response[65]; most studies show that Lassa virus infection of dendritic and peripheral blood mononuclear cells does not result in significant secretion of proinflammatory cytokines, upregulation of costimulatory molecules or significant T-cell proliferation. Absent or diminished inflammatory cytokine responses (including TNFα, IL-8 and IFN IP-10) are often noted in both in vitro and in vivo experiments and have been correlated with a poor outcome in humans. In contrast, early and strong cytokine and cellular immune responses correlated with survival in monkey models and in case reports on humans. The lack of an immune response may reflect active Lassa virus-induced downregulation induced, at least in part, by counter-action of the type I IFN response by Lassa virus. Based on data from guinea pig models, cardiac inotropy may be directly or indirectly inhibited from a yet-to-be-identified soluble mediator in the serum. Disseminated intravascular coagulopathy does not appear to be part of the pathogenesis of Lassa fever, although this finding bears confirmation.

There is considerable sequence heterogeneity of Lassa viruses across West Africa, with four recognized lineages: three in Nigeria and one in the area comprising Sierra Leone, Liberia, Guinea and the Ivory Coast. There is also considerable genetic heterogeneity within lineages, especially in Nigeria. Field and laboratory data suggest variation in virulence among the various lineages and strains of Lassa virus, although systematic strain classifications based on virulence have not been possible. Interestingly, strains isolated from pregnant women and infants were benign in guinea pigs, suggesting that host factors such as immunosuppression play a significant role in human disease. There is evidence that three human genes, including *LARGE*, *DMD* and *IL-21*, have undergone positive selection in populations in endemic areas for Lassa fever in Nigeria, suggesting a protective effect.[66]

Based on the few cases noted to date, the pathogenesis of Lujo HF appears to be very similar to that of Lassa fever.

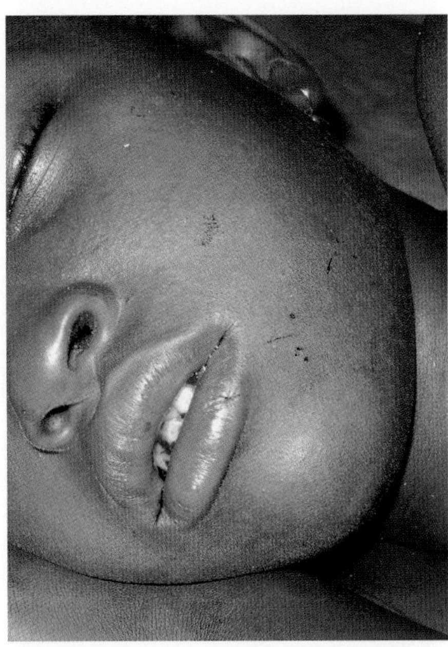

Figure 16.8 Facial swelling and mild gum bleeding in Lassa fever. *(Photo by Donald Grant.)*

CLINICAL FEATURES

A long-standing mystery of Lassa fever is the apparent extreme range of clinical severity. Up to 80% of Lassa virus infections are mild or asymptomatic, although this finding bears repeating with newer more sensitive and specific diagnostic assays. Case fatality in symptomatic persons is often in the range of 25%. The reasons for the considerable variation of clinical severity are unknown, but may relate to heterogeneity in the virulence of infecting Lassa virus strains, route and dose of inoculation, genetic predisposition, underlying co-infections and/or premorbid conditions (such as malaria, malnutrition and diabetes) or misclassification of reinfection as new infection due to waning of antibody.

Pharyngitis is common and may be particularly severe in Lassa fever, sometimes with an exudate that has led to misdiagnosis of streptococcal pharyngitis. A morbilliform or maculopapular skin rash almost always occurs in fair-skinned persons but, for unclear reasons, rarely in persons with black skin. Swelling in the face and neck and bleeding and to a lesser degree conjunctival injection, are particularly specific signs but are not very sensitive – seen in less than 20% of cases (Figures 16.8 and 16.9). Lassa fever is one of the viral HFs with the lowest likelihood of clinically discernible haemorrhage – less than 20%, most often consisting of mild epistaxis and oozing from the oral mucous membranes and, in the late stages, venepuncture sites. Central nervous system manifestations may also be seen in the late phases, with virus isolated from the cerebrospinal fluid of some but not all patients and without apparent correlation between disease severity and virus or antibody titre. The cellular and chemistry profile in cerebrospinal fluid is usually normal.

Fatal disease is occasionally seen in persons who have already cleared Lassa virus from the blood and produced a strong IgM antibody response. The pathogenesis of these unusual cases is poorly understood but may relate to persistent Lassa virus sequestered in the central nervous system, perhaps facilitated by an immunocompromised state in some patients with HIV/AIDS, severe malnutrition or diabetes. In one unusual case, Lassa virus was isolated from the CSF, but not the blood, of a patient with encephalopathy after the febrile stage of disease. Other cases with sudden deterioration after apparent stabilization may involve acute complicating events, such as pericardial tamponade.

Lassa fever is particularly severe in pregnancy, with Lassa virus found at high concentrations in placenta and fetal tissues. Anasarca has been described in a single report of children with Lassa fever (termed the 'swollen baby syndrome') but may have been related to aggressive rehydration. One instance of polyserositis with pleural and pericardial effusions and ascites 6 months after infection was reported. Lassa virus could not be recovered from the effusion fluid, but lymphocytes and high levels of antibody were noted, suggesting an immune-mediated mechanism.

Sensorineural deafness is the only recognized permanent sequela of Lassa fever. It is reported to occur in as many as 25% of cases, although this seems like a significant overestimate from our experience in West Africa over the last 15 years. Deafness typically presents during convalescence and is unassociated with the severity of the acute illness or level of viremia, suggesting an immune-mediated pathogenesis. Deafness may be uni- or bilateral and is permanent in approximately two

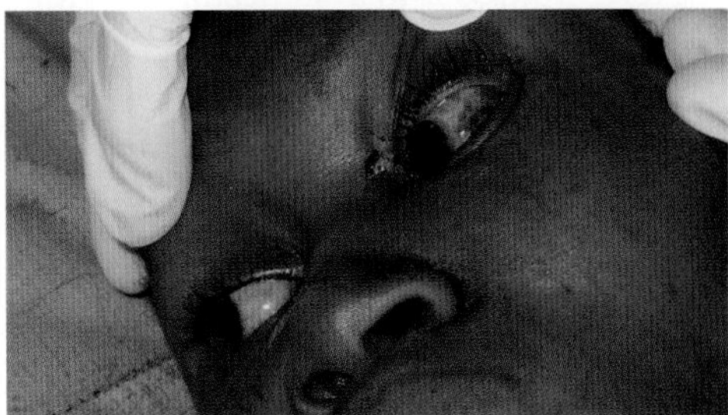

Figure 16.9 Conjunctival infection in Lassa fever. *(Photo by Donald Grant.)*

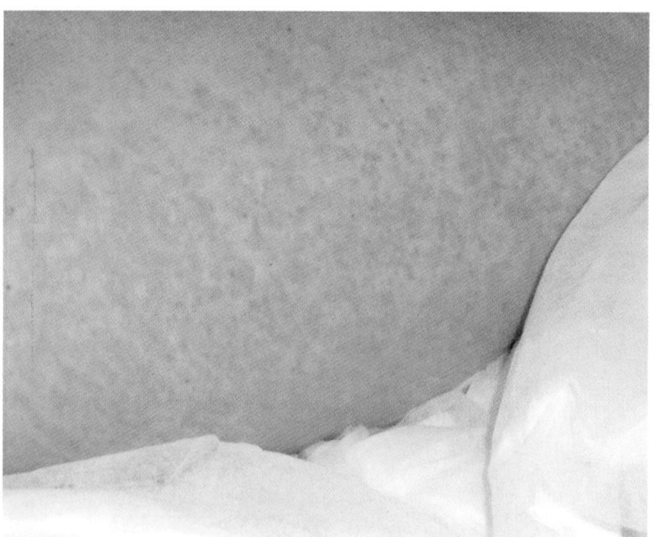

Figure 16.10 Maculopapular rash in Lujo haemorrhagic fever. *(Photo by TH Dinh.)*

thirds of cases. Auditory patterns resemble idiopathic nerve deafness.

The clinical features of Lujo HF are similar to Lassa fever. In the limited series of five cases reported to date, key features included prominent facial oedema, pharyngitis and diffuse macular rash with shock, depressed consciousness and convulsions in fatal cases (Figure 16.10). Bleeding was not a prominent feature.

DIAGNOSIS

Although ELISA has been the traditional mainstay of diagnosis, RT-PCR is becoming an increasingly valuable tool and can detect Lassa virus in over 80% in the first 10 days of illness.[67] Sequence heterogeneity of Lassa virus across West Africa has traditionally posed a challenge to PCR-based diagnostics due to primer–target mismatch but recent development of assays targeting conserved portions of the genome may have resolved this problem. Post-mortem diagnosis through immunohistochemistry does not appear to be as reliable for Lassa fever as for some of the other viral HFs, although it was helpful in the diagnosis of Lujo HF..

MANAGEMENT AND TREATMENT

Intravenous ribavirin has been shown to decrease mortality in severe Lassa fever from 55% to 5% when begun within the first 6 days of illness and should be given to all patients with this disease.[20] There is still benefit, albeit less, after 6 days. Convalescent plasma has been used in Lassa fever with apparent benefit, but is only efficacious if it contains a high titre of neutralizing antibody, which is not uniformly the case even in survivors. Furthermore, animal studies suggest that a close antigenic match between the infecting Lassa virus of the donor and recipient is required for the treatment to be effective. The infrequency of bleeding in Lassa fever relative to most other viral HFs might make it a logical candidate for trials with activated protein C. Statin drugs, which appear to have immunomodulatory, anti-inflammatory, antimicrobial and vasculature-stabilizing properties, were included in the successful treatment of a case of Lujo HF along with the antioxidant and free radical scavenger N-acetylcysteine.

PREVENTION

Post-exposure Prophylaxis

Post-exposure prophylaxis with oral ribavirin should be considered for persons with high-risk exposures following the guidelines described above.[21,22]

Vaccines

A number of experimental vaccine platforms are being explored. The recombinant vesicular stomatitis virus platform is perhaps the most promising, providing 100% protection after a single dose in a monkey model.[68]

Reservoir Control

Measures to prevent contact with rodents are important in control of Lassa fever. Since multimammate rats often colonize human dwellings, prevention is best achieved by improving 'village hygiene', including eliminating unprotected storage of garbage, foodstuffs and water and, when possible, plugging holes that allow rodents entry into homes.[1] Rodent trapping or poisoning is generally not thought to be an effective long-term control strategy because animals from surrounding fields will likely soon recolonize the area.

New World Arenavirus Diseases: South American Haemorrhagic Fevers

The New World Arenavirus Complex is divided into three major clades: A, B and C.[69] Five arenaviruses are known to cause natural infection and viral HF, all belonging to clade B. Although there may be subtle differences among the syndromes produced by these five viruses, they are usually grouped and referred to simply as the 'South American HFs'. Each virus is named after its place of first finding, with the disease name generally named after the country (Figure 16.3). Junin virus, the aetiological agent of Argentine HF, was identified in 1958 after a new disease emerged in the Argentine pampas. Annual outbreaks have been noted since then, with progressive extension of the endemic area and increase in the population at risk. Bolivian HF was first described in 1959 in Bolivia's Beni Department and the aetiological agent, Machupo virus, identified in 1964. Community outbreaks of Bolivian HF continued during the 1960s and were brought under control, in part, by rodent trapping. There were then no reported cases for decades, followed by sporadic cases and small outbreaks reported again in the 1990s and continuing through the time of this writing. An outbreak of viral HF in the Portuguesa State, Venezuela, in 1989 originally thought to be dengue HF, eventually was attributed to a new arenavirus named Guanarito. Outbreaks of Venezuelan HF have been reported every 4–5 years since then, suggesting some cyclic climatic or social influence. Sabiá virus was isolated from a fatal case of viral HF in Sao Paulo State, Brazil, in 1990. Since then, only two cases have been identified, both from laboratory infection. A second arenavirus, named Chapare, was discovered in Bolivia in 2003 after a small outbreak of viral HF near Cochabamba. Cases have not been noted since but surveillance is limited.

EPIDEMIOLOGY

Like Old World arenaviruses, New World arenaviruses are maintained in rodents and spread to humans via exposure to rodent excreta.[1,59] The reservoirs of Junin and Guanarito viruses are generally found in rural areas, often in agricultural lands. Consequently, the highest risk of Argentine and Venezuelan HFs is among agricultural workers. Incidence may vary considerably with variations in rodent population densities that may relate to both climatic changes and human-induced habitat perturbation. Although cases can be seen throughout the year, incidence is usually highest at times of peak agricultural activity: March–June in Argentina and November–January in Venezuela. The reservoir for Machupo virus is primarily a household pest. Although Bolivian HF may be seen throughout the year, incidence is usually increased during the dry season (June–August), sometimes with family and community clusters. The reservoirs for Sabiá and Chapare viruses are unknown, but are presumed to be rodents.

New World arenaviruses appear to be less transmissible between humans than their Old World counterparts, although human-to-human transmission of Machupo virus has been reported in both community and nosocomial settings. Only one family cluster of Argentine HF is described, with the index case presenting with atypical skin lesions that may have facilitated transmission.

CLINICAL FEATURES

The clinical syndrome of South American HF is generally similar to that of the Old World arenaviruses, although bleeding and central nervous system manifestations are thought to occur more frequently, especially in Argentine HF. Characteristic signs and symptoms included flushing of the face, neck and upper chest; enanthem over the soft palate with petechiae and small vesicles; gum bleeding; petechiae in the axillae, upper chest and arms; enlarged cervical lymph nodes; fine tremor of the hands and tongue; moderate ataxia; cutaneous hyperesthesia; and decreased deep tendon reflexes and muscle tone (Figures 16.11 and 16.12). Sore throat is frequently reported in Venezuelan HF.

PATHOGENESIS AND PATHOLOGY

The pathogenesis of the New World arenavirus infection is thought to be similar to that of their Old World counterparts. A notable exception is the increased frequency of bleeding in South American HF. An acute transitory immunodeficiency after illness has also been noted.

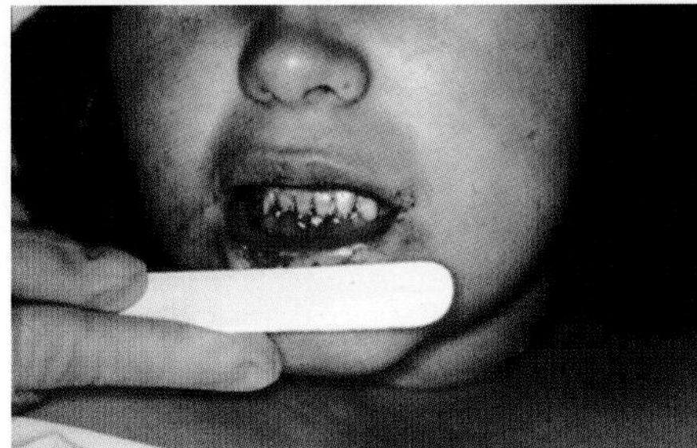

Figure 16.11 Gum bleeding in Argentine haemorrhagic fever.

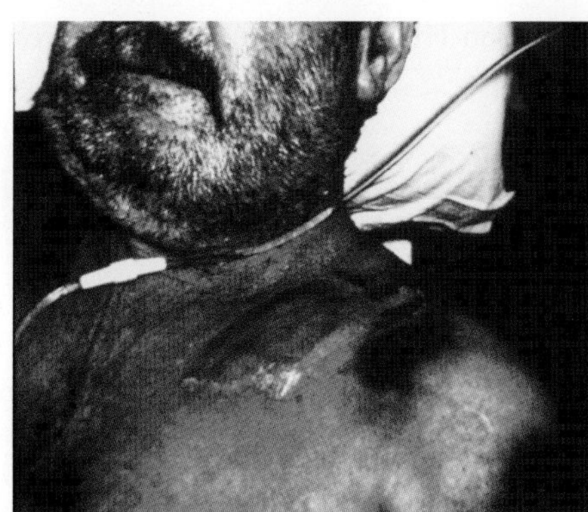

Figure 16.12 Petechial rash in Argentine haemorrhagic fever.

DIAGNOSIS

South American HF should be suspected in persons with a compatible clinical syndrome in endemic areas, especially in those with rural agricultural exposures. Laboratory diagnostic assays employed are similar to those used for the other arenaviruses.

MANAGEMENT AND TREATMENT

Transfusion of appropriately titred immune plasma within the first 8 days of illness reduces the mortality of Argentine HF from 15–30% to less than 1%.[70] Treatment after this time is not effective. However, this therapy has been associated with a convalescent-phase neurologic syndrome characterized by fever, cerebellar signs and cranial nerve palsies in 10% of those treated. Ribavirin appears to be efficacious in the treatment of the South American HFs although randomized trials have not been performed.

PREVENTION

Post-exposure Prophylaxis

Immune plasma is indicated as post-exposure prophylaxis for high-risk exposures to Junin virus, substituting oral ribavirin following the guidelines described above when immune plasma is not available or when the exposure was to one of the other New World arenaviruses.[21,70]

Vaccine

A live attenuated vaccine called Candid No.1 decreases the morbidity and mortality of Argentine HF and may also protect against Bolivian HF, although it does not appear to cross-protect against other arenaviruses.[71] The vaccine is generally not available or approved, however, outside of Argentina and even within Argentina supplies are insufficient to cover the population at risk.

Reservoir Control

Trapping and other rodent control measures in and around houses have contributed to stemming epidemics of Bolivian HF in villages. This approach is not feasible for control of Argentine

HF and Venezuelan HF, however, for which the reservoirs are widespread in fields.[1]

Bunyavirus Diseases: Haemorrhagic Fever with Renal Syndrome and Hantavirus Pulmonary Syndrome

Hantaviruses comprise a genus of the Bunyaviridae family.[59,72] Over 20 pathogenic hantaviruses are currently recognized (Table 16.6). Hantaviruses are taxonomically and clinically divided into Old World (i.e. Asia, Europe and Africa) and New World (i.e. the Americas) groups akin to the Arenaviruses described above. One Old World *Hantavirus*, Seoul, is now found virtually worldwide because its reservoir, the common Norway rat, has spread globally through transport on ships.

EPIDEMIOLOGY

Hantaviruses have been identified on every continent except Antarctica. The pathogenic hantaviruses are maintained in rodents, again with a tight reservoir–virus pairing like arenaviruses (Table 16.6). Transmission between rodents is horizontal through biting. Transmission to humans is through exposure to infected excreta. With the exception of Seoul virus, for which the rodent host is common in urban settings, Hantavirus reservoirs are rural rodents and disease is highest in persons exposed in rural areas, usually during outdoor occupational or recreational activities. Prevalence of exposure in humans varies greatly from region to region, from zero (0) to as high as 40% among some rural indigenous populations in South America. Although there appears to be a relationship between outbreaks in humans, rodent population density, proportion of infected rodents and climatic factors, such as El Niño effects, the precise nature of the relationship is complex and remains to be fully elucidated. Person-to-person transmission has been documented only for Andes virus, a New World hantavirus found in South America (Tables 16.1 and 16.6).

CLINICAL FEATURES

Hantaviruses have the longest incubation periods of any of the viral HFs, ranging up to 7 weeks, although 2–4 weeks is typical. Two distinct syndromes are recognized: Old World hantaviruses cause HF with renal syndrome, a term coined in 1983 to integrate various previously recognized febrile syndromes entailing haemostatic and renal disturbances, including 'Korean HF', 'nephropathia epidemica' and others. New World hantaviruses cause HPS, a disease first recognized in the USA in 1993 and across the Americas since. While these clinical distinctions generally hold true, elements of both syndromes may occasionally be seen and the pathogenicity and degree to which the classic syndromes manifest themselves may vary considerably depending upon the specific infecting virus.

TABLE 16.6 Hantaviruses Known to be Human Pathogens

Hantavirus	Reservoir Common Name (Scientific Name)	Disease	Geographic Distribution
Old World Viruses			
Amur	Korean field mouse (*Apodemus peninsulae*)	HFRS	Far eastern Russia
Dobrava-Belgrade	Yellow-necked field mouse (*Apodemus flavicollis*)	HFRS	Balkans, European Russia
Hantaan	Striped field mouse (*Apodemus agrarius*)	HFRS	China, Korea, Russia
Puumala	Bank vole (*Myodes glareolus*)	HFRS	Europe, European Russia
Saaremaa	Striped field mouse (*Apodemus agrarius*)	HFRS	Northern Europe
Seoul	Norway or Brown rat (*Rattus norvegicus*)	HFRS	Worldwide
New World Viruses			
Anajatuba	Fornes colilargo (*Oligoryzomys fornesi*)	HPS	Northern Brazil
Andes	Long-tailed colilargo (*Oligoryzomys longicaudatus*)	HPS	Southwestern Argentina, Chile
Araraquara	Hoary-tailed akodont (*Bolomys lasiurus*)	HPS	Southern Brazil
Bayou	Marsh oryzomys (*Oryzomys palustris*)	HPS	Southeastern United States
Bermejo	Chacoan colilargo (*Oligoryzomys chacoensis*)	HPS	Northern Argentina, southern Bolivia
Black Creek Canal	Hispid cotton rat (*Sigmodon hispidus*)	HPS	Southeastern United States (Florida)
Castelo dos Sonhos	Brazilian pygmy rice rat (*Oligoryzomys utiaritensis*)	HPS	Central Brazil
Central Plata	Yellow Pygmy rice rat or Flavescent colilargo (*Oligoryzomys flavescens*)	HPS	Uruguay
Choclo	Fulvous colilargo (*Oligoryzomys fulvescens*)	HPS	Panamá
Hu39694	Yellow Pygmy rice rat or Flavescent colilargo (*Oligoryzomys flavescens*)	HPS	Argentina
Juquitiba	Black-footed Pygmy rice rat or Black-footed colilargo (*Oligoryzomys nigripes*)	HPS	Southeastern Brazil
Laguna Negra	Little laucha or small vesper mouse (*Calomys laucha*)	HPS	Paraguay, Bolivia
Lechiguanas	Yellow Pygmy rice rat or Flavescent colilargo (*Oligoryzomys flavescens*)	HPS	Central Argentina
New York	White-footed deer mouse (*Peromyscus leucopus*)	HPS	Northeastern United States
Orán	Long-tailed colilargo (*Oligoryzomys longicaudatus*)	HPS	Northwestern Argentina
Río Mamoré	Small-eared Pygmy rice rat (*Oligoryzomys microtis*)	HPS	Amazon Basin of Brazil and contiguous lowlands of Peru, Bolivia and Paraguay
Sin Nombre	North American deer mouse (*Peromyscus maniculatus*)	HPS	Canada, United States

HFRS, haemorrhagic fever with renal syndrome; HPS, hantavirus pulmonary syndrome.
Controversy exists for some viruses regarding whether they constitute distinct species and whether the rodent listed above is the definitive reservoir.

Haemorrhagic Fever with Renal Syndrome. HF with renal syndrome caused by the prototype virus, Hantaan, is classically divided into five progressive phases: prodrome, hypotension, oliguria/renal failure, diuresis and convalescence. However, in clinical practice, phases may overlap or be completely absent, especially when other viruses such as Seoul and Puumala are the culprits, in which bleeding is much less common and mortality much lower. Liver involvement is frequent in Seoul virus infection.

Disease starts with a prodrome of abrupt onset of high fever and constitutional symptoms lasting 3–7 days. The fever then begins to abate and the patient enters the hypotensive phase, often with accompanying confusion, nausea, vomiting and worsening back pain. Around 15% of patients progress to severe shock with some fatalities at this stage. Plasma extravasation usually results in haemoconcentration and urinary concentration (Table 16.4). The platelet count reaches its nadir and the WBC count increases markedly, often above 30 000/μl. Radiological exams of the abdomen may show retroperitoneal oedema and haemorrhage.

A period of oliguria and renal failure follows the hypotensive phase, with the usual complications of uraemia and electrolyte abnormalities. Although platelets begin to rise, bleeding may be troublesome during this stage. Gastrointestinal bleeding and haematuria are characteristic. Low-grade DIC is common. Fluid resorption from third spaces may lead to high-output cardiac failure and pulmonary oedema, especially if the patient is overhydrated. Dialysis is often needed. Finally, after 2–7 days of oliguria, a period of diuresis ensues, sometimes reaching several litres of daily urine output that may cause electrolyte abnormalities and dehydration.

Complications include kidney rupture, right atrial haemorrhage and arrhythmias and retroperitoneal and intracranial haemorrhage, which may cause acute and chronic abnormalities of pituitary hormone secretion if the bleeding involves the pituitary gland. A urine-concentrating defect may persist for as long as 3 months. Recovery is usually complete, although an association between hypertensive chronic renal failure and antibodies to Seoul virus has been reported.

Hantavirus Pulmonary Syndrome. HPS typically begins with the gradual onset of fever and constitutional symptoms lasting 3–5 days, sometimes with prominent gastrointestinal complaints. Pharyngitis, rhinorrhea, cough, tachypnea and rash are usually absent and may help distinguish HPS from influenza and other upper respiratory illnesses. Pulmonary symptoms then abruptly ensue, with worsening shortness of breath, tachypnea and cough, which may be productive. Arterial desaturation may be noted on oximetry or blood gas analysis. Rales are typically noted but objective signs of pulmonary oedema may still be absent. The chest X-ray may be normal, show subtle signs of increased pulmonary vascular permeability, such as peribronchial oedema and Kerley B lines or show marked alveolar infiltrates and pleural effusions. Findings may be asymmetrical.

Deterioration in the patient's pulmonary status may then rapidly occur, with progressive hypoxia culminating in severe pulmonary oedema requiring intubation in two-thirds of patients. The high degree of pulmonary capillary permeability may result in copious, highly proteinaceous endotracheal secretions, the content of which resembles serum. Impaired cardiac inotropy is a key and dangerous component of the disease. Systemic vascular resistance is typically elevated, cardiac index decreased and pulmonary wedge pressure normal or even low. The cardiogenic shock is often refractory to fluid administration, inotropic and pressure support and independent of the management of the pulmonary component of the disease, death often coming in the form of electromechanical dissociation. Severe metabolic acidosis and lactate levels above 4 mmol/L confer a poor prognosis. Bleeding signs and DIC have been reported, but are uncommon. HPS is generally a very acute disease, with most deaths occurring within 48 hours of admission. Survivors usually have no long-term sequelae.

Anecdotal observations suggest some variation in clinical manifestations depending on the specific infecting hantavirus. Persons infected with some South American hantaviruses may more commonly manifest conjunctival congestion, head and neck suffusion, haemorrhage and renal impairment, the latter especially seen with infection with *Andes* and *Lechiguanas* viruses in Argentina.

PATHOGENESIS AND PATHOBIOLOGY

The pathogenesis of hantavirus infection is thought to be similar to that of other viral HFs, with particularly severe involvement of the renal and pulmonary vasculature in HF with renal syndrome and HPS, respectively.[59] In HPS, viral antigen is primarily detected in pulmonary capillary endothelial cells. Pathological findings include serous pleural effusions and severe oedema of the lung with mild-to-moderate numbers of hyaline membranes, normal pneumocytes and, in contrast to infectious pneumonias, absence of acute inflammatory cells. Myocarditis, hepatic necrosis, renal medullary lesions and thrombosis of small vessels may be noted. In contrast to other viral HFs, the immune response may play a detrimental role in HPS, indicated by the frequent clearance of viremia prior to onset of the most severe phases of disease.

DIAGNOSIS

Hantavirus infection should be suspected in persons with a compatible clinical syndrome who are at risk of exposure to rodent excreta, especially in rural areas where hantaviruses are known to be endemic. Detection of IgM antibody by ELISA and/or nucleic acid by RT-PCR are the typical diagnostic means, with sequencing of PCR products to identify the specific infecting virus. Hantaviruses are difficult to isolate in cell culture.

MANAGEMENT AND TREATMENT

Ribavirin has been shown to reduce mortality in HF with renal syndrome if administered within 4 days of onset.[73] Two clinical trials of ribavirin for HPS were inconclusive due to limitations in the studies' design and statistical power, although the trends did not suggest benefit.[74] One problem is that the nonspecific early presentation of HPS often results in delayed diagnosis, precluding early administration of ribavirin when it might logically be assumed to be most effective. To circumvent this problem, a protocol has been approved in Argentina, where cases are often seen in clusters, for early administration of ribavirin to high-risk contacts of confirmed HPS cases who develop a febrile syndrome. The use of adjunctive steroids is also being examined in South America.

PREVENTION

Patient Isolation, Personal Protective Equipment and Nursing Precautions

Patient isolation and viral HF precautions should be implemented in patients with exposures in Argentina and Chile if Andes virus infection is suspected.

Vaccines

A vaccine for HF with renal syndrome is available in parts of Asia but the efficacy has not been extensively evaluated and the vaccine is not generally licensed or available outside these regions.[75] The vaccine is based on hantaviruses found in Asia and is unlikely to protect against those found in Europe or the Americas.

Reservoir Control

Because almost all hantavirus reservoirs are rural sylvatic rodents which cannot and should not be exterminated, control measures focus on avoiding human exposure to rodent excreta through rodent-proofing houses and avoiding sites of occupational or recreational exposure such as abandoned cabins or wood piles.

Bunyavirus Diseases: Rift Valley Fever

Rift Valley fever virus belongs to the *Phlebovirus* genus of the family Bunyaviridae. The virus was first isolated in Kenya in 1930 following an outbreak of 'enzootic hepatitis' in sheep in the East Africa's Rift Valley. Sporadic disease is seen throughout Africa and the Arabian Peninsula, but large outbreaks are most common in Africa, especially in east Africa, sometimes resulting in tens of thousands of infections in humans and hundreds of thousands of infections, spontaneous abortions and deaths in livestock.

EPIDEMIOLOGY

Rift Valley fever virus is maintained in a cycle between domestic ruminants (i.e. livestock, such as cattle, buffalo, sheep, goats and camels) and zoophilic flood-water breeding *Aedes* mosquitoes, with *Culex* mosquitoes sometimes serving as vectors during epizootics.[76] The virus may provoke abortions in pregnant animals with heavy mortality in newborns and is thus a major agricultural concern. Epizootics generally occur in 5–15-year cycles and follow droughts broken by heavy rains. Transovarial transmission in *Aedes* is thought to be responsible for virus maintenance during interepidemic periods.

Transmission of Rift Valley fever virus to humans occurs through direct contact with the blood and tissues of infected animals, especially during parturition, by mosquito bite and rarely through ingestion of unpasteurized infected milk. Farmers, abattoir workers and veterinarians are at particular risk. With the exception of needle stick injuries, human-to-human transmission has not been documented. Patient isolation is therefore not warranted, although patients should be protected from mosquito bites to curtail transmission.

PATHOGENESIS AND PATHOLOGY

The liver is a major target organ in HF, with histopathological examination showing moderate focal or midzonal coagulative necrosis.[77] Necrosis in the ventricular myocardium, fibrin thrombi in the glomeruli and small intertubular vessels of renal medulla in the kidneys and mild depletion of lymphocytes from white pulp and the deposition of eosinophilic amorphous fibrin-like material in red pulp cords in the spleen may be seen. An IFN-α response may play a significant role in mitigating disease.

CLINICAL FEATURES

Most human Rift Valley fever virus infections are asymptomatic or cause a mild and nonspecific illness with fever, headache, myalgia and sometimes photophobia. Severe disease occurs in a minority of infected persons and may include hepatitis, encephalitis and HF. Mortality though is high in persons with hepatitis and HF. Retinitis is a late complication of Rift Valley fever infection. Illness may be biphasic, with a brief amelioration before worsening symptoms. There are generally no sequelae in survivors, with the exception of occasional optic retinopathy resulting in vision loss.

DIAGNOSIS

Rift Valley fever should be suspected in persons with a compatible clinical syndrome, especially those with exposures to livestock in Africa. Disease in livestock, especially abortions, is usually a clue that Rift Valley fever virus is circulating. Single human cases are rarely detected.

MANAGEMENT AND TREATMENT

Although ribavirin has in vitro activity against Rift Valley fever virus, the drug is considered contraindicated after some patients treated in Saudi Arabia in 2000 succumbed to late-onset encephalitis, although the association with ribavirin is not clear. There are no controlled studies for the use of immune plasma for Rift Valley fever patients.

PREVENTION

Vaccine

A live-attenuated virus vaccine based on the Smithburn strain of Rift Valley fever virus leads to long-term immunity in sheep and goats, but not cattle.[78,79] This vaccine is associated with abortion in a small proportion of pregnant animals, which often creates significant resistance to its use among farmers. A killed vaccine was developed for use in cattle, but repeated doses are required, again discouraging use by farmers. A formalin inactivated cell culture-derived vaccine (TSI-GSD-200) is efficacious in humans but is not widely available and requires yearly boosters.

Bunyavirus Diseases: Crimean-Congo Haemorrhagic Fever

Crimean-Congo HF virus is a member of the genus *Nairovirus* within the family Bunyaviridae.[80] The virus was first discovered in 1944 in Crimea on the southern coast of Ukraine and recognized in 1969 as the same virus that caused an outbreak of illness in the Democratic Republic of the Congo.

Crimean-Congo HF virus is found across Africa, the Balkans, the Middle East and western Asia (Figure 16.4).

EPIDEMIOLOGY

Crimean-Congo HF virus is maintained in small mammals such as hares, between which the virus is spread by ticks, primarily of the *Hyalomma* species. Humans are infected either by tick bites or by exposure to contaminated blood or excreta of the reservoir animals. Ticks also spread Crimean-Congo HF virus to large mammals, including cattle, sheep and ostriches, whose transient and asymptomatic viraemia puts farmers, abattoir workers and veterinarians at risk. Nosocomial human-to-human transmission occurs frequently if universal precautions are not maintained.

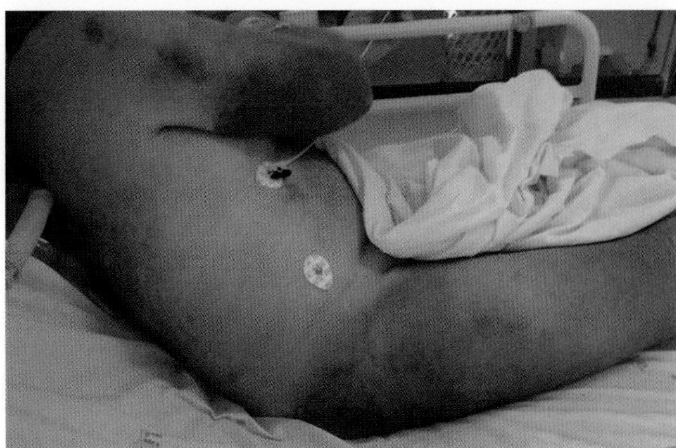

Figure 16.13 Extensive ecchymosis in Crimean-Congo haemorrhagic fever. *(Photo by Freak Bester.)*

PATHOGENESIS AND PATHOLOGY

Hepatocellular necrosis is present in all cases, frequently associated with haemorrhage, cell loss and eosinophilic changes of hepatocytes with formation of Councilman bodies.[81] Histological changes are not pathognomonic. Disseminated intravascular coagulopathy is an early and central event in the pathogenesis.

CLINICAL FEATURES

The incubation period may vary from as short as 1 day following tick bite transmission up to 11 days after other modes of inoculation.[82] Symptom onset is typically abrupt. Patients may undergo sharp changes of mood over the first two days, with feelings of confusion and aggression. Neck pain and stiffness, sore eyes and photophobia may be noted. By day 2–4, patients may exhibit lassitude, depression and somnolence and have a flushed appearance with infected conjunctivae or chemosis. Hepatomegaly with right upper quadrant tenderness may be discernible, as well as lymphadenopathy and enanthema and petechiae of the throat, tonsils and buccal mucosa. A petechial rash appears on the trunk and limbs by days 3–6 of illness and may be followed rapidly by the appearance of large bruises and ecchymoses, especially in the antecubital fossae, upper arms, axillae and groin (Figure 16.13). Internal bleeding, including retroperitoneal and intracranial haemorrhage, may occur. Severely ill patients develop hepatorenal and pulmonary failure from about day 5 onwards, with progressive drowsiness, stupor and coma. Jaundice may be seen during the 2nd week of illness. During the first 5 days of illness any of the following clinical laboratory values are highly predictive of a fatal outcome: leucocyte count $\geq 10 \times 10^9$/L; platelet count $\leq 20 \times 10^9$/L; AST $\geq$200 U/L; ALT $\geq$150 U/L; APTT $\geq$60 seconds; and fibrinogen $\leq$110 mg/dL. Leucopenia does not have the same poor prognostic connotation as leucocytosis at this early stage and all clinical laboratory values may be grossly abnormal after day 5 of illness without necessarily being indicative of a poor prognosis. Asthenia, conjunctivitis, slight confusion and amnesia may persist for months after acute disease.

DIAGNOSIS

Crimean-Congo HF should be suspected in persons with a compatible clinical syndrome (especially if bleeding is present) and likely exposure to ticks, animals or patients in endemic areas. African tick bite fever and other rickettsial infections are major considerations in the differential diagnosis (Table 16.3). Thrombocytopenia and elevated aspartate and alanine transferases are consistent findings in Crimean-Congo HF and the absence of these on successive blood draws should suggest an alternative diagnoses.

MANAGEMENT AND TREATMENT

Ribavirin has in vivo activity against Crimean-Congo HF and is often administered in both IV and oral forms to patients with the disease with apparent benefit. However, randomized controlled trials have not been performed.[79,83,84] Limited studies, but no placebo controlled trials, have suggested that immune plasma administered early in the course of illness may be efficacious. Platelet transfusion is often beneficial in patients with platelets counts of <50 000 and bleeding. Empiric doxycycline treatment for rickettsial infection should be considered until the diagnosis of Crimean-Congo HF can be confirmed.

PREVENTION

Post-exposure Prophylaxis

Post-exposure prophylaxis with oral ribavirin should be considered for persons with high-risk exposures following the guidelines described above.[21]

Vaccine

There is presently no vaccine for Crimean-Congo HF.[85]

Reservoir and Vector Control

Prevention of Crimean-Congo HF is achieved by controlling ticks through acaricides treatment of livestock and use of protective materials by abattoir workers and other animal workers to prevent contact with blood of viraemic animals.

Acknowledgements

The authors thank Irma Latsky, Cecilia Gonzales and Claudia Guezala for assistance in preparing the manuscript.

REFERENCES

1. Bond NG, Moses LM, Peterson AT, et al. Environmental aspects of the viral hemorrhagic fevers. In: Friis R, editor. Praeger Handbook of Environmental Health. Santa Barbara: Praeger; 2012. p. 133–61.
19. Levy MM, Dellinger RP, Townsend SR, et al. The Surviving Sepsis Campaign: results of an international guideline-based performance improvement program targeting severe sepsis. Crit Care Med 2010;38(2): 367–74.
26. CDC and WHO. Infection control for viral haemorrhagic fevers in the African health care setting. Atlanta: Centers for Disease Control and Prevention; 1998.
44. Towner JS, Sealy TK, Ksiazek TG, et al. High-throughput molecular detection of hemorrhagic fever virus threats with applications for outbreak settings. J Infect Dis 2007;196(Suppl. 2):S205–12.
72. Macneil A, Nichol ST, Spiropoulou CF. Hantavirus pulmonary syndrome. Virus Res 2011; 162(1–2):138–47.

Access the complete references online at www.expertconsult.com

Rabies

MARY J. WARRELL

KEY POINTS

- Domestic dogs are the dominant rabies reservoir and are the origin of 99% of human infection.
- Human encephalitis due to dog rabies virus has always been fatal.
- A bite from a bat anywhere in the world should be considered as a possible risk of *Lyssavirus* infection.
- Human rabies, especially the paralytic form, is a hidden disease. Patients have been misdiagnosed as dying of cerebral malaria or drug intoxication.
- The combination of pre-exposure and post-exposure booster vaccination has proved 100% successful in preventing human rabies.
- Post-exposure treatment is always urgent.
- There is no antiviral agent effective against rabies.
- Patients bitten by bats in the Americas have recovered from rabies encephalitis, but there are no known survivors of dog rabies virus infection. Rabies viruses in American bats are different from other *Lyssavirus* types and seem to be less pathogenic.
- Compassionate palliative care is the recommended management of rabies patients except for those infected by a bat in the Americas, in which case intensive care treatment may be appropriate.

Epidemiology

Rabies is a widespread infection of certain mammal species, which is occasionally transmitted to man. Transmission of the infection from dogs' saliva was known to the Egyptians at the time of the Pharaohs, and in China from the fifth century BC. Louis Pasteur's work in the 1880s demonstrated that rabies was an infection of the central nervous system.

LYSSAVIRUS TYPES

Rabies virus is a species of the genus *Lyssavirus* (Gk: *lyssa*, rage/frenzy) of the large family of Rhabdoviridae (Gk: *rhabdos*, rod). There are seven genotypes: rabies genotype 1 and rabies-related viruses genotypes 2–7 (Table 17.1).[1–3] All but one have caused fatal infection in man (see below). The lyssaviruses are divided into two phylogroups. Phylogroup II is less pathogenic in terrestrial mammals.

An alternative classification is for 12 *Lyssavirus* species, which include the seven genotypes (above) and five bat lyssaviruses identified in the last 20 years,[4] and new types are still emerging for example Ikoma and Bokeloh viruses. West Caucasian Bat virus is likely to be assigned to a new Phylogroup III.

Other rhabdoviruses which very rarely cause disease in humans are: the vesicular stomatitis viruses, *Chandipura*, *Piry* and *Le Dantec* viruses.[5]

GEOGRAPHICAL DISTRIBUTION

Rabies and rabies-related lyssaviruses are enzootic in mammals almost worldwide. Areas free of lyssaviruses are where there is no infection in terrestrial mammal species and there are no bats, as in Antarctica or where thorough surveillance has shown no evidence of bat rabies. The risk of introduction of the infection by animal migration, infiltration or importation is universal.

Global surveillance is so poor that the WHO no longer lists countries where rabies is reported. Areas considered to be free of rabies in terrestrial mammals (i.e. excluding bats) include: Antarctica, Australia, New Zealand, Papua New Guinea, Japan, Hong Kong Islands, Singapore, Peninsula Malaysia, Sabah, Sarawak; some islands in the Indian Ocean; many Pacific islands, e.g. Solomon Islands, Fiji, Samoa and Cook Islands; Iceland, Ireland, UK, France, Belgium, Luxembourg, the Netherlands, Austria, Switzerland, Germany, Finland, Sweden, Norway (except the Svalbard Islands), Denmark, Spain, Portugal, the Mediterranean islands and some Caribbean islands (e.g. Barbados, Bahamas, Jamaica, St Lucia, Martinique and Antigua).

However in the UK, along with other Western European countries and Australia, rabies-related lyssaviruses are found in bats. As there is no surveillance of bats in many countries, the risk of human infection from bats should be considered global.

The rabies virus is enzootic in separate cycles of transmission within dogs and wild mammal reservoirs. Infection sometimes spills over to other species, including humans and domestic mammals, which might then become vectors and transmit to man. Strains of virus from different species and locations can be identified by genetic sequence analysis or by antigenic typing using a panel of monoclonal antibodies. The enzootic in domestic dogs is of most importance to man[6], and is the cause of more than 99% of human rabies cases (Figure 17.1). The pattern of sylvatic (wildlife) rabies shows great geographical variation (Figure 17.2). The prevalence of rabies in reservoir mammal species is influenced by: altering mammal habitats, as in deforestation forcing vampire bats to roost near villages; movement of refugee populations; disruption caused by war; animal vaccination campaigns and a high mortality in dog owners from HIV infection, resulting in packs of ownerless dogs in southern Africa.[7] Knowledge of current local epizootics enables the prevention of human rabies fatalities. The distribution of dominant reservoir species is summarized in Table 17.2.

TABLE 17.1 Classification of genus *Lyssavirus* of the Rhabdoviridae

Genotype	Source	Known Distribution
***Lyssavirus* Phylogroup I**		
1 Rabies virus	Dog, fox, mongoose, raccoon, skunk, **all bats in the Americas**	Widespread
4 *Duvenhage*	Insectivorous bat, e.g. *Nycteris thebaica* Fruit bats	South Africa, Zimbabwe, Kenya (very rare)
5 European bat *Lyssavirus*	1a Bats, e.g. *Eptesicus serotinus*	Denmark, Germany, Netherlands, Russia, Poland, France, Hungary Czech Republic
	1b Bats, e.g. *Eptesicus serotinus*	Netherlands, France, Spain
6 European bat *Lyssavirus*	2a *Myotis dasycneme* bats	Netherlands
	Myotis daubentonii bats	UK (and Ukraine in other bat sp.)
	2b *Myotis daubentonii* bat	Switzerland, Finland, Germany (rare)
7 Australian bat *Lyssavirus*	Flying foxes (*Pteropus* sp.) Insectivorous bats	Australia
NEW *LYSSAVIRUS* SPECIES		
Irkut	*Murina leucogaster* bat	Siberia, China
Aravan[a]	*Myotis blythi* bat	Kyrgyzstan
Khujand[a]	*Myotis mystacinus* bat	Tajikistan
Phylogroup II		
3 *Mokola*	Shrews (*Crocidura* spp.), cats	Southern Africa, Nigeria, Cameroon, Ethiopia (rare)
2 Lagos bat virus	Bats, cats	Africa
NEW *LYSSAVIRUS* SPECIES		
Shimoni virus[a]	*Hipposideros commersoni* bat	Kenya
Phylogroup III		
West Caucasian bat virus[a]	*Miniopterus schreibersi* bat	Russia

Shaded area viruses have NOT been detected in man.
[a]Single isolates only.

INCIDENCE OF HUMAN RABIES

In endemic tropical areas, especially where dogs are the reservoir, the true incidence of human rabies is unknown because of under-reporting or lack of published figures. Estimates for Asia and Africa include an annual mortality of 55 000, with an incidence of $1.4/10^5$ population, but under-reporting is suspected. There is a high mortality, 12 700 (99% CI 10 000 to 15,500) furious cases/year, in India[8] and also in Bangladesh and Pakistan. A survey in Cambodia indicated mortality of 5.8 deaths/year/10^5 population, which is 15 times the official figures.[9] Human deaths from dog rabies in southern China have been rising recently, reaching 3300 cases in 2007. Dog rabies persists in 10 Latin American countries: Bolivia, Brazil, Colombia, Cuba, El Salvador, Guatemala, Haiti, Mexico, Peru and Venezuela.[10] Human mortality from outbreaks of vampire bat rabies is reported in the Amazonian regions of Peru and Ecuador. In the USA, where sylvatic rabies is endemic, there have been 31 deaths in 10 years since 2000, an average of 3 cases/year. A total of 74% were indigenous infections, and 96% (22 of 23) of these were due to insectivorous bat rabies viruses. A study of 61 fatalities from bat rabies in North America showed that 55% reported a bat bite or had direct contact with a bat, but 34% of patients had no known association with bats whatsoever.[11] Recent European data show an average of 6 deaths annually, the great majority are in Russia and the Ukraine.

Imported human rabies is easily missed, but over 20 years, 42 rabies deaths were imported mostly from Asia or Africa, into Europe, the USA and Japan, and none were reported in Canada, Australia and New Zealand.[12]

TRANSMISSION OF INFECTION

Animal Contact

Humans are usually infected by virus-laden saliva, inoculated during the bite of a rabid dog. Inoculation of rabies virus into a wound or on to a mucous membrane may result in infection. This includes contamination of an unhealed lesion. Intact skin

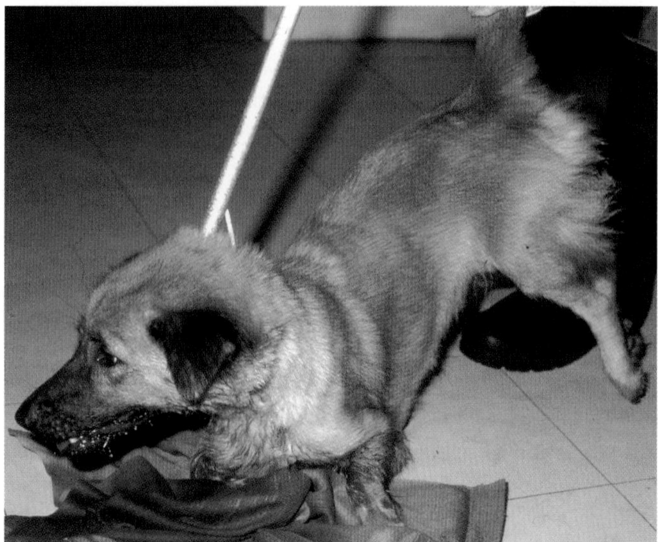

Figure 17.1 Domestic dog with paralytic rabies in Bangkok. Paralysis of fore limbs and drooling of saliva. *(Copyright D. A. Warrell.)*

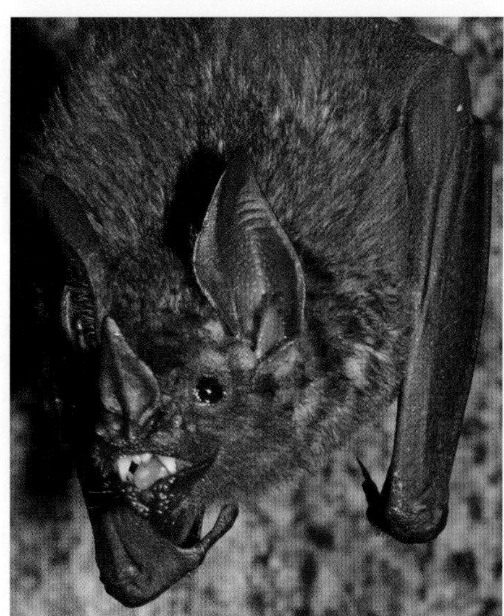

Figure 17.2 Short-tailed leaf-nosed bat (*Carollia perspicillata*) one of several rabies reservoir bat species in South America. *(Copyright © D. A. Warrell.)*

is a barrier against viral entry. The chance of developing rabies following exposure is revealed by data from the pre-vaccine era (see page 205).

Human-to-Human

There are old anecdotal reports of infections from contact with human saliva, kissing, biting, sexual intercourse, breast-feeding and eating infected meat, but these routes remain unproven in man. Viraemia has not been detected.[13]

Transmission has occurred through *grafting of infected corneas*. Six virologically proven cases followed transplants from donors with unsuspected rabies. In Texas and in Germany, mysterious encephalitis killed a total of seven *organ transplant* recipients. Liver, kidney, pancreas and even an iliac artery graft transmitted rabies virus from two donors aged 20 and 26 years old, who both died of undiagnosed neurological disease. Subsequent histories elicited a previous bat bite in the USA and contact with a dog in India.[14–17] Two cornea transplant recipients were given rabies post-exposure prophylaxis and remain healthy.

Transplacental infection occurs in animals, and a Turkish woman and her 2-day-old infant died of virologically confirmed rabies. This is exceptional. Many mothers with rabies have been delivered of healthy babies.

Other Routes

Two rabies infections resulted from inhaled aerosols of 'fixed' virus in laboratory accidents.[18,19] Two more people were possibly infected by inhalation of aerosolized virus in bat-infested caves, but direct bat contact was not excluded.[20] Butchering dogs or cats is another source of rabies, but consuming the cooked rabid meat did not cause infection.[21]

Inactivation

Rabies virus is rapidly inactivated by heat. At 56°C the half-life is less than 1 minute, but at 37°C it is prolonged to several hours in moist conditions. At 4°C, there is little loss after 2 weeks.

The lipid coat is disrupted by detergents or a 1% soap solution. Other virucidal agents include iodine solutions (1 : 10 000 available iodine), 45% ethanol and 1% benzalkonium chloride, but phenol is not so effective.

VIRUS AND PATHOGENESIS[22]

The bullet-shaped rabies virion (Figure 17.3) measures 180 × 75 nm, and contains a single strand of negative-sense RNA encoding five proteins. The genome combines with a nucleoprotein, a phosphoprotein and RNA polymerase to form a helical coil. This viral core, the ribonucleoprotein complex, is covered by a matrix protein and then by glycoprotein bearing

TABLE 17.2 Distribution of Important Reservoir Species of Rabies Genotype 1 and Other Lyssaviruses

Species	Distribution
Africa	
Domestic dog	Widespread dominant vector
Black-backed jackals (*Canis mesomelas*)	Zambia, Zimbabwe, Namibia
Yellow mongoose (*Cynicitis penicillata*)	South Africa
Fruit bats and insectivorous bats	South, West and Eastern Africa
Americas	
Arctic fox (*Alopex lagopus*)	North-west Canada, Alaska
Striped skunk (*Mephitis mephitis*)	Central and north-eastern USA, California, central southern Canada
Raccoon (*Procyon lotor*)	Eastern-USA and Texas
Fox	Texas and eastern USA
Coyote (*Canis latrans*)	Southern Texas
Insectivorous bats	North and South America
Domestic dog	Widespread Mexico, Central and parts of South America
Vampire bat (*Desmodontidae*)	Southern Texas, Mexico, Trinidad and Tobago, Central America and northern South America to Argentina, Chile
Mongoose (*Herpestes* species)	Puerto Rico, Grenada, Cuba, Dominican Republic
Asia	
Domestic dog	Widespread dominant vector
Wolf	Iran, Iraq, Afghanistan
Europe and Middle East	
Fox	Widespread from Eastern Europe to Russian Federation, Middle East
Arctic fox (*Alopex lagopus*)	Northern Russia
Raccoon dog (*Nycterentes procyonoides*)	Baltic states, Russia, Poland, Ukraine
Wolf	Russian Federation
Dog	Turkey, Afghanistan, Israel, countries of the Middle East, Russian Federation
Insectivorous bats	Across Europe Russia
Australia	
Fruit bats (flying foxes) (*Pteropus* spp.)	Northern and eastern coastal regions
Insectivorous bats	

All rabies virus, genotype 1, except for shaded areas (see Table 17.1).

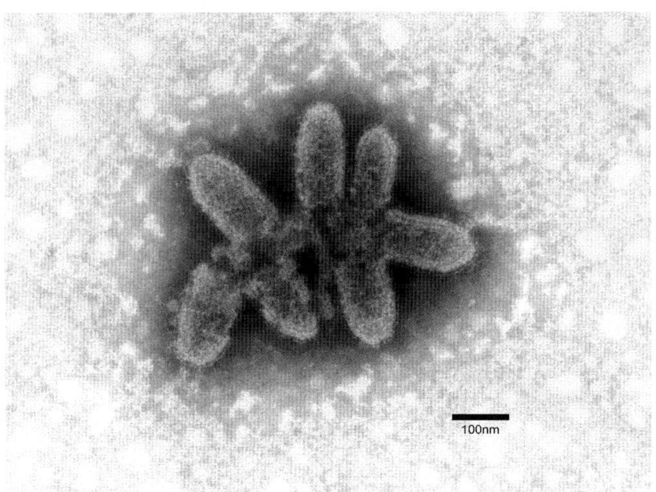

Figure 17.3 Negatively stained electron micrograph of a clump of bullet-shaped rabies virions. *(Courtesy of ©VLA EM Unit, Weybridge, UK.)*

trimeric club-shaped spikes (Figure 17.4), which project outward through a host cell-derived lipid bilayer.[23–24]

The extraordinary journey of rabies virions along nerves up to the brain, and then outward to many organs, is gradually being unravelled. It usually begins with the bite of a rabid animal inoculating virus-laden saliva through the skin, often into muscle. Experiments show that viral replication can occur locally in striated muscle, or mucous membrane, before neuronal invasion. The virus attaches to several types of cell receptors experimentally. At neuromuscular junctions, infection may involve specific binding to the post-synaptic nicotinic acetylcholine receptor in close proximity to the pre-synaptic axon terminal. The mechanism by which the rabies virus crosses the synaptic cleft to enter the axon is unknown, but the neural cell adhesion molecule is the most likely receptor on the pre-synaptic membrane, leading to cell entry by glycoprotein-dependent endocytosis. The route of infection may be different following superficial inoculation by a bat bite.

Once inside a neuron, the virus moves centripetally carried by strictly retrograde axonal transport. There is evidence that vesicles containing intact virions are loaded onto dynein molecular motors moving along microtubules.[25] Viral glycoprotein-vesicle binding may be via the p75 neurotrophin receptor. The rabies virus replicates in the cell body, protein synthesis occurs also in dendrites, and the virus acquires an envelope when passing through the cell membrane. Transsynaptic transmission to the adjacent axon terminal continues as the virus ascends through the motor nerve pathway eventually reaching the brain. Progression can be halted by sectioning nerves or by microtubule inhibitors, such as colchicine.

Intraneuronal viral replication occurs on a massive scale in the brain. The classical Negri bodies are cytoplasmic inclusions consisting largely of accumulated rabies RNAs, nucleoprotein and phosphoprotein. They function as viral factories. The often minimal histopathological changes do not account for the gross neuronal dysfunction, but there is evidence of viral influence on the expression of host genes, disrupting normal functions including altering neurotransmitter activity.

The rabies virus remains virtually confined to neurons as centrifugal dissemination progresses via autonomic and peripheral nerves. The virus has been isolated from human skeletal and cardiac muscle, skin, lung, kidney, adrenal, lachrymal and, of course, salivary glands.[13] Rabies antigen is found in neuronal

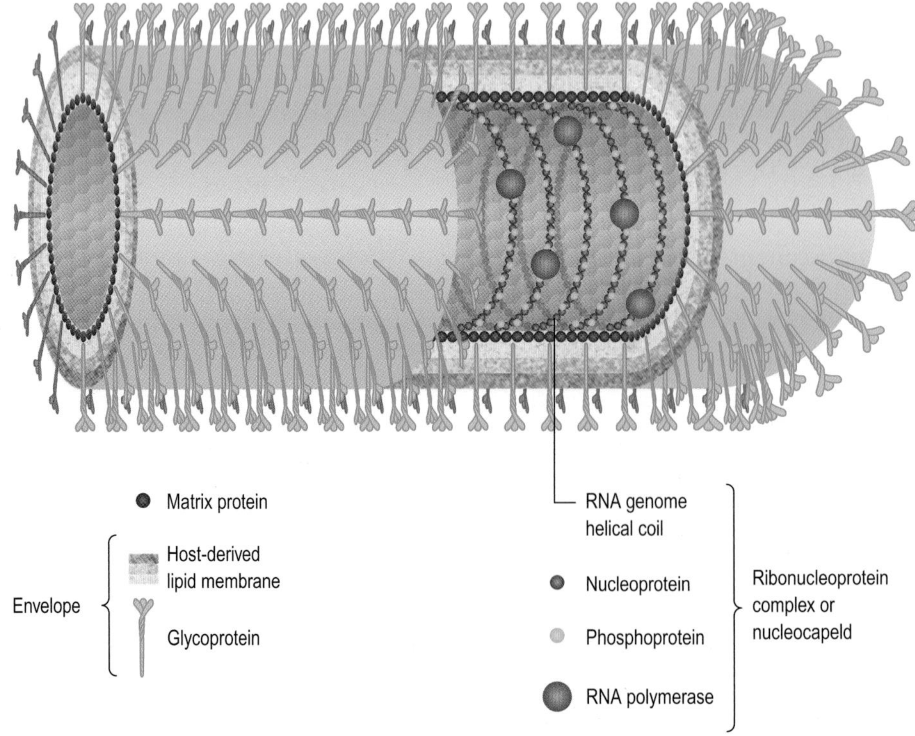

Figure 17.4 Diagram of rabies virion.

tissue in most of these areas and around the gastrointestinal tract.[26]

In contrast to events in neurons, virus replication in acinar cells of the salivary glands produces large amounts of extracellular virus. Although there is no evidence of viraemia, rabies virus is shed in human lachrymal and respiratory tract secretions and possibly in urine and in milk.

Pathology

Cerebral congestion and a few petechial haemorrhages are usual findings in rabies encephalitis, but not gross cerebral oedema. A lymphocytic perivenous infiltrate is common, and neutrophils are occasionally seen, perhaps only early in the disease. Eosinophilic cytoplasmic inclusions, Negri bodies are found in 75% of patients, most frequently in large neurons of the hippocampus, Purkinje cells of the cerebellum and medulla.

Neuronophagia, microglial reaction, foci of demyelination and perineural infiltration (Babès' nodules) also occur. The brain stem and spinal cord are predominantly affected, but changes are often widespread. Involvement of the limbic system causes aggressive behaviour and enables transmission from a vector species to another host. A meningeal reaction is common in children, and in paralytic disease the spinal cord is most severely affected. The extent of the histopathological change varies from complete disruption of neuronal structure and axonal degeneration of peripheral nerves following intensive care,[27] to an absence of any inflammation or degeneration. Extraneural pathology includes focal degeneration of salivary glands, liver, pancreas, adrenal medulla and lymph nodes, and also interstitial myocarditis.

Immunology

RESPONSE TO INFECTION

Following a rabid bite, no immune response is detectable in unvaccinated subjects before encephalitis has developed. Rabies antibody is found first in serum then in cerebrospinal fluid (CSF) at least a week after the onset.[28] Neutralizing antibody may rise to a high level if life is prolonged. Specific rabies IgM antibody is occasionally present, but is unhelpful in diagnosis as it does not appear early and can also be present in postvaccinal encephalitis if following Semple or other vaccine of nervous tissue origin.[29]

There is little evidence of lymphocyte-mediated responses to encephalitis in man. Pleocytosis is observed initially in only 60% of patients, with a mean leucocyte count of $75/mm^3$. Very low levels of interferon have been found in the serum and CSF of about 30% of patients with rabies encephalitis.

The intraneural virus evades immunological surveillance until a late stage of the disease. At the site of inoculation, some virus is briefly exposed, but once within the CNS virions and their antigens are hidden. During the final centrifugal phase of infection, when extracellular virus is produced, rabies antigens are expressed on cell membranes but if an immune response is induced, it is too late to combat the overwhelming infection.

Animal models show suppression of both adaptive and innate immune responses, especially the inhibition of interferon production. Clearance of rabies virus from the CNS is related to the presence of neutralizing antibody, immune T and B lymphocytes and other immune effectors in the brain. Survival following attenuated rabies infection is associated with expression of viral glycoprotein, minimal neuronal apoptosis and a high titre of neutralizing antibody.[22]

RESPONSE TO VACCINE

The best available measure of immunity after vaccine treatment is the level of glycoprotein-induced neutralizing antibody, which usually appears 7–14 days after starting a primary vaccine course. The amount of antibody needed for protection against rabies in man cannot be determined, but the World Health Organization (WHO) recommends that a minimum neutralizing antibody level of 0.5 IU/mL should be attained to demonstrate unequivocal seroconversion.[30] The production of neutralizing antibody following rabies vaccine is influenced genetically. A relatively delayed, lower response occurred in 3–10% of vaccinees.[31] Increasing age (over 50 years) and immunosuppression including HIV infection, also impair antibody production.

The role of cell-mediated immunity in protection against disease is not clear but priming of CD4 lymphocyte memory cells is important. A small amount of interferon may be induced briefly following a first dose of rabies vaccine, but it is very unlikely to afford significant protection in man.

Clinical Features

INCUBATION PERIOD

The interval between inoculation and the onset of symptoms is between 20 and 90 days in at least 60% of cases,[32] but it has varied from 4 days to 19 years.[33] It is reported to be over a year in up to 6%, but a subsequent exposure may be difficult to exclude. In general, the nearer the bite is to the head, the shorter the incubation period.

PRODROMAL SYMPTOMS

Itching or paraesthesia at the site of the healed bite wound are the only specific prodromal symptoms, occurring in about 40% of patients. The wide range of nonspecific features include: fever, headache, myalgia, fatigue, sore throat, gastrointestinal symptoms, irritability, anxiety and insomnia. The disease progresses to either furious or paralytic rabies encephalomyelitis, usually within 1 week.[34]

FURIOUS RABIES

The familiar presentation of 'furious rabies'[34,35] is probably the most common in humans. Malfunction of the brain stem nuclei, limbic system, reticular activating system and higher centres results in the characteristic hydrophobic spasms. This is a reflex contraction of inspiratory muscles provoked by attempts to drink water, and later, through conditioning, even the sound or mention of water, and also sometimes by draughts of air (aerophobia), touching the palate, bright lights or loud noises.

Intense thirst forces patients to try to drink. They may have a tight feeling in the throat, the arm trembles, and jerky spasms of the sternomastoids, diaphragm and other inspiratory muscles lead to a generalized extension, sometimes with convulsions and opisthotonos (Figure 17.5). There is an associated

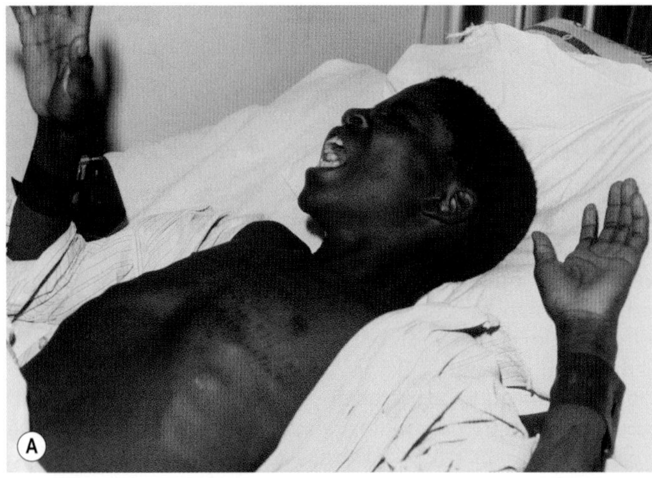

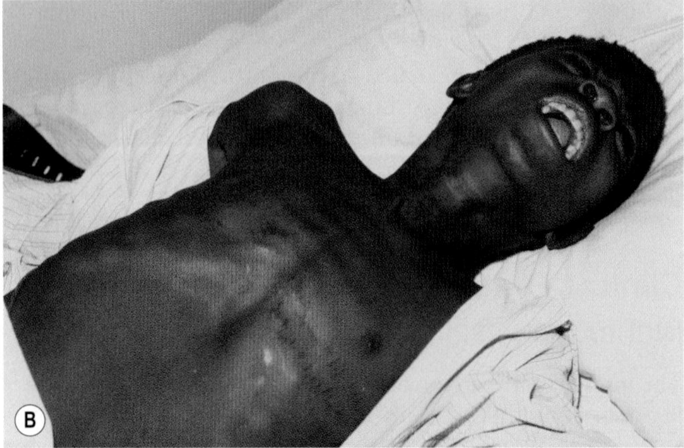

Figure 17.5 Progression of a hydrophobic spasm associated with terror in a Nigerian boy with furious rabies. (A) Note the powerful contraction of the diaphragm (depressing the xiphisternum) and sternocleidomastoid muscles. (B) The episode terminates in opisthotonos. *(Copyright © D. A. Warrell.)*

inexplicable feeling of terror which occurs during the first episode, and is not a learned response. Respiratory or cardiac arrest following a hydrophobic spasm is fatal in one-third of cases.

Episodes of excitation, aggression, anxiety or hallucinations are interspersed with periods of calm lucidity, during which no neurological abnormality may be detectable and patients realize their appalling predicament. Other features include cardiac arrhythmias, myocarditis, respiratory disturbances (e.g. cluster breathing), meningism, lesions of cranial nerves III, VII and IX, abnormal pupillary function, muscle fasciculation, autonomic stimulation with lacrimation, salivation, labile blood pressure and temperature and rarely increased libido, priapism and spontaneous orgasms. Low cerebral oxygen uptake suggests irreversible brain damage. Coma eventually ensues, with flaccid paralysis, and the agonizing illness rarely lasts more than a week without intensive care.

PARALYTIC RABIES

Less common than furious rabies, paralytic or 'dumb' rabies may be missed, unless there is a high level of suspicion. Paralytic disease is characteristic of vampire bat-transmitted rabies and it is common following infections by other American bat viruses, attenuated viruses,[18,19,36] and perhaps after post-exposure vaccination.

Prodromal symptoms are followed by paraesthesia or hypotonic weakness, commonly starting near the site of the bite and spreading cranially. Fasciculation or piloerection may be seen. The ascending paralysis results in constipation, urinary retention, respiratory failure and inability to swallow. Flaccid paralysis, especially of proximal muscles, is associated with loss of tendon and plantar reflexes, but sensation is often normal. Hydrophobic spasms may occur in the terminal phase and death ensues after 1–3 weeks.[34]

RABIES-RELATED VIRUS INFECTIONS

All *Lyssavirus* genotypes[3,7] (Table 17.1) have caused human deaths, except for genotype 2: *Lagos bat virus. Mokola* virus, genotype 3 Phylogroup II, is the only rabies-related virus not found in bats. Its main reservoir host is unknown, but it has been found in shrews and other rodents, which may infect cats and dogs. *Mokola* has been isolated from rabies-vaccinated cats, which is to be expected, as there is no serological cross-reaction with Phylogroup I lyssaviruses. It is less pathogenic than rabies and may have caused fatal encephalitis in a Nigerian child, while another recovered from pharyngitis and probably a febrile convulsion, but neither were typical of clinical rabies. A laboratory worker recovered from an accidental *Mokola* infection.[37] *Duvenhage* virus is named after the first of three patients who were bitten by bats in Africa and died of rabies-like *Duvenhage* encephalitis.

European insectivorous bats harbour *European bat Lyssavirus* genotypes 5 (*EBLV-1*) and 6 (*EBLV-2*), and each is subdivided into subtypes *a* and *b* (Table 17.1).[1] Five human infections from bats have been reported in Europe.[38] Two Russian girls died of rabies following bat bites. In 1985, a Swiss zoologist bitten by a bat from an unknown source died in Finland of furious rabies-like encephalitis, due to *EBLV-2b*. In 2002, a bat conservationist in Scotland, UK, died from encephalitis caused by *EBLV-2a*. A Ukrainian died from infection including hydrophobia after a bat bite. A similar case occurred in China the same year. Irkut virus caused a death in Russia.

In Australia in 1996, flying foxes (fruit bats, genus *Pteropus*) were discovered to harbour the *Australian bat Lyssavirus* (genotype 7),[39] which has caused a rabies-like fatal illness in three people. *Lyssavirus* antibodies, some related to genotype 7, have been reported in bats in the Philippines, Cambodia, Thailand, Bangladesh and China. In Europe, *EBLV*-seropositive bats with PCR-positive saliva indicate that bat infections are not always fatal. There is no evidence of chronic infection or virus excretion in bats.

Differential Diagnosis

Rabies should be suspected if inexplicable neurological, psychiatric or laryngopharyngeal symptoms occur in those who have been to an endemic area. The animal contact may have been forgotten or unnoticed. The differential diagnoses include the following:[34]

- Tetanus, another wound infection, has a short incubation period, usually less than 15 days. The muscle rigidity is constant, without relaxation between spasms. The CSF is always normal

- Intoxications with drugs acting on the CNS, poisons and even delirium tremens could be confused with rabies. Rabies has been misdiagnosed as recreational drug abuse
- Guillain–Barré syndrome may present as paralytic rabies, and very rarely follows rabies tissue culture vaccine treatment
- Post-vaccinal encephalitis (see below), an allergic response to nervous-tissue-containing rabies vaccine, can be clinically indistinguishable from paralytic rabies
- Other viral encephalomyelitides, including Japanese encephalitis, poliomyelitis and treatable *Cercopithecine herpesvirus* (B virus) encephalomyelitis from a monkey bite, should be considered
- Paralytic rabies has been misdiagnosed as cerebral malaria in children
- Rabies phobia is a hysterical response, usually very soon after a bite, with aggressive behaviour and an excellent prognosis.

DIAGNOSIS

Laboratory investigations are likely to be normal initially, except for a mild pleocytosis. A variety of nonspecific EEG changes are reported. CT and MRI scans may be normal throughout, but nonspecific MRI changes have been seen especially in brainstem, or basal ganglia regions, and possibly in the spinal cord in paralytic disease. Confirmation of rabies infection is useful to prevent further investigation and supportive treatment of patients with predominantly paralytic or atypical signs, to test the brains of potentially rabid biting mammals and as surveillance among neurological patients and dogs.

Intravitam Confirmation of Human Rabies Encephalitis

The diagnosis of rabies can be made by virus isolation, rapid identification of antigen or, in unvaccinated people, antibody detection.

Isolation of Rabies Virus. Culture of the virus is most successful during the first week of illness from saliva, throat, tracheal or eye swabs, brain biopsy samples, CSF and possibly centrifuged urine.[28] Viraemia has not been detected. The method of inoculation of suckling mice yields results in 1–3 weeks, but tissue culture isolation in murine neuroblastoma cells takes about 2 days.

Antigen Detection. Rabies diagnosis by a variety of methods of polymerase chain reaction (RT-PCR) tests on saliva, CSF and skin biopsy is only possible in a few laboratories, which usually use their own protocols.[40] In remote areas, testing is possible if three saliva samples collected on different days are stored frozen for a retrospective PCR test at a distant reference laboratory.[41]

A direct immunofluorescent antibody (IFA) test rapidly identifies antigen in frozen sections of skin biopsies taken from a hairy area, usually the nape of the neck. Rabies-specific immunofluorescence appears in nerve twiglets around the base of hair follicles.[42] Careful controls of specificity are needed, but this method is 60–100% sensitive.[29,43] False positives have not been reported. The corneal smear test is too insensitive to be useful and false positives have occurred.

Antibody Detection. In unvaccinated patients, rabies seroconversion often occurs during the 2nd week of illness and is diagnostic,[28] but many remain seronegative at death. In vaccinated people, very high levels of antibody in the serum, and especially in the CSF, suggest the diagnosis.[44,45]

Postmortem Diagnosis in Humans

All the methods mentioned above may confirm the diagnosis postmortem, especially if the clinical illness was very short. Virus isolation from secretions is usually unsuccessful after 2 weeks of illness, but culture of brain tissue should be possible post mortem, even if the IFA staining is negative. Samples can be obtained without a full postmortem examination. Brain necropsies are taken with a Vim–Silverman or other long biopsy needle via the medial canthus of the eye, through the superior orbital fissure or an occipital approach through the foramen magnum. Cerebral malaria and other encephalitides may also be diagnosed from these specimens.

Retrospective rabies diagnosis from formalin-fixed brain specimens is possible by trypsin digestion and labelled antibody staining with immunofluorescent, enzymatic or in situ hybridization methods.

DIAGNOSIS IN THE BITING MAMMAL

If laboratory facilities are available, suspect rabid animals should be killed immediately and their brains tested for rabies infection. Observation in captivity is potentially dangerous and uncertain. Ideally, samples of hippocampus, brain stem and cerebellum should be tested, but brain specimens can be obtained from dogs without craniotomy via the occipital foramen.[46] Direct immunofluorescent antibody (IFA) staining of acetone-fixed impression smears takes 2–3 hours and is the usual method of diagnosis. It is about 98% sensitive compared with viral culture by the mouse inoculation test. The IFA test is unreliable for detecting rabies-related viruses. An alternative not requiring a fluorescent microscope is an American method using light microscopy, the direct rapid immunohistochemical test. Commercial enzyme immunodiagnostic kits are produced for antigen detection in brain tissue suspensions, although less sensitive than the IFA test, they may be useful for decomposing samples. No single test should be relied upon to make this important diagnosis. Virus isolation should ideally be attempted on all IFA test-negative samples.

Rabies, or rabies-related viruses from different vector species or geographical areas, can be differentiated by genetic sequence analysis or monoclonal antibody typing.

RECOVERY FROM RABIES

Ten patients are reported to have survived clinical rabies encephalitis. The diagnoses were based on rabies neutralizing antibody in the serum and CSF. Virus antigen was identified in a single patient.

One patient claimed to have recovered completely, received a nervous tissue vaccine following a dog bite. Post-vaccinal encephalitis is a possible alternative diagnosis.[47] Four further patients, given pre- or post-exposure tissue culture vaccines, survived months or years with profound neurological impairment: a microbiologist who inhaled fixed rabies virus,[19] two boys in Mexico and a girl in India bitten by dogs.

A sixth patient, a boy bitten by a bat in the USA 40 years ago, was given post-exposure prophylaxis with duck embryo vaccine. He completely recovered from encephalitis after intensive care treatment.[44]

The first unvaccinated patient to survive rabies, a teenager in Milwaukee, USA, is now leading an independent life following intensive care and antiviral therapy.[45] The induction of coma and nonspecific antiviral treatments have become known as the Milwaukee protocol. A boy bitten by a vampire bat in Brazil was given post-exposure vaccination but developed encephalitis. Rabies virus was isolated, he was treated with intensive care and has survived 3 years with neurological deficits. Two final remarkable unvaccinated patients in the USA had very low levels of rabies antibody in serum and CSF: one teenager visited a cave containing a large bat population and recovered from a relatively mild neurological illness;[48] the other was an 8-year-old girl who had had contact with feral cats but her rabies antibody level did not rise and so the diagnosis is open to question. She had brief intensive care and recovered in a month.

To summarize, five survivors of infection by a virus of canine origin did not recover. Two patients bitten by insectivorous bats in the USA recovered, and one infected by a vampire bat has some deficits. Two patients with possible insectivorous bat rabies recovered.

Although bat rabies viruses of the Americas are classical rabies genotype 1, they have a different pattern of infection to the dog rabies strains, experimentally.[49] Silver-haired bat rabies virus infection is slower to evolve and does not induce apoptosis in the brain of experimentally infected mice.[50] Genotype 1 rabies bat viruses of the Americas are genetically separate from dog rabies strains. Recovery was only seen in patients infected by American bats, or where the source was uncertain. Their symptoms were of paralytic rabies, so they had no damaging hydrophobic spasms, and neutralizing antibody was detected early in the infection. The evidence suggests that American bat rabies is less pathogenic in man.

Management and Complications

Rabies remains a fatal infection, although rare recoveries have been reported (see above). Intensive care therapy can prolong life for 3–4 weeks, occasionally for months and exceptionally for years (see above).

During this time, complications arise in every system. Cardiac arrhythmias are controlled by pacing, and respiratory failure requires ventilation. Full barrier nursing of the unconscious patient is needed, with specific treatment for likely complications such as convulsions, fluctuating blood pressure, pneumonia, pneumothorax, cerebral oedema, hyper- or hypopyrexia, diabetes insipidus, inappropriate antidiuretic hormone secretion and haematemesis from stress ulceration.[34]

Treatment with hyperimmune serum and several antiviral agents, including intrathecal tribavirin (ribavirin) and interferon-α, have not been effective and the success claimed for the Milwaukee protocol, a regimen of sedation and multiple antiviral drugs in a girl infected by bat rabies in the USA, has not been confirmed in >20 patients infected with canine or bat rabies viruses.[51] No antiviral or other therapeutic agent has proved effective against rabies virus experimentally.

IS INTENSIVE CARE TREATMENT JUSTIFIED?

No-one is known to have recovered from encephalitis due to dog rabies virus, so attempts to treat are not appropriate.

However, intensive care therapy should be considered for patients infected by American bats who are at an early stage in the disease, in patients vaccinated before the onset of symptoms or if rabies antibody is present. There is no evidence that the Milwaukee protocol has any advantage over standard intensive care treatment. Otherwise, patients with suspected rabies should be admitted to hospital and given compassionate care with adequate doses of sedatives and analgesics to relieve their agonizing symptoms. We must wait for new antiviral methods to prove effective in animals.

Prevention

CONTROL OF ANIMAL RABIES

The optimal method of protecting man from rabies infection or associated financial loss varies greatly in different endemic areas. The species of vector, its prevalence and interaction with man dictate whether vaccination of animals and perhaps elimination of the virus is possible, appropriate and economically feasible.

Canine Rabies

Human rabies deaths in developing countries would be almost abolished if dog rabies were eliminated. The control of rabies in areas where dogs are the reservoir species requires: epidemiological surveillance; laboratory diagnostic facilities; education of the population about the disease; publicity for the campaign, and effective vaccination of dogs, cats and humans.[52]

The size of a population of stray dogs depends on available food and shelter. Attempts at control by killing dogs result in an increased reproduction rate and rapid restoration of numbers. There has been an impressive reduction in the number of local human cases following vector control campaigns, including vaccination, dog population control and removal of food and shelter by clearing street rubbish. Canine rabies vaccines are usually parenteral inactivated tissue culture products. Oral vaccination is only possible with a live virus. Although a poxvirus recombinant is immunogenic, there is as yet no safe way of distributing oral vaccine to stray dogs. Contraceptive methods for dogs include surgical sterilization, hormone depot injections and new contraceptive vaccines. Mass rabies vaccination campaigns, aimed at immunizing 80% of dogs, have eliminated canine infection in Japan and Taiwan, and from densely populated urban areas of Argentina, Brazil and Peru. Despite localized successes, there has been no evidence of a significant change in the overall incidence of animal rabies in most tropical endemic areas of Africa and Asia. The results of ambitious trials aimed at controlling or even eliminating dog rabies in selected areas of Africa and South-east Asia are awaited.

Sylvatic (Wildlife) Rabies

Active control is not attempted for some reservoir species, owing to the low rate of transmission to other mammals or lack of effective methods. Insectivorous bats in North America and Europe are examples and simple measures are used to prevent contact with man. In contrast, where infection of domestic animals and humans is likely, as with fox rabies, campaigns for population control and vaccination have been mounted. Some inaccessible animals are vaccinated orally.

Trapping, gassing, poisoning and hunting are generally inefficient means of population reduction. Oral fox vaccine campaigns have been successful. Live attenuated rabies virus vaccine disguised in baits has been distributed first by hand, then by aircraft over European countries. After 30 years of repeated campaigns, terrestrial rabies has been eliminated from the whole of Western Europe. Oral fox vaccination is continuing in the Balkans and Eastern Europe. In North America live vaccinia recombinant vaccine expressing rabies glycoprotein is used to control rabies in raccoons, coyotes and grey foxes. Skunks have a poor response, so new recombinant vaccines are being developed. In Latin America, vampire bat rabies is a major cause of death in cattle, with disastrous economic consequences. Specific control methods include bovine vaccination or treatment with anticoagulants, diphenadione or warfarin, to which bats, but not cattle, are highly sensitive. Anticoagulant or vaccine paste can be smeared on the backs of a few bats, and after they return to the roost it is licked off by other bats.

RABIES PROPHYLAXIS IN HUMANS

Although prophylaxis is usually given post-exposure as an emergency procedure after possible inoculation of the virus, there are immunological, practical and financial advantages in immunizing people at risk of infection in advance by pre-exposure vaccination.

Post-exposure Prophylaxis

This treatment is needed after suspected contact with rabies virus through an open wound or mucous membrane (Figure 17.6). Intact skin is a barrier against infection. Post-exposure treatment is aimed at killing or neutralizing rabies virus in a wound before it enters a nerve ending. Once within the nervous system, virions are apparently inaccessible to immune attack and disease is inevitable. Post-exposure treatment has three components: wound treatment, active immunization and passive immunization with rabies immune globulin.

Assessing the Risk of Rabies Infection

Knowledge of the local epidemiology of rabies vectors, the circumstances of the animal bite or contact and the health and behaviour of the animal, all contribute to assessment of the risk of exposure to rabies. An unprovoked attack by an unvaccinated sick animal indicates a high risk, but so does contact with a paralysed or unusually tame wild mammal. Unusual contact with a bat is a potential risk even if a wound is not visible. Vaccinated animals have also transmitted rabies. In endemic areas, strenuous efforts should be made to have the biting animal put down and its brain examined for rabies. If the animal has escaped or there is any doubt, post-exposure prophylaxis should be given, irrespective of the length of time since the bite. The official WHO recommendations[53] are summarized in Table 17.3.

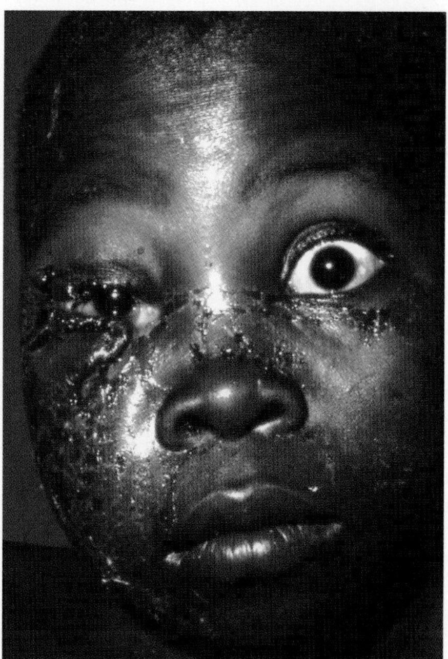

Figure 17.6 Facial bites inflicted by a rabid dog in Nigeria. *(Copyright © D. A. Warrell.)*

Wound Treatment. Immediate cleaning of the wound or site of contact with a rabid animal is imperative by scrubbing all wounds with concentrated soap solution or detergent and copious running water for 5 minutes or more. If possible, swab with a virucidal agent: iodine solutions or 40–70% alcohol.[54] Concentrated quaternary ammonium compounds (at least 1% benzalkonium chloride) are effective against rabies but they are

TABLE 17.3 Recommended Criteria for Post-Exposure Treatment

Type of Exposure	Criteria	Action[a]
No exposure[b]	Touching animals or licks on intact skin	No treatment
Minor exposure (WHO Category II)	Nibbling (tooth contact) with uncovered skin, or minor scratches or abrasions without bleeding	Start vaccine immediately
Major exposure (WHO Category III)	Single or multiple bites or scratches that break the skin, or licks on broken skin, or licks or saliva on mucosae, or physical contact with bats	Immediate rabies immunoglobulin and vaccine
Severe exposure (WHO Category III)	Bites on the head, neck, hands or multiple bites	Immediate rabies immunoglobulin is mandatory with vaccine

[a]For all cases: stop treatment if the dog or cat remains healthy for 10 days; stop treatment if animal's brain proves negative for rabies by appropriate investigation; exposure to rodents, rabbits and hares seldom, if ever requires specific anti-rabies prophylaxis.
[b]This is 'WHO Category I', but that name is misunderstood as implying some risk and might lead to unnecessary treatment. This scheme is a modification of WHO recommendations.[53]

neutralized by soap and are not generally recommended.[55] Energetic wound cleaning may require local or even general anaesthesia. Suturing should be delayed or avoided to prevent inoculation of virus deeper into the tissues.

Tetanus prophylaxis may be required, and other bacterial infections associated with mammal bites may be treated with antibiotics, e.g. *Pasteurella multocida* is usually sensitive to ampicillin, tetracycline and co-trimoxazole.

Active Immunization: Vaccine Treatment. All current human rabies vaccines contain inactivated whole virus which has been grown on a variety of substrates, usually in tissue culture. Fibroblast grown human diploid cell vaccine (HDCV) was introduced 40 years ago. Two vaccines are now widely exported: a purified chick embryo cell vaccine (PCECV) Rabipur® or RabAvert® manufactured in Germany or India, and a French purified vero cell vaccine (PVRV) Verorab®. A vial of PVRV contains 0.5 mL, whereas other vaccines are 1 mL/vial. A purified duck embryo vaccine (PDEV) Vaxirab®, originally made in Switzerland is now produced in India. Tissue culture vaccines are also made, mainly for local use, in India, Japan and Russia. Chinese vaccines are being exported.

The only rabies vaccines fulfilling WHO criteria are PCECV, PVRV, HDCV and for intramuscular (IM) use only, PDEV.

Post-exposure Vaccine Regimens for Tissue Culture Vaccines (Table 17.4)[53,56,57]

Intramuscular Regimens

The *standard intramuscular (IM) 5-dose (Essen) regimen* is as follows:

- Days 0, 3, 7, 14 and 28: one vial IM into the deltoid (or anterolateral thigh in children, but never the gluteal region).

An *alternative method* is a *2–1-1 IM (Zagreb) regimen*:

- Day 0: 2 IM doses (deltoids)
- Days 7 and 21: 1 IM one vial (deltoid).

A total of 4 doses, but the antibody level is likely to fall more rapidly.

Intradermal Regimens.[57,58] The prohibitive cost of IM treatment may be reduced using less vaccine injected intradermally (ID), taking advantage of the dermal antigen presenting dendritic and Langhans cells which facilitate antigen transfer to local lymph nodes. T cells are thereby activated more efficiently and rapidly than after IM inoculation. Multiple site ID doses have proved immunogenic and economical. The distribution of sites is designed to stimulate different groups of lymph nodes. Sharing vials of vaccine is economical and vaccine should not be wasted. Opened ampoules must be kept in the refrigerator and used within 8 hours. Any left over can be used as pre-exposure ID vaccination for relatives or others. A new syringe and needle must be used for each patient with strict aseptic precautions.

Two post-exposure ID regimens were approved by the WHO in 1997: an eight-site regimen and a two-site regimen.

The *eight-site ID economical regimen.* This method is only practical with vaccines of 1 mL/vial, PCECV and HDCV. Although recognized as the most immunogenic,[59] it is inconvenient and cannot be used with 0.5 mL/vial vaccines. It is therefore now replaced by the 4-site regimen which is exactly the same as the 8-site method but uses half the number of injection sites and twice the vaccine dose per site. Unlike the 8-site method, it can be used economically with all the vaccines.

The *4-site ID regimen.*[57] The dose per ID site for this regimen depends on the volume per vial. For PVRV (0.5 mL/vial) the ID dose is 0.1 mL/site, and for PCECV or HDCV (1.0 mL/vial) the equivalent ID dose is 0.2 mL/ site. If injecting 0.2 mL ID proves difficult, the needle is withdrawn and the remainder injected into an adjacent area.

- Day 0: a whole vial of vaccine is used in giving four ID injections of 0.1/0.2 mL approx., depending on the vaccine (deltoids and suprascapular or thighs)
- Day 7: two ID sites 0.1/0.2 mL (deltoids)
- Day 28: one ID site 0.1/0.2 mL (deltoid).

This regimen is as immunogenic as the ‘gold standard’ 5 dose IM regimen.[60] Less than 2 IM doses of vaccine are needed if vials are shared, a 60% reduction of the IM regimen. Only three visits (days 0, 7 and 28) are required, the same timing as the pre-exposure course. Injecting a whole vial of vaccine divided between ID sites on day 0, with no sharing is more practicable for use in small clinics, and gives the best chance of survival to patients who default. Accidental subcutaneous instead of ID injection should not impair the immunogenicity because a whole vial is used on the first crucial day. Furthermore, half the

TABLE 17.4 Rabies Vaccine Regimens

Regimen	Route	Days of Injection Superscript = Number of Injection Sites						Total Number of Vials of Vaccine
Pre-Exposure	IM or ID[a]	0		7		21	→28	IM 3 or ID 0.3/0.6
Post-Exposure[b]								
IM 5 dose	IM	0	3	7	14		28	5
IM 4 dose	IM	0^2		7		21		4
2-site ID	ID[a]	0^2	3^2	7^2			28^2	<2
4-site ID	ID[c]	0^4[d]		7^2			28	<2
Post-Exposure if Previous Vaccine								
IM 2 dose	IM	0	3					2
4-site ID	ID[a]	0^4						1 or 0.4 mL

[a]ID dose is 0.1 mL/site with all vaccines.
[b]Rabies immune globulin also given on day 0 with all regimens.
[c]Volume of ID dose is 0.2 mL/site with PCECV and HDCV, 0.1 mL/site with PVRV.
[d]Using whole vial of vaccine, divided between 4 sites. See text for details.

dose is immunogenic in trial conditions. This indicates a wide margin of safety even in inexperienced hands.

The *2-site ID economical regimen*[61] consists of:

- Days 0, 3, 7 and 28: two ID injections (deltoids).

The ID dose for many years depended on the vaccine volume per vial, 0.1/0.2 mL/site. The WHO then declared that the ID dose must be 0.1 mL/site for all products. The dose of vaccines of 1 mL/vial is therefore halved, with the result that some countries demand higher potency vaccine batches for use with this regimen.

The manufacturer's instructions should be followed for all other vaccines.

Post-exposure Treatment for those who have had Previous Vaccination. Wound care and booster doses of vaccine are still vital and urgent. Provided that a full pre- or post-exposure course of one of the recommended vaccines (Table 17.4) has been given, or if at least 0.5 IU/mL of rabies neutralizing antibody has been documented following any other treatment, a short booster course vaccine is given and no passive immunization required. Otherwise, a full course of vaccine and rabies immune globulin are advised. Two booster regimens are recommended:

A *two dose IM regimen*, vaccine is given on days 0 and 3.

A *4-site ID single day regimen*, four ID 0.1 mL doses of vaccine given on deltoid and thigh ares. This is as immunogenic as the IM regimen.[62,63] A whole dose of vaccine of 0.5 mL/vial is used. With 1 mL/vial vaccines, sharing a vial with precautions (see above) is economical in clinics treating more than one patient a day. Vaccine must not be wasted; any remainder can be also used as pre-exposure immunization. Otherwise, it is more practical, and safer in inexperienced hands, to recommend using a whole ampoule of any vaccine divided between 4 ID sites (deltoids and suprascapular or thighs) on a single day.

Side-effects of Tissue Culture Vaccines. Minor local reactions occur in 2–74% of vaccinees, and include pain, erythema, swelling, aching and paraesthesia. Multiple-site ID injections cause local itching in 7–64% in different studies. Mild systemic reactions, reported by 3–40% of vaccines, consist of influenza-like symptoms, headache, fever, malaise, myalgia, nausea, dizziness or a rash.

Booster doses of HDCV, usually about a year after previous treatment, have caused systemic allergic reactions in 6% of American vaccinees. After 3–13 days, urticaria, rash, angio-oedema and arthralgia appear, but always respond promptly to symptomatic treatment.

Extremely rare neurological illness following HDCV is either Guillain–Barré-like (in four patients) or local limb weakness (in two patients). PCECV has also been implicated in two neurological illnesses. Recovery is usually rapid, and none has been fatal.[64,65]

Rabies vaccines have been used widely in pregnancy without problems.

Nervous Tissue Vaccines (NTVs). Although they are being phased out, these homogenates of infected animal brains are still in use in some countries in Asia, Africa and South America. Sheep brain Semple vaccine, first produced in 1911, is used in Pakistan. Seven to 14 daily injections are given subcutaneously (SC) over the anterior abdominal wall; a large area able to accommodate the 2–5 mL doses of vaccine. Fuenzalida's suckling mouse brain vaccine is used in parts of South America and Africa. The potency of NTVs is variable, and treatment failures occur. They should not be used for pre-exposure prophylaxis. Although post-vaccinal encephalitis is a serious complication, post-exposure treatment is urgent, so if it is the only vaccine available, treatment can be started and changed to tissue culture vaccine at any time.

Post-vaccinal Encephalomyelitis following Nervous Tissue Vaccines.[47] This is an inflammatory, demyelinating, autoimmune response due to sensitization by myelin and other neural antigens contained in the vaccine. Estimates of its incidence vary with different products, but the frequency is up to 1:220 recipients of Semple vaccine, with a mortality rate of 3%. Symptoms usually appear within 2 weeks of starting the course, but may not appear until 2 months later. Suckling mouse brain vaccines have a lower complication rate (1:8000 to 1:27 000) but peripheral nervous system signs, such as Guillain–Barré-like syndrome, frequently predominate and are fatal in 22% of cases.

A wide variety of neurological signs include polyneuritis often involving limbs, transverse myelitis, ascending paralysis and meningoencephalitis. It can be clinically identical to paralytic rabies. Corticosteroid therapy (e.g. prednisolone 40–60 mg/day) is conventional, and cyclophosphamide in addition has been suggested. No further nervous tissue vaccine must be given, but the course completed with a tissue culture vaccine. Recovery often occurs within 2 weeks and is usually complete, but neurological deficits can persist.

Passive Immunization. *Rabies immune globulin (RIG)* provides passive protection by neutralizing virus in a wound in the interval before vaccine-induced antibody appears, 7–10 days after starting a primary post-exposure course.

The efficacy of RIG treatment combined with rabies vaccine has been proved by animal studies and natural experiments when wolves have bitten groups of people in Iran[66] and China.[67] The mortality from head wounds was reduced fivefold by the addition of immune serum to vaccine treatment.[68]

A dose of 40 IU/kg of *equine RIG* or 20 IU/kg of *human RIG* should ideally accompany every primary post-exposure vaccine course, but it is essential following severe bites: that is, on the head, neck or hands, and multiple or deep bites. RIG is infiltrated around the wound if anatomically possible, and any remaining injected IM at a site remote from the vaccine, but not into the gluteal region. RIG given days or even hours before the first vaccine dose impairs the immune response.[69] Increasing the dose of RIG may reduce the immunogenicity of the vaccine. RIG is prohibitively expensive and is unobtainable in large areas including many entire countries of Asia and Africa.

A large study showed an incidence of reactions to equine and human RIG of 1.8% and 0.09%, respectively, and serum sickness occurred in 0.72% and 0.007% of recipients.[70] An intradermal skin test does not predict anaphylaxis or most other reactions and it is no longer recommended.[53] Adrenaline (epinephrine) should be at hand in case of anaphylaxis.

Efficacy of Post-exposure Prophylaxis

The untreated mortality from rabid animal bites depends on the part of the body affected and the severity of the bite. Data from the pre-vaccine era give an estimate of the chance of infection from suspect rabid dogs. The mortality from multiple bites on the head was 60–80%, from a single facial bite 30%, and from bites on the hand 15–67%. In India, the overall mortality from proven rabid dog bites was 35–57% but no information on wound treatment was given in these studies.

If wound treatment, tissue culture vaccine and RIG are given on the day of the bite in the correct manner, prophylaxis is virtually 100% effective. Nevertheless, patients are known to have died of rabies despite receiving these vaccines.[71] This mortality has been attributed to human or circumstantial failure to deliver optimum treatment, and not to reduced antigen content or other failure of tissue culture vaccines.

Possible reasons for failure of post-exposure prophylaxis are as follows:

1. Any delay in starting treatment increases the chance of the rabies virus entering neurons before the immune response is generated. The mortality following head wounds from Iranian rabid wolves doubled if vaccine was delayed beyond 8 days.[68] Treatment is urgent, and it is never too late to begin. Vaccine and RIG should be used even if the bite occurred months before.
2. Wound cleaning is omitted or inadequate.
3. Errors in the timing, dose or delivery of vaccine. For example failure to complete the course or injecting vaccine into the gluteal area.
4. Failure to give rabies immune globulin or to infiltrate the wound, especially with severe exposure.
5. A poor immune response to vaccine due to chronic disease (e.g. HIV infection, cirrhosis) or immunosuppressive drugs (e.g. steroids).

Rabies genotype 1 viruses show a high degree of homology with the strains used in vaccine production, but there is great antigenic diversity within the genus. Vaccine efficacy against other genotypes is related to their proximity on the genetic tree.[2] Australian bat *Lyssavirus* and genotype 6, EBLV2, are close to genotype 1, and vaccines have some effect against all Phylogroup I. There is no protection afforded against Phylogroup II lyssaviruses.

Pre-exposure Prophylaxis

No deaths from rabies have been reported in anyone who has had pre-exposure treatment and booster injections after exposure. Pre-exposure prophylaxis[53,56] is advisable for anyone likely to be in contact with a rabid animal. This may include veterinarians, animal handlers, laboratory staff, zoologists, wildlife enthusiasts, health workers, residents of and travellers to endemic areas where dogs are the dominant vector species. The duration of travel has been a criterion for vaccination, but half of exposures to a risk of rabies occurred in the first 10 days in visitors to Thailand.[72] The need for prophylaxis depends on an assessment of risk of contact with a possibly rabid animal at the destination, in view of the traveller's intended activities.

A pre-exposure vaccine course is three doses of one of the recommended vaccines (Table 17.4), given IM on days 0, 7 and 28. The third dose may be advanced towards day 21 if short of time. An economical alternative is ID injections of 0.1 mL at the same intervals.[53,57] If the injection is too deep, withdraw the needle and repeat the procedure. A separate syringe must be used for each patient, and other precautions when sharing vaccine vials (see above). Chloroquine taken as malaria prophylaxis is immunosuppressive to ID primary vaccination, so give by the IM route. Vaccinees must keep a record of their immunization. If there is no time for a complete course before travelling, start vaccination. Having had any vaccine will increase chances of survival if exposed to rabies, but if the course is incomplete full post-exposure treatment will be needed.

A booster dose 1–2 years after the primary course increases the persistence of antibody to 10 years in 96% of people in a study of IM treatment.[73] Although the titre of antibody falls more rapidly after ID than IM inoculation, the response to a booster dose is similar, whatever the original route. Confirmation of seroconversion is unnecessary unless immunosuppression is suspected. Booster doses may be given intradermally or intramuscularly at intervals depending on the risk of infection. Boosters are not necessary if the rabies neutralizing antibody level is at least 0.5 IU/mL.

Laboratory staff handling rabies virus should have a serology test or booster injection every 6 months, but others may require booster doses after 2–10 years according to their risk of exposure. Travellers who will have rapid access to vaccine if exposed need not have further immunization, and in the USA no boosters are given at all. However, if medical resources will be unreliable, booster vaccination may be advisable before departure, if 3–5 years have elapsed since the last dose. It is always preferable to have an antibody test before repeat vaccination as most people will have persistent antibody, and not need vaccine.

REFERENCES

3. Nel LH, Markotter W. Lyssaviruses. Crit Rev Microbiol 2007;33:301–24.
13. Helmick CG, Tauxe RV, Vernon AA. Is there a risk to contacts of patients with rabies? Rev Infect Dis 1987;9:511–18.
22. Schnell MJ, McGettigan JP, Wirblich C, et al. The cell biology of rabies virus: using stealth to reach the brain. Nat Rev Microbiol 2010;8(1): 51–61.
34. Warrell DA. The clinical picture of rabies in man. Trans R Soc Trop Med Hyg 1976;70: 188–95.
57. Warrell MJ. Current rabies vaccines and prophylaxis schedules: preventing rabies before and after exposure. Travel Med Infect Dis 2012;10: 1–15.

Access the complete references online at www.expertconsult.com

18

Rotavirus and Other Viral Diarrhoea

NIGEL A. CUNLIFFE | ROGER I. GLASS | OSAMU NAKAGOMI

KEY POINTS

- Rotavirus, norovirus, sapovirus, enteric adenovirus and astrovirus are established aetiological agents of acute gastroenteritis across all age groups in all settings.
- Rotavirus is the single most important pathogen associated with severe dehydrating gastroenteritis in infants and young children worldwide.
- Norovirus causes sporadic and epidemic disease in adults and children.
- All gastroenteritis viruses infect the epithelial cells of the intestinal mucosa, causing acute, non-inflammatory watery diarrhoea mostly of less than 1 week duration.
- Aetiological diagnosis requires the detection of either specific antigens of each virus with immunologic assays, or the presence of the viral genome with molecular assays or visualization of virus by electron microscopy.
- Treatment is primarily supportive and consists of rehydration and restoration of electrolyte balance.
- Two live, oral, attenuated vaccines, Rotarix and RotaTeq, have been developed to prevent global morbidity and mortality due to rotavirus infection.
- Both rotavirus vaccines are entering childhood immunization schedules following successful clinical trials in representative populations worldwide, with early evidence of substantial impact.

Introduction

The gastrointestinal tract is the commonest portal of entry for a variety of pathogens, including viruses, but not all of these viruses are causally associated with diarrhoeal disease. Among the viruses that infect enterocytes, or at least use them as a portal of entry, there are two major groups. The first group comprises those viruses that cause systemic infections after entering into the body through the gastrointestinal tract, and diarrhoea, if ever present, is not a major feature of infection. This group includes many enteroviruses, including poliovirus and coxsackieviruses, hepatitis A and E viruses and some adenoviruses. The second group comprises viruses that infect the upper small intestine and cause non-inflammatory diarrhoea. There are currently five established gastroenteritis viruses affecting humans, i.e. *Rotavirus*, *Norovirus*, *Sapovirus*, Human *Astrovirus*, and *Human Adenovirus F* (formerly called group F adenovirus).

Rotavirus

Human rotavirus was discovered in 1973 on thin-section electron microscopy of duodenal biopsies from a child with acute gastroenteritis.[1] Virus particles were subsequently identified in large numbers in faeces by direct negative-stain electron microscopy[2] and significant antibody titre rises were demonstrated between acute and convalescent sera from diarrhoeal children by using immune electron microscopy.[3] The virus was named rotavirus because of its characteristic wheel-shaped (*rota* = Latin for wheel) morphology on electron microscopy (Figure 18.1).

EPIDEMIOLOGY

Virtually all children are infected with rotavirus at least once by the age of 3–5 years, whether they live in developing or developed countries. However, the consequences of infection are markedly different according to geographic location, with over 95% of deaths due to rotavirus diarrhoea occurring in the developing countries of the Indian subcontinent, sub-Saharan Africa and Latin America (Figure 18.2).[4–6] Rotavirus diarrhoea occurs at an earlier age in children in developing countries than in children in developed countries (Figure 18.3). The median age of children hospitalized with rotavirus diarrhoea in many African and Asian counties is 6–9 months, and up to 80% are less than 1 year old. In contrast, the median age in developed countries is 13–16 months and the highest proportion of cases occurs in the 2nd year of life.[7,8] In temperate countries, rotavirus infections peak in the winter and early spring, with fewer cases detected at other times. In tropical countries, rotavirus infections characteristically occur throughout the year, although more cases are typically observed in the cooler and drier months. Although the mode(s) of transmission of rotavirus are not completely understood, person-to-person spread of rotavirus by the faecal–oral route is likely to play a central role.

In both developing and developed countries, rotavirus is the major cause of severe gastroenteritis requiring hospitalization. It was estimated that, from 1986 to 1999, a median of 22% (range 17–28%) of acute diarrhoea cases in children less than 5 years of age were due to rotavirus[4] but this proportion nearly doubled from 2000 to 2004 to 39% (range 29–45%),[5] related in part to the widespread application of more sensitive detection methods, and to a decrease in the proportion of gastroenteritis caused by bacterial pathogens. The annual global mortality due to rotavirus diarrhoea among children less than 5 years of age has been estimated as 453 000 in the pre-rotavirus vaccine era, with rotavirus accounting for 37% of all diarrhoea deaths and 5% of all-cause deaths in children under 5 years of age.[9] The Democratic Republic of Congo, Ethiopia, India, Nigeria, and

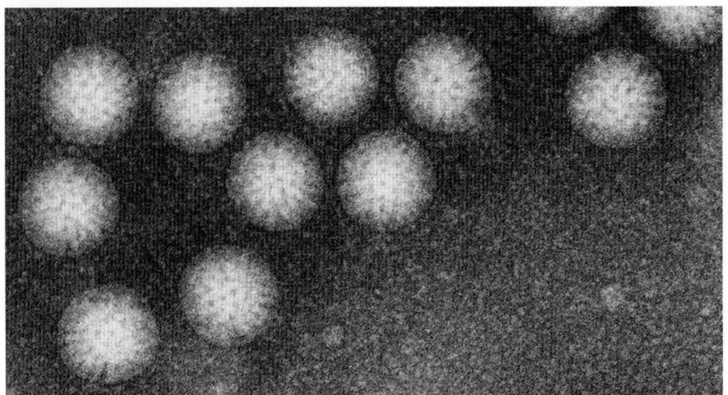

Figure 18.1 Negative-stain electron micrograph of rotavirus (×200 000).

Pakistan accounted for more than half of all rotavirus deaths, with India alone accounting for 22% of deaths.[9]

VIROLOGY

Rotavirus is a genus within the family *Reoviridae*, and within the genus there are seven groups (A–G), each of which represents a separate species, e.g. *Rotavirus A*, *Rotavirus B*, etc.[10] Only group A, B and C rotaviruses are established human pathogens. Group A rotavirus has the greatest medical importance and, unless mentioned otherwise, the word rotavirus usually infers Group A rotavirus. Group B rotavirus infection is rare and affects both adults and children, causing both outbreaks and sporadic infections, primarily in China, India and Bangladesh.[11,12] Group C rotaviruses tend to affect older children than do group A rotaviruses, and up to one-third of adult humans have serological evidence of infection with Group C rotavirus.[13,14]

By conventional negative-stain electron microscopy, rotavirus has a characteristic double capsid appearance measuring approximately 75 nm in diameter (Figure 18.1), but cryo-electron microscopic studies demonstrated that the rotavirus virion comprises a triple-layered capsid with 60 spikes protruding from its surface, making its overall diameter nearly 100 nm. The outermost layer (outer capsid) consists of two proteins, VP4 and VP7, each of which independently serves as a neutralization antigen (Figure 18.4). The serotype defined by the VP4 protein is called the P type, for protease-sensitive protein (because VP4 is proteolytically cleaved into VP8* and VP5*), and the serotype defined by the VP7 protein is called the G type, for glycoprotein. The middle capsid consists of the most abundant viral protein, VP6, which is the major protein against which non-neutralizing antibodies are raised during infection. The core or the innermost layer consists of VP2, a scaffolding protein, and inside this layer are VP1 (viral RNA-dependent RNA polymerase) and VP3 (guanyltransferase), which is present in association with the 11 segments of double-stranded genomic RNA. In addition to these five structural proteins, there are six non-structural proteins (NSPs), each of which is encoded by a single genome segment, except for NSP5 and NSP6 (encoded by RNA segment 11), which carry out various functions during replication and morphogenesis. NSP4 is a chaperone protein enabling the subviral particle to acquire the outer capsid proteins VP4 and VP7 during the later phases of viral morphogenesis. NSP4 also acts as a viral enterotoxin, causing diarrhoea in newborn mice.[15–17]

Rotavirus genomic RNA can be extracted directly from clinical specimens and separated by polyacrylamide gel electrophoresis (PAGE). With this, two major RNA migration patterns are recognized in which genome segments 10 and 11 of long RNA pattern viruses migrate faster than do those of short RNA pattern viruses (Figure 18.5).[18] The precise migration pattern is

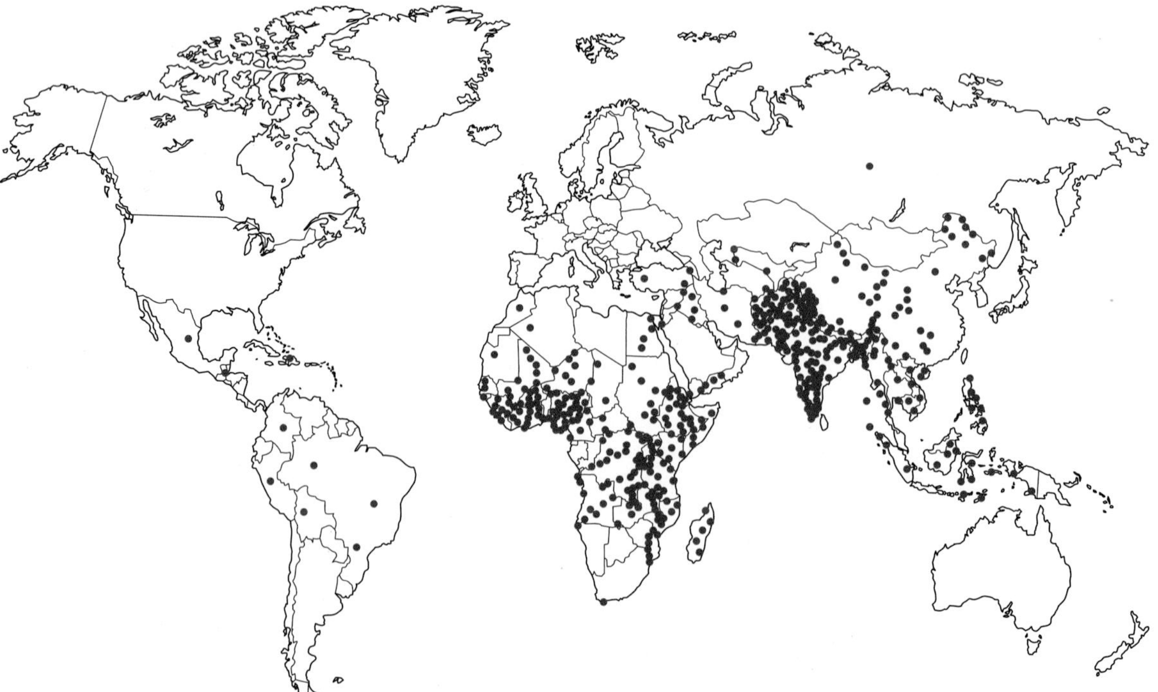

Figure 18.2 Map of global distribution of rotavirus mortality in children less than 5 years of age. Each dot represents 1000 deaths. *(Reprinted from Parashar UD, Gibson CJ, Bresse JS, et al. Rotavirus and severe childhood diarrhea. Emerg Infect Dis 2006;12:304–6.)*

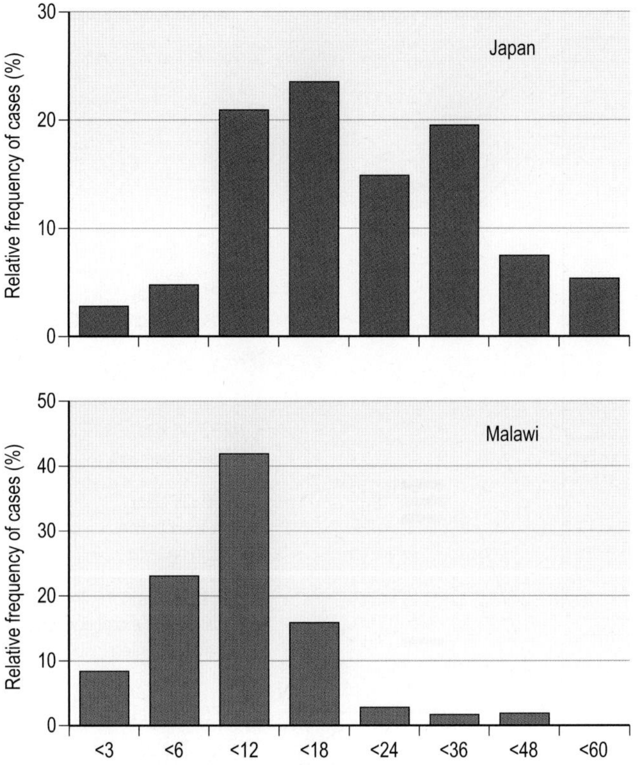

Figure 18.3 Two contrasting patterns of age distribution of rotavirus diarrhoea occurring in Malawi (as an example of a developing country) and in Japan (as an example of a developed country). *(Data from Nakagomi T, Nakagomi O, Takahashi Y, et al. Incidence and burden of rotavirus gastroenteritis in Japan as estimated from a prospective sentinel hospital study. J Infect Dis 2005;192 (Suppl 1):106–10. and Cunliffe NA, Ngwira BM, Dove W, et al. Epidemiology of rotavirus infections in children in Blantyre, Malawi,1997–2007. J Infect Dis 2010;202:S168–74.)*

characteristic for each rotavirus strain and is called an 'electropherotype', which was extensively applied in molecular epidemiological studies, until the use of genotyping and sequencing methods became more widespread.[19]

The serotype is the most important antigenic determinant of rotavirus and is defined by serological assays. However, serological typing methods have been largely replaced by molecular typing (genotyping). In addition to VP7 (G) and VP4 (P) genotyping, a nucleotide sequence-based, complete genome classification system has recently been introduced for rotavirus classification;[20] the genome of individual rotavirus strains is given the complete descriptor of Gx-P[x]-Ix-Rx-Cx-Mx-Ax-Nx-Tx-Ex-Hx. Of these 11 genotypes, the G and P genotypes have been extensively investigated because of their importance in protective immunity. There are thus far 26 G genotypes and 35 P genotypes reported among human and animal rotaviruses, but the G and P type combinations (Figure 18.6) detected in human rotaviruses are mostly limited to G1P[8], G2P[4], G3P[8], G4P[8] and G9P[8].[21,22] However, G12 strains have now emerged across the world,[23] and G8 strains with either P[6] or P[4] account for a significant proportion of human rotavirus strains in Africa.[24,25] Such genetic diversity is generated by frequent reassortment of the genome segments and interspecies transmission of rotaviruses between humans and animals.[26–28]

PATHOGENESIS

Rotavirus exclusively infects the mature differentiated villous enterocytes of the small intestine. Rotavirus attaches to its cellular receptors (sialoglycoprotein and integrins) via the VP4 protein. The minimum infective dose is as low as 10^2–10^3 virus particles in adult volunteers.[29] Progeny virus is produced after 10–12 h, and released in large numbers into the intestinal lumen ready to infect other cells. The pathogenesis of rotavirus diarrhoea includes both malabsorptive and secretory components.[30] Malabsorption may be consequent upon damage to mature absorptive enterocytes resulting in malabsorption of nutrients, electrolytes and water; virus-induced downregulation of the expression of absorptive enzymes; and functional changes in tight junctions between enterocytes leading to paracellular leakage. Biopsies show atrophy of the villi and mononuclear cell infiltrates in the lamina propria. Secretory mechanisms include those mediated by activation of the enteric nervous system and the effect of NSP4, the latter being via activation of cellular Cl^- channels, leading to increased Cl^- and consequently water secretion. Rotavirus infection was previously thought to be limited to the intestine, but rotavirus causes viraemia for at least a short period in the acute phase of infection in immunocompetent infants as well as in experimentally infected animals.[31] The clinical significance of this systemic spread of rotavirus remains unclear.

IMMUNITY

In general, one or more episodes of rotavirus infection confer protection against subsequent moderate or severe rotavirus diarrhoea but not against asymptomatic reinfection or mild diarrhoea. Furthermore, infection with one serotype generally provides serotype-specific (homotypic) protection, and repeated infections lead to partial cross-serotype (heterotypic) protection. These beliefs are supported by the findings of a cohort study in Mexico, where children who had experienced one, two or three episodes of rotavirus diarrhoea had adjusted relative risks of experiencing a further attack of rotavirus diarrhoea of 0.23, 0.17 and 0.08, respectively, and of asymptomatic rotavirus infection of 0.62, 0.40 and 0.34, respectively.[32] However in a cohort study in Vellore, India, while protection against moderate or severe disease increased with successive infections it was only 79% after three infections and no evidence of homotypic protection was demonstrated, indicating that immune protection following natural infection may vary by location.[33] In the Indian study, multiple infections were common, with only 30% of all identified infections being primary. Immunity following natural rotavirus infection is believed to be mediated by both humoral and cell-mediated immune responses.[34] Rotavirus-specific immunoglobulin (Ig) A antibodies on the enteric mucosal surface are thought to be the primary mediator of protective immunity. Cellular immunity is considered to be important in the resolution of rotavirus infection and appears to be cross-protective between the different G serotypes.[35]

Protection of neonates against rotavirus infection appears to be mediated by transplacentally acquired maternal antibody[36,37] and by antibodies and other factors in breast milk.[38] However, a study in Bangladesh showed that hospitalized children with rotavirus diarrhoea were more likely to be breast-fed than were children with diarrhoea due to other infectious agents.[39] Rotavirus infection in neonates often results in asymptomatic infection and

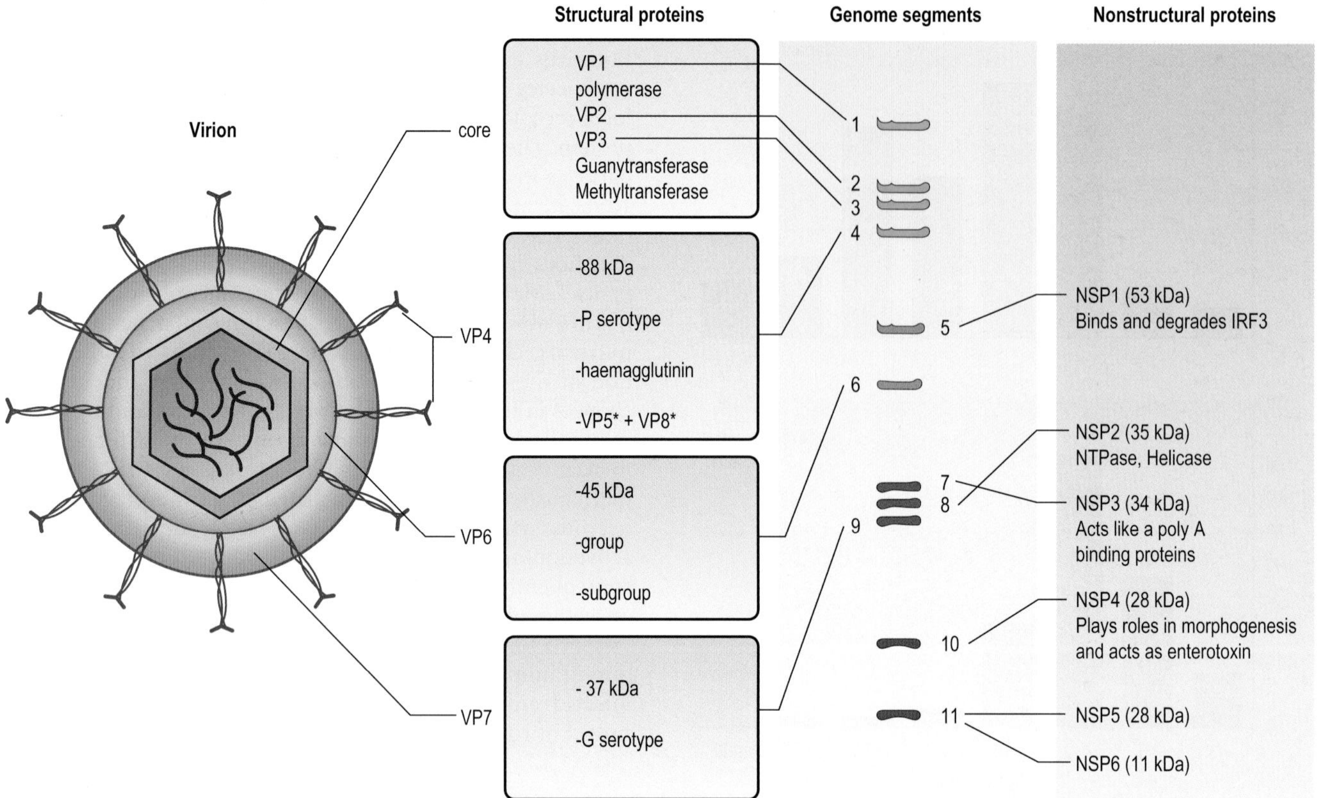

Figure 18.4 Schematic diagram showing the relationships between the structure of the rotavirus virion and the genomic double-stranded RNA segments. IRF3, interferon regulatory factor 3; NTPase, nucleotide triphosphatase.

rotavirus can therefore circulate silently in neonatal units. Neonatal strains are often unusual and can infect even in the presence of high titres of transplacental antibody from the mother. Asymptomatic neonatal infections may induce protection against subsequent severe rotavirus gastroenteritis.[40] Finally, it is increasingly recognized that otherwise healthy adults can experience rotavirus diarrhoea and elderly people can develop severe rotavirus gastroenteritis as their immunity wanes.[41,42]

CLINICAL FEATURES

The outcome of rotavirus infection varies from asymptomatic, through mild short-lived watery diarrhoea, to an overwhelming gastroenteritis with dehydration leading to death. The onset of symptoms is abrupt after a short incubation period of 1–2 days. Fever, vomiting and watery diarrhoea are seen in the majority of infected children and last for 2–6 days. Rotavirus diarrhoea tends to be more severe than that due to other common enteropathogens.[43] Extraintestinal manifestations during rotavirus gastroenteritis, including encephalopathy, have captured attention since rotavirus viraemia was reported.[44] It is not possible to distinguish rotavirus gastroenteritis from other viral causes of diarrhoea solely on clinical grounds.[45] The stools are usually watery or loose, and are seldom blood-stained. In severe cases, the cause of death is dehydration, which can be hypo- or hypernatraemic and is often associated with metabolic acidosis. Underlying conditions such as malnutrition may be a risk factor for a more severe disease outcome. Rotavirus does not appear to produce more severe disease in HIV-infected infants.[46,47]

DIAGNOSIS

Large numbers of rotavirus particles (up to 10^{11}/g of faeces) are excreted during the acute phase of infection. Children with severe diarrhoea excrete more virus than do children with less severe diarrhoea.[48] Rotavirus can be detected in stool specimens by a number of techniques, including electron microscopy, PAGE, antigen detection assays, RT-PCR and virus isolation. Electron microscopy remains a valuable diagnostic tool since it is a catch-all technique that will also detect other potential viral enteropathogens. PAGE is a convenient diagnostic tool for the detection of rotavirus RNA extracted directly from stool specimens (Figure 18.5). The assay also allows detection of non-group A rotaviruses, which fail to react in most antigen detection assays. PAGE is a relatively simple technique with high specificity for rotavirus (100%) and reasonable sensitivity (80–90%), and can be performed in tropical countries relatively cheaply.[49] It has the added advantage of providing epidemiological information because the electrophoretic migration pattern of the 11 segments of the double-stranded RNA genome is specific to each rotavirus strain.[18,50]

Antigen detection tests are currently the most widely used assays for rotavirus infection in diagnostic laboratories and include enzyme-linked immunosorbent assays (ELISAs), and immunochromatographic assays.[51] The sensitivity and specificity of the majority of these tests are generally high (90–95%) but they are designed to detect only group A rotaviruses. Detection of viral genome by RT-PCR is predominantly a research tool which provides information on the genotypes of the circulating strains[52–54] and the duration of viral shedding in stool

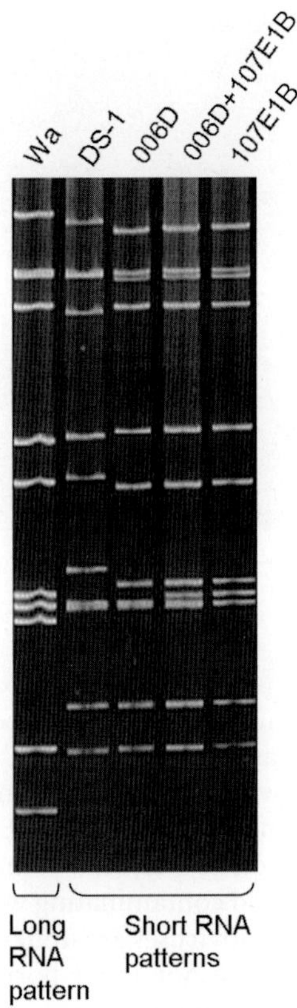

Figure 18.5 Separation of rotavirus genomic RNA into 11 bands by polyacrylamide gel electrophoresis. Two RNA patterns, long and short, are represented by prototype strains Wa and DS-1, respectively. Strains 006 and 107E1B have similar but distinct RNA electropherotypes. The differences in migration of segments 7, 8 and 9 are clearly demonstrated by co-electrophoresis in which RNAs from both 006 and 107E1B were loaded on the same lane. *(Adapted from Nakagomi T, Gentsch JR, Das BK, et al. Molecular characterization of serotype G2 and G3 human rotavirus strains that have an apparently identical electropherotype of the short RNA pattern. Arch Virol 2002;147: 2187–95.)*

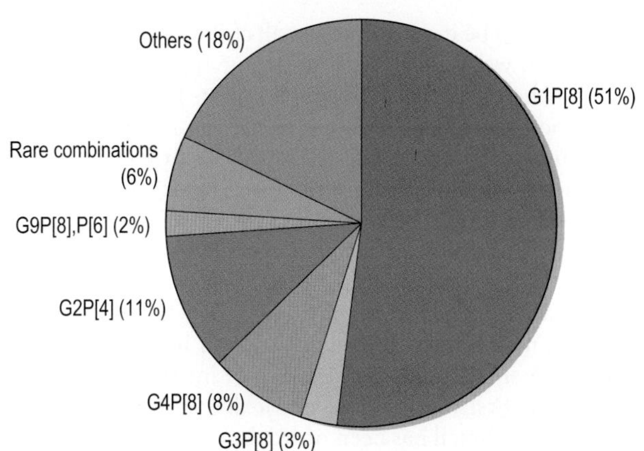

Figure 18.6 Relative frequencies of rotavirus genotypes detected globally among human rotaviruses over the period 1994–2003. *(Adapted from Gentsch JR, Laird AR, Bielfelt B, et al. Serotype diversity and reassortment between human and animal rotavirus strains: implications for rotavirus vaccine programs. J Infect Dis 2005;192(Suppl 1):146–59.)*

which can be prolonged.[55,56] Group A and group C rotaviruses can be isolated in cell culture but viral culture is limited to research purposes.

MANAGEMENT

The mainstay of management consists of assessment of dehydration and replacement of lost fluid by oral rehydration with fluids of specified electrolyte and glucose composition, together with administration of zinc in children over age 6 months and where the prevalence of malnutrition is high.[57] Intravenous rehydration therapy is indicated for patients with severe dehydration, shock or reduced levels of consciousness. Human or bovine colostrum and hyperimmune human serum immunoglobulin have been used to manage chronic rotavirus infection in immunocompromised children. Administration of probiotics such as *Lactobacillus casei* GG also appears beneficial. The antiprotozoal drug nitazoxanide was shown to decrease the median duration of rotavirus gastroenteritis by 44 hours in a randomized double-blind placebo-controlled trial in Egyptian children.[58] As an adjunct to oral rehydration, the antisecretory agent racecadotril reduces diarrhoea duration and stool volume in children with acute gastroenteritis.[59]

PREVENTION AND CONTROL

Since virtually all children will have experienced rotavirus infection by the age of 3–5 years in both developing and developed countries, it is clear that hygiene and sanitation practices are not sufficient to prevent the spread of rotavirus infection within the community. Thus, prevention of severe rotavirus gastroenteritis by vaccines remains the only practical preventive measure.[60] The first licensed rotavirus vaccine, a rhesus monkey rotavirus-based tetravalent human reassortant vaccine (RotaShield®), was withdrawn after this live, oral vaccine was associated with the development of intestinal intussusception in approximately 1 : 10 000 vaccine recipients in the USA, with intussusception cases occurring disproportionately in those infants who received their first dose of vaccine at over three months of age.[61,62] These unfortunate events stimulated the further development and testing of two additional live, oral rotavirus vaccines, Rotarix® (GlaxoSmithKline Biologicals) and RotaTeq® (Merck & Co.). Rotarix® is a monovalent, human rotavirus vaccine of serotype G1P1A[8] administered as a two-dose schedule, whereas RotaTeq® is a pentavalent, bovine–human reassortant vaccine comprising types G1, G2, G3, G4 and P[8] and is given in a 3-dose schedule.[63] Both vaccines were found to be safe in large, phase III clinical trials, each involving more than 60 000 infants and were 85–95% efficacious in preventing severe gastroenteritis due to rotavirus.[64,65] In countries that have introduced rotavirus vaccine into their childhood immunization programmes, hospitalizations due to rotavirus gastroenteritis have dramatically fallen.[66,67] Evidence of an indirect effect of rotavirus vaccines has been presented from the USA and other settings, with reduced incidence of disease in children too old to have been vaccinated and in adults.[66,67]

Both vaccines have recently been evaluated in clinical trials in Africa and Asia, where efficacy against severe rotavirus gastroenteritis was lower than previously experienced in other settings (50–75%), with poorer countries generally having lower efficacy (e.g. 50% in Malawi).[68–70] The reason for reduced efficacy in low-income countries is not yet known, but other live, oral vaccines against polio and cholera are known to be less efficacious in developing countries.[71,72] Despite more modest efficacy in low-income countries, the high burden of rotavirus disease led the WHO to issue a recommendation that rotavirus vaccines should be incorporated in all childhood immunization programmes worldwide, with a strong recommendation for countries where diarrhoeal disease accounts for more than 10% of childhood mortality.[73] Because of the age-related occurrence of intussusception, the WHO recommended that the first dose of vaccine should be administered by 15 weeks of age and that the full course should be completed by 32 weeks of age.[73]

An early indication of the major public health benefit that rotavirus vaccination can bring has been demonstrated in Mexico, where diarrhoea mortality has fallen since the introduction of Rotarix into its childhood immunization programme.[74] A small increase in the risk of intussusception noted following the first vaccine dose in Mexico and after the second vaccine dose in Brazil has been noted, but the risk is outweighed by the number of diarrhoea deaths that will be prevented.[75] A re-evaluation of the risk/benefit ratio of rotavirus vaccination, in particular the impact of vaccination on severe disease in high mortality settings, has led to a WHO recommendation that the age restrictions on immunization be removed but that surveillance for intussusception should be implemented to monitor vaccine safety.[76] Additional assessments should include examination of the impact of rotavirus vaccination on rotavirus epidemiology including the distribution of rotavirus strains. Early studies suggested an increase in prevalence of G2P[4] strains following Rotarix introduction in Brazil, but it remains unclear whether this results from immune pressure secondary to vaccine use or natural fluctuation in strain types.[77] Continuous global strain surveillance is required to address this question.[78]

Enteric Adenovirus

Adenovirus is an unenveloped DNA virus with an icosahedral capsid measuring 70–75 nm in diameter (Figure 18.7). Its genome comprises double-stranded linear DNA of 33–45 kbp. Taxonomically, human adenoviruses that primarily cause diarrhoea are classified as species *Human adenovirus F* (formerly called group F) within the genus *Mastadenovirus*, family *Adenoviridae*. Within *Human adenovirus F*, more often referred to as 'enteric adenovirus', two serotypes 40 and 41 are distinguished based upon virus neutralization assays. These enteric adenoviruses account for approximately 5% of cases of infantile diarrhoea, occurring most often in children under 2 years of age without a clear seasonality.[79] However, it was reported that enteric adenoviruses were detected in as many as 20% of hospitalized children in northern Taiwan.[80] Enteric adenoviruses are spread from person-to-person by the faecal–oral route. Adenoviruses were found contaminating water in poor sanitary settings,[81] but these adenoviruses are unlikely to be enteric adenoviruses. No food-borne nor water-borne spread of enteric adenoviruses has been documented.

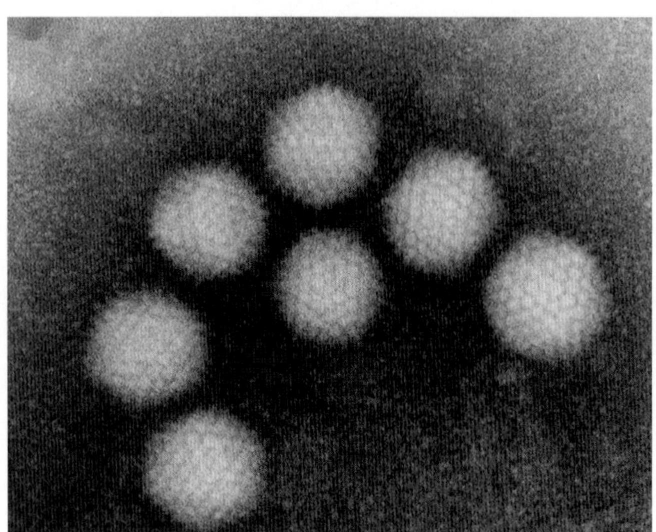

Figure 18.7 Negative-stain electron micrograph of enteric adenovirus (×200 000).

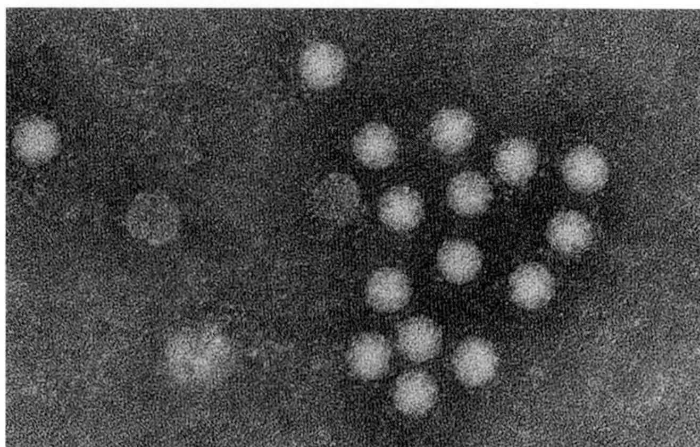

Figure 18.8 Negative-stain electron micrograph of astrovirus (×200 000).

The clinical features of enteric adenovirus gastroenteritis do not differ from those of rotavirus but the duration of diarrhoea tends to be longer in adenovirus infection than in rotavirus infection.[82,83] Other than gastroenteritis, adenovirus is implicated as a cause of idiopathic intussusception in infants.[84,85] These adenoviruses are of serotypes 1, 2, 3 and 5, and rarely of 40 or 41 (enteric adenoviruses).

The diagnosis of adenovirus infection is by visualization of characteristic virions in stool specimens under the electron microscope; demonstration of adenovirus antigens in stool by ELISA or immunochromatography or by detection of the genome by PCR which has much higher sensitivity.[80]

Treatment of adenovirus diarrhoea is by managing dehydration. There is neither a specific therapeutic intervention nor an available vaccine.

Astrovirus

Human astrovirus, a species in genus *Mamastrovirus*, family Astroviridae, has an unenveloped virion measuring 28–30 nm in diameter with a characteristic star shape 'stamped' on its surface, a five- or six-pointed star with an electron-dense centre (*astron* = Greek for a 'star') (Figure 18.8). Its genome is positive-sense single-stranded RNA approximately 7 kb in length, which encodes an RNA polymerase (ORF1a), a serine protease (ORF1b) and three capsid proteins (ORF2). While astrovirus was first described in humans in 1975, astrovirus can infect a variety of animal species.

There are eight serotypes of *Human astrovirus* with serotype 1 the most frequently detected.[86] Other serotypes can cause outbreaks of food-borne infections and there appears to be more diversity in developing countries.[87] More recently, however, a greater number of astroviruses in human stool have been found far beyond the eight serotypes of *Human astrovirus*;

while their association with disease has yet to be established, there are five additional novel astroviruses, MLB1, MLB2, VA1, VA2 and VA3, described on the basis of phylogenetic analysis.[88] Astrovirus infections predominate in young children aged between 4 months and 4 years, and account for between 2% and 10% of cases of diarrhoea in children. The disease tends to be milder and more frequently encountered in community-based studies.[89] One such study in Mexico estimated the incidence of astrovirus gastroenteritis to be 0.1 episodes/child per year.[90] Seroepidemiological studies have demonstrated that more than 90% of children in the USA will have experienced astrovirus infections by the age of 6–9 years.[91] Astrovirus has been detected in all countries where sufficiently sensitive detection methods have been used. In temperate countries it shows a similar seasonal distribution to rotavirus but peaks earlier.

Astrovirus is transmitted faeco–orally either directly or by ingestion of food. It infects the upper small intestine but the mechanism of diarrhoea is not known. The features of the illness are similar to those of rotavirus but may be milder and its duration is 4–5 days on average. However, in Bangladesh, astrovirus was found to be associated with prolonged diarrhoea.[87]

Diagnosis used to be solely by electron microscopy, but this is now being replaced by more sensitive and easy-to-perform ELISA or by detection of the genome by RT-PCR. Treatment is by managing dehydration. There is no vaccine available and little is known of immunity to infection, other than that children with immunodeficiency syndromes excrete the virus for long periods.[92]

Norovirus

VIROLOGY

Genus *Norovirus*, of which *Norwalk virus*[93] is the type species, belongs to the family *Caliciviridae*. Norovirus has an unenveloped virion with icosahedral symmetry, measuring 27–35 nm in diameter with a feathery-ragged outline (Figure 18.9). Its genome is positive-sense, single-stranded RNA, approximately 7 kb in length, with a stretch of poly A sequence at its 3′ terminus.[94] The genome contains three ORFs, of which ORF2 encodes VP1, a 59 kDa protein, on which the antigenicity of a virus strain is expressed. Since neither animal model nor cell culture systems are available to test the infectivity of norovirus other than human volunteers, serotypes of Norovirus have not been established. The genome of norovirus exhibits a great diversity and there are more than 30 genotypes that are distributed into five genogroups (GI–GV)[95] of which human noroviruses cluster into GI, GII and GIV.[96]

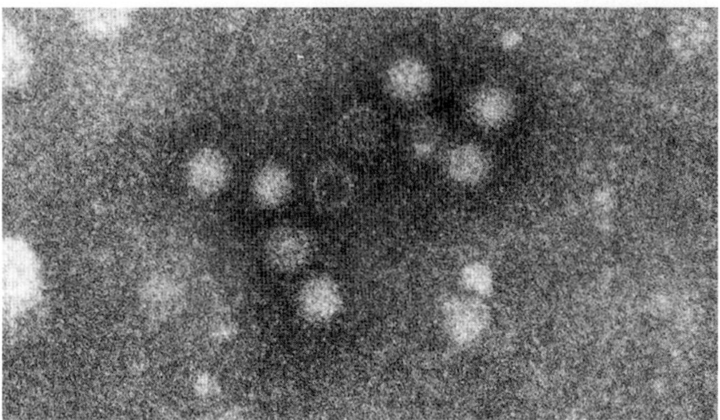

Figure 18.9 Negative-stain electron micrograph of norovirus with a feathery-ragged outline (×200 000).

EPIDEMIOLOGY

Norovirus spreads faeco–orally from person to person and from contaminated food and water; the respiratory route has also been suggested from epidemiological observations that aerosolized saliva or vomitus can be the source of infection.[97] In temperate countries, norovirus gastroenteritis tends to show winter seasonality. Norovirus was initially thought solely to cause epidemic gastroenteritis limited to older children and adults, but it is the cause of gastroenteritis in four epidemiological settings. These include: (1) Epidemic food-borne gastroenteritis that affects a large number of otherwise healthy adults over a short period of time; the illness usually resolves spontaneously without sequelae. (2) Sporadic gastroenteritis in the community.[98] (3) Healthcare-associated infections occurring in semi-closed settings such as hospital wards and residential homes resulting in often prolonged illness with increased severity. (4) Infantile diarrhoea in both developing and developed countries.[99] In a study in Finnish children, norovirus was responsible for 20% of gastroenteritis cases.[100] Similarly, in Iraq,[101] Libya,[102] and Brazil,[103] norovirus was detected in 30%, 18%, 15%, of diarrhoeal children less than 5 years of age, respectively. Norovirus is now the most common virus detected in children with acute gastroenteritis seeking medical attention in the US, where rotavirus vaccine has been part of the childhood immunization programme since 2006.[104]

CLINICAL FEATURES

Norovirus causes an illness with an abrupt onset of vomiting, diarrhoea and abdominal pain following an incubation period of 1–2 days. The illness is generally mild and fever rarely exceeds 38°C. Recovery follows within 1–3 days, but excretion of norovirus into stool lasts longer, sometimes up to 4 weeks. Approximately half of those infected with norovirus remain asymptomatic.

DIAGNOSIS

Similar to other viral gastroenteritis cases, diagnosis is based on the detection of virus in stool specimens. Historically, immune-electron microscopy was used to detect norovirus particles in stool specimens obtained in the acute phase of the illness. However, the diagnosis of norovirus gastroenteritis is now most commonly undertaken by sensitive, real-time PCR assays with genogroup-specific Taqman probes that provide both virus detection and quantification.[105] When the amount of virus is abundant, this will be followed by qualitative RT-PCR to amplify the end of ORF1 and the first part of ORF2 and subsequent sequencing to determine the genotype of a strain. In practice, a web-based genotyping tool is conveniently used (see: http://www.rivm.nl/mpf/norovirus/typingtool). Although much less sensitive than these molecular-based assays, commercial antigen detection kits have been developed; immune-chromatography, in particular, allows diagnosis at the point of care. While the specificity of such immunoassays is close to 100% for those norovirus genotypes to which antibodies used in the kit are raised, diagnostic accuracy in practice may be lower because of the antigenic diversity likely to be encountered.

IMMUNITY

Short-term homologous immunity (against the infecting strain) appears to follow an episode of norovirus gastroenteritis. However, great antigenic diversity permits repeated illness with different norovirus strains. It was noticed in early challenge studies with volunteers that there are individuals with natural resistance against some strains of norovirus. Recent progress in understanding the relationships between norovirus and histo-blood group antigens has partly solved this mystery.[106] Norovirus appears to use ABO and Lewis blood group antigens expressed on the mucosal surface of the enterocytes as viral receptors; thus, non-secretors, in whom such antigens are not expressed on the intestinal mucosa, are resistant to norovirus infection.[107] Recent studies propose an evolutionary model in which the most prevalent GII.4 noroviruses persist by altering histo-blood group antigen binding targets as well as changing epitopes surrounding the binding pocket over time.[108]

TREATMENT AND PREVENTION

There is no specific therapy. Vaccines using virus-like particles are under clinical development.

Sapovirus

Genus *Sapovirus* (the type species *Sapporovirus* was found in Sapporo, Japan[109]), within the family *Caliciviridae*, has an unenveloped virion with icosahedral symmetry, measuring 30–35 nm in diameter, with characteristic cup-like depressions (*calyx* = Greek for a 'cup', hence, *calici*[110]), on its surface (Figure 18.10). Negative-stain electron microscopy reveals characteristic particle morphology with cup-like depressions, often described as the 'Star of David' (Figure 18.10). Its genome is positive-sense, single-stranded RNA of approximately 7 kb in length with a stretch of poly A sequence at its 3′ terminus. Unlike norovirus, sapovirus encodes the capsid protein contiguous with the large non-structural polyprotein (ORF1). The junction that corresponds to ORF1 and ORF2 of norovirus consists of a one- or four-nucleotide overlap between the stop codon of ORF1 and the first AUG codon of ORF2. This creates a −1 frameshift. The 3′ end of ORF1 encodes a single polypeptide of 62 kDa.

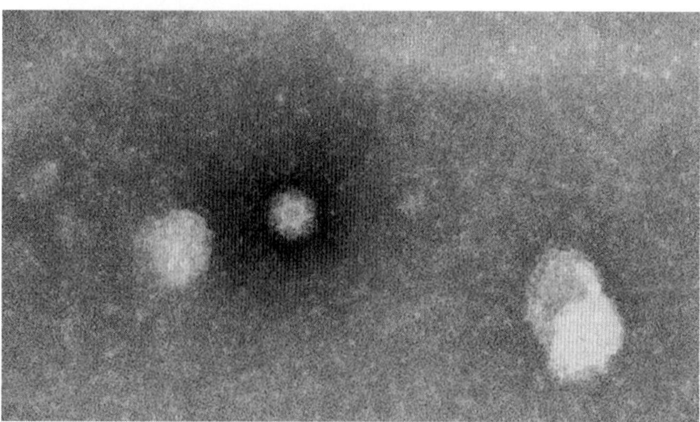

Figure 18.10 Negative-stain electron micrograph of a sapovirus with the classical 'Star of David' morphology (×200 000).

Illness due to sapovirus tends to predominantly occur in young children, and virtually all children appear to have experienced infection by sapovirus by the age of 5 years. Sapovirus gastroenteritis may occur year-round, although it seems to occur more frequently in winter. Sapovirus accounts for approximately 5% of cases of infantile diarrhoea[111,112] and is distributed globally. Sapovirus rarely causes outbreaks of food-borne gastroenteritis.

Sapovirus spreads faeco-orally and infects, and causes predominantly diarrhoea in infants and young children. Protective immunity appears to follow infection, since adults rarely get sapovirus gastroenteritis.

While a typical calicivirus-like morphology under the electron microscope strongly suggests the presence of sapovirus, the definitive diagnosis needs to be made based on either antigen detection or identification of the sapovirus genome by RT-PCR.[106]

Treatment is by management of dehydration. There is neither specific antiviral chemotherapy nor a vaccine available.

Other Viruses

A number of other viruses, including coronavirus[113] torovirus,[114] picobirnavirus[115,116] pestivirus,[117] Aichi virus[118] and bocavirus[119] have been detected in stool specimens of patients with acute gastroenteritis. Their clinical and epidemiologic significance as aetiological agents of diarrhoea is being investigated.

REFERENCES

9. Tate JE, Burton AH, Boschi-Pinto C, et al. WHO-coordinated Global Rotavirus Surveillance Network. 2008 estimate of worldwide rotavirus-associated mortality in children younger than 5 years before the introduction of universal rotavirus vaccination programmes: a systematic review and meta-analysis. Lancet Infect Dis 2012;12:136–41.
33. Gladstone BP, Ramani S, Mukhopadhya I, et al. Protective effect of natural rotavirus infection in an Indian birth cohort. N Engl J Med 2011;365: 337–46.
68. Madhi SA, Cunliffe NA, Steele AD, et al. Effect of human rotavirus vaccine on severe gastroenteritis in African infants. N Engl J Med 2010; 362:289–98.
74. Richardson V, Hernandez-Pichardo J, Quintanar-Solares M, et al. Effect of rotavirus vaccination on death from childhood diarrhea in Mexico. N Engl J Med 2010;362:299–305.
99. Glass RI, Parashar UD, Estes MK. Norovirus gastroenteritis. N Engl J Med 2009;361:1776–85.

Access the complete references online at www.expertconsult.com

19

Respiratory Viruses and Atypical Bacteria

PAUL S. McNAMARA | H. ROGIER VAN DOORN

KEY POINTS

- Viral and atypical pathogens can cause most clinical manifestations of respiratory disease, but some are associated with particular clinical conditions.
- Clinical disease from the common cold to severe lower respiratory tract infection with systemic dissemination.
- Pathogens generally have a global distribution but prevalence and disease burden often vary seasonally.
- Spectrum of pathogens from established endemic human-adapted viruses to emerging highly pathogenic viruses from animal reservoirs with pandemic threat.
- Severe disease can occur in all age groups but young children, the elderly and the immunocompromised are generally more at risk for severe disease.
- Bacterial and viral co-infection is increasingly being recognized as we test for more pathogens.
- There is a real clinical need to develop vaccines against the commonest viral and atypical bacterial pathogens.

Introduction

Acute respiratory infections are the most frequently occurring illnesses in all age groups globally. Although infections are usually limited to the upper respiratory tract and generally cause mild, self-limiting illnesses, a small percentage progress to the lower respiratory tract, where they can cause potentially life-threatening conditions, such as bronchiolitis and pneumonia.

Annually, 450 million cases of pneumonia are recorded, of whom 4.2 million die (7% of the world's yearly total annual deaths). Young children and the elderly are at particular risk, especially in developing countries: 151 million of 156 million reported episodes of childhood pneumonia are in the developing world. Pneumonia is responsible for about 17% of all deaths in children aged less than 5 years, of which more than 70% occur in sub-Saharan Africa and South-east Asia. In 2008, 1.6 million children under 5 died of pneumonia.[1–3]

Pneumonia is also a major cause of morbidity and mortality at the other end of the age spectrum. The annual incidence of pneumonia in elderly, non-institutionalized patients is between 25 and 44 per 1000 population; up to four times that of patients younger than 65.[4]

The most important aetiological agents of severe lower respiratory illness include bacteria such as *Streptococcus pneumoniae* and *Haemophilus influenzae* type b, and viruses such as respiratory syncytial virus and influenza virus. Bacteria are the main causes of pneumonia, and generally have a higher case fatality rate, although this may change with the widespread introduction of *H. influenzae* type b and pneumococcal conjugate vaccines, which could lead to viruses becoming much more prominent causes of respiratory disease. Viruses are the predominant cause of bronchiolitis and exacerbations of asthma and episodic viral wheeze. These clinical syndromes overlap considerably and are often difficult to tell apart.

The clinical manifestations of infection depend not only on the particular agent but also on the individual patient. Pre-existing structural changes to the respiratory tract caused by congenital malformations or damage from previous episodes of infection or trauma, as well as the circumstances of the individual (immunocompromise, malnutrition, poverty, overcrowding, sanitation, pollution, etc.), profoundly affect outcome.

Aetiology

Confirming the presence of a virus will often identify the cause of an illness, although multiple infections can and do occur and there is evidence of viral shedding in healthy individuals post-infection or asymptomatically. In this section, the commonest viruses associated with acute respiratory infection are described. Also mentioned are some organisms found in the respiratory tracts of clinically normal individuals (especially children), for which clinical relevance is as yet unclear, and likewise those recently discovered viruses that have no associated clinical syndrome.

DNA VIRUSES

Adenoviruses

There are 52 different serotypes of human adenovirus, belonging to six different species (A–F). Only about one-third of these are associated with symptomatic illness: species B, C and E are associated with respiratory tract infections, whereas species D causes large epidemics of infective conjunctivitis and species F (serotype 41–42) is associated with infectious diarrhoea. Infections with species B serotypes 3, 7 and 21 are associated with bronchiolitis obliterans, a post-infectious condition characterized by persistent airways obstruction secondary to peribronchiolar fibrosis.[5]

Adenovirus infections are common, have a worldwide distribution and occur throughout the year. Respiratory infections are frequent during childhood, tend to be self-limiting and induce serotype-specific immunity. Outbreaks of adenoviral respiratory infections can occur in closed communities such as day-care centres, boarding schools and especially, among military recruits.[6] Adenoviruses are unusual in that prolonged asymptomatic carriage (up to 2 years in some cases) may occur in the tonsils of children. Thus, the clinical significance of adenoviruses isolated from the throats of children must be interpreted with caution.

Bocavirus

Human bocavirus, a member of the *Parvoviridae* family, was discovered in 2005 in nasopharyngeal aspirates from children with respiratory tract infections.[7] Although suspected, establishing its role as a respiratory pathogen has been difficult for several reasons. First, human bocavirus is not related to any known human respiratory pathogen. Second, it is commonly detected with other respiratory viruses, which have established pathogenic potential. Third, detection may simply reflect asymptomatic persistence or prolonged viral shedding, since other human parvoviruses also show this capacity. It has been suggested that human bocavirus may be reactivated or produce a transient asymptomatic super-infection triggered by the presence of another replicating respiratory agent.

Several studies have shown an association between human bocavirus detection and acute respiratory symptoms, and viral DNA has been detected in the blood of children with both respiratory symptoms and human bocavirus in respiratory specimens. However, definitively establishing a causal relationship will require further study.[8]

RNA VIRUSES

Orthomyxoviridae – Influenza

The influenza viruses, especially influenza virus A, are the most variable of the respiratory viruses. Their pandemic potential and the unpredictability of their emergence is a continuous cause for concern.

There are three genera: influenza virus A, B and C. Influenza virus C only rarely causes (mild) disease in humans and will not be further discussed. Influenza A viruses are subtyped based on their two surface antigens: hemagglutinin (HA; H1–H16) and neuraminidase (NA; N1–N9), which are responsible for host receptor binding/cell entry and cleavage of the HA-receptor complex to release newly formed viruses, respectively. Key amino acids in these proteins, especially in HA, are associated with host specificity and transmissibility.

Aquatic birds are the natural reservoir of influenza A viruses, harbouring all possible subtypes. A selection of subtypes has established endemicity among a range of land and water mammals (e.g. humans, pigs, horses, seals). Currently, H3N2 and H1N1 are endemic among humans. At the time of writing, circulating H1N1 is the lineage that caused a pandemic of mild influenza in 2009 (see below), called H1N1-pdm09. Influenza virus B is almost exclusively a human pathogen also causing yearly seasonal epidemics, with rare reports of infection in dogs, cats, swine and seals.

Both influenza virus A and B exhibit 'antigenic drift'. This phenomenon occurs when the surface antigens of the virus gradually change, progressively and directionally, to escape immunological pressure from the host species. Yearly epidemics of influenza virus A and B are caused worldwide by these drift variants, and contribute to mortality (an estimated 250–500 000 every year) in the elderly, and in those with pre-existing conditions such as chronic cardiopulmonary or renal disease, diabetes, immunosuppression or severe anaemia ('acute on chronic').

New lineages of influenza virus A emerge every few decades through re-assortment of gene segments in animal hosts infected with two different viruses ('antigenic shift') resulting in global pandemics with varying severity due to the absence of immunity in the human population (1918 Spanish flu: H1N1, 40–100 million deaths; 1957 Asian flu: H2N2, 2 million deaths; 1968 Hong Kong flu: H3N2, 500 000 deaths; 2009 H1N1-pdm09, 15 000 deaths).[9] After such an introduction, the new virus usually becomes the dominant circulating lineage of influenza A. One exception was the pandemic of mild influenza among patients under 20 following the reintroduction (after 20 years of absence when H2N2 became dominant) of H1N1 in the human population in 1977; possibly caused by an escape from a research laboratory. Another exception was the introduction in 2009 of a novel lineage of H1N1 influenza virus A, most likely from pigs, in North America, causing a pandemic of relatively mild influenza (with an estimated 15 000 deaths) and generating massive attention from both the public health communities and the general public, and replacing (only) the 1977 H1N1 lineage. Between the 2009 pandemic and the time of writing, H1N1-pdm09 and H3N2 influenza virus A have been co-circulating with influenza B viruses and continue to cause yearly seasonal epidemics worldwide. The timing, extent and direction of either 'drift' or 'shift' have so far been completely unpredictable. With no animal reservoirs to provide such new antigens, shift does not occur in influenza B and thus major epidemics do not occur.

Sporadic dead-end human infections of animal, especially avian, viruses are known to occur and have caused concern regarding pandemic potential. Seal H7N3 and avian H7N7 and H9N2 viruses have caused conjunctivitis and – mostly – mild influenza-like illness in patients in close contact with infected seals or birds.[10] In 2011 there were reports of sporadic human-to-human transmission of porcine H3N2 viruses causing mild influenza-like illness.[11] In contrast, H5N1 avian influenza viruses have consistently caused severe human respiratory illness, in Asia and North Africa, with a mortality of over 50% (Figure 19.1). Highly pathogenic H5N1 viruses were first detected in birds in 1996 in China. Transmission to 18 humans occurred in Hong Kong, six of which were fatal. During the next 6 years, no human or animal cases were recorded. In 2003, the virus re-emerged in China. Since then it has become panzootic among poultry and wild birds and, at the time of writing, has caused 573 sporadic infections (336 fatal) in humans,[12] most of whom reported close contact with wild birds or domestic poultry. The disease presents as a rapidly progressive viral pneumonia with

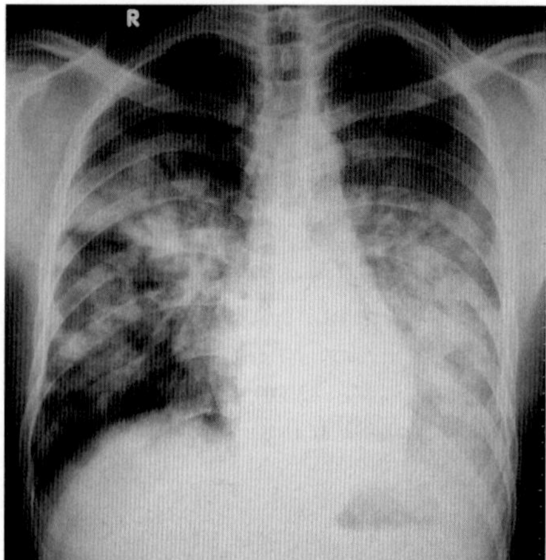

Figure 19.1 A chest X-ray of a 32-year-old man admitted to a Vietnamese hospital on Day 5 of his illness with pneumonia caused by H5N1 avian influenza. Respiratory support on intensive care was initially needed but the patient responded well to oseltamivir.

severe leucopenia and lymphopenia, progressing to ARDS (acute respiratory distress syndrome) and multi-organ dysfunction that fail to respond to standard antibiotic therapy for pneumonia. Early diagnosis and treatment with oseltamivir are associated with a better prognosis.

Despite ferret-transmission models showing that only five mutations are required to enable transmission of virulent virus,[13] their worldwide presence for many years, the huge human–animal interface in Asia and suspected small-scale human-to-human transmission in family clusters, no efficient or sustained human-to-human transmission of H5N1 viruses has yet been recorded.[14]

At the time of writing (April 2013), another avian influenza virus (H7N9) is causing - as yet only - sporadic zoonotic transmission events to humans in China, with no recorded sustained human-to-human transmission. In contrast to H5N1 this virus does not cause disease in wild or domestic birds, making it more difficult to contain. Over a period of 2 months more than 100 cases have been identified. The case fatality rate is around 20 % and elderly people are most affected. This again highlights the unpredictability of these events and the continuously changing threats posed by influenza A viruses. The continued zoonotic transmission of these avian viruses does not imply that they will inevitably lead to another pandemic. However, the unusual severity of H5N1 and H7N9 disease in humans is a continuous cause for concern, because one cannot assume that the acquisition of human-to-human transmissibility (if ever) will be associated with a loss of virulence (as is usual). Irrespective of whether or not this pandemic threat becomes reality, it is clear that avian H5N1 (and H7N9) viruses have already had a significant impact on the global poultry industry and on human economic and social wellbeing and thus ultimately on human health.

Picornaviridae

Rhinoviruses. Virology and clinical textbooks and virtually all web-based information sources describe the 99 serotypes of human rhinovirus (HRVs) as the most frequent cause of the common cold, in both the developed and the developing world. Although the common cold is considered a trivial illness, it is an important disease worldwide in terms of morbidity and economic impact.

In addition to causing the common cold, there is now convincing evidence that HRVs play a significant role in causing lower respiratory symptoms. HRVs can replicate in the lower airways and do appear to play a critical role in causing exacerbations of asthma and other chronic lung diseases. They can also drive the infant immune system towards the asthmatic phenotype, and cause episodes of bronchiolitis and pneumonia that require hospitalization.[15]

Until a few years ago, only two groups of HRVs (A and B) were recognized, but sequencing of HRVs led to the discovery of a third species (HRV-C) in 2006, with distinct structural, biological and possibly also clinical features.[16,17]

Other *Picornaviridae*. The over 100 serotypes of enterovirus (coxsackie A and B viruses, echoviruses and enteroviruses 68–71) are mainly transmitted by the oral–faecal route but can be transmitted by respiratory droplets. Enteroviruses are a major cause of aseptic meningitis in children and adults, but are also associated with common cold, herpangina in children and large epidemics of acute haemorrhagic conjunctivitis and hand, foot and mouth disease. Similarly, parechoviruses are another common cause of aseptic meningitis, but are also implicated as frequent causes of (mild) respiratory illness.

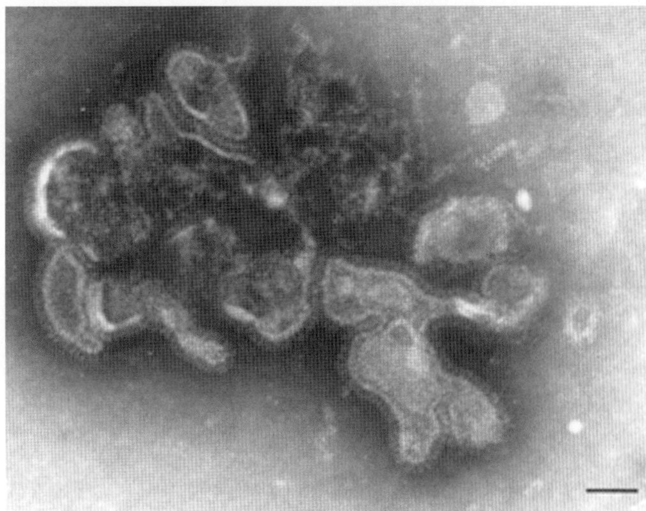

Figure 19.2 Negative stain electron micrograph of human respiratory syncytial virus (bar = 100 nm). *(Original image kindly provided by Professor CA Hart; reproduced from original in British Medical Bulletin; McNamara PS, Smyth RL. The pathogenesis of respiratory syncytial virus disease in childhood. Br Med Bull 2002;61(1):13–28.)*

Paramyxoviridae

Respiratory Syncytial Virus (RSV). This virus is distributed worldwide and is found wherever it has been sought. It is the leading cause of bronchiolitis and the most commonly detected virus in children under 2 years of age hospitalized for lower respiratory infection (Figure 19.2). It is estimated that half of all children are infected during the first year of life, and that by 3 years of age all have experienced at least one infection. Immunity following primary infection does not prevent secondary or subsequent infections, caused by both antigenic differences and failure of RSV to induce (persistent) neutralizing antibodies. In temperate regions, large seasonal epidemics occur annually over cold winter months, but this seasonality is more variable in the tropics (see below). Two subtypes (A and B) have been described and may co-circulate, with one usually predominating in any given year. No obvious differences in disease severity or pathogenesis have been documented between these two subtypes.[18,19]

RSV causes a substantial but variable LRTI disease burden in tropical countries. In a population-based study of infants in Kenya, it was found that RSV was common; approximately 36% of infections led to LTRI, 23% were severe and 3% of infected children were hospitalized.[20] RSV was also the most commonly detected respiratory pathogen in hospitalized children in Vietnam.[21] More recently, it has become clear that RSV causes significant morbidity in the elderly as well as in infants.[22]

Human Metapneumovirus (hMPV). This virus was discovered in 2001.[23] The disease it causes, its distribution and seasonality are very similar to those of RSV. It also has two subtypes and causes infections in children under 2 years old and in the elderly. Retrospective serology, has shown that this is not a new human pathogen, but has been around for a long time.[24]

Parainfluenza Viruses (PIV). There are four species of parainfluenza virus: PIV1–4. PIV1–3 are major causes of lower respiratory tract infections in infants, young children, the immuno-compromised, the chronically ill, and the elderly. PIV1 and 2 typically cause alternating biennial fall epidemics of croup, a high-pitched barking cough in children 2–4 years of age. PIV3 infections occur mainly in the first two years of life. Bronchiolitis and pneumonia are the most common clinical presentations. Only RSV causes more lower respiratory tract infections in neonates and young infants. Both in temperate and tropical regions, there is dissociation between the peaks of activity of PIV3 and RSV/hMPV. Host defence against PIV is mediated largely by humoral immunity to the two surface antigens, but repeated infections are often needed before protection develops.[25]

Rubeola Virus – Measles. There are a number of reasons why measles is often not recognized as a major cause of lower respiratory tract infections. Children with measles may not always be admitted to a general paediatric ward, the aetiology may be attributed to a super infecting pathogen rather than to measles, and some patients with measles (especially when immunocompromised) will fail to develop the typical rash. In patients who do not manifest the typical clinical features, clinical diagnosis of measles is difficult and specific laboratory diagnostics will most likely not be requested and performed. Where the diagnosis has been actively sought in developing countries, measles was found to be a major cause of lower respiratory tract infection, accounting for 6–21% of its morbidity and 8–50% of its mortality.[26] Radiographic evidence of pneumonia is common, also in clinically uncomplicated measles. The effects of the virus on the respiratory tract can be direct (giant cell pneumonitis), in any part of the respiratory tract, or indirect. The latter includes the suppressive effects of the virus on the host immune system, stores of vitamin A and overall nutritional status. All of these may lead to an increased risk of super-infection with other (viral or bacterial) pathogens. Measles pneumonitis can be especially severe in immunocompromised patients.[27]

Nipah Virus. Human Nipah virus infection was first recognized in a large outbreak of 276 reported cases in peninsular Malaysia and Singapore from September 1998 through May 1999. Most patients had contact with sick pigs. Patients presented primarily with encephalitis; 39% died. Large fruit bats of the genus *Pteropus* are the natural reservoir of Nipah virus.

In the 10 years following, no further human cases were noted in Malaysia, but annual human outbreaks have been reported in Bangladesh from May to December. The clinical presentation is dominated by respiratory symptoms and the case fatality has been over 70%.

The most frequently implicated route of infection is ingestion of fresh date palm sap. Date palm sap is harvested from December through March, particularly in west central Bangladesh. A tap is cut into the tree trunk and sap flows slowly overnight into an open clay pot. Infrared camera studies have confirmed that *Pteropus giganteus* bats frequently visit the trees, lick the sap during collection, thus transmitting infection. Humans can also become infected through direct contact with bat secretions, contact with domestic animals that become infected by eating partially eaten bat-saliva-laden fruit or infected date palm sap, or by human-to-human transmission through infected saliva.[28]

Coronaviridae

Coronaviruses. Human coronavirus (HCoV) strains 229E and OC43 have been long recognized as the second main cause of the common cold (10–25%). More recently, two other viruses associated with similar presentation were detected in humans: NL63 and HKU1. These four viruses are ubiquitous and regularly detected in respiratory specimens of a small proportion (1–10%) of children hospitalized with acute respiratory disease in many parts of the world. Infection with these human coronaviruses may present as an upper respiratory tract infection, asthma exacerbation, acute bronchiolitis, pneumonia, febrile seizures and also as croup (especially NL63). Reinfection is common due to rapidly decreasing antibody levels.

SARS-Coronavirus. In 2002–2003, a novel severe form of pneumonia of unknown aetiology emerged in Guangdong, China and was named severe acute respiratory syndrome (SARS). After smouldering for several months, the disease then spread to Hong Kong and rapidly across the world, facilitated by international air travel and a few so-called 'super-spreaders', with most notable outbreaks in Hong Kong and Toronto, Canada. Of affected cases, 21% were healthcare workers.

The rapidly identified culprit, SARS coronavirus, is thought to have jumped to humans in live animal markets in Guangdong. The precursor virus is present in wild *Rhinolophus* bats.[29] Civet cats and other small mammals sold as delicacies in wet markets provided a reservoir and amplifier for the virus and the opportunity for adaptation to humans.

The epidemic of SARS with 8096 cases and 744 deaths in 29 countries across five continents started in November 2002 and came to an end in July 2003. Few sporadic community- and laboratory-acquired infections including limited person-to-person transmission have been recorded since.[30]

SARS was characterized by fever and myalgia rapidly progressing to a respiratory syndrome of cough, dyspnoea followed by acute respiratory distress syndrome. Mortality was significantly lower in children.

SARS is primarily spread by the respiratory route, but oral–faecal transmission has also been implicated. Why the SARS epidemic did not continue to spread is subject to much speculation. Explanations may include the fact that SARS is most infectious in a later stage of infection, allowing for timely containment, and an extraordinary worldwide public health effort to control spread.[31]

With the new interest in coronaviruses, more and more closely related coronaviruses from distantly related animals have been discovered, many of which were the result of recent interspecies jumping. Coronaviruses are implicated as a likely candidate for future outbreaks of zoonotic diseases, and - indeed - a novel coronavirus (EMC) is currently associated with sporadic transmission to humans in the middle-east.

New World Hantaviruses

Hantavirus pulmonary syndrome (HPS) is a rare but important cause of severe respiratory illness in the North and South American continents. It was first recognized in May 1993 during an outbreak of severe, and frequently fatal, respiratory disease in the four corners region of the USA, where the four states Arizona, Colorado, New Mexico and Utah abut.[32] The causative agent was found to be a Hantavirus and was later named *Sin Nombre* virus. The natural host was found to be the deer mouse,

Peromyscus maniculatus, the local population of which had recently increased rapidly. The Hantaviruses are transmitted to humans by inhalation of aerosolized dried excreta. Closely related viruses have since been isolated in North (e.g. New York, Bayou, Black Creek Canal viruses) and South (e.g. Andes virus) Americas, with different rodent hosts but all associated with HPS. These viruses all belong to the same Hantavirus genus as those causing haemorrhagic fever with renal syndrome (HFRS) in the Old World: Hantaan, Seoul and Puumala viruses. Both HFRS and HPS have a similar febrile prodrome with thrombocytopenia and leucocytosis. In HPS, the key differences are that the capillary leakage which follows is localized to the lungs and that, with *Sin Nombre* virus, renal dysfunction is minimal. There was no evidence of human-to-human transmission in this outbreak, but there is evidence that some of the South American Hantaviruses causing HPS may be transmitted between humans in a nosocomial setting.[33]

Herpesviruses

Varicella pneumonitis can occur as a severe complication of chickenpox or in the absence of classical symptoms. It occurs more commonly in adults, an estimated 1:400, and can be life-threatening if it occurs during pregnancy or in immunocompromised patients. Although relatively rare, radiographical abnormalities of the lungs without respiratory symptoms are reported in more than 15% of adults with chickenpox.[34]

Pneumonitis can also rarely occur as a complication of cytomegalovirus or Epstein–Barr virus mononucleosis.[27] Cytomegalovirus is an opportunist pathogen in immunocompromised patients in whom it can cause serious or even fatal respiratory complications. It is more important as an opportunist pathogen of transplant recipients (especially bone marrow transplants) than those immunocompromised through AIDS. Perinatal cytomegalovirus infection may occasionally present as pneumonitis in the newborn.

Atypical Bacteria Associated with the Virology Laboratory

The diagnosis of atypical bacteria has traditionally been undertaken in virology laboratories, because these agents cause syndromes that overlap partially with viral respiratory infection and they were diagnosed serologically before the polymerase chain reaction was added to our diagnostic arsenal (see below). They do not cause the typical clinical picture of lobar pneumonia caused by *Streptococcus pneumoniae* and other bacteria, hence the name 'atypical'. These include: *Mycoplasma pneumoniae, Chlamydophila pneumoniae* and *psittaci* and *Coxiella burnetii*. The related *Legionella* bacteria are also discussed here.

Mycoplasma pneumoniae is an important cause of upper respiratory tract infection and bronchitis/pneumonia, usually as sporadic infections or outbreaks through human-to-human transmission among families or in closed environments. In the developed world, it has the highest attack rates among 5–20-year-olds and it is one of the major causes of pneumonia in young adults. A wide spectrum of extra-pulmonary manifestations and post-infectious syndromes has been described, but fall beyond the scope of this book. The chest radiographical patterns of *Mycoplasma* pneumonia are nonspecific and variable and can be indistinguishable from those of bacterial and viral pneumonia.[35] Systematic data from tropical areas are scarce, but its distribution is worldwide.[36]

Chlamydophila are obligate intracellular bacteria. *Chlamydophila pneumoniae* is a common human respiratory pathogen and causes a similar clinical picture to *Mycoplasma*. It is frequently isolated from animals, but their role in transmission is unclear and spread is thought to be human to human. Serosurveys also show worldwide distribution for this bacterium.[37] *Chlamydophila psittaci* is the causative agent of psittacosis, a (rare) zoonotic infection related to exposure to birds which usually presents with fever, headache and myalgia and sometimes causes pneumonia.[38]

Coxiella burnetii causes Q-fever. It is an obligate intracellular bacterium with a spore stage, making it highly resistant to environmental conditions. Humans are infected by aerosol inhalation and develop an acute febrile illness that is either self-limiting or develops into pneumonia or less frequently, endocarditis or a systemic chronic syndrome. Cattle, sheep and goats are the main reservoirs and when infected, shed bacteria in urine, faeces, milk and especially when giving birth. Placentas contain high concentrations of bacteria and people exposed to these are at risk. Given the environmental resilience of this organism, less direct contact with infected animals/placentas may also cause disease. There is no human-to-human spread.[39]

Legionella bacteria are naturally occurring aquatic bacteria. These may grow to high concentrations in warm water, e.g. in cooling towers, heaters and drinking water plumbing, especially when associated with free-living amoebae. Aerosolization and inhalation of *Legionella pneumophila* may lead to (outbreaks of) a self-limited febrile illness called Pontiac fever or a more severe systemic illness with pneumonia called Legionnaires' disease.[40] *Legionella* and *Coxiella* belong to the same family of bacteria, and both are associated with a syndrome of long-lasting post-infectious fatigue.

These bacteria are under-reported in most parts of the world. However, as they are usually susceptible to macrolides/azalides, tetracyclines and fluoroquinolones, it is important that they are diagnosed and treated. The methods of choice to detect these pathogens revolve around nucleic acid amplification techniques on respiratory specimens. A rapid urinary antigen test is available for detection of *Legionella pneumophila*. Detection of *Mycoplasma* specific IgM is useful in acute settings. *Mycoplasma* and *Legionella* can also be cultured, but this may take 1–2 weeks. Detection of seroconversion may provide a diagnosis retrospectively or in chronic disease, and may be useful for epidemiologic purposes.

Empiric treatment protocols for uncomplicated pneumonia usually consist of penicillins, such as amoxicillin with or without clavulanic acid, and do not cover these bacteria. However, most severe pneumonia treatment protocols do tend to include antimicrobial agents such as macrolides that cover these organisms. For any pneumonia of unknown aetiology that does not respond to empiric treatment, adding antimicrobial agents that cover atypical bacteria, is recommended.

CO-INFECTION

With advanced molecular diagnostic techniques (see below), it is now possible to rapidly and simultaneously detect multiple pathogens within biological samples. In recent years, multiplex reverse-transcription PCR has changed our understanding of the viral causes of respiratory illness, and doubtless newer technologies such as 16S rRNA gene sequencing will have a similar effect on how we view bacterial causes over the coming years.

The challenge with these technological advances will be in interpreting the data in a meaningful way for clinicians.

Viral Co-infection

Over the last 5 years, there has been an increase in the number of studies using multiplex RT-PCR to investigate pathogen prevalence in acute respiratory infection. Most of these have been in pre-school children in whom getting respiratory samples (particularly nasopharyngeal aspirates) is routine and relatively easy. In some studies, viruses and atypical bacteria have been detected in over 80% of samples, detection rates much higher than in studies using traditional culture techniques.[41] However, as has been mentioned, these studies should be interpreted with some caution. Pathogens such as Bocavirus and Adenovirus persist for weeks and sometimes months after acute infection and thus their significance during an acute episode, especially when detected with other pathogens, may be uncertain.

This increase in reported prevalence has been mirrored by an increase in the rates of viral co-infection (or probably more accurately, co-detection). In recent studies, two or more viral pathogens have been found in up to 44% of upper respiratory samples from young children with acute respiratory infection.[21,41–45] Co-infection rates appear to vary depending on age, country and living conditions, as well as the number of pathogens tested (Table 19.1). Some of the highest viral detection and co-infection rates have been reported in pre-school children from low-income families living in Brazil, Vietnam and Jordan.[21,41,42] A number of groups has suggested co-infection as a risk factor for severe disease. However, there is no real consensus in the literature supporting this premise, which is perhaps not surprising given that most of the published studies have investigated very different populations and looked for different numbers of pathogens (Table 19.1).

Bacterial Co-infection

For some conditions, a link between viral and bacterial infection is well established. For instance, data reassessed from the influenza pandemics of 1918, 1957 and 1968 suggest that most deaths during these periods were due to secondary bacterial pneumonia, approximately four weeks after the acute infection.[47] Overall, however, the significance of contemporaneous bacterial and viral co-infection in acute respiratory infection is difficult to assess, particularly if analysis is limited to upper airway secretions. While it is often inferred that viral pathogens detected in the upper airways are also in the lower airways of children with chest symptoms, the same cannot be said for bacteria where upper airway detection is as likely to be due to asymptomatic nasopharyngeal carriage.

However, in studies where lung aspirates have been obtained from children with clinical signs of severe pneumonia, both viral and bacterial pathogens can be detected. In a study from the Gambia on 74 children with community-acquired pneumonia, one-third of the 45 with pneumococcal pneumonia, had RSV infection.[48] In contrast, in children from Malawi with a high prevalence of HIV, only 9% of those with pneumococcal infection had a viral co-infection (the commonest being with adenovirus).[49] It is also worth considering, that in the UK, one-fifth of infants with severe RSV bronchiolitis have bacteria in their lower airways at the time of intubation and length of time spent ventilated correlates to bacterial carriage.[50]

Clinical Syndromes

Most viruses and atypical bacteria can cause most clinical manifestations of acute respiratory infection, but some viruses are associated with particular clinical presentations; RSV with bronchiolitis, Adenovirus B3, 7 and 21 with bronchiolitis obliterans, and PIV1-2 with croup.

Infections confined to the upper respiratory tract cause symptoms such as rhinitis, coryza and cough and are for the most part mild, with the exception of croup, which although uncomfortable and distressing, is more severe but not normally fatal. In practice, acute lower respiratory tract infection accounts for most of the serious disease burden. Infections normally start in the upper respiratory tract and then spread to the lower airways, where the effects can be extensive and are rarely confined to one lobe or even one lung. This is in marked contrast with pneumococcal pneumonia. Common lower respiratory tract manifestations of viral or atypical bacterial infections are: bronchiolitis, pneumonia and asthma/episodic viral wheeze.

TABLE 19.1 Viral Atypical Bacterial Prevalence Detected Using Multiplex PCR in Children Presenting to Hospital with Acute Respiratory Infection

	India[44]	Jordan[42]	Hong Kong[46]	Nepal[45]	Brazil[41]	Vietnam[21]	Kenya[43]
Year published	2007	2008	2009	2009	2011	2011	2010
Age (years)	<5	<5	<5	<3	<5	<13	<12
Total number patients in study	301	326	475	629	407	309	759
In-patient (%)	45%	100%	100%	100%	52%	100%	100%
Co-infection rate	7	25	4	1	40	20	7
hRSV	20	43	8	14	37	24	34
hRV	–	11	4	–	19	4	–
AdV	–	37	5	–	25	5	4
Influenza A and B	3	1	11	7	3	17	6
PIV	16	0	9	10	8	7	8
CoV	–	1	4	–	3	8	10
Human Metapneumovirus	4	3	1.5	1	10	7	3
HBoV	–	18	–	–	19	16	2
Mycoplasma Pneumoniae	–	0	2	–	10	–	–
Chlamydophila Pneumoniae	–	5	0	–	1	–	–
PCR negative	65	22	53	70	15	28	44

BRONCHIOLITIS

RSV is the commonest cause of bronchiolitis and is detected in 43–74% of cases.[51] Upper respiratory tract symptoms usually precede lower respiratory tract involvement by a few days. Dyspnoea, subcostal recession and feeding difficulties characterize lower respiratory tract infection. In bronchiolitis, wheeze may be present with a prolonged expiratory phase and crackles.[52] Air trapping results in a rapid respiratory rate, a palpable spleen and liver and a typical radiographic pattern of hyperinflation with diffuse interstitial markings and peribronchial thickening. Segmental atelectasis is often seen. Bronchiolitis may lead to acute respiratory failure with severe bronchospasm, moderate to severe hypoxia and carbon dioxide retention. Apnoea tends to occur in infants under 2 months of age and often in those born prematurely. Supportive measures are still the mainstay of treatment for bronchiolitis. Symptoms associated with clinically significant bronchiolitis (particularly RSV) are not limited to the acute episode, with many children wheezing for years afterwards.

Two key risk factors for getting bronchiolitis are age (<6 months) and exposure to tobacco smoke (particularly antenatally).[52] Other factors increasing the risk of getting more severe disease include male gender, prematurity, an underlying heart or lung condition and never having been breast-fed. Also, poverty, living in a crowded environment and having siblings who attend school or child-care increase the risk of getting bronchiolitis.

PNEUMONIA

Cases of viral pneumonia generally occur during seasonal epidemics of influenza and RSV, and are normally preceded by upper respiratory tract infection.[53] Whereas symptoms of bacterial pneumonia include a rapid onset of fever, rigors, malaise, cough and dyspnoea, symptoms of viral pneumonia tend to be of slower onset and while including cough and dyspnoea, are just as likely to present with rhinitis and wheezing. Biomarkers of sepsis such as white-blood cell count, C-reactive protein and procalcitonin are often normal, and chest radiograph findings likely to show bilateral interstitial infiltrates rather than lobar changes. Children with viral pneumonia respond slowly or not at all to antibiotics in marked contrast to those with bacterial pneumonia. Similar to bronchiolitis, risk factors for severe disease include household smoking and cessation of breast-feeding before 6 months, poverty, malnutrition, HIV and other immunosuppressive disease.

ASTHMA/EPISODIC VIRAL WHEEZE

The asthma epidemic experienced by developed countries over the past three decades is now being mirrored in developing countries as they become more urbanized. Environmental factors appear to be a key factor behind these changes in prevalence.[54] Global associations which positively correlate with asthma symptom prevalence include Gross National Product, *trans*-fatty acids, paracetamol, and women smoking, whereas inverse associations include a diet with food of plant origin, pollen, immunizations, tuberculosis notifications, air pollution, and men smoking.[54]

There is clinical overlap between childhood asthma and episodic viral wheeze. In both conditions, cases tend to be preceded by a viral URTI 1–2 days before wheeze develops.[55] Episodic viral wheeze is a series of discreet episodes of respiratory distress characterized by wheeze occurring in pre-school children, whereas asthma later develops into a chronic disease with exacerbations of sudden deterioration in airway function, day-to-day variation in airway function and fixed or persistent airway obstruction.[56] In developed countries, one-third of children with episodic viral wheeze as a young child go on to develop atopic asthma.[57] Rhinovirus appears to be a particularly common viral cause of asthma exacerbations (especially Rhinovirus C) but other viruses commonly isolated include RSV, hMPV and PIVs.

Epidemiology

Overall, the viruses that cause acute respiratory infection worldwide are the same (Table 19.1), but there are local variations, particularly during outbreaks of unusual organisms (Nipah virus in Bangladesh and India). In temperate parts of the world, there is a clear seasonal pattern in the prevalence of viral respiratory tract infection, with peaks occurring over the cold, winter months. In tropical regions, where average temperature is higher and seasonal temperature change less, variations in prevalence are still seen. This has been best demonstrated for RSV. Strong RSV seasonal patterns, which correlate with rainfall, have been found in Vietnam,[21] India,[58] Papua New Guinea,[59] North-East Brazil,[41] Kenya and the Gambia.[60,61] A possible explanation for this is that children tend to be kept indoors during the rainy season, and the resultant crowding in damp, humid environments prolongs viral survival and encourages spread. This is probably not the whole story however, as in some parts of the world, RSV activity shows no pattern at all (Taiwan[62]), or peaks during the summer months when ambient temperatures are highest (Hong Kong[63]).

Similar patterns are found for influenza virus infection.[64] Thus, for studies large enough to detect such variations, influenza activity peaks in India, North-East Brazil and Senegal, during the months with the highest rainfall and humidity. Similar seasonal variations have also been described for hMPV and PIVs. In contrast, rhinovirus, adenovirus and bocavirus infection appears, for the most part, to be endemic throughout the year. One recent study in North-East Brazil reported peaks in *Mycoplasma pneumoniae* infection that were unrelated to the rainy season.[41] In this study, the authors found that at its peak *Mycoplasma pneumoniae* infection accounted for 17% of hospitalized pneumonia cases in pre-school children, a finding with clear implications for management, given that current treatment guidelines for pneumonia in this age group do not include macrolide/quinolone antibiotics.

Diagnoses

Epidemiological characteristics, patient history, clinical features and accompanying signs and symptoms may give some clues in establishing the diagnosis of specific viral agents, but clinical syndromes are nonspecific and overlap considerably. Aetiological diagnosis can only reliably be made by detection of live virus, viral antigens or nucleic acids in respiratory or other specimens and to a lesser extent by (retrospective) detection of (a rise in) specific antibodies.

There are three main reasons for providing an aetiological diagnosis of viral respiratory infections: to aid clinical management (specific therapy, stopping antibiotic therapy, infection control); to monitor routine virus activity in the community (epidemiology, e.g. vaccine strain selection for influenza); or for research purposes.

Rapid diagnosis of viral respiratory infections (i.e. in less than 3 hours) has been shown to reduce antibiotic use and to be cost-effective.[65] In addition, such confirmation of the cause is useful in hospital infection control (e.g. in cohorting similar cases) and, occasionally, in deciding whether to use antiviral drugs in selected high-risk patients (see below). Equally, making a rapid diagnosis in an outbreak situation (e.g. of influenza), may justify the use of antiviral medications to limit disease spread.

Diagnosis for some respiratory infections is achievable within 2–3 hours using techniques such as antigen detection (see below). However, these techniques are not universally available, even in hospitals in the developed world, mainly because they are labour- and expertise-intensive. Commercially available point-of-care diagnostic tests, usually lateral flow assays in 'kit format', are available for the diagnosis of influenza virus A and B and for RSV. They are however, expensive, and while they have adequate positive and negative predictive value of infection during influenza epidemics, they can have poor predictive values during periods of low influenza activity.[66]

The increasing need to accurately detect avian influenza H5N1 is best done by sensitive molecular methods (e.g. RT-PCR) because other techniques are less sensitive and virus culture necessitates biosafety level 3 facilities. This is driving reference laboratories, especially in developing countries where H5N1 disease sporadically occurs, to invest in these newer technologies. In time, this will hopefully allow molecular tests for multiple respiratory pathogens (Multiplex PCR) to be undertaken in these same laboratories. However, these methods remain resource- and expertise-intensive and need regular quality control exercises. Microarray techniques that have the potential to detect multiple pathogens in a single test are in development. These methods have enormous potential to increase our understanding of viral (and bacterial) epidemiology.

METHODS OF VIRAL DIAGNOSIS

Laboratory diagnosis of respiratory virus infections depends on the demonstration of either virus or viral components in the patient at the acute stage of the illness, or subsequently an immune (serological) response to the virus.

Demonstration of Virus

There are several approaches to this that include demonstration of: (1) viral antigens by immunofluorescence or enzyme immunoassays;[67] (2) viral infectivity by growth in cell culture; or (3) viral nucleic acid by various techniques. Details of the techniques are not given here, but the advantages and disadvantages of each are indicated in Table 19.2. When setting up a diagnostic laboratory, its purpose should be clearly thought out. If the catchment population is very large, the number of specimens may also be large and the advantages of automation (e.g. in machine-based nucleic acid amplification or enzyme immunoassays) may be significant. Most specimens are likely to come from hospitalized patients because of the practical difficulties in collecting and delivering specimens from the community. Virology specimens are perishable and must be delivered to the laboratory without delay. The quality of the specimen is paramount to obtaining meaningful results. It is easier to take a bad specimen than a good one, and close cooperation with the laboratory will help to raise the positivity rate.

Demonstration of an Immune Response

This, at present, means demonstrating an antibody response in the serum to the stimulus provided by the virus. Seeking responses in cellular immunity or antibody in other body fluids remain research techniques only.

For a valid diagnosis, a convalescent specimen of serum (usually taken after at least 2 weeks) is needed but may

TABLE 19.2 Advantages and Disadvantages of Various Techniques of Virus Diagnosis

Technique	Advantages	Disadvantages
Immunofluorescence	Rapid, i.e. same day Allows assessment of specimen quality Sensitive and specific in experienced hands	Labour-intensive Requires experienced observer(s) Requires high-quality reagents Obtaining good specimens requires skill, determination and persistence evidence of shedding of some viruses in healthy
Enzyme immunoassay	Rapid, available in point-of-care format (~30 min) for some viruses Suitable for large numbers Can be semi-automated Detects incomplete virus particles	No feedback on specimen quality Requires high-quality reagents Automated equipment expensive Difficult to assess results at threshold of positivity Relevance of detection of viral antigens not always clear
Culture	Provides more virus for further analysis Confirms presence of replicating/infective virus Generally regarded as the gold standard	Expensive and a continuing expense Labour-intensive Not as sensitive as nucleic acid amplification, some viruses difficult to isolate or cannot be cultured Mixed infections pose problems Requires high-quality reagents to identify isolates
Detection of nucleic acid by amplification ([RT-] PCR and others)	Sensitive and specific Can detect virus in the presence of antibody Allows assessment of specimen quality Allows for multiplexed assays, random PCR-based array tests in development	Expensive Requires vigilance against false-positive results Labour- and skill-intensive Relevance of detection of viral nucleic acids not always clear

be difficult to collect. This is particularly true with children. Nevertheless, unless an antibody response can be demonstrated (seroconversion or a rising titre) some uncertainty over the validity of the result will remain. An alternative is to demonstrate an IgM-class response but this suffers from the twin disadvantages that IgM antibodies (and thus the corresponding results), are relatively non-specific compared to IgG, and such tests are not routinely available for all viruses.

Treatment

Supportive care with fluids and oxygen remain the mainstay of treatment for most respiratory viral infections. For some individuals, respiratory support on high-dependency units or intensive care is needed. Extracorporeal membrane oxygenation (ECMO) is sometimes required to maintain oxygen saturation in individuals with severe viral pneumonia.

The Adamantanes (amantadine and rimantadine) were options for prevention (in outbreaks within closed communities of high-risk individuals) and less convincingly, for treatment of influenza virus A infections.[68] However, these therapies have now become obsolete as H3N2 resistance to them has been increasing since 2003, and H1N1-pdm09 and most avian H5N1 viruses are completely resistant.

Neuraminidase inhibitors such as oseltamivir (Tamiflu), zanamivir (Relenza) and peramivir (Rapiacta), which inhibit the viral enzyme neuraminidase in both influenza virus A and B, are effective for treatment and prophylaxis of influenza. In the 2007/2008 influenza season an influenza virus A H1N1 lineage emerged that was naturally resistant against oseltamivir, and soon became the dominant lineage worldwide. This was a cause for serious concern, but in 2009 the oseltamivir-susceptible H1N1-pdm09 virus replaced the resistant lineage.

For treatment of uncomplicated influenza, neuraminidase inhibitors have to be given within 48 hours of onset for apparent clinical benefit. For severe influenza, influenza in the immuno-compromised, and avian influenza, benefit can still be found if these drugs are administered after 48 hours and so treatment should not be withheld in these cases. They are expensive and are best used on those most at risk of serious illness – those at the extreme ends of life. While both zanamivir (given by inhaler) and oseltamivir (given orally) can be used for prophylaxis against H5N1 influenza disease, the systemically active oseltamivir is the preferred option for treatment given the potential for dissemination of H5N1 beyond the respiratory tract. However, experience with human cases of H5N1 avian influenza has shown that resistance may develop rapidly and may be a major problem in widespread prophylactic or therapeutic use.

Ribavirin is a purine nucleoside analogue that is believed to interfere with viral nucleic acid function. It is expensive, difficult to deliver and teratogenic (therefore potentially toxic to both patient and treating team). Systematic reviews have failed to show any convincing evidence for its use in either acute bronchiolitis or in more severe disease.[69] Given the high cost, safety concerns, challenges in delivery and weakness of trial data, ribavirin is generally reserved for use with immunocompromised children in a PICU setting. Ribavirin may have some effect in influenza but evidence to support its use is minimal. It has also been used in Hantavirus pulmonary syndrome but, again, the evidence of efficacy is minimal.

Cidofovir is available for severe adenovirus infections, but causes severe side-effects and needs to be administered simultaneously with probenecid.

Intravenous acyclovir and oral valacyclovir are effective in the treatment of varicella or herpes simplex infections of the respiratory tract in the immunocompromised patient. It should also be used in an immunocompetent patient (usually an adult) with varicella pneumonia. Ganciclovir and foscarnet are useful in cytomegalovirus infection in the immunosuppressed, but a detailed discussion of this problem is beyond the scope of this chapter.

In many parts of the world (especially South-east Asia), antibiotics are extensively used to treat any form of mild respiratory illness. Although there may be some benefit to the use of antibiotics in preventing secondary bacterial sinusitis, otitis media or pneumonia, over-the-counter availability of antibiotics, self-medication or medication by untrained pharmacy workers should be strongly discouraged because of the selection and subsequent spread of resistant pathogens and of (multidrug) resistant commensal bacteria in oral and intestinal flora.

Prevention

With the cells of the target organ immediately accessible to viruses, it is proving difficult to produce effective vaccines to respiratory tract viruses.[70] Other than in measles, which has a systemic phase, vaccines have had only limited success. In the tropics, even the measles vaccine has limitations as much of this virus' impact is during infancy, when existing vaccines lack effectiveness at inducing immunity in the presence of passive maternal antibody.

Yearly influenza vaccination is recommended in many countries for persons at high risk (e.g. patients with underlying heart, respiratory or immunocompromising diseases, patients on dialysis, the elderly) and contains antigens from two current influenza A virus subtypes (H3N2 and H1N1-pdm09) and from influenza virus B. The constituents are modified annually for each hemisphere as the prevalent strains 'drift and shift' (see above). The conventional influenza vaccine is formalin-killed egg-grown virus and has provided useful protection, particularly in the elderly and those with pre-existing lung damage in whom even minimal protection may be enough to prevent death. An alternative approach of a live attenuated vaccine containing cold-adapted influenza strains has shown some efficacy and such vaccines are also available.

The possible emergence of an H5N1 avian strain adapted to man has stimulated research into new ways to produce vaccines (e.g. using reverse genetics or a disabled adenovirus as a vector for influenza antigens) and for new antiviral drugs. Currently (at time of writing), H5N1 vaccines are licensed for use in the USA and the EU, but these are not available in endemic countries.

Earlier attempts at production of formaldehyde inactivated RSV vaccine were associated with more severe forms of disease in vaccinees. Prevention of RSV, severe measles and varicella in susceptible (immunocompromised or severely malnourished) contacts may also be achieved by passive immunization. Monoclonal antibodies such as Palivizumab provide some protection to RSV infection in vulnerable infants (e.g. premature babies), but it is very expensive and administration is in the form of monthly intramuscular injections over the RSV season.[71]

Normal human gamma globulin is effective in preventing/attenuating measles if administered within 3 days of contact. For the prophylaxis of varicella, high-titre varicella-zoster human immune globulin (ZIG) must be used. Maximum protection (from severe disease, but not from infection) follows administration within 48 hours of contact, but some benefit may accrue if given within 10 days of exposure.

Summary

Respiratory viral disease, like diarrhoeal disease, is a major cause of morbidity and mortality in the developing world and has significant economic consequences. Much respiratory disease, particularly in childhood, is either totally due to viruses or is virus-initiated, with similar organisms found in tropical and temperate regions. Viral and atypical bacterial epidemiological data are incomplete everywhere (but more so for the poorer parts of the world) and come mostly from hospitalized patients.

RSV is a universal childhood pathogen found everywhere. The numbers of virologically confirmed diagnoses each year in hospitalized children in the Newcastle and Tyneside area in the UK (population about 1 million) and from Hong Kong island (population about 0.7 million) are remarkably similar: 500–600 and 500–700 cases, respectively. There are likely to be many more RSV cases in the larger cities of Asia and South America, in overcrowded environments where the potential for severe disease will be exacerbated by malnutrition, air pollution, poor sanitation, minimal medical care, etc.

A new pandemic of influenza A (similar to the one that swept the world in 1918/1919) could be a major health problem of the future, but when and if this will happen is unknown. We have learnt from the 2009 pandemic that pandemics can be mild, but there is still fear of H5N1 crossing the species barrier and causing a pandemic with a high case fatality rate. Current preparative measures, such as 'stockpiling' oseltamivir and vaccine development, may help to reduce its impact.

There is a very real clinical and economic need to develop effective treatments and vaccines against the common causes of viral and atypical bacterial respiratory disease but this will require an enormous commitment of resources.

REFERENCES

2. Black RE, Cousens S, Johnson HL, et al. Global, regional, and national causes of child mortality in 2008: a systematic analysis. Lancet 2010;375(9730):1969–87.
21. Do AH, van Doorn HR, Nghiem MN, et al. Viral etiologies of acute respiratory infections among hospitalized Vietnamese children in Ho Chi Minh City, 2004–2008. PLoS One 2011;6(3):e18176.
41. Bezerra PG, Britto MC, Correia JB, et al. Viral and atypical bacterial detection in acute respiratory infection in children under five years. PLoS One 2011;6(4):e18928.
43. Berkley JA, Munywoki P, Ngama M, et al. Viral etiology of severe pneumonia among Kenyan infants and children. JAMA 2010;303(20):2051–7.
70. Gillim-Ross L, Subbarao K. Emerging respiratory viruses: challenges and vaccine strategies. Clin Microbiol Rev 2006;19(4):614–36.

Access the complete references online at www.expertconsult.com

20 Viral Exanthems

FLOR M. MUNOZ

KEY POINTS

- Viral infections remain an important cause of morbidity and mortality worldwide.
- The skin is a common site where viral diseases are manifested.
- Most viruses cause characteristic exanthems and can be diagnosed clinically.
- In patients with immune deficiencies, such as HIV/AIDS, or conditions where the cellular immune response is impaired, the clinical presentation and severity of these viral exanthems could be atypical or enhanced.
- Diagnosis can be confirmed with available laboratory methods, particularly molecular detection techniques.
- Specific antiviral treatment is not widely available and emerging antiviral resistance poses new challenges.
- Safe and effective vaccines reduce the morbidity and mortality associated with viral infections in susceptible populations.

Introduction

Viruses are classified based on their genome as RNA or DNA viruses, and grouped in families with distinct virion morphology, genome structure, or replication strategy.[1] Medically important RNA and DNA viruses that result in skin manifestations in children and adults and the diseases they cause are described in Tables 20.1 and 20.2.

RNA Viruses Causing Cutaneous Disease

Several RNA viruses cause skin manifestations in humans. Measles, rubella and enteroviruses are discussed in this chapter. Diseases due to other RNA viruses are described elsewhere.

MEASLES

Epidemiology

Measles remains a leading cause of child mortality worldwide. Measles is one of the most prevalent infectious diseases of the tropics, and probably the most serious of the acute childhood febrile exanthematous illnesses. In 2011, 243 308 cases were reported to the WHO, mostly from Africa, South-east Asia and the Western Pacific regions (Figure 20.1).[2] The WHO estimates that 164 000 people died of measles in 2008, with the majority of these deaths occurring in children under 5 years of age and more than 95% occurring in developing countries.[3] Recent outbreaks in industrialized countries have been associated with low immunization coverage. However, great progress in measles control has been made in resource-poor countries through improved measles-control efforts, including measles vaccination and case-based surveillance.

Pathogenesis and Pathology

The causative agent is a single-stranded RNA virus with pleomorphic appearance on electron microscopy (100–300 nm in size); it consists of two components: an outer envelope with short projections and an inner nucleocapsid of RNA and a glycoprotein. There is only one strain and no known antigenic variation; alterations in virulence worldwide are due to underlying host and environmental factors. The virus grows slowly in human and monkey cell cultures forming intranuclear inclusion bodies, which differentiate it from other paramyxoviruses.

Humans are the only host. Measles is highly contagious; approximately 90% of susceptible individuals will contract the disease after contact with a case. Transmission is by direct contact with secretions from the respiratory tract or by droplet spread. Patients are infectious only in the early stages, when virus can be isolated from the throat. Transplacental spread does not seem to occur.

In tropical countries, epidemics occur during the dry season when festivals and gatherings of people usually take place. In large cities, measles is endemic throughout the year; in smaller towns, childhood epidemics tend to occur every 2–3 years.

Pathogenesis

Infection begins in the upper respiratory tract, bronchial epithelial cells and pulmonary macrophages; following amplification in regional lymph nodes, the virus spreads (via leucocytes, particularly monocytes) to cells of the reticuloendothelial system (thymus, spleen, lymphatic tissue) and other target organs including the skin, conjunctivae, lung, gastrointestinal tract, liver, kidney and genital mucosa. Virus replication occurs in epithelial and endothelial cells, as well as monocytes and macrophages, producing the appearance of large multinucleate giant cells. Viraemia occurs 4–5 days before the appearance of the rash, and abates within 24–48 hours. The typical measles rash is caused by infection of the dermal endothelial cells followed by spread into the overlying epidermis, focal keratosis and edema, with accumulation of epithelial giant cells and mononuclear cells around the blood vessels. Koplik's spots, the characteristic enanthem in the oral mucosa of patients with measles is pathologically similar, affecting the local submucosal glands. In the respiratory and gastrointestinal tracts, there is local inflammation followed by exfoliation of dead epithelial cells.

TABLE 20.1 RNA Viruses and Typical Disease with Cutaneous Manifestations

Family	Virus	Cutaneous Disease
Paramyxovirus	Measles	Measles (Rubeola)
	Mumps	Mumps
	Retroviruses HIV-2, HIV-2	AIDS dermatitis
Picornavirus	Enterovirus	Hand-foot-mouth disease, exanthems
	Coxsackie viruses	
	Echoviruses	
Togavirus	Rubivirus	Rubella (German measles)
Flavivirus	Arboviruses	
	Mosquito-borne	
	Dengue virus	Dengue
	Yellow fever virus	Yellow fever
	West Nile virus	West Nile encephalitis
	Japanese encephalitis virus	Japanese encephalitis
	Tick-borne	Tick-borne encephalitis
	Tick-borne encephalitis virus	
Arenaviruses	Guanarito virus Lassa virus	Haemorrhagic fever
	Machupo virus	
	Junin virus	
Filoviruses	Marburg virus	Haemorrhagic fever
	Ebola virus	

TABLE 20.2 DNA Viruses and Typical Disease with Cutaneous Manifestations

Family	Virus	Cutaneous Disease
Pox viruses	Variola	Smallpox
		Monkey pox
		Cowpox
		Tanapox
		Molluscum contagiosum
Herpesviruses	Herpes simplex virus (HSV) type 1	Orofacial herpes
	Herpes simplex virus (HSV) type 2	Genital herpes
	Varicella zoster virus (VZV)	Varicella (chickenpox) Zoster (shingles)
	Cytomegalovirus (CMV)	Exanthem, mucositis
	Epstein-Barr virus (EBV)	Exanthem, Infectious mononucleosis
	Human herpesvirus (HHV)	
	HHV-6	Roseola (exanthem subitum)
	HHV-7	Roseola
	HHV-8	Kaposi sarcoma
Adenoviruses	Adenovirus	Exanthem
Papovavirus	Human papilloma virus (HPV)	Skin and mucosal warts
Parvoviruses	Parvovirus B-19	Erythema Infectiosum (5th disease)

Immunity acquired after recovery from measles infection is lifelong. Clearance of the virus requires both antibody- and cell-mediated responses. IgM antibodies appear simultaneously with the rash, peak at 10 days and disappear after 1 month; IgG antibodies peak after resolution of symptoms and decrease slowly over time. IgG antibodies transferred from mother to infant transplacentally last for the first few months of life. During measles infection and several weeks after recovery, the production of antibodies and cellular immune responses to new antigens are impaired. The immunosuppressive effects of measles have significant consequences in patients living in tropical countries where malnutrition, vitamin A deficiency, and

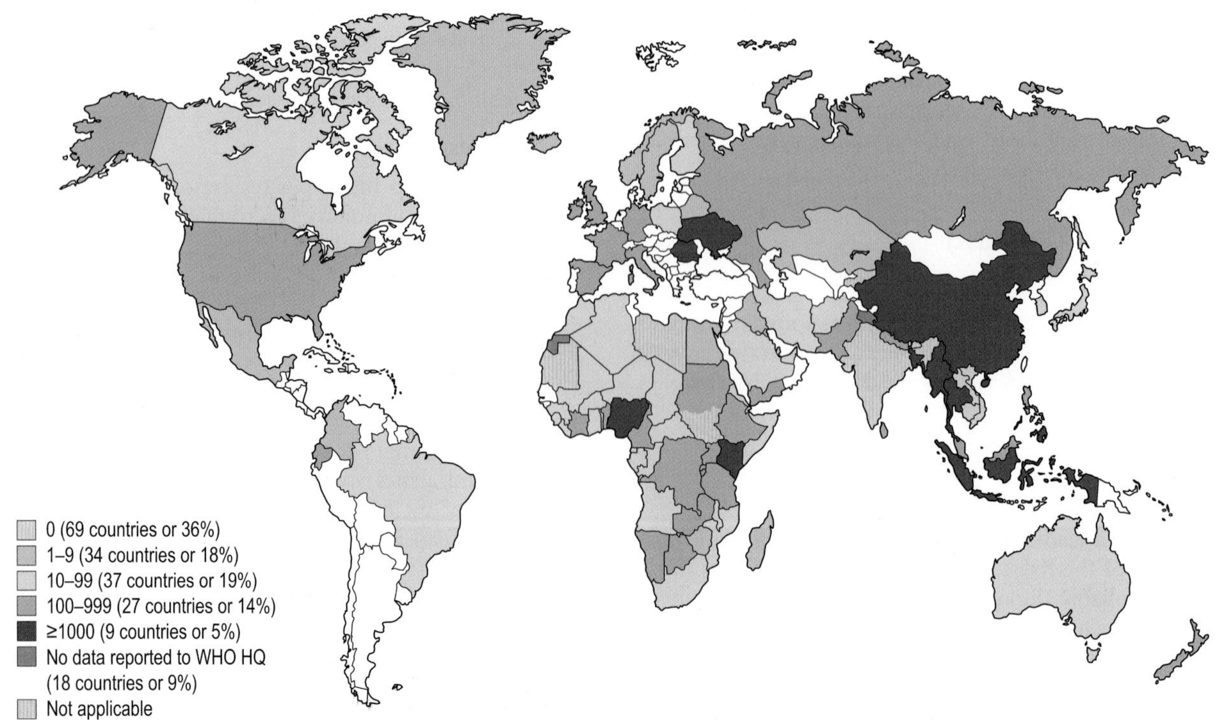

Figure 20.1 Reported cases of measles to the World Health Organization (WHO) from August 2011 to February 2012. (Source: *WHO.*)

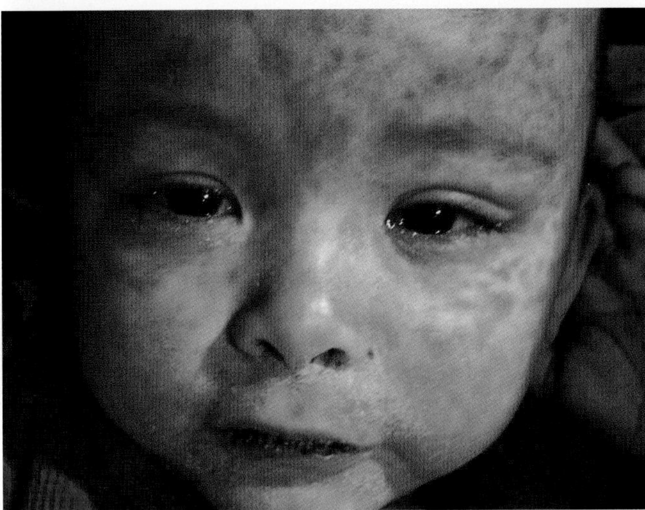

Figure 20.2 Child with measles coryza, conjunctivitis and rash. *(Courtesy of Stephen Thacker, MD.)*

other infectious diseases such as HIV/AIDS and tuberculosis are prevalent, resulting in increased morbidity and risk for mortality.

Clinical Features

The clinical signs and symptoms of measles develop after an incubation period of 10–14 days. The initial prodromal phase lasts 3–4 days with high fever and prominent coryza, followed by severe conjunctivitis and cough (Figure 20.2). Within 3 days of onset (and typically 24 h before the rash appears), Koplik's spots can be visualized as bright red spots with a small white centre on the buccal mucous membrane. A maculopapular rash appears first on the forehead and neck, spreading to the trunk and extremities over 3–4 days (Figure 20.3). The skin lesions at first reddish and maculopapular later become dark and brown. In dark skin they may appear deep red or purple. The rash lasts for a total of 5–6 days, followed by severe desquamation. This may lead to patchy depigmentation and, occasionally, boils. Haemorrhagic measles with a purpuric rash and bleeding from mucous membranes is rare and carries a very high mortality rate.

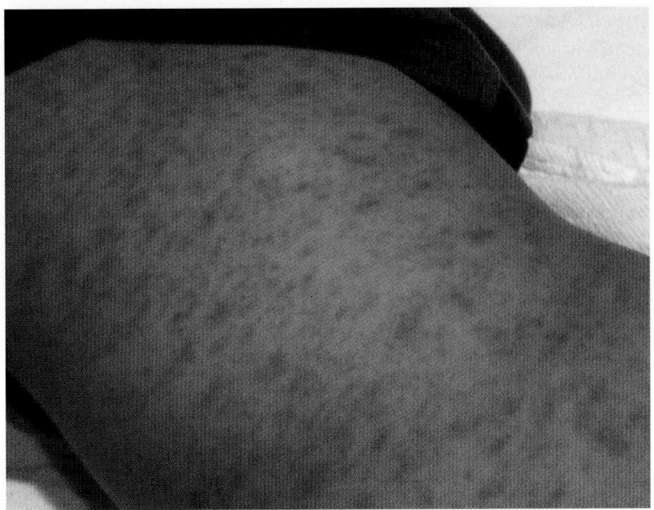

Figure 20.3 Measles exanthema. *(Courtesy of Stephen Thacker, MD.)*

Complications

Measles is self-limited, with full recovery in most cases. However, measles infection can have a major impact on a child's health and development. Associated morbidity includes difficulty sucking and eating due to mucosal lesions which aggravates or precipitates states of malnutrition (marasmus, kwashiorkor), otitis media and mastoiditis, laryngitis or laryngotracheobronchitis (croup), severe bronchopneumonia or giant cell pneumonia with respiratory failure, diarrhoea leading to dehydration and malabsorption, severe conjunctivitis and blindness, meningoencephalitis and seizures, gangrene of the extremities, and intercurrent infections (herpetic disease) or worsening or pre-existing illnesses due to associated immune-suppression. Measles is one of the most common causes of blindness in the tropics given that conjunctivitis and vitamin A deficiency are associated with corneal perforation and permanent blindness.[4] Death often results from respiratory and neurological complications. In tropical populations with high levels of malnutrition and limited access to medical care, the case fatality rate is estimated to be about 10%, but may be higher during outbreaks.[3,5]

Encephalitis. Acute encephalitis occurs in 1 of every 1000 cases. The onset is usually 4–7 days after the appearance of the rash, and is characterized by fever, irritability, meningismus, generalized seizures and coma. The cerebrospinal fluid shows moderate pleocytosis and high protein concentration. The mortality rate can be as high as 10–15% and one-quarter of affected children are left with a permanent neurological deficit. This phenomenon probably has an immunological basis, as shown by the histological changes, perivascular cuffing, demyelination and gliosis.

Subacute Sclerosing Panencephalitis (SSPE). This rare complication is caused by a persistent viral infection within the brain. It usually manifests 5–10 years after wild-type virus infection, and has a slow degenerative course, starting with personality changes and deterioration of intellect, and progressing to a state of decerebrate rigidity and seizures. Very high levels of antibody to measles virus are present in cerebrospinal fluid.

Diagnosis

A clinical diagnosis is made with the recognition of the typical signs and symptoms of fever, cough, conjunctivitis, coryza, Koplik's spots in the mouth, and a morbilliform rash. Other infections with dermatological manifestations that are often mistaken for measles include Group A streptococcal disease (scarlet fever), tick-borne and louse-borne disease, meningococcaemia, rubella, adenovirus or enterovirus infection and infectious mononucleosis.

Laboratory confirmation is made with a positive measles IgM antibody titre, which is detectable up to 1 month after the onset of the rash, a significant rise in measles IgG antibody concentration in paired acute and covalescent serum samples, or by isolation of measles virus or detection of measles RNA PCR in nasopharyngeal secretions, throat samples, blood or urine.[6] Genotyping of viral isolates facilitates the evaluation of transmission patterns, including the importation of viruses into different countries, as well as the differentiation of infection with wild-type virus from vaccine virus.

During the prodromal phase large multinucleate (giant) cells can be visualized in stained smears of sputum, urine, or Koplik's spots on the buccal mucosa. Immunofluorescent staining of cells may demonstrate measles antigen in smears from the nasopharynx or Koplik's spots.

Management

There are no antivirals specific for the treatment of measles. Nutrition and good hydration should be maintained. Antibiotics are indicated when otitis media, bacterial pneumonia and secondary skin infections are present. Temperature control may reduce the occurrence of febrile convulsions.

The WHO recommends treatment with vitamin A for all children with acute measles, regardless of which country or environmental conditions they live in because treatment with at least two doses of vitamin A is associated with decreased morbidity and mortality in developing countries.[4] Vitamin A should be given once daily for 2 days, with dosing calculated based on the child's age: 50 000 IU for infants younger than 6 months of age, 100 000 IU for infants 6–11 months of age, and 200 000 IU for children ≥12 months of age. A third dose is recommended 2–4 weeks later in children with clinical evidence of vitamin A deficiency.[6]

Prevention

Measles is a notifiable disease. Contact and air-borne precautions are recommended for patients with measles for 4 days after the onset of the rash, or until resolution of the illness for immunocompromised patients. Both passive immunization with human immunoglobulin and active immunization with a live attenuated vaccine are highly successful.

Passive Immunization. Passive immunization with human immune globulin (0.25 mL/kg given intramuscularly, maximum 15 mL) is effective to prevent or reduce the severity of measles in susceptible individuals if given within 6 days of exposure. In immunocompromised patients the dose of immune globulin should be 0.5 mL/kg (max. 15 mL). Persons who are not vaccinated or unable to receive measles vaccine, infants, pregnant women and the immunocompromised receive the greatest benefit from human immune globulin. HIV-exposed or -infected children and adolescents should receive a 0.5 mL/kg dose of immune globulin, regardless of their immunization status. Intravenous immune globulin (IVIG) preparations also contain measles antibody.

Active Immunization. In countries with high endemicity and associated mortality, routine measles vaccination of infants is recommended, along with mass immunization campaigns. Low measles vaccination coverage rates are associated with outbreaks. A reduction of measles mortality by 95% from 2000 to 2015 is the goal of the Measles Initiative, an effort supported by WHO, UNICEF, the American Red Cross, the CDC and the United Nations Foundation. In the first 10 years, vaccination campaigns and surveillance worldwide have resulted in important reductions in measles deaths in children.

Measles vaccine is prepared with a live attenuated strain of the virus that is grown in chicken embryo cell culture. The measles vaccine is available individually or as part of combination vaccines containing live attenuated mumps, measles and rubella (MMR), sometimes with varicella virus (MMRV). Single and combination measles vaccines are highly efficacious. Almost 100% of children vaccinated with 2 doses of vaccine will have protective immunity if the first dose is given after 12 months of age. Maternal antibody transferred transplacentally may inhibit vaccine efficacy up to the age of 6–12 months. However, in areas of high endemicity, the first dose is usually given at 9 months of age and vaccination at 6 months, despite a lower seroconversion rate, is used in areas and situations of high risk, such as during outbreaks. According to the WHO, in 2010, approximately 85% of the world's children received one dose of measles vaccine by their first birthday.[3] Ideally, children who receive the first dose in the first year of life should receive two additional doses, separated by a minimum of 4 weeks after their first birthday.

The measles vaccine is safe in most children. Uncommon side-effects may include transient fever of moderate severity, a mild rash, and transient thrombocytopenia. Febrile seizures may occur in predisposed children, but encephalitis is a rare complication.

Asymptomatic and not severely immunocompromised HIV-positive children may receive measles vaccine because the risk of acquiring wild virus disease outweighs the risks of the vaccine. Severely immunocompromised HIV infected persons, patients with immune deficiencies that increase the severity of viral infections, persons with previous hypersensitivity reactions to vaccination and pregnant women should not receive measles vaccine. Human immunoglobulin should be combined with measles vaccine in exposed malnourished children.

RUBELLA (GERMAN MEASLES)

Rubella is a mild, self-limited viral illness of childhood. The clinical importance of rubella lies in the potentially disastrous consequences of infection in early pregnancy leading to severe congenital malformations (congenital rubella syndrome).

Epidemiology

Rubella is an endemic disease of worldwide distribution, although in countries where routine childhood immunization schemes include rubella vaccine, the incidence of this disease has been reduced significantly and cases occur only sporadically in unvaccinated populations. In most tropical countries where rubella vaccine is not administered routinely, epidemics may occur in cycles every 6–9 years. Unvaccinated persons are susceptible to infection through adulthood.

Pathogenesis and Pathology

Rubella virus is an enveloped icosahedral RNA virus of approximately 60 nm of diameter that is easily inactivated by extremes of pH and heat, ultraviolet light, formalin, lipid solvents and trypsin. Transmission occurs via the air-borne route, by person-to-person contact as humans are the only host. The incubation period from exposure to development of fever is 14–21 days. Similar to measles, viraemia occurs before the onset of the rash, and immunity develops as the rash appears. A person with rubella remains infectious from 7 days before the onset of rash to 4–5 days afterwards, but generally is less infectious than a measles patient. Direct viral infection and immune-mediated responses are thought to contribute to the rubella exanthem.

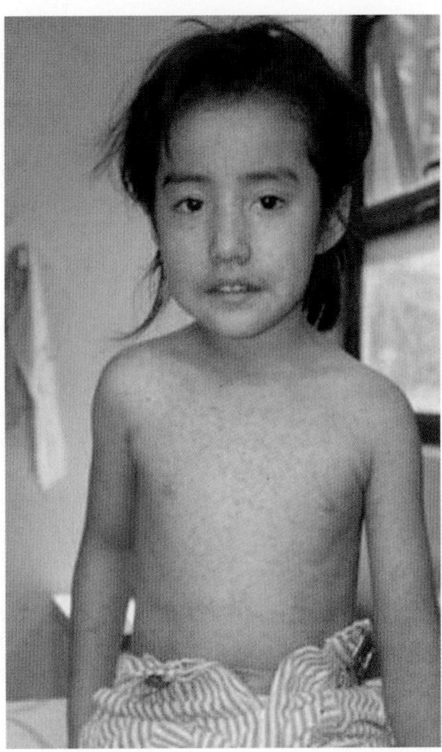

Figure 20.4 School-aged child with rubella, exanthem and cervical lymphadenitis.

Clinical Features

Many cases of rubella are subclinical or mild. Patients may develop a fever with mild pharyngitis and conjunctivitis. A maculopapular skin rash appears on the 2nd or 3rd day, spreading from the face and behind the ears to the rest of the body (Figure 20.4). The fever typically resolves with the appearance of the rash. A skin rash may not be present in all cases and thus, the diagnosis may be difficult. The macules do not coalesce into one another and fade with no or only minimal desquamation in 4–5 days. Characteristic suboccipital, posterior auricular and cervical lymphadenopathy may appear before the rash and last for 5–8 days, along with generalized adenopathy and rarely splenomegaly. Painful joints of the hands and feet and polyarthritis are more common in young adults than in children, providing a clue to the diagnosis of congenital rubella in an infant born to a young woman with these symptoms. Adults may also have a prodrome of fever, malaise and anorexia, absent in children.

The differential diagnosis of a rubelliform skin exanthem includes measles, parvovirus infection, enterovirus infection, scarlet fever (group A streptococcus), staphylococcal or streptococcal toxic shock syndrome and drug reactions.

Complications

Complications of rubella include: thrombocytopenia, encephalitis, mild hepatitis and arthralgia/polyarthritis. In most cases, transient thrombocytopenia lasting from 1 to 3 weeks, to several months may be found, particularly in children. Haemorrhage in vital organs such as the brain and kidney may occur in association with the thrombocytopenia and possibly vascular damage. Thrombocytopenic purpura has been reported in association with childhood rubella infection. Encephalitis is rare, occurring in 1 in 5000 cases, particularly adults. Severity is variable from self-limited with no long-term sequelae to potentially fatal. Arthritis and arthralgia are also more common in adults, particularly women, and usually involves the fingers, wrists and knees. Although most cases resolve without resulting in chronic arthritis, the course may be prolonged for several weeks.

CONGENITAL RUBELLA SYNDROME

Rubella infection during pregnancy results in viraemia and fetal infection. The effects on the fetus are more severe if infection occurs in the 1st trimester of gestation, when the risk of transmission is also higher (up to 85% risk), but deleterious effects occur with infection later in pregnancy as well, including long-term developmental and cognitive deficits. Fetal death, pre-term delivery and prematurity, and congenital anomalies are associated with rubella infection in pregnant women. The main defects caused by rubella in the fetus are a triad of: (1) ophthalmologic manifestations (cataracts, glaucoma, retinopathy and microphthalmia); (2) neurological manifestations, particularly sensorineural deafness, but also mental retardation and behavioural disorders; and (3) heart anomalies (patent ductus arteriosus, ventricular septal defect (VSD), pulmonary artery stenosis or tetralogy of Fallot). Affected newborns also have a generalized infection which, together with the anatomic defects, constitutes the congenital rubella syndrome. Clinical manifestations may include: low birth weight, growth retardation, hepatosplenomegaly, hepatitis, jaundice, thrombocytopenia, anaemia, interstitial pneumonitis and radiolucent lesions in the metaphysis of long bones. Severe anaemia and thrombocytopenia result in the characteristic 'blueberry muffin' rash, erythematous maculopapular lesions associated with dermal hematopoiesis, along with petechia and ecchymoses. These clinical manifestations are indistinguishable from the illness caused by congenital CMV infection. Severely affected infants have a poor prognosis for survival. Survivors, and even infants who appear 'normal' at birth after maternal infection, may suffer from long-term complications and associated morbidities, including blindness, deafness, seizures, progressive encephalopathy, thyroid disorders and diabetes.[7]

Diagnosis

The diagnosis is clinical in most cases of post-natal rubella. A positive IgM antibody titre can be detected by the 5th day of the illness. IgG antibody seroconversion or a fourfold rise in titre in acute and convalescent sera is also diagnostic. Rubella virus can be isolated from nasal or throat specimens or detected using PCR. In pregnant women, recent infection is diagnosed by detection of rubella-specific IgM antibodies in serum or detection of the virus by PCR. False-positive IgM results may occur with other viral co-infections or a positive rheumatoid factor. Immune status and exposure history are therefore important considerations to establish the diagnosis of rubella infection in pregnancy.

Infants with congenital rubella syndrome have detectable IgM antibodies in the first month of life, although not always present at birth. A persistent or increasing concentration of rubella-specific IgG antibodies in the first several months of life is also diagnostic of congenital rubella. Furthermore, these infants have prolonged viral activity and shedding and may have positive cultures from blood, urine, cataract and respiratory specimens in the first year of life.

Management

Treatment is symptomatic and supportive. Children with rubella should avoid contact with pregnant women. Serological testing (IgG and IgM) should be done in exposed pregnant women. Women infected in the 1st trimester of gestation are best advised to terminate the pregnancy. Those who find this unacceptable may be given passive immunization with intramuscular immunoglobulin, which may reduce viral replication and viraemia, theoretically decreasing the probability of fetal infection. Rubella is a notifiable disease.

Prevention

Rubella vaccine is a live attenuated preparation of the virus, found typically in combination with measles and mumps vaccine (MMR). The vaccine is efficacious and results in protective immunity in more than 90% of children vaccinated at or after one year of age. Vaccine recommendations vary significantly worldwide from routine vaccination in childhood, to vaccination of adolescent females only, to rubella vaccine not being part of the immunization schedule. Pregnant women and people with immune deficiencies should not receive rubella vaccine. As for measles, asymptomatic and not severely immunocompromised patients with HIV infection may be vaccinated.

ENTEROVIRUSES

The non-polio enteroviruses, coxsackieviruses and echoviruses cause a variety of illnesses often associated with fever and exanthems. More recently, enterovirus serotype 71 has been recognized as a cause of central nervous disease with cutaneous manifestations in many parts of the world.

Epidemiology

Enterovirus infections are very common and endemic worldwide, with outbreaks occurring in limited geographic locations and populations such as schools and healthcare institutions. Young children experience the highest attack rates and severity of disease. Enteroviruses typically cause summer time respiratory, gastrointestinal and central nervous system illnesses, but seasonality is less evident in tropical regions, where infections may occur year round and infections are more frequent when poor hygiene and overcrowding living conditions exist.

Pathogenesis and Pathology

The enteroviruses are exclusive human pathogens traditionally classified as Group A and B coxsackieviruses, echoviruses and numbered enteroviruses. Based on genetic similarity, they are grouped into four species, as human enteroviruses A, B, C and D. Transmission occurs from person to person by the respiratory route or through faecal–oral contact, and from a mother to her infant in the immediate postpartum period.

The severity of the diseases caused by enteroviruses varies with the patient's age and immune status, but also by the specific virus and serotype. Newborns, young children and patients with humoral and combined immune deficiencies are at greatest risk for invasive disease and complications. Most infections result in self-limited, nonspecific febrile illnesses, but viraemia and involvement of other organs such as brain, heart, lungs, and liver may occur.

Clinical Features

The exanthems seen in enteroviral infections are not a cause of morbidity per se, but represent a clinical clue to the diagnosis of enteroviral disease.

Hand-foot-mouth disease associated with coxsackie A16 is the enterovirus infection with the most characteristic exanthem. Other enteroviruses associated with hand-foot-mouth disease include coxsackie viruses A4, A5, A6, A7, A9, A10, A24, B2 to B5, echovirus 18 and enterovirus 71. Preschool and school-aged children often present with moderate fever for 1–2 days, sore throat or mouth, and in some cases difficulty eating due to the presence of mucosal vesicular lesions that ulcerate in the tongue, soft palate and buccal mucosa. At least two-thirds of patients concomitantly develop tender erythematous papulovesicular lesions in the palms and soles, occasionally extending to the extremities, gluteal and perineal regions. These lesions may appear similar to those caused by herpes or varicella viruses, but in hand-foot-mouth disease the lesions have a characteristic distribution and are always associated with oral lesions. Viruses can be isolated from these lesions, indicating direct viral invasion of dermal and epidermal cells, as well as a localized inflammatory and immune response. Other enteroviruses associated with herpetiform exanthems are coxsackievirus A9 and echovirus 11, causative agents of viral myopericarditis and aseptic meningitis. The vesicular skin lesions in these patients are similar to those seen in hand-foot-mouth disease, but are found on the head, trunk and extremities, and are not associated with oral lesions.

Other exanthems associated with enterovirus infections are much less characteristic and do not allow to discern a specific a etiologic diagnosis based on their clinical features alone. Based on their appearance, enterovirus exanthems are classified as morbilliform (or rubelliform), roseoliform and petechial (a fourth type being herpetiform, as described above).

Morbilliform exanthems appear as fine maculopapular lesions resembling rubella, starting on the face and spreading to the neck, trunk and extremities during the febrile phase of the illness. The lesions are small (<2–3 mm in diameter), not pruritic, and do not desquamate. Unlike patients with rubella, patients with enterovirus do not typically have coryza, conjunctivitis, or lymphadenopathy. Echovirus 9, which causes aseptic meningitis, is the serotype most frequently associated with a morbilliform rash, while infection with echoviruses 2, 4, 11, 19, 25 and coxsackievirus A9 have also been reported to cause a similar rash. The presence of generalized skin lesions, occasionally including the palms and soles, in an infant with aseptic meningitis is a clue to the diagnosis of enterovirus infection (Figure 20.5).

Echovirus 16 causes a roseola-like illness distinct from human herpesvirus (HHV)-6 associated roseola only by the timing of appearance of the rash, which in echovirus 16 is simultaneous with the fever. The lesions are maculopapular, non-pruritic, and distributed mainly on the face and upper part of the chest, without involving the extremities. The rash resolves in 1–5 days with the resolution of the fever. Coxsackie B1 and B5, and echovirus 11 and 25 can also cause this roseoliform rash.

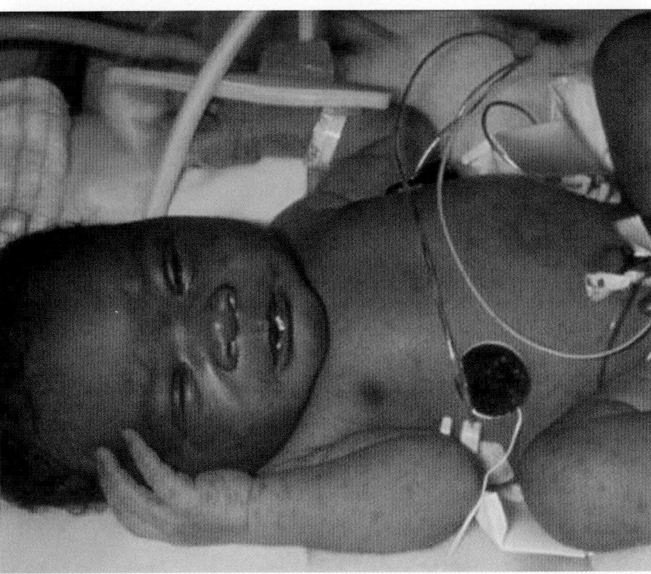

Figure 20.5 Infant with enterovirus infection and generalized maculopapular exanthem that involves palms and soles.

Coxsackieviruses A9 and A16, and echovirus 9 may cause exanthems with petechial and purpuric lesions, and urticariform lesions.

Diagnosis

In addition to recognition of the enterovirus clinical syndromes, the most sensitive method to confirm the diagnosis of enterovirus infection is by PCR in cerebrospinal fluid, blood, stool or rectal, urine and respiratory (throat, respiratory secretions) specimens. Isolation of enterovirus in cell culture is limited by poor growth or no growth of most serotypes in vitro.

Management and Treatment

Treatment is symptomatic and supportive, as no specific antiviral is available. In life-threatening infections such as neonatal enterovirus, viral myocarditis, enterovirus 71 neurological disease, and enterovirus meningoencephalitis in immunocompromised patients, administration of intravenous immunoglobulin has been used in an attempt to modify the disease and improve survival, but the effectiveness of this intervention is unproven.

Prevention

Vaccines are not yet available to prevent non-polio enterovirus infection, including enterovirus 71, although research is ongoing. Patients with humoral and combined immunodeficiencies may benefit from IVIG administration. Given the risk of transmission through the respiratory and gastrointestinal tracts, hand washing is the most important measure to prevent enterovirus infection.

DNA Viruses Causing Cutaneous Disease

DNA viruses are likely to be associated with cutaneous manifestations. Poxviruses, herpesviruses, cytomegalovirus (CMV), Epstein–Barr virus (EBV) and papillomaviruses cause well described exanthems in otherwise healthy hosts with illnesses that vary in severity from benign and self-limited to sometimes fatal. In immunocompromised hosts the skin lesions may be atypical and severe, often life-threatening. Most DNA viruses characteristically establish persistent or latent infections that can reactivate in both immunocompetent and immunocompromised hosts. Treatment of these viral infections is challenging. Antivirals with specific activity against some of these agents are available and new agents are under development (Table 20.3).[8]

DISEASES DUE TO POX VIRUSES

Orthopoxviruses

Orthopoxviruses belonging to the family of Poxviruses that infect humans are *variola* (smallpox), *vaccinia*, monkey pox and cowpox. Poxviruses are large (200–450 nm in size), brick- or ovoid-shaped double-stranded DNA viruses that are especially adapted to epidermal cells.[9] Variola virus, the cause of small pox is the only one that affects humans exclusively, the others are zoonotic infections. Poxvirus infections may be localized to the skin or disseminated. The initial site of infection may be the skin, a mucosal surface, or the respiratory tract. The virus then spreads through regional lymphatics to cause viraemia and involvement of the reticuloendothelial system with secondary viraemia. The typical pock skin lesions result from direct viral infection of the skin. Antibodies directed against a member of the orthopoxviruses can provide cross-protection against other species. Although no specific antiviral treatment is available, certain compounds, such as cidofovir and ribavirin, have in vitro activity against all pox viruses, and other agents are under evaluation. Drugs active against herpes virus, particularly acyclovir, are not active against pox viruses.

Smallpox

Smallpox is a formerly devastating, severe, febrile illness characterized by an extensive, profuse, vesicular rash, high transmissibility, and a high mortality rate (10–75%). Survivors were left with severe disfiguring scars. The skin lesions varied from focal to generalized and flat to vesicular and hemorrhagic. Seven to 14 days after exposure to infected respiratory secretions or lesions cases would develop high fever, headache, backache, vomiting and prostration, followed by centrifugal (more prominent in face and extremities) maculopapular, then vesicular and pustular rash that involved the palms and soles. Resolving lesions dried up after 2 weeks and formed a scab that sloughed off, leaving a scar. Human smallpox virus was one of the most contagious (secondary attack rates ranging from 30% to 80%) and fatal of viral infections. In 1980, the WHO declared that smallpox had been eradicated globally, highlighting the success of mass vaccination programs with a highly effective vaccine, search and identification of new cases, and containment interventions. The fact that humans were the sole hosts of this virus also contributed to its elimination. In 2008, smallpox again became a concern to both physicians and the general public given suggestions that it could be used as a bio-weapon in current global conflicts.

Monkey Pox

Epidemiology. Monkey pox was first described in 1958 in captive Asiatic monkeys, but it is only found naturally in Africa,

TABLE 20.3 Antiviral Agents Available for the Treatment of Viruses Associated with Exanthems

Virus and Disease	Antivirals Recommended for Treatment	Other Treatment Options
RNA VIRUSES		
Measles	None	Supportive Vitamin A once daily for 2 days <6 months of age: 50 000 IU 6–11 months: 100 000 IU ≥12 months: 200 000 IU Vitamin A once in 2–4 weeks for children with clinical evidence of Vitamin A deficiency Ribavirin (in vitro activity, but not approved for routine treatment)
Rubella	None	Supportive
Enterovirus (EV)	None	Supportive Intravenous immunoglobulin (IVIG) in life-threatening neonatal infection, myocarditis, EV 71 neurological disease, and chronic EV meningoencephalitis in immunocompromised patients
DNA VIRUSES		
Poxviruses (smallpox, monkey pox, cowpox) Tanapox	None	Supportive Cidofovir (in vitro activity, used in severe disease, but not approved for routine treatment)
Molluscum contagiosum	Cidofovir (IV or topical) (immunocompromised)	Physical destruction Curettage Cryotherapy (liquid nitrogen) Electrodesiccation (laser) Surgical removal Chemical agents (podophyllin, cantharidin, tretinoin, silver nitrate, iodine, potassium hydroxide, liquefied phenol, 25–50% trichloroacetic acid) Immune modulators Cimetidine (PO) Imiquimod (Topical)
Herpes simplex virus (HSV-1, HSV-2)	Acyclovir (IV/PO) Valacyclovir (PO) Famciclovir (PO) Topical penciclovir Topical ophthalmic agents (1% trifluridine, 0.1% iododeoxyuridine, 3% vidarabine)	Foscarnet (in vitro activity, used for acyclovir-resistant strains) Cidofovir (in vitro activity, used for acyclovir-resistant strains)
Varicella zoster virus (VZV)	Acyclovir (IV/PO) Valacyclovir (PO) Famciclovir (PO)	Foscarnet (in vitro activity, used for acyclovir-resistant strains) Varicella zoster immunoglobulin Intravenous immunoglobulin (IVIG)
Epstein–Barr virus	None	Supportive
Cytomegalovirus (CMV)	Ganciclovir (IV) Valganciclovir (PO) Foscarnet (IV) Cidofovir (IV)	CMV immune-globulin
Human Herpesvirus (HHV-6, 7, 8)	None	Supportive
Adenovirus	Cidofovir (IV) (immunocompromised)	Supportive
Human Papillomavirus (HPV)	Cidofovir (IV) (immunocompromised)	Physical destruction Curettage Cryotherapy (liquid nitrogen) Electrodesiccation (laser) Surgical removal Chemical agents (tretinoin, podophyllin, cantharidin) Immune modulators Cimetidine (PO) Intralesional interferon-α
Parvovirus B-19	None	Supportive Intravenous immune globulin (severe cases)

primarily in remote villages in Central and West Africa, near tropical rainforests. The first human case was recognized in Zaire in 1970. Since then, more than 200 cases have been reported, mainly in Zaire (now Democratic Republic of Congo), but also in Liberia, Nigeria, Ivory Coast, Cameroon, Sierra Leone and most recently, in Sudan. In 2003, human cases were diagnosed in the USA, as a result of global commerce of exotic pets, with rodents playing a role as potential reservoirs, although this is the only time monkey pox has occurred outside of Africa.[10,11]

It is not known whether the primary maintenance hosts are chimpanzees, other primates or small mammals. Most patients give a clear account of contact with monkeys which they have caught and/or eaten. Most cases occur during the dry season and children are affected more than adults.

Pathology and Pathogenesis. The monkey pox virus is morphologically indistinguishable from variola. In culture, the pocks on chick chorioallantoic membrane are slightly larger and more haemorrhagic than those caused by variola. Unlike variola, monkey pox virus is pathogenic in rabbits, and has a higher temperature ceiling for growth. It grows readily in green monkey and rodent cell cultures.

Humans are infected by direct contact with blood, body fluids, or skin lesions of infected animals or by droplet spread via the respiratory tract. The disease is not readily transmitted from person to person, but secondary cases have been recorded as a consequence of contact with respiratory secretions, skin lesions or infected fomites. The attack rate is 10% in susceptible individuals in close contact with a primary case, in contrast to smallpox infection in which it was 20%. Little tertiary spread occurs, and epidemics are not a feature.

The pathogenesis is similar to that of smallpox, with an incubation period of about 12 days (range 5–17 days), viraemia and dissemination to organs and skin. The smallpox-like rash evolves over 2–4 days, followed by complete recovery after 2–3 weeks. Only rarely does human monkey pox result in death (<10% of cases). There is well-defined immunity to reinfection, and complete cross immunity with variola and vaccinia. Monkey pox has never been reported to occur in an individual vaccinated for smallpox.

Clinical Features. The clinical manifestations of monkey pox can be divided into two stages. The onset is abrupt with a prodromal illness lasting 2–5 days characterized by fever, severe headache, myalgias, back pain, prostration and characteristically, marked lymphadenopathy, particularly cervical, submandibular and sublingual. On the 3rd to 5th days, the exanthem appears; this consists of a single crop of discrete papules, more abundant on the face and extremities than on the trunk (Figure 20.6). The soles of the feet and palms are usually involved. The papules form pustules which become umbilicated and are covered with crusts which separate after about 10 days, leaving small scars. The number of lesions varies from a few to several thousand, affecting the oral mucosa (in 70% of cases), genitalia (30%), conjunctivae (20%) and the cornea. Resolution of the illness takes 2–3 weeks. Mild atypical cases occur in which there may be fewer than 10 lesions, separation of the crusts occurring by the 5th day. Complications include keratitis, encephalopathy, secondary bacterial skin infection, gastrointestinal disease, and airway obstruction due to severe lymphadenopathy. The differential diagnoses include smallpox, chickenpox, measles, bacterial skin infections, scabies, syphilis and drug reactions.

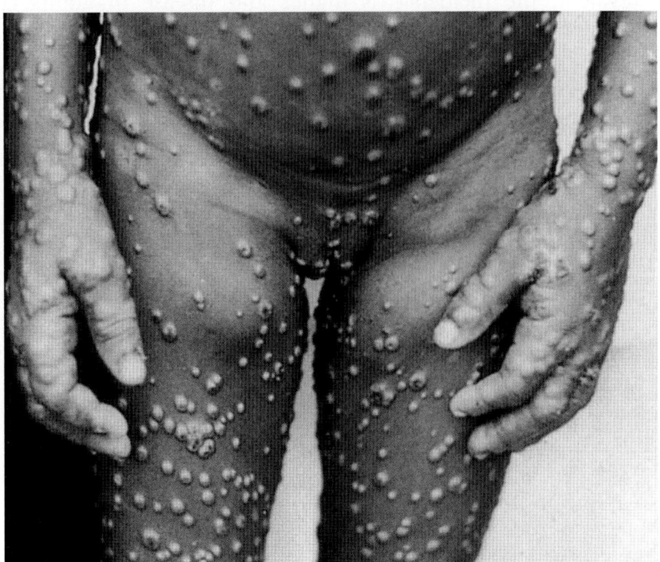

Figure 20.6 Monkey pox, with characteristic inguinal and femoral lymphadenopathy.

Diagnosis. The diagnosis is based on clinical findings, epidemiology and a history of contact with monkeys. Lymphadenopathy is an important distinguishing feature from smallpox. A definitive diagnosis can be achieved by identification of the virus by PCR, electron microscopy, isolation in cell culture, antigen detection tests and antibody detection by ELISA.

Management. Treatment is symptomatic and supportive.

Prevention. Previous smallpox vaccination is protective in most persons. During outbreaks, contact precautions are important to prevent spread. Animal-to-human exposure can be prevented through awareness of the illness and source of infection, appropriate handling of sick animals and animal products, and complete cooking of products for human consumption.

Cowpox

Cowpox is a rare zoonotic infection resulting from occupational exposure with infected cows and other animals such as cats, elephants, and rats. Cases have been reported in restricted geographic locations in Europe and its bordering regions of Asia. Unlike smallpox and monkey pox, the exanthem of cowpox is localized in the hands (fingers) and face, and two-thirds of patients have only a single lesion. The lesion is initially macular and very painful, becomes papular, vesicular and pustular with associated surrounding edema and erythema, and crusts into a black scab before leaving a permanent scar. Other concomitant symptoms include fever, malaise and regional lymphadenitis owing to lymphatic and viremic dissemination. Children and immunocompromised hosts have a more severe illness. Complete resolution takes several weeks, up to 3 months. Definitive diagnosis can be made by identification of the virus in vesicle fluid or extracts of crusts by PCR or electron microscopy, or isolation of the virus on chorioallantoic membrane or specific cell lines.

OTHER POX VIRUSES

Other pox viruses that infect humans include Parapox virus, Tanapox, and Molluscum contagiosum. Parapox is a zoonosis acquired through contact with infected cattle, goats or sheep, and presents clinically similarly to cowpox, with localized papulovesicular lesions at the site of inoculation, which is usually a break in the skin. The lesions can ulcerate (e.g. human form infection) or become nodular due to granuloma formation (e.g. milker's node lesions).

Tanapox

Tanapox virus is not an Orthopoxvirus; with the Yabapox virus, it forms a distinct subgroup of pox viruses, the Yatapox viruses. Humans are incidental hosts.

Epidemiology. Tanapox was first described in 1957 and 1962 in epidemics temporally associated with flooding in the lower Tana River of Kenya. Serological surveys have shown continuing transmission to humans in the area. Human infections have since been recorded in the forest area of Zaire (Democratic Republic of Congo). Tanapox is restricted to Eastern and Central Africa, although a few cases have been reported in travelers returning from the area to Europe and the USA.

The primary maintenance hosts are unknown; many monkeys, especially vervet (*Cercopithecus aethiops*) are susceptible, and are common in endemic areas.

Epidemiological studies suggest that the virus is transmitted from monkeys to humans by a mosquito or arthropod intermediary. Tanapox infections demonstrate a seasonal variation that coincides with the activity of local arthropods. Rare cases of transmission to humans after direct contact with a primate have been described. There is no evidence of direct person-to-person spread.

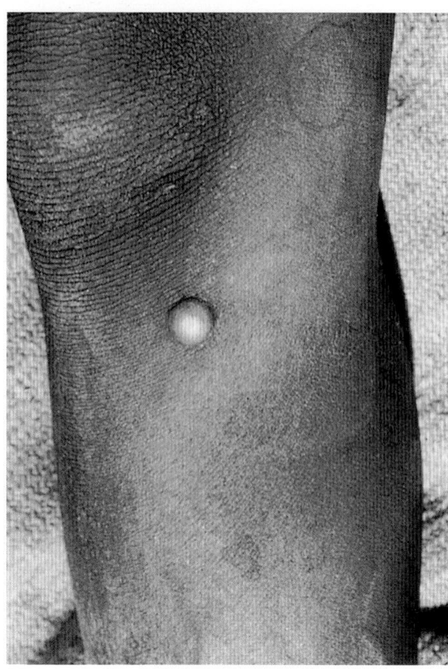

Figure 20.7 Tanapox. Solid pock containing firm whitish material.

Pathology. A Yaba-like virus causes tanapox in humans. The initial site of infection is the skin, through an insect bite or an area of skin breakdown. Pathology is limited to the epidermis where the pock lesions form. There are few or no destructive changes. Hypertrophied epidermal cells containing acidophilic inclusion bodies predominate; cellular infiltration is mild, and the dermis remains intact. Infection likely results in lifelong immunity. Antibodies that develop in infected individuals and monkeys persist for some years. There is no cross-immunity with *vaccinia*; recently vaccinated individuals can develop the disease.

Clinical Features. The illness is usually mild and self-limited, with full recovery within 6 weeks. The incubation period is unknown. Onset is abrupt with fever lasting 2–4 days, accompanied in some cases by severe headache, backache and prostration. The fever and localized pruritus precede the appearance of one or two (no more than 10 lesions have been reported) pock-like lesions on the skin. Initially macular, lesions become papular and indurated. They never proceed to pustule formation, rather, over a period of about 2 weeks they become elevated nodules that appear umbilicated with firm centres or ulcerated (Figure 20.7). The surrounding skin also becomes indurated and erythematous, and regional lymphadenopathy can be appreciated. The pocks occur mainly on exposed surfaces, particularly the extremities, and less commonly on the face, neck and trunk. Recovery takes place over several weeks; no scars are left and there are no residual complications.

Diagnosis. Tanapox can be distinguished by its unique geographic distribution, the larger size and small number of lesions, which characteristically are firm, solid nature and lack postulation, and the benign course of the illness. The virus can be seen in lesion material by electron microscopy or identified by molecular methods as the genome has been sequenced. It can be isolated by culture in cell lines such as green monkey kidney or Vero cells, and is clearly distinguished by antigenic structure from orthopoxviruses.

Management. Specific treatment is not required as lesions are self-limited.

Molluscum Contagiosum

Molluscum contagiosum is a benign, self-limited papular infection of the skin in otherwise healthy hosts. Immunocompromised individuals may experience more severe disease that is difficult to treat.

Epidemiology. Molluscum is an exclusive disease of humans, with a worldwide distribution. It is more common in young children who may acquire the infection in nursery or school.[12] Molluscum frequently affects young sexually active adults and immunocompromised individuals. In areas where HIV/AIDS is prevalent, the incidence is higher and disease in adults is observed.

Pathogenesis and Pathology. There are four subtypes of molluscum contagiosum viruses differentiated by restriction endonuclease digests, but the clinical disease they cause is indistinguishable. Infection is acquired by direct contact or autoinoculation. The incubation period is variable and usually prolonged, weeks to months. The infected cells in the lower layer of the epithelium proliferate, vacuolate, enlarge and protrude above the skin surface as pearly, umbilicated lesions. The central cavity of the lesion contains white, cheesy material with infectious vacuolated cells. Accumulation of molluscum inclusion bodies in the cytoplasm causes compression of the nucleus to the periphery of the cell, leading to rupture and infection of adjacent cells. The viral genome encodes cell products involved in the pathogenesis and evasion of immune mechanisms, such as apoptosis inhibitors. No or very little surrounding inflammatory responses are noted.

Clinical Features. The lesions occur isolated or in groups, usually on the face, arms or near the genitalia, and their

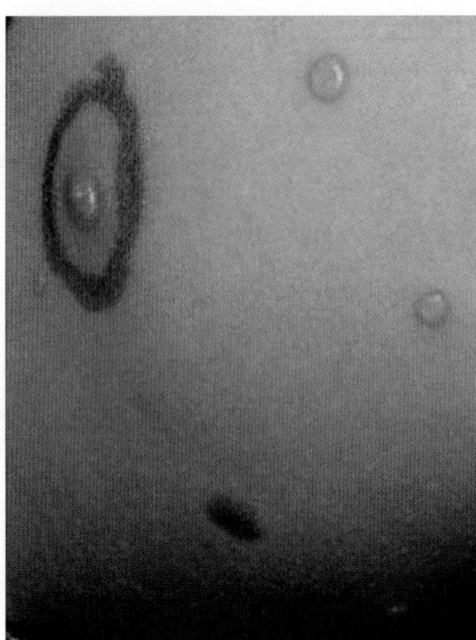

Figure 20.8 Molluscum contagiosum with mild surrounding erythema and characteristic flesh-coloured umbilicated lesions.

appearance is characteristic. Initially they appear as a small papule, 2–5 mm in diameter, flesh-coloured or pearly appearing, with a smooth surface that is often umbilicated (Figure 20.8). A whitish material can be easily expressed from some lesions.

In immunocompetent individuals, the lesions are self-limiting and regress spontaneously with time (6–12 weeks). Only a few scattered lesions are usually seen in a circumscribed location. The number of lesions in HIV positive individuals can exceed 100, and coalesce forming large plaques with many smaller lesions ('agminate form'). In some cases, molluscum infection can induce localized dermatitis known as molluscum dermatitis. Lesions in HIV-positive individuals and patients with impaired cell-mediated immunity do not usually resolve spontaneously, persisting for months or even years.

Diagnosis. The diagnosis of molluscum contagiosum is clinical. However, HIV-positive patients may have other lesions of similar appearance, such as those caused by cryptococcosis, cutaneous pneumocystosis and other infectious disorders. Solitary lesions may resemble other entities (e.g. pyogenic granuloma, keratoacanthoma and basal cell carcinoma). A biopsy will confirm the characteristic histopathology of molluscum lesions or exclude more serious conditions. Molluscum contagiosum does not grow in standard tissue cultures, but it can be seen by electron microscopy in lesion material, or identified by PCR.

Management. Most patients do not require specific treatment as the lesions resolve spontaneously. Treatment of persisting lesions is by physical means, including cryotherapy, curettage, electrosurgery, topical keratolytic preparations such as cantharidin, podophyllin, tretinoin, iodine, salicylic acid, liquefied phenol, silver nitrate, potassium hydroxide and 25–50% trichloroacetic acid. These methods have variable efficacy and they can be very painful and may lead to scarring and discoloration of the skin.[13] Topical treatment with 3% cidofovir cream or suspension, or immune modulation with oral cimetidine or topical imiquimod has been reported to be efficacious in some cases. Combinations of these therapies are often employed. Marked improvements are now being observed in patients receiving highly active antiretroviral therapy (HAART).[14]

HUMAN HERPESVIRUSES

All herpesviruses are large (150–250 nm) enveloped double-stranded DNA viruses that have the property of remaining latent in viable form within host cells after primary infection. Herpesviruses reactivate from the latent state to produce recurrent disease, often with mucocutaneous manifestations.[15] Human herpesviruses have a worldwide distribution and are usually transmitted through close contact with infected lesions, secretions, or mucosal surfaces, or by vertical transmission from mother to infant. Humans are the only host of the viruses described here.

Herpes Simplex Viruses (HSV)

Herpes simplex virus type 1 (HSV-1) and type 2 (HSV-2) cause a variety of clinical illnesses that affect persons of all ages and can be severe in the immunocompromised.

Clinical Syndromes Due to HSV Type 1 (Usually Orofacial)

1. Gingivostomatitis: vesicles or ulcers in and around gums and mouth
2. Ocular herpes: keratoconjunctivitis with vesicles or ulcers on eyelids, conjunctiva, cornea
3. Meningoencephalitis.

Clinical Syndromes Due to HSV Type 2 (Usually Anogenital)

1. Balanoposthitis: vesicles or ulcers on prepuce and glans penis
2. Vulvovaginitis: vesicles or ulcers on vulva and vaginal mucosa
3. Anoproctitis: vesicles or ulcers around the anal skin and in the anus.

Other Herpetic Infections with Cutaneous Manifestations

1. Neonatal herpes infection. Primary genital infection in the mother (usually HSV-2, but HSV-1 may also cause neonatal infection) transmitted to the newborn passing through the birth canal at delivery results in a serious systemic infection manifested in the neonatal period in three distinct clinical forms: mucocutaneous disease with typical herpetic vesicular lesions usually appearing in areas of skin trauma, central nervous disease with necrotizing meningoencephalitis and seizures, and disseminated disease with multiorgan involvement and sepsis-like manifestations including pancytopenia, hepatosplenomegaly and shock. When present, cutaneous vesicular lesions provide a clue to the diagnosis (Figure 20.9). The fatality rate is high even in treated patients. If untreated, isolated mucocutaneous disease may progress to involve the central nervous system or disseminate. In utero infection is rare, but potentially devastating.
2. Herpetic 'whitlow' is the term given to herpes simplex lesions on fingertips. This may occur from inoculation from a primary oral or genital herpes, or occupational exposure with affected patients. The lesion, which tends to recur periodically at the initial site of infection, presents with painful vesicles filled with serous exudate and

surrounded by erythema. Regional lymphadenopathy may be noted.

3. Eczema herpeticum or Kaposi's varicelliform eruption. This is a superinfection of eczematous skin by herpes simplex, seen mainly in young children.

Primary HSV Infection

Primary infection with HSV, when the virus is encountered for the first time, may be asymptomatic or present with clinical manifestations depending on the site of infection. Exposure of the skin or mucosal surfaces with HSV results in infection of epithelial cells and local replication. The basic pathological lesions are cutaneous or mucocutaneous vesicles or ulcers with a surrounding area of erythema. The virus then spreads to other skin areas, local ganglial and neuronal tissue via migration through peripheral sensory nerves. Viraemia results in spread to other organs and potentially life-threatening disease.

Latency. Following a primary mucocutaneous infection, HSV enters nerve endings underlying the skin lesion and travels through peripheral nerves to ganglion cells in the anatomic region of the original infection. HSV then enters a latency stage in the ganglia for days to years.

Reactivation can occur as a result of immunosuppression, physical or emotional stress, fever (e.g. orofacial herpes is common in patients with lobar pneumonia and malaria), skin trauma, menstruation, fatigue or exposure to ultraviolet light. During reactivation, HSV is transmitted back to the primary mucocutaneous site via efferent nerves, causing the reappearance of vesicular lesions. Reactivation may recur sporadically throughout life. The frequency of reactivation varies with the type of HSV, the initial site of infection, and the immune status of the host.

Primary HSV Infections in HIV-infected Individuals. Persistent and recurrent herpetic infections are one of the most common clinical manifestations of HIV infection.[16] Importantly, prior HSV infection increases the risk of acquisition of HIV via alteration of epithelial barriers and by localizing CD4+ cells, the primary target of HIV, to the ulcers. It is hypothesized that antigenic stimulation of mucosal sites by reactivation of HSV can potentially increase HIV-1 replication on mucosal surfaces. Therefore prevention and treatment of HSV infections could significantly impact the epidemiology of HIV.

Most HIV-positive patients have clinical manifestations of HSV infection in the course of their disease, and these tend to be more severe and persistent than in immunocompetent hosts. In HIV-positive individuals, primary infections may be life-threatening, or may manifest as chronic ulcerative mucocutaneous lesions, verrucous plaques or hyperplastic nodules. Painful and often deep, these chronic ulcers usually present around the mouth, perianal or genital areas. Other manifestations include herpetic infection of the cornea, tracheobronchial tree, oesophagus, lung, pericardium, liver and brain.

Diagnosis of HSV Infections. Clinical characteristics and laboratory testing aid in the diagnosis of herpetic infections. HSV grows readily in tissue culture causing a distinct cytopathic effect within 2–5 days of inoculation. Identification of HSV DNA by PCR provides a more rapid, sensitive and specific diagnosis. These methods also permit subtyping of the virus. HSV can be identified from a variety of samples, including: vesicular fluid (which can be obtained by placing a small needle into the vesicle and aspirating), scrapings from the base of the lesions, tissue biopsy, blood leukocytes, cerebrospinal fluid and mucosal secretions, including conjunctiva.

The differential diagnosis of HSV includes all causes of vesicular exanthems and ulceration. Ulcerated lesions can mimic: (a) aphthous ulcers; (b) cytomegalovirus (CMV) ulcers; (c) drug reactions, (d) opportunistic atypical mycobacterial infections, (e) fungal infections and (f) traumatic ulcers. Verrucous-appearing lesions can mimic such entities as warts and epithelial neoplasms.

Treatment of HSV Infections. Acyclovir, famciclovir and valacyclovir are effective for the treatment of mucocutaneous and systemic HSV infections. Treatment with topical preparations of acyclovir and other compounds that can be applied to the eye is also available. Antiviral drugs are rarely required in superficial mucocutaneous infections in an immunocompetent individual.

VARICELLA–ZOSTER VIRUS INFECTIONS

Varicella (chickenpox) and zoster (shingles or herpes zoster) are different diseases caused by the same virus. Varicella is a primary illness, whereas zoster is a reactivation disease.

Varicella (Chickenpox)

Chickenpox is a systemic infection with a characteristic vesicular rash. The primary infection usually occurs in young children and is always symptomatic. In the majority of cases, the illness is benign and recovery is complete, but it may be severe and fatal in infants infected in the first 2 weeks of life, in adults and in immunocompromised hosts.

The incubation period for chickenpox is 12–24 days, averaging 15–18 days. Transmission is by person-to-person contact with vesicular lesions, or by air-borne spread of respiratory secretions. The infectious period is usually 1–2 days before and up to 6 days after the appearance of the rash. Shedding may be prolonged in immunocompromised patients.

Clinical Features. Children present with low-grade fever, malaise, anorexia and a rash. Adults have more severe symptoms. The characteristic exanthem is the presence of lesions in different stages of evolution, including macules, papules, vesicles, and ulcers that scab with a dark crust. The lesions are pruritic and may leave a scar after healing. Lesions appear in waves with new lesions appearing as the older ones evolve (cropping). Successive crops of lesions are smaller and eventually fail to develop as immunity is established. Lesions appear most densely on the trunk and face; the hands and feet are relatively spared. Lesions may affect the conjunctivae, buccal mucosa, intestinal mucosa, and lungs. In immunosuppressed individuals (post-transplantation, corticosteroid therapy, HIV/AIDS), primary chickenpox infection may cause a serious clinical disease with extensive cutaneous and systemic manifestations. Haemorrhagic varicella is typically associated with other complications.

An important complication of chickenpox is secondary bacterial infection with *Staphylococcus aureus* or *Streptococcus pyogenes* (Group A streptococcus). These may sometimes progress to cellulitis, erysipelas, sepsis, or toxic shock syndrome, causing significant morbidity and mortality even in previously healthy hosts. This may be an important problem in tropical countries where contamination is more likely to occur.

Other complications include viral dissemination to cause central nervous system manifestations such as ataxia or encephalitis, which are more frequently seen in children, or varicella pneumonitis, a potentially life-threatening complication in adults. Systemic disease may also result in disseminated intravascular coagulation, and multiorgan involvement, particularly abnormal renal and hepatic function.

Newborns are at greatest risk of disseminated disease and fatal varicella when exposed at the time of birth to a mother with primary chickenpox infection with onset of the rash within 5 days prior to 2 days after delivery. The absence of passively transferred maternal antibodies and relative immaturity of the infant's immune system accounts for the elevated risk of perinatal varicella.

Diagnosis. The diagnosis of chickenpox is mostly by clinical examination and identification of the characteristic lesions and exposure history, particularly in perinatal varicella where maternal lesions are present (Figure 20.9). Confirmation can be made by PCR or tissue culture of material from vesicular lesions or scrapings of the base of the lesion, tissue biopsy, or cerebrospinal fluid. Other methods include direct immunofluorescent antibody and serologic tests.

Management and Treatment. Chickenpox is a self-limited illness and most patients recover without specific treatment. The decision to use antiviral therapy is based on the immune status of the host and the duration and extent of the infection, since viral replication is limited to the first 38–72 hours of the illness. Otherwise, healthy children do not require treatment. Patients with certain conditions that may increase their risk of complications, such as adolescents and adults, persons receiving chronic steroid or aspirin treatment, and secondary contacts may benefit from treatment. Oral acyclovir may reduce the duration of fever and active rash (from 6.5 to 5.7 days). Other oral antivirals for adults include famciclovir and valacyclovir. Aspirin (acetylsalicylic acid) should not be used for reduction of fever, or analgesia because of an association with Reye syndrome. Intravenous acyclovir is recommended for immunocompromised hosts, however, asymptomatic or not severely immunocompromised HIV-positive patients can be treated with oral agents. Secondary bacterial infections are common and thus antibiotics with anti-staphylococcal and anti-streptococcal activity must be used.

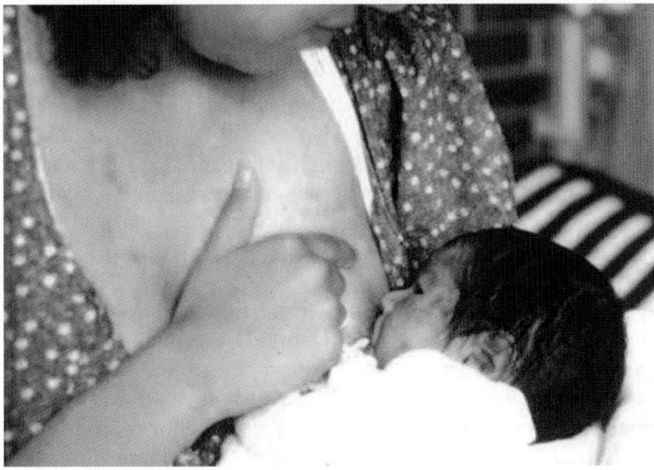

Figure 20.9 Maternal and neonatal varicella showing lesions in mother and infant. *(Courtesy of Gerardo Cabrera-Meza, MD.)*

Administration of varicella-zoster immunoglobulin (VZIG) or intravenous immunoglobulin (IVIG) within 96 hours of exposure may prevent or reduce the risk of complications in exposed high-risk patients such as persons with no previous immunity who are pregnant or immunocompromised, newborns and premature infants.

A live attenuated varicella vaccine is safe and highly effective. Unfortunately, it might not be widely available in developing countries. Routine administration of varicella vaccine has resulted in a significant decrease in the incidence of varicella and it complications in the USA.

Shingles or Zoster

Varicella-zoster virus (VZV) produces lifelong latency and reactivates usually later in life, causing 'shingles', which presents as a painful vesicular rash with a dermatomal distribution. In persons who have had chickenpox, the virus remains dormant usually in the dorsal root ganglia, until reactivation, at which time it travels down the nerve to manifest the typical cutaneous lesions of zoster (shingles) along the distribution of one or two dermatomes served by a dorsal root ganglion. The mechanism of reactivation is unclear, although contributing factors include stress, ageing, underlying malignancy and immunosuppression.

Clinical Features. Patients with herpes zoster typically experience a prodromal phase of varying severity, which may manifest as pain, numbness, tingling and/or itching in a localized region of the body. This is commonly followed by the appearance of erythematous maculopapular lesions that rapidly evolve into an eruption of vesicles in a specific dermatomal distribution, multiple dermatomes, or on any part of the body, including eyes and mucosal surfaces (Figure 20.10). Vesicles may coalesce to form bullae before gradually resolving over 1–2 weeks. Although rare in children, zoster may be seen in children infected with HIV (Figure 20.11). Zoster generally appears within 2–7 years of HIV seroconversion, most commonly during the asymptomatic phase. In these and other immunocompromised patients, shingles is more severe and more difficult to treat, leaving serious scarring.

Complications of zoster include ophthalmic zoster resulting in conjunctivitis and blindness. The risk of post-herpetic neuralgia (persistence of pain for months or years) tends to increase with age but not with immunosuppression. Complications in immunocompromised individuals include dissemination over large areas of the skin with possible secondary infection, potentially fatal pulmonary involvement, and encephalitis. Zoster also tends to have a higher rate of recurrence (5–23%) in HIV-infected individuals, compared with less than 5% in immunocompetent hosts. Verrucous plaques can also occur in zoster; these are chronic and often resistant to therapy with aciclovir.

Zoster is usually diagnosed clinically and elicits a history of previous varicella infection. Confirmatory tests are similar to those for varicella. Tzanck smear with the presence of

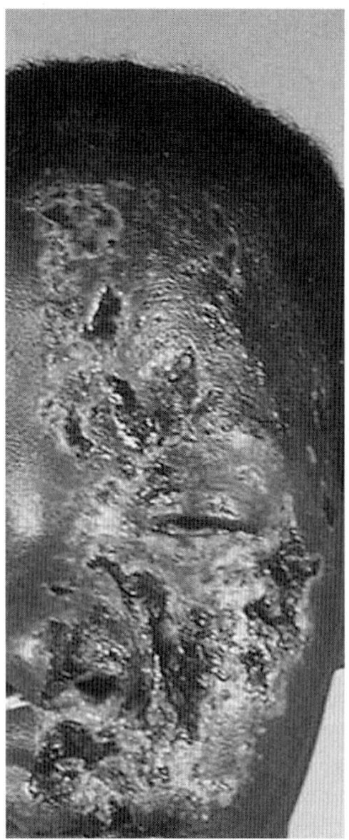

Figure 20.10 Multidermatomal herpes zoster in a patient with AIDS.

multinucleated giant cells can help diagnose HSV or VZV but cannot distinguish between HSV-1, HSV-2 and VZV. Acyclovir, famciclovir and valacyclovir can be used for the treatment of zoster. Foscarnet is reserved for acyclovir-resistant VZV strains. Post-herpetic neuralgia can be treated symptomatically with topical analgesic agents such as capsaicin. Other modalities that may be effective include the use of amitriptyline, carbamazepine, nerve blocks, lidocaine and fentanyl patches.

EPSTEIN–BARR VIRUS

Epstein–Barr virus (EBV) typically causes infectious mononucleosis or 'glandular fever' and is associated with other specific disorders including Burkitt lymphoma (most commonly seen in Central Africa), nasopharyngeal carcinoma (most frequent in South-east Asia), B- or T-lymphocyte lymphomas (Hodgkin's and non-Hodgkin's) involving the central nervous system, post-transplant lymphoproliferative disease (particularly in liver and heart transplant patients), X-linked lymphoproliferative disorders, and gastric carcinoma as well as other epithelial malignancies. HIV-infected patients and immunocompromised hosts are at greater risk for these diseases.

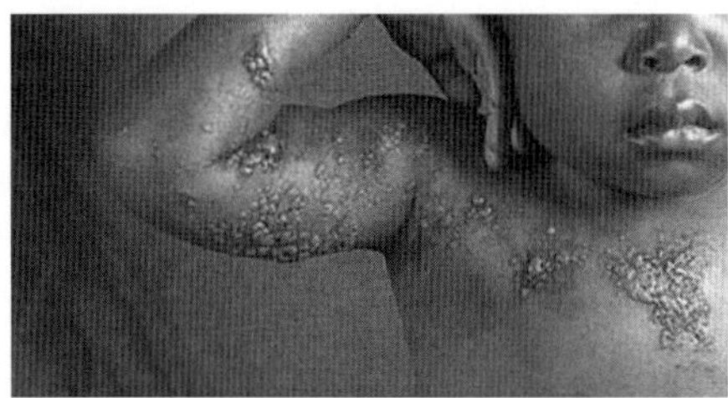

Figure 20.11 Herpes zoster in an HIV-positive child with typical dermatomal distribution.

Primary EBV infection begins in oropharyngeal epithelial cells where EBV virions replicate and from there disseminate through lymphatics and blood into other organs. Infectious mononucleosis presents as a self-limited febrile illness with fever, pharyngitis, lymphadenopathy which may be prominent, hepatosplenomegaly, and peripheral blood atypical lymphocytosis. The course may be protracted and other complications such as hepatitis, central nervous system involvement, and bone marrow suppression can ensue. In addition to epithelial cells, salivary gland duct cells, B cells, T cells, natural killer (NK) cells, macrophages/monocytes, smooth muscle cells and endothelial cells may become infected. The EBV-infected B cells express various EBV-associated antigens that are the target molecules recognized by the host immune response. When the immune surveillance system fails, reactivation of EBV-infected B cells occurs with subsequent polyclonal proliferation and dissemination of EBV to other tissues.

Cutaneous Manifestations of EBV Infection

In immunocompetent hosts, the cutaneous manifestations of infectious mononucleosis may include a petechial skin rash (due to thrombocytopenia) or macular lesions appearing after the use of ampicillin (not an allergic reaction).[17] A diffuse erythematous macular rash may be seen in some patients with infectious mononucleosis who do not receive ampicillin. Gianotti–Crosti syndrome, also known as acrodermatitis of childhood, consists of pruritic pink-red papules or papulovesicles on the extensor surface of the extremities, cheeks and buttocks that follows typical symptoms of infectious mononucleosis. Histologically, these lesions show lymphocytic vasculitis, spongiotic or lichenoid changes, red blood cell extravasations and papillary dermal oedema. The mucocutaneous manifestations of EBV in HIV-infected patients with moderate to advanced immunodeficiency include oral hairy leukoplakia (OHL), which manifests as whitish plaques on the inferolateral margins of the tongue. The surface of the plaques may be smooth, corrugated or folded with thick hair-like projections. Lesions of OHL can mimic other mucous membrane lesions such as tobacco-associated leukoplakia and candidiasis. Lesions caused by OHL cannot be dislodged by a tongue depressor. They are asymptomatic and cause few problems; however, they occasionally become verrucous and may lead to dysphagia. OHL must be distinguished from candidiasis by the absence of hyphae in a microscopic examination of scrapings. Lesions caused by OHL can also mimic tobacco-associated leukoplakia, squamous cell carcinoma, condyloma acuminatum, genital ulcers, lichen planus, white sponge nevus, leukokeratosis oris, mucous patches of syphilis and aphthous ulcers.

Diagnosis

Diagnosis is made by serology. Detection of IgM antibodies directed to the viral capsid antigen (VCA) is diagnostic. Once infection is established, IgG antibodies to the viral capsid antigen remain positive for life. Antibodies to the nuclear antigen develop with resolution of the illness and when present are indicative of a previous (past) infection with EBV. A monospot test to detect heterophile (IgM) antibodies (Paul-Bunnell) may be useful, as it is commonly available, but its sensitivity is variable and the test is unreliable in children younger than 4 months of age. Molecular methods using PCR may detect EBV DNA in peripheral blood mononuclear cells.

Management

Treatment is supportive; no specific antiviral treatment is available. Reduction of immunosuppressive treatments might be beneficial in some patients. Cytotoxic agents and immunomodulators are used in patients with EBV-associated lymphoproliferative disorders.

CYTOMEGALOVIRUS

Human cytomegalovirus (CMV) is a ubiquitous virus that infects most people during childhood or adolescence. Most infections are self-limited and mild, and involve the upper respiratory tract in immunocompetent hosts. CMV remains latent in the infected individual and can reactivate during periods of immunosuppression. Reinfection with other strains of CMV is also possible. Transmission is by person-to-person contact with infected secretions or receipt of blood products. Sexual transmission has been considered a possible route of infection.

Congenital CMV occurs when pregnant women acquire primary CMV infection during pregnancy and the fetus is infected in utero. The spectrum of disease of congenital CMV varies according to the time of infection during pregnancy from asymptomatic infection to a devastating syndrome that may be indistinguishable from congenital rubella and includes intrauterine growth retardation, anatomic defects (microcephaly, intracerebral calcifications), sensorineural hearing loss, retinitis, hepatitis, hepatosplenomegaly, bone marrow suppression with purpura, and sepsis-like syndrome. Congenital CMV has significant implications for affected infants who might have a shortened life, or important sequelae such as deafness, blindness and mental retardation, and for society.

HIV-infected persons and those who are immunocompromised, particularly those receiving immunosuppressive therapy for cancer or after transplantation, are at greater risk for complications from new-onset CMV infection or reactivation. Up to 90% of patients with AIDS develop acute active CMV infection at some point during their illness; it is one of the most common opportunistic viral infections in patients with AIDS, particularly when CD4 counts drop below 100 cells/mm^3. Clinical manifestations include retinitis, gastroenteritis, hepatitis, pneumonia, oesophagitis, colitis and encephalitis.

Cutaneous Manifestations

CMV viraemia is usually followed by infection of the vascular endothelium of every organ, skin lesions, vasculitis and ulceration of mucosal surfaces.[18] Three patterns of vascular injury are associated with CMV; leukocytoclastic vasculitis, necrotizing lymphocytic vasculitis, and pauci-inflammatory cell injury with luminal thrombosis.[19] Cutaneous lesions of CMV include:

1. Macular rash
2. Localized and diffuse ulcers, particularly in areas contiguous to mucosae
3. Palpable purpuric or necrotic papules
4. Petechiae
5. Vesicular, bullous and generalized morbilliform eruptions
6. Keratotic verrucous lesions
7. Hyperpigmented indurated plaques
8. Generalized bullous toxic epidermal necrolysis-like eruption associated with CMV hepatitis.

Infants with congenital CMV may present with a combination of petechiae, purpuric and maculopapular lesions similar to those seen in congenital rubella syndrome.

Diagnosis

Cutaneous manifestations of CMV infection are not distinctive enough to allow the diagnosis to be made on clinical grounds alone. Identification of the virus in the blood or affected organs confirms the diagnosis. CMV can be isolated in cell culture from urine, respiratory secretions, saliva, vaginal and cervical secretions, semen, stool, peripheral blood leukocytes, cerebrospinal fluid, tissues and other body fluids. Identification of CMV DNA by PCR is particularly helpful in tissue specimens and cerebrospinal fluid. Quantification of viral load can be obtained with this method. Another available assay is the direct antigenaemia test, which consists of the direct detection of CMV antigen in nuclei of peripheral blood leucocytes using monoclonal antibodies directed against the CMV lower matrix protein pp65 (UL83). The test is also able to quantify the number of pp65-positive cells, thus providing an estimate of viral burden. Quantitative PCR and the antigenaemia assay are the most rapid and reliable tests for the diagnosis of CMV disease in both patients with AIDS and organ transplant recipients.

The diagnosis of cutaneous CMV can also be established histologically. Cytomegalic intranuclear inclusions, CMV antigens or CMV DNA detected in skin biopsy specimens may be helpful to diagnose CMV infection.

Management

The usual treatment for clinical disease caused by CMV is intravenous ganciclovir. Cidofovir, foscarnet and fomivirsen are also approved for the treatment of CMV retinitis in patients with AIDS. An oral formulation of ganciclovir, valganciclovir is available for prophylaxis in high-risk patients.

HUMAN HERPESVIRUSES 6 AND 7

HHV-6 and HHV-7 are prevalent in humans with a tropism for CD4+ lymphocytes. Primary infection with HHV-6 results in exanthema subitum (roseola or sixth disease) in young children, a nonspecific febrile illness often associated with seizures which presents with a diffuse, nonspecific macular rash is noted when the fever resolves, and a characteristic flushed or erythematous appearance of the face. The exanthem resolves over a few days with complete resolution of the illness. Other clinical associations made with this virus include an infectious mononucleosis-like illness and drug-induced hypersensitivity syndrome. More recently, HHV-6 has been recognized as an opportunistic pathogen in patients with HIV infection and in transplant recipients, causing fever, a maculopapular skin rash, malaise and visceral involvement such as hepatitis and encephalitis. HHV-6 has also been implicated in graft versus host disease and various malignancies. HHV-7 infection occurs later in life with clinical manifestations, similar to those of HHV-6 and accounts for repeat cases of roseola and probably pityriasis rosea.[19] Diagnosis by PCR is the most sensitive and specific. There is no specific treatment, although ganciclovir has been used in immunocompromised patients with severe HHV-6 infection.

HUMAN HERPESVIRUS 8

This herpesvirus was first discovered in 1994 and was named Kaposi's sarcoma-associated herpesvirus because it was found in almost 100% of Kaposi's sarcomas from patients with AIDS. This virus is now commonly referred to as human herpesvirus 8 (HHV-8) and has subsequently been found in peripheral blood mononuclear cells of patients with Kaposi sarcoma, in classical and in other forms of Kaposi sarcoma, in lymphomas in HIV-positive patients, and patients with multicentric Castleman disease. Kaposi sarcoma lesions evolve from an initial purpuric macule or patch, to plaques, nodules or small angiomas or hematomas, and in some cases ulceration. HHV-8 DNA has also been detected in patients with pemphigus vulgaris, pemphigus foliaceus, carcinoma and lymphoma. In Africa, paediatric Kaposi sarcoma is a type of cancer that is commonly seen in children with or without HIV infection. Primary infection consists of a febrile illness and a macular rash that mimics purpura, as reported in areas that are endemic, including Africa, the Middle East and Mediterranean countries. Diagnosis can be made by PCR, immunohistochemistry and immunofluorescence methods. There is no specific antiviral treatment.

ADENOVIRUS

Adenoviruses are non-enveloped, double-stranded DNA viruses grouped into six species (A–F), of which distinct serotypes are associated with clinical syndromes including acute respiratory tract illness, conjunctivitis, gastroenteritis, and hemorrhagic cystitis among others. Adenovirus infections occur at all ages, worldwide, with no clear seasonality. Some serotypes cause severe disseminated disease in otherwise healthy hosts, while immunocompromised hosts are at risk for severe and potentially fatal adenovirus infection. Cutaneous manifestations of adenovirus occur in the context of systemic disease and may include a nonspecific maculopapular rash, petechial or purpuric lesions, and conjunctivitis.

PAPOVAVIRUSES

Human Papillomavirus

Human papillomavirus (HPV) causes cutaneous and mucosal lesions and is associated with epithelial and genital malignancies.[20] Papillomaviruses are non-enveloped, icosahedral, double-stranded DNA viruses approximately 55 nm in diameter. Among more than 100 known species of papillomaviruses, human papillomaviruses are exclusive human pathogens found in all regions of the world. Infection is common in children, occurs at all ages, and is often subclinical or persistent with a prolonged period of latency. Immunocompromised hosts are at greater risk to develop clinical manifestations and more severe disease.

Cutaneous Manifestations. HPV is transmitted by direct contact with infected secretions or lesions and result in cutaneous or mucosal disease, depending on the type of epithelium they infect. Cutaneous HPV cause skin warts, which vary in size and number and usually resolve spontaneously. Mucosal HPV species cause venereal warts and condyloma acuminatum, the most common manifestations of genital HPV infection. HPV are directly associated with cervical, vaginal, vulvar, rectal and perianal cancer. Newborns exposed to HPV in the birth canal can develop laryngeal or respiratory papillomatosis with obstructive symptoms. Immunocompromised individuals have an increased risk and incidence of HPV infection and disease.[21] Penile and perianal warts are twice more common in HIV-positive men than in individuals with a normal immune system. The incidence of genital warts in HIV-positive women has been reported to be increased by as much as 10-fold. Giant condyloma acuminata (also known as Buschke–Lowenstein tumour), epithelial pre-malignant lesions and frankly malignant disease are more frequently seen in HIV-infected individuals. These lesions are increased in number and severity and are difficult to treat. Many recur after treatment. Invasive cervical cancer, which is closely associated with oncogenic HPV, is considered an AIDS-defining illness in HIV-positive women. Cervical cancer is the second most common cancer killer of women worldwide.

Diagnosis. Cutaneous and anogenital warts are diagnosed clinically. Detection of viral nucleic acid (DNA or RNA) by PCR is diagnostic in tissue and cytology samples.

Management. The optimal treatment for warts that do not resolve spontaneously is unknown. Depending on their size, extent and location, warts can be treated with topical agents (podophyllin, salicylic acid, tretinoin), cryotherapy with liquid nitrogen, and laser or surgical excision. High recurrence rates of warts are common in both HIV-positive and non-HIV patients. Immunomodulators such as intralesional interferon-α and topical imiquimod are available for the treatment of genital warts and are often used in combination with other methods. Cidofovir is a broad-spectrum antiviral agent with activity against all human herpes viruses and HPV. Effective virus-like particle vaccines are available to prevent infection by common HPV types associated with genital warts and cervical cancer. While these vaccines are licensed and administered to adolescent girls and boys in several industrialized countries, the vaccine may not be accessible in regions of the world where HIV is endemic and its impact would be greatest.

PARVOVIRUS INFECTIONS

Human Parvovirus B19

Parvovirus B19 is a non-enveloped, single-stranded DNA virus that infects precursors of red blood cells in humans. The cutaneous manifestations of human parvovirus B19 infection include a reticular or lace-like erythematous centrifugal rash that moves peripherally from the trunk to the extremities in association with the 'slapped cheek' appearance noted in children with erythema infectious or fifth's disease; a painful petechial and purpuric eruption in a 'glove and stocking' distribution that includes palms and soles known as purpuric gloves and socks syndrome (PPGSS), and a febrile illness with a rubelliform or purpuric rash distinct from the typical rash of erythema multiforme. Other cutaneous findings include vasculitis, erythema nodosum, vesiculo-pustular eruptions, a lupus erythematosus-like syndrome, pityriasis lichenoides and scleroderma.[22] These clinical manifestations are typically associated with viraemia and other systemic symptoms including fever, malaise, respiratory symptoms, and sometimes arthralgias. The dermatopathology of parvovirus B19 infection suggests that tissue injury is a result of viral invasion and the host immune response, including delayed-type hypersensitivity, antibody-dependent cellular immunity directed at antigenic targets in the epidermis and endothelium, and circulating immune complexes in the setting of leucocytoclastic vasculitis. Most illnesses caused by parvovirus B19 are self-limited, but complications including persistent or chronic anemia, pure red cell aplasia and transient aplastic crises are more likely to occur in immunocompromised hosts.

REFERENCES

4. Huiming Y, Chaomin W, Meng M. Vitamin A for treating measles in children. Cochrane Database Syst Rev 2005;(4):CD001479.
8. Dropulic LK, Cohen JI. Update on new antiviral under development for the treatment of double stranded DNA virus infections. Clin Pharmacol Therapeut 2010;88(5):610–19.
9. Diven DG. An overview of poxviruses. J Am Acad Dermatol 2001;44(1):1–16.
14. Rodgers S, Leslie KS. Skin infections in HIV infected individuals in the era of HAART. Curr Opin Infect Dis 2011;24(2):124–9.
19. Chisholm C, Lopez L. Cutaneous manifestations caused by Herpesviridae: A review. Arch Pathol Lab Med 2011;135(10):1357–62.

Access the complete references online at www.expertconsult.com

21 Virus Infections of the Nervous System

TOM SOLOMON

KEY POINTS

- Viruses can affect any part of the nervous system.
- Some viruses occur only in the tropics, particularly those which are arthropod-borne.
- For others, which are found worldwide, there are specific issues around diagnosis and management in the tropics.
- The lumbar puncture is the single most useful investigation for patients with suspected viral central nervous system infections, supported by cerebrospinal PCR testing for some viruses and detection of IgM antibody for others.
- While some pathogens are nearly eradicated, e.g. poliovirus, others such as enterovirus 71 are growing in importance.
- People with HIV are especially susceptible to some viral CNS pathogens.

Summary

HERPES SIMPLEX VIRUS TYPES 1 AND 2

- Herpes simplex virus (HSV) type 1 is transmitted by droplet spread and causes encephalitis.
- HSV type 2 is more likely to be transmitted via the genital route and cause meningitis.
- The incidence of HSV1 in the tropics is thought to be the same as elsewhere.
- HSV2 also causes neonatal encephalitis.
- HSV encephalitis is treated with aciclovir. Its role in HSV meningitis is less clear.

VARICELLA ZOSTER VIRUS

- Varicella zoster virus (VZV) causes chickenpox during primary infection, which is associated with acute neurological syndromes, especially cerebellitis.
- The virus reactivates later in life, especially in the elderly or immunocompromised, to cause a range of central nervous system (CNS) and peripheral nervosus system presentations, including shingles, stroke and small vessel vasculitis.
- The CNS syndromes are treated with high-dose aciclovir with or without corticosteroids.

EPSTEIN–BARR VIRUS

Epstein–Barr virus (EBV) can cause:

- Acute primary CNS infections, as part of infectious mononucleosis
- Primary CNS lymphoma especially in HIV and other immunocompromised states
- EBV is also often detected in the CSF of patients with other CNS infections and may contribute to severe disease
- Diagnosis is by PCR detection in the CSF
- Primary CNS lymphoma is treated with methotrexate or other combinations of chemo- and radiotherapy
- There is no vaccine.

CYTOMEGALOVIRUS

- Cytomegalovirus infection is very common, either acquired in utero or subsequently, through saliva or sexual contact.
- Clinically important infection occurs in two major groups – those infected congenitally and those that are immunocompromised.
- Congenital infection can result in a syndrome with severe multi-organ involvement, including encephalitis.
- In the immunocompromised, especially those with HIV, CMV causes encephalitis, retinitis and radiculitis.
- A pleocytosis with neutrophil predominance is characteristic; occasionally a ventriculitis is seen.
- Treatment is with ganciclovir, its pro-drug valganciclovir or foscarnet.

MEASLES VIRUS

- Measles viruses can cause:
  - Acute measles encephalitis, which presents as an acute disseminated encephalomyelitis (ADEM) days to weeks after measles
  - A sub-acute 'inclusion body' encephalitis several months after infection, in the immunocompromised
  - Sub-acute sclerosing panencephalitis (SSPE), many years after the original infection.
- ADEM occurs in approximately one per 10 000 measles cases.
- There is no specific treatment for any form of measles encephalitis, though various therapies have been tried for SSPE.

NIPAH VIRUS

- The first outbreak of Nipah virus was in Malaysia in 1998, with subsequent smaller outbreaks in Bangladesh and neighbouring India.
- The virus causes respiratory symptoms and acute encephalitis, in humans and pigs.

- Late presentations of Nipah, months after viral exposure, have also been described.
- Transmission is directly from fruit bats (the natural hosts) and also between humans.
- Pathologically there is neuronal damage, perivascular inflammation, vasculitis and infarcts.
- There is no treatment or vaccine.

MUMPS VIRUS

- Mumps virus causes acute parotitis and in approximately 5% of cases aseptic meningitis; deafness and encephalitis also occur.
- Mumps is preventable with live attenuated vaccines, which are used in most developed and one quarter of developing countries.

ENTEROVIRUS 71 AND OTHER NON-POLIO ENTEROVIRUSES

- The enteroviruses include: polioviruses (see below), coxsackieviruses, echoviruses and newer enteroviruses such as enterovirus 71.
- The non-polio enteroviruses can cause exanthemas (rashes), enanthemas (eruptions in the mouth) and other systemic manifestations, as well as neurological disease, most commonly aseptic meningitis.
- Enterovirus 71 is responsible for large outbreaks of hand, foot and mouth disease, with aseptic meningitis and encephalitis, especially in Asia. A severe form of brainstem encephalitis is associated with cardiac dysfunction and pulmonary oedema.
- Parechoviruses constitute a newly formed genus in the family Picornaviridae and include the former echoviruses 22 and 23; they cause aseptic meningitis in young children.
- Intravenous immunoglobulin is used for severe enterovirus 71 disease.
- There are no vaccines for any of the non-polio-enterovirus. During outbreaks of enterovirus 71, social distancing measures are used to reduce spread.

POLIOMYELITIS

- The three serotypes of poliovirus cause paralytic poliomyelitis, which may include brainstem encephalitis.
- Vaccination with trivalent live attenuated vaccine has eradicated the disease from much of the world, but Pakistan, Afghanistan, Nigeria, among other countries, continue to have cases.

HUMAN T-LYMPHOTROPIC VIRUS TYPE 1

- Human T-lymphotropic virus type 1 (HTLV-1) associated myelopathy, also known as tropical spastic paraparesis, is a chronic non-remitting spastic paraparesis caused by (HTLV-1).
- HTLV-1 is transmitted by breast-feeding (the most common route), blood transfusion, needle sharing and sexual intercourse.
- The virus also causes adult T-cell leukaemia-lymphoma in some people.
- There are no antiviral drugs; treatment is supportive, aimed at minimizing disability.
- There is no vaccine. Prevention is by safe sexual practices and screening of blood products.

HUMAN IMMUNODEFICIENCY VIRUS

- As well as secondary neurological infections, HIV can cause aseptic meningitis, as part of a primary seroconversion illness, and chronic cognitive impairment.
- Cognitive disease, called HIV-associated neurocognitive disorder, ranges from asymptomatic impairment detected on neuropsychological testing, through mild neurocognitive disorder to full blown HIV-associated dementia.
- Patients with HIV-associated neurocognitive disorder have memory difficulties, slowness of thought and of movement.
- Other causes of cognitive impairment must be excluded.
- Good control of HIV viral load in the blood and probably also the CNS, is thought to be key to preventing neurocognitive disorder. Choice of drugs with better CNS penetrance may be important.

PROGRESSIVE MULTIFOCAL LEUKOENCEPHALOPATHY

- Progressive multifocal leukoencephalopathy (PML) is caused by JC virus and BK virus, polyomaviruses that cause no other disease in human.
- The viruses are common but only cause disease in those with immunosuppression, especially advanced HIV disease.
- PML presents with a progressive dementia and white matter change on MRI, with no mass effect or gadolinium enhancement.
- There is no established antiviral treatment; those with HIV are treated with combination antiretroviral drugs.

PRION DISEASES

- Prion diseases are progressive fatal neurodegenerative diseases with transmissible properties that affect animals and humans.
- CJD is sporadic or familial.
- Variant CJD is associated with ingestion of meat containing prion protein from cattle with bovine spongiform encephalopathy.
- Kuru was described in Papua New Guinea and caused by ingestion of brain and offal.
- There is no treatment.

Introduction

All parts of the neuraxis, including the brain, spinal cord and nerves, can be infected by viruses. Some of the most important viruses to infect the central nervous system (CNS) are covered in separate chapters, including rabies (Chapter 17) and the arthropod-borne viruses (arboviruses), such as Japanese encephalitis (Chapter 14). This chapter focuses on other important viral causes of CNS infection. Broadly speaking, viruses can be considered according to their route of entry into the body, whether they are DNA or RNA, whether they cause acute or chronic infections and whether they primarily affect the brain, spinal cord, meninges or nerve roots. Some viruses are particularly important in the tropics; others are important globally, but may pose specific diagnostic and treatment challenges in a tropical setting. In this introductory section the viral causes of CNS infection are considered as a whole, before subsections on each of the important pathogens. At the end of the chapter, prion diseases, which are caused by infectious proteins rather than viruses, are considered.

EPIDEMIOLOGY

Viral brain infections occur across the globe, but their epidemiology varies with a number of factors, in particular climate, vaccination rates, HIV incidence and poverty (Table 21.1). Arthropod-borne viral diseases, such as the flavivirus, Japanese encephalitis and the alphavirus Western equine encephalitis, only occur in climates where the temperature will support viral replication in the extrinsic (mosquito) part of the cycle.[1]

TABLE 21.1 Viral CNS Infections

Groups	Viruses	Geography[a]	Comments
Herpes viruses (family: Herpesviridae)			
	Herpes simplex virus type 1	Sporadic, global	Most commonly diagnosed sporadic encephalitis
	Herpes simplex virus type 2	Global, important in people with HIV	Causes meningitis (esp. recurrent); Meningoencephalitis occurs in the immunocompromised or in neonates
	Varicella zoster virus type 1	Increased importance in areas with high HIV prevalence	Acute cerebellitis, stroke syndromes, vasculitis
	Epstein–Barr virus	Increased importance in areas with high HIV prevalence	Encephalitis during infectious mononucleosis; Drives primary CNS lymphoma
	Cytomegalovirus	Increased importance in areas with high HIV prevalence	Encephalitis in neonates and the immunocompromised; with retinitis, radiculitis; ventriculitis
	Human herpes virus 6 and 7	Global	Febrile convulsions in children (after roseola); Encephalitis in immunocompromised adults
Enteroviruses (family: Picornaviridae)			
	Enterovirus 70	Outbreaks in India in the past	Epidemic haemorrhagic conjunctivitis, with CNS involvement
	Enterovirus 71	Especially important in southeast Asia	Epidemic hand, foot and mouth disease, with aseptic meningitis, brainstem encephalitis, myelitis
	Poliovirus	Persists in a few countries of Asia and Africa	Myelitis
	Coxsackieviruses, Echoviruses, Parechovirus	Global	Mostly aseptic meningitis
Paramyxoviruses (family: Paramyxoviridae)			
	Measles virus	Important in areas with low vaccination rates	Causes acute post-infectious encephalitis, sub-acute encephalitis and sub-acute sclerosing panencephalitis
	Mumps virus	Important in areas with low vaccination rates	causes meningitis more than encephalitis
Retroviruses (family: Retroviridae)			
	Human immunodeficiency virus	Global, but especially important in Africa and Asia	Acute meningitis or encephalitis during seroconversion, HIV-associated neurocognitive disorder
	Human T lymphotropic virus type 1	Especially important in Caribbean, Japan	
Polyomavirus			
	JC/BK viruses	Global	Progressive multifocal leukoencephalopathy in the immunocompromised
Others (rarer causes)			
	Influenza viruses, Adenovirus, Parvovirus B19, Lymphocytic choriomeningitis virus, Rubella virus		
Zoonotic viruses			
	Rabies, other Lyssa viruses	Africa, Asia, parts of Americas	Rabid dogs, cats, Daubenton's bats in UK
	Other Lyssa viruses	Localized to different geographical areas	
	Nipah virus	Malaysia, Bangladesh	Transmitted in faeces of fruit bats
Arboviruses (most are also zoonotic)			
Flaviviruses (family: Flaviviridae)			
	West Nile virus	Africa, parts of Asia, southern Europe, Americas, Australia	North America, Southern Europe, associated with flaccid paralysis, Parkinsonian movement disorders
	Japanese encephalitis virus	Asia, Pacific	Asia, associated with flaccid paralysis, Parkinsonian movement disorders

TABLE 21.1 Viral CNS Infections—cont'd

Groups	Viruses	Geography[a]	Comments
	Tick-borne encephalitis	Northern Europe, Northern Asia	Travel in Eastern Europe, former USSR; tick bite; upper limb flaccid paralysis
	Dengue	All countries between tropics of Cancer and Capricorn	Causes fever, arthralgia, rash and haemorrhagic disease, occasional CNS disease
Alphaviruses (family: Togaviridae)			
	Western, Eastern and Venezuelan equine encephalitis virus	Americas	Found in the Americas; encephalitis of horses and humans
	Chikungunya	Africa, Asia, Pacific, Australia, Southern Europe	Asia Pacific
Bunyaviruses			
	Lacrosse virus	America	Encephalitis in children in America
Coltiviruses			
	Colorado tick fever	America	
Vesiculoviruses			
	Chandipura virus	India	Outbreaks in India

[a]Approximate locations of most important disease activity.

However, for many of these viruses, the factors governing whether outbreaks will occur in a particular year are poorly understood. Recent modelling studies have shown a complex interplay of temperature, rainfall and possibly climate change.[2,3] Many of the viruses that cause CNS infections are now vaccine-preventable; hence encephalitis caused by measles, mumps, polio and rabies virus are now rare or non-existent in many industrialized settings, while they still cause disease in countries with limited vaccination programmes. The HIV incidence of a particular region has a bearing on other viral CNS infections: disease caused by herpes viruses, particularly Epstein–Barr virus (EBV) and cytomegalovirus (CMV) are more common in people with HIV; HIV can also affect the clinical presentation – for example herpes simplex virus (HSV) encephalitis has more of an indolent presentation in those with marked immunocompromise. JC virus (named after the first patient from whom it was isolated) causing progressive multifocal encephalitis (PML) is extremely rare outside the context of HIV. Many of the viruses to have emerged in recent years are zoonotic, occurring naturally in animal cycles and then spilling over into humans. Nipah, which first occurred in Malaysia in the late 1990s is a good example of this, having spread from bats to pigs to humans.[4,5] However, one of the biggest changes in the epidemiology of CNS infections in Malaysia in recent years has been the emergence of enterovirus 71; this is transmitted directly between humans and causes large outbreaks of hand, foot and mouth disease, with associated systemic and CNS complications.[6] Most emerging viruses, including enterovirus 71, are RNA viruses, which have a more rapid rate of evolution than DNA viruses. Poverty has a large impact on almost all the diseases described above; much of this influence is through a lack of vaccination, but some of it is through the incidence of HIV.

There are few good epidemiological studies examining the incidence of encephalitis. In non-outbreak situations the incidence has been reported to range from 0.07–12.6 cases per 100 000 population.[7] During outbreaks it may be much higher, e.g. up to 40 per 100 000 children in some outbreaks of Japanese encephalitis.[8] For viral meningitis there are even fewer studies of the incidence and causes in tropical settings, possibly because of the relative unimportance of this syndrome compared to bacterial meningitis or viral encephalitis. However, studies have tended to show that enteroviruses and HSV type 2 are common, as they are in Western settings; in addition, those viruses, which are better known for causing large outbreaks of encephalitis, e.g. polioviruses or JEV, also contribute to the meningitis burden.[9] Importantly, HIV can present with aseptic meningitis as part of a seroconversion illness.[10,11]

PATHOGENESIS AND PATHOLOGY

Entry into the CNS

The pathogenesis of viral CNS infections is best thought of by considering how the virus enters the body and subsequently the nervous system and then the relative contributions of viral replication and host response in causing the damage. For example, HSV type 2 is usually sexually transmitted and is thought to enter the nervous system via sacral nerves to cause meningitis; whereas HSV type 1's postulated transmission via the olfactory nerves may explain its predisposition to cause a fronto-temporal lobe encephalitis. Arboviruses are injected through the skin by blood-sucking insects or ticks, while enteroviruses are transmitted primarily via the faeco–oral route; although these are very different routes of entry into the body, both enteroviruses and arboviruses cause a viraemia, before crossing the blood–brain barrier into the nervous system. This may partially explain the overlap in some of the clinical syndromes they cause – particularly affecting the brain stem and anterior horn cells of the spinal cord, which have a very good vascular supply. RNA viruses tend to cause CNS disease during the primary infection.[12] In contrast DNA viruses, such as the herpes viruses, can cause disease during primary infection or they may lie dormant and become pathogenic through later reactivation: for EBV and CMV reactivation is particularly associated with advanced HIV disease and other immunocompromised states. In recent years it has become clear that encephalitis which appears to be mediated by anti-neuronal antibodies, for example anti NMDA or voltage-gated potassium channels N-methyl D aspartate.

The Blood–Brain Barrier and Host Response

For most viral CNS infections, the blood–brain barrier plays a key role, not only because of its function in keeping pathogens out, but also because it controls the influx of inflammatory and immune cells which fight infection. Viruses may use a range of routes to cross the blood–brain barrier and enter the CNS: transmission of free viral particles through or between the vascular endothelial cells is probably important for arboviruses; for HIV carriage across the barrier within leukocytes, the 'Trojan horse' mechanism, is characteristic. Some viruses such as rabies and HSV type-1, enter peripheral nerves and then are carried centripetally to the CNS.

Uncontrolled inflammation leads to vasogenic oedema (i.e. fluid leakage across blood vessels), which compounds cytotoxic oedema (within damaged cells) and ultimately causes swelling and raised intracranial pressure. Swelling is especially harmful in the brain because it lies in a fixed vault, the cranium, with little room for expansion and shift. Many viruses, including HSV, the arboviruses and the enteroviruses infect the neurones themselves and are thought to cause direct damage through cytolysis or by inducing apoptosis. However, for some viruses infection of the non-neuronal glial cells is more important. For example, HIV infects microglial cells (the CNS equivalent of macrophages) and possibly astrocytes (which have a structural as well as immunological role) causing a chronic cytokine release which ultimately affects neuronal function leading to HIV dementia.[13] JC virus infects and destroys the oligodendrocytes (which produce the myelin sheaths surrounding neurones); thus the pathogenesis is characterized by a loss of CNS white matter, with little inflammation. Rabies is peculiar in that the immune response occurs very late in disease, while for VZV infection and inflammation of the vascular endothelium is the major pathogenic process leading to vasculitis.[14]

The host response to infection consists of innate and adaptive immune processes, both in the periphery, where the infection first occurs and within the CNS itself. There has been much interest in recent years in the innate responses of neurons to viral invasion, mediated through toll-like receptors.[15] Adaptive responses include the production of specific antibody, which may be able to clear virus from infected cells without cytolysis and killing of virally infected cells by CD8-positive cytotoxic T cells. Antibody can mediate intracellular viral killing, without destroying the infected neurones, may be a more appropriate approach to protection from viral CNS infections, given that neurones are non-renewable![16] Additional neuronal damage may occur because cytokines released by inflammatory cells cause apoptosis in uninfected cells, so-called 'bystander' cell death.[17]

CLINICAL FEATURES

The clinical presentation of a viral CNS infection reflects the anatomical location of the infection and the speed of onset. Thus infection of the meninges causes meningitis, infection of the brain parenchyma itself is encephalitis (from the Greek *encephalon* = brain); when the spinal cord is involved it is described as myelitis (Greek *myelos* = marrow); radiculitis describes infection and inflammation of the nerve roots. These terms are sometimes joined to reflect the multiple sites which may be involved, hence meningoencephalitis, meningoencephalomyelitis and sometimes, even radiculomeningoencephalomyelitis!

Although, strictly speaking, these are pathological terms which should only be used when there is histological confirmation, for practical purposes clinical case definitions are used, though to some extent these are a bit arbitrary. For viral infections we distinguish meningitis (signs of meningism, but normal consciousness) from encephalitis (when there is alteration in consciousness); but in bacterial CNS disease, the same distinctions are not used: patients with bacterial *meningitis* often have altered consciousness, but the term 'bacterial meningoencephalitis' is rarely used. For HIV, terms are used differently again. There is not normally the classical perivascular infiltration of inflammatory cells seen in the acute viral encephalitides, but rather chronic diffuse infiltration of monocytes and macrophages, with multinucleate giant cells. Pathologically, this is HIV encephalitis; in the past the term HIV encephalitis was also used for the clinical syndrome of altered cognitive function associated with HIV, but that is now known as HIV-associated neurocognitive disorder.

The other viruses that present with chronic infection and dementia are JC virus, which causes PML and measles. The presentations of measles virus infection of the CNS can range from acute viral encephalitis, to sub-acute encephalitis seen in the immunocompromised, to a chronic dementing illness, sub-acute sclerosing panencephalitis (SSPE), which presents many years after the initial measles infection. EBV can cause an acute meningitis or encephalitis as part of the infectious mononucleosis illness, but is more often associated with lymphoma in people with HIV; CMV is also seen in those with advanced HIV, where it characteristically causes a radiculitis.

Severe headache is one of the most common features of any acute viral CNS infection, be it meningitis or encephalitis. It is often described as the worst headache the patient has ever experienced. In encephalitis headache is typically associated with a febrile prodrome and soon followed by altered consciousness. However, in approximately 10% of patients with encephalitis, fever may not be apparent; the proportion of patients without fever is even higher for viral meningitis, especially that due to enterovirus.[18,19]

Altered consciousness, the cardinal feature of acute viral encephalitis, may take the form of behavioural changes, which are sometimes mistaken for psychiatric illness, disorientation or confusion. There are often associated seizures, particularly in children, which tend to prompt more rapid referral to hospital and initiation of treatment. Movement disorders, including tremors, dyskinesias and even choreoathetosis, occur if the basal ganglia are involved, for example in arboviral encephalitis. There are few pathognomonic indicators as to the cause of a viral CNS infection, the exception being hydrophobia which is seen in rabies.

Lower motor neurone weakness and fasciculations indicate damage in the anterior horn cells of the spinal cord; this is seen for some of the arboviruses – particularly tick-borne encephalitis – and also in the paralytic form of rabies.[20]

There may be clinical features outside the CNS which point to particular diagnoses. Mucocutaneous disease occurs in some enterovirus infections and for HIV there are often peripheral clues such as lymphadenopathy.

DIAGNOSIS

The lumbar puncture is the single most important investigation for diagnosing any CNS infection. It should be performed in all patients with a suspected CNS infection unless there are contraindications. Typically, there is a moderate pleocytosis of a few dozen cells, predominantly lymphocytes, with a normal CSF to blood glucose ratio. However, there are exceptions. For example an early lumbar puncture may show no pleocytosis, especially in children and the glucose ration is sometimes marginally low.

The diagnosis of viral CNS infections presents some particular challenges. At its most simplistic, infections are diagnosed by detecting the virus itself or by detecting a specific immune response, indicating that infection has occurred. Originally, virus detection was achieved by culturing the virus in specific cell lines, eggs or even weanling mice; or by showing viral antigen is present, e.g. in nasopharyngeal aspirates. More recent approaches include nucleic acid detection, through the polymerase chain reaction (PCR) and measurement of soluble viral antigen, e.g. non-structural proteins released by flaviviruses.[21] Whereas PCR requires specific primers for specific infections, in modern high-throughput sequencing approaches, which are used as research tools, any nucleic acid in a sample is amplified and then bioinformatics techniques are used to determine whether this includes anything that might be a pathological organism.[22]

Antibody detection is especially useful for diagnosing acute viral infections, such as those caused by arboviruses. In the past, there has been a whole range of antibody detection tests, such as the haemagglutination inhibition and the complement fixation assay, which were rather nonspecific. Neutralization tests, such as the plaque reduction neutralization assay, are more specific and show that a sample contains antibody which actually neutralizes the virus in question; however they are laborious to perform and require specialized laboratories that can culture virus. More recently, ELISAs for immunoglobulin (Ig)M and IgG have become popular; typically IgM is raised early in an acute viral infection and IgG rises subsequently. Some of these ELISA assays have now been developed into simple bedside kit formats.[23]

Antibody detection methods are less useful for CNS infections caused by reactivation of a latent infection, for example HSV or CMV: showing that a patient has IgG antibody against a virus in the serum does not tell you whether this reflects previous exposure or active disease. Immunoblot methods to detect antibody in the CSF can be helpful, but are underused.[24]

Although we now have many tools for diagnosing viral infections, the challenge comes in knowing how to use and interpret the tests. The gold standard, showing that a patient has CNS inflammation pathologically, culturing the virus from that sample and detecting an appropriate immune response to the infection, is rarely achieved, because pathological material is not often obtained. For acute CNS infections caused by arthropod-borne viruses we therefore take PCR detection of virus in the CSF and/or detection of specific IgM antibody in the CSF as a good enough proxy. However, CSF is not always available; and so IgM antibody detection in the serum is often taken as a surrogate of this; in the context of a patient presenting with an acute CNS syndrome, this approach is probably reasonable;[25] though one must bear in mind that many viruses of interest may cause an acute peripheral infection only, which could be coincidental to the real cause of CNS disease. Enteroviruses present a different set of problems. Serological tests are not usually helpful because enterovirus infections are common and there is cross reactivity between them. Virus detection in the CSF by PCR is possible for viruses which cause meningitis, such as ECHO 30, but not for others, notably EV71 which is rarely detected in CSF.[26] Enteroviruses may also be detected in the vesicles of hand, foot and mouth disease or throat swabs or in the stool, but coincidental carriage is common, especially in the stool, making interpretation difficult.[27]

For viruses that cause chronic infections, including the herpes viruses, serological tests are far less useful, as explained above. PCR detection in the CSF is taken as indicative of CNS infection for some viruses, such as HSV;[28] for others the interpretation may be problematic; e.g. EBV may be coincidentally carried into the CSF in lymphocytes during another infection. The recognition that dual infection may occur makes interpretation of results even more challenging.[29]

MANAGEMENT AND TREATMENT

The initial approach to the patients with a suspected viral CNS infection is similar to that for any acute CNS infection, namely stabilizing the patients, treating any complications of infection such as seizures and raised intracranial pressure, considering antimicrobial and adjunct treatments and ultimately thinking about rehabilitation.

Stabilizing the patient with viral encephalitis in the tropics may be especially challenging. Although traditionally people have advised fluid restriction in those with CNS infection, by the time they come to hospital many patients are markedly dehydrated; this is because they may have been ill for many days, with little fluid intake, compounded by vomiting. Recent data on sepsis suggest that fluid boluses increase the mortality in critically ill children with infection in resource-poor African settings.[30] Our current practice is to cautiously rehydrate adults and children with suspected CNS infections that are dry.[26,31]

In addition to clinically overt seizures, some patients may have subtle motor status epilepticus, in which there is seizure activity in the brain, but the only clinical signs are subtle twitching of a digit or around the eye or mouth. In many tropical settings, where facilities for ventilation on intensive care are limited, clinicians have to be extra cautious in their use of sedating anticonvulsant drugs. Where there is a strong suspicion of raised intracranial pressure mannitol and other osmotic diuretics are often used. The little data available suggest that any relief they give may only be temporary.[32] Other common complications to look for and treat are secondary pneumonias and urinary tract infections.

There are few antiviral drugs available for CNS infections (Table 21.2). Although in Western industrialized settings any patient with suspected encephalitis is given aciclovir, in the context of a large outbreak of an arboviral encephalitis this may not be sensible; the real challenge then becomes identifying a patient who may have treatable HSV encephalitis, among the many who do not. Cerebral imaging may be helpful in this context.

Steroids are sometimes used in acute viral encephalitis when there is marked oedema and brain shift. They were assessed in a small trial of Japanese encephalitis, but there was no evidence of benefit.[34] In VZV encephalitis they are often given, because much of the damage is thought to be post-viral. For enterovirus 71 infection, intravenous immunoglobulin is used. Although no RCTs have been performed, there is good circumstantial evidence supporting its use.[26] Some simple measures employed during the acute infection can reduce the risks of sequelae in those that survive the acute illness. Gentle physiotherapy to the joints can reduce the risk of contractures and keen attention is needed to avoid bed sores. Simple guides to rehabilitation are available on the Web.[35]

TABLE 21.2 Treatment Options in Viral Encephalitis

Acute Viral Encephalitis	
Herpes simplex virus	Aciclovir
Varicella zoster virus (including cerebellitis)	Aciclovir plus corticosteroids
Human herpes virus-6	Ganciclovir, foscarnet
Rabies	Ketamine[a], amantadine, ribavirin
Sub-Acute/Chronic Encephalitis	
In the immunocompromised	
Varicella zoster virus	Aciclovir
Cytomegalovirus	Ganciclovir, foscarnet, cidofovir
Measles inclusion body encephalitis	Ribavirin
Enterovirus	Pleconaril, specific immunoglobulin
Progressive multifocal leukoencephalopathy in HIV patients	Combined antiretroviral therapy (cART), cidofovir
In the immunocompetent	
Sub-acute sclerosing panencephalitis	Interferon-α (intraventricular), ribavirin inosiplex
Progressive multifocal leukoencephalopathy	Consider cytosine arabinoside
Progressive rubella panencephalitis	Plasma exchange

[a]Considered experimental, may be effective for bat-borne rabies virus.
Acute disseminated encephalomyelitis presents acutely; the others typically present with a sub-acute encephalitis. Many of these treatments are unproven, experimental, or only appropriate in certain patients.
Modified from: Boos J, Esiri MM. Viral encephalitis in humans. Washington DC: ASM Press; 2003.[33]

PREVENTION

For those diseases where vaccines are available, e.g. polio, Japanese encephalitis, measles, mumps and tick-borne encephalitis, this is the mainstay of prevention. There are issues in some areas around which vaccines should be included in the expanded programme on immunization (EPI) and to make decisions better information on incidence and disease burden is needed; whether rabies vaccine should be included in the EPI in some countries is under debate. For rabies there is also the peculiar situation where, in addition to control of stray dogs, vaccination of dogs may be one of the best ways to prevent human disease.[36]

For the arthropod-borne viruses where there is no vaccine such as Eastern equine encephalitis virus and West Nile virus, prevention is through vector control and personal protection against bites. Clearly, any measures which protect against HIV also have a big impact on the risk of subsequent viral CNS infections

Herpes Simplex Virus Types 1 and 2

EPIDEMIOLOGY

Herpes simplex viruses (HSV) types 1 and 2 are among eight herpes viruses in the *Herpesviridae* family that cause disease in humans (Table 21.3). They are DNA viruses that following primary infection can become latent only to reactivate later. HSV-1 and 2, along with VZV, are alpha herpes viruses and infect neurones; EBV is, like HHV-8, a gamma herpes virus that becomes latent in B cells; CMV is a beta herpes virus and like HHV-6 and -7 is thought to become latent in T lymphocytes.

Herpes viruses are ubiquitous, being found across the globe. HSV-1 predominantly causes encephalitis in people of all ages, while HSV-2 causes meningitis in adults and encephalitis in neonates. HSV-1 is transmitted by droplet spread; herpetic lesions around the mouth are the main source, but in addition, studies have shown up to 10% of adults and children are asymptomatic excretors of HSV in their saliva.[38] Those in lower socio-economic groups become infected younger, but by the fourth decade approximately 90% of people are positive to HSV-1 serologically.

HSV-2 is predominantly transmitted via the genital route. It is responsible for most genital ulcer disease worldwide, although the proportion due to HSV-1 is increasing. HSV-2 incidence increases with age, number of sexual partners and is greater among women than men.[39] Epidemiological studies show that HSV-2 prevalence is disproportionately high among people infected with HIV, making it a particular problem in parts of Africa.[40] Advanced HIV is associated with increased risk of persistent ulcers, but also higher rates of subclinical viral shedding, which both increase the risk of HSV-2 transmission.[41]

CNS Disease Caused by HSV

HSV-1 is the most commonly diagnosed cause of viral encephalitis in Western industrialized nations, with an annual incidence of one in 250 000–500 000.[42] Some 90% of these cases are due to HSV-1, but about 10% are HSV-2. There is a bimodal distribution of cases of HSV-1 encephalitis, with one-third of cases occurring in those less than 20 years old and one half in those aged 50 years or more. This is thought to reflect primary HSV-1

TABLE 21.3 Herpes Viruses that Infect the Nervous System

Viruses	Characteristics
Alpha herpes viruses	Become latent in nerves
Herpes simplex virus type 1	Typically infects oral mucosa and causes encephalitis
Herpes simplex virus type 2	Typically infects genital mucosa and causes meningitis
Varicella zoster virus	Transmitted in droplet spread
Beta herpes viruses	Thought to become latent in monocytes and T lymphocytes
Cytomegalovirus	Retinitis, encephalitis, radiculitis
Human herpes virus 6	Meningoencephalitis; recurrent febrile seizures; chromosomal integration
Human herpes virus 7	Meningoencephalitis; recurrent febrile seizures
Gamma herpes viruses	Become latent in B cells
Epstein–Barr virus	Meningoencephalitis during infection mononucleosis; Drives CNS lymphomas in the immunosuppressed
Human herpes virus 8	Causes Kaposi's sarcoma in HIV patients

Modified from: Solomon T. Encephalitis and infectious encephalopathies. In: Donaghy M, editor. Brain's Diseases of the Nervous System. 12th edn. Oxford: Oxford University Press; 2009. p. 1355–428.[37]

infection in younger patients and reactivation of latent virus in older people. HSV encephalitis has been reported from Africa and Asia, where the incidence is thought to be similar to the rest of the globe.[43–45]

The neurological syndromes caused by HSV-2 include meningitis, encephalitis, particularly in neonates, lumbosacral radiculitis and meningitis, especially recurrent meningitis. HSV-2 is now considered to be responsible for most cases of what was previously called Mollaret meningitis, a recurrent meningitis with large friable cells in the CSF, probably activated macrophages. Up to one-third of patients presenting with primary genital herpes have clinical findings consistent with meningeal involvement, including headache, photophobia and meningismus.

In neonates, HSV infections occur in about one in 3000–10 000 live births,[46] causing serious morbidity and mortality and leaving many survivors with permanent sequelae. Although both HSV-1 or -2 can cause neonatal infection, HSV-2 is more common and has a worse outcome.[47] Neonatal HSV infection is acquired intra-uterine, perinatally or postnatally, when the virus is acquired from someone involved with child-care. Perinatal infection is most important, accounting for about 85% of infections.

PATHOGENESIS AND PATHOLOGY

Primary infection with HSV-1 occurs via the oral mucosa where the virus may give ulcers or be asymptomatic. Following primary infection the virus travels centripetally along the trigeminal nerve to cause latent infection of the trigeminal ganglion. More than two-thirds of patients with HSV-1 encephalitis have antibody present at the start of the illness indicating that their illness is due to reactivation of latent virus rather than a primary infection. However, encephalitis can also occur as a result of primary infection, especially in children or even secondary infection with a different virus strain.[48] Recently, specific deficiencies in Toll-like receptor-3 and related pathways involved in generation of interferons in response to viral infection, have been linked to development of HSV encephalitis in a few families.[49,50]

Pathologically in HSV encephalitis, the damage principally affects the limbic system and nearby structures. Thus the temporal lobes are most often affected, along with the inferior frontal, parietal and occasionally occipital lobes; deeper structures include the amygdala, hippocampus, insular cortex and cingulate gyrus. The damage is often bilateral, but usually more marked on one side. Initially there is swelling, inflammation and congestion, with petechial or larger haemorrhages, which may proceed to frank necrosis and liquefaction (Figure 21.1). Although it is clear that viral replication in the limbic system is critical, what is less clear is how and when the virus reaches here. Postulated mechanisms include spread from the olfactory bulbs and tracts, reactivation of latent virus in the trigeminal ganglion and spread from here or reactivation of virus that had already established latency within the brain itself.[52]

HSV-2 infection occurs via the genital mucosa. The virus is thought to become latent in the sacral plexus and reactivate from there. The pathogenesis of recurrent HSV-2 meningitis is poorly understood, but immune-mediated pathology has been postulated.[53] Neonatal HSV infection is most commonly acquired from the birth canal during delivery. However, in utero infection can also occur, via the placenta or through retrograde spread through ruptured or seemingly intact membranes.[54]

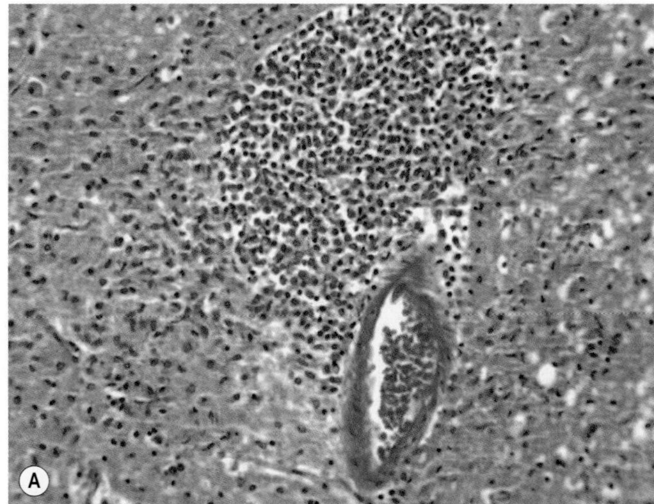

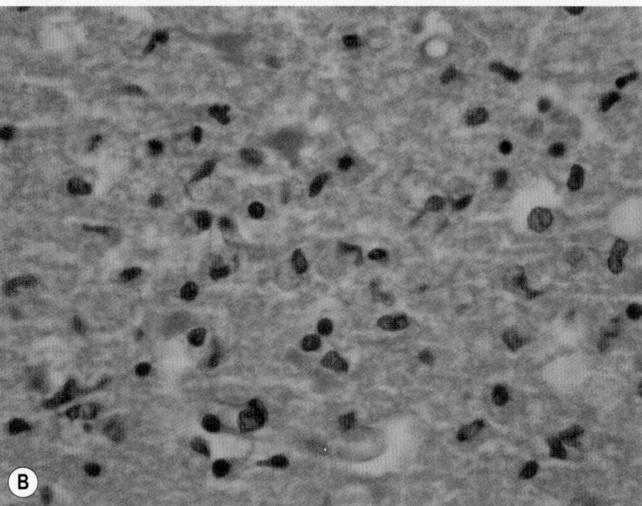

Figure 21.1 Histopathological changes in herpes simplex virus encephalitis. (A) Intense perivascular inflammatory infiltrate consisting of activated microglia, macrophages and lymphocytes (H&E staining, x620). (B) High-power view showing microglia and dead neurons with nuclear dissolution (karyolysis) and hypereosinophilia within the cytoplasm retaining the original pyramidal contour (H&E, x640). *(Pictures from Solomon T, Hart IJ, Beeching NJ. Viral encephalitis: a clinician's guide. Practical neurology 2007;7:288–305, courtesy of Dr Daniel Crooks.)*[51]

CLINICAL FEATURES

HSV-1 encephalitis classically presents as an acute flu-like prodrome, developing into an illness with high fever, severe headache, nausea, vomiting and altered consciousness, often associated with seizures and focal neurological signs. Of 93 adults, 85 (91%) with HSV-1 encephalitis in one study were febrile on admission.[55] Disorientation (76%), speech disturbances (59%) and behavioural changes (41%) were the most common features and one-third of patients had seizures.[55] Alterations in higher mental function include lethargy, drowsiness, confusion, disorientation and coma. With the advent of CSF PCR more subtle presentations of HSV-1 encephalitis have been recognized.[56]

HSV meningitis presents with a fever and meningism. Genital lesions are present in approximately 85% of patients with primary HSV-2 meningitis and generally precede the onset of CNS symptoms by about 7 days. In neonates, HSV can cause localized disease of the skin, eyes and mouth, CNS disease or disseminated disease, which may involve the CNS. Approximately one-third of neonates with HSV infection has CNS involvement, which usually presents in the 2nd or 3rd week of life. About two-thirds of cases have cutaneous vesicles at some stage during the illness. Initially, there may be no obvious CNS manifestations, but subsequently, there may be lethargy, irritability, poor feeding, focal or generalized seizures, a swollen fontanelle and tremors.[57]

DIAGNOSIS

HSV meningitis and encephalitis are diagnosed most often by PCR detection of virus in the CSF. This test has sensitivity above 90% and specificity approaching 100%. False negatives are rare, but occur when the CSF is taken very early in the illness or late when viral nucleic acid has cleared. For example, CSF PCR for HSV between days 2 and 10 of illness has overall sensitivity and specificity of >95% for HSV encephalitis in immunocompetent adults.[58]

If the CSF sample is negative for HSV, but the sample was taken in the first few days of illness, it should be repeated. If a patient has presented late and PCR is negative, then testing CSF for HSV-specific antibody can be helpful. In neonatal HSV encephalitis, detection of HSV in the blood can also be useful. Prior to the availability of PCR brain biopsy was used and it still has a role when the diagnosis is uncertain.

Even if neonates only have features of mucocutaneous or systemic HSV, they should still undergo lumbar puncture examination, because there may be CNS infection, without obvious clinical features of CNS disease. Approximately 25% of infants with HSV of the skin, eye and mouth and 90% of those with disseminated HSV have HSV DNA in their CSF.[54] In recurrent HSV meningitis, Mollaret cells may be seen in the CSF; these large friable cells with faintly staining vacuolated cytoplasm, are now thought to be activated macrophages. They are also seen occasionally in other CNS infections.

The CSF opening pressure is usually mildly elevated in HSV meningitis and encephalitis and there are typically tens to hundreds of cells/mm^3, predominantly lymphocytes, with a moderately elevated protein and normal glucose ratio; in children, especially young children, there may be no pleocytosis.[58,59]

In HSV encephalitis, computer tomography scans may be normal if performed early or there may be subtle swelling of the fronto-temporal region with loss of the normal gyral pattern. Subsequently, there is hypodensity and there may be high signal change if haemorrhagic transformation occurs (Figure 21.2). Magnetic resonance imaging (MRI) shows characteristic high signal changes on T2-weighted images in the fronto-temporal regions, which may also involve the parietal areas (Figure 21.2).[51] Changes are typically bilateral but asymmetrical. Diffusion-weighted MRI may be especially useful for demonstrating early changes (Figure 21.3).[51,60] In neonatal HSV encephalitis, in addition to the classical temporal lobe changes, abnormalities there may be multifocal, brainstem or cerebellar abnormalities.[61]

An EEG usually shows nonspecific diffuse high-amplitude slow waves of encephalopathy, but can be useful to look for subtle motor seizures. Periodic lateralized epileptiform discharges were once thought to be diagnostic of HSV encephalitis, but have since been seen in other conditions.[62]

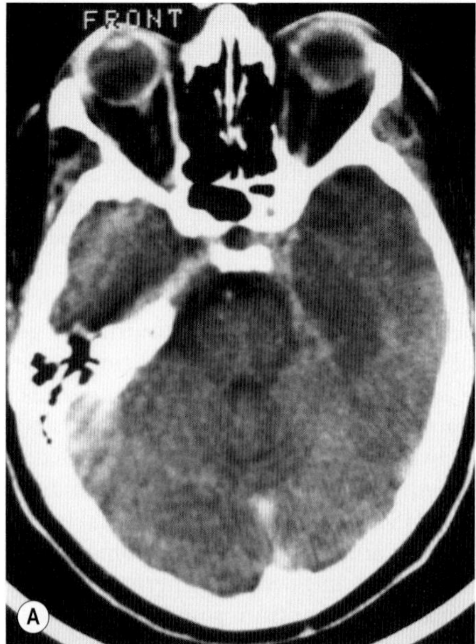

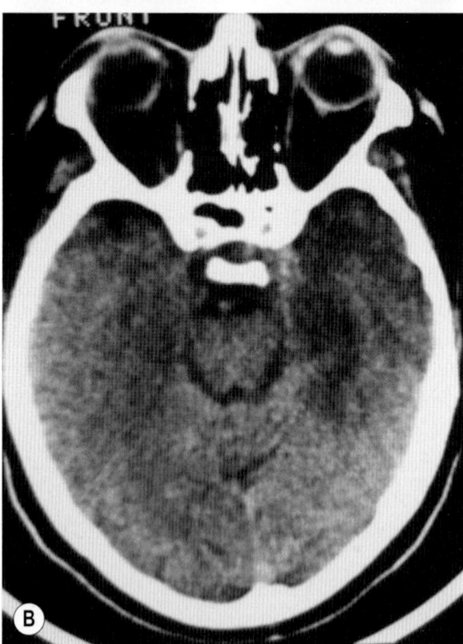

Figure 21.2 Computed tomography scan in HSV encephalitis. This scan, 1 week into the illness, shows (A) a low-density area in the left temporal lobe, with swelling and some contrast enhancement and (B) the same patient 4 days later, with more marked changes. *(Photos: T Solomon, from Solomon T, Hart IJ, Beeching NJ. Viral encephalitis: a clinician's guide. Practical Neurology 2007;7:288–305.)*[51]

MANAGEMENT AND TREATMENT

Aciclovir should be administered intravenously as soon as there is a strong clinical suspicion of HSV encephalitis. Most patients that present with an encephalopathy do not have HSV encephalitis and so our practice is to perform CSF examination, with or without imaging as soon as possible, to help decide whether encephalitis is likely.[51] Although the randomized placebo-controlled trials were for 10 days of treatment, most give 14 or 21 days because of cases of apparent relapse. Recent studies suggest ongoing inflammation may make an important contribution to relapse.[63] Our practice is to examine the CSF again after 2–3 weeks of treatment and continue aciclovir if virus is detected.[58,59] Aciclovir is also given empirically to infants with

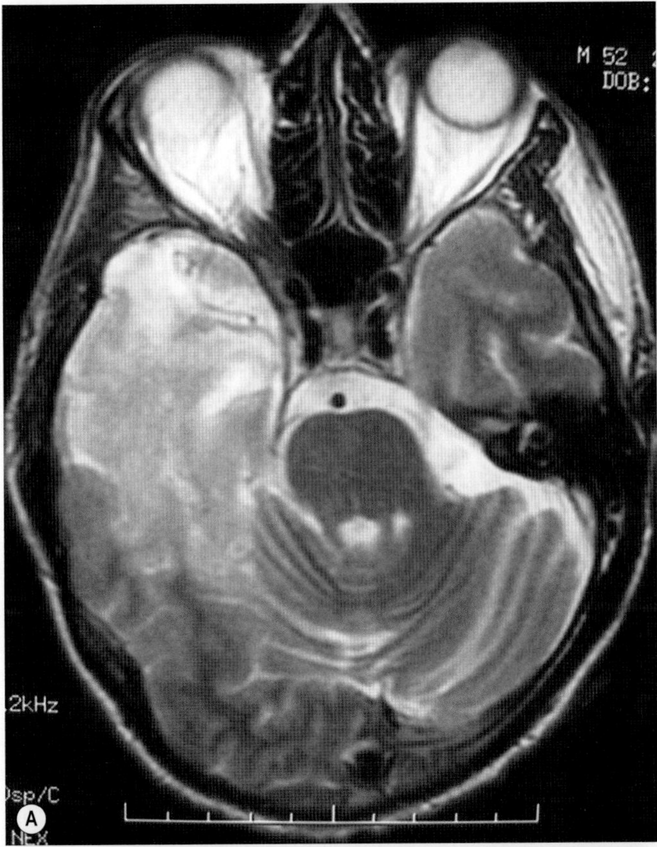

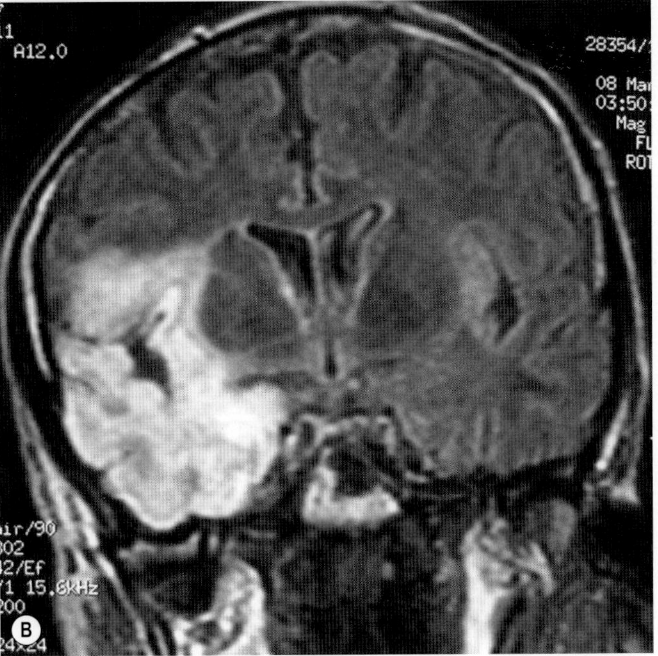

Figure 21.3 T2-weighted MRI brain scan in HSV encephalitis. Coronal (A) and sagittal (B) sections show right temporal lobe hyperintensity and swelling. *(Photos: T Solomon, from Solomon T, Hart IJ, Beeching NJ. Viral encephalitis: a clinician's guide. Practical Neurology 2007;7:288–305.)*[51]

clinical features suggestive of HSV infection including mucocutaneous vesicles, seizures, lethargy or sepsis. In other clinical scenarios, such as CSF pleocytosis in a neonate who is otherwise well, some argue that aciclovir should not be started until there is virological confirmation.[64]

In parts of the tropics, where there are resource limitations and other causes of encephalitis are more common, judicious use of aciclovir may be especially important. For example, in much of Asia, large outbreaks of Japanese encephalitis occur, while in large parts of Asia and sub-Saharan Africa, HIV-associated CNS infections and cerebral malaria are common. In practical terms this may mean that during an outbreak of Japanese encephalitis in a recourse-poor part of Asia, aciclovir is not given to all patients, but only those where the clinical pattern and imaging make Japanese encephalitis seem unlikely. Although not formally examined in efficacy trials, oral therapy with the prodrug valacyclovir achieved adequate aciclovir concentrations in the CSF of patients with HSV encephalitis and may be an acceptable early treatment for suspected HSE in resource-limited settings.[65] Corticosteroids are sometimes used to control inflammation, especially if there is lots of swelling on imaging, but their role has not been assessed in randomized trials. Seizure control and other supportive measures may also be needed, as described above.

The role of aciclovir in acute HSV-2 meningitis is less certain. While it might be argued that it makes sense virologically and isolated case series support this approach, HSV meningitis is generally self-limiting and there are risks associated with prolonged intravenous treatment. Some clinicians' practice is to give valacyclovir prophylaxis to patients who have had recurrent HSV-2 meningitis in the hope of preventing further episodes. However, a recent placebo-controlled trial giving 0.5 g of valacyclovir twice daily for 1 year showed no benefit; indeed in the year following cessation of the drug, the treatment group had more frequent episodes than the placebo group, possibly due to a rebound phenomeneon.[66]

PREVENTION

There are no vaccines for HSV-1 or HSV-2. Neonatal HSV infection is prevented by managing infants born to mothers with active HSV genital lesions.

Varicella Zoster Virus

EPIDEMIOLOGY

Varicella zoster virus is a double-stranded DNA virus. Primary infection causes a diffuse vesicular rash known as chickenpox (varicella). The virus becomes latent in sensory dorsal root ganglia and then reactivates later in life to cause shingles – a painful vesicular eruption usually in the distribution of a single dermatome – and CNS syndromes. The varicella and shingles were linked epidemiologically in the early 1900s when it was noted that chickenpox developed in children exposed to adults with shingles;[67] some 50 years later, it was demonstrated that both conditions are caused by the same virus.[68] Acute cerebellitis and a more diffuse encephalitis are the most common neurological complications of primary infection with VZV. VZV reactivation is associated with a much wider range of complications including encephalitis, stroke syndromes and a small vessel vasculitis, cranial neuropathies and myelitis (Table 21.4).

Most primary infection with VZV occurs via respiratory droplet spread from children with chickenpox, but virus shed at the time of shingles can also be infectious. In temperate regions, most people acquire infection with VZV during childhood or early adulthood; typically more than 95% are

TABLE 21.4 Neurological Complications of Varicella Zoster Virus

Complications of acute infection (varicella)
Cerebellitis
Acute encephalitis

Complications of viral reactivation (zoster)
Cranial neuropathies
- Ramsay Hunt syndrome
- Herpes zoster ophthalmicus
- Trigeminal neuronitis
- Optic and oculomotor neuropathies/retinitis
- Mononeuritis of other cranial nerves
- Polyneuritis cranialis

Stroke syndromes
- Herpes zoster ophthalmicus with delayed contralateral hemiparesis
- Cervical zoster with posterior circulation infarcts
- Granulomatous angiitis of the basilar artery

Encephalitis syndromes
- Encephalitis
- Diffuse small/medium vessel arteritis

Myelitis

Modified from: Boos J, Esiri MM. Viral Encephalitis in Humans. Washington DC: ASM Press; 2003.[33]

seropositive by the age of 20.[69] In tropical countries, varicella occurs mainly among young adults. Infections in adults and those under 1 year old are more likely to result in severe disease, including neurological disease. The risk of shingles increases with age and occurs at some stage in up to 20% of the population. Shingles and CNS complications are more likely to occur in those with underlying malignancy or immunocompromised states. Similarly the neurological complications of chickenpox are more often seen in children with immunocompromise who tend to have prolonged illness.

Acute cerebellar ataxia is the most common neurological complication of chickenpox, occurring in approximately 1 per 4000 cases of chickenpox.[70] In one series of 57 children with neurological complications of chickenpox, one half had cerebellitis and made a good recovery; 40% had a diffuse encephalitis and worse outcomes.[71] Acute encephalitis or cerebritis is a rare complication of chickenpox, with an incidence of about 1–2 per 10 000 cases. The incidence is higher in adults over 20 or infants less than 1 year.

PATHOGENESIS AND PATHOLOGY

Chickenpox is highly contagious and most infections with VZV are acquired through droplet spread from the nasopharyngeal secretions of someone infected. Direct cutaneous contact with vesicle fluid from a skin lesion can also lead to transmission. Replication in local lymph nodes is followed by primary viraemia, seeding in the reticuloendothelial system and then secondary viraemia, at which stage, skin lesions develop. Cell free virus in the skin is thought to infect nerve endings and migrate along sensory axons to establish latency in neurons within the regional ganglia.

The CNS syndromes associated with VZV emergence from latency appear to be primarily caused by immune-mediated reactions to the virus, rather than viral replication itself.[72] However, viral replication may occur at a low level, particularly in immunocompromised patients and may contribute to the pathogenesis. Pathological studies in VZV encephalitis have shown diffuse oedema, perivascular infiltration of mononuclear cells, demyelination and occasionally focal haemorrhage.

VZV vasculopathies are thought to be due to viral replication in cerebral arteries, either during primary infection or reactivation; this can be unifocal or multifocal and result in ischaemic strokes, haemorrhage or dissection. Pathologically, a granulomatous inflammatory process in the wall of the thrombosed vessel is seen and in some cases there is evidence of viral replication in the adventitia or smooth muscle of the vessel wall. Viral particles have also been seen in endothelial cells. The delay in the development of the stroke syndrome is postulated to represent the time it takes for the virus to spread from the trigeminal ganglion along the branches of the ophthalmic division of the trigeminal nerve to the cerebral arteries.

CLINICAL FEATURES

Neurological Complications of Chickenpox

Neurological complications of primary infection usually follow the onset of the rash by a few days to a week, though they can occur before the rash and very occasionally, may not be associated with rash at all.[73] In the acute cerebellar syndrome, ataxia is typically accompanied by headache, vomiting and lethargy; there may also by fever, nystagmus, slurred speech and neck stiffness. In more diffuse chickenpox encephalitis, there is headache, fever, vomiting, reduced consciousness and seizures. Other CNS complications associated with chickenpox include myelitis, aseptic meningitis, strokes and rarely choreoathetosis, facial nerve palsy and Guillain–Barré syndrome.[14]

Neurological Complications of VZV Reactivation

There is a wide range of neurological syndromes associated with VZV reactivation. Although they can occur at any age, they are more common in the elderly, those with advanced HIV disease or with other immunocompromised states, particularly if cell-mediated immunity is impaired. Thus, patients with leukaemia and lymphoproliferative disorders are vulnerable and especially patients that have bone marrow suppression before transplant. Importantly, these syndromes may occur without any cutaneous evidence of zoster – thus being equivalent to the zoster sine herpete originally described for the pain of shingles without the rash. Segmental zoster paresis is weakness of muscles supplied by a single nerve root or nerve, is probably under-reported and probably reflects damage in the anterior horn or motor roots[74] (Figure 21.4).

VZV Cranial Neuropathies and Brainstem Encephalitis

Ramsay Hunt syndrome is the classical cranial neuropathy associated with VZV reactivation. There is zoster over the auricle or in the ear canal, associated with facial pain and a facial palsy. However, there may be extension of the rash to other areas supplied by the trigeminal nerve or extension of the nerve dysfunction to ipsilateral cranial nerves; this often includes the VIIIth nerve, but may also involve cranial nerves V, VI, IX or X. The term 'Ramsay Hunt plus' has been applied to such syndromes. Alternatively, VZV may cause single or multiple cranial neuropathies in the absence of a vesicular rash. Involvement of the VII nerve alone is thought to be due to compression of the nerve fibres as they pass through the

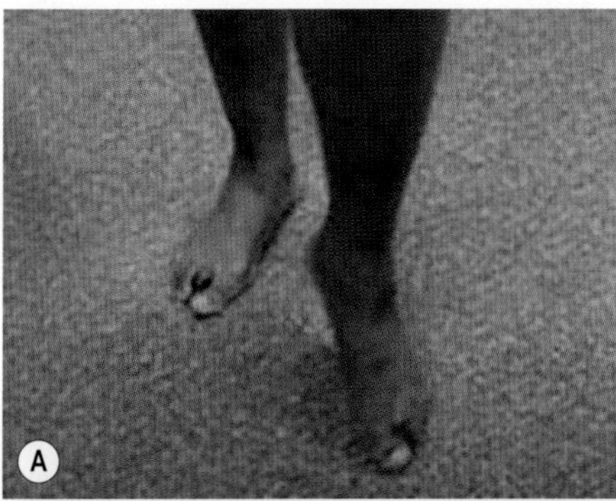

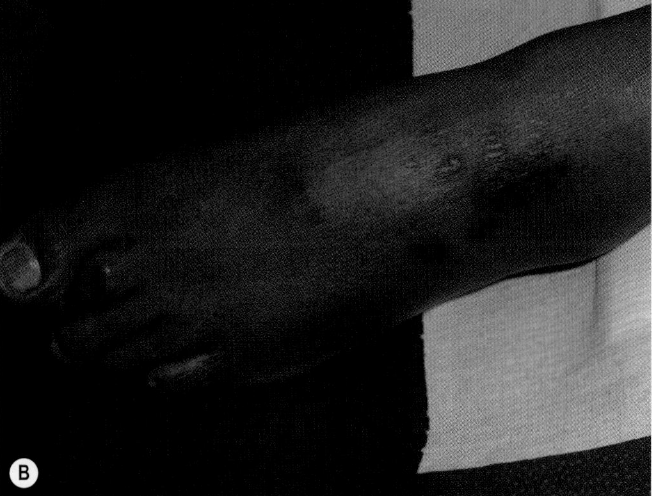

Figure 21.4 Segmental zoster paresis. An HIV-positive man with shingles in the left L5 dermatome and associated foot drop (note that in the left foot a normal heel strike is replaced by a toe drop). *(Photos T Solomon.)*

inflamed geniculate ganglion, but this has not always been demonstrated pathologically and more widespread involvement of other cranial nerves suggests extension of the inflammatory process to the brainstem.

VZV Vasculopathy and Vasculitis

A delayed contralateral hemiparesis following herpes zoster ophthalmica was the first recognized VZV stroke-related syndrome, being described in immunocompetent elderly people.[75] A similar VZV vasculopathy syndrome appears to be an important cause of stroke in children. In these groups, major arteries are affected. Vascular syndromes in the posterior circulation, including pontine infarcts, have been reported following zoster in a C2 distribution. Typically, contralateral hemiplegia occurs 8 weeks (range 8 days to 6 months) after the rash. A small (or sometimes medium) vessel vasculitis occurs in immunocompromised patients, particularly those with HIV or organ transplant recipients. It has a sub-acute presentation with headache, fever, hemiplegia, aphasia, visual field defects, altered consciousness and seizures.[76] There is often no herpetic rash, though patients may have had the rash weeks or months previously.

VZV Encephalitis and Myelitis

Prior to the arrival of HIV, VZV encephalitis was very rare. Typically, it followed a VZV rash by 1–3 weeks and tended to occur in the elderly or those with malignancies. However, it has been recognized as an important cause of encephalitis in patients with HIV. In both patient groups, it may occur in the absence of a rash. It can be especially difficult to diagnose VZV encephalitis because there is not always fever or seizures and there may not be a CSF pleocytosis.[77] Myelitis is a rare complication of shingles, occurring in less than 1:1000 cases. It most often follows thoracic zoster, with neurological features occurring 1–2 weeks after the onset of the rash. However, it can occur in the absence of a rash. There is unilateral motor and posterior column dysfunction, which may evolve to paraplegia with bladder and bowel involvement. Immunocompromised patients, particularly those with HIV, are at increased risk.

DIAGNOSIS

In acute cerebellar ataxia caused by VZV, the CSF may be normal or show a moderate lymphocytic pleocytosis, with slightly elevated protein and normal glucose ratio. VZV has not been isolated from such cases, but can be detected by PCR, with intrathecal production of anti-VZV antibodies in the CSF. An EEG shows slowing in approximately 20% of patients. On computer tomography scanning of patients with chickenpox encephalitis there may be oedema and MRI may show grey or white matter abnormalities. CSF examination shows a typical viral picture.

The diagnosis of VZV cranial neuropathy can be confirmed by isolating virus from vesicles or by showing a rise in antibody titres in the serum; alternatively virus may be detected in the CSF by PCR or there may be anti-VZV antibodies.

In stroke syndromes secondary to VZV, the CSF usually shows a pleocytosis with elevated protein and digital subtraction angiography or magnetic resonance angiography can demonstrate segmental restrictions of flow. Virus cannot be isolated from the CSF, though it has on occasion been detected by PCR and has also been found in cerebral arteries.

MRI of patients with VZV vasculitis shows multiple ischaemic and haemorrhagic infarcts of different sizes in the cortex and subcortical grey and white matter; there may also be demyelination. When these lesions are predominantly in the white matter the MRI changes are reminiscent of progressive multifocal leukoencephalopathy, though they are smaller and more discrete. In VZV myelitis MRI shows abnormal signal at the level of the lesion. The diagnosis is confirmed by PCR detection of virus or anti-VZV antibodies in the CSF.

MANAGEMENT AND TREATMENT

Shingles is treated with antiviral treatment to speed resolution of skin lesions and the acute neuritis.[78] Whether such treatment also reduces the chance of post herpetic neuralgia is unclear.[79] Although the evidence is limited, for VZV cranial neuropathies most would recommend treatment with aciclovir (intravenously or orally) for up to 14 days, with or without corticosteroids,[80] especially if it can be started within a few days of symptom onset.[81] In addition, early use of amitriptyline significantly reduces post-herpetic neuralgia.

VZV cerebellitis is usually self-limiting, requiring no treatment and resolving within 1–3 weeks, though it may continue for several months. The relative contribution of viral cytopathology and immunologically mediated demyelination is not clear. The cerebellar syndrome is usually benign and only requires supportive care.

VZV encephalitis, stroke and vasculitis are usually treated with aciclovir and steroids although there are no randomized studies in any of these conditions.[73] Typical regimens include 2 weeks treatment of aciclovir 10–15 mg/kg, with corticosteroids. If patients are deteriorating at this stage or the CSF still has detectable virus, many recommend continuing treatment.[72,82,83] Approximately 5–10% of encephalitis cases are fatal.

PREVENTION

A live attenuated vaccine has been used in the USA since 1995, leading to a significant reduction in morbidity and mortality. It is also universally recommended in Canada and is being used increasingly in Europe, but has not yet been used much in the developing countries.[84]

Epstein–Barr Virus

EPIDEMIOLOGY

Epstein–Barr virus (EBV) is a double-stranded DNA herpes virus that can cause CNS disease as part of a primary infectious mononucleosis illness or by reactivating to drive primary CNS lymphomas, principally in people with HIV. In addition, recent data suggest co-infection with EBV may contribute to the pathogenesis of other CNS infections, such as bacterial meningitis. The controversial issue of EBV's role in the pathogenesis of multiple sclerosis[85] will not be discussed here.

Infection with EBV is ubiquitous. Serological studies show 90–95% of adults have been exposed. The majority of infections are asymptomatic, particularly in infants and young children. Older children and young adults can develop infectious mononucleosis. Neurological complications of acute EBV infection are reported in 1–18% of patients with infectious mononucleosis and include encephalitis, meningitis, transverse myelitis, cranial and peripheral neuropathies and radiculopathies.[86,87]

EBV leads to primary CNS lymphoma in 2–6% of patients with HIV, which is at least 1000 times higher than in the general population.[88] In an autopsy series of HIV-infected patients, lymphoma is reported in up to 10%.[89] EBV is commonly detected in patients with other CNS infections, especially in the immunocompromised. In one study from the USA 60 (7%) of nearly 900 CSF samples tested from unselected patients were EBV positive and one quarter of these had another pathogen detected, most of whom were immunocompromised;[29] the pathogens included CMV in patients who all had lymphoma, JC virus detected in patients with PML, VZV, *Streptococcus pneumonia* and other microbes. In a study from Malawi, EBV was detected in the CSF of more than 50% of HIV-positive patients with bacterial meningitis.[90]

PATHOGENESIS AND PATHOLOGY

EBV is secreted in saliva and transmitted through intimate contact ('kissing disease'). Epithelial and B cells in the lymphoid tissue of the oropharynx become infected and the virus is disseminated to the rest of the body, including the CNS, via the lymphoreticular system. Lytic infection of epithelial cells results in production of virions. Infection of B cells results in latent infection, which later can become reactivated to release virus.

Autopsies from fatal cases of EBV encephalitis show there is perivascular lymphocytic infiltration, which may include atypical lymphocytes, parenchymal oedema and microglial proliferation.[91] Viral DNA and protein are not often seen in brain biopsies, which is thought to reflect the fact that this is primarily an immune-mediated encephalitis.[92] In HIV patients, primary CNS lymphoma is almost always associated with EBV; the virus is thought to 'drive' the replication of malignant B cell clones. Lymphoma is more common in patients with low CD4 counts, typically <50/μL.

The significance of EBV when detected in the CSF of patients with other infections is not clear. Because it is carried in lymphocytes anyway, there is the concern that it might simply be latent virus carried across into the CSF by lymphocytes recruited to fight a different infection. However, in HIV-positive patients with bacterial meningitis and EBV detected, mortality was associated with increased EBV CSF load, suggesting this is pathogenic reactivation; the effects of EBV on the inflammatory process are postulated to be the mechanism by which viral reactivation leads to increased mortality.[90]

CLINICAL FEATURES

Aseptic meningitis occurring during primary EBV infection is clinically indistinguishable from that caused by other viruses, although pharyngitis and lymphadenopathy may be a clue that this is infectious mononucleosis. Encephalitis also often follows the typical pattern of viral encephalitis, with headache seizures and altered behaviour or consciousness. Any area of the brain can be involved, but cerebellitis is common, causing cerebellar ataxia. Although encephalitis most often happens 1–3 weeks after infectious mononucleosis, it can occur before or during the acute febrile illness and occasionally occurs without any features of infectious mononucleosis.[93]

EBV-driven primary CNS lymphoma can present with a variety of focal or non-focal signs and symptoms. The clinical presentation may be characterized by confusion, lethargy, memory loss, hemiparesis, aphasia, with focal neurology and in approximately 15% seizures that have usually been present for less than three months. The sub-acute onset of 2–8 weeks can be helpful in distinguishing lymphoma from other space-occupying lesions, particularly toxoplasma, which typically presents more acutely.

DIAGNOSIS

The cardinal investigation is detection of EBV DNA in the CSF by PCR. In primary infection, detection of the virus in the CSF is always likely to be significant. In situations where people have been infected previously and reactivation of latent virus is thought to be the driving mechanism, e.g. suspected CNS lymphoma or EBV co-infection, then interpretation of PCR results can be more difficult. In these scenarios, quantification of the viral load and comparison with viral load in the blood can help determine whether the EBV detected is likely to be significant. For example, many patients with HIV may have low levels detected, but in a patient with suspected lymphoma and high CSF viral titre, this suggests local viral replication in the CNS. The detection of mRNA from the EBV lytic cycle confirms that virus is replicating, but this is not normally available in routine diagnostic practice.[29]

In aseptic meningitis and encephalitis caused by EBV, the CSF profile is similar to that from other causes. An EEG in encephalitis may show slowing, with sharp wave activity and periodic discharges in patients with seizures. Imaging in encephalitis shows high signal changes on T2 weighted scans and FLARE images localizing the site of parenchymal damage.

In lymphoma, CSF examination may also reveal malignant cells. In terms of imaging, lymphoma typically causes a single lesion or several adjacent lesions; these may be anywhere in the brain parenchyma but are commonly peri-ventricular; typically there is moderate oedema and homogeneous contrast enhancement throughout the mass (Figure 21.5). In contrast, other space-occupying lesions in HIV, such as toxoplasma and

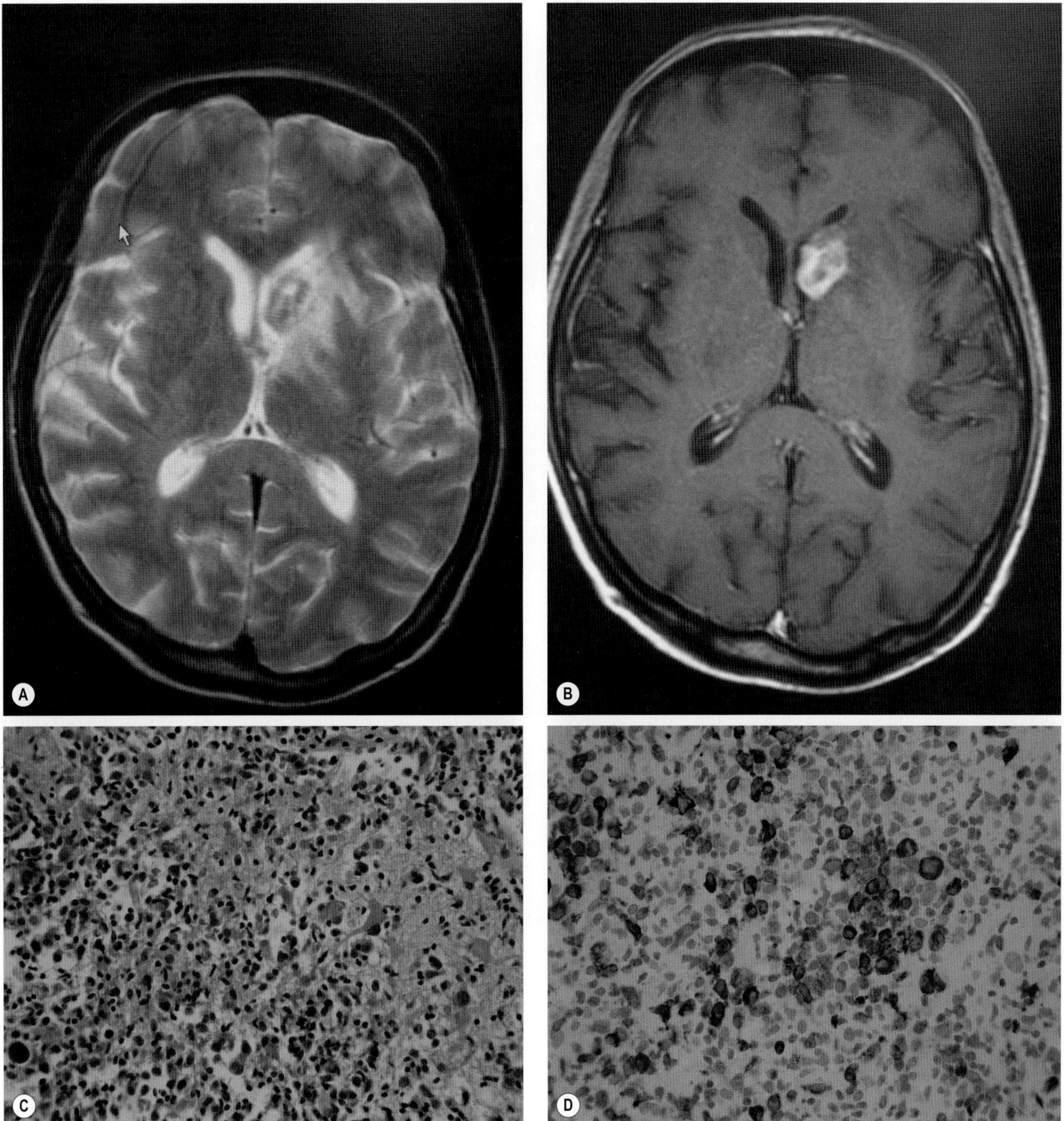

Figure 21.5 Epstein–Barr virus driven primary CNS lymphoma. (A) Transient spin echo (TSE) and (B) T1-weighted gadolinium enhanced. Magnetic resonance images from an HIV-positive man with primary CNS lymphoma. The H&E histology stain (C) showed an abnormal infiltrate and the stain with a lymphocytic marker (D) confirms this is a non-Hodgkin's lymphoma.

tuberculomas, typically have ring enhancement.[94] Thallium SPECT (single-photon emission computed tomography) scanning is also being investigated as a means of improving the diagnostic capabilities for primary CNS lymphoma.[95] It may prove especially useful in combination with CSF PCR for EBV.[96] The definitive diagnosis is made by biopsying the lesion, with a stereotactic brain biopsy. Typically this is only performed in patients who have had a treatment trial for toxoplasma, but not improved.

MANAGEMENT AND TREATMENT

There is no specific treatment for the acute CNS complications of infectious mononucleosis. Ganciclovir is a nucleoside analogue that has some efficacy against EBV, though it is not used in routine clinical practice. In HIV patients with EBV-driven primary lymphoma, the first priority is to ensure they are on optimal antiretroviral treatment. Options for treatment of the lymphoma include high-dose methotrexate, rituximab, corticosteroids and whole-brain irradiation. The optimum treatment is not known and clinical practice varies.[97] Ganciclovir has been used experimentally and found to reduce EBV viral load, whether this was associated with prolonged survival is unclear.[98]

PREVENTION

There are no vaccines available for EBV.

Cytomegalovirus

EPIDEMIOLOGY

Cytomegalovirus (CMV) is named after the cytopathic effect which it produced in cell culture. It is a double-stranded DNA beta herpes virus, which, like other herpes viruses, becomes latent in cells. Humans are the only hosts for the virus, with the age and incidence of infection depending on socioeconomic circumstances. The virus crosses the placenta and can be acquired congenitally or during delivery. It is also excreted in saliva and urine, so much transmission occurs during childhood in nurseries and schools. Those not infected in childhood become infected as adults, through kissing and sexual intercourse. Infection thus occurs earlier in those from poor socioeconomic backgrounds and in developing countries, with virtually 100% of adults infected; in contrast in developed countries approximately 60% of adults are infected.[99]

Congenital CMV

CMV is the most widespread viral cause of congenital infection in humans and is a leading cause of congenital infection in the developed world. Approximately 2% of infants born in the USA are estimated to be congenitally infected.[100] In Africa, the estimated incidence rate of congenital CMV infection ranges from 1.4% in Ivory Coast[101] to 14% in The Gambia.[102] Less than 5% of those infected in utero are symptomatic, although a proportion of those who are well at birth develop problems later.

CMV in the Immunocompromised

Patients whose immune system is suppressed are particularly at risk of developing CMV infection, both primary and reactivated and this often involves the CNS. It is an especially important problem in transplant recipients and people with HIV (Drew 1988). Immunosuppressed transplant recipients can develop CMV disease either because they were already infected (endogenous disease) or because the transplanted organ is infected (exogenous disease). The latter are more severe.

Almost all adults with HIV are co-infected with CMV. In children, co-infection with HIV can have important impact on disease progression (see below). Although CMV is primarily associated with immunosuppression, it is becoming recognized increasingly as a pathogen in immunocompetent individuals, causing CNS or gastrointestinal disease.[103,104]

PATHOGENESIS AND PATHOLOGY

CMV infection causes inclusion bodies with the typical 'owl's eye' appearance in affected tissues. In infants the lungs, kidneys and liver are affected. In the brain, CMV can infect astrocytes, neurons, oligodendroglia, cells of the monocyte-macrophage lineage and capillary endothelia.[105] There is focal necrosis of neuronal tissue with microglial nodules (accumulation of macrophages and microglial cells). In CMV periventriculitis, there is inflammation of the ependymal lining and nearby periventricular tissue.[106] At autopsy CMV is detected in the CNS of 15–76% of people who died with severe HIV disease.[107–109]

CLINICAL FEATURES

The clinical features depend on the age at which individuals become first infected or their immune status if they are already affected. Infants infected transplacentally are severely affected with high morbidity and mortality. Those affected during childhood are usually asymptomatic. When adults are infected for the first time, there may be an infectious mononucleosis-like syndrome with abnormal lymphocytes, splenomegaly and impaired liver function, but without pharyngitis. A similar syndrome can occur if infection is acquired through blood transfusion.

Congenital CMV

Cytomegalic inclusion disease affects many organs and the infant may have low birth weight, hepatosplenomegaly, jaundice, thrombocytopenia, choroidoretinitis and encephalitis with microcephaly. This leads to mental retardation, seizures, spasticity and deafness. Early trimester infections are more likely to result in CNS complications although these CNS complications tend to be mainly chronic rather than acute.[110] When asymptomatic infected infants are followed-up, neurological defects are found as they get older; up to 20% have problems, including lower IQs, behavioural disorders, minor in-coordination, defects in perceptual skills and neural deafness.

CMV in the Immunocompromised

Primary infection in the immunocompromised is usually symptomatic with persistent pyrexia which may last for weeks and is often fatal if bacterial or fungal infection supervenes. In some, disease may be limited to or accompanied by, severe choroidoretinitis.

Clinically, adults with CMV have a sub-acute or chronic encephalitis with confusion, disorientation, lethargy and occasionally seizures.[111] In those with HIV, the features are often not distinguishable from HIV-associated dementia itself (see below). However, polyradiculopathy or retinitis may be a clue that CMV is contributing to an HIV patient's neurological status. Interestingly, one study in Malawian adults with HIV found no increased incidence of CMV retinitis.[112]

A lumbosacral radiculopathy with pain and paraesthesia in a saddle distribution, which may spread to involve the lower limbs and sphincters is another common presentation of CMV CNS infection in adults and also occasionally in children;[113] CMV retinitis may precede or follow these syndromes. Brainstem encephalitis, space-occupying lesions and myelitis due to CMV have also been described.

Studies in HIV-infected children have shown that CMV may affect HIV disease progression independent of CD4 count or HIV viral load.[114] Those co-infected with CMV have a higher risk of progression of HIV and death than those with HIV infection alone, independent of plasma HIV RNA levels.[105] By 18 months there is also a higher incidence of impaired brain growth or progressive motor deficits among children infected with HIV and CMV compared with those infected only with HIV.

DIAGNOSIS

Traditionally, CMV infection was demonstrated histologically by showing the cytomegalic inclusion bodies with their characteristic intranuclear 'owl's-eye' appearance in infected organs or alternatively by virus isolation from saliva or urine. Serological diagnosis is based on demonstrating fourfold elevation in IgG antibody titres, though in the severely immunocompromised, such a rise may not occur; alternatives include IgM detection with an enzyme immunoassay. Antigen detection methods have also been developed and are useful for monitoring transplant recipients,[115] but PCR of CMV DNA is now the most common and popular means of viral detection in both blood and CSF.[116] In the blood, there may be issues over whether virus detected is clinically significant, but the advent of quantitative PCR has helped with this.[117,118]

In infants with congenital CMV, periventricular calcification is commonly seen on X-ray and on brain scanning with ventricular dilatation. In adults with CMV infection, there is often nothing specific about brain imaging.[119] A distinct syndrome of ventriculoencephalitis caused by CMV in advanced HIV disease is characterized by simultaneous retinitis or other organ disease, mental change, large ventricles and periventricular enhancement on imaging, with CSF pleocytosis. The pleocytosis is characteristically neutrophilic, rather than lymphocytic.

MANAGEMENT AND TREATMENT

The introduction of highly active antiretroviral therapy (HAART) has provided a means of reconstituting the immune system of those with HIV/AIDS in such a way as to allow CMV infection to be controlled. In doing so, HAART has done much to reduce the mortality rate associated with CMV disease in such patients. Despite this, response to treatment in these patients remains suboptimal.

If CMV disease develops, intravenous ganciclovir is recommended as initial therapy and continued in a maintenance fashion, with its prodrug valganciclovir, which can be discontinued should CD4 count remain above 100 cells/mm^3 for 6 months.[120] The development of encephalitis, despite treatment with antiviral drugs for CMV at other sites has been reported.[121,122]

Both ganciclovir and valganciclovir can cause bone marrow suppression. The alternative is foscarnet, but this should be limited to ganciclovir-resistant cases due to the high level of toxicity associated with the drug and its intravenous mode of administration. The nucleoside analogue cidofovir may also have a role.[120]

PREVENTION

Although vaccines are in development, none is yet available. In transplant recipients who are CMV negative before transplantation, efforts are made to ensure they receive organs from transplant-negative donors, where possible.

Measles Virus

EPIDEMIOLOGY

Measles virus is an RNA virus (family, Paramyxoviridae; genus, *Morbillivirus*) spread by droplets and is highly infectious. Before the development of an effective vaccine, 99% of the population had been affected by the age of 20 and as shown by serological studies. In Western industrialized countries the incidence is now greatly reduced, though there are still sporadic cases and outbreaks, chiefly because not everyone is immunized. Worldwide, measles is a significant cause of morbidity and mortality. Although it is hard to get precise figures, in 2000 there were an estimated 31–39.9 million cases worldwide, with an estimated 733 000–777 000 deaths, making measles the fifth most common cause of death in children under 5 years of age.[123]

Measles virus causes three distinct CNS syndromes. The first is acute measles encephalitis, which occurs within from a few days to a few weeks after the onset of the rash and which pathologically fits the pattern of a post- or para-infectious acute disseminated encephalomyelitis (ADEM). Some authors treat these as two distinct presentations, considering acute encephalitis when the rash is still apparent different from the post-infectious encephalitis weeks after the rash has gone, but most consider them as points on a spectrum. The incidence of acute measles encephalitis is around 1 in 1000 cases and increases with increasing age. Measles ADEM accounts for about 95% of cases of measles CNS disease.

The second syndrome is a sub-acute 'inclusion body' measles encephalitis, which occurs in the immunocompromised and presents several months after the acute illness; it is thought to affect approximately 1 in 10 immunocompromised people that develop measles. Inclusion body measles encephalitis is typically seen in children who have had lymphocytic leukaemia and received therapy for this. However, it can also occur in lymphoma, renal transplantation and people with HIV.

Third, sub-acute sclerosing panencephalitis (SSPE) presents in the immunocompetent patients, many years after measles infection; the incidence is about 1 per million cases. It seems to be more common in those that developed measles age less than 2 or who had a severe measles infection and is 3–4 times more common in boys than girls, for reasons unknown. All racial groups are affected by SSPE, but it seems that there is a higher incidence around the eastern Mediterranean area and in Arabs.

Interestingly, even in uncomplicated measles subclinical CNS infection seems to be common, as judged by the fact that 30% of measles patients have a CSF pleocytosis and 50% have EEG abnormalities.

PATHOGENESIS AND PATHOLOGY

Measles is an antigenically stable virus and the development of most neurological complications is thought to be due to variations in host susceptibility, age and immune status, rather than to viral properties. However, there is evidence that the virus found in cases of sub-acute sclerosing panencephalitis (SSPE) differs from wild virus because it is has a deficient M protein, one of the virus-specific structural proteins. Antibody to M protein is low, while the antibody response to N and P proteins is particularly robust.

Pathologically, measles encephalitis is similar to other viral post-infectious forms of acute disseminated encephalomyelitis with perivenous demyelination, gliosis, perivascular cuffing and in more severe cases, a frank haemorrhagic leuco-encephalitis. The pathogenesis is thought to be similar to that of experimental allergic encephalomyelitis – an autoimmune demyelinating disease triggered by measles.

In inclusion body measles encephalitis, there are inflammatory changes seen throughout the brain and eosinophilic inclusions have been identified in the nuclei of neurons.

The factors underlying the development of SSPE are poorly understood. Current thinking is the virus enters the CNS at the time of the acute measles infection, probably by infection of cerebral capillary endothelium – measles virus containing immune complexes have been found in blood vessel wall.[124] It is then thought to mutate to a less invasive and more persistent form, which has defective coding for M protein;[125] the persisting viral infection is then thought to trigger an immune-mediated response which is responsible for the widespread demyelination. At autopsy, in SSPE, there is neuronal degeneration, gliosis, proliferation of astrocytes, perivascular cuffing, lymphocytic and plasma cell infiltration and demyelination. SSPE is occasionally seen in children who never had measles, including those that were vaccinated, possibly reflecting subclinical measles infection.[126]

CLINICAL FEATURES

In acute measles encephalitis, there is febrile illness with onset of altered consciousness. Sometimes this occurs as part of the acute measles illness, with rash still present, sometimes a few weeks after the acute infection. Clinically, there may be convulsions and abnormal movements and paresis.[127] Approximately 15% of patients die and more than 50% have serious neurological sequelae.

In inclusion body measles encephalitis, there is lethargy, mental confusion, seizures and myoclonus, progress relentlessly to death in a few months.[128,129] The diagnosis should thus be considered in any immunosuppressed child that develops seizures. Other causes of seizures in this patient group, including extension of the leukaemia to the CNS, haemorrhagic complications of leukaemia, complications of radio- or chemotherapy and other opportunistic infections must be ruled out. EEG, CSF and brain imaging show normal findings or nonspecific changes only.

SSPE typically occurs in children age 8–10 years and on average 7 years after the acute measles illness. Some 90% of cases occur before the age of 16. The onset is insidious with behavioural change, emotional lability and impaired school performance, progressing to clumsiness, cognitive defects, ataxia, myoclonus and seizures. Often, psychiatric illness is considered before the diagnosis is made.

The onset of myoclonic jerks, which start focal but become generalized, heralds the second stage of the disease. They become frequent and repetitive and correlate with the giant complexes seen on EEG.[130] Pyramidal and extra-pyramidal signs with dystonia and dyskinesia appear. There is inexorable progression to a vegetative state with dementia, decortication and decerebration. Rarely, this may be interrupted by remission and exceptionally by stabilization of the disease. Progression is highly variable. Death may occur within weeks of onset, about half die within a year and most die within 2 years.[131]

DIAGNOSIS

In acute measles encephalitis, the MRI scan findings are similar to ADEM from other causes; typically T2-weighted images show widely distributed, multifocal high signal in both cerebral hemispheres with swelling of the cortex and bilateral, symmetrical involvement of the putamen and caudate nucleus. Detection of virus in the CSF is rare, but the diagnosis is usually confirmed by IgM with or without IgG antibody detection in the serum.

The diagnosis of inclusion body measles encephalitis can be hard to establish because antibody titres are low or absent, reflecting immune suppression. Brain biopsy may be necessary, revealing the characteristic, eosinophilic inclusions in the nuclei of neurons.

In SSPE, once myoclonus has developed the EEG shows high-voltage stereotyped slow-wave complexes, often synchronous with clinical myoclonus (Figure 21.6). CT and MR brain scans are not diagnostic and may show white matter change and atrophy. CSF examination is most useful and demonstrates great elevation of the gamma globulin fraction of the protein content due to the presence of measles antibody which is found in high concentration. PCR is reported to be useful.

MANAGEMENT AND TREATMENT

For acute measles encephalitis, when the presentation is consistent with ADEM, most would recommend high-dose corticosteroids. In inclusion-body measles encephalitis there is no established treatment but ribavirin was associated with recovery in one report.[129] A range of therapies has been tried for SSPE. Inosiplex (Isoprinosine) has both immune-modulating and antiviral properties that are dose-dependent and may be beneficial.[132] Interferon-alpha has been administered systemically, intrathecally and intraventricularly.[133] Ribavirin has been given in combination with inosiplex and/or interferon alpha, with apparent benefit.[134,135]

Nipah Virus

EPIDEMIOLOGY

Nipah virus is an enveloped negative-strand RNA paramyxovirus (genus, *Henipavirus*; family, Paramyxoviridae) that first appeared in Malaysia and Singapore in 1998–1999, when it caused disease in humans and pigs.[136] More than 250 people were affected with more than 100 deaths.[137] It has caused subsequent outbreaks in Bangladesh from 2001 to 2004,[138] and neighbouring West Bengal, India in 2001. Typically, there are a few dozen people affected each time. Nipah virus

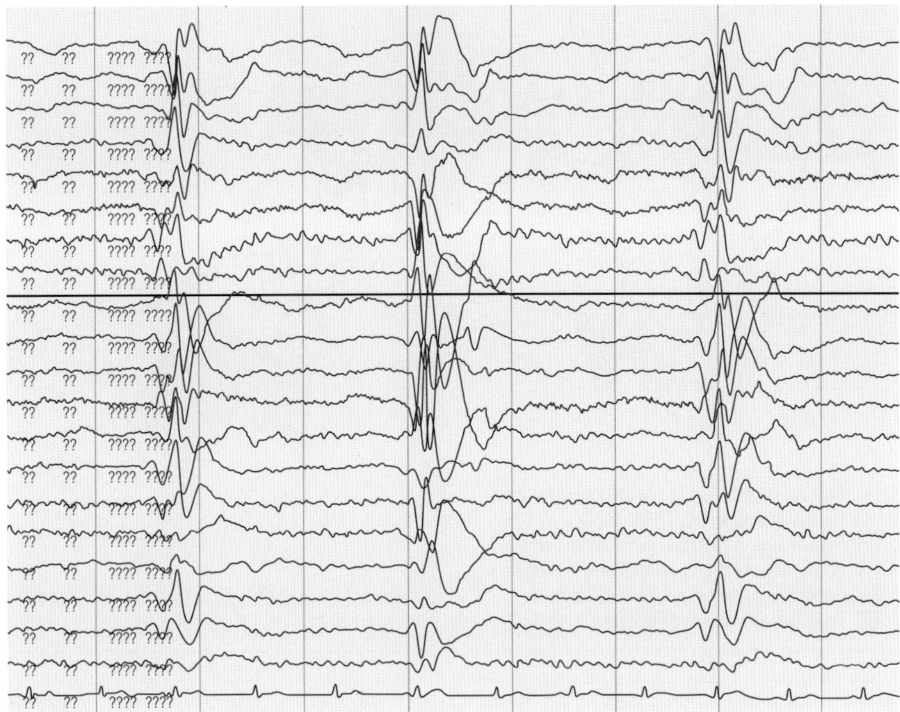

Figure 21.6 Sub-acute sclerosing panencephalitis (SSPE) caused by measles virus. An electroencephalogram from a 17-year-old boy with SSPE showing the characteristic widespread large-amplitude rhythmic slow waves every 3 seconds on a low-amplitude background.

is related to Hendra virus, which caused disease in horses and their handlers in Australia in 1994 and in sporadic cases since then.

The natural reservoir for Nipah virus is 'flying fox' fruit bats (genus *Pteropus*) (Figure 21.7),[139] with both virus detection and serological evidence for infection. Serological evidence of Nipah virus infection has subsequently been found in 23 species of bats from 10 genera in regions as widely spread as Yunan and Hainan Island in China, Cambodia, Thailand, India, Madagascar and Ghana in West Africa (Figure 21.8).

The virus is excreted in bat urine. In the original Malaysian outbreak, pigs became infected, possibly through eating fruit which had been contaminated by bats or directly from bat urine. The virus was excreted in pig urine, saliva and respiratory secretions, which is how humans, principally pig farmers, their families and abattoir workers, become infected. Cats, dogs and other domestic animals can also be affected. In the Bangladesh outbreaks humans become ill with no associated disease in animals and so they are thought to have been infected directly from bats. Drinking date palm sap (juice) which had been contaminated by bat droppings or saliva has been implicated.[140] In addition human-to-human transmission has been documented in Bangladesh.[141]

PATHOGENESIS AND PATHOLOGY

Humans become infected with Nipah virus by inhalation of respiratory secretions from pigs or humans, from bat excreta and possibly by ingestion of the virus in contaminated date juice. Pathologically endothelial damage and vasculitis are seen in the brain parenchyma, along with nuclear inclusions similar to those of other paramyxovirus infections, such as measles. Widespread microinfarcts are seen, thought to be caused by

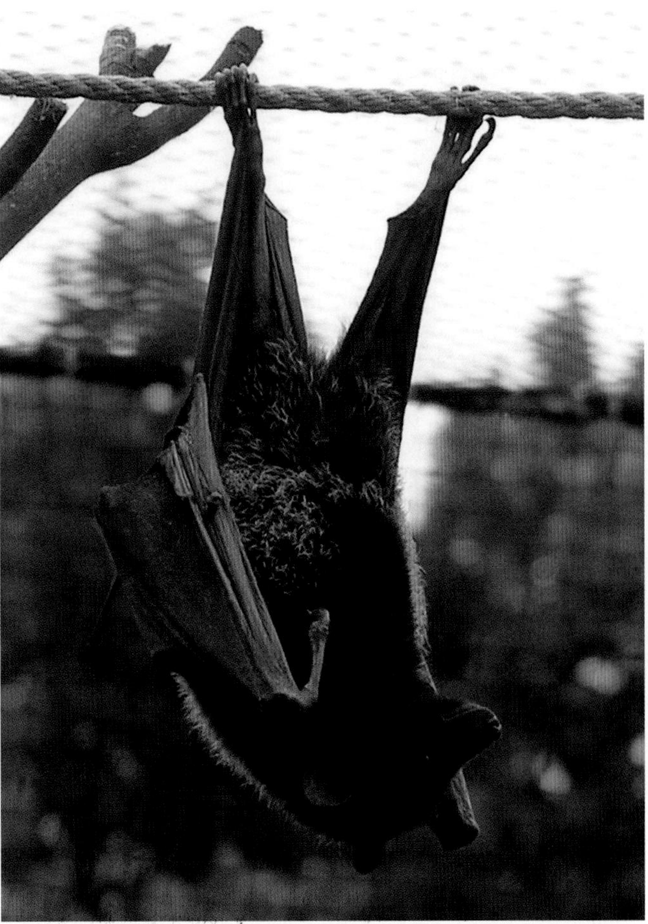

Figure 21.7 The flying fox fruit bat, the natural reservoir for Nipah virus. *(From http://commons.wikimedia.org/wiki/File:Bristol.zoo.livfruitbat.arp.jpg.)*

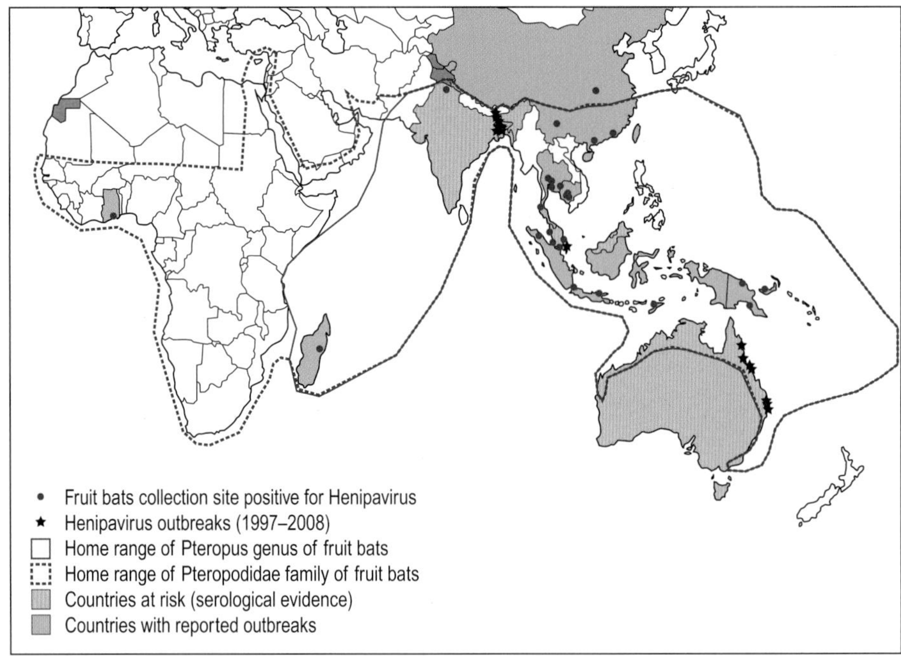

Figure 21.8 Geographic distribution of Nipah virus. The map shows outbreaks caused by Nipah or Hendra viruses, countries with serological evidence of transmission and the distribution of fruit bats of the Pteropodidae family. *(Image modified from http://www.who.int/csr/disease/nipah/en/index.html.)*

vasculitis-induced thrombosis. In addition direct neural invasion occurs.[142]

CLINICAL FEATURES

Human infection with Nipah virus causes an encephalitis characterized by a reduced level of consciousness, myoclonus, areflexia and hypotonia.[5] A smaller number of patients may present with atypical pneumonia with chest radiographs showing diffuse interstitial infiltrates. The incubation period ranges from 7 to 40 days. About one third of patients have meningism and generalized seizures occur in about 20%. Myoclonus typically involving the diaphragm, arms and neck is also seen. In addition there may be cerebellar dysfunction, tremors and areflexia. In more severe cases there is brainstem involvement, characterized by pinpoint, unreactive pupils, abnormal oculocephalic reflexes, tachycardia and hypertension.

Several reports have shown that patients who originally had mild or asymptomatic infections can present with encephalitis several months after the exposure.[143,144] Clinically and immunologically these cases are reminiscent of sub-acute sclerosing panencephalitis caused by the paramyxovirus, measles virus.[5,143] In the Malaysian outbreak, the mortality was approximately 35%, but in Bangladesh it has been more than 70%.

DIAGNOSIS

There may be mild thrombocytopenia and elevated liver function tests. In the CSF, there is usually pleocytosis, with lymphocyte predominance. Because Nipah virus is a Biosafety level 4 pathogen, culture is not routinely attempted. The diagnosis is confirmed by IgM capture ELISA or PCR. MRI shows increased signal intensity in the cortical white matter. Typically there are small lesions in the subcortical and deep white matter, with surrounding oedema.

MANAGEMENT AND TREATMENT

There is no treatment or vaccine, though ribavirin has been used in some cases. Because of the risk of nosocomial transmission, appropriate precautions should be taken, especially if patients are ventilated.

PREVENTION

There is no vaccine for Nipah virus. Preventive measures are aimed at stopping pig infection, human infection from infected animals and human-to-human transmission.[145] Routine cleaning and disinfection of pig farms is thought to be important, as is animal surveillance – part of a 'one health' approach.[146] Farmers need to be wary of the 'barking pig' with respiratory symptoms. If an outbreak in pigs is suspected, the animals should be culled and carcasses disposed of, in a safe manner. Those handling sick animals should wear personal protective equipment.

Education of humans about the risk factors is important. In particular the need to boil freshly collected date-palm juice and to wash and peel fruit. Gloves and protective equipment should be worn when caring for people with suspected Nipah virus infection.

Mumps Virus

EPIDEMIOLOGY

Mumps is a viral infection which primarily affects the parotid glands to cause swelling, but which also causes neurological disease, especially meningitis. The virus is a single-stranded negative-sense RNA virus (family, Paramyxoviridae; genus *Rubulavirus*) transmitted by direct contact or via air-borne droplets from the upper respiratory tract of infected people. The incidence has decreased considerably in Western industrialized nations, since the live attenuated vaccine was introduced; but there are still outbreaks in those who are susceptible because they were not vaccinated. Vaccines are used less in developing countries, where more mumps and mumps meningitis is seen. Approximately 1 in 6000 mumps virus infections results in encephalitis and it was the most common cause of encephalitis in the USA, when mumps was at its peak in the 1960s. Hearing loss due to cochlear nerve involvement is also a relatively common complication.

PATHOGENESIS AND PATHOLOGY

The virus is acquired via the respiratory route and presumed to replicate in the upper respiratory mucosa before invading the parotid gland to give parotitis. Viral spread to distant organs, including the pancreas, gonads, myocardium, breast, kidneys and CNS, is thought to occur during a viraemia. The incubation period is approximately 2 weeks and viral shedding occurs mostly during this interval, peaking approximately 3 days before parotitis develops and decreasing in the first few days of symptoms.[147]

CLINICAL FEATURES

Symptomatic disease is twice as frequent in males as females and neurological involvement three times more common, for reasons that are not known. Studies have shown that more than 50% of individuals with mumps parotitis have a CSF pleocytosis,[148] but most of these people do not have clinical symptoms of meningitis. Clinical meningitis is reported for 4–6% of people with mumps parotitis, typically 4–10 days into the illness.[149] But in some patients, the meningitis precedes the parotitis by up to a week and others develop mumps virus meningitis with no parotid disease at all; this has been reported up to 50% in some series.[150] In most cases, the clinical features of mumps meningitis are typical for those of other viral meningitides, with fever, headache, vomiting and neck stiffness. However, occasionally orchitis or pancreatitis may be a clue that a case of meningitis is due to mumps virus. Bradycardia, lethargy and anaemia are also reported.

Patients with mumps encephalitis typically have fever, altered consciousness, seizures and weakness.[151] As many as one-third of encephalitis patients present without parotitis; as a result, the absence of parotitis does not exclude the diagnosis of mumps. Hearing loss usually comes on abruptly, but may be more gradual; it is sometimes associated with vestibular symptoms, such as nystagmus.[152]

DIAGNOSIS

In CNS disease due to mumps virus, a lumbar puncture typically reveals 10–500 leukocytes/mm^3, though there may be several thousand. There is usually a CSF lymphocytosis, but up to 25% may have polymorphonuclear predominance. The protein is often mildly elevated and up to 30% of patients may have a slightly reduced glucose ratio, which may be more common than for other viral meningitides. The symptoms usually resolve in 3–10 days, though the CSF abnormalities may persist for weeks.

The diagnosis of mumps virus infection is most often confirmed serologically, by detection of IgM antibody in a single serum sample using an ELISA or by showing a fourfold rise between acute and convalescent serum using complement fixation tests, haemagglutination inhibition assays or neutralizations tests.[153] IgM antibody can also be detected in the CSF in mumps meningitis. Virus can be isolated in the saliva from 2–3 days before the onset of parotitis to about 5 days after. It can also be detected by culture or PCR of CSF during the first 3 days of meningeal symptoms.[154] An elevated serum amylase may suggest mumps infection.

MANAGEMENT AND PREVENTION

There is no specific antiviral treatment for mumps or its neurological complications, but antipyretics are given usually. Live attenuated mumps vaccine is used routinely in most Western industrialized nations, but only about one quarter of developing countries.[155]

Enterovirus 71 and Other Non-polio Enteroviruses

EPIDEMIOLOGY

Enteroviruses belong to the *Enterovirus* genus in the Picornaviridae family. The genus includes polioviruses, coxsackieviruses, echoviruses and newer enteroviruses. Echoviruses (enteric cytopathic human orphan) were so-named as their relationship to human disease was unknown originally. Echoviruses 22 and 23 were subsequently reclassified in the new genus *Parechovirus* within the family Picornaviridae and so are no longer considered to be enteroviruses.

Aseptic meningitis is the most common neurological manifestation of the non-polio enteroviruses, though they can also cause encephalitis and acute flaccid paralysis. Enteroviruses are spread via the faeco–oral route, particularly among children, though for some, particularly enterovirus 71, respiratory spread has also been implicated. For enterovirus 70, which causes acute haemorrhagic conjunctivitis and acute flaccid paralysis, there is direct transmission to the eye from fingers or fomites (inanimate objects). In any part of the world, each enterovirus 'season' is usually dominated by only a few serotypes, the predominant ones cycling with varying periodicity.

Enterovirus 71 causes hand, foot and mouth disease, with associated aseptic meningitis and encephalitis. The virus was first isolated, in California, USA, in 1969, with subsequent small outbreaks of encephalitis and aseptic meningitis in different locations across the globe. In 1997, a large outbreak of enterovirus 71 in Sarawak, Malaysia, heralded the start of a series of large outbreaks across the Asia-Pacific region,[156] with an estimated 1.5 million people affected in Taiwan in 1988.[6] Many countries in the region have experienced cyclical epidemics that occur every 2–3 years. There has been rapid evolution of subgenotypes of enterovirus 71 during these outbreaks, with some suggestion that the new subgenotypes have greater epidemic potential.[156] Young children are predominantly affected, suggesting that older people have immunity already. Large outbreaks seem to occur when there is a new cohort of susceptible children. Outside the Asia-Pacific region, enterovirus 71 has continued to circulate at a low level in Africa, Europe and the USA.

PATHOGENESIS AND PATHOLOGY

Enteroviruses are thought to replicate in the lymphoid tissue of the oral mucosa. Following a mild viraemia the virus enters the CNS, by means which are not completely certain.[156] Pathologically in enterovirus 71, there is perivascular cuffing with inflammatory cells and neuronophagia, especially in the grey matter of the spinal cord and medulla oblongata.

There is some evidence that strain virulence determinants have a role in the pathogenesis of severe enterovirus 71 disease; specifically different subgenus groups may alter in their potential to cause neurological disease.[157,158] Dual infection with an adenovirus was also been implicated in one outbreak in Sarawak.[159] Host factors are also important. A lack of partial cross-protective immunity from previous outbreaks is thought to explain why young age is a risk factor for severe disease. One genetic study in Taiwan reported that HLA-A33 is associated with increased susceptibility to enterovirus 71 infection;[160] while another found that enterovirus 71 patients with meningoencephalitis had a higher frequency of G/G genotype at position 49 of exon 1 in the *CTLA4* gene, than those without meningoencephalitis and controls.[161] The gene is an important regulator of T-cell cytotoxicity, with a role in the regulation of an immune response.

The aetiology of the fulminant pulmonary oedema, which characterizes severe enterovirus 71 encephalitis, is unclear and has been the cause of some controversy; inflammation in the vasomotor centre of the medulla is postulated to lead to severe systemic and pulmonary hypertension, thus causing neurogenic pulmonary oedema; a cytokine storm, increased permeability of the pulmonary vasculature and cardiac dysfunction may also contribute (Figure 21.9). Although a frank viral myocarditis does not occur, cardiac dysfunction is seen on echocardiogram and cardiac specific troponin 1 can be elevated. Cardiotoxicity of elevated catecholamines or perhaps dysfunction caused by specific cytokines may be the cause.[162]

CLINICAL FEATURES

The non-polio enteroviruses are associated with a wide spectrum of clinical manifestations. These include exanthemas (skin rashes), enanthemas (lesions on the oral mucosa),

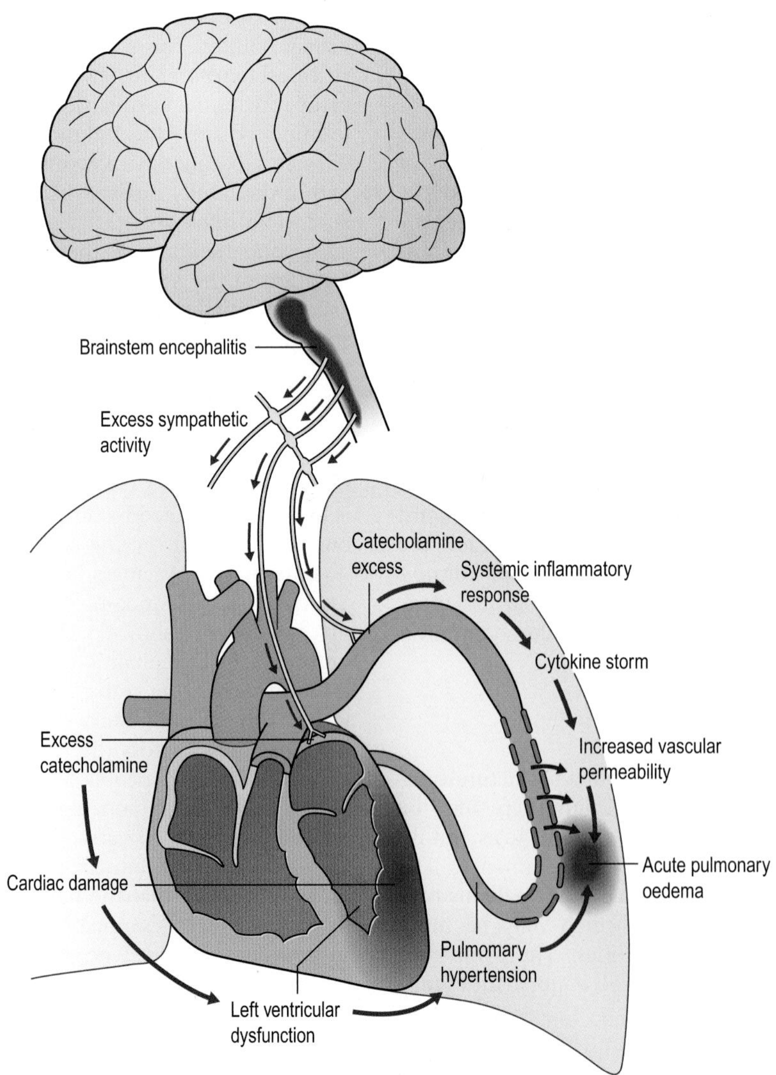

Figure 21.9 The postulated pathogenesis of enterovirus-71-associated acute pulmonary oedema.

conjunctivitis, respiratory infections, myocarditis, pericarditis, pleurodynia (intercostals muscle inflammation and pain), aseptic meningitis, encephalitis and acute flaccid paralysis. Some of these illnesses are associated with many different enteroviruses, but others are characteristic of particular groups or serotypes. Aseptic meningitis is the most common neurological manifestation.[19]

In older children enterovirus meningitis is typically biphasic with a nonspecific febrile prodrome followed by a brief remission before fever returns with symptoms of meningeal involvement. Nonspecific features include vomiting, anorexia, rash, diarrhoea, cough, pharyngitis and myalgia.[163] Neck stiffness and headache are present in adults and children old enough to report it; photophobia and febrile seizures are common.

Enterovirus 70

Enterovirus 70 infection is characterized by acute haemorrhagic conjunctivitis followed two to five weeks later by acute flaccid paralysis.[164] This is typically in adults and presents with a mild febrile illness followed by radicular pain, paraesthesia and asymmetrical flaccid paralysis, with bulbar paralysis in 50% of cases.[165] Coxsackievirus A24 is a less common cause of acute haemorrhagic conjunctivitis.

Enterovirus 71

Enterovirus 71 causes both neurological disease and mucocutaneous disease.[26] The latter most commonly presents as hand, foot and mouth disease or herpangina. Hand, foot and mouth disease is a common childhood exanthema that is characterized by a brief, generally mild, febrile illness with papulovesicular rash on the palms and soles and multiple oral ulcers (Figure 21.10). In *Herpangina*, there is febrile illness with multiple oral ulcers that predominantly affect the posterior of the oral cavity, including the anterior pharyngeal folds, uvula, tonsils and soft palate. Coxsackievirus A16 is also a common cause of hand, foot and mouth disease but is not normally associated with neurological complications. Other features of hand, foot and mouth disease include upper respiratory tract infection, gastroenteritis and nonspecific viral rashes.

Enterovirus 71 encephalitis is a brainstem encephalitis which is sometimes accompanied by severe cardiorespiratory symptoms, similar to those associated with poliomyelitis; there is

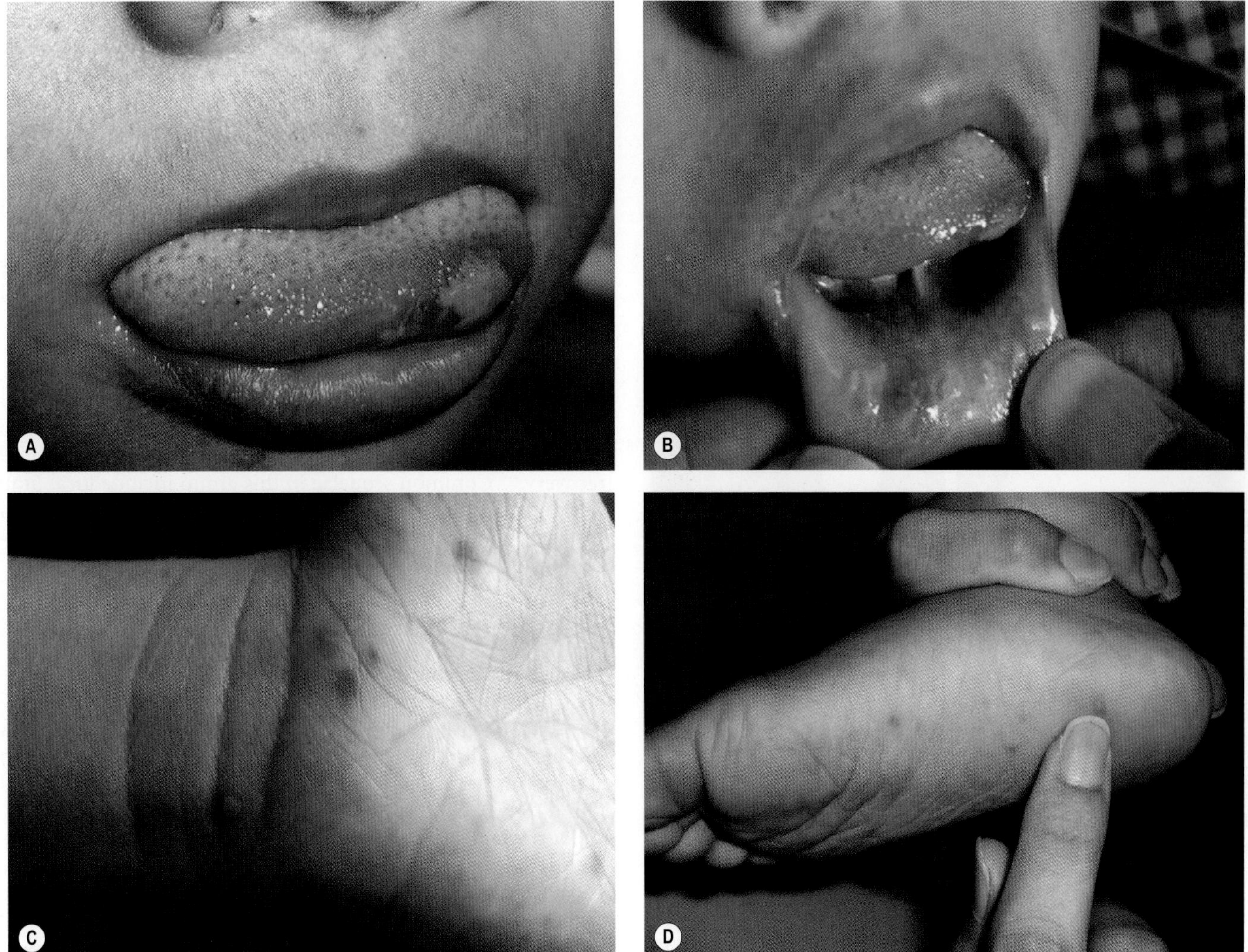

Figure 21.10 Mucocutaneous lesions in enterovirus 71 hand, foot and mouth disease. Ulcers on (A) the tongue and (B) inside the lip and vesicular and macular lesions on (C) the wrists and (D) the soles of children with enterovirus 71. *(Photo T Solomon, from Ooi MH, Wong SC, Lewthwaite P, et al. Clinical features, diagnosis and management of enterovirus 71. Lancet neurology 2010;9:1097–105.)*[26]

acute and rapidly progressing cardiorespiratory failure, which presents as shock and pulmonary oedema or haemorrhages. Myoclonic jerks are seen more often in enterovirus 71 than in other enteroviruses and can be an early indicator of neurological involvement, particularly in the brainstem. Acute flaccid paralysis in enterovirus 71 infection may be due to poliomyelitis-like anterior horn cell destruction (anterior myelitis), Guillain–Barré syndrome or transverse myelitis.[166]

Enterovirus infections in the neonatal period are usually severe and systemic. Thus, in addition to meningitis, echoviruses will often cause hepatic failure, while coxsackie viruses cause myocarditis; other complications include encephalitis and necrotizing enterocolitis.[19] The mortality in neonates may be as high as 10%. Maternal illness is often reported at the same time, but the question of whether the infection can be acquired transplacentally is unresolved. Parechovirus is another common cause of aseptic meningitis in younger children.

DIAGNOSIS

In the majority of cases, the CSF examination will reveal a lymphocytic pleocytosis of between 100 and 1000 cells,[163] though polymorphonuclear cells may predominate in the first 1–2 days and occasionally, there is no pleocytosis, particularly in young infants. Mild elevation of protein is common. The glucose ratio is usually normal, but may be mildly reduced.[163] When the brainstem is involved there may be high signal in the pons and medulla (Figure 21.11).[167]

Traditionally, enterovirus meningitis has been diagnosed by isolating virus from the CSF, throat or stool.[168] More recently, reverse transcriptase and real-time PCR have begun to replace culture.[169,170] Virus detection in the throat or stool is more likely to be positive, but because these are not sterile sites, detection from here could represent recent coincidental infection from a virus that is still being shed. Shedding from the throat continues for about one week after infection, but from the rectum it may continue for several weeks. Interestingly, for enterovirus 71, virus is rarely detected in the CSF and vesicles and the throat are more useful.[171]

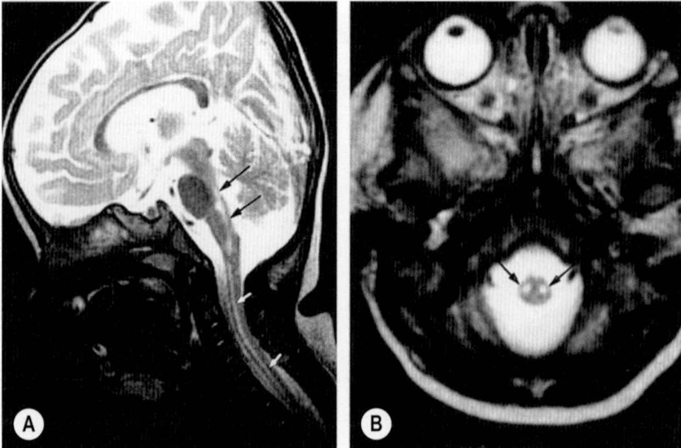

Figure 21.11 MRI changes in enterovirus-71-associated encephalomyelitis. T2-weighted images of a child aged 10 months with brainstem encephalitis showing high signal in (A) the posterior portion of the pons and medulla (dark arrows) and anterior cervical cord (white arrows) on a sagittal section; and (B) in the two anterior horns of the cervical cords (white arrows) on an axial section. *(Modified from Shen WC, Chiu HH, Chow KC, et al. MR imaging findings of enteroviral encephalomyelitis: an outbreak in Taiwan. Am J Neuroradiol 1999;20:1889–95 with permission of the American Society of Neuroradiology.)*[167]

MANAGEMENT

Pleconaril has broad activity against most enteroviruses, but not enterovirus 71. Although in phase III clinical trials oral pleconaril reduced symptoms of aseptic meningitis, particularly headache, by approximately two days, compared with placebo controls, it is not routinely used in this group.[172] Pleconaril has also been used in patients with chronic enterovirus due to agammaglobulinaemia, enterovirus myocarditis, poliovirus vaccine-associated paralysis and neonatal infection.

Severe enterovirus 71 infection is treated with intravenous immunoglobulin. The drug was first used during the large outbreaks of enterovirus 71 in Asia in the late 1990s, on the presumptive basis that it would neutralize the virus and have non-specific anti-inflammatory properties. Retrospective comparisons of patients who did and did not receive immunoglobulin suggest a benefit from this treatment if given early,[173] and analysis of cytokine profiles showed reductions in concentrations of some pro-inflammatory cytokines in patients with encephalitis. Although no randomized controlled trials have been performed, intravenous immunoglobulin has become standard treatment for severe enterovirus 71 disease. Milrinone, a cyclic nucleotide phosphodiesterase inhibitor used in the treatment of congestive heart failure, has been given to children with enterovirus 71-induced pulmonary oedema with some apparent benefit, but further studies are needed.[174]

Careful fluid management is essential in children with severe enterovirus 71 encephalitis, shock and pulmonary oedema and ionotropic support is often needed, ideally guided by central venous pressure measurement.

The prognosis for children with enterovirus meningitis is generally good with most making a good recovery in less than a week. Although the short-term recovery is good, several controlled long-term studies suggest that children who had neurological enterovirus disease in early life develop cognitive, developmental and language abnormalities.[175] In contrast, only a quarter with severe enterovirus 71 brainstem encephalitis and fulminant cardiorespiratory failure make a full neurological recovery.[176] Common sequelae in this group include focal limb weakness and atrophy, swallowing difficulties requiring nasogastric feeding, central hypoventilation, facial nerve palsies, seizures and psychomotor retardation.

PREVENTION

There is no vaccine against enterovirus 71 or any of the non-polio enteroviruses. Vaccines in development include inactivated whole-virus, live attenuated, subviral particle and DNA vaccines. An inactivated vaccine based on C4 genogroup with aluminium adjuvant was recently evaluated in humans and found to be well tolerated with high immunogenicity.[177]

During enterovirus 71 outbreaks, social distancing measures are used. These include closing nurseries and schools. Disease surveillance for hand, foot and mouth disease, with appropriate virological support to establish the cause, is now implemented in many Asian countries. Health education focuses on personal hygiene and good sanitation, including frequent hand washing, proper disposal of soiled nappies and disinfection of soiled surfaces with chlorinated (bleach) disinfectants.

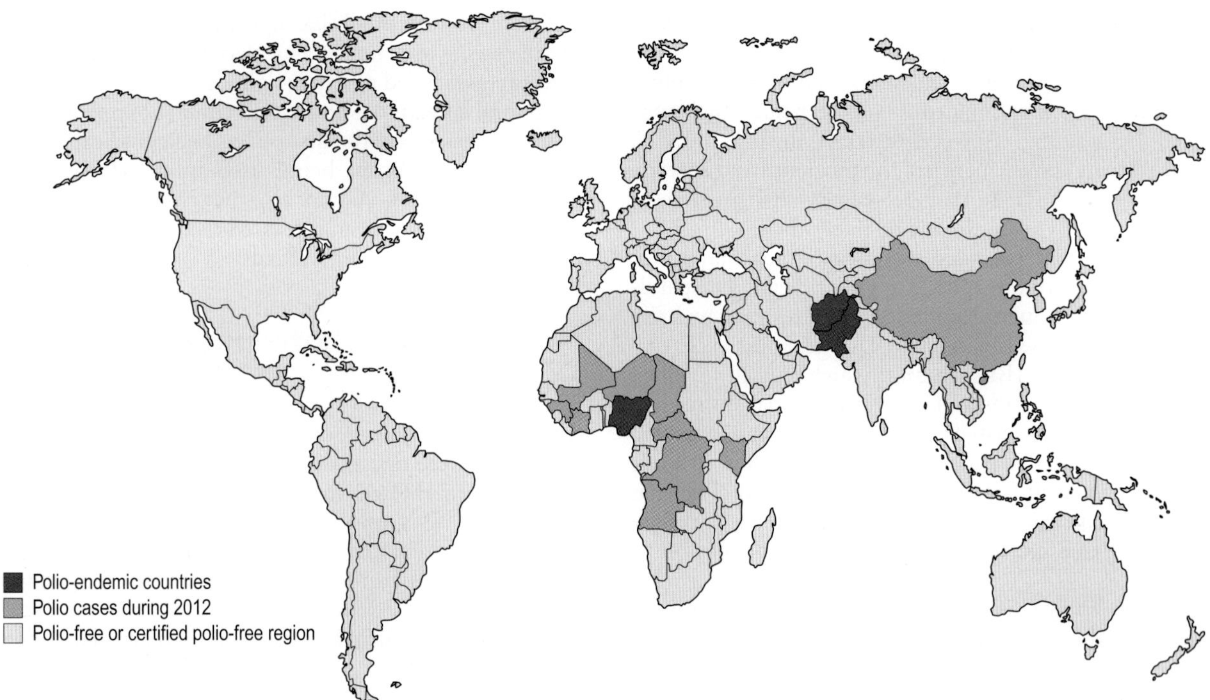

Figure 21.12 Map showing countries with endemic (red) and imported (orange) polio cases, 2012. (*Source: WHO.*)

Poliomyelitis

EPIDEMIOLOGY

The term poliomyelitis is derived from the Greek *polio* meaning 'grey' and *myelos* meaning 'marrow or spinal cord' and describes the pathological lesions that affect the grey matter in the anterior horn of the spinal cord. The earliest record of a withered shortened leg with the characteristic appearance of poliomyelitis is an Egyptian stele of the eighteenth dynasty (1580–1350 BC).

Poliomyelitis is caused by one of the three serotypes of poliovirus, which is a single-stranded RNA virus belonging to the *Enterovirus* genus of the family Picornaviridae.[178] Type 1 is epidemiologically the most important. Polioviruses are carried in the human gastrointestinal tract and transmitted via the faeco–oral route. Humans are the only natural hosts and reservoir. Before the late nineteenth century, polio was predominantly a sporadic disease, which mostly affected children under 5 years old. Subsequently, there were large epidemics in Europe and the USA, especially in older children.

In temperate regions, infection tends to occur in late summer and autumn, whereas there is year-round disease in tropical regions. Following the development of the inactivated and live attenuated polio vaccines and their widespread, use the epidemiology has changed considerably. In 1988, when the World Health Assembly announced the target of polio eradication by 2000, the number of cases was approximately 350 000 annually, across 25 countries. Although the target was not achieved, by 2001 there were only 483 confirmed cases. However, there have been several setbacks in subsequent years, e.g. in 2004, there were 1255 confirmed cases from 16 countries. With more aggressive vaccination campaigns and major funding, by 2011 just 650 cases were reported and Pakistan, Afghanistan and Nigeria were the only countries never to have been polio-free. Although Angola, Chad and Democratic Republic of the Congo were previously polio-free re-importation of wild polio virus resulted in transmission being re-established, while nine other countries were affected by outbreaks (Figure 21.12).[179] In 2012, spread of polio from Pakistan to China, which was declared polio free in 2000, highlighted the risk of rebound if the disease is not finally eradicated.[180]

PATHOGENESIS AND PATHOLOGY

After ingestion, virus replicates in the gut wall and adjacent deep lymph nodes before spreading to the reticuloendothelial system resulting in viraemia. Entry into the CNS is thought to be direct spread from the bloodstream and possibly from muscle up peripheral nerves to the CNS. Destruction of neurons is accompanied by an inflammatory infiltrate of polymorphonuclear leukocytes, lymphocytes and macrophages. Primarily the grey matter of the anterior horns of the spinal cord and the motor nuclei of the pons and medulla are affected.[181]

CLINICAL FEATURES

Infection with poliovirus can result in one of six syndromes: inapparent infection with no symptoms, which is common in young children; a mild febrile illness only, known in older literature as 'abortive' poliomyelitis; a viral meningitis syndrome, 'non-paralytic' poliomyelitis; 'paralytic poliomyelitis', which is the classic flaccid paralytic syndrome which may be spinal or bulbar; and 'encephalitis', which is rare. Estimates of the ratio of apparent to inapparent infections vary from 1 in 60 to 1 in 1000.

Paralytic poliomyelitis occurs in 0.1% of all poliovirus infections. In children there is typically a biphasic course.[182] Initially, there is a nonspecific febrile illness lasting 1–3 days that coincides with a viraemia. Following this the patients may be asymptomatic for 2–5 days, before developing the fever, headache, malaise, vomiting and neck stiffness. In older patients, there is often spontaneous muscle pain, which may be relieved by walking. However exercise during the first 3 days of the second phase increases the incidence and severity of paralytic disease.[183] There may be sensory changes such as localized cutaneous hyperaesthesia and paraesthesias. After 1–2 days there is frank paralysis and weakness, which may range from a single portion of one muscle to quadriplegia. The paralysis is flaccid and although deep tendon reflexes may be brisk transiently, they soon become absent. The weakness is characterized by its asymmetrical distribution, which typically involves the legs more than the arms and proximal muscles more than distal ones. The weakness usually reaches a maximum over 2–3 days and stops when the patient becomes afebrile.[182] Muscle wasting commences and fasciculations are prominent. Paralysis of the bladder, which is usually associated with leg paralysis, occurs in about one quarter of adults, but is uncommon in children.

In bulbar poliomyelitis there is paralysis of the muscles innervated by the lower cranial nerves, particularly the ninth and tenth, resulting in dysphagia, nasal speech and occasionally dyspnoea.[178] Its frequency has been reported as 5–35% and it is more common in adults.[184] Rarely the medullary respiratory and vasomotor centres may be affected leading to irregular respiratory patterns, respiratory failure, circulatory collapse, cardiac dysrhythmias and (neurogenic) pulmonary oedema.[185]

DIAGNOSIS

There is typically a CSF pleocytosis, often with elevated polymorphonuclear cells, a slightly elevated protein and normal glucose ratio. Polioviruses can usually be isolated from throat secretions during the 1st week of illness and from faeces subsequently. Virus is rarely isolated from the CSF in patients with paralysis.

MANAGEMENT AND TREATMENT

Bed rest is advised for patients with paralysis, because of the risk that movement exacerbates the disease. Physiotherapy should be initiated once the progression of paralysis has ceased. Patients with respiratory failure receive positive pressure ventilation, which has replaced the 'iron lung' tank respirators which were used in the past.

PREVENTION

In the 1950s, a formalin inactivated vaccine was developed by Salk and a live attenuated vaccine by Sabin and their usage was associated with a dramatic decline. The oral polio vaccine is a mixture of live attenuated poliovirus types 1, 2 and 3. Although the target of global eradication by 2000 was not achieved, there is hope that with the current final push, polio will be eradicated. The challenges have included difficulty immunizing in areas of ongoing conflict, poor compliance with immunization because of mistrust in some communities, natural disasters disrupting infrastructure and issues over financing the programme. Despite this, there is still hope that ultimately the wild-type virus will be eradicated.[179]

There is a very small risk (approx. 1 case per 2 million doses) of the vaccine reverting to a virulent form to cause poliomyelitis (vaccine-associated paralytic poliomyelitis) in a recipient; or via faeco–oral spread to a household contact of a recipient. Hence, in some areas where the disease has been eradicated inactivated vaccine is once again being used more widely. Those with immunodeficiency should also be given inactivated vaccine because they too have an increased risk of reversion to virulence and long-term shedding of virus.

Human T-Lymphotropic Virus Type 1

EPIDEMIOLOGY

Although descriptions of tropical spastic paraparesis in the Caribbean were first published in 1956,[186] its association with antibodies to HTLV-I in serum and CSF was not recognized until 1985.[187] A group in Japan called the condition HTLV-1 associated myelopathy but it was soon realized that tropical spastic paraparesis and HTLV-1 associated myelopathy were the same disease.

HTLV-I is a retrovirus (family, Retroviridae) thought to infect 10–20 million people worldwide, as estimated by seroprevalence studies. However, the virus is associated with disease in only approximately 2% of those infected.[188] Seroprevalence increases with age and women are nearly twice as likely to be infected as men; this gender difference is thought to reflect the relative efficiency of sexual transmission from male to female. Because women are more likely to be infected with the virus, they are also more likely to develop myelopathy.

The virus is primarily transmitted by breast-feeding, although spread via blood transfusion, sharing of needles and sexual intercourse also occurs. Cases tend to cluster in familial or geographically discrete groups. The virus is endemic in southern Japan, the Caribbean, South America, the Melanesian islands, Papua New Guinea, the Middle East and central and southern Africa. Seroprevalences range from 3 to 5% in Trinidad and up to 30% in parts of southern Japan.[189] In the USA and Europe, the prevalence rates are less than 1%.

PATHOGENESIS AND PATHOLOGY

HTLV-1 is a retrovirus (family Retroviridae; genus *Deltavirus*) which, like HIV, infects CD4 T cells; after reverse transcription, its DNA becomes incorporated into the DNA of the host cell thus making a provirus. However, whereas HIV eventually destroys the cells it infects, HTLV-1 causes them to proliferate, hence leading to leukaemia in some patients.

Interestingly, HTLV-1 associated myelopathy is more likely when HTLV1 is acquired via blood transfusion, whereas HTLV1 acquired through breast feeding is more likely to be associated with adult T-cell leukaemia-lymphoma. Low levels of viral DNA in peripheral blood mononuclear cells occur in asymptomatic infection while higher levels correlate with symptomatic disease. The host response includes antibody production and development of cytotoxic T cells. These cells, plus CD4 T cells are part of the perivascular inflammatory infiltrate contributing to the myelitis. Neuronal damage is caused by release of inflammatory cytokines, rather than direct viral invasion of neurones.[190] Risk factors for development of myelopathy include high proviral load and certain polymorphisms in the interleukin (IL)-10 promoter and in the IL28B gene.

CLINICAL FEATURES

HAM is a chronic progressive myelopathy characterized by bilateral pyramidal tract involvement giving lower limb weakness, especially proximally, spasticity and generalized hyperreflexia.[191] There may also be minor sensory changes, especially tingling, pins and needles, burning paresthesias and loss of vibration sense. There is often bladder dysfunction and lower-back pain, which radiates into the legs. Bladder dysfunction may take the form of nocturia, urinary frequency and incontinence. Impotence is common and constipation occurs later. Cognitive function is normal and cranial nerves and upper limbs are usually unaffected.

The onset of HTLV-1 associated myelopathy is insidious, a median 3 years after infection with the virus; but it may be as soon as 4 months or as late as 30 years. Although sometimes the disease reaches a plateau phase after the initial onset, a continuous slow progression is the norm. In one large series with more than 100 patients in Martinique, the median time from disease onset to use of one walking stick was 6 years and to use of a wheelchair was 21 years.[192] More rapid progression is associated with higher viral load, older age of onset, especially over 65 and acquisition of virus via blood transfusion. The disease is sometimes seen in children and tends to have a more rapid progression in this group.

DIAGNOSIS

At lumbar puncture, CSF examination reveals a low-level lymphocytosis in approximately one-third of cases, with mildly elevated protein concentration. Anti-HTLV-I antibodies are detectable in the CSF with a high CSF/serum ratio. Virus can be cultured from CSF lymphocytes and proviral DNA detected by PCR. On magnetic resonance imaging there may be atrophy of the cervical or thoracic cord with or without white matter lesions in the subcortical and periventricular regions. Neurophysiologic studies may reveal evidence of posterior column dysfunction as well as a peripheral neuropathy.

The original rather broad description and diagnostic criteria produced by WHO in 1985 for HTLV-1 associated myelopathy have since been refined into three levels of ascertainment: definite, probable and possible, based on neurological features, serological findings, detection of HTLV-1 DNA in the serum and exclusion of other causes.[191] The diagnosis is confirmed by detecting antibodies to HTLV-1 or detecting proviral DNA.

An enzyme-linked immunosorbent assay is the most frequently used screening test, with western blotting used for confirmation; western blotting can distinguish between infection with HTLV-I and the related but less pathogenic HTLV-II. PCR-based testing to detect proviral DNA in peripheral blood mononuclear cells is an alternative diagnostic test, which can also differentiate HTLV-I from HTLV-II and provide quantification of proviral load in the blood. Viral detection in the CSF has also been proposed as an additional diagnostic test.[193]

MANAGEMENT AND TREATMENT

There is no established antiviral therapy for HTLV-1 associated myelopathy, even though antiretroviral regimens have shown some promise for HTLV-1 associated adult T-cell leukaemia-lymphoma. The combination of the nucleoside analogue reverse transcriptase inhibitor zidovudine, with IFN-α, has been used with some success in patients with adult T-cell leukaemia-lymphoma. In this group, others have tried lamivudine, another nucleoside analogue reverse transcriptase inhibitor, with unclear results. Lamivudine, with or without zidovudine, has been examined in a small number of patients with HAM; although proviral load in the blood is reduced, this does not seem to be associated with a consistent improvement in neurological function.[194] In a small open-label trial, interferon-β showed some benefit in clinical and immunological parameters. In a recent non-randomized study, interferon-α reduced viral load, altered immunological parameters and appeared to have an effect on neurological function.[195] In some case series, but not others, corticosteroids appeared to be beneficial. The anabolic steroid danazol was also reported to be helpful. There have been no randomized studies.

PREVENTION

Screening of blood donors, promotion of safe sex and reduction of needle sharing reduce the spread of HTLV-1. Breast-feeding of infants is also discouraged for those who are HTLV-1-positive.[196]

Human Immunodeficiency Virus

EPIDEMIOLOGY

As well as causing secondary complications in the CNS (described in Chapter 10), HIV, which is in the family Retroviridae, genus *Lentivirus*, directly invades the nervous system to cause an acute seroconversion meningoencephalitis and a more chronic cognitive impairment. This section will discuss these manifestations.

A mild seroconversion illness, with fever, headache, malaise and lymphadenopathy is thought to occur when most people acquire HIV,[197] though in the majority, the cause is not recognized at the time. Aseptic meningitis is less common, occurring in up to 10% of patients[198] and in a small minority of these there is also encephalopathy.

HIV-associated dementia, also known as AIDS dementia complex, was first described in those with advanced HIV. It consists of a combination of acquired limitations in cognitive abilities (attention or concentration, processing speed, abstraction, memory, speech or visual-spatial skills) plus abnormalities in motor function or changes in emotional or behavioural functioning. The patient is fully conscious, but the overall symptoms cause significant impairment in work or activities of daily living. While the incidence of this severe syndrome has decreased markedly in the era of antiretroviral drugs, moderate and mild forms of HIV-associated neurocognitive disorder, also known as HAND, are recognized increasingly.[13] In some series, as many as 30–40% of people with HIV are reported to have mild HIV-associated neurocognitive disorder.[199] However, there is controversy around this issue, particularly around what constitutes mild HIV-associated neurocognitive disorder.[200]

PATHOGENESIS AND PATHOLOGY

HIV enters brain at the time of the primary HIV infection. It is carried across the blood–brain barrier by monocytes and lymphocytes in a 'Trojan horse' mechanism. On crossing the barrier, monocytes may become activated perivascular macrophages. HIV replicates in these cells, as well as in microglia and astrocytes. This chronic viral replication results in secretion of neurotoxic cytokines. In addition, the excitatory neurotransmitter glutamate is released, which is also neurotoxic at high levels. Collectively the neurotoxins produce neuronal damage so although there is not direct viral invasion of neurons, this indirect damage is thought to lead to cognitive impairment.[13]

Various host factors also appear to contribute to the development of HIV-associated neurocognitive disorder; these include genetic predisposition, such as an association with apolipoprotein E e4 alleles (as in Alzheimer's disease) and a polymorphism in a gene encoding the potent chemotactic protein MCP-1. There is also synergy with other causes of dementia, such as insulin resistance, other metabolic disorders, ageing and vascular disease. Indeed vascular risk factors appear to be more strongly associated with cognitive impairment than markers of HIV disease severity, such as plasma HIV RNA level. Nadir CD4 count may also be a risk for cognitive impairment,[201] and HIV subtype and drug resistance may be important. HAND is more common in those that use stimulant drugs, such as methamphetamine and cocaine or have hepatitis C virus infection.

CLINICAL FEATURES

The clinical features of aseptic meningitis, which occurs as part of an acute HIV seroconversion illness, are similar to other forms of viral meningitis, with fever, headache and meningism. However, there may be other clinical clues to suggest this is HIV disease, in particular a generalized rash, sore throat, oral or genital ulcers and lymphadenopathy. The syndrome usually occurs 2–4 weeks after HIV infection. The differential includes infectious mononucleosis due to EBV, though it is unusual for this to cause a rash.

The chronic effects of HIV on the brain range from mild behavioural disorders, which may be difficult to distinguish from those in any other chronic illness, such as depression, anxiety and sleep disturbances, to HIV-associated neurocognitive disorder. This disorder is sub-divided into asymptomatic neurocognitive impairment, mild neurocognitive disorder and HIV-associated dementia. Diagnosis of HIV-associated neurocognitive disorder requires acquired impairment in at least two cognitive abilities. For the diagnosis of asymptomatic neurocognitive impairment, the impairment does not interfere with daily function; the interference is mild for mild neurocognitive disorder and severe for HIV-associated dementia. In advanced HIV dementia, there is a frontal subcortical dementia with a slowness in mental alacrity (bradyphrenia) and slowness of movement (bradykinesia) with memory difficulties. In addition, patients experience impaired saccadic eye movements, marked difficulty with smooth limb movement (especially in the lower extremities), dysdiadochokinesia, hyperreflexia and frontal release signs such as grasp, root, snout and glabellar reflexes.[202]

DIAGNOSIS

Aseptic meningitis due to HIV seroconversion is diagnosed when there is a high viral load or positive p24 viral antigen, in a patient with appropriate clinical features. Viral loads are typically 100 000 copies/mL and HIV antibody tests are negative or indeterminate. Loads less than 10 000 copies/mL should raise the suspicion of false positives and patients should be retested. In the CSF there is pleocytosis, typically tens to hundreds of lymphocytes per μL. This is in contrast to the very minor CSF pleocytosis (typically <20 cells/μL), which is often seen in patients with established HIV who have no clinical features of meningism. Virus can often be detected in the CSF by PCR or culture though this is not done in routine clinical practice. A positive test should be confirmed with antibody testing, though it may take several weeks for this to become positive.

The diagnosis of HAND depends on exclusion of other causes of cognitive impairment and neuropsychological testing to help classify the disease. Because detailed testing takes time and is not available in many parts of the world where HIV occurs, screening tests have been developed, such as the International HIV Dementia Scale.[203] Other tools include the ACTG (AIDS Clinical Trials Group) Longitudinal Linked Randomized Trial (ALLRT) Neurocognitive Screen, which consists of connect-the-dot tests and digit-symbol comparison tests.[204] A CSF examination, serological studies and brain imaging, will exclude most other causes of cognitive impairment, including progressive multifocal leukoencephalopathy, tuberculosis, neurosyphilis and toxoplasmosis. Cerebral imaging shows atrophy.

MANAGEMENT AND TREATMENT

As with other forms of HIV seroconversion illness, patients with seroconversion meningitis are highly infectious to others, because of their high viral loads. This underscores the public health importance of diagnosing the condition. There is no specific treatment for HIV seroconversion meningitis, though there is debate about whether early antiretroviral treatment improves prognosis overall.[205]

In HIV-associated neurocognitive deficit there is no specific treatment. Patients with advanced disease should be on combined antiretroviral therapy. Some patients who are not already on antiretroviral drugs do improve cognitively once the drugs are started. Antiretrovirals with better penetrance into the CNS are recommended, including zidovudine, stavudine, lamivudine, abacavir, nevirapine, indinavir, though it is unclear whether they do actually lead to reduced CSF viral loads and improved cognition (see below). Control of vascular risk factors such as hypertension and hypercholesterolaemia are important.

PREVENTION

The measures to prevent aseptic meningitis as part of an HIV seroconversion illness are the same as those for prevention of HIV infection itself (Chapter 12). To reduce the chances of developing severe HIV-associated neurocognitive deficit, good control of HIV viral load through antiretroviral drugs appears to be important. Measures to prevent mild disease are less clear. Choice of drug with better CNS penetration may be important. The CNS Penetration Effectiveness Score ranks antiretroviral regimens based on chemical properties of the drugs, data on CSF concentrations and antiretroviral effectiveness in various clinical studies of neurocognitive dysfunction. Regimens with high scores are recommended for those with HIV-associated dementia. In one study, a low score was associated with an increased chance of detecting HIV RNA in the CSF, although the score explained only 12% of the variance in viral loads.

There is some suggestion that strong suppression of viral load in the serum may be equally important in controlling CSF viral load and ultimately controlling HIV-associated neurocognitive disorder.[206] Polymorphisms of transporter drugs at the blood–brain barrier may have a critical role in controlling drug concentrations within the CNS. Low drug concentrations may allow the development of resistance phenotypes. Control of other risk factors for dementia, for example vascular risk factors, may also be important.

Progressive Multifocal Leucoencephalopathy

EPIDEMIOLOGY

Progressive multifocal leucoencephalopathy (PML) is caused by a papovavirus. These are DNA viruses named after the major subvarieties of virus: *pa*pilloma, *po*lyoma and the *va*cuolating viruses. The most common is JC, although a related BK virus also causes some cases. Both are named after the initials of the first patient from whom they were isolated. These viruses are unusual in that they cause no systemic disease, PML is the only clinical presentation.

Seroepidemiological studies show that exposure to JC virus is ubiquitous among adults of all races across the globe. Seroconversion takes place during childhood and does not result in disease unless the subject becomes immunocompromised. PML was a very rare disease, associated with a range of immunocompromised conditions, such as sarcoidosis, carcinomatosis, organ transplantation and immunosuppressive drug regimens. However it has become more common in the era of HIV: in one series 3% of all AIDS cases examined at autopsy had PML.[207] Recently, 'biological' immunosuppressive drugs such as the humanized monoclonal antibody to alpha4 integrin, natalizumab or to CD20 on B cells, rituximab[208] have been found to cause PML.[208,209] In patients with multiple sclerosis, the overall risk of PML with natalizumab therapy is estimated to be approximately 2.1 per 1000. The risk is increased with the duration of natalizumab therapy, prior immunosuppressant treatment and seropositivity for anti-JC virus antibodies prior to natalizumab treatment.

Interestingly, although many other opportunistic infections and tumours of the brain have decreased significantly since the availability of highly active antiretroviral therapy (HAART) for HIV infection, the incidence of PML remains virtually unchanged.[210] However, HAART has had an impact on the clinical presentation and diagnosis. For example, it is not uncommon for patients with HIV infection on HAART to have clinical and radiological features of PML, but without virus detected in the CSF; for this reason it has been proposed that such patients be considered 'possible PML'.[211]

In addition, PML has been shown to develop in HIV-infected patients shortly after the introduction of HAART, despite a recovery of the immune system. Therefore, PML may, in some cases, be another manifestation of the immune reconstitution inflammatory syndrome.[212]

PATHOGENESIS AND PATHOLOGY

The kidney is the site of latent JCV infection. It is thought that when the immune system is suppressed, JC virus enters the circulation and travels to the brain, lung and lymphoreticular system.[213] In the brain the oligodendrocytes become loaded with virus, with resultant cell destruction which leads to the breakdown of the myelin sheath and to the patchy demyelination which is so characteristic of the condition. An alternative hypothesis is that PML is due to reactivation of latent, previously non-pathogenic JC virus infection in the brain. For example, evidence of JC virus DNA was found in oligodendroglia and astrocytes of elderly patients who had no evidence of PML.[214]

The pathology of PML is characteristic. JC virus produces a lysing infection of oligodendroglia, which become large and spherical and have big inclusions. Astrocytes alter and show changes which are seen in malignancy. Inflammatory change is absent or minimal. There are multiple foci of white matter demyelination which coalesce as they enlarge. These are scattered throughout the cerebral hemispheres, cerebellum and brainstem and their location determines the clinical features.

CLINICAL FEATURES

The clinical features of PML are determined by the area of the brain which is involved. The onset is insidious and often difficult to recognize, even in retrospect, especially when it occurs in the evolution of an established predisposing disease. The most common symptoms and signs are mental disturbance and impairment of awareness and of consciousness. Multiple enlarging, but not space-occupying, lesions of white matter give rise to hemiparesis, parietal syndromes, visual pathway upset, pseudobulbar palsy, cortical blindness, dementia and seizures; less commonly the white matter of the brainstem and cerebellum is affected with ataxia, nystagmus and bulbar palsies. Raised intracranial pressure is seldom a problem and headache is uncommon.

DIAGNOSIS

Brain imaging reveals widespread, multiple and often confluent, non-enhancing white matter lesions that are not space-occupying and have no mass effect or oedema. CSF examination is usually unremarkable or it may show a slight pleocytosis and some rise of the protein content. It is now possible to detect and quantify JC virus in CSF and this may correlate with survival rates.[215] High viral load of JC virus in the CSF is the norm. It may be necessary to resort to brain biopsy to diagnose PML and also to exclude other pathologies such as lymphoma and other infection in patients with HIV. The characteristic pathological changes can usually be seen with light microscopy and virus particles can be seen with the electron microscope. A variety of immunocytological techniques and PCR can be used to demonstrate JC virus in tissue samples.

MANAGEMENT AND TREATMENT

Treatment of PML remains difficult.[216] In HIV-positive patients, combined antiretroviral therapy is the only effective treatment for PML. It probably acts indirectly by suppressing HIV replication and thus allowing the immune system to keep JCV replication under control. The mortality rate of PML is now between 30% and 50% of patients during the first 3 months, although some patients stabilize and survive for many years. Survival of PML for more than 1 year has increased from 10% before the HAART era to approximately 50% of cases. Nevertheless, PML continues to occur in patients receiving HAART. It makes sense for HIV patients with PML to be on treatment regimens which include drugs with good blood–brain barrier penetration. Favourable prognostic factors include starting HAART at PML diagnosis in patients previously naive to antiretroviral agents and a CD4 cell count greater than 100 cells/μL. However, as oligodendrocytes destroyed by JCV are not replaced in the central nervous system (CNS), PML survivors are often left with devastating neurological sequelae.

For HIV-negative patients who are on immunosuppressive drugs for malignancy, stopping or reducing the immunosuppressive drugs is an option that may be beneficial. Cidofovir, which had looked promising in vitro and in animal models for treating PML was shown not to be effective in HIV-positive patients in clinical trials. Other failed candidate drugs for PML in HIV-positive patients include IFN-α2B and cytosine arabinoside and steroids. Interestingly, however, the latter was clearly active in decreasing JCV replication in vitro and may have helped stabilize seven out of 19 HIV-negative patients (36%) with PML in a retrospective study,[217] despite significant bone marrow toxicity. Therefore, cytosine arabinoside should be considered in HIV-negative patients with PML. Other potential therapies which have theoretical and in vitro evidence of support, but no supporting evidence from randomized controlled trials include the serotonin reuptake inhibitor, mirtazapine and the antimalarial, mefloquine.

For patients with multiple sclerosis who develop PML during natalizumab therapy, the drug should be stopped and plasma exchange considered to remove any circulating drug.

PREVENTION

In most patients with PML, there is no means of prevention. However, for patients with multiple sclerosis in whom natalizumab is being considered, the risks of PML are assessed before starting natalizumab by considering whether a patient has anti-JC virus antibody indicating they have been infected with the virus and whether they have had prior immunosuppressant treatment; both of which are risk factors for developing the disease.[218]

Prion Diseases

EPIDEMIOLOGY

The prion diseases or transmissible spongiform encephalopathies are progressive neurodegenerative diseases with transmissible properties that affect animals and humans. They are rare, affecting approximately one person per million per year. The term 'prion' was coined by Prusiner in 1982 and referred to a *pro*teinaceous *in*fectious particle that he believed to be the agent which caused scrapie, a prion disease of sheep, recognized in Scotland for hundreds of years.[219]

Kuru is a prion disease described in Papua New Guinea since the 1950s; epidemiological studies linked the disease to the practice of cannibalism, particularly exposure to brain and offal of infected carcasses. The prion disease, bovine spongiform encephalopathy was first described in British cattle in the 1980s and thought to be caused by feeding them on scrapie-infected feed derived from sheep. Creutzfeldt–Jacob disease (CJD) has been recognized in humans since the 1920s, with variant CJD occurring since the 1990s and caused by ingestion of meat contaminated with bovine spongiform encephalopathy.[220] To date, less than 180 cases of variant CJD have been reported worldwide, the vast majority in the UK.[221] There is also a familial form of CJD. More important Iatrogenic forms of CJD follow insertion of infected graft material such as dura mater or cornea, injection of growth hormone from human cadavers or use of inadequately sterilized neurosurgical instruments. Fatal familial insomnia and Gerstmann, Straüssler, Scheinker syndrome are very rare autosomal dominant inherited prion diseases, the latter characterized by dementia with ataxia. The incubation periods of prion disease are long, ranging from 2 years for iatrogenic cases to years or even decades for kuru.[222]

PATHOGENESIS AND PATHOLOGY

Prion diseases result from neuronal accumulation of a misfolded isoform of the prion protein, which is a glycoprotein with unknown function. Once an abnormal prion protein is present in the brain, it replicates by an autocatalytic mechanism, whereby it binds to the endogenous protein and converts it to the misfolded isoform. The abnormal protein can arise spontaneously, be ingested in diseases such as kuru or variant CJD or be experimentally injected. Probable transmission of vCJD in blood products has been demonstrated.[223] The coding gene for prion protein is located on the short arm of chromosome 20 and the longer of its two exons contains the entire transcribed 253 codon region of the gene. Most cases of sporadic CJD are homozygous for a common PrP protein polymorphism. Approximately 90% of CJD patients are homozygous for either methionine or valine at codon 129, compared with 50% of non-affected individuals. The different subtypes of CJD appear to relate to the genotype at codon 129, homozygosity for methionine or valine or heterozygosity and the electrophoretic mobility of the prion protein.[221] Nearly 100% of cases of variant CJD are homozygous for methionine at this position.

The abnormal forms of prion protein accumulate in the brain in amyloid plaques.[224] Pathologically there are widespread changes throughout the neuraxis, with neuronal loss in all layers of the cortex, astrocytic proliferation and marked spongiform changes particularly in the deeper cortical layers. There is little demyelination. Spongiform change precedes neuronal loss and is due to the appearance of vacuoles within the cytoplasm of the neurophil. There is virtually no inflammatory change. Amyloid plaques are found within the extracellular space, particularly in the cerebellar cortex.[225]

CLINICAL FEATURES

The classical triad of features in CJD is dementia, ataxia and myoclonus. The initial symptoms are nonspecific and variable and no different from other forms of dementia with forgetfulness, fatigue, cognitive disturbance, depression, personality disorder, behavioural upset, derangement of sleep, weight loss and malaise. However they rapidly progress and about 70% of all sporadic cases are dead within 6 months. Myoclonus appears at any stage of the disease and is highly suggestive of the diagnosis; an exaggerated startle response is characteristic. The Brownell–Oppenheimer variant presents with a cerebellar syndrome, while the Heidenhaim form presents with dyspraxia, agnosia and cortical blindness.

The age of onset for CJD is between 60 and 70 years for sporadic cases, whereas it is less than 50 years in familial cases.

Patients with variant CJD have a much younger age of onset, typically teenagers and young adults, present with psychiatric problems with behavioural changes, develop ataxia and cerebellar dysfunction early and have a longer disease duration. Kuru is characterized by gait and truncal ataxia, dysarthria, tremor and titubation, usually with retention of intellect. Cerebellar deterioration becomes increasingly evident with disruption of eye movements and increasing disability, the appearance of pyramidal and extra-pyramidal signs and various forms of movement disorder, but not myoclonus. Emotional lability, generalized muscle wasting and paralysis supervene and lead rapidly to death.[226]

DIAGNOSIS

The differential is broad and includes other forms of sub-acute encephalopathy and dementia. However, prion disease should be high in the differential for any rapidly progressive dementia, especially if there is myoclonus. A definite diagnosis of CJD requires pathological confirmation. According to the World Health Organization criteria, a case is probable if there is progressive dementia with no alternative diagnosis, there are at least two of the following four clinical features: myoclonus, visual or cerebellar disturbance, pyramidal or extrapyramidal dysfunction and akinetic mutism; and there is a typical EEG or a positive CSF 14–3-3 assay (for patients in whom the duration to death is less than 2 years).[227]

Investigations to exclude other forms of dementia include B_{12}, thyroid function tests, HIV and syphilis serology and tests for anti-thyroid antibodies to exclude Hashimoto's encephalopathy. In addition paraneoplastic antibodies for limbic encephalitis (anti-Ri antibodies) and for a cerebellar syndrome (anti-Yo antibodies) should be considered, as well as investigations for possible vasculitis (erythrocyte sedimentation rate, C-reactive protein and autoantibodies), especially in patients under 55 years. A heavy metal screen, copper and caeruloplasmin (to exclude Wilson's disease in younger patients) and investigations for Whipple's disease may be appropriate.

Imaging of the brain should be carried out to exclude other pathology and to look for characteristic features of CJD.[221] These include high signal intensities in the putamen and caudate nuclei on T2 and proton dense weighted images in many causes of sporadic and familial CJD. Diffusion-weighted MRI may be useful for early diagnosis.[221]

The EEG shows diffuse slow waves and in sporadic CJD, often has rhythmic and periodic bursts of high-amplitude bi- and triphasic periodic sharp wave complexes which may be synchronous with myoclonus. CSF examination is important to rule out other treatable causes; there may be a minor elevation of total protein and 14–3-3 protein may be detectable.[228]

MANAGEMENT AND TREATMENT

No treatment has been demonstrated to be effective to limit the progression of prion diseases which are universally fatal. Symptomatic treatment is given for seizures, spasticity and myoclonus and is generally ineffective.

PREVENTION

Prion diseases related to ingestion of contaminated food, namely variant CJD and kuru, have declined once the association was recognized and public health interventions established. Because of the infectious nature of prion diseases, staff treating such patients must take strict precautions. Prions are resistant to standard disinfecting agents and so special precautions are necessary. Guidelines exist for the disposal of specimens and surgical instruments and for necropsy. People suspected of suffering from prion diseases should not donate blood and they are not suitable as donors for organ transplantation. If a hereditary form of prion disease is confirmed, genetic counselling should be offered.

REFERENCES

1. Whitley RJ, Gnann JW. Viral encephalitis: familiar infections and emerging pathogens. Lancet 2002;359:507–13.
5. Goh KJ, Tan CT, Chew NK, et al. Clinical features of Nipah virus encephalitis among pig farmers in Malaysia. N Engl J Med 2000;342: 1229–35.
6. Ho M, Chen ER, Hsu KH, et al. An epidemic of enterovirus 71 infection in Taiwan. Taiwan Enterovirus Epidemic Working Group. N Engl J Med 1999;341:929–35.
12. Griffin DE. Immune responses to RNA-virus infections of the CNS. Nat Rev Immunol 2003;3:493–502.
13. Letendre S. Central nervous system complications in HIV disease: HIV-associated neurocognitive disorder. Top Antivir Med 2011;19: 137–42.
26. Ooi MH, Wong SC, Lewthwaite P, et al. Clinical features, diagnosis and management of enterovirus 71. Lancet Neurol 2010;9:1097–105.
29. Weinberg A, Bloch KC, Li S, et al. Dual infections of the central nervous system with Epstein-Barr virus. J Infect Dis 2005;191: 234–7.
54. Kimberlin DW. Neonatal herpes simplex infection. Clin Microbiol Rev 2004;17:1–13.
58. Solomon T, Michael BD, Smith PE, et al. Management of suspected viral encephalitis in adults – Association of British Neurologists and British Infection Association National Guidelines. J Infect 2012;64:347–73.
59. Kneen R, Michael BD, Menson E, et al. Management of suspected viral encephalitis in children – Association of British Neurologists and British Paediatric Allergy, Immunology and Infection Group national guidelines. J Infect 2012;64:449–77.
66. Aurelius E, Franzen-Rohl E, Glimaker M, et al. Long-term valacyclovir suppressive treatment after herpes simplex virus type 2 meningitis: a double-blind, randomized controlled trial. Clin Infect Dis 2012;54:1304–13.
72. Gilden DH, Kleinschmidt-DeMasters BK, LaGuardia JJ, et al. Neurologic complications of the reactivation of varicella-zoster virus. N Engl J Med 2000;342:635–45.
73. Hausler M, Schaade L, Kemeny S, et al. Encephalitis related to primary varicella-zoster virus infection in immunocompetent children. J Neurolog Sci 2002;195:111–16.
87. Connelly KP, DeWitt LD. Neurologic complications of infectious mononucleosis. Pediatr Neurol 1994;10:181–4.
97. Gerstner E, Batchelor T. Primary CNS lymphoma. Expert Rev Anticancer Ther 2007;7: 689–700.
99. Kelly M BLA, Cartwright K, Ajdukiewicz K, et al. Prevalence of HSV, EBV and CMV in the Cerebrospinal Fluid of Adults with Clinically Suspected Bacterial Meningitis in Malawi [abstract]. London: Meningitis Research Foundation Annual Meeting; 2009.
104. Rafailidis PI, Mourtzoukou EG, Varbobitis IC, et al. Severe cytomegalovirus infection in apparently immunocompetent patients: a systematic review. Virology J 2008;5:47.
122. Kovacs JA, Baseler M, Dewar R, et al. Increases in CD4 T Lymphocytes with intermittent courses of Interleukin-2 in patients with human immunodeficiency virus infection. A preliminary study. N Engl J Med 1995;332: 567–75.
127. Johnson RT, Griffin DE, Hirsch RL, et al. Measles encephalomyelitis – clinical and immunologic studies. N Engl J Med 1984;310: 137–41.
130. Yaqub BA. Sub-acute sclerosing panencephalitis (SSPE): early diagnosis, prognostic factors and natural history. J Neurol Sci 1996;139: 227–34.

145. WHO. Nipah virus. Health Section of the Secretariat of the League of Nations. Wkly Epidemiol Rec 2011;86:451–5.
155. Galazka AM, Robertson SE, Kraigher A. Mumps and mumps vaccine: A global review. Bull World Health Organ 1999;77:3–14.
156. Solomon T, Lewthwaite P, Perera D, et al. Virology, epidemiology, pathogenesis and control of enterovirus 71. Lancet Infect Dis 2010;10:778–90.
157. McMinn PC. An overview of the evolution of enterovirus 71 and its clinical and public health significance. FEMS Microbiol Rev 2002;26:91–107.
176. Huang CC, Liu CC, Chang YC, et al. Neurologic complications in children with enterovirus 71 infection. N Engl J Med 1999;341: 936–42.
179. Centers for Disease C, Prevention. Progress toward interruption of wild poliovirus transmission – worldwide, January 2011–March 2012. MMWR 2012;61:353–7.
183. Russell WR. Paralytic poliomyelitis: the early symptoms and the effect of physical activity on the course of the disease. BMJ 1949;1:465.
191. De Castro-Costa CM, Araujo AQ, Barreto MM, et al. Proposal for diagnostic criteria of tropical spastic paraparesis/HTLV-I-associated myelopathy (TSP/HAM). AIDS Res Hum Retroviruses 2006;22(10):931–5.
192. Olindo S, Cabre P, Lezin A, et al. Natural history of human T-lymphotropic virus 1-associated myelopathy: a 14-year follow-up study. Arch Neurol 2006;63:1560–6.
199. Heaton RK, Clifford DB, Franklin Jr DR, et al. HIV-associated neurocognitive disorders persist in the era of potent antiretroviral therapy: CHARTER Study. Neurology 2010; 75:2087–96.
203. Sacktor NC, Wong M, Nakasujja N, et al. The International HIV Dementia Scale: a new rapid screening test for HIV dementia. AIDS 2005;19:1367–74.
213. Houff SA, Major EO, Katz DA, et al. Involvement of JC virus-infected mononuclear cells from the bone marrow and spleen in the pathogenesis of progressive multifocal leukoencephalopathy. N Engl J Med 1988;318: 301–5.
218. Kappos L, Bates D, Edan G, et al. Natalizumab treatment for multiple sclerosis: updated recommendations for patient selection and monitoring. Lancet Neurol 2011;10:745–58.
220. Will RG, Ironside JW, Zeidler M, et al. A new variant of Creutzfeldt-Jakob disease in the UK. Lancet 1996;347:921–5.
226. Gajdusek DC, Zigas V. Degenerative disease of the central nervous system in New Guinea; the endemic occurrence of kuru in the native population. N Engl J Med 1957;257:974–8.

Access the complete references online at www.expertconsult.com

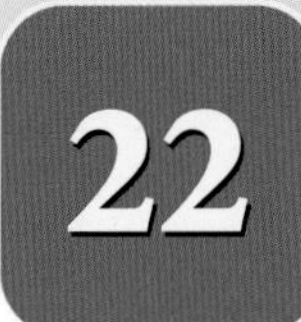

Tropical Rickettsial Infections

DANIEL H. PARIS | NICHOLAS P. J. DAY

KEY POINTS

- *Rickettsia* and *Orientia* are obligate intracellular bacteria.
- Ticks, fleas, mites and lice transmit *Rickettsia* and *Orientia* to humans and are both vectors and major reservoirs of these pathogens.
- Humans are dead-end hosts and play no role in the rickettsial/oriential life-cycles rickettsial/oriential life-cycles (with exception of *R. prowazekii* in epidemics).
- Due to lack of awareness and difficulties in diagnostics, rickettsial diseases are responsible for a substantial proportion of undiagnosed febrile illnesses in humans in many parts of the tropics.
- All forms of typhus due to *Rickettsia* and *Orientia* are treatable (with tetracyclines).
- There is currently no effective vaccine available (exception: a low-virulence live-attenuated strain of *R. prowazekii* was evaluated during the Second World War, but in 14% of recipients caused illness).
- Scrub typhus is the most common tropical rickettsial disease across South-east Asia and adjoining regions. Sporadic cases have been described in Africa and South America.
- The major differential diagnoses of 'typhus-like illness' with similar clinical presentation and geographical distribution, include: dengue, leptospirosis, typhoid, melioidosis, malaria and chikungunya fever.
- Scrub typhus and murine typhus are the two dominant forms of typhus in the tropics and together are the leading causes of undifferentiated febrile illness in many regions of South-east Asia.

Introduction

Tropical rickettsioses are a diverse group of zoonotic infectious diseases caused by obligate intracellular bacteria grouped in the family Rickettsiaceae, a member of the order *Rickettsiales*, within the α-Proteobacteria class. The order *Rickettsiales* harbours two families: the Anaplasmataceae and Rickettsiaceae, which together include six genera: *Rickettsia*, *Orientia*, *Ehrlichia*, *Anaplasma*, *Neorickettsia* and *Wolbachia*.[1] These organisms are non-flagellated, small coccobacilli located freely (not bound by a vacuole) within the cytoplasm of host cells. They are usually transmitted to humans by arthropods – ticks, fleas, lice and/or mites – in which they may be maintained by transovarial transmission.

Coxiella spp. belong to the class γ-Proteobacteria, the order *Legionellales* and the family Coxiellaceae, with its single genus, *Coxiella*. These bacteria enter the host cell by phagocytosis and remain and replicate within the phagosome until the cell dies.

A modern classification based on whole-genome analysis divides the species of the genus *Rickettsia* into four groups: spotted fever group (*R. rickettsii*, *R. conorii* and others); typhus group (*R. prowazekii* and *R. typhi*); an ancestral group (*R. bellii* and non-pathogenic *R. canadensis*) and the recently formed transitional group (*R. akari*, *R. australis* and *R. felis*). Ongoing investigations of a variety of non-arthropod vector hosts (including non-haematophagous insects, amoebae and leeches) have identified many novel *Rickettsia* clades, pointing to an ecologically diverse and complex evolutionary history.[2]

Causative agents responsible for human rickettsial disease in the tropics are:

- *Orientia tsutsugamushi*, which causes scrub typhus, a rickettsiosis widespread in Asia, the islands of the western Pacific and Indian Oceans and in foci in northern Australia
- The typhus group (TG) of the genus *Rickettsia*, containing *R. prowazekii*, the agent of classic epidemic or louse-borne typhus, and *R. typhi*, which causes murine or flea-borne typhus. *R. prowazekii* is the only pathogen among various rickettsial species with the acknowledged capacity to maintain persistent subclinical infection in convalescent patients, which can later manifest as recrudescent typhus or Brill–Zinsser disease
- The spotted fever group (SFG) *Rickettsia*, containing a large and ever-increasing number of species, mostly transmitted from rodents and other vertebrate hosts by ticks
- The transitional group rickettsiae, with *R. australis*, *R. akari* and emerging group of *R. felis* and *R. felis*-like rickettsiae (transmitted by ticks, mites, fleas)
- *Coxiella burnetii*, the cause of Q-fever, which is considered a typhus-like illness. Q-fever will be covered in this chapter, although *C. burnetii* has recently been transferred to the γ-Proteobacteria order *Legionellales*
- The members of the Anaplasmatacae family, which the genus *Ehrlichia* (family: Anaplasmataceae), which includes the genera *Anaplasma*, *Ehrlichia*, *Wolbachia* and *Neorickettsia*. Although only limited data exist, these rickettsioses are considered emerging diseases.

Typhus remains a substantially under-recognized disease entity, particularly in Asia, where up to 28% of malaria-negative fevers can be attributed to rickettsial infections.[3–5] Scrub typhus, caused by *Orientia tsutsugamushi*, and murine typhus caused by *Rickettsia typhi* are the two main rickettsial disease groups in South-east Asia, although cases of spotted fever rickettsiosis have also been described.[6–9] Together, they probably represent the most frequent neglected but treatable infections in the world. In South-east Asia alone, an estimated 1 million cases of scrub typhus occur yearly, which based on available mortality rates, translates into approximately 50 000–80 000 deaths per year.[10]

Although rickettsial infections are an important cause of 'fever of unknown origin' (FUO), and increasing numbers of returning travellers have fevers attributable to rickettsial infections, robust epidemiological data on typhus remain very limited, especially from Africa and South America. Although some rickettsioses are distributed worldwide (e.g. Q-fever, murine typhus), diseases are usually associated with a specific area. Rickettsial agents are associated with arthropods, which require their preferred environmental conditions, biotopes and hosts to act as vectors, reservoirs and/or amplifiers of the organisms, which in turn determines their geographic distribution and consequently, define the areas of risk for contracting a particular rickettsial illness. Most rickettsioses are therefore geographic diseases. However, these geographical boundaries may be influenced by the dynamics of climate and environmental changes, and should be adapted in the light of new discoveries. *Orientia chuto* sp. nov. was recently discovered in the United Arabic Emirates (UAE), well beyond the expected geographical range for scrub typhus. Reports of febrile cases from Chile and Africa[11–14] with possible scrub typhus suggest that the disease could be distributed around the tropical/subtropical belt rather than confined to Asia.

African tick-bite fever (ATBF) is caused by a spotted fever group Rickettsia *(R. africae)* and is transmitted by cattle ticks (of the *Amblyomma* genus). *R. africae* has been detected by PCR in many African countries, including Niger, Mali, Burundi, Sudan and recently, Senegal, and in most countries of equatorial and southern Africa and often affects visitors to these regions.[15,16] Epidemic louse-borne typhus is still present in foci of low socio-economic standards found in the highlands of northern and eastern Africa, in Eastern Europe, and also in the mountainous regions of Central America, north-western South America, southern Asia, and southern Africa.[17–19]

Rickettsial diseases account for approximately 1.5–3.5% of febrile illnesses in travellers and can be life-threatening.[20] From published accounts the vast majority of travel-associated cases of imported rickettsial illnesses are murine typhus (*R. typhi*), Mediterranean spotted fever (*R. conorii*), African tick-bite fever (*R. africae*) or scrub typhus (*O. tsutsugamushi*).[21–23]

There are no vaccines currently available against any tropical rickettsioses. Prevention is mainly focused on avoiding an arthropod bite. Currently, the best method to prevent tick, louse, flea and chigger bites is to apply DEET (N,N-diethyl-m-toluamide) insect repellent to exposed skin and treat clothing with permethrin, which kills arthropods on contact. Bites may also be limited by covering exposed body parts (i.e. wearing long trousers tucked into boots). People staying in infested or endemic areas should be advised to check their bodies routinely for the presence of arthropods. If any mites, ticks, fleas and/or lice are found, seeking professional advice for arthropod removal and initiation of adequate baseline/follow-up diagnostics should be prioritized (Figure 22.1, Table 22.1).

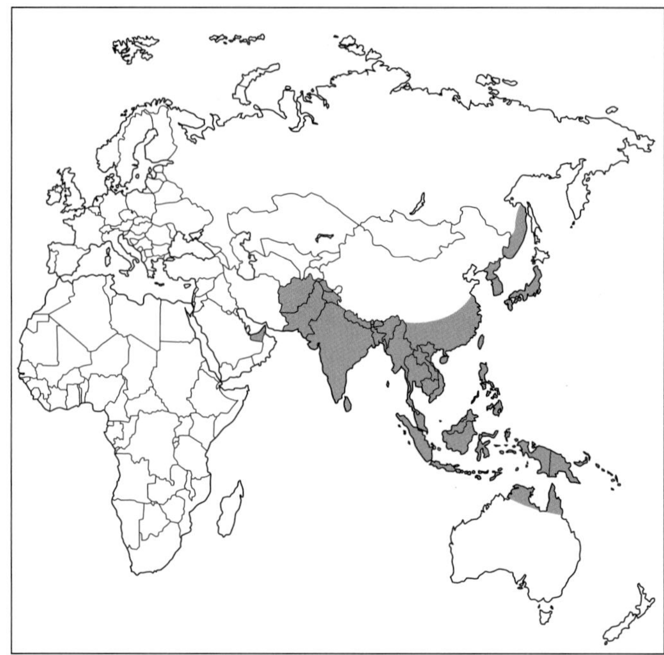

Figure 22.1 Map of the scrub typhus endemic geographical regions. Reports of scrub typhus-like cases from Africa (Cameroon) and South America (Chile) suggest that the disease could be distributed around the tropical/subtropical belt rather than confined to Asia. The primary vectors for the described regions are given in Table 22.1.

HISTORY

The major milestones in our understanding of typhus and typhus-like diseases, their causative agents and their transmission modes are summarized in Table 22.2.

The term 'typhus' initially referred to a wide spectrum of undefined infections causing a particular clinical syndrome, but over the last two centuries, its usage has become more restricted as our knowledge of the causes of these illnesses has expanded, and it now refers only to those caused by *Rickettsia.*

Ancient Accounts

Hippocrates in 460 BC used the term *typhus*, meaning 'smoke', to describe the 'confused state of the intellect – a tendency to stupor' associated with high fevers.[24] His first book *L'epidemion*, contains descriptions of typhus as a febrile, exanthematic illness associated with nervous symptoms.[25] In an account of the plague of Athens in 430–425 BC his contemporary colleague Thucydides describes what could be 'classical' epidemic typhus, although recently measles and smallpox have also been considered possible causes.[26,27]

The earliest concise accounts consistent with epidemic typhus underline its later association with times of crises, wars and famine in the fifteenth century. In 1492, during the civil wars in Granada (Andalusia, Spain), six times more people were killed from this 'febrile eruption' termed *Tabardillo* (Spanish 'red cloak') than in battle. Reports from missionaries in Mexico in the sixteenth century speak of millions of native Indians in the highlands dying of Tabardillo.[28] Typhus was particularly associated with siege-warfare where high population density and poor hygiene led to epidemics in the besieged population, e.g. during the French Imperial Army's siege of Naples in 1494.[25,29]

In 1546, Girolamo Fracastoro – Fracastorius (1478–1553)- differentiated 'plague' from 'typhus' for the first time in *De contagione et contagiosis morbis* ('On Contagion and Contagious Diseases').[30] During outbreaks in armies, ships and prisons measures such as the burning of clothes, changing of bedding and the introduction of crude quarantine measures

TABLE 22.1 Worldwide Distribution of Tropical Rickettsioses

Location by Continent	Vectors	Disease	Agent	Specific Areas	Risk of Exposure
AFRICA	**TICKS**				
	Rhipicephalus sanguineus	Mediterranean spotted fever	*Rickettsia conorii*	Mediterranean area (Algeria, Tunisia, Morocco, Libya, Egypt, Israel, Turkey) Kenya, Somalia, Central African Republic, Zimbabwe and South Africa	Urban (2/3) and rural (1/3)
	Amblyomma sp.	African tick-bite fever	*R. africae*	Sub-Saharan Africa	Rural area. Safaris
	Hyalomma marginatum	Unnamed	*R. aeschlimmanii*	Morocco, Zimbabwe, South Africa	
	Dermacentor marginatus[a]	Tick-borne lymphadenopathy (TIBOLA)	*R. slovaca*	Morocco[a]	
	Dermacentor marginatus[a]	Unnamed	*R. raoultii*	Morocco[a]	
	Rhipicephalus sanguineus[a]	Unnamed	*R. massiliae*	Morocco[a]	
	R. muhusamae[a]			Mali[a], Central African Republic[a]	
	H. truncatum[a]	Unnamed	*R. sibirica mongolotimonae*	South Africa, Algeria, Nigeria[a]	
	Ixodes ricinus[a]	Unnamed	'*R. monacensis*'	Morocco[a], Tunisia[a]	
	FLEAS				
	Xenopsylla cheopis (rat flea)	Murine typhus	*R. typhi*	Ubiquitous. High prevalence	Contact with rats and rat fleas
	Ctenocephalides felis, C. canis, X. cheopis, Pulex irritans (human flea)[a]	Flea-borne spotted fever	*R. felis*	Tunisia, Algeria, Egypt, Senegal, Kenya	
	LICE				
	Pediculus humanus corporis	Epidemic typhus	*R. prowazekii*	Ethiopia, Burundi, Rwanda, Uganda, Algeria	Civil war, refugee camps, lack of hygiene in cold or mountainous areas
AMERICAS	**TICKS**				
	Dermacentor andersoni (wood tick), D. variabilis (American dog tick), Amblyomma americanum (lone-star tick), A. maculatum, A. cajennense and Haemaphysalis leporispalustris (rabbit tick)	Rocky Mountain spotted fever	*R. rickettsii*	Central America (Mexico, Panama, Costa Rica), South America (Brazil, Colombia)	Rural areas *Note: rabbit ticks do not bite humans but maintain infection in rabbits, as a reservoir for transmission to human-biting ticks*
	Amblyomma triste	Unnamed	*R. parkeri*	Brazil, Argentina, Uruguay, Peru, Chile	
	Amblyomma spp.	African tick-bite fever	*R. africae*	West Indies	Rural areas
	Amblyomma spp.	Unnamed	*R. parkeri*	Brazil	
	FLEAS				
	Xenopsylla cheopis (rat flea)	Murine typhus	*R. typhi*	Ubiquitous	Contact with rats and rat fleas
	Ctenocephalides felis (cat flea)[a], *C. canis, et al.*	Flea-borne spotted fever	*R. felis*	Mexico, Brazil, Peru	
	LICE				
	Pediculus humanus corporis	Epidemic typhus	*R. prowazekii*	Peru and Andes	Lack of hygiene in mountainous areas
ASIA	**TICKS**				
	Rhipicephalus sanguineus	Indian tick typhus	*R. conorii indica*	India. Suspected in Thailand, Korea, Laos and Sri Lanka	
	Ixodes granulatus	Flinders Island spotted fever	*R. honei* (TT118)	Thailand, Australia	

Continued on following page

TABLE 22.1 **Worldwide Distribution of Tropical Rickettsioses—cont'd**

Location by Continent	Vectors	Disease	Agent	Specific Areas	Risk of Exposure
	Ixodes ovatus	Oriental or Japanese spotted fever	*R. japonica*	Japan[b]	Agricultural activities, bamboo cutting
	Dermacentor taiwanensis *Haemaphysalis longicornis* *Haemaphysalis flava*				
	Ixodes ovatus,[a]	Unnamed	*R. helvetica*	Japan[b] Suspected in Thailand, Laos	
	I. persulcatus,[a] *I. monospinus*[a]				
	Hyalomma asiaticum[a]	Lymphangitis-associated rickettsiosis	*R. sibirica mongolotimonae*	China (Inner Mongolia)[a,b]	
	Dermacentor nuttalli, D. marginatus	North-Asian tick typhus	*R. sibirica sibirica*	Northern China, former USSR (Asian republics, Siberia), Armenia, Pakistan	
	Haemaphysalis concinna				
	Dermacentor silvarum	Far-Eastern tick-borne	*R. heilongjiangii*	North-eastern China	
	Unknown	*Unnamed*	*'R. kellyi'*	India	
			R. monacensis	Republic of Korea	
	FLEAS				
	Xenopsylla cheopis (rat flea)	Murine typhus	*R. typhi*	Ubiquitous	
	Ctenocephalides felis (cat flea)[a]	Flea-borne spotted fever	*R. felis*	Thailand, Laos, China, Cambodia, Indonesia, Rep. of Korea	
	TROMBICULID ACARINS				
	Leptotrombidium spp.	Scrub typhus	*Orientia tsutsugamushi*	Asia-Pacific region from Korea to Papua New Guinea and Queensland, Australia, and from Japan to India and Pakistan	Rural activities Agricultural activities Soldiers in the field
			Orientia sp. nov. *chuto*	United Arabic Emirates	
	LICE				
	Pediculus humanus corporis	Epidemic typhus	*R. prowazekii*	China. India (Kashmir)	Civil war, refugee camps, lack of hygiene in cold or mountainous areas
	HOUSE MOUSE MITE				
	Liponyssoides sanguineus	Rickettsialpox	*R. akari*	Korea[c]	
AUSTRALIA	**TICKS**				
	Unknown	Flinders Island spotted fever	*R. honei*	Flinders Island, north-eastern Australia	
	Ixodes holocyclus	Queensland tick typhus	*R. australis*	North-eastern Australia	
	FLEAS				
	Xenopsylla cheopis (rat flea)	Murine typhus	*R. typhi*	Ubiquitous	Contact with rats and rat fleas
	C. felis, C. canis, X. cheopis, et al	Flea-borne spotted fever	*R. felis*	Ubiquitous	
	TROMBICULID ACARINS				
	Leptotrombidium spp.	Scrub typhus	*Orientia tsutsugamushi*	Northern Territory and Western Australia, Queensland, Australia	Rural activities Agricultural activities Soldiers in the field

[a]Suspected by detection of the pathogen in the relevant arthropod.
[b]Although not included in tropical areas, Japan and China are included as relevant to tropical travel medicine.
[c]Isolated from voles (*Microtus fortis pelliceus*).

TABLE 22.2 Historical Chronology of Milestones – the Gradual Dissection of the 'Typhus' Entity

Year	Important Findings	Comments	References
460 BC	Hippocrates defines typhus – as 'fever with a confused state of the intellect – a tendency to stupor'.		24
430 BC	Thucydides and Hippocrates first describe epidemic typhus cases.		26
313 BC	First clinical accounts of '*Tsutsugamushi disease*' in the '*Zhouhofang*', a Chinese clinical manual.	Description of regional vector mites, no linkage to transmission	151
15th century	Epidemic typhus and murine (endemic) typhus (*Tabardillo*) rages in Europe.	No distinction made between different forms of typhus	28
1485–1551	The five epidemics known as the 'English Sweat' occur in UK.	Probably relapsing fever (*Borrelia recurrentis*)	222,223
1546	Girolamo Fracastoro – Fracastorius (1478–1553) differentiates 'typhus' from 'plague' in '*De contagione et contagiosis morbis*'.	'Contagiousness' – epidemiological observations on transmission of germs	30
Early 1700s	Typhus = Typhoid and Typhus and 'Relapsing Fever'	Era of differential diagnostic confusion!	224–227
1734	John Huxham makes the first clinical distinction between epidemic typhus and typhoid fever in the UK.	Typhus = 'slow nervous' fever Typhoid = 'putrid malignant' fever	224
1760	Boisier de Sauvages in Montpellier creates the clinical term '*Typhus exanthematique*' for epidemic typhus.	Based on clinical appearance of the characteristic skin rash	228
1762	James Lind (1716–1794) promotes hygienic measures during typhus outbreaks to reduce mortality.	Limes for prevention of scurvy (scorbut), burning of clothes after outbreaks	32,31
1810	Hakuju Hashimoto first describes a *tsutsuga* (disease, harm, noxious) resembling typhus, in the Niigata prefecture	The basis of the name '*Tsutsugamushi* disease'	54,229
1812–1813	Napoleon suffers the greatest loss of troops to epidemic typhus (and Trench Fever).		33,34
1837	William W. Gerhard (1809–1872) first distinguishes enteric fevers (i.e. typhoid) from rickettsial fevers (i.e. typhus).	Post-mortem hyperplastic nodules in Peyer's patches	255
1843	Craigie and Hendersen differentiate 'relapsing fevers' clinically and pathologically from (epidemic) typhus	Post-mortem observations in autopsies	226,231
1858	Charles Murchison epidemiologically emphasizes the contagious nature of typhus – association of 'epidemics' with poor hygienic standards		232
1878	First account of *Tsutsugamushi* disease from Japan to be published in Europe by Theobald Palm.	Reported as 'Shima-mushi', or 'Island insect disease'	53
1898	Brill's Disease – an outbreak of atypical typhus, what Brill called 'abortive-typhoid in New York and Zinsser ...		233,234
1906	Howard T. Ricketts and Russel M. Wilder discover the causative agent and transmission vector (wood tick) of Rocky Mountain spotted fever (RMSF)		36
1908	Schüffner describes 'Pseudo-typhoid' in Sumatra (which later was revealed to be *Tsutsugamushi* disease)	Suspected mite transmission	235
1909	Charles J.H. Nicolle discovers the transmission of epidemic typhus by the human body louse.	Nobel Prize received by C.J.H Nicolle in 1928	35,236
1910	Howard T. Ricketts first discovers Rickettsiae in the blood of epidemic typhus patients in Mexico ('*Tabardillo*'), together with Russel M. Wilder.	Ricketts dies of epidemic typhus in Mexico	39
1916	Rocha Lima first describes Rickettsiae as intracellular microorganisms	*R. prowazekii* – named after Ricketts and Prowazek (epidemic typhus)	37
1910	Smithson describes a 'sporadic' form of typhus, in Australia.	Later revealed as scrub typhus or *Tsutsugamushi* disease	237
1910	Conor and Bruch describe 'Fievre Boutonneuse' in Tunis.	Later revealed as Mediterranean spotted fever (MSF)	42
1911	McNaught describes 'Para-typhoid' in South Africa, with suspected tick transmission.	Later revealed to be two forms; MSF and African tick typhus	45,47
1913	McKenchie describes a typhus-like illness in the Kumaon Region, N-India (Himalayan foothills)	unpublished, reviewed by Megaw 1921 – 'Megaw's tick bite' in 1916	62
1916	Weil and Felix first describe the diagnostic serum agglutination for typhus, based on the *Proteus vulgaris* strain called '*Proteus* OX19'	Diagnostic breakthrough	59
1922	Hone describes a new form of typhus in Australia (OX19 positive)	Later revealed as *R. honei*, a spotted fever group Rickettsia	238
1923	Maxcy and Havens describe murine typhus as an endemic form of sporadic typhus	Hypothesis that fleas are vectors	61
1924	Fletcher distinguishes scrub from murine typhus	Based on the Weil-Felix test using *Proteus* OX19 and OXK	57
1924	Kingsbury visits Malaysia and introduces a new strain of *Proteus mirabilis* 'OXK' for Weil-Felix serological test to diagnose rickettsial diseases	OXK allows separation of 'urban/shop' and 'rural' typhus	58
1926	Fletcher and Lesslar describe co-existence of *Tsutsugamushi* disease and scrub typhus in Malaya		239,240

Continued on following page

TABLE 22.2 Historical Chronology of Milestones – the Gradual Dissection of the 'Typhus' Entity—cont'd

Year	Important Findings	Comments	References
1926	Fletcher and Lesslar create the term 'tropical typhus'	Defined as non-contagious or 'sporadic' typhus-like fevers	57
1928	Scrub typhus is *Tsutsugamushi* disease	Based on entomological, cross-immunity and clinical criteria	52,58,239,241
1930	Nagayo demonstrates *Rickettsia tsutsugamushi* for the first time inside cells	Localization in the Descemet's membrane of rabbit eyes	56
1931	Dyer proves Maxcy right – *R. typhi* of murine typhus is transmitted by rat fleas	Dyer isolates *R. typhi* from rat fleas (*X. cheopis*)	50
1945	'Operation Tyburn' – first mass-production of scrub typhus vaccine	Based on Burmese strains, did not work in Malaya	242
1947	Discovery of Chloromycetin (chloramphenicol), a derivative from *Actinomyces* bacteria	Cured chick embryos infected with Rickettsia	69
1948	Smadel demonstrates chloramphenicol as effective chemotherapy for scrub typhus	Volunteer studies with naturally infected chigger inoculation	71,243
1959–1975	Vietnam Conflict – scrub typhus is one of the major causes of fevers of unknown origin (FUO) especially among soldiers working in the 'bush'		74
1997	Epidemic typhus re-emerges dramatically in Burundi	Epidemic affects approx. 100 000 refugees of Rwanda	18,19
2000s	Reemergence of scrub in Maldives, Palau, etc.	Possibly de novo emergence	244–246
2010–2011	Endemic region for scrub typhus increases to include UAE and Chile		14

were found to be very effective in reducing mortality, promoting the understanding of the 'epidemic' and 'contagious' notion of this disease.[31,32]

In 1812, Napoleon's Grande Armée of 422 000 men was reduced over 42-fold to 10 000 during his invasion of Russia and subsequent retreat, with the vast majority dying from typhus rather than combat.[33] In 2006, *R. prowazekii* and *Bartonella quintana* DNA was demonstrated by PCR methods in clothes and dental pulp of corpses excavated in mass graves near Vilnius, Lithuania.[34]

The 'Dissection' of Typhus and Creation of Rickettsiology

In the nineteenth century, the ill-defined entity of 'typhus' was dissected into a triad of typhus, typhoid and relapsing fevers – based on refinement of clinical syndromes into 'exanthematic fevers', 'abdominal or enteric fevers' and 'recurrent fevers', as well as new postmortem pathological findings.

A major breakthrough came in 1909 when Charles Nicolle demonstrated that the body louse *Pediculus humanis corporis* was the vector of epidemic typhus[35] – for which he received the Nobel Prize in 1928. Howard Taylor Ricketts in 1910 first described rickettsial organisms in the blood of typhus patients in Mexico, and in infected lice and their faeces.[36] The Brazilian Henrique da Rocha Lima officially described the organism and proposed the name *Rickettsia prowazekii* to honor Howard Taylor Ricketts and Stanislaus von Prowazek, who had both recently died from typhus acquired during their research efforts.[37]

Epidemic Typhus. Also known as louse-borne typhus, this form caused large epidemics in the First World War in Serbia, Poland, Eastern Germany and Mesopotamia, and in the Second World War in the Balkans, Naples, Russia and Germany, and especially in the concentration camps at Belsen, Auschwitz and Buchenwald.

Rocky Mountain Spotted Fever (RMSF). The first reports of typhus in North America date from before the arrival of Europeans. According to historical accounts of Indian tribes in Montana, certain forest areas were avoided in spring because 'people got ill there'. Later accounts of pioneers in the 1890s describe a febrile disease associated with certain wilderness trails known as 'trail fever'.[38]

Between 1906 and 1909, Ricketts discovered RMSF by demonstrating the infectious organism in patient blood, describing its transmission to guinea pigs and rhesus monkeys, and by characterizing the induced immune response.[39] He discovered that the wood tick *D. andersoni* was the vector, making RMSF the first bacterial disease proven to be transmitted by an arthropod.[36] Ricketts, followed-up by demonstrating the wood tick was capable of transmitting the 'agent' vertically from one generation of ticks to the next.[40] In 1908, McCalla performed the only recorded human transmission experiments in RMSF, by transmission to healthy volunteers through feeding of a tick taken from a patient with RMSF.[41]

Mediterranean Spotted Fever (MSF). In 1910, Conor and Bruch described a new form of spotted fever in Tunis, North Africa:[42] It was first named 'macular fever' or 'boutonneuse fever', due to its papular rather than macular rash, and it was associated with an inoculation eschar.[43,44] It is caused by *Rickettsia conorii*, which is transmitted to humans by the bite of the dog tick, *Rhipicephalus sanguineus*. This disease, later to be called Mediterranean spotted fever (MSF), was soon reported from around the whole Mediterranean basin, and also from India, the Black Sea, the Middle East and South Africa.

African Tick-bite Fever. In 1911, McNaught reported an anomalous form of 'paratyphoid' occurring in South Africa, consisting of fever and a profuse rash in patients reporting having been bitten by ticks prior to the onset of symptoms.[45,46] By the1930s, it was thought that two spotted fever group (SFG) rickettsioses occurred in South Africa. One was 'boutonneuse fever' caused by *Rickettsia conorii* and transmitted by ticks from dogs in urban areas, and the other was tick-bite fever, a milder disease caused by a different SFG *Rickettsia* and transmitted by ticks (*Amblyomma hebraeum*) of cattle and game in rural areas.[47] The causative agent was initially named *R. conorii* var. *pijperi* and was not to be named *R. africae* until 1992.[48]

Murine Typhus. Flea-borne (murine) typhus (*Rickettsia typhi*) had been described in Mexico in 1570 by Bravo, and the complicating myocarditis was to kill Ricketts there in 1910. It was recognized as a separate disease from louse-borne epidemic typhus by several groups, and was termed 'endemic typhus'. However, the final bacteriological separation from *R. prowazekii* did not occur until Maxcy proposed rodents and their fleas as the potential reservoirs and vectors in 1928; a hypothesis confirmed in 1931 by Dyer who isolated *Rickettsia* from rat fleas (*Xenopsylla cheopis*) in Baltimore.[49,50] The agent of murine typhus was initially termed *R. mooseri*, but renamed *R. typhi* in 1945.[51]

Scrub Typhus. Scrub typhus, or Japanese river fever, was known in Japanese folklore to be associated with the jungle mite or chigger, termed 'tsutsugamushi' in Japanese (*tsutsuga* = disease, harm, noxious and *mushi* = bug). The term 'Tsutsugamushi disease' has been in use since 1810 to describe these fevers, but is not the only term used by the Japanese. Theobald Palm brought the first account of this disease to Europe in 1878, referring to 'Shima-mushi' ('Island-insect') disease (Figure 22.2).[52–54]

A detailed report by Kawamura highlighted the severity of this disease, with the mortality in the Niigata prefecture (1903–1920) reaching 41.4% in 1917.[55] Although advances in understanding the ecology, vector, clinical disease and epidemiology of *Tsutsugamushi* disease had been made before the beginning of the First World War, the first scientific evidence of the causative agent came in 1930, when Nagayo and colleagues demonstrated the pathogenic rickettsiae in experimentally infected rabbits.[56]

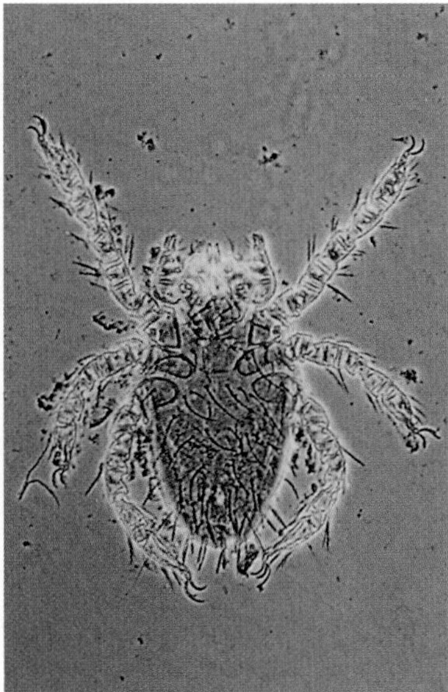

Figure 22.2 Larval mites transmit the *O. tsutsugamushi* from rodent to humans when they come into accidental association with mite-infected terrain. The mites act as reservoirs since transovarial transmission of the *Rickettsia* occurs. (x 80) *(Reproduced from Peters W and Pasvol G (eds). Tropical Medicine and Parasitology, 5th edition, Mosby, London 2002, image 39.)*

The Emergence of 'Tropical Typhus'

In the 1900s the term 'tropical typhus' was used for non-contagious fevers in the Asian British colonies, especially India and the Malay states, where expatriate military personnel encountered a vast array of 'tropical fevers'.[57,58]

In 1916, Weil and Felix introduced a new diagnostic test for typhus, based on the positive agglutination of *Proteus vulgaris* (OX19) serum from patients with all forms of typhus except scrub typhus.[59] In 1924, Dr AN Kingsbury unknowingly introduced a *Proteus mirabilis* strain (instead of OX19) to Malaya, and suddenly strong agglutinations were seen for scrub typhus sera and weak reactivities for other typhus forms. The ability of this antigen, termed OXK (K = Kingsbury), to identify two contrasting typhus forms – agglutination of the conventional *Proteus* OX19 but not OXK and vice versa – led to the differentiation of 'scrub' from 'murine typhus'. Thus, the OXK strain, albeit originating in England, not only became the cornerstone of 'scrub typhus' diagnostics – but also led to the discovery of flea-borne murine typhus in Malaya.[57,60]

The South-east Asian form of scrub typhus resembled Tsutsugamushi disease from Japan so closely in many ways – clinically, ecologically and entomologically – that these two diseases, originally thought to be allopatric, were described as co-existing within the same endemic area in the Malay States.[49,61] Cross-immunization and inoculation tests with agents from Sumatra, Australia and Japan finally proved the two diseases to be the same, with identical immunological reactivities and Tsutsugamushi disease and scrub typhus were unified into a single entity.[50]

These important discoveries required refinement of the hitherto ill-defined term 'tropical typhus' and led Sir John Megaw (UK medical adviser to the India Office) to propose a new classification: 'The Typhus Group of Fevers', which distinguished between 'epidemic' and 'non-epidemic' forms and contained the vector-associated subgroups 'tick-typhus', 'mite-typhus' and 'flea-typhus' to which an 'unknown-vector' subgroup was added later (Figure 22.3).[62,63]

'Typhus Fevers' and the Second World War

Scrub Typhus. The major infectious disease that dominated the Second World War in Asia was scrub typhus. Its impact on immunologically naive Allied troops between 1942 and 1945 resulted in 18 000 cases and 639 deaths (4.0%), as well as an estimated 20 000 cases in Japanese troops.[64,65] The Second World War had a major impact on scrub typhus research, which led to improvements in diagnostics, prevention, epidemiology, clinical management and entomological understanding of transmission and greatly intensified the search for effective vaccines and for therapeutic drugs.

The successful immunization of the cotton rat (*Sigmodon hispidus*) against *R. prowazekii*, with the induction of neutralizing complement-fixing antibodies, triggered a major initiative to develop a scrub typhus vaccine. This classified project, named 'Operation Tyburn', produced over 300 000 doses of vaccine designed for use in the Burmese theatre in the Second World War by the 'Scrub Typhus Research Laboratory' at Imphal, India.[66] As field trials were complicated by troop movements in Burma, the vaccine (based on Burmese strains of

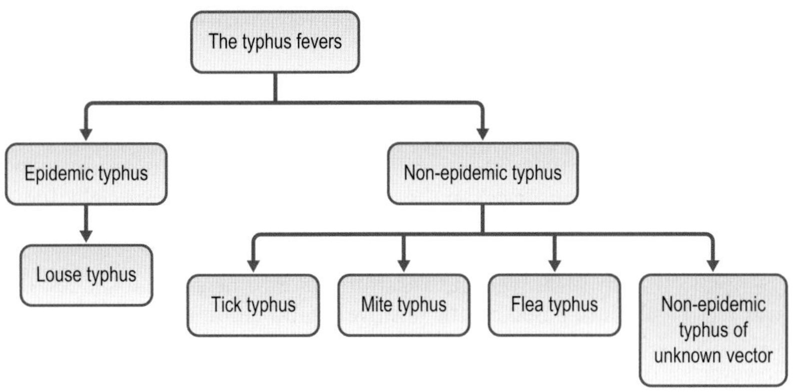

Figure 22.3 Diagram of the first attempt to classify Typhus fevers, based on their vectors. *(Table taken from Megaw J. Typhus Fevers in the Tropics. BMJ 1934;2:244–6.)*

O. tsutsugamushi) was evaluated in troops based in Malaya, where it provided insufficient protection against scrub typhus. In view of the concomitantly discovered heterogeneity of strain-dependent antigens, and the lack of cross-immunity among them, it was concluded in the late 1960s that effective protection against scrub typhus could probably not be achieved via vaccination.[65]

Murine Typhus. During the Second World War, murine typhus occurred as sporadic cases in troops. Of the 787 murine typhus cases reported in US troops, 497 were from within the USA, mostly in the southeast, and 34 were in the China-Burma-India (CBI) theatre of operations.[67] Fifteen deaths were recorded in the US army, of which 14 fatal cases were contracted overseas (fatality rate of 19 per 1000). The Second World War recorded 104 epidemic typhus cases (no deaths) in American troops, and the incidence of flea-borne typhus actually exceeded that of louse-borne typhus in the US Army.[64,68]

In the post-war era, a critical breakthrough came with the discovery of chloramphenicol (Chloromycetin) in 1947 by Ehrlich and colleagues.[69] Chloramphenicol, derived from an *Actinomyces* species (*Streptomyces venezuelae*), was found to be effective in killing *R. prowazekii* in chick embryos and in the treatment of 'flea-typhus' in America. In 1948, Joseph Smadel performed the famous clinical studies in human volunteers with scrub typhus infected by mites from different hyperendemic areas in Malaya, Burma and New Guinea, where he demonstrated within days that chloramphenicol was a highly effective treatment for patients with rickettsial diseases.[70–72]

The Vietnam Conflict

In December 1972, the Armed Forces Epidemiology Board reported that when malaria and other identifiable diseases were excluded, 20–30% of the remaining FUOs in the Vietnam conflict were attributable to scrub typhus and approximately 10–15% to murine typhus.[68] Unlike the high fatality rates of troops during the Second World War, scrub typhus caused no known American deaths during the Vietnam conflict.[73] But serological data from reports of the 9th Medical Laboratory from 1969 showed that scrub typhus was the primary cause of FUOs (18%), followed by amoebiasis (17%) and murine typhus (15%). Thus scrub typhus and murine typhus were responsible for approximately one-third of FUOs.[74] Generally, most scrub typhus cases occurred among artillery and infantry personnel based in the field, and most murine cases were reported from support troops in urban areas.[75] The report also suggests that due to clinical and diagnostic limitations the frequency of scrub typhus among US and indigenous forces in Vietnam was under-reported and its significance seriously underestimated.[76]

PATHOGENESIS AND IMMUNITY

Rickettsiae replicate in the salivary glands of ticks and mites, from which they are then inoculated into the epidermis or dermis of the skin during vector feeding. The early innate immune responses and dissemination pathways remain incompletely understood. Presumably rickettsial dissemination occurs via direct haematogenous and lymphatic spread, involving recirculating infected tissue monocytes or dendritic cells from the inoculation site. The hallmark of the disease is a vasculitis-like systemic disease, as the pathogens invade and proliferate within vascular endothelial cells (ECs) lining small and medium-sized blood vessels, the major target cells of rickettsial infection. The mechanisms of host defence are not completely understood, although cell-mediated immunity plays a crucial role in controlling infection.[77–79]

Rickettsia *spp.*

SFG and TG rickettsiae grow mainly in endothelial cells and to a lesser extent in macrophages.[80] SFG organisms spread rapidly from cell to cell and usually accumulate intracellularly in significantly lower numbers than typhus group rickettsiae. They achieve intracellular mobility by polymerizing actin at a unipolar tail to propel them forward through the cytosol of cells, from cell to cell, and avoid phagolysosomal fusion upon cellular entry to divide by binary fission as naked bacteria in the cytosol (Figure 22.4).[81,82]

Cellular injury in endothelial cells occurs through lipid peroxidation via production of reactive oxygen species in response to rickettsial infection which as a consequence affects vascular permeability resulting in fluid imbalance and oedema of vital organs.[83,84]

Typhus group rickettsiae lack directional actin polymerization and tend to accumulate within the cytoplasm until cell lysis. *R. prowazekii* does not stimulate actin-based mobility and *R. typhi* exhibits only erratic mobility. Typical coagulation changes at the perturbed endothelial interface in SFG and TG infections demonstrate an 'endothelial' profile with expression of thrombomodulin, and release of von Willebrand factor, expression of tissue factor, secretion of plasminogen activator inhibitor and production of platelet-activating factor. However, disseminated intravascular coagulation occurs rarely even in lethal cases and is not a common feature of rickettsioses.[85,86]

Based on mouse studies, *Rickettsia* spp. are recognized by dendritic cells through TLR4 receptors, which then induce a

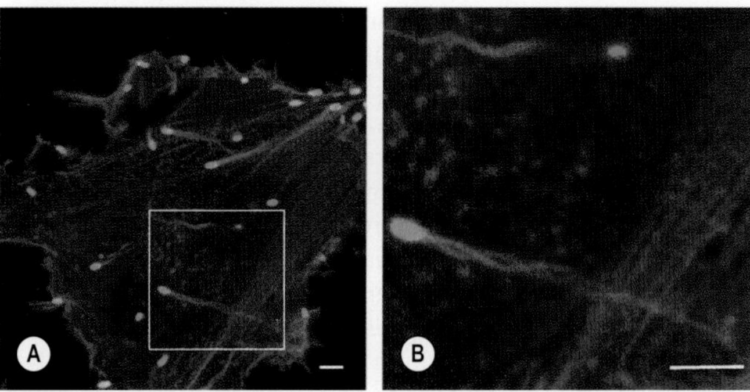

Figure 22.4 Rickettsiae use directional actin polymerization to propel themselves through cytoplasm of host cells. *R. rickettsii* showing long actin tails that are frequently comprised of multiple, twisting, distinct F-actin bundles. F-actin is stained red and intracellular bacteria are stained green in this laser scanning confocal microscopy image. *(Taken from Van Kirk LS, Hayes SF, Heinzen RA. Ultrastructure of Rickettsia rickettsii actin tails and localization of cytoskeletal proteins. Infect Immun 2000;68:4706–13.)*

vigorous proinflammatory response, activate NK cells and lead to generation of a subsequent antigen-specific immunity.[87,88] Immunity to *rickettsiae* spp. is mediated by T-lymphocytes, both CD4 and CD8 T-cells secrete proinflammatory cytokines, which activate endothelial cells, macrophages and hepatocytes to produce reactive oxygen species and kill rickettsiae.[89,90] CD8 lymphocytes destroy infected host cells via their perforin-dependent mechanism, which is controlled by MHC class-I-dependent cytotoxic T lymphocyte activity.[78,79,91] Studies in guinea pigs and BALB/C mice on adoptive transfer of immune spleen cells, cytotoxicity and natural killer cells have demonstrated the importance of cell-mediated immunity (CMI) in protection from murine typhus and that CMI can mediate heterologous protection.[92–98] Human post-mortem and mouse studies provide strong evidence for the endothelial cell as the target cell of *R. typhi*, and the critical importance of CMI for controlling typhus infections.[99,100]

Orientia *Spp.*

O. tsutsugamushi can infect a broad spectrum of cells in vitro, however in humans there is only limited evidence in vivo of infection of ECs, DCs, macrophages, polymorphonuclear leucocytes (PMNs) and lymphocytes.[101–103] The bacterium uses host fibronectin interactions with the 56-kDa type-specific antigen (TSA56) for attachment, then invades host cells via induced phagocytosis, enters a phagosome out of which a proportion of organisms escape into the cytoplasm. *O. tsutsugamushi* replicate via binary fission in the cytoplasm, as like TG rickettsiae they lack directional actin polymerization.[104] They tend to accumulate within the cytoplasm and form groups of budding *Orientia* on the cell surface after 2–3 days of incubation. The host cell membrane surrounds the protruding bacteria and the released bacteria covered by host cell membrane may either infect neighbouring cells directly by fusion of membranes, or the surrounding host cell membrane may be lost leaving naked *Orientia* to invade other cells (Figure 22.5).[105,106]

Recent investigations suggest that the pathophysiology of *Orientia* infection differs from that of endothelium-targeting SFG or TG rickettsiae. A study of soluble adhesion molecule levels in patients with scrub typhus showed that mononuclear cell activation was more prominent than endothelial activation when compared to endothelial-tropic murine typhus.[107] In a large cohort of scrub and murine typhus patients in vivo coagulation activation, with high plasma concentrations of TATc and sTF, was found to be prominent, and related to a strong pro-inflammatory response in scrub typhus, whereas in murine typhus changes in coagulant and fibrinolytic pathways were suggestive of endothelial cell perturbation.[86] These data suggest that although late-stage endothelial infection is common in both diseases, the in vivo pathogenic mechanisms of *R. typhi* and *O. tsutsugamushi* differ in the early phase of infection and may contribute to disease differentiation. Although vascular endothelial cells have been shown to be major target cells of *O. tsutsugamushi* infection, resulting in primary cytopathic destruction of the endothelium of blood vessels causing a vasculitis responsible for end organ damage in severe disease, these data are based on post-mortem examinations and animal studies and contrast with in vivo findings in early disease.[101,108,109] Histological studies in eschars have described perivascular collections of mononuclear cells, including lymphocytes, plasma cells, and macrophages in humans as well as in cynomolgus monkeys.[110,111] In skin biopsies of eschars in scrub typhus, *O. tsutsugamushi* was located within dermal dendritic cells (DDCs) and tissue monocytes.[103] Activated DDCs, such as dermal

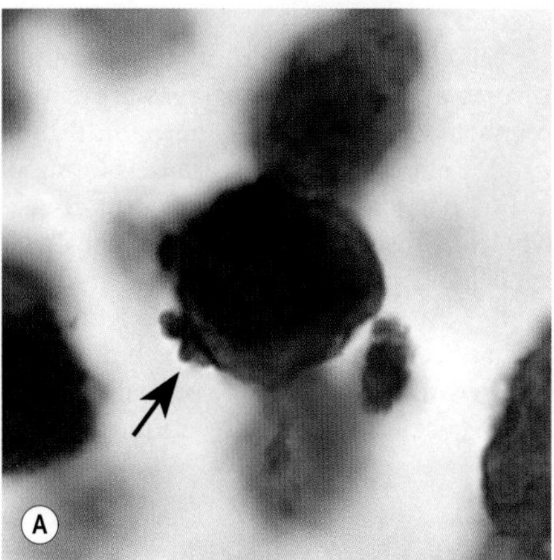

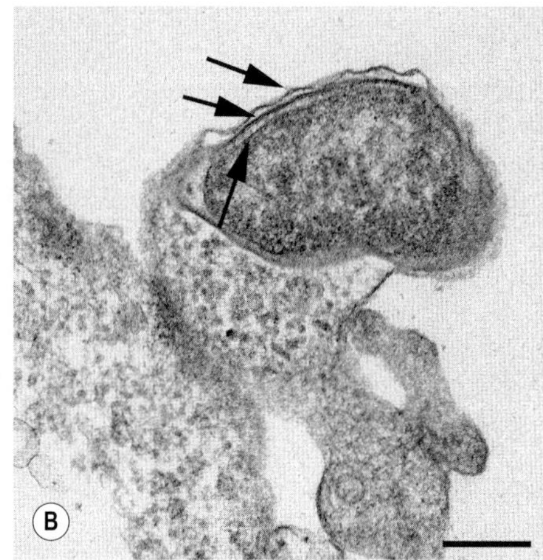

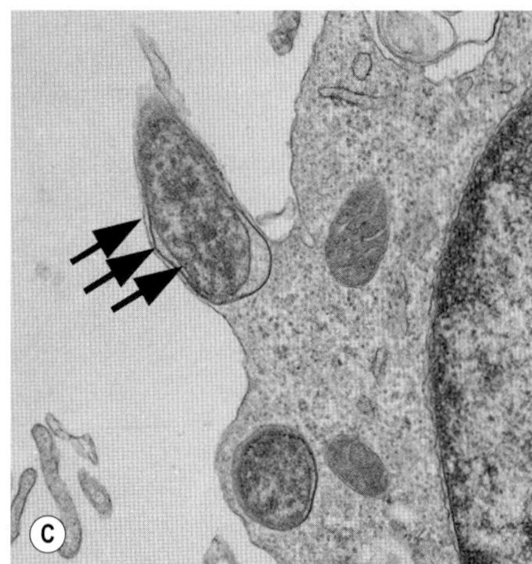

Figure 22.5 Budding of *O. tsutsugamushi* on the cellular surface (arrow), with three distinct membranes visible in the EM images (arrows): two outer membranes derived from *O. tsutsugamushi* and one from the host cell. (Magnification ×1000; panel A).

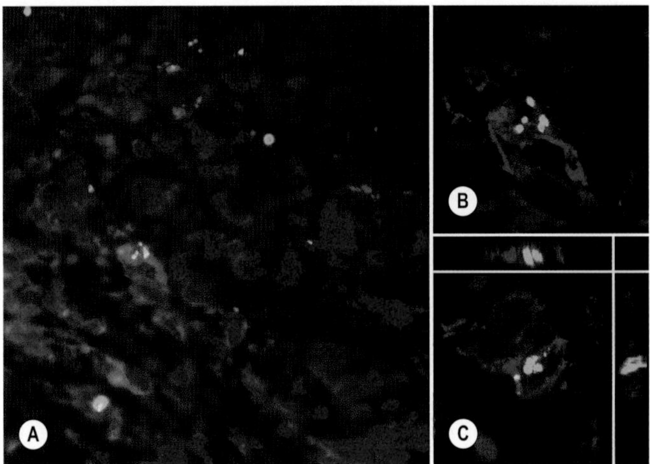

Figure 22.6 Multiple intracellular *O. tsutsugamushi* within antigen presenting cells (APCs) in the superficial dermis. APCs are characterized by MHC class II receptor (HLADR) positivity and are associated with intracellular *O. tsutsugamushi* in admission samples of an eschar from a patient with acute scrub typhus. APCs in red, *O. tsutsugamushi* in green. Panels B and C are laser scanning micrographs, with a 3D reconstruction of intracytosolic *O. tsutsugamushi* in panel C.

Langerhans cells, can recirculate from skin to lymph nodes and represent a potential route of intracellular spread away from the eschar site. Intracellular infection of APCs also has the potential to interfere with downstream host immune responses via immunomodulatory effects (Figure 22.6).

As TLRs are important for innate immunity to rickettsiae, NLR proteins are involved in innate immune mechanisms to *Orientia* infection. During *O. tsutsugamushi* infection, NOD1 senses an *Orientia* component in ECs and activates the downstream production of proinflammatory cytokines and NK activation[112] to develop adaptive immunity. A Type-1 cell-mediated immunity and IFN-γ production of T cells in response to *O. tsutsugamushi* antigen is essential for immune protection against infection, and the cell-mediated immunity (CMI) is central in heterologous protection across different strains in inbred mice.[98,113–115] In mouse models, resistance to infection can be transferred via T cells for spotted fever group,[116] scrub typhus group,[117] and typhus group *Rickettsia*.[95] Although CMI was shown to be essential for immune protection against *O. tsutsugamushi* in mice, heterologous protection was transient.[113,118] Similarly, immunological studies in human volunteers revealed that homologous immunity to a single strain lasted up to a year, but heterologous protection (to other than the inoculated strain) waned within 2 months.[119]

The immunopathophysiological knowledge gaps in these diseases are substantial and achieving a better understanding of major immunogenic antigens, the temporal immune response dynamics in vivo, and the mechanisms limiting the duration of heterologous protection are prerequisites for the development of an effective vaccine for rickettsial diseases.

Coxiella burnetii

Compared with other obligate intracellular bacterial pathogens, such as *Chlamydia* and *Rickettsia* spp., *C. burnetii* is metabolically complex with far less genome reduction. Thus, relative to these bacteria, the adaptation of *C. burnetii* to an obligate intracellular lifestyle appears to be a relatively recent evolutionary event.[120]

In *C. burnetii* pathogenesis, one must take into account phase variants of the agent. Following internalization by the host target cells (monocytes/macrophages),[121] *C. burnetii* replicates in the resulting phagosome, a large parasitophorous vacuole (PV), that acquires lysosomal characteristics with acidic pH, hydrolases and cationic peptides.[122] This is where the pathogen differentiates in a biphasic developmental cycle resulting in two alternate forms; a non-replicating, small cell variant (SCV) form, and the dominant replicating, large cell variant (LCV) form.[123] SCV to LCV morphogenesis occurs during a lag phase (approx. 2 days), after which an exponential replication of LCV occurs (approx. 4 days), when LCV differentiate back to SCV. The SCV, with its highly condensed chromatin, is considered the environmentally stable form of *C. burnetii*,[120] while its intracellular large cell variant has adapted to survival in the harsh conditions of phagolysosomes, which enables the long-term survival and persistence of *C. burnetii* in monocytes/macrophages.

The virulent forms of *C. burnetii* attach to monocytes via the αv β3 integrins alone, whereas the avirulent forms require αv β3 integrins and the complement C3 receptor as well.[124] Host factors, such as immunosuppression, underlying disease,[125] and the level of cell-mediated immunity,[126] play critical roles in the outcome of infection. *C. burnetii* has the ability to induce persistent infections both in humans and animals.[127] Chronic Q-fever is typically associated with patients who are immunocompromised and/or who have pre-existing heart valve defects, and most commonly presents as endocarditis.[121]

Host control of *C. burnetii* is mediated primarily by activated monocytes/macrophages via the production of reactive oxygen and nitrogen intermediates exerting potent antimicrobial activities.[128] The capability of *C. burnetii* to survive within these cells is associated with downregulation of macrophage responses and induction of suppressor factors. Defective phagosome maturation and impaired *C. burnetii* killing have been observed in patients with chronic Q-fever.[129]

In vitro studies with monocytes have shown that increases in interleukin-10 levels support *C. burnetii* replication in monocytes, and high IL-10 plasma levels in patients are associated with deficient killing of *C. burnetii* in monocytes and favour the development of chronic Q-fever.[130]

As an obligate intracellular pathogen residing in a lysosome-like compartment in phagocytes, *C. burnetii* presents a challenge to immunologists. Despite its intracellular niche, passive immunization with antiserum provides complete protection against *C. burnetii* infection.

In murine models, cell-mediated immunity is absolutely required for control of primary infection, as T cells are critical for IFNγ and TNFα-mediated clearance of *C. burnetii*. B- and NK-cell deficiencies do not affect clinical disease development or bacterial clearance but particularly the absence of B-cells increases the severity of histopathological changes.[131,132] However, the precise mechanisms of immunity to *C. burnetii* remain to be determined.[133] Although an efficacious whole cell vaccine against Q-fever has been developed, the mechanisms by which this vaccine provides protection are only partially understood and unfortunately its use is limited by reactions in sensitized individuals.

Ehrlichia *and* Anaplasma *spp.*

***Ehrlichia* Spp.** *E. chaffeensis* targets monocyte/macrophages and DCs, and replicates within cytoplasmic membrane-bound vacuoles to form microcolonies, called *morulae*, that contain one to over 400 organisms. Infection of the host cell involves dense-cored Ehrlichiae expressing certain 'tandem repeat proteins' (TRPs) on their surface, which have important roles in the binding and entry process (particularly TRP120). Ehrlichiae binding to the host cell occurs through membrane receptors, such as E- and L-selectin and other glycosylphosphatidylinositol-anchored proteins located in caveolae (tiny indentations in the cell surface membrane) that trigger receptor-mediated endocytosis.[134,135]

Ehrlichiae live in endosomes and can inhibit their maturation and fusion with lysosomes.[136] They can modulate host cell gene expression via DNA-binding and other effector proteins, which are secreted through the vacuole membrane into the host cell cytosol. A wide range of immuno-modulating effects include the inhibition of apoptosis of infected cells, manipulation of innate immune defence mechanisms, suppression of reactive oxygen species (ROS) production, suppression of specific cytokines which activate macrophages, and cellular signalling associated with cell-mediated immune responses.[135]

Murine models have revealed that CD4 and CD8 T type 1 lymphocyte responses, IFN-γ, TNF-α, and antibodies, play roles in protective immunity, while a weak CD4 T-helper response, overproduction of TNFα, and very high IL-10 are associated with toxic-shock-like mortality.[137]

The mechanisms by which *E. chaffeensis* causes tissue damage and disease manifestations remains unknown. Patients with *E. chaffeensis* infection present with a low bacterial burden in blood and tissues. An initial flu-like illness can progress rapidly to a severe multisystem disease with toxic-shock-like syndrome, meningitis, or ARDS.[137] While immunocompromised patients react with significant necrosis of liver, spleen and other reticulohistiocytic organs associated with high bacterial burden (*morulae*), this is not the case in immunocompetent patients, where the pathogen is often difficult to find and necrosis is rare.[138] Lesions include perivascular cuffs containing mononuclear-histiocytic infiltrates and granuloma formation (which is associated with successful control of infection), often with apoptotic lymphocytes in tissues and blood.[139] These findings of both discrepant bacterial load and tissue damage are suggestive that host immunopathogenic mechanisms play a role in the disease process.[140]

***Anaplasma* spp.** In the pathogenesis of anaplasmosis in cattle, the *A. marginale* major surface proteins (MSPs) play a crucial role in the host–pathogen interactions, and include adhesion proteins and MSPs from multigene families that undergo antigenic change and selection which contributes to maintenance of persistent infections.[141] Cattle that survive acute infection develop persistent infections characterized by cyclical low-level rickettsaemia.[142] Persistently infected or 'carrier' cattle have lifelong immunity and, upon challenge-exposure, do not develop clinical disease.

In humans, the pathogenesis of human granulocytic anaplasmosis (HGA) is not well understood and while early investigations associated increased disease severity with high pathogen loads, the current evidence points more towards immunopathogenic mechanisms to be responsible for disease manifestations.[143] The hallmark of infection reflecting a direct pathogen-mediated cytolytic injury, is leukopenia, particularly neutropenia as *A. phagocytophilum* infects almost exclusively neutrophils in vivo. However, many more neutrophils are affected than actually infected, suggestive that additional mechanisms are in play.[144] *A. phagocytophilum* also has multiple mechanisms to subvert neutrophil antimicrobial responses.[145] The clinical and histopathological features in patients with severe disease suggest macrophage activation and haemophagocytosis; whether these mechanisms lead to human disease remains unclear.[146] An imbalance between cytotoxic lymphocyte activation and suppression of cytotoxic responses raises the question whether disease severity relates more to microbial or genetically determined diversity of the human immune and inflammatory response.[143]

Scrub Typhus

EPIDEMIOLOGY

Scrub typhus is an important and widespread cause of febrile illness in rural areas of Asia and northern Australia. The disease is caused by *Orientia tsutsugamushi* (formerly *Rickettsia tsutsugamushi*), and contracted via the bite of the larval stage (chigger) of several species of trombiculid mite of the genus Leptotrombidium ('chiggers'). Infected mites are characteristically found in discrete foci called 'mite islands', which can occur in a wide range of vegetation types from scrub (tall-growing coarse grass) and primary forest to gardens, beaches, paddy fields, bamboo patches and oil palm or rubber estates. The obligate intracellular bacterium *O. tsutsugamushi* is maintained transovarially in the mite population and in rodents on which the larval stage of the mite normally feeds. Humans are accidental hosts. Serological and molecular strain characterization has revealed dramatic phenotypic and genotypic diversity across Asia and recently a new species, *O. chuto*, has been described in the UAE.[13,147]

CLINICAL DESCRIPTION

Scrub typhus presents as a systemic vasculitis-like infection, although much about the pathogenesis remains unknown. Symptoms usually occur between 6 and 10 days after the mite bite. The presenting features are typically fever, generalized or regional lymphadenopathy, a macular or maculopapular rash, severe headache and myalgia. Muscle tenderness is minimal or absent. Nausea and vomiting, diarrhoea, constipation, conjunctival suffusion and reversible sensorineural deafness can also occur. A painless papule occurs at the bite site, prior to other disease symptoms, that later ulcerates, and transforms into a black crust or 'eschar' in a variable proportion of patients. Variability in the thoroughness of the physical examination explains some of this variability, although other factors remain to be investigated (immunological, bacterial virulence, etc.) (Figure 22.7).

Complications include jaundice, meningoencephalitis, myocarditis, interstitial pneumonia leading to ARDS, and renal failure.[148,149] Animal experiments suggest that disease severity may vary widely with the strain of bacteria or the species of chigger transmitting.[113,150] In the pre-antibiotic era, mortality rates as high as 42% were reported, and the disease still carries a significant risk of death in rural areas where effective treatment is unavailable or delayed.[151]

Immunity to scrub typhus following overt disease is remarkably short-lived, lasting only a few months, and is highly

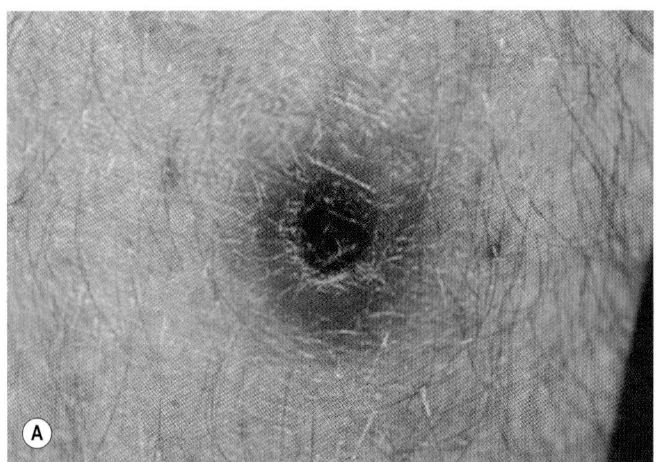

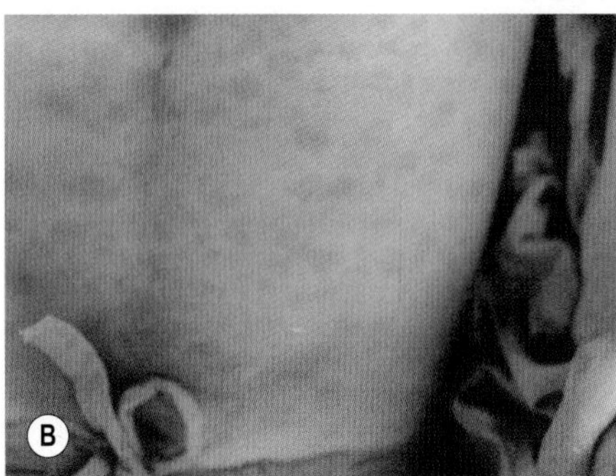

Figure 22.7 Eschar and skin rash of scrub typhus in an American soldier during the Vietnam conflict. Images from the US Army Medical Department, Office of Medical History (1982). *(Taken from Barret OJ, Stark FR. Rickettsial Diseases and Leptospirosis. Internal medicine in Vietnam, Vol II, Infectious Diseases. Office of the Surgeon General and Center of Military History. Washington DC: Dept. of the Army; 1982. p. 75–90.)*

strain-specific, so that heterologous protection is insufficient to protect from infection with different strains.[119,152]

DIAGNOSIS

The 'gold standard' diagnostic tests for scrub typhus are the immunofluorescent assay (IFA) and indirect immunoperoxidase test (IIP) based on cell-culture-derived *O. tsutsugamushi* antigens, applied to paired admission and convalescent samples.[153–155] These tests are not standardized across laboratories and are usually unavailable in poor tropical areas. They are, however, superior to the old Weil–Felix test (based on detection of antibodies cross-reactive to antigens of the OX-K strain of the unrelated bacteria *Proteus mirabilis*).[156]

Anti-*O. tsutsugamushi* IgM- and IgG-based rapid diagnostic tests have been developed but have not been adequately evaluated in the field.[157] Enzyme-linked immunosorbent assays (ELISA) similarly use cell culture-derived *O. tsutsugamushi* antigens or recombinant proteins to detect *Orientia*-specific antibodies. ELISAs have the benefit of performing multiple tests at one time, are inexpensive, sensitive, specific and reproducible (Figure 22.8).[158]

Polymerase chain reaction methods detecting different gene targets of *O. tsutsugamushi* have been developed but, despite the high sensitivities and specificities, are not standardized or in

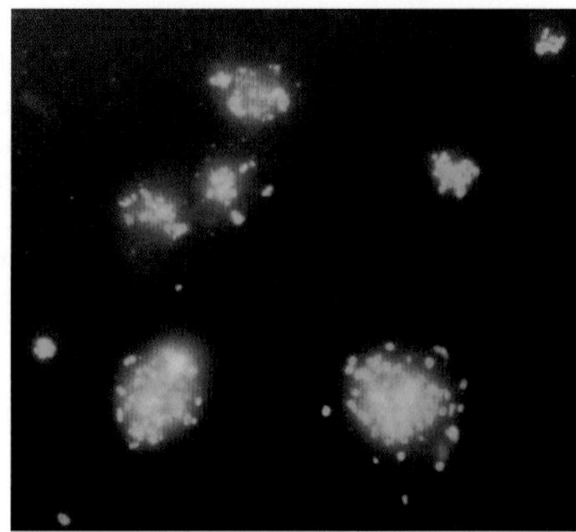

Figure 22.8 Immunofluorescence image of *Orientia tsutsugamushi* (stained bright apple green) cultured in vitro in Vero cell monolayers.

widespread use as yet. Target genes include the 47 kDa, 56 kDa, 16S rRNA and *groEL* genes.[159–162]

O. tsutsugamushi can be cultured from blood, though this takes several weeks and requires special tissue culture techniques and a BioSafety Level 3 facility. Samples taken from eschars have been shown to be useful for both PCR-based[163] or immunohistochemical diagnosis[111] upon admission, due to high bacterial loads.

DIFFERENTIAL DIAGNOSIS

A list of diseases causing 'typhus-like illness' should be considered:

- *Typhus* (SFG, TG and/or STG) – distinguished only by specific serological tests with acute and convalescent samples (IFA, IIP, ELISA, RFD) or PCR assays tests, same treatment for all
- *Malaria* – by stained blood films, antigen detection assays
- *Arbovirus infections* (e.g. dengue, chikungunya) – by serological methods (NS1, IgM, IgG assays). The dengue rash is finer and more erythematous than scrub typhus and often accompanied by marked thrombocytopenia
- *Leptospirosis* – by PCR (full blood) or culture (blood, CSF)
- *Relapsing fever* (lice or ticks) – demonstration of *Borrelia* in blood smears, serology or PCR
- *Meningococcal disease* – by blood and CSF cultures
- *Typhoid* – by blood and bone marrow cultures
- *Viral fevers* – with macular rash, for example Epstein–Barr virus, infectious mononucleosis, and primary HIV infection, distinguished serologically.

Prevention

Scrub typhus can be partly prevented or controlled by wearing protective clothing, by treatment of clothing with repellents or acaricides, application of DEET, etc. to exposed areas of the skin, when walking in terrain of endemic areas. Scrub typhus remains easily treatable (see below), though to date, no sufficiently protective vaccine has been developed.

Treatment

Scrub typhus is very responsive to treatment with appropriate antibiotics, which should be given empirically if the diagnosis is suspected. Unless contraindicated, doxycycline is the standard treatment with an adult oral dose of 100 mg twice daily for 7 days.

Tetracycline 500 mg every 6 hours for 7 days may also be used. Azithromycin (1000–500 mg on the first day followed by 500–250 mg daily for 2 days) is an effective alternative,[164] and has been shown to be effective in a single-dose treatment.[165] Azithromycin is particularly useful if tetracyclines are contraindicated, such as in pregnancy.[166] Trials of shorter courses are underway for both doxycycline and azithromycin-based regimens.

Chloramphenicol is an alternative to the tetracyclines (500 mg every 6 hours in adults or 50–75 mg/kg per day in children for 7 days), although side effects need to be considered. Roxithromycin, telithromycin and rifampicin have also been used successfully. Fluoroquinolones have been associated with treatment failures and intrinsic resistance despite good in vitro activity and should not be used for treatment of scrub typhus.

Typhus Group

MURINE TYPHUS

Epidemiology

Murine typhus, also known as flea-borne typhus or endemic typhus, is a flea-borne rickettsiosis caused by *R. typhi*. The Oriental rat flea *Xenopsylla cheopis* is the principal vector and rodents, mainly *Rattus norvegicus* and *R. rattus*, act as reservoirs.[50] In suburban areas of the USA, the cat flea, *Ctenocephalides felis*, can act as the principal vector.[167] People become infected when flea faeces containing *R. typhi* contaminate the fleabite site and lead to scratching and self-inoculation of skin. There is no eschar associated with murine typhus. Rubbing contaminated fingers into the conjunctival membrane or inhalation of dried faeces are also potential infection routes. Murine typhus has a worldwide distribution and although cases are regularly documented from the USA, Mexico and Europe, murine typhus is usually under-recognized in tropical regions. Serological surveys suggest a higher prevalence in coastal urban areas, probably due to higher population densities of rats and their ectoparasites. Murine typhus has no seasonality and occurs all year round. Exposure to rat fleas is linked to exposure to rats, and high endemicity tends to occur in areas with large rat populations (Figure 22.9).

Clinical Description

Murine typhus is a usually mild disease with nonspecific signs and symptoms. The incubation period is 7–14 days and at presentation the classic triad of fever, headache and skin rash is observed in less than 15% of cases. The skin rash is usually non-pruritic, macular, or maculopapular; starting on the trunk and then spreading peripherally, sparing the palms and soles; lasting up to 4 days; and occurring, on average approximately 1 week after the onset of fever; is often transient or difficult to observe in the early onset of fever (in less than 50% of patients 3–5 days after fever).[167–169] Nausea, vomiting, abdominal pain, diarrhoea, jaundice, myocarditis, confusion, seizures and renal failure have been reported, but serious neurological, renal and other complications are rare. Eschars do not occur in murine typhus, and generalized lymphadenopathy is significantly less common than in scrub typhus, making these clinical features useful for distinguishing the two diseases in areas of Asia where they co-exist.[5] Mortality is low, around 1–2% with antibiotic treatment, and even without treatment the disease is usually a self-limiting illness lasting 7–14 days.

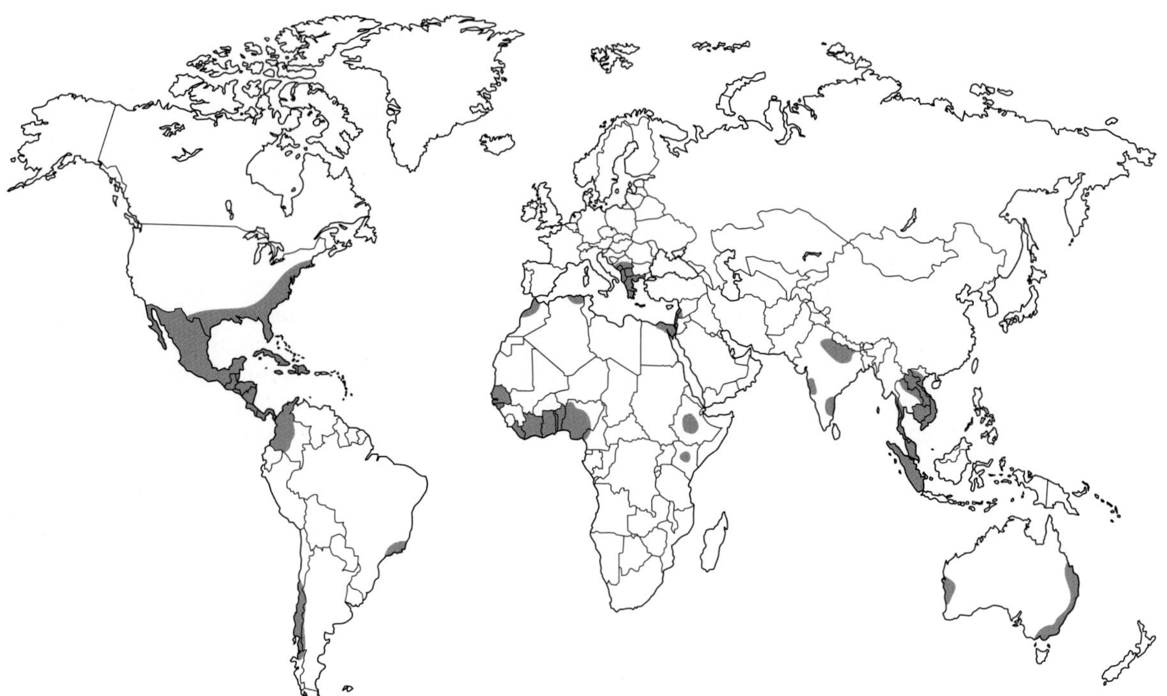

Figure 22.9 Geographical distribution of murine (flea-borne) typhus. *(Courtesy of the Department of Entomology, London School of Hygiene and Tropical Medicine.)*

Diagnosis

The definitive diagnostic test is serology by IFA on paired admission and convalescent samples. Cross-absorption of sera and Western blotting can be used to differentiate infections when false positives occur due to cross-reactivity with antigens from other bacteria. Anti-*R. typhi* IgM-based rapid diagnostic tests have shown relatively good specificity but low sensitivity and thus unfortunately have limited utility for admission diagnosis.[170] PCR-based molecular methods have been devised for detecting TG organisms (either individually or combined for *R. prowazekii* and *R. typhi*).[171] In vitro culture using vero (green monkey kidney cells) or L929 (mouse fibroblasts) cell lines is mainly a research, rather than a diagnostic tool, as sensitivity is low and BSL3 laboratory facilities are required.

Differential Diagnosis

The same range of diseases causing 'typhus-like illnesses' as discussed above should be considered.

Prevention

Prevention of murine typhus aims at reducing human contact with rodents and their fleas:

- Domestic and peri-domestic rodent and shrew control
- Proofing of grain and other food stores against rodents
- The wearing of protective clothing by garbage workers
- Hygienic measures in refugee camps or high population densities.

Treatment

The drug of choice is doxycycline in both non-pregnant adults (100 mg 12-hourly orally or intravenously) and children (4 mg/kg daily, divided 12 hourly up to a maximum of 100 mg per dose). The usual recommended duration of treatment is 7 days, but shorter courses may well be as effective. Chloramphenicol and azithromycin can be used as alternatives, and may be useful in pregnancy and uncomplicated cases, but treatment failures have been reported and data are limited.[247]

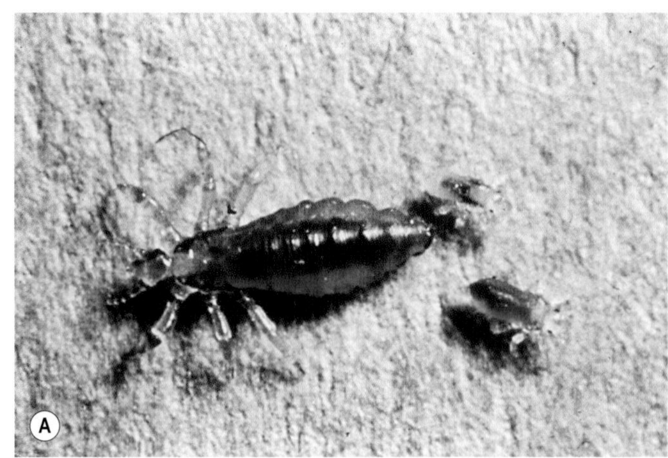

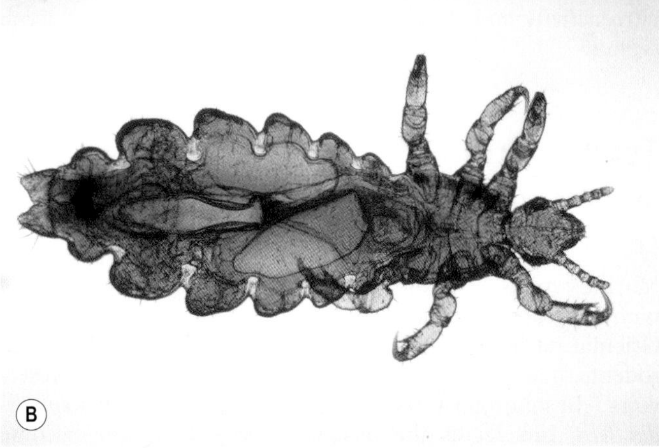

Figure 22.10 Human body louse (*Pediculus humanus corporis*). *(A: Image taken from the World Health Organization and the Public Health Image Library of the Centers for Disease Control and Prevention, image 5289. B: From Centers for Disease Control and Prevention [CDC], Atlanta, GA. CDC Public Health Image Library, image 377.)*

EPIDEMIC TYPHUS

Epidemiology

Epidemic typhus, caused by *R. prowazekii*, once considered among the most dangerous of arthropod-borne diseases, remains a potential public health threat as demonstrated by the recent typhus epidemics in Ethiopia, Burundi, Russia and Peru and sporadic cases reported recently from North Africa and France.[172] Louse infestation appears to become more prevalent worldwide, associated with a decline in social and hygienic conditions provoked by civil unrest and economic instability, hence epidemic typhus (as well as relapsing fever – *Borrelia* spp. spirochetes and trench fever – *Bartonella quintana*) should still be considered a potential health risk in tropical countries, particularly in environments such as refugee camps in cooler mountainous areas.[173]

Transmission of *R. prowazekii* to humans occurs via the infected human body louse (*Pediculus humanus corporis*), and *R. prowazekii* is transmitted to people by infected louse faeces (in which *R. prowazekii* survives for weeks), through aerosols (thought to be the main route of infection for health workers attending patients) or by skin auto-inoculation, following scratching. In contrast to the other vectors of rickettsial diseases, the bacteria are not transmitted vertically in lice and humans are the major reservoir, though sporadic cases have been reported through contact with the flying squirrel *Glaucomys volans* in the USA (Figure 22.10).[174]

Clinical Description

After an incubation period of 10–14 days, patients develop malaise and non-specific symptoms before the abrupt onset of signs including fever, headache and myalgia. Other common signs include nausea or vomiting, coughing and epistaxis. Meningoencephalitis is a common complication in severe cases, with meningism, tinnitus, deafness, and altered consciousness ranging from mild confusion through agitated delirium and coma. Diarrhoea, pulmonary involvement, myocarditis, splenomegaly and conjunctivitis may also occur. Most patients (20–80%) develop a skin rash that classically begins on the trunk of the body and spreads to the limbs. It may be macular, maculopapular or petechial and may be difficult to detect on darker skin tones. The overall mortality rate is around 20%, rising to 60% in the malnourished and aged, though with appropriate antibiotic treatment mortality may be reduced to approximately 4%. Recrudescence of epidemic typhus unrelated to louse infestation, or Brill–Zinsser disease, can appear many years/decades after the acute disease and has milder symptoms.

Diagnosis

The gold standard diagnosis of epidemic typhus is serologically by IFA, though Western blot combined with cross-adsorption tests are required to differentiate it from murine typhus. The Weil–Felix test (based on cross-reactivity with the *Proteus vulgaris* OX-19 antigen) is even less specific and should not be used. *R. prowazekii* can be cultured in Vero and L929 cells, using fresh blood or skin biopsy samples. Recently, quantitative real-time PCR assays specific for *R. prowazekii* have been developed.[175]

Treatment

In suspected cases, antibiotics should be given prior to confirmation of the diagnosis. The following antibiotic regimens are considered effective: doxycycline 100 mg daily (4 mg/kg daily for children), in two divided doses if possible, for 3 days; tetracycline 300–500 mg 6-hourly (children 50 mg/kg daily, divided 6-hourly) orally or intravenously; or chloramphenicol 500 mg to 750 mg 6-hourly (children 75 mg/kg divided 6-hourly) orally or intravenously for 7 days.

In outbreak situations, a single 200 mg dose of doxycycline is usually effective.

Prevention

Louse eradication (e.g. in refugee camps) is the most important preventive measure and is essential in the control of outbreaks. Since body lice live only in clothing, the simplest method of delousing is to remove and then destroy or wash and boil all clothing. Dusting of all clothing with 10% DDT, 1% malathion or 1% permethrin is also a rapid and effective method of killing body lice and reduces the risk of re-infestation.

Rickettsial Spotted Fevers

The spotted fevers are caused by a large and expanding number of rickettsial species, all of which are transmitted by ticks. Ticks are not only vectors but also reservoirs maintaining the organisms via vertical transmission of the currently known spotted fever group rickettsiae. Ecologic characteristics of the tick are keys to the epidemiology of each tick-borne disease. For example, the brown dog tick *Rhipicephalus sanguineus*, which is the vector of *R. conorii*, lives in dog-specific environments (kennels, farms and human houses) and has a low affinity for humans. Cases of Mediterranean spotted fever are sporadic in endemic areas and most cases are encountered in urban areas.[176] In contrast, *Amblyomma hebraeum*, which are heavily infected vectors of *R. africae* in southern Africa, emerge from their habitats and actively attack animals, particularly ruminants. They also feed readily on people that enter their biotopes, so cases of African tick-bite fever often occur as grouped cases among subjects entering the bush (e.g. during a safari) and people can suffer several tick bites simultaneously.[177]

CLINICAL PRESENTATION

The clinical symptoms of spotted fever group rickettsioses begin 6–10 days after the arthropod bite and typically include fever, headache, muscle pain, rash, local lymphadenopathy and a characteristic inoculation eschar ('tache noire') at the bite site.

An eschar is present in only a proportion of patients and thus is an unreliable finding. African tick-bite fever is characterized by the occurrence of multiple inoculation eschars and grouped cases (as in safari tourists or cross-country runners), as numerous highly infected *Amblyomma* ticks may attack and bite many people in several places at the same time.[178] In contrast, in Mediterranean spotted fever due to *R. conorii*, a single eschar is common (although multiple eschars have been described), because of the low likelihood of the tick biting people and a low rate of infection of the ticks. The rash is usually a petechial skin eruption, beginning as blanching erythematous macules (especially in RMSF around the wrists and ankles) and progressing to maculopapular lesions often associated with pustules or vesicles involving the trunk and sometimes the palms and soles. Despite the spotted fever appelation, a rash can be absent in a substantial proportion of patients, i.e. 'unspotted' or 'spotless' spotted fever (>50% of ATBF cases) (Figure 22.11).[179–181]

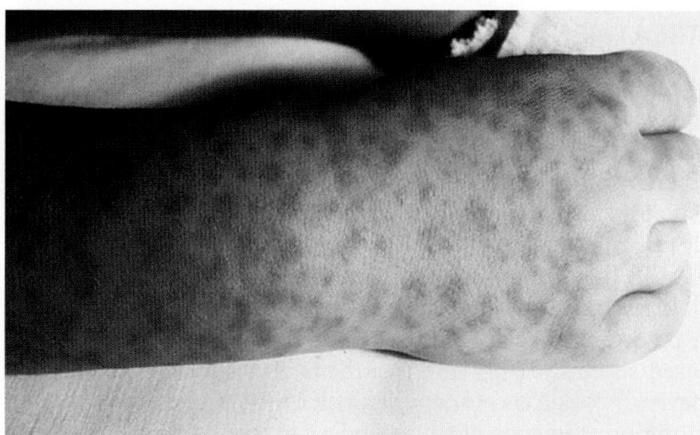

Figure 22.11 Typical skin rash in Rocky Mountain spotted fever (RMSF). *(Image from the Hardin Library for the Health Sciences, University of Iowa.) E-link:* http://hardinmd.lib.uiowa.edu/cdc/1962.html.)

Spotted fever group rickettsioses range from mild to severe and fatal diseases. African tick-bite fever is common in tropical regions, but no deaths or severe complications have been reported to-date, whereas the mortality rate from Mediterranean spotted fever may range from 3.2–32%.[176]

DIAGNOSIS

The development of new diagnostic molecular, immunological and serological tools has led to a dramatic increase in spotted fever rickettsial species now known to cause human disease. IFA remains the gold standard technique, basing definitive diagnosis on seroconversion and fourfold increase of specific antibodies on paired admission and convalescent samples. In specialist centres, a panel of antigens is used for testing for a range of possible SFG pathogens and cross-adsorption assays or PCR-based techniques are often required to identify to the species level, as cross-reactivity within the SFG, between the SFG and the TG, and with other unrelated pathogens is a common problem.

Low bacterial loads in blood and the transient rickettsaemic phase pose difficulties for antigen-based diagnostics, however immunodiagnosis on blood and skin biopsies can be of value, as can in vitro culture of the pathogen. Quantitative real-time PCR (qPCR) assays targeting the 17 kDa and *gltA* genes[160] at the genus level and the *ompA* and *ompB* genes for species-specific SFG rickettsiae[182] have been developed and are under prospective evaluation in the clinical setting.

TREATMENT

The treatment of choice for spotted fever rickettsioses is 100 mg doxycycline twice daily for 1–7 days depending on the severity of the disease. Doxycycline is safe and appropriate as initial therapy of children with suspected RMSF (and other SFG rickettsioses). Unfortunately there is an unjustified fear of toxicity leading to hesitancy to use Doxycycline as empiric therapy for RMSF. In children and pregnant women, macrolides including josamycin (50 mg/kg per day in children or 3 g/day in adults), roxithromycin, clarithromycin and azithromycin have all been used successfully for the treatment of Mediterranean spotted fever,[248,249] as has chloramphenicol. Chloramphenicol is a good antibiotic but considered secondary to tetracyclines due to side effects and inferior outcomes.[247,250]

Rocky Mountain Spotted Fever (RMSF)

Rocky Mountain Spotted Fever (RMSF), due to *R. rickettsii*, is a potentially life-threatening infection. Following its original description in the Rocky Mountain states of northwest USA in the late nineteenth century and the demonstration of the organism in its tick vector by Ricketts in 1906, RMSF has since been recognized as an important cause of illness throughout the USA, especially now in the southeastern and south-central states and on the eastern seaboard. RMSF has been described in Canada and in tropical regions of Mexico, Colombia and Brazil, especially in the area of Sao Paulo, where it is known as Brazilian spotted fever. An eschar at the site of the tick bite is usual and the illness is otherwise very similar to RMSF (Figure 22.12).

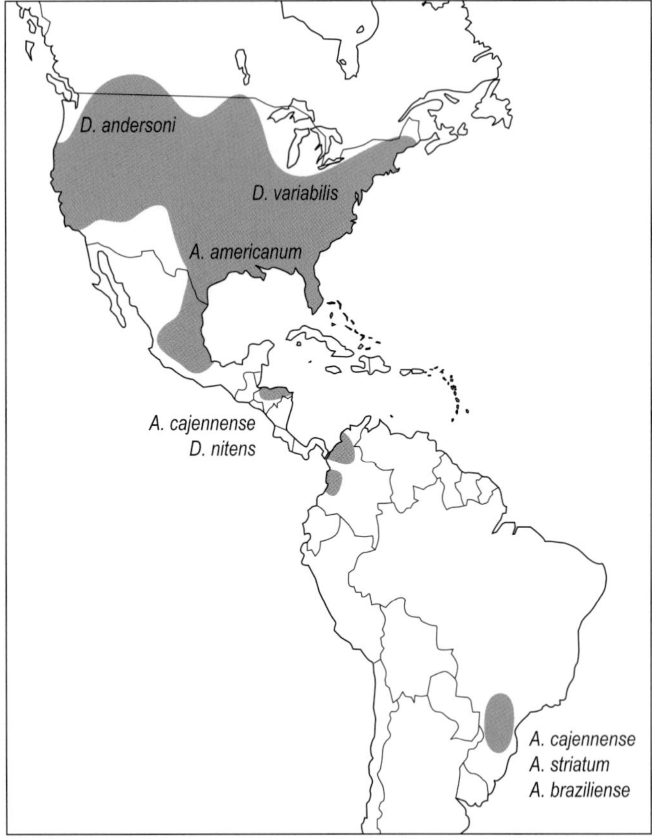

Figure 22.12 Geographical distribution of Rocky Mountain spotted fever (*R. rickettsii*). (*Courtesy of the Department of Entomology, London School of Hygiene and Tropical Medicine.*)

Transovarial transmission of rickettsiae occurs in ixodid ticks, which to current knowledge represent the main reservoir, although this has been challenged.[176,183] *Dermacentor andersoni* ticks normally live on goats, sheep, badgers, lynx and black bears, and their larvae on squirrels. *Dermacentor variabilis* and *Amblyomma* spp. ticks live on domestic dogs, rabbits, foxes, opossums, gophers and racoons, and their larvae on field mice.

Mediterranean Spotted Fever (MSF)

Mediterranean spotted fever (MSF), caused by *R. conorii*, was first described over a century ago in Tunis, followed by reports along the Mediterranean Basin.[42] However, the clinical severity and epidemiological distribution of this disease are changing, and an increasing number of regions have been reporting MSF cases, such as recently described in Algeria, Malta, Cyprus, Slovenia, Croatia, Kenya, Somalia, South Africa, and in areas surrounding the Black Sea (Turkey, Bulgaria and Ukraine).[176] Reports of severe cases of MSF are also increasing with complications, including renal, neurological, cardiac, phlebitis and retinal complications and reporting of case-fatality rates of up to 32% in the Mediterranean area.[184,185]

African Tick Bite Fever (ATBF)

African tick bite fever, caused by *R. africae*, has recently emerged as one of the most common causes of flu-like illness in international travellers to sub-Saharan Africa. ATBF should now be considered along with malaria, typhoid fever, and other tropical fevers when assessing febrile returnees from this region.[178,186] ATBF is a mild illness and is usually characterized by fever, lymphadenopathy and multiple eschars. No serious complications or fatal cases have been described. Most recently, *R. africae* has been found in ticks collected from humans and birds in Oceania (New Caledonia, Vanuatu).[187] The vectors are *Amblyomma* ticks; mainly *A. hebraeum* and *A. variegatum* in sub-Saharan Africa and parts of the eastern Caribbean and *A. loculosum* in Oceania.

Rickettsialpox

Rickettsialpox is a spotted fever that produces a vesicular skin eruption. It is caused by *R. akari*, which is transmitted by *Liponyssoides sanguineus*, a mite that lives on house mice (*Mus musculus or domesticus*) and field mice (one of several species of mice in genus *Apodemus*). Foci of this infection are known to exist in the eastern USA,[188] Central and South Africa,[189] Crimea,[190] Korea,[191] Ukraine and Costa Rica. As a result of increased awareness following the terror attacks on New York City in 2001, 34 cases of rickettsialpox were then diagnosed there over an 18-month period.[188]

R. akari is serologically more closely related to *R. australis* and *R. felis* than to *R. conorii* and *R. rickettsii*.[192,193] After an incubation period of 7–10 days, an eschar is present at the inoculation site in 90% of cases. Fever and general symptoms are as in other forms of typhus. The rash appears rapidly and consists of sparse macules and papules that become vesicular before crusting and fading. The differential diagnoses include chickenpox, monkey pox, primary HIV infection and secondary syphilis.

Rickettsialpox can be distinguished from other rickettsial infections by specific agglutination but not by group antigen serology. Treatment is as for other forms of typhus. Preventive measures should be directed at rodent control and efficient garbage clearance.

Q-fever

HISTORY AND EPIDEMIOLOGY

Q-fever is a zoonotic infection caused by *Coxiella burnetii*, usually acquired occupationally by the ingestion or inhalation of virulent organisms from infected mammals, mostly goats, sheep and cattle and their products.

C. burnetii has a worldwide geographical distribution and is an important cause of abortion in domestic goats and cattle. *C. burnetti* can infect a variety of hosts, including humans, ruminants (cattle, sheep, goats), pets and, rarely, reptiles, birds and ticks. It is a sturdy and highly infectious organism, which can survive in the environment for weeks and a single or very few organisms are sufficient to cause disease.[194] Humans are exposed to the disease due to animals shedding the organism in faeces, urine, milk, and products of conception. Particularly parturient products contain large numbers of bacteria that become aerosolized after drying and remain virulent for months.[195] Infection can also be acquired via ingestion or direct skin penetration. Infective dust can be spread by winds over long distances and result in human cases. Q-fever is primarily an occupational disease among farmers, abattoir workers and veterinarians. Human-to-human transmission is extremely rare.[196]

Q-fever was named by Derrick in 1937 as 'Query fever' before the causative organism was discovered (and not after Queensland, Australia, where he discovered it). This initially temporary name has persisted, despite the discovery and naming of the causative agent *C. burnetii*. The disease has also been known as 'Balkan grippe', 'Red River fever' (Zaire) and 'Nine Mile fever' (from a creek in the Rocky Mountains).

C. burnetii, is a 0.3–0.7 μm long, pleomorphic, Gram-negative coccobacillus and has a worldwide distribution. Phylogenically, the bacterium was reclassified from the order Rickettsiales to *Legionellales* in the gamma group of Proteobacteria on the basis of the sequence of its 16S rRNA.[194] It is an obligate intracellular bacterium that is highly adapted to reside, survive and replicate within a fully formed, acidic eukaryotic phagolysosome. A spore stage exists, which explains its particular resistance to heat and drying. *C. burnetii* undergoes phase variation: the virulent phase I exists in nature and in laboratory animals and the avirulent phase II develops due to chromosomal deletions following repeated passage of phase I bacteria in embryonated chicken eggs.[197]

CLINICAL DESCRIPTION

The presentation of Q-fever is extremely variable: infection can lead to asymptomatic seroconversion, acute disease (ranging from a flu-like syndrome to severe pneumonia), or chronic disease (manifesting mainly as endocarditis).[195]

Acute Q-fever is usually mild, with asymptomatic seroconversion occurring in 50–60% of infected individuals. A self-limited febrile syndrome occurs most frequently in symptomatic patients, but in more serious cases hepatitis, pneumonitis ('atypical' pneumonia) and prolonged fever may develop.[196]

Chronic Q-fever represents the development of the acute disease in predisposed hosts. It mainly presents as endocarditis (up to 80%) in patients with underlying heart valve lesions or, more rarely, as vascular aneurysms, graft infections, chronic bone infections or pseudotumours of the lung.[194]

DIAGNOSIS

Signs and symptoms are nonspecific and the diagnosis of Q-fever relies mainly on serology.[195] Indirect immunofluorescence (IF) is the reference method for serological diagnosis.[198] Enzyme immunoassay (EIA) and complement fixation (CF) tests are also in routine use.[199] Significant titres may take 3–4 weeks to appear, so treatment should be started as soon as a clinician suspects the disease to be present.[200]

In an apparent paradox, antibodies to the phase II organism are high in acute disease, and antibodies to the phase I organism are raised in chronic disease.[200] For acute Q-fever, a fourfold rise in paired sera gives the highest specificity. Although sufficiently elevated single IF tests also have good specificity, there is considerable variation in cut-off titres used, which might be explained by regional differences in background positivity.[200] Recent re-evaluation of the current positive predictive value of serologic analysis for endocarditis suggested a phase I (virulent bacteria) IgG cut-off titre of ≥1600 in France.[201]

Although PCR seemed promising, the sensitivity of serum PCR is too low for clinical use. Serum contains few intracellular organisms, and use of buffy coat specimens may increase test sensitivity.[202] However, PCR is highly sensitive on tissue samples such as heart valves, which have higher numbers of bacteria.[203]

DIFFERENTIAL DIAGNOSIS

Q-fever should be distinguished from:

- Typhoid (blood and bone marrow culture)
- Atypical pneumonia (e.g. viruses, *Mycoplasma pneumoniae, Chlamydia pneumoniae, Chlamydia psittaci* – appropriate serological methods)
- Viral hepatitis (serology)
- Other viral infections (e.g. Epstein–Barr, HIV and cytomegalovirus – appropriate serology)
- Brucellosis and Lyme disease (serology)
- Leptospirosis (muscle tenderness, polymorphonuclear leucocytosis – isolation or PCR)
- Miliary tuberculosis (chest radiography and tuberculin testing)
- Other causes of bacterial endocarditis (blood cultures).

TREATMENT

No antibiotic is bactericidal against *C. burnetii*. The first-line treatment for early uncomplicated Q-fever is as for the typhus and rickettsial spotted fevers – with doxycycline, although some resistant strains have been found.

The treatment of choice for acute Q-fever is doxycycline 100 mg 12-hourly for 14 days.

Life-long antibiotic treatment has been recommended for endocarditis, but 18 months of doxycycline (100 mg, twice daily) and hydroxychloroquine (200 mg, three times daily) are sufficient for native valves and 24 months for prosthetic valves.[204,205] Chloroquine raises the pH in the phagolysosome, increasing the efficacy of doxycycline.[206] Chloroquine levels between 0.8 mg/L and 1.2 mg/L and doxycycline levels over 5 mg/L are associated with the best response. Most patients treated with this regimen have photosensitivity, and regular heart and eye examinations are needed.[205]

Treatment should continue until IgA and IgG antibodies to phase I antigen fall below 1:200 although targets of 1:800 for IgG and 1:50 for IgA have also been recommended.[205]

Q-fever during pregnancy is treated with co-trimoxazole until delivery, and serology to detect recrudescence is needed in subsequent pregnancies.[207] A year of doxycycline and chloroquine after delivery may prevent recrudescence. Mothers should be advised that both *C. burnetii* and doxycycline are excreted in breast milk.[180]

PREVENTION AND CONTROL

Aerosol dissemination of *C. burnetii* is difficult to prevent because adequate control of the disease in domestic animals is nearly impossible. Milk should be pasteurized.

A vaccine against Q-fever has been used in Australia for agricultural and abattoir workers, veterinarians, etc., according to the National Q-fever Management Program. A vaccine may currently be available at the US Army Medical Research Institute of Infectious Diseases (USAMRIID), Fort Detrick, Frederick, MD, USA.

Neorickettsia

Neorickettsia are obligate intracellular bacteria of the order *Rickettsiales*, family, Anaplasmataceae. This family also includes tick-borne *Anaplasma*, *Ehrlichia* and *Wolbachia* symbionts of arthropods and filaria. The zoonotic cycle of *N. sennetsu* encompasses infecting trematodes that parasitize fish. Vertebrates that eat uncooked fish containing infected flukes may be either definitive or incidental hosts.

Rickettsia sennetsu infection was reported for the first time in 1954 from the Japanese island of Kyushu as a mononucleosis-like infectious disease with fever, weakness, anorexia, generalized lymphadenopathy, hepatosplenomegaly and peripheral blood mononucleosis with atypical lymphocytes. The disease was called 'Sennetsu fever', from the Japanese for infectious mononucleosis, and had an incubation period of ~14 days.[208,209] The causative agent isolated from patients' peripheral blood, lymph nodes, and bone marrow was subsequently renamed *Ehrlichia sennetsu* and more recently *Neorickettsia sennetsu*.[210]

Neorickettsia are obligate intracellular bacteria closely related to *Ehrlichia* and *Anaplasma* and, unlike *Rickettsia*, grow in host membrane–lined cytoplasmic vacuoles.[211]

Neorickettsia species can have complex cycles with infection of trematodes, the cercariae of which may infect snails and aquatic insects,[212] which again are ingested by fish, mammals and birds. *N. helminthoeca* can infect flukes and canids, causing salmon poisoning disease in dogs in the USA,[213] whereas *N. risticii* causes Potomac horse fever in North America and Europe and is probably transmitted by trematodes of snails, insects, bats and swallows.[214] In humans, they infect mostly mononuclear phagocytes (Figure 22.13).

Sennetsu was shown to be transmissible to mice and then to humans in Japan. The consumption of raw grey mullet (*Mugil cephalus*, a diadromous fish) has been associated with a sennetsu-like illness, and when *N. sennetsu* was cultured from the blood of these patients, the infection was linked to eating raw fish.[215] The disease has been documented in Japan, peninsular Malaysia and most recently in the Lao PDR (linked to the climbing perch '*Anabas testudineus*'), where raw fish and fermented fish paste are commonly eaten.[216]

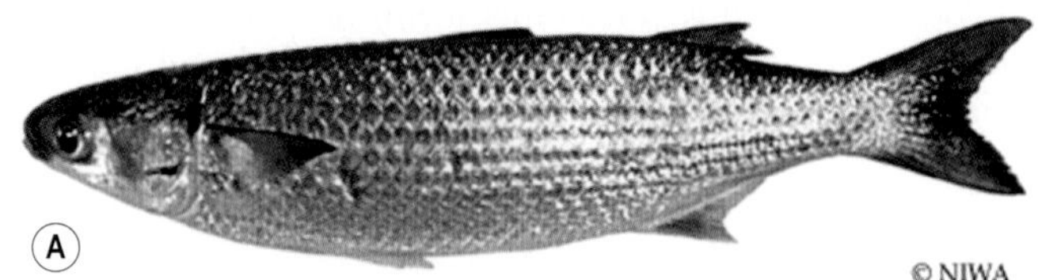

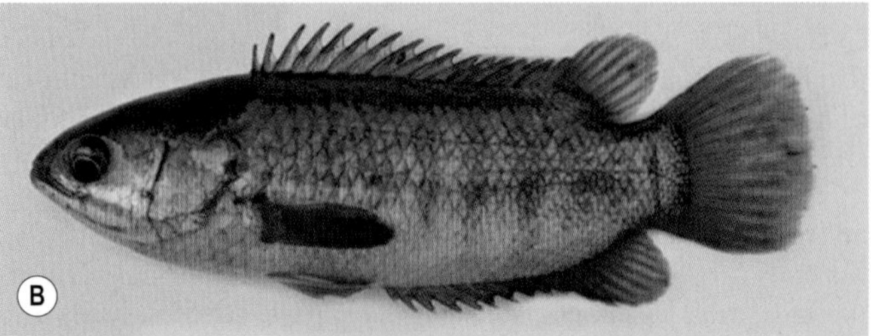

Figure 22.13 The grey mullet '*Mugil cephalus*' (A) and the climbing perch '*Anabas testudineus*' (B), are associated with the transmission of *N. sennetsu*, the causative agent of Sennetsu disease. *(A: Image taken from* www.nabis.govt.nz. *Copyright © NIWA. B: Image taken from* http://www.bdfish.org. *Photo credit: Balaram Mahalder.)*

Treatment consists of doxycycline orally 2×100 mg/day usually for 7–14 days, but at least until 3 days after defervescence. Most patients defervesce after 36–48 hours.

Rickettsioses in Travel Medicine

Rickettsial diseases are increasingly being recognized among international travellers.[186] A recent study of ~7000 returnees with fever as the major reason for seeking medical care found that 2% of these could be shown to be caused by rickettsioses and that 20% of these patients are hospitalized.[217] With more than 350 reported cases, African tick bite fever has emerged as the most important rickettsiosis in travel medicine, notably in travellers to sub-Saharan Africa,[186] where the number of such cases exceeds that of typhoid or dengue.[218] In a recent investigation comprising 280 international travelers reported with a rickettsial illness acquired abroad within the GeoSentinel surveillance Network during 1996–2008, 231 (82.5%) had spotted fever (SFG) rickettsiosis; 16 (5.7%) scrub typhus; 11 (3.9%) Q-fever; 10 (3.6%) typhus group (TG) rickettsiosis; 7 (2.5%) bartonellosis; 4 (1.4%) indeterminable SFG/TG rickettsiosis and 1 (0.4%) human granulocytic anaplasmosis.

A total of 197 (87.6%) SFG rickettsiosis cases acquired in sub-Saharan Africa were associated with higher age, male gender, travel to southern Africa, late summer season travel, and travel for tourism. More than 90% of patients with rickettsial disease were treated with doxycycline, 43 (15.4%) required hospitalization and four had a complicated course, including one fatal case of scrub typhus encephalitis acquired in Thailand.[22]

A delay in diagnosis and the common practice of prescribing β-lactam antibiotics as empirical therapy may result in life-threatening complications or permanent disability in some infected travellers.[219] Thus, a high index of suspicion is advisable when encountering a patient with fever and constitutional symptoms after having returned from an endemic area. All age groups are at risk for rickettsial infections during travel to endemic areas. Due to an incubation period of up to

14 days for most rickettsial diseases, tourists may not necessarily experience symptoms during their trip, and onset may coincide with their return home or develop within a week of returning.[13]

For prevention, weekly 200 mg doses of doxycycline can prevent scrub typhus and possibly other rickettsioses, and may thus be a valuable option for backpackers, trekkers and other visitors at high risk.[220,221] However, African tick bite fever has been reported in safari travellers despite the concomitant use of tetracycline hydrochloride as malaria prophylaxis.[186] Protective clothing should be advised for travellers to sub-Saharan Africa on safari and hunting trips, and topical repellents, such as DEET, should be used on exposed skin; notably, frequent application is required because of the short-lasting effect against the ticks that transmit African tick bite fever.

Scrub typhus is endemic to the Asia-Pacific, including south-central Russia, India, Sri Lanka and also the Arabian Peninsula in Western Asia. Most travel-acquired cases of scrub typhus occur during visits to rural areas in endemic countries for activities such as camping, hiking, or rafting, but urban cases have also been described.

Flea-borne rickettsioses caused by *R. typhi* and *R. felis* are widely distributed throughout the tropics and subtropics, and especially in port cities and coastal regions with high rodent populations. Humans exposed to flea-infested cats, dogs, and peri-domestic animals while travelling in endemic regions or entering areas infested with rats are at highest risk. Murine typhus has been reported among travellers returning from Asia, Africa and southern Europe and has also been reported from Hawaii, California and Texas in the USA.

Ehrlichiosis is most commonly reported in the southeastern and south-central USA, Europe and Asia, but also in Brazil, Panama and Africa.

Anaplasmosis occurs worldwide. Known endemic regions include the USA, Europe, China, Russia and Korea.

Sennetsu fever occurs in Japan, Malaysia, Laos and possibly other parts of Asia. Sennetsu fever can be contracted from eating raw infected fish.

REFERENCES

64. Zarafonetis CJD. The Typhus fevers. In: Coates Jr JB, Havens Jr WP, editors. Internal Medicine in World War II. Vol II. Washington, DC: Office of the Surgeon General, Dept. of the Army; 1963. Chapter VI Scrub Typhus.
70. Smadel JE, Woodward TE, Ley HL, et al. Chloromycetin in the treatment of scrub typhus. Science 1948;108:160–1.
86. Paris DH, Chansamouth V, Nawtaisong P, et al. Coagulation and inflammation in scrub typhus and murine typhus – a prospective comparative study from Laos. Clin Microbiol Infect 2012;18:1221–8.
147. Kelly DJ, Fuerst PA, Ching W-M, et al. Scrub typhus: the geographic distribution of phenotypic and genotypic variants of *Orientia tsutsugamushi*. Clin Infect Dis 2009;48(Suppl 3): S203–30.
155. Blacksell SD, Bryant NJ, Paris DH, et al. Scrub typhus serologic testing with the indirect immunofluorescence method as a diagnostic gold standard: a lack of consensus leads to a lot of confusion. Clin Infect Dis 2007;44: 391–401.

Access the complete references online at www.expertconsult.com

23

Sexually Transmitted Infections (Excluding HIV)

JOHN RICHENS | PHILIPPE MAYAUD | DAVID C. W. MABEY

KEY POINTS

- Sexually transmitted infections (STIs) are a major cause of morbidity in developing countries.
- STIs, especially those which cause genital ulceration, facilitate the sexual transmission of HIV.
- Syndromic management of STIs enables symptomatic cases to be treated immediately, preventing onward transmission.
- Many people with an STI have no symptoms. There is a need for more accessible screening tests to identify individuals with asymptomatic gonorrhoea or chlamydial infection in particular.
- Syphilis in pregnancy remains a major cause of stillbirth and neonatal mortality.
- New point of care serological tests for syphilis facilitate screening of pregnant women in health facilities without access to a laboratory.
- *Neisseria gonorrhoeae* is resistant to most antibiotics in many countries. Antimicrobial resistance should be monitored to inform national treatment guidelines.
- Effective vaccines are available for the types of human papilloma virus commonly associated with cervical cancer.
- Innovative strategies are needed for STI control in high-risk groups.

Introduction

Sexually transmitted infections (STIs) are among the most common reasons for seeking medical care in developing countries, accounting for ≥10% of medical consultations in some parts of Africa.[1] Nevertheless, and in spite of their serious consequences (particularly for women and children) and extensive evidence that they facilitate the transmission of human immunodeficiency virus (HIV) through sexual contact,[2] they have often been accorded low priority by medical professionals and health planners. The consequent lack of good facilities for their management has led many patients with these conditions to seek treatment outside the formal health sector, with inadequate treatment regimens leading to increasing antimicrobial resistance among sexually transmitted pathogens. Because so few statistics are available for patients treated outside the formal health sector, the extent of the problem continues to be underestimated.

Epidemiology of Sexually Transmitted Diseases

Certain broad generalizations can be made about the epidemiology of sexually transmitted diseases (STIs). Clearly, they are diseases of the sexually active, although mother-to-child transmission also occurs. None of the sexually transmitted agents described in this chapter has an epidemiologically significant non-human reservoir. They are more common among young adults, among single people of both sexes, and among those who travel. Although no sexually active individual is immune, certain groups can be identified, whose behaviour places them at higher risk than others. Such groups include sex workers and their clients, bar workers, adolescents, the military, truck drivers and sailors.

The behaviour of STIs within populations, as with other infectious diseases, can be predicted if information is available about the proportion of individuals who are susceptible to infection, the average efficiency of transmission per contact, the rates of contact between infected and uninfected persons and the average duration of infection. This is commonly expressed as the basic reproductive number (R_0), i.e. the average number of new cases arising from one infected person, with the equation $R_0 = \beta \times c \times d$, where β = the transmission efficiency, c = the rate of partner change and d = the duration of infection. The viral STIs which are persistent, maintain themselves with ease, whereas some bacterial STIs such as chancroid, which are usually short-lived and require high rates of partner change to maintain themselves, can be brought under control relatively easily. Each of these factors is amenable to public health intervention, e.g. improving access to treatment, promoting delay in sexual debut and the use of barrier methods of contraception.

Accurate STI prevalence figures are not routinely available for any developing country, but much useful information has been gathered during limited surveys of antenatal women.[3] In a large research study in rural Uganda, a community-based survey of adults aged 15–59 years found the prevalence of syphilis to be 10%, of gonorrhoea 1.6% and of chlamydial infection 3%. A total of 24% of women had *Trichomonas vaginalis* infection, and 51% had bacterial vaginosis.[4] Box 23.1 shows a number of factors which may explain the higher incidence and prevalence of STIs in developing compared with industrialized countries. Lack of access to effective treatment probably explains much of the difference in the case of the curable STIs.

The relative importance of certain STIs is much greater in developing countries. For example, chancroid remains a cause of genital ulceration in African countries but has almost disappeared from Europe. Sporadic outbreaks among impoverished communities in North America in the 1980s suggest that this

BOX 23.1 FACTORS CONTRIBUTING TO THE HIGH INCIDENCE OF STIs IN DEVELOPING COUNTRIES

1. Demographic factors (high proportion of population are young adults)
2. Rural–urban migration with breakdown of traditional customs
3. Prostitution
4. Lack of adequate medical services
5. High prevalence of antibiotic-resistant strains of *Neisseria gonorrhoeae, Haemophilus ducreyi*
6. Polygamy.

has more to do with socioeconomic factors than with climate. Donovanosis (granuloma inguinale) is highly prevalent in certain parts of Papua New Guinea, India and South Africa but appears to be rare outside these areas. The lack of reliable and cheap diagnostic tests for the three classical 'tropical STIs' – chancroid, donovanosis and lymphogranuloma venereum (LGV) – has hindered attempts to study their epidemiology.

Because of the lack of adequate diagnostic and treatment facilities for STIs in many developing countries, complications are commonly seen, particularly among women and children. Pelvic inflammatory disease (PID), due in the majority of cases to gonorrhoea or chlamydial infection, is a frequent cause of admission to gynaecology wards in Africa.[5] Ectopic pregnancy as a sequela of PID is up to three times as common in Africa as in Europe, and tubal infertility, another common sequela, is widespread, with up to 20% of women affected in some regions of Africa.[6] The incidence of carcinoma of the cervix linked to the persistence of oncogenic HPV genotypes is extremely high in many developing countries. Some 2–3% of infants born in some African cities develop gonococcal ophthalmia neonatorum. Congenital syphilis has been an important cause of hospital admission among infants aged less than 3 months in Lusaka, Zambia,[7] and a more recent study in Tanzania showed that syphilis was responsible for 50% of all stillbirths.[8]

Table 23.1 lists organisms transmissible by sexual contact and the diseases they cause. In this chapter, only those responsible for major morbidity in developing countries will be considered further.

TABLE 23.1 Sexually Transmitted Infections in Humans

	Agent	Disease
STIs Producing Genital Lesions		
Viruses	Herpes simplex virus	Genital herpes, disseminated and neonatal herpes infection
	Human papilloma virus	Genital warts, juvenile laryngeal papillomatosis, squamous carcinoma in anogenital area
	Molluscum contagiosum virus	Molluscum contagiosum
Bacteria	*Neisseria gonorrhoeae*	Gonococcal infections of urethra, epididymis, pharynx, rectum, conjunctiva, upper genital tract of women, disseminated gonococcal infection
	Chlamydia trachomatis, serotypes D–K	As for gonorrhoea, except for disseminated infection; also infantile pneumonia and reactive arthritis
	Chlamydia trachomatis, serotypes L1,2,3	Lymphogranuloma venereum
	Ureaplasma urealyticum	Non-gonococcal urethritis
	Mycoplasma genitalium	Urethritis, cervicitis and pelvic infection
	Haemophilus ducreyi	Chancroid
	Treponema pallidum	Syphilis
	Gardnerella vaginalis and anaerobes	Bacterial vaginosis
	Klebsiella (formerly Calymmatobacterium) granulomatis	Donovanosis (granuloma inguinale)
Fungi	*Candida albicans*	Genital candidiasis
Protozoa	*Trichomonas vaginalis*	Trichomoniasis
Arthropods	*Phthirus pubis*	Pediculosis
	Sarcoptes scabiei	Scabies
Infections Which can be Sexually Transmitted but Which do not Generally Produce Genital Lesions		
Viruses	Hepatitis viruses	Hepatitis A to D
	Cytomegalovirus (CMV)	CMV infections of newborn and immunosuppressed
	HIV	Acquired immune deficiency syndrome
	HTLV-1	Tropical spastic paraparesis T-cell leukaemia/lymphoma
Bacteria	*Shigella* spp.	Shigellosis
	Campylobacter spp.	Campylobacter enteritis
	Salmonella spp.	Salmonellosis
	Group B streptococcus	Neonatal sepsis
Protozoa	*Giardia lamblia*	Giardiasis
	Cryptosporidium spp.	Cryptosporidiosis
	Entamoeba histolytica	Amoebiasis[a]
Helminths	*Enterobius vermicularis*	Enterobiasis
	Strongyloides stercoralis	Strongyloidiasis
	Trichuris trichiura	Trichuriasis

[a]Occasionally produces anogenital ulceration in tropical countries.
Source: World Health Organization.

Control of STIs

Strategies for the control of STIs include primary and secondary prevention, and, in the case of bacterial and protozoal infections, improving access to curative treatment. Primary prevention is health education given to young people before they are exposed to the risk of STIs, emphasizing the importance of delaying the onset of sexual activity, limiting the number of their sexual partners, and using condoms to reduce risk. Secondary prevention refers to health education given to individuals with STIs, aimed at reducing the risk to their sexual partners, and the likelihood of their becoming reinfected.

Improved case management, in which accessible, affordable and effective treatment is made available to patients with symptomatic STIs, is a cornerstone of STI control. Effective treatment should be given at the first visit, to reduce onward transmission and the likelihood of complications. The treatment of sexual partners of STI patients is also of critical importance for STI control. Since many STIs are asymptomatic, especially in women, screening programmes can play an important role in STI control, e.g. screening of pregnant women is an important strategy for the prevention of congenital syphilis. Effective control of STIs cannot be achieved by health ministries in isolation. Coordinated multisectoral interventions which attempt to address broader societal issues that allow STIs to thrive (e.g. migrant labour and prostitution) also need to be tackled vigorously.[9]

STIs and HIV Infection

There is no doubt that STIs, by causing inflammation and ulceration of the genital tract, facilitate the transmission of HIV infection through sexual contact.[2] Ulcerative STIs, in particular, increase both the infectivity of HIV-positive individuals, and the susceptibility of HIV negatives, by a factor of 10–100 per sexual exposure.[10] Gonococcal and chlamydial infections have been shown to increase the shedding of HIV at the cervix, and gonorrhoea to increase the shedding of HIV in seminal fluid.[11] An intervention trial in Tanzania showed that the incidence of HIV infection was reduced by 40% following the introduction of improved case management of STIs, using the syndromic approach, in rural health centres, although the effect of improved STI management upon HIV transmission has been less clear in other trials (Chapter 15).[12] These studies have given renewed impetus to STI control programmes.

History-taking and Examination in the STI Clinic

It is not possible to provide a good clinical service for STIs unless one gains the confidence of the patient(s). This requires privacy and the avoidance of a moralistic attitude.

It is usually possible to take a history and examine a patient with an STI in 10 minutes. When taking a history, the following information should be collected:[13]

1. The nature and duration of the symptoms
2. The nature of any treatment already taken for this condition
3. A sexual history, which should indicate when and with whom the patient has had sexual intercourse. This information is essential in order to attempt contact tracing and/or partner notification. Information about the type of sexual activity and condom use will assist in examination, collection of specimens and preventive counselling
4. Past medical history and history of previous STIs and HIV testing
5. History of drug allergy
6. In female patients a menstrual and obstetric history should be taken.

STI patients should always be counselled concerning risk reduction, including the promotion of condom use; the importance of compliance with the full course of treatment if directly observed single-dose treatment is not given; and the importance of referring sexual contacts for treatment.

The examination should be carried out in private in a good light. After examination of the mouth and palms, patients should be exposed from the umbilicus to the knees. The skin of the abdomen, groins and perineum should be examined in particular for evidence of scabies and pediculosis, and the inguinal glands palpated. In males the penis should be inspected, after retraction of the foreskin in uncircumcised patients. If a urethral discharge is not apparent, evidence of urethritis can be sought by milking the urethra forward and examining the meatus for discharge. The scrotum should be palpated for evidence of epididymitis. Female patients should be examined in the lithotomy position. The lower abdomen should be palpated for evidence of PID (masses and/or tenderness) and, after inspection of the vulva, a vaginal speculum should be passed. The cervix should be examined and the speculum then slowly withdrawn while the walls of the vagina are examined. Bimanual examination is used to identify pelvic masses and/or tenderness. The presence of pain on moving the cervix (cervical excitation tenderness) suggests the presence of PID. In both sexes the perianal skin should also be inspected, and proctoscopy may be performed to check for rectal infections.

The laboratory investigations requested will depend on the facilities available. In general, they should be selected on the principle that a patient with one STI is also at increased risk of other STIs; that is, they should not be limited to tests designed to identify the cause of the present symptoms. All patients with an STI should be offered screening for syphilis and HIV after suitable pre-test discussion.

In settings where laboratory diagnosis is not feasible, the World Health Organization (WHO) recommends syndromic management, in which patients with a syndrome such as urethral discharge or genital ulcer are treated for all the likely causes of that syndrome. Even when laboratory diagnosis is available, syndromic management has the advantage that treatment is given at the first visit, rather than relying on the patients to return for their results. Effective syndromic treatment depends on knowledge of local disease patterns and antimicrobial susceptibilities; a laboratory is required to monitor these, preferably in each country or province. WHO syndromic treatment flowcharts for eight common STI syndromes are shown in Figure 23.1.[14] The advantages and disadvantages of syndromic management are shown in Box 23.2. The flowchart for vaginal discharge is the least satisfactory, as many women with this complaint are not suffering from an STI. This not only leads to over-treatment, but can also jeopardize relationships if such women are asked to refer their partners for STI treatment.

BOX 23.2 ADVANTAGES AND DISADVANTAGES OF SYNDROMIC MANAGEMENT OF STIs

ADVANTAGES
- Simple
- Rapid
- No laboratory required
- Treatment given at first visit, preventing complications and further transmission
- Simplifies reporting and supervision

DISADVANTAGES
- Leads to over-treatment, especially in women
- May lead to problems with partner notification, especially in women who are told they have an STI when they do not
- Only symptomatic STIs treated.

Diseases Causing a Genital Discharge

URETHRAL DISCHARGE IN MALES

Urethritis in males is either gonococcal, non-gonococcal or of mixed aetiology; the presence of gonococci is easily demonstrated by Gram stain. When the Gram stain is negative, the presence of >5 polymorphs per high-power field is accepted as evidence of non-gonococcal urethritis. In most developing countries, the majority of cases presenting to hospital are gonococcal. Up to 50% of cases of non-gonococcal urethritis are due to *Chlamydia trachomatis*; a proportion of the remaining cases are associated with *Mycoplasma genitalium*,[15–18] and a small percentage may harbour *Trichomonas vaginalis* or adenovirus.[19] According to the WHO syndromic management guidelines,

Text continued on page 302.

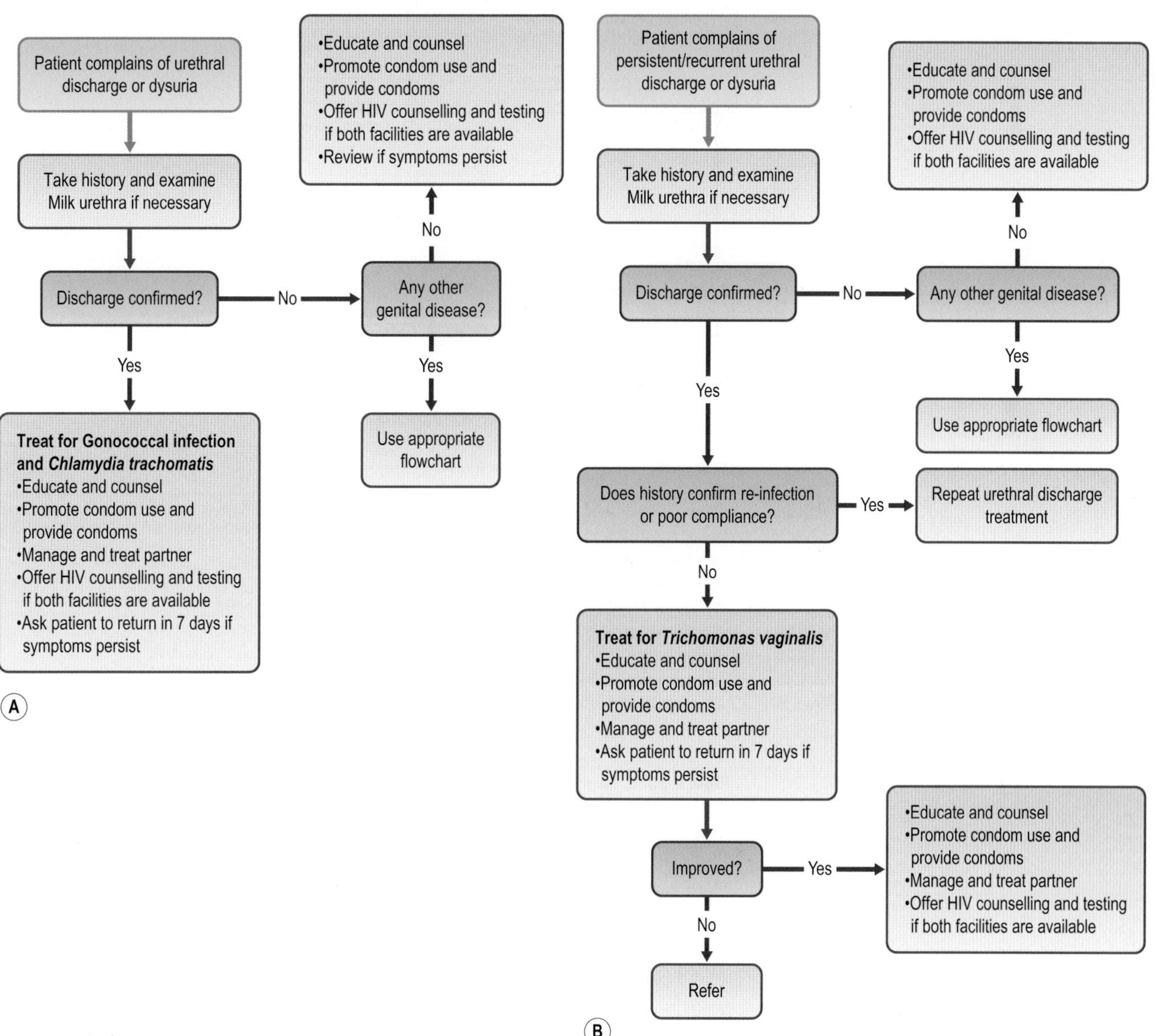

Figure 23.1 WHO flowcharts for the management of common STI-associated syndromes. (A) Urethral discharge. (B) Persistent urethral discharge in men *(WHO 2003.)*

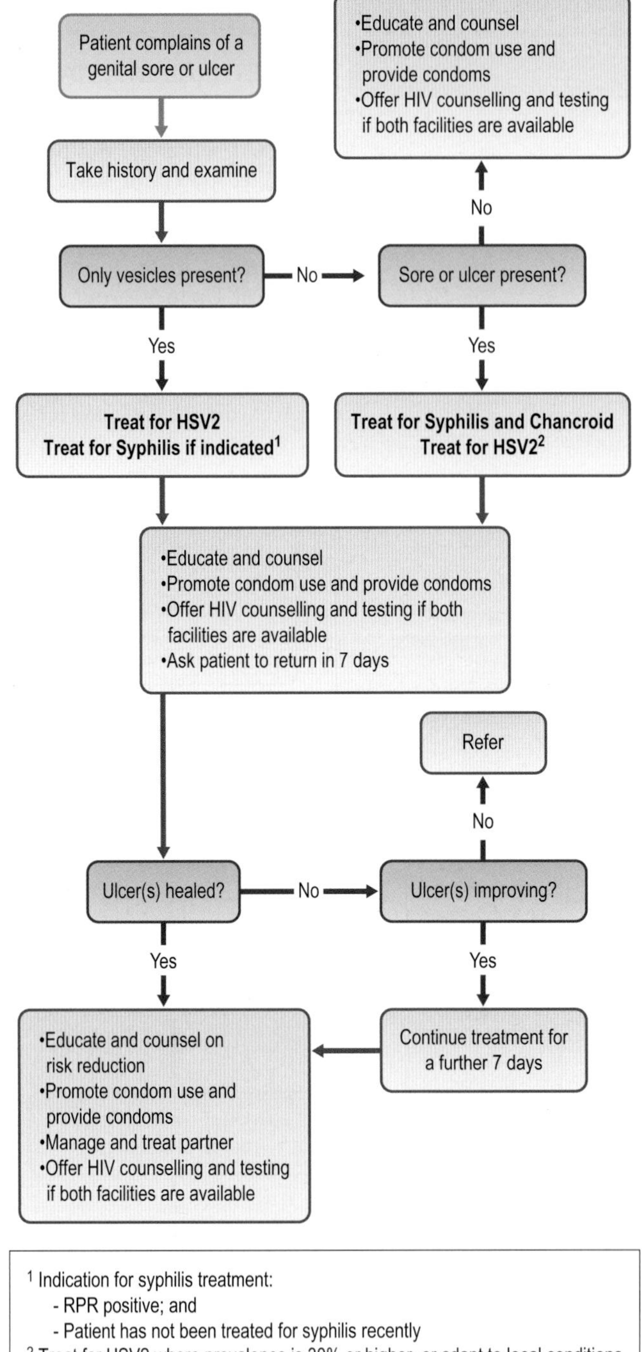

Figure 23-1, cont'd (c) Genital ulcer

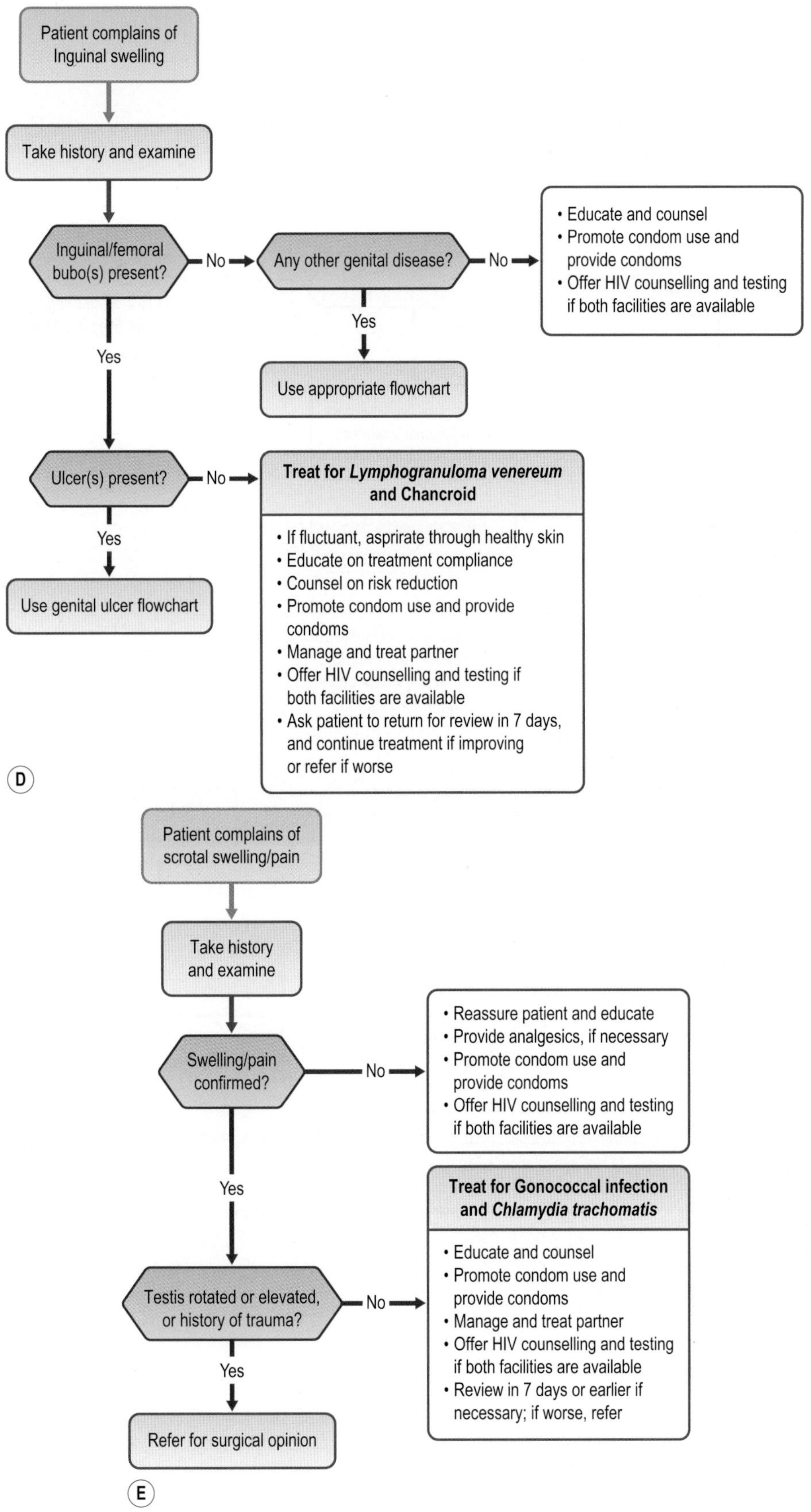

Figure 23-1, cont'd (D) Inguinal bubo, (E) Scrotal swelling

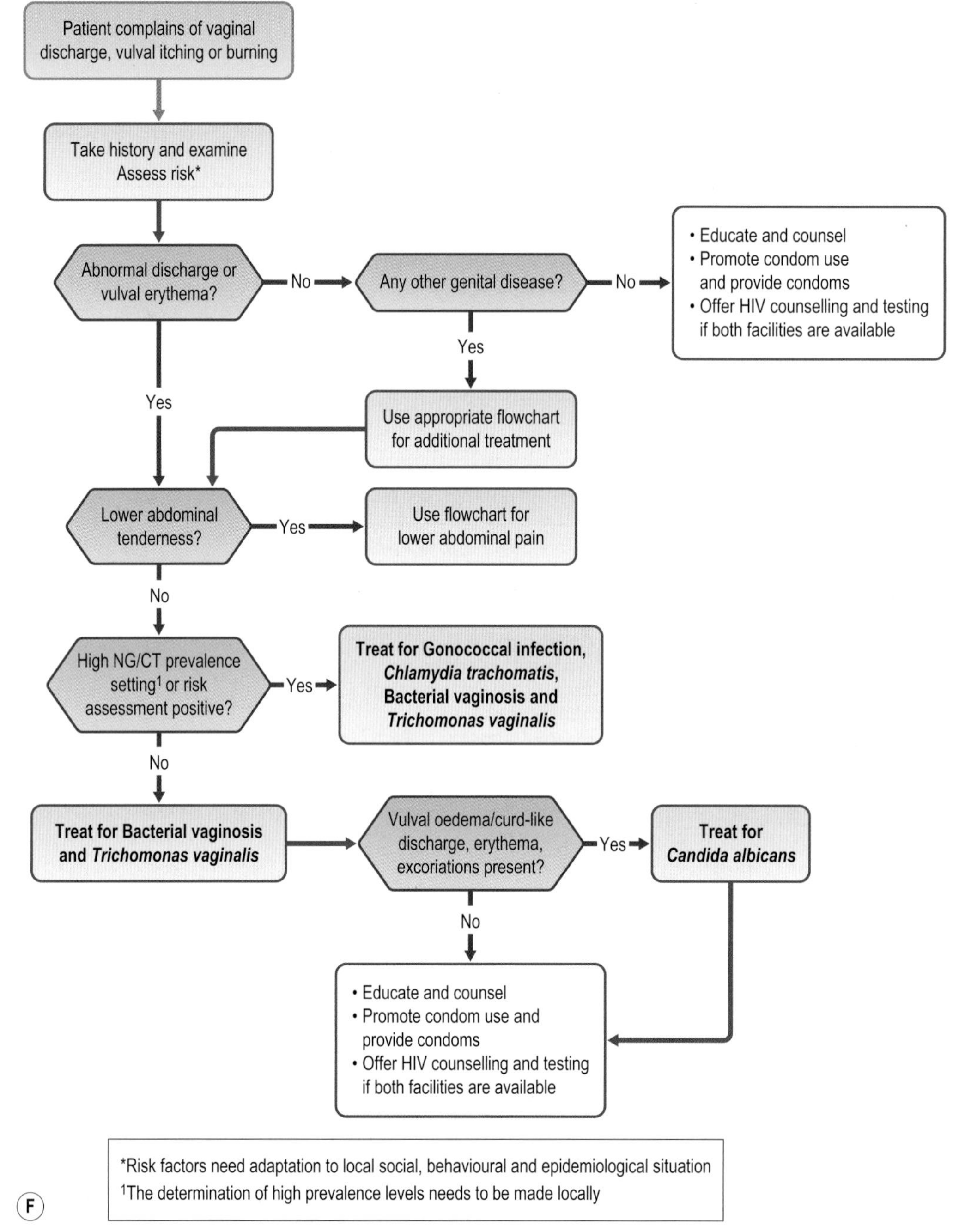

Figure 23-1, cont'd (F) Vaginal discharge

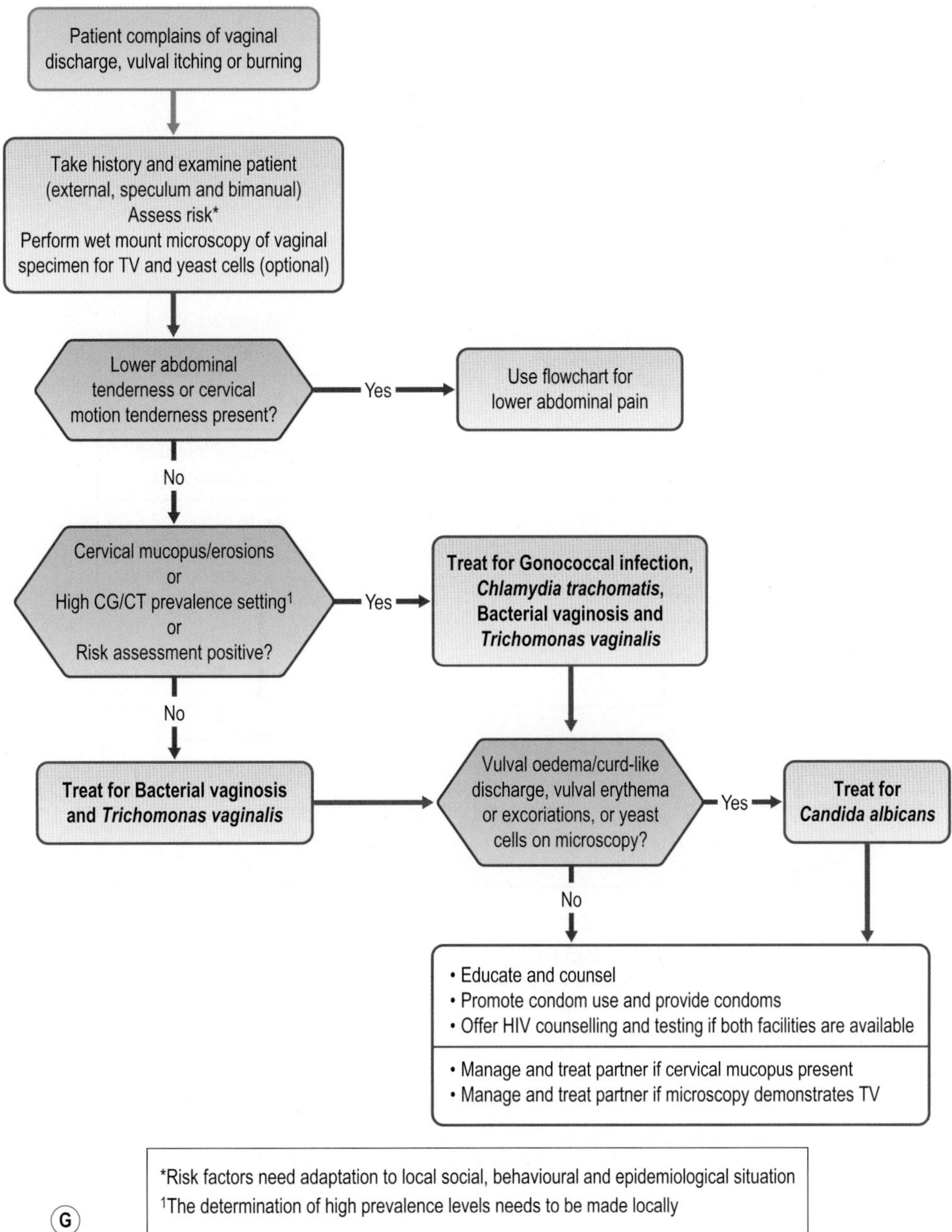

Figure 23-1, cont'd (G) Vaginal discharge: bimanual and speculum, with or without microscope

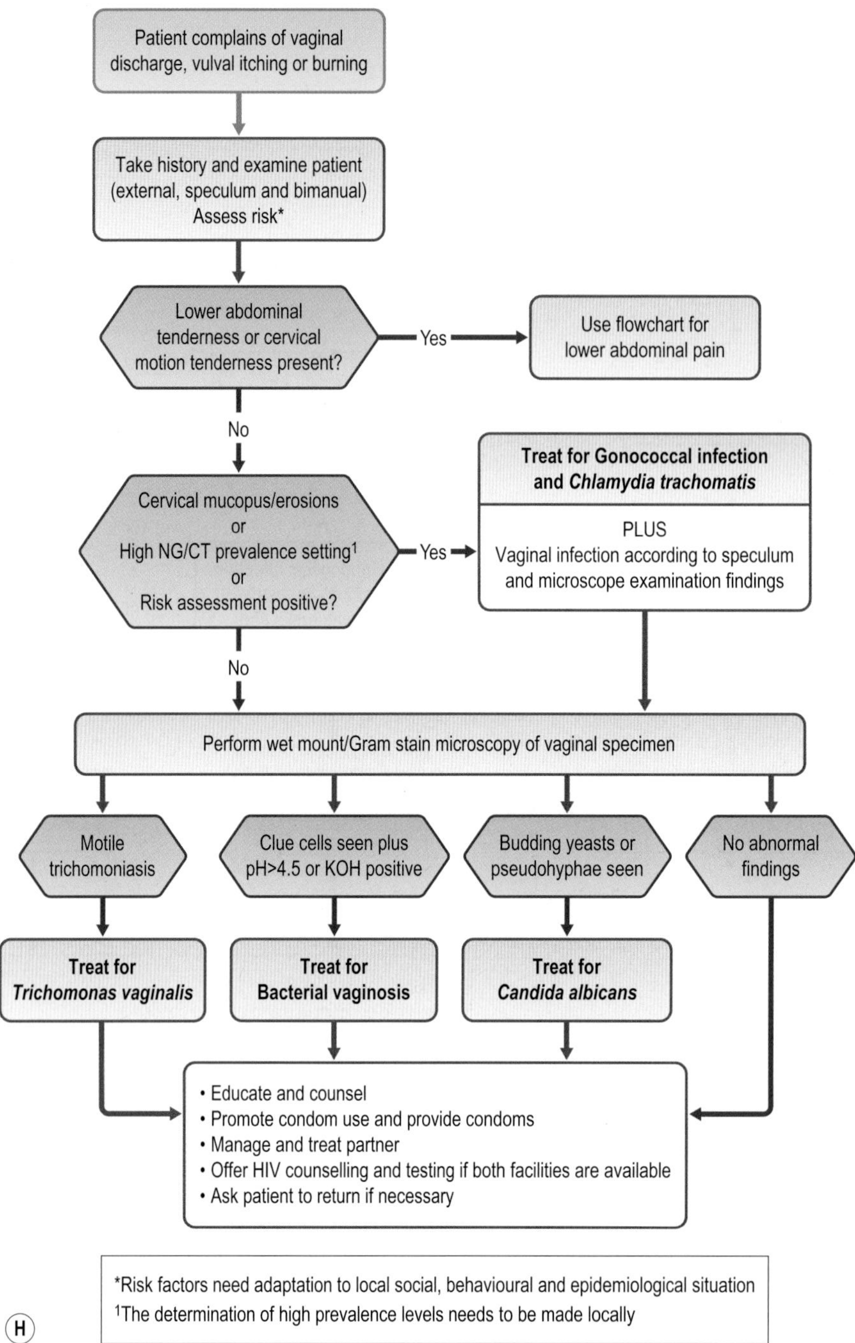

Figure 23-1, cont'd (H) Vaginal discharge: bimanual, speculum, with microscope. KOH, potassium hydroxide OR (amine detection)

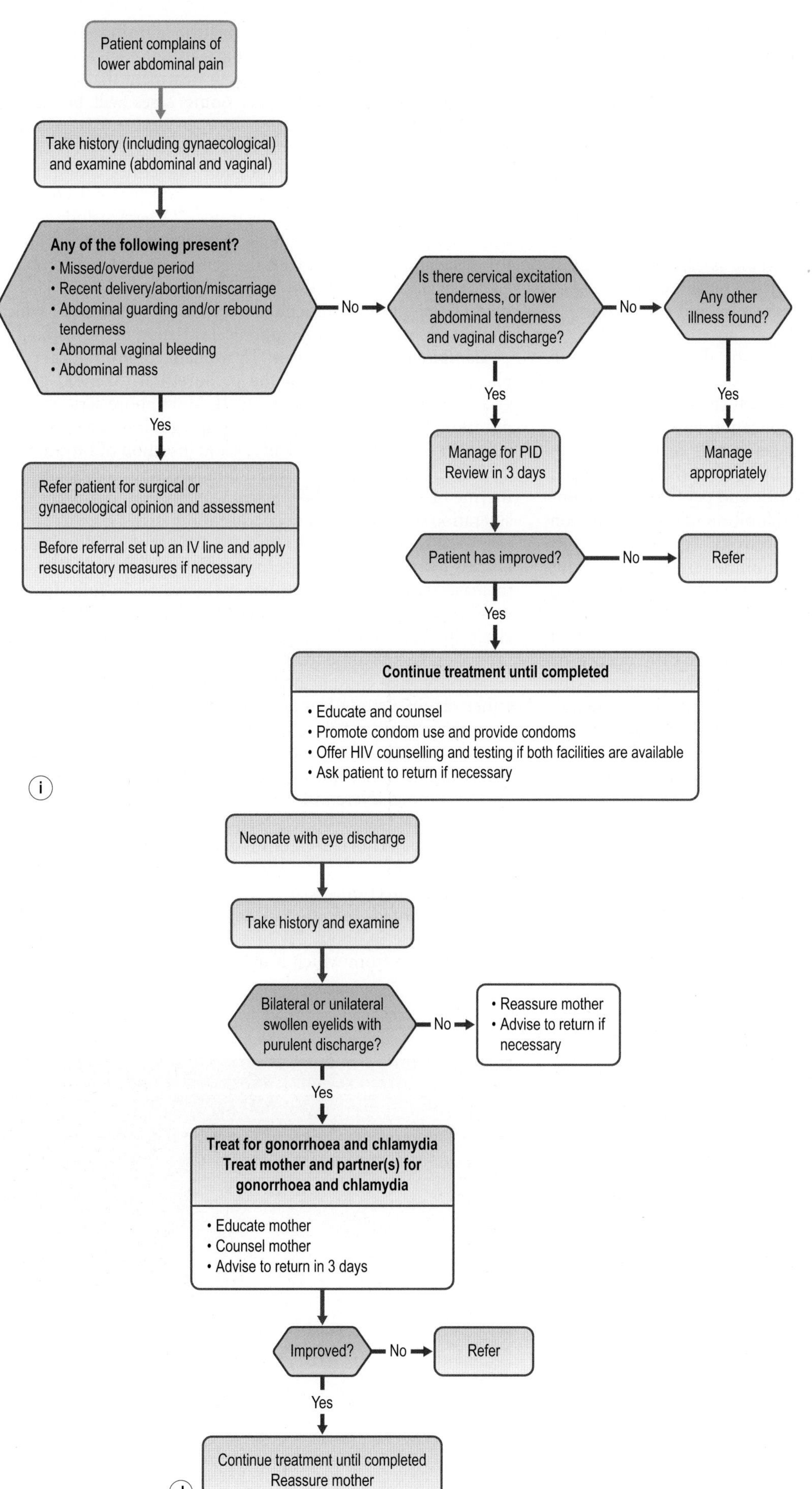

Figure 23-1, cont'd (I) Lower abdominal pain, (J) Neonatal conjunctivitis. PID, pelvic inflammatory disease

men with urethral discharge should be treated for both gonorrhoea and chlamydial infection (this will also cover most cases of *Ureaplasma* and *Mycoplasma* infection). Cases in which it is possible to exclude gonorrhoea by microscopy of a Gram stain can be treated for chlamydial infection alone.

GONORRHOEA

Gonorrhoea is the most prevalent bacterial STI in the tropics. The causative organism, *Neisseria gonorrhoeae*, a Gram-negative oval diplococcus found only in human, is especially adept at colonizing the epithelial surfaces of the male and female urogenital tract, conjunctiva, pharynx, rectum and synovium.

Pathogenesis. Virulence is conferred by the presence of pili which mediate adherence, sufficient to withstand hydrodynamic forces within the urethra, and which also inhibit uptake by phagocytes. Invasion and multiplication have been demonstrated in mucus-secreting non-ciliated cells of the Fallopian tubes. No specific toxins produced by *N. gonorrhoeae* have been identified but the lipo-oligosaccharide and peptidoglycan components have been implicated in inhibition of ciliary function and the genesis of synovitis, respectively. *N. gonorrhoeae* is highly adept at avoiding the host immune response. The pilus antigens, the protein designated Por (formerly protein I, PI) and the lipo-oligosaccharide are all capable of antigenic variation sufficient to permit repeated reinfection of the same host within a short period. Antibodies to Rmp (formerly PIII) do not fix complement and can block bactericidal, complement-fixing antibodies to the lipo-oligosaccharide. The bacteria produce an IgA_1 protease which may impair the host mucosal immune response. The mucosal immune response to infection is characterized by the production of IgA, IgM and IgE, which can inhibit adherence and facilitate opsonization. These responses have been demonstrated in both infected and non-infected exposed contacts of infected individuals. Strains responsible for disseminated gonococcal infection have been shown to be less susceptible to killing by human serum, are less chemotactic to neutrophils and elicit greater amounts of blocking antibody.

Clinical Features. The risk of contracting gonorrhoea after a single exposure is about 20% for males and probably higher for females. Typically men develop symptoms after a 2–5-day incubation period, with 90% of symptomatic infections manifesting within 14 days. Asymptomatic infections are frequent in women – up to 80% of infections are detected in contacts of symptomatic partners. Community-based studies from Tanzania have indicated much higher levels of asymptomatic gonorrhoea in males than previously recorded (about 85%).[20]

Symptomatic uncomplicated infections in males typically manifest as a thick, yellow urethral discharge. In symptomatic females, vaginal discharge or dysuria are the major symptoms. Accompanying symptoms include a variable degree of meatal itching, burning, dysuria, frequency and oedema. Infections of the pharynx and rectum (mostly asymptomatic) can result from orogenital and genito–anal sexual contact. In females the rectum is easily infected by contamination from an infected vaginal discharge. Gonococcal infection may present as vulvovaginitis in children infected by sexual abuse or by infected fomites.

Complications in Men. In males, spread of the infection to the epididymis, usually unilaterally, is the most common complication (20% of patients not receiving antibiotics). Acute epididymitis has initially to be distinguished from acute torsion. Because it is often difficult to establish an aetiological diagnosis, sexually active males should be given treatment that is effective for gonorrhoea and chlamydia. Some cases will be due to mumps virus infection, and in older men Gram-negative bacilli from the urinary tract may be responsible.

The older literature on gonorrhoea describes a number of complications seldom encountered in industrialized countries but which may still be seen in the tropics.[21] These include abscess and fistula formation resulting from spread of infection to various glands associated with the genitourinary tract (prostate, glands of Tyson, Littré, Cowper). Ultimately, these may lead to urethral stricture, a difficult complication to manage, which appears to show marked geographical variation in the tropics.[22,23]

Complications in Women. In women, common local complications are infections of the paraurethral (Skene's) glands and Bartholin's glands (Figure 23.2). Much more serious complications may ensue when infection spreads into the uterus and fallopian tubes. Abortion, delivery and insertion of intrauterine devices are risk factors for ascending infection. Intermenstrual uterine bleeding in sexually active women should prompt consideration of a possible gonococcal endometritis. Further spread may lead to acute complications such as acute salpingitis and abscess formation or long-term problems of chronic PID, and increased risk of ectopic pregnancy (increased 10-fold after one episode of salpingitis). Acute salpingitis has to be differentiated clinically from ectopic pregnancy (pregnancy test, ultrasonography) and acute appendicitis (laparoscopy).

Sterility may complicate both overt and silent infection in either sex. In a study from central Africa, fallopian tube occlusion was present in 83% of infertile women.[24] Acute salpingitis has been estimated to produce sterility in 17% of patients, the risk rising with multiple episodes of infection, in older patients and with more severe inflammation. Gonorrhoea in pregnancy has been associated with low birth weight,[25] premature rupture of membranes, chorioamnionitis and postpartum upper genital tract infection.[26] There is also a higher risk of disseminated gonococcal infection.

Disseminated Infection. Disseminated gonococcal infection may arise in about 2% of patients with gonorrhoea. The local infection from which it originates is often asymptomatic.

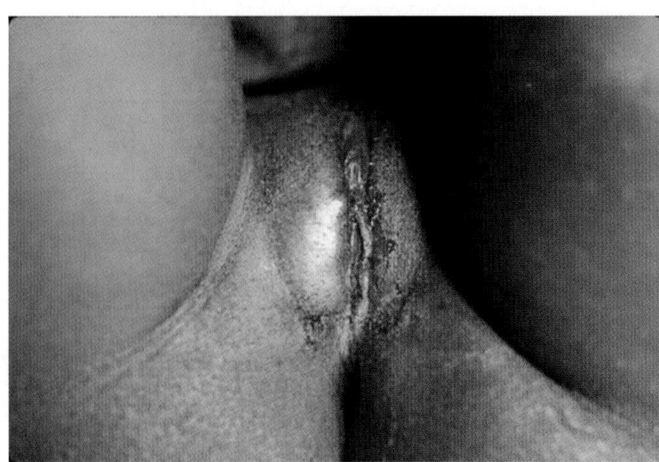

Figure 23.2 Acute bartholinitis due to gonorrhoea. *(Courtesy of D. Mabey.)*

It manifests most often as an asymmetric oligoarthritis with a predilection for knees, ankles and large and small joints of the upper limb. Tenosynovitis occurs frequently. The skin lesions (classically the tender necrotic pustule, but many other forms also occur) often noted in white skins are rare in dark-skinned patients. Gonococcal arthritis accounts for as much as 20% of acute arthritis in young adults in the tropics.[27] It has to be differentiated from other septic arthritides, and in particular from reactive arthritis, which is also often sexually acquired. Rarer manifestations of disseminated gonococcal infection include endocarditis and meningitis. A total of 7 days therapy with an extended-spectrum cephalosporin is recommended.

Ocular Gonococcal Infections. Ocular gonococcal infection in adults, which is presumed to follow autoinoculation with a contaminated finger in most cases, is a common and potentially blinding complication in developing countries.[28] It presents as an acute purulent conjunctivitis which may progress rapidly to corneal perforation in the absence of adequate systemic and topical antimicrobial treatment.

Ophthalmia Neonatorum. Ophthalmia neonatorum is defined as an acute conjunctivitis occurring in the first month of life. The high prevalence of infection with *N. gonorrhoeae* and *C. trachomatis* among pregnant women in many tropical countries is reflected in a correspondingly high incidence of ophthalmia neonatorum, which occurs in 30–50% of children born to infected mothers if prophylaxis is not administered.

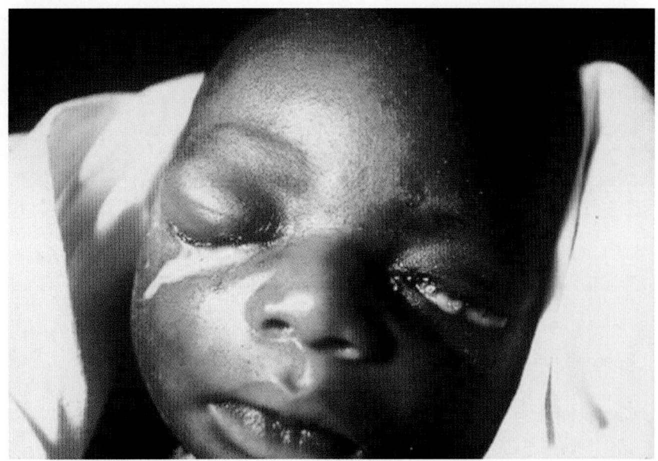

Figure 23.3 Gonococcal ophthalmia in a 7-day-old neonate. *(Courtesy of D. Mabey.)*

Ophthalmia neonatorum usually presents as an acute bilateral purulent conjunctivitis (Figure 23.3). Gonococcal infections frequently present in the first week and can lead to blindness. The diagnosis can often be made by microscopy (Gram stain for gonorrhoea, Giemsa-stain for chlamydial inclusions). Cultures should be made when possible. Systemic and topical treatment (Table 23.2) should be administered to the

TABLE 23.2 Recommended treatment for STIs[a]

Disease	First-line Antibiotics	Alternative Antibiotics	Notes
Gonorrhoea	Cefixime 400 mg×1 *OR* Ceftriaxone 250 mg IM×1 *OR* Spectinomycin 2 g IM ×1		Presumptive treatment for chlamydia co-infection is recommended. Disseminated infections require daily treatment for 1 week. Resistance to cephalosporins is starting to emerge.[29]
Gonococcal ophthalmia	Ceftriaxone 50 mg/kg IM ×1	Spectinomycin 25 mg/kg IM ×1 or kanamycin 25 mg/kg IM ×1	Special precautions need to be taken to avoid nosocomial spread of infection.
Chlamydia	Doxycycline 100 mg twice daily for 1 week *OR* Azithromycin 1 g×1	Erythromycin 500 mg four times daily for 7 days	Amoxicillin has been validated for use in pregnant women. Azithromycin is recommended for pregnant women by WHO
Chlamydial ophthalmia	Erythromycin syrup 50 mg/kg per day divided in 4 doses for 14 days		
Early syphilis	Benzathine penicillin 2.4 MU IM ×1	Doxycycline 100 mg twice daily for 14 days *OR* Procaine penicillin 1.2 MU IM daily×10	Strains of *T. pallidum* with resistance to azithromycin have been reported in some parts of the world. Extended courses of penicillin are needed for late or complicated syphilis. Doses of benzathine are usually given half into each buttock.
Late syphilis	Benzathine penicillin 2.4 MU IM once weekly×3		
Early congenital syphilis	Procaine penicillin 50 000 units/kg IM daily for 10 days		
Chancroid	Ciprofloxacin 500 mg twice daily for 3 days *OR* Ceftriaxone 250 mg IM ×1 *OR* Azithromycin 1 g×1	Erythromycin 500 mg 4 times daily for 7 days	Fluctuant inguinal buboes may require needle aspiration or incision and drainage.

Continued on following page

TABLE 23.2 **Recommended treatment for STIs[a]—cont'd**

Disease	First-line Antibiotics	Alternative Antibiotics	Notes
Lymphogranuloma venereum	Doxycycline 100 mg twice daily for 21 days	Erythromycin 500 mg 4 times daily for 21 days	Treatment failure reported following use of azithromycin for rectal LGV
Donovanosis	Azithromycin 500 mg daily or 1 g weekly Doxycycline 100 mg twice daily	Erythromycin 500 mg twice daily Ciprofloxacin 500 mg twice daily Tetracycline Co-trimoxazole	Treatment should be continued until lesions have re-epithelialized.
Trichomoniasis	Metronidazole 2 g×1	Tinidazole 2 g×1	Higher doses of metronidazole may be required to overcome resistance in some cases
Bacterial vaginosis	Metronidazole 2 g×1 or 4–500 mg twice daily for 5–7 days	Clindamycin 2% cream 5 g daily for 7 days	Treatment of sexual partners is not indicated.
Candidiasis	Clotrimazole 500 mg×1 *OR* Fluconazole 150 mg×1 *OR* Econazole 150 mg *OR* clotrimazole 200 mg daily for 3 days	Nystatin	Treatment of sexual partners is not indicated.
Genital herpes (first episode)	Aciclovir 200 mg five times daily for 5–10 days	Valaciclovir 500 mg twice daily for 5 days *OR* Famciclovir 250 mg three times daily for 5 days	Topical therapy is less effective than the oral route. Aciclovir treatment is less useful during recurrent episodes. If used, it needs to be started <24 h after the onset of lesions.
Genital herpes (recurrent episodes)	Aciclovir 200 mg five times daily for 7 days *OR* Aciclovir 400 mg three times daily for 7 days	Valaciclovir 500 mg twice daily (or 1 g once daily) for 7 days *OR* Famciclovir 125 mg twice daily for 7 days	
Genital herpes (suppression)	Aciclovir 400 mg twice daily	Valaciclovir 0.5–1 g daily *OR* Famciclovir 125 mg twice daily	
Genital warts (self-treatment)	Podophyllotoxin Imiquimod 5% cream		
Genital warts (provider treatment)	10–25% podophyllin Cryotherapy with liquid nitrogen	80–90% trichloroacetic acid Surgical excision or electrosurgery	
Non-gonococcal urethritis	Doxycycline 100 mg twice daily for 7 days *OR* Azithromycin 1 g×1	Erythromycin 500 mg twice daily for 14 days	Treatment with metronidazole 2 g or azithromycin 1 g can be used in patients not responding to their first treatment.
Pelvic inflammatory disease (PID)	Treatment for gonorrhoea plus doxycycline 100 mg twice daily plus metronidazole 400 mg twice daily for 2 weeks	Clindamycin 900 mg IV 8-hourly plus gentamicin 1.5 mg/kg IV 8-hourly	Treatment for gonorrhoea may be omitted in low prevalence settings where a culture has been taken. Intravenous treatment is indicated for more severe cases and is continued for 3 days after improvement and then followed with oral doxycycline for 14 days.
Epididymitis	Treatment for gonorrhoea and treatment for *Chlamydia*	Ciprofloxacin 500 mg twice daily for 10 days Ofloxacin 200 mg twice daily for 7–14 days	Above the age of 40 epididymitis is less likely to be caused by STIs and treatment for other pathogens such as *E. coli* with ciprofloxacin or ofloxacin may be indicated. Severe cases may require intravenous antibiotics.
Genital scabies	Permethrin 5% *OR* Malathion 0.5%	Benzyl benzoate 25% *OR* Ivermectin 200 μg/kg repeated after 2 weeks	Ivermectin has proved useful in treatment of patients with crusted scabies.
Pediculosis	Malathion 0.5% *OR* Permethrin 1% *OR* Phenothrin 0.2% *OR* Carbaryl 0.5 and 1%		If the eyelashes are involved a 10 min application of permethrin 1% lotion with the eyes closed can be used.

[a]These recommendations are drawn from STI Treatment Guidelines published by the World Health Organization (2003, revised 2008), Centers for Disease Control and Prevention (2010) and the British Association for Sexual Health and HIV (most recent updates 2010–12).

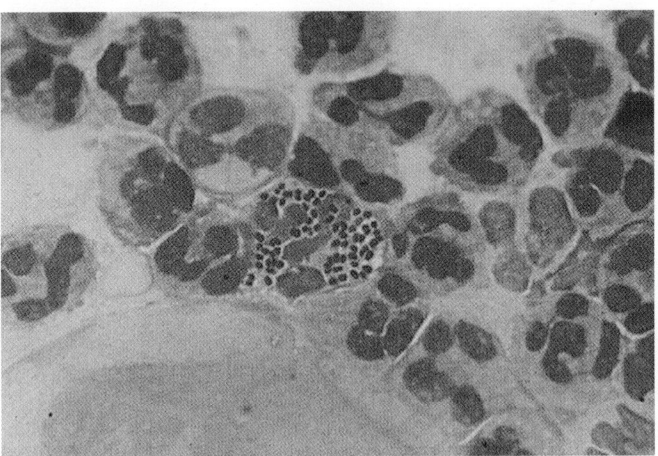

Figure 23.4 Appearance of *Neisseria gonorrhoeae* in a Gram-stained smear of urethral discharge.

neonate, and the mother and her sexual partner(s) should also be treated.[29]

The use of ocular prophylaxis in countries where the prevalence of gonorrhoea in antenatal women exceeds 1% is highly cost-effective. The high prevalence of antibiotic-resistant strains of *N. gonorrhoeae* poses a problem for ocular prophylaxis but one trial has demonstrated that 2.5% povidone-iodine was as effective as 1% silver nitrate in preventing chlamydial and gonococcal ophthalmia.[30]

Laboratory Diagnosis. The diagnosis of gonorrhoea traditionally rests on the isolation of *N. gonorrhoeae*, which remains essential if determination of antibiotic susceptibility is required. This is not feasible in many health facilities in the tropics. The demonstration of Gram-negative diplococci in urethral smears (Figure 23.4) has a sensitivity and specificity of >95% for the diagnosis of gonorrhoea in symptomatic males, but both sensitivity (<50%) and specificity are considerably lower in females, where culture is the method of choice. In disseminated infection, specimens from joints, blood or skin lesions give a rather poor yield and the organism may be isolated more readily from the genital tract.

When cultures are to be made, the sites for swabbing should be determined by the history and examination findings. In males, it is best to obtain a urethral specimen by insertion and rotation of a swab in the urethra for 5 s. For women, the ectocervix should be wiped clean and a swab should be inserted into the cervical os and rotated for 10 s. Rectal swabs are best obtained through a proctoscope. *N. gonorrhoeae* is a delicate organism, highly susceptible to drying, and prompt inoculation of media and careful adherence to recommended laboratory technique is important to maximize isolation rates.

Nucleic acid amplification tests (NAAT) for gonorrhoea are being used increasingly. They have superior sensitivity to culture. In men, urine and urethral samples show comparable sensitivity and, in women, endocervical and vaginal swabs (but not urine) show comparable sensitivity. NAATs can also be used on rectal and pharyngeal specimens.

Treatment. Gonorrhoea is treated ideally with a single dose of supervised oral treatment (Table 23.2). The dose administered should give a serum level of at least three times the minimum inhibitory concentration for ≥8 h. Throughout the tropics an increasing proportion of isolates of *N. gonorrhoeae* show both plasmid- and chromosomally mediated resistance to penicillin, tetracyclines, and quinolones.[31] WHO recommendations for the treatment of uncomplicated gonorrhoea are shown in Table 23.2. A test of cure should be recommended if resources permit, prioritizing suspected treatment failure, pharyngeal infections or when first-line treatment has not been used.

Treatment of contacts should extend to all individuals exposed within 2 weeks of the onset of symptoms in the index case and within 4 weeks of diagnosis of asymptomatic infected individuals. Many clinicians offer blind treatment for chlamydial infection to all patients with gonorrhoea. In the UK in 2009, *Chlamydia* was identified in 35% of heterosexual males and 41% of females with gonorrhoea.

Prevention. The major obstacle to the control of gonorrhoea is the large reservoir of asymptomatic or clinically nonspecific infections in women and the difficulty of establishing the diagnosis in women. The greatly increased cost of effective treatment for resistant gonorrhoea is an added burden for tropical countries. Given these constraints it is more appropriate to direct resources to condom promotion and other safe sex messages than to costly strategies to increase case-finding and treatment. The development of vaccines for gonorrhoea has been hindered by the antigenic variation manifest by the organism.

CHLAMYDIAL INFECTIONS

The demonstration in 1909 of chlamydial inclusions in cervical scrapings from the mother of an infant with inclusion conjunctivitis and in urethral scrapings from her male partner laid the basis for our understanding of genital chlamydial infections, but it was not until it became possible to isolate *Chlamydia trachomatis* in tissue culture in 1965 that the extent of the morbidity due to this organism became clear.

Epidemiology. *C. trachomatis* is the most prevalent sexually transmitted bacterial pathogen in industrialized countries,[32] and appears to be at least equally prevalent in developing countries (Box 23.1). Studies in industrialized countries have shown that genital chlamydial infection is more prevalent in younger age groups, even after taking account of differences in sexual activity, implying that some degree of protective immunity may develop after natural infection.

Aetiology. *C. trachomatis* is a Gram-negative bacterium which is an obligate parasite of eukaryotic cells. The genus *Chlamydia* has a unique developmental cycle. The metabolically inert infectious elementary body has a rigid cell wall and is adapted for extracellular survival. It appears to infect preferentially columnar epithelial cells, by which it is actively taken up. After entering the host cell it differentiates over a number of hours to the metabolically active reticulate body, which divides by binary fission until an intracellular inclusion is formed, which may contain several thousand organisms. The cycle is completed when reticulate bodies condense to form elementary bodies, which are released from the inclusion after lysis of the host cell.

A number of serotypes of *C. trachomatis* have been identified by the microimmunofluorescence test.[33] Serotypes A–C cause ocular infection in trachoma-endemic areas, whereas serotypes D–K cause genital tract infections worldwide. Serotypes L1, L2 and L3 are more invasive both in vitro and in vivo, and cause lymphogranuloma venereum (LGV). The *C. trachomatis* genome contains genes homologous with those coding for virulence factors in other bacteria, including a cytotoxin gene, genes encoding a type III secretion pathway and a protease, proteasome-like activity factor (CPAF), which is secreted into the host cell cytoplasm, where it interferes with the assembly and surface expression of HLA molecules and inhibits apoptosis.[34] A recent study has identified genetic variations in six genes of *C. trachomatis* that are associated with increased virulence in a primate model.[35]

Pathology. The pathological hallmarks of infection with *C. trachomatis* are: (1) the subepithelial lymphoid follicle; and (2) fibrosis and scarring. The latter may progress for months and years even in the absence of chlamydial organisms demonstrable by conventional means. The host immune system is believed to play an important part in the pathogenesis of chlamydial infections, and studies of gene expression at the site of infection have shown the importance of innate immune pathways in the scarring process. Case–control studies have identified polymorphisms in several immune response genes associated with the development of scarring following ocular *C. trachomatis* infection.[36,37]

Clinical Features. The clinical spectrum of disease due to chlamydial infection is similar to that seen in gonococcal infection. Although, in general, chlamydial infections are less likely than gonococcal to cause severe symptoms, they are more likely to cause serious sequelae, particularly in women.[38]

In males, chlamydial infection causes urethritis and, in a proportion of cases, epididymo-orchitis. It is possible that urethral stricture is a late sequela of chlamydial urethritis.

In females, chlamydial cervicitis is often asymptomatic. Sometimes patients will complain of vaginal discharge, and the finding of a mucopurulent discharge at the cervical os is suggestive of chlamydial or gonococcal cervicitis. Ascending infection of the female genital tract may lead to endometritis, salpingitis or PID and this is facilitated by trauma to the cervix, e.g. during childbirth, insertion of an intrauterine device or termination of pregnancy. Because the symptoms of chlamydial PID are often mild, patients may present only when the sequelae of irreversible damage to the Fallopian tubes (infertility, ectopic pregnancy) become apparent. Infection may track to the right upper quadrant, giving rise to a perihepatitis with characteristic adhesions between the liver capsule and peritoneum (Curtis–FitzHugh syndrome).

In both sexes, a sexually acquired reactive arthritis has been described as a sequel of chlamydial infection. This may involve both large and small joints and be accompanied by enthesitis and skin lesions (circinate balanitis and keratodermia blennorrhagica).

Some 30% of infants born to infected mothers become infected. In the majority of cases the only consequence of this is a self-limiting conjunctivitis presenting within the first 2 weeks of life, but occasionally chlamydial ophthalmia is more severe and if it persists it may give rise to conjunctival scarring. A small proportion of infected infants develop chlamydial pneumonitis, presenting usually between the ages of 6 weeks and 3 months with a paroxysmal cough and tachypnoea in the absence of fever. Rales may be heard on clinical examination, and a chest radiograph often reveals extensive bilateral pulmonary infiltrates with hyperinflation. There is characteristically a raised serum total IgG and IgM, and a mild eosinophilia.[39]

Diagnosis. Nucleic acid amplification tests (NAATs), such as the polymerase chain reaction (PCR) are now the gold standard for the diagnosis of genital chlamydial infection. Several are on the market, but they are expensive, and require expensive equipment as well as careful laboratory practice. NAATs are more sensitive than antigen detection tests or isolation, the sensitivity of which is only approximately 70%.[40] This means that the type of specimen taken is less critical. Whereas for culture and antigen detection it was essential to collect intra-urethral or endocervical samples, NAATs give good results in first-catch urine samples or self-administered vaginal swabs.

Serology has no place in the diagnosis of uncomplicated chlamydial infections, with the exception of the more invasive LGV, but may be helpful in the diagnosis of suspected PID and is the method of choice for the diagnosis of neonatal chlamydial pneumonia. Serological tests may cross-react with the highly prevalent respiratory tract pathogen, *Chlamydia pneumonia*, but a serological assay targeting antibodies to a plasmid-encoded protein of *C. trachomatis*, pg3, appears to be more specific than other assays.[41]

Management. *C. trachomatis* remains sensitive to tetracyclines and macrolides, and single-dose treatment with azithromycin is effective in uncomplicated chlamydial infection (Table 23.2).[42]

VAGINAL DISCHARGE

The three most prevalent causes of vaginal discharge are *Candida albicans, Trichomonas vaginalis* and bacterial vaginosis. *Neisseria gonorrhoeae* and *Chlamydia trachomatis*, which infect the endocervix rather than the vagina, are less commonly associated with symptomatic discharge. Unfortunately, it is not possible to distinguish reliably between these infections on clinical grounds, although the presence of mucopurulent discharge at the cervical os has been proposed as a marker of gonococcal or chlamydial infection. A wet preparation made from a swab collected from the posterior fornix, examined with a phase-contrast microscope, can usually distinguish between candidiasis, trichomoniasis and bacterial vaginosis. Sexual transmission is not considered important in vulvovaginal candidiasis and bacterial vaginosis, and treatment of sexual partners of affected women has not been shown to help women who develop repeated episodes of these infections.

Vulvovaginal Candidiasis

Candida albicans can be isolated from the vagina of up to 50% of sexually active women, the majority of whom are asymptomatic. Although sexual transmission may occur, the gastrointestinal tract has also been implicated as a source of infection. Symptomatic disease is associated with an increase in the number of yeasts present in the vagina; factors which predispose to this are pregnancy, antimicrobial therapy, oral contraceptive use, immunosuppression (e.g. HIV-related) and glycosuria. It has also been suggested that tight, poorly ventilated nylon underclothing, by increasing perineal moisture, may predispose to symptomatic disease.

The cardinal clinical features of vulvovaginal candidiasis are pruritus vulvae and vaginal discharge. The discharge is typically whitish, with curd-like plaques adhering to the vaginal wall, and does not smell. There may be erythema and/or oedema of the vulva and vaginal walls.

The diagnosis can be made on a wet preparation made from the vaginal discharge, the sensitivity of which can be increased by adding 10% potassium hydroxide. Typical mycelia and yeast cells are seen. For the treatment of vulvovaginal candidiasis, see Table 23.2.

Trichomoniasis

Trichomonas vaginalis has been found in the vagina of up to 30% of antenatal clinic attenders in certain African centres. Studies in the USA have shown that its prevalence is higher among women with many partners, and that it can be isolated from a high proportion of male contacts of infected women, suggesting that transmission is primarily through sexual contact. In males, most infections are believed to be asymptomatic and self-limiting, although occasionally it may give rise to urethritis. Studies using more sensitive diagnostic techniques have shown substantially higher rates of infection in males in developing countries.[43]

Up to 75% of women attending STI clinics with *T. vaginalis* infection complain of vaginal discharge. Pruritus vulvae, dyspareunia and dysuria are also common symptoms. On examination, a profuse yellow-green frothy discharge is typically noted. The vulva and vaginal walls may be excoriated and erythematous in severe cases, and punctate haemorrhages may be seen on the cervix.[44]

The diagnosis can be made on a wet preparation collected from the posterior fornix. Under phase contrast, increased numbers of polymorphonuclear leucocytes are usually seen, and motile flagellated parasites, slightly larger than polymorphonuclear leucocytes, are present. Compared with culture, direct microscopy is less than 80% sensitive, so that culture or PCR diagnosis should also be performed when available. For the treatment of trichomoniasis, see Table 23.2.

Bacterial Vaginosis

Bacterial vaginosis is a syndrome in which a malodorous vaginal discharge is associated with characteristic changes in the vaginal bacterial flora. There is a massive increase in numbers of anaerobes, *Gardnerella vaginalis* and *Mycoplasma hominis*, such that protective lactobacilli are no longer predominant. Bacterial vaginosis is common among women of reproductive age, reaching prevalences of 50% in women of black race in some studies. It is considered to be an endogenous, rather than a sexually transmitted infection and symptomatic episodes have been linked to menstruation, presence of an intrauterine contraceptive device and genital douching.

The discharge of bacterial vaginosis is typically homogeneous and white-grey, and associated with increased vaginal pH (>4.5). The characteristic fishy smell (due to amines release) is more easily detectable after the addition of a drop of 10% potassium hydroxide (KOH) (to help define in the flowcharts) to a drop of discharge on a slide. Bacterial vaginosis has been shown to be associated with adverse pregnancy outcome (premature labour, chorioamnionitis and postpartum endometritis).[45] And, more recently, with HIV acquisition and transmission. BV in pregnancy has been associated with second trimester miscarriage and pre-term delivery in a minority of infected women but the value of screening and treating BV in all pregnant women has not been established.

The microbiological diagnosis of bacterial vaginosis can be made on Gram stain of a vaginal swab, according to Nugent's criteria, in which a score is given depending on the relative proportion of lactobacilli and Gram-negative rods and coccobacilli.[45a] A simplified version of Nugent's criteria put forward by Ison and Hay is gaining in popularity and is easier to use than the criteria of Nugent. Essentially, this classifies the flora as either normal (predominantly lactobacilli), mixed flora or BV (clue cells observed).[46] For the treatment of bacterial vaginosis, see Table 23.2.

ANAL DISCHARGE

Anorectal infections with gonorrhoea and *Chlamydia* commonly present in homosexual/bisexual men and transgender individuals with anal discharge, bleeding and tenesmus. Less commonly lymphogranuloma venereum, herpes simplex virus and syphilis cause proctitis and rectal specimens should be tested for these infections when feasible. In clinics where homosexual men attend for screening it is generally advised that specimens for gonorrhoea and *Chlamydia* screening are obtained from the pharynx and rectum in addition to urethral or urine screening.

Diseases Causing Genital Ulceration

CHANCROID

Chancroid, or soft sore, was first distinguished from the hard chancre of syphilis by Ricord in 1838. In 1889, Ducrey, in Naples, showed that the inoculation of material from chancroidal ulcers into the skin of the forearm caused ulceration which could be serially passaged, and identified the causative organism which now bears his name. The development of defined solid media for the isolation of *Haemophilus ducreyi* in the 1970s enabled detailed epidemiological studies of chancroid to be carried out for the first time.[47,48]

Epidemiology

Chancroid is an important cause of genital ulceration in Africa. Before the HIV epidemic it accounted for more than 60% of genital ulcers seen in hospital, but in the 1990s hospital-based studies in several countries found that the proportion of ulcers due to *Herpes simplex* had increased, and that the proportion due to chancroid had decreased correspondingly.[49] Although generally rare in industrialized countries, there have been several well-documented outbreaks in North America since the 1970s. Characteristic features of these outbreaks have been a high male-to-female case ratio, the involvement of prostitutes and the low socioeconomic status of the populations affected. A study in Nairobi investigated the role of asymptomatic females in the transmission of the disease and concluded that they were of little importance.[50] Studies among Australian soldiers during the Vietnam War suggest that chancroid is more common among uncircumcised than circumcised males.[51]

The prevalence of chancroid is high among commercial sex workers in the cities of Africa (Figure 23.5), as is the prevalence of HIV infection. Prospective studies among both males and females at high risk of HIV infection in Nairobi have suggested that chancroid significantly increases the risk of transmission of HIV via heterosexual contact, either by increasing infectivity,

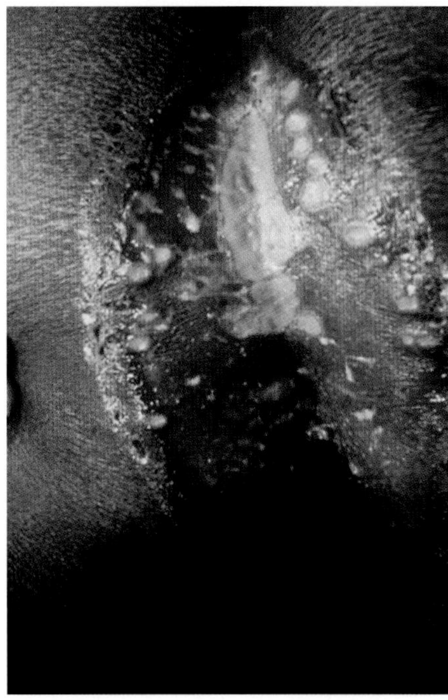

Figure 23.5 Extensive perianal ulceration resulting from a *Haemophilus ducreyi* infection in a sex worker. *(Courtesy of D. Mabey.)*

susceptibility or both.[52,53] The unusually high rates of partner change required to sustain the transmission of chancroid make it a tempting target for local disease control campaigns and suggest that, compared to other STIs, it presents a relatively easy target for global elimination.[54]

Aetiology

Chancroid is caused by *Haemophilus ducreyi*, a small facultatively anaerobic Gram-negative bacillus which requires haemin (X factor), reduces nitrate to nitrite and forms typical streptobacillary chains on Gram stain. It is a fastidious organism which will only grow on enriched media and grows best at 30–33°C in an atmosphere of 5% carbon dioxide.

Pathogenesis

Histopathologically, chancroidal ulcers contain three distinct zones: a superficial zone consisting of necrotic tissue, fibrin and numerous bacteria; an intermediate zone showing oedema and new vessel formation; and a deep zone containing a dense infiltrate of neutrophils and plasma cells with fibroblastic proliferation.

Studies involving the inoculation of human volunteers have improved our understanding of the pathogenesis of chancroid.[55] The application of *H. ducreyi* to the human forearm does not produce a lesion unless the skin is traumatized. There is some evidence that virulent strains are relatively resistant to phagocytosis by human polymorphonuclear leucocytes and to complement-mediated killing by normal human and rabbit serum. An isogenic mutant lacking a receptor for haemoglobin showed reduced virulence in humans.[56] Two toxins have been characterized: one is a cell-associated haemolysin, similar to those produced by *Proteus mirabilis*, toxic to human foreskin fibroblasts but not to HeLa cells in tissue culture. The other is a soluble toxin, homologous to the cytolethal distending toxin produced by a number of enteric organisms, which is toxic to

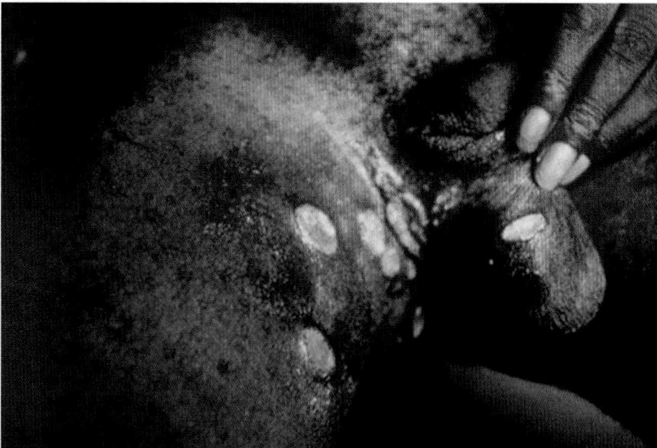

Figure 23.6 Chancroid: multiple soft painful ulcers. *(Courtesy of D. Mabey.)*

a variety of cell lines.[57] The suppurating lymphadenopathy of chancroid is notable for the large number of neutrophils and small number of bacilli present.

Clinical Features

After an incubation period of 3–7 days, a papule appears at the site of inoculation which soon ulcerates. The typical ulcer of chancroid (Figure 23.6) is painful and soft, has a purulent base with an undermined edge, and bleeds on contact. Multiple ulcers are commonly present, and there is painful inguinal lymphadenopathy (Figure 23.7) in some 50% of cases, often unilateral. Atypical presentations are, however, common, and even in experienced hands chancroid cannot reliably be distinguished from primary syphilis on clinical grounds.[58] Herpes simplex, LGV and donovanosis must also be considered in the differential diagnosis of chancroid. Chancroid may cause extensive local destruction (Figure 23.8), particularly in HIV-infected individuals who may fail to respond to antimicrobial treatment, but the infection does not disseminate.

Diagnosis

Gram stain of smears obtained from ulcers has been advocated in the past for the diagnosis of chancroid, but this lacks both

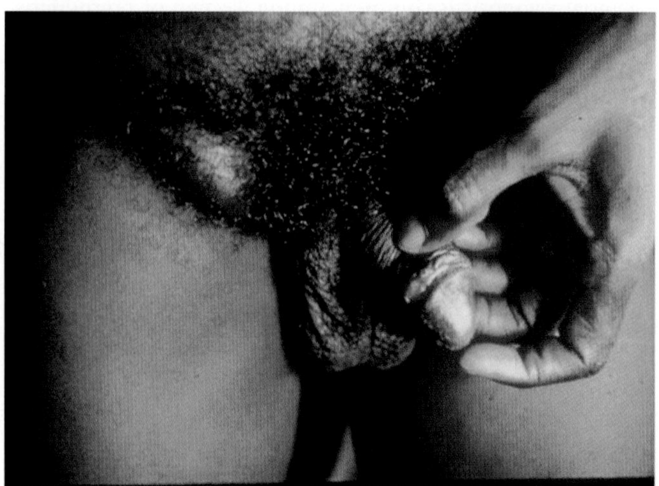

Figure 23.7 Chancroid: ulcer of corona accompanied by a painful bubo. *(Courtesy of D. Mabey.)*

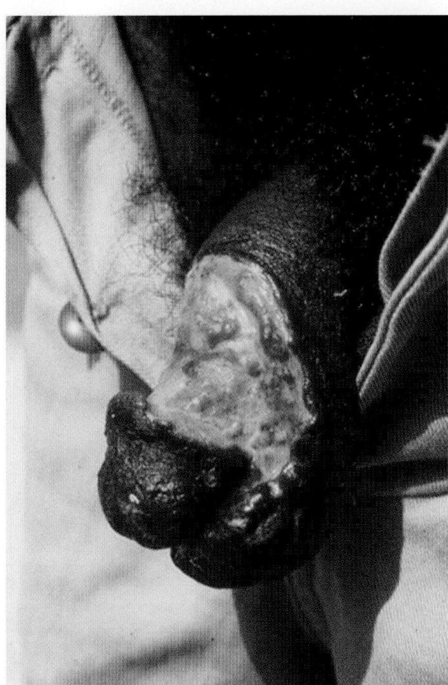

Figure 23.8 Phagedenic chancroid: destructive ulcer of penile shaft. *(Courtesy of D. Mabey.)*

sensitivity and specificity. Preferred methods for the laboratory diagnosis of chancroid are now either isolation of *H. ducreyi* from the ulcer or the use of NAATs. Swabs for culture should be taken from the ulcer base or its undermined edge and plated directly on appropriate blood-containing media enriched with fetal calf serum and Vitox and made selective with vancomycin. For optimal rates of isolation, media made up from both GC agar and Mueller–Hinton agar base should be inoculated. Plates should be incubated for at least 72 h in an atmosphere of 5% carbon dioxide at 33°C. *H. ducreyi* is identified by its typical colonial morphology (colonies are difficult to break up and can be moved intact across the surface of the agar), Gram stain and inability to ferment sugars.

Management

Chancroidal ulcers should be kept clean and dry, with regular washing in soapy water. Ciprofloxacin 500 mg daily for 3 days by mouth, ceftriaxone 500 mg as a single intramuscular dose or azithromycin as a single 1 g oral dose are all effective (see Table 23.2). Longer courses of treatment may be required in HIV-positive patients.

SYPHILIS

History

Syphilis, a young shepherd boy, was the eponymous hero of a Latin poem written in 1530 by the Italian G. Fracastorio. He succumbed to an apparently new disease which had swept across Europe a few years earlier in the wake of the French army's retreat from Naples. The timing of this epidemic led to the suggestion that syphilis had been brought back from the New World by Columbus and his men in 1493. An alternative hypothesis put forward by E. H. Hudson, a physician working in the 1930s in Mesopotamia (now Iraq), was that syphilis originated as an endemic infection of childhood (yaws) in the hot humid tropics, and that venereal transmission only became important when living standards improved sufficiently to prevent transmission in childhood giving rise to long-lasting immunity. This so-called unitarian hypothesis is supported by recent evidence of very close DNA homology between *Treponema pallidum* and the organism causing yaws, *T. pertenue* (recently re-classified as *T. pallidum* subsp. *pertenue*).[59,60] Studies in animal models do however demonstrate different tissue tropisms between *pallidum* and *pertenue* strains of *T. pallidum*.[61] Although syphilis in all its clinical aspects had been described in detail by nineteenth-century physicians, notably Hutchinson in Britain and Fournier in France, it was not until 1905 that the causative organism, *T. pallidum*, was first identified by Schaudinn and Hoffman; in 1906, Wasserman described the first serological test for the diagnosis of syphilis. Investigation of the *T. pallidum* genome is yielding important insights into the extraordinary survival capability of *T. pallidum* following human infection.[62]

Epidemiology

The incidence of syphilis has declined steadily for most of the twentieth century in Western Europe and North America, with the exception of a brief rise during and immediately after each world war. Since the mid-1990s there were notable increases in syphilis among men who have sex with men in many developed countries.

There are no reliable incidence figures for developing countries. Seroprevalence surveys have shown high rates of positivity among antenatal clinic attenders and in the general population in many African countries.[3,63] The relative rarity of late syphilis in parts of Africa where early syphilis is common has led to speculation that the disease has become more common in recent years, perhaps reflecting loss of herd immunity following the mass treatment campaigns against endemic treponemal disease in the 1950s and 1960s.

Transmission by sexual contact requires exposure to moist mucosal or cutaneous lesions; experiments in the rabbit suggest that an inoculum of some 50 organisms is sufficient to initiate infection. The rate of transmission from an infected partner is approximately 30%.

Aetiology

Syphilis is caused by *T. pallidum*, one of a small group of treponemes (of the order *Spirochaetales*) pathogenic to man. It cannot be distinguished morphologically from the agents responsible for yaws and pinta (*T. pallidum* subsp. *pertenue* and *T. carateum*, respectively). It is a spiral organism 6–15 mm in length and 0.15 mm in width, visible by light microscopy only under conditions of dark-field illumination, and cannot be grown on artificial media. In tissue culture and in animal models it divides slowly, with a replication time of approximately 30 h. The cell wall of *T. pallidum* is remarkable for a very low density of outer membrane proteins, which probably contributes to the organism's ability to persist in its host for lengthy periods. It is highly susceptible to drying.

Pathogenesis

T. pallidum has not been shown to produce either exotoxins or endotoxins. Following experimental infection in the rabbit, *T. pallidum* begins to replicate once it has passed through the epithelium. An initial polymorphonuclear leucocyte response at the lesion is soon replaced by an infiltrate of T and

B lymphocytes. The primary chancre also contains mucoid material, mainly hyaluronic acid and chondroitin sulfate, which may modulate the host immune response. Both circulating *T. pallidum*-specific T cells and specific antibody can be found in the majority of cases of primary syphilis. At the same time as these are first noted, the number of organisms in the lesion decreases and the ulcer begins to heal, suggesting that the immune system is controlling the infection.

The appearance of secondary lesions some weeks later, due to the dissemination of organisms and circulating immune complexes, indicates that this is not the case. Secondary syphilis coincides with the emergence of an antigenically distinct new strain which is no longer susceptible to antibodies directed at the infecting strain.[62] Much of the pathology of secondary syphilis may be immune complex mediated. High levels of anti-treponemal antibody are present in the circulation, but cell-mediated immune responses are depressed.

Eventually cell-mediated immune responses to *T. pallidum* are restored as the lesions are brought under control, leading to the latent stage. Follow-up studies in the pre-penicillin era showed that relapse of infectious secondary lesions occurred in up to 25% of cases. The organism can survive in the body for many years thereafter, causing tertiary lesions characterized by the presence of a small number of organisms and a lymphocytic host response giving rise to an endarteritis.

Clinical Features

After an incubation period of 10–70 days (median 21 days), a primary chancre (Figure 23.9) develops at the site of inoculation. The chancre is typically painless, indurated, with a clean base and a raised edge, and does not bleed on contact. There is usually only a single lesion; in the male it is most commonly on the glans, the foreskin, the coronal sulcus or the shaft of the penis, and in the female on the cervix or vulva. The primary chancre is often accompanied by inguinal lymphadenopathy; the glands are characteristically hard (the 'bullet bubo' of Hutchinson) and painless.

The primary chancre generally resolves spontaneously over several weeks. Between 3 and 6 weeks after its first appearance, the features of secondary syphilis appear. The rash of secondary syphilis may take many forms: papular, macular or pustular; annular lesions are not uncommon. It often desquamates, but in moist areas of the body (e.g. perineum, axilla) soft raised

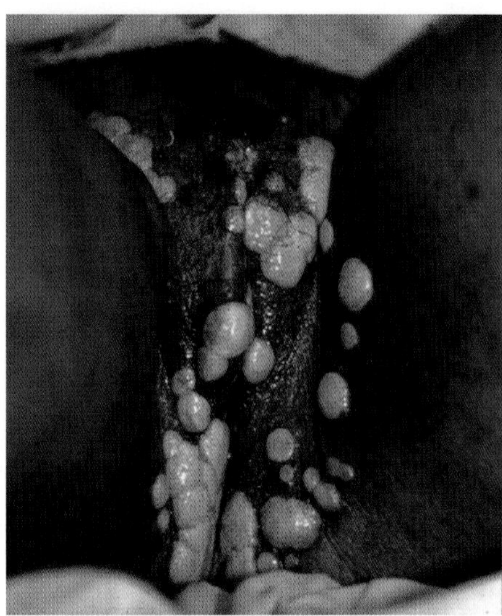

Figure 23.10 Secondary syphilis: condylomata lata. *(Courtesy of J. Richens.)*

condylomata lata may be seen (Figures 23.10, 23.11). It generally affects the palms (Figure 23.12) and soles, and does not itch. The mucous membranes may be involved, with mucous patches or oral ulceration sometimes in the form of the characteristic 'snail track' ulcer. In addition to its cutaneous manifestations secondary syphilis may cause systemic illness (fever, malaise), generalized lymphadenopathy, nephritis, hepatitis, meningitis or uveitis.

The lesions of secondary syphilis generally resolve after several weeks, although relapses commonly occurred in the pre-antibiotic era. In the absence of adequate treatment the patient then enters the latent stage of the disease, and is liable to develop tertiary syphilis at some time in the future.

The lesions of tertiary syphilis fall into three categories: the gumma, cardiovascular disease and central nervous system disease. The classic Oslo study of untreated syphilis, in which some 1400 patients were followed for up to 50 years, found that the most common manifestation was the gumma, a painless 'punched out' ulcer with little or no inflammatory reaction, which developed in 15%: 70% were cutaneous, 10% involved bone and rarely the viscera were involved. Most cases occurred in the first 15 years following infection. Cardiovascular lesions

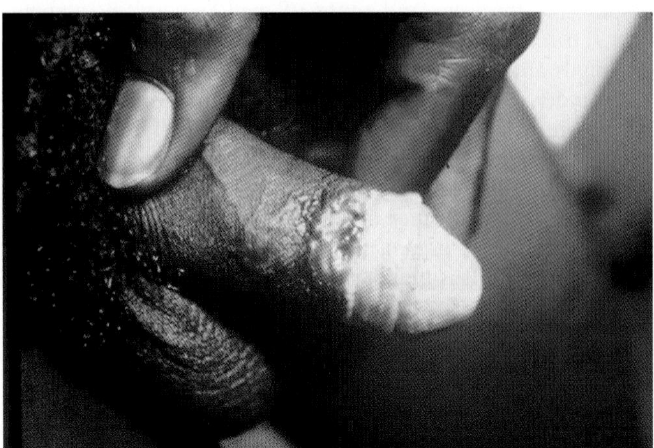

Figure 23.9 Syphilis: primary chancre. *(Courtesy of D. Mabey.)*

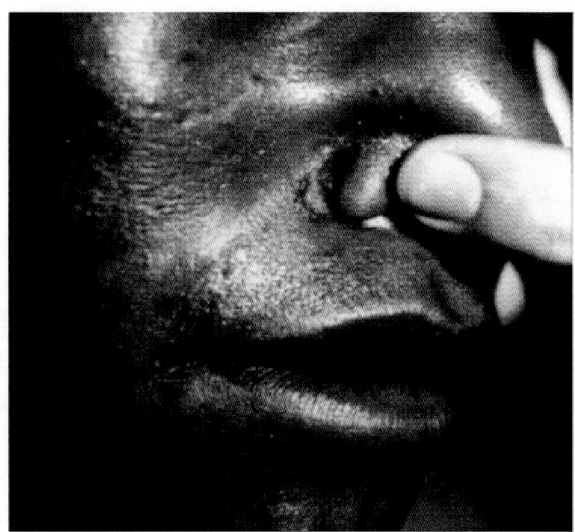

Figure 23.11 Secondary syphilis: condyloma abutting on ala nasi. *(Courtesy of J. Richens.)*

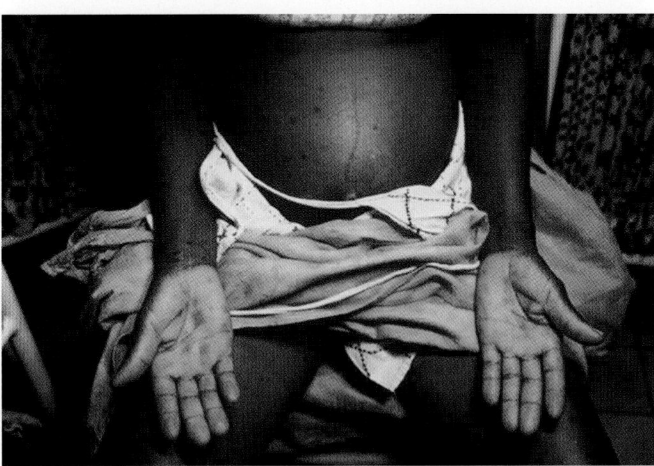

Figure 23.12 Secondary syphilis: typical palmar rash. *(Courtesy of D Mabey.)*

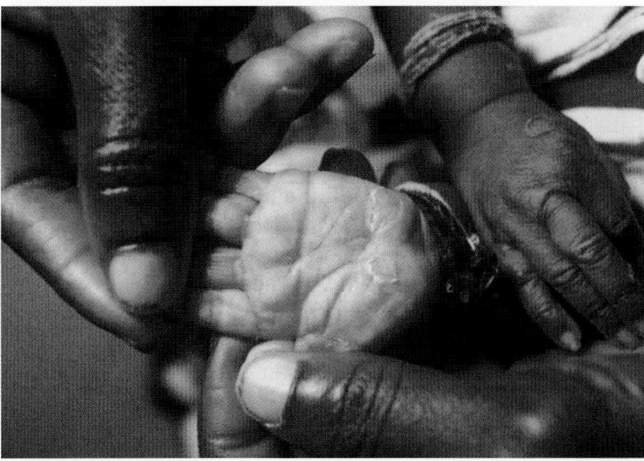

Figure 23.14 Congenital syphilis in a 3-month-old infant: desquamating lesion of palm. *(Courtesy of D. Mabey.)*

(aortitis, aortic valve disease or coronary ostial occlusion) were seen in 15% of males and 8% of females, with onset typically 30–40 years after infection. Neurological manifestations were seen in 9% of males and 5% of females, with meningovascular disease typically occurring after 15–20 years and tabes dorsalis or general paresis after 20–30 years.[64] The Tuskegee study of untreated black Americans showed similar results. It is therefore surprising that tertiary syphilis, and in particular neurosyphilis, appears rather uncommon in Africa in spite of the high incidence of early syphilis.

Notable variations in the clinical expression of syphilis have been described in patients co-infected with HIV. These include multiple primary lesions, overlap of primary and secondary phases and early development of gummatous lesions.[65]

Congenital Syphilis

Early Congenital Syphilis

Pregnant women with untreated early or latent syphilis are liable to give birth to congenitally infected infants. The risk is highest among those with primary or secondary syphilis during pregnancy, and diminishes as the duration of latent syphilis increases. Studies conducted in the pre-antibiotic era found that untreated early syphilis in the mother led to stillbirth in 25% of cases, neonatal death in some 15% of cases and a syphilitic infant in about 40% of cases. Corresponding figures for untreated late syphilis were 12%, 9% and 2%.[66] A recent study in Tanzania found that 25% of pregnant women with active syphilis (RPR titre >1:4) delivered a stillbirth, 33% a low birth weight and 20% a premature infant.[8]

Signs of congenital syphilis in the neonate include a bullous rash (Figure 23.13), anaemia, jaundice and hepatosplenomegaly. The infant is often small for dates and may have feeding difficulties. The prognosis is poor in infants with signs of congenital syphilis at birth. More commonly, the syphilitic infant appears normal at birth, and presents in the first 3 months of life with: failure to thrive; a rash which resembles that of secondary syphilis, with desquamation usually involving the palms (Figure 23.14) and soles; persistent nasal discharge (sometimes blood-stained); and anaemia or hepatosplenomegaly (Figure 23.15). Periostitis of the long bones, with or without metaphyseal abnormalities, is radiologically evident in more

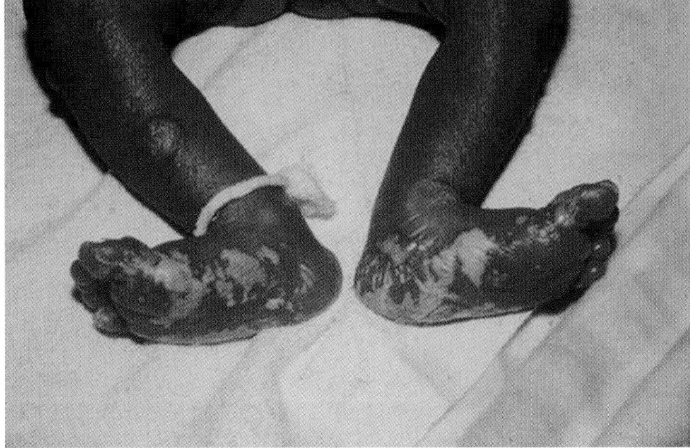

Figure 23.13 Congenital syphilis in a neonate: bullous lesions of feet. *(Courtesy of D. McGregor.)*

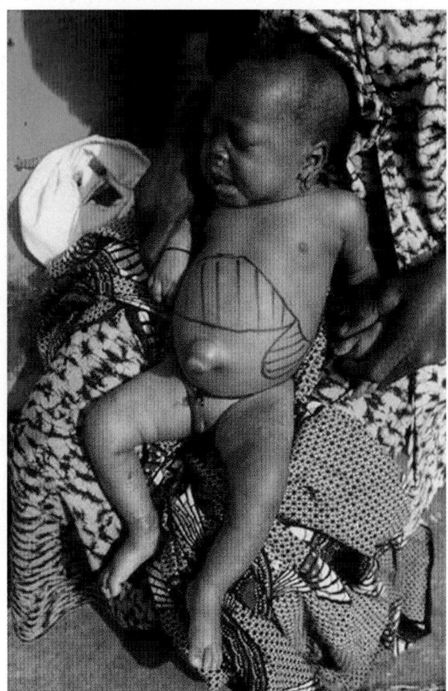

Figure 23.15 Congenital syphilis in a 3-month-old infant: hepatosplenomegaly. *(Courtesy of D. Mabey.)*

than 90% of cases, and may present clinically as pseudoparalysis of one or more limbs. The prognosis is very much better in those presenting in the postnatal period.[7]

Late Congenital Syphilis

Late congenital syphilis in the child or adolescent corresponds to tertiary syphilis in the adult, although the cardiovascular system is seldom involved. Manifestations include bony and dental abnormalities (skull bossing, Hutchinson's teeth) and inflammatory lesions of the cornea (interstitial keratitis) and joints (Clutton's joints). Eighth nerve deafness is commonly seen, and symptomatic neurosyphilis may occur, corresponding to tabes dorsalis or general paresis in the adult. In view of the high incidence of early congenital syphilis in many African cities, late manifestations of the disease are surprisingly rare in Africa.

Diagnosis

Clinically, it may not be possible to distinguish a syphilitic primary chancre from other causes of genital ulceration. In most parts of Africa, herpes and chancroid are the most important differential diagnoses, but in areas where donovanosis is prevalent, this should also be considered. The primary chancre should also be distinguished from LGV, herpes and non-venereal causes of genital ulceration. Secondary syphilis may resemble a variety of other skin conditions, but rashes which do not itch and affect the palms and soles should be considered syphilitic until proved otherwise. Early congenital syphilis in the neonatal period may be confused with perinatally acquired herpes simplex on account of the bullous rash, or with other intrauterine infections causing hepatosplenomegaly, anaemia and jaundice (e.g. cytomegalovirus, toxoplasmosis, rubella).

Dark-field Microscopy. *T. pallidum* may be demonstrated by dark-field microscopy in fluid from ulcerated or moist lesions of early syphilis, or in bulla fluid from lesions of early congenital syphilis. It can be distinguished from other spirochaetes that may be present under the foreskin by its characteristic shape and motility. Dark-field microscopy is likely to be negative in patients who have applied antiseptics to the lesion or taken antibiotics.

Serological Diagnosis. Two categories of test are available for the serological diagnosis of syphilis: non-treponemal or reagin tests (e.g. Venereal Disease Research Laboratory (VDRL), rapid plasma reagin (RPR)), and treponemal tests (*T. pallidum* haemagglutination (TPHA) or particle agglutination assays (TPPA), fluorescent treponemal antibody test (absorbed) (FTA)), and the new point-of-care tests. The reagin tests are useful for monitoring the response to treatment because they exhibit a falling titre after successful therapy, but they may give false-positive reactions in subjects with other chronic infections. The treponemal tests generally remain positive for life, and cannot therefore distinguish between a current and a past infection. They are more specific than the reagin tests but cannot distinguish between sexually acquired and endemic treponemal infections such as yaws. The new point-of-care tests are simple to perform, and do not require electricity or laboratory equipment.[67]

Management

T. pallidum remains fully sensitive to penicillin. Because it is a slowly dividing organism it is necessary to ensure adequate circulating penicillin levels for at least 10 days. Recommended treatment regimens are shown in Table 23.2. A single dose of benzathine penicillin remains the mainstay of treatment for early syphilis in all patients including those with pregnancy and HIV despite demonstrably lower concentrations in the cerebrospinal fluid.[68] Epidemiological treatment is recommended for sexual contacts. A single 2 g dose of azithromycin has recently been validated as a useful oral alternative to benzathine penicillin in early syphilis but the emergence of macrolide resistance in syphilis may limit the usefulness of this option in the future.[69,70]

Early congenital syphilis should be treated with procaine penicillin 50 000 units/kg IM daily for 10 days. If compliance is considered unlikely, benzathine penicillin 50 000 units/kg IM as a single dose may be given, although this does not give therapeutic levels in the cerebrospinal fluid. The mother and her sexual partner(s) should be investigated and treated appropriately. If possible, infants should be followed up after 6 months to ensure that the RPR or VDRL test has reverted to negative.

Prevention

Congenital syphilis can be prevented by serological screening of pregnant women at antenatal clinics. Experience in Tanzania has shown that in a developing country setting, this is only successful if serological tests are performed in the clinic and treatment given immediately.[71]

LYMPHOGRANULOMA VENEREUM

Lymphogranuloma venereum (LGV) is also known as lymphogranuloma inguinale, lymphopathia venereum, tropical or climatic bubo and Durand–Nicolas–Favre disease.

Epidemiology

The epidemiology of LGV is not well-defined, owing to the lack of a sensitive and specific diagnostic test. The classical form of LGV is largely confined to the tropics, where in most places it accounts for only a small proportion of patients with STIs. The disease is seen more often in men than women. Since 2004, there has been a dramatic rise in LGV presenting with proctitis among homosexual HIV-positive males in Europe.[72]

Aetiology

LGV is caused by the invasive L1, L2 and L3 strains of *Chlamydia trachomatis.*

Pathology

The characteristic pathological features are a thrombolymphangitis and perilymphangitis with proliferation of the endothelial cells of the lymphatics. In the lymph nodes prominent migration of neutrophils leads to characteristic stellate abscess formation.

Clinical Features

The disease is important, chiefly as a cause of bubo. When a sexually active adult presents with an inguinal bubo not associated with genital ulcer, LGV is an important diagnosis to consider. The initial event in infection, occurring 3–30 days after exposure, is typically a small, painless, usually herpetiform ulcer of the genitalia which may pass unrecognized and resolves spontaneously. It is thought likely that some patients develop asymptomatic infections of the urethra and cervix. The second

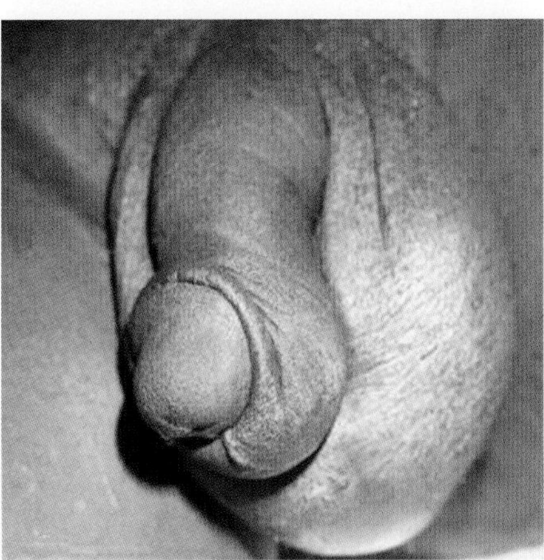

Figure 23.16 Lymphogranuloma venereum: elephantiasis in long-standing case. *(Reproduced with permission from: Arya OP, Osoba AO, Bennett FJ. Tropical Venereology. Edinburgh: Churchill Livingstone; 1980.)*

phase of the illness is the development of increasingly painful lymphangitis and lymphadenitis, accompanied by fever and malaise. The infected nodes (bilateral in a third of cases) coalesce into a matted mass which may project outwards below or above the inguinal ligament to give the classical 'groove sign'. The nodes are liable to rupture, forming multiple sinuses. Untreated, the disease may cause extensive lymphatic damage, resulting in elephantiasis of the genitalia (Figure 23.16). The combination of elephantiasis with skin breakdown sometimes seen in late cases is referred to as esthiomene. An additional characteristic feature in long-standing cases is the development of fenestrations in the labia.

In women and homosexual men, the disease may present as an acute proctocolitis which, in a proportion of cases, leads to abscess formation, fibrosis, fistula and rectal stricture.[73] A number of cases have been misdiagnosed as having inflammatory bowel disease which has overlapping histological features.

Diagnosis

Since the resurgence of LGV in Europe, a useful array of new tests has been developed. Widely used protocols for diagnosis now start with an initial generic NAAT test for *C. trachomatis*, followed by a second PCR targeting LGV-specific DNA or alternatively amplification of the *omp*1 gene followed by restriction enzyme digestion to identify LGV serovars in specialist laboratories.[74,75] Older serological tests show cross-reaction with other serovars of *C. trachomatis*, and with other species of *Chlamydia*, e.g. the prevalent respiratory tract pathogen *C. pneumoniae*.

Treatment

The drugs recommended for treatment of acute cases are of the tetracycline or macrolide groups, as for other chlamydial infections, but for a longer duration (21 days) (Table 23.2). There are reports that suggest doxycycline is superior to azithromycin in the treatment of rectal infections. Benefit in late cases, e.g. with rectal stricture, is slight. Plastic surgery may be of benefit in cases with extensive elephantiasis or deformity. Aspiration of buboes through adjacent healthy skin is usually advised.

DONOVANOSIS

Synonyms are granuloma inguinale, granuloma venereum. It is important not to confuse this disease with lymphogranuloma venereum (see above) or to confuse Donovan bodies (see below) with Leishman–Donovan bodies (leishmaniasis). The disease was first recognized in India, where Donovan observed the bodies that bear his name in an oral lesion of the disease. Sir Patrick Manson did much to promote awareness of the disease by devoting a chapter to 'ulcerating granuloma of the pudenda' in the first edition of this textbook.

Epidemiology

Endemic areas are localized to a few specific areas of the tropics. The most important of these are currently India, Papua New Guinea (PNG), Brazil and eastern parts of South Africa. The disease is strongly associated with prostitution and low socio-economic status. Major epidemics of donovanosis have been reported from PNG but are unlikely to be seen again. Outside PNG, the highest recently reported incidence of donovanosis has been in Durban, South Africa, where 16% of genital ulcers in men were due to donovanosis.[76] There is strong evidence that the disease is sexually transmitted in most patients. The risk of transmission to partners appears to be lower than for other STIs. Perinatal transmission is rare.

Aetiology

The disease is caused by a poorly characterized, encapsulated, Gram-negative coccobacillus, previously called *Calymmatobacterium granulomatis*, recently re-classified as a *Klebsiella* on the basis of ribosomal RNA sequences.[77] It is an intracellular parasite that can be grown in tissue culture.[78]

Pathology

The disease primarily attacks the skin. The bacteria are carried to inguinal nodes, where they occasionally cause a suppurating periadenitis ('pseudobubo') but more often they escape to produce ulcers in the overlying skin. The key histological features are: (1) epithelial hyperplasia; (2) a dense dermal infiltrate of plasma cells and (3) scattered large macrophages containing clusters of Donovan bodies. Donovan bodies stain poorly with haematoxylin and eosin but with Giemsa they typically display a capsule and bipolar densities which give a characteristic closed safety-pin appearance.

Clinical Features

The first manifestation, appearing after a 3–40-day incubation period, is usually a small papule, which ruptures to form a granulomatous lesion that is characteristically pain free, 'beefy-red' in colour, bleeds readily on contact and is often elevated above the level of the surrounding skin. The lesion has to be differentiated from other forms of genital ulcer. Most likely to cause confusion are chancroid,[79] condylomata lata, ulcerated warts and squamous carcinoma. Untreated, the ulcers slowly extend (Figure 23.17), particularly along skin-folds towards the groins (Figure 23.18) and anus. Special features are extra-genital lesions (mostly neck and mouth); cervical lesions (resemble carcinoma or tuberculous cervicitis); involvement of uterus; tubes and ovaries (hard masses, abscesses, 'frozen pelvis',

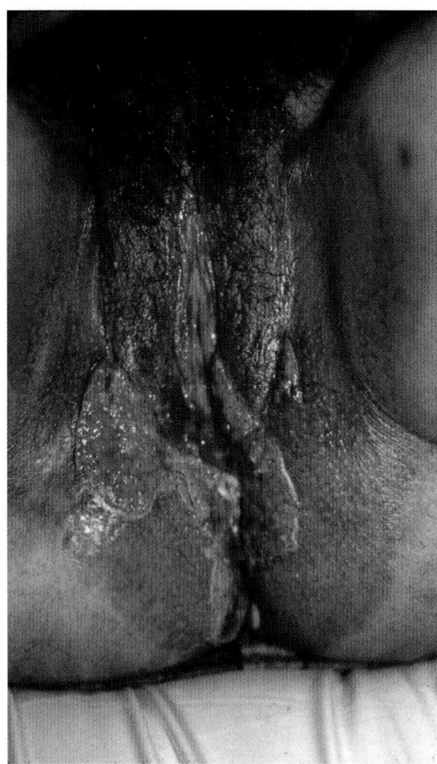

Figure 23.17 Donovanosis: slowly extending painless ulceration. *(Courtesy of J. Richens.)*

hydronephrosis) and rare cases of haematogenous dissemination to lung, liver, spleen and bone. Complications include rapid extension of lesions secondarily infected with fusospirochaetal organisms, scarring (in some populations very prominent), elephantiasis and the development of squamous carcinoma.[80]

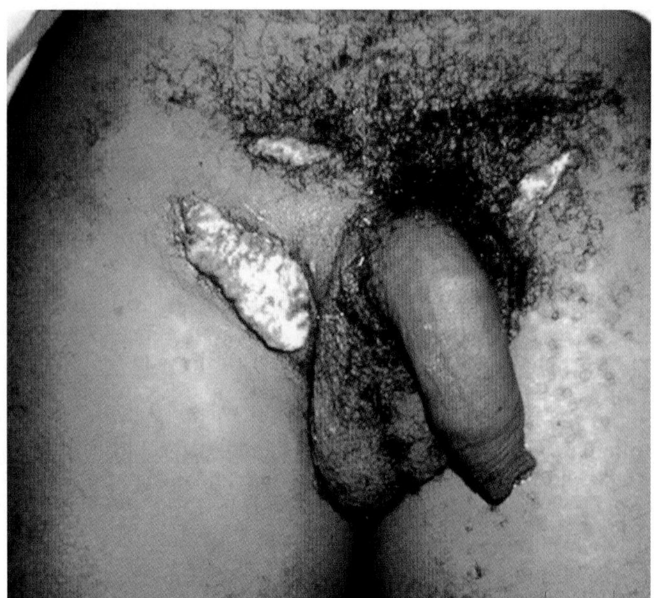

Figure 23.18 Donovanosis: lesion extending along inguinal fold. *(Courtesy of J. Richens.)*

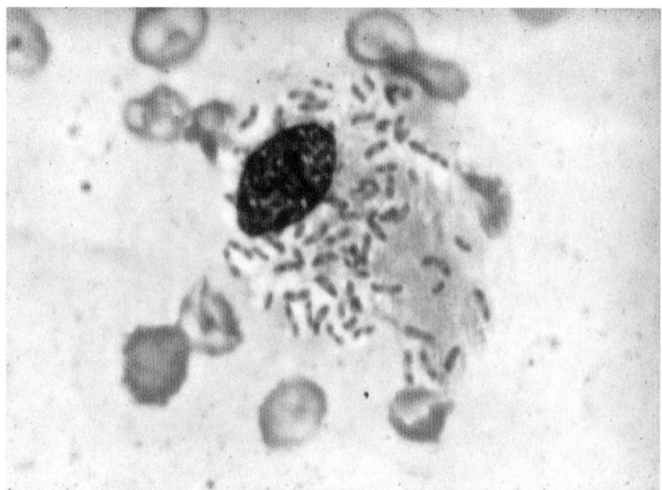

Figure 23.19 Donovan bodies: Giemsa-stained smear from genital ulcer demonstrating intracellular organisms with bipolar densities.

Diagnosis

The diagnosis requires the demonstration of intracellular Donovan bodies (Figure 23.19) in either biopsy material (best stained with silver stains or Giemsa) or smears taken from active areas which can be stained by Giemsa or Leishman-stains. For collection of specimens, a recommended technique is to thoroughly clean the lesions of surface debris, detach one to three 3–5 mm pieces of tissue by punch or snip biopsy, and then prepare a smear from one piece, followed by air-drying and fixation in 95% ethanol and fixing the remaining tissue in 10% formalin for histology.[81]

Management

The bacteria respond to many broad-spectrum antibiotics active against Gram-negative bacilli.[80] The most widely used in recent years have been azithromycin, doxycycline, co-trimoxazole and erythromycin. Fluoroquinolones have also been shown to be of value, but experience in Australia suggests that azithromycin is the most useful treatment.[82] Treatment should be continued until lesions have resolved and, if possible, a little longer to reduce the risk of relapse. Plastic surgical procedures are required in some patients. Epidemiological treatment of contacts exposed within 40 days of the onset of symptoms in the index case may be recommended (Table 23.2).

GENITAL HERPES

Genital herpes is an ulcerative STI caused principally by herpes simplex virus type 2 (HSV-2) and to a lesser extent by herpes simplex virus type 1 (HSV-1), the usual cause of oral herpes. In the past genital herpes accounted for a lower proportion of patients attending clinics with genital ulcers in the tropics than in developed countries, but this pattern has changed dramatically in the last 20 years, particularly in areas with high HIV incidence. Several epidemiological, biological and modelling studies support the role of HSV-2 in fuelling the HIV epidemic in many parts of the world,[83–86] and vice-versa (Chapter 15). HIV is known to profoundly influence the clinical features, duration and response to treatment of HSV-2.[87] Prior infection with HSV-1 infection, which is almost universal

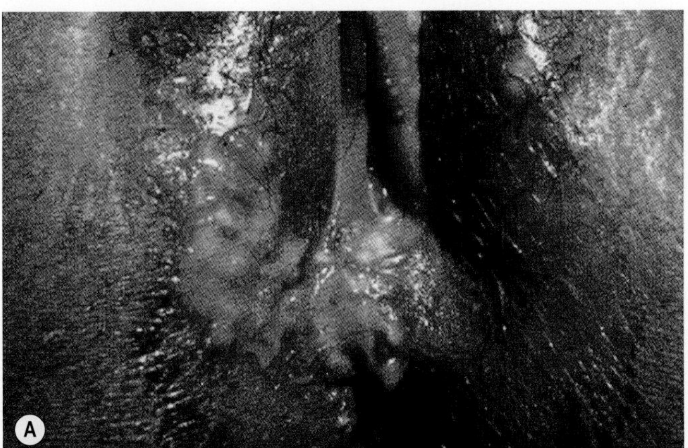

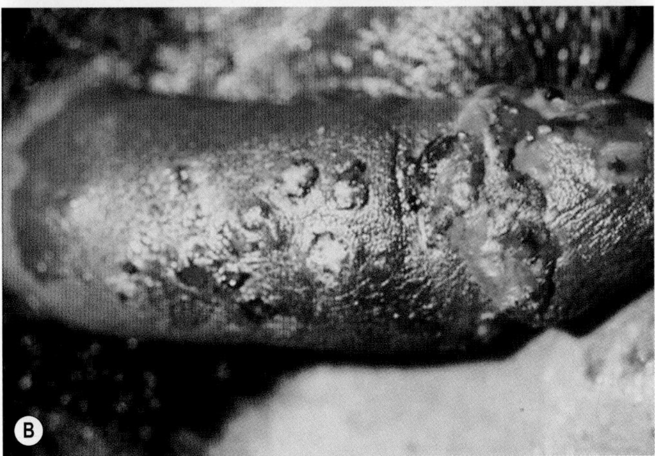

Figure 23.20 Recurrent genital herpes: cluster of small painful ulcers of corona sulcus (Courtesy P. Mayaud).

by the age of puberty in many developing countries, reduces the severity and frequency of clinical recurrences in HSV-2 infection.

Clinical Features

The clinical picture is highly characteristic in many cases (in the absence of immune suppression), with its localized clusters of vesicles, which break down to form ulcers (Figure 23.20), crust over and then resolve. Sites of involvement include the external genitalia, neighbouring skin, the urethra and cervix (both endocervix and ectocervix), pharynx and rectum. Tender lymphadenopathy may occur. During the primary attack, the virus ascends the peripheral nerves to local ganglia, where a latency is established, which is liable to be interrupted by periodic recurrences for the remainder of the patient's life. The primary attack is notably more severe than subsequent episodes, with lesions covering a wider and more symmetric area. HSV-2 causes substantially more severe primary disease than HSV-1 and is followed by more frequent relapse. The complications of genital herpes include a sacral radiculomyelopathy which may manifest with constipation and retention of urine as well as shooting pains down the legs. Other complications include aseptic meningitis, extragenital lesions and disseminated herpes. In pregnant women, recurrences and dissemination are more frequent and premature delivery may complicate primary attacks. Severe and intractable ulceration due to HSV-2 occurs in patients immunosuppressed by HIV.

Diagnosis

Clinical diagnosis alone is often sufficient. Genital herpes has to be distinguished from other STIs that cause painful genital ulcer and from non-infectious conditions such as Behçet's syndrome and Crohn's disease. The definitive diagnosis rests on viral isolation. Kits for antigen detection are available commercially, and DNA amplification tests have been successfully used to identify HSV-2 in symptomatic and asymptomatic shedders. Serological diagnosis is only of value in a primary attack.

Management

Specific treatment can rarely be offered in the tropics; nonetheless patients require explanation, reassurance and advice, just as elsewhere (Table 23.2). Patients need to be instructed to keep the lesions clean and dry. They should be told that the disease is likely to recur and that they will transmit the infection to others if they have sexual intercourse while they have lesions. Aciclovir has been shown to be of value in ameliorating symptoms of the primary attack, treatment of infected neonates and adults with immunosuppression or disseminated disease. Continuous prophylactic (suppressive) therapy has been found useful in ameliorating and preventing clinical recurrences in patients particularly troubled by recurrent disease. Recent studies have demonstrated that periods of asymptomatic shedding commonly occur in short bursts (a few hours) several times a day, and quite intermittently and that this shedding can only be suppressed (albeit imperfectly) by antiviral agents at high doses.[88]

In view of the role of HSV-2 in enhancing HIV acquisition and transmission, and influencing HIV disease progression, a number of randomized trials have been conducted in the last 10 years. Disappointingly, these trials were unable to demonstrate an impact of HSV-2-suppressive therapy with acyclovir at standard doses on HIV acquisition among HSV-2-infected HIV-seronegative men who have sex with men (MSM) and high-risk women;[89,90] and on HIV transmission in HIV-serodiscordant couples,[91] although an impact was noted on HIV-disease progression.[92] However, a number of smaller treatment trials have confirmed the role of HSV-2 in increasing HIV replication, viral loads and genital shedding in both women[93–96] and men.[97] It is plausible that higher dosages of existing[98] or new and more efficacious antiherpetic drugs such as helicase-primase inhibitors[99] or an effective therapeutic HSV-2 vaccine[100] would be required to have any notable impact on HSV-2 replication, and thereby on HIV. This field of research has opened up new avenues to better understand the biology and immunological control of HSV-2.[101,102]

Herpes in Pregnancy

Transmission from mother to child occurs in 50% of cases with a primary attack at term, is much lower in patients with recurrences (about 1%) and occasionally occurs as a result of asymptomatic viral shedding by the mother at term. Neonatal herpes carries a 60% mortality, which has changed little with the introduction of aciclovir. The presence of first-episode herpetic lesions of the cervix at term is an indication for caesarean section, although this operation does not fully protect against infection developing in the neonate. Aciclovir can be used in late pregnancy to reduce viral shedding among women recently diagnosed with herpes and as an alternative to caesarean for women who fear having a recurrence at term.

HUMAN PAPILLOMAVIRUSES AND GENITAL WARTS

Epidemiology

In developed countries, genital infection with the human papillomavirus (HPV) is the most common viral STI and is four times as frequent as genital herpes. Using the most sensitive diagnostic methods, infection can be demonstrated in as many as 40% of sexually active women.[103] In the tropics, particularly in Africa, HPV infections are common (12–34% of women tested)[104,105] and cervical carcinoma is one of the commonest cancers of women.[106]

Aetiology

HPVs are small DNA viruses which can cause a range of diseases from simple skin warts, to genital warts and anogenital cancers. Based on DNA homologies, over 75 different HPV genotypes have been characterized from mucosal and cutaneous sites. Of the several anogenital HPV types identified, about 15 genotypes including HPV-16, 18, 31, 33, -35 and others have oncogenic potential and are associated with genital cancers (i.e. from the cervix, vulva, vagina, penis and anus), while HPV-6 and -11, which have a lower potential for causing neoplasia, are more closely associated with exophytic (as opposed to flat) lesions of the genitalia (genital warts) and, rarely, with the development of respiratory papillomas in children born to infected mothers.

Pathology

The virus infects the basal layer of differentiating squamous epithelium and produces a pathognomonic large, clear, perinuclear zone known as koilocytotic atypia. Full assembly of viral particles is confined to the more superficial layers of the epithelium. Most HPV infections are asymptomatic and cleared within a few months to 1 year. Persistence of oncogenic types is aetiologically linked with the development of neoplasia. Factors such as HIV-associated immunosuppression and other cofactors such as smoking and prolonged hormonal contraception promote carcinogenic development.[107]

Clinical

The lesions produced by HPV vary from the well-known soft, fleshy, vascular condylomata acuminata with their frond-like appearance (Figure 23.21) to papular warts which resemble those seen on other parts of the body, pigmented and non-pigmented papules and leucoplakia. Warts may sometimes grow in the urethra. Recent research has shown that many patients have subclinical HPV infections that can only be visualized by simple inspection or colposcopy (with magnifying lenses) after application of 5% acetic acid and/or Lugol's iodine (VIA/VILI technique). In pregnancy, in immunosuppressed patients and in the presence of genital discharges, there is a tendency for warts to grow rapidly. The lesions showing the greatest similarity to genital warts are lesions of molluscum contagiosum, condylomata lata of secondary syphilis, and anal skin tags. Laryngeal papillomas have been reported in infants born to mothers with genital warts at delivery.

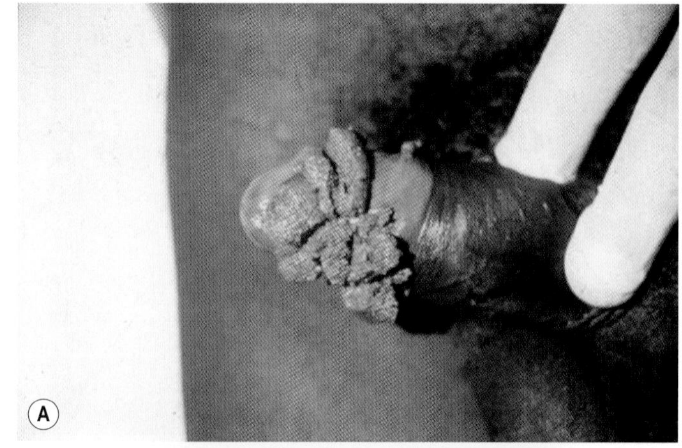

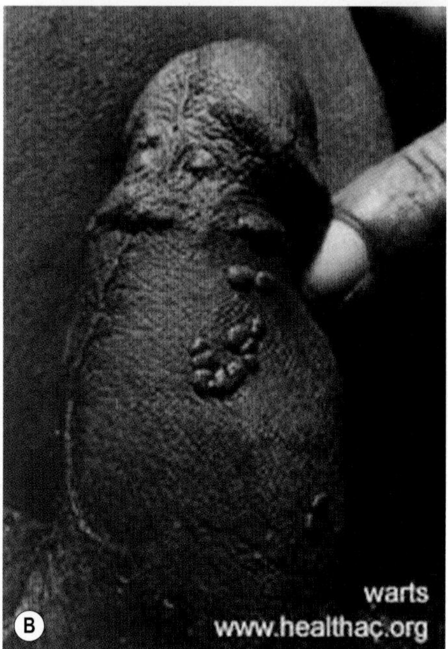

Figure 23.21 Genital warts: condylomata acuminata caused by human papillomavirus. *A. Courtesy P. Mayaud; (B, From* www.healthac.org*)*

Diagnosis and Management

Condylomata acuminata are diagnosed clinically, but can be confused with condylomata lata of secondary syphilis, *Molluscum contagiosum* and, occasionally, verrucose forms of donovanosis. Biopsy confirmation of the diagnosis of condylomata acuminata warts is optional.

Cervical cytology, where available, is recommended for female patients and female contacts in order to detect progression of lesions to cervical intraepithelial neoplasia. Biopsy collected during colposcopy can confirm the presence of cervical intraepithelial neoplasia (CIN).

Treatment is generally reserved for macroscopic lesions because subclinical infections show high spontaneous regression rates and also show a strong tendency to relapse with currently available forms of treatment. Specific treatment for warts includes treatment with trichloroacetic acid and the traditional application of 20% podophyllin (maximum 0.5 mL) once or twice weekly.[108] Cure rates with podophyllin, at 50%, are not very satisfactory. Care is needed to avoid burning normal skin, which can be protected with glycerine. Podophyllin should be washed off after 4 h and is contraindicated in pregnant women. Larger warts can be removed with cryotherapy or diathermy. More modern treatments include the application of 5-fluorouracil cream, self-treatment with podophyllotoxin or imiquimod, and carbon dioxide laser treatment. Relapse rates of the order of 30% are seen with all forms of treatment. Persistent cervical lesions and suspicious lesions should be excised surgically. The advent of highly effective vaccines against HPV[109] has raised the prospect of bringing cervical carcinoma under control across the world.[110]

STI Control Programmes

The important components of an STI control programme are: (1) gathering of information, e.g. STI morbidity surveillance, special surveys on the aetiology of genital ulcer in a particular area, data on antibiotic sensitivities of local strains of *Neisseria gonorrhoeae* and *Haemophilus ducreyi*; (2) provision of management guidelines; (3) training programmes; (4) provision of healthcare to patients with STIs wherever they may present; (5) coordinated programmes of education about STIs for patients and the general public; and (6) management and supervision of the programme. Each of these will be discussed in more detail.

Information Gathering

Morbidity surveillance in the tropics is often incomplete and unreliable. Given the rudimentary facilities available in many centres, it is often best to record numbers of patients by syndrome (ulcer, discharge, etc.) rather than by specific diagnosis. High-quality reporting from a few representative sentinel sites may be more useful than unreliable reports collated from the whole country. When possible, special surveys should be undertaken periodically, such as studies of the prevalence of gonorrhoea, chlamydial infection and syphilis in antenatal mothers. Statistics on ophthalmia neonatorum, congenital syphilis, PID, ectopic pregnancy and infertility may be useful for impressing upon health planners the full extent of STI morbidity.

Standard Management Guidelines for STIs

When a reasonable amount of information is available about the picture of STIs in a country and the antibiotic sensitivity patterns of local isolates, it is possible to draw up rational guidelines for local use, based on those recommended by the World Health Organization.[14] These guidelines can be tailored to different levels of the health system according to the availability of supporting laboratory tests and drugs. They can be conveniently set out as flow charts or algorithms in pocket manuals which are supplied to all health workers who need to manage STIs. In view of the constantly changing pattern of antibiotic sensitivities of *N. gonorrhoeae* and *H. ducreyi*, it is important that guidelines are reviewed and revised at 3–4-yearly intervals.

Training

The high incidence of STIs in tropical populations makes it important for all health workers to acquire the basic skills to manage patients appropriately according to standard guidelines, to prevent ophthalmia neonatorum and congenital syphilis, and to promote the following health education messages which are important in STI prevention:

- Reduction of the number of sexual partners
- Avoidance of sex with high-risk partners
- Use of condoms for protection against STIs
- Knowledge of the symptoms, sequelae and transmissibility of STIs
- Avoidance of sexual contact when symptoms are present
- Knowledge of what AIDS is and how HIV is transmitted
- Obtaining proper treatment promptly for STI symptoms
- Ensuring that the patients' contacts are treated whether they have symptoms or not.

Provision of Services for Patients with STIs or at High Risk for STIs

The aim should be to maximize coverage and access of STI services for men and women and to have a way of referring problem cases. Costs to patients should be kept as low as possible and confidentiality safeguarded. Specialist STI clinics are valuable where the volume of patients is high, but in general, the provision of specialist clinics for the treatment of STIs, which has been successful in controlling these diseases in certain industrialized countries, is neither appropriate nor feasible in most developing countries, where patients with STIs should be managed at the primary healthcare level. Family planning and antenatal clinics provide opportunities for STI control activities which tend to be underutilized at present.

Special services should be provided for groups at higher risk of STIs. Outreach programmes for sex workers or truck drivers have been introduced in several countries of the developing world. These programmes rely on the interaction with individuals who have privileged access to the target populations such as 'peers' or 'gate-keepers'. Services can be provided through static or mobile clinics and STI care can be combined with other reproductive health or HIV prevention and care interventions. Experience in many sub-Saharan African settings has shown that such services can result in a large reduction in HIV and STI prevalence and incidence among sex workers as well as among their clients and sexual partners.[111,112]

Education Programmes

The appropriate content for education messages has been described above. These messages must be expressed in a sensitive manner after widespread consultation and careful pre-testing before they are disseminated by health workers, through posters and by the media. It is particularly important to target schoolchildren, sex workers and patients attending for treatment of STIs. Interest has recently focused on the use of peer educators to encourage people to listen to health messages. Condom promotion is of particular importance and the social marketing of condoms has shown promise in many countries.

Supervision and Management of STI Control Activities

It is important for programmes of STI and HIV control to be fully integrated because of their many shared objectives. The delegation of much routine STI treatment and control to the primary healthcare level is unlikely to succeed, unless the morale and commitment of healthcare workers responsible for treating patients with STIs are maintained by regular supportive visits by programme managers.

REFERENCES

8. Watson-Jones D, Changalucha J, Gumodoka B, et al. Syphilis in pregnancy in Tanzania. I. Impact of maternal syphilis on outcome of pregnancy. J Infect Dis 2002;186(7):940–7.
63. Chico RM, Mayaud P, Ariti C, et al. Prevalence of malaria and sexually transmitted and reproductive tract infections in pregnancy in sub-Saharan Africa: A systematic review. JAMA 2012;307(19):2079–86.
67. Mabey D, Peeling RW, Ballard R, et al. Prospective, multi-centre clinic-based evaluation of four rapid diagnostic tests for syphilis. Sex Transm Infect 2006;82(Suppl 5):v13–6.
86. Van de Perre P, Segondy M, Foulongne V, et al. Herpes simplex virus and HIV-1: deciphering viral synergy. Lancet Infect Dis 2008;8(8):490–7.
91. Celum C, Wald A, Lingappa JR, et al. Acyclovir and transmission of HIV-1 from persons infected with HIV-1 and HSV-2. N Engl J Med 2010;362(5):427–39.
109. Koutsky LA, Ault KA, Wheeler CM, et al. A controlled trial of a human papillomavirus type 16 vaccine. N Engl J Med 2002;347(21):1645–51.

Access the complete references online at www.expertconsult.com

24

Bacterial Enteropathogens

GAGANDEEP KANG | C. ANTHONY HART | PAUL SHEARS

KEY POINTS

- The principal bacterial agents of diarrhoeal diseases are *Vibrio cholerae*, *Salmonella* spp., *Shigella* spp., *Campylobacter* spp. (especially *C. jejuni*) and a variety of enteropathogenic *Escherichia coli* strains, including the enterotoxigenic ETEC strains that are the main agents of travellers' diarrhoea.
- *H. pylori* causes acute and chronic non-autoimmune gastritis and is probably the commonest bacterial infection of mankind. Long-term infections cause up to 60% of gastric carcinomas and intestinal mucosa-associated lymphoid tumours (MALTomas).
- *Escherichia coli* is the major aerobic component of the normal intestinal flora. Most strains are commensals, but some pathotypes cause diarrhoeal disease. Over time, five different mechanisms have been described: enteropathogenic *E. coli* (EPEC); enterotoxigenic *E. coli* (ETEC); enteroinvasive *E. coli* (EIEC); enterohaemorrhagic *E. coli* (EHEC); and enteroadhesive or enteroaggregative *E. coli* (EAEC or EAggEC).
- Campylobacters can produce both inflammatory diarrhoea and non-inflammatory diarrhoeas and are associated with Guillain-Barré syndrome. Data on *Campylobacter* infection in tropical areas is limited, partly because of the difficulty of isolating the organism with limited laboratory facilities.
- Cholera is characterized by severe watery diarrhoea leading to dehydration, electrolyte imbalance and hypovolaemia, with a mortality ranging from less than 1 to 40%. In the past decade, devastating epidemics of cholera have occurred in Angola, Ethiopia, Zimbabwe, Pakistan, Somalia, Sudan, Vietnam and Haiti.
- Dysentery has been a disease of poor and crowded communities throughout history and continues to be a major cause of morbidity and mortality in the tropics. *Sh. dysenteriae* and *Sh. flexneri* are responsible for most infections in the tropics. Shigellosis occurs both endemically and as epidemics.
- The wide diversity of organisms that may cause infections of the gastrointestinal tract and the differences in symptoms complicate accurate surveillance and diagnosis, especially in developing countries with limited access to modern laboratory procedures.

Introduction

Diarrhoeal diseases represent a major health problem in developing countries and are also a high risk to travellers who visit these countries. There is a high death toll from diarrhoeal disease estimated at about 2 million deaths per year.[1] Most of these deaths occur in children under 5 years of age. A rate of 3.2 episodes of diarrhoea/year per child has been reported, but can be higher in some settings. In addition to acute illness, repeated infections can lead to acute or chronic malnutrition and consequent effects on physical and mental development of children that may eventually translate into impairment of human fitness and productivity in adults.[2] Moreover, outbreaks of cholera, shigellosis and typhoid fever most often occur in resource-poor countries, adding to the burden of disease among the most vulnerable subpopulations.

The wide diversity of organisms that may cause infections of the gastrointestinal tract and the differences in symptoms complicate accurate surveillance and diagnosis, especially in developing countries with limited access to modern laboratory procedures. Among the principal bacterial agents of diarrhoeal diseases are *Vibrio cholerae* (cholera), a variety of *Salmonella* spp. and of *Shigella* spp., the agents of shigellosis (bacterial dysentery), *Campylobacter* spp. (especially *C. jejuni*) and a variety of enteropathogenic *Escherichia coli* strains, including the enterotoxigenic ETEC strains that are the main agents of travellers' diarrhoea. Bacterial diarrhoeas can also be caused by a variety of bacterial pathogens such as *Staphylococcus aureus*, *Clostridium perfringens*, *Clostridium difficile* or *Klebsiella*. In addition, infections may not result in gastroenteritis, for example, *Salmonella typhi* causes typhoid fever and *Helicobacter pylori* is associated with a range of symptoms from gastritis to malignancies.

In the gastrointestinal tract, bacteria that make up the normal flora are present from shortly after birth. The number of bacteria increases distally, with bacteria found in the stomach and small intestine in low numbers (10^2–10^4 colony forming units [cfu]/mL) which are usually transient(s) and the lower ileum and colon containing large numbers of bacteria (~10^{12} cfu/mL). In disease, the detection of the causative agent can be difficult and has led to several approaches to laboratory diagnosis and the assessment of causality. In this chapter, bacteria causing disease in the gastrointestinal tract are reviewed, pathogens that enter through the gut but have their major disease manifestations outside the gut, as in *Salmonella typhi* infections, are covered elsewhere.

Helicobacter pylori

Since the beginning of the 1900s, histopathologists have described spiral bacteria in the stomach. In 1983, Warren and Marshall were able to grow the bacterium originally named *Campylobacter pyloridis* and finally designated *Helicobacter pylori*.[3] It is now accepted that *H. pylori* causes acute and chronic non-autoimmune gastritis and is probably the commonest bacterial infection of mankind. It is responsible for up to 80% of gastric and 95% of duodenal ulcers. In 1994, the International Agency for Research on Cancer classified *H. pylori* as a grade 1 carcinogen, the only bacterial agent of cancer. Long-term infections of 30–40 years cause up to 60% of gastric carcinomas. It is also associated with intestinal mucosa-associated lymphoid tumours (MALTomas).

Epidemiology

Infection with *H. pylori* is present all over the world.[3] In developed countries, approximately 10% of healthy individuals under 30 years of age have serological evidence of infection and this rises to 60% in those over 60. In developing countries, infection is highly prevalent and is acquired at a younger age. For example, in the Gambia, 46% of those under 5 years and in Peru, 48% of children under 12 years had evidence of infection.[4,5] In most developing countries, virtually 100% are seropositive by early childhood.[6] Infection is usually acquired in the first 5 years of life but improving hygienic and socioeconomic conditions in some developing countries have led to a decreased rate of acquisition. Humans are the major reservoir for *H. pylori*. The bacterium has been grown or its genome detected in saliva, dental plaque, vomitus, gastric juice and faeces.[7] The relative importance of different modes of transmission are unclear. Person-to-person spread via endoscopes, pH electrodes or nasogastric feeding tubes has been documented. Close contact clearly promotes spread, e.g. families of infected children have a higher incidence of infection, as have those who are occupationally exposed.[8,9] Family clusters of infection are related to socioeconomic status[10] and infection is readily transmitted between siblings.[11] The faecal–oral route is the most likely mode of spread and *H. pylori* DNA and antigen have been detected in faeces. Inter-oral spread has also been proposed, with the oral cavity considered a permanent reservoir of *H. pylori*.[12] The domestic fly (*Musca domestica*) can become colonized by *H. pylori* and *H. pylori* DNA has been detected in houseflies from three continents.[13] This raises the possibility of fly contamination of food leading to food-borne infection. *H. pylori* does not grow in foods but does survive in a cool, moist and non-acidic environment. Water-borne spread has also been suggested as a major route in developing countries.[5] Finally, some animal species, including the macaque, sheep and pig, have been shown to harbour *H. pylori*, suggesting the possibility of zoonotic spread.[7] A number of other *Helicobacter* species have been detected in a variety of animals, but only *H. heilmannii* is found in the human stomach.

Microbiology

H. pylori is a sinusoidal Gram-negative bacterium, 3.5 μm long by 0.5–1 μm in diameter (Figure 24.1), with a smooth surface and four to six sheathed flagella with terminal bulbs. The bacterium produces a urease and is well adapted to living beneath the mucous layer attached to the surface of gastric enterocytes. *H. pylori* is fastidious and slow-growing. It requires enriched selective media for isolation from clinical specimens. Growth is optimal at 37°C under humidified microaerophilic conditions in 10% carbon dioxide and takes 4–6 days.

Pathogenesis

A causal association has been demonstrated for antral non-autoimmune (type B) gastritis both in adults and in children.[3,14,15] There is also a strong association between *H. pylori* and peptic ulceration. Infection can be established with

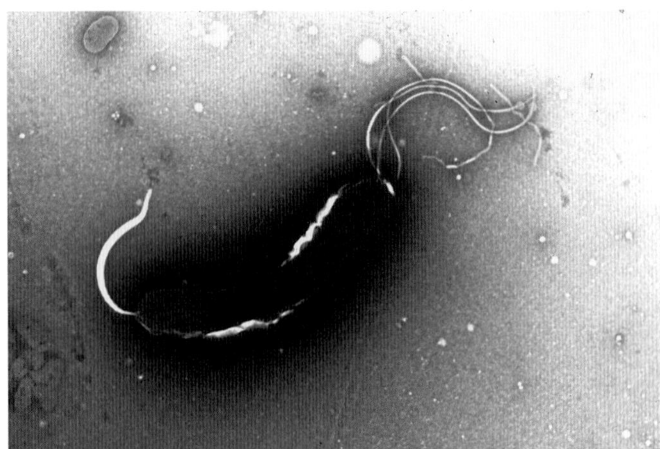

Figure 24.1 Negative-stain electron micrograph of *Helicobacter pylori* showing sheathed flagella with a terminal bulb.

doses of between 10^5–10^9 cfu. *H. pylori* is able to survive an acidic gastric pH to penetrate the mucus covering the gastric epithelial cells, where it can exist free or attach to the epithelial cells (Figure 24.2). The bacterium's spiral morphology and flagella are important for pathogenesis.[9] *H. pylori* makes an enzyme, urease, which breaks down urea to ammonia which helps to neutralize the acidic pH, a cytotoxin which causes vacuolation (Vac A), and a protease which hydrolyses mucus and other factors which stimulate gastric acid secretion. Recently it has been found that strains of *H. pylori* that have a 40 kb pathogenicity island called the *cag* pathogenicity island (PAI) are more likely to produce inflammation. The *cag* PAI region encodes a secretion system (type IV) that transports a protein, cag, across both bacterial membranes and injects it into host cells. Cag, also encoded in the PAI, induces the secretion of pro-inflammatory cytokines.[16] CagA interacts with the tumour suppressor apoptosis-stimulating protein of p53-2 (ASPP2), promoting p53 degradation. The pathogenesis of MALToma production appears to involve chronic antigenic stimulation and elimination of *H. pylori* is associated with cure of the lymphomas.

Infected individuals mount a systemic and local humoral immune response to the bacterium. The immune response to

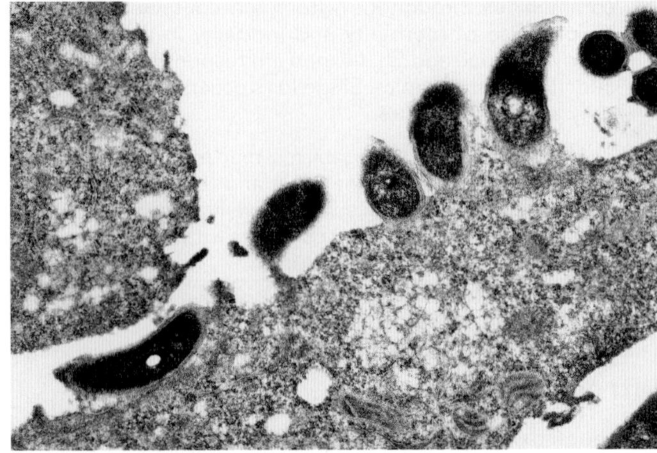

Figure 24.2 Thin-section electron micrograph of *H. pylori* intimately attached to a gastric enterocyte.

Helicobacter pylori is multifaceted, involving responses that are both protective and damaging to the host. The innate and the adaptive immune responses lead to damaging inflammatory responses, but these responses may fail, allowing for persistence of infection.[17]

Pathology

Examination of biopsies in antral gastritis reveals *H. pylori* in close apposition to the gastric mucosa, which shows an infiltrate with mono- and polymorphonuclear leukocytes. *H. pylori* and evidence of inflammation may also be found in areas of gastric metaplasia in the oesophagus (Barrett's oesophagus) or duodenum. Duodenal ulceration is associated with chronic antral gastritis. *H. pylori* can be detected in both antrum and duodenal ulcer tissue, but it will not colonize the duodenum except in areas of duodenal metaplasia.[18]

Clinical Features

Although a large proportion of infections are asymptomatic, chronic epigastric pain is common in infected individuals. In sub-Saharan Africa, non-ulcerous dyspepsia and duodenal ulcer are the most common causes of epigastric pain.[19] Infection with *H. pylori* was found in 88% of adult Malawians undergoing gastroscopy for chronic epigastric pain. Other features associated with *H. pylori* gastritis include nausea, vomiting and flatulence. Similar features may also be seen in children with *H. pylori* infection.[15]

Diagnosis

Specific diagnosis may be reached by invasive or non-invasive techniques (Table 24.1).

Invasive Techniques. Endoscopic biopsies from the antrum, duodenal ulcer(s) or other areas of potential colonization are examined by culture and histology and for urease activity. Two biopsy specimens from the antrum are sufficient to detect *H. pylori*.[19] Histological samples may be stained by Giemsa, silver impregnation or acridine orange for detection of *H. pylori*.

For culture, biopsy specimens are either rolled on the surface of an appropriate culture medium (e.g. brain–heart infusion-enriched Columbia blood agar incorporating Skirrow's antibiotics) or homogenized and similarly applied. In tropical countries it is advisable to incorporate an antifungal such as amphotericin B into the medium. A '1 minute' urease test, in which the biopsy is immersed in a urea (10% deionized water) solution containing a pH indicator (phenol red), has proved highly sensitive and specific.[19]

Non-invasive Techniques. Detection of antibody to *H. pylori* in serum or saliva is possible using an enzyme-linked immunosorbent assay (ELISA). Such tests have proved highly sensitive[14,15] but the specificity is variable, since it is possible to detect antibody in those who are no longer infected.[19]

Breath tests which involve administering [^{13}C] urea and measuring the release of the isotope in the patient's breath have been useful but require the availability of the isotope and are expensive. They depend upon the presence of *H. pylori* urease, which hydrolyses the urea with release of $^{13}CO_2$. Antigen-capture ELISAs have been developed for detection of *H. pylori* in stool. It has proved sensitive and specific[20] and is useful as a test of cure. It is rapid and easy to carry out and in the case of monoclonal antibody-based tests, is at least equivalent to the urea breath test[21] but is infrequently used in developing countries because of the cost.

Management and Treatment

In developing countries, non-ulcer dyspepsia may not be treated other than by symptomatic management. *H. pylori* is susceptible in vitro to a wide range of antimicrobials, including ampicillin, quinolones, cephalosporins, nitroimidazoles and macrolides, but all fail as monotherapy in vivo. Current recommendations for first-line empirical therapy in areas with low clarithromycin resistance are clarithromycin containing regimens with proton pump inhibitors with and without amoxicillin or metronidazole and where resistance is high, bismuth-containing quadruple therapy.[21] Unfortunately, resistance of *H. pylori* to metronidazole is increasing. In cases of failure, levofloxacin is used, but levofloxacin resistance is also reported.[21]

Complications

In Gambian children, an association between *H. pylori* and chronic diarrhoea and malnutrition has been described.[4] *H. pylori* gastritis was associated with protein-losing enteropathy in South African children.[22] Co-infection with *H. pylori* and *Vibrio cholerae* 01 was found frequently in Peruvian children and elderly adults, suggesting that hypochlorhydria induced by acute and chronic *H. pylori* infection might increase susceptibility to cholera.[23] Finally, epidemiological studies have suggested a link between current infection with *H. pylori* and atherothrombogenesis.[24]

TABLE 24.1 Invasive and Non-Invasive Tests for the Diagnosis of *H. pylori* Infection

Test	Sensitivity (%)	Specificity (%)	Cost	Comment
Non-Invasive				
Antibody detection – ELISA	84–95	80–95	+	Can be used for proof of cure
Antibody detection – rapid	60–75	88–92	+	Can be used for proof of cure
Stool antigen detection	90–100	92–95	++	Becomes rapidly negative after therapy
^{13}C breath test	90–96	99	+++	Needs specialized equipment
^{14}C breath test	90–96	99	+++	Needs specialized equipment
Invasive				
Histology	80–90	93–100	+++	Takes time
Culture	75–90	100	+	Takes 3–4 days
Urease	85–95	99	+	Rapid test
Gram or other stain	75–90	80–90	+	Rapid but not ideal
PCR	95–100	95–99	+++	Very sensitive, takes 4–5 hours

TABLE 24.2 *Escherichia coli* and Gastroenteritis

Pathogenicity Type	Site of Action	Associated Serogroups	Pathogenicity Genes/ Products	Acute or Chronic Diarrhoea	Antibiotic Therapy Needed
ETEC	Small bowel (secretory)	O6, O8,O15, O2O, O25, O128, O139, O148, O153, O159	CFA, LT, ST	Acute	No
EIEC	Large bowel (inflammatory)	O28, O29, O124, O136, O143	*ipa*, *ial*, EIEC	Acute	Not usually
EPEC	Small bowel (osmotic)	O55, O86, O111, O119, O125, O126, O127, O128, O142	LEE (EspA, intimin, Tir)	Chronic	Yes
EHEC	Large bowel (inflammatory)	O26, O111, O118, O138, O157	LEE, EHEC, VT1, VT2	Acute	No
EAggEC	Large bowel (inflammatory)	O44, O111, O126 *but* most are non-groupable	EAggEC adhesin, EAST-1	Acute and chronic	Yes

CFA, colonization factor antigen; EAST, EAggEC heat-stable toxin; *ipa* and *ial*, invasion-associated loci; LEE, locus of enterocyte effacement; LT, heat-labile toxin; ST, heat-stable toxin; Tir, translocatable intimin receptor; VT, vero (or Shiga-like) toxin.

Prevention and Control

Infection with *H. pylori* is ubiquitous throughout the world. Until more is known about the mode of spread, pathogenesis and immunity, prevention and control are impossible. The decrease in infection in children in developed countries suggests that improving socioeconomic and hygienic conditions should decrease the burden of infection. While no vaccines are currently licensed; new treatments/regimens have been shown to increase the eradication rates.[25]

Escherichia coli

Escherichia coli is the major aerobic component of the normal intestinal flora (~10^7 cfu/mL). Most strains are commensals, but some pathotypes cause diarrhoeal disease. The strains of *E. coli* causing diarrhoea were originally called enteropathogenic *E. coli* (EPEC), but over time five different mechanisms have been described: EPEC, enterotoxigenic *E. coli* (ETEC), enteroinvasive *E. coli* (EIEC), enterohaemorrhagic *E. coli* (EHEC) and enteroadhesive or enteroaggregative *E. coli* (EAEC or EAggEC).

E. coli was first described as a cause of gastroenteritis by its association with outbreaks of diarrhoea in infants.[26,27] This was done by showing that all infants were excreting strains of *E. coli* with the same O or somatic antigen. Different O antigens were associated with the different enteropathogenetic mechanisms of *E. coli* (Table 24.2) and while O serogrouping was used to classify EPEC until the 1980s, more recently molecular methods have been used to classify the diarrhoeagenic *E. coli.*

ENTEROTOXIGENIC *E. COLI* (ETEC)

Epidemiology

ETEC have been described worldwide, but with higher rates in some developing countries. In addition, they are a major cause of traveller's diarrhoea. In community-based studies in Bangladesh, ETEC were responsible for 15–20% of cases of diarrhoea.[28] In hospital-based studies, ETEC are a common bacterial cause of gastroenteritis. ETEC infections occur throughout the year but are most common in the wet season. Spread is by the faecal–oral route, either directly or indirectly via food or water. Infants are at particular risk at weaning. The infective dose is high (10^6–10^{10} cfu). In a recent review focusing on ETEC epidemiology with regard to toxin and colonization factor antigen (CFA) production, 60% of isolates expressed heat-labile toxin (LT) either alone (27%) or in combination with the heat-stable toxin (ST, 33%). CFA/I-expressing strains were common in all regions (17%), as were ETEC expressing CFA/II (9%) and IV (18%). There is a marked variation in toxins and CFs across regions and populations.[29]

Pathogenesis

ETEC colonize the small intestine and elaborate one heat-labile toxin (LT) or heat-stable toxin (ST) or both. ETEC colonize the small intestine by means of adhesive fimbriae or pili called colonization factor antigens or CFAs (Figure 24.3), which bind to specific receptors on the enterocyte surface. The bacteria then release their toxins. LT is a subunit toxin with a structure and mode of action similar to cholera toxin. Subunit B binds to GM_1 ganglioside on the enterocyte surface and allows subunit A to activate adenylate cyclase inside the enterocyte. The raised intracellular cyclic AMP concentration causes active C1– secretion from villous crypt cells. The net effect is that a large fluid load enters the colon and a voluminous watery stool is produced. ST is a low-molecular-weight protein that activates guanylate cyclase. This results in secretion of fluid and electrolytes into the intestinal lumen. There are no specific histopathological changes to be seen in the small-intestinal mucosa and no

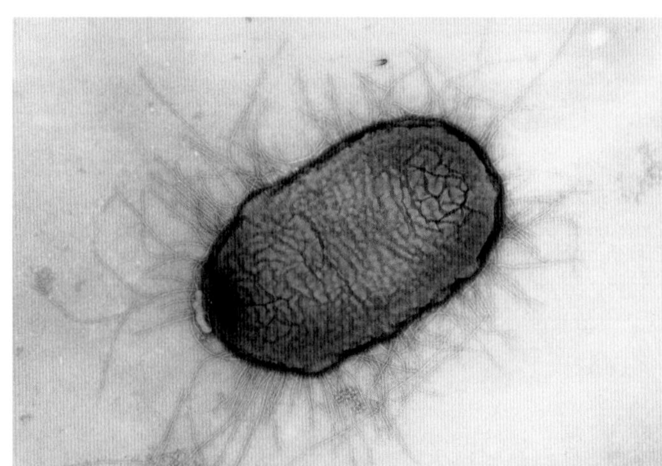

Figure 24.3 Negative-stain electron micrograph of an enterotoxigenic *E. coli* covered with fimbriae.

evidence of inflammation. The genes encoding fimbriae, LT and antibiotic resistance are carried on plasmids in ETEC.

Clinical Features

The incubation period is 1–2 days, with anorexia, vomiting and abdominal cramps in 25% of patients. The diarrhoea is explosive, voluminous and watery, up to 10 times a day. The illness is self-limiting and usually lasts 1–5 days in well-nourished persons, but up to 3 weeks in malnourished children. Dehydration is the major complication, which, in a study in Bangladesh, was seen in 46% of adults and 16% of children.[28]

Diagnosis

Specific diagnosis depends upon culture of *E. coli* from faeces and detection of pathogenicity genes (CFA, LT, ST) by PCR, or their gene products by ELISA, immunoprecipitation or bioassay. Even though molecular methods are becoming more available,[30] ETEC diagnosis in developing countries is rarely done outside of research studies.

Treatment

The mainstay of treatment is the assessment of dehydration and replacement of fluid and electrolytes. Administration of antibiotics has been shown to shorten the course of illness and duration of excretion of ETEC in adults in endemic areas and in traveller's diarrhoea. The antibiotic used depends upon susceptibility patterns in the particular geographical region. Currently, the antibiotics of choice are currently fluoroquinolones or azithromycin, with an emerging role for rifaximin. Oral rifaximin, a semisynthetic rifamycin derivative, is an effective and well-tolerated antibacterial for the management of adults with non-invasive traveller's diarrhoea. Rifaximin was significantly more effective than placebo and no less effective than ciprofloxacin in reducing the duration of diarrhoea. While rifaximin is effective in patients with *E. coli*-predominant traveller's diarrhoea, it appears ineffective in patients infected with inflammatory or invasive enteropathogens.[31]

Prevention

Antibodies against the LT and major CFs of ETEC provide protection against LT-producing ETEC expressing homologous CFs. Oral inactivated vaccines consisting of toxin antigen and whole cells, i.e. the licensed recombinant cholera B subunit (rCTB)-WC cholera vaccine Dukoral and candidate ETEC vaccines have been developed. In different trials, the rCTB-WC cholera vaccine provided high (85–100%) short-term protection. An oral ETEC vaccine consisting of rCTB and formalin-inactivated *E. coli* bacteria expressing major CFs has been shown to be safe, immunogenic and effective against severe diarrhoea in American travellers but not against ETEC diarrhoea in young children in Egypt. A modified ETEC vaccine consisting of recombinant *E. coli* strains overexpressing the major CFs and a more LT-like hybrid toxoid called LCTBA, have been developed and are being tested.[32]

ENTEROINVASIVE *E. COLI* (EIEC)

EIEC produce inflammatory diarrhoea by invading and killing colonic enterocytes (Figure 24.4). They resemble shigellae in O antigens, in being non-motile and have similar pathogenicity genes on a large plasmid that encode surface proteins mediating invasion into cells. Infection is less common than shigellosis.

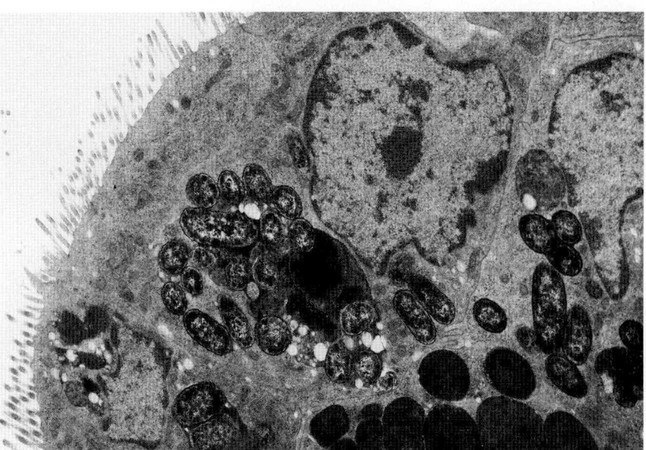

Figure 24.4 Thin-section electron micrograph of colonic enterocytes showing enteroinvasive *E. coli* that have invaded into the cells.

For example, EIEC were responsible for 4.2% of episodes of endemic diarrhoea in children in Thailand and shigellae for 23%.[32] Infection is uncommon in children under 1 year old but can be a cause of traveller's diarrhoea. The clinical features of EIEC infection are similar to those of shigellae. Diagnosis is by stool culture and detection of EIEC pathogenicity genes by DNA hybridization or PCR.[30] Antimicrobial chemotherapy is usually not indicated and no vaccine is currently available for prevention.

ENTEROPATHOGENIC *E. COLI* (EPEC)

In the early 1970s, when the pathogenesis of ETEC and EIEC had been defined, it became apparent that a large number of the classical O serogroups did not elaborate LT or ST, nor were they invasive. However, they were able to produce diarrhoea in volunteers.[33] Since these were the original classical O serogroups that caused outbreaks of infantile diarrhoea, they were termed enteropathogenic *E. coli*. EPEC were originally defined by serogroups. However, it became clear that serogroup/serotype designation over-diagnosed EPEC. Subsequently, they were defined by their characteristic localized adherence pattern in tissue-cultured cells. Currently, they are identified mainly based on the presence of specific virulence genes.[34]

Epidemiology

The first infections with EPEC were described in the UK and the USA in the 1940s and 1950s in epidemics of infantile diarrhoea. They are now considered a cause of sporadic disease in young children. EPEC has also been associated with traveller's diarrhoea. Transmission is by the faecal–oral route, either directly or in food or water. The infective dose appears to be low ($<10^4$ cfu).

Pathogenesis

EPEC have an unusual pathogenetic mechanism, in that they synthesize, secrete and insert their own receptor into host cell membranes. The ingested EPEC adhere to the mucus overlying the small-intestinal enterocytes using fimbriae. On contact with enterocytes, pathogenicity island (called the locus of enterocyte effacement: LEE)-associated genes are activated. This induces the formation of a type III secretion system that delivers effector molecules across both bacterial membranes and through a

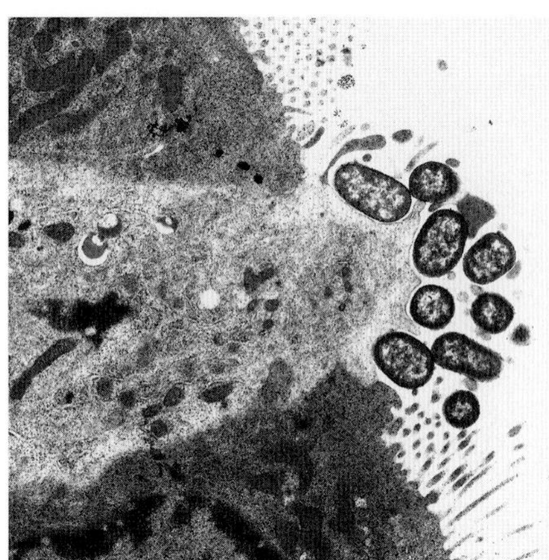

Figure 24.5 Thin-section electron micrograph of duodenal mucosa showing loss of brush border and intimately attached enteropathogenic *E. coli* (attaching/effacement).

pilus-like structure into the enterocyte.[35] Secreted effectors include Tir (translocatable intimin receptor), which becomes inserted in the enterocyte membrane. This has affinity for intimin, a surface protein on the EPEC, which then mediates the intimate attachment of EPEC to the enterocyte surface.[36] The brush border is lost with a flattening of the surface and re-arrangement of enterocyte cytoskeleton to form a cup or pedestal where the bacterium is attached, an attaching effacing lesion (Figure 24.5). Although the process is maximal in the small intestine, it can occur throughout the gastrointestinal tract. The net result is that large areas for absorption of nutrients are lost. In addition, because the disaccharidase enzymes are integral proteins in the microvillous membrane, levels of these enzymes are markedly depressed.[37] The disaccharides sucrose, lactose and maltose in the diet must be hydrolysed for monosaccharides to be absorbed. Because of loss of the brush border, the disaccharides cannot be cleaved and are thus not absorbed. They pass to the colon and cause a non-inflammatory osmotic diarrhoea, although in some cases there also appears to be a secretory component.

Clinical Features and Diagnosis

EPEC tend to produce severe and prolonged diarrhoea, which may remit and relapse. There is initially vomiting, with fever and profuse diarrhoea with mucus but no blood. Fatality rates in early epidemics ranged from 30% to 50%, but with oral rehydration and antibiotic therapy mortality rates have decreased to less than 8%.[38]

Diagnosis was previously made by stool culture on semi-selective media such as MacConkey agar followed by serogrouping on non-mucoid lactose fermenting colonies identified to be *E. coli* with specific antisera. Recently, serogrouping has been replaced by a combination of culture and molecular methods to identify specific genes. Recent epidemiological studies indicate that atypical EPEC (aEPEC) is more prevalent than typical EPEC (tEPEC) in both developed and developing countries and that aEPEC is important in both paediatric endemic diarrhoea and diarrhoeal outbreaks.[34]

Treatment and Prevention

The initial treatment is rehydration. Because the diarrhoea can be prolonged, enteral or parenteral nutrition and antibiotics may be indicated.[39] Resistance to most antibiotics has been observed in EPEC and probiotics have been suggested to restore gut health. A vaccine is not currently available for prevention of infection.

ENTEROHAEMORRHAGIC *E. COLI* (EHEC)

EHEC were first described in 1983, when they were linked to cases of haemorrhagic colitis and haemolytic–uraemic syndrome.[40,41] Infections were caused by a newly recognized serogroup, *E. coli* O157. Subsequently, a number of other *E. coli* O serogroups and other coliforms (*Enterobacter cloacae* and *Citrobacter freundii*), have been recognized to cause similar disease in humans. The recognition of the production of specific cytotoxins by EHEC, led to additional terms, such as verocytotoxin producing *E. coli* (VTEC) or Shiga toxin producing *E. coli* (STEC).

Epidemiology

Infections with EHEC were initially described in industrialized countries, where they cause outbreaks of infection usually as the result of the consumption of incompletely cooked beef or pork, or following contact with animals such as in petting zoos.[42] EHEC can be part of the normal enteric flora of cattle, pigs, sheep, goats, cats and dogs, in which they cause no disease.

Symptomatic infections are not as frequently reported from developing countries,[43] except in specific settings, such as large outbreaks of haemorrhagic colitis caused by EHEC associated with animal contamination of open water supplies in drought-affected areas in Swaziland and in Cameroon.[44,45] However, because the infective dose is low ($<10^2$ cfu), person-to-person spread also occurs.

In 2011, large outbreaks of haemolytic-uraemic syndrome in Europe drew attention to an unusual strain of EAHEC O104:H4 as an emerging *E. coli* pathotype that is endemic in Central Africa and has spread to Europe and Asia. EAHEC strains have evolved from enteroaggregative *E. coli* by uptake of a Shiga toxin 2a (Stx2a)-encoding bacteriophage. Except for Stx2a, no other EHEC-specific virulence markers including the locus of enterocyte effacement are present in EAHEC strains. EAHEC O104:H4 colonizes humans through aggregative adherence fimbrial pili encoded by the enteroaggregative *E. coli* plasmid. The aggregative adherence fimbrial colonization mechanism substitutes for the locus of enterocyte effacement functions for bacterial adherence and delivery of Stx2a into the human intestine, resulting clinically in haemolytic-uraemic syndrome.[46]

Pathogenesis

EHEC produce attaching effacement, limited to the terminal ileum and colon and similar genes to those in the EPEC LEE pathogenicity island. In addition, they release one or both of the toxins originally named verocytotoxins (VT) 1 and 2. These toxins are now called Shiga-like toxins (SLT) 1 and 2; they inhibit protein synthesis and are cytotoxic.[47] They are subunit toxins that bind to globoside receptors (the P-blood group antigen) on cells. The receptors are more densely expressed on renal endothelial cells and in children. In the colon they kill enterocytes, leading to an inflammatory haemorrhagic colitis. If they enter the systemic circulation, they can damage renal endothelial cells and precipitate the haemolytic–uraemic syndrome.

Clinical Features

Haemorrhagic colitis presents with abdominal cramps and watery diarrhoea that is followed by a haemorrhagic discharge resembling a colonic bleed. There is rarely an accompanying fever. Haemolytic-uraemic syndrome (HUS) is one of the commonest, if not the most common, cause of acute renal failure in childhood in industrialized countries. It has also been reported from developing countries, but is less frequent even though EHEC are more common in HUS than shigellae.[48] HUS presents with acute renal failure, thrombocytopenia, coagulopathy and evidence of microangiopathic haemolytic anaemia. With peritoneal dialysis, the fatality rate falls from 50% to less than 10%.

Diagnosis

The first strains of *E. coli* associated with haemorrhagic colitis and HUS were of serogroup O157; and sorbitol non-fermenters. Thus, serogrouping and sorbitol MacConkey agar are used to diagnose infections. However, other serogroups (Table 24.1) are also implicated. The toxins SLT1 and SLT2 are transferable between bacteria on promiscuous bacteriophages. Thus, specific diagnosis depends upon detection of SLT or its genes (by DNA hybridization or PCR) or of EHEC plasmid encoded fimbrial adhesin genes.[30] Excretion of EHEC beyond the period of diarrhoea is short-lived. For retrospective diagnosis it is possible to detect serum antibody to SLT.[49]

Treatment and Prevention

The treatment of haemorrhagic colitis is essentially treatment of dehydration. Antibiotics have no role and in some cases (as with *Sh. dysenteriae* 1) may increase the risk of complications.[50] For haemolytic–uraemic syndrome, peritoneal dialysis is the most important intervention. No vaccine is currently available. Prevention requires meticulous attention to food safety and to high levels of hygiene where contact with animals, particularly ruminants, is expected.

ENTEROAGGREGATIVE *E. COLI* (EAGGEC OR EAEC)

EAggEC are the most recently discovered pathogenic group.[51] As well as sporadic cases, outbreaks of EAggEC-caused diarrhoea have been described. EAggEC is a cause of acute diarrhoeal illness among children residing in both developing and developed regions, adults and persons with HIV infection residing in developing regions and travellers to developing regions in both developing and industrialized regions. The definition of EAggEC is the ability of the microorganism to adhere to epithelial cells such as HEp-2 in a very characteristic 'stacked-brick' pattern. Although many studies searching for specific virulence factor(s) unique for this category of DEC have been published it is still unknown why the EAggEC cause persistent diarrhoea. The gold standard for identification of EAggEC includes isolation of the agent and an adherence assay using tissue culture, *viz.* HEp-2 cells.

EAggEC strains are relatively heterogeneous and limited numbers of studies that examined the independent roles of the many putative EAggEC virulence genes in acute diarrhoeal illness have led to no firm conclusions regarding class-wide pathogenetic mechanisms. Molecular targets used for diagnosis by PCR include aaf, aggR, aaiC and aatA.[52]

EAggEC can cause both acute and persistent diarrhoea. In a survey of EAggEC infection in India, the most notable clinical features were fever, vomiting, overt blood in the stool and a mean duration of diarrhoea of 17 days.[53] Although not all EAggEC infections result in symptomatic illness, the most commonly reported symptoms are watery diarrhoea with or without blood and mucus, abdominal pain, nausea, vomiting and low-grade fever. Electron microscopy of infected small- and large-intestinal mucosa, from children between 3 and 190 months, cultured with several different EAggEC strains, reveals bacteria in a thick mucus layer above the intact enterocyte brush border. In the colon, EAggEC elicits inflammatory mediators and produces cytotoxic effects such as microvillus vesiculation, enlarged crypt openings and increased epithelial cell extrusion. Numerous putative virulence factors, a yersiniabactin system, a complex carbohydrate-specific lectin, enterotoxins and cytotoxins have been identified.[54]

One of the major difficulties in identifying the mechanism of pathogenesis for EAggEC is the diversity and the heterogeneity of EAggEC strains. No virulence factor has been identified as common to all EAggEC strains. EAggEC pathogenesis is therefore a complex host–pathogen interaction that involves host genetic susceptibility, heterogeneity of virulence among EAggEC strains and the amount of bacteria ingested by the infected host.

Campylobacter jejuni

The genus *Campylobacter* is a major cause of gastroenteritis in both developed and developing countries. Although *C. fetus* was recognized as an opportunist pathogen as early as 1947, the full role of *Campylobacter* species as major enteric pathogens was not realized until appropriate selective media were devised.[55]

A related genus, *Arcobacter* (principally *A. butzleri*), is increasingly recognized as an enteropathogen with similar pathogenic potential to *Campylobacter*.[56]

Epidemiology

Although *C. jejuni* continues to be the leading cause of bacterial gastroenteritis in humans worldwide, advances in molecular biology and the development of innovative culture methodologies have led to the detection and isolation of a range of under-recognized and nutritionally fastidious *Campylobacter* spp., including *C. concisus*, *C. upsaliensis* and *C. ureolyticus*. These emerging *Campylobacter* spp. have been associated with a range of gastrointestinal diseases, particularly gastroenteritis, inflammatory bowel disease and periodontitis. Over 90% of cases of *Campylobacter* gastroenteritis are associated with *C. jejuni*.

All *Campylobacter* spp. can be normally present in the gastrointestinal tract of domestic and wild animals and birds, which act as the major reservoir for infection. *C. lari*, in particular, can be part of the normal intestinal flora of birds. Campylobacters can survive for 2–5 weeks in cow's milk or water kept at 4°C but they do not multiply. Infection is spread faeco-orally, human-to-human or animal-to-human, either directly or indirectly in food and water.

- *Animal-to-human.* Close contact with animals increases the risk of infection
- *Human-to human.* Transmission may occur from infected individuals or from convalescent carriers, especially young

children. Epidemics of infection can occur in nurseries or paediatric wards

- *Food*. Contamination can occur during preparation of food from the animal's intestinal content(s) or by incomplete cooking
- *Milk*. Consumption of raw unpasteurized milk is strongly associated with illness, as is contamination of bottled milk following attack by birds[57]
- *Water*. Excreta from wild and domesticated animals can contaminate surface water and water-borne transmission is important in developing countries.

The incubation period is 2–5 days with an infective dose of 500 cfu. The median duration of excretion of *C. jejuni* following cessation of diarrhoea is 2–3 weeks. Infection is most common in those under 1 year old, with a decrease in attack rate with increasing age. Data on *Campylobacter* infection in tropical areas are limited, partly because of the difficulty of isolating the organism with limited laboratory facilities. Its prevalence has been shown from studies in India, Egypt and southern Africa.[58–60] *Campylobacter* infection has been associated with Guillain–Barré syndrome, an autoimmune polyneuropathy affecting the peripheral nervous system.[61]

Bacteriology

Campylobacters are Gram-negative bacteria with a single polar flagellum (Figure 24.6). They are spiral or bent rods, 0.2–0.5 μm in diameter and 1.5–3.5 μm long. They are thermophilic and will grow at 42°C but prefer a microaerophilic atmosphere. *C. jejuni* can hydrolyse hippurate, which distinguishes it from *C. coli* and *C. lari*. *C. coli* is sensitive to nalidixic acid but *C. lari* is resistant. All can be cultivated on simple media, but isolation can be facilitated with the use of antibiotics, oxygen quenching agents or a low oxygen atmosphere.[61]

Pathogenesis

Campylobacters can produce both inflammatory diarrhoea and non-inflammatory diarrhoeas. How Campylobacters cause diarrhoea is unclear but it does involve attachment to the intestinal mucosa and is also dependent on motility by means of flagella.[61] Other factors include iron acquisition, invasion of enterocytes and possibly toxin production.

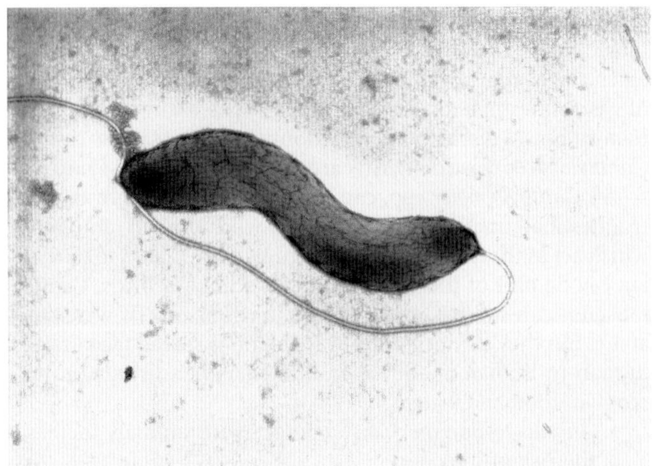

Figure 24.6 Negative-stain electron micrograph of *Campylobacter jejuni*.

Immunity to infection appears to be acquired following one or more infections, but duration of immunity is unknown. Following infection, serum and secretory antibodies to *Campylobacter* flagella, enterotoxin, lipopolysaccharide and other surface antigens that are involved in attachment are produced. In developing countries, antibodies are acquired in early life[62,63] – perhaps because of continuous exposure from animals. This higher exposure may account for greater asymptomatic infection and the lower prevalence of disease in adults in developing countries compared with developed countries. In a small proportion of those infected, usually the immunocompromised, bacteria translocate from the intestinal lumen, causing bacteraemia. In Guillain-Barré syndrome, the pathogenesis is due to a form of molecular mimicry, where *Campylobacter* contains ganglioside-like epitopes in the lipopolysaccharide moiety that elicit autoantibodies reacting with peripheral nerve targets.

Pathology

In the more severe dysentery-like illness, inflammatory infiltrates into the lamina propria and crypt abscesses can be seen in the rectal, colonic and terminal ileal mucosa.

Clinical Features

In developing countries, *Campylobacter* enteritis is generally less severe than that in developed countries. It is more likely to be of the non-inflammatory type, without fever or bloody diarrhoea.[63] However, severe bloody diarrhoea resembling bacillary dysentery can occur and also occurs in travellers acquiring infection in developing countries. In general, diarrhoea is self-limiting and resolves in 2–7 days.

Disseminated infection can occur and predisposing factors include: malnutrition, hepatic dysfunction, malignancy, diabetes mellitus, renal failure and immunosuppression. Extraintestinal and rare forms of infection include: asymptomatic bacteraemia, meningitis, deep abscesses and cholecystitis. Reactive arthritis may follow campylobacteriosis enteritis in genetically susceptible individuals (HLA-B27). *Campylobacter* enteritis is one of the commonest precipitating causes of Guillain–Barré syndrome.

Diagnosis

The features of *Campylobacter* infection are not sufficiently distinctive to make a clinical diagnosis. Examination of faecal smears by Gram stain or dark-field microscopy can provide a rapid presumptive diagnosis. Where laboratory facilities are not optimal, this may be the best diagnostic tool. However, the basis of specific diagnosis is isolation of the bacteria from faeces. *Campylobacter* spp. will grow on most basal media, especially if lysed blood is incorporated. Common media include Columbia Blood Agar base, Butzler's medium and Preston medium. In order to make the media selective, antibiotics such as trimethoprim are incorporated.[64] More recently, a blood-free medium containing charcoal, cefoperazone and amphotericin B has been developed. Culture is usually at 42°C (to inhibit gut commensals) and in a microaerophilic atmosphere. Culture plates and swabs should be kept out of the light prior to use since *Campylobacter* spp. are rapidly killed by free radicals generated by ultraviolet irradiation.

Treatment

Severe watery diarrhoea is treated by adequate rehydration. Cases of severe dysentery or disseminated infection will need antimicrobial chemotherapy. *C. jejuni* is usually sensitive to erythromycin, but increased resistance has been reported and quinolones such as ciprofloxacin may be required.

Prevention and Control

There is no vaccine for prevention of infection; thus, non-specific methods for prevention such as improvements in sanitation, provision of clean potable water and good food hygiene are important.[61]

Yersinia enterocolitica

The genus *Yersinia* comprises *Y. pestis*, the cause of plague, *Y. pseudotuberculosis* and *Y. enterocolitica*. Yersiniosis is a food-borne illness that has become more prevalent in recent years due to human transmission via the faecal–oral route and prevalence in farm animals. Yersiniosis is primarily caused by *Yersinia enterocolitica* and less frequently by *Yersinia pseudotuberculosis*.

Epidemiology

Although *Yersinia* infection is said to have a worldwide distribution, it is found much more commonly in temperate zones than in the tropics. Even in temperate countries, infection is more prevalent in colder climates and is more common in winter.[65] In most surveys of acute diarrhoeal disease where *Y. enterocolitica* was sought, it was either absent, or present in less than 1% of cases.[66] However, cases of generalized infection have been recorded in South Africa and other studies have shown infection in West Africa and Ethiopia.[67–69]

The reservoir for *Y. enterocolitica* is a variety of animal species, including birds, frogs, fish, snails, oysters and most mammals. The organism is excreted in faeces from pigs and cattle and can persist in lakes, streams, soil and vegetables. Patient-to-patient spread is rare except by blood transfusion. The incubation period is 1–11 days and bacteria are excreted for 14–97 (mean 42) days.

Bacteriology

Y. enterocolitica is a small Gram-negative rod with peritrichous flagella. It will grow on simple media and is lactose non-fermenting on MacConkey agar. It is psychrophilic and isolation from clinical samples often involves a cold enrichment step. O serogrouping is used to subdivide strains. The human pathogenic strains most frequently isolated worldwide belong to serogroups O:3, O:5,27, O:8 and O:9.

Pathogenesis

Pathogenic strains of *Y. enterocolitica* carry a large plasmid that encodes surface proteins and lipopolysaccharides mediating cell attachment, resistance to phagocytosis and serum resistance. *Yersinia* adhesion A protein (YadA) mediates mucus and epithelial cell attachment and, in concert with invasin, promotes host cell invasion. Induction of YadA expression is coordinated with the upregulation of Yops (*Yersinia* outer membrane proteins). Chromosomal genes (*inv*, *ail*: attaching invasion locus) encode the ability to invade epithelial cells. The Yops are translocated through a host-cell docked *Yersinia* secretion protein F needle, directly into the targeted host cells. The YopB and YopD proteins form a pore in the host cell plasma membrane, allowing for translocation of the effector proteins. YadA elicits an inflammatory response in epithelial cells by inducing mitogen-activated protein kinase-dependent IL-8 production and by contributing to the resulting intestinal inflammatory cascade.[70] Although *Y. enterocolitica* produces a toxin similar to LT, its role in pathogenesis is unclear. *Y. enterocolitica* invades ileal enterocytes and M cells in Peyer's patches, where it multiplies. This produces an inflammatory diarrhoea. Bacteria may pass to local lymph nodes and subsequently produce systemic disease.

In addition to disease produced directly by *Y. enterocolitica*, there are a number of autoimmune phenomena which present in a proportion of patients after initial infection. These include: erythema nodosum, reactive arthropathy, Reiter's syndrome and glomerulonephritis. In addition, there is a linkage with thyroid disorders, in that patients with Hashimoto's thyroiditis have high titres of *Y. enterocolitica*-agglutinating antibodies and that the surface of *Y. enterocolitica* has receptors for thyroid-stimulating hormone.

Clinical Features

Most symptomatic infections are in children under 5 years of age.[65] Characteristically, clinical features consist of diarrhoea, low-grade fever and abdominal pain. The diarrhoeic stool will be frankly blood-stained in a quarter of cases. Nausea, vomiting, headache and pharyngitis are minor presentations. The abdominal pain may be present alone or with mild diarrhoea and is often termed the pseudoappendicular syndrome. Infection may spread elsewhere to produce bacteraemia, peritonitis, hepatic, renal and splenic abscesses, pyomyositis and osteomyelitis.[65,68] These are more likely to occur in patients who are immunocompromised or who have iron overload – as in haemochromatosis.[67] The extraintestinal manifestations are more likely to occur in adults, as are the autoimmune phenomena. Of those with reactive arthritis, 80% are of HLA-B27 histocompatibility type.

Diagnosis

Y. enterocolitica can be isolated from stool, appendix, mesenteric lymph nodes, blood and other focal sites of infection, using simple media. Strategies for isolation include MacConkey agar incubated at 25–30°C for 48 hours or selective media such as cefsulodin–irgasan–novobiocin (CIN) agar at 37°C. For isolation from food or water, cold enrichment in phosphate-buffered saline for up to 4 weeks at 4°C prior to plating on to CIN agar greatly increases the yield of both pathogenic and non-pathogenic *Yersinia* spp. Speciation is obtained by biochemical tests and it is noteworthy that all non-pathogenic *Y. enterocolitica* have pyrizinamidase activity. Pathogenic *Y. enterocolitica* all possess the virulence plasmid. For retrospective diagnosis, serology using ELISA, whole cell agglutination, or complement fixation tests can be performed. They can be difficult to interpret and cross-reactions, for example *Y. enterocolitica* 0:9 with *Brucella abortus*, *E. coli*, *Morganella morganii* and *Salmonella* spp., do occur. The specificity of the test can be improved by detecting a greater than fourfold increase in titre between acute and convalescent sera.

Treatment and Control

Gastrointestinal infections are usually self-limiting and do not merit antimicrobial therapy. Nonetheless, fluoroquinolones or

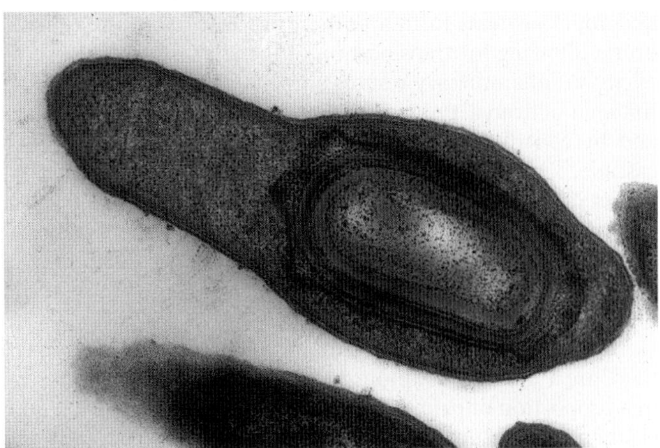

Figure 24.7 Thin-section electron micrograph of *Clostridium perfringens* showing its endospore.

third-generation cephalosporins, the best therapeutic options, are warranted to treat enterocolitis in compromised hosts and in patients with septicaemia or invasive infection, in which the mortality can be as high as 50%.[71]

Clostridium spp.

Clostridia are anaerobic sporing Gram-positive rods (Figure 24.7). Two species, *Cl. perfringens* and *Cl. difficile*, are associated with diarrhoeal disease.

CLOSTRIDIUM PERFRINGENS

Two forms of diarrhoeal disease are associated with *Cl. perfringens* (formerly *welchii*). The first is a food-poisoning illness due to ingestion of *Cl. perfringens* type A or the enterotoxin it produces. Although this is a common cause of food poisoning in industrialized countries, it produces mild, short-lived disease and is extremely uncommon in the tropics. *Cl. perfringens* type C, in contrast, is common in certain areas of the tropics and produces severe necrotic enteritis.

Epidemiology

Cl. perfringens type C has been implicated in enteritis necroticans (Darmbrand) seen in malnourished individuals in Northern Europe after the Second World War and 'pigbel' in the highlands of Papua New Guinea. A similar disease has been described in Uganda, Malaysia, Thailand, Indonesia, China and, more recently, in India.[72–75]

Infection can occur sporadically but also in epidemics.[72–74] It occurs at any age but is more likely to present as acute toxic or acute surgical problems in children under 10 years old. In Papua New Guinea, pigbel is associated with large 'pig feasts' that occur every 3–10 years. Infection is more common in males than females; whether this represents a true difference in susceptibility is unclear. *Cl. perfringens* type C can be found in the human normal intestinal flora, in pig excreta and in soil.

Pathogenesis

The enteric toxins of *Cl. perfringens* share two common features: (1) they are all single polypeptides of modest (approx. 25–35 kDa) size, although lacking in sequence homology and (2) they generally act by forming pores or channels in plasma membranes of host cells. These enteric toxins include *Cl. perfringens* enterotoxin (CPE), which is responsible for the symptoms of a common human food poisoning and acts by forming pores after interacting with intestinal tight junction proteins. Two other *Cl. perfringens* enteric toxins, epsilon-toxin (a bioterrorism select agent) and beta-toxin, cause veterinary enterotoxaemias when absorbed from the intestines; beta- and epsilon-toxins then apparently act by forming oligomeric pores in intestinal or extra-intestinal target tissues. The action of a newly discovered *Cl. perfringens* enteric toxin, beta2 toxin, has not yet been defined but precedent suggests it might also be a pore-former.[76]

Since *Cl. perfringens* type C can be found as part of the normal intestinal flora, it is considered that host-dependent factors are also involved in pathogenesis. First, the bulk of the normal anaerobic flora is found in the large bowel and one hypothesis is that overgrowth of *Cl. perfringens* type C in the jejunum might be related to development of disease. A more attractive hypothesis links malnutrition and type of diet with disease. The β toxin is readily inactivated by intestinal proteases. Protein deficiency decreases intestinal protease levels; in addition, the sweet potato, which is a staple diet in highland Papua New Guinea, contains heat-stable trypsin inhibitors. Thus, consumption of meat contaminated by *Cl. perfringens* type C or its β toxin in an individual with low intestinal protease activity due to malnutrition or dietary protease inhibitors would allow the toxin to produce intestinal damage.[74,76]

Pathology

Gross pathology shows patchy segmental acute ulcerative necrosis of the jejunum and, to a lesser extent, the ileum, caecum and colon. This may rapidly progress to segmental gangrene with gas in the mucosa, mesentery or lymph nodes. Microscopically, the intestinal wall shows separation of the mucosa from the submucosa, with large denuded areas covered with a pseudomembrane of dead enterocytes and infiltrating neutrophils and red blood cells. Healing occurs with fibrosis and strictures and adhesions may form later.

Clinical Features

Pigbel varies in severity from mild diarrhoea to a rapidly fatal necrotizing enteritis, with high mortality (up to 85%). The incubation period is approximately 48 hours after the feast but can vary from 24 hours to up to a week.

Disease has been classified into four main presentations.[72] Type I (acute toxic) presents with fulminant toxaemia and shock. Type II (acute surgical) presents as mechanical and paralytic ileus, acute strangulation, perforation and peritonitis. Type III (subacute surgical) presents later, with complications of mild type II. Finally, type IV (mild or trivial) presents with mild diarrhoea but may rarely progress to type III. Type I disease occurs most commonly in young children and has the highest mortality (85%). Type II disease has a 42% mortality; type III, 44% mortality; and type IV is never fatal. In type II and type III disease, a palpable segment of thickened intestine may be found. The stool will contain blood and pus cells and there is a neutrophil leukocytosis in peripheral blood. The differential diagnosis includes: acute causes of inflammatory diarrhoea, peritonitis, acute abdominal obstruction, acute pancreatitis, acute amoebic colitis and sickle cell crises.

Diagnosis

Cl. perfringens can be cultured from faeces, peritoneal fluid or other infected sites by plating on to neomycin blood agar and incubating anaerobically. *Cl. perfringens* type C is differentiated from other *Cl. perfringens* by serological techniques, including immunofluorescence and type C antibody-coated silica beads.[77] Interpretation of results can be difficult since *Cl. perfringens* type C is also found in normal individuals. Detection of antibodies to the toxin can be useful in reaching a diagnosis in survivors.

Treatment

Acute resuscitation is by fluid and electrolytes intravenously, together with bowel decompression by restricting oral intake and nasogastric intubation. Antibiotics will be needed if there is extraintestinal spread of the organism (e.g. peritonitis) and metronidazole, ampicillin, chloramphenicol or penicillin should be of value. Administration of *Cl. perfringens* type C antiserum is also beneficial. Surgical intervention will be necessary if there is persisting obstruction, increasing signs of toxaemia, or signs of peritonitis or of strangulation. There is some evidence that early surgical intervention can decrease mortality.

Prevention

Active immunization with a toxoid prepared from *Cl. perfringens* type C toxins has decreased the incidence of pigbel in children in the past.[78]

CLOSTRIDIUM DIFFICILE

Cl. difficile is the cause of antibiotic-associated colitis and of pseudomembranous colitis. In adults, a clinical prediction rule found the best signs to be: significant diarrhoea ('new onset of more than three partially formed or watery stools per 24 hour period'), recent antibiotic exposure, abdominal pain, fever (up to 40.5°C) and a distinctive foul stool odour. The bacteria release toxins that can cause bloating and diarrhoea, with abdominal pain, which may become severe. Symptoms of *Cl. difficile* infection often mimic some flu-like symptoms and can mimic disease flare in patients with inflammatory bowel disease-associated colitis. *Cl. difficile* infections (CDI) are the most common cause of pseudomembranous colitis and in rare cases this can progress to toxic megacolon, which can be life-threatening. The bacterium can be found worldwide but its role as a cause of diarrhoeal disease in developing countries is probably underestimated. The new hypertoxin-producing BI/NAP1/O27 strain of *Cl. difficile* is thus far confined to developed countries.[79] Of all patients treated for CDI, 20% relapse and 65% of those experiencing a second relapse become chronic cases.

Pathogenic *Cl. difficile* strains produce several known toxins. The most well-characterized are enterotoxin (*Cl. difficile* toxin A) and cytotoxin (*Cl. difficile* toxin B), both of which are responsible for the diarrhoea and inflammation seen in infected patients, although their relative contributions have been debated. Toxins A and B are glucosyltransferases that target and inactivate the Rho family of GTPases. Toxin B (cytotoxin) induces actin depolymerization by a mechanism correlated with a decrease in the ADP-ribosylation of the low molecular mass GTP-binding Rho proteins. Another toxin, binary toxin, has also been described, but its role in disease is not yet fully understood.[80]

Current recommendations include metronidazole for treatment of mild to moderate CDI and vancomycin for severe CDI. Results from small clinical trials suggest that nitazoxanide and teicoplanin may be alternative options to standard therapies, whereas rifaximin has demonstrated success in uncontrolled trials for the management of multiple recurrences.[81] Anecdotal reports have also suggested that tigecycline might be useful as an adjunctive agent for the treatment of severe complicated CDI. Fidaxomicin, a macrocyclic antibiotic, has a narrow spectrum of activity against Gram-positive anaerobes and is bactericidal against *Cl. difficile*. It has no activity against Gram-negative bacteria. Fidaxomicin has minimal activity against *Bacteroides* species, which may be advantageous in maintaining colonization resistance and protecting the gastrointestinal tract from colonization by *Cl. difficile*.[82] A vaccine is being developed targeted at closed communities, hospitals and those patients needing prolonged antibiotic therapy.[83]

The cornerstone of prevention is appropriate contact precautions and strict hand hygiene. Other important approaches are effective cleaning and antibiotic stewardship.[84]

Aeromonas and *Plesiomonas*

These two genera within the Vibrionaceae family are both aquatic microorganisms and can be readily isolated from fresh and salt water, fish, soil and food. Today, the genus *Aeromonas* is regarded not only as an important disease-causing pathogen of fish and other cold-blooded species but also as the aetiological agent responsible for a variety of infectious complications in both immunocompetent and immunocompromised persons.[85]

AEROMONAS HYDROPHILA

Epidemiology

A. hydrophila has been associated with gastroenteritis in many countries throughout the world. In tropical countries, it can be isolated from healthy as well as diarrhoeic individuals. In Thailand, *Aeromonas* spp. were isolated from 9% of cases of gastroenteritis and were second in importance only to ETEC.

Microbiology

The genus *Aeromonas* encompasses three motile species which cause disease in humans: *A. hydrophila*, *A. caviae* and *A. sobria*. A fourth, non-motile species, *A. salmonicida*, is a fish pathogen and will not grow above 30°C. They are oxidase-positive and will grow on most simple media. *Aeromonas* produces a wide range of extracellular factors including: proteases, elastases, esterases, DNAse, haemolysins, cytotoxins and enterotoxins.

Pathogenesis

Aeromonas is associated with both inflammatory and non-inflammatory diarrhoea. It possesses both fimbrial and non-fimbrial adhesins for attachment to the intestinal mucosa. *Aeromonas* produces two types of flagella, a constitutively expressed polar flagellum (Pof) and multiple inducible lateral flagella (Laf). Pof produces swimmer cells in liquid environments, while Laf induces swarming motility on solid medium surfaces. *Aeromonas* produces biofilms, which are regulated by

TABLE 24.3 Classification of *Shigella* Serotypes

Species	No. of Serotypes	Glucose	Mannitol (Fermentation)	Lactose
Sh. dysenteriae	10	+	–	–
Sh. flexneri	6	+	+	–
Sh. boydii	15	+	+	–
Sh. sonnei	1	+	+	Late

quorum sensing. Once established in the gastrointestinal tract, aeromonads can apparently produce diarrhoea by elaboration of enterotoxigenic molecules, causing enteritis, or by invasion of the gastrointestinal epithelium, producing dysentery or colitis.

Clinical Features

Based upon frequency, *Aeromonas* clinical infections fall into four broad categories, namely: (1) gastrointestinal tract syndromes, (2) wound and soft tissue infections, (3) blood-borne dyscrasias and (4) a miscellaneous category which includes a myriad of less frequently encountered ailments and infectious processes. Gastroenteritis associated with *Aeromonas* spp. can vary from acute watery diarrhoea with fever to chronic dysentery with fever and abdominal cramps.[85]

Diagnosis

Aeromonas can be isolated from faeces using selective media such as ampicillin blood agar. Prior enrichment in alkaline peptone water increases the sensitivity of isolation. Since *Aeromonas* spp. can be isolated from normal individuals, isolation does not prove causation. For the future, it may be necessary to detect pathogenicity factors (toxins, adhesins or invasiveness) to link isolation with the disease in a particular patient.

Treatment

Rehydration is usually the only intervention needed. If infection becomes disseminated or there is chronic dysentery, antimicrobials such as fluoroquinolones might be of benefit.

PLESIOMONAS SHIGELLOIDES

This bacterium has been associated with food-borne (usually fish) gastroenteritis in Mali and India and there has even been a case of snake-to-human transmission.[86–88]

Shigellosis (Bacillary Dysentery)

Dysentery has been a disease of poor and crowded communities throughout history and continues to be a major cause of morbidity and mortality in the tropics. Dysentery bacilli were first demonstrated by Shiga in 1898 and subsequent studies showed that four species, *Shigella dysenteriae*, *Sh. flexneri*, *Sh. boydii* and *Sh. sonnei*, were responsible for the disease described as bacillary dysentery. *Sh. dysenteriae* and *Sh. flexneri* are responsible for most infections in the tropics. A recent review of the literature for 1990–2009 indicates that ~125 million shigellosis cases occur annually in Asia, of which ~14 000 are fatal.[89] Shigellosis occurs both endemically and as epidemics.

Bacteriology

Shigella species are members of the Enterobacteriaceae and are aerobic, Gram-negative, non-motile bacilli. In pure growth, *Shigella* spp. are readily cultured on non-selective media, but for isolation from clinical specimens, selective media such as MacConkey and xylose lysine deoxycholate (XLD) are necessary. They are typically non-lactose-fermenting, lysine-decarboxylase-negative and do not produce gas from glucose. The exceptions are *Sh. sonnei*, which ferments lactose slowly and *Sh. flexneri* 6 and *Sh. boydii* 13, which produce gas from glucose. *Sh. dysenteriae*, *Sh. flexneri* and *Sh. boydii* are each divided into a number of serotypes (Table 24.3).

Serotype (O) antigens are located on the outer polysaccharide chains of the lipopolysaccharide component of the cell wall. *Shigella* spp. are non-motile and do not possess H antigens. For epidemiological studies, serotypes may be subdivided by molecular methods such as the enterobacterial repetitive intergenic sequence-based polymerase chain reaction (ERIC-PCR) typing or the current standard for the typing of Shigella, pulsed field gel electrophoresis (PFGE).[90]

Pathogenesis

Shigella dysentery is characterized by invasion of the colonic mucosa, local spread of the infecting organism and death of intestinal epithelial cells. In a proportion of cases, extraintestinal complications occur, including seizures, hyponatraemia and hypoglycaemia, septicaemia, Reiter syndrome, encephalopathy and the haemolytic–uraemic syndrome. Interaction of *Shigella* with epithelial cells includes contact of bacteria with the cell surface and release of Ipa proteins through a specialized type III secretion. A complex signaling process involving activation of small GTPases of the Rho family and c-src causes major rearrangements of the cytoskeleton, thereby allowing bacterial entry by macropinocytosis. After entry, shigellae escape to the cell cytoplasm and initiate intracytoplasmic movement through assembly of actin filaments caused by bacterial surface protein IcsA, which binds and activates a protein inducing actin nucleation. Actin-driven motility promotes efficient colonization of the host cell cytoplasm and rapid cell-to-cell spread via protrusions that are engulfed by adjacent cells in a cadherin-dependent process. Bacterial invasion turns infected cells to strongly pro-inflammatory cells through sustained activation of nuclear factor-kappaB. A major consequence is interleukin (IL)-8 production, which attracts polymorphonuclear leukocytes (PMNs). On transmigration, PMNs disrupt the permeability of this epithelium and promote its invasion by shigellae. At the early stage of infection, M cells of the follicle-associated epithelium allow bacterial translocation. Subsequent apoptotic killing of macrophages in a caspase 1-dependent process causes the release of IL-1β and IL-18, which accounts for the initial steps of inflammation.[91] A number of pathogenic factors and their genetic determinants have been described. Invasion is associated with specific outer membrane proteins that are encoded on a plasmid (extrachromosomal) DNA of size 220 kb. Strains not containing these plasmids have been shown to be non-virulent. *Sh. dysenteriae* 1 produces a toxin, Shiga toxin (Stx). Stx inactivates ribosomal RNA, inhibiting protein synthesis and leads to cell death. Stx is composed of A and B subunits, the genes being chromosomally located and is the same as SLT1 and SLT2 produced by EHEC. The cytotoxic effects of *Shiga* toxin are involved both in the haemorrhagic intestinal manifestations and in the haemolytic–uraemic syndrome.

Pathology and Immunology

The characteristic pathology is an acute, locally invasive colitis, ranging from mild inflammation of the mucous membranes of the distal colon to severe necrosis of much of the large bowel. Sigmoidoscopy reveals a red, bleeding mucosa with patches of necrotic membrane, which may separate to leave ulcerated areas. The inflammatory process may extend through the submucosa to the muscle layer. In severe cases, complete healing may not occur, resulting in fibrous tissue formation and persistent ulceration. Bacteraemia is uncommon in *Shigella* infection, but is a probable risk factor for increased mortality.[92] Circulating endotoxin is likely to play an important role in the systemic manifestations of *Shigella* infection. In *Sh. dysenteriae* 1 infections, Shiga toxin exerts both enterotoxic effects, through specific glycolipid binding sites and is responsible for the haemolytic–uraemic syndrome. Infection with *Shigella* spp. leads to both local (gut) immunity and the production of circulating antibodies. Circulating antibodies are directed against the O (lipopolysaccharide) antigens and have been shown to be serotype-specific.

Epidemiology

Man is the only natural host for infection by *Shigella* spp. Infection is by ingestion, the infective dose being as low as 10–100 bacteria for *Sh. dysenteriae*. The incubation period is 1–5 days. Shigellosis occurs as an endemic disease in conditions of crowding, poor sanitation and inadequate water supply and is primarily a disease of poor disadvantaged communities in the tropics.

Endemic shigellosis is largely a paediatric disease, most cases occurring in children below 10 years of age. In a recent review of data from Asia, the median frequency of *Shigella* spp. isolation from diarrhoea cases in the community in children 0–4 years of age was 4.4%, while at facilities it was 6.6% and in older individuals it was 4.0% in the community and ~11.6% in facilities.[90] Routes of infection include direct person-to-person transmission (from cases or asymptomatic excreters) and transmission via contaminated water or food. The evidence for person-to-person transmission in endemic areas of the tropics comes from a number of community studies that show a high frequency of secondary household cases in the family of an index case, but no differences between families with cases and control families in relation to water or food supply.[93] In epidemics of *Sh. dysenteriae* 1, person-to-person transmission is also more common than point-source food or water outbreaks. Though occasional water-borne epidemics have been described, a seasonal pattern of shigellosis is seen in most endemic areas. In Bangladesh, peak transmission rates occur at the beginning of the monsoon season, with a second, lower peak in the winter season.[94]

Clinical Features

Shigellosis may vary from relatively mild watery diarrhoea to severe dysentery with intestinal and extraintestinal complications. In severe cases, the onset is abrupt, with tenesmus, fever and frequent passage of bloody, mucoid stools. The degree of dehydration may be considerably less than in other diarrhoeas, though stool frequency may be as many as 30 times per day. Diarrhoea is often accompanied by fever, headache and malaise. Intestinal complications include toxic megacolon, perforation and a protein-losing enteropathy. Electrolyte imbalance may arise – in particular, prolonged hyponatraemia. *Sh. dysenteriae* and *Sh. flexneri* infections may result in a number of extraintestinal complications. Haemolytic–uraemic syndrome occurs particularly with *Sh. dysenteriae* 1 and can develop 7–10 days after the onset of disease. Convulsions may occur with infections caused by all species of *Shigella*, particularly in children. They may occur before diarrhoea begins and are usually accompanied by a rising fever. Encephalopathy and hemiplegia have been reported.[95]

Diagnosis

In many parts of the tropical world, the diagnosis and subsequent management of *Shigella* infections occur in the absence of laboratory facilities. While clinical algorithms (Figure 24.8) have been used to aid in the differential diagnosis of dysentery symptoms, the more general case definition of 'acute diarrhoea with visible blood in the stools' is the clinical case definition recommended for surveillance.[96] Laboratory isolation and identification of *Shigella* spp. is necessary to confirm the

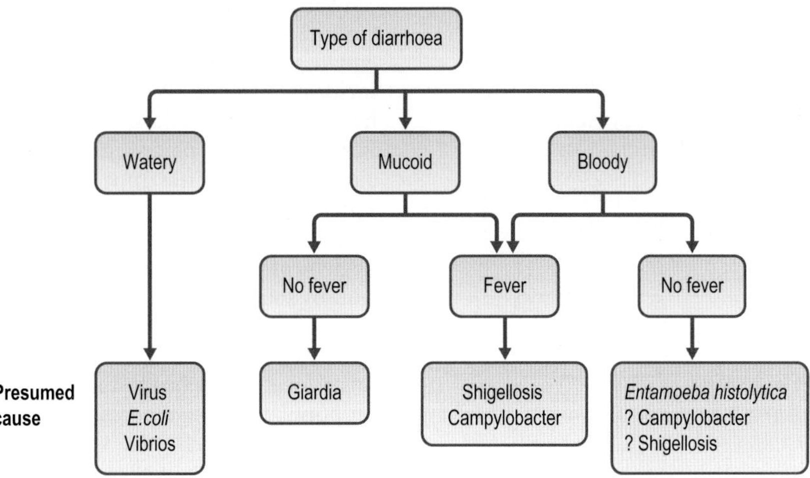

Figure 24.8 Clinical algorithm in the differential diagnosis of diarrhoea.

diagnosis and to enable antimicrobial sensitivities to be determined.

Shigellae survive poorly in ambient temperatures in the tropics and if the stool specimens cannot be cultured within a few hours of collection, they should be placed in transport medium and stored at +4°C. Cary–Blair medium and buffered glycerol saline (BGS) are the recommended transport media. In the investigation of epidemics, it is more useful to collect specimens from a small number of patients who fit the clinical case definition and to ensure that these specimens are transported and processed appropriately. For molecular approaches, new transport technique (DNA/RNA Protect™, Sierra Diagnostics Inc., Sonora, CA, USA) permits detection of *ipaH* from stool specimens held for prolonged periods at room temperature.[97]

Figure 24.9 shows the WHO guidelines for the culture of specimens for isolation and identification of *Shigella* spp. Faecal specimens or rectal swabs should be cultured overnight on MacConkey medium and a more selective medium such as xylose lysine deoxycholate (XLD) agar. Shigellae appear as pale, non-lactose-fermenting colonies on MacConkey medium and as pink colonies on XLD. Suspect colonies are incubated overnight on Kligler iron agar (KIA) and motility indole urea (MIU) medium. Table 24.4 shows the typical reactions of *Shigella* spp. in these composite media. Positive isolates may be typed by slide agglutination using the appropriate *Shigella* antisera. Antimicrobial sensitivities should be determined using a disc diffusion method. It is essential that a standardized technique is used and the Kirby Bauer-based CSLI (formerly NCCLS) methodology is recommended.[98]

TABLE 24.4 Reactions of *Shigella* spp. on Kligler Iron Agar (KIA) and Motility Indole Urea (MIU) Medium

Bacterium	Urea	Slant	Butt	H_2S	Gas	Motility	Indole
E. coli	–	A	A	–	+	(+)	D
Sh. dysenteriae	–	K	A	–	–	–	D
Sh. flexneri	–	K	A	–	–[a]	–	D
Sh. boydii	–	K	A	–	–[b]	–	D
Sh. sonnei	–	K	A	–	–	–	–

A, acid (yellow) reaction; K, alkaline (red) reaction; +, positive reaction; –, negative reaction; d, different biochemical types.
[a]Some *Sh. flexneri* serotype 6 gas (+).
[b]Serotypes 13 and 14 gas (+).

Management

The management of cases of shigellosis requires appropriate rehydration and electrolyte therapy, antimicrobial treatment and the management of complications. Dehydration is rarely severe; oral rehydration is usually sufficient to restore water and electrolyte imbalances. High-risk patients include children less than 5 years of age, patients who are dehydrated or seriously ill when first seen and older children and adults who are malnourished. Effective antimicrobial therapy will shorten the duration of illness and is particularly necessary in severe cases. Resistance of *Shigella* spp. to commonly used antimicrobial agents is an increasing problem in many tropical countries and data on local sensitivities are essential if effective treatment is to be implemented.

Resistance of *Sh. dysenteriae* to ampicillin, co-trimoxazole and chloramphenicol is now widespread and nalidixic acid is the first-line drug of choice where resistance is not wide spread. Resistance to nalidixic acid is increasing, leaving only fluoroquinolones such as ciprofloxacin and ofloxacin and pivmecillinam as effective oral therapies. Several clinical trials have demonstrated the efficacy of short courses of fluoroquinolones being effective.[99] Unresolved issues remain over the use of fluoroquinolones in children. The importance of local sensitivity data cannot be over-emphasized.

Maintaining adequate levels of nutrition in patients is an essential component of management, particularly in children, who may already be malnourished. Studies in Bangladesh have shown the value of supportive nutrition in the outcome of children with shigellosis.

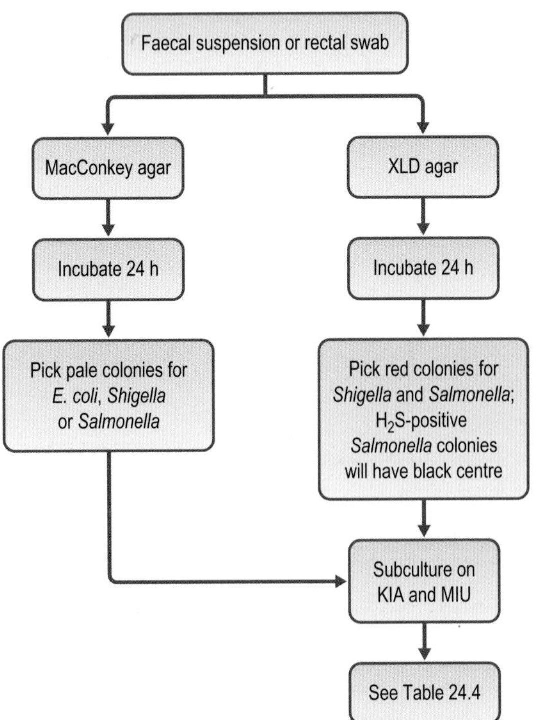

Figure 24.9 Culture protocol for isolation of *Shigella* spp.

Prevention and Control

Shigellosis is primarily a disease of crowded and usually poor communities, living in an environment characterized by inadequate sanitation and often polluted water. In the long term, the incidence of shigellosis will be reduced only by improved public health and the alleviation of poverty. Since most transmission is from person to person, improvements in water supply quality alone may have little impact. Most studies show that increased water quantity and general improvement in the level of hygiene reduce the incidence of diarrhoeal disease. Improvement in hygiene at the household level, particularly through the provision of soap for hand washing, has been shown to reduce the transmission of shigellosis. In epidemics of shigellosis, coordinated action is necessary at the local and regional level in diagnosis, local public health interventions and possibly restrictions on population movements, markets, religious gatherings, etc.

There are no effective vaccines against shigellosis, although current approaches include (1) live attenuated deletion mutants based on rational selection of genes that are key in the

TABLE 24.5 The First Six Cholera Pandemics

Pandemic	Date	Indian Sub-Continent	South-East Asia	Middle East	Europe	North Africa	East Africa	America
First	1817–1823	+	+	+	–	–	+	–
Second	1826–1837	+	+	+	+	+	+	+
Third	1842–1862	+	+	+	+	+	+	+
Fourth	1865–1875	+	+	+	+	+	+	+
Fifth	1881–1896	+	+	+	+	+	+	+
Sixth	1899–1923	+	+	+	+	–	+	–

pathogenic process and (2) conjugated detoxified polysaccharide parenteral vaccines, or more recently conjugated synthetic carbohydrates. Some of these approaches have already undergone phase I and II clinical trials with promising results, but important issues have also emerged, particularly the discrepancy between colonization and immunogenic potential of live attenuated vaccine candidates depending upon the population concerned, particularly in endemic areas.[100] For the foreseeable future, however, prevention of morbidity and mortality caused by shigellosis will depend on public health interventions and effective and timely case management.

Vibrio cholerae

Cholera occurs endemically in many areas of the tropics, particularly in South and South-east Asia and Africa. In 1991, cholera appeared in Latin America for the first time in the twentieth century. A cholera-like disease was described by early Indian, Greek and Chinese writers, but it is uncertain whether the disease had spread beyond the Indian subcontinent before the nineteenth century. From 1817 to 1923 there were six pandemics of cholera, spreading extensively from its natural home in the Gangetic plain and delta (Table 24.5). The seventh pandemic of cholera, which began in 1961, is described under Epidemiology (see below).

Bacteriology

In 1883, Koch demonstrated the bacterial cause of cholera during a visit to Egypt and subsequent work defined the species *Vibrio cholerae*. Vibrios are comma-shaped, aerobic Gram-negative bacteria which have a characteristic darting movement (Figure 24.10). They are oxidase-positive and ferment sucrose and glucose but not lactose. Vibrios possess both flagellar and somatic antigens. The species *V. cholerae* is divided into many serovars, according to somatic antigens. Until the appearance of *V. cholerae* serotype O139 in 1992, *V. cholerae* O1 was the only serotype responsible for cholera. Other serovars with different O antigens may cause a diarrhoea-like illness but are not associated with epidemic cholera. There are two biotypes of *V. cholerae* O1: classical and El Tor. Table 24.6 summarizes their characteristic properties. *V. cholerae* El Tor was first isolated from pilgrims at the El Tor quarantine station in Sinai in 1906. Until 1961, the El Tor biotype was isolated only in Sulawesi, Indonesia and had caused four localized epidemics between 1937 and 1958. The classical and El Tor biotypes are each divided into three serotypes: Ogawa, Inaba and Hikojima. *V. cholerae* O139 is related to the El Tor biotype.

V. cholerae does not form spores and is killed by heating at 55°C for 15 minutes and by phenolic and hypochlorite disinfectants. It can survive in saline conditions at low temperatures for up to 60 days and may survive in aquatic environments for extended periods in a non-cultivable state. *Vibrio cholerae* is often associated with zooplankton and shellfish in water and it can use chitin as a carbon and nitrogen source. In water, *V. cholerae* enter a viable but non-culturable form, also called active but non-culturable or conditionally viable environmental cells.[101] Excluding seafoods, *V. cholerae* survives for only a limited time on foodstuff, although contaminated food may act as a vehicle for transmission. In fish and shellfish, *V. cholerae* may survive from 2 to 5 days at ambient temperatures, a property often associated with food-related outbreaks.

TABLE 24.6 Differentiating Properties of Classical and El Tor Biotypes of *Vibrio Cholerae* 01

	Classical	El Tor
Chicken cell haemagglutination	–	+
Voges–Proskauer test	–	+
Polymyxin B sensitivity	Sensitive	Resistant

Pathogenesis and Immunity

Cholera is characterized by severe watery diarrhoea leading to dehydration, electrolyte imbalance and hypovolaemia, with a mortality ranging from less than 1 to 40%.

There is a wide spectrum of severity and mild and asymptomatic cases may occur. *V. cholerae* is non-invasive;

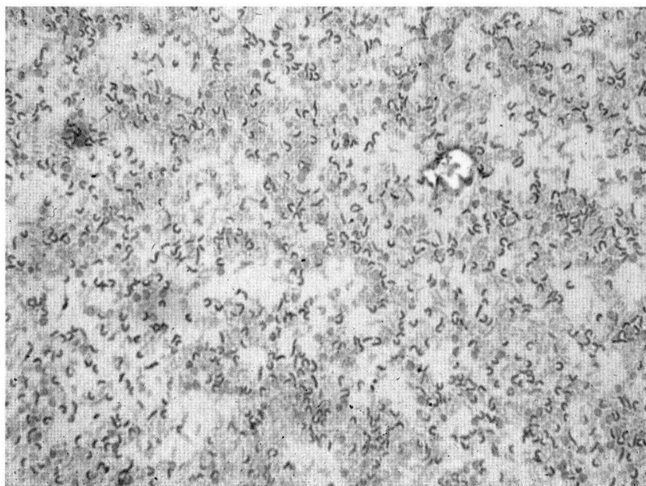

Figure 24.10 Gram stain of *V. cholerae* showing typical comma-shaped bacilli.

pathogenesis is due to an enterotoxin that causes excessive fluid and electrolyte loss. Bacteria that survive gastric acid reach the small intestine and elaborate cholera toxin, the major virulence factor for pathogenic strains. Cholera toxin consists of one A subunit associated with five B subunits. The B subunit pentamer binds to the ganglioside GM1 on eukaryotic cells and the A subunit is translocated intracellularly, where it activates adenylate cyclase and raises intracellular cyclic AMP. This leads to chloride secretion through the apical chloride channel and secretory diarrhoea. The second major virulence factor of pathogenic strains of *V. cholerae* is the toxin-coregulated pilus, a colonization factor whose expression is regulated in parallel to cholera toxin.

The genes for cholera toxin are encoded within the genome of a filamentous bacteriophage, the CTX phage. The classical and El Tor strains have different versions of this bacteriophage, which can insert at one or two attachment sites in the genome depending on the biotype. The bacterial cell surface receptor for CTX phage is the toxin-coregulated pilus, which is encoded within the vibrio pathogenicity island (VPI-1). Virulence in *V. cholerae* evolved with sequential acquisition of VPI-1 followed by the CTX phage and all pandemic strains of El Tor have two vibrio pathogenicity islands.

VPI-1 and VPI-2 are additional toxins and factors known to be involved in cholera pathogenesis include Zonula occludens toxin (Zot), which increases the permeability of the small-intestinal mucosa by affecting the structure of the intercellular tight junctions and the accessory cholera exotoxin (Ace) which increases transmembrane ion transport.

Immunity to both cholera toxin and bacterial surface antigens follows natural infection. Most studies of immune response have measured serum vibriocidal antibodies which have been shown to be mainly against LPS antigens. In a study of cholera index patients and their household contacts containing both O1 or O139 index cases, it was shown that circulating IgA levels for anti-LPS, anti-TcpA (TcpA being the major TCP pilus subunit) and anti-cholera toxin B-subunit (CTB) can be correlated with protection from O1 infection and that circulating anti-TcpA IgA correlates with protection from O139, whereas circulating IgG showed no such correlations.[102] Anti-TcpA responses could, therefore, be helpful to the generation of cross-O1/O139 protection and IgA may be important to protection from natural cholera infection.

Epidemiology

Man is the only known natural host of *V. cholerae*. Transmission is by ingestion, through contaminated water or food. The infective dose is high, up to 10^{11} bacteria being required. The incubation period ranges from a few hours to 5 days.

Serological studies have shown that, both in endemic areas and during outbreaks, for each symptomatic case there may be from 5 to 40 infected but asymptomatic or mildly symptomatic cases. Contamination of water or food may thus occur from symptomatic cases or asymptomatic, transient carriers. Most are free from infection within 2–3 weeks and there have been few examples of persistent carriage.

V. cholerae O1 can survive for weeks to months in the natural aquatic environment, but there is uncertainty whether this occurs only in relation to frequent contamination by infected persons, or whether *V. cholerae* O1 truly survives as an environmental bacterium. Studies have described the occurrence of 'non-culturable' dormant strains, which may persist for long periods in natural aquatic environments.[101] Change from the dormant to a culturable form may be influenced by environmental factors influencing toxin regulatory genes.

There are important epidemiological differences between classical and El Tor *V. cholerae*. For El Tor, the ratio of carriers to cases may range from 30 : 1 to 50 : 1, compared with 5 : 1 for classical. El Tor can also survive for longer periods in the environment. These factors give El Tor an epidemiological advantage in the spread of the disease, which has occurred in the seventh pandemic and has contributed to the displacement of the classical type by El Tor. Only in parts of southern Bangladesh has the classical biotype persisted beyond the 1980s.[103]

The seventh pandemic of cholera began in 1961, originating on the island of Sulawesi in Indonesia. The pandemic strain was *V. cholerae* O1 El Tor and it spread rapidly to countries of South-east Asia. Between 1963 and 1969 the pandemic spread to the Indian subcontinent, displacing the classical biotype and by 1970 had reached the Middle East. The pandemic entered Africa by two routes, in West Africa, probably by a returning traveller and from the Arabian peninsula, through Djibouti into East Africa. By 1978, most countries of central and southern Africa were affected. The final stage of the pandemic was the arrival of cholera in the South American continent in January 1991, the first time that cholera had entered the continent since the fifth pandemic in the 1880s.

V. cholerae O139 was first isolated in south India in 1992. It was designated O139 as it did not agglutinate with O1 antisera, nor with antisera to any of the 137 other known, non-cholera-producing serotypes of *V. cholerae*. During 1992–1994, *V. cholerae* O139 spread to Bangladesh, where for some time it was the dominant serotype.[101] In the past decade, devastating epidemics of cholera have occurred in Angola, Ethiopia, Zimbabwe, Pakistan, Somalia, Sudan, Vietnam and Haiti.[104] In Haiti, following the earthquake, cholera appeared in 2010, affecting over 275 000 individuals with over 2000 fatalities. Genomic sequence analysis identified the source of the strain as a UN contingent from South Asia.[105]

Recent seventh pandemic strains have been described that have the classical CTX phage instead of the El Tor CTX phage, or a variant of the El Tor CTX phage encoding the B subunit of cholera toxin that occurs in classical V cholerae O1 strains.[106] These variant El Tor strains have largely replaced the earlier El Tor strains and might be associated with more severe diarrhoea.

Clinical Features

The clinical picture of infection with *V. cholerae* O1 may range from mild diarrhoea to severe dehydration with death occurring within hours. In most cases there is progress from the onset of diarrhoea to shock in 4–12 hours, with death following in several days if adequate management is not instituted. The symptoms are a reflection of the severe dehydration, electrolyte loss and metabolic acidosis. Hypovolaemia and hypotension lead to impaired consciousness and to renal failure. Hypoglycaemia may occur, particularly in children. Electrolyte loss leads to hyponatraemia and hypokalaemia. The latter may result in ileus, muscle weakness and cardiac arrhythmias.

Diagnosis

In epidemics, the diagnosis of cholera may be made presumptively on clinical and epidemiological grounds. The WHO clinical case definition for suspected cholera, or 'acute watery diarrhoea', is 'a patient 5 years of age or older, who develops acute watery diarrhoea with or without vomiting', with the caveat that it is in an area where cholera is likely to occur. Laboratory diagnosis may be required when sporadic cases occur and when an extensive outbreak requires confirmation and typing of the aetiological agent. Dark-field microscopy of faecal specimens may show the characteristic darting movement of the vibrios. Inhibition of movement by addition of diluted O1 antisera to the slide will provide strong evidence that *V. cholerae* O1 is the causative agent. To confirm the diagnosis, specimens need to be cultured on a selective medium, such as thiosulphate citrate bile salt sucrose (TCBS) agar. Specimens should be transported from the field in alkaline peptone water or Cary–Blair transport medium and kept cool. *V. cholerae* O1 yields yellow, oxidase-positive colonies after overnight incubation on TCBS, which may be confirmed by slide agglutination with specific antiserum. In outbreak investigations, isolates should be sent to a reference laboratory for biotyping and serotyping. Sensitivity to tetracycline and other antimicrobial agents should be performed on a selected number of isolates. Where detailed epidemiological data are required, molecular methods have been used to distinguish different strains.[106]

Case Management

The successful management of cholera cases relies on adequate and appropriate rehydration and restoration of electrolyte balance. Except in the most severe cases, oral replacement solutions may be used. Oral solutions are based on the role of glucose enhancing the active uptake of sodium and water. As glucose is rarely available in rural areas, sucrose and rice-water-based solutions have been used with success.[105] The volume of replacement will depend on the degree of dehydration and the rate of continuing fluid loss. The compositions of oral and intravenous rehydration solutions are given in Table 24.7. WHO guidelines provide detailed protocols for rehydration and fluid maintenance.[107] Severe dehydration is characterized by 10% loss of body weight, lethargy or impaired consciousness, hypovolaemic shock and acidosis. In such patients, rapid intravenous rehydration is necessary, using a large-bore needle and multiple sites if necessary, aiming to restore normal hydration and acid–base balance within 2–3 hours. Of the losses, 50% should be replaced in the first 30–45 min, at a rate of 30 mL/kg, requiring 1–2 L in adults. Rehydration should then be slowed to 1 L per 30–45 min until normal hydration is achieved. Once rehydration is achieved, the maintenance phase requires the replacement of continuing stool losses. In the severely ill patient, this may require continuing intravenous therapy for some time, but in most cases oral rehydration using WHO or other rehydration solution is appropriate. Fluid replacement should be in the ratio of 1.5 volumes of oral fluid for each volume of stool. For children, this will be 100–200 mL per stool passed. In adults, in the recovery stage, fluid can be given as required. Moderate dehydration, characterized by 5% loss of body weight, clinical dehydration (poor skin turgor etc.) but no acidosis or shock, requires oral or intravenous rehydration initially, followed by oral maintenance. In adults, 2–4 L of ORS may be required in the first 4 hours to ensure rehydration. Potential complications in severely ill patients on presentation and during intravenous therapy include renal failure, hypoglycaemia, particularly in children and in prolonged dehydration, hypokalaemia and ileus and pulmonary oedema during rapid intravenous therapy when the metabolic acidosis has not been corrected, which is more likely when normal saline alone is used for rehydration. Hypokalaemia may occur during the maintenance phase, but should be uncommon if potassium-containing oral fluids are used.

Antimicrobial agents have been shown to shorten the period of diarrhoea and the amount of fluid loss. Tetracycline and doxycycline are the drugs of choice in adults where strains are sensitive, but the increasing occurrence of resistant strains limits their usefulness. Co-trimoxazole and furazolidone have been used, but antibiotics are secondary to the importance of early rehydration. Single-dose azithromycin is the preferred therapy in children.[105]

TABLE 24.7 Composition of Rehydration Solutions

Solution	Composition (mmol/L)				
	Na	Cl	K	Bicarbonate	Glucose
Ringers	130	109	4	28	0
Dhaka	133	98	13	48	0
WHO ORS	90	80	20	30	111
Reduced osmolarity ORS	50	40	20	30 citrate	111

Prevention and Control

Cholera is transmitted by the faecal–oral route through the contamination of water or food. Hence, public health measures to improve water and sanitation are essential for long-term control. The management of outbreaks is based on interrupting transmission, appropriate control and management of cases and contacts and effective surveillance. In most cholera outbreaks the source and routes of transmission are not obvious and general sanitary measures will need to be imposed. These may include chlorination of water supplies, boiling of water at household level and construction and maintenance of temporary latrines. Action will need to be taken to control the cleanliness of markets and the postponement of festivals and gatherings. Adequate, though basic, sanitation facilities must be made for disposal of faeces from cases during treatment.

The most appropriate group for chemoprophylaxis is household contacts of cases. The relatively high carriage rate of *V. cholerae* in this group has been described previously. Assuming strains are sensitive, tetracycline or doxycycline may be used in adults. For doxycycline, a single oral dose of 300 mg is adequate. The formerly used killed whole cell vaccines, given parenterally, have no useful role to play in the management or prevention of cholera: individual protection does not exceed 50–60%; vaccination does not reduce excretion of vibrios and is likely to give a false sense of security to both the affected population and the authorities during outbreaks.

Effective surveillance is an essential component of cholera control. Active reporting of suspected cases in areas previously uninfected, with appropriate bacteriological confirmation, will allow the early introduction of the control measures described above. At the international level, systematic reporting of cases to WHO and its collaborative bodies will help to coordinate the international response and limit spread between countries.

Cholera Vaccines

While the formerly used killed whole cell vaccine given parenterally was of only limited efficacy, new oral vaccines have been developed. The principle of these vaccines is to give an oral vaccine providing somatic (O antigen) with and without B subunit toxin immunity in the gut. Cholera vaccines are given orally, have an excellent safety profile and target induction of mucosal immunity. Two oral killed vaccines, prequalified for use by WHO, are licensed and commercially available. Dukoral (whole cell, recombinant B subunit) contains several biotypes and serotypes of *V. cholerae* O1 supplemented with 1 mg per dose of recombinant cholera toxin B subunit. Shanchol (Shantha Biotechnics-Sanofi Pasteur, India) contains several biotypes and serotypes of *V. cholerae* O1 and *V. cholerae* O139 without toxin B subunit. Shanchol is the bivalent vaccine that is internationally available; mORCVAX (VaBiotech, Vietnam) is the locally produced Vietnamese version of this vaccine.[105,109]

The vaccines are administered as 2 or 3 doses depending on age. The vaccines provide 60–85% protective efficacy for 2–3 years, although protection among young children is shorter. There is some evidence of herd protection when vaccine coverage rates are high.[108,109]

Several live attenuated oral cholera vaccines have also been developed, including CVD 103-HgR, Peru-15 and others. These genetically modified vaccine strains do not express cholera toxin. These vaccines have been shown to be safe and immunogenic in volunteer studies, but CVD 103-HgR failed to show protection in a field study in an endemic setting. Peru-15 is safe and immunogenic in different age groups in Bangladesh, but has not yet been tested in field studies.[105]

NON-CHOLERA VIBRIOS

Vibrio spp. other than *V. cholerae* O1 and O139 may cause diarrhoeal diseases in the tropics but are rarely associated with extensive outbreaks. Five species have been associated with diarrhoeal diseases: *V. cholerae* non-O1, *V. parahaemolyticus, V. fluvialis, V. hollisae* and *V. mimicus*. Among *V. cholerae* O1 strains, some have been isolated that are non-toxigenic but cause diarrhoea. They have been isolated from 1–3% of patients admitted to the cholera hospital in Dhaka, Bangladesh. *V. parahaemolyticus* is principally associated with seafoods. *V. fluvialis* has been implicated in an outbreak of diarrhoeal disease in Bangladesh. Few data are currently available on the prevalence of these vibrios in most tropical countries.

Bacteroides fragilis

Bacteroides fragilis is the only strain of *Bacteroides* spp. associated with diarrhoeal disease. Toxin-producing strains of *B. fragilis*, termed enterotoxigenic *Bacteroides fragilis* (ETBF), are an established cause of diarrhoeal disease in humans. The clinical syndrome associated with ETBF diarrhoeal disease consists of abdominal pain, tenesmus and inflammatory diarrhoea.

ETBF strains have a conjugative transposon containing a pathogenicity island with a distinct virulence gene encoding a 20-kDa metalloprotease toxin called the *B. fragilis* toxin or BFT (also known as fragilysin). BFT is secreted and is detectable in stool. Three subtypes of BFT (BFT-1, BFT-2 and BFT-3) have been identified, with BFT-1 expressed by about two-thirds of ETBF isolated around the globe followed by BFT-2 (25%) and BFT-3 (~10% and mostly identified in South-east Asia). BFT stimulates the cleavage of intercellular adhesion protein E-cadherin on colonic epithelial cells, resulting in increased human colon permeability and activates nuclear factor-kappa B signalling, resulting in proinflammatory cytokine secretion by colonic epithelial cells.[110]

In an observational study of children and adults with acute diarrhoeal illnesses in Dhaka, Bangladesh,[111] ETBF was identified to cause a clinical syndrome with marked abdominal pain and nonfebrile inflammatory diarrhoea in both children (age >1 year) and adults. Faecal leukocytes, lactoferrin and proinflammatory cytokines [interleukin (IL)-8, tumour necrosis factor-α] as well as systemic and faecal anti-BFT responses (IgA, IgG) increased rapidly in ETBF-infected patients. ETBF have also been identified as a cause of travellers' diarrhoea.

Laribacter hongkongensis

This recently described bacterium is a cause of gastroenteritis and traveller's diarrhoea.[112] Although first described in Hong Kong, cases of infection have occurred in mainland China, Japan, Switzerland, Cuba and Tunisia. This bacterium is found in freshwater fish and infection is associated with consumption of improperly cooked fish or poor hygiene in kitchens where raw freshwater fish are handled. It can cause either a watery (80% of cases) or bloody (20%) diarrhoea. Treatment is by rehydration. It is susceptible to fluoroquinolones, co-amoxiclav and aminoglycosides, but resistant to all cephalosporins, mediated by a β-lactamase.

REFERENCES

1. Black RE, Cousens S, Johnson HL, et al. Child Health Epidemiology Reference Group of WHO and UNICEF. Global, regional and national causes of child mortality in 2008: a systematic analysis. Lancet 2010;375(9730):1969–87.
2. Guerrant RL, Kosek M, Moore S, et al. Magnitude and impact of diarrhoeal diseases. Arch Med Res 2002;33:351–5.
30. Platts-Mills JA, Operario DJ, Houpt ER. Molecular diagnosis of diarrhea: current status and future potential. Curr Infect Dis Rep 2012;14(1):41–6.
77. Abubakar I, Irvine L, Aldus CF, et al. A systematic review of the clinical, public health and cost-effectiveness of rapid diagnostic tests for the detection and identification of bacterial intestinal pathogens in faeces and food. Health Technol Assess 2007;11(36):1–216.
84. Dubberke E. Strategies for prevention of *Clostridium difficile* infection. J Hosp Med 2012;7(Suppl 3):S14–17.

Access the complete references online at www.expertconsult.com

25 *Salmonella* Infections

NICHOLAS A. FEASEY | MELITA A. GORDON

KEY POINTS

- Both typhoidal and non-typhoidal pathovars of *Salmonella* are important causes of invasive bacterial disease globally.
- Typhoid fever caused by *S. typhi* and *S. paratyphi* remains common across South and South-east Asia, and a vaccine against emerging increases in *S. paratyphi* is an important priority.
- Non-typhoidal Salmonellae (e.g. *S. typhimurium* and *S. enteritidis*) have emerged as one of the commonest causes of invasive bacterial disease among adults with HIV, and children with malaria, malnutrition and HIV in sub-Saharan Africa. There is no existing vaccine, and this is a priority area.
- Non-typhoidal Salmonellae also cause enterocolitis and diarrhoeal disease globally.
- Emerging antimicrobial resistance among typhoidal and non-typhoidal Salmonellae is an important global problem, including resistance to cephalosporins and fluoroquinolones.

Bacteriology

The genus *Salmonella* is part of the family of Enterobacteriaceae. Its taxonomy has been revised and has the potential to confuse. It comprises two species, *Salmonella bongori* and *Salmonella enterica*, the latter of which is divided into six subtypes: enterica, salamae, arizonae, diarizonae, houtenae and indica.[1,2] The taxonomic group contains more than 2500 serovars, defined on the basis of the somatic O (lipopolysaccharide) and flagellar H antigens (Kaufmann–White scheme).[1] The full name of a serovar is given as, for example, *Salmonella enterica* subsp. *enterica serovar Typhimurium*, but can be abbreviated to *Salmonella Typhimurium*. Further differentiation of strains may be achieved by antibiogram and by supra- or subgenomic techniques such as pulsed field gel electrophoresis (PFGE), multi-locus sequence typing (MLST) and increasingly by whole genome sequencing (WGS) in order to assist clinico-epidemiological investigation.

On the basis of host preference and disease manifestations in man, the Salmonellae have historically been clinically categorized as invasive (typhoidal) or non-invasive (non-typhoidal Salmonellae or NTS):

- *Typhoidal strains*: *S. typhi*, *S. paratyphi A*. These serotypes are exclusively host-restricted to humans and cause an invasive and bacteraemic illness known as typhoid or enteric fever, in which diarrhoea rarely plays a major role.
- *Non-typhoidal Salmonellae (NTS)*: These have a much broader host-range, including humans and many vertebrate animals. Infection in immunocompetent individuals is usually confined to the bowel, presenting as acute enterocolitis causing diarrhoea. Transmission is often zoonotic or related to industrialized methods of food production, reflecting the broad host-range. In at-risk immunocompromised individuals, however, NTS strains may cause severe invasive disease, and the most dramatic instance of this has been an epidemic of severe invasive NTS (iNTS) disease in sub-Saharan Africa, associated with immune compromise secondary to malaria, malnutrition and the HIV pandemic.[3] The thousands of serovars of enterica subspecies account for most human and vertebrate animal infections, and are grouped on the basis of sharing of a common O antigen. Examples of commonly occurring groups of enterica subspecies serotypes are given in Table 25.1.

Different NTS pathovars are, however, thought to have different intrinsic levels of invasiveness and pathogenicity in humans,[4] and the somewhat arbitrary distinction between typhoidal and non-typhoidal pathovars breaks down in a setting with immunocompromised hosts.[5]

KEY PATHOGENIC MECHANISMS OF INVASIVE AND DIARRHOEAL *SALMONELLA* DISEASE

The ability to invade epithelial cells, and then to survive in an intracellular niche in the reticulo-endothelial system, are both key pathogenic capabilities for Salmonellae causing systemic, invasive disease.

Epithelial Invasion

The target of *Salmonella* invasion is the microfold or M cell[6] but the bacteria must cross the epithelial layer to achieve this. Salmonellae invade the intestinal epithelial cells by a complex mechanism that includes triggering active rearrangements, formation of membrane ruffles, and phagocytosis of the bacterium into the cells. The ruffling–internalization process is controlled by a type III secretion system encoded by genes found in the *inv* locus (containing genes *inv A–H*).[7] These genes are located on *Salmonella* Pathogenicity Island 1, SPI-1. SPI-1 activity is downregulated after a few hours of invasion and the type III secretion system encoded on SPI-2 is activated.[8] An alternative, paracellular route of invasion involving dissemination via sampling by CD18+ cells such as dendritic cells has also been described.[9,10]

Intracellular Survival

Salmonella serotypes that cause enteric fever must be able to survive and replicate within the host macrophage system so that

TABLE 25.1 **Some Examples of Commonly Occurring *Salmonella* Serotypes and the Groups to Which They Belong**

Group	Serotype
A	*S. paratyphi A*
B	*S. paratyphi B*
	S. stanley
	S. saintpaul
	S. agona
	S. typhimurium
C	*S. paratyphi C*
	S. cholerae-suis
	S. virchow
	S. thompson
D	*S. typhi*
	S. enteritidis
	S. dublin
	S. gallinarum

they may establish a systemic infection.[8] Once there, they are shielded from the effect of human immunity, but to do this they must overcome the nutrient-poor environment within the macrophage and defeat its bactericidal mechanisms.[11] *Salmonella* genes necessary for survival inside macrophages are constituents of a two-component response regulator termed phoP/phoQ. Genes activated by this phoP/phoQ are known as *pag* genes, of which *pag A–C* have been characterized. The *pag* genes are expressed within the macrophage phagosome and are required to promote intracellular replication of *Salmonella*.[12] Conversely, the phoP repressed genes switch off in the phagosome and include components of the SPI-1. Mutants that are phoP null or with constitutive expression of phoP have defective virulence, suggesting that proper timing of switching on and off of these mechanisms is critical in ensuring successful invasion and survival.

A second pathogenicity island, SPI-2, activated within the phagosome, translocates bacterial effector proteins from the phagosome into the macrophage cytosol, and prevents killing by evading the NADPH oxidative burst.[8,13] SPI2 mutants have a virulence defect characterized by reduced intracellular replication.[14]

The Vi capsular polysaccharide antigen, which is exclusively expressed by *S. typhi*, requires expression of both viaA together with viaB in SPI7. Vi masks LPS, reducing inflammatory response, and prevents opsonization and phagocytosis of the organism,[15] but its expression is unstable and non-essential for pathogenesis.

Mechanisms of Diarrhoeal Disease

NTS provoke an intense mucosal inflammatory response with polymorph neutrophil infiltration, which enables them to out-compete the gut microbiome,[16–18] and produce diarrhoea which facilitates their ultimate transmission. Observations in experimental animals of an enteropathy with water and electrolyte transport defects suggest the existence of secretory mechanisms.[19] Production of prostaglandin-like secretagogues and other mediators by the inflammatory tissues and toxin production by the organisms have been suggested. Salmonellae produce an enterotoxin and a cytotoxin. The enterotoxin activates adenylate cyclase and has some physicochemical characteristics in common with cholera toxin but limited antigenic homology.

Typhoid and Paratyphoid Fevers or Enteric Fever

Typhoid fever was so named because its symptoms and signs resembled typhus. The confusion between the two was resolved only with the publication in 1850, of William Jenner's book *On the Identity or Non-Identity of Typhoid and Typhus Fevers*.[20]

EPIDEMIOLOGY

Typhoid and paratyphoid fevers are endemic at high incidence (<100/100 000 p.a.) in the Indian subcontinent, South-east and South-central Asia, and at medium incidence (10–100/100 000 p.a.) in the rest of Asia, Africa and Central and South America.[21,22] Although the overall ratio of disease caused by *S. typhi* to that caused by *S. paratyphi* is about 10:1, the proportion of *S. paratyphi* infections is increasing in some parts of the world.[23]

TRANSMISSION

Typhoid is an exclusively human disease and the organisms that are responsible for infection are transmitted through food or water contaminated with the faeces of a patient or carrier. It is thus common in overcrowded conditions, including informal settlements and refugees camps, and poor human sanitation plays a major role in disease transmission. Raw fruit and vegetables are important vehicles in some countries where human faeces are used as a fertilizer or where contaminated water is used to make fruit look attractive in the market.

PATHOGENESIS

Natural infection in enteric fever occurs by ingestion, followed by penetration through the intestinal mucosa. Disease production is dependent on several factors: number of organisms swallowed; state of gastric acidity; and possession of Vi antigen by the organisms. The infecting dose of *S. typhi* needs to be large to produce illness in healthy individuals. In volunteer studies in the 1960s, a dose of 10^9 organisms administered with 30 mL milk to partially protect from stomach acid induced disease in 95% subjects, but a dose of 10^3 did not cause invasive disease. The infecting dose resulting in a 50% attack rate was 10^7 organisms.[24] A larger infecting dose shortened the median incubation period (range 5–9 days), but did not affect the severity or pattern of subsequent disease. Possession of Vi capsular antigen is linked with increased infectivity: Vi antigen-positive strains caused illness more commonly than non-Vi variants in healthy volunteers.[24] Gastric acidity is an important defence against enteric infections, and gastric hypoacidity from any cause (e.g. antacids, H_2 antagonists and proton-pump inhibitors) will likely reduce the infective dose required for invasive disease. Also, the infective dose may be reduced if it is delivered in food where the organisms are protected from gastric acid. Once in the small intestine, the organisms penetrate rapidly through the intestinal mucosa. Organisms multiply in the lumen for a short period and stools can be culture-positive during the first 4 days of the incubation period, but early stool positivity does not

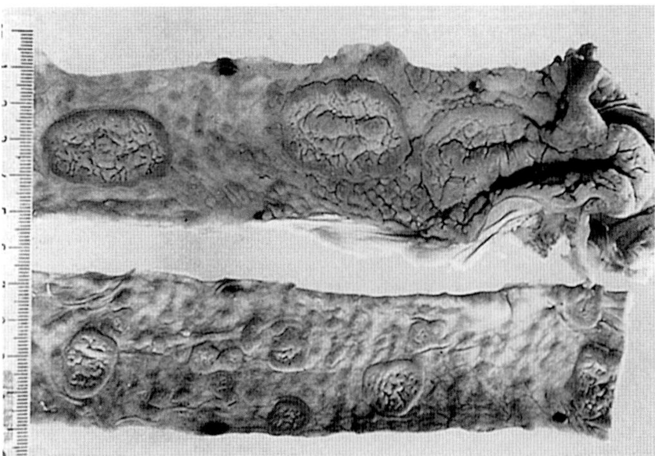

Figure 25.1 Typhoid ulceration of the small intestine. *(Courtesy of the Wellcome Tropical Institute Museum (WTIM).)*

correlate with development of invasive disease in volunteer studies, and invasive disease could occur without early stool culture becoming positive.[24]

From the submucosa, invading bacteria are taken up by macrophages, and the organisms travel to mesenteric lymph nodes. After a brief period of multiplication here, the organisms enter the bloodstream via the thoracic duct (causing a transient primary bacteraemia) and are transported to the liver and spleen. After a period of further intracellular multiplication at these sites, huge numbers of organisms enter the bloodstream, marking the onset of clinical illness (secondary bacteraemia). During this secondary bacteraemia, which continues for the greater part of the illness, metastatic infection is widespread, and the involvement of the gallbladder and Peyer's patches in the lower small intestine have important clinical significance. The gallbladder is probably infected via the liver and the resultant cholecystitis is usually subclinical. The infected bile renders stool cultures positive. Pre-existing gallbladder disease predisposes to chronic biliary infection, leading to chronic faecal carriage. Long-term biliary carriage also carries an increased risk of gallbladder cancer.[25,26]

Invasion of the Peyer's patches may occur during primary luminal infection, or during the secondary bacteraemia either by metastatic infection or by contact with infected bile. The Peyer's patches become hyperplastic, with infiltration of chronic inflammatory cells. Later, necrosis of the superficial layer leads to formation of irregular, ovoid ulcers along the long axis of the gut (Figure 25.1). If an ulcer erodes into a blood vessel, severe haemorrhage results. Transmural perforation leads to peritonitis.

MECHANISMS OF IMMUNITY

Production of humoral antibody appears to play little role in recovery from acute infection, as the patient often continues to deteriorate, despite the appearance of O, H and Vi antibodies. Cell-mediated immunity is probably the key factor in recovery. Investigation of the transcriptomic host immune response during acute disease and convalescence has provided insights into this process.[27] Although Vi polysaccharide is non-essential for pathogenesis, the ability of Vi antibody to prevent infection is demonstrated by the efficiency of Vi antigen polysaccharide and, more recently, conjugate vaccines. The lack of Vi expression by some clinical Typhi strains, and its absence in Paratyphoid pathovars remains a problem for vaccine strategy. Protection afforded by the live oral Ty21a, however, which does not contain Vi antigen, indicates a role for other polysaccharide or protein antibodies. Local gut innate and acquired immunity is probably important in preventing infection and re-infection. Specific secretory IgG and IgA antibodies have been demonstrated in gut.[28]

In the endemic countries, enteric fevers have the highest prevalence in children and adolescents, adults having acquired substantial immunity through previous exposure(s). The highest levels of endemicity are associated with prevalence among children in the 1st year of life, reflecting earlier subclinical exposure and earlier development of immunity in the general population.[21,22]

It is particularly intriguing that conditions of immune compromise do not appear to make individuals more susceptible to typhoid fever.[5] Indeed, epidemiological evidence suggests that HIV may reduce the risk of typhoid fever.[29,30]

CLINICAL MANIFESTATIONS

The incubation period of typhoid fever varies with the size of the infecting dose and averages from 10 to 20 (range 3–56) days. In paratyphoid fever it ranges from 1 to 10 days.

The duration of illness in untreated cases of average severity is usually 4 weeks. In the first week, the features are nonspecific, with headache, malaise and a rising remittent fever. Constipation and a mild non-productive cough are common. During the second week, the patient looks toxic and apathetic with sustained high temperature. The abdomen is slightly distended and splenomegaly is common. While rose spots, crops of 2–4-mm-diameter pink papules which fade on pressure, are a hallmark of typhoid, they have been found to be uncommon in some series[31] and are difficult to detect in dark-skinned individuals. Rose spots may also occur in iNTS and shigellosis. The spots are caused by bacterial embolization and rose-spot cultures may be positive, although this is rarely performed.

Historical, classical accounts of the third week describe how the patient may become progressively more unwell, with development of continuous high fever and a delirious confusional state. Abdominal distension becomes pronounced, with scanty bowel sounds and ileus, or diarrhoea may occur, with liquid, foul green–yellow stools. The patient is likely to become obtunded and hypotensive and crackles may develop over the lung bases. Death may occur at this stage from overwhelming toxaemia, myocarditis, intestinal haemorrhage or perforation. Convalescence is often lengthy. Untreated, the mortality is historically described as approximately 20%, but with the use of antibiotics neither this disease evolution nor death are common (<1%).[32]

Variation in the clinical picture is common, and mild and unapparent infections are frequent. Diarrhoea may occur even during the first week[33] and young children may present with a high fever and febrile convulsion(s). Chronic or recurrent fever with bacteraemia may occur in association with concurrent schistosomiasis, as Salmonellae are able to survive attached to the adult helminth's tegument, protected from the body's defences.[33]

The diagnosis of typhoid fever, particularly in the developing world, is usually made on clinical grounds. The symptoms sometimes mimic other common illnesses, such as malaria, sepsis with other bacterial pathogens, tuberculosis, brucellosis, tularaemia, leptospirosis and rickettsial disease. Viral infections such as dengue, acute hepatitis and infectious mononucleosis are also included in the differential diagnosis.[34]

Relapse

A relapse typically occurs a week or so after stopping therapy, but occurrence after 70 days has been reported. The blood culture is positive again, even in the presence of high serum levels of H, O and Vi antibodies, and rose spots may reappear. A relapse is generally milder and shorter than the initial illness. The incidence of relapse after treatment with fluoroquinolones (1.5%) or broad-spectrum cephalosporins (5%) is lower than after treatment with chloramphenicol, trimethoprim-sulfamethoxazole and ampicillin.[35] Rarely, second or even third relapses may occur.

Complications

Extra-intestinal infectious complications can occur and recognition of these can prevent a delay in diagnosis.[36]

INTESTINAL

The two most serious complications of enteric fever are intestinal haemorrhage and perforation, which result from erosion at the Peyer's patches separate during the late second or early third week of the illness. Clinical signs of haemorrhage are a sharp fall in body temperature and blood pressure, and sudden tachycardia. The blood passed per rectum is usually bright red but may be altered if intestinal stasis is present. Sometimes there may not be any passage of blood – when frank ileus is present.[37]

Management of haemorrhage is conservative, with volume expansion and transfusion unless there is evidence of perforation, when surgery is indicated.

Typhoid perforation often occurs on a background of a tender or already-distended abdomen with scanty bowel sounds, making recognition of perforation difficult.[38,39] The clinician must be alert for worsening of pain, changes in the daily abdominal examination, deepening of a sepsis syndrome, and seek evidence of free abdominal fluid on ultrasound examination or air under the diaphragm on an erect CXR.

After resuscitation, the treatment of choice for typhoid perforation is surgical intervention, although conservative management with nasogastric suction, antibiotic therapy directed against anaerobes and Enterobacteriaceae, and general supportive care will reduce the mortality to 30%.[40,41] Most surgeons prefer simple closure of perforation with drainage of the peritoneum, and reserve small-bowel resection for patients with multiple perforations. Early diagnosis, appropriate fluid resuscitation and rapid, simple surgery, are the key to lower mortality. The prognosis is clearly related to the time elapsed between perforation and surgery.

Liver, Gallbladder and Pancreas

Mild jaundice may occur in enteric fever and may be due to hepatitis, cholangitis, cholecystitis or haemolysis. Biochemical changes indicative of hepatitis are common during the acute stage.[42] Liver biopsy in such cases often shows cloudy swelling, balloon degeneration with vacuolation of hepatocytes, moderate fatty change and focal collection of mononuclear cells – 'typhoid nodules' (Figure 25.2). Intact typhoid bacilli can be seen at these sites. Pancreatitis has also been reported.[43]

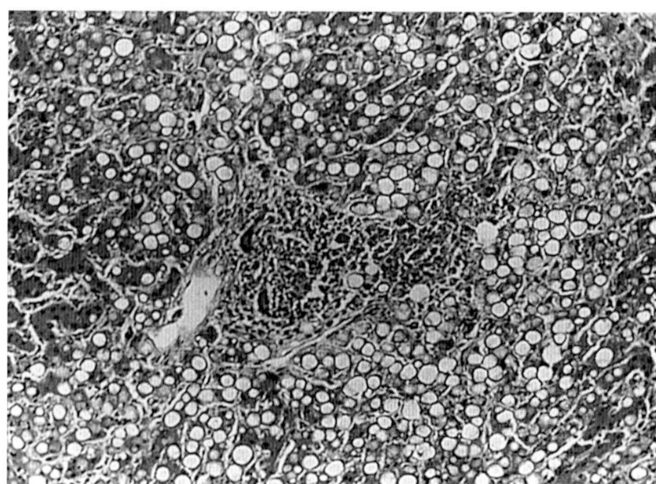

Figure 25.2 Typhoid nodule in portal tract of liver. *(Courtesy of WTIM.)*

Cardiorespiratory

Toxic myocarditis and endocarditis occur in 1–5% of cases and represent a significant cause of death in endemic countries.[41] Both occur in severely ill patients and are characterized by tachycardia, weak pulse and heart sounds, hypotension and electrocardiographic abnormalities. Respiratory symptoms, such as cough and mild bronchitis, occur in 11–86% of cases[41] and bronchopneumonia or lobar consolidation may develop rarely.

Neurological

A toxic confusional state, characterized by disorientation, delirium and restlessness, is characteristic of late-stage typhoid but occasionally these and other neuropsychiatric features may dominate the clinical picture from an early stage.[36] Facial twitching or convulsion(s) may be the presenting feature; sometimes, paranoid psychosis or catatonia may develop during convalescence.[44] Meningism is not uncommon, but bacterial meningitis caused by *S. typhi* is a rare complication. Encephalomyelitis may develop and the underlying pathology may be that of demyelinating leukoencephalopathy.[45] Rarely, transverse myelitis, polyneuropathy or cranial mononeuropathy may develop.

Haematological and Renal

Subclinical disseminated intravascular coagulation occurs commonly in typhoid fever; this rarely manifests as haemolytic–uraemic syndrome.[46] Haemolysis may also be associated with glucose 6-phosphate dehydrogenase (G6PD) deficiency. Immune complex glomerulitis has been reported and IgM immunoglobulin, C3 and *S. typhi* antigen can be demonstrated in the glomerular capillary wall.[47] Nephrotic syndrome may complicate chronic *S. typhi* bacteraemia associated with urinary schistosomiasis.[47]

Musculoskeletal and Other Systems

Skeletal muscle characteristically shows Zenker's degeneration (a hyaline degeneration of muscle fibres), particularly affecting the abdominal wall and thigh muscles; clinically evident polymyositis may occur.[48]

Metastatic localization may occur in almost any organ/system, and involvement of bones, joints, meninges, endocardium, spleen and ovary have all been reported.[48]

In general, the illness caused by paratyphoid A infection is somewhat milder than in typhoid fever and complications are less frequent.[49]

LABORATORY FINDINGS

Mild leukocytosis may develop initially, but, with disease progression, leucopenia and neutropenia commonly develop. Even in uncomplicated cases, low-grade normocytic anaemia, mild thrombocytopenia, modestly elevated serum transaminases and mild proteinuria are common.

DIAGNOSIS

The definitive diagnosis of enteric fever requires isolation of the organism from blood or bone marrow.[32] Isolation from stool or urine provides strong presumptive evidence only in the presence of a characteristic clinical picture.

Blood and Bone Marrow Culture

The definitive diagnosis of typhoid is by the isolation of the organism from a sterile site. Isolation of the organism from the stool is useful information but may be a false positive due to long-term carriage. Thus, in patients with suspected typhoid, blood or bone marrow cultures should be performed. Modern automated systems rapidly detect the presence of the organism, but non-automated methods also have a high diagnostic yield.

In untreated patients, blood cultures are usually positive in about 60–80% of cases, usually early in the course of disease.[32] The number of viable organisms/mL is low, a median of 1 bacteria per mL of blood, so at least 5–10 mL of blood should be taken to increase the sensitivity of blood culture.[50] A success rate of about 80–90% is obtained from bone marrow culture, where the viable bacterial load becomes higher as disease progresses.[32,51,52] Prior antibiotic therapy makes positive blood culture less likely but the bone marrow culture often remains positive in the face of antibiotic therapy.[53] A high yield (60%) has also been reported from rose-spot cultures in such a situation.[53]

Faecal and Urine Cultures

With modern techniques, faecal cultures are often positive even during the first week, though the percentage positivity rises steadily thereafter. Urine cultures are positive less often.

Serology

The traditional Widal test measures antibodies against flagellar (H) and somatic (O) antigens of the causative organism. In acute infection, O antibody appears first, rising progressively, later falling and often disappearing within a few months. H antibody appears a little later but persists for longer. Rising or high O antibody titre generally indicates acute infection, whereas raised H antibody helps to identify the type of enteric fever. However, the Widal test has many limitations. Many small local laboratories offer Widal testing with little quality control. Raised antibodies may have resulted from previous typhoid immunization or earlier infection(s) with Salmonellae sharing common O antigens with *S. typhi* or *S. paratyphi*. In endemic countries, the population has higher H antibody titres. This is a particular problem in developing countries, as cross-reactivity with NTS and numerous other pathogens and/or past exposure to *S. typhi* mean that the Widal test lacks specificity. Moreover, some patients show a poor or negligible antibody response to active infection. Vi antibody is often raised during acute infection and persists afterwards during chronic carriage. However, its use as a screening test for the carrier state is limited because of the frequency of false positives and false negatives.[54]

Newer Diagnostic Methods

Newer tests that directly detect IgM or IgG antibodies to a wide range of specific *S. typhi* antigens have been developed, such as Typhidot and Tubex. Some of these tests have been adapted to a simple dipstick technique using whole bacteria antigens to detect IgM antibody and may be of benefit in situations where a laboratory is not available.[55] While they compare favourably with the Widal test, none of them performs as well as blood culture.[56] Furthermore, antimicrobial susceptibility testing cannot be performed, nor can molecular epidemiological work. Their use should currently be confined to outbreak situations, where pretest probability of typhoid is high.[55] Urinary Vi antigen ELISAs and PCR-based assays are under development,[56,57] but have not yet reached the point where they are ready for deployment as rapid-diagnostic tests.

CARRIER STATE IN ENTERIC FEVER

Faecal Carrier

Volunteer challenge studies[24] demonstrate that the stool is positive initially for a few days, reflecting initial replication in the gut, then often becomes negative. Stool shedding then recommences with secondary GI infection of the bile and Peyer's patches, and coincides with the peak of illness. Most individuals have stopped shedding *S. typhi* in the stool by weeks 3–6 after infection, but 1–3% become chronic carriers, with shedding which may be intermittent. Antibiotic treatment of the initial illness does not completely prevent chronic carriage, but some agents are more effective in reducing subsequent carriage than others – fluoroquinolones are most effective, followed by fourth generation cephalosporins, and both are superior to the older agents such as chloramphenicol or beta-lactam. Chronic carriage once established may be treated with prolonged fluoroquinolone treatment. Underlying gallbladder or biliary disease is a major cause of chronic carriage, and should be sought with ultrasound (transabdominal or endoscopic) and treated surgically or endoscopically as appropriate. Chronic carriage is associated with an increased risk of gall bladder cancer. Tracing and treatment of chronic carriage is an effective preventative strategy in low-prevalence areas, but not in areas of very high incidence.

Urinary Carrier

In the absence of urinary tract pathology, persisting urinary carriage is rare after the third month, Urinary schistosomiasis is probably the commonest global cause of chronic urinary carriage.

MANAGEMENT

Patients should be managed with attention to adequate handwashing and safe disposal of faeces and urine. They should receive attention to nutrition and correction of fluid and electrolyte imbalance. Antibiotic therapy is essential and should begin empirically if the clinical suspicion of an enteric fever is strong. Patients should also be monitored for complications, particularly changing abdominal signs, and for clinical relapse. Convalescence is often lengthy. In non-endemic countries, patients who work in the food industry or in health care, residential care or childcare should be kept under bacteriological surveillance after clinical recovery until three consecutive negative faecal and urine cultures are obtained, to comply with local regulations relating to carriers.

Choice of Antimicrobial Agents in Enteric Fever

Patterns of drug resistance amongst Salmonellae are continually changing and it is important for clinicians to be aware of local susceptibility patterns especially in settings where diagnostic microbiology facilities are unavailable. Sadly, this information is often lacking in regions with the highest burden of disease. The choice of antibiotic and the dose chosen are crucial to the treatment of the acute infection, the prevention of secondary transmission and chronic carriage. The best clinical response in typhoid and paratyphoid is achieved with the highest ratio of the Cmax:MIC. The antibiotics should be used at the maximum dose recommended. There are very few data on the use of combination antibiotic therapy in enteric fever.

Emergence of Multi-resistant Typhoid Fever

Like other Gram-negative pathogens, *S. typhi* has a propensity to evolve resistance to antimicrobials rapidly. Plasmid-mediated resistance to chloramphenicol, ampicillin and co-trimoxazole emerged rapidly in the late 1980s in the Indian subcontinent and parts of South-east Asia. This led to the increasing use of fluoroquinolones in the management of typhoid, which are superior in efficacy even for fully susceptible strains. A decline in the use of the older three agents has led to the beginning of a re-emergence of chloramphenicol-susceptible *S. typhi*. Meanwhile, reduced susceptibility and poorer clinical response to the older fluoroquinolones (Ciprofloxacin and ofloxacin) has emerged in South and South-east Asia, predominantly through chromosomal mutations on the gyrA gene. This has left azithromycin as the treatment of choice for empirical management of typhoid where reduced susceptibility to quinolones is common. Plasmid-mediated resistance to cephalosporins through production of extended-spectrum beta-lactamases has also been described although this remains relatively uncommon. Increasing resistance in strains of *S. paratyphi* A have been seen in travellers to the Indian subcontinent, again mediated through *gyrA* mutations in the quinolone resistance determining region of the chromosome.[58] As with *S. typhi*, plasmid mediated quinolone resistance is uncommon.

Ciprofloxacin and Other Fluoroquinolone Drugs. Fluoroquinolones have proved to be highly effective in the treatment of typhoid and paratyphoid fevers, and are the treatment of choice for both fully susceptible and MDR strains in areas where there is not yet established fluoroquinolone resistance. They are superior to chloramphenicol even for fully susceptible strains.[59,60] Defervescence occurs in 3–5 days; convalescent carriage and relapses are rare (<2%).[32] Ciprofloxacin and ofloxacin, both 4-quinolone drugs, are probably equally effective.[61] The dose of ciprofloxacin and ofloxacin is 20 mg/kg daily for 5–7 days, and 2–3 day short courses of ofloxacin have been successfully trialled.[62] If vomiting or diarrhoea is present, the drug should be given intravenously. Fluoroquinolones are now recommended for the treatment of illness in children where the benefits of treatment outweigh the small risks of musculoskeletal adverse effects. The new-generation fluoroquinolone gatifloxacin has proved successful in treating typhoid and paratyphoid even in regions with reduced susceptibility to the older-generation fluoroquinolones. It should not be used in elderly patients or those with diabetes, but in the predominately young individuals who typically suffer from typhoid it is effective, safe and affordable.

Third-generation Cephalosporins. Cefotaxime, ceftriaxone and cefoperazone have good in vitro activity against *S. typhi* and other Salmonellae. Although they have an acceptable efficacy in the treatment of typhoid fever, they are less efficacious with a longer time to clinical response than the fluoroquinolones against susceptible strains.[60] Only intravenous formulations are available. Cefotaxime is given 1 g three times daily (in children: 200 mg/kg daily in divided doses) for 14 days. Ceftriaxone, 2 g/daily in adults, has the advantage of only requiring a single dose daily. The oral third-generation cephalosporins, cefixime, should not be used in typhoid or paratyphoid fever. Note that second-generation cephalosporins do not penetrate well intracellularly, are associated with a high recurrence rate, and are not appropriate for the treatment of typhoid fever either orally or intravenously.

Azithromycin. Azithromycin is a macrolide antibiotic that achieves high tissue concentrations but low serum concentrations because of its unique pharmacokinetic properties. The antibiotic is concentrated within cells, making it ideal for the treatment of infection by an organism with an intracellular lifestyle. It is at least as efficacious as chloramphenicol and fluoroquinolones, and more efficacious in populations with drug-resistant strains, and is considered the most appropriate first-line treatment in areas where clinically important fluoroquinolone resistance is established among *S. typhi* strains.[63] Azithromycin should be used at 20 mg/kg per day for 7 days.

Chloramphenicol, Ampicillin, Amoxicillin and Co-trimoxazole. Chloramphenicol was introduced in 1948, and proved to be remarkably effective in the treatment of enteric fever. Although it now has a much-reduced role globally, it still has a limited role in low-resource areas where resistance is not established and other agents are not available. It produces clearance of fever in 3–5 days. The recommended adult dose is 500 mg every 4 hours until defervescence, then 6-hourly for a total course of 14 days. The oral route has superior bioavailability to parenteral administration, and should be used if possible. The intravenous route is preferable to the intramuscular route, as the latter gives unsatisfactory blood levels and may delay fever clearance. The disadvantages of chloramphenicol are: the 14-day treatment course, a higher relapse rate than modern agents (5–15%), particularly when treatment courses are shortened, more secondary transmission, the rare marrow toxicity and aplastic anaemia;[64] and global emergence of resistant strains of *S. typhi*. Although cheap, it is clinically inferior to fluoroquinolones even in susceptible strains.

Although ampicillin is inferior to chloramphenicol, its close relative amoxicillin is at least as effective as chloramphenicol in respect of fever clearance time and relapse rate (4–8%).[64] It is usually given orally four times daily for 14 days. Co-trimoxazole is also as effective as chloramphenicol, and is given orally 960 mg twice daily. None of these drugs should now be regarded as first-line therapy for typhoid and paratyphoid fever.

Corticosteroid Therapy

High-dose dexamethasone (initially 3 mg/kg body weight, followed by eight doses of 1 mg/kg 6-hourly) was shown to reduce mortality in severely ill patients with depressed levels of consciousness or shock as adjunctive treatment with chloramphenicol,[65] but there is no evidence supporting its use with more modern agents such as fluoroquinolones, third generation cephalosporins or azithromycin.

Management of Chronic Carriers

Prolonged courses of amoxicillin or co-trimoxazole may be effective, but the failure rate is high if there is chronic gallbladder disease. Ciprofloxacin (750 mg twice daily) and norfloxacin (400 mg twice daily) have been much more effective, with cure rates of 78% and 83%, respectively.

Cholecystectomy should be performed if clinically indicated, but is not always successful, because of persisting hepatic infection. Chronic urinary carriers should be investigated for urinary tract abnormalities, including schistosomiasis.

PROGNOSIS

Early antibiotic therapy has transformed a previously life-threatening illness of several weeks' duration with a mortality rate approaching 20% into a short-lasting febrile illness with negligible mortality. The high mortality rates which continue to be reported from some endemic countries are undoubtedly related to delayed diagnosis and/or inappropriate treatment.

PREVENTION

In endemic countries, the most cost-effective strategy for reducing the incidence of enteric fever is the institution of public health measures to ensure safe drinking water and sanitary disposal of excreta. The effects of these measures are long lasting and will also reduce the incidence of other enteric infections which are a major cause of morbidity and mortality in those areas. In the absence of such a strategy, mass immunization with typhoid vaccines at regular intervals will also reduce the incidence of infections considerably, and has been recommended by WHO since 2008.[66] The typhoid vaccines currently in use are described in Box 25.1. The need to administer multiple oral doses of Ty21a has led to attempts to develop single-dose oral vaccines. Phase I and II clinical trials have been successful in a number of these novel typhoid fever vaccines.[75,76]

Vi vaccines are generally regarded as ineffective against *S. paratyphi* A, B and C, as these serotypes lack the Vi antigen.[68] Multiple-antigen or live oral vaccines, including Ty21a, offer potential for protection against Vi-negative typhoidal *Salmonella* strains.

BOX 25.1 TYPHOID VACCINES CURRENTLY IN USE

Vi CAPSULAR POLYSACCHARIDE ANTIGEN VACCINE

This is a single parenteral dose vaccine from the Merieux Institute. Observed overall protection rates of 75% in Nepal,[67] 64% in South Africa[68] and 70% in China[69] compare favourably with the efficacy of the killed vaccine and it has the advantage of minimal side-effects. Re-vaccination is necessary every 3 years to maintain protection. It is not suitable for children under 18 months of age, as polysaccharide antigens evoke a weak antibody response. The Vi vaccine can be given simultaneously with other vaccines relevant for international travellers.[70]

Vi-CONJUGATE VACCINE

Re-vaccination using the Vi vaccine does not elicit a booster effect because the immune response against polysaccharides does not involve T cells. To overcome this limitation, the Vi vaccine has been conjugated to a non-toxic recombinant *Pseudomonas aeruginosa* exotoxin A was recently evaluated in Vietnam and shown to have 91.5% protective efficacy. This vaccine is suitable for children.[71] Other conjugate Vi vaccines such as Vi-CRM(197) conjugated to a modified diphtheria toxin are also in development and clinical trials.[72]

LIVE ATTENUATED VACCINES

An oral vaccine containing live chemically attenuated *S. typhi* Ty21a strains in an enteric-coated capsule is commercially available. It is well tolerated and an overall protective efficacy of 67–80% has been demonstrated for up to 7 years after three doses given on alternate days. There is also evidence of indirect protection (herd immunity), possibly due to the vaccine causing significant reduction in excretion of virulent *Salmonella* and fewer temporary carriers.[73] Ty21a does not carry Vi, and is likely to provide some cross-protection against other invasive *Salmonella* pathovars including Paratyphi. A four-dose schedule, which appears to give better protection,[74] is preferred in the USA. However, only 42% efficacy was recorded in Indonesia, suggesting that the vaccine may not be as effective in areas where exposure is intense.[23] Other genetically modified live oral vaccines are in development.

Typhoid vaccination is recommended for travellers to highly endemic areas in Asia and Africa. However, the protection is partial and travellers should be made aware of this and encouraged to pay close attention to personal, food and water hygiene.

Non-typhoidal *Salmonella* (NTS) Infections

NTS are a major public health problem worldwide. In industrial settings a wide range of non-typhoidal serovars predominantly cause self-limiting enterocolitis, with low associated mortality and invasion to cause bacteraemia or metastatic complications being an occasional consequence. In contrast, in the developing world, especially sub-Saharan Africa (SSA), NTS are a frequent cause of invasive disease, sepsis and death (Figure 25.3).[29] In SSA, invasive NTS disease shows a bi-modal age distribution, with a peak of bacteraemia in children under the age of 3 with malaria or malnutrition or HIV, and a second peak in adults with advanced HIV.[77,78] *S. typhimurium* and *S. enteritidis* are the commonest serovars isolated in this setting, although other spp. are also reported.

NTS infection is facilitated by compromise of innate barriers to infection, such as a reduction in gastric acidity. Infection is more likely to be invasive and systemic in those who are

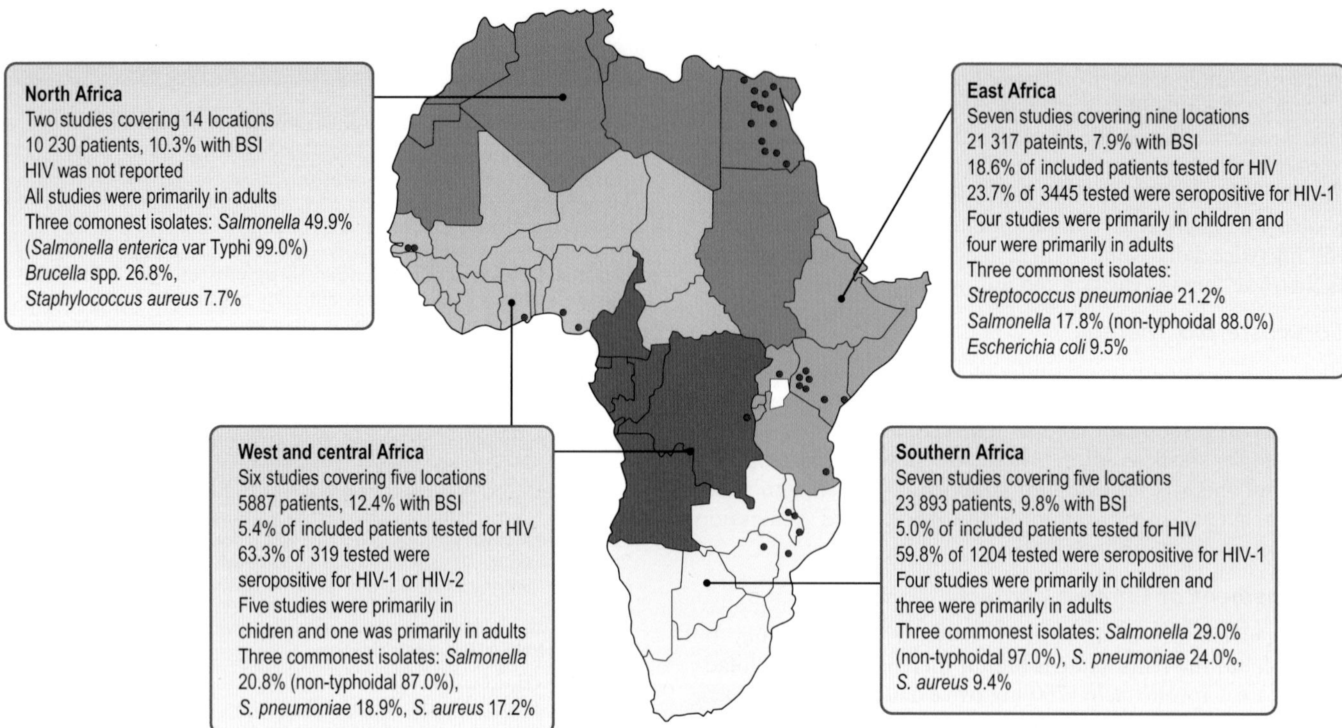

Figure 25.3 Map of Africa showing results of a meta-analysis of studies investigating the cause of bloodstream infection in febrile adults and children in Africa. BSI bloodstream infection. *(From Reddy EA, Shaw AV, Crump JA. Community-acquired bloodstream infections in Africa: a systematic review and meta-analysis. Lancet Infect Dis 2010; 10:417–432.)*

immunocompromised, and individuals with structural abnormalities in organs or tissues are most at risk of focal suppurative complications.

Salmonella transmission is frequently epidemic. Outbreaks of NTS diarrhoeal disease in the community and in institutions are common, caused by a range of *Salmonella* serotypes, and penta-resistant *S. typhimurium* DT104 caused an international zoonotic epidemic of diarrhoeal disease in Europe and North America in the 1990s.[79] In Africa, local epidemics of invasive NTS disease caused by *S. typhimurium* and *S. enteritidis* have been documented,[80,81] and epidemic transmission and microevolution of *S. typhimurium* pathovars has been demonstrated right across the African continent, apparently fuelled by the emergence of antimicrobial resistance to chloramphenicol and by the HIV pandemic.[3]

EPIDEMIOLOGY

NTS infection is usually acquired by ingestion of contaminated foods. Factors which have contributed to the emergence of NTS infections as a public health problem in developed countries include the adoption of large-scale intensive farming methods for rearing food animals and the industrialization of food production and distribution.[82]

In contrast to the typhoidal strains, which are human-restricted, NTS have a broad vertebrate host range and are widely distributed in the animal kingdom. Domestic animals, notably cattle, pigs and poultry, are frequent excretors and many wild animals may be infected. A variety of household pets such as dogs, cats, birds and reptiles are potential, albeit rare, sources of human infection. There is also an increasing appreciation of the specific mechanisms which NTS have evolved to enable attachment to and thus growth on a diverse array of fruit (i.e. tomatoes) and vegetables (spinach, jalapeno peppers and beansprouts), however it is as yet unclear how important of this is to the epidemiology of NTS.[83]

In addition to the intensive farming of food-animals, the use of bulk-imported infected animal feeds has contributed to the spread of NTS. The extensive and poorly controlled use of antimicrobials in farm animals has been proposed as a cause of the rising incidence of drug-resistant Salmonellae, although recent studies questioned the direction in which resistance mechanisms flow.[84] Carcasses of infected animals may become contaminated during evisceration and infection spreads to other non-infected carcasses during large-scale storage. Similarly, inadequately cooked meat or precooked food contaminated by raw meat in the kitchen are important vehicles of transmission. *Salmonella* may survive deep freezing, and adequate thawing is essential before cooking.

Fresh shell hen eggs infected through vertical transmission continue to be an important source of *S. enteritidis* infection, although since 1999 most infections in the UK have been associated with eggs imported from abroad.[85] Unpasteurized milk is a recognized source in some countries. Industrial processing of fruit and vegetables may also play a role in NTS outbreaks, specific examples including chilies, basil and tomatoes. Manufacturing processes have led to contamination of the ingredients used to make chocolate and thus chocolate-associated outbreaks.

In recent years, there has been a decrease in NTS infections in the UK and this has been attributed to vaccination in poultry with consequent reduction in *S. enteritidis* isolations, and to improvements in the microbiological quality of food, the 'farm to fork' approach.[86]

In developing countries, the epidemiological pattern is likely to be very different, as large-scale rearing of food animals is not common and food production is less industrialized. Transmission mechanisms are poorly understood in less industrialized settings, and remain the biggest gap in our knowledge. There is a critical shortage of diagnostic microbiology facilities in Africa, but the high-quality bacteraemia studies that have been performed indicate that iNTS are the most common cause of blood stream infection in the sub-Saharan region,[29] and are associated with malaria, malnutrition and HIV among children, and with HIV in adults. There is currently sparse information about the prevalence of *Salmonella* diarrhoeal disease in Africa; it may cause 2–5% of cases of diarrhoea in children. The high prevalence of invasive NTS disease in SSA is not reflected in Asia, where typhoidal strains remain the commonest cause of invasive *Salmonella* disease.[22,87] Whole genome sequencing studies of invasive *S. typhimurium* from Africa suggest that the emergence of a novel pathovar (MLST type ST313), has been facilitated by the HIV pandemic and the emergence of antimicrobial resistance, and that this pathovar may have evolved genome-restriction that is typically seen in more human-restricted, invasive Salmonellae.[3,81]

Pathogenesis

The size of the infecting dose influences the outcome of *Salmonella* exposure. Limited experimental evidence in volunteers suggested that an infecting dose of 10^5 is required to cause clinical illness.[4] The rarity of water borne outbreaks of NTS suggests the importance of a large infecting dose that can usually be found only in food following multiplication. The size of the infecting dose is influenced by the infectivity of the organism and host factors such as age, immune status, underlying debilitating disease or stress factors, and the physiological state of the stomach and upper small intestine at the precise time of intake of the organism. Gastric acidity is a significant barrier to enteric infection. Hypoacidity increases the susceptibility to infection, and proton pump inhibitors are a significant risk factor for *Salmonella* diarrhoea.[88] The low levels of contamination in some chocolate-associated outbreaks suggest certain foods may shield the pathogen from gastric acid, facilitating their safe transit beyond the stomach.

A number of immune defects have been identified in HIV that increase susceptibility to iNTS disease, including depletion of IL-17-producing cells from the gut,[89] dysregulation and attenuation of pro-inflammatory cytokine responses,[90] and dysregulated production of anti-LPS antibodies that may paradoxically prevent humoral killing of intravascular NTS organisms (Figure 25.4).[91]

Virulence of the Organism

Although any serotype can cause invasive disease, some appear more invasive in healthy humans than others. Invasive disease associated with underlying immune compromise is generally associated with a lower frequency of diarrhoea.[92,93] *S. choleraesuis* and *S. dublin* are particularly notable as relatively invasive serovars in the human host.[4,94] Ultimately, however, the clinical syndrome produced by NTS infection results from the way in which both host and pathogen interact; as an example, the HIV pandemic has created an ecological niche among immunocompromised individuals in Africa which favours systemic NTS disease, and to which *S. typhimurium* pathovar ST313 appears to be especially well adapted.[3,81] The factors governing the virulence potential of the different serovars are only just beginning to be understood, thanks in part to rapid advances in genomic, transcriptomic and proteomic methods.

CLINICAL MANIFESTATIONS

There is wide variation in both the pattern and severity of disease that may be caused by NTS pathovars, from acute enterocolitis (most common) to invasive blood stream infection, meningitis and other metastatic extraintestinal suppurative infections. These clinical patterns are determined both by the pathovars and by the immune status of the patient. The incubation period is usually between 12 and 48 hours, but longer incubation periods have been reported.

Acute Enterocolitis

This is the preferred term to describe the acute diarrhoeal illness caused by NTS, because both the small and predominantly the large intestine are involved in the disease process. The illness begins with nausea and sometimes vomiting, often associated with malaise, headache and fever, followed by cramp-like abdominal pains and diarrhoea. Initially, the stools are of large volume and watery without visible blood or mucus; later, the volume may decrease and blood or mucus appear, indicating development of colitis. The severity of diarrhoea is quite variable, from a mild attack of several loose stools for a day to voluminous watery stools every half hour or so over several days, leading to dehydration. The elderly, the very young, and those with underlying immunosuppression (HIV, diabetes, haematological or solid malignancy, cirrhosis or renal impairment, steroid or other immunosuppressive treatment, transplant patients) are most prone to develop secondary bacteraemia, and may paradoxically have less intestinal inflammation and less severe diarrhoea disease.[5]

More severe cases develop a frank infective colitis, with the passage of blood-stained liquid stool containing pus. This may be associated with pain and tenderness, and the clinician must be alert to the risks of colonic dilatation or perforation. Barium enema is not diagnostically helpful, and sigmoidoscopy with biopsy is the initial investigation of choice – bowel preparation is usually unnecessary. Sigmoidoscopy shows mucosal oedema, granular, erythematous mucosa, friability with mucosal contact bleeding, or ulceration. Colonic involvement is usually continuous but may show skip lesions or rectal sparing. Occasionally, ileal involvement may be the predominant feature, with pain and tenderness localized over the right lower abdomen; this may be misdiagnosed as appendicitis.

Histological changes are predominantly in the colon, with occasional 'backwash' ileitis but no Peyer's patch involvement.[95] Histological features include capillary dilatation in the mucosa and submucosa, with focal collections of polymorphonuclear leukocytes in the lamina propria. In others there may also be a diffuse increase in chronic inflammatory cells in the lamina propria. Crypt abscesses are common and typical, but crypt architecture is usually normal with a normal goblet cell population; however, in severe cases, crypt distortion with mucus depletion may occur and distinction from inflammatory bowel disease is difficult, in which case repeat sigmoidoscopy and histology is useful at 6–8 weeks to establish chronicity.

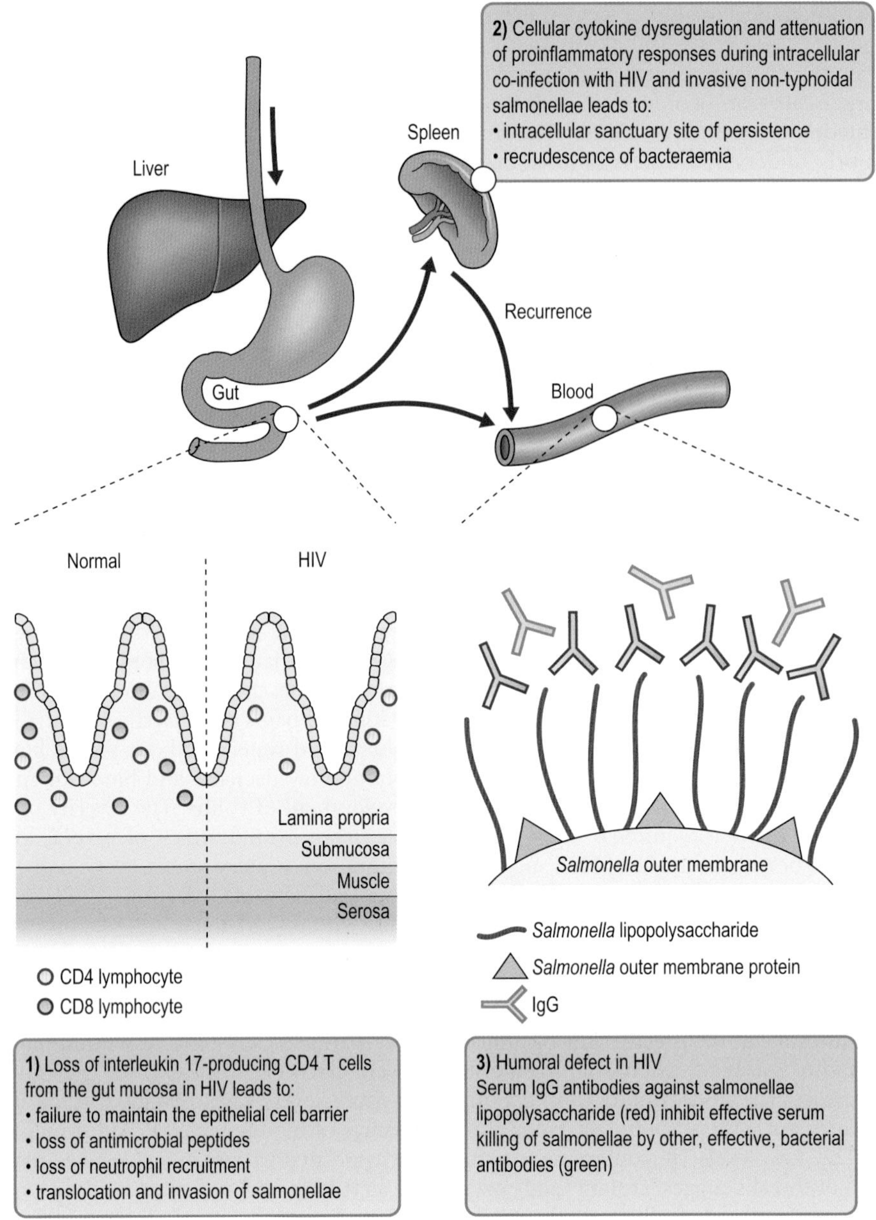

Figure 25.4 Three key defects that contribute to the pathogenesis of invasive non-typhoidal Salmonellae in HIV-positive people.

Blood Stream-Infection and Systemic Disease

Globally, bacteraemia is a common manifestation of NTS infection, especially in sub-Saharan Africa. Its frequency is especially dependent on host immunity, with HIV infection, falciparum malaria and malnutrition being especially important predisposing risk factors for iNTS. Recurrent *Salmonella* sepsis was one of the first reported AIDS-defining illnesses and a first episode of iNTS is now a WHO stage IV AIDS-defining condition. Invasive NTS (iNTS) is a particular problem in sub-Saharan Africa where the HIV epidemic coincides with malnutrition and endemic malaria.[78] As malaria incidence has fallen at some locations, corresponding decreases in iNTS disease have also been noted.[96] The serotypes most commonly associated with iNTS in sub-Saharan Africa are *S. typhimurium* and *S. enteritidis*, rather than NTS serovars that are more 'classically' invasive in industrialized settings, but other serovars including *S. concorde*, *S. isangi*, *S. bovismorbificans* and *S. dublin* are also reported.

iNTS disease in SSA is associated with high mortality of 20–25% in most recent reports.[80] Presentation is frequently with either a primary bacteraemic illness which frequently has no obvious clinical focus (fever and sepsis), or an illness which may be reminiscent of typhoid fever (high fever, hepatosplenomegaly and paucity of diarrhoea). Abnormalities in the lung are common, often caused by co-infections with TB or *Streptococcus pneumoniae* (Figure 25.5). Relapse of bacteraemia is common in HIV-infected adults unless antiretrovirals are urgently initiated. In one study from the pre-ART era, 45% of HIV-infected adults who survived a primary episode of iNTS had bacteraemic relapse within 2–8 months.[97]

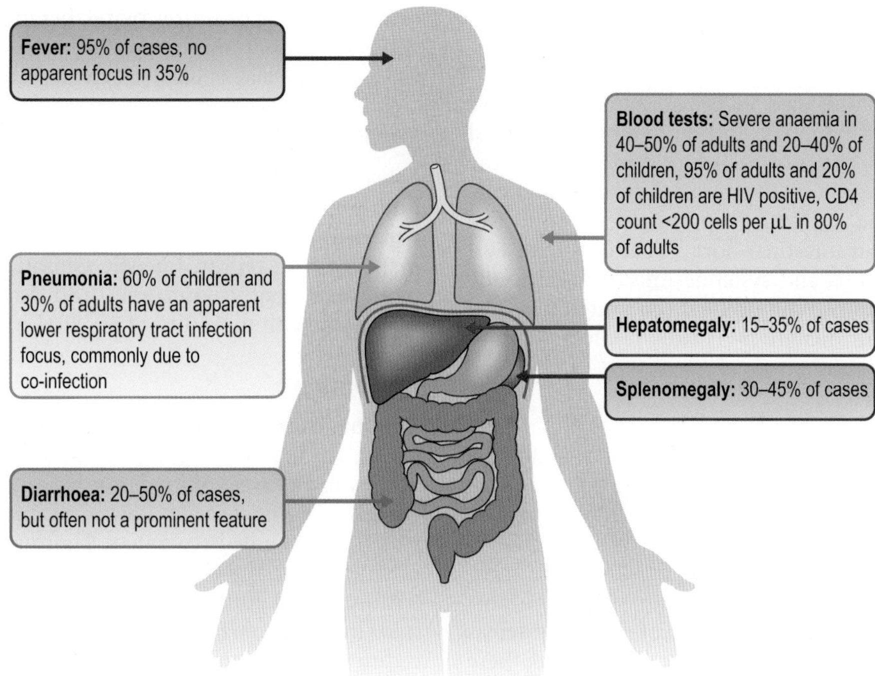

Figure 25.5 Clinical features of invasive non-typhoidal *Salmonella* disease in adults and children in Africa.

Salmonella meningitis predominantly occurs in neonates and children under 3 years of age, and reports of high incidence have come from a number of the developing countries, with high associated mortality.

Individuals with underlying structural abnormalities are likely to develop focal suppurative *Salmonella* complications. Sickle cell anaemia with resultant avascular necrosis from crises is a strong risk factor for *Salmonella* osteomyelitis or septic arthritis. *Salmonella* infection accounts for most cases of aortic and other endovascular infections in the elderly. Atherosclerotic aneurysms of the abdominal aorta or iliac vessels, or prosthetic valves and grafts may all be infected. Patients with chronic schistosomiasis are prone to suffer from recurrent bacteraemia from *Salmonella* organisms harboured on the tegument of the helminth in the bloodstream.[98] Abnormalities of the biliary or renal tract may be a focus for *Salmonella* infections. There may also be focal or suppurative disease in the lungs, endocardium, liver, spleen and ovaries. Soft tissue localization can also occur.[48]

Reactive Arthritis

Sterile synovitis may follow *Salmonella* infection, particularly in HLA-B27-positive individuals. The symptoms usually develop 1–2 weeks after the acute infection. Any joint may be affected, although the knees and ankles are most frequently involved. Occasionally, there is migratory polyarthritis, resembling acute rheumatic fever, or bilateral proximal interphalangeal joint involvement, as in rheumatoid arthritis. Acute iridocyclitis may complicate the picture.

Carrier State

Adults recovering from *Salmonella* infection usually continue to excrete the organism(s) for 4–8 weeks; infants and the elderly may excrete for longer periods. Chronic carriage beyond 1 year occurs in fewer than 1% of cases.

DIAGNOSIS

Diagnosis of *Salmonella* enterocolitis requires either faecal isolation or PCR. Where available, blood cultures should be done in all severely ill patients with enterocolitis. Inflammatory bowel disease or other causes of colitis such as ischaemic colitis should be suspected if bloody diarrhoea persists beyond 2 weeks despite the use of an appropriate antibiotic (e.g. ciprofloxacin). Sigmoidoscopic and barium contrast study findings are not discriminatory at this stage, but rectal biopsy is often helpful as features of ulcerative colitis (crypt architectural distortion and prominent goblet cell depletion) or other types of colitis may be present. When such a distinction is not possible, the patient should be treated with prednisolone and antibiotics continued. In those who respond promptly, the diagnostic dilemma can be resolved only by a repeat biopsy after 6 weeks. In primary *Salmonella* colitis the rectal biopsy histology usually returns to normal by this time, but this is quite uncommon in ulcerative colitis.

As has been stated, iNTS may present with non-focal sepsis and in sub-Saharan Africa, all febrile patients or patients suspected of having sepsis should have a blood culture where available, irrespective of the result of malaria film. As in typhoid, the number of viable bacteria in blood is not high (median 1 CFU/mL)[99] so at least 10 mL blood should ideally be sampled, although this may not be realistic in children. At the time of writing, rapid-diagnostic tests are under development,[100] but do not yet out-perform conventional culture. Systemic or focal co-infections with other invasive bacterial pathogens or *Mycobacterium tuberculosis* are relatively common.[97]

MANAGEMENT

Enterocolitis

Most patients with uncomplicated *Salmonella* enterocolitis have a short-lasting, self-limiting illness and require only increased fluid intake. Antibiotics have not been found to influence the clinical illness and may prolong the duration of intestinal carriage, possibly due to the antibiotics suppressing the protective effects of the commensal intestinal flora.[101] Patients with evidence of both enterocolitis and systemic infection, especially with circulatory compromise should be given antibiotics. The complication of colonic dilatation usually resolves without surgery.

iNTS

Antibiotics are definitely indicated in patients with confirmed sepsis and/or metastatic infection(s) and the same classes of antimicrobials described in the management of *S. typhi* may be effective against iNTS. The absolute incidence of iNTS disease is unknown, but meta-analysis shows that iNTS is the most common cause of bacteraemia in sub-Saharan Africa[29] and this must be reflected in empirical management of suspected sepsis among febrile admissions in this setting. As with *S. typhi*, there is much geographical variation in the prevalence of the resistant strains and, where possible, decisions on empirical therapy should be based on local susceptibilities.

Antimicrobial resistance among iNTS has spread rapidly across Africa in the last decade,[3] with emergence of plasmid-mediated resistance to chloramphenicol, co-trimoxazole and amoxicillin, therefore empirical management of sepsis should include a third generation cephalosporin or fluoroquinolone. In South Africa iNTS are frequently both ESBL-producing and fluoroquinolone-resistant and carbapenems or azithromycin may be required. In Northern African countries and other parts of the developing world, iNTS is thought to be a less common cause of bacteraemia. Azithromycin is potentially a useful agent in the management of iNTS, but no clinical end-point studies of the optimal management of iNTS have been performed. A 10–14-day course of effective antimicrobial therapy if iNTS is confirmed or suspected is appropriate, in view of the high rate of recurrence in immunocompromised individuals. Urgent commencement of antiretroviral therapy (ART) in HIV-infected patients is important, irrespective of and without waiting for a CD4 count. Delay is likely to favour relapse.

Focal Infection

Salmonella infection of the aorta generally requires surgical intervention and infected grafts should be replaced if the patient will tolerate the procedure. Septic arthritis may be successfully managed with repeated needle aspiration combined with antibiotic treatment.[102] Outcomes from *Salmonella* meningitis are very poor, with mortality of 50–80% in children and adults.[103]

Prevention

The main control measures in industrialized settings are directed at maintaining high standards of hygiene in slaughterhouses and all areas of food preparation and distribution – both commercial and private. Raw meat and cooked food must be stored and handled separately. Thorough cooking of raw meat after adequate thawing is essential. Eggs should be boiled for 5 minutes and liquid egg for commercial use should be pasteurized. In developing countries, adequate infection control procedures are essential in paediatric hospitals if the problem of endemic *Salmonella* spp. cross-infection is to be controlled.[104,105] Asymptomatic excretors who are handlers of unwrapped food meant for consumption without further cooking or reheating should be free of infection before returning to work. Others may do so or return to school once their diarrhoea has settled, provided their hygiene standards are adequate.

These factors are undoubtedly less relevant in the African context, from where there is epidemiological and genomic evidence to suggest that iNTS Typhimurium ST313 has become human host-adapted and therefore that transmission from human to human may be important.[81,106] Here, protection of susceptible hosts through early diagnosis and treatment of HIV, prevention of mother-to-child transmission of HIV, improved nutritional standards and malaria control interventions are critical to prevention of iNTS. There is current interest in developing iNTS vaccines for use to protect against invasive disease in Africa, based on LPS conjugates, protein antigens or attenuated live strains,[107] but they remain in research and development.

REFERENCES

3. Okoro CK, Kingsley RA, Connor TR, et al. Intracontinental spread of human invasive *Salmonella* Typhimurium pathovariants in sub-Saharan Africa. Nat Genet 2012;44(11):1215–21.
14. Figueira R, Holden DW. Functions of the *Salmonella* pathogenicity island 2 (SPI-2) type III secretion system effectors. Microbiology 2012;158(Pt 5):1147–61.
78. Feasey NA, Dougan G, Kingsley RA, et al. Invasive non-typhoidal *Salmonella* disease: an emerging and neglected tropical disease in Africa. Lancet 2012;379(9835):2489–99.
84. Mather AE, Matthews L, Mellor DJ, et al. An ecological approach to assessing the epidemiology of antimicrobial resistance in animal and human populations. Proc Biol Sci 2012;279(1733):1630–9.
100. Tennant SM, Zhang Y, Galen JE, et al. Ultra-fast and sensitive detection of non-typhoidal *Salmonella* using microwave-accelerated metal-enhanced fluorescence ('MAMEF'). PLoS One 2011;6(4):e18700.

Access the complete references online at www.expertconsult.com

26 Pneumococcal Disease

NEIL FRENCH

KEY POINTS

- *Streptococcus pneumoniae* is the most important bacterial cause of pneumonia and meningitis globally, responsible for an estimated 1 million deaths annually in children alone.
- The risk of pneumococcal disease is substantially increased by HIV infection in adults and children.
- Pneumococcal conjugate vaccines are highly protective against pneumococcal serotypes included in the vaccine and reduce the transmission of these serotypes through reduction of nasopharyngeal carriage.

Introduction

Streptococcus pneumoniae, the pneumococcus, is a ubiquitous human respiratory bacterial pathogen, well known for its association with pneumonia and meningitis. It causes disease in all age groups, particularly at the extremes of infancy and old age and is a major cause of morbidity and mortality in the tropics.[1] The pneumococcus is the leading cause of acute lower respiratory tract infections which are an important cause of death and the principal cause of global morbidity assessed in disability adjusted life years. In addition, the epidemiology of pneumococcal infection in many regions of the tropics has been profoundly altered by the interaction of the pneumococcus with the human immunodeficiency virus (HIV) leading to much increased disease burden. Antibiotic resistance among pneumococci continues to evolve and this threatens to undermine the basic principles of affordable management.

Set against these concerns conjugate vaccine technology has the potential to dramatically alter the burden of pneumococcal disease globally. However, widespread vaccine-based control of pneumococcal disease will take some time to be achieved and the pneumococcus will continue to be a leading public health and clinical problem for the foreseeable future.

Epidemiology

No significant animal reservoir of infection exists and pneumococcal transmission is a consequence of human contact and an inescapable fact of human life. The overwhelming majority of human–bacteria encounters will result in asymptomatic nasopharyngeal carriage, which will persist for days or months. In only a few of these human–bacteria interactions will clinical disease develop – by local mucosal spread to the sinuses, middle ear or bronchial tree. Rarely, the bacteria will invade tissue to produce bacteraemia, meningitis and other metastatic infections.

Young children and elderly adults are typically at greatest risk of serious pneumococcal infection. However, in regions of high HIV prevalence invasive disease has become a feature of young adults. Males have higher rates of disease than females at all ages and this is a consistent phenomenon in geographically and historically diverse reports. Pneumococcal infections also show seasonality. In the temperate regions of the globe, infection rates increase during the winter months and decline in the summer. In the tropics rates of disease rise and fall at different times of the year and while these fluctuations show a relationship to rainfall and humidity, these relationships are not consistent in different regions. As such the observed climate relationships may have more to do with spread of respiratory viruses (co-factors for colonization and disease) as a consequence of human mobility rather than climate parameters *per se*.

Pneumococci can be sub-typed by determining the seroreactivity of their bacterial polysaccharide capsule against a set of standard antisera – so-called serotypes. More than 90 serotypes have been identified although this number is set to increase with more extensive global surveillance and improved discriminatory techniques. Serotyping has been used as a tool for epidemiological surveillance and although molecular methods offer more detailed and differential measures, serotype determination remains relevant as it is an important determinant of virulence and thus clinical phenotype.[2] The predominant serotypes causing disease vary by age and by region[3] with some notable for causing serious disease in adults (serotype 3), while other serotypes are associated with multiple antibiotic resistance (6B, 14, 19F and 23F).[4]

Molecular methods have taken over as the tools of choice for epidemiological studies as they are more objective than conventional serotyping, have greater discriminatory power and can identify capsular shifts. This occurs when a pneumococcus changes its capsular type but retains its basic genotype. This behaviour has been known about for some time but is accelerated by the use of conjugate vaccines and allows pneumococci to escape the immune responses created by these vaccines. Multilocus sequence typing (MLST) has been used to track the global spread of drug-resistant pneumococci and open access libraries of MLST types exist. Whole genome sequence analysis (WGS) is likely to take over as the preferred method. In the case of WGS the ability to derive serotype and MLST type from gene analysis, infer relationships over time and space, investigate recombination and count individual genes makes this a particularly powerful tool for studying patterns and mechanisms of transmissibility and virulence.[5–7]

EPIDEMIOLOGY OF CARRIAGE

Nasopharyngeal carriage is critical to the maintenance and spread of pneumococci. Evidence from several sites in the tropics would suggest that early colonization is more intense than that found in developed countries. Point prevalence studies in infants and children throughout the tropics have recorded high rates of carriage, typically 60–80% and very often with multiple serotypes. These rates fall in older children and adults when 20% carriage rates are more typical. Nevertheless, these rates are still higher than those found in age-matched populations in the developed world. Defects in the mucosal immune response may contribute to these higher rates of carriage and this is demonstrable in HIV-infected children and adults. A further explanation is that there is continued high exposure to pneumococci at all stages of life.[8,9] The serotypes carried in the nasopharynx tends to be different to that causing invasive disease, with different capsular types having different invasive potential. Serotype 1 is rarely identified as a carried type but is the second most frequent cause of invasive disease on the African continent.

CHILDHOOD EPIDEMIOLOGY

Serious manifestations of pneumococcal disease are highly prevalent in paediatric populations across the tropics. *S. pneumoniae* is a leading blood culture isolate from most reported bacteraemia studies in infants and children globally, although notably infrequent in reports from Asia. Community-based incidence data from Africa consistently report high rates of disease. Studies from Soweto in South Africa,[10] The Gambia[11] and coastal Kenya[12] measured rates of invasive disease in under 5s of 130, 240 and 111 per 100 000 child years, respectively, rates several-fold higher than those in the developed world (*cf* 20 per 100 000 child years in the UK in under 5s). Peak rates are found in infants, and in The Gambia, rates in this group exceeded 500 per 100 000 child years. Moreover, rates of pneumococcal pneumonia are significantly higher and a major contributor to childhood morbidity.[13] Meningitis is the most lethal of the clinical syndromes associated with pneumococcal infection. In the African meningitis belt, pneumococcal meningitis has taken over as the leading cause of outbreaks following the successful introduction of meningococcal vaccination.[14,15]

The explanation for these high rates of disease is undoubtedly multifactorial. Low birth weight, poor nutrition, micronutrient and vitamin deficiencies, increased pneumococcal exposure and smoke exposure have all been implicated, although the relevant contribution of each probably differs by region. In a formal case-control study in The Gambia, overcrowding, parental education and occupation showed no clear association with risk but passive smoking, cooking indoors and preceding illness were significant risk factors.

Acute otitis media is the most frequent manifestation of pneumococcal disease in children in the developed world but little is known about its epidemiology in the developing world. Hearing impairment and chronic suppurative ear problems are a frequent finding in children in the tropics and the long term consequences of this in terms of failure of language skills and education are poorly understood. The pneumococcal-attributable contribution to acute and subsequent chronic ear disease remains to be established. Prevention of acute pneumococcal otitis media is not currently a priority for pneumococcal vaccine strategies in the developing world. With more data on disease burden priorities may change.

ADULT EPIDEMIOLOGY

Limited community-based incidence rates of pneumococcal disease exist for adult populations in the tropics. Little of this is properly stratified by age and the additional disease burden in the elderly is not well characterized. The best available estimates would suggest rates between 20 and 300 cases of invasive (bacteraemia and/or meningitis) pneumococcal disease per 100 000 adult years.[16] The lower-level estimates are similar to the rates of invasive disease in elderly populations in the UK. In otherwise healthy adults, bacteraemia complicates pneumonia in about one-quarter of cases; thus the rates of pneumococcal pneumonia may be four times greater.

In west Africa severe outbreaks of pneumococcal meningitis occur mimicking meningococcal disease and are associated with high case-fatality. These outbreaks are a consequence of specific pneumococcal strains, typically serotype 1, to which there is only limited immunity.

The higher rates of pneumococcal infection in otherwise fit and well adults particularly in sub-Saharan Africa, compared with adults in the developed world, is incompletely understood. Environmental and social factors are believed to play a leading part and it is perhaps important to note the similarities in rates of disease today in the tropics to those measured in the industrialized world in the 1920s and 1930s.[17] Host genetic factors are also believed to be important. Studies in the USA have found rates of pneumococcal infection to be higher among African-Americans than European-Americans, a finding incompletely accounted for by social and environmental confounding. The dynamics of carriage and the intensity of exposure to serotypes not previously encountered may also contribute to disease rates. Pneumococcal disease is more likely to occur when an individual is exposed to a new pneumococcal serotype, and this will happen more frequently in an environment of intense transmission. This was an important factor in the epidemics of pneumococcal disease in South African gold miners, which drove the initial studies of pneumococcal vaccination, and outbreaks in crowded conditions continue to be described.

The use of tobacco in the developing world, a predisposing factor for invasive pneumococcal disease in the industrialized world, is on the increase. The increased burden of other non-communicable diseases such as diabetes and cardiovascular disease will also contribute to the risk of pneumococcal disease.

HIV-ASSOCIATED PNEUMOCOCCAL DISEASE

HIV increases the risk of pneumococcal pneumonia by between 6–20 times and bacteraemia 10–100 times compared with age-matched HIV-uninfected individuals. Even with optimal antiretroviral therapy HIV-infected adults remain at significantly elevated risk of disease.[18,19] Community-based incidence data from East Africa have recorded rates of invasive disease in HIV-infected adults between 1700 to 4200 per 100 000 person years.[16] Rates of disease show a strong association with HIV-related immunosuppression; higher rates at lower CD4+ T-cell counts. Furthermore re-infection rates are extremely high, up to 25 000/100 000 person years.[20] In African countries with generalized HIV epidemics, invasive pneumococcal disease in an adult has a positive predictive value for HIV co-infection of between 80–95%. As in adults, HIV increases the risk of pneumococcal disease in children although in relative terms this effect is smaller given the high background rate of disease in this group.

Pathogenesis and Pathology

Microbiology. *Streptococcus pneumoniae* is a Gram-positive bacterium, which grows in chains in liquid media, but is more characteristically seen as pairs in clinical specimens. The term lanceolate is used to describe this paired appearance, the organisms appearing egg-shaped with their flatter ends opposed. A source of H_2O_2 is required for growth and consequently pneumococci grow better in the presence of catalase. In the diagnostic laboratory this is usually achieved by growing the organism in the presence of blood on a blood agar or heated blood agar (chocolate agar) plate. They grow best at 37°C (growth range 25–40°C) in the presence of 5–10% CO_2, conditions which can be achieved in a candle-extinction jar. Horse blood is typically used in media preparation. When this is not readily available sheep or goat blood provides a suitable alternative. Human or cow blood is best avoided, not only for the infection risks associated with handling human blood products, but growth may be suboptimal. Liquid media appropriate for use in manual blood culture systems to recover pneumococci are nutrient broth, tryptone soya broth and brain-heart infusion broth. For further information on media and reagent preparation relevant to laboratory practice in the developing world, see Cheesbrough.[21]

On a blood agar plate, pneumococci form colonies that are usually opaque, 1–2 mm in diameter with central umbilication which are surrounded by a characteristic green zone (α-haemolysis) as a result of the action of an exotoxin, pneumolysin, producing a pigment from haemoglobin. Production of a polysaccharide capsule by the bacteria is responsible for the opaque appearance. Colonies may appear mucoid if the bacteria produce large quantities of capsule. Failure to produce a significant capsule leads to the growth of transparent colonies. These phenotypic characteristics may be important in pathogenesis (see below). Pneumococci readily undergo autolysis and death, and this explains the umbilicated characteristics of the colonies, with the centre of the colony collapsing. This characteristic may hinder diagnosis. Pneumococci grown in liquid media will produce turbidity that may then clear on further culture in as little as 16 hours. Although less of a problem with modern continually monitored blood culturing systems, laboratories using manual systems need to time visual inspections and subculturing to avoid this pitfall. A zone of 'haemolysis' above the sedimented red cells in a manual system will provide additional evidence of bacterial growth.

Pneumococci must be differentiated from other α-haemolytic Streptococci by demonstrating sensitivity to Optochin (ethyl hydrocupreine, a quinine derivative, once used for therapy but withdrawn because of toxicity) and solubility when cultured after exposure to bile salts. Antibiotic sensitivity testing should be performed when available. This is particularly crucial for managing meningitis when knowledge of penicillin sensitivity is key to appropriate therapy (see below). Penicillin sensitivity is best assessed with a 1 μg oxacillin disc. Not only are oxacillin discs more stable and storage-friendly than low-strength penicillin discs, they are also relatively precise in predicting reduced susceptibility to penicillin (zone diameter ≤19 mm). Accurate determination of the susceptibility characteristics of pneumococci will require measurement of the minimal inhibitory concentration (MIC) by a broth or agar dilution method or the use of a graduated antibiotic-impregnated plastic strip, E-test® (AB Biodisk, Sweden). Serotyping of pneumococci is unnecessary for routine clinical diagnostic work, but may be performed for epidemiological surveillance. The Quellung reaction is the classical standard method for this. A suspension of pneumococci is incubated with capsular-type-specific antiserum and methylene blue for 10 min. If there is recognition of the capsule by the anti-serum present, the resultant capsular–antibody complex leads to a change in the refractive index of the capsule that stands out and contrasts (often referred to as swelling) against the methylene-blue-stained intracellular contents. A phase-contrast microscope is needed to correctly view these changes and a positive control should be available for comparison as the reactions are often difficult to assess. A commercially available latex agglutination kit for serogrouping the major pneumococci greatly simplifies this task but does not provide factor typing and therefore does not obviate the need for performing the Quellung reaction.

Bacterial Anatomy and Physiology. The membranous and external structures of the pneumococci are made up of a triple-layered cell membrane, cell wall and a polysaccharide capsule (Figure 26.1). Nested within this are a range of cell surface proteins. These structures confer the principal mechanisms underlying the pathogenicity and virulence of the bacteria. Exotoxin production is more limited than in other streptococcal species, and tissue damage as a consequence of pneumococcal infection is believed to be primarily the consequence of the inflammatory response triggered by cell wall and capsular components.

The cell wall is made up of a combination of peptidoglycan bound covalently to teichoic acid which protrudes deep into the capsule. This is the C-polysaccharide and is unique (with the exception of a few *Viridans* streptococci) to the pneumococcus. C-polysaccharide activates complement either by the alternative pathway or by the classical pathway in the presence of anti-C-polysaccharide antibody and also leads to the production of inflammatory cytokines.

The pneumococcal capsule is formed from the polymerization of oligosaccharides, which are bound to the bacterial cell wall. Permutations in the monosaccharides used in the production of the oligosaccharide macro-molecules leads to antigenic diversity. Genetic control of capsule production depends on the use of several genes combined into a single translational unit,[5] but importantly bacteria may possess or acquire additional capsule-related genes and thus can change their capsular characteristics. This process occurs naturally, but is accelerated under vaccine-induced immune pressure.

The polysaccharide capsule is critical to the organism's virulence and in the absence of type-specific opsonizing antibodies the capsule blocks phagocytosis. The mechanism by which the capsule does this is not clear. It is probably in part related to its ability to cover and hide cell wall bound complement and immunoglobulin which would otherwise act as opsonins and thereby prevent phagocytosis. Other cell surface components have been identified and are likely to play a role in pathogenesis.[22] A comprehensive review of current knowledge about these proteins is beyond this text. However among them are specific proteins which are of interest as vaccine or therapeutic targets. These include pneumococcal surface antigen A (PsaA), which protects pneumococci from oxidative stress; pneumococcal surface protein A (PspA), which interferes with complement activation; histidine triad proteins (PhtD A-D), which are zinc-binding proteins; and pilus proteins (RrgA-C), which modulate adherence of pneumococci to host cells.

Pneumolysin and autolysin (LytA) are exotoxins, which contribute to virulence. The former is cytotoxic for phagocytic and respiratory epithelial cells and is proinflammatory by activating complement. Some strains possess non-cytolytic

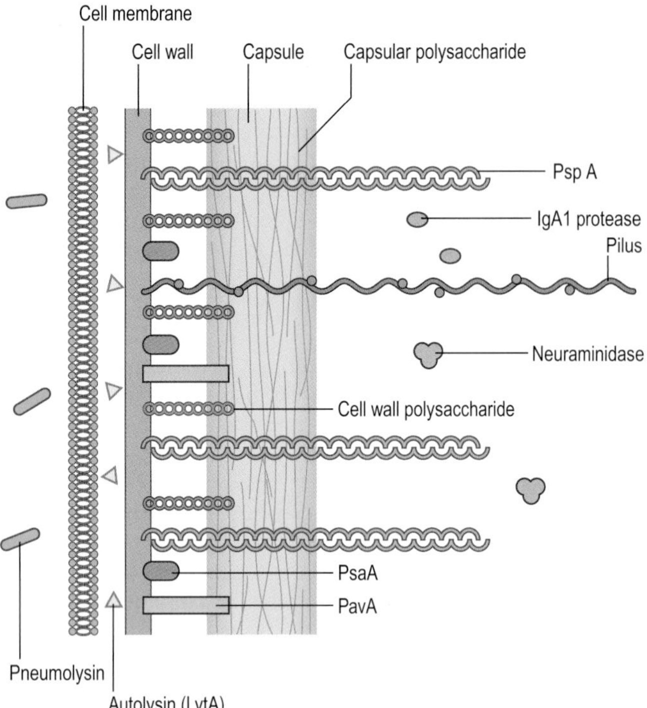

Figure 26.1 Schematic structure of pneumococcal cell membrane, wall and capsule. Pneumococcal surface protein A (Psp A), one of several choline-binding proteins, protrudes through the capsule and may act to stabilize the capsular structure and inhibits complement activation through the alternative pathway. PsaA is genetically and antigenically conserved across most capsular serotypes. It protects the bacteria from oxidative stress. PavA is an adhesin that binds fibronectin. Neuraminidase is an enzyme that cleaves cell surface components to expose cell surface receptors and aid adhesion. Autolysin (LytA) is a lytic enzyme linked to the release on intracellular contents in particular pneumolysin, a cytolytic exotoxin. IgA1 protease disrupts IgA1 subtype immunoglobulin. The pneumococcal pilus is an arrangement of several protein sub-units and mediates bacterial adherence, although it is not present in all pneumococci. Cell wall polysaccharide consists of teichoic acid, peptidoglycan and phosphorylcholine. When bound to a lipid molecule it is able to extend into the lipid-rich cell membrane and is then known as the Forssmann or F-antigen.

mutants and still remain virulent. Autolysin is involved in cell wall remodelling and plays a part in the release of pneumolysin from within the cell. Other bacterial components, of which there are now many identified and studied, also contribute to virulence/pathogenicity but their role in human disease awaits clarification.

Host Susceptibility. For pneumococcal disease to develop several critical events must take place. The bacteria must gain entry to the nasopharynx (or rarely to the female genital tract in the case of primary pneumococcal peritonitis) and adhere to the epithelial cells. Subsequently it must spread to susceptible anatomical sites, i.e. sinuses, middle ear, bronchial tree, reproduce freely and finally may breach endothelial surfaces and invade the bloodstream and other distant sites. In broad terms the host defends itself against pneumococcal mucosal infection by preventing mucosal attachment and spread, using the mucociliary system that lines the respiratory tract and adaptive mucosal immune responses. Defence against invasive disease is critically dependent on the presence of opsonizing anti-capsular antibodies and a functioning phagocytic system. A list of conditions predisposing to pneumococcal infection is shown in Table 26.1.

Anatomical Defences. The immature development of the Eustachian tube and the inability to clear secretions and bacteria from the middle ear are believed to underlie the susceptibility of young children to otitis media. Similarly, other factors which interfere with mucociliary function will predispose to infection: cigarette smoking; smoke inhalation from poorly ventilated fires; and preceding viral infection leading to direct destruction of ciliated epithelium in the upper respiratory mucosa. In addition viral infections may upregulate the mucosal expression of ligands improving mucosal attachment. This may be particularly relevant for allowing access of more virulent pneumococcal serotypes, which may have a decreased capacity for carriage but a high propensity for invasion once attached. Furthermore, inflammatory changes, mucus hyper-secretion and the subsequent post-nasal drip which often accompanies 'colds and flu' will predispose to aspiration of pneumococci through the larynx and into the bronchial tree.

Mucosal Immune Response. Innate and adaptive immune system responses contribute to prevention of carriage or spread of pneumococci across mucosal surfaces. Lactoferrin, lysozyme and lactoperoxidase are components of the innate immune system and act by binding and opsonizing pneumococci for clearance by mucosally associated phagocytes. C-reactive protein (CRP) and mannose binding lectin (MBL) are other agents of the innate immune response which appear to act both systemically and also at the mucosal level to opsonize pneumococci. Polymorphisms in the genes encoding MBP are associated with invasive pneumococcal disease and have been described in African populations. It has been postulated that the evolutionary persistence of CRP is a direct consequence of its ability to protect against pneumococcal disease.

Pattern recognition receptors including the transmembrane toll like receptors (TLR) and the cytosolic NOD receptors are now recognized as of importance in recruiting inflammatory cells and modulating the immune response in defence against pneumococcal infection. They are of therapeutic interest as nonspecific stimulation may enhance clearance and improve outcome from pneumococcal infection or co-stimulation may improve vaccine responses. Products are in active development for this purpose.

Both humoral and cellular components of the adaptive immune response are implicated in protection against pneumococcal disease, with increasing evidence of the pivotal role played by the cellular system at the mucosal level.[23–25] CD4+ T cells, particularly those secreting IL17, are critical to controlling pneumococcal colonization of the nasopharynx. These T-cell responses develop to a range of pneumococcal proteins and the breadth of the responses increases during early childhood. Subsequent exposure to pneumococci during adulthood acts to maintain and boost these responses. Increased pneumococcal colonization in HIV-infected adults is in part explained by the loss of these responses.

Antibodies have also been shown to modulate colonization. Secretory IgA, the predominant human immunoglobulin at the upper respiratory mucosal surface, has the ability to prevent binding of pneumococci (and possibly neutralizes pneumolysin) and opsonizes bacteria for phagocyte recognition. Of the two IgA isotypes IgA2 is the most important as it is resistant to an IgA protease secreted by the pneumococcus that is able to disrupt IgA1. Animal studies have confirmed the defensive

TABLE 26.1 Conditions that Predispose to Pneumococcal Infection in the Tropics by Mechanism of Susceptibility

	Increased Exposure	Reduced Mucosal Clearance[a]	Anatomical Defects	Defective Antibody	Complement Deficiency	Phagocyte Dysfunction	Comments
Important							**Common Condition or Strong Association with Risk**
HIV infection		(X)		X			Debility interferes with respiratory secretion clearance in late stages
Sickle cell disease				X	X	X	
Infancy and ageing	(X)		X	X			High carriage rates in siblings of infants leads to increased exposure
Alcoholism		X				X	
Chronic chest disease		X	X			X	Tuberculosis, asthma and bronchiectasis
Malnutrition		X		X			
Diabetes						X	
Liver cirrhosis			X			X	
Smoking/air pollution[b]		X				X	Mucociliary interference and direct toxicity on alveolar macrophages
Poverty	X						Overcrowding and usually co-existent nutritional deficiencies
Less Important							**Less Common Condition or Weak Association with Risk**
Kidney disease				X	X		
Lymphoproliferative disease				X			
Visceral leishmaniasis (and other parasitic infections)				X	X	X	Complex immune defects and abnormalities of splenic function

[a]By virtue of immobility, bed-ridden or defective mucociliary action.
[b]Includes biomass fuel use.

properties of IgA. The importance of IgA in the overall scheme of protection against pneumococci in humans remains unclear, however. Selective deficiencies of IgA are not clearly associated with pneumococcal infection and are believed to be uncommon in non-Caucasian populations. Moreover, pneumococci may use cleaved IgA to assist with attachment and translocation across the mucosa.

Serum IgG is associated with protection against colonization after-pneumococcal conjugate vaccination but not the clearance of established colonization. Vaccine-serotype colonization is markedly reduced in the immediate post-vaccine period in direct relation to the peak level of serum IgG achieved.[26] To what extent this reduction is directly a result of IgG and/or associated IgA production at the mucosal surface is unclear. Nevertheless, this impact on colonization is the primary reason for the major herd protection achieved with these vaccines. Whether IgG plays a role in natural protection against nasopharyngeal colonization is less clear. However, it is the critical opsonin in the alveolus and increases the ability of the alveolar macrophage to clear pneumococci from this location.

Systemic Immune Response. Critical to protection against invasive disease is the presence of capsule-specific opsonizing antibodies and an intact phagocytic cell system in the liver and particularly the spleen.

The central role of serum in protection was identified in the late nineteenth century, when protection could be achieved in animal models by the infusion of immune serum. In the 1920s, further discoveries led to the realization that the antibody conferring protection was directed against the pneumococcal capsule. Subsequently, passive vaccination or serum therapy using serotype-specific antisera formed the basis of early therapeutic successes in treating pneumococcal disease. Recent studies have confirmed the association between low levels/decreased activity of capsule-specific IgG and risk of disease. Unfortunately, the absolute level of capsule-specific immunoglobulin in isolation is not a wholly reliable predictor of protection or susceptibility.

Diseases that lead to underproduction of immunoglobulins are associated with an increased risk of pneumococcal disease. This is perhaps most dramatic in the primary and acquired hypogammaglobulinaemias, in which repeated episodes of otitis, sinusitis, pneumonia and invasive disease occur. The high rates of invasive pneumococcal disease in early childhood are in part related to underproduction of an IgG isotype, IgG2, the principal isotype contributing to anti-capsular antibodies in adults. An IgG2 response is produced when derivatives of the complement factor C3, which is an important opsonin of pneumococcal polysaccharide, binds a co-receptor on the B cell (complement receptor 2:CR2:CD21) in association with B-cell receptors binding polysaccharide. Importantly, children under 2 years of age do not adequately express complement receptor 2 on B-cells, and consequently little IgG produced is of the IgG2 isotype.

Deficient capsule-specific IgG production underpins the increased susceptibility of HIV-infected individuals to pneumococcal disease. Massive and progressive B-cell destruction is a feature of uncontrolled HIV infection. HIV has a selective preference for destruction of B cells which use the VH3 family of genes to produce their immunoglobulin heavy chain variable regions. In healthy adults, it is B cells expressing antibodies of this VH3 idiotype that make up the majority of those active against pneumococci. Thus HIV destroys the humoral immune response that protects against pneumococcal infection. No other HIV-associated immune defect has been clearly shown to be linked to risk of disease, although carriage of pneumococci increases with decreasing CD4 count and this appears to be linked to changes in cellular response at the mucosal level.

Malnutrition, old age, diabetes, malignancy, chronic pulmonary disease, chronic liver disease including alcohol-related disease and renal failure are associated with pneumococcal disease.[27] Although impaired immunoglobulin production to a greater or lesser extent is a feature of these conditions, other factors play a part in increasing susceptibility, e.g. impaired cough reflex, immobility, phagocyte defects, presence of ascites and orthostasis.

In addition to immunoglobulin, complement will also opsonize pneumococci. *In vitro* studies confirm the value of complement in stimulating phagocytosis of pneumococci and as mentioned above complement is able to modulate B-cell responses to polysaccharides. Gram-positive organisms are able to resist the effects of the terminal membrane attack complex (C5–C9); consequently, it is the early complement factors that are implicated in defence. Perhaps surprisingly, there are few reports of specific complement deficiency states associated with pneumococcal infection, although the increased risk of disease in nephrotic syndrome is believed to be due to hypocomplementaemia as a consequence of deposition and consumption of the early complement factors in the kidneys.

Once opsonized, pneumococci must be removed from circulation and killed by phagocytes. Polymorphonuclear leukocytes and macrophages in the liver and spleen undertake this task. Surprisingly, primary defective functioning of phagocytes either by chemotaxis or impaired oxidative killing is not associated with increased rates and severity of pneumococcal disease, although neutropenic individuals are at greater risk. Likewise individuals who lack a spleen (following splenectomy) or are functionally asplenic (homozygous sickle cell disease) suffer high rates of pneumococcal disease which is in part due to the reduction in phagocytic function, although other factors including abnormal antibody production and loss of the critical marginal zone of the spleen, contribute to increased susceptibility. Other phagocytic defects occur as a result of variation in phagocyte-expressed Fc receptors, particularly FcγRIIa. These have been associated with increased susceptibility to respiratory infections in children. However, the importance of polymorphisms in these receptors and risk of pneumococcal disease in African or Asian populations remains to be established.

Clinical Features

PNEUMONIA

Pneumonia is the most important presentation of pneumococcal disease by virtue of its frequency, accounting for 80–90% of all pneumococcal disease in adults, and its significant mortality. In the pre-antibiotic era case-fatality was 40–50%. In the antibiotic era case-fatality in adults of 10% remains typical for bacteraemic disease.[28] Delayed presentation as a consequence of compromised health-seeking behaviour through poverty or lack of access to health care, markedly influences case-fatality rates. Mortality rates in children were similarly high but early access to antibiotic therapy dramatically improves outcome from pneumococcal pneumonia and mortality rates of 1–2% are achievable, but not necessarily typical. A clear understanding of the presentation, management and expected outcome of pneumonia is essential knowledge for basic healthcare provision in the tropics.

Clinical Presentation

Presentation is typically acute with a 2- or 3-day history of cough, fever, dyspnoea and purulent sputum production. A more prolonged course may occur if the pneumonia has been partially treated or if there is underlying chronic chest disease, in particular tuberculosis. Other symptoms, which may be prominent include: haemoptysis, the classic 'rusty sputum,' is characteristic when present (the pigmentary effect of exotoxins on haemoglobin) but infrequent; pleuritic chest pain; headache, often severe and associated with meningism without confirmed meningitis; and diarrhoea, which may occasionally be the primary presenting complaint and lead to confusion with acute gastroenteritis.

Patients appear unwell and will be tachycardic and tachypnoeic. Cyanosis if present indicates more severe disease but is difficult to assess in individuals with black skin. Chest signs of consolidation (dullness to percussion, bronchial breathing and aegophony) or more commonly coarse inspiratory crackles consistent with retained secretions are usually heard on auscultation. A pleural rub may also be present and does not necessarily predict complicated pleural disease. Diagnostic confusion may occur if the presentation is hyperacute with abrupt onset of rigors, when malaria, other bacterial septicaemic illness or fulminant viral illness may then head the list of differential diagnoses. Presentations with acute psychosis, confusion, hypothermia, jaundice and abdominal pain can occur and may lead to diagnostic confusion.

The presentation, recognition and assessment of pneumonia in children are detailed in Chapter 80.

Investigations

Pneumonia is confirmed by finding consolidation in a lobar, segmental or sub-segmental distribution on chest radiography. Chest radiography is not a requirement when the clinical presentation is clear but will often resolve diagnostic confusion (Figure 26.2). Radiographic features in children may be less clear-cut but even small changes in lung parenchyma would be consistent with a diagnosis of pneumonia.

Confirmation of a pneumococcal aetiology can be made definitively by the recovery of pneumococci from blood culture or from a transthoracic needle lung aspirate. This latter technique has proved a safe and valid technique in both adults and children when aspiration is performed on consolidated

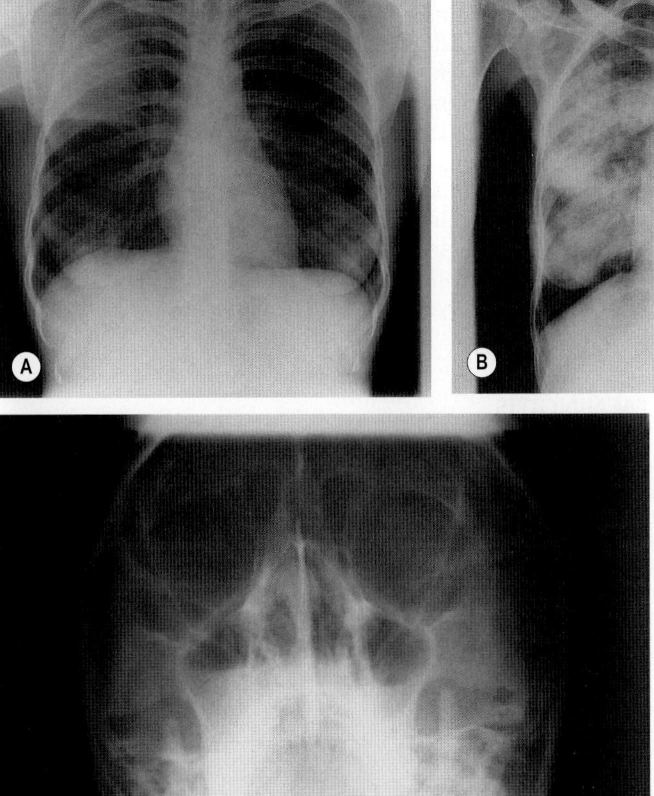

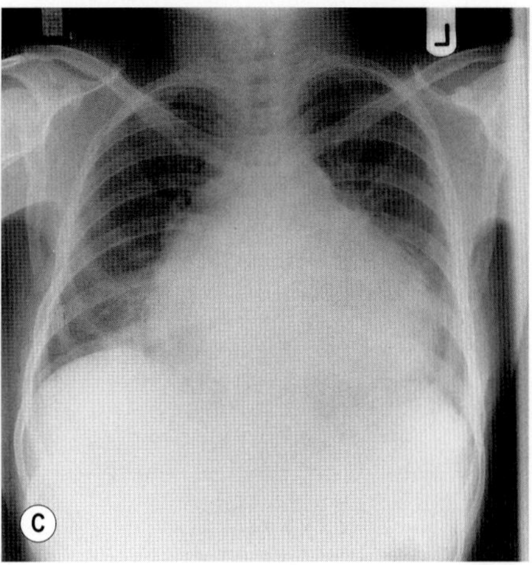

Figure 26.2 Radiographic appearances of pneumococcal disease: (A) Classical right upper lobe pneumococcal pneumonia in a 32-year-old HIV-infected Kenyan woman; (B) bilateral pulmonary consolidation particularly in the right lung as a consequence of a *S. pneumoniae/M. tuberculosis* co-infection in a 26-year-old HIV-infected Kenyan woman; (C) pneumococcal pericarditis and pericardial effusion in a 34-year-old Ugandan male of uncertain HIV status; (D) bilateral maxillary sinus fluid levels in a 28-year-old HIV-infected Kenyan with pneumococcal bacteraemia and no pulmonary focus.

pulmonary tissue using a small-gauge needle. Sputum is often the most readily available clinical specimen. Interpretation of Gram stain examination and culture results require some caution. Pneumococci carried in the nasopharynx may contaminate expectorated sputum specimens and lead to a false-positive diagnosis. Macroscopic examination of a sputum sample should reveal purulent material (yellow/green mucus). Gram-positive diplococci in association with 10–20 pus cells and no epithelial cells per high-powered field (×100 oil immersion objective) provides good supporting evidence of pneumococcal aetiology. Examination of the sputum for acid- and alcohol-fast bacilli should be performed because of the frequent co-existence of tuberculosis with pneumococcal pneumonia. Commercial kits for the identification of pneumococcal capsular polysaccharide in blood or urine are available. They have variable sensitivity, particularly in regions of intense carriage and in HIV infection, and are usually an unjustifiable cost for basic diagnostic laboratories. Serological tests have no place in routine clinical practice at present. Newer techniques based on polymerase chain reaction may find a place in diagnosis in the future. Quantitative assessment of pneumococcal carriage in the nasopharynx or pneumococcal DNA in blood have been shown to have diagnostic value in pneumococcal disease, but significant shifts in simplifying molecular technology will be needed to make these assays available in resource-limited settings.

Subsidiary investigations including white cell counts, arterial blood gases, electrolyte measurements and liver function tests are not particularly helpful in establishing a diagnosis, but may be used as measures of severity.

Differential Diagnosis

When respiratory symptoms and signs are lacking pneumococcal pneumonia may need to be differentiated from a wide range of febrile conditions. When a diagnosis of pneumonia is established, the primary differential is from other infectious agents of pneumonia, and occasionally typhoid or amoebic liver abscess (right-sided effusion). Making a definitive diagnosis of these infections is in many ways more difficult than pneumococcal disease. Many are not readily identifiable (e.g. chlamydial, mycoplasma, rickettsial, viral) or investigations are difficult to interpret (i.e. Gram-negative organisms in sputum). Tuberculosis is the most critical differential diagnosis to consider. It may present as an acute pneumonic illness or as a co-infection with the pneumococcus. *M. tuberculosis* may be implicated in 5–15% of adult community acquired pneumonia (CAP) in sub-Saharan Africa, the association being particularly important in HIV-infected adults. Ziehl–Neelsen staining of sputum samples will help in making the diagnosis, however between 20–50% of cases of *M. tuberculosis* infection presenting acutely will require mycobacterial culture to establish a diagnosis. When TB co-infection exists, response to antibiotics may be initially satisfactory. Follow-up and a high index of suspicion for TB should be maintained. Poor response to antibiotics, pleural effusions, cavitation of lung lesions, cervical or other giant lymphadenopathy or incomplete resolution of pneumonia at follow-up should raise the suspicion of *M. tuberculosis* infection.

Management and Therapy

With overcrowded in-patient facilities, the threshold for admission to hospital will be towards more severe disease and an

TABLE 26.2 Associations of Severe Disease and Poor Outcome in Pneumonia

	Severity Grading
Demographic Features	
Age >55	A
Consultation of traditional healer	A
Increasing distance from health centre	B
Recent migration/refugee camps	B
Clinical Features	
Confusion	B
Diastolic blood pressure <60 mmHg	A
Respiratory rate >30 breaths/min	A
Pulse rate >120 beats/min	A
Cyanosis	B
Extra-pulmonary infection	B
Jaundice	B
Reduced body mass index/wasted	B
Investigations: If Available at Initial Assessment	
Multilobar disease	B
White cell count <4000 cells/μL	A
White cell count >18 000 cells/μL	B
Investigations: If Available During Therapy	
Co-infection with tuberculosis	B
Pneumococcal bacteraemia	B

This table represents a summary of information from several sources. Factors are graded as A – strongly associated with severe disease and death (five times or greater risk of death if present) and B – moderately associated (less than 5 times or poorly quantified increased risk of death). No validated scheme to determine the need for hospital admission or use of parenteral antibiotics exists, however the presence of ≥2 grade A factors, ≥3 grade B factors should lead to hospital admission if available. Such an approach will be sensitive for identifying severe disease but will lack specificity.

assessment of suitability for out-patient oral therapy or the need for in-patient parenteral therapy is required. Indicators of poor outcome are listed in Table 26.2. Further indicators of the suitability of oral therapy involve an assessment of gastrointestinal signs and symptoms and microbial factors. Vomiting or profuse diarrhoea are relative contraindications to oral therapy as antibiotic absorption may be impaired.

In addition to antimicrobial therapy, other supportive treatment should be initiated. Supplemental oxygen, preferably monitored with blood gases or peripheral saturation measurements, should be provided when hypoxia is present. Maintenance of appropriate hydration (with IV fluids if necessary) and clearance of respiratory secretions may also be necessary. The latter will be achieved by changing posture, suctioning and nebulized saline to prevent desiccation of respiratory and pharyngeal secretions. Assisted ventilation will be necessary when respiratory muscle fatigue develops, heralded by a rising partial pressure of CO_2 and more latterly altered conscious level, blood pressure instability and decreasing respiratory effort.

Complications

Pneumococcal pneumonia may be complicated by metastatic spread of infection and empyema. Osteomyelitis, arthritis, endocarditis, suppurative pericarditis and other localized infections are unusual. Empyema complicates 2–3% of pneumonic episodes and may be more common with particular strains of pneumococci particularly serotype 1. Inadequate or sub-therapeutic antibiotic therapy may predispose to this complication. Management of pleural effusions/empyema should be active from the outset to avoid the late sequelae of chronic empyema. Pleural fluid should be examined. Parapneumonic effusions may be left while infected effusions/empyema should be drained. Differentiating between the two may be problematic. Biochemical measures can assist in determining the likelihood of infection (low pH, low glucose and high lactate dehydrogenase), but macroscopic appearance and microscopy will provide broad indicators of infection, the presence of bacteria being a clear indicator of infection. If empyema is diagnosed, drainage of fluid/pus by use of a chest drain or at least with a needle and syringe should be performed, with the intention of removing as much fluid/pus as possible.

MENINGITIS

Meningitis is the most lethal syndrome associated with pneumococcal infection and high rates of serious complications are present in survivors. Case fatality in children admitted to hospital has been measured in excess of 60% and similar rates are recorded in adults.[29,30] These rates are substantially higher than those seen in the developed world. It is unlikely that the difference is wholly down to type of therapy but more to timing of therapy. It is likely that late presentation and poor access to health care extending the time to first antibiotic from the onset of symptoms is a major determinant of this poor outcome.

Clinical Presentation

Pneumococcal meningitis follows the typical pattern of headache and fever in association with neck stiffness, progressive alteration in conscious level and features of disseminated sepsis, with symptoms evolving over 12–48 hours. Preceding or concurrent pneumonia is also common. Difficulties in diagnosis arise when neck stiffness is absent, which may be associated with advanced disease, infancy, old age and immunosuppression, and the diagnosis may be missed or confused with cerebral malaria.

Investigations

Examination of cerebrospinal fluid (CSF) is essential to confirm the diagnosis. CSF findings will show the characteristics of a bacterial infection, polymorphonuclear leukocyte pleocytosis, raised protein, low sugar and a Gram stain demonstrating Gram-positive lanceolate diplococci. White cell counts can, however, be low in the immunosuppressed or those with overwhelming infection. In such circumstances Gram stain evidence of bacteria is usually found. In the absence of a confirmatory Gram stain or following antibiotic therapy, it may be possible to detect pneumococcal antigen in CSF to provide a rapid diagnosis. Definitive proof of pneumococcal aetiology relies on culture and laboratory characterization. In the absence of evidence of pneumococcal aetiology, empiric therapy should always include an agent effective against pneumococci. In laboratories able to perform sensitivity testing, this should be performed on all isolates from CSF as reduced susceptibility to penicillin is critically important in determining therapy for meningitis (see below).

The risks of performing a lumbar puncture must be balanced against the value of the information obtained. However only basic laboratory equipment is required to perform a CSF examination (microscope, counting chamber, slides, Gram stain) and this will often rapidly establish an aetiological diagnosis. The presence of a focal neurological deficit (present in 20% of cases of bacterial meningitis), altered conscious level (>60% of cases), papilloedema (<1% of cases), seizures (30% of cases) and suppurative ear disease should necessitate a reconsideration of the need for lumbar puncture, but are not absolute contraindications.

Differential Diagnosis

This includes other forms of bacterial meningitis (see Chapter 27), the meningococcus being the most important; falciparum malaria; rickettsial infections; relapsing fever; leptospirosis; viral meningo-encephalitis; and cryptococcal meningitis. Tetanus, hypertensive crisis, poisoning and sub-arachnoid haemorrhage may also need to be considered. Differentiation relies on CSF examination. Blood cultures should also be performed on all cases of suspected meningitis. Bacterial growth will occur within 24 hours and this is a particularly valuable investigation when lumbar puncture is contraindicated.

Management and Therapy

Therapy for meningitis should be started as soon as the diagnosis is considered. A lumbar puncture should be performed (see above for safety considerations) as soon as possible after commencement of antibiotic therapy and should not delay the receipt of antibiotics. Parenteral therapy is obligatory and should be continued for at least 10 days. In addition to antimicrobial agents other supportive therapy will be needed. These are aimed at treating the complications of bacteraemia with intravenous fluids and supplemental oxygen if available; preventing the complications of immobility by good nursing care; and minimizing the rise in intracranial pressure by nursing in a head-up position. High-dose corticosteroids are recommended for the treatment of pneumococcal meningitis based on clinical trial findings from Europe. However, two large trials from Malawi in children and adults do not support this approach in settings where HIV is prevalent and where presentation may be delayed.[31,32] Glycerol given as an oral agent has also been suggested for use in children[33] but has not shown any benefit in adult meningitis.[34]

Complications

Outcome following pneumococcal meningitis is poor. In survivors convalescence may be prolonged and residual neurological deficit and disability are common, notably deafness, stroke and blindness. Subdural collections may occur in children but are infrequent in adults.

OTHER SYNDROMES

The pneumococcus is associated with several other common syndromes, notably sinusitis, otitis media and conjunctivitis. In the immunocompromised the sinuses may act as a source of bacteraemia and meningitis. Acute otitis media is predominantly a complication of children, for anatomical and other reasons outlined above in the section on susceptibility. It is likely that much acute otitis media in the tropics passes unnoticed in the large burden of febrile disease. Uncommon presentations include pericarditis, arthritis, osteomyelitis, mediastinitis, endocarditis, pyomyositis, brain abscess and peritonitis (specifically young women and alcoholics).

SPECIAL SITUATIONS

Human Immunodeficiency Virus. HIV infection dramatically increases susceptibility to pneumococcal infection and particularly invasive disease, with disease risk increased at lower WHO clinical stage or CD4 T-cell counts. The general management of acute pneumococcal disease should be unaffected by HIV-status. However, HIV testing should be recommended to any adult presenting with pneumococcal disease/pneumonia in sub-Saharan Africa. In those who are HIV-infected, serious bacterial infections constitute a WHO clinical stage 3 criterium and antiretroviral therapy is recommended for these individuals.

Sickle Cell Disease. Fulminant pneumococcal sepsis is a feature of sickle cell disease.[35] The most serious infections occur in the under-5s and commonly present as a septicaemic illness. The features of infarction that will accompany the infective episode may confuse presentation. Presumptive therapy of a sick sickle cell child with infection should include anti-pneumococcal therapy as a priority. Adrenal failure/Waterhouse–Friderichsen syndrome is a recognized complication and steroid support may be necessary.

Antimicrobial Therapy

Antibiotic therapy is considered obligatory in the treatment of invasive pneumococcal disease and pneumococcal pneumonia, although it is recognized that occult and self-limited bacteraemia in children can occur. Penicillins continue to be the agents of choice for managing pneumococcal disease (Table 26.3). However, the expanding problem of penicillin-resistant pneumococci is beginning to threaten the simplicity of this approach.

In 1973, pneumococci with a reduced susceptibility to penicillin were first reported from South Africa. During the 1990s increasing resistance to penicillin among pneumococci has been steadily emerging and continues to evolve throughout most parts of the globe. The clinical impact of resistance to penicillin in pneumococci is highly dependent on the clinical syndrome. There is little clinical evidence of an adverse impact of resistance on pneumococcal pneumonia, but a very significant impact on the outcome of meningitis. Pneumococci that need a concentration of penicillin ≥0.1 mg/L to inhibit growth (minimal inhibitory concentration or MIC) cannot be treated with penicillin if causing meningitis, while pneumococci requiring concentrations of up 2 mg/L can be treated with penicillin if causing pneumonia. Penicillin penetration into the CSF (an active process across the blood–brain barrier) is poor, making effective penicillin levels unachievable in this compartment.

Penicillin exerts its antibacterial action by covalently binding and inhibiting enzymes involved in the production of cell wall peptidoglycans – penicillin-binding proteins (PBP). Six PBPs with decreased affinity for binding penicillin have been identified and occur as a result of genetic transformations after acquiring DNA from other streptococcal species carried in the nasopharynx. The consequence of these alterations is a graduated increase in the concentration of penicillin required to achieve inhibition of growth or killing of the bacteria. With the widespread and often unregulated use of antibiotics, penicillin-resistant pneumococcal clones have become widespread. The 'Spanish' 23F clone for instance has been found in every continent. Penicillin-resistant pneumococci are frequently multi-drug-resistant. Penicillin, co-trimoxazole, macrolide and

TABLE 26.3 Antimicrobial Therapy for Pneumococcal Infections

		Penicillin Sensitive		Penicillin Resistance	
		Adult	Child	Adult	Child
Pneumonia and/or Bacteraemia	Parenteral	BZP 600 mg 6-hourly	BZP 50–100 mg/kg per day[a]	BZP 1.2 g–2.4 g 4-hourly	BZP 100–300 mg/kg per day[b]
	Oral	AXL[c] 250–500 mg 8-hourly	AXL125–250 mg 8-hourly	AXL 1 g 6–8-hourly	AXL 90 mg/kg per day in 3 divided doses
Meningitis[d]	Parenteral	BZP 1.8 g 4–6-hourly	BZP 100–300 mg/kg per day[b]	CFX[e] 2 g 6-hourly *OR* CHL 50–100 mg/kg in 4 divided doses[f]	CFX 200 mg/kg per day in 2–4 divided doses *OR* CHL 25–100 mg/kg per day in 4 divided doses[g]
Sinusitis and Otitis media	Oral	AXL 500 mg 8-hourly	AXL 80–90 mg/kg per day in 3 divided doses		

The decision to treat an infection as penicillin-resistant may be based on known sensitivity testing or local knowledge and suspicion. Failure of response to first-line therapy over 48 hours should stimulate a reconsideration of the diagnosis, a search for localized infection/abscess and the possibility of antimicrobial resistance. Parenteral therapy may be discontinued after 48 hours in the presence of a response. Continuation therapy should complete at least 7 days of treatment for uncomplicated pneumonia and 10 days for uncomplicated meningitis. In the event of penicillin allergy, a third-generation cephalosporin (10% cross-sensitivity) or chloramphenicol should be used as a parenteral alternative. Erythromycin or chloramphenicol offer oral alternatives. BZP, benzylpenicillin; AXL, amoxicillin; CFX, cefotaxime; CHL, chloramphenicol.

[a]In neonates up to 7 days old, 50 mg/kg in 2 divided doses; in infants 1–4 weeks, 75 mg/kg in 3 divided doses and other children 100 mg/kg 4–6 divided doses.

[b]In neonates up to 7 days old, 100 mg/kg in 2 divided doses; in infants 1–4 weeks 150 mg/kg in 3 divided doses and other children 300 mg/kg 4–6 divided doses.

[c]Ampicillin may be substituted given 6-hourly.

[d]Dosages used for meningitis are appropriate for managing peritonitis, pericarditis, arthritis and other body cavity infections combined with suitable drainage of pus.

[e]Other third-generation cephalosporins may be substituted such as ceftriaxone 2 g 12-hourly.

[f]100 mg/kg dose should be reduced to 50 mg/kg as soon as clinical response established.

[g]In neonates up to 14 days old, 25 mg/kg in 4 divided doses; in infants 2 weeks–1 year 50 mg/kg in 4 divided doses and other children 50–100 mg/kg in 4 divided doses – 100 mg/kg dose should be reduced to 50 mg/kg as soon as clinical response is established.

chloramphenicol resistance is commonly found in the same pneumococcal clone making empiric selection of effective therapy potentially difficult. Genetic material conferring resistance to these other agents is found in the same translational elements encoding for the altered PBPs.

The scale of antibiotic resistance in pneumococci in the tropics is unclear and based on information from only a few centres. Penicillin resistance appears at its greatest in South-east Asia where up to 60% of clinically relevant pneumococci are resistant with 80% of these isolates with MICs >2 mg/L. As locally available sensitivity testing tends to be unavailable, national surveillance and guidelines take on great importance to inform the appropriate use of antimicrobials at the district-level hospitals and clinics.

For uncomplicated bloodstream infections and pneumonia, penicillin remains the antimicrobial of choice. A single intravenous bolus of 5 megaunits (MU) of penicillin (3.0 g of Benzylpenicillin) will achieve a serum and pulmonary concentration of penicillin above 4 mg/L for 4–5 hours post-dose in an adult. Thus four daily doses of 5 MU penicillin will provide effective coverage of all but the most resistant pneumococci. Moreover, a 4 MU bolus followed by a continuous infusion of 24 MU of penicillin over 24 hours will achieve a steady serum concentration of 20 mg/L – a concentration in excess of the highest MIC yet reported for pneumococci. Thus, the approach to the management of pulmonary and bloodstream infections in regions where penicillin resistance is recognized, should be an increase in the dose of penicillin and/or an adjustment in the dosing schedule.

Therapy for meningitis and other body cavity infections where antibiotic penetration is decreased needs to be altered if penicillin resistance is considered or known to be present. Increased penicillin dosing will be insufficient. CSF concentrations of penicillin are usually between 1–5% of serum levels and maintaining a concentration above the MIC for at least 40% of the dosing interval (a figure required for therapeutic success with β-lactams in animal studies) is unachievable. When available, a third-generation cephalosporin should be used as the initial therapy of meningitis, and modified on the basis of sensitivity testing. In the absence of cephalosporins, chloramphenicol may be appropriate to use. Local sensitivity knowledge will assist with these decisions. Other agents with anti-pneumococcal activity which have been used to treat penicillin-resistant pneumococcal meningitis include; carbapenems (e.g. meropenem), glycopeptides (e.g. vancomycin), oxazolidinones (e.g. linezolid) and rifampicin. These agents are expensive and less readily available than cephalosporins and with the exception of Rifampicin, none are included in the WHO essential drugs list. Rifampicin is widely available as a combination tablet with other antituberculous drugs but more difficult to find as a single agent and resistance rapidly develops when used alone. The aminoglycosides gentamicin and streptomycin, should not be used as single agents as achievable tissue concentrations are below the MICs of even the most sensitive organisms.

Prevention

Prevention of pneumococcal disease and pneumonia in children by the use of pneumococcal protein conjugate vaccine is now an important part of the international agenda for health improvement. Studies from Africa[36,37] have demonstrated the efficacy of these vaccines and with routine use falls in the burden of pneumococcal disease and its attributable mortality are expected.

POLYSACCHARIDE VACCINE

These vaccines have been available in some form for the past 90 years. The current formulations contain capsular polysaccharides from the 23 commonest disease-causing pneumococcal serotypes. The efficacy of these vaccines is debatable and while they have been used widely in North America and Europe, use of the vaccine elsewhere and particularly in the tropics has been very limited. The vaccine provides protection against invasive pneumococcal disease in immunocompetent adults particularly in settings of epidemic pneumococcal spread but has not been shown to be effective in immunocompromised groups. The vaccine has never been shown to convincingly reduce pneumonia. The vaccine is not used in infants. Thus current recommendations for use of the vaccine in the tropics are somewhat limited but extend to individuals with sickle cell disease, or other causes of functional or anatomic asplenia. Use of the vaccine in HIV-infected adults in Africa is not recommended.[38]

PROTEIN CONJUGATE PNEUMOCOCCAL VACCINE

The development of protein conjugate vaccines (PCV) was driven by the ineffectiveness of polysaccharide vaccines in young children and an understanding that by attaching the polysaccharide to a polypeptide 'carrier' the vaccine becomes T-cell-dependent. T-cell-dependent responses are present from birth, unlike responses to pure polysaccharide. With T-cell involvement not only does the vaccine become immunogenic in infants there is also the production of functionally competent, affinity-matured antibodies and the creation of long-lived memory B-lymphocytes.

These vaccines have now been shown to be highly efficacious in African trials, preventing pneumonia, invasive disease and mortality; they work in HIV-infected children; and they create herd protection. This latter effect is so large that more pneumococcal disease has been prevented through this mechanism than directly by the vaccine recipients. Vaccine-serotype invasive disease has now almost disappeared from the USA.[39,40]

Vaccines are now being introduced widely, with several African nations including PCV in their EPI schedule.[41] Whether these vaccines will be more or less effective in Africa than in the developed world, remains to be seen. The major concern is the extent of non-vaccine serotype replacement that may occur. In the USA, non-vaccine serotype disease has increased but the effect to date has not significantly offset the net benefit of vaccine except in HIV-infected adults. In this group decreases in vaccine serotype disease through indirect benefits of vaccine have been completely offset by non-vaccine serotype replacement. This effect will be larger in regions of high HIV prevalence but whether this will limit the overall programmatic benefits of vaccine or durability of effect is doubtful. A further concern has been uncertainties over efficacy of specific serotypes within the conjugate vaccines, particularly serotypes 3 and 1. No proof of efficacy exists at present, although this should be forthcoming in the near future, but there is clearly a difference in individual serotype efficacy within these vaccines. However, it is the economics of vaccination that is likely to be the major problem going forward. Conjugate vaccines are relatively expensive (current GAVI price for Africa is of the order of $7 per dose) and large-scale and continuous donor support will be necessary to allow developing country governments to continue their introduction.

Conjugate vaccines are efficacious in adult populations and in particular in HIV-infected adults. Policies for the use of pneumococcal conjugate vaccines in adult populations remain to be established. With the potential for indirect effects from paediatric vaccine programmes, it may well be that widespread introduction of infant vaccination will have the same effect as direct vaccination of high-risk adults. But where disease risk and funding exist, it seems likely that PCV will be an appropriate part of disease prevention.

OTHER VACCINE CANDIDATES

Concerns over the high production costs of conjugate vaccines and their serotype-specific limitations have led the search for other vaccine candidates. Several pneumococcal peptides are under investigation and a whole cell. A capsulate killed vaccine. They are attractive because they may work independent of capsular serotype and/or may be significantly easier to produce. Several of these candidates have reached human studies, but it is unclear as to which, if any, will become viable pharmaceutical products.[42]

CHEMOPROPHYLAXIS

The use of penicillin prophylaxis (oral phenoxymethylpenicillin 125–250 mg twice daily or intramuscular benzathine penicillin 1.2 MU 4 weekly) is recommended for the prevention of pneumococcal disease in sickle cell disease (SCD) and in individuals without a spleen. Prophylaxis should continue at least up until the age of 5 years in SCD and for a minimum of 5 years post-splenectomy. More prolonged prophylaxis may be beneficial as the true morbidity and mortality of late pneumococcal sepsis in these conditions is uncertain. The increasing prevalence of penicillin-resistant pneumococci may decrease the value of this approach in the future. Alternative agents for prophylaxis include erythromycin or azithromycin.

Co-trimoxazole is recommended by the WHO for HIV-infected individuals (adults and children). This recommendation is based strongly on studies from Côte D'Ivoire and Zambia that showed the benefits of this approach at reducing several morbid end-points including presumed bacterial pneumonia. Discontinuation of co-trimoxazole prophylaxis after successful initiation of ART is an area of research interest, but at present therapy is recommended life-long.

ANTIRETROVIRAL THERAPY

Antiretroviral therapy reduces rates of primary and recurrent pneumococcal disease in HIV-infected adults although rates of disease remain substantially higher than in the HIV-uninfected and thus other prophylactic strategies will still be needed.

REFERENCES

1. O'Brien KL, Wolfson LJ, Watt JP, et al. Burden of disease caused by *Streptococcus pneumoniae* in children younger than 5 years: global estimates. Lancet 2009;374:893–902.
19. Klugman KP, Madhi SA, Feldman C. HIV and pneumococcal disease. Curr Opin Infect Dis 2007;20:11–15.
37. Cutts FT, Zaman SM, Enwere G, et al. Efficacy of nine-valent pneumococcal conjugate vaccine against pneumonia and invasive pneumococcal disease in The Gambia: randomised, double-blind, placebo-controlled trial. Lancet 2005;365:1139–46.
38. World Health Organization. 23-valent pneumococcal polysaccharide vaccine. WHO position paper. Wkly Epidemiol Rec 2008;83:373–84.
41. World Health Organization. Pneumococcal conjugate vaccine for childhood immunization – WHO position paper. Wkly Epidemiol Rec 2007;82:93–104.

Access the complete references online at www.expertconsult.com

27

Bacterial Meningitis

MATTHIJS C. BROUWER | DIEDERIK VAN DE BEEK

KEY POINTS

- Bacterial meningitis is a medical emergency with high mortality and morbidity.
- Vaccinations against *Haemophilus influenzae* type b (Hib), *Streptococcus pneumoniae* and *Neisseria meningitidis* have reduced the incidence, but their availability is still limited.
- Outside the neonatal period *Streptococcus pneumoniae* and *Neisseria meningitidis* are the most common pathogens.
- Neonatal meningitis is mostly caused by *Streptococcus agalactiae, Escherichia coli* and *Listeria monocytogenes.*
- Cerebrospinal fluid (CSF) examination is warranted in all patients with suspected bacterial meningitis.
- The diagnosis is confirmed by typical CSF abnormalities, CSF Gram stain, CSF culture and/or CSF polymerase chain reaction (PCR).
- Early antibiotic treatment improves outcome.
- Adjunctive dexamethasone therapy has been shown to be beneficial in high-income countries, but in low-resource countries, no adjunctive therapy has been proven effective.

Introduction

Bacterial meningitis is a medical emergency that is common in many areas of the tropics. The epidemiology varies with geographical and climatic conditions, with age, with rate of HIV infection and other causes of immunosuppression, and with the availability of vaccines (Tables 27.1, 27.2). The epidemiology has substantially changed in the past 25 years after the introduction of vaccines against *Haemophilus influenzae* type b, *Streptococcus pneumoniae* and *Neisseria meningitidis*, although only recently have these vaccinations reached populations in research-poor settings, where the incidence is highest.[1] Currently, two pathogens cause most cases outside the neonatal period: *Streptococcus pneumoniae* and *Neisseria meningitidis.*[2,3] Neonatal meningitis may also be caused by these organisms but other bacteria such as *Escherichia coli*, *Streptococcus agalactiae* (Group B streptococcus) and *Klebsiella pneumoniae* tend to predominate. The relative importance of *H. influenzae*, pneumococci and meningococci outside the neonatal period varies according to country; for example, in humid low-lying regions *S. pneumoniae* and *H. influenzae* predominate, whereas in dryer regions, e.g. the meningitis belt of sub-Saharan Africa, the meningococcus causes vast spreading epidemics.[4] Bacterial meningitis has a high mortality, and carries a high risk of neurological sequelae.

Neonatal Meningitis

With improvements in, and the more widespread availability of neonatal intensive care, neonates of increasing prematurity have a chance of survival. The premature neonate is not only immature in terms of pulmonary, alimentary and renal function but is also an immunocompromised host. This means that the neonate, and especially the premature neonate, is at increased risk of infection. Neonates with bacterial meningitis often present with nonspecific signs and symptoms.[5] Neonatal bacterial meningitis is usually part of a syndrome of neonatal sepsis.[6]

GEOGRAPHY

The incidence of neonatal meningitis varies according to region and standard of medical care. In the USA and other industrialized countries, the incidence is estimated at 0.3 cases per 1000 live births.[7] In reports from India, Pakistan and Guatemala, the incidence varies from 0.8 to 6.1 per 1000 live births.[8] A study in a large district hospital in Kenya shows the number of children admitted with neonatal meningitis has remained stable for the past 20 years.[9]

EPIDEMIOLOGY

Common causative microorganisms of neonatal meningitis during the first week of life are *S. agalactiae*, *E. coli* and *Listeria monocytogenes.*[10–12] Late-onset neonatal meningitis occurs between the first week of life and 2–3 months of age and may be caused by a wide variety of species, including staphylococci, *L. monocytogenes*, and Gram-negative bacilli.[1,11,12] *S. agalactiae* is the most common cause in both industrialized and developing countries, but incidence varies considerably: *S. agalactiae* causes 66% of neonatal meningitis cases in the USA, 35–89% in Durban (South Africa) and 30% in Malawi and Kenya.[13,14] The incidence of *S. agalactiae* meningitis in neonates has recently decreased in the USA, since pregnant woman are given antimicrobial prophylaxis when rectovaginal colonization by the pathogen is shown in the 35–37th weeks of pregnancy.[15] In some regions in Africa, *Klebsiella* spp. and *Salmonella* spp. are the most important pathogens.[13] For example, non-typhoidal *Salmonellae* accounted for 33% of cases of neonatal meningitis in Malawi.[16] The classical bacterial pathogens, *S. pneumoniae*, *H. influenzae* and *N. meningitidis* can also cause neonatal meningitis. Finally, in endemic areas unusual pathogens such as *Burkholderia pseudomallei* can be identified in neonatal meningitis.[17]

TABLE 27.1 Aetiology of Acute Meningitis

Purulent	Lymphocytic
NEONATAL	
Group B streptococcus	Herpes simplex virus
Listeria monocytogenes	Enteroviruses
Escherichia coli	Mumps virus
Klebsiella pneumoniae and other coliforms	
Salmonella spp.	
Pseudomonas aeruginosa	
Candida albicans	
OLDER INDIVIDUALS	
Neisseria meningitidis	*Mycobacterium tuberculosis*
Haemophilus influenzae	*Leptospira* spp.
Streptococcus pneumoniae	*Treponema pallidum*
Streptococcus suis	*Borrelia* spp.
Salmonella spp.	Enteroviruses
Listeria monocytogenes	Mumps virus
Burkholderia pseudomallei	Arthropod-borne Togaviruses
Naegleria fowleri	Adenovirus
Anaerobes, such as:	Lymphocytic choriomeningitis virus
Fusobacterium necrophorum	Human immunodeficiency virus

PATHOGENESIS

In cases of early-onset neonatal meningitis, the child becomes colonized by the pathogen during birth, which then translocates to produce bacteraemia. Bacteria can then cross the blood–brain barrier and cause meningitis. In cases where infection presents within the first 48 hours of life, the bacteria have been acquired from the birth canal or maternal perineum. Risk factors for infection in these children include premature rupture of membranes, maternal fever, positive vaginal group B streptococcus culture, prematurity, clinical asphyxia in the neonate, and an Apgar score of less than 3 at 1 min.[10] The premature neonate has defects in both humoral and cell-mediated immunity that predispose it to serious infection. For example, the neonate's phagocytes do not work efficiently and the activity of the complement cascade is only 50% of that of adults. At birth, the neonate's own IgM production is 20% of adult levels, of IgG is 5% of adult levels and IgA production begins at birth. Thus, the neonate also has defects in humoral immunity, and especially in the tropics where placental malaria, HIV-infection and maternal hypergammaglobulinaemia independently impair transplacental transfer of antibodies.[18]

CLINICAL FEATURES

The early signs of meningitis in premature neonates are often indistinguishable from those of septicaemia. The signs of septicaemia in premature neonates are not specific to infections; for example, in one series of 139 episodes of septicaemia, fever was present in only six episodes.[6] Signs that suggest neonatal meningitis, such as bulging fontanelle, stiff neck, convulsions of opisthotonos, are uncommon. For example, 17% of neonates with meningitis present with a bulging fontanelle, 33% with opisthotonos, 23% with neck stiffness and 12% with convulsions.[19–23] Thus to diagnose neonatal meningitis will require a high index of suspicion and part of the investigation of suspected neonatal septicaemia should include examination and culture of cerebrospinal fluid (CSF).

TABLE 27.2 Aetiology of Chronic Meningitis

Bacteria	Fungi	Parasites
Mycobacterium tuberculosis	*Cryptococcus neoformans*	*Toxoplasma gondii*
Brucella spp.	*Histoplasma capsulatum*	Cysticercosis
Treponema pallidum	*Coccidioides immitis*	
Borrelia burgdorferi	*Candida albicans*	
Neisseria meningitidis	*Actinomyces israelii*	

DIAGNOSIS

Clinical scoring methods have been devised to predict neonatal sepsis including meningitis in newborns in developing countries but their sensitivity and specificities are not ideal.[24] CSF examination can provide the definitive diagnosis by lumbar or ventricular puncture and is essential in the diagnostic work-up of a neonate with suspected meningitis. However, negative results do not rule out neonatal meningitis.[19] In a cohort study of 9111 neonates at an estimated gestational age of ≥34 weeks, 10% of the 95 neonates with culture-proven meningitis had fewer than three leukocytes per mm^3 in the CSF.[19] The median CSF leukocyte count was low (six cells per mm^3; range, 0–90 000). For culture-proven meningitis, CSF white blood cell (WBC) counts of more than 21 cells per mm^3 had a sensitivity of 79% and a specificity of 81%. CSF glucose concentrations varied from 0 to 11 mmol/L or 0–198 mg/dL (median, 1.1 mmol/L or 20 mg/dL), and protein concentrations varied from 0.4 to 19.6 g/L (median, 2.7 g/L); culture-proven meningitis was not diagnosed accurately by CSF glucose or by protein.[19] Gram staining of CSF can be helpful in the diagnosis of neonatal meningitis, but a negative CSF Gram stain does not rule out the disease. One review reported a sensitivity of 60% for Gram staining for showing bacteria in the CSF of neonates.[25] Latex agglutination is a diagnostic test that has been utilized for the aetiological diagnosis of bacterial meningitis, providing results in less than 15 minutes. Tests for detection of bacterial antigens are available for *S. agalactiae*, *S. pneumoniae*, *N. meningitidis*, *H. influenzae* and *E. coli*. Although the reported sensitivities are high, several studies showed that latex agglutination tests had no additional value next to standard tests.[1] Polymerase chain reaction (PCR) has proven its incremental value next to Gram stain and CSF culture in identifying the causative microorganism, especially in patients who received antibiotic treatment before lumbar puncture was performed.[1] Broad-range PCR can be used to detect the most common microorganisms in one test, and has been reported to have adequate sensitivity and excellent specificity, although this has not been validated for neonatal meningitis.[26–28] Although PCR techniques evolve rapidly, the availability is still limited, especially in developing countries. Culture remains the gold standard but will take up to several days to turn positive. It also has the advantage that it will provide information on the antimicrobial susceptibility of the pathogen.

MANAGEMENT

Neonates with meningitis may require elective ventilation and circulatory support but the mainstay of therapy is administration of antibiotics that achieve therapeutic levels in CSF (Tables

TABLE 27.3 Empiric Antibiotic Treatment for Bacterial Meningitis Based on Clinical Subgroup

Clinical Subgroup	Initial Therapy (Daily Dose [Dosing Interval])[a]	Predominant Bacteria
Neonates – early onset[b]	Ampicillin (150 mg/kg/day [8 hours]), plus gentamicin (5 mg/kg/day [12 hours]) or cefotaxime (100–150 mg/kg/day [8–12 hours])	*S. agalactiae, E. coli, L. monocytogenes*
Neonates – late onset[c]	Ampicillin (200 mg/kg/day [6–8 hours]), plus gentamicin (7.5 mg/kg/day [8 hours]) or cefotaxime (150–200 mg/kg/day [6–8 hours])	*L. monocytogenes, S. agalactiae,* Gram-negative bacilli
Infants, Children and Adults	Cefotaxime (8–12 g/day [4–6 hours] or ceftriaxone (4 g/day [12 hours]) plus ampicillin (12 g/day [4 hours]) plus vancomycin (30–60 mg/kg/day [8–12 hours])[d]	*S. pneumoniae, N. meningitidis*
Elderly and Immunocompromised	Cefotaxime (8–12 g/day [4–6 hours]) or ceftriaxone (4 g/day [12 hours]) plus ampicillin (12 g/day [4 hours]) plus vancomycin (30–60 mg/kg/day [8–12 hours])[d]	*S. pneumoniae, N. meningitidis, L. monocytogenes*

[a]Dosages recommended in patients with normal renal function.
[b]Within the 1st week of life.
[c]Between the 1st and 6th weeks of life.
[d]Vancomycin should be added in regions with cephalosporin resistance to pneumococci.
Adapted from Molyneux E, Nizami SQ, Saha S, et al. 5 versus 10 days of treatment with ceftriaxone for bacterial meningitis in children: a double-blind randomised equivalence study. Lancet 2011;377:1837–45.

27.3, 27.4). Because there is a large range of potential pathogens, initial antibiotic therapy must cover as wide a spectrum as possible. Guidelines advise empirical therapy for neonatal meningitis consisting of ampicillin, gentamicin and cefotaxime.[1,29] The use of gentamicin to cover neonatal meningitis due to Gram-negative bacteria has been debated, as CSF concentrations are usually only minimally above the MIC.[11,25] The general recommendation for the addition of gentamicin has been based on data from in vitro studies, which showed synergistic activity in antimicrobial killing.[11,25,29] After the pathogen has been identified and the antimicrobial susceptibility pattern has been established, the antibiotic regimen can be augmented (Table 27.5). Intrathecal administration of aminoglycoside in young children with Gram-negative meningitis results in high CSF concentrations,[30,31] but a study of intrathecal versus intravenous gentamicin in 117 infants with Gram-negative meningitis showed no clinical benefit.[32] Furthermore, a randomized controlled trial of intraventricular versus systemic gentamicin found a significantly higher mortality in the patients receiving intraventricular therapy (43% versus 13%).[33] Instillation of gentamicin directly into the ventricles is therefore not recommended for therapy of neonatal bacterial meningitis. One non-randomized clinical trial evaluated the effect of adjunctive dexamethasone in neonatal meningitis and did not identify a clinical benefit.[34,35] Corticosteroids do not have a role in managing neonatal meningitis.

TABLE 27.4 Penetration of Antibiotics Into Cerebrospinal Fluid

Antibiotic	Serum Level in CSF (%)	Therapeutic Level
PENICILLINS		
Penicillin	2–6	+
Ampicillin	10	+
CEPHALOSPORINS		
Cephalothin	1–5	±
Cefuroxime	5–10	+
Cefotaxime	10–25	+
Ceftazidime	20	+
Ceftriaxone	5–10	+
AMINOGLYCOSIDES		
Gentamicin	10–30	–
Netilmicin	20–25	–
OTHERS		
Sulphadiazine	50–80	+
Sulfamethoxazole	25–30	±
Trimethoprim	30–50	+[a]
Tetracycline	25	+
Chloramphenicol	90	+
Ciprofloxacin	5–20	+[b]

[a]Not effective against *N. meningitides*.
[b]Not effective against *S. pneumoniae*.

PROGNOSIS

The prognosis of neonatal meningitis is generally poor. Most of the 5 million neonatal deaths each year are in developing countries and over 40% of these result from sepsis.[24] A meta-analysis of studies on neonatal meningitis showed that mortality from neonatal meningitis in developing countries is estimated to be 40–58%, against 10% in developed countries.[13] The mortality rates associated with neonatal meningitis vary according to the gestational age. Thus, meningitis in neonates of extremely low birth weight (<1000 g) is associated with mortality rates of up to 80%, and that in neonates of very low birth weight (<1500 g) is 10–20% in developed countries.[36] In less well developed countries, the mortality rates vary with gestational age from 46% to 90%.[20–22] Another important risk factor for poor outcome is infection caused by Gram-negative organisms.[5,11,37] Acute complications include hydrocephalus, subdural effusions, deafness and blindness. Ventriculitis complicates Gram-negative bacillary meningitis in particular (70% of cases) and can make therapy very difficult. Outcome in survivors of neonatal meningitis has not been extensively studied in developing countries. In the UK, a follow-up study of 1584 children showed that 5% had severe neuromotor disabilities 5 years after neonatal meningitis.[38] Hearing difficulties occurred in 25%, behavioural problems in 12% and speech and language problems in 16%.[38] A recent study from Senegal in 65 surviving children that suffered from bacterial meningitis in the first 3 years of life showed that 70% suffered from major sequelae: almost half had problems with activities of daily living and were not attending school.[39]

TABLE 27.5 Specific Antibiotic Therapy for Bacterial Meningitis Based on Causative Microorganism

Microorganism	Standard Therapy	Alternative Therapies
HAEMOPHILUS INFLUENZAE		
β-Lactamase negative	Ampicillin	Cefotaxime; ceftriaxone; cefepime; chloramphenicol; aztreonam; fluoroquinolone
β-Lactamase positive	Cefotaxime or ceftriaxone	Cefepime; chloramphenicol; aztreonam; fluoroquinolone
β-Lactamase negative amoxicillin resistant (BLNAR)	Cefotaxime or ceftriaxone plus meropenem	Cefotaxime or ceftriaxone plus fluoroquinolone
NEISSERIA MENINGITIDIS		
Penicillin MIC <0.1 μg/mL	Penicillin G or ampicillin	Cefotaxime or ceftriaxone; chloramphenicol
Penicillin MIC 0.1–1.0 μg/mL	Cefotaxime or ceftriaxone	Chloramphenicol; fluoroquinolone; meropenem
STREPTOCOCCUS PNEUMONIAE		
Penicillin MIC <0.1 μg/mL	Penicillin G or ampicillin	Cefotaxime or ceftriaxone
Penicillin MIC 0.1–1.0 μg/mL	Cefotaxime or ceftriaxone	Meropenem; cefepime
Penicillin MIC ≥2.0 μg/mL; or cefotaxime or ceftriaxone MIC >1.0 mg/mL	Vancomycin plus cefotaxime or ceftriaxone	Cefotaxime or ceftriaxone plus moxifloxacin

Adapted from Brouwer MC, Tunkel AR, van de Beek D. Epidemiology, diagnosis, and antimicrobial treatment of acute bacterial meningitis. Clin Microbiol Rev 2010;23:467–92 and Tunkel AR, Hartman BJ, Kaplan SL, et al. Practice guidelines for the management of bacterial meningitis. Clin Infect Dis 2004;39:1267–84. With permission of Oxford University Press.

PREVENTION

Prevention of neonatal meningitis can be difficult, first because so many different pathogens may be involved and second, the premature neonate is an immunocompromised host. For prevention of *S. agalactiae* sepsis, two strategies have been investigated. Given the factors that increase the risk of early-onset group B streptococcal disease, several studies demonstrated that the intravenous or intramuscular injection of antimicrobial agents in colonized women is highly effective in reducing neonatal colonization with group B streptococcus.[40] Current CDC guidelines recommend the universal screening of all pregnant women for rectovaginal colonization at 35–37 weeks' gestation and the administration of antimicrobial prophylaxis to carriers.[41] One study demonstrated that the prevalence of early-onset group B streptococcal disease decreased from two cases per 1000 live births in 1990 to 0.3 cases per 1000 live births in 2004, following the institution of these recommendations.[42] Since screening efforts were instituted in the 1990s, the USA has experienced an 80% reduction in early-onset group B streptococcal disease.[14,15] This approach however does not work for other pathogens and will be difficult to implement in developing countries. A second strategy for prevention of neonatal meningitis is vaginal irrigation with chlorhexidine prior to delivery, which has been shown to decrease the incidence of neonatal group B streptococcal sepsis in Sweden and in Malawi.[43,44] In the Malawi study, 6968 women giving birth to 7160 babies received either manual cleansing of the birth canal with chlorhexidine or no intervention. Infants born to mothers that received the intervention were less likely to be admitted for neonatal sepsis (7.8 vs 17.9 per 1000 live births, $p<0.001$), had a lower overall mortality rate (28.6 vs 36.9 per 1000 live births, $p<0.06$), and were less likely to die from infectious causes (2.4 vs 7.3 per 1000 live births, $p<0.005$).[44] A recent randomized controlled trial in South Africa however, did not show a beneficial effect.[45] Further studies of this intervention in different settings are needed before definitive conclusions can be drawn on its use.

Non-neonatal Meningitis

Outside the neonatal period *N. meningitidis* and *S. pneumoniae* are responsible for 85% of cases of acute bacterial meningitis.[2,3,46,47] The remaining cases are due to a variety of bacteria, including: *L. monocytogenes*, *H. influenzae*, and both *Salmonella typhi* and non-typhoidal *Salmonellae*. In areas with a high rate of HIV infection, *S. pneumoniae* causes most cases but meningitis due to *Salmonella* spp. also frequently occurs.

GEOGRAPHICAL ASPECTS

Acute bacterial meningitis is found throughout the world but the relative contribution of the main pathogens varies considerably. The reasons for this variation are not completely understood. The reported incidence of bacterial meningitis in Europe and the USA is reported to be 1.4–2.6 per 100 000 population per year.[2,48] In the meningitis belt of sub-Saharan Africa (Figure 27.1), epidemics of meningococcal meningitis can occur with 2-14-year cycles. During epidemics, the incidence rises to over 400 cases/100 000 population per year but even between epidemics, the endemic rate is often over 50 cases/100 000 per year.[49] These cases are most often due to group A meningococci. Occasionally, group C meningococci can cause epidemics but more recently groups W135, X and Y have emerged in various countries in the belt.[50] The meningitis belt currently includes Tunisia and Algeria to the north and Somalia, Kenya, Tanzania, Zambia, Uganda and Rwanda to the east and south.[4] Over the last 20 years, epidemics have also been reported from Angola, Namibia, Mozambique, the south of the Democratic Republic of Congo (DRC: previously Zaire) and Botswana (Figure 27.2). A common feature for the occurrence of epidemics is the 300–1100 mm mean annual rainfall isohyets. Thus, climatic changes may govern the distribution of the meningitis belt. In contrast, in certain parts of Africa such as in the Congo basin of DRC[51–54] and in temperate industrialized countries epidemics with group A meningococci are rarely reported. In low-lying regions such as DRC pneumococci are the major meningeal pathogens in all

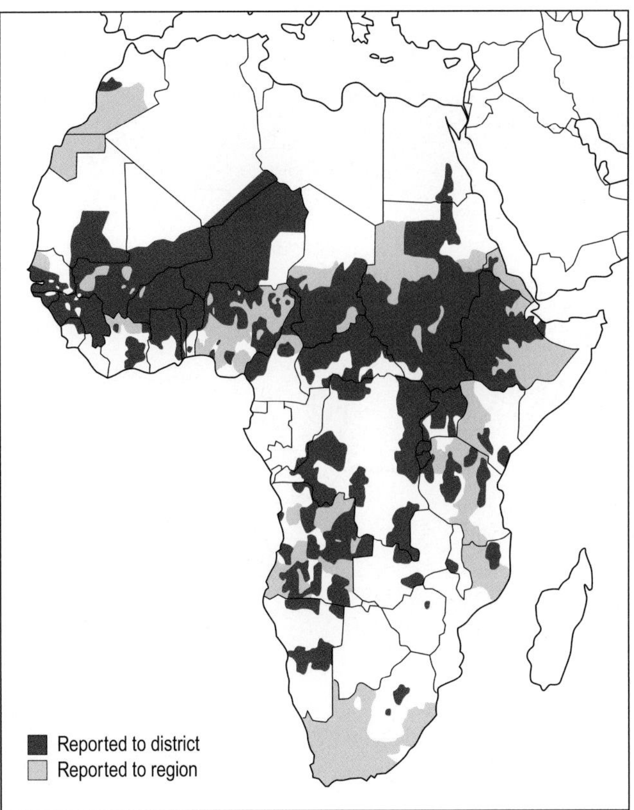

Figure 27.1 'The classical meningitis belt' of sub-Saharan Africa where epidemics occur in 2–14 year cycles and the districts affected by epidemics in the twentieth century.

age groups. *H. influenzae* is responsible for cases of meningitis in children under 5 years old in all regions of the world where the conjugate vaccine is not routinely used.[55] *N. meningitidis* is able to produce epidemics spreading through many parts of the world.[49,56] For example, a clone of group A *N. meningitidis* (III-1) produced an epidemic of disease in China in the 1970s which spread to Nepal and India in 1982, causing an epidemic in 1983–1984. The same clone was responsible for epidemics in New Delhi (1985) and Pakistan (1985). It was then brought by *hadjis* to Mecca in 1987 (Figure 27.3). Clone III-1 was then disseminated throughout the world by *hadjis* returning home. In the African meningitis belt, it initiated a wave of epidemics in 1988 but in other areas such as Europe and USA, despite up to 11% of returning pilgrims being carriers, it rarely caused secondary cases. However, epidemics in 2004 and 2005 have been due to serogroup W135 and with this, secondary cases did occur when pilgrims returned to Europe.[57] Although in Africa, epidemic meningococcal disease occurs in the dry season this is not the sole determinant. Person-to-person spread of the meningococcus occurs as readily throughout the year and it is thought the seasonality of disease is related to increased invasiveness. This may reflect an effect of the dust storms, extreme dryness and heat on the host's mucosal defences.[4,49,56]

EPIDEMIOLOGY

Classically, *S. pneumoniae*, *N. meningitidis* and *H. influenzae* were the most important causative microorganisms in bacterial meningitis, but after the introduction of the *H. influenzae* type b vaccine, this pathogen has virtually disappeared from

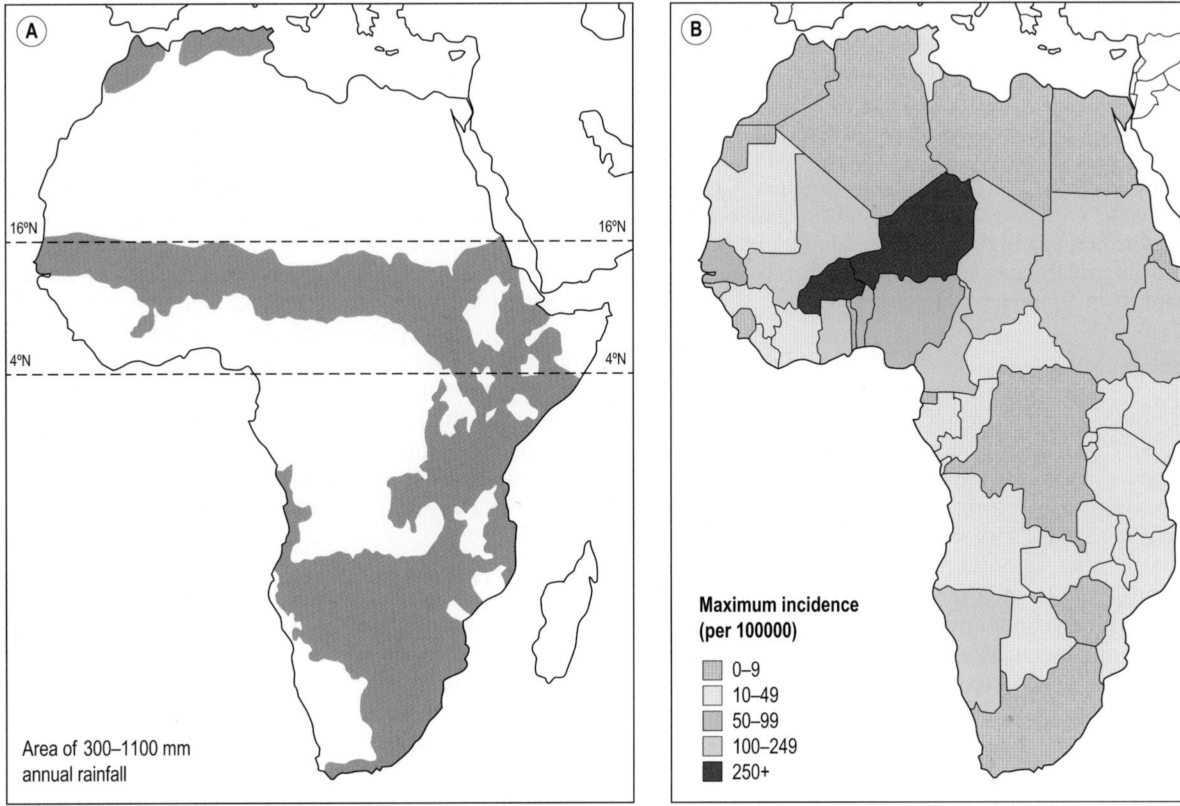

Figure 27.2 (A) Area of 300–1100 mm annual rainfall. (B) Maximum rates of meningococcal meningitis reported to WHO 1980–1999.

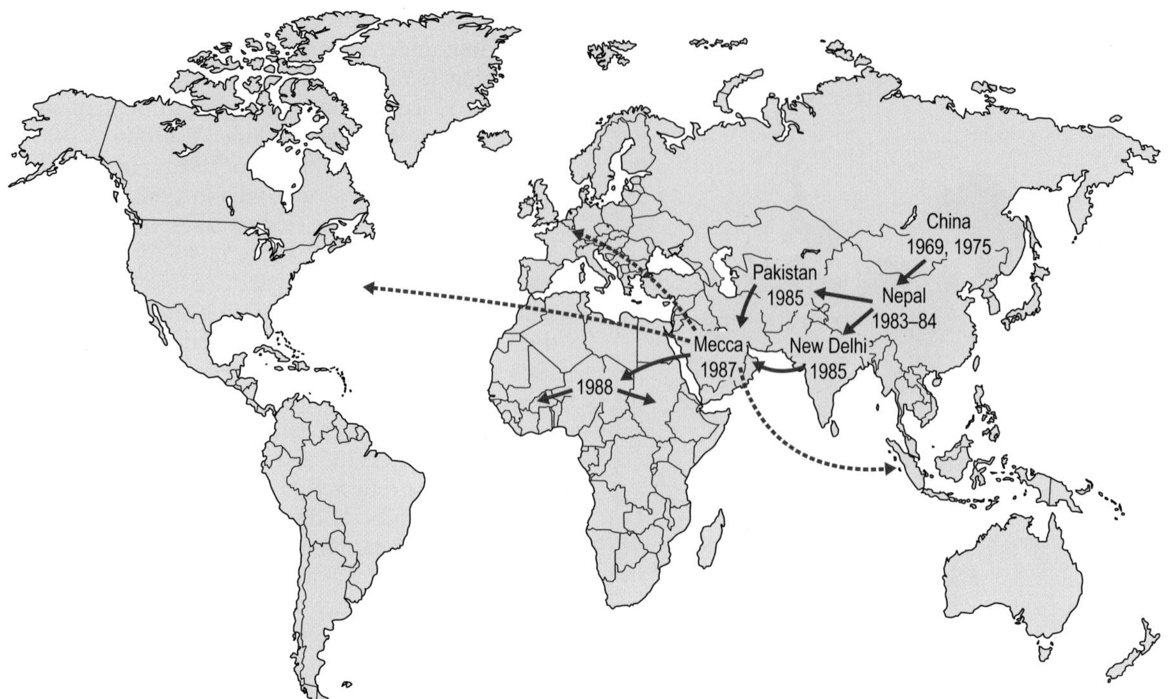

Figure 27.3 Intercontinental spread of clone III-1 of group A *N. meningitidis*.

countries where vaccination has been implemented.[1] Recent studies show that both in developed and developing countries in both adults and children beyond the neonatal age, the most common pathogen is *S. pneumoniae*.[3,58,59] Depending on the region and vaccination status *H. influenzae* type b and *N. meningitidis* are the second most commons cause. In southeast Asia, *Streptococcus suis* is an important cause of meningitis, that can be transmitted to from pigs to humans by close contact.[60,61] *L. monocytogenes* meningitis is mostly found in immunocompromised patients and the elderly.[62] The bacterium is principally spread by contaminated food and can cause small epidemics. Bacterial meningitis due to other *Streptococcus pyogenes*, *S. agalactiae*, *Staphylococcus aureus* and aerobic Gram-negative bacteria, such as *Klebsiella* spp. and *Acinetobacter baumannii*, occur infrequently and are usually associated with specific risk factors, such as endocarditis in *S. aureus* meningitis.[1]

PATHOGENESIS

Invasive disease by *S. pneumoniae* and *N. meningitidis* is preceded by nasopharyngeal colonization. Asymptomatic colonization of pneumococci and meningococci occurs in up to 100% and 18%, respectively, of the normal population.[63–65] There is evidence to suggest that the risk of disease is greatest in the period immediately after colonization. Bacteria in the nasopharynx then translocate to enter the circulation. The bacteria localize in the pia and arachnoid maters and cause an inflammatory response in the meninges and cerebrospinal fluid. The presence of capsule allows bacteria to survive longer in the circulation and meninges. Various components of the bacterial cell surface, such as teichoic acid in pneumococci, lipopolysaccharide (endotoxin) in meningococci and *H. influenzae* and peptidoglycan in all of them, induce secretion of a variety of factors such as tumour necrosis factor (TNF), interleukins 1 and 6 (IL-1, IL-6), eicosanoids and platelet activating factor (PAF). This results in potentiation of inflammation, further activation of neutrophils, further complement activation and increased permeability of the blood–brain barrier. This can then produce cerebral vessel thrombosis and vasculitis, cerebral oedema, intracranial hypertension and cerebral infarction. Finally, the activated neutrophils consume large amounts of glucose and oxygen and deprive neuronal tissues of these essential components, driving the brain into anaerobic respiration and production of lactate which is also neurotoxic.[66]

The risk of infection by pneumococci and meningococci after nasopharyngeal colonization has been associated with variation in the host genetic make-up. Patients with recurrent or familial meningitis or sepsis due to *S. pneumoniae* or *N. meningitidis* are often found to have rare mutations that cause a substantial increase in susceptibility to infection.[67] These mutations are mostly founding genes coding for the innate immune system (the complement system, and toll-like receptor signalling pathway).[67] A genome-wide association study has shown that genetic variation in complement factor H decreases the risk of meningococcal disease.[68] Genetic risk factors for increased susceptibility to bacterial meningitis have not been identified yet, but may present targets for new therapies.

PATHOLOGY

The pathological features of acute bacterial meningitis are similar for each of the pathogens. The principal feature is of a purulent exudate in the subarachnoid space which often damages the pia mater and the underlying superficial cortex. There is cerebral small vessel vasculitis and both arterial and venous thrombosis with neuronal damage and superficial encephalitis. There may also be damage to cranial and spinal nerves as they traverse the subarachnoid space.

CLINICAL FEATURES

Early diagnosis and rapid initiation of appropriate therapy are vital in the treatment of patients with bacterial meningitis. A systematic assessment of the sequence and development of early symptoms in children and adolescents with meningococcal disease (encompassing the spectrum of disease from sepsis to meningitis) before admission to the hospital showed that classic symptoms of rash, meningismus, and impaired consciousness develop late in the pre-hospital illness, if at all.[69] Early signs before admission in adolescents with meningococcal disease were leg pain and cold hands and feet.

Bacterial meningitis is often considered but may be difficult to recognize. The clinical presentation of a patient with bacterial meningitis may vary depending on age, underlying conditions and severity of illness. Clinical findings of meningitis in young children are often minimal and in childhood bacterial meningitis and in elderly patients' classical symptoms such as headache, fever, nuchal rigidity and altered mental status may be less common than in younger and middle-aged adults.[1,70] In a prospective study on adults with bacterial meningitis, the classic triad of signs and symptoms consisting of fever, nuchal rigidity and altered mental status was present in only 44% of the patients.[2] Certain clinical features may predict the bacterial cause of meningitis. Predisposing conditions like ear or sinus infections, pneumonia, immunocompromise, and dural fistulae are estimated to be present in 68–92% of adults with pneumococcal meningitis.[58,71] Rashes occur more frequently in patients with meningococcal meningitis, and have a reported sensitivity between 63–80% and specificity between 83–92%.[72]

Nuchal rigidity, Kernig's sign, and Brudzinski's sign were shown to have a low diagnostic sensitivity for the diagnosis of bacterial meningitis.[73,74]

DIFFERENTIAL DIAGNOSIS

Meningitis can be missed in its early stages, especially in children when there may be only subtle signs of meningism. It should be considered in any child with febrile convulsions or in patients suddenly becoming confused. Similar clinical features may be seen in cerebral malaria, typhus, relapsing fever and cerebral tumours. Viral, fungal or tuberculous meningitis may also present in a similar fashion. Examination of CSF will help to differentiate bacterial meningitis from the rest.

COMPLICATIONS

Bacterial meningitis is often complicated by neurologic and systemic complications, including cerebral infarctions, hydrocephalus, septic shock, multi-organ failure and respiratory failure.[2,75,76] Focal neurologic abnormalities occur in half of the episodes during admission and seizures are found in one in six episodes.[77] The high rate of complications results in substantial mortality rates. Recent data from randomized controlled trials in Malawi show mortality rates of 49% and 55% in adults in the placebo groups.[47,78] Mortality in children in the meningitis belt region is also high: 33–41% of children died in studies in Angola and ~30% of children died in a study in Malawi.[3,79,80] Risk factors for mortality were impaired consciousness, severe dyspnoea and seizures.[80] The mortality rates outside Africa are substantially lower: a study in Vietnamese adults showed a mortality rate of 10%, while studies from the Netherlands and the USA showed rates between 15% and 21%.[2,48,59] In a paediatric trial in several South-American countries, the mortality rate was 12%.

Hearing loss is the most important sequela of bacterial meningitis and occurs in 15–25% of children and adults with bacterial meningitis.[3,81–83] Long-term follow-up studies in developed countries have shown that neurocognitive defects frequently occur in survivors of bacterial meningitis. This results in learning disabilities in children and cognitive slowness in adults.[84,85] The rate of mortality and neurological sequelae differs per causative microorganisms. In general, pneumococcal meningitis has the highest mortality and risk of sequelae, while meningococcal meningitis has a low mortality.[2,59] *H. influenzae* has been known to cause a high rate of hearing loss in children.[83]

Meningococcal Disease

Although the mortality from meningococcal meningitis is relatively low, its mortality in the meningitis belt is higher during endemic periods and the early stages of an epidemic, with the lowest mortality occurring at the end of an epidemic. In addition, if infection is complicated by septicaemia it can prove rapidly fatal. The meningococcus continuously blebs off part of its outer membrane (Figure 27.4). Approximately 25% of the lipid in the outer membrane is lipo-oligosaccharide (LOS). This is a powerful endotoxin, and release of endotoxin produces activation of clotting and complement factors, activation of neutrophils and macrophages, with release of IL-1 (endogenous pyrogen), and TNF vasculitis. This can result in profound shock and bleeding from capillaries. On the skin this produces petechiae, purpura and ecchymoses which together with adrenal haemorrhage constitute the Waterhouse–Friderichsen syndrome. The onset of disease is sudden, with fever and progression through shock, purpura and coma, and death can be rapid (as fast as 2 hours). It is important to distinguish meningococcal meningitis from meningococcal meningitis with septicaemia or septicaemia alone,[86] since the management and progression of the two differ. The proportion of cases of meningococcal disease with a septicaemic component appears to be significantly lower in the meningitis belt. For example, only 4 of 112 (4%) cases of

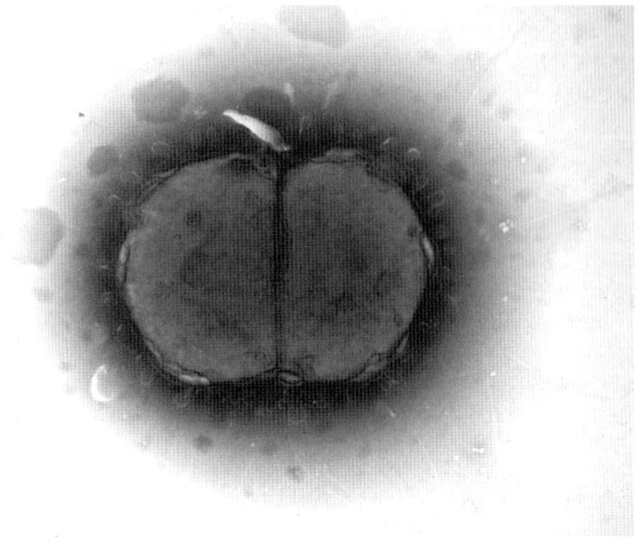

Figure 27.4 Transmission electron micrograph of *N. meningitidis* showing pili and loss of the outer membrane by 'blebbing'.

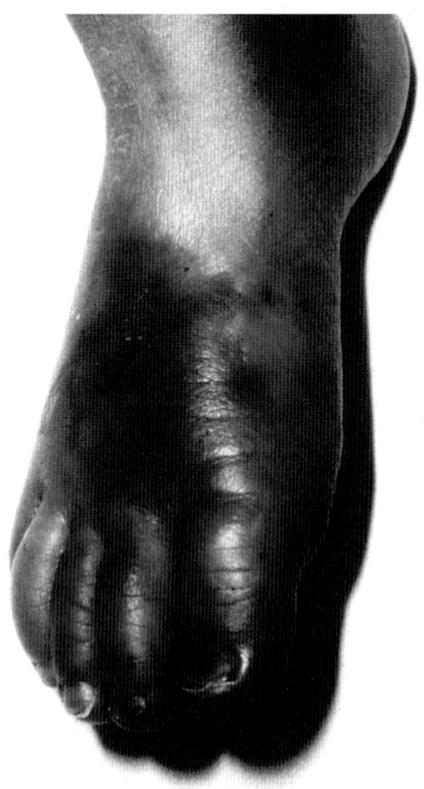

Figure 27.5 An African child with meningococcal septicaemia.

meningococcal disease had septicaemia in one study in Sudan[87] and only 11 cases of septicaemia out of 329 cases of meningococcal disease (3.3%) in Malawi.[4] A similarly low incidence of meningococcal septicaemia (5%) was observed in Nigeria.[88] By contrast, only 19% of cases of meningococcal disease on Merseyside had no septicaemic component and in tropical countries outside the African meningitis belt over two-thirds of cases have a septicaemic component at presentation.[86] Whether this difference represents a true difference in susceptibility to meningococcal septicaemia, or is a reflection of the difficulties of recognizing a petechial rash on dark skin (Figure 27.5), or patients in Africa with septicaemia are dying prior to reaching hospital, is unclear. However, the former seems more likely.[4] Complications of meningococcal septicaemia include gangrene of the skin and extremities and arthritis, which can be purulent or immunologically mediated.

DIAGNOSIS

The definitive diagnosis of bacterial meningitis depends upon examination of CSF (Table 27.6). The CSF is usually turbid due to the presence of large numbers of neutrophils and yellow due to high protein content. However, in early infection, low cell counts (<200/mm^3) may cause the CSF to appear clear. A high CSF neutrophil count and protein concentration and low CSF glucose reflect the extent of inflammation and indicate a poorer prognosis. A prediction model based on 422 patients with bacterial or viral meningitis showed that individual predictors of bacterial meningitis consisted of a glucose concentration of <0.34 g/L (1.9 mmol/L), a ratio of CSF glucose to blood glucose of <0.23, a protein concentration of >2.2 g/L, or a white cell count of >2000 cells/mm^3.[89] However, lower CSF protein (>0.5 g/L) and neutrophil count (>100/mm^3) thresholds are

TABLE 27.6 Cerebrospinal Fluid in Meningitis

	Normal	Bacterial Meningitis	Aseptic Meningitis
Volume (mL)	40–120	–	–
Appearance	Clear	Turbid	Clear to opalescent
Pressure (mmH_2O)	<180–200	Raised	Normal
Protein (g/L)	0.15–0.4	0.5–20.0	0.5–1.0[b]
Mononuclear cells (×10^6/L)	0–5	Can be raised	15–500
Neutrophils (×10^6/L)	0	100–200 000	<100
Glucose (mmol)[a]	2.2–3.3	0–2.2	2.2–3.3

[a]Must be compared with serum glucose concentration.
[b]In tuberculous meningitis, the CSF protein is usually high and glucose low.

also indicative of bacterial meningitis.[90] The majority of patients presenting with community-acquired bacterial meningitis have CSF parameters characteristic of bacterial meningitis.[1] However, low CSF white blood cell counts do occur, especially in patients with septic shock and systemic complications.[72,91] Experimental pneumococcal meningitis studies also showed a relationship between a large bacterial CSF load, a lack of response of CSF leukocytes, and intracranial complications,[92] probably indicating excessive bacterial growth and a lack of a CSF leukocyte response.

A specific aetiological diagnosis can be obtained rapidly by examining a Gram-stained smear of centrifuged CSF deposits. This will provide a specific diagnosis in 50–90% of cases, depending on the causative microorganism.[1] CSF culture will take 18–24 hours but has the advantage of being relatively cheap and providing data on the antimicrobial susceptibility of the bacterium. Blood culture, if facilities are available, is a useful adjunct to diagnosis and is positive in 40–80% of cases.[1] PCR was shown to be a valuable addition in the diagnosis of bacterial meningitis. The sensitivities of multiplex PCR for CSF from 409 bacterial meningitis patients in Burkina Faso (diagnosed by either CSF culture, latex agglutination test, PCR or Gram stain) were: 72% for *H. influenzae*; 61% for *S. pneumoniae*; and 88% for *N. meningitidis*, with specificities of 95%, 95% and 97%, respectively.[27] In this study, the incremental value of PCR next to culture, Gram stain and latex agglutination was high: 29 (43%) of 68 patients with *H. influenzae* meningitis; 43 (27%) of 162 with pneumococcal meningitis; and 66 (37%) of 179 with meningococcal meningitis were diagnosed with only PCR.[27] The availability of PCR is however limited.[82]

A study in Kenya estimated that the diagnosis of acute childhood bacterial meningitis is likely to be missed in about one-third of cases in the absence of adequate and reliable laboratory support.[93]

MANAGEMENT

Antibiotic Treatment

When bacterial meningitis is suspected, empirical treatment should be initiated as soon as possible, as early antibiotic treatment has been shown to improve outcome in bacterial meningitis (Table 27.3).[94,95] The regimen of the empirical antibiotic treatment depends on local epidemiology (specifically the antibiotic resistance patterns of local causative microorganisms) and the patient's age and comorbid conditions.[1,29,96] The efficacy of antimicrobial chemotherapy depends upon the penetration of the antibiotic into CSF (Table 27.4) and the susceptibility of the infecting microorganism. Resistance to penicillin and 3rd generation cephalosporins in *S. pneumoniae* is an increasing problem in both the developed and developing world.[1] Chloramphenicol resistance is also a concern in developing countries, where chloramphenicol is often used as first-line therapy for patients with bacterial meningitis. Therefore, the recommended regimen for bacterial meningitis with unknown cause consists of vancomycin and a 3rd generation cephalosporin.[1,29,96] However, as vancomycin is expensive and rarely available in developing countries with, monotherapy with 3rd generation cephalosporins is currently the most common regimen in the regions.[82] Rifampicin has been suggested as an alternative when vancomycin is not available, but this drug is vital for tuberculosis treatment, and increased use of rifampicin in bacterial meningitis could result in rifampicin-resistant tuberculosis.[82] Therefore, widespread use of rifampicin is not recommended for bacterial meningitis. During epidemics of meningococcal meningitis, uncomplicated meningococcal disease can be treated effectively with one intramuscular dose of ceftriaxone or oily chloramphenicol.[97,98] However, the WHO recommends at least 5 days of therapy in non-epidemic situations, in patients who are younger than 24 months of age, or if fever, coma, or convulsions last for more than 24 hours.[98] When the causative microorganism has been identified, the antibiotic treatment can be augmented according to the susceptibility patterns (Table 27.5). If a cerebral abscess is suspected, antibiotic treatment should also cover anaerobes.

Adjunctive Therapies

The role of adjunctive therapy with dexamethasone has been debated. A European trial showed a beneficial effect on mortality in adults with bacterial meningitis, and meta-analysis showed a decreased risk of hearing loss in children with bacterial meningitis.[35,99] However, studies in Malawi, Vietnam and South America did not find a beneficial effect of dexamethasone, although the Vietnam trial did show benefit in patients with confirmed bacterial meningitis.[47,59,83,100] A recent Cochrane meta-analysis showed that in both children and adults, adjunctive dexamethasone is beneficial in high-income countries, but is ineffective in low-income countries.[35]

Adjunctive glycerol is a hyperosmolar agent used to decrease intracranial pressure, which has been evaluated in three trials on bacterial meningitis.[78,83,101] Trials in Finland and several South American countries showed potential benefit in children treated with glycerol.[83,101] A recent trial in adults performed in Malawi however, was stopped early because of increased mortality in patients treated with glycerol.[78] Therefore, currently glycerol can not be advised in the treatment of bacterial meningitis in adults. The evidence for standard treatment with glycerol in children is not strong enough and should first be studied in other populations. Adjunctive treatment with high-dose paracetamol has been studied in a randomized controlled trial in Angola, but did not show a beneficial effect.[79] In all, no adjunctive treatment has been shown to be effective in African countries so far.

CHEMOPROPHYLAXIS

Chemoprophylaxis is used to prevent secondary cases of meningococcal meningitis in household contacts of an index case. Most trials of chemoprophylaxis use eradication of nasopharyngeal carriage of meningococci as their endpoint and demonstrate benefit. It has been shown that 10% of patients presenting with meningococcal meningitis in Nigeria were secondary cases.[102] Two strategies have been employed. In the first, phenoxymethyl-penicillin or amoxicillin is given as pre-emptive therapy for 7 days. The rationale for this is that most secondary cases occur in the first week after contact.[103] This will not affect nasopharyngeal carriage nor will it prevent secondary cases after therapy has ceased. The second strategy aims to eradicate nasopharyngeal carriage. Antibiotics that are effective in eradicating susceptible nasopharyngeal meningococci include sulphadiazine, minocycline, rifampicin, ciprofloxacin or ceftriaxone.[104]

VACCINATION

The major decrease in burden of disease from bacterial meningitis has come from the introduction of vaccines against *H. influenzae* type b, *S. pneumoniae* and meningococci. The acidic capsular polysaccharides of each of the three bacteria are highly immunogenic and vaccines are available for all of them. The problem in using polysaccharide antigens is that they are T cell-independent antigens, which means that the antibody response is predominantly IgM and IgG2 and immunological memory is poor. Therefore, conjugated vaccines have been developed that result in a strong immunological response and memory.

H. influenzae

The capsular polysaccharide of *H. influenzae* (b) (Hib) is polyribitol phosphate. The problem of poor immunogenicity of the capsular antigen has been overcome by conjugating it to a diphtheria or tetanus toxoid protein. This significantly improves the quantity and duration of antibody response, even in those under 2 years old.[1] The Hib vaccine can be given together with the triple (diphtheria, pertussis, tetanus) vaccine with no deleterious effects. Routine immunization of infants in The Gambia with Hib conjugate vaccine reduced the annual incidence of Hib meningitis from over 200/100 000 children aged younger than 1 year (1990–1993) to 0/100 000 in 2002, and from 60 to 0 in children <5 years old. Currently, almost 90% of countries have introduced the *H. influenzae* type b vaccine (www.gavialliance.org), resulting in a >95% reduction of cases.[1,55]

The Hib vaccine was also found to eliminate oropharyngeal carriage and thus provides herd immunity.

S. pneumoniae

Studies demonstrated that of the serotypes isolated from the cerebrospinal fluid (CSF) of patients with pneumococcal meningitis, 74–90% represented serotypes contained in the 23-valent pneumococcal polysaccharide vaccine. This vaccine is recommended for the prevention of bacteraemic pneumococcal disease in certain high-risk groups (e.g. splenectomized patients), even though the efficacy of the vaccine in the prevention of pneumococcal meningitis has never been proven. It has been assumed that the overall efficacy against pneumococcal meningitis was about 50%.[105,106] Because children less than 2 years of age have the highest rate of invasive pneumococcal disease and the 23-valent vaccine has no proven efficacy in this age group, pneumococcal conjugate vaccines were developed in which capsular polysaccharides were conjugated to carrier proteins. An initial multicentre, controlled, double-blind study examined the efficacy of the heptavalent pneumococcal conjugate vaccine administered in 4 doses to 37 868 infants and children.[107] For fully vaccinated children, the overall efficacy was 97.4% for the prevention of invasive pneumococcal disease caused by pneumococcal serotypes in the vaccine. Introduction of the 7-valent vaccine resulted in the lower incidence of pneumococcal meningitis, from 1.13 cases to 0.79 cases per 100 000, but there was an increase in meningitis caused by serotypes (specifically 19A, 22F and 35B) not included in the vaccine.[108] The World Health Organization has recommended the inclusion of the heptavalent pneumococcal conjugate vaccine in national immunization programmes, but only 26 of 193 World Health Organization member states have introduced this vaccine into their national immunization programmes for children so far.[109] Countries that have introduced vaccination are primarily high-income countries with relatively few childhood deaths. There is a strong need for the development of immunization programmes in poor countries to reduce morbidity and mortality.[110] Surveillance studies of serotypes causing invasive pneumococcal disease in developing countries have also demonstrated that the current 7-valent pneumococcal vaccine would not cover all serotypes causing invasive disease and have suggested that wider coverage would be provided by the 10-valent or 13-valent pneumococcal conjugate vaccines.[1] The introduction of these vaccines into these vulnerable populations is a crucial, but expensive, step to reduce the burden of bacterial meningitis. A step forward has recently been made in Rwanda and The Gambia, where the 7-valent pneumococcal vaccine was introduced into the childhood immunization schedule.[111,112]

N. meningitidis

As a result of the success of conjugate vaccines against invasive disease caused by *H. influenzae* type b and *S. pneumoniae*, conjugate vaccines against specific serogroups of *N. meningitidis* were developed. Implementation of monovalent serogroup C meningococcal conjugate vaccine in the UK resulted in a decrease in incidence by more than 90%, while carriage was reduced by 66%.[113–115] A quadrivalent meningococcal conjugate vaccine containing serogroups A, C, Y, and W-135 was recommended in the USA for all persons aged 11–18 years.[1] Further surveillance data are needed, however, to determine the effectiveness of these vaccines in preventing meningococcal meningitis. A monovalent vaccine against serogroup A meningococci, which causes most cases in the meningitis belt will be introduced in African countries in the coming years.[115] The group B meningococcal capsule is a homopolymer of N-acetylneuraminic acid and is a self-antigen found on human neuronal glycoproteins and glycolipids. Therefore, there is no group B capsular vaccine. By using genomic material from the serogroup B meningococcus, a combination of immunogenic meningococcal genes was combined in a multicomponent group B meningococcal vaccine. This vaccine was recently shown to result in adequate serum bactericidal activity in a phase 2b/3 trial performed in Chile.[116] Further clinical studies are needed to prove the vaccines efficacy before it can be recommended for routine use.

REFERENCES

1. Brouwer MC, Tunkel AR, van de Beek D. Epidemiology, diagnosis, and antimicrobial treatment of acute bacterial meningitis. Clin Microbiol Rev 2010;23:467–92.
5. Saez-Llorens X, McCracken GH Jr. Bacterial meningitis in children. Lancet 2003;361:2139–48.
48. Thigpen MC, Whitney CG, Messonnier NE, et al. Bacterial meningitis in the United States, 1998–2007. N Engl J Med 2011;364:2016–25.
82. Scarborough M, Thwaites GE. The diagnosis and management of acute bacterial meningitis in resource-poor settings. Lancet Neurol 2008; 7:637–48.
96. van de Beek D, de Gans J, Tunkel AR, et al. Community-acquired bacterial meningitis in adults. N Engl J Med 2006;354:44–53.

Access the complete references online at www.expertconsult.com

28

Brucellosis

NICK J. BEECHING | M. MONIR MADKOUR

KEY POINTS

- Brucellosis is a zoonosis. Elimination of human disease depends on the prevention and control of animal infections.
- In endemic settings, brucellosis typically affects rural pastoralist communities with inadequate access to healthcare and preventive education.
- There is often a history of illness in the family, occupational exposure or travel from an endemic area.
- The clinical features are protean, most commonly presenting as nonspecific fever, accompanied by musculoskeletal problems in almost half of patients.
- The most important differential diagnosis is tuberculosis, especially in localized infections.
- The diagnosis should be confirmed by prolonged cultures (when available) of blood or other sterile fluids, e.g. joint aspirates or by serological tests.
- The microbiology laboratory should be warned if brucellosis is suspected, both to optimize testing strategies and to reduce the significant risk of laboratory-acquired infection.
- Treatment regimens should include at least two antimicrobial agents for 6 weeks minimum, in order to prevent relapse. Aminoglycoside-containing regimens are superior.
- More prolonged treatment with a triple antimicrobial combination may be required for complicated infections.

Introduction

Brucellosis is a systemic infection caused by intracellular bacteria of the genus *Brucella* transmitted from animals to humans (zoonosis). *Brucella* species are classified according to their preferred animal host, and four species, each comprising several biovars, are traditionally recognized in humans: *B. melitensis* (goats, sheep and camels), *B. abortus* (cattle), *B. suis* (pigs) and *B. canis* (dogs). There have been occasional human infections with novel species from marine mammals (*B. pinnipedialis*) and in association with prosthetic implants (*B. inopinata*).[1–3] The organisms may survive in unpasteurized white soft goat cheese for up to 8 weeks and die within 60–90 days in cheese that has undergone lactic acid fermentation. Freezing dairy products or meat does not destroy the organisms but they are killed by pasteurization and boiling. The organisms are shed in animal urine, stool and products of conception, and remain viable in soil for 40 days or more.

Epidemiology

The true global incidence of human brucellosis is difficult to determine. In many countries, brucellosis is not considered a notifiable disease; however, more than 500 000 new cases of brucellosis every year are reported to the World Health Organization.[2,4] In the USA, only 4–10% of cases are recognized, probably related to the illegal importation of unpasteurized dairy products. The distribution of brucellosis is worldwide, but there is a high prevalence in certain geographical areas in the Mediterranean region, Indian subcontinent, Mexico and Central and South America, with new foci being recognized in Asia and Polynesia.[3] *B. melitensis* is the most common cause of brucellosis in the world. Worldwide, the incidence of human and animal brucellosis is increasing while eradication of the disease in animals has been achieved in only 17 countries. Factors contributing to the rising incidence are the recent expansion of animal industries with a lack of scientific and modern methods of animal husbandry. Other factors include traditional eating habits, standards of personal and environmental hygiene, methods of processing milk and its products, and the rapid movement of animals, both locally and internationally. Control and eradication programmes in animals are expensive and difficult to implement.[5] With the ease of modern travel, patients may contract the disease while visiting endemic countries.

In endemic areas brucellosis affects predominantly male and younger age groups, and is typically a problem of rural pastoralists with poor access to healthcare. Late presentations and underdiagnosis are common due to lack of awareness and of diagnostic facilities.[6–8] Traditionally, farm animals considered as pets are kept in close proximity to humans, and childhood disease indicates its endemicity in the community (Figure 28.1). In countries where brucellosis is controlled in animals, human brucellosis is mostly an occupational disease (including hunting feral animals) or related to travel to or immigration from endemic areas.

Mode of Transmission

Ingestion of untreated dairy products, raw meat, liver or bone marrow is a common route of infection through the gastrointestinal tract. Inhalation of the organisms is the most frequent route as an occupational hazard among herdsmen, dairy-farm workers, workers in meat-processing factories and laboratory workers. Penetration by pieces of bone or intact or abraded skin is a route of infection among abattoir workers.

Accidental autoinoculation or conjunctival splashing of live brucella vaccine during animal vaccination is well recognized

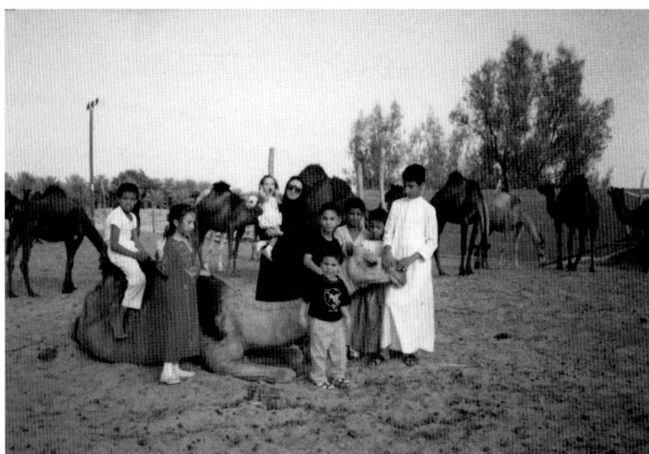

Figure 28.1 Animal contact. Children in endemic areas are seen playing with camels and in the backyards of houses.

among veterinarians. Transplacental transmission, transmission via breast-milk feeding, blood transfusion or marrow or organ transplantation, and sexual transmission are recognized in humans, although rare.

Microbiology

Brucella spp. are small, non-encapsulated, non-motile, non-spore-forming, Gram-negative, aerobic bacilli. The complete sequencing of the *B. abortus* genome was accomplished in 2001, followed by *B. melitensis* and *B. suis* in 2002, with rapid subsequent progress for other species.[9,10] Extended culture for up to 6 weeks using biphasic culture media (solid and liquid) or with the Castañeda bottle (incubated at 37°C with and without an atmosphere of carbon dioxide) are commonly used, as cultures are rarely positive before 7–10 days and may take several weeks. Automated culture systems (e.g. BACTEC) are more sensitive and usually positive within 7 days, but should be retained for 3 weeks. Bone marrow culture may rarely be required.[10] Identification of *Brucella* species and biotypes can be achieved by their taxonomic characteristics. The taxonomic characteristics of *Brucella* species and biovars are differentiated by their carbon dioxide requirements; ability to use glutamic acid, ornithine, lysine and ribose; hydrogen sulphide production; growth in the presence of thionine or basic fuchsin dyes; agglutination by antisera directed against certain lipopolysaccharide epitopes and by susceptibility to lysis by bacteriophage. PCR-based restriction fragment length polymorphism (PCR-RFLP) assay and 16S rRNA-based fluorescence in situ hybridization assay are tools for the molecular diagnosis and identification of *Brucella* species and biotypes.

Pathogenesis

The pathogenesis that is involved in the survival and replication of *Brucella* inside host macrophages remains relatively unknown. Significant advances have recently been made in understanding the mechanisms of *Brucella* intracellular survival, particularly in the field of the virulence factors. Full identification and characterization of the bacterial and host molecules involved in the biogenesis of the replicative vacuole and other factors has not yet been achieved.[11,12]

Immunity against *Brucella* infection involves antigen-specific T-cell activation and humoral responses. *Brucella* does not bear classic virulence factors and its lipopolysaccharide pathogenicity is not typical. The virulence factors implicated in the interaction between *Brucella* and the host have been identified. Recent genomic studies of *Brucella* have identified genes implicated in the virulence of the organisms that modify the processes of phagocytosis, phagolysosome fusion, cytokine secretion and apoptosis. One virulence factor of *Brucella* is an analogue of the Vir B system. It consists of a type IV secretion system potentially responsible for the injection of toxins into the cytoplasm of infected cells.[13]

Shortly after its entry through the mucosa, polymorphonuclear leukocytes and activated macrophages migrate to the site of access. The initial response is not antigen or organism specific and is therefore an innate immunity. It involves γδ T cell (Vγ9Vδ2), natural killer (NK) cell and CD4 and CD8 T-cell activation. Lipopolysaccharides on the surface of *Brucella* are recognized by these cells, which deliver signals to activate macrophages and facilitate phagocytosis of bacteria. Activated γδ T cells may provide the initial production of γ-interferon (IFNγ), TNF-α and other cytokines, which become cytotoxic for *Brucella*-infected monocytes and the bacteria, impairing their intracellular survival. The majority of brucellae are rapidly eliminated by phagolysosome fusion. Intracellular killing mechanisms in the macrophages are initiated with the help of cytokines secreted by T-helper cells. Macrophages activate the secretion of TNF-α which initiates a complex cascade of host defence mechanisms, leading to the production of hydrolytic enzymes and the peroxide-halide system. This mechanism is also known as 'oxidative-burst' or 'oxygen-based killing'.

The remaining bacteria survive in *Brucella*-containing compartments in which rapid acidification takes place. The *Brucellae* resist killing by oxidative-burst by using the myeloperoxide–hydrogen peroxide–halide system. Bacteria enter the macrophages through a particular structure found in the macrophage, lipid rafts or lipid microdomain. This is considered as the key for bacterial survival in infected macrophages. *Brucella* requires smooth lipopolysaccharides (S-LPS) to avoid the bactericidal arsenal of macrophages.

Reports indicate that an immune defect occurs during the invasive phase of infection. The disease is associated with an impaired Th1 immune response and defective T-cell proliferation, NK cell cytotoxic activity and IFNγ production. *Brucellae* were found to resist lysosome-mediated killing and phagosome acidification. Trafficking of the *Brucella*-containing phagosomes within macrophages and lack of fusion with the lysosome occurs but its mechanism is not yet understood.

Brucellae multiply in the endoplasmic reticulum of macrophages without affecting host cell integrity. The organisms are then released by induced cell necrosis and lysis. The virulence strategies of *Brucella* will determine the survival or death of infected macrophages. *Brucellae* protect infected cells from death by apoptosis in a mechanism that utilizes IFNγ or TNF-α. In the early stage of infection, *Brucellae* increase the activation of the cAMP/PKA pathway which regulates a variety of mechanisms that favour *Brucella* infection by preventing host cell elimination and rendering macrophages resistant to apoptosis.[14,15]

After entry to the human body and being taken by local tissue lymphocytes, *Brucellae* are later transferred through lymphatics to regional lymph nodes, then via the bloodstream to all organs of the body, particularly the reticuloendothelial system. The localization process of the organisms in body organs may be associated with inflammatory cellular infiltrates with or without granulomatous formation, caseation, necrosis or even abscess formation. Specific antibody production as a host response to *Brucella* occurs early after infection. In the first week of infection, IgM against lipopolysaccharide appears in the serum. One week later, IgG and IgA appear, and peak during the 4th week. The appearance of the anti-LPS antibodies plays a limited role in the host defence response against infection, yet it plays a very important role in the diagnosis of the disease.

Clinical Features

The incubation period of brucellosis is about 1–3 weeks but may extend up to several months.[7] Rarely brucellosis presents as a focal infection, years after exposure. Brucellosis is a disease of protean manifestations that may simulate other febrile illnesses. History of travel to endemic areas should be obtained, as well as the patient's occupational and recreational history. The onset of symptoms may be sudden (1–2 days) or gradual (1 week or more). Brucellosis presents as a febrile illness, with or without localization to particular body organs. *Brucella* infection is classified according to whether or not the disease is active (i.e. history, clinical features, and significantly raised *Brucella* agglutinins with or without positive blood cultures) and whether or not there is localized infection in body organs. Evidence of active disease and the presence of localization have a significant impact on the recommended treatment regimen and its duration. Classification of brucellosis as acute, subacute, chronic, serological, bacteraemic or mixed types serves no purpose in diagnosis and management. The term 'active brucellosis with/without localization' is recommended. The most frequent symptoms noted in the clinic of one of the authors (MM) are summarized in Table 28.1 and are mirrored in reports of *B. melitensis* infections in other countries.[7] The fever has no distinctive pattern that could differentiate it from other febrile illnesses. It usually shows diurnal variation, being normal in the morning and high in the afternoon and evening. Chills or rigors with profuse sweating may simulate malaria. Patients with brucellosis commonly look deceptively well and, less frequently, may look acutely ill, resembling enteric fever. If left untreated, the fever may 'undulate' over several weeks or more. Physical signs (Table 28.1) may be lacking despite the multiplicity of symptoms, but hepatosplenomegaly may occur in up to 25% of patients without other localized clinical features.

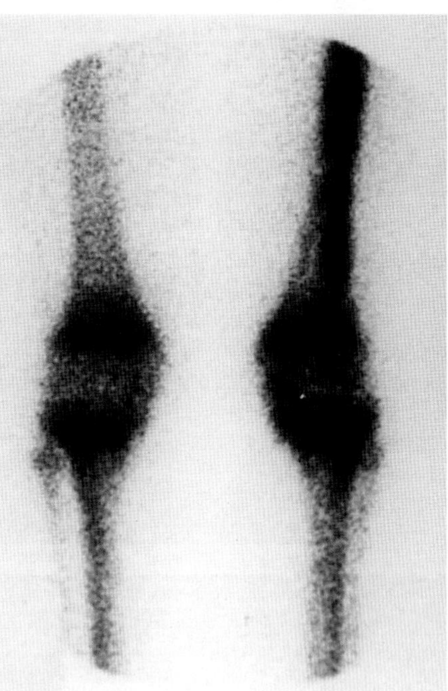

Figure 28.2 Brucellar arthritis and osteomyelitis. Scintigram showed increased uptake in the osseous components of the left knee and the distal half of the left femur.

TABLE 28.1 History, Symptoms and Signs in 500 Patients with *B. melitensis* Infection Who Attended the Clinic of One of the Authors (MM)

	n	(%)
HISTORY		
Animal contact	368	73.6
Raw milk/cheese ingestion	350	70
Raw liver ingestion	147	29.4
Family history	188	37.6
SYMPTOMS		
Fever	464	92.8
Chills	410	82.0
Sweating	437	87.4
Body aches	457	91.4
Lack of energy	473	94.6
Joint pain	431	86.2
Back pain	431	86.2
Headaches	403	80.6
Loss of appetite	388	77.6
Weight loss	326	65.2
Constipation	234	46.9
Abdominal pain	225	45.0
Diarrhoea	34	6.8
Cough	122	24.4
Testicular pain (of 290 males)	62	21.3
Skin rash	72	14.4
Sleep disturbances	185	37.0
SIGNS		
Ill-looking	127	25.4
Pallor	110	22.0
Lymphadenopathy	160	32.0
Splenomegaly	125	25.0
Hepatomegaly	97	19.4
Arthritis	202	40.4
Spinal tenderness	241	48.0
Epididymo-orchitis (of 290 males)	62	21.3
Skin rash	72	14.4
Jaundice	6	1.2
CNS abnormalities	20	4.0
Cardiac murmur	17	3.4
Pneumonia	7	1.4

Localizations

The most common localization is to the musculoskeletal system, in which case it must be distinguished from tuberculosis, as the latter is usually more destructive and requires appropriate therapy. Septic monoarthritis may occur as a result of haematogenous spread and localization of *Brucella* to the synovium or via direct extension from neighbouring brucellar osteomyelitis (Figure 28.2). Joints affected include the knee, hip,

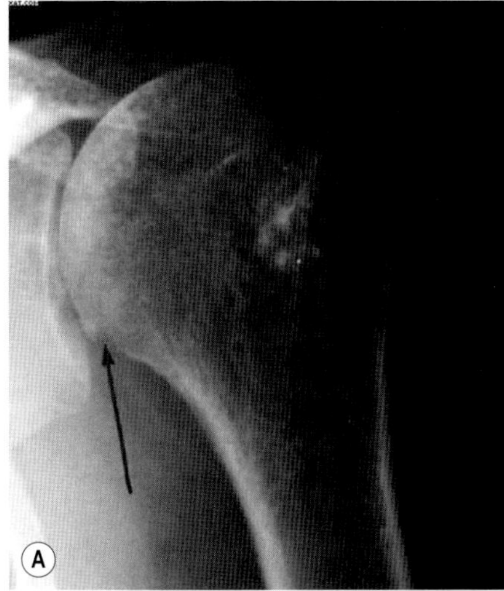

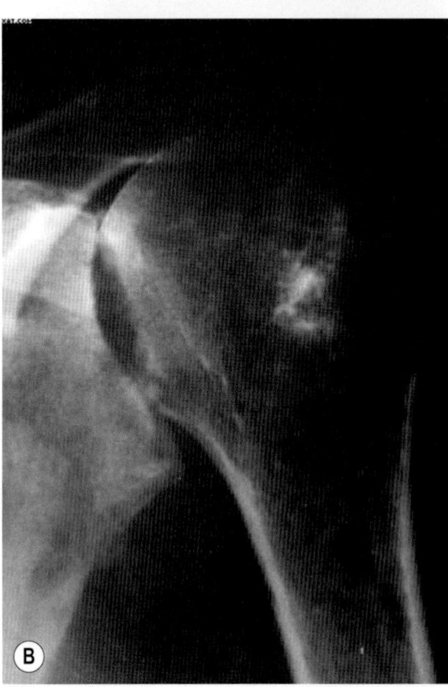

Figure 28.3 Destructive brucellar arthritis. (A) Frontal film of the shoulder joint showing diffuse cartilage loss in the glenohumeral joint. (B) Film taken 6 months later.

sternoclavicular, sacroiliac and shoulder or the sternum (Figures 28.3–28.6). Joint destruction with loss of function may occur if not diagnosed and treated early. In the spine, localization of infection starts at the superior end-plate anteriorly, an area of rich blood supply. The infection may either regress and heal or progress to involve the entire vertebra, intervertebral disc and adjacent vertebrae and rarely is associated with paravertebral abscess formation. Brucellar spondylitis may involve single or, less frequently, multiple sites, and rarely causes sufficient damage to compromise the spinal cord. The lumbar spine, particularly L4, is the most frequent site (Figure 28.7). Plain radiography may help to differentiate brucellar spondylitis from tuberculous spondylitis (Figure 28.8). Extraspinal brucellar osteomyelitis is rare and may affect the femur, tibia, humerus or the manubrium sterni (Figures 28.2 and 28.6). Bursitis, tenosynovitis and subcutaneous nodules may rarely occur. The

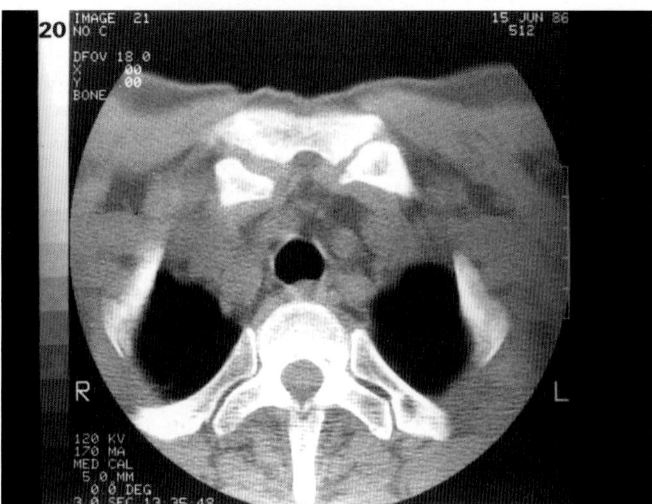

Figure 28.4 Destructive brucellar arthritis. High-resolution CT showing marked cartilage loss and sternoclavicular erosions in the left sternoclavicular joint.

peripheral white cell count is normal in brucellar septic arthritis and spondylitis. The total white cell count in the synovial fluid ranges from 400–40 000/mm^3 with 60% polymorphonuclear cells; glucose may be reduced and culture may be positive in about 50% of the cases.

Cardiovascular localization may include endocarditis, myocarditis, pericarditis, aortic root abscess (Figure 28.9), myotic aneurysms, thrombophlebitis and pulmonary embolism. Patients who live in endemic areas and have what has been labelled as 'culture-negative infective endocarditis' should have their blood culture extended for a period of up to 6 weeks. Respiratory symptoms are common, but, because they are usually mild, clinicians tend to overlook them. A "flu-like" illness with sore throat and mild dry cough is a common feature.

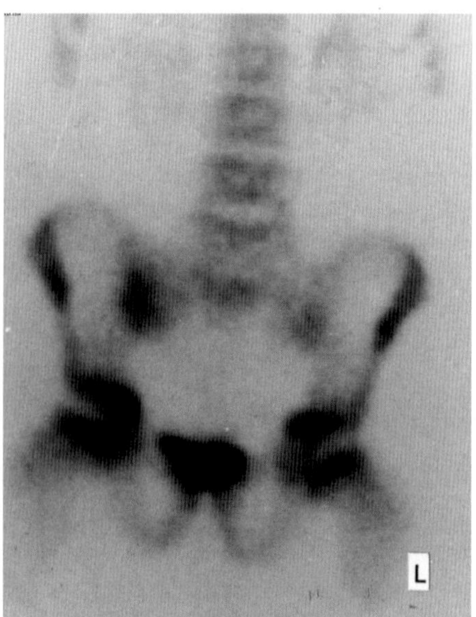

Figure 28.5 Brucellar sacroiliitis. There is increased uptake in the right sacroiliac joint which can be noted on the anterior view of the scintigram.

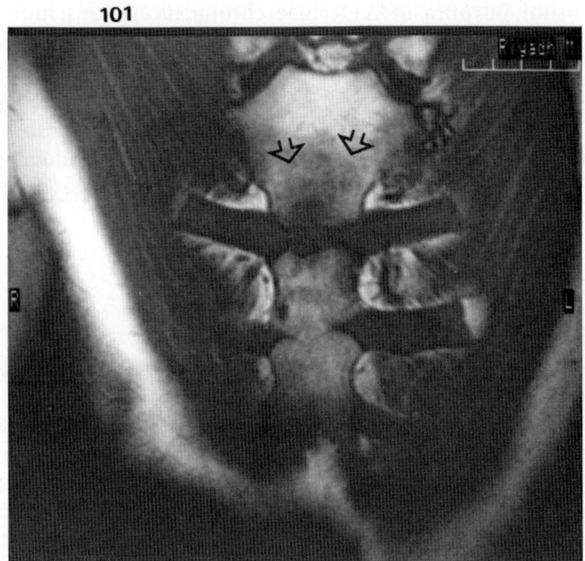

Figure 28.6 Brucellar osteomyelitis. MRI of the sternum, coronal cut, T1-weighted image, showing an area of patchy decreased signal intensity in the lower half of the manubrium.

Other rare foci of infection include hilar and paratracheal lymphadenopathy; pneumonia, with solitary or multiple nodular lung shadowing or even with abscess formation; soft tissue miliary shadowing; pleural effusion; empyema; and mediastinitis.

Gastrointestinal infections are usually mild and are rarely a presenting feature of the disease. They include tonsillitis, and hepatitis with mild jaundice (either nonspecific or granulomatous with suppuration and abscess formation). Splenic abscess formation is rare. Mesenteric lymphadenopathy with abscess formation, cholecystitis, peritonitis, pancreatitis and ulcerative colitis have been described. The liver transaminases, alkaline phosphatase, and serum bilirubin may be mildly raised.

Genitourinary localizations may be the presenting feature of brucellosis. The most common in both children and adults is unilateral or bilateral epididymo-orchitis, and may be confused with mumps or tuberculosis. Men can develop prostatitis and

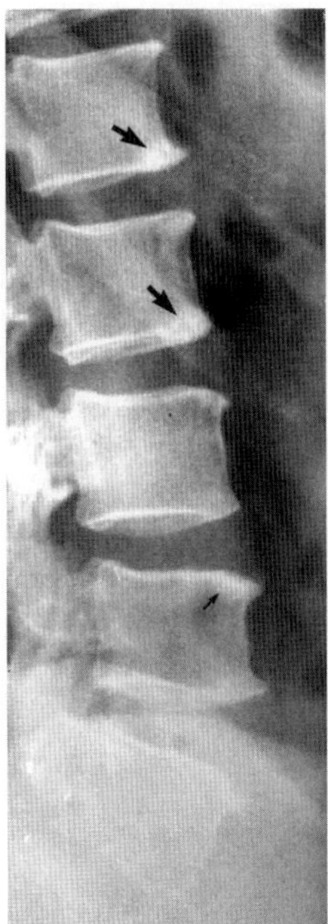

Figure 28.7 Early brucellar spondylitis. There is sclerosis at the anterior aspect of the superior end-plate of L4. Similar areas are seen in the inferior end-plates of L1 and L2. Note the normal disc spaces.

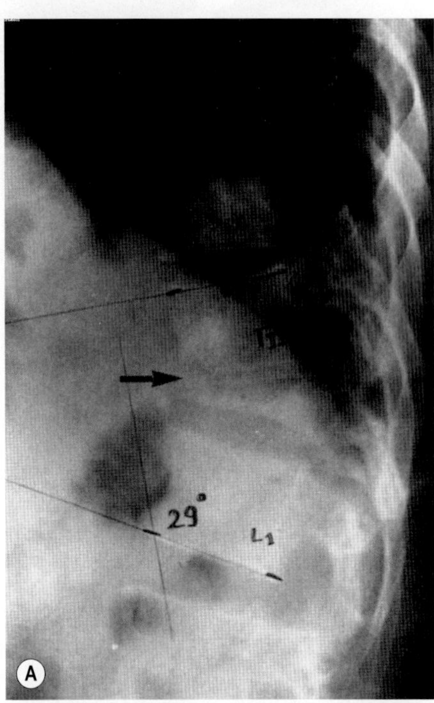

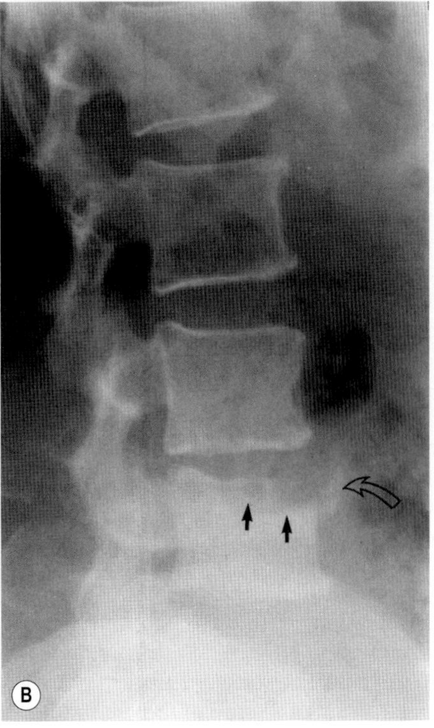

Figure 28.8 Comparative image features of plain radiography of tuberculous (A) and brucellar (B) spondylitis.

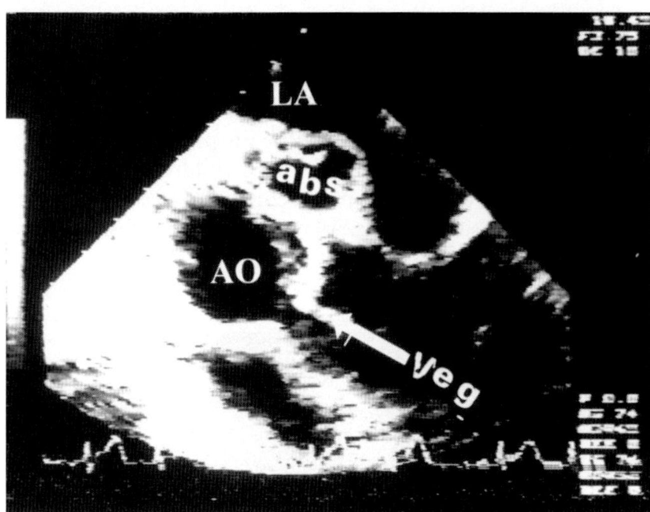

Figure 28.9 Brucellar aortic root abscess and aortic valve vegetation demonstrated in this horizontal transoesophageal endocardiography view.

seminal vesiculitis, and women dysmenorrhoea, amenorrhoea, tubo-ovarian abscesses, chronic salpingitis, and cervicitis. Acute nephritis or acute pyelonephritis-like features, renal calcifications, and calyceal deformities may occur. Renal granulomatous lesions with abscess formation, with caseation and necrosis may occur, as may cystitis and posterior urethritis.

Urine culture may be positive in about 50% of patients with brucellosis. *Brucella* organisms have been isolated from semen during investigation of possible sexual transmission. Granulomatous myositis and rhabdomyolysis may occur rarely.

Neurobrucellosis is uncommon but serious. It includes meningoencephalitis, multiple cerebral or cerebellar abscesses, ruptured mycotic aneurysm, cranial nerve lesions, transient ischaemic attacks, hemiplegia, myelitis, radiculoneuropathy and neuritis, Guillain–Barré syndrome, a multiple-sclerosis-like picture, paraplegia, and sciatica. Frank psychiatric features of brucellosis are probably no more frequent than those observed and caused by other infections. However, prolonged mild depression and lethargy have a significant adverse effect on productivity, and often only become apparent to the patient when they resolve after treatment. Neurobrucellosis may be caused by direct blood-borne invasion by *Brucella* organisms, pressure from destructive spinal lesions, vasculitis, or an immune-related process. In meningoencephalitis the cerebrospinal fluid (CSF) pressure is usually elevated and the fluid may look clear, turbid or, rarely, haemorrhagic; the protein content and number of cells (predominantly lymphocytes) are raised, while glucose may be reduced or normal. *Brucella* organisms may be cultured from CSF. *Brucella* agglutinins in CSF are usually raised but occasionally may not be detected.

In endemic areas, the outcome of pregnancy in humans is similar to that in animals; this includes normal delivery of healthy infants, abortion, intrauterine fetal death, premature delivery, or retention of the placenta and other products of conception, as well as transmission to infants through breast milk.[16,17] Skin manifestations are uncommon. They include maculopapular eruptions and contact dermatitis, particularly among veterinarians and farmers assisting animal parturition. Other dermatological manifestations include erythema nodosum, purpura and petechiae, chronic ulcerations, multiple cutaneous and subcutaneous abscesses, vasculitis, superficial thrombophlebitis and discharging sinuses. Direct splashing of live *Brucella* vaccine into the eyes may cause conjunctivitis. Keratitis, corneal ulcers, uveitis, retinopathies, subconjunctival and retinal haemorrhages, retinal detachment, and endogenous endophthalmitis with positive vitreous cultures are well documented.

Diagnosis

Definite diagnosis of brucellosis requires the isolation of the organism from the blood, body fluids or tissues, but serological methods may be the only tests available in many settings[7,10,18] Positive blood culture yield ranges between 40% and 70% and is less commonly positive for *B. abortus* than *B. melitensis* or *B. suis*. Identification of specific antibodies against bacterial lipopolysaccharide and other antigens can be detected by the standard agglutination test (SAT), rose Bengal, 2-mercaptoethanol (2-ME), antihuman globulin (Coombs') and indirect enzyme-linked immunosorbent assay (ELISA). SAT is the most commonly used serological test in endemic areas. An agglutination titre of ≥1 : 160 is considered significant in non-endemic areas and ≥1 : 320 in endemic areas.

Due to the similarity of the O. polysaccharide of *Brucella* to that of various other Gram-negative bacteria (e.g. *Francisella tularensis, E. coli, Salmonella* Urbana, *Yersinia enterocolitica, Vibrio cholerae, Stenotrophomonas maltophilia*) the appearance of cross-reactions of class M immunoglobulins may occur. The inability to diagnose *B. canis* by SAT due to lack of cross-reaction is another drawback. False-negative SAT may be caused by the presence of blocking antibodies (the prozone phenomenon) in the α2-globulin (IgA) and in the α-globulin (IgG) fractions. Dipstick assays are new and promising, based on the binding of *Brucella* IgM antibodies, and found to be simple, accurate and rapid. ELISA typically uses cytoplasmic proteins as antigens. It measures IgM, IgG and IgA with better sensitivity and specificity than the SAT in most recent comparative studies.[19] The commercial Brucellacapt test, a single-step immunocapture assay for the detection of total anti-*Brucella* antibodies, is an increasingly used adjunctive test when resources permit. PCR is fast and should be specific. Many varieties of PCR have been developed (e.g. nested PCR, real-time PCR and PCR-ELISA) and found to have superior specificity and sensitivity in detecting both primary infection and relapse after treatment.[20] Unfortunately, these have yet to be standardized for routine use, and some centres have reported persistent PCR positivity after clinically successful treatment, fuelling the controversy about the existence of prolonged chronic brucellosis.[21] Other laboratory findings include normal peripheral white cell count, and occasional leucopenia with relative lymphocytosis. The serum biochemical profiles are commonly normal.

Treatment

Treatment of brucellosis is still far from ideal, the major problem being identification of the most practical and affordable double or triple antimicrobial combination to prevent relapse, which is very common after treatment with single agents.[4] However, antimicrobial resistance is rarely a clinical problem, relapse usually being related to inadequate duration and/or combinations of therapy. There is still poor agreement about optimal regimens in many settings, current debates being well summarized in an expert Consensus statement[22] and two meta-analyses.[23,24]

Two classical regimens recommended by the WHO – a combination of doxycycline plus streptomycin (DS) or of doxycycline plus rifampicin (DR) – have been used all over the world, as out-patient management, for many years and have remained effective. As both streptomycin and rifampicin are active against *Mycobacterium tuberculosis*, tuberculosis must be excluded as the cause of the patient's illness before these agents are used. Regimens containing doxycycline are more efficient, with fewer therapeutic failures and relapses, than other regimens. Doxycycline (preferred to other tetracyclines) is the most effective agent for the treatment of brucellosis. Doxycycline has increased activity in the acidic environment of the phagolysosomes in the macrophages. The streptomycin-containing regimen is slightly more efficacious in preventing relapses, as rifampicin reduces doxycycline levels in the serum. Doxycycline is given in an oral dose of 100 mg 12-hourly for 6 weeks. Streptomycin is administered intramuscularly, in a single daily dose of 15 mg/kg for 2–3 weeks. Rifampicin is used in a single oral daily dose of 600–900 mg for 6 weeks. Patients with localizations such as spondylitis, endocarditis, neurobrucellosis and abscess formations in body organs may require hospitalization for possible surgery and triple antibiotics (doxycycline, aminoglycoside and rifampicin) should be used for a longer period of up to 6 months. Urgent valve replacement or drainage of abscesses may also be required with antibiotics. The overall therapeutic failure and relapse rates with DS and DR regimens range between 3% and 10% in research studies and may be double this in less controlled healthcare settings. The parenteral administration of aminoglycoside, nephrotoxicity and ototoxicity require adequate monitoring in the healthcare system. Monotherapy has been abandoned by most physicians because of the unacceptably high rates of therapeutic failure and relapses, although this view has been challenged recently.[24]

Alternative aminoglycoside-containing regimens have been used over the past 2 decades and are now preferred to streptomycin, with the additional advantage that they are not clinically active against *M. tuberculosis*. Both gentamicin and netilmicin have been used, administered intramuscularly or intravenously as a single daily dose of 5 mg/kg for 10–14 days, together with doxycycline 100 mg 12-hourly for 45 days. This combination of gentamicin plus doxycycline has been found to be as effective as the DS regimen. A longer duration of gentamicin plus doxycycline (GD) or netilmicin plus doxycycline (ND), for at least 14 days, followed by doxycycline alone for a further 30–60 days, is associated with less therapeutic failure and a lower relapse rate than a regimen containing aminoglycoside for only 7 days. Regimens comprising co-trimoxazole in an oral dose of 2 tablets (480 mg each), twice daily for 2 months plus doxycycline (CD) or plus rifampicin (CR), have been used. The efficacy of the CD regimen is better than that of the CR regimen.[25] In endemic areas, tuberculosis and/or leprosy may also be common and the use of rifampicin may be restricted to avoid the emergence of resistance.

Quinolones (ciprofloxacin or ofloxacin) have been used in several inadequately powered clinical studies in patients without disease localization, and the overall findings have been disappointing, with inferiority of combinations both to treat infection and to prevent relapse.[23] However, the conclusion that they should not be used in first-line regimens, despite their favourable side-effect profile, has been challenged in the more recent meta-analysis.[24] The antimicrobial activities of quinolones are decreased in the acidic environment of phagolysosomes in macrophages. Quinolones may have some role, particularly to replace doxycycline or rifampicin whenever toxicity occurs. They may be used in a second-line regimen for patients who fail to respond or, possibly, who develop relapse after using another regimen. Ofloxacin, in an oral dose of 400 mg 12-hourly, or ciprofloxacin, in an oral dose of 500 mg 12-hourly, can be used in combination with doxycycline or rifampicin for 6 weeks.[12]

Azithromycin is a macrolide (azalide subclass) rapidly distributed into tissue and cells, particularly phagocytes. The acidic phagolysosomal environment within macrophages attenuates its antibacterial activities. Results showed high rates of therapeutic failure and relapses when used in a regimen for *B. melitensis* infection. Children less than 8 years of age with brucellosis are treated with co-trimoxazole plus rifampicin (CR). Rifampicin can be given orally or intravenously as a single dose of 10–20 mg/kg per day. Co-trimoxazole is used as an intravenous infusion of 36–54 mg/kg per day in two divided doses. Paediatric suspension is used orally in a dose of 240 mg/mL 12-hourly. The optimum duration of therapy for children has not yet been established in comparative prospective trials.

Doxycycline is approved and used in the USA for the treatment of Rocky Mountain spotted fever in infants and young children. In Italy, infants and young children with brucellosis were treated with oral minocycline 2.5 mg/kg in combination with intravenous rifampicin 10 mg/kg (both given 12-hourly) for 3 weeks: this regimen did not cause dental defects and was found to be very effective.[26] Pregnant women with brucellosis are usually treated with co-trimoxazole plus rifampicin (CR).[16,17] Patients with renal impairment should be carefully monitored for serum urea, creatinine and aminoglycoside levels. If such facilities are not available, then the DR regimen should be utilized.

Monitoring of the response to treatment is based on improvement of symptoms (within 14 days) and signs (within 2–4 weeks) after commencing antibiotics. Therapeutic failure is considered if there is no clinical improvement 14 days after commencing antibiotics till the end of therapy. Serological follow-up tests are not the ideal tools for monitoring response to treatment. The titres may not decrease or may even rise further if the patient develops a Jarisch–Herxheimer reaction with initial worsening of symptoms a few days after starting treatment. In the first 3 months after completion of treatment, SAT may show a decrease in titre to less than 1:320 in only 8.3% of patients, and 28.6% of cured patients continue to have a titre of 1:320 or higher 2 years after completion of successful treatment. Patients receiving doxycycline in the treatment regimen are more likely to have serological cure than those not receiving such. Relapse is considered if clinical features recur and the agglutination titre rises with or without positive blood culture 1 year (usually in the first 3–6 months) after completion of treatment. In endemic areas, where the re-exposure risk is persistent, reinfections may be difficult to differentiate from relapses.

Some authors recommend screening all household members of a brucellosis patient, as other family members are often found to have undiagnosed infection which requires treatment.[27,28]

Prognosis and Prevention

The mortality of the disease in 1909, as recorded in the British Army and Navy stationed in Malta, was 2%. The most frequent cause of death was endocarditis. Recent advances in antibiotics and surgery have been successful in preventing death due to endocarditis.

Prevention of human brucellosis can be achieved by eradication of the disease in animals by vaccination and other veterinary control methods such as testing herds/flocks and slaughtering animals when infection is present. This requires prolonged commitment and financial support at the highest levels of government, with strong cooperation between both animal and public health authorities. Currently, no effective vaccine is available for humans.

Boiling milk before consumption or using it to produce other dairy products is protective against transmission via ingestion. Changing traditional food habits of eating raw meat, liver or bone marrow is necessary but difficult to implement. Patients who have had brucellosis should probably be excluded indefinitely from donating blood or organs.

Exposure of diagnostic laboratory personnel to *Brucella* organisms remains a problem in both endemic settings and when brucellosis is unknowingly imported by a patient.[29] After appropriate risk assessment, staff with significant exposure should be offered post-exposure prophylaxis (PEP) and followed up serologically for 6 months.[30] Recent published experience confirms that prolonged and frequent serological follow-up consumes significant resources without yielding much information, and is burdensome for the affected staff, who often fail to comply.[31] The side-effects of the usual recommended regimen of rifampicin and doxycycline for 3 weeks also reduce treatment adherence. As there is no evidence that PEP with two drugs is superior to monotherapy, British guidelines now recommend PEP with doxycycline alone for 3 weeks and a less onerous follow-up protocol.

REFERENCES

3. Pappas G. The changing *Brucella* ecology: novel reservoirs, new threats. Int J Antimicrob Agents 2010;36(Suppl 1):S8–S11.
7. Franco MP, Mulder M, Gilman RH, et al. Human brucellosis. Lancet Infect Dis 2007;7:775–86.
10. Al Dahouk S, Nöckler K. Implications of laboratory diagnosis on brucellosis therapy. Expert Rev Anti Infect Ther 2011;9:833–45.
23. Skalsky K, Yahav D, Biishara J, et al. Treatment of human brucellosis: systematic review and meta-analysis of of randomised controlled trials. BMJ 2008;336:701–4.
31. Sam C, Karunakaran R, Kamarulzaman A, et al. A large exposure to *Brucella melitensis* in a diagnostic laboratory. J Hosp Infect 2012; 80:321–5.

Access the complete references online at www.expertconsult.com

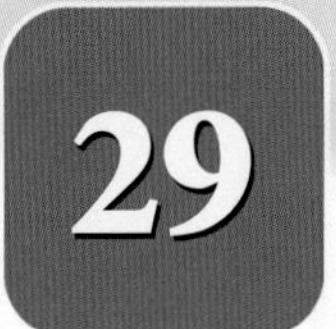

Noma, Actinomycosis and Nocardia

M. LEILA SROUR | VANESSA WONG | SARAH WYLLIE

KEY POINTS

Noma

- Noma is an opportunistic infection of unclear aetiology, causing devastating orofacial gangrene, afflicting primarily malnourished children living in poor rural villages.
- Noma is a neglected disease, under-reported and unknown by most health workers.
- Acute noma has an untreated mortality rate of ~70–90%, with the majority of patients having no access to treatment.
- Noma survivors suffer from disfigurement, functional impairment and disabling social stigma.[1–3]
- Noma is an indicator of extreme poverty and severely inadequate public health systems.[2,4]
- Noma is called 'The Face of Poverty', because the disease primarily occurs in extremely poor communities and the survivors are often severely disfigured.[2]
- *Noma*, also known as *cancrum oris*, originates from the Greek word 'to devour' or 'graze'.

Actinomycosis

- Actinomycosis is a rare, chronic, slowly progressive disease caused by filamentous Gram-positive anaerobic bacteria from the *Actinomycetaceae* family.
- Actinomyces are commensals that normally reside in the oropharynx, gastrointestinal tract and urogenital tract and can become pathogenic when the mucosa is breached.
- The disease is classified by anatomical location with oro-cervicofacial disease being the most common, followed by thoracic and abdominopelvic.
- It generally presents with a densely fibrotic 'wooden' mass that spreads unhindered by tissue fascial planes, invades local structures and can lead to the formation of sinus tracts, which may spontaneously heal and recur.
- The infection can mimic other conditions including malignancy and tuberculosis.
- Treatment is normally with long-term antibiotics, usually penicillin-based agents, but surgery may be needed.

Nocardia

- *Nocardiae* are environmental, aerobic, Gram-positive bacteria which appear on microscopy to be branching and beaded (see Figure 29.5).
- *Nocardiae* are primarily opportunistic pathogens causing pulmonary, cutaneous or neurological infection.
- *Nocardia* spp. are easy to culture in vitro, however accurate speciation requires referral to a reference laboratory.
- Molecular technology has identified over 90 species of *Nocardiae*, of which about a third are currently associated with human disease. *Nocardia abscessus, N. asteroides, N. brasiliensis, N. cyriacygeorgica, N. farcinica, N. nova, N. transvalensis* are most commonly reported as causing human disease.
- Co-trimoxazole or amoxicillin-clavulanate are used as first-line treatment.

Noma

LEILA SROUR

EPIDEMIOLOGY

The majority of reported noma patients are children 1–7 years of age in sub-Saharan Africa in the 'noma belt' stretching across West Africa to central Sudan. Until recently, there have been few reports from Asia.[5] WHO (1998) estimated a worldwide incidence of 140 000 cases per year, survival rate of 10–30%, at least 100 000 childhood deaths annually and 770 000 survivors with severe sequelae.[1,6] The disease may be much more frequent than reported in poor countries throughout the world.[1–6] Many cases are not discovered due to weak healthcare systems, lack of knowledge about the disease, the stigma and neglect. Children often die without diagnosis or treatment or their deaths being recorded.[2,4] The 'paradox of noma' is that when countries develop sufficient public health resources to recognize and report noma cases, the economic and health development usually allows the disease to disappear.[2] Noma was common in the West until the twentieth century, when economic progress, adequate nutrition and public health services improved and noma almost disappeared. Noma recurred in the Second World War concentration camps.[2] Noma can occur in children and adults with immunosuppression, including patients with AIDS.[7]

PATHOGENESIS

Risk factors are chronic malnutrition, lack of exclusive breastfeeding, vitamin deficiencies, poor oral hygiene, viral infections, especially measles and HIV, poor sanitation and living in close proximity to livestock.[1,2,4,8] The pathogenesis of noma remains unclear. It appears to result from an interaction of severe malnutrition, intraoral infections and compromised immunity. Noma may be preceded by a febrile illness, especially measles, herpes, malaria or acute necrotizing stomatitis. Overgrowth of periodontal bacteria breaks the resistance of the child's weakened immune system. Microbiological samples of children with acute noma have grown *Fusobacterium necrophorum*, *Prevotella intermedia*, spirochetes, *Staphylococcus aureus* and others. However, their importance in the actual tissue destruction remains uncertain.[1,2,7,9–13] Chronic immunostimulation in severely malnourished children results in uncontrolled production of cytokines and other inflammatory mediators. The rapid destruction of tissues suggests an immunopathological reaction between mouth flora and the immune system.[1,3,11–13]

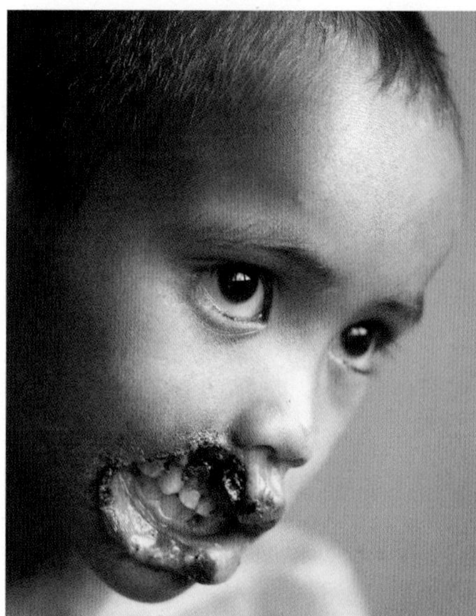

Figure 29.1 Acute noma of the lip and cheek in a 6-year-old child. *(Photograph taken by Bryan Watt, In: M. Leila Srour, Bryan Watt, Bounthom Phengdy, Keutmy Khansoulivong, Jim Harris, Christopher Bennett, Michel Strobel, Christian Dupuis, and Paul N. Newton, 'Noma in Laos: Stigma of Severe Poverty in Rural Asia', American Journal of Tropical Medicine and Hygiene, 78(4), 2008.)*

CLINICAL FEATURES

Acute Noma

Poor chronically malnourished children, living in rural areas with inadequate sanitation, who have mouth ulcers, often recovering from another infection like measles or malaria, may develop noma. The noma lesion begins with inflammation of the gingiva or the inside of the cheek. Severe, painful swelling of the cheek, halitosis and excessive salivation are common, accompanied by fever and anorexia. At this stage, medical treatment and nutritional support can significantly reduce mortality, but this acute stage of noma only lasts a few days, so the window of intervention is very short.[1,2,8,13]

Untreated, noma progresses to involve the lip and cheek with extensive intraoral destruction (Figure 29.1). A gangrenous lesion develops rapidly with a black necrotic centre. Soft tissue, bone and teeth are lost. The gangrene can spread to the nose, eye or the other side of the face. Most children suffer and die from complications such as pneumonia and septicaemia associated with severe malnutrition.[1,2,4,8]

Sequelae of Noma

The survivors slough the dead tissue and may develop secondary infections. Healing occurs with contraction of scar tissue, leaving holes and varying degrees of facial disfigurement, trismus, incontinentia oris, speech and dental problems (Figure 29.2). Disfigurement, functional impairment and difficulties with speech and chewing, result in isolation and psychological scarring. Survivors may be hidden for years before seeking medical treatment.[1,2,4,5]

DIAGNOSIS

Noma is diagnosed clinically. Few diseases look like noma. Other ulcerative lesions such as leishmaniasis, malignant oral lesions, syphilitic lesions and leprosy rarely occur in children. Facial swelling, foul-smelling discharge and the rapid development of orofacial gangrene define the acute disease. Survivors present with various degrees of facial disfigurement and disability and may be distinguished from patients with congenital deformities, including cleft lip and trauma, by their history.[1,2,9,14]

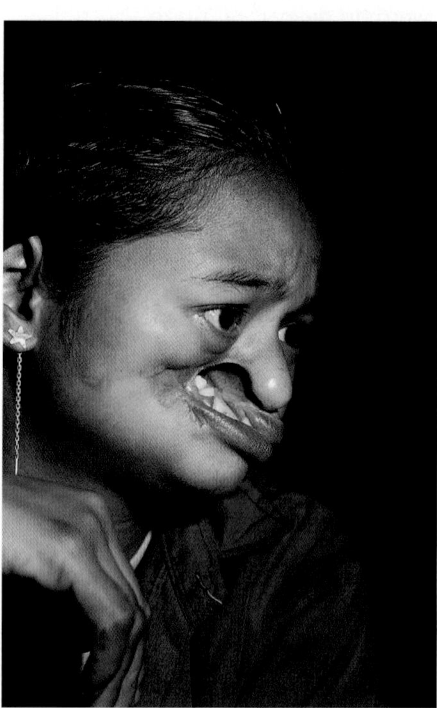

Figure 29.2 A 16-year-old survivor with sequelae of acute noma at 4 years of age. *(Photograph taken by Bryan Watt, In: M. Leila Srour, Bryan Watt, Bounthom Phengdy, Keutmy Khansoulivong, Jim Harris, Christopher Bennett, Michel Strobel, Christian Dupuis, and Paul N. Newton, 'Noma in Laos: Stigma of Severe Poverty in Rural Asia', American Journal of Tropical Medicine and Hygiene, 78(4), 2008.)*

MANAGEMENT AND TREATMENT

There is little information on the optimum therapy of acute noma, due to the 'paradox of noma' (above), but nutritional support, antibiotics and topical treatment appear to be helpful. Commercial nutritional formulas can be used or local foods including eggs, milk, soy products and peanuts, liquefied and fed orally or enterally. Penicillin/cloxacillin and metronidazole have been used to treat the suspected aerobic and anaerobic oropharyngeal bacteria but the optimum antibiotic therapy remains unclear. Concomitant malaria, intestinal parasites, tuberculosis and vitamin deficiencies should be looked for and treated.[1,2,15] Dead tissue may be debrided, without further surgery during the acute phase. Physiotherapy is important to prevent contractures of the mouth.[1]

The reconstructive surgical management of sequelae in noma survivors is complex. Treatment should be postponed for at least 1 year after acute noma. Improving the nutritional status of the patient before and after surgery is likely to improve outcome. Surgical treatment consists of excision of all scar tissue, correction of trismus and closure of tissue defects with local, pedicled or free flaps. Surgery cannot restore normal appearance but can significantly improve the patient's appearance and their life.[2,16,17]

PREVENTION

However, the most important intervention is the prevention of noma, through poverty reduction and strengthening health systems, especially in remote rural areas. It is likely that early recognition, diagnosis and treatment can significantly reduce mortality. The elimination of extreme poverty, improving prenatal care, promotion of exclusive breast-feeding, immunizations, food security and improved nutrition for the poorest children can hopefully lead to the eradication of noma.[1,2,4–6,8]

Actinomycosis

VANESSA WONG

EPIDEMIOLOGY

Actinomyces are opportunistic pathogens that can infect anyone.[18] An accurate estimate of incidence of the disease is difficult, since there is a lack of recent data, particularly in developing countries; a prevalence of 1 case per 630 000 admissions was reported in the 1970s.[19] More recently, the Department of Health in the UK reported that 0.0006% of hospital consultations (71 in total) were for actinomycosis in England between 2002 and 2003.[20] Men are three times more likely to be infected than women,[21,22] the exception being pelvic actinomycosis which predominately affects women with a history of intrauterine contraceptive device (IUCD) use. Although the disease can affect immunocompromised individuals, most reported cases are in immunocompetent people.[18,23]

PATHOGENESIS AND PATHOLOGY

Resulting from normal commensals of the human oropharynx, gastrointestinal tract and urogenital tract actinomycosis is predominantly an endogenous infection.[24] However, there have been a few reports of human bite wounds resulting in exogenous spread of the organism.[25] A breach of the mucosal barrier allows the bacteria to invade local tissues and spread.

The first species described was *A. bovis* in 1877, which, although not a cause of human disease, was isolated from masses on the jaw of cattle. Over 30 species have been identified since, with *A. israelii* being the most common human pathogen. Less common species include *A. naeslundii, A. meyeri, A. viscosus, A. odontolyticus, A. turicensis, and A. radingae.*[24,26]

These bacteria are rarely isolated alone from clinical specimens, but are found with other normal commensals such as *Aggregatibacter actinomycetemcomitans*, fusobacteria, staphylococci, streptococci or *Enterobacteriaceae.*[26] For treatment purposes, it is important to note that many of these bacteria are pathogens in their own right. Animal studies have also suggested that some species are able to aid actinomyces in establishing an infection by inhibiting host defences, although exact roles in this co-pathogenicity mechanism remain unclear.[27]

CLINICAL FEATURES

Actinomycosis is classified into clinical forms according to the anatomical site infected: orocervicofacial, thoracic, abdominopelvic, central nervous system, musculoskeletal and disseminated.

Orocervicofacial

Orocervicofacial actinomycosis is the commonest form of the disease and comprises approximately 50% of all reported cases.[21] It has been associated with poor dentition, dental manipulation or oral trauma. Presentations include fever and a chronic swelling of the soft tissue in the perimandibular region described as 'lumpy jaw'. Lesions can become firm and woody with a bluish appearance and develop chronically discharging sinuses. They are generally painless, but can be tender. Regional lymphadenopathy is typically absent in early stages of the disease. Direct extension into bone, muscle, and the central nervous system has also been reported.[28]

Thoracic

Thoracic actinomycosis accounts for 15–20% of cases.[21,29] Infection commonly follows aspiration of oropharyngeal secretions or a foreign body, but it can also occur after oesopharyngeal perforation, local spread from orocervicofacial and abdominal infection or from haematogenous spread.[24] The clinical picture is one of chronic pneumonia with fever, cough, shortness of breath and chest pain, as well as haemoptysis and weight loss.[30] Complications can include pleural effusion, mediastinal invasion, rib destruction and empyema necessitans. Invasion of the myopericardium is an understandably fatal but thankfully rare complication commonly resulting in pericarditis, with myocarditis and endocarditis occurring less frequently.[31,32]

Abdominopelvic

About 20% of all cases of actinomycosis involve an abdominal organ.[21] The commonest precipitating event is acute appendicitis, particularly with perforation, which accounts for 65% of cases.[33] Predisposing factors include gastrointestinal perforation, previous surgery, neoplasia and foreign body ingestion. Diagnosis is challenging because the patients often present with nonspecific symptoms of fever, weight loss, and vague abdominal pain.[34] Although patients may present with a palpable right iliac fossa mass, there may be little to give away underlying disease on clinical examination; the majority of cases are actually diagnosed postoperatively.

Cases of pelvic actinomycosis have been recognized in patients with a history of prolonged IUCD use (>2 years), although the disease can still occur in the absence of an IUCD.[34,35] Patients typically complain of fever, vaginal discharge, pelvic or abdominal pain and weight loss.

Rare Presentations of Disease

Central nervous system infection is normally a result of haematogenous spread or direct extension from orocervicofacial infection. The commonest clinical manifestation is brain abscess; meningoencephalitis, actinomycoma, subdural empyema and epidural abscess occur less frequently.[36] Musculoskeletal infections can arise from spread from neighbouring tissues (which accounts for the majority of cases), local trauma or haematogenous spread.[37] The commonest sites of infection are the facial bones, particularly the mandible because of its proximity to the buccal mucosa which allows direct access when breached. Reports of actinomycosis involving joint prostheses have been described.[38] Despite the possibility of haematogenous spread from an established infection at any site, disseminated disease has become exceptionally rare since the development of antibiotics.

LABORATORY DIAGNOSIS

Histopathology

Microscopic examination showing filamentous rod-shaped organisms and sulphur granules on tissue staining is highly suggestive of actinomycosis. The filamentous bacteria can be visualized using a Gram (Figure 29.3), Gomori methenamine-silver or Giemsa stains. Sulphur granules are actually clumped colonies of organisms that can be observed on staining with haematoxylin and eosin (Figure 29.4).[23] However, granules may not always be seen in the specimen; they are also not specific to actinomycosis with several other conditions yielding sulphur granules, such as nocardiosis, chromomycosis, eumycetoma and botryomycosis.[24] Another histopathology technique often utilized is a species-specific conjugated antibody, which detects bacteria in tissue, even after fixation with formalin.[39]

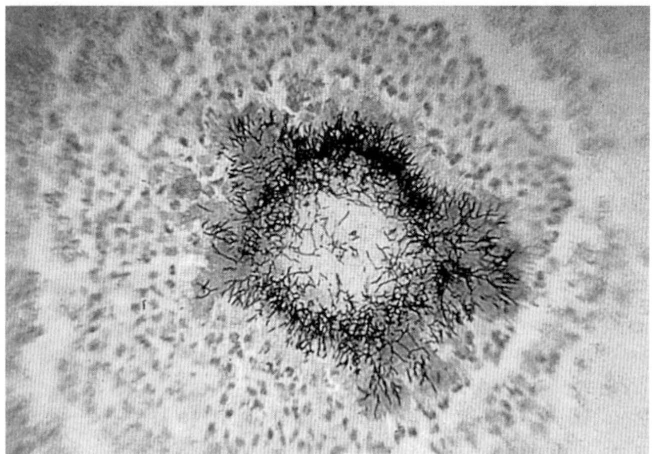

Figure 29.3 Actinomyces stained with Gram stain, revealing typical central Gram-positive branching bacteria.

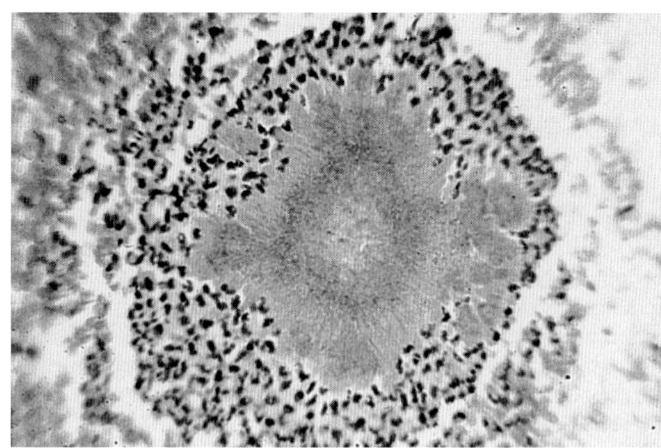

Figure 29.4 Sulphur granules stained with haematoxylin and eosin.

Microbiology

A definitive diagnosis of actinomycosis is made on isolating the organism from a clinical specimen such as pus, tissue or sulphur granules. However, culturing the organism can be exceedingly difficult for a number of reasons, including previous antibiotic treatment.[19] Microscopy of the specimen using a Gram stain may be more sensitive than culture if the patient has received antibiotics. Actinomyces are slow-growing organisms that can be cultured on selective media at 37°C in anaerobic conditions for up to 2–3 weeks.[23] Commercial biochemical kits have made speciation easier and quicker, although the accuracy of these kits has been reported to be poor compared to conventional tests.[40] Serological assays are also available, but not widely used because of the lack of accuracy. Molecular techniques, including 16s rRNA sequencing, have been developed for more rapid and accurate identification, but these are mainly used in research or reference facilities.[41,42]

MANAGEMENT AND TREATMENT

Actinomyces are susceptible to a wide range of antimicrobials. Historically, penicillin has been the drug of choice. Patients are treated with high doses of intravenous penicillin G over 2–6 weeks, followed by oral penicillin V for 6–12 months.[22] Although a prolonged course of antibiotics is generally advocated this traditional course may not be necessary for all patients. The current approach is to tailor treatment to the individual, the exact regimen depending upon a number of factors including the site of infection, severity of disease, performance of any surgical intervention, and the patient's response. Furthermore, patients must be monitored clinically and radiologically with regularity to ensure complete resolution of the disease.

Lessons from clinical experience have shown that alternatives to penicillin include tetracycline, doxycycline, minocycline, clindamycin and erythromycin (the safe option in pregnancy).[21,43–45] There is little clinical evidence available on the newer β-lactam agents except for case reports of infections treated successfully with ceftriaxone, piperacillin, imipenem and meropenem.[46–49]

It is important to be aware that in vitro antibiotic susceptibility testing does not always correlate with clinical efficacy. However metronidazole, aminoglycosides, oxacillin, dicloxacillin and cephalexin exhibit reduced in vitro activity against actinomyces, suggesting that they should not be used.[50]

The initial therapeutic regimen should be broad, taking into account other pathogens that may also be present at the site of infection. A reasonable first-line treatment consists of a β-lactam such as amoxicillin and a β-lactamase inhibitor such as clavulanate, which provides cover against potential β-lactamase producers including *S. aureus* and *Enterobacteriaceae*.[22]

Surgical resection may also be appropriate in some cases, particularly if extensive necrotic tissue, sinus tracts or fistulae are present. Surgery has also been used to control symptoms such as haemoptysis in thoracic disease.[22,23] Shorter courses of antibiotics have been used in combination with surgical drainage.

PREVENTION

Given the rarity of actinomycotic infection, there is little known about effective preventive measures. However, it seems logical that improving dental hygiene could prevent orocervicofacial actinomycosis associated with poor dentition.

Nocardia

SARAH WYLLIE

EPIDEMIOLOGY

Nocardia spp. are found in the environment worldwide and are especially associated with decaying vegetation. The organism was first isolated by Edmond Nocard, a French veterinarian, from a case of bovine lymphadenitis in 1888.[51]

In tropical countries, they cause cutaneous abscesses or chronic subcutaneous infections (mycetoma) as a result of traumatic inoculation of organisms into superficial abrasions.[52] Other clinical presentations are more likely to be associated with immunosuppression.

PATHOGENESIS AND PATHOLOGY

Infection usually occurs by inhalation of the bacteria and pneumonia is the most common illness. Direct inoculation of the skin or sclera of the eye can also cause disease. Nocardiosis or disseminated infection occurs as a result of invasion from a primary source and causes secondary abscesses in other organs, particularly the brain. Cell-mediated immunity is crucial to containing the infection and a variety of immune-compromising conditions such as organ transplantation, malignancy, advanced HIV disease, long-term corticosteroid use, diabetes mellitus or treatment with other immunosuppressants such as chemotherapy agents and immunomodulatory drugs have all been reported to increase the risk of invasive disease.[53,54] Invasive infection may occur despite antibacterial prophylaxis with co-trimoxazole. Risk of pulmonary infection is increased in those with pre-existing pulmonary disease such as chronic obstructive pulmonary disease and alveolar proteinosis or in those with respiratory insult from near-drowning. Around one-half of nocardial pneumonias will disseminate. Central venous catheters have been reported as a source for *Nocardia* bloodstream infection.[55]

CLINICAL FEATURES

Primary Cutaneous Nocardiosis

This presents as a nodule, ulcer or abscess at the site of inoculation of the organism. There may be secondary lesions along the course of the lymphatic drainage system and local lymphadenopathy is common. Primary cutaneous infection is commonly caused by *Nocardia brasiliensis* and may resolve spontaneously. It is primarily seen in tropical countries.[52] Alternative diagnoses include subcutaneous mycoses and atypical mycobacterial infection.

Mycetoma (Madura Foot)

Mycetoma is a chronic infection involving the skin, subcutaneous tissues and deeper tissues including bone as a result of traumatic inoculation by a variety of bacteria and fungi. It is commonly seen on the hands and feet but may also affect other parts of the body. Over half of the reported infections are caused by actinomycetes, of which *Nocardia brasiliensis* is the most common.

Pulmonary Nocardiosis

Pneumonia caused by nocardial infection may be indistinguishable from other pneumonias, but should be suspected in any prolonged pneumonia that does not respond to empirical treatment and in anyone who is at increased risk due to immunosuppression. Pulmonary tuberculosis is a common differential diagnosis. Chest radiographs often show infiltrates or cannonball lesions. A pleural effusion may be present which is exudative in nature. There may be local spread from the lower respiratory tract to the pericardium and mediastinum causing pericarditis and mediastinitis respectively. A positive nocardial culture is not always associated with clinical disease and in some patients with chronic lung conditions it may represent normal colonizing flora.[51]

Ocular Nocardiosis

Nocardial infection of the eyes may cause keratitis, scleritis and endophthalmitis. It usually presents following a traumatic injury to the eye or after ophthalmic surgery.

Disseminated Nocardiosis

Haematogenous spread to other organs is common in the immunocompromised patient and may occur in the absence of pulmonary signs and symptoms. The central nervous system is the organ most commonly affected in nocardiosis. Infection of the central nervous system presents with localized cerebral abscesses without meningeal involvement. Clinical presenting features are headache, fever, and focal neurological deficits such as seizures and cranial nerve palsies. The differential diagnosis includes other infective causes of cerebral abscess and malignancy.

LABORATORY DIAGNOSIS

The most useful diagnostic test is a Gram stain of a clinical specimen (sputum, pus, bronchial washings or tissue). This may reveal the characteristic Gram-positive branching and beaded bacilli (Figure 29.5). Nocardiae may be more readily visualized

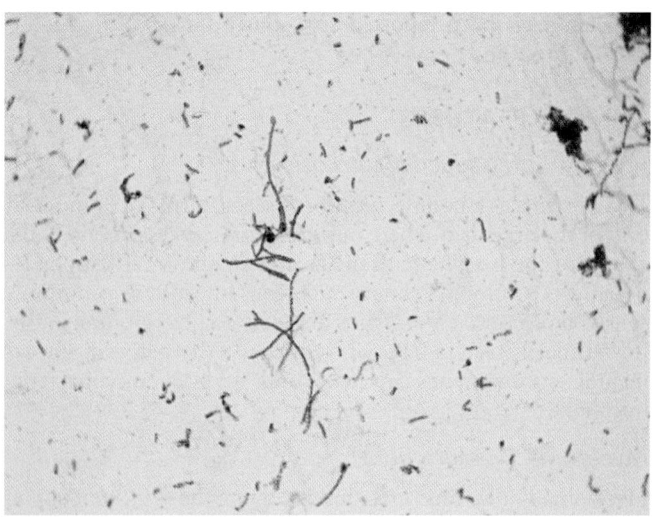

Figure 29.5 Nocardia stained with Gram stain, revealing characteristic Gram-positive branching and beaded bacilli. *(Photograph taken by C Walker, Portsmouth NHS Trust.)*

with the use of the modified acid-fast stain which uses a weaker acid such as 1% sulphuric acid as the decolourizing agent.[51] A positive result with the modified acid-fast stain helps to distinguish *Nocardia* species from *Streptomyces* species or other members of the aerobic actinomycetes. Colonies of *Nocardia* spp. typically grow within 48–72 hours on most routine bacteriological mediums when incubated aerobically, but may take up to 14 days to appear. Colonial morphology is variable, some are pigmented e.g. *N. brasiliensis* typically has a yellow colonial colouration, and some have aerial hyphae.

Molecular techniques such as analysis of 16SrRNA gene sequences are required for identification of the infecting species.[56] Alternative gene targets such as *secA1* may also be used to facilitate accurate identification. These molecular tests are carried out in reference laboratory facilities.[57]

Antimicrobial susceptibility testing is carried out either by broth microdilution as recommended by the Clinical and Laboratory Standards Institute or by E-test.[58,59] The recommended primary antimicrobials for susceptibility testing are amikacin, amoxicillin-clavulanic acid, ceftriaxone, ciprofloxacin, clarithromycin, imipenem, linezolid, minocycline, trimethoprim-sulfamethoxazole and tobramycin.[51,60]

MANAGEMENT AND TREATMENT

Drainage of pus from abscesses and surgical debridement of infected tissue facilitates resolution of infection in combination with antibacterial chemotherapy. Co-trimoxazole, a mixture of sulfamethoxazole and trimethoprim, is commonly used first-line, especially for pulmonary nocardiosis and mycetoma. Co-trimoxazole is well absorbed orally and has excellent penetration into most tissue compartments including the central nervous system. Minocycline or amoxicillin-clavulanate can be used in patients who are unable to tolerate sulphonamides.[61]

Disseminated infection is usually treated with two antibacterial agents such as a combination of imipenem and amikacin. Isolates causing disseminated infection should be tested for antimicrobial susceptibility. Linezolid has good oral bioavailability, tissue penetration and activity against *Nocardia* spp., however haematological side-effects often limit the longer-term use of this agent.[62] Duration of treatment of nocardial infection depends on the burden of infection and the host's immune function, but is usually prescribed for several months.

PREVENTION

Wearing adequate footwear and cleaning of cutaneous cuts in high-risk areas should help prevent mycetoma.

REFERENCES

1. Enwonwu CO, Falkler WA Jr, Phillips RS. Noma (cancrum oris). Lancet 2006;368(9530):147–56.
4. Ziegler J. Human Rights Council Resolutions: Right to Food 'The Tragedy of Noma. Human Rights Council Advisory Committee. August 2009. Online. Available: http://axisoflogic.com/artman/publish/Article_63958.shtml
18. Acevedo F, Baudrand R, Letelier LM, et al. Actinomycosis: a great pretender. Case reports of unusual presentations and a review of the literature. Int J Infect Dis 2008;12(4):358–62.
22. Brook I. Actinomycosis: diagnosis and management. South Med J 2008;101(10):1019–23.
51. Brown-Elliot BA, Brown JM, Conville PS, et al. Clinical and laboratory features of the *Nocardia* spp. based on current molecular taxonomy. Clin Microbiol Rev 2006;19(2):259–82.

Access the complete references online at www.expertconsult.com

30 Bartonellosis, Cat-scratch Disease, Trench Fever, Human Ehrlichiosis

EMMANOUIL ANGELAKIS | DIDIER RAOULT

KEY POINTS

- A single *Bartonella* species can cause either acute or chronic infection or either vascular proliferative or suppurative manifestations.
- *Bartonella* species cause long-lasting intra-erythrocytic bacteraemia in their mammalian reservoir.
- People usually become infected with *Bartonella* species incidentally.
- People are the only proven hosts for *B. quintana.*
- The clinical situations caused by *Bartonella* species are so different that the approach to treatment must be adapted to each species and clinical situation.
- The diagnosis of infections due to *Bartonella* spp. is difficult because of the fastidious nature of the bacteria and the nonspecific clinical manifestations.

Introduction

Bartonella species are Gram-negative bacilli or coccobacilli belonging to the α2 subgroup of *Proteobacteria* and are closely related to the genus *Brucella* and *Agrobacterium* on the basis of 16S rDNA gene comparison.[1] Until 1990, the genus *Bartonella* contained only two species: *B. bacilliformis*, the agent of Carrion's disease and *B. quintana* the agent of trench fever. In 1993, Brenner and colleagues[2] proposed that previously designated *Rochalimaea* species be united with the genus *Bartonella* and renamed *B. quintana*, *B. vinsonii*, *B. henselae* and *B. elizabethae.* This reclassification also resulted in the transfer of these organisms from the family *Rickettsiaceae* to the family *Bartonellaceae*, which included *B. bacilliformis*, and removed the family *Bartonellaceae* from the order *Rickettsiales*. In 1995, Birtles and colleagues[3] proposed the unification of the genus *Grahamella* with the genus *Bartonella*, which resulted in five additional *Bartonella* species: *B. talpae*, *B. peromysci*, *B. grahamii*, *B. taylorii*, and *B. doshiae*. In effect, these reclassifications eliminated the previous genera *Rochalimaea* and *Grahamella*. The genus now comprises *B. bacilliformis* and additional, recently described species (Table 30.1).

Depending on the level of host adaptation, *Bartonella* infections in the reservoir host range from an asymptomatic or subclinical (most animal-specific species) to clinical manifestations with low morbidity and limited mortality (such as human-specific *B. quintana* infections), or even to life-threatening disease, such as severe haemolytic anaemia associated with the human-specific infection by *B. bacilliformis*. People usually become infected with *Bartonella* species incidentally, as the organisms are normally found in the reservoir hosts of *Bartonella* species. *Bartonella* species cause long-recognized diseases, such as Carrion's disease, trench fever and cat-scratch disease (CSD), and more recently recognized diseases, such as bacillary angiomatosis (BA), peliosis hepatis (PH), chronic bacteraemia, endocarditis, chronic lymphadenopathy and neurological disorders. A remarkable feature of the genus *Bartonella* is the ability of a single species to cause either acute or chronic infection and either vascular proliferative or suppurative manifestations.

Bacteriology

Members of the genus *Bartonella* are short, pleomorphic, Gram-negative rods that are fastidious, aerobic and oxidase-negative organisms within the α2 subgroup of the class *Proteobacteria.* They have a close evolutionary homology with members of the genera *Brucella*, *Agrobacterium* and *Rhizobium*. *B. bacilliformis* and *B. clarridgeiae* have flagella, which in the case of *B. bacilliformis* facilitates erythrocyte invasion.[4] Polar structures resembling fimbriae have been observed on *B. tribocorum*. Other *Bartonella* spp., such as *B. henselae*, appear to lack flagella.[4] Based upon in-vitro studies using human umbilical vein endothelial cells, *B. henselae* is internalized by an actin-dependent invasome-mediated mechanism of cellular invasion.[5] Because no distinguishing phenotypic characteristics have been described for *Bartonella* spp., their identification and phylogenetic classification have been mainly based on genetic studies. Many DNA regions and encoding gene sequences have been used in genetic studies, including the 16S rDNA gene; the 16S-23S rRNA intergenic spacer region (ITS); the citrate synthase gene (*gltA*); the heat shock protein gene (*groEL*); the genes encoding the PAP31 and 35-kDa proteins; and the cell division protein gene (*ftsZ*). According to La Scola and colleagues,[6] the gltA, gro EL, rpoB, fts Z and ITS genes have all good discriminating power, with a discriminatory power (DP) ranging from 92.6% to 94.4%. The gene with the highest discriminating power appears to be ribC, which has a DP of 86.5%.

Epidemiology of *Bartonella* Species

The mode of transmission for many novel *Bartonella* spp. remains elusive or essentially unstudied, and only three *Bartonella* spp. are known to infect and replicate in the digestive tract of their respective vectors: *B. quintana* in body lice; *B. henselae* in cat fleas; and, more recently, *B. schoenbuchensis* in the deer ked (deer fly).[7] The role of ticks in transmission of *Bartonella* spp. is suspected and supported by direct or indirect evidences.[8–10] *Bartonella* spp. have a natural cycle that contains a reservoir host

TABLE 30.1 **Infections Caused By *Bartonella* Species**

Bartonella Species	First Cultivation	Reservoir Host/Vector	Human Disease(s)
B. alsatica	Wild rabbit (*Oryctolagus cuniculus*)	Rabbit	Endocarditis, lymphadenopathy
B. australis	Grey kangaroo (*Macropus giganteus*)		
B. bacilliformis	Human	Human/sandfly	Carrion's disease: Oroya fever and verruga peruana
B. birtlesii	Mouse (*Apodemus* spp.)	Rat	
B. bovis (*B. weissii*)	Cow	Cow	
B. capreoli	Roe deer (*Capreolus capreolus*)	Ruminant	
B. chomelii	Domestic cattle (*Bos taurus*)		
B. clarridgeiae	Cat	Cat/Cat flea	Cat-scratch disease
B. coopersplainsensis	Mottle-tailed rat (*Rattus leucopus*)		
B. doshiae	Woodland mammal (*Microtus agrestis*)	Rat	
B. durdenii	Squirrel		
B. elizabethae	Endocarditis patient	Rat	Endocarditis, neuroretinitis
B. grahamii	Woodland mammal (*Clethrionomys glareolus*)	Rat, insectivore	Neuroretinitis
B. henselae	Cat	Cat/Cat flea	Cat scratch disease, endocarditis, bacillary angiomatosis, bacillary peliosis, Parinaud's oculoglandular, neuroretinitis, osteomyelitis, arthropathy, bacteraemia with fever
B. koehlerae	Domestic cat	Cat	Endocarditis
B. melophagi			
B. peromysci	Mouse (*Peromyscus* spp.)	Mice	
B. phoceensis	Wild rat (*Rattus norvegicus*)		
B. queenslandensis	Grassland melomys (*Melomys* spp.)		
B. quintana	Human	Human/body louse	Trench fever, endocarditis, bacillary angiomatosis
B. rattiaustraliensis	Tunney's rat (*Rattus tunneyi*)		
B. rattimassiliensis	Rat (*Rattus norvegicus*)		
B. rochalimae	Human		Bacteraemia, fever, splenomegaly
B. schoenbuchensis	Wild roe deer (*Capreolus capreolus*)	Ruminant/deer ked	
B. silvicola	Bat		
B. talpae	Mole	Mole	
B. tamiae	Human		Febrile illness
B. taylorii	Woodland mouse (*Apodemus* spp.)	Rat	
B. tribocorum	Wild rat (*Rattus norvegicus*)		
B. vinsonii arupensis	Cattle rancher	Dog, rodent/ticks	Bacteraemia with fever
B. vinsonii berkhoffii	Valvular endocarditis dog	Dog/ticks	
B. vinsonii vinsonii	Vole (*Microtus pennsylvanicus*)	Vole/vole ear mite	
B. volans	Squirrel		
B. washoensis		Ground squirrel	Myocarditis
B. weissii	Domestic cat	Deer, elk, beef, cattle	

and a vector that transmits the bacteria from the reservoir hosts to new susceptible hosts. There is apparently a species-specific association between *Bartonella* species and their animal hosts or vectors.[11,12] All *Bartonella* species appear to be associated mainly with a mammalian host. Natural *Bartonella* infections begin with the inoculation of the bacteria, and this is usually associated with the feeding of the arthropod vector. Differences in the clinical presentations of individuals with primary infections may be due to several factors. After the primary infection, which might or might not be symptomatic, an asymptomatic chronic bacteraemia occurs in the natural mammalian host. The host is then a competent reservoir from which an arthropod vector can become infected with *Bartonella*. Although the geographic distributions of the *Bartonella* species may reflect the geographic distributions of their hosts or of their vectors, the knowledge related to vector transmission of *Bartonella* organisms is very incomplete.

Pathogenicity of *Bartonella* Species

Bartonella spp. cause long-lasting intraerythrocytic bacteraemia in their mammalian reservoir (Figure 30.1).[13] Some *Bartonella* spp. appear to be restricted to cause intraerythrocytic infection in a single mammalian species, e.g. *B. bacilliformis* in humans or *B. henselae* in domestic cats, while other species have several, but typically closely related mammalian reservoir hosts, e.g. *B. bovis* or *B. schoenbuchensis* infecting various ruminant hosts, such as roe deer, red deer, mule deer, elk and cattle.[14] Besides erythrocytes, endothelial cells represent another major target cell type for *Bartonella* within their mammalian hosts. Animal models of intraerythrocytic infection have been established for several *Bartonella* with data for the characteristics and course of intraerythrocytic bacteraemia to be similar for all these models.[15–18] As a result, 5 days after an intravenous inoculation with plate-grown *B. tribocorum*, large numbers of bacteria were released from the primary niche into the bloodstream.[15,19] In the bloodstream *B. tribocorum* adhere to mature erythrocytes, indicating that bacteria become competent for erythrocyte interaction during colonization of the primary niche. After adhesion to erythrocytes *B. tribocorum* invade and replicate intracellularly until a critical density is reached. The number of intracellular bacteria remains static for the remaining lifespan of the infected erythrocytes, which is indistinguishable from that of uninfected erythrocytes.[15] During this intraerythrocytic

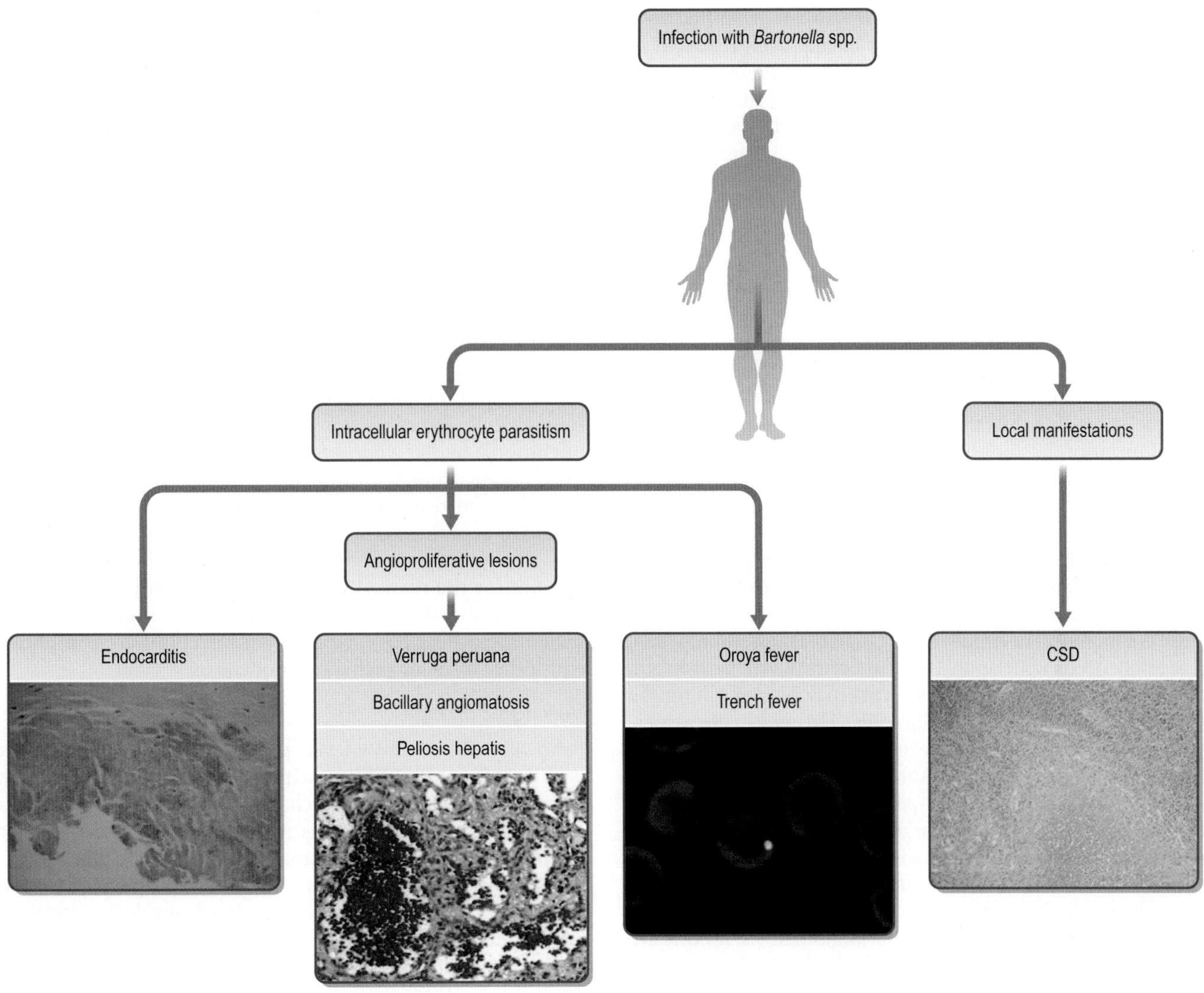

Figure 30.1 *Bartonella* species clinical syndromes.

bacteraemia, antibodies are unlikely to function against infected erythrocytes, as the lifespan of these cells is similar to that of uninfected erythrocytes.[15,16] In rats, the intraerythrocytic bacteraemia caused by *B. tribocorum* subsides spontaneously after approximately 10 weeks,[15] whereas a similar duration of bacteraemia is observed in other experimental models of *Bartonella* infection.[20]

Infections by *Bartonella Bacilliformis*

B. bacilliformis is the causative agent of Carrion's disease, also known as bartonellosis, Oroya fever, and verruga peruana and was the first infectious agent of the genus *Bartonella* to be formally described as a species.

Transmission of *Bartonella bacilliformis*

The vector implicated in the transmission of *B. bacilliformis* is a female sandfly (*Lutzomyia* sp.).[21] Sandflies were implicated as vectors as early as 1764, but this was not demonstrated until the Battistini experiment was done. He was the first to establish direct transmission of *B. bacilliformis* by sandfly feeding. Twenty-three sandflies were released within an enclosure and allowed to feed on a rhesus monkey. Within 18 days, blood cultures became positive for *B. bacilliformis*. The species of *Lutzomyia* used in this study is unknown.[21,22] Direct proof of transmission of *Bartonella* spp. by a tick was reported by Noguchi in 1926,[23] who described experimental transmission of *B. bacilliformis* to monkeys by *Dermacentor andersoni*. In this study, ticks were allowed to feed on infected monkeys for 5 days. After removal, partially engorged ticks were placed on healthy monkeys in which disease then developed. This study showed that ticks could acquire and transmit the bacteria but did not demonstrate their vector competence or transtadial transmission throughout the tick's life cycle. Outbreaks continue to occur in *B. bacilliformis* endemic and *Lutzomyia verrucarum* non-endemic areas, leading to implications that other *Lutzomyia* sandflies or other arthropods can serve as potential vectors. In Peru, the main vector species is *L. verrucarum*. In Peru, Ellis and co-workers[11] demonstrated that 1% of 104 wild-caught *Lutzomyia peruensis* (Shannon) contained *B. bacilliformis* by PCR analysis.[24] There is no known animal reservoir for bartonellosis. It was believed that the limited geographic distribution of *L. verrucarum* was responsible for the apparent limited geographic distribution, with most cases having been reported in arid areas at 500–3000 m above sea level in the Peruvian Andes between south-western Colombia and central Peru.[13] However, recent events have demonstrated that bartonellosis can occur outside the recognized verruga zone, in areas where *L. verrucarum* is not the dominant sandfly species.[24] The disease has a seasonal transmission, with most cases reported in the months of January to June, when rainfall is greatest.[25]

PATHOGENESIS

When *B. bacilliformis* gains access to the human circulatory system, it disseminates from the point of inoculation by passive means. Motility conferred by lophotrichous flagella may contribute to spreading, but the importance of this appendage in host colonization has not been conclusively demonstrated.

Large numbers of organisms may be seen in the cytoplasm of cells lining blood vessels and lymph channels and in reticuloendothelial cells in lymph nodes, liver, spleen, bone marrow, kidneys, adrenals and pancreas. At the end of the incubation period, the primary or erythrocytic invasive phase of the disease occurs. Most commonly, only a few cells are parasitized and the disease is subclinical or mild without anaemia. Less often, severe disease may occur with up to 100% of erythrocytes parasitized, and compact masses of bacillary forms may be seen filling the cytoplasm of capillary endothelial cells. This is usually associated with sudden onset of fever, chills, severe haemolytic anaemia and a high mortality. Autopsy shows gross changes of acute haemolytic anaemia with pallor and jaundice. The liver, spleen and lymph nodes are enlarged mainly because of swollen reticuloendothelial cells which show engorgement with fragments of red cells and *B. bacilliformis* organisms. The bone marrow is usually hyperplastic.

In *verruga peruana*, as in bacillary angiomatosis, lesions are comprised of proliferating endothelial cells, bacteria and mixed infiltrates of macrophages/monocytes and polymorphonuclear neutrophils whereas the bacteria are presenting as aggregates both surrounding and within endothelial cells, indicating that the vascular endothelium represents a target tissue for intra- and extracellular colonization in vivo.[26] These vasoproliferative lesions indicate a chronic inflammation. An acute inflammatory reaction triggered by the *Bartonella*-infected endothelium may be crucial for initiating chronic inflammation. In general, an acute inflammatory response is thought to induce a mediator cascade that activates the endothelium, resulting in the release of proinflammatory chemoattractants and the sequential establishment of receptor–ligand interactions between the activated endothelium and circulating polymorphonuclear eutrophils.[19]

CLINICAL MANIFESTATIONS

Oroya Fever

Oroya fever is the acute or haematic phase of Carrion's disease. The epidemiological cycle of Oroya fever begins when *L. verrucarum* transmit *B. bacilliformis* to susceptible people during feeding. The majority of infected people are children or young adults.[13] Although primary infections can be asymptomatic, Oroya fever can develop when organisms enter erythrocytes.[27] After an incubation period of 3 weeks (range, 2–14 weeks), the disease may be manifested by insidious onset of mild fever, headache, anorexia and malaise lasting from 2 days to 1 week, or longer. *B. bacilliformis* invades up to 80% of erythrocytes and produces their massive haemolysis, which results in severe haemolytic anaemia, the major symptom of Oroya fever.[19] Less commonly, the onset may be abrupt with high fever, shaking chills, copious sweating and rapidly developing anaemia with marked pallor of the skin, mild scleral icterus, hepatosplenomegaly and generalized lymphadenopathy. Headache, vertigo, stupor and delirium may be present. These patients may have severe weakness, tachycardia and flow heart murmurs. A chronic asymptomatic bacteraemia which may last for up to 15 months usually follows, and *B. bacilliformis* may be transmitted to sandflies that feed on patients during this time.[13] Approximately one-third of patients present with opportunistic infections due to non-typhoid *Salmonellas*, sepsis by *Shigella dysenteriae*, *Enterobacter*, *Pseudomonas aeruginosa*, *Staphylococcus aureus*, pneumonia by *Pneumocystis jiroveci* or reactivation of tuberculosis, toxoplasmosis, and histoplasmosis.[28] Mortality rates can be high in untreated patients, reaching 85%, especially if infections are complicated with other diseases such as salmonellosis.[29] There are genetic variants of *B. bacilliformis* that might account for the marked variability in mortality and morbidity seen in outbreaks.[30] Mortality rates can be high in untreated patients, reaching 85%, especially if infections are complicated with other diseases such as salmonellosis.[29]

Verruga Peruana

Following acute Oroya fever, patients usually develop angioprolific cutaneous disease within 1–2 months; the 'verruga peruana'. Verruga peruana is characterized by the appearance of pleomorphic nodular lesions mainly over the arms and legs, although the face and trunk may be involved.[31] Lesions vary in size and number and may appear as red or purple papules a few millimetres in diameter to pedunculated, sessile or plaque-like lesions several centimetres across. New lesions may arise for up to 6 months in untreated patients.[31] Commonly, this eruptive phase adopts three patterns: a miliary eruption, with multiple and widely distributed lesions 2–3 mm in diameter; a nodular eruption, characterized by a few eruptions 8–10 mm in diameter; and a 'mular' eruption, a unique, large, deep-seated lesion.[31] This eruptive phase clinically resembles Kaposi's sarcoma or bacillary angiomatosis (BA). However, it has a low morbidity and there are no reports of mortality.[31] As in BA, lesions are characterized by lobular proliferations, atypical endothelial cells forming both relatively solid sheets as well as small, well-formed vessels with patent lumens. Lesions are also typically infiltrated by neutrophils indicating a chronic inflammatory process.[26] The most common symptoms are bleeding of the wart, fever, malaise and arthralgias. The bacteria can be isolated from patients' blood cultures and can be observed in blood films indicating that patients are sometimes bacteraemic.

Trench Fever

Trench fever, also known as 5-day fever or quintana fever, is a manifestation of initial infection with *B. quintana*. Detailed descriptions of the disease were first reported in infected troops during the First World War.

Transmission of *Bartonella quintana*

Pediculus humanus humanus has been the identified vector of *B. quintana* for several decades. Lice infected with *B. quintana* appear to remain so until they die, although their lifespan apparently does not decrease. *P. humanus corporis* lives in clothes and is associated with poverty and lack of hygiene. In a research of 930 homeless persons, that took place in Marseille, lice infestation was present in 22% and was associated with hypereosinophilia.[32] Pediculosis (lice infestation) is transmitted by contact with clothes or bedding. *B. quintana* multiplies in the louse's intestine and is transmitted to humans by faeces through altered skin.[33] Body lice usually feed 5 times a day and inject biological proteins with their bites, including an anaesthetic that provokes an allergic reaction and leads to pruritus and scratching, which facilitates the faecal transmission of *B. quintana*, and persistent *B. quintana* bacteraemia facilitates its spread by lice.[34] Historically, infection with *B. quintana* was thought to be limited to people with human body louse exposure. However, recently *B. quintana* was identified in head lice from homeless children in Nepal;[35] in head lice from homeless adults in San Francisco;[36] and in head lice nits from homeless people.[37] *Ctenocephalides felis* appears to be a potential vector for *B. quintana*[38] and it is possible that the cat fleas can maintain infection with *B. quintana* and transmit the organism among cats, which can subsequently transmit *B. quintana* to people via a bite or scratch.[39] Recently, the understanding of the epidemiology of *B. quintana* as an emerging source of human infection has changed as *B. quintana* was isolated from a non-human research primate (*Macaca fascicularis* Raffles) and from dogs with endocarditis.[22] Moreover, the bacterium was detected in cat fleas[38] and in cat dental pulp,[40] which suggests bacteraemia in cats, and has been isolated in a patient who owned a cat and sought treatment for chronic adenopathy.[41] *B. quintana* was also detected in *Pulex irritans* (Linnaeus) removed from a pet *Cercopithecus cephus* (Linnaeus) monkey in Africa.[42]

PATHOGENESIS

Trench fever is characterized by intracellular erythrocyte parasitism of *B. quintana* (Figure 30.2), the proportion of which varies between 0.001% and 0.005%.[43] Bacteria can also be seen either extracellularly, in mature erythrocytes or in erythroblasts.[44] This intracellular erythrocyte parasitism can probably preserve the pathogens for efficient transmission by body lice, protect *B. quintana* from the host immune response, and contribute to decreased antimicrobial efficacy. This immune evasion might explain the frequent relapses seen after antibiotic treatment of such patients.

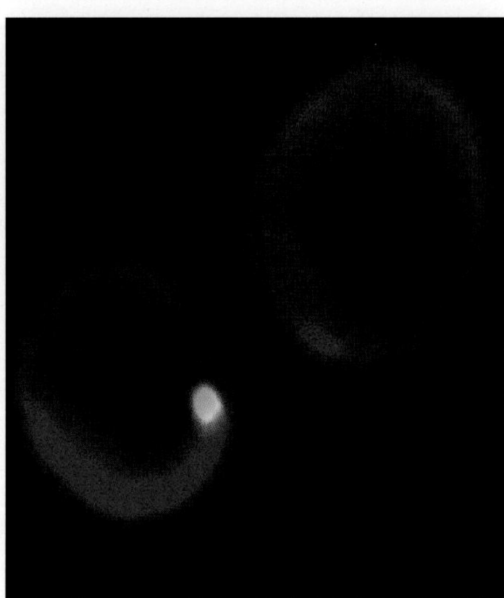

Figure 30.2 Intracellular erythrocyte parasitism of *B. Quintana*.

Bartonella endocarditis causes significant destruction of the valvular cusps which is characterized by mononuclear cell inflammation, extensive fibrosis, large calcification and small vegetation.[45] Lepidi and colleagues identified that more than half of the patients with *Bartonella* endocarditis had pre-existing valvular disease that could lead to the development of degenerative changes, especially fibrosis, calcification and chronic inflammation, independent of the infective process.[45] The bacteria are seen extracellularly in dense immunopositive clusters mainly included in vegetations and intracellularly in neutrophil and macrophage cytoplasms.[46] Patients with *Bartonella* endocarditis have a higher death rate and undergo valvular surgery more frequently than patients with endocarditis caused by other pathogens.[47]

Trench Fever

Clinical manifestations may range from asymptomatic infection to severe, life-threatening illness. After an incubation period of 2–3 weeks, there is a sudden onset of fever that lasts 1–3 days and is associated with headache, shin pain and dizziness.[48] Often there is tachycardia, marked conjunctival injection in 95% of subjects, myalgia, arthralgia and severe pain in the neck, back and legs, especially the tibia (shinbone fever). Several crops of erythematous macules or papules measuring 1 cm or less on the abdomen, chest and back may occur in 70–80% of patients. Symptoms are most severe during the initial episode, diminishing with each subsequent attack except bone pain, especially in the shins, which usually grows more severe with each attack. Although fatal cases have not been reported, the disease may persist for 4–6 weeks and result in prolonged disability. Relapses may occur years later and in some cases, there may be bacteraemia with no clinical signs. Persistent bacteraemia has long been also associated with *B. quintana* infection and Kostrzewski showed that *B. quintana* was present in the blood of trench fever patients up to 8 years after initial infection.[49]

Endocarditis

Bartonella bacteraemia may result in endocarditis mostly in people with existing heart valve abnormalities. The most common identified agents of *Bartonella* endocarditis are *B. quintana*, followed by *B. henselae*.[50] *B. quintana* endocarditis mostly develops in persons without any previous valvular injuries; known risk factors are alcoholism, homelessness and body lice infestation. *B. henselae* endocarditis patients frequently have a previous valvulopathy, and disease is associated with cat bites or scratches and cat flea exposure. However, sporadic cases of endocarditis have been also associated by *B. koehlerae*, *B. vinsonii* subsp. *berkoffii*, *B. vinsonii* subsp. *arupensis*, *B. elizabethae* and *B. alsatica*.[51] Patients with endocarditis tend to have pre-existing heart valve disease that promotes the development of infective endocarditis, and in some cases, a definite risk factor for infection specifically with *Bartonella* is present. Patients appear to have chronic, blood culture-negative endocarditis; fever is usually present (90%), a vegetation is usually observed on echocardiography (90%) and >90% of patients require valvular surgery.[47]

Cat-scratch Disease

B. henselae was discovered a quarter of a century ago as the causative agent of cat-scratch disease (CSD), a clinical entity described in the literature for more than half a century.

Transmission of *Bartonella henselae*

Cats are the main reservoir of *B. henselae*, and the bacterium is transmitted between cats by the cat flea (*Ct. felis*).[52] However, epidemiological data do not support efficient transmission from cat to human via *Ct. felis*[52] and most case series of CSD patients report that symptoms developed after the individual received a scratch.[53] The transmission of *B. henselae* from cat to human via a scratch is nevertheless a rare event, considering the number of pet cats and the frequency of cat scratches and bites inflicted by these pets. Experimentally, *B. henselae* was transmitted by transferring fleas from bacteraemic cattery cats to specific-pathogen-free (SPF) cats.[54] Fleas were placed on the kittens and within 2 weeks, four of the five kittens were found to be bacteraemic with *B. henselae*. In this study, it was not established whether *Ct. felis* served as both a mechanical and biologic vector; however, cat fleas can become infected and support the replication of *B. henselae* following ingestion of a blood meal from an infected cat.[55] Bartonellae are visible in dissected flea guts and can be cultured from flea faeces up to 9 days after fleas were fed infected blood.[55] The presence of *Ct. felis* is essential for the maintenance of *B. henselae* infection within the cat population[54] and it has been shown that the flea infestation is more frequent in bacteraemic than in non-bacteraemic cats and this association is even stronger when evaluating only pet cats.[56] Cats reported to have been infested with fleas during the preceding 6 months were also more likely to be seropositive than cats without fleas during the same period.[57] It is proposed that the higher seroprevalence of *B. henselae* in the pet cat population in warm, humid climates than in the cats in cold, dry climates is explained because *Ct. felis* is more common in warmer climates.[56] This is explained because the environmental conditions of temperature and relative humidity are the two most important factors for the successful reproduction, development and survival of fleas.[58] As a result, cats have more fleas during the summer and autumn months than in the other two seasons.[59] In conclusion, CSD is a seasonal infection that starts in September and finishes in April with a peak in December, which may be explained by both seasonality of the birth of cats and by the activity of their fleas.[60]

PATHOGENESIS

Transmission of *Bartonella* to humans by cat scratch or bite can result in a wide range of clinical symptoms, ultimately determined by the status of the immune system of the infected individual. Immunocompetent individuals develop most commonly CSD, a self-limiting but long-lasting swelling of the lymph node(s) draining the primary site of infection. *B. henselae*, *B. alsatica* and *B. quintana* are the causative agents of CSD.[61–63] The presence of *B. henselae* in the skin papule was first proposed by Margileth et al. who identified that the primary inoculation site and the lymph nodes of patients with CSD contained the same small Gram-negative bacilli.[64] Lin and colleagues, by the use of immunohistochemical stain, found that *B. henselae* existed in the cytoplasm of histiocytes within the granulomatous lesions in nine lymph nodes and one skin biopsy of patients with CSD.[65] Avidor and co-workers identified the presence of *B. henselae* in the inflammatory papules and pustules of two patients with CSD.[66] *B. henselae* was identified in the scalp eschars of patients with SENLAT (scalp eschar and neck lymphadenopathy after tick-bite)[10] and recently live *B. henselae* were identified in the primary inoculation site of three patients after a cat scratch was identified.[67] In the next 1–2 weeks following organism inoculation, there appears a self-limiting regional lymphadenitis in the lymph nodes that drain the area. At this stage, immunopathogenesis is assumed to play an important role, as *B. henselae* is infrequently grown from the lymph nodes of humans and *B. henselae* has been isolated from only a few patients with CSD.[63,68] In experimental models in mice, *B. henselae* was eliminated within a few days to 1 week after systemic (intraperitoneal or intravenous) infection.[69] Vermi and colleagues proposed that *B. henselae*-infected dendritic cells locally produce cytokines (interleukin (IL)-10) and chemokines (CXCL13) that contribute to the formation of the characteristic B cell and neutrophil-rich CSD granulomata.[70] Kunz and colleagues observed in mice that *B. henselae*-induced lymphadenopathy resulted from immune cell recruitment and enhanced B-lymphocyte proliferation.[69] Lymphadenopathy may sometimes last for months, and in a few cases can be prolonged for as long as 12–24 months.

Immunodeficient patients are at risk for bacillary angiomatosis, which manifests as cutaneous angiogenic lesions. The mechanism by which *B. henselae* induces angiogenesis is not fully understood and it is believed that *Bartonella* modulates host or target cell cytokines and growth factors, which leads to angiogenesis. When *Bartonella* adheres to or is phagocytozed by macrophages, these cells secrete vascular endothelial growth factor (VEGF). It is thought that *Bartonella* adhesin A is crucial for the secretion of VEGF and other proangiogenic cytokines.[71]

CLINICAL MANIFESTATIONS

Typical Cat-scratch Disease

Typical cat-scratch disease (CSD) is usually a self-limiting regional lymphadenitis. In most immunocompetent patients, a round, red-brown, non-tender papule develops in the scratch line after 3–10 days (Figure 30.3). In the next 1–2 weeks, one or

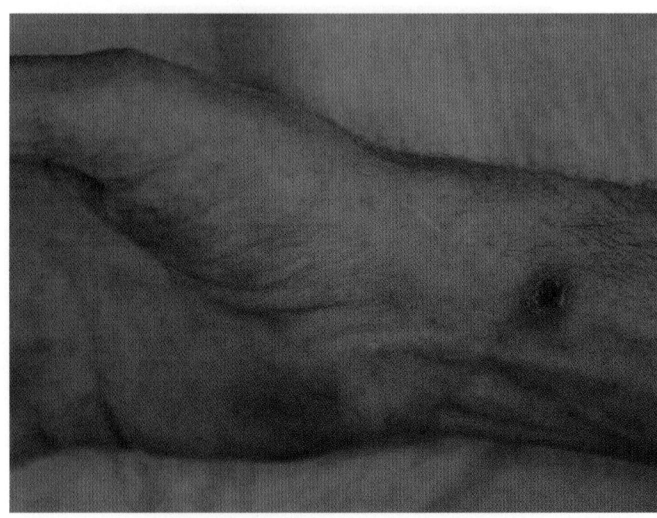

Figure 30.3 Papule in the scratch line.

more regional lymph nodes that drain the area gradually enlarge, reaching a maximal size of several centimetres or more in 2–3 weeks. Lymphadenitis usually regresses in size over a period of weeks or months, but in 10% of patients may become suppurative.[13] Lymphadenopathy is seen in all patients with typical CSD, and 85% of patients have only a single node involved.[72] Lymphadenopathy occurs most frequently in the axillary and epitrochlear nodes (46%), head and neck (26%) and the groin (17.5%).[72] Complications such as rash, hepatosplenomegaly, lytic bone lesions and deep lymphadenitis can occur in 5% of patients, most often in children.[13] Most patients with typical CSD remain afebrile and are not ill throughout the course of their disease. Lymphadenitis can last for 2–3 months. Some cases are more severe and more protracted, lasting up to several months, and many are so mild they remain unsuspected and undiagnosed.

Atypical Cat-scratch Disease

Atypical cat-scratch disease (CSD) occurs in a minority of cases (5–14%) with most patients suffering from severe systemic symptoms, reflecting a disseminated infection.[72,73] Patients with atypical CSD have prolonged fever (>2 weeks), myalgia, arthralgia-arthropathy, malaise, fatigue, weight loss, splenomegaly and Parinaud's oculoglandular syndrome.[52] Parinaud's oculoglandular syndrome appears to be the most common ocular complication of CSD, affecting approximately 5% of symptomatic patients. Parinaud's oculoglandular syndrome occurs when *B. henselae* bacilli are inoculated onto the conjunctiva of the patient, resulting in conjunctivitis and local adenopathy. Typical symptoms include foreign body sensation, unilateral eye redness, serous discharge and increased tear production. On examination, patients present with a necrotic granuloma with ulceration of the conjunctival epithelium and regional lymphadenopathy that affects the preauricular, submandibular or cervical lymph nodes.[74] The granuloma typically disappears after several weeks, without scarring.[72] Encephalopathy and neuroretinitis appear to be another less common manifestation of CSD with two-thirds of patients suffering from neuroretinitis having past evidence of infection by *B. henselae*. Other *Bartonella* spp. related with retinitis are *B. quintana*, *B. grahami*, *B. claridgeiae* and *B. elizabethae*. Retinitis is typically stellar. The onset of neurological complications varies from a few days to 2 months after the onset of lymphadenopathy. These complications tend to occur more often in older school-age children, and include encephalopathy, headache, malaise, lethargy lasting for 1 to several weeks, acute episode of left hemiplegia, optic disk oedema and macular star formation, loss of vision with central scotoma and glaucoma.[75]

Bacillary Angiomatosis and Peliosis Hepatis

Bartonella spp. have the ability to cause vasoproliferative lesions, a process of pathological angiogenesis resulting in the formation of new capillaries from pre-existing ones. These typical vasoproliferations are evident by lesions of the skin called bacillary angiomatosis (BA), which are caused by *B. quintana* and *B. henselae* and by a cystic form in liver and spleen called peliosis hepatis (PH) which is caused only by *B. henselae*. Skin lesions are manifested by gradual appearance of numerous brown to violaceous or colourless vascular tumors of the skin and subcutaneous tissues.[1] They may number from a few to several hundred and vary in size from a few millimetres to several centimetres.[1] Skin lesions are very similar to those reported for verruga peruana and three morphologically distinct cutaneous lesions have also been described.[1,31] BA has been most often reported in AIDS patients, less frequently in patients with other causes of immunosuppression and exceptionally in immunocompetent patients.[76] The potentially systemic nature of BA is reflected by involvement of brain, bone, lymph node, bone marrow, skeletal muscle, conjunctiva and mucosal surfaces of the gastrointestinal and respiratory tracts.[25] PH affects solid internal organs with reticuloendothelial elements and mostly the liver in which PH is defined as a vascular proliferation of sinusoidal hepatic capillaries resulting in blood-filled spaces, but the spleen, the abdominal lymph nodes and the bone marrow may also be involved.[52]

Diagnosis

The diagnosis of infections due to *Bartonella* spp. is difficult because of the fastidious nature of the bacteria and the non-specific clinical manifestations. Diagnostic techniques for *Bartonella*-related infections include: culture of the pathogen; detection of organisms in lymph nodes by immunofluorescence; molecular techniques, including PCR amplification of *Bartonella* spp. genes; and serologic analysis.

SPECIMEN COLLECTION

Different specimens are useful for the diagnosis of *Bartonella*-related infections, especially serum, blood and biopsy specimens. These specimens should be sampled as soon as possible after the onset of the disease. The diagnosis could also be made by the detection of *Bartonella* in various arthropods (xenodiagnosis), including ticks, lice and fleas. Ticks collected for use in attempts to isolate *Bartonella* spp. should be kept alive in a box which retains moisture prior to testing or they may also be frozen. The arthropod can be disinfected with iodinated alcohol and then be crushed in medium before being inoculated onto a shell vial for culture or being processed using molecular methods.[77]

CULTURE

The most widely used methods for isolation are direct plating into solid media, blood culture in broth and co-cultivation in cell culture. Generally, for the culture of *Bartonella* sp. either axenic media supplemented with sheep/horse blood agar[78] or cell cultures are used.[41] *Bartonella* sp. can be grown on blood agar at 37°C in a 5% CO_2 atmosphere except for *B. bacilliformis* that should be grown at 30°C. Primary isolates are typically obtained after 12–14 days, although an incubation period of up to 45 days may be necessary. The bacterial colonies are translucent to opaque in white or cream colour and sizes range from 1 to 3 mm in diameter.

The culture of *Bartonella* spp. in eukaryotic cells is reported to be more sensitive and more rapid for the growth of bacteria as compared to blood agar plates. Lysis centrifugation has been shown to enhance the recovery of *Bartonella* species as well as sample congelation from blood. Primary isolates are typically obtained after 12–14 days, although an incubation period of up to 45 days may be necessary.[79] The centrifugation-shell vial technique using ECV 304 human endothelial cell monolayers has been performed for culturing *Bartonella* sp. from samples of heparinized blood, cardiac valves, skin biopsies, lymph nodes or osteomedullar biopsies.[80]

MOLECULAR ASSAYS

Bartonella species can be detected from blood and tissues by using polymerase chain reaction (PCR). Various tissues may be used, including lymph node, cardiac valve, skin and liver. Althoug-embedded tissues may also be used for PCR-based assay. The current target genes used for the detection and identification of *Bartonella* species are the citrate synthase gene (*gltA*); the 16S RNA gene; the 16S-23S rRNA *ITS*; the 60-kDa heat-shock protein (*groEL*); and the *pap31* gene. Although these methods are highly specific, their sensitivity may vary according to the type of samples, and we recently proved that in cases of negative 16 S rDNA PCR, an infection by CSD agent is not excluded given the low sensitivity of eubacterial PCR.[61] Thus, the current strategy for the diagnosis of *Bartonella* infections is to use two different target genes (e.g. ITS gene and *pap31*), and if the results are discordant, to use a third gene (*groEL*).[61]

SEROLOGICAL ASSAYS

A more practical means of laboratory diagnosis is serology for *Bartonella* antibodies, because it avoids invasive sample collection, use of specialized equipment and techniques, and long incubation periods. Immunofluorescence assay (IFA) is the reference method to diagnose *Bartonella* infection and immunoglobulin G titres >1:50 indicate *Bartonella* infection, whereas titres >1:800 predict endocarditis.[81] Cross-reactions have been reported between *Bartonella* spp. and *Coxiella burnetii* or *Chlamydia pneumoniae*.[82] Western blot and cross-adsorption resolve this problem and can be used to determine the species involved.[83] Detection of *Bartonella* spp. using specific antibodies has been achieved in various cases. Visualization of microorganisms by the Whartin–Starry stain in valve tissues is a classic criterion for the histological diagnosis of infective endocarditis.

TABLE 30.2 Treatment of *Bartonella* Syndromes

Disease	Treatment	Duration
Typical CSD	No recommendation	
	Azithromycin (10 mg/kg) on day 1 and (5 mg/kg) per day on days 2–5	5 days
	Doxycycline (100 mg PO or intravenously (IV) twice daily) with rifampin (300 mg PO twice daily)	5 days
Neuroretinitis	Doxycycline (100 mg PO or IV twice daily) with rifampin (300 mg PO twice daily)	4–6 weeks
Hepatosplenic CSD	Rifampin (20 mg/kg per day) alone or with gentamicin or trimethoprim-sulfamethoxazole	4–6 weeks
Bacillary angiomatosis	Erythromycin (500 mg four times daily)	3 months
	Doxycycline (100 mg PO or IV twice daily) with rifampin (300 mg PO twice/day)	3 months
Peliosis hepatis	Erythromycin (500 mg four times daily)	4 months
	Doxycycline (100 mg PO or IV twice daily) with rifampin (300 mg PO twice/day)	
Trench fever	Gentamicin (3 mg/kg/day for 2 weeks) and doxycycline (200 mg/day for 4 weeks)	6 weeks
Endocarditis	Doxycycline (100 mg) 2 times daily orally for 6 weeks and gentamicin (3 mg/kg/day) in 1 intravenous daily dose for 14 days	8 weeks
Carrion's disease	Ciprofloxacin 500 mg PO	10 days
	Chloramphenicol 500 mg PO or IV and another antibiotic (a β-lactam is preferred)	10 days
Verruga peruana	Rifampin 10 mg/kg/day	14–21 days

IMMUNOHISTOCHEMISTRY

Immunological detection has been reported directly in the lymph nodes for patients suffering from cat-scratch disease (CSD); for patients with peliosis hepatis (PH); in red blood cells of bacteraemic homeless people; in cardiac valves and in cutaneous biopsies. On immunohistochemical tests, *Bartonella* species are observed in proliferating endothelial cells localized in the upper reticular dermis in patients with bacillary angiomatosis (BA).[46] Lepidi and co-workers have developed autoimmunohistochemistry, which is a peroxidase-based method with the patient's own serum as the source of antibodies directed against the aetiological microorganism for the diagnosis of infective endocarditis.[46] The rate of detection of bacteria by autoimmunohistochemistry was significantly higher than that by culture but was similar to that by PCR.[46]

Treatment

The various clinical manifestations and localizations of *Bartonella* spp. explain why a single treatment for all *Bartonella*-related diseases has not been found, and the approach to treatment must be adapted to each species and clinical situation (Table 30.2).[13] In addition, limited clinical studies exist with a standard case definition, culture confirmation, rigidly defined disease outcomes and patients with similar host defences. Clinical information about *Bartonella* treatment is mostly based on case reports with a very limited number of subjects.

CAT-SCRATCH DISEASE

Typical cat-scratch disease (CSD) is a self-limited illness that resolves within 2–6 months, and usually does not respond to therapy and management consists of treatment with analgesics for pain and prudent follow-up. However, many cases report the effectiveness of antibiotics for the treatment of typical, uncomplicated CSD.[84–86] Large painful lymph nodes can be removed surgically and in cases of long-lasting lymphadenopathy patients should be reassured that the adenopathy is benign and that it will probably subside spontaneously within 2–4 months.[86]

TRENCH FEVER-ENDOCARDITIS

Before the discovery of antibiotics, aspirin was the most effective drug for the pain caused by trench fever.[1] Foucault and co-workers reported that chronic *B. quintana* bacteraemia should be treated with a combination of doxycycline (200 mg PO daily for 28 days) and gentamicin (3 mg/kg of body weight IV once daily for 14 days).[87,88] Patients with chronic bacteraemia should be carefully evaluated for endocarditis, because the presence of this complication will necessitate a longer duration of therapy and closer monitoring. Raoult and colleagues found that patients receiving an aminoglycoside were more likely to recover fully ($p = 0.02$), and those treated with aminoglycosides for at least 14 days were more likely to survive than those with shorter therapy duration ($p = 0.02$).[89] Patients with suspected or proved *Bartonella* endocarditis should be treated with doxycycline 100 mg twice daily orally for 6 weeks in combination with gentamicin 3 mg/kg per day in 1 intravenous daily dose, for 14 days.[34]

OROYA FEVER

Before the antibiotic era, the treatment for Oroya fever was blood transfusion, but the effectiveness of this treatment was poor and the mortality rate was high.[1] Ciprofloxacin for 10 days is the recommended treatment for adults and children over age 6 years, without complications.[31] If a complication occurs during the acute phase, and the patient is not pregnant, then the treatment would be ciprofloxacin and ceftriaxone or ceftazidime for 10 days.[31] If the symptoms do not retreat within 72 hours after beginning the antibiotic treatment, a complication should be suspected.

VERRUGA PERUANA

Streptomycin (15–20 mg/kg per day for 10 days) was the traditional treatment for verruga peruana. However, its use is problematic, especially in children, so since the mid-1970s, rifampin has become the drug of choice for treatment of eruptive-phase bartonellosis.[1]

Prevention

As the cycle of the *Bartonella* spp. in nature remains unclear, likely predisposing epidemiological factors also remain uncertain, and thus it remains difficult to establish valid recommendations for the prevention of *Bartonella*-induced illnesses. For trench fever, the role of the human body louse (*Pediculus corporis*) as a vector and potential reservoir of *B. quintana* has often been proposed.[79,90] Transmission of *B. quintana* by this vector is also suspected in homeless people suffering from bacteraemia[91] and endocarditis.[41] People infested with body lice should bathe and use a pediculicide such as permethrin lotion, shampoo or powder on the hair-covered areas of the body. Clean clothes must be provided and old clothes, bedding, towels, etc. incinerated or washed and dried using the hot cycle of the washing machine and dryer. There is now both epidemiological and microbiological evidence for the involvement of domestic animals in the life cycles of *Bartonella* spp. Cat fleas live on both cats and dogs and are best controlled by fumigating areas where cats and dogs live. Also, veterinary advice should be sought about effective topical insecticides for cats and dogs in the household. Rather than depriving people of their cats, which often play an important role in improving the quality of life of patients, measures should be taken to prevent situations arising where scratches or bites are likely to occur. Sandflies can be controlled by spraying the environment with long-acting insecticides. Individual protection depends on avoiding exposed biotopes at night and the use of insect repellents N,N-diethyl-m-toluamide (DEET) or mosquito nets treated with permethrin/deltamethrin.

Human Ehrlichiosis

Ehrlichiosis and anaplasmoses are caused by bacteria within the family Anaplasmataceae. These diseases have been known for a long time in veterinary medicine but have been identified only recently in human medicine. Four pathogens have been recognized in humans: *Neorickettsia sennetsu* (formerly *Ehrlichia sennetsu*) the agent of glandular fever reported during the 1960s in Japan, *Ehrlichia chaffeensis* causing human monocytic ehrlichiosis, *Ehrlichia ewingii* causing granulocytic ehrlichiosis and *Anaplasma phagocytophilum* causing human granulocytic anaplasmosis.[92]

BACTERIOLOGY

The evolutionary relationships determined by 16S ribosomal RNA gene (*rrs*) and *groESL* comparisons indicate that *Ehrlichia* and *Anaplasma* spp., share a common ancestor with other obligate intracellular pathogens such as *Wolbachia, Neorickettsia, Orientia* and *Rickettsia*.[93] Agents of human tick-borne ehrlichiosis are small (approx. 0.4–1.5 μm), obligately intracellular Gram-negative bacteria that replicate in membrane-bound compartments inside host granulocytes (*E. ewingii*) or mononuclear phagocytes (*E. chaffeensis* and *E. canis*).[93] Ehrlichiae replicate within the host vacuoles forming microcolonies called morulae, derived from the Latin word 'morus' for mulberry.[94] All *Ehrlichia* species pathogenic for humans can be cultivated in cell culture except *E. ewingii*.[93] *Ehrlichia* have the characteristic Gram-negative cell wall structure, but lack important cell membrane components including lipopolysaccharide and peptidoglycan.[95] However, the ehrlichial cell wall is rich in cholesterol, which is derived from the host cell and appears to be important for ehrlichial survival and entry into mammalian cells.

EPIDEMIOLOGY

The dominant zoonotic cycle of *E. chaffeensis* involves a reservoir of many persistently infected white-tailed deer (*Odocoileus virginianus*) and the tick vector, *Amblyomma americanum* (lone-star tick), prevalent throughout south-east and south-central USA.[92] *E. chaffeensis* has been found in 5–15% of *A. americanum* ticks in 14 American states.[96] There is a lower prevalence of *E. chaffeensis* in nymphal ticks than adults.[97] Other reservoirs such as dogs and coyotes and other tick vectors including *Ixodes pacificus, Ixodes ricinus, Haemophysalis yeni, Amblyomma testudinarium, Amblyomma maculatum* and *Dermacentor variabilis* may also have a limited role in human transmission.[93] *Ehrlichia ewingii* was exclusively a canine pathogen until a series of human cases of *E. ewingii* infection were described in 1999.[98] Similar to *E. chaffeensis*, *E. ewingii* is transmitted by the lone-star tick.[92] The epidemiology of *E. ewingii* remains poorly defined due to the lack of a specific serological assay for this organism and the absence of a dedicated reporting system for this infection. Most infections reported to date have occurred in patients with HIV,[98,99] or who were immunosuppressed following organ transplantation.[100]

Human monocytotropic ehrlichiosis (HME) was first described in 1986, and now more than 2300 cases have been reported to the US Centers for Disease Control and Prevention (CDC) in the past 19 years.[93] *E. chaffeensis* resides primarily in south-eastern, south-central and mid-Atlantic USA, where *A. americanum*, is endemic.[101] Most cases reported to the CDC are from Missouri, Oklahoma, Tennessee, Arkansas and Maryland.[101] Active surveillance in endemic areas has suggested rates of HME of 100–200 cases per a population of 100 000.[93] The true incidence of human infection with *E. chaffeensis* is likely to be much higher, as two-thirds of the infections are either asymptomatic or minimally symptomatic.[93] A seroprevalence study found that 20% of the children residing in endemic areas had a detectable antibody to *E. chaffeensis*, without prior history of clinical disease.[102,103]

PATHOGENESIS

In vertebrate hosts, *E. chaffeensis* infects predominantly mononuclear phagocytic cells. The most frequently infected blood cells are monocytes, however, infections in other cell types have been described, including lymphocytes, atypical lymphocytes, promyelocytes, metamyelocytes and band and segmented neutrophils.[94] Although *E. chaffeensis* appears capable of inhabiting other phagocytic cells (e.g. granulocytes), it is likely that mononuclear phagocytes maintain the productive infection.[104] Infected cells typically contain only 1 or 2 morulae, although as many as 15 have been observed in leukocytes of immunosuppressed patients.[93]

CLINICAL MANIFESTATIONS

Within 1–2 weeks (median, 9 days) following exposure to an infecting tick, patients experience a prodrome characterized by malaise, low-back pain or gastrointestinal symptoms or may develop sudden onset of fever (often >39°C). The main clinical signs reported are fever (98%); malaise (30 to 80%); headache (77%); myalgias (65%); vomiting (36%); cough (25%); and neurological signs with changes in mental status (20%).[96] A skin rash that involves the trunk and extremities, and less commonly the face, occurs in 12–36% of patients and is more common in children (67%). Although age (>60 years) is an independent risk factor for severe or fatal human monocytic ehrlichiosis in some studies, many severe or fatal cases have been described in apparently healthy children or young adults. These also occur in immunocompromised patients.[96]

DIAGNOSIS

In endemic areas, the disease should be suspected in all patients presenting with fever, headache, elevated liver transaminases, thrombocytopenia and leucopenia, even if there is no history of tick attachment.

Occasionally, diagnoses can be made when morulae are seen in monocytes in Romanowsky-stained peripheral blood smears, buffy coat preparations or CSF. Various cell lines have been used, including a canine histiocytic line (DH82), a human monocytic leukaemia line (THP-1), HEL-22 cells (fibroblast-like cells), Vero cells and a human promyelocytic leukaemia cell line (HL-60).[105] Detection of ehrlichial DNA/RNA in peripheral blood is probably the best method to diagnose HME in the acute phase. Most often, this is with primers that amplify a section of the 16S rRNA gene.[105]

Most diagnoses are made using the indirect IFA. Many diagnoses are made retrospectively with convalescent phase sera, as relatively few patients (30%) seen in the acute phase of human monocytic ehrlichiosis have reactive antibodies.[106] Immunoblotting procedures have higher specificity than the indirect microimmunofluorescence antibody assay but are generally only available in research laboratories.

TREATMENT AND PREVENTION

Doxycycline (4 mg/kg per day in 2 divided doses; maximum, 100 mg/dose) has become the antimicrobial agent of choice, even in children.[105] In patients allergic to doxycycline, tetracycline (25 mg/kg per day in 4 divided doses; maximum, 500 mg/dose) or rifampin (20 mg/kg per day given in 2 divided doses; maximum, 600 mg) are acceptable alternatives[105] Antimicrobial therapy should be continued for at least 3 days after the patient becomes afebrile, with the minimum course being between 5 and 10 days.

Avoidance of tick-infested areas is the first line of defence in preventing cases of human ehrlichiosis. If the use of protective clothing is not practical, insect repellents containing DEET can be used.

REFERENCES

1. Rolain JM, Brouqui P, Koehler JE, et al. Recommendations for treatment of human infections caused by *Bartonella* species. Antimicrob Agents Chemother 2004;48(6):1921–33.

13. Jacomo V, Kelly PJ, Raoult D. Natural History of *Bartonella* infections (an exception to Koch's postulate). Clin Diagn Lab Immunol 2002;9(1):8–18.

19. Dehio C. Molecular and cellular basis of *Bartonella* pathogenesis. Annu Rev Microbiol 2004;58:365–90.

33. Raoult D, Roux V. The body louse as a vector of reemerging human diseases. Clin Infect Dis 1999;29:888–911.

52. Bass JW, Vincent JF, Person DA. The expanding spectrum of *Bartonella* infections: II. Cat scratch disease. Pediatric Infectious Disease Journal 1997;16(2):163–79.

Access the complete references online at www.expertconsult.com

31 Anthrax

EDWARD EITZEN

KEY POINTS

- *Bacillus anthracis* (anthrax) is a Gram-positive rod-shaped organism that forms hardy spores and inhabits the soil. The spore form may survive for decades in the soil under the right environmental conditions.
- In nature, anthrax is primarily a disease of herbivores, grazing animals such as cattle that ingest the organism.
- Humans may be infected by three main potential routes of exposure: by dermal contact, by ingestion and by inhalation. Three types of disease are produced by these routes, respectively: cutaneous anthrax, oropharyngeal or gastrointestinal anthrax and inhalational anthrax.
- Cutaneous disease is by far the most common human form and is fairly easily treated with antibiotics. Gastrointestinal and inhalational anthrax cases are often very severe and have a high case-fatality rate, but may be cured if treated early and aggressively with antibiotics and intensive supportive care.
- Anthrax is widely considered to be a key potential agent of biological warfare and bioterrorism by the aerosol route.

Epidemiology

Anthrax, derived from the Greek for coal or carbuncle, and the middle English *anthrax* for a 'malignant boil', occurs worldwide in animals, especially in Africa, Asia and in south-eastern Australia. Domestic herbivores (cattle, sheep, goats, and horses) or wild animals become infected when they ingest infective *B. anthracis* spores while grazing in contaminated areas or by eating contaminated feed or meat. Ingested spores are transformed in vivo into the vegetative bacilli that cause disease. When the animal dies, the contaminated carcass and infectious fluids re-contaminate the environment. Some geographic areas become endemic, where numerous animal cases have occurred, such as in the American Midwest and Southwest, where cattle were raised and driven to market over and over. Soil in these areas may be heavily spore-contaminated. The organism may be spread in the environment as fomites by insects or on the legs of vultures that have fed on contaminated carcasses.

Human cases occur when humans are exposed to infected animals or animal products, including hair and wool, meat, hides, carcasses and bone. The majority of human cases are cutaneous and associated with dermal exposure; more rarely gastrointestinal cases are caused by ingestion of contaminated meat and inhalational cases by inhalation of spores. In developed countries, cases tend to be sporadic and relatively rare, but in the developing world, large outbreaks can occasionally occur such as the one seen in Zimbabwe from 1978 to 1980, with an estimated 6000–10 000 cases. Inhalational anthrax has been referred to historically as 'wool-sorters' disease' because it had a propensity to occur in industrial settings where spore-contaminated animal hides were handled. In 1957, five cases of inhalational anthrax occurred in a plant in Manchester, New Hampshire, culminating in four deaths. However, inhalational disease is relatively rare – only 18 cases were reported in the USA in the twentieth century. In the 1800s, a number of cases occurred in the Bradford district of Britain, where a number of animal hair factories were located.

Anthrax is also often mentioned prominently as a potential agent of biowarfare and bioterrorism. In the 1950s and 1960s, both the USA and the former Soviet Union developed anthrax as a biological weapon, as have other countries such as Iraq, more recently. An accidental release of air-borne anthrax spores from a bioweapons production facility in the town of Sverdlovsk (now Ekaterinburg) in the former USSR (now Russia) in April of 1979, caused at least 66 deaths in persons downwind of the factory. In the autumn of 2001, a perpetrator mailed anthrax-laced letters to several high-profile sites along the East Coast of the USA, causing 22 cases of disease (11 inhalational and 11 cutaneous), five deaths among the inhalational cases, and contamination of newsrooms, congressional office buildings and postal facilities.

Pathogenesis and Pathophysiology

Anthrax is caused by a large, aerobic, non-motile, Gram-positive rod that forms spores under certain environmental conditions. The spores are relatively resistant to heat, desiccation and ultraviolet light exposure, especially in soil. The vegetative bacilli form grey-white colonies on growth media; colonies which have a ground-glass appearance. Most isolates are non-haemolytic. Many different strains of anthrax exist and there is genetic diversity even within strains.

The pathology produced by *Bacillus anthracis* is related to a number of virulence mechanisms. These include the anti-phagocytic capsule of the vegetative organism, encoded on a plasmid called pX02, and several toxins encoded on another plasmid called pX01. Included among these are protective antigen (PA), lethal factor (LF) and oedema factor (EF).

After exposure to anthrax spores, macrophages engulf the spores and carry them into the lymphatics, where they germinate into vegetative Gram-positive rod-shaped bacilli. The toxin-producing bacilli multiply and, after cytolysis, enter the bloodstream and are carried throughout the body. The bacilli release protective antigen (B subunit) and oedema and lethal factors (A subunits). PA combines with oedema factor to form oedema toxin; likewise lethal factor and PA combine to form lethal toxin. EF is a calcium- and calmodulin-dependent adenylate cyclase, whereas LF is a zinc-dependent metalloprotease. PA forms a heptameric structure after attaching to anthrax toxin receptors on cell surfaces – this structure functions to facilitate endocytosis of bound lethal factor and oedema factor into cells, followed by translocation of the toxins into endosomes. The toxins are released inside the cell and mediate increases of cyclic AMP with alterations of cell water homeostasis (EF), impairment of neutrophil function (EF), and inhibition of other pathways involving immune function and signal transduction, as well as cytolysis and release of proinflammatory mediators and lysosomal enzymes (LF). Full virulence of the anthrax organism requires the presence of the antiphagocytic capsule and all three toxin components. The anthrax toxins themselves may also cause significant alterations in peripheral vascular function and direct deleterious effects on myocardial and renal function thus contributing directly to the pathogenesis of severe anthrax disease. It has recently been demonstrated that there is human genetic variation in cellular sensitivity to anthrax toxins because of differences in genetic expression of several host cell surface proteins that function as receptors for the PA-LF and PA-EF toxins. In 254 people studied, the cells of three persons were virtually insensitive to the toxins, whereas the cells of some were hundreds of times more sensitive than those of others.

In inhalational anthrax, spores are carried to the perihilar and mediastinal lymph nodes, where they germinate and the organisms multiply rapidly, producing a haemorrhagic thoracic lymphadenitis, mediastinitis and pleural effusions. Septicaemia and toxaemia then occur and microbiological concentrations of bacilli in blood and body fluids can become very high. Overwhelming infection leads to sepsis, spreads to other organ systems, impairs ventilatory function, acidaemia and ultimately death. Inhalational anthrax has been said to have an 80–100% case-fatality rate, however with modern intensive supportive care and aggressive antibiotic treatment, 45% of inhalational anthrax patients in the 2001 mail attacks survived.

Clinical Features

Clinical features of anthrax depend on the route of exposure to the organism. The most common clinical form of the disease is *cutaneous anthrax*, due to dermal exposure, accounting for 95% of all cases. Cutaneous anthrax tends to occur in areas where the skin is abraded or cut, allowing penetration and localized infection. After 1–5 days, a small erythematous papule develops at the site of inoculation and develops into a vesicle containing fluid, serosanguineous in nature, in 1–2 more days. The vesicle then ruptures and a necrotic ulcer forms centrally; the central ulcer may also be surrounded by smaller peripheral vesicles. The ulcer then evolves into a central black eschar of 1–3 cm diameter over a week or so. The eschar finally separates after 1–2 more weeks, leaving a scar. The lesion is often surrounded by oedema that in some cases may be extensive, and patients often have fever, malaise and headache. The skin lesion is characteristically non-pruritic and non-purulent. The timing and progression of the skin lesion may not be changed significantly by antibiotic therapy. Mortality of cutaneous anthrax is less than 5% with adequate antibiotic treatment, and sepsis is rare.

Gastrointestinal anthrax results from the consumption of contaminated meat and is extremely rare. Ingestion of spores results in a full-blown haemorrhagic gastroenteritis. Signs and symptoms may include fever, abdominal pain that may be severe, haematemesis, bloody diarrhoea, hypovolaemia and prostration. Intestinal obstruction or perforation and ascites may occur. Sepsis is common and the case fatality rate is high, at 25–75%. There is also a rare *oropharyngeal* form of disease associated with spore ingestion. This form presents with severe sore throat, neck swelling, adenopathy, and dysphagia. Tonsillar or pharyngeal pseudomembrane formation and respiratory compromise may occur.

Inhalational anthrax results from inhalation of infectious spores that are usually from 1 to 5 microns (μm) in size. The estimated LD50 calculated from animal studies is 8000–10 000 spores, although, because of host factors, a much smaller spore dose may cause infection and death in some individuals. The small spore size allows penetration of the agent deep into the lungs and into the terminal bronchioles and pulmonary alveoli. Pulmonary macrophages take up the spores and they migrate to the perihilar and mediastinal lymph nodes where the spores germinate and form vegetative bacilli. Localized mediastinal and nodal infection occurs and bacilli are released into the bloodstream, causing toxaemia and septicaemia. Animal studies have revealed that bacilli and toxins appear in the bloodstream late on day 2 or on day 3, after aerosol challenge. Spread to other organ systems such as the CNS occurs. After an incubation period of 1–6 days, patients with the inhalational form of the disease develop fever, malaise and fatigue, often with chest discomfort and a non-productive cough; headache, drenching sweats, nausea and vomiting, myalgias and confusion may also occur. These manifestations may last 2–3 days, sometimes followed by a brief period of symptomatic improvement. These early phases are then followed by sudden deterioration, with severe respiratory distress, dyspnea and stridor, diaphoresis and cyanosis. Chest radiographs at this stage may reveal significant mediastinal widening and often, pleural effusions that may be haemorrhagic. Pneumonic infiltrates or consolidation may be seen on chest X-ray or CT scan but actual bronchoalveolar pneumonia is rarely found on autopsy. Sepsis, shock and death typically occur within 24–36 hours of clinical deterioration. Haemorrhagic meningitis is present in about 50% of cases of inhalational anthrax. Mortality in inhalational anthrax is very high: 80–90% if untreated. Even with aggressive intravenous antibiotic treatment and intensive supportive care, mortality is still almost 50% (5 out of 11 patients died in the 2001 anthrax mail attacks). Survivors may have significant sequelae for months or even years.

Differential diagnosis of cutaneous anthrax may include cutaneous diphtheria ulceroglandular tularemia, localized rickettsial infection after a tick-bite, bubonic plague, bacterial infection such as *Staphylococcus aureus* or *Streptococcus pyogenes*, and necrotizing arachnidism (spider envenomation). Oropharyngeal anthrax may be confused with diphtheria clinically. Inhalational anthrax would usually only be suspected clinically with potential occupational exposure or in a known bioterrorism attack. A high index of suspicion by an astute clinician is critical to the diagnosis. The inhalational form might be confused with other forms of severe respiratory disease, pneumonia, septicaemia and meningitis.

Clinical and Laboratory Diagnosis

Inhalational anthrax is initially a clinical diagnosis requiring a high index of suspicion. Recent history of occupational exposure or a bioterrorism attack is helpful. In such a historical setting, a severe infectious illness with respiratory compromise and widening of the mediastinum with or without pleural effusions on chest radiograph should be considered pathognomonic. Pleural fluid or CSF is often bloody. Fever, tachycardia, hypotension and hypoxaemia with elevated alveolar-arterial oxygen gradient may be present.

Clinical laboratory features may include an elevated leukocyte count, neutrophilia, elevated transaminases, metabolic acidosis and elevated creatinine.

Definitive laboratory diagnosis can involve a number of tests. Gram-staining of infected fluids or blood may reveal numerous Gram-positive rods in high concentration. The gold standard and most sensitive test is still classical microbiological culture of the organism from skin lesion aspirate, blood, pleural fluid or cerebrospinal fluid. Standard blood culture should show growth within 24 hours. Colonies are non-haemolytic on 5% sheep blood agar and are tyrosine deaminase negative.

Several other tests are useful in the reference laboratory. These include IFA with microscopy, ELISA, gamma-phage sensitivity, electro-chemiluminescence and nucleic acid amplification (PCR).

Pathology may also be helpful. Examination of punch biopsy specimens from a skin lesion may reveal the characteristic rod-shaped organisms. Postmortem pathological findings may include thoracic haemorrhagic lymphadenitis, haemorrhagic necrotizing mediastinitis and haemorrhagic meningitis.

Management and Treatment

Management and treatment of the different clinical forms of anthrax is complex and depends on: the potential route(s) of exposure; infectious dose to which exposed; host immunocompetence; age; possibility of pregnancy; severity of illness and other factors. All the nuances of management and antibiotic treatment are beyond the scope of this chapter and the reader should refer to more comprehensive, definitive references for consensus treatment recommendations, including antibiotic options and dosages.

Cutaneous anthrax in a setting where there is no risk of inhalational infection and no immune compromise may involve treatment with only 7–10 days of antibiotics. Oral penicillin, ciprofloxacin and doxycycline are the antibiotic options. Consensus recommendations call for ciprofloxacin or doxycycline until penicillin sensitivity is proven. A total of 60 days of treatment is recommended if there has been risk of aerosol exposure and the possibility of retained spores in the lung.

Antibiotic options for inhalational anthrax also include penicillin, ciprofloxacin and doxycycline. Antibiotics should be started immediately if the disease is suspected. Patients treated early, before severe disease develops, are more likely to survive. Penicillin was the classic treatment historically, as most natural strains are sensitive, however concerns about penicillin resistance or bioengineered resistant strains have prompted a recommendation for initial treatment with IV ciprofloxacin, especially in the setting of a suspected bioterrorism attack, until antibiotic sensitivities are determined. In patients with inhalational anthrax following the 2001 attacks, there was clinical information to suggest that patients treated with two or more antibiotics active against *B. anthracis* were more likely to survive. Thus, consensus recommendations in the wake of those attacks suggested that two or more antibiotics with in vitro activity should be used initially. In addition to ciprofloxacin (and other fluoroquinolones) and doxycycline, antibiotics with in vitro activity against *B. anthracis* include clindamycin, rifampin, imipenem, aminoglycosides, chloramphenicol, vancomycin, cefazolin, tetracycline, linezolid and the macrolides. Even in patients with full-blown inhalational anthrax who recover, antibiotic treatment for 60 days (switch to oral treatment after clinical recovery) due to the possibility of retained un-germinated spores in the lung, is recommended. Consideration of CNS penetration of antibiotics through the blood–brain barrier may be important in cases where anthrax meningitis is present.

Intensive supportive care in the ICU is critically important for inhalational anthrax patients. Antibiotics may sterilize the blood after a few doses, yet in patients where antibiotic therapy is begun after clinical deterioration, the outcome is usually poor. Ventilatory support, maintenance of adequate perfusion and oxygenation, and fluid management are all very important. Newer therapies that may be available, including anthrax immune globulin (AIG) and monoclonal antibody treatments against anthrax toxins, may be important for enhanced survival.

Prevention

Prevention of anthrax poisoning involves either prevention of exposure in occupational settings or immunization. In high-risk settings, immunization is preferred. In the USA, there is one FDA-licensed anthrax vaccine – Anthrax Vaccine Adsorbed (AVA, trade name BioThrax) – produced by a company called Emergent Biosolutions (formerly know as Bioport Corporation). This vaccine is a protective antigen-based product and works by stimulating antibodies to PA, thus inhibiting the ability of EF and LF toxins to enter human cells. It is given intramuscularly (IM) in the deltoid muscle in a five-dose series at 0 and 4 weeks, with three more injections at 6, 12 and 18 months. If risk of exposure continues, yearly boosters are recommended. Although there has been some resistance to use of AVA in some groups at risk (postal workers after 9/11 and a very small percentage of military recipients), it has been shown to be a generally safe and effective vaccine with relatively mild side-effects such as erythema and swelling at the injection site. Next-generation recombinant-PA vaccine candidates are under development but thus far none are licensed in the USA.

In the setting of a suspected bioterrorism event, those suspected of aerosol exposure to anthrax should receive post-exposure prophylaxis (PEP). PEP consists of 60 days of oral antibiotics, usually ciprofloxacin or doxycycline, with or without vaccination with AVA. Although animal studies have shown that 30 days of antibiotics in combination with anthrax immunization during the same period protects against inhalational anthrax after antibiotic cessation, the official recommendation has been 60 days of antibiotics, regardless of whether the patient receives AVA immunization, due to concern about retained viable spores in the lungs that might still germinate after the end of PEP antibiotic therapy. Patient compliance with 60 days of antibiotics may be poor, especially in well-feeling individuals, and close monitoring of those with potential aerosol exposure for onset of fever or other characteristic symptoms is important.

BIBLIOGRAPHY

Inglesby TV, O'Toole T, Henderson DA, et al. Anthrax as a biological weapon. Updated recommendations for management. Consensus statement. JAMA 2002;287(17):2236–52.

Meselson M, Guillemin J, Hugh-Jones M, et al. The Sverdlovsk anthrax outbreak of 1979. Science 1994;266:1202–8.

Plotkin SA, Brachman PS, Utell M, et al. An epidemic of inhalation anthrax, the first in the twentieth century. I. Clinical Features. Am J Med 1960;29:992–1001.

Purcell BK, Worsham PL, Friedlander AM. Anthrax. In: Dembek ZF, Lenhart MK, Lounsbury DE, et al, editors. Medical Aspects of Biological Warfare. Textbooks of Military Medicine. Washington: Borden Institute; 2007. p. 69–90.

Scott GM. Anthrax. In: Cook GC, Zumla AI, editors. Manson's Tropical Diseases. Philadelphia: Saunders/Elsevier; 2009. p. 1109–12.

Access the complete references online at www.expertconsult.com

32 Tetanus

C. LOUISE THWAITES | LAM MINH YEN

KEY POINTS

- Tetanus is a disease characterized by skeletal muscle stiffness and spasm. In severe cases, there is autonomic nervous system disturbance producing cardiovascular instability.
- Tetanus can be prevented by vaccination. Neonatal tetanus can be prevented by maternal vaccination during pregnancy.
- Tetanus is caused by a potent neurotoxin produced by the bacterium *C. tetani*. This results in skeletal muscle spasm and cardiovascular instability, which if untreated are often fatal.
- Diagnosis is clinical, although there are no defined clinical criteria.
- Treatment consists of antitoxin, muscle relaxants, cardiovascular and respiratory support and immunization.

Epidemiology

Tetanus causes an estimated 100 000 deaths each year. Tetanus is now primarily confined to developing countries as a consequence of inadequate immunization. Some 60% of tetanus deaths occur in neonates and children under the age of 5. In 2010, an estimated 19.3 million children did not complete their primary immunization course and only 68% of pregnant women were fully vaccinated.[1] Although the global incidence of tetanus has fallen, as worldwide vaccination coverage has improved, the World Health Organization has repeatedly failed to meet its deadlines for tetanus elimination and the disease remains an important global health concern.[2]

The causative agent of tetanus, *Clostridium tetani* is a ubiquitous organism, present in the soil and in human and animal faeces. Neonatal tetanus usually arises from contamination of the umbilical stump. Infection is linked to delivery on unclean surfaces, traditional midwifery practices such as cutting the umbilical cord with bamboo and applying soil, cow dung, clarified butter or even engine oil to the umbilical stump. Ritual surgery such as ear-piercing or circumcision may also cause infection. Even after maternal immunization, the infant is still at risk in many countries, as malaria and HIV reduce placental transfer of protective antibody. Antibody titres may also be low in other conditions such as post-chemotherapy and may warrant re-immunization.[3]

In children and adults, lacerations to feet and hands are common injuries associated with tetanus.[4] Otitis media is an important portal for the disease in children. Tetanus arising from injections (either therapeutic medical or drug abuse) carries an especially poor prognosis, as does tetanus arising from other internal sites of infection.

In the developed world, tetanus is rare: in 2010, there were nine cases in the UK. Similarly, US data from 2000–2008 show an average 0.1 cases per million population/year. Most cases occur in the elderly – a group at increased risk due to declining protective antibody levels. However, recent studies have shown that younger people are also vulnerable, due to missed immunizations or additional risk factors. Outbreaks have occurred in drug users – the exact reasons for this remain unclear, but it appears that many had incomplete vaccination or used a high-risk administration method known as 'skin popping'. Heroin users are known to be particularly at risk from tetanus. Heroin is sometimes mixed with quinine, which causes local necrosis, thus a favourable environment for *C. tetani* multiplication as well as its low pH facilitating toxin entry into nerves.

Pathology and Pathophysiology

C. tetani is a strictly anaerobic Gram-positive bacillus and is found in soil and animal faeces (Box 32.1). When subjected to adverse conditions, rounded terminal spores are formed: this gives the classical 'drumstick' appearance to the bacillus, although this is not always seen (Figure 32.1). *C. tetani* is described as Gram-positive, but from cultures more than 24 hours old, it is readily decolourized and thus can appear to be Gram-negative. It is motile by means of numerous flagella and when cultured on blood agar, this results in swarming, giving a film with a feathery margin on the surface of the agar. Increasing the concentration of agar in the medium will inhibit swarming. Discrete colonies are flat, translucent and show a narrow zone of haemolysis.[5]

The biochemical activity of *C. tetani* is limited. In general, it does not ferment sugars, although some strains will ferment glucose. Gelatin is slowly hydrolysed but other proteins used in laboratory tests are not digested. Indole is produced slowly, but not hydrogen sulphide. Neither lecithinase nor lipase is produced. Gas–liquid chromatography of broth culture extracts reveals the major bacterial products to be acetic, butyric and propionic acids.

Antibiotics to which the bacilli of *C. tetani* are susceptible include penicillin, erythromycin, clindamycin, tetracycline, chloramphenicol and metronidazole. The spores are very resistant to many physical and chemical agents. Spores may survive in boiling water for several minutes or longer (although they are destroyed by autoclaving at 121°C for 15–20 min), and they can survive desiccation, most household disinfectants and marked changes in pH. Spores are commonly found in soil from all areas of the world, and the organism may be found in animal and human faeces, although isolation rates have varied widely.[6]

BOX 32.1 FEATURES OF *C. TETANI*

- Strictly anaerobic Gram-positive spore-forming rod
- Spores are very resilient and widespread in soil, dust, and faeces throughout the world
- Produces a potent neurotoxin, tetanospasmin, which causes tetanus
- Sensitive to penicillin, metronidazole, tetracycline and erythromycin.

C. tetani requires low oxygen tensions for germination and multiplication. In well-oxygenated healthy tissue, germination does not occur and spores are removed by phagocytes. However, if spores are inoculated into damaged tissue, along with adjuvants such as soil, faeces, chemical substances or other bacteria, local oxygen tensions are lowered and favourable conditions are created for germination and vegetative growth.

Only toxin-producing strains of *C. tetani* are capable of causing disease. The toxin is a potent neurotoxin, encoded on a 75 KB plasmid, and produced as a single chain (molecular mass 150 kDa) which undergoes post-translational cleavage to form one heavy and one light chain linked by a disulphide bond. The entire amino acid sequence has been determined and is similar to that of the botulinum toxins, but as botulinum toxins are not transported into the central nervous system, they produce a different clinical picture.

Tetanus toxin enters the nervous system from adjacent muscle. It may also be disseminated to distant sites via the lymphatics and the blood. Neuronal internalization results from binding of the carboxy terminal of the heavy chain to predominantly neuronal gangliosides – hence the neurospecificity of the toxin. The toxin then undergoes retrograde axonal transport from the periphery followed by trans-synaptic transition to presynaptic nerves, where it exerts its effects. The toxin light chain is a zinc-dependent metalloprotease which cleaves the vesicle-associated membrane protein 2, VAMP-2 (or Synaptobrevin).[7] This protein is a key component of the SNARE (soluble N-ethylmaleimide-sensitive factor attachment protein receptors) complex responsible for endocytosis and release of

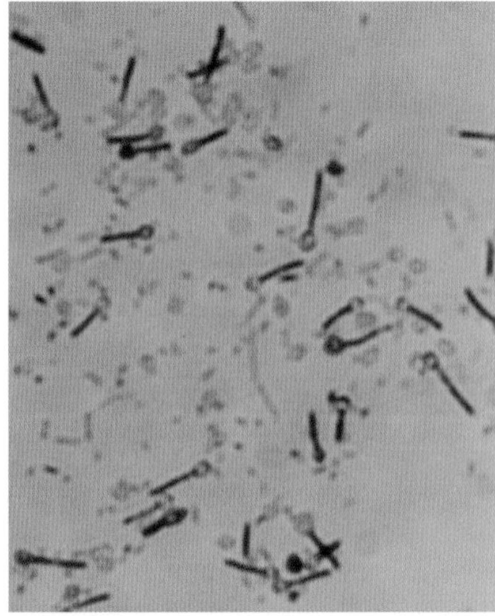

Figure 32.1 *C. tetani. (Courtesy of J. Campbell.)*

neurotransmitter. By this mechanism, tetanus toxin blocks the release of neurotransmitter. The toxin acts as a presynaptic inhibitor at many neuronal sites including the neuromuscular junction, but its principal effect is on the γ-aminobutyric acid (GABA) inhibitory interneurones, normally responsible for inhibition of motor neurones. Reduced inhibition at this site results in disinhibited motor neurone discharge, which gives rise to characteristic features of muscle rigidity and spasms. Muscle groups with the shortest neuronal pathways are affected first – hence trismus and dysphagia are common early symptoms.

Disinhibition of the autonomic nervous system also occurs and results in uncontrolled sympathetic and parasympathetic discharge. Tetanus toxin is able to enter adjacent neurones and spread within the CNS. Animal experiments with radiolabelled toxin show transportation of toxin within the brain stem. The effects of toxin here may explain the cardiovascular, respiratory and temperature disturbances seen in severe cases of the disease.

Clinical Features

Signs and symptoms of tetanus result from the actions of the neurotoxin within the central nervous system. Disinhibition of motor nerves results in increased muscle tone and symptoms of muscle stiffness and aches. Increasing disinhibition gives rise to skeletal muscle spasm – the characteristic feature of tetanus. The rate of symptom progression varies but is generally faster in more severe disease and can be used for prognosis (Table 32.1). There is an initial asymptomatic period after inoculation with *C. tetani* termed the incubation period (commonly 7–10 days). This is followed by a period of increasing symptoms, eventually resulting in muscle spasm – the period of onset (approx. 24–72 hours). Common early symptoms are trismus (lockjaw), muscle stiffness, back pain and general myalgia. Signs can sometimes be confined to muscles adjacent to the site of the wound (local or cephalic tetanus) but usually involve the whole body (generalized tetanus).

In very mild forms of tetanus, muscle stiffness and pain may be the only symptoms. However, most patients will progress to experience spasms. Spasms are phasic amplifications in muscle tone, varying in intensity and duration from brief twitches to prolonged contractions. They are most pronounced during the first 2 weeks of the disease. Spasms occur spontaneously or as a result of stimuli such as loud noises, bright lights or physical manipulation. Spasms have been reported to cause vertebral fractures or tendon avulsions but this is very rare. Facial muscle involvement results in the characteristic facial appearance of the 'risus sardonicus' or 'sardonic smile' (Figure 32.2). Involvement of muscles of the back and neck produces opisthotonos (Figure 32.3). Particularly serious are spasms involving the respiratory muscles which, if frequent or prolonged, may result in death due to asphyxia. Laryngeal spasm involving the vocal cords usually occurs without warning relatively early in the course of the disease and can result in acute airway obstruction. Aspiration is a particular problem in tetanus, occurring as a consequence of the combination of excessive secretions and inability to swallow due to pharyngeal muscle rigidity. Together, these factors explain why hypoxia is a common feature in those presenting with moderate to severe tetanus.

The advent of mechanical ventilation has led to a reduction in mortality from respiratory failure, but in doing so has

TABLE 32.1 Tetanus Severity Score (TSS), Calculated from the Total of Individual Section Scores

		Score
Age	≤70 years	0
	71–80 years	5
	>80 years	10
Time from 1st symptom to admission	≤2 days	0
	3–5 days	–5
	>5 days	–6
Difficulty breathing on admission	No	0
	Yes	4
Co-existing medical conditions[a]	Fit and well	0
	Minor illness or injury	3
	Moderately severe illness	5
	Severe illness not immediately life-threatening	5
	Immediately life-threatening illness	9
Entry site[b]	Internal or injection	7
	Other (including unknown)	0
Highest systolic blood pressure recorded during 1st day in hospital (mmHg)	≤130	0
	131–140	2
	>140	4
Highest heart rate recorded during 1st day in hospital (bpm)	≤100	0
	101–110	1
	111–120	2
	>120	4
Lowest heart rate recorded during 1st day in hospital (bpm)	≤110	0
	>110	–2
Highest temperature recorded during 1st day in hospital (°C)	≤38.5	0
	38.6–39	4
	39.1–40	6
	>40	8

[a]Defined according to ASA Physical Status Scale.
[b]'Internal' site includes postoperative/postpartum or open fractures; 'injection' include intramuscular, subcutaneous or intravenous injections.

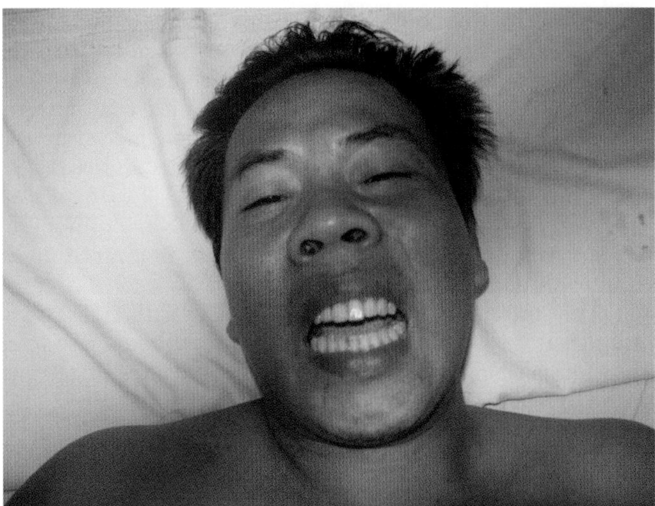

Figure 32.2 Facial spasm causing appearance of 'Risus Sardonicus'.

unmasked another major cause of mortality: the syndrome of autonomic overactivity. This usually becomes apparent during the second week of the illness and typically takes the form of sustained labile hypertension and tachycardia, accompanied by pyrexia and profuse sweating. Circulating catecholamines are raised, even compared with critically ill patients with other diseases and adrenaline is particularly elevated, indicating the involvement of the adrenal medulla.[8] Occasionally, the opposite occurs: bradyarrhythmias, refractory hypotension and even cardiac arrest. This is usually a pre-terminal event.

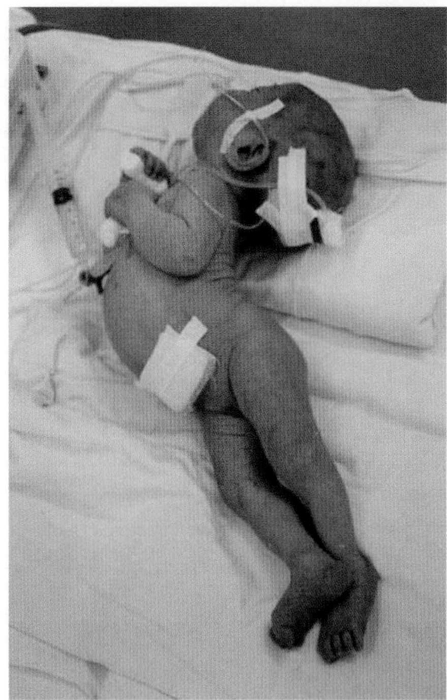

Figure 32.3 Opisthotonos.

Autonomic system dysfunction commonly affects the gastrointestinal system, resulting in excessive production of secretions, gastric stasis or diarrhoea. The syndrome is also associated with acute renal failure. This occurs in the absence of rhabdomyolysis and is characteristically non-oliguric.

Diagnosis

Tetanus is a clinical diagnosis based on the presence of clinical features and the absence of proper immunization. Isolation of *C. tetani* from a wound is supportive but not diagnostic and the bacterium is difficult to culture. In many cases, no entry wound can be found.

The differential diagnosis includes strychnine poisoning, which may closely mimic tetanus. Strychnine is a competitive antagonist of the inhibitory neurotransmitter glycine, which results in presynaptic disinhibition, leading to hyperreflexia, severe muscle spasms and convulsions. There is usually a history of ingestion and symptoms may begin within 30 minutes; toxicological tests of urine, serum or gastric contents can confirm the diagnosis.

Dystonic reactions to phenothiazines may simulate trismus and may cause spasms of the back resembling opisthotonos. However, the abnormality rapidly disappears after administration of anticholinergic agents.

Treatment

Management of tetanus is essentially supportive. It involves three main strategies: to prevent further toxin release; to neutralize any unbound toxin; and to minimize effects of

BOX 32.2 TREATMENT OF TETANUS

- Neutralize unbound antibody with antitoxin – consider using intrathecal administration
- Eradicate *C. tetani* using antibiotics (metronidazole) and clean/debride wound
- Establish and maintain a secure airway – tracheostomy or endotracheal intubation if experienced
- Control muscle spasms using muscle relaxants or neuromuscular blocking agents
- Stabilize autonomic effects using sedation, fluids, inotropes or magnesium sulphate as indicated
- Full course of immunization.

already-bound toxin, while maintaining the airway and adequate respiration (Box 32.2).

Prompt debridement of the wound is essential to prevent further multiplication and toxin release of *C. tetani*. Metronidazole is the antibiotic of choice (adult dose of 400 mg rectally or 500 mg IV every 6 hours for 7 days). Penicillin is still widely used, although patients treated with metronidazole have fewer spasms and require less sedation than those treated with penicillin. Penicillin is similar in structure to GABA, and although it does not readily cross the blood–brain barrier, in high doses, it can act as a central GABA competitive antagonist, thus exacerbating the effects of tetanus toxin.

Unbound toxin should be neutralized with antitoxin. Historically, equine anti-tetanus serum has been used, but it is associated with a high incidence of anaphylactic reactions. In many countries it has now been replaced by the human tetanus immune globulin (HTIG). Much debate has centred on the best route of administration of antitoxin. Results of animal experiments almost 100 years ago suggested that intrathecal administration of antitoxin may be superior and recent work has once again suggested that intrathecal immunoglobulin (50–1500 IU HTIG) may indeed reduce progression to more severe disease and reduce hospital stay and length of mechanical ventilation in both adults and neonates.[9]

Good nursing care is crucial to the outcome of patients with tetanus. All patients should be nursed in quiet, dark rooms to minimize provoked spasms. Frequent turning is necessary to prevent the development of pressure sores, although truncal rigidity of the patients makes this difficult. Patients who are unable to swallow will require a nasogastric tube. Close attention should be paid to fluid balance as tetanus patients have greatly increased insensible fluid losses. Up to 3.5 L/day of insensible losses may occur, especially in the presence of autonomic dysfunction.

Benzodiazepines are the mainstay of treatment in mild to moderate tetanus. As inhibitors of an endogenous inhibitor at the GABAA receptor they oppose the effects of tetanus toxin on the GABA-ergic neurones. Diazepam is the most commonly used although its long half-life, and those of its metabolites, may cause prolonged effects. It can be given orally in mild cases, or intravenously in more severe disease.[10] Doses up to 100 mg/h have been reported, and up to 200 mg/day is common. Intravenous infusion of midazolam may be a preferred option by virtue of its shorter half-life, although prolonged use will still lead to accumulation. The anaesthetic agent propofol has been used to provide sedation and additional muscle relaxation. It is non-cumulative and has a short duration of action, making it an attractive adjunct.

If spasms persist despite benzodiazepine therapy, then paralysis and mechanical ventilation should be instituted. Non-depolarizing muscle relaxants, with minimal cardiovascular effects, are the muscle relaxants of choice. Older agents, such as pancuronium, may exacerbate autonomic instability. Tracheostomy is the usual means of securing the airway, allowing ventilation and secretion clearance. Patients with laryngeal spasm may require urgent tracheostomy. For this reason all tetanus patients should be nursed under close supervision with appropriately skilled personnel at hand to deal with any emergencies.

Tetanus literature contains many reports of the use of other agents used to treat spasticity: dantrolene has been used to reduce spontaneous muscular spasms, but it is potentially hepatotoxic if used for prolonged periods. The GABAB agonist baclofen has also successfully suppressed spasticity.

In patients with autonomic instability, the usual manifestation is a tachycardia accompanied by hypertension. First-line therapy in this situation has been intravenous or intramuscular morphine. It inhibits sympathetically mediated vasoconstriction and induces peripheral arteriolar vasodilatation by inhibiting central sympathetic discharge. Other opioid agents with shorter half-lives have also been reported to be beneficial, although no randomized controlled trials have been performed. Peripheral beta-adrenoceptor blockade alone is usually insufficient to gain satisfactory cardiovascular control in severe cases of tetanus. The relatively long duration of action of most agents has been associated with subsequent refractory hypotension and cardiac arrest. The combined α- and β-blocker labetalol may confer some advantages, but its duration of action is still too long to be a useful alternative. The short-acting β-blocker, esmolol, however, has been used successfully. Peak effects are observed within 6–10 minutes of injection, and have almost completely disappeared after 20 minutes. Chlorpromazine, clonidine and epidural bupivacaine have all been used with success in the past. Recent interest has surrounded magnesium sulphate – a vasodilator and muscle relaxant that offers the potential to control both muscle spasms and autonomic instability. An initial series reported such benefits that the authors suggested it as an alternative to benzodiazepines as a first-line agent, however a larger randomized controlled trial has not shown such convincing benefits, although it does indeed appear to have beneficial effects in controlling spasms and reducing autonomic instability.[11]

Hypotension may be treated by head-down positioning, noxious stimulation or inotropic agents. Bradyarrythmias require atropine.

Finally, the amount of toxin circulating in natural disease is insufficient to provoke an immunizing antibody response. Therefore all patients should receive a full course of tetanus toxoid to prevent recurrences.

Prevention

The prevention of tetanus depends on primary immunization and the thorough management of wounds in those people who have not been immunized or whose immune status is thought to be inadequate. In addition, health education and improved socioeconomic conditions are important, e.g. the use of aseptic techniques in the management of the umbilical cord and the provision of adequate protective footwear.

Tetanus toxoid is produced by formaldehyde treatment of the toxin (plain toxoid). Although it is a relatively good immunogen, the duration of antibody response is much improved by adsorption with aluminium hydroxide as an adjuvant. It may be given alone, or preferably in combination with diphtheria toxoid. Tetanus toxoid is considered very safe, even in immunocompromised individuals.

The WHO recommends a 6-part primary immunization programme, with 5 childhood doses (3 under 1 year and boosters aged 4–7 years and 12–17 years), with one further dose in adult life, e.g. first pregnancy or military service.

In the UK, the first dose is given at 2 months of age, followed by the second and third doses at 4-week intervals. Adsorbed toxoid is available in combination with diphtheria toxoid and pertussis vaccine (DTP) for use in these immunization schedules of young children. Two booster doses of tetanus and diphtheria toxoids (DT) are given at 3–5 years of age and at 13–18 years old. In the USA, an initial four-dose schedule is recommended with intervals of 4–8 weeks between the first three doses and the fourth dose 6–12 months later. A booster is given at 4–6 years old and again 10 years later. In the USA, advice is to give additional booster doses of adsorbed tetanus toxoid every 10 years. However, in the UK, advice is that five doses (primary course plus two boosters) are sufficient and additional booster doses are not recommended unless a tetanus-prone wound occurs.

Neonatal tetanus may be prevented by immunization of women during pregnancy. In women with incomplete or unknown vaccination history, two or preferably three doses of adsorbed toxoid should be given, with the last dose at least 2–4 weeks prior to delivery. Immunity is passively transferred to the fetus and the antibodies will remain long enough to protect the baby during the neonatal period. Special care should be taken to ensure those with HIV or living in malaria-endemic areas receive a full course of vaccination.

Prevention of tetanus also depends on the effective management of wounds. It is most important that wounds are thoroughly cleaned, all foreign material removed and non-viable tissue debrided. Particular attention should be given to tetanus-prone wounds. These include puncture wounds, burns, animal and human bites, wounds contaminated with soil or faeces and any wound where treatment is delayed. These wounds should not be sutured: packing, frequent inspection and delayed primary closure is preferable. Antibiotic chemoprophylaxis is of secondary importance to good surgical management and immunoprophylaxis. When indicated, a long-acting penicillin can be given. If the wound is infected with β-lactamase-producing staphylococci, an appropriate alternative antibiotic such as erythromycin or flucloxacillin should be used.

A history of previous immunization should be sought, as this will determine the exact type of immunoprophylaxis to be given. If the patient has received a full course or a booster of tetanus toxoid within 10 years, a further dose is not required. If the last dose was more than 10 years previously, a further dose should be given. Where there is doubt about previous immunization or a full course was never completed, a full course of adsorbed tetanus toxoid should be commenced.

Passive immunization with HTIG (250 units) should also be given for tetanus-prone wounds occurring in people with inadequate immunization status (i.e. incomplete, unknown or a booster more than 10 years previously). Even where immunization is adequate (the last dose within 10 years) a dose of HTIG may be given if the risk of developing tetanus is high. If HTIG is not available, equine antiserum (1500 units) is an alternative. Very high-risk wounds are those with heavy soil or faecal contamination, extensive burns or where foreign material or necrotic tissue cannot be removed. In these cases, or if more than 24 hours have elapsed, the dose of HTIG should be doubled to 500 units and a further dose may be given after 4 weeks if the wound is still not clean or healed. Both toxoid and immunoglobulin can be given at the same time provided that separate injection sites are used.

REFERENCES

2. Roper MH, Vandelaer JH, Gasse FL. Maternal and neonatal tetanus. Lancet 2007;370(9603):1947–59.
4. Thwaites CL, Yen LM, Nga NT, et al. Impact of improved vaccination programme and intensive care facilities on incidence and outcome of tetanus in southern Vietnam, 1993–2002. Trans Roy Soc Trop Med Hyg 2004;98(11):671–7.
5. Brook I. Current concepts in the management of *Clostridium tetani* infection. Expert Rev Anti Infect Ther 2008;6(3):327–36.
9. Kabura L, Ilibagiza D, Menten J, et al. Intrathecal vs. intramuscular administration of human antitetanus immunoglobulin or equine tetanus antitoxin in the treatment of tetanus: a meta-analysis. Trop Med Int Health 2006;11(7):1075–81.
10. Okoromah CN, Lesi FE. Diazepam for treating tetanus. Cochrane Database Syst Rev 2004(1):CD003954.

Access the complete references online at www.expertconsult.com

33

Plague

MINOARISOA RAJERISON | MAHERISOA RATSITORAHINA | VOAHANGY ANDRIANAIVOARIMANANA

KEY POINTS

- The plague bacterium *Yersinia pestis* is maintained by rodents and their fleas. Humans are incidental hosts and are extremely susceptible to plague infection.
- Human plague cases mainly occur in remote areas where the disease is endemic and where people live in unsanitary conditions. The rapidly progressing, serious illness in humans can be treated with antibiotics ensuring full recovery when detected early enough. However, resistant strains are an increasing problem.
- Current plague vaccines have not been proven to be an approach that can effectively prevent plague outbreaks. Vaccination is of little use during human plague outbreaks, since a month or more is required to develop a protective immune response. Plague is always a medical emergency. In some circumstances (to be determined according to IHR decision tree), it can also be considered as a public health emergency.
- Suspected plague patients with evidence of pneumonia should be placed in isolation and managed under respiratory droplet precautions; for all other suspected plague cases, standard patient-care precautions should be used.

Epidemiology

During the course of human history, three plague pandemics have been recorded. The first pandemic, also known as the Justinian's plague, originated in Egypt in approximately 540 AD. The second pandemic referred to as the 'Black Death' was introduced into Sicily in 1347 AD. It was estimated that up to one-third of the European population was killed during this epidemic. The third pandemic started in the Chinese province of Yünann, reached Hong Kong and Canton in 1894 and Bombay in 1898. The vast trading network by steamships and railways has favoured the spread of the disease via its rodent host throughout the world. The constant colonization of new geographic areas allows the establishment of stable enzootic foci (particularly in endemic countries in Africa, Asia and the Americas).

Today, endemic foci still persist in Africa, Asia and the Americas. During the 10 years from 1999 to 2009, over 24 000 human cases were reported to the World Health Organization (WHO) by 20 countries.[1] The African region accounted for more than 96% of the total cases, with 35% of the world's reported cases from Madagascar. In 2009, a considerable drop in the annual incidence was recorded for the Democratic Republic of Congo and Madagascar, which had been the most affected countries in Africa (Figure 33.1).

Plague is now classified as a re-emerging disease, since several outbreaks have reappeared after decades of silence in areas within countries such as Madagascar, India, Algeria, Libya and Peru.

Plague is a flea-borne zoonosis and maintained in nature through transmission between fleas and their rodent hosts. The universal flea, *Xenopsylla cheopis* is the main vector in the plague cycle and found in most foci representing a high risk for transmission to humans.

Rodent species and their susceptibility to plague differ considerably depending on the geographical location of the focus. The great gerbil (*Rhombomys opimus*), for example, represents the major source of human plague in Central Asia and in the desert regions of Kazakhstan. This species is resistant to plague, whereas black-tailed prairie dog (*Cynomys ludovicianus*) hosts in the north of the USA are highly susceptible. In Madagascar, the susceptible *Rattus rattus* is the main reservoir of plague.[2]

Plague is seasonal in most endemic countries, depending on environmental characteristics (altitude, temperature, humidity, rainfall, etc.). In Madagascar, the plague season in the central highlands (altitude >800 m) extended from October to April, which correlates with the rainy tropical summer season, while in the port city of Mahajanga, on the west coast, the human cases are recorded mostly between July and November, which is characteristically a dry and cool season.[3] Plague seems to be correlated to climate and in Central Asia, plague among great gerbils has been found to be positively correlated with wetter summers and warmer springs.

Pathogenesis and Pathology

PATHOGENESIS

Within the *Enterobacteriaceae* family, the genus *Yersinia* is composed of environmental species, a fish pathogen, two enteropathogenic species (*Yersinia enterocolitica* and *Yersinia pseudotuberculosis*) and the plague bacillus *Y. pestis*. It has been demonstrated that *Y. pestis* has evolved from *Y. pseudotuberculosis* only within the last 20 000 years. Although these two species share a high degree of homology at the genomic level, they differ radically in their pathogenicity and transmission. Indeed, *Y. pestis* has caused three pandemics, including millions of deaths, whereas *Y. pseudotuberculosis* only causes a mild enteric disease that rarely leads to death.[4]

Plague remains primarily a disease of rodents and their associated fleas. Distinct subsets of genes are differentially expressed during the *Y. pestis* life cycle and are regulated by temperature. While in the insect, *Y. pestis* expresses the hms chromosomal gene required for biofilm formation, essential for blocking of flea proventriculus. To promote the colonization of flea midgut, phospholipase D encoded by the 100 kb pFra plasmid, is needed.

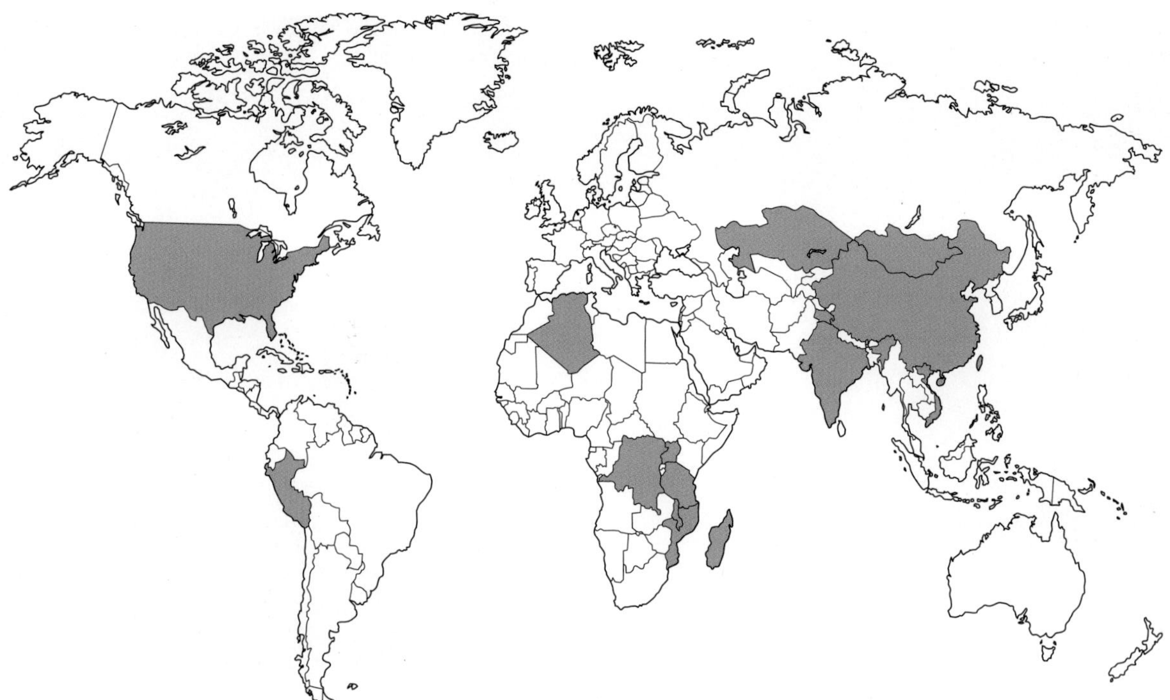

Figure 33.1 Countries that notified cases of human plague to WHO, 2002–2005.[2]

Once in the mammalian host (a temperature shift from <26 to 37°C), the pPst plasmid (9,5 kb) encodes a plasminogen activator that facilitates the dissemination of *Y. pestis* from the inoculation site. Another virulence factor encoded by pFra plasmid is the fraction 1 (F1) capsular antigen which is a highly immunogenic protein involved in the ability of *Y. pestis* to prevent phagocytosis by macrophages. However, *Y. pestis* strains lacking F1 antigen expression have also been reported to be virulent. Moreover, a 70 kb- pCD1 plasmid common to all three *Yersinia* pathogen species encoded the type III secretion system (T3SS) and the associated effector proteins, generally designated as *Yersinia* outer proteins (Yops) and the LcrV allowing the bacteria to circumvent the host immune system.

PATHOLOGY

In nature, fleas feeding on a septicaemia host, prior to its death, become infected. The infected flea transmits *Y. pestis* to mammals during subsequent blood meals via an early phase (blockage/biofilm-independent) mechanism and/or by a blockage/biofilm-dependent mechanism. Shortly after entering the mammal, *Y. pestis* infects macrophages that serve as transport for the bacteria to regional lymph nodes. Within the lymph nodes, they multiply to high levels resulting in the characteristic swollen buboes that become necrotic and haemorrhagic; a sign that the host immune response failed to respond. The bacteria then leave the lymph node and spread via the bloodstream to the liver and spleen to initiate septicaemia. During the course of bubonic plague, the lungs can become infected leading to secondary pneumonic plague. Transmission between humans or non-human primates via respiratory droplets causing primary pneumonic plague is almost 100% fatal without prompt and appropriate treatment.

Clinical Features

BUBONIC PLAGUE

In humans, plague most commonly presents in the bubonic form of the disease, which is mostly associated with the bite of an infectious flea or rarely with direct contact with infectious bodily fluids or tissue of a host. Symptoms appear after an incubation period of 2–6 days but occasionally longer, with acute and very rapid onset of nonspecific symptoms, including high fever (38–40°C), malaise, headache, muscle aches, and sometimes nausea and vomiting. At the same time, or within 24 hours, the patient notices buboes characterized by severe pain, swelling and marked tenderness. A patient suffering from bubonic plague is distinguishable from patients with other lymphadenitis by the absence of cellulitis (caused by injury or toothache), by the rapid onset of symptoms and by the rapid decline of the patient's condition.

The lymph node responsible for draining the area proximal to the site of infection is affected and a bubo develops. There is surrounding oedema and the overlying skin is warm and reddened. At days 2 or 3 of the onset of symptoms buboes of the size of a bean (in 35% of cases) or slightly larger are easy to identify by palpation. Palpation at this stage is usually painful or very uncomfortable for the patient, who also limits movement, pressure, and stretching around the bubo; even contact with clothes is very painful.

On day 5 or 6 without effective antimicrobial treatment, bubonic plague may progress to an increasingly toxic state of fever, tachycardia and lethargy leading to prostration, agitation and confusion and, occasionally, convulsions and delirium. Failure of the body to filter out and kill the bacteria in the lymph node allows haematogenous spread and invasion of peripheral organs. Progression to this systemic stage of disease, termed septicaemic plague, is marked by a mortality

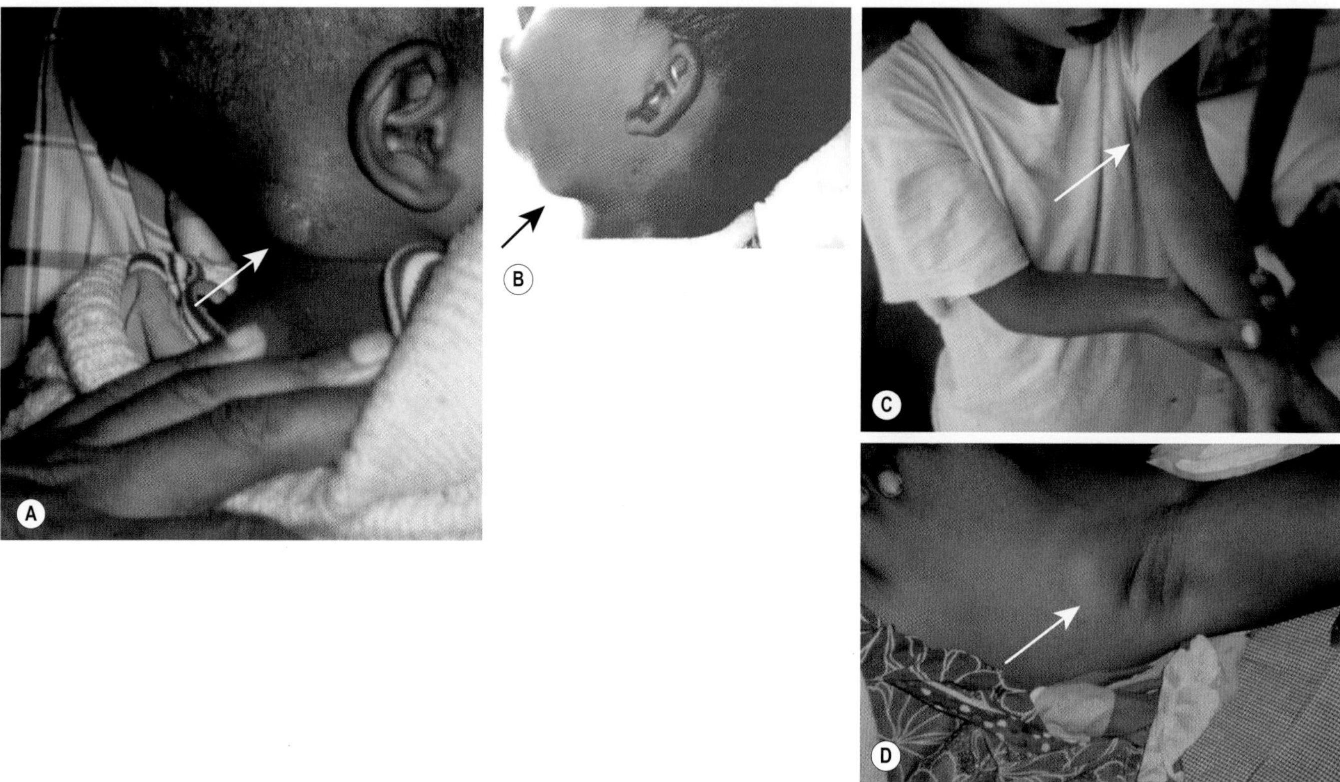

Figure 33.2 Children's bubo localization: (A) cervical, (B) under chin, (C) forearm, (D) arm.

rate of 90%. The terminal stage of bubonic plague is secondary pneumonic plague: *Y. pestis* colonizes the lung via the bloodstream.

When an appropriate course of antibiotics is given at the early stages of the disease, the patient usually responds quickly and fever disappears followed by the other systemic manifestations over 2–5 days, although buboes often remain enlarged and tender for a week or more after treatment.

In Madagascar, about 92% of reported cases are bubonic plague with a common localization of inguinal and femoral buboes. In most villages, people walk barefoot and often have open wounds which could be infected with environmental pathogens. Upper body sites may be relatively more involved in children (Figure 33.2). The location of the primary bubo often suggests the place of source of infection. In cases where patients are exposed to flea bites while sleeping (human dwellings invaded by plague-infected rats and rat fleas), localization to the upper or lower torso is evocative. Inguinal buboes suggest that infection occurred in the lower extremities, during field activities for instance. Axillary buboes suggest upper extremity inoculation, through handling of infected animal tissues for example.

Differential diagnoses include streptococcal or staphylococcal lymphadenitis, infectious mononucleosis, cat-scratch fever, lymphatic filariasis, tick-borne typhus, among others. Due to the high prevalence of tuberculosis in Africa, TB lymphadenitis (especially at the cervical area) should also be considered for differential diagnosis but the onset is not so rapid. Involvement of intra-abdominal lymph nodes may mimic appendicitis, acute cholecystitis, enterocolitis or other intra-abdominal surgical emergencies.

SEPTICAEMIC PLAGUE

Septicaemic plague is always fatal if not treated. This clinical form is usually secondary to bubonic plague but can be clinically inaugural (bubo misdiagnosed or deep node). In the acute stages of bubonic plague, intermittent bacteraemia typically occurs and may lead to sepsis. The presence of rapidly replicating plague bacilli in the bloodstream initiates a self-perpetuating immunological cascade typically linked to host response to severe injury. The host response may result in a wide spectrum of pathological events including disseminated intravascular coagulopathy, multiple organ failure, and adult respiratory distress syndrome. Disseminated intravascular coagulation can lead to haemorrhages in the skin and sometimes results in acral cyanosis and tissue necrosis. Metastatic infections of other organ systems may occur including: plague pneumonia, plague meningitis, plague endophthalmitis, hepatic or splenic abscesses, or generalized lymphadenopathy. The clinical presentation does not differ from other septicaemia and differential diagnosis depends on the laboratory investigations.

PNEUMONIC PLAGUE

Pneumonic plague is a highly virulent form of plague with an incubation period from a few hours to 2–3 days. As few as 1 day after inhalation, the patient starts showing severe symptoms of pneumonia and could be dead the next day. Clinical presentation does not differ from pneumonia of other origins; however, a rapid course and high lethality are indicative of pneumonic plague.

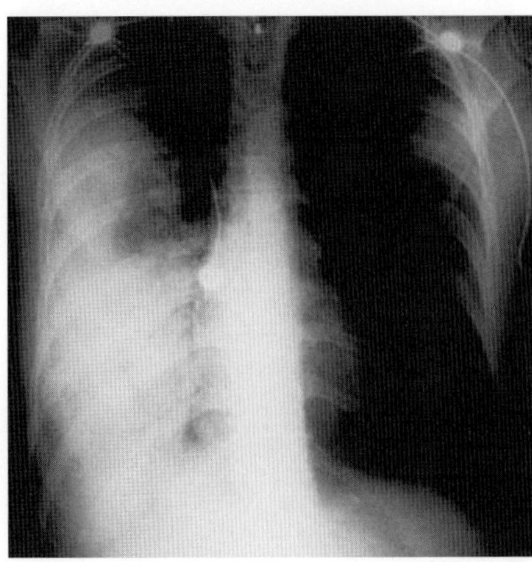

Figure 33.3 Chest radiograph of a patient who has primary plague pneumonia, showing extensive infiltrates in the right middle and lower lung fields. *(From Cohen J, Powderly WG, Opal S. Infectious Diseases. 3rd ed. St Louis: Mosby; Copyright © 2009 with permission from Elsevier.)*

Secondary plague pneumonia results from haematogenous spread of *Y. pestis* to the lungs, usually due to untreated or advanced infection of an initial bubonic or septicaemic form. A patient has usually been acutely ill for several days prior to lung invasion. Many patients die before they develop a well-advanced pneumonia. Those who do not die may be so sick that their cough reflex lacks the strength to produce finely aerosolized droplets. Consequently, during the early stages of disease, the risk of transmission is high.

Primary pneumonic plague is a rare but often fatal form of *Y. pestis* infection that results from direct inhalation of bacteria and is potentially transmissible from person-to-person and has the potential for propagating epidemics. The onset of pneumonic plague is most often sudden (with chills, fever, headache, body pains, weakness, dizziness, and chest discomfort) (Figure 33.3). Sputum is mucoid at first, rapidly develops blood specks, and then becomes uniformly pink or bright red and foamy. Tachypnoea and dyspnoea are present on the second day of illness, but pleuritic chest pain is not. Signs of consolidation are rare, and rales may be absent.

This form of the infection evolves rapidly, spreads more easily from person to person, and is far more deadly, killing 100% of those who do not receive the appropriate antibiotics soon after exposure.

Diagnosis

According to the revised International Health Regulations that came into effect in June 2007, any event that may constitute a public health emergency of international concern, such as the occurrence of plague in an area not known to be endemic, requires to be reported to the WHO.

Although, *Y. pestis* can be identified by different methods in the laboratory (Figure 33.4), it remains a challenge in remote locations where human cases of plague are often reported. Biological samples for diagnosis of bubonic, pneumonic and septicaemic plague are, respectively, bubo aspirate, sputum and blood. Postmortem samples (lung or liver puncture) can also be diagnosed.

Smears from these specimens are usually assessed by microscopy where the plague bacterium appears as bipolar 'closed-safety pin', with Wayson rather than with Gram staining. The organism can also be identified by direct fluorescence assay using an antibody directed against the F1 antigen, a capsular antigen expressed predominantly at 37°C. Therefore, samples that have been refrigerated for more than 30 hours of cultures that were incubated at temperatures less than 35°C or samples from fleas will be negative.

The bacteriological identification method remains the reference test for the diagnosis of plague. This confirmation technique requires at least 7 days of culture. *Y. pestis* grows on most laboratory routine culture media. *Y. pestis* colonies are visible after 48 hours of incubation with an optimum temperature between 25°C to 29°C. In broth culture (e.g. brain heart infusion), *Y. pestis* appears as clumps of cells at the bottom of the tube. Conventional biochemical identification systems and a specific bacteriophage lysis test may be used for identification and culture confirmation of *Y. pestis* isolates respectively. Characteristically, *Y. pestis* is oxidase-negative, catalase-positive, urea-negative, indole-negative and lactose-negative.

Serology by passive haemagglutination or enzyme-linked immunosorbent assay (ELISA) may be used as confirmation tests if the pathogenic agent could not be isolated. These immunological approaches required two serum samples from the patient (acute and convalescent sera). Antibodies against the F1 antigen usually appear 1 week after the onset of symptoms. A 4-fold rise in titre of paired samples is confirmatory for *Y. pestis*. Recently, rapid diagnostic tests (RDT) for the detection of plague anti-F1 antibodies in a range of reservoir species have been developed and evaluated. This is of great interest for the surveillance of reservoirs and active foci and for plague diagnosis.

RDT for detecting F1 antigen based on the use of monoclonal antibodies to the F1 antigen of *Y. pestis* have been developed, produced and evaluated in field conditions in Madagascar. This RDT is suitable for a wide range of clinical specimens (bubo aspirate, sputum, serum and urine) and has shown an excellent sensitivity and a great specificity compared to bacteriology and ELISA methods. This simple, rapid and easy-to-use method is of key importance for health workers located in remote sites. Indeed, its development and commercialization have contributed to better case-management and surveillance in Africa. The availability of such a test in other countries with endemic plague is expected to have a similar impact.[5]

The use of molecular tools is common in research laboratories. Polymerase chain reaction (PCR) for the F1-specifying *cafI* gene or PCR for the *Y. pestis*-specific *pla* gene is also available for diagnosis of *Y. pestis* infection. However, they are either not used routinely or still need to be evaluated under field conditions.

Management and Treatment

Human plague usually manifests in two main clinical forms: bubonic and pneumonic plague.

The patient case-management must be performed by health workers once the diagnosis of plague is suspected. Moreover, laboratory confirmation tests should be initiated. Early antibiotic therapy remains essential soon after biological sample collection. The key to successful treatment of human plague relies on prompt diagnosis and rapid administration of appropriate

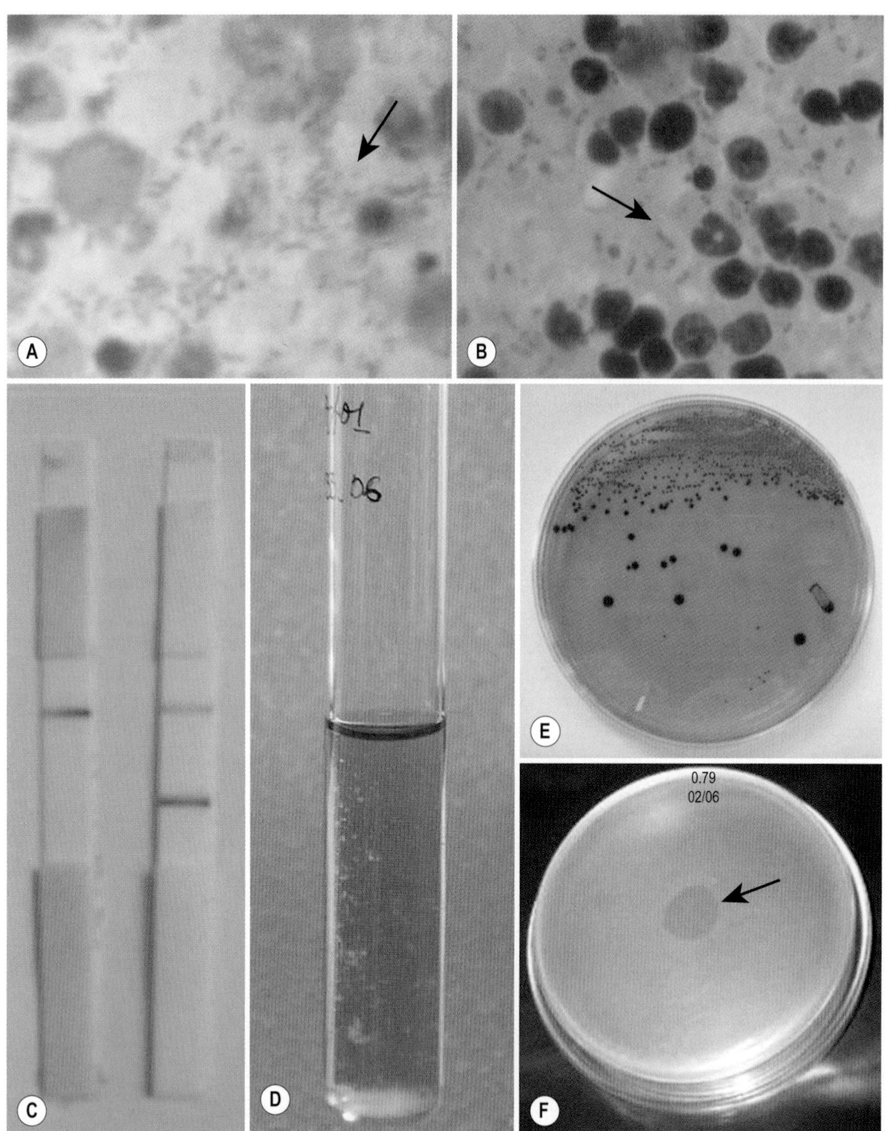

Figure 33.4 Plague diagnostic tools (A,B) Gram and Wayson stain, respectively, with bipolar appearance of coccobacilli. (C) Rapid test for antigen F1 detection – left: Negative, right: Positive. (D) Culture on BHI broth: medium clear with some flakes on the tube wall and some clumps at the bottom. (E) *Y. pestis* on selective medium 72 hours old. (F) Confirmation of *Y. pestis* isolated by bacteriophage lysis: a clear lysis area in the middle.

treatments. Effective antibiotic therapy consists of administration of drugs at a sufficient dose for at least 10 days and considerably contributes to the reduction of the case fatality rate worldwide. Aminoglycosides (streptomycin and gentamicin), chloramphenicol and tetracycline are the reference antibiotics for the treatment of plague.

According to the recommendation of the plague control programme in Madagascar, the treatment protocol combines two drugs: injection of streptomycin in the first 4 days and oral sulfamethoxazole-trimethoprim for 6 days from the third day onwards (Table 33.1). The dosage depends on the age of the patient.

TABLE 33.1 Plague treatment

Antibiotics	Dose Per Day	Number of Daily Dose	Days of Treatment
Bubonic plague – Adult			
Streptomycin	3 g, IM	6 (every 4 h)	Day 1–day 2
	2 g, IM	2 (every 12 h)	Day 3–day 4
Sulfamethoxazole/trimethoprim	3 g 40 mg/kg (6 tablets), PO	2	Day 3–day 8/10
Pneumonic plague – Adult			
Streptomycin	4 g, IM	8 (every 3 h)	Day 1–day 2
	3 g, IM	6 (every 4 h)	Day 3–day 4
	2 g, IM	2	Day 5–day 8/10
Chemoprophylaxis – Adult			
Sulfadoxine (Fanasil)	500 mg (3–4 tablets), PO	1	Day 1

AMINOGLYCOSIDES: STREPTOMYCIN AND GENTAMICIN

Streptomycin is regarded as the most effective antibiotic against *Y. pestis* and the drug of choice for plague treatment, particularly for the pneumonic form. The usual dose is 30 mg/kg per day (up to a total of 2 g/day) in repeated doses by intramuscular route.

Gentamicin has been proven to be effective and can be used to treat human plague cases if the use of streptomycin is contraindicated.

CHLORAMPHENICOL

Chloramphenicol can be used as an alternative to aminoglycosides in the treatment of plague. The recommended dosage is 50 mg/kg per day in repeated doses administered by parenteral or oral route for 10 days. Chloramphenicol can be used in association with aminoglycosides.

TETRACYCLINE

This group of antibiotics is bacteriostatic but effective in the treatment of patients with bubonic plague. The dosage should be progressive, ranging from 15 mg/kg per day at the start of the antibiotic treatment (not to exceed 1 g in total) to reach 25–50 mg/kg per day (up to a total of 2 g/day). The overall treatment lasts for 10 days.

ALTERNATIVE TREATMENT

Sulfonamides may be indicated to treat human plague but some studies reported higher mortality, increased complications and a prolonged treatment duration compared with streptomycin, tetracycline or chloramphenicol. Sulfadiazine (Adiazine, 4–6 g/day) or late-sulfonamides such as sulfalene (Kelfizine) or sulfadoxine (Fanasil, single injection of 2 g in adults; 0.5–1 g in a child) are also suitable. Sulfamethoxazole-trimethoprim (Bactrim, 6 tablets per day) is also effective. Fluoroquinolones such as ciprofloxacin, showed promising results against *Y. pestis* in vitro and in animals, however no studies have yet reported its use in human plague treatment.

Other classes of antibiotics (penicillin, cephalosporin, macrolides) are ineffective or have produced adverse effects in the treatment of plague and must be prohibited in case of human plague.

Prevention

Prophylaxis is indicated to prevent the occurrence of *Y. pestis* infection for those in close contact with pneumonic plague patients or in direct contact with *Y. pestis*. Current preventive measures are sulfonamides, tetracyclines or chloramphenicol.

A mortality rate of 7.5% was recorded by the WHO during the period 1999–2009. Additionally, the re-emergence of the disease and the possible use of the plague bacterium as a bioterrorism agent raise the urgent need to develop a safe and effective vaccine against plague. Protection against pneumonic plague is of paramount importance to prevent epidemic spread.

Two types of plague vaccine are currently used in various parts of the world. The live-attenuated vaccine, usually related to EV76, retains virulence and is not commercially available for use in humans at present. The existing killed-whole-cell vaccine (KWCV) based on a heat-killed bacteria have been shown to be protective against bubonic plague but not effective for the pneumonic form of the disease. Adverse effects and short duration of protective immunity of these vaccines have encouraged researchers to improve the development of new vaccines essentially based on the combination of two virulence factors, the Fraction 1 (F1) and V (virulence) proteins, expressed in recombinant form.

The recombinant plague vaccine, comprising rF1 + rV antigens in alhydrogel, has been assessed successfully during a phase I trial in humans. Phase II clinical trials have subsequently demonstrated safety and immunogenicity for either the rF1–V or rF1 + rV formulations.[6]

REFERENCES

1. WHO. Human plague: review of regional morbidity and mortality, 2004-2009. Wkly Epidemiol Rec 2010;85:37–48.
2. WHO. International meeting on preventing and controlling plague: the old calamity still has a future. Wkly Epidemiol Rec 2006;81:278–84.
3. Gage KL, Kosoy MY. Natural history of plague: perspectives from more than a century of research. Annu Rev Entomol 2005;50:505–28.
4. Chanteau S. Atlas de la peste à Madagascar. Paris: Institut Pasteur; 2006.
5. Chauvaux S, Dillies MA, Marceau M, et al. In silico comparison of *Yersinia pestis* and *Yersinia pseudotuberculosis* transcriptomes reveals a higher expression level of crucial virulence determinants in the plague bacillus. Int J Med Microbiol 2011;301:105–16.
6. Chanteau S, Rahalison L, Ralafiarisoa L, et al. Development and testing of a rapid diagnostic test for bubonic and pneumonic plague. Lancet 2003;361:211–16.
7. Williamson D, Oyston PC. The natural history and incidence of *Yersinia pestis* and prospects for vaccination. J Med Microbiol 2012;61(Part 7):911–18.

34 Melioidosis

DAVID A. B. DANCE

KEY POINTS

- Melioidosis is the name used to describe any infection of humans and a wide range of other animals caused by the saprophytic environmental bacterium *Burkholderia pseudomallei*.
- The disease is increasingly recognized as an important indigenous infection in many tropical and sub-tropical regions, but is probably greatly under-diagnosed.
- This increasing recognition, including travel-associated cases, along with its potential as a biological weapon, has seen a surge of interest in the disease in recent years.
- Diagnosis usually requires isolation of the causative organism from clinical samples: available serology and molecular diagnostic tools lack sensitivity and specificity.
- Clinical manifestations are highly variable, but melioidosis is most frequently associated with community-acquired sepsis and pneumonia, with abscess formation, especially in lungs, liver, spleen, prostate and parotid, being common.
- It is an opportunist pathogen, particularly strongly associated with diabetes mellitus, chronic renal and lung disease, but not HIV infection, although up to 20% of cases may have no known underlying predisposition.
- The diagnosis should be considered in anyone with compatible symptoms, particularly those with a predisposing condition, who has ever visited an endemic area because of the potential for long periods of latency.
- Treatment requires long courses of antibiotics, initially an intensive parenteral phase with either ceftazidime or a carbapenem, followed by an oral eradication phase with co-trimoxazole or co-amoxiclav, although both relapses and reinfection may occur.
- There is currently no available vaccine, so prevention depends on minimizing contact with environmental organisms: fortunately person-to-person spread is very rare.

Epidemiology

GEOGRAPHIC DISTRIBUTION

Melioidosis was originally identified by Whitmore and Krishnaswami in Burma, in 1911.[1] It is widely endemic in South and South-east Asia, especially Thailand, and northern Australia, although it is unevenly distributed within these areas.[2,3] The reasons for its focal distribution are poorly understood, but probably relate to climatic and environmental factors that favour the persistence and proliferation of the organism in soil and surface water.[4] Sporadic cases have also been reported in the Americas, the Caribbean and sub-Saharan Africa, although the true incidence in these areas is unclear because of a lack of laboratory facilities and clinical awareness.[2,3,5–8] During the 1970s, a unique epizootic also occurred in France.[2,3,5] A map of the worldwide distribution is shown in Figure 34.1.

PREVALENCE, INCIDENCE AND SEASONALITY

In northeast Thailand, the average annual incidence was estimated as 4.4/100 000 between 1987 and 1991, when *B. pseudomallei* accounted for almost 20% of community-acquired septicaemia.[9] More recently, the incidence increased between 1997 and 2006 to 21.3/100 000, and melioidosis is now the third most common cause of death from infectious diseases in North-east Thailand after human immunodeficiency virus and tuberculosis.[10]

The disease is highly seasonal, some 75–85% of cases presenting during the rainy season,[3,6,9,11–13] and clusters have been reported in association with severe weather events such as typhoons.[12] In northern Australia, where in some places melioidosis is the commonest cause of fatal community-acquired bacteraemic pneumonia, the average annual incidence is 19.6/100 000, although rates as high as 41.7/100 000 have been reported during years experiencing intense wind and rain associated with tropical cyclones.[3,13]

IMPORTANT ASSOCIATIONS

In endemic areas, *B. pseudomallei* is readily isolated from soil and surface water.[4] Melioidosis is most common in people who have close contact with soil and water (e.g. rice farmers in Thailand, Aboriginals in Australia), although in most cases the precise mode of acquisition is unclear. It is usually assumed that the majority of infections result from inoculation, although inoculation events can only be identified in 5–22% of cases.[3,9,13] Occasional cases follow immersion in, or aspiration of, fresh water, such as occurred during the Asian tsunami of 2004.[3,14] Mounting evidence suggests that inhalation is a more important mode of acquisition than previously thought, especially during severe weather events.[11,12] Other recent outbreaks have been traced to contaminated potable water supplies and contaminated disinfectants or detergents.[3] Iatrogenic and laboratory-acquired infections have occurred occasionally,[2,3] but transmission through direct contact with infected humans or animals, including transplacental transmission and mother-to-infant spread via breast milk, has been described only rarely.[2,3]

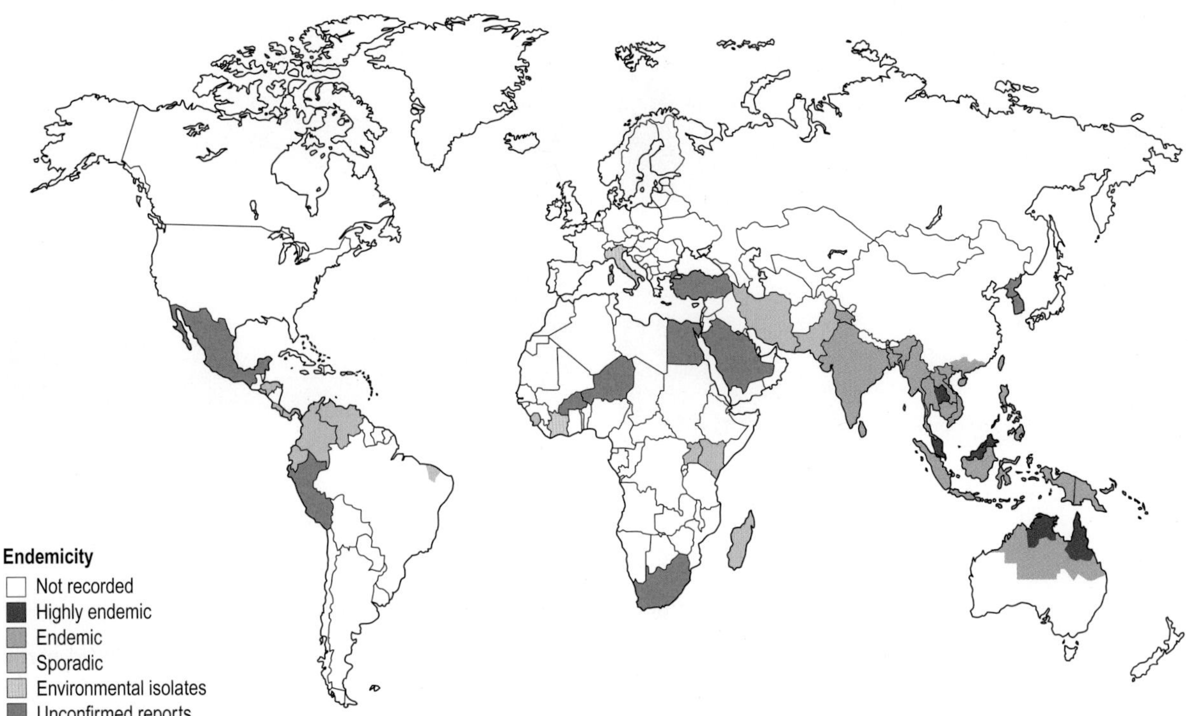

Figure 34.1 Map of the global distribution of melioidosis. *(From Currie BJ, Dance DA, Cheng AC. The global distribution of Burkholderia pseudomallei and melioidosis: an update. Trans R Soc Trop Med Hygiene 2008;102(Suppl 1):S1–4.)*

When a specific exposure can be identified, the incubation period is usually 1–21 days (mean 9 days).[3] However, *B. pseudomallei* has the unusual ability to remain latent for periods of up to 62 years,[15] which has given rise to the nickname 'Vietnamese time-bomb'. The proportion of seropositive persons who are latently infected is unknown. The seasonal nature of the disease, however, suggests that most cases result from recent exposure to the organism in the environment and only 4% of cases in Australia are thought to represent recrudescent latent infections.[3,13]

Although severe melioidosis may occur in apparently normal individuals, 60–90% of cases have underlying diseases, most frequently diabetes mellitus or chronic renal failure.[3,5,6,13,16,17] Steroid therapy, alcohol abuse and liver disease, chronic lung disease (including cystic fibrosis), cardiac failure, kava consumption, malignant disease, thalassaemia, chronic granulomatous disease and pregnancy may also predispose to melioidosis but, surprisingly, infection with HIV does not appear to.[3,5,6,13,16,17] Recrudescence of latent infection also usually occurs at times of intercurrent stress.[18]

Pathogenesis and Pathology

The result of exposure to *B. pseudomallei* in the environment varies markedly from person to person, ranging from asymptomatic seroconversion (the commonest outcome) to fulminant sepsis and death. Which route is followed in any individual depends on a balance between the size and route of the inoculum and the virulence of the infecting strain on the one hand, and the host response on the other. This topic has been comprehensively reviewed.[3,5,6,17,18] A range of bacterial factors, including an antiphagocytic polysaccharide capsule, quorum sensing mechanisms, a type III secretion system associated with intracellular growth and spread, bacterial components such as lipopolysaccharide, flagella, pili, secreted products (e.g. protease, lipase, lecithinase, various toxins) and a siderophore ('malleobactin') have all been associated with virulence,[3,5,6,17] but the relative contributions of individual virulence factors to the disease process have not been well characterized. The ability of the organism to survive and grow intracellularly or become metabolically inactive within granulomas probably contributes to the recalcitrant and persistent nature of the infection.[18] On the host side, innate immune mechanisms, macrophage and neutrophil function, and both cellular and humoral responses probably all play a role in defence against the organism.[3,5,17,19] An exaggerated host response may also be damaging.[3,5,17]

Clinical Features

AGE/SEX/RACIAL GROUP

All age groups can develop melioidosis but incidence peaks between 40 and 60 years. The male:female ratio is 1.4:1 in Thailand[9] and 2.3:1 in Australia[13] but from 2.8–7.2:1 in Singapore,[20] probably reflecting differences in exposure to soil and water between different populations. The disease disproportionately affects the Aboriginal population in Australia[13] and Malays in Malaysia[21] but it is unclear whether this reflects any intrinsic inter-ethnic differences in susceptibility as opposed to simply greater exposure to environmental organisms. There are certainly considerable inter-species and inter-strain differences in susceptibility in other animals.

Clinical Presentations

The variable course and manifestations have made it difficult to develop a satisfactory clinical classification of melioidosis.

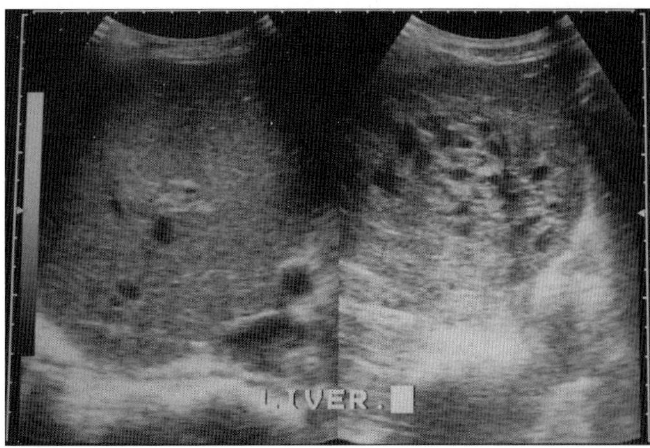

Figure 34.2 Ultrasound of liver showing multiple abscesses in a patient with septicaemic melioidosis. (© *Professor S.J. Peacock.)*

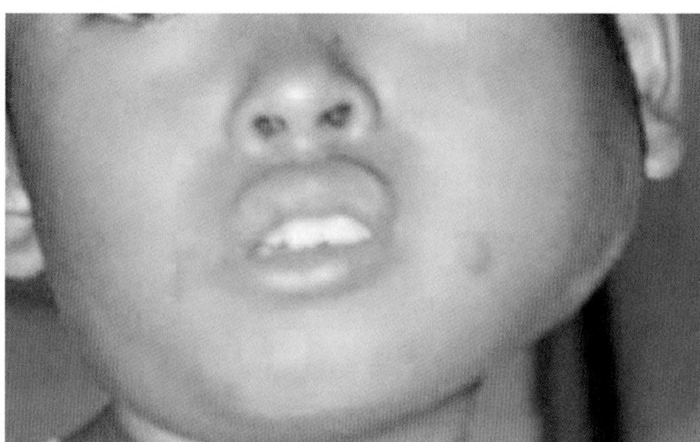

Figure 34.4 Parotid abscess in a patient. (© *Professor N. J. White.)*

Since 60–70% of the population in endemic areas have antibodies to *B. pseudomallei* by the age of 4 years,[22] yet few acquire clinically apparent melioidosis, the majority of infections are presumably mild or asymptomatic. Seroconversion has been associated with a flu-like illness.[23] Some of the more common clinically apparent forms are described below.

SEPTICAEMIC MELIOIDOSIS

Some 46–60% of cases of culture-positive melioidosis are bacteraemic, and the majority of these are clinically septicaemic.[3,5,13,24] Patients usually have a short history (median 6 days; range 1 day to 2 months) of fever and rigors.[24] Approximately half have evidence of a primary focus of infection, usually pulmonary or cutaneous.[3,5,13,21,24] A reduced level of consciousness, jaundice and diarrhoea may also be prominent features. Deterioration is often rapid, with the development of widespread metastatic abscesses, particularly in the lungs, liver (Figure 34.2), spleen (Figure 34.3) parotid (Figure 34.4) and prostate, and metabolic acidosis with Kussmaul's breathing. Mycotic aneurysms are being recognized with increasing frequency.[25] Cutaneous or subcutaneous abscesses occur in approximately 10% of cases.

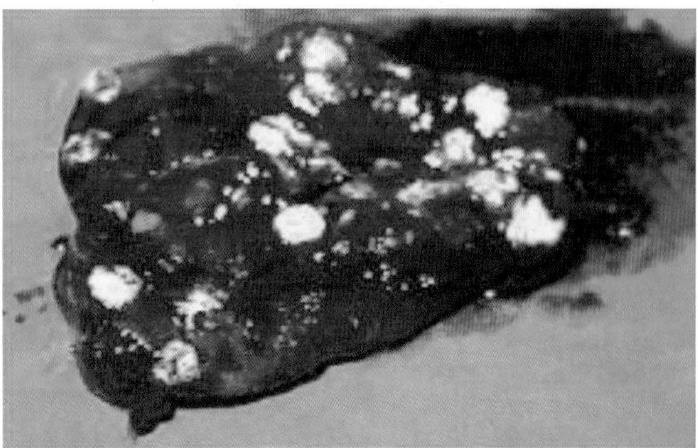

Figure 34.3 Spleen removed from a patient with chronic melioidosis showing multiple abscesses. (© *Professor N. J. White.)*

LOCALIZED MELIOIDOSIS

The lung is the most common site for localized melioidosis,[13] causing pneumonia with a tendency to cavitate. Any lung zone may be affected, although there is a predilection for upper lobe involvement.[26]

Localized *B. pseudomallei* infection may occur in any organ. Well described forms include: cutaneous and subcutaneous abscesses, suppurative parotitis, lymphadenitis, osteomyelitis and septic arthritis, liver and/or splenic abscesses, cystitis, pyelonephritis, prostatic abscesses, epididymo-orchitis, keratitis, meningoencephalitis, mastitis/breast abscess and brain abscesses.[3,5,13]

GEOGRAPHICAL VARIATIONS

For reasons that have yet to be explained, parotitis in children is common in Thailand but not Australia. Hepatosplenic abscesses are also commoner in Thailand than Australia, whereas prostatic abscesses and neurological melioidosis are reported more frequently from Australia than Thailand.[3,5,13]

Differential Diagnosis

With such variable manifestations that it has been nicknamed 'the remarkable imitator', the range of differential diagnoses of melioidosis is very wide, and varies considerably from patient to patient depending on the site of infection. Common differentials in acute severe cases include any bacterium causing community-acquired septicaemia, pneumonia or abscesses, particularly *Staphylococcus aureus*. Chronic pulmonary cases must be distinguished from tuberculosis and anaerobic lung abscesses, and hepatic cases from mixed bacterial or amoebic liver abscesses.

COMPLICATIONS

Septicaemic melioidosis may progress to full-blown septic shock with all the features of the systemic inflammatory response syndrome, although there is some evidence that *B. pseudomallei* lipopolysaccharide is intrinsically less toxic than that of other Gram-negative bacteria.[27] Established septic shock is associated with a high mortality rate (50% in Australia despite optimal supportive treatment).[13] Localized complications of pulmonary melioidosis include pneumothorax, empyema and purulent pericarditis, whilst parotitis may rarely cause facial nerve palsy.

Diagnosis

MICROBIOLOGY

B. pseudomallei is an irregularly staining, oxidase-positive, motile Gram-negative bacillus, which sometimes exhibits marked bipolarity microscopically. It grows readily on most routine culture media, often forming rugose colonies, although a wide range of variation is seen,[28] and gives off a sweet earthy smell. Other important characteristics include arginine dihydrolase and gelatinase activity, growth at 42°C, the ability to use a wide range of carbon and energy sources, and intrinsic resistance to aminoglycosides, polymyxins and the early β-lactams, but susceptibility to co-amoxiclav. The species is antigenically homogeneous, but a number of molecular techniques, most usefully multilocus sequence typing, can distinguish between isolates.[3,6] The genome has been sequenced and comprises two chromosomes of 4.07 and 3.17 megabase pairs, associated with core and accessory function respectively, with a high proportion of genomic islands.[3,6,29] *Burkholderia mallei*, the causative agent of glanders, appears to be a clone of *B. pseudomallei* that has lost genetic material in association with adaptation to equine hosts. Another closely related but avirulent soil organism, *Burkholderia thailandensis*, has proved useful for the study of *B. pseudomallei* virulence determinants.[17]

Melioidosis should be considered in any patient who has ever visited an endemic area who presents with septicaemia and/or abscesses, especially if they have a strongly associated predisposing condition such as diabetes. It is difficult to make a clinical diagnosis with confidence. A failure to defervesce on empirical treatment with penicillin and gentamicin, a combination often used to treat patients with septicaemia in the tropics, is useful supporting evidence, but usually the diagnosis depends on the isolation of *B. pseudomallei*, the detection of its antigens or nucleic acid, or the presence of specific antibodies. Microscopy of pus, sputum or urine may reveal bipolar or unevenly staining Gram-negative rods, but this appearance is not specific for *B. pseudomallei*. The most useful rapid diagnostic tool is immunofluorescence on pus or secretions, but this is only available in certain centres.[30] Numerous PCR assays for *B. pseudomallei* have been developed and some have shown promise in small-scale evaluations,[3,6,31] but none is in widespread use.

The organism should be sought in blood, pus, urine, sputum or any other specimen indicated by the patient's clinical presentation. Isolation of *B. pseudomallei* from any site can be taken as evidence of melioidosis as asymptomatic carriage has not been reported. The laboratory should be notified when melioidosis is suspected, since selective techniques increase the isolation rate,[3,5,6] and the organism may be overlooked or discarded as a contaminant by the unwary. Ashdown's medium is widely used in endemic areas, although commercial *B. cepacia* medium is more likely to be available outside endemic areas and compares favourably with other media designed to grow *B. pseudomallei*.[32] The organism is also classified as a 'hazard group 3' pathogen and needs to be handled in appropriate laboratory containment because of the potential for infection among laboratory staff, although this has occurred only rarely.

An oxidase-positive Gram-negative rod that is resistant to aminoglycosides and colistin/polymyxin but susceptible to co-amoxiclav should be assumed to be *B. pseudomallei* until proved otherwise. Commercial identification kits such as the API 20NE usually identify the organism correctly[33] but may give misleading results,[6] so possible isolates should ideally be sent to a Reference Laboratory by those who rarely encounter the organism. A latex agglutination test using a monoclonal antibody to the 200 kDa extracellular polysaccharide is also useful for screening suspect colonies.[33]

There is no standard assay for serodiagnosis of melioidosis. An indirect haemagglutination (IHA) test, using a crude mixture of poorly characterized antigens, is the test most widely used in endemic areas, although many other assays have been described. Most tests have disappointing sensitivity and specificity, particularly in endemic areas where background seropositivity rates are high.[3,5,6] A commercial immunochromatographic test produced in Australia gave variable results in field evaluations and is no longer available.[3,6] Serology may be useful in patients from non-endemic areas, in whom a single IHA titre of >1 : 40 at presentation is suggestive of melioidosis. In patients from endemic areas, only a rising or very high titre in a patient with a compatible illness can be taken as presumptive evidence of melioidosis.

HAEMATOLOGY AND BIOCHEMISTRY

Initial investigations in patients with severe melioidosis usually reveal anaemia, a neutrophil leukocytosis, coagulopathy and evidence of renal and hepatic impairment, although these are really just indicators of severe systemic sepsis. Plasma or serum concentrations of CRP and other inflammatory markers may sometimes be useful in monitoring treatment, but can be misleading.[34]

RADIOLOGY

An abnormal chest radiograph is found in 80% of melioidosis patients, the most common pattern being widespread, nodular shadowing (Figure 34.5). More chronic forms include a

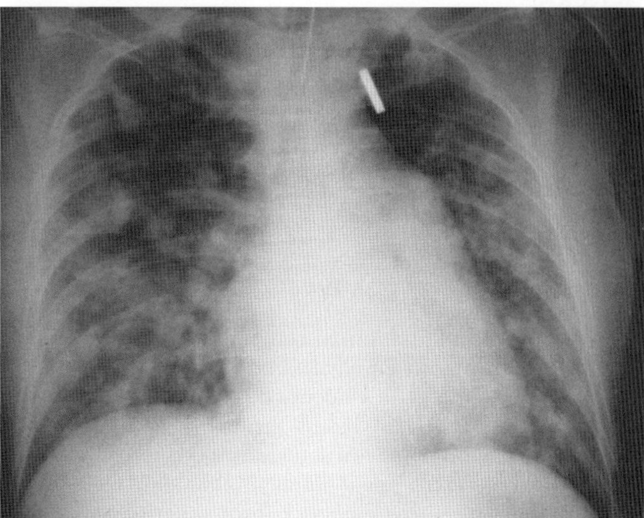

Figure 34.5 Septicaemic melioidosis. Widespread nodular shadowing representing blood-borne pneumonia. *(© Professor N. J. White.)*

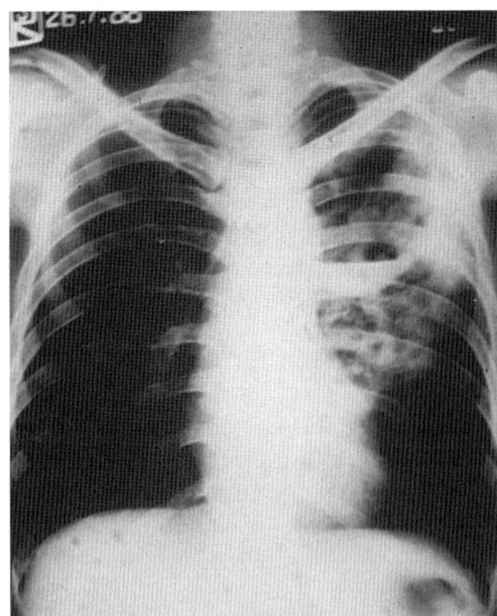

Figure 34.6 Cavitating pneumonia in melioidosis, with an air–fluid level.

cavitating pneumonia accompanied by profound weight loss, which is often confused with tuberculosis or lung abscess (Figure 34.6). Abdominal imaging (either ultrasound or CT scan), which should be undertaken routinely in all patients, may show liver and/or splenic abscesses (Figures 34.2 and 34.3), or prostatic abscesses in men.[13,35]

BIOPSY

The microscopic appearance of lesions is not pathognomonic and forms a spectrum from abscess to granuloma depending on the duration of the illness and the response of the individual. Multinucleate giant cells, often containing 'globi' of bacteria, in a background of acute necrotizing inflammation, are a characteristic feature.[36]

Management and Treatment

GENERAL

Patients with septicaemic melioidosis require aggressive supportive treatment, with particular attention to correction of volume depletion and septic shock, respiratory and renal failure, and hyperglycaemia or ketoacidosis. Severe cases should ideally be managed in an intensive care unit. Abscesses should be drained surgically whenever possible in both disseminated and localized disease.

ANTIMICROBIAL THERAPY

Several prospective randomized comparisons of antimicrobial therapy for melioidosis have been undertaken over the past 20 years, resulting in a good evidence base for treatment, which has been summarized in recent reviews.[3,5,6,37] The standard approach to chemotherapy of severe disease is to use at least 2 weeks of parenteral treatment initially, followed by 12–20 weeks of oral 'eradication' therapy to reduce the risk of relapse. Although susceptible in vitro to many third generation cephalosporins, ceftazidime is the preferred drug within this class. Retrospective non-comparative observations suggest that mortality is higher with cefotaxime than ceftazidime. Mild cases may be treated with oral drugs alone. Preferred regimens are given in Table 34.1. Co-amoxiclav and cefoperazone-sulbactam have also been used for parenteral treatment, but experience is more limited. In the past, combinations of oral agents (e.g. co-trimoxazole plus doxycycline) have been used for the eradication phase, but clinical experience over several years in Australia combined with an as yet unpublished clinical trial undertaken in Thailand suggests that co-trimoxazole alone is effective. In vitro resistance to co-trimoxazole, which can only reliably be determined by 'E-test', is not uncommon, but it is not known whether this increases the risk of relapse or should alter the choice of treatment.[6,38] Oral co-amoxiclav is associated with a higher risk of relapse than co-trimoxazole-containing regimens[39] and so should only be used when co-trimoxazole is contraindicated.

Encouraging results using G-CSF for adjunctive treatment of melioidosis septic shock were reported in an uncontrolled study from northern Australia,[3,6] but this did not achieve

TABLE 34.1 Preferred Regimens for Antimicrobial Therapy for Melioidosis

Agent	Dose
ACUTE PARENTERAL PHASE (AT LEAST 2 WEEKS AND LONGER IF PERSISTENT FEVER, UNDRAINED ABSCESSES, ETC.)	
Ceftazidime	50 mg/kg/dose (up to 2 g) every 8 h or 6 g per day by continuous infusion after a 2 g bolus
or	
Meropenem	25–40 mg/kg/dose (up to 2 g) every 8 h
1. Consider addition of co-trimoxazole at doses below for patients with deep-seated infection involving the brain, prostate, or other 'privileged' sites, given by IV infusion over 30–60 min, nasogastric, or oral, as appropriate.	
2. Switch to meropenem indicated if patient condition worsens on ceftazidime, e.g. organ failure, development of a new focus of infection during treatment, or if repeat blood cultures remain positive.	
ORAL ERADICATION PHASE (12–20 WEEKS)	
Co-trimoxazole	Children 8/40 mg/kg/dose orally twice daily up to 320 mg/1600 mg Adults >60 kg: 2×160/800 mg (960 mg) tablets twice daily 40–60 kg: 3×80/400 mg (480 mg) tablets twice daily <40 kg: 1×160/800 mg (960 mg) or 2×80/400 mg (480 mg) tablets twice daily
or	
Amoxicillin-clavulanate (for infection with co-trimoxazole-resistant isolates or patients in whom co-trimoxazole is contraindicated)	Children 20/5 mg/kg per dose up to 1000 mg/250 mg three times a day Adults >60 kg: 3×500 mg/125 mg tablets three times a day <60 kg: 2×500 mg/125 mg tablets three times a day

Note: Adjust doses as necessary in renal impairment.

statistical significance in a prospective randomized trial in Thailand, although patients treated with G-CSF survived longer, potentially allowing physicians to 'buy time'.[40]

Even with optimal antibiotic treatment, the mortality of severe melioidosis is 14% in Australia and 40% in Thailand, death within the first 48 hours of hospital admission being common.[3,5,6,13] In those who recover, the response to therapy is often slow (median time to resolution of fever 9 days).[5,24] The mortality rate is low in those with no underlying disease (2% in Australia),[13] and paradoxically diabetics have a lower overall mortality than non-diabetics in Thailand, possibly related to the anti-inflammatory activity of glibenclamide.[41] Poor prognostic features include hypotension, absence of fever, leucopenia, azotaemia, abnormal liver function tests, high level or persistent bacteraemia, raised levels of a range of pro-inflammatory cytokines, and positive urine or sputum cultures.[3,5,6,42] Follow-up blood cultures should routinely be performed weekly until negative, but follow-up cultures of other sites is not necessary unless the patient shows clinical signs of treatment failure or relapse.[16,42] Relapse occurs in 6–10% overall, and is commoner in those with disseminated infections who receive less than 12 weeks of treatment.[13,16,43] Reinfection also appears to occur in 1–3.4% of survivors followed-up for long periods of time.[13,43] Antibiotic resistance may develop occasionally during the course of treatment, although this is rare (<1%) with β-lactams. A form of β-lactam resistance associated with treatment failure resulting from gene deletion and characterized by the development of auxotrophs that can only be isolated on certain media has recently been described and may be difficult to detect.[44]

Prevention

No *B. pseudomallei* vaccine has been developed for human use, although experimental vaccines are under investigation.[45] Guidelines for the use of prophylaxis following laboratory exposure have been developed,[46] but there is limited evidence of its efficacy.[3] Prevention is thus limited minimizing contact with *B. pseudomallei* in the environment, particularly by 'at-risk' individuals such as diabetics, the removal of point sources and adequate chlorination of water supplies. The risk of cross-infection appears to be very low, but cases should be nursed in isolation in non-endemic areas and where facilities are available.

REFERENCES

3. Cheng AC, Currie BJ. Melioidosis: epidemiology, pathophysiology, and management. Clin Microbiol Rev 2005;18:383–416.
5. White NJ. Melioidosis. Lancet 2003;361:1715–22.
6. Peacock SJ. Melioidosis. Curr Opinion Infect Dis 2006;19:421–8.
13. Currie BJ, Ward L, Cheng AC. The epidemiology and clinical spectrum of melioidosis: 540 cases from the 20 year Darwin prospective study. PLoS Negl Trop Dis 2010;4:e900.
16. Limmathurotsakul D, Peacock SJ. Melioidosis: a clinical overview. Br Med Bull 2011;99:125–39.
17. Wiersinga WJ, van der Poll T, White NJ, et al. Melioidosis: insights into the pathogenicity of *Burkholderia pseudomallei*. Nature Rev Microbiol 2006;4:272–82.

Access the complete references online at www.expertconsult.com

35

Diphtheria

TRAN TINH HIEN | NICHOLAS J. WHITE

KEY POINTS

- Diphtheria is a disease caused by the bacteria *Corynebacterium diphtheriae*. Some strains of *C. ulcerans* (and very rarely *C. pseudotuberculosis*) may produce diphtheria toxin and the illness caused may present as clinical diphtheria.[1–3] It can cause respiratory symptoms or non-respiratory forms that affect other parts of the body, including the skin. The word diphtheria originates from the term 'diphtherite', which has a Greek root meaning skin or hide, and refers to the leathery appearance of the characteristic pharyngeal membrane.[4]
- The disease is caused by the local effects of destructive infection (usually in the nasopharynx) and the distal effects of diphtheria toxin on the heart, peripheral nerves and kidneys. Death results from airways obstruction, myocarditis or polyneuritis.
- Diphtheria has declined dramatically in affluent countries over the past 80 years,[5,6] but it remains an important disease in many parts of the tropics and there has been a recent resurgence of the disease in the West. Between 1990 and 1999, over 158 000 cases and 4000 deaths were reported in the countries of the former Soviet Union. Since 2002 *C. ulcerans* has been more commonly reported than *C. diphtheriae* in the UK and France. These infections are usually acquired from raw milk and/or contact with farms and farm animals or close contact with companion animals and pets (cow, goat, cat and dog).
- The increasing incidence in the illness has resulted in the expansion of the notification criteria of the E-CDC and US-CDC for diphtheria to include infection caused by *Corynebacterium diphtheriae* and *C. ulcerans.*
- This increase in the number of clinical cases of diphtheria also highlights the need to maintain vaccination coverage in the population above the 95% as recommended by the World Health Organization. Approximately 100 years ago, 1% of all medical publications were on diphtheria. Now there is very little clinical research on diphtheria. Most new developments are in vaccine formulations.

Bacteriology

The diphtheria bacillus was first grown in pure culture by Loeffler in 1884. The causative organism, *C. diphtheriae* is a non-motile, non-capsulated, non-spore-forming aerobic bacillus. Although it is described as Gram-positive, it is easily decolourized during the staining procedure and may appear Gram-negative. On microscopy, *C. diphtheriae* exhibits considerable pleomorphism, ranging from the classical club shape to long slender bacilli. The arrangement of organisms on a smear often resembles Chinese letters. The presence of metachromatic granules when stained by Loeffler's methylene blue or Albert's stain is characteristic, although this should not be relied upon for identification.

C. diphtheriae grows well on blood agar, but tellurite blood agar (Hoyle's medium) is recommended as this inhibits other respiratory flora and allows the characteristic colonial morphology of the three biotypes (gravis, intermedius and mitis) to develop.[7] Although, as the name implies, toxigenic gravis strains are generally associated with more severe disease, in vitro mitis strains often produce more toxin than gravis or intermedius strains. Toxin production is very dependent on the composition of the growth medium. The iron content is particularly important. Young organisms produce more toxin than older organisms, and thus increased toxin production is associated with rapid growth. The association between biotype and severity is not constant. *C. diphtheriae* is further identified by biochemical reactions: acid is produced from glucose and maltose but only very rarely from sucrose; urea is not hydrolysed. The gravis biotype ferments starch.[8] Simple screening tests have been developed for identification of the pathogenic corynebacteria, which do not produce pyrazinamide, but do produce cystinase (seen as a brown halo around colonies, when cystine is incorporated into modified Tinsdale's agar).[9]

Pathogenesis

The potentially lethal effects of diphtheria in humans are caused by an exotoxin. The toxigenicity of *C. diphtheriae* depends on the presence of a tox$^+$ phage (α lysogenic β-phage) which induces the organism to produce toxin. Harmless non-toxigenic strains of *C. diphtheriae*, lacking the tox$^+$ β-phage, can be converted to pathogenic toxigenic strains by infection with a lysogenic phage (in vitro). This process may also occur in vivo.[10]

Toxin production by corynebacteria is usually detected by Elek's test[8] or guinea pig inoculation, but recently enzyme immunoassays have been developed which are cheaper and easier.[11] Diphtheria toxin can also be produced by *C. ulcerans* and this has resulted in clinical diphtheria.[12]

Diphtheria exotoxin is a 62 000 Da polypeptide, which includes two segments: the active toxin moiety (A) and the binding (B) segment, which binds to specific receptors on susceptible cells. The binding B portion attaches to the cell membrane, allowing the active A portion to enter the cells where it catalyses a reaction that inactivates the transfer RNA (tRNA) translocase 'elongation factor 2' (EF-2), in eukaryotic cells. This factor is essential for reactions that transfer triplet codes from messenger RNA to amino acid sequences via tRNA. Thus EF-2 inactivation stops synthesis of the polypeptide chains. The diphtheria toxin affects all human cells, but the most profound effects are on the myocardium (myocarditis), peripheral nerves (demyelination) and kidneys (acute tubular necrosis).

Epidemiology

The only known reservoir for *C. diphtheriae* is the human. Diphtheria spreads from person to person, either from acute cases or from asymptomatic carriers. The principal modes of spread are by respiratory droplets or direct contact with secretions from the respiratory tract or exudate from infected skin. Fomites and dust are not important vehicles of transmission, but the organism can resist drying and may be isolated from floor dust in a ward or a room in which an infected patient is being nursed. Epidemics have been caused by milk contaminated by a human carrier. Some patients become carriers and continue to harbour *C. diphtheriae* for weeks or months, or rarely, for a lifetime.

The incidence of diphtheria in the Western world has decreased in the last 50–75 years (152 cases per 100 000 population in 1920 to 0.002 per 100 000 in 1980 in the USA). In 2008, 47 cases were reported across the EU. Of these, 62% were reported by Latvia. Although diphtheria is a rare disease in the EU, the indigenous transmission of the disease persists in certain countries and suggests that epidemic diphtheria remains a potential threat to the EU. Therefore, high vaccination coverage must be maintained, adult booster coverage increased, and epidemiological surveillance and laboratory capacity preserved despite the small number of cases.[13] As diphtheria began to decline before the immunization programmes were instituted, and epidemics have occurred even in well immunized populations,[14] it seems that there are additional undefined factors contributing to the low incidence of diphtheria in affluent countries. Although there has been a great decline in the disease in wealthy countries (such that most physicians in these countries have never seen a case of diphtheria), the disease is still a significant problem in many developing countries.

Clinical Manifestations of Acute Infection

Diphtheria is predominantly a disease of childhood.[15,16] After an incubation period of 2–5 days, diphtheria presents in a variety of different forms depending upon the location of the pseudomembrane. The grey-white membrane is the hallmark of the infection. It is caused by the destructive effects of the toxin on epithelial cells. The membrane is composed of a coagulum of leukocytes, bacteria, cellular debris and fibrin. It is adherent to underlying tissues and bleeds if pulled away. In clinical practice, the disease can be divided into groups as follows: cutaneous, nasal, faucial, tracheolaryngeal and malignant diphtheria. Faucial diphtheria is the most common, whereas cutaneous diphtheria is relatively rare in endemic areas; however, where the disease is rare, cutaneous diphtheria is relatively more common.

ANTERIOR NASAL DIPHTHERIA

The principal symptom is nasal discharge (100%). This is usually unilateral, thin at first, then purulent and bloody with excoriations of the nostril and skin above the upper lip. Nasal diphtheria is relatively common in infancy. It is often mild, except when nasopharyngeal or faucial forms co-exist.

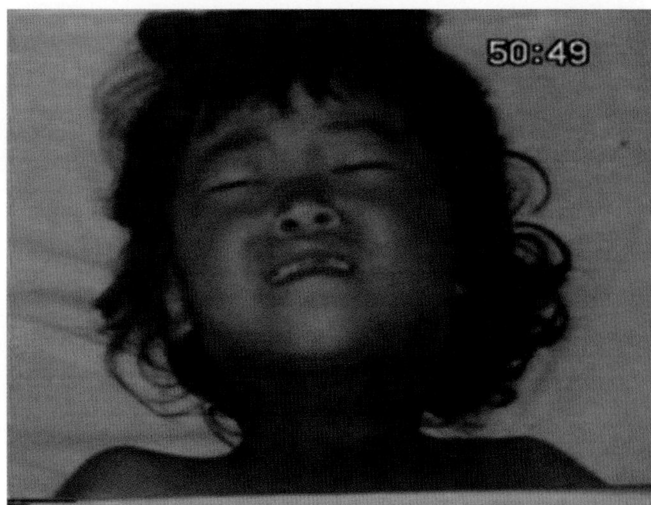

Figure 35.1 Swollen neck with enlarged lymph nodes.

FAUCIAL DIPHTHERIA

This is the most common form of diphtheria. The onset is usually slow, with moderate fever, malaise and sore throat (80%). Other symptoms may include nausea, vomiting and painful dysphagia. There is typically a patch or patches of greyish-yellow adherent membrane with a surrounding dull red inflammatory zone on one or both tonsils. At the beginning of the illness, diphtheria can look like any type of tonsillitis, with only a small spot of membrane on one tonsil. The membrane may then extend to the uvula, soft palate, oropharynx, nasopharynx or larynx. The lymph nodes in the neck are enlarged and painful, and the neck may be slightly swollen (Figure 35.1). The fetor of diphtheria is characteristic and was once one of the four criteria for clinical diagnosis (membrane, fetor, lymphadenitis, oedema).[5]

TRACHEOLARYNGEAL DIPHTHERIA

Diphtheria of the larynx is usually secondary to faucial diphtheria (85%). Occasionally, there is no membrane on the pharynx at all. The initial symptoms include moderate fever (75%) with hoarseness (100%), unproductive cough and dyspnoea. Obstruction of breathing by the expanding membrane and associated oedema occurs gradually over about 24 hours. Sometimes the membrane detaches, causing acute respiratory obstruction. The severely affected child appears frightened and agitated, but is quiet, sweating and ominously cyanotic. The accessory muscles of respiration are used, with retraction of supraclavicular, substernal and intercostal tissues on inspiration. Without a tracheostomy the child will suffocate and die.

MALIGNANT DIPHTHERIA

This is the most severe form of diphtheria. The onset is more acute than in other forms. The patient becomes rapidly 'toxic', with high fever, rapid pulse, low blood pressure and cyanosis. Usually, extension of the membrane is more rapid, spreading from the tonsils to the uvula, then creeping forward across the hard palate, up the nasopharynx, or sometimes down the nostrils. Cervical adenitis and oedema produce the classical 'bull neck' appearance. The patient may bleed from the mouth, nose and skin. Cardiac involvement with heart block occurs earlier, within a few days from the onset. More than 50% of malignant diphtheria cases are fatal, and this high mortality rate has changed little with treatment.

CUTANEOUS DIPHTHERIA

Skin infections with *C. diphtheriae* are now more common than nasopharyngeal disease in the West. This particularly affects vagrants and alcoholics living in unhygienic conditions. The clinical features range from a simple pustule to a chronic non-healing ulcer with a grey, dirty, membrane. Toxic complications from these infections are infrequent, and when they do occur, are more likely to manifest as neuritis than myocarditis.

OTHER SITES

Occasionally, clinical infections with *C. diphtheriae* may occur in other sites, such as ears, conjunctiva or vagina. Swabs of ear discharge from otitis media may occasionally grow *C. diphtheriae* but toxic manifestations are rare.

Toxic Complications

Severe diphtheria is a terrible disease. Even if patients survive the acute destructive phase of the infection, they are likely to die from the remote effects of the toxin. Patients recovering from diphtheria may die suddenly up to 8 weeks following the acute disease. The most prominent toxic complications of diphtheria are myocarditis and neuritis. The risk and the severity of toxin damage correlate with the extent of the pseudomembrane and the delay in administration of antitoxin. The frequency of cardiac involvement following laryngeal and malignant diphtheria is 3–8-fold higher than for tonsillar diphtheria, and 2–3-fold higher if antitoxin is given 48 hours or more from the onset of disease.

MYOCARDITIS

Overall, approximately 10% of patients with diphtheria develop myocarditis, although two-thirds of patients with severe infection will have some evidence of cardiac involvement. Myocarditis can be predicted on admission by the extent of the pseudomembrane, and is almost invariable if there is a bull neck.[16–19] The first evidence of cardiac toxicity usually occurs in the second week of illness. Clinical signs include soft heart sounds, a gallop rhythm, and less commonly signs of congestive heart failure. Incompetent murmurs may develop as the ventricles dilate. The mortality rate associated with diphtheritic myocarditis is approximately 50%. Echocardiography shows dilated, poorly contracting ventricles. Electrocardiographic (ECG) abnormalities are more common than clinical signs of myocarditis and include frequent supraventricular and ventricular ectopics, bursts of tachyarrhythmia, broadening of the QRS complex, ST and T wave changes, varying degrees of heart block, and bradyarrhythmias.[18–20] The loss of anterior R waves or the development of complete heart block is an ominous sign. Patients with bundle branch block and complete heart block have a very high mortality rate (more than 80%). Levels of cardiac enzymes (creatine phosphokinase MB, myoglobin and troponin) rise in proportion to the degree of cardiac damage.[19] Although early reports suggested that diphtheria might cause conduction disturbances to arise after recovery, this has not been confirmed in recent series.

NEUROPATHY

Neurotoxicity is evident in 10–20% of cases. As with myocardial damage, the extent and severity of nervous system involvement is determined by the extent and severity of the primary (usually) oropharyngeal infection. The exotoxin causes segmental degeneration of the myelin sheath and in severe cases, degeneration of the axon cylinder. Polyneuritis is uncommon in mild diphtheria but occurs in approximately 7–10% of moderate and severe cases. Neurological complications develop late, usually between 3 and 8 weeks after the onset of local symptoms, and often when other severe manifestations are resolving. Paralysis of the soft palate is a characteristic and early manifestation of neuropathy. It does not occur with cutaneous diphtheria and therefore probably results from local toxin spread in the oropharyngeal tissues.[17,18] This results in a nasal voice and regurgitation of ingested fluids through the nose. Later, blurred vision may occur because of paralysis of the muscles of accommodation together with paralysis of the pharynx, larynx and respiratory muscles. The IXth and Xth cranial nerves are most commonly affected, followed by the VIIth nerve, and the nerves to the external ocular muscles (III, IV and VI).[19] Quadriparesis is common, and death from respiratory failure may result either from paralysis of the respiratory muscles or paralytic closure of the larynx. Limb weakness occurs in about half of those with neuropathy. Sensory deficit affects proprioception in particular. Autonomic dysfunction is common, and sudden hypotension may occur between the fourth and seventh weeks of disease. The evolution of the neurological deficit is often asynchronous such that cranial nerve deficits may be improving while peripheral nerve deficits worsen. In comparing diphtheria with Guillain–Barré syndrome (GBS), diphtheric polyneuropathy is much more likely than GBS to have a bulbar onset, to lead to respiratory failure, to evolve more slowly, to take a biphasic course, and to cause death or long-term disability. In a recent series of adults with diphtheria from Latvia, 41% of those with limb weakness still could not work at their 1-year follow-up. Antitoxin seems ineffective in preventing neuropathy if administered after the second day of diphtheritic symptoms.[21–24]

OTHER COMPLICATIONS

Less common complications of diphtheria include acute tubular necrosis, disseminated intravascular coagulation, endocarditis and secondary pneumonia. The overall mortality rate of diphtheria is approximately 5–10%, with relatively higher rates in infancy and old age.

Diagnosis

In many parts of the world, especially in developing countries, diphtheria is still a common disease. It should be considered in any patient with the following symptoms: tonsillitis and/or pharyngitis with pseudomembrane, hoarseness and stridor,

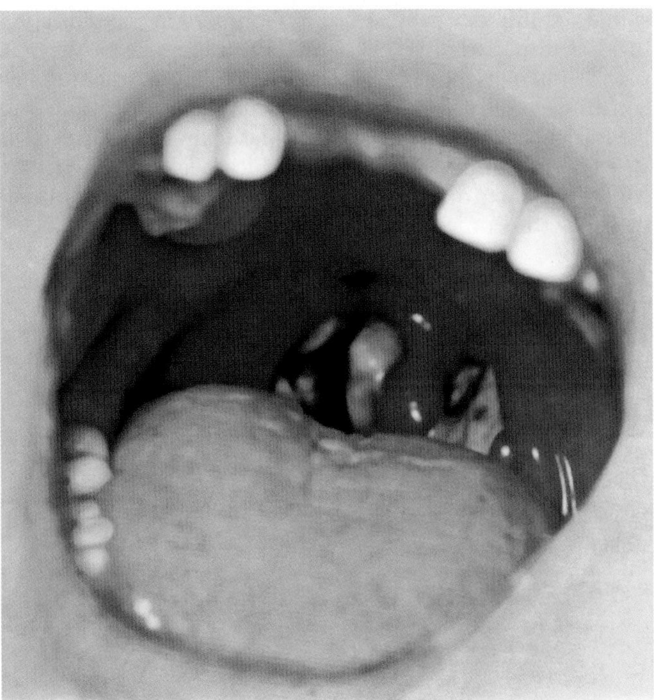

Figure 35.2 Tonsillar diphtheria. *(Courtesy of Franklin H. Top, MD, Professor and Head of the Department of Hygiene and Preventive Medicine, State University of Iowa, College of Medicine, Iowa City, IA; and Parke, Davis & Company's* Therapeutic Notes. *In: Kliegman R, et al, editors. Nelson Textbook of Pediatrics. 19th ed. Saunders, Copyright © 2011, with permission from Elsevier.)*

cervical adenopathy or cervical swelling (bull neck), unilateral bloody nasal discharge or paralysis of the palate. Direct smears of infected areas of the throat are often made, but these are unreliable. The diagnosis is confirmed by isolation and identification of *C. diphtheriae* from infected sites, but cultures are often negative, particularly if the patient has received antibiotics before admission to hospital. The differential diagnosis includes streptococcal or viral pharyngitis and tonsillitis, and Vincent's angina. Common and sometimes tragic errors are to diagnose tonsillar diphtheria (Figure 35.2) as infectious mononucleosis, or a case of 'bull neck' (malignant diphtheria) as mumps. If possible, cardiac enzymes or troponin should be monitored along with the electrocardiogram to anticipate myocardial dysfunction and conduction disturbances.

Management

Emergency tracheostomy should be performed to anticipate or relieve respiratory obstruction in laryngeal diphtheria.[25,26] The procedure must not be delayed until the patient develops cyanosis. Agitation and the use of the accessory respiratory muscles are indications for immediate tracheostomy. As the mortality rate of diphtheria increases with delay in antitoxin administration, treatment with diphtheria antitoxin should be started on clinical suspicion, without waiting for definitive laboratory confirmation. The dose of antitoxin depends on the site of primary infection, the extent of pseudomembrane, and the delay between the onset and the antitoxin administration: 20 000–40 000 units for faucial diphtheria of less than 48 hours' duration, or cutaneous infection; 40 000–80 000 units for faucial diphtheria of more than 48 hours' duration, or laryngeal infection; 80 000–100 000 units for malignant diphtheria (bull neck, toxic state). Adrenaline (epinephrine) should be available to cope with rare anaphylactic reactions to the antitoxin.

Antibiotics will stop toxin production and prevent further spread of organisms in the host. *C. diphtheriae* is susceptible to a variety of antibiotics including penicillin, cephalosporins, erythromycin and tetracycline. In a randomized comparison in Vietnam, the use of penicillin was associated with shorter fever clearance (median 27 hours) compared with 46 hours for erythromycin recipients and, whereas there was no penicillin resistance, 27% of the *C. diphtheriae* isolated were resistant to erythromycin.[27] The recommended antibiotic treatment regimen is therefore penicillin G, 50 000 units/kg daily in 4 divided doses, with erythromycin, parenterally or orally, 5 mg/kg four times daily as an alternative for penicillin-allergic patients. Antibiotic susceptibility should be checked when cultures are positive. Erythromycin is considered to be more effective in eliminating the carrier state, although there are limited data to support this.

Bed rest is recommended during the acute phase, but there is no proof of its benefit. Close electrocardiographic monitoring is indicated, particularly after the first week, to detect early signs of cardiac involvement. Angiotensin-converting enzyme inhibitors (captopril) have been used in patients, but there have been no randomized trials. If there is high-grade or complete heart block, then temporary pacing should be performed, although again there have been no large trials to determine whether these measures influence outcome. One study has suggested that carnitine may be beneficial by decreasing the incidence of myocarditis,[28] but additional evidence of its efficacy is required. The administration of corticosteroids may benefit laryngeal diphtheria by reducing swelling,[29] but otherwise is of no benefit.[30]

Insertion of a temporary pacemaker is indicated in complete heart block with bradycardia, although the mortality remains high.[31,32]

Prevention

Diphtheria is readily preventable by vaccine administration. This is included in the triple vaccine: diphtheria, tetanus and pertussis vaccine (DTP) or the quintuple diphtheria, tetanus, pertussis, polio and Hib vaccine. The recommended primary course of immunization of children aged up to 7 years consists of three doses: the first at 6–8 weeks of age, the second at 3 months and the third at 4 months. A booster dose of diphtheria, tetanus, pertussis, and polio (dTaP/IPV or DTaP/IPV) vaccine is given between 40 months and 5 years of age. A final immunization with diphtheria, tetanus, polio (Td/IPV) vaccine is given between 13 and 18 years of age. If primary immunization is delayed until 7 years of age, or is interrupted, a series of three doses of tetanus and diphtheria toxoid adsorbed (DT ads), which contains less diphtheria toxoid than DTP, should be completed, giving the second dose 4–8 weeks after the first, and the third 6–12 months later. Immunity wanes over time; decennial booster doses are required to maintain protective antibody levels. Large populations of older adults may be susceptible to diphtheria in developed countries as well as in developing countries. Research continues into combination vaccines and the intranasal delivery route. Patients with diphtheria should receive active immunization after recovery. Close contacts should be screened for *C. diphtheriae* with throat swab culture.

If the immunization status is unclear, they should be treated with an appropriate antibiotic if culture positive, and receive primary immunization according to their age. Immunity following immunization can be assessed by means of the Schick test. A standardized sterile diluted filtrate from a culture of *C. diphtheriae* (the Schick test toxin) is injected intradermally (0.2 mL) into the flexor surface of the left forearm. An equal volume (0.2 mL) of heat-inactivated filtrate (Schick test control) is injected intradermally into the right forearm. The injection sites are inspected after 24–48 hours and again at 5–7 days. A lack of inflammation indicates adequate antitoxic immunity. Sometimes nonspecific reactions (pseudoreactions) occur, but these are usually equal in both arms (i.e. toxin and control elicit an equal inflammatory reaction). Schick-negative patients are either resistant to disease or, with gravis and intermedius strains, they may sometimes develop mild disease.

REFERENCES

1. European Centre for Disease Prevention and Control. Online. Available: http://ecdc.europa.eu/en/healthtopics/diphtheria.
2. CDC. Notes from the field: Respiratory diphtheria-like illness caused by toxigenic *Corynebacterium ulcerans* – Idaho, 2010. MMWR 2011;60(3):77.
15. Hong NT, Phu VT, Hien TT. A study of 2597 cases of diphtheria treated at Cho Quan Hospital during 10 years (1976–85). Annual Scientific Report of Cho Quan Hospital, Vietnam; 1985:65–78.
26. Rakhmanova AG, Lumio J, Groundstroem K, et al. Diphtheria outbreak in St. Petersburg: clinical characteristics of 1860 adult patients. Scand J Infect Dis 1996;28:37–40.
32. Dung NM, Kneen R, Kiem N, et al. Treatment of severe diphtheritic myocarditis by temporary insertion of a cardiac pacemaker. Clin Infect Dis 2002;35:1425–9.

Access the complete references online at www.expertconsult.com

36

Endemic Treponematosis Including Yaws and Other Spirochaetes

JUAN C. SALAZAR | NICHOLAS J. BENNETT

KEY POINTS

Endemic Treponematoses

- The endemic treponemal infections are chronic, primarily cutaneous infections with characteristic epidemiological and clinical findings (Table 36.1). They are pinta, yaws and endemic syphilis (bejel).
- The causative agent of pinta is named *Treponema carateum*, that of yaws *Treponema pallidum* subsp. *pertenue*, and that of endemic syphilis *Treponema pallidum* subsp. *endemicum*. They are impossible to distinguish from each other using conventional serological or morphological criteria.
- The organisms themselves are helical, motile spirochaetes that lack the lipo-polysaccharide (LPS) of typical Gram-negative bacilli. They are approximately 0.1–0.2 micrometers (µm) in width and about 10 µm in length, with periplasmic flagellum running the length of the organism.
- Prior to the era of antibiotic use, endemic treponematoses were widespread through areas of South America, Africa, Indonesia and Papua New Guinea. Global eradication campaigns in the1940s, coordinated by the World Health Organization (WHO) and with the help of UNICEF and local governments, resulted in dramatic reductions in the incidence and prevalence of infection worldwide.[1,2]
- The most recent global data available are from 2010 (Figure 36.1 – WHO map of worldwide endemic treponematoses).
- The microbiology of the endemic treponemes has been hampered by the difficulty of readily obtaining specimens for investigation – although the causes have been given specific taxonomic identifiers, in reality the diagnosis is made on the basis of the clinical presentation rather than through the identification of a specific organism.
- Historically, there has been considerable debate and dispute as to whether the different clinical manifestations were indeed due to different species of *Treponema* or demographic or environmental differences, but DNA sequencing and restriction-fragment length polymorphisms (RFLP) do exist between the various species.[3–7]
- The recommended treatment for all treponemal infections is a single dose of intramuscular penicillin.

Lyme Disease (Lyme borreliosis)

- Lyme disease (LD), one of the most commonly reported vector-borne illnesses in the USA and Europe,[8] is a tick-borne, multi-system, infectious disorder caused by the spirochaetal bacterium *Borrelia burgdorferi*.[9,10]
- Despite increased public awareness, the disease has continued to increase in endemic areas and has spread geographically in the Northern hemisphere, paralleling the distribution of its primary vector, *Ixodes ricinus* complex, and the explosive growth in the white-tailed deer population.[11]
- Most cases occur from June through August, when nymphal ticks feed and humans in the Northern hemisphere are most likely to engage in outdoor activities.[8]
- If treated appropriately, the prognosis is excellent;[12,13] however, if untreated, spread of the bacterium may give rise to a wide range of clinical manifestations, most commonly involving the central nervous system, joints and heart.[14]
- Physicians and other medical care providers, particularly those in non-endemic areas, need to appreciate the focal geographic distribution of the disease when considering the diagnosis.

Pinta (Mal De Pinta, Carate, Enfermedad Azul)

The name *Pinta* is from the Spanish word for 'painted', an appropriate description of the appearance of the skin of affected individuals. Pinta is a solely cutaneous disease, with no systemic effects whatsoever. The colour of the lesions can vary, from dark brown or even black through red, grey or white. The pale patches are due to loss of melanin within the skin, and the degree of depigmentation can vary within lesions and with time, generally becoming more apparent as the infection progresses over several years.

EPIDEMIOLOGY

Pinta is associated with the tropical countries of Central and South America, predominantly among those living in poverty.[15] It has also been reported from the Caribbean. It was typically found in the low-lying river basins of Brazil, Colombia, Ecuador, Mexico, Peru and Venezuela and was rarely encountered at

TABLE 36.1 Clinical Characteristics, Geographic Distribution and Treatment of Pinta, Yaws and Endemic Syphilis

Disease	Organs Affected	Age	Geography	Treatment
Pinta	Skin only, hyper- and hypo-pigmented patches	Any age, commonly children and young adults	(Presumed eradicated) Low-lying areas and river basins of Central and South America, and the Caribbean	Penicillin 1.2 million Units IM once (600 000 Units for children under 10 years) Alternatives: Tetracycline 500 mg PO 4× daily for 15 days (250 mg for ages 8–15 years), erythromycin, azithromycin
Yaws	Skin (papules, papilloma, ulcers), bone, cartilage – late destructive lesions of face and joints in a minority	Young children	Endemic in Papua New Guinea, the Solomon Islands and Vanuatu in the Western Pacific region, and Indonesia and Timor-Leste in South-east Asia	
Endemic syphilis	Skin, bone, cartilage (rarely heart, brain, eyes). Late disease common, thought to be autoimmune	Pre-pubescent children	Isolated areas of the Arabian Peninsula and the southern border of the Sahara Desert. Rarely found in Asia and India.	

higher elevations.[16] Cases have also been reported from Argentina, Bolivia, Chile, the Dominican Republic, Honduras and Nicaragua. Pinta may have been eradicated as part of the worldwide efforts against endemic treponemal infections: the last reported case was in an Austrian traveller from Cuba in 1999. If it still exists it is in isolated areas. It was at one point considered endemic in South America, with hundreds of thousands of cases occurring annually in the early 20th century. Pinta is more common in young adults and children, but can occur at any age. It does not have a predilection for either sex, and the racial mix of patients mimics the local racial proportions. Pinta is associated with poverty, crowded living conditions and poor hygiene – probably due to its mode of transmission through broken skin (see below).

PATHOGENESIS

Pinta is caused by *Treponema carateum*, which causes infection by entering the body through breaks in the skin.[17] Pinta is not known to be acquired through vertical or blood-borne transmission. There has been no confirmed association with insect vectors, although this has been proposed as a possible mode of transmission. Infection is limited to the dermal and epidermal tissues, even after systemic dissemination. In primary and secondary lesions there are large numbers of organisms and a proliferative infiltrate of plasma cells, lymphocytes and Langerhans cells. Regional lymphadenopathy may develop in draining lymph nodes. Blood vessels in the affected areas remain normal, unlike in the secondary lesions of syphilis where they may exhibit proliferative changes. The primary and secondary lesions are highly infectious, containing large numbers of organisms, and direct contact with these lesions is the primary mode of transmission to uninfected individuals. In tertiary lesions the numbers of organisms decline until they are no longer detectable, and concomitantly there is loss of skin pigment until the skin becomes completely achromic.[18] There may also be loss of hair follicles and sweat glands. The changes typically occur at different rates in different lesions,

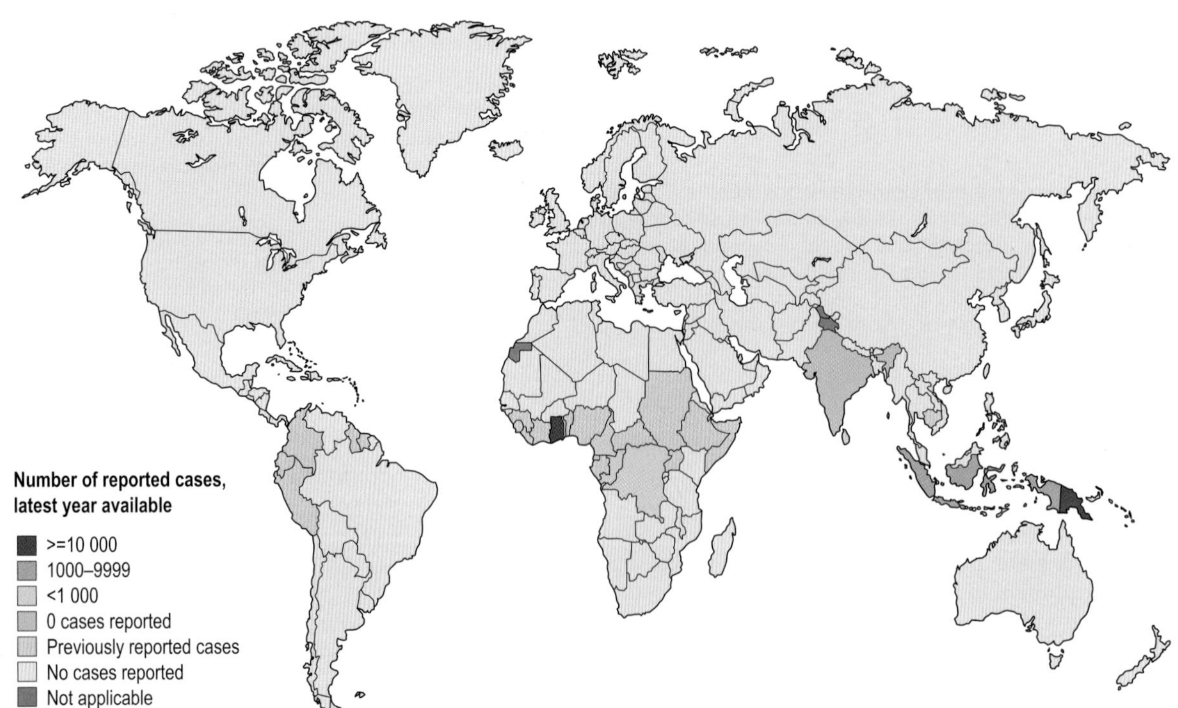

Figure 36.1 Geographic distribution of the endemic treponematoses as of 2010. *(Reproduced with permission from WHO.)*

and even within lesions, leading to a polychromatic appearance.

CLINICAL FINDINGS

The characteristic clinical findings are single or multiple areas of hyper-pigmented and depigmented skin, but the specific appearance varies with the clinical stage of infection.[17] Lesions at different stages may co-exist.[15] The incubation period from exposure to clinical findings is typically 2–3 weeks, but may be as short as a few days or as long as 2 months. Primary lesions are small erythematous papules that may appear scaly or indurated. Over the course of a few months they grow in size and may coalesce. They become more pigmented initially and may have raised margins. Regional lymphadenopathy may be apparent. Some primary lesions will self-resolve, but in other cases they may persist for several months or years.

Secondary lesions, called pintids, appear after several months and may co-exist with the primary lesions. They initially start as small scaly erythematous papules and can occur on any area of the skin, as they are due to dissemination of the organism rather than direct inoculation. Pintids generally get darker with time. Sun exposure seems to have an effect on the colour of the lesions, with darker lesions being seen in areas of greater sun exposure. Lesions on the legs are usually shades of brown.

The tertiary stage is characterized by depigmentation of the skin, and can occur as early as 3 months from the start of infection (Figure 36.2). It usually begins after several years, and is a slowly progressive loss of skin colour similar to that seen in vitiligo. In Cuba, there is an association with hyperkeratosis of the soles of the feet with this stage of infection. Because the lesions are relatively nonspecific, especially early on, they may be confused with skin diseases that are also characterized by scaly, hyperkeratotic, hyperpigmented or hypopigmented lesions. Psoriasis, parapsoriasis, lichen planus, vitiligo, ochronosis or leprosy may be considered in the differential diagnosis.[17]

DIAGNOSIS

Diagnosis is based upon detection of a treponemal organism from lesions in the appropriate clinical setting. There are no specific laboratory tests to definitively identify *T. carateum* from other treponemes. There are no isolates available for analysis with modern molecular techniques due to the fact that the disease has declined so much, therefore it may never be known how the organism differs genetically from other treponemes.

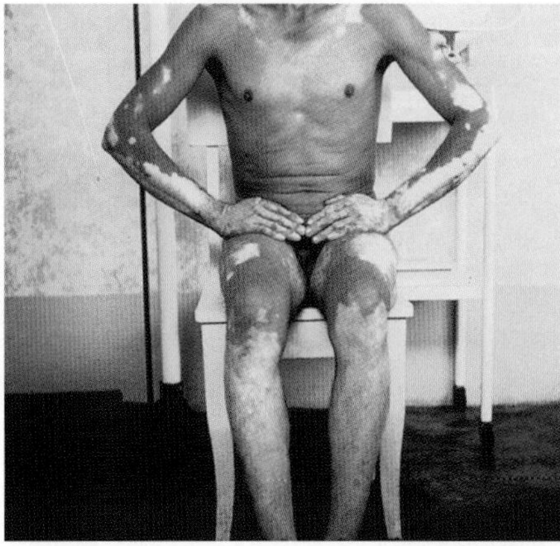

Figure 36.2 Depigmented lesions of pinta. *(Reprinted from Peters W, Pasvol G. Atlas of Tropical Medicine and Parasitology. 6th edn. Elsevier; 2006. p. 330, Copyright © 2007, with permission from Elsevier.)*

MANAGEMENT AND TREATMENT

The treatment of choice is penicillin (see below). Because Pinta is limited to cutaneous manifestations the medical prognosis of infected individuals is excellent. However, the social stigma associated with the appearance of the disease may force some individuals away from the support of mainstream society into situations they are less able to seek and obtain medical treatment for their infection.

Yaws (Frambesia, Pian, Buba, Bouba)

Yaws is a transmissible treponemal disease of the tropics, which is typically acquired early in childhood and characterized by relapsing/remitting cutaneous lesions that result in local destruction of the tissues and subsequent permanent damage.[17] Clinically yaws may be confused with any of the other endemic treponemes, as the clinical manifestations overlap to some degree. Early lesions may apparently resolve, but late disease causes long-term damage to skin, bones and cartilage and can result in significant life-long disfiguration. Ulcerative skin and mucosal lesions are susceptible to secondary bacterial infection. Destructive lesions may resemble those seen in tertiary venereal syphilis, mucocutaneous leishmaniasis, leprosy or rhinoscleroma.

EPIDEMIOLOGY

In 1995, the WHO estimated fewer than 500 000 cases worldwide from an initial peak of 50 million cases, but there have been no reliable global statistics available since 1990. Yaws is found in rural areas of tropical countries and has been reported from Africa, South America, South-east Asia, the Caribbean and Pacific islands.[19] There was a 95% reduction in the number of infections with an eradication campaign between 1952 and 1964, but rates have risen in some countries in recent decades as attention has been diverted elsewhere.[20,21] Attempts by the World Health Organization to restart the programs in the 1970s and 1980s failed in part due to delegation of the programme to local health services rather than relying on the large resources of the WHO and UNICEF, who had led the initial eradication efforts.

In 2008, the World Health Organization reported that yaws remained endemic in Papua New Guinea, the Solomon Islands and Vanuatu in the Western Pacific region, and Indonesia and Timor-Leste (known also as East Timor) in South-east Asia.[19] In 2005, cases were reported from the Democratic Republic of Congo, an area previously thought to have eradicated the infection, and this was supported by a serological survey reported in 2009.[22] About one-third of school children examined on the island of Tanna in Vanuatu in 2008 had skin lesions consistent with yaws, although only 33–60% of possible or probable clinical cases had positive serological tests.[23] In contrast, India has continued surveillance and treatment efforts, and has reported no new cases since 2004.[24] The WHO has called yaws 'a forgotten disease', despite the fact that it is amenable to possible eradication.

Yaws is normally seen in young children and is associated with crowding and unhygienic conditions.[7] Transmission is from close contact with the infected lesions of another individual through a break in the skin. The typical entry sites are the lower legs, head, face and mouth. The disease is usually acquired in childhood and is probably not transmissible by the time the host reaches adolescence, as sexual and vertical transmissions do not occur. There is no apparent predilection for males or females. Yaws seems to provide immunity to re-infection in humans, and may also provide cross-protection to *T. pallidum* subsp. *pallidum* and *endemicum*.

The possible isolation of *T. pallidum* subsp. *pertenue* from West African monkeys, and positive serological tests in these animals, suggests that they may act as a reservoir for the agent in this area, although this has not been confirmed.[25] Yaws has also been described in gorillas, where it has negative effects on their health.[26]

PATHOGENESIS

T. pallidum subsp. *pertenue* enters the host through breaks in the skin, typically in the lower leg. The primary site of infection demonstrates lymphocytic infiltrates, plasma cells, macrophages and hyperkeratosis. There is often adenopathy of the draining lymph nodes and both the primary lesion and the regional lymph nodes contain numerous organisms. Dissemination occurs throughout the body and secondary sites of infection are seeded in the skin, bones and cartilage. Chronic inflammatory changes at these sites are similar to those seen at the initial site of infection, but vascular changes are unusual in cutaneous yaws. Primary and secondary lesions will regress with treatment or with successful immune control.

CLINICAL FINDINGS

Similar to Pinta, yaws is primarily a cutaneous disease initially, with findings of relapsing and remitting skin lesions and later destruction of deeper tissues.[27] The incubation period is between 9 days and 3 months, but is typically about 3 weeks. A primary lesion, a raised papule that enlarges to become a papilloma with hyperkeratosis, is known as a 'mother yaw' and may be several centimetres across (Figure 36.3). With time it gradually ulcerates and then heals, leaving a hypopigmented patch of skin with hyperpigmented margins. There may be regional adenopathy associated with this early lesion.

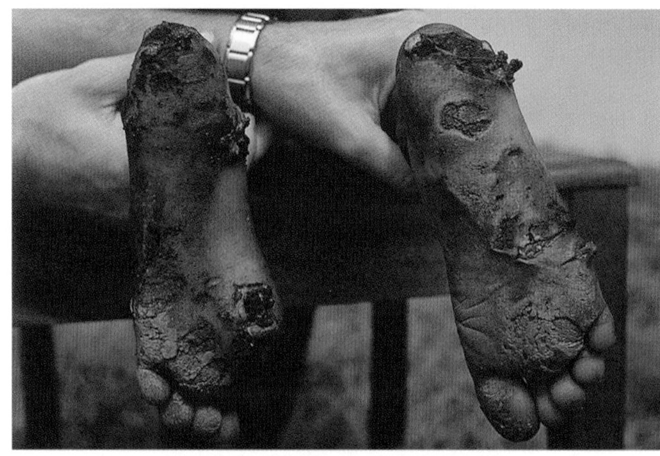

Figure 36.4 Indeterminate yaws: plantar hyperkeratosis (crab yaws). *(Reprinted from Peters W, Pasvol G. Atlas of Tropical Medicine and Parasitology. 6th edn. Elsevier; 2006. p. 329, Copyright © 2007, with permission from Elsevier.)*

Secondary lesions appear around the time that the mother yaw heals, but may appear several weeks before to several months after the initial lesion has healed. Secondary lesions may appear on the mucous membranes, in the long bones as periosteitis, osteitis and osteomyelitis although they are non-destructive at this stage. Hyperkeratosis of the skin may be painful, especially when it occurs on the feet and results in fissuring, and may result in a peculiar gait where the affected individual is forced to walk on the sides of their feet to reduce the pressure on their soles – a condition known as 'crab yaws' (Figure 36.4). The lesions on mucous membranes may be papules, or more resembling condylomata lata. If they do not fade spontaneously they may form 'daughter yaws' or 'satellite secondaries' – which are approximately 1–3 cm in diameter, and appear as lobular or granulated circular patches (Figures 36.5–36.7). They are reddish-yellow in colour and ooze a yellow discharge, which crusts to form a black scab. Untreated

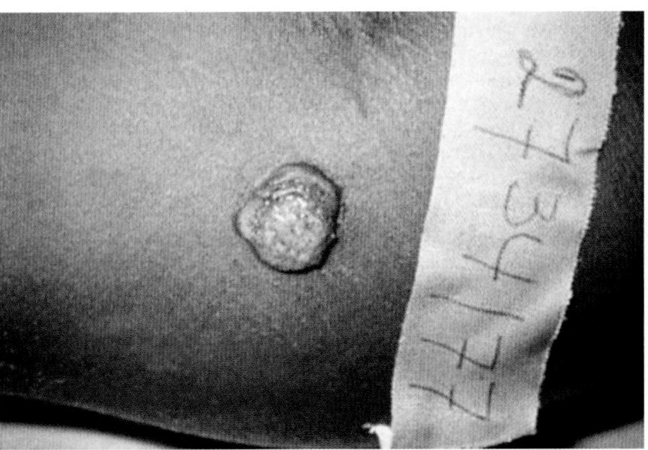

Figure 36.3 Yaws: initial lesion 'mother yaw'. *(From Perine PL, Hopkins DR, Niemel PLA, et al. Handbook of Endemic Treponematoses. Geneva: World Health Organization; 1984.)*

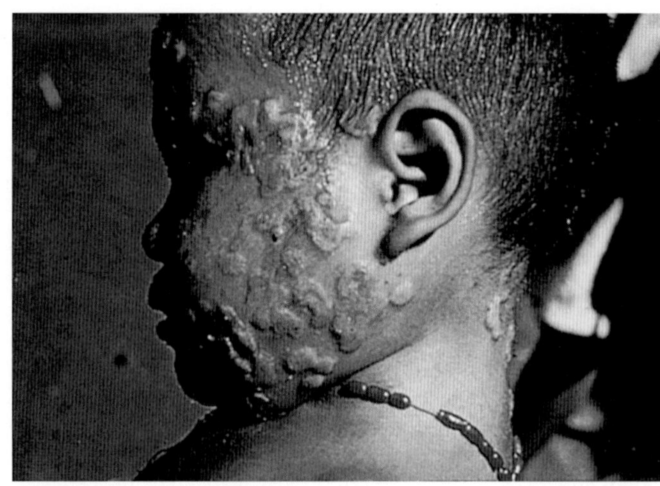

Figure 36.5 Cutaneous early yaws: papillomas. *(Courtesy of C. J. Hackett.)*

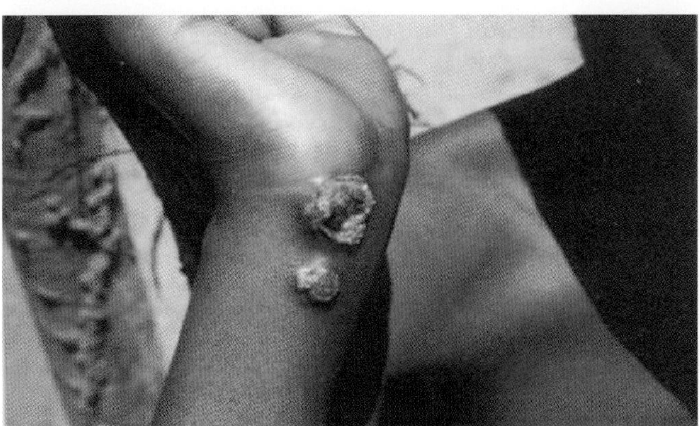

Figure 36.6 Early yaws papillomata over the wrist. *(Reprinted from Lal S, Dhariwal AC, Yaws, Pinta, and Endemic Syphilis. In: International Encyclopedia of Public Health, p. 651–7, Copyright © 2008, with permission from Elsevier Inc.)*

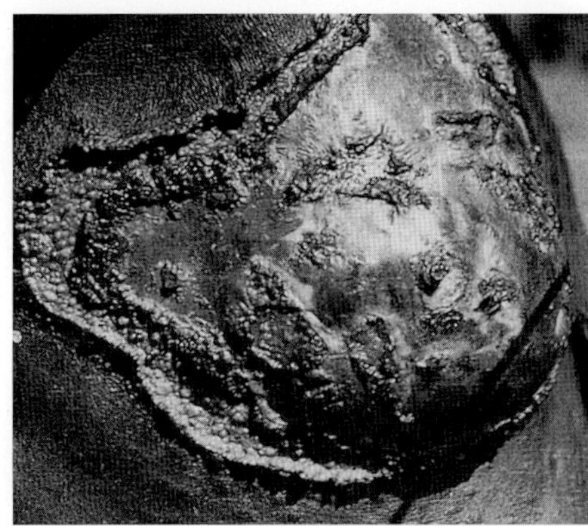

Figure 36.8 Late yaws: gumma of the right breast. *(Courtesy of C. J. Hackett.)*

secondary lesions are eventually controlled by the immune response, which involves both humoral and cellular components, at least in an animal model.[28] Some lesions may persist for several months and occasionally are complicated by secondary bacterial infections that may impair healing, otherwise there is usually little to no scarring of secondary yaws.

The disease then goes into a state of clinical latency, but relapses occur in many patients, usually several times over a period of 3–5 years. The mechanisms for late disease and recurrence from clinical latency may be due to failure of the immune response, hypersensitivity reactions, or antigenic variation in the organism. Simple recurrences from latency may resolve spontaneously. The number of organisms in secondary lesions tends to decrease over time and with each recurrence. Late disease occurs in a minority of patients (approx. 10%) after several years of clinical latency without outbreaks, and is characterized by gummatous (Figure 36.8) and destructive lesions in the cartilage and bone, with periosteitis, nodular or non-nodular osteomyelitis (Figure 36.9) or periarticular granulomatous nodules. Late disease, if it occurs, persists for the life of the patient. Significant clinical manifestations include rhinopharyngitis mutilans, known colloquially as 'gangosa' (Figure 36.10), which is a terribly disfiguring destructive process of the skin and bones of the central face; painful hyperkeratosis of the palms and soles of the feet (Figure 36.4); saber tibiae (Figure 36.11) and a progressive hypertrophic osteitis disease of the frontal processes of the maxillae, known as 'goundou' (Figure 36.12). Goundou was last reported in 1989.[29]

DIAGNOSIS

Yaws is caused by *T. pallidum* subsp. *pertenue*. Diagnosis is based upon detection of a treponemal organism from typical lesions in the appropriate clinical setting. With the exception of real-time PCR amplification of specific treponemal DNA sequences,[7] there are no specific laboratory tests to definitively identify

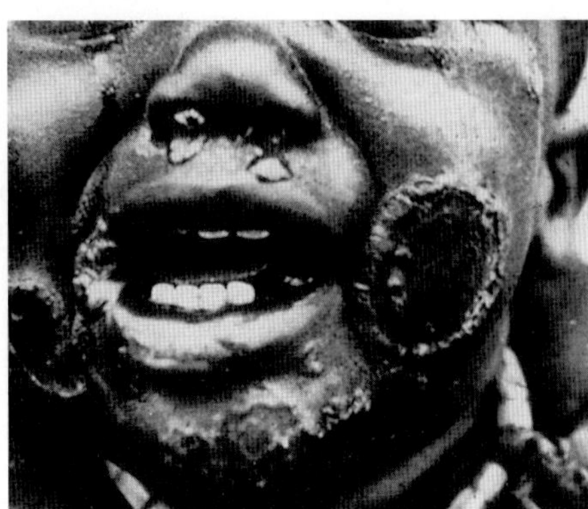

Figure 36.7 Cutaneous early yaws: papillomas. *(Courtesy of C. J. Hackett.)*

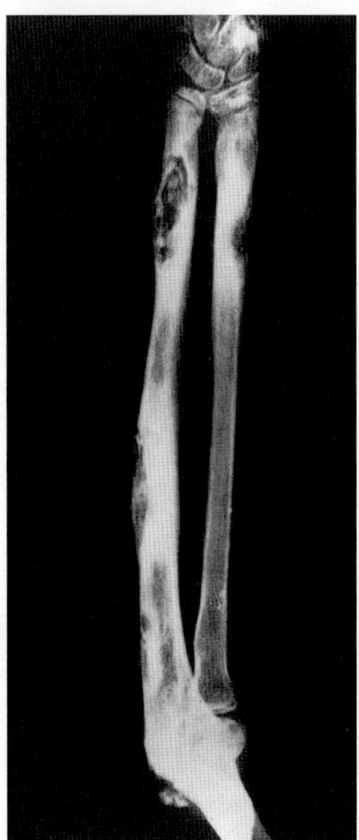

Figure 36.9 Late yaws: gummatous osteitis of radius and ulna. *(Courtesy of C. J. Hackett.)*

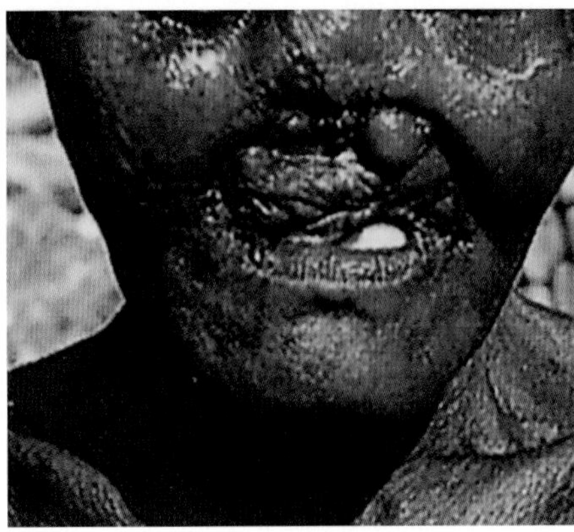

Figure 36.10 Late yaws: gangosa. *(Reprinted from Peters W, Pasvol G. Atlas of Tropical Medicine and Parasitology. 6th edn. Elsevier; 2006. p. 330, Copyright © 2007, with permission from Elsevier.)*

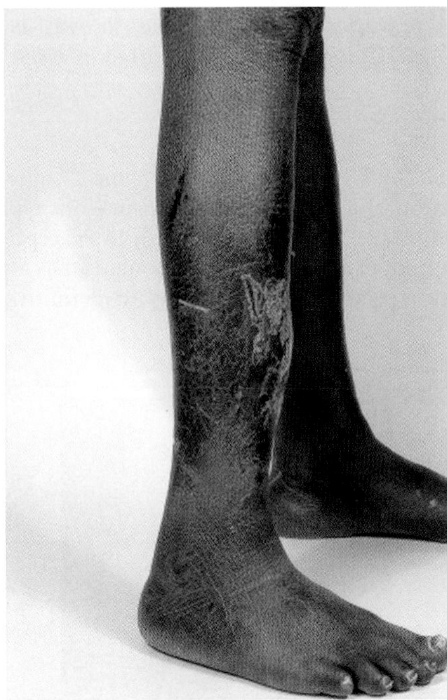

Figure 36.11 Late yaws: sabre tibia. *(By courtesy of R.A. Marsden, MD, St George's Hospital, London, UK., Reprinted from McKee's Pathology of the Skin. 4th edn. Grayson, Wayne, p. 760–895, Copyright © 2012, with permission from Elsevier Ltd.)*

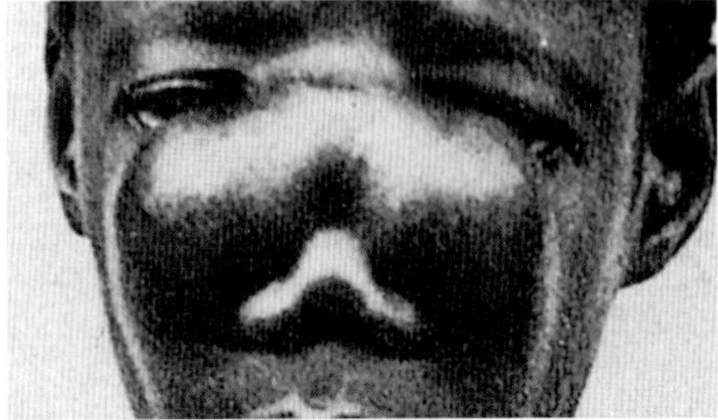

Figure 36.12 Early yaws: goundou. *(Courtesy of C. J. Hackett.)*

T. pallidum subsp. *pertenue* from other treponemes. Isolates available for genetic analysis have confirmed it as a distinct organism from *T. pallidum* subsp. *pallidum* and *endemicum*, the causes of venereal and endemic syphilis respectively.[3] Animal models exist for yaws and can be used to distinguish treponemal organisms – rabbits and hamsters developed lymphadenopathy and cutaneous lesions that differ in distribution, form and number from those seen in models of syphilis.

MANAGEMENT AND TREATMENT

Intramuscular penicillin is the drug of choice for treating yaws. Untreated, yaws is not a benign infection, but its effects are limited to the potentially severe disfiguration and pain that can occur as a result of the destructive lesions of late disease. Even the bony abnormalities rarely lead to fractures. Contractures can occur as a result of lesions close to joints. One particularly important complication requiring adjunct antimicrobial treatment is that of secondary bacterial infections in exposed bone or damaged skin, which aside from leading to further damage and scarring may also cause significant problems in their own right.

Recently, a clinical trial of single-dose azithromycin compared to IM penicillin in 250 children in Papua New Guinea proved to be effective in treating yaws[30] and has the advantage of not requiring refrigeration of the drug, unlike penicillin. It also facilitates mass drug administration with oral antimicrobials for other endemic parasitic diseases. A new approach towards yaws eradication was proposed by the WHO in March of 2012, requiring total community treatment in areas of seropositivity until there are zero clinical cases.[31]

Endemic Syphilis (Bejel, Njovera, Siti, Dichuchwa)

Endemic syphilis, caused by *T. pallidum* subsp. *endemicum*, is a disease acquired in early childhood. It typically affects children living in dry and arid regions in the African continent and the Arabian Peninsula. The worldwide eradication efforts of the mid-twentieth century led to a dramatic reduction in cases, but some remnants remain.[21] Of the three endemic treponemes it has the highest rate of long-term morbidity among infected individuals.

EPIDEMIOLOGY

Endemic syphilis currently exists as isolated endemic foci in some areas of the Arabian Peninsula,[32] and the southern border of the Sahara Desert, an area known as the Sahel region, where it occurs in semi-nomadic tribes.[15] Outbreaks were described in the 1970s and 1980s throughout Africa. It is rare in Asia, India and other countries where it was once known, due to the effectiveness of mass treatment campaigns.[21] It is associated with conditions of poor hygiene and over-crowding which favor transmission of the organism. Transmission is often via the oral route, through contaminated eating, drinking, or food preparation utensils. Saliva can spread the infection via contaminated fingers or direct mouth-to-mouth contact. Examples have been described of nursing mothers developing a primary lesion on a breast from a nursing infant who is infected. Unlike the high rates of mother-to-child transmission of *T. pallidum* in gestational syphilis, congenital transmission does not occur in endemic syphilis. Infection is typically seen in pre-pubescent children with an equal sex distribution. The role of insect vectors is probably limited to causing breaks in the skin which become routes by which an infection may occur.

PATHOGENESIS

Infection typically occurs through the oral mucosa, but there may not be sufficient inoculum to result in a noticeable primary lesion.[33] If one does occur, it manifests as a chronic inflammatory response which appears as a papule or ulcer. Lymphocytes, macrophages and plasma cells are found at the site. A similar response is seen in the regional lymph nodes, and organisms may be found in lymph nodes within just a few hours of infection. The incubation period from infection to the appearance of a primary lesion is approximately 3 weeks. Regardless of whether a primary lesion occurs, systemic dissemination leads to widespread infection via the circulation. The typical sites for secondary lesions are the oral mucosa, skin, bone, axillary and anogenital regions. A similar lymphocytic inflammatory response is seen, along with vascular changes such as perivascular cuffing.

Untreated lesions heal over a period of 6–9 months as a result of immune responses involving both humoral and cellular arms, and the infection enters a period of clinical latency.[34,35] Late disease is thought to be due to hypersensitivity responses rather than a direct effect of the organism, and infectiousness during this phase of the infection is a matter of debate. Experiments using inbred hamsters suggest resistance to re-infection and cross-protection to *T. pallidum* subsp. *pallidum* and *T. pallidum* subsp. *pertenue.*[36]

CLINICAL FINDINGS

In terms of the appearance of the lesions, endemic syphilis more closely resembles venereal syphilis than the other endemic treponemes.[37] There is not usually a primary lesion, but if one does appear they are a painless ulcer or papule, usually in the oropharynx, occurring approximately 3 weeks after exposure (10–90 days) (Figure 36.13). They may not heal for several years. After a further 3–6 months, secondary lesions appear which may be indistinguishable from those of secondary syphilis (disseminated papules).[38] Common forms of secondary lesions are: relatively painless oropharyngeal ulcers involving the tongue, lips, palate and tonsils; angular stomatitis or papules; condylomata similar to those of secondary syphilis (Figure 36.14); and annular papilloma patches. Regional lymphadenopathy is common, including cervical adenopathy with oropharyngeal involvement. The larynx may be affected and lead to hoarseness of the voice.[39]

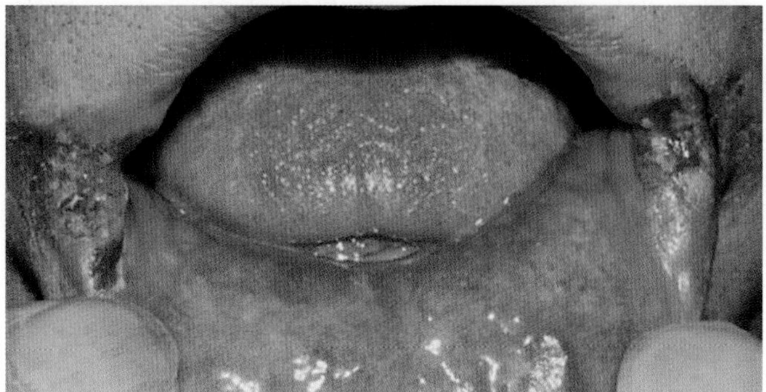

Figure 36.13 Early endemic syphilis: mucus papules of the oral mucosa of the lip. *(From Kinghorn GR. Syphilis. Medicine 1995;24:64–8, with permission of The Medicine Group (Journals) Ltd.)*

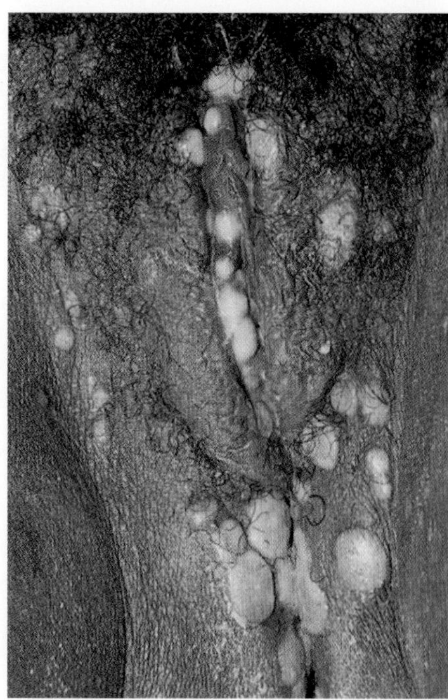

Figure 36.14 Secondary syphilis: moist papules. *(Reprinted from Lynch PJ and Edwards L, Genital Dermatology (Fig. 9.3), Churchill Livingstone.)*

Tertiary disease is common and occurs in most patients, typically in the later teenage years and in early adulthood.[37] Lesions resemble tertiary venereal syphilis or late yaws. Destructive bony lesions and ulcerations of the skin and nasopharynx may lead to severe disfigurement similar to gangosa in late yaws. Periosteitis of the long bones of the legs is the most common bony manifestation, and is painful. Synovitis and periarticular disease can also occur. Unlike tertiary venereal syphilis, neurologic, ocular, and cardiac disease is rare, and tends to be mild if it does occur.[40]

A number of dermatological diseases should be considered in the differential diagnosis. Secondary lesions can be confused with those of the other endemic treponemal diseases, as well as eczema, mycoses, psoriasis, leprosy, perlèche and condylomata acuminata. Oral lesions may resemble those of herpes simplex virus (although gingivostomatitis due to herpes simplex is usually extremely painful). Tertiary lesions may resemble those of yaws or malignant skin tumours, and the destructive facial appearances in particular may mimic those seen in gangosa, venereal syphilis, mucocutaneous leishmaniasis, rhinoscleroma or leprosy.

DIAGNOSIS

Diagnosis is based upon detection of a treponemal organism from lesions in the appropriate clinical setting. There are no specific laboratory tests to definitively identify *T. pallidum* subsp. *endemicum* from other treponemes. Isolates available for genetic analysis have confirmed it as a distinct organism from *T. pallidum* subsp. *pertenue*, the cause of yaws and *T. pallidum* subsp. *pallidum*, the cause of venereal syphilis.[3,4,6] Animal models do exist in rabbits and hamsters, and the various endemic treponemes causing yaws, endemic syphilis and venereal syphilis can be distinguished based upon the distribution, form and number of lesions and affected lymph nodes.

MANAGEMENT AND TREATMENT

Penicillin is the drug of choice for treatment of endemic syphilis (see below). As with all the endemic treponemes, the morbidity associated with untreated endemic syphilis is largely due to the destructive and disfiguring nature of the late lesions, and the negative effects on the individual in terms of social ostracization and a resulting loss of support and access to medical care. Bony lesions can be painful enough to severely affect the patient's quality of life and ability to work.

General Points

DIAGNOSIS

The diagnosis of the endemic treponemes is based upon the clinical appearance as well as attempts to detect the organisms from biopsies of the lesions. The treponemes usually require dark-field microscopy to detect due to their narrow width (0.1–0.2 μm), and this technique might not be available in resource-poor settings. Under dark field microscopy of fresh specimens, motile organisms might be visible. The organism stains poorly with conventional laboratory techniques but can be identified using direct fluorescent antibody (DFA) techniques or silver stains. Molecular techniques using DNA amplification or sequencing have been developed.[7,41,42]

Serological testing is composed of non-treponemal tests such as the reactive plasma reagin (RPR) or Venereal Disease Research Laboratory (VDRL) tests, as well as treponemal-specific antibody tests such as fluorescent-treponemal-antibody absorption (FTA-ABS). These tests are identical to those used to diagnose venereal syphilis and cannot be used to distinguish the endemic treponemes from each other or from venereal syphilis. As with venereal syphilis, treatment of the endemic treponemes is associated with at least a twofold decline in the titre of the RPR antibody level. Care must be taken to avoid misdiagnosis due to false-positive cross-reactions.[43] In Pinta seroconversion may not occur for several months after the appearance of the initial lesion, whereas in yaws and endemic syphilis patients usually test positive within a month.

MANAGEMENT, TREATMENT AND PREVENTION

Treatment of the endemic treponemal disease is almost universally successful. Clinical recurrences are usually due to reinfection. Pinta takes the longest time to respond to therapy, and hypopigmented lesions may never recover their natural skin colour. Primary and early secondary lesions may take up to 6 months to disappear, and it is not uncommon for late secondary lesions to take up to a year to heal completely. Yaws is rendered non-infectious in a few days and complete healing of early lesions takes only 7–10 days. Later lesions may respond more slowly – severe lesions may require surgery. The response of endemic syphilis to therapy is similar to that of yaws.

The drug of choice is intramuscular benzathine penicillin G. For patients older than 10 years of age with clinically active disease, latent disease or close contacts of known cases, 1.2 million units as a single dose is effective. For children younger than 10 years of age the dose is 600 000 units. Reports of resistance are unusual and may actually represent reinfection or problems with drug administration or refrigeration.

Alternative therapies that have been tried include: oral penicillin, tetracycline and azithromycin. Tetracycline at a dose of 500 mg orally, 4 times a day for 15 days, is considered a reasonable alternative for adults who are allergic to penicillin. Children aged 8–15 years may receive half the dose. Children under the age of 8, or pregnant women, should not receive tetracycline due to its adverse effects on tooth development. Erythromycin may be effective, as it has been used successfully to treat syphilis, at a dose of 8–10 mg/kg 4 times daily up to a total daily dose of 1 g. A recent clinical trial of a single dose of azithromycin was successful in treating yaws.[30] The major advantage of these alternative therapies is the lack of a need to refrigerate the antibiotic.

Penicillin has been the mainstay of eradication, along with improvements in living conditions and sanitation. The WHO guidelines recommend mass treatment of a population where seroprevalence exceeds 10%. For places with seropositive rates of 5–10% all patients, close contacts, and all children under 15 years of age are treated. For places with seropositive rates of under 5% all patients, close contacts, and household members are treated. This approach has been remarkably effective. In 2012 the WHO updated their recommendations for Yaws eradication, to treat all people in areas of seropositivity until there are no longer any clinical cases."

Lyme Disease (Lyme Borreliosis)

EPIDEMIOLOGY

Lyme disease (Lyme borreliosis) is a tick-borne, complex, multisystem infection caused by the spirochetal bacterium *Borrelia burgdorferi*. The disease affects adults and children living in temperate zones of the Northern Hemisphere. Since first identified in Connecticut in the 1970s,[44] LD has become the most prevalent arthropod-transmitted infection in the USA and Europe.[8] In 2011, most cases of LD in the USA were reported several Northeastern and Midwestern states (Connecticut, Delaware, Massachusetts, Maryland, Minnesota, New Hampshire, New Jersey, New York, Pennsylvania, Rhode Island, Virginia and Wisconsin, see: http://www.cdc.gov/lyme/stats/chartstables/incidencebystate.html). In Europe, the highest incidence of the disease is seen in Slovenia, Austria and the Netherlands (206, 135 and 103 per 100 000, respectively).[45] *B. burgdorferi*, also has been isolated from hard ticks collected from other geographic locations[46] including countries in Asia[47] and Northern Africa. Despite isolated reports, there is little evidence that LD is a significant problem in the tropics or in the Southern hemisphere.

PATHOGENESIS

The Bacterium

Phylogenetic analyses have led to the division of LD spirochaetes into several species, collectively referred to as *B. burgdorferi* sensu lato. Three genospecies predominate as human pathogens, *B. burgdorferi* sensu stricto in the USA and Western Europe,[48] and *Borrelia garinii* and *Borrelia afzelli.* in Eurasia.[48] *B. burgdorferi's* genomic features,[49] as well as its unique molecular architecture,[50] are considered to play seminal roles in how the the bacterium is transmitted from ticks to humans and how it triggers innate and adaptive immune responses in its human host.

Enzootic Cycle

B. burgdorferi is transmitted by ticks of the *Ixodes ricinus* complex.[51,52] *I. scapularis* (Figure 36.15), *I. ricinus*, and *I. persulcatus* are the principal vectors in the northeastern USA, Europe and Asia, respectively. *Ixodes* ticks have a 2-year life cycle with four life-stages: egg, larva, nymph and adult. They feed only three times, once at each non-egg life-stage.[53] Ticks are born uninfected, and only become infected with *B. burgdorferi* after feeding upon an infected animal. Naïve larvae acquire the spirochete by feeding on an infected reservoir host, typically a rodent (e.g. *Peromyscus leucopus*, the white-footed mouse), and, after molting to the nymphal stage, transmit the pathogen when they feed on an uninfected host. Nymphal ticks are believed to be responsible for the majority of human infections, although adult ticks are capable of transmitting the pathogen.[54] Nymphs, which have the highest infection rates, nymphs quest during the summer months when humans are most likely to be outdoors.

The Immune Response

In humans the initial entry of spirochaetes into the dermis induces a robust local inflammatory response that within a few days becomes manifest as an expanding annular rash, commonly known as erythema migrans (EM).[14] The spirochaetes also migrate outwards from the feeding site and downward towards the dermal microvasculature, en route to disseminating hematogenously.[55] The ensuing local inflammatory response, which is amplified as *B. burgdorferi*-specific T cells are primed in draining lymph nodes, enter the circulation, and traffic back to the inflamed site. The immunohistological pattern of EM is

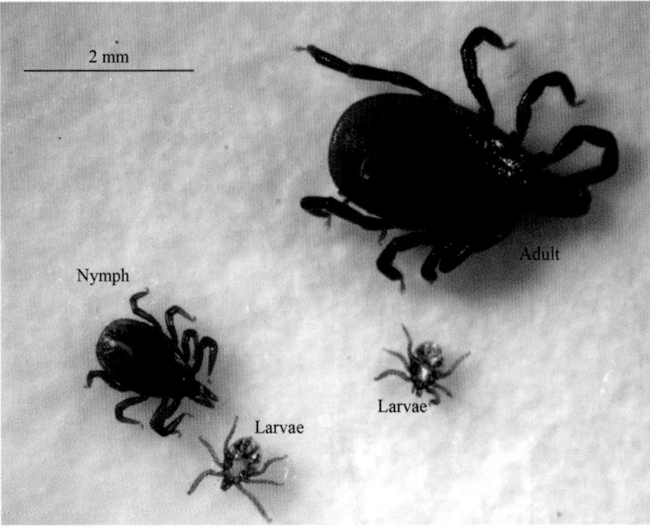

Figure 36.15 *Ixodes scapularis* pass through four developmental stages: eggs, larvae, nymphs and adults. The larvae, nymph and female adult are shown here prior to feeding. *(Courtesy of Star Dunham-Emms.)*

characterized by a dense dermal immune cellular inflammatory infiltrate composed of lymphocytes, neutrophils, monocytes and macrophages, as well as activated dendritic cells (DCs).[56,57] Activation of local and recruited dermal innate immune cells present in EM lesions very likely occurs as soon as these cells come into contact with the bacterium, which ultimately results in transcription and secretion of a wide array of pro- and anti-inflammatory cytokines, chemokines and inflammatory mediators.[56,58] Not surprisingly, this stage of the disease is also frequently accompanied by systemic symptoms, including myalgia, arthralgia, and fever. Since *B. burgdorferi* lacks orthologues of known exotoxins, or the specialized secretory machinery required for the delivery of noxious molecules into host cells,[49] it is well accepted that both local (skin) and systemic clinical manifestations of Lyme disease are the consequence of innate and co-evolving adaptive humoral and cellular immune responses to the spirochaete. Paradoxically, while these responses induce tissue damage, they are critical for the eradication of the bacterium.

Innate Immune Recognition

For several years, most efforts to understand how *B. burgdorferi* initiates innate immune cell activation in tissues were focused chiefly on the pro-inflammatory attributes of isolated spirochaetal lipoproteins,[59–66] while less was done to define the mechanisms underlying immune recognition of live spirochaetes. The emphasis on Borrelial lipoproteins (BLPs) as innate immune agonists first emerged from the discovery that spirochaetes express an abundance of these molecules,[49,67] many on their outer membrane, and that the Borrelial cell envelope lacks the potent Gram-negative proinflammatory glycolipid, lipopolysaccharide (LPS).[49,68] Unlike LPS, which signals through TLR-4 and CD14,[69] lipoproteins signal through TLR1/2 heterodimers[61,64,70–72] in a CD14-dependent manner.[63,73,74] The use of synthetic lipopeptides and recombinant proteins proved unambiguously the role of lipoproteins as *bona fide* innate immune agonists.[75–77] Collectively, these prior studies led investigators to conclude somewhat prematurely that innate immune cell activation in LD occurred predominantly, if not exclusively, through the interaction of spirochaetal lipoproteins with CD14 and TLR1/2 at the cell surfaces of monocytes, macrophages and DCs. The finding that experimentally infected mice deficient in CD14,[74,78] TLR2,[65,79] or in the TLR adapter protein MyD88,[80] developed similar or even more severe arthritis and carditis than their wild-type counterparts, confirmed that intact spirochaetes have to employ PRRs other than TLR2 and CD14 to induce inflammation. In line with this idea, phagocytosed live *B. burgdorferi* is capable of inducing a more robust and diversified and complex inflammatory response in human peripheral blood mononuclear cells (PBMCs) than can be achieved by cell plasma membrane TLR1/2 stimulation in response to individual Borrelial lipoproteins.[81–83] There is now a substantial body of evidence that innate immune responses to the LD spirochaete are fundamentally different when *B. burgdorferi* is phagocytosed and degraded,[81–83] from those initiated by individual spirochaetal PAMPs at the monocyte/macrophage plasma membrane. Indeed, the phagosome appears to be the single location where all of the spirochaetal pathogen-associated molecular patterns (PAMPs) (e.g. lipoproteins and nucleic acids) can be made available for sampling by pattern recognition receptors, including TLR2 and several endosomal TLRs (TLR7, TLR8 and TLR9).[84,85]

Adaptive Immunity

IgG and IgM antibodies to the spirochaete develop slowly and are directed against an array of spirochetal proteins flagellin B (FlaB) and p66, OspC (25 kDa) VlsE, fibronectin-binding protein (BBK32), FlaA (37 kDa), BmpA (39 kDa), and decorin-binding protein A (DbpA).[87–90] These antibodies have bactericidal activity[91,92] and they also can passively protect animals against inoculation with in vitro cultivated spirochaetes.[93] The presence of diverse antibody responses in patients with late manifestations of disease[94] provides evidence that spirochaetes can persist despite high titres of circulating antibodies.

T-cell-mediated adaptive immune responses to the spirochaete are also likely to be directly involved in control of bacterium in the skin and other tissues.[55] While the antigenic specificities of the circulating $CD4^+$ T cells remains an open question, these uncertainties do not detract from the notion that antigen-specific T cells recruited to infected sites become activated and contribute to tissue pathology. Limited work in humans,[95] corroborated by studies in mice,[96,97] suggests that *B. burgdorferi* infection also can prime $CD8^+$ T cells. Since *B. burgdorferi*, as an extracellular pathogen, is taken up by phagocytosis,[98] priming of $CD8^+$ T cells would have to occur by some form of cross-presentation. Presumably peptides presented in the context of class I MHC molecules at the site of inflammation could lead to activation of primed lymphocytes.

CLINICAL MANIFESTATIONS

Dermatologic Manifestations

Erythema migrans is the most common manifestation of Lyme disease in Europe and in the USA.[12,99] The primary lesion develops at the site of tick inoculation, within 7–14 days of the initial tick bite.[100,101] Primary EM can be located anywhere but, in adults, it is most commonly found below the waist.[102] It is well known that only a fraction of patients (14-32%) presenting with EM recall a tick bite.[102] To distinguish EM from the transient and more localized inflammatory reactions that often develop following an insect bite, the CDC designated 5 cm as the minimum lesion diameter required for clinical diagnosis (Figure 36.16). While this size criterion has improved the specificity of clinical diagnosis, it must be emphasized that bona fide EM lesions can be less than 5 cm, particularly when detected shortly after tick detachment. EM is traditionally described as an expanding, annular, erythematous skin lesion with central clearing, the so-called classic 'bull's eye rash'.[94] Rapid expansion is a key characteristic of EM and is thought to reflect the speed at which spirochaetes migrating away from the bite site are trailed by the local inflammatory response. EM-associated constitutional symptoms can vary from none to mild to moderate flu-like symptoms consisting of arthralgia, malaise, fatigue, headache, and low-grade fever and chills.[100,102] Patients can be spirochaetaemic and have low-grade fever, arthralgias and malaise without developing EM.[103] Regional lymphadenopathy is the most common physical finding associated with EM in both Europe and North America.

Borrelial lymphocytoma and acrodermatitis chronicum atrophicans (ACA), are associated with *B. burgdorferi* infection in Europe. Borrelial lymphocytoma may occur concurrently with the acute infection or months later.[104] Borrelial lymphocytomas generally appear as solitary, bluish-red nodules on the ear lobes and in the nipple areas of children or genital areas of adults.[105] Histopathologically, it is characterized by a dense lymphocytic infiltrate in the dermis or subcutaneous tissue that can be difficult to differentiate from lymphoma. Both *B. afzelii* and *B. garinii* have been associated with lymphocytoma, while *B. burgdorferi* sensu stricto has not. Acrodermatitis chronicum atrophicans (ACA) is a very late manifestation of Lyme disease, typically developing 10 years after the onset of untreated infection.[55,104] Occurring throughout northern, central, and eastern Europe, ACA is primarily associated with *B. afzelii* infection.[106,107] Initially the skin lesions are distinguished by the presence of inflammation and oedema; however erythema is not always seen and in fact relatively normal-appearing skin may be present, but swelling of soft tissue is characteristic. Early ACA can have an appearance similar to the acute oedematous phase of scleroderma. With time, the lesions eventually become atrophic or sclerotic. ACA typically involves the distal extremities and less commonly the trunk, sparing the face, palms, and soles.

Nervous System Manifestations (Neuroborreliosis)

Early nervous system involvement is usually manifested by the involvement of cranial and/or peripheral nerves or nerve roots and/or meningitis. Initial studies of North American patients with untreated EM found that approximately 15% developed meningitis or cranial neuritis within the first 3 months after presentation.[108,109] It is now believed that early neurologic involvement is much more common in Europe than in the USA, reflecting the high prevalence of infections by neurotropic genospecies other than *B. burgdorferi* sensu stricto, particularly *B. garinii*.[110] Although late disseminated *B. burgdorferi* infection has been purportedly associated with a variety of nervous system abnormalities, the neurologic entities generally accepted as being associated with late Lyme disease are encephalomyelitis, encephalopathy, and axonal polyneuropathy;[94,111] all of these are now considered to be rare. Peripheral nerve involvement in late Lyme disease is an axonopathy that may be distributed symmetrically or asymmetrically and in some cases resemble polyneuritis multiplex.[112] Patients with this entity complain of paraesthesia and hyperaesthesia and have abnormal nerve conduction studies. In Europe, peripheral neuropathy can be found in association with ACA but it rarely if ever occurs in patients without ACA.[113]

Cardiac Manifestations

Lyme carditis, a rare complication of LD, is usually manifested by acute conduction defects, typically heart block proximal to the Bundle of His, that resolve with antimicrobial therapy.[114,115] Although chronic myocarditis and dilated cardiomyopathy have been reported in the European literature,[116,117] *B. burgdorferi* infection is not associated with these forms of cardiac disease in North America.[118,119] It is interesting to note that the predominance of heart block syndromes correlates with the propensity of spirochaetes to localize to the connective tissue at the base of the heart in the experimental mouse model.[120,121]

LYME ARTHRITIS

Lyme arthritis is a monoarticular or oligoarticular large joint arthritis characterized by episodes of joint inflammation with

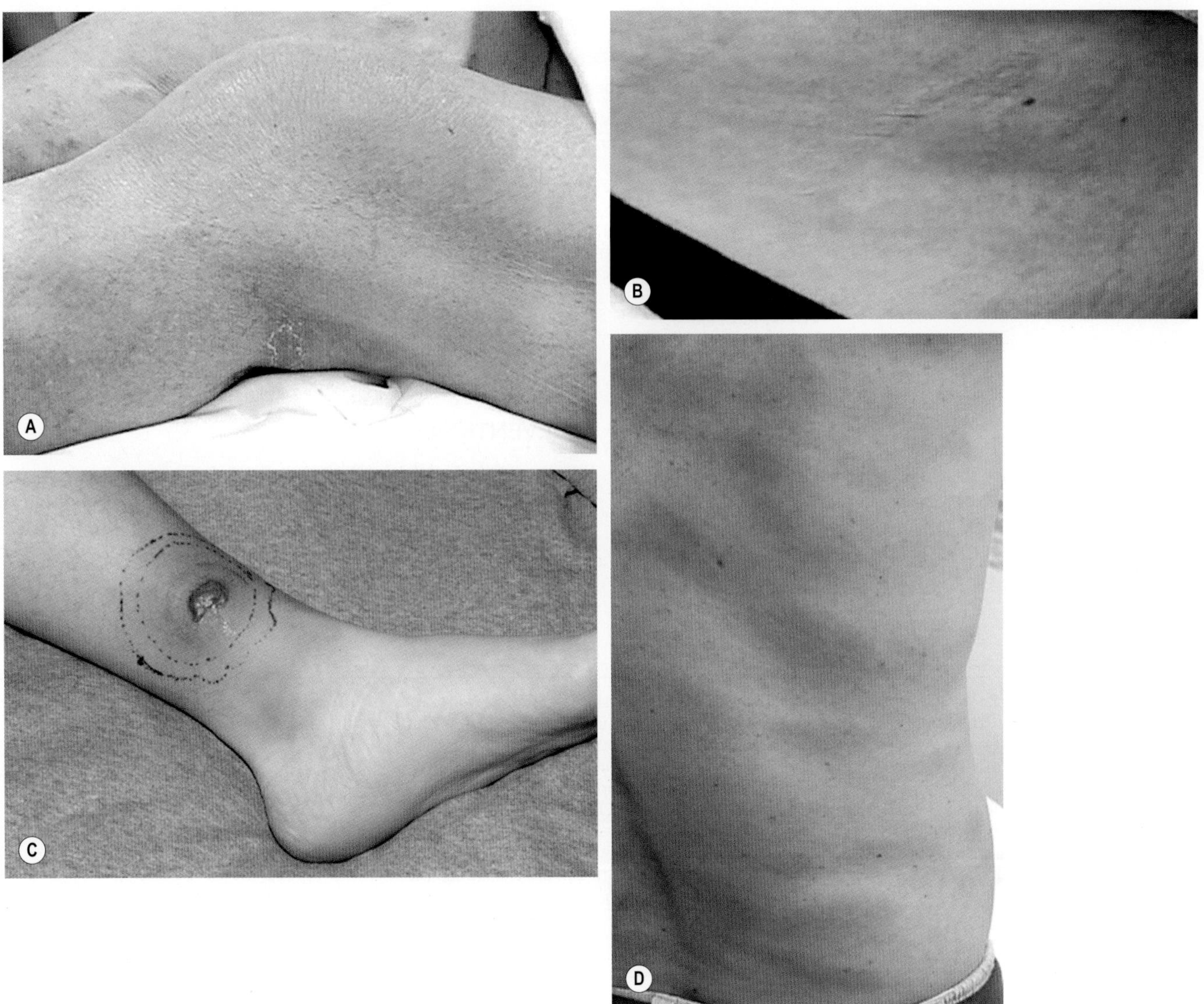

Figure 36.16 Erythema Migrans (EM) lesions: (A) Large EM expanding centrally and anteriorly from popliteal tick bite schar in elderly woman. (B) EM lesion over left iliac crest with surrounding centripetal rings consistent with classic target lesion. (C) Ulcerated and necrotic atypical EM lesion. Black lines demarcate area of reseeding erythema following 24 hours of antibiotic therapy in a young man with a recent history of a tick bite. (D) Multiple EM lesions over upper and lower back. *(From Samuels & Radolf, Borrelia: Molecular Biology, Host Interaction and Pathogenesis, Copyright Caister Academic Press 2010.)*

swelling large effusions and surprisingly little pain; the knee is by far the most commonly affected joint.[8,94] The percentage of individuals who develop arthritis as a complication of Lyme disease is now less than 10%.[103,122] Physicians must therefore be cautious in making a diagnosis of Lyme arthritis.

DIAGNOSIS

Because approximately half of patients with EM do not mount detectable antibody responses to the pathogen, lack of seroreactivity cannot be used to rule out the diagnosis of EM.[94] Seroreactivity increases substantially following therapy for EM,[105,123] indicating that killing of the bacterium enhances processing of spirochaetal antigens. By one month, the majority of patients have detectable antibodies.[90,94] Accordingly, clinical manifestations caused by the dissemination of spirochaetes are, for the most part, accompanied by seroreactivity.[94] It is important to note that IgG antibodies can be present for life and cannot be used alone as evidence of active infection. While assays using whole-cell lysates are less affected by strain variability and the heterogeneity in patient responses than those using single antigens, they can yield false-positives due to the presence of cross-reactive, background antibodies. This problem has been circumvented by the development of the two-tiered testing algorithm in which immunoblotting is used to confirm serological reactivity by ELISA.[90]

MANAGEMENT AND TREATMENT

The Infectious Disease Society of America (IDSA) and its counterpart in Europe have issued comprehensive guidelines for the diagnosis and management of this infection (Table 36.2).[12]

TABLE 36.2 Lyme Disease Treatment

Clinical Disease	Recommended Treatment
Early localized disease (erythema migrans)	Amoxicillin 50 mg/kg/day (max. dose 1.5 g) divided into THREE doses If older than 8 years then Doxycycline 100 mg/dose TWICE daily for 14 days. Alternative – Cefuroxime 30 mg/kg/day in TWO divided doses (max. dose 1 g a day)
Early disseminated disease (multiple erythema migrans, facial nerve palsy)	Same regimen as for early localized disease, but for 21–28 days
Late disseminated disease (arthritis)	Same regimen as for early localized disease, but for 28 days
Recurrent arthritis, carditis, meningitis, encephalitis	IV Ceftriaxone 50 mg/kg (max. dose 1 g) ONCE daily for 28 days. Alternative – Penicillin, 300 000 U/kg/day IV, divided every 4 hours (max. dose 20 million U/day) for 14–28 days. A repeat course of oral therapy can be considered for recurrent arthritis

Doxycycline (100 mg twice per day), amoxicillin (500 mg 3 times per day), or cefuroxime axetil (500 mg twice per day) for 14 days (range, 10–21 days for doxycycline and 14–21 days for amoxicillin or cefuroxime axetil) is recommended for the treatment of adult patients with early localized or early disseminated Lyme disease associated with erythema migrans.[12]

PREVENTION

The best currently available method for preventing infection with *B. burgdorferi* and other *Ixodes* species-transmitted pathogens is to avoid exposure to vector ticks. Measures recommended to reduce the risk of infection include the use of both protective clothing and tick repellents.

REFERENCES

2. Antal GM, Causse G. The control of endemic treponematoses. Rev Infect Dis 1985;7(Suppl. 2):S220–6.
3. Cejkova D, Zobanikova M, Chen L, et al. Whole genome sequences of three *Treponema pallidum* ssp. *pertenue* strains: yaws and syphilis treponemes differ in less than 0.2% of the genome sequence. PLoS Negl Trop Dis 2012;6(1):e1471.
15. Engelkens HJ, Vuzevski VD, Stolz E. Nonvenereal treponematoses in tropical countries. Clin Dermatol 1999;17(2):143–52.
19. Asiedu K, Amouzou B, Dhariwal A, et al. Yaws eradication: past efforts and future perspectives. Bull World Health Organ 2008;86(7):499–499A.
51. Radolf JD, Caimano MJ, Stevenson B, et al. Of ticks, mice and men: understanding the dual-host lifestyle of Lyme disease spirochaetes. Nat Rev Microbiol 2012;10(2):87–99.

Access the complete references online at www.expertconsult.com.

37

Leptospirosis

WIRONGRONG CHIERAKUL

KEY POINTS

- Leptospirosis is caused by eight pathogenic *Leptospira* species, which have many mammalian animals as reservoirs. Humans are accidental and dead-end hosts, who contact directly or indirectly with *Leptospira*-contaminated water or animal products.
- Many infections in endemic areas are asymptomatic or oligosymptomatic.
- Clinical manifestations are those of a nonspecific acute febrile illness. Complications such as cholestatic jaundice, aseptic meningitis, acute renal injury, haemorrhage especially in the lung and myocarditis can occur and lead to a fatal outcome. Overall mortality is less than 10%.
- Clinical diagnosis is important but nonspecific. Laboratory diagnosis is not practical for patient care, but very important for epidemiology, since both culture and serology take a relatively long time.
- Differential diagnoses are dengue and other haemorrhagic fevers, malaria, scrub typhus, hepatitis, yellow fever, Hantavirus (both HPS and HFRS), enteric fever and other bacterial sepsis, especially in patients with severe complications.
- Antibiotic treatment should be given as early as possible. Doxycycline is the drug of choice in uncomplicated cases; penicillin, doxycycline, ceftriaxone and cefotaxime are efficacious alternatives in severe cases.
- No effective human vaccine available, protection from contact is crucial. Weekly doxycycline chemoprophylaxis in very high-risk groups is also effective.

Introduction

Leptospirosis is a worldwide zoonotic disease caused by pathogenic *Leptospira* species. The disease presents in both tropical and temperate zones. The major reservoirs of the organisms are cattle, horses, canines and rodents. Humans are accidentally infected through contact with contaminated water. The symptoms range from mild or asymptomatic to severe fatal illness. The severe illness, characterized by febrile illness with jaundice, acute renal injury and bleeding, is recognized as Weil's disease, though many different local names have been used such as Fort Bragg, mud, swamp and sugar cane fevers. Specific treatment with antibiotics is valuable at all stages of the illness and prevents development of severe disease. In severely ill patients, intensive care supportive treatment is crucial.

Causative Agents

Molecular biology studies have led to major advances in our understanding of *Leptospira* spp. during the past decade. *Leptospira* are spiral bacteria (spirochaete) in the family of Leptospiraceae. There are eight pathogenic, seven non-pathogenic *Leptospira* species, and five intermediate species with unknown ability for causing disease. *Leptospira interrogans* and *L. borgpetersenii* are the two most common species causing diseases in human and animals. The schematic classification of the organisms is shown in Figure 37.1.

The old phenotypic classification of *Leptospira*, based on serology using the cross-agglutination absorption test (CAAT) is still in use. Approximately 250 pathogenic serovars, grouped by related antigenicity into 24 serogroups, have been identified to date. The concept of a serovar is complicated and may fail to define epidemiologically important strains. Serovars of the same serogroup may distribute between different species identified by DNA-DNA hybridization (Table 37.1).[1,2] The current recommendation for *Leptospira* nomenclature is using species name followed by the term 'serovar' and serovar name with initial capital letter and non-italic, e.g. *Leptospira interrogans* serovar Autumnalis.

The whole genomes of two pathogenic (*L. interrogans* and *L. borgpetersenii*) and a non-pathogenic species (*L. biflexa*) have been sequenced. *L. interrogans* has 35–41% GC content in two circular chromosomes of approximately 4 Mb and 300 Kb in size. *L. borgpetersenii* has a smaller genome (3.9 Mb) and a larger proportion of pseudogenes (20%), compared with *L. interrogans*. This may impair the ability of *L. borgpetersenii* to survive in the external environment, and so require direct contact between hosts to maintain the transmission cycle.[3,4]

Recent developments in molecular typing have characterized relationships between pathogenic strains and assisted outbreak investigation and epidemiology. Several typing techniques have been developed. One is the sequence-based approach, multilocus sequence typing (MLST). Using MLST the major outbreak of leptospirosis in Thailand during 1996–2000 was shown to have been caused by one successive clone, strain type (ST) 34 of *L. interrogans* serovar Autumnalis. (MLST has been used to create a standard global database for typing and mapping strains of *Leptospira*, see: http://leptospira.mlst.net).[5]

Life Cycle and Transmission

A wide range of mammalian species, including rodents, cattle, pigs, domestic and wild animals, are the major reservoirs and carriers, whereas humans are mostly accidental and dead end hosts. The infecting organism is sustained naturally by chronic infection of the renal tubules of maintenance hosts after primary

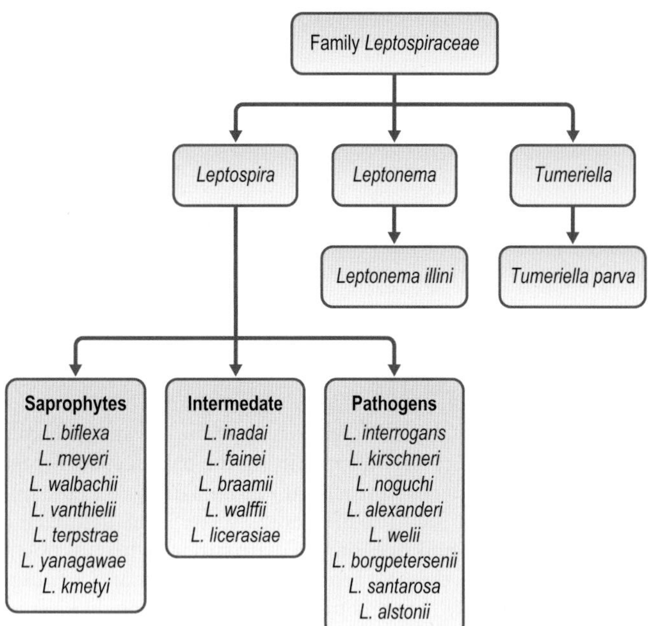

Figure 37.1 Classification of *Leptospira.*

infection. The organisms are usually transferred from animal to animal by direct contact. The maintenance hosts or carriers can excrete *Leptospira* in their urine for long periods of time or for their entire lives. Leptospires survive weeks or months in moist and warm soil, stagnant water at neutral or slightly alkaline pH. Humans are infected via direct contact with infected animal urine, animal abortion products or most commonly through indirect contact with infected urine-contaminated water. The oral route of transmission had been reported in water-borne fatal outbreaks in Portugal, Greece, Russia, Italy and India,.[2,6,7] Breast milk transmission may occur.[8] Sexual and vertical transmission in humans occurs rarely.

Humans at risk for leptospirosis are those with occupational exposure. These include farmers, fishermen, miners, animal slaughterers, veterinarians, sewage and canal workers, sugar cane workers, soldiers, etc. Special events and activities clearly related to the diseases are recreational water sports, including triathlon, canoeing and white-water rafting, and natural disasters, such as hurricanes, floods, etc. Laboratory-acquired infection may occur when dealing with high concentrations of organisms in culture.

Epidemiology

The true global burden is largely unknown both in human and animals. Leptospirosis occurs in tropical, subtropical and temperate regions. The disease is often under-recognized and neglected because of the difficulties confirming the diagnosis. Furthermore many infections in endemic areas are asymptomatic or oligosymptomatic. The six highest incidences reported are from the Indian Ocean and Caribbean Sea islands (Seychelles, Trinidad and Tobago, Barbados, Jamaica, Costa Rica and Sri Lanka). Countries in South-east Asia, except Thailand and Singapore, have no official incidence data, so the true incidence is unknown.[9]

The Leptospirosis Burden Epidemiology Reference Group (LERG) set up by World Health Organization (WHO) is trying to assess the global burden of human leptospirosis, and thereby hopefully, will inform rational deployment of effective control and preventive measures.[10] According to the second report of LERG in 2010, the median global incidence of human leptospirosis, excluding outbreak cases, was five cases per 100 000 population. The incidence by WHO regions from highest to lowest were Africa, Western Pacific, America, South-east Asia, and Europe, with the median (range) of 95.5 (62.8–160.2), 66.4 (1.1–975.0), 12.5 (0.1–306.2), 4.8 (0.3–7.3) and 0.5 (0.1–15.8) cases/100 000 population, respectively. There were no data available from the Eastern Mediterranean in this report.[11]

Leptospira serovars show specific, but not exclusive, host preferences. For example, *L. borgpetersenii* serovar Hardjo predominates in farm animals especially cattle, *L. interrogans* serovar Canicola circulates mainly in dogs. The incidence of leptospirosis is seasonal in several countries, mostly related to rainfall.

Pathogenesis, Pathology and Immunology

After skin or mucosal penetration, the organisms cross the tissue barriers through intercellular junctions. Leptospires can be detected in the bloodstream shortly after penetration into the body, and from some organs within three days after infection. Leptospires are rarely observed within host cells. However, they can reside transiently within cells while crossing cell barriers. The organisms can evade host immune response during the initial phase of infection through unclear mechanisms. They are resistant to the alternative pathway of complement activation and acquire complement factor H and related fluid-phase regulators through ligands such as leptospiral endostatin-like A (LenA) proteins.[12] Recent data show that pathogenic leptospires can bind human plasminogen (PLG), and plasmin activity on the bacterial surface interferes with complement C3b and IgG deposition, therefore decreasing opsonization of the organisms.[13] Lipopolysaccharide (LPS) of pathogenic leptospires can activate Toll-like receptor 2 (TLR2) but not TLR4 pathway, and activate the production of pro-inflammatory cytokines mediating inflammation and damaging end-organ tissues.[14]

Comparison of putative pathogenicity factors with the saprophyte, *L. biflexa* has identified several pathogenic processes. These can be divided into three components; *adhesins* (proteoglycans, LenA, 36 kDa outer surface membrane protein, 24 and 21 kDa laminin binding protein (Lsa24, Lsa21), Leptospiral immunoglobulin-like proteins (Lig A, Lig B and Lig C proteins); *evasion of natural defences or phagocytosis*; and *resistance to complement* as described above. Unlike other Gram-negative bacteria, the lipopolysaccharides (LPS) of leptospires cause minor endotoxicity, while leptospiral outer membrane lipoproteins (OMPs), such as Lip32, Loa22 play a major role as virulence factors.[15]

Although the early phase of the disease does not cause much inflammation, hepatocellular and tubular damage can occur. Liver pathology ranges from no appreciable changes, unicellular damage with oedema, to spotty necrosis surrounded by mononuclear cells without hepatocyte ballooning or swelling. Complete liver cell necrosis is not unusual. Kupffer cells and sinusoidal lining cells may show swollen cytoplasm. Biliary stasis with bile droplets in hepatocytes and bile thrombi in the canaliculi is prominent in the centrolobular areas, with

TABLE 37.1 Number of *Leptospira* Serovars in the Serogroups Distributed Among *Leptospira* Species

Species	Serogroup: Andaman	Australis	Autumnalis	Ballium	Bataviae	Canicola	Celledoni	Codice	Cynopteri	Djasiman	Grippotyphosa	Hebdomadis	Holland	Hurstbridge	Icterohaemorrhagiae	Javanica	Lyme	Louisiana	Manhao	Mini	Panama	Pyrogenes	Pomona	Ranarum	Sarmin	Sejroe	Semaranga	Shermani	Tarrossovi	Undesignated
PATHOGEN GROUP																														
L. interrogans		9	10		5	11				4	3	2			14			1	1	2		8	4	1	1	12				
L. kirschneri		1	5		1	3			1	1	4	2			5								3							
L. noguchii		5	1		2					1								3			2	1	2					1	1	
L. borgpetersenii		1	1	6	1		2					4				9				1		2				9			7	
L. welii							3					1			1	3			2	1		1			1	1			3	
L. santarosai			1		5				3		1	7				3				4		7	2		3	6		3	12	
L. alexanderi												2				1			2	1										
L. alstonii																								1						1
INTERMEDIATE GROUP																														
L. wolffii																														1
L. licerasiae														1																
L. inadai						1									1	1	1		2									1	1	
L. fainei														1																
L. broomii																														1
SAPROPHYTE GROUP																														
L. kmetyi																													1	
L. wolbachii								1																						
L. meyeri																1				1				1		1	1			
L. biflexa	1																										1			
L. vanthielii													1																	
L. terpstrae															1															
L. yanagawae																											1			

Adapted from Cerqueira, GM and Picardeau, M. 2009, by permission of Elsevier.

biliary capillary microvilli disappearance and distortion, indicating cholestastis.[16] Renal pathology is mainly tubulointerstitial nephritis. In severe cases, tubular necrosis and medullary tubular cell desquamation can occur. Glomeruli contain exudates and inflammatory cell infiltration, but are usually spared.[17] Primary injury of the proximal convoluted tubules is regarded as the hallmark of renal pathology, especially affecting sodium and water transportation.[18] Recently developed *in situ* hybridization assays and immunohistochemistry suggest that cell membrane damage in both the liver and kidney may be important in pathogenesis.[19]

Vasculitis is a prominent feature of leptospirosis. Endothelial damage and increased capillary fragility lead to internal organ haemorrhage. Disseminated intravascular coagulation (DIC) is not obvious in the pathology in fatal cases. However, with new definitions and sensitive markers for detection of DIC, patients with leptospirosis do have significantly elevated fibrinogen, D-dimer, thrombin-antithrombin III complexes, and prothrombin fragment 1,2. Using DIC scores, defined by the DIC scientific subcommittee of the International Society of Thrombosis and Haemostasis, overt DIC was evident in nearly half of patients.[20] Fatal bleeding usually occurs in the lung, with fibrin aggregation suggestive of adult respiratory distress syndromes (ARDS) in nearly 60% of fatal cases. Capillary lesions characterized by swollen endothelial cells with an increase in pinocytotic vesicles and haemorrhagic pneumopathy with septal capillary lesions were present.[21]

Clinical Features

The average incubation period is 5–14 days, with a range of 2–30 days.[22] The clinical spectrum is extremely broad; ranging from subclinical or asymptomatic, mild insignificant, self-limited symptoms, to severe fatal manifestations. A substantial proportion of people in endemic areas infected with leptospirosis may have subclinical disease evidenced only by serology. Leptospirosis is an important cause of acute undifferentiated fever. In the Seychelles, 37% and 9% of screened people had past and recent infections respectively, though none of them reported any recognizable symptoms of leptospirosis.[23] The reasons for protean manifestations are unclear. There were some reports of serovar-specific presentations and serovar-related severity, such as serovar Icterohaemorrhagiae and hepatorenal syndrome (pulmonary haemorrhage and renal failure), serovar Copenhageni and uveitis, serovar Bataviae with neurological preference.

The classical manifestation of leptospirosis has been described as 'biphasic' pattern, an early nonspecific leptospiraemic phase lasts for a week followed by an immune phase with complications during the second week of illness. This biphasic course of leptospirosis dictates the selection of specimens for laboratory diagnosis, since it describes the phase of leptospires and the immunologic response in human hosts. The fever too may be biphasic.[24] Complications such as jaundice, acute renal injury, haemorrhage, especially pulmonary haemorrhage, aseptic meningitis, myocarditis, shock, occur early during the course of illness. Direct invasion of leptospires and the host-response cause organ damage although specific immune responses may not be measurable until the second week of illness. Certain distinctive complications, such as uveitis, usually occur as a late complication months later, sometimes without detectable clinical symptoms during the acute infection.

The majority of patients are mild, self-limited 'flu-like' symptoms and may not seek medical attention. A small proportion of patients present with sudden onset of febrile illness and non-specific symptoms, such as headache, myalgia, backache, abdominal pain, conjunctival suffusion, chills, diarrhoea, anorexia, transient rash, cough, sore throat, etc. Myalgia can be mild or severe accompanied by muscle tenderness and elevated muscle enzyme (creatinine phosphokinase; CPK) levels in serum. Hepatomegaly may develop, but splenomegaly is unusual. Severe leptospirosis is a multi-system disease. Nearly 60% of patients develop the following complications during the course of illness.

HYPOTENSION

Shock is a common presenting sign of leptospirosis, and may occur in 45% of patients. This results from several factors, including hypovolaemia from low fluid intake compounded by increased capillary permeability and vasodilatation from high fever, microvascular dysregulation, inflammatory responses to the high levels of bacteraemia, and low cardiac output from myocarditis and dysrhythmias. The majority of shocked patients will response to fluid replacement and low-dose inotropic agents, but in severe myocarditis and patients with sepsis-like syndrome, the prognosis of profound shock is poor.

HEPATIC DYSFUNCTION

Jaundice is a notable feature of severe leptospirosis. The proportion of patients with jaundice was reported as ranging widely from less than 20% up to more than 70%. Extreme elevations of bilirubin may occur. Jaundice in leptospirosis is associated with cholestasis rather than hepatocellular damage, reflected by a characteristic dissociation between the slight elevations in transaminase and alkaline phosphatase concentrations despite the exceedingly high bilirubin levels. The prothrombin time may be slightly prolonged. Severe hepatic necrosis and fatal liver failure does occur rarely. Jaundice usually appears on days 3–6 (up to 9 days) after the onset of illness, and is not associated with pruritus. Haemolysis may also contribute to the degree of jaundice. Liver enlargement can be prominent in severe cases.

RENAL COMPLICATIONS

Renal involvement is an important manifestation of severe leptospirosis. In mild cases, the only abnormal findings are in the urinary sediment. These include albuminuria, microscopic haematuria, pyuria and the presence of granular casts in freshly examined urine. Renal impairment may be attenuated by dehydration from low fluid intake and high fever. Therefore, careful supportive treatment is very important. Presenting symptoms can be non-oliguric, oliguric or anuric in severe cases. Renal insufficiency commonly occurs together with jaundice, and is usually evident within the first 3–4 days of illness, followed by a rapid rise of plasma urea and creatinine often requiring renal replacement therapy. Hyperkalaemia from acute renal injury can occur, but hypokalaemia due to impairment of sodium transporters in the proximal tubules and spared function of the distal tubules is more common. The polyuric phase may develop after 10–18 days, and the serum creatinine begins to fall at the end of the second week and normalizes within 3–5 weeks after the onset of illness as in other causes of acute tubulointerstitial nephritis. Renal injury from leptospirosis is never permanent.

PULMONARY COMPLICATIONS

Pulmonary involvement occurs in 20–70% of cases. This is mostly mild and often overlooked, but can be serious, leading to death. The severity of the pulmonary involvement is unrelated to liver dysfunction. The most common symptom is cough, with or without secretions. Blood-tinged sputum or obvious haemoptysis may occur. Abnormal radiological findings are found in more than half of patients despite the absence of respiratory symptoms. Many different abnormalities can be found, including localized lesions such as lobar, confluent, or patchy infiltrations, or diffuse reticulonodular or interstitial infiltration. Pulmonary haemorrhage usually presents with nodular or patchy infiltration, and sometimes with localized confluent consolidation, isolated interstitial infiltration is uncommon. Pulmonary oedema with cardiomegaly due to volume overload or congestive heart failure from myocarditis and diffuse ground glass appearance without cardiomegaly reflecting ARDS are both observed and sometimes are difficult to distinguish. This fatal complication can occur as early as 2–3 days after onset of fever. Pulmonary haemorrhage can be minimal or severe diffused leading to respiratory failure and is the leading cause of fatal outcome.

CARDIAC AND VASCULAR COMPLICATIONS

Cardiac involvement in leptospirosis is relatively common but often goes unnoticed. The most common finding is slight PR interval prolongation on the electrocardiogram (ECG), although other more severe conduction abnormalities may occur. Atrial fibrillation is the most common dysrhythmia. Fatal arrhythmias such as ventricular tachycardia seldom occur. These ECG changes and arrhythmias usually resolve after treatment. Myocarditis, pericarditis, aortitis, arteritis of coronary and cerebral arteries and vasculitis have been reported, and may contribute to an unfavourable outcome.

OCULAR COMPLICATIONS

Conjunctival suffusion is prominent in patients with leptospirosis, and subconjunctival haemorrhage is a common sign. Subconjunctival haemorrhage is found more frequently compared with patients with scrub typhus (which commonly coexists in endemic areas of East Asia), whereas red eyes happen equally in both diseases. More serious complications to the eyes are vitreous oedema or haemorrhages, and retinal haemorrhages which occur as early complications, or uveitis and anterior iridocyclitis as late complications, which may lead to permanent disturbance of vision.

NEUROLOGICAL COMPLICATIONS

Several forms of central nervous system involvement have been reported. The most common neurological complication is aseptic lymphocytic meningitis which occurs in 11–25% of patients. Patients usually present with severe headache, photophobia and nuchal rigidity accompanying the onset of fever. *Leptospira* can be isolated from cerebrospinal fluid (CSF) within 5 days after onset of fever. The usual findings are a raised CSF opening pressure, raised protein with normal CSF glucose level and lymphocytic pleocytosis. The CSF is culture negative for fungi or other aerobic bacteria. Thus the main differential diagnosis is viral meningitis. Seizure is rare and usually occurs late after the onset of other complications.

Other uncommon reported neurological manifestations include encephalomyelitis, polyneuropathies, Guillain–Barré syndrome, mononeuritis multiplex, cranial or peripheral nerve palsies. Patients may present with a psychiatric syndrome characterized by mania, or may have mood instability as a rare complication which may persist for years.

BLEEDING DIATHESES

Besides pulmonary haemorrhage, abnormal bleeding may be observed in other areas, such as gastrointestinal bleeding, epistaxis, gum bleeding, vaginal bleeding, and skin bleeding presenting as petechiae or ecchymoses. Bleeding in vital organs with fatal sequelae have been reported in the adrenal glands and subarachnoid space. The mechanism of bleeding is unclear, but several factors contribute. These include thrombocytopenia, capillary endothelial damage, and coagulation defects resulting from hepatic dysfunction, consumptive coagulopathy and DIC.

OTHER COMPLICATIONS

Patients with serositis may occasionally present with severe abdominal pain and peritonism. Sometimes the abdominal pain is severe and indistinguishable from appendicitis, acute cholecystitis or cholangitis, especially in jaundiced patients, leading to unnecessary intra-abdominal surgery. Acute pancreatitis has been reported rarely, although serum amylase may be raised in up to 60% of patients with severe disease due to renal impairment. Leptospirosis in pregnancy may result in abortion, postpartum haemorrhage and intrauterine fetal death. Congenital leptospirosis occurs rarely. Other rare complications include erythema nodosum, life-threatening rhabdomyolysis associated with renal failure, and reactive arthritis.

These complications appear in variable proportions and can overlap. Weil's disease was first described by a German doctor, Professor Adolf Weil, in 1886 in four patients with a febrile illness together with severe nervous symptoms, hepatosplenomegaly, jaundice and signs of renal disease which recovered rapidly. Nowadays, the term 'Weil's syndrome' usually refers to the extremely severe form of leptospirosis, characterized by the combination of jaundice, renal dysfunction, and haemorrhagic diathesis, especially pulmonary haemorrhage. This syndrome occurs in less than 10% of patients and carries a mortality rate of 5–40%. Overall mortality of patients hospitalized with leptospirosis varies among countries and series reports, and usually does not exceed 10%.

Laboratory Findings

Anaemia is a prominent finding especially in severe cases, partly due to blood loss and haemolysis. White blood cell count can be normal (50%) or elevated with the median WBC count around $10–11 \times 10^9$/L and more than 80% neutrophil, with elevation of erythrocyte sedimentation rate and C-reactive protein concentrations. White blood cell counts higher than 13 000/mm^3 are associated with poorer outcomes. The bleeding, prothrombin and activated partial thromboplastin times can be prolonged in 50% of patients. Thrombocytopenia, a platelet count $\leq 100 \times 10^9$/L, occurs in 40–60% of patients. Thrombocytopenia is an indicator of severe disease and risk of bleeding.

Differential Diagnosis

Acute febrile illness accompanied by jaundice and renal failure should always include leptospirosis in the differential diagnosis. A history of either indirect exposure to possible contaminated water or direct contact with animals occupationally or recreationally increases the probability of the diagnosis. Many patients from the same community presenting with similar symptoms within a short period of time alerts to the likelihood of an outbreak and intervention may be needed to minimize the number of severe and fatal cases. However, the symptoms and signs of leptospirosis are not specific and can mimic many other acute febrile illnesses in endemic areas.

In patient with marked jaundice, viral hepatitis has to be excluded. Biliary tract infection may mimic leptospirosis especially in patients with severe upper abdominal pain. Since the disease is found worldwide, the list of differential diagnoses is broad and may differ among different geographical areas. Table 37.2 shows the differential diagnosis of leptospirosis according to symptoms and regions. Of these, rickettsioses, especially scrub typhus, carries the same clinical spectrum and geographical distribution of the disease and completely overlaps with leptospirosis in Asia-Oceania. There have been several reports of co-infections from the South-east Asia regions. Sepsis is difficult to rule out in patients with severe forms, and co-infections can also occur. *Hantavirus*, which cause haemorrhagic fever with renal syndrome and is associated with rodent exposure, has similar epidemiology and clinical manifestations as leptospirosis. In addition, dual infection of leptospirosis and *Hantavirus* has been reported.

Diagnosis

The clinical diagnosis of leptospirosis cannot be certain because of the nonspecific symptoms and signs which overlap with those of other common febrile diseases. In endemic areas, awareness should be raised during the rainy season. In some circumstances, such as natural disasters with fresh water exposure, health care workers should be alert for outbreaks. A definite diagnosis of leptospirosis is based on the isolation of *Leptospira* from clinical specimens (mainly from blood or CSF), or a positive microscopic agglutination test (MAT), both of which are laborious and not widely available.

ISOLATION OF PATHOGENIC *LEPTOSPIRA*

Although *Leptospira* can survive in some commercial aerobic bacteria culture bottles, the recommended media used for isolation is the semi-solid Ellinghausen, McCullough, Johnson, and Harris (EMJH) medium. Cultures are usually kept at 28–30°C without CO_2 incubation. It may take 2–3 weeks for *Leptospira* to multiply to detectable densities. Cultures should be examined weekly by dark field microscopy. This technique is not routine practice in a standard microbiological laboratory.

Recently, a new solid medium called LVW agar was developed. It can increase the growth rate of *Leptospira*. Using this

TABLE 37.2 Differential Diagnosis of Leptospirosis According to Symptoms and Regions

Clinical Symptoms	Europe	North America	South America	Africa	Asia-Oceania
Acute febrile illness	Enteric fever Chikungunya (severe joint pain) Tularemia (skin lesion) Relapsing fever (sporadic-Middle East)	Rickettsioses RMSF (rash) Epidemic typhus Ehrlichosis Relapsing fever (sporadic)	Malaria Rickettsioses Spotted Fever Group (skin lesions) Epidemic typhus Enteric fever Bartonellosis Tularemia (skin lesion) Brucellosis Schistosomiasis Dengue fever Acute American trypanosomiasis Relapsing fever (sporadic)	Malaria Dengue fever Schistosomiasis Chikungunya (severe joint pain) Acute African trypanosomiasis Relapsing fever (sporadic) Rickettsioses Epidemic typhus Spotted Fever Group (skin lesions)	Malaria Rickettsioses Scrub typhus (eschar) Murine typhus Spotted Fever Group (skin lesions) Enteric fever Dengue fever Chikungunya (severe joint pain)
Acute febrile illness with haemorrhage	Meningococcaemia	*Hantavirus* (HFRS) DHF	Meningococcaemia Yellow fever (vaccination) *Hantavirus* (HFRS) DHF Junin virus Machupo virus Sabia virus Guanarito virus	Meningococcaemia Yellow fever (vaccination) DHF *Hantavirus* (HFRS) Lassa fever Rift Valley fever Ebola Marburg viruses	Meningococcaemia DHF
Acute febrile illness with pulmonary involvement	Influenza	Influenza *Hantavirus* (HPS) SARS	Influenza *Hantavirus* (HPS)	Influenza *Hantavirus* (HPS)	Influenza SARS Melioidosis Rickettsioses

DHF, Dengue haemorrhagic fever; HPS, Hantavirus pulmonary syndrome; HFRS, haemorrhagic fever with renal syndrome; SARS, severe acute respiratory syndrome; RMSF, Rocky Mountain spotted fever.

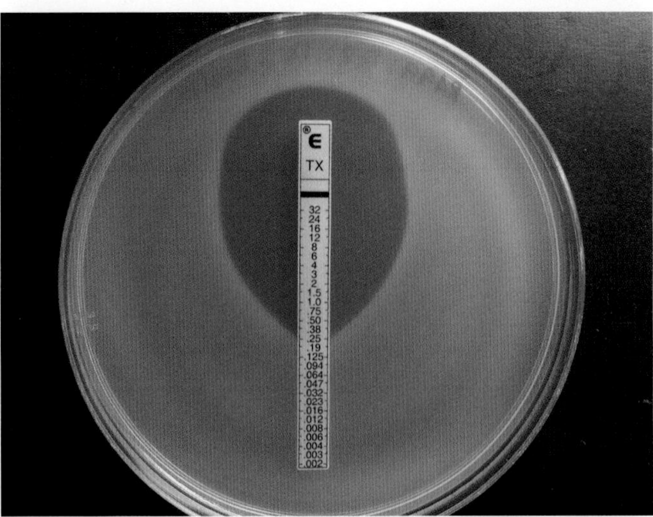

Figure 37.2 E-test of *Leptospira* performed on a novel LVW solid agar. *(Courtesy of Vanaporn Wuthiekanun.)*

novel agar, simple antimicrobial susceptibility testing, using the E-test can provide clear cut-offs and easy-to-read minimal inhibitory concentrations (MIC) of antimicrobials currently recommended for treatment (Figure 37.2). The novel LVW agar may open a new era in the clinical practice for diagnosis and rapid antimicrobial susceptibility testing of leptospirosis.[25]

Isolation of leptospires should be performed from blood or CSF of untreated patients who present not later than 5 days after onset of illness. Antibiotic pre-treatment substantially decreases the yield of the isolation. Isolation from urine is less useful, since leptospiruria usually occurs during the second week in which antibiotics have been given and antibodies are readily detectable. The acidity of the urine reduces the sensitivity of culture.

SEROLOGY TESTS

The gold standard serological test is MAT. The test is serovar-specific and useful for epidemiological studies. It detects mixed IgG and IgM. The MAT test is considered positive if there is either a fourfold rise of the convalescent titre compared to the acute titre, or there is a titre of more than or equal to 1:400 in single or paired sera. This may not be useful for patient care, since the diagnosis is usually obtained late. The test can be performed to a reliable standard in only a few places. New simplified confirmatory methods are urgently needed.

Several other serological tests have been developed and used in many places, although the sensitivity, specificity and accuracy of the tests are generally unsatisfactory. All of these tests are non-serovar-specific, so they have no epidemiological usefulness, and are used for screening purposes only. Examples of these tests are the immunochromatographic test (ICT) or cassette test, microcapsule agglutination test (MCAT), and latex agglutination test (LA).

MOLECULAR METHODS

Standard PCR diagnostics are not available for leptospirosis. PCR methods using various target genes have been developed. Real time PCR may be a good candidate for future confirmatory tests.

Management and Treatment

Leptospira are broadly sensitive to many antibiotics; however the efficacy of antibiotic treatment has been confirmed in only small series. Because of the biphasic course of the disease, the usefulness of antibiotic treatment has been doubted when given in the second immune phase. There are insufficient randomized controlled trial data to provide clear evidence on the efficacy of treatment at different stages of the infection. There have been seven randomized controlled trials; four trials with 403 patients compared an antibiotic with placebo or no intervention. Penicillin shortened the fever time, times to normalization of creatinine level and hospitalization in a small randomized, placebo-controlled trial even late in the course of disease in Thailand, but showed a non-significant trend to reduction in mortality in Brazil when given after 4 days of illness. Despite these uncertainties effective treatment should be given in every patient as soon as possible at any stage of the disease. The recommended drugs and doses are shown in Table 37.3. All regimens, except 3-day azithromycin, should be given for 7 days. Penicillin, cefotaxime and ceftriaxone can be switched to oral amoxicillin if patients improve and can tolerate oral drug treatment.

Oral doxycycline remains the drug of choice in uncomplicated cases of leptospirosis. Alternative choices for patients with

TABLE 37.3 Treatment of Leptospirosis

	Drug	Dose	Route of Administration	Adverse Effect and Remarks
Uncomplicated leptospirosis	Doxycycline	100 mg (2 mg/kg) twice daily	Oral	Take with meal to prevent GI irritation Avoid strong sunlight exposure to prevent photosensitivity
	Amoxycillin	1 g (20 mg/kg) twice daily	Oral	
	Azithromycin	1 g (20 mg/kg) initially then 500 mg (10 mg/kg) once daily	Oral	
Moderate and severe complicated leptospirosis	Doxycycline	200 mg (4 mg/kg) initially then 100 mg (2 mg/kg) 12 hourly	Infused in 30 minutes	Not available in many countries
	Penicillin G Sodium	1.5 mU (30 000 U/kg) 6 hourly	Intravenous	Hypersensitivity precaution
	Ceftriaxone	1 g (20 mg/kg) once daily	Intravenous	
	Cefotaxime	1 g (20 mg/kg) 6 hourly	Intravenous	

hypersensitivity and pregnant or lactating woman are oral amoxicillin or azithromycin. In severe cases, penicillin, doxycycline, ceftriaxone and cefotaxime have similar efficacy. However, in South-east Asia, the use of doxycycline or a cephalosporin in combination with doxycycline are recommended because scrub typhus co-infection is common.

Supportive care in severely ill patients is critical in leptospirosis. Careful fluid resuscitation should be given in patients with hypovolaemic shock. Inotropic drug administration should be given to patients with refractory shock despite effective fluid replacement. Haemodialysis should be started early in patients with hypercatabolic renal injury. Daily haemofiltration or dialysis may be needed in some patients, and renal replacement should be continued until clear improvement. Bleeding precautions are needed; however, routine use of proton-pump inhibitors and H2 blockers is not recommended and should be used with caution, especially in patients who are intubated, as they may increase the occurrence of ventilator-associated pneumonia. Respiratory support is mandatory in patients with respiratory failure either from ARDS or severe pulmonary haemorrhage. Ventilation should be supervised in the intensive care unit care to maintain adequate oxygenation. The use of high-dose steroids is not indicated and may be harmful predisposing to superimposed bacterial infections.[26]

Prevention and Control

People at risk of exposure and people living in endemic areas should be informed about the disease and the risks. The education of people at risk and awareness of healthcare workers enable early detection and treatment. Reducing rodent populations in housing and working areas may reduce the risk of exposure. However, the disease circulates mainly in mammals other than rodents. Immunization of domestic farm animals and pets reduces the overall risks to humans significantly. The use of personal protective measures such as long boots, gloves and protective clothing are recommended and should be emphasized in all workers at risk.

Chemoprophylaxis is recommended in people at particularly high risk. Doxycycline is effective for prevention when given at 200 mg weekly during high-risk exposure. The main adverse effect is gastrointestinal irritation causing vomiting, so the drug should be administered with food.[27] Human serovar-specific, short-term protective vaccines are available in China, Cuba, France and Russia. The efficacy of the vaccines in other areas have never been evaluated. Genome sequencing of all pathogenic *Leptospira* species may provide the opportunity to identify new vaccine candidates which ultimately aim to protect against all eight pathogenic *Leptospira* species.[10]

REFERENCES

1. Cerqueira GM, Picardeau M. A century of Leptospira strain typing. Infect Genet Evol 2009;9(5):760–8.
10. Hartskeerl RA, Collares-Pereira M, Ellis WA. Emergence, control and re-emerging leptospirosis: dynamics of infection in the changing world. Clin Microbiol Infect 2011;17(4): 494–501.
15. Cinco M. New insights into the pathogenicity of leptospires: evasion of host defences. New Microbiol 2010;33(4):283–92.
25. Wuthiekanun V, Amornchai P, Paris DH, et al. Rapid isolation and susceptibility testing of Leptospira spp. using a new solid medium, LVW agar. Antimicrob Agents Chemother 2013; 57(1):297–302.
27. Brett-Major DM, Lipnick RJ. Antibiotic prophylaxis for leptospirosis. Cochrane Database Syst Rev 2009;(3):CD007342.

Access the complete references online at www.expertconsult.com.

38 Fungal Infections

RODERICK J. HAY

KEY POINTS

Dermatophytosis

- This is common.
- It is confined to the skin or structures derived from it.
- Tinea capitis is common in children, tinea pedis and corporis in adults.
- Where laboratory diagnosis is not available, it is still useful to know which fungi cause dermatophyte infections in the patient's country of origin.
- For localized lesions, topical antifungals, terbinafine or azoles, such as clotrimazole, are effective.
- For extensive infections or nail and hair disease, griseofulvin, terbinafine or itraconazole, are necessary.

Superficial candidosis

- This is common in mouth or vulvovaginal infections.
- It may indicate diabetes mellitus or HIV infection.
- In tropical areas, non-*albicans Candida* species which are fluconazole-resistant, may cause infections of mouth or vagina.

Scytalidium infections

- These are common tropical pathogens.
- They mimic dermatophyte infections.
- They respond poorly to most antifungal agents.

Malassezia yeast infections

- These are common tropical infections, such as pityriasis versicolor.
- Seborrhoeic dermatitis may be an early sign of HIV/AIDS.

Mycetoma

- This is caused by actinomycetes (actinomycetomas), treatable with antibiotics or fungi (eumycetomas), which respond poorly to chemotherapy.
- It is usually painless but discharging sinuses are typical.
- Key to diagnosis is the demonstration of small particles or grains in the sinus discharge.

Chromoblastomycosis

- This is seen in tropical areas with high annual rainfall.
- It is present with large wart-like lesions.
- It responds to itraconazole or terbinafine.

Sporotrichosis

- Infection leads to a single granuloma or a chain of inflammatory nodules along a lymphatic.
- Trauma after contact with plant materials, such as straw or cats, may be sources of infection.
- Histology may not show the organisms, as very few are present in the lesions.
- It responds to a saturated solution of potassium iodide, itraconazole or terbinafine.

Cryptococcosis

- An infection caused by two species: *Cryptococcus neoformans* and *C. gattii*.
- *C. neoformans* infection is commonest in areas where HIV is endemic – *C. gattii* occurs in patients without HIV infection in the tropics.
- Often it has nonspecific presentations with fever and malaise, sometimes headache.
- Meningitis, fungaemia and skin lesions often occur.
- Diagnosed by antigen test, microscopy (India ink or Nigrosin stain) or culture.
- Treatment is amphotericin B plus flucytosine or fluconazole.

Introduction

The fungi are recognized causes of disease in all parts of the world. The commonest of the infections caused by these eukaryotic organisms are superficial, and include diseases such as dermatophytosis or ringworm and candidosis. However, extensive, deforming and potentially fatal deep or systemic fungal infections can also occur.[1] Fungal cells are similar to animal cells but are characterized by the presence of a polysaccharide-based cell wall. There are two principal types of fungi: the yeasts, single cells which reproduce by a process of bud formation to give rise to single daughter cells; and the mycelial or mould fungi, which form chains of contiguous cells, hyphae. Some fungi, the dimorphic fungi, exist as either yeasts or mycelia at different stages of their life cycles. Examples of dimorphic organisms include most of the major respiratory pathogens such as *Histoplasma capsulatum* and *Coccidioides immitis*. The formation of specialized reproductive structures or spores (conidia) is also typical of fungi, although this usually only occurs under laboratory conditions. Fungi can cause human disease in a number of different ways, through the production of toxins, sensitizing antigens (allergens) or by the invasion of tissue. Invasive diseases caused by fungi are known collectively as the mycoses: the superficial, subcutaneous or systemic mycoses.

The distribution of mycoses is affected by a number of factors: the presence of the organisms in the environment, host immunity, frequency and route of exposure and the use of invasive or immunosuppressive medical technology. These influence the spread of fungal disease in the tropics as well as in temperate climates. The main superficial mycoses are common in the tropics. The subcutaneous infections, which occur through implantation of pathogenic organisms via injury, are largely confined to the tropics and subtropics. The main systemic mycoses due to respiratory pathogens such as *Histoplasma capsulatum* also occur in the tropics, while systemic opportunistic infections caused by organisms such as *Aspergillus* are probably more common in temperate areas when there is a greater use of therapeutic immunosuppression.

Superficial Mycoses

Superficial infections caused by fungi are common in all environments, particularly the tropics. While, on occasions, this is due to the existence of endemic foci of specific species such as the causes of tinea imbricata or tinea capitis, there is also a real increase in prevalence of certain infections. Factors such as climate, humidity of the skin surface and the PCO_2 concentration may all affect the expression of these diseases.

The main superficial infections are dermatophytosis or ringworm, superficial candidosis and pityriasis (tinea) versicolor (Box 38.1). However, other conditions such as foot infections caused by *Scytalidium dimidiatum* as well as the hair shaft infections, white and black piedra, and tinea nigra are also seen. Otomycosis, a superficial infection of the external auditory meatus, is also common. Oculomycosis, in particular mycotic keratitis, occurs in both temperate as well as tropical environments but poses a frequent and difficult management problem in the tropics (see Ch. 67).

DERMATOPHYTOSIS

The dermatophyte or ringworm fungi are common causes of superficial infections.[2] They can invade epidermis but remain confined to the stratum corneum or the hair shaft or nail plate. There are three pathogenic genera of dermatophyte in humans:

BOX 38.1 SUPERFICIAL MYCOSES

- Dermatophytosis (ringworm, tinea)
- Superficial candidosis (thrush)
- *Malassezia* infections: pityriasis versicolor, *Malassezia* folliculitis, seborrhoeic dermatitis
- *Scytalidium* infections
- Less common: tinea nigra, white piedra, black piedra, alternariosis, onychomycosis due to mould fungi
- Otomycosis
- Keratomycosis.

Trichophyton, Microsporum and *Epidermophyton*. These organisms normally cause exogenous infections originating from outside the human host. There are three main sources: other humans, animals or soil, known respectively as anthropophilic, zoophilic or geophilic.

Epidemiology

In most tropical countries, dermatophytoses are common.[3–7] The main types of infection seen are tinea corporis, tinea cruris and tinea capitis. Tinea pedis is considered to be less common in many parts of the tropics. However, there are several features of the epidemiology of foot infections which may be relevant.[8] Occlusion of the feet with shoes or socks predisposes to clinical infection, although a higher proportion of the populace may have asymptomatic infections of their soles. In areas of the tropics where there is industrial activity, such as in the mining or petroleum industries, the incidence of foot infections may be much higher. There are a number of different organisms which can cause this type of infection, ranging from dermatophytoses to *Candida* or *Scytalidium* species, Gram-negative bacteria and erythrasma, a Gram-positive bacterial infection.[9] For instance, in eastern Saudi Arabia there is a higher rate of *Candida* infection in the toe-web spaces than dermatophytosis.[10] Populations of organisms on the feet, particularly those affecting the interdigital spaces, may vary from time to time and one may replace another to cause infection; the term 'dermatophytosis complex' has been coined to describe this phenomenon.[9]

Pathogenesis

The fungi invade after adhering to stratum corneum cells and producing keratinases or proteases such as subtilisins. Factors which encourage fungal invasion include increased environmental humidity and CO_2 content, both of which may occur in a tropical environment and in the presence of occlusion. Less is known about those factors which determine human susceptibility; generally it is thought that most individuals are susceptible to infection.[11] The presence of medium chain length fatty acids in sebaceous material may, however, prevent hair shaft invasion by dermatophytes in post-pubertal children. There is evidence that susceptibility to tinea imbricata may be mediated via an autosomal recessive gene.[12] In addition, patients with persistent treatment-unresponsive dermatophytosis affecting the palms and soles are significantly more likely to be atopic than others.[13] Resistance is largely mediated via non-specific factors such as an increase in epidermal turnover, epidermally derived peptides or by activation of T-cell-mediated immunity. Patients with HIV infection, for instance, although not apparently showing an increased incidence of infection, may have clinically atypical and extensive lesions.[14]

Laboratory Diagnosis

Clinical diagnosis of dermatophytosis is not completely reliable and it can be confirmed by demonstrating the organisms in skin scrapings or hair or nail samples taken from lesions.[2,15] Scrapings are generally best removed with a scalpel from the edge of lesions. They are mounted in 5–10% potassium hydroxide and are then microscopically examined. The organisms are seen in scrapings as chains of cells forming hyphae. In addition, they grow on mycological media such as Sabouraud's agar and their gross and microscopic morphology are used to distinguish the different species. At present molecular techniques play little part in their diagnosis.

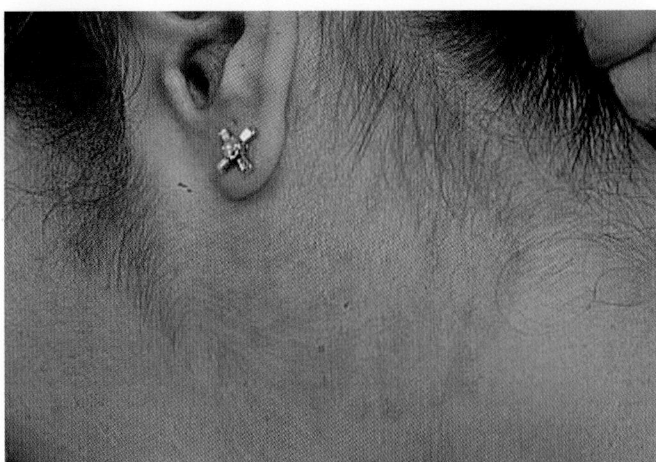

Figure 38.1 Tinea corporis due to *Trichophyton rubrum.*

Clinical Features

The normal term for dermatophytosis is 'tinea', followed by the Latin for the appropriate part of the body affected (tinea *capitis*, head; tinea *cruris*, groin, etc.).

Tinea Corporis. This presents with a scaly and itchy rash affecting the trunk or proximal limbs. The typical lesion is a circular scaling patch with some central clearance, but it may be difficult to see (Figure 38.1). However, in many lesions the main abnormalities, scaling or papule/pustule formation, are seen at the edge where an intact or broken rim can just be made out. Tinea corporis lesions may be very large and affect a wide area on the back and chest. In patients with HIV the symptoms and signs may be altered considerably, with extensive or follicular forms being seen in some patients.[16]

Tinea imbricata is a specific type of tinea corporis caused by the fungus *Trichophyton concentricum.*[17] It is endemic in remote and humid tropical areas in the West Pacific and parts of Malaysia, India, Brazil (Amazonas) and Mexico. Lesions are characterized by the development of multiple concentric rings of scales which may cover a large area of the body from childhood (Figure 38.2). Other patterns include diffuse desquamation with large scales and lichenification. This infection is notoriously difficult to eradicate from patients who are living in endemic areas.

Localized tinea corporis responds to one of the azole antifungals such as clotrimazole or econazole or topical terbinafine. Whitfield's ointment is also effective but slower. Oral therapy is generally needed for extensive disease or tinea imbricata; the main choices are griseofulvin, itraconazole or terbinafine.

Tinea Capitis. Tinea capitis or scalp ringworm is endemic in many developing countries. It can be caused by either anthropophilic or zoophilic fungi.[18] Generally in rural areas anthropophilic organisms are more common and this is true for large areas of India, Latin America and Africa.[19] By contrast, in the Middle East and in some South American countries, particularly in cities, zoophilic infections are being seen more frequently, usually caused by *Microsporum canis.* The difference between the two types is in their transmission, with those originating from human sources being more easily transmitted from child to child, causing small or large epidemics of disease. In many communities in Africa, for instance, scalp ringworm is endemic.[20–22] There is also evidence of a change over time with an increase in the incidence of *T. tonsurans* infections in Africa and Brazil.

Tinea capitis is an infection generally confined to prepubertal children. With most anthropophilic fungi the infections present insidiously with diffuse or circumscribed areas of hair loss. Scaling may be minimal and hairs are broken at scalp level, leaving a swollen black dot in the hair follicle (Figure 38.3). More scaly types resemble seborrhoeic dermatitis, but highly inflammatory lesions (kerion) are occasionally seen. The course of disease is indolent but lesions normally clear at puberty. The zoophilic organisms are generally more inflammatory, and scaling with hair loss is obvious. Lesions are often quite itchy and inflammatory crusts cover the lesions. Children (and adults) may carry the organisms without clinical lesions.[23,24] Adult tinea capitis, although rare, may be seen in HIV-positive patients.

Favus is a specific form of scalp ringworm caused by *Trichophyton schoenleinii.* It is found mainly in isolated pockets in parts of North, East and South Africa, the Middle East and South America. The infection is characterized by the formation of large matted crusts – scutula – over the scalp. This infection is usually recognized by the local population as distinct from

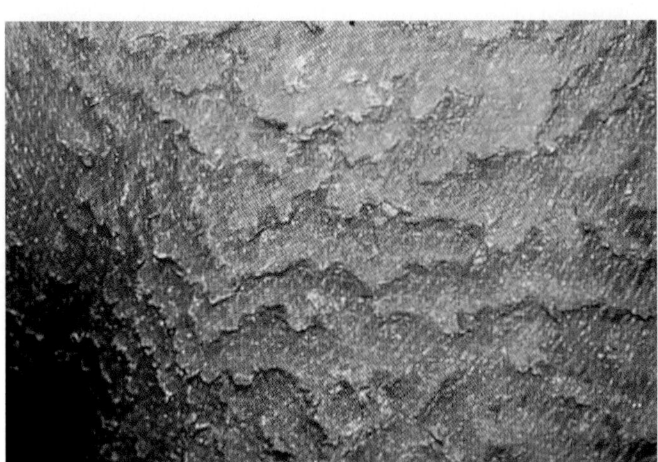

Figure 38.2 Tinea imbricata.

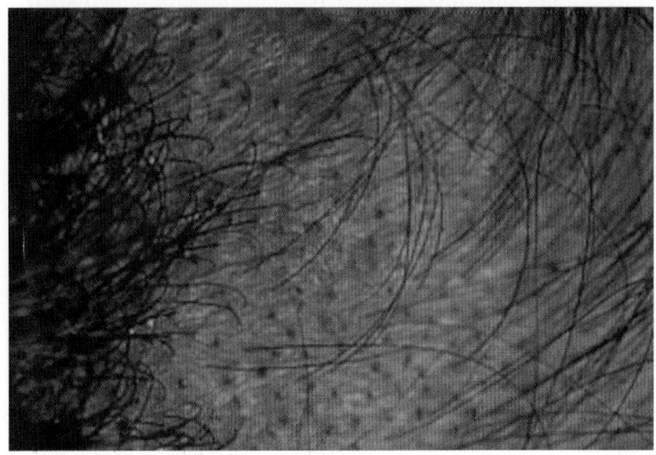

Figure 38.3 Scalp ringworm (tinea capitis) due to *Trichophyton violaceum* showing the 'black dot' appearance.

other forms of tinea capitis. Hairs are often retained until late in the course of the disease but their loss may be permanent.

The diagnosis of this infection can be confirmed by examining scrapings from the patient's scalp and by culture.[25] Some causes of dermatophytosis affecting hairs, e.g. *Microsporum* species, produce greenish fluorescence in scalp hairs under a filtered ultraviolet (Wood's) light.

The best treatment for dermatophytosis affecting the scalp is oral; topically applied drugs are seldom effective.[22] Griseofulvin in a dose of 10–20 mg/kg daily is the least costly agent.[26,27] The normal duration of therapy is 6–8 weeks. However, in some cases, it is possible to use a single dose of 1 g daily, which can be given under supervision to large numbers of children in a school.[18] Terbinafine and itraconazole are also effective, the latter showing particular activity against tinea capitis due to *Trichophyton* species.

Tinea Cruris. Dermatophytosis affecting the groin – tinea cruris – is common in most tropical countries. It is almost always caused by anthropophilic species of dermatophytes, mainly *Trichophyton rubrum* and *Epidermophyton floccosum.* Sometimes these infections may appear to reach epidemic proportions in certain groups such as soldiers or prisoners. The usual lesion is an itchy rash with a raised border extending from the groin down the upper thigh, and on occasions into the natal cleft. In women it may extend around the waist area. Treatment with topically applied antifungal creams such as clotrimazole or miconazole or half-strength Whitfield's ointment works well in most cases.[28]

Tinea Pedis. Dermatophytosis affecting the feet is very common in most temperate climates; although less common in developing countries, it none the less occurs. The most common sites of infection are the interdigital spaces or the soles. The main symptoms are itching and occasionally pain. There may be erosions affecting web spaces. If there are severe erosive changes, particularly if there is greenish discoloration of the area, Gram-negative bacteria such as *Pseudomonas* species may be implicated. Other possibilities include *Candida* and *Scytalidium* species or erythrasma, a bacterial infection caused by *Corynebacterium minutissimum. Scytalidium* infections which are indistinguishable from those due to *T. rubrum* are encountered frequently in West Africa.

The usual treatment for toe-web dermatophytosis is a topically applied antifungal. Good results can be obtained with a range of compounds including Whitfield's ointment, azoles such as clotrimazole or miconazole or terbinafine. For infections of the sole requiring treatment, oral therapy with griseofulvin, terbinafine or itraconazole is preferable.

Onychomycosis. Nail plate invasion caused by dermatophytes is common in temperate countries, where it may affect up to 15% of the population. The prevalence of this infection in the tropics is lower. It normally occurs together with sole or web-space infections and is most common in the toe-nails. The usual causes are anthropophilic fungi such as *Trichophyton rubrum.* The affected nails become thickened and opaque; distal erosion of the nail plate occurs in long-standing cases (Figure 38.4).[29] Superficial invasion of the nail plate caused by dermatophytes, such as *T. interdigitale* or moulds such as *Acremonium* or *Fusarium* species, is seen more frequently in the tropics.[30] This is called superficial white onychomycosis. Therapy is difficult, with few nail infections responding to topical antifungals, although in the early stages some will clear with tioconazole or amorolfine nail solutions. The cheapest oral treatment, griseofulvin, is associated with a high relapse rate when toe-nails are involved. It may have to be used for 12–18 months. Other oral drugs, terbinafine (250 mg daily)[31] or itraconazole (400 mg daily for 1 week/month × 3),[32] produce higher recovery rates in shorter periods (3 months). They are more expensive than griseofulvin.

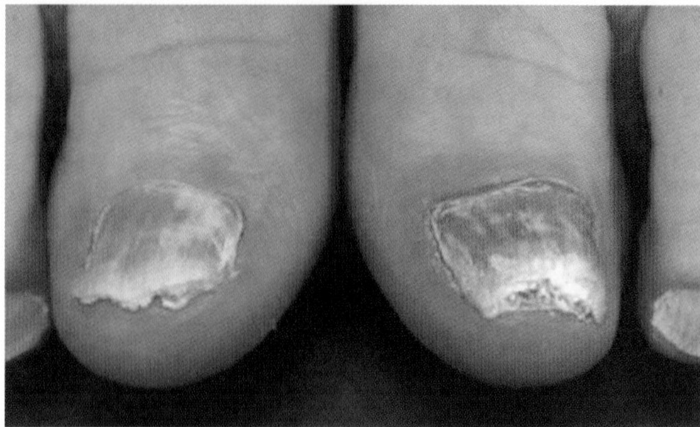

Figure 38.4 Onychomycosis due to a dermatophyte.

SUPERFICIAL CANDIDOSIS

Superficial infections due to *Candida* species are common in a tropical environment and include oral and vaginal as well as skin infections.[33] The principal pathogen is *C. albicans*, although other species such as *C. tropicalis*, *C. parapsilosis*, *C. krusei* and *C. glabrata* may also cause human infections. The disease is seen worldwide, although some clinical varieties such as interdigital candidosis are more common in warm climates.

Epidemiology

Candida albicans is a normal commensal of the mouth, gastrointestinal tract and vagina. Carriage rates vary but 15–60% of normal individuals have commensal carriage in the mouth. Somewhat lower percentages have colonization of the gastrointestinal tract or vagina.[34] Candidosis is seen in association with diabetes mellitus (groins, vagina), obesity (interdigital) and HIV/AIDS (oropharyngeal).

Survival of the organisms in these sites depends on a variety of factors, including their ability to adhere to mucosal cells and compete with commensal bacteria. Factors which disturb this balance favour either elimination or growth and subsequent invasion by the organism. These can usually be explained logically. For instance, use of antibiotics eliminates other members of the commensal flora of the mouth and bowel and allows *Candida* to invade. Depression of either T lymphocyte or neutrophil-mediated immunity allows the organisms to grow and invade following inhibition of normal control mechanisms. The main exception is vaginal candidosis, where most women with this common infection have no detectable predisposition.

Clinical Features

The main clinical forms of superficial disease are oropharyngeal, vaginal and cutaneous candidosis. In addition, chronic

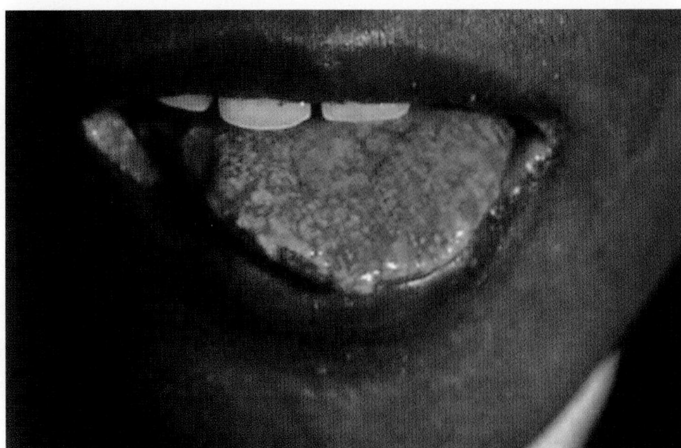

Figure 38.5 Oral candidosis.

mucocutaneous candidosis is a condition which may appear as a rare chronic infection in predisposed patients. Systemic candidiasis will be discussed elsewhere.

Oropharyngeal Candidosis. Oral infection is seen in all countries, particularly in infants, the elderly and immunocompromised patients, including those with HIV infection.[35] It occurs in breast-fed and bottle-fed infants and may be a complication of malnutrition, in which it can affect the reintroduction of feeding because of soreness of the mouth. Oropharyngeal candidosis is a common and early manifestation of the development of advanced HIV infection.

There are a number of different clinical types of oropharyngeal candidosis.[36,37] These are largely distinguished by their chronicity and clinical appearances. Acute pseudomembranous candidosis presents with white plaques on the epithelium that are inflamed and easily detached. The scattered nature of these appearances is suggestive of the speckling on a thrush's breast, hence its common name 'thrush'. This may present as an acute infection in infants, the elderly or in patients who are immunocompromised, such as those with HIV infection. In the last group and in patients with chronic mucocutaneous candidosis the condition is often persistent and refractory to therapy – chronic pseudomembranous candidosis (Figure 38.5).

In some individuals plaques are not formed but the mucosal surface appears red and glazed – acute erythematous candidosis, also known as acute atrophic oral candidosis. This may occur in HIV-positive patients.[37,38] In patients presenting with inflammatory changes and oral discomfort associated with dentures, persistent erythema associated with *Candida* is a common feature – chronic erythematous candidosis. In smokers, chronic candidosis may have additional features such as the appearance of irregular white plaques, which cannot be detached, on the tongue and other areas of the mouth – chronic plaque-like candidosis. Any of the above changes can be accompanied by splitting at the corners of the mouth (angular cheilitis), which in these cases may be due to *Candida* infection. This is an important and common sign of candidosis.

In most patients the main focus of infection is the buccal mucosa, but in severely infected individuals there is involvement of the tongue or pharynx, as well as the oesophagus. Oesophageal candidosis is mainly seen in patients with AIDS (see Ch. 12), leukaemia or chronic mucocutaneous candidosis. While it may present with retrosternal pain on swallowing, it is often asymptomatic. Secondary oral infection due to *Candida* may occur in patients with epithelial abnormalities such as hyperkeratosis or ulceration due to lichen planus, pemphigus and other conditions such as oral submucous fibrosis.

Vaginal Candidosis. Vaginal *Candida* infection is normally caused by *C. albicans*, although other *Candida* species such as *C. glabrata* or *C. tropicalis* have also been cultured.[33] While it can occur in pregnant women or diabetic persons, one of the features of this condition is that there is usually no underlying abnormality to be found. Severely immunocompromised women do not usually show a higher frequency of persistent vaginal infections than appropriate control groups.

The main clinical forms of vaginal candidosis are similar to those seen in the oral mucosa, most commonly an acute (pseudomembranous or erythematous) form.[34] However, chronic relapsing or persistent vaginal candidosis and secondary vaginal candidosis can all occur.[39] The symptoms of the acute types vary from a creamy discharge to itching and dyspareunia. Recurrent infections are unfortunately common and occasionally they are persistent. The clinical appearances are varied but the main variations are the presence or absence of soft white plaques (thrush). Secondary candidosis may occur in those with underlying mucosal disease such as pemphigoid, lichen planus or Behçet's syndrome.

***Candida* Intertrigo.** The skin is only indirectly involved in vaginal infection when there is spread of infection to the vulva and the perineum. In this case a prominent red rash in the groin and on the upper surface of the thighs may appear, together with satellite pustules and papules. The same can occur in other sites such as beneath the breasts and around the umbilicus. In some cases there is no underlying skin abnormality, although groin candidosis in males and females is more common in diabetic subjects. Eczema or psoriasis affecting the skin flexures may be accompanied by secondary candidosis.

Interdigital Candidosis. Infection of the finger or toe-web spaces by *Candida* is more common in hot climates. It may be the most common type of foot infection in army groups in the tropics. Lesions are white with soggy-looking skin which is superficially eroded. *Candida* may be a secondary invader of interdigital dermatophytosis. Lesions between the fingers are mainly seen in women and a relationship between repeated washing and cooking has been suggested; it is also more common in the overweight.

***Candida* Infection and Nappy Dermatitis.** Nappy rash in infants is a form of irritant eczema, which is often secondarily infected with, among other organisms, *C. albicans*. The presence of yeasts may be suspected by the appearance of satellite pustules and this is confirmed by culturing the organisms from swabs of the area.

Candidosis of the Nails. Paronychias are acute or chronic infections of the nail folds caused by *Candida* species such as *C. albicans* or *C. parapsilosis*.[40] These are common in the tropics. They occur in patients who are likely to immerse their hands frequently in water or whose occupations involve cooking. In addition to swelling of the nail fold, pain and intermittent

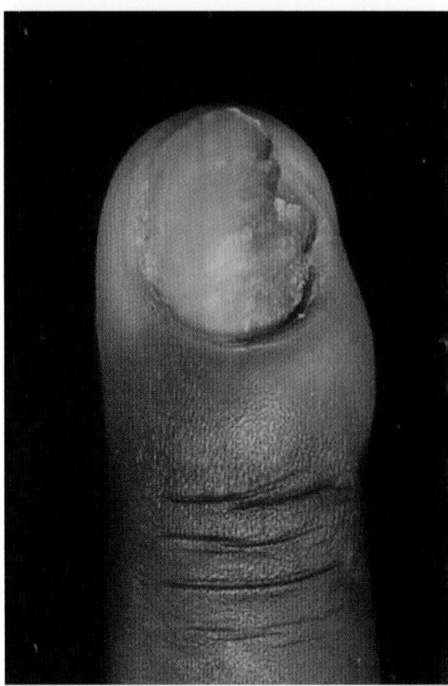

Figure 38.6 Chronic *Candida* paronychia.

discharge of pus, the lateral border of the nail may be undermined with onycholysis (Figure 38.6). Other causes of paronychia are staphylococcal and Gram-negative bacterial infections. The latter often co-exist with *Candida* species. However, in many chronically affected patients this disease is complicated by irritant dermatitis and eradication of the organisms alone will not effect recovery.

Chronic Mucocutaneous Candidosis. The rare syndrome of chronic mucocutaneous candidosis (CMC) usually presents in childhood or infancy with oral, nail and cutaneous candidosis which recurs despite treatment.[41] Other chronic skin infections such as warts (papilloma viruses) and dermatophytosis may also appear. An adult form also exists.

The oral lesions are usually of the chronic pseudomembranous or plaque types. The skin may be covered with crusted plaques particularly where the infection has spread to the face or scalp. The fingernail changes involve the nail plates, nail folds and periungual skin, all of which may be severely damaged.

A large number of immunological abnormalities have been described in association with this condition but with few exceptions these have been found to change with time and therapy. In most cases infection forms part of the autoimmune polyendocrinopathy, candidiasis and ectodermal dystrophy syndrome with associated hypoadrenalism or hypoparathyroidism; the common defect is a mutation in the autoimmune regulator (AIRE) genes. Extensive immunological investigation of children with CMC is not necessary unless they have very extensive infections or a history suggestive of abnormal responses to other infections, such as chickenpox or severe staphylococcal boils. Here it is worth excluding functional leucocyte abnormalities, such as chronic granulomatous disease, although such patients usually have a history of internal infection. With the exception of bronchiectasis most patients with CMC do not have internal disease, although the most severely affected patients may later develop systemic infections such as tuberculosis. It is also worth screening all cases for the endocrinopathy.

Laboratory Diagnosis

The diagnosis of superficial candidosis can be confirmed by direct microscopy (see Dermatophytosis, above) of skin scrapings or swabs. Both yeasts and hyphae can be seen. *Candida* species can be distinguished on culture by assimilation and fermentation reactions.[15]

Treatment

Candida infections respond well to a range of antifungals available in cream, vaginal tablet or oral pastille forms.[27] These include the polyene antifungals such as amphotericin B or nystatin and azole drugs (econazole, clotrimazole, ketoconazole, miconazole). Patients with AIDS may respond poorly to topical therapy and orally absorbed antifungals, such as fluconazole 100–200 mg daily),[42] ketoconazole (200–400 mg daily)[43] or itraconazole (100–200 mg daily),[44] given intermittently are used. Prolonged use of ketoconazole and fluconazole in AIDS patients may give rise to drug resistance although this is less common where highly active antiretroviral therapy (HAART) is available. Patients with infections due to *C. glabrata* and *C. krusei* are usually resistant to fluconazole.

SCYTALIDIUM INFECTIONS

Scytalidium dimidiatum, a plant pathogen found in the tropics and subtropics, and *S. hyalinum*, which has only been isolated from humans, cause infections of the skin which mimic the dry-type infections caused by *Trichophyton rubrum*.[45] These infections have mainly been reported in immigrants from tropical areas to temperate countries, although infection in the tropics may be more common than previously believed.[46] Studies from Nigeria, for instance, have suggested that this is a common infection in both dermatological outpatients and industrial groups such as mine workers. Infections have been reported from West and East Africa, India and Pakistan, Thailand, Hong Kong and several countries in Latin America.

The infection presents with scaling of soles and palms and cracking between the toe-webs (Figure 38.7). Nail dystrophy is common and onycholysis without significant thickening is often seen; some patients have nail fold swelling. The clinical

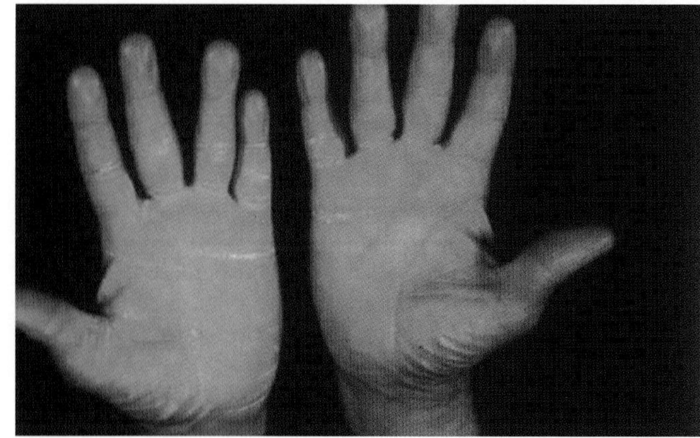

Figure 38.7 Palm infection caused by *Scytalidium*. This mimics dermatophytosis.

features of *S. dimidiatum* and *S. hyalinum* infections are indistinguishable.

It is important to recognize these infections because they are common in some areas and do not respond to most antifungal drugs. The laboratory diagnosis follows similar lines to that used in dermatophytosis – skin scrapings and culture.[47] The appearance of these fungi in skin scrapings is characteristic as they are sinuous and irregular. They do not grow on media containing cycloheximide.

Treatment of these infections is difficult. Nail disease does not respond to any of the antifungal agents. Responses of skin infection have been recorded with a number of compounds such as Whitfield's ointment, econazole or terbinafine, although relapse is common.

Malassezia *Yeast Infections*

The *Malassezia* (lipophilic) yeasts are skin-surface commensals which have also been associated with certain human diseases, the most common of which are pityriasis versicolor, *Malassezia* folliculitis and seborrhoeic dermatitis and dandruff.[48] In addition these organisms rarely cause systemic infections, usually in neonatal infants receiving intravenous lipid infusions. There are a number of *Malassezia* species which are oval or round yeasts and their distribution on the skin surface differs. The formation of short stubby hyphae by round yeasts on the skin surface is a feature of the development of pityriasis versicolor.

Pityriasis Versicolor. The pathogenesis of pityriasis versicolor is still ill understood. The disease occurs in young adults and older individuals but is less common in childhood.[49] Pityriasis versicolor is a common disease in otherwise healthy patients and there is no evidence of immunosuppression in these groups. However, it has also been associated with Cushing's syndrome and immunosuppression associated with organ transplantation, but not with HIV. The infection is very common in the tropics and incidence rates of over 70% have been reported in some studies. Generally this disease is associated with warm climates and sun exposure.

The rash consists of multiple hypo- or hyperpigmented, occasionally red, macules which are distributed across the upper trunk and back; with time these coalesce. The lesions are asymptomatic and scaly. The hypopigmented lesions may be confused with vitiligo but here there is complete loss of pigmentation. The presence of scaling and partial loss of pigment is, however, typical of pityriasis versicolor.

Lesions can also be highlighted by shining a Wood's light on the area. They fluoresce with a yellowish light, although this is generally a weak response and complete darkness as well as a powerful light source are necessary. Alternatively, scrapings from the lesions will show the characteristic organisms, which consist of clusters of round yeasts closely associated with short stubby hyphae. These are normally viewed in 10% potassium hydroxide-treated mounts, although the addition of Parker ink to the potassium hydroxide is an easy stain to apply and it highlights the fungi well. This infection is usually caused by *Malassezia globosa.*

***Malassezia* Folliculitis.** A second condition associated with *Malassezia* yeasts is an itchy folliculitis on the back and upper trunk which often appears after sun exposure usually in teenagers or young adult males. Lesions are itchy papules and pustules which are often widely scattered on the shoulders and back. The condition has to be distinguished from acne as it does not respond to the same range of treatments.

Seborrhoeic Dermatitis. Lipophilic yeasts of the genus *Malassezia* are part of the normal skin flora and therefore any evidence that they are either directly or indirectly implicated in the pathogenesis of common skin diseases such as dandruff (scalp scaling) or seborrhoeic dermatitis is difficult to assess. However, these yeasts are found in large quantities in the scales of seborrhoeic dermatitis and dandruff. Most patients with seborrhoeic dermatitis or dandruff respond to treatment with azole antifungal agents and this coincides with the disappearance of the yeasts. Seborrhoeic dermatitis is one of the earliest and most consistent abnormalities seen in patients with HIV infection[50] but it is also common in perfectly healthy individuals.

The main clinical feature of seborrhoeic dermatitis is the appearance of erythema, together with greasy scales in the scalp, eyebrows and eye lashes, in the nasolabial folds, behind the ears and over the sternum.

Management

Treatment of *Malassezia* infection can usually be accomplished using topical azole antifungals such as clotrimazole (cream) or ketoconazole (cream or shampoo). Oral therapy with ketoconazole or itraconazole is also effective. Cheaper alternatives include selenium sulphide (1–2%) or 20% sodium hyposulphite solution. In the case of seborrhoeic dermatitis, topically applied azole antifungals will produce significant improvements; other possibilities include topical tar-based preparations and corticosteroids.

RARER SUPERFICIAL INFECTIONS

White piedra is a chronic infection of the hair shafts caused by a yeast, *Trichosporon ovoides.*[51] It is generally sporadic and rare and the infection is mainly seen in genital hair. It may also affect the axilla and scalp. The lesions are soft yellowish nodules around the hair shafts.[52] This disease can be seen in temperate and tropical areas. It is usually asymptomatic and is noticed on routine inspection. Trichomycosis axillaris, in which hairs in the axillae are covered with a soft yellowish coating, is caused by a bacterial infection associated with excessive sweating. It is generally easily controlled with an antiperspirant.

Black piedra caused by *Piedraia hortae* is a rare asymptomatic infection confined to the tropics. Here, scalp hairs are surrounded by a dense black concretion containing spores, thus forming a small nodule.[53] The disease has been reported in both humans and apes.

Tinea nigra is an infection of palmar or plantar skin caused by a black yeast, *Phaeoannellomyces werneckii.* It is mainly seen in the tropics but can present in Europe and the USA. The main differential diagnosis is an acral melanoma as it presents as a flat pigmented mark on the hands or feet. If the lesion is scraped with a glass slide or scalpel it can be shown to be scaly. Lesions are usually solitary. The presence of pigmented hyphae in skin scrapings is typical. Tinea nigra responds to a variety of treatments including Whitfield's ointment and azole creams.

Alternaria species cause a rare form of skin granuloma, often presenting with ulceration in normal or immunocompromised patients. The lesions are most often located over exposed sites such as the dorsum of the hands. It has been seen in patients with AIDS.

A variety of different fungi, such as *Fusarium*, *Aspergillus* and *Pyrenochaeta*, also occasionally cause onychomycosis. *Acremonium* and *Fusarium* species, in particular, are sometimes associated with superficial nail-plate invasion (superficial white onychomycosis) in the tropics.

Otomycosis

Otomycosis or otitis externa caused by fungi is seen in most tropical areas. The most common cause is *Aspergillus niger*,[54] which forms a dense mat in the external auditory meatus, with loss of hearing and serous secretion. This can be removed carefully through an auroscope.

Subcutaneous Mycoses

Subcutaneous fungal infections are mainly confined to the tropics and subtropics (Box 38.2). While they are seldom common, their diagnosis and management are difficult and it is important to establish the correct diagnosis. These infections are generally caused by direct introduction of organisms through the skin into the dermis or subcutaneous tissues and for this reason they are often called 'mycoses of implantation'. They generally remain confined to their site of introduction, only spreading locally; however, there are rare examples where the infection disseminates beyond this area to affect distal sites. In addition, the disease sporotrichosis has both a subcutaneous and a systemic form, in the latter instance the infection spreading from a primary pulmonary focus.

BOX 38.2 SUBCUTANEOUS MYCOSES

- Mycetoma
- Chromoblastomycosis (chromomycosis)
- Phaeohyphomycosis
- Sporotrichosis
- Lobomycosis
- Subcutaneous mucormycosis
  - due to *Basidiobolus*
  - due to *Conidiobolus*.

MYCETOMA

Mycetoma (Madura foot) is a chronic subcutaneous infection caused by actinomycetes or fungi in which the organisms form into aggregates (called grains), attracting an inflammatory response in the deep dermis and subcutaneous tissue and leading to the development of draining sinuses communicating with the overlying skin and causing osteomyelitis.[55] Those mycetomas caused by actinomycetes are called actinomycetomas; those caused by fungi, eumycetomas (mycotic mycetomas) (Table 38.1).

TABLE 38.1 Causes of Mycetoma

Organism	Colour of Grain	Common Distribution
FUNGI		
Madurella mycetomatis	Black	Africa, Middle East, India
M. grisea	Black	Central and South America, Caribbean
Scedosporium apiospermum	White/yellow	Anywhere, USA and Europe
Fusarium or Acremonium spp.	White/yellow	Anywhere
Aspergillus nidulans	White/yellow	Sudan, elsewhere
Neotestudina rosati	White/yellow	Africa
ACTINOMYCETES		
Actinomadura madurae	White/yellow	Africa, Middle East, elsewhere
A. pelletieri	Red	Africa, India, elsewhere
Streptomyces somaliensis	White/yellow	Africa, Middle East, elsewhere
Nocardia spp.	Small white/yellow	Americas, elsewhere

Epidemiology

Mycetoma is seen in the tropics or subtropics.[55,56] It is more often seen in semi-desert or desert areas. The main regions for this infection are Mexico, Central and northern South America, Africa, the Middle East and India. Cases are reported less frequently in the Far East, e.g. Thailand. The main causes of mycetoma, together with their main endemic areas are shown in Table 38.1. As a general principle, the main causes of mycetoma in Mexico and Central America are *Nocardia* species,[57] whereas in most African countries and the Indian subcontinent *Madurella mycetomatis* is the most common cause. The causes of mycetoma are generally classified according to organism, namely fungi (eumycetoma) or actinomycetes (actinomycetoma), and by grain colour – black, red or pale, e.g. red grain actinomycetoma is an infection caused by *Actinomadura pelletieri*. Many of the fungi isolated from pale grain eumycetomas are sterile moulds which can only be identified using genetic techniques.

Pathogenesis

Mycetoma is more common in males than females and generally affects adults. It is also mainly seen in agricultural workers, although this is not invariable. The majority of patients appear to have no predisposing illness. There is evidence that the organisms are spread from the environment via a penetrating injury such as thorn implantation. The fungal causes of mycetoma have been isolated from plants, plant debris and soil; *Nocardia* species have been isolated from soil. Mycetoma organisms possess mechanisms that aid survival in the human host allowing them to evade immune defences. Some of the mechanisms of adaptation include the deposition of intra- or extracellular melanin, cell wall thickening and immunomodulation.[58]

Clinical Features

The earliest sign of a mycetoma is the appearance of a small symptom-free dermal or subcutaneous swelling.[55,56] It is difficult to give an accurate estimate of incubation periods as few patients give a history of a penetrating injury. However, it may take several years before the first sign of disease is seen. With time this slowly enlarges and sinuses appear on the surface of the nodule (Figure 38.8). Pain may occur prior to rupture of sinuses on to the skin surface which in the early stages heal up. Chronically discharging sinuses are formed in well-established lesions and there is considerable woody swelling affecting the site, accompanied by deformity.

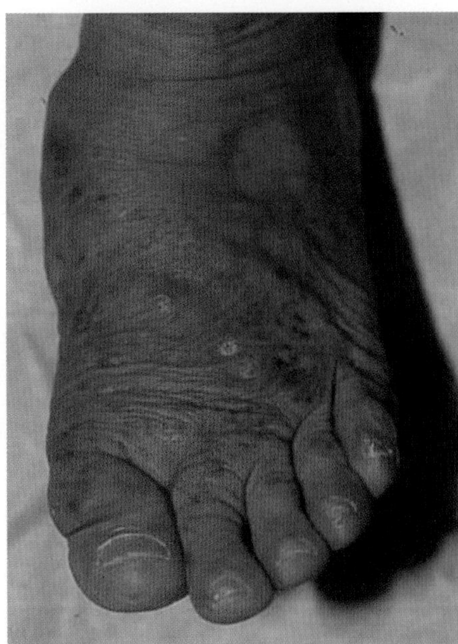

Figure 38.8 Mycetoma affecting the foot due to *Madurella grisea*.

The main areas affected are those subject to trauma such as the feet, lower legs and hands. *Nocardia* species are prominent among causes of lesions on the chest and back; *Streptomyces somaliensis* is the most common cause of head and neck lesions. Dissemination is rare, although some infections may become very extensive and spread widely over a limb. The only threat to life is where they involve the skull.

Radiological changes include cortical thinning or hypertrophy, periosteal proliferation and lytic lesions.[59] Magnetic resonance imaging (MRI) is the most accurate method of delineating the extent of lesions.

Differential Diagnosis

Mycetomas may be mistaken for osteomyelitis caused by bacteria or actinomycosis. Actinomycosis is an infection caused by *Actinomyces israelii, A. bovis* or other actinomycetes such as *Arachnia propionica*. These infections are usually located close to the sites where the organisms can be carried, such as the oral cavity, chest, and within the abdominal cavity, around the caecum.

Laboratory Diagnosis

The laboratory diagnosis of mycetoma depends on the demonstration of grains of the organisms.[60] These are generally obtained by opening a sinus where there is a small amount of pus beneath the skin surface, using a sterile needle. The grains can usually be seen with the naked eye in the pus and blood coming from the sinus tract. They can be processed as follows:

- Direct microscopy. Grains are mounted in 5–10% potassium hydroxide (Figure 38.9). They are gently squashed. As a general rule if the filaments can be seen with the ×40 objective the cause is a fungus. However, if these are not visible the cause is likely to be an actinomycete.
- Grains can be taken directly from sinuses for histology and embedded after formalin fixation.[61] The appearance of many grains is typical in haematoxylin and eosin stained sections and the use of special fungal stains such as periodic acid–Schiff or methenamine silver is not strictly necessary.
- Grains can be cultured on a variety of media and the appearances of the fungi or actinomycetes are typical, although a specialist laboratory will be needed for their identification.
- If grains cannot be obtained by this method a deep and wide biopsy is necessary and the specimen submitted for histology and culture.

A main aim of laboratory diagnosis is to separate fungal and actinomycete causes because the treatment of each is different.

Management

The treatment of mycetoma depends on knowing whether the cause is an actinomycete or a fungus.[62] The actinomycetes respond to a variety of antibiotics such as sulphonamides and sulphones or co-trimoxazole. For many infections it is advisable to use a second drug such as rifampicin or streptomycin. Alternatives include amikacin, ciprofloxacin and imipenem for difficult cases. Several weeks of treatment may be required.

Treatment of eumycetomas is more difficult. About 40–50% of infections due to *Madurella mycetomatis* respond to an azole such as ketoconazole 200–400 mg daily, itraconazole (200–400 mg daily) or voriconazole (400 mg daily). Therapy may need to be continued for over a year. Although surgery remains an option, the most effective operation is amputation and if the patient is not incapacitated by the infection, which is often the case, removal of a limb, for instance, may result in greater disability where facilities for artificial limbs and rehabilitation are poor. Generally mycetomas are only slowly progressive and are seldom life-threatening. It may be better for the patient to receive no operative treatment in these circumstances.

CHROMOBLASTOMYCOSIS

There are a number of fungal infections which are caused by pigmented (dematiaceous fungi).[63] Generally, these organisms contain visible melanin or secrete extracellular melanin into the environment. Many other fungi that are not visibly pigmented also contain melanin. The production of melanin is of importance as it allows the fungi to withstand environmental changes

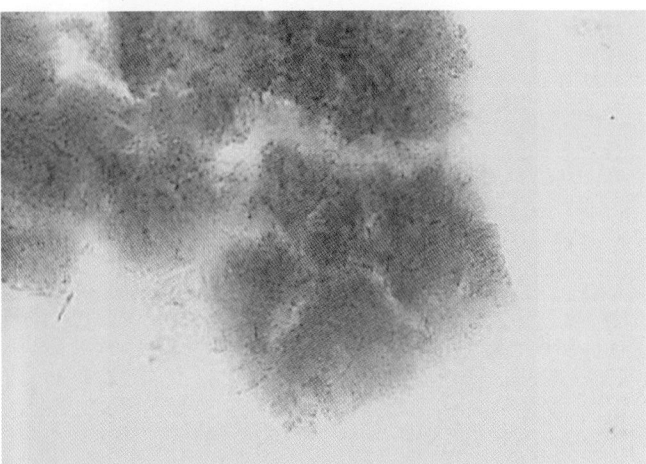

Figure 38.9 Direct microscopy in potassium hydroxide (10%) of a black grain eumycetoma (×40).

such as drought, heat or cold. There are a number of different infections caused by dematiaceous fungi but the most common is chromoblastomycosis (chromomycosis).

Epidemiology and Pathogenesis

Chromoblastomycosis is a chronic infection caused by pigmented fungi which form specialized cells, muriform or sclerotic cells, in tissue.[64] It involves the dermis and epidermis where a variety of pathological changes occurs, ranging from pseudoepitheliomatous hyperplasia to granuloma formation. The organisms which cause this infection are found in the natural environment in plant debris or forest detritus. The main range of chromoblastomycosis involves the tropics and subtropics and the incidence of infection is highest in countries with a high rainfall. The disease is mainly seen in countries of central and northern South America, parts of Africa, particularly the east coast of southern Africa, the Far East, Japan and the West Pacific.[63] The infection is most common in males and in agricultural workers. The main causes are *Fonsecaea pedrosoi* and *Cladophialophora carrionii*, but other fungi also cause this infection.

Like mycetoma there is no evidence of underlying predisposition in those with chromoblastomycosis. The infection is believed to gain entry via an abrasion, although there are no animal models of the infection to establish this as the chief mode of entry.

Clinical Features

The hallmark of chromoblastomycosis is warty proliferation of the skin. The early lesions are small nodules or papules which slowly enlarge.[65,66] They become raised and verrucose and adjacent nodules amalgamate to form a complex of warty growth (Figure 38.10). Other lesions are flatter and plaque-like and extend slowly, sometimes healing with central scarring. Cystic and mycetoma-like lesions are also seen. The lesions are asymptomatic, although with necrosis of keratin there is often an unpleasant smell associated with them. Long-standing lesions can cause considerable local swelling and rarely squamous carcinomas can develop.

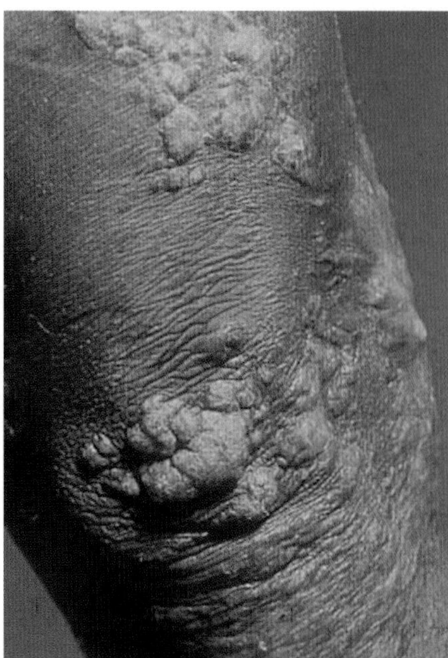

Figure 38.10 Chromoblastomycosis.

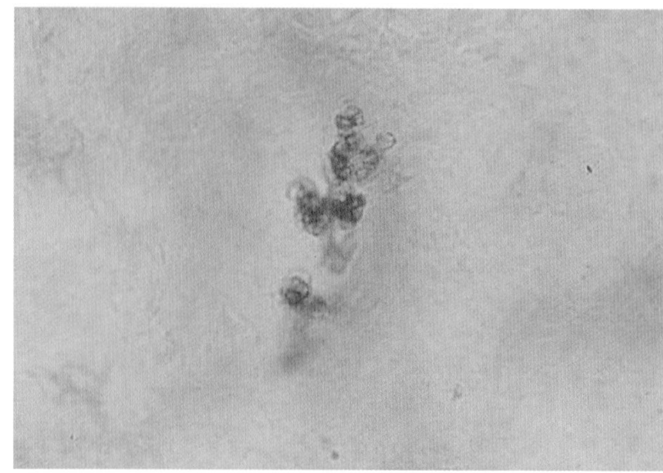

Figure 38.11 Direct microscopy in potassium hydroxide (10%) of a skin scraping from a case of chromoblastomycosis showing the muriform cells (×40).

The main sites affected are those on peripheral locations such as hands, feet and lower legs. The infection spreads locally and bloodstream dissemination is very rare. Occasionally, deep infections with the same organism have been reported.

Differential Diagnosis

The changes of chromoblastomycosis are typical, although there are some features which may be confused with other diseases. For instance, early lesions may resemble other warty conditions such as papilloma virus infections or tuberculosis verrucosa. In extensive chromoblastomycosis the chronic changes may superficially resemble mossy foot secondary to lymphoedema or podoconiosis. However, in the latter conditions the changes are diffusely distributed over the skin surface.

Laboratory Diagnosis

The process of identification of chromoblastomycosis follows standard mycological lines:

- Direct microscopy of skin scrapings. These should be taken from the surface of lesions. The pigmented muriform cells with transverse septa can be seen in potassium hydroxide-treated specimens (Figure 38.11).
- Biopsy. The histopathology of chromoblastomycosis is characteristic. The epidermis shows pseudoepitheliomatous hyperplasia with some attempt at transepidermal elimination of fungi. The latter can also be seen as pigmented cells in granulomas or neutrophil abscesses.
- Culture. Although the organisms grow readily on conventional mycological media, they are black moulds, which are difficult to identify. Often it is necessary to send cultures to specialist laboratories.[67] However, the diagnosis can be made on histopathological grounds alone and species identification does not alter treatment.

Management

Generally surgical excision is inadvisable unless the lesion is very small as the infection may spread within the scar. The commonly used drugs are itraconazole (100–400 mg daily) or terbinafine (250 mg daily). A combination of terbinafine and itraconazole or flucytosine is probably most successful in late and extensive cases. A further approach to therapy is the use of local heat applied from heat-retaining gels or pocket handwarmers. The heat must be enough to be comfortable when applied to the skin.

PHAEOHYPHOMYCOSIS

Phaeohyphomycosis is another infection due to pigmented fungi of different species in the skin. Cases are diffusely distributed through most tropical countries but are not common. Generally the infection presents with large cysts around the lower or upper limbs and these can mimic ganglia or Baker's cysts.[67]

The organisms are implanted from the environment and in some of these cysts there are fragments of plant material. Each cyst is surrounded by a fibrous capsule but contains palisading granulomas and a necrotic centre. The fungi are present as irregular mycelial fragments whose pigmentation may be very variable and sometimes it is necessary to use specific fungal stains. Occasionally, this form of infection is seen in immunocompromised patients, particularly those receiving systemic corticosteroids. The treatment is excision.

SPOROTRICHOSIS

Sporotrichosis, the infection caused by the dimorphic fungal pathogen *Sporothrix schenckii*, is widely distributed through the tropical world.[68] It may present either as a cutaneous infection or on occasions as a deep mycosis (see below). Extensive disseminated cutaneous infections are seen in patients with AIDS.[69]

Epidemiology and Pathogenesis

Sporotrichosis is seen in central and southern USA but the main foci of infection are in Mexico, Central and South America, Africa and Japan. Scattered cases are seen in the Far East and Australia. The organism is a member of an extensive group of soil and plant fungi, the *Sporothrix* and *Sporotrichum* species. But *Sporothrix schenckii*'s ability to invade animals is unique, as is its dimorphism whereby it exists as a mould at room temperature and in the environment but as a yeast in animal tissue.[68] More recently it has been suggested that the genus Sporothrix should be divided into different species – *Sporothrix albicans, Sporothrix brasiliensis, Sporothrix globosa, Sporothrix luriei, Sporothrix mexicana* and *S. schenckii* on the basis of molecular characteristics; but the clinical value of this classification has not been assessed. Exposure to infection is usually sporadic, although small outbreaks of infection have been described in certain occupational groups, such as florists, packers, plant workers, fishermen and armadillo hunters. There are also focal areas where the disease appears to be hyperendemic in Guatemala,[70] Mexico, Brazil, Peru and South Africa. In South Africa, contamination of pit props has been reported to cause disease in mine workers, whereas in Brazil there has been a recent large outbreak of infection in cats and humans.

Sporotrichosis affects both males and females and can also infect children and infants.

Clinical Features

There are a variety of different clinical forms of sporotrichosis.[71,72] Some infections appear to resolve spontaneously, although the frequency of this occurrence is unknown. Certain patients develop fixed lesions which are usually solitary ulcerated granulomas on exposed sites, including the face. Small satellite lesions frequently develop around the edge of these. Ulcers enlarge slowly. A second form of cutaneous sporotrichosis is called lymphangitic because the infection spreads from a primary granuloma or ulcer along the course of local lymphatics. Secondary lesions formed along the lymphatic path may discharge or ulcerate. Other forms of infection may mimic chronic leg ulcers and lupus vulgaris. Disseminated deep lesions of sporotrichosis may affect other body sites such as the joints, lungs and meninges.[73] While most of these patients do not have major underlying conditions, alcoholism or diabetes are seen in some. In patients with HIV infection, these infections may spread to involve multiple skin sites with large numbers of ulcers or nodules.[71]

Differential Diagnosis

Leishmaniasis may resemble either of the two principal forms of sporotrichosis. Atypical mycobacterial infection, particularly those due to *Mycobacterium marinum*, may cause similar changes along draining lymphatics.

Laboratory Diagnosis

Sporotrichosis differs from the other subcutaneous mycoses in that culture is the most reliable mode of diagnosis because there are few organisms present in lesions and these may be difficult to find.[68]

- *Direct microscopy* seldom has a role to play although it may be used to screen for amastigotes of *Leishmania* species.
- *Culture. Sporothrix schenckii* grows well on Sabouraud's agar and will form characteristic spores. Samples from swabs, curettings and biopsies are all suitable. They should be taken from the edge of lesions.
- *Biopsy*. The histopathology shows a mixed granulomatous and polymorphonuclear response. Organisms are very sparsely scattered in this infiltrate, although some are surrounded by a refractile eosinophilic halo called an asteroid body.

Management

The classical treatment for sporotrichosis is potassium iodide made up in a saturated solution. The starting dose is 1–2 mL given three times daily and increased drop by drop to a maximum of 4–6 mL three times a day. The slow increase is necessary because of the unpleasant taste and the possibility of symptoms of iodism: nausea, dry mouth, altered taste, swollen salivary glands. The normal duration of therapy is at least 2 months and often up to 4 months. Itraconazole is effective in doses of 100–200 mg daily: terbinafine 250–500 mg daily is an alternative; amphotericin may be needed for disseminated disease infection.

SUBCUTANEOUS INFECTION DUE TO CONIDIOBOLUS AND BASIDIOBOLUS

Subcutaneous mucormycosis (phycomycosis) comprises two separate diseases: those caused by *Basidiobolus* and *Conidiobolus*.[74] Generally the clinical features of these infections are distinct, as are their epidemiology and age prevalence.

Subcutaneous mucormycosis due to *Conidiobolus* (conidiobolomycosis, rhinoentomophthoromycosis) is uncommon but is found in different tropical areas of the West Indies, South

America, Africa and Southern India.[75,76] The causative organism is usually *C. coronatus*, a fungus which is an insect pathogen. The usual focus of infection is within the nasal cavity and the infection spreads from the turbinates to involve the subcutaneous tissues of the face and neck with a hard painless swelling. The deformity may be severe. This infection is seen mainly in adults.

Subcutaneous mucormycosis is also caused by *Basidiobolus* (subcutaneous phycomycosis, basidiobolomycosis). The usual cause of this infection is *B. ranarum*, a pathogen of amphibians and reptiles. The site of infection is usually confined to the limb girdles or proximal limbs.[77,78] It is mainly seen in Central, East and West Africa but is reported from elsewhere and chiefly infects children. Once again the swelling is deforming and has a woody consistency.

In both diseases, the histology is similar, with a dense infiltrate of eosinophils in the subcutis and large strap-like hyphae contained in granulomas.

The treatment is either ketoconazole or itraconazole, although saturated potassium iodide can be used.

TABLE 38.2 Systemic Mycoses

Mycosis	Organism
ENDEMIC RESPIRATORY INFECTIONS	
Histoplasmosis	*Histoplasma capsulatum var. capsulatum*
African histoplasmosis	*H. capsulatum var. duboisii*
Blastomycosis	*Blastomyces dermatitidis*
Coccidioidomycosis	*Coccidioides immitis*
Paracoccidioidomycosis	*Paracoccidioides brasiliensis*
Infection due to *Penicillium marneffei*	*P. marneffei*
OPPORTUNISTIC INFECTIONS	
Systemic candidosis	*Candida albicans, C. tropicalis, C. glabrata*, etc.
Aspergillosis	*Aspergillus fumigatus, A. flavus, A. niger*
Cryptococcosis	*Cryptococcus neoformans*
Mucormycosis	Species of *Absidia, Rhizopus* and *Rhizomucor*
Infection due to *Pneumocystis jirovecei* (see Ch. 39)	
OTHERS: INFECTIONS DUE TO *FUSARIUM, TRICHOSPORON*	

LOBOMYCOSIS

Lobomycosis is a rare infection, seen in Central and South America, caused by *Lacazia loboi*, a fungus which has not been cultured to date.[79] The infection is seen in subcutaneous tissues and presents with plaques and keloid-like scars. The only treatment is excision. The epidemiology of the infection is unusual as it is seen mainly in remote areas[80] and the same infection has also been seen in sea or freshwater dolphins. Rarely squamous carcinomas may develop in long-standing lesions.

Systemic Mycoses

The systemic mycoses are fungal infections that involve deep organs. While some, often referred to as the endemic mycoses, affect healthy individuals, others are opportunistic infections which occur in patients with some underlying predisposition. In recent years systemic mycoses, such as cryptococcosis and histoplasmosis, have become prominent as secondary complications in patients with HIV infection, although it is of interest that not all systemic mycoses have increased in this population. Generally in most developed countries the opportunistic infections are more common but in many tropical areas the endemic systemic fungal infections are seen more frequently although often these are HIV-related.

ENDEMIC SYSTEMIC MYCOSES

The main endemic mycoses are shown in Table 38.2. The usual route of entry of all organisms in this group is the lung, although direct implantation into the skin after an accident is also possible. Each disease has a defined endemic area and their pathogenesis is similar. The majority of people exposed to infection are merely sensitized to the organism detectable by intradermal testing or antibodies (the asymptomatic form). In some patients there is a primary illness which appears to follow massive exposure to the organisms (the acute pulmonary form). Chronic pulmonary forms of these diseases may also occur and they closely resemble pulmonary tuberculosis. Dissemination from the primary lung focus may also take place. It may be a rapid event followed by widespread infiltration of organs (acute disseminated form). The infection in such cases progresses rapidly and the disease may be fatal unless treatment is instituted. Acute disseminated forms are most likely to occur in patients who are immunosuppressed (HIV, lymphoma) but may also be seen in infants and others. More slowly progressive forms also occur and have to be monitored carefully (chronic disseminated forms). While generally they only spread slowly, in some situations they may begin to disseminate. In some infections, histoplasmosis and coccidioidomycosis for example, disseminated and pulmonary forms do not generally coexist. Primary cutaneous infections following cutaneous inoculation are rare and generally follow laboratory or post-mortem room accidents.

Histoplasmoses

The classification of histoplasmosis in man is somewhat complicated. There are two main types.[81] The first, sometimes called classical or small form histoplasmosis, is caused by *Histoplasma capsulatum* var. *capsulatum*. This is a dimorphic fungus whose yeast phase forms are those present in tissue. The disease is endemic throughout much of the world, with the exception of Europe, and presents with pulmonary and disseminated infection affecting the lungs, reticuloendothelial system and mucosal surfaces. The yeast forms seen in tissue are small (2–4 mm in diameter). It will be referred to hereafter as histoplasmosis (Box 38.3). The second form, African or large-form histoplasmosis caused by *H. capsulatum* var. *duboisii*, only occurs in Africa.[82] The yeasts found in tissue are large (12–20 mm) and the main signs of infection follow dissemination to lymph nodes, skin and bones. The organisms isolated from both are identical in

BOX 38.3 HISTOPLASMOSIS

- Infection caused by *Histoplasma capsulatum*
- In tropics it is often an HIV/AIDS-related infection
- May present with non-specific signs and symptoms, e.g. fever and weight loss, multiple skin papules
- Responds well to amphotericin B and/or itraconazole.

culture but can be differentiated by molecular genetic techniques and are regarded as variants of a single species, *H. capsulatum*.

Epidemology. The organism can be found in soil or areas where large numbers of birds or bats have roosted, including barns, caves and under the eaves of houses. There is no association with any one particular bat species in the tropics. The endemic areas include parts of the USA, West Indies, Central and South America, Africa, India and the Far East.[81] Apart from the USA the endemic areas with the highest incidence of new infections occur in Central and South America. It is thought that bird or bat excreta provides the necessary milieu for growth of organisms present in the environment, although bats can also be infected. Exposure in man is usually sporadic, although occasionally the disease is seen in groups of exposed patients such as cave explorers or farm workers.

Pathogenesis. Defence against *H. capsulatum* is largely by cell-mediated responses. The organism is about 2–4 mm in diameter and can be taken up by macrophages. The infection may therefore be prolonged in individuals with defective T lymphocyte-mediated responses, including those with HIV infection.

Clinical Features. The majority of patients who acquire histoplasmosis remain asymptomatic, the only sign of past exposure being a positive intradermal histoplasmin test which is read after 48 hours. This test is used for studying the epidemiology of infection but has little value as a diagnostic procedure because it only indicates exposure and many patients with active infection may have negative results.

The acute pulmonary form of histoplasmosis often follows exposure to a site containing numerous *Histoplasma* spores such as a cave. Patients develop an acute febrile illness 10–14 days after exposure. There is cough, chest pain, uveitis, joint pains and, in some cases, erythema multiforme. Radiologically, there is often diffuse mottling and in some cases hilar enlargement (Figure 38.12). Normally, spontaneous recovery occurs and no treatment is given except supportive measures. However, very rarely in some patients the disease progresses and disseminates.

Some patients may be found on routine imaging to have solitary or multiple asymptomatic pulmonary nodules, which are biopsied for diagnosis. These are then found to contain

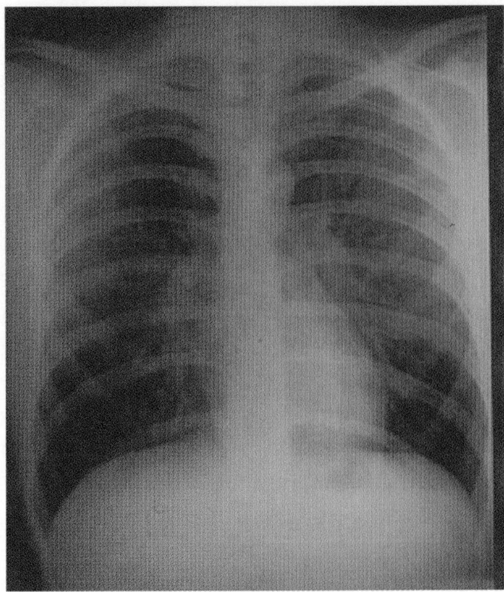

Figure 38.12 Acute pulmonary histoplasmosis.

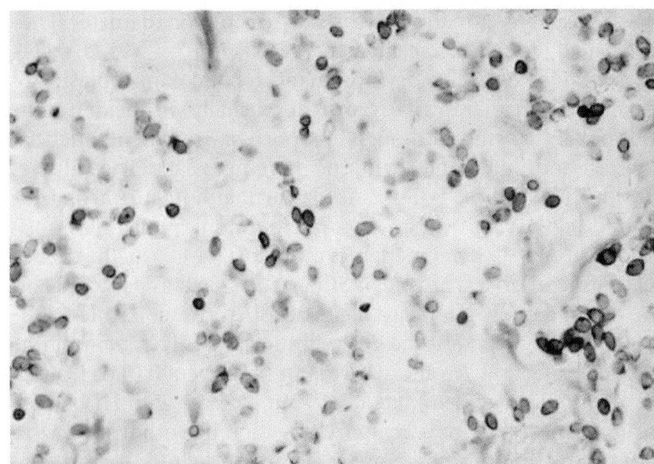

Figure 38.13 *Histoplasma capsulatum* in a lung lesion. Gomori (methenamine silver) (GMS ×100).

Histoplasma yeasts (Figure 38.13). Once again therapy is not necessary. A second type of chronic pulmonary disease produces focal consolidation and cavitation, usually in one or both apices, seen on radiography. This closely resembles pulmonary tuberculosis. The main symptoms, such as cough, chest pain and haemoptysis, are also similar. In the early stages some recovery can occur but later in established cases there is slow progression of the inflammatory lesion to involve other lung areas. This form of histoplasmosis is not often seen in the tropics.

Acute disseminated histoplasmosis affects the bone marrow and lymph glands as well as the liver and spleen.[83] Patients present with fever, weight loss, malaise and hepatosplenomegaly. Diffuse pulmonary infiltrates and small skin papules and ulcers can also occur. This type of histoplasmosis will progress to death if unchecked. Acute forms of disseminated histoplasmosis are seen in patients with HIV infection.[84,85] In the latter groups the symptoms may be nonspecific (weight loss and fever), although some clues such as hepatosplenomegaly or multiple skin lesions (nodules, papules, ulcers) may be seen. A more indolent type of disseminated histoplasmosis is seen in otherwise healthy individuals. They usually present with either oral ulceration or hypoadrenalism. Adrenal involvement should be investigated in such patients. Chronic disseminated histoplasmosis may present years after the patient has left an endemic area. The oral ulcers are persistent and painful. Laryngeal involvement, meningitis and endocarditis can also occur.

Laboratory Diagnosis. The organisms of *H. capsulatum* are very small and difficult to visualize by direct microscopy but they can sometimes be seen in bone marrow or blood smears stained with Giemsa. They can be grown readily from sputum or other sources such as bone marrow in appropriate cases. Blood cultures are sometimes positive in patients with HIV infection. The organisms grow as moulds at room temperature and yeasts at 37°C. The identification of primary cultures is confirmed by molecular testing using standard probes or the exoantigen test. Serology has a useful role in diagnosis. There are complement fixation tests for histoplasmosis as well as an immunodiffusion test, both of which use standardized reagents. These tests can be used in diagnosis and as a guide to prognosis. The detection of circulating *Histoplasma* antigen is of particular value in HIV-positive patients. Histopathology is also useful.

Histoplasmas are small oval yeasts up to 5 mm in diameter. They are usually found intracellularly.

Management. The asymptomatic forms of histoplasmosis do not require therapy. Therapy is also usually withheld in acute pulmonary forms, although supportive treatment such as bedrest and fluids may be given where necessary. The value of antifungals in these types is not known, although itraconazole would be the main choice. Chronic pulmonary histoplasmosis and chronic disseminated histoplasmosis are usually treated with itraconazole. The role of other azoles such as posaconazole in this infection is not as yet established. Itraconazole (200–400 mg daily) can also be given in more rapidly disseminating types of infection. An alternative is amphotericin B (0.6–1.0 mg/kg daily) in the disseminated types. In patients with HIV infection it is necessary to use suppressive therapy with itraconazole after induction of remission with amphotericin B; if antiretrovirals are commenced, long-term treatment can be cautiously withdrawn after 4–6 months.

African Histoplasmosis

African histoplasmosis, as the name suggests, is confined to Africa. It is caused by *H. capsulatum* var. *duboisi*, which resembles the other variant but forms larger yeasts in tissue.[82] The infection is not common but occurs in Central and West Africa south of the Sahara and north of the Zambezi River. It is only rarely seen in HIV-positive patients. The ecological source of this fungus is unknown. It is thought that, as with the other type of histoplasmosis, it gains entry through the lungs.

The patient usually presents with focal disease affecting the skin, bone or a lymph gland. Alternatively multiple sites may be affected, including the gastrointestinal tract, lungs and other mucosal surfaces. This form is more rapidly progressive.

The disease is diagnosed by the presence of large oval yeasts (8–14 mm) seen in direct microscopy or histopathological examination of biopsied lesions. The organism can be isolated in culture. Serology is generally negative. The main agents are itraconazole, ketoconazole or even amphotericin B.

Blastomycosis

Blastomycosis is a systemic fungal infection caused by *Blastomyces dermatitidis*, a dimorphic fungus.[86] The disease is mainly found in the USA and Canada but cases have also been seen in Africa, India and the Middle East. As with histoplasmosis the main portal of entry is via the respiratory tract. Yeast phase organisms cause disease.

Epidemiology and Pathogenesis. *B. dermatitidis* has only occasionally been isolated from the natural environment, usually in North America and in sites where there is a risk of flooding, such as river banks.[87] The organism has not been isolated from such sources in Africa and its ecological niche here is unknown. Cases have been described from a variety of African countries from the north (e.g. Algeria) to Namibia.[88] The largest number of cases has been seen in Zimbabwe. It is not clear whether the disease differs in different geographic areas, but in African cases the principal signs of the disease are those of disseminated infection affecting the bone or skin. There is also evidence that the organisms from African and US sources are antigenically and genetically different although morphologically identical. Other cases have been detected in the Middle East,[89] India[90] and Europe. It is not more frequent in patients with HIV/AIDS.

Clinical Features. The main clinical features of infection follow a somewhat similar pattern to those seen with histoplasmosis.

It is likely that subclinical exposure occurs in endemic areas. There is an uncommon acute pulmonary form of the infection which presents with acute respiratory symptoms – cough, pleuritic pain and fever. This is most often seen in children and has not been described in the tropics.[86]

The chronic pulmonary type of blastomycosis presents with focal consolidation and cavitation in the chest with symptoms of cough, fever and weight loss. This may be confused radiologically with pulmonary tuberculosis. Unlike histoplasmosis this may coexist with disseminated lesions of blastomycosis. Disseminated blastomycosis is most often seen in the tropics. The main sites of dissemination are the skin and bones. Skin lesions may be ulcers, abscesses, granulomas or crusted plaques which heal with scar formation. The bones involved are principally axial skeletal bones, such as vertebrae, and spinal cord compression may occur as a result of this infection. Dissemination also occurs in the immunocompromised patient.[91]

Laboratory Diagnosis. The diagnosis of this infection is based on direct microscopy at suitable sites as well as sputum and culture. *B. dermatitidis* is a dimorphic fungus, which grows as a mould at room temperature but as a yeast at 37°C. Histological changes of blastomycosis are typical as the yeasts produce a characteristic broad-based bud.

Management. Therapy of blastomycosis involves the use of either itraconazole (200–400 mg daily) or intravenous amphotericin B (0.6–1.0 mg/kg daily).

Coccidioidomycosis

This infection is cause by *Coccidioides immitis* or *C. posadasii*, which are soil organisms, geographically confined to semi-desert areas of the New World.[92] The infection consists of a respiratory disease which may spread to other sites. Coccidioidomycosis may affect both healthy and immunocompromised patients.

Epidemiology and Pathogenesis. This infection is seen mainly in a geological zone known as the lower Sonoran life zone, where there is a low annual rainfall and a characteristic vegetation including cacti and creosote bushes. The disease is confined to the semi-desert areas of the New World in the USA, Central America (Honduras, Guatemala), Colombia, Venezuela, Argentina and Paraguay. The infecting form is an arthrospore which is inhaled but transforms in the host into a spore-like structure, the spherule. This is a large 50–80 μm diameter spore containing small endospores which are released by rupture of the spherule; they can develop into further spores.

Clinical Features. Infection follows inhalation. In the endemic area, a significant proportion of the populace appear to be subclinically sensitized, e.g. up to 70%.[93] The primary infection, when it is symptomatic, may present with fever, weight loss, cough and chest pains. Arthralgia, conjunctivitis and erythema nodosum or erythema multiforme may all develop. The radiological changes vary from minimal focal consolidation to pleural effusion to massive hilar adenopathy. This clinical type is usually self-resolving, although progression is much more likely in Native Americans, Black Americans or Mestizos.

Pregnant women are also at risk from dissemination. An extensive pneumonia may follow infection in patients with depressed T lymphocyte function, such as those who have received organ transplants. Chronic pulmonary nodules or cavitation may also occur.[92] The latter is characteristically thin-walled on radiography. Dissemination is also seen. Dissemination of coccidioidomycosis often affects the joints or meninges, but skin and other organs may also be affected. Skin changes include ulcers and granulomas as well as warty papules and nodules. Meningitis is a chronic process which clinically mimics tuberculous infection. In patients with HIV infection, prolonged pneumonia and disseminated infections can both occur.[94]

Laboratory Diagnosis. The diagnosis depends on the identification of spherules in smears, biopsies or sputum as well as on the growth of the organism. *Coccidioides* is a white mould fungus which is easily spread by aerosol: the two species can only be distinguished by molecular genetic techniques. It is a potential laboratory hazard and laboratory staff should be forewarned if this is a diagnostic possibility. There are also a number of useful serological tests (complement fixation, immunodiffusion and immunoelectrophoresis).

Management. The treatment of coccidioidomycosis has been changing in recent years, with an increasing reliance on the use of itraconazole and fluconazole. Intravenous amphotericin B is an alternative. Posaconazole may also prove to be an effective therapy. The disease often relapses and the responses of widely disseminated infection and meningitis to these treatments are often poor.

Paracoccidioidomycosis

Paracoccidioidomycosis (also called South American blastomycosis) is a systemic fungal infection which is confined to Central and South America.[95] It causes a range of pulmonary and systemic symptoms but is a sporadically occurring infection caused by the dimorphic fungus *Paracoccidioides brasiliensis*. Yeast phase organisms can be found in tissue.

Epidemiology and Pathogenesis. The main areas where this disease is present are Colombia, Venezuela, Ecuador, Brazil and Argentina, but other South and Central American countries may be involved. Skin testing reveals that the distribution of sensitization in the community is patchy, and seldom more than 25% have positive skin tests. Both sexes may be sensitized but this infection is more common in men than women. The process of transformation from hyphal (environmental) phase to yeast phase *P. brasiliensis* is partly regulated by an intracytoplasmic oestrogen receptor. The natural source of the organism is probably soil.

Clinical Features. The presence of a small group of healthy individuals in an endemic area with positive skin test reactions suggests that there is a subclinical form of this disease.[96] The main clinical types are named after those parts of the body predominantly affected, such as pulmonary, lymphonodular, mucocutaneous or mixed. In chronic pulmonary infection there is often widespread and extensive infiltration followed by severe fibrosis. There is also dissemination to other sites such as the oral or nasal mucosa or lymph nodes.[97] These are the mucosal (mucocutaneous) or lymphatic forms, respectively, but the most common variety is a mixed type where there are multiple foci of infection. Usually all are only slowly progressive and infection is virtually confined to males. On mucosal surfaces this infection produces large erosions and ulcers, less commonly warty papules. While in most patients paracoccidioidomycosis is an indolent infection, an aggressive widespread form of disease occurs occasionally in younger patients. Paracoccidioidomycosis is rare in patients with HIV infection.

Laboratory Diagnosis. The infection is diagnosed by demonstrating presence of the characteristic yeast forms in sputum, smears or biopsies. These yeasts form multiple buds, often appearing around the periphery of a parent cell. The organism is a dimorphic fungus which can be isolated in culture. At room temperature it grows as a mycelial form and has to be converted on enriched agar into the yeast phase at 37°C. Immunodiffusion and complement fixation tests are also available.

Management. The main treatments are itraconazole (100–200 mg daily) or ketoconazole (200 mg daily), but intravenous amphotericin B is an alternative. The latter may be necessary in the widespread aggressive forms of infection.

Infection Due to Penicillium Marneffei

P. marneffei is a fungus which is a pathogen of bamboo rats of the genus Canomys found in China and South-east Asia. It causes a disease which grossly resembles histoplasmosis in both otherwise healthy and immunocompromised patients.[98,99] It is common in HIV-positive patients. The endemic areas extend from parts of Malaysia through Thailand to Myanmar and Assam and north to South China, Taiwan and Hong Kong. Infections are commoner after the rains and it is assumed that the main portal of entry is the lung.

The main sites affected are the lungs, skin, liver, spleen and bone marrow. Most patients have disseminated disease although occasionally the infection is localized. Skin lesions occur in about 60% of cases with HIV and consist of umbilicated papules, small ulcers of nodules. They are very prominent on the face.

The organisms resemble *Histoplasma* species but do not form buds, individual cells being divided by septa. Cells may also be curved. The organism has a characteristic appearance in culture and often produces a diffusible red pigment.

The main therapeutic agents used are itraconazole or amphotericin B. In HIV-positive patients the initial treatment is amphotericin B followed by long-term suppressive treatment with itraconazole. Itraconazole can be withdrawn with caution after 4–6 months in patients who commence antiretrovirals

SYSTEMIC OPPORTUNISTIC PATHOGENS

In industrialized countries they are a major problem in severely ill patients, particularly those with neutropenia and those receiving solid organ or bone marrow transplants. They are also seen in intensive care units. In addition to these, some infections such as cryptococcosis are present in patients with HIV infection. In the tropics less attention has been paid to some of these opportunists, such as candidosis and aspergillosis, with some important exceptions;[100] by contrast, cryptococcosis is recognized to be a common and increasingly important problem everywhere. For more detailed information on these infections the reader is referred to other texts.[101]

Systemic Candidosis

Systemic *Candida* infections occur in a variety of patients, particularly those who are neutropenic, such as leukaemia patients, those who have received major surgery and patients receiving long-term intravenous feeding. The importance of these infections in the tropics is largely unknown. Their management is discussed elsewhere.[101]

Aspergillosis

Aspergillosis is a disease caused by species of the genus *Aspergillus*, principally *A. fumigatus, A. flavus* and *A. niger*. There are a number of different clinical syndromes caused by these fungi, which occur in temperate and tropical climates alike. Aspergilli are well-recognized causes of allergic pulmonary disease, either when inhaled as spores (extrinsic asthma) or when growing within airways where, in susceptible individuals, they may cause a form of intrinsic asthma known as allergic bronchopulmonary aspergillosis.[102] The latter causes reversible bronchoconstriction in the early stages but thereafter irreversible pulmonary damage may occur. This type of disease has been recorded in India, among other tropical areas. A form of aspergillosis seen in tropical areas is the development of a fungus ball or aspergilloma in patients with pulmonary cavitation, usually secondary to tuberculosis.[103] This fungus ball may elicit an inflammatory response and in a minority of patients (15%) will cause severe haemoptysis.[104] The other mode of pathogenesis by *Aspergillus* is through invasion of tissue. This is mainly a problem in the severely neutropenic patient. However, there is one invasive *Aspergillus* syndrome which is mainly seen in the tropics: invasive *Aspergillus* granuloma.

Invasive *Aspergillus* granuloma of the paranasal sinuses is a slowly progressive infection affecting the sinuses, orbit and brain.[101,105] It is seen mainly in Africa and the Middle East and in most patients is caused by *A. flavus*. The patient presents with headache, nasal obstruction and orbital swelling with, in some cases, proptosis. In later stages invasion of the brain may ensue. On radiography a mass can be seen in the maxillary or ethmoid sinuses with erosion of the bones of the base of the skull and orbit. These changes can be confirmed with computed tomography. If MRI is available the infiltrated area contains a typically dense mass. If the lesions are biopsied the main change is a hard granulomatous mass with fibrosis. Scattered fungal fragments can be seen in giant cells, using specific stains, and the organism can be isolated in culture. Serology (immunodiffusion) is often positive. The main differential diagnosis consists of other *Aspergillus*-related illnesses. The presence of an intrasinus mass without bone erosion may be due to an aspergilloma or dense colonization with aspergilli. In this instance presence of the organism may not be of pathological significance. Aggressive paranasal sinus invasion may also occur in neutropenic patients.

The main treatment for paranasal *Aspergillus* granuloma is surgical removal of as much of the tumour as is possible, followed by long-term therapy with itraconazole (200–400 mg daily). This may have to be extended for 6–24 months and, if available, serology is a helpful way of monitoring. An alternative therapeutic option is amphotericin B but long-term therapy is not possible with this drug. There are no reports as yet of experience with voriconazole, now a first-line therapy for other forms of aspergillosis.

Mucormycosis

Fungi belonging to the genera *Absidia, Rhizopus* and *Rhizomucor*, and less commonly, other genera, may cause an aggressive paranasal, pulmonary or disseminated infection in predisposed groups such as diabetic or neutropenic patients as well as traumatic victims of natural disasters such as mud slides.[106] This infection, known as mucormycosis, is seen in temperate as well as tropical countries and may cause the rapid demise of a patient unless there is prompt surgical intervention and treatment with intravenous amphotericin B. It may also present with orbital cellulitis or as a necrotizing wound infection. In malnourished children it may cause a necrotizing gastrointestinal infection.

Treatment with amphotericin B combined, where possible, with surgical debridement offers the best chance of recovery.

Cryptococcosis

Cryptococcosis is a systemic infection caused by an encapsulated yeast fungus, *Cryptococcus neoformans* and *Cryptococcus gattii*. Its distribution is worldwide and it generally presents with meningitis or some other manifestation of extrapulmonary dissemination. While it may cause disease in otherwise healthy individuals, it is also a pathogen of patients with defective T lymphocyte function, such as patients with HIV, lymphoma or solid organ transplant recipients.

Epidemiology and Pathogenesis. *Cryptococcus neoformans* causes disease in immunocompromised patients including those with HIV infection, and is found in most countries. Its ecological niche appears to be soil or areas where there are large amounts of pigeon excreta, from which this fungus can be isolated. The presumed route of entry is via inhalation.[107] *Cryptococcus gattii* is seen mainly in tropical areas and generally occurs in healthy individuals. It has been reported from Africa, the Far East, Papua New Guinea and Australia. This organism is found in the environment in debris from certain species of *Eucalyptus*.[108] In addition to the differences in distribution there are possible differences in their clinical behaviour apart from the predilection of *C. neoformans* for patients with HIV infection.[109] In *gattii* infections, mass lesions, e.g. lung, appear to be more common.

Subclinical sensitization occurs in the general population. Infection rates in the tropics appear to be variable, even in patients with HIV infection. However, cryptococcal infection is one of the commonest opportunistic infections in HIV-infected individuals in both Africa and Asia and is a major cause of death. There have been estimates of up to 500 000 deaths annually in sub-Saharan Africa.

Cryptococcus has a number of important virulence determinants such as its capsule which is antiphagocytic, melanin and the ability to grow best at 37°C. Gene disruption studies also show that phospholipase and urease production are involved in pathogenicity. The activation of a T-cell response with production of cytokines such as interferon-γ and interleukin Il-2 are critically important in activation of an effective immune response. Antibody production, e.g. to capsular polysaccharide is probably an additional element in the immune response. Raised intracranial pressure commonly occurs and may contribute to poor outcomes.

Clinical Features. Cryptococcal infection may present with pulmonary infection – cough, chest pain and fever.[108] However, pulmonary lesions are more often present as an incidental, and symptomless, finding in a patient with other manifestations of cryptococcosis. The common presentation of this infection in the non-HIV-positive patient is with chronic meningitis, although headache and neck stiffness may not be severe, other signs such as confusion, drowsiness, photophobia and cranial nerve palsies may be seen. In patients with HIV infection, the symptoms of meningitis may be less prominent and fever may be the main clinical sign, together with malaise and tiredness.[110] Cryptococcaemia is common and other signs of dissemination such as papular or ulcerative skin lesions, lytic bone deposits and prostatitis may be found.

Laboratory Diagnosis. The laboratory diagnosis of cryptococcosis is straightforward. It depends on the demonstration of the organism(s) by staining smears, cerebrospinal fluid (CSF) or sputum with Indian ink (Figure 38.14) or nigrosin. The capsule surrounding the organism displaces the opaque stain and the surrounding clear halo seen with the microscope is typical of *Cryptococcus*. This is usually positive in HIV-positive patients. The organism can be cultured readily on conventional mycological media such as Sabouraud's agar, although it may take 3–12 days for the yeasts to be recognizable. Sources of culture material include CSF, sputum and biopsies.[111,112] In patients with HIV infection, blood cultures may also be positive. CSF findings classically demonstrate high lymphocyte counts with raised protein but the CSF can be normal in advanced HIV infection.

The quickest method of diagnosis is the use of the antigen detection test, which employs antibody-sensitized latex particles or an enzyme-linked immunosorbent assay test. Both are used to detect capsular antigen in serum or CSF. The tests are specific and the ELISA or latex tests will produce a positive response in 30 minutes. Titres of anticapsular antibody are high in both serum and CSF in HIV-positive patients, e.g. in excess of 1 : 1000. It can also be used to follow the course of therapy. Newer lateral flow antigen detection assays are becoming available which are cheaper and can be used at the bedside. Biopsy material will also show the large yeast cells using periodic acid-Schiff or Grocott stains; the mucicarmine stain is specific for cryptococcal capsule, which it stains pink.

CT or MRI scans where available may occasionally demonstrate cryptococcomas although it is important to recognize that other diseases such as lymphoma may cause CNS lesions in HIV-infected patients.

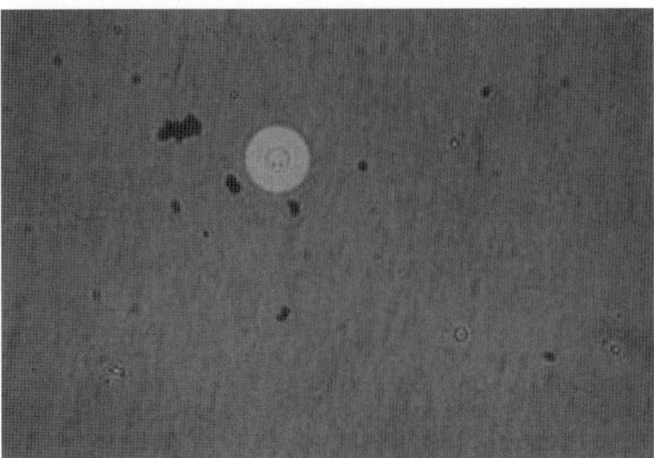

Figure 38.14 Cryptococcal cell in CSF (India ink ×100).

Management. The therapy of choice in the non-HIV patient is a combination of intravenous amphotericin B (0.4–0.8 mg/kg daily) and flucytosine (120–150 mg/kg daily divided in 4 doses). The response in most patients is good but therapy may have to be continued for 4–6 weeks, and sometimes longer. The treatment of patients with HIV infection is more complex. The usual strategy is to start with a period of induction therapy followed by long-term suppression to prevent relapse until immune reconstitution occurs following antiretroviral therapy. At present the best choice of drugs is still unclear. Higher doses of amphotericin (0.7–1.0 mg/ kg daily) appear to be most effective, ideally in combination with flucytosine for 2 weeks, followed by consolidation therapy with fluconazole (400–800 mg daily) for 6–8 weeks followed by suppressive therapy with fluconazole at 200 mg daily.[113] If amphotericin is not available, fluconazole may also be used to produce remission on its own at doses of 800–1200 mg daily. Management of raised intracranial pressure by regular lumbar punctures may also be important in improving outcomes. The optimum timing to start antiretrovirals after a new diagnosis of cryptococcal infection is not known – most clinicians defer until 2–6 weeks after antifungal therapy has started. Cryptococcal IRIS is increasingly being recognized as a problem in a small proportion of patients. If patients are receiving antiretrovirals, long-term suppressive therapy can be withdrawn after a year when the CD4 count is higher than 200/μL. The mortality in developing countries remains high particularly where there is evidence of a high infective burden at the outset of treatment.[114] This has led to suggestions that screening patients by using antigen detection may be a cost-effective way of identifying infection at an early stage.

OTHER MYCOSES

Other opportunistic infections with fungi are seen in different countries and are not specifically associated with the tropics. Again they usually occur in the neutropenic patient. They include infection with *Trichosporon*, *Fusarium* and *Bipolaris* species. These diseases are generally uncommon, but carry a high mortality.

Oculomycosis

Infections of the eye caused by fungi are regularly seen in the tropics (see also Ch. 67). Generally, they involve the cornea and follow contamination of a traumatic external injury (keratomycosis).[115] The chief causes in the tropics are filamentous fungi of the genera *Fusarium*, *Aspergillus*, *Curvularia*, *Acremonium* and *Penicillium*. Less commonly, yeasts such as *Candida* species are implicated. Patients usually present with pain in the eye and photophobia. There is often an obvious ulcer, although it may be necessary to demonstrate this with slit-lamp microscopy. The ulcer may be covered with slough and with small satellite ulcers around the edge. Surrounding chemosis and a hypopyon may also be present. If the condition is not treated, severe intraocular infection followed by glaucoma, blindness and perforation of the globe will occur. Scrapings from the ulcer will readily show the presence of fungal hyphae and these can then be isolated on Sabouraud's medium. It is very important to establish the presence of fungi in such cases of keratitis because their management is very different from that used for bacteria.

Intensive application of antifungal drops such as econazole, clotrimazole or natamycin every few hours is advised. Oral itraconazole or voriconazole may help in some infections although it is seldom useful where *Fusarium* is involved. Mechanical debridement may also be useful in some cases. Keratomycosis is a preventable cause of blindness if recognized and treated as soon as possible.

REFERENCES

1. Anaissie EJ, McGinnis MR, Pfaller MA. Clinical Mycology. 2nd ed. London: Churchill Livingstone Elsevier; 2009.
18. HPA Tinea capitis in the United Kingdom. A report on its diagnosis, management and prevention. Online. Available: www.hpa.org.uk/web/HPAwebFile/HPAweb_C/1194947321499 (Accessed 26 Aug 2011).
33. Edwards JE. *Candida* species. In: Mandell GL, Bennett JE, Dolin R, editors. Principles and Practice of Infectious Diseases. 5th ed. Philadelphia: Churchill Livingstone; 2000. p. 2656–74.
81. Kauffman CA. Histoplasmosis: a clinical and laboratory update. Clin Microbiol Rev 2007; 20:115–32.
107. Chirianni A, Esposito V. HIV-related Cryptococcal meningitis in resource-limited settings. HIV Ther 2010;4:567–76.

Access the complete references online at www.expertconsult.com.

39 *Pneumocystis jirovecii* Infection

ROBERT F. MILLER | SARAH R. DOFFMAN

KEY POINTS

- *Pneumocystis jirovecii* is the cause of *Pneumocystis* pneumonia (PCP).
- In North America and in Europe, PCP remains a common AIDS-defining presentation in those unaware of their HIV serostatus.
- PCP also occurs in medically immunosuppressed (HIV-uninfected) patients.
- In Africa and other developing world environments, PCP occurs in up to 39% of (sputum AFB smear-negative) hospitalized HIV-infected adults with respiratory symptoms.
- The presentation of PCP, with progressive dyspnoea and non-productive cough and radiological appearances are nonspecific.
- The 'gold standard' diagnostic test is demonstration of the organism, using histochemical stains, in a respiratory sample (induced sputum or bronchoscopic alveolar lavage fluid).
- Molecular diagnostic tests have a higher sensitivity but poorer specificity compared to traditional diagnostic methods.
- Co-trimoxazole (trimethoprim-sulfamethoxazole) is the treatment of first choice for PCP, regardless of disease severity. Clindamycin with primaquine is used as second-line therapy for adults.
- Adjunctive corticosteroids should be given to those with PaO_2 <9.3 kPa and are associated with improved outcomes in HIV-infected patients.
- The optimal timing for initiating ART following treatment of PCP in HIV-infected patients is unclear.

Introduction

Different species of the ascomycetous fungus *Pneumocystis* asymptomatically infect a wide range of mammalian hosts and may cause a pneumonia, known as PCP (from PneumoCystis Pneumonia). In humans, *Pneumocystis* pneumonia is caused by *Pneumocystis jirovecii* (previously called *Pneumocystis carinii*).[1]

Pneumocystis was first described by Chagas, in 1909, but it was not until 1951 that it was identified as a human pathogen, being the cause of 'plasma cell interstitial pneumonitis', which occurred in premature and malnourished children, especially among those in orphanages. During the 1960s and 1970s *Pneumocystis* pneumonia occurred largely in children with congenital defects of the immune system and in both children and adults with acquired immune defects secondary to malignancy or its treatment. As organ transplantation developed, it became apparent that *Pneumocystis* pneumonia was associated with the immunosuppression used to prevent organ rejection. In 1981, clusters of *Pneumocystis* pneumonia in previously healthy men precipitated a search for underlying immunosuppression and subsequently the acquired immune-deficiency syndrome (AIDS) was defined.[2,3] Introduction of prophylaxis and combination antiretroviral therapy (ART) in the 1990s led to a marked reduction in incidence of *Pneumocystis* pneumonia among HIV-infected populations with access to these interventions.[4,5] *Pneumocystis* pneumonia remains a significant health problem among patients with solid organ and haematological malignancy, solid organ and bone marrow transplants and autoimmune disease, as well as those receiving 'disease-modifying' agents such as tumour necrosis factor (TNF)-α inhibitors as treatment for inflammatory and malignant conditions (Table 39.1).[6]

Epidemiology and Mode of Transmission

Most patients who develop *Pneumocystis* pneumonia have abnormalities of T lymphocyte function or numbers; rarely *Pneumocystis* pneumonia occurs in patients with isolated B cell defects and in persons without underlying immunosuppression.[6] Irrespective of the nature or intensity of the underlying immunosuppression, glucocorticoid therapy is an independent risk factor for development of *Pneumocystis* pneumonia in non-HIV immunosuppressed individuals.[6]

Before the introduction of prophylaxis, attack rates for *Pneumocystis* pneumonia in adults with organ transplants varied from 4–10% following renal transplantation to 16–43% after heart or heart–lung transplantation (Table 39.1).[6]

The CD4+ T lymphocyte count is used in HIV-infected patients to determine the risk of *Pneumocystis* pneumonia in an individual and also when to start prophylaxis (see below).[7] The CD4+ T lymphocyte count may also be useful in determining the risk of *Pneumocystis* pneumonia in non-HIV-infected immunosuppressed patients.[6]

Pneumocystis pneumonia remains a common AIDS-defining diagnosis in Europe, North America and Asia, but is largely confined to patients unaware of their HIV status at presentation and to those who are non-compliant with or intolerant of prophylaxis and antiretroviral therapy.[5,7]

Pneumocystis pneumonia, although increasingly recognized in some developing world settings,[8–10] has until recently been regarded as uncommon in HIV-infected patients in Africa, by contrast with the high incidence reported in developed countries in the early stages of the HIV epidemic. Data from Africa examining the significance of *Pneumocystis* pneumonia among

TABLE 39.1 Patients at Risk of Developing *Pneumocystis* Pneumonia, Unless Prophylaxis Is Given

General Medical Patients Receiving
Prednisolone ≥20 mg OD for >4 weeks, if patient has underlying immunosuppressive disorder or COPD
TNF-α inhibitors, especially if also receiving corticosteroids[a] or other intensive immunosuppression
Corticosteroids[a] and a steroid sparing agent, e.g. methotrexate or azathioprine
Cancer Patients Receiving
Corticosteroids[a] and cyclophosphamide
Corticosteroids[a]
Alemtuzumab during and for ≥2 months after treatment and until CD4 count is >200 cells/μL
Temozolomide and radiotherapy, until CD4 count is >200 cells/μL
Fludarabine and T cell-depleting agents, e.g. cladribine, until CD4 count is >200 cells/μL
Any anti-leukaemia therapy
HIV-Positive Patients
With a history of *Pneumocystis* pneumonia
With a CD4 count of <200 cells/μL
With oropharyngeal candida, irrespective of CD4 count
Rheumatology Patients with 'Granulomatosis and Angiitis' Receiving
Cyclophosphamide, especially if also receiving corticosteroids[a]
Transplant Patients
For ≥180 days after allogenic stem cell transplantation
For 3–6 months after autologous peripheral blood stem cell transplantation
For ≥6–12 months after solid organ transplantation
Patients with Primary Immunodeficiency
Severe combined immunodeficiency
Idiopathic CD4 T-lymphocytopaenia
Hyper-IgM syndrome

OD, per day; COPD, chronic obstructive pulmonary disease; TNF, tumour necrosis factor.

[a]Corticosteroids = prednisolone ≥16–20 mg OD for >4 weeks (or equivalent dose of other corticosteroid).

Reproduced from Carmona EM, Limper AH. Update on the diagnosis and treatment of *Pneumocystis* pneumonia. Ther Adv Respir Dis 2011;5:41–59.

adult patients with HIV infection are conflicting. Differences in patient selection criteria, difficulties in diagnosing *Pneumocystis* pneumonia or true geographical variation in the prevalence of *Pneumocystis* might in part account for such differences.[11] More recently, studies from Central, East and North Africa show that between 11% and 39% of sputum AFB 'smear-negative' HIV-infected adults hospitalized with respiratory symptoms, have *Pneumocystis* pneumonia.[12–14]

In HIV-infected infants (especially 2–6 months of age), *Pneumocystis jirovecii* is a common cause of severe pneumonia and is often associated with poor outcomes.[15] Routine cotrimoxazole prophylaxis strategies for HIV-infected and -exposed infants in high-HIV-prevalence countries has improved outcomes considerably in this group.

Based on its morphology and lack of response to antifungal drugs, *Pneumocystis* was previously regarded taxonomically as a protozoan. *Pneumocystis* is now known to be an ascomycetous fungus.[1] *Pneumocystis* cannot be reliably cultured in vitro. *Pneumocystis* from humans and other mammalian host species shows antigenic, karyotypic and genetic heterogenicity. Cross-infection with *Pneumocystis* among different host species has not been achieved, inferring host specificity and that *Pneumocystis* infection in humans is not a zoonosis. Lower levels of genetic diversity are seen among isolates of human-derived *Pneumocystis* than occur among *Pneumocystis* derived from different mammalian hosts.[1]

The majority of healthy children and adults have antibodies to *Pneumocystis*, suggesting that primary exposure occurs in early childhood and that *Pneumocystis* pneumonia in an immunosuppressed individual might arise by reactivation of this often asymptomatic latent infection.[1] This hypothesis is challenged by several observations: first, the failure to find *Pneumocystis* in bronchoalveolar lavage fluid or autopsy lung tissue from the majority of immune-competent individuals and second, the observation that low levels of *Pneumocystis*-specific DNA are detectable in a minority of HIV-positive patients with CD4+ T lymphocyte counts lower than 200 cells/μL who present with respiratory episodes but who have confirmed alternative diagnoses. *Pneumocystis* pneumonia in humans is now thought to arise by *de novo* infection from an exogenous source; identification of different *Pneumocystis* genotypes in patients with recurrent *Pneumocystis* pneumonia supports this hypothesis. Molecular data also suggest that transmission of *Pneumocystis* from infected patients to susceptible immunocompromised individuals may occur,[16,17] although there are insufficient data to support routine isolation of patients with suspected or proven *Pneumocystis* pneumonia. *Pneumocystis*-specific DNA may be detected in respiratory samples from patients without clinically-apparent *Pneumocystis* pneumonia who have minor levels of immunosuppression induced by HIV infection, non-HIV-infected patients receiving long-term glucocorticoid therapy and also immune-competent individuals with chronic pulmonary disease.[18,19] These observations suggest that asymptomatic carriage or 'colonization' by *Pneumocystis* may occur.[18–21]

Pathogenesis

Pneumocystis is inhaled and having evaded upper airways defences, deposits in the alveoli where it attaches to type I pneumocytes. The organism is rapidly eliminated by coughing in healthy individuals but may reside in the lungs of individuals with minor immunocompromise (e.g. bronchiectasis) for several days or weeks, i.e. causing 'colonization'; in the immunodeficient host, *Pneumocystis* pneumonia will develop.

Pathology

Pulmonary infection with *Pneumocystis* is characterized by an eosinophilic foamy intra-alveolar exudate that is associated with a plasma cell interstitial infiltrate. Two forms of *Pneumocystis* may be identified morphologically. Thick-walled cystic forms (6–7 μm in diameter), each containing 4–8 sporozoites, occur freely within the alveolar exudate (Figure 39.1). The exudate itself consists largely of thin-walled, irregularly shaped, single nucleated trophic forms (2–5 μm in diameter). Hypertrophy of type II alveolar cells, indicative of tissue repair is often seen. With severe disease diffuse alveolar damage and interstitial fibrosis may occur. Uncommonly, granulomatous inflammation, formation of cavitary lesions and pneumatoceles may be

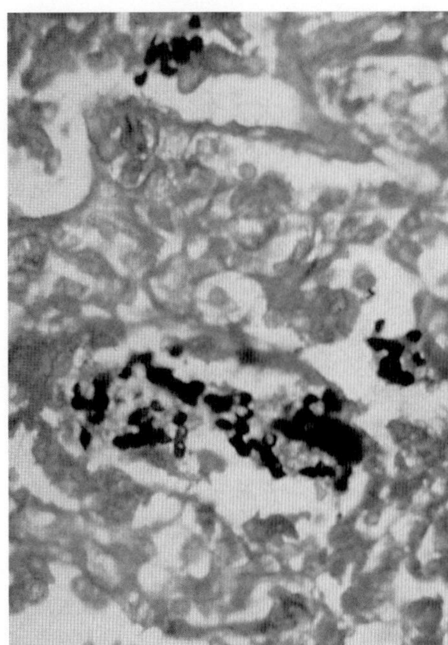

Figure 39.1 Transbronchial biopsy showing cystic form of *Pneumocystis jirovecii* (Grocott's methenamine silver; ×200).

seen. Rarely, *Pneumocystis* infection may extend beyond the alveoli and extrapulmonary pneumocystosis involving liver, spleen or gut is described.

TABLE 39.2 Presentation of *Pneumocystis* Pneumonia

Typical Features		Atypical Features
SYMPTOMS		
Progressive exertional dyspnoea over days or weeks		Sudden onset of dyspnoea over hours
Cough: non-productive or productive of mucoid sputum		Cough productive of purulent sputum
Tachypnoea		Pleuritic chest pain
Inability to take in a deep breath, not due to pleuritic pain		Haemoptysis
Fever ± sweats		
SIGNS		
Normal breath sounds or fine end-inspiratory basal crackles		Signs of focal consolidation, pleural effusion or wheeze
INVESTIGATIONS		
Chest radiograph		
Normal *or* perihilar haze		Early presentation
Bilateral interstitial shadowing *or* alveolar-interstitial changes *or* 'white out' (marked alveolar consolidation)		Later presentation
Arterial blood gases		
PaO_2	$PaCO_2$	
Normal	Normal or hypocarbia	Early presentation
Hypoxaemia	Normal or hypercarbia	Later presentation

Reproduced from Malin AS, Miller RF. *Pneumocystis carinii* pneumonia: presentation and diagnosis. Rev Med Microbiol 1991;3:80–7.

Clinical Manifestations

Clinical presentation is non-specific. Patients typically present with progressive exertional dyspnoea, a non-productive cough and fever of several days' or weeks' duration, which is often associated with chest tightness. A productive cough should raise suspicion for a bacterial infection. Haemoptysis is not a feature. Among patients immunosuppressed by HIV infection, symptoms are usually of longer duration than among medically immunosuppressed patients.[22] Auscultation of the chest is usually normal; rarely, fine inspiratory crackles may be heard (Table 39.2).[23] The clinical features in infants and children may be subtle but can also be difficult to distinguish from other causes of severe pneumonia. PCP should always be considered in any HIV-infected child with respiratory symptoms, particularly in children aged under 6 months or children with significant hypoxia.

Diagnosis

NON-INVASIVE INVESTIGATIONS

Chest Radiology

In early pneumonia, the chest radiograph may be normal; diffuse perihilar interstitial infiltrates are seen with later presentation or more severe disease (Figure 39.2). These appearances may progress to diffuse bilateral air space (alveolar) consolidation resembling pulmonary oedema (Figure 39.3).[23] With delayed presentation or untreated severe disease, there may be confluent alveolar shadowing ('white out') throughout both lungs, with sparing of the costophrenic angles and apices. The chest radiographic appearances in *Pneumocystis* pneumonia may change rapidly from being normal at presentation to markedly abnormal over a period of only 2–3 days. Atypical radiographic features include cystic air space and pneumatocele formation, unilateral consolidation, lobar infiltrates, nodules,

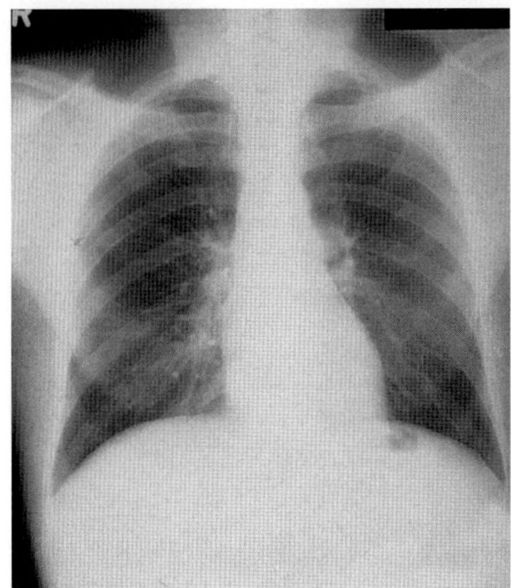

Figure 39.2 Chest radiograph showing perihilar shadowing in a patient with early *Pneumocystis* pneumonia.

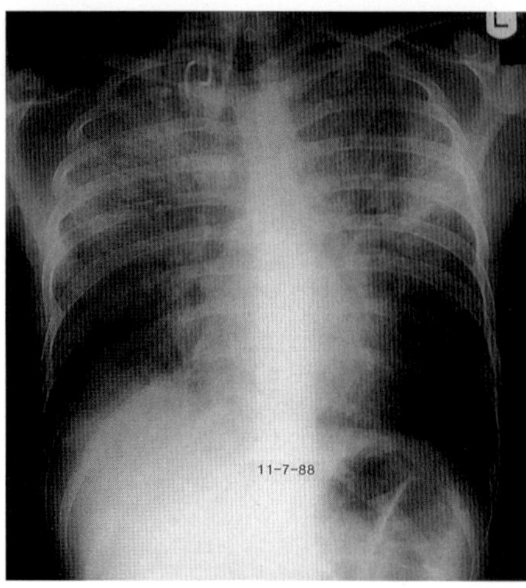

Figure 39.3 Chest radiograph showing extensive bilateral shadowing in a patient with severe *Pneumocystis* pneumonia.

mediastinal lymphadenopathy, pleural effusions and upper zone infiltrates resembling tuberculosis (Figure 39.4).

Although the chest radiograph is a sensitive way of detecting *Pneumocystis* pneumonia, it is nonspecific; these typical and atypical radiographic appearances may also occur in other fungal, mycobacterial and bacterial infections and in non-infectious conditions, such as pulmonary Kaposi's sarcoma and nonspecific interstitial pneumonitis.

With treatment, improvements in the chest radiographic appearances are not usually apparent for 7–10 days. After treatment and clinical recovery, some radiographs remain abnormal for many months in the absence of symptoms; others show residual fibrosis or post-infectious bronchiectasis.

High-resolution Computed Tomography

This may be useful in the symptomatic patient with a normal or equivocal chest radiograph. Patches of 'ground glass' shadowing are typical for *Pneumocystis* pneumonia, but also occur in cytomegalovirus or fungal pneumonia and in occult alveolar haemorrhage (Figure 39.5).

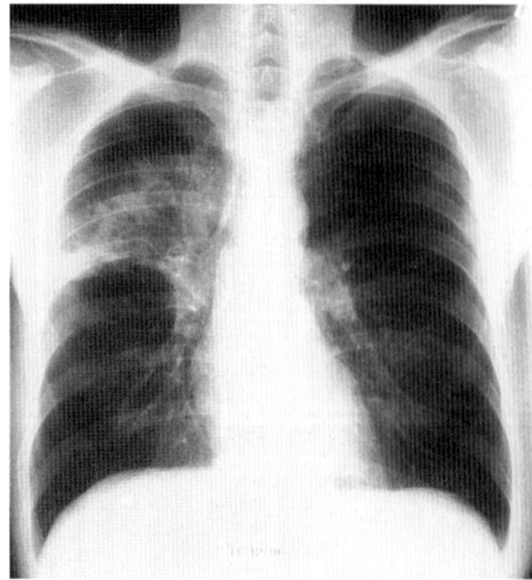

Figure 39.4 Chest radiograph showing atypical appearances of upper lobe consolidation, mimicking tuberculosis, in a patient with *Pneumocystis* pneumonia.

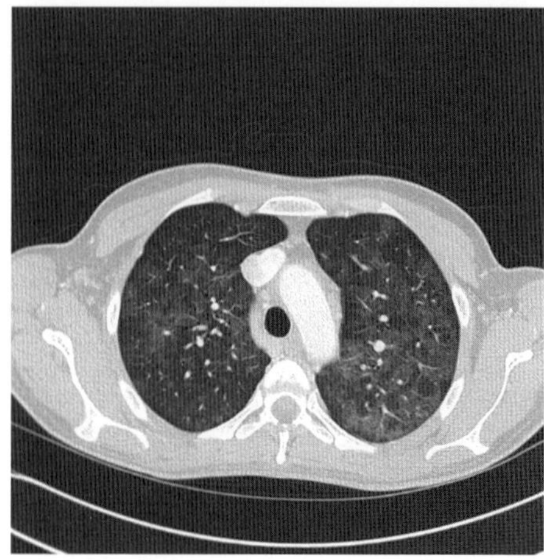

Figure 39.5 CT scan showing widespread 'ground glass' shadowing, typical of *Pneumocystis* pneumonia.

Arterial Blood Gases

In patients presenting early with *Pneumocystis* pneumonia, even though the arterial oxygen tension (PaO_2) may be normal or near normal, low arterial $PaCO_2$ levels (indicating hyperventilation) are often present. With progression of *Pneumocystis* pneumonia hypoxaemia may occur. The alveolar–arterial oxygen gradient ($A–aO_2$) may be calculated, if arterial blood gas analysis is done. The $A–aO_2$ gradient is widened in over 90% of patients with *Pneumocystis* pneumonia, but this finding, although suggestive, is nonspecific as both hypoxaemia and a widened $A–aO_2$ gradient may also occur in bacterial and mycobacterial infections, nonspecific interstitial pneumonitis and in pulmonary Kaposi's sarcoma.

Exercise Oximetry

In immunosuppressed patients with respiratory symptoms, normal or near-normal chest radiographs and normal resting PaO_2 values, exercise-induced arterial desaturation is a sensitive and specific method of detecting *Pneumocystis* pneumonia. A normal exercise test (with no desaturation) virtually excludes the diagnosis.

Serum Lactate Dehydrogenase

An elevated serum lactate dehydrogenase (LDH) level is highly suggestive of *Pneumocystis* pneumonia in an HIV-infected patient with sub-acute respiratory symptoms.[4,24] However, an elevated serum LDH is nonspecific, as it is also found in other pulmonary diseases, including pulmonary embolism, nonspecific interstitial pneumonitis, fungal, bacterial and mycobacterial pneumonia, as well as in extra-pulmonary disease, such as multicentric Castleman disease and lymphoma.

Serum (1,3) ß-D-Glucan

Serum (1,3) ß-D-glucan (BG) is a cell wall component of all fungi, including *Pneumocystis*. Serum BG levels are higher among patients with *Pneumocystis* pneumonia (both HIV-infected and uninfected), when compared with symptomatic patients who have alternative diagnoses. Using a cut-off of 100 pg/mL, this assay has 100% sensitivity and 96.4% specificity for diagnosis of *Pneumocystis* pneumonia.[25] As serum BG levels are also raised in patients with other fungal infection, e.g.

disseminated *Histoplasmosis*, the BG assay cannot be used to non-invasively diagnose *Pneumocystis* pneumonia, nor can it be used to monitor treatment response in those with confirmed *Pneumocystis* pneumonia, as, despite clinical recovery, reduction in BG levels is both delayed and unpredictable.

S-Adenosylmethionine

Pneumocystis was thought to be unable to metabolize S-adenosylmethionine (SAM or Adomet), as it lacks SAM synthetase and so 'scavenges' this from the human host. Thus, it was hypothesized that patients with *Pneumocystis* pneumonia might have low serum/plasma SAM levels. While some studies have shown that measurement of plasma SAM levels enables clear discrimination between *Pneumocystis* and other (e.g. bacterial, mycobacterial) causes of pneumonia among HIV-infected patients, other studies have shown SAM levels overlap.[4,26] Thus, this assay lacks diagnostic utility.

INVASIVE INVESTIGATIONS

Sputum Induction

Pneumocystis is rarely identified in spontaneously expectorated sputum. Induced sputum, obtained by inhalation of an aerosol of hypertonic saline is a useful screening technique. The success rate for this technique varies considerably between centres. Deployment of an experienced nurse or physiotherapist to supervise the procedure increases the success rate. The sensitivity varies widely among different patient populations and healthcare facilities; a negative result for *Pneumocystis* from sputum induction should prompt referral for bronchoscopy.

Fibreoptic Bronchoscopy

Fibreoptic bronchoscopy with bronchoalveolar lavage (BAL) has a diagnostic yield of 90% or greater for detection of *Pneumocystis* pneumonia.[4,27] Transbronchial biopsy adds little additional diagnostic information, yet is associated with a higher rate of complications, including pneumothorax and haemorrhage. Treatment should never be deferred pending results of bronchoscopy in a patient with suspected *Pneumocystis* pneumonia as significant clinical deterioration may occur. The yield for diagnosis of *Pneumocystis* from BAL fluid is not reduced for up to 14 days after starting specific anti-*Pneumocystis* therapy among HIV-infected persons: the diagnostic yield falls rapidly in those with transplant- or chemotherapy-associated immune suppression and BAL is rarely positive after 5 days or more of specific therapy.

Surgical Lung Biopsy

Both open and video-assisted thorascopic (VATS) lung biopsy are still occasionally performed in immunosuppressed patients with diffuse pneumonia and negative results from two or more bronchoscopies and in patients whose clinical course is at variance with findings from induced sputum or BAL fluid.

HISTOCHEMICAL DIAGNOSIS

Pneumocystis cannot be cultured and so diagnosis of *Pneumocystis* pneumonia is by microscopic visualization of the organism in respiratory specimens such as BAL fluid or induced sputum. Stains either stain the wall of the cystic form (e.g. methenamine silver, toluidine blue O and cresyl violet) or stain the nuclei of both trophic and cystic forms (e.g. Diff-Quik or Wright–Giemsa). Immunofluorescence using *Pneumocystis*-specific monoclonal antibodies is more sensitive than histochemical stains, but is more expensive and requires specific laboratory expertise.

MOLECULAR DETECTION TESTS

Detection of *Pneumocystis*-specific DNA using the polymerase chain reaction in BAL fluid and induced sputum is superior to histochemical staining for diagnosis of *Pneumocystis* pneumonia.[28–30] *Pneumocystis* DNA may also be detected in oropharyngeal wash (OPW) samples (obtained by gargling normal saline). However, *Pneumocystis* DNA can also be found in samples (BAL fluid, induced sputum or OPW) from immunosuppressed patients with respiratory symptoms, who do not have *Pneumocystis* pneumonia but who have a confirmed alternative diagnosis and who are colonized with *Pneumocystis*; thus reducing the specificity of molecular detection assays.[28,29,30] In HIV-negative immunosuppressed patients, the negative predictive value for PCR detection on BAL fluid is high, thereby effectively ruling out PCP as a cause of the respiratory presentation. Further research is needed in order to determine whether a specific quantitative DNA 'cut-off' can be used to discriminate between *Pneumocystis* colonization and pneumonia.

EMPIRICAL THERAPY

Empirical therapy for HIV-infected patients presenting with symptoms, chest radiographic and arterial blood gas abnormalities typical of *Pneumocystis* pneumonia is used in healthcare settings that lack diagnostic facilities. This strategy is appropriate if the patient with a CD4 <200 (or stigmata of immune suppression, such as oral hairy leukoplakia, cutaneous Kaposi's sarcoma) has typical radiological abnormalities, is not receiving *Pneumocystis* prophylaxis or ART and has a low probability of other (opportunistic) infections (e.g. tuberculosis).[27]

Treatment

An assessment of the severity of the pneumonia, using the history, examination findings, results of arterial blood gas estimations and the chest radiograph (Table 39.3), will enable decisions to be made about choice of therapy; some drugs are unproven or ineffective in severe disease.[7] Severity stratification also identifies patients who will benefit from adjunctive glucocorticoids (see below). Patients with glucose 6-phosphate dehydrogenase deficiency should not receive co-trimoxazole, dapsone or primaquine as they increase the risk of haemolysis.

Therapy

CO-TRIMOXAZOLE

High-dose co-trimoxazole (100 mg/kg daily of sulfamethoxazole and 20 mg/kg daily of trimethoprim) given in 2–4 divided doses orally or intravenously is first choice therapy for *Pneumocystis* pneumonia of all grades of severity.[7] In HIV-infected

TABLE 39.3 Grading of Severity of *Pneumocystis* Pneumonia

	Mild	Moderate	Severe
Clinical features	Increasing exertional dyspnoea ± cough and sweats	Dyspnoea on minimal exertion, occasional dyspnoea at rest, fever ± sweats	Dyspnoea at rest, tachypnoea at rest, persistent fever, cough
Arterial blood gas (room air)	PaO_2 normal, SaO_2 falling on exercise	PaO_2 = 8.1–11 kPa	PaO_2 <8.0 kPa
Chest radiograph	Normal or minor perihilar infiltrates	Diffuse interstitial shadowing	Extensive interstitial shadowing ± diffuse alveolar shadowing ('white out'), sparing costophrenic angles and apices

SaO_2, arterial oxygen saturation, measured with a *transcutaneous oximeter*.
Reproduced from Miller RF, Mitchell DM. *Pneumocystis carinii* pneumonia. Thorax 1992;47:305–14.

patients, treatment is given for 21 days because shorter courses are associated with treatment failure. In patients with other causes of immunosuppression, shorter courses (e.g. 14–17 days) are often given.[6] In patients with moderate or severe disease, cotrimoxazole is given intravenously for the first 7–10 days, then orally; in patients with mild disease oral co-trimoxazole may be given throughout.[7] There is a lack of evidence to support use of oral co-trimoxazole in severe PCP, but it is frequently the only therapeutic option outside of North America and Europe. Adverse reactions to co-trimoxazole, which are usually first evident at 6–14 days of treatment, are common and include neutropenia and anaemia in up to 40% of patients, rash in 25%, fever in over 20% and abnormal liver function in approximately 10%.[31]

Co-administration of folic or folinic acid does not reduce or prevent haematological toxicity and may be associated with increased therapeutic failure. Dose reduction of co-trimoxazole, to 75% of the dose given above, is associated with a reduced toxicity profile but may be associated with reduced efficacy. It is not clear why there is such a high frequency of adverse reactions to co-trimoxazole in patients immunosuppressed by HIV infection compared with patients immunosuppressed by other causes, but it may be due to HIV-induced changes in acetylator status, accumulation of toxic metabolites such as hydroxylamines or to glutathione deficiency.

ALTERNATIVE THERAPY

Several other treatments are available if co-trimoxazole is not tolerated by the patient or if treatment fails (Table 39.4).[7,32,33]

Clindamycin with Primaquine

This combination was originally only used to 'salvage' patients with mild and moderately severe *Pneumocystis* pneumonia who failed to respond to co-trimoxazole or pentamidine. It is now used as an alternative therapy in patients with pneumonia of all grades of severity. Clindamycin 450–600 mg four times daily with primaquine 15 mg daily (by mouth) are used. Higher doses of primaquine confer no therapeutic advantage and are associated with a greater risk of methaemoglobinaemia. Treatment is for 21 days regardless of the type of underlying immunosuppression. Clindamycin is usually given intravenously for the first 7–10 days, then orally in moderate and severe disease; the treatment may be given orally throughout in patients with mild disease. Clindamycin-primaquine is as effective as co-trimoxazole or dapsone-trimethoprim (see below) when given as initial treatment for patients with *Pneumocystis* pneumonia of mild and moderate severity and is superior to intravenous pentamidine when used in patients intolerant of, or who are failing treatment with, co-trimoxazole.[32,33] Almost two-thirds of patients develop a rash and approximately 25% develop diarrhoea. If diarrhoea occurs during clindamycin-primaquine therapy, analysis of stool for detection of *Clostridium difficile* is indicated.

Dapsone with Trimethoprim

In patients with mild or moderately severe *Pneumocystis* pneumonia, the combination of dapsone (100 mg/day) and trimethoprim (20 mg/kg daily) is as effective as co-trimoxazole (doses as above) and is better tolerated.[7] Rash, nausea and vomiting and asymptomatic methaemoglobinaemia (due to dapsone) are the major side-effects with this combination. Approximately 50% of patients develop mild hyperkalaemia (<6.1 mmol/L), which is due to trimethoprim. This combination has not been shown to be effective in severe disease.

Atovaquone

Atovaquone 750 mg twice daily orally for 21 days, is less effective than either oral high-dose co-trimoxazole or intravenous pentamidine for treatment of mild and moderate severity *Pneumocystis* pneumonia, but is better tolerated than either drug. It

TABLE 39.4 Treatment of *Pneumocystis* Pneumonia

	Mild	Moderate	Severe
First choice	Co-trimoxazole	Co-trimoxazole	Co-trimoxazole
Second choice	Clindamycin–primaquine	Clindamycin–primaquine	Clindamycin–primaquine
Third choice	Dapsone–trimethoprim or Atovaquone	Dapsone–trimethoprim or Atovaquone	IV Pentamidine
Fourth choice	IV Pentamidine	IV Pentamidine	–
Adjunctive glucocorticoids	Unproven benefit	Yes	Yes

is ineffective in patients with severe pneumonia.[7] Common adverse reactions include rash, nausea and vomiting and constipation. Absorption of the drug from the gastrointestinal tract is variable; taking the suspension with food may increase its absorption.

Parenteral Pentamidine

Intravenous pentamidine is now rarely used in mild and moderately severe disease because of its toxicity profile and because other less toxic treatments have equivalent efficacy.[7,32] It continues to be used in patients with severe pneumonia. It is given at a dose of 4 mg/kg daily, by intravenous infusion for 21 days. Compared with high-dose co-trimoxazole, intravenous pentamidine is of almost equivalent efficacy but has a greater toxicity profile. Up to 60% of patients receiving pentamidine develop nephrotoxicity, which usually manifests as an isolated increase in the serum creatinine level; approximately half develop leucopenia. Hypotension and nausea/vomiting both occur in up to 25% of patients. Hypoglycaemia occurs in approximately 20% of patients. There are no therapeutic advantages to combining high-dose co-trimoxazole and intravenous pentamidine and this combination has a much higher toxicity profile.

Caspofungin

Caspofungin is an echinocandin that inhibits (1,3)-β-D-glucan synthase and is effective against *Aspergillus* and *Candida* spp. Case reports and small case series show that caspofungin monotherapy or combination therapy may be effective in patients with *Pneumocystis* pneumonia who are not responding to or tolerating first-line therapy. Caspofungin has not been prospectively evaluated against TMP-SMX or other regimens as first-line therapy.

Nebulized Pentamidine

This form of therapy has no role in the treatment of *Pneumocystis* pneumonia.

Corticosteroids

Adjunctive therapy with glucocorticoids for patients with moderate and severe *Pneumocystis* pneumonia has been shown to reduce the likelihood of respiratory failure (by half) and death (by one-third) in HIV-infected patients.[7] In the non-HIV-infected immunosuppressed population, adjuvant steroids reduce the duration of time on mechanical ventilation and overall time in the intensive care unit. Corticosteroids probably act by reducing the body's intrapulmonary inflammatory response to *Pneumocystis*. It is recommended that glucocorticoids are given to HIV-infected patients with proven or suspected *Pneumocystis* pneumonia who have a PaO_2 <9.3 kPa or $A - aO_2$ >4.7 kPa (both measured while the patient is breathing room air). No specific recommendations exist for non-HIV-infected patients, but the above criteria are often used in clinical practice.

Corticosteroid treatment should begin at the start of specific anti-*Pneumocystis* therapy. Clearly, in some patients treatment will begin on a presumptive basis and it is necessary to confirm the diagnosis as soon as possible. Several regimens have been used, the most common being oral prednisolone 40 mg twice daily for 5 days, thereafter 40 mg once daily for days 6–10 and then 10 further days of 20 mg daily.[7] Intravenous methylprednisolone may be given at 75% of these doses; alternatively, higher doses may be given for a shorter period of time, such as methylprednisolone 1 g once daily for 3 days and 0.5 g on days 4–6, followed by oral prednisolone 80 mg once daily reducing to zero over 17 days.[7] There is no evidence that adjunctive corticosteroids are of benefit in patients with mild *Pneumocystis* pneumonia.

PAEDIATRIC TREATMENT

Therapeutic options for the treatment of *Pneumocystis* pneumonia in children and adults are similar to those in adults (Table 39.5). The evidence base for the use of corticosteroids in severe disease in children is more limited than in adults but corticosteroids should be given in severe disease using the same criteria as for adults.

GENERAL MANAGEMENT

Patients with mild *Pneumocystis* pneumonia may be treated with oral co-trimoxazole as out-patients under close supervision of a physician. All patients with moderate and severe *Pneumocystis* pneumonia should be treated in hospital with intravenous co-trimoxazole or with clindamycin with primaquine and adjunctive corticosteroids. Patients not responding by 5–7 days or deteriorating before this time, should be switched to alternative therapy.[33]

TABLE 39.5 **Therapeutic Options for the Treatment of *Pneumocystis* Pneumonia in Children**

Drug	Infant and Child Dosage
Trimethoprim-sulfamethoxazole (TMP-SMX) (drug of first choice)	TMP: 15–20 mg/kg per day, PO or IV, divided into 4 doses SMX: 75–100 mg/kg per day, PO or IV, divided into 4 doses
Pentamidine	4 mg/kg per day intravenously
Atovaquone	3–24 months of age: 45 mg/kg per day, PO, divided into 2 doses 1–3 months and over 24 months: 30 mg/kg per day, PO, divided into 2 doses (maximum daily dose 1500 mg)
Dapsone plus trimethoprim	Dapsone: 2 mg/kg per day (maximum 100 mg), PO, once daily Trimethoprim: 15 mg/kg per day, PO, divided into 3 doses
Primaquine plus clindamycin	Primaquine: 0.3 mg/kg per day (maximum 30 mg), PO, once daily Clindamycin: 40 mg/kg per day, IV, divided into 4 doses (no paediatric data for this regimen)

Adapted from Gigliotti F. Pneumocystis jiroveci infection. In: Long SS, et al, editors. Principles and Practice of Pediatric Infectious Disease. 4th ed. With permission from Elsevier.

All hypoxaemic patients with *Pneumocystis* pneumonia should receive supplemental oxygen therapy via a tight-fitting face mask in order to maintain the PaO_2 ≥8.0 kPa. If an inspired oxygen concentration of 60% fails to maintain the PaO_2 ≥8.0 kPa, referral to the ICU for mechanical ventilation should be considered. The prognosis of patients with severe *Pneumocystis* pneumonia with respiratory failure has improved in recent years, as a consequence of general improvements in ICU management of respiratory failure.[34–36] Most centres would mechanically ventilate HIV-infected adults with a first- or second-episode of *Pneumocystis* pneumonia, who deteriorate despite appropriate anti-*Pneumocystis* therapy (including adjunctive corticosteroids) and who develop respiratory failure and those who rapidly deteriorate following bronchoscopy.

Despite clear evidence showing a survival advantage among patients with mild *Pneumocystis* pneumonia who commence ART early (at 12–14 days after initiation of anti-*Pneumocystis* therapy), the optimal time to start ART in patients with severe *Pneumocystis* pneumonia remains uncertain.[7,37]

Prognosis

Several clinical and laboratory features have been shown to predict a poor outcome among HIV-infected patients with *Pneumocystis* pneumonia. Prognostic factors at presentation include, increasing patient age, lack of knowledge of HIV status, presentation with a second or subsequent episode of *Pneumocystis* pneumonia, evidence of poor oxygenation (PaO_2 <7.0 kPa or A–aO_2 = 4.0 kPa), marked chest radiographic abnormalities, peripheral blood leukocytosis (white blood cell count >10.8×10^9/L), a low haemoglobin (<12 g/dL), a low serum albumin concentration (<35 g/L) and raised serum lactate dehydrogenase (LDH) enzyme levels (>300 IU/L). After admission and investigation, identification of co-morbidity, e.g. non-Hodgkin's lymphoma, the presence of pulmonary Kaposi's sarcoma or a co-pathogen or neutrophilia >5% in BAL fluid and elevated serum LDH enzyme levels (that do not fall despite treatment), need for mechanical ventilation and/or development of a pneumothorax are also predictive of a poor outcome.[38–40] It is not surprising, given the diversity of underlying causes of immune suppression, that host-related risk factors have not been as clearly defined among HIV-uninfected adults with *Pneumocystis* pneumonia.

Chemoprophylaxis

With progressive immunosuppression and falls in CD4+ T lymphocyte counts, HIV-infected individuals are at increased risk of developing *Pneumocystis* pneumonia. Primary prophylaxis, to prevent a first episode of *Pneumocystis* pneumonia, is given when the CD4+ T lymphocyte count falls below 200 cells/μL or the CD4 total lymphocyte ratio is <1:5, to patients with HIV-related constitutional symptoms such as unexplained fever of 3 weeks or more in duration or oral candida regardless of CD4 count and to patients with other AIDS-defining diagnoses, such as Kaposi's sarcoma.[7] Secondary prophylaxis is given in order to prevent a recurrence. In individuals immunosuppressed by other causes, prophylaxis is given to those with high attack rates for *Pneumocystis* pneumonia (Table 39.1).[7] Specific recommendations justify use of prophylaxis among 'at-risk' non-HIV-infected adults with medical/iatrogenic immune suppression.[6]

Co-trimoxazole 960 mg once daily is the first-choice regimen for both primary and secondary prophylaxis.[7] Lower doses, 960 mg three times weekly or 480 mg once daily, may be equally effective and have fewer side-effects. Co-trimoxazole may also protect against bacterial infections, reactivation of cerebral toxoplasmosis and malaria in endemic settings. Rash, with or without fever, occurs in up to 20% of patients. Desensitization should be attempted in those unable to tolerate co-trimoxazole. Alternatively, other less effective agents may be used for prophylaxis. These include nebulized pentamidine, 300 mg once per month, via a Respirgard II nebulizer (once per fortnight in HIV-infected patients with a CD4+ T lymphocyte count <50 cells/μL), dapsone 100 mg daily, dapsone 50 mg daily with pyrimethamine 75 mg once weekly (pyrimethamine may protect against cerebral toxoplasmosis) and leucovorin 25 mg once weekly or dapsone 200 mg with 75 mg pyrimethamine and 25 mg leucovorin (all once weekly) or atovaquone, 750 mg twice daily, with or without pyrimethamine 75 mg daily and leucovorin 25 mg daily.[7]

STOPPING PROPHYLAXIS

The widespread availability and uptake of combination antiretroviral therapy (ART) in North America, Europe and Australasia has been associated with marked reductions in incidence of many opportunistic infections, including *Pneumocystis* pneumonia, hospital admissions and mortality from HIV infection.[5] In most patients, within a few weeks of starting ART, there are rapid decreases in plasma HIV RNA and, in parallel, increases in CD4+ T lymphocyte counts. The US Public Health Service/Infectious Disease Society of America recommend that primary prophylaxis against *Pneumocystis* pneumonia may be discontinued in HIV-infected patients who respond to ART with an increase in CD4 lymphocyte counts to above 200 cells/μL, sustained for at least 6 months.[7] Many of these patients will also have a reduction in HIV RNA to below the limit of detection. Withdrawal of secondary prophylaxis may be carried out, using these criteria. If, despite ART, the CD4 lymphocyte count falls to below 200 cells/μL and/or the HIV RNA 'load' rises, then prophylaxis should be re-instituted using the criteria for primary prophylaxis. Clearly, close patient monitoring is needed to detect any such changes rapidly.[7]

PROPHYLAXIS IN CHILDREN

Co-trimoxazole prophylaxis has been shown to improve survival in children aged 1–14, at least in part due to a reduction in *Pneumocystis* pneumonia.[41] *Pneumocystis* is a major common cause of pneumonia and death in HIV-infected infants and since 2006, WHO have recommended the routine use of cotrimoxazole prophylaxis in HIV-exposed infants in resource-poor settings. Prophylaxis should commence 4–6 weeks after birth and continue until breast-feeding has stopped and HIV infection has been excluded. In HIV-positive infants, cotrimoxazole should be continued until the age of 5, when it should be reconsidered.[42] Despite the challenges of scaling up this approach, the strategy has led to a decline in *Pneumocystis* infection as a cause of pneumonia and along with the expansion of paediatric ART, considerable improvement in outcomes for HIV-infected infants and children.[43]

REFERENCES

4. Huang L, Cattamanchi A, Davies JL, et al. on behalf of the International HIV-associated opportunistic pneumonias (IHOP) study; the lung HIV study. Proc Am Thorac Soc 2011;8: 294–300.
6. Carmona EH, Limper AH. Update on the diagnosis and treatment of *Pneumocystis* pneumonia. Ther Adv Respir Dis 2011;5:41–59.
7. Kaplan JE, Benson C, Holmes KH, et al; Centers for Disease Control and Prevention (CDC); National Institutes of Health; HIV Medicine Association of the Infectious Diseases Society of America. Guidelines for prevention and treatment of opportunistic infections in HIV-infected adults and adolescents: recommendations from CDC, the National Institutes of Health and the HIV Medicine Association of the Infectious Diseases Society of America. MMWR Recomm Rep 2012;58(RR-4):1–207; quiz CE1–4.
19. Morris A, Norris KA. Colonization by *Pneumocystis jiroveci* and its role in disease. Clin Microbiol Rev 2012;25:297–317.
33. Benfield T, Atzori C, Miller RF, et al. Second-line salvage treatment of AIDS-associated *Pneumocystis jirovecii* pneumonia: a case series and systematic review. J Acquir Immune Defic Syndr 2008;48:63–7.

Access the complete references online at www.expertconsult.com

40 Tuberculosis

GUY THWAITES

KEY POINTS

- Tuberculosis is caused by *Mycobacterium tuberculosis* and *Mycobacterium bovis* and, rarely, *Mycobacterium africanum* and *Mycobacterium canettii*.
- *M. tuberculosis* is transmitted between humans by the inhalation of infectious droplets aerosolized by coughing individuals with pulmonary tuberculosis.
- Some 9 million people suffer from tuberculosis worldwide each year and nearly 2 million people die from the disease; India and China have the greatest number of people with the disease, although parts of southern Africa have the highest incidence, driven by the strong association between HIV infection and tuberculosis.
- *M. tuberculosis* infection classically causes necrotizing granulomatous inflammation, which can control the infection and lead to prolonged asymptomatic infection (latent tuberculosis), or fail to control the infection and result in pulmonary (80%) or extra-pulmonary disease (20%) (active tuberculosis).
- Active tuberculosis typically presents over weeks or months with fever and weight loss and symptoms specific to the organ(s) affected. Pulmonary tuberculosis classically results in apical infiltrates seen on chest radiography, with cavitation. Young children (<5 years) and all immune-suppressed individuals (e.g. HIV infection) are at high risk of disseminated extra-pulmonary tuberculosis, including miliary and meningeal tuberculosis which are often fatal without prompt anti-tuberculosis chemotherapy.
- The diagnosis of latent tuberculosis requires the absence of symptoms and signs of active tuberculosis and the demonstration of T-cell-mediated immune reactivity to *M. tuberculosis* antigens, either by the intra-dermal injection of purified protein derivative (PPD) (e.g. the Mantoux skin test) or, more recently, the interferon gamma release assays (IGRAs) performed on peripheral blood.
- The diagnosis of active tuberculosis is dependent on demonstrating the presence of *M. tuberculosis* in a specimen from an affected tissue (e.g. sputum, tissue biopsy, cerebrospinal fluid). Microscopy, following Ziehl Neelsen staining of the specimen and culture have been used for more than a century; rapid molecular methods (e.g. Xpert MTB/RIF test) can detect specific *M. tuberculosis* nucleic acid sequences, including those which confer rifampicin resistance, in clinical specimens within 2 hours.
- The treatment of latent tuberculosis prevents the development of active tuberculosis and is the core tuberculosis control strategy for some countries (e.g. the United States). Latent infection with drug-susceptible *M. tuberculosis* can be treated with 6–9 months of isoniazid; 3 months of isoniazid and rifampicin is safe and effective in HIV-uninfected individuals.
- The treatment of active tuberculosis requires combination drug therapy for at least 6 months: a 4-drug 'intensive' phase followed by a 2-drug 'continuation' phase. Longer courses are required for drug-resistant tuberculosis, especially if the bacteria are resistant to the two most active anti-tuberculosis drugs, isoniazid and rifampicin (multidrug resistance).
- Tuberculosis can be prevented by reducing transmission and reducing the numbers of patients with latent infection who develop active disease. Transmission can be interrupted by identifying infectious cases early, treating them promptly, isolating them from others while they remain infectious and the wearing of masks by patients and staff. The development of tuberculosis can be reduced by BCG vaccination and the treatment of latent infection.

Epidemiology

PRINCIPLES OF TUBERCULOSIS TRANSMISSION

Tuberculosis is an infectious disease caused by members of the *Mycobacterium tuberculosis* complex of bacteria. The complex is formed by several closely related sub-species which have plagued human and animal populations for thousands of years. The human-adapted species, which cause tuberculosis, include *M. tuberculosis*, *M. africanum*, *M. bovis* and *M. canettii*; animal-adapted species include *M. microti* (voles), *M. caprae* (goats), *M. pinnipedii* (seals) and *M. mungi* (mongooses) and rarely cause human disease. *M. africanum* causes up to one-quarter of tuberculosis cases in some parts of West Africa and *M. canettii* is a rare cause of tuberculosis in people from the Horn of Africa. This chapter, however, will deal exclusively with *M. tuberculosis* and *M. bovis*, which cause the overwhelming majority of human tuberculosis.

M. tuberculosis only infects humans and is transmitted by individuals with pulmonary disease; their coughing expels droplets of respiratory secretions containing the bacteria into the surrounding air, which can be inhaled to infect others. Much of the current understanding of the air-borne transmission of tuberculosis comes from a classical series of experiments performed by Richard Riley and others in the 1950s.[1,2] Riley designed a ward for patients with tuberculosis in which the air from each room was ducted into cages containing around 150 guinea pigs (which are naturally highly susceptible to *M. tuberculosis* infection). Each month, the animals were tested for new *M. tuberculosis* infection by assessing their intradermal reactivity to purified protein derivative (PPD) of the bacteria. Those found to be reactive were culled and dissected to confirm the pathological changes of infection (see Pathology and Pathogenesis, below).

Over the first 2 years of the experiment, approximately half of the guinea pigs became infected with *M. tuberculosis*. The infection rate varied from 0 to 10 animals each month; or one infection every 10 days on average. The infectiousness of the ward patients appeared to vary substantially, but those with untreated pulmonary tuberculosis and one adult with tuberculous laryngitis, were responsible for the majority of guinea pig infections. By calculating the volume of air breathed by 150 guinea pigs over 10 days they estimated that there was on average one 'quantum' of tuberculosis infection in about 12 000 cubic feet of air.

These findings are critical to understanding the transmission and epidemiology of tuberculosis. They introduced and validated the theory of droplet-generated air-borne transmission of tuberculosis. Long-range aerosol transmission of infectious agents is only possible if the infected droplets are sufficiently small to remain air-borne for long periods. The dispersal of these small droplets, often called 'droplet nuclei', are dependent on their size and the airflow patterns, which carry them (Figure 40.1). Riley's experiments supported the premise that the likelihood of transmission increased with the concentration of infectious droplet nuclei and the volume of air inhaled. As discussed further below, this has great significance to control measures for preventing tuberculosis transmission, especially in healthcare settings. Their findings also indicated that the infectiousness of patients with tuberculosis was highly variable, but untreated and by extension undiagnosed, patients carry the greatest risk to their contacts.

The relevance of this seminal work to current tuberculosis epidemiology was reinforced by a remarkable recent repetition of the same experimental design in a tuberculosis hospital in Peru, complete with rooftop guinea pigs.[3,4] Unlike Riley and his colleagues, these investigators were able to study the impact of HIV and drug resistance on transmission. Over 18 months, 292 rooftop guinea pigs were exposed to the ducted air from 118 patients with tuberculosis (97 were HIV-infected). Monthly testing found 159 guinea pigs became infected, but just as Riley observed, there was substantial variation in the rate of infection over time. The HIV-positive patients with pulmonary tuberculosis produced a mean of 8.2 infectious quanta per hour, compared with 1.3 reported by Riley; but average monthly patient infectiousness varied from 0–44 infectious quanta per hour. Indeed, 8.5% of the patients were responsible for 98% of the guinea pig infections and three patients with inadequately

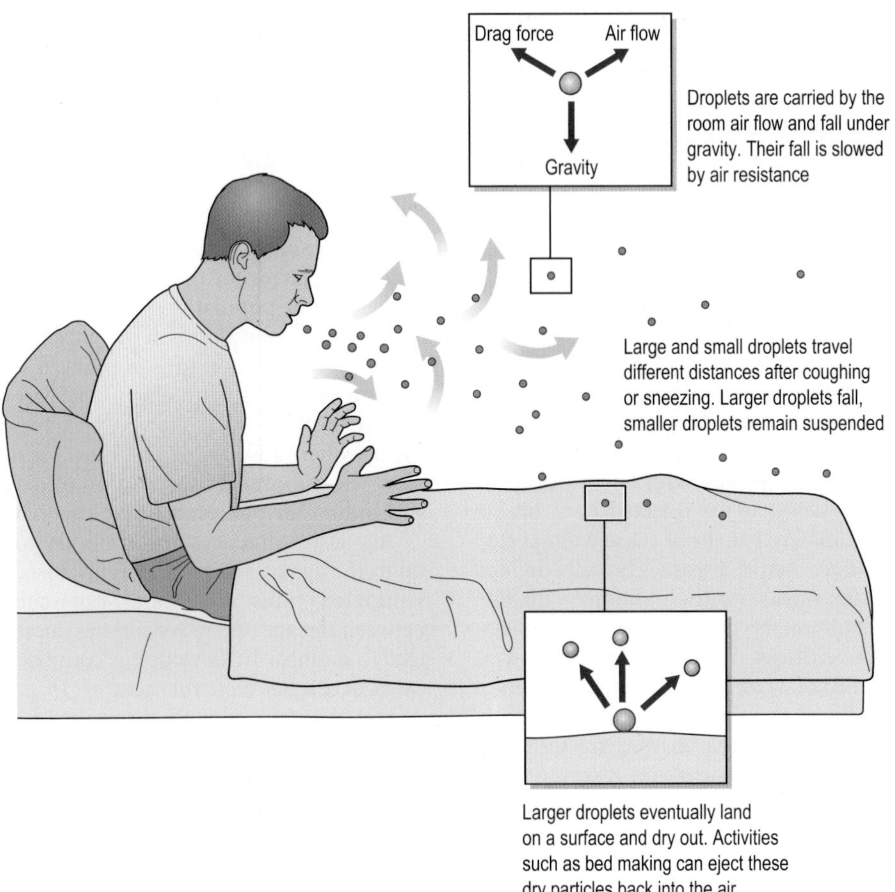

Figure 40.1 Dynamics of air-borne transmission of infectious agents such as *M. tuberculosis* by droplet suspension. *(Taken from: Tang, JW et al. Journal of Hospital Infection 2006; 64:100–114.)*

TABLE 40.1 **Risk Factors for Active Tuberculosis Infection: Relative Risk, Prevalence and Population Attributable Risk in the 22 Highest-Burden Countries**

Risk Factor	Relative Risk for Active Tuberculosis (Range)	Weighted Prevalence in Total Population	Proportion of Cases in Population Attributable to Risk Factor
HIV infection	8.3 (6.1–10.8)	1.1%	7.3% (5.2–9.6)
Malnutrition	4.0 (2.0–6.0)	17.2%	34.1% (14.7–46.3)
Diabetes mellitus	3.0 (1.5–7.8)	3.4%	6.3% (1.6–18.6)
Heavy alcohol use (>40 g/day)	2.9 (1.9–4.6)	7.9%	13.1% (6.7–22.2)
Smoking	2.6 (1.6–4.3)	18.2%	22.7% (9.9–37.4)
Indoor pollution	1.5 (1.2–3.2)	71.1%	26.2% (12.4–61.0)

treated multi-drug-resistant tuberculosis were responsible for 90% of transmissions. The same investigators also confirmed Riley's premise that enhanced ventilation would reduce tuberculosis transmission by showing that natural ventilation (opening windows) of pre-1950 hospital wards reduced the infectiousness of ward air far more effectively than the mechanical ventilation of wards built in the last two decades.[5] These findings have very significant practical applications for countries trying to control the transmission of drug-resistant tuberculosis among highly susceptible patients with HIV in busy hospitals with limited resources.

In the late nineteenth and early twentieth centuries *M. bovis* caused around a quarter of all human cases of tuberculosis.[6] *M. bovis* is transmitted to humans from infected cattle through the ingestion of contaminated dairy products, although *M. bovis* can also be transmitted between people through the inhalation of infectious droplet nuclei, especially among immunosuppressed individuals. Pasteurization has largely removed the risk of animal-to-human transmission, alongside case detection with PPD skin tests and slaughter of infected animals. Today, in countries with these practices in place, 1–2% of all human tuberculosis cases are caused by *M. bovis*. In regions with limited access to these preventative measures, this route of transmission remains an important public health problem.

M. TUBERCULOSIS INFECTION AND DISEASE

As with many infectious diseases, the number of people suffering from *M. tuberculosis* disease is a small fraction of the total number infected. Estimates of the number infected have conventionally been calculated by intradermal reactivity to PPD. Reactivity is taken to represent exposure with latent infection: one in three people are believed to be infected or 2 billion people worldwide. Approximately 1 in 10 of these will develop active disease in their lifetime.[7] Active disease is broadly divided into three categories: sputum smear-positive pulmonary disease; sputum-smear-negative pulmonary disease; and extrapulmonary disease. Smear-positive disease is defined by demonstration of acid-fast bacilli (AFB) of *M. tuberculosis* within a clinical specimen by microscopy. From an epidemiological perspective, individuals with sputum smear-positive disease are the most important, as they represent infectious cases and are responsible for the majority of tuberculosis transmission; although as Riley demonstrated, infectiousness is extremely variable. The WHO and International Union against Tuberculosis and Lung Disease (IUTLD), hold the detection and treatment of sputum smear-positive cases to be a fundamental tenet of tuberculosis control[8,9] (see below).

RISK FACTORS FOR TUBERCULOSIS

There are two broad categories of risk for tuberculosis: environmental and biological. Environmental risk factors determine the intensity and duration of exposure of an individual to others with infectious tuberculosis. Prominent among this group are residence in prisons, nursing homes, homeless shelters and hospitals. High transmission rates and well-documented outbreaks have been reported in all of these institutions. However, sustained physical proximity is not the only reason these environments present special risk. Their populations frequently possess numerous biological reasons for increased susceptibility to tuberculosis. Alcohol dependence, intravenous drug use and human immunodeficiency virus (HIV) infection are common biological risk factors shared by the homeless and those in prison. Other important biological risk factors, often shared by those in nursing homes or hospitals, are diabetes mellitus, corticosteroid therapy, gastrectomy, end-stage renal disease, silicosis and malnutrition. More recently, tobacco smoking has been shown to be a major risk factor for disease and death from pulmonary tuberculosis, particularly in India. Table 40.1 presents the relative risks, prevalence and population attributable risk of the major risk factors for tuberculosis in the 22 countries with the highest tuberculosis burden.[10] These figures demonstrate that although HIV is the strongest individual risk factor for the development of active tuberculosis, its impact on the population relative to other risk factors is dependent upon its prevalence in the population. In populations with high HIV prevalence, such as parts of southern Africa, the proportion of cases attributable to HIV are much higher than that shown in Table 40.1. However, in regions such as India and China, where HIV is currently less prevalent, these data underscore the important contribution of diabetes mellitus, smoking and indoor air pollution to the tuberculosis epidemic.

Age also influences susceptibility to tuberculosis. Children up to the age of 5 years are highly susceptible, especially to disseminated tuberculosis and tuberculous meningitis. Those between the age of 5 years and the onset of puberty appear relatively resistant. In developing countries the great majority of cases occur between the ages of 15 and 59 years. Surveys in several countries show that more males than females are diagnosed with tuberculosis but it is not clear whether this is caused by gender-related differences, lifestyle factors such as smoking, or the ability to access healthcare.

TUBERCULOSIS GLOBAL EPIDEMIOLOGY

In the early twentieth century tuberculosis declined among the richer nations. In 1900, the incidence of tuberculosis in the USA

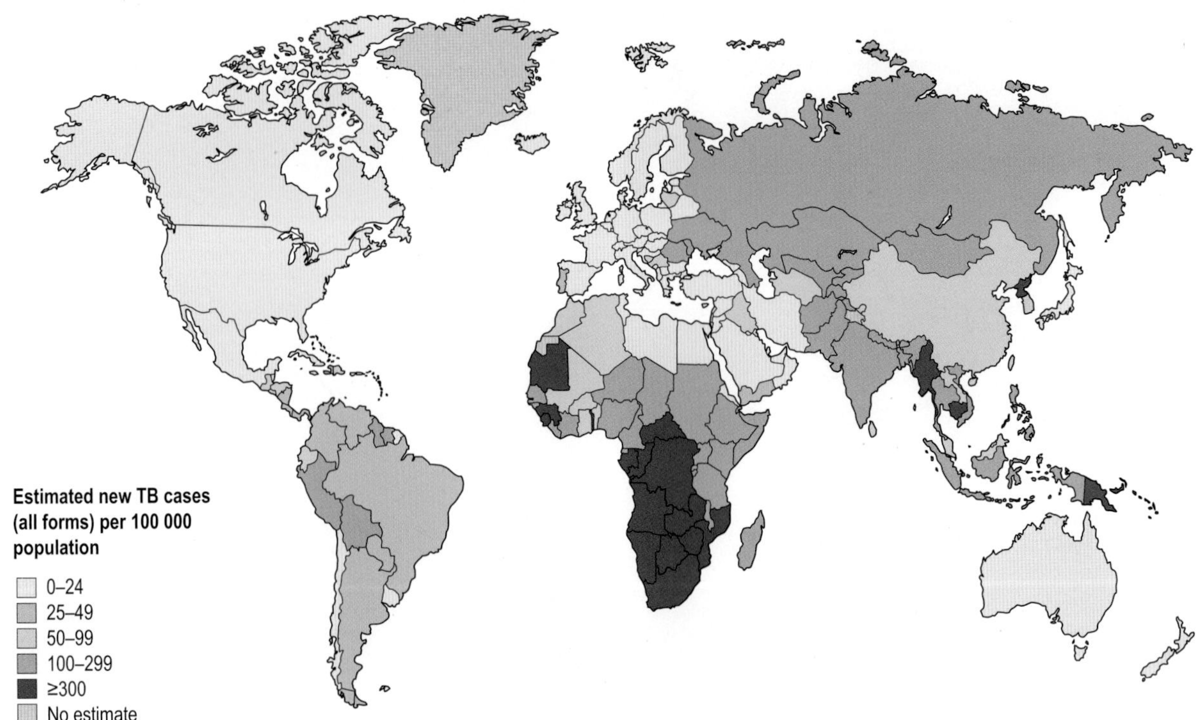

Figure 40.2 Estimated worldwide tuberculosis incidence rates according to the WHO in 2010. (Source: *WHO*.)

was approximately 250 per 100 000, with a death rate >100/100 000. By 1973, the incidence had fallen to 15/100 000, with a death rate of <2/100 000. These figures fuelled enormous optimism, famously encapsulated in 1969 by William Stewart, Surgeon General to the United States, when he suggested it was, 'time to close the book on infectious disease'.

Unfortunately, the figures for the rest of the world told a different story. In 1995, the WHO published an overview of the global impact of tuberculosis.[11] They estimated that one in three people was infected with the tubercle bacillus and that in 1990, there were approximately 8 million new cases of active tuberculosis and 2.6 million deaths. The most recent WHO global tuberculosis control report estimated that in 2010, there were 8.8 million new cases of tuberculosis worldwide (range 8.5–9.2 million) and 1.45 million deaths from the infection. Globally, the absolute numbers of new tuberculosis cases began to fall from a peak in around 2006/2007. In addition, tuberculosis mortality has been falling from a peak of around 3 million in the late 1990s. These new figures are encouraging, although they disguise great regional variation. A map showing the WHO estimates of incidence of tuberculosis in different countries is provided in Figure 40.2. Twenty-two high-burden countries account for 81% of all the estimated cases worldwide. Southern Africa has the highest incidence of the disease (>300 cases/100 000 population), but 59% of all cases occurred in Asia compared with 26% in Africa. The five countries with the largest number of incident cases were India (2.0–2.5 million); China (0.9–1.2 million); South Africa (0.4–0.59 million) and Pakistan (0.33–0.48 million).

Globally, the prevalence of tuberculosis (the number of active cases of disease in a population at any given time) has been falling since 1990, despite the rise in the numbers of new cases up to 2006. This paradox may be explained by an increasing global population (around 1% per annum) and the high mortality in those with new tuberculosis cases infected with HIV.

IMPACT OF HIV ON GLOBAL EPIDEMIOLOGY

HIV infection increases the risk of *M. tuberculosis* reactivation from 1 in 10 to 1 in 3 and increases the likelihood of progressive disease after new infection with *M. tuberculosis*. A cohort study in a South African gold mine found the risk of tuberculosis doubled within the first year of HIV infection; by 11 years from HIV seroconversion almost half the miners had had active tuberculosis.[12]

The HIV epidemic has had an enormous impact on the global epidemiology of tuberculosis. The WHO estimated that of the 34 million people infected with HIV in 2009, approximately 15 million are co-infected with tuberculosis.[13] Of the 8.8 million new cases of tuberculosis in 2010, 1.3 million (13%) were infected with HIV. The HIV prevalence in new tuberculosis cases varies considerably by geographical region, but Africa accounted for 82% of all HIV-associated tuberculosis (Figure 40.3).

Highly active antiretroviral therapy (HAART) for HIV reduces risk of tuberculosis by up to 90%, although risk does not decrease until after 3 months of therapy and never equates to HIV-uninfected individuals.[13] HAART has great potential to change the current epidemiology of HIV-associated tuberculosis, although it remains uncertain whether enhanced HAART delivery alone will control tuberculosis in this vulnerable group. Other measures, such as enhanced case detection and the

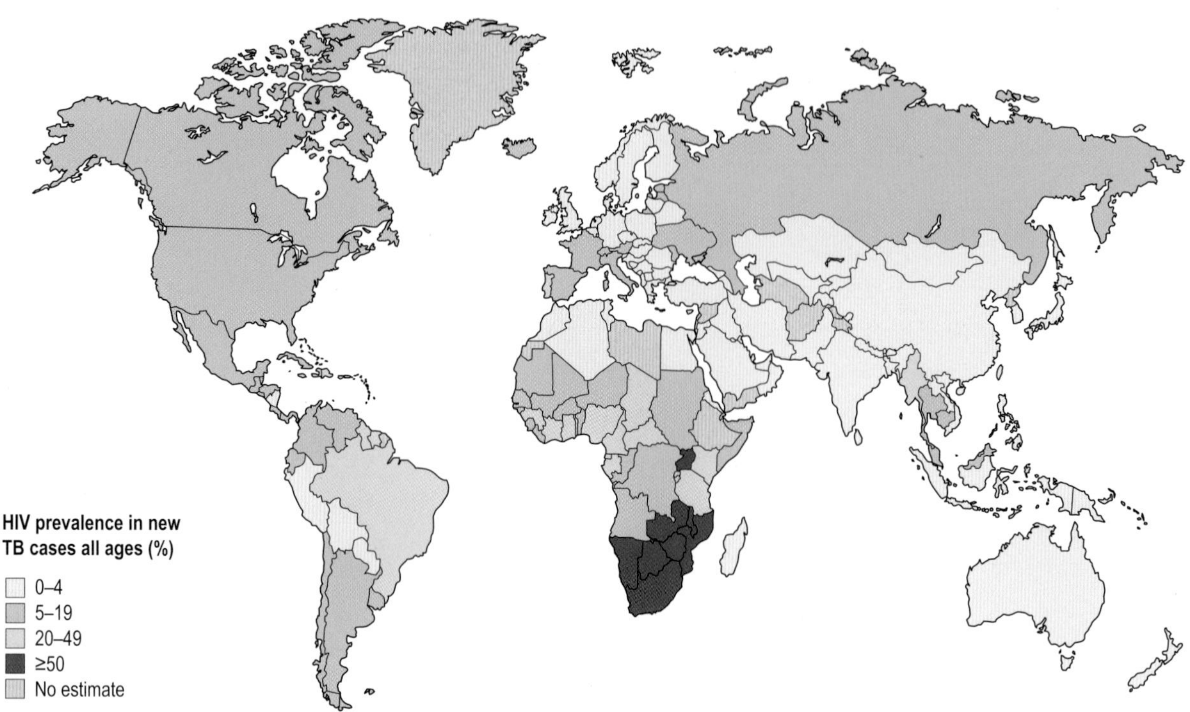

Figure 40.3 WHO estimates of worldwide prevalence of HIV infection in new cases of tuberculosis in 2010. (Source: *WHO.*)

treatment of latent infection, are likely to be required and will be discussed in more detail below.

IMPACT OF DRUG RESISTANCE ON GLOBAL EPIDEMIOLOGY

Combination anti-tuberculosis chemotherapy renders most patients with pulmonary tuberculosis non-infectious within 2 weeks, provided the bacteria are susceptible to the first-line drugs (see Management and Treatment of Tuberculosis, below). If the bacteria are resistant to rifampicin and isoniazid, the essential components of first-line therapy, the infection is termed multi-drug resistant (MDR). First-line therapy is no longer effective against these bacteria and the disease and its transmission continue unabated until second-line drugs are started. This global problem is compounded by the inability of most laboratories to perform drug-susceptibility testing; even if they can it takes at least 8 weeks to get the results; and second-line drugs may not be available, are more toxic and less effective than the first-line drugs. These issues are discussed at greater length later in this chapter. When MDR *M. tuberculosis* acquires additional resistance to fluoroquinolones and one of the injectable second-line drugs (e.g. amikacin, kanamycin, capreomycin), it is termed extensively drug resistant (XDR) and is even harder to treat.

Over the last decade, the uninterrupted disease progression and transmission of MDR and XDR tuberculosis has had a substantial impact on the global epidemiology of tuberculosis. The WHO estimated that in 2008, there were 390 000–510 000 new cases of MDR tuberculosis worldwide, representing around 4% of all cases.[14] These numbers continue to rise every year. Half of all MDR cases occur in China and India. Approximately 100 000 new cases of MDR tuberculosis emerge in China each year, with rates of 5.7% among all new tuberculosis cases and 25.6% among those previously treated. These figures are extremely challenging to the country's tuberculosis control programme, responsible for their diagnosis and treatment. The situation in other regions, however, is much worse: in north-west Russia, for example, one in four cases of tuberculosis are MDR.

In 2006, a report from South Africa awoke the world to the devastating potential impact of XDR on tuberculosis epidemiology.[15] Over a 14-month period from January 2005, drug susceptibility testing was performed on 475 *M. tuberculosis* isolates obtained from a single, government-sponsored tuberculosis treatment programme in rural KwaZulu Natal. The prevalence of MDR and XDR tuberculosis among culture-confirmed cases, was 39% and 6%, respectively. All of the patients with XDR were infected with HIV, more than half had never been treated for tuberculosis before and nearly 70% of them had been recently admitted to the local hospital. Furthermore, the genotypes of 85% of the XDR strains were identical. These findings strongly suggested recent nosocomial transmission was responsible for many of the XDR cases. The report stated that 52 of the 53 patients with XDR tuberculosis died after a median 16 days from diagnosis. The report shook the tuberculosis community, exposing a systematic failure of public health with far-reaching implications for tuberculosis control programmes worldwide. It underscored the importance of preventing MDR/XDR generation through the appropriate use of the first- and second-line drugs, its timely detection and treatment and the prevention of transmission in the very places patients with tuberculosis depend upon for diagnosis and treatment. The strong link between XDR and HIV infection and the extraordinarily high and rapid case-fatality provoked metaphors of the 'perfect storm' and sent an unambiguous message that more needed to be done to control the two infections. In 2008, 5.4% of MDR cases were XDR and eight countries reported XDR in more than 10% of their MDR isolates. Six of these countries were in central Asia or Eastern Europe.

Finally and inevitably, totally drug-resistant (TDR) tuberculosis was first reported in 2009 among 15 patients in Iran[16] and has subsequently been reported in India.[17] In these cases, *M. tuberculosis* was resistant to all first- and second-line drugs in clinical use in these countries and was, therefore, untreatable.

OTHER IMPORTANT INFLUENCES ON GLOBAL EPIDEMIOLOGY

The dynamics of tuberculosis epidemiology are complex and as control programmes worldwide have struggled to contain the epidemic, so new influences on tuberculosis transmission have been sought.[18] The influence of bacterial and host genetic variation on the disease and its transmission remains poorly defined. Various clinical and epidemiological studies have reported *M. tuberculosis* strains from the East Asian/Beijing lineage are associated with increased drug resistance and more severe disease, with enhanced transmission and spread compared with other strains. Human genetic variability may also influence tuberculosis epidemiology, with susceptibility to *M. tuberculosis* altered by polymorphisms in genes responsible for the innate (e.g. macrophage protein SLC11A1, nitric oxide synthase pathways) and adaptive immune response (e.g. interleukin-12 and interferon-γ axis). The effect sizes of these polymorphisms are modest (odds ratios <3) but they may be important determinants of disease if the gene is common and the population large with a high burden of tuberculosis. There are also likely to be interactions between host and bacterial genetic polymorphisms which will determine the outcome of infection with *M. tuberculosis*, but large studies are required to delineate these and few have been performed.

Epidemics of non-infectious diseases, such as diabetes mellitus, are having an increasing influence on tuberculosis epidemiology. Diabetes mellitus triples the risk of contracting tuberculosis; its rapid rise in India, for example, could have a potentially catastrophic effect. Paradoxically, the rise in diabetes mellitus is linked to increasing affluence and the economic drivers of urbanization. It is unclear, at present, how the mass movement from rural to city dwelling will influence tuberculosis epidemiology in countries like India and China. Greater wealth and easier access to medical services may aid tuberculosis control, but the benefit could be overcome by the rising prevalence of diabetes mellitus and the increased age of the population. Adults over 45 years of age have the highest incidence of lung tuberculosis. In China, for example, the average age of new cases of tuberculosis has risen in those older than 55 years, but fallen in those under 25 years. This is an important finding which may be explained by urban migration of the young, increasing HIV infection in that group, or possibly the spread of new and more virulent strains of *M. tuberculosis*.

Pathology and Pathogenesis

The seventeenth century post-mortem observations of Franciscus Sylvius, Professor of anatomical medicine at Leiden in the Netherlands, were the first to describe the profusion of nodules within the organs of patients with *phthisis* (Greek for 'wasting') and refer to them as 'tubercles'. Then, in 1821, the French physician Laennec recognized that all the diverse clinical forms of 'tubercle' were a single disorder,[19] although his thesis only gained complete acceptance with the discovery of the causative agent of 'tuberculosis' by Robert Koch in 1882.[20]

TABLE 40.2 Granulomatous Disorders Which Can Mimic Tuberculosis

Infectious Causes	Non-Infectious Causes
Leprosy	Sarcoid
Bartonellosis	Crohn's disease
Brucellosis	Wegener's granulomatosis
Actinomycosis	Churg–Strauss syndrome
Syphilis	Rheumatoid arthritis
Yersinia enterocolitis	Granuloma annulare
Histoplasmosis	Foreign bodies (e.g. beryllium, lipids, urate, silicon, tattoo dye, talc, drugs)
Coccidiomycosis	
Blastomycosis	
Cryptococcosis	
Schistosomiasis	
Leishmaniasis	

'Tubercles' are formed by granulomas, which are aggregates of immune cells, predominantly macrophages. Granulomas develop in tissues as an immune response to a variety of infectious and non-infectious stimuli (Table 40.2). Thus, although granulomatous inflammation is the hallmark of tuberculosis, the diagnosis can only be confirmed with accompanying isolation of the pathogen (Diagnosis of Tuberculosis, below).

TUBERCULOSIS PATHOLOGY: THE GRANULOMA

For much of the last 100 years, the granuloma has been seen as benefiting the host, walling off the bacteria from surrounding tissues and so limiting its ability to spread and cause disease.[21] The classical microscopic appearance is of macrophages and occasional neutrophils surrounding a central necrotic core; circumscribing the macrophages is a cuff of lymphocytes (both T- and B-cells) which are contained within a rim of fibroblasts (Figure 40.4). The bacteria are found within the macrophages or the central necrotic debris, an environment considered to be hypoxic. The lesions vary in size from 1 mm to >2 cm, the largest being clearly visible macroscopically and often radiographically as nodules. Considerable variety in tuberculosis granuloma architecture has been described, although the significance to disease pathogenesis remains uncertain.[22] Some granulomas have no necrotic centre, are formed predominantly of macrophages with a few peripheral lymphocytes and are usually associated with active disease (rather than latent infection). In these lesions, the bacteria are contained within the macrophages. Alternatively, fibroblasts can predominate, with few macrophages and little necrosis; these fibrotic granulomas are more commonly associated with latent infection and few bacteria. It is increasingly recognized that tuberculous granulomas are extremely heterogeneous, with their size, structure and cellular consistency changing independently over time, especially during anti-tuberculosis chemotherapy.

Studying the formation and dynamics of tuberculous granulomas in humans is extremely difficult. Therefore, various animal models have been used to better understand the interactions between *M. tuberculosis* and the host's immune cells

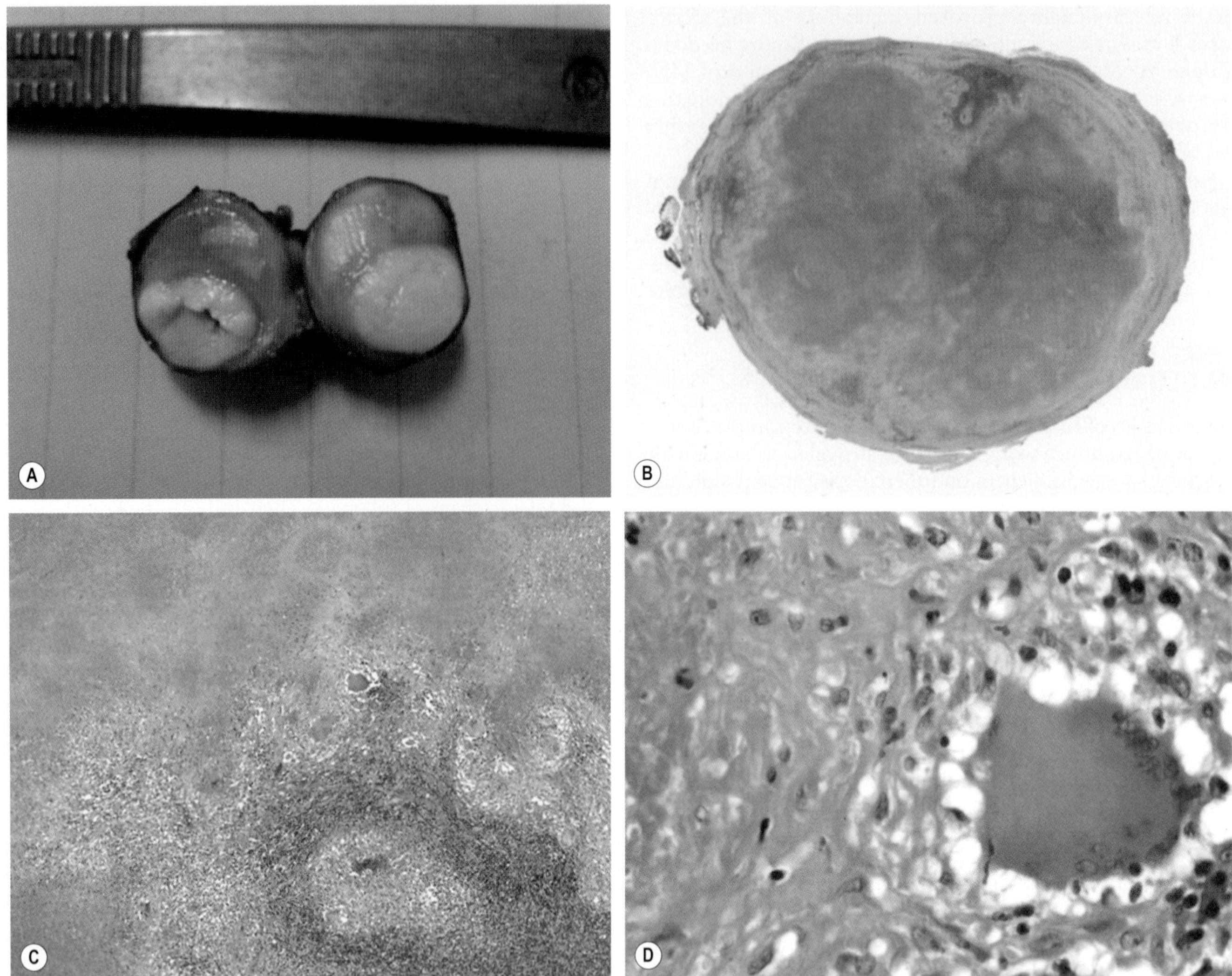

Figure 40.4 Granulomatous lymphadenopathy caused by *M. tuberculosis*. (A) Excision of enlarged cervical lymph node with cross-section showing well-defined caseous material within the node. (B) Whole mount of cross-section of node stained by H&E showing replacement of most the central part of the node by caseous necrosis. (C) Magnification x40 of H&E-stained section of node demonstrating caseous necrosis with a surrounding cuff of granulomatous inflammation composed of epithelioid macrophages, lymphocytes and Langhans' multinucleated giant cells. (D) Magnification x400 (H&E stain) showing a Langhans' multinucleated giant cell with its horseshoe-shaped arrangement of nuclei adjacent to some caseous necrosis. *(By kind permission of Mr Roger Webb, Consultant Maxillofacial Surgeon and Dr Jon Salisbury, Consultant Histopathologist, King's College Hospital, London, United Kingdom.)*

leading to granuloma formation. Important new insights have recently been obtained using zebra fish larvae infected with *M. marinum*, a mycobacterium which shares some key virulence determinants with *M. tuberculosis* (most notably the RD1 virulence locus) and induces granulomatous inflammation in fish.[23,24] Uniquely, the model enables both macrophages and bacteria to be tracked in vivo as granulomas are formed following infection. Contrary to prior assumptions, the model suggests granulomas facilitate early mycobacterial growth and dissemination. Uninfected macrophages are actively recruited to granulomas where they are productively infected and then disseminate to infect surrounding tissues. These findings suggest that in early infection, before the induction of T-cell-mediated immunity, mycobacteria subvert the host's granulomatous response to augment their own replication and dissemination. Whether the same occurs following human infection with *M. tuberculosis* remains to be confirmed.

TUBERCULOSIS PATHOGENESIS: INITIAL HOST AND BACTERIAL INTERACTIONS

The first stage of *M. tuberculosis* infection is the phagocytosis of the inhaled bacilli by the alveolar macrophage. The bacteria reside within the newly formed phagosome and must resist a variety of host defence mechanisms.[25] A superoxide burst generated by an NADPH complex occurs early in phagocytosis, although the impact on *M. tuberculosis* is unclear, as mice with macrophages that lack the burst are not more susceptible to *M. tuberculosis* infection. The acidification of the phagosome following lysosome fusion and acquisition of lysosomal hydrolases is a critical host defence mechanism. Unimpeded, the pH within the newly formed phagolysosome falls rapidly to around 4.8–5.0, inducing potent antimicrobial activity. *M. tuberculosis*, however, blocks phagolysosomal acidification, arresting the pH at around 6.2 and thereby enabling its survival. How the bacteria do this is not clear, but a number of bacterial factors have been implicated, including components of the lipid-rich cell wall of *M. tuberculosis*.

Whether the macrophage succeeds in killing the phagocytosed bacteria is determined by its innate, genetically determined, ability to kill *M. tuberculosis*; the degree to which its antimicrobial activity has been upregulated by other immune cells (e.g. T-lymphocytes) and cytokines (e.g. interferon-γ); and the virulence of the infecting bacteria. Therefore, some infections are terminated early through the actions of macrophages alone. In others, infected macrophages recruit other macrophages and, according to the zebra fish model,[24] a nascent granuloma is formed which becomes the focus for the recruitment, infection and dissemination of the bacteria. In humans, this initial infection is termed the *primary focus* or, in the older literature, the *Ghon focus*.

Various lines of evidence suggest tumour necrosis factor-alpha (TNF-α) is an essential cytokine in the early control of *M. tuberculosis* infection. Patients with autoimmune disorders given monoclonal antibody therapy directed against TNF-α become uniquely susceptible to tuberculosis, with disruption of the granuloma architecture suggesting the cytokine is critical to granuloma integrity and function.[26] Conversely, TNF-α is also cited as a major factor in host-mediated destruction of infected tissue. Small concentrations of TNF-α given to animals previously exposed to *M. tuberculosis* result in substantial tissue necrosis. The yin and yang of TNF-α in tuberculosis pathology is poorly understood, although recent work using the zebra fish model has illuminated some of the mystery.[27] A polymorphism in a gene encoding the leukotriene A4 hydrolase enzyme has been found to influence tuberculosis susceptibility in both zebra fish and humans by causing either excessive or inadequate TNF-α. Zebra fish at both poles of the inflammatory response (minor and major allele homozygotes) were unable to control mycobacterial replication within granulomas, whereas those fish with intermediate TNF-α response (the heterozygotes) controlled the infection. The phenotype of the homozygous fish could be changed to that of the heterozygotes through the respective addition or inhibition of TNF-α. Furthermore, adjunctive corticosteroids (see Management and Treatment of Tuberculosis, below) were only found to benefit major allele homozygous adult humans (hyperinflammatory) with tuberculous meningitis, suggesting, for the first time, a pharmacogenomic approach to anti-tuberculosis treatment.

TUBERCULOSIS PATHOGENESIS: PRIMARY PROGRESSIVE DISEASE

As the primary pulmonary infection progresses some bacilli are transported to the regional lymph nodes (the mediastinal, paratracheal and, occasionally, the supraclavicular nodes), where secondary lesions may develop. The combination of the primary focus and regional lymphadenopathy is termed the *primary* or *Ghon complex*, which may be detectable by plain chest radiography. Symptoms are uncommon at this stage. In around 5% of those infected, primarily children under 5 years and immune-suppressed adults (e.g. with HIV infection), primary tuberculosis progresses rapidly to symptomatic clinical disease (so-called 'primary progressive tuberculosis'). The primary pulmonary infection expands to involve large areas of the lung and can progress to widespread tuberculous pneumonia with tissue destruction and high mortality. Alternatively, primary foci at the lung periphery can rupture into the pleural cavity, causing tuberculous empyema. The bacteria disseminate freely; diseased mediastinal lymph nodes may rupture into the pericardial cavity, causing tuberculous pericarditis, or into a bronchus, causing a spreading endobronchial infection. Enlarged mediastinal lymph nodes may, particularly in young children, press on the major bronchi, causing partial or total obstruction and pulmonary collapse (Figure 40.5). Haematogenous dissemination commonly accompanies primary progressive tuberculosis, with involvement of the bones (especially the spine), kidneys and the brain.

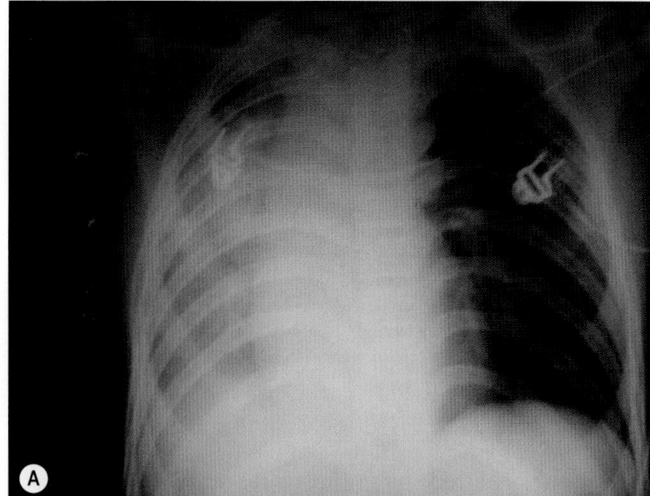

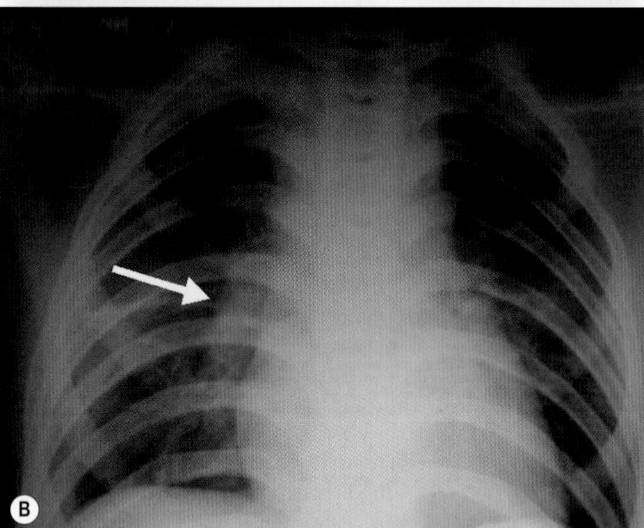

Figure 40.5 Chest radiography of primary tuberculosis causing right hilar lymph node enlargement (white arrow, B) and right middle lobe pulmonary collapse (A).

TUBERCULOSIS PATHOGENESIS: LATENT INFECTION AND POST-PRIMARY DISEASE

In the majority (95%), the primary infection is controlled with the induction of specific T-cell-mediated immunity. CD4 T-cells specific for mycobacterial peptides appear approximately 2 weeks after the initial infection and enhance *M. tuberculosis* macrophage killing by secreting interferon-γ. T-cell-activated macrophages also produce cytokines interleukin 1-beta and TNF-α that promote granuloma formation and enhance bacterial killing. Over time the tuberculous granuloma evolves, becoming more fibrotic; it may even subsequently calcify; but bacilli are able to persist within these dormant lesions and also possibly in surrounding normal tissue, for years or decades without causing symptoms. The nature of these 'persisters' has generated much speculation as they are the key to understanding 'latent' and subsequent 'post-primary' tuberculosis.[28] Some researchers postulate that they are truly dormant until reactivated by a 'wake-up call', while others suggest that they replicate continuously, albeit slowly, but are destroyed by immune mechanisms at roughly the same rate. Current opinion favours the later hypothesis, with bacteria cycling into more active phases dependent on the heterogenous, granuloma-dependent restraint exerted on the bacteria by the host immune response.[22]

In individuals with so-called 'latent tuberculosis', there is a 5–10% lifetime risk the bacteria will reactivate to cause 'post-primary' tuberculosis. The distinction between primary and post-primary tuberculosis has traditionally depended upon whether disease occurred before or after 5 years from the initial infection. This rather arbitrary definition is only useful if all post-primary disease is considered to be consequent to endogenous reactivation of latent bacilli. Studies using bacterial genotyping have shown that in high tuberculosis prevalence regions a high proportion of adults with presumed post-primary pulmonary disease actually have recent reinfection with a different strain of *M. tuberculosis*. This is especially true of those with HIV infection.

Despite the hazards of distinguishing primary from post-primary tuberculosis clinically, there are important pathological differences between the two disease entities. For reasons that remain obscure, post-primary pulmonary tuberculosis most frequently involves the lung apices.[29] The infection is also more commonly associated with extensive tissue damage and lung cavitation.

For many years it was hypothesized that cavitation was the result of a robust T-cell-mediated immunity: a delayed-type hypersensitivity reaction to exposed tuberculoproteins causing caseous necrosis that coalesces to form cavities.[30] More recently, it has been argued that the fibrillar collagens that provide the lung's tensile strength are highly resistant to enzymatic degradation and can only be cleaved by collagenases (matrix metalloproteinases) induced by *M. tuberculosis* infection.[31] Despite the mechanistic uncertainty, extensive pulmonary cavitation can result in arterial invasion and massive haemoptysis, pneumothorax with broncho-pleural fistulae and contiguous spread to the mediastinum (the pericardium, for example), pleura and vertebral column.

TUBERCULOSIS PATHOGENESIS: EXTRA-PULMONARY DISEASE

Tuberculosis most commonly affects the human lung, but some of the most devastating clinical consequences of the disease result from the ability of *M. tuberculosis* to spread from the lung to other organs. The trafficking of bacteria from the initial site of infection – the pulmonary alveolus – to regional lymph nodes and elsewhere has two conflicting consequences. First, it facilitates the presentation of *M. tuberculosis* antigens within the regional lymph nodes, essential for the development of a protective T-cell-mediated immune response. Second, it results in the dissemination of bacteria from the lung to other organs and result in extra-pulmonary tuberculosis (see below).[32]

M. tuberculosis infects other organs via the bloodstream. Nearly 100 years ago, the blood of patients with miliary tuberculosis (disseminated tuberculosis of multiple organs) was found to contain viable bacteria. In the 1930s, Rich and McCordock showed that the development of tuberculous meningitis was dependent upon an initial bacteraemia to seed the brain.[33] Meningitis ensued when the resulting cerebral granuloma (or 'Rich foci') released bacteria into the subarachnoid space. Studies in mice have indicated that haematogenous dissemination occurs early in the infection, before the infection has been controlled by the adaptive immune response. In humans, this explains why those with impaired T-cell responses (e.g. HIV-infected) are particularly susceptible to disseminated disease and why those whose T-cell response has been primed with BCG vaccination are protected against disseminated tuberculosis.

HIV AND THE PATHOLOGY OF TUBERCULOSIS

Advanced HIV infection induces extreme susceptibility to tuberculosis, which indicates HIV impairs critical components of the normal effective immune response to *M. tuberculosis* infection. The consequences of HIV infection on the pathology of tuberculosis vary, dependent upon the degree of immune suppression. Patients with CD4+ counts >200 cells/μL have relatively preserved cellular immune responses and develop granulomas similar to those found in HIV-infected individuals. With progressive immune suppression and the decline of CD4+ T cells, cell-mediated immune responses are attenuated and granulomatous inflammation is disordered. Intracellular killing of mycobacteria by macrophages is compromised and the numbers of bacteria increase. The caseous centres may enlarge centrifugally and coalesce. Finally, in the late stages of AIDS, when peripheral CD4+ counts are <50 cells/μL, there can be almost entire abrogation of the granulomatous response. Disseminated anergic tuberculosis develops, which is often only detected at autopsy. Indeed, in one autopsy study performed in Kenya before the advent of antiretroviral therapy, occult disseminated tuberculosis was present in more than half of HIV-infected adults at death. Granulomas did not form; caseous necrosis was replaced by suppuration, coagulative necrosis and large amounts of apoptotic debris. Large numbers of mycobacteria were present within macrophages and in the necrotic areas.

Given the microscopic findings associated with HIV-associated tuberculosis, it is hypothesized that HIV infection increases susceptibility to *M. tuberculosis* infection by impairing an effective granulomatous immune response.[34] The mechanisms are ill-defined. HIV infection reduces the numbers of CD4+ lymphocytes associated with the granuloma and CD8+ cells may be distributed throughout the granuloma, rather than be restricted to the periphery. In addition to reducing the absolute numbers of CD4+ T-cells, which, as discussed above, are critical to controlling *M. tuberculosis* infection, HIV also appears to reduce the activity of the remaining CD4+ cells to produce less interferon-γ, TNF-α and IL-12. These cytokines activate the full macrophage effector functions against *M. tuberculosis*. HIV may also directly infect and affect macrophage function. Macrophages taken from HIV-infected people are more susceptible to *M. tuberculosis* infection and less likely to undergo apoptosis. Apoptosis may be advantageous to the host, as bacteria within apoptotic bodies are consumed by other macrophages, limiting the opportunity for bacteria to disseminate. HIV may also disrupt the acidification of the phagolysosome and so assist *M. tuberculosis* survive within the macrophage.

Clinical Tuberculosis

The clinical manifestations of tuberculosis are legion, as almost any organ can be affected, but they are primarily dependent upon the age and immune status of the sufferer. In the very young (<3 years) and in those with depressed cell-mediated immunity of any cause (e.g. HIV infection), haematogenous dissemination with multiple organ involvement is common. In immune-competent individuals older than 8 years, so-called 'adult-type' disease predominates; classically involving the lungs with apical cavitation. In low-prevalence settings, where there is minimal respiratory transmission, a greater proportion of cases have extra-pulmonary disease. These cases most commonly occur in immigrants from high tuberculosis prevalence regions; their disease is assumed to represent reactivation of latent infection acquired in their country of origin. They illustrate the importance to disease pathogenesis of the early and usually asymptomatic, bacillaemia accompanying primary infection.

The symptoms and signs of tuberculosis are dependent on the organs affected, but they generally evolve over weeks and sometimes months. They are accompanied with nonspecific abnormalities in laboratory investigations, including an elevated erythrocyte sedimentation rate (ESR), anaemia of chronic disease, hypoalbuminaemia, hyponatraemia and mildly deranged liver function tests. The total peripheral white cell count is usually normal, although a modest leucocytosis can occur with a monocytosis. As with many granulomatous diseases, tuberculosis can cause a modest hypercalcaemia.

TUBERCULOSIS IN CHILDREN

The burden of tuberculosis in children is substantial, but has not, until recently, received the same attention as adult disease.[35] This may be because childhood disease was considered mild, was hard to diagnose and quantify and did not generally contribute to tuberculosis transmission. However, the HIV epidemic, in particular, has prompted a reappraisal. It has long been appreciated that the incidence of childhood disease is directly linked to the numbers of infectious adults and thereby provides an unhappy measure of the effectiveness of tuberculosis control programmes. In sub-Saharan Africa, where the HIV epidemic has led to a large increase in adult tuberculosis, particularly among younger adults and women of a childbearing age, the exposure of very young children to *M. tuberculosis* has substantially increased. A recent study from South Africa reported 10% of children aged 3–4 months had been exposed to *M. tuberculosis*[36] and an autopsy study in Zambia suggested tuberculosis equalled bacterial pneumonia as the major cause of death in HIV-infected and -uninfected children.[37] Consequently, in many settings struggling to cope with the current tuberculosis epidemic, the burden of disease in children is substantial.

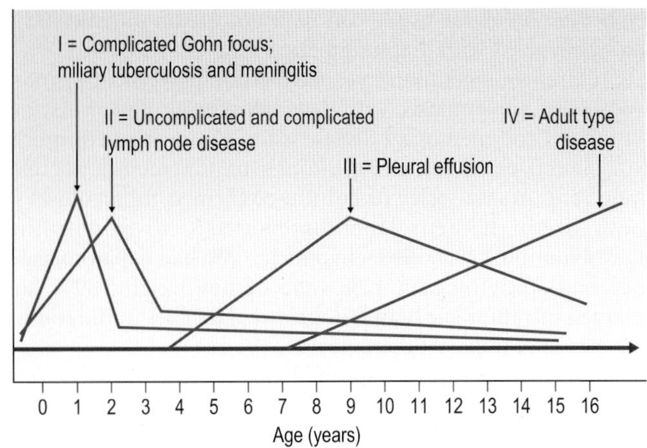

Figure 40.6 Childhood tuberculosis: age profile of different disease manifestations following primary infection.

The clinical presentation of tuberculosis in children is often nonspecific and differs from the patterns seen in adults. There is a clear and well-described pattern of disease according to age (Figure 40.6 and Table 40.3).[38] Intrathoracic lymphadenopathy is the commonest disease manifestation of primary infection acquired before 5 years of age. Descriptions of tuberculosis in the pre-chemotherapeutic era reported 50–60% of children had hilar lymphadenopathy (detected by plain chest radiographs) following primary infection, but only around 40% experienced symptoms. Of these, two-thirds had a cough and one-third had a fever. Primary infection can leave residual radiographic evidence: haematogenous seeding of lung apices can result in fibronodular scarring (Simon's foci) and hilar lymph nodes can calcify; if they do so in combination with a calcified Ghon focus it is called Ranke's complex.

The younger the child, the higher the risk of the disease progressing. The lymph nodes can enlarge to cause major airway obstruction; or they can rupture into an airway and the material may be aspirated to cause a progressive, destructive pneumonia. Intense localized pneumonia may undergo central necrosis with formation of pneumatoceles (thin-walled tension cysts within the pneumonic process). Broncho- or

TABLE 40.3 Patterns of Tuberculosis Following Primary Pulmonary Infection by Age Group

Age at Primary Infection	Consequence of Infection	Proportion (%)
<2 years	No disease	50–70
	Pulmonary disease	10–30
	Miliary/meningitis	2–10
2–10 years	No disease	95–98
	Pulmonary disease	2–5
	Miliary/meningitis	<0.5
>10 years	No disease	80–90
	Pulmonary disease	10–20
	Miliary/meningitis	1

trachea-oesophageal fistula can develop; or the phrenic nerve can be involved with diaphragmatic palsy.

Children younger than 3 years old are at high risk of primary progressive tuberculosis with haematogenous dissemination. Lymphatic and meningeal disease is the commonest complication; pleural, peritoneal and genitourinary tuberculosis are relatively rare. A case-series of culture-confirmed tuberculosis in South African children <3 months reported 57% were coughing at presentation; 82% were tachypnoeic; 66% had hepatomegaly; 53% had splenomegaly; 42% were of low weight; 89% had enlarged intrathoracic lymph nodes on plain chest radiographs; and 26% had miliary tuberculosis.[39]

Adult-style disease occurs in those 8 years and over. The posterior apical segments of the upper lobes, right more than left and the superior segments of the lower lobes are most commonly affected. Cavities form as the disease advances. Tuberculous pleural effusions are rare in children <3 years old (occurring in <10% of cases), but around 25% of young adolescents with tuberculosis develop effusions. In the majority, these are sterile, lymphocyte-rich, straw-coloured effusions and considered immune-mediated rather than directly attributable to infection. Purulent tuberculous empyema is rare in children. Pericardial tuberculosis can result from haematogenous seeding or from rupture of a necrotic sub-carinal lymph node into the pericardial space.

CONGENITAL TUBERCULOSIS

Congenital tuberculosis is very rare, occurring when a mother with active tuberculosis transmits the infection to her child in utero or during delivery.[40] Transplacental infection can occur before delivery; alternatively the baby may aspirate or swallow contaminated amniotic fluid. Recognizing infection in the newborn is difficult as symptoms and signs may be minimal or even absent. Symptoms, if they occur, usually develop 2–3 weeks after birth. The commonest clinical signs are hepatosplenomegaly (75%), respiratory distress (75%), fever (50%), lymphadenopathy (40%), abdominal distension (25%) and papular skin lesions (15%). Transplacental infection typically causes primary hepatic tuberculosis and the infant presents with hepatomegaly, jaundice, fever and failure to gain weight. Respiratory infection leads to extensive lung involvement, often with respiratory distress and diffuse nodular opacities on chest X-ray. Diagnostic criteria have been proposed to help distinguish true congenital infection from infection occurring after birth.[41] Tuberculous lesions appear in the neonate in the first week of life; a primary hepatic complex is typical of transplacental infection. Macro- and microscopic evidence of endometrial or placental tuberculosis should be present; and respiratory transmission after birth should be excluded.

Neonatal tuberculosis is characterized by numerous bacilli in the lungs and/or liver with relatively little cellular reaction. Mortality is as high as 50% and anti-tuberculosis therapy should be commenced on suspicion of the disease, probably with adjunctive corticosteroids.

PULMONARY TUBERCULOSIS IN ADULTS

Pulmonary tuberculosis accounts for approximately 80% of all forms of tuberculosis in adults. The disease is usually slowly progressive, causing weeks, if not months, of gradually worsening symptoms. Rapidly progressive disease does occur, particularly in some racial groups believed to be more susceptible to the disease[42] and in immune-suppressed individuals. Patients usually present with symptoms of cough (70–90%), fever (15–50%) and weight loss (50–75%); blood is reported in the sputum (haemoptysis) of around one–third. Massive haemoptysis is an uncommon but potentially fatal complication of advanced disease, occurring when large vessels in cavity walls become aneurysmal (Rasmussen's aneurysms) and rupture. Before the advent of chemotherapy around 5% of patients with pulmonary tuberculosis died from pulmonary haemorrhage.

The physical examination of those with pulmonary tuberculosis is often unremarkable: the wasted, *phthisical* characteristics noted by the Greeks may not be present in early disease. Respiratory system examination is frequently normal (it is harder to elicit physical signs from the affected lung apices than the middle and lower lobes) and extra-pulmonary signs may be few. Digital clubbing only occurs in longstanding disease and regional lymphadenopathy and enlargement of liver and spleen are rare. Fever is present in around 70%; it is most likely to be absent in the elderly.[43]

Despite the limited physical signs, plain chest radiography reveals the characteristics and extent of the disease (Figure 40.7). The classical appearances are reticulonodular shadowing, with or without cavities, in the apical and posterior segments of the right upper lobe, apicoposterior segments of the left upper lobe, or superior segments of either lobes. The cavities usually have irregular walls; air–fluid levels are uncommon. There may be associated volume loss, particularly in advanced disease. These classical findings, however, are absent in around a third.

Alternatively, patients may have lower zone involvement (~5%), miliary tuberculosis (~5%) or enlarged intrathoracic lymph nodes and/or isolated nodules. Endobronchial tuberculosis is an important but unusual subset of pulmonary tuberculosis, which also results in 'atypical' chest X-ray findings. It is caused by peribronchial lymphadenitis with invasion and destruction of the bronchus, which can lead to stenosis and fistula formation. Bronchial constriction can produce wheeze and a barking cough. It is an important cause of lower lung zone pulmonary tuberculosis.

EXTRA-PULMONARY TUBERCULOSIS IN ADULTS

The proportion of patients with extra-pulmonary tuberculosis has risen over the last 40 years in the USA and other wealthy countries for reasons that are poorly defined. HIV infection is an important component of this change, as it increases the risk of haematogenous dissemination of *M. tuberculosis*. In affluent countries, the burden of disease now falls among racial and ethnic minorities and recent immigrants.

Haematogenous dissemination of *M. tuberculosis* can result in infection of any organ (see Figure 40.8). Commonly affected are the brain, the kidneys, the bones and the cervical lymph nodes that drain the pulmonary vessels. In the USA in 2010, there were 11 182 cases of tuberculosis reported to the Centers for Disease Control and Prevention (CDC), Atlanta: 78% were pulmonary 22% were extra-pulmonary.[44] The commonest extra-pulmonary cases reported were pleural (16%), lymph node (40%), bone or joint (10%), genito-urinary tract (5%), meningeal (6%) and peritoneal (6%).

The clinical manifestations of extra-pulmonary tuberculosis are as diverse as the organs it can affect. However, nonspecific

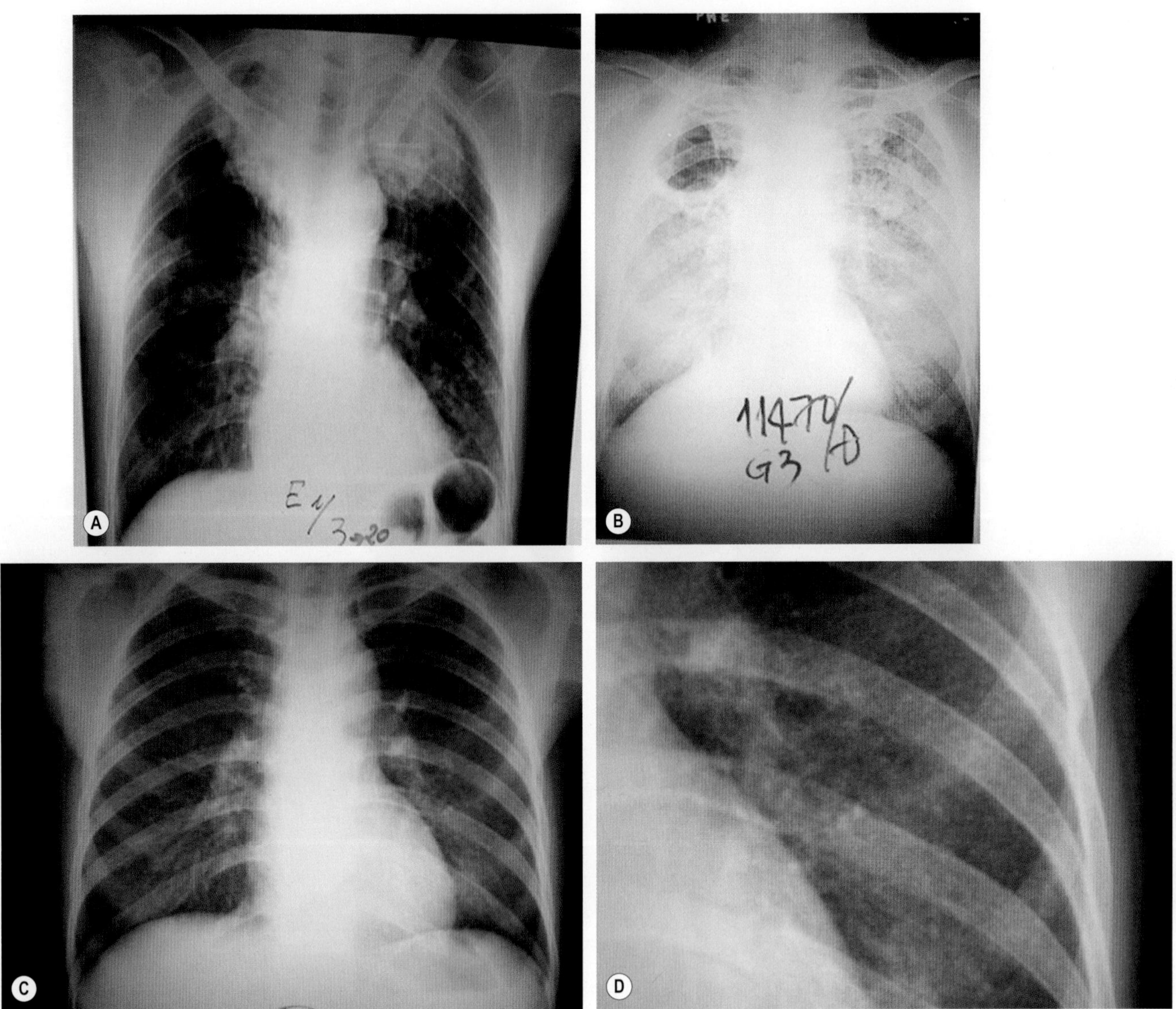

Figure 40.7 Chest radiographic appearance of pulmonary tuberculosis. (A) Bilateral apical fibro-nodular changes (left more extensive than right). (B) Dissemination nodular changes throughout both lung fields (miliary pattern) with a large right apical cavity. (C) Faint, diffuse, nodular pattern throughout both lung fields (miliary tuberculosis). (D) Enlarged view of left lung field of (C), demonstrating the diffuse nodules which are easily missed without close inspection.

clinical presentations, difficulty in obtaining adequate diagnostic samples and the paucity of bacilli causing disease, all serve to make the extra-pulmonary tuberculosis a major clinical challenge.

MILIARY (HAEMATOGENOUSLY DISSEMINATED) TUBERCULOSIS

Miliary tuberculosis is a descriptive radiological diagnosis which has historically depended upon a plain chest radiograph showing numerous 1–2 mm well-defined nodules scattered throughout both lung fields (see Figure 40.7). To those who first described these appearances 100 years ago, the nodules looked like millet seeds. Each 'seed' represents a granuloma and marks the point where a single bacterium, carried within the bloodstream, has settled to infect the lung. Miliary tuberculosis is, therefore, the consequence of a heavy and sustained bacteraemia. Extra-pulmonary involvement is almost invariable, with the liver, spleen, bone marrow and brain most commonly involved. On occasions, 'miliary' tuberculosis occurs without the classical chest X-ray appearances; so-called 'cryptic' disseminated tuberculosis. Newer imaging modalities, such as computerized tomography (CT), have helped enormously in these circumstances as they can reveal profusions of nodules too small to be detected by plain X-ray or unsuspected in other internal organs (Figure 40.9). Indeed, new imaging techniques have challenged the old chest X-ray-dependent definition of 'miliary' tuberculosis and the disease may be better described as 'haematogenously disseminated' tuberculosis, whether or not the lung is involved.

Constitutional symptoms such as fever, malaise and weight loss, predominate in the clinical presentation of miliary tuberculosis. A dry cough occurs in around two-thirds and fever is documented in 80–90%.[45] Rarely, the pulmonary disease is so

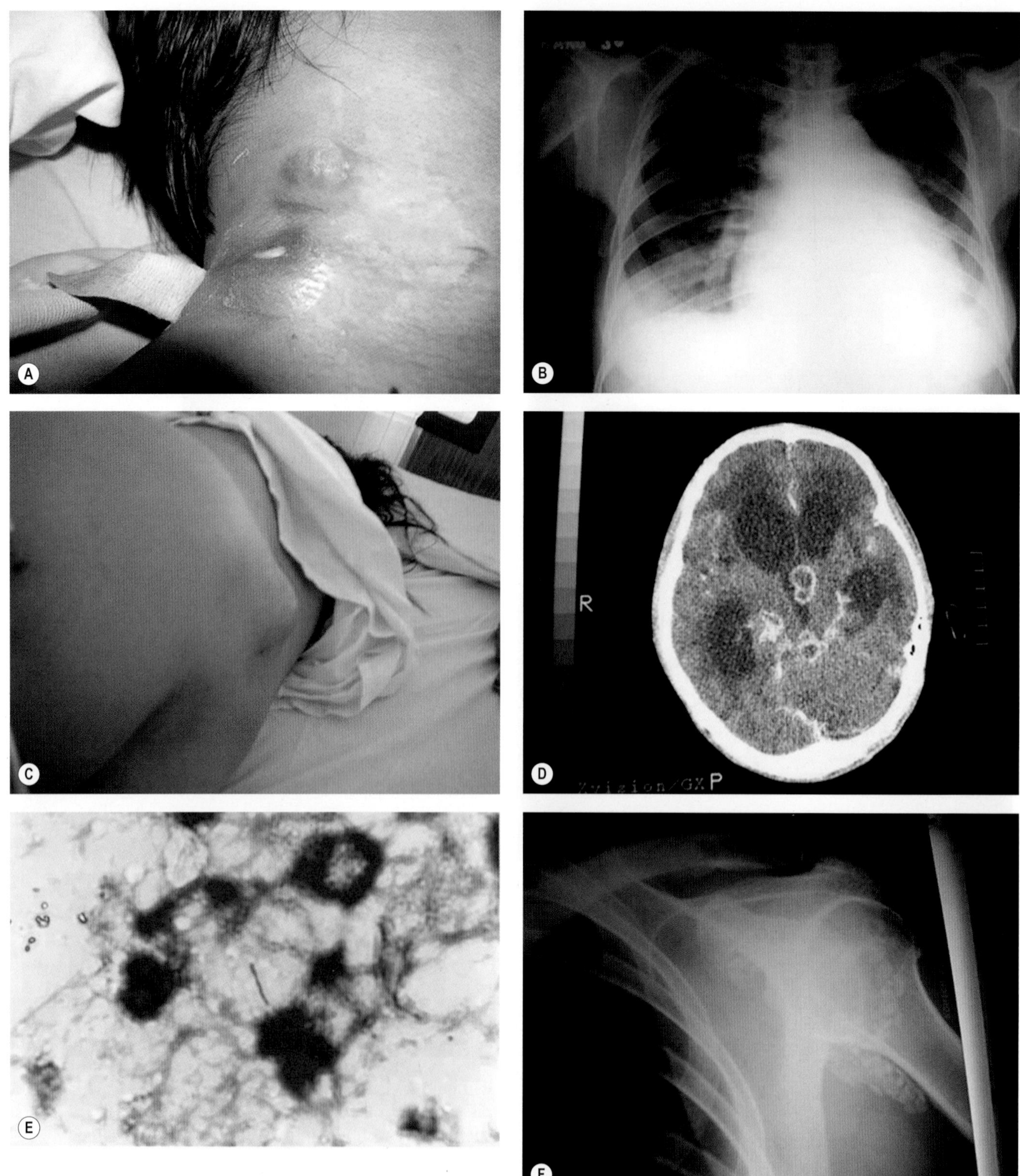

Figure 40.8 Extra-pulmonary tuberculosis. (A) Enlarged posterior cervical chain tuberculous lymphadenopathy with fistula formation and scrofuloderma. (B) Chest radiograph showing globular enlargement of the cardiac shadow secondary to effusive tuberculous pericarditis. (C) Lumbar spine gibbus secondary to Pott's disease (tuberculous vertebral osteomyelitis). (D) Contrast-enhanced brain computerized tomography of an adult with tuberculous meningitis demonstrating enlarged ventricles and multiple ring-enhancing tuberculomas. (E) Single acid-fast bacillus seen in the cerebrospinal fluid from a patient with tuberculous meningitis. (F) Plain radiograph of left shoulder demonstrating multiple calcified lymph nodes from previous *M. tuberculosis* infection.

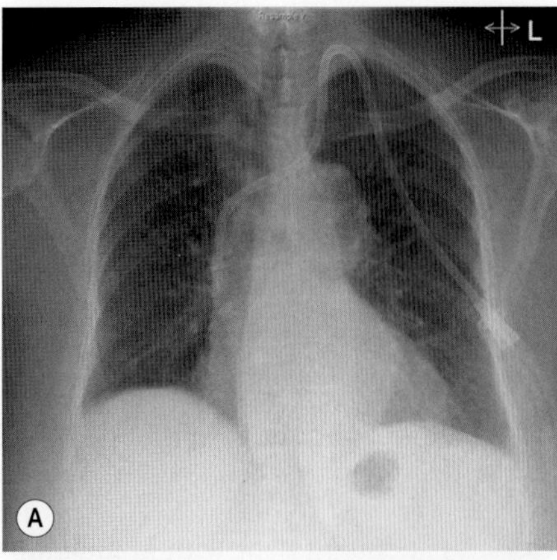

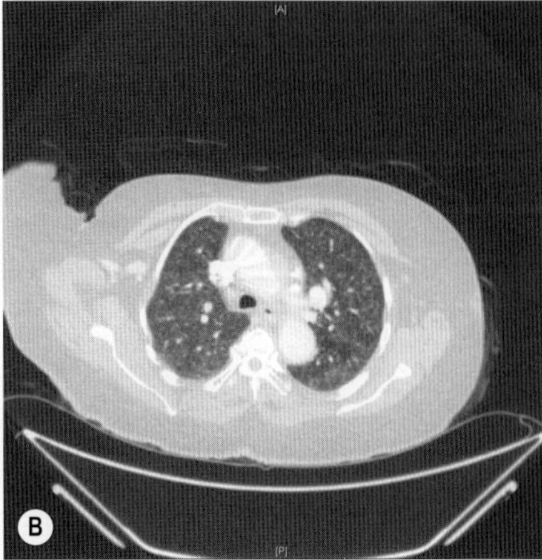

Figure 40.9 Enhanced sensitivity of computerized tomography over plain chest radiography for the diagnosis of pulmonary tuberculosis. (A) Chest radiograph: reported as normal. (B) CT chest with contrast demonstrating diffuse micro-nodular changes consistent with miliary tuberculosis.

extensive it causes acute respiratory distress which can be exacerbated by starting anti-tuberculosis chemotherapy. Extra-pulmonary involvement should be carefully sought, particularly meningitis, which manifests as headache and vomiting followed by confusion and coma (see below). Involvement of liver and spleen with their enlargement occurs in 30–50% and 20%, respectively. Generalized lymphadenopathy is rare, except in the context of HIV infection. Haematogenous seeding of the choroid can result in visible nodules in 5–20% of cases by ophthalmoscopy (chorioid tubercles), which represents one of the few clinical findings with high specificity for disseminated tuberculosis. Papular and macular skin rashes occur rarely, indicating cutaneous dissemination.

Laboratory investigations provide nonspecific confirmation of a chronic multi-system inflammatory disorder. Fifty percent of patients with miliary tuberculosis are anaemic. Leucopenia and leucocytosis occur with equal frequency, although around 80% with miliary tuberculosis are lymphopenic, rising to nearly 100% if the bone marrow has been infiltrated.[46] Rarely, leukaemoid reactions are reported. Abnormal liver function tests, usually with moderate elevations in transaminases, occur in more than half and indicate hepatic infection.

CENTRAL NERVOUS SYSTEM TUBERCULOSIS

Central nervous system tuberculosis takes two major forms: tuberculous meningitis and tuberculoma.[47] Tuberculous meningitis causes progressive confusion and coma, with death if treatment is not started sufficiently quickly. It should be considered a medical emergency, mandating rapid diagnosis and treatment. Tuberculoma are well-defined, granulomatous, space-occupying lesions, which can occur anywhere in the central nervous system, but most commonly above the cerebral tentorium. Their clinical manifestations depend upon their anatomical location, but an isolated seizure secondary to an intra-cerebral lesion is the commonest presentation. Tuberculomas are not immediately life-threatening unless they rupture and release bacteria into the subarachnoid space to cause tuberculous meningitis.

The clinical features of tuberculous meningitis are variable and nonspecific. The features have been extensively described in a multitude of case reports and clinical series and are similar to many sub-acute and chronic meningoencephalitides.[48] The patient's description of the variety of symptoms is often unhelpful to the diagnosis. One case series reported that on admission to hospital, only 28% complained of headache, 25% were vomiting, 13% reported fever and 2% described the classical meningitic symptoms of photophobia and neck stiffness.[49] However, accurate determination of the duration of symptoms is essential: tuberculous meningitis nearly always presents with more than 5 days of preceding symptoms and this is a useful way of distinguishing it from acute pyogenic bacterial meningitis.

The neurological manifestations of tuberculous meningitis are numerous and varied.[47] Their nature and diversity can be predicted from the site of disease and the pathogenesis. Basal meningeal adhesions can result in cranial nerve palsies (particularly II, III, IV, VI, VII) or constriction of the vessels resulting in stroke. Cerebral infarction occurs in approximately 30% of cases, commonly in the internal capsule and basal ganglia, causing a range of problems from hemiparesis to movement disorders. Obstruction of CSF flow leads to raised intracranial pressure, hydrocephalus and reduced conscious level. Seizures occur in around 30% of children and less than 5% of adults with tuberculous meningitis and may be caused by hydrocephalus, infarction, tuberculoma, oedema and hyponatraemia due to inappropriate anti-diuretic hormone secretion. The diagnosis of spinal tuberculous meningitis should be considered in those presenting with root pain, with either spastic or flaccid paralysis with loss of sphincter control. Approximately 10% of those with tuberculous meningitis will have concomitant spinal cord involvement, which is frequently overlooked.

PLEURAL TUBERCULOSIS

Tuberculosis is the commonest cause of pleural effusions in young adults in tuberculosis-endemic regions and pleural tuberculosis constitutes around 20% of all extra-pulmonary tuberculosis.[50] There are three pathological subtypes of tuberculous pleural effusion. The first most commonly accompanies primary infection in children and represents an immune-mediated hypersensitivity reaction. The fluid is straw-coloured and sterile. Similar effusions can accompany miliary tuberculosis and are frequently bilateral and present alongside pericardial and peritoneal effusions. The second subtype represents reactivation of a lesion seeded to the pleura during the primary bacteraemia. These effusions are usually unilateral, rarely larger than 1 litre and present relatively acutely with pleuritic chest pain, breathlessness and fever; 70% present with less than 4 weeks of symptoms and around 30% with an illness of less than 1 week.[51] A pleural rub is heard in around 20% of cases. Tuberculous empyemas represent the third subtype of pleural tuberculosis. These are caused by the sudden rupture of an infected lymph node releasing caseous tuberculous material into the pleural space. Symptoms are marked, with acute pleuritic chest pain and high swinging fever. The infection can erode the chest wall with development of a fluctuant chest wall mass and, ultimately, a sinus to the skin draining tuberculous pus.

GENITOURINARY TUBERCULOSIS

Haematogenous dissemination of *M. tuberculosis* is responsible for tuberculosis of the kidney, bladder, prostate, epididymis and fallopian tubes. The rest of the urogenital tract can become infected by the passage of bacteria from these infected organs (e.g. kidney infection can result in ureteric tuberculosis and fallopian infection may lead to vaginal tuberculosis). Urogenital tuberculosis more commonly occurs in older adults and there is a male predominance. Before anti-tuberculosis chemotherapy 4–8% of those with lung tuberculosis also had involvement of the renal tract.

Renal tuberculosis typically presents late with advanced disease because the early stages cause few symptoms and evades diagnosis.[52] A sterile pyuria may be the only clinical feature early in infection. As the infection progresses, renal colic can occur secondary to papillary necrosis and parenchymal granulomas can coalesce to cause irregularly enlarged kidneys. Both kidneys are involved in around 30% of cases. Calcification within the parenchyma, or as calculi within the collecting system, is a presenting feature in around one half, reflecting the delays in diagnosis. Late in the disease the calcification can occur in a lobar distribution and result in end-stage renal failure with so-called 'auto-nephrectomy'.

Infection can spread down the renal tract to involve the ureters and bladder. Ureteric tuberculosis causes multiple strictures and eventual calcification can result in a 'pipe-stem' appearance on plain radiography. The bladder can be infected either through the passage of infected urine or by haematogenous seeding. The infection causes urinary frequency, dysuria, haematuria and pyuria and the thickened bladder wall mimics transitional cell carcinoma.

In men, the epididymis, because of its rich blood supply, is the commonest part of the genital tract affected by tuberculosis. The main symptoms are pain and swelling, with a craggy, irregular epididymis found on examination. The disease is usually unilateral. There is a strong association between the presence of epididymal and renal tuberculosis.

In women, the fallopian tubes are involved in around 90% of those with genital tuberculosis. The infection is commonly bilateral and tends to affect the abdominal rather than the uterine ends of the tubes; if left untreated the infection spreads into either the peritoneum or the uterine cavity to cause peritonitis or endometritis respectively. Fallopian tuberculosis manifests clinically as chronic lower abdominal pain, irregular vaginal bleeding and infertility.

MUSCULOSKELETAL TUBERCULOSIS

Approximately 5–10% of all tuberculosis involves bone and/or joints and the incidence increases with age. The spine is the commonest site affected, followed in decreasing order by hip, knee, sacroiliac joint, shoulder, elbow and ankle. Of all bone and joint tuberculosis, 75% involves the spine, hip or knee. In young children and the immune-suppressed any bone or joint can be affected, including the small bones of the hands and feet.[53]

Percival Pott (1714–1788) was the first to describe spinal tuberculosis, or Pott's disease as it became known and the benefit of surgery in treating the resulting paraplegia. In one-half of cases, the disease affects the lower thoracic and upper lumbar spine; the cervical spine is affected in around one-quarter of cases.[54] Patients present with gradual onset of back pain as the infection typically erodes the anterior vertebral end-plate of two adjacent vertebrae. The result is a wedge collapse with intervening disc destruction, although the discs are spared early in the disease. The disease can manifest clinically as a kyphosis with a bony step or 'gibbus'. Complications include epidural abscess formation and cord compression. Bilateral fusiform paraspinal abscess can occur as pus dissects tissue planes (Figure 40.10). Cord compression with muscle weakness and loss of bladder and bowel control is the most serious complication and occurs in up to 30% of patients.

Tuberculous arthritis generally occurs as a consequence of metaphyseal infection crossing the epiphyseal plate. Ultimately, both the synovium and the periarticular bone are involved. Transphyseal spread is characteristic of tuberculosis and rarely occurs in pyogenic bacterial infections. A single joint is involved in 90% of cases, typically the hip or knee and presents with slowly progressive pain, swelling and loss of function. Radiographic features include joint effusion, lytic lesions, joint space narrowing and periosteal new bone formation. Rarely, patients with miliary/disseminated tuberculosis, or long-standing untreated pulmonary tuberculosis, suffer from a reactive symmetrical polyarthritis (Poncet's disease), which particularly affects the small joints. The condition is considered to be an immunological phenomenon; bacteria cannot be cultured from the joints.

Tuberculous osteomyelitis is less common than arthritis and, because it occurs as a consequence of bloodstream seeding of bone, is often multi-focal and presents in different stages of progression. It more commonly affects the bones of the extremities, including the small bones of the hands and feet. The clinical features include localized bony pain, swelling and, in more advanced cases, sinus tract formation. On rare occasions, tuberculosis can cause a dactylitis, with cyst-like cavities within the phalanges and accompanying soft tissue swelling.

Tuberculosis of tendons is rare, resulting from either contiguous or haematogenous spread. The tendon and/or synovium become thickened and infiltrated and the tendon may rupture. Secondary involvement of synovial bursas occurs rarely. Muscle tuberculosis is extremely rare and usually only affects severely immune-suppressed patients with contiguous spread from an infected bone or joint.

LYMPH NODE TUBERCULOSIS

Lymph node enlargement is a characteristic feature of tuberculosis. The involvement of peripheral lymph nodes, particularly

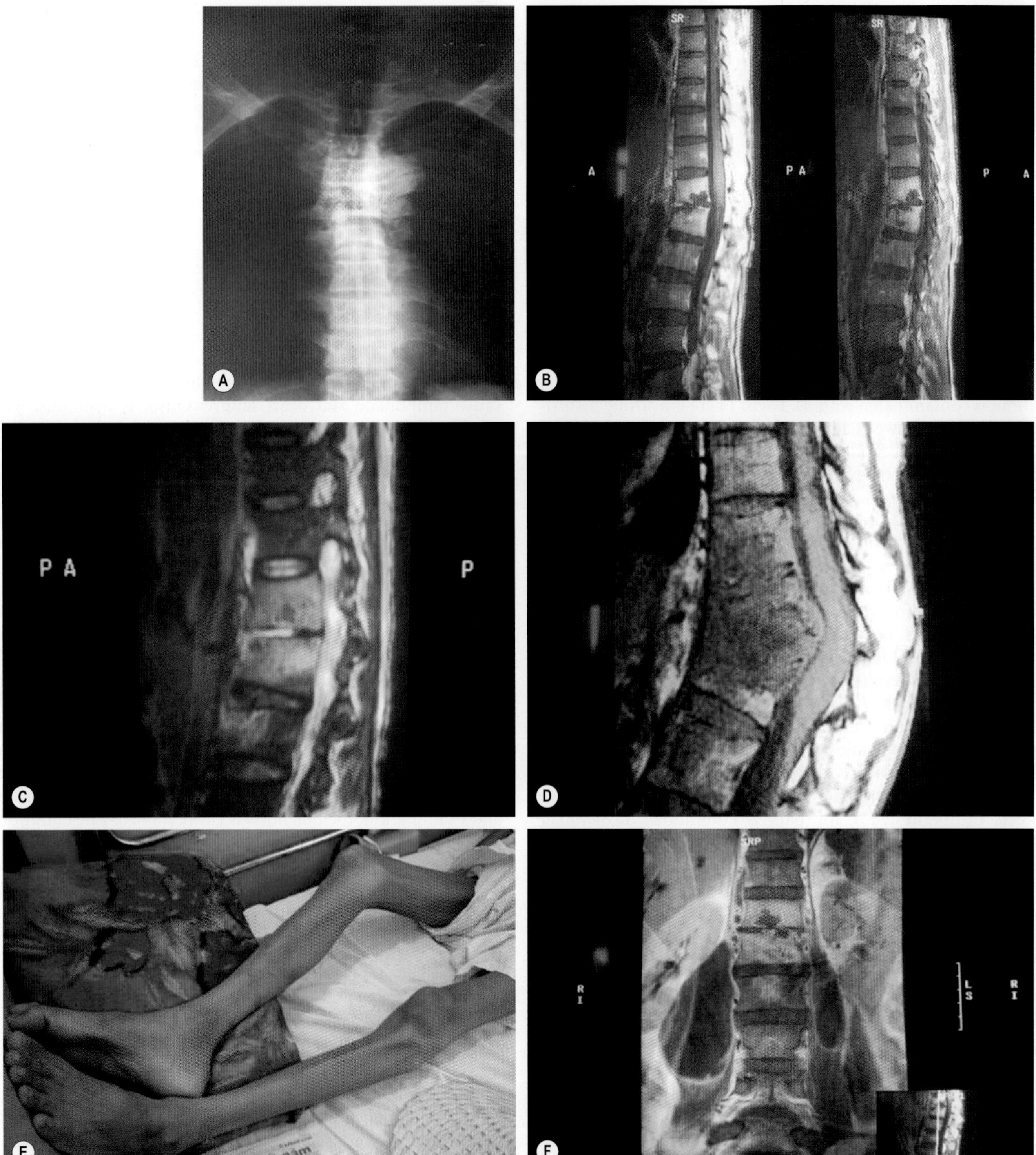

Figure 40.10 Tuberculous vertebral osteomyelitis (Pott's disease). (A) Plain radiograph showing gross destruction and displacement of thoracic vertebrae. (B) T1-weighted MRI scan of the thoracic spine showing lytic lesions in two adjacent thoracic vertebrae with anterior wedge collapse of the lower vertebra. (C) T2-weighted MRI scan of the same lesion shown in (B). (D) T2-weighted MRI scan showing gross destruction of three lumbar vertebrae with impingement on the cord. (E) Bilateral wasting of both legs secondary to extensive spinal tuberculosis (see images in (F). (F) T1-weighted MRI showing destruction of two lumbar vertebrae and large, bilateral, fusiform paraspinous abscesses.

of the cervical chain, is the commonest form of extra-pulmonary tuberculosis, representing 35% of all cases. Enlargement is typically indolent, unilateral and painless; more than one node is usually affected, matted together by inflammation. Without treatment, the nodes can undergo necrosis and liquefaction, forming a cold abscess that may eventually rupture to from a sinus. Unlike other forms of extra-pulmonary tuberculosis, constitutional symptoms are mild or absent.

ABDOMINAL TUBERCULOSIS

Abdominal tuberculosis encompasses disease of any intra-abdominal organ and any part of the gastrointestinal tract from mouth to anus. Solid organs are involved through haematogenous dissemination, whereas the gastrointestinal tract is affected either through the ingestion of infected lung secretions, by contiguous invasion from infected lymph nodes, or through dairy products contaminated with *M. bovis*. There is a strong historical association between advanced pulmonary tuberculosis and gastrointestinal tuberculosis, reflecting the importance of swallowing infectious respiratory secretions to the pathogenesis of this disease.

The clinical manifestations of abdominal tuberculosis are protean, dependent upon the organs involved.[55,56] Ulceration, stricture, perforation and fistula formation are the cardinal pathological features of gastrointestinal tuberculosis, with additional complications dependent upon which segment of the bowel is involved. For example, serious bleeding may complicate gastric and colorectal tuberculosis, whereas malabsorption more commonly results from small bowel infection. Jejunoileal and ileocaecal tuberculosis is the commonest part of the bowel to be affected by tuberculosis, occurring in 50–70% of all forms of abdominal tuberculosis. The commonest symptom is abdominal pain, which is reported by 90% of patients; if the disease is luminal the pain may be colicky; if the infection affects the peritoneum, the pain is continuous. Ileojejunal/caecal tuberculosis typically presents with days or weeks of colicky abdominal pain, borborygmi and vomiting. Examination may reveal a mass in the right lower quadrant. The most common complication is sub-acute intestinal obstruction, although acute-on-chronic abdominal pain may indicate perforation. In India, tuberculosis is the second commonest cause of bowel perforation to typhoid. Tuberculous perforations are usually single and proximal to a stricture. Isolated colonic disease presents with pain, change in bowel habit and bleeding (in 70%). The disease is multifocal in one-third with diffuse ulceration mimicking ulcerative colitis.

The intra-abdominal solid organs are involved in around 20% of patients with abdominal tuberculosis; especially in those at high risk for haematogenously disseminated tuberculosis, i.e. young children and HIV-infected adults. Hepatic, pancreatic and splenic tuberculosis often accompany miliary tuberculosis, as do multiple peritoneal tubercle deposits. Enlarged intra-abdominal lymph nodes typically accompany this form of the disease.

PERICARDIAL TUBERCULOSIS

Tuberculous pericarditis is commonest in the 3rd to 5th decades of life and currently accounts for around 10% of all hospitalized patients with heart failure in Africa. Its incidence is increased with HIV infection, which also lowers the age of sufferers.

Following the haematogenous seeding of the pericardium. there are four pathological stages:

1. Fibrinous exudate develops within the pericardium, containing large numbers of neutrophils, relatively abundant bacteria and loosely formed granulomas.
2. The exudate increases in volume and becomes serosanguineous, with a shift from neutrophils to lymphocytes and monocytes.
3. The exudate/pericardial effusion is absorbed, granulomas mature with caseation and the pericardium thickens with accompanying fibrosis.
4. On-going fibrosis leads to pericardial constriction.

These pathological stages explain the clinical manifestations of the diseases. Three clinical forms are recognized: effusive, effusive-constrictive and constrictive pericarditis.[57] Effusive disease accounts for 80% of all cases and is characterized by the gradual accumulation of pericardial fluid which may eventually cause tamponade and heart failure. Onset is insidious, with nonspecific symptoms including fever and weight loss. Chest pain, cough and breathlessness are common, although they are rarely as marked as in acute viral or pyogenic bacterial pericarditis. The frequency of the various accompanying physical signs have been estimated from case series,[58] and include: cardiac percussion dullness and/or hepatomegaly in 95%; pulsus paradoxus and raised JVP in 85%; a sinus tachycardia in 80%; ascites in 70%; peripheral oedema in 25%; and a friction rub in 20%. Around 5% of patients present with effusive-constrictive pericarditis, with some features of effusive disease together with signs suggestive of pericardial constriction. The diagnosis is made by persistent elevation of right atrial pressures despite drainage of the effusion.

Constrictive pericarditis is found in around 15% of patients at diagnosis and complicates 20% of all patients with tuberculous pericarditis, despite anti-tuberculosis chemotherapy. The clinical features are highly variable and without a careful history and examination, the diagnosis is easily missed. The commonest clinical signs are of an elevated JVP with hepatomegaly, ascites and peripheral oedema.[58] A pericardial knock and sudden inspiratory splitting of the second heart sound are specific, but relatively insensitive physical signs (each found in 20–30% of cases).

CUTANEOUS TUBERCULOSIS

Cutaneous tuberculosis is rare, representing less than 1% of all cases of tuberculosis, but has a bewildering number of forms.[59] These can be divided according to whether they are directly attributable to infection or represent an immunological reaction to tuberculosis elsewhere in the body. Lesions attributable to infection can be classified according to whether they result from haematogenous spread or from contiguous infection and the number of bacteria present within the lesion (see Table 40.4).[60]

The commonest forms of cutaneous tuberculosis are scrofuloderma and lupus vulgaris. Scrofuloderma occurs when the skin overlying a tuberculous lymph node becomes infiltrated with *M. tuberculosis*. The neck, axillae, chest wall and groins are the commonest sites. Lupus vulgaris results from haematogenous seeding of the skin and the face is the commonest site affected. It causes a slowly enlarging plaque with an elevated verrucose border; the centre of the lesion is said to resemble 'apple jelly' and may ulcerate.

TABLE 40.4 The Classification of Cutaneous Tuberculosis

Number of Bacteria Associated with Skin Lesion	Pathogenesis	Disease Type	Clinical Appearance
Multi-bacillary	Direct inoculation	Chancre	Painless papulonodule; can ulcerate
		Orificial tuberculosis	Nodules; painful punched out ulcers
	Contiguous spread	Scrofuloderma	Nodule over affected node; can ulcerate
	Haematogenous	Miliary tuberculosis	Profuse pinpoint papules
		Gumma	Nodule
	Direct inoculation (re-exposure)	Tuberculous Verrucosa cutis	Papule or verrucous plaque with soft centre
Paucibacillary	Haematogenous	Lupus vulgaris	Varied appearances from plaque, to nodular to ulcerative; classical 'apple jelly' appearance
No bacteria	Immune mediated/hypersensitivity reactions (usually active tuberculosis in other organs)	*The tuberculids:*	
		Lichen scrofulosorum	Perifollicular lichenoid papules
		Erythema induratum of Bazin	Indurated/ulcerated nodules of calf
		Phlebitic tuberculid	Non-ulcerating nodules
		Papulonecrotic tuberculid	Small papules; can crust/ulcerate

Less common forms of cutaneous tuberculosis include macules and papules associated with miliary tuberculosis, which typically present on the trunk. Skin and soft tissue gumma can also result from bacteraemia. Direct inoculation of the skin can lead to tuberculous chancres; these tend to occur in laboratory workers or in children living with infectious adults and are most commonly found on the hands, face and feet. Occasionally, in patients with prior *M. tuberculosis* infection, inoculation of bacteria into the skin produced a painless, solitary verrucose plaque, usually on a hand or foot, known as tuberculosis verrucosa cutis.

Breast tuberculosis is not conventionally considered with cutaneous tuberculosis, but is here as it often presents with skin changes.[61] The commonest form is a nodular, well-circumscribed, painless mass that gradually expands and may ulcerate. It may be mis-diagnosed as breast cancer. Occasionally, bloodstream dissemination may lead to multiple lesions with enlarged and matted draining lymph nodes in the axilla.

The diversity of cutaneous tuberculosis caused by immunological reactions, rather than direct infection, is especially challenging to non-dermatologists. Known as the tuberculids, they are a spectrum of related and overlapping clinicopathological entities driven by tuberculin hypersensitivity. Active tuberculosis is usually evident elsewhere in the body and the lesions typically resolve with successful anti-tuberculosis chemotherapy.

The more common tuberculids are papular necrotic and nodular tuberculid, erythema induratum of Bazin, lichen scrofulosorum and nodular granulomatous phlebitis. Papular necrotic tuberculid is characterized by multiple symmetrical papules with umbilicated and sometimes necrotic centres. They usually occur on the extensor areas of extremities in young adults and children with active tuberculosis and are associated with phlyctenular conjunctivitis, another type of hypersensitivity reaction discussed in more detail below (ocular tuberculosis). Erythema induratum (of Bazin) is a tuberculosis-associated panniculitis which results in nodules on the backs of calves. It is different from erythema nodosum, which typically affects the shins and has a broad range of infectious and non-infectious precipitants. Lichen scrofulosorum is an eruption of multiple miniature follicular or parafollicular lichenoid papules, which cluster on the trunk. It is more common in young children, 30% of whom will not have active tuberculosis elsewhere.

OCULAR TUBERCULOSIS

M. tuberculosis may infect the eyes by direct invasion, inoculation or haematogenous spread. The eyes can also be affected by hypersensitivity reactions, most commonly phlyctenular conjunctivitis, which presents with conjunctival inflammation, photophobia, tearing and blepharospasm.

Between 1% and 5% of all cases of tuberculosis may have ocular involvement of some sort; this rises to 10–20% in those with disseminated disease and possibly even to 75% in young children with tuberculous meningitis.[62] Almost any part of the eye can be affected: a uveitis, retinitis, optic neuropathy, endophthalmitis, scleritis, keratitis, conjunctivitis and dacrycystitis are all well-described. However, posterior uveitis is the commonest manifestation, typically with choroid involvement. Choroid tubercles are apparent as greyish-yellow nodules with indistinct margins on ophthalmoscopy and usually occur in groups of less than five. Untreated, they can expand to form tuberculomas and result in retinal detachment and blindness. A review of 92 patients with tuberculous eye disease reported 34% had choroid tubercles with or without inflammatory signs, 27% had a choroiditis/choroidoretinitis, 24% had a vitritis, 13% had a iridocyclitis/anterior uveitis and 11% had a panuveitis.[63]

HIV-ASSOCIATED TUBERCULOSIS

The risk of active tuberculosis increases as peripheral numbers of CD4 T-lymphocytes fall secondary to HIV infection. However, even those with relatively well-preserved CD4 counts are at greater risk of tuberculosis than HIV-uninfected individuals.[13] Clinical presentation also changes with declining CD4 counts: patients with very low counts (<100 cells/μL) are more likely to have nonspecific presenting symptoms and extrapulmonary disease, often involving more than one organ. Approximately 50% of adults with HIV have extra-pulmonary disease and 10% and have disseminated disease (commonly with central nervous system involvement) compared with 15% and 1%, respectively, in HIV-uninfected adults.[64] Granulomatous inflammation in affected tissues becomes less prominent in patients with low CD4 counts (it may even be absent in those with the most advanced HIV) and mirrors a rise in the bacterial tissue burden. These features explain why the presenting features of tuberculosis in HIV-infected individuals may be nonspecific; why classical cavitatory lung disease is relatively rare; and why severe disseminated disease with detectable mycobacteraemia is common. The high incidence of tuberculosis on starting ART emphasizes the need for pre-ART tuberculosis screening and effective identification of those most at risk of developing disease (see below).

The advent of antiretroviral therapy (ART) has led to some important changes in the clinical presentation of HIV-associated tuberculosis. There is a high incidence of active tuberculosis in the first 3 months of starting ART, which has been especially well-documented in tuberculosis-endemic regions of sub-Saharan Africa.[65] It is suggested that ART has a number of effects during this period, which may explain the increased incidence.[66] First, ART may shorten the time for asymptomatic tuberculosis to become symptomatic; a phenomenon which has been termed 'unmasking'. Second, it may increase the rapidity of initial onset of tuberculosis symptoms. And third, it may heighten the intensity of clinical manifestations. In all these circumstances it is proposed that the disease be referred to as 'ART-associated tuberculosis'.[67]

A subset of patients with ART-associated tuberculosis present with immune reconstitution inflammatory syndrome (IRIS). IRIS is believed to be caused by dysregulated recovery of pathogen-specific immune responses during the initial months of ART. This leads to the development of unusual and overtly inflammatory clinical manifestations, most commonly in association with mycobacterial, cryptococcal and cytomegalovirus infections. A recent systematic review and meta-analysis of 1699 cases of IRIS in 13 103 patients starting HAART calculated the crude incidence of IRIS in those with any previously diagnosed AIDS-defining illness was 38% (95% confidence intervals 27–49%).[68] In those previously diagnosed with tuberculosis, the incidence was 16% (10–25%).

Case definitions for tuberculosis-associated IRIS have been proposed:[67] patients must have had a diagnosis of tuberculosis before starting HAART and must have made an initial response to treatment. The reaction must have occurred within 3 months of HAART initiation and be accompanied by at least one major criteria (new/enlarging lymph nodes; new/worsening radiological features and/or central nervous system involvement and/or serositis) or two minor criteria (new/worsening constitutional symptoms and/or respiratory symptoms and/or abdominal pain with either peritonitis, organomegaly or intra-abdominal lymphadenopathy). An alternative explanation, such as drug resistance, opportunistic infection or poor adherence must be excluded.

Patients who start HAART with CD4 counts <50 cells/μL are at the greatest risk of developing IRIS.[68] Tuberculosis IRIS occurs in 10–40% of patients with HIV/tuberculosis co-infection; the median interval from initiation of HAART to the onset of tuberculosis IRIS is 2–4 weeks.[69] The risk of tuberculosis IRIS is also related to bacterial load: the risk is highest in those in whom HAART is started soon after anti-tuberculosis chemotherapy and if the patient has disseminated extra-pulmonary disease.

The commonest clinical manifestations of tuberculosis IRIS are fever with accompanying lymph node enlargement, or new or worsening lung infiltrates or pleural effusions.[70] Granulomatous hepatitis, central nervous system involvement with new or enlarging tuberculomas and new or recurring tissue cold abscesses are also well-reported.[71]

Diagnosis of Tuberculosis

GENERAL PRINCIPLES

The consequences of *M. tuberculosis* infection vary from lifelong, asymptomatic infection to severe, disseminated disease with multiorgan involvement and rapid death. For many decades these diverse manifestations were simplified for clinical purposes to either 'latent' or 'active' tuberculosis, dependent on the presence or absence of symptoms and the results of standard diagnostic tests. For most patients worldwide nothing has changed: management algorithms and treatment guidelines still depend on the physician determining in which of these two groups the patient belongs.

By definition, all patients with latent tuberculosis are asymptomatic. As described above, latent infection follows primary (usually pulmonary) infection but the host's adaptive immune response has controlled the infection, arresting bacterial replication and its pathological consequences. Viable bacteria are present, usually in the lung and sometimes in other organs seeded during the bacteraemia accompanying primary infection, but their very low numbers and diverse locations have meant that their direct detection does not, at present, form the basis of a diagnostic test. Instead, the diagnosis of latent tuberculosis depends on detecting the host's immunological response to *M. tuberculosis*. The long-held assumption is that the presence of a detectable immune response signifies the presence of viable bacteria. The methods for detecting this response have not altered substantially over the last 100 years.

Robert Koch was the first to produce 'tuberculin', or the purified protein derivative (PPD) of *M. tuberculosis* and made the now famous error of believing it represented a therapeutic rather than diagnostic immunological reagent. Charles Mantoux, however, understood its diagnostic value and, in the early 1900s, refined the technique of intra-dermal injection of tuberculin. The consequent delayed-type hypersensitivity reaction in those infected with *M. tuberculosis*, causing measurable skin induration, has formed the basis of latent tuberculosis diagnosis ever since.

More recently, tuberculin skin tests have been joined by two blood tests – the interferon gamma release assays (IGRAs) – which assess the immune response to *M. tuberculosis* by quantifying the release of interferon gamma from either whole blood (the QuantiFERON-TB Gold) or peripheral blood mononuclear cells (T-SPOT.TB) in response to challenge with a panel of specific *M. tuberculosis* antigens. The role of the tuberculin skin test and IGRAs in the diagnosis of latent and active tuberculosis is discussed in greater detail below.

Unlike latent tuberculosis, the diagnosis of 'active' tuberculosis is dependent on demonstrating the presence of *M. tuberculosis* at the site of disease. Tuberculosis can affect almost any tissue in the body; therefore the physician must first identify the organ(s) affected and second, determine how best to isolate *M. tuberculosis* from them. The former relies on taking a careful history, examining the patient and selecting the appropriate radiological investigations; the latter on taking the right diagnostic specimen and subjecting it to the right laboratory tests. The art of tuberculosis diagnosis rests within these choices. Sadly, for most clinicians, the science of tuberculosis diagnosis has not advanced beyond the stain invented by Ziehl and Neelsen 120 years ago to visualize bacteria using light microscopy.

DIAGNOSIS OF LATENT TUBERCULOSIS

Over the last century, the standard diagnostic test for latent tuberculosis has been the tuberculin skin test. The test has two principal forms: the Mantoux and Heaf tests. The Mantoux test requires the intradermal injection of PPD into the dorsal aspect of the forearm. After 48–72 hours, the transverse diameter of any palpable induration (not the erythema) is measured. In the UK and USA, an induration diameter of ≥5 mm to 1 international unit (IU) of PPD and of ≥10 mm to 5 IU PPD are, respectively, regarded as positive. For the purpose of diagnosis, smaller reactions are usually regarded as negative, although they do not exclude tuberculosis because immune suppression (e.g. HIV infection, immune modulating drugs) and, paradoxically, active tuberculosis may suppress the response. Conversely, a positive reaction does not necessarily indicate *M. tuberculosis* infection. False-positive reactions may be due to prior BCG vaccination, or exposure to cross-reacting environmental mycobacteria. However, a reaction of 15 mm or more strongly suggests *M. tuberculosis* infection. Misleading results may also occur through faulty storage of the PPD or, much more commonly, poor technique.

The Heaf test employs a spring-loaded 'gun' which drives six needles into the skin of the dorsal aspect of the forearm through a drop of undiluted PPD. The method is technically easy and the results are less operator-dependent, but it is necessary to autoclave the gun between use in order to avoid transmission of blood-borne viruses. Some guns have detachable magnetic heads which can be autoclaved separately. The practice of dipping the head in alcohol and flaming it is unsafe.

Like the Mantoux, the Heaf test is read at 48–72 hours and the reaction is scored as 5 grades: grade 0 is no reaction; grade I is at least 4 discrete papules; grade II is confluent papules forming a ring; grade III is a disc of induration <10 mm; and grade IV is a disc of induration >10 mm or vesicular formation. Grades III and IV correspond to a Mantoux reaction of ≥15 mm and are regarded as strong evidence of *M. tuberculosis* infection. Grade II corresponds to a Mantoux reaction of 10–14 mm and indicates probable infection.

Two commercial IGRA blood tests have entered clinical practice over the last decade: the T-SPOT.TB test (Oxford Immunotech, Abingdon, UK) and the QuantiFERON-TB Gold in tube (Cellestis Ltd, Carnegie, Australia). These have now been extensively tested in many different clinical situations, including in children and those infected with HIV.[72,73] The major advantage of these tests is that the antigens used are specific to *M. tuberculosis* and are not present in *M. bovis*; therefore, unlike the tuberculin skin test, prior BCG vaccination does not give false-positive results. Both tests appear to perform equally well, although there are some data to suggest the T.SPOT.TB may be less affected by immune suppression than the QuantiFERON-TB Gold or skin test.[74] A meta-analysis of all clinical studies performed up to 2007 concluded that IGRAs were at least as sensitive as the tuberculin skin test for the diagnosis of latent *M. tuberculosis* infection, but more specific.[75] Two more recent meta-analyses performed on data from children and HIV-infected individuals have reported that IGRAs are of equivalent sensitivity to skin tests, but concluded that skin tests and IGRAs have sub-optimal sensitivity for the diagnosis of latent tuberculosis in these patient populations.[74,76] The authors suggest there is no clear evidence that IGRAs should replace skin tests and the decision to use IGRAs should depend upon logistical considerations and the resources available.

DIAGNOSIS OF ACTIVE TUBERCULOSIS

The diagnosis of active tuberculosis is challenging regardless of the setting and laboratory resources available. It requires the physician to link the patient's symptoms and signs, which are frequently nonspecific, with compatible disease pathology and isolate *M. tuberculosis* from the affected tissues. The diagnostic approaches for the commonest forms of tuberculosis are provided in Table 40.5.

Imaging is an essential component of the diagnostic process: all patients with suspected tuberculosis should have a chest X-ray. Active pulmonary tuberculosis may be suggested by infiltrates, cavities, nodules and effusions (Figure 40.7) and mandate submission of respiratory specimens (e.g. sputum) for microbiological examination. Approximately 50% of patients with extra-pulmonary tuberculosis will have an abnormal chest X-ray, although the abnormalities may include residual evidence of the primary infection with a calcified Ghon focus or apical scarring. High-resolution computerized tomography, when available, is substantially more sensitive than chest X-ray at detecting tuberculous lung parenchymal disease and may also reveal disease in other organs.

Extra-pulmonary tuberculosis is particularly hard to diagnose primarily because the affected tissues usually contain very few bacteria. There are two key principles to successful diagnosis. First, when possible, biopsy affected tissue. The diagnostic yield from affected tissue is higher than that of associated fluid (e.g. pus or effusion) and the histological examination of tissue provides important supportive diagnostic information. Second, the more tissue or associated fluid submitted for laboratory examination the greater the likelihood of isolating *M. tuberculosis*. The best-documented proof of this diagnostic principle is in the diagnosis of tuberculous meningitis: the diagnostic yield from <2 mL of cerebrospinal fluid (CSF) is less than 40%, whereas it increases to around 80% if >8 mL of CSF are carefully examined.[77] These two core diagnostic principles apply regardless of whether the laboratory can only perform microscopy, or whether they have the best available molecular assays and culture techniques.

ZIEHL–NEELSEN (ZN) STAIN AND *M. TUBERCULOSIS* CULTURE

For most of the world, the diagnosis of active tuberculosis still depends upon a 120-year-old test. Only recently have new diagnostic assays been developed, some of which are beginning to be used in the resource-limited laboratories of tuberculosis-endemic regions and will be discussed below. The stain developed by Franz Ziehl (1857–1926) and Friedrich Neelsen (1854–1894) in 1882 has many drawbacks, but is considered to have sufficient diagnostic sensitivity and specificity to detect those with the most infectious forms of tuberculosis. The ZN stain of sputum for the diagnosis of active, infectious pulmonary tuberculosis has, therefore, formed the basis of global tuberculosis control programmes for many years.

The ZN stain depends upon the 'acid-alcohol fast' biological properties of *M. tuberculosis*. Paul Ehrlich first elucidated these properties in 1882[78] and they were developed into a test by Ziehl and Neelsen. Neelsen introduced the use of the dye basic fuchsin

TABLE 40.5 Summary of Clinical Presentation, Imaging and Principlal Methods of Diagnosis for the Commonest Forms of Tuberculosis

Type of Tuberculosis	Typical Localizing Clinical Features	Imaging	Diagnostic Procedures/ Specimens	Comment
Pulmonary	Productive cough, chest pain, haemoptysis	Apical infiltrates, nodules and cavities on chest X-ray/high-resolution CT	Expectorated sputum Induced sputum Bronchoscopy with bronchoalveolar lavage (BAL) Gastric aspirates	Sensitivity of ZN stain ~50% and culture ~70%; Xpert RIF MTB ~70% sensitive. Diagnostic yield from induced sputum as good as BAL; gastric washings less sensitive
Pleural	Chest pain, dyspnoea, dry cough	Unilateral effusion on chest X-ray	Pleural fluid Pleural biopsy	<30% sensitivity of ZN stain of pleural fluid; diagnostic yield of pleural biopsy greater
Intrathoracic lymph node	Dry cough, dyspnoea	Enlarged, often necrotic, mediastinal lymph nodes on chest X-ray or CT	Endobronchial ultrasound (EBUS) biopsy Mediastinoscopy with biopsy Open biopsy	EBUS, where available, diagnostic procedure of choice
Superficial lymph node	Cervical, axillary, or inguinal mass(es)	Ultrasound reveals numbers and size of nodes affected (often multiple)	Fine needle aspirate Core biopsy	Yield from biopsy greater than fine needle aspirate but increased risk of sinus formation following biopsy
Miliary/ disseminated	Dry cough, cachexia	Numerous, bilateral nodules on chest X-ray or CT, similar appearances by CT in liver, spleen, kidney and brain	Early morning urine Bone marrow biopsy Induced sputum/BAL Mycobacterial blood culture Lumbar puncture Liver biopsy	Multiple tests may be required. Highest yield from induced sputum and BAL, followed by liver biopsy. Always consider concurrent meningitis
Meningitis	Headache, vomiting, confusion progressing to coma, cranial nerve palsies, hemiplegia	Basal meningeal enhancement and hydrocephalus on CT/ MRI brain	Lumbar puncture	Diagnostic yield dependent on volume of CSF: submit >8 mL when possible. Negative microbiology/PCR never rules out diagnosis; empiric therapy often required
Vertebral	Back pain, gibbus, hemi/paraplegia	Lytic destruction of ventral portion of vertebra with anterior wedge collapse. Soft tissue paraspinous collections common	Bone/tissue biopsy	Diagnostic yield 50–70%
Renal	Loin pain, sterile pyuria	Enlarged kidneys, sometimes with parenchymal calcification	Early morning urine Renal biopsy	Consider concurrent involvement of fallopian tubes/epididymis
Pericardial	Dyspnoea, abdominal and ankle swelling	Globular heart on chest X-ray, or pericardial calcification	Pericardiocentesis Pericardial biopsy	Low diagnostic yield from both microbiology and histology; empiric therapy often required
Abdominal	Abdominal pain, change in bowel habit, ascites, palpable abdominal mass	Nodular deposits on peritoneum by CT Strictures and ulceration by barium studies	Ascitic tap Laparoscopic peritoneal biopsy Terminal ileum biopsy Abdominal lymph node biopsy	Diagnosis difficult because protean manifestations. Low yield from ascitic fluid; take directed biopsy of affected tissue when possible

and found that tubercle bacilli were identifiable from nearly all other species of bacteria by their ability to resist decolouration with weakly acidified alcohol.[79] He observed that the red-stained bacilli were easier to visualize with the background counter-stained with methylene blue (Figure 40.11). Small variations on this method exist, but the principles remain unchanged today.

The demonstration of acid-fast bacilli (AFB) in the sputum/fluid/tissue of a patient suspected of tuberculosis is the primary diagnostic method for much of the world. There are, however, some important limitations to the method. First, the sensitivity of a direct sputum smear is no more than 50–60%. Optimal sensitivity is achieved by examining at least 3 specimens and concentrating the specimen by centrifugation after the addition of a mucolytic agent. Second, it is impossible to tell the species of *Mycobacterium* apart by microscopy. Other *Mycobacterium* (e.g. *Mycobacterium kansasii*) can cause pulmonary disease, or can contaminate respiratory specimens without causing disease. Only culture of the *Mycobacterium* will allow a full identification and confirm the diagnosis of tuberculosis.

More recently, fluorescence microscopy using the auramine-rhodamine stain has improved the speed and ease of microscopy. The staining principles are exactly the same, except the auromine-rhodamine -stained bacilli fluoresce when excited with UV light. The bacilli are easier to see than by ZN stain and

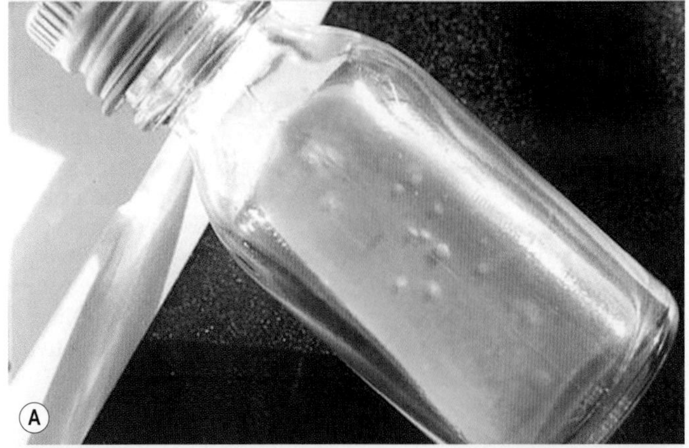

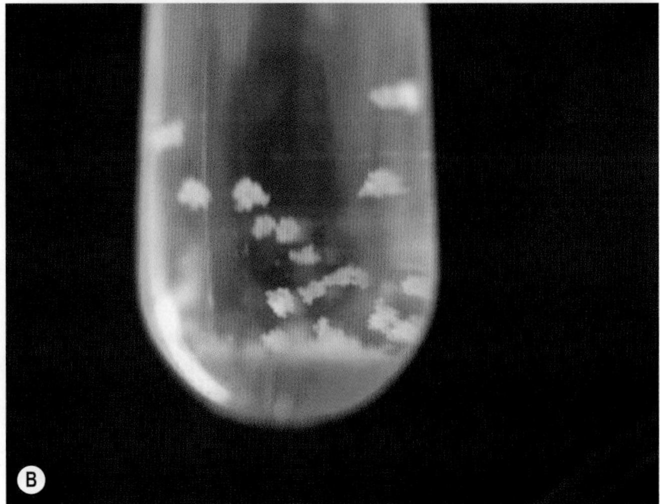

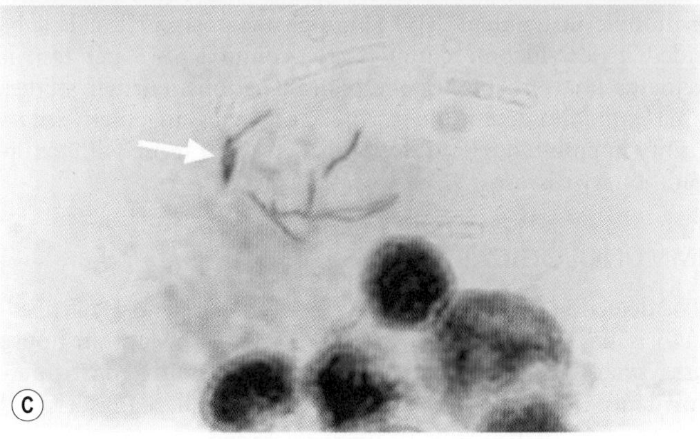

Figure 40.11 Diagnostic microbiology of *M. tuberculosis*. (A) Creamy, breadcrumb-like colonies of *M. tuberculosis* on Lowenstein Jensen media after incubation at 37°C for 4 weeks. (B) Colonies of *M. tuberculosis* adherent to the Mycobacterium Growth Indicator Tube (MGIT) after incubation at 37°C for 2 weeks. (C) Ziehl–Neelsen stain of cerebrospinal fluid showing numerous acid-fast bacilli.

slides can be quickly and effectively screened under low magnification. However, when few bacilli are present (e.g. in CSF), fluorescing debris can be mistaken for bacilli and a confirmatory ZN stain should always be performed.

Confirmation of infection with *M. tuberculosis* can only be made by culture, but as Robert Koch found, *M. tuberculosis* does not grow well on conventional media. Koch eventually found the bacilli grew well on slopes of coagulated blood serum and subsequently many different culture media have been devised. The solid media used most widely are egg-based (Lowenstein–Jensen, Figure 40.11) and agar-based (Middlebrook's 7H10 or 7H11). Liquid media (Middlebrook's 7H9 or Kirchner's media) are less selective but especially useful when culturing specimens other than sputum, when the chances of contamination with other bacteria or fungi are low.

Simple growth characteristics allow the preliminary laboratory identification of *M. tuberculosis*. The early bacteriologists recognized that cultivable mycobacteria could be divided into 'rapid growers' (growth on egg-media within 5 days) and 'slow growers'. *M. tuberculosis* and most other pathogenic mycobacteria are 'slow growers': they take between 4 and 8 weeks to produce significant colonies on egg-based solid media. *M. tuberculosis* grows best at 37°C, is non-pigmented and demonstrates characteristic 'cords' of bacilli when stained by ZN, but the formal identification rests on an array of confirmatory tests, or more recently by nucleic acid probes. It is not within the scope of this chapter to review these methods, but they are time-consuming and difficult and are usually only performed by experienced technicians in reference laboratories. For these reasons, in many settings, the culture and identification of *M. tuberculosis* remains impossible and tuberculosis diagnosis rests upon the result of the ZN stain alone.

MOLECULAR DIAGNOSTIC METHODS: NUCLEIC ACID AMPLIFICATION

The lack of diagnostic sensitivity and specificity of conventional microbiology and the time required to culture and identify the organism, have led to the development of nucleic-acid-based amplification tests. In the early 1980s the polymerase chain reaction (PCR) became the first molecular method to amplify DNA sequences and was widely expected to revolutionize the diagnosis of infectious diseases. But the early promise was not fulfilled and commercial assays based on PCR were generally less sensitive than culture and were never capable of leaving resource-rich laboratories.

Line-probe assays, which detected the bacteria and the genetic mutations associated with rifampicin-resistance within 48 hours, represented a major breakthrough; but these tests remained the preserve of the reference laboratory. The WHO endorsed line-probe assays in 2008, but they failed to represent a global solution to the inadequacies of conventional smear and culture. They are expensive and can only be reliably performed on smear-positive specimens.

The GeneXpert platform was initially launched in 2004 for the rapid detection of anthrax bacillus by PCR-based technology. It integrated sample prep, amplification and detection in a single tube and took approximately 100 minutes to obtain a result. The Xpert MTB/RIF cartridge (Cepheid Inc., Sunnyvale, CA, USA), which detects rifampicin-resistant or -susceptible *M. tuberculosis*, took a further 4 years to develop but represented a major advance in tuberculosis diagnostics. The result is a fully automated, enclosed (and therefore safe) real-time PCR, which required no special skills or lab to perform and gives a result in 120 minutes.[80]

The Xpert MTB/RIF test is performed in a single, enclosed, plastic cartridge. It uses molecular beacon technology to detect specific sequences within a 192 base-pair (bp) segment of DNA, amplified by a hemi-nested, real time-PCR. Five different nucleic acid hybridization probes are used in the same multiplex reaction; these span the entire 81 bp core region of the *rpoB* gene. Each probe is complementary to a different target sequence within the *rpoB* gene and is labelled with a differently coloured fluorophore. As a consequence, the test provides concurrent detection of both *M. tuberculosis* and the presence or absence of the genetic mutations known to confer rifampicin resistance. The test also gives a semi-quantitative estimate of bacillary concentration in the specimen: either high, medium, low, or very low. The results are available in around 120 minutes, with less than 15 minutes of hands-on time.[80]

Xpert MTB/RIF is able to detect a minimum of 4.5 genome copies in a sample. This translates to around 131 colony-forming units (CFU)/mL of sputum (95% confidence intervals 106–176 CFU/mL). By comparison, the limits of detection of standard ZN stain and liquid media culture are around 10 000 CFU/mL and 10–100 CFU/mL, respectively. Therefore, Xpert MTB/RIF performs with equivalent sensitivity to culture, but within 2 hours, also confirms the identity of the organism and its susceptibility to rifampicin. Furthermore, because it is performed within an enclosed cartridge, its use does not mandate special biosafety precautions. Indeed, it is probably much safer than performing ZN stain and culture.

The seminal clinical evaluation of Xpert MTB/RIF was reported in 2010.[81] The study enrolled 1730 symptomatic patients in Peru, Africa and India with chronic cough: 40% were HIV-infected and 46% had been previously treated for tuberculosis. Three 1.5 mL specimens of sputum were submitted by each patient, two of which were cultured and one was subjected to ZN stain and Xpert MTB/RIF. Xpert MTB/RIF detected *M. tuberculosis* in 98% of all smear positive specimens and 73% of smear-negative -(culture-positive) specimens. The latter figure rose to 90% if three specimens were tested. The specificity of the test was greater than 99%. In addition, the test correctly identified 98% of rifampicin-resistant and -sensitive isolates, respectively.

Additional studies have been reported examining the use of Xpert MTB/RIF in children, extra-pulmonary tuberculosis and in 'real life' non-specialist laboratories. A study on South African children examined the performance of Xpert MTB/RIF on induced sputum from 452 children and found that two Xpert tests identified 76% of culture-positive specimens, whereas ZN stain identified 38% of positive specimens.[82] The specificity of Xpert MTB/RIF was 98.8%.

The data on the use of Xpert MTB/RIF for the diagnosis of extra-pulmonary tuberculosis are more limited and further studies are required to delineate the use of the test in particular forms of tuberculosis, e.g. meningitis. However, used on a wide variety of extra-pulmonary samples (including CSF) the diagnostic sensitivity is reported at around 75% and the specificity approaching 100%. A study from India of 546 patients with diverse forms of extra-pulmonary tuberculosis found Xpert MTB/RIF was positive in 96% of smear-positive specimens and 64% of smear-negative specimens.[83] An unpublished study in Vietnamese adults with suspected tuberculous meningitis found the sensitivity of Xpert MTB/RIF performed on CSF was 61% (43/71) against clinical diagnostic criteria, with 100% specificity (Professor Jeremy Farrar, pers comm).

The true worth of Xpert MTB/RIF will only become apparent when it has been extensively tested in programmatic, rather than research settings. So far, one study has been performed assessing its use in non-specialist laboratories.[84] Xpert MTB/RIF and ZN stain were compared on sputum from 6648 adults from six different countries with cough for longer than 2 weeks. Culture for *M. tuberculosis* was performed in a centralized laboratory. The sensitivity of Xpert MTB/RIF was 90% compared with 67% for ZN stain; 98% of smear-positive samples-were positive by Xpert MTB/RIF compared with 77% of smear negative samples. For patients with smear-negative sputum, Xpert MTB/RIF reduced the time-to-treatment from median 56 days to 5 days. The study provides powerful evidence for the utility of Xpert MTB/RIF outside of specialist laboratories, but it also unearthed a significant problem with the assay. The sensitivity for the detection of rifampicin resistance was 97%, but the specificity was 96%. This indicates a small but significant problem with false-positive rifampicin resistance results, which may lead to the inappropriate starting of expensive, toxic second-line anti-tuberculosis drugs. The importance of this problem will vary according to the prevalence of MDR tuberculosis in which the test is being used. If the prevalence of MDR tuberculosis is >15% then the positive predictive value (PPV) of a positive rifampicin-resistant Xpert MTB/RIF is >90%; however, if the prevalence of MDR tuberculosis is <5% then the PPV falls to <70%. This is, therefore, an important technical problem with the assay and will need to be resolved before widespread implementation of the assay.

In summary, Xpert MTB/RIF represents a huge advance in the diagnosis of active tuberculosis and one which should help clinicians and patients worldwide. WHO endorsed the assay in 2010 and, in 2011, strongly recommended it should be used as the *initial* diagnostic test in individuals suspected of MDR-tuberculosis or HIV-associated tuberculosis. There are issues that remain to be resolved, as outlined above. In addition, the cost of the instrument remains high (around US$17 500 for the 4-module instrument) and although the cost per test is subsided in low-income countries to around US$18 per test, it remains unaffordable for the poorest nations. Further studies are required to determine its cost effectiveness together with its utility in children, HIV-infected patients and those with extra-pulmonary disease.

IMMUNOLOGICAL ASSAYS

The detection of antibodies in serum for the diagnosis of tuberculosis has a long and checkered history.[85,86] Many in-house assays have been described, often with excellent diagnostic performance in preliminary studies done on small, highly selected groups of patients. None of these assays has gone on to make a major impact on tuberculosis diagnostics. Indeed, a systematic review and meta-analysis of the data available on the use of commercial diagnostic serological tests concluded that none of the assays improved upon the ZN stain.[87] In 2011, the WHO advised that none of the commercial point-of-care diagnostic tests currently available should be used for the diagnosis of tuberculosis.

The role of IGRAs in the diagnosis of active, rather than latent tuberculosis, has been a source of on-going controversy. A recent meta-analysis of data from studies which have examined the utility of IGRAs for the diagnosis of active pulmonary tuberculosis in low- and middle-income countries concluded that neither IGRAs nor skin tests have diagnostic value for active tuberculosis.[88] A total of 27 studies were included in the analysis and data from 590 HIV-uninfected and 844

HIV-infected patients. In HIV-infected patients, the pooled estimates of sensitivity were 76% for T-SPOT.TB test and 60% for the QuantiFERON-TB Gold in tube. The diagnostic specificity was low for both: 52 and 50%, respectively. Whether IGRAs are any better at predicting the development of active tuberculosis compared to skin tests also remains a moot point. A systematic review and meta-analysis of 15 studies, with a combined sample size of 26 680 individuals and median follow-up of 4 years, found IGRA-positive and skin test positive people were at much the same risk for developing active tuberculosis. The incidence rates ratios were 2.1 for IGRA and 1.6 for skin test.[89] The identification of a biomarker which better predicts the progression from latent to active tuberculosis represents one of the 'holy grails' of current tuberculosis research.[90]

There are some data, however, which indicate that the use of IGRAs on site-specific lymphocytes (e.g. from BAL, pleural fluid or CSF) may be useful in the diagnosis of active disease of those sites.[86] To date, the most promising findings have been with the use of BAL and pleural fluid.[91] In those unable to expectorate, the combination of IGRA on BAL lymphocytes and a ZN stain on induced sputum identified more than 90% of patients with culture-confirmed disease.[92]

IGRAs appear to be less useful in the diagnosis of tuberculous meningitis. A limited number of studies suggest large volumes of CSF are require to ensure there are sufficient numbers of lymphocytes to enable the assay to work (5–10 mL) and that indeterminate results are common.[93,94] In addition, whether blood or CSF are used in the assay, around 30–40% have a false-negative result. Given the fatal consequences of a tuberculous meningitis missed diagnosis, this is a crucial limitation. Until more supportive data become available, CSF IGRA cannot be recommended for the routine diagnosis of tuberculous meningitis.

URINARY LIPOARABINOMANNAN

Lipoarabinomannan is a heat-stable major cell wall constituent of *M. tuberculosis,* which is excreted in the urine of some patients with tuberculosis. It can be detected using a simple sandwich ELISA, using polyclonal antibodies and was first developed as a commercial 'MTB ELISA' test (Chemogen Inc.) and subsequently marketed as the 'Clearview TB ELISA' (Inverness Medical Innovations). The first field evaluations were promising, reporting a sensitivity of 80% and specificity of 99% for smear-positive pulmonary tuberculosis.[95] Subsequent investigations, however, were disappointing with much lower sensitivity (<10%) and variable specificity, particularly in HIV-uninfected people. Nevertheless, more recent studies suggest the sensitivity of the test increases with advancing immune suppression and it may have a role in combination with smear and Xpert MTB/RIF in those with advanced HIV.[96] Given these patients are often smear-negative and are at high risk of dying, the detection of urinary lipoarabinomannan may prove especially useful, but more studies are required to delineate its role.

DETECTION OF DRUG-RESISTANT *M. TUBERCULOSIS*

Ever since the late 1940s, when tuberculosis became a treatable disease, drug susceptibility testing (DST) of the bacteria has remained the preserve of the reference laboratory. A variety of phenotypic methods on solid media are used, including the 1% proportion, absolute concentration and resistance ratio methods.[97] All these methods are laborious and slow and results are issued to clinicians 2–3 months after the original diagnostic specimens were sent.

In most parts of the world, DST is only performed if the patient has failed first-line therapy (still smear-positive at the end of 2 months of 4-drug standard treatment). Only at this point are bacteria cultured and sent to the specialist regional laboratory for conventional DST. As the test results are awaited those with MDR tuberculosis will continue to transmit their bacteria to their contacts.

While this situation was tolerable when the prevalence of drug-resistant organisms was very low, the rise of MDR tuberculosis over the last decade – there are now more than 500 000 cases each year worldwide – means conventional DST methods are unacceptably slow and inaccessible. The development of affordable tests capable of rapidly detecting drug-resistant *M. tuberculosis* is a global priority.[98]

Currently available DST methods are summarized in Table 40.6. These tests can be divided into phenotypic and genotypic; the advantage of the former being they do not require knowledge of the underlying mechanisms of resistance. The phenotypic methods include various commercial liquid media systems, including the Bactec Mycobacterial Growth Indicator Tube (MGIT) system and MBBacT. These cut the time-to-results from 6–12 weeks for solid media to 3–4 weeks, but they are expensive, require the organism to be accurately identified by other methods and are prone to contamination with other bacteria or fungi.

The microscopic observation drug susceptibility (MODS) assay is an elegant solution to many of the problems posed by the conventional liquid and solid media methods. Pre-prepared decontaminated sputum is inoculated into small wells containing liquid growth media. Some of the wells contain media with known concentrations of rifampicin, isoniazid, streptomycin and ethambutol. The plate is incubated for a few days then each well is examined using an inverted light microscope. *M. tuberculosis* grows in unique cords in liquid media, which can be observed without special stains. Therefore, the presence of cords in the well signifies that the specimen contains *M. tuberculosis*; if there is bacterial growth in the wells containing a drug it signifies that the organism is resistant to that drug. Thus, in 9–12 days, MODS will identify *M. tuberculosis* in a specimen and give concurrent information regarding its drug susceptibility. This method has been proven to be at least as good as the gold-standard solid media methods.[99] MODS, along with the nitrate reductase assay and the calorimetric redox indicator (see Table 40.6), were endorsed by the WHO in 2010 for DST. Other phenotypic methods, such as those based on reporter bacteriophages, are in development, but have yet to be trialled outside of specialist research laboratories.

Genotypic resistance tests have the great advantage of speed, with results available within 24 hours. They rely, however, on an understanding of the genetic mechanisms of resistance. Rifampicin resistance testing is especially amenable to genetic testing as almost all the mutations which confer rifampicin resistance are contained within a well-defined segment of the *rpoB* gene. Thus, when these mutations are detected (e.g. by the LIPA or Xpert MTB RIF tests) they are strongly predictive of phenotypic rifampicin resistance. The genetic mechanisms of resistance for the other anti-tuberculosis drugs are more

TABLE 40.6 **Current Laboratory Methods for the Detection of Drug-Resistant *M. Tuberculosis***

Method	Drug Resistance Tested	Turn-Around Time from Time Diagnostic Specimen Submitted	Comment
Conventional solid media assays (1% proportion, absolute concentration, resistance ratio)	All drugs	2–3 months	Slow, technically laborious and demanding, expensive
Mycobacterial growth indicator tube (MGIT)	All drugs	18–28 days	Fully automated, must identify species, expensive
Microscopic observation drug susceptibility (MODS)	Rifampicin and isoniazid	4–21 days	Low cost, simple, safe, but requires trained staff and inverted light microscope
Colorimetric redox indicators	Rifampicin and isoniazid	7 days after primary isolation	Low cost, simple methods, but not validated from direct clinical specimen (only from primary culture)
INNO-LIPA Rif	Rifampicin only	6–48 hours	Commercial, reliable, good performance on smear positive samples, but not validated on smear negative and requires trained staff
Genotype MTBDR and MTBDR-Plus	Rifampicin and isoniazid	6–48 hours	Good performance in smear positive, less good if smear negative, high sensitivity for rifampicin, around 80% sensitivity for isoniazid resistance
Xpert MTB/RIF	Rifampicin only	1.5–2 hours	Rapid, safe, fully automated, performs well on both smear positive and negative specimens

complex (see Table 40.7). For example, around 80% of isoniazid-resistant strains contain mutations in the genes *inhA* and *katG*, but the genes responsible for the remaining 20% of isoniazid-resistant strains are diverse and poorly characterized. Therefore, genetic tests for isoniazid resistance are less predictive.

SPECIAL DIAGNOSTIC CHALLENGES: PAEDIATRIC, EXTRA-PULMONARY TUBERCULOSIS AND MENINGITIS

Children with tuberculosis provide a particular diagnostic challenge because they generally do not develop cavitatory lung tuberculosis amenable to diagnosis by ZN stain of sputum. Indeed, many children with respiratory tuberculosis do not produce sputum; therefore alternative methods for examining respiratory specimens have been developed. Several studies have shown that the diagnostic yield from induced sputum is as good as, if not better than, BAL.[100] Yet, there are problems with performing induced sputum safely and protecting others from infectious aerosols and it is not a procedure which can be performed in young children.

The examination and culture of gastric washing have long been used as an alternative; respiratory secretions are continually being swallowed and therefore can be sampled from the stomach. The diagnostic yield from gastric washing is probably no more than 30%, but it is a relatively simple, safe and cheap technique.

More recently, the string test – previously used for diagnosing upper gastrointestinal parasites – has been developed for tuberculosis diagnosis in children and adults. Patients swallow a capsule with string attached, which is taped to the side of the patient's mouth and stops the capsule passing beyond the duodenum. The capsule is left in situ for around 4 hours, during which time the string is contaminated with swallowed respiratory secretions. Upon withdrawal the string is examined and cultured for *M. tuberculosis*. There are limited current data, but it appears that the string test may be as sensitive as induced sputum and safer/easier to perform.[86]

Intrathoracic lymph node tuberculosis represents a common diagnostic challenge in children and adults. Making a tissue diagnosis of isolated intrathoracic nodal disease was, until recently, a serious challenge that required biopsies taken either by mediastinoscopy or open surgery. Endobronchial ultrasound (EBUS)-guided aspiration of mediastinal lymph nodes has transformed this approach. A recent study of 156 consecutive patients with a clinical diagnosis of intrathoracic tuberculous lymphadenitis reported EBUS confirmed the diagnosis in 94% of patients, either through positive histology (86%) or culture (47%).[101]

Superficial lymph tuberculosis can be diagnosed by aspiration using a 22 or 23 gauge needle. Slides are prepared for cytology and the residual material in the needle and syringe is rinsed directly into a liquid mycobacterial culture medium. A prospective study of 200 South African children showed that in high-risk populations, fine needle aspiration of lymph nodes using a combination of cytomorphology, autofluorescence and ZN staining provided a rapid and definitive diagnosis of tuberculosis.[102] The study compared fine needle aspiration against gastric aspirates and induced sputum and found fine needle aspiration gave positive results in 61% of children versus 39% for any of the other tests.

The diagnosis of miliary/disseminated tuberculosis may require a multi-faceted approach with a range of specimens taken to optimize diagnostic yield. Patients with miliary tuberculosis rarely produce sputum, therefore induced sputum and/or gastric washes are useful. More invasive sampling may also be indicated, depending upon the available expertise. Liver and bone marrow biopsy may be particularly helpful. A study of 109 South African adults with disseminated tuberculosis found bone marrow examination was diagnostic in 19 of 22 (86%) patients and in 100% (10/10) of those selected for liver biopsy.[103] Early morning urine should also be examined and cultured; it is positive in less than 20% of patients with miliary tuberculosis, but it is a simple and safe test.

Patients with miliary tuberculosis often have concurrent meningitis and require rapid investigation and treatment. Tuberculous meningitis should be managed as a medical emergency; delays in starting treatment are intimately associated with death or severe neurological sequelae.[47] Cerebrospinal fluid (CSF) examination is an essential component of diagnosing tuberculous meningitis. The typical findings are of 50–1500 white cells (/mm^3), which may vary from being predominantly (up to 90%) neutrophils to all lymphocytes. The CSF protein is typically raised from 50–250 mg/dL and the ratio of CSF : plasma glucose is <50% in 95% of patients. The diagnostic yield from ZN stain and culture is dependent upon the volume of CSF submitted and the care with which it is examined. Repeated meticulous examination of large (>10 mL) volumes of CSF has been shown to yield bacteria from almost all patients.[104] In reality, most laboratories see bacteria in CSF in less than 10% of patient and culture is positive in 30–50%. Performing commercial PCR-based assays on CSF has been shown to be around 50% sensitive and nearly 100% specific. The Xpert MTB/RIF assay may be marginally more sensitive (around 60%) and gives valuable, rapid information concerning rifampicin susceptibility, but better tests are still required. Importantly, a negative ZN stain, culture or PCR/Xpert MTB/RIF should never be used to rule out the possibility of tuberculous meningitis. In many cases, due to the inadequate currently available diagnostic methods, anti-tuberculosis treatment should be started empirically on the basis of compatible clinical features.

Management and Treatment of Tuberculosis

BACKGROUND AND PRINCIPLES

There was no effective treatment for tuberculosis until 1944. The Greeks and the Romans advocated fresh air and rest: factors they believed could redress the imbalance of the humors causing the disease. Two thousand years later, belief in the therapeutic effect of clean air remained and led to the development of the tuberculosis sanatoria. Hermann Brehmer is credited with opening the first European 'Kurhaus' for tuberculous patients in 1859, inspiring Edward Trudeau to develop a similar institution in the USA at Saranac Lake in 1875. By 1942, there were nearly 100 000 sanatorium beds in the USA and similar numbers in the European Alps, providing fashionable retreats for the tuberculous middle and upper classes. They inspired some (notably Thomas Mann, who wrote *The Magic Mountain* in 1924 after his experiences in a sanatorium in Davos, Switzerland), but cured none. However, institutionalizing tuberculosis allowed physicians to experiment with alternative treatments on large numbers of individuals. Some of the methods developed were at best misguided and at worst dangerous and deforming. Pulmonary collapse therapy, either by pneumothorax, phrenic crush, or pneumoperitoneum, led the way, regardless of the lack of evidence for its therapeutic effectiveness.

The chemotherapeutic era began with the inspiration from a soil microbiologist from the Ukraine and a biochemist from Sweden. Selman Waksman was born in the Ukraine and emigrated to the USA in 1910. By the 1930s, he was studying the mechanisms of action of fungal enzymes found in the soil and driven by the possibility of a soil microbe that could kill *M. tuberculosis*. In 1943, Waksman's laboratory discovered that *Streptomyces griseus* produced a substance that inhibited the growth of a wide range of bacteria, including *M. tuberculosis*. They named the substance *Streptomycin*.

Jorgen Lehmann, a Dane working in Sweden, approached the same problem from a different perspective. In 1941, a single page report appeared in the journal *Science* that showed salicylate greatly increased the oxygen uptake of *M. tuberculosis*.[105] Lehmann reasoned that alteration of the salicylate molecule might inhibit *M. tuberculosis* metabolism and believed the para-amino salt of salicylate was most likely to work. In 1944, despite difficulties with production, Lehmann showed that *para-amino salicylic acid* (PAS) inhibited growth of *M. tuberculosis* in vitro and was capable of reducing disease in both guinea pigs and humans.

The assessment of these two drugs for the treatment of tuberculosis was a defining moment in medicine. The need for a rapid, authoritative, unbiased assessment was recognized as paramount. The methodology chosen – the random assignment of control and experimental treatment regimens – would become the cornerstone of clinical research. The British Medical Research Council (MRC) performed the first of such trials, comparing streptomycin with bed rest for acute progressive bilateral pulmonary tuberculosis.[106] This study showed that over 6 months, streptomycin reduced mortality and improved bacteriological and radiological cure rates. However, resistance to streptomycin developed in 35/41 patients and after 5 years of follow-up, the deaths in the streptomycin group (53%) were only slightly less than in controls (63%). Urgent strategies were required to overcome the problem of resistance and in 1948, the MRC started a trial comparing streptomycin alone, PAS alone and the two in combination. It demonstrated unequivocally that combined therapy reduced the risk of acquisition of resistance.[107]

Consistent and complete cures only became reality in 1952, with the addition of isoniazid to these two drugs. Although the curative power of this three-drug regimen was recognized quickly by some, it took some years to become universally accepted. There was a reasonable basis for scepticism: data from randomized trials were slow to appear and conclusive evidence of the efficacy of all three drugs in combination did not become available until 1964.[108]

At least 12 months of treatment were required for sustained cure with these regimens. The advent of ethambutol led to its exchange with PAS (which caused frequent side-effects) and a better-tolerated regimen, but reductions in treatment length only became possible with the addition of rifampicin. Rifampicin-containing regimens were tested in three different durations of chemotherapy: 6, 9 and 12 months.[109] The trial demonstrated that a sustained cure was possible with 9 months of treatment and the term 'short-course chemotherapy' was invented.[110]

A series of trials performed by the MRC in East and Central Africa defined the limits of 'short-course chemotherapy' and demonstrated that complete cure could be achieved with 6 months.[111] They discovered that pyrazinamide (a drug that was discarded initially due to fears of hepatic toxicity), in combination with rifampicin and isoniazid, showed powerful sterilizing activity with rapid conversion to smear-negative sputum. After further trials in Hong Kong, Singapore, Madras and Algeria, it was shown that the best results were achieved using an 'intensive' phase of 2-months rifampicin, isoniazid and pyrazinamide, followed by a 'continuation' phase of 4-months rifampicin and isoniazid. Thioacetazone or ethambutol could replace rifampicin in the continuation phase, but treatment should be extended by 2 months. The mechanisms of action of the first-line drugs and the ways in which *M. tuberculosis* can become resistant to their effects, are presented in Table 40.7.

TABLE 40.7 Mechanisms of Action and Modes of Resistance for First-Line Anti-Tuberculosis Drugs

Drug	Mechanism of Action	Mechanism of Resistance	Mutation Locus (Prevalence Among Resistant Strains)
Streptomycin	Inhibition of protein synthesis by binding to 30S subunit of ribosomes	(i) Mutations of 30S subunit binding site (ii) Possible changes in cell permeability to drug	*rpsL* (ribosomal protein subunit 12) (60%) *rcs* (16S ribosomal RNA) (25%)
Ethambutol	Inhibits biosynthesis of cell wall, in particular arabinogalactan (AG) + lipoarabinomannan (LAM)	Mutation in gene encoding arabinosyl transferase causing increased AG+LAM	*embAB* (50%)
Isoniazid	Uncertain. Pro-drug activated by *M. tuberculosis* catalase peroxidase (KatG) inhibits mycolic acid synthesis	Uncertain. Multiple possible .mechanisms and loci	*KatG* (50%) *InhA* (25%) *ahpC* (15%) *kasA* (unknown)
Rifampicin	Inhibits RNA polymerase preventing mRNA production	RNA polymerase subunit B mutation prevent drug binding	*rpoB* (98%)
Pyrazinamide	Unknown. Bacterial pyrazinamidase converts to active pyrazinoic acid	Unknown	*pncA* (unknown)

By the late 1970s, the best drug combinations and the duration of treatment required, had been worked out. Then, in 1986, the tuberculosis trials units of the MRC closed. In 40 years, they had delineated all of the measures necessary for successful tuberculosis control, the optimal drug regimens and the importance of directly observed therapy. Two subsequent events suggest the closure of these units was premature. The first was predictable: the increasing prevalence of drug resistance and resulting treatment failures. The second, the arrival of HIV, was not predictable, although by 1986 there was already clear evidence that tuberculosis and HIV had a special relationship.

RECOMMENDED ANTI-TUBERCULOSIS TREATMENT REGIMENS

Table 40.8 summarizes the doses of the first-line anti-tuberculosis drug recommended by the WHO and the Infectious Diseases Society of America (IDSA).[112,113] The WHO recommends the same 6-month regimen for the treatment of all patients with tuberculosis, regardless of disease site or HIV status: rifampicin, isoniazid, pyrazinamide and ethambutol for the first 2 months, followed by rifampicin and isoniazid for 4 months. A 5-month continuation phase of isoniazid and ethambutol has been demonstrated to be less effective than 4 months of isoniazid and rifampicin.[114]

The IDSA provide more nuanced recommendations with advice to extend the continuation phase in some circumstances, while acknowledging the limited supporting evidence for so doing. They recommend a 3-month extension (9 months total treatment) for patients with extensive lung cavitation and bacteria cultured from their sputum after the first 2 months of treatment. They advise extending the duration of treatment if any one of the three key drugs – rifampicin, isoniazid and pyrazinamide – cannot be used. In addition, many experts, including the authors of the IDSA guidelines, recommend tuberculous meningitis should be treated for 9–12 months given the severity

TABLE 40.8 Recommended Regimens of First-Line Anti-Tuberculosis Drug Treatment of Adults and Children

	RECOMMENDED DOSE			
	DAILY		3-TIMES-A-WEEK	
	Dose (mg/kg Body Weight)	Maximum (mg)	Dose (mg/kg Body Weight)	Maximum (mg)
ISONIAZID				
Adults	5	300	10	900
Children	10–15	300		
RIFAMPICIN				
Adults	10	600	10	600
Children	10–20	600		
PYRAZINAMIDE				
Adults	25	2000	35	
Children	15–30	2000		
ETHAMBUTOL				
Adults	15		30	
Children	15–20	1000		
STREPTOMYCIN				
Adults	15	1000	15	1000
Children	20–40	1000		

Based on current WHO and USA guidelines.

of the disease and poor penetration of many of the drugs into the brain.[48]

In the intensive phase, daily regimens are probably more effective than three-times-a-week regimens, particularly when there is a risk of isoniazid resistance and/or the patient is immune-compromised. Daily regimens are strongly advised for disseminated tuberculosis, tuberculous meningitis and those with advanced untreated HIV infection. Three-times-weekly regimens lend themselves to directly observed therapy (DOT) and are effective in the continuation phase of treatment, provided they are well supervised. In those with chronic kidney disease requiring dialysis, three-times-weekly regimens are preferred as they are associated with reduced drug-related toxicity.[115]

Tablets using fixed-dose combinations are recommended by the WHO as they have equivalent efficacy and safety to single drugs[116] and are easier to take and may improve adherence. It is, however, important to ensure patients receive the right mg/kg dose for each drug contained within the tablet. For example, patients over 90 kg may need to take extra pyrazinamide when prescribed some of the 3-drug fixed dose tablets. Conversely, splitting tablets for children is a common source of dosing error. Paediatric syrups for rifampicin and isoniazid are manufactured, but are not widely available in resource-poor settings. Syrups may ease administration to children but are easily over- and under-dosed, therefore they must be used with adequate supervision. Prescribing errors are common and, if perpetuated over several months of treatment, can have severe consequences, including treatment failure, on-going transmission and the development of drug resistance. Physicians must ensure they prescribe the right drugs at the right dose for the right length of time; tuberculosis would be far better controlled than it is today had these principles been adhered to in the past.

MONITORING THERAPY

Anti-tuberculosis therapy should be monitored for effectiveness and toxicity. The latter will be discussed below. When treating pulmonary tuberculosis, the WHO recommends sputum should be examined for AFB at the end of the intensive phase, although evidence suggests the test is a poor predictor of relapse, treatment failure and drug resistance. If bacteria are seen at 2 months, the WHO advises repeating the test after a further month of treatment without changing the anti-tuberculosis drug regimen.[113] If bacteria remain visible in the sputum, they should be cultured and drug susceptibility tests performed. It should be noted (see above) that by conventional methods, the results of these tests will not return for 2–3 months, by which time the patients will have completed 6 months of first-line therapy. This system of monitoring therapy and the delayed selection of those most likely to have drug-resistant bacteria, has attracted strong criticism.[98] Delayed drug susceptibility testing is a pragmatic approach, given most tuberculosis control programmes in resource-poor settings have limited access to these tests, but it leaves those with multi-drug-resistant tuberculosis undetected and untreated for many months, with the potential for on-going transmission and the generation of further resistance.

If a patient fails therapy (defined by positive sputum microscopy by 6 months) or the disease relapses after the end of treatment, the WHO recommend re-treatment with five drugs for 2 months (the original four drugs plus streptomycin); four drugs for 1 month (streptomycin stopped) and a further 5 months of isoniazid, rifampicin and ethambutol. The effectiveness of this re-treatment regimen in practice is dependent on whether the treatment failure/relapse was due to drug resistance or the failure to prescribe or adhere to an appropriate first-line drug regimen. Thus, the early detection of drug resistance is essential; blind re-treatment of multi-drug-resistant tuberculosis with the above standard re-treatment regimen is unlikely to lead to cure and risks generating resistance to ethambutol, streptomycin and pyrazinamide. There is a 'golden rule' to tuberculosis treatment: never add a single drug to a failing regimen; always add at least two, preferably three drugs, while trying to determine, as quickly as possible, the drug susceptibility of the infecting organism.

Monitoring therapy in extra-pulmonary tuberculosis is more difficult as the serial assessment of bacterial numbers at the disease site is rarely possible. In addition, symptoms may worsen after the start of treatment, before they improve. These so-called 'paradoxical' treatment reactions are often seen during the treatment of lymph node and central nervous system tuberculosis. The lymph nodes enlarge, becoming inflamed and painful; or intracerebral tuberculomas expand, causing focal neurological deficit or reduced consciousness. If these reactions occur in HIV-infected individuals it is called IRIS, although the pathogenesis of both reactions is likely to be similar.

Paradoxical treatment reactions commonly occur between 20 and 60 days into therapy and although they can result in marked symptoms, they are rarely life-threatening. They can, however, be hard to distinguish from the progressive treatment failure associated with primary drug-resistant tuberculosis. Unlike paradoxical reactions, drug-resistant treatment failure does not present following a period of clinical improvement; and paradoxical reactions usually have a marked inflammatory component to their presentation. Adjunctive corticosteroids can help reduce the symptoms of paradoxical reactions, whereas they will cause enhanced disease progression in those with drug-resistant infection. Repeat diagnostic sampling with re-culture is frequently required to address the dilemma.

ADVERSE REACTIONS TO ANTI-TUBERCULOSIS DRUGS

Approximately 9 million people take first-line anti-tuberculosis therapy each year. The majority do so without suffering significant adverse reactions to the drugs. There are, however, well-described reactions to each of the first-line drugs which are summarized in Table 40.9. In general, the drugs are safe and well-tolerated. With the exception of streptomycin, all can be given safely to pregnant and breast-feeding mothers.

Some of the adverse reactions are preventable. For example, isoniazid can cause vitamin B6 deficiency through excess excretion of the vitamin in the urine. Supplementation with vitamin B6 (pyridoxine) is recommended by the WHO in all those at higher risk of B6 deficiency, including those with HIV, malnutrition, pregnancy, chronic alcoholism and chronic liver or kidney failure.[113] When possible, all patients receiving isoniazid should receive pyridoxine to prevent the consequences of deficiency, which include peripheral neuropathy, seizures, cheilitis, conjunctivitis and sideroblastic anaemia. Other reactions require careful monitoring; chief among these are the hepatic reactions caused by pyrazinamide, rifampicin or isoniazid, or the retrobulbar optic neuritis caused by ethambutol.

TABLE 40.9 Adverse Reactions to First-Line Anti-Tuberculosis Drugs

Drug	Common	Rare	Neurological
Isoniazid	Hepatitis	Haemolytic anaemia Aplastic anaemia Sideroblastic anaemia Agranulocytosis Lupoid reactions Arthralgia Gynaecomastia	Peripheral neuropathy Convulsions Optic neuritis Mania/psychosis
Rifampicin	Hepatitis Thrombocytopenia Fever	Haemolytic anaemia Acute renal failure	Headaches Confusion Drowsiness
Pyrazinamide	Hepatitis Anorexia Flushing Arthralgia Hyperuricaemia	Gout Photosensitivity	
Ethambutol	Arthralgia	Hepatitis Rash	Retrobulbar neuritis Peripheral neuropathy Confusion
Streptomycin	Vertigo Deafness Acute renal failure		Neuromuscular block

The presenting ocular symptoms of ethambutol toxicity vary among affected individuals, but usually occur weeks or months into treatment.[117] Toxicity is much more likely in those taking high doses (>25 mg/kg per day) or if the patient has renal impairment. The risk of optic neuritis in those with normal renal function taking the standard 15 mg/kg per day dose is less than 1%. Patients with toxicity may complain of bilateral progressive painless blurring of vision or decreased colour perception. Central vision is most commonly affected, though other visual field loss has also been described. Some individuals may be asymptomatic with abnormalities detected only by vision tests, hence most authorities recommend colour vision testing with Ishihara charts before and during ethambutol therapy. The drug should be stopped if there is any suggestion of toxicity; the effects are reversible in most but not all.

Hepatic toxicity is the most important serious anti-tuberculosis drug-related adverse event and is more common in old age, malnutrition, alcoholism, HIV infection and chronic hepatitis B and C infection. It generally occurs in the first month of therapy and many physicians will monitor liver function tests weekly for the first 2–3 weeks of therapy. The drugs may need to be stopped or reduced to prevent hepatic failure, but it is uncertain when this should be done. Low-grade liver enzyme abnormalities are extremely common following the start of therapy and most resolve spontaneously. Some authorities recommend stopping isoniazid, rifampicin and pyrazinamide immediately if the serum transaminases rise above five times normal, or if the bilirubin rises above normal. Others recommend stopping isoniazid alone if the transaminases rise above three times normal and stopping all drugs if serum albumin falls or the prothrombin time increases. There is a striking lack of evidence for most of these statements. In most forms of tuberculosis a short period without treatment does not affect outcome, but treatment interruptions are an independent risk factor for death from tuberculous meningitis. Therefore, for meningitis and other severe forms of tuberculosis the threshold for stopping should probably be higher and other drugs, not liable to cause hepatitis (e.g. streptomycin, ethambutol, moxifloxacin), should be started if rifampicin and/or isoniazid cannot be given.[48]

A randomized controlled trial of gradual versus immediate reintroduction of the standard drug regimen following drug-induced hepatitis in pulmonary tuberculosis reported significantly fewer hepatitis recurrences when the drugs were reintroduced gradually.[118] Importantly, pyrazinamide was omitted from the former, but not the latter, treatment group, suggesting this drug may be responsible for recurring hepatitis.

The WHO do not recommend a threshold for AST/ALT above which anti-tuberculosis drugs should be stopped, but advise stopping all drugs if there is clinical evidence of hepatitis (nausea, vomiting, abdominal pain, jaundice).[113] They suggest re-introducing drugs one at a time: first rifampicin, then isoniazid, then pyrazinamide. If the hepatitis was a severe reaction and the patient tolerates the two most active agents, rifampicin and isoniazid, then many physicians would not re-introduce the pyrazinamide, but prefer to treat for longer (at least 12 months) with the other agents.

ADJUNCTIVE CORTICOSTEROIDS

Ever since tuberculosis became a treatable disease in the late 1940s, it has been recognized that response to antimicrobial therapy is slow and that the disease and its consequences result from a persistent inflammatory response. Equally long-standing is the related hypothesis that adjunctive corticosteroids will attenuate the inflammatory response and so improve clinical outcomes. It is an attractive hypothesis, but it has eluded many attempts to prove it correct.

The first trials of adjunctive corticosteroids were performed in the early 1950s for the treatment of tuberculous meningitis. These studies were too small to confirm or refute a beneficial clinical effect, but they indicated corticosteroids depressed the inflammatory response within the CSF and might speed recovery. It would take a further 50 years before these early promising results were supported by data from adequately powered trials.

TABLE 40.10 **Adjunctive Corticosteroid Regimens Used in the Treatment of Tuberculous Meningitis and Associated with Improved Outcome**

Trial Setting and Year of Publication	Egypt (1991)	South Africa (1997)	Vietnam (2004)	
Number of subjects	280	141	545	
Age of subjects	Children and adults. 60% <14 years (median 8 years)	<14 years	>14 years	
MRC Grade	All grades	Grade II and III	Grade I	Grade II and III
Drug	Dexamethasone	Prednisolone	Dexamethasone	Dexamethasone
Time	Dose/route	Dose/route	Dose/route	Dose/route
Week 1	12 mg/day IM (8 mg/day if <25 kg)	4 mg/kg/day[b]	0.3 mg/kg/day IV	0.4 mg/kg/day IV
Week 2	12 mg/day IM (8 mg/day if <25 kg)	4 mg/kg/day	0.2 mg/kg/day IV	0.3 mg/kg/day IV
Week 3	12 mg/day IM (8 mg/day if <25 kg)	4 mg/kg/day	0.1 mg/kg/day oral	0.2 mg/kg/day IV
Week 4	Reducing over 3 weeks to stop[a]	4 mg/kg/day	3 mg total/day oral	0.1 mg/kg/day IV
Week 5		Reducing dose to stop[c]	Reducing by 1 mg each week	4 mg total/day oral
Week 6				Reducing by 1 mg each week

[a]Dexamethasone tapered to stop over 3 weeks: exact regimen not published. [b]Route of administration not published. [c]Prednisolone tapered to stop over unspecified time: regimen not published.

Two key trials performed in South African children[119] and Vietnamese adults[120] provided the strongest evidence to date that adjunctive corticosteroids (either prednisolone or dexamethasone) improve survival from tuberculous meningitis. The most recent Cochrane meta-analysis of all trial data concluded corticosteroids reduce death and disability from tuberculous meningitis and should be given to children and adults with the disease.[121] Whether HIV-infected patients with tuberculous meningitis benefit from adjunctive corticosteroid remains uncertain, but there is no evidence these patients are harmed by this intervention. The relative effectiveness of different corticosteroid regimens has not been studied, but the regimens used in the trials which have demonstrated benefit are given in Table 40.10. The WHO and IDSA recommend adjunctive corticosteroids for all patients with tuberculous meningitis.[112,113]

Whether adjunctive corticosteroids improve outcome in patients with other forms of tuberculosis has been hard to confirm. Two trials published in the *Lancet* in the late 1980s examined whether corticosteroids reduced the need for open drainage in effusive percarditis[122] or surgical pericardectomy for constrictive pericarditis.[123] The trials found adjunctive prednisolone (60 mg/day for 4 weeks, reducing to stop over next 7 weeks) reduced the need for drainage but had no impact on the need for pericardectomy. A 10-year follow-up of the patients enrolled in these trials found that the prednisolone group had lower all-cause mortality.[124] A single trial has been published examining whether prednisolone benefitted HIV-infected patients with tuberculous pericarditis and found that the effusion resolved faster and fewer patients died in the corticosteroid arm.[125] The WHO and IDSA recommend all patients with tuberculous pericarditis should be given adjunctive corticosteroids, although they acknowledge the benefit may be most apparent in those with effusive disease.

For all other forms of tuberculosis, there is insufficient evidence to recommend the routine use of adjunctive corticosteroids. In general, trials in pulmonary and pleural tuberculosis have suggested patients' symptoms may resolve faster with the addition of corticosteroids but there is no effect on longer-term outcomes. Consistent with the data for pericarditis, it appears that corticosteroids may reduce the symptoms associated with acute inflammation and effusions, but have no impact on the longer-term fibrotic complications. There are anecdotal data which indicate corticosteroids improve survival in those with severe disseminated tuberculosis with adult respiratory distress syndrome (ARDS) and many physicians use them in this circumstance. In addition, corticosteroids are probably effective at reducing the size of tuberculous lymph nodes or relieving airway obstruction during endobronchial tuberculosis.

DRUG-RESISTANT TUBERCULOSIS

M. tuberculosis resistant to isoniazid and/or streptomycin is the most frequently encountered resistance pattern worldwide, present in up to 40% of isolates in some populations. Isolated streptomycin resistance rarely impacts on outcome because the other agents counter its effect and streptomycin has been largely superseded by ethambutol in first-line treatment.

Isoniazid resistance, however, probably does reduce the effectiveness of conventional first-line regimens and warrants changes in the treatment, although there are limited data on the effectiveness of alternative regimens. The picture is complicated by low- and high-level isoniazid resistance among strains. Standard isoniazid dosing (5 mg/kg) result in plasma concentrations which easily exceed the minimal inhibitory concentration of bacteria with low-level isoniazid resistance and the impact on clinical outcome is probably minimal. High-level resistance is far more likely to have a detrimental impact on clinical outcome and some adjustment of the standard regimen is probably required. The WHO recommends three-times-weekly regimens should be avoided in all those with isoniazid resistance because there is evidence that the risk of acquiring additional rifampicin resistance is higher if intermittent regimens are used.[113] The IDSA recommends using rifampicin, ethambutol and pyrazinamide throughout the continuation phase of treatment for isoniazid-resistant tuberculosis.[112] Limited evidence suggests there is no need to extend treatment beyond 6 months if this regimen is used; some experts extend treatment to 9 months in these circumstances. For example, guidelines

TABLE 40.11 Potential Regimens for the Treatment of Tuberculosis Caused by Drug-Resistant Organisms

Pattern of Resistance	IDSA Recommendation	UK NICE Recommendation	Comments
Isoniazid ± streptomycin	6REZ ± Fluoroquinolone (if severe disease)	2RZSE/7RE (if susceptible to S) *OR* 2RZE/10RE	Studies suggest limited impact of isoniazid resistance on outcome as long as pyrazinamide used for 6 months. Fluoroquinolones may improve outcome in severe disease, e.g. meningitis
Rifampicin monoresistance	9HZE+ injectable agent *OR* 12HZE	2HZE/16HE	Injectable agent, e.g. streptomycin or amikacin, or a fluoroquinolone, for first 2 months may improve outcomes in more severe disease
Isoniazid + rifampicin (MDR)	6ZE (if not resistant) + fluoroquinolone + injectable agent + another agent (see Table 40.12) Stop injectable at least 4 months after culture conversion	As for IDSA	Regimens should be tailored to individual susceptibility patterns when possible. Intensive phase of 6 months with an injectable agent, followed by 12–18 months continuation phase with at least 3 agents. Surgery should be considered
Isoniazid + rifampicin + fluoroquinolone + injectable agent (XDR)	At least 5 drugs tailored to susceptibility tests with at least one injectable (e.g. capreomycin) and a 4th generation fluoroquinolone (e.g. moxifloxacin)	As for IDSA	As for MDR

Based on the recommendations made by the IDSA and UK NICE.
R, rifampicin; H, isoniazid; Z, pyrazinamide; E, ethambutol. Number preceding, number of months of treatment with drug combination.

published in the UK recommend 9–12 months of treatment with rifampicin/ethambutol in the continuation phase.[126] Table 40.11 summarizes the potential treatment regimens for drug-resistant tuberculosis.

Patients with multi-drug-resistant tuberculosis (MDR-TB) (defined as resistance to *at least* rifampicin and isoniazid) are considered incurable with conventional regimens and, until recently, were left untreated in many countries. Extremely drug-resistant tuberculosis (XDR) (defined as resistance to *at least* rifampicin and isoniazid *and* a fluoroquinolone *and* an injectable agent) is an increasing problem and even harder to treat. A panel of other 'second-line' anti-tuberculosis drugs are used in these circumstances (see Table 40.12), but they are generally less effective than the first-line drugs, are associated with greater toxicity and the regimens have not been subject to any randomized controlled clinical trials. A meta-analysis of 33 cohort studies including data from more than 8000 cases of MDR tuberculosis showed that overall treatment success was 62% (95% confidence intervals 58–67%).[127]

Despite the lack of controlled-trial data, widely accepted principles underpin the treatment of MDR/XDR tuberculosis in both children and adults.[128,129] They are as follows: use at least

TABLE 40.12 Group Classification of Second-Line Drugs Used to Treat MDR Tuberculosis and Their Important Adverse Reactions

Group	Drugs	Daily Dose (adults)	Important Adverse Reactions
1. First-line oral agents: use both if possible	Pyrazinamide	30 mg/kg	Hepatitis
	Ethambutol	15–25 mg/kg	Optic neuritis
2. Injectable agents: use one	Kanamycin	15 mg/kg	Ototoxicity and nephrotoxicity
	Amikacin	15 mg/kg	Ototoxicity and nephrotoxicity
	Capreomycin	15 mg/kg	Ototoxicity and nephrotoxicity
	Streptomycin	15 mg/kg	Ototoxicity and nephrotoxicity
3. Fluoroquinolones: use one	Moxifloxacin	7.5–10 mg/kg	
	Levofloxacin	15 mg/kg	
4. Oral bacteriostatic second-line agents: if <4 agents used from groups 1–3 add at least 2 from this group (at least 5 drugs in total)	Para-aminosalicylic acid	150 mg/kg	Nausea, hypothyroidism
	Cycloserine/Terizidone	15 mg/kg	Psychosis/low mood
	Ethionamide	15 mg/kg	Nausea and vomiting
	Protionamide	15 mg/kg	Nausea and vomiting
5. Agents with an unclear role: only use if <4 drugs from all other groups	Clofazimine	100 mg	Nausea, vomiting, skin discolouration
	Linezolid	600 mg twice daily	Thrombocytopenia, neuropathy
	Amoxicillin/clavulanate	875/125 twice daily	Hypersensitivity, diarrhoea
	Thioacetazone	150 mg	Rash/severe hypersensitivity
	Imipenem/cilastatin	500–1000 mg four times daily	Rash, diarrhoea, seizures
	High-dose isoniazid	10–15 mg/kg	Confusion, seizures, neuropathy
	Clarithromycin	500 mg twice daily	Diarrhoea

four drugs certain to be effective; do not use drugs for which there is a possibility of cross-resistance, e.g. rifabutin/rifampicin; and do not use unsafe drugs or drugs of uncertain provenance. The drugs are chosen from five groups (Table 40.12) in a hierarchical selection process, with the most active (in groups 1–3) chosen first. Tailor the regimen according to the results of susceptibility tests. For regimens containing fewer than four drugs from groups 1–4; use at least two from group 5. Sometimes as many as seven drugs are needed, particularly if treating XDR tuberculosis. Whenever possible, seek expert help when treating MDR/XDR tuberculosis.

Treatment of MDR/XDR tuberculosis takes 18–24 months. The intensive phase is defined by the duration of injectable agent and should last at least 6 months, or at least 4 months after bacteria can no longer be cultured from the sputum conversion. Close monitoring is required during treatment of MDR/XDR tuberculosis to ensure adherence, manage adverse reactions to the drugs (Table 40.11) and document response to therapy. Patients often require substantial medical and psychological support to help them complete 18–24 months of daily therapy. The continuation phase should last at least 18 months after culture conversion. Surgery may be helpful when the disease is sufficiently localized and less than four drugs are available.

NEW DRUGS AGAINST TUBERCULOSIS

The discovery of new drugs against tuberculosis faltered after the introduction of rifampicin in 1963. For the next two decades, the anti-tuberculosis drug arsenal was considered well-stocked, the disease was being successfully treated worldwide, resistance was not believed to be a major problem and the impetus to develop new drugs slowed to a stop. The complacency of this approach was rudely exposed in the late 1980s and early 1990s by the emergence of HIV, the rise of MDR *M. tuberculosis* and the realization that current diagnostic and treatment strategies would not bring the burgeoning global tuberculosis epidemic under control.

The situation invigorated governments and funding agencies, leading to substantial increases in tuberculosis research funding and, in particular, renewed efforts to find novel anti-tuberculosis agents. As a result, the once-dry anti-tuberculosis drug pipeline now contains a trickle of new agents.[130] The drugs which have reached clinical testing are summarized in Table 40.13. Some of the agents – rifapentine and the fluoroquinolones – are in phase III testing and the results of large randomized controlled trials defining their role in standard therapy (e.g. the REMOX TB trial and OFLOTUB studies) will be available by mid-2014. Others – TMC207 (bedaquiline) and OPC-67683 (delamanid) – have reached phase II testing, but data from controlled trials examining their efficacy in the treatment of MDR suggest both these agents have considerable promise.[131,132] These drugs have novel mechanisms of action and retain their activity against MDR *M. tuberculosis*. There is, therefore, grounds for cautious optimism that anti-microbial chemotherapy will remain a highly effective intervention against tuberculosis, but it is tempered by the difficulty of defining the role of new agents within multi-drug combinations for a disease in which clinical success is best measured a year or more after the start of treatment. It may be another decade before we know the full value of TMC207 and OPC-67683. The role of agents just entering the pipeline will not become apparent for many years after that, unless innovative trial designs and accurate early biomarkers of treatment success are developed.

SURGERY FOR TUBERCULOSIS

Surgery was a major component of the treatment of pulmonary tuberculosis before the advent of chemotherapy. Various techniques were used to collapse affected parts of the lungs, the theory being that collapse reduced the oxygenation of the tissue which was detrimental to the bacteria. Highly effective drug treatments rendered these procedures rapidly redundant and for many years, thoracic surgery was not required for the treatment of pulmonary tuberculosis. MDR/XDR tuberculosis has forced a reappraisal of the role of surgery in therapy.[133] The aim of surgery is to remove a large, focal burden of heavily infected, necrotic lung tissue. The indications for surgical resection in MDR/XDR tuberculosis are based on expert opinion and observational studies. They are as follows:

- Persistently positive smear or culture despite best available anti-tuberculosis chemotherapy
- High risk of relapse (based on drug resistance profile and severity of disease)
- Localized lesion amenable to resection
- Complication of tuberculosis, including localized bronchiectasis, empyema and aspergilloma
- Sufficient drug treatment available to enable postoperative healing/cure
- Sufficient cardiopulmonary reserve to tolerate lung resection.

In some patients with XDR-TB, there may be insufficient active drugs and surgery may be the only hope of cure. The preoperative work-up should include chest radiography and CT to precisely define the extent of the disease and to plan the surgical procedure; bronchoscopy is often used to rule out endobronchial tuberculosis, contralateral disease and malignancy. Lung function tests and echocardiography are performed to assess cardiorespiratory reserve. A muscle-sparing posterolateral thoracotomy is the most frequent surgical approach with subsequent pneumonectomy, lobectomy, segmentectomy and wedge resection all described. The surgeon must balance removal of sufficient diseased lung against the preservation of adequate postoperative pulmonary reserve. Controversy surrounds the need for bronchial-stump reinforcement to prevent bronchopulmonary fistula formation; many surgeons perform restricted dissection of the peribronchial tissue to promote bronchial stump healing. The most common complications of surgery are prolonged air leak, empyema with or without bronchopulmonary fistula, bronchopulmonary fistula alone, infection, bleeding and respiratory insufficiency. Success rates from case series vary considerably, but rates of postoperative culture conversion (from positive to negative) and a generally favourable outcome were reported in 50–100% of cases.[133]

There has been a long-standing role for surgery in other forms of tuberculosis, most notably tuberculous meningitis and pericarditis. Obstructive hydrocephalus is a common complication of tuberculous meningitis and requires the urgent placement of a ventricular–peritoneal shunt.[48] Communicating hydrocephalus may be initially managed with diuretics (furosemide and acetazolamide) but if these fail, a shunt is required. Corticosteroids do not appear to influence the incidence or progression of tuberculous meningitis-associated hydrocephalus.

TABLE 40.13 New Drugs Against Tuberculosis Currently in Clinical Testing

Drug	Class	Mechanism of Action	Stage of Clinical Testing	Comment
Rifapentine	Rifamycin	Inhibits bacterial protein synthesis	Phase III	Half-life 10–15 h (rifampicin is 2–3 h). Trials published >10 years ago showed once weekly dose associated with relapse and development of rifamycin resistance (especially in HIV-infected). Recent trial (published 2011) suggests 3 months weekly rifapentine + isoniazid is effective treatment for latent tuberculosis.
Moxifloxacin	Fluoroquinolone	Inhibits bacterial DNA replication	Phase III	Phase II RCT showed moxifloxacin sterilized sputum faster if used instead of ethambutol, but not if replaced isoniazid. REMOX TB – a global phase III study – investigates whether moxifloxacin can shorten standard therapy to 4 months; it will report in 2014.
Gatifloxacin	Fluoroquinolone	Inhibits bacterial DNA replication	Phase III	Reports of associated dysglycaemia have hampered its development (it is no longer licensed in many markets). However, may be just as effective as moxifloxacin. Large phase III RCT (OFLOTUB study) will complete shortly, which will determine whether gatifloxacin can reduce standard therapy to 4 months.
TMC 207 (Bedaquiline)	Diarylquinoline	Inhibits bacterial ATP synthase	Phase II	Potent bactericidal activity. Phase II RCT in MDR tuberculosis showed it significantly enhanced sterilizing activity over first 8 weeks of conventional treatment.
OPC-67683 (Delamanid)	Nitroimidazopyran	Uncertain. May inhibit synthesis of cell wall ketomycolates and may inhibit bacterial respiration by donating nitric oxide during enzymatic nitro-reduction	Phase II	MIC 10× lower than related drug PA-824. Uncertain, yet, whether this translates into greater clinical efficacy. Recent phase II RCT in MDR tuberculosis demonstrated it significantly enhanced 8-week sputum sterilization when added to conventional regimen.
PA-824	Nitroimidazopyran	Uncertain: similar to OPC-67683.	Phase I	Limited human data; early bactericidal activity studies suggest dose escalation beyond 200 mg/day does not improve activity and higher doses associated with renal impairment.
Linezolid	Oxazolidinone	Inhibit protein synthesis	Phase II	Low MIC against *M. tuberculosis* (0.125–1.0 µg/mL); therefore often used off-label in treatment of MDR tuberculosis. Side-effects (bone marrow suppression, optic/peripheral neuropathy) limits long-term use.
PNU-100480 (Sutezolid)	Oxazolidinone	Inhibit protein synthesis	Phase I	Hopefully, less toxic than linezolid. Human data currently limited to safety and tolerability and pharmacokinetic studies.
AZD-5847 (Posizolid)	Oxazolidinone	Inhibit protein synthesis	Phase I	Hopefully, less toxic than linezolid. Human data currently limited to safety and tolerability and pharmacokinetic studies.
SQ109	1,2-ethylenediamine (Ethambutol analogue)	Inhibits cell-wall formation by inhibition of trehalose monophosphate transferase	Phase I	No cross-resistance with ethambutol. Currently undergoing safety and tolerability studies.

Surgical intervention may also be required for the treatment of tuberculous pericarditis. The role of routine pericardiotomy at the outset was studied in a trial of 122 adults randomized to open complete pericardiotomy, or as required percutaneous pericardiocentesis.[122] Open pericardiotomy did not significantly reduce the need for subsequent pericardectomy for constriction, nor did it reduce the risk of death. Constrictive pericarditis occurs in 20–50% of patients with effusive tuberculous pericarditis, despite anti-tuberculosis drugs or adjunctive corticosteroids. Open surgical pericardectomy is indicated for all patients with calcific constrictive pericarditis, or those with on-calcific constriction with persistent or worsening constriction despite 6–8 weeks of anti-tuberculosis treatment.[134]

Vertebral tuberculosis (Pott's disease) can result in cord compression requiring urgent surgical decompression. Whether surgery benefits a wider group of patients with vertebral tuberculosis has been the subject of on-going controversy. A Cochrane meta-analysis of all available trial data up to 2005 (331 patients in total randomized within two trials) concluded there was no evidence routine surgery helped improve long-term outcomes.[135] However, surgery may be require if there is large abscess formation or there is severe kyphosis (>60°), or the kyphosis is likely to heal leading to severe deformity. Some authorities recommend children younger than 7 years with three or more affected vertebral bodies in the dorsal or dorsolumbar spine are likely to have progressive kyphosis and surgical correction is required.[54]

HIV-ASSOCIATED TUBERCULOSIS

Patients co-infected with HIV and *M. tuberculosis* present special problems in clinical management. Adverse drug events are more common and standard regimens may be less efficacious. In particular, regimens that do not contain rifampicin have a high frequency of failure and relapse.[136] Antiretroviral therapy introduces new problems when used in combination with anti-tuberculosis drugs: many antiretroviral drugs interact with the rifamycins and immune reconstitution following the start of antiretroviral therapy can cause paradoxical clinical worsening of tuberculosis.

As advised by the WHO, the priorities in the management of HIV-associated tuberculosis are to treat the tuberculosis, give *Pneumocystis jiroveci* prophylaxis with co-trimoxazole and start HAART.[113] HIV-infected patients should receive daily treatment with a rifamycin-based anti-tuberculosis drug regimen whenever possible.[137] Less frequently administered regimens, especially those given twice weekly, have been associated with the development of rifamycin resistance in those with CD4 cells <100/μL and should be avoided. Those with drug-susceptible tuberculosis should receive the same 6-month regimen as recommended for HIV-uninfected patients. Some experts believe those with advanced HIV infection and extensive tuberculosis should receive longer than 6 months, but supportive data are lacking. A 9–12-month regimen is recommended for the treatment of central nervous system tuberculosis.[48]

Drug interactions and adverse reactions require careful consideration in HIV-infected patients. Rifampicin interacts with protease inhibitors (PIs), non-nucleoside reverse transcriptase inhibitors (NNRTIs), chemokine (C-C motif) receptor 5 (CCR5) antagonists and antimicrobials such as fluconazole. Rifabutin is a less potent inducer of hepatic CYP450 and may be used as an alternative to overcome some of these difficulties. A summary of the important interactions between rifamycins and the agents of HAART is provided in Table 40.14. Rash, fever and hepatitis are common side effects of anti-tuberculosis drugs, NNRTIs and co-trimoxazole and can, therefore, lead to difficult management decisions. Determining the cause of the reaction may be impossible without serial withdrawal of the individual drugs. The NRTIs ddI and d4T both cause peripheral

TABLE 40.14 Summary of the Important Interactions Between Rifamycins and Antiretroviral Drugs

Antiretroviral Class	Combination	Comments
Non-nucleoside reverse transcriptase inhibitors (NRTIs)	Rifampicin + efavirenz	Rifampicin causes a 20–30% reduction in efavirenz concentrations. The preferred combination of many authorities. Use efavirenz 800 mg/day if >60 kg; 600 mg/day if <60 kg. If possible, measure efavirenz plasma concentrations after 2 weeks.
	Rifampicin + nevirapine	Widely used combination in resource-poor settings, although nevirapine concentrations reduced by 20–50% by rifampicin. May need to increase nevirapine dose, but increased risk of nevirapine hypersensitivity. If possible, define dose by measuring drug concentrations.
	Rifabutin + efavirenz	Efavirenz induces metabolism of rifabutin: increase rifabutin dose to 450 mg/day
	Rifabutin + nevirapine	Can probably be given together without alteration of dose of either drug. Nevaripine may increase concentrations of rifabutin by up to 20%; may be increased risk of rifabutin toxicity
Protease inhibitors (PIs)	Rifampicin + unboosted PI	Do not use. Rifampicin causes 75–95% reduction in concentration of PIs, with exception of ritonavir.
	Rifampicin + boosted PI	Not recommended because of complexity of interaction and increased hepatic toxicity
	Rifabutin + unboosted PI	Reduce rifabutin to 150 mg daily and increase dose of unboosted PI
	Rifabutin + boosted PI	Ritonavir boosts concentration of other PI and inhibits metabolism of rifabutin. Reduce rifabutin to 150 mg three times a week
Integrase inhibitors	Rifampicin + elvitegravir	Do not use
	Rifampicin + raltegravir	Rifampicin reduces trough concentrations of raltegravir by 60%. Best avoided if other combinations available.
	Rifabutin + elvitegravir	Do not use
	Rifabutin + raltegravir	Current limited data suggest both drugs can be used together at standard doses.
Entry inhibitors	Rifampicin + maraviroc	Maraviroc concentrations reduced by rifampicin; may need to double dose of maraviroc, especially if used with efavirenz
	Rifampicin + enfuvirtide	Not recommended.
	Rifabutin + maraviroc	No predicted clinically significant interaction: use standard doses of both drugs
	Rifabutin + enfuvirtide	No data. Not recommended

Based on the British HIV Association 2011 guidelines.

neuropathy, with additive toxicity when used with isoniazid. All patients taking HAART and isoniazid should take preventative daily 10 mg pyridoxine.

The WHO recommends that the first-line HAART regimen contains one non-nucleoside reverse transcriptase inhibitor (NNRTI) and two nucleoside reverse transcriptase inhibitors (NRTIs). These drugs are efficacious, relatively inexpensive, have generic and fixed-dose formulations, do not require a cold chain and preserve the protease inhibitors for second-line regimens. The WHO recommends either efavirenz or nevirapine as the NNRTI, although the use of rifampicin/nevirapine has been associated with increased likelihood of virological failure when compared with rifampicin/efavirenz. For this reason, most physicians prefer efavirenz over nevirapine for rifampicin-based tuberculosis treatment. However, because of concerns related to teratogenicity, efavirenz should not be used in women of child-bearing potential without adequate contraception, nor should it be used for women who are in the first trimester of pregnancy. Nevirapine can be used in pregnancy. The WHO's preferred NRTI backbone is zidovudine (AZT) or tenofovir disoproxil fumarate, combined with either lamivudine (3TC) or emtricitabine (FTC). The NRTIs do not have clinically significant interactions with rifampicin or rifabutin.

If a boosted protease inhibitor is required to treat HIV, a rifabutin-based anti-tuberculosis regimen is recommended. If rifabutin is not available, the use of rifampicin and a boosted antiretroviral regimen containing lopinavir or saquinavir with additional ritonavir dosing is recommended, but this regimen should be closely monitored and is only recommend if other combinations are unavailable.

The timing of HAART initiation in those who present with tuberculosis has been the subject of debate for some years. Three landmark randomized controlled trials were published in October 2011 addressing this question.[138–140] These trials found the initiation of HAART early in treatment (within 2 weeks) reduced mortality, especially in those with the most advanced disease (CD4 count <50 cells/μL). Early HAART was associated with an increased incidence of IRIS, although this was rarely life-threatening. A single-centre trial from Vietnam examined the same question but only in those with tuberculous meningitis and found early HAART did not confer any benefit on mortality but was instead associated with an increased risk of adverse events.[141] Therefore, the current data suggest HIV-infected patients with pulmonary tuberculosis probably benefit from starting HAART within 2 weeks of starting anti-tuberculosis treatment, particularly if they have advanced immune suppression. The benefit may not extend to other forms of tuberculosis.

Finally, as discussed above, those starting HAART are at risk of IRIS. Evidence from one randomized controlled trial has suggested adjunctive prednisolone speeds recovery from IRIS.[70] A total of 110 patients were randomized to 4 weeks of prednisolone (1.5 mg/kg per day for 2 weeks then 0.75 mg/kg per day for 2 weeks) or placebo; those given prednisolone were discharged from hospital faster and their symptoms resolved quicker. There are anecdotal reports supporting the use of other agents, including non-steroidal anti-inflammatory drugs, pentoxifylline, montelukast, thalidomide and hydroxychloroquine.[142] Recurrent aspiration of abscesses/lymph nodes can also be useful in selected patients. Interrupting HAART may be necessary in those with life-threatening IRIS, but should be avoided when possible.

Prevention

BCG VACCINE

More than 100 million people receive the live-attenuated Bacillus Calmette–Guérin (BCG) vaccine each year. The vaccine was created by Albert Calmette and Camille Guérin working at the Institute Pasteur in Lille, France, more than 90 years ago. It was first administered in 1921 and since then its efficacy in preventing tuberculosis has been evaluated by many clinical trials in different parts of the world. These trials have demonstrated that BCG confers consistent protection against disseminated tuberculosis in infants and, in particular, tuberculous meningitis.[138] BCG also provides protection against leprosy.

The protective effect of BCG against pulmonary tuberculosis, however, is highly variable. Meta-analysis of trial data has found BCG provides, on average, around 50% protection from all forms of tuberculosis, but the figure varies from none at all to around 80% protection.[143] The degree of protection appears to fall with proximity to the equator, an observation attributed to prior exposure to environmental non-tuberculous mycobacterial species. Such exposure may reduce BCG's effectiveness by a number of mechanisms; they include inducing a level of protective immunity that BCG cannot further enhance; effectively 'vaccinating' against BCG and preventing its replication and successful 'immunization'; and, possibly, inducing a tissue-damaging immune response to *M. tuberculosis* that BCG vaccination is unable to attenuate. Other factors, such as genetic variation between strains of the vaccine, may also account for the varied efficacy of BCG.

BCG is given by intradermal injection or, in neonates, percutaneously by means of multi-puncture devices. Complications, such as abscess formation, may follow the accidental administration by deep cutaneous or intramuscular injection, or the intradermal injection of vaccine prepared for percutaneous use, which contains many more bacilli than the intradermal preparation.

Normally, BCG vaccination causes a small papule to develop within 10–14 days; in some cases a shallow ulcer forms but usually heals within 6–12 weeks. At least 3 months should elapse between BCG vaccination and administration of yellow fever, measles, rubella, mumps and smallpox vaccines and no vaccination should be given in the same arm for 4 months.

BCG vaccination is safe, if properly given, and complications are uncommon. Local adverse reactions usually occur at a rate of 0.1–0.5/1000 and serious, disseminated complications occur at a rate of less than one in a million. Local complications include necrotic lesions due to excessive delayed hypersensitivity reactions, subcutaneous abscesses, lymphadenopathy (mostly axillary) and keloid scar formation. Hypersensitivity reactions usually occur within a few days of vaccination and are more frequent in revaccinated subjects and in those who are tuberculin-positive. The risk of keloid scarring is reduced by giving the injection in the skin overlying the insertion of the deltoid muscle. Injections higher up the arm are much more likely to lead to keloid scarring. Local abscesses usually appear between 1 and 5 months after vaccination or even later. Lymphadenopathy occurs in the drainage area of the vaccinated site, usually the axilla, although cervical lymphadenopathy may occur if the vaccine is given in the upper deltoid region. Transient lymphadenopathy is common after percutaneous vaccination of neonates. Disseminated BCG disease is a very rare complication of BCG vaccination with a high mortality. It tends to occur in severely immune-suppressed children, either with advanced HIV infection or an occult congenital immune-deficiency. Genetic mutations in the IL-12/interferon-γ pathways have been strongly associated with disseminated environmental mycobacterial infection, including with BCG.[144]

Specific treatment may be required if the reactions are serious. Local hypersensitivity reactions usually resolve spontaneously and, although topical steroids are often prescribed, there is no clear evidence that they are effective. Local abscesses may resolve after aspiration, but if they recur, isoniazid, 6 mg/kg body weight daily to a maximum of 300 mg for 1 month is usually curative. Local lymphadenitis usually resolves spontaneously; antimicrobial therapy has little effect and surgery should only be used if the nodes are grossly enlarged or if there is suppuration and sinus formation. More serious disease, such as osteitis and disseminated infection, requires treatment with standard anti-tuberculosis therapy, although BCG, in common with all *M. bovis* strains, is innately resistant to pyrazinamide.

NEW VACCINES AGAINST TUBERCULOSIS

There is an urgent need for a better vaccine than BCG. To date, 12 new potential vaccines have entered early clinical testing.[145] Two different strategies have emerged: either to replace BCG with a new and improved vaccine, or to boost the protective effect of BCG.[146] An example of the first strategy is the vaccine candidate VMP 1002, which includes listeriolysis secretion to enhance antigenic escape from the phagolysosome and induce cross-priming of protective CD8 T-cells. This vaccine is currently being investigated in a phase IIa trial in South Africa.

Vaccines which employ the BCG 'booster' approach are a little further on in their clinical development. They can either be given immediately after BCG in infancy, or during adolescence when the protective immunity of neonatal BCG may be waning. These vaccines either induce immunity via protein-adjuvant conjugates, or through recombinant viral vectors. Examples of the former included M72 (being developed by Glaxo-Smith Kline) currently in phase IIa studies; and Hybrid I/HyVAC IV, a fusion protein created from ESAT6 and Ag85 which is currently in phase I testing. There are two recombinant viral vectors in phase II safety and efficacy testing. The Aeras 402/Ad35-85B-TB10.4 uses a replication deficient adenovirus to deliver the antigens Ag85A, Ag85B and TB10.4. This vaccine is currently undergoing phase II safety and efficacy testing in HIV-infected adults in South Africa. The Oxford modified vaccinia virus expressing Ag85A (MVA85A) is at a similar stage in development.

PREVENTING TUBERCULOSIS BY TREATING LATENT INFECTION

The identification and treatment of those with latent tuberculosis is an effective way to prevent active tuberculosis. Indeed, in the USA, where BCG vaccination is not used, it forms the basis for their tuberculosis control programme. In all patients, however, the risks of treatment (primarily hepatoxicity) must be judged against the benefits.

Randomized clinical trials have demonstrated treating latent tuberculosis reduces the risk of developing future active tuberculosis by at least 50%. The duration of this protective effect varies dependent upon the patient's likelihood of reinfection and progression to active disease. Protection for nearly 20 years has been reported in young, fit patients living in low tuberculosis prevalence regions, whereas protection may last only a few months in HIV-infected individuals living in tuberculosis-endemic regions with high transmission. Thus the treatment of latent tuberculosis infection in the USA is a far more effective tuberculosis control measure than in many parts of sub-Saharan Africa.

The major risk of treating latent infection is the development of drug-related hepatitis. Overall, the risk of severe hepatitis from 6-months isoniazid monotherapy is 0.3–0.5%. The risk increases with age, if more than one anti-tuberculosis drug is used, or the patient is co-infected with hepatitis B or C and/or HIV. Therefore, many authorities do not advocate the treatment of latent tuberculosis in adults over 35 years of age (except in high-risk groups) and combination therapy is not advised for HIV-infected individuals and for those with pre-existent liver disease.[147]

There are a number of different regimens used for the treatment of latent tuberculosis, all with equivalent efficacy. The most widely used is 6–9 months of daily isoniazid. The USA favours 9 months; the UK 6 months; neither regimen has been associated with increased isoniazid resistance. Much longer durations have been advocated in those repeatedly exposed to *M. tuberculosis*. Three months of rifampicin and isoniazid appears to be as effective as 6–9 months isoniazid in low tuberculosis prevalence settings and is more likely to be completed; but dual therapy is not recommended for those with HIV due to an increased risk of hepatitis and the potential for interactions with anti-retroviral drugs (see above). Six months of rifampicin monotherapy is also an effective regimen, especially when infection with isoniazid resistant *M. tuberculosis* is known or suspected.

For a while, the USA used a combination of isoniazid and pyrazinamide, but this resulted in a number of fatal hepatitis reactions and was withdrawn. Recently, trials have demonstrated the effectiveness and high rate of adherence and completion of a once-weekly regimen of isoniazid and rifapentine (a new, long-acting rifamycin) and recent guidance from the USA supports the use of this regimen in HIV-uninfected and -infected individuals.[148]

There are no recommended drug regimens for the treatment of suspected latent MDR tuberculosis. Other than those at very high risk of progression (e.g. infants and profoundly immune-suppressed adults), the recommended approach is 'watchful waiting': warn patients of the early symptoms of tuberculosis, perform follow-up chest X-rays and ensure they are investigated and appropriately treated if signs of disease occur. In those highly susceptible to developing active disease, early empirical therapy should be considered, with a regimen defined by the drug susceptibility of the contact's isolate.

Special care needs to be taken with young children in close contact with adults with infectious respiratory tuberculosis. For neonates, UK guidelines recommend giving 3 months of isoniazid immediately, then performing a skin test/IGRA.[126] If the skin test is positive (>6 mm), or the IGRA positive, the child should be investigated for active disease. If these tests are negative, the child should be given a further 3 months of isoniazid. For children aged 4 weeks to 2 years, the guidelines recommend starting isoniazid and arranging a skin test/IGRA, if the contact is close and prolonged. If these tests are positive, treat with isoniazid for 6 months unless there is evidence of active disease. If the skin test/IGRA is negative, re-test after 6 weeks. If it is still negative, stop the isoniazid and BCG vaccinate.

THE TREATMENT OF LATENT INFECTION IN HIV-INFECTED PATIENTS

A recent meta-analysis of 12 trials, including a total of 8578 randomized participants, examined the efficacy of treating latent tuberculosis in HIV-infected individuals.[149] Overall, preventive therapy was associated with a lower incidence of active tuberculosis (RR 0.68, 95% CI 0.54–0.85). This benefit was restricted to individuals with a positive tuberculin skin test (RR 0.38, 95% CI 0.25–0.57) and not found in those with a negative skin test (RR 0.89, 95% CI 0.64–1.24). Efficacy was similar for all regimens (regardless of drug type, frequency or duration of treatment). However, compared with isoniazid monotherapy, multi-drug regimens were much more likely to require discontinuation due to adverse effects. It is uncertain whether CD4 count influences response to latent tuberculosis therapy.[150]

While there is strong evidence that the treatment of latent tuberculosis prevents progression to active disease in HIV-infected individuals, there are many barriers to its implementation as a global tuberculosis control strategy. The requirement for a skin test prior to treatment represents a formidable obstacle for those tuberculosis control programmes with few resources. In addition, protection may last no longer than 2–4 years and it is unclear what should be done once protection ends. The degree of protection is also influenced by immune reconstitution by antiretroviral drugs. There are some data which indicate a combination of antiretroviral treatment and isoniazid may be more effective than either alone in controlling tuberculosis. Therefore, to be most effective, HIV and tuberculosis treatment programmes require coordinated delivery; this remains a distant goal for many countries.

PREVENTION OF TUBERCULOSIS IN HEALTHCARE WORKERS

Healthcare workers in tuberculosis-endemic regions are at high risk of contracting tuberculosis as they are subject to frequent and repeated exposure to *M. tuberculosis*. A prospective study of medical students and interns from Peru reported a 10–15-fold increased risk of developing active tuberculosis compared with the general population.[151] The risk of infection among healthcare workers is particularly high for those involved in aerosol-inducing procedures, such as induced sputum, bronchoscopy, intubation and autopsy.

Reducing exposure to tuberculosis in settings with few resources is challenging but a number of simple measures can reduce transmission. As discussed above, improved natural ventilation by opening windows and doors has been shown to substantially reduce tuberculosis transmission in clinics and wards. Such methods are most effective in older hospitals with large open wards, big windows and high ceilings. In addition, several reports have suggested that patients with suspected pulmonary tuberculosis should be encouraged to cough hygienically, dispose of tissue and sputum safely and wear a surgical mask.[152] Patients with drug-susceptible tuberculosis should be considered infectious until they have adhered to and completed 2 weeks of appropriate anti-tuberculosis therapy. Those with MDR-TB may be infectious for many weeks and should be considered so until bacteria are neither seen nor cultured from sputum.

Masks/respirators are effective at preventing tuberculosis transmission.[153] A simple surgical mask is reported to decrease the risk of contracting tuberculosis 2.4-fold, but will only provide protection for a few hours or until they get wet. A High Efficiency Particulate Air (HEPA) filter mask (FFP 2/3 or N95) reduces risk 17.5-fold; a cartridge respirator 45.5-fold; and Powered Air Purifying Respirators (that require electricity for charging and regular maintenance) 238-fold. FFP 2/3 and N95 masks are the most widely used and cost between US$1.5–4.5 per mask. They must be the correct size and be tightly fitted to be effective.

In the UK, current guidelines recommend that staff only need to wear facemasks if a patient has suspected or proven multi-drug-resistant tuberculosis or during aerosol-generating procedures.[126] In the USA the CDC, however, advise wearing N95 masks during any contact with patients with suspected tuberculosis, regardless of resistance.[112] It is impractical to apply these recommendations to settings with few resources and high prevalence of tuberculosis, although the use of surgical masks may represent an affordable alternative. Modelling studies that followed the recent XDR tuberculosis outbreak in South Africa concluded that hospital transmission of XDR tuberculosis could be reduced by improving natural ventilation, decreasing admissions of infectious patients or reducing their time spent as inpatients, staff wearing HEPA masks and coughing patients wearing surgical masks and more rapid testing and diagnosis.[154]

GLOBAL TUBERCULOSIS CONTROL MEASURES

Performance targets for the global control of tuberculosis were first formulated during the 44th World Health Assembly in 1991. They aimed for a case detection rate of at least 70% and a treatment cure rate of 85% by 2000; modelling suggested that if these goals were achieved there would be a 5–10% yearly decline in the prevalence and incidence of tuberculosis worldwide. In 1993, the WHO declared tuberculosis was a global emergency and launched the directly observed treatment, short course (DOTS) strategy for tuberculosis control. DOTS placed the detection and treatment of sputum-smear-positive, infectious cases of tuberculosis at the centre of the global WHO tuberculosis control programme for the next decade. Each country was required to perform a quarterly cohort analysis and report all their data each year to the WHO. Between 1995 and 2008 the global case detection rate of sputum-smear-positive tuberculosis rose from 15% to 61% and the treatment success rate from 77% to 87%, respectively. Over the same period, DOTS is estimated to have averted around 6 million deaths and cured around 36 million people from tuberculosis. However, it was also estimated that, in 2008, 39% (or 1.6 million people) of all smear-positive cases were not reported; only 7% with MDR-TB were detected and treated; and only 7% of those with TB/HIV received antiretroviral therapy. DOTS was failing as a global tuberculosis control measure because of rising HIV co-infection and the inability of many developing countries to deliver the strategy.

In 2006, in response to the worsening global tuberculosis epidemic, the new STOP TB Strategy and the Global Plan to Stop TB (2006–15) were launched. The goals of the Stop TB Partnership were to reduce the global burden of tuberculosis (prevalence and mortality) by 50% by 2015 compared with

1990 levels and eliminate tuberculosis as a public health problem by 2050. These ambitious aims were combined with the UN's Millennium Development Goal (MDG) 6, which was to halt and begin the reversal of national, regional and global tuberculosis incidence by 2015. The international community recognized that to achieve these ambitious targets would require a substantial increase in resources. Success would require a new focus on controlling the HIV-associated and drug-resistant tuberculosis epidemic and improving weak health systems and engagement with private healthcare providers and communities.[155] Further emphasis on HIV-associated tuberculosis was provided by the WHO's '3Is strategy': standing for 'Intensified case finding', 'Isoniazid preventive treatment' and 'Improved infection control'. Thus, the early identification and successful treatment of individual patients remained at the core of the control strategy, but its delivery would require dedicated health system strengthening with a special emphasis on the management of those infected with HIV.

Has there been any progress since the launch of these initiatives 5 years ago? According to WHO figures, the worldwide incidence of tuberculosis peaked in 2004; but it is falling by less than 1% per year. Globally, the absolute numbers of new tuberculosis cases began to fall from a peak in around 2006/2007 and tuberculosis mortality has been falling from a peak of around 3 million in the late 1990s. However, even if the Stop TB plan were to be implemented in full, it is estimated that the incidence of tuberculosis will still be 100 times the elimination target in 2050. Urgent action is needed by governments to properly fund their tuberculosis control programmes and for the wealthier nations to support these efforts. In addition, tuberculosis control would be greatly improved with an effective vaccine, a cheap point-of-care diagnostic test and substantially shorter treatment regimens. These remain elusive goals for researchers and, for the foreseeable future, the diagnosis and treatment of tuberculosis will remain an essential clinical skill for all doctors.

REFERENCES

9. Arnadottir T. Tuberculosis and Public Health. Policy and Principles in Tuberculosis Control. Paris: International Union Against Tuberculosis and Lung Disease; 2009.
14. WHO. Multi-drug and Extensively Drug Resistant Tuberculosis: 2010 Global Report on Surveillance and Response. Geneva: World Health Organization; 2011.
112. Treatment of tuberculosis. MMWR Recomm Rep 2003;52(RR-11):1–77.
113. WHO. The Treatment of Tuberculosis Guidelines. 4th ed. Geneva: World Health Organization; 2010.
137. Pozniak AL, Coyne KM, Miller RF, et al. British HIV Association guidelines for the treatment of TB/HIV coinfection 2011. HIV Med 2011; 12(9):517–24.

Access the complete references online at www.expertconsult.com.

41 Leprosy

STEPHEN L. WALKER | STEPHEN G. WITHINGTON | DIANA N. J. LOCKWOOD

KEY POINTS

- *Mycobacterium leprae* infection is curable.
- Most patients with leprosy are diagnosed clinically.
- Multi-drug therapy – rifampicin, dapsone and clofazimine – is freely available.
- Leprosy nerve damage is a major cause of disability.
- Early diagnosis with monitoring of nerve function is essential to minimize the disabling complications of leprosy.

Introduction

Leprosy is a chronic granulomatous disease caused by infection with *Mycobacterium leprae*. It is characterized by infection of skin and nerves and associated immunological damage. Nerve damage is responsible for repeated ulceration and paralysis affecting hands, feet and eyes. Globally, leprosy is an important cause of physical disabilities, affecting people in their most productive stage of life. The disability and related social stigma associated with leprosy and its complications result in significant barriers to full participation in society, and in considerable socioeconomic burden to those affected, and society as a whole.

Epidemiology

A total of 228 474 new cases of leprosy were reported to WHO in 2010, from 130 countries; the vast majority occurring in South and South-east Asia, South America and Africa. The countries that reported the most new cases were: India, Brazil, Indonesia, Democratic Republic of Congo, Ethiopia and Nigeria.[1]

The global registered prevalence of leprosy (the number of cases registered for treatment) has decreased markedly since 1985, when around 5.4 million were on treatment registers. Interpretation of prevalence and incidence trends is, however, complicated by significant reductions in the duration of treatment, the widespread updating of treatment registers, and large-scale public health campaigns. In addition, recent changes in health system management of leprosy, particularly the integration of leprosy into general health services in many countries, notably India, have necessitated a major simplification of guidelines for diagnosis and treatment, and a decreased focus on leprosy. Over 14 million people have been cured of leprosy since 1985; however, a significant proportion of these have ongoing disability as a result of leprosy-related nerve damage. An estimated 3 million people are living with leprosy-related physical impairments and disabilities and the associated stigma.

DISTRIBUTION

Leprosy occurs at all ages, with incidence rates peaking in young adulthood. Disability due to leprosy is associated with increasing age at diagnosis. Males are more commonly diagnosed with leprosy than women in many, though not all countries, often in the ratio of 2:1. Since the diagnosis of leprosy is highly sensitive to operational issues involved in case finding, decreased access for women to health information and health services needs to be considered as a possible explanation for the sex ratio observed. The development of clinical leprosy is associated with poverty, though it can affect people of every socioeconomic status. Leprosy had virtually disappeared from some historically endemic regions, such as Northern Europe, prior to the era of effective chemotherapy; the reasons for this are unclear.

INCIDENCE AMONG CONTACTS

Most newly diagnosed patients do not have a history of contact with an affected person and most of those in close contact with leprosy-affected people will not develop leprosy. Nevertheless, attack rates for contacts are higher than in the surrounding population, 5–10 times higher in contacts of multibacillary index cases (who have multiple lesions corresponding to more bacilli as in Figure 41.1), and 2–4 times higher in paucibacillary cases. There appears to be a gradient in susceptibility depending on how physically or socially close the contact is, along with a weak genetic effect that is independent of physical distance.[2]

TRANSMISSION

Mycobacterium leprae was first identified by Armauer Hansen in specimens from Norwegian patients in 1873.[3] Humans are the reservoir of *M. leprae*. People with untreated lepromatous leprosy may harbour billions of organisms per gram of tissue, which are shed from nasal mucosa. Non-lepromatous cases have a lower bacillary load located intracellularly. The carriage of *M. leprae* by healthy subjects in nasal mucosa may also play a role in the transmission of leprosy. Rates of population nasal carriage of *M. leprae* DNA based on PCR studies are much higher than registered prevalence rates of leprosy.[4] The natural occurrence of disease due to *M. leprae* in wild, nine-banded armadillos is associated with human disease in parts of the Americas.

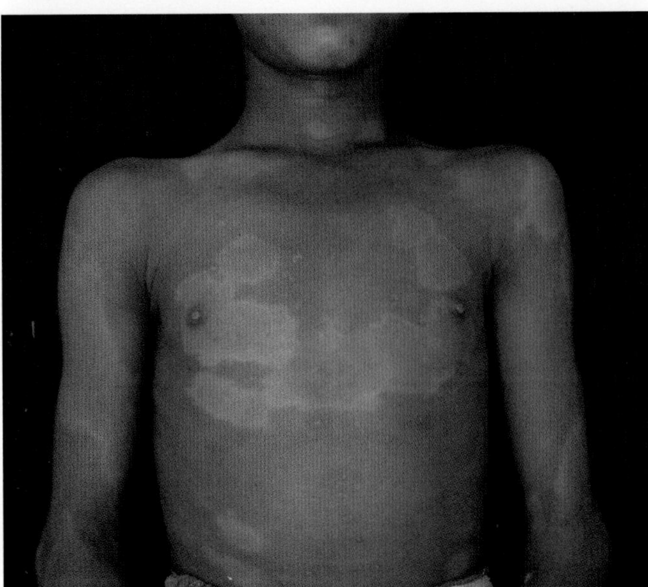

Figure 41.1 Multiple lesions of multibacillary leprosy.

PORTAL OF EXIT

Nasal secretions are believed to be the main portal of exit of *M. leprae*, while the role of desquamating skin is less certain. Large numbers of viable organisms can be detected in the nasal secretions of those with untreated lepromatous leprosy. By contrast, despite the presence of a large number of bacilli in deeper layers of the skin, it has generally proved difficult to detect acid-fast bacilli in desquamating epithelium of such patients, although Job and co-workers have reported *M. leprae* in more superficial layers.[5]

VIABILITY OUTSIDE THE HOST

M. leprae is known to survive for many days and possibly months under optimal conditions of high humidity and low sunlight.

PORTAL OF ENTRY

The portal of entry for *M. leprae* is uncertain but the only seriously considered sites are the upper respiratory tract and skin. Rees and McDougall succeeded in experimentally infecting immunodeficient mice through aerosols containing *M. leprae* and the nasal route is generally thought to be most important.[6] It is hypothesized that after a brief bacteraemic phase, the organism settles in the lymph node and from there migrates to the skin and nerves. Experimental models and clinical examples of transmission through the skin have, however, also been reported.[7]

INCUBATION PERIOD

The incubation period for leprosy is both difficult to define and extremely variable. The incubation period for tuberculoid leprosy varied between 2.9 and 5.3 years and between 9.3 and 11.6 years for lepromatous disease in US military personnel exposed for relatively short periods of time.[8,9] However, the incubation period has been as long as 30 years in other individuals.

HOST SUSCEPTIBILITY

Host susceptibility plays a significant role in the development of clinical leprosy. Various genes and regions in the human genome have been linked to or associated with susceptibility to leprosy per se or with a particular type of leprosy. These include HLA DR2 and the *Taq1* polymorphism of the vitamin D receptor gene, Alleles in the *PARK2* and *PACRG* region on chromosome 6 are associated with susceptibility to leprosy in Vietnamese and Brazilian patients.[10,11] PARK2 is expressed by both Schwann cells and macrophages. It is a ubiquination E3 ligase. However, this finding was not reproduced in a study of six single nucleotide polymorphisms in these regions in Indian patients.[12]

Microbiology

Mycobacterium leprae is an acid-fast bacillus closely resembling *Mycobacterium tuberculosis*. Organisms may be identified in stained biopsies, smears of nasal secretions or, more commonly, from slit-skin smears. Bacilli are occasionally present in large clumps known as globi. It is thought that only the few solid staining organisms are viable, while the vast majority of organisms, which show patchy staining and fragmented morphology, are non-viable. The proportion of solidly staining organisms (known as the Morphological Index or MI) is often around 4–5% in untreated lepromatous leprosy patients.

GROWTH CHARACTERISTICS

Mycobacterium leprae is extremely fastidious in regard to growth requirements and is yet to be successfully cultured on artificial media. It can be grown in laboratory mice using Shepard's hind footpad inoculation method. Antibiotic sensitivities are determined through the ability of the organism to grow in mice fed different concentrations of antibiotics. The organism generation time is extremely long, around 14 days on average, thus the determination of antibiotic sensitivity takes several months.

The nine-banded armadillo (*Dasypus novemcinctus*), in addition to being a natural host for *M. leprae*, has become the principal source of the organism for immunological and biochemical research. The animal's low body temperature makes for ideal incubation conditions for *M. leprae*.

GENOME

The genome of *M. leprae* in comparison with *M. tuberculosis* reveals an extreme case of reductive evolution. The genome of *M. leprae* is over 25% smaller than *M. tuberculosis*, amounting to a reduction of 1200 protein sequences. Less than half of the genome contains functional genes, and whole metabolic pathways together with their regulatory circuits have been eliminated.[13] This is likely to explain the organism's extreme generation time and inability to grow in vitro.

Pathogenesis

IMMUNOLOGY

The clinicopathological manifestations of leprosy are determined by the host immunological response to *M. leprae*. The natural history of leprosy is characterized by much higher rates of infection than clinical disease. A protective immune response

TABLE 41.1 Clinical and Immunological Spectrum of Leprosy

	Tuberculoid	Borderline	Lepromatous
Immunological Classification	(TT)	(BT) ↔ (BB) ↔ (BL)	(LL)
Cell-mediated immune response	Strong	Intermediate and unstable	Weak
Antibody production	Low or absent	Variable	Prominent
T cell and cytokine response	Th1 pattern		Th2 pattern
M. leprae presence in lesions	Not detected	Variable	Large numbers
Histological appearance	Epithelioid granulomas	Mixed	Foamy macrophages
Skin lesions	Few asymmetrical lesions, definite loss of sensation	Variable number and type of lesions	Usually many lesions, more symmetrical, less sensory loss in lesions
Leprosy reactions	Type 1 reactions may occur	Type 1 common; ENL less common	ENL reactions not uncommon

ENL, erythema nodosum leprosum.

in leprosy is dependent on cell-mediated immunity to kill *M. leprae*. Humoral antibodies are produced in response to various antigens of *M. leprae*, and are abundant in lepromatous leprosy but do not contribute to elimination of the organism. The ability to produce and develop cell-mediated immunity determines whether clinical leprosy develops, heals spontaneously or evolves into one of the clinico-pathological subtypes. With appropriate cell-mediated immune response, spontaneous resolution of early leprosy occurs. Single lesion leprosy typically resolves without treatment in the majority of cases.[14] Individuals who develop leprosy cell-mediated immunity are strong in tuberculoid leprosy but weak or absent in lepromatous leprosy (Table 41.1). Dendritic cells appear to be the most efficient antigen-presenting cells, and cell membrane antigens from *M. leprae* may be the most immunogenic, resulting in enhanced lymphocyte activation in tuberculoid leprosy compared with normal subjects.[15]

The innate immune system appears to play a role in leprosy nerve and skin involvement. Toll-like receptor 2 (TLR2) and a TLR2–TLR1 heterodimer receptor have been shown to be crucial in the process of recognizing mycobacterial lipoproteins and generating an appropriate Th1 response. These receptors are more strongly expressed in skin lesions from tuberculoid patients than those with lepromatous leprosy.[16]

Pathology

HISTOPATHOLOGICAL CLASSIFICATION OF THE SKIN

Leprosy can be classified as tuberculoid (TT), borderline tuberculoid (BT), borderline borderline (BB), borderline lepromatous (BL) and lepromatous leprosy (LL) types, as in Table 41.1.

EARLY CHANGES

The earliest indication of skin infection with *M. leprae* is the multiplication of bacilli within the fixed cells of the dermis. Early invasion of nerves by *M. leprae* produces focal damage at blood vessels near their site of entry into the nerves. Bacteria spread centripetally along the fine fibres of cutaneous nerves and proliferate within Schwann cells, which then burst, releasing bacteria into endoneural spaces, where they are engulfed by histiocytes.

INDETERMINATE LEPROSY

The earliest visible skin lesion in the natural history of leprosy is the indeterminate stage of infection. It is most commonly observed early in the course of infection in children in whom the type and level of immune resistance to *M. leprae* have not yet been fully determined. This stage may last for months, may spontaneously resolve, or may progress to tuberculoid, borderline or lepromatous leprosy, depending on the host immune response to the infection. Histology shows foci of inflammatory cellular exudates, mainly around the finest nerve fibres in dermal plexuses (perineural paravascular inflammation), consisting of lymphocytes and histiocytes predominantly, with or without scarce acid-fast bacilli.

TUBERCULOID LEPROSY

An appropriate cell-mediated immune response generated through initial interaction between bacteria and dermal histiocytes results in a shift from indeterminate leprosy towards the tuberculoid pole of the leprosy immunological spectrum. Histologically, this is recognized by the transformation of histiocytes into groups of epithelioid cells, which may coalesce to form giant cells. Well-circumscribed foci of these cells in the dermis are often surrounded by a zone of lymphocytes, and known as epithelioid granulomata. Granulomatous cords follow the lines of neurovascular bundles (Figure 41.2). Efficient mycobacterial phagocytosis and antigen presentation results in an effective Th1 immune response of cell-mediated type, and hence few, if any, recognizable acid-fast bacilli are seen histologically. Nerve bundles become swollen by proliferation of Schwann cells, which develop into epithelioid cells.

LEPROMATOUS LEPROSY

In lesions of lepromatous leprosy macrophages proliferate and may become foamy because of an abundance of poorly processed mycobacterial lipid material but a failure of phospholipase activity results in inadequate antigen processing. Lymphocytes are scanty. In fully developed lepromatous disease chronic inflammatory tissue with bacteria-filled cells dominates the dermis (Figure 41.3), while the subepidermal zone of the dermis is clear of infiltrate.

Histoid leprosy is a rare nodular form of lepromatous leprosy. The histopathological features consist of well-formed

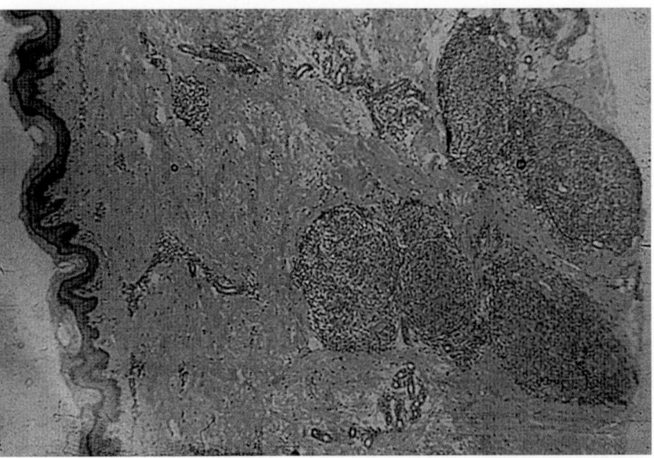

Figure 41.2 Granulomas in the dermis of tuberculoid leprosy (high power). *(Courtesy of the late S. G. Browne.)*

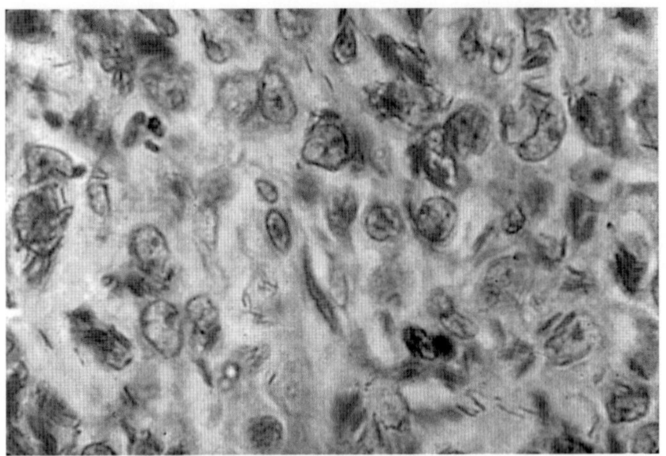

Figure 41.3 Lepromatous leprosy infiltrate throughout the dermis with *M. leprae*. *(Courtesy of the late S. G. Browne.)*

lesions, spindle-shaped, polygonal and foamy histiocytes, and a large number of solid staining acid-fast bacilli.

BORDERLINE LEPROSY

Histologically, borderline leprosy shows features intermediate between those of lepromatous and tuberculoid leprosy. An inflammatory reaction is seen in the superficial layers of the dermis, consisting of small round cells, histiocytes and clumps of epithelioid cells but without giant cells. Borderline leprosy is immunologically unstable, with potential for sharp upgrading towards the tuberculoid pole of the spectrum (known as a Type 1 or reversal reaction) or a more gradual drift to the lepromatous pole, sometimes referred to as downgrading.

PATHOLOGY OF NERVE DAMAGE

M. leprae's propensity for nerve damage is based on its unique tendency to invade Schwann cells. A 21-kDa histone-like protein of *M. leprae*, known as LBP21, and phenoglycolipid-1 antigen (PGL-1) bind to the extracellular matrix protein laminin-2. Direct cytotoxicity of T cells activated by Schwann cell

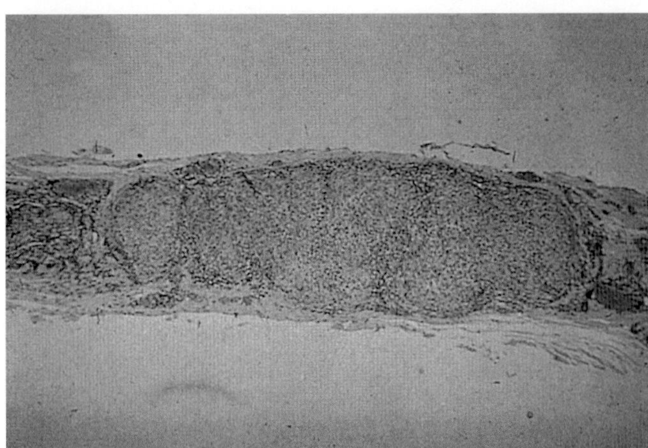

Figure 41.4 Tuberculoid granulomas in a nerve. *(Courtesy of the late S. G. Browne.)*

processing and presentation of *M. leprae* proteins and peptides to MHC Class II-restricted CD4+ Th1 cells[17] in turn leads to inflammatory damage to the nerve as an innocent bystander. Nerves may become difficult to recognize, and occasionally nerves undergo caseation. Fibrosis is common, and a mixture of myelinated fibre loss and remyelination, as well as axonal degeneration and regeneration can be observed. Peripheral nerves are commonly involved in tuberculoid leprosy. Autonomic nerves may also be involved.

Different pathologies contribute to the development of nerve damage.[18,19] Inflammation is promoted by the presence of mycobacterial antigens in nerve lesions and the action of pro-inflammatory cytokines The entry of *M. leprae* into Schwann cells generates an immune response determined by the type of leprosy that the patient has. TLRs are involved in immunological interactions between the host and *M. leprae.*[16] Schwann cell killing through the activation of TLR2 by *M. leprae* has been shown in vitro. The histological characteristics of inflammation of peripheral nerves in leprosy are similar to the spectrum of responses described in the skin (Figures 41.4 and 41.5). In tuberculoid disease, granulomatous inflammation develops at sites of infection, including the endoneurium, and may destroy

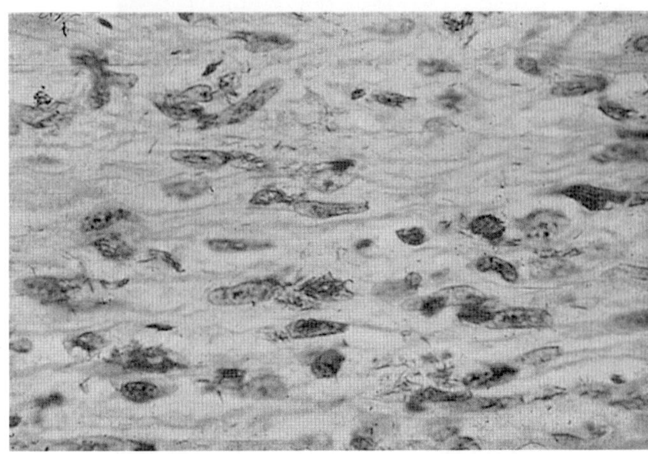

Figure 41.5 Nerve lesions (high power) of lepromatous leprosy. *(Courtesy of the late S. G. Browne.)*

infected nerve fibres. In lepromatous disease, prolific bacterial growth occurs inside Schwann cells and endoneural macrophages.[20] Persisting mycobacterial antigens (both protein and glycolipid) have been identified in nerves by Shetty[21,22] and these contribute to chronic ongoing neural inflammation.

Pro-inflammatory cytokines such as TNF-α have been detected in nerve lesions and these also promote nerve damage.[23] TGF-β, a downregulatory cytokine, was also detected in these biopsies.[24] TNF-α was detected in the serum in the weeks before a new nerve-damaging event.[25] *M. leprae* can also deregulate MAP kinases and the high and medium weight monofilament proteins which could contribute to structural nerve damage.[26,27]

These processes produce Wallerian and axonal damage at the tuberculoid end of the spectrum.[28,29] In lepromatous leprosy demyelination occurs. However, this is often a late event. Patients with lepromatous leprosy can have a very high bacterial load but relatively little inflammation. Further damage leads to fibrosis and the creation of an empty matrix.

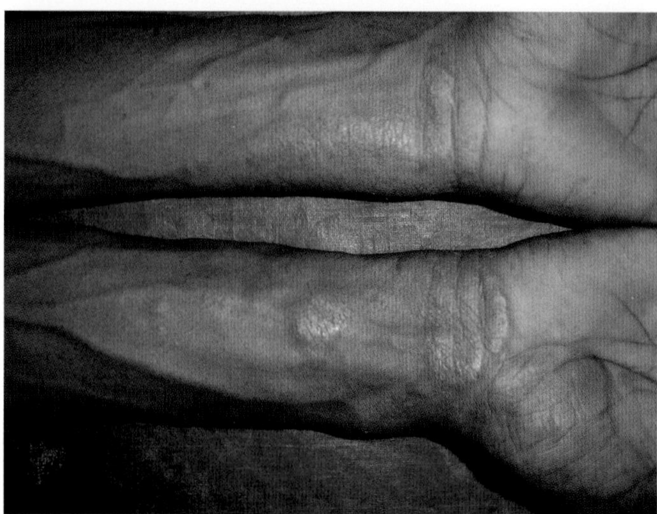

Figure 41.7 Plaques of borderline tuberculoid leprosy.

Clinical Manifestations

SYMPTOMS AND SIGNS: THE CARDINAL SIGNS

The presence of the cardinal signs of leprosy: skin lesions with definite sensory loss or thickened peripheral nerves or the demonstration of *M. leprae* on slit-skin smears or on histology of tissue (skin or nerve) is diagnostic.

Skin

Lesions can be found anywhere on the body. The most common sites are the face, buttocks (Figure 41.6) and extremities. Palms and soles are not spared, but lesions are rare in the scalp, axillae and groin. Sensory loss within skin lesions is a typical feature of leprosy, tested usually by light touch and/or pin prick. Early skin lesions may be rather poorly defined hypopigmented or erythematous macules. Sensation in these early stages may be unaltered.

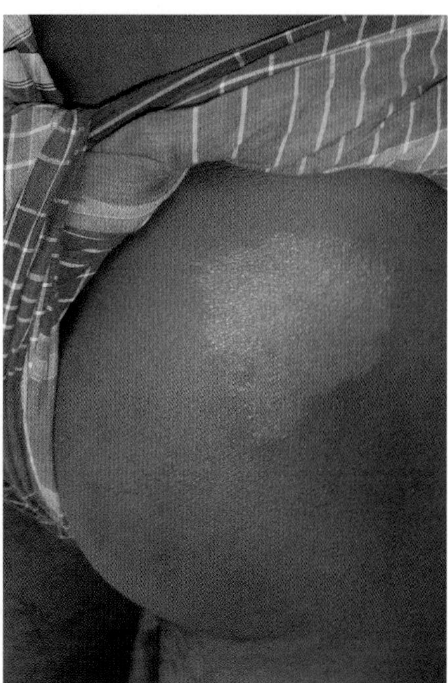

Figure 41.6 Patch of tuberculoid leprosy on buttock.

TT leprosy is characterized by a single or very few lesions. These are macules or plaques with well-defined edges. In dark skin hypopigmentation predominates over the erythema or copper colour more usually seen in lighter skin. The lesions are frequently anaesthetic. The anaesthesia is due to destruction of dermal sensory and autonomic nerve fibres. Anaesthesia may not be present in facial lesions. Involvement of autonomic fibres is often marked and results in dry lesions with a tendency to scale due to loss of sweating. Hairs are reduced in number or may be completely absent. The TT form carries a good prognosis and lesions will often self-heal. A few small 'satellite' lesions may be seen alongside a tuberculoid plaque. Thickened cutaneous nerves may also be palpated in the vicinity of the lesions and the edge of lesions should be palpated to detect such cutaneous nerves.

Individuals with BT leprosy have similar lesions to those with TT leprosy but the margins of lesion are less pronounced and less infiltrated. BT lesions tend to be more numerous and larger (Figures 41.1 and 41.7). TT lesions tend to heal before enlarging to greater than 10 cm, whereas BT lesions may involve a large part of a limb or the trunk. The BT lesions of an affected individual may vary in size and shape.

BB leprosy is very unstable immunologically. Patients may have macular or papular or plaque-like skin lesions or even a combination. Larger lesions may have a geographic appearance and some lesions have an ill-defined outer margin with a well-defined ('punched-out') anaesthetic inner margin. These annular lesions are a characteristic form of BB leprosy.

BL leprosy usually starts with a few macular lesions which become more widespread and symmetrically distributed. The macules become progressively more infiltrated. Papular and nodular lesions may develop and are more defined than those seen in LL. Skin lesions at the lepromatous (BL/LL) end of the spectrum may not have demonstrable sensory loss.

Lepromatous disease may be present for many years before diagnosis. The early skin changes are widely and symmetrically distributed macules. They are poorly defined with mild hypopigmentation and erythema. Flesh-coloured or occasionally erythematous papules and nodules may be present. The skin if left

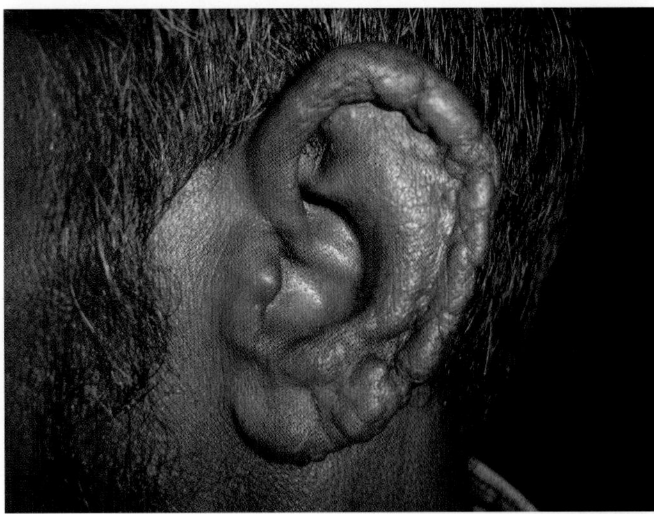

Figure 41.8 Nodular changes in ear lobe in lepromatous leprosy.

untreated thickens due to dermal infiltration giving rise to the 'leonine facies'. A variety of morphologies of skin lesions are seen, including macules, papules, nodules and plaques (infiltrations). Sometimes all of these may be present at the same time in advanced disease. Hair is lost from affected skin, notably from eyelashes and eyebrows (superciliary and ciliary madarosis, respectively). *M. leprae* have been demonstrated in hair follicles located in the dermal papilla and the outer root sheath during anagen and telogen in untreated lepromatous patients. The ears should always be carefully examined by close inspection and palpation. The earlobes are more constantly affected than any other part of the body, and appear thickened quite early in the course of the disease, later becoming nodular (Figure 41.8).

Nerves

Leprosy affects peripheral mixed nerves and cutaneous nerves. The most common peripheral nerves affected, in order of frequency, are the posterior tibial, ulnar, median, lateral popliteal (common peroneal), facial and radial nerves. The trigeminal nerve, especially the ophthalmic branch, may also be affected, causing loss of corneal sensation. Enlargement of involved nerves at particular sites, notably the ulnar nerve at the elbow and the lateral popliteal at the head of the fibula, is characteristic of leprosy and requires training and practice to detect reliably. Cutaneous nerve thickening usually affects small nerves adjacent to leprosy skin lesions. Particular regional cutaneous nerves may also be enlarged, notably the greater auricular nerve and radial cutaneous nerve. Sensory loss is usually more prominent than motor function loss.

Subjective symptoms of paraesthesiae, hyperaesthesiae and hyperalgesia may signal sensory nerve function impairment, though frequently the impairment of light touch, temperature or pain sensation develops 'silently'. Loss of position sense, vibration sense and tendon reflexes is rare. Motor nerve function impairment also often develops with associated muscle wasting and resulting deformities (Figure 41.9), such as claw hand (ulnar nerve), drop foot (common peroneal nerve) and facial palsy (facial nerve) are all too frequent complications. Autonomic nerve involvement may be signalled by mild oedema of the hands and feet, which later may become dry, puffy and cyanosed. In approximately 5% of cases, there are no skin lesions, and these patients are classified as having pure neural leprosy.

Affected nerves in *tuberculoid leprosy* are thickened, often irregularly, and associated sensory, motor or autonomic nerve function may be impaired. Sensory disturbances are most common. Motor changes are shown by muscle weakness or wasting and should always be examined for in the face, the intrinsic muscles of the hand and the dorsiflexors of the foot. It is rare for the dorsiflexors of the wrist to be affected, as the radial nerve is less commonly affected.

Nerve thickening and associated impairment occurs more slowly in *lepromatous leprosy* than in other forms of leprosy but may involve multiple nerves. As with skin involvement, nerve thickening tends to be bilateral and symmetrical. Glove and stocking loss of sensation is common in established lepromatous leprosy.

Nerve involvement can very often be demonstrated in *borderline leprosy*. Symptoms such as paraesthesiae and hyperalgesia often precede the clinical detection of skin lesions. Nerves are involved asymmetrically.

Peripheral sensory nerve damage may present with trophic skin ulcers, due to a lack of self-protection from burns, sharp object trauma and repetitive minor trauma. Ulcers are most common on the plantar aspect of the feet over pressure areas – toes, metatarsal heads, heel and lateral foot border. Ulcers also occur on the fingers and palm, often due to burns. Repetitive minor injury results in gradual absorption and shortening of digits of fingers and toes. Trophic ulcers also occur on anaesthetic patches if they occur at trauma-prone sites, e.g. on buttocks or elbows.

Eyes

The anterior portion of the eye is primarily involved in leprosy. The cornea, iris and lens can all be directly infiltrated by *M. leprae*. Lagophthalmos (Figure 41.10), the failure of eyelid closure due to facial nerve damage, leads to exposure keratitis and predisposes to corneal trauma. Reduced or absent corneal sensation due to involvement of the ophthalmic branch of the trigeminal nerve causes corneal ulceration and scarring.

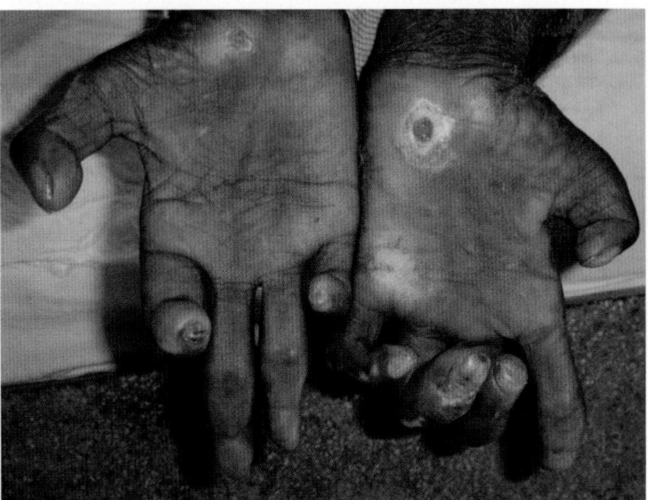

Figure 41.9 Typical leprosy hand deformities: ulnar claw, 'ape thumb' and pressure ulceration.

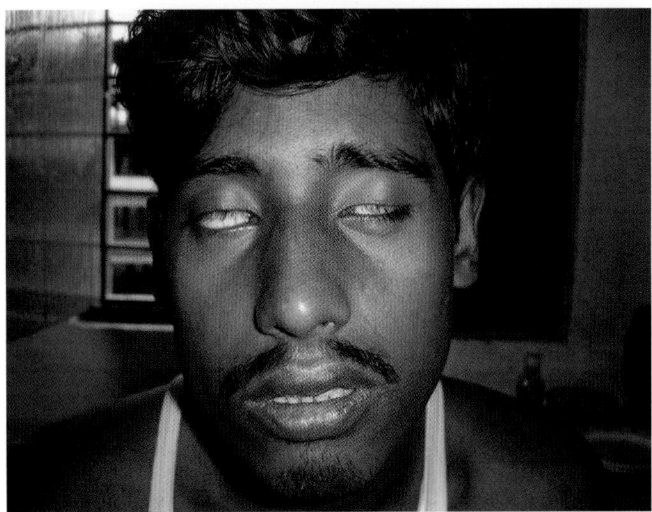

Figure 41.10 Lagophthalmos due to leprosy.

Iridocyclitis occurs as part of the erythema nodosum leprosum (ENL, Type 2 reactions) in lepromatous leprosy and may be an acute or chronic process. Acute iridocyclitis is signalled by pain, photophobia and a red eye. Untreated, it may become chronic and the development of posterior synechiae leads to a small irregular pupil. A more insidious form of chronic iridocyclitis also occurs in lepromatous leprosy. Slit-lamp examination shows 'flare' (cloudiness of aqueous fluid) and cells in the anterior chamber. Later, iris atrophy develops and a regular pinpoint pupil without posterior synechiae formation. Cataract formation is also increased in lepromatous leprosy. Chronic iridocyclitis is a common cause of cataract as is the use of long-term systemic steroids for leprosy reactions.

Mucous Membranes

Mucous membranes are frequently involved in lepromatous leprosy, especially in the upper respiratory tract. Nasal discharge, possibly blood-stained, and nasal stuffiness may occur. Examination reveals hyperaemia and swelling of the mucosa. Nasal septal ulceration may progress to perforation, cartilage destruction, and nasal bridge collapse causing the characteristic 'saddle-nose' deformity. Laryngeal involvement is a very rare and serious complication characterized by hoarse cough, husky voice and stridor.

Bones

Extensive bony changes in the hands and feet occur for a variety of reasons. Repeated trauma due to anaesthesia, secondary infection with resultant osteomyelitis, and sensory loss may lead to the development of Charcot joints, disuse due to paralysis and contractures and generalized osteoporosis.

Reticuloendothelial System

Enlargement of lymph nodes may occur, and occasionally one or more nodes become swollen and inflamed as part of a leprosy reaction or more commonly in response to secondary infection of ulcers. Lymphoedema, especially of the lower legs, may occur. Spleen, liver and bone marrow may also be invaded by *M. leprae* in lepromatous leprosy.

BOX 41.1 THE THREE CARDINAL SIGNS OF LEPROSY

- Hypopigmented or erythematous skin lesions showing definite reduction in sensation *or*
- Enlarged and clinically impaired nerves at sites characteristic of leprosy *or*
- Acid-fast bacilli in slit-skin smears.

Testes

Infertility and gynaecomastia may result from testicular invasion by *M. leprae* and resulting testicular atrophy in lepromatous leprosy. The orchitis of ENL is a significant cause of testicular dysfunction.

Kidneys

Renal involvement in lepromatous leprosy occurs rarely, but is probably under-diagnosed. Glomerulonephritis, interstitial nephritis, pyelonephritis, and renal amyloidosis have been described. The latter appears to be related to the severity and frequency of ENL, in which disseminated antigen-antibody immune complex deposition occurs.

Diagnosis

Early diagnosis and treatment of leprosy are essential to minimize disability. Delay in diagnosis has been associated with a significant increase in nerve damage at diagnosis.

Leprosy is primarily a clinical diagnosis based on the cardinal signs (Box 41.1).

CLINICAL CLASSIFICATION FOR TREATMENT

Leprosy classification has been simplified to counting the number of skin lesions. Individuals with up to five leprosy skin lesions are classified as having *paucibacillary* (PB) disease, while those with six skin lesions or more are classified as having *multibacillary* (MB) disease (Table 41.2). It has been shown that more than 60% of MB cases are slit-skin smear negative in an Indian cohort of patients.

BODY CHARTING

A clear 'body-map' showing the site and size and type of skin lesions, sites of nerve enlargement, and any nerve impairment due to leprosy is an invaluable aid to clinical diagnosis and ongoing management. It provides an important baseline against which future improvement or deterioration, particularly the possibility of relapse, can be measured.

Peripheral Nerve Function Assessment

Peripheral nerve trunks should be formally examined for enlargement and for loss of function at diagnosis and on a

TABLE 41.2 WHO Classification of Leprosy

Paucibacillary (PB) Leprosy	Multibacillary (MB) Leprosy
Five skin lesions or less	Six skin lesions or more

regular basis thereafter, to detect any deterioration. It is important that all patients suspected of having leprosy should have their nerves carefully palpated for enlargement and tenderness. Voluntary muscle testing using the MRC grading system should be performed. Sensation is commonly tested using a ball-point pen in the field and with graded monofilaments in specialist departments. Nerve conduction studies are the most sensitive test of nerve function but are not used routinely.

Laboratory

SLIT-SKIN SMEARS AND THE BACTERIOLOGICAL INDEX

Slit-skin smears are obtained by scraping fluid from a 2–4 mm depth of pinched blood-free skin, using the edge of the disposable scalpel blade turned perpendicularly and reversed after slitting the skin. This fluid is then smeared onto a microscope slide; 1% acid alcohol is used to decolourize an initial stain, which is usually carbol fuchsin, and counterstained with methylene blue. Bacterial load is determined through quantitative microscopy of slit-skin smears under the ×100 oil immersion lens. The results are expressed in a logarithmic scale called the Bacteriological Index (BI), which ranges from 1+ (1–10 bacilli per 100 high-power fields) to 6+ (>1000 bacilli per single high-power field). The use of smears requires training of skilled personnel, laboratory infrastructure and adequate finances.

Most patients with leprosy will have a negative slit-skin smear. Nevertheless, a positive test is diagnostic and very helpful for those with early lepromatous disease in whom cardinal clinical signs are often not present. Many recommend 2–4 sites for skin smears, at least one being from a skin lesion, if present, and from routine sites such as the earlobes.

BIOPSY

Skin biopsy may be required to confirm the diagnosis in the absence of a cardinal sign of leprosy. It is also useful in confirming alternative diagnoses. The most active (red, infiltrated and/or enlarging) part of a lesion, usually the edge is most suitable for biopsy. The tissue should be stained with haematoxylin and eosin (H&E) and the Fite (or Ziehl–Neelsen) stain for acid-fast bacilli. If a nerve biopsy is required, a thickened cutaneous nerve rather than a peripheral nerve is selected because of the potential for complications.

RESEARCH DIAGNOSTICS

Serology

Anti-phenolic glycolipid-1 antigen (PGL-1) antibodies correlate with bacterial load. Positive anti-PGL-1 serology is a predictor of nerve function impairment.[30]

Polymerase Chain Reaction (PCR)

PCR detection of *M. leprae* DNA is not routinely used in the diagnosis of leprosy. The relevance of identification of *M. leprae* DNA in specimens has to be determined by correlation with the clinical findings. In tuberculoid disease, positivity rates will be much lower than lepromatous cases and the absence of *M. leprae* DNA does not exclude the diagnosis of leprosy.[31]

DIFFERENTIAL DIAGNOSIS

Skin

Leprosy can manifest itself in a wide variety of skin lesions and the differential diagnosis of leprosy-like skin lesions is therefore correspondingly wide. Careful sensation testing, recognition of the presence or absence of associated features of leprosy, such as enlarged cutaneous or peripheral nerves, and exclusion of other skin conditions are needed to establish a diagnosis.

Pityriasis versicolor is a common cause of hypopigmented oval skin lesions particularly in tropical regions. The lesions are usually smaller, have a superficial scale and are often noted in flexural areas. Vitiligo causes depigmentation rather than hypopigmentation. Other common skin lesions that may be confused with leprosy include dermatophyte infection, psoriasis, lichen planus. Filarial disease, with its tendency to lower limb ulceration, may occasionally be confused with leprosy. Cutaneous leishmaniasis, particularly diffuse cutaneous and post kala-azar dermal leishmaniasis, may closely resemble the nodular lesions of lepromatous leprosy, but sensation is intact, and demonstration of amastigotes in skin smears from lesions will establish the diagnosis.

Blastomycosis may produce skin lesions similar to leprosy. Syphilitic and yaws skin lesions may closely resemble the maculae of leprosy but sensation is intact. The VDRL reaction alone cannot always be depended upon, as false-positive reactions are not uncommon in lepromatous leprosy.

The early lesions of mycosis fungoides can be mistaken for nodular leprosy. Lupus vulgaris and other mycobacterial skin lesions may resemble leprosy lesions but sensation is intact. Cutaneous sarcoidosis, granuloma annulare, and granuloma multiforme can resemble tuberculoid leprosy but there is no sensory loss and no nerve thickening and the histological appearances are different.

Scleroderma, localized or diffuse, may be confused with the infiltrative plaques of leprosy but biopsy will help to differentiate.

Nerves

Enlarged nerves have a narrow differential diagnosis. Neurofibromatosis may cause enlarged nerves at multiple sites, but not particularly in the characteristic sites and nerves affected by leprosy. Peripheral nerve impairment is not as common as in leprosy. Some forms of hereditary sensory neuropathy, notably familial hypertrophic interstitial neuritis (Déjérine–Sottas disease), may cause confusion because of thickening of peripheral nerves, together with sensory and motor nerve impairment. The differential diagnosis of diffuse peripheral polyneuropathy in the absence of enlarged nerves is very broad. The syndromes of mononeuropathy and mononeuritis multiplex also have a wide potential range of differential diagnoses. Plantar anaesthesia leading to trophic ulceration can occur in diabetes, tabes dorsalis, alcohol-related neuropathy, familial sensory radicular neuropathy, primary amyloidosis, and many other causes of peripheral neuropathy. Polyneuritic leprosy affecting the hands must be differentiated from syringomyelia, in which differential sensory loss occurs – loss of pain and temperature sensation, but preservation of light touch.

Neuropathy due to trauma of the ulnar nerve or brachial plexus or a cervical rib may cause confusion, but history and radiological examination are generally conclusive. Nerve entrapment syndromes such as meralgia paraesthetica causing anaesthesia of the anterolateral region of the thigh, and pressure injury to exposed nerves such as the lateral popliteal (common peroneal) nerve following prolonged sleep or intoxication may also cause confusion.

Treatment

CHEMOTHERAPY OF LEPROSY WITH MULTI-DRUG THERAPY (MDT)

The WHO has recommended MDT since 1982 and it is highly effective in treating infection with *M. leprae*. PB leprosy is treated with rifampicin and dapsone for 6 months, while MB leprosy is treated for 12 months with rifampicin, dapsone and clofazimine. Monotherapy is to be avoided in order to prevent the emergence of resistance. Chemotherapy of leprosy has been standardized globally by WHO to allow for simplified treatment regimens for decentralized prescription (Table 41.3). Blister packaging for better treatment adherence and worldwide donor funding of leprosy treatment have facilitated huge improvements in availability of treatment and successful completion rates.

RIFAMPICIN

Rifampicin is the key bactericidal component of all leprosy chemotherapy regimens. A single dose of rifampicin can reduce the number of viable bacilli to undetectable levels within a few days, with killing rates measured in excess of 99.9% after 1 month. Standardized WHO regimens employ a *monthly* dose of rifampicin.

Rates of resistance in reported series and in clinical practice remain low. Rifampicin resistance in leprosy is rare. Mutations in the *rpoB* gene, which encodes the β-subunit of RNA polymerase, lead to high-level resistance to rifampicin in *M. leprae*.[32] Leprosy treatment depends heavily on rifampicin and so contraindication to the drug requires significant modification of treatment. At least one bactericidal drug such as ofloxacin should be added to the treatment regimen.

Occasional cases of renal failure, thrombocytopenia, influenza-like syndrome and hepatitis are reported due to rifampicin. Rifampicin characteristically produces a reddish-brown colour in urine, sputum and sweat. The effect of oral corticosteroids given to treat reactions does not appear to be diminished by monthly rifampicin.

DAPSONE

Dapsone is a synthetic sulphone, similar to the sulphonamide drugs, targeting dihydropteroate synthase, a key enzyme in bacteria. Despite early reports of widespread resistance following monotherapy, dapsone remains very useful in combination with rifampicin in WHO MDT regimens for leprosy. Its main role in paucibacillary leprosy is probably to prevent the emergence of rifampicin-resistant organisms. In combination with clofazimine, dapsone is bactericidal, though not as powerful as single-dose rifampicin.

Dapsone is inexpensive and major adverse effects are uncommon. Dapsone hypersensitivity syndrome is characterized by an exfoliative dermatitis, fever and hepatitis which may be life-threatening. Dapsone hypersensitivity typically develops after 4–6 weeks of treatment and patients must be warned to stop the drug and seek urgent medical attention if symptoms develop. Mild haemolytic anaemia is common following dapsone treatment and rarely warrants change of therapy, but severe haemolysis occurs in patients with glucose-6-phosphate dehydrogenase deficiency and dapsone should be avoided in these patients. Agranulocytosis has rarely been reported due to dapsone.

CLOFAZIMINE

Clofazimine is an aminophenazone dye whose mechanism of action is not yet fully elucidated and may be multifactorial. Clofazimine is useful in combination with dapsone and rifampicin for the treatment of MB leprosy, and reports of resistance are very rare. An increased booster monthly dose of clofazimine is added to the daily dosage in the WHO MDT regimen to achieve target total monthly dosage. The pharmacokinetics of clofazimine are complex, including a very long half-life. In the dosage employed in the WHO MDT regimen for MB leprosy, clofazimine is relatively non-toxic. Increased pigmentation of the skin, particularly within skin lesions, is common but it clears within 6–12 months after stopping treatment. Higher doses (200–300 mg daily) of clofazimine are used for their immunomodulatory effect in the control of recurrent ENL reactions. In higher doses, clofazimine produces more significant skin pigmentation and occasionally is accompanied by severe gastrointestinal side-effects, which may mimic an acute abdomen, through crystal deposition in the intestinal tract.

OFLOXACIN

Ofloxacin is a fluoroquinolone antibiotic with anti-leprosy activity. Ofloxacin has a long half-life and is given as a single daily dose. Side-effects include nausea, diarrhoea and other gastrointestinal complaints, and skin rash may occur. A variety of central nervous system complaints have been reported,

TABLE 41.3 **Standard WHO Multi-Drug Therapy (MDT) for Leprosy**

Multibacillary Leprosy		**Paucibacillary Leprosy**	
The Recommended Standard Adult[a] Regimen is:		The Recommended Standard Adult[a] Regimen is:	
Rifampicin	600 mg once a month, supervised	Rifampicin	600 mg once a month, supervised
Dapsone	100 mg daily, self-administered	Dapsone	100 mg daily, self-administered
Clofazimine	300 mg once a month, supervised, and 50 mg daily, self-administered		
Duration	12 months	Duration	6 months

[a]Children should receive appropriately reduced doses of the above drugs.

including insomnia, headaches, dizziness, nervousness and hallucinations.

MINOCYCLINE

Minocycline is the only member of the tetracycline group which has demonstrated significant bactericidal activity against *M. leprae*. Adverse effects include gastrointestinal upset, photosensitivity, and dizziness. Administration to children and pregnant women is not recommended.

OTHER ANTIBIOTICS

Clarithromycin in combination with minocycline was shown to be highly bactericidal against *M. leprae* in lepromatous patients. Rifabutin and a variety of fluoroquinolones are active against *M. leprae*.

PREGNANCY AND LACTATION

Standard WHO MDT regimens have been used safely in pregnancy, however, ofloxacin and minocycline should be avoided. Small quantities of anti-leprosy drugs are excreted through breast milk but there are no reports of adverse effects as a result apart from mild discolouration of infants due to clofazimine.

CO-INFECTION WITH HIV OR TUBERCULOSIS

The response of patients with HIV co-infection to standard leprosy treatment is similar to that of other leprosy patients and does not require modification. Patients suffering from both leprosy and tuberculosis require standard antituberculosis therapy in addition to MDT for their leprosy. Rifampicin must be given in the dosage and frequency required for tuberculosis.

RELAPSE

Relapse is defined as the appearance of new leprosy skin lesions with an associated increase in bacterial index after completion of MDT. Relapse after MDT therapy for leprosy is uncommon. Studies of large series have generally reported relapse rates of less than 0.5% after at least 5 years of follow-up in paucibacillary leprosy treated with 6 months of WHO PB MDT and in multibacillary leprosy treated with 2 years of WHO MB MDT. Prospective studies of relapse rates after 12 months MB MDT for multibacillary disease are still lacking. The requirement for a negative bacterial index on slit-skin smear prior to discontinuing MDT therapy has been discarded in favour of fixed duration therapy both because of practical difficulties with skin smears and the continued decline in bacterial index post MDT discontinuation in the vast majority of patients. Patients who relapse after MDT usually respond to a further course of MB MDT.

Distinguishing relapse from late Type 1 reaction can be complicated and a definite rise in bacterial index on skin smear is usually required to confirm relapse in lepromatous cases. In doubtful cases, trial of steroid therapy is useful to help distinguish reaction from relapse.

Leprosy Reactions

Leprosy reactions are a major cause of the disability and morbidity associated with leprosy. They may occur before, during or after successful completion of MDT. The treatment of reactions is a key aspect of the management of leprosy. It is important that patients are taught to recognize the early signs and symptoms of reactions and to report promptly for treatment. Health workers should be trained to diagnose and treat or refer patients with reactions as appropriate. In addition to appropriate treatment of the reaction MDT should be started in newly diagnosed leprosy patients or continued in those who are already taking it.

TYPE 1 REACTIONS

Immunology

Type 1 reactions are delayed hypersensitivity reactions that occur predominantly in borderline forms of leprosy.[33] *M. leprae* antigens have been demonstrated in the nerves and skin of patients experiencing Type 1 reactions. The antigens were localized to Schwann cells and macrophages.[22] Human Schwann cells express TLR-2.[34] *M. leprae* infection may lead to the expression of MHC II on the surface of the cells and this may give rise to antigen presentation which triggers CD4 lymphocyte killing of the cell mediated by cytokines such as TNF-α.[35]

Clinical Features

Type 1 skin reactions typically begin as redness, swelling, warmth and, occasionally, tenderness arising suddenly within existing leprosy skin lesions (Figure 41.11). Occasionally, new skin lesions that were not previously apparent are 'unmasked' through the upgrading in cell-mediated immune responses characteristic of Type 1 reactions. These reactions are most common in the first few months following institution of antibiotic therapy for leprosy, but can occur before and after treatment. Generalized swelling of hands, feet and ankles may also accompany the more localized changes within leprosy skin lesions. Associated damage to involved nerves is another common manifestation of Type 1 reactions. Nerves affected by Type 1 reactions typically show an abrupt loss of function, often in the absence of other manifestations of inflammation.

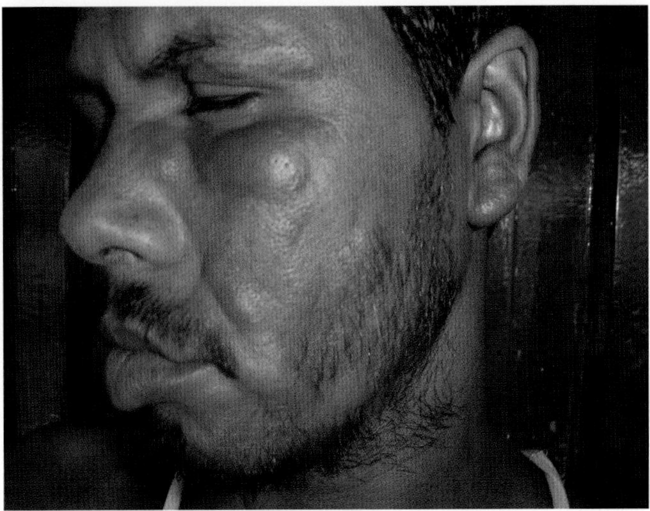

Figure 41.11 Borderline leprosy skin lesions in Type 1 reaction.

Erysipelas resembles borderline tuberculoid leprosy in reaction, but the presence of fever and the absence of sensory deficits differentiate these two conditions.

Treatment

Type 1 reactions are treated with a reducing course of oral prednisolone usually for a period of 6 months. Some patients may require further courses of prednisolone and if adverse effects occur steroid-sparing agents such as azathioprine are used. Physical treatments are often used in conjunction with corticosteroids in the case of neuritis, including rest, splinting, physiotherapy, and occasionally surgical decompression of nerves.

Nerve damage that has been present for longer than 6 months does not respond to corticosteroid therapy.

ERYTHEMA NODOSUM LEPROSUM (ENL, TYPE 2 REACTIONS)

Immunology

ENL reactions in the skin and elsewhere are considered an immune complex disease, with resultant granulocyte attraction and complement activation. Th2 cytokine activation is characteristic of Type 2 reactions with selective dynamic increases in IL-6, IL-8, and IL-10 mRNA, alongside persistent increases in IL-4 and IL-5 mRNA in lesions.

Pathology of ENL

Vasculitis is a major pathological event in ENL. There may also be infiltration of neutrophils and increased T cell activity. Neutrophils are the pathological hallmark of ENL but are not always present.

Clinical Features

ENL is a systemic disorder affecting many organ systems. ENL skin reactions are characterized by crops of subcutaneous nodular lesions, which may occur at any body site, but rarely on the face. When severe, these lesions may ulcerate and become pustular. ENL occurs in approximately 50% of individuals with lepromatous leprosy and is characteristically associated with a systemic inflammatory response including fever, tachycardia and malaise. Other organ systems may be involved and ENL may cause lymphadenitis, orchitis, uveitis, osteitis, arthritis and dactylitis. ENL reactions are frequently recurrent and in some patients may persist for years.

ENL may be mistaken for folliculitis, for other forms of erythema nodosum and panniculitis. Febrile neutrophilic dermatoses such as Sweet's syndrome should also be considered. Some leprosy workers advocate the taking of slit-skin smears in all cases of suspected erythema multiforme. Carefully taken skin smears will be positive for acid-fast bacilli in ENL.

Treatment

ENL reactions vary in severity, duration and organ involvement. Severe ENL, often accompanied by neuritis, should be treated with prednisolone. ENL reactions are frequently recurrent following reduction in steroid therapy and continue for years after completion of MDT. Thalidomide in doses of up to 400 mg/day is the most effective agent for the treatment of ENL but its use is limited because of its teratogenic effects.

High-dose clofazimine (200–300 mg/day in adults) is used in those with recurrent ENL reactions in an attempt to reduce the dose of corticosteroids. The total duration of high-dose clofazimine therapy should not exceed 12 months.

LUCIO'S PHENOMENON

A rare variant of lepromatous skin infiltration was described by Lucio and Alvarado in Mexico in 1852. The entire skin is diffusely infiltrated with no discrete lesions seen. These patients may experience 'Lucio's phenomenon' characterized by painful, purpuric, ulcerating patches of skin lesions. It is often fatal.

NEURITIS AND SILENT NEUROPATHY

Neuritis is present if an individual has any of the following: spontaneous nerve pain, paraesthesia, tenderness, or new sensory or motor impairment. It indicates inflammation in the nerve. Nerve pain, paraesthesia or tenderness may precede nerve function impairment, which, if not treated rapidly and adequately, becomes permanent.

Silent neuropathy is the phenomenon of nerve function impairment occurring in the absence of symptoms of inflammation and as a result the patient may be unaware of it. Regular examination of the peripheral nerves is required to detect the problem.

The treatment of neuritis and silent neuropathy is with prednisolone as for Type 1 reactions.

LEPROSY AND HIV

It was feared that HIV infection would increase the risk of developing leprosy, the risk that leprosy will present as lepromatous, or the dually infected people would have worse leprosy prognosis. None of these fears have been confirmed. The skin lesions in HIV/leprosy co-infected patients with low circulating CD4 counts had normal granuloma formation with numerous intralesional CD4 cells. With the use of antiretroviral therapy leprosy patients have been reported with BT leprosy and also with increased rates of Type 1 reactions. Leprosy has been reported presenting as immune reconstitution disease among HIV patients starting antiretroviral treatment. Treatment of a leprosy patient with concurrent HIV infection does not differ from that of an uninfected leprosy patient and reactions should be managed with corticosteroids or thalidomide as appropriate.

Prevention of Disability and Management of Complications

The early detection of deterioration in nerve function and the rapid introduction of corticosteroid therapy are essential to minimize nerve damage and thus prevent disability.

EYE COMPLICATIONS

Iridocyclitis is an important cause of blindness in leprosy and should be treated promptly with mydriatics and topical steroids. Patients with lagophthalmos require eye protection by use of goggles or sunglasses. Frequent use of artificial tear-drops during the day and ointments or oily drops at night is also useful to prevent exposure keratitis.

PARALYSIS

Joints affected by paralysed muscles should be kept mobile to prevent fixed flexion deformities. Surgical intervention for lagophthalmos, foot drop and claw hands and toes is available in some centres. Tendons are transferred from innervated muscles and reattached to enable the performance of actions affected by paralysis. This requires specific, multidisciplinary expertise including substantial physiotherapy intervention before and after surgery.

TROPHIC ULCERS

Prevention and management of ulceration on sensory-impaired skin, particularly on the plantar aspect of anaesthetic feet, is an ongoing issue for many people affected by leprosy, long after MDT therapy has been discontinued. Trophic ulceration in leprosy resembles that in diabetes, and patients can benefit from advances in diabetic ulcer management. Appropriate self-care is critical, combining modifications to life-style and daily activities with regular self-examination plus soaking and cleaning in water, and scraping off callus formation. Use of simple oils to help retain moisture is very helpful in dry skin with little autonomic nerve supply. Wearing of appropriate, well-fitting footwear, modified as necessary with appropriate insoles, or specially moulded to fit damaged feet is very important. The need to distribute weight over the plantar surface of damaged feet has encouraged the use of multi-cellular rubber in shoe insoles or sandal soles.

Anaesthetic hands need to be protected from damage associated with the actions of daily living. In addition to cleaning and appropriate bandaging, the key ingredient to healing of leprosy-related ulcers is rest, just as overuse in the absence of perception of pain is the cause of ulceration. Antibiotics and debridement may be required in deeper ulcers, or where cellulitis, osteomyelitis or tenosynovitis have ensued. Gram-positive organisms usually predominate, though mixed infections are common and relatively broad-spectrum antibiotics may sometimes be required. Plantar ulcers may be improved using local superficial flaps.[36]

NEUROPATHIC FEET

Neuropathic bone disintegration in those with advanced nerve damage due to leprosy is difficult to treat. Initial management is by immobilization in a non-weight-bearing cast. Orthopaedic intervention through arthrodesis of talar and subtalar joints may be required in advanced cases of joint destruction.

NEUROPATHIC PAIN

Neuropathic pain is an increasingly recognized complication of leprosy. It has been reported to be as high as 20% in treated patients and is associated with persistent nerve enlargement.

REHABILITATION AND ADVOCACY

Physiotherapy and occupational therapy have an important role to play in the rehabilitation of those with physical impairments due to leprosy. Groups of leprosy-affected people have been particularly successful in maintaining physical and emotional wellbeing. Community-based rehabilitation programmes that are not leprosy-specific have the further advantage of addressing the stigma attached to the disease in appropriate ways. In many countries people affected by leprosy have formed associations that campaign for improved equality for their members.

Prognosis

Long-term prognosis in leprosy is good, as evidenced by the low relapse rates documented above. Early mortality is rare, confined generally to those with severe sepsis from untreated ulcers, and occasionally in those with severe drug reactions, particularly to dapsone. Nevertheless, leprosy patients are exposed to increased mortality risks due to its indirect and ongoing effects, approximately two to four times higher than in the general population.

Despite high cure rates, physical impairments due to leprosy are common in MB cases, where diagnosis is delayed, and in those with manual occupations. Social stigmatization due to leprosy remains one of the most unfortunate aspects of the disease, though there is wide anecdotal evidence of considerable mitigation of stigma through the successful and widespread implementation of MDT therapy and social mobilization programmes.

Prevention

BCG vaccine provides protection against leprosy in all the locations where it has been studied but this effect varies.[37] The protection is thought to be greatest for close contacts.

Single-dose rifampicin chemoprophylaxis reduces the risk of leprosy in close contacts compared to placebo but this effect is not sustained. The protective effect of BCG and rifampicin appears to be additive.[38] Socioeconomic improvements in nutrition, housing and sanitation may also help reduce the risk of acquiring leprosy.

Elimination

The 1991 World Health Assembly resolved to 'eliminate leprosy as a public health problem' – defined as reducing prevalence below one case per 10 000 population by 2000. The effort accompanying this resolution, the use of MDT, and possibly the widespread use of BCG vaccination, led to a marked reduction of prevalence. Transmission however continued and substantial numbers of new cases are still being detected. The use of the word 'elimination' in the resolution led to a perception that leprosy was about to disappear, and resulted in a reduction in resources for leprosy research and control. Furthermore, leprosy-endemic countries felt pressure to reduce the numbers of cases that they reported. India probably attained the elimination target by under-reporting of cases which was achieved by stopping active case finding and household contact tracing. Recent surveys in India have found substantial numbers of undiagnosed cases. In the latest WHO 'Strategic Plan for Leprosy' 'elimination' was replaced by 'reducing leprosy burden'; this term encompasses both the burden of disease and the burden of disability, as leprosy is one of the main infectious causes of disability worldwide.

REFERENCES

8. Fine PE. Leprosy: the epidemiology of a slow bacterium. Epidemiol Rev 1982;4:161–88.
16. Krutzik SR, Ochoa MT, Sieling PA, et al. Activation and regulation of Toll-like receptors 2 and 1 in human leprosy. Nat Med 2003;9: 525–32.
18. Scollard DM. The biology of nerve injury in leprosy. Lepr Rev 2008;79:242–53.
22. Lockwood DN, Colston MJ, Khanolkar-Young SR. The detection of *Mycobacterium leprae* protein and carbohydrate antigens in skin and nerve from leprosy patients with type 1 (reversal) reactions. Am J Trop Med Hyg 2002;66:409–15.

Access the complete references online at www.expertconsult.com

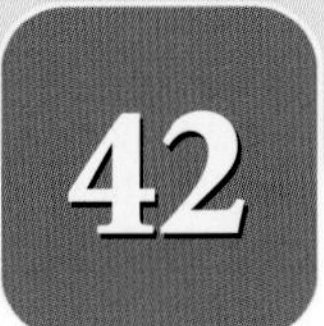

Mycobacterium ulcerans Disease

THOMAS JUNGHANSS | ROCH CHRISTIAN JOHNSON | GERD PLUSCHKE

KEY POINTS

- *Mycobacterium ulcerans* disease ('Buruli ulcer', BU) is the most common mycobacterial disease in humans after tuberculosis (see Chapter 40) and leprosy (see Chapter 41).
- *M. ulcerans* disease mainly affects children, and is stigmatizing, disfiguring and disabling if not treated early.
- Sub-Saharan Africa carries the main burden of disease, but it also occurs in Asia, the South Pacific and Latin America.
- Active early case detection and treatment are key to improving outcome.
- *M. ulcerans* disease can be treated effectively with antibiotics, particularly when treated early.
- The potential development of drug resistance needs to be carefully observed.
- In addition to specific treatment, patients require wound care and, in advanced disease, skin grafting.
- Patients with advanced disease in particular require nutritional and psychological support, physiotherapy and reconstructive surgery.
- Sooner or later after the initiation of antimycobacterial treatment, healing frequently stops or deteriorates for some time (so-called 'paradoxical reaction'). A major challenge is to distinguish this from secondary bacterial infections and specific treatment failure (which is rare).
- Prevention is limited since the modes of transmission which could be targeted are still unclear.

Epidemiology

GEOGRAPHICAL DISTRIBUTION

Buruli ulcer (BU) is prevalent in countries with a hot and humid climate. It has been reported in over 30 countries around the world. Endemic foci are geographically circumscribed around aquatic ecosystems (rivers, lakes, artificial or natural wetlands, irrigation systems). Table 42.1 presents a summary of the countries in which BU has been reported. Figure 42.1 shows the global distribution of BU in 2011 according to the WHO.

MOLECULAR EPIDEMIOLOGY AND TRANSMISSION

M. ulcerans has evolved from the aquatic dwelling *M. marinum*.[1] By acquisition of a virulence plasmid (pMUM), a progenitor of *M. ulcerans* has gained the unique property of producing a polyketide-derived macrolide toxin termed mycolactone.[2] Adoption of pMUM was most likely the key event in the emergence of *M. ulcerans*, constituting a population bottleneck that led to the development of a new species with a highly clonal population structure. Subsequent reductive evolution is indicative for the adaptation to more stable niches[1] and has led to the development of at least three mycolactone-producing mycobacterial lineages considered as different *M. ulcerans* ecotypes.[3] Two of these lineages have been isolated from human BU lesions. The ancestral lineage comprises haplotypes from Asia, South America and Mexico[4] and causes only sporadic disease in humans. In contrast, focal incidence rates in BU endemic areas of Africa and Australia, where the disease is caused by the classical lineage, can be >1/1000 per year. Disease isolates from different African countries are genetically nearly identical. However, by whole genome sequencing, a small number of single nucleotide polymorphisms (SNPs) can be identified.[5,3] SNP-based fine typing of isolates has demonstrated that localized clonal expansion is leading to the development of local clonal complexes in individual BU-endemic areas.[6,3]

Since BU-endemic areas are typically associated with slow-flowing or stagnant water bodies, it is generally assumed that infection takes place through trauma of the skin or insect bites from an environmental reservoir present in the aquatic ecosystems. Both biotic components, such as biofilms and aquatic invertebrate species are being considered as potential vectors and/or reservoirs. Recent findings from a BU-endemic area in Victoria (Australia) have implicated mosquitoes as vectors[7–10] and possums as an animal reservoir.[11] So far, a similar mammalian reservoir has not been identified in BU-endemic regions of Africa. Molecular epidemiological studies have revealed an extremely focal transmission of individual *M. ulcerans* haplotypes,[6] which excludes transmission by insect species that fly over large distances or infection from *M. ulcerans* containing biofilms in the river water. While there is no published evidence for direct person-to-person transmission of *M. ulcerans*, it remains to be analysed whether contamination of an environmental reservoir with *M. ulcerans* from chronic ulcers plays a role in local transmission.

SURVEILLANCE, PREVALENCE AND DETECTION

The true prevalence of BU in the various countries in which it is endemic is not known. The annual number of reported cases of BU, which increased in the early and mid-1990s to about 10 000 new cases per year, has stabilized more recently at about 5000 new cases per year according to the WHO data. Although underreporting is suspected in some countries, the cumulative number of BU cases in the African region at the end of 2008 was estimated to be 60 000.[12]

TABLE 42.1 Countries in Which BU Has Been Reported

Regions	Countries
Africa	Angola, Benin, Burkina Faso, Cameroon, Congo, Côte d'Ivoire, Democratic Republic of Congo, Gabon, Ghana, Guinea, Equatorial Guinea, Kenya, Liberia, Nigeria, Sierra Leone, Uganda, Sudan, Togo and Central African Republic
Latin America	Brazil, French Guyana, Mexico, Peru, Suriname
Asia	China, Japan
South Pacific	Australia, Indonesia, Kiribati, Malaysia, Papua New Guinea, Sri Lanka

The detection of cases is influenced by operational factors such as the efficacy of a country's health system.

EPIDEMIOLOGY AND SURVEILLANCE: BENIN AS AN EXAMPLE

In Benin, as in most endemic countries in Africa, the health system is structured in three levels. At the national level, BU control activities are organized by a National Control Program. The intermediate level, composed of regional hospitals and public health authorities, provides integrated supervision of all diseases. Activities are implemented at the operational/district level. There are five BU referral, detection and treatment facilities, 'Centre de Dépistage et de Traitement de l'Ulcère de Buruli (CDTUB)', distributed across the main endemic regions of Benin. The health workers at these facilities have considerable experience in diagnosing and treating BU patients. As with other endemic diseases such as Guinea worm, tuberculosis and leprosy, the detection of BU cases relies heavily on community-based surveillance teams comprising two village volunteers, called 'relais communautaires'. The team of the 'relais communautaires' is complemented by one or two teachers ('focal points') and is supervised by the health workers of the nearest health facility. This team is responsible for detecting and referring patients to the CDTUBs, as well as follow-up. At each CDTUB, a trained nurse registers each case on the BU 02 form developed by WHO. To facilitate and expedite the reporting of cases, the form has been developed into a triplicate register. Each quarter, the completed first sheet is sent to the national program. The second sheet is sent to the regional authorities and the third is kept at the health facility. At the national level, data are computerized for analysis and mapping. Each year, a training workshop for the team is held before the start of the first campaign. Feedback is also provided annually by the national programme at a review meeting attended by the heads of all treatment centres (CDTUBs) and other partners involved in BU activities in Benin. The CDTUBs perform quarterly data analyses which they feed back to the teams. At the same time, refresher workshops are conducted and new team members are trained. With this system in place, from 1 January 2003, to 31 December 2010, a total of 7139 new and recurrent cases of BU were reported and treated in Benin. The number of reported cases per year increased steadily from 1997, reached a peak of 1200 cases in 2007 and decreased continuously thereafter, to 572 in 2010.[13] The geographical distribution of BU cases is shown in Figure 42.2A. The distribution of the disease is very focal. In the Lalo district (one of the most endemic districts in Benin), for example the overall prevalence of BU is 88.9 cases per 10 000 inhabitants. When we consider only active cases, the prevalence is 18.9 cases per 10 000 inhabitants. This exceeds by far the threshold of more than 1 case per 10 000 inhabitants set

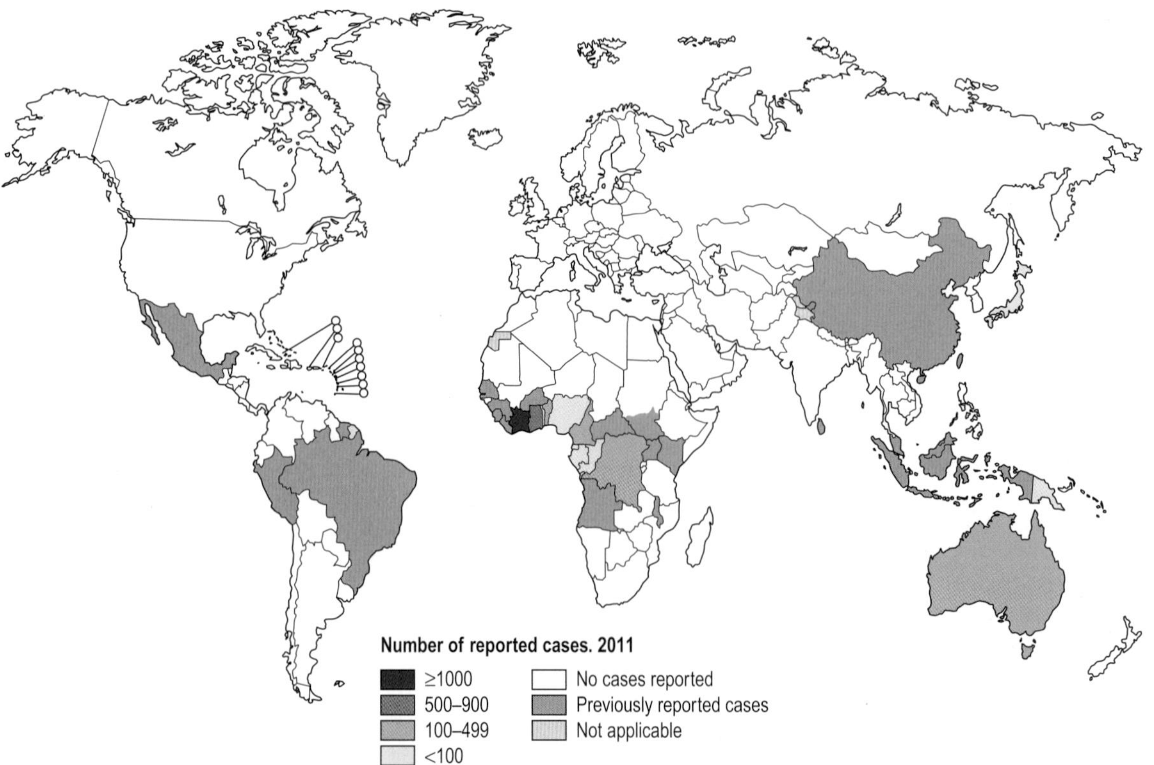

Figure 42.1 The distribution of BU by country as of 2011. Imported BU is occasionally diagnosed in the USA, Canada and Europe http://apps.who.int/neglected_diseases/ntddata/buruli/buruli.html.

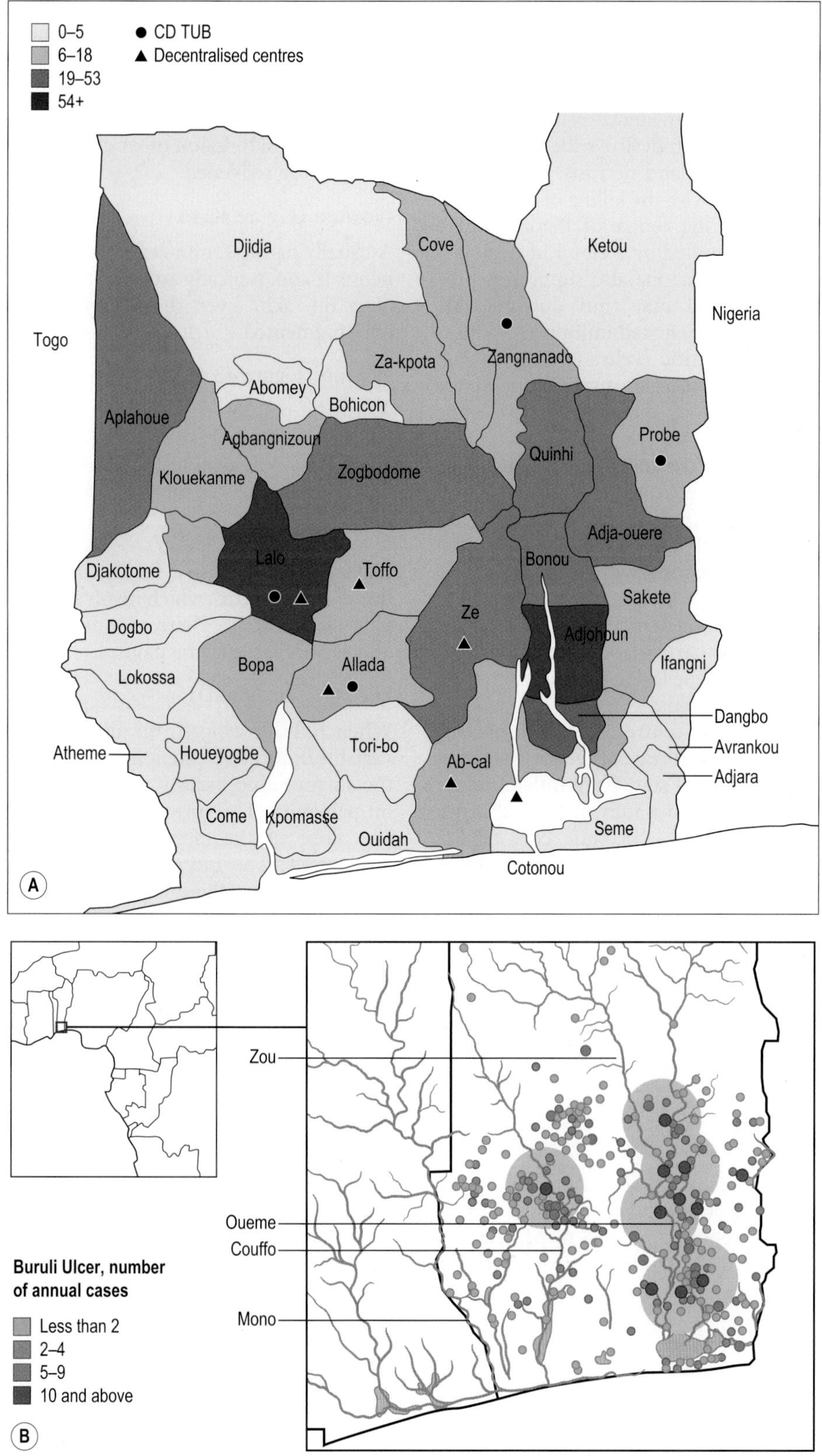

Figure 42.2 (A) BU distribution in Benin at department level. (B) BU distribution in Benin at village level.

by WHO for diseases to be considered a public health issue. Within a given district, the prevalence varies from one subdistrict to another. In the district of Lalo, the most endemic subdistrict Ahomadégbé recorded 249 cases per 10 000 inhabitants. This continues to the village level, as shown in Figure 42.2B, where the majority of cases occur within a very few kilometres along the Couffo and Oueme rivers. At the same time, it appears that very few cases occur along the Mono river, suggesting possible environmental and behavioural factors in the epidemiology of BU.[14]

Pathogenesis and Pathology

M. ulcerans mostly causes indolent necrotizing skin lesions harbouring large clusters of extracellular bacilli within areas of coagulative necrosis. Pathogenesis is mediated primarily by the macrolide toxin mycolactone,[15] which destroys the host tissues at the site of infection by apoptosis and necrosis. Strong local immunosuppression is associated with the killing of infiltrating inflammatory cells attracted to the centre of lesions, where mycobacterial clusters are surrounded by a cloud of mycolactone. At low concentrations mycolactone also suppresses production of certain cytokines and may thus downregulate systemic innate and adaptive cell-mediated immune responses in circulating leukocytes, dendritic cells and lymphoid organs.[16,17] Due to the diffusible nature of mycolactone, tissue destruction usually extends beyond those areas with large numbers of mycobacteria.

BU is primarily an infection of the subcutaneous fat tissue. Tissue destruction spreads laterally from the initial infection focus with multiplication of *M. ulcerans*. Necrosis of the dermis eventually leads to ulceration, which may be a late event, leading to the development of plaque lesions with extended tissue destruction prior to ulceration. *M. ulcerans* grows optimally at temperatures below the core body temperature (29–33°C), favouring infection of the skin, in particular on the limbs. Nevertheless, some patients develop bone lesions subjacent to their skin lesions or metastatic osteomyelitis.

Neutrophil debris found in the centre of BU lesions may represent the remains of an acute infiltrate at the early stage of infection.[18] Otherwise, the absence of significant inflammatory infiltration is one of the hallmarks of a fully developed active BU lesion.[19] At the periphery of the necrotic core of BU lesions, interaction of phagocytes with AFBs and intracellular *M. ulcerans* can be observed, and in resolving BU lesions in particular, granulomatous inflammation can be found. Under antibiotic treatment, massive infiltration of lesions and development of ectopic organized lymphoid tissue is observed (Figure 42.3).[20] Frequent seroconversion of healthy individuals living in areas in which BU is endemic, indicates that minor *M. ulcerans* infections may often heal by themselves in an early stage.[21,22]

Clinical Features

The first clinical descriptions of BU possibly date back to the late nineteenth century in the Congo. Patients with a 'new mycobacterium in man' were reported in 1948 by MacCallum and colleagues from Australia.[23] The name is derived from the Buruli district in Uganda, from where many of the early cases were reported.[24]

Most cases (around 75%) are children of 15 years of age or younger, and most lesions (around 80%) are located on the extremities.[25] Genetic susceptibility has been suggested[26] but has still to be validated more broadly.

BU MANIFESTATIONS AT THE LEVEL OF THE SKIN

At the level of the skin, BU manifests as papules, nodules, plaques, oedema or ulcers. Definitions of these skin conditions, in particular size ranges, vary between dermatology textbooks. A standardized description is important for comparison between studies, and therefore, we follow the definitions of the WHO BU Working Group,[27,28] as follows:

Papule

A usually painless, non-tender, sometimes itchy, raised, palpable intradermal skin lesion of <1 cm in diameter. The surrounding skin may be reddened.

Nodule (Figure 42.4A)

A usually painless, non-tender, sometimes itchy, firm, subcutaneous lesion, typically attached to the skin, of 1–2 cm in diameter; the skin over the lesion may be discoloured, often hypopigmented.

Plaque (Figure 42.4B)

A usually painless, non-tender, discoloured, well-demarcated, elevated, indurated lesion of >2 cm in diameter with irregular edges. The skin around the lesion is often also discoloured, in dark-skinned people mostly hypopigmented.

Oedema (Figure 42.4C)

Diffuse, often extensive, firm, usually non-pitting swelling with ill-defined margins, which involves part or all of a limb or other part of the body. There may be changes in colour over the affected area. It may be painful.

Ulcer (Figure 42.4D)

When fully developed, the ulcer has undermined edges and variable induration extending from the margin of the ulcer into the surrounding healthy skin, usually with good demarcation on palpation. The surrounding skin may also be oedematous. The floor of the ulcer may have a white, cotton-wool-like appearance. The ulcer is painless or minimally painful and odourless unless there is secondary bacterial infection. When there is more than one ulcer and the ulcers are close together, they often communicate beneath the skin surface, which may appear intact.

BU MANIFESTATIONS BEYOND THE LEVEL OF THE SKIN

Osteitis/Osteomyelitis

M. ulcerans infection near bones can lead locally to osteitis or can progress to osteomyelitis. Rarely, systemic osteomyelitis occurs, most likely through haematogenous spread.

Disseminated Disease

Multiple lesions of the skin disseminated across the body with or without osteomyelitis (distant from local lesions). In principle, the individual lesions exhibit the same characteristics as listed above.

Differential Diagnosis

The early skin manifestations, i.e. papules, nodules and (small) plaques, are entirely unspectacular and unspecific. The early ulcers fare a bit better with some pathognomonic features (see above). Long-standing advanced disease in patients in a region endemic for BU is comparably easy to diagnose, but this is not the disease stage which people exposed to *M. ulcerans* should reach. The differential diagnosis of the different manifestations of BU is never complete. The selection

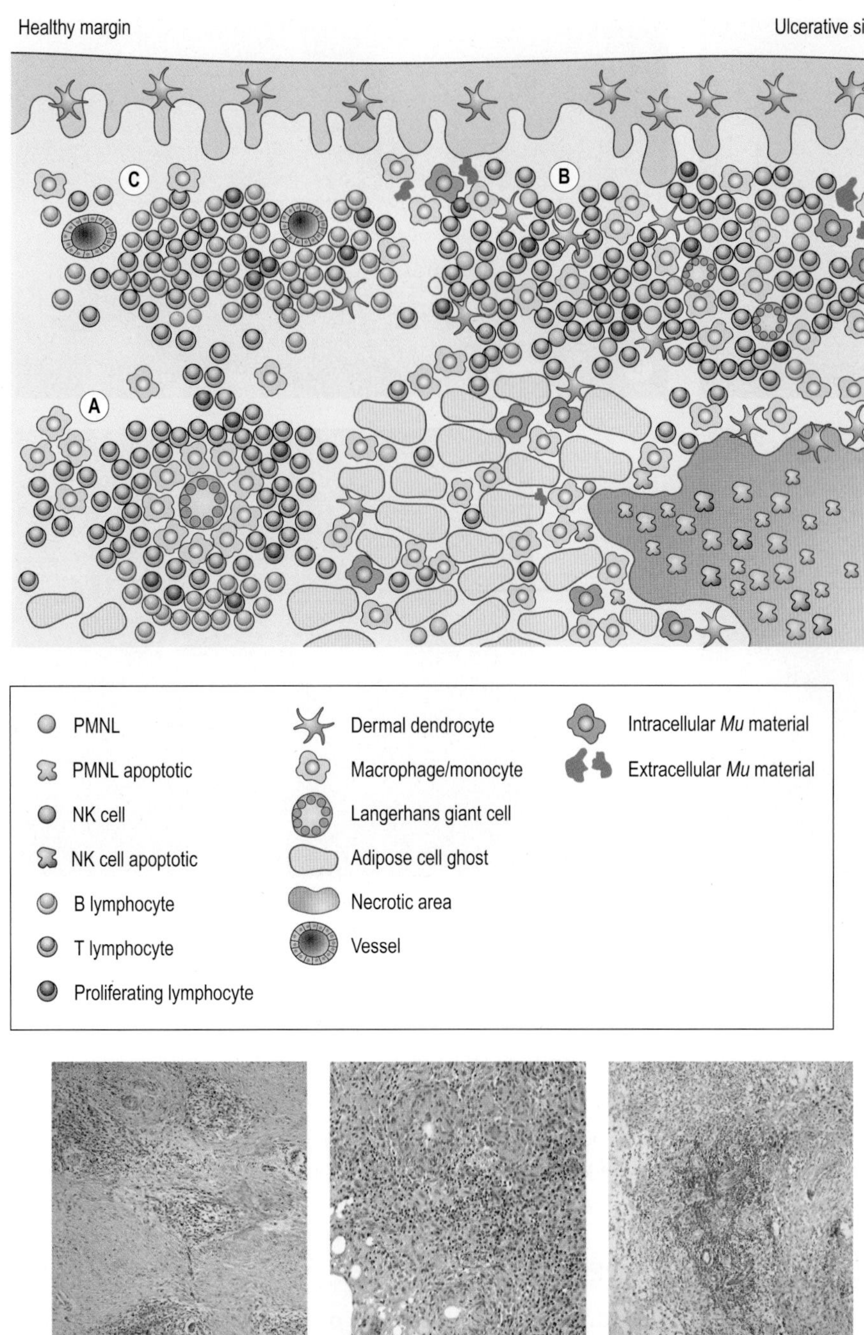

Figure 42.3 Three major types of cellular infiltration can be distinguished in antibiotic-treated BU patients (Schütte et al. 2007; copyright PLoS Negl Trop Dis). Upper part: schematic overview of cellular infiltration patterns and distribution of mycobacterial material. Lower part: three types of cellular infiltration are documented with HE. (A) Granuloma formation in the connective tissue (×640). (B) Diffuse heterogeneous cellular infiltration of the connective and adipose tissue (×6100). (C) Follicle-like lymphocyte focus adjacent to vessels (×640).

presented in the list below is based on: (1) the expected frequency of diagnoses and (2) overlap of diagnoses in regions in which BU is endemic. For easier orientation, the differential diagnoses are grouped under mycobacterial, bacterial, viral, parasitic and mycotic infections and nutritional, genetic and other disorders.

PAPULE

The differential diagnoses of papules are, by and large, those of nodules, complicated by the fact that the differentiation between clinically relevant and irrelevant lesions is even more difficult at sizes <1 cm. The clinical course will usually tell, and if the patient can be followed-up reliably and at short intervals, it is justified to wait and observe to avoid overdiagnosis and overtreatment of BU and other conditions which require treatment.

NODULE

Mycobacterial Infections

- Cutaneous tuberculosis (lupus vulgaris, scrofuloderma)
- Atypical mycobacteriosis
- Leprosy

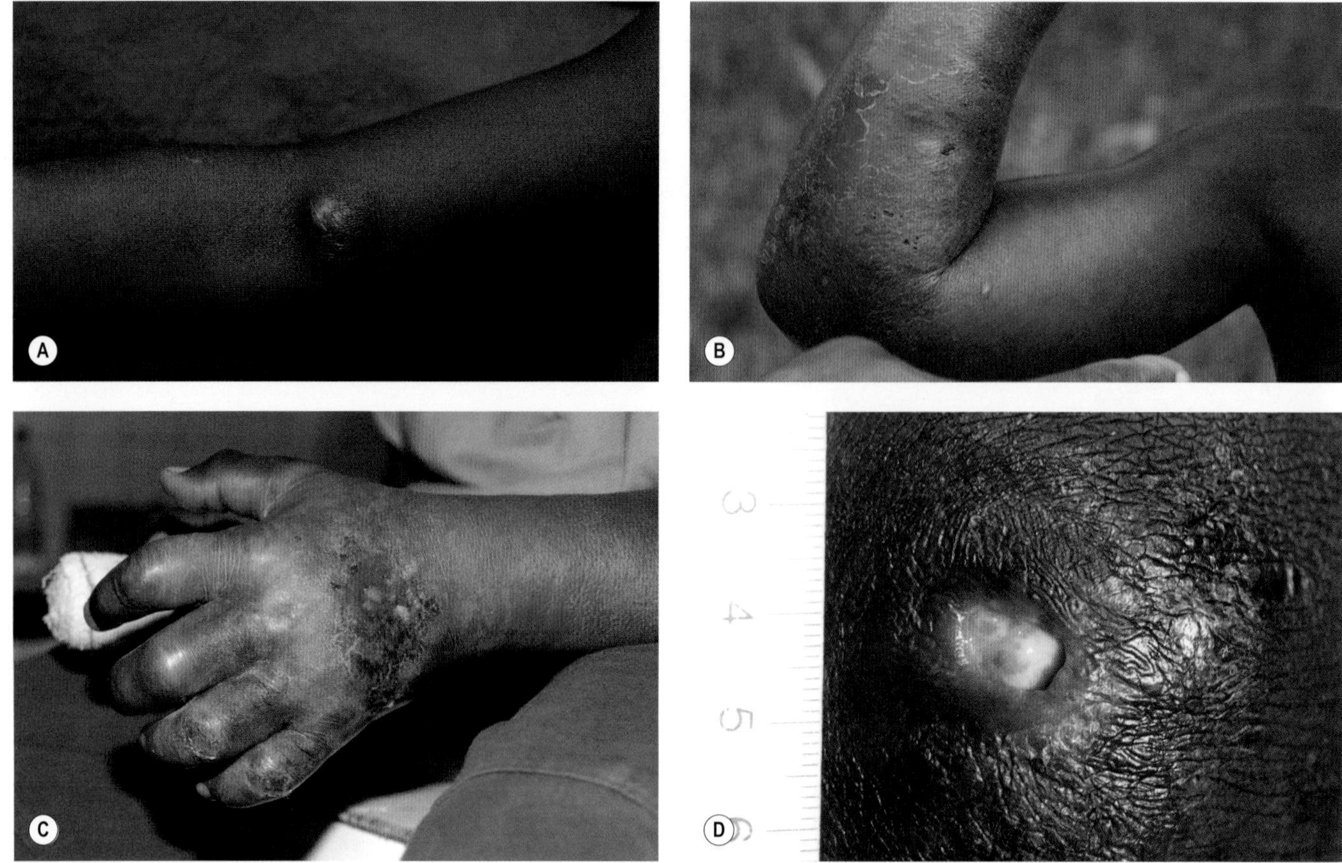

Figure 42.4 The four major skin manifestations of active *M. ulcerans* disease. (A) Nodule. (B) Plaque. (C) Oedema. (D) Ulcer. For a description of the lesions, see text. *(Photographs: Bayi/Vogel/Junghanss.)*

Bacterial Infections

- Furuncle
- Subcutaneous abscess
- Yaws
- Noma
- Actinomycosis (Madura foot)

Parasitic Infections

- Onchocerciasis nodule (onchocercoma)
- Early (muco)-cutaneous leishmaniasis
- Myiasis

Other Disorders

- Lymph node
- Sebaceous cyst
- Dermoid cyst
- Lipoma
- Joint ganglion

PLAQUE

Mycobacterial Infections

- Cutaneous tuberculosis (lupus vulgaris)
- Leprosy

Bacterial Infections

- Cellulitis/erysipelas

Mycotic Infections

- Tinea (e.g. ringworm)

Other Disorders

- Psoriasis
- Skin lymphomas
- Sarcoidosis

OEDEMA

The differential diagnosis of oedema of the skin is endless. Important to note is that oedema in BU is almost exclusively asymmetric, differentiating it from cardiac oedema and oedema due to venous insufficiency. In BU, oedema is often combined with induration of the skin and with an extended plaque, which – sooner or later – ulcerates. Acute forms of oedema must be differentiated from chronic lymphoedema. The latter can be caused by lymphatic filariasis, but patients with extended BU can also develop lymphoedema when damage to the subcutaneous tissue is extensive and circular.

ULCER

Mycobacterial Infections

- Cutaneous tuberculosis (fistulae of deep lymphadenitis or osteomyelitis, lupus vulgaris, scrofuloderma)
- Atypical mycobacterial ulcers
- Leprosy

Bacterial Infections

- Bacterial ulcer [ulcerated staphylococcal abscess, ulcerated streptococcal skin infections (erysipelas), secondary bacterial infection of skin trauma]
- Cutaneous diphtheria
- Late treponematosis, including yaws and tertiary syphilis (gumma)
- Fistulae of deep lymphadenitis or osteomyelitis
- Noma
- Actinomycosis (Madura foot)

Parasitic Infections

- (Muco)-cutaneous leishmaniasis
- Amoebiasis (late complication of amoebic liver abscess)

Mycotic Infections

- Ulcerated mycosis (e.g. sporotrichosis)

Genetic Disorders

- Skin ulcers in sickle-cell disease

Other Disorders

- Burns
- Ulcerated insect, spider or snake bites (including secondary bacterial infections)
- Tropical (phagedenic) ulcer
- Venous ulcers (often associated with varicose veins)
- Arterial ulcers (often associated with diabetes, hypertension, smoking)
- Pyoderma gangrenosum
- Leukocytoclastic vasculitis
- Ulcerated skin tumours/malignancies (e.g. melanoma, Kaposi's sarcoma)
- Ulcerated gout tophi
- Immune reconstitution syndrome with skin lesions, e.g. in AIDS patients

CLASSIFICATION AND STAGING OF *MYCOBACTERIUM ULCERANS* DISEASE

Various classifications of *M. ulcerans* disease have been suggested. None can serve all purposes. WHO currently defines three categories as a basis for treatment recommendations:[28]

- Category I: a single lesion ≤5 cm in diameter including the indurated areas defined by palpation
- Category II: a single lesion 5–15 cm in diameter including the indurated areas defined by palpation
- Category III: a single lesion >15 cm in diameter including the indurated areas defined by palpation, multiple lesions, lesions at critical sites (eye, breast and genitalia), osteomyelitis.

Publication of this classification coincided with the 'Provisional guidance on the role of specific antibiotics in the management of *Mycobacterium ulcerans* disease (Buruli ulcer)'.[28] The decision to introduce antibiotic combination therapy into the clinical management of BU required specification of assignment to surgery, antibiotic treatment or a combination of both, which is currently based on the WHO categories I–III. The rationale for including lesions at critical sites (eye, breast and genitalia) into category III is driven by the idea of terminating specific pathology conservatively and limiting the need for surgery as much as possible.

Creating categories mainly on the basis of size has one major drawback. Not rarely, large skin defects have evolved to near termination of specific disease activity. In these cases, size is not a problem with regard to specific antimycobacterial treatment but rather general wound management and definite wound closure. Inspection and assessment of the wound margins is therefore very important. In some instances only 'pockets' of ongoing *M. ulcerans* infection are found (see Figure 42.5C), whereas the greater part of the ulcer has already healed, though not yet closed due to the sheer size of the defect or secondary problems, in particular secondary bacterial infection or paradoxical reaction.

For the same reasons, for clinical trials a more differentiated classification system may be required which has less variability within categories.

An earlier WHO classification[27] had divided BU into non-ulcerative (nodules/papules, plaques, oedema, disseminated, mixed), ulcerative (early and late ulcerative, involvement of organs, e.g. eye, osteomyelitis, mixed) and post-ulcerative disease (scars with and without sequelae, e.g. contracture, deformity, loss of limb, eye, mixed).

In general classifications systems and in particular the categories of criteria employed have to be adapted to the specific purpose. For the complex pathology of BU, there is no single classification which can serve all purposes. For purely descriptive purposes, a morphological classification of lesions should follow dermatologically well-defined categories, i.e. papule – nodule – plaque – oedema – ulcer (see above). BU-specific features should then be added on, e.g. undermined edges, cotton wool appearance of the base of an ulcer.

A different approach is the classification which describes stages in the evolution of the disease from early to late and finally healed stages. This pathway is still controversial. With more intense interdisciplinary research, pathways are currently elucidated primarily by correlating clinically well-defined phenotypes with carefully described immunohistopathological changes over time. In addition to the natural pathway, it is important to understand treatment-induced modulations, in particular the so-called paradoxical reaction.

A third, and for clinical purposes, very important classification captures the severity of disease on the basis of clinically recognizable manifestations and assigns treatment approaches accordingly. Here, it is particularly important to differentiate pathology which is driven by *M. ulcerans* infection from common problems of wounds independent of the cause. As discussed above, the size of the ulcer, currently still the most common manifestation in patients reporting at most African treatment centres, does not seem to be a decisive criterion for the degree of specific disease activity but is so for wound complications and management problems in general, which are independent of the cause and increase with size. The challenges of large skin and subcutaneous tissue defects are the control of secondary bacterial infection and closure by skin grafting and reconstructive techniques.

A clinically pragmatic approach (Box 42.1) supported by data from ongoing interdisciplinary research is to distinguish:

- Localized *M. ulcerans* disease manifestations:
  - *(Highly) active*. Nodules (Figure 42.4A), plaques (Figure 42.4B) and oedema (Figure 42.4C) which break down within a short time and ulcerate (possibly accelerated

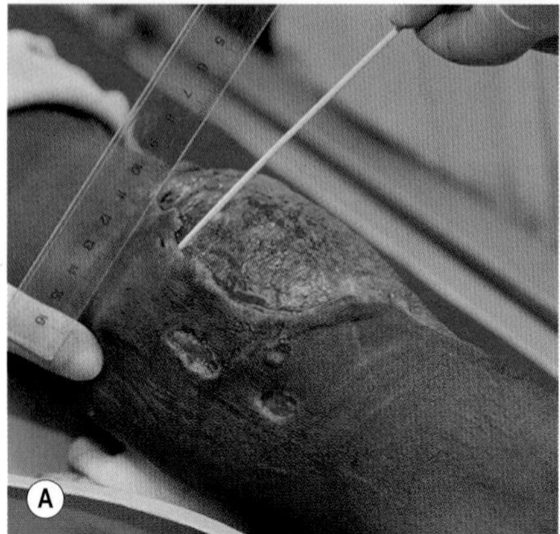

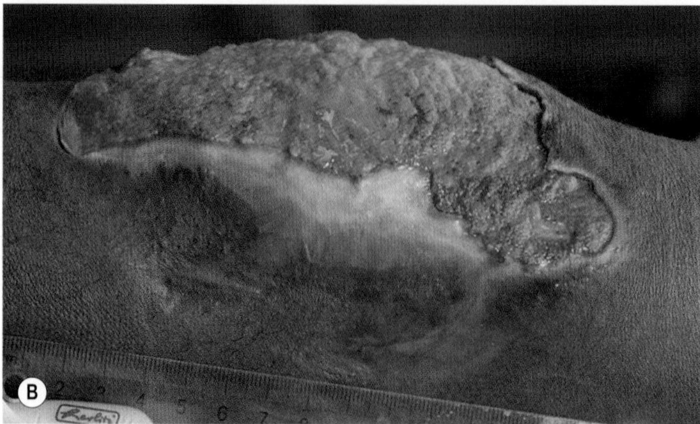

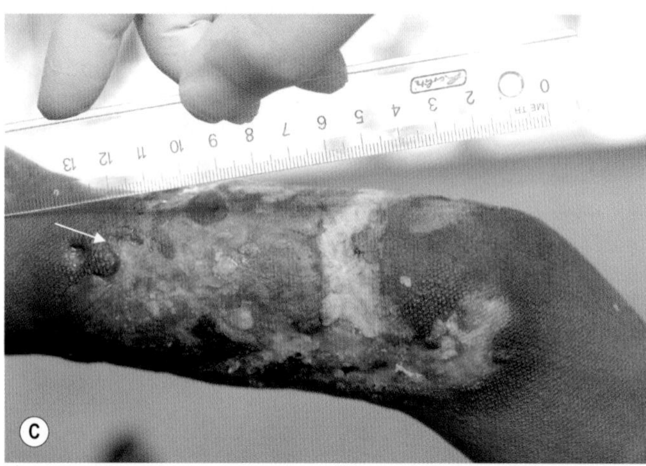

Figure 42.5 Extended lesions with mixed active–inactive manifestations of the margin: active ulcers with undermined edges and surrounding induration alternating with healed margin segments (scarring). (A) Large ulcer with wide undermined edges connected subcutaneously to 'satellite' lesions on the medial side (A) and scarring (healing) on the lateral side (B) of the ulcer. (C) Small active ulcer with surrounding induration (arrow) at the proximal end of the extended lesion with a mostly scarred (healed) margin. *(Photographs: Bayi/Vogel/Junghanss.)*

BOX 42.1 SIGNS ON WHICH CLINICAL JUDGEMENT SHOULD BE BASED

- Specific signs of *M. ulcerans*-driven disease activity: induration, oedema and discolouration of the skin which has not yet broken down (ulcerated); acceleration and increase in the size of the ulceration under antimycobacterial treatment (paradoxical reaction).
- Signs of general wound complications independent of the cause: size and site of the skin and subcutaneous tissue defect, with the corresponding risk of secondary bacterial infection, contractures, deformities and loss of function.

by antimycobacterial therapy), and ulcers with undermined edges and circular induration (Figure 42.4D) which (rapidly) increase in size (possibly accelerated by antimycobacterial therapy)
  - *Mixed active–inactive*. Often very extended lesions with mixed active–inactive manifestations of the margin: active segments of ulcers with undermined edges and surrounding induration alternating with healing/healed margin segments (frequently scarring) (Figure 42.5)
  - *Inactive*. Complete epithelialization (small lesions) or closure of lesions by scarring with or without contractures and deformities (Figure 42.6).
- Disseminated *M. ulcerans* disease manifestations:
  - Multiple lesions, osteomyelitis (distant from local lesion). In principle, the individual lesions exhibit the same characteristics as listed under 'localized *M. ulcerans* disease manifestations' above.

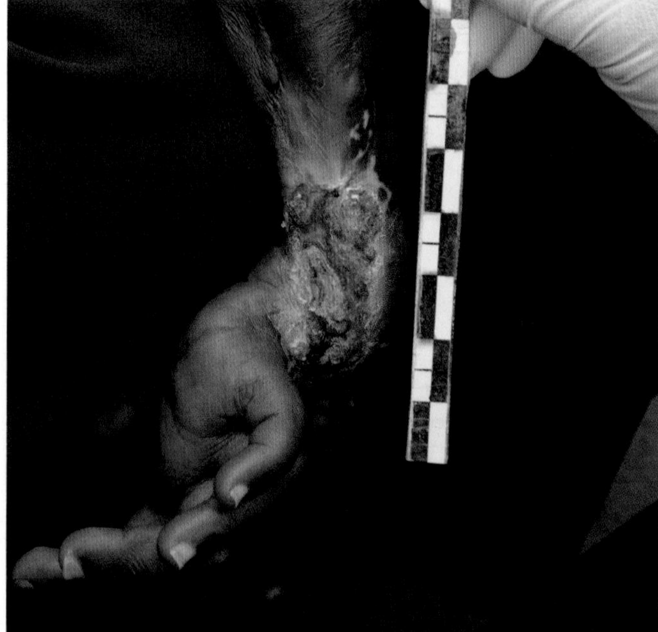

Figure 42.6 Inactive lesion with scarring and contractures leading to deformities and loss of function. *(Courtesy of Markus Schindler, Section Clinical Tropical Medicine, University Hospital, Heidelberg.)*

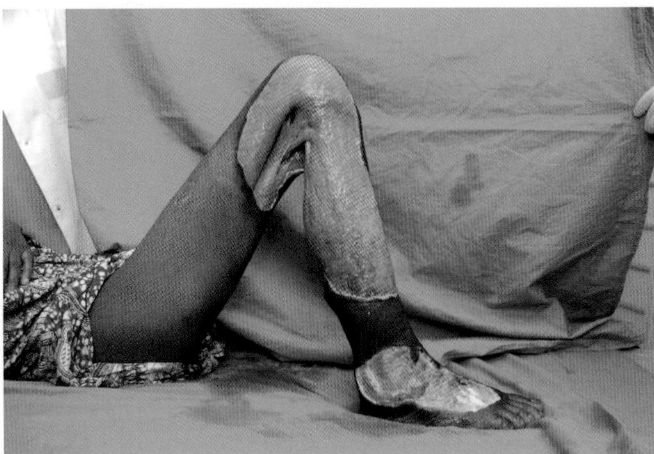

Figure 42.7 Extended *M. ulcerans* disease: complete loss of the skin and subcutaneous tissue above the level of the muscular fascia on the upper and lower leg after rifampicin/streptomycin combination therapy and debridement. The leg is ready for skin grafting. The patient made a good recovery including mobilization of the contractures after physiotherapy. *(Photograph: Bayi/Vogel/Junghanss.)*

- Treatment-associated manifestations:
  - So-called 'paradoxical reaction' (for details, see below).
- Recurrence:
  - As in the other mycobacterial diseases, recurrence is a problem and requires attention both in clinical practice and as an important endpoint in clinical trials. A recurrent case is defined as: a patient with previous BU-specific treatment who presents with a lesion at the same or a different site within one year of the end of the last treatment.
- Non-BU-specific problems:
  - Two major problems require particular consideration:
    - Extent (Figure 42.7) and site (Figure 42.5A, 42.6, 42.7) of the skin and subcutaneous defects and
    - Secondary bacterial infection (Figure 42.8).

PARADOXICAL REACTION

BU lesions frequently deteriorate sooner or later after initiation of antimycobacterial therapy. This is a phenomenon which has long been recognized in leprosy and tuberculosis and has been defined as transient worsening and/or appearance of disease-specific lesions under appropriate treatment with or without initial improvement.

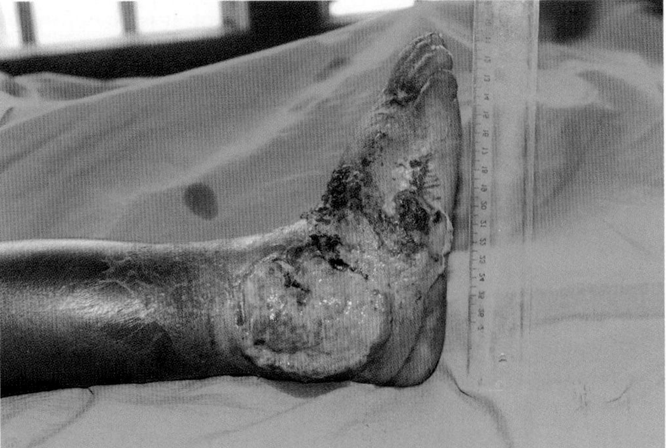

Figure 42.8 Extended *M. ulcerans* disease of the lower leg with an extended ulcer, oedema and a wide area of infiltration. Heavy secondary bacterial infection was present upon referral from the community to the district hospital. *(Photograph: Bayi/Vogel/Junghanss.)*

In tuberculosis paradoxical reactions are more common and severe in HIV-positive individuals who are also on highly active antiretroviral therapy. In these cases, the underlying mechanism of the paradoxical reaction may be an immune reconstitution inflammatory syndrome (IRIS). However, paradoxical reactions also occur in patients who are not immunocompromised; here the exact mechanisms are not well understood. In a substantial proportion of Ghanaian patients under antimycobacterial treatment Nienhuis and colleagues observed an increase in lesion size and non-ulcerative lesions that ulcerated before healing set in, while in some cases new lesions appeared. These effects culminated towards the end of the 8-week period of drug treatment.[30] In BU the definition of paradoxical reaction includes the enlargement of ulcers, accelerated progression of non-ulcerated plaques and oedemas to ulcerative lesions, and the emergence of new lesions during chemotherapy. Mycolactone causes massive immune suppression in BU lesions and practically all BU patients develop vigorous local immune responses during antimycobacterial chemotherapy.[19] Based on their histopathological work, Ruf and colleagues showed that neither ulceration of plaque lesions during antimycobacterial treatment[18] nor the appearance of 'new' lesions emerging many months after completion of antimycobacterial treatment which heal without additional specific therapy[31,32] represent failures of the antimycobacterial treatment.

In many patients massive infiltration of lesions and the development of atopic lymphoid tissue is not interfering with wound healing. Therefore, strong local immune responses are a good marker of the success of antimycobacterial treatment associated with the killing of *M.ulcerans* and the corresponding decline in mycolactone secretion. These vigorous immune responses are not necessarily associated with complications. In patients being treated for BU, it is therefore difficult to differentiate between deterioration resulting from a local immune reconstitution inflammatory syndrome[29] and deterioration resulting from other causes, such as secondary infections.

The understanding, definition and diagnosis of the paradoxical reaction are of paramount importance for two reasons:

- In clinical practice, paradoxical reactions need to be differentiated from lesions which are non-responsive or show a delayed response to antimycobacterial treatment. The two possible scenarios should trigger entirely different therapeutic responses.
- In clinical trials, the paradoxical reaction complicates and blurs the definition and observation of antimycobacterial therapy-specific study endpoints.

Diagnosis

SPECIFIC DIAGNOSIS

There is still urgent need for a simple, specific and highly sensitive point-of-care laboratory diagnostic method. In areas in which BU is endemic, the disease is often diagnosed by experienced health workers based only on clinical findings (see above). Where available, a laboratory diagnosis by a reference laboratory is frequently used to confirm the clinical diagnosis after initiation of treatment. Clinical specimens analysed

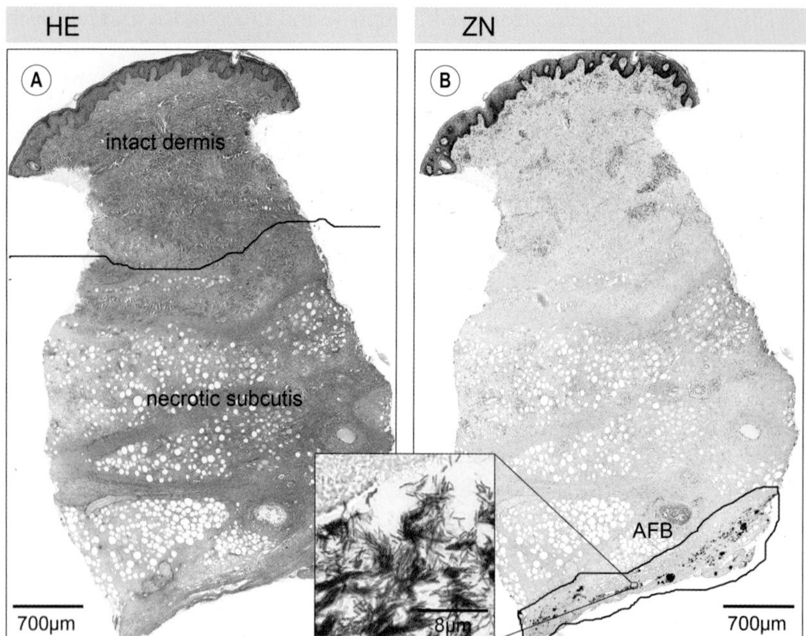

Figure 42.9 Histological sections of a punch biopsy from a BU plaque lesion stained either with H&E or Ziehl–Neelsen (counterstain methylene blue) (ZN). While epidermis and dermis are still relatively intact, deeper tissue layers are necrotic and oedematous. Fat cell ghosts and minimal infiltration limited to the surrounding of a few remaining partially intact blood vessels are characteristic hallmarks of BU. A band of extracellular acid-fast bacilli (AFB) is found in a deep layer of the necrotic subcutis. *(Taken from: Ruf MT, Sopoh GE, Brun LV, et al. Histopathological changes and clinical responses of Buruli ulcer plaque lesions during chemotherapy: a role for surgical removal of necrotic tissue? PLoS Negl Trop Dis 2011a;5:e1334.)*

include punch biopsies, swabs from the undermined edges of ulcerative lesions and fine needle aspirates (FNAs) from closed lesions. Four confirmatory laboratory methods are currently used:[33]

- Microscopic examination of FNAs or smears from the undermined edges of ulcers after staining of the bacilli with the Ziehl–Neelsen or auramine O acid-fast stain. While this is the only simple point-of-care diagnostic method currently available, its sensitivity is unfortunately limited (40–60%), since *M. ulcerans* is distributed focally in the affected tissue.
- Detection of *M. ulcerans* DNA by polymerase chain reaction (PCR). Because of its high sensitivity and specificity, PCR targeting the *M. ulcerans* specific insertion sequence IS*2404* has developed into the most commonly used method. It can be performed with FNAs and swabs from ulcers as well as tissue biopsies. Both conventional PCR and real-time PCR are used by reference laboratories. For conventional PCR in particular, strict adherence to the three-room principle is required to avoid contamination of samples with amplicons leading to false-positive results.
- Histopathological analysis of tissue biopsies. Analysed samples should include all levels of the skin and subcutaneous tissue down to the fascia. Characteristic histopathological features include epidermal hyperplasia, vasculitis, contiguous coagulative necrosis of the subcutaneous tissue, fat cell ghosts and a remarkable lack of inflammatory infiltration. Advanced lesions often show calcification. After Ziehl–Neelsen staining, clusters of extracellular AFB may be found. These are typically located in deeper layers of the necrotic adipose tissue, but may not be found in punch biopsies or smaller excisions due to the uneven distribution of the bacilli (Figure 42.9).
- Culture of *M. ulcerans*. The extremely slow-growing *M. ulcerans* can be cultured at temperatures between 29 and 33°C on standard mycobacteriological media. With this method the sensitivity is also only about 40% for cultures from FNA and swab samples. It can be higher for tissue biopsies, but with all types of samples mycobacterial colonies usually appear only after >8 weeks of incubation.

General diagnostics regularly required in the course of the management of BU patients:

- Laboratory tests should be performed as appropriate (haematology, biochemistry)
- For patients on rifampicin and streptomycin, the same precautions apply as for antituberculosis treatment
- If involvement of bones is suspected, including osteomyelitis, a radiological work-up needs to be performed
- Secondary bacterial infection, in particular systemic infection, requires bacterial culturing and resistance testing.

Management and Treatment

The outcome of the clinical management and the demands on healthcare services are determined by the disease stage at which the patient seeks and finds help. This is complicated by the fact that the features of very early disease manifestations are unspecific and often pass unnoticed by the patient. It is, therefore, of paramount importance in endemic regions to incorporate BU into health education and to establish surveillance in the affected communities. A further hurdle to early health-services-based treatment is stigmatization and the fact that patients frequently consult traditional healers first and may remain with them until their suffering becomes unbearable.[34,35]

For decades, BU has not received the attention this devastating disease deserves. With the lack of sensitive and specific diagnostic tools available at the community level a substantial degree of uncertainty remains when deciding on treatment. Confirmatory tests demand high laboratory standards and training (see above).

Surgery dominated the clinical management of BU for decades because other options failed or were not rigorously pursued. In poor rural communities surgery was not well accepted by patients and health services and thus not effective to control the disease. Limiting factors were the high demands on infrastructure and resources, the risks and trauma involved, long hospitalization times and an inverse correlation between the size of excisions and relapse rates.

With a *Mycobacterium* as the causative agent it was tempting to explore antituberculous drugs, which could be implemented much more easily than surgery. Looking back on two decades of studies, two major bottlenecks are obvious: there was a lack of funds for clinical trials on a scale and at standards necessary to produce convincing evidence for or against the use of various combinations of antituberculous drugs and antibiotics, and it turned out to be difficult to define criteria for the endpoint 'cure' for the specific part of the treatment directed against *M. ulcerans*. The same applied for other treatment candidates, e.g. thermotherapy.[36] It is not easy to determine on clinical grounds when specific treatment can confidently be stopped and only general wound management has to continue to finally achieve closure of the skin defect. With increasing insight into the dynamics of BU wounds it becomes clear that a period of 'worsening', the so-called 'paradoxical reaction', after initiation of specific treatment is often inescapable (see above). As soon as specific therapy directed against *M. ulcerans* is effectively completed, the post-specific therapy healing process and the requirements for definite wound closure follow the general rules for wound management.

An additional component which complicates the determination of treatment efficacy needs to be remarked upon, i.e. the spontaneous cure rate.[37] From patients treated with clofazimine, which is most probably not active against *M. ulcerans*, and patients treated with placebo[38] we may gain a vague idea of the spontaneous healing rate, which could be significant. This is also reflected by observations in the community which are highly suggestive of a proportion of spontaneously healed BU lesions.

ANTIMYCOBACTERIAL DRUG COMBINATION THERAPY

Before the 'Provisional guidance on the role of specific antibiotics in the management of *Mycobacterium ulcerans* disease (Buruli ulcer)' was issued in 2004,[28] various attempts had been made to explore the use of antimycobacterial drugs to treat BU.[38–40] The comparison of rifampicin plus dapsone versus placebo by Espey and colleagues in 41 subjects in the Cote d'Ivoire, 30 of whom completed the trial, illustrates several common pitfalls in clinical BU trials and weaknesses of the earlier studies.[40] The endpoint for assessing healing was defined as a change in the size of the lesion between enrolment and completion of treatment (2 months). Independent of the fact that the results of this study are flawed by a range of problems, including significantly different median sizes of the lesions of the treatment and the placebo group (26.2 cm^2 vs 4.8 cm^2) due to differential loss to follow-up, it demonstrates two common problems of clinical BU trials. These are the timing and the means of assessment of the endpoint 'healing' (see section on 'Paradoxical reaction', above) and the failure to distinguish between the endpoint which evaluates the effect of the specific BU therapy and the endpoint, which assesses definite closure of the skin defect.

Etuaful and colleagues launched another attempt with a pilot study in Ghana carried out in 2001/2002. A total of 21 patients with laboratory-confirmed nodules and plaques were treated with rifampicin (10 mg/kg) and streptomycin (15 mg/kg) for 2 (five patients), 4 (three patients), 8 (five patients) or 12 weeks (three patients). Five patients received no treatment. The lesions of the patients who received no treatment were excised at enrolment, while the lesions of patients who received treatment were excised after the completion of drug therapy. The lesions of the five patients who received no treatment and the five patients who received 2 weeks of drug therapy were culture-positive after excision. All others were negative. The authors concluded that combination therapy for more than 4 weeks kills *M. ulcerans* in human tissue and that a clinical trial for early *M. ulcerans* disease is justified.[41]

This study was followed by a case series of Chauty and colleagues from 2003/2004 in Benin. Of 215 patients who were classified as treatment successes, 102 patients were treated exclusively with oral rifampicin (10 mg/kg) and intramuscular streptomycin (15 mg/kg), once daily for 8 weeks and 113 patients with at least 4 weeks of rifampicin and streptomycin, as well as surgical excision and skin grafting. With regard to long-term follow-up (1 year after completion of treatment), 208 of the 215 patients were available, of whom three had a recurrence.[42]

The evaluation of evidence available at the time presented at the 6th and 7th WHO Advisory Meetings on Buruli Ulcer in 2003[43,44] and 2004,[45,46] respectively, and further elaborated at an International Workshop on the Management of Buruli Ulcer held in Yaoundé, Cameroon in 2004 prompted the issuing of the 'Provisional guidance on the role of specific antibiotics in the management of *Mycobacterium ulcerans* disease (Buruli ulcer)'.[28]

A large clinical trial followed, recruiting patients between 2006 and 2008 in Ghana and comparing oral rifampicin (10 mg/kg) plus intramuscular streptomycin (15 mg/kg) for 8 weeks (n = 76; R/S group) with rifampicin plus streptomycin for 4 weeks followed by rifampicin plus oral clarithromycin (7.5 mg/kg) for 4 weeks (n = 75; R/S-C group) in patients with lesions with a diameter of <10 cm. All lesions were confirmed by PCR. The primary endpoint was defined as healing of lesions 1 year after the start of drug treatment without recurrence and extensive surgical debridement. 73 patients (96%) in the R/S group and 68 (91%) in the R/S-C group had healed lesions at 1 year. No recurrence was observed. Three patients had vestibulotoxic events.[47]

The clinical efficacy of the combination therapy of oral rifampicin (10 mg/kg) and intramuscular streptomycin (15 mg/kg) once daily for 8 weeks was further confirmed by a case series (n = 160 PCR-confirmed cases) that recruited patients between 2006 and 2007 in Ghana.[48]

Chauty and colleagues further explored a purely oral treatment regimen of rifampicin (10 mg/kg) plus clarithromycin (12 mg/kg) once daily for 8 weeks in 30 patients with PCR-confirmed disease with lesions with a diameter of <10 cm in 2007–2009 in Benin. Nine patients had non-ulcerative lesions, while 11 patients had ulcerative lesions. The primary endpoint was healing at 1 year with no recurrence 1.5 years after the start of drug treatment. In all patients, the wound had closed by 1 year, and there were no relapses after 1.5 years. A majority of the non-ulcerative lesions required additional surgery. Interestingly, three patients had extensive surgery and in none were there persisting viable mycobacteria. As discussed above, the need for surgery is not at all necessarily associated with persistence of specific disease activity. Therefore the need for extensive surgery or an increase in lesion size are not suitable as endpoints for the assessment of efficacy of the BU-specific treatment component in the management of skin and subcutaneous tissue defects induced by *M. ulcerans*.[49]

The development of drug resistance needs to be carefully observed. Resistant strains were found after rifampicin monotherapy in experimentally treated mice.[50]

THERMOTHERAPY

M. ulcerans grows best at 30–33°C and not above 37°C. This property was explored for therapeutic purposes by Meyers and colleagues in eight patients from Zaire in the 1970s. A temperature of approximately 40°C maintained in the ulcerated area for a mean duration of 68 days led to cure in all treated patients. There was no evidence of local recurrence during follow-up periods of up to 22 months.[36] Further investigation was hampered by the lack of a heat application device suitable for countries in which BU is endemic. In 2007, a cheap phase change material device, widely used in commercial pocket heat pads, which is rechargeable in hot water and non-toxic, was explored in a prospective observational single-centre proof-of-principle trial in Cameroon in six laboratory-reconfirmed patients with ulcerative lesions. They received between 28 and 55 days of local thermotherapy. The patients were completely mobile during the well-tolerated heat application. In patients with smaller ulcers, wounds healed completely without further intervention. Patients with large defects had skin grafting after successful heat treatment. One and a half years after completion of treatment, all patients were relapse-free.[51] A clinical trial is ongoing in Cameroon to test the device in a larger number of patients.

Within a few years antituberculous combination therapy has gained substantial support through formal clinical trials and observational studies in West Africa and Australia.

It has further become clear that the treatment and healing process falls into three phases (Box 42.2), with an intervening phase of a so-called paradoxical reaction of variable severity between phase 1 and 2.

Phase 1 of the Treatment and Healing Process

On the basis of the above reviewed evidence WHO recommends in its new version of the treatment guidelines the following standard regimens for specific BU therapy:[54,55]

- Oral rifampicin (10 mg/kg) and intramuscular streptomycin (15 mg/kg) once daily for 8 weeks (contraindicated in pregnancy). Maximum daily doses for rifampicin and streptomycin need to be obeyed. Patients need to be carefully monitored for side effects.
- Oral rifampicin (10 mg/kg) once daily plus oral clarithromycin (7.5 mg/kg) twice daily for 8 weeks (pregnant women). Maximum daily doses for rifampicin and clarithromycin need to be obeyed. Patients need to be carefully monitored for side effects.

Modifications currently in use in Australia are acknowledged. Potential development of drug resistance needs to be carefully monitored (see above).

Local thermotherapy appears to be a well-tolerated and effective alternative to treat local disease, but requires confirmation by the trial currently being conducted in a large group of patients and further feasibility studies in the community.[51]

Papules and small nodules can be excised with primary closure. It must be decided in the individual case if accompanying antimycobacterial combination therapy or, possibly, local thermotherapy is of additional value to prevent recurrence.

Phase 1 needs to be accompanied by rigorous wound management (see below) and optimal hygienic conditions as well as nutritional support. Debridement of non-viable, contaminated or infected tissue is essential (Ia level of evidence).[52] Good wound management includes good pain management!

BOX 42.2 TREATMENT AND HEALING PROCESS

- *Phase 1*: specific antimycobacterial therapy leading to killing of the mycobacteria. General wound management including debridement of non-viable, contaminated or infected tissue is essential.
- *Intervening phase*: worsening of the lesions (ulceration of non-ulcerative lesions and increase in size of already established ulcers; appearance of new lesions) – the so-called 'paradoxical reaction' requiring intensified wound management, often with additional debridement.
- *Phase 2*: definite wound healing phase including skin grafting where needed following on from completion of specific treatment and subsidence of the 'paradoxical reaction'.
- *Phase 3*: restoration of function including physiotherapy and reconstructive surgery where needed.

BOX 42.3 WOUND MANAGEMENT

There is no easy answer to the provision of optimal wound management adapted to the conditions that continue to prevail in resource-poor healthcare settings. Perfect hygiene is a must in order to avoid repeated setbacks.

- The absolute minimum requirements are clean dressing rooms, sufficient amounts of clean water, sterile dressing material and clean bandages, antiseptics, sterile physiological sodium chloride solution to keep the wound moist and an autoclave to sterilize instruments and materials which come into contact with open wounds.
- In case of systemic bacterial infections, the standard antibiotics must be available.
- Debridement of non-viable, contaminated or infected tissue is essential (Ia level of evidence).[52]
- Good wound management includes good pain management and nutritional support.
- Training staff in wound management is essential and very rewarding, since it is of immediate use for all areas in health posts and hospitals. Wound management is a sorely neglected field in all countries with limited resources.

Guidance can be found in the WHO publication 'Wound and lymphoedema management'. *WHO. Wound and lymphoedema management. In: Macdonald JM, Geyer MJ, editors. WHO/HTM/NTD/GBUI/2010.1. World Health Organization; 2010.*

The Intervening Phase

This phase is of variable intensity and intervenes in a large proportion of patients sooner or later after the initiation of drug treatment with a peak incidence towards the end of the specific therapy.[30] The major challenge is to distinguish this from specific treatment failure (which is very rare) and from secondary bacterial infection, in particular erysipelas.

Good wound management is particularly important during this phase, including debridement of non-viable, contaminated or infected tissue.

Phase 2 of the Treatment and Healing Process

After successful completion of specific treatment and after the effects of the 'paradoxical reaction' have subsided, longer periods of straightforward wound management follow (Box 42.3).

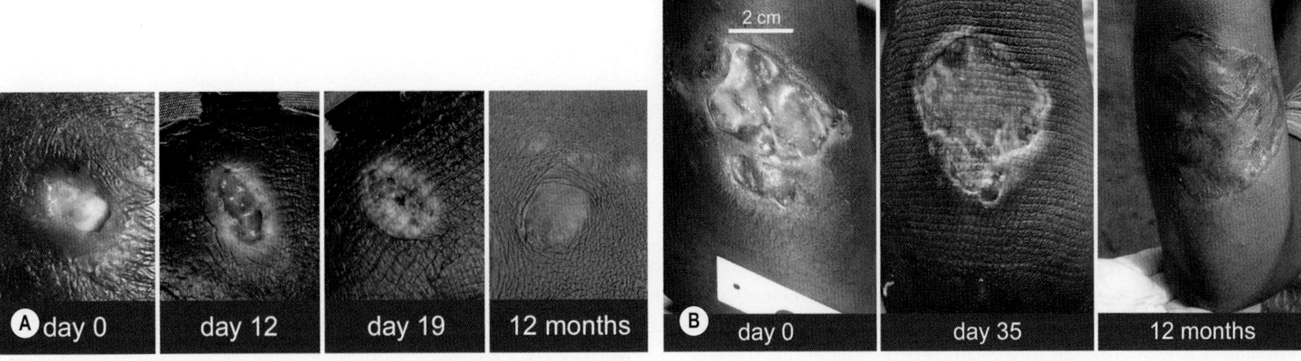

Figure 42.10 Primary healing of a small ulcer with scarring (A) and healing of a large ulcer which required skin grafting for closure (B). Both cases were treated with local thermotherapy. *(Taken from Junghanss T, Um Boock A, Vogel M, et al. Phase change material for thermotherapy of Buruli ulcer: a prospective observational single centre proof-of-principle trial. PLoS Negl Trop Dis 2009;3:e380.)*

Small wounds close with a stable scar; in large wounds or wounds in critical sites, skin grafting is often required (Figure 42.10). The guidelines for wound management should be carefully followed. In settings with well-established and functioning health services, this is routine. In resource-poor settings, in which most cases have to be treated, this phase is critical, and initial success of the specific treatment phase is often jeopardized by intervening secondary bacterial infection.

Phase 3 of the Treatment and Healing Process

Restoration of function needs to be established as soon as possible, in particular of limbs, where most lesions occur. Physiotherapy is absolutely essential, but again, in most regions where patients require help, physiotherapy is not available or not well developed. This problem is even more severe when reconstructive surgery is needed.

Useful WHO documents for the recording and reporting of BU cases and clinical management can be found at:

- http://www.who.int/buruli/control/forms_2/en/index.html
- http://www.who.int/buruli/information/publications/en/index.html.

Prevention

The mode(s) of transmission of BU are still unclear. This hinders the development of recommendations for prevention of infection.[53] Bacille Calmette–Guérin vaccination may convey some short-term protection from the disease. Research to develop a vaccine is still in its early stages.

REFERENCES

20. Schütte D, Um-Boock A, Mensah-Quainoo E, et al. Development of highly organized lymphoid structures in Buruli ulcer lesions after treatment with rifampicin and streptomycin. PLoS Negl Trop Dis 2007;1:e2.
33. WHO. Buruli ulcer. Diagnosis of *Mycobacterium Ulcerans* Disease. In: Portaels F, Johnson P, Meyers WM, editors. WHO/CDS/CPE/GBUI/2001.4. Geneva: World Health Organization; 2001. (under revision: http://www.who.int/buruli/information/publications/en/index.html).
47. Nienhuis WA, Stienstra Y, Thompson WA, et al. Antimicrobial treatment for early, limited *Mycobacterium ulcerans* infection: a randomised controlled trial. Lancet 2010;375:664–72.
54. WHO. Buruli Ulcer. Management of *Mycobacterium ulcerans* disease. A manual for health care providers Buntine and Crofts (eds). World Health Organization; 2001. (under revision: http://www.who.int/buruli/information/publications/en/index.html).
55. WHO. Treatment of *Mycobaterium ulcerans* disease (Buruli ulcer): guidance for health workers. World Health Organization; 2012. http://www.who.int/iris/bitstream/10665/77771/1/9789241503402_eng.pdf

Access the complete references online at www.expertconsult.com

Malaria

NICHOLAS J. WHITE

KEY POINTS

- Malaria is a protozoan infection of red blood cells transmitted by the bite of a blood-feeding female *anopheline* mosquito.
- It is the most important parasitic disease of humans and often the most common cause of fever in the tropics.
- Human malaria infections are caused by *Plasmodium falciparum*, *P. vivax*, *P. malariae*, *P. ovale* and also by the simian parasite *P. knowlesi*.
- Malaria is prevalent across the tropical world. In Africa, *P. falciparum* predominates, whereas in many parts of Asia and the Americas *P. vivax* is more common.
- Malaria is diagnosed by microscopy of suitably stained thick and thin blood smears or by rapid diagnostic tests, which detect parasite antigens in the blood.
- The clinical manifestations of malaria are fever, anaemia and splenomegaly. Most deaths result from *P. falciparum* infections which may cause coma (cerebral malaria), acidosis, severe anaemia, renal dysfunction and pulmonary oedema.
- Treatment of uncomplicated malaria is with artemisinin combination treatments which combine the rapidly acting and rapidly eliminated artemisinin compounds with more slowly eliminated antimalarial drugs. *P. vivax*, *P. malariae*, *P. ovale* and *P. knowlesi* may also be treated with chloroquine.
- *P. vivax* and *P. ovale* malaria also require treatment with primaquine to eliminate the persistent liver forms (hypnozoites) which cause relapse of the infection.
- The key elements of malaria control are effective drug treatment, deployment of insecticide-treated bed nets and where appropriate indoor residual insecticide spraying, supplanted in some areas by intermittent preventive treatments and mass chemoprevention given to all the target population.
- The main threats to malaria control are increasing antimalarial drug resistance and increasing insecticide resistance. There is currently no available malaria vaccine.

Introduction

Malaria is the most important parasitic disease of man. The malaria parasite is a mosquito-transmitted protozoan. *Plasmodia* are sporozoan parasites of red blood cells transmitted to animals (mammals, birds, reptiles) by the bites of mosquitoes. Protozoan parasites of the phylum Apicomplexa contain three genetic elements: the nuclear and mitochondrial genomes characteristic of virtually all eukaryotic cells and a 35-kilobase (kb) circular extrachromosomal DNA. This encodes a vestigial plastid (the apicoplast) that is an evolutionary homologue of the chloroplasts of plant and algal cells. Four species of the genus *Plasmodium* infect humans preferentially and the simian parasite *P. knowlesi* is an important cause of human malaria in parts of South-east Asia. Occasional infections with other errant primate malarias may also occur.[1] Parasites very similar to those infecting humans are found in African great apes. The individual characteristics of the four species of human malaria parasites are shown in Table 43.1. Almost all deaths and severe disease are caused by *P. falciparum*. In phylogenetic terms, this parasite is closest to the avian malarias (*P. lophurae*, *P. gallinaceum*), but it is now clear that *P. falciparum* has co-evolved with its human host through several evolutionary bottlenecks and was not a recent acquisition from birds as once thought. The three 'benign' malarias, *P. vivax*, *P. ovale* and *P. malariae*, all lie closer together on the evolutionary tree near the other primate malarias. It has recently been discovered that '*P. ovale*' comprises two sympatric non-recombining parasite species tentatively termed *P. ovale wallikeri* and *P. ovale curtisi*.[2] Severe disease with these species is relatively unusual, although occasionally patients will die from rupture of an enlarged spleen and they reduce birth weight which predisposes to neonatal death. Full genome sequences are now available for hundreds of *P. falciparum* and *P. vivax* isolates and many of the other *Plasmodia*. The remarkably AT-rich *P. falciparum* genome is approximately 23 Mb in size and encodes about 5300 genes on 14 chromosomes.

History

Malaria, or ague as it was commonly known, has been described since antiquity. Hippocrates is usually credited with the first clear description among occidental writers: In *Epidemics*, he distinguished different patterns of fever and in his *Aphorisms*, he describes the regular paroxysms of intermittent fever. In Europe, seasonal periodic fevers were particularly common in marshy areas and were frequently referred to as 'paludial' (L. *palus*, marshy ground; Fr. *paludisme*). In the early nineteenth century miasmatic influences were believed to cause a variety of diseases. Malaria was thought by Italian writers to be caused by the offensive vapours emanating from the Tiberian marshes. The word 'malaria' comes from the Italian and means literally 'bad air'. Indeed the cause of the seasonal periodic fevers was a continuous source of debate until the late nineteenth century. The work of Meckel, Virchow and Frerichs had established that the dark malaria pigment (mistakenly thought to be melanin) observed in the blood of some patients with periodic fever resulted from the destruction of red blood corpuscles. This same pigment caused the characteristic grey discoloration of the internal organs in patients dying from this disease. In the

TABLE 43.1 **Human Malaria Parasites**

	P. falciparum	*P. vivax*	*P. ovale*	*P. malariae*	*P. knowlesi*
Exoerythrocytic (hepatic) phase of development (days)	5.5	8	9	15	?7
Erythrocytic cycle (days)	2	2	2	3	1
Hypnozoites (relapses)	No	Yes	Yes	No	No
Number of merozoites per hepatic schizont	30 000	10 000	15 000	2000	
Erythrocyte preference	Young RBCs but can invade all ages[a]	Reticulocytes	Reticulocytes	Old RBCs	All ages
Maximum duration of untreated infection (years)	2	4	4	40	?

[a]Parasites causing severe malaria are not selective in red cell invasion.

1870s, medicine slowly moved towards the germ theory of disease, following the pioneering work of Koch. In 1879, Edwin Klebs and Corrado Tommasi-Crudelli reported the identification of a bacterial cause of malaria. Recovery of the 'organism', *Bacillus malariae*, from patients with malaria was confirmed by several influential Italian physicians and pathologists – and similar reports began to appear in the USA. It was not surprising, therefore, that the report of a French Army surgeon working in Algeria, claiming that malaria was caused by a parasite, was treated initially with some scepticism. On 20 October 1880 (in a later publication he gives the date as 6 November), Charles Louis Alphonse Laveran was examining the fresh blood of a patient with ague and observed moving bodies (he was probably watching gametocyte exflagellation), which he surmised correctly were parasites of the red blood cells. The transmissibility of the infection in blood was proved 4 years later by Gerhardt, but the route of natural infection was not discovered until the next decade. Following the suggestion of Patrick Manson, a young Scottish physician in the Indian Medical Service, Ronald Ross, began to investigate the possibility that malaria could be transmitted by mosquitoes. In 1897, after many months of failure, he reported the presence of pigmented bodies in the gut of a certain species of brown 'dapple winged' mosquito fed on patients with malaria. He speculated that these might represent the parasite stage in the mosquito (he was in fact describing the oocysts) but, because of difficulties in obtaining these 'unusual' mosquitoes and his transfer to Calcutta, he was unable to characterize the complete life cycle, i.e. transmission from human to mosquito to human. After many years of study, Ross finally proved the existence of the complete life cycle involving a mosquito in the malaria of canaries. He identified the anopheles mosquito as the vector of human malaria, although by the time Ross finally had the opportunity to demonstrate *Plasmodium falciparum* sporogony in *anopheline* mosquitoes in Sierra Leone, Bignami and his colleagues, following the pioneering work of Grassi, had succeeded in infecting a healthy volunteer with *P. falciparum* from mosquito bites in Rome. Both Laveran and Ross received Nobel Prizes for their respective discoveries.

Understanding of the biology of malaria was further advanced by a third Nobel-prize winning discovery. In 1883 the Viennese psychiatrist Julius Wagner–Jarregg became interested in the relationship between fever and mental illness. Between 1888 and 1917 he experimented on a number of methods of inducing fever to treat patients with 'general paralysis of the insane' (GPI is a form of neurosyphilis). On 14 June 1917 he inoculated blood from a soldier with tertian fever into two patients with GPI. So began the era of malariatherapy of neurosyphilis. This became standard practice throughout the world until the introduction of penicillin 30 years later. Malaria became the most studied infection of humans. Overall, at a time when GPI accounted for 10% of all mental hospital inpatients in Europe, malaria therapy gave approximately 30% of patients a full and 20%, a partial remission of this debilitating and ultimately lethal infection.

Until the nineteenth century, malaria was found in northern Europe, North America and Russia – and transmission in parts of southern Europe was intense. Since then it has been eradicated from these areas and the number of cases in the Middle East, China and parts of Asia and South America has fallen, but elsewhere in the tropics there was a resurgence of the disease. Between 1970 and 2000 the number of cases worldwide and the number of deaths steadily increased. This rising death toll was not a result of failing health systems as the number of deaths from many other infectious diseases fell. It resulted from increasing resistance of the *anopheline* vector to insecticides and of the parasite to the antimalarial drugs that were deployed.

Life Cycle

PRE-ERYTHROCYTIC DEVELOPMENT

Infection with human malaria begins when the feeding female *anopheline* mosquito inoculates plasmodial sporozoites at the time of feeding. The small motile sporozoites are injected during the phase of probing as the mosquito searches for a vascular space before aspirating blood. In most cases, relatively few sporozoites are injected (approx. 8–15), but up to 100 may be introduced in some instances. Most sporozoites come from the larger salivary ducts and represent only a small fraction of the total number in the salivary gland. After injection, they enter the circulation, either directly or via lymph channels (approx. 20%) and rapidly target the hepatic parenchymal cells. Within approximately 45 minutes of the bite all sporozoites have either entered the hepatocytes or have been cleared. Each sporozoite bores into the hepatocyte and there begins a phase of asexual reproduction. This stage lasts on average between 5.5 (*P. falciparum*) and 15 days (*P. malariae*) before the hepatic schizont ruptures to release merozoites into the bloodstream (Table 43.2). In some instances, the primary incubation period can be much longer. In *P. vivax* and *P. ovale* infections a proportion of the intrahepatic parasites do not develop, but instead rest inert as sleeping forms or 'hypnozoites', to awaken weeks or months later and cause the relapses which characterize infections with these two species.[3] During the pre-erythrocytic or hepatic phase

TABLE 43.2 Malaria Incubation Periods in Malaria Therapy and Volunteer Studies

	Prepatent Period (Days)	Incubation Period (Days)
P. falciparum	11.0±2.4	13.1±2.8
P. vivax	12.2±2.3	13.4±2.7
P. malariae	32.7[a]	34.7[a]
P. ovale	12.0	14.1

Values are mean±SD.

[a]These data are taken from artificially induced malaria data in Boyd (1948); naturally acquired infections are considered to have an incubation period of between 13–28 days.

of development considerable asexual multiplication takes place and many thousands of merozoites are released from each ruptured infected hepatocyte. However, as only a few liver cells are infected, this phase is asymptomatic for the human host.

ASEXUAL BLOOD-STAGE DEVELOPMENT

The merozoites liberated into the bloodstream closely resemble sporozoites. They are motile ovoid forms which invade red cells rapidly. The process of invasion involves attachment to the erythrocyte surface, orientation so that the apical complex (which protrudes slightly from one end of the merozoite and contains the rhoptries, the micronemes and dense granules) abuts the red cell and then interiorization takes place by a wriggling or boring motion inside a vacuole composed of the invaginated erythrocyte membrane. Once inside the erythrocyte the parasite lies within the erythrocyte cytosol enveloped by its own plasma membrane and a surrounding parasitophorous vacuolar membrane. The attachment of the merozoite to the red cell is mediated by attachment of one or more of a family of erythrocyte binding proteins, localized to the micronemes of the merozoite apical complex, to a specific erythrocyte receptor. In *P. vivax* and *P. knowlesi* this is related to the Duffy blood group antigen Fy^a or Fy^b. The absence of these phenotypes in West Africans, or people who originate from that region, has been suggested to explain their proven resistance to infection with *P. vivax* and the absence of *vivax* malaria in West Africa. But early malariatherapy observations and recent epidemiological studies in continental Africa and Madagascar show that *P. vivax* can infect Duffy-negative individuals, so there are probably multiple invasion pathways. For *P. falciparum* the reticulocyte-binding protein homologue 5 (PfRh5) is indispensable for erythrocyte invasion. Basigin (CD147, EMMPRIN) has been identified as the erythrocyte receptor of PfRh5 and shown to be essential for the invasion of multiple strains.[4] The merozoite protein EBA 175, a member of the 'Duffy binding like' (DBL) superfamily of genes encoding ligands for host cell receptors is also clearly important. This binds to sialic acid and the peptide backbone of the red cell membrane sialoglycoprotein glycophorin A. Other sialic-acid-dependent and -independent pathways of invasion also occur indicating considerable reserve in the invasion system. Binding is linked to activation of a parasite actin motor which provides the mechanical energy for the invasion process. The red cell surface receptors for *P. malariae* and *P. ovale* are not known.

During the early stage of intraerythrocytic development (<12 hours) the small 'ring forms' of the four parasite species appear similar under light microscopy. The young developing parasite looks like a signet ring or, in the case of *P. falciparum*, like a pair of stereo-headphones, with darkly staining chromatin in the nucleus, a circular rim of cytoplasm and a pale central food vacuole. Parasites are freely motile within the erythrocyte. As they grow they increase in size logarithmically and consume the erythrocyte's contents (most of which is haemoglobin). With this increase in size the *P. falciparum* parasitized erythrocyte becomes spherical and less deformable. Proteolysis of haemoglobin within the digestive vacuole releases amino acids which are taken up and utilized by the growing parasite for protein synthesis, but the liberated haem poses a toxic threat. Freed from its protein scaffold haem is highly reactive and readily oxidizes to the ferric form. Toxicity is avoided by spontaneous and protein-facilitated dimerization to an inert crystalline substance, haemozoin. Non-polymerized haem exits the food vacuole but is then degraded in the cytosol by glutathione. Excess non-polymerized haem overwhelms the defence mechanism and is toxic. The digested products, mainly the brown or black insoluble pigment haemozoin, can be readily seen within the digestive vacuole of the growing parasite. To obtain amino acids and other nutrients and to control the electrolytic milieu in the infected erythrocyte the parasite inserts specific transporters and other proteins in the red cell membrane. These and other disruptions make the red cell more permeable. The *P. falciparum* infected erythrocyte becomes progressively less elastic and deformable and more spherical as the parasite grows.

At approximately 12–14 hours of development *P. falciparum* parasites begin to exhibit a high-molecular-weight strain-specific variant antigen, *Plasmodium falciparum* erythrocyte membrane protein 1 (*Pf*EMP1) on the exterior surface of the infected red cell which mediates attachment to vascular endothelium. This is associated with knob-like projections from the erythrocyte membrane. Expression increases towards the middle of the cycle (24 hours). These 'knobby' or K+ red cells then progressively disappear from the circulation by attachment or 'cytoadherence' to the walls of venules and capillaries in the vital organs. This process is called 'sequestration'. The other three 'benign' human malarias do not cytoadhere in systemic blood vessels and all stages of development circulate in the blood-stream.

As *P. vivax* grows it enlarges the infected red cell, which in contrast to *P. falciparum*, leads to an increase in deformability as the parasite matures. Red granules known as Schuffner's dots appear throughout the erythrocyte. Similar dots are also prominent in *P. ovale*, which also distorts the shape of the infected erythrocyte (hence its name). *P. malariae* produces characteristic 'band forms' as the parasite grows. It is usually present at low parasitaemias. When humans are infected with the potentially lethal monkey malaria *P. knowlesi* it is often mistaken for *P. malariae* under light microscopy.[1] High parasitaemias (over 2%) are usually caused by *P. falciparum* or *P. knowlesi*. Approximately 36 hours after merozoite invasion (or 54 hours in *P. malariae*) repeated nuclear division takes place to form a 'segmenter' or schizont (the term 'meront' is etymologically more correct). Eventually the growing parasite occupies the entire red cell which has become spherical, depleted in haemoglobin and full of merozoites. This then ruptures; so that between 6 and 36 merozoites are released, destroying the remnants of the red cell. Following *P. falciparum* schizogony the residual cytoadherent erythrocyte membrane and associated malaria pigment often remains attached to the vascular endothelium for many hours. The released merozoites rapidly reinvade other red cells and start a new asexual cycle. Thus the infection expands logarithmically at approximately 10-fold per cycle. Only a sub-population of erythrocytes can be invaded, determined largely by red cell age. *P. vivax* can invade red cells for up to 2 weeks after emergence from the bone marrow. In Thailand, *P. falciparum* parasites causing severe malaria showed unselective invasion and had a greater multiplication potential at high densities than those which caused uncomplicated malaria. The asexual life cycle is approximately 24 hours for *P. knowlesi*, 48 hours for *P. falciparum*, *P. vivax* and *P. ovale* and 72 hours for *P. malariae*.

SEXUAL STAGES AND DEVELOPMENT IN THE MOSQUITO

After a series of asexual cycles in *Plasmodium falciparum*, a subpopulation of parasites develops into sexual forms (gametocytes) which are long-lived and motile. These are the stages which transmit the infection. The process of gametocytogony takes about 7–10 days in *P. falciparum* but only 4 days in *P. vivax* which begins gametocytogenesis immediately in the blood stage infection. Thus there is an interval of approximately 1 week between peak asexual and sexual stage parasitaemia in acute *falciparum* malaria. There is no delay with *P. vivax* so symptomatic *P. vivax* infections are more likely to present with patent gametocytaemia before treatment (and therefore to transmit) than acute *P. falciparum* infections. The male-to-female gametocyte sex ratio for *P. falciparum* is approximately 1 : 4, although each male gametocyte can produce up to 8 microgametes each capable of individual fertilization. Following ingestion in the blood meal of a biting female *anopheline* mosquito, the male and female gametocytes become activated in the mosquito's gut.[5] The male gametocytes undergo rapid nuclear division and each of the eight nuclei formed associates with a flagellum (20–25 μm long). The motile male microgametes then separate and seek the female macrogametes. Fusion and meiosis then take place to form a zygote. For a brief period the malaria parasite is diploid. Within 24 hours the enlarging zygote becomes motile and this form (the ookinete) penetrates the wall of the mosquito mid-gut (stomach) where it encysts (as an oocyst). This spherical bag of parasites expands by asexual division to reach a diameter of approximately 500 μm, i.e. it becomes visible to the naked eye. During the early stage of oocyst development there is a characteristic pigment pattern and colour that allows speciation (it was this that caught the eye of its discoverer, Ronald Ross, in 1894), but these patterns become obscured by the time the oocyst has matured to contain thousands of fusiform motile sporozoites. The oocyst finally bursts to liberate myriads of sporozoites into the coelomic cavity of the mosquito. The sporozoites then migrate to the salivary glands to await inoculation into the next human host during feeding. The development of the parasite in the mosquito is termed sporogony and takes between 8 and 35 days depending on the ambient temperature and species of parasite and mosquito. The longevity of the mosquito is a critical factor in determining its vectorial capacity (see above).

MOLECULAR GENETICS

Inheritance in *Plasmodium* is similar to that in other eukaryotes. Haploid and diploid generations alternate. A large number of individual genes were cloned and sequenced on the long and winding (and as yet unfinished) road towards the development of a malaria vaccine and in the past few years the entire genomes of several hundred malaria parasites have been sequenced. *P. falciparum* has approximately 5300 genes in its 14 chromosomes and extrachromosomal elements compared with the 31 000 of its natural host. Codon composition is extremely biased to adenine and thymine in *P. falciparum* but more evenly balanced in the other malaria parasite genomes. There appear to be some groupings of genes related to function. For example, the genes encoding the merozoite surface proteins are grouped. The many genes encoding the variant red cell surface antigens (*var* and *rif* families), which contribute to the antigenic diversity necessary for the parasite to elude the host immune system, are also located close to each other near the telomeres. The *var* gene product, the variant surface protein which mediates cytoadherence (*Pf*EMP1) appears to be the main antigen determining the parasite population structure during chronic *falciparum* malaria infections. Variation in surface antigenicity results from the activation of different *var* genes. This switching occurs at different rates, some of which exceed 2% per asexual cycle. It has been suggested that the diversity of these immunodominant variant repeat sequences interferes with the selection of high-affinity antibody responses and perpetuates low-affinity responses in malaria. This 'confusion of the immune response' delays the development of effective immunity. Immune selection also provides the selective pressure to maintain diversity in T- and B-cell epitopes through a high frequency of non-synonymous base mutations during the asexual development of malaria parasites. At a larger scale, genetic changes resulting in drug resistance have had a profound effect on the malaria parasite population structure with the progeny of drug-resistant parasites originating in South-east Asia sweeping across India and then spreading across Africa.[6]

The mechanisms maintaining genetic diversity within the parasite genome are many and complex. Some of the polymorphic antigens identified are encoded by single gene copies in the haploid genome. These polypeptide antigens are characterized by tandem repeat sequences. Unequal crossing over during recombination can generate completely different sequences of these repeats. As these repeat sequences are also antibody targets, their variation provides further antigenic diversity.

Epidemiology

Malaria infects approximately 5% of the world's population and causes over six hundred thousand deaths each year. Most of these deaths are in African children. Malaria (both *P. falciparum* and *P. vivax*) also contributes to neonatal mortality by reducing birth weight.

DISTRIBUTION

Malaria is found throughout the tropics (Figure 43.1). In Africa, *P. falciparum* predominates, as it does on the island of New Guinea and in Haiti, whereas *P. vivax* is more common in Central and parts of South America, North Africa, the Middle East and the Indian subcontinent. The prevalence of both species is approximately equal in other parts of South America, South-east Asia and Oceania. *P. vivax* is rare in West Africa (but is common in the horn of Africa, whereas *P. ovale* is common only in West Africa. *P. malariae* is found in most areas, but is

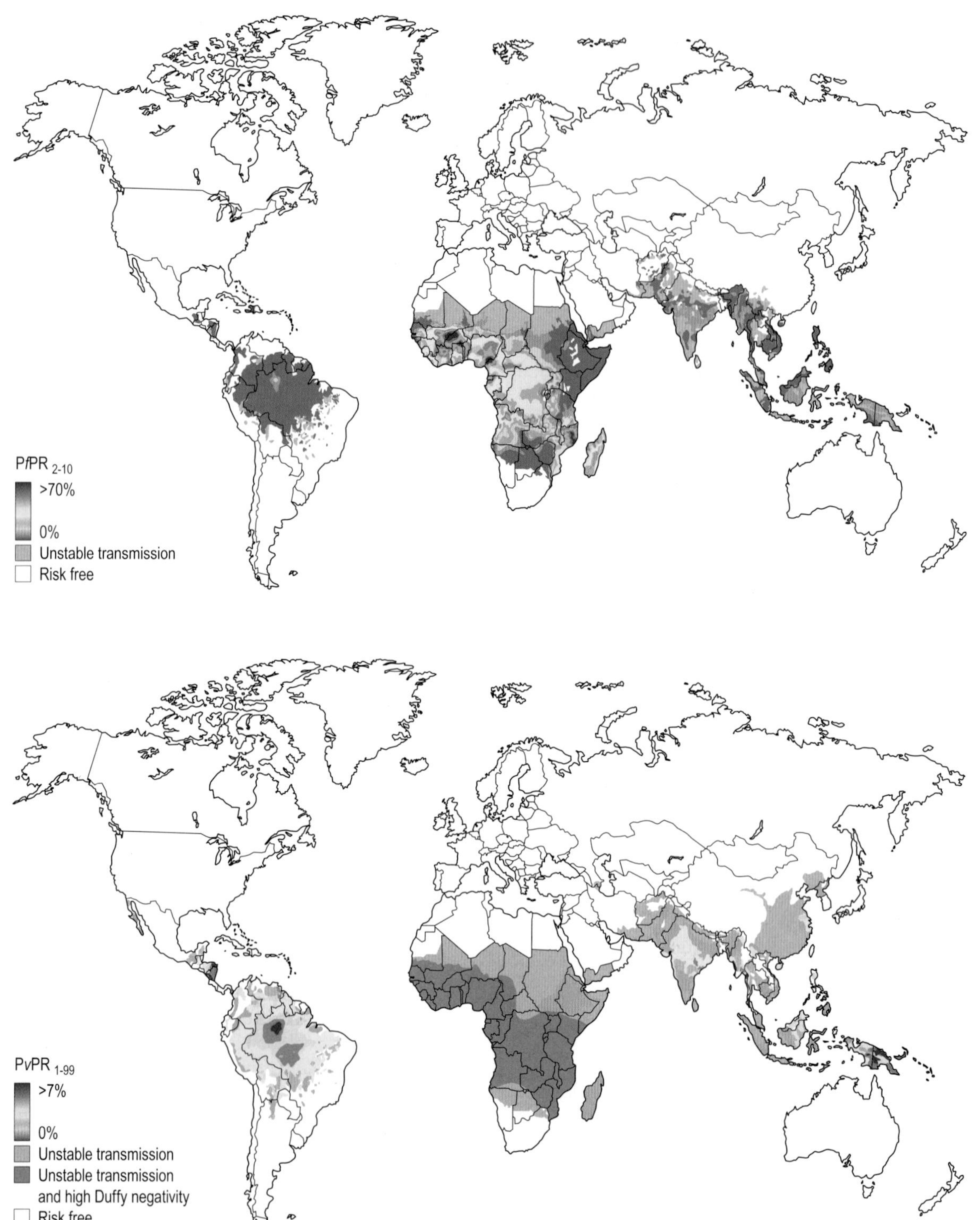

Figure 43.1 Global distribution of *Plasmodium falciparum* and *Plasmodium vivax* malaria. Upper panel shows the model-based geostatistical point (MBG) estimates of the *Plasmodium falciparum* annual mean parasite rate *Pf*PR2–10 (defined as the predicted proportion of 2–10-year-olds with patent parasitaemia) for 2010 within the spatial limits of stable *P. falciparum* malaria transmission.[40] Lower panel shows equivalent estimates of the *Plasmodium vivax* annual mean parasite rate (*Pv*PR1–99).[41] Note this prediction is for all age groups (1–99). *P. vivax* is rare in areas with a high prevalence of Duffy (blood group) negativity.

relatively uncommon outside Africa. Malaria was once endemic in Europe and northern Asia and was introduced to North America, but it has been eradicated from these areas. In South and South-east Asia, Oceania and South America *P. vivax* relapses at frequent regular intervals (of 3 weeks if rapidly eliminated antimalarial drugs are given). In North and Central America, Europe, North Africa, the Middle East, parts of North India, central China and North Korea *P. vivax* has (or had) a different relapse periodicity; after the initial illness the first relapse is 8–10 months later. In Northern Europe and Northern Russia the interval between inoculation and first illness was 8–10 months (*P. vivax* hibernans).[3]

THE MOSQUITO VECTOR

Malaria is transmitted by some species of *anopheline* mosquitoes. Malaria transmission does not occur at temperatures below 16°C, or above 33°C, and at altitudes >2000 m because development in the mosquito (sporogony) cannot take place. The optimum conditions for transmission are high humidity and an ambient temperature between 20°C and 30°C. Although rainfall provides breeding sites for mosquitoes, excessive rainfall may wash away mosquito larvae and pupae.

The epidemiology of malaria is complex and may vary considerably even within relatively small geographic areas. In low-transmission settings small foci of much higher transmission sustain malaria and confound elimination efforts. Malaria transmission to man depends on several interrelated factors. The most important pertain to the *anopheline* mosquito vector and in particular its longevity. As sporogony (development of the sporozoite parasites in the vector) takes over a week (depending on ambient temperatures), the mosquito must survive for longer than this after feeding on a gametocyte-carrying human, if malaria is to be transmitted. Macdonald gave the following formula for the likelihood of infection based on the sporozoite rates, i.e. the proportion of *anopheline* mosquitoes with sporozoites in their salivary glands.

$$S = \frac{P^n ax}{ax - \log_e P}$$

where P = the probability of mosquito survival through 1 day; n = the duration, in days, of the extrinsic cycle of the parasite in the mosquito; a = average number of blood meals on man per day and x = the proportion of bites infective to man. The probability of a mosquito surviving n days is given by:

$$\frac{P^n}{-\log_e P}$$

The inoculation rate, or the mean daily number of bites (h) received by sporozoite-bearing mosquitoes is given by:

$$h = mabs$$

where m = *anopheline* density in relation to man and b = proportion of bites that are infectious. The reproductive rate of the infection (r) or the number of secondary cases resulting from a primary case is then given by:

$$r = \frac{ma^2bP^n}{-z\log_e P}\left(1 - \frac{ax}{ax - \log_e P}\right)$$

where z is the recovery rate, or the reciprocal of the duration of human infectivity. This is usually estimated at 80 days for *P. falciparum* in a non-immune subject, i.e. $z = 0.0125$. The term:

$$1 - \frac{ax}{ax - \log_e P}$$

refers to the proportion of *anopheline* mosquitoes 'not yet infected'. When transmission is very low (i.e. x approaches 0) then the basic reproductive rate (r_0) reduces to:

$$r_0 = \frac{ma^2bP^n}{-z\log_e P}$$

Thus, as a general approximation, malaria transmission is directly proportional to the density of the vector, the square of the number of times each day that the mosquito bites man and the tenth power of the probability of the mosquito surviving for 1 day. The model described by MacDonald has certain theoretical limitations (it has been refined in recent years to accommodate these), but it does illustrate certain fundamental points of practical relevance to control or eradication programmes. Vector longevity in determining transmission is clearly of central importance and focuses control measures on the adult mosquito. At very high levels of transmission there is considerable reserve in the system and large reductions in transmission reduce malaria by a negligible amount (e.g. a reduction in transmission of 90% from 300 infectious bites per year to 30 bites/year will make very little difference to the prevalence of malaria) – but as r_0 approaches the critical value of 1 (below which the disease dies out), small reductions in r_0 have very large effects on the amount of malaria. Thus, malaria is potentially very vulnerable in low-transmission settings. Control programmes can be very effective in these circumstances and can eradicate malaria – as indeed they did in Europe where r_0 was certainly low in many areas, drug treatment was freely available, and the vector rested inside houses and could be attacked with residual insecticides. Vectors differ considerably in their natural abundance (particularly with season of the year), feeding and resting behaviours, breeding sites, flight ranges, choice of blood source (many *anopheline* vectors also bite animals), and vulnerability to environmental conditions and insecticides.

There is also considerable variation in the ability of different anopheline mosquito species to transmit malaria (the vectorial capacity). There are nearly 400 species of *anopheline* mosquitoes and many are species complexes. Confusingly, the taxonomy continually changes as differences within species complexes are characterized and molecular genetics reveals their phylogeny. Approximately 80 *anopheline* species can transmit malaria, 66 are considered natural vectors, and about 45 are considered important vectors. Each vector has its own behaviour patterns, and even within a species these can vary between geographic areas and can change with selection pressures (such as insecticide use). For example in South-east Asia mosquitoes of the *Anopheles dirus* complex are an important cause of 'forest and forest fringe' malaria. They breed in the tree collections of water and are consequently vulnerable to deforestation, or too little or too much rainfall, but they are very difficult to attack with insecticides. *A. sundaicus* and *A. epiroticus* are found near the coast as they breed in brackish water. Human biting times vary considerably within the species complexes. *A. stephensi*, the principal vector in the Indian subcontinent, breeds in wells or stagnant water and can be controlled by treating breeding sites with insecticides or polystyrene balls. The most effective malaria vectors (such as the *A. gambiae* complex in Africa) are hardy, long-lived, naturally occur in high densities and bite humans frequently. Malaria is often seasonal, coinciding with the rainy season which provides water for mosquito breeding and increased humidity favouring mosquito survival. Other factors, which are not well understood, also influence mosquito populations and lead to fluctuations in the prevalence of malaria.

THE HUMAN HOST

The behaviour of man also plays an important role in the epidemiology of malaria. There must be a human reservoir of viable gametocytes to transmit the infection. In areas of high transmission infants and young children are more susceptible to malaria than the more immune older children and adults.

Parasite densities are higher and gametocytaemia is detected more frequently in children. In endemic areas the relative contributions to overall transmission of the younger age group, who have higher parasite densities, become ill more often and are therefore more likely to receive drugs, versus the older asymptomatic individuals who have lower parasite densities and also immunity and are less likely to receive antimalarial treatment, is unclear. The endemicity of malaria is best defined by the entomological inoculation rate (EIR), or number of infectious mosquito bites received per person per year (although this is difficult to measure accurately), but is defined traditionally in terms of the spleen or parasite rates in children aged between 2 and 9 years.

- Hypoendemic: spleen rate or parasite rate 0–10%
- Mesoendemic: spleen or parasite rate 10–50%
- Hyperendemic: spleen or parasite rate 50–75% and adult spleen rate is also high
- Holoendemic: spleen or parasite rate over 75% and adult spleen rate low. Parasite rates in the 1st year of life are high.

In areas which are holoendemic or hyperendemic for *P. falciparum*, such as much of tropical Africa or coastal New Guinea, people are infected repeatedly throughout their lives. There is considerable morbidity and mortality during childhood. In The Gambia, where people were infected once each year on average (a relatively low figure for the African continent), malaria was estimated to cause 25% of deaths between 1 and 4 years of age. The effects of insecticide-treated nets on death rates in children (average reduction in all-cause mortality in children under 5 years old of approximately 20%) across sub-Saharan Africa is further testament to the impact of malaria on child survival. But eventually, if the child survives, a state of 'premunition' is achieved where infections cause little or no problems to the host. Thus a form of immunity develops which is sufficient to control, but not prevent, the infection. The slow rate at which premunition is acquired may be a function of age. Non-immune adults entering an area of intense transmission acquire premunition more rapidly than children. *Falciparum* malaria infections are more severe in pregnancy, particularly in primigravidae, and appears to be augmented by iron supplementation.

It is difficult to be precise about how many people die each year from malaria, as the disease is most prevalent where health services are lacking. But in recent years a considerable effort has gone into deriving estimates of the global burden of disease.[7] It is widely quoted that 90% of the deaths from malaria in the world are in African children, but recent studies suggest that the burden of malaria in Asia may have been underestimated.[8] It has also been claimed that there is a large and previously unrecognized mortality from malaria in older adults, but this is misleading and reflects the lack of specificity of the verbal autopsy approach to ascertaining cause of death. The setting up of standardized demographic surveillance systems in many malaria-endemic areas has resulted in more accurate data and more accurate measurement of the impact of interventions.

CLINICAL EPIDEMIOLOGY

Babies develop severe malaria relatively infrequently (although, if they do, the mortality is high). The factors responsible for this apparent protection include passive transfer of maternal immunity and the high haemoglobin F content of the infants' erythrocytes which retards parasite development. In holoendemic areas the baby is inoculated repeatedly with sporozoites during the first 6 months of life, but the blood stage infection is seldom severe. People may receive up to three infectious bites per day. In this epidemiological context the main clinical impact of *falciparum* malaria is to cause severe anaemia in the 1–3-year age group (Figure 43.2). With less intense or more variable or unstable transmission the age range affected by severe malaria extends to older children and cerebral malaria becomes a more prominent manifestation of severe disease.[9] Although mortality falls with decreasing transmission intensity, it remains substantial until the EIR falls well below one. In hyperendemic and holoendemic areas indigenous adults never develop severe malaria, unless they leave the transmission area and return years later (and even then malaria is seldom life-threatening). Immunity is constantly boosted and effective premunition prevents parasite burdens reaching dangerous levels. Nearly all infections in adults are asymptomatic. In terms of the mathematical models presented earlier, an index of malaria transmission stability is given by $al\text{-}log_eP$; values of >2.5 indicate stable transmission.

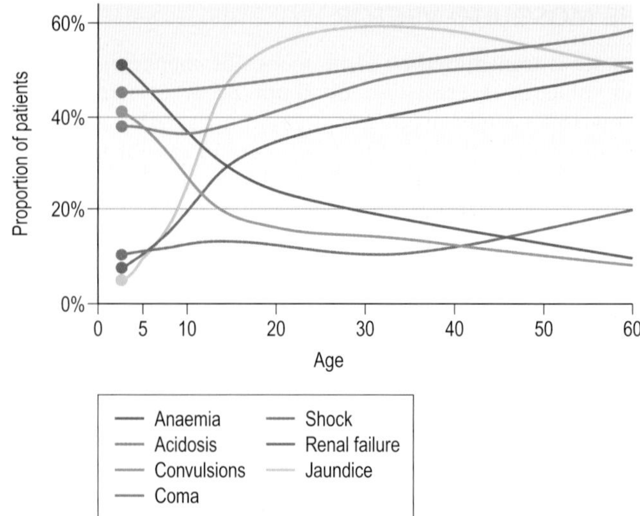

Figure 43.2 Relationship between age and the clinical presentations of severe falciparum malaria at different levels of malaria transmission.

Where transmission of malaria is low, erratic, markedly seasonal, or focal, symptomatic infections are more common. A state of premunition is often not attained. Symptomatic disease occurs at any age and cerebral malaria is a prominent manifestation of severe disease at all ages. This is termed 'unstable' malaria. Epidemics with high mortality may occur. In many areas the transmission of malaria varies considerably over short distances and severe disease is common when non-immune individuals enter these areas (e.g. woodcutters in South America and South-east Asia where malaria is of the 'forest fringe' type, or highland refugees in Burundi descending into malarious lowlands).With declining malaria as malaria control efforts are successful the clinical epidemiology of malaria changes and older children and adults are increasingly likely to develop symptomatic illness.

Malaria is usually a 'rainy season disease' coinciding with increased mosquito abundance. In some areas parasite rates (i.e. the proportion of people with positive blood smears) are relatively constant throughout the year, but the majority of cases still do occur during the wet season. Deforestation, population migration and changes in agricultural practice have profound effects on malaria transmission. Urban malaria is becoming an increasing problem in many countries. Malaria can also behave as an epidemic disease carrying a high mortality. Epidemics are caused by migrations (i.e. introduction of susceptible hosts), the introduction of new vectors, or changes in the habits of the mosquito vector or the human host. Epidemics have occurred in North India, Sri Lanka, South-east Asia, Ethiopia, Madagascar, Brazil (when the formidable African vector *A. gambiae* was inadvertently imported from Africa in the 1930s) and more recently in Burundi and KwaZulu Natal, where drug resistance was also a contributory factor.

Increasing international air travel and worsening antimalarial drug resistance have led to an increase in imported cases of malaria in tourists, travellers, and immigrants. With the recent exception of some of the former Soviet republics in East Europe and West Asia, this has not led to the reintroduction of malaria to areas from where it had earlier been eradicated (although the vector, and thus the potential, remains). Imported malaria is often misdiagnosed, leading to delays in treatment and severe presentations of *falciparum* malaria are not uncommon. Malaria may also be transmitted by blood transfusion, transplantation, or through needle-sharing among intravenous drug addicts.

GENETIC FACTORS PROTECTING AGAINST MALARIA

In 1949, JBS Haldane suggested that people who were heterozygous for red cell abnormalities such as thalassaemia or sickle cell disease might be protected against malaria. This, he said, would explain the high gene frequencies for the haemoglobinopathies in tropical areas and their rarity in colder climates. A state of 'balanced polymorphism' would exist, whereby the loss of the disadvantaged homozygotes would be offset by the survival advantage in heterozygotes. There is now good evidence from detailed epidemiological studies that this hypothesis is correct. The greatest protection is conferred by sickle cell trait and Melanesian ovalocytosis. These patients' cells resist parasite invasion (in the case of sickle cell trait under low oxygen tensions) and once invaded the AS cells sickle readily, facilitating their clearance by the reticuloendothelial system. *P. falciparum*-infected red cells containing haemoglobins S and C show reduced cytoadherence because of reduced presentation of the ligand *Pf*EMP1. The protective effect conferred by the thalassaemias or glucose-6-phosphate dehydrogenase (G6PD) deficiency (which share a geographical distribution with malaria) is generally weaker. The main protection is against severe malaria (Hb AS, CC, AC, AE, homozygous and heterozygous alpha thalassaemia, G6PD deficiency).[10]

The mechanism of protection in many of these haemoglobinopathies, and how they interact with each other, is still incompletely understood.[11] The rate of decline of haemoglobin F in the 1st year of life is slower in α- and β-thalassaemia heterozygotes. Erythrocytes containing high haemoglobin F concentrations do not support parasite growth well. But studies from Vanuatu indicate that children with α-thalassaemia actually have more malaria (both *P. falciparum* and *P. vivax*) in the early years of life than their 'normal' counterparts suggesting a complex interaction between malaria species and haemoglobin chain synthesis. Melanesian ovalocytic erythrocytes both resist invasion by malaria parasites and provide a hostile intraerythrocytic ionic milieu for development. Haemoglobin E heterozygotes (HbAE) are haematologically almost normal and these individuals are susceptible to *falciparum* malaria but appear to be protected against severe malaria. Parasite multiplication at high densities is reduced. G6PD deficiency reduces parasite densities in *P. vivax* infections.[12]

Apart from the well-established protection conferred by polymorphisms in the genes encoding haemoglobin, a large and confusing array of other polymorphisms associated with protection and susceptibility to malaria have been reported. In some cases a polymorphism has been associated with protection in one study and susceptibility in another! Three different TNF promoter polymorphisms appear independently to be associated with severe malaria; Gambian children homozygous for the TNF-308A allele were at a sevenfold increased risk of dying or recovering with neurological sequelae. Although this association was confirmed in East Africa it was not found in two independent studies in Asia. TNF-238A was associated independently with severe anaemia and TNF-376A with susceptibility to cerebral malaria. A single nucleotide polymorphism in the inducible nitric oxide synthase gene promoter region was associated with severe anaemia in Gabon. Separate case–control studies on genetic polymorphisms in CD36 and ICAM-1, the two major receptors for *P. falciparum* cytoadherence have given conflicting results. The CD36 polymorphism protected from severe malaria in one study but increased the risk in the other. An African ICAM-1 polymorphism predisposed to cerebral malaria in Kenya, was neutral in The Gambia, and protected in Gabon. In some of these associations the possibility of linkage cannot be ruled out (i.e. the polymorphic gene lies close to another gene which is causally associated with the observed effect). For example the MHC III region, where the TNF promoter polymorphisms are located, contains a remarkably high density of genes with probable immune functions. The contribution of epistasis, which is the interaction between genes, to malaria susceptibility and resistance has been underappreciated. This makes interpretation of genetic associations very difficult and probably explains many of the inconsistencies described above.

Pathology

EXPANSION OF THE INFECTION

When the hepatic schizonts rupture, they liberate approximately 10^5–10^6 merozoites into the circulation (i.e. the product of 5–100 successful sporozoites). These invade passing red cells immediately. In non-immune subjects the multiplication rate in *P. falciparum* usually approximates 10 per cycle (i.e. >50% efficiency) but may reach twenty-fold per cycle during the expanding phase of the infection (Figure 43.3). For the first few cycles the host is unaware of the brewing infection. On average, parasites are detectable in the blood by microscopy on the 11th day after sporozoite inoculation (the diligent microscopist can detect 20–50 parasites/μL reliably on Giemsa-stained thick films). At this stage the host may still feel well, or may complain of vague non-specific symptoms of malaise, headache, myalgia, weakness or anorexia. On average the fever begins 1–2 days later, but in some cases fever precedes detectable parasitaemia. The rise in parasite count is logarithmic initially, with a rising sine wave pattern of parasitaemia in

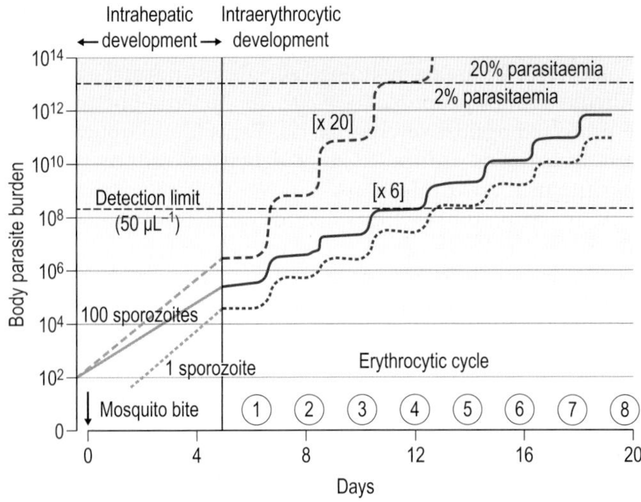

Figure 43.3 Logarithmic expansion of malaria infections in vivo. The body burden represents the total number of parasites in the body following infection of an adult of 50 kg. In falciparum malaria the infection rapidly reaches a lethal burden at high multiplication rates unless restrained. Maximum recorded multiplication rates are approximately ×20/cycle in vivo.

falciparum malaria, but in most cases the parasite expansion terminates abruptly to limit the infection at a parasitaemia of 10^4–10^5/uL (Figure 43.3). Only *P. falciparum* and *P. knowlesi* have the capacity for untrammelled multiplication and parasitaemias may exceed 50% in some cases. Several factors converge to limit parasite multiplication. The host mobilizes specific and nonspecific immune defences (particularly in the spleen). The parasite schizonts are also damaged by high fevers. The availability of suitable red cells is exhausted: *P. vivax* and *P. falciparum* prefer younger red cells and *P. malariae* prefers older cells. Interestingly whereas *P. vivax* shows invasion restricted to only 13% of the red cell population and *P. falciparum* causing uncomplicated malaria to 40%, *P. falciparum* parasites causing severe malaria in South-east Asia show unrestricted invasion. Thus the untreated infection increases exponentially, then the rate of expansion decelerates rapidly, parasitaemia fluctuates, settles around a plateau, then declines and continues for several weeks to several years at low levels before finally being eliminated. Although natural infections often contain two or more genetically different parasite strains, development tends to be relatively synchronous from the outset. Further synchronization takes place in untreated infections in non-immune subjects, such that merogony ('sporulation') takes place within 1–2 hours. This is associated with fever and rigors (the 'paroxysm'). Although one 'brood' predominates, in *P. falciparum* there is often at least one minor 'brood' or subpopulation cycling 24 hours out of phase with the major brood.

The periodicity of malaria is enshrined in the terminology of the fever pattern. *P. malariae* has a 72-hour life cycle and in untreated infections the paroxysm occurred on the 4th day (using the Greek system of 'inclusive reckoning' the previous paroxysm is considered to occur on day 1). This is termed 'quartan malaria'. The other malarias are termed tertian (fever on the 3rd day; 48-hour asexual cycle). *P. falciparum* often synchronized to a daily fever spike (quotidian fever), presumably caused by two broods of approximately equal size oscillating 24 hours out of phase, or failed to synchronize at all. The classic descriptions of malaria symptomatology derive largely from detailed clinical observations made in the late nineteenth and early twentieth centuries, the experience with artificial infections in early chemotherapy trials, studies conducted by the military, and the extensive use of malaria therapy in the treatment of neurosyphilis. These observations were usually made on non-immune adults. In malaria therapy patients with neurosyphilis were artificially infected, by mosquito bite or transfusion and the infection with *P. falciparum* or *P. vivax* was left untreated so that the patient experienced recurrent high fevers, or if symptoms were severe, was judiciously titrated with quinine. Nowadays, these characteristic fever charts with regular fever spikes are seen rarely because malaria is treated promptly. It was also apparent from these studies and later animal experiments that some strains of *P. falciparum* and *P. vivax* were more virulent than others. For example, the now extinct European strains of *P. falciparum* were notorious. The virulence factors of malaria parasites have not been characterized fully, but include multiplication capacity, cytoadherence and rosetting ability, the potential to induce cytokine release, antigenicity, and antimalarial drug resistance.

PARASITE BIOMASS

Malaria is readily diagnosed from the blood film stained with a Romanowsky dye. In the benign malarias (where sequestration is considered not to occur) the number of parasites in the body may be estimated simply by multiplying the parasitaemia by the estimated blood volume. In *P. falciparum* infections the microscopist can see only the first third of the asexual life cycle. In the second two thirds the parasitized cells are sequestered in the capillaries and venules. As a consequence, there may be large discrepancies between the number of parasites in the peripheral (circulating) blood and the number of parasites in the body (the parasite burden) (Figure 43.4). This has often puzzled and mis-led clinicians; some patients appear to tolerate high parasitaemia with little adverse effects, whereas others die with low

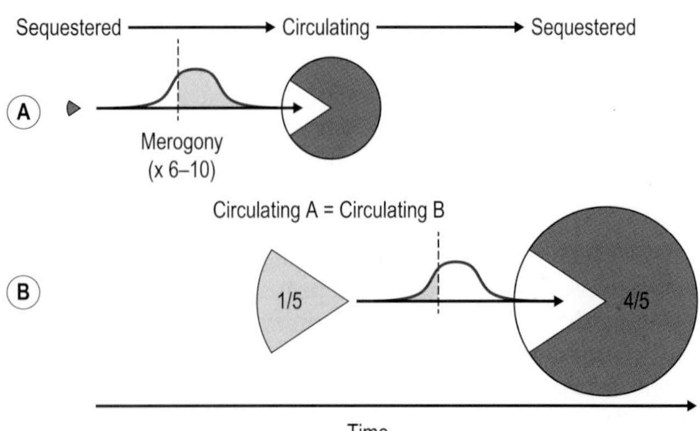

Figure 43.4 The problem of assessing the parasite burden from the peripheral parasitaemia in *P. falciparum* malaria. Sequestration hides the parasites causing harm. Two patients (A and B) have the same parasitaemia. In patient A, most of the parasites are circulating and only a few from the previous cycle have yet to undergo merogony (schizont rupture). In patient B, most of the parasites have already sequestered and only 20% of the biomass still circulates. There are over 60 times more parasites in patient B than in patient A. The clue lies in the stage distribution (shown crossing the hatched lines) of the circulating parasites which will be more mature in patient B.

parasite counts. The clue to the discrepancy lies both in the immune status of the host and in the stage of development of parasites on the peripheral blood smear. A predominance of more mature parasites indicates that a greater proportion is sequestered and carries a worse prognosis for any parasitaemia than a predominance of younger forms. Two patients with the same peripheral parasitaemia may have as much as a one-hundred-fold difference in the total number of parasites in the body. The presence of intraneutrophilic phagocytosed malaria pigment (in more than 5% of neutrophils) also reflects the degree of previous schizogony and is also a valuable prognostic index. Measurement of proteins released by the parasite such as *Pf*HRP2 provide a good method of assessing this hidden pathogenic sequestered biomass.[13] In synchronous *P. falciparum* infections the peripheral blood parasite numbers fall at the time of sequestration and rise abruptly at the time of merogony (when a predominance of tiny rings are seen). The other explanation for the ability to tolerate high parasitaemias without apparent adverse effects relates to the development of 'antitoxic' immunity. The host adapts to repeated infection by producing less cytokines for a given quantum of parasites (see below). Eventually a state is reached where infections are asymptomatic. This is called premunition.

IMMUNITY

The precise mechanisms controlling malaria infections are still incompletely understood. It was apparent from the era of malaria therapy for neurosyphilis, that a strain-specific immunity developed which protected against rechallenge with the same parasite strain, but did not protect from challenge with a different strain. Effective immunity, as distinct from premunition, may be reached when there has been exposure to all local strains of malaria parasites. This is difficult to quantify as there is still no good in vitro correlate of either antitoxic or strain-specific immunity to malaria. In controlling the acute infection nonspecific host defence mechanisms and the later development of more specific cell-mediated and humoral responses are both important. Protective antibodies inhibit parasite expansion by agglutinating merozoites and through cooperation with the monocyte-macrophage series by binding to parasitized erythrocytes and then activating these cells' Fc receptors. Non-specific effector mechanisms include non-opsonic phagocytosis via direct binding to monocyte-macrophage CD36, pro-inflammatory cytokine release, and the activation of phagocytic cells (including neutrophils) to release toxic oxygen species and nitric oxide, both of which are parasiticidal. The reaction of these oxygen intermediates with lipoproteins produces lipid peroxides. These are more stable cytotoxic molecules and are unaffected by antioxidants. There is also augmentation of splenic clearance function: both filtration and Fc receptor-mediated phagocytosis are increased. *P. falciparum*-infected erythrocytes are more rigid and more opsonized than uninfected red cells as they express both host- and parasite-derived neoantigens on the erythrocyte surface. However, the parasite proteins expressed on the red cell surface undergo antigenic variation,[14] and this is instrumental in avoiding complete immune clearance and sustaining the untreated infection. The systemic and splenic monocyte-macrophage series appear to be the most important immune effector cells in the direct attack on parasitized erythrocytes and merozoites, although neutrophils may also play a role.

THE IMMUNE RESPONSE

Following natural infection there is a transient humoral response to sporozoite antigens; sporozoite antibodies decline, with a half-life of 3–4 weeks. In areas of high transmission sporozoite antibody levels tend to plateau between 20 and 30 years of age and do not correlate with premunition. Cytotoxic T-cell immune responses cannot be directed against the blood-stage parasite as red cells do not express human leukocyte (HLA) antigens, but the pre-erythrocytic liver stages of the parasite are vulnerable to T cell attack. Several lines of experimental evidence in animal malarias and the observation that certain HLA types are relatively protected from severe malaria, indicate that class 1 restricted CD8(+) T-cells play an important role in immunity. There is evidence supporting a role for both alpha-beta and gamma-delta CD4+ cells in the immune response to malaria.

Strain-specific immunity to the asexual blood-stage parasites develops slowly during natural untreated infections, but it then provides good protection against rechallenge. However, parasite populations are diverse and cross-strain protection is initially weak or negligible. The development of immunity in endemic areas may represent the gradual acquisition of a repertoire of immunological memory for the range of local parasites. This involves strain transcending immunity sufficient to ameliorate disease (antitoxic immunity) and a more strain-specific immunity which protects from or attenuates the infection. The immune response to malaria is clearly very complex and the relative importance of humoral and cellular immunity in man has not been defined clearly. Infusion of hyperimmune serum to patients with acute malaria can reduce or eliminate parasitaemia mainly through opsonization and activation of phagocytic and cytotoxic effector functions by cytophilic IgG antibodies and augmentation of ring-form infected erythrocyte clearance. Immune serum also reduces parasite multiplication by agglutinating merozoites. In addition to the role of cellular immunity in preventing preerythrocytic development, the relatively weak but definite increase in malaria severity in patients living in endemic areas with the acquired immune deficiency syndrome (HIV-AIDS) suggests that CD4+ cells do play a significant role in modulating the severity of *falciparum* malaria.

Pathophysiology

The pathophysiology of malaria results from destruction of erythrocytes, the liberation of parasite and erythrocyte material into the circulation, and the host reaction to these events. *P. falciparum* malaria-infected erythrocytes sequester in the microcirculation of vital organs, interfering with microcirculatory flow and host tissue metabolism.

TOXICITY AND CYTOKINES

For many years malariologists hypothesized that parasites contained a toxin which was liberated at schizont rupture and caused the symptoms of the paroxysm. No toxin in the strict sense of the word has ever been identified, but malaria parasites do induce release of cytokines in much the same way as bacterial endotoxin. A glycolipid material with many of the properties of bacterial endotoxin is released on meront rupture. This material is associated with the glycosylphosphatidylinositol anchor which covalently links proteins including the malaria parasite surface antigens to the cell membrane lipid bilayer. This activates host inflammatory responses in macrophages by signalling through toll-like receptor (TLR) 2 and to a lesser extent TLR 4. Malaria-antigen-related IgE complexes also activate cytokine release. The limulus lysate assay, a test of endotoxin-like activity, is often positive in acute malaria. These products of malaria parasites and the crude malaria pigment which are released at schizont rupture, induce activation of the cytokine cascade in a similar manner to the endotoxin of bacteria. But they are *considerably* less potent. For example an *E. coli* bacteraemia of 1 bacterium/mL carries an approximate mortality of 20% whereas in *falciparum* malaria only parasite densities of well over 10^9/mL produce such a lethal effect. Clearly compared with bacteria, malaria parasites are notable for their lack of toxicity! Cells of the macrophage-monocyte series, gamma/delta T cells, alpha/beta T cells, CD14+ cells and endothelium are stimulated to release cytokines in a mutually amplifying chain reaction. Initially tumour necrosis factor (TNF), which plays a pivotal role, interleukin (IL)-1 and gamma interferon are produced and these in turn induce a cascade of other 'pro-inflammatory' cytokines including IL-6, IL-8, IL-12, IL-18. These are balanced by production of the 'anti-inflammatory' cytokines notably IL-10 and related cytokines. Inflammatory cytokines are responsible for many of the symptoms and signs of the infection, particularly fever and malaise. Plasma concentrations of cytokines are elevated in both acute *vivax* and *falciparum* malaria. In established *vivax* malaria, which tends to synchronize earlier than *P. falciparum*, a pulse release of TNF occurs at the time of schizont rupture and this is followed by the characteristic symptoms and signs of the 'paroxysm', i.e. shivering, cool extremities, headache, chills, a spike of fever and sometimes rigors followed by sweating, vasodilatation and defervescence. For a given number of parasites *Plasmodium vivax* is a more potent inducer of TNF release than *P. falciparum*, which may explain its lower pyrogenic density.

Whether pro-inflammatory cytokines contribute directly to the pathology of severe malaria remains uncertain. Cytokine concentrations in the blood fluctuate widely over a short period of time and are high in both *P. vivax* and *P. falciparum*; indeed some of the highest TNF concentrations recorded in malaria occur during the paroxysms of synchronous *P. vivax* infections. Nearly all the TNF measured in these assays is bound to soluble receptors; there is usually little or no bioactivity. Nevertheless, in most series there is a positive correlation between cytokine levels and prognosis in severe *falciparum* malaria. Acute malaria is associated with high levels of most cytokines but the balance differs in relation to severity. IL-12 and TGF-β 1, which may regulate the balance between pro- and anti-inflammatory cytokines, are higher in uncomplicated than severe malaria. IL-12 is inversely correlated with plasma lactate – a measure of disease severity. IL-10, a potent anti-inflammatory cytokine, increases markedly in severe malaria but, in fatal cases, does not increase sufficiently to restrain the production of TNF. A reduced IL-10/TNF ratio has also been associated with childhood malarial anaemia in areas of high transmission. All this points to a disturbed balance of cytokine production in severe malaria.

The first studies to associate elevations in plasma cytokine levels with disease severity focussed on TNF and cerebral malaria and led to the suggestion that TNF played a causal role in coma and cerebral dysfunction. Genetic studies from Africa indicated that children with the (308A) TNF2 allele, a polymorphism in the TNF promoter region, had a relative risk of 7 for death or neurological sequelae from cerebral malaria.[15] This finding was not confirmed in studies from South-east Asia. A separate polymorphism in this region which affects gene expression was associated with a fourfold increased risk of cerebral malaria. On the other hand the clinical studies in cerebral malaria with anti-TNF antibodies and other strategies to reduce TNF production, reported to date have shown no convincing effects other than reduction in fever. Cytokines do play a causal role in the pathogenesis of cerebral symptoms in murine models of severe malaria, but these models are clinically and pathologically unlike human cerebral malaria. There is no direct evidence that systemic release of TNF or other cytokines causes coma in humans (although mechanisms involving local release of nitric oxide and other medicators within the central nervous system and consequent inhibition of neurotransmission can be hypothesized). In a large prospective study in adults with severe malaria, elevated plasma TNF concentrations were associated specifically with renal dysfunction and TNF levels were actually lower in patients with pure cerebral malaria than those with other manifestations of severe disease. Severe malarial anaemia has been associated with a different TNF promoter polymorphism (238A; odds ratio 2.5). Taken together these suggest some role for TNF and other cytokines in severe disease, not encephalopathy per se, but the extent to which this is the cause or an effect of severe disease remains to be determined.

Cytokines are probably involved in placental dysfunction, suppression of erythropoiesis and inhibition of gluconeogenesis, and they certainly do cause fever in malaria. Tolerance to malaria, or premunition, reflects both immune regulation of the infection and also reduced production of cytokines in response to malaria ('antitoxic immunity'). Cytokines upregulate the endothelial expression of vascular ligands for *P. falciparum*-infected erythrocytes, notably ICAM-1 and thus promote cytoadherence. They may also be important mediators of parasite killing by activating leukocytes and possibly other cells, to release toxic oxygen species, nitric oxide, and by generating parasiticidal lipid peroxides and causing fever. Thus, whereas high concentrations of cytokines appear to be harmful, lower levels probably benefit the host.

SEQUESTRATION

Erythrocytes containing mature forms of *P. falciparum* adhere to microvascular endothelium ('cytoadherence') and thus disappear from the circulation. This process is known as sequestration (Figure 43.5).[14] The simian malaria parasites *P. coatneyi* and *P. fragile* infecting rhesus monkeys also sequester, but this does not occur to a significant extent with the other human malaria parasites. Sequestration is thought to be central to the pathophysiology of *falciparum* malaria. The mechanics of cytoadherence are similar to leukocyte endothelial interactions. Tethering (the initial contact) is followed by rolling and then firm adherence (stasis). Once adherent, the parasitized cell remains stuck until schizogony and even afterwards the residual membranes (and often the attached pigment body) remain attached to the vascular endothelium. Rolling is probably the rate-limiting factor determining cytoadherence.

Blood is a complex mixture of deformable cells suspended in plasma proteins, electrolytes, and a variety of small organic molecules. Its effective viscosity changes nonlinearly under the

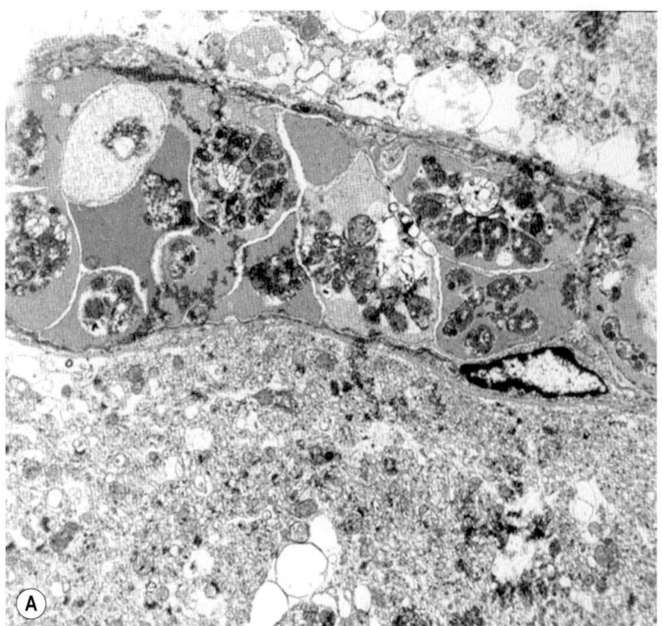

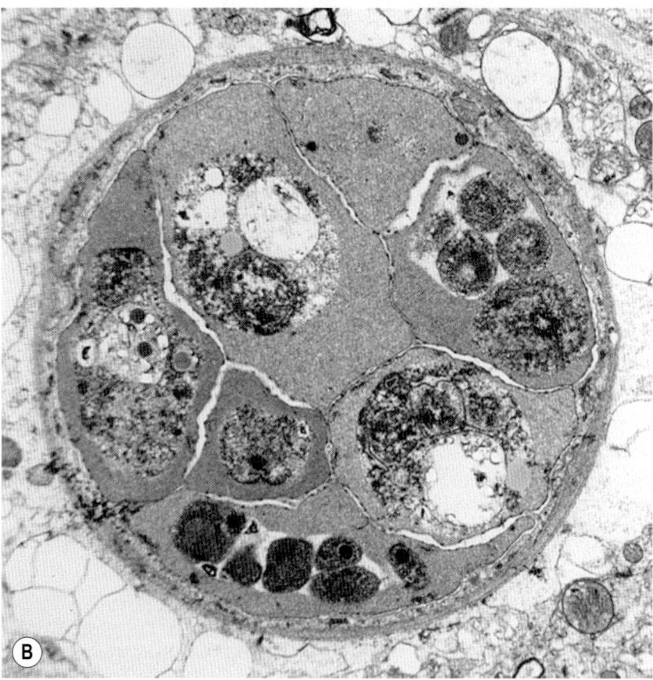

Figure 43.5 Two electron micrographs (×4320) showing densely packed parasitized erythrocytes sequestered in cerebral venules of a fatal case of cerebral malaria. Note that even when no intracellular parasite is seen, electron dense deposits are evident on the cell membranes indicating the red cell does contain a parasite, but that its body has been missed in the section. The packing of red cells is much tighter than in normal conditions. *(Courtesy of Emsrii Pongponratn.)*

different shear rates encountered in the circulation (non-Newtonian behaviour). Only at haematocrits <12% (i.e. severe anaemia) do red blood cell suspensions exhibit Newtonian behaviour. Under experimental conditions changes in haematocrit over the range commonly encountered in severe malaria (venous haematocrit, 10–30%; capillary values are lower) have major effects on cytoadherence. Rolling increased fivefold as haematocrit rose from 10% to 20% and cytoadhesion rose 12-fold between 10% and 30%. Over this range, the viscosity of blood approximately doubles and so if shear stress is held constant, shear rates fall by approximately half allowing greater time for contact between cells and endothelium. The higher the haematocrit, the more cells roll along the endothelial surface and so a higher proportion of these adhere to the vascular endothelium.

Once infected red cells adhere, they do not enter the circulation again, remaining stuck until they rupture at merogony (schizogony). Under febrile conditions cytoadherence begins at approximately 12 hours after merozoite invasion and reaches 50% of maximum between 14–16 hours. Adherence is essentially complete in the second half of the parasites' 48-hour asexual life cycle. As a consequence, whereas in the other malarias of man mature parasites are commonly seen on blood smears, these forms are rare in *falciparum* malaria and often indicate serious infection. It was thought that ring-stage-infected erythrocytes do not cytoadhere at all, but pathological and laboratory studies show that that they do, although much less so than more mature stages. Ring-form-infected parasites are also concentrated in the spleen and placenta, raising the intriguing possibility that the entire asexual cycle could take place away from the peripheral circulation. Sequestration occurs predominantly in the venules of vital organs. It is not distributed uniformly throughout the body, being greatest in the brain, particularly the white matter, prominent in the heart, eyes, liver, kidneys, intestines and adipose tissue, and least in the skin. Even within the brain the distribution of sequestered erythrocytes varies markedly from vessel to vessel, possibly reflecting differences in the expression of endothelial receptors. Cytoadherence and the related phenomena of rosetting and autoagglutination lead to microcirculatory obstruction in *falciparum* malaria (Figure 43.6). The gross microcirculatory obstruction caused by cytoadherent erythrocytes has recently been clearly visualized in vivo using polarized light imaging (in the buccal and rectal microcirculations) and by high-resolution fluorescein angiography of the retinal circulation.[17,18]

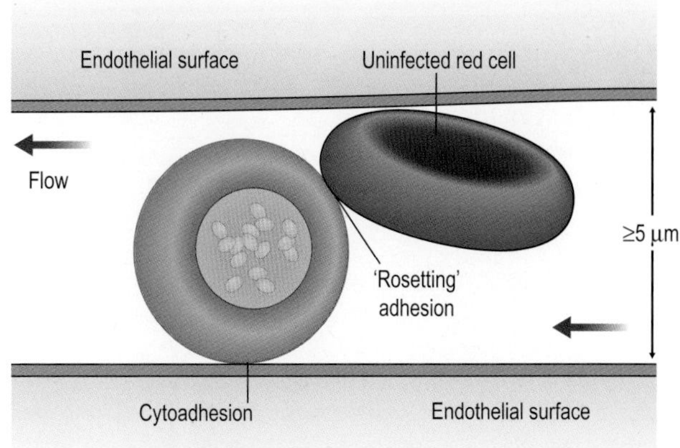

Figure 43.6 Uninfected red cells must squeeze past the static rigid, spherical cytoadherent parasitized erythrocytes to maintain flow. This is compromised by the reduced deformability of uninfected red cells in severe malaria and the intererythrocytic adhesive forces that mediate rosetting.

The consequences of microcirculatory obstruction are activation of the vascular endothelium, endothelial dysfunction, together with reduced oxygen and substrate supply, which leads to anaerobic glycolysis, lactic acidosis and cellular dysfunction.

CYTOADHERENCE

Cytoadherence is mediated by several different processes.[14] The most important parasite ligands are a family of strain-specific, high-molecular-weight parasite-derived proteins termed *P. falciparum* erythrocyte membrane protein 1 or PfEMP-1. These variant surface antigen (VSA) proteins (molecular mass 240–260 kDa) are encoded by *var* genes, a family of ~60 genes distributed in three general locations within the haploid genome: either immediately adjacent to the telomere, close to a telomeric *var* gene, or in internal clusters. Each parasitized red cell expresses the product of a single gene, a process which is tightly controlled at the transcriptional level and varies between different parasites and different PfEMP-1 genes. PfEMP-1 is transcribed, synthesized and stored within the parasite and, beginning at around 12 hours of development, it is then exported to the surface of the infecting erythrocyte. There it is apposed by an electrostatic interaction through the membrane to a submembranous accretion of parasite-derived knob-associated histidine-rich protein (KAHRP), which is in turn anchored to the red cell via the cytoskeleton protein ankyrin. These accretions cause humps or knobs on the surface of the red cell (Figure 43.7) and these are the points of attachment to vascular endothelium. The protuberances are not essential for cytoadherence. A small subpopulation of naturally occurring parasites do not induce surface knobs and parasites can be selected in culture which are knob negative (K-) but still cytoadhere. However, natural parasite isolates are nearly always knob positive (K+). PfEMP-1 proteins protrude from the red cell surface offering several Duffy binding-like (DBL) domains each capable of binding to particular vascular 'receptors'. Analysis of multiple PfEMP-1 sequences has revealed common antigenic determinants in the DBL-1α domain, a constituent of the so-called 'head structure' common to all PfEMP-1 variants, that is involved in the formation of rosettes and in cytoadherence.[19] PfEMP-1 expression is greatest in the middle of the asexual cycle. PfEMP1 is an important adhesin and also appears to be a major antigenic determinant for the blood stage parasite, although two other variant proteins encoded by different gene families have been identified – the *Rifins* and the *Surfins*. Their function is uncertain.

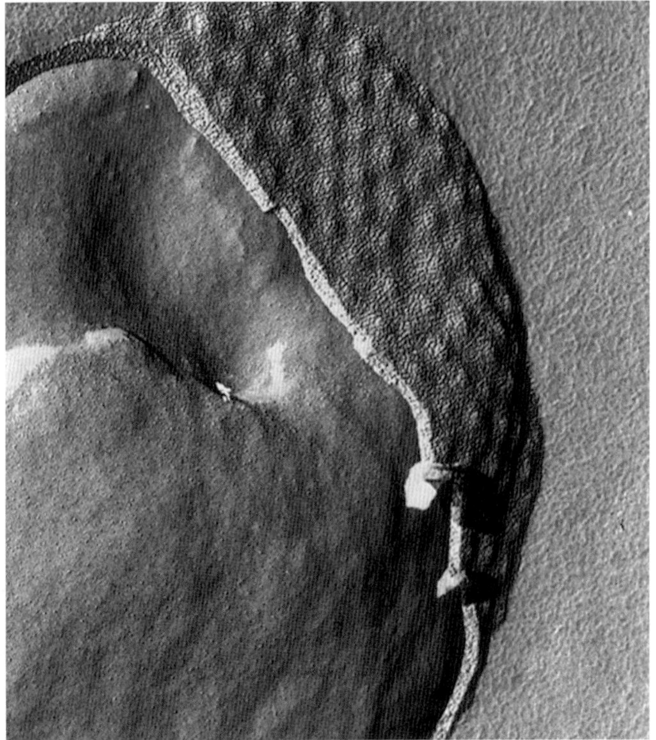

Figure 43.7 Freeze fracture electron micrograph of the membrane of a red cell containing mature *P. falciparum* showing regularly spaced knobs. *(Courtesy of David Ferguson.)*

In addition, proteins expressed only on the younger ring stage infected red cells have also been identified in parasite lines which subsequently develop a chondroitin-sulphate A binding phenotype which could play a role in ring stage cytoadherence.

As in other protozoal parasites the immunodominant surface antigen undergoes antigenic variation to 'change its coat' and avoid immune-mediated attack. Each *P. falciparum var* gene appears to have different rates of switching on and off, with a net result that the infecting parasite population 'switches' to a new variant of PfEMP1 at an average rate of about 2% per asexual cycle in culture although this may be considerably higher in vivo. Interestingly, the PfEMP-1 gene expressed shows some dependence on previous variant expression, reflecting the effects of host immune response on parasite antigenic variation.

In the chronic phase of untreated infections this antigenic variation results in small waves of parasitaemia approximately every 3 weeks. A protein similar to PfEMP-1 named sequestrin (molecular mass 270 kDa) has been identified on the surface of infected red cells using anti-idiotypic antibodies raised against one of the putative vascular receptors CD36 (see below). The protein MESA may also be partially expressed on the surface of the red cell and has been suggested as a contributor to cytoadherence. The central role of parasite-derived proteins in cytoadherence is not accepted by all. It has been suggested that cytoadherence is mediated by altered red cell membrane components such as a modified form of the red cell cytoskeleton protein band 3 (the major erythrocyte anion transporter, also called *Pf*alhesin). In culture, most *P. falciparum* parasites lose the ability to cytoadhere after several cycles of replication. In vivo, cytoadherence may be modulated by the spleen. This has been shown in *Saimiri* monkeys infected with *P. falciparum*. Parasitized erythrocytes do not cytoadhere in splenectomized monkeys. Rare patients who have had a splenectomy develop *falciparum* malaria and in some of these all stages of the parasite are seen in peripheral blood smears.

P. vivax generally does not cytoadhere but recent studies indicate significant adhesion to chondroitin sulphate A – the main receptor for placental cytoadhesion. *Plasmodium vivax* also has a variant subtelomeric multigene family called *vir*. Its subcellular localization and function has been unclear although there is recent evidence it might mediate attachment to ICAM-1.

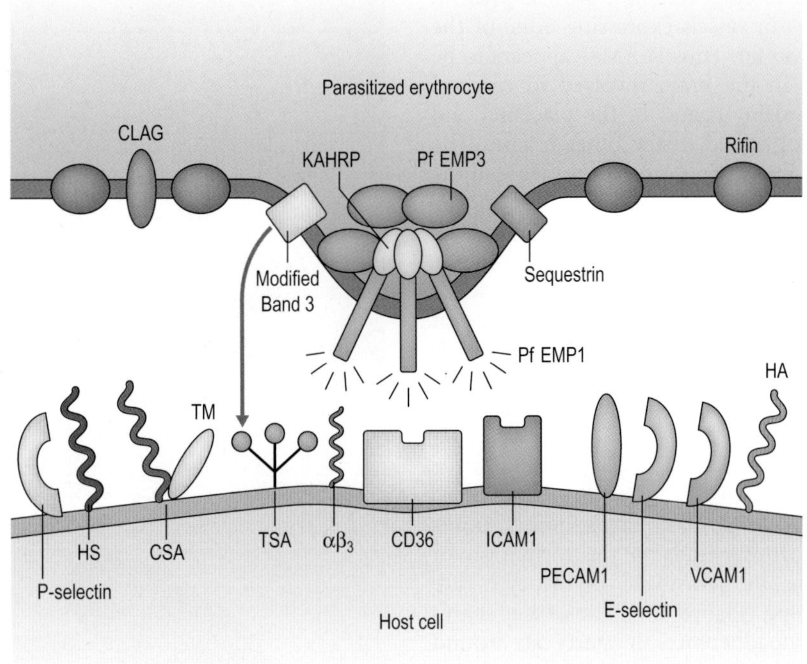

Figure 43.8 Schematic representation of cytoadherence in *falciparum* malaria. On the red cell side (above) the principal ligand is the variant antigen *Plasmodium falciparum* erythrocyte membrane protein 1 (*Pf*EMP1). This is expressed on the surface of 'knobs' which protrude from the red cell surface. It is anchored beneath to the knob-associated histidine-rich protein (KAHRP) and stabilized by *Pf*EMP3. The *rifin* and CLAG gene products are not directly involved in adhesion but CLAG does appear to be required for cytoadherence. Parasite-modified band 3 (the major anion transporter) contributes to adhesion probably by binding to thrombospondin (TSA). Sequestrin is a distinct parasite-derived protein also mediating adhesion. The ring stage adhesion (not shown) is distinct from *Pf*EMP1 and expressed in the first third of the asexual cycle. On the vascular endothelial side many molecules facilitate adhesion by binding *Pf*EMP1. The most important is the cellular differentiation antigen: CD36. Intercellular adhesion molecule 1 (ICAM1) is important particularly in the brain, elsewhere it synergizes with CD36. Chondroitin sulphate A (CSA) attached to thrombomodulin (TM) is very important for placental sequestration. The other identified adhesion molecules are vascular cell adhesion molecule 1 (VCAM1), E-selectin, platelet endothelial cell adhesion molecule 1 (PECAM1), $\alpha\beta_3$ integrin, heparan sulphate (HS) and P-selectin.

VASCULAR ENDOTHELIAL LIGANDS

A number of different cell adhesion molecules expressed on the surface of vascular endothelium have been shown to bind parasitized red cells (Figure 43.8). The interaction between these proteins and the variant surface adhesin of the parasitized red cell is complex. The property of cytoadherence can be studied in vitro with cells expressing the potential ligands on their surface (e.g. human umbilical vein/dermal microvascular or cerebral endothelial cells or transfected COS cells) or with the immobilized purified candidate ligand proteins. Probably the most important of these proteins is the leukocyte differentiation antigen CD36; nearly all freshly obtained parasites bind to CD36. Binding is increased at low pH (<7.0) and in the presence of high calcium concentrations. CD36 is constitutionally expressed on vascular endothelium, platelets and monocytes/macrophages but is usually not present on the surface of cerebral vessels, although it has been suggested that parasitized erythrocytes could bind via CD36 to platelets adherent to cerebral vascular endothelium. Endothelial activation causes exocytosis of intracellular Weibel–Palade bodies, containing bioactive molecules which include von Willebrand factor (vWF) and angiopoietin-2. Ultralong vWF multimers may mediate cytoadherence and sequestration by binding activated platelets which express CD36. Concentrations of ADAMTS13, which cleaves and inactivates UL-vWF, are low in patients with severe malaria. The intercellular adhesion molecule (ICAM-1 or CD54), which is also the receptor for rhinovirus attachment, appears to be the major cytoadherence receptor in the brain. ICAM-1, but not CD36, is upregulated by cytokines (notably TNFα) and provides a plausible pathological scenario whereby cytokine release enhances cytoadherence. At physiological shear rates (i.e. those likely to be encountered in the human microcirculation) the binding forces (c.10^{-10}N) are similar for CD36 and ICAM-1. For both, the forces of attachment are lower than those required for detachment, which suggests post-attachment alterations to increase adhesion. Binding to the two ligands is synergistic. Thrombospondin (a natural ligand for CD36) will also bind to some parasitized red cells (probably to modified band 3). Other proteins including VCAM-1, PECAM/CD31, E-selectin and the integrin alpha-beta3 have also been shown to bind in some circumstances. P-selectin has been shown to mediate rolling. The relative importance of these molecules and their interactions in vivo is still not clear. Chondroitin sulphate A (CSA) appears to be the major receptor for cytoadherence in the placenta. Binding to CSA is mediated by a particular PfEMP1 (*var*2CSA) which gives hope for a specific vaccine against malaria in pregnancy. Thus the placenta selects a parasite subpopulation expressing this epitope. Antibodies which inhibit parasitized red cell cytoadherence by binding *var*2CSA are generally present in multigravidae in endemic areas, but not primigravidae which probably explains why the adverse effects of pregnancy on birth weight are greatest in primigravidae.

Other as yet unidentified vascular receptors are also present, as sequestration also occurs in vessels expressing none of the potential ligands identified so far. Thus ICAM-1 appears to be the major vascular ligand in the brain involved in cerebral sequestration, CSA is the major ligand in the placenta, and CD36 is probably the major ligand in the other organs. The relationship between cytoadherence, measured ex vivo and the severity of infection or clinical manifestations has been inconsistent between studies. This is not particularly surprising as all parasitized erythrocytes cytoadhere. Severity is related to the number of parasites in the body and the distribution of cytoadherence within the vital organs. The relative importance of parasite phenotype and the various potential vascular ligands in the pathophysiology of severe *falciparum* malaria and the precise role of the spleen still remains to be determined.

ROSETTING

Erythrocytes containing mature parasites also adhere to uninfected erythrocytes. This process leads to the formation of 'rosettes' when suspensions of parasitized erythrocytes are viewed under the microscope (Figure 43.9). Rosetting shares some characteristics of cytoadherence. It starts at around 16 hours of asexual life cycle development (slightly after cytoadherence begins) and it is trypsin-sensitive. But parasite species which do not sequester do rosette and unlike cytoadherence, rosetting is inhibited by certain heparin subfractions and calcium chelators. Furthermore, whereas all fresh isolates of *P. falciparum* cytoadhere, not all rosette. Rosetting is mediated by attachment of a specific subgroup of PfEMP1 adhesins (with red cell binding mediated by the N-terminal DBL1α_1 domain) to the complement receptor CR1, heparan sulphate, blood group A antigen and probably other red cell surface molecules. Attachment is facilitated by serum components including Complement factor D, albumin and IgG anti-band 3 antibodies. The protective effect of group O against severe malaria is thought to result from reduced rosetting. The forces required to separate a rosette are approximately five times greater than those required to separate cytoadherent cells, although shearing forces may still be effective in disrupting rosettes in vivo. When known rosetting parasite lines (K+R+) were perfused through the rat mesocaecum, an ex vivo model for the study of vascular perfusion, they caused significantly more microvascular obstruction than isolates which cytoadhered but did not rosette (K+R−). Rosetting has been associated with severe malaria in some studies but not in others. It has been suggested that rosetting might encourage cytoadherence by reducing flow (shear rate), which would enhance anaerobic glycolysis, reduce pH and facilitate adherence of infected erythrocytes to venular endothelium. Rosetting tends to start in venules and this could certainly reduce flow. The adhesive forces involved in rosetting could also impede forward flow of uninfected erythrocytes as they squeeze past sticky cytoadherent parasitized red cells in capillaries and venules (Figure 43.6). The mechanical obstruction or 'static hindrance' would be compounded by the lack of deformability of the adherent parasitized red cells and circulating unparasitised red cells.

AGGREGATION

Platelet-mediated aggregation of parasitized erythrocytes is mediated via platelet CD36 and is associated with disease severity. Aggregation could also contribute to vascular occlusion.

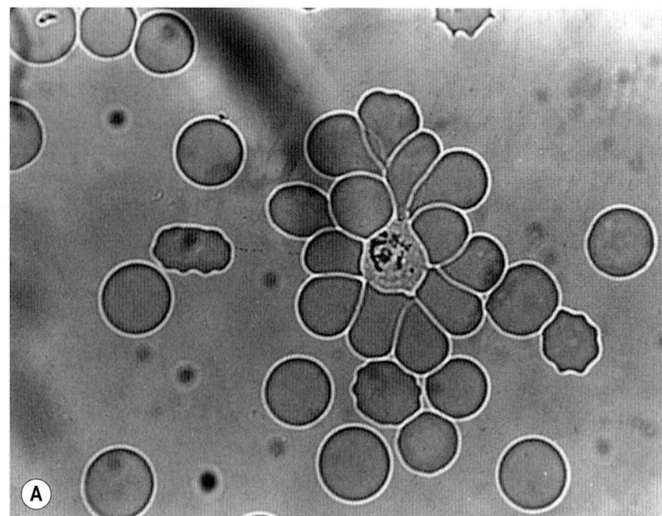

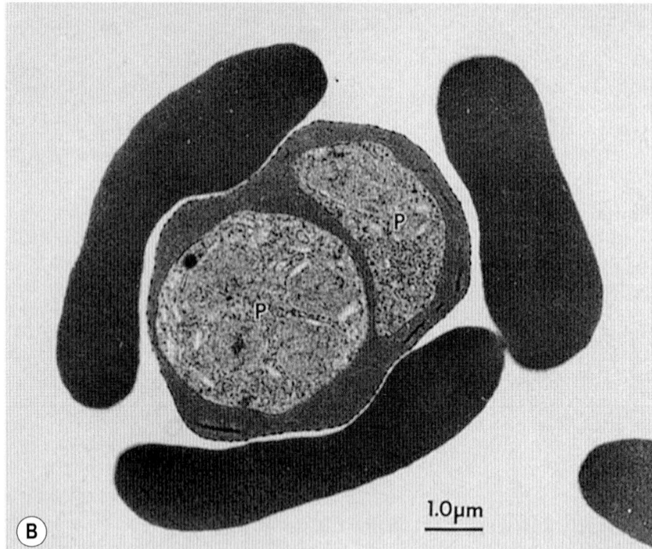

Figure 43.9 Rosetting. (A) Uninfected red blood cells bind to a *P. vivax*-infected erythrocyte. (B) Transmission electron micrograph of a rosette around a *P. falciparum*-infected erythrocyte. *(A, Courtesy of Rachanee Udomsangpetch. B, Courtesy of David Ferguson.)*

RED CELL DEFORMABILITY

As *Plasmodium vivax* matures inside the erythrocyte, the cell enlarges and becomes more deformable. *Plasmodium falciparum* does exactly the opposite; the normally flexible biconcave disc becomes progressively more spherical and rigid. The reduction in deformability results from reduced membrane fluidity, increasing sphericity and the enlarging and relatively rigid intraerythrocytic parasite. Infected red cells are less filterable than uninfected cells. It has been argued that sequestration is an adaptive response to escape splenic filtration. However, reduced deformability alone cannot account for microvascular obstruction as it would lead to obstruction at the mid-capillary (i.e. the smallest internal diameter in the vasculature) and could not explain sequestration in venules. Loss of uninfected red cell deformability has been recognized as a major contributor to disease severity and outcome. Increased erythrocyte rigidity measured at the low shear stresses encountered in capillaries and venules is correlated closely with outcome in severe malaria, and when assessed at the shear rates encountered on the arterial side and importantly, in the spleen, reduced red cell deformability also correlates with anaemia.

IMMUNOLOGICAL PROCESSES

The contribution of immune processes to the pathology of human malaria remains uncertain. It has been suggested that severe malaria, and in particular cerebral malaria, results from specific immune-mediated damage. This is unlikely. Confusion arises when the term cerebral malaria is applied equally to human disease and to neurological dysfunction in animal models infected with unusual parasites. Neuropathology in rodent models does result from immune-mediated damage, but human cerebral malaria has very different pathology and very different responses to interventions. In rapidly fatal cerebral malaria there is intense parasitized red cell sequestration, but relatively few leukocytes are found in or around the cerebral vessels in fatal cases, although recent pathological studies have shown more host leukocyte and particularly platelet accumulation in the cerebral vasculature of African children who died from cerebral malaria compared to the findings in South-east Asian adults.[16,20] The degree of host leukocyte response depends on the stage of infection and is less than that seen in other organs such as the kidney or lung, which may relate to the immunologically privileged state of the cerebral parenchyma. When leukocytes are seen they are often fulfilling their housekeeping role of clearing away residual cytoadherent membranes and pigment. There is little pathological evidence in man for widespread cerebral vasculitis in cerebral malaria although there is undoubted endothelial activation, and recent studies have shown evidence for intraparenchymal responses including widespread astroglial activation, evidence of blood–brain barrier leakage, and axonal injury.

Although some glomerular abnormalities have been noted in fatal malaria the clinical and pathological findings suggest that acute tubular necrosis, and not acute glomerulonephritis, is the cause of renal dysfunction. The pathogenesis of pulmonary oedema is uncertain – as it is for the adult respiratory distress syndrome in other conditions – but it is unlikely to involve a specific immune-mediated process. Thus despite the enormous intravascular antigenic load in malaria, with the formation and deposition of immune complexes and variable complement depletion, there is little evidence of a specific immunopathological process in severe falciparum malaria.

While innate immune responses are very important in controlling malaria, acute infections are associated with malaria antigen-specific unresponsiveness. This selective paresis is one of the factors contributing to the slow development of an effective and specific immune response in malaria. Acute malaria is characterized by non-specific polyclonal B-cell activation. There is a reduction in circulating T cells with an increase in the γ/δ T-cell subset, but other T-cell proportions are usually normal. Although residents of hyperendemic or holoendemic malarious areas have hypergammaglobulinaemia, most of this antibody is not directed against malaria antigens. In non-immune individuals, the acute antibody response to infection often comprises mostly IgM or IgG2, isotypes which are unable to arm cytotoxic cells and thus kill asexual malaria parasites. These observations have led to the suggestion that malaria induces an immunological 'smoke-screen' with broad-spectrum and non-specific activation that interferes with the orderly development of a specific cellular immune responses and immune memory. In severe malaria there is evidence of a broader immune suppression, with defects in monocyte and neutrophil chemotaxis, reduced neutrophil and monocytic phagocytic function (which may result from ingestion of malaria pigment), and a tendency to bacterial super-infection. In the nephrotic syndrome associated with chronic *P. malariae* infections, malaria antigen and immune complexes can be eluted from the kidney, indicating an immunopathological progress in this condition. But why some children are affected but the majority are not remains unresolved.

VASCULAR PERMEABILITY

There is evidence of a mild generalized increase in systemic vascular permeability in severe malaria. Focal perivascular and intraparenchymal oedema is seen in the brain in 70% of fatal cases. In the past it was suggested that cerebral malaria resulted from a marked increase in cerebral capillary permeability, which led to brain swelling, coma and death. The imaging studies conducted to date indicate that, although there may be some increases in brain water, as might be expected given the widespread venular and capillary obstruction, and some patients do develop cerebral oedema (particularly agonally), the majority of adults and children with cerebral malaria do not have substantial cerebral oedema (Figure 43.10). However, the role of raised intracranial pressure in cerebral malaria still remains unclear. Whereas 80% of adults have opening pressures at lumbar puncture which are in the normal range (<200 mm CSF), 80% of children have elevated opening pressures (>100 mm CSF: the normal range is lower in children) and intracranial pressure may rise transiently to very high levels. Uncontrolled epileptic seizure activity increases cerebral metabolism thereby increasing the imbalance between energy demand and limited supply (because of microvascular obstruction) and may cause brain swelling. Some patients with cerebral malaria die from acute respiratory arrest with neurological signs that are compatible with brain stem compression. But these signs are also common and may persist for many hours in survivors. The elevation in CSF opening pressure is usually not great (in general, it is much lower than in bacterial or fungal meningitis) and there is no difference between these lumbar puncture opening pressures in surviving children and fatal cases. Studies of computerized tomography (CT) or magnetic resonance imaging (MRI) have generally shown brain swelling in cerebral malaria (compatible with an increased intracerebral blood volume resulting from sequestration), sometimes discrete focal areas of oedema (particularly in white matter) or abnormal areas of signal attenuation in severe cases, but usually not generalized cerebral oedema. MRI studies show abnormal T2 signal intensity; and diffusion-weighted abnormalities in the cortical, deep gray and white matter structures. Focal abnormalities evident on MRI do not conform to arterial vascular distributions.[21]

Where generalized cerebral oedema has been reported it has sometimes been inferred from brain swelling on CT and could have resulted from increased intracerebral blood volume. Immunohistochemical studies on autopsy brain tissues indicate focal disruption of specialized endothelial cell tight junctions and endothelial activation in areas of intense sequestration, but clinical investigations have also failed to detect major alterations in blood–brain barrier permeability. Thus, raised intracranial

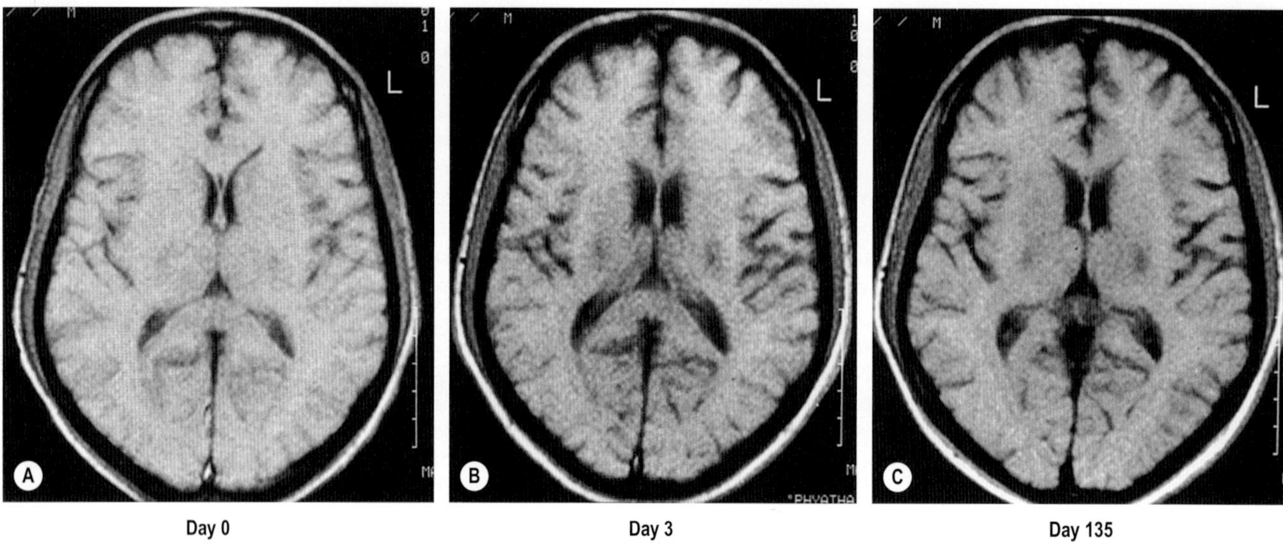

Figure 43.10 (A) T1-weighted magnetic resonance imaging (550/25 TR/TE) of the brain in a 28-year-old man with cerebral malaria. (B) Following recovery of consciousness showing shrinkage. (C) 135 days later the brain is normal. There was no evidence of cerebral oedema on T2-weighted images. The acute swelling was interpreted as representing increased intracerebral blood volume.

pressure probably arises mainly from an increase in cerebral blood volume. Any contribution of increased permeability is likely to be small. The increased cerebral blood volume results from the addition of the circulating blood required to maintain cerebral perfusion and the considerable sequestered static biomass of intracerebral parasitized erythrocytes. Children may be particularly vulnerable as after the skull sutures have fused, as there is less space for cranial expansion than in adults. The relationship between intracerebral pressure and volume is non-linear (i.e. once the brain has expanded to fill the skull, only small further increases in volume cause large increases in intracranial pressure). The possibility that a sudden rise in intracranial pressure accounts for some deaths cannot be excluded.

PATHOGENESIS OF COMA

Coma in severe malaria is called cerebral malaria. Although several factors may contribute to impaired consciousness in severe malaria (seizures, hypoglycaemia) there is a syndrome of diffuse but reversible encephalopathy which is characteristic of malaria and is not seen in other infections. The cause of coma is not known. There is undoubtedly an increase in cerebral anaerobic glycolysis with cerebral blood flows that are inappropriately low for the arterial oxygen content, increased cerebral metabolic rates for lactate and increased CSF concentrations of lactate, but these changes which reflect impaired perfusion, do not provide sufficient explanation for coma. Presumably the metabolic milieu created adjacent to the sequestered and highly metabolically active parasites and their attachment to the activated cerebral vascular endothelium interferes with endothelial and blood–brain barrier function. But how this then interferes with neurotransmission is not known. Cytokines increase production of nitric oxide, a potent inhibitor of neurotransmission, by leukocytes, smooth muscle cells, microglia and vascular endothelium through induction of the enzyme nitric oxide synthase. Inducible nitric oxide synthase expression is increased in the brain in fatal cerebral malaria. Thus, local synthesis of nitric oxide could be relevant to the impairment of consciousness. Local release of haemoglobin and haem depletes nitric oxide (NO) causing endothelial dysfunction. L-arginine (an NO precursor) concentrations are low and asymmetric dimethylarginine levels (an inhibitor of NO synthase) are increased in patients with severe malaria. Reversible axonal dysfunction has recently been shown in neuropathological studies and this probably plays an important role in central nervous system dysfunction. Coma in malaria is not caused by raised intracranial pressure. There has been considerable interest in the mechanism of coma and attempts to reverse it. But it should be remembered that the brain in cerebral malaria has a compromised blood supply and waking a patient from coma may result in an increased cerebral metabolic demand. Coma in cerebral malaria could be neuroprotective.

ACUTE KIDNEY INJURY

There is renal cortical vasoconstriction and consequent hypoperfusion in severe *falciparum* malaria. In patients with acute kidney injury (AKI) renal vascular resistance is increased. The renal injury in severe malaria results from acute tubular necrosis. The oxygen consumption of the kidneys is reduced in AKI and it is not improved by dopamine-induced arteriolar vasodilatation and consequent increase in renal blood flow suggesting a fixed injury. Acute tubular necrosis presumably results from renal microvascular obstruction and cellular injury consequent upon sequestration in the kidney and the filtration of nephrotoxins such as free haemoglobin, myoglobin and other cellular material. AKI always recovers fully in survivors. Significant glomerulonephritis is very rare. The role of systemic and local cytokine release and altered regulation of renal microvascular flow is uncertain. Massive haemolysis compounds the insult in blackwater fever complicating malaria and haemoglobinuria may itself lead to renal impairment. AKI also occurs in young children with severe malaria and levels of blood urea are important independent prognostic indices, but established acute renal failure requiring renal replacement is almost exclusively confined to older children and adults.

PULMONARY OEDEMA

Despite intense sequestration in the myocardial vessels, the heart's pump function is remarkably well preserved in severe malaria. Pulmonary oedema in *falciparum*, *vivax* and *knowlesi* malaria results from a sudden increase in pulmonary capillary permeability that is not reflected in other vascular beds. The pulmonary capillary wedge pressure is usually normal and the pressure threshold for the development of pulmonary oedema is relatively low. The cause of this increase in pulmonary capillary permeability is not known, although the presence of sequestered PRBC and host leukocytes in pulmonary capillaries may have a role in causing pulmonary capillary endothelial cell dysfunction.

FLUID SPACE AND ELECTROLYTE CHANGES

Haemodynamic studies in adults clearly point to microvascular and not macrovascular dysfunction as the primary circulatory abnormality in severe malaria. Following rehydration the plasma volume is increased in moderate and severe malaria. In most adults total body water and extracellular volume are normal. Plasma renin activity, aldosterone and antidiuretic hormone concentrations are elevated, reflecting an appropriate activation of homeostatic mechanisms to maintain adequate circulating volume in the presence of general vasodilatation and a falling haematocrit. Mild hyponatraemia and hypochloraemia are common in severe malaria, but serum potassium concentrations are usually normal. Occasionally hyponatraemia is severe. Studies in Kenyan children indicate inappropriate antidiuretic hormone (arginine vasopressin) secretion in two-thirds of cases. There has been much recent debate whether children with severe malaria are hypovolaemic and fluid-depleted. When measured directly in Gabonese children total body water was either normal or slightly reduced arguing against dehydration, whereas studies in Kenyan children suggested there may be benefit from infusions of colloid, particularly albumin solutions. However a definitive multicentre study in African children was stopped early because of increased mortality in those receiving vigorous crystalloid or albumin fluid loading.[22]

ANAEMIA

The pathogenesis of anaemia is multifactorial. It results from the obligatory destruction of red cells containing parasites at merogony, the accelerated destruction of non-parasitized red cells that parallels disease severity, and it is compounded by bone marrow dyserythropoiesis. In severe malaria anaemia develops rapidly; the rapid haemolysis of unparasitized red cells is the major contributor to the decline in haematocrit. Bone marrow dyserythropoiesis persists for days or weeks following acute malaria and reticulocyte counts are usually low in the acute phase of the disease. The cause of the dyserythropoiesis is thought to be related to intramedullary cytokine production. Serum erythropoietin levels are usually elevated, although in some series it has been suggested that the degree of elevation was not sufficient for the degree of anaemia. In *falciparum* malaria the entire red cell population (i.e. both infected and uninfected red cells) becomes more rigid. This loss of deformability correlates with disease severity and outcome and, when measured at the high shear rates encountered in the spleen, with the degree of resulting anaemia. The mechanism responsible has not been identified, although there is evidence in acute malaria for increased oxidative damage which might compromise red cell membrane function and deformability.[23] In simian malarias there is evidence of an inversion of the erythrocyte membrane lipid bilayer in uninfected erythrocytes, but this has not been studied in man. The role of antibody (i.e. Coombs'-positive haemolysis) in anaemia is unresolved. The majority of studies to date do not show increased red cell immunoglobulin binding in malaria, but in the presence of a lowered recognition threshold for splenic clearance, this might be difficult to detect. The splenic threshold for the clearance of abnormal erythrocytes, whether because of antibody coating or reduced deformability, is lowered.[23] Thus, the spleen removes large numbers of relatively rigid cells causing shortened erythrocyte survival, particularly in severe malaria. This is unaffected by corticosteroids. The spleen also fulfils its normative function of removing damaged intraerythrocytic parasites from red cells (particularly following treatment with an artemisinin derivative and returning the 'once parasitized' red cells back to the circulation by a process of 'pitting'.[23] These erythrocytes then have reduced survival and so following successful treatment of hyperparasitaemia may result in a delayed haemolytic anaemia.

In the context of acute uncomplicated malaria the anaemia is worse in younger children and those with protracted infections. Loss of unparasitized erythrocytes accounts for approximately 90% of the acute anaemia resulting from a single uncomplicated infection. Iron deficiency and malaria often coincide in the same patient and in some areas routine iron supplementation following malaria promotes recovery from anaemia.

COAGULOPATHY AND THROMBOCYTOPENIA

There is accelerated coagulation cascade activity with accelerated fibrinogen turnover, consumption of antithrombin III, reduced factor XIII and increased concentrations of fibrin degradation products in acute malaria. In severe infections, the antithrombin III, protein S and protein C are further reduced and prothrombin and partial thromboplastin times may be prolonged. In occasional patients (<5%), bleeding may be significant. The coagulation cascade is activated via the intrinsic pathway. Intravascular thrombus formation is observed rarely at autopsy in fatal cases and fibrin deposition is sparse and platelets are strikingly unusual in adults, in contrast to paediatric cases.

Thrombocytopenia is common to all the human malarias and is caused by increased splenic clearance. Thrombocytopenia is associated with high levels of IL-10 and appropriately raised concentrations of thrombopoietin (a key growth factor for platelet production). Plasma concentrations of macrophage colony stimulating factor are high, which stimulate macrophage activity and may increase platelet destruction. Platelet turnover is increased. The role of platelet-bound antibody in malarial thrombocytopenia is controversial. There has been evidence of platelet activation in some studies, but not others. Erythrocytes containing mature parasites may activate the coagulation cascade directly and cytokine release is also procoagulant. The high plasma levels of P-selectin found in severe malaria may derive from platelets, but could also come from vascular

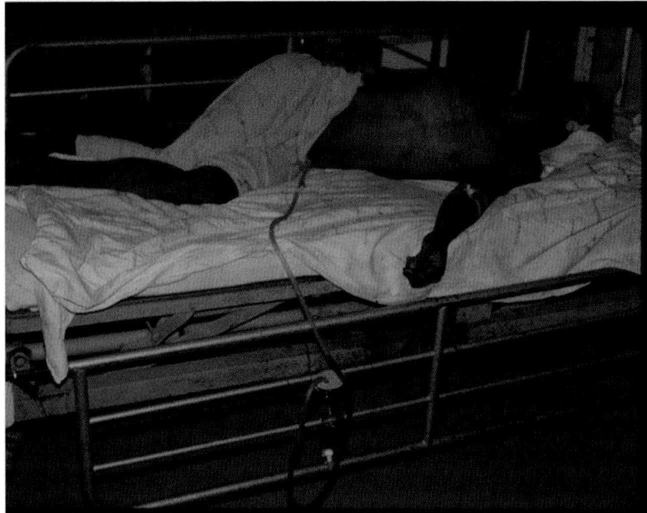

Figure 43.11 Blackwater fever and cerebral malaria. A 22-year-old male with severe malaria and massive haemolysis.

endothelium, as plasma concentrations of other endothelial-derived proteins (thrombomodulin, E-selectin, ICAM-1, VCAM-1) are also elevated. It was suggested in the past that disseminated intravascular coagulation (DIC) is important in the pathogenesis of severe malaria, but detailed prospective clinical and pathogenesis studies have refuted this. Coagulation cascade activity is directly proportional to disease severity, but hypofibrinogenaemia resulting from DIC is significant in less than 5% of patients with severe malaria and lethal haemorrhage (usually gastrointestinal) is very unusual.

BLACKWATER FEVER

This is a poorly understood condition (Figure 43.11), in which there is massive intravascular haemolysis and the passage of 'Coca-Cola'-coloured urine. Historically, this was linked to frequent quinine self-medication in expatriates living in malarious areas and indeed blackwater fever almost disappeared from Africa during the 'chloroquine' era from 1950 to 1980 but has since reappeared. Blackwater (urine) occurs in four circumstances: (1) when patients with G6PD deficiency take oxidant drugs (e.g. primaquine or sulphones), irrespective of whether they have malaria or not; (2) occasionally when patients with G6PD deficiency have malaria and receive quinine treatment; and (3) in some patients with severe *falciparum* malaria who have normal erythrocyte G6PD levels irrespective of the treatment given (4) when people who are exposed to malaria self-medicate frequently with quinine (or structurally related drugs). In severe malaria, rates of blackwater in Asian patients are similar whether the patients receive quinine or an artemisinin derivative. How quinine causes blackwater in these last three situations is not known, as it is not an oxidant drug. G6PD-deficient red cells are particularly susceptible to oxidant stress as they are unable to synthesize adequate quantities of NADPH through the pentose shunt. This leads to low intraerythrocytic levels of reduced glutathione and catalase and consequent alterations in the erythrocyte membrane and increased susceptibility to organic peroxides. Blackwater fever may be associated with acute renal failure, although in the majority of cases renal function remains normal.

THE SPLEEN

There is considerable and rapid splenic enlargement in malaria, mainly as a result of cellular multiplication and structural change and an enhanced capacity to clear red cells from the circulation both by Fc receptor-mediated (immune) mechanisms and by recognition of reduced deformability (filtration).[23] The increased filtration of the spleen and the reduced deformability of the entire red cell population results in the rapid development of anaemia in severe malaria. The spleen may also modulate cytoadherence. It plays a central role in limiting the acute expansion of the malaria infection by removing parasitized erythrocytes and this has led to the suggestion that a failure to augment splenic clearance sufficiently rapidly may be a factor in the development of severe malaria. Characteristic changes to the immuno-architecture of the spleen are seen during infection which may reflect a central role for dendritic cells in orchestrating specific immune responses.

The spleen is capable of removing damaged intraerythrocytic parasites and returning the once infected red cells to the circulation (a process known as 'pitting'), where they have shortened survival. This is an important contributor to parasite clearance following antimalarial drug treatment (particularly treatment with artemisinin derivatives).

GASTROINTESTINAL DYSFUNCTION

Abdominal pain may be prominent in acute malaria. Minor stress ulceration of the stomach and duodenum is common in severe malaria. The pattern of malabsorption of sugars, fats and amino acids suggests reduced splanchnic perfusion. This results from both gut sequestration and visceral vasoconstriction. Gut permeability is increased and this may be associated with reduced local defences against bacterial toxins, or even whole bacteria in severe disease. Antimalarial drug absorption is remarkably unaffected in uncomplicated malaria, except for those drugs which have fat- (i.e. food-) dependent absorption (atovaquone, lumefantrine).

LIVER DYSFUNCTION

Jaundice is common in adults with severe malaria and there is other evidence of hepatic dysfunction, with reduced clotting factor synthesis, reduced metabolic clearance of the antimalarial drugs and a failure of gluconeogenesis which contributes to lactic acidosis and hypoglycaemia. Nevertheless, true liver failure (as in fulminant viral hepatitis) does not occur. There is sequestration in the hepatic microvasculature and, although many patients with acute *falciparum* malaria have elevated liver blood flow values, in very severe infections liver blood flow is reduced. In adults, liver blood flow values <15 mL/kg per minute are associated with elevated venous lactate concentrations, which suggests a flow limitation to lactate clearance and thus a contribution of liver dysfunction to lactic acidosis. Direct measurements of hepatic venous lactate concentrations in severe malaria confirm that the hepatosplanchnic extraction ratio is inversely correlated with mixed venous plasma lactate (i.e. hyperlactataemia is associated with reduced liver clearance of lactate). There is no relationship between liver blood flow and impairment of antimalarial drug clearance. Jaundice in malaria appears to have haemolytic, hepatic and cholestatic components. Cholestatic jaundice may persist well into the recovery period. There is no residual liver damage following malaria.

ACIDOSIS

Acidosis is a major cause of death in severe *falciparum* malaria both in adults and children. This has been considered to be mainly a lactic acidosis, although ketoacidosis (and sometimes salicylate intoxication) may predominate in children and the acidosis of renal failure is common in adults. In severe malaria the arterial, capillary, venous and CSF concentrations of lactate rise in direct proportion to disease severity. Acid–base assessment or venous lactate concentrations four hours after admission to hospital are very good indicators of prognosis in severe malaria. In bacterial sepsis, there is also hyperlactataemia, but, unless there is profound shock, the lactate–pyruvate ratio is usually less than 15. This indicates that hypermetabolism is the source of lactate accumulation. In severe malaria the pathogenesis is different; lactate–pyruvate ratios often exceed 30 reflecting tissue hypoxia and anaerobic glycolysis. Lactic acidosis results from several discrete processes: the tissue anaerobic glycolysis consequent upon microvascular obstruction; a failure of hepatic and renal lactate clearance; and the production of lactate by the parasite. Hypovolaemia is usually not a major contributor to lactic acidosis. Mature malaria parasites consume up to 70 times as much glucose as uninfected cells and over 90% of this is converted to L+lactic acid (plasmodia do not have the complete set of enzymes necessary for the citric acid cycle). Interestingly, up to 6% of the lactic acid appears as D-lactate, but this does not contribute materially to the acidosis. However calculations based on glucose and lactate turnover in man indicate that the majority of the lactic acid produced in malaria derives from host rather than parasite sources. Lactate levels also rise after generalized convulsions. Lactate turnover in both adults and children with severe malaria is increased approximately three-fold compared with values obtained in healthy adults. Studies in children using stable isotope techniques indicate that increased lactate production (resulting from anaerobic glycolysis) rather than reduced clearance is the main cause of lactate accumulation, although in adults reduced clearance is certainly a contributor. Hyperlactataemia is associated with hypoglycaemia and is accompanied by hyperalaninaemia and elevated glycerol concentrations reflecting the impairment of gluconeogenesis through the Cori cycle. Lactate, glutamine and alanine are the major gluconeogenic precursors. There is evidence for the presence of another, as yet unidentified strong organic anion, in acidotic patients with severe malaria, which is the major contributor to acidosis.

Triglyceride and free fatty acid levels are also elevated in acute malaria and plasma concentrations of ketone bodies are raised in patients who have been unable to eat. Ketoacidosis may be prominent in children. In severe malaria, there is dysfunction of all organ systems, particularly those with obligatory high metabolic rates. The endocrine glands are no exception. Pituitary–thyroid axis abnormalities result in the 'sick euthyroid' syndrome and also parathyroid dysfunction. Mild hypocalcaemia is common and hypophosphataemia may be profound in the very seriously ill. By contrast, the pituitary–adrenal axis appears normal in acute malaria.

HYPOGLYCAEMIA

Hypoglycaemia is associated with hyperlactataemia and shares the same pathophysiological aetiology: an increased peripheral requirement for glucose consequent upon anaerobic glycolysis (the Pasteur effect), the increased metabolic demands of the febrile illness, and the obligatory demands of the parasites which use glucose as their major fuel (all of which increase demand); and a failure of hepatic gluconeogenesis and glycogenolysis (reduced supply). Hepatic glycogen is exhausted rapidly: stores in fasting adults last approximately 2 days, but children only have enough for 12 hours. Healthy children have approximately three times higher rates of glucose turnover compared with adults, but in severe malaria turnover is increased by more than 50% (to values five times higher than those in adults with severe malaria). The net result of impaired gluconeogenesis, limited glycogen stores and greatly increased demand results in a hypoglycaemia in 20–30% of children with severe malaria. In patients treated with quinine, this is compounded by quinine-stimulated pancreatic β-cell insulin secretion. Hyperinsulinaemia is balanced by a reduced tissue sensitivity to insulin, which returns to normal as the patient improves. This probably explains why quinine-induced (hyperinsulinaemic) hypoglycaemia tends to occur after the first 24 hours of treatment, whereas malaria-related hypoglycaemia (with appropriate suppression of insulin secretion) is often present when the patient with severe malaria is first admitted. Hypoglycaemia contributes to nervous system dysfunction and in cerebral malaria is associated with residual neurological deficit in survivors.

PLACENTAL DYSFUNCTION

Pregnancy increases susceptibility to malaria. This is probably caused by a suppression of systemic and placental cell-mediated immune responses. There is intense sequestration of *P. falciparum*-infected erythrocytes in the placenta, local activation of pro-inflammatory cytokine production and maternal anaemia. This leads to cellular infiltration and thickening of the syncytiotrophoblast and placental insufficiency with consequent fetal growth retardation. Illness close to term also results in prematurity. In areas of intense transmission a malaria attributable reduction in birth weight (circa 170 g) is confined to primigravidae. There is no convincing evidence that malaria causes abortion or stillbirth in this context. With lower levels of transmission (i.e. less immunity) the risk extends to other pregnancies and there is a propensity to develop severe malaria with a high incidence of fetal death. *Plasmodium vivax* also reduces birth weight (by about two-thirds the amount caused by *P. falciparum*), which questions the primary role of extensive sequestration in the pathogenesis of placental insufficiency. Malaria in early pregnancy may cause abortion.

BACTERIAL INFECTION

Patients with severe malaria are vulnerable to bacterial infections, particularly of the lungs and urinary tract (following catheterization). Postpartum sepsis is also common. Spontaneous bacterial septicaemia is an important complication of severe malaria. This is relatively unusual in adults (probably <1% of cases) but is much more common in young children. There is undoubtedly considerable overlap between sepsis (both pneumonia and septicaemia) and malaria in endemic areas. The difficulty is one of diagnosis; where transmission is high and parasitaemia is common in children, it may be difficult or impossible to distinguish bacterial infections with *coincident* parasitaemia from infections complicating malaria. The blood smear is sensitive but not specific for malaria as the cause of the illness, whereas blood culture is insensitive in the diagnosis of bacteraemia. Recent studies suggest that plasma *Pf*HRP2 concentrations may be a useful discriminant. Non-typhoid *Salmonella* septicaemias are an important complication of otherwise uncomplicated *falciparum* malaria in African children. Malaria predisposes young children to systemic non-typhoidal *Salmonella* infections which are a major cause of septicaemia in sub-Saharan Africa, particularly where HIV-AIDS is prevalent.

Histopathology

As the benign human malarias are rarely fatal there is relatively little information available on the histopathology of these infections. Unfortunately, this is not the case for *P. falciparum* malaria. In fatal malaria, the microvasculature of the vital organs is packed with erythrocytes containing mature forms of the parasite. There is abundant intra- and extra-erythrocytic pigment and organs such as the liver, spleen and placenta may be grey-black in colour. Sequestration is not uniformly distributed; it tends to be greatest in the brain and heart followed by the gut, kidney, adipose tissue, liver, lungs and least of all in bone marrow and skin. There is remarkably little extravascular pathology in malaria.

BRAIN

If the patient dies from the acute infection, the brain is commonly mildly swollen with multiple small petechial haemorrhages throughout the white matter. Different architectural types of haemorrhage are seen; simple petechial, zonal ring haemorrhages, and Durck's granulomata. Haemorrhages are less prominent in the grey matter. Large haemorrhages or infarcts are rare. There is usually no evidence of tentorial or foramen magnum herniation. Capillaries and venules are distended and packed with erythrocytes containing mature forms of the parasite (whereas these are seen rarely in peripheral blood smears) (Figure 43.5). This sequestration is particularly prominent in the white matter, although the tissue is much less vascular than the grey matter. The degree of cerebral sequestration and the intensity of erythrocyte packing is greater in cerebral malaria than in fatal malaria in which the patient was not comatose. A large quantity of intra- and extra-erythrocytic pigment is evident. In the white matter, accumulations of glial cells are seen surrounding haemorrhagic foci (Durck's granuloma) where vessels appear to have been occluded by a mass of parasitized cells and then ruptured. At a microvascular level, there is considerable variation in the intensity of sequestration between vessels, with each vessel having a discrete age distribution of parasite maturity. At the ultrastructural level the erythrocytes are seen to be packed closely together and the infected red cells are adherent to the vascular endothelium by attachment of knob-like surface projections to the endothelial surface. In adults occasional fibrin strands are seen but there is a striking absence of platelets and usually only focal leukocyte aggregation, i.e. there is no evidence of thrombus formation or vasculitis. In children there is more fibrin deposition and platelets can be seen. On immunofluorescent staining malarial antigens may be seen on the endothelial basement membrane, but the significance of this observation is uncertain (i.e. does it reflect pathology in vivo or an agonal artefact?). In some cases there are only a few, or no parasites in the cerebral vessels. This occurs when death was several days after parasite clearance, or the diagnosis was incorrect. Secondary neuropathological changes include widespread astroglial activation and nonspecific signs of neuronal stress response. Axonal injury and consequent dysfunction correlate with premortem coma and this provides a plausible mechanism whereby the parasitized erythrocyte, remaining within the vascular space, can reversibly affect neurological function.

HEART AND LUNGS

Despite intense sequestration in the myocardial microvasculature the heart is remarkably normal, although petechial epicardial haemorrhages are common and in anaemic patients the heart is commonly pale and dilated. As in all other organs, extravascular pathological changes are rare. In adults the lungs often show evidence of pulmonary oedema, although this may be patchy. Hyaline membrane formation suggests leakage of proteinaceous fluid. There is moderate sequestration and leukocyte aggregates are more prominent than in the brain. There may be secondary bacterial pneumonia. Pathophysiological studies in *P. vivax* infections suggest pulmonary vascular sequestration but as yet there is no pathological confirmation of this.

LIVER AND SPLEEN

The liver is generally enlarged and may be black from malaria pigment. There is congestion of the centrilobular capillaries with sinusoidal dilatation and Kupffer cell hyperplasia. Sequestration of parasitized erythrocytes is associated with variable cloudy swelling of the hepatocytes and perivenous ischaemic changes, and sometimes centrizonal necrosis. In adults, hepatic glycogen is often present despite hypoglycaemia. In uncomplicated malaria the liver histology is often normal. The spleen is often dark or black from malaria pigment, enlarged, soft and friable. It is full of erythrocytes containing mature and immature parasites. There is evidence of reticular hyperplasia and architectural reorganization. The soft and acutely enlarged spleen of acute lethal infections contrasts with the hard fibrous enlargement associated with repeated malaria.

KIDNEYS

The kidneys are often slightly swollen. In adults there are commonly tubular abnormalities consistent with ischaemia, including acute tubular necrosis and tubular epithelial cell regenerative change. There is patchy sequestration, particularly in the glomerular capillaries, although this is less than that seen in cerebral capillaries. Occasional mesangial and endothelial cell proliferative changes are seen. Leukocyte sequestration is similar to that in the lung and more marked than in the brain. Immunofluorescence and electron microscopic studies show minimal immunoglobulin deposition on the glomerular capillary basement membranes, but the changes are not those of a primary immune complex-mediated glomerulonephritis.

ALIMENTARY TRACT

Upper gastrointestinal bleeding from erosions may occur in severe malaria. There is intense sequestration in the gut and visceral ischaemia may explain the acute abdominal pain that sometimes occurs in severe malaria. Despite this, drug absorption is often remarkably normal.

BONE MARROW

Dyserythropoietic change is prominent in all the acute malarias. Bone marrow macrophages contain pigment and erythrophagocytosis may be seen. Iron is usually plentiful. The platelet and white cell series are usually normal.

PLACENTA

The placenta may be black from malaria pigment even if the mother is asymptomatic throughout pregnancy. Large numbers of mature *P. falciparum* parasites are seen on crush smears, although the peripheral blood smear may be negative. This is not seen in *P. vivax* infections. There is often trophoblastic thickening, macrophage infiltration, pigment deposition and perivillous fibrin deposition. Active infection is associated with basement, membrane thickening, fibrinoid necrosis and syncytial knots. Chronic infection is associated with marked mononuclear cell infiltration.

Laboratory Diagnosis

Malaria is diagnosed by microscopic examination of the blood. It is not a clinical diagnosis.

Thick and thin blood films are made on clean, grease-free glass slides (Figure 43.12). Having written the patient's name, time and date, the glass slide can be cleaned by breathing on the surface and wiping with a clean cloth. The patient's finger should be cleaned with alcohol, allowed to dry and then the side of the finger tip should be pricked with a sharp sterile lancet or

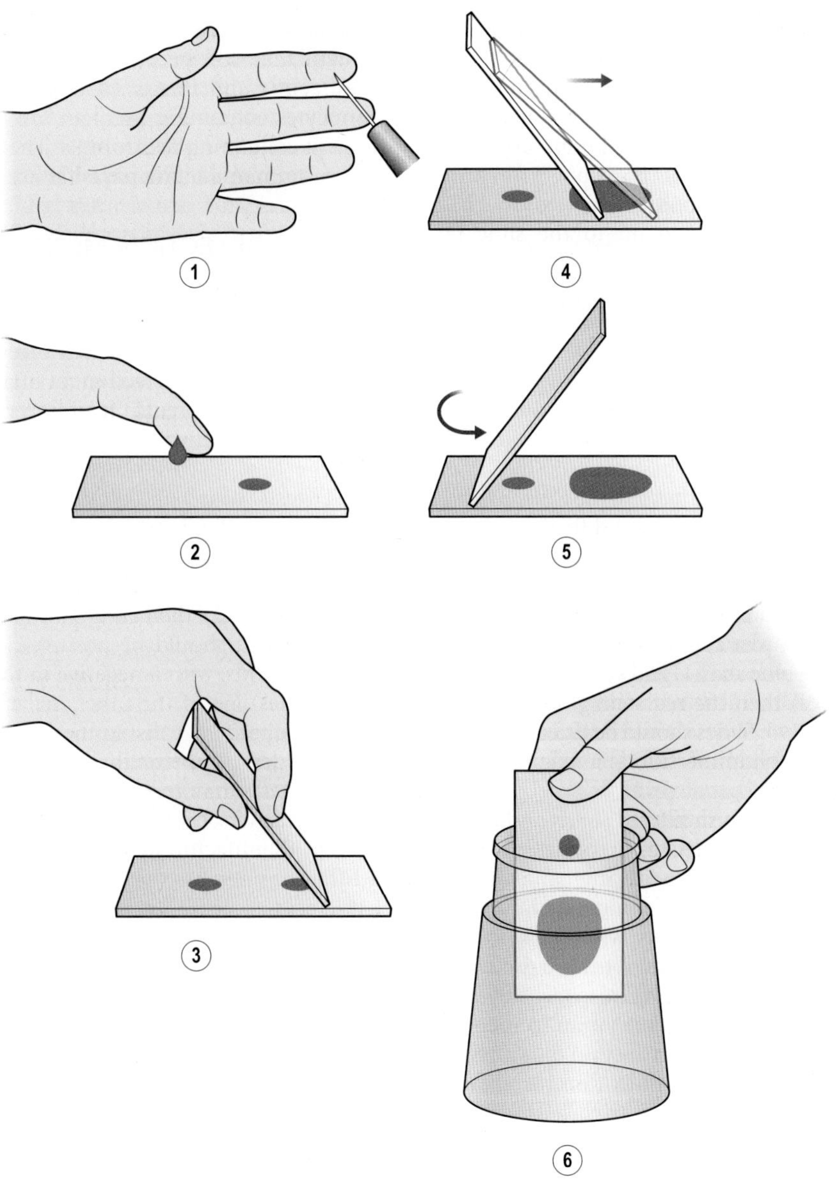

Figure 43.12 Making a peripheral blood smear.

needle. Two drops of blood are placed at one end of the slide. The thin film is made immediately by placing the *smooth* leading edge of a second (spreader) slide in the central drop of blood, adjusting the angle (less blood – more acute) and, while holding the edges of the slide, smearing the blood with a swift and steady sweep along the surface. If the blood drop is too large, the spreader slide should be dunked in the drop, then 'jumped' to the slide surface carrying a smaller amount of blood – and then smeared. Making good thin films requires some practice. Anaemic blood smears poorly. The thick film should be stirred in a circular motion with the corner of the second slide until clotting takes place. The thick film must be of uneven thickness, but it should be possible to read the hands, but not the figures, of a watch face through the film.

INTRADERMAL SMEARS

Chinese researchers have shown that smears from intradermal blood may contain more mature forms of *P. falciparum* than the peripheral blood. This is considered to allow a more complete assessment of severe malaria. The intradermal smears may also be positive or may show pigment containing leukocytes after the blood smear is negative. In terms of diagnostic sensitivity the intradermal smear is similar to the bone marrow (i.e. slightly more sensitive than peripheral blood). The smears are taken (Figure 43.13) from multiple intradermal punctures with a 25G needle on the volar surface of the upper forearm. The punctures should not ooze blood spontaneously, but sero-sanguinous fluid can be expressed on to the slide by squeezing.

STAINING AND READING

The thick film should be dried thoroughly otherwise it may wash away during staining. The thin film is then fixed in anhydrous methanol (taking care *not* to fix the thick film). Giemsa's stain buffered to a pH of 7.2 makes the best malaria slides, but for optimum results the stain should be left on the slide for 30 min. Field's stain is quicker, but the thin and thick films are treated differently. The thin film is immersed in the red stain (Field's B) for 6 seconds (s), then gently washed off for 5 s; then immersed in the blue stain (Field's A) for 3–4 s and then gently washed off (5 s). The reverse order applies to the thick film: the slide is first immersed in the blue stain (Field's A) for 5 seconds, then gently washed off (5 s) then the red stain (Field's B) for 5 s, then gently washed off (5 s). Slides should be dried in a slide rack before examining under oil immersion at a magnification of ×1000.

Best results are obtained with fresh filtered stains and anhydrous methanol for fixing the thin film. Use of repeatedly reused stain, full of precipitates and particles, with methanol left to absorb atmospheric water and a poorly maintained fungus-infected microscope (familiar to all of us who work in the tropics) makes accurate parasite counting a lot more difficult.

Before going to oil immersion on the microscope, the slide should be scanned briefly under low magnification to identify the best area for detailed examination. For the thin film, the tail of the film should be examined; for the thick film the area of optimum thickness and staining and least artefact is chosen. The thick film is approximately 30 times more sensitive than the thin film, although sensitivity and specificity depend to a great extent on the experience of the microscopist, the quality of the slides, stains and microscope and the time spent examining the slide. Artefacts are common and often confusing. Speciation of malaria at the trophozoite stage is easier on the thin film, although gametocytes and schizonts are more likely to be seen on the thick film. The thin film is more accurate for parasite counting. The number of parasitized red cells per 1000 red cells should be counted. If there are two parasites in one red cell, this is counted as one. At low parasitaemias (<5/1000 on the thin film) the thick film should be counted; the number of parasites per 200, or preferably 500 white cells is noted. These figures can then be corrected by the total red cell and white cell counts to give the number of parasites per unit blood volume (μL). If the white count is not available then the count is assumed to be 8,000 μL. An alternative is to count all parasites in a fixed volume of blood. In severe malaria parasitaemias are usually high and the stage of parasite development should be assessed on the thin film. The proportion of asexual parasites containing visible pigment (i.e. mature trophozoites and schizonts) should be counted. The presence of pigment in neutrophils and monocytes should also be noted and counted. In patients who have already received antimalarial treatment, pigment may still be present in leukocytes after clearance of parasitaemia and this is an important clue to the diagnosis. Monocytes containing pigment are cleared more slowly than pigment containing neutrophils. The morphological characteristics of human malaria parasites are given in Table 43.3.

ANTIGEN DETECTION METHODS

The introduction of simple, rapid, sensitive, highly specific and increasingly affordable dipstick or card tests for the diagnosis of malaria has been a major advance in recent years. These are based on antibody detection of malaria-specific antigens in blood samples; currently histidine-rich protein 2 (*Pf*HRP2), parasite lactate dehydrogenase (which is antigenically distinct from the host enzyme) and aldolase. Current *Pf*HRP2 and *Pf*LDH tests, based on colour reactions, provide a diagnostic sensitivity for *P. falciparum* similar to trained microscopists. Many tests also include 'pan-malaria' antibody which detects all malaria species or a specific *P. vivax* LDH or aldolase antibody.[24] The cards or sticks then carry two band colour reactions plus a control (which should be positive). Thus a positive test with these two bands, with a negative in the *Plasmodium falciparum* test, signifies one of the other malaria species (or *P. vivax* for the specific tests) is causing the infection. This part of the test usually is less sensitive than good microscopy. The antigen detection tests may remain positive in patients with persistent gametocytaemia. There are now many different tests from many different manufacturers, based on several different antibodies and the considerable variability between them in performance characteristics has been reduced as a result of regular WHO evaluations (see: http://www.who.int/malaria/publications/atoz/9789241502566/en/index.html). Most current tests are based on *Pf*HRP2. These tests are the least expensive, simplest to perform and the most robust under tropical conditions. Variability in the diagnostic sensitivity of *Pf*HRP2-based tests also results from sequence diversity in the gene encoding *Pf*HRP2 and consequent variability in the number of antigenic repeats. Because *Pf*HRP2 is cleared very slowly from the blood, these tests may remain positive for up to a month after the acute

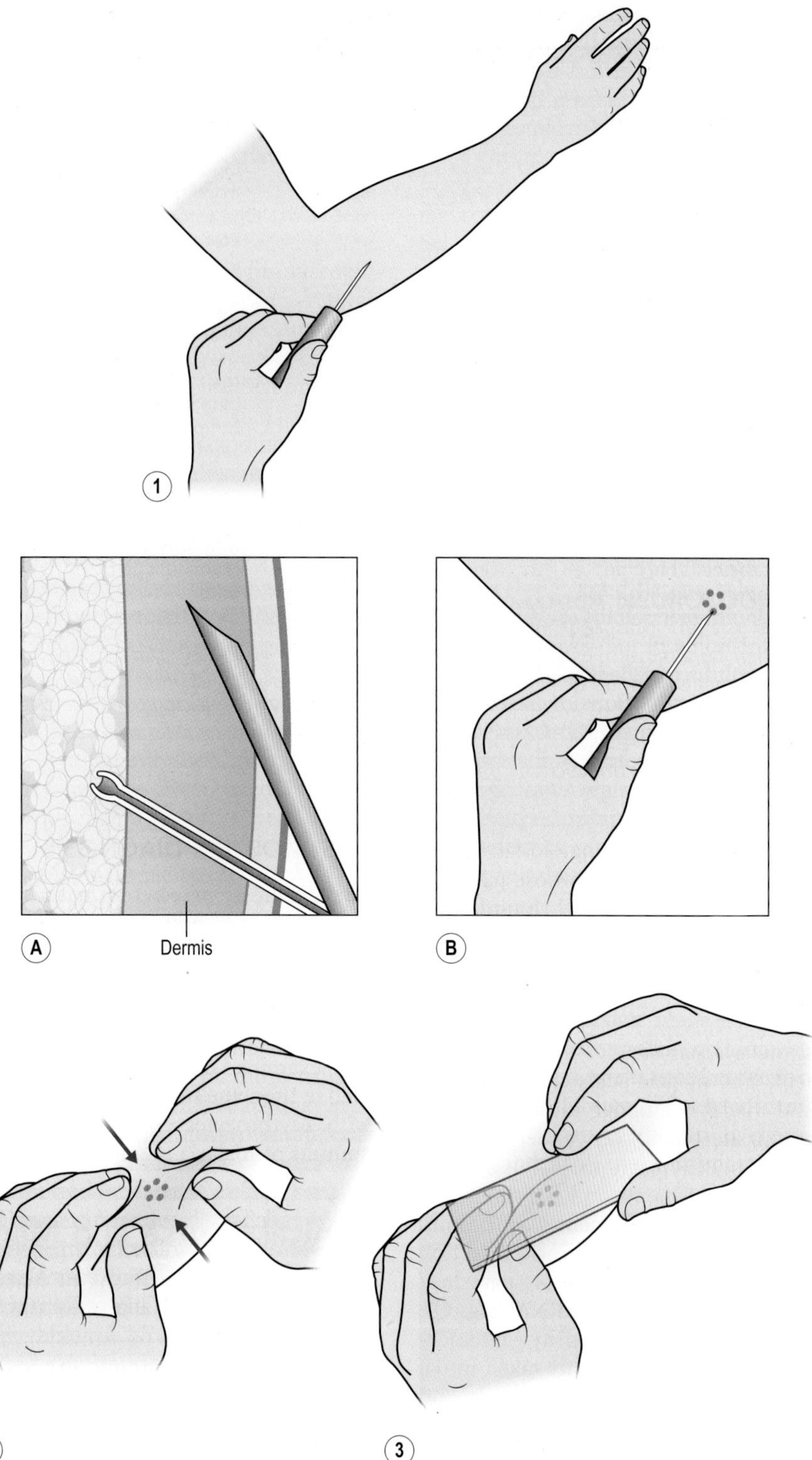

Figure 43.13 Making an intradermal smear.

infection, particularly if the original parasitaemia was high. This is a disadvantage in areas where transmission is high and infections frequent, but is very useful in the diagnosis of severely ill patients who have received previous antimalarial treatment. Their parasitaemia may have cleared but the *Pf*HRP2 test will remain strongly positive. In contrast *Pf*LDH is cleared rapidly from blood and so the test becomes negative within days of treatment. *Pf*HRP2 is present in parasitized erythrocytes but it is also secreted into plasma and plasma concentrations (which can be assessed semi-quantitatively from the intensity of the colour reaction) are a valuable guide to the parasite biomass and thus severity. The *Pf*HRP2 test has proved useful in detecting mixed *P. falciparum* and *P. vivax* infections where the former was not evident microscopically. False-positive tests may occur

TABLE 43.3 **Morphological Characteristics of Human Malaria Parasites**

	P. falciparum	*P. vivax*	*P. ovale*	*P. malariae*
Asexual parasites	Usually only ring forms seen. Fine blue cytoplasm oval, circular, comma- shaped or occasionally thick band forms. squeezed to the edge of the cell (appliqué form). One or two chromatin dots. Parasitaemia may exceed 2%	Irregular large fairly thick rings becoming very pleomorphic as the parasite matures. One chromatin dot	Regular dense ring enlarges to compact blue mature trophozoite. One chromatin dot Low parasitaemia usual	Dense thick rings, maturing to dense round trophozoites Rectangular or band-form trophozoites Pigment associated with rings and trophozoites. Large red chromatin dot or band. Low parasitaemia usual
Meronts (Schizonts)	Rare in peripheral blood. 8–32 merozoites, dark brown-black pigment	Common. 12–18 merozoites, orange brown pigment	8–14 merozoites, brown pigment	8–10 merozoites, black pigment
Gametocytes	Banana-shaped. Male: light blue. Female: darker blue. Red-black nucleus with few scattered blue-black pigment granules in cytoplasm	Round or oval. Male: round, pale blue. Female: oval, dark blue. Triangular nucleus, few orange pigment granules	Large round dense blue like *P. malariae*, but prominent James' dots. Brown pigment	Large oval-shaped. Male: pale blue. Female: dense blue. Large black pigment granules
Red cell changes	Normal size. As parasite matures cytoplasm becomes pale, the cells become crenated, and a few small red dots appear over the cytoplasm (Maurer's clefts)	Enlarged. Pale red Schüffner's dots increase in number as parasite matures	Cells become oval with tufted ends. Prominent James' dots	Normal size and shape. No red dots

Note. Multiple invasion is often quoted as a feature of falciparum malaria. This is simply a function of higher parasite densities. At any given density multiple invasion is over three times more frequent with *P. vivax* compared with *P. falciparum*. *P. knowlesi* resembles *P. falciparum* in the first 8 hours of asexual development, then begins to resemble *P. malariae* when older.

in patients with high concentrations of rheumatoid factor and false negatives have been reported in patients whose parasites have a rare antigenically variant form of *Pf* HRP2 (found occasionally in South America).

OTHER TECHNIQUES

Unlike mature red cells, malaria parasites contain DNA and RNA and malaria pigment. The nucleic acids can be stained with fluorescent dyes and visualized under ultraviolet light microscopy, or, with appropriate filters, seen under ordinary light and they can be amplified in PCR reactions. PCR is increasingly used in epidemiological assessments and is particularly useful in identifying parasite species in low-density infections. qPCR detection on 1 mL blood samples can reach detection thresholds 1000 times lower than the blood smear (10 parasites/mL). Quantitative assessment of gametocyte mRNA (e.g. QT NASBA) allows accurate quantitation of low-density gametocytaemia. In the QBC™ technique blood samples are taken into a specialized capillary tube containing acridine orange stain and a float. Under high centrifugal forces (14 000 g) the infected erythrocytes, which have a higher buoyant density than uninfected cells, become concentrated around the float. Using a modified lens adaptor (Paralens™) with its own light source, the acridine orange fluorescence from malaria parasites can be visualized through an ordinary microscope. Although slightly more sensitive than conventional light microscopy, it does not give parasite counts or speciation with accuracy and it is relatively expensive. It is useful for screening large numbers of blood samples rapidly. Detection of malaria antibody can be useful in some circumstances, such as confirmation of earlier infection and in epidemiological assessment of transmission intensity, but has no place in acute diagnosis.

POSTMORTEM DIAGNOSIS

The diagnosis of cerebral malaria postmortem can be confirmed from a brain smear. A needle aspirate or biopsy is obtained through the superior orbital foramen or the foramen magnum. A smear of grey matter is examined after staining the slide in the same way as for a thin blood film. Capillaries and venules are identified under low magnification microscopy and then examined under high magnification (×1000). If the patient died in the acute stage of cerebral malaria, the vessels are packed with erythrocytes containing mature parasites and a large amount of malaria pigment.

Clinical Course and Management

The clinical manifestations of malaria are dependent on the premorbid immune status of the host. In areas of intense *P. falciparum* malaria transmission, asymptomatic parasitaemia is usual in adults (premunition). Severe malaria never occurs in this age group: it is confined to the first years of life and becomes progressively less frequent with increasing age. In Africa before recent strengthening of control measures the average age of children admitted to hospital with severe malaria was 3 years and peak mortality was in the third year of life. The rate at which age-specific acquisition of premunition occurs is proportional to the intensity of malaria transmission. In areas with a constant high-level *P. falciparum* transmission (e.g. average infected *anopheline* biting frequencies of daily up to monthly), severe malaria occurs predominantly between 6 months and 3 years of age; milder symptoms are seen in older children and adults are usually asymptomatic and have low parasitaemias. Malaria is common in pregnancy, but is asymptomatic (although anaemia may be severe). The birth weight of babies born to primigravidae is reduced significantly. Spleen rates are high (>50%) in children between 2 and 9, corresponding with the epidemiological terms hyperendemic and holoendemic malaria. Severe anaemia in young children is the most common presentation of severe *falciparum* malaria in these circumstances. With lower or more seasonal or unstable transmission patterns the age distribution of severe malaria shifts upwards, severe malaria is seen in older children as well and cerebral malaria becomes the most prominent manifestation. Spleen rates in children are lower than 50%. With even lower or more sporadic patterns of transmission and when non-immunes travel to endemic areas, symptomatic disease is seen at all ages. Although severe anaemia is a common presentation in children on the island of New Guinea where transmission of *P. vivax* is very high, other manifestations of severe malaria do not occur commonly with *P. vivax*, *P. ovale*, or *P. malariae*. Nevertheless, the acute infection in a non-immune patient is still serious and debilitating. With more intense exposure a state of premunition is also reached with these infections.

INCUBATION PERIOD

In most cases of *falciparum* or *vivax* malaria the incubation period is approximately 2 weeks (Figures 43.14 and 43.15). Primary incubation periods can be long, particularly if the infection is suppressed by partially effective chemoprophylaxis. Most tropical strains of *P. vivax* had similar incubation periods to *P. falciparum*, but strains from cooler countries often had extremely long incubation periods. The primary infection began 8–12 months after sporozoite inoculation to coincide with the short summer-time mosquito breeding season in these cold countries. These strains of *P. vivax* (*P. vivax* var *hibernans*) acquired in northern and eastern Europe, Russia, central and northern China, may now be extinct.[3] The incubation period (time from sporozoite inoculation to fever) is prolonged by ineffective antimalarial treatment or prophylaxis – both of which reduce the effective multiplication rate. The durations of the prepatent and incubation periods are also strongly influenced by previous exposure, i.e. 'immunity'. Effective immunity both reduces effective multiplication, which prolongs the prepatent period and raises the threshold at which symptoms occur (premunition), which prolongs the incubation period. In *vivax* malaria the symptom threshold is raised disproportionately in immune individuals, i.e. the gap between the prepatent and incubation periods widens.

MIXED SPECIES INFECTIONS

The incidence of mixed species infections is always underestimated. Even with sensitive PCR detection methods, which reveal a much higher rate than microscopy, mixed infections are underestimated. In simultaneous infections with *P. falciparum* and *P. vivax*, the former suppresses the latter and the primary *vivax* malaria infection may not appear until several weeks later. Sometimes the reverse occurs and *P. vivax* suppresses *P. falciparum*. In sub-Saharan Africa *P. falciparum* commonly occurs together with *P. malariae* or *P. ovale*. In many areas outside Africa *P. falciparum* and *P. vivax* are both common and co-existent infections are frequent but, because of mutual suppression, the incidence is considerably underestimated. In Thailand, approximately 30% of patients with *P. falciparum* malaria will have a subsequent symptomatic infection with *P. vivax* within 2 months of their primary *falciparum* malaria, without further exposure to malaria infection.[25] In Myanmar, the figure is 50%. The converse (*P. vivax* malaria with undiagnosed coincident *P. falciparum* infection) occurs in

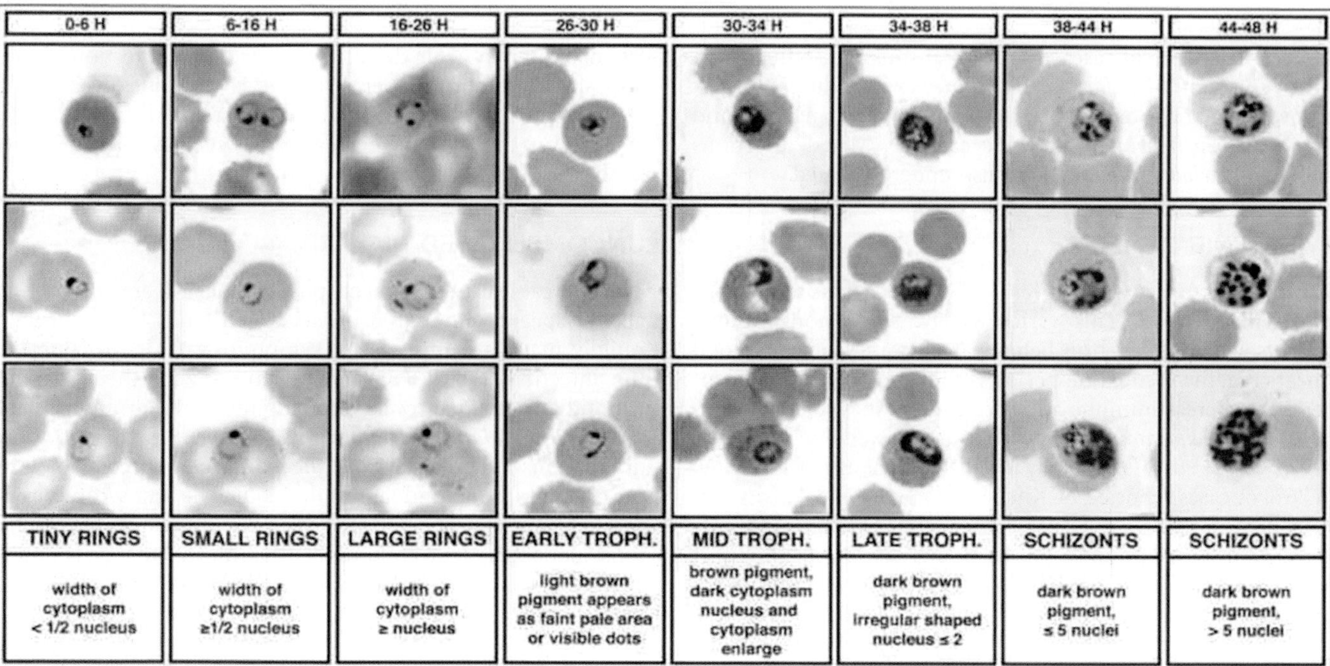

Figure 43.14 Asexual life cycle of *Plasmodium falciparum* with approximate ages of development. After some 13–16 hours of development the parasitized erythrocytes start to adhere to the vascular endothelium lining the capillaries and venules.

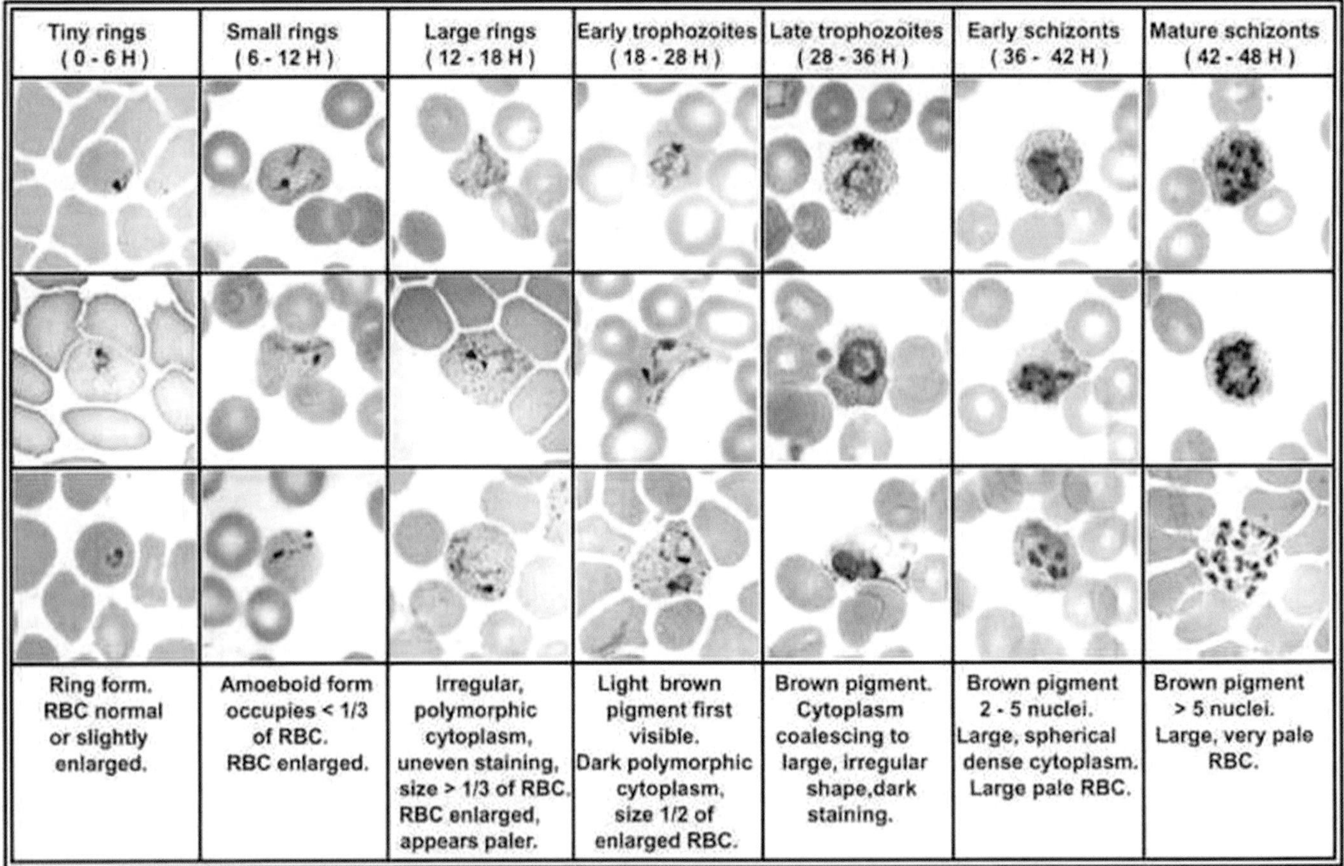

Figure 43.15 Asexual life cycle of *Plasmodium vivax* with approximate ages of development.

approximately 8% of cases. In a low transmission setting coincident infection of *P. falciparum* with *P. vivax* reduces the risk of severe malaria fourfold,[26] reduces the degree of anaemia, and reduces *P. falciparum* gametocyte carriage. Mixed infections with *P. malariae* and *P. ovale* are also underestimated.

PYROGENIC DENSITY

The parasitaemia at which fever (>37.3°C) occurs is termed the 'pyrogenic density'. This varies widely: some non-immune patients will become febrile before parasites are visible on blood smears (i.e. the incubation period is shorter than the prepatent period), whereas immune adults can sometimes tolerate up to >10,000 *P. falciparum* parasites/μL without fever. The pyrogenic density for *P. vivax* is generally lower than that of *P. falciparum*; in 76% of cases reported by Kitchen, the pyrogenic density was <100 parasites/μL. In *P. falciparum* infection average pyrogenic densities in non-immunes can be as high as 10 000/μL, but it must be remembered that less than half the life cycle circulates in *falciparum* malaria. The parasites in the blood smear are the circulating parasites in the generation subsequent to that which underwent pyrogenic merogony and they are therefore an underestimate of the total parasite burden. The pyrogenic density is a marker of immunity. High pyrogenic densities indicate premunition and a lower risk of severe disease. There are less data on pyrogenic densities in *P. malariae* infections, but it appears that they are higher than for *P. vivax*; values over 500/μL were found in 38% of Boyd's cases. There are limited data on *P. ovale*, but the available evidence suggests a pyrogenic density similar to *P. vivax*.

UNCOMPLICATED MALARIA

The clinical features of uncomplicated malaria are common to all five species although *P. vivax*, which tends to synchronize rapidly, may cause more severe symptoms early in the course of the infection and *P. knowlesi* infections with their 24-hour (quotidian) asexual cycle can rapidly develop into severe malaria. *P. malariae* and possibly *P. ovale* both have a more gradual onset than *P. vivax*. *P. falciparum* is unpredictable: the onset ranges from gradual to fulminant. The first symptoms of malaria are nonspecific and resemble influenza. Headache, muscular ache, vague abdominal discomfort, lethargy, lassitude and dysphoria often precede fever by up to 2 days. The temperature rises erratically at first, with shivering, mild chills, worsening headache and malaise, loss of appetite and sometimes abdominal discomfort. Children are irritable, lethargic and anorexic. If the infection is left untreated the fever in *P. vivax* and *P. ovale* regularizes to a 2-day cycle (tertian) and *P. malariae* fever spikes occur every 3 days (quartan pattern).

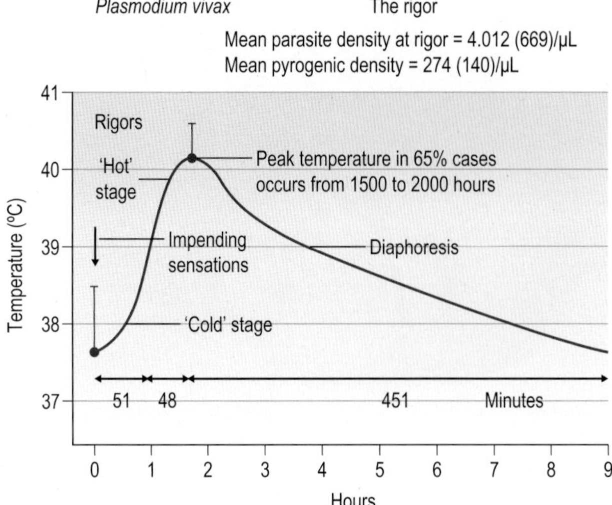

Figure 43.16 The rigor of *P. vixax* malaria. True rigors are rare in *P. falciparum* malaria. In infections with the other three human malaria parasites rigors occur when the parasite population has synchronized sufficiently. *(The time course of signs and symptoms is taken from Kitchen & Puttnam: J Natl Malaria Soc 1946;5:57–78.)*

P. falciparum remains erratic for longer and may never regularize to a tertian pattern. These terms derive from the Greek practice of 'inclusive reckoning', in which the beginning of the fever is considered day 1. Thus, a tertian fever recurs every 3rd day and a quartan fever every 4th day, with intervals of 2 and 3 days, respectively. Some infections consist of two broods cycling 24 hours out of phase and in these there is a daily fever spike (quotidian fever). Even more complex fever patterns are described in detail in the early literature.

The classical malaria fever charts (which graced earlier editions of this textbook) and the teeth-chattering rigors and profuse sweats that characterized the 'paroxysm' (Figure 43.16), are relatively unusual today as malaria therapy of neurosyphilis has been long abandoned (penicillin is more effective and more pleasant) and symptomatic infections are treated as soon as they are diagnosed. In a true paroxysm, the temperature usually rises steeply from a normal or slightly elevated level to exceed 39°C. As the temperature begins to rise there is intense headache and muscular discomfort. The patient feels cold, clutches at blankets and curls up shivering and uncommunicative (the chill). There is peripheral vasoconstriction and often 'goose-pimples'. Within minutes, the limbs begin to shake and the teeth chatter and the temperature climbs rapidly to a peak (usually between 39°C and 41.5°C). The rigor usually lasts 10–30 min, but can last up to 90 min (Figure 43.16). By the end of the rigor, there is peripheral vasodilatation and the skin feels hot. A profuse sweat then breaks out. The blood pressure is relatively low and there may be symptomatic orthostatic hypotension. The patient feels exhausted and may sleep. Defervescence usually takes 4–8 hours. Paroxysms with rigors are more common in *P. vivax* and *P. ovale* than in *P. falciparum* or *P. malariae* malaria. They may herald a relapse, or occur after several days of more chaotic fever in primary infections with these two malaria species. True rigors are unusual in naturally acquired *falciparum* malaria. As the infection continues the spleen and liver enlarge and anaemia develops and the patient loses weight. If no treatment is given the natural infection stabilizes for several weeks or months and then gradually resolves.

The duration of illness is proportional to the level of immunity and differs between the parasite species. Mild abdominal discomfort is common in malaria and rarely patients may appear to have an 'acute abdomen'. Either constipation or diarrhoea may occur. In some areas, watery diarrhoea is a prominent manifestation. However, there is usually no difficulty distinguishing malaria from gastroenteritis. A dry cough is relatively common but is not prominent. However, the respiratory rate may be raised, particularly in children and this can give rise to diagnostic confusion in primary healthcare facilities where respiratory rate is used as the only criterion for the diagnosis of acute respiratory infection. On chest examination there is no evidence of consolidation or effusion, but in an endemic area the clinical distinction between early pneumonia and severe malaria in young children can be very difficult. In routine clinical practice in malarious areas of the tropics, malaria is the most common cause of fever in children and is the most likely diagnosis in a febrile patient with no obvious respiratory or abdominal abnormalities. In travellers returning from such areas, any fever must be considered to be malaria unless proved otherwise. In semi-immune patients low-grade fever may be the only complaint in malaria. In tropical practice, malaria is so common that it must be excluded in any febrile patient.

RELAPSE

Both *P. vivax* and *P. ovale* have a tendency to relapse after resolution of the primary infection. Relapse, which results from maturation of persistent hypnozoites in the liver, must be distinguished from recrudescence of the primary infection because of incomplete treatment. *P. falciparum* is the usual cause of recrudescent infections and these tend to arise 2–4 weeks following treatment (but this can be as long as 10 weeks following treatment with slowly eliminated drugs). Relapses occur weeks or months (or even years) after the primary infection. The proportion of cases relapsing and the intervals between relapses vary between strains and depends on the size of the inoculum and the intensity or previous exposure. The pattern of relapse is also determined by the geographic origin of the infection. For example, over 50% of *P. vivax* infections in Thailand relapse whereas in most of India the proportion is closer to 20%.[3] The subtropical *P. vivax* has an interval usually of 8–10 months between primary illness and relapse whereas tropical strains have frequent relapses at short intervals (3–6 weeks depending on the drugs used). In Patrick Manson's famous experiment, conducted in September 1900, he infected his 23-year-old son with *P. vivax*, through mosquitoes sent by rail from Rome to London. His son became ill with 'double tertian fever', but was treated with quinine and recovered fully. In June 1901 (i.e. 9 months later), he suddenly became ill again with *vivax* malaria; a relapse interval of 9 months. In recent years, a relapse interval of 6 weeks has been quoted widely for tropical *Plasmodium vivax* but this is an artefact of the use of chloroquine which suppresses the first relapse (which would otherwise emerge at 3 weeks). The symptoms of a relapse start more abruptly than in the primary infection as the infection is more synchronous. They may begin with a sudden chill or rigor.

MALARIA IN PREGNANCY

Malaria (all species) in early pregnancy causes abortion. In areas of intense transmission the principal impact of *falciparum* malaria in pregnancy is an increased incidence of anaemia and a reduction in birth weight (approx. 170 g on average) of babies born to primigravidae. Thus, a greater proportion of babies have low birth weights (<2.5 kg). Low birth weight is a major risk factor for infant death. Malaria reduces birth weight mainly by intrauterine growth retardation (IUGR). In high transmission areas, malaria may also cause prematurity. In low transmission areas, prematurity is caused by symptomatic malaria close to term, not earlier in the pregnancy. The net result is an increased risk of neonatal death. In high transmission areas despite intense sequestration of *P. falciparum* parasites in the placenta, the mothers are usually asymptomatic, although they are more likely to be anaemic. In areas with lower levels of malaria transmission (mesoendemic or hypoendemic) symptomatic disease occurs and pregnant women are at an increased risk of severe *falciparum* malaria, particularly in the 2nd and 3rd trimesters. In low transmission areas, the adverse effects of malaria on birth weight extend to the first three pregnancies (and in non-immunes, to all pregnancies). Again anaemia is common and there is an increased risk of developing severe malaria. Anaemia itself is a risk factor for maternal mortality; moderate anaemia (Hb 4–8 g/dL) carrying a relative risk of 1.35 and severe anaemia (Hb <4 g/dL) a risk of 3.5. If a pregnant woman does develop severe malaria, fetal loss is common and the maternal mortality is very high. The mortality of cerebral malaria in pregnancy is approximately 50%, compared with 15–20% in non-pregnant adults. Acute pulmonary oedema and hypoglycaemia are particular complications of severe malaria in pregnancy. The baby is commonly stillborn. The clinical features of uncomplicated *vivax*, *ovale* or *malariae* malaria are similar to those of uncomplicated *P. falciparum*. *P. vivax* infections also increase anaemia and they reduce birth weight by approximately 100 g. In contrast to *P. falciparum*, *vivax* malaria affects multigravidae more than primigravidae. If a mother delivers with acute malaria bloodborne transmission to the newborn is not uncommon, but this often resolves spontaneously. Nevertheless, babies must be observed closely for congenital malaria and malaria considered in the differential diagnosis of neonatal fever or anaemia.

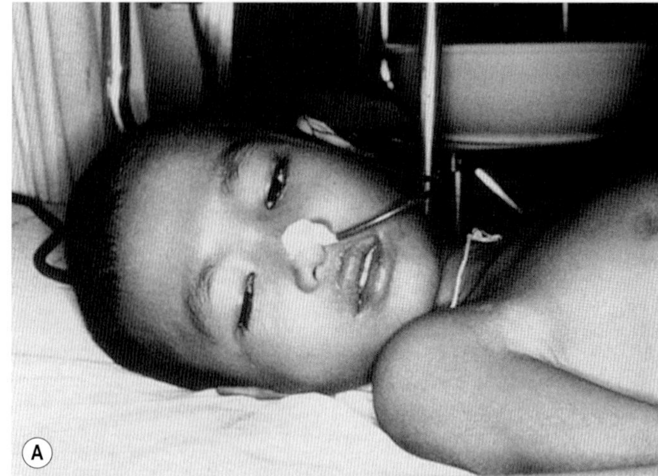

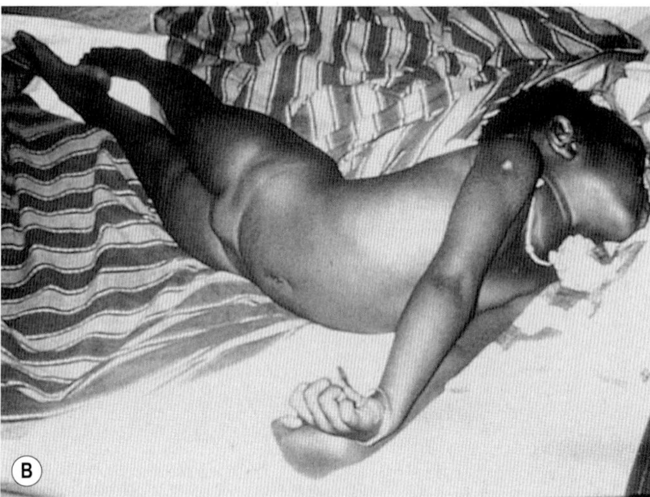

Figure 43.17 A 6-year-old Thai boy with cerebral malaria. His father was admitted at the same time with cerebral malaria – both survived. (B) A 3-year-old Gambian girl with cerebral malaria and opisthotonos. *(Courtesy of Jane Crawley.)*

MALARIA IN CHILDREN

The majority of childhood malaria infections (Figure 43.17) present with fever and malaise and respond rapidly to antimalarial treatment. Severe *falciparum* malaria is rare in infancy, although when it does occur the mortality is high. In young children the progression of *falciparum* malaria can be rapid. Generalized seizures are associated with fever, but they are more common in *P. falciparum* than *P. vivax* malaria, even in the absence of other signs of cerebral involvement. This suggests that cerebral sequestration causes significant pathology even in conscious patients. Coma, convulsions, acidosis, hypoglycaemia and severe anaemia are common presenting features of severe malaria in childhood. At the bedside, the presence of respiratory distress (acidotic breathing) or deep coma defines children at high risk of dying. These two clinical syndromes account for the majority of lethal infections. In areas of intense transmission profound anaemia is the usual manifestation of severe malaria and this occurs mainly in the 1–3-year age group. Severe malaria is rare in older children in high transmission settings. In areas of lower, less stable transmission cerebral malaria becomes a predominant manifestation of severe disease and the age range shifts upwards. Jaundice and pulmonary oedema are unusual in young children and renal failure requiring dialysis or haemofiltration is very rare (a significant difference compared with adults). As a consequence iatrogenic overhydration is less of a problem than in adults, although intravenous fluid administration must still be carefully supervised in small children. Dehydration is more common but rapid fluid loading is potentially lethal. In cerebral malaria seizures occurs frequently, particularly in the <3-year age group and should be treated promptly. Hypoglycaemia is common, occurring in up to 30% of children with severe malaria and is often accompanied by lactic acidosis. The blood glucose should be checked frequently and, where possible, continuous intravenous infusions of 5% or 10% dextrose given as a preventive measure.

In general children tolerate the antimalarial drugs better than adults and their symptoms resolve more quickly. The temptation to estimate body weight by 'eye' should be resisted and all children should be weighed if possible so that the doses of antimalarial drugs can be given on a mg/kg basis. Although administration of drugs adjusted to surface area is theoretically preferable, antimalarial doses have been devised on the basis of body weight. Children with acute malaria vomit readily, particularly if the temperature is high. Oral antimalarial treatment is more likely to be retained if it is palatable and the child is cool and calm before drug administration. In busy tropical clinics, only a minority of patients can be admitted to hospital and many children with moderately severe malaria have to be treated on an outpatient basis. It was common practice to administer a single dose of parenteral quinine and to send the patient home with the remainder of the oral regimen and to give the parents advice to return if the child deteriorated further. In this situation there is a danger of significant iatrogenic hypotension if the child is kept upright (e.g. on the mother's back). If possible, the child should be observed for at least 2 hours following parenteral drug administration and reassessed before discharge.

The diagnosis of severe malaria in children living in malaria-endemic areas may be difficult. As a positive blood smear is common in apparently healthy children, finding malaria parasites in the blood of a sick child does not necessarily mean the child has severe malaria. Fever and rapid laboured breathing could be pneumonia even if the blood smear is positive. The obtunded child might have meningoencephalitis and the shocked child might be septicaemic despite positive blood smears. The net result is that severe malaria in children tends to be overdiagnosed.

MALARIA AND HIV

When the enormity of the HIV epidemic in Africa was first recognized it was thought that malaria and HIV infection did not interact significantly. This is not true. While asymptomatic HIV infection has little impact on malaria, with increasing immunosuppression in HIV-AIDS immune control of malaria is impaired. There is an increasing risk of parasitaemia, increasing risk of illness, and in low transmission settings an increased risk of severe malaria. HIV infection compounds malaria-associated reduction in birth weight. Therapeutic responses to antimalarial treatment are impaired so treatment failure rates are increased and preventive therapies less effective. Drug interactions between antiretrovirals and antimalarials have not been studied in sufficient detail yet. Where sulfadoxine-pyrimethamine is effective, then prophylaxis against opportunistic infections with trimethoprim-sulfamethoxazole will protect from malaria also.

SEVERE MALARIA

Death from acute *P. vivax*, *P. ovale* or *P. malariae* infections is very rare. Occasionally, already debilitated patients, or those with another disease process may succumb and fatal haemorrhage may follow a ruptured spleen (either traumatic or spontaneous), but these events are uncommon. Severe anaemia may follow repeated *P. vivax* infections and is an important presenting feature in children in high transmission settings. Pulmonary oedema carries a better prognosis in *vivax* than in *falciparum* malaria but can be lethal. There have been many case reports of 'cerebral *vivax* malaria'. Some of these may have been misdiagnoses, but there are several recent reports of severe *Plasmodium vivax* infections from Indonesia, India and South America. In low transmission settings the case-specific risk of developing severe malaria with *vivax* malaria is substantially lower (>100 fold) than with *falciparum* malaria and even in high transmission settings it is over ten times lower. The simian parasite *P. knowlesi* is potentially lethal, capable of producing fulminant disease with the rapid development of anaemia, acidosis, pulmonary oedema and acute kidney injury as the major manifestations. Coma does not occur.

Falciparum malaria is the major cause of death from malaria. The progression to severe disease can be rapid. In young children presenting with cerebral malaria a history of less than 1 day's illness is common. Although undernutrition is associated with an increased risk of clinical malaria and anaemia in high transmission settings, cerebral malaria is rare in severe malnutrition and often seems to strike down the healthiest people. The great malariologist, Ettore Marchiafava, noted over 100 years ago how common severe malaria was in the 'hale and hearty' Italian shepherds who descended from the malaria-free mountains to the malarious valleys every autumn. In adults, patients with severe malaria usually have a history of being ill for several days before admission to hospital.

Definitions of severe *falciparum* malaria are useful for clinical and epidemiological purposes. Definitions were proposed by working groups convened by the World Health Organization (WHO) in 1986, 1990 and 2000 and they are currently being revised.[27] In severe malaria, there is often evidence of multiple vital organ dysfunction and more than one of the above criteria are fulfilled (Table 43.4A,B). Strictly defined severe malaria has a mortality of approximately 10% in children and 15% in adults but this depends on the degree of vital organ dysfunction. Of the various major criteria severe anaemia (Hb<5 g/dL) carries a much better prognosis than evidence of severe cerebral, renal or metabolic dysfunction. Physicians should not worry unduly about definitions or semantics. They should treat *any patient about whom they are worried* as having severe malaria, even if they do not fall clearly into one of the above categories.

CEREBRAL MALARIA

This may be defined strictly as unrousable coma (i.e. there is a non-purposeful response or no response to a painful stimulus) in *falciparum* malaria. This is usually a Glasgow Coma Score of <11 or in young children a Blantyre Coma Score of <3. In practice, any patient with altered consciousness should be treated for severe malaria. Although cerebral malaria is the most prominent feature of severe *falciparum* malaria, some patients with ultimately lethal infections never lose consciousness until they die. In cerebral malaria the onset of coma may be sudden, often following a generalized seizure, or gradual, with initial drowsiness, confusion, disorientation, delirium or agitation, followed by unconsciousness. Extreme agitation is a poor prognostic sign in *falciparum* malaria. The length of the prodromal history is usually several days in adults, but in children can be as short as 6–12 hours. A history of convulsions is common.

On examination the patient is febrile and unrousable. There may be some passive resistance to head flexion, but the board-like rigidity of meningitis is not found and there are no other signs of meningeal irritation. There may be anaemia, which in some cases, particularly children, may be profound. Conversely jaundice is relatively unusual in children but common in adults. Signs of bleeding are unusual and indicate a poor prognosis. The patient is usually warm, dry and well perfused peripherally, with a low-normal blood pressure and a sinus tachycardia. Skin perfusion is variable. Poor capillary refill (refill time >2 s) is a serious prognostic sign in children. Intermittent 'goose-pimples' are common in association with cutaneous vasoconstriction. Sustained hyperventilation is a poor prognostic sign as it

TABLE 43.4A **1990 WHO Definition of Severe Malaria**

1. Cerebral malaria – unrousable coma not attributable to any other cause in a patient with falciparum malaria. The coma should persist for at least 30 min (1 hour in the 2000 definition) after a generalized convulsion to make the distinction from transient postictal coma. Coma should be assessed using the Blantyre Coma Scale in children or the Glasgow Coma Scale in adults (see Table 43.14).
2. Severe anaemia – normocytic anaemia with haematocrit <15% or haemoglobin <5 g/dL in the presence of parasitaemia more than 10 000/μL. Note that finger prick samples may underestimate the haemoglobin concentration by up to 1 g/dL if the finger is squeezed. If anaemia is hypochromic and/or microcytic, iron deficiency and thalassaemia/haemoglobinopathy must be excluded. (These criteria are rather generous; and would include many children in high transmission areas. A parasitaemia of >100 000/μL might be a more appropriate threshold).
3. Renal failure – defined as a urine output of <400 mL in 24 hours in adults, or 12 mL/kg in 24 hours in children, failing to improve after rehydration, and a serum creatinine of more than 265 μmol/L (>3.0 mg/dL). (In practice for initial assessment, the serum creatinine alone is used).
4. Pulmonary oedema or adult respiratory distress syndrome.
5. Hypoglycaemia – defined as a whole blood glucose concentration of <2.2.mmol/L (40 mg/dL).
6. Circulatory collapse or shock – hypotension (systolic blood pressure <50 mmHg in children aged 1–5 years or <70 mmHg in adults), with cold clammy skin or core-skin temperature difference >10°C. (The more recent review declined to give precise definitions, but noted the lack of sensitivity or specificity of core-peripheral measurements.) Capillary refill time is not mentioned but recent studies indicate this simple test provides a good assessment of severity.
7. Spontaneous bleeding from gums, nose, gastrointestinal tract, etc. and/or substantial laboratory evidence of DIC. (This is relatively unusual.)
8. Repeated generalized convulsions – more than two observed within 24 hours, despite cooling. (In young children, these may be febrile convulsions, and the other clinical and parasitological features need to be taken into account.) Clinical evidence of seizure activity may be subtle (e.g. tonic clonic eye movements, profuse salivation, delayed coma recovery).
9. Acidaemia – defined as an arterial or capillary pH<7.35 (note temperature corrections are needed as most patients are hotter than 37°C; add 0.0147 pH unit per degree Celsius (°C) over 37°C), or acidosis defined as a plasma bicarbonate concentration <15 mmol/L or a base excess >10. (Operationally the clinical presentation of 'respiratory distress' or 'acidotic breathing' is focussed upon in the 2000 recommendations. Abnormal breathing patterns are a sign of severity indicating severe acidosis, pulmonary oedema or pneumonia).
10. Macroscopic haemoglobinuria – if definitely associated with acute malaria infection and not the result of oxidant antimalarial drugs in patients with erythrocyte enzyme defects such as G6PD deficiency. (This is difficult to ascertain in practice: if the G6PD status is checked following massive haemolysis, the value in the remaining red cells may be normal even in mild G6PD deficiency. This part of the definition is not very useful.)
11. Postmortem confirmation of diagnosis. In fatal cases a diagnosis of severe falciparum malaria can be confirmed by histological examination of a postmortem needle necroscopy of the brain. The characteristic features, found especially in cerebral grey matter, are venules/capillaries packed with erythrocytes containing mature trophozoites and schizonts of *P. falciparum*. (These features may not be present in patients who die several days after the start of treatment, although there is usually some residual pigment in the cerebral vessels.)

The 2000 recommendations also included the following (Table 43.4B)

12. Impairment of consciousness less marked than unrousable coma. (Any impairment of consciousness must be treated seriously assessment using the Glasgow Coma Scale is straightforward, but the Blantyre Scale needs careful local standardization particularly in younger children.)
13. Prostration: Inability to sit unassisted in a child who is normally able to do so. In a child not old enough to sit, this is defined as an inability to feed. This definition is based on examination not history. Prostration alone, without other signs of severity, carries a relatively low mortality.
14. Hyperparasitaemia – the relation of parasitaemia to severity of illness is different in different populations and age groups, but in general very high parasite densities are associated with increased risk of severe disease, e.g. >4% parasitaemia is dangerous in non-immunes, but may be well tolerated in semi-immune children. In non-immune children studied in Thailand a parasitaemia ≥4% carried a 3% mortality (30 times higher than in all uncomplicated malaria) but in areas of high transmission values much higher may be tolerated well. Whatever the circumstances a parasitaemia ≥20% indicates severe malaria.

The following were not considered criteria of severe malaria:

Jaundice – detected clinically or defined by a serum bilirubin concentration >50 μmol/L (3.0 mg/dL). This is only a marker of severe malaria when combined with evidence of other vital organ dysfunction such as coma or renal failure).

Hyperpyrexia – a rectal temperature above 40°C in adults and children is no longer considered a sign of severity.

TABLE 43.4B **Outline Classification of Severe Malaria in Children (WHO 2000)**

GROUP 1

Children at immediately increased risk of dying who require parenteral antimalarial drugs and supportive therapy

Prostrated children (prostration is the inability to sit upright in a child normally able to do so, or to drink in the case of children too young to sit)

- Prostrate but fully conscious
- Prostrate with impaired consciousness but not in deep coma
- Coma (the inability to localize a painful stimulus)

Respiratory distress (acidotic breathing)

- Mild – sustained nasal flaring and/or mild intercostal indrawing (recession)
- Severe – the presence of either marked indrawing (recession) of the bony structure of the lower chest wall or deep (acidotic) breathing

GROUP 2

Children who, though able to be treated with oral antimalarial drugs, require supervised management because of the risk of clinical deterioration, but who show none of the features of group 1 (above)

Children with a haemoglobin level <5 g/dL or a haematocrit <15%

Children with two or more convulsions within a 24-h period

GROUP 3

Children who require parenteral treatment because of persistent vomiting but who lack any specific clinical or laboratory features of groups 1 or 2 (above).

indicates metabolic acidosis if the chest is clear on clinical examination, or pneumonia or pulmonary oedema if it is not. The liver and spleen are commonly enlarged, but soft. Massive splenomegaly is not found. There is no lymphadenopathy and no rash. The clinical features are usually of a symmetrical encephalopathy. Focal signs are unusual. On examination of the nervous system the gaze is usually normal or divergent (but there is no evidence of extraocular muscle paresis) (Figure 43.13). The pupils are usually mid-size and equally reactive. The fundus should be examined carefully. Five distinct funduscopic abnormalities have been observed; retinal whitening, retinal haemorrhages, focal whitening of vessels, papilloedema and cotton wool spots.[17] This retinopathy is highly specific for *falciparum* malaria and is more easily seen using indirect ophthalmoscopy. Papilloedema is unusual and is a sign of poor prognosis, as is retinal oedema. Retinal haemorrhages are common. The haemorrhages, which rarely affect the macula, are often flame- or boat-shaped and may have a pale centre resembling Roth spots. The retinal vessels should be examined for a very characteristic segmental whitening that probably reflects intense sequestration with red cells containing little haemoglobin and mature parasites. High-resolution digital imaging retinal angiography shows irregular vascular lining in some vessels and obstruction reflecting cytoadherence.[17] In adult patients, the corneal reflexes are usually preserved but in children with deep coma they may be lost (a poor prognostic sign). It is important to examine the eyes carefully to exclude the rapid repetitive jerky movements that indicate seizure activity. There may be forced jaw closure with repetitive spontaneous teeth grinding (bruxism). The jaw jerk is sometimes brisk and there is often a pout reflex. Other frontal release signs are very unusual. Cranial nerve abnormalities are rare. Tone may be increased, decreased or normal. Likewise the reflexes can be brisk or depressed. The abdominal reflexes are invariably absent, the cremasteric reflexes often preserved and the plantar responses extensor in approximately half the patients. Patients may exhibit phasic increases in tone with extensor posturing of the decorticate (arm flexed, legs extended), or more usually, decerebrate (arms and legs extended) types. The back may arch as in opisthotonos, with sustained, usually upward and lateral, ocular deviation. The posturing is commonly associated with noisy hyperventilation. Generalized or sometimes focal seizures may occur. The duration of coma varies considerably but overall is shorter in children (average 1 day) than in adults (average 2–3 days). Clinical evidence for seizure activity may be very subtle (e.g. tonic clonic eye movements without limb movement) and in some children there are no signs despite electroencephalographic evidence. Aspiration pneumonia is a potentially lethal sequel.

Untreated cerebral malaria is probably nearly always fatal. The overall mortality of treated cerebral malaria obviously depends on the referral practices and medical facilities available, but in reported studies with quinine treatment averaged 15% in children and 20% in adults (but up to 50% in pregnancy). Some series reported lower mortalities, but in these the definition of cerebral malaria has been more 'generous', i.e. they have included patients who were prostrated, obtunded or delirious but not unrousable. Treatment with artesunate reduces this mortality by between one-fifth (children) and one-third (adults). Hospitals acting as secondary or tertiary referral centres often experience higher mortalities as they see a residue of more severe patients. The later the patient is referred, the higher the mortality. In the Vietnam War, the mortality from acute *falciparum* malaria was higher in soldiers who had returned to the USA than it was in Vietnam. Obviously the diagnosis was made much more rapidly in Vietnam where physicians were well aware of malaria, than in the USA, where they were not.

CONVULSIONS

Seizures are common, particularly in young children. They are associated with *falciparum* malaria even in uncomplicated infections. In the majority of cases the child recovers uneventfully following one or two generalized convulsions, but some patients do not recover consciousness rapidly (<30 min) and may remain unrousable (cerebral malaria). In some cases the cause of the protracted coma is status epilepticus. Focal seizures may also occur, but they are less common. Aspiration pneumonia is a common and preventable sequel to grand mal seizures. Repeated grand mal seizures in cerebral malaria are associated with residual neurological sequelae.

POST-MALARIA NEUROLOGICAL SYNDROMES AND DEFICITS

In approximately 1–3% of adults and 10–23% of children there is a clinically obvious persistent neurological deficit following cerebral malaria (Figure 43.18). In children, this is associated with preceding profound and protracted coma, anaemia and prolonged and repeated convulsions. In a retrospective study from Kenya, multiple seizures were associated with persistent motor deficits, malnutrition, hypoglycaemia and seizures with subsequent language deficits and deep coma with cognitive impairment. In The Gambia hypoglycaemia was not a risk factor for neurological deficit. About 10% of children have demonstrable language deficit following cerebral malaria. There is also an increased risk of epilepsy following severe malaria in childhood. As severe malaria and seizures associated with malaria are so common in children, subtle but significant psychomotor impairment is of tremendous importance to tropical countries.[28] It is often difficult to distinguish a pre-existing neurological condition 'revealed' by symptomatic malaria from a malaria-induced condition, but it is becoming increasingly clear

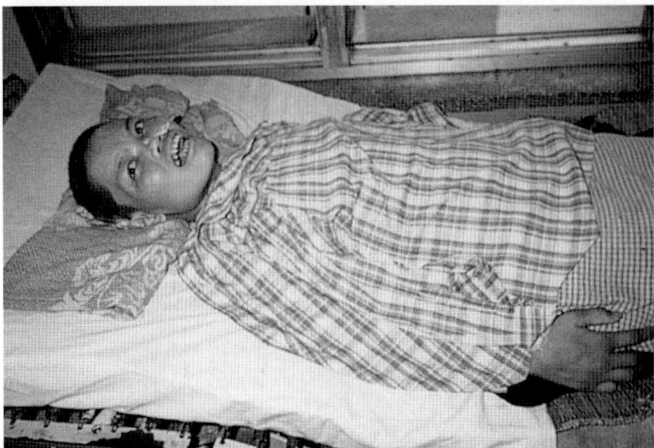

Figure 43.18 Permanent global residual neurological deficit following prolonged hypoglycaemia in a 33-year-old Vietnamese woman who had cerebral malaria in pregnancy. She had received intravenous quinine but despite parenteral glucose administration became repeatedly hypoglycaemic.

that subtle but important neurocognitive deficits may follow recovery from cerebral malaria, particularly in children. The long-term prognosis of these has not yet been established.

In approximately 60% of severe cases with residual neurological deficit, there is a hemiparesis with variable hemisensory deficit and sometimes hemianopia. Cortical blindness, diffuse cortical damage, tremor and occasionally isolated cranial nerve palsies may occur. Many of these substantial deficits recover rapidly and by 6 months only 4% of survivors have clinically obvious neurological abnormalities.

Rarely patients who recover from cerebral malaria may lapse into coma again, usually after a period of 1–2 days when they are rousable. In this condition the CSF protein may be elevated (200–300 mg/dL) and there is sometimes an increase in CSF lymphocytes. There may be residual neurological deficit on recovery. A variety of other late neurological complications may occur following recovery from cerebral malaria. These include psychosis, encephalopathy, Parkinsonian rigidity and tremor, a fine tremor and cerebellar dysfunction. These post-malaria neurological syndromes (PMNS) may also rarely follow uncomplicated malaria and could account for some of the cases previously attributed to mefloquine or chloroquine neurotoxicity. On the other hand there appears to be a strong interaction between mefloquine and cerebral malaria such that 5% of patients who receive mefloquine after severe malaria develop PMNS (a risk 10–50 times higher than following mefloquine treatment of uncomplicated malaria). Mefloquine should therefore not be used following cerebral malaria. The conditions are self-limiting, but very distressing and usually resolve over several days, or sometimes 1–2 weeks. The syndrome of cerebellar ataxia occurring 2–3 weeks after acute uncomplicated malaria appears to be relatively common in Sri Lanka. It too is usually self-limiting with recovery over a few weeks.

ACUTE KIDNEY INJURY

In some adult patients with severe malaria, acute oliguric renal impairment and other vital organ dysfunction is present on admission, whereas in others renal dysfunction becomes evident as the patient recovers from the acute phase of severe disease. In the fulminant presentation, there is a high incidence of associated hepatic dysfunction and metabolic acidosis and pulmonary oedema is the usual terminal event. The blood pressure is normal. Jaundice is common and there may be a bleeding tendency. There may be slight proteinuria, but the urine sediment is unremarkable. The subacute presentation carries a better prognosis. The patient may be oliguric but is rarely anuric. The serum creatinine rises over a period of days until either dialysis is required because of hyperkalaemia or uraemic complications such as bleeding, pleural or pericardial effusions, encephalopathy or intractable vomiting, or there is gradual resolution with an increase in urine output. In the subacute presentation of acute renal impairment parasitaemia may have cleared following antimalarial treatment before the patient is referred to hospital. Although AKI is a common complication of malaria in adults living in areas of low or unstable transmission and elevated blood urea is an important manifestation of severe malaria in children, it is very unusual for children to require renal replacement therapies. AKI is also associated with haemoglobinuria in patients with massive haemolysis (see Blackwater Fever, below).

METABOLIC ACIDOSIS

The main clinical indication of metabolic acidosis is laboured hyperventilation with increased inspiratory effort (often termed respiratory distress) and a clear chest on auscultation (Kussmaul's breathing). This usually results from accumulation of organic acids including lactic acid, but ketoacidosis may be present in children. There is a wide anion gap. Hypovolaemia must be corrected but recent evidence suggests that this does not play a major role in causing acidosis. In areas where aspirin is still used widely salicylate intoxication should be considered. Acidosis may be associated with renal failure in adults, but in the acute infection there is also a lactic acidosis. There may be a temporary worsening of lactic acidosis following grand-mal seizures, but the outlook for persistent acidosis is poor. Although blood pressure and tissue perfusion are usually adequate initially, hypotension commonly ensues.

BLACKWATER FEVER

The sinister reputation of blackwater fever derives from the high mortality (20–30%) documented in Europeans and Asians working in colonial Africa in the first half of the twentieth century. However the passage of black or dark-brown-red urine (blackwater) is often not associated with significant renal impairment. Blackwater is usually transient and resolves without complications, but in severe cases AKI may develop. This behaves as acute tubular necrosis. Blackwater results from massive haemolysis. In some patients myoglobinuria may also be present. Transfused blood is also rapidly haemolysed. The mortality is highest when blackwater fever is associated with severe malaria and other evidence of vital organ dysfunction. Patients with blackwater fever and severe anaemia often have a slate-grey appearance and their plasma may be red (haemoglobinaemia).

ACUTE PULMONARY OEDEMA

Hyperventilation or Kussmaul's breathing (sometimes termed respiratory distress) is a poor prognostic sign in malaria. In the tachypnoea associated with high fever, breathing is shallow compared with the ominous laboured hyperventilation associated with metabolic acidosis, pulmonary oedema or bronchopneumonia. Acute pulmonary oedema (acute respiratory distress syndrome) may develop at any time in severe *falciparum* malaria. It is particularly common in pregnant women, but rare in children. In some cases malaria ARDS may be difficult to distinguish clinically from pneumonia. The heart sounds are normal. The central venous pressure and pulmonary artery occlusion pressures are usually normal, the cardiac index is high and systemic vascular resistance is low. This points to an increase in capillary permeability (unless the patient has been overhydrated). The chest radiograph shows increased interstitial shadowing and a normal heart size.

HYPOTENSION

The majority of patients with severe malaria are febrile, with a high cardiac output, a low systemic vascular resistance and a low-normal blood pressure. They are usually warm and well perfused. Patients with severe disease may develop sudden hypotension and become shocked. This was called 'algid malaria'.

In a proportion of cases there is bacterial septicaemia, but in the majority blood cultures are subsequently negative. In children poor capillary refill is a valuable prognostic sign. Shock usually responds temporarily to saline infusion and inotropes, but pulmonary oedema may be provoked if too much saline is given. The mortality is high. Orthostatic hypotension is common in acute uncomplicated malaria. It is associated with impaired reflex cardioacceleration and is worsened by the quinolone antimalarial drugs. Rarely symmetrical peripheral gangrene can be associated with severe *falciparum* malaria. This does not appear to result from disseminated intravascular coagulation, but the role of red cell and platelet agglutination and vascular obstruction have not been characterized.

HYPOGLYCAEMIA

Hypoglycaemia is either asymptomatic in severely ill patients, or presents as a further deterioration in the level of coma. It is a sign of poor prognosis. In severe malaria, the usual signs of sweating and increased sympathetic nervous system activity are commonly absent or indistinguishable from the signs of malaria. Hypoglycaemia occurs in approximately 8% of adults and up to 30% of children with cerebral malaria. It is often recurrent in quinine-treated patients. The clinical response to glucose is usually disappointing. In pregnant women with quinine-stimulated hyperinsulinaemic hypoglycaemia, the clinical features of hypoglycaemia are usually evident and the patient responds dramatically to glucose. Hypoglycaemia can often be prevented by infusion of 10% dextrose but frequent monitoring is still necessary.

ANAEMIA

The degree of anaemia and the rate at which it develops in malaria varies enormously. The haemoglobin concentration may fall by up to 2 g/dL each day. Anaemia is a particular problem in children, where profound anaemia may lead to sudden death. These complications are particularly likely with haemoglobin concentrations below 5 g/dL (15% haematocrit) and the risk rises steeply below 4 g/dL. Some patients appear to tolerate severe malarial anaemia relatively well. These patients usually have an underlying chronic anaemia and have adapted by increasing oxygen carriage (right-shifted oxygen dissociation curve). Thus it is both the absolute haemoglobin concentration and the magnitude of the fall that determine the clinical consequences. In the past a syndrome of malaria-associated anaemic congestive heart failure was often diagnosed and was managed by fluid restriction and often very cautious blood transfusion. It is now clear that the majority of these children with severe anaemia, rapid deep breathing and low blood pressure are acidotic and need quite the opposite treatment; intravenous rehydration and urgent blood transfusion.

PERSISTENT FEVER

Patients with severe malaria may have persistent fever after parasite clearance. Although a proportion of cases have an identifiable chest or urinary tract infection, or in children blood cultures may grow *Salmonella* spp., the majority of cases have no clear explanation and the fever eventually resolves in a few days without further treatment.

Laboratory Findings

There is a progressive normochromic normocytic anaemia. The white count is usually normal, but may be raised in very severe malaria and very occasionally there is a leucoerythroblastic picture. There is slight monocytosis, lymphopenia and eosinopenia, with reactive lymphocytosis and eosinophilia in the weeks following the acute infection. The platelet count is reduced in all acute malarias, usually to around 100 000/μL, but thrombocytopenia is profound in some cases. Thrombocytopenia alone does not usually cause serious bleeding and does not indicate severe malaria. Fibrinogen levels are usually elevated – a reduction indicates significant consumption (DIC). The fibrin degradation products are elevated. There is evidence of increased coagulation cascade activity through intrinsic pathway activation with antithrombin III depletion that is proportional to disease severity and there may be prolongation of the prothrombin and partial thromboplastin times. Polymorphonuclear leucocyte elastase levels are elevated in severe infection, suggesting neutrophil activation.

The C-reactive protein, orosomucoid (α1-acid glycoprotein), procalcitonin and fibrinogen levels are raised and immunoglobulin levels rise while albumin falls. Cytokine levels are raised in acute malaria and there is an increase in urinary neopterin. There may be mild hyponatraemia but the potassium is remarkably normal, unless there is severe acidosis, although it may fall during the recovery phase from severe malaria. The plasma bicarbonate is often reduced and the anion gap widens in proportion to the acidosis. The serum creatinine and blood urea may be raised, with often marked elevations in adults and an increased urea to creatinine ratio. Total and conjugated bilirubin are often elevated in adults, the transaminase concentrations are often raised and there may also be slight elevation of the hepatic alkaline phosphatase concentration. In children the 5-nucleotidase is raised in proportion to disease severity. Creatinine phosphokinase, myoglobin and plasma urate levels are elevated in adults and children with severe malaria. The serum calcium may be low and hypophosphataemia may be profound in severe infections. Hypoglycaemia may occur and in the absence of quinine treatment this is accompanied by elevated ketones, raised plasma lactate and alanine and low insulin levels. Lactate levels in arterial or venous blood, or CSF, are elevated and blood bicarbonate is reduced in proportion to disease severity.

CEREBROSPINAL FLUID

The pressures in adults and children are similar, averaging approximately 160 mm CSF. But because the normal range in children is lower (<100 mm) most values in children are elevated. The CSF is usually normal in cerebral malaria, but moderately raised concentrations of protein are common (sometimes up to 200 mg/dL). There may be up to 10 cells/μL and on occasions up to 50 are seen (all lymphocytes). The CSF lactate concentration is raised in cerebral malaria and the glucose may be slightly low relative to blood. If the patient is deeply jaundiced the CSF may appear yellow.

PROGNOSTIC FACTORS

The prognostic factors listed in Table 43.5 reflect vital organ dysfunction and the magnitude of the parasite burden. They are

TABLE 43.5 Laboratory Indicators of a Poor Prognosis in Severe Malaria

BIOCHEMISTRY	
Hypoglycaemia	<2.2 mmol/L
Hyperlactataemia	>5 mmol/L
Acidosis	Arterial pH <7.3, venous plasma HCO_3 <15 mmol/L
Serum creatinine	>265 µmol/l[a]
Total bilirubin	>50 µmol/L
Liver enzymes	sGOT (AST) >3 upper limit of normal sGPT (ALT) >3 upper limit of normal 5-Nucleotidase ≠
Muscle enzymes	CPK ≠ Myoglobin ≠
Urate	>600 µmol/L
HAEMATOLOGY	
Leucocytosis	>12 000/µL Severe anaemia (PCV <15%)
Coagulopathy	Platelets <20 000/µL Prothrombin time prolonged >3 s Prolonged partial thromboplastin time Fibrinogen: <200 mg/dL
PARASITOLOGY	
Hyperparasitaemia	>100 000/µL – increased mortality[b] >500 000/µL – high mortality[b] >20% of parasites are pigment-containing trophozoites and schizonts >5% of neutrophils contain visible malaria pigment

PCV, packed cell volume; sGOT (AST), serum glutamic oxaloacetic transferase (aspartate aminotransferase); sGPT (ALT), serum glutamic pyruvic transaminase (alanine aminotransferase); CPK, creatine phosphokinase.

[a]This is the criterion for adults. Less elevated values are found in children with severe malaria.

[b]These refer to thresholds in non-immune adults. The thresholds are much higher in children in endemic areas.

not absolute and in fatal cases several factors usually co-exist. Some of the apparently poor prognostic factors can have a benign explanation. Hyperventilation (deep laboured breathing; respiratory distress) is usually a bad sign (indicating metabolic acidosis, pulmonary oedema, or pneumonia), but shallow tachypnoea can result from high fever alone (the tidal volume is lower). Upper gastrointestinal bleeding in cerebral malaria may also occur spontaneously. The prognostic implications of severe anaemia depend on the rate at which the haematocrit falls, the co-existing parasitaemia and metabolic abnormalities (particularly acidosis) and the stage of the infection. If anaemia develops gradually then even haemoglobin values <7 g/dL (packed cell volume <20%) can be surprisingly well tolerated as there is time for homeostatic adaptations such as the right shift in the oxygen dissociation curve, the increase in cardiac index and the fall in systemic vascular resistance. Hypotension is a poor prognostic sign only when associated with poor tissue perfusion, as evidence by cool peripheries and poor capillary refill. Patients, particularly children, with acute malaria often have very low blood pressures but they are warm and well perfused. The biochemical measures are in general proportional to severity, but individual abnormalities can have other explanations. For example, hypoglycaemia carries a fivefold higher mortality in severe malaria, but in pregnant women treated with quinine hypoglycaemia may occur in uncomplicated infections because of quinine-stimulated hyperinsulinaemia. The concentration of lactate in venous or arterial blood or CSF is linearly proportional to the severity of disease. In terms of predictive prognostic value the admission venous bicarbonate concentration has the best sensitivity and specificity and it is available widely. Persistent acidosis with low plasma bicarbonate and elevated plasma lactate four hours after admission indicates a poor prognosis. Although deep jaundice is often a bad sign, some adult patients develop a profound cholestatic jaundice without other evidence of vital organ dysfunction. Parasitaemia has traditionally been used as a measure of severity since the classic studies of Field and colleagues in Kuala Lumpur. They established that *P. falciparum* parasite counts over 100 000/µL were associated with an increased risk of dying and that the mortality of a count over 500 000/µL was 50%. The distribution of parasite counts in severe malaria is shifted to higher parasitaemias in children living in areas of intense transmission, compared with non-immune adults. For example, parasite counts over 200 000/µL are not uncommon in ambulant semi-immune children who are mildly ill, whereas parasitaemias in this range are usually associated with severe disease in non-immune adults (Table 43.6). The sensitivity and specificity of parasitaemia alone as a prognostic indicator are limited, but can be improved by staging parasite development (more mature parasites – worse prognosis) and noting the number of polymorphonuclear neutrophil leukocytes which contain pigment (>5% – poorer prognosis). For any parasitaemia the prognosis is worse if >20% of parasites contain visible pigment and better if >50% of parasites are at the tiny ring stage. In severe malaria, if >5% of neutrophils contain visible pigment the prognosis is worse. Recent studies indicate that measurement of *Plasmodium falciparum* Histidine Rich protein2 (PfHRP2) in plasma or serum can be used to estimate the sequestered parasite biomass in severe malaria.

Antimalarial Drug Treatment

Extracts of the plant qinghao (*Artemesia annua*), known as qinghaosu, have been used in traditional medical practice in China for over two millennia. In AD340 Ge Hong described use of qinghao infusions for the treatment of fever in the famous *Handbook of Emergency Treatments*. Thereafter, qinghao is mentioned frequently in the Chinese materia medica as a treatment for agues. Antimalarial drug discovery has often been linked to war. With the growing conflict in Vietnam in the 1960s Ho Chi Minh sought assistance from the Chinese leadership in combating malaria threatening his troops. Chinese scientists examined both synthetic and traditional medicine treatments. The antimalarial properties of qinghaosu were rediscovered in 1971 when extracts of the plant were shown to have activity against experimental rodent malaria. On the other side of the world another medicinal plant came to medical attention during the reign of the Count of Cinchon as Viceroy of Peru between 1628 and 1629 (Figure 43.19). Legend has it that the Viceroy's wife, the Countess, was afflicted by ague in Lima. She was a well-known and popular figure and news of her illness spread inland. It eventually reached Lloxa where a Spaniard was in governorship. He knew of a local remedy obtained from the bark of a tree and sent it to the ailing Countess. The therapeutic result was excellent; she improved rapidly and was so impressed that she ordered the bark in quantity and dispensed it to the poor of Lima who commonly suffered from the dangerous tertian

TABLE 43.6 Severe Manifestations of *P. falciparum* Malaria in Adults and Children

Prognostic value[a]			Frequency[a]	
Children	Adults		Children	Adults
		CLINICAL MANIFESTATIONS[b]		
+	(?)	Prostration	+++	+++
+++	++	Impaired consciousness	+++	++
+++	+++	Respiratory distress (acidotic breathing)	+++	++
+	++	Multiple convulsions	+++	+
+++	+++	Circulatory collapse	+	+
+++	+++	Pulmonary oedema (radiological)	±	+
+++	++	Abnormal bleeding	±	+
++	+	Jaundice	+	+++
+	+	Haemoglobinuria	±	+
		LABORATORY FINDINGS		
+	+	Severe anaemia	+++	+
+++	+++	Hypoglycaemia	+++	++
+++	+++	Acidosis	+++	++
+++	+++	Hyperlactataemia	+++	++
±	++	Hyperparasitaemia	++	+
++	++	Renal impairment	+	+++

[a]On a scale from + to +++ ; ± indicates borderline prognostic value or infrequent occurrence.
[b]Anuria and hypothermia (core temperature <36.5°C) are also poor prognostic signs.

fevers. The pulverized bark became known as 'los polvos de la Condeca' or the Countess's powder and Linnaeus subsequently named the tree from which the bark was obtained 'Cinchona' in honour of the Countess. Sadly, the detective work of one AW Haggis, reported in 1941, has shown that 'the fabulous story of the Countess of Cinchon' is almost certainly a romantic fable. Nevertheless, it is likely that the bark was introduced to Europe by the Fathers of the Society of Jesus around the time of the story, or even earlier (*c.*1630) and was widely promoted in Europe by the Jesuit Cardinal Juan de Hugo. For these reasons it became known as Jesuit's bark. Not everyone was convinced by the new remedy and when in 1653 Archduke Leopold of Austria relapsed 1 month after being cured of double quartan fever, his personal physician Jean-Jacques Chifflet began a bitter polemic on the merits of the bark, which was to last for 200 years. Much of the dispute stemmed from the fact that many considered all fevers had the same cause and clearly not all responded to Jesuit's bark. It was probably Torti in 1712 who first stated that the bark was 'specific solely for the ague'.

Another source of debate and one that is still active today, was dosage. Sir Robert Talbor [Talbot] was one of the few physicians who was not afraid to give the bark in large and repeated doses and when he cured the Dauphin (the son of Louis XIV) with his *remede anglais* his fame spread far and wide. He subsequently treated Charles II of England successfully with the same medicament. Others were less enthusiastic. Many

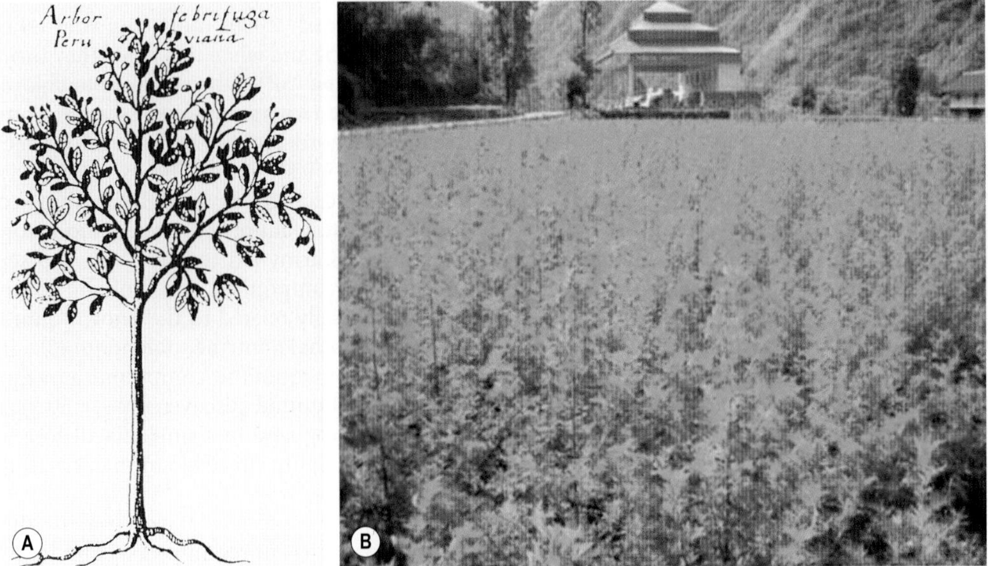

Figure 43.19 (A) The 'Arbor febrifuga Peruviana'. 'In the district of the city of Loja, diocese of Quito, grows a certain kind of large tree, which has a bark like cinnamon, a little more coarse and very bitter: which ground to powder is given to those who have fever and with only this remedy, it leaves them' *(A, Bernabe Cobo S. J. Historia del Nuevo Mundo; 1582–1657.) (B) Qinghao (Artemisia annua) plantation in China.*

Protestants believed the bark to be a poison disseminated by the Jesuits. The dose–response question was clarified in 1768 by Lind, who demonstrated clearly that in order to get best results the bark should be given in full doses as soon as the disease was diagnosed (advice that has stood the test of time).

In 1820, the French chemists Pierre Pelletier and Joseph Caventou isolated the alkaloid quinine from cinchona bark. Purification of the various cinchona alkaloids allowed standardization of dosage. Adequate doses could now be given in relatively small amounts of pure drug, but by the middle of the nineteenth century enormous doses (up to 100–150 grains over 2 days) were being prescribed. Toxicity was common and the popularity of the medicine fell. Gradually, however, the diagnosis of agues and the prescription of Cinchona alkaloids became more rational and logical. The new colonial powers recognized the importance of Cinchona and improved methods of horticulture resulted in better yields of the alkaloids from the cultivated trees. The Dutch took the lead and vast plantations of high-yielding *Cinchona ledgeriana* were started in the East Indies (principally in Java).

Laveran, having identified haematozoa as the cause of paludism, later concluded that quinine cured the disease by killing the newly discovered parasites. This theory encountered considerable resistance in the years immediately following its publication. In 1880 Bacelli described the intravenous method of administering quinine (although there is evidence that this route had been used for 50 years before that). Laveran considered intravenous injection to be dangerous, giving rise to both local and general complications and was only justified in 'the most grave and pernicious disease'. He also confirmed the earlier observations of Thomas Willis (1659) that cinchona cured the acute attacks of ague, but did not prevent relapses and also appeared to have no effect on crescents (gametocytes of *P. falciparum*). The eminent Italian malariologists subsequently showed that quinine prevented asexual blood-stage development but could not stop sporulation of formed segmenters (meronts).

In England in 1856, William Henry Perkin accidentally discovered analine purple (mauve) while attempting to synthesize quinine from coal tar products. Thus began the synthetic dye industry. Later in Germany, the antimicrobial properties of those newly discovered aniline dyes were investigated. In 1890 Ehrlich showed that methylene blue had antimalarial activity against *P. cathemerium* in canaries, but the dye proved disappointing in clinical practice (although it is now undergoing a resurgence of interest) and structural modifications did not lead to compounds with improved activity. During the Great War (1914–1918), whole armies were immobilized in the Balkans because of malaria and there were heavy losses in Mesopotamia, East Africa and the Jordan Valley. The British and French armies used quinine extensively and despite frequent objections to the bitter medicament, many lives were saved. The military and strategic importance of antimalarial drugs stimulated much research immediately after the war. In the early 1920s the resurgent German chemical industry again focused its attention on new antimicrobial compounds. The first synthetic antimalarial was discovered in 1924 originating from attempts to combine chemically the properties of quinine and methylene blue. This was an 8-aminoquinoline compound, plasmoquine, also known as pamaquine or plasmochin, a precursor of primaquine. Plasmoquine was followed by the acridine compound mepacrine (atebrine, quinacrine) in 1932 and the structurally related 4-aminoquinoline, chloroquine, in 1934. Initially, chloroquine was rejected as being too toxic for human use and the research team at Bayer were asked to produce a safer compound. They then produced 3-methylchloroquine (Sontoquine) but, despite clinical studies, these compounds were generally unavailable at the outbreak of the Second World War.

Armies fighting in tropical theatres of war usually lose more men to malaria than bullets. At the outset of the Second World War, the Allies knew their position was precarious in the tropics as most of the world's Cinchona was grown in Java and this was vulnerable to Japanese invasion. They embarked upon a tremendous combined research effort into the development and evaluation of new antimalarials. This led to the rediscovery of chloroquine and the development of primaquine. An entirely separate line of research in the UK led to the discovery in 1945 of the antimalarial biguanides, proguanil and subsequently chlorproguanil. These compounds were later shown to inhibit the plasmodial enzyme dihydrofolate reductase (DHFR). Researchers at the Wellcome Research Laboratories synthesizing purine analogues developed the antimitotic compound 6-mercaptopurine (and later azathioprine) and in 1952 discovered the antiprotozoal DHFR inhibitor pyrimethamine. This same line of Nobel Prize winning research later developed trimethoprim, which has considerably greater affinity for bacterial DHFR (but also inhibits the plasmodial enzyme) and also allopurinol, acyclovir and zidovudine (AZT).

By the early 1950s, the 4-aminoquinolines, chloroquine and to a much lesser extent amodiaquine, had become the treatment of choice for all malaria throughout the world. Pyrimethamine was also used in treatment and chloroquine, pyrimethamine and proguanil were used for prophylaxis. Primaquine was given to prevent relapses of *P. vivax* and *P. ovale*. The Cinchona alkaloids were little used outside Francophone Africa and, with the discontinuation of quinine, blackwater fever became a rarity. This was the heyday of the malaria eradication era and with the tremendous successes in Europe and North America and many urban areas of the tropics, interest in the development of new antimalarial drugs waned rapidly. But eradication in the tropics failed and in the 1960s antimalarial drug resistance emerged as a major threat.

Until the early 2000s most countries relied on chloroquine to treat malaria and when this failed they turned to sulfadoxine-pyrimethamine (SP). But resistance to chloroquine emerged at the end of the 1950s simultaneously in Colombia and the Thai–Cambodian border and over the next four decades spread across the entire tropical world. The expanding tide of antimalarial drug resistance, together with the looming conflict in Vietnam and the manifest failure of the eradication programme prompted a massive US army-led research effort to screen and test new antimalarial compounds. Most of the compounds developed were structurally related to the known quinoline antimalarials (mefloquine, halofantrine, tafenoquine). In the 1980s, the hydroxynaphthaquinone compound atovaquone (a modification of a compound discovered over 50 years ago) was combined with proguanil in a single fixed-dose formulation which is a safe and highly effective antimalarial, but is very expensive to manufacture.

It is the Chinese who have given us the most important antimalarial drugs in recent years. Four are related to quinoline antimalarials; lumefantrine (formerly known as benflumetol), pyronaridine, piperaquine and naphthoquine and all are active against multi-drug-resistant malaria. By far the most important development in malaria treatment in recent years has been the Chinese rediscovery and development of the drugs related to artemisinin (qinghaosu). They are structurally unrelated to existing antimalarials, rapidly effective, well tolerated and safe. After an inordinate delay in gaining global recognition, artemisinin-based combination treatments (ACTs) are now recommended by the World Health Organization as first-line treatment for all uncomplicated *falciparum* malaria and parenteral artesunate is the treatment of choice for severe malaria. There have been more clinical trials on artemisinin and its derivatives than any other antimalarial drugs.

Between the 1960s and the 1990s there was very little research on new antimalarial drugs by the international pharmaceutical industry. In recent years, increased international funding and the formation of public–private partnerships has lead to a resurgence of research and development. There is now the 'healthiest' pipeline for new antimalarials in living memory and over 15 new antimalarials are in various stages of development.

ANTIMALARIAL DRUG RESISTANCE

In the last two decades of the twentieth century, the global death toll from malaria rose while the mortality from other infectious diseases (with the notable exception of HIV-AIDS) generally fell. This was attributed directly to drug resistance. *Plasmodium falciparum* has now developed resistance to all classes of antimalarial drugs including the artemisinin derivatives. The other human malarias are generally more sensitive to antimalarial drugs than *P. falciparum*, although resistance of *P. vivax* to antifols is widespread. Significant chloroquine resistance has now also developed in *Plasmodium vivax* in many locations. Quinine resistance in *P. falciparum* was first reported from Brazil in 1910, but has never been high grade and has not compromised use of the drug. Within years of the introduction of the antifols proguanil and pyrimethamine, resistance was noted in both *P. falciparum* and *P. vivax* which certainly did compromise use of these drugs, but antimalarial resistance was not treated seriously until chloroquine resistance in *P. falciparum* developed almost simultaneously in South-east Asia and South America at the end of the 1950s. The selection of resistance may have resulted from the misguided use of chloroquine (and pyrimethamine) impregnated salt in an attempt to control malaria by mass prophylaxis. During the 1970s, chloroquine resistance in *P. falciparum* spread from South-east Asia and South America and fuelled the resurgence of *falciparum* malaria in the tropics. By the early 1980s chloroquine was no longer effective in many countries and the first ominous reports of resistance from the east coast of Africa appeared. Since then chloroquine resistance spread remorselessly across Africa and today few countries in the tropics (such as those north of the Panama Canal) are unaffected. Pyrimethamine resistance has also worsened rapidly and the synergistic combination with sulphonamides (SP; sulphadoxine-pyrimethamine) is no longer effective in much of East Asia, Southern and Central Africa and South America. The importance of transcontinental spread of resistance in *P. falciparum* has been highlighted by recent molecular epidemiological studies which confirm that both the chloroquine resistance and the SP resistance that have wreaked such havoc in Africa, originated in South-east Asia.[6]

South-east Asia and in particular Cambodia and Thailand have traditionally had the world's most drug-resistant malaria

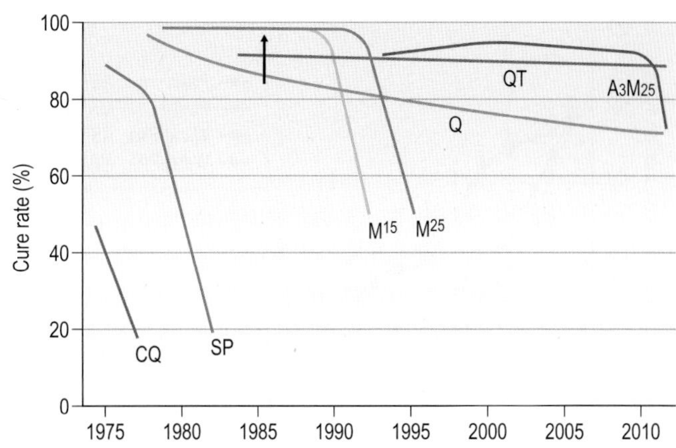

Figure 43.20 Antimalarial resistance at its most severe; the decline in antimalarial drug efficacy against *P. falciparum* malaria on the western border of Thailand. Chloroquine (CQ) and sulphadoxine-pyrimethamine (SP) were no longer effective by the beginning of the 1980s. Quinine (Q) efficacy declined slowly. Mefloquine (M) was introduced in November 1984 (arrow), at a dose of 15 mg/kg combined with SP–although SP was already useless by then. Resistance to mefloquine developed rapidly despite tight control over its use. A 7-day quinine-tetracycline regimen (QT) remained effective, but the introduction of artesunate-mefloquine (artesunate 12 mg/kg over 3 days, combined with 25 mg/kg mefloquine split dose) in 1994 led to a remarkable reversal of the resistance trend. This regimen remained over 90% efficacious until 2010, after which efficacy declined sharply coincident with the increasing prevalence of artemisinin-resistant parasites.

parasites and events there act as harbingers of the development of resistance elsewhere (Figure 43.20). Chloroquine resistance spread throughout the region in the 1960s and 1970s and SP fell rapidly to resistance in the early 1980s. In 1984 mefloquine replaced quinine as the treatment of choice for *falciparum* malaria in Thailand. This was the first country in which mefloquine was used widely. It was introduced in combination with sulfadoxine and pyrimethamine in order to delay the onset of resistance. However, since 1988 mefloquine resistance developed rapidly in Thailand and adjacent Cambodia and western Burma and later in Vietnam, while sensitivity to quinine declined very gradually. By 1994 high-level mefloquine resistance had developed in some areas with early treatment failures in 10% of cases. On the western border of Thailand, the combination of artesunate, given for 3 days and high-dose mefloquine (25 mg/kg) was introduced. Despite the fact that *P. falciparum* there was already mefloquine-resistant, this proved remarkably effective. In the subsequent 15 years cure rates remained over 90%. Following deployment of the ACT there was an improvement of mefloquine sensitivity and there was a marked decline in the incidence of *falciparum* malaria. Unfortunately, resistance to the artemisinins has emerged in western Cambodia. By 2007 there was increasing evidence of reduced susceptibility and by 2009 there was unequivocal proof[29] (Figure 43.21). Resistance has also either spread or emerged independently on the Thailand–Myanmar border and in southern Vietnam. Resistance is manifest by considerable slowing in the rate of parasite clearance following artemisinin treatment. This has now begun to compromise the efficacy of ACTs, particularly artesunate-mefloquine. Cure rates on the western border of Thailand have fallen from over 90% to less than 70% in the past 2 years. Up to date information on all aspects of antimalarial drug resistance is freely available on the internet (http://www.wwarn.org).

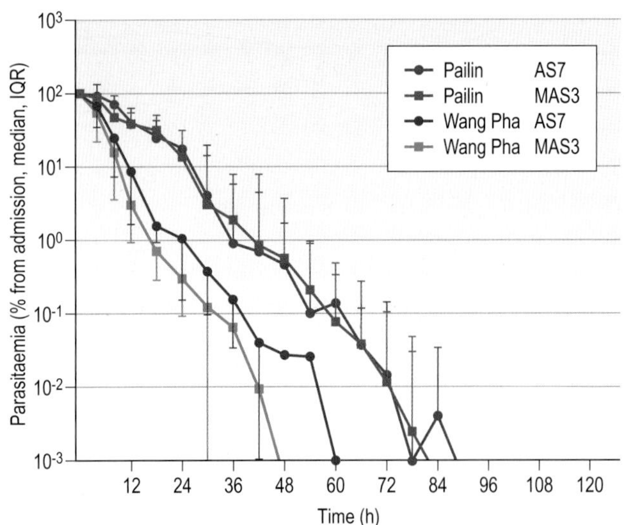

Figure 43.21 Artemisinin-resistant *P. falciparum* malaria; parasite clearance profiles in Western Cambodia (Pailin) where resistance was established and Western Thailand (Wang Pha) following artesunate monotherapy (AS7) and mefloquine–artesunate (MAS3).[29]

ANTIMALARIAL TREATMENT

In general, the antimalarial drugs are more toxic than antibacterials, i.e. the therapeutic ratio is narrower, but serious adverse effects are rare. The available antimalarials fall into three broad groups: the aryl aminoalcohol (quinoline-related or quinoline-like) compounds (quinine, quinidine, chloroquine, amodiaquine, mefloquine, halofantrine, lumefantrine, piperaquine, pyronaridine, primaquine, tafenoquine); the antifols (pyrimethamine, proguanil, chlorproguanil, trimethoprim); and the artemisinin compounds (artemisinin, dihydroartemisinin, artemether, artemotil, artesunate). Of these, the artemisinin drugs have the broadest time window of action on the asexual malarial parasites, from ring forms to early schizonts, and they produce the most rapid therapeutic responses. It is the unusual ring stage activity which explains their rapidity of action and their life-saving benefit in severe malaria and it is this property which is lost in resistant parasites. Several antibacterial drugs also have antiplasmodial activity, although in general their action is slow and they are used in combination with the antimalarial drugs. Those used are the sulphonamides and sulphones, tetracyclines, clindamycin, macrolides and inadvertently, chloramphenicol. Fosmidomycin is an active antimalarial antibiotic under investigation. Significant resistance has been reported to the sulphonamides but not the other classes of antibiotics (although macrolide resistance is readily induced in the laboratory). Drugs which are active against sensitive *P. falciparum* are also active against the other malaria species.

Antimalarial Pharmacodynamics

The principal effect of antimalarial drugs in the treatment of uncomplicated malaria is to inhibit parasite multiplication (by stopping parasite development). The untreated infection can multiply at a maximum rate given by the average number of viable merozoites per mature schizont (100% efficiency). In non-immunes multiplication is often relatively efficient with multiplication rates of 6–20/cycle (30–90% efficiency). Antimalarials exerting their maximum effects (Emax) will convert this to a negative figure from −10 to −10 000, thus reducing parasite numbers by between 10- and 10 000-fold per cycle. The Emax is the maximum effect, which is the effect represented at the top of the sigmoid dose–response or concentration–effect relationship. Drugs differ in their Emax; for example the artemisinins often produce a 10 000-fold reduction per asexual cycle, whereas antimalarial antibiotics such as tetracycline or clindamycin may achieve only at most a 10-fold parasite reduction per cycle (Figure 43.22). The lowest blood or plasma concentration of antimalarial drug which results in Emax can be considered a minimum parasiticidal concentration or MPC. Parasite reduction appears to be a first-order process throughout. This means that provided that the MPC is exceeded then a fixed fraction of the population is removed each successive asexual cycle. Patients with acute malaria may have up to 10^{12} parasites in the circulation. Even with killing fractions per cycle of 99.99% it will take at least three life cycles (6 days) to eradicate all the parasites. Thus antimalarial treatment must usually provide therapeutic drug concentrations for 7 days (covering four cycles) to effect a cure. For rapidly eliminated drugs this means the course of treatment must be 7 days (Figure 43.23). Treatment responses are always better in patients with some immunity. In endemic areas this means that the worst treatment results are seen in young children.

In the treatment of severe malaria the antimalarial drug activity on the different stages of parasite development is also important as the object of treatment is to stop parasite maturation, particularly from the less pathogenic circulating ring forms to the more pathogenic cytoadherent stages. The drugs used for the treatment of severe malaria all act predominantly in the middle third of the life cycle when there is the greatest increase in parasite synthetic and metabolic activity. The antifols act later on the forming schizont, but none of the drugs will prevent rupture and reinvasion once the meront (schizont) has formed (the widely used term schizontocidal is therefore

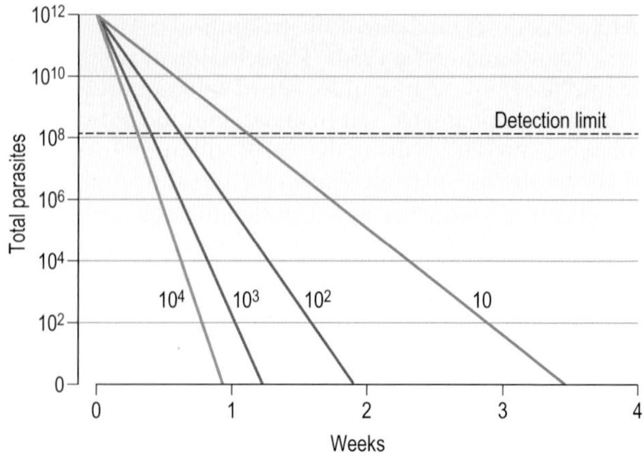

Figure 43.22 Pharmacodynamics. The effects of different rates of parasite killing on the elimination of the malaria infection. The individual parasite biomass is given on the vertical axis. 10^{12} parasites corresponds to about 2% parasitaemia in an adult who is not anaemic. The artemisinin derivatives achieve the highest parasite reduction rations (PRR: 10^4 per asexual cycle) and eradicate the infection in 6–8 days. Most of the other antimalarials achieve PRR values of 10^2–10^3 per cycle. The antimalarial antibiotics alone (e.g. doxycycline) have PRR values of approximately 10 and take 3 weeks to cure malaria if used alone (which they clearly should not be!).

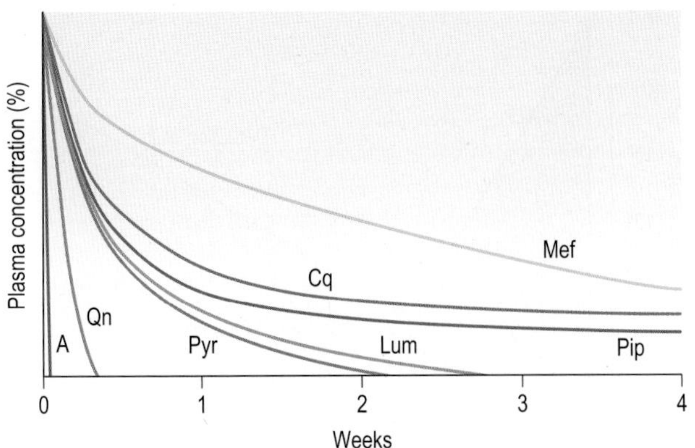

Figure 43.23 Pharmacokinetics. A comparison of the elimination profiles of the antimalarial drugs (normalized to the initial peak concentration). A, artemisinin and derivatives; Qn, quinine/quinidine; Pyr, pyrimethamine; Lum, lumefantrine; Cq, chloroquine; Mef, mefloquine; Pip, piperaquine.

incorrect). Young rings are also relatively drug-resistant (particularly to quinine and pyrimethamine). The artemisinin compounds have the broadest time window of antimalarial action and the most rapid in vivo activity. These compounds and to a lesser extent chloroquine, prevent maturation of ring stages inducing accelerated clearance and reducing subsequent cytoadherence (whereas quinine does not). The life-saving benefit of artesunate over quinine in severe malaria results largely from the additional killing of circulating ring stage parasites which are thereby prevented from maturing and sequestering. Quinine does not do this.

MODE OF ACTION AND MECHANISMS OF RESISTANCE

Resistance means that there is a shift to the right in the dose–response (concentration–effect) relationship. Higher concentrations of drug are required to achieve parasite killing. The shape of the relationship may also change and the maximum effect lowered.

Antifols and Sulphas

Pyrimethamine and the antimalarial biguanides interfere with folic acid synthesis, in the parasite by inhibiting the bifunctional enzyme dihydrofolate reductase – thymidylate synthase (DHFR). Sulphonamides act at the previous step in the synthetic pathway by inhibiting dihydropteroate synthase (DHPS). There is marked synergy in antimalarial activity between the two classes of compounds. Resistance to proguanil and pyrimethamine in *P. falciparum* and *P. vivax* were reported within a few years of their introduction. DHFR resistance is associated with point mutations in the DHFR gene which lead to reduced affinity (100–1000 times less) of the enzyme complex for the drug. The first mutation is usually at position 108 of *Pf*DHFR (serine to asparagine) and the corresponding position 117 of *Pv*DHFR. This has little clinical relevance for treatment initially, but then in *P. falciparum*, mutations arise at positions N51I and C59R conferring increasing levels of in vivo resistance to pyrimethamine. Infections with triple mutants are relatively resistant but some therapeutic response is usually seen. The stage is then set for the acquisition of a fourth and devastating mutation at position 164 (isoleucine to leucine). In *Plasmodium vivax* a similar sequence of events occurs with sequential acquisition of mutations in *Pv*DHFR conferring increasing antifol resistance. The I164 L mutation renders the available antifols completely ineffective against *Plasmodium falciparum* malaria. This mutation is prevalent in parts of SE Asia and South America and has been reported in East Africa. Interestingly mutations conferring moderate pyrimethamine resistance do not necessarily confer cycloguanil resistance and vice versa. For example, mutations at position 16 (alanine to valine) plus serine to threonine at 108 confer high-level resistance to cycloguanil but not pyrimethamine.[5] In general the biguanides (cycloguanil, chlorcycloguanil) are more active than pyrimethamine against the resistant mutants (and they are more effective clinically too), but they are ineffective against parasites with the *Pfdhfr* I164L mutation.

The marked synergy with sulphonamides and sulphones is very important for the antimalarial activity of sulphapyrimethamine or sulphone-biguanide combinations. Sulphonamide and sulphone resistance also develops by progressive acquisition of mutations in the gene encoding the target enzyme DHPS (which is a bifunctional protein with the enzyme PPPK). Specifically in *Plasmodium falciparum* altered amino acid residues associated with reduced antifol susceptibility have been found at positions 436, 437, 540, 581 and 613 in the DHPS domain. Parasites with DHPS mutations nearly always have DHFR mutations as well. The addition of the 540 to the 437 mutation is associated with particularly high failure rates. *Plasmodium falciparum* parasites with 'quintuple mutations' (*Pfdhfr* S108N, N51I and C59R and *Pfdhps* A437G, K540E) are now widespread in tropical countries and are associated with high SP treatment failure rates and poor responses to the artesunate SP combination. The *Pfdhps* 581 and 631 mutations are also increasingly prevalent. They do not occur in isolation, but always on top of an initial mutation (usually alanine to glycine at 437) and confer additional resistance.

Quinolines and Related Drugs

The mode of action of the quinoline antimalarials has been a source of controversy for years. These drugs are weak bases and they concentrate in the acid food vacuole of the parasite, but this in itself does not explain their antimalarial activity. Chloroquine intercalates DNA, but only at concentrations (1–2 mmol/L) much higher than required to kill parasites (10–20 nmol/L). Chloroquine binds to ferriprotoporphyrin IX, a product of haemoglobin degradation and thereby chemically inhibits haem dimerization. This is an essential defence mechanism for the parasite to detoxify haem and inhibition of this process provides a plausible explanation for the selective antimalarial action of these drugs. Chloroquine also competitively inhibits glutathione-mediated haem degradation, another parasite detoxification pathway. Chloroquine resistance is associated with reduced concentrations of drug in the acid food or digestive vacuole. Both reduced influx and increased efflux have been implicated. The resistant parasites lose chloroquine from the digestive vacuole 40–50 times faster than drug-sensitive parasites. This efflux mechanism is similar to that found in multidrug-resistant (MDR) mammalian tumour cells. The first efflux mechanism to be characterized was the ATP-requiring transmembrane pump, *P. glycoprotein*. These unmutated *Pfmdr1* genes are found in increased copy numbers in most quinine-, mefloquine- and lumefantrine-resistant *P. falciparum* parasites, whereas point mutations in codons 86 (N86Y) and also 184 (Y184F) and 1246 (D1246Y) have been related to chloroquine and amodiaquine resistance. Amplification of *Pfmdr* is the main contributor to mefloquine and lumefantrine resistance. Transfection studies confirm a role for *Pfmdr* in mediating resistance to chloroquine and mefloquine. Thus lumefantrine and amodiaquine, the two most widely used partner drugs in Africa provide opposite selection pressures on *Pfmdr* so deployment of both together would be expected to slow the emergence of resistance at this locus. But the critical discovery has been the association of point mutations in CRT (a food vacuolar membrane protein thought to have a transporter function), with chloroquine resistance. The central role of a *PfCRT* mutation resulting in a change in coding from lysine to threonine at position 76 gene in mediating chloroquine resistance has been shown unequivocally in the laboratory by transfection studies and in epidemiological studies where therapeutic responses are predicted by this single polymorphism. In several regions where chloroquine resistance was prevalent, a reversion to wild-type PfCRT in parasite populations has been associated with a return of chloroquine susceptibility.[30] PfCRT also plays an important role in amodiaquine and quinine resistance. From an epidemiological standpoint multiple unlinked mutations probably contribute to chloroquine resistance, modifying the central role of CRT. It is likely that other contributors to quinoline resistance remain to be discovered.

The chloroquine efflux mechanism in resistant parasites can be inhibited by a number of structurally unrelated drugs: calcium channel blockers, tricyclic antidepressants, phenothiazines, cyproheptadine, antihistamines, etc. whereas mefloquine resistance is reversed by penfluridol, which does not reduce chloroquine efflux. This gave hope that chloroquine resistance might be reversed in clinical practice. Initial evaluations were uniformly disappointing, but studies in Nigerian children given chloroquine together with very high doses of chlorpheniramine, did indicate significantly improved efficacy against chloroquine-resistant *falciparum* malaria. In general antimalarial drug resistance to mefloquine, quinine, lumefantrine and halofantrine is linked. Within a particular geographic area there is a reciprocal relationship; increasing mefloquine resistance is associated with increasing susceptibility to chloroquine.

Atovaquone

Atovaquone interferes with parasite mitochondrial electron transport and it also depolarizes the parasite mitochondria thereby blocking cellular respiration. High levels of resistance result from single point mutations in the gene encoding cytochrome *b*. This gene is encoded on a small extrachromosomal plastid-like DNA-containing organelle (the apicoplast), which is phylogenetically of algal origin. Resistance mutations arise frequently in vitro and in vivo (Figure 43.24).

Artemisinin and Derivatives

The mechanism of action of the artemisinin drugs remains uncertain. Initially it was thought to involve cation (mainly the ferrous ion) mediated generation of carbon-centred free radicals which alkylate critical proteins. Parasiticidal activity is certainly dependent on the integrity of the peroxide bridge and can be blocked by the iron chelator desferrioxamine.

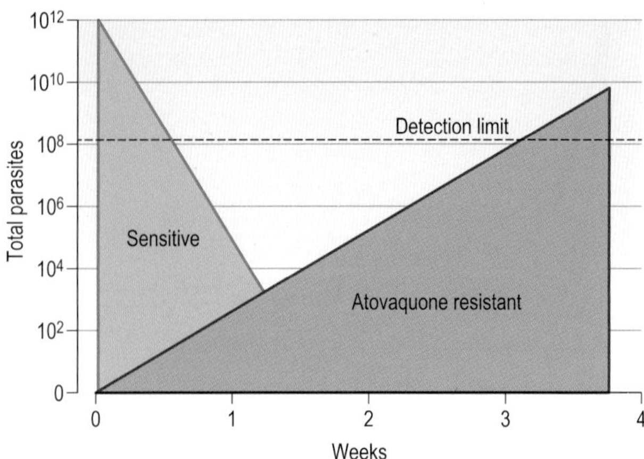

Figure 43.24 The de novo emergence of high-level resistance. Following atovaquone (only) treatment highly resistant recrudescent infections emerged in one-third of patients. This represented untrammelled growth of a single starting parasite; a per parasite mutation frequency of 1 in 10^{12}.

THE EMERGENCE AND SPREAD OF ANTIMALARIAL DRUG RESISTANCE

Antimalarial drug resistance is a major threat to health in the tropics. The development of resistance can be divided into the relatively rare event giving rise to resistance de novo and the subsequent spread of resistance among the parasite population. Malaria parasites do not acquire resistance genes by lateral transfer from other parasites. Resistance arises from spontaneous chromosomal point mutations or gene duplications which are independent of drug selection pressure. Once formed, these more resistant mutants have a survival advantage in the presence of antimalarial drugs. Several factors encourage the development of resistance. These are the intrinsic frequency with which the genetic changes occur, the degree of resistance conferred by the genetic change (pharmacodynamics), the proportion of all transmissible infections which are exposed to the drug, the drug concentration profile (pharmacokinetics), the pattern of drug use and the immunity profile of the community. Resistant parasites will be selected when parasites are exposed to subtherapeutic drug concentrations (i.e. concentrations which would eradicate most sensitive infections but not infections with the resistant mutants). Thus, non-immune patients infected with large numbers of parasites who receive inadequate treatment (either because of poor drug quality, adherence, vomiting of an oral treatment, etc.) are a potent source of de novo resistance. This emphasizes the importance of correct prescribing and good adherence to prescribed drug regimens, particularly in patients with heavy parasite burdens in slowing the emergence of resistance.

The emergence of resistance is slower in high transmission areas, because background immunity eliminates the majority of infections and so clears resistant mutants and stops them being transmitted. The spread of resistant mutant parasite is facilitated by the use of drugs with long elimination phases which provide a 'selective filter', allowing infection by the resistant parasites while the residual antimalarial activity prevents infection by sensitive parasites. Slowly eliminated drugs such as mefloquine (T1/2 β 2–3 weeks) or chloroquine (T1/2 β 2 months) persist in blood and provide such a selective filter for months after drug administration (Figure 43.23). The selection

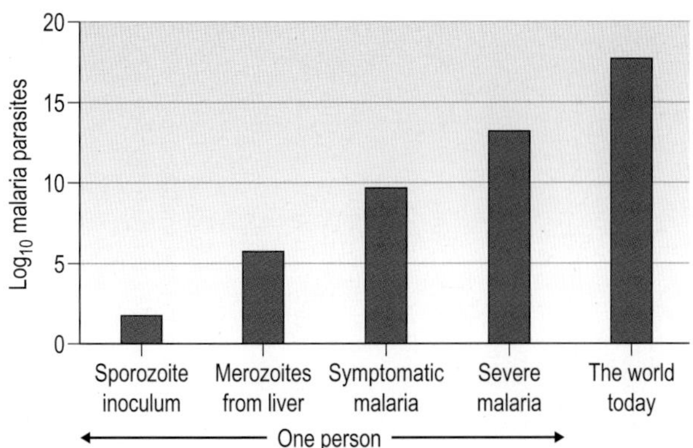

Figure 43.25 The logarithmic distribution of malaria parasites. There are probably between 10^{16} and 10^{18} parasites in the world today. The day after tomorrow, there will be another 10^{16}–10^{18}!

pressure can be enormous. In Africa approximately 250 000 kg or 170×10^6 adult treatment doses of chloroquine were consumed annually. Thus in many parts of the continent the majority of the population had chloroquine in the blood at any time.

The emergence of resistance can be prevented by the use of combinations of drugs with different mechanisms of action and therefore different drug targets. The same rationale underlies the current treatment of tuberculosis, leprosy, HIV infections and many cancers. If two drugs are used, which do not share a common mode of action and therefore the parasite develops different mechanisms of resistance to them, then the per-parasite probability of developing resistance to both drugs is the product of their individual per-parasite probabilities. For example, if the per-parasite probabilities of developing resistance to drug A and drug B are both 1 in $10,^{12}$ then a simultaneously resistant mutant will arise spontaneously every 1 in 10^{24} parasites (Figure 43.25). The lower the de novo per-parasite probability of developing resistance, the greater the delay in the emergence of resistance. However, this powerful approach has several limitations. If not everyone receives the combination and some patients only receive one of the components, then resistance can arise (emphasizing the importance of achieving high coverage when these drugs are deployed). Mutual protection works only if the both drugs are always present together, but in current ACTs there is a considerable pharmacokinetic mismatch such that the slowly eliminated partner drug is present for days or weeks unprotected by the artemisinin component. This will enhance the spread of resistance. Combinations are also more expensive. But the increased cost is outweighed by the longer-term benefits. Another effective approach to delaying the spread of resistance is to deploy different drugs with different resistance mechanisms at the same time. With this 'multiple first-line treatment' approach the fitness disadvantage incurred by resistance mechanisms is exploited. At present there are a number of important, but unanswered, practical questions concerning resistance. We do not know the relative importance of all the factors which contribute and therefore the optimum strategy to prevent resistance.

QUININE

Quinine is a bitter powder obtained from the bark of the Cinchona tree. It is widely used as a flavouring (tonic water, bitter lemon) and it is an effective treatment for night cramps, as well as for malaria. Contrary to widespread belief quinine is not antipyretic. Quinine is usually formulated as the dihydrochloride salt for parenteral administration and as the sulphate, bisulphate, dihydrochloride, ethylcarbonate, hydrochloride or hydrobromide salts for oral administration. Unlike the other antimalarials and somewhat confusingly, quinine doses are usually prescribed as weights of salt rather than base (the different salts have different base contents). Quinine acts principally on the mature trophozoite stage of parasite development. It does not prevent sequestration or further development of formed meronts and does not kill the pre-erythrocytic or sexual stages of *P. falciparum*.

Pharmacokinetics

Quinine is well absorbed after oral or intramuscular administration both in adults and children (Table 43.7). Peak levels are usually reached within 4 hours (more rapidly if the intramuscular injections are diluted) (Figure 43.23). In acute malaria the total apparent volume of distribution (Vd) is contracted and systemic clearance reduced in proportion to disease severity. As a result blood concentrations are higher in uncomplicated malaria than in healthy subjects and highest in severe malaria. The elimination half-life is approximately 18–20 hours in cerebral malaria, 16 hours in uncomplicated malaria and 11 hours in health. In children and pregnant women the apparent volume of distribution is relatively smaller and elimination is more rapid. Malnutrition reduces both Vd and clearance similar to malaria. Quinine is a base and is bound principally to the acute phase plasma protein α1-acid glycoprotein. Plasma protein binding is increased in malaria from approximately 75–80% in healthy subjects to over 90% in severe malaria. Red cell concentrations vary between one-third and one-half of corresponding plasma concentrations and concentrations in breast milk and cord blood are approximately one-third of those in plasma. The therapeutic range has not been well defined but total plasma concentrations of between 8 and 15 mg/L are certainly safe and effective. Toxicity is increasingly likely with plasma concentrations over 20 mg/L (free quinine >2 mg/L). Approximately 80% of the administered drug is eliminated by hepatic biotransformation, principally via CYP 3A4 and also CYP 3A5 and the remaining 20% is excreted unchanged by the kidney. Although systemic clearance is reduced in severe malaria, this 80 : 20 proportion is preserved. The principal metabolite 3-hydroxyquinine is biologically active, contributing approximately 10% to antimalarial activity, but more in renal failure where it accumulates. The other more polar metabolites are either much less active, or inactive as antimalarials.

Toxicity

Minor adverse effects are common with quinine but serious toxicity is remarkably rare in the treatment of malaria. Allergic reactions (thrombocytopenia, haemolysis, rash, haemolytic-uraemic syndrome) are all rare in malaria treatment. Quinine is extremely bitter and therefore unpleasant to take and regularly produces a symptom complex known as 'cinchonism'. This comprises tinnitus, reversible high-tone hearing impairment, nausea, dysphoria and often vomiting. As a consequence compliance with the 7-day regimens required for cure is poor. Quinine predictably prolongs depolarization in skeletal and cardiac muscle and this is the main contributor to the prolongation of the QTc interval on the electrocardiograph by

TABLE 43.7 Pharmacokinetic Properties of the Antimalarial Drugs

Drug	Absorption: Time to Peak (hours)		Oral Dose (mg/kg)	Peak Plasma Level (mg/L)	Binding (%)	V_d/f (L/kg)	Clearance/f (mL/kg/min)	$T_{1/2}\beta$ (hours)	Comments
	PO	IM							
UNCOMPLICATED MALARIA									
Quinine	6	1	10	8	90	0.8	1.5	16	Protein binding increased. Vd and clearance further reduced in severe malaria. Rate of IM absorption proportional to concentration of injectate
Quinidine	1	–	10	5	85	1.3	1.7	10	
Chloroquine	5	0.5	10	0.12	55	10–1000	2.0	30–60 days	Concentrated in red cells, white cells and platelets Kinetics unaffected by disease severity
Desethylamodiaquine			30					11 days	Almost all antimalarial activity after oral administration of amodiaquine is provided by this metabolite
Piperaquine	6		55	0.15	>98	728	23	28 days	Lower exposure in young children 1–2 weeks after dosing
Pyronaridine	6		36	0.18	96	90	13	13 days	Shorter elimination half-life in children ~ 10 days
Mefloquine	17	–	25	–	>98	20	0.35	14 days	(+) RS enantiomer concentration higher, and (–)SR enantiomer lower, in whole blood than plasma
Halofantrine	15	–	8	0.9	>98	–	7.5	113	Metabolized to active desbutyl metabolite which is eliminated more slowly. Absorption increased by fats
Lumefantrine	6	–	9	3.5	>98	2.7	3.0	86	Very variable bioavailability; absorption dependent on coadministration of fat
Pyrimethamine	4	41	1.25	0.5	94	–	0.33	87	Concentrations in 2–5-year-old children lower than in older children and adults
Chlorproguanil	4	–	2.0	0.1	75	30	20	35	Mainly a prodrug for active triazine metabolite chlorcycloguanil, which is eliminated more rapidly
Atovaquone	6	–	15	5	99.5	6	2.5	30	Absorption increased by fats
Artesunate	1.5	0.5	4	0.5	–	0.15	50	0.75	Rapidly hydrolysed in the stomach to dihydroartemisinin. (DHA). Very little artesunate in blood after oral administration
Artemether	2	3–18	4	1.5	95	2.7	54	1	Erratic absorption after intramuscular administration. Rapidly metabolized to after oral administration to DHA
Dihydroartemisinin	4		4		70			1	Absorption very formulation dependent.
The pharmacokinetic properties of chloroquine, lumefantrine, artemether, artesunate, atovaquone and proguanil in late pregnancy are significantly altered so that plasma concentrations are approximately half those in non-pregnant adults. Pyrimethamine and sulfadoxine plasma concentrations in young children are approximately half those in older children and adults for the same administered dose.									
HEALTHY SUBJECTS									
Primaquine	3	–	0.6	0.15	–	3	6	6	Active metabolites not well characterised
Proguanil (Chloroguanide)	3	–	3.5	0.17	75	24	19	16	Mainly a prodrug for active triazine metabolite cycloguanil, which is eliminated more rapidly
Pyrimethamine	4	–	0.3	0.35	–	2.9	0.4	85	–

approximately 10% at therapeutic concentrations. The effect is greater in children under 2 years of age. This can be used as a pharmacodynamic measure of toxicity. These antiarrhythmic effects are qualitatively different to the QT prolongation with quinidine, which results from delayed repolarization (JT prolongation) and can, under some circumstances, be proarrhythmic. Significant conduction or repolarization abnormalities are rare and iatrogenic dysrhythmias are extremely uncommon. Quinine, like the other quinoline antimalarials, exacerbates malaria-induced orthostatic hypotension, but iatrogenic supine hypotension is rare. Blindness, resulting from retinal ganglion cell toxicity, and deafness are common following self-poisoning, but very rare in malaria treatment. Perhaps the most important toxic effect of quinine is its stimulatory action on the pancreatic β-cell. This causes hyperinsulinaemic hypoglycaemia. It is particularly common in pregnant women but may occur in any severely ill patient, particularly if intravenous glucose solutions are not given. Contrary to popular opinion, quinine does not induce premature labour at therapeutic doses. Quinine is rarely associated with a variety of allergic reactions, notably immune thrombocytopenia and rarely the haemolytic-uraemic syndrome. Various skin reactions are associated with quinine. Pruritus, skin flushing and urticaria are the commonest manifestations of quinine hypersensitivity. Other rashes, reported rarely, have included photosensitivity, cutaneous vasculitis, lichen planus and lichenoid photosensitivity. Granulomatous hepatitis has been reported occasionally.

Blackwater fever is undoubtedly associated with quinine use, but the underlying pathophysiological mechanism is still not understood. Incorrect or non-sterile administration of intramuscular quinine is associated with tetanus and this carries a very high mortality.

Concerns over quinine cardiovascular toxicity in severe malaria are generally exaggerated in comparison to the dangers of undertreatment and tend to arise from units in temperate countries managing occasional elderly travellers with imported malaria. Quinine is certainly potentially lethal if given by intravenous injection, but iatrogenic hypotension is very unusual when quinine is given by rate-controlled infusion. Severe malaria is a potentially lethal condition. Antimalarial treatment is the only intervention proven to reduce mortality. Undertreatment may cause death – but physicians usually blame the malaria infection in a fatal case and seldom ascribe death to their use of inadequate doses of quinine. On the other hand cardiovascular complications are readily ascribed to the treatment rather than the fulminant disease. Large studies in endemic countries have confirmed the safety of quinine in severe malaria. It is essential that patients receiving this drug achieve therapeutic concentrations of quinine in their blood within hours of reaching a treatment facility.

Use

Parenteral quinine should be given by rate-controlled intravenous infusion in either 0.9% saline, 5% or 10% dextrose or by deep intramuscular injection to the anterior thigh. It should *never* be given by intravenous injection (as it causes potentially lethal hypotension). The initial doses (mg/kg) in children and pregnant women are the same as in non-pregnant adults, although in areas with resistant parasites it has been recommended that the dose be increased in children to 15 mg salt/kg from day 4 to day 8 to prevent recrudescent infection. In severe malaria, treatment should begin with a loading dose so that therapeutic levels are reached as quickly as possible. If adequate treatment has been given before referral to hospital (i.e. >15 mg/kg in the preceding 24 hours) the loading dose is unnecessary. But if there is any doubt at all, or lower doses have been given, then the full loading dose should be given. In severe malaria quinine doses should be reduced by one-third to one-half after 48 hours if there is no clinical improvement, or if there is acute renal failure. This prevents blood concentrations accumulating to toxic levels. Intramuscular quinine is painful and sclerosant if given undiluted (300 mg/mL). It should be diluted in sterile water 1:3 to 1:5 and given to the anterior thigh, never the buttock (to avoid the risk of sciatic nerve damage), using strict aseptic technique. Oral quinine is given in a dose of 10 mg salt/kg three times daily for 7 days (shorter courses are less effective) combined with either doxycycline or clindamycin.

CHLOROQUINE

Chloroquine is a 4-aminoquinoline. It is formulated as sulphate, phosphate and hydrochloride salts and is prescribed in weights of base content. Various liquid formulations are available for paediatric use. Chloroquine can be given by intravenous infusion, intramuscular or subcutaneous injection, orally, or by suppository. Chloroquine acts mainly on the large ring-form and mature trophozoite stages of the parasite. It produces more rapid parasite clearance than quinine but is slower than artemisinin derivatives. Chloroquine is also used in the treatment of hepatic amoebiasis and for some collagen-vascular and granulomatous diseases, notably rheumatoid arthritis (where hydroxychloroquine is preferred).

Pharmacokinetics

Chloroquine has complex pharmacokinetic properties with an enormous Vd (resulting from extensive tissue binding) and a very long elimination phase (Table 43.7). The terminal elimination half-life is 1–2 months. As a consequence, the blood concentration profile during malaria is determined mainly by distribution rather than elimination processes. Chloroquine is well absorbed by mouth. Chloroquine is approximately 55% bound to plasma proteins. The principal metabolite of chloroquine, desethylchloroquine, has approximately equivalent antimalarial activity. This is of relevance to prophylactic, but not therapeutic efficacy.

Toxicity

Chloroquine is generally well tolerated. Oral chloroquine may induce nausea or dysphoria and visual disturbances. Orthostatic hypotension may be accentuated. Pruritus is particularly troublesome in dark-skinned patients and may be dose limiting. Itching is described as a widespread prickling sensation mostly affecting the palms, soles and scalp which starts within 6–24 hours and may last for several days. It can be very distressing. Antihistamine treatment is not usually very effective. Very rarely chloroquine may cause an acute and self-limiting neuropsychiatric reaction. In prophylaxis cumulative doses over 100 g (>5 years prophylaxis) are associated with an increased risk of retinopathy. Retinal signs include a pale optic disc, arteriolar narrowing, peripheral retinal depigmentation, macular oedema, retinal granularity and oedema and retinal pigmentary changes consisting of a circle of pigmentation and central pallor; the so-called 'doughnut' or 'bull's eye' macula.

Reversible corneal opacities can be seen in 30–70% of rheumatology patients within a few weeks of high-dose treatment. Half are asymptomatic but others may complain of photophobia, visual halos around lights, and blurred vision. Residents on long-term chloroquine prophylaxis should probably have regular ophthalmological checks after taking the drug for 5 years, or if they experience any visual loss. Myopathy is rare at the doses used in antimalarial prophylaxis. Less common cutaneous side effects include lightening of skin colour, various rashes (photoallergic dermatitis, exacerbation of psoriasis, bullous pemphigoid, exfoliative dermatitis, pustular rash), skin depigmentation (with long-term use) and hair loss. In self-poisoning, chloroquine produces hypotension, arrhythmias and coma and is commonly lethal. It has been suggested that diazepam is a specific antidote, but recent studies do not support a specific role for this drug above good haemodynamic and ventilatory support.

Use

Chloroquine is still the drug of choice for sensitive malaria parasites although ACTs are used increasingly. Chloroquine is therefore used widely for *P. vivax*, *P. malariae* and *P. ovale*, but except in a very few areas has been replaced for *P. falciparum* treatment. The time-honoured oral chloroquine regimen of 25 mg base/kg spread over 3 days (10, 10, 5 or 10, 5, 5, 5 mg/kg at 24-hour intervals) can be condensed into 36 hours of drug administration. There is no role today for parenteral chloroquine. Chloroquine is considered safe in pregnancy and in young children.

AMODIAQUINE

Amodiaquine is a 'Mannich base' 4-aminoquinoline with a similar mode of action to chloroquine. It is more active against resistant isolates of *P. falciparum* and is combined with artesunate as an ACT. Amodiaquine is still effective against *falciparum* malaria in parts of South America, western and central Africa and a few parts of Asia, but resistance has increased. Amodiaquine is best given in the newly developed fixed-dose coformulation given as artesunate-amodiaquine 4/10 mg/kg daily for 3 days.

Pharmacokinetics

Oral amodiaquine undergoes extensive first-pass metabolism by intestinal and hepatic CYP 2C8 to the biologically active metabolite desethylamodiaquine. The metabolite exerts the principal antimalarial activity. The parent compound has an elimination half-life of approximately 10 hours but desethylamodiaquine, like chloroquine, is extensively distributed and eliminated slowly with an estimated terminal half-life of about 10 days. There are no parenteral formulations commercially available, although a structurally similar compound, amopyraquine, is available for intramuscular administration in some countries.

Toxicity

Prophylactic use of amodiaquine is associated with an unacceptably high incidence of serious toxicity. Approximately 1 in 2000 patients develop agranulocytosis. Serious hepatotoxicity also occurred at an estimated rate of 1:15 000. Agranulocytosis results from bioactivation to a reactive quinoneimine metabolite. Simple modifications to the chemical structure prevent formation of this metabolite and in theory produce a much safer compound. The incidence of these serious reactions is certainly lower when amodiaquine is used in treatment, although precise estimates of the risk are still lacking. In general artesunate-amodiaquine is well tolerated. Unusual fatigue has been prominent in some series. Case reports in the literature have documented rare neurological problems such as protruding tongue, intention tremor, excess salivation and dysarthria in four African patients following amodiaquine treatment. In two patients, these signs occurred on reexposure to the drug. There is one case report of amodiaquine use over use over 1 year, resulting in yellow pigmentation of skin and mucosae, the development of corneal and conjunctival inclusion bodies and retinopathy. Minor adverse effects are similar to those of chloroquine, although pruritus is less of a problem and although it is still has an unpleasant taste, children find the drug more palatable.

MEFLOQUINE

Mefloquine is a fluorinated 4-quinoline methanol compound used for the treatment of multi-drug-resistant *falciparum* malaria. It has two asymmetric carbon atoms and is used clinically as a 50:50 racemic mixture of the erythroisomers. These have equal antimalarial activity but very different pharmacokinetic properties. The parasiticidal action is similar to that of quinine. Mefloquine is very insoluble in water. It is available as tablets, which should be kept dry. There are no parenteral or paediatric liquid formulations. A fixed-dose co-formulation with artesunate in a 2:1 ratio has been developed and registered.

Pharmacokinetics

Mefloquine is moderately well absorbed, extensively distributed and slowly eliminated (Table 43.7). It is highly (>98%) bound to plasma proteins. Mefloquine is cleared principally by hepatic biotransformation to inactive metabolites. The apparent volume of distribution and clearance of the (+)RS enantiomer is four to six times higher than for the (−)SR enantiomer. The overall terminal elimination half-life is approximately 3 weeks in healthy subjects and 2 weeks in malaria (Figure 43.23). The absorption of mefloquine is reduced in the acute phase of illness and bioavailability of the higher 25 mg/kg dose is improved by dividing it (e.g. giving 15 mg/kg initially and 10 mg/kg 8–24 hours later, or 8 mg/kg per day for 3 days) or in combination with artesunate delaying mefloquine administration until the 2nd day of treatment. Splitting the dose also reduces the incidence of acute adverse effects. Blood concentrations are higher in malaria than in healthy subjects and are reduced in diarrhoea (probably by interruption of enterohepatic recycling). Mefloquine clearance is increased in pregnancy. The pharmacokinetics in adults and children are similar. Co-administration with artesunate results in a more rapid recovery from malaria which enhances the oral bioavailability of doses after the first. Although blood concentrations are higher with split dosing early vomiting is reduced. The new fixed-dose coformulation is given as artesunate-mefloquine 4/8 mg/kg daily for 3 days.

Toxicity

Nausea, vomiting, dizziness, weakness, sleep disturbances and dysphoria are relatively common with mefloquine. Although children are more likely to vomit immediately after receiving mefloquine, and this was a significant problem when the drug was used alone, they otherwise tolerate the drug better than adults. The fixed-dose combination is associated with less early vomiting than administration of the loose tablets (possibly because of the lower mefloquine dose on day 1). Women, in particular, commonly complain of dizziness and dysphoria for up to 4 days after receiving mefloquine treatment. Mefloquine exacerbates malarial orthostatic hypotension. The main serious adverse effect of mefloquine is the development of acute but self-limiting neuropsychiatric reactions (convulsions, psychosis, encephalopathy). The incidence of these is approximately 1:10 000 when used as a prophylactic, but higher with treatment (1:1000 in Asian patients, 1:200 in Caucasians or Africans) and 1:20 following severe malaria. For these reasons mefloquine should not be given following severe malaria. In one large study from Thailand mefloquine treatment in pregnancy was associated with a four-fold increased risk of stillbirth, although this effect was not seen in women exposed before conception (who would have had residual drug levels during early foetal organogenesis). This effect was not seen in the other large study experience with mefloquine in pregnancy in Malawi. The overall experience of mefloquine use over two decades suggests that mefloquine is safe in pregnancy.

Use

Mefloquine is used for the oral treatment of uncomplicated multi-drug-resistant *falciparum* malaria. It is given in combination with artesunate 4 mg/kg per day for 3 days. The usual dose is approximately 25 mg base/kg and should be split (15 mg/kg stat. followed by 10 mg/kg 8–24 hours later, or in a fixed-dose combination at 8 mg/kg per day for 3 days). A single dose of 15 mg base/kg alone was widely used in semi-immune patients, but there is theoretical evidence that this leads more rapidly to resistance and it is no longer recommended. If the patient vomits the dose should be repeated (full dose if vomiting within 30 min, half dose 30–60 min, no further dose if after 1 hour). Mefloquine is used for antimalarial prophylaxis at a dose of approximately 4 mg base/kg once weekly for both adults and children.

HALOFANTRINE

Halofantrine is a 9-phenanthrene methanol. It has one asymmetric carbon atom and is used as a racemate. The enantiomers have equal antimalarial activity. Halofantrine is intrinsically more potent than quinine or mefloquine, but unfortunately it is associated with rare but potentially lethal ventricular tachycardias which have rightly curtailed its use. It is available as tablets and a suspension for paediatric use. As there are several much safer alternatives, halofantrine should be withdrawn.

Pharmacokinetics

Halofantrine is poorly and erratically absorbed. Furthermore, absorption appears to be 'saturable', i.e. with individual doses over 8 mg/kg no increment in blood concentrations occurs (Table 43.7). Absorption is increased markedly by coadministration with fats. Halofantrine is extensively distributed and cleared largely by hepatic biotransformation. It is bound principally to lipoproteins in the plasma. The terminal elimination half-life is about 1–3 days in healthy subjects and approximately 4 days in patients with malaria. There is significant first-pass metabolism to a biologically active desbutyl metabolite. This is eliminated more slowly (T1/2 3–7 days) than the parent compound and undoubtedly contributes significantly to antimalarial activity (and cardiotoxicity).

Toxicity

Halofantrine is very well tolerated subjectively, but it carries a significant risk of sudden death, presumably resulting from ventricular tachyarrhythmias. Halofantrine slows atrioventricular conduction and produces the 'quinidine effect' on myocardial repolarization reflected in a significant dose-related prolongation of the electrocardiograph QT interval. This is increased by previous treatment with mefloquine. This dangerous effect is a property of both halofantrine and its desbutyl metabolite. Diarrhoea may be provoked by high halofantrine doses. There are no data for pregnancy, so halofantrine should not be used.

Use

Halofantrine is only available for oral use. When used at standard doses (8 mg/kg given three times at 6–8-hour intervals and repeated 1 week later in non-immune patients), in patients with a normal resting electrocardiogram, halofantrine was considered safe and effective in areas with fully sensitive malaria parasites. In multi-drug resistant areas, higher total doses are required for high cure rates, but these are associated with an unacceptable risk of cardiotoxicity. Halofantrine should not be used to treat recrudescent infections following mefloquine treatment as the cardiac effects are potentiated.

PYRIMETHAMINE

Pyrimethamine is a dihydrofolate reductase (DHFR) inhibitor. It is now used only together with long-acting sulphonamides such as sulfadoxine (as SP) and sulfalene in fixed-dose combinations which considerably potentiate its activity. SP is not a combination, in the 'resistance prevention' sense. The mechanism of action of the two drugs is linked, so although they do provide some mutual protection, they do not protect each other from resistance to the extent unrelated drugs would. SP has been used to treat chloroquine-resistant *falciparum* malaria, but in many areas high-level SP resistance has developed. *Plasmodium vivax* is also often resistant. There is an intramuscular formulation of SP but this should not be used to treat severe malaria. The DHFR inhibitors inhibit development of the mature trophozoite stage of the asexual parasite, in addition to having pre-erythrocytic and sporontocidal activities. Pyrimethamine is also used for the treatment of toxoplasmosis.

Pharmacokinetics

Pyrimethamine is well absorbed following oral administration and is eliminated over several days (Table 43.7) (T 1/2 3 days; the companion sulfadoxine T 1/2 is 7 days), allowing single-dose treatment (Figure 43.23). Dose recommendations were devised originally in adults. A recent large study has shown that the pharmacokinetic properties of both pyrimethamine and sulfadoxine are altered significantly in children (aged 2–5 years) who have larger Vd and oral clearance values and consequently blood concentrations that are approximately half those in adults. This suggests that dose recommendations in this important age group may have been too low. Studies in pregnancy have shown conflicting results with some studies showing lower concentrations than in non-pregnant adults. Following intramuscular injection pyrimethamine absorption is as rapid as after oral administration but blood concentrations are lower and more variable, which suggests incomplete intramuscular bioavailability.

Toxicity

Pyrimethamine is very safe and well tolerated. Occasionally megaloblastic anaemia, neutropenia or thrombocytopenia may develop in patients with pre-existing folate deficiency. The toxicity of the widely used combinations with long-acting sulphonamides (sulfadoxine, sulfalene) or sulphones (dapsone) is almost entirely related to the sulpha components. A long list of possible adverse effects has been reported with sulphonamides. These include: (1) rare gastrointestinal toxicity: glossitis, stomatitis, pancreatitis, salivary gland enlargement and pseudomembranous colitis; (2) cutaneous toxicity: exfoliative dermatitis, toxic epidermal necrolysis, urticaria, photosensitivity, cutaneous vasculitis, erythema nodosum, lichen planus, pruritus and hair loss; (3) CNS: dizziness, ataxia, benign intracranial hypertension, aseptic meningitis, hearing loss, tinnitus, reversible peripheral neuropathy; (4) renal effects: proteinuria, haematuria, acute interstitial nephritis, crystalluria (older sulphas – not generally associated with sulfadoxine); (5) haematological; thrombocytopenia, antibody-mediated haemolysis, neutropenia and (6) drug fever. The sulphones commonly cause methaemoglobinaemia, cause haemolytic anaemia in G6PD deficiency and also rarely cause blood dyscrasias.[31] Severe reactions occurred in about 1:7000 subjects receiving sulfadoxine-pyrimethamine prophylaxis (mortality was 1:18 000). The risk with treatment use is almost certainly much lower, but there are no precise estimates.

Use

Combinations of pyrimethamine with long-acting sulphonamides (SP) should not be used for prophylaxis, whereas the sulphone combination, which appears to be safer (at a once-weekly dose), is used occasionally for prophylaxis but not treatment. Pyrimethamine alone is no longer prescribed as an antimalarial. SP is given in a single oral dose ensuring that this contains a minimum of 1.25 mg/kg of pyrimethamine. This should be combined with a 3-day course of artesunate (4 mg/kg per day) to improve treatment efficacy. This is well tolerated, inexpensive and effective where efficacy of SP remains high (cure rates >80%). SP is regarded as safe in pregnancy. Studies from Africa indicate that administration of SP at least three times during pregnancy (at intervals ≥1 month) has a beneficial effect on maternal anaemia and pregnancy outcome (birth weight). HIV-positive women need SP more frequently for the same effect. This approach has now been extended to infancy and possible incorporation in EPI programmes. Whether other drugs are as good as SP in IPT, whether the findings in high transmission settings apply also to low transmission settings, whether artesunate should be added and what to do when resistance develops, all remain to be determined. Across the Sahel where malaria transmission is intense over 3–4 months each year it is now recommended that monthly treatment courses of amodiaquine and SP should be given to children aged between 3 and 59 months at monthly intervals, beginning at the start of the transmission season, to a maximum of 4 doses during the malaria transmission season (provided both drugs retain sufficient antimalarial efficacy). This is termed 'seasonal malaria chemoprevention'.

PROGUANIL/CHLORPROGUANIL

Proguanil (chloroguanide) and the dichlorobiguanide chlorproguanil are considered the safest of all antimalarials. Both compounds are mainly prodrugs for the active triazine metabolites cycloguanil and chlorcycloguanil. The metabolites are DHFR inhibitors. The parent compounds do possess weak antimalarial activity, probably by affecting mitochondrial electron transport.

Pharmacokinetics

Proguanil and chlorproguanil are well absorbed by mouth reaching peak concentrations in approximately 4 hours and are converted rapidly to the triazine metabolites (Table 43.7). These in turn are metabolized to the inactive metabolites chloro- and dichlorophenylbiguanide, respectively. As the parent compounds are eliminated more slowly than the metabolites the profile of antimalarial activity resulting from the cyclic metabolites is determined by the parent drug distribution and elimination. The T1/2 of proguanil has been reported as approximately 16 hours in healthy subjects and 13 hours in malaria. Recent population pharmacokinetic studies in malaria with a more sensitive assay report an estimated chlorproguanil terminal elimination half-life of 35 hours. Interestingly, the pharmacokinetic properties of chlorproguanil, chlorcycloguanil and dapsone are not affected by malaria. Approximately 3% of Caucasian and African populations, but up to 20% of Orientals, fail to convert the parent compounds to their active metabolites. In some parts of Micronesia the prevalence is even higher. This is related to a genetic polymorphism in the 2C19 subfamily of the cytochrome P450 mixed-function oxidase system. The conversion of proguanil to the active metabolite is reduced in pregnancy.

Toxicity

The antimalarial biguanides and chlorproguanil-dapsone are very well tolerated. The biguanides occasionally cause mouth ulcers and at high doses abdominal discomfort. Hair loss has been reported. Two patients with renal failure, in whom the drugs presumably accumulated, developed pancytopenia following prophylactic administration of proguanil. The toxicity of chlorproguanil-dapsone results from the dapsone component. The main concern is haemolysis in patients who are G6PD-deficient. Methaemoglobinaemia is also common. In large-scale evaluations chlorproguanil-dapsone caused potentially dangerous anaemia in African children and led to its withdrawal as an antimalarial drug. Rare idiosyncratic reactions of sulphones (like sulphonamides) include leukopenia and agranulocytosis, cutaneous eruptions, peripheral neuropathy, psychosis, toxic hepatitis, cholestatic jaundice, nephrotic syndrome, renal papillary necrosis, severe hypoalbuminaemia without proteinuria, an infectious mononucleosis-like syndrome, and minor neurological and gastrointestinal complaints.

Use

Proguanil has been used as a prophylactic taken once daily (3 mg/kg), often in combination with chloroquine. Chlorproguanil-dapsone has been withdrawn as a treatment of uncomplicated *falciparum* malaria because of haemolytic toxicity. The treatment doses of proguanil used are 5–8 mg/kg per day (in combination with atovaquone).

ATOVAQUONE-PROGUANIL

This highly active hydroxynaphthaquinone antimalarial drug is active even against multi-drug-resistant *falciparum* malaria. The speed of therapeutic response is similar to that with mefloquine and slower than that with artemisinin derivatives. Originally atovaquone alone was developed, but high-level resistance developed in approximately 30% of treated patients. This suggested that the point mutations in *cyt b*, which conferred resistance, occurred at an approximate frequency of 1 in 10^{12} parasites. The fixed combination with proguanil proved much more effective producing cure rates of nearly 100% and emergence of resistance in less than 1:500 treated patients. It is this combined formulation (Malarone®), which is registered both for prophylaxis and treatment use in many countries. Nevertheless it must be considered vulnerable and for treatment use in endemic areas should ideally be combined with an artemisinin derivative. This creates a highly effective and well-tolerated artemisinin based combination treatment. Interestingly it is the parent compound proguanil which is the important contributor to antimalarial efficacy, as atovaquone-proguanil is equally effective against highly antifol-resistant parasites and also in individuals unable to convert proguanil to cycloguanil. Unfortunately, the very high cost of atovaquone synthesis makes this drug largely unaffordable in tropical countries.

Pharmacokinetics

Atovaquone is similar to halofantrine and lumefantrine in that oral absorption is augmented considerably by fats (Table 43.7). Elimination is slower in patients of African origin (T1/2 70 hours) than in Oriental patients (T1/2 30 hours). There are no significant interactions with proguanil or artesunate. Concentrations of both components are reduced by almost one half in late pregnancy Atovaquone is eliminate.

Toxicity

The combination is really very well tolerated. Atovaquone-proguanil may cause vomiting in some patients. The adverse effects otherwise are similar to those of proguanil.

Use

Atovaquone-proguanil is becoming established as a safe, effective and expensive antimalarial prophylactic for travellers – as it is effective everywhere. The adult prophylactic dose is one tablet (atovaquone 250 mg proguanil 100 mg) daily with food. The treatment dose is 15–20/6–8 mg/kg per day for 3 days, which corresponds to an adult dose of 4 tablets per day. It is equally efficacious and well tolerated in young children. The triple combination with artesunate is well tolerated and highly effective against multidrug-resistant *falciparum* malaria and should be given if this drug is used in endemic areas. Artesunate-atovaquone-proguanil has been evaluated in pregnant women failing other treatments. It was well tolerated and effective, although plasma levels of all components were reduced suggesting that a higher dose would be needed. For treatment use cost has been a major barrier to its use and its use is almost exclusively confined to the treatment of imported malaria in temperate countries and in very limited deployments against artemisinin-resistant *falciparum* malaria in Eastern Thailand.

PRIMAQUINE

Primaquine is an 8-aminoquinoline used mainly for its actions against the hypnozoites of *P. vivax* (to prevent relapse) and the gametocytes of *P. falciparum* (to prevent transmission). Primaquine has significant liver stage pre-erythrocytic activity against all the malarias (which accounts for its prophylactic efficacy) and it also has significant activity against asexual stage parasites of *P. vivax*, *P. malariae* and *P. ovale*. Thus, the radical treatment of *vivax* and *ovale* in infections, where primaquine is combined usually with chloroquine, is a combination treatment which should provide mutual protection against resistance.

Pharmacokinetics

Primaquine is well absorbed after oral administration. It is cleared by hepatic biotransformation with an elimination half-life of 8 hours to the more polar biologically inactive metabolite carboxyprimaquine, which is eliminated more slowly. Metabolism via cytochrome P450 biotransformation produces several other metabolites. It is not clear which of these highly reactive metabolites mediates the biological effects of primaquine.

Toxicity

Nausea, headache, vomiting and abdominal pain or cramps are relatively common particularly if higher doses of primaquine (>30 mg) are taken on an empty stomach. Taking primaquine with food considerably improves tolerability. At an adult dose of 15 mg mild abdominal pain was reported in 3% of US servicemen and 22.5 mg produced abdominal symptoms in 12% which required treatment in 3%. In general adult doses of 30 mg base are well tolerated if taken with food. Mild diarrhoea, chest pain, weakness, visual disturbances and pruritus occur occasionally. Significant methaemoglobinaemia (>10%) such that the patient appears cyanosed occurs in less than 10% of adult patients receiving ≤22.5 mg/day. The principal toxicity of primaquine is oxidant haemolysis. This may result from oxidant species induced by the phenolic metabolite 5-hydroxyprimaquine. This is the most serious side-effect in individuals with glucose 6 phosphate dehydrogenase (G6PD) deficiency, other enzyme deficiencies (e.g. glutathione synthetase) that counter oxidant stress, and several haemoglobinopathies (e.g. Hb Zurich, Hb Torino). Although haemolytic toxicity first recognized in the 1920s with plasmoquine, it was not until the early 1950s that the sex-linked G6PD deficiency was discovered. The severity of haemolysis is related to the degree of G6PD deficiency and the primaquine dose. Haemolysis is, therefore, generally less severe in the African (A^-) form. In such patients, haemolysis tends to be self-limiting but in some of the Asian variants and the Mediterranean type haemolysis may be severe. There are a large number of different G6PD genotypes and there is considerable phenotypic variation within the genotypes. This makes generalizations about the risks of haemolysis difficult. Essentially all subjects who are G6PD deficient (<30% of normal activity) will haemolyse following primaquine administration to an extent determined by the degree of deficiency and the dose and duration of treatment. Fortunately because primaquine is eliminated rapidly haemolysis is self-limiting if the drug is stopped. There is insufficient information on the relationship between genotype, red cell G6PD concentrations and haemolytic tendency with primaquine. Haemolysis may be exacerbated by concurrent infections, liver disease (altered primaquine metabolism), renal impairment (delayed excretion) and co-administration of other drugs with haemolytic potential, e.g. sulphonamides. Primaquine is contraindicated in pregnancy.

Use

Radical curative activity depends on the total dose administered and this is limited by adverse effects. Primaquine is given once daily in a dose of 0.25–0.5 mg base/kg (adult doses 15–30 mg) together with food. The higher dose is now recommended for tropical 'strains' and the usual course of treatment for the radical treatment of *vivax* and *ovale* malaria is 14 days. Shorter courses with higher doses have also proved effective (30 mg twice daily for 7 days). In particular, there is no evidence that the previously recommended 0.25 mg base/kg per day for 5-days is effective. There is no evidence for adverse interactions with other antimalarial drugs but this has been little studied. In patients with mild G6PD deficiency a once weekly dose of 0.6–0.8 mg/kg (adult dose 45 mg) is given for 8 weeks. For *P. falciparum* gametocytocidal activity a single dose of 0.5–0.75 mg base/kg is recommended although recent evidence suggests that a single 0.25 mg base/kg dose gives maximal transmission blocking activity with less haemolysis in G6PD-deficient patients. For prophylaxis the adult dose evaluated has been 30 mg daily taken with food. This has been remarkably well tolerated. In most *vivax*-endemic areas G6PD deficiency is prevalent but testing is not available and there is no consensus on how primaquine should be used in these circumstances. If significant haemolysis occurs primaquine should be stopped and the patient observed. Transfusion is rarely necessary except when there is severe deficiency.

TAFENOQUINE

Formerly known as etaquine or WR 238605, this slowly eliminated 8-aminoquinoline was developed by the US army. It is currently undergoing phase III trials in antimalarial prophylaxis and for the radical treatment of *vivax* malaria. Tafenoquine has a terminal elimination half-life of approximately 2 weeks. Tafenoquine is more efficacious and better tolerated than primaquine, although it still causes oxidant haemolysis in G6PD-deficient subjects.

METHYLENE BLUE

Methylene blue was first shown to have antimalarial activity by Gutthman and Ehrlich over 100 years ago. Recently interest has been rekindled in this well-established dye and studies completed showing antimalarial activity in vivo and gametocytocidal activity against *P. falciparum* in vitro.

QINGHAOSU (ARTEMISININ)

Qinghaosu or artemisinin is a sesquiterpene lactone peroxide extracted from the leaves of the shrub *Artemesia annua* (Qinghao). Four derivatives are used widely: the oil-soluble methyl ether artemether (or the very similar compound artemotil formerly known as arteether), the water-soluble hemisuccinate derivative artesunate and dihydroartemisinin (DHA). A semisynthetic derivative artemisone and fully synthetic trioxalone compounds (OZ 277; arterolane and OZ 439) with similar modes of action are under development. Artesunate, artemether and artemotil are all synthesized from DHA and they are

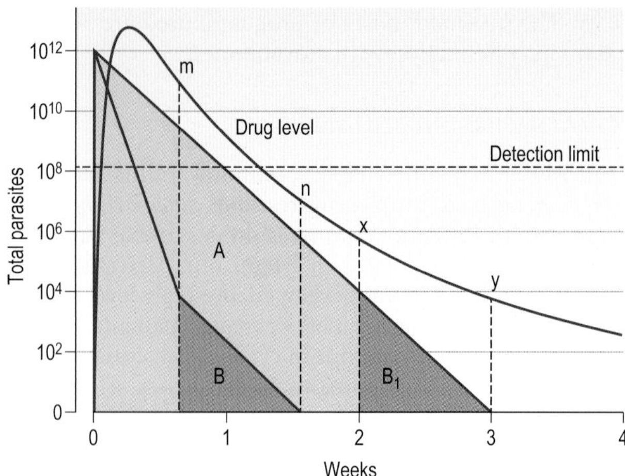

Figure 43.26 Artemisinin combination treatment. The effects of adding a 3-day course of artesunate to high-dose (25 mg/kg) mefloquine on malaria parasite killing in an area of pre-existing mefloquine resistance (e.g. in Thailand). The parasite burden is relatively high in the example (corresponding to about 2% parasitaemia). Without the artesunate the parasitaemia declines 100-fold per asexual cycle and is eliminated finally in 3 weeks. If artesunate is added for 3 days, covering two asexual cycles, then the parasite biomass is reduced 10^8-fold leaving a maximum residuum of only 10^5 parasites remaining (and usually much fewer) for the high concentrations of mefloquine to remove (B). This offers a hundred-million-fold lower opportunity of selecting a resistant parasite. Note that without artesunate the corresponding number of parasites (B1) 'see' much lower concentrations of mefloquine (from x to y, compared with m to n) and have therefore an increased risk of recrudescing.

converted back to it within the body (Figure 43.26). Artemisinin itself is available in a few countries. It is 5–10 times less active than the derivatives and is not metabolized to DHA. These drugs are the most rapidly acting of known antimalarials and they have the broadest time window of antimalarial effect (from ring forms to early schizonts). They produce more rapid parasite clearance than other antimalarial drugs and they have proved to be very safe in clinical practice. They are simply the best drugs for severe malaria (Figure 43.27). In a large randomized controlled trial in severe malaria, conducted in four Asian countries, artesunate reduced the mortality of severe malaria by 35% compared with quinine. Most of these patients were adults (n=1461; of whom 202 were children). In a subsequent trial, the largest ever conducted in severe malaria, conducted in 5425 African children, artesunate reduced mortality by 22.5% (Figure 43.28).[32] There were no serious adverse effects. Artesunate reduced the incidence of hypoglycaemia, convulsions and neurological deterioration and importantly did not increase the incidence of neurological sequeale. These are very large mortality reductions and they have established artesunate as the treatment of choice for severe malaria. Later investigations based on estimation of the parasite biomass using plasma PfHRP2 suggested that some of this difference between the mortality reduction in Asia and that in Africa (35% vs 22.5%) might be explained by overdiagnosis of severe malaria in African children, i.e. that some children fulfilling the definition of severe malaria die from another pathological process – most likely sepsis.[13] In *falciparum* malaria the artemisinin derivatives also effectively prevent progression to severe disease. For example in western Thailand a parasitaemia over 4% without vital organ dysfunction carries a 3% mortality (i.e. 30 times higher than uncomplicated malaria but less than one fifth that of severe

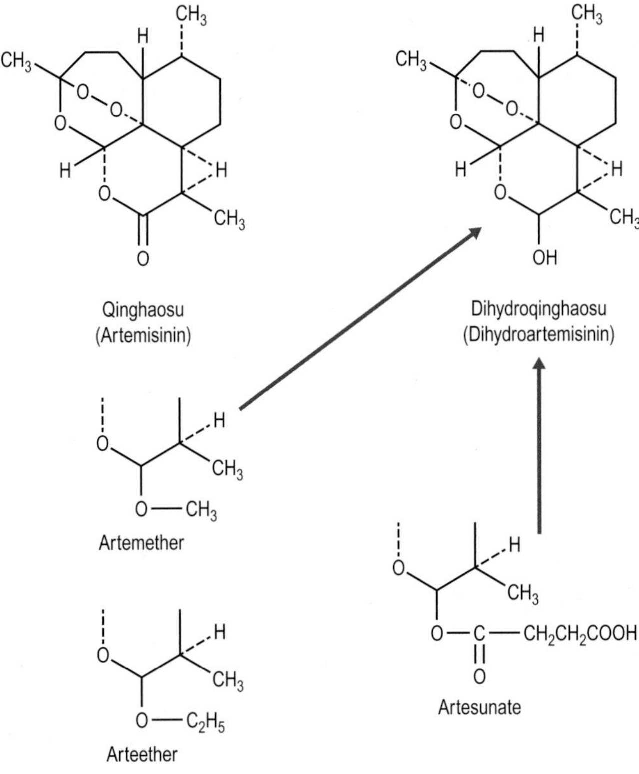

Figure 43.27 Qinghaosu: the parent compound artemisinin and the three derivatives. The oil-soluble ethers, artemether and artemotil (arteether) and the water-soluble artesunate are all converted in vivo to a common biologically active metabolite dihydroartemisinin. The peroxide bridge in the sesquiterpene structure is essential for antimalarial activity.

malaria). In this context, oral artesunate produces considerably superior therapeutic responses compared with an intravenous quinine loading dose. This property of rapidly stopping parasite development and thereby arresting progression of the infection also prevents development of severe malaria. Before the recent definitive studies of artesunate trials in severe malaria were conducted mainly with artemether. In randomized controlled trials which together enrolled nearly 2000 patients, intramuscular artemether was associated with a significantly lower mortality in South-East Asian adults when compared with quinine, but there was no significant difference in African children. Artemether was not associated with more rapid clinical responses (fever clearance, coma recovery) but it did accelerate parasite clearance. But artemether (or artemotil) were not the best drugs to have chosen. Although they are highly effective in vitro, in vivo these oil-based intramuscular injections were found to be slowly and erratically absorbed – particularly in the most severely ill patients. This pharmacokinetic disadvantage countered the intrinsic pharmacodynamic advantage of this drug class. The water-soluble artesunate by contrast is reliably and rapidly absorbed following intramuscular injection, and can be given intravenously. In a recent large randomized comparison of artesunate versus artemether conducted in Vietnam there was a borderline mortality advantage to artesunate. Thus artesunate is better than artemether, which is in turn better than quinine in the treatment of severe malaria.

Most deaths from severe malaria take place in or near home and far from facilities capable of providing injections. Rectal formulations of artemisinin and artesunate have been developed for community use as treatments for patients suspected of having severe malaria, who are febrile and unable to take

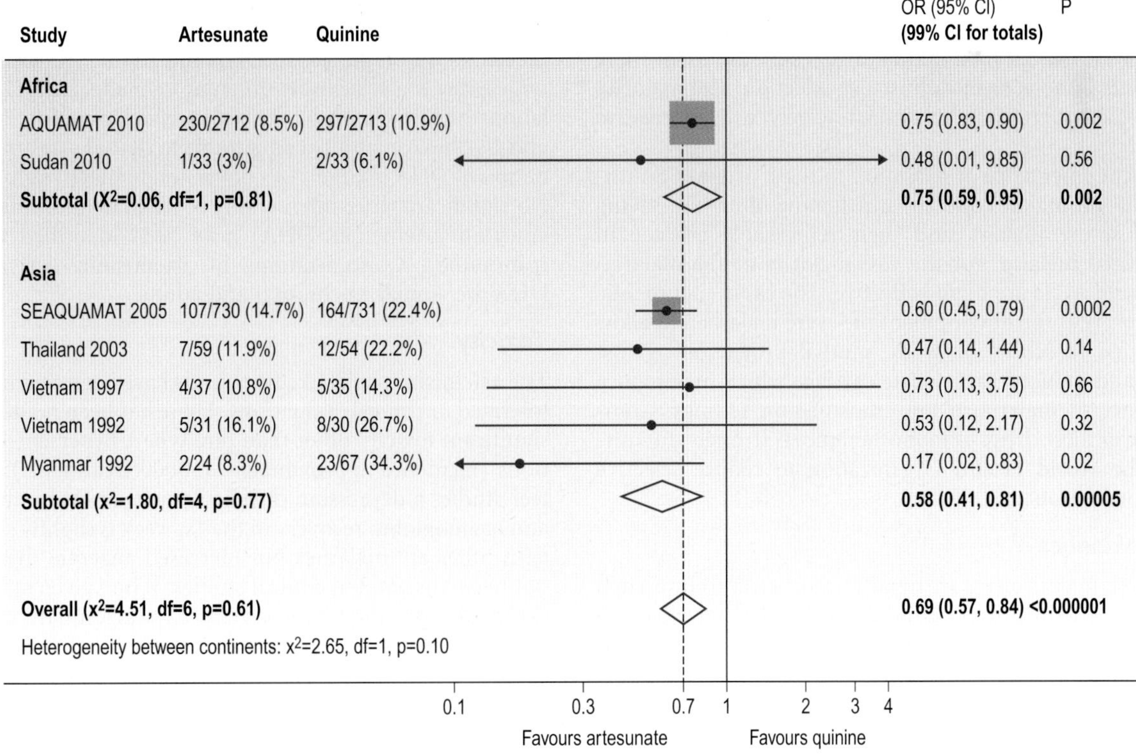

Figure 43.28 Forest plots from individual patient data analyses of randomized trials comparing parenteral artesunate versus the standard quinine loading dose regimen in severe falciparum malaria. These show a highly significant difference between artesunate and quinine. Artesunate reduced mortality by 35% in adults and by 22.5% in children.

TABLE 43.8 Dosage for Rectal (Rectocap) Artesunate Initial (Pre-Referral) Treatment in Children (Aged 2–15 Years) and Weighing at Least 5 kg

Weight (kg)	Age	Artesunate Dose (mg)	Regimen (Single Dose)
5–8.9	0–12 months	50	One 50-mg suppository
9–19	13–42 months	100	One 100-mg suppository
20–29	43–60 months	200	One 100-mg + one 50-mg suppository
30–39	6–13 years	300	Three 100-mg suppositories
>40	>14 years	400	One 400-mg suppository

medications by mouth. A rectal formulation of artesunate was evaluated in a very large multicentre trial, conducted in Ghana, Tanzania and Bangladesh (Table 43.8). Preferral administration of rectal artesunate reduced the mortality of children under 5 years with malaria who could not tolerate oral treatment by 25%.[33]

In clinical studies in uncomplicated *falciparum* malaria the artemisinin derivatives provide both more rapid parasite and fever clearance than with other treatments and also reduce gametocyte carriage and thus transmission. Concerns over their neurotoxic potential, revealed in animal studies, have not been confirmed in large and detailed clinical, neurophysiological and pathological studies. Indeed their remarkable safety, efficacy and lack of adverse effects have led to widespread unregulated use and the manufacture of fake products.

Artemisinin is available as capsules of powder or as suppositories. Artemether is formulated in peanut oil and arteether in sesame seed oil, for intramuscular injection and in capsules or tablets for oral use. Artesunate is formulated either as tablets, in a gel enclosed in gelatin for rectal administration (called a Rectocap™), or as dry powder of artesunic acid for injection, usually supplied with an ampoule of 5% sodium bicarbonate. The powder is dissolved in the sodium bicarbonate, to form sodium artesunate and then diluted in 5% dextrose or 'normal' saline for intravenous or intramuscular injection. The majority of clinical data pertain to the most widely used derivative artesunate.

The recent emergence of resistance to these drugs in Southeast Asia is of major concern, threatening their life-saving benefit in severe malaria and their remarkable efficacy in uncomplicated malaria. For the vast majority of the malaria-affected world ACTs are highly effective. The rapid therapeutic responses prevent the development of severe malaria and allow earlier return to school or work, mutual protection against resistance and reduced gametocyte carriage which may reduce the incidence of malaria in low transmission settings. Community use of these drugs as monotherapies is strongly discouraged by the World Health Organization to reduce selective pressure for resistance.

Pharmacokinetics

The artemisinin derivatives are rapidly absorbed and eliminated (Table 43.7). Artemisinin is cleared by metabolic conversion to inactive metabolites. It is a potent inducer of its own metabolism. Artesunate, artemether and artemotil are converted to the active metabolite dihydroartemisinin, which has an elimination half-life of approximately 45 min. Parenteral artesunate is hydrolysed rapidly at neutral pH and this is accelerated by plasma esterases. Artemether and artemotil are converted by hepatic biotransformation. Although they are by far the most rapidly eliminated of the antimalarial drugs, because of their broad stage specificity of action they are highly effective when given once daily. Unlike some antibiotics it is not necessary to exceed the MIC throughout the dosing interval for antimalarial drugs (after all it is only necessary to kill each parasite once!). After oral or parenteral administration artesunate is hydrolysed rapidly (by stomach acid and esterases in plasma and erythrocytes) and most of the antimalarial activity results from the DHA metabolite. Oral absorption is rapid and bioavailability is approximately 60%. Rectal bioavailability is more variable; following administration of the Rectocap™ bioavailability averages 50% (although rates of absorption vary widely). As for quinine there is a contraction in the volume of distribution and reduced clearance in acute malaria, which increases blood concentrations. There is also be a malaria-related inhibition of intestinal and hepatic first pass metabolism (by glucuronidation) which improves oral bioavailability. After oral administration artemether is absorbed rapidly, but is converted more slowly (via CYP 3A4) to DHA, although the metabolite still accounts for the majority of antimalarial activity. In contrast after intramuscular administration absorption of artemether and artemotil (arteether) is slow and erratic. Peak concentrations are often not reached for many hours. Following intramuscular administration of artemether concentrations of the parent compound exceed those of the active DHA metabolite. In some patients with severe malaria absorption may be inadequate. Oral formulations of DHA contain excipients which promote absorption and give bioavailability comparable to that of artesunate. Elimination of DHA is largely by conversion to inactive glucuronides. No significant drug interactions other than autoinduction (art emisinin>artemether>DHA) have been identified with these compounds. Concentrations of artemisinin derivatives and DHA are similar in children and adults.

Toxicity

The artemisinin-related compounds have been remarkably well tolerated in clinical evaluations. There has been no documented significant toxicity other than rare type 1 hypersensitivity reactions (incidence approximately 1:3000 treatments). In volunteer studies a depression of reticulocyte counts has been noted and haemoglobin recovery in the 1st week is slightly slower than with other antimalarials but increased anaemia thereafter has not been observed in clinical studies. When given at high doses (≥6 mg/kg per day) over several days artesunate causes self-limiting neutropenia. Following treatment of hyperparasitaemia a haemolytic anaemia may be seen resulting from shortened survival of once-parasitized red cells. In animal studies the artemisinin derivatives are much less toxic than the quinoline antimalarials. The principal toxicity in animals has been an unusual dose-related selective pattern of neuronal cell damage affecting certain brain stem nuclei. This is related to the pharmacokinetic properties of the drug. Neurotoxicity is related to protracted

TABLE 43.9 **Antimalarial Drug Doses in Severe Malaria**

Hospital	Health Clinic	Rural Health Clinic
Intensive care unit (ICU) Artesunate 2.4 mg/kg stat. by IV injection followed by 2.4 mg/kg at 12, and 24 hours then daily if necessary	No intravenous infusions possible As for hospital ICU: artesunate can also be given by IM injection	No injection facilities Artesunate Rectocap: 10 mg/kg daily Artemisinin suppository 20 mg/kg at 0 and 4 hours, then daily
IF ARTESUNATE UNAVAILABLE		
Artemether 3.2 mg/kg stat. by IM injection followed by 1.6 mg/kg daily		
IF ARTESUNATE AND ARTEMETHER UNAVAILABLE		
Quinine dihydrochloride 20 mg salt/kg infused over 4 hours. Maintenance dose: 10 mg salt/kg infused over 2–8 hours at 8-hour intervals	Quinine dihydrochloride 20 mg salt/kg diluted 1:2 with sterile water given by split injection into both anterior thighs. Maintenance dose: 10 mg/kg 8-hourly	

General points: Infusions can be given in 0.9% saline, 5% or 10% dextrose/water. Infusion rates for quinine should be carefully controlled. Oral treatment should start as soon as the patient can swallow reliably enough to complete a full course of treatment. A full course of artemisinin combination treatment should be given.

exposure related to sustained blood concentrations, as follows intramuscular administration of the oil-based artemether and arteether. Much less neurotoxicity is seen following oral administration or intravenous artesunate because the drug levels are not sustained. Extensive clinical neurophysiological and, to a lesser extent, pathology studies have failed to show any evidence of neurotoxicity or cardiotoxicity in clinical use. Initial animal studies also suggested effects on the electrocardiographic QT interval (ventricular repolarization) but this was probably secondary to neurotoxicity. These drugs do not affect the heart in clinical use. The main concern over their use relates to early pregnancy. In experimental animals exposure during a critical time window in early pregnancy causes fetal loss as a result of inhibition of erythropoiesis. Whether this effect could produce fetal developmental abnormalities in primates and therefore could be teratogenic in clinical use in the treatment of malaria was of great concern. Prospective clinical studies in over 1000 exposed pregnancies, including over 100 1st trimester exposures is reassuring to date.[26] Indeed, given their superior efficacy over other drugs and the harmful effects of malaria illness comparative trials with ACTs in the 1st trimester are being undertaken. These drugs are still not recommended for the treatment of uncomplicated *falciparum* malaria in early pregnancy (1st trimester), unless there are no effective alternatives, but this may change. There is now confidence in their safety in the 2nd and 3rd trimesters and ACTs should be used – although higher dosages or longer courses may be needed for optimum efficacy. Thus overall no adverse effects on the pregnancy or infant development have been seen in prospective studies.

Use

In severe malaria, artesunate is given by intravenous or intramuscular injection. The doses are 2.4 mg/kg given at 0, 12, 24 hours, then daily.[34] Artemether and artemotil (arteether) are given by intramuscular injection to the anterior thigh. The dose of artemether is 3.2 mg/kg initially followed by 1.6 mg/kg daily (Table 43.9). The artesunate Rectocap is used in a dose of 10 mg/kg per day until parenteral or oral treatment can be given (Table 43.8). For oral treatment fixed-dose ACTs are preferred (Table 43.10). If used alone, the artemisinin derivatives should be given in a 7 (not 5)-day course, but this should be combined with doxycycline or clindamycin where possible. The initial oral

TABLE 43.10 **Oral ACT Dosing Schedules**

ARTEMETHER-LUMEFANTRINE[a]

Age (years)	Body weight (kg)	Number of Artemether-lumefantrine tablets per dose (twice daily for 3 days)
<3	5–14	1
3–9	15–24	2
9–14	25–34	3
>14	>34	4

ARTESUNATE-AMODIAQUINE, ARTESUNATE-SP, ARTESUNATE-MEFLOQUINE

Age (years)	Number of Artesunate 50 mg tablets per dose (Daily for 3 days)	Number of Amodiaquine 153 mg tablets per dose (Daily for 3 days)	Number of Sulfadoxine-Pyrimethamine 25/500 mg tablets (single dose)	Number of Mefloquine 250 mg tablets (Daily for 3 days)
½ to 1	½	½	½	¼
1–6	1	1	1	½
7–13	2	2	2	1
>13	4	4	3	2

These are dosage guides, but adjusting tablets on the basis of weight is preferable.
[a]The drug should be taken with food or milk.

dose is 4 mg/kg followed by 2 mg/kg per day. Dose restrictions are not necessary in renal failure or with liver disease. The artemisinin derivatives are safe in infants and children. Until more information is available as a policy of caution they should not be used in the 1st trimester of pregnancy (although there is no evidence of harm), but should be used in the 2nd and 3rd trimesters. These drugs should be used for the treatment of severe malaria in pregnancy at any gestational age as they save lives and they are safer than quinine.

ARTEMISININ COMBINATION TREATMENTS

The ACTs are rapidly effective and generally reliable treatments. The artemisinin derivatives induce a rapid resolution of fever and illness. This may improve absorption of the combination partner (mefloquine, lumefantrine). While present in the blood (usually 3 days) they also protect the partner drug from the emergence of resistance and they reduce gametocyte carriage. The partner drug then removes the relatively few parasites remaining after the 3-day course of treatment (a hundred million times less than when treatment started) and also protects the artemisinin derivative from resistance (Figure 43.27). But once the artemisinin derivative has been eliminated the partner compound is no longer 'protected' and may then select for resistance. Thus, provided the partner is effective and full doses are absorbed protection of the artemisinin component from resistance is complete, whereas protection of the partner drug is incomplete. WHO currently recommends five ACTs; artesunate-amodiaquine, artesunate-sulphadoxine–pyrimethamine (in areas where prevalent malaria parasites are a sensitive to the partner drugs) and artesunate-mefloquine, artemether-lumefantrine and dihydroartemisinin-piperaquine which can be used everywhere.[34]

ARTEMETHER-LUMEFANTRINE

Formerly called benflumetol, lumefantrine was developed by Chinese scientists. It is now available only in a fixed tablet combination with artemether. Each tablet contains artemether 20 mg and lumefantrine 120 mg. This is the most widely used ACT in the world accounting for approximately 70% of all use. Artemether-lumefantrine is very effective against multi-drug-resistant *falciparum* malaria and it is remarkably well tolerated.

Pharmacokinetics

Lumefantrine is lipophilic and hydrophobic (Table 43.7). Its absorption is dose-limited and is considerably augmented by taking the drug together with food (a 16-fold increase with a fatty meal). Only a small amount of fat is required. Dose-finding studies with soya milk showed 36 mL (equivalent to 1.2 g fat) were required to produce 90% of maximum absorption. The absorption of lumefantrine is reduced in the acute phase of malaria, but then increases considerably as symptoms resolve and the patient starts to eat. Absorption is capacity limited so increasing the current dose does not provide a corresponding increase in the amount of drug absorbed. This means the drug cannot be given once daily. Lumefantrine is metabolized to a desbutyl metabolite (principally by CYP 3A4) which has greater antimalarial activity but contributes relatively little to overall antimalarial effect. The elimination half-life is 3–4 days. As a result it provides a shorter duration of post-treatment prophylaxis compared with more slowly eliminated drugs such as mefloquine and piperaquine. This results in earlier recurrences and less suppression of *P. vivax* relapses. The pharmacokinetic properties of lumefantrine are similar in adults and children. The principal pharmacokinetic variable which correlates with therapeutic response is the area under the plasma concentration-time curve (AUC). The plasma or whole blood level on day 7 after starting treatment is a good surrogate of the AUC for this and other slowly eliminated antimalarials. Plasma concentrations of both drug components are reduced by approximately half in pregnancy so the current dose regimen is insufficient for optimum cure rates in this important patient group.

Toxicity

This combination is remarkably free of adverse effects. Concerns about possible cardiotoxicity have been refuted by careful studies. Lumefantrine is not cardiotoxic.

Use

There is now extensive experience with artemether-lumefantrine from all parts of the malaria-affected world attesting to safety and efficacy. The treatment course initially recommended was 1.5/ 9 mg/kg (adult dose 4 tablets) given at 0, 8, 24 and 48 hours. This was effective in patients with background immunity, but cure rates in non-immune patients with multi-drug-resistant infections were approximately 80%. Increasing the regimen to 6 doses (i.e. twice daily on each day) resulted in >95% cure rates and this regimen has proved effective across the world. Where it has been assessed, adherence to this regimen has been relatively good. The patient should be encouraged to take the drug with food or a small amount of milk. Several studies suggest artemether-lumefantrine is safe in the 2nd and 3rd trimesters of pregnancy, although more information is needed and dose optimization is required. A paediatric formulation has been developed.

PYRONARIDINE

Structurally a relative of amodiaquine, pyronaridine has been developed and used in China. It is active against multidrug-resistant *Plasmodium falciparum* malaria[35] and, like many drugs in this class, it is extensively distributed and slowly eliminated. Originally pyronaridine was deployed as an enteric-coated formulation for monotherapy (which had poor oral bioavailability) and was given in a 3-day course of 1200 mg or 1800 mg (adult dose) over 5 days. Pyronaridine has been developed as the tetraphosphate and now registered as a fixed co-formulation with artesunate in a 3 : 1 dose ratio. The efficacy of artesunate-pyronaridine against all malaria tested to date has been excellent.

Pharmacokinetics

There are few data on the pharmacokinetics of pyronaridine in the public domain. In phase II clinical trials on the pharmacokinetics, clinical and safety outcome of artesunate-pyronaridine carried out in 16 patients in Uganda with acute *falciparum* malaria indicated a large apparent volume of distribution and a long elimination phase. The latest assessment of the terminal elimination half-life of pyronaridine is approximately 10–13 days. Pyronaridine is concentrated in red blood cells.

Toxicity

Although generally well tolerated, there remains some concern over the potential of pyronaridine for hepatotoxicity. This is being addressed in Phase IV trials.

Use

Artesunate-pyronaridine is highly effective against all malarias, including multi-drug-resistant *falciparum* malaria.

PIPERAQUINE

Also developed in China this bisquinoline compound and its hydroxy-derivative are active against multidrug-resistant *Plasmodium falciparum*.[36] Piperaquine replaced chloroquine in China as first-line treatment for *falciparum* malaria in 1978 and was used until 1994. Over 200 tonnes were dispensed. Resistance reportedly developed, but reversed after piperaquine was discontinued. In recent years, piperaquine has been developed as a fixed combination with dihydroartemisinin. The currently available formulation contains 40 mg of dihydroartemisinin and 320 mg of piperaquine (as the phosphate) per tablet and is given in an adult dose of 3 tablets/day (equivalent to approx. 2.3/16 mg/kg, once daily for 3 days. It is relatively inexpensive (adult doses currently just over US$1). This combination is registered, endorsed by the World Health Organization and used increasingly. The combination is well tolerated and effective everywhere.

Another combination artemisinin-piperaquine (as the base) is also available in some areas.

Pharmacokinetics

Oral dihydroartemisinin absorption is very dependent on the formulation and excipients. In current formulations, it is reliably and rapidly absorbed. Piperaquine is more slowly absorbed. It is extensively distributed and very slowly eliminated. The pharmacokinetic properties are similar to those of chloroquine. Absorption is slightly increased by fats. Latest estimates for the terminal elimination half-life are approximately 1 month. Young children have lower plasma concentrations than adults, particularly 1–2 weeks after drug administration and therefore need a higher mg/kg dose than adults. As with other slowly eliminated antimalarials the day 7 plasma or blood concentration is a valuable predictor of efficacy.

Toxicity

Piperaquine is safer than chloroquine. It is generally very well tolerated. Dosing is limited by abdominal discomfort. Apart from rare urticarial reactions to DHA occasional abdominal discomfort and diarrhoea have been reported in clinical trials which may have resulted from piperaquine. Although piperaquine does slightly prolong the electrocardiogram QT interval (approximately similar in magnitude to chloroquine) it is safer than chloroquine in experimental animals and there is no clinical evidence for cardiovascular toxicity. No serious adverse effects have been reported.

Use

Large trials in many countries attest to an excellent efficacy and safety profile. DHA-piperaquine has already established itself as an important antimalarial. It is effective against drug-resistant *falciparum* and *vivax* malaria. When measured adherence has been excellent. Recent studies also indicate good efficacy and excellent tolerability in African children. The long period of post-treatment prophylaxis conferred by the slowly eliminated piperaquine is both an advantage in preventing reinfections and suppressing *P. vivax* relapses, but also increases the selection pressure on resistance.

ANTIBACTERIALS WITH ANTIMALARIAL ACTIVITY

The antibacterials which act on protein or nucleic acid synthesis often have significant antimalarial activity. But they are not sufficiently active to be used alone to treat malaria. The sulphonamides and sulphones inhibit plasmodial folate synthesis by competing for the enzyme dihydropteroate synthetase. The sulphonamides and sulphones are usually used in combination with pyrimethamine or the antimalarial biguanides with which they are synergistic. Trimethoprim is also an antifol; it has good antimalarial activity and shares resistance profiles with pyrimethamine. The tetracyclines are consistently active against all species of malaria. Doxycycline is the most widely used both for prophylaxis and treatment. Clindamycin is as effective as the tetracyclines and has the advantage that it can be used in children and pregnant women. The macrolides are active in vitro but are generally disappointing in vivo. Azithromycin is more active and has been evaluated both in prophylaxis and treatment. Rifampicin has a weak antimalarial effect in vivo. Chloramphenicol has antimalarial activity but this has not been well characterized. The fluoroquinolones have some activity but, despite one promising sentinel report, subsequent clinical experience has proved uniformly disappointing. Fosmidomycin has good antimalarial activity and is under investigation. These drugs all act relatively slowly and they are therefore used in combination with more rapidly acting agents.

ANTIMALARIAL DRUG INTERACTIONS

Antimalarial drug interactions have not been well characterized. Mefloquine, halofantrine, quinidine and quinine are structurally similar and may compete for blood and tissue binding sites. Cardiotoxicity is assumed to be additive and significant only for halofantrine, where there is a potentially dangerous interaction with mefloquine. It has been recommended that mefloquine should not be given to people also receiving quinine to avoid adverse cardiovascular effects, but no interaction has been demonstrated. Inducers of CYP 3A4 such as rifampicin, ritonavir boosted lopinavir and anticonvulsant drugs accelerate the clearance of quinine and mefloquine resulting in lower drug levels (and a greater chance of treatment failure). There is no evidence that the structurally dissimilar antimalarials interact. Use of artesunate together with mefloquine improves the tolerance and absorption of mefloquine presumably by curing malaria more rapidly. Similarly, the absorption of lumefantrine improves as the patient recovers. There are several potential or proven interactions with antiretroviral drugs usually resulting in reduced antimalarial exposure. For example nevirapine reduces oral artemether and DHA exposure. On the other hand protease inhibitors may increase quinine exposure. Amodiaquine has a toxic interaction with efavirenz resulting in hepatotoxicity.

There are many reports of synergy or antagonism between antimalarial drugs based on isobolograms drawn from in vitro observations. These are often used to justify a particular choice of antimalarial combination but, for the most part, the results are irrelevant to the clinical use of the drugs. Only when synergy or antagonism is extreme, such as the marked synergy between sulphadoxine and pyrimethamine, is this relevant clinically. There are no cases of marked antagonism between the available antimalarial drugs.

Treating Malaria

In severe malaria, parenteral artesunate should be given. Rectal formulations of artemisinin or its derivatives (particularly artesunate) offer the possibility of starting treatment in the home or village before referring to the hospital or health centre (Tables 43.8–43.11). Rectal artesunate should become much more widely available in the next few years. For uncomplicated *falciparum* malaria artemisinin-based combination treatments (ACTs) are now recommended as first-line treatment everywhere. WHO currently recommends one of five ACTs. The choice of partner drug depends on local patterns of sensitivity and cost. For the treatment of *P. vivax*, *P. malariae*, *P. ovale* malaria chloroquine can still be relied upon in many areas although high-level resistance is now well established in Indonesia, Micronesia and the island of New Guinea and there are increasing reports of low-level resistance from many parts of Asia and South-America.

ASSESSMENT OF THE THERAPEUTIC RESPONSE

Generally understood and standardized definitions of antimalarial drug treatment responses are important for epidemiological purposes and helpful in therapeutic decision making. The definitions of severe malaria and treatment failure and the methods of assessing the therapeutic response have all undergone changes in recent years. In uncomplicated malaria the immediate therapeutic response is usually assessed by the parasite and fever clearance rates or times. WHO definitions of treatment failure are shown in Table 43.12.

Fever Clearance Times (FCT), Parasite Clearance Rates and Times (PCT)

The FCT is the interval from beginning antimalarial treatment until the patient is apyrexial. This is easier said than read! Fever does not come down linearly – it often fluctuates erratically. The method and site of measurements should be standardized and the use of antipyretics documented. One approach is to record when temperature first falls below 37.5°C (FCTa) and then when the temperature falls and remains below 37.5°C for 24 hours (FCTb).

The PCT is the interval between beginning antimalarial treatment and the first negative blood slide. The accuracy of the measurement depends on the frequency with which blood slides are taken and the quality of microscopy. The PCT is directly proportional to the admission parasitaemia. The time taken for parasitaemia to fall to half of the admission value (PCT50) and to fall to 10% of the admission value (PCT90) is also a useful comparative measure. In assessing artemisinin responses measurement of the parasite clearance half-life is recommended – this is derived from the slope of the log-linear

TABLE 43.11 Treatment of Uncomplicated Malaria

FIRST-LINE DRUGS FOR ENDEMIC AREAS

MALARIA	DRUG TREATMENT
Known chloroquine sensitive *P. vivax*, *P. malariae*, *P. ovale*, *P. knowlesi*, or *P. falciparum*[a]	Chloroquine 10 mg base/kg stat. followed by 5 mg/kg at 12, 24 and 36 h; or 10 mg/kg at 24 h, 5 mg/kg at 48 h or Amodiaquine 10–12 mg base/kg/day for 3 days
Sensitive *P. falciparum* malaria[a] or *P. vivax*, *P. malariae*, *P. ovale* or *P. knowlesi*[a]	Artesunate 4 mg/kg/day for 3 days + sulfadoxine 25 mg/kg + Pyrimethamine 1.25 mg/kg (SP) single dose *or* Artesunate 4 mg/kg/day for 3 days + Amodiaquine 10 mg base/kg/day for 3 days as FCT
All including multi-drug resistant *P. falciparum* malaria or *P. vivax*, *P. malariae*, *P. ovale*, or *P. knowlesi*	Artemether-lumefantrine 1.5/9 mg/kg twice daily for 3 days with food *or* Artesunate 4 mg/kg/day + mefloquine 8 mg/kg/day for 3 days in FCT *or* Dihydroartemisinin-piperaquine 2.5/20 mg/kg/day for 3 days

FCT: Fixed dose combination treatment. In low transmission settings a single dose of primaquine 0.25 mg base/kg should be added to all falciparum malaria treatments and given with the first dose of ACT, except to infants and pregnant women.

SECOND-LINE TREATMENTS

Artesunate 2 mg/kg daily (initial dose may be 4mg/kg) plus either: (a) tetracycline 4 mg/kg four times daily *or* (b) doxycycline 3 mg/kg once daily *or* (c) clindamycin 10 mg/kg twice daily for 7 days

Quinine 10 mg salt/kg three times daily plus *either:* (a) tetracycline 4 mg/kg four times daily *or* (b) doxycycline 3 mg/kg once daily *or* (c) clindamycin 10 mg/kg twice daily for 7 days

Atovaquone-proguanil 20/8 mg/kg once daily for 3 days with food.

RADICAL TREATMENT

After screening for G6PD deficiency patients with tropical *P. vivax* malaria should also be given primaquine 0.5 mg base/kg daily and patients with temperate (long latency) strains or *P. ovale* infections should be given 0.25 mg base/kg all for 14 days to prevent relapse. In mild G6PD deficiency 0.75 mg base/kg should be given once weekly for 8 weeks. Primaquine should not be given in severe G6PD deficiency or to young infants or pregnant women.

GENERAL POINTS

Pregnancy: Artemisinin derivatives are currently not recomended in the 1st trimester. Halofantrine, primaquine, and tetracycline should not be used at any time in pregnancy, and sulfadoxine should not be used very near to term (if alternatives are available).

Vomiting is less likely if the patient's temperature is lowered before oral drug administration.

Short courses of artesunate or quinine (<7 days) alone are not recommended.

In renal failure the dose of quinine should be reduced by one-third to one-half after 48 hours, and doxycycline but not tetracycline should be prescribed.

The doses of all drugs are unchanged in children and pregnant women.

None of the tetracyclines or doxycycline should be given to pregnant women or children under 8 years of age

[a]All ACTs are highly effective against *P. vivax*, *P. malariae*, and *P. ovale*, with the exception of combinations containing SP, as resistance to SP is widespread in *P. vivax*.

TABLE 43.12 **WHO Definitions of Antimalarial Treatment Failure in Uncomplicated Falciparum Malaria**

Treatment Outcome	Symptoms and Signs
Early treatment failure	Development of danger signs or severe malaria on days 1–3 in the presence of parasitaemia Parasitaemia on day 2 higher than the day 0 count irrespective of axillary temperature Parasitaemia on day 3 with axillary temperature of ≥37.5°C Parasitaemia on day 3 of ≥25% of count on day 0
Late treatment failure	
Late clinical failure	Development of danger signs or severe malaria after day 3 in the presence of parasitaemia, without previously meeting any of the criteria of early treatment failure Presence of parasitaemia and axillary temperature of ≥37.5°C (or history of fever) on any day from day 4 to day 28, without previously meeting any of the criteria of early treatment failure
Late parasitological failure	Presence of parasitaemia on any day from day 7 to day 28 and axillary temperature of <37.5°C, without previously meeting any of the criteria of early treatment failure or late clinical failure
Adequate clinical and parasitological response	Absence of parasitaemia on day 28 irrespective of axillary temperature without previously meeting any of the criteria of early treatment failure, late clinical failure or late parasitological failure.

phase of parasite decline (a parasite clearance estimator is freely available at http://www.wwarn.org). In areas with fully sensitive parasites, mean values are less than 4 hours.

In vivo Testing of Antimalarial Drug Efficacy

The World Health Organization now recommends that antimalarial drug treatment policy should aim for cure rates of at least 95% and that there should be consideration of policy change if failure rates exceed 10%. Frequent assessment of antimalarial drug efficacy is therefore needed to monitor antimalarial drug resistance and inform policy. In comparative studies, the groups should reflect the population affected by malaria. Too many trials have been conducted in older children or adults in highly endemic areas. These groups have significant background immunity, little or no symptoms and a high rate of self-cure. Drug efficacy is therefore overestimated. The analysis should be age stratified if there is a wide age range included in the study. It is very important that patients, parents or guardians truly understand that participation in a drug trial is voluntary and give informed consent. Ideally pre-treatment with another antimalarial drug is an exclusion criterion, but in some areas this is very common, in which case, such patients should be included provided details are taken and preferably a baseline blood level is taken.

Design of Trials

An adequate sample size is required. For example with a sample size of 60 studied patients and six treatment failures, the 95% confidence interval around the 90% cure rate is 82.4–97.6%. This study is too small as it leaves too much uncertainty as to the true cure rate in the population. In the past antimalarial drug trials have been powered to detect differences between drugs – usually with 95% confidence and 80% power. This is a 'superiority' trial. But conducting such trials is increasingly difficult with cure rates over 90% (as they should be) because of the exponential increase in the sample size required. The higher the standard treatment's cure rate, the more difficult it is to demonstrate conclusively a small difference in favour of a new treatment. An alternative approach is the non-inferiority trial which aims to show that an experimental treatment is 'not worse' than the active control (i.e. current treatment) by more than a specified amount – the equivalence margin (often denoted δ). The null hypothesis being tested is that there *is* a difference between the two groups (i.e. it is the opposite to that in conventional superiority trials) and it is greater than the δ. The main limitation is that confounders introduced in a poorly conducted trial which affect both groups and are unrelated to differences in the efficacy (or toxicity) of the trial regimens, can obscure significant differences. In a superiority trial this might lead to a failure to disprove the null hypothesis – i.e. failure to show difference – but in a non-inferiority trial the direction is opposite; a false rejection of the null hypothesis and conclusion of non-inferiority. This emphasizes the importance in antimalarial drug trials of avoiding errors in drug allocation and administration, poor adherence, errors in end-point ascertainment (for antimalarial efficacy this refers particularly to identification of recrudescence) and loss to follow-up.

Blinding is often used to avoid bias in comparative trials although it is often difficult in antimalarial drug assessments because of differences in treatment regimens and the difficulties in masking the taste of the drugs. Compared with superiority trials, blinding does not protect against bias as well in non-inferiority trials because a biased investigator wishing to show non-inferiority can simply give all patients similar results! Analysis of non-inferiority trials requires a calculation of the difference between the failures rates in the treatment groups and a calculation of the confidence interval around this difference using appropriate methods and 'effective' sample sizes.

In antimalarial drug trials, data should be entered on a case record form. Baseline clinical and demographic details should be recorded and, at a minimum, the parasitaemia counted and haemotocrit measured. In well-equipped sites, parasite culture to correlate the in vivo response with in vitro susceptibility can also be performed. A baseline whole blood sample (or blood spot on filter paper) should be stored for parasite genotyping. Molecular typing of *Plasmodium falciparum* (usually by assessment of size polymorphisms in fragments of the genes encoding MSP1, MSP2 and GLURP) has considerably improved the accuracy of drug trials conducted in endemic areas. The genotype(s) of infections recurring within the follow-up period is compared with those in the initial isolate. If the same genotype is found the infection is considered a recrudescence (i.e. a treatment failure). A different genotype indicates a newly acquired infection. The method is not foolproof; genotypes may be difficult to ascribe in mixed infections (which are usual in high transmission settings) and resistant infections might be subpatent on admission and therefore be considered erroneously as a new infection when they subsequently recrudesce. But genotyping is a considerable advance which allows community-based studies to be conducted in endemic areas. For studies of slowly eliminated drugs, taking a blood level measurement at day 7 in all patients helps to interpret treatment failures (i.e. whether they resulted from drug resistance or low blood concentrations). For many drugs, simple filter paper whole blood assays are now available.

Antimalarial treatment should be observed and adverse effects recorded. The patients should be followed daily until parasite clearance, then at weekly intervals. The rate of resolution of anaemia is a sensitive measure of the treatment response. The haemoglobin or haematocrit should be measured each time a parasite count is performed in therapeutic assessments. Four weeks is the minimum follow-up duration for rapidly eliminated drugs and 6 weeks is the minimum for drugs with intermediate or long terminal elimination half-lives. At least 90% follow-up at 4 weeks should be aimed for and sample sizes adjusted for likely 'drop-out' rates. The appearance of *P. vivax*, *P. malariae* or *P. ovale* malaria requires chloroquine treatment. Whether such patients should be excluded from the analysis in a *falciparum* malarial trial depends on the level of chloroquine resistance in *P. falciparum* and needs to be decided before the trial.

Interpretation of Trials

In antimalarial drug trials two or more groups of patients are followed for a prespecified time after different antimalarial treatments. The cure rates, which means the proportions of patients who reach the end of this follow-up period without recrudescence of the infection, are compared. In the past, antimalarial treatment efficacy was usually assessed on a particular day (often day 14 or day 28 after starting treatment), so only patients followed to that day were included in the analysis. This is often referred as a *'per-protocol' (PP) analysis*. But in most trials, there are patients who do not complete the follow-up period, yet these patients do contribute useful information before they leave the trial and this can and should be used. If such a patient did not fail (i.e. remained aparasitaemic) when last observed, that patient's data are said to be 'censored' at the time they were last followed up. The appropriate analysis for such data is *survival analysis* which deals explicitly with censored values. Patients with different follow-up periods cannot be treated the same way – someone who is followed-up for longer has a greater chance of being recorded as treatment failure than another patient followed up for a shorter time. Failure rates should be estimated using the Kaplan–Meier method. This is now endorsed by the recent WHO recommendations for antimalarial resistance monitoring which suggest use of life tables (i.e. survival analysis) in analysing in vivo studies. The *'intention to treat' (ITT) analysis* which includes all missing patients or indeterminate values as treatment failures should be reported also, but it should not be the primary endpoint of a study as it overestimates the true failure rates.

Severe Malaria Trials

In addition to parasite and fever clearance the rate of clinical recovery in survivors should be assessed. In unconscious children the Blantyre Coma Scale (BCS) is most widely used and in adults the Glasgow Coma Score (GCS) should be measured. If possible these should be assessed 4–6-hourly and the times to reach BCS scores of 3, 4 and 5 and GCS scores of 8, 11 and 15 recorded. The time to drink, sit, walk and leave hospital should also be documented. The changes in venous lactate, venous bicarbonate and plasma or serum urea or creatinine can also be followed and used as measures of the therapeutic response.

In Vitro Antimalarial Drug Susceptibility Testing

Both in vivo and in vitro assessments of antimalarial efficacy are needed to guide treatment recommendations and planning of policy. *P. falciparum* can be cultured relatively easily in vitro, whereas the other malaria parasites are more difficult to grow ex vivo. Short-term culture of *P. falciparum* over one cycle requires only simple sterile culture media, a candle jar and an incubator. Short-term culture of *P. vivax* is also relatively easy with modifications to the conditions. Antimalarial drug susceptibility can be tested by measuring the inhibition by different concentrations drugs of parasite maturation to the schizont stage, the degree of inhibition of radio-labelled ^{3}H-hypoxanthine uptake or sybr green nucleic acid staining, or the synthesis of parasite-specific lactate dehydrogenase or histidine-rich protein 2. The PfLDH and PfHRP2 tests require only an ELISA reader and have the additional advantage of being possible at low parasite densities. These are useful epidemiological tools, but they do not predict the clinical response to treatment in an individual because they do not reflect differences between people in antimalarial pharmacokinetics, immunity or stage of disease.

Patient Management

In many tropical countries 'malaria' is synonymous with 'fever'. Antimalarial drugs are self-administered on a vast scale. Where possible, a definite species diagnosis should be obtained by microscopy examination of the blood smear or use of a suitable rapid antigen-based diagnostic test (RDT). If there is any doubt, *Plasmodium falciparum* infection should be assumed. The management of malaria depends very much on the health facilities available and the endemicity of disease, i.e. the likely immune status of the patient. For example, in areas of intense transmission infants and young children are often parasitaemic. Distinguishing malaria from other infections as the cause of fever may be difficult or impossible and so all febrile parasitaemic children must be treated for malaria unless there is an evident alternative diagnosis. In these settings asymptomatic parasitaemia is also common in older children and adults, but in these age groups fever is more likely to be the result of some other infection. On the other hand fever may precede detectable parasitaemia in non-immune adults or young children. The blood film should be rechecked in suspected cases. 'Blood smear-negative malaria' is a common diagnosis in the tropics – but one to be avoided. Other infections are more likely. If the patient has a sub-patent parasitaemia and no signs of severity it is safe to wait, seek other causes for the symptoms and repeat the blood smears at 12–24-hour intervals. In severely ill patients antimalarial treatment should be started immediately in full doses, but other diagnoses sought. Patients may remain unconscious or develop renal failure after parasite clearance, but there is usually a clear history of previous treatment and malaria pigment may still be found in monocytes in peripheral blood or intradermal smears and the *Pf*HRP2 dipstick will be positive. If the temperature is high on admission (>38.5°C) then symptomatic treatment with oral antipyretics (paracetamol, not aspirin) and tepid sponging brings symptomatic relief and may also reduce the likelihood that the patient vomits the oral antimalarials. This is particularly important for young children who are less likely to have a seizure and more likely to tolerate oral antimalarials when their temperature has been lowered and they are quiet and calm. Unfortunately, there are no paediatric formulations for some of the ACTs. For young children large pills should be crushed and given as a suspension in a small volume of sweet drink or milk when treating young children. A disposable syringe (*without* the needle!) may be used to draw up and give an accurate volume of the suspension into the child's mouth.

P. VIVAX, P. OVALE OR *P. MALARIAE*

Although *P. vivax*, *P. ovale* or *P. malariae* rarely kill, the disease can be moderately severe, requiring initial parenteral treatment. Occasional patients with *vivax* malaria do develop vital organ dysfunction and these should be treated as for severe *falciparum* malaria. More usually oral treatment with chloroquine (Table 43.11) leads to resolution of the fever within 2–3 days. The total dose is usually 25 mg base/kg. The initial dose is 10 mg base/kg and this is followed at 12-hour intervals with subsequent doses of 5 mg/kg or the dose is divided as 10, 10, 5 mg/kg on days 0, 1 and 2, respectively. ACTs are a highly effective alternative (with the exception of artesunate – SP in some areas). Resistance to SP is widespread and high-level resistance to chloroquine in *P. vivax* is now a significant problem on the island of New Guinea and in parts of Indonesia. These infections respond to piperaquine or mefloquine containing ACTs. *Plasmodium vivax* responds to antimalarial drugs similarly to *Plasmodium falciparum*. After screening for G6PD deficiency a full radical course of primaquine should be given to all patients with *P. vivax* or *P. ovale* to prevent relapse. The incidence of relapse varies considerably by geographic region and transmission intensity. The efficacy in preventing relapse is determined by the total dose of primaquine taken. The 5-day regimens widely used on the Indian subcontinent were insufficient. The recommended dose is 0.5 mg base/kg per day for 14 days although the lower dose of 0.25 mg base/kg per day is reliably effective against long latency temperate strains. Primaquine is often considered unnecessary if the patient is going to return immediately to a highly endemic area, although the risk–benefit assessment for use in children in Asia (where G6PD deficiency is common) has not been made. Primaquine should not be given to pregnant or lactating women or infants or patients with known severe variants of G6PD deficiency. If mild variants of G6PD deficiency are known or likely then primaquine can be given in a dose of 0.75 mg/kg (45 mg) once weekly for 8 weeks. Primaquine does have significant activity against the asexual blood stages of *P. vivax* and this may mask chloroquine resistance in combined treatment, but may also protect against chloroquine resistance in areas with sensitive parasites.

P. KNOWLESI MALARIA

This should be treated in the same way as acute *falciparum* malaria with ACTs or artesunate for severe malaria. *P. knowlesi* is sensitive to chloroquine.

P. FALCIPARUM MALARIA

In endemic areas uncomplicated *falciparum* malaria is treated on an outpatient basis in the same way as the other malarias. In temperate countries imported cases should usually be hospitalized. The choice of drugs will depend on the local pattern of resistance where the infection was acquired. Because of the propensity for *P. falciparum* infections to kill, careful assessment of severity is most important. There is obviously a distribution of severity from asymptomatic parasitaemia to fulminant lethal malaria. In practice any patient who is unable to take oral medication will require parenteral treatment and careful observation and any impairment of consciousness should be treated seriously. The progression to cerebral malaria can be rapid, particularly in young children.

MANAGEMENT OF SEVERE *P. FALCIPARUM* MALARIA

Severe malaria is a medical emergency.[27] (See Table 43.13 for immediate clinical management.) The airway should be secured in unconscious patients, an intravenous infusion should be started and other resuscitation measures taken. A rapid clinical assessment of the degree of dehydration and the intravascular volume should be made. Vital signs and capillary refill time should be recorded. Particular attention should be paid to the respiratory pattern and any signs of respiratory distress (laboured deep breathing, flaring of the alar nasae, intercostal or substernal retraction) should be noted. The patient should be weighed or weight assessed so that the antimalarials can be given on a body weight basis (for adults, a simple method is for the stretcher-bearers to stand on bathroom scales with and without, the patient). Immediate measurements of blood glucose (stick test), haematocrit, parasitaemia (parasite count, stage of development and proportion of neutrophils containing malaria pigment) and renal function (blood urea or creatinine) should be taken. The degree of acidosis is an important determinant of outcome; the plasma bicarbonate or venous lactate should be measured if possible (lactate rapid stick tests are now available). Arterial or capillary blood pH and gases should be measured in patients who are unconscious, hyperventilating, or shocked. Blood should be taken for cross-match and later (if available) full blood count, platelet count, clotting studies, blood culture and full biochemistry. Parenteral antimalarial treatment should be given as soon as possible. Where there are adequate nursing facilities the antimalarial drugs should be given by intravenous infusion. There is no specific treatment for severe malaria other than antimalarial drugs. These are potentially life-saving and so it is very important that the dosing is correct (the first dose is by far the most important). Artesunate should be given by intravenous or intramuscular injection and artemether by intramuscular injection only. If quinine is used a full loading dose (20 mg dihydrochloride salt/kg) should be given to all patients unless there is a clear history of adequate pretreatment. Quinine is compatible with saline or dextrose solutions. It should *never* be given by bolus intravenous injection. In African children with severe malaria sepsis usually cannot be excluded reliably and so empirical broad-spectrum antibiotics should be given from the outset until a bacterial infection can be excluded.

The assessment of fluid balance is critical in severe malaria. In children there is not a consensus as to optimum fluid management. Some children are clearly 'dry 'on admission and need rehydration but rapid fluid loading has proved clearly harmful. Urgent blood transfusion is required for severely anaemic (haematocrit <15%) acidotic children, but the role of colloids otherwise remains controversial. In adults there is a thin dividing

TABLE 43.13 **Immediate Clinical Management of Severe Manifestations and Complications of Falciparum Malaria**

Manifestation/Complication	Immediate Management[a]
Coma (cerebral malaria)	Maintain airway, place patient on his or her side, exclude other treatable causes of coma (e.g. hypoglycaemia, bacterial meningitis); avoid harmful ancillary treatment such as corticosteroids, fluid loading, mannitol, heparin and adrenaline; intubate if necessary.
Hyperpyrexia	Administer tepid sponging, fanning, cooling blanket and antipyretic drugs.
Convulsions	Maintain airways; treat promptly with intravenous or rectal lorazepam, diazepam or intramuscular paraldehyde.
Hypoglycaemia (blood glucose concentration of <2.2 mmol/L)	Check blood glucose, correct hypoglycaemia and maintain with glucose-containing infusion.
Severe anaemia (haemoglobin <5 g/100 mL or packed cell volume <15%)	Transfuse with screened fresh whole blood.
Acute pulmonary oedema[b]	Prop patient up at an angle of 45°, give oxygen, give a diuretic, stop intravenous fluids, intubate and add positive end-expiratory pressure/continuous positive airway pressure if hypoxaemic
Acute kidney injury	Exclude pre-renal causes, check fluid balance and urinary sodium; if in established renal failure start haemofiltration or haemodialysis, or if unavailable, peritoneal dialysis. The benefits of diuretics/dopamine in acute renal failure are not proven.
Spontaneous bleeding and coagulopathy	Transfuse with screened fresh whole blood (cryoprecipitate, fresh frozen plasma and platelets if available); give vitamin K injection.
Metabolic acidosis	Exclude or treat hypoglycaemia, hypovolaemia and septicaemia. If severe start haemofiltration or haemodialysis.
Shock	Suspect septicaemia, take blood for cultures; give parenteral antimicrobials, correct haemodynamic disturbances.

[a]It is assumed that appropriate antimalarial treatment will have been started in all cases.
[b]Prevent by avoiding excess fluid administration.

line between overhydration which may precipitate pulmonary oedema and underhydration which may contribute to shock or precipitate or worsen acidosis and renal impairment. Careful and frequent evaluations of the jugular venous pressure, peripheral perfusion, venous filling, skin turgor and urine output should be made. Where there is uncertainty over the jugular venous pressure and if nursing facilities permit, a central venous catheter may be inserted and the pressure (CVP) measured directly and maintained between 0 and 5 cm. However, recent studies shows that the CVP correlates poorly with other haemodynamic indices and is thus a poor guide to fluid replacement. If the venous pressure is elevated (usually because of over-enthusiastic fluid administration) and the patient becomes breathless they should be nursed with the head at 45° and if necessary intravenous frusemide given. Acidotic breathing or respiratory distress, particularly in severely anaemic children may indicate hypovolaemia and requires prompt rehydration and, if available, urgent blood transfusion. Convulsions should be treated promptly with intravenous or rectal lorazepam (or if unavailable diazepam or midazolam) or intramuscular paraldehyde. The role of prophylactic anticonvulsants is unresolved (see below).

When these immediate measures have been completed a more detailed clinical examination should be conducted, with particular note of the level of consciousness and record of the coma score. Several coma scores have been advocated. The Glasgow Coma Scale (GCS) is suitable for adults and the simple Blantyre modification (BCS) is readily performed in children (Table 43.14). Unconscious patients must have a diagnostic lumbar puncture to exclude bacterial meningitis. The opening pressure should be recorded and the rise and fall with respiration noted. The CSF should be sent for microscopy examination, culture and measurement of glucose, lactate and protein. Subsequent clinical observations should be as frequent as possible and should include vital signs, with an accurate assessment of respiratory rate and pattern, assessment of the coma score and urine output. The blood glucose should be checked, using rapid stick tests every four hours if possible, until recovery of consciousness. These stick tests may overestimate the frequency of hypoglycaemia so laboratory confirmation may be necessary. Important milestones on the road to recovery are the time to recover consciousness (GCS 15 or BCS 5), time to drink and times to sit unaided and walk.

CEREBRAL MALARIA

When managing a patient who is unconscious with severe malaria, the physician must exclude, as far as possible, continuous seizure activity and hypoglycaemia as the cause. Both are more common in children than in adults. Many adjuvant therapies have been suggested, based on the prevailing pathophysiology hypotheses of the time. These include heparin, low-molecular-weight dextran, urea, high-dose corticosteroids, aspirin, prostacyclin, pentoxifylline (oxpentifylline), desferrioxamine, anti-TNF antibody, cyclosporine, hyperimmune serum, mannitol, albumin and saline fluid loading. Unfortunately none has proved to be beneficial and many have proved harmful. None of these adjuvants should be used. The cornerstone of management is good intensive care and prompt appropriate antimalarial treatment.

Prophylactic phenobarbitone prevents seizures in cerebral malaria. But the role of prophylactic anticonvulsants is uncertain since a large double-blind trial in Kenyan children with cerebral malaria (and no access to mechanical ventilation) showed a doubling of mortality in children receiving a single prophylactic intramuscular injection of phenobarbitone (20 mg/kg). Mortality was increased in children who received three or more doses of diazepam (i.e. had recurrent treated seizures), which suggests a possible interaction between these two drugs and points to respiratory depression as the lethal

TABLE 43.14 Coma Scales to Assess Levels of Consciousness in Adults and Children

The Blantyre Coma Scale for Children		The Modified Glasgow Coma Scale for Adults	
	Score[a]		Score[b]
BEST MOTOR RESPONSE		**BEST MOTOR RESPONSE**	
Localizes painful stimulus[c]	2	Obeys commands	5
Withdraws limb from pain[d]	1	Localizes pain	4
Nonspecific or absent response	0	Flexion to pain	3
		Extension to pain	2
		None	1
VERBAL RESPONSE[e]	2	**VERBAL RESPONSE**	
Appropriate cry	1	Oriented	5
Moan or inappropriate cry	0	Confused	4
None		Inappropriate words	3
		Incomprehensible sounds	2
		None	1
EYE MOVEMENTS		**EYE OPEN**	
Directed (e.g. follows mother's face)	1	Spontaneously	4
Not directed	0	To speech	3
		To pain	2
		Never	1

[a]Total score can range from 0 to 5; 2 or less indicates 'unrousable coma'.
[b]Total score can range from 3 to 14; 'Cerebral malaria defined by GCS <11; Unrousable coma' reflects a score of <9.
[c]Painful stimulus: rub knuckles on patient's sternum.
[d]Painful stimulus: firm pressure on thumbnail bed with horizontal pencil.
[e]Not readily assessed in preverbal children.

effect. Thus the standard loading dose of phenobarbitone is contraindicated unless the patient can be ventilated. Some physicians give a smaller dose of phenobarbitone in unconscious patients, others do not give any seizure prophylaxis and rely on treatment. The safety and effectiveness of phenytoin, fosphenytoin and other anticonvulsants is not well characterized. Although approximately 80% of children with cerebral malaria have moderately elevated pressures at lumbar puncture (whereas in adults 80% of pressures are in the normal range) and some children have very high pressures, use of the osmotic agent mannitol proved harmful in a recent trial conducted in adults. Those factors known to exacerbate raised intracranial pressure such as uncontrolled seizures and hypercapnoea should be treated promptly. Specific management includes care of the unconscious patient, careful fluid balance, rapid treatment of convulsions, treatment of hyperpyrexia and early detection and treatment of other manifestations or complications of severe malaria.

Hypoglycaemia should be suspected in any patient who deteriorates suddenly and this should be treated empirically if glucose stick tests are unavailable. Supervening bacterial infections are common, particularly chest infections and catheter-related urinary tract infections and spontaneous septicaemia may occur occasionally. Bacteraemia is much more common in African children than in adults or children studied in South-East Asia. There is undoubtedly diagnostic overlap between severe malaria and bacterial septicaemia with incidental parasitaemia, but there is also a genuine predisposition to septicaemia in severe malaria. If not already given empirical broad-spectrum antibiotics should be given to any patient who deteriorates suddenly and in whom hypoglycaemia has been excluded. Aspiration pneumonia commonly follows generalized seizures. Patients should be nursed on their sides and turned frequently. Most children will recover consciousness within 2 days and most adults within 3 days. Rarely adults may remain unconscious for as long as 10 days. With longer periods of coma complications such as pressure sores and secondary infections become increasingly likely.

FLUID BALANCE

Children with severe malaria may be dehydrated, but renal failure and pulmonary oedema are extremely unusual in young children. A common mistake is to be too cautious in giving blood to an anaemic acidotic child for fear of precipitating 'congestive failure'. Anaemic congestive failure is uncommon and that respiratory distress in these children represents metabolic acidosis not pulmonary oedema. The acidosis is aggravated by severe anaemia and sometimes hypovolaemia. However the concept that hypovolaemia is an important cause of death has been challenged by the clear demonstration that fluid loading with either crystalloid or colloid increases mortality. This argues for a more cautious approach to fluid resuscitation in children as well as adults. In approximately 50% of adults admitted with severe malaria there is evidence of renal impairment. In the majority of these there will be a transient period of oliguria, followed by uncomplicated recovery, but a minority will progress to established acute tubular necrosis. A polyuric phase is unusual. Adults with severe malaria are very vulnerable to fluid overload and the physician treads a narrow path between underhydration and thus worsening renal impairment and overhydration, with the risk of precipitating pulmonary oedema. Following admission patients should be rehydrated carefully with 0.9% (normal) saline or other isotonic electrolyte solutions. Thereafter the daily fluid requirements will depend on urine output (plus diarrhoea) and insensible losses, which can be considerable in febrile patients nursed in hot environments. Water and glucose are provided by 5% or 10% dextrose solutions. Hypoglycaemic patients will often require 10% dextrose infusions after a bolus glucose correction. It is not possible to generalize on initial fluid requirements as these can vary from deficits of several litres, to patients who are admitted oliguric and unconscious on a saline infusion and are well hydrated with a slightly elevated jugular venous pressure. Each patient's requirements should be assessed individually. If there is no CVP line it is well worth spending some time establishing clearly the level of the jugular venous pressure. If blood glucose is <4 mmol/L then 10% glucose should be started following saline replacement; if it is <2.2 mmol/L then hypoglycaemia should be treated immediately (0.3–0.5 g/kg of glucose). The fluid regimen must also be tailored around infusion of the antimalarial drugs. Artesunate and artemether are simple injections but quinine infusions must be rate-controlled. Some physicians prefer to put the 24-hour quinine maintenance dose in one 500 mL bottle of 0.9% saline or 5% dextrose water and infuse this at constant rate, while adjusting fluid balance as necessary through a separate piggy-backed line. It is rarely necessary to give potassium or other electrolyte supplements in the acute phase. Many patients will require blood transfusion. The exact criteria for transfusion will depend on blood availability, but in general if the haematocrit falls below 20% then blood should be given, although in high transmission settings this would necessitate too many transfusions. The lower threshold of 15% haematocrit is often used. In adults with severe malaria where there is a greater danger of precipitating pulmonary oedema, transfusion of packed cells may be indicated. In practice, if blood is allowed to sediment in a bag or bottle, only the cells can be given. If the patient is volume overloaded the transfusion should be stopped, or continued very slowly, adding frusemide (0.3 mg/kg) to each unit.

ACUTE KIDNEY INJURY

If the patient remains oliguric (<0.4 mL of urine/kg per hour) despite adequate rehydration and the blood urea or creatinine are rising or already high, then fluids should be restricted to replace insensible losses only. Dialysis or haemofiltration renal replacement therapies (RRT) should be started early when there is evidence of multiple organ dysfunction. There is no evidence that use of dopamine and loop diuretics prevents the progression of renal failure. Renal impairment is hypercatabolic in the acute phase of the disease and once conventional indications for RRT have been reached (i.e. metabolic acidosis, uraemic complications, volume overload, or less commonly hyperkalaemia) the patient may deteriorate quickly. An electrocardiogram should be performed if acute renal failure is suspected and an immediate blood potassium measurement is unavailable. If there are signs of hyperkalaemia (peaked T waves, widening of the QRS complex) then calcium and glucose plus insulin, should be given immediately. The tempo of disease is faster in patients with acute disease and multiple organ dysfunction and RRT should be started earlier than in those whose renal failure develops *after* other acute manifestations have resolved. Haemofiltration or haemodialysis are preferable to peritoneal dialysis. Haemofiltration is associated with a considerably more rapid resolution of biochemical abnormalities and a lower mortality than peritoneal dialysis. Despite the coagulopathy associated with severe malaria bleeding problems are unusual. After the initial outlay for the pumps and balance haemofiltration is also less expensive, although well-trained nursing care is essential. When there is no alternative to peritoneal dialysis the addition of hypertonic dextrose to the peritoneal dialysate can be used to remove excess fluid and also to provide glucose in hypoglycaemic cases. The efficiency of peritoneal dialysis often improves after the first 24 hours. Reduced peritoneal clearance is thought to be related to sequestration in the peritoneal microvasculature during the acute phase. Peritonitis (cloudy dialysis effluent) is relatively common if dialysis is continued for more than 72 hours. The dose of quinine should be reduced by between one-third and one-half on the 3rd day of treatment. Tetracycline is contraindicated, but doxycycline can still be given. The median time to recovery of urine flows (>20 mL/kg per 24 hours) is 4 days. The overall prognosis and rate of recovery is better in oliguric than in anuric cases (Figure 43.29).

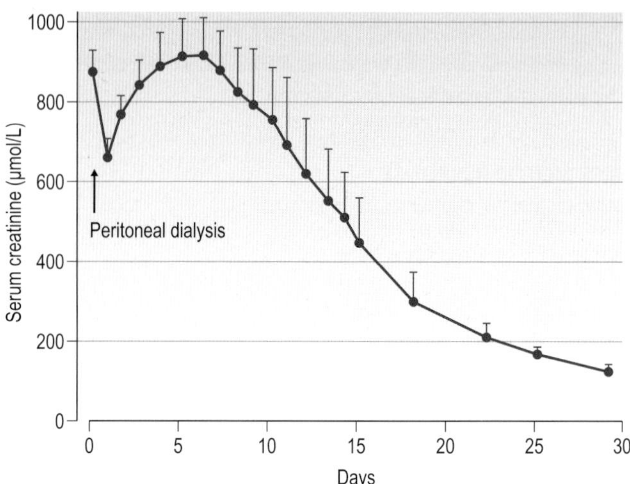

Figure 43.29 Recovery from malaria acute renal failure. This results from acute tubular necrosis. Many patients will not become oliguric, despite a rising serum creatinine in the first few days of hospitalization and can be managed conservatively. *(From Trang et al. Clin Infect Dis 1992;15:874–880.)*

Patients with blackwater fever should be managed in the same way as other patients. Parenteral antimalarial treatment should continue. The preventative or therapeutic role of urinary alkalinization has not been evaluated yet. Blood transfusion is often needed but the increase in haematocrit is often less than predicted because of the brisk haemolysis of the transfused cells. If the patient is volume overloaded, but needs blood, then dialysis or haemofiltration must be given first to create enough vascular 'space' for the blood. Packed cells should be given and the transfusion administered as slowly as possible.

ACUTE PULMONARY OEDEMA

This grave manifestation of severe malaria commonly co-exists with acute renal failure. The differential diagnosis includes pneumonia, if there are abnormal chest signs and metabolic acidosis, if the chest is clear. Frothing at the mouth does not necessarily mean acute pulmonary oedema. In children, it is often hypersalivation resulting from continuous seizures. Tachypnoea is a serious sign in malaria; occasionally it results from high fever alone, in which case breathing is shallow, but more usually there is noisy hyperventilation with use of accessory muscles of respiration, intercostal recession and flaring of the nostrils. Patients with acute pulmonary oedema should be nursed upright and given oxygen and the right-sided filling pressures should be reduced with whichever treatments are available (loop diuretics, opiates, venodilators, venesection, haemofiltration, dialysis). The right-sided pressure should be reduced to the lowest level compatible with an adequate cardiac output. Positive pressure ventilation should be started if the patient becomes hypoxic.

HYPOGLYCAEMIA

There should be a low threshold for suspecting hypoglycaemia. There may be no signs of hypoglycaemia in a patient already unconscious with cerebral malaria. Ideally, blood glucose should be checked 4-hourly while patients are unconscious. Hypoglycaemia should be treated by slow intravenous injection of 0.5–1 mL/kg of 50% dextrose water and prevented by administering a 10% dextrose infusion at 1–2 mg/kg per hour. Quinine-stimulated hyperinsulinaemia may be blocked by somatostatin or its synthetic analogue, if available (they seldom are!). If possible, serum potassium should be checked frequently in hypoglycaemic patients receiving quinine and hypertonic dextrose solutions.

ACIDOSIS

Hypovolaemia should be corrected although recent evidence suggest that this is not a major contributor to acidosis. The circulatory status is more difficult to assess in children than in adults. But in many cases the acidosis persists despite adequate blood pressure, adequate capillary refill and warm peripheries and normal jugular venous pressure. Although acidosis may result from acute renal failure, ketonaemia and even salicylate poisoning, in most cases lactic acidosis is a significant contributor to the wide anion gap. Venous, arterial and CSF concentrations of lactate rise in proportion to disease severity and in contrast to sepsis, they are associated with an increased lactate–pyruvate ratio (often >30) indicating anaerobic glycolysis. Lactic acid accumulation is buffered initially, but decompensation often occurs in severe malaria. The role of sodium bicarbonate in the treatment of metabolic acidosis has declined from established practice to the controversial. Now most authorities either do not give sodium bicarbonate at all, or give it once only in very severe acidosis (e.g. pH <7.15). The pyruvate dehydrogenase activator dichloroacetate has proved promising in preliminary clinical trials, but its role in treatment remains to be defined. Haemofiltration or haemodialysis may be used to control acidosis.

BLEEDING

Patients with cerebral malaria may have haematemesis or a bloody nasogastric aspirate because of acute gastric erosions. The incidence of upper gastrointestinal bleeding has declined since the discontinuation of high-dose corticosteroids in cerebral malaria. The role of prophylactic antacids, H2 blockers, sulfacrate or proton pump inhibitors has not been studied specifically in severe malaria. Less than 5% of patients with severe malaria develop clinically significant DIC. These patients should be given fresh blood transfusions and vitamin K.

BACTERIAL SUPERINFECTION/CONTINUED FEVER

The treatment of suspected septicaemia will depend on local antimicrobial susceptibility patterns, bearing in mind that *Salmonellae* may be implicated. Patients with secondary pneumonia should be given empirical treatment with a third-generation cephalosporin, unless admitted with clear evidence of aspiration, in which case penicillin or clindamycin is adequate. Children with persistent fever despite parasite clearance may also have a systemic *Salmonella* infection, although in the majority of cases of persistent fever after parasite clearance no other pathogen is identified. Urinary tract infections are common in catheterized patients. Antibiotic treatments should depend on likely local antibiotic sensitivity patterns. Sustained high fever in the acute phase of severe malaria is a poor prognostic sign. Continued fever after parasite clearance is common; antibiotic treatment is only indicated if the patient becomes severely ill or there is a definite focus of infection.

TREATMENT OF RECRUDESCENT INFECTIONS

Treatment failure within 14 days of receiving an ACT is very unusual. Thus the majority of treatment failures occur more than 2 weeks after treatment. In many cases failures are not recognized because patients presenting with malaria are not asked whether they have received antimalarial treatment within the preceding 1–2 months. Recurrence of malaria can be the result of a reinfection, a recrudescence (i.e. failure) or, a relapse malaria due to *P. vivax* and *P. ovale*, although relapses do not appear within 14 days of the primary infection. In an individual patient it is initially not possible to distinguish recrudescence from reinfection. Wherever possible, treatment failure must be confirmed parasitologically – preferably by blood slide examination, as the HRP2-based stick tests may remain positive for weeks after the initial infection even without recrudescence. Treatment failures may result from drug resistance, poor adherence or unusual pharmacokinetic properties in that individual. It is important to determine from the patient's history whether he or she vomited previous treatment or did not complete a full course. Recurrence of fever and parasitaemia more than 2 weeks after treatment (either recrudescence or new infection), can be retreated with the first-line ACT. If it is a recrudescence, then the first-line treatment should still be effective in most cases. This simplifies operational management and drug deployment. However, reuse of mefloquine within 28 days of first treatment is associated with an increased risk of neuropsychiatric sequelae and, in this particular case, second-line treatment should be given. If there is a further recurrence, then malaria should be confirmed parasitologically and second-line treatment given. The following second-line treatments are recommended by WHO, in order of preference:[34]

- Alternative ACT known to be effective in the region
- Artesunate plus tetracycline or doxycycline or clindamycin (7 days)
- Quinine plus tetracycline or doxycycline or clindamycin (7 days).

The alternative ACT has the advantages of simplicity, familiarity and, where available, coformulation to improve adherence. The 7-day quinine regimens are not well tolerated and adherence is likely to be poor if treatment is not observed.

Malaria in Pregnancy

SEVERE MALARIA

Pregnant women in the 2nd and 3rd trimesters are more likely to develop severe malaria than other adults, often complicated by pulmonary oedema and hypoglycaemia. Fetal death and premature labour are common. The role of early caesarean section for the viable live fetus is unproven, but recommended by many authorities. Obstetric advice should be sought at an early stage, the paediatricians alerted and the blood glucose checked frequently. Hypoglycaemia should be expected and is often recurrent if the patient is receiving quinine. Artesunate is safer and more effective. The antimalarial drugs should be given in full doses. Severe malaria may also present immediately following delivery. Postpartum bacterial infection is a common complication in these cases. *Falciparum* malaria has also been associated with severe mid-trimester haemolytic anaemia in Nigeria. This often requires transfusion, in addition to antimalarial treatment and folate supplementation.

UNCOMPLICATED MALARIA

Symptomatic malaria in pregnancy requires hospitalization where possible. Premature labour may occur and pregnant women receiving quinine are liable to develop hypoglycaemia. Chloroquine, pyrimethamine, proguanil, mefloquine, quinine and the sulphonamides are considered safe in pregnancy. Amodiaquine has been widely used but not well documented. The artemisinin derivatives are safe in the 2nd and 3rd trimesters, but there is still some uncertainty in the 1st trimester, where they are currently not recommended. There is increasing confidence in the safety of artemether-lumefantrine and some preliminary experience with atovaquone-proguanil and dihydroartemisinin-piperaquine indicating that these drugs are also safe. The tetracyclines and primaquine are contraindicated. As a consequence the five first-line ACTs are recommended for the treatment of *falciparum* malaria in the 2nd and 3rd trimesters. Quinine (10 mg salt/kg three times daily for 7 days) is still the treatment of choice for *falciparum* malaria in the 1st trimester but it is poorly tolerated and low adherence leads to high treatment failure rates. The artemisinin derivatives and quinine should both be combined with clindamycin (10 mg/kg twice daily) to increase cure rates. Treatment failure rates are higher in pregnant women than in non-pregnant adults for any antimalarial regimen. Pharmacokinetic studies indicate that blood concentrations of the artemisinin derivatives, lumefantrine, atovaquone and proguanil are all significantly reduced in late pregnancy, so current dose recommendations may not be optimal. Data on sulfadoxine-pyrimethamine are variable and both mefloquine and piperaquine pharmacokinetics are not significantly altered. Close follow-up of pregnant women is essential. Women in malarious areas should be encouraged to attend weekly antenatal clinics where blood smears and haematocrit can be checked, in addition to routine obstetric assessment.

Prevention

PROPHYLAXIS

If effective in the area and safe, antimalarial prophylaxis should be given during pregnancy. Chloroquine (5 mg base/kg per week) is generally still very effective in preventing *P. vivax*. *P. ovale* and *P. malariae*. Unfortunately, *P. falciparum* is usually present at the same time and nearly always resistant. In areas where *P. falciparum* is still sensitive to antifols daily proguanil (3.5 mg/kg per day) is safe and effective. There have been some concerns over mefloquine in treatment use, although there is no significant evidence of an increased stillbirth risk when used as prophylaxis. Primaquine and doxycycline are contraindicated. Preliminary evidence suggests that atovaquone-proguanil is safe.

INTERMITTENT PREVENTIVE TREATMENT (IPTp)

Studies conducted in high transmission areas of Africa have shown that administration of treatment doses of sulfadoxine-pyrimethamine (SP) two or three times during pregnancy was associated with reduced placental parasitization, reduced anaemia and increased birth weight. IPTp with SP has been increasingly adopted but since the original studies were conducted resistance has worsened considerably in Africa compromising efficacy. A review of available information suggests continuing efficacy in many areas but has led to revised recommendations that IPTp SP should be given more frequently (maximum monthly). Alternative drugs are under evaluation.

BREAST-FEEDING

Nearly all the antimalarial drugs appear in breast milk, but the actual amounts excreted are small. Primaquine should be avoided, pending further information, but otherwise there seems no reason to discourage breast-feeding in women receiving antimalarial drugs.

Malaria in Children

Although maternal malaria is very common, congenital malaria is surprisingly rare given the high frequency with which placental smears are positive in endemic areas and the not infrequent finding of parasites in cord blood smears. Nevertheless, it may occur with any of the four human malarias. Congenital *falciparum* malaria is seldom severe. Congenital *P. vivax* or *P. ovale* infections do not require radical treatment as there are no pre-erythrocytic stages in the baby.

Severe malaria is relatively uncommon in the first 6 months of life, although when it does occur the mortality is high. In young children malaria presents as a febrile illness without focal signs. In *P. falciparum* infections, convulsions are an important complication in the first 3 years. They are twice as common as in *P. vivax* malaria, despite similar fever profiles. The progression to cerebral malaria in young children can be very rapid. Recovery is also rapid compared with adults. In areas of intense transmission, severe anaemia in the 1–3-year age group is the principal manifestation of severe *falciparum* malaria and may also occur with repeated *vivax* infections. A comparison of the relative frequencies of complications in adults and children is shown in Table 43.15.

Children receive the brunt of malaria's assault on humans. Most of the deaths from malaria are in children and most of those are in Africa. Malaria is also an important cause of morbidity, failure to thrive and probably increased susceptibility to other infections. Whether cerebral malaria, malaria-associated convulsions, or the debilitating effects of repeated weakening febrile illnesses and anaemia cause developmental or intellectual retardation needs to be determined. There is evidence for learning difficulties in children who have had seizures in malaria and in cerebral malaria survivors. In general children tolerate the antimalarial drugs better than adults. In severe malaria fluid

TABLE 43.15 Relative Incidence of Severe Falciparum Malaria Complications

	Non-Pregnant Adults	Pregnant Women	Children
Anaemia	+	++	+++
Convulsions	+	+	+++
Hypoglycaemia	+	+++	+++
Jaundice	+++	+++	+
Renal failure[a]	+++	+++	–
Pulmonary oedema	++	+++	±

[a]Requiring renal replacement. Elevated blood urea common in children with severe malaria.

balance is also easier as renal failure is very unusual. However, the difficulties of providing adequate nursing in the tropics, of obtaining intravenous access and the small volumes of intravenous fluid required often mean that antimalarial drugs are given by the intramuscular or suppository routes. Children may deteriorate very rapidly in severe malaria. Sudden death is common in cerebral malaria but, if the child survives, recovery is more rapid than in adults. Iron deficiency is common in tropical countries, protects against malaria, yet commonly coexists with malaria. In general, the benefits of iron supplementation in iron deficiency, both on short-term anaemia and long-term neurocognitive development, outweigh the risks. Routine iron supplementation has not been recommended following the results of a large carefully controlled study from Pemba, Tanzania in which the risks of death or severe illness of providing routine iron plus folic acid supplementation (in doses similar to those recommended by WHO) to young children exposed to high rates of malaria infection outweighed any immediate benefits.[37] However these conclusions have been disputed and this remains a controversial area.

Malaria with Limited Resources

Many patients with malaria are either untreated or treated inadequately by self-medication. In many countries the private sector is the main source of antimalarial treatment. Fake or substandard drugs are common and incomplete treatment courses are often sold. Education of the public and the private commercial vendors is vitally important. Coherent and efficient schemes for the purchase and distribution of quality-assured drugs are needed. In order to slow the pace of antimalarial resistance it is essential that whoever gives antimalarial treatment (parent, relative, village health worker, shop assistant) ensures a full course of treatment is administered.

Most patients with severe malaria are not admitted to hospital; they are treated at home or at rural health clinics. Most deaths from malaria occur in or near home. Where intravenous infusions cannot be given, intramuscular administration is acceptable for quinine or the artemisinin derivatives. It is essential that sterile technique is adhered to fully. Artesunate suppositories are simple and effective alternatives to parenteral administration and as a pre-referral treatment they have been shown to reduce the mortality of children (under 5 years) with malaria who cannot take oral medication by 25%.Where injections or suppositories are not possible then oral, or, if a tube is available, nasogastric instillation should be attempted, pending transfer of the patient.

Prevention

INSECTICIDE-TREATED BED NETS

The chances of being bitten by a malaria-infected female *anopheline* mosquito can be reduced considerably by simple measures. Covering exposed skin surfaces and remaining indoors or under a net at peak biting times will obviously reduce exposure. For example, most mosquitoes feed at night so sleeping indoors under insecticide (permethrin, deltamethrin)-treated bed nets reduces morbidity and mortality in malarious areas. A single impregnation of a cotton or nylon mosquito net will provide protection for 1 year. Nylon tends to retain permethrin and deltamethrin better than cotton. The impregnated bed nets (ITN) can be washed and can tolerate small tears or holes without markedly reducing the protective effects. Now 'long-lasting impregnated nets' (LLIN) have been developed which retain insecticidal activity for many years. These are more expensive but may be cost-effective. At the time of writing four types of LLINs have full endorsement and nine have interim endorsement by the WHO Pesticide Evaluation Scheme. The benefits conferred by bed-nets depend greatly on the biting habits of the mosquito, the size and constitution of the nets, whether they are impregnated with insecticide, the number of nets being used in the village and a variety of sociological factors that determine actual use of the nets in practice. The much lower protective efficacy of unimpregnated bed-nets is variable and depends very much on the way in which they are used (Do they have holes? Are they tucked under the mattress?, etc.). These considerations are relatively unimportant for ITNs. Many ITN studies have been conducted and these give an overall estimated all-cause child mortality reduction of 20% for their use in Africa. As a consequence many countries have taken up ITN programmes as an important component of their antimalarial strategy. In recent years, the proportion of people who sleep under an ITN has risen substantially with increased subsidized deployment. Currently 289 million LLINs have been deployed in sub-Saharan Africa, enough to cover 76% of the 765 million people at risk of malaria. Impregnation of household curtains, hammocks, clothing, or even cattle has been shown to reduce malaria. It has been assumed that ITNs work mainly through personal protection, but their mass insecticidal effect may be more important in some contexts. Thus the protection afforded by sleeping without a net in a village where ITNs are used extensively, may be greater than sleeping under an ITN in a village where no-one else uses them.

Impregnated nets are effective throughout Africa but do not work in some areas (notably parts of South-east Asia), because of different human and mosquito behaviour. Obviously if malaria is contracted by vectors which bite in the early evening or early morning away from human habitation then ITNs are not going to be very effective.

REPELLENTS

Other simple preventive measures, including the application of permethrin or deltamethrin to clothing or the use of insect repellents such as diethyltoluamide (DEET) on exposed skin surfaces, are also effective and need not be prohibitively expensive. DEET is generally very safe, including in pregnancy. Coconut oil and DEET 'soap bar' preparations are available which are cheap, stable and readily applied. Houses can be mosquito-proofed by using wire-mesh grilles over windows and designed in such a way as to discourage mosquito ingress. All these measures reduce the chances of an infection, but they do not eliminate it.

CHEMOPROPHYLAXIS

Although the early colonists devised many ingenious methods of taking quinine regularly (including 'Indian tonic water'), they were generally neither pleasant nor fully effective. Quinine (a poor prophylactic) was relied upon by armies and colonists until after the Great War. The subsequent discovery of mepacrine (quinacrine, atebrine) in 1934 gave the militaries an efficacious, albeit rather toxic, prophylactic which prevented malaria effectively during the Second World War. However, it was the introduction of chloroquine, the antimalarial biguanides and subsequently pyrimethamine after the war, that finally brought safe and effective antimalarial prophylaxis. The DHFR inhibitors (pyrimethamine, proguanil, chlorproguanil), primaquine and atovaquone all inhibit parasite development in the liver (pre-erythrocytic activity). They are sometimes called causal prophylactics. Chloroquine and mefloquine inhibit asexual blood-stage development but they do not prevent development of the liver stages. Thus the parasites emerge from the liver but cannot multiply in the red cells. Drugs with this action are called suppressive prophylactics. These drugs also have gametocytocidal activity against *P. vivax*, *P. malariae* and *P. ovale*, but not *P. falciparum*. Atovaquone–proguanil, doxycycline and primaquine have been added to the list of antimalarial prophylactics. Each is active against resistant *P. falciparum* but each must be taken daily. Antimalarial prophylaxis must be taken regularly to ensure therapeutic (i.e. suppressive) antimalarial concentrations are maintained. Recommendations vary considerably depending on risk, prevalence and drug resistance. Up-to-date recommendations are easily obtained on the internet (see, e.g.: http://www.who.int). Increasing drug resistance in recent years has meant that many prophylactic drugs can no longer be relied upon, particularly in areas of multiple drug resistance such as South-east Asia and South America.

The recommended prophylactic drug regimens are shown in Table 43.16. When prescribing antimalarial prophylaxis to travellers, it is important to emphasize that no antimalarial is completely effective and that a febrile illness could still be malaria. It is essential that prophylaxis is taken regularly and for most drugs continued for 4 weeks after leaving the transmission area. The need to take the drugs for a month after leaving the transmission area is to 'catch' any parasites acquired shortly before departure when they leave the liver. But drugs acting on the liver stages (atovaquone-proguanil, primaquine) can be stopped immediately. This is a particular advantage for travellers visiting a malarious area for a short time. It is prudent to begin prophylaxis 1 week before departing for a malarious area so that tolerbility to the drug regimen can be assessed and therapeutic concentrations are present on arrival. In anglophone countries, chloroquine is prescribed weekly, but in francophone countries it is given once daily (this is theoretically preferable). Mefloquine and pyrimethamine-dapsone are taken once a week and proguanil, atovaquone-proguanil, primaquine and doxycycline daily. Amodiaquine, quinine, sulfadoxine-pyrimethamine and the artemisinin drugs should not be used for prophylaxis.

In situations where the risk of infection is low, or there are no effective antimalarials available, or there is brief repeated exposure to intermediate or high transmission (e.g. aircrews), travellers can be advised to carry a treatment course of antimalarial drugs with them. If they become ill and there are no medical facilities for malaria diagnosis and treatment, the treatment course is self-administered.

TABLE 43.16 Antimalarial Chemoprophylaxis[a]

	Weight Adjusted Dose for Children	Adult Dose
CHLOROQUINE-SENSITIVE MALARIA		
Chloroquine[b]	5 mg base/kg weekly *or*	300 mg base
	1.6 mg base/kg daily	100 mg base
and/or		
Proguanil	3.5 mg/kg daily	200 mg base
CHLOROQUINE-RESISTANT MALARIA		
Mefloquine[c]	5 base/kg/weekly	250 mg base
or		
Doxycycline[d]	1.5 mg/kg daily	100 mg
or		
Primaquine	0.5 mg base/kg daily with food	30 mg base
or		
Atovaquone-proguanil	4/1.6 mg/kg daily	250/100 mg

For current World Health Organization recommendations, see http://www.who.int.

[a]Detailed local knowledge of *P. falciparum* antimalarial drug susceptibility and malaria risk should always be obtained.

[b]Chloroquine should not be taken by people with a history of seizures, generalized psoriasis or pruritus previously on chloroquine.

[c]Mefloquine is not recommended for babies <3 months of age. Mefloquine should not be taken by people with psychiatric disorders, epilepsy, or those driving heavy vehicles, trains, aeroplanes, etc. or deep-sea diving.

[d]Doxycycline may cause photosensitivity. Use of sunscreens is recommended.

The use of antimalarial prophylaxis by the inhabitants of malarious areas remains controversial. It is generally agreed that pregnant women should take antimalarial prophylaxis if there is a significant risk of malaria, but that other adults should not. Chloroquine, pyrimethamine and proguanil are all considered safe in pregnancy, but are now largely ineffective against *P. falciparum*. Mefloquine is now considered safe. Tetracyclines and primaquine are contraindicated in pregnancy and atovaquone-proguanil has not been evaluated sufficiently. The use of antimalarial prophylaxis by children living in an endemic area has been shown to reduce mortality; in The Gambia administration of pyrimethamine and dapsone (Maloprim) in the 1–4-year age group reduced mortality by 25%. Despite the reduction in mortality, a reduction in the incidence of clinical attacks of malaria and anaemia, improved nutrition and, in older children, a decrease in absenteeism from school, this practice has not been generally adopted, largely because of concerns that widespread deployment of chemoprophylaxis would encourage the spread of drug-resistant parasites and/or inhibit the development of naturally acquired immunity to malaria.

INTERMITTENT PRESUMPTIVE TREATMENT IN INFANCY (IPT_I) AND CHILDHOOD (IPT_C)

Following the success of IPT in pregnancy, the strategy of providing a treatment dose of antimalarials to all infants in high transmission settings at the time of EPI immunizations (given at 2, 3 and 9 months of age) was developed. The two drugs evaluated mainly have been SP and amodiaquine. The main benefit demonstrated has been a reduction in the incidence of clinical attacks of malaria and anaemia. The protection is for approximately once a month after administration so it is incomplete with current regimens. The evidence whether protection extends to the second year of life as once claimed is conflicting. This is important as the majority of deaths occur after the first year of life. The benefits have been greatest in areas of high stable transmission. Predictably the benefits have been lower in areas of lower seasonal transmission where the major impact of malaria is after the first year of life, but studies in such areas (Senegal and Mali) showed that IPT given to older children during the malaria transmission season was remarkably effective in preventing malaria. Use of chemoprevention in older children is likely to be most effective in areas where a high level of malaria transmission is concentrated in a short period of the year. This has now been demonstrated conclusively and monthly administration of amodiaquine and sulphadoxine-pyrimethamine (seasonal malaria chemoprevention: SMC) is now recommended during the 3–4 rainy season months across the Sahel.[38] It is estimated that in areas suitable for SMC, there are 39 million children under 5 years of age, who experience 33.7 million malaria episodes and 152 000 childhood deaths from malaria each year. Tens of thousands of deaths can therefore be prevented using effective SMC. Obviously widescale use of prophylaxis, IPT or SMC will encourage the selection of resistance, although modelling studies to date are moderately reassuring. Another concern is that highly effective interventions such as prophylaxis together with ITN deployment might so reduce exposure that the acquisition of effective immunity was delayed, thereby increasing vulnerability to severe malaria at an older age. Again the available evidence is reassuring, but more information is needed on these important issues.

ADVERSE EFFECTS OF CHEMOPROPHYLAXIS

Adverse effects are a very important determinant of adherence to antimalarial prophylaxis regimens. As those taking the drugs prophylactically are healthy subjects, their tolerance of adverse effects is much lower than in treatment of malaria (where the patient often ascribes side-effects to the disease and takes the drugs only for a brief period). About 20% of patients taking prophylactic antimalarial drugs report some adverse effects. These are usually minor and do not require a change in prophylaxis. Nausea is the most common side effect. Chloroquine causes pruritus in dark-skinned subjects. Dizziness, dysphoria and sleep disturbances are particularly associated with mefloquine, visual disturbances with chloroquine, and photosensitivity and monilia with doxycycline. The risks of neuropsychiatric reactions or seizures are approximately 1 : 10 000 and appear similar for mefloquine and chloroquine. There has been much televised publicity over the CNS adverse effects of mefloquine. Minor, but debilitating, CNS effects are reported more commonly in travellers taking mefloquine than in other groups of subjects. Mefloquine prophylaxis should not be offered to subjects with epilepsy, psychiatric disorders, or to subjects in whom any CNS disturbances could have disastrous consequences such as pilots, coach drivers etc. Primaquine (0.5 mg/kg per day) is well tolerated if taken with food. It should not be given to subjects who are G6PD deficient or who are pregnant. On an empty stomach primaquine (0.5 mg base/kg) causes abdominal discomfort. Atovaquone-proguanil is remarkably well tolerated (similar adverse effects to proguanil alone) and highly effective.

Progress Towards a Malaria Vaccine

There are no vaccines for parasitic diseases of humans. Despite considerable effort and expense (worldwide funding has run at US$70–100 million/year), a generally available and highly effective malaria vaccine is still unlikely in the near future. The original goals of a vaccine producing sterile immunity (like the polio or yellow fever vaccines) without natural boosting are now considered unrealistic. The path of vaccine development has proved long and strewn with pitfalls, but there has been progress. Research has concentrated on all stages of the parasite life cycle: the sporozoite, the liver stage, the asexual blood stage and the gametocyte. Vaccines directed against the sporozoites and pre-erythrocytic liver stage are most advanced. The most effective vaccine produced to date was produced 40 years ago and consisted of irradiated sporozoites. This approach has been reactivated and an irradiated sporozoite vaccine is under development. Indeed there are numerous vaccines in various stages of development. By far the leading synthetic candidate, the result of 20 years development, is called RTS,S.[39] The RTS,S/AS01 vaccine is a hybrid construct of the hepatitis B surface antigen fused with a recombinant antigen derived from part of the circumsporozoite protein (the protein coat of the sporozoite). Keys to the success of the vaccine are the immunogenic polymeric nature of RTS,S particles and the proprietary adjuvant AS01. In the first large double-blind efficacy trial conducted in Mozambique, about 2000 children one to 4 years of age were assigned to receive 3 doses of either RTS,S or a control vaccine. The primary end point was the time to the first episode of symptomatic *P. falciparum* malaria during a 6-month surveillance period; the vaccine's efficacy in preventing clinical malaria was 29.9%. Of the 745 children in the RTS,S group 11 had at least one severe episode of malaria, compared with 26 of 745 children in the control group, a 58% protection against severe disease. However, the target population is younger children. In a large, multicentre phase 3 trial of RTS,S/AS01 15 460 children in two age categories: 6–12 weeks and 5–17 months – were enrolled. In the older group vaccine efficacy was 56% against all clinical malaria infections and 47% against severe malaria during a 12-month follow-up period. In the younger group vaccine efficacy against clinical malaria assessed in 6537 infants was 31% in the per-protocol population and efficacy against severe malaria was 26% in the intention-to-treat population.[38] Decisions on whether to deploy this vaccine are expected in 2015. For the development of a blood-stage vaccine, work has concentrated on the different merozoite surface antigens (MSP1, MSP2, MSP3), the ring-infected erythrocyte surface antigen (RESA) and, to a lesser extent, proteins associated with the rhoptries and the parasitophorous vacuole. Transmission blocking vaccines directed against *P. falciparum* gametocytes and vaccines against *P. vivax* sporozoite are also under development.

Chronic Complications of Malaria

Malaria is a major cause of chronic ill health in the tropics, particularly in childhood. Repeated attacks of malaria cause anaemia, failure to thrive and probably also contribute to vulnerability to other infections and retard educational development. Chronic malaria is associated with certain specific syndromes.

QUARTAN NEPHROPATHY

The nephrotic syndrome, with albuminuria, hypoalbuminaemia, oedema and variable renal impairment, is common in the tropics. Repeated or continuous *P. malariae* infection is associated with childhood nephrotic syndrome in West Africa and Papua New Guinea. In the past, quartan nephropathy was also described in eastern Asia. It has disappeared from countries where *P. malariae* has been eradicated, such as Guyana, where Giglioli first described the relationship between malaria and nephrosis. This strong epidemiological association has been supported by pathological studies, although it is not known why certain individuals develop quartan nephropathy whereas the majority of those infected with *P. malariae* do not. The other species of malaria are also suspected of causing occasional glomerulonephritis, but the evidence is less convincing than for *P. malariae*.

Pathology

Quartan nephropathy is a chronic soluble immune complex nephropathy. Renal biopsy reveals a variety of abnormalities. There is commonly thickening of the subendothelial aspect of the basement membrane, giving rise to a double contour of argyrophilic fibrils. The changes are segmental initially. The capillary lumens narrow and become obliterated. On electron microscopy the basement membrane is irregularly thickened with lacunae of electron-dense material. Immunofluorescent study shows IgG and IgM along the capillary walls. In two-thirds of cases this is accompanied by C3 and other complement components. Coarse granular deposits with IgG3 are more common than fine granular or linear staining, which is more associated with IgG2 and a poor response to cytotoxic therapy. In acute disease *P. malariae* antigens are demonstrable in approximately one-third of cases, but these are not evident in long-standing nephrosis. The severity of the glomerulonephritis is usually graded: <30% glomeruli involved, grade I; 30–75% glomeruli involved + tubular atrophy, grade II; and >75% of glomeruli involved, with extensive tubular pathology, grade III. Very occasionally, adults develop a proliferative glomerulonephritis. This is not seen in children.

Clinical Features

The pattern of renal involvement varies from asymptomatic proteinuria to full-blown nephrotic syndrome. Oedema, ascites or pleural effusions are usual presenting features. Anaemia and hepatosplenomegaly are common and many patients have fever on admission. The blood pressure is usually normal; the urinary sediment may show granular or hyaline casts in addition to proteinuria, but haematuria or red cell casts are rare. The disease usually progresses inexorably to renal failure over 3–5 years. Spontaneous remission is rare. Antimalarial treatment does not prevent progression and corticosteroids are usually ineffective. Some cases respond to cytotoxic therapy.

HYPER-REACTIVE MALARIAL SPLENOMEGALY

This is also known as the tropical splenomegaly syndrome. It occurs where transmission of malaria is intense and has been reported throughout the tropics. The highest incidence of hyper-reactive malarial splenomegaly (HMS) yet reported is in the Upper Watut Valley of Papua New Guinea, where 80% of adults and older children have large spleens. Genetic factors undoubtedly also play a role because within a malarious area the geographical distribution of HMS does not follow closely that of malaria transmission. In Ghana, 1st-degree relatives have a four times higher incidence of HMS than age- and location-matched controls.

Pathology

There is gross splenomegaly with normal architecture and lymphocytic infiltration of the hepatic sinusoids with Kupffer cell hyperplasia. The massively enlarged spleen leads to hypersplenism with anaemia, leukopenia and thrombocytopenia. There is polyclonal hypergammaglobulinaemia with high serum concentrations of IgM. High titres of malaria antibodies and a variety of autoantibodies (antinuclear factor, rheumatoid factor) are usually present. The hypergammaglobulinaemia is believed to result from polyclonal B-cell activation in the absence of adequate numbers of CD8+ suppressor T-cells, which have been removed by an antibody-dependent cytotoxic mechanism. Cell-mediated immune responses are otherwise normal. Immunoglobulin gene rearrangements have been demonstrated in a sub-group of patients with HMS. This indicates clonal lymphoproliferation and the potential for progression to malignant lymphoma or leukaemia.

Clinical Features

Most patients present with abdominal swelling and a dragging sensation in the abdomen. The malaria blood slide is usually negative. HMS commonly presents in pregnancy. The large, hard spleen is vulnerable to trauma. Acute left-sided abdominal pain suggests splenic infarction. The liver is also enlarged. Anaemia is often symptomatic and associated with pancytopenia (hypersplenism) and there is an increased susceptibility to bacterial infections. The long-term prognosis of HMS is not good, with an increased mortality from infection. HMS appears to be a pre-malignant condition developing into lymphoma in some patients.

Treatment

The enlarged spleen usually regresses over a period of months with effective antimalarial prophylaxis. Most experience has been gained with chloroquine and mefloquine. The liver also returns to normal and the IgM levels fall. Treatment is required for the duration of malaria exposure. Splenectomy is only recommended if there is an unequivocal failure of prophylaxis given for at least 6 months and there is severe hypersplenism.

Lymphoma

In some countries, Burkitt's lymphoma is the most common malignancy of childhood. It is an uncontrolled proliferation of B lymphocytes and is associated with Epstein–Barr (EB) virus infections and malaria. The epidemiological association between malaria and Burkitt's tumour is very strong. EB virus infections are widespread in the tropics and in most countries over 80% of children have serological evidence of infection by the age of 3 years. Normally, progression of EB virus in B lymphocytes is controlled by virus-specific cytotoxic T-cells (the atypical mononuclear cells of infectious mononucleosis). This EB virus cytotoxic T-cell response is decreased significantly during acute malaria and there is increased proliferation of EB virus-infected lymphocytes. This may predispose to malignant transformation. In areas of high stable transmission there is attenuated immune responsivity to EB virus in children between 5 and 9 years of age – the range of peak Burkitt's lymphoma incidence.

In Ghana prospective studies of HMS and splenic lymphoma with villous lymphocytes suggest that a proportion of patients with HMS develop lymphoma. The prognosis is poor.

Malaria Control

In his classic work on the prevention of malaria, Ronald Ross (1910) noted that in approximately 550 BC, Empedocles rid the Sicilian town of Selinus from a pestilence by draining the nearby marshes. Hippocrates (400 BC) knew that stagnant water and marshlands were unhealthy and that people living nearby would have enlarged spleens. The principles of drainage and landfill to control disease have continued since Roman times. The early attempts at joining the Atlantic and Pacific oceans were thwarted by disease, of which malaria was a major contributor, but during the final building of the Panama Canal, malaria was almost eradicated from the Canal zone by a vigorous combination of felling, drainage, house screening, pesticide use and antimalarial drugs (quinine). In recent years the practices of vector control have evolved and environmental management and modification have come to the fore, both for disease control and for agricultural and other economic purposes. This is a complex and multidisciplinary field. Only a brief outline of the various approaches to malaria control will be described here. There are three main arms to malaria control; vector control through use of insecticides, deployment of insecticide treated bed-nets (or other treated materials) and use of effective drugs.

WATER-LEVEL MANAGEMENT

The oldest method of vector control – drainage – remains the most cost-effective, particularly in relatively dry areas where there is a high ratio of population to standing water. The practical aspects of drainage are beyond the scope of this book. Water-level management to flush out mosquito breeding areas and to provide a hostile aquatic environment for mosquito egg and larval development, is an alternative to drainage. Changing water salinity or allowing organic matter pollution may also reduce vector populations. As always, major alterations to the environment should not be undertaken lightly: short-term benefits may be offset by long-term problems.

HUMAN BEHAVIOUR

Mosquitoes cannot fly far; most *anopheline*s cannot fly more than 4 km and in general they remain within 2 km of their breeding sites. Of course they can be blown further and occasionally they take plane journeys and deliver malaria around airports in other countries. If humans do not live near breeding sites, the chances of infection are reduced. Many vectors bite inside houses and the design and protection offered by the dwelling are important determinants of malaria risk. Wire-mesh screens and other mosquito-proofing measures are effective but expensive and may also reduce ventilation. Where domestic species of *anopheline*s exist (e.g. *A. stephensi* in India), water jars, tanks or containers should be closed to prevent mosquito access.

Simple measures such as introducing polystyrene balls to float on top of well water may be remarkably effective. The use of mosquito-proof bed-nets prevents human–vector contact, but they are considerably more effective in preventing malaria when impregnated with insect repellents or insecticides. Pyrethroid insecticide (permethrin, deltamethrin)-impregnated nylon nets are best and now long-lasting nets have been developed which retain activity for many years. Insecticide-treated durable wall linings are currently under evaluation.

IMAGOCIDES

Although chemical agents, such as the larvicide Paris green and pyrethrum insecticides, had been widely used for vector control before the Second World War, the discovery of 2,2-bis-(*p*-chlorophenyl)-1,1,1-trichloroethane (DDT), with excellent activity against the adult mosquito (imagocidal activity), was a major advance in malaria control. DDT had residual imagocidal activity, which pyrethrum did not. It could be sprayed on the interior of houses and would kill or deter mosquitoes for many months afterwards. DDT, along with two other chlorinated hydrocarbon residual insecticides, gamma benzene hexachloride (γ-HCH) and dieldrin, were the principal weapons in the campaign to eradicate malaria and they had a tremendous impact on health and development in the tropics. Imagocides can be classified into three general categories.

Pyrethrins and Pyrethroids

The naturally occurring compounds are light-sensitive and unstable, but the synthetic pyrethroids (permethrin, deltamethrin) are both highly toxic to mosquitoes and stable, giving good residual activity. A single point mutation (resulting in phenylalanine or serine for leucine at position 1014) in the gene encoding a voltage-gated sodium channel protein is associated with pyrethroid and DDT resistance. Known as the pyrethroid knock down resistance (*kdr*) mutation, it has been found at several different locations, but predominantly in *A. gambiae* in West and South Africa. The mechanisms implicated in pyrethroid resistance include metabolic resistance based on elevated levels of cytochrome P450 as well as mutations in the target site, the *kdr* mutations. Insecticide resistance is spreading and may represent a serious threat to the efficacy of impregnated bed-nets and vector control.

Chlorinated Hydrocarbons (DDT, γ-HCH, Dieldrin)

These are widely used as water-dispersible powders which form an aqueous suspension suitable for spraying. Resistance, human toxicity and ecological concerns have restricted the use of DDT in recent years. This valuable insecticide was vastly overused in the agricultural sector. Use in disease control was relatively small in comparison. But a global ban threw the baby out with the bathwater and threatened disease control in some areas where DDT was the only affordable and effective insecticide. Fortunately, the ban has been relaxed for vector-borne disease control. Used appropriately, DDT is still a very valuable malaria control tool (e.g. in Kwazulu Natal where pyrethroid resistant but DDT sensitive *A. funestus* caused an epidemic in the late 1990s which was terminated by combined insecticide (DDT) spraying and artemether-lumefantrine deployment. Dieldrin is now considered too toxic to humans and it is no longer used.

Anticholinesterases

These comprise the organophosphorus compounds (malathion, fenitrothion) and the carbamates (propoxur, trimethacarb, bendiocarb). Although resistance to the organophosphates has limited use in some areas, these compounds are still distributed widely. Malathion is the cheapest and most widely used. The anticholinesterases pose a potential health hazard to spraying teams, despite their wide therapeutic ratios.

General Principles

Imagocides are also classified either by their portal of entry to the body of the mosquito, or to the method of application. Residual insecticides are applied as a deposit on to surfaces where the mosquitoes will rest (e.g. walls, ceilings). Space sprays fill the air with a mist or fog of insecticide. The choice of insecticide and application method will be determined by the sensitivity and behaviour of the local vectors and the nature of the environment. The *anopheline* mosquito vectors have countered these chemical assaults by changing their behaviour (resting and feeding preferences) and evolving resistance to the insecticides. This has had drastic consequences: reduced effectiveness; the necessity for more expensive replacements (to which resistance has also developed in some species); a disinclination of the chemical industry to invest further in a difficult and often unprofitable field; and as a consequence an inability of impecunious governments to pay for the new insecticides. Over 50 vector species are resistant to one or more of the organochlorine insecticides, over ten are resistant to the organophosphates and pyrethroid resistance is spreading. Most important, *A. gambiae s. l.*, the dominant vector in Africa, has developed resistance to organochlorine insecticides in many areas. In Central America, *A. albimanus* has developed multiple insecticide resistance. In India the major vectors, *A. culicifacies* and *A. stephensi*, have become resistant to the organochlorines and malathion. Indoor residual spraying (IRS) is a major component of malaria control where *anopheline* vectors are susceptible. The number of people protected by IRS in the Africa region increased from 13 million in 2005 to 75 million in 2009, representing approximately 10% of the population at risk.

LARVICIDING

With the problems besetting use of residual imagocidal insecticides, there has been renewed interest in methods of larval control in recent years. These include environmental and water manipulation to prevent creation of mosquito breeding sites, the use of larvivorous fish and bacterial toxins and the application of chemical agents. Mineral oils were the first larvicides to be employed and diesel oil is still used today. Many of the imagocidal compounds described above are also used for larvicides. However, the organochlorines were highly effective but are no longer recommended because of their adverse environmental impact and the development of resistance. The organophosphorus compounds are used widely and are relatively safe; for example, compounds such as temephos are safe to warm-blooded animals and fish and can be used to treat potable water.

OVERALL APPROACH

The objectives of a malaria control programme will depend on the prevailing epidemiological situation, the availability of resources and feasibility. One size definitely does not fit all! The first priority is the reduction of malaria mortality by making available facilities, personnel, diagnostics and drugs for diagnosis and effective treatment. Then activities should focus on reducing malaria morbidity (such programmes should focus on malaria in childhood and malaria in pregnancy) and rely on use of effective drugs and vector control. In low transmission settings epidemics need to be anticipated. Having 'secured' the situation, it is also necessary to secure those areas free from malaria to prevent re-establishment of the infection. Finally and in a carefully planned and multifaceted programme, work to eliminate the disease should begin.

The Millennium Development Goals set a target of reducing the mortality of children under 5 years of age by two-thirds and halting and reversing the spread of malaria, by the end of 2015. Substantial resources have been made available to tropical countries for malaria control through the Global Fund for AIDS, TB and Malaria and other national and international donor agencies. This has resulted in substantial reductions in malaria morbidity and mortality. Estimated mortality has fallen by about one third over the past decade. The current global economic downturn and the emergence of resistance to insecticides and the artemisinin drugs represent a serious threat to these achievements.

REFERENCES

10. Taylor SM, Parobek CM, Fairhurst RM. Haemoglobinopathies and the clinical epidemiology of malaria: a systematic review and meta-analysis. Lancet Infect Dis 2012;12:457–68.
13. Hendriksen IC, Mwanga-Amumpaire J, von Seidlein L, et al. Diagnosing severe *falciparum* malaria in parasitaemic African children: a prospective evaluation of plasma PfHRP2 measurement. PLoS Med 2012;9:e1001297.
24. Wilson ML. Malaria rapid diagnostic tests. Clin Infect Dis 2012;54:1637–41.
35. Croft SL, Duparc S, Arbe-Barnes SJ, et al. Review of pyronaridine anti-malarial properties and product characteristics. Malar J 2012;11:e270.
41. Gething PW, Elyazar IR, Moyes CL, et al. A long neglected world malaria map: *Plasmodium vivax* endemicity in 2010. PLoS Negl Trop Dis 2012;6(9):e1814.

Access the complete references online at www.expertconsult.com

44

Babesiosis

PETER L. CHIODINI

KEY POINTS

- *Babesia* infect red blood cells causing haemolytic anaemia.
- Most human babesiosis cases are due to *Babesia microti* species complex or to *B. divergens* but other species, some newly described, are now emerging, especially in the USA.
- Previous splenectomy is a major risk factor.
- Clinical features of babesiosis are nonspecific, so the diagnosis may be unsuspected for some time.
- Co-infection with babesiosis and Lyme disease results in a more severe and longer illness than either infection alone.
- *Babesia* seen in a blood film may be misdiagnosed as malaria parasites.
- Blood-transfusion-transmitted babesiosis is a significant problem in highly endemic areas.
- *Babesia divergens* treatment consists of exchange blood transfusion plus quinine and clindamycin.
- *Babesia microti* is treated with atovaquone plus azithromycin or with quinine plus clindamycin.

Introduction

Babesia spp. are protozoan parasites of domestic and wild animals. They are members of the phylum Apicomplexa, order Piroplasmida, family Babesiidae.

The *Babesias* infecting humans come from four different clades:[1]

- *Babesia microti*, a small *Babesia*, itself existing as a species complex
- Other small *Babesias* including *Babesia duncani*
- Small *Babesias* including *Babesia divergens*, which despite being small are related to the large *Babesias*
- Large *Babesias* infecting ungulates, including the KO1 strain.

B. microti can no longer be regarded as a single species, but exists as a worldwide species complex consisting of three subclades, one containing zoonotic isolates.[2,3] As phylogenetic analyses based on molecular criteria develop further, more new *Babesia* species are likely with further revision of the taxonomy of this genus.

Most human cases of babesiosis are due to *Babesia microti* species complex or to *B. divergens*, but with increasing recognition of human cases, other species, some of them newly described, have been found to infect humans.

Babesia duncani n.sp., formerly known as WA1, was isolated from a patient in Washington State, USA.[4,5] Parasites from cases of human babesiosis in California, USA, known as CA1–CA4, are closely related to WA1 on molecular criteria.[4] A *Babesia divergens*-like parasite, MO1, was isolated from a fatal case of babesiosis in Missouri, USA,[6] and another *B.-divergens*-like parasite, unrelated to WA1, was recorded from Washington state.[7] EU1, a previously uncharacterized *Babesia* distinct from *Babesia divergens* and closely related to *B. odocoilei*, a parasite of white-tailed deer was described from Italy and Austria[8] and has since been identified as *B. venatorum*, which normally infects roe deer[1]. A *Babesia microti*-like organism has caused human infection in Taiwan.[9] *B. caucasica* has also been reported to infect humans, but Hoare[10] considered it to be synonymous with *B. bovis*. There is one case reportedly due to *B. canis.*[11]

Life Cycle

Human babesiosis is a zoonosis acquired by tick bite when individuals accidentally interact with the natural life cycle of the parasite. Humans represent dead-end hosts for *Babesia* spp.

BOVINE BABESIAS

Sporozoites are injected into the bloodstream by tick bite and penetrate erythrocytes. In contrast to the malaria life cycle, no tissue stage has ever been demonstrated for *B. bovis* or *B. divergens*. Within the erythrocyte the parasites vary in appearance, being oval, round or pear-shaped.

Ring forms, especially, may be confused with malaria parasites, especially *Plasmodium falciparum*. However, *Babesia* does not form pigment and does not cause alterations in red cell morphology or staining, such as the Maurer clefts of *P. falciparum*, the Schüffner dots of *P. vivax*, or the James dots of *P. ovale*. *Babesia* multiplies in the red cell by budding (*Plasmodium* by schizogony). Release of daughter parasites is followed by reinvasion of fresh erythrocytes and further asexual multiplication.

Some of the sporozoites injected by the tick vector follow a different path of intraerythrocytic development, growing slowly and 'folding' to form accordion-like structures, thought to be gametocytes[12] that are destined to undergo further development in the tick vector.

Within the gut of the tick the accordion-like stage is able to resist digestion and eventually fuses with another, to form a zygote. Further development outside the intestine occurs in a variety of tissues, the salivary glands and ovaries being especially important for transmission.

Sporozoites in tick salivary glands are injected into the mammalian host at the next blood meal. Transovarial transmission of *B. bovis* also takes place so that newly hatched larvae are already infected. Trans-stadial transmission to nymph and then to adult stages can then take place.

BABESIA MICROTI

In the small mammal host of *B. microti*, sporozoites from the tick vector first enter lymphocytes and undergo merogony, the daughter parasites then enter erythrocytes.[12] There is no published report of this intralymphocytic stage in human *B. microti* infections. The presence of schizogony in lymphocytes of its vertebrate host is one of the factors which has led Uilenberg to conclude that *B. microti* is not a *Babesia* and could logically be called *Theileria microti*.[13] Until the taxonomic issue is further clarified, this chapter will continue to refer to *Babesia microti*.

B. microti do not undergo transovarial transmission,[12] but once a larva has become infected from a mammalian host it is able to pass on the infection trans-stadially to the nymph.

Epidemiology

Human infection follows tick bite or, rarely, blood transfusion or transplacental/perinatal infection. Each *Babesia*–vector–mammalian host system has its own characteristics, and the ecology and bionomics of the vector tick define the pattern of risk for the human population.

EUROPEAN CASES

Approximately 40 cases of human infection with bovine *Babesias*, usually *B. divergens*, have been reported in Europe since 1957.[2,14,15] European cases reportedly due to *B. microti* and to *B. canis* have also been recorded.[11] The vector of *B. divergens* is *Ixodes ricinus* and that of *B. microti* in UK is *I. trianguliceps*, in contrast to the situation in the USA where *B. microti* is transmitted by *I. dammini*. A total of 84% of European cases of *B. divergens* infection had previous splenectomy.[16] However, *B. divergens* infection, confirmed by PCR, was found in an immunocompetent adult patient in France, making the point that in Europe this parasite can also cause illness in previously healthy individuals.[15]

There is an association of human *B. bovis* infection with exposure to land grazed by infected cattle.

NORTH AMERICAN CASES

The USA reports the highest number of human babesiosis cases. *B. microti* accounts for the great majority and is endemic in the Northeast and upper Midwest.[1,17–19] *B. duncani* is found in Washington State and California[1,5] and human infection with parasites resembling *B. divergens* has been reported from Missouri, Kentucky and Washington State.[1]

B. microti infects the mouse *Peromyscus leucopus*, the preferred host for the larva of *I. dammini*. Nymphs of this tick feed either on *Peromyscus* or on the deer, *Odocoileus virginianus*, which does not appear to be susceptible to *B. microti*. Adult *I. dammini* prefer to feed on *Odocoileus*. Humans appear to become infected via nymphs and the peak month for transmission is June, which coincides with their active feeding period. There have been at least 100 cases of transfusion-transmitted babesiosis in the USA, 12 of them fatal,[20] raising significant concern regarding blood transfusion safety. The vector for *B. microti* in North America is *I. dammini*, which is also the vector for *Borrelia burgdorferi*, the causative agent of Lyme disease. Co-infection of the same patient can occur and, in such cases, there are more symptoms and greater duration of illness than in patients with either infection alone.[21,22] Co-infection with *Babesia* should be considered in any Lyme disease patient who complains of marked "flu-like" symptoms or has unexplained splenomegaly, anaemia or thrombocytopenia or who fails to respond to appropriate antimicrobial treatment for Lyme disease.[23]

B. microti in North America can infect previously healthy individuals with intact spleens. The infection is more severe in splenectomized individuals. Benach and Habicht[24] studied common risk factors for babesiosis in 17 patients. They found no association with a particular blood group. Age was an important risk factor. The presence of a significant medical history (including splenectomy, cancer, cancer therapy, autoimmune disease, endocrinopathy and previous parasitic disease) was noted in 10 of the 17 cases. The mean age of patients with a significant medical history (47.7 years) was significantly lower than of those who were previously healthy (63.4 years). *B. microti* infection has been reported in human immunodeficiency virus (HIV)-positive patients, in whom persistent parasitaemia and severe disease have occurred.[25,26]

OTHER GEOGRAPHICAL REGIONS

Human babesiosis has also been reported from Australia (*B. microti*),[27] Taiwan and Japan (*B. microti*-like),[1,9] and Korea (currently named only as KO1 strain).[1]

Pathology

Haemolytic anaemia, jaundice due to unconjugated hyperbilirubinaemia, frank haemoglobinuria and acute renal failure due to acute tubular necrosis are all features of *B. bovis* infection in splenectomized individuals.[28] Thrombocytopenia may occur.[29]

B. microti infection also results in haemolytic anaemia, which may last for several days to a few months.[30] Its presence in splenectomized as well as spleen-intact patients indicates that hypersplenism alone cannot explain the haemolytic anaemia. Scanning electron microscopy of human blood infected with *B. microti* has revealed substantial damage to the erythrocyte membrane, with protrusions, inclusions and perforations evident, suggesting that red cell destruction is parasite-mediated.[31] C3 and C4 levels were suppressed in acute *B. microti* infections.[32] Thrombocytopenia and raised levels of liver enzymes occur in severe cases.[33] *B. microti* infection has been reported to cause a false-positive Monospot test.[34]

There is no evidence that parasite sequestration contributes to the pathogenesis of severe multiorgan failure in human babesiosis.[35]

Shaio and Lin[36] demonstrated elevated TNF-α, IFN-γ and IL-2, but not IL-4 or IL-10 in a patient with acute *B. microti* infection. E-selectin, VCAM-1, and ICAM-1 levels were also elevated and, like the cytokines, fell back to normal after successful treatment. Krause and co-workers[37] feel that excessive production of TNF and other proinflammatory cytokines plays a major part in causing the symptoms of babesiosis.

The spleen plays a critical role in protection against *Babesia* infection, as shown by the predominance of splenectomised individuals in case series of *B. divergens* infection and the association of splenectomy with severe *B. microti* cases. Immunity to babesiosis depends upon humoral and cellular factors.

Homer and colleagues regarded the humoral component of limited importance, the role of antibodies being restricted to the brief period after the parasites have entered the bloodstream but not yet become intracellular.[30] On the other hand, Vannier and Krause[1] point out the critical role of B cells in resolving *B. microti* infection in individuals with diminished cellular immunity and suggest that they also help to clear this parasite in immunocompetent patients. T cells also play a major part in developing immunity to *Babesia*. CD4+ T helper cells are regarded as the subpopulation mainly responsible, via their production of IFN-gamma which promotes macrophage-mediated killing of intracellular parasites and antibody synthesis by B cells.[1,30] Shaoi and Lin[36] found a marked increase in natural killer cells in the acute phase in a patient with acute *B. microti* infection which returned to normal in the post-treatment convalescent phase and suggested that cytokine-mediated natural killer cell cytotoxicity is also involved in the immunopathogenesis of human babesiosis.

Clinical Features

BABESIA BOVIS/DIVERGENS

The incubation period varies from 1 to 4 weeks. The patient may feel vaguely unwell at first, but by the time the diagnosis has been made is usually very ill, with fever, prostration, myalgia, jaundice, anaemia and haemoglobinuria. Nausea, vomiting and diarrhoea may also occur.[28] Hepatomegaly, signs of pulmonary oedema, and oliguric renal failure may develop. Finding an operation scar gives a clue to previous splenectomy. Infection is sometimes unsuspected and, given the fulminant nature of this condition, may not be confirmed until after the patient has died or the diagnosis is considered to be *P. falciparum* malaria when intraerythrocytic parasites are seen in the blood film. Other misdiagnoses include leptospirosis and viral hepatitis. Thus, for the diagnosis to be made early, babesiosis should be considered in the differential diagnosis of any splenectomized patient in whom exposure to tick bites is a possibility.

BABESIA MICROTI

Most human infections are subclinical.[38] Where clinical illness develops, the incubation period is 1–3 weeks, occasionally up to 6 weeks, for tick-transmitted infections and 6–9 weeks for post-transfusion cases. The illness usually begins gradually, with anorexia and fatigue, plus fever (without periodicity), sweating, rigors and generalized myalgia. Physical examination may reveal only fever, but may also show mild splenomegaly and sometimes mild hepatomegaly.[19] In a series of 34 patients with severe babesiosis requiring hospitalization, 41% developed complications which included the adult respiratory distress syndrome, disseminated intravascular coagulation, congestive heart failure and renal failure. Complicated babesiosis was more often associated with the presence of haemoglobin concentrations <10 g/dL.[33]

Given the nonspecific nature of the clinical findings, human infection with *B. microti* cannot be diagnosed with certainty on clinical grounds alone. In a series of patients with severe babesiosis, the average time from onset of symptoms to diagnosis was 15 days.[33] A history of tick bite is helpful but is not elicited in most cases.[24] However, public knowledge of Lyme disease, which shares the same vector with *B. microti* in the USA, can raise awareness of tick-transmitted diseases. The relatively localized geographical distribution of human *B. microti* infections in the USA means that local physicians may become very aware of the infection but it may be missed by those practising in non-endemic areas in other countries.

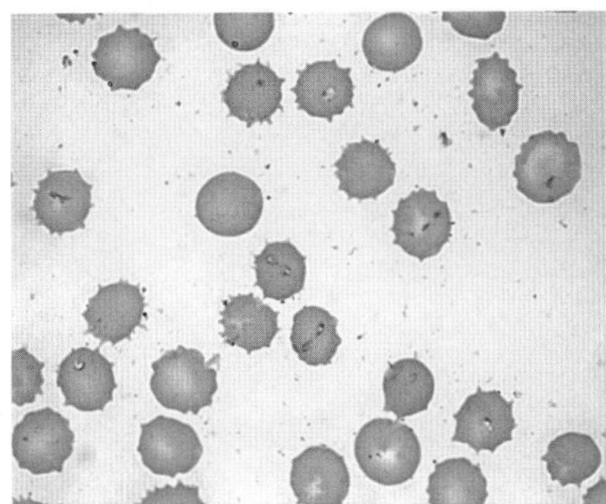

Figure 44.1 Human infection with *Babesia divergens*.

Laboratory Diagnosis

Definitive diagnosis depends upon finding parasites on blood film examination. The use of the polymerase chain reaction (PCR) is increasing and serodiagnosis is also helpful. Hamster inoculation is very seldom indicated.

BLOOD FILM EXAMINATION

Babesia bovis/divergens (Figure 44.1)

B. divergens was separated from *B. bovis* as a result of the predominance of paired forms, diverging at a wide angle of up to 180°, situated on the periphery of the red cell.[10] *B. divergens* is smaller (0.4×1.5 µm) than *B. bovis* (2.4×1.5 µm). However, the parasites are pleomorphic and their size can vary depending upon the host they infect.[10] *B. bovis* and *B. divergens* are pear-shaped, oval or round, and may exist in pyriform pairs. In fulminant human cases, *B. divergens* takes the form of rings, loops, clubs, rods, pyriform and amoeboid shapes. Occasional divergent forms are seen. There may be one to eight parasites per red cell. A 70% parasitaemia has been reported from a fatal case.[28] The 'Maltese cross' form is unique to *Babesia* among members of the Apicomplexa, but in its absence it may be very difficult to distinguish young ring forms of *Plasmodium* spp., especially *P. falciparum*. The absence of pigment cannot be relied upon as young rings of *Plasmodium* spp. do not exhibit pigment. If cultured in vitro, *P. falciparum* will develop pigment, but *Babesia* will not. *Babesia* is smaller than malaria parasites, and in some of the larger rings there is a white vacuole, instead of the pink vacuole containing erythrocyte stroma seen in malaria. *Babesia* does not form schizonts.

Babesia microti

In *Babesia microti* (Figure 44.2), ring, rod-shaped, pyriform, amoeboid and 'Maltese cross' forms are seen.[10] In heavy infections different stages may be noted in the same red cell. Intraerythrocytic stages measure approximately 2×1.5 µm. In very high parasitaemias extracellular merozoites with plentiful cytoplasm may be found singly or as a syncytial structure.[31]

Peak parasitaemia varies between less than 1% to approximately 10%[19] but a splenectomized patient who was also taking systemic steroids developed a *B. microti* parasitaemia of 85%.[31]

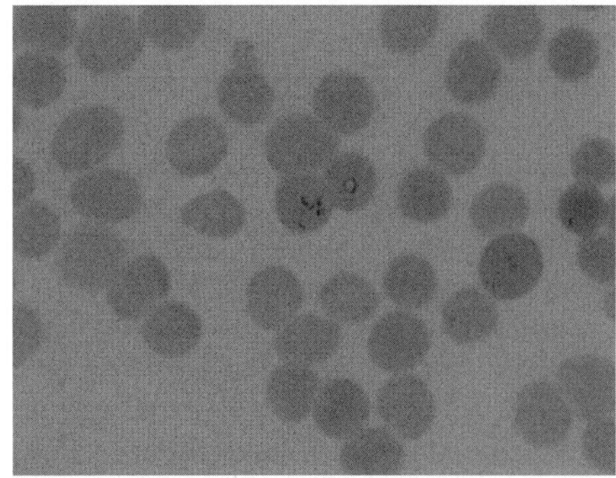

Figure 44.2 Human infection with *Babesia microti.*

OTHER LABORATORY FINDINGS

Babesia bovis/divergens

Anaemia, leukocytosis, haemolysis, unconjugated hyperbilirubinaemia and raised blood urea levels are found. Reticulocytosis occurs in response to the haemolytic anaemia. Frank haemoglobinuria may occur.[28]

Babesia microti

Anaemia may be mild to moderately severe, ranging from 5.8 to 11.6 g/dL in one series.[17] Plasma haptoglobin levels are usually be reduced and the reticulocyte count increased, supporting the view that most of the anaemia is due to haemolysis. Total white blood cell counts are low or normal and there may be thrombocytopenia.[19]

Mean and differential lymphocyte counts and percentages of B lymphocytes and levels of T lymphocytes with the immunoglobulin (Ig) G Fc receptor are raised in acute infection. Polyclonal hypergammaglobulinaemia is found. Levels of serum IgG, IgM and C1q binding are significantly increased; C3 and C4 levels and haemolytic activity are reduced in acute-phase sera.[32]

There may be a mild increase in serum glutamic oxaloacetic transaminase (aspartate aminotransferase), alkaline phosphatase and bilirubin concentrations.[10]

ELECTRON MICROSCOPY

This technique is not helpful for routine diagnosis of human babesiosis but may provide useful confirmation of the nature of the infection. Transmission electron microscopy of *B. microti* from a splenectomized patient also receiving systemic steroids showed considerable pleomorphism. All developmental stages were seen in both reticulocytes and mature erythrocytes. The same study identified convoluted cells with many free ribosomes, thought to represent an early gametocyte stage.[31]

SERODIAGNOSIS

The indirect fluorescent antibody test (IFAT) is available for bovine *Babesia* and for *B. microti*. However, serology should not be seen as an alternative to blood film examination, especially in view of the fulminant nature of bovine *Babesia* infection in splenectomized patients. Demonstration of parasites in a blood film provides unequivocal proof of current infection. Some *B. microti* infections may have low-level or transient parasitaemia,[38] and serology, with PCR testing of seropositive individuals,[30] has a useful part to play in establishing the diagnosis. Ruebush et al.[38] defined individuals with IFAT titres to *B. microti* of 64 or greater as seropositive. In patients with acute *B. microti* infection, IFAT titres were greater than or equal to 1 in 1024, and fell to 1 in 256 or 1 in 64 over 8–12 months. The possibility of cross-reaction with antimalarial antibody must be borne in mind when serological results are interpreted. The *B. microti* IFAT has a reported 88–96% sensitivity and 90–100% specificity.[39] A brief report describing an IgG ELISA for the detection of antibody to *B. microti* has been published. This assay has a reported sensitivity of 95.5% and specificity of 94.1% compared with the *B. microti* IFAT.[40] An immunoblot is also available.[41]

POLYMERASE CHAIN REACTION (PCR)

PCR for *B. microti* with a reported limit of detection of approximately three merozoites/100 μL has been developed.[42] Real-time PCR for *B. microti* has been reported to detect as few as 100 gene copies in 5 μL of whole blood, making it more sensitive than light microscopy.[43] PCR is deployed increasingly to confirm infection in antibody-reactive individuals and to monitor the response to treatment.[30]

ANIMAL INOCULATION

This is not used for routine diagnosis of individual cases, but *B. microti* from human cases can be isolated in hamsters,[19] and *B. divergens* from a fatal human case was successfully passaged to gerbils and to a splenectomized calf.[28]

Clinical Course and Management

BABESIA BOVIS/DIVERGENS

If untreated, infection of splenectomized humans with bovine *Babesias* leads to fulminant illness and death. Specific treatment is based upon anecdotal case reports. Diminazene (Berenil) is active against *Babesia* in animals and was used in a case of human *B. divergens* infection, but the patient died.[44] Successful treatment of *B. divergens* (5% parasitaemia) in a splenectomized patient with pentamidine plus co-trimoxazole has been recorded.[44] The veterinary compound imidocarb was used successfully in the treatment of two cases of human infection with *B. divergens*.[45] Quinine and chloroquine plus pyrimethamine have proven ineffective.[28] Brasseur and Gorenflot[46] reported successful treatment of three cases with massive exchange blood transfusion (2–3 blood volumes) followed by intravenous clindamycin and oral quinine.

Atovaquone is effective against *B. divergens* in vitro.[47] In the absence of data from randomized controlled trials, current therapy should consist of exchange blood transfusion plus intravenous clindamycin and intravenous or oral quinine, depending upon the patient's condition.

BABESIA MICROTI

In most instances, patients suffer a mild illness from which they recover spontaneously. Recovery may be prolonged, with several months of fatigue and malaise.[19] Where treatment is required, oral quinine 650 mg every 8 h plus clindamycin 300–600 mg intravenously or intramuscularly every 6 h (adult doses) for 7–10 days has been regarded as the treatment of choice,[11,48] although it is not universally effective.[49] Paediatric dosage is oral quinine 25 mg/kg per day and intravenous or intramuscular clindamycin 20 mg/kg per day. Krause et al.[50] compared atovaquone 750 mg every 12 h plus azithromycin 500 mg on day 1 and 250 mg daily thereafter for 7 days with clindamycin 600 mg every 8 h and quinine 650 mg every 8 h for 7 days; all drugs being given orally. Atovaquone plus azithromycin proved to be as effective as clindamycin plus quinine and had fewer adverse reactions. The authors recommended that atovaquone plus azithromycin be considered for the treatment of non-life-threatening babesiosis in immunocompetent adult patients and in others who could not tolerate clindamycin and quinine.[50] Weiss et al.[51] reported the successful use of azithromycin 12 mg/kg per day and atovaquone 40 mg/kg per day in neonates, without toxic effects, and had used a higher dose of azithromycin (600 mg/day) in combination with atovaquone (750 mg twice daily) in adults. They reported that the 600 mg daily dose of azithromycin led to earlier resolution of fever and rapid clearance of parasites from the blood.[51] The Infectious Diseases Society of America states that higher doses of azithromycin (600–1000 mg/day adult doses) may be used for immunocompromised patients with babesiosis.[52] Ranque[53] suggested that a trial of atovaquone plus clindamycin should be performed.

Chloroquine is ineffective. Diminazene was used in one case and the patient recovered but developed neurological complications resembling the Guillain–Barré syndrome.[54] Artesunate has activity against *B. microti* in vitro and in mice.[55]

Whole blood or red cell exchange transfusion has produced a rapid and substantial fall in parasitaemia and its use as an adjunct to chemotherapy should be considered in severely ill patients with high parasitaemia.[56]

Prevention

There is no vaccine licensed for human use. Prevention of human babesiosis depends upon avoidance of tick bite: avoidance of tick habitats; wearing appropriate clothing to cover the lower part of the body; use of insect repellent (e.g. diethyltoluamide and permethrin-impregnated clothing); and prompt removal of ticks found on the person. The number of transfusion-transmitted babesiosis cases in the USA has caused considerable concern, such that regional screening in highly endemic areas, e.g. the Northeast and upper Midwest, is under active consideration.[20] A laboratory-based donor screening programme using IFAT-based antibody detection and real time PCR has been shown to be feasible in operational transfusion practice and able to detect *B. microti*-infected units.[57]

REFERENCES

1. Vannier E, Krause PJ. Human Babesiosis. N Engl J Med 2012;366:2397–407.
20. Leiby DA. Transfusion-transmitted *Babesia* spp.: Bull's-eye on Babesia microti. Clin Microbiol Rev 2011;24:14–28.
22. Martínez-Balzano C, Hess M, Malhotra A, et al. Severe babesiosis and *Borrelia burgdorferi* co-infection. QJM 2012;PMID:22685248.
43. Teal AE, Habura A, Ennis J, et al. A new real-time PCR assay for improved detection of the parasite *Babesia microti*. J Clin Microbiol 2012;50(3):903–8.
57. Young C, Chawla A, Berardi V, et al; the Babesia Testing Investigational Containment Study Group. Preventing transfusion-transmitted babesiosis: preliminary experience of the first laboratory-based blood donor screening program. Transfusion 2012;52(7):1523–152.

Access the complete references online at www.expertconsult.com

45

Human African Trypanosomiasis

CHRISTIAN BURRI | FRANÇOIS CHAPPUIS | RETO BRUN

KEY POINTS

- Human African trypanosomiasis (HAT) (or sleeping sickness) is caused by two subspecies of the protozoan parasite *Trypanosoma brucei*. *T.b. gambiense* causes the chronic form in Central and West Africa and represents >95% of all cases while *T.b. rhodesiense* is responsible for a more acute form of the disease in East and Southern Africa. Different species of tsetse flies (*Glossina* spp.) transmit the parasites while taking a bloodmeal, but only about 1 in 1000 flies carries a mature trypanosome infection.
- By the late 1990s approximately 25 000 new cases were reported per year, while estimates of the number of new cases actually reached over 300 000 per year. In the meantime, increased control measures led to a substantial decline in the number of new reported cases to just below 10 000 (98% due to *T.b. gambiense*) in 2009 and an estimated number of cases of 30 000. Nevertheless, areas with high disease prevalence ('hot spots') and areas without surveillance ('blind spots') still remain.
- Perivascular inflammation is the main feature observed in the brain of patients during the neurological (second) stage of *T.b. gambiense* HAT. The inflammatory lesions spare the cerebral cortex, where neurons are well preserved, which contrasts with cortical lesions observed in neurosyphilis. As potentially reversible inflammatory lesions predominate over irreversible destruction of tissues, partial or full recovery of neuropsychiatric symptoms follows HAT treatment. Demyelinization and atrophy are only observed in the terminal stage of the illness.
- Whereas *T.b. gambiense* HAT is a slowly evolving disease, *T.b. rhodesiense* HAT is usually an acute febrile illness with a faster clinical evolution. Exceptions to this rule do occur. Individual and geographical variations in the clinical presentation have been described in both forms of the disease, most likely due to a combination of parasite and host genetic factors.
- The diagnosis of *T.b. gambiense* HAT still follows the pathway: screening, diagnostic confirmation, and staging. Suspected cases detected by serological methods (usually the card agglutination test for trypanosomiasis, CATT) undergo parasitological confirmation by investigation of the blood and/or lymph and if positive, examination of the CSF for staging. *T.b. rhodesiense* is usually directly detected in the blood. However, rapid diagnostic screening tests and molecular assays requiring only simple technology are under development and may significantly change diagnostics in the near future.
- Over the past decade, substantial achievements in the chemotherapy of the disease were made and hence, the recommendations for treatment in this edition differ substantially from the older editions. Nifurtimox-eflornithine combination therapy (NECT) was included into WHO's 'Essential Medicines List' in 2009 and replaces melarsoprol as first-line treatment for second-stage *T.b. gambiense* HAT. No replacement was yet found for the treatment of second-stage *T.b. rhodesiense*, but the abridged treatment regimen for melarsoprol was recommended in 2009.
- The disease can be kept under control by: (1) passive and active surveillance of the population and identification of patients, followed by treatment and (2) by tsetse fly control using insecticides, traps and release of sterile males. The main challenge is to sustain such control measures, despite a low prevalence of patients. With new diagnostic tools and safe and effective drugs, elimination of HAT appears achievable.

Biology of the Parasite and the Vector

T. brucei subspecies trypanosomes of the subgenus *Trypanozoon* are morphologically indistinguishable. However, since the 1970s, much research has been undertaken to identify biochemical and molecular markers that better define clinical disease and epidemiology. The problems that these extensive studies have addressed are the identity and potential infectivity to humans of trypanosomes circulating in domestic and game animals, and those isolated from *Glossina*.

The morphology of *T. brucei* is described by Hoare (Figure 45.1).[1] Parasites are pleomorphic, extracellular in the blood, lymph and tissues, and vary in length from 12 to 42 μm; they have a small subterminal kinetoplast and a free flagellum. Parasite multiplication is impaired by specific antibodies produced by the host, resulting in a decrease in the parasitaemia. However, some parasites escape the immune response by antigenic variation, a mechanism that enables the trypanosomes to produce a surface coat composed of another glycoprotein.[2] The result is a fluctuating parasitaemia with multiple progressive pathological changes, which vary in pattern and intensity with different parasite strains and hosts.

T. brucei organisms are infective to laboratory animals: inoculation of infective material from human, animal reservoir and *Glossina* produces infection in a range of laboratory animals. *T.b. rhodesiense* can be propagated only in the multimammate rat (*Mastomys natalensis*), the thicket rat (*Grammomys* spp.)[3] or

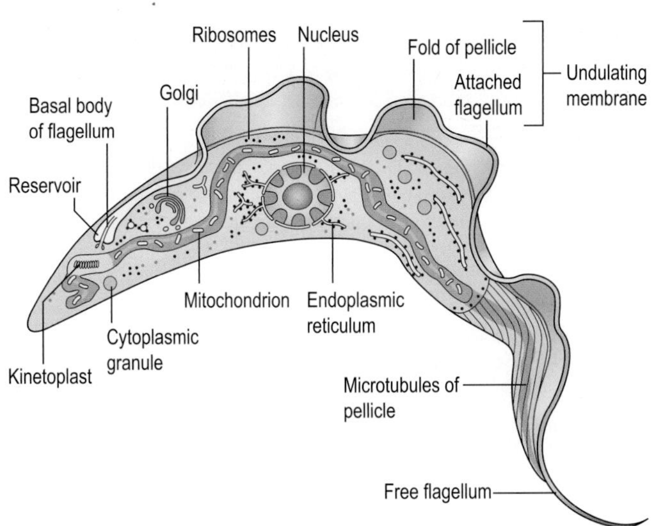

Figure 45.1 Morphology of *Trypanosoma brucei*. *(Reproduced with permission from Apted FIC. Treatment of Human Trypanosomiasis (Chapter 36). In: Mulligan HW, editor. The African trypanosomiasis. London: Allen & Unwin Ltd.; 1970. p. 684–710.)*

in mice with severe combined immune deficiency (SCID).[4] For isolation purposes, infected patients' blood can be cryopreserved in the field using, e.g. the cryomedium Triladyl® and liquid nitrogen.[5] In the laboratory the frozen blood sample can be thawed and injected into a susceptible rodent for propagation.[6]

It is generally recognized that *T.b. brucei* is the animal infective form of the subgenus *Trypanozoon*, which is not infective to humans because of its sensitivity to human serum. *T.b. brucei* is lysed by human serum; this is associated with high-density lipoprotein molecules, which are trypanocidal.[7] Today, PCR methods are available which make use of the *T.b. rhodesiense* specific SRA (serum resistance associated) gene[8] or the *T.b. gambiense* specific TgsGP gene.[9]

The analysis of parasite populations using modern technologies reveals the diversity and complexity of the trypanosomes infective to humans. The problem of understanding the relationships between different populations has been compounded by the demonstration that *T. brucei* can hybridize in *Glossina* in the laboratory.[10] It has also been shown that human serum resistance can be passed on from a parent to the offspring of a cross *T.b. rhodesiense* x *T.b. brucei*.[11] Neither the frequency of hybridization in the wild nor its significance for the epidemiology and patterns of drug resistance are yet known. PCR analysis of mobile genetic elements[12] and the use of microsatellite markers[13] are new technologies which will help to distinguish different strains of *T. brucei* across all three subspecies and notably among *T.b. gambiense*, which is the least genetically variable *T. brucei* subspecies.

T. brucei subspecies are transmitted to mammalian hosts by the bite of tsetse flies (*Glossina* spp.). A tsetse fly becomes infected when taking a bloodmeal on an infected mammalian host. A complex developmental cycle in the fly ends with the infective metacyclic form in the lumen of the salivary glands (Figure 45.2). This process may take 3–4 weeks. Metacyclic trypanosomes are injected into the skin of the mammalian host during the feeding process. Development in the tsetse fly involves a series of changes in the morphology and biochemistry of the parasite. Several factors play key roles in these changes: lectins present in *Glossina* midgut and haemolymph, the presence of *Rickettsia*-like organisms, and molecular signals that influence parasite transformation, establishment and maturation.[14] Knowledge of the parasite–vector interactions could eventually lead to novel control strategies to interrupt transmission.

The possibility of mechanical (non-cyclical) transmission by biting insects or *Glossina* has been suggested, although there is only circumstantial evidence to support the idea. Mechanical transmission has been suggested as the reason for the clustering of cases in a household or where cases are found outside the normal range of *Glossina*.

Epidemiology

OVERVIEW

Sleeping sickness is endemic only in areas where *Glossina* species (tsetse flies) are found. The ecological limit of *Glossina* distribution is approximately a line from 14°N from Senegal in the West to 10°N in Southern Somalia in the East, and 20°S corresponding to the Northern fringes of the Kalahari and Namibian Deserts.[15] The distribution of *Glossina* is determined by climatic factors (temperature and humidity) through its effects on

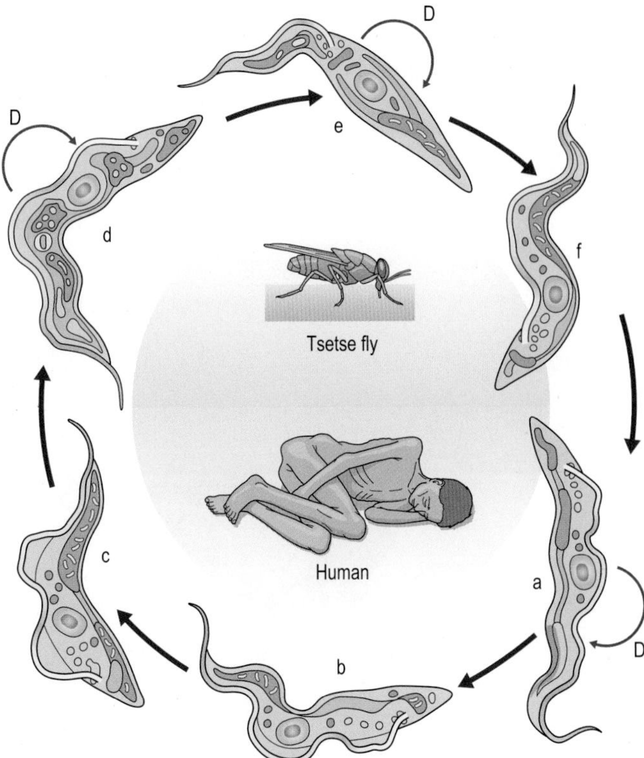

Figure 45.2 Cycle of *T. brucei* spp. showing the different morphological forms in the human and in the tsetse fly. In the blood and lymphatic system of humans: (a) slender; (b) intermediate and (c) short stumpy forms are present. Stumpy forms differentiate in the fly midgut to (d) procyclic forms, then to (e) epimastigote forms and finally in the salivary glands to (f) infective metacyclic forms. Bloodstream forms (a–c) and metacyclic forms are covered by the variable surface glycoprotein (VSG) coat. D indicates the capability to undergo cell division. *(Reproduced from Brun R. Sleeping sickness in Africa; on the rise again. Karger Gazette 1999;63:5–7, with permission from Karger, Basel.)*

vegetation. It is anticipated that satellite technology will be of increasing use in defining fly distribution in relation to habitats.[16] Comparison of such images over time will, in association with geographical information system (GIS) techniques, be of value in predicting tsetse distribution in relation to changes in environment. Rogers and Williams[17] examined how GIS can contribute to studies of human and animal trypanosomiasis and how data from meteorological satellites help to understand the spatial distribution of vectors and disease.

There are over 20 species of *Glossina* and a number of subspecies, most of which are capable of acting as vectors of trypanosomes that cause human sleeping sickness (as well as animal disease). The tsetse flies are separated into three groups, of which two groups are mainly responsible for the transmission of sleeping sickness: the *palpalis* group transmitting *T.b. gambiense*, which is responsible for the chronic form of the disease; and the *morsitans* group transmitting *T.b. rhodesiense*, which causes a more acute disease. The major vectors for the two forms of disease are listed in Table 45.1. The current distribution of sleeping sickness in Africa is shown on the map in Figure 45.3. Jordan[18] provides a summary of *Glossina* biology and control.

Sleeping sickness is endemic in over 200 known foci in 36 countries and *Glossina* spp. infest approximately 10 million km^{1} or about one-third of the African continent.

In the late 1990s, the WHO had not only emphasized the recrudescence of the disease but also the dramatic lack of awareness about the disease situation. The resulting under-surveillance had led to reporting of approximately 25 000 new cases per year while estimates of the infection level reached over 300 000 new cases.[19] In the meantime, control measures could increase significantly due to higher political stability in several affected countries, the commitment of several non-governmental organizations to combat the disease; and the investments of governments in large-scale bilateral projects. The WHO played a crucial role through reinforcing networks and advocacy, and particularly through a partnership with two major pharmaceutical companies who allowed the provision of the treatments for free. As a consequence, during the past 10 years, surveillance activities have increased, leading to a substantial decline in the number of new cases.[20–28] The reported number of cases in 2009 was just below 10 000 (98% due to *T.b. gambiense*) and the new estimated number of actual cases was 30 000.[26] In view of this significant progress, various organizations and authors recommended to launch an elimination programme for sleeping sickness.[26,29–31] To reach this goal, the continued efforts in the development of safer drugs, preferably oral, and simpler and more reliable diagnostic tests will be key, as this will allow implementing the treatment also in primary health care facilities. The main challenge will be to maintain awareness, strengthen surveillance and sustain efforts to achieve the goal of elimination. It must not be forgotten, that neglecting the disease will inevitably lead to a new resurgence.

TABLE 45.1 Major Vectors of *T.b. gambiense* and *T.b. rhodesiense* and Geographical Distribution

Vector	Geographical distribution
T.b. GAMBIENSE	
G. PALPALIS PALPALIS, G. PALPALIS GAMBIENSIS	Angola, Benin, Burkina Faso, Cameroon, Central African Republic, Congo, Democratic Republic of the Congo, Gabon, Gambia, Ghana, Guinea, Guinea-Bissau, Ivory Coast, Liberia, Mali, Nigeria, Senegal, Sierra Leone, Togo
G. TACHINOIDES	Benin, Burkina Faso, Cameroon, Central African Republic, Chad, Ethiopia, Ghana, Guinea, Ivory Coast, Mali, Niger, Nigeria, Sudan, Togo
G. FUSCIPES QUANZENSIS, G. FUSCIPES MARTINII	Angola, Congo, Democratic Republic of the Congo
G. FUSCIPES FUSCIPES	Cameroon, Central African Republic, Chad, Congo, Democratic Republic of the Congo, Sudan, Uganda
T.b. RHODESIENSE	
G. MORSITANS MORSITANS, G. MORSITANS CENTRALIS	Angola, Botswana, Burundi, Malawi, Mozambique, Rwanda, Tanzania, Zambia, Zimbabwe
G. PALLIDIPES	Burundi, Ethiopia, Kenya, Malawi, Mozambique, Rwanda, Sudan, Tanzania, Uganda, Zambia, Zimbabwe
G. SWYNNERTONI	Kenya, Tanzania
G. FUSCIPES FUSCIPES	Ethiopia, Kenya, Tanzania, Uganda

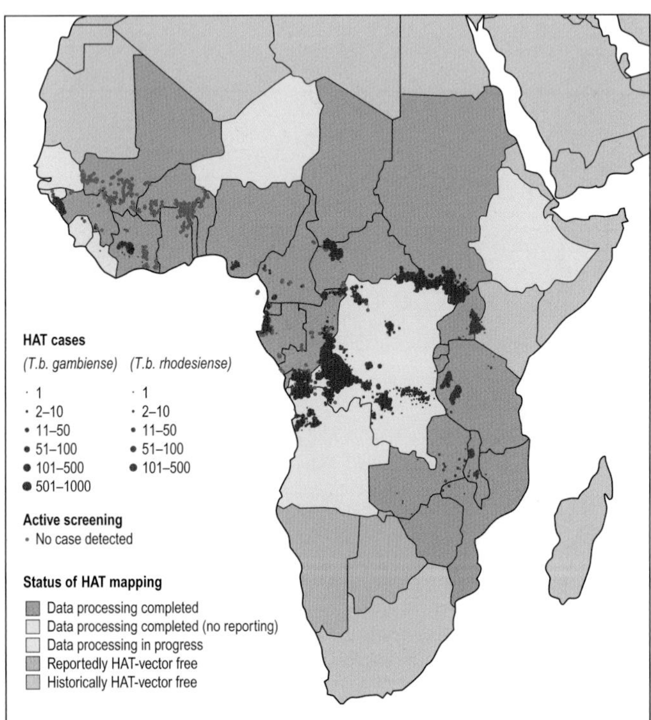

Figure 45.3 Distribution of human African trypanosomiasis. *(Reproduced with permission from WHO. Control and surveillance of African trypanosomiasis. Geneva: WHO; 1998. p. 1–114.)*

T.B. GAMBIENSE DISEASE

T.b. gambiense is endemic throughout West and Central Africa, and is frequently associated with foci of infection, areas where prevalence is often tenfold higher. Transmission of *T.b. gambiense* is associated with particular sites, usually near riverine

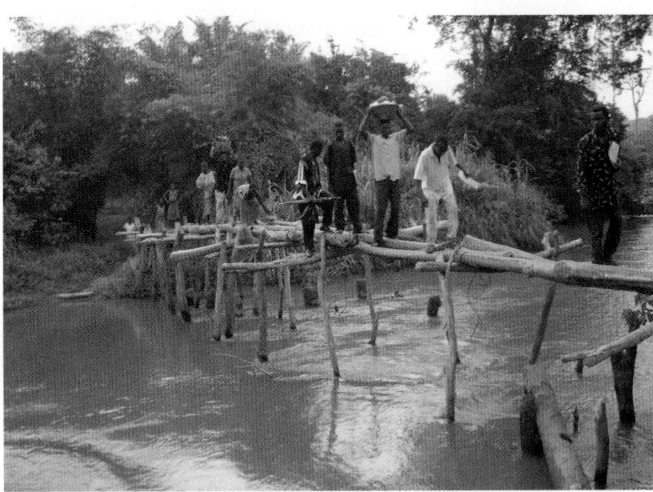

Figure 45.4 Typical place of transmission of *T.b. gambiense* where human–fly contact is high; habitat of *G. palpalis*. (*Source: Christian Burri (Swiss Tropical and Public Health Institute): Kikongotanga, Democratic Republic of the Congo.*)

vegetation, river crossings, water collection points, washing sites and villages adjacent to rivers or lakes (Figures 45.4 and 45.5). *T.b. gambiense* transmission is 'site associated', and intense transmission was considered to occur, particularly at the end of the dry season, when contact between humans and *G. palpalis* was most frequent. Flies require regular blood meals and humans are always available at these particular sites. In more humid forest regions, however, *G. palpalis* distribution is more widespread and human–fly contact is less intense. Once infected, a fly can transmit trypanosomes each time it bites; hence a single infected tsetse fly could infect many individuals at a particular site.

The most recent categorization of *T.b. gambiense* places this organism in a particular strain group comprised of six zymodemes (stocks with characteristic isoenzyme profiles). There are, however, chronic infections of humans from the Ivory Coast, the most sampled area, which are now placed in the Bouaflé strain group and which belong to the same zymodeme as stocks isolated from a range of wild and domestic animals.[32] Classical *T.b. gambiense* strains (termed 'type 1') cannot be propagated in laboratory rodents nor be transmitted by *morsitans* group tsetse flies. There is also a second type of *T.b. gambiense* circulating in Central and West Africa (termed 'type 2'), which shares characteristics with *T.b. rhodesiense* such as developing high parasitaemias in laboratory rodents and being transmitted by *morsitans* group tsetse flies. Information on the animal reservoir of *T.b. gambiense* is scarce and consists of the examination of a few animals. Pigs, dogs and cattle but also the game animal species kob (*Kobus kob*) and hartebeest (*Alcelaphus buselaphus*) have been found infected with *T.b. gambiense*. A study in Cameroon examined 164 wild animals by PCR and found 8% (rodents, antelopes, monkeys and carnivores) infected with *T.b. gambiense*.[33]

Recent decades have seen a considerable increase in our understanding of the complex interrelationships of the subgenus *Trypanozoon*. Earlier studies were handicapped by a lack of methods for parasite isolation and identification. Isoenzyme analysis and molecular methods have provided a strong base for future detailed epidemiological studies, particularly using PCR, to identify the strain group based on small amounts of parasite material from humans, mammals or *Glossina*.

T.B. RHODESIENSE DISEASE

T.b. rhodesiense is the causative agent of the acute form of sleeping sickness. It is distributed from Uganda in the northern part of East Africa to Zimbabwe in the south. Recent biochemical and molecular studies have identified two main strain groups associated with acute sleeping sickness, Zambezi and Busoga, the strain groups representing the southern and northern limits of distribution, respectively. Zambezi strains from Zambia and Malawi are often less virulent than the Busoga strain group from Uganda and Tanzania.[34,35]

Sleeping sickness is endemic throughout eastern and south-eastern Africa, and humans are infected by the bite of *Glossina* spp. associated with woodland savannah habitats (Figure 45.6).

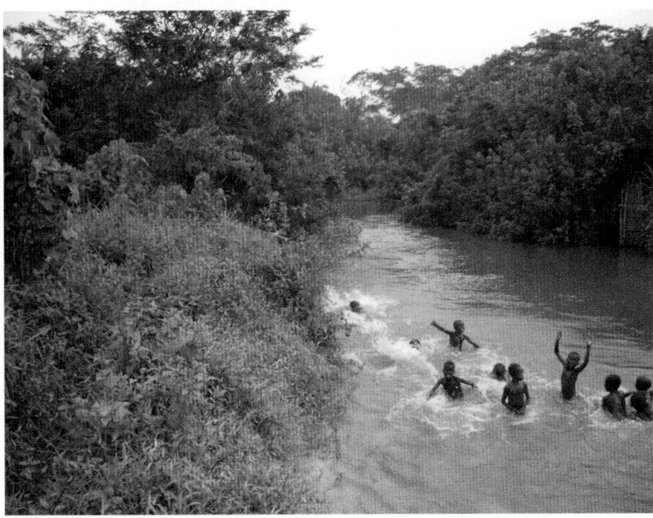

Figure 45.5 Typical place of transmission of *T.b. gambiense* where human–fly contact is high; habitat of *G. palpalis*. (*Source: Christian Burri (Swiss Tropical and Public Health Institute): Kikongotanga, Democratic Republic of the Congo.*)

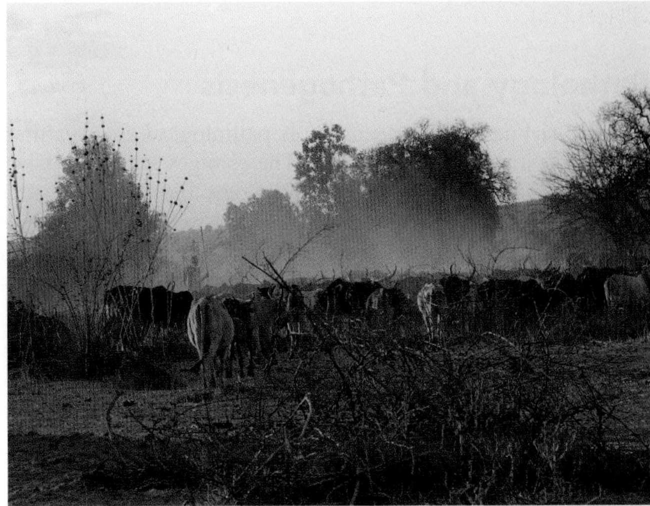

Figure 45.6 Typical place of transmission of *T.b. rhodesiense*; habitat of *G. morsitans*. (*Source: Irene Küpfer (Swiss Tropical and Public Health Institute): Urambo District, Tanzania.*)

The *morsitans* group, particularly *G. pallidipes* and *G. swynnertoni*, as well as *G. morsitans* itself, are the vectors; these species are preferentially bovid feeders and are not attracted to humans. Savannah *Glossina* spp. therefore feed on humans only when other hosts are not available. In Uganda also the *palpalis* group species *G. fuscipes* is a main vector for *T.b. rhodesiense*. The classical view of the epidemiology of *T.b. rhodesiense* trypanosomiasis is that specific groups of people are more at risk of becoming infected – usually those whose activities or occupations bring them into more frequent contact with *Glossina*. Examples of such groups are honey gatherers, fishermen, game wardens, poachers and firewood collectors. *T.b. rhodesiense* is a zoonosis; the known reservoir hosts are domestic animals such as cattle, sheep and goat, and a variety of game animals including carnivores.[36] The difference between *T.b. brucei* and *T.b. rhodesiense* is the sensitivity or resistance to human serum. Responsible is the serum resistance-associated gene, which is co-expressed with the variant surface antigen in *T.b. rhodesiense* stocks.[8,37,38]

Epidemics of acute disease have been observed over many decades, but most recently in Busoga, Uganda. This epidemic involved around 8000 cases per year in the mid-1980s but could be brought under control through a combination of intense surveillance, diagnosis and treatment, and vector control. The epidemic in Busoga was believed to be caused by a change in the agriculture of the area when cotton and coffee production ceased and the land was not cultivated, allowing the weed *Lantana camara* to become abundant. This shrub provided a suitable habitat for *G. f. fuscipes* to invade Busoga from the lakeside. A similar invasion of *G. f. fuscipes* occurred in Alego, Kenya,[39] and was associated with an earlier epidemic. In both of these epidemics cattle have been involved as reservoir hosts.[40,41] Detailed analysis of zymodemes has allowed the characterization of these parasites into the strain group Busoga, with a smaller number of isolates belonging to the Zambezi strain group which is more characteristic of Zambia. *G. f. fuscipes* flies can be found in peridomestic situations in East Africa, associated with cattle and pigs as a reservoir. This situation parallels peridomestic populations of West African riverine flies where, in humid areas, peridomestic *palpalis* group flies are associated with domestic pig populations living close to or within villages.[42]

Pathology and Pathogenesis

Sleeping sickness produces multiple pathological changes that involve most organs and systems. The changes are progressive and their anatomy, histology, physiology, biochemistry and immunology have been described extensively. The damage results from a complex interplay of parasite and host factors.

PATHOLOGY

A local inflammatory response with oedema and infiltration by macrophages and lymphocytes occasionally occurs in the skin at the site of infection, leading to a clinical lesion called a chancre. Trypanosomes are present in the chancre and can be detected by fine-needle aspiration. They then spread through the lymphatic and venous vessels to the haematolymphatic system. Lymph nodes become enlarged and infiltrated by lymphocytes and mononuclear cells.[43] The parasites can be found in the fluid obtained by lymph node puncture. The spleen and liver can be enlarged, but not massively. In the spleen, there is proliferation of the reticuloendothelium, congestion at the periphery of the splenic sinuses and often focal necrosis with macrophages and ingested red corpuscles; in the liver, infiltration with mononuclear cells in the periportal tracts, occasionally leading to granulomas, are prominent features.

Parasites multiply in the lymph and blood, as well as in extravascular tissues. In the initial stage of the illness, tissues that are most frequently involved are the skin, the skeletal muscles, the serous membranes of the pericardium, pleurae and peritoneum and the heart.[44] Microscopically, interstitial infiltration of mononuclear cells and vasculitis are observed. The heart is very heavily affected in *T.b. rhodesiense* infection, with a pancarditis involving all layers of the heart. Histologically, there is a marked interstitial infiltration with plasma and morular cells, with destruction of muscle fibres and fibrosis.

Invasion of the central nervous system (CNS) occurs weeks to months (*T b. rhodesiense*) or months to years (*T.b. gambiense*) after initial infection. The second stage of the illness is, by convention, defined by the appearance of trypanosomes or mononuclear inflammatory cells in the cerebrospinal fluid (CSF). The parasite entry into the CNS is mediated by both parasite- and host-derived factors, and does not result from simple diffusion as a consequence of a breakdown of the blood–brain barrier.[45,46]

The pathological changes in the human brains of *T.b. gambiense* and *T.b. rhodesiense* infected patients are similar.[47] Macroscopically, signs of leptomeningitis and granular ependymitis are seen. Signs of oedema may occur. Microscopically, a non-specific inflammatory cell infiltration in the leptomeninges and perivascularly, predominantly in the white matter, is the most prominent finding. In the white matter, there is proliferation of astrocytes and microglial cells, and an infiltration by Mott's morular cells that contain IgM in large intracellular vacuoles and that most likely derive from plasma cells. Morular cells can be observed in other CNS chronic infections such as syphilis and tuberculosis, but in smaller numbers. The location in the brain of the predominant white matter lesions correlates with the main clinical features.[48] Perivascular inflammation can also occur in cranial and spinal nerve roots, and in peripheral nerves. The inflammatory lesions spare the cerebral cortex, where neurons are well preserved, which contrasts with cortical lesions observed in neurosyphilis. As potentially reversible inflammatory lesions predominate over irreversible destruction of tissues, partial or full recovery of neuropsychiatric symptoms is observed after HAT treatment. Demyelinization and atrophy are observed in the terminal stage of the illness.

Blood homeostasis becomes significantly disturbed. Anaemia is common. Leukocytosis or leucopenia can occur and lymphocytosis is usually present, including occasional plasmocytes. Sleeping sickness is commonly associated with minor haemorrhages and multiple petechiae, although life-threatening bleeding is uncommon. Thrombocytopenia, when present, is more intense in *T.b. rhodesiense* infection, where it is occasionally associated with coagulopathy, including cases of disseminated intravascular coagulation.[49]

IMMUNOPATHOLOGY AND PATHOGENESIS

The variant surface glycoprotein (VSG) coat covering the membrane of African trypanosomes protects them from lytic factors in human plasma and allows them to escape the host immune reaction.[50] The VSG coat determines the antigenic phenotype of the parasite and protects invariant constituents of the outer membrane from the immune system. Each parasite genotype contains a repertoire of around 1000 different VSG genes. At any time, only a single VSG gene is actively transcribed.

The invasion of the brain by trypanosomes and the subsequent brain dysfunction observed in second-stage HAT is due to a complex and only partially understood interplay of parasite- and host-derived factors, as recently reviewed.[46]

Clinical Features

T.b. gambiense and *T.b. rhodesiense* HAT differ in many respects (Table 45.2), including clinical presentation. Whereas *T.b. gambiense* HAT is a slow-evolving disease, *T.b. rhodesiense* HAT is usually an acute febrile illness with a faster clinical evolution. Exceptions do occur, i.e. acute disease in *T.b. gambiense* and slow-evolving illness in *T.b. rhodesiense* HAT. Inter-individual and inter-geographical variations in the clinical presentation have been described in both forms of the disease, most likely due to a combination of parasite and host genetic factors.[51]

T.b. GAMBIENSE

T.b. gambiense infections run a chronic course from infection to extensive nervous system involvement and the classical picture of sleeping sickness.[52] The duration of first- and second-stage illness has recently been estimated by Checchi et al.[53] The mean first-stage duration was 526 days, with 3% of patients expected to remain in stage 1 for more than 5 years. The mean duration of second stage was corrected to a mean of 252 days (95% confidence interval: 171–399) by the same authors. Only

TABLE 45.2 Differences between *T.b. gambiense* and *T.b. rhodesiense* Sleeping Sickness

	West African (*T.b. gambiense*)	East African (*T.b. rhodesiense*)
Parasite	*T.b. gambiense*	*T.b. rhodesiense*
Main vectors	*G. palpalis* group	*G. morsitans* group
Main habitat	Near water	Savannah, cleared bush
Highest incidence	Central African Republic, Congo (DRC), South Sudan, North Uganda	South-east Uganda, Tanzania
Main reservoir	Humans, pig, dog	Antelope and cattle
Disease type	Chronic (years)	Acute (months)
Parasitaemia	Low	Moderate
Diagnosis	Lymph node aspiration, blood (concentration methods)	Blood
	CSF (lumbar puncture)	CSF (lumbar puncture)
Serology	CATT	None
TREATMENT		
First stage	Pentamidine	Suramin
Second stage	Eflornithine and Nifurtimox	Melarsoprol
Alternative treatment	Melarsoprol	(Melarsoprol and Nifurtimox)
Disease control	Active case search & Tsetse trapping	Tsetse trapping

Adapted after Pepin J. African Trypanosomiasis. In: Strickland GT, editor. Hunter's Tropical Medicine and Emerging Infectious Diseases. 8th edn. Philadelphia: Saunders; 2000. p. 643–54.

three patients with infection duration of more than 8 years have been reported. There is recent evidence that self-resolving first-stage infections can occur, at least with West African parasite strains,[54] but asymptomatic or mildly asymptomatic chronic carriage has not been demonstrated. The vast majority of patients therefore evolve from first to second stage and death in the absence of treatment.[55] Whereas some symptoms and signs are clearly associated with first (e.g. high fever) or second stage (e.g. neuropsychiatric disorders), none can be considered pathognomonic and staging predominantly relies on the examination of CSF (see below).

Systemic Symptoms and Signs

The incubation period is not known with precision as most infections occur in residents who experience tsetse bites, sometimes on a daily basis. The time between infection and the appearance of systemic symptoms (e.g. fever) lies in the range of weeks or months. The initial trypanosomal chancre, when present, can occur only days after the tsetse bite. The lesion consists of a tense, painful and itchy nodule that develops at the site of the infecting tsetse bite. It can be confused with a furuncle but does not suppurate, and spontaneously disappears in 1–2 weeks. In a case series that included a sizeable proportion of Europeans, 22% (19/84) presented with a chancre,[56] but the chancre is very rarely observed in endemic areas where lesions are generally considered as common insect bites, and where patients present at later disease stages.[57]

Systemic symptoms and signs are more common and marked during first-stage illness but also occur during the second stage. In addition, advanced disease is often associated with superimposed bacterial infections (e.g. pneumonia, meningitis) or other concomitant infections (e.g. malaria) that may contribute to fever and other symptoms. Fever is irregular, remittent, varying over a 24-hour period or in cycles of several days. It may be accompanied by fatigue, general malaise, anorexia and myalgia. It is more pronounced during the initial stage of the illness, marking the host's invasion by the parasite and the onset of immune response. It was observed on hospital admission in only 16% of 2505 patients with second-stage HAT in a multicentre study (Table 45.3).[58]

A circinate or serpiginous macular erythematous rash, often referred to as trypanosomal rash or trypanids, occasionally occurs on the trunk and proximal aspects of extremities, sometimes coalescing into large plaques. The rash is evanescent, fading in one place and reappearing in another over a period of several weeks. It is nearly impossible to detect on dark skin and has mainly been described in European patients, where it has been reported in up to 50% of cases.[56] Pruritus is a common finding in both stages but is more frequent and generalized during the second stage, when it affects around 50% of patients.[58] Concomitant conditions such as scabies and filariasis can contribute to the itching. Non-inflammatory oedema of the face and, more rarely, of extremities, is occasionally observed during the first stage.

Local or generalized enlargement of lymph nodes is a cardinal sign that must be systematically looked for, in practice by cervical palpation. When present, the degree of clinical suspicion of HAT is increased and lymph nodes can be punctured for diagnostic confirmation purpose. The latero-posterior cervical and supraclavicular groups are most commonly involved (Winterbottom sign) (Figure 45.7), but enlarged lymph nodes can be found elsewhere. Winterbottom was a British medical

TABLE 45.3 Typical Symptoms and Signs of Second-Stage *T.b. gambiense* Sleeping Sickness

Symptoms and Signs	(%)
Headache	78.7
Sleeping disorder	74.4
Adenopathy	56.1
Generalized pruritus	51.1
Splenomegaly[a]	42.5
Motor weakness	34.8
Hepatomegaly[a]	25.5
Malnutrition	25.2
Unusual behaviour	24.7
Disturbed appetite	22.9
Walking difficulties	21.7
Tremor	21.0
Fever	16.1
Speech disorder	13.4
Abnormal movements	10.5

[a]Information only available of 504 patients.

Compiled data from 2541 second-stage sleeping sickness patients from different countries and settings who were treated in multinational drug utilization study on an abridged treatment for melarsoprol (IMPAMEL II). Adapted from Blum J, Schmid C, Burri C. Clinical aspects of 2541 patients with second-stage human African trypanosomiasis. Acta Trop 2006;97(1):55–64.

officer in charge of examining 'candidates' for the slave trade on the African coast. Individuals with cervical lymph nodes were considered as unfit, as they would likely die of sleeping sickness during travel or be unable to work. Lymph nodes are painless, soft (but get harder as the illness evolves), moveable, and of variable size. They are detected in both disease stages in various (34–85%) proportions of patients.[58] Splenomegaly and, less frequently, hepatomegaly, can also be found in a variable proportion of patients in both stages but organ enlargement is not massive.

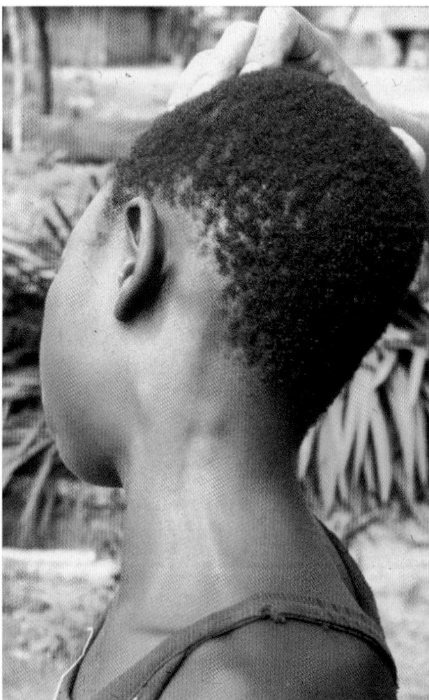

Figure 45.7 Winterbottom's sign; enlarged cervical lymph nodes in a patient with *T.b. gambiense* infection. (*Source: Johannes Blum (Swiss Tropical and Public Health Institute); Vanga, Democratic Republic of the Congo.*)

The mononuclear infiltration of the heart, first perivascular then becoming interstitial, can lead to myocarditis and more rarely to pancarditis, but these conditions are rarely clinically apparent, or detected, in *T.b. gambiense* HAT patients.[59] Whereas some symptoms (e.g. dyspnoea) and laboratory findings (pro-brain natriuretic peptide) consistent with decreased ventricular function were more frequent in HAT patients than in healthy controls, no patient received treatment for congestive heart failure in a cohort of 60 second-stage patients.[60] Recent ECG studies showed that the mean QTc interval was significantly longer in both first- and second-stage patients (421 and 423 ms, respectively) compared with healthy controls (403 ms), and was considered as prolonged in 11–12% of patients, but ominous prolongation (>500 ms) appears to be very rare. Other major ECG alterations in both disease stages were repolarization changes (35%) and low voltage (20–30%), which suggest some degree of pericarditis.[61] The presence of pericardial involvement is also supported by an echocardiographic study that showed pericardial effusion in 12% of 25 patients.[62]

Whereas symptoms consistent with hypothyroidism (e.g. lethargy, cold intolerance, peripheral oedema) or adrenal insufficiency (i.e. fatigue, hypotension, anorexia) are common in *T.b. gambiense* HAT patients, none of 60 Congolese patients with second-stage illness were diagnosed with hypothyroidism or adrenal insufficiency in a recent study.[63] These findings contrast with observations made in animal and human *T.b. rhodesiense* trypanosomiasis. Amenorrhea, loss of libido and impotence with decreased oestradiol and testosterone levels are found in at least 50% of patients and are likely to be of central origin (hypophyseal-subthalamic involvement).[64,65]

Neuropsychiatric Symptoms and Signs

Nonspecific neurological or psychiatric symptoms such as headaches and mood or behavioural changes are commonly found in both the first and second stages, but their intensity and persistence increase as the illness evolves. Once parasites cross the blood–brain barrier and invade the central nervous system (second stage), the clinical manifestations are partly explained by the predominant location of the brain lesions, e.g. sleep disturbances from involvement of supraoptic nuclei. It must be emphasized that neuropsychiatric symptoms and signs are absent or mild/moderate in the majority of second-stage patients at time of diagnosis,[66] unless access to diagnosis is severely impaired and therefore delayed (e.g. geographical remoteness, conflict areas).

Sleep disturbances are another clinical hallmark of the illness, giving it its common name, sleeping sickness. Some degree of sleep disturbance (nocturnal insomnia, daytime sleep) is not an uncommon complaint in first-stage patients, but the frequency and intensity of these symptoms increase in second-stage patients (Table 45.3), in whom it was correlated with duration of illness and the numbers of white cells in the CSF.[58] This is not hypersomnia, as the total duration of sleep is normal. Patients have frequent sleep episodes of short durations during both day and night caused by a dysregulation of the circadian rhythm of the sleep/wake cycle. Somnographic studies confirmed that a fragmentation of the sleeping patterns, characterized by the occurrence of sleep-onset rapid eye movements (SOREM), rather than an inversion of sleep, is characteristic for sleeping sickness.[67]

Disorders of tone and mobility, and abnormal movements are common features in advanced disease, reflecting the localization of lesions in the diencephalon and superior mesencephalon. Motor weakness and walking difficulties are common symptoms and signs. Signs of extra-pyramidal disorders are sometimes predominant, with Parkinson-like rigidity and paratonia. Abnormal movements can be athetoid or choreic, predominantly involving the distal portions of the upper extremities. Cerebellar involvement can be suspected in patients with ataxia and abnormal gait. A diffuse fine tremor or resting myoclonus can also be observed, with or without other motor disorders. Hemiplegia is rare, and is usually associated with very advanced stage.[68]

Mental disorders are a key disease feature that can start early in the course of the illness (first stage), and that may lead to the wrong diagnosis of primary psychiatric illness.[69] Common presentations are mood disorders with irritability or indifference, aggressive or antisocial behaviour, hyperactive or apathic attitudes, depression and/or delirium with hallucinations. Dementia does not develop until the terminal stage of the illness. Considering the wide spectrum of clinical presentations, any mental disorder should lead physicians to search for HAT in all patients who stayed, even years earlier, in endemic areas.

In the terminal stage, severe disturbances of consciousness, dementia and sometimes epilepsy are present, leading to incontinence, coma, cachexia, bed sores, bacterial infections (e.g. aspiration pneumonia) and death (Figure 45.8).

Most neuropsychiatric disturbances are reversible with antitrypanosomal treatment, including sleep alterations.[70] This correlates with the predominance of potentially reversible inflammatory lesions observed in histopathology. The improvement observed during hospitalization continues after discharge from hospital but various degrees of irreversible sequelae may nevertheless occur, especially if the disease has been diagnosed and treated at an advanced stage. Sequelae may be subtle, such as delayed sexual maturity or decreased school performance, as observed in children with second-stage HAT treated with melarsoprol.[71] The medium- and long-term neuropsychiatric outcome of second-stage patients treated with eflornithine, with or without nifurtimox, is yet unknown.

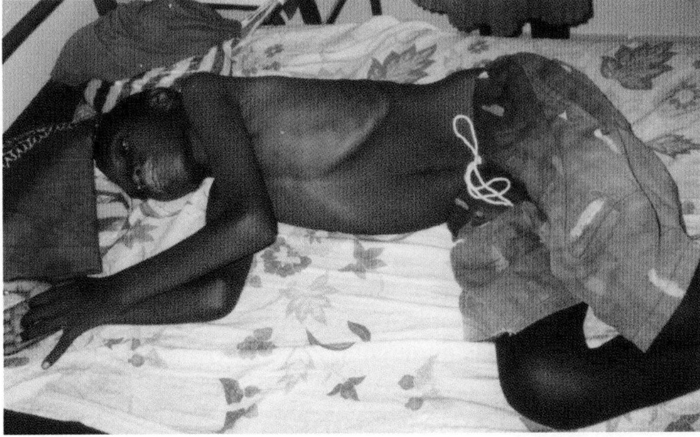

Figure 45.8 Patient with advanced second-stage *T.b. gambiense* infection. (Source: *Christian Burri (Swiss Tropical and Public Health Institute); Viana, Angola.*)

Specific Groups

Children. The clinical presentation is overall comparable in both children and adults. The prevalence and the detection of trypanosomes in cervical lymph nodes are less frequent in preschool children than in older children and adults.[72] Most symptoms and signs are seen with similar frequencies in first- and second-stage children, including sleep disturbances.[72–74]

Travellers. The clinical presentation of *T.b. gambiense* HAT in travellers (or expatriates) has been recently reviewed and compared with immigrants from endemic countries.[75] In travellers, the incubation time is shorter (<1 month in 75%), whereas chancre (47%), trypanosomal rash (33%) and splenomegaly (60%) are more often reported. Neuropsychiatric symptoms and signs are less frequently observed in travellers but this may be biased by earlier access to diagnosis.

HIV co-infected patients. HIV prevalence was not higher in HAT patients than in healthy controls in several West and Central African countries, suggesting that HIV infection does not predispose people to an increased risk of HAT.[76–78] The potential impact of HIV infection – or other causes of immunosuppression – on the clinical presentation of HAT has not been studied.

T.b. RHODESIENSE

The diversity of clinical presentations appears to be even more pronounced with *T.b. rhodesiense* than with *T.b. gambiense* infection. The spectrum of disease severity ranges from a chronic disease pattern, including reports of possible asymptomatic infections,[79] in southern endemic countries (e.g. Malawi, Zambia), to the 'typical' acute form observed in northern endemic countries (e.g. Uganda). The clinical presentation may even differ between sites in the same country, e.g. in Uganda.[80] Trypanosomes isolated from Uganda and Malawi showed to be of different genotypes and induced different immune response.[35]

Systemic Symptoms and Signs

The incubation period is not known with accuracy in residents from endemic regions but appears short (weeks) in areas where the clinical presentation is acute and long (months) in areas where the disease is more chronic. The initial trypanosomal chancre clinically looks similar to the lesion seen in *T.b. gambiense* infection (see above), but is more frequently observed.[75] Fever is seen on hospital admission in various proportions of both first-stage and second-stage patients. Headaches, diffuse muscle pain and joint pain are reported by the vast majority (>90%) of patients. Oedema of the face and legs has been reported in 20–43% of patients.[81,82] Patients may complain of pruritus, especially in the second stage of the illness. Lymphadenopathy has been reported in a very wide range of proportions in both disease stages, from 10% in Tanzania to 86% in Kenya.[81,83] Enlarged lymph nodes are mainly found in submandibular, inguinal and axillary regions. Hepatomegaly and splenomegaly are also reported in various proportions and predominate in foci where patients have a chronic disease course including a prolonged first stage.[80]

Perimyocarditis can be severe and seems to play an important part in the clinical course and fatal outcome, with histopathological examinations showing myocardial degeneration and interstitial haemorrhage.[84] In contrast, clinical symptoms and signs of heart failure are rarely described and do not appear to be prominent in large published case-series. Cardiac involvement may contribute to some nonspecific signs commonly reported in *T.b. rhodesiense*-infected patients such as leg oedema and hepatomegaly. There are scarce data on ECG findings, which appear to be similar to those described in *T.b. gambiense* HAT.[85]

Neuropsychiatric Symptoms and Signs

Neuropsychiatric features are comparable to those described above with *T.b. gambiense* infections, but the evolution towards coma and death is faster in *T.b. rhodesiense* HAT. Sleep disturbances, abnormal movements, alteration in gait, tremor, unusual behaviour, and aggressiveness are reported with variable frequencies depending on geographical locations.[80,81] Neuropsychiatric disturbances are associated with second-stage illness but some alterations (e.g. sleep and gait disturbances, tremor) have also been described in patients with first-stage illness in Uganda.[80]

Specific Groups

Children. Apart from a case report,[86] there is no specific description of *T.b. rhodesiense* HAT clinical features in children.

Travellers. *T.b. rhodesiense* HAT in travellers is an acute febrile illness with short (<3 weeks) incubation time as recently reviewed.[75] Trypanosomal chancre (>80%) and rash (~30%) are more frequently seen in travellers than in residents and can be observed in both disease stages. Signs of myopericarditis with conduction abnormalities have been reported, including various degrees of atrioventricular blocks, as well as clinical features of severe sepsis with disseminated intravascular coagulopathy and renal or multiorgan failures. In contrast, neuropsychiatric disorders such as sleep disturbances are rare findings in travellers.

HIV co-infected patients. Clinical features in HIV-negative and HIV-positive patients with *T.b. rhodesiense* HAT appear similar, but only a few co-infected patients ($n=16$) have been studied.[81]

Diagnosis

The diagnosis of *T.b. gambiense* HAT usually follows the pathway: screening, diagnostic confirmation and staging. Suspected cases detected by serological methods (usually the card agglutination test for trypanosomiasis, CATT) undergo parasitological diagnosis by investigation of the blood and/or lymph and, in case of a positive result, examination of the CSF follows for stage determination.[87] *T.b. rhodesiense* is usually directly detected in the blood.

IMMUNOLOGICAL METHODS

Field diagnosis of infections with *T.b. gambiense* relies on the initial screening with the card agglutination test for trypanosomiasis (CATT/*T.b. gambiense*) in most endemic areas. The test is a cheap and quick serologic test that has been widely used since it was developed in 1978.[88] The basis is a reagent composed of stained freeze-dried trypanosomes of selected variable antigen types (VATs), which can be obtained from the Institute of Tropical Medicine, Antwerp, Belgium. The CATT is an agglutination test of high sensitivity and specificity, and is easy to perform in the field. A drop of heparinized whole blood is mixed with a drop of the reagent on a card and, in the presence of specific antibodies, the trypanosomes in the reagent will agglutinate. It is inexpensive and results are obtained within 5 min.[19] Use of the CATT has considerably increased the detection rate in active surveys compared with the sole use of parasitological methods. No such test exists presently for *T.b. rhodesiense*, but parasite detection in the blood is much easier in this form of the disease. The specificity of the CATT can be further improved when performed on plasma or serum or when the plasma/serum is titrated. However, to date, there is no consensus about the cut-off. Confirmatory diagnosis by parasitological methods remains the gold standard. If the treatment decision is based on the CATT dilution, the epidemiological situation has to be considered and a stage determination must be performed to prevent patients from being unnecessarily exposed to drugs with a high risk for severe adverse drug reactions.[89–91]

Alternative tests, such as the LATEX/*T.b. gambiense* test, have been developed as a field alternative to the CATT.[92] The test is based on the combination of three purified variable surface antigens coupled with suspended latex particles. The test procedure is similar to CATT, including the use of a similar rotator. Compared with CATT, the LATEX/*T.b. gambiense* showed a higher specificity (96–99%) but a lower or similar sensitivity (71–100%) in recent field studies conducted in several Western and Central African countries.[87] Further evaluation is needed before it can be recommended for routine field use. For laboratory use, other methods, such as immunofluorescence (IF), indirect haemagglutination (IHA), enzyme-linked immunosorbent assay (ELISA) and different PCR methods, have been suggested.

MOLECULAR METHODS

Different PCR assays have been developed; but none of them has been validated for diagnostic purposes.[87,93] In a 2-year longitudinal study, a PCR test was evaluated in sleeping sickness patients in the Democratic Republic of the Congo.[94] For diagnostic purposes, the outcome was very positive with a sensitivity of 88.4% and a specificity of 99.2%, while for treatment follow-up, the test did not perform as expected. Loop-mediated isothermal amplification (LAMP) of trypanosome DNA is a new technique under investigation. It is fast and does not require expensive equipment since the PCR is done at a constant temperature.[95,96] It can be expected that a test kit will soon enter the market, which will facilitate diagnosis as well as follow-up of treated patients.

Simple and inexpensive methods will be required to allow the future diagnosis of sleeping sickness in primary healthcare facilities. Several methods are currently under investigation, and one of them, a simple molecular dipstick for visualization of PCR products, has undergone Phase I evaluation.[97]

PARASITOLOGICAL METHODS

As mentioned above, serological diagnosis of a trypanosome infection alone does not justify treatment because of the relative

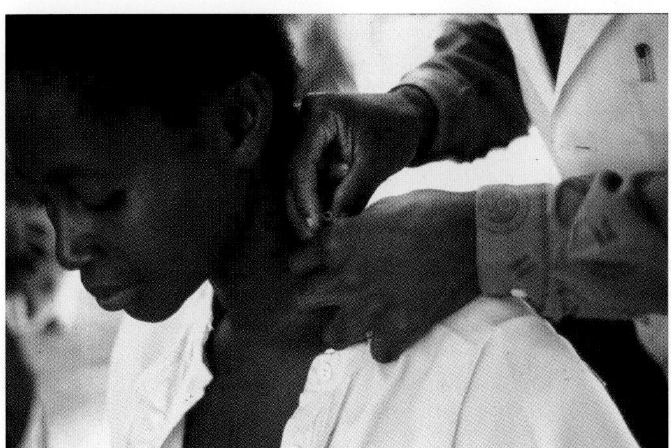

Figure 45.9 Lymph node aspiration for diagnosis. (Source: *Johannes Blum (Swiss Tropical and Public Health Institute); Vanga, Democratic Republic of the Congo.)*

toxicity of all drugs in use. Therefore, the detection of the parasite is of great importance. The body fluids that are most commonly examined for the presence of trypanosomes are blood, lymph node aspirate (Figure 45.9) and CSF. Trypanosomes may also be detected in bone marrow aspirates and ascites fluid.

- Techniques used for diagnosis in blood:
  - Blood films (thin, thick or wet) can be used for direct detection of trypanosomes. Wet blood films are used for the detection of motile trypanosomes, whereas thin and thick blood films are fixed in methanol and stained with Giemsa.
  - Concentration methods increase the chances for detection of the parasite because the parasitaemia, especially in *T.b. gambiense* infections, is usually very low.
  - The microhaematocrit centrifugation technique (m-HCT)[98] is based on microscopic examination of the buffy coat zone of blood cells using a low-power objective (×10 or ×20) following centrifugation in microhaematocrit capillaries. This method is used widely in the field.
  - The miniature anion-exchange centrifugation technique (m-AECT)[99] is based on the detection of trypanosomes in the eluate after the passage of infected blood through an anion-exchange (diethylaminoethyl cellulose) column followed by centrifugation. This method has proven to be more sensitive under field conditions than any other method.
- For analysis of the lymph:
  - A wet preparation of the aspirate from enlarged lymph nodes is examined at a magnification of ×400.[19]

A new simple method using fluorescence microscopy after acridine orange staining was developed by FIND Diagnostics (www.finddiagnostics.org) and Carl Zeiss. The sensitivity and ease of performance are much better than the standard bright field microscopy and field validation studies are underway.[100]

In vivo inoculation of biological material from humans, animal hosts or vectors into susceptible animals has been used to detect trypanosomes. Mice and rats are used for detecting *T.b. rhodesiense*, whereas immunosuppressed *Mastomys natalensis*, suckling rats or SCID (severe combined immunodeficient) mice should be used for *T.b. gambiense*.[6]

Determination of the Stage of the Disease

Chemotherapy, especially the use of melarsoprol for second-stage disease, bears the risks of adverse drug reactions. Today, treatment decision follows the staging and therefore, a correct determination of the stage is crucial before commencing treatment. Examination of the CSF is used to determine the stage of the disease. Parasites can sometimes be seen during white cell counting, but detection after concentration by centrifugation is substantially more sensitive.

The criteria for second-stage infection are: either trypanosomes detected in the CSF and/or a raised leukocyte count of >5 cells/mm^3.[19] A small-scale investigation indicated that infections of up to 20 cells/mm^3 may be treated with the first-stage drug pentamidine with only a minor increase in the relapse rate.[101] Other investigations have indicated however, that the cut-off should rather be maintained at 5 cells/mm^3. In one study, the risk of treatment failure in patients with a CSF leukocyte count of 6–10 cells/mm^3 was more than three times higher than in those with a count of 0–5 cells/mm^3.[25] In another investigation, patients with cell counts of 11–20 cells/mm^3 had 7.1 times higher odds for relapse than patients with a lower cell count (95% confidence interval 1.4–36).[102] An increased protein content of the CSF was formerly used as an additional criterion for staging, but due to the frequent lack of materials, variability of the results and the lesser predictive value compared with white blood cell counting, this method has been abandoned.[103]

The CSF of second-stage HAT patients contains high levels of immunoglobulins, especially IgM. An increased CSF IgM level has thus long been considered by some authors as a strong potential marker of second-stage HAT. A LATEX agglutination test for IgM in CSF (LATEX/IgM) has been designed for field use and was evaluated with CSF samples from patients from different countries.[104] It was found that CSF end titres obtained by the LATEX/IgM paralleled the IgM concentrations determined by light scatter measurement and ELISA. At a cut-off value of ≥1 : 8, the sensitivity and specificity of LATEX/IgM for intrathecal IgM were 89% and 93%, respectively.

Sleep–wake recordings may become another useful tool to detect CNS involvement and second-stage disease. In a small-scale investigation, the 24-hour distribution of sleep–wake, the altered sleep structure, sleep onset REM sleep periods (SOREM) and the EEG morphological alterations of first- and second-stage patients, were recorded. The sleep–wake cycle and sleep structure were totally disrupted in second-stage patients; these alterations being alleviated by treatment with melarsoprol. However, similar alterations were also observed in some first- or 'intermediate'-stage patients (5–20 cells/mm^3). More work is required to fully understand the influence of the disease on the sleep structure.[70]

Differential Diagnosis

Owing to the many clinical variations of sleeping sickness, it is difficult to describe a 'typical' case of the disease; differential diagnosis is therefore be of unusual importance. In first-stage human African trypanosomiasis, other causes of protracted febrile illness such as malaria, typhoid fever and viral hepatitis should be considered. The prominent lymphadenopathy can be suggestive of mononucleosis or tuberculous

TABLE 45.4 **Treatment of *T.b. gambiense* and *T.b. rhodesiense* Sleeping Sickness**

	West African (*T.b. gambiense*)	East African (*T.b. rhodesiense*)
FIRST STAGE		
Endemic countries	According to National legislation or guidelines	
Other countries	Pentamidine (pentamidine isethionate) 4 mg kg^{-1} body weight at 24 hourly intervals for 7 days IM (IV infusion)	Suramin Test dose of 4–5 mg kg^{-1} body weight at day 1, followed by five injections of 20 mg kg^{-1} body weight every 7 days (e.g. day 3, 10, 17, 24, 31). The maximum dose per injection is 1 g
SECOND STAGE		
Endemic countries	According to National legislation or guidelines	
Other countries	NECT 200 mg/kg of eflornithine IV as a short infusion every 12 hours for 7 days; combined with nifurtimox 5 mg/kg orally every 8 h for 10 days	Melarsoprol 2.2 mg kg^{-1} body weight IV at 24-hourly intervals for 10 days

lymphadenitis. In second-stage disease, syphilitic meningomyelitis, cerebral tumour, cerebral tuberculosis, HIV-associated cryptococcal meningitis and chronic viral encephalitis must be considered.

Management and Treatment

For a summary on the treatment options, refer to Table 45.4.

OVERVIEW

Sleeping sickness received major attention from the colonial administrations when it was perceived to be a threat to the native population and the expatriates living in Africa and hampered the exploitation of whole regions. Drug research was innovative in the early to mid-twentieth century and was performed by very prominent researchers, e.g. Paul Ehrlich[105] and Louise Pearce.[106] The interest in the disease however, dwindled after the decolonization of the African countries and the resulting decreased economic interest, and the new authorities set their focus on other priorities. Over the past half a century, human African trypanosomiasis has become one of the most neglected diseases as its prevalence has resurged. Despite intense basic research on trypanosomes, no safe drugs have been put forward.[107] All substances developed in the first half of the twentieth century had major disadvantages; either they were very toxic (melarsoprol) or they were fairly tolerable but did not cross the blood–brain barrier (suramin, pentamidine). The latter disadvantage meant that different drugs were needed for treatment of the first and second stages, making lumbar punctures essential to discriminate first- and second-stage disease and to follow-up the patients after treatment. First-stage sleeping sickness is still treated with pentamidine (*T.b. gambiense*) and suramin (*T.b. rhodesiense*) and, until very recently, the first-line treatment of second-stage disease was melarsoprol.

However, over the past decade, substantial developments in the chemotherapy of the disease have been made and hence, the recommendations for treatment here differ very much from older editions of this book.

In the 1980s, an antineoplastic drug, eflornithine, received increasing attention for its antitrypanosomal activities[108] and the compound was eventually registered by the US FDA for this indication in 1990.[109] However, the use of the drug remained limited to emergency interventions of a few NGOs, mainly because of its very complex administration requiring sophisticated logistics and nursing care and initially, due to its high costs (Figure 45.10); nor is eflornithine active against *T.b. rhodesiense*.[110] At the same time, nifurtimox, developed for Chagas disease, was used in experimental settings, mainly to treat melarsoprol-refractory cases. The compound had only very limited activity when used as a monotherapy and it also led to significant adverse drug reactions.[108] However, the availability of different compounds raised the interest of scientists with regard to combination therapy. Many combinations of registered and experimental compounds were tested on animals.[111]

In the mid-1990s, the pharmacokinetics of melarsoprol were finally elucidated[112] and allowed the possibility of one abridged regimen for treatment of second-stage sleeping sickness with melarsoprol, instead of the various empirically derived complex schemes. The new schedule, recommended by the 27th International Scientific Council for Trypanosomiasis Research and Control (ISCTRC) in 2003[113] as standard treatment for

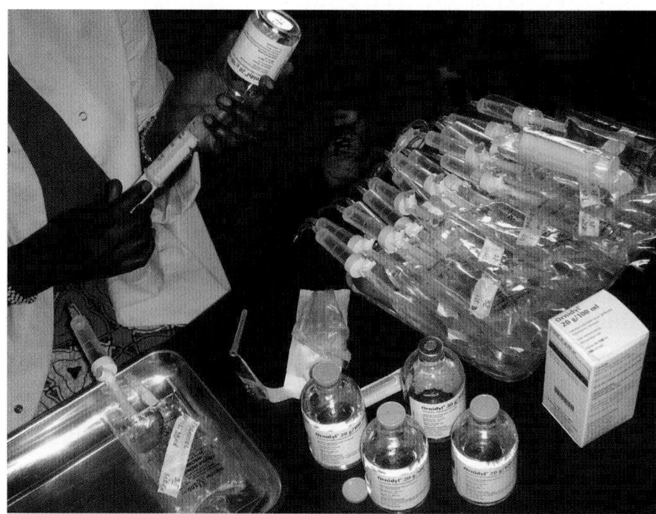

Figure 45.10 Preparation of eflornithine. (*Source: François Chappuis (Médecins sans Frontières Switzerland); Banda, Democratic Republic of the Congo.)*

second-stage *T.b. gambiense* HAT, reduced the treatment duration from 25–36 to 10 days. The new scheme had not only a major socioeconomic advantage because of the shorter hospitalization and drug saving, but also the IMPAMEL programme (improved application of melarsoprol) comprised the first large-scale clinical trial on HAT executed according to good clinical practice (GCP), and thus demonstrated the feasibility of modern clinical development in Africa. The abridged melarsoprol regimen however, could not be regarded as a complete breakthrough, since the frequency of the major adverse drug reactions remained significant. Encephalopathic syndromes continued to occur in 5–10% of patients treated with melarsoprol and resulted in death in 10–50% of those in whom encephalopathy developed.

At the end of the last century, the treatment of sleeping sickness was in decline: the availability of the drugs was threatened, either by increasing price (pentamidine), halted production (eflornithine) or planned cessation of production (nifurtimox, suramin and melarsoprol),[114] and there was an increasing number of cases refractory to melarsoprol.[115,116]

In a landmark effort, the World Health Organization (WHO) initiated a network in 1999 to ensure availability and affordability of antitrypanosomal drugs. The exercise resulted in 2001, in renewable contracts with two manufacturers: Aventis (now Sanofi) and Bayer, who committed themselves to manufacturing and free donation of the essential drugs to treat HAT, for distribution by the WHO.[117] Those contracts not only significantly improved access to treatment, but were also one of the elements to trigger a new era of research. Several trials assessing combinations of eflornithine, melarsoprol and nifurtimox were conducted. In all trials, the efficacy was better with combination therapy compared with monotherapy. However, combinations containing melarsoprol continued to result in very high frequencies of severe adverse drug reactions[118,119] and were rapidly abandoned. In a multi-centre trial, nifurtimox–eflornithine combination therapy (NECT) was initiated in the Republic of Congo and the DRC, and the results were compared with the standard eflornithine therapy.[120] NECT reduces the number of infusions from 56 to 14; it shortens hospitalization time by one-third and reduces the total amount of eflornithine by half.[121] Based on these favourable trial results, NECT was included for treatment of second-stage *T.b. gambiense* HAT into WHO's Essential Medicines List (EML) in May 2009.[122] NECT can be considered a milestone improvement but the complexity of its application still restricts the use in second-stage disease. Lumbar puncture for diagnostic staging is therefore still required.

A breakthrough in the treatment of *T.b. rhodesiense* however, is not in sight. The only substantial progress made in the past 60 years has been the recommendation of the abridged treatment regimen for melarsoprol by the ISCTRC in 2009, based on the last trial of the IMPAMEL programme.[123]

TREATMENT OF FIRST-STAGE DISEASE

Trypanocidal drugs that do not sufficiently cross the blood–brain barrier to reach adequate drug levels in the CNS are limited to the first stage of the disease. Drugs able to cure second-stage disease were for a long time too toxic for use against the first stage, and the new first-line treatment NECT is still too complex to be used against first stage. Therefore, treatment of the first stage remains restricted to pentamidine and suramin.

Pentamidine

Pentamidine, introduced in 1940, became the drug of choice for first-stage *gambiense* sleeping sickness. Cure rates are 93–98% and have not decreased over the decades.[19] Failures in *rhodesiense* sleeping sickness, have been reported to be quite frequent,[124] but no recent results are available.

Today, all national sleeping sickness programmes follow a schedule of daily injections of 4 mg/kg of pentamidine isethionate for 7 days. For treatment of sleeping sickness, the drug is usually given as deep intramuscular injection, because of the frequent occurrence of hypotension after intravenous application. A bolus injection must be avoided and infusions should last 60–120 minutes. An abridged schedule of three injections is currently being studied, but no information is yet available.

Generally, pentamidine is well tolerated, although minor adverse reactions are common.[125] Immediate adverse drug reactions include hypotension in about 10% of the patients, with dizziness, sometimes collapse and shock; after intravenous injection, the frequency of hypotensive reactions can be as high as 75%. Other adverse drug reactions occasionally observed are nausea and/or vomiting, and pain at the injection site. Sterile abscesses or necrosis may occur at the intramuscular injection site. Systemic reactions reported include azotaemia due to a nephrotoxicity, leucopaenia, abnormal findings in liver function tests, hypoglycaemia and hyperglycaemia. Precipitation of diabetes is a rare event.[126]

The maximum plasma levels in patients treated for *T.b. gambiense* with 10 intramuscular injections of pentamidine methanesulfonate are generally reached within 1 hour after injection and vary extensively (214–6858 ng/mL). The median plasma concentration after the last dose is about five times higher than after the first. The median half-life associated with the first, second and third phase of elimination is 4 minutes, 6.5 hours and 512 hours, respectively.[127] Pentamidine is converted to at least seven primary metabolites by the cytochrome P-450-dependent oxygenases in rat liver homogenates and rat liver microsomes.[128]

The mode of action of pentamidine is unknown. Binding to nucleic acids, disruption of kinetoplast DNA, inhibition of RNA editing in trypanosomes and inhibition of messenger RNA trans-splicing have all been suggested.[129]

Due to the high potency of pentamidine and the low drug levels detected in the CSF,[127] the use in 'intermediate-stage' patients (up to 10 or 20 WBC/mm^3 in CSF) was suggested.[101] The resulting efficacy in respective studies is equivocal.[23,25,130] Hence, the use of pentamidine for patients with 5–20 cells/mm^3 should not be generally recommended, but should be restricted to areas where melarsoprol is still in use and thus the risk for severe adverse drug reactions remains very high, and where a very good adherence to follow-up and rapid access to rescue treatment is guaranteed.

Suramin

Suramin was introduced in 1920 in Germany for the treatment of trypanosomiasis. It is effective against the first stage of both forms of the disease, but pentamidine is generally preferred today for treatment of *T.b. gambiense*.

The most commonly used dosage regimen consists of a test dose of suramin 4–5 mg/kg body weight on day 1, followed by five injections of 20 mg/kg body weight of suramin every 7 days (e.g. days 3, 10, 17, 24, 31).[19] The maximum dose per injection is 1 g. Suramin is injected intravenously after dilution in distilled water.

Some degree of renal impairment is common, but nephrotoxicity is usually mild and reversible.[124] The first symptoms are albuminuria, then cylindruria and haematuria. Regular urine checks during the course of treatment are therefore recommended. Other adverse drug reactions reported are early hypersensitivity reactions such as nausea, urticaria and circulatory collapse. Exfoliative dermatitis and haemolytic anaemia, peripheral neuropathy and bone marrow toxicity with agranulocytosis and thrombocytopenia may occur. Pruritus is more frequent with concomitant filariasis, due to the effect of suramin on adult worms.

About 99.7% of the drug is bound to plasma proteins (e.g. albumin, globulins, fibrinogen), which places suramin in the class of the most extensively bound drugs. Suramin has one of the longest half-lives of all drugs given to humans. In patients with HIV/AIDS who were given suramin once weekly for 5 weeks, the drug accumulated during the time of administration and then diminished, with a half-life of 44–54 days;[131] in patients with onchocerciasis, the terminal half life was 92 days.[132] Total plasma levels remained above 100 μg/mL for several weeks. The volume of distribution was 38–46 L, and total clearance was <0.5 mL/min.[131] The renal clearance contributed essentially to the removal of the drug from the body.

Suramin non-specifically inhibits numerous enzymes, including: 1-α-glycerophosphate oxidase; glycerol-3-phosphate dehydrogenase; RNA polymerase and kinases; thymidine kinase; dihydrofolate reductase; hyaluronidase; urease; hexokinase; fumarase; trypsin; reverse transcriptase and the receptor-mediated uptake of low-density lipoprotein by trypanosomes. Suramin is taken up by trypanosomes by pinocytosis, as a plasma protein-bound complex.[133] The accumulation of suramin in trypanosomes was hypothesized to be one of the reasons for the differential toxicity between the host and the parasite.

TREATMENT OF SECOND-STAGE DISEASE

For over 50 years, the organo-arsenical drug, melarsoprol (Arsobal®, Sanofi), developed in 1949, was the only option for treatment of second-stage disease. In May 2009, the nifurtimox-eflornithine combination therapy (NECT) was included, for treatment of second-stage *T.b. gambiense* HAT, into WHO's Essential Medicines List (EML)[122] and therefore melarsoprol should now be restricted to treatment of infections caused by *T.b. rhodesiense* and for cases relapsing after treatment of *T.b. gambiense* infection with NECT.

Eflornithine

In 1990, the US Food and Drug Administration (FDA) had approved eflornithine (α-difluoromethylornithine; DFMO, Ornidyl® Sanofi) for the treatment of *gambiense* sleeping sickness.[109] Eflornithine resulted in significantly fewer deaths and severe adverse events than did 10 days of therapy with intravenous melarsoprol. No evidence of increased death or relapse rates within 12 months after the completion of eflornithine treatment was found. However, the use of eflornithine as monotherapy is very complicated. The lack of trained medical staff in many remote healthcare centres and the insufficient financial and logistic capacities in most endemic countries hampered the universal implementation of eflornithine. The introduction of a combination with nifurtimox (NECT) mitigated those difficulties (see below).

Adverse drug reactions under eflornithine treatment are frequent and similar to those of other cytotoxic drugs. They increase with the duration of treatment and the severity of the general condition of the patient. The most frequent adverse effects are bone marrow toxicity (anaemia, leucopenia, thrombocytopenia) in 25–50% of treated patients. Gastrointestinal symptoms such as nausea, vomiting and diarrhoea are observed in about 10%, alopecia, usually towards the end of the treatment, is seen in about 5–10%, and neurological symptoms such as convulsions in 7% of treated patients. Generally, adverse drug reactions of eflornithine are reversible after the completion of the treatment course. The drug arrests embryonic development in mice, rats and rabbits; the excretion into breast milk is unknown.[134]

After low oral doses (5–10 mg/kg), peak plasma concentrations are reached within 1.5–6 hours. The mean half-life is 3.3 hours and the volume of distribution in the range of 0.35 L/kg. Renal clearance is about 2 mL/min per kg (after intravenous application) and accounts for more than 80% of drug elimination. Bioavailability of an orally administered 10 mg/kg dose was estimated at 54%. Eflornithine produces CSF: plasma ratios of between 0.13 and 0.51.[135]

Eflornithine acts by inhibiting the trypanosomal enzyme ornithine decarboxylase (ODC), which catalyses the conversion of ornithine to putrescine, the first and rate-limiting step in the synthesis of putrescine and the polyamines spermidine and spermine.[136] Polyamines are involved in nucleic acid synthesis, contribute to the regulation of protein synthesis and are essential for the growth and multiplication of all eukaryotic cells.[137] Trypanosomes are more susceptible to the drug than human cells, possibly because of the slow turnover of this enzyme in *T.b. gambiense*.[136] The rapid turnover of ODC is responsible for the innate resistance of *T.b. rhodesiense* to eflornithine.[138]

Nifurtimox

Nifurtimox (Lampit®; Bayer) is a drug that was introduced in the late 1960s for use in patients with Chagas disease.[139] The drug is not registered for use in sleeping sickness, and its use was restricted to the compassionate treatment in combination with other trypanocidal drugs of patients not responding to melarsoprol and is now a component of NECT. Nifurtimox was tested empirically in HAT case series during the 1970s and 1980s, with conflicting results.[119] These evaluations differed in treatment regimens and evaluation criteria, making them difficult to compare. For treatment schedules, see below and Table 45.4.

Nifurtimox is not well tolerated, and only about one-third of the patients remain free of adverse drug reactions[140] but normally, adverse drug reactions are not severe, very rarely fatal and dose-related.[141] Gastrointestinal disturbances with nausea, abdominal pain and vomiting are frequent, and neurological adverse reactions with generalized convulsions, tremor or agitation may occur. The development of peripheral polyneuropathy and generalized skin reactions are seen occasionally. All adverse reactions are rapidly reversible after discontinuation of the drug.

In healthy human volunteers given a single oral dose of 15 mg/kg nifurtimox, average peak plasma levels of 751 (range 356–1093) ng/mL were reached within 2–3 hours. The drug has an apparent volume of distribution of about 755 L (approx.

15 L/kg) and a high apparent clearance of 193 L/h (about 64 mL/min per kg). Nifurtimox is quickly eliminated with an average plasma elimination half-life of 3 (range 2–6) hours.[142]

The mechanism of action of nifurtimox is not completely elucidated. Its trypanocidal action may be related to its ability to undergo partial reduction to form chemically reactive radicals, causing the production of superoxide anions, hydrogen peroxide and hydroxyl radicals. These free radicals may react with cellular macromolecules and cause membrane injury, enzyme inactivation, damage to DNA and mutagenesis.[143]

Melarsoprol

The use of melarsoprol is associated with a high frequency of severe adverse drug reactions, including an encephalopathic syndrome, which occurs in 5–10% of treated cases, and which is fatal for about 10–50% of those affected.[19,144] In several foci of Angola, the Democratic Republic of the Congo (DRC), Southern Sudan and Uganda, treatment failures have reached levels of 30%. Several parasite strains isolated from relapse cases lack the P2 transporter, which has been described to import melarsoprol into the parasite.[145] However, so far the demonstration of parasite resistance in the field has been hampered by difficulties in retrieving *T.b. gambiense* isolates from patients for investigation.

Due to the lack of efficient alternatives, melarsoprol remains the first-line treatment for second-stage *T.b. rhodesiense* HAT. In 2009, the abridged schedule was recommended by the 30th Meeting of the International Scientific Council for Trypanosomiasis Research and Control (ISCTRC), as the standard regimen.[123]

NECT: Nifurtimox-Eflornithine Combination Therapy

To overcome the precarious treatment effects of melarsoprol, a combination of the existing drugs was suggested. A preliminary clinical trial combining melarsoprol and nifurtimox indicated the potential usefulness of this approach.[146] A further trial conducted in Omugo, Uganda was designed to compare three different combination treatment regimens: melarsoprol-nifurtimox, melarsoprol-eflornithine and nifurtimox-eflornithine. For ethical reasons, the enrolment was suspended after about one-third of the planned recruitment, as high fatality rates and toxicity were observed in the melarsoprol-nifurtimox arm. An intention-to-treat analysis yielded cure rates of 44.4% for melarsoprol-nifurtimox; 78.9% for melarsoprol-eflornithine and 94.1% for nifurtimox-eflornithine.[119]

Subsequently, a multi-country trial of NECT was carried out to compare standard eflornithine therapy with an empirically established abridged regimen consisting of 200 mg/kg of eflornithine IV as a short infusion every 12 hours for 7 days, combined with nifurtimox 5 mg/kg orally every 8 h for 10 days. This regimen reduces the number of infusions from 56 to 14 and the treatment duration from 14 to 10 days.[120,121,147] The reduction from four to two daily applications of eflornithine was based on the argument that the short half-life of eflornithine might be balanced by the long-lasting pharmacodynamic effect on trypanosomes, explained by the long time (18–19 h) needed by *T.b. gambiense* to replenish their ornithine decarboxylase after inhibition by eflornithine[147] and that a previous combination trial using standard dose eflornithine with nifurtimox had resulted in a very low relapse rate.[119] The relapse after 18 months of follow-up among the 286 patients enrolled was 5.7% under eflornithine and 1.4% under NECT treatment (intention to treat population). Adverse events were frequent in both groups; 41 (28.7%) patients in the eflornithine group and 20 (14.0%) in the NECT group had major (grade 3 or 4) reactions, but the proportion of patients with major (grade 3–4) drug-related adverse events was lower in the NECT group than in the eflornithine group (20/143 [14.0%] vs 41/143 [28.7%]; $p=0.002$). Neurological events were the leading cause (seizures and coma); gastrointestinal disorders were expectedly very frequent; but major events were very rare. The overall mortality observed within 30 days of treatment was lower under NECT treatment (3/143 [2.1%] vs 1/143 [0.7%]; $p=0.622$), which is very low compared with the average fatality rates under melarsoprol, of 5–6%.[121]

NECT has large operational advantages over the eflornithine monotherapy: it is easier to administer, reduces the amount of drug, staff and logistic resources, requires a significantly shorter hospital stay and it may be speculated to have a positive effect against development of drug resistance. Based on those advantages and the favourable results of the trials conducted so far, NECT was included for treatment of second-stage *T.b. gambiense* HAT into WHO's Essential Medicines List (EML), in May 2009.[122]

The current challenge is the implementation of the new treatment. This effort is supported by a currently ongoing field study (NECT-FIELD) to assess the effectiveness of the NECT treatment under real conditions, learn about the limitations of its use in very rural settings and to optimize its use and logistics.[148] A total of 630 patients including 100 children and 40+ pregnant women were enrolled for the study and it was due to reach the end of the 2 years follow-up at the end of 2012.[149]

A complete set of studies conducted on chemotherapy of second-stage HAT has recently been summarized in a report by the Cochrane Collaboration.[150]

New Developments

As a result of increased efforts in the identification of targets, and high throughput as well as whole cell screening, a number of new drug targets and several compounds with promising activity have been identified. So far, drug target validation and lead identification and optimization has proved to be difficult but nevertheless, successful. Currently, there are only a few molecules in pre-clinical and two in clinical development for the treatment of HAT.

The most advanced new drug candidate is fexinidazole, which belongs to the nitroimidazole class of compounds that has previously shown activity against trypanosomes.[151] The molecule was re-discovered during an extensive compound mining effort undertaken by the DNDi since 2005, to explore new and old nitroimidazoles as drug leads against human African trypanosomiasis.[152] The compound proved to be orally active against *T.b. gambiense* and *T.b. rhodesiense* in animal studies and had an excellent safety profile. Since it penetrates the blood–brain barrier, it could be effective in both stages of sleeping sickness. In September 2009, the first in-human Phase I study was initiated.[153] Some authors have expressed concerns about potential cross-resistance between nifurtimox and fexinidazole. Trypanosome strains selected for resistance to fexinidazole were 10-fold more resistant to nifurtimox than their parents.[154] The implications of this finding will have to be further explored during the development process. Fexinidazole entered Phase II clinical trials in the third quarter of 2012.

Besides fexinidazole, a novel class of boron-containing molecules, benzoxaboroles, is being explored to yield another clinical candidate against sleeping sickness. Several members of this class proved to be very potent against *T.b. gambiense* and *T.b. rhodesiense in vitro* and *in vivo*. Pharmacokinetic analysis in rodents and primate models shows that oxaboroles are highly bioavailable and readily cross the blood–brain barrier, which makes them potential candidates for treatment of second-stage disease. One candidate, SCYX-7158, is about to enter the clinical phase of development.[155–157]

In 2008, the development of a new medicine against first-stage HAT, DB289 or pafuramidine maleate, failed. After extensive Phase I (healthy volunteers) and Phase II testing (proof of concept in patients), a pivotal Phase III trial was initiated in August 2005 and its follow-up ended in mid-2009. A total of 273 patients were enrolled in four centres in the DRC and in one centre each, in Angola and South Sudan. All patients completed the assigned drug regimen of pafuramidine, 100 mg bid, oral for 10 days or pentamidine 4 mg/kg IM for 7 days. The safety profile of pafuramidine appeared to be very inconspicuous; ALT and AST elevations were much more frequently recorded and only reached Grades 2 and 3 elevation under pentamidine therapy. The per protocol efficacy at the 12-month follow-up was 89% for pafuramidine and 96% for pentamidine, respectively. However, during an additional Phase I trial designed to provide supportive safety data for the registration of pafuramidine, the development programme was placed on hold by the US FDA to allow the investigation of unexpected liver toxicity. Subsequently, five subjects of the same healthy volunteer study developed renal failure approximately 8 weeks post-treatment, that required medical intervention. Re-examination of the Phase III sleeping sickness data identified three subjects who had developed glomerulonephritis or other nephropathies post-pafuramidine treatment; two of these events may retrospectively be considered possibly related to pafuramidine. No patient in the pentamidine group was reported to have renal problems. The clinical development programme for pafuramidine was discontinued at this time.[158] A number of other diamidine compounds are further pursued and showed high activities in mouse models.[159] Aza-analogues of pafuramidine and its parent diamidine achieved the cure of a monkey model mimicking first stage (oral application) and also second stage (IM application).[151]

TREATMENT FOLLOW-UP

All patients should be monitored for 2 years, with lumbar punctures performed every 6 months.[160] In the absence of trypanosomes visualized in CSF, blood or lymph nodes, first-stage patients should be considered to have relapsed if they present at any examination with a white cell count >20 cells/mm^3. In second-stage cases, a relapse is suspected if the CSF white cell count is ≥50 cells/mm^3, and has doubled since the previous examination, or 20–49 cells/mm^3 with recurrence of symptoms. In case of equivocal results, the patient should be seen again after 1–2 months. A relapse is confirmed if trypanosomes can be found in the CSF at any follow-up examination.[161] There is no analytical method for distinguishing between relapse and reinfection. Based on the current knowledge retreatment should be attempted with melarsoprol, with or without nifurtimox.

The 2-year follow-up period is very difficult to implement in practice due to low adherence to follow-up visits, notably related to patients' reluctance to undergo repeated lumbar punctures. A prospective study conducted in DRC showed that patients with ≤5 cells in CSF at the 6-month post-treatment visit were at low risk of later relapse and can safely be considered as cured.[162] This new follow-up schedule – also called 5–50–20 – may allow shortening follow-up to 6 (in the majority of patients) to 12 months.

Prevention and Disease Control

Individual prophylaxis aims at preventing contact with tsetse flies or being bitten by them. Tsetse flies occur in foci and are bound to certain types of vegetation (e.g. *Lantana* sp.) or to water (e.g. along rivers in gallery forests). Such 'hot spots' should be avoided, thus reducing the risk of contact with the flies. The use of repellents may be considered but it is known that their protection is limited. Tsetse flies like to follow large moving objects such as cars. When passing through an area infested by tsetse flies, it is recommended to close the windows of the vehicle to prevent the insects from entering. Tourists normally do not come across tsetse flies, unless they travel up country or to national parks in East Africa.

Control of HAT relies on identification and treatment of patients who also act as reservoirs of the parasites, and on control of the insect vector. Infected persons may remain almost asymptomatic for long periods before they develop signs of sleeping sickness but they always represent a threat by harbouring the trypanosomes. Therefore, the most important control measure for *T.b. gambiense* trypanosomiasis is active case-finding, followed by treatment of the infected subjects. Populations of endemic areas (foci) with a prevalence of >1% should be examined once a year by mobile teams (Figure 45.11). In areas with a prevalence <1%, active case detection may be maintained with a reduced periodicity.[19] The use of the CATT has become a routine tool, and its increased sensitivity over lymph node aspiration has partially made up for the lower participation of the population today, compared with that in colonial times. CATT-positive patients should be subjected to the diagnostic path described above. However, the parasitological methods have a limited sensitivity and therefore do not allow all HAT patients with a positive screening result to be confirmed parasitologically and receive treatment. One option is to examine these serologically suspected individuals at regular intervals (e.g. every 3 months) for 1–2 years, but compliance

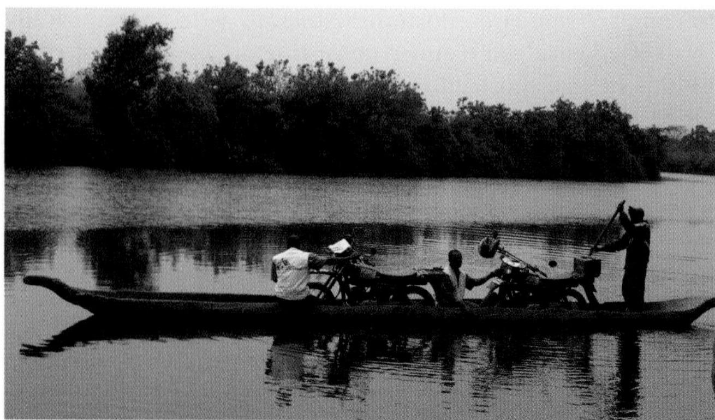

Figure 45.11 Active screening team. (Source: *Pierre Havouis (Médecins sans Frontières); near Ango, Democratic Republic of the Congo.)*

with this procedure is usually low. A more promising option is to determine a subgroup of serologically suspected individuals at high risk of being infected with *T.b. gambiense* and to treat them. It was suggested to treat all serologically suspected individuals with a CATT end titre of ≥1 : 16, when the prevalence of HAT in the investigated population is sufficiently high. It remains an open question which prevalence threshold should be chosen for this approach, but it should probably be no less than 1%.[87] However, the risk of unnecessary treatment should also be considered, and thus other factors such as poor access to care and the absence of concentration methods for the parasitological diagnosis, may positively influence the decision to perform titration of serum and treat individuals with a CATT end titre of ≥1 : 16.

Vector control is the second powerful tool in the control of HAT. At the time of the colonial powers, spraying of insecticides was a common measure to reduce the fly density. After DDT became banned, based on environmental considerations, synthetic pyrethroids were used as ultra-low-dose aerial spraying, as pour-on for cattle or to impregnate targets.[163] The use of traps is still an effective way to reduce the number of tsetse flies. There are several types of traps. They are made of blue and black (most attractive colours for tsetse flies) cloth, which can be treated with insecticides.[160,164,165] Tsetse flies of the *morsitans* group can be further attracted by host odours or the components acetone, octanol and phenols, while flies of the *palpalis* group are more responsive to visual stimuli.[166] Such traps can be produced and maintained through community participation, a system that proved to be highly effective as long as it is sustained. In 2001, the Pan African Tsetse and Trypanosomiasis Eradication Programme (PATTEC) was launched with the support of affected African nations and international organizations. The goal is to eliminate tsetse flies and African trypanosomiasis of humans and domestic animals, mainly by tsetse eradication measures. Traps and aerial spraying should reduce the tsetse populations and the use of the sterile insect technique (SIT) will eventually lead to elimination of tsetse flies in a given area. Proof of this concept is the eradication of *Glossina austeni* from Unguja, one of the islands of Zanzibar.[167] SIT has to be employed for each tsetse species occurring in an area, by releasing sterile male flies in excess of the number of normal males. Isolated foci can best be tackled one by one in a process that can finally lead to the elimination of the disease in 20–30 years from now.[163]

REFERENCES

15. Brun R, Blum J, Chappuis F, et al. Human African trypanosomiasis. Lancet 2010;375:148–59.
28. Simarro PP, Diarra A, Ruiz Postigo JA, et al. The human African trypanosomiasis control and surveillance programme of the World Health Organization 2000–2009: the way forward. PLoS Neglect Trop Dis 2011;5(2):e1007.
58. Blum J, Schmid C, Burri C. Clinical aspects of 2541 patients with second-stage human African trypanosomiasis. Acta Trop 2006;97(1):55–64.
87. Chappuis F, Loutan L, Simarro P, et al. Options for field diagnosis of human African trypanosomiasis. Clin Microbiol Rev 2005;18(1):133–46.
151. Brun R, Don R, Jacobs RT, et al. Development of novel drugs for human African trypanosomiasis. Future Microbiol 2011;6(6):677–91.

Access the complete references online at www.expertconsult.com

46

American Trypanosomiasis: Chagas Disease

CARLOS FRANCO-PAREDES

KEY POINTS

- Chagas disease (CD), or American trypanosomiasis, is a zoonotic tropical disease caused by the flagellate protozoan parasite *Trypanosoma cruzi* (*T. cruzi*). Most infections occur through vector-borne transmission by triatomine insects in endemic areas, but can also occur through blood transfusion or organ transplantation, vertically from mother to infant, more rarely by ingestion of food or liquid contaminated with *T. cruzi*; or accidents among laboratory personnel who work with live parasites.
- Since its discovery in Brazil by Carlos Chagas in 1909, the lack of effective vaccines, optimal chemoprophylaxis, or evidence-based chemotherapy to control CD, continues to place this disease as one of the most important historical public health challenges in the Americas.
- Approximately 7.6 million people are currently infected with CD, according to the most recent estimates. The disease is endemic in Mexico, Central and South America. Rare cases of CD attributed to local vector-borne transmission have been reported in the USA, although there may be a greater burden of disease than previously realized. CD is currently considered a global parasitic infection due to the increasing migration of populations from highly endemic areas to non-endemic settings; and from rural to peri-urban and urban settings. However, due to the current global economic recession there has been some reverse migration to endemic areas.
- CD is considered as a neglected tropical disease because of its substantial impact in terms of premature mortality and its associated disability.
- After exposure to the parasite, a minority of patients will develop an acute syndrome of 4–8 weeks' duration. Roughly 30–40% of infected patients will subsequently develop the cardiac and/or digestive forms of chronic CD, usually 10–30 years after the initial exposure.
- Chagas heart disease (CHD) is the most common aetiology of cardiomyopathy in Latin America, and a major cause of cardiovascular death among middle-aged individuals in endemic areas. It manifests as three major syndromes that often co-exist in the same patient: arrhythmia, heart failure and thromboembolism. Chronic CD in the gastrointestinal tract leads mostly to megaoesophagus or megacolon. Reactivation disease can occur in immunocompromised patients producing dermatological manifestations, myocarditis and/or meningoencephalitis.
- In CHD, arrhythmias are very common and of different types, frequently associated with, and may cause, palpitations, dizziness, syncope and sudden cardiac death (SCD). Frequent, complex PVCs, including couplets and runs of NSVT, are a common finding. 24-hour heart failure is often a late manifestation of CHD. It is usually biventricular with a predominance of left-sided failure at initial stages and of right-sided failure in more advanced disease. Systemic and pulmonary embolisms arising from mural thrombi in the cardiac chambers are quite frequent. Sudden cardiac death is the main cause of death in patients with CHD, accounting for nearly two-thirds of all deaths, followed by refractory heart failure and thromboembolism.
- In patients with high suspicion of chronic CD or in those with a compatible clinical syndrome, because parasitaemia is scarce, the presence of IgG antibodies against *T. cruzi* antigens needs to be detected by at least two different serological methods (usually enzyme-linked immunosorbent assay, indirect immunofluorescence or indirect haemagglutination), to confirm the aetiological diagnosis.
- Antitrypanosomal drug treatment is always recommended for acute, congenital and reactivated *T. cruzi* infection (most frequently in patients co-infected with HIV) and for chronic *T. cruzi* infection in children up to 18 years old. In adults, treatment is currently recommended for those up to 50 years of age with serologic evidence of *T. cruzi* infection, based on recent data suggesting that a course of antitrypanosomal treatment delays progression of cardiomyopathy and improves overall outcomes. There is no evidence that antitrypanosomal treatment affects the progression of gastrointestinal CD.
- Persistence of parasites and the accompanying chronic inflammation is the basis for the pathology in CHD. Thus, unless demonstrated otherwise by the ongoing randomized controlled trial (BENEFIT), benznidazole or nifurtimox should be offered to patients <50 years old with presumably long-standing indeterminate *T. cruzi* infections or even with mild to moderate disease.
- Medical treatment of CHD is clinically relevant. Amiodarone markedly reduces the frequency and complexity of ventricular arrhythmias and has been shown to reduce mortality in the only two randomized trials that included Chagasic patients. Because mild segmental LV wall motion abnormalities are predictors of deterioration of ventricular function during follow-up, the use of an ACE inhibitor is also highly recommended. Finally, whether administration of a beta-blocker (to prevent further myocardial damage and death) and either aspirin or warfarin (to prevent thromboembolism) should be considered, remains an open and challenging question.

Epidemiology

Trypanosoma cruzi is endemic in South, Central and parts of North America (also Mexico and possibly South Texas). Historically, the disease disproportionately affected mostly underserved individuals because transmission of *T. cruzi* infection occurred mainly in rural areas where humans live in poorly constructed dwellings and in close contact with potential vectors (Figure 46.1).[1–3] However, rural-to-urban and international migrations have changed the epidemiology of CD affecting peri-urban, urban, endemic and non-endemic areas alike. As a result of dynamic changes in the affected populations and the coordinated efforts of endemic countries to interrupt vectorial and transfusional transmission, the prevalence and incidence of the disease are decreasing.[4,5] In the 1980s the overall prevalence of *T. cruzi* infection was estimated to reach 17 million cases in 18 endemic countries, with 100 million people at risk.[3] Multinational vector control programmes and compulsory blood-bank screening achieved enormous success in the 1990s, decreasing the incidence of new infections (700 000 cases per year in 1983) by 70% and the number of annual deaths by approximately 50%, and by eradicating transmission of *T. cruzi* by the main domiciliary vector species, *Triatoma infestans*, from three endemic countries (Uruguay in 1997; Chile in 1999; and Brazil in 2006).[3] According to the most recent estimates, there are currently 7.6 million people infected with *T. cruzi* in Latin America.[6] Although precise estimates documenting the total burden of cardiac involvement with *T. cruzi* are not available, it could be assumed that 20–30% of the 7.6 million infected individuals are or will potentially develop chronic heart disease or gastrointestinal complications.[7] CHD, in turn, is thought to represent the principal cause of cardiac morbidity and mortality among young adults in endemic countries, with at least 21 000 deaths each year. Additionally, because of the constant influx of immigrants from disease-endemic countries, CD is becoming an important health issue in North America and many parts of Europe, Japan and Australia, where a growing number of individuals are suspected to be infected.[4,6] Yet, the recent global economic downturn has caused an inverse migration of native populations to endemic countries, and thus recent estimates may be shifting.

Pathogenesis and Pathology

Vector-borne transmission involves transmission of the infective form of the parasite (the metacyclic trypomastigotes) to humans by the excreta of the triatomine insect through mucous membranes or through breaks in the skin.[3] Trypomastigotes then invade local host cells where they differentiate into amastigotes and multiply within the cell. When the cell is swollen with amastigotes, they transform back into trypomastigotes by growing flagellae. The trypomastigotes lyse the cells, invade adjacent tissues, and spread via the lymphatics and bloodstream to distant sites. The cycle is completed when a reduviid bug becomes infected by ingesting blood from an infected host.[1,3]

During the initial phase of infection, the abundance of parasites associated with the acute phase of *T. cruzi* infection argued in favour of the parasite's direct implication in the tissue damage and myocarditis observed during this stage of the disease.[7,8] Shortly afterwards, demonstration of myocytolysis of non-parasitized cardiomyocytes led to the implication of parasite-directed cellular immune-mediated inflammatory damage. This immune-mediated damage, associated with large numbers of amastigotes in cardiac myocytes, translates into hyaline degeneration of muscle fibres, coagulation necrosis of myocytes and surrounding tissues as well as involvement of the epicardium and pericardium.[1] Cellular and possibly humoral immune responses elicited by the parasite eventually control the acute infection but fail to completely eliminate the parasite.[7] A variably long asymptomatic phase then ensues, where factors such as the parasite strain, the parasite load during the acute phase, the quality of the immune response, and the presence or absence of reinfection all might influence the course of chronic disease.[7,8] Regarding the pathogenesis of the interstitial fibrosis, myocytolysis and ongoing lymphocytic infiltration observed in the chronic phase of CD, the paucity of parasites in cardiac tissue probably reflects the use of insensitive histological techniques in past decades.[2,5] In recent years, more powerful and sensitive methods of parasite detection, such as immunohistochemistry and polymerase chain reaction (PCR) have demonstrated a higher frequency of *T. cruzi* antigens or parasite DNA in chronic lesions.[5] The spectrum of outcomes of patients infected with *T. cruzi* is varied and probably stems from intrinsic genetic differences of both the parasite and the host, and perhaps even the likelihood of ongoing infection in highly endemic areas. Evidence exists for multiple hypotheses to explain the aetiology of chronic cardiac lesions implicating the parasite directly, the immune reaction to the parasite and autoimmunity elicited either directly by the parasite (mimicry) or indirectly (bystander activation).[7,8] The end-product of these lesions is varying degrees of necrosis, neuronal damage, microvascular damage and fibrosis. The contributing role of each mechanism to the pathogenesis of CHD is a whole other topic of debate.

There is evidence of both functional and anatomical parasympathetic neuronal damage in Chagasic patients.[8] Patients with CD lack the tonic inhibitory parasympathetic action on the sinus node and thus the chronotropic mechanism to respond to changes in blood pressure or venous return. Neuronal loss is thought to occur during the acute stage of the disease; the extent of neuronal damage however, does not correlate with disease stage.[8] Therefore, despite possible contributions of parasympathetic impairment to the impact of CHD (i.e. increasing vulnerability to malignant arrhythmias and sudden death or accentuating existing contraction abnormalities that can culminate in cardiac chamber dilatation), cardiac dysautonomia is unlikely to explain the main pathogenic mechanism underlying CHD.[5,8]

In addition to the neuronal damage, microcirculatory changes leading to ischaemia have also been implicated in the pathogenesis of chronic CHD. Diffuse collapse of intramyocardial arterioles has been observed in the hearts of chronically infected patients.[1] Occlusive platelet thrombi in small epicardial and intramural coronary arteries and increased production of cytokines and mediators that promote vasospasm and platelet aggregation have been demonstrated in experimental models of CD.[5] Clinically, despite consistently normal epicardial coronary arteries on coronary angiography, reversible perfusion defects on stress-induced myocardial perfusion scintigraphy that correlate with ischaemia and abnormal coronary flow regulation, have been shown in patients with CHD.[5,8]

As mentioned above, tissue damage caused directly by the parasite or possibly by the immune response elicited by it, has been postulated to underlie and potentiate the aggression to

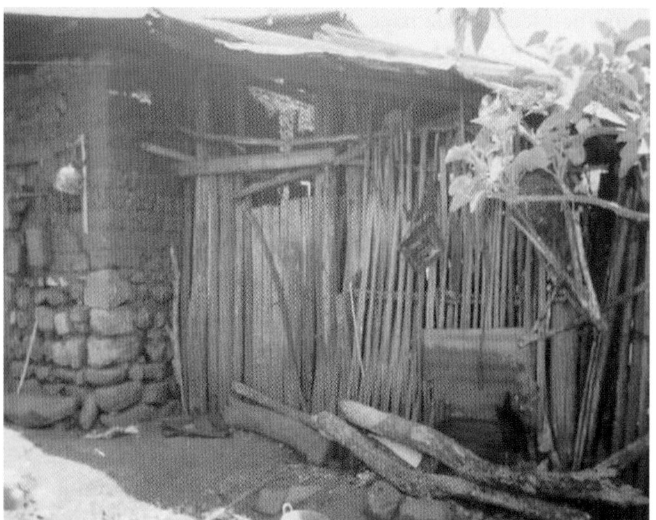

Figure 46.1 Poorly constructed house in an endemic area for Chagas disease in rural Honduras.

cardiac myocytes and neurons.[5] The inflammatory infiltrate in chronic Chagasic cardiomyopathy has a predominance of macrophages, CD8+ and CD4+ lymphocytes (in a 2 : 1 ratio) and in some instances has been shown to correlate with more advanced stages of the disease. Persistence of parasites and antigens is thought to be involved in recruitment of *T. cruzi*-specific CD8+ T lymphocytes which predominate in the myocardial infiltrate of chronic myocarditis.[8] The cytokine profile associated with this myocarditis is also shifted toward Th1 cytokines so that elevated INF-γ levels and decreased IL-10 levels may potentially perpetuate an existent, ongoing inflammatory process. However, the exact mechanism responsible for the turning point from immunoprotection to immune-mediated aggression leading to irreversible tissue damage remains elusive: not only is parasite persistence true for both symptomatic and asymptomatic patients, but presence of the parasite in heart tissue does not always correlate with inflammation.[5,7]

Autoimmunity has also been postulated as a plausible aetiology for the chronic myocarditis observed in *T. cruzi*-infected patients.[5] Several *T. cruzi* antigens that cross-react with cardiac and non-cardiac host components have been identified, but only some have been shown to have functional activity. Among these, attention has focused on antibodies that cross-react with cardiac myosin and the immunodominant *T. cruzi* antigen B13 initially because they were detected in 100% of patients with chronic Chagasic cardiomyopathy in contrast to 14% of asymptomatic infected individuals, and later because T-cell clones derived from lesions of chronic CHD were found to be simultaneously reactive to cardiac myosin heavy chain and the B13 *T. cruzi* protein. Opponents to the molecular mimicry theory with specific relevance to anti B13-cardiac myosin cross-reactive antibodies and derived cellular autoimmunity contend that these antibodies do not bind to intact myocytes, are not unique to *T. cruzi* infection, are present in asymptomatic patients without heart lesions, and that myosin autoimmunity is not essential for cardiac inflammation in experimental models.[7] Arguing against autoimmunity developing as a result of parasite-specific immune responses, antigen exposure after tissue damage may also sensitize autoreactive T cells to self-antigens given a proinflammatory environment. The question, therefore, is not whether autoimmunity is present, but whether it is a primary cause or merely a contributing factor to the pathogenesis of chronic myocarditis.[5] Further evidence is required from experiments to prove an association between the development of similar cardiac lesions with transfer of autoantibodies and/or autoreactive cells to susceptible hosts.[1,7,8]

In summary, although the effects of both autonomic and microvascular disturbances in CHD may play an important role in potentiating and perpetuating cardiac muscle damage, persistent inflammation in the setting of continuous antigenic stimulation is perhaps the common pathway for tissue damage. Multiple mechanisms seem to explain this chronic inflammation (including anti-parasite immunity and possibly autoimmunity), which are not necessarily mutually exclusive.[7,8] The course to progression to chronic CHD and other forms of the disease has been suggested to be related to genetic properties of both host and parasite. However, the molecular mechanisms underlying tissue tropism and the initial trigger or determinant of the course of chronic disease are not yet known.

Clinical Features

ACUTE CHAGAS DISEASE

Acute myocarditis as evidenced by autopsy studies probably occurs in ~100% of patients with acute CD.[1,5] However, there is an enormous discrepancy between autopsy findings and clinical data. Acute infection is asymptomatic in approximately 90–95% of cases; and even in symptomatic patients, acute Chagasic myocarditis is diagnosed in only 1–40% of them (Figure 46.2).[1] Findings on cardiac auscultation may include tachycardia (not always proportional to the degree of fever), cardiac

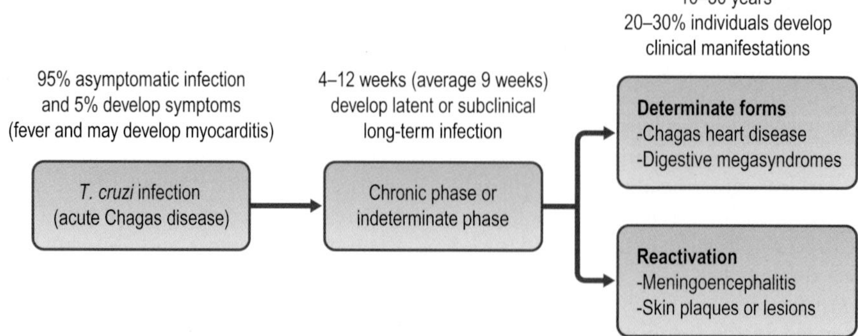

Figure 46.2 Clinical stages of Chagas disease.

murmurs and muffled heart sounds. The principal electrocardiographic (ECG) alterations are 1st-degree atrioventricular block, low QRS voltage, and primary T-wave changes.[2] A chest radiograph may show variable degrees of cardiomegaly, and pericardial effusion is the most frequently reported echocardiographic abnormality. Death in the acute phase occurs occasionally (in 5–10% of the symptomatic patients) as a result of congestive heart failure (due to severe myocarditis) and/or meningoencephalitis.[1,2] After the acute phase, most patients return to a normal or near normal myocardial status but some (30%) then chronically develop a fibrosing myocarditis.

CHRONIC CHAGAS HEART DISEASE

Cardiac involvement is the most frequent and most severe manifestation of chronic CD[1,2,5] (Table 46.1). Transition from the indeterminate form to the cardiac form of chronic CD is usually manifested by the appearance of ECG changes such as incomplete or complete right bundle branch block (RBBB), left anterior fascicular block (LAFB), minimal ST-T changes, and monomorphic premature ventricular contractions (PVCs) mostly in asymptomatic or oligosymptomatic patients.[9] As the disease advances, associated intraventricular conduction defects (usually RBBB with LAFB), polymorphic PVCs (Figure 46.3), bradyarrhythmias, high-grade atrioventricular blocks, q-waves, nonsustained or sustained ventricular tachycardia and ultimately atrial flutter or fibrillation may ensue.[9] Symptoms such as palpitations, atypical chest pain, presyncope, syncope, dyspnoea on exertion and oedema are usually observed throughout the course of CHD. Findings on physical examination vary according to the stage of the disease and the presence of conduction system abnormalities.[1,9] They include: cardiac rhythm irregularities; displaced point of maximal impulse; gallop rhythms; a loud second heart sound implying pulmonary hypertension; mitral or tricuspid regurgitation murmurs; an increase in the systemic venous pressure with liver enlargement and oedema; and borderline low systolic blood pressure with a reduced radial pulse implying systolic dysfunction. On echocardiogram, diastolic dysfunction usually precedes systolic dysfunction, potentially allowing for early detection of cardiac involvement in CD.[9] Characteristic echocardiographic findings include: apical aneurysms (Figure 46.3), which are reported in 8.5–55% of cases (depending on the stage of the disease and the method of detection, i.e. if postmortem, at echocardiography or angiography); segmental left ventricular (LV) contractile abnormalities (more commonly at the posteroinferior wall); and reduced LV systolic function.[10] Echocardiographic evidence of impaired LV function as characterized by increased LV systolic dimension, reduced LV ejection fraction, presence of segmental or global LV wall motion abnormality and/or an LV aneurysm is the most common and consistent independent predictor of death. Other important clinical and non-invasive adverse prognostic indicators, which not surprisingly reflect and parallel the degree of myocardial dysfunction, include advanced functional class (NYHA III/IV), cardiomegaly, and non-sustained ventricular tachycardia on 24-hour ECG monitoring (Figure 46.4).[10]

The clinical course of CHD is diverse and difficult to predict, with some patients remaining asymptomatic lifelong, despite electrocardiographic and/or echocardiographic evidence of the disease; some presenting with signs, symptoms and complications of progressive heart failure or advanced cardiac arrhythmias; and others dying unexpectedly without prior symptoms.[9] Currently, several staging systems of CHD are available (Table 46.2). They can help to identify patients at different degrees of risk, facilitate choices among treatment alternatives and aid patient counselling.[5,9,10] Most systems classify patients into four or five stages, based on their functional capacity, ECG findings and the presence or absence of heart enlargement and/or systolic dysfunction on echocardiogram. Progression of disease to more advanced stages has been estimated to occur in 10% of patients over a follow-up period of 3–10 years.[10] Another important aspect of staging derives from its prognostic information: mortality of individuals at early stages of CHD is not significantly different from that of the general population. However, life expectancy of patients with symptomatic and advanced CHD stages (involving systolic dysfunction and/or cardiomegaly), is less than 30% at 5 years and their overall prognosis is worse when compared with patients with dilated cardiomyopathies of other aetiologies.[5,10] Systemic and pulmonary embolism arising from mural thrombi in the cardiac chambers is relatively frequent. Although the brain is by far the most common clinically recognized site of embolisms (followed by limbs and lungs), at necropsy, embolisms are found more frequently in the lungs, kidneys and spleen. CD is an independent risk factor for stroke in endemic areas.[1,9] Mortality in CHD is due to sudden cardiac arrest in 55–65% of patients, congestive heart failure in 25–30% of patients and thromboembolic phenomena in 10–15%.[1,5,9]

TABLE 46.1 Clinical Manifestations of Chronic Chagas Heart Disease

HEART (MYOCARDIAL) FAILURE
Diastolic dysfunction initially
Isolated left heart failure in the early stages of cardiac decompensation
Biventricular with a predominance of right-sided failure in advanced stages
ARRHYTHMIAS
Ventricular extrasystoles
Non-sustained and sustained ventricular tachycardia
Bradyarrhythmias
Ventricular fibrillation
Atrial fibrillation/flutter
CONDUCTION ABNORMALITIES
Sick sinus syndrome
Complete and incomplete right bundle branch block
Left anterior fascicle block
Bifascicular and trifascicular blocks
1st, 2nd and 3rd degree AV blocks
THROMBOEMBOLIC PHENOMENA
Brain (most frequent)
Lungs, kidneys, spleen, extremities
APICAL ANEURYSM
Found in 52% in autopsy series
More frequent in men, 80% in the LV apex
SUDDEN CARDIAC DEATH
Ventricular fibrillation (most frequent)
Bradyarrhythmias
Rupture of apical aneurysm (rare)

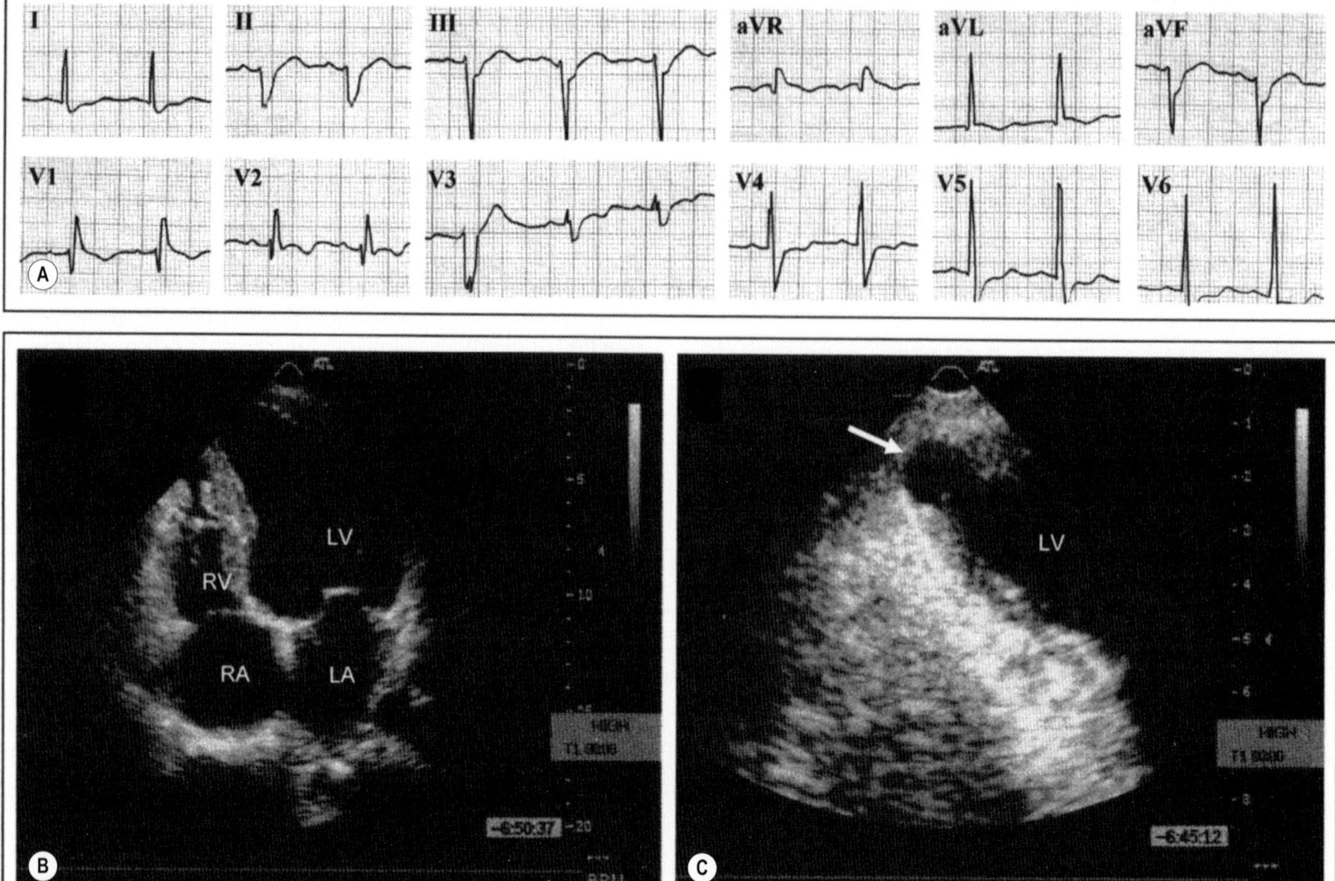

Figure 46.3 (A) 12-lead ECG showing the three most frequent abnormalities in Chagas heart disease in a man from rural Brazil: right bundle branch block, left anterior fascicular block, and a premature ventricular contraction (lead V3). (B) Transthoracic echocardiogram recorded at the four chambers apical view showing slightly diminished left ventricular systolic function and mildly dilated left ventricle. (C) Two chamber apical view showing more clearly a characteristic digitiform left ventricular apical aneurysm (arrow). *(From Rassi Jr A, Rassi A, Franco-Paredes C. A Latin American man with palpitations, dizziness, episodes of non-sustained ventricular tachycardia, and apical aneurysm. PLoS Neglect Trop Dis 2011;5(2):e852.)*

CHRONIC CHAGAS GASTROINTESTINAL DISEASE

Approximately 30% of patients with long-term *T. cruzi* infection may develop digestive megasyndromes due to injury to the enteric nervous system including both excitatory and inhibitory innervation impairments (Table 46.3).[1,11] Gastrointestinal manifestations of CD include salivary glands, oesophagus, lower oesophageal sphincter, stomach, small bowel, colon, gallbladder or the biliary tract beng affected. Salivary gland hypertrophy and sialorrhoea are present in many patients with CD associated with vomiting and regurgitation in Chagasic achalasia. In this sense, Chagasic achalasia and its consequence of Chagasic megaoesophagus are common findings in CD that can lead to severe malnutrition (Figure 46.5). Delayed gastric emptying has been described in patients with CD but megastomach is extremely rare. Small bowel bacterial overgrowth may occur associated with slowing of the interdigestive migrating motor complex. A major cause of gastrointestinal morbidity and mortality is megacolon that may lead to severe constipation and fecal impaction.[11]

OTHER CLINICAL MANIFESTATIONS

Among some immunosuppressed hosts such as HIV-infected individuals and transplant recipients, reactivation of infection and de novo infection (including transmission with transplanted organs among transplant patients) have been reported.[1,12] With reactivation in HIV-positive patients, myocarditis has been reported in up to 45% of cases.[12] Reactivation of CD among heart transplant patients has been estimated to occur in approximately 30% of cases. However, not all these cases are accompanied by florid symptoms or diagnosed by endomyocardial biopsy and therefore, the true incidence of myocarditis with reactivation is difficult to estimate. Acute *T. cruzi* infection can also result as a consequence of donor-related transmission, which has been reported after kidney, heart, liver and multi-organ transplants. Involvement in this setting can range from asymptomatic parasitaemia that easily responds to treatment without further complications to severe, fulminant disease despite therapy (including death directly attributable to Chagasic myocarditis). Approximately 1 in 20 *T. cruzi* infections in pregnant women is passed vertically to the unborn fetus.[1] In

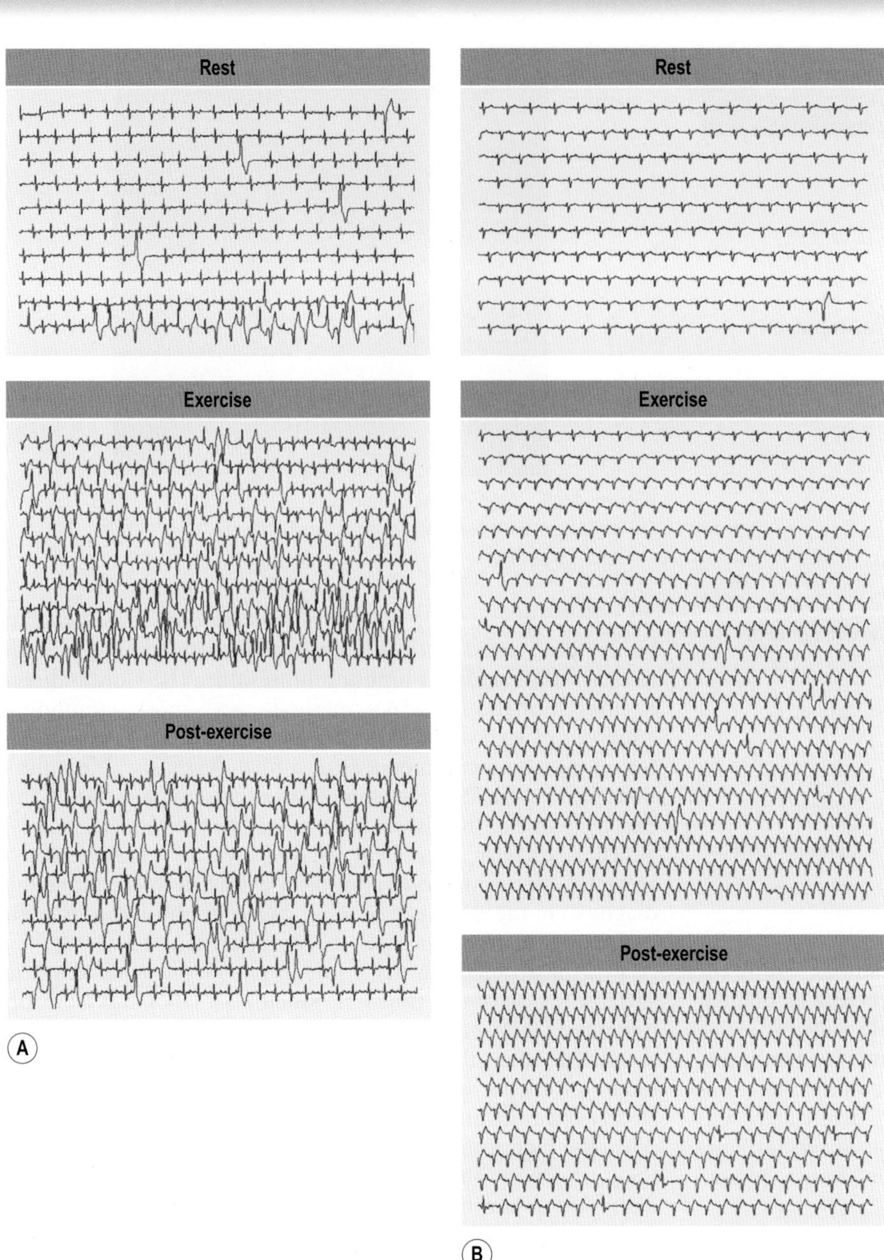

Figure 46.4 Exercise testing performed and recorded in a man from rural Brazil during the last hour of Holter monitoring: (A) Control exercise showing frequent premature ventricular complexes, couplets, and short runs of nonsustained ventricular tachycardia. (B) Exercise testing after administration of amiodarone (400 mg/day), showing a significant reduction in the number of premature ventricular complexes and couplets, and a complete abolition of episodes of nonsustained ventricular tachycardia. *(From Rassi Jr A, Rassi A, Franco-Paredes C. A Latin American man with palpitations, dizziness, episodes of non-sustained ventricular tachycardia, and apical aneurysm. PLoS Neglect Trop Dis 2011;5(2):e852.)*

congenitally infected infants, the most common symptoms, which may be apparent at birth or develop within weeks after delivery, are hypotonicity, fever, hepatosplenomegaly and anemia. Other findings include prematurity and low birth weight. In utero infections are also associated with abortion and placentitis. Serious manifestations, including myocarditis, meningoencephalitis and pneumonitis, are uncommon, but carry a high risk of death.[1,5] Finally, reactivation of latent CD may present with dermatological manifestations including indurated erythematous plaques with necrosis, erythematous papules and nodules, panniculitis or skin ulcers.[13] Some of these lesions may resemble erythema migrans due to Lyme disease borreliosis.

Diagnosis

Diagnosis of acute myocarditis relies on demonstration of the parasite and/or anti-*T. cruzi* IgM in a patient with the correct epidemiological background and clinical picture. IgM serology assays are not widely available in developing countries and not standardized, so diagnosis is usually performed by visualizing the trypomastigotes in fresh blood smears, thick drop preparations or buffy coat smears.[1,2,5] The level of parasitaemia diminishes to almost undetectable levels by the 6th–10th weeks of infection, making parasite identification in peripheral blood extremely difficult at this time. Diagnosis could also be attempted by haemoculture on specialized media (which has improved sensitivity over direct examination) or xenodiagnosis (which involves detecting the parasite by infecting lab-reared triatomine bugs directly or indirectly with the patient's blood). However, even considering only congenital CD, haemoculture is rarely performed for the diagnosis of acute infection since it requires a specialized laboratory and personnel and is usually not widely available. Indirect parasitological tests are of limited value in the diagnosis of acute CD, as they can take more than 1 month to obtain the results.

TABLE 46.2 Classifications or Staging Systems for Chagas Heart Disease

FIRST STAGE: INDETERMINATE FORM

No evidence of heart involvement by:
- ECG and CXR (Stage 0 KC)
- ECG, echocardiogram, and signs of CHF (Stage IA MLAC)
- ECG, echocardiogram, CXR and NYHA functional class (Stage A-ACC/AHA)

SECOND STAGE: CHD WITHOUT SIGNS OR SYMPTOMS OF HEART FAILURE

Evidence of structural heart disease by:
- ECG ± CXR (Stage I-II KC)
- ECG ± echocardiogram (Stage A-B2 BCC)
- Echocardiogram ± ECG (Stage IB-II MLAC)
- ECG (Stage B A-ACC/AHA)

THIRD STAGE: COMPENSATED CHD

Incorporate clinical symptoms:
- Compensated CHF (Stage C BCC)
- NYHA II-III (Stage C A-ACC/AHA)

FOURTH STAGE: OVERT, REFRACTORY OR ADVANCED CHD

Includes:
- Stage III from the KC and the MLAC
- Stage D from the BCC and the A-ACC/AHA classification

Modified from Hidron A, Vogenthaler N, Santos-Preciado JI, et al. Cardiac involvement with parasitic infections. Clin Microbiol Rev 2010;23(2):324–49. Kuschnir Classification (KC), the Brazilian Consensus classification (BCC), the modified Los Andes classification (MLAC), and the classification incorporating AAC/AHA Staging (A-AAA/AHA).

A diagnosis of CHD should be suspected among young or middle-aged patients who present with a segmental or dilated cardiomyopathy of unknown aetiology if within endemic areas or within the right epidemiological context.[2] It should be remembered that CHD presents years after the initial infection and therefore patients who migrated to non-endemic areas are still at risk of developing cardiac compromise. Given the low and probably intermittent parasitaemia in the chronic phase,

TABLE 46.3 Extracardiac Manifestations of Chagas Disease

CENTRAL NERVOUS SYSTEM
- Meningoencephalitis
- Meningitis
- Encephalitis

DERMATOLOGIC
- Infiltrating plaques or erythematous plaques
- Erythematous papules and nodules
- Panniculitis
- Skin ulcerations

GASTROINTESTINAL
- Salivary gland hypertrophy and sialorrhea
- Delayed gastric emptying
- Achalasia-like syndrome
- Megaoesophagus
- Dysmotility of small bowel
- Small bowel bacterial overgrowth
- Megacolon
- Megagallblader and megacholedochus

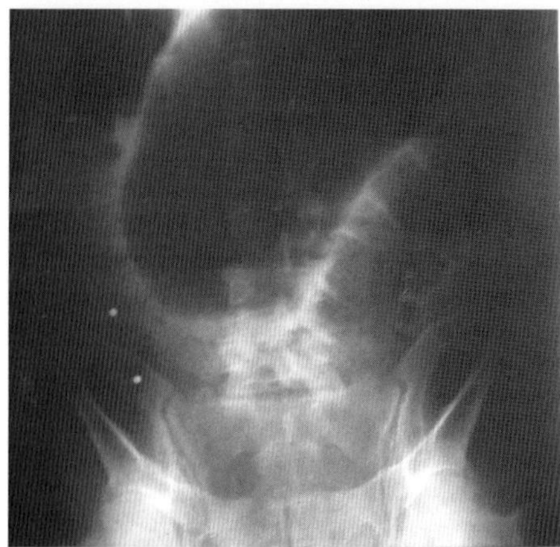

Figure 46.5 Abdominal radiograph demonstrating dilated loops of colon (megaoesophagus) in a 49-year-old male in Santa Cruz, Bolivia.

diagnosis relies on serologic methods by detecting IgG that binds to *T. cruzi* antigens. Enzyme-linked immunosorbent assay (ELISA), indirect immunofluorescence (IIF) and indirect haemagglutination (IHA) methods are most commonly employed. Two positive tests using any of the three conventional techniques are recommended for a final diagnosis.[5] Identification of the parasite by haemoculture or xenodiagnosis in the chronic phase of the disease is hampered by their low sensitivity, which is directly dependent on the level of parasitaemia.[1,5] However, these methods may have a role in confirming the diagnosis in the rare cases of serologically doubtful results or in evaluating treatment failures at specialized centres.

PCR-based methods using one of two target sequences (the variable region of the minicircle kinetoplast DNA and a 195-bp reiterated DNA sequence of the parasite) have achieved higher sensitivities than that of xenodiagnosis and haemoculture. The major problems with PCR-based techniques are the lack of standardization and commercial availability of assays for *T. cruzi*, the high level of complexity required and the reliance of their sensitivity on the level of parasitaemia (which is low by definition in chronic disease). PCR is therefore still considered among non-conventional methods and is recommended only as an adjunct in specialized centres to confirm parasitaemia in congenital *T. cruzi* infection (since in this context its sensitivity seems to be greater than microscopic examination) or for the evaluation of antiparasitic drug therapy. However, a single or even repeated negative post-treatment PCR result does not necessarily mean parasitological cure.[1,5] They are only indicative of the absence of parasite DNA at those moments. The value of PCR lies mainly in the positive results they yield that usually reflects treatment failure. Whether assessment of parasite load by quantitative real-time PCR will correlate with the impact of trypanocidal treatment on parasitological cure or resistance, as well as on disease evolution, should be a matter for further investigation. A multinational effort among 26 expert laboratories from 16 countries is currently evaluating the sensitivities and specificities among 48 reported PCR-based assays to detect *T. cruzi* DNA. This is a crucial step towards standardizing this molecular methodology to be incorporated into clinical decision-making in the near future.[14]

The initial evaluation of the newly diagnosed patient with chronic *T. cruzi* infection includes a complete medical history and physical examination, and a resting 12-lead electrocardiogram. Asymptomatic patients with a normal ECG have a favourable prognosis and should only be followed up annually or biannually.[2,10] Patients with ECG changes consistent with CHD should undergo a routine cardiac evaluation, including ambulatory 24-h Holter monitoring (complemented with an exercise test whenever possible) to detect arrhythmias and assess functional capacity, chest radiography and 2D echocardiography to assess ventricular function, and other cardiologic tests as indicated.[2] Based on the results of these tests, it is possible to risk-stratify individual patients and implement appropriate therapy.[10]

Management and Treatment

ANTITRYPANOSOMAL THERAPY

Treatment has been recommended for all cases of acute and congenital infection, reactivated infection, and in early chronic CD (particularly children/adolescents <18 years), based on evidence of shortening of the disease's clinical course, cure of infection or reduction of parasites.[2,15–18] For infected adults without advanced cardiomyopathy up to age 50 years, aetiological treatment should generally also be offered.[2,5,18] The rationale for these recommendations stems from evidence of slowing of the progression of cardiomyopathy. In a recent observational trial, 566 chronically infected adults (30–50 years of age) without heart failure were assigned, in alternating sequence, to benznidazole or no treatment.[16] After a median follow-up of 9.8 years, fewer treated patients had progression of disease or developed ECG abnormalities. Negative seroconversion was more frequent in treated patients. Another recently published controlled study including 111 patients (17–46 years of age) with chronic CD and a normal electrocardiogram, showed similar favourable results with benznidazole over a mean follow-up of 21 years.[16] For those over the age of 50 years, aetiological treatment is considered optional, because of the lack of any available data. A multi-centre, randomized, placebo-controlled trial of benznidazole enrolling 3000 patients with mild to moderate CHD and 18–75 years of age is currently underway, and should help clarify treatment decisions in this population.[17]

In contrast, aetiological treatment is contraindicated during pregnancy and in patients with severe renal or hepatic insufficiency, and it should generally not be offered to patients with advanced Chagasic cardiomyopathy or megaoesophagus with significant impairment of swallowing.[15,16] A more controversial issue is prophylactic treatment for transplant patients: some authors have recommended it for patients with Chagasic cardiomyopathy who undergo cardiac transplantation to prevent disease reactivation, while others recommend it for all infected donors pre-transplant and for their respective recipients post-transplant. For chronic CD, cure is documented when previously positive serologic tests turn negative, usually years or decades after treatment.

Only two drugs, benznidazole and nifurtimox, are recommended for treatment of CD. Of the two, benznidazole (a nitroimidazole derivative) has been more extensively investigated in clinical studies and is better tolerated overall.[15,16] Adverse reactions such as generalized or, sometimes, localized allergic dermatitis occurs in approximately 20–30% of patients and consists of pruritic and non-bullous polymorphous erythematous rashes, often followed by desquamation. Severe exfoliative dermatitis can occur and should lead to prompt discontinuation of treatment. Another adverse effect, which occurs in approximately 5–10% of patients, most commonly late in the treatment course, is a dose-dependent peripheral sensitive neuropathy, affecting mainly the distal parts of the lower limbs; it also should prompt cessation of treatment. Rare serious adverse events include leukopaenia with granulocytopaenia or agranulocytosis (sometimes followed by fever and tonsillitis), and thrombocytopenic purpura. Additional reported side effects include nausea, vomiting, anorexia, weight loss, insomnia, loss of taste and onycholysis. Nifurtimox, a nitrofuran compound, can be associated with gastrointestinal side effects in 30–70% of patients as well as central and peripheral nervous system toxicity. Both compounds are better tolerated by children allowing for increased dosage regimens. Individuals younger than 12 years of age should be treated with benznidazole orally at a dose of 10 mg/kg per day in 2 divided doses for 60 days; nifurtimox is an alternative in those younger than 10 years, at a dose of 15–20 mg/kg per day orally in 3–4 divided doses for 90 days or at a dose of 12.5–15 mg/kg per day orally in 3–4 divided doses for 90 days among those 11–16 years of age. Individuals 12 years of age and older should be treated with benznidazole at a dose of 5–7 mg/kg per day in 2 divided doses for 60 days. Nifurtimox is recommended at a dose of 8–10 mg/kg per day in 3–4 divided doses for 90 days. Both drugs are contraindicated in pregnancy.[2,18]

MEDICAL TREATMENT

Treatment of heart failure in patients with CHD should follow specific treatment targeted at each stage, according to current guidelines for heart failure of other aetiologies.[9] An important exception is the use of beta-blockers, which should be used with caution in CHD due to a higher incidence of atrioventricular conduction defects and associated bradyarrhythmias. Cardiac transplantation has been performed with good results for patients with advanced CHD but may not be available or accessible in all countries where this disease is endemic. Although not tested in randomized controlled clinical trials, amiodarone has been associated with a survival advantage in case–control studies among patients with ventricular tachycardia and has therefore been proposed for management of patients with sustained and non-sustained ventricular tachycardia.[1] However, treatment with amiodarone has been associated with pulmonary, cardiac, thyroid, liver, ocular, skin, central nervous system and genitourinary toxicities so that treatment needs to be individualized. Pacemaker implantation is the recommended treatment for severe bradyarrhythmias and advanced conduction abnormalities. The role of cardioverter-defibrillator implantation and cardiac resynchronization, however, are not well established in CHD. Finally, anticoagulation has been advocated for patients with atrial fibrillation, previous thromboembolic phenomena or an LV aneurysm with thrombus.[1,9]

There is no evidence that antiparasitic treatment affects the progression of gastrointestinal CD.[11,18] Decisions to treat a patient with gastrointestinal dysfunction should be guided on evidence of cardiac disease, to prevent its progression. Antiparasitic treatment may be cumbersome to administer to patients if they have a digestive megasyndrome such as in the case of megaoesophagus due to dysphagia or decreased intestinal absorption. Surgical management of megasyndromes is crucial for improving quality of life, and in the case of megaoesophagus to enable the ability to provide oral antiparasitic treatment and other medications if indicated to decrease progression of heart disease.[18]

Prevention

Most *T. cruzi* infections can be prevented by decreasing vectorial transmission, improving blood product screening and detecting and treating transplacental transmission. Multinational programmes involving the endemic countries have achieved enormous success in decreasing both the prevalence and incidence of CD by following several operational stages. The tools for interrupting transmission are based on implementation of vector control activities such as insecticide spraying, housing improvements and education as well as strengthening implementation of policy for use and screening of blood products for transfusion.[3] All initially reactive donations are re-tested in duplicate using the same screening test; donations testing repeatedly reactive have confirmatory testing by the radioimmunoprecipitation assay (RIPA).[6] Continued surveillance is also important to consolidate and maintain the success achieved.

For individuals travelling to endemic areas, compliance with general food and water precautions is advised to prevent the extremely rare occurrence of food-borne CD. More importantly, travellers should avoid sleeping in poorly constructed houses or consider sleeping in insecticide-impregnated bed nets. However, the protective efficacy of insecticide-treated materials in reducing CD transmission and eliminating the vector population has yet to be demonstrated. Finally, no vaccine for CD is currently available. However, the Slim Initiative for Antipoverty Vaccine Development, a private–public partnership has recently gathered a group of experts and key players in Latin America to develop preventive and therapeutic vaccines against *T. cruzi* infection.

REFERENCES

1. Rassi Jr A, Rassi A, Marin-Neto JA. Chagas disease. Lancet 2010;375:1388–402.
2. Bern C, Montgomery SP, Herwaldt B, et al. Evaluation and treatment of Chagas disease in the United States: a systematic review. JAMA 2007;298:2171–81.
3. Miles MA, Feliciangeli MD, Rojas de Arias A. American trypanosomiasis (Chagas disease) and the role of molecular epidemiology in guiding control strategies. BMJ 2003;326:1444–8.
17. Marin-Neto JA, Rassi Jr A, Morillo CA, et al. Rationale and design of a randomized placebo-controlled trial assessing the effects of etiologic treatment in Chagas' cardiomyopathy: the BENznidazole Evaluation For Interrupting Trypanosomiasis (BENEFIT). Am Heart J 2008;156:37–43.
18. Bern C. Antitrypanosomal therapy for chronic Chagas' disease. N Engl J Med 2011;364;26:2527–34.

Access the complete references online at www.expertconsult.com

47

Leishmaniasis

MARLEEN BOELAERT | SHYAM SUNDAR

KEY POINTS

- The leishmaniases are poverty-related parasitic diseases transmitted by sandflies. Up to 20 *Leishmania* species are pathogenic for humans. The outcome of infection depends on the host as well as on the *Leishmania* species and ranges from asymptomatic carriership to fatal disease. Leishmaniases are differentiated into three clinical syndromes: visceral leishmaniasis (VL), cutaneous leishmaniasis (CL) and mucocutaneous leishmaniasis (MCL).
- Every year, there are close to 2 million new cases of leishmaniasis around the world. VL causes an estimated 500 000 cases per year mostly in the Indian subcontinent, East Africa and Brazil. CL is common in South America, Africa and Asia and is also regularly seen in travel clinics around the world. MCL is restricted to South America.
- About 70 species of sandflies can transmit *Leishmania*. They belong to the genus *Phlebotomus* in the Old World (Europe, Asia and Africa) and *Lutzomyia* in the New World (Americas). For certain *Leishmania* species, dogs, rodents or other wild mammals act as a reservoir (zoonotic transmission cycle). For others, humans are the main reservoir (anthroponotic cycle). Transmission without the intervention of a sandfly vector is possible but very rare.
- Parasites of the genus *Leishmania* are flagellate protozoa. They replicate in the macrophages of a mammal host as amastigotes, a stage without flagellum. When picked up by the sandfly they transform into promastigotes, with flagellum. The three clinical syndromes are caused by different species: VL is caused by *L. infantum* or *L. donovani*; CL by *L. major*, *L. tropica* and other species and MCL mainly by *L. braziliensis* and *L. panamensis*.
- VL, also called kala-azar, is the most severe of the three syndromes and is usually fatal if not treated. The disease is slowly progressive and characterized by protracted fever and hepatosplenomegaly evolving to cachexia, with anaemia, leukopenia and thrombocytopenia, and polyclonal hypergammaglobulinaemia. Up to 9 out of 10 infections remain asymptomatic. Post-kala-azar dermal leishmaniasis (PKDL) is a late complication of VL and manifests as a chronic macular, papular or nodular rash.
- The clinical manifestations of CL are chronic, painless ulcers or nodules. MCL is characterized by chronic and very destructive lesions in the mouth and nose. Diffuse cutaneous leishmaniasis (DCL) and leishmaniasis recidivans are special manifestations of CL.
- The definite diagnosis of leishmaniasis requires the demonstration of the amastigote form of the parasite. In VL, amastigotes can be found in spleen aspirates, bone marrow or other tissues. Rapid diagnostic tests, based on antibody detection, are used for diagnosis in primary care settings. Antigen detection techniques are under development. In CL and MCL, amastigotes can be found in Giemsa-stained smears of tissue scrapings, fine-needle aspirations or punch biopsies.
- Until recently, antimonials were the mainstay of leishmaniasis treatment. However, drug resistance has emerged, particularly in VL in India. After intensive clinical research in recent years, alternative drug regimens are now available for VL: miltefosine, paromomycin, (liposomal) amphotericin B and combination regimens. Treatment options for PKDL, CL and MCL are still unsatisfactory.

Epidemiology

INCIDENCE AND PREVALENCE

Leishmaniases are a group of vector-borne diseases caused by the *Leishmania* parasite. The estimated number of new cases of leishmaniasis is close to 2 million per year. More than 350 million people live in areas with *Leishmania* transmission[1] and cases are reported from 98 countries in South America, Africa, southern Europe and Asia. The disease is poverty-related and is one of the '*Neglected Tropical Diseases*'.[2] Leishmaniases are often classified by their geographical location, namely in the Old World (Europe, Asia and Africa) or in the New World (Americas).

At least 20 species of the genus *Leishmania* are pathogenic for humans. They lead to a spectrum of pathology ranging from latent infections over localized skin ulcers to fatal systemic disease. Three main clinical syndromes are distinguished: visceral, cutaneous and mucocutaneous leishmaniasis.[3]

Visceral leishmaniasis (VL) is fatal if not treated and causes an estimated 500 000 human cases and over 50 000 deaths worldwide each year. Close to 90% of these cases occur in the Indian subcontinent, East Africa and Brazil.[4] Incidence rates of VL documented in prospective studies in endemic communities in East Africa and Asia vary between 2 and 14 per 1000 inhabitants per year. However, as transmission occurs in discrete foci, incidence rates observed in small communities cannot necessarily be extrapolated to larger areas. Anthroponotic transmission of *L. donovani* prevails in East Africa and the Indian subcontinent – usually in a cycle of recurring outbreaks – while zoonotic transmission of *L. infantum* causes more sporadic

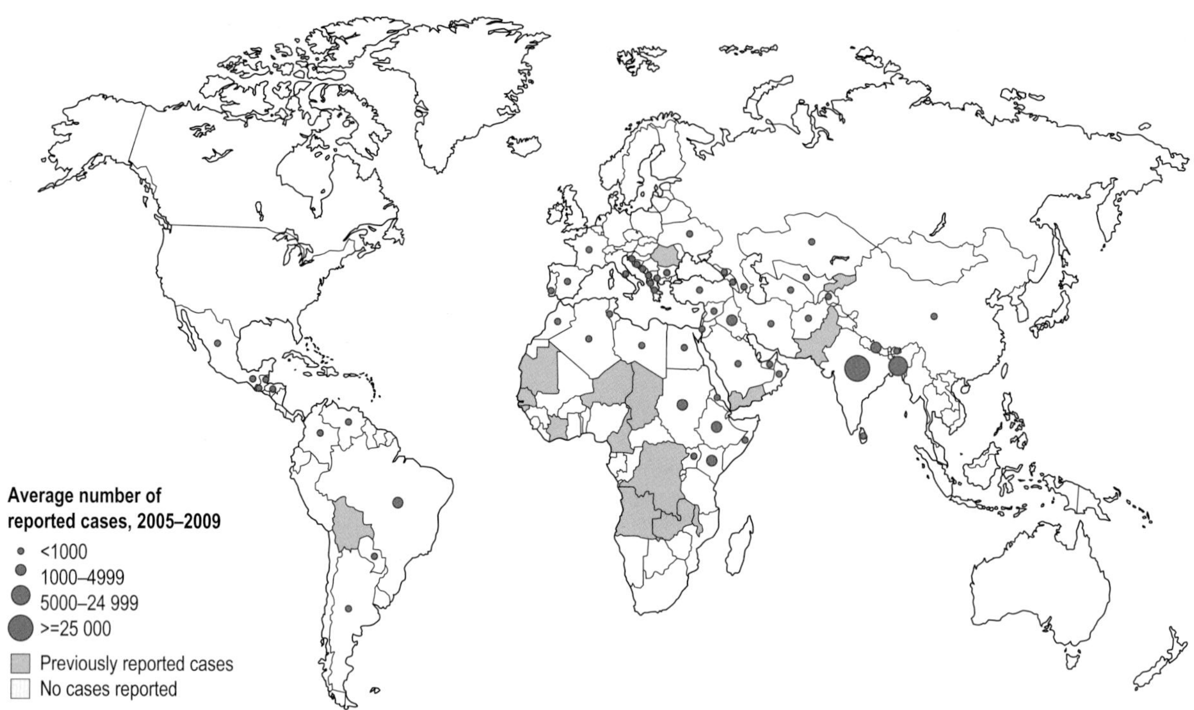

Figure 47.1 Distribution of visceral leishmaniasis, worldwide, 2009. (Source: *World Health Organization. Working to overcome the global impact of neglected tropical diseases. First WHO report on neglected tropical diseases. P 93.)*

cases of VL in the Mediterranean Basin, the Middle East, Central Asia, China and South America (Figure 47.1).

Cutaneous leishmaniases (CL) are reported from 77 countries and are commonly seen in travel clinics around the world.[5] Some 90% of the estimated 1.5 million annual cases occur in Afghanistan, Algeria, Brazil, Colombia, Iran, Pakistan, Peru, Saudi Arabia and Syria (Figure 47.2). Because of the lifelong scars CL is feared in endemic areas, especially by young women. CL can be anthroponotic or zoonotic.[6,7] Old World CL occurs typically in open semi-arid or even desert regions, while in the New World it used to be associated with forests, but peri-urban areas are now increasingly affected.

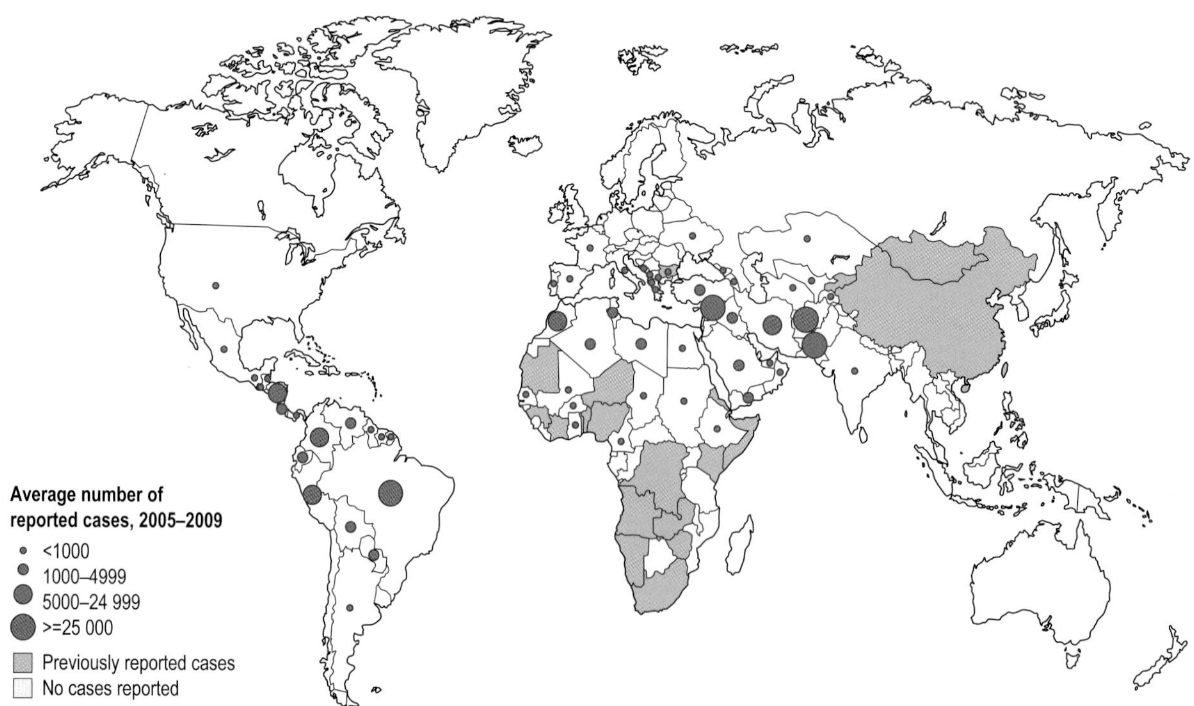

Figure 47.2 Distribution of cutaneous leishmaniasis, worldwide, 2009. (Source: *World Health Organization. Working to overcome the global impact of neglected tropical diseases. First WHO report on neglected tropical diseases. P 93.)*

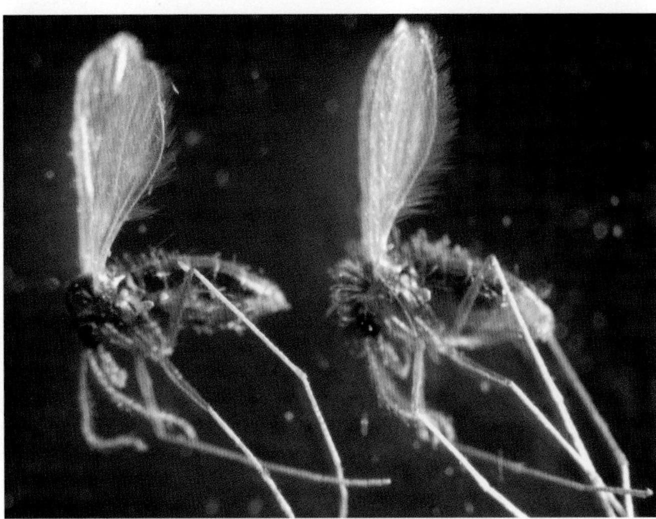

Figure 47.3 Blood-fed *P. argentipes* sandflies. *(Courtesy of S. Sundar.)*

Reported incidence rates are in the range of 1–10 per 10 000 per year, usually with marked space–time clustering. A 5-year prospective study of CL in an endemic area of Brazil documented an annual incidence of disease of 8 per 1000 inhabitants and a prevalence of 15%.[7]

Mucocutaneous leishmaniasis (MCL) is restricted to South America and is a rare complication of CL occurring in less than 5% of cases. It is a severely mutilating disease usually leaving highly disfiguring scars and can lead to fatal complications. In the above cited cohort, it occurred in 2.7% of patients with primary lesions after a median of 6 years after the initial CL. Mucosal involvement is also possible in CL and VL in the Old World.

*HIV/*Leishmania *Co-infection*

HIV/*Leishmania* co-infection was initially reported from southwestern Europe, mainly from Spain, Italy, France and Portugal.[8] After the first case report in 1985, a total of 1911 cases had been reported by 2001.[9] A total of 70% were intravenous drug users. VL was observed in 3–7% of persons with HIV and up to 70% of adult VL cases were HIV-infected.[9] Thanks to the introduction of antiretroviral therapy in 1997, the incidence of HIV/*Leishmania* co-infection has decreased in Europe, with only 241 new cases reported between 2001 and 2006.[10]

Cases of HIV/*Leishmania* co-infection are now reported from 35 countries. In Asia and Africa, the incidence of co-infection remains low, with the exception of Ethiopia where in some centres, up to 30% of VL patients are co-infected with HIV.[11] Co-infection with cutaneous species has remained rare with the exception of outbreaks of visceralizing *L. major* in HIV-co-infected persons in Western Africa (Burkina Faso).

TRANSMISSION

Leishmaniases are transmitted through the bite of a sandfly (Figure 47.3). Very exceptionally, transmission occurs congenitally,[12] during transfusion,[13] organ transplant[14,15] or in laboratory accidents.[16] Transmission of *L. infantum* in HIV-co-infected patients in Spain became dissociated from the sandfly vector and the dog reservoir: it was established that intravenous drug users transmitted leishmaniasis by sharing non-sterile needles.[17,18] In CL, mere skin contact with the active lesion is innocuous; infection requires inoculation of material from active sores, a principle exploited in the ancient practice of 'leishmanization'.

Vector

Sandflies (Diptera: *Psychodidae, Phlebotominae*) are small, hairy insects of 2–4 mm length (Figure 47.3). Of the around 1000 known species, 70 are proven vectors of *Leishmania*; they belong to the genera *Phlebotomus* and *Lutzomyia*. The vector competence of a certain sandfly species for a certain *Leishmania* species is remarkably specific and is linked to polymorphism of the lipophosphoglycan on the surface membrane of the parasite. During daytime, sandflies rest in cool, dark, sheltered places such as corners of houses, cracks and crevices in walls, rodent burrows, rock crevices and termite hills. At and after dusk they become active and can fly small distances. Both sexes feed on plant sugars, but the females need a blood meal to lay eggs. Larval development takes 30–60 days and takes place in moist microhabitats rich in organic matter. The precise localization of breeding sites of many sandfly species remains unknown, and this is a major hindrance for control.

The insect can transmit *Leishmania* to a mammalian host 7–10 days after an infected meal. The mammalian host is infectious to the sandfly as long as parasites persist in the circulating blood or in the macrophages of the dermis. Even after clinical recovery, humans may remain infectious for sandflies, especially in nodular post-kala-azar dermal leishmaniasis (PKDL).[19] It is still uncertain whether asymptomatic infected humans play a role in transmission, although it has been demonstrated that asymptomatic dogs are infectious.

Reservoir

Most leishmaniases are zoonoses. Various mammals are responsible for the long-term maintenance of *Leishmania* in nature.[20]

Domestic dogs are the main reservoir of zoonotic VL caused by *L. infantum* and commonly develop a generalized, fatal form of the disease (Figure 47.4). Nonetheless, more than 50% of infected dogs remain asymptomatic. These asymptomatic carrier dogs can infect sandflies. Wild carnivores such as foxes (*Vulpes* sp.), crab-eating foxes (*Cerdocyon thous*), jackals (*Canis aureus*), wolves (*C. lupus*) and raccoon dogs (*Nyctereutes procyonoides*) can also carry *L. infantum* and could be ancestral hosts.

Wild animals are the main reservoir host for other *Leishmania* species in the Old World. Various rodent species and hyraxes are reservoirs of CL. The great gerbil (*Rhombomys optimus*) in the arid regions of Central Asia and the Fat Sand Jird (*Psammomys obesus*) in the Near East and North Africa maintain *L. major* transmission. Hyraxes are the main reservoir hosts of *L. aethiopica* in Ethiopia and Kenya.

In the New World, the sylvatic reservoirs of CL and MCL include mammals of the forest canopy, such as sloths (*Choloepus didactylus* and *Bradypus tridactylus* for *L. guyanensis* and *C. hoffmani* for *L. panamensis*); ground-level rodents such as the spiny rat (*Proechimys guyanensis* and *P. cuvieri*) for *L. amazonensis*; the climbing rat (*Ototylomus phyllotis*) for *L.*

Links to published literature about the distribution of the leishmaniases can be found on: http://apps.who.int/tools/geoserver/www/ecomp/index.html (Accessed 2 Jan 2011).

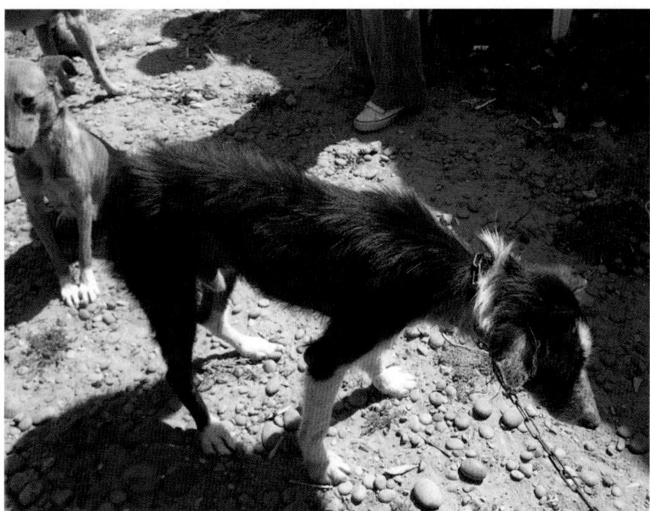

Figure 47.4 Dog with visceral leishmaniasis in Morocco. *(Courtesy of A. Petavy.)*

mexicana; the paca (*Cuniculus paca*) for *L. lainsoni*; and the armadillo (*Dasipus novemcinctus*) for *L. naïffi*.

For other species such as *L. donovani* or *L. tropica*, there is no known animal reservoir and transmission involves only sandflies and humans.

DISEASE BURDEN BY REGION AND RISK FACTORS

Old World Visceral Leishmaniasis

VL is caused by *L. donovani* in large parts of East Africa and in South Asia. In these regions, VL has caused devastating epidemics in the past. The first reported outbreak, initially attributed to 'virulent malaria', occurred in 1824 in Jessore (now Bangladesh). VL claimed a high death toll when it spread over the Ganges plain in Bengal territory and into Assam. Between 1892 and 1898, one-third of the population of Nowgong district in Assam died.[21] Between 1918 and 1923, a further 200 000 people died of VL in Assam and in the Brahmaputra valley. The next epidemic appeared in 1944. After extensive insecticide spraying in the 1950s by the malaria eradication campaign, VL incidence declined in India only to reappear in the 1970s – after cessation of the spraying. Between 1984 and 1994, a VL epidemic in the Western Upper Nile province in Sudan caused an estimated 100 000 deaths in a community of 280 000 people.[22] Forced migration due to the civil war was a major factor in transmission, and the poor nutritional status of the population contributed to the high mortality rates.

The densely populated Ganges/Brahmaputra basin spanning North-East India, South-East Nepal and Central Bangladesh accounts for nearly two-thirds of the world's VL cases. Figure 47.5 shows the cases of VL notified in the state of Bihar, India since the 1970s. These figures are an underestimate, as there are 5–8 unreported cases for every officially reported case.[23] Many people with VL seek treatment in the private sector and are never noted. Moreover, because of the geographical clustering of VL, the country-aggregated figures do not reflect the real importance of the disease in affected communities, where it can lead to a vicious cycle. VL affects the poorest of the poor, such as daily wage labourers or subsistence farmers.[24] They are at higher risk to contract leishmaniasis and to die from it, while the disease itself leads to further impoverishment through catastrophic health expenditure, income loss, and death of wage earners.

Around the Mediterranean Basin, where VL is endemic as a zoonosis caused by *L. infantum*, there are an estimated 4500 human cases each year, of which 700 occur in Southern Europe.[25] In the past, VL was essentially a paediatric disorder, but this epidemiological pattern has changed in recent years because of the HIV epidemic.

New World Visceral Leishmaniasis

In South America VL used to be a rural disease affecting children but in recent years, it is increasingly becoming a peri-urban disease linked to migration of poor rural families to major cities. Poor environmental hygiene in these settings contributes to increased risk. The VL disease burden is not exactly known because most countries lack effective surveillance systems.[26] Between 1990 and 2006 Brazil declared a total of 50 060 clinical VL cases. This number accounts for 90% of all reported VL cases in the Americas, but is subject to substantial underreporting. Moreover, ratios of 8–18 incident asymptomatic infections for each incident clinical case were described in Brazil. Risk factors for progression to disease include malnutrition, genetic factors and HIV co-infection.

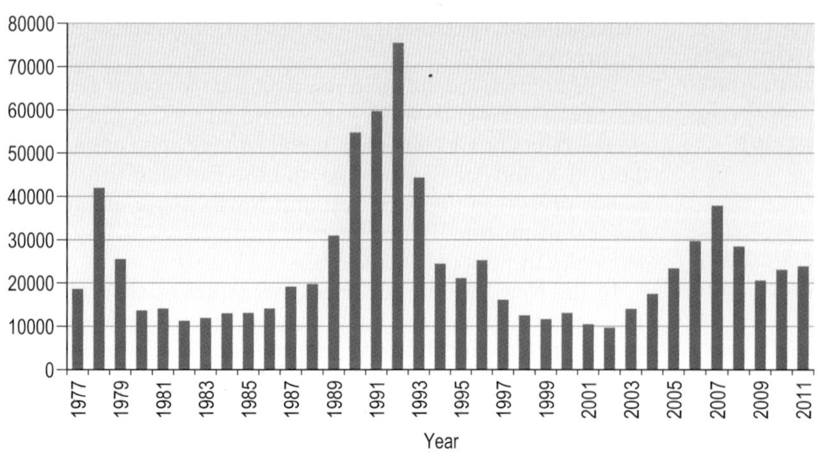

Figure 47.5 Trend of visceral leishmaniasis in Bihar since the 1970s. *(Adapted from data provided by Ministry of Health, India.)*

Old World Cutaneous Leishmaniasis

CL caused by *L. major* is the most common form; it occurs in Northern Africa, the Middle East, Central Asia and limited areas of South-east Asia (Pakistan, India). *L. tropica* has a more restricted distribution in the north-eastern Mediterranean basin, the Middle East, Central Asia and parts of South-east Asia (Pakistan, India). *L. aethiopica* is only found in Ethiopia, Kenya and Uganda and causes CL as well as a severe disseminated form, called diffuse CL.

Epidemics of CL caused by *L. tropica* occurred in war-stricken Kabul, Afghanistan, in the 1990s, followed by large outbreaks in refugee camps in Pakistan.

New World Cutaneous Leishmaniasis

L. braziliensis is the most widespread pathogen causing CL in South America, followed by *L. guyanensis* (Amazon region), *L. panamensis* (Panama and Colombia), *L. peruviana* and *L. mexicana* (Mexico and Belize). Where CL was in the past mostly a sporadic occupational disease related to rubber tapping, military operations, road constructions, etc. in the jungle, it now regularly leads to outbreaks when immunologically naïve populations infringe on areas of sylvatic transmission in a context of deforestation and migration.

Mucocutaneous Leishmaniasis

MCL is a rare complication of CL in the New World presenting in less than 5% of CL cases several years after cure. Bolivia, Brazil and Peru report most of the MCL cases. Initially it was believed that only *L. braziliensis* caused this syndrome. The current concept is that most New World *Leishmania* species can cause MCL, depending on host immune response and parasite strain among other factors.[27] In the Old World, *L. donovani* as well as other species may cause mucosal lesions, especially in elderly or immunosuppressed people.

Pathogenesis and Pathology

CAUSATIVE AGENT

The *Leishmania* parasite is a protozoan belonging to the family *Trypanosomatidae* in the order of the *Kinetoplastida*. These are unicellular flagellated organisms with a typical 'kinetoplast', i.e. a DNA-containing mass in their single, large mitochondrion. *Leishmania* parasites have two forms: the amastigote in the mammalian host and the promastigote form in the insect vector. Amastigotes are oval bodies about 2–6 μm in size containing a nucleus and a kinetoplast. They replicate intracellularly in the macrophages of the mammalian host. In the gut of the insect vector the parasite develops into a slender flagellated promastigote form (about 15–30 μm by 2–3 μm).

Since the original description of the genus by Ross,[28] at least 20 pathogenic species have been identified. Though these species are morphologically indistinguishable, they can be differentiated by iso-enzyme analysis[29,30] or molecular methods.[6,31] Lainson and Shaw divided the genus into two subgenera: *Leishmania sensu strictu* and *Viannia*.[32] The distribution of the subgenus *Viannia* is restricted to the New World. Table 47.1 gives an overview of the *Leishmania* species found in humans.

The genus *Leishmania* can be divided broadly into viscerotropic (*L. donovani, L. infantum*) and dermatotropic species (roughly all other). Exceptions to this include: (i) *L. infantum*, which has a dermatotropic enzymatic variant causing sporadic cases of CL in the Mediterranean Basin and (ii) *L. tropica* and *L. amazonensis*, which can occasionally cause visceralizing disease in immunocompetent persons. New World dermatotropic species are known for their secondary mucosal spread, but, there are also sporadic cases of mucosal involvement caused by Old World dermatotropic species. Even patients with visceral disease and PKDL may develop mucosal lesions in the mouth, nose or on the genitals. Atypical presentations are most commonly observed in HIV-co-infected patients (see below).

PARASITE LIFE CYCLE

In nature, *Leishmania* parasites are alternatively hosted by a sandfly vector as promastigotes – evolving from a procyclic to an infective metacyclic stage – and by a mammalian host in the intracellular amastigote form (Figure 47.6). When an infected female sandfly bites a mammal, the metacyclic promastigotes are regurgitated from the sandfly gut and deposited directly into the bite wound with some sandfly saliva. This sandfly saliva

TABLE 47.1 *Leishmania* Species Found in Humans

Subgenus	L. (Leishmania)	L. (Leishmania)	L. (Viannia)	L. (Viannia)
Old World	*L. donovani* *L. infantum*	*L. major* *L. tropica* *L. killicki*[a] *L. aethiopica*		
New World	*L. infantum*	*L. infantum* *L. mexicana* *L. pifanoi*[a] *L. venezuelensis* *L. garnhami*[a] *L. amazonensis*	*L. braziliensis* *L. guyanensis* *L. panamensis* *L. shawi* *L. naïffi* *L. lainsoni* *L. lindenbergi* *L. peruviana* *L. colombiensis*[b]	*L. braziliensis* *L. panamensis*
Principal tropism	Viscerotropic	Dermotropic	Dermotropic	Mucotropic

[a]Species status is under discussion.
[b]Taxonomic position is under discussion.
Source: World Health Organization. Control of the Leishmaniases. Geneva: WHO press. WHO Technical Report Series 2010;949:1–186. Reproduced with permission.

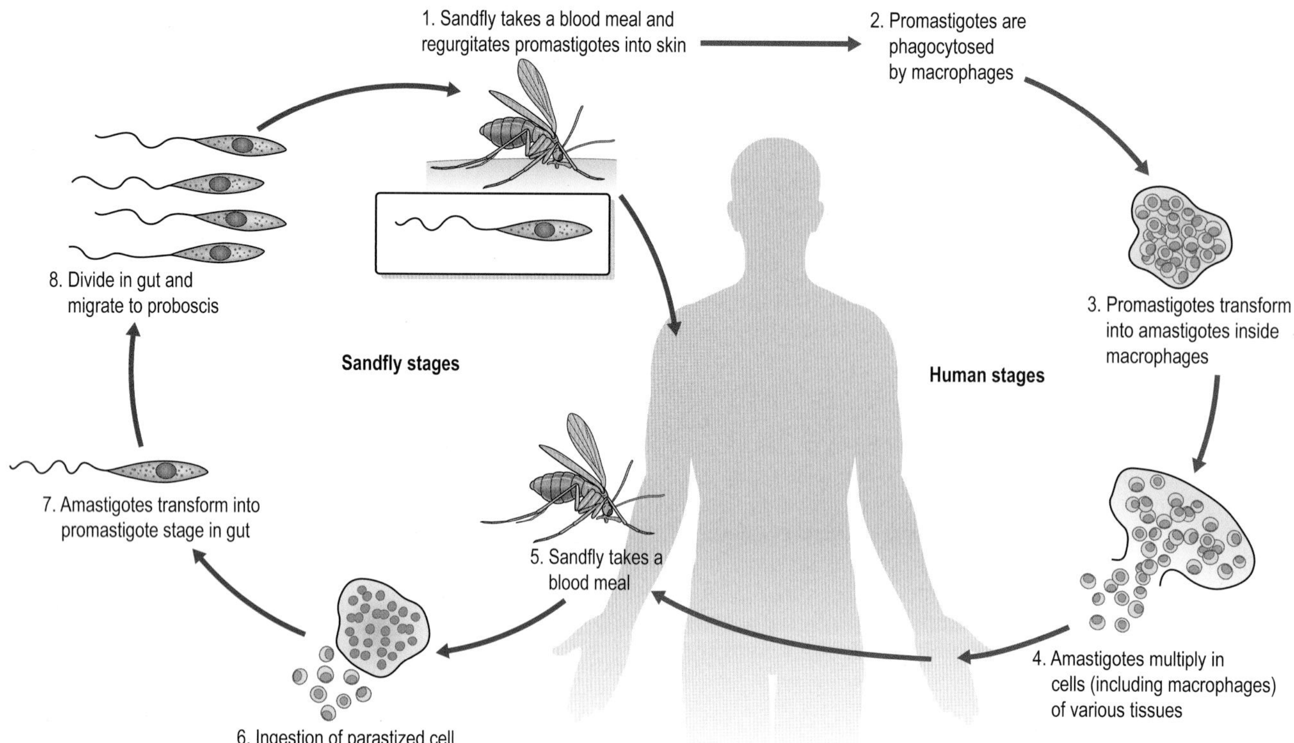

Figure 47.6 Life cycle of *Leishmania* parasites. *(Reprinted from the Lancet Infectious Diseases, from Reithinger R, Dujardin JC, Louzir H, et al. Cutaneous leishmaniasis. Lancet Infect Dis 2007;7:581–96. With permission from Elsevier.)*

enhances infectivity.[33] In the skin the promastigotes escape lysis through complement activation because of certain surface membrane components – mainly lipophosphoglycan and glycoprotein 63 (gp63) – but they are phagocytized by macrophages. Low pH and mammalian body temperature then induce differentiation of promastigotes into amastigotes with the capacity to survive the extreme hostile intracellular macrophage environment. They multiply by simple division until the macrophage eventually lyses and the parasites are released and infect other phagocytes. When another female sandfly later bites the same mammal, these infected macrophages can be ingested with the blood meal. The amastigote parasites will transform into promastigotes in the sandfly and multiply in the midgut (*Leishmania* subgenus) or in the hindgut and midgut (*Viannia* subgenus). The parasites then migrate to the anterior part of the sandfly gut where they transform into free-swimming metacyclic promastigotes, ready for inoculation when the insect bites its next victim.

PATHOGENESIS

The clinical outcomes of *Leishmania* infection depend on the infecting species as well as on host genetic factors and host immune status. These factors decide whether *Leishmania* parasites will reside in the skin, causing CL, or migrate to draining lymph nodes to become established in the mononuclear phagocyte system, primarily the spleen, bone marrow and liver to cause life-threatening VL.[34] However, even in the latter case, the majority of *L. infantum* and *L. donovani* infections remain asymptomatic in immunocompetent individuals.[35] After cure of a clinical episode intracellular infection is probably lifelong as viable residual parasites are known to persist in macrophages.

Visceral Leishmaniasis

VL is a disease of the mononuclear phagocytic system. It commonly affects the spleen, liver, lymph nodes and bone marrow, but other organs (intestine, lung, skin) may also become involved. Marked hepatosplenomegaly is characteristic. In immunosuppressed patients and in advanced cases, all body organs are involved. The histological aspects are organ-specific but can be summarized as reticuloendothelial hyperplasia, with marked proliferation of macrophages and plasma cells, and heavy parasitism of haematopoietic organs (Figure 47.7A,B). The most striking sign for the pathologist are probably the granulomata caused by the proliferation of activated macrophages, as parasites could easily be missed if pathology slides are only examined at ×400 magnification and in cases of light infection. Suppression of erythrocyte, thrombocyte and leukocyte cell lines leads to pancytopenia in the most severe and advanced cases.

The presence of amastigotes within macrophages is the hallmark of *Leishmania* infection. Amastigotes thrive and replicate within the phagolysosomes and seem to be protected from lytic enzymes by their dense surface coat. However, macrophages can be stimulated to kill the parasites. Studies in mouse models revealed that the production of interleukin (IL)-12 by antigen-presenting cells (APCs) and interferon (IFN)-γ by T cells is required for control of the parasites and development of

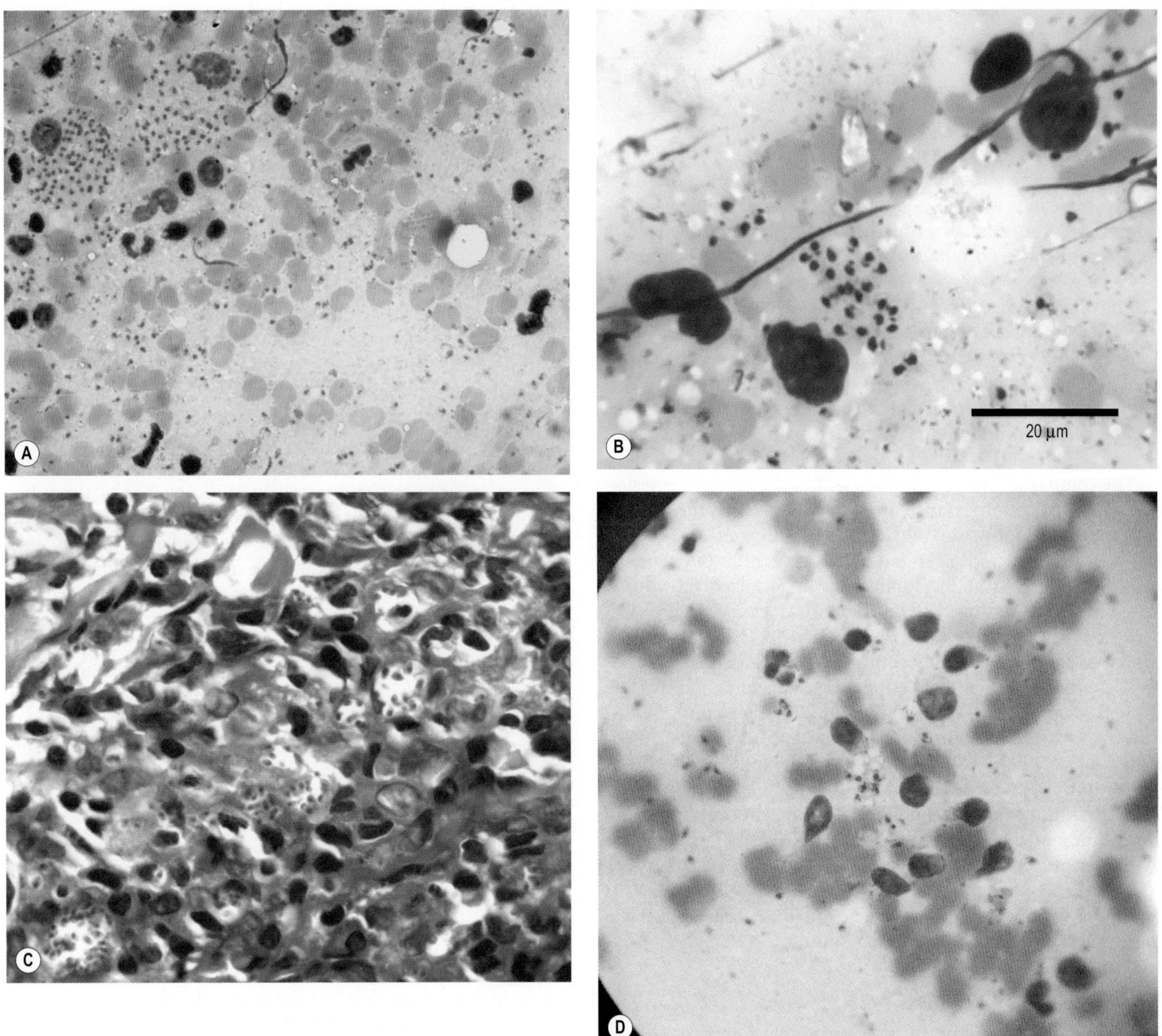

Figure 47.7 Histopathology of leishmaniasis. Amastigotes have an oval form and an eccentric nucleus. Occasionally, the kinetoplast is visible as a condensation within the amastigote at the opposite side of the nucleus. Other conditions in which conglomerates of microorganisms, all of the same size, may be visible include histoplasmosis and cryptococcosis. (A,B) Spleen aspirates from an Ethiopian patient with visceral leishmaniasis showing amastigotes in macrophages and in the intercellular space. (C) Skin biopsy from a Peruvian patient with cutaneous leishmaniasis. (D) Skin smear from an Ethiopian patient with diffuse cutaneous leishmaniasis. *(Courtesy of (A,B,D) C. Yansouni. (C) F. Bravo, Instituto de Medicina Tropical Alexander von Humboldt).*

acquired resistance.[36–38] In human VL the immune response is not polarized in a strict Th1 and Th2 dichotomy. There is increased production of multiple cytokines and chemokines, primarily pro-inflammatory, as indicated by the elevated plasma levels of IL-1, IL-6, IL-8, IL-12, IL-15, IFN-γ and tumour necrosis factor (TNF)-α, with elevated levels of IFN-γ mRNA in affected tissues, such as the spleen and bone marrow.[39] On the other hand there are high levels of regulatory suppressive cytokines, like IL-10, that have primarily suppressive effects on immune function, targeting multiple activation and antigen presentation pathways of macrophages and dendritic cells. Based on clinical and experimental studies, IL-10 is believed to trigger many of the immunologic defects in VL.[40]

Human VL is associated with high levels of anti-leishmanial antibodies. Apart from being useful as diagnostic markers, the immunologic role of these anti-leishmanial antibodies is still unclear. Although T cells appear to be the main source of IL-10 during the early stages of disease, the evolution of high antibody titres and immune complex formation in VL might drive higher IL-10 production by macrophages and other cells as well, contributing to the progressive decline in the immune status of VL patients and to the fatal outcome in untreated cases.

Cutaneous Leishmaniasis

The common, localized, self-healing CL lesions are characterized by an epidermal and dermal infiltrate consisting of histiocytes containing amastigotes, lymphocytes and plasma cells (Figure 47.7C). The histological patterns of the two special, non-healing forms of CL show diffuse granulomas containing large numbers of macrophages full of amastigotes and almost no lymphocytes in DCL (Figure 47.7D) and hypersensitive tuberculoid granulomas with many Langhans giant cells with small numbers of lymphocytes and plasma cells in leishmaniasis recidivans.

The cytokine pattern in patients with CL reveals a mixed Th1 and Th2 response. The presence of *Leishmania*-specific T cells with Th1-like cytokine production profile is associated with mild disease (self-healing) whereas predominant Th2 activity is associated with the non-healing form. IFN-γ plays a role in the healing process while IL-4 is associated with the persistence of lesions.[41]

The cellular immune responses within the cutaneous lesion are of primary importance in the outcome of the disease and vary depending on the causative pathogen. CD4+ and CD8+ T cells, macrophages and B cells constitute the majority of infiltrating cells at the lesion site. In localized CL caused by *L. braziliensis*, the mRNA of the Th1 cytokine IFN-γ is expressed abundantly while the mRNA of Th2 cytokines is expressed more weakly.[42] By contrast, in CL caused by *L. mexicana*, there is minimal intralesional mRNA expression of IL-2, IL-3, IL-4 and IL-5, whereas IL-6, IL-10, IFN-γ and TNF-α mRNA is expressed abundantly.[43] In cutaneous lesions caused by *L. major*, there is high IFN-γ, IL-10 and IL-12 mRNA expression.

IL-10 inhibits the macrophage-activating effect of IFN-γ and contributes to disease progression.[44] IL-10 is reported to be mainly produced by monocytes and CD4+CD25+ regulatory T cells. The role of regulatory T cells in human leishmaniasis is not yet clear; however, the frequency of these cells appears to increase with the duration of the lesion.

Mucocutaneous Leishmaniasis

The exact pathogenesis of mucocutaneous leishmaniasis (MCL) is still unclear, although it is believed that host genetic factors play a role. The initial lesion in MCL develops in a similar way to that of CL. After the skin lesion has healed, the infection remains dormant for a variable period of time, from weeks to several years. Mucocutaneous involvement usually starts on the nasal mucosa, on the anterior cartilaginous part of the nasal septum. It appears as a small-sized hyperaemic inflammatory granuloma that rapidly evolves to an ulcer.[45] The nasal septum is invaded, perforated and destroyed. Lesion biopsies show an intense inflammatory reaction, dominated by lymphocytes and macrophages with few or no parasites. This is associated with acute vasculitis and coagulative necrosis of the walls of the small blood vessels. The most severe part of the lesion usually lies in the deep nasal mucosa.

The immunopathogenesis involves hyperactive specific T-cell immune responses with an exuberant lymphoproliferation.[46,47] There is production of high levels of pro-inflammatory cytokines, such as IFN-γ and TNF-α, as well as a decreased ability of IL-10 and TGF-β to modulate this response. This dominant Th1 pro-inflammatory response is responsible for tissue destruction.[48]

Clinical Features

VISCERAL LEISHMANIASIS

Signs and Symptoms

VL is the most severe clinical form of leishmaniasis and is usually fatal if not treated. The incubation period is thought to be 2–6 months, ranging between 10 days and 2 years. Longer incubation periods are possible when asymptomatically infected persons harbouring a few dormant intracellular parasites develop full-blown clinical disease many years after infection because of immunosuppressive therapy or co-infections as HIV. VL patients present symptoms and signs of a chronic systemic infection (fever, fatigue, weakness, loss of appetite and weight) and of parasite invasion of the mononuclear phagocyte system (enlarged lymph nodes, spleen and liver). The triad of enlarged spleen, fever and pancytopenia is strongly suggestive of VL but is not always present (Figure 47.8). At disease onset fever is moderate to high, usually associated with rigor and chills and may be intermittent and irregular. With passage of time there is resolution of fever, but it usually recurs somewhat less severely after a few days or weeks. Fatigue and weakness are worsened by anaemia, which is caused by the chronic inflammatory state, the destruction of erythrocytes in the enlarged spleen (hypersplenism), and sometimes by bleeding. Anaemia is often severe and may result in congestive heart failure and its associated features such as tachycardia, hepatomegaly and pedal oedema. Splenomegaly is almost always present. It is firm, smooth, mobile and painless. The spleen grows steadily over time and may eventually extend down into the right hypochondrium. Hepatomegaly due to VL is less frequent and develops later. The liver is usually slightly enlarged and painless.

Diarrhoea is frequently reported and may be caused by ulcerations of the digestive mucosa and associated amoebic or bacterial infections. Pulmonary involvement is often due to secondary infection, and bacterial pneumonia is quite frequent as is tuberculosis. Episodes of bleeding are possible, usually epistaxis and more rarely bleeding from gums, purpura, petechiae and menorrhagia. Symptoms and signs of superimposed bacterial infections (e.g. pneumonia, diarrhoea, otitis media, tuberculosis) may confuse the clinical picture.

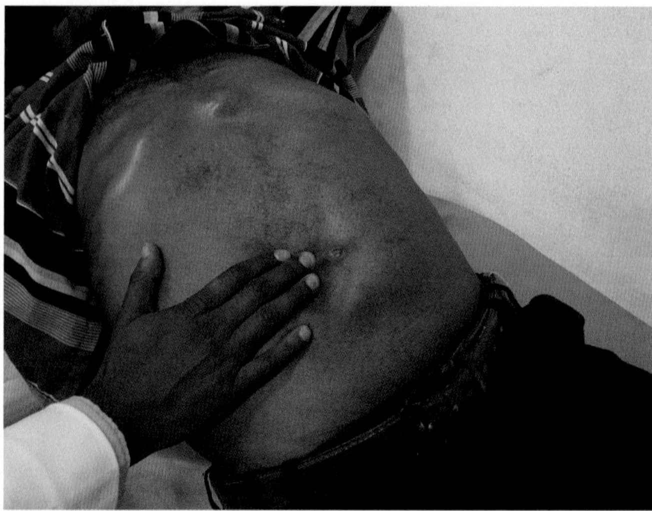

Figure 47.8 Splenomegaly in an Ethiopian patient with visceral leishmaniasis. *(Courtesy of C. Yansouni.)*

This clinical presentation of VL is similar in the various endemic areas but some differences do occur, e.g. enlarged lymph nodes are frequent in Sudanese patients but are rarely found in Indian VL.[49,50] Hyperpigmentation, a feature of chronic untreated VL, which probably led to the name of 'kala-azar' ('black fever', in Hindi), has only been described in VL patients from the Indian subcontinent, though it is rarely seen now.

Clinical Biology

Anaemia is the major and most frequent haematological sign and is generally of the normochromic, normocytic type. Haemoglobin levels are usually around 7–10 g/dL but can decrease down to 4 g/dL. Leukopenia (1–3000/mm^3 with neutropenia is often observed and can lead to many associated infections. Platelets are frequently decreased. Profound thrombocytopenia (below 40 000/mm^3) and alterations of hepatic coagulation factors can result in severe haemorrhages. The simultaneous decrease of the three cell lines corresponds to the classical sign of 'pancytopenia'. The inflammatory syndrome causes an elevated erythrocyte sedimentation rate (ESR) and an increase of C-reactive protein (CRP). The plasma protein profiles are disturbed, with low albumin levels and hypergammaglobulinaemia (up to 20 g/L) corresponding to overproduction of polyclonal immunoglobulins, mainly IgG. The presence of mono-, bi- or pancytopenia, systemic inflammation or polyclonal hypergammaglobulinaemia (detected by the formol gel test), reinforce the clinical suspicion but are not sufficiently specific to confirm VL. Therefore, *Leishmania*-specific laboratory tests are required to confirm VL (see below).

Evolution

The disease evolves slowly over many months or even years, and in the endemic areas, patients often receive appropriate care only very late in the disease process. As the disease advances, patients gradually lose weight and splenomegaly may become massive, causing abdominal distension and pain, sometimes increased by hepatomegaly. The typical pattern is that of an extremely wasted patient with a protuberant abdomen. Ascites is considered a late sign of bad prognosis, sometimes associated with oedema and pleural effusion. Wasting progressively evolves into cachexia, and if no treatment is given, the spontaneous evolution is fatal in over 90% of cases. Death is usually caused by superimposed infections, severe anaemia or haemorrhages.

Special Clinical Forms

Asymptomatic and Subclinical Infections. Not every infected individual develops disease, and there is a spectrum from asymptomatic infection over subclinical disease to the full-blown VL syndrome.[51] Subclinical or mild forms of visceral disease were described in a Brazilian study[52] as well as in veterans of Operation Desert Storm.[53] Epidemiological surveys showed that asymptomatic and subclinical forms are frequent.[54,55] The prevalence of asymptomatic infections of *L. infantum* varied between 0.6% and 71% in endemic areas.[54] In prospective studies, the ratio of incident asymptomatic infections to clinical cases varied from 2.4:1 in Sudan;[56] 4:1 in Kenya;[57] 5.6:1 in Ethiopia;[58] 6:1[59] to 18:1 in Brazil;[52] 4:1 in Bangladesh[60] or 8.9:1 in India and Nepal.[55]

Post Kala-Azar Dermal Leishmaniasis (PKDL). Post kala-azar dermal leishmaniasis (PKDL) is a chronic rash and a complication of VL, mostly seen in areas where *L. donovani* is endemic, i.e. in Asia (India, Nepal and Bangladesh) and in East Africa (Ethiopia, Kenya and Sudan). The skin lesions usually appear several months to years after treatment in patients who are otherwise well. PKDL can sometimes develop concomitantly with the VL episode or in patients with no history of VL.[61] In East Africa, the interval between VL and PKDL is short. PKDL has been described in 50–60% of Sudanese VL patients within weeks to a few months after treatment with antimonials. In the Indian subcontinent PKDL takes longer to develop and is less frequent. In Bangladesh, 10% of VL patients had developed PKDL 3 years after treatment with antimonials, and in India, 5–10% after an interval of 6 months to 4 years. PKDL due to *L. infantum* is rare but has been reported among HIV/*Leishmania* co-infected patients treated with antimonials. The frequency of PKDL varies from country to country for reasons that are not entirely clear, though the nature of the treatment of the initial VL episode seems to play a role. Incomplete or inadequate treatment and treatment with antimonials are risk factors. It is uncommon following treatment with amphotericin B.

PKDL lesions range from hypopigmented maculae over papulae to nodules. (Figure 47.9). A mixed maculo-nodular form is often observed. The lesions usually start on the face and expand to other parts of the body. Exposure to sunlight may be an important factor in its pathogenesis as the distribution of lesions mirrors the clothing pattern. Three grades of severity are used to describe PKDL in East-Africa. In grade one the

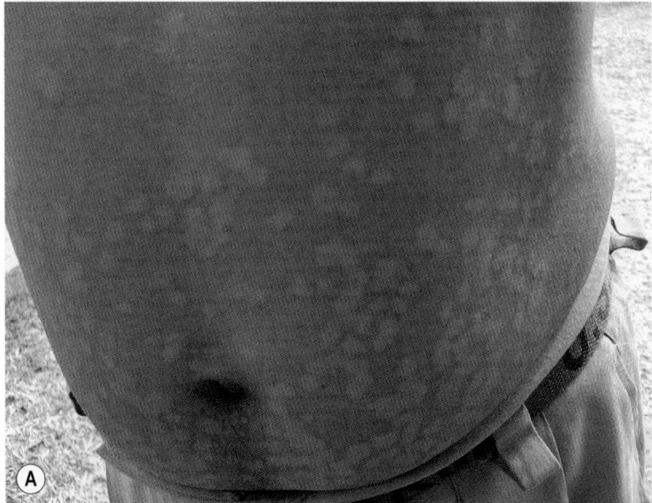

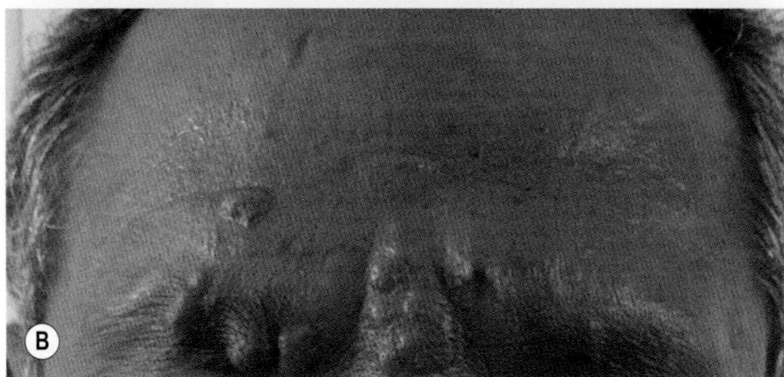

Figure 47.9 Post-kala-azar dermal leishmaniasis in patients from Nepal. (A) Hypopigmented maculae on the abdomen. (B) Nodular rash on the face. *(Courtesy of S. Uranw.)*

maculo-papular or nodular rash occurs mainly on the face with no or very few lesions on the chest and arms. Grade two is defined as a rash covering most of the face and extending to the chest, back, upper arms, and upper legs, gradually diminishing distally, with only few lesions on the forearms and lower legs. Grade three is defined as a rash covering most parts of the body, including hands and feet. In grade three, crusting, ulceration, sloughing, scaling, and spreading to the mucosa of the lip (cheilitis) and the palate may occur. The nodular forms of PKDL are believed to play a role as an inter-epidemic reservoir in the anthroponotic transmission cycle.

CUTANEOUS LEISHMANIASES

Signs and Symptoms

CL (known also as Oriental sore, Aleppo boil, Bouton de Biskra, Baghdad boil, or uta) usually starts at the place of the insect bite as a papule that gradually enlarges to a nodule, remaining red but painless (Figure 47.10). Very slowly, the central part necrotizes and when the crust falls off, it leaves an ulcer with an indurated edge (Figure 47.10C). This well-defined, firmly infiltrated border is very typical for CL and is helpful in the differential diagnosis. The whole process takes several weeks (1–3 months) to reach its final size, usually in the range of 0.5–10 cm in diameter. The aspect can then be that of a large, open, wet sore with a healing granuloma in the floor of the lesion (especially seen in New World CL with *L. mexicana*, *L. guyanensis* and *L. braziliensis*, but also in *L. major*), or that of a more dry and squamous lesion (*L. tropica*, *L. peruviana*) (Figure 47.10B). Flat plaques or hyperkeratotic lesions are also seen in Old World CL while a nodular aspect with little inflammation suggests infection by *L. donovani*, *L. infantum* or *L. aethiopica* (Figure 47.10A). The lesion can sometimes be surrounded by smaller daughter papules (Figure 47.11). CL lesions are normally painless. Bacterial superinfection may lead to suppuration or erythematous painful borders. CL may present as multiple lesions, depending on the number of infecting bites (Figure 47.10E).

CL is not usually associated with systemic signs or symptoms, but lymphangitic dissemination does occur. At palpation one detects a lymphangitic cord, regularly enlarged with small round and painless nodules, containing parasites. Lymphangitic dissemination is mainly reported with *L. guyanensis*, *L. panamensis*, *L. braziliensis* and *L. major*. The differential diagnosis of nodular or ulcerated lesions with nodular lymphangitis includes: sporotrichosis, nocardiosis, *Mycobacterium marinum*, anthrax and tularemia.

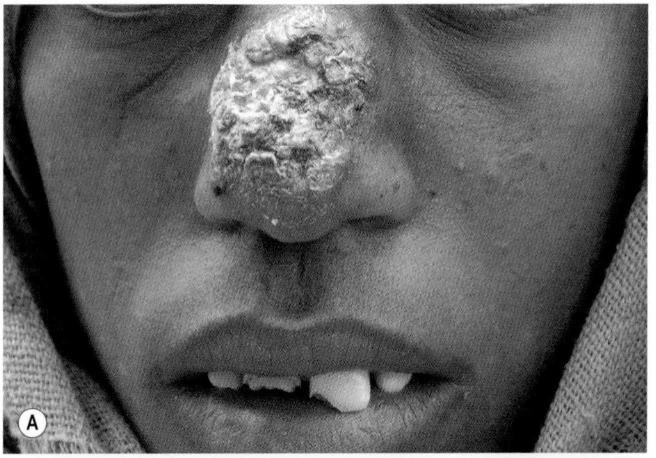

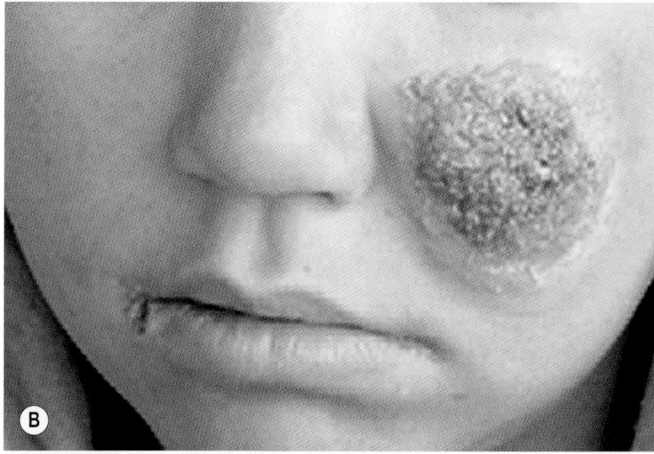

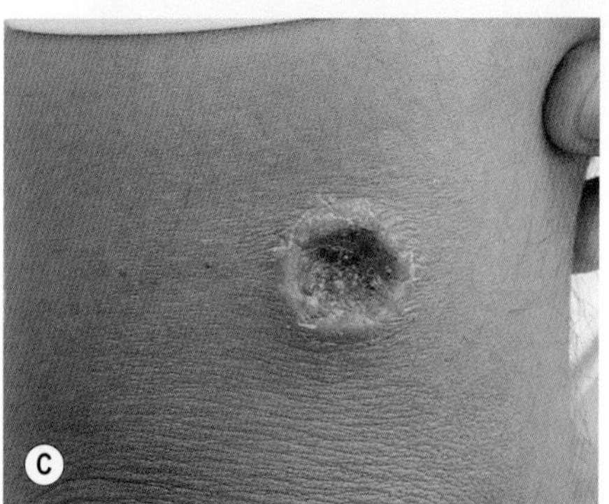

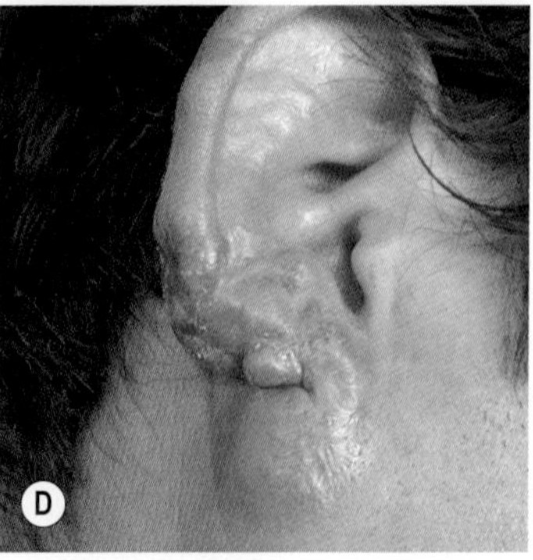

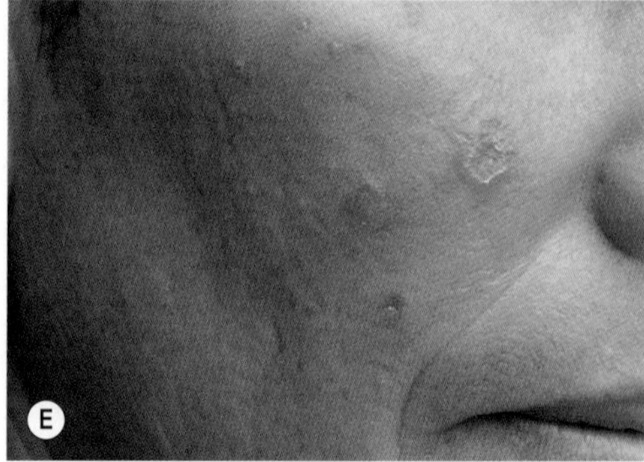

Figure 47.10 Typical lesions of cutaneous leishmaniasis (A) Old World cutaneous leishmaniasis. Ulcer with hyperkeratosis in a patient from Ethiopia. (B) Old World cutaneous leishmaniasis. Large ulcer caused by *L. tropica* in Kabul, Afghanistan. (C) New World cutaneous leishmaniasis. Peruvian patient with a painless lesion that appeared 1 month after a stay in the Amazon region. Typical ulcer with elevated and indurated edges. (D) New World cutaneous leishmaniasis. Peruvian patient with a destructive lesion of the pinna of the ear. Disease duration: 2 months. Such lesions are sometimes called 'chiclero's ulcer', because they were common among workers who harvested rubber ('chicle') from the tropical forest. (E) New World cutaneous leishmaniasis (Peru). Patients often present with multiple lesions. *((A) Courtesy of C. Yansouni. (B) Reprinted from the Lancet Infectious Diseases, from Reithinger R, Dujardin JC, Louzir H, et al. Cutaneous leishmaniasis. Lancet Infect Dis 2007; 7:581–596. With permission from Elsevier. (C–E) Courtesy of Instituto de Medicina Tropical Alexander von Humboldt).*

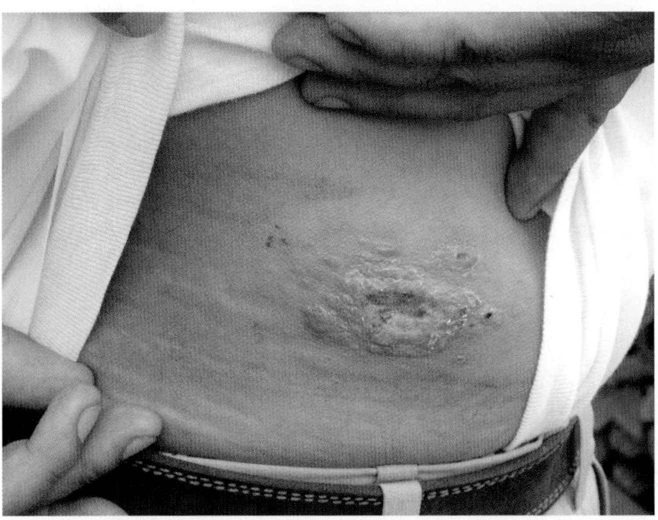

Figure 47.11 Satellite papules. In this patient from Peru, a large lesion is surrounded by smaller daughter papules. *(Courtesy of Instituto de Medicina Tropical. Alexander von Humboldt)*

Evolution

Whatever the clinical type of lesion, the evolution is chronic and leads most often to spontaneous cure, after a time span that depends on the species, from a few months to a few years. Very often, healing leads to disfiguring scars, pinkish or whitish on pale skin and hyperpigmented on dark skin.

L. major usually produces self-healing lesions, but sometimes causes severely inflamed ulcers that heal in 4–6 months. CL by *L. tropica* is usually more chronic with lesions taking more than a year to heal. In its most severe form, leishmaniasis recidivans (see below), it is very difficult to treat. In the New World, *L. mexicana* usually produces relatively benign lesions but some locations such as the external ear (chiclero's ulcer) are very hard to treat and can lead to partial amputation of the auricle (see Figure 47.10D).

Special Clinical Forms

Diffuse Cutaneous Leishmaniasis. Diffuse CL (DCL) is a particularly severe form of CL first described in Venezuela.[62] It is a rare manifestation caused by *L. aethiopica* in the Old World, and by *L. amazonensis* and occasionally *L. mexicana* in the New World in patients with a specific defect in cell-mediated immunity. The disease is thought to be an anergic variant of localized CL. The patients have a negative Leishmanin Skin Test[63] but high titres of *Leishmania*-specific antibodies in serum. DCL is characterized by multiple, slowly progressive nodules or plaques without ulceration, involving almost the entire skin surface (Figure 47.12). These lesions are very rich in parasites. Lepromatous lepra is the main differential diagnosis, as the patient may have a 'leonine' facies. The histopathology of the DCL lesion is characteristic, with a homogeneous epidermal and dermal infiltrate of vacuolated macrophages full of *Leishmania* amastigotes.

During the development of this condition, there is no ulceration, nor mucosal or visceral involvement, but a slow constant aggravation by successive relapses, interrupted with phases of remission. This form never cures spontaneously and is resistant to therapy by classical anti-leishmanial drugs. In HIV/*Leishmania* co-infection, DCL has been reported due to other species, such as *L. braziliensis*,[64] *L. major*,[65] *L. infantum*[66] and *L. donovani*.[67]

Leishmaniasis Recidivans. Leishmaniasis recidivans is a chronic form of leishmaniasis, due essentially to *L. tropica* in the Old World and occasionally to *L. braziliensis* in the New World. The lesion is usually located on the face. At 1–2 years after the acute lesion has healed, new papules and nodules appear at the margin of the scar. The typical lesion consists of a central, healed part surrounded by a peripheral, constantly enlarging and active part (Figure 47.13). The presentation mimics that of lupus vulgaris. The lesion contains a small

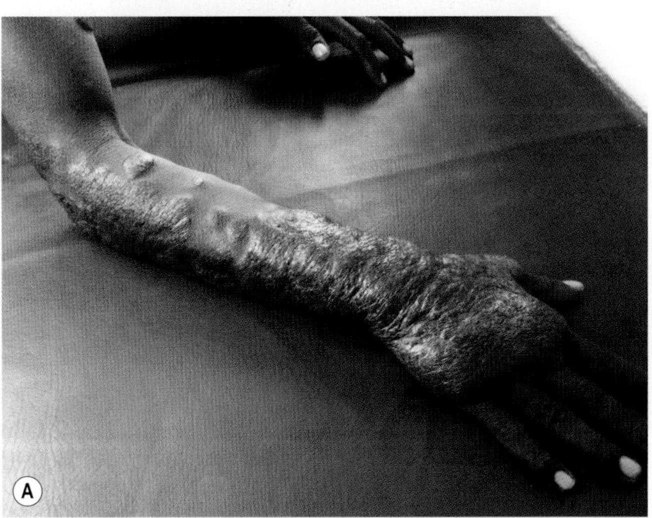

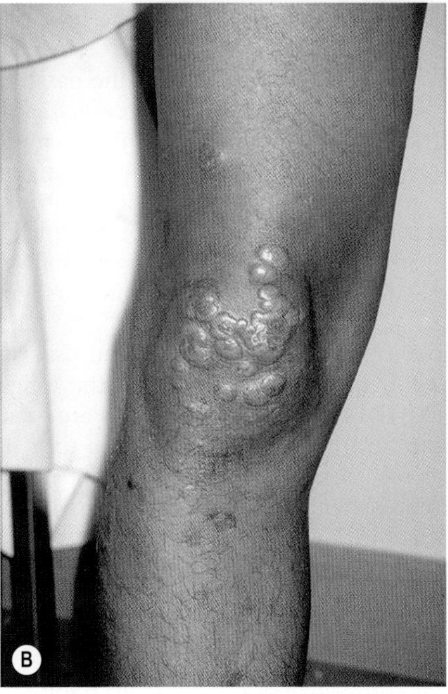

Figure 47.12 Diffuse cutaneous leishmaniasis caused by *L. aethiopica*. (A) Patient from Ethiopia; disease duration: three years. (B) Multiple lesions on the knee. *((A) Courtesy of C. Yansouni. (B) Copyright © Illustrated Lecture Notes in Tropical Medicine. Institute Tropical Medicine Antwerp.)*

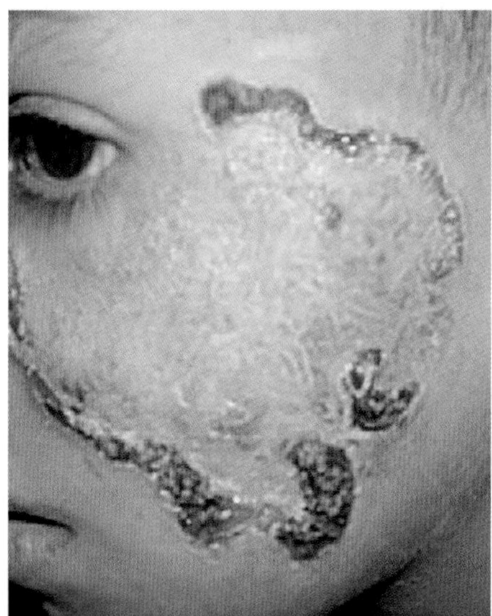

Figure 47.13 Leishmaniasis recidivans caused by *L. tropica* in Kabul, Afghanistan. A central, healing part of the lesion is surrounded by a peripheral, active zone. *(Reprinted from the Lancet Infectious Diseases, from Reithinger R, Dujardin JC, Louzir H, et al. Cutaneous leishmaniasis. Lancet Infect Dis 2007;7:581–96. With permission from Elsevier.)*

number of parasites and corresponds to an exaggerated cell-mediated immune response.

MUCOCUTANEOUS LEISHMANIASIS

MCL, also named 'espundia', is caused by *L. braziliensis* and other New World species. It evolves in two stages: a primary cutaneous lesion followed after a variable time of latency by mucosal lesions, either by metastatic or local spread.[45] As the mucosal involvement usually starts on the nasal mucosa, the patient first suffers from nasal congestion which causes discomfort at night. Epistaxis can also be the initial symptom. In this early stage congestion and oedema of the nasal pyramid can be observed (Figure 47.14A). The nasal lesion evolves to an ulcer, and leads to perforation of the nasal septum which is generally considered pathognomonic for MCL in endemic regions. The nose becomes flattened and weighed down, a sign known as 'tapir nose'.

The oral mucosa is affected later. The mucosae of palate and lips are most frequently involved while the tongue remains intact (Figure 47.14B). The palatal lesions are granulomatous and extensive, and reach the velum where they produce the classical 'Escomel cross'. The lip lesions are inflamed and ulcerated, sometimes extending to the external part, with frequent tissue destruction (Figure 47.14C). A palatal perforation can occur in the later stages.

Laryngeal extension is at first infiltrative and manifests as dysphonia and metallic cough. If the lesion becomes granulomatous, it can cause obstruction of the respiratory tract, with possible fatal consequences due to acute respiratory distress. Dysphagia and the ensuing malnutrition are also severe consequences for the patient.

In the advanced stage, widespread tissue necrosis results in disfiguring mutilations. The nose and lips can totally disappear at which point the nasal and oral cavity connect into a single hole. The sociopsychological consequences for the patient are dramatic and often lead to suicide. Death can also occur because of pulmonary superinfection or acute respiratory obstruction. When treated and cured, patients often exhibit disfiguring retractile scar tissue.

Lesions of MCL are painless and this helps in making the differential diagnosis which includes paracoccidiomycosis and cancer.

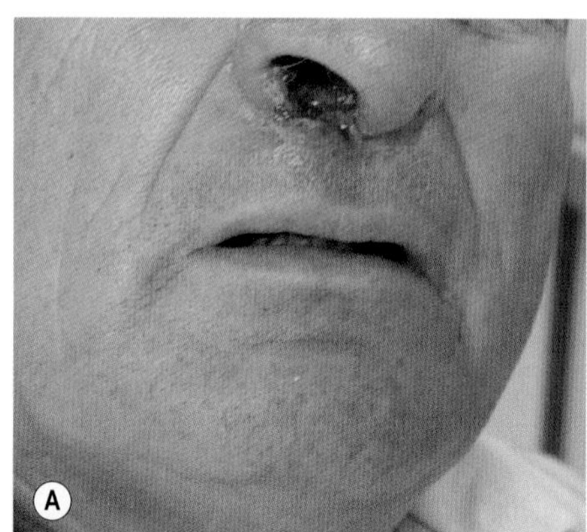

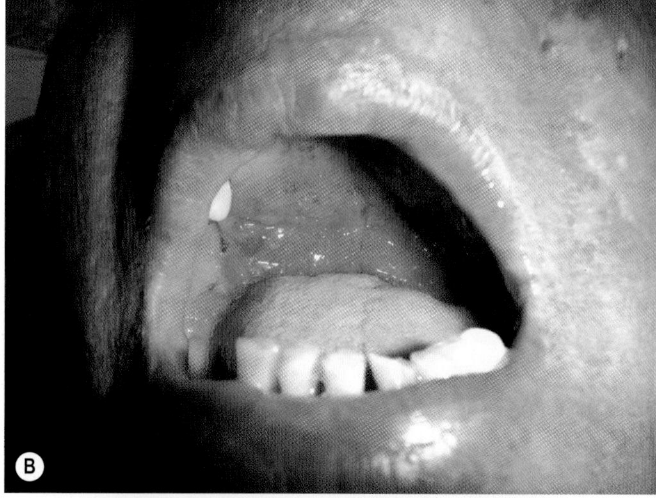

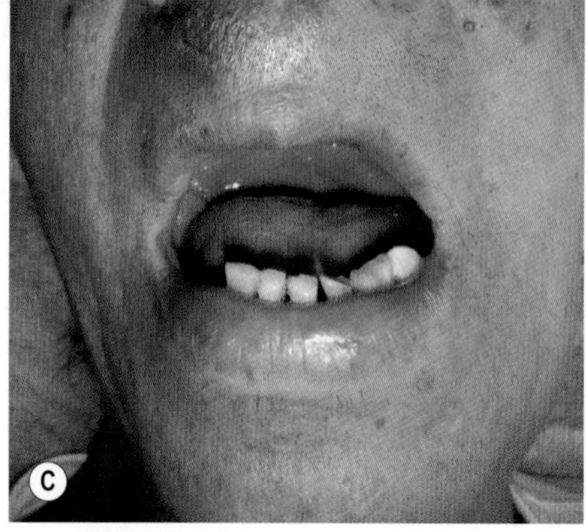

Figure 47.14 Mucocutaneous leishmaniasis in patients from Peru. (A) Early lesion involving mainly the nasal mucosa. (B,C) Later, the lesion also affects the oral mucosa, palate and lips. *(Courtesy of Instituto de Medicina Tropical Alexander von Humboldt*

LEISHMANIASIS AND IMMUNOSUPPRESSION

Leishmaniasis has emerged as a common and serious opportunistic infection of HIV and this changes the clinical picture. The broad distinction in viscerotropic and dermatotropic species described above is even less valid in co-infection. Visceralizing disease has been reported for *L. major*, *L. mexicana* and *L. braziliensis* in HIV-co-infected patients. Atypical presentations are most frequent in patients with low CD4 counts. They include cutaneous, mucosal, digestive or pulmonary disease with parasites present in lung, pleura, oesophagus, stomach, duodenum, jejunum, colon, rectum and skin.[9] In visceral disease HIV-infected patients have a lower frequency of splenomegaly than HIV-negative individuals and a greater frequency and degree of leukopenia, lymphocytopenia, and thrombocytopenia. Almost all co-infected patients relapse after VL treatment.[68]

Diagnosis

The demonstration of parasites in tissue samples from bone marrow, spleen and lymph nodes (for VL); from mucocutaneous lesions (MCL); or skin lesions (PKDL and CL) establishes the diagnosis of leishmaniasis. This method requires invasive sampling and a skilled laboratory technician, and generally lacks sensitivity, except for spleen aspiration in VL. Sensitivity can be increased by inoculating biphasic media, such as Novy-Nicolle-McNeal, or by inoculating laboratory animals. In practice, in low-resource settings, diagnostic options are often limited. Each of the clinical syndromes poses its own diagnostic challenges as explained below.

VISCERAL LEISHMANIASIS

Clinical presentation combined with epidemiological context and nonspecific biological parameters lead to a suspicion of VL, but confirmation of the diagnosis by parasitological or serological methods is essential before deciding to treat. WHO has established a clinical case definition that is a useful starting point for a diagnostic algorithm: in an endemic area, any case with fever of more than 2 weeks, splenomegaly and/or weight loss is suspected of having VL and should be further investigated.[69]

Demonstration of Parasites

Visualization of the amastigote form of the parasite by microscopic examination of aspirates from lymph nodes, bone marrow or spleen is the classical confirmatory test for VL. In spite of their invasiveness, the aspiration of bone marrow from the sternum or the iliac crest and spleen aspiration are the most commonly used techniques. Lymph node aspiration is safe and simple but is only relevant in regions where lymphadenopathy is a frequent sign in VL patients as in Sudan. Collected material is smeared onto a microscope slide and stained with a Romanowsky-type stain, such as Giemsa, Wright's, or May Grünwald-Giemsa stain. Amastigotes – though usually inside mononuclear phagocytes – are frequently seen extracellularly in smears. The nucleus and kinetoplast characteristically stain purple and their clear demonstration confirms suspected objects as *Leishmania* parasites. They are not seen in any of the other causes of small 2–6 µm intra-leukocytic oval bodies with which *Leishmania* amastigotes may be confused, including *Histoplasma capsulatum*, *Penicillium marneffei* and, occasionally, granules in normal immature leukocytes in the bone marrow. The specificity of direct smear microscopy is high, but the sensitivity varies, being higher for spleen (93–99%) than for bone marrow (53–86%) or lymph node (53–65%) aspirates.[70] The accuracy of microscopic examination is influenced by the parasite load, by the skills of the laboratory technician and the quality of the reagents. Spleen aspiration is complicated by life-threatening haemorrhage in ~0.1% of procedures and therefore requires strict precautions and considerable technical expertise, as well as facilities for nursing surveillance, blood transfusion and surgery.[71]

The sensitivity of parasite detection techniques can be increased by culture or by using molecular techniques such as PCR (see below). Culture allows for parasite species identification and drug sensitivity testing, by isoenzyme electrophoresis, monoclonal antibodies or specific probe hybridization. Guidelines for *Leishmania* culture can be found in Evans et al.[72] *Leishmania* cultures are incubated at 24–26°C. The parasite develops a mobile promastigote stage and grows slowly with a doubling time of about 48–72 hours. Animal inoculation into the golden hamster, one of the most susceptible laboratory animals, is an alternative to in vitro cultivation but is not really practical for clinical diagnosis. In general, in low-resource settings a good quality parasitological diagnosis is often not available at primary care level.

Immunological Diagnosis

Several *host antibody-detection* tests have been developed for VL and have been evaluated in different endemic settings with variable results. Tests based on indirect fluorescence antibody testing (IFAT), enzyme-linked immunosorbent assay (ELISA), counter-current immuno-electrophoresis, indirect haemagglutination, and immunoblot techniques have shown good to high diagnostic accuracy in most studies but are poorly adapted to field settings.[73–75] Few techniques are relatively easy to use in field conditions: direct agglutination test (DAT), rK39 immunochromatographic test (rK39 ICT), dot-ELISA and the Fast Agglutination Screening Test (FAST).

The first antibody detection test for VL that could be used in field settings was the DAT, a semi-quantitative test that uses relatively little equipment. Increasing dilutions of patient's serum or blood are mixed with stained killed *L. donovani* promastigotes on microtitre plates.[76] If specific antibodies are present, agglutination is visible after 18 hours with the naked eye. It has been widely used, more recently in a lyophilized format.[77] As the DAT requires multiple pipetting and has a relatively long turn-around time (24 h) it is not very user-friendly. The rK39 ICT detects antibodies against rK39, a 39-amino-acid repeat that is part of a kinesin-related protein in *L. chagasi* and conserved in the *L. donovani* complex. The DAT as well as the rK39 ICT were found to have high sensitivity and specificity in a meta-analysis[78] and were recommended for clinical practice. Many rK39 ICTs are easy to perform, rapid (10–20 min), cheap, give reproducible results, and can therefore be used for early diagnosis in peripheral health centres. They improve patients' access to care in poor rural areas where most VL patients live.

All serological tests suffer from two limitations. First, specific antibodies remain detectable up to several years after cure.[79]

Therefore, a relapse episode of VL cannot be diagnosed by serology. Second, a significant proportion of healthy individuals living in endemic areas with no history of VL are positive for anti-leishmanial antibodies owing to asymptomatic infections. Antibody-based tests must therefore always be used in combination with a standardized clinical case definition for VL diagnosis. Other drawbacks include the lower sensitivity of antibody detection techniques in HIV-coinfection, and in the case of rK39, a lower sensitivity in East-Africa and Brazil compared to the Indian subcontinent.

The Leishmanin skin test (LST) or Montenegro test measures the delayed-type hypersensitivity reaction by the injection of *Leishmania* antigen (Leishmanin) intradermally into the forearm. After 48–72 hours, the induration is measured; an induration of at least 5 mm is considered positive. The LST is typically negative in active VL because of the anergic state of the patients. After successful treatment it will turn positive in 80% of VL patients after 6 months. The LST has little diagnostic value in active VL but it may be useful for epidemiological studies as it reveals a state of asymptomatic infection. There are some supply issues; LST is not commercially available and is produced by several research institutes. Its production requires culture and fixation of – preferably – a local species of *Leishmania* and therefore lacks standardization.

Detection of Parasite Products

In theory, antigen detection tests that mirror disease activity should be more specific than antibody-detection tests and can potentially distinguish active from past infections. A latex agglutination test detecting a heat-stable, low-molecular-weight carbohydrate antigen in the urine of VL patients showed good specificity but only low to moderate sensitivity in East Africa and the Indian subcontinent (40–80%).[80] In HIV/*Leishmania* co-infected persons sensitivity seems more adequate, due to their higher parasitaemia. This urine-based latex agglutination test detects only active patients and turns negative after a successful treatment response. It was therefore used with some success as a prognostic marker in HIV/*Leishmania* co-infected persons. Unfortunately, the current test format employs boiled urine and interpretation is quite subjective. Further work is needed to improve its sensitivity, reproducibility and feasibility.

Quantitative and Qualitative Detection of Parasite DNA

PCR can be performed on a wide range of clinical samples such as tissue aspirates, blood, urine and even buccal swabs. The clinical benefit of PCR in the diagnosis of VL is not yet fully demonstrated – with the notable exception of HIV/*Leishmania* co-infection (see below). PCR is probably the most sensitive and specific test for *Leishmania* infection today and its ability to determine the species is an important advantage over other techniques. Nonetheless, in endemic areas PCR positivity alone cannot be taken as a proof of active VL disease because a substantial proportion of asymptomatic healthy individuals will test PCR positive.[81] In one study, 58% of 81 healthy individuals from around Marseilles, France were found positive for *L. infantum* with real-time quantitative PCR.[82] PCR results should therefore always be interpreted in conjunction with the clinical and biological data. Recent advances in real-time quantitative PCR hold promise for the use of this technique as a way to discriminate asymptomatic from symptomatic infection[82] and to monitor clinical progression under treatment.[83]

Various DNA targets for amplification have been identified – with a notable lack of standardization.[84] The cost of reagents as well as the technology needed for DNA extraction and/or amplicon detection limit the use of PCR for routine VL diagnosis to well-equipped laboratories.

CUTANEOUS LEISHMANIASIS

The clinical spectrum of CL is broad and the differential diagnosis includes a variety of other skin conditions such as leprosy, staphylococcal or streptococcal infections, mycobacterial ulcers, sporotrichosis and other mycoses, cancer, sarcoidosis and tropical ulcer. As the clinical presentation of CL lacks specificity and treatment is costly, cumbersome and/or toxic, diagnostic confirmation is required.

Demonstration of Parasites

Parasitological diagnosis remains the reference standard in CL diagnosis, because of its high specificity. Material for parasitological diagnosis can be obtained by scraping, fine-needle aspiration or biopsy of lesions. Scraping is performed at the bottom and edges of the ulceration by means of a scalpel with a curved blade. The scraping material should be sufficiently abundant to cover at least half the slide. Using local anaesthetic considerably reduces the discomfort of the procedure for the patient. Bloodless scraping, which facilitates microscopic examination, can be obtained by using a local anaesthetic that contains 1–2% adrenaline (epinephrine) (generally contraindicated for lesions on extremities, genitals and cartilaginous structures) or by pinching the lesion between thumb and finger (until blanching). The 2–4 mm skin biopsy obtained by punch provides more abundant material (an advantage when parasites are scarce) and facilitates the search for alternative diagnoses by culture (e.g. mycobacteria, fungi) and histopathological examination. Moreover, impression smears from the biopsy can be done, stained and examined. The material obtained by any of these methods can be used for microscopic examination, culture and molecular diagnostic techniques. Microscopic examination of Giemsa-stained material is often the only available method at primary, secondary or tertiary healthcare level in endemic areas. Culture of the parasite on simple media (e.g. Novy-Nicolle-McNeal medium) allows for species identification and characterization. The detection of parasite nucleic acids by molecular diagnosis, essentially by PCR-based methods, improves the diagnostic sensitivity and allows for identification of the *Leishmania* species.[85–87] This is particularly useful in regions where several *Leishmania* species – with various clinical outcomes and responses to treatment – co-exist. Both culture and molecular-based diagnosis require substantial laboratory infrastructure and a wealth of technical expertise, limiting their use to reference laboratories.

Immunological Diagnosis

CL caused by *L. major* or *L. tropica* does not usually lead to a detectable antibody response. The LST evaluating the cell-mediated response against *Leishmania* spp. usually is positive and may remain so for life. For this reason, the LST fails to distinguish between past and present infections.

MUCOCUTANEOUS LEISHMANIASIS

The diagnosis of MCL should be suspected in patients with typical mucosal lesions and a history of CL with one or more visible scar(s), or more rarely with concomitant CL. Other diseases such as allergic rhinitis, paracoccidioidomycosis or other deep mycoses, cancrum oris, leprosy and sarcoidosis may mimic early or advanced MCL. Confirmation of the diagnosis is difficult, as it is more difficult to obtain samples than in CL. The lesions bleed on contact and anaesthesia is difficult to administer. Furthermore, parasites are scarce in mucosal lesions because of the strong local immune reaction. Therefore, the search for parasites in mucosal samples – obtained by scraping or biopsy – by microscopic examination or by culture has low sensitivity. Positive serology (e.g. IFAT, ELISA) or LST increase the clinical suspicion. The demonstration of parasites' nucleic acids by PCR has proved to be a more sensitive tool.

POST-KALA-AZAR DERMAL LEISHMANIASIS (PKDL)

In the endemic areas of South Asia or East Africa, diagnosis of PKDL is mainly clinical and based on typical skin lesions in persons reporting a previous kala-azar episode. Diagnosis may be more difficult when it occurs in patients without previous history of VL. The diagnosis can be confirmed by finding parasites in skin lesion samples obtained by biopsy or scraping of skin slit, but the sensitivity of these techniques is rather low (20–40%). *Leishmania* amastigotes are more frequently observed in nodular lesions. More sensitive techniques – immunohistochemistry, culture and PCR – can be performed in well-equipped laboratories. Serological tests are of limited value as persons with a past episode of VL will test positive in antibody detection tests for many months and years. Such tests can be helpful though when the previous history of VL is uncertain. Histopathology sections of the dermis show various patterns. The dermis is infiltrated by lymphocytes and macrophages but plasma cells are scanty or absent. The main differential diagnosis of PKDL is leprosy.

HIV/*LEISHMANIA* CO-INFECTION

The diagnosis is essentially parasitological as HIV co-infected VL patients have few circulating antibodies. While clinical manifestations in HIV-infected VL patients without severe immunosuppression are similar to those in immunocompetent patients, atypical clinical features can be found in patients with a low CD4 T-cell count (<200/mL). In the latter group, physicians may order investigations for VL even in the absence of classical signs (e.g. in people without splenomegaly). A substantial proportion of HIV-VL patients may present with other opportunistic infections that complicate the clinical diagnosis. The parasite load is high and parasites may be found in unusual sites, especially in severely immunosuppressed patients. Therefore, the sensitivity of microscopic examination, culture or PCR in blood (plain blood or buffy coat) or blood marrow aspirates is higher than in immunocompetent VL patients. *Leishmania* parasites can occasionally be found in biopsies from the skin, gastrointestinal tract or lungs. Limited data also showed high sensitivity of the latex agglutination test in the urine of HIV co-infected VL patients. In contrast, the sensitivity of serological tests is decreased in co-infected patients, but study results are equivocal and depend on several factors such as test format, geographical region and level of immunosuppression. Increased sensitivity can be obtained by using a sequential combination of different serological tests, e.g. rK39 ICT followed by DAT as suggested in Ethiopia.[88]

Management and Treatment

Management of leishmaniasis is complex and depends upon the clinical syndrome and the causative organism. There are only a few anti-leishmanial drugs and their efficacy varies according to the species and region of infection. *L. donovani* for example, does not respond to drugs in the same way in the Indian subcontinent and in East Africa. Some patients relapse within 6 months to 1 year irrespective of the regimen used. Particularly in HIV-co-infected individuals, relapse is very common. In recent years, intensified research efforts have led to significant changes in the therapeutic approach to VL. We first give an overview of anti-leishmanial drugs and then discuss the specific management of the three clinical syndromes.

PRODUCTS AND DEVICES

Pentavalent Antimonials

The first to report the use of trivalent antimonials (also known as tartar emetic) for the treatment of MCL was Vianna in 1912. Later Cristina and di Cariona used it against VL in Sicily as did Rogers in India in 1915.[89] In the Assam epidemics, tartar emetic was used with great success but the adverse effects were severe. The development of less toxic pentavalent antimonials by Brahmachari in 1920 subsequently led to the synthesis of sodium stibogluconate (SSG) in 1945.

Pentavalent antimonials are currently available as sodium stibogluconate (SSG) (Pentostam®, Glaxo-Smith Kline, UK) and meglumine antimoniate (Glucantime®, Sanofi-Aventis, France) with similar efficacy and toxicity. The products differ by the strength of the Sb^V solution: meglumine antimoniate solution contains 8.1% of Sb^v (81 mg Sb^V/mL) and sodium stibogluconate contains 10% Sb^v (100 mg Sb^V/mL). The effectiveness of a generic form of SSG (Albert David, India) was equivalent to the branded product.[90–92]

Antimonials act by their toxic effect on the parasite after reduction of Sb^V to Sb^{III} but also indirectly by restoring the host cell's defence mechanisms.[93] Sb^{III} profoundly disturbs the parasite's unique thiol redox metabolism by increasing thiol efflux and inhibiting trypanothione reductase. The indirect effect explains why antimonials fail to adequately cure patients without an intact T-cell-dependent immune response (such as patients with AIDS). Antimonials have poor oral absorption and are therefore administered by the parenteral route. They are rapidly excreted by the kidneys.

The current WHO recommendation on antimonial use in VL (in areas with no resistance) is to administer a dose corresponding to Sb^V 20 mg/kg per day for 30 days through the intramuscular (IM) or intravenous (IV) route – either by slow infusion (over 5–10 min) or by slow injection with a fine needle. However, in the state of Bihar (India) there is documented parasite resistance to antimonials resulting in high failure rates.[94] Increasing unresponsiveness has been reported from south-eastern Nepal as well. Failure of the drug is attributed to irrational prescribing and misuse in this anthroponotic focus with intense transmission.[95] In other parts of the world, antimonials continue to be effective. The recommended dosage for systemic antimonial treatment in CL and MCL is 20 and 30 days respectively at 20 mg/kg per day.[1,96]

Intralesional treatment of meglumine antimoniate is widely used in CL but has only been validated for *L. tropica*. The technique requires the skills of a specialized medical professional. Doses of 0.5–5 mL per session are injected into the base and margins of the lesion to produce complete blanching. Injections are given daily, every other day or weekly for up to 8 infiltrations or until healing of the lesion. A major drawback of the procedure is that it is rather painful and causes too much discomfort to be used in small children. Adding anaesthesia in the syringe is of no use as the added volume increases the pain. The combination of local infiltration of antimonials with cryotherapy was superior to each treatment alone.[97]

Antimonials are rather toxic drugs and systemic treatment leads to frequent side-effects such as anorexia, vomiting, nausea, abdominal pain, a metallic taste in the mouth, arthralgia, myalgia, acute pancreatitis especially in HIV-co-infected patients, hepatitis and cardiac arrhythmias. Prolongation of a corrected Q-T interval (>0.5 s) in an electrocardiogram is an ominous sign and can culminate into ventricular arrhythmias and death. Patients <2 or >45 years with signs of advanced VL and/or severe malnutrition are at higher risk of death during antimonial therapy.[22,98] Patients should be closely monitored through serum chemistry, complete blood counts and electrocardiography. The quality of the drug should be strictly assured as the literature describes that substandard drugs may cause fatal cardiotoxicity.[99,100]

Amphotericin B Deoxycholate

Amphotericin B is a polyene antibiotic with antifungal and anti-leishmanial activity. Amphotericin B binds irreversibly to ergosterols in the membrane of the *Leishmania* parasite causing pores that leak ions and subsequent cell death.[101]

Amphotericin B deoxycholate is formulated as a colloidal suspension (Fungizone®, Bristol Myers Squibb), which is administered as a slow (6–8 h) IV infusion in a dose of 0.5–1 mg/kg for 15–20 infusions either daily or on alternate days. It has consistently shown very high cure rates in VL (approximately 97%). A major limiting factor is the almost universal occurrence of infusion reactions like high fever with rigor and chills, and thrombophlebitis. Severe adverse events may also occur and include myocarditis, severe hypokalaemia, renal dysfunction and even death. Therefore, it requires prolonged hospitalization, proper hydration, potassium supplementation and close monitoring, thus precluding its use in most peripheral health facilities.

Lipid Formulations of Amphotericin B

The incorporation of amphotericin B into phospholipid vesicles (liposomes) and/or cholesterol esters facilitates the uptake of the drug by the macrophages. This targeted drug delivery system leads to a better therapeutic index. Three lipid formulations of amphotericin B are commercially available: amphotericin B lipid complex (Abelcet®; ENZON Pharmaceuticals Inc.); amphotericin B cholesteryl sulfate complex, also called amphotericin B colloidal dispersion (Amphocil; Sequus Pharmaceuticals); and liposomal amphotericin B (L-Amb) (AmBisome®; Gilead Sciences). The latter is the form evaluated in most clinical trials for leishmaniasis and is registered in the USA and Europe for this indication.

Liposomal amphotericin B is administered as an intravenous infusion over 2 hours. Mild infusion reactions (fever, chills, and rigor) and back pain occur in some patients; transient nephrotoxicity or thrombocytopenia is occasionally seen.

The efficacy of L-Amb against VL varies according to region and species. In Europe a total dose of 18–21 mg L-Amb cures almost every immunocompetent patient.[102] Experience in Africa is not so extensive. The excellent safety profile of the drug allowed for trials of shorter regimens at a higher dose. In a phase III trial in India, a single dose of 10 mg/kg cured 95.7% of VL patients. Similarly in Europe, two doses of 10 mg/kg cured 97.5% of immunocompetent children.

Until recently, the high cost of L-AmB precluded its use in resource-poor settings. However, in 2007, WHO successfully negotiated a preferential pricing scheme with the company for its use in VL in developing countries and more recently a donation scheme has been announced. This opens up the prospect for using L-AmB in countries where it was hitherto unaffordable.[103]

Miltefosine

Miltefosine and other alkyl phospholipids such as ilmofosine and edelfosine were originally registered for the treatment of metastasis of mammary carcinomas but were abandoned due to severe gastrointestinal toxicity.[104] Miltefosine was later developed as the first orally effective anti-leishmanial agent[105] and registered to treat VL in adults and children in India, Nepal and Bangladesh. In a phase IV trial, the final cure rate was 82% by intention-to-treat and 95% by per-protocol analysis, with only three deaths out of 1132 patients.[106] Data on miltefosine use in East Africa are restricted to one study conducted in northern Ethiopia, where it was found to be as safe and effective as sodium stibogluconate among HIV-negative patients and safer, but less effective, among HIV-co-infected patients.[107] Recommended doses are 50 mg daily for 28 days for adults weighing <25 kg, and 100 mg daily for 28 days for those who weigh >25 kg. For children below 12 years, the dose is 2.5 mg/kg per day for 28 days. It should always be taken after meals and in divided doses, if multiple capsules are prescribed. Oral miltefosine has also been evaluated in CL and MCL. Its efficacy was low in Iran in *L. major* lesions, though it induced healing in a small cohort (without control group) of Dutch soldiers returning from Afghanistan.[108] The effectiveness of miltefosine in CL due to *L. braziliensis* varies from country to country.[109–111] With 4 or 6 weeks of miltefosine in MCL, about 70% of patients were cured.[112]

Adverse effects include mild to moderate vomiting in 40% and diarrhoea in 20% of patients. More severe adverse events including hepatotoxicity and renal insufficiency occur in up to 1.5% of patients.[113] As miltefosine is teratogenic, it is contraindicated in pregnancy. Women of child-bearing age should strictly observe contraception for the duration of therapy and a further 3 months because of its long half-life. The long half-life (around 150 h) explains also that parasite resistance can easily be induced in vitro.[114] Because of this risk of drug resistance, adherence to treatment is very important. Unfortunately, the long duration of the regimen and the many adverse events are not facilitating good compliance.

Paromomycin

Paromomycin (formerly known as aminosidine) is a wide-spectrum antibiotic belonging to the class of aminoglycosides. It is effective against *Leishmania, Entamoeba* and *Cryptosporidium*. After its anti-leishmanial activity was discovered in the 1960s, its clinical development remained erratic. Its efficacy in VL was demonstrated in several phase II studies in India and Africa[115,116] but the manufacturers stopped to invest in the further development of the drug. Eventually, in 2006, a phase III trial in India led to the first registration of paromomycin for VL[106] in a dose of 11 mg/kg base IM for 21 days (*Note*: paromomycin base 11 mg is approximately equivalent to paromomycin sulfate 15 mg). It is today included in the essential drug lists of WHO, India, Nepal and Bangladesh and is produced by Gland Pharma Ltd., Hyderabad, India. Paromomycin is the cheapest anti-leishmanial compound available today: a treatment course for an adult costs about US$15. There is no significant nephrotoxicity or ototoxicity, but in 6% of the patients, hepatic enzymes became elevated.[106]

In Africa, the efficacy of paromomycin for VL was unsatisfactory; this treatment should not be used as monotherapy.[117,118] A combination regimen of paromomycin with antimonials for 17 days was superior to SSG alone and safer (see below).

Several topical formulations of paromomycin have been developed for the treatment of CL with variable results. A meta-analysis of 14 trials concluded that paromomycin ointment is effective when it is combined with methylbenzethonium chloride (PM 15%/MBC 12% applied twice daily for up to 20 days) and could be a therapeutic option in selected cases of Old World CL.[119] The topical aminoside ointment (paromomycin and gentamycin) developed by the Walter Reed Institute was superior to placebo in a randomized controlled trial.[120]

Sitamaquine

Sitamaquine, an orally active 8-aminoquinoline analogue, was effective in animal models[121] and in phase II clinical studies in Brazil,[122] Kenya[123] and India,[124] but is nephrotoxic. Because the therapeutic index was too small, its clinical development has now been stopped.

Pentamidine

Pentamidine, an aromatic diamidine, was previously used as a second-line treatment of antimonial-resistant VL in India. At present, it is only available as the isethionate salt for human use (Pentacarinat®, Sanofi-Aventis). Pentamidine may cause severe side effects such as insulin-dependent diabetes mellitus, hypoglycaemia and unexplained shock. Moreover, its efficacy for VL in India has progressively declined to cure rates of approximately 70%. Therefore, it is not used anymore for VL. In CL due to *L. guyanensis* and *L. panamensis* in the Northern Amazon basin, short courses of pentamidine (four doses of 4 mg/kg IM or slow IV injections on alternate days) are used under strict precautions.[125]

Other Drugs

IFN-γ alone or in combination with antimonials has been tested in clinical trials with contradicting results and is no longer used in the treatment of leishmaniasis.

Ketoconazole, itraconazole and fluconazole have been used in CL in different parts of the world with varying response.

Combination Therapy for VL

Combination therapy for VL has been advocated for several reasons: (1) it could delay the emergence of resistance if drugs with different modes of action and mechanisms of resistance are used;[126] (2) it could reduce treatment duration and cost and (3) it could enhance treatment efficacy especially in complicated cases such as the HIV-co-infected. Several combinations are in clinical development in the Indian subcontinent and in East Africa. In a phase II clinical trial in India, a single dose of L-AmB (3.75–5.0 mg/kg) followed by miltefosine for 7–14 days produced a high cure rate of >95%.[127] In a recent randomized controlled phase III trial in India, three combination regimens were compared with conventional amphotericin B treatment: (a) a single injection of 5 mg/kg liposomal amphotericin B on day 1 followed by 7 days of 50 mg oral miltefosine or by (b) 10-days of 11 mg/kg IM paromomycin; and (c) co-administration of miltefosine and paromomycin for 10 days. The efficacy of the three combination regimens was similarly high with cure rates above 97%.[128] In Sudan, a trial of the co-administration of 11 mg/kg paromomycin base IM with 20 mg/kg SSG IM for 17 days showed a high efficacy.[129]

Devices for Local CL Treatment

Thermotherapy. Dermatotropic species such as *L. major, L. tropica*, and *L. mexicana* are thermosensitive: amastigote replication is inhibited at higher temperatures. Topical heat therapy with an FDA-approved device (Thermomed, Thermosurgery Technologies, Inc, Phoenix AZ, USA) was effective in controlled trials of CL caused by *L. tropica* in Afghanistan[130] and by *L. major* in Iraq.[131] One or two applications of localized heat (50°C for 30 seconds) are applied to the lesion under local anaesthesia. The drawback of the method is that it causes a 2nd-degree burn with initial increase in lesion size and blistering, oozing and erythema. The device is expensive but portable and battery-operated which are advantages when used in the field.

Cryotherapy. Cryotherapy is performed by repeated topical applications of liquid nitrogen preferably with a spray device (and not a cotton swab) to obtain a bleaching of about ten seconds, up to 2 mm outside the lesion margin. The procedure is repeated weekly for up to 6 weeks. If it is applied too deeply it can lead to permanent hypopigmentation. Cryotherapy was more than 95% effective in Egypt, Israel and Jordan, but less effective than intralesional antimonials in Turkey.

TREATMENT

Visceral Leishmaniasis

For the past 70 years, VL therapy was based on pentavalent antimonials, with amphotericin B and pentamidine as second-line drugs. The past decade has brought the approval of miltefosine, paromomycin, and liposomal amphotericin B. These drugs largely increase the therapeutic options, but their efficacy varies geographically and not all products have been evaluated to the same degree in every region. In 2010 WHO issued specific, evidence-based recommendations for every geographic region (Box 47.1). The best therapeutic option seems to be a regimen based on liposomal amphotericin B[102] or a combination regimen. In case of non-response, the best rescue treatments are

BOX 47.1 RECOMMENDED TREATMENT REGIMENS FOR VISCERAL LEISHMANIASIS, RANKED BY PREFERENCE

ANTHROPONOTIC VISCERAL LEISHMANIASIS CAUSED BY *L. DONOVANI* IN BANGLADESH, BHUTAN, INDIA AND NEPAL

1. Liposomal amphotericin B: 3–5 mg/kg per daily dose by infusion given over 3-5-day period up to a total dose of 15 mg/kg (A) by infusion or 10 mg/kg as a single dose by infusion (A).
2. Combinations (co-administered) (A)
   - liposomal amphotericin B (5 mg/kg by infusion, single dose) plus miltefosine (daily for 7 days, as below)
   - liposomal amphotericin B (5 mg/kg by infusion, single dose) plus paromomycin (daily for 10 days, as below)
   - miltefosine plus paromomycin, both daily for 10 days, as below.
3. Amphotericin B deoxycholate: 0.75–1.0 mg/kg per day by infusion, daily or on alternate days for 15–20 doses (A).
4. Miltefosine: for children aged 2–11 years, 2.5 mg/kg per day; for people aged ≥12 years and <25 kg body weight, 50 mg/day; 25–50 kg body weight, 100 mg/day; >50 kg body weight, 150 mg/day; orally for 28 days (A).
   or Paromomycin: 15 mg (11 mg base) per kg body weight per day intramuscularly for 21 days (A).
5. Pentavalent antimonials: 20 mg Sb5+/kg per day intramuscularly or intravenously for 30 days in areas where they remain effective: Bangladesh, Nepal and the Indian states of Jharkhand, West Bengal and Uttar Pradesh (A).

VISCERAL LEISHMANIASIS CAUSED BY *L. DONOVANI* IN EAST AFRICA (ETHIOPIA, ERITREA, KENYA, SOMALIA, SUDAN AND UGANDA) AND YEMEN

1. Combination: pentavalent antimonials (20 mg Sb5+/kg per day intramuscularly or intravenously) plus paromomycin (15 mg [11 mg base] per kg body weight per day intramuscularly) for 17 days (A).
2. Pentavalent antimonials: 20 mg Sb5+/kg per day intramuscularly or intravenously for 30 days (A).
3. Liposomal amphotericin B: 3–5 mg/kg per daily dose by infusion given over 6–10 days up to a total dose of 30 mg/kg (B).
4. Amphotericin B deoxycholate: 0.75–1 mg/kg per day by infusion, daily or on alternate days, for 15–20 doses (A).
5. Miltefosine orally for 28 days at dosage as above (A).

VISCERAL LEISHMANIASIS CAUSED BY *L. INFANTUM*: MEDITERRANEAN BASIN, MIDDLE EAST, CENTRAL ASIA, SOUTH AMERICA

1. Liposomal amphotericin B: 3–5 mg/kg per daily dose by infusion given over a 3–6 days period, up to a total dose of 18–21 mg/kg (B).
2. Pentavalent antimonials: 20 mg Sb5+/kg per day intramuscularly or intravenously for 28 days (B).
3. Amphotericin B deoxycholate: 0.75–1.0 mg/kg per day by infusion, daily or on alternate days for 20–30 doses, for a total dose of 2–3 g (C).

Source: WHO Technical Report Series 949. Control of the leishmaniasis. WHO, Geneva, 2010.[1] Regimens are ranked based on a review of the evidence with (A) at least one randomized controlled trial, (B) trials without randomization, (C) expert committees and (D) expert opinion without conclusive studies.

conventional amphotericin B deoxycholate infusions or liposomal amphotericin B at higher doses.

Many VL patients are very ill when they are diagnosed, especially in East Africa. Dehydration, renal or hepatic dysfunction, anaemia and consequent cardiac decompensation, hypoproteinaemia with ascites and oedema, and concurrent infections are seen as complications of VL. Supportive treatment is important and all patients should be properly hydrated and given nutritional supplements. Many may need a blood transfusion and treatment of concomitant infections such as tuberculosis, pneumonia and diarrhoea. Patients responding to treatment become afebrile in 4–5 days; and the other clinical symptoms and biological parameters slowly normalize. Complete regression of splenomegaly may take several months. Circulating antibodies will persist for a long time (usually 6–8 months) and are not useful to monitor prognosis. An initial cure can be declared if there is clinical improvement at the end of treatment. If the patient is clinically well 6 months after treatment, this can be taken as an indicator of definite cure.

Cutaneous Leishmaniasis

Treatment of localized CL depends on the type and extent of the lesion(s), the species as well as the geographical region. Three options exist: no, local or general treatment, but clinical evidence is limited and choice should always be based on the individual risk/benefit ratio for the patient. As bacterial superinfections are common it is important to apply wound cleaning and dressing.

Old World CL. Mild, rapidly healing forms of CL due to *L. major* can remain untreated if the patient wishes, as many lesions will have spontaneously healed at 6 months.[132,133] Local wound care and careful clinical follow-up may thus suffice in a majority of immunocompetent patients with small (<5 cm) and few (<4) lesions, and if their location is not potentially disfiguring or disabling (i.e. on face, hands, feet, joints).

For more severe *L. major* lesions as well as for CL due to *L. tropica*, local treatment is recommended. The options are local infiltration with antimonials, topical paromomycin treatment, topical heat – and cryotherapy or combinations of these (see above). Systemic treatment with antimonials was often used in the past but is now discouraged because of its relative toxicity and as there is no convincing evidence of its clinical benefit compared to topical treatment.[134] A placebo-controlled trial on the efficacy of systemic meglumine antimoniate in CL due to *L. major* in Algerian children failed to show an effect.[132] In Afghanistan, (*L. tropica*) cure rates were significantly higher in patients treated with intralesional antimony than in those treated with systemic antimony.[130]

Little data support the use of oral drugs (azoles or miltefosine).[134,135] Oral fluconazole was more efficient than placebo in Saudi Arabia (*L. major*[136] but was inconstantly effective in a cohort of French travellers (*L. major* MON-25, and *L. infantum*).[133] Itraconazole was more effective than placebo in one small Indian trial (*L. tropica*),[134] but not in Iran (*L. major*).[137–139] In conclusion, systemic treatment in Old World CL should only be used if local therapy has failed or in severe cases (more than four lesions, lesions in the face or other complex lesions).

New World CL. New World CL tends to be more severe and to last longer than Old World CL. Self-healing is less common and as there is a risk of evolution to MCL specific treatment is recommended. Unfortunately the evidence base is not yet very large except for *L. braziliensis*, and therefore the risk/benefit ratio has to be evaluated in every individual patient. There is only very limited experience with local treatment.

Thermotherapy was effective in Colombia and Guatemala. Topical paromomycin was effective against CL caused by *L. mexicana*, *L. panamensis* and *L. braziliensis*. Systemic treatment with antimonials is the treatment of choice for all species except for *L. guyanensis*. More than ten randomized trials have confirmed their efficacy. The usual dose is 20 mg/kg for 20 days, and as opposed to VL, the drug is quite safe in patients with CL, though minor side-effects might occur.

Pentamidine isethionate is the drug of choice for *L. guyanensis* infections in French Guyana and Surinam and as second-line drug for *L. panamensis* infection in doses of 2 mg/kg IM/IV infusion, on alternate days to a total of seven injections (see above). For New World CL, ketoconazole 600 mg daily for 4 weeks demonstrated comparable efficacy to a course of sodium stibogluconate in the treatment of *L. panamensis* infection (76% cure rate for ketoconazole versus 68% for sodium stibogluconate)[140] and also showed efficacy against *L. mexicana*, but not against *L. braziliensis* in Guatemala.[141] In contrast, little evidence supports the use of itraconazole to treat New World CL.[142]

Diffuse Cutaneous Leishmaniasis

Once established, DCL is resistant to treatment. Systemic pentavalent antimonials can improve the clinical evolution temporarily. Pentamidine showed some efficacy but with high doses close to toxicity. A combination of paromomycin and antimonials gave good results in two Ethiopian patients. There is an urgent need for new treatment regimens for DCL, although the low number of patients will not facilitate their evaluation.

Mucocutaneous Leishmaniasis

Treatment of mucosal lesions should be as early as possible to avoid extension. MCL treatment outcome depends on the location of the lesions. High cure rates are observed if these are limited to the nose and mouth. Evaluation of the treatment response is based on clinical criteria and follow-up visits are needed every 6 months at least up to 1 year after treatment. Reported cure rates with systemic antimonials range from 30% to 90%. The currently recommended dosage is 20 mg Sb^{v}/kg per day for 30 days. A combination with oral pentoxifylline was more effective than antimonial monotherapy in a randomized trial. There is more limited evidence about the other options: amphotericin B deoxycholate and its lipid formulations, pentamidine and miltefosine.

Post-Kala-Azar Dermal Leishmaniasis (PKDL)

PKDL in the Indian subcontinent requires prolonged treatment. In the past, more than 4 months of SSG were given. More recently, good results were obtained in a small series of patients with 12 weeks of miltefosine[143] or amphotericin B deoxycholate (60 infusions over 3 months).[144] In East Africa by contrast, the majority of the patients heal spontaneously; only the most severe cases require treatment; and if so, 2 months of SSG is considered adequate.[61] More clinical evidence on PKDL treatment is urgently needed.

HIV/Leishmania Co-infection

Antiretroviral treatment has improved survival in HIV/*Leishmania* co-infection and prevents the development of clinical VL in asymptomatically co-infected patients. However, when clinical VL occurs in HIV-infected patients it does not respond well to the classical anti-leishmanial drugs, with incomplete cure and frequent relapses.[10] In immunocompromised patients, the side-effects of anti-leishmanial drugs are more frequent and severe than in immunocompetent patients, and a full-course of antimonials is generally considered too toxic for use in co-infected patients. L-Amb is the drug of choice and is given in a total dose of 40 mg/kg (4 mg/kg on days 1–5, 10, 17, 24, 31 and 38). In the treatment of relapse, miltefosine induced a (often transient) remission in 64% of patients.[145] An immune reconstitution syndrome can be observed in VL[10,146] and in CL.[147]

The high frequency of relapses is the most salient feature in the treatment of HIV/*Leishmania* co-infection. In a patient not on antiretroviral therapy, VL almost always relapses within one year, but this can be partially prevented with secondary prophylaxis regimens. Numerous schemes have been proposed: monthly injections of antimonial, twice-monthly injections of L-Amb,[148,149] or of pentamidine, daily allopurinol or itraconazole. All these protocols need to be validated. Secondary prophylaxis is usually withdrawn when the CD4 cell count has been maintained above 200 cells/mL for more than 6 months. In co-infected patients suffering multiple relapses, splenectomy can restore haematological parameters and reduce the need for blood transfusions, but it does not protect from relapses.[150]

Prevention and Control

Strategies for prevention and control of leishmaniasis face the very complex and diverse ecology of leishmaniasis transmission. Many different animals can act as reservoir hosts and a multiplicity of sandfly vectors have distinct behaviour patterns. In 2010, a WHO Expert Committee described no less than 12 distinct nosogeographical entities and defined control strategies for each of them. As there is currently no vaccine for human use, the ways to protect individuals from contracting the infection include avoiding intrusion in natural zoonotic foci and protecting oneself against sandfly bites with repellents and other devices. VL control aims at interrupting the transmission cycle of the parasite and eventually to eliminate the disease. Control strategies can target the vector, the animal reservoir in case of zoonotic disease, and/or the pool of infectious people by active case detection and treatment. Effective control of the disease often seems to hinge upon a combination of these methods.[151]

There are historical examples of effective leishmaniasis control programmes. Visceral leishmaniasis was one of the major parasitic diseases in China before the creation of the People's Republic in 1949. From the areas north of the Yangtze river, about 530 000 cases were reported in 1951.[152] Between 1950 and 1958, a nationwide control campaign (mass treatment of patients, killing of infected dogs, and use of insecticides) brought the disease under control in the plains where the anthroponotic form had reigned. Transmission could, however, not be stopped in the mountainous and desert region where sporadic cases of zoonotic transmission continue to be reported till today.[152]

Bihar in India also controlled a large anthroponotic VL epidemic in the 1970s through a combination of active case detection and treatment in the community and residual spraying in the houses.[153,154] Unfortunately, the epidemic came back in the mid-1980s. Recurring cycles with inter-epidemic periods of about 15 years are now observed. In 2005, the governments of

Bangladesh, Nepal and India signed a memorandum of understanding to eliminate VL by 2015. They aim to achieve an annual incidence of less than 1 per 10 000 at district level.

Control of zoonotic disease is usually not easy or even not feasible as, e.g. in the New World where almost all the leishmaniases are sylvatic. Even clearing forest may not reach the objective, as various *Leishmania* species have proved to be remarkably adaptable to environmental degradation. *L. braziliensis* survived the deforestation of eastern Brazil.

VACCINE

Today, no vaccine is available for use in humans but candidate vaccines are in development for VL and CL.[155] The fact that self-healing CL with *L. major* usually leads to benign lesions as well as lifelong protection from reinfection was known since ancient times. People in Asia and the Middle East inoculated exudate from active sores into the buttocks of children to spare them the development of disfiguring CL scars in the face. The first true vaccines containing live *L. major* promastigotes exploited the same principle. They were empirically used in the Central Asian republics of the former USSR, Israel and in Iran for more than 60 years.[156,157] 'Leishmanization' as the procedure was known is now discontinued mainly for safety reasons. Vaccines containing killed promastigotes mixed with BCG as adjuvant failed to protect against VL[158] or CL.[159] Second-generation vaccines, which consist of attenuated parasites, recombinant molecules or parasite DNA mixed together in a cocktail vaccine, and recombinant organisms carrying leishmanial genes are in development. Three vaccines are registered for use in dogs: two in Brazil and one in Europe. Their impact on the transmission to humans in zoonotic VL has not yet been firmly established.

SANDFLY CONTROL

Sandfly control methods include chemical control, environmental management and personal protection measures. To be effective, a vector control strategy should involve more than one method. These methods should be well adapted to the behaviour of a specific vector, because this behaviour differs widely between species. Without detailed knowledge of vector species, its habitat, resting sites, flight range, and seasonality, such a strategy is bound to fail.

Destruction of Breeding Sites

The breeding sites of only a few sandfly species are known: rodent burrows for *P. papatasi* and *P. duboscqi* are the best example. The destruction of these burrows, combined with both reservoir and vector elimination was an efficient control method in Central Asia.[160] Replacement of traditional mud or straw houses with plastered brick houses has also been adopted as a vector control strategy in Bihar, India.

Insecticide Spraying

Insecticide residual spraying (IRS) of houses and animal shelters is used in the Indian subcontinent where the vector (*P. argentipes*) is restricted to the intra- and peri-domiciliary area. The evidence on its effectiveness is largely circumstantial. Following the malaria eradication campaign in the 1950s that used large-scale insecticide spraying (DDT) VL almost completely disappeared from the Indian sub-continent. Unfortunately, VL re-emerged when spraying campaigns were discontinued. A community trial in India showed that after two rounds of DDT spraying in one village, no *P. argentipes* were found during the peak vector season; in contrast, a large number of these sandflies were collected in the unsprayed comparison village.[161]

Many classes of insecticide can be used in IRS including organochlorines (e.g. DDT), organophosphates (e.g. malathion), carbamates (e.g. propoxur) and synthetic pyrethroids (e.g. deltamethrin and lambda-cyhalothrin). Resistance to DDT has been reported from India. The choice of insecticide has to be strictly regulated at the national level and an insecticide rotation plan has to be developed as part of an integrated vector management policy.

IRS is pointless if the vector is not peri-domestic as in Sudan where transmission takes place mainly outside the villages in *Acacia* sp. and *Balanites aegyptiaca* woodlands,[162] and where activities such as wood cutting and shepherding expose people to sandflies.[163] Similarly, IRS alone may have a limited impact on zoonotic leishmaniasis. In Brazil IRS is used to control the *L. infantum* vector in combination with other strategies such as reservoir control (see below).[26]

Insecticide-treated Materials

Pyrethroid-impregnated bed nets and other treated materials have shown their efficacy in field trials for the prevention of CL.[164,165] There is limited evidence that insecticide-treated bed nets (ITNs) also provide protection against VL. Case–control studies conducted in Bangladesh and Nepal showed that sleeping under a (non-impregnated) bednet during the warm months was a protective factor against VL.[166,167] However, a large randomized controlled trial in Nepal and India testing the efficacy of long-lasting ITNs to prevent *L. donovani* infection and VL failed to show an additional protective effect in villages were large proportion of households used untreated nets.[168,169] Depending on sleeping traditions of the population and biting habits of the local vector, other insecticide-impregnated materials should be evaluated (e.g. curtains, blankets).[165] There is no strong evidence that using clothes treated with insecticide (e.g. soldiers' uniforms) protects individuals against sandfly bites and reduces the risk of leishmaniasis.

Repellents may be an alternative for personal protection against sandfly bites. However, as for insecticide-treated clothes there is limited evidence on their efficacy to prevent leishmaniasis. The use of repellents as a long-term public health intervention in endemic regions may be difficult as they require repeated applications (i.e. protection lasts for a maximum of 10 hours). Nevertheless, insect repellents may be the only option in regions where *Leishmania* transmission occurs outdoors. The efficacy of repellents combined with other vector control tools (i.e. ITNs) should be further explored.

RESERVOIR CONTROL

In zoonotic VL, the control of the animal reservoir remains a challenge.[170] Dogs are the main reservoir of *L. infantum* in zoonotic VL in the Mediterranean Basin and in South America. Despite some evidence from experimental studies showing a decreased incidence of VL in both dogs and children following serological screening of dogs and killing of seropositive animals,[171] the efficiency and acceptability of this strategy is increasingly debated[170] and has failed to control VL in Brazil. Culled dogs are quickly replaced by fully susceptible young pets and these maintain *Leishmania* transmission.

Test-and-treat strategies have been recommended without convincing evidence on their impact. Treating infected dogs may not be an effective control measure as relapses are frequent, and because despite clinical cure, dogs can recover infectivity weeks after treatment.[172] Deltamethrin-treated dog collars protect against *Leishmania* infection in dogs and when treated collars were applied to all dogs in endemic villages in Iran the risk of infection in children was also reduced.[173] Unfortunately, using dog collars is not very sustainable as a public health intervention as they need to be replaced every 6 months and dogs tend to lose them rapidly. In Europe, no particular measures are taken at veterinary public health level but insecticide-treated collars and spot-on insecticides are commonly used to protect individual dogs against sandfly bites in endemic areas. Ultimately the best strategy would be to vaccinate the dogs if its effectiveness to reduce transmission is demonstrated.

If the reservoirs are peri-domestic species such as the fat sand jird, reservoir of *L. major* in North Africa, their elimination (i.e. using rodenticides or destruction of borrows) could be an effective control measure. However when the *Leishmania* cycle is maintained by sylvatic reservoirs (i.e. the climbing rat for *L. mexicana*) there are no effective methods to control them.

CASE DETECTION AND MANAGEMENT

Untreated VL and PKDL patients act as a reservoir of parasites and contribute to disease transmission in anthroponotic VL areas (i.e. in *L. donovani* endemic regions in the Indian subcontinent and in East Africa). Mathematical modelling suggests that asymptomatic carriers may contribute to transmission but currently there is no treatment available safe enough to justify its use in otherwise healthy persons. In anthroponotic transmission areas there are almost no other options to control the disease than early case detection and treatment given the absence of a vaccine and the limited effectiveness of vector control in many places. Another very good reason to promote early case detection is that treatment outcome is worse in patients with advanced VL disease. In Sudan, adult patients with severe anaemia, malnutrition and a long duration of disease had a high risk of dying during treatment.[98] Early diagnosis and treatment is thus important for the individual patient as well as for the community and is therefore considered to be an essential component of VL control.[174,175]

The VL elimination initiative that was launched in 2005 by the governments of India, Nepal and Bangladesh, opted for a case finding and treatment strategy based on the rK39 ICT as diagnostic tool and miltefosine as first-line drug. In regions where antimonials remain effective, they continue to be widely used, but their toxicity profile requires reconsideration of this policy. Programmes now have the choice between single-dose L-Amb or one of the combination regimens, though more evidence from large pragmatic trials is required before these can be adopted. Since 2011 L-Amb has been made available under a donation scheme for low-resource settings.

The detection and treatment of PKDL patients is also likely to be beneficial for control, as they are thought to be an important source of transmission. The feasibility, impact and cost of a strategy for PKDL management should be properly evaluated.

In zoonotic disease, control usually targets the animal reservoir (see above). But since the emergence of HIV/*Leishmania* co-infection, early human case detection and treatment has also become important in *L. infantum* areas given the potential for human-to-human transmission.

Acknowledgements

The authors are indebted to J. Dedet and F. Pratlong who wrote the chapter in the previous edition. They wish to thank P. Desjeux, B. Ostyn, A. Picado, K. Verdonck and C. Yansouni who provided excellent comments and support for the writing of this revision, as well as A.M. Trooskens for her work on the references.

All pictures taken in Peru belong to the collection of the Instituto de Medicina Tropical Alexander von Humboldt, Leishmaniasis unit headed by Prof. Dr. Alejandro Llanos-Cuentas. They were taken resp. by F. Bravo, K. Verdonck and C. Yansouni. The clinical pictures from Nepal were taken by S. Uranw in the Centre for Tropical Diseases at the B.P. Koirala Institute of Health Sciences, courtesy of Prof. Dr. S. Rijal.

REFERENCES

1. World Health Organization. Control of the Leishmaniases. Geneva: WHO Press. WHO Technical Report Series 2010;949:1–186.
3. Chappuis F, Sundar S, Hailu A, et al. Visceral leishmaniasis: what are the needs for diagnosis, treatment and control? Nat Rev Microbiol 2007; 5:873–82.
6. Reithinger R, Dujardin JC, Louzir H, et al. Cutaneous leishmaniasis. Lancet Infect Dis 2007;7: 581–96.
10. Alvar J, Aparicio P, Aseffa A, et al. The relationship between leishmaniasis and AIDS: the second 10 years. Clin Microbiol Rev 2008;21: 334–59, table.
40. Nylen S, Sacks D. Interleukin-10 and the pathogenesis of human visceral leishmaniasis. Trends Immunol 2007;28:378–84.

Access the complete references online at www.expertconsult.com

48 Toxoplasmosis

MELBA MUÑOZ-ROLDAN | MARKUS M. HEIMESAAT | OLIVER LIESENFELD

KEY POINTS

- *Toxoplasma gondii* is a protozoan parasite with worldwide distribution most commonly acquired by either ingestion of water or food contaminated with the oocyst stage of the parasite excreted from members of the cat family, or by consumption of undercooked or raw meat containing tissue cysts.
- Pathological changes in affected organs such as lymph nodes, eye, brain and the fetus most likely are caused directly by the parasite and by the strong T-helper-cell 1 response; immunosuppression (i.e. AIDS, transplantation) results in reactivation and uncontrolled parasite replication.
- Clinical manifestations are driven by pathological changes in affected organs and range from asymptomatic in the majority of acutely infected subjects to cervical lymphadenitis and retinochoroiditis; encephalitis results from reactivation in immunocompromised hosts while transmission during pregnancy causes congenital toxoplasmosis.
- Diagnosis of past infection is established using detection of *T. gondii*-specific IgG antibodies while IgM (and IgA) antibodies allow diagnosis of acute infection in immunocompetent hosts; direct detection in body fluids or tissues using PCR or (immuno)histopathology is required for the diagnosis in immunocompromised hosts.
- Primary infection with *T. gondii* in immunocompetent subjects typically does not require antiparasitic treatment, while treatment in immunocompromised subjects always requires antiparasitic treatment that is based on inhibitors of folate synthesis including the combination of pyrimethamine and sulfadiazine; leucovorin is added to the combination therapy to substitute the hosts foline synthesis.
- Prevention strategies include avoidance of infection with the parasite using education on sources of infection and sanitary measures (primary prevention); antiparasitic prophylaxis prevents reactivation in immunocompromised hosts and transmission of the parasite to the fetus in pregnant women (secondary prevention).

Introduction

Toxoplasma gondii is an obligate intracellular protozoan able to infect a wide variety of animal species and humans. The parasite exists in three stages: *oocysts*, the product of sexual recombination in the intestine of members of the feline family, *tachyzoites*, the invasive, rapidly replicating intracellular stage of the parasite, and *bradyzoites*, the slowly replicating stages found in cysts in latently infected hosts. *T. gondii* infects up to a third of the world's population by ingestion of contaminated water and food containing oocysts, or by the consumption of raw or undercooked meat containing tissue cysts. *T. gondii* crosses the intestinal, the placenta and the blood–brain barriers, and persists in its latent form in the central nervous system and muscle tissue. Both the cellular and humoral arms of the immune system control primary infection but cellular immune mechanisms, i.e. adequate T-helper-1 cell responses, are essential to prevent reactivation of infection. Signs and symptoms of primary infection range from flu-like syndrome to lymphadenopathy and retinochoroiditis; infection is mostly asymptomatic in pregnant women but can lead to severe birth defects or intrauterine death in the fetus. In immunocompromised patients, i.e. those with AIDS and following organ transplantation, reactivation of latent infection may present as toxoplasmic encephalitis. Whereas serum or intraocular antibody responses are useful to detect primary infection, direct detection of the parasite allows the definitive diagnosis of reactivated infection. Treatment of infection is based on combination therapy with agents active against folic acid synthesis, i.e. pyrimethamine and sulfadiazine. Primary prevention can be achieved by avoidance of contaminated food and water; secondary prevention (of reactivation) in immunocompromised hosts is achieved by antiparasitic prophylaxis and/or reconstitution of the immune status.

Epidemiology

Toxoplasma gondii is an obligate intracellular protozoan that belongs to the phylum Apicomplexa, subclass *coccidia*. The parasite can be found in nature in different forms.[1] *Oocysts* are the product of the parasite's sexual cycle in the intestine of all members of the cat family and release infectious sporozoites. *Tachyzoites* are asexual forms that invade host cells, and the cysts which contains *bradyzoites, the* dormant stage of the parasite in tissues. The *T. gondii* genome is haploid, except during the stages of its sexual division in cats, and contains approximately 8×10^7 base pairs.

Members of the cat family are definite hosts of the parasite; parasites complete the sexual cycle resulting in the production of oocysts in the intestines of cats (Figure 48.1).[2] During acute infection, several million oocysts (10×12 μm in size) are shed in the faeces of felines for 7–21 days. Following sporulation (between 1 and 21 days), sporozoites are released and may infect new hosts when ingested, giving rise to the tachyzoite stage.

Tachyzoites (2–4 μm wide and 4–8 μm long) are crescentic or oval and are rapidly multiplying obligate intracellular stages of the parasite (Figure 48.1). Tachyzoites enter all nucleated cells by active penetration and form a cytoplasmic vacuole. Following repeated replication, host cells are disrupted and tachyzoites

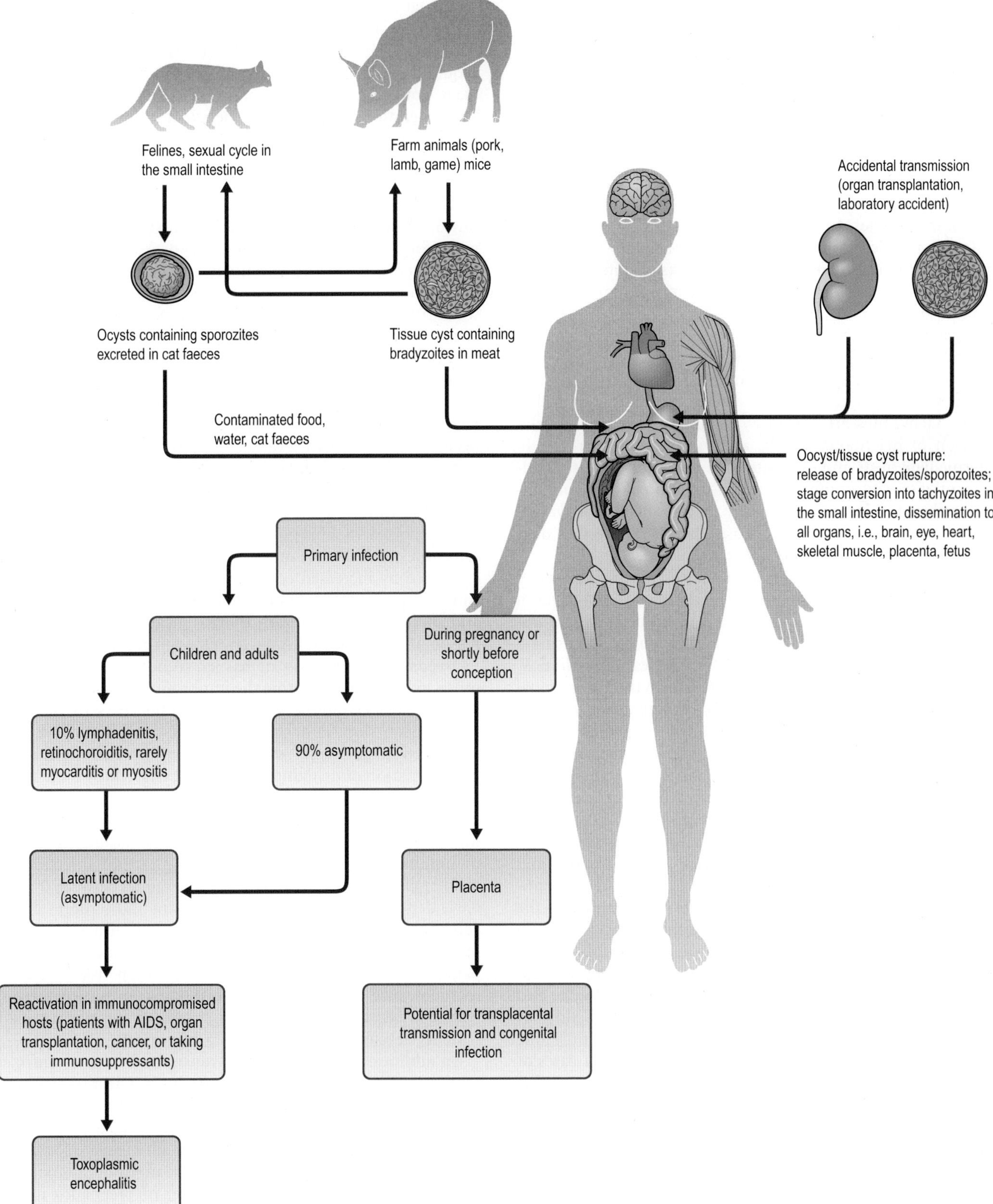

Figure 48.1 Life cycle of *T. gondii* and clinical manifestations of toxoplasmosis. *(With permission from Montoya JG, Liesenfeld O. Lancet 2004;363:1965–76.)*

invade neighbouring cells. The tachyzoite form causes a strong inflammatory response and tissue destruction and is therefore responsible for clinical manifestations of the disease. Under the pressure of the immune system, tachyzoites are transformed into bradyzoites that form cysts.

Bradyzoites persist inside cysts for the life of the host (Figure 48.1). Bradyzoites are morphologically identical to tachyzoites but multiply slowly, express stage-specific molecules and are functionally different. Tissue cysts containing between hundreds and thousands of bradyzoites are found in brain, skeletal and heart muscles. In immunocompromised patients bradyzoites are released from cysts, transform back into tachyzoites, and cause reactivation of the infection. Cysts are infective stages for intermediate and definitive hosts via consumption of muscle or brain tissue.

Ingestion of *T. gondii* cysts or oocysts is the natural route of infection. After ingestion, cysts (or oocysts) are disrupted and the bradyzoites (or sporozoites) are released into the intestinal lumen where they rapidly enter cells and multiply as tachyzoites. Tachyzoites are spread by disruption of infected cells, invasion of neighbouring cells and via the blood stream. In intermediate hosts and extraintestinal tissues of the cat, development of specific immunity causes formation of cysts containing bradyzoites. Immunodeficiency may result in reactivation of latent infection and severe disease whereas re-infection does not appear to cause clinically apparent disease.

Molecular analysis has revealed that *T. gondii* consists of three clonal lineages designated types I, II, and III that differ in virulence and epidemiological pattern of occurrence.[3] Strain-specific peptides allow for typing of *T. gondii* strains using a patient's serum.[4] In Europe and North America, *T. gondii* possesses a simple population genetic structure; the three clonal lineages (referred to as Types I, II, or III) dominate the majority of human infections. Severity of human congenital disease appears to be associated with non-Type II infections while DNA sequencing data identified a diversity of recombinant and atypical strains associated with the incidence and severity of disease in patients with AIDS and ocular toxoplasmosis in the USA, Central and South America. A higher prevalence of recombinant strains has also been identified in Central and South America, suggesting a greater diversity of parasite genotypes than previously envisaged. *T. gondii* was identified as the source of an unusual outbreak of toxoplasmosis in a village with 33 inhabitants in Surinam.[5] Eleven cases of toxoplasmosis occurred; eight patients without immunodeficiencies presented with multivisceral involvement resulting in one death. Two lethal cases of congenital toxoplasmosis were observed. Molecular analysis demonstrated that identical isolates of only one atypical strain were responsible for at least 5 of the 11 cases of toxoplasmosis in the outbreak; the atypical genotype of this strain was found to be unrelated to the three known main lineages and seems to be related to a number of cases of severe toxoplasmosis observed in immunocompetent adults in neighbouring French Guiana.[6] While the source of infection could be formally established the severity of outbreak of toxoplasmosis suggest an environmental contamination linked to the forest-based cycle of infection involving wild felids and their prey in the Amazon rainforest.

In Europe, however, Type II strains account for 70–80% of human infections, the majority of congenital cases (85%) among pregnant women, and ocular toxoplasmosis cases in France.

Sexual recombination between two distinct and competing clonal lines of the parasite most likely drove natural evolution of virulence in *T. gondii*; direct oral transmission, a recently acquired evolutionary change in the life history of *T. gondii*, likely contributed to widespread expansion of Toxoplasma.[7] The generation of specific gene-deficient strains of *T. gondii* and the ongoing sequencing of the Toxoplasma genome (see: http://ToxoDB.org/) will provide further insight into the immunopathogenesis of infection with *T. gondii*.

Humans become infected with *T. gondii* after ingestion of raw or undercooked meat containing tissue cysts, or contaminated food and water containing oocysts excreted in the faeces of infected cats (Figure 48.1).[1] In a recent study in the USA, infection by ingestion of oocysts was reported to be the major source of infection based on the detection of sporozoite-specific antibodies. Seroprevalence of *T. gondii* rises with age, does not vary between genders, and is lower in cold regions, hot and arid areas, and at high altitudes.[8] Global epidemiologic surveillance for infection with *T. gondii* is limited, however; a few studies have shown that the seroprevalence of *T. gondii* infections have been steadily falling in several countries over the past decades.[9] Eating and hygiene habits can give rise to seroprevalence differences worldwide; while the overall seroprevalence of *T. gondii* is 22.5% in the USA. Seroprevalences of more than 50% have been reported in Europe (Figure 48.2). An increased rate of infection in rural areas in the second half of the year has been explained by increased consumption of fresh vegetable in the summer, prolonged indoor contact with cats later in the year, and increased consumption of raw meat during the holiday season at Christmas followed by a sharp drop in January.

Exposure to infected cats has led to outbreaks of toxoplasmosis in humans, indicating the importance of oocyst excretion by cats. Socioeconomic status also influences seroprevalence and transmission. Poor socioeconomic conditions have been associated with several outbreaks of toxoplasmosis through contamination of drinking water by oocysts, which is the major route of transmission under these conditions.[10] Blood transfusion or organ transplantation from an infected to an uninfected individual may transmit the parasite and may causes infections in immunocompromised patients. The rate of infections in solid organ transplant patients typically ranges between 0% and 0.6% depending on the type of transplant and seroprevalence/geographical region; the rate is highest in heart transplant patients. Patients with haematological malignancies, especially patients with Hodgkin's disease, are at a high risk to develop recrudescence of the infection. Among organ transplantation patients, heart, lung, kidney, and bone marrow transplant patients develop toxoplasmosis at a higher rate.

In addition, *T. gondii* can be transmitted from an infected mother to the fetus during pregnancy.[1,11] The prevalence of congenital toxoplasmosis ranges from one to 10 per 10 000 live births in Europe and North America. Whereas early maternal infection (1st and 2nd trimester) may result in severe congenital toxoplasmosis and death of the fetus in utero or spontaneous abortion, infection in the 3rd trimester of pregnancy usually results in normal-appearing newborns. However, infected newborns if untreated can later develop retinochoroiditis and/or mental abnormalities. Importantly, the overall frequency of subclinical infection in newborns with congenital toxoplasmosis is as high as 85%. The occurrence of congenital transmission depends on the time when the pregnant woman acquired the infection. Whereas infections around the time of conception

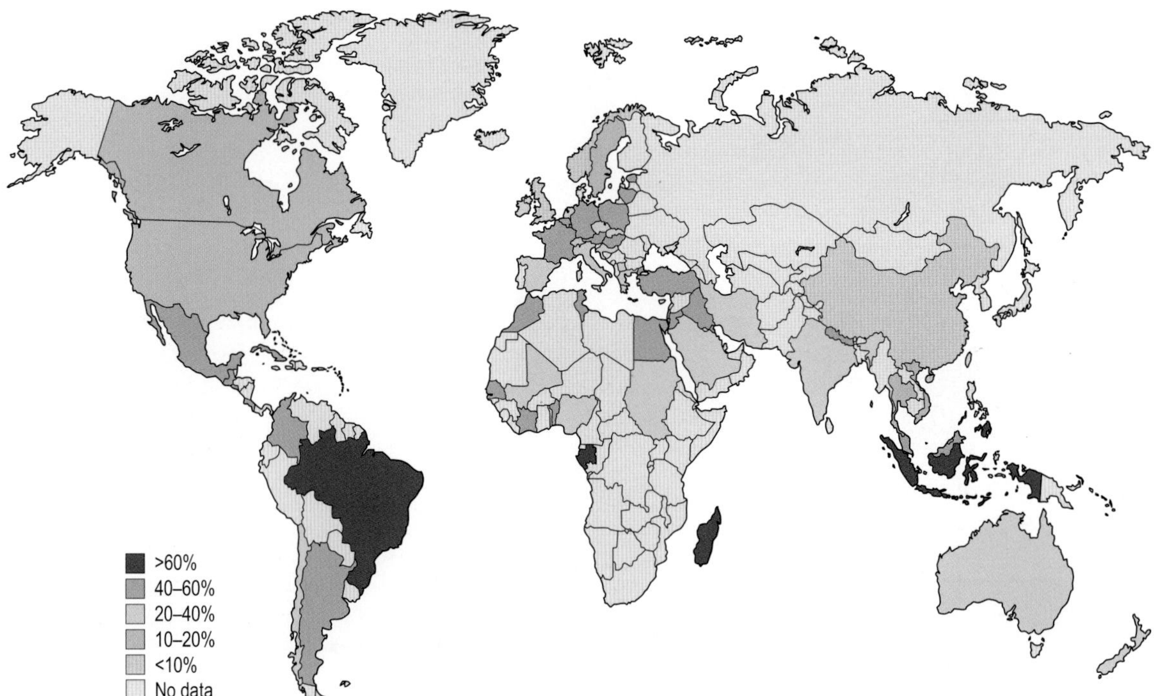

Figure 48.2 *T. gondii* seroprevalence rates worldwide in females of reproductive age or pregnant. *(Modified from Pappas G, et al. Int J Parasitol 2009;39:1385–94.)*

and within the first 2 weeks of gestation do not result in transmission in most cases, infections in the last trimester result in 60% transmission frequencies. Treatment aimed to prevent vertical transmission should be given within 3 weeks after infection but since most of the infections are asymptomatic, prevention of congenital toxoplasmosis is difficult to achieve. General population seroprevalence is an important factor to predict the infection risk of a woman during pregnancy. In a population with low seroprevalence, the overall risk for infection is low due to the low rate of environmental and/or food contamination with *T. gondii*, however; the low percentages of immune individuals results in an increased risk of primary infection during pregnancy with the risk of congenital transmission. On the other hand, in a population with high seroprevalence, the chances of women acquiring primary infection during pregnancy are lower due to the past exposure to *T. gondii*. However, those individuals who have not been exposed to the parasite are at increased risk for primary infection during pregnancy due to the presence of *T. gondii* in the environment and food supply.

The incidence of TE among human immunodeficiency virus (HIV)-infected individuals correlates directly with the prevalence of *T. gondii* antibodies among the general HIV-infected population, the degree of immunosuppression (best measured by the CD4+ cell count), the immunological response to antiretroviral drugs, and the use of effective prophylactic treatment regimens against development of TE.[1,12,13] AIDS-associated TE and toxoplasmosis involving other organs almost always are due to reactivation of a latent infection. It is estimated that 20–47% of AIDS patients who are infected with *T. gondii* but are not receiving antitoxoplasmic prophylaxis or antiretroviral drugs will develop TE. Even before the emergence of AIDS, TE had been recognized as a cause of incapacitating disease and death among immunocompromised patients, especially in patients whose underlying disease or therapy caused a deficiency in cell-mediated immunity. Reductions in TE incidence and mortality have been observed in AIDS cohort after introduction of HAART.[14,15]

From the beginning of the human immunodeficiency virus (HIV) epidemic, toxoplasmosis has been an indicator for AIDS. Estimated HIV-associated toxoplasmosis hospitalizations increased between 1993 and 1995, but then dropped. The rate of HIV-associated toxoplasmosis hospitalizations among all HIV-related hospitalizations decreased from 1993 to 2008; however, hospitalizations dropped little after 2000, implying an antiretroviral therapy failure or late diagnosis of some HIV-infected individuals. Patients developing toxoplasmic encephalitis in the post-HAART era typically did not receive HAART or had not taken HAART adequately. In addition, concurrent diagnosis of TE and HIV appears to be significantly more often in the post-HAART compared to the pre-HAART era.

Pathogenesis and Pathology

The immunological status of the individual is one of the most important factors in the course of infection in humans. Other important factors include the inoculum size, the genetic background of the individual and the virulence of the parasite.[16] Following active invasion of the parasite into the host cell, *T. gondii* induces the formation of a parasitophorous vacuole containing secreted parasite proteins but excluding host proteins that would promote phagosome maturation and subsequently lysosome fusion. *T. gondii* has developed powerful mechanisms to modulate its host cells and generates latent infections by evading the host's immune system.[16–18]

Following host cell invasion, the parasite replicates rapidly, disrupts the host cell and disseminates via the bloodstream throughout the host. *T. gondii* has the ability to cross the blood–brain barrier and form cysts in the brain (Figure 48.3). In

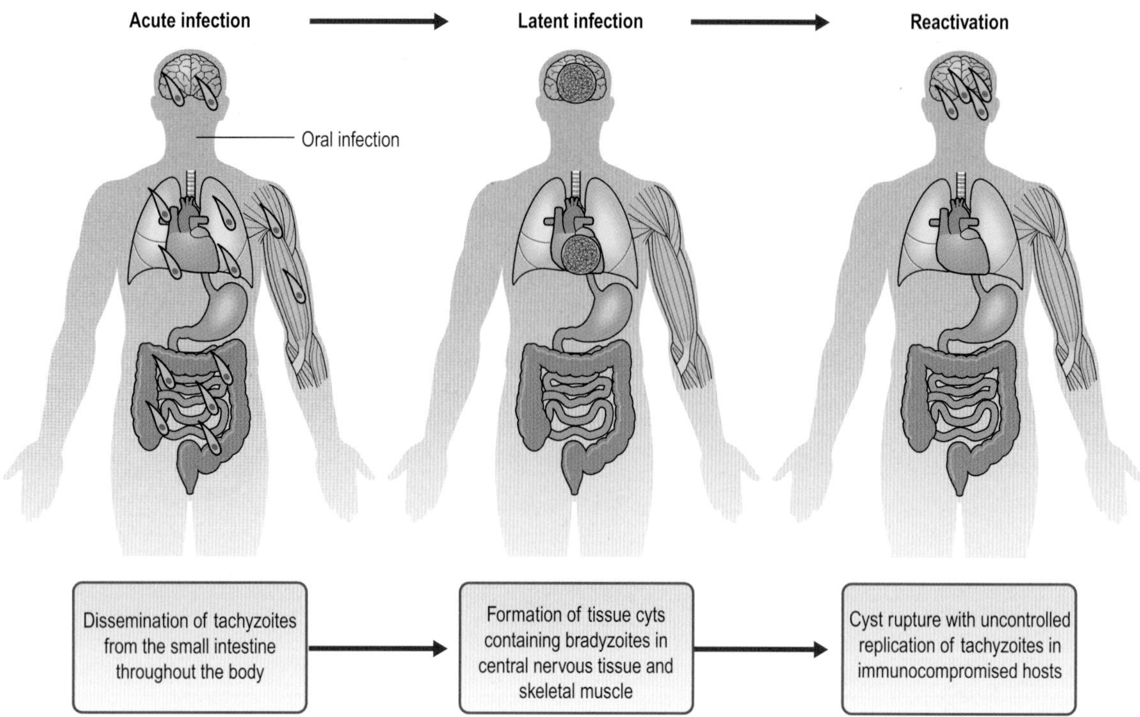

Figure 48.3 Stages of infection with *T. gondii* in humans.

addition, the parasite can localize not only in skeletal and heart muscle but also in the retina and the placenta. Dendritic cells are likely candidates as the key cells that traffic the parasite throughout the body ('Trojan Horse'). This hypothesis is supported by murine models of infection and by in vitro studies where parasites preferentially infect and replicate inside of monocytes and dendritic cells. In addition, infection of dendritic cells increased their migratory capacity.

T cells, macrophages, and type 1 cytokines (IFN-γ, IL-12) are crucial for control of *T. gondii* infection. Adoptive transfer experiments in murine models proved that T cells are essential for control of *T. gondii* infection; CD8+ T cells are primarily responsible for this resistance, although significant protection is also conferred by CD4+ T cells. The costimulatory molecules CD28 and CD40 ligand are pivotal for the regulation of IL-12 and IFN-γ production in response to the parasite. *T. gondii* infection of antigen-presenting cells, such as dendritic cells and macrophages, causes upregulation of the counterreceptors for CD28 and CD40L, CD80/CD86 and CD40, respectively. Binding of CD80/CD86 to CD28 enhances production of IFN-γ by CD4+ T cells. In addition, binding of CD40L to CD40 triggers IL-12 secretion, which enhances production of IFN-γ. The relevance of CD40L in the immune response to *T. gondii* is supported by reports of TE and disseminated toxoplasmosis in children with congenital defects in CD40L signaling (i.e., hyper-IgM syndrome). More recent studies have shown that expression of CD40L is defective on CD4+ T cells from HIV-infected patients. This deficiency may play a role in defective IL-12/IFN-γ production associated with HIV infection.

Cytokine and chemokine production results in the accumulation and activation of inflammatory cells leading to clearance of the invading parasites. Numerous studies have emphasized the antimicrobial role of IFN-γ, however; IFN-γ plays a dichotomous role in the host: as a mediator of severe hyper-inflammation and as an anti-parasite effector. INF-γ combined with TNF activates professional phagocytic cells, such as macrophages to produce high levels of reactive nitrogen intermediates that are involved in the control of parasite replication. CD8+ T cells, capable of lysing infected host cells play a major role as effector lymphocytes against the parasite, whereas CD4+ T cells are important to regulate immune responses to *T. gondii*. In addition, counter-regulatory mechanisms are simultaneously induced by the parasite. *T. gondii* triggers production of anti-inflammatory cytokines including IL-10 and TGF-β that inhibit IFN-γ production and impair macrophage activation. The role of B-lymphocytes and antibody production has not been studied in great detail. Within 2 weeks after infection IgG, IgM, IgA and IgE antibodies against the parasite can be detected; IgA production on mucosal surfaces seems to confer protection against reinfection. Extracellular tachyzoites are lysed by specific antibodies in the presence of complement. In mice, humoral immunity results in limited protection against less virulent strains of *T. gondii*, but not against virulent strains.

Among others, the genotype of the parasite appears to impact the pathogenesis of infection. Type I, but not Types II and III strains, are highly virulent to mice while the association between strain type and severity of disease in humans is not yet fully understood. Infections in mice indicate that different strains of *Toxoplasma* encode and differentially secrete polymorphic effector proteins that specifically target critical pathways of the host pro-inflammatory response (e.g. ROP5, ROP16, ROP18, GRA15) critically impacting the development of protective immunity.[19,20] It is likely that *T. gondii* genotype effector mechanisms also regulate the induction of host responses in humans. Recent work examining congenital infections in the USA has shown that non Type II serotype correlates with prematurity and severity of disease.[21] In Europe, Type II strains account for ~80% of human infections and the majority of

TABLE 48.1 Rates of Congenital Transmission and Risk of Congenital Infection in Offspring

Gestational Age at Maternal Seroconversion (Weeks)	Risk of Congenital Infection		Development of Clinical Signs in Infected Off-Spring	
	(%)	95% CI	(%)	95% CI
13	6	3–9	61	34–65
26	40	33–47	25	18–33
36	72	60–81	9	4–17

Modified after Montoya JG, Remington JS. Clin Infect Dis 2008;47:554–66.

congenital cases (85%) among pregnant women (Table 48.1). In contrast, atypical and Type I-like strains are increasingly associated with severe forms of ocular toxoplasmosis in the USA. While *T. gondii* non-reactive and Type II serotypes were recently found to predominate in German patients with ocular toxoplasmosis, non-reactive serotypes were associated with more serious, recurrent ocular toxoplasmosis. Defining the population structure of *T. gondii* will have important implications for transmission, immunogenicity and pathogenesis, and the association of specific genotypes with severity and/or frequency of recurrences of infection will allow for improved and personalized management of patients.

Pathological changes also depend on the specifics of infection with the parasite (Table 48.2). Whereas primary infection in immunocompetent hosts most often goes unnoticed, toxoplasmic lymphadenitis occurs in a minority of subjects and is characterized by distinctive and often diagnostic histopathological changes in the lymph nodes: follicular hyperplasia and irregular clusters of epithelioid histiocytes invading the margins of the germinal centres are observed.[1]

In patients with toxoplasmic encephalitis resulting from reactivation of latent infection in the central nervous system, affected organs include the grey and white matter of the brain, retinas, lungs, heart, and skeletal muscle. The presence of multiple brain abscesses is the most characteristic feature of toxoplasmic encephalitis. CT or MRI scans of the brain may show single or in the majority of cases multiple foci of enlarging necrosis and microglial nodules. In the areas around the abscesses, oedema, vasculitis, haemorrhage, and cerebral infarction secondary to vascular involvement also may be present. Toxoplasmic encephalitis has a propensity to involve the basal ganglia, but it is also found scattered throughout the brain at the grey matter–white matter junction. In congenital toxoplasmosis microcephaly, microphthalmia, hydranencephaly, hydrocephalus secondary to aqueduct stenosis, porencephalic cyst, and periventricular calcification are found. Periaqueductal and periventricular vasculitis and necrosis are pathognomonic of toxoplasmosis. Necrosis of the brain is most intense in the cortex and basal ganglia. The necrotic areas may calcify and lead to striking radiographic findings suggestive but not pathognomonic of toxoplasmosis. Hydrocephalus may result from obstruction of the aqueduct of Sylvius or foramen of Monro. Tachyzoites and tissue cysts may be seen in and adjacent to necrotic foci, near or in glial nodules, in perivascular regions, and in cerebral tissue uninvolved by inflammatory change. Immunodeficient patients who develop pulmonary toxoplasmosis may also show interstitial pneumonitis, necrotizing pneumonitis, consolidation, pleural effusion, or emphysema. Pneumonitis is associated with fibrinous or fibrinopurulent exudates and alveolocytes may harbour tachyzoites. At autopsy, histopathological evidence of multiorgan involvement by the parasite has been observed in organ transplant patients with TE. The organs most commonly involved are brain, heart, and lungs, but many other organs, including eyes, liver, pancreas, adrenal, and kidney, may harbour the parasite.

Eye infections (retinochoroiditis) are characterized by severe inflammation and necrosis; the extent of inflammation and necrosis is dependent on the immune status of the patient.[22] In

TABLE 48.2 Overview of Clinical Presentations, Associated Symptoms, Pathological Changes, and Differential Diagnoses of Infection with *T. Gondii*

Clinical Feature (Host Immune Status)	Signs and Symptoms	Pathology	Differential Diagnosis
Lymphadenitis (immunocompetent)	Absent (90% of cases); rarely fever, malaise, night sweats, hepatosplenomegaly, lymphadenopathy	Follicular hyperplasia, irregular clusters of epithelioid histiocytes invading the margins of the germinal centres	Hodgkin's disease, mononucleosis, cat scratch fever, lymphoma, leukaemia
Toxoplasmic encephalitis (immunocompromised)	Hemiparesis, personality changes, aphasia, seizures, weakness, sensory abnormalities	Multiple brain abscesses, foci of enlarging necrosis, microglial nodules	Multifocal leukoencephalopathy, fungal and mycobacterial infection
Retinochoroiditis (immunocompetent and immunocompromised)	Ocular pain, loss of visual acuity, scotoma, photophobia	Necrotizing retinitis at the posterior pole and inner layer (frequently unilateral)	CMV retinitis, syphilis, infection with herpes simplex or varicella zoster
Congenital toxoplasmosis (immunocompetent mothers)	Microcephaly, blindness, epilepsy, psychomotor or mental retardation	Necrosis of cortex and basal ganglia, hydrocephalus, periaqueductal and periventricular vasculitis	Infection with herpes simplex virus, CMV, rubella virus

primary ocular toxoplasmosis, a unilateral focus of necrotizing retinitis is present at the posterior pole in more than 50% of cases. The area of necrosis usually involves the inner layers of the retina and is described as a white-appearing lesion surrounded by retinal oedema.

Clinical Features

Whereas immunocompetent individuals in most cases develop asymptomatic infections (*Toxoplasma infection*), symptomatic infection (toxoplasmosis) presents as lymphadenopathy and/or retinochoroiditis in up to 10% of cases of primary infection accompanied by unspecific flu-like symptoms including fever, malaise, night sweats, myalgias, sore throat, and maculopapular rash. Toxoplasmosis may also present as congenital infection in fetuses and newborns of mothers with primary infection during pregnancy, and as TE or disseminated disease in immunocompromised patients with reactivation of latent infection.

ACUTE INFECTION

Clinical manifestations of acute toxoplasmosis in an immunocompetent individual resemble in many cases those observed in patients with infectious mononucleosis or CMV infection, but acute toxoplasmosis probably causes no more than 1% of 'mononucleosis' syndromes. Lymph nodes are usually tender, discrete and may remain enlarged for up to 6 weeks. *T. gondii* has been estimated to cause 3–7% of clinically significant lymphadenopathy. Retroperitoneal or mesenteric lymphadenopathy may produce abdominal pain. In most cases the clinical diagnosis of acquired toxoplasmosis is challenging because none of the clinical presentations is distinctive. Differential diagnosis of toxoplasmic lymphadenitis also includes lymphoma, cat-scratch disease, sarcoidosis, tuberculosis, tularaemia, and leukaemia. Symptoms typically resolve within a few months. Other manifestations including myocarditis, polymyositis, pneumonitis, hepatitis or encephalitis are extremely rare in otherwise immunocompetent individuals, and may be associated with specific atypical parasite strains and/or host factors, especially in tropical regions (see above).

Recent reports have suggested a potential link of *Toxoplasma* seropositivity with a number of neuropsychiatric disorders such as epilepsy and schizophrenia.

REACTIVATED INFECTION IN IMMUNOCOMPROMISED INDIVIDUALS

Immunocompromised patients with defects in T-cell-mediated immunity, such as those receiving corticosteroids or cytotoxic drugs, patients with haematological malignancies, organ transplant recipients, or those with AIDS are at high risk for developing toxoplasmosis from reactivation of latent infection; immunomodulatory TNF-blocking therapies have been reported to result in reactivation of infection with *T. gondii* in rare cases.[23] Immunocompromised patients may also acquire primary infection that presents as disseminated disease (sepsis). In contrast to immunocompetent patients, toxoplasmosis is fatal in immunocompromised individuals if not recognized and treated early. Clinical manifestations of toxoplasmosis in AIDS patients commonly reflect involvement of the central nervous system, i.e. TE, the eye (retinochoroiditis), and the lung (pneumonitis). Disseminated infection with multiple-organ involvement is not unusual and clinical manifestations in many cases do not reflect the extent and severity of the disseminated infection. The most common clinical manifestation of toxoplasmosis is encephalitis, which occurs when the CD4+ cell count is below 200 cells/μL. In the era before the introduction of antiparasitic prophylaxis and later the introduction of highly active antiretroviral therapy (HAART), TE was the most common infectious manifestation of AIDS in the central nervous system; however, the incidence of TE decreased significantly after the broad use of trimethoprim/sulfamethoxazole (TMP-SMX) prophylaxis for *P. jiroveci* pneumonia. HAART TE is rarely observed in patients receiving appropriate care for HIV infection; demographic, clinical and laboratory characteristics do not appear to differ markedly between patients developing TE before or after the introduction of HAART. In patients with HAART showing CD4+ counts at sustained levels greater than 200 cells/μL for 3–6 months, prophylaxis regimens can be discontinued safely.[13,15] Clinical findings of TE include altered mental state, seizures, weakness, cranial nerve disturbances, sensory abnormalities, cerebellar signs, meningismus, movement disorders and neuropsychiatric manifestations (Table 48.3). In about 75% of cases, the most common manifestation is the sub-acute onset of focal neurologic abnormalities such as hemiparesis, personality changes or aphasia. The characteristic presentation usually has a subacute onset with focal neurological abnormalities in up to 89% of patients. However, symptoms may appear abruptly with seizures or cerebral haemorrhage in 15–25% of cases. Table 48.3 summarizes the baseline characteristics of HIV-infected individuals with TE together with their signs and symptoms. The differential diagnosis of TE includes central nervous system lymphoma, progressive multifocal leukoencephalopathy and cerebral infection with cytomegalovirus, *Cryptococcus neoformans*, *Aspergillus fumigatus* and *Mycobacterium tuberculosis*. In addition, some patients might show neuropsychiatric symptoms, such as paranoid psychosis, dementia, anxiety and agitation.

TABLE 48.3 Baseline Characteristics and Clinical Signs and Symptoms in Patients with Toxoplasmic Encephalitis

Parameter	Value
Baseline Characteristics	
Sex (% males)	86
Age (mean, SD)	40 ± 9.5
CD4 cell count (median, IQR /10^6/L)	27 (9–62)
Positive *T. gondii* serology	97%
Prophylaxis for toxoplasmosis	32%
Suggestive signs on brain imaging	98%
Signs and Symptoms	
Fever	59%
Headache	55%
Seizures	22%
Focal signs	70%
Motor-sensory defects	49%
Cranial nerve palsies	12%
Ataxia, aphasia, hemianopsia	15%
Cerebellar signs	10%
Diffuse neuropsychiatric signs	15%
Coma, lethargy	5%
Other neurological signs	8%

Modified after Raffi F, et al. AIDS 1997;11:177–84.

Spinal cord involvement can occur and manifests as motor or sensory disturbances of single or multiple limbs, bladder or bowel dysfunctions or both, and local pain. Patients may present with a clinical syndrome resembling a spinal cord tumor. Toxoplasmosis can also be manifested as retinochoroiditis, pneumonitis or multiorgan disease accompanied by acute respiratory failure and signs of septic shock. Pulmonary disease due to toxoplasmosis has been reported in patients with AIDS, and can be diagnosed by the detection of the parasite in BAL fluid. Extrapulmonary disease may be present in about 50% of cases with toxoplasmic pneumonitis. The differential diagnosis of toxoplasmic pneumonitis includes *Pneumocystis jirovecii* pneumonia and infection with *Mycobacterium tuberculosis*, *Cryptococcus neoformans*, *Coccidioides immitis* and *Histoplasma capsulatum*.

Retinochoroiditis is the second most common presentation of toxoplasmosis in immunocompromised patients characterized by ocular pain and loss of visual acuity. Necrotizing lesions, in some cases multifocal or bilateral, are found in funduscopic examination. Furthermore, vitreal inflammation can often accompany necrotizing lesions and 10% of the individuals with toxoplasmic retinochoroiditis might show involvement of the optic nerve. Toxoplasmic retinochoroiditis in AIDS patients has been associated with concurrent TE in 63% of patients. The differential diagnosis includes CMV retinitis, syphilis, infection with herpes simplex virus, varicella zoster virus or fungi.

Clinical manifestations are similar in patients with different causes of immunosuppression, i.e. solid organ transplantation. The majority of (seronegative) patients develop primary infection within 6 months of transplantation presenting with fever; respiratory and neurological symptoms; disseminated disease is observed in less than 25% of patients. Patients with solid organ transplants develop toxoplasmosis, most commonly as a result of acquiring *T. gondii* infection through the transplanted organ when the organ of a seropositive donor is given to a seronegative recipient. Toxoplasmosis can also result from reactivation of a previously acquired infection in the recipient regardless of the serologic status of the donor due to the transplantation-accompanying immunosuppressive therapy. The latter scenario is especially important in bone-marrow transplant recipients. Fever is often the first manifestation in transplant recipients, followed by clinical signs referable to the brain and lungs.

OCULAR TOXOPLASMOSIS IN IMMUNOCOMPETENT INDIVIDUALS

Toxoplasmic retinochoroiditis results from congenital or postnatally acquired acute infection or recurrence.[1,11,24] Age is one of several host factors that are believed to influence severity of ocular toxoplasmosis and a more severe disease has been observed at the extremes of age. The retina is the primary site of *T. gondii* infection in the eye and infection with *T. gondii* is one of the most frequently identified causes of uveitis. Toxoplasmosis is responsible for more than 85% of posterior uveitis cases in southern Brazil, in which 9.5% of seroconverters and 8.3% of seropositive patients without ocular involvement developed typical lesions during 7 years of follow-up. Factors including the host and parasite genetics, or the environment dictate the duration and intensity of ocular toxoplasmosis. Recurrences are frequent, occurring in 79% of patients followed for more than 5 years in one study, with a median time to recurrence of 2 years; lesions were more common in the eye originally involved and may be more common after cataract extraction. In contrast, patients who present with toxoplasmic retinochoroiditis in the setting of acute toxoplasmosis are more often older than 30, they most often have unilateral involvement, and the eye lesions usually spare the macula and do not present with associated old scars.

The choroid, vitreous and anterior chamber can frequently be compromised. Retinochoroiditis, usually bilateral, typically affects the posterior pole of a single eye but lesions might also be solitary, multiple or satellite to a pigmented retinal scar. Ocular disease in patients with acute toxoplasmosis can also be detected by active lesions present as grey-white focuses of retinal necrosis with adjacent choroiditis, vasculitis, haemorrhage and vitreitis and these lesions are frequently unilateral. In contrast, more aggressive bilateral or multifocal disease is found in elderly or immunocompromised patients. Focal necrotizing retinitis can initially appear in the fundus as a yellowish white, elevated cotton patch with indistinct margins, usually on the posterior pole. Furthermore, the choroid can be secondarily inflamed, accompanied by increased intraocular pressure and an intense secondary iridocyclitis may also be present. Presence of active retinal lesions with severe vitreous inflammatory reaction can cause the classic 'headlight in the fog' appearance. Recurrent lesions mostly occur at the borders of chorioretinal scars, and might be found in clusters. Panuveitis may accompany retinochoroiditis.

Individuals who develop with retinochoroiditis as a late sequela of congenital infection are more frequently in their second and third decades of life. In these cases the hallmarks of retinal disease include bilateral disease, old retinal scars, and involvement of the macula.

Acute retinochoroiditis may produce symptoms of blurred vision, scotoma, pain, photophobia, and epiphora. Involvement of the macula results in the impairment or a loss of central vision. As inflammation resolves, vision improves, frequently without complete recovery of visual acuity. In most cases, toxoplasmic retinochoroiditis is diagnosed by ophthalmologic examination, and empirical therapy directed against the organism often is initiated based on clinical findings and serologic test results.

T. gondii retinochoroiditis may resemble posterior uveitis of tuberculosis, syphilis, leprosy, or ocular histoplasmosis syndrome. Atypical clinical manifestations of toxoplasmic retinochoroiditis have been reported most commonly in elderly and in immunodeficient individuals, and include multiple foci of active retinitis, acute retinal necrosis syndrome (vitritis, peripheral retinitis, retinal vasculitis), significant intraretinal haemorrhage, or an absence of ophthalmoscopically visible chorioretinal scarring.

CONGENITAL TOXOPLASMOSIS

T. gondii can be transmitted to the fetus when the parasite enters the fetal circulation by infection of the placenta in women who acquire primary infection during gestation.[25] However, in very rare cases persistent parasitaemia in immunocompetent women infected shortly before pregnancy, reactivation of latent toxoplasmosis in HIV-infected mothers, and reinfection with a different parasite strain in an immune mother during pregnancy have been described to result in congenital infection.

Whereas fetal infection may result in natural abortion, early detection of the infection acquired during the gestation and rapid initiation of treatment is often associated with favourable outcomes. Initial manifestations at birth are not only strongly influenced by the time during gestation when infection was acquired but also involve host and parasite genetics. The frequency of transmission and severity of congenital toxoplasmosis are inversely related. The likelihood of fetal infection increases with gestational age (close to zero around the time of conception, up to 10% at the end of the 1st trimester, 30–54% at the end of the 2nd trimester, and more than 60% in the 3rd trimester); the likelihood of severe fetal disease manifestations decreases at the same time.

Importantly, manifestations of clinical disease might not be apparent at birth and complications develop later in life. Congenital toxoplasmosis caused by atypical parasite genotypes appears to be more severe than that caused by typical genotypes. Atypical genotypes are also associated with more severe ocular disease in children with congenital toxoplasmosis in Brazil and Europe. Congenital infection can appear at different time points after birth and show different levels of severity in the newborn. Toxoplasmosis can be manifested early as a neonatal disease; second, as a mild or severe disease occurring in the first months of life; third, as sequelae of a previously undiagnosed infection later during infancy or childhood. A wide spectrum of clinical manifestations of congenital toxoplasmosis can be observed in infected newborns. Most signs and clinical presentations are nonspecific and may mimic disease due to organisms such as herpes simplex virus, CMV, and rubella virus. The classic triad of retinochoroiditis, hydrocephalus, and cerebral calcification is seldom observed. General signs include retinochoroiditis, strabismus, blindness, epilepsy, psychomotor or mental retardation, anaemia, jaundice, rash, petechiae due to thrombocytopenia, encephalitis, pneumonitis, microcephaly, intracranial calcification and nonspecific illness. Children with subclinical disease at birth may develop retinal disease by the time they are adolescents in more than 82% of the cases. Children who had generalized or neurological signs at birth, if left untreated or treated for only 1 month, have a >85% chance of developing mental retardation; 81% seizures; 70% motor difficulties; 60% severe vision loss; 33% hydro- or microcephalus; 14% hearing loss, and only 11% are normal.

Frequently, the initial manifestation of congenital toxoplasmosis is retinochoroiditis, which appears at a mean age of 3.7 years. Some children develop unilateral blindness, whereas others have no loss of visual function. Neurological sequelae include delayed psychomotor development, microcephaly, and seizure disorder minor cerebellar signs. A study from the Netherlands reported that five of nine congenitally infected, untreated children followed for up to 14 years developed retinochoroiditis. Information from prospective studies suggests that early instigation of specific therapy in infants with congenital infection but without clinical signs markedly reduces untoward sequelae. Transmission of the parasite to the fetus has rarely been observed in HIV-infected pregnant women. The course of congenital infection appears to be accelerated in HIV-infected newborns; HIV-infected newborns fail to thrive, develop fever, hepatosplenomegaly, retinochoroiditis and seizures. Most children have multiorgan involvement including CNS, cardiac, and pulmonary disease.

Small intestinal immunopathology following oral infection with tissue cysts of *T. gondii* has been described in susceptible laboratory mice caused by local overproduction of Th1-type cytokines (cytokine storm).[16,26] The immunopathogenesis of this pathology resembles that of inflammatory bowel disease in humans, i.e. Crohn's disease. Interestingly, similar clinical syndromes have frequently been described in a large variety of animal species.

Diagnosis

The diagnostic approach to infection with *T. gondii* depends on the clinical presentation and patient's immune status.[1,27] Indirect detection – widely used in immunocompetent patients – is achieved by serological methods, whereas direct detection is commonly performed in immunocompromised patients by isolation of the parasite, demonstration of the organism by polymerase chain reaction and/or demonstration in tissue sections by histology. The presence of IgG antibodies is further used to indicate immune protection against primary infection in pregnant women prior to or early in pregnancy, and to identify those immunocompromised patients at risk for reactivation of latent infection. A variety of serological tests including the Sabin–Feldman dye test, the immunofluorescent antibody test, enzyme-linked immunosorbent assay (ELISA), and IgG avidity test are used for the detection of IgG antibodies that arise within 1–2 weeks after infection and persist for the life of the individual. Tests for the avidity (functional affinity) of IgG antibodies have become standard to determine the time of infection (recent or distant). The IgM ELISA and IgM immunosorbent agglutination assay (ISAGA) detect IgM antibodies that arise within the first week of infection, rapidly rise to later decrease and disappear at highly variable rates. A negative IgM test result essentially rules out recently acquired infection. Combinations of serological tests allow a better assessment of the stage of infection. Local antibody production in the eye has been used successfully for the diagnosis of ocular toxoplasmosis.

DIRECT DETECTION

Quantitative PCR amplification of multi-copy genes of *T. gondii* in body fluids and tissues has successfully been used to diagnose congenital, ocular, cerebral and disseminated toxoplasmosis. The sensitivity of PCR depends on the appropriateness of sample handling, shipping and storage conditions, particular technique used for amplification and detection of PCR products and by prior use of anti-*T.-gondii*-specific drugs. PCR has enabled the early diagnosis of congenital infection in the fetus from amniotic fluid, thereby avoiding the use of more invasive procedures on the fetus. Peripheral blood, cerebrospinal fluid and urine have been used to assist in the diagnosis of congenital toxoplasmosis in the newborn. Parasite detection by PCR in vitreous or aqueous fluid establishes the diagnosis in patients with atypical retinal lesions, suboptimal responses to anti-*Toxoplasma* therapy, or in immunocompromised patients. Blood (buffy coat), and affected body fluids including bronchoalveolar lavage, cerebrospinal, pleural, ascitic, peritoneal or ocular fluids, bone marrow aspirate, and tissues have been used to detect parasite DNA; however, a positive PCR result in brain tissue will not differentiate between parasite DNA associated with toxoplasmic encephalitis or parasite DNA (in cysts) in dormant infections. Isolation of the parasite can be performed by mouse inoculation or inoculation in cell cultures using any human tissue or body fluid. Detection of tachyzoites in tissue sections and body fluid (e.g. BAL, CSF) by direct staining or immunostaining during primary acute infection or during reactivation establishes the diagnosis of toxoplasmosis.

Management and Therapy

INFECTION IN THE IMMUNOCOMPETENT HOST

Toxoplasmic Lymphadenitis

Toxoplasmic lymphadenitis in immunocompetent adults and children is most often diagnosed by characteristic histological changes in lymph node biopsies and a panel of serological tests (IgG, IgM, IgG avidity).[28] Most patients do not require treatment with antiparasitic drugs unless symptoms are severe or persistent. If required, treatment is usually administered for 2–4 weeks, followed by reassessment of the patient's condition. The combination of pyrimethamine, sulfadiazine, and folinic acid for 4–6 weeks is the most common drug combination used (Table 48.4).

Maternal and Fetal Infection

Tests for IgG and IgM antibodies should be obtained before or early in pregnancy as screening tools since the absence of IgG antibodies prior to or early in pregnancy identifies women at risk for primary infection during pregnancy.[29] IgM antibodies may indicate primary infection but are known to persist in a significant percentage of women; negative results in test for IgM antibodies during the first two trimesters essentially rule out a recently acquired infection unless sera are obtained so early that an IgM antibody response is not yet detectable. Confirmatory testing performed at reference laboratories (using a battery of tests including dye test and differential agglutination test, IgM, IgA and IgE ELISA) helps to determine the time of infection, while communication of results and their correct interpretation has been shown to decrease the rate of unnecessary abortions. The presence of high-avidity (functional affinity) antibodies within the first 3–4 months of pregnancy allows ruling out an infection acquired during pregnancy.[30] The definitive diagnosis of acute *Toxoplasma* infection or toxoplasmosis during pregnancy requires demonstration of a rise in titres in serial specimens (either conversion from a negative to a positive titre or a significant rise from a low to a higher titre). However, without systematic screening during pregnancy these serial results are not available. Therefore, treatment of women with suspected or confirmed acute acquired infection using spiramycin is recommended before 18 weeks of gestation to reduce the frequency of fetal infection.[25] It has been estimated that

TABLE 48.4 **Antiparasitic Treatment of Infection with *T. Gondii***

	Drug	Dosage	Duration
Acute infection	No antiparasitic treatment[a]		
Acute infection in pregnancy before 18 weeks' gestation[b]	Spiramycin	3 g daily in 3 divided doses without food	Until term or until fetal infection is documented
Documented fetal infection (after 17 weeks' gestation)[b]	Pyrimethamine	Loading dose of 50 mg every 12 hours for 2 days, followed by 50 mg per day	Until term
	plus sulfadiazine	Loading dose of 75 mg/kg, followed by 50 mg/kg every 12 hours (max. 4 g daily)	Until term
	plus folinic acid	5–20 mg daily	During and for 1 week after pyrimethamine therapy
Congenital toxoplasmosis in the infant	Pyrimethamine	Loading dose of 1 mg/kg every 12 hours for 2 days, then 1 mg/kg daily for 2–6 months, then this dose every Monday, Wednesday, Friday	1 year
	plus sulfadiazine	50 mg/kg every 12 hours	1 year
	plus folinic acid	10 mg 3 times weekly	During and for 1 week after pyrimethamine therapy
	Prednisolone[c]	1 mg/kg daily (in the morning)	Until resolution of signs and symptoms
Toxoplasmic retinochoroiditis in adults	Pyrimethamine	Loading dose of 200 mg, then 50–75 mg daily	Usually 1–2 weeks after resolution of symptoms
	plus sulfadiazine	Oral 1–1.5 g every 6 hours	Usually 1–2 weeks after resolution of symptoms
	plus folinic acid	5–20 mg 3 times weekly	During and for 1 week after pyrimethamine therapy
	Prednisone[c]	1 mg/kg daily (in the morning)	Until resolution of signs and symptoms
Acute/primary therapy of TE in patients with AIDS	Pyrimethamine	Oral 200 mg loading dose, then 50 to75 mg daily	At least 4–6 weeks after resolution of signs and symptoms (see text)
	plus folinic acid	Oral, I.V., or I.M. 10–20 mg daily (up to 50 mg daily)	During and for 1 week after pyrimethamine therapy
	plus sulfadiazine	Oral 1–1.5 g every 6 hours	[d]
	or clindamycin	Oral or I.V. 600 mg every 6 hours (up to I.V. 1200 mg every 6 hours)	[d]

[a]If signs or symptoms are severe or persist, pyrimethamine/sulfadiazine and leucovorin are initiated.
[b]Practises vary widely between centres.
[c]When cerebrospinal protein is ≥1 g/dl and when active retinochoroiditis threatens vision.
[d]Duration of treatment as for pyrimethamine in patient with TE.
Modified after Montoya and Liesenfeld. Lancet 2004;363:1965–76.

spiramycin reduces the incidence of vertical transmission by approximately 60%; the efficacy of spiramycin is under debate since the design of studies performed to date has not permitted a definitive conclusion. Therapy should be initiated as soon as possible after diagnosis of recently acquired maternal infection using spiramycin (for 1st and early 2nd trimesters) or pyrimethamine/sulfadiazine (for late 2nd and 3rd trimesters) for women with suspected or confirmed acute *T. gondii* infection acquired during gestation (Table 48.4). Maternal infection does not in all cases result in fetal infection. Therefore, suspected or established maternal infection acquired during gestation (based on ultrasonography or serology) must be confirmed by prenatal diagnosis of fetal infection using PCR on amniotic fluid; the sensitivity of PCR ranges from 60% to 99% and is highest after 16 weeks of infection. In case of a negative PCR result, spiramycin is continued throughout pregnancy, or is followed by a 4-week course of pyrimethamine plus sulfadiazine at 17 weeks' gestation. In case of a positive PCR result or very highly probable infection of the fetus (i.e. acquisition of the maternal infection in late 2nd or 3rd trimesters), treatment is continued throughout pregnancy and consists of pyrimethamine/sulfadiazine (in some countries pyrimethamine/sulfadiazine and spiramycin regimens are alternated). Prenatal treatment with pyrimethamine/sulfadiazine reduces the sequelae of disease in the newborn. Folinic (not folic) acid is added to reduce bone marrow suppression observed with pyrimethamine therapy; careful monitoring for haematotoxicity is mandatory. Ultrasound should be performed at least monthly until term if the initial examination revealed no abnormalities; the presence of hydrocephalus has been used as an indication for termination of the pregnancy.

Since up to 85% of newborns will have no signs or symptoms of congenital toxoplasmosis at birth, serology is commonly performed for the diagnosis in all newborns born to mothers who acquire their primary infection during gestation. *Toxoplasma*-specific IgG antibodies in the newborn may reflect maternal and/or the newborn's own antibodies. However, detection of IgG antibodies after 1 year of life is establishing the diagnosis since maternally transferred IgG antibodies decline and disappear within 6–12 months. The combination of highly sensitive tests for IgM (ISAGA or ELISA) and IgA (ELISA) identifies up to 75% of infected newborns. In newborns with suspected congenital toxoplasmosis with positive IgG but negative IgM and IgA tests results, IgG/IgM Western blots of mother–infant pairs should be used.

Tests for the direct demonstration of *T. gondii* (PCR, cell culture, mouse inoculation) in cerebrospinal fluid, blood, and urine can be combined with ophthalmological testing, radiological studies, and examination of cerebrospinal fluid to aid in the diagnosis of congenital disease.[11] Treatment of the newborn throughout the first year of life consists of the combination of pyrimethamine/sulfadiazine and has proven effective; folinic acid is always added to the regimen to avoid bone marrow toxicity (Table 48.4). Drug levels and effects on bone marrow should be monitored at pre-determined time points throughout therapy. The presence of IgG antibodies at the end of the first year of life typically confirms the diagnosis of congenital infection while the absence of IgG antibodies throughout the first year of life rules out infection; however, antiparasitic treatment may render antibodies undetectable.

Retinochoroiditis

The ophthalmologist typically makes the decision to treat active toxoplasmic retinochoroiditis based on results of eye examination that reveal characteristic lesions rather than based on results of antibody tests. In adults the distinction between recurrences of congenital infection with the parasite and postnatally acquired infection is often impossible. Low titres of IgG but not IgM antibody are present in patients with active retinochoroiditis due to reactivation of congenital infection. Patients with retinochoroiditis due to postnatally acquired disease more frequently have serological test results consistent with a recently acquired infection. Most ophthalmologists would recommend treatment if severe inflammatory responses and/or proximity of retinal lesions to the fovea or optic disk are observed. The combination of pyrimethamine, sulfadiazine, and prednisone is the most commonly used regimen (Table 48.4); clindamycin or trimethoprim/sulfamethoxazole (TMP/SMX) have also been used with favourable clinical results. Because toxoplasmic retinochoroiditis can be self-limited in immunocompetent individuals, many clinicians may not treat small, peripheral retinal lesions that are not immediately vision-threatening. Long-term intermittent treatment of recurrent toxoplasmic retinochoroiditis with TMP/SMX significantly reduced the frequency of recurrence. If ophthalmological examination does not provide characteristic retinal lesions, or suboptimal treatment responses are observed, detection of an abnormal *T. gondii*-specific antibody response in ocular fluids compared with serum (Goldman–Witmer coefficient) and/or detection of parasite DNA by PCR have proven helpful to establish the diagnosis.

INFECTION IN THE IMMUNOCOMPROMISED HOST

Toxoplasma Encephalitis

Generalized Infection. Physicians caring for severely immunocompromised patients (i.e. bone marrow transplant or AIDS patients) should have a baseline *Toxoplasma* IgG test result available for their patients. Transplant patients who are more likely to acquire their *T. gondii* infection via the allograft need to have the donor and the recipient tested for a baseline *Toxoplasma* IgG test (i.e. heart, lung, heart-lung, kidney transplant patients). The setting of a seropositive donor (D+)/seronegative recipient (R–) represent the highest risk for disease in these patients. TMP/SMZ prophylaxis is highly effective in this setting. Recipients from D–/R–, D–/R+ or D+/R+ pairs rarely develop toxoplasmosis. When reactivated (cerebral) toxoplasmosis is suspected treatment must be started independent of the diagnostic evaluation; direct tests for detection of the parasite rather than antibody-based tests should be used to establish the diagnosis in combination with neuroimaging studies such as computed tomography (CT) or magnetic resonance imaging (MRI) of the brain and/or spinal cord. A clinical and radiological response to specific anti-*T. gondii* therapy supports the diagnosis of CNS toxoplasmosis. Patients with cerebral toxoplasmosis usually improve more than 50% of their baseline neurological examination by days 7–10. The most commonly used and successful regimen is the combination of pyrimethamine/sulfadiazine and folinic acid administered for up to 4–6 weeks after resolution of signs and symptoms (Table 48.4). Clindamycin can be used instead of sulfadiazine in patients intolerant to TMP/SMZ. TMP/SMZ appears to be equivalent to pyrimethamine/sulfadiazine. The role of other drugs in combination with pyrimethamine, including atovaquone, clarithromycin, azithromycin, or dapsone is less well established.

After treatment of the acute phase, maintenance treatment (secondary prophylaxis) must be instituted. This is usually accomplished with the same regimen used in the acute phase but at half doses. Currently, maintenance therapy should be continued for the life of the patient or until the underlying immunosuppression has ceased. In patients with AIDS, secondary prophylaxis is generally discontinued when the patient's CD4 count has returned to above 200 cells/mm^3 following initiation of HAART and the HIV PCR peripheral blood viral load has been controlled for at least 6 months.

Prevention

Primary prevention is the strategy of choice in seronegative patients in order to avoid ingestion of the parasite. Therefore, public health measures should be key to attempt to diminish the burden of disease in humans and animals since the infection is acquired through ingestion of undercooked meat containing tissue cysts or food or water contaminated with oocysts. Epidemiological studies can help to identify the main sources of infection and to determine the focus of preventive education. In Europe, inadequately cooked or cured meat was identified as the main risk factor for infection whereas undetected contamination of food and water by oocysts most frequently caused human infections in North America.

Primary prophylaxis using TMP/SMX has proven effective in seropositive immunocompromised patients (e.g. patients with AIDS) or seronegative recipients of organ transplants from seropositive donors (e.g. heart transplant patients).

Secondary prevention is employed to prevent transmission from the acutely infected mother to her fetus using spiramycin and in immunocompromised patients following treatment of reactivated toxoplasmosis (maintenance therapy).

There are wide differences in public health policies to prevent congenital infection; however, data regarding the efficacy of such policies are lacking. Systematic serological screening of all pregnant women is common practice in a rather small number of countries. The uncertainty regarding the incidence of congenital infection, its cost-effectiveness, the significant problems with sensitivity and specificity of serological tests and the most recent studies suggesting lack of spiramycin efficacy have hampered attempts to implement screening programmes in a number of countries. Neonatal screening programmes have been successfully performed as a less costly alternative compared with systematic screening of pregnant women.

An effective vaccine against *T. gondii* infection in humans continues to be a desirable but elusive target. Only the attenuated live S48 strain of the parasite has been licensed for its use in sheep in Europe and New Zealand.

REFERENCES

1. Montoya JG, Liesenfeld O. Toxoplasmosis. Lancet 2004;363:1965–76.
2. Tenter AM, Heckeroth AR, Weiss LM. *Toxoplasma gondii*: from animals to humans. Int J Parasitol 2000;30:1217–58.
8. Robert-Gangneux F, Darde ML. Epidemiology of and diagnostic strategies for toxoplasmosis. Clin Microbiol Rev 2012;25:264–96.
16. Munoz M, Liesenfeld O, Heimesaat MM. Immunology of *Toxoplasma gondii*. Immunol Rev 2011;240(1):269–85.

Access the complete references online at www.expertconsult.com

49 Intestinal Protozoa

PAUL KELLY

KEY POINTS

- Pathogenic intestinal protozoa produce disease by infecting the small or large intestine, or both.
- Intestinal protozoa are found in highest prevalence in developing countries, where they are responsible for a substantial burden of disease.
- Health impacts vary with age: the small intestinal protozoa *Giardia intestinalis* and *Cryptosporidium* spp. have their major impact in children, while the large bowel pathogen *Entamoeba histolytica* infects all age groups with its most profound effects in adults.
- Understanding of epidemiology of intestinal protozoan infection is constantly evolving: new species are identified and taxonomy revised using molecular genetics.
- Some of the protozoa, particularly *Cryptosporidium* and *Isospora belli*, have a greatly increased morbidity in immunodeficiency states, whereas the severity of disease due to giardiasis and amoebiasis is little affected.
- As yet, there is no candidate vaccine for any of the intestinal protozoa.
- Chemotherapy is not straightforward and many cases are difficult to treat.

Introduction

This chapter deals with human intestinal protozoan infections, which are found worldwide in both developing countries and the industrialized world. Although the microsporidia have now been reclassified as fungi, they are dealt with in this chapter, as there are many common themes with disease caused by true protozoa.

The Sarcodina (Amoebae)

The subphylum Sarcodina is characterized by organisms that move by pseudopodia or by locomotive protoplasmic flow without discrete pseudopodia; flagella, when present, are usually restricted to developmental or other temporary stages. Most species are free living, such as *Acanthamoeba* and *Naegleria*. However, many species such as *Entamoeba histolytica*, *E. dispar*, *E. coli*, *E. hartmanni*, *E. gingivalis*, *Dientamoeba fragilis*, *Endolimax nana* and *Iodamoeba bütschlii* have been definitely established as parasites or commensals of humans. All inhabit the large intestine, except *E. gingivalis*, which is found in the mouth.

ENTAMOEBA HISTOLYTICA

Amoebiasis, the infection caused by the parasitic protozoan, *E. histolytica*, is a worldwide cause of much morbidity and mortality. The history of its understanding spans a century, and is an interesting story. Fedor Löch in St Petersburg in 1875,[1] first described the clinical and autopsy findings of a case of fatal dysentery and identified the amoeba. Although he was able to infect a dog with this organism, he was not able to mimic the disease produced in his patient and failed to recognize the relationship. In 1890, William Osler[2] reported the case of a young man who contracted dysentery and developed an hepatic abscess that led to his death. One year later, Councilman and Lafleur[3] conducted a detailed study of patients with amoebic dysentery and hepatic abscess. They confirmed the pathogenic role of amoebae and created the terms 'amoebic dysentery' and 'amoebic liver abscess'. Schaudinn[4] differentiated *E. histolytica* from *E. coli* in 1903. In 1913, Walker and Sellards[5] definitively established the pathogenicity of *E. histolytica* by feeding cysts to volunteers. Brumpt[6] in 1925 was the first to suggest that the differences in symptomatology and in the global distribution of invasive amoebiasis were due to the presence of two species of amoeba, morphologically indistinguishable one from another, but with different pathogenic potential. He suggested the term *E. dysenteriae* for the pathogenic amoeba and *E. dispar* for the non-pathogenic amoeba. Because Brumpt was unable to distinguish morphologically between the two proposed species and because there was growing evidence that cysts obtained from asymptomatic carriers could produce experimental infection, his explanation gained little support. It regained favour only after Sargeaunt and associates[7,8] were able to distinguish pathogenic strains of *E. histolytica* from non-pathogenic strains on the basis of isoenzyme typing. Since then, many other markers that allow the discrimination between both groups have been identified. In 1993, Diamond and Clark,[9] using biochemical, immunological and genetic evidence for distinguishing pathogenic from non-pathogenic strains of *E. histolytica*, re-described *E. histolytica* Schaudinn, 1903, formally separating it from *E. dispar* Brumpt, 1925. In 1997, a World Health Organization (WHO) expert committee endorsed the separation of pathogenic and non-pathogenic strains into two separate species.[10,11] It is now emerging that a third morphologically identical species, *E. moshkovskii* (also known as the Laredo strain), has also been confusing the understanding of amoebiasis for many years, and now with use of molecular-based tools, the epidemiology of amoebiasis is gradually becoming clearer.

Epidemiology

E. histolytica has a worldwide distribution and is endemic in most countries with low socioeconomic conditions. Before the separation of the 'non-pathogenic strains' into a different species, it was estimated that approximately 480 million people, or 12% of the world's population, were infected and 40 000–110 000 persons died anually.[12] In endemic areas, it is now clear that *E. dispar* is by far the more prevalent species. The risk of asymptomatic carriers of *E. histolytica* developing invasive disease is estimated at about 10%.[13] In Europe and North America, where invasive amoebiasis is rare, almost all infections previously ascribed to *E. histolytica* were in fact due to *E. dispar*. When these data are taken into account, it is more likely that less than 10% of the 480 million infections (approx. 40–50 million people) are infected with *E. histolytica*, whereas the rest have infections with *E. dispar* or *E. moshkovskii*.

Infection occurs via the faecal–oral route, food and drink becoming contaminated through exposure to human faeces. Food-borne outbreaks of disease are due to unsanitary handling of food and its preparation by infected individuals. Therefore, it is not surprising that prevalence is high in places where human faeces are used for fertilizer. Cyst carriers are the main reservoir of infection. Epidemics occur when raw sewage contaminates water supplies. Sexual transmission can also occur. Recognized high-risk groups include travellers, immigrants, migrant workers, immunocompromised individuals, individuals in mental institutions, prisons and, possibly, children in day-care centres. Severe infections occur in very young children, pregnant women, the malnourished and individuals taking corticosteroids. Patients with AIDS do not have an increased risk of severe infection. Recent attempts to re-write the epidemiology of amoebiasis, using molecular tools to distinguish *E. histolytica* from *E. dispar*, suggest that generalizations will be difficult and the relative frequency of these two amoebic infections will differ in different populations. In Australia the ratio of *histolytica* to *dispar* was 1 : 13,[14] but in Mexico it was 1.5 : 1,[15] and in Brazil all identifiable samples were *E. dispar*.[16]

An interesting recent attempt to define genetic risk factors for amoebiasis has demonstrated excess risk (about fourfold) conferred by the Q223R mutation in the leptin receptor gene.[17] Undoubtedly, new patterns of genetic susceptibility will emerge.

Pathogenesis

The complete life cycle of *E. histolytica* consists of four consecutive stages: the trophozoite, precyst, cyst and metacyst. The cyst is resistant to gastric acid, and on ingestion it passes into the small intestine. The amoeba within the cyst becomes active in the neutral or alkaline environment of the small intestine. The cyst wall is digested, probably by the digestive enzymes within the lumen of the gut. The encysted amoeba becomes very active and each of the four nuclei in the emerging *E. histolytica* undergoes one round of division, thus forming eight amoebae, smaller than the trophozoites seen in the colon, from a single cyst. They are carried into the caecum where they complete their maturation. They multiply by binary fission, the nucleus dividing by modified mitosis. As the amoebae pass down the colon they become dehydrated and assume a spherical shape known as a precyst. A thin cyst wall is secreted, forming an unripe cyst. Two mitotic divisions occur, resulting in a cyst that contains four nuclei. They are evacuated in the stool and discharged into the environment. Cysts remain viable and infective for several days in faeces and water, but are easily killed by desiccation.

E. histolytica has the capacity to destroy almost all tissues of the human body. The intestinal mucosa, the liver and, to a lesser extent, the brain and skin are affected most commonly. Even cartilage and bone can be eroded by *E. histolytica* trophozoites. Several virulence factors have been identified, such as adhesion molecules, contact-dependent cytolysis, proteases, haemolysins and phagocytic activity.

To produce damage, trophozoites must first colonize the colon. The presence of bacteria is essential for colonization as they provide an environment with low oxygen tension and probably supply other metabolic needs. Trophozoites then penetrate through the mucus layer and adhere to the host cells. *E. histolytica* enhances mucus secretion, alters its composition and depletes goblet cells of mucin, thereby making epithelial surfaces more vulnerable to invasion. The parasite also induces the expression of cathelicidin, an antimicrobial peptide to which *E. histolytica* is resistant through its cysteine protease,[18] which reduces competition. Once the mucus barrier has been broken down, *E. histolytica* reaches the luminal surface of enterocytes and initially produces a contact-dependent focal and superficial epithelial erosion. Trophozoites adhere to colonic mucins and host cells through the N-acetyl-d-galactosamine-inhibitable lectin, a 260-kDa protein also known as the Gal/GalNAc adherence lectin, composed of a 170-kDa and a 35/31-kDa subunit. The 170-kDa subunit is immunologically similar to the integrins.[19] Other molecules are involved in adhesion including a 220-kDa lectin, a 112-kDa adhesin and a surface lipophosphoglycan. The first contact of the trophozoite with the immune system is through the epithelial intestinal cells. *E. histolytica* stimulates human intestinal epithelial cells to secrete interleukin (IL)-8 and tumour necrosis factor (TNF)α.[20,21] Neutrophils are rapidly recruited and activated in response to the proinflammatory cytokine IL-8. Cell infiltration around invading amoebae leads to rapid lysis of inflammatory cells followed by tissue necrosis.

The primary pathogenetic event is host cell death: *E. histolytica* is well named. There are four steps in this pathway;[22]

- Lectin-mediated contact
- Calcium influx
- Tyrosine dephosphorylation
- Caspase 3 activation leading to the final steps of apoptosis.

The Gal/GalNAc adherence lectin is not directly cytotoxic but it is required for cytolysis as target cell lysis is reduced in the presence of galactose. Furthermore, a monoclonal antibody against the heavy subunit is capable of partially inhibiting cytolysis without blocking adherence. It has been suggested that cell lysis is produced through the channel-forming peptides of *E. histolytica* (amoebapores). Three isoforms have been identified, amoebapores A, B and C, which are present in a ratio of 35 : 10 : 1, with the genes showing 35–57% deduced amino acid sequence identity.[23] Like other pore-forming peptides, amoebapores are readily soluble but are capable of changing rapidly into a membrane-inserted stage. Oligomerization occurs by formation of a channel through the plasma membrane, allowing the passage of water, ions and other small molecules, and thus lysing the target cell. The presence of pore-forming activity in the non-pathogenic *E. dispar*, although 60% less potent, suggests that the primary function of amoebapores is to destroy phagocytosed bacteria.

During the invasion to deeper layers of the mucosa, trophozoites must lyse surrounding cells and degrade the extracellular matrix. Contact of trophozoites with the extracellular matrix induces the formation of adhesion plaques, containing actin filaments, vinculin, a-actinin, tropomyosin and myosin I. Binding to the extracellular matrix occurs through a 37-kDa fibronectin-binding protein and a 140-kDa integrin-like receptor, inducing a sustained rise of intracellular calcium concentration needed to reorganize the trophozoite cytoskeleton to form the adhesion plaque. In the absence of calcium, adhesion is poor. Contact of trophozoites with the extracellular matrix also induces the release of cysteine proteases and the content of electron-dense granules, which includes collagenase, two proteases and at least 25 other polypeptides. The array of cysteine proteases secreted by the trophozoite also degrades host defence molecules such as IgA, LL-37 and complement proteins.

Amoebae probably spread from the intestine to the liver through the portal circulation. The presence and extent of liver involvement bears no relationship to the degree of intestinal amoebiasis, and these conditions do not necessarily coincide. It is thought that liver damage is not caused directly by the amoebae but rather by the lysosomal enzymes of lysed polymorphonuclear neutrophils (PMNs) and monocytes that accumulate around the parasite. During experimental infection, hypocomplementaemic and leukopaenic animals demonstrate reduced amoebic-induced liver damage when compared with normal animals. In severe cases, especially in patients treated with corticosteroids, amoebic trophozoites can be found in virtually every organ of the body, including the brain, lungs and eyes.

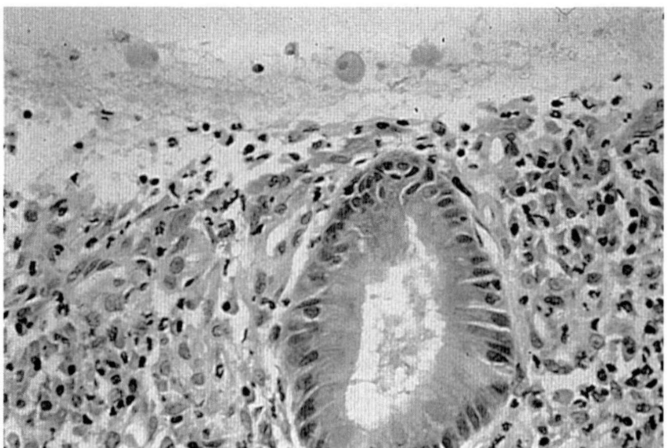

Figure 49.1 Colonic mucosa showing superficial ulceration with amoebic invasion, (H&E; ×400). *(Courtesy of Paola Domizio, Department of Morbid Anatomy, St Bartholomew's Hospital, London.)*

Clinical Features

The clinical spectrum of *E. histolytica* infection ranges from an asymptomatic carrier state or acute colitis, to fulminant colitis with perforation. Asymptomatic cyst carriage of *E. histolytica* is well documented. The majority will clear the infection spontaneously. An epidemiological study in a semirural area in South Africa showed that 90% of asymptomatic carriers of pathogenic *E. histolytica* zymodemes cleared the infection within a year; the remaining 10% developed amoebic colitis.[13]

Intestinal Amoebiasis (Table 49.1)**.** The onset is insidious, except in fulminating cases, with abdominal discomfort, loose motions or frank diarrhoea, not necessarily with blood or excessive mucus. In more severe cases, the stools rapidly become bloodstained with mucus. Tenesmus occurs in half of the patients and is always associated with rectosigmoid involvement. Constitutional symptoms are not prominent. On physical examination tenderness may be localized anywhere in the lower abdomen but is usually over the caecum, transverse colon or sigmoid. Rectosigmoidoscopy and colonoscopy of mild or moderate cases usually reveals the presence of small ulcers (3–5 mm in diameter) which most frequently involve the caecum and rectum but may be scattered throughout the colon and are especially numerous in the region of the flexures. The ulcers are initially superficial with hyperaemic borders and a necrotic base covered with a yellowish exudate. There is normal mucosa between sites of invasion. However, diffuse inflammation has also been described, making firm diagnosis on gross appearance difficult. On rare occasions involvement of the blood vessels at the base of the ulcer may produce brisk bleeding. More rarely, an ulcer may perforate leading to peritonitis. Extensive inflammatory polyposis has been demonstrated as a complication of amoebic colitis and this may be a source of confusion with idiopathic inflammatory bowel disease. Acute amoebic dysentery must be differentiated from bacterial colitis caused by *Shigella* spp., *Salmonella* spp., *Campylobacter jejuni*, enteroinvasive and enterohaemorrhagic *Escherichia coli*, *Yersinia enterocolitica* and *Balantidium coli*.

TABLE 49.1 **Symptoms and Findings in Acute Amoebic Colitis**

	(%)
Symptoms	
Duration of symptoms (weeks)	
0–1	48
2–4	37
>4	15
Diarrhoea	100
Dysentery	99
Abdominal pain	85
Low back pain	66
Physical Findings	
Fever	38
Abdominal tenderness	83

From Adams EB, MacLeod IN. Invasive amebiasis. I. Amebic dysentery and its complications. Medicine 1977;56:315–23.

In surgical specimens ulcers look flat and oval in shape, without induration of the underlying bowel wall. Histologically, there is nonspecific diffuse inflammation around the superficial ulcerations. As the disease advances, the classically described flask-shaped ulcers with undermined edges are formed. The lamina propria is infiltrated by plasma cells, lymphocytes, neutrophils and eosinophils. There is oedema and focal haemorrhage. The infiltrate also involves the surface epithelium, and frequently there is an overlying exudate within which trophozoites may be found (Figure 49.1).

Fulminant colitis is the result of confluent ulceration and necrosis of the colon. The clinical picture is virtually indistinguishable from that of fulminant ulcerative colitis. The bowel is dilated, particularly in its transverse portion. The patient is extremely febrile and toxic, and shows signs of hypovolaemia and electrolyte imbalance. Despite the severity of the illness, amoebae may not be readily recovered from the stools of these patients. Surgical specimens reveal extensive areas of necrosis within which some patches of intact hyperaemic mucosa are found.

An amoeboma, or amoebic granuloma, may result from repeated invasion of the colon by *E. histolytica*, complicated by pyogenic infection. Amoebomas may be found anywhere in the colon but are more frequent at the caecum (40%) and rectosigmoid junction (20%). These mass lesions are often mistaken for malignancy and may occasionally be palpable.

TABLE 49.2 Symptoms and Findings in Amoebic Liver Abscess

	(%)
Symptoms	
Duration of symptoms (weeks)	
<2	37–66
2–4	20–40
4–12	16–42
>12	5–11
Pain	90
Diarrhoea and/or dysentery	14–66
Weight loss	33–53
Cough	10–32
Dyspnoea	4
Physical Findings	
Localized tenderness	80–95
Enlarged liver	43–93
Fever	75–98
Rales, rhonchi	8–47
Localized intercostal tenderness	40
Epigastric tenderness	22
Swelling over the liver	10
Jaundice	10–25
Laboratory Findings	
Increased bilirubin	10–25
White blood cell count >10×10^{9}/L	63–94
Raised transaminases	26–50
Raised alkaline phosphatase	38–84
Increased erythrocyte sedimentation rate	81

Amoebic Liver Abscess (Table 49.2). This is the most common extraintestinal form of invasive amoebiasis. Amoebic abscesses may be found in all age groups, but are 10 times more frequent in adults than in children, and are more frequent in males than in females. They are more common in the poorest sectors or urban populations. Approximately 20% of patients have a past history of dysentery. About 10% of patients have diarrhoea or dysentery at the time of diagnosis of amoebic liver abscess. The parasite can be detected in faeces by standard microscopy in less than 50% of cases, though recent molecular tests have increased this substantially (see below). The onset of symptoms is usually abrupt, with pain in the upper abdomen and high fever. The pain is intense and constant, radiating to the scapular region and right shoulder; it increases with deep breathing or coughing, or when the patient rests on the right side. When the abscess is localized on the left lobe, pain occurs on the left side of the abdomen and may radiate to the left shoulder. Localized tenderness in the region of the abscess, most commonly at the lower right intercostal spaces, is frequent even in the absence of diffuse liver pain. Fever is present in most cases; it varies between 38°C and 40°C, frequently in spikes but sometimes constant over several days, with rigors and profuse sweating. Anorexia, weight loss, nausea, vomiting and fatigue may all be present. On physical examination the cardinal sign of amoebic liver abscess is painful hepatomegaly. Digital pressure will often produce intense pain in the liver region. On palpation the liver is soft and smooth. Hepatomegaly may not be detected in patients with amoebic abscess of the dome of the liver because the enlargement is upward. Mild jaundice is quite common, but severe obstructive jaundice is rare. Amoebic abscess and cirrhosis may coexist, so a hard liver does not exclude the diagnosis. Movement of the right side of the chest and diaphragm is restricted and there is hypoventilation of the right lower lobe of the lung. The presentation may be so abrupt that it can be confused with an acute surgical abdomen.

Lesions are usually single and most are found in the right lobe of the liver. The incidence of amoebic abscess of the left lobe ranges from 5% to 21%. The liver abscess has a thin capsular wall with a necrotic centre composed of a thick fluid, an intermediate zone of coarse stroma and an outer zone of nearly normal tissue. Typically, abscess fluid is odourless, resembling 'chocolate syrup' or 'anchovy paste', and bacteriologically sterile, although secondary bacterial invasion may occur. Microscopic examination of the abscess fluid reveals granular eosinophilic debris with no or few cells; amoebae tend to be located at the periphery of the abscess, and in fact the term 'abscess' is a misnomer as the 'pus' is better described as liquefied liver (Figure 49.2). Liver abscesses may heal, rupture or disseminate. The mortality rate has been estimated to be around 0.2–2.0% in adults and up to 26% in children.

Peritoneal Amoebiasis. This is caused by the rupture of a hepatic liver abscess or, less frequently, by perforation of the caecum. It is characterized by a sudden increase in abdominal pain, frequently generalized, which resembles that of septic peritonitis. A plain abdominal radiograph usually reveals the presence of free air in the peritoneal cavity. In some instances the perforation may be localized.

Pericardial Amoebiasis. Pericardial involvement is the most serious complication of an amoebic liver abscess. It occurs in less than 1% of all amoebic liver abscesses, especially of the left lobe. Although there may be a presuppurative stage that is associated with a sterile effusion, perforation of the abscess into the pericardium is usually followed by progressive tamponade or the sudden development of shock. Although the mortality rate from pericardial involvement has decreased from more than 90% to less than 40%, it is still frequently necessary to perform open drainage because of the development of loculations and thickened pericardium.

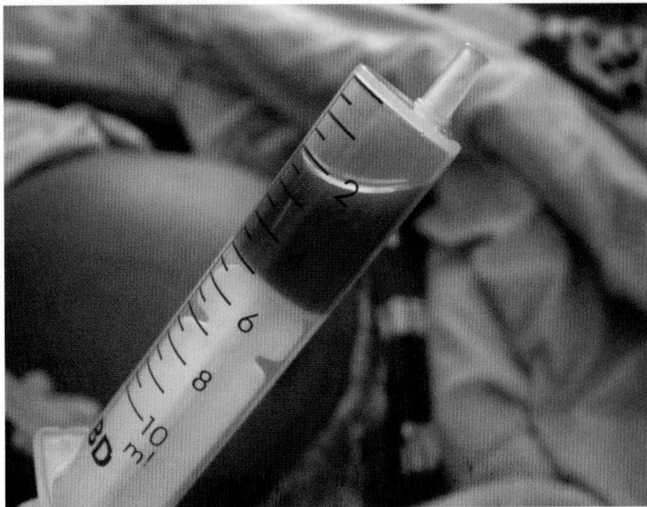

Figure 49.2 'Pus' aspirated from amoebic liver abscess in a recent case in Zambia.

Pleuropulmonary Amoebiasis. Invasion of the pleural cavity or the lung parenchyma is most commonly due to extension from a liver abscess and occurs in less than 1% of those with amoebic dysentery,[24] in 3% of all autopsies on people dying from amoebiasis and in 15% of patients with liver abscess. Haematogenous spread is rare. The first clinical symptoms are those of the liver abscess, followed by severe pain in the lower chest, often radiating to the right shoulder. There may be dyspnoea and non-productive cough. Broncho-hepatic fistulas are characterized by expectoration of large amounts of dark brown material. Superimposed bacterial infections are common.

Cerebral Amoebiasis. Cerebral involvement has been documented in 1.2–2.5% of patients who have amoebiasis at autopsy, but in less than 0.1% of patients whose cases are reported in studies of large clinical series. Although the symptoms of cerebral amoebiasis depend on the site and size of the lesion, as many as 50% of patients may have abrupt onset of symptoms and die from cerebellar involvement or rupture within 12–72 hours.

Genitourinary Amoebiasis. Renal amoebiasis, a rare complication of amoebic liver abscess, is thought to occur by rupture of a hepatic abscess, haematogenous spread from lesions in the liver or lungs, or extension through the lymphatics. Patients who have renal amoebiasis usually respond well to aspiration and medical therapy. Genital lesions also occur infrequently and are usually caused by fistulas from a liver abscess or rectocolitis. Typically, lesions are painful punched-out ulcers with profuse discharge. Medical treatment is usually sufficient for resolution of the lesions.

Cutaneous Amoebiasis. This results from perforation of an abscess or intestine into the skin. It may also develop from surgical wounds infected secondarily with an internal amoebic lesion or in the perineal–genital area. Histologically, there is ulceration with extensive necrosis in the base, pseudoepitheliomatous hyperplasia at the margins, and a non-specific inflammatory infiltrate extending into the deep dermis and subcutaneous tissues beneath the ulcer base.

Diagnosis

Microbiology. The time-honoured diagnostic test is stool microscopy. However, this requires fresh stool and a high degree of skill on the part of the microscopist, and it is insensitive as wet mount preparations will be positive in only 10% of cases.[25] But it remains true that the gold standard of diagnosis is the finding of haematophagous trophozoites (i.e. trophozoites which have phagocytosed red blood cells) as this is seen only with *E. histolytica*. In fresh isolates, *E. histolytica* can move as fast as 5 µm per second. Trophozoites move by means of pseudopodia, cytoplasmic protrusions that may be formed at any point on the surface of the organism. The precyst amoebae are colourless, round or oval cells that are smaller than the trophozoite but larger than the cyst. They may be distinguished by a rounded single nucleus, absence of ingested material and lack of a cyst wall.

While cysts in stool are strongly suggestive of amoebiasis, their presence does not confirm that they are pathogenic and cysts of *E. dispar* and *E. moshkovskii* are morphologically indistinguishable. The cysts are round or oval, slightly asymmetrical hyaline bodies, 10–16 mm in diameter, with a smooth, refractive, non-staining wall about 0.5 mm thick. The immature cyst has a single nucleus, about one-third of its diameter, whereas the mature infective cyst contains four smaller nuclei, rarely more.

Stool Antigen and Molecular Tests. There are at least five commercially available test kits for detection of *E. histolytica* antigens in stool samples.[26,27] The stated sensitivities and specificities of these kits all exceed 90%, but compared against the rather insensitive 'gold standard' of axenic culture. However, if molecular techniques are used as the gold standard, the sensitivity and specificity fall to 62.5% and 96.5%, respectively.[27] We are then faced with an old dilemma: what is the 'gold standard', against which these other tests should be evaluated? Is it useful to detect ever less intense infections at the expense of cost and laboratory time? There is no easy answer to this, though statistical analyses may help,[28] but there is an emerging consensus that the antigen tests are useful screening tests, and in the context of a clinical picture which is compatible with clinical amoebiasis they can be relied upon to confirm a diagnosis with sufficient usefulness to permit therapy. The big breakthrough in molecular diagnosis has been the advent of simple DNA extraction techniques using miniature separation columns which allow DNA to be separated from the large number of PCR inhibitors in faeces, such as bile salts. Multiplex panels of diagnostic tests can be run on small samples and the next few years will see the emergence of established protocols for this approach.

Blood Tests – General. In mild cases of colitis, laboratory tests are normal. Leucocytosis is present in severe disease. About 75% of patients with amoebic liver abscesses have a white blood cell count $>10\times10^9$/L. Eosinophilia is not associated with extraintestinal amoebiasis. Anaemia is common, particularly in patients who have chronic amoebic liver abscesses. The level of alkaline phosphatase is raised in more than 75% of patients, particularly in those with long-standing disease. Levels of transaminases may be increased in 50% of cases, especially in patients with acute disease or complications. The levels of transaminases usually return to normal soon after therapy is initiated, although alkaline phosphatase concentration may remain raised for several months.

Blood Tests – Specific. Serology is very useful in the diagnosis of amoebiasis, particularly in non-endemic areas. A specific antibody response is present in 85–95% of patients with invasive disease, but in endemic areas many patients with recent infection, or with asymptomatic infection, will also have positive serology. Virtually all known serological tests have been employed to detect anti-amoebic antibody, including immunofluorescent antibody tests, indirect haemagglutination assays (IHAs), radio-immunoassay, countercurrent immunoelectrophoresis and enzyme-linked immunosorbent assays (ELISAs). ELISAs are the most sensitive and for all intents and purposes do not give false-negative results in patients with amoebic liver abscesses.[26] The results of serological tests may be negative in patients who present acutely and should be repeated in 5–7 days. Serological responses measured by agar gel diffusion, countercurrent immunoelectrophoresis and ELISA usually become negative within 6–12 months, although they may persist for more than 3 years. However, results of IHAs may remain positive for more than 10 years after clinical and parasitological cure, even in the absence of reinfection. Therefore these tests should be interpreted with caution as antibody may be present for prolonged periods, and in areas of high endemicity a high prevalence of seropositivity already exists. Clinical laboratories should interpret serological tests in the light of local epidemiology.

Radiology and Endoscopy. In the acutely ill patient, the first investigation should be a plain abdominal radiograph to check for colonic dilatation. If this is present, surgery must be considered (the criteria for intervention are exactly the same as in acute severe ulcerative colitis) and further imaging investigations are unwise until it is clear that the situation is resolving. Endoscopically, ulcers are initially shallow but may deepen and assume a 'collar-button' or flasked-shaped appearance. Radiological changes in the colon seen by double-contrast barium studies consist of mucosal oedema, haustral blunting and ulceration, usually localized to one part of the colon.

Amoebomas manifest as an intraluminal mass, an annular lesion or irregularity of the bowel wall with lack of normal distensibility. Differential diagnosis with carcinoma may be difficult; rapid disappearance of the lesion after treatment favours the diagnosis.

In patients with hepatic involvement, plain radiography of the thorax may reveal elevation of the right hemidiaphragm, pleural reaction obscuring the right costophrenic angle. Radiologically, unruptured abscesses do not show a fluid level, and calcification of the liver parenchyma is rare. Ultrasonography, the most important investigation of all in suspected hepatic amoebiasis, typically reveals a round or oval hypoechoic area that is contiguous to the liver capsule and without significant wall echoes (Figure 49.3). Computed tomography and magnetic resonance imaging are also sensitive studies for demonstrating amoebic liver abscesses (Figure 49.4). More than 80% of patients who have symptoms of an abscess for more than 10 days have a single lesion of the right lobe of the liver, while 50% of patients who present acutely may have multiple lesions. Abscesses resolve slowly and may increase in size during the first few weeks after therapy, even with successful treatment. The ultrasonographic abnormalities resolve within 6 months in two-thirds of the patients with amoebic liver abscess; however, 10% remain abnormal for more than 1 year after treatment. The differential diagnosis includes pyogenic liver abscess, gallbladder disease and sepsis.

Management

Two classes of drugs are used in the treatment of amoebic infections. Luminal amoebicides, such as diloxanide furoate and iodoquinol, act on organisms in the intestinal lumen and are not effective against organisms in tissue. Tissue amoebicides, such as metronidazole, tinidazole, nitazoxanide, dehydroemetine and chloroquine, are effective in the treatment of invasive amoebiasis but less effective in the treatment of organisms in the bowel lumen (Table 49.3).

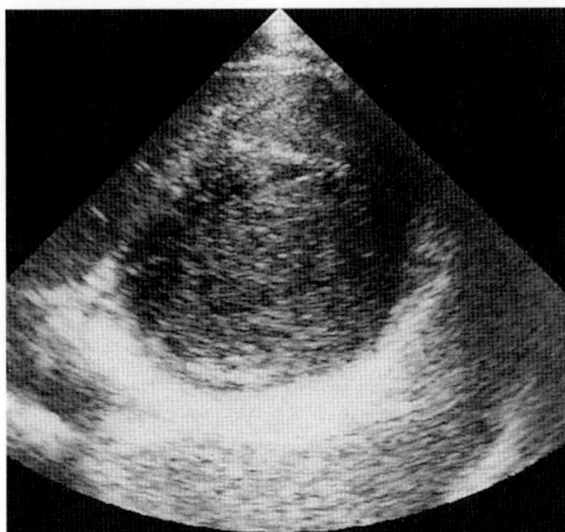

Figure 49.3 Liver ultrasonogram demonstrating an amoebic hepatic abscess. *(Courtesy of Alison McLean.)*

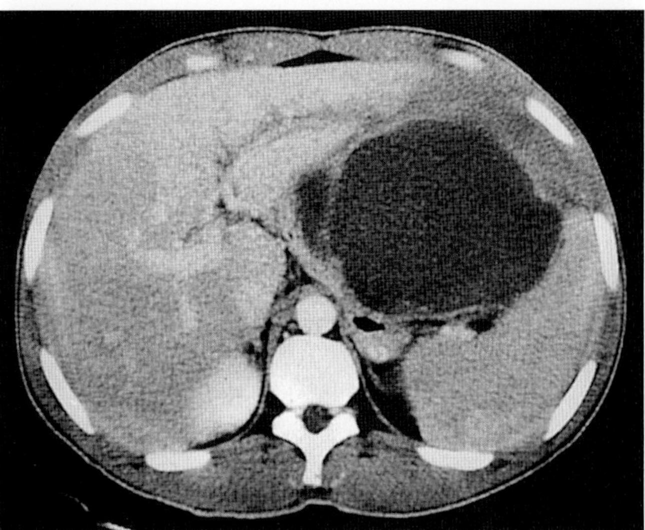

Figure 49.4 Computed tomogram of the liver demonstrating a left lobe amoebic abscess. *(Courtesy of Alison McLean.)*

Asymptomatic patients do not necessarily require treatment. However, intuitively a clinician may feel it wise to treat confirmed cases of *E. histolytica* but not *E. dispar* infection in order to prevent secondary transmission. There is no evidence to guide this decision. Metronidazole or tinidazole are the drugs of choice for amoebic colitis as they are very effective against the trophozoite; however, they have little effect on the cyst and therefore treatment should be followed by a luminal agent such as diloxanide furoate. Other imidazole compounds such as ornidazole or secnidazole may be used, and nitazoxanide has also been evaluated for therapy.

Liver Abscess. Metronidazole or tinidazole followed by diloxanide furoate is the treatment of choice. The potential cardiovascular and gastrointestinal adverse effects of dehydroemetine and emetine limit their use, and they are used only as second-line treatment. Higher relapse rates are associated with chloroquine than with other therapeutic agents. Aspiration of the abscess is advisable in specific situations (Box 49.1). Surgery should be reserved for patients with rupture of the abscess, with bacterial superinfection, or when an abscess that needs

BOX 49.1 INDICATIONS FOR ASPIRATION OF AMOEBIC LIVER ABSCESS

FORMAL INDICATIONS

- To rule out a pyogenic abscess, particularly with multiple lesions
- As adjunct to medical therapy (no response after 72 hours)
- If rupture is believed to be imminent
- Abscess in the left lobe where the risk of rupture is increased

POSSIBLE INDICATIONS

- To reduce the period of disability (further trials are necessary to confirm this indication)

TABLE 49.3 **Treatment of Amoebiasis**

	Drug/s	Adult Dosage	Paediatric Dosage (mg/kg daily)
Asymptomatic Intestinal Carrier			
1st choice	diloxanide furoate	500 mg 3 times a day ×10 days	20 (divided in 3 doses ×10 days)
2nd choice	paromomycin	25–30 mg/kg daily in 3 doses ×7–10 days	25–30 (divided in 3 doses ×7–10 days)
	OR		
	iodoquinol	650 mg 3 times a day ×20 days	20–40 (divided in 3 doses ×20 days)
Intestinal Infection			
1st choice	metronidazole followed by	750–800 mg 3 times a day ×10 days	35–50 (divided in 3 doses ×10 days)
	diloxanide furoate[a]	500 mg 3 times a day ×10 days	20 (divided in 3 doses ×10 days)
	OR		
	tinidazole followed by	2 g/day ×2–3 days	50–60 (×3 days)
	diloxanide furoate[a]	500 mg 3 times a day ×10 days	20 (divided in 3 doses ×10 days)
	OR		
	nitazoxanide followed by	500 mg bd ×10 days	100 mg bd (age 1–3 years) 200 mg bd (age 4–11 years)
	diloxanide furoate[a]	500 mg 3 times a day ×10 days	20 (divided in 3 doses ×10 days)
2nd choice	paromomycin	25–30 mg/kg daily in 3 doses ×7–10 days	25–30 (divided in 3 doses ×7–10 days)
Amoebic Liver Abscess			
1st choice	metronidazole followed by	750–800 mg 3 times a day ×10 days	35–50 (divided in 3 doses ×7–10 days
	diloxanide furoate[a]	500 mg 3 times a day ×10 days	20 (divided in 3 doses ×10 days)
	OR		
	tinidazole followed by	2 g/day ×3–5 days	50–60 (×5 days)
	diloxanide furoate[a]	500 mg 3 times a day ×10 days	20 (divided in 3 doses ×10 days)
2nd choice	dehydroemetine followed by	1–1.5 mg/kg daily (max. 90 mg/day) IV ×5 days	1 (×10 days maximum)
	diloxanide furoate[a]	500 mg 3 times a day ×10 days	20 (divided in 3 doses ×10 days)

[a]Paromomycin or iodoquinol may be used as an alternative to diloxanide furoate.

drainage cannot be approached percutaneously for anatomical reasons.

Prevention

The control of invasive amoebiasis could be achieved through improvement of living standards and the establishment of adequate sanitary conditions in countries where the disease is prevalent. Methods of attack should aim at: (1) the community, through the improvement of environmental sanitation including water supply, adequate disposal of faeces, food safety and health education to prevent faecal–oral transmission; and (2) the individual, through early detection and treatment in cases of infection and disease.

Cysts remain viable and infective for several days in faeces and may survive in soil for at least 8 days at 34–38°C, and for 1 month at 10°C. They also remain infective in fresh water, sea water, sewage and wet soil. Cysts survive for up to 45 minutes in faecal material lodged under the fingernails but are killed within 1 minute by desiccation on the surface of the hands. Amoebic cysts are destroyed by exposure to 200 parts per million of iodine, 5–10% acetic acid, and heating at a temperature above 68°C. They can be removed from water by sand filtration but are not killed by the quantity of chlorine ordinarily used to purify water; therefore chlorination alone cannot prevent epidemics originating from faecal contamination of water. In places where purification of water supplies is inadequate, boiling for 10 minutes will kill all cysts. Household water treatment strategies using filtration will undoubtedly reduce transmission.

There is no vaccine available against amoebiasis.[29] Several antigens of *E. histolytica* have been developed as possible immunogens. These have different degrees of purity and are used in conjunction with a variety of adjuvants. As yet these have been tried only in animal models. Individual chemoprophylaxis for travellers is not indicated because the possibility of acquiring the infection has been shown to be very low (0.3%).

ENTAMOEBA DISPAR (FORMERLY KNOWN AS NON-PATHOGENIC *E. HISTOLYTICA*)

E. dispar is the most frequently found *Entamoeba* both in humans and primates. It is morphologically identical to *E. histolytica* and is its closest genetic relative in the genus. Unlike *E. histolytica, E. dispar* does not cause disease in humans. However, there is some evidence to suggest that *E. dispar* is capable of inducing focal surface erosion of the colonic mucosa without invading the submucosa or causing ulcers. Although up to 20% of *E. dispar* infections may lead to seropositivity for standard immunodiagnosis of *E. histolytica*, the antibody levels during *E. dispar* infection never approach those seen with *E. histolytica*. Infection is asymptomatic and does not require treatment.

Several biological differences have been described between *E. dispar* and *E. histolytica*, but none of them fully explains why *E. dispar* is unable to produce invasive disease. *E. dispar* produces less protease, does not bind to target cells as strongly and is less cytotoxic, has a thinner glycocalyx, higher surface charge and has less phagocytic activity than *E. histolytica*. In vitro, *E. dispar* is less likely to be lysed by complement.

ENTAMOEBA MOSHKOVSKII ('*E. HISTOLYTICA*-LIKE' AMOEBAE)

E. moshkovskii was originally isolated from sewage in Moscow and subsequently reported in many parts of the world. *E. moshkovskii* is described as morphologically indistinguishable from *E. histolytica* but is isolated from free-living sources, usually in the sediment of sewage-polluted waters. Similar amoebae have been isolated from humans and were grouped under the name of '*E. histolytica*-like amoebae'. The best known of these is the 'Laredo' strain. Numerous studies revealed differences between these strains and true *E. histolytica*, including a lack of serological cross-reactivity, dissimilar DNA base composition and distinctive isoenzyme profiles. Recently, analysis of the small subunit rRNA gene has suggested that these amoebae are strains of *E. moshkovskii* and are not closely related to *E. histolytica*. This amoeba has a wide temperature tolerance, multiplying at 10–37°C. It is highly resistant to amoebicidal drugs.

ENTAMOEBA COLI, POLECKI AND HARTMANNI

These non-pathogenic amoebae are of note only because they are frequently found in stool samples submitted for diagnosis. As yet, there is no convincing evidence that they can cause symptoms.

ENDOLIMAX NANA

Endolimax nana is a cosmopolitan and common intestinal amoeba of humans, primates and pigs which can be confused with *E. histolytica*. *Endolimax nana* is non-pathogenic. The trophozoites are small (6–15 µm in diameter). Movement is by pseudopodia but this fails to produce directional locomotion. The cysts are 8–10 µm in diameter and have a refractile cyst wall. The details of nuclear structure and the appearance of the cytoplasm closely resemble those of *Iodamoeba bütschlii*.

IODAMOEBA BÜTSCHLII

Iodamoeba bütschlii is the most common amoeba of swine, and the pig was probably its original host. It is also frequently found in humans and monkeys. Trophozoites vary greatly in size, ranging from 6 to 20 µm in diameter. The cytoplasm contains one or more glycogen mass(es) that may be seen after iodine staining, as well as bacteria, yeasts and debris; red blood cells are never ingested. Cysts of *I. bütschlii* are 8–15 µm in diameter, commonly ovoidal or irregularly pyriform in shape. The cysts are distinctive in preparations stained with iodine because of the constant presence of the large, sharply outlined and dense glycogen-containing vacuole. *I. bütschlii* is non-pathogenic; only exceptionally has the presence of this parasite been linked to symptomatic infection in humans.

The Mastigophora (Flagellates)

GIARDIA INTESTINALIS

Giardia intestinalis (syn. *lamblia, duodenalis*) is the most common human protozoan enteropathogen and there is good evidence to indicate that infection with this parasite can cause both acute and chronic diarrhoea. Intestinal malabsorption may be severe, such that chronic infection in children may be associated with retardation of growth and development. Our knowledge of this parasite has expanded rapidly since it was first cultured in the 1970s, but many aspects of its biology and interactions with its mammalian hosts remain unanswered. There is no unifying explanation for the diverse clinical spectrum seen in giardiasis, which ranges from asymptomatic carriage to persistent diarrhoea with malabsorption. As yet no classical virulence factors have been identified and thus a clear explanation of pathogenesis is lacking. In addition, despite extensive investigation in animal models and to some extent during human infection, the key immunological determinants for clearance of acute infection and the development of protective immunity remain only partially defined. There is now good evidence that this infection is a zoonosis that can be transmitted through domestic water supplies; control within the environment is therefore an important public health issue.

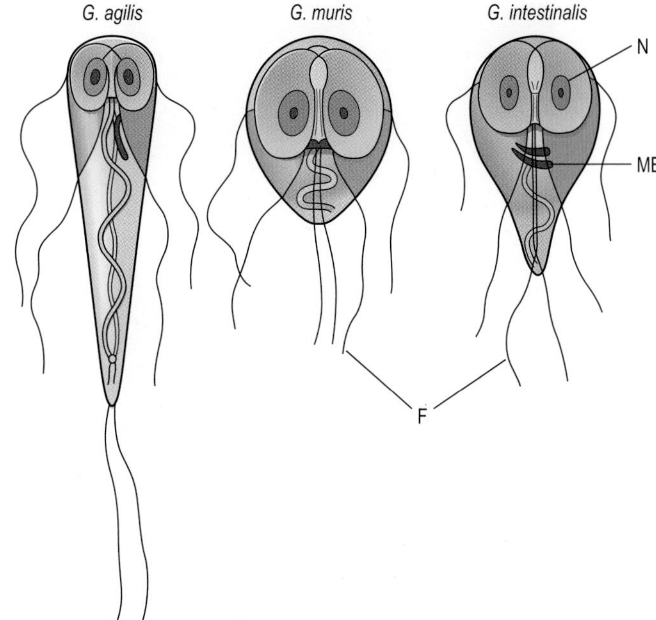

Figure 49.5 *G. agilis, G. muris* and *G. intestinalis*. N, nucleus; MB, median body; F, flagellum.

Epidemiology

The life cycle of *Giardia* is simple, involving the ingestion of cysts in contaminated water or food or through direct person-to-person contact, infection being initiated with as few as 10 to 100 cysts. Excystation occurs in the proximal small intestine where the trophozoite (Figures 49.5, 49.6) multiplies. The cycle is completed when encystation occurs in the distal small intestine and colon, and cysts are excreted again into the environment in faeces at a concentration of approximately 150 000–20 000 cysts per gram of faeces. Molecular genetic approaches have shown that human *Giardia* isolates may be subdivided into two major genotypes, which are now often referred to as assemblages A and B, though there are many subtypes within these assemblages. The implications for epidemiology of this molecular insight have not as yet been fully explored, but a few studies are available to date. These suggest that the ratio of assemblages A:B varies from 1:41 in Malaysia[30] and 9:43 in Brazil[31] to 9:11 in Cuba[32] and in Italy[33] - all were Assemblage A. In two of these studies, from Cuba[33] and Malaysia,[31] assemblage B was more likely to be associated with diarhoea.

Age-specific prevalence, not necessarily resulting in disease, rises throughout infancy and childhood, declining only in adolescence. In the industrialized world, prevalence varies between 2% and 5%, although within these low-prevalence areas there may be localized regions of higher prevalence. Undernutrition may increase the susceptibility to infection, as indicated by a

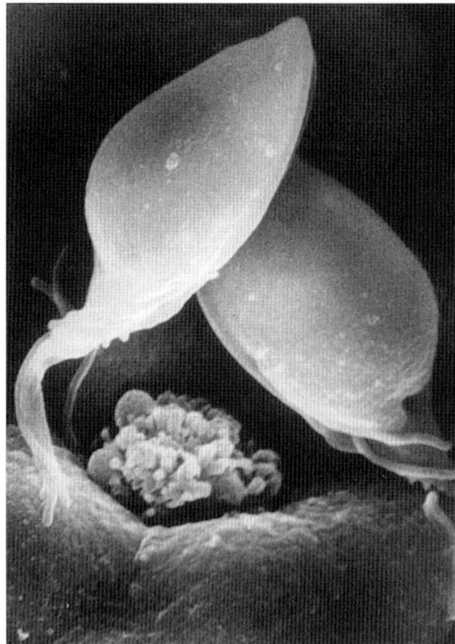

Figure 49.6 Scanning electron micrograph showing two *G. intestinalis* trophozoites.

study in Gambian children with chronic diarrhoea and malnutrition of whom 45% had giardiasis compared with only 12% of healthy age- and sex-matched controls.[34]

Giardiasis is well recognized to occur in travellers, although overall it accounts for no more than 5% of cases of traveller's diarrhoea. However, 30% of travellers to the former Soviet Union were positive for *Giardia* in one study and more than 40% of Scandinavian visitors to St Petersburg acquired the infection.[35] Travelling within the USA may be hazardous for visitors to national parks and ski resorts if they drink the apparently clean surface water.

Individuals with hypogammaglobulinaemia or agammaglobulinaemia are at risk of chronic giardiasis, and patients with IgA deficiency, but individuals with HIV and AIDS do not seem to be at particularly increased risk of developing symptomatic disease. These observations are consistent with the view that secretory immunity in the intestinal lumen is more important for clearance than cell-mediated responses within the intestinal mucosa.

A key factor in transmission of giardiasis is the ability of the cyst to survive for long periods in a suitable environment outside the host. Surface water in many parts of the world, including North America and Europe, is contaminated with *Giardia* cysts, which are not inactivated by chlorination alone. Interruption of the ancillary water purification procedures can lead to contamination of municipal water supplies and has been shown to account for many of the reported epidemics of water-borne giardiasis. Water-borne transmission has also been shown to occur in swimming pools. Despite these epidemics, water-borne transmission probably represents a relatively small proportion of the total infections worldwide. Food has also been shown to be a vehicle for transmission of giardiasis, although again this is probably a relatively uncommon route of transmission.

Direct person-to-person spread by faecal–oral transmission certainly accounts for the high prevalence of giardiasis in day-care centres, schools and residential institutions, where prevalence may be as high as 35%. Person-to-person spread is also known to occur as a result of sexual contact.

Pathogenesis

The pathogenesis of giardiasis is complex and multifactorial.[36] Major contributors to pathogenesis include epithelial remodelling (increased turnover, increased apoptosis), reduced barrier function, brush border (microvillous) effacement, increased transit, bile salt metabolism, and inhibition of pancreatic enzymes.

Giardia attaches to the intestinal epithelium, probably by a variety of mechanisms, although it seems likely that the ventral disc plays a major part, either by flagella-generated hydrodynamic forces beneath the disc or by direct disc movement mediated by its contractile proteins, particularly those in the peripheral regions of the disc. *Giardia* also possesses a mannose-binding surface lectin that appears to exist as a prolactin in the cytoplasm and is activated by trypsin. Experiments in attachment models using mammalian intestinal epithelial cells or culture cell lines suggest that both disc and lectin-mediated mechanisms are important, at least in vitro.

In human giardiasis the full spectrum of abnormalities of villous architecture (Figure 49.7) has been described, ranging from normal to subtotal villous atrophy. A majority of infected individuals have relatively mild abnormalities of villous architecture, with associated crypt hyperplasia. Infections in experimental models produce similar changes but, as in human infection, the abnormalities are generally mild. Ultrastructural abnormalities such as shortening and disruption of microvilli are apparent, especially at the point of ventral disc attachment, where microvillus effacement is obvious. This brush border damage is associated with reduction in disaccharidase activity. In animal models, diarrhoea is at its peak when disaccharide activities are most profoundly reduced. However, other mechanisms of epithelial cell damage operate. Work in tissue culture cell lines has shown that *Giardia* trophozoites induce localized condensation of F-actin and loss of peri-junctional α-actinin, and tight junction changes have been associated with alterations in claudin. These cytoskeletal rearrangements could account for

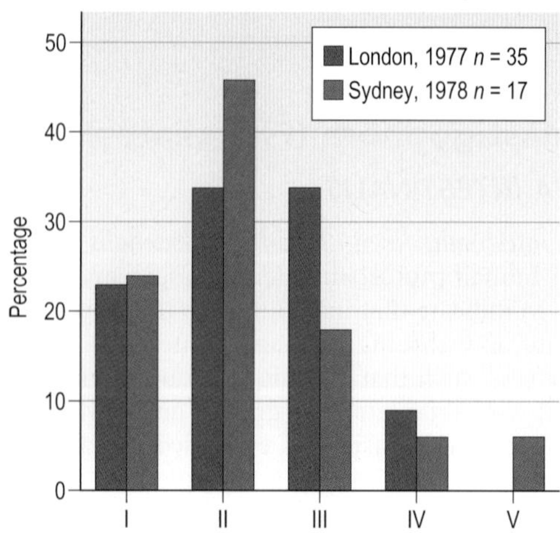

Figure 49.7 Percentage of patients with giardiasis with normal (I), mild (II), moderate (III) and severe (IV) partial villous atrophy, and subtotal villous atrophy (V).

early changes in epithelial cell function. There is also evidence to suggest that *Giardia* trophozoites produce cytopathic substances that might be responsible for this disruption of epithelial structure and function.

There is increasing evidence to suggest that T-cell activation within the intestinal mucosa can produce villous atrophy.[37] This mechanism also operates in graft-versus-host disease and in coeliac disease. Giardiasis has been associated with increased numbers of aerobic and/or anaerobic bacteria in the upper small intestine of the indigenous Indian population or in travellers to the Indian subcontinent. Bacterial overgrowth can produce architectural abnormalities in the small intestine similar to those seen in giardiasis and thus may have a role in the pathogenesis of mucosal damage. Bile salts have an important role in the life cycle of *Giardia*. There is evidence to suggest that the organism takes up bile salts during growth by an energy-requiring active transport process, possibly involving a membrane carrier. Although the precise metabolic advantages to the parasite have not been defined, a secondary effect of this process could be the depletion of intraluminal bile salt, thus impairing micellar solubilization of dietary fats and at the same time inhibition of pancreatic lipase, which is dependent on bile salts for full expression of hydrolytic activity. *Giardia* trophozoites are also able to inhibit trypsin and lipase activity in vitro. The precise mechanisms by which the organism achieves this have not been established, although it seems likely that this may relate to a direct effect of parasite-derived proteinases on the secreted pancreatic proteins.

Until specific virulence factors have been identified it is unlikely that the relative importance of these mucosal and luminal mechanisms in pathogenesis will be established. At present it seems reasonable to assume that the process is multifactorial, involving a combination of varying degrees of mucosal injury combined with disruption of the luminal phases of digestion and absorption.

Clinical Features

The most common form of giardiasis is asymptomatic carriage. This is common in highly endemic areas in the developing world, although it also occurs in Europe and North America. Such individuals appear to suffer no ill effects from the parasite, although there have been no systematic studies of the subclinical impact of such an infection. It is unclear whether asymptomatic infections relate to carriage of 'non-pathogenic' strains or whether the host is able to maintain parasite numbers at a level below expression of clinical disease without complete clearance of the infection. It does not seem likely that all of the differences in clinical features in human giardiasis can be attributed to parasite assemblage.

Acute giardiasis has been well characterized in individuals travelling from areas of low to high endemicity. Symptoms usually begin within 3–20 (mean 7) days of arrival within a high-risk area and in the vast majority recovery occurs within 2–4 weeks. In up to 25% of travellers with giardiasis, symptoms may persist for 7 weeks or more. Diarrhoea is the major symptom and is usually watery initially but subsequently develops the features of steatorrhoea, often associated with nausea, abdominal discomfort, bloating and weight loss. Although giardiasis is self-limiting in the majority of healthy immunocompetent individuals, a proportion goes on to have persistent diarrhoea, usually with features of steatorrhoea. Weight loss can be profound, with losses of 10–20% of the usual or ideal body weight. In symptomatic patients with persistent diarrhoea, 50% will have biochemical evidence of fat malabsorption and possibly of other nutrients, including vitamin A and vitamin B_{12}. Secondary lactase deficiency is well recognized to occur in human giardiasis and in experimental models, and patients may take many weeks to recover even after clearance of the parasite.

Complications of Giardiasis. A series of hospital-based studies has clearly shown the potential of giardiasis to impair growth and development in infants and young children. This is a highly selected population, biased towards more severely affected children, and thus gives no indication as to the impact of giardiasis in the community. Several studies from Central America and West Africa suggest that giardiasis does have an independent inhibitory effect on child growth, but it is difficult to arrive at firm conclusions because within these populations many other factors contribute to undernutrition and impaired development, and a definitive demonstration of the size of the effect on child growth is awaited. Protein-losing enteropathy is a rare occurrence in giardiasis but has been described in children in West Africa and may contribute to undernutrition.

Diagnosis

Many of the same issues apply to diagnosis of giardiasis as apply to diagnosis of amoebiasis. Clinically, giardiasis is often suggested by a typical history which often includes a period of recent foreign travel. The main differential diagnoses include other causes of intestinal malabsorption such as tropical sprue and coeliac disease. Other infective causes of persistent diarrhoea include strongyloidiasis, cryptosporidiosis, microsporidiosis and cyclosporiasis. Many clinicians treat giardiasis empirically with a nitroimidazole derivative, even without achieving a firm microscopic diagnosis.

Microbiology. *Giardia* cysts and occasionally trophozoites are detected in faecal specimens by light microscopy, which continues to be the gold standard for the diagnosis of giardiasis. Faecal specimens are examined, either fresh or fixed with polyvinyl alcohol formalin, and then stained with trichrome or iron haematoxylin. Cyst detection can be improved by concentration techniques using formalin-ethyl acetate or zinc sulphate. Examination of multiple faecal specimens increases the chances of making a positive diagnosis, with up to 70% of positive stools detected following examination of a single faecal specimen, rising to 85% when at least three separate stool specimens are examined. Trophozoites are usually found only in freshly passed watery diarrhoea. Trophozoites can also be detected microscopically in duodenal fluid and, although overall this technique has a lower sensitivity than faecal microscopy, it does complement the latter, in that some patients with negative stool microscopy will have a positive duodenal aspirate. Trophozoites may also be detected in histological sections collected endoscopically (Figure 49.8) or by endoscopic brush cytology.

Faecal Antigen ELISA. Antigen tests come in two main formats: ELISAs and rapid strip tests. Generally, these tests offer simplicity and they save time, but their sensitivity is not much higher than microscopy, anywhere between 44% and 82%.[38,39] Specificity is generally high, over 95%. False-positives are almost always reported in these assays and the interpretation of these findings is difficult.

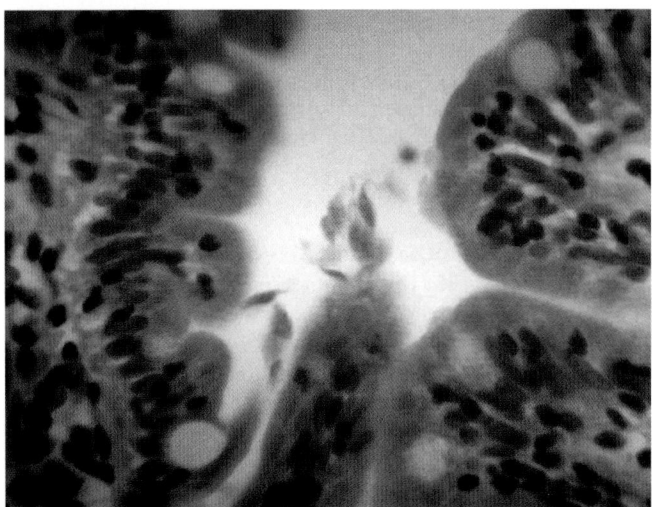

Figure 49.8 *Giardia* trophozoites seen in histological section from a Zambian patient with diarrhoea.

Serology. Anti-*Giardia* IgG titres are not helpful in diagnosis because they are commonly found to be increased in non-infected individuals in endemic areas. Anti-*Giardia* IgM titres are usually increased only in infected individuals and have been shown to be useful in a research setting for detecting individuals with acute giardiasis in endemic areas such as India and The Gambia. Sensitivity and specificity decrease in children with persistent diarrhoea, in some of whom anti-*Giardia* IgM titres persist for several months.

DNA-Based Techniques. Stool-based PCR diagnosis is emerging as the leading diagnostic test for *Giardia* as it is incorporated into multiplex systems such as multiplex PCR[40,41] and multiplex PCR detection using beads conjugated to DNA probes and analysed on a Luminex multi-channel analyser.[42] Taking advantage of the advances in DNA extraction techniques, these tests have a sensitivity which is very high. It remains to be seen whether the clinical significance of the lowest infectious burdens merits the extra investment in these techniques.

Management

In many healthy immunocompetent individuals giardiasis is a self-limiting illness, with the parasite being eradicated by host defence mechanisms without specific treatment. Administration of an anti-giardial drug will generally reduce the severity of symptoms and the duration of the illness. Although symptomatic patients with giardiasis are generally offered antimicrobial chemotherapy, the question as to whether asymptomatic patients, particularly those in an endemic area, should be treated continues to be discussed. Since the development of in vitro culture techniques for *Giardia* isolates, methods have been developed to assess drug sensitivity. However, the precise relationship between indices of drug susceptibility in vitro and the subsequent behaviour of the drug in vivo has not been clearly established. Treatment failures do occur and it is thought that at least some of these episodes are related to drug resistance.

Four classes of drugs are commonly used to treat giardiasis (Table 49.4): the nitroimidazole derivatives, nitazoxanide, the acridine dyes such as mepacrine, and the nitrofurans such as furazolidone. Nitroimidazole derivatives are probably the drugs of choice, particularly when used as short-course regimens. Mepacrine has a similar efficacy but is generally less well tolerated. Furazolidone has a lower efficacy but is popular for the treatment of giardiasis in childhood as it has relatively few adverse effects and is available as a suspension.

A variety of other chemotherapeutic agents has been assessed in vitro and some have also been used in the clinical setting. The benzimidazole drugs appear to have some anti-giardial activity, which almost certainly relates to their ability to inhibit cytoskeletal function. Albendazole has been shown to have anti-giardial activity in vitro and recent clinical trial data support its value in human infection. Other drugs such as sodium fusidate, d- and dl-propranolol, mefloquine, doxycycline and rifampicin have all been shown to have anti-giardial activity, although the majority have not been subjected to rigorous evaluation in clinical practice.

Prevention

It seems highly unlikely that *Giardia* spp. will ever be eliminated from the environment, as cysts can survive for weeks or months outside the host in water or a moist environment and it is now well established that surface water in many parts of the world is contaminated with *Giardia* cysts. This reservoir could potentially maintain the animal reservoir of *Giardia*, which is increasingly thought to be another potential source of human infection. Despite vigilance about water quality, it is vital to ensure that contaminated surface water collecting grounds are appropriately treated before water enters the public water supply. Attention to personal hygiene in order to break the faecal–oral cycle is also important, particularly in residential institutions and day-care centres.

There is compelling evidence that breast-feeding protects against giardiasis; this can be partly attributed to passive immunization. Whether active immunization in the form of a vaccine is feasible, or even appropriate, continues to be evaluated. Parenteral immunization with adjuvants can protect experimental animals from challenge with *G. intestinalis*, and the epidemiological evidence in humans that protective immunity does

TABLE 49.4 Drug Treatment of Giardiasis

	Efficacy		
Drug	Adults	Children	(%)
Metronidazole	2 g (single dose) daily ×3 days *OR* 400 mg three times daily ×5 days	15 mg/kg per day (max. 750 mg) ×10 days	>90
Tinidazole	2 g single dose	50–75 mg/kg single dose	>90
Nitazoxanide	500 mg twice daily ×3 days	1–3 years: 100 mg twice daily ×3 days 4–11 years: 200 mg every 12 hours ×3 days	
Mepacrine (quinacrine)	100 mg three times daily ×5–7 days	2 mg/kg three times daily ×5–7 days	>90
Furazolidone	100 mg four times daily ×7–10 days	2 mg/kg three times daily ×7–10 days	>80

eventually develop, probably over a number of years, suggests that immunological approaches to prevention are feasible. However, it is unclear as to why the development of protective immunity following natural infection appears to require repeated exposure to the organism. It is possible that this is related, at least in part, to the variable antigenic profiles of different isolates. In addition, it is known that the expression of certain *Giardia* antigens can vary during both experimental and human infection, thus providing a way in which the organism may evade the host immune response. Failure to mount an antibody response to *Giardia* heat shock antigen in children with chronic diarrhoea in The Gambia suggests that impaired response may also be a factor. Clearly all of these issues need to be taken into account in planning a vaccine development strategy.

Studies in experimental models and limited studies in human giardiasis have made it possible to attribute essential roles to the immune system in the eradication of acute infection and to determine, at least in part, the determinants of persistent infection in an otherwise immunocompetent host. There is increasing evidence to suggest that immunological factors are important in protecting mammalian hosts from reinfection, and thus the development of protective immunity. It seems unlikely that a single infection provides long-lasting protective immunity because age-specific prevalence increases throughout childhood and into early adolescence, suggesting that multiple exposures to the parasite are required before protection is achieved.

DIENTAMOEBA FRAGILIS

According to morphological and molecular evidence, *Dientamoeba fragilis* is now considered to be an aberrant trichomonad flagellate, not an amoeba. Infection with this organism may be associated with gastrointestinal symptoms, such as diarrhoea and abdominal pain, but most cases are asymptomatic.[43] *D. fragilis* is a small (6–12 µm) cosmopolitan parasite. Only trophozoites are known; they can be differentiated from other intestinal amoebae by the presence of two nuclei in the majority of them. However, around 30–40% of organisms are mononucleate and may be confused with *Blastocystis hominis*, which is more common. Trichrome stains should always be performed. Culture is possible and the parasite can be differentiated by its distinct isoenzyme profile. Polymerase chain reaction (PCR)–restriction fragment length polymorphism analysis of its ribosomal genes suggests the presence of two genetically distinct forms.[44] Further studies are needed to determine whether there is a correlation between these genetic groups and virulence.

NON-PATHOGENIC FLAGELLATES

There are a number of other flagellates found in humans that do not appear to cause disease. *Trichomonas hominis* is commonly found in faeces of individuals living in the developing world. Only the trophozoite form is recognized; it varies from 5 to 14 µm in length. There is a single nucleus, anterior to which are basal bodies from which arise three to four flagella. *Chilomastix mesnili* occurs as both cysts and trophozoite and is larger than *Trichomonas hominis*, being usually 10–15 µm in length, although it may occasionally be as large as 20 µm. The trophozoite has a large spiral longitudinal cleft anteriorly and an anterior single nucleus. Basal bodies at the anterior pole of the nucleus give rise to three anterior flagella, two fibrils that support the margins of the longitudinal cleft (the mouth), and a fourth flagellum which moves within the longitudinal cleft. There are no cytoskeletal elements, the parasite maintaining its shape by a pellicle. The cyst is pear-shaped and approximately 18 µm in length. Internal structures are apparent in the stained cyst in which one or two nuclei may be observed. Rare non-pathogenic flagellates include *Embadomonas intestinalis* and *Enteromonas hominis.*

The Ciliophora

Members of this class are all relatively large in size and covered by short hair-like organelles called cilia, which give the organism its motility. They have two nuclei, one somatic and one germinal. Reproduction is by binary fission, although conjugation does occur when nuclear material is exchanged between parasites. The only ciliate that is pathogenic to humans is *Balantidium coli.*

BALANTIDIUM COLI

Balantidium coli is the largest and probably least common protozoan pathogen of humans.[45] It can cause a severe life-threatening colitis which is potentially avoidable by appropriate antibiotic therapy. Fatalities are almost invariably due to diagnostic imprecision.

Epidemiology

The parasite is found in northern and southern hemispheres, although it is most commonly reported in tropical and subtropical regions, particularly Central and South America, Iran, Papua New Guinea and the Philippines. Prevalence is usually less than 1%, although higher rates are reported in hyperendemic areas and some residential institutions. *B. coli* is found in many mammals other than humans, particularly pigs and monkeys. Swine appear to be the most important animal reservoir for human disease, although enteric disease does not seem to occur in this host. The largest reported epidemic of balantidiasis, involving 110 persons, resulted from gross contamination of ground and surface water supplies by pig faeces after a severe typhoon. Communities that live in close association with swine tend to have increased prevalence of the disease because carriage by pigs in endemic areas has been estimated to be 40–90%.

Pathogenesis

The trophozoite is able to invade the distal ileal and colonic mucosa to produce intense mucosal inflammation and ulceration. The mechanisms involved are not clearly understood, although it is considered that the motile trophozoite is able to penetrate the mucosa and submucosa, and even in some instances the muscle layers of the colon. Invasion is thought to be facilitated by the enzyme hyaluronidase, produced by the parasite. The resulting inflammation may be mediated partly by other products liberated by the parasite and possibly by recruitment of mucosal inflammatory cells, particularly neutrophils.

Clinical Features

In many respects the illness produced by infection with *B. coli* closely resembles amoebic colitis. Clinical presentation occurs in three forms: (1) the asymptomatic carrier state, most commonly seen in persons in institutional care and possibly accounting for up to 80% of all infections; (2) acute and acute fulminant colitis; and (3) chronic infection. In the acute form, diarrhoea with blood and mucus begins abruptly and may be associated with nausea, abdominal discomfort and marked weight loss. Proctosigmoidoscopy reveals inflammatory changes, including discrete ulceration, although the rectum is not invariably involved. The illness can progress rapidly, accompanied by fever and prostration, and lead to death, usually due to peritonitis from colonic perforation. A protracted course with intermittent diarrhoea but only occasional blood in the stools is typical of the chronic form of the disease. A few cases of balantidial appendicitis have been reported.

Diagnosis

The benchmark diagnostic test is stool microscopy. *B. coli* exists as a trophozoite (usually found in stools of acute infection) and cysts, which become more apparent in chronic infection or asymptomatic carriers. The trophozoite is oval in shape, about 17 µm long and 15 µm wide. In its favoured host, the pig, trophozoites may reach 200 µm in length, when they can be seen with the aid of a hand lens or in some cases with the naked eye. The trophozoite is covered with cilia which propel the organism through the fluid contents of the intestinal lumen. At the anterior end of the trophozoite there is a cytostome (a mouth) leading into the cytopharynx, which extends approximately one-third of the body length. Posteriorly there is a cytopyge (anus). *B. coli* forms a large spherical cyst which may reach 60 µm in diameter. Cysts can survive outside the mammalian host for several weeks in moist conditions but are rapidly destroyed in hot, dry conditions. Infection is usually transmitted by the cyst.

Management

The most commonly used treatment is tetracycline 500 mg four times daily for 10 days. The parasite is also sensitive to bacitracin, ampicillin, metronidazole and paromomycin. Surgery may be required in fulminant disease, as in amoebiasis, although a conservative approach should be taken wherever possible.

Prevention

As *Balantidium coli* is a zoonosis, prevention strategies have not been well-defined, apart from general hygiene measures to prevent infection from pigs. No vaccine is available.

The Coccidia

CRYPTOSPORIDIUM SPP.

The current taxonomy of the genus *Cryptosporidium* is in rapid evolution,[46] and this makes the literature difficult to read at the current time as new species and genotypes are constantly being defined and renamed. Importantly, the distinction between *C. parvum* and *C. hominis* now seems secure, and as these account for the vast majority of human infections, we will only deal with these. The life cycle of these Apicomplexa parasites is complex (Figure 49.9) but for the history and taxonomy of this interesting genus the reader is referred to Fayer (2010).[46]

Epidemiology

Cryptosporidiosis (the infection due to *Cryptosporidium* spp.) is now recognized to represent a substantial threat to HIV-infected individuals, with a lifetime risk of infection of around 10%, but it is also responsible for substantial outbreaks of

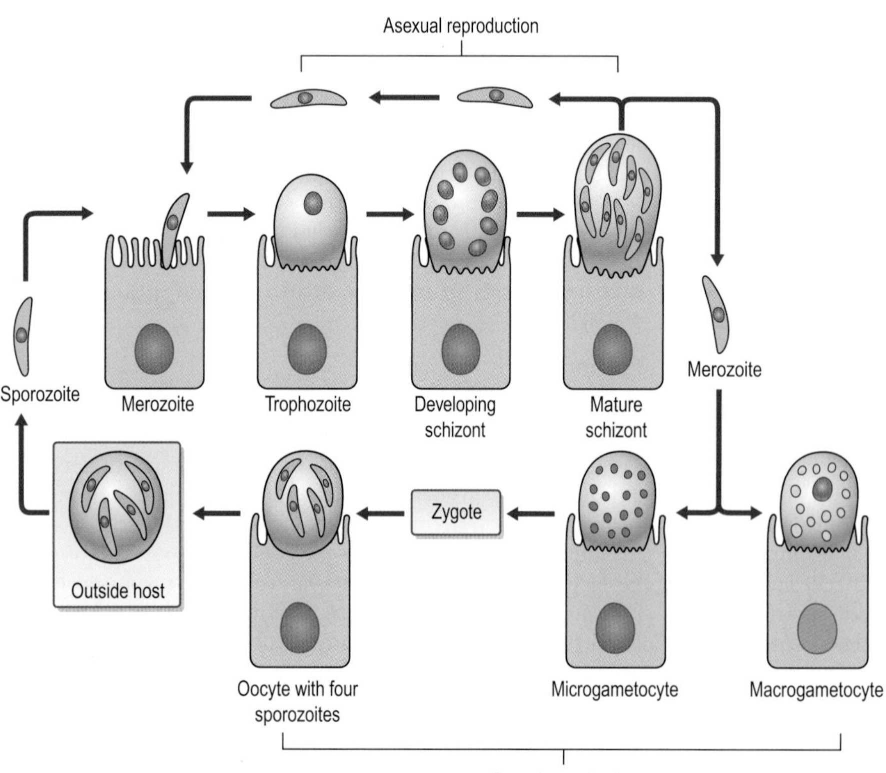

Figure 49.9 Life cycle of *C. parvum/hominis.*

water-borne diarrhoea in the immunocompetent, and for diarrhoea in travellers and in children.

Immunocompetent Individuals. Substantial evidence has accumulated implicating *Cryptosporidium* spp. in outbreaks of water-borne diarrhoea and in stable endemic childhood diarrhoea among the poor of the developing world. Travellers' diarrhoea may result from infection with this parasite. The evidence for the water-borne nature of the infection comes from epidemics that have occurred along water distribution patterns and the finding that oocysts can be detected in the water supply by filtration of large volumes through 1-μm pores. Chlorination of water at usual levels fails to inactivate oocysts. It is probably this resistance to chlorination that allowed transmission to 70 cases following contamination of a swimming pool in the UK, and in a similar outbreak reported from California. As cryptosporidiosis is a common pathogen in calf and lamb diarrhoea, it is probably a zoonosis, transmitted in surface run-off water contaminated by calf faeces. There is an emerging consensus that *C. hominis* is an exclusively human pathogen, whereas transmission of *C. parvum* is predominantly zoonotic in industrialized countries but largely anthroponotic in developing countries.[47,48] However, in a direct comparison of cryptosporidiosis in farm animals and farm workers, there was evidence of zoonotic transmission in Zambia.[49] Cryptosporidiosis can also be food-borne.[50]

Cryptosporidiosis is an important contributor to childhood diarrhoea, with a prevalence among children with diarrhoea of 1–3% in the industrialized world and 4–17% in developing countries. In the developed world cryptosporidiosis is found in outbreaks clustered around day-care nurseries. In a careful prospective study in Guinea-Bissau, cryptosporidia were found in 6.1% of patients with acute (<2 weeks) diarrhoea and in 15% of those with chronic diarrhoea, with a relative mortality in children with cryptosporidial diarrhoea in the first year of life of 2.9%.[51]

Insight into the transmission and pathobiology of the infection arises from the report of an outbreak of cryptosporidiosis in Denmark in 1990.[52] The setting was an infectious disease ward with a mixed population of HIV-seropositive and -seronegative patients; the index case was a demented seropositive man with cryptosporidial diarrhoea who contaminated an ice machine with faeces. None of the 73 HIV-seronegative inpatients became infected, but 18 (32%) of 57 HIV-positive patients developed infection, 17 of whom had AIDS. The mean incubation time was at least 13 days.

Immunodeficient Individuals. Cryptosporidiosis first came to prominence as a problem in the context of AIDS, to the extent that chronic cryptosporidial diarrhoea is a case-defining diagnosis for AIDS. The course of the illness is variable and depends largely, but not entirely, on the degree of immune deficiency, as measured by the CD4 cell count in the peripheral blood, as demonstrated by studies performed before antiretroviral therapy became widely available.[53] Table 49.5 gives a summary of studies that have examined relative contributions of protozoal infection to AIDS-related diarrhoea. Infections other than protozoa have been described, particularly salmonellae, shigellae and, in Africa, *Strongyloides stercoralis*. The contribution of viruses to the diarrhoea is uncertain at present. Differences in the proportions of specific infections found in patients in Africa and in patients in developed countries may reflect the more advanced stage of immune deficiency in the latter group before death, as well as the overall prevalence of the infection in the environment.

TABLE 49.5 Summary of Studies of Prevalence of Protozoa in HIV-related Diarrhoea in Different Geographical Areas

	Percentage of Cases in which Protozoan Identified	
	Africa and Caribbean[a]	Industrialized countries[b]
C. parvum	27	12
I. belli	13	0.5
Microsporidia	5[c]	27[d]
G. intestinalis	2	5
E. histolytica	2	5

[a]Means of 11 studies from Haiti, Zaire, Uganda, Burundi, Zambia and Mali.
[b]Means of 15 studies from UK, USA, France, Germany, Holland and Australia.
[c]Only two studies included a search for microsporidia.
[d]Some of these studies were of selected patients and the prevalence is raised artefactually.

Pathogenesis

Human studies on the distribution of infection are limited, but it can occur anywhere in the intestine with a predominance of ileal and caecal infection.[54] Electron microscopy of the infection shows that the presence of the trophozoites leads to destruction of the microvilli (Figure 49.10), which is associated with a reduction in disaccharidase activity.[55] Detailed ultrastructural work in a guinea pig model of infection shows the initial event to be attachment of the sporozoite to the microvillus, followed by invagination of the protozoan into an envelope of host cell origin. Subsequently, the parasite induces conformational changes in the host membrane, which eventually breaks down with the formation of a 'feeder organelle' by which the parasite communicates directly with host cytoplasm.

Cryptosporidial infection has been associated with increased numbers of mitotic figures in the crypts and with villous atrophy. In the normal human intestine, cell maturation takes

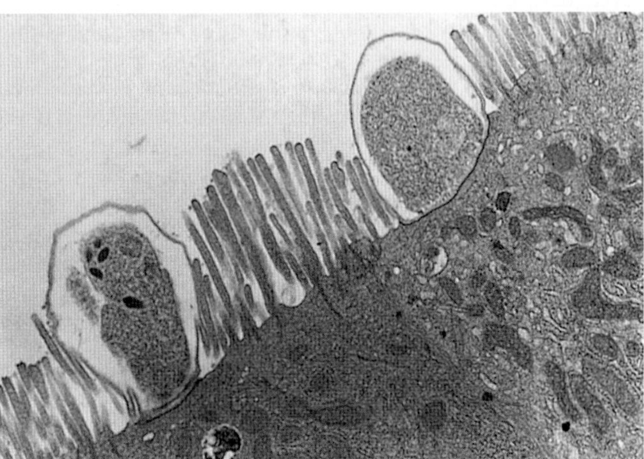

Figure 49.10 Transmission electron micrograph of *Cryptosporidium* trophozoites in distal duodenal mucosa. The trophozoites occupy an intracellular but extracytoplasmic position (×20000). *(Courtesy of Graham McPhail.)*

place during migration up the crypt and along the length of the villus. This process is accompanied by the change from a crypt cell generating net water and salt secretion to a villous cell with net salt and water absorption. Maturation is also accompanied by the synthesis of a normal complement of brush-border enzymes, including disaccharidases, lipases and alkaline phosphatase. According to this 'enterocyte immaturity hypothesis', the repopulation of the villus with immature enterocytes leads to the failure of digestion and absorption seen in many protozoal small bowel parasitoses.

It has been assumed that, because some conspicuous individuals have high sodium and water losses in stool, often quoted at up to 20 L/day, the principal mechanism of diarrhoea must be a cholera-like jejunal secretory state: 'diarrhoea in the human appears to be mostly due to hypersecretion of fluid and electrolytes from the proximal small intestine into the gut lumen'. Animal perfusion studies in a neonatal piglet model of cryptosporidiosis do not support this hypothesis; nor do studies in humans using a jejunal perfusion technique, though electrolyte absorption is impaired.[56] It has been suggested that ileal malabsorption of bile salts may have a role in the pathogenesis of the diarrhoea. A series of elegant studies recently, using cholangiocytes as a model of infection, have showed that apoptosis is an important part of the pathogenesis of the infection.[57]

Clinical Features

Early reports considered the infection in the context of AIDS as 'unremitting, profuse diarrhoea lasting for months', but this is an oversimplification. The clinical picture of infection is variable, and there is variation in disease severity even after accounting for the degree of immune deficiency by blood CD4 cell count. It is now established that even patients with AIDS may carry heavy parasite burdens asymptomatically, and in the community asymptomatic infection is commoner than symptomatic infection.[58] In the last decade, the introduction of antiretroviral therapy has had a dramatic and positive impact on HIV-infected individuals, but although the number of patients with severe, chronic cryptosporidiosis has fallen, cases still do occur especially in Africa.

In AIDS, a substantial proportion of patients present with diarrhoea, abdominal cramps and vomiting. About 8% of patients in London had fulminant diarrhoea, with collapse and severe dehydration due to the passage of high volumes of diarrhoea. The majority of patients in this study had stool volumes of 500–1500 mL/24 hours, with stool frequency of 2–10 per day.[59] There is no way of clinically distinguishing patients with cryptosporidiosis from those with any other chronic diarrhoeal illness. The natural history of the infection in Europe is that of a remitting and relapsing diarrhoea, but some patients do get diarrhoea every day. In a series of patients in Lusaka, Zambia, the median duration of diarrhoea at presentation with cryptosporidiosis was 5 months, with 60% admitting to intermittent diarrhoea (unpublished observations). Patients in all areas of the globe show considerable wasting as AIDS progresses, but it is difficult to discern how much can be attributed to any particular infection. There is certainly anorexia in AIDS, and oral and oesophageal candidiasis exacerbate the problem.

Some patients may also develop involvement of the biliary tract, an infectious form of sclerosing cholangitis, sometimes associated with cholecystitis. This may also occur in microsporidiosis or due to cytomegalovirus, or it may be impossible to identify a cause. The disorder usually occurs in patients with advanced AIDS and chronic diarrhoea and is associated with progressive right upper quadrant abdominal pain. The patients tend to have had other opportunistic infections by this stage of the HIV infection. Biochemical tests of hepatic damage usually show raised serum levels of alkaline phosphatase and γ-glutamyltransferase in the absence of jaundice. This complication of AIDS-related cryptosporidiosis is much less common than it used to be in the 1980s.

In children, cryptosporidiosis causes diarrhoeal disease which is usually self-limiting. However, in developing countries it is associated with malnutrition and increased mortality in children in developing countries. Longitudinal studies in Guinea-Bissau have demonstrated that cryptosporidiosis precedes the development of growth failure.[60] In malnourished children with persistent diarrhoea in Zambia, cryptosporidiosis was associated with higher mortality independent of HIV infection.[61]

Diagnosis

Current diagnostic methods in most laboratories around the world rely heavily on the identification of the oocysts in faeces, though again the parasite is often detectable in histological sections of intestinal biopsies (Figure 49.11). Three staining methods are in common use: auramine staining, modified Ziehl–Neelsen staining and immunofluorescence using monoclonal antibodies to oocysts. These techniques are relatively insensitive. The threshold of reliable (100%) detection was found to be 10 000 cysts/g in watery stool, but in formed stool thresholds were 50 000/g by immunofluorescence and 500 000/g by acid-fast staining.[62]

ELISAs that incorporate anti-oocyst antibodies to detect cryptosporidial antigen in faeces have been developed, and rapid strip tests are also available. In a head-to-head comparison of seven diagnostic assays,[63] the least sensitive was the modified Ziehl-Neelsen stain, followed by auramine-phenol fluorescence microscopy and then immunofluorescence microscopy. The ELISA format tests were all similar in sensitivity to the auramine-phenol procedure. One commercial ELISA test does not distinguish between *Giardia* and *Cryptosporidium* antigens, and this author is not convinced of its usefulness.

The performance of multiplex PCR assays is encouraging and this approach is emerging as a leading diagnostic technique. For large numbers of samples it is more efficient than microscopy.[40–42]

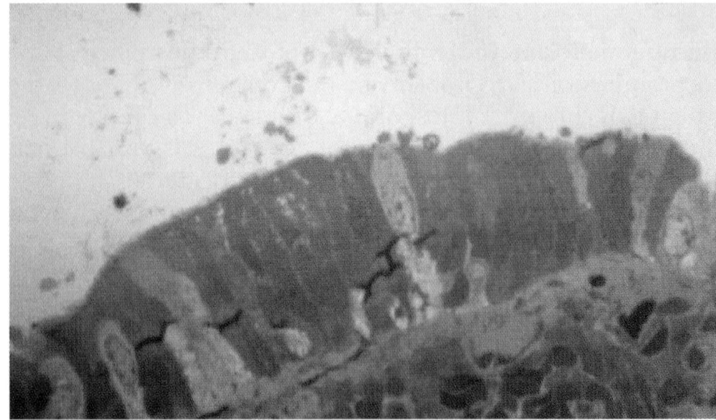

Figure 49.11 *Cryptosporidium* trophozoites and schizonts seen in duodenal biopsy section from a Zambian patient with diarrhoea; semi-thin section stained with toluidine blue.

Management

There is no effective treatment that will eradicate cryptosporidial infection in all cases. Several controlled trials have now confirmed that nitazoxanide is effective against *Cryptosporidium* spp. in well-nourished and malnourished HIV-uninfected children.[64–66] A 3-day course is effective: children under 4 years receive 100 mg twice daily and those over 4 years 200 mg twice daily, orally. A Cochrane review suggests that none of the treatments evaluated was consistently effective in immunocompromised adults or children, but the number of trials available for inclusion in the meta-analysis was small.[64] New agents are on the horizon,[67] but experience shows that there is a wide gap between in vitro efficacy and efficacy proven in randomized controlled trials. The most important aspect of treatment is fluid and electrolyte replacement with oral rehydration solutions, although intravenous therapy may be necessary. Symptomatic treatment with codeine phosphate or powerful opiates should be given readily, according to resources, and nutritional support is probably beneficial.

Prevention

Immunocompromised individuals should ideally boil all drinking water and avoid swimming in public water. Children in tropical environments should ideally be given boiled water to drink. Chlorination does not confer protection against cryptosporidiosis. Household water treatment strategies based on filtration probably offer the best realistic means of reducing transmission.[68] Unfortunately, solar disinfection (SODIS) which has high efficacy against enteric bacteria and other protozoa that cause diarrhoea, does not seem to be effective against *Cryptosporidium* spp.[69] Intensive handwashing reduces diarrhoeal disease in HIV-infected adults, and *Cryptosporidium* may possibly be one of the agents against which this is effective, though the study which demonstrates this was probably underpowered.[70] There is no immediate prospect of effective immunization against the infection.

Prevention of nosocomial or laboratory-acquired infection requires strict attention to containment and generous washing of any contaminated areas. Disposables should be used where possible. The oocysts are resistant to many disinfectants, but are reliably inactivated by boiling, freezing, drying and 3% hydrogen peroxide.

ISOSPORA BELLI

This coccidian was first described in 1915 but has received much less attention in the world literature than cryptosporidia, probably because of its comparative rarity in the developed world. It has recently attracted interest because of its identification in patients with AIDS. The infective form of the parasite is the oocyst, which releases sporozoites, leading to a small bowel infection. The parasite there takes up an intracellular location and undergoes merogony and sporogony.

Epidemiology

The route of transmission of the parasite is not established but faecal–oral spread seems likely. Infection is uncommon in the developed world, as reflected by the prevalence in European and North American patients with AIDS (compared with Africans) shown in Table 49.5. A survey of over 55 000 stool specimens in Chile over a 10-year period revealed only 452 (0.8%) positives. In Paris, in a series of 3500 patients from the tropics studied before the HIV pandemic, only five (0.1%) cases of isosporiasis were found, but more recent data from an HIV clinic in Paris reveal that imported isosporiasis is now a significant problem, and treatment failures are common. The contrast between Europe and Africa is very striking, with isosporiasis the commonest infection in Zambian AIDS patients in our clinics for many years.[71]

Pathogenesis

Isosporiasis is associated with mild to a subtotal villous atrophy. This is seen in patients with AIDS, but was also reported before the HIV pandemic. Inflammatory cells and eosinophils are seen in the lamina propria. Understanding of the pathogenesis of isosporiasis is very limited indeed, but may be similar to cryptosporidiosis.

Clinical Features

As with cryptosporidiosis, isosporiasis leads to a self-limiting diarrhoea in the immunocompetent, and to chronic diarrhoea in the immunocompromised. The illness in the apparently immunocompetent may be prolonged, extending to 20 years, in one report. There is little evidence regarding the frequency with which isosporiasis spontaneously remits in patients with AIDS. In AIDS, isosporiasis is associated with watery diarrhoea, cramping abdominal pain and nausea, wasting and dehydration.[72]

Diagnosis

Diagnosis rests on stool examination using wet preparations and modified Ziehl–Neelsen acid-fast stained smears. The oocysts appear oval, larger than cryptosporidial oocysts (20–30 μm); some oocysts are sporulated before leaving the host and have two easily identified sporoblasts. The oocysts fluoresce with the phenol auramine stain under ultraviolet light. The parasites may also be recognized in small bowel biopsies, visible within enterocyte cytoplasmic vacuoles under electron microscopy and light microscopy.

Management

Treatment with oral co-trimoxazole (sulfamethoxazole 800 mg and trimethoprim 160 mg) four times daily for 10 days eliminated the parasite from stool in most cases, with an interruption in diarrhoea.[73] Unfortunately, this was followed by relapse in 50%, usually within 12 weeks. Re-treatment was usually effective. Prophylactic co-trimoxazole may be necessary. Pyrimethamine-sulphonamide combinations are probably also effective, but no good clinical trial data support this assertion. There is little information on the regimen of choice for those who are intolerant of sulphonamides.

SARCOCYSTIS SPECIES

Infection with this coccidian, formerly known as *Isospora hominis*, is uncommonly recognized. The parasite is similar to *I. belli* in its biology, but the life cycle requires alternating infection of intermediate hosts, such as cattle and pigs, and definitive hosts, such as humans. In one European study, the infection was present in 0.4–1.5% of all stool specimens. The infection has not so far been recognized in AIDS. Biopsy specimens may show an eosinophilic infiltrate. Sporocysts are recognized in stool with the same stains as are used for isosporiasis, but the cysts are smaller (15×10 μm). It is likely that improved molecular diagnostic techniques for these uncommon food-borne parasites[74] will make epidemiology clearer,[75] but for the moment they are better known to veterinary pathologists than physicians.

CYCLOSPORA CAYETANENSIS

During the mid-1980s a new intestinal pathogen was identified in the stools of individuals with persistent diarrhoea; these were initially known as cyanobacterium-like bodies. It has subsequently become evident that this organism is a member of the coccidia, of the genus *Cyclospora*. The organism was tentatively named *Cyclospora cayetanensis*.[76]

Epidemiology

Cyclospora spp. were first identified in individuals with a history of foreign travel and those infected with HIV. Seasonal outbreaks were described in Nepal among foreign residents and travellers, and a small outbreak has been reported in medical staff in a Chicago hospital. Since these initial observations, a more detailed study in Nepal has revealed new information about the infection. As yet the global prevalence of the infection is unknown, although a prevalence of 4–7% has been reported in foreign residents in Nepal, with peak prevalence rates occurring during the warmer months with higher rainfall. *Cyclospora* diarrhoea has now been described in the Americas, the Caribbean, Africa, Bangladesh, South-east Asia, Australia, England and Eastern Europe. The incubation period is quite short, ranging from 1 to 7 days. Transmission appears to be by the faecal–oral route, with water being the most important vehicle. The first waterborne outbreak in the USA was reported in 1995. However, in 1996 a major outbreak of cyclosporiasis was investigated in the USA which was found to be due to the ingestion of Guatemalan raspberries.[77] Several further outbreaks have been documented in the USA and Canada, which again were thought to be associated with the consumption of berries. In a recent study of travellers, cyclosporiasis was as common as cryptosporidiosis (3%).[78]

Pathogenesis

The mechanism by which this organism produces diarrhoea has not been clearly established. However, the organism takes up an intracellular location within enterocytes, and histological examination of small intestinal biopsies has demonstrated mild reduction in villous height, with associated mucosal inflammation and increased numbers of intraepithelial lymphocytes. No specific virulence factors have yet been identified. *Cyclospora* diarrhoea has been associated with the development of the Guillain–Barré syndrome.

Clinical Features

There is increasing epidemiological evidence that *C. cayetanensis* is responsible for persistent diarrhoea in both immunocompetent and immunocompromised individuals. Diarrhoea can last for 1–8 weeks and may be associated with abdominal pain, nausea, vomiting and anorexia. Abdominal gas and bloating are also commonly associated features. In prolonged infection weight loss can be profound. Other than the persistence of symptoms there are no specific features that can distinguish *Cyclospora* diarrhoea from other causes of persistent diarrhoea.

Diagnosis

Oocysts can be detected in stool by light microscopy and can be induced to sporulate in the presence of 5% potassium dichromate solution. Cyst concentration techniques can be used to increase the chances of cyst identification and typical features of the *Cyclospora* spp. can be detected by transmission electron microscopy. Parasites can also be detected in small intestinal biopsies by transmission electron microscopy. Differential diagnosis includes other parasitic infections such as giardiasis, cryptosporidiosis, microsporidiosis and tropical sprue. A careful search for these parasites in faeces and in small intestinal biopsies is required to identify these infective agents. As with other protozoa, molecular diagnosis is becoming possible.[79]

Management

The treatment of choice for *C. cayetanensis* infection is trimethoprim–sulfamethoxazole (TMP-SMX) (160–800 mg twice daily for 7 days).[80] This results in the eradication of infection in more than 90% of individuals; continuation of treatment for a further 3 days will cure the majority of remaining patients. Ciprofloxacin is less effective but is suitable for patients who cannot tolerate TMP-SMX.[81]

Prevention

Epidemiological studies suggest that the major vehicle for the transmission of *Cyclospora* spp. oocysts is water. Travellers should be advised to heed the usual advice regarding the drinking of tap water in tropical and subtropical climates. As yet there are no data on the susceptibility of sporocysts to chlorination, although it is likely that, like other members of the protozoa, this is an unreliable way of inactivating cysts. However, boiling water for 10 minutes should lead to their destruction. TMP-SMX is effective for chemoprophylaxis but is usually indicated only in immunocompromised patients who experience frequent reinfections or in those who fail to clear the infection following the standard treatment regimen. There are no vaccines, though the availability of a veterinary vaccine for *Eimeria tenella* infection[82] demonstrates that there is no biological reason why a vaccine could not be developed for this or indeed any of the coccidia.

The Microspora

Microsporidia fall into the phylum Microspora.[83] Known to be parasites of vertebrates and invertebrates for many years, it is only since the HIV epidemic that they have been found to infect humans. Two species cause intestinal disease in humans: *Enterocytozoon bieneusi* and *Encephalitozoon intestinalis*. These organisms have been reclassified as Fungi.[84] Microsporidia are obligate intracellular spore-forming organisms with a wide range of hosts. Infection is acquired via the spore. Following ingestion, the spore extrudes a polar tube, through which sporoplasm is passed, infecting any enterocytes penetrated by the tube. This infection of the enterocyte is followed by proliferation by binary fission (merogony), with the meront in an intracytoplasmic position, surrounded by a simple membrane. Merogony overlaps with sporogony, which leads to the development of spores which are about 1.5×0.9 μm in size, and are shed in the faeces.

ENTEROCYTOZOON BIENEUSI

Infection in humans had not been reported before the syndrome of AIDS-related diarrhoea was recognized, but various microsporidia infect other species of vertebrates and invertebrates. Since the first report, many cases have been identified, and microsporidial infection is prominent among those infections to which the HIV-infected individual is susceptible.

Epidemiology

The prevalence of infection with microsporidia in studies of patients with AIDS diarrhoea is shown in Table 49.5. It is important to note that different diagnostic tools were used and that some of the patient series were subject to selection. There are a few reports of the infection in patients without HIV infection, but overall there is little information on the epidemiology of microsporidiosis. Infection has been diagnosed in immunocompromised organ transplant recipients, and in one child with a congenital thymic immunodeficiency. Early data from longitudinal studies of intestinal infection in Lusaka, Zambia, indicate that microsporidiosis can affect both HIV-seropositive and HIV-seronegative adults, although persistent diarrhoea is more likely in patients with advanced immunodeficiency. There is now evidence that microsporidiosis is a common infection of Ugandan children, with negative consequences for growth.[85]

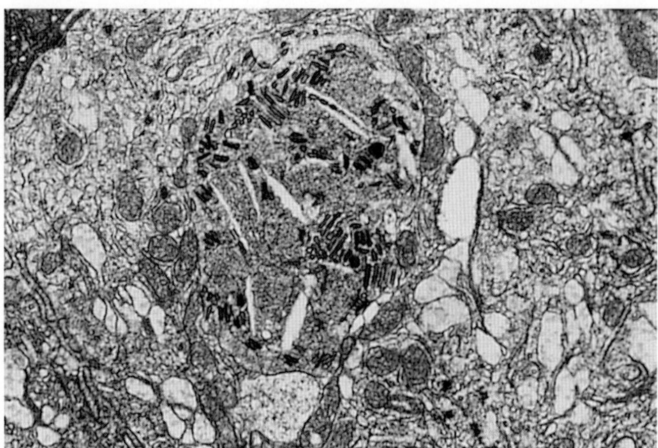

Figure 49.12 Meront of *Enterocytozoon bieneusi*, showing EDDs (×20 000). *(Courtesy of Graham McPhail.)*

Pathogenesis

Morphological studies of biopsies of infected small bowel reveal multiple meronts and sporonts in the host cell, often around the nucleus. Cells thus infected are apparently healthy at first, but the development of the later stages of sporogony is associated with enterocyte degeneration, vacuolation and loss of the brush border. These cells are subsequently sloughed off into the lumen, where the spores are liberated after cytolysis. Adjacent uninfected cells are not apparently damaged. Infection of enterocytes with microsporidia is seen only on the villi, not in the crypts. Villous atrophy occurs, possibly through increased enterocyte loss. It is not known whether adjacent spread of infection occurs from cell to cell. There is no synchrony of life cycles among different organisms parasitizing the same cell. Infection is confined to the small bowel, principally from the distal duodenum to the ileum. Studies in patients have demonstrated diminished d-xylose absorption compared with patients with AIDS-related diarrhoea without microsporidiosis, but serum vitamin B_{12} concentrations were not reduced.

Clinical Features

E. bieneusi infection is most frequently diagnosed in patients with AIDS and persistent diarrhoea. Among 38 HIV-seropositive patients with the infection, the mean duration was 7 months and only one did not have diarrhoea.[86] Most series do not report any asymptomatic infections. The volume of the diarrhoea is variable, and is associated with anorexia, nausea and crampy abdominal pain. This is probably true of all forms of AIDS-related diarrhoea. There are several reports in the literature of a sclerosing cholangitis-like syndrome, indistinguishable from that associated with cryptosporidiosis.

Diagnosis

The original and gold standard technique for diagnosis is electron microscopy of small bowel biopsies. Early meronts are recognized by the paler appearance of the cytoplasm relative to that of the host cell (Figure 49.12). The hallmark of the late meront or sporont is the development of the characteristic electron-dense polar tube, which has about 5–7.5 coils. Other characteristics include the presence of electron-lucent inclusions (ELIs) and electron-dense discs (EDDs). Spores are identifiable by their intensely osmophilic walls. Light microscopic diagnosis of histological sections of small bowel biopsy material is possible using careful scanning of sections stained with Giemsa, Brown–Brenn or Unna blue. Biopsies obtained from the distal duodenum are perfectly adequate, and either light or electron microscopy provides a more sensitive diagnostic tool than stool examination. Again, molecular diagnosis is now possible.[79]

Management

Albendazole is the treatment of choice, but fumagillin has also been found to be effective. The problem with fumagillin is its toxicity and there is an urgent need for better drugs. Albendazole inhibits microtubule formation, and thus reduces cell division and possibly polar tube action. The usual dose is 400 mg twice daily for 4 weeks, but there is evidence that *E. bieneusi* responds much less satisfactorily than *E. intestinalis.*

ENCEPHALITOZOON SPP.

Unlike *Enterocytozoon bieneusi*, *Encephalitozoon* spp. are widespread among other vertebrates. *Encephalitozoon cuniculi* is the best known, and differs from *Enterocytozoon bieneusi* in that all stages lie within a parasitophorous vacuole, and it does not cause enteropathy. Five human cases have been recorded, three with neurological disorders, one with hepatitis and one with peritonitis in a patient with AIDS. However, serological testing for *Encephalitozoon cuniculi* indicates that exposure to this microsporidian may in fact be quite common.

Another microsporidian, *Encephalitozoon intestinalis*, has been reported in patients with AIDS in developed countries and in Africa. The first case was of chronic diarrhoea due to an organism resembling, but distinct from, *Encephalitozoon cuniculi*. Subsequently, it has become apparent that this microsporidian is capable of dissemination, leading to an interstitial nephritis. The microsporidia may be found in lamina propria macrophages, and free spores can be found in the renal vasculature and portal vein. The spores are then shed in the urine. One of the characteristics of this organism is its development within a parasitophorous vacuole which is septated. For this reason, it was originally given the name *Septata intestinalis.* Most series report that it is less common in patients with AIDS and persistent diarrhoea than *E. bieneusi*, but it is more sensitive to albendazole.

REFERENCES

22. Ralston KS, Petri WA. Tissue destruction and tissue invasion by *Entamoeba histolytica*. Trends Parasitol 2011;27:253–62.
26. Fotedar R, Stark D, Beebe N, et al. Laboratory diagnostic techniques for *Entamoeba* species. Clin Microbiol Rev 2007;20:511–32.
29. Bethony JM, Cole RN, Guo X, et al. Vaccines to combat the neglected tropical diseases. Immunol Rev 2011;239:237–70.
41. ten HR, Schuurman T, Kooistra M, et al. Detection of diarrhoea-causing protozoa in general practice patients in The Netherlands by multiplex real-time PCR. Clin Microbiol Infect 2007;13:1001–7.
63. Chalmers RM, Campbell BM, Crouch N, et al. Comparison of diagnostic sensitivity and specificity of seven *Cryptosporidium* assays used in the UK. J Med Microbiol 2011;60:1598–604.

Access the complete references online at www.expertconsult.com

50

Pathogenic and Opportunistic Free-living Amoebae: Agents of Human and Animal Disease

GOVINDA S. VISVESVARA

KEY POINTS

- Since their recognition as potential human pathogens, free-living amoebae have become increasingly important during the last decade.
- *Acanthamoeba* spp. are agents of chronic granulomatous amoebic encephalitis, cutaneous and disseminated infections in principally immunocompromised persons and keratitis in immunocompetent persons.
- *Balamuthia mandrillaris* is the only species in the genus causing acute and granulomatous amoebic meningoencephalitis in both immunocompetent and immunocompromised people, particularly in persons with solid organ transplantation.
- *Naegleria fowleri* causes acute and fulminating meningoencephalitis in children and young adults with a history of recent exposure to warm fresh water resulting almost always in death in 7–10 days.
- *Sappinia pedata* is commonly found in soil contaminated with faeces of elk, bison, cattle and decaying vegetation has caused central nervous system infection in a single individual who recovered after surgical intervention and therapy.

Introduction

Members of the genera *Acanthamoeba*, *Balamuthia* and *Naegleria* are free-living, mitochondria-bearing, non-parasitic, eukaryotic amoebae that are capable of causing devastating infections in humans and other animals.[1–8] They are also called amphizoic amoebae because they exist as free-living organisms in nature and occasionally invade the host and live as parasites.[9] In addition to these three genera, one case of human infection with the genus *Sappinia* has been described.[10,11] Since their recognition as potential human pathogens, these free-living amoebae have become of increasing importance during the last decade.

The concept that the free-living amoebae can cause human infections was first developed by Culbertson and colleagues when, in 1951, they isolated an amoeba, now known as *Acanthamoeba culbertsoni*, from an uninfected monkey kidney cell culture used as control during the production of poliomyelitis vaccine. They observed plaques or cleared areas in the cell culture, which they believed was due to an unknown simian virus. When an aliquot of the cell culture was inoculated into experimental animals including monkeys, guinea pigs and mice the animals developed symptoms of meningoencephalitis and died. Culbertson et al. hypothesized that such infections might also occur in humans.[12]

Several species of *Acanthamoeba* cause a chronic infection of the central nervous system (CNS) called granulomatous amoebic encephalitis (GAE). It also disseminates into other organs including skin, lungs, nasal areas, and kidneys. Typically, such infections occur in immunocompromised hosts, including patients with human immunodeficiency virus (HIV)/acquired immune deficiency syndrome (AIDS).[1,2,4–8] Additionally, *Acanthamoeba* causes a vision-threatening infection of the eye, *Acanthamoeba* keratitis.[13–15] *Balamuthia* also causes GAE in both immunocompetent and immunocompromised individuals and disseminates into other organs including skin, sinus, lungs, kidneys, spleen and liver[1,2,4–8] In contrast, *Naegleria* causes an acute and fulminant primary amoebic meningoencephalitis (PAM) in children and young adults in apparent good health.[1,3,5,6,8,15,16]

Acanthamoeba

BIOLOGY AND TAXONOMY

In 1913, Puschkarew isolated an amoeba from dust and named it *Amoeba polyphagus*. Page re-described this amoeba as *Acanthamoeba polyphaga*.[17] The well described *Acanthamoeba castellanii* that occurred as a contaminant in a yeast culture plate was isolated by Castellani in 1930.[18]

Life Cycle of Acanthamoeba

The life cycle of *Acanthamoeba* includes a trophozoite and a cyst stage.

The amoeboid stage measures ~14–50 μm in diameter and is characterized by the presence of spine-like projections, termed acanthopodia from the surface of the body. It is uninucleate and the nucleus has a centrally placed, large, densely staining nucleolus. The cytoplasm is finely granular with numerous mitochondria, ribosomes, food vacuoles, and a contractile vacuole. In its environmental niche it feeds on bacteria and divides by binary fission. The amoebae differentiate into cysts when food supply becomes scarce or when environmental conditions change. Cysts are double-walled, range in size from 10–25 μm, and possess an outer wrinkled ectocyst and an inner stellate, polygonal, oval or round endocyst. The endocyst contains cellulose. Pores or ostioles are formed at the junction of the ecto- and endocysts.[17] When favourable conditions return, the dormant cyst converts into a trophozoite. *Acanthamoeba* spp. occur worldwide and have been isolated from a variety of environmental samples including soil, fresh, brackish and seawater, bottled mineral water, water faucet taps, filters of heating, ventilating and air conditioning units, cooling towers of electric and nuclear power plants, humidifiers, Jacuzzi tubs, hydrotherapy baths in hospitals, dental irrigation units, dialysis machines, home aquaria, dust in the air, bacterial, fungal and mammalian cell cultures, eye wash irrigation units, contact lens paraphernalia, ear discharge, pulmonary secretions, swabs obtained from nasopharyngeal mucosa of patients with respiratory complaints as well as healthy individuals, maxillary sinus, mandibular autografts, stool samples, and any moist environment where a bacterial food source is available for growth.[1,2,5–8] Since acanthamoebae have occurred as contaminants of tissue cultures, they have been mistaken for viruses.[19]

The classical taxonomic classification of Protozoa consisted of four groups: Sarcodina (amoebae); Mastigophora (flagellates); Sporozoa (most spore-forming parasitic protozoa); and Infusoria (ciliates). Recently, the International Society of Protozoologists abandoned the classical taxonomy and created a new system based on modern morphological approaches, biochemical pathways and molecular phylogenetics.[20] According to this new schema, the Eukaryotes have been classified into six clusters or 'Super Groups' namely: Amoebozoa, Opisthokonta, Rhizaria, Archaeplastida, Chromalveolata and Excavata. *Acanthamoeba* and *Balamuthia* are included under Super Group Amoebozoa (Acanthamoebidae); *Naegleria fowleri* under Super Group Excavata (Heterolobosia, Vahlkampfiidae) and *Sappinia* under Super Group Amoebozoa (Flabellinea, Thecamoebidae).[20]

In the genus *Acanthamoeba*, more than 24 species were created based on the morphology and size of trophozoites and cysts and included in three different groups.[2,6,7,9,21,22] Group 1 consists of those species that have large trophozoites with cysts ranging in size from 16–30 μm. Group 2 includes by far the largest numbers of species with cysts measuring around 18 μm or less. Group 3 also consists of species with cysts measuring 18 μm or less but have subtle differences in the cyst morphology. Since morphology of cysts varies based on the culture methods employed it is considered unreliable, therefore non-morphologic methods, especially molecular characteristics based on the sequencing of the18S rRNA gene, are considered more accurate for identifying and defining phylogenetic relationships of *Acanthamoeba*.[23,24] Currently, 18 genotypes (T1–T18) of *Acanthamoeba* have been established based on sequence differences.[23–27]

Acanthamoeba spp. can be easily cultivated on non-nutrient agar plates coated with bacteria such as *Escherichia coli* or *Enterobacter aerogenes*. The amoebae feed on bacteria, multiply, and colonize the plates within a few days and encyst when almost all of the food is consumed.[28] Cysts are resistant to adverse physical and chemical conditions and remain viable for a long time. For example, cysts of *Acanthamoeba* spp. belonging to many different genotypes survived desiccation for more than 20 years.[29] *Acanthamoebae* can be maintained in the laboratory indefinitely by periodically cutting out a small piece of agar containing trophozoites and/or cysts and transplanting it onto a fresh agar plate coated with bacteria. Hence the agar plate method is the recommended technique for the isolation and maintenance of *Acanthamoeba* from clinical specimens such as brain, lungs, skin, nasal tissues and corneal scrapings, and environmental samples. Additionally, *Acanthamoeba* spp. can also be cultured on axenic cultures, mammalian cell cultures as well as a chemically defined medium. Isolates from GAE cases grow optimally at 37°C whereas isolates from keratitis cases grow better at 30°C consistent with their superficial location.[28]

GRANULOMATOUS AMOEBIC ENCEPHALITIS

Clinical Features and Diagnosis

Several species of *Acanthamoeba* (e.g. *A. castellanii, A. culbertsoni, A. hatchetti, A. healyi, A. polyphaga, A. rhysodes, A. astronyxis, A. lenticulata* and *A. divionensis*) are known to cause GAE, an insidious and chronic infection of the CNS which might span from several weeks to months.[1,2,5,8] *Acanthamoeba* GAE cases are increasing in number particularly in organ transplant recipients in addition to patients with HIV/AIDS or persons who are chronically ill, diabetic, or are otherwise debilitated and with compromised metabolic, physiologic or immunologic integrity.[30–61] GAE cases may occur at any time of the year and have no relation to seasonality or exposure to freshwater. The portal of entry may vary because of the ubiquity of *Acanthamoeba* in the environment. For example it might enter the body: (a) through the skin and cause infection; (b) via the nasal sinuses since trophozoites and/or cysts of *Acanthamoeba* have been isolated from dust in the air and the nasal mucosa of healthy and hospitalized persons.[61–64] In one case, amoebae were also found in a biopsy of a perforated gastric ulcer, suggesting an oral route.[65] The prodromal period of *Acanthamoeba* GAE is unknown and several weeks or months might elapse before the disease becomes apparent. The common clinical symptoms consist of headache, stiff neck, and mental state abnormalities as well as nausea, vomiting, low-grade fever, lethargy, cerebellar ataxia, visual disturbances, haemiparesis, seizures and coma. Facial palsy with facial numbness resulting in facial asymmetry is often seen. Chronic skin ulcers, abscesses, or erythematous nodules are also seen in some HIV/AIDS patients.[1,2,5–8] Several cases with skin ulcers without CNS involvement have also been reported.[1,2,5–8,46,50]

Amoebae are occasionally found in the CSF.[53,56,61] CSF examination in general, reveals lymphocytic pleocytosis with mild elevation of proteins and normal or slightly depressed glucose. Computerized tomography (CT) scans of the brain show either patchy or large areas of hypodensity abnormality mimicking a single or multiple space-occupying mass. Magnetic resonance imaging (MRI) shows diffuse leptomeningeal enhancements involving cerebrum, the cerebellum, basilar cisterns and middle fossa or may show multiple, ring-enhancing lesions in the brain.[66] Cerebral hemispheres are often oedematous, with extensive haemorrhagic necrosis involving the temporal, parietal, and occipital lobes. Finally hydrocephalus develops, leading to brain herniation and death. Brainstem, cerebral hemispheres and cerebellum may show areas of haemorrhagic infarcts. Histopathologic examination at biopsy/autopsy reveals multinucleated giant cells along with trophozoites and/or cysts of *Acanthamoeba* in the cerebral hemispheres, brain stem, midbrain, cerebellum, and basal ganglion (Figure 50.1).[1,2,5–8] Additionally, blood vessels are cuffed by polymorphonuclear leukocytes (PMN) and trophozoites and cysts. Although *Acanthamoeba* can be identified by haematoxylin and eosin (H&E) staining; it can also be mistaken for macrophages and necrotic epithelial cells. Immunohistochemical stains for CD68 and pancytokeratin might help in excluding macrophages and necrotic keratinocytes. Since *Balamuthia* also produces cysts that are

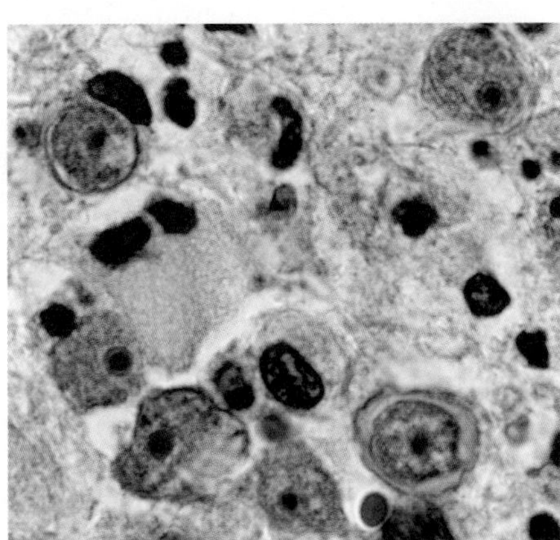

Figure 50.1 CNS section with *Acanthamoeba* trophozoites and cyst. (A, H&E, ×100; B, H&E, ×1000).

morphologically similar to *Acanthamoeba* in the H&E-stained tissue sections immunohistochemical techniques are necessary to differentiate *Acanthamoeba* from *Balamuthia*.[1,2,5–8,67] PCR and real-time PCR are also used in the identification of *Acanthamoeba*.[68,69] A multiplex real-time PCR assay that detects all three free-living amoebae is used currently at the Centers for Disease Control and Prevention (CDC).[68]

In addition to causing infections in humans, *Acanthamoeba* spp. also cause infections of the CNS of animals including gorillas, monkeys, dogs, sheep, cattle, horses, and kangaroos as well as birds, reptiles, amphibians, fish and even invertebrates.[1,2,5–8,70–73] The pathogenic potential and virulence of *Acanthamoeba* isolates is usually determined by intranasal inoculation of young mice.[1,2,5–8] The animals develop ruffled fur, aimless wandering, partial paralysis and die in 1–4 weeks following inoculation.[74]

ACANTHAMOEBA KERATITIS (AK)

Clinical and Laboratory Diagnostic Methods

AK is a painful vision-threatening infection that may lead to ulceration of the cornea, loss of visual acuity, and eventually blindness and enucleation.[1,2,5–8,13,14] AK is characterized by: inflammation of the cornea; severe ocular pain and photophobia; lacrimation; a characteristic 360° or paracentral stromal ring infiltrate; recurrent breakdown of corneal epithelium; and a corneal lesion refractory to the commonly used antibiotics. AK is often misdiagnosed as dendritic keratitis due to herpes simplex.[1,2,5–8] Unlike GAE, AK occurs in immunocompetent individuals following corneal trauma[75,76] or due to contact lens (CL) wear and using contaminated CL solutions or CL cases.[13,14,77,78] Once established in the CL case, amoebae proliferate and can migrate from the lens surface to the corneal surface. Amoebae adhere to the corneal surface probably because of the presence of specific receptors on the surface, and the presence of calcium ion.[79] Once attached, they infiltrate the stroma and cause tissue necrosis.[13,14] The trophozoites differentiate into cysts in the presence of commonly used antibiotics. Because the cysts are resistant to these agents, they survive the course of therapy and when the antibiotics are withdrawn, the cysts convert into trophozoites and cause further problems. In the early stages, *Acanthamoeba* invades and destroys the anterior cornea and the trophozoites and cysts are seen interspersed with the polymorphonuclear leukocytes (PMN). During later stages, ulceration, descemetocele formation and perforation of the cornea occur.

Definitive diagnosis is made upon microscopic examination of stained (H&E, calcofluor white or immunofluorescence) slides, or PCR of corneal scrapings or biopsies or cultivation of *Acanthamoeba* from infected tissue.[75–82] Recently, confocal microscopy has been used as a diagnostic tool.[81] Although as many as 18 sequence types (T1–T18) have been described, amoebae belonging to sequence type T4 has been identified predominantly from AK cases.[81,82]

The first cases of AK were described from the UK and the USA.[75,80] Jones et al.[75] reported in 1973, a case of AK in a south Texas rancher with a history of trauma to his right eye. An increase in the numbers of AK reported in 1985 in contact lens wearers[77] resulted in a study by CDC which revealed that a major risk factor for AK was the use of contact lenses and that the patients with AK were significantly more likely than controls to use homemade saline solution instead of commercial solution.[78] A recent CDC investigation on a national increase in the AK cases, identified an association with a specific multipurpose contact lens solution[82] probably because of the inefficiency of the solution in killing *Acanthamoeba* cysts.[83]

Pathogenesis

Acanthamoeba uses several different pathogenic mechanisms to cause damage to cornea or brain tissues. When co-cultured with hamster cornea *Acanthamoeba* undergoes morphological changes and ingests bits and pieces of host cells by phagocytosis.[84] Additionally, acanthamoebae secrete enzymes including phospholipases, cysteine proteinases, metalloproteinases and plasminogen, which lyse the host cells and thus facilitate spread of amoebae.[85–88] Other studies using rabbit corneal epithelium have shown that mannose, but not other sugars, inhibits binding of *Acanthamoeba* trophozoites to the epithelial cells. The initial process of invasion occurs when a 136-kDa mannose-binding protein on the surface of the amoeba adheres to mannose glycoproteins on the surface of the epithelial cells facilitating the invasion and destruction of the corneal stroma.[14,79,86] Further, *Acanthamoeba* trophozoites when co-cultured with microglial cells produce a variety of interleukins (IL-1α and β, and tumor necrosis factor).[88,89] The interleukins together with macrophage might play a role in the destruction of *Acanthamoeba*. The macrophage-mediated killing is probably contact-dependent.[3,13,14,79,86] Additionally, the neutrophils might release lysosomal enzymes and reactive oxygen intermediates including hypochlorite and hydrogen peroxide after activation by the complement thereby killing the amoebae.[90] However, in the immunosuppressed individual, due to the lack of T-lymphocytes and macrophages and impairment of cell-mediated immunity, acanthamoebae are able to proliferate and damage the CNS and other tissues.[1,2,5–8]

Immunology

It is quite likely that humans develop antibodies to *Acanthamoeba* because of its ubiquity.[87,91–95] Whether this natural antibody results in protective immunity against infection is unknown. Previous studies have shown that antibodies to *Acanthamoeba* exist in sera of healthy soldiers as well as hospitalized patients in Czechoslovakia, adults and children from New Zealand, and patients hospitalized for respiratory problems.[1,2,5–8,93] Antibodies to *Acanthamoeba* have also been demonstrated in patients who developed GAE and/or skin infections. Antibodies to *Acanthamoeba* in patients with AK have also been detected by a variety of techniques including gel diffusion, immunofluorescence and enzyme-linked immunosorbent assay (ELISA).[1,2,5–8,92] Another study using an ELISA test found that Hispanic Americans had lesser ability to develop antibodies to *Acanthamoeba* compared with other groups of Americans.[95]

Management

Most cases of GAE have been identified only at autopsy. However, a few patients have survived after therapy with multiple antimicrobial agents including pentamidine, itraconazole, 5-fluorocytosine, rifampin, cotrimaxazole and miltefosine.[31,32,46,48,50,53,57–60] Cutaneous ulcers in two of these patients were cleansed with topical application of chlorhexidine and ketoconazole cream.[46,50] Other drugs used in the treatment include fluconazole, ketoconazole or itraconazole.[1,2,5–8] No single drug has been effective in clearing an infection. Voriconazole, a triazole compound has been used recently to clear skin ulcers in a patient recovering from lung transplantation.[46] This was possible because in vitro testing on four clinical isolates found it to be inhibitory even at a concentration of 5 μg/mL.[96] In vitro studies have shown that miltefosine, a hexadecylphosphocholine, has amoebicidal activity[60,96] and it has been used both orally and topically to treat successfully a GAE patient in Austria.[60] Currently, treatment of GAE patients include pentamidine isethionate IV 4 mg/kg body weight/24 hours; sulfadiazine 500 mg daily, pyrimethamine 50 mg once a day; voriconazole 200 mg twice a day and miltefosine along with topical application of chlorhexidine and miltefosine.

Treatment of AK also included a combination of drugs including clotrimazole, ketoconazole, miconazole, itraconazole, paromomycin, polymyxin B, propamidine isethionate, dibromopropamidine isethionate (Brolene®), neomycin along with debridement of the cornea and penetrating keratoplasty.[1,2,5–8,13,14] Brolene® has been used in conjunction with neomycin for treating AK. It may be accompanied by drug toxicity and the amoebae might develop resistance.[97,98] Medical cure has recently been achieved with the use of either polyhexamethylene biguanide (PHMB) or chlorhexidine gluconate along with neomycin.[99,100] Currently, the drugs of choice for AK are 0.02% chlorhexidine digluconate in 0.9% physiological saline and 0.1% propamidine isethionate (Brolene®) given hourly around the clock for the first 72 hours. Thereafter, it is given every two hours during the day for 4 weeks followed by 3-hourly during the day for 4 weeks and every 4 hours during the day for another 4 months. Some patients have also been cured with the use of PHMB in conjunction with propamidine isethionate and neomycin.[14]

Endosymbionts. *Acanthamoeba* spp. harbour human pathogenic bacterial endosymbionts. For example: *Legionella* spp., *Francisella tularensis*, *Mycobacterium avium*, *Burkholderia*, *Vibrio cholerae*, *Listeria monocytogenes*, *Helicobacter pylori*, *Afipia felis* and *Escherichia coli* serotype O157 have been identified as endosymbionts.[101] *Acanthamoeba* infected with *Legionella*-like bacteria has been isolated from soil samples.[102] Both *M. avium* and *Legionella* have been found to survive within *Acanthamoeba* cysts.[103,104]

Prevention

No method is available for the prevention of *Acanthamoeba* GAE. However, AK can be controlled by educating lens wearers to: (a) remove CLs before any activity involving contact with water, including showering, using a hot tub, or swimming; (b) wash hands with soap and water and dry before handling CLs; (c) clean CLs according to the manufacturer's guidelines, including using fresh cleaning or disinfecting solution each time lenses are cleaned and stored; (d) store reusable lenses in the proper storage case, clean as directed and replace the case at least every 3 months.

Balamuthia mandrillaris

BIOLOGY

The isolation of *Balamuthia mandrillaris*, initially described as leptomyxid amoebae, from the brain of a pregnant mandrill baboon that died in the San Diego Wildlife Park, and subsequent development of rabbit antiserum against it, enabled the detection of the several non-*Acanthamoeba-Naegleria* cases as due to *B. mandrillaris*.[105,106] *Balamuthia* trophozoites are pleomorphic and are larger (12–60 μm in length) than either *Acanthamoeba* or *N. fowleri*. *Balamuthia* exhibits two types of locomotion; in one type it moves by typical amoeboid locomotion in cultures. In the second type it exhibits a spider-like locomotion on extended leg-like pseudopodia when feeding on tissue culture.[105,106] It has a cyst stage but lacks a flagellate stage. The cyst is spherical, and ranges in size from 12 to 30 μm, with a mean of 15 μm. The cyst wall appears as double-layered under light microscopy, but is actually three-layered when examined with the electron microscope. It has an outer thin and irregular ectocyst, a thick endocyst and a middle amorphous fibrillar mesocyst. Both trophozoites and cysts are uninucleate and contain a large centrally placed nucleolus. Binucleate trophozoites are occasionally seen. Occasionally, the nucleus, especially in tissue sections of infected patients, may have more than one nucleolus.[105,106] *B. mandrillaris* was initially identified as a leptomyxid amoeba because it resembles, especially in the cyst stage, many features that are typical to the amoebae included in the family leptomyxidae.[107] However, molecular sequencing revealed that this amoeba was different from the leptomyxids but was related to *Acanthamoeba*.[108,109] According to the new taxonomic schema therefore *Balamuthia* is classified with *Acanthamoeba*, and is placed in the family Acanthamoebidae, Amoebozoa.[20]

B. mandrillaris will not grow on bacteria although it has been shown to ingest fluorescently labelled, heat-killed bacteria.[110] However, it grows well on tissue culture monolayers such as monkey kidney, human lung fibroblasts, rat glial cells, and human brain microvascular cells.[105,106,111–114] Therefore, *Balamuthia* amoebae have been routinely isolated from CSF and brain and skin tissue using mammalian cell cultures. The amoebae feed on the cell monolayer and destroy it within a short time. Amoebae maintained on tissue culture cells cause a cytopathic effect (CPE) on the cell culture but lose their ability to cause CPE if maintained in axenic medium for a long period.[111]

GRANULOMATOUS AMOEBIC ENCEPHALITIS

Clinical Features and Diagnosis

Balamuthia causes a slow, insidious and chronic disease like that caused by *Acanthamoeba* and may develop over a period of time from about 2 weeks to 2 years. Infections with *Balamuthia* have occurred in immunocompromised hosts, including HIV/

AIDS patients and immunocompetent individuals.[1,4–6,8] Infections with *B. mandrillaris* have been documented from all over the world.[114–152] Cases have occurred in children,[115,117,122,124,128,135,139,142,144,151,152,153] as well as older persons.[1,4–6,8] The disease has occurred in humans over a wide age range from 0.8 years to >50 years. Most of the young who developed the disease have had no obvious risk factors and have reportedly been in good health. Children infected with *Balamuthia* developed facial skin lesions and/or rhinitis/sinusitis,[141,145] or otitis media.[122,151] With few exceptions,[119,128,129,135–137,143] all individuals who developed GAE have died.

Symptoms

The disease is insidious and chronic in most cases. However, in the recent transplant transmitted cases, infections manifested within 3 weeks.[137,138] In most cases the common symptoms include headache, meningismus, nausea, vomiting, low-grade fever, lethargy, myalgia, visual disturbances, facial nerve palsy, ataxia, weight loss, haemiparesis and seizures leading to, over a period of several months to 2 years,[106,124,144,145] coma and death due to increased intracranial pressure and/or brain herniation.[1,4–6,8] CSF shows lymphocytic pleocytosis typically with less than 500 cell/mm^3, increased protein, increasing from normal (15 to 45 mg/dL) to over 1000 mg/dL, but near- or below-normal levels of glucose.[115–118,122–124,127,128,139] Differential diagnoses include neurotuberculosis, neurocysticercosis, bacterial abscess, viral or bacterial encephalitis, acute disseminated encephalomyelitis, leptomeningitis, and brain tumour. Rarely, *Balamuthia* amoebae have been isolated from the CSF.[113,137] However, *Balamuthia* mitochondrial DNA has been demonstrated in CSF by PCR.[154]

Neuroimaging

Although CT scans are unremarkable, MRI scans show single or multiple lesions of low density with peripheral ring enhancement and mass effect.[66,155] Single lesions may be seen initially but may develop into multifocal lesions as the disease progresses.[66] MRIs of two surviving patients showed changes in cranial lesions following recovery. The lesions came to be enclosed by calcified walls which, in turn, were surrounded by oedematous areas.[4,128,155] With time, the lesions regressed in size and the oedematous areas resolved. One patient, a 5-year-old child, showed no gross neurologic deficits but the other survivor, a 60+-year-old man, had significant neurological deficits.[128]

In addition to the typical CNS infection *Balamuthia* causes disseminated infections and spreads to skin, nasal sinuses, lungs, pancreas, liver, adrenals, kidneys and uterus.[1,4–6,8] In many disseminated cases skin lesions on the trunk and limbs occur a few months before CNS symptoms appear.[4,116,119,128,129,140,141,143] In Peruvian cases, neurological signs appear 1 month to 2 years (average 5–8 months) after skin ulcers develop.[119] The skin ulcers usually occur in the form of an erythematous plaque of rubbery to hard consistency and are located on the nose, cheeks, trunk and/or the limbs.[119] It is likely that the initial portal of entry is the skin or the lower respiratory tract and haematogenous dissemination to CNS occurs subsequently.

Immune Response

Since *Balamuthia* causes chronic infection it elicits a humoral response. In the early stages of infection, IgM, and later an IgG, response occur.[156–160] Despite the elevated levels of these antibodies, the infection progresses insidiously. In several patients that survived the infection serum antibody dropped from 1:256 to 1:64 after a few months or years.[137] In a Western blot assay, positive human sera reacted strongly with electrophoresed antigens around 25, 40, 50, and 75 kDa. Incidentally, antigens around 40 kDa detected by human serum were not recognized by hyperimmune rabbit serum.[158] Huang et al.[159] identified both IgM and IgG antibodies in the sera of healthy individuals in Australia. Schuster et al.[156] screened 290 individuals with encephalitis by *Balamuthia* antibodies and found seven cases (2%) by IFA with titres of ≥1:128. All of these cases were positive by immunohistochemical staining and/or by PCR. Kiderlen et al.[160] found elevated levels of anti-*Balamuthia* antibodies in 19% (11/59) of German blood donors, 92% (23/25) of persons involved in a primate project in West Africa and all West Africans belonging to traditional farming and hunting communities.[160] and concluded that the high-titred antibody to *Balamuthia* is probably the result of exposure to either *Balamuthia* or some other antigenically similar free-living amoebae.

Pathology, Pathogenesis and Epidemiology

B. mandrillaris may cause both a granulomatous as well as an acute meningoencephalitis.[67] Gross pathology reveals an oedematous brain often with evidence of uncal and tonsillar herniation. Pathologic examination revealed a spectrum from acute inflammation consisting primarily of neutrophils to granulomatous inflammation.[67] In some cases, acute inflammatory infiltrates were seen in the subarachnoid spaces and meninges, suggesting a possible route of infection via olfactory mucosa.[67,131] Generally, in most cases however, haemorrhagic necrosis in the midbrain, thalamus, brainstem, cerebral hemispheres and cerebellum[8] are seen. In some cases, amoebae infiltrated blood vessels provoking vasculitis and thrombosis.[4,8,115,123,127,139] The amoebae with two or more nucleoli (Figure 50.2) were difficult to identify and can be mistaken for macrophages in areas of the CNS where there is intense inflammation and necrosis.[67] Immunofluorescence, PCR and real-time PCR assays using primer sets of 230-bp and 1075-bp in length have been used in diagnosis.[68,161,162]

Balamuthia rapidly destroys the tissue culture by active phagocytosis probably by producing feeding cups.[114]

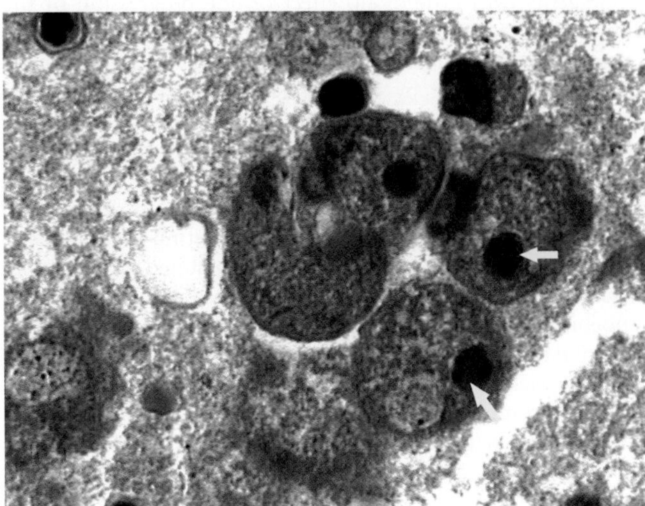

Figure 50.2 *Balamuthia mandrillaris* in a CNS section (H&E ×1000). Note: *Balamuthia* trophozoite with multiple nucleoli. Arrows at cysts.

Additionally, the amoebae cause the mouse macrophage cells to swell and apparently rupture and the destruction of feeder cells was contact-dependent.[111] Separation of amoebae from target cells by a semipermeable membrane reduced or prevented destruction, as did lysates of the amoebae and inhibitors of actin polymerization (cytochalasin B, latrunculin and an algal toxin). In another study *Balamuthia* was shown to penetrate the cells and lie quiescent for several hours before exiting the cell.[163] Another possible mechanism is the production of metalloproteases, enzymes which function both intra- and extracellularly.[164] The proteases destroy the extracellular matrix (collagen, elastin and plasminogen) that hold brain cells together and facilitate penetration into the brain parenchyma. Additionally, other enzymes – lipase, phospholipase A and lysophospholipase A – may also be involved.[4,164] *Balamuthia* stimulates IL-6 production in the host.[4] The release of IL-6 causes alterations in the blood–brain barrier facilitating movement of leukocytes (and perhaps *Balamuthia*) across the blood–brain barrier.[4]

In the USA, *Balamuthia* infection has occurred disproportionately in Hispanic Americans. Almost one half of the cases have occurred in Hispanics, although they comprise little more than 30% of the population. Possibly Hispanics are either genetically predisposed or other factors such as lifestyle, socioeconomic status, travel background, access to clean water and availability of medical services may have played a role.[165]

Balamuthia GAE has also been reported in animals, particularly those in zoological parks.[1,4,5,162,166] An animal model for the study of *Balamuthia* GAE has been made using both the SCID (severe combined immuno deficient) and immunocompetent mice.[167–169]

The environmental niche of *Balamuthia* amoebae is not well established. They have been isolated only a few times from soil[170,171] and dust[172] samples, although their DNA has been identified in a variety of environmental samples, including water.[173] Therefore, contamination of a wound while gardening[128,129] or inhalation of dust in the environment[4,116] or exposure to fresh dirty water[162] are probably sources of infection and spread via a haematogenous route to the brain and other organs.

Management

Until recently, most of the individuals infected with *Balamuthia* were treated empirically with antibacterial, antifungal, or antiviral agents with little or no effect on the progression of the disease. In vitro studies have shown that pentamidine and propamidine isethionate at a concentration of 1 μg/mL inhibit growth of amoebae by 82% and 80%, respectively.[112] The drugs were amoeba static but not amoebicidal. Other drugs including macrolides, antibiotics, azoles, gramicidin, polymyxin B, trimethoprim, sulfamethoxazole, and a combination of trimethoprim-sulfamethoxazole did not have any appreciable effect on *Balamuthia*.[112] A recent in vitro testing of miltefosine revealed that concentrations of 40 mM inhibited growth of all isolates and caused rapid lysis of amoebae and the minimal amoebicidal concentration (MAC) was 75 mM. Voriconazole did not have any activity at all on the *Balamuthia* trophozoites.[95] Several patients have recovered from this infection[128,129,135–138,143] following combination or sequential antimicrobial therapy. A 60+-year-old man was treated with 5-fluorocytosine (flucytosine; 2 g every 6 hours PO), fluconazole (400 mg/day), pentamidine isethionate (4 mg/kg per day IV), and sulfadiazine (1.5 g every 6 hours PO) and clarithromycin (500 mg/day).[128] A 5-year-old-girl was treated with clarithromycin (14 mg/kg per day) and flucytosine (~110 mg/kg per day), fluconazole (14 mg/kg per day), thioridazine (1 mg/kg per day), and pentamidine (1 mg/kg per day).[128] An 80-year-old woman from Australia was treated with IV pentamidine, oral azithromycin, oral itraconazole, oral sulfadiazine, and oral flucytosine after surgical excision of the lone cerebral lesion. Pentamidine was removed because of toxicity but the four oral drugs were continued for 7 months.[129] Recently, a transplant-transmitted patient was successfully treated with: fluconazole 400 mg IV twice a day; pentamidine 380 mg IV daily; sulfadiazine 150 mg four times a day; flucytosine 2000 mg PO daily and miltefosine 150 mg PO daily[137] and a Peruvian patient recovered after fluconazole 400 mg IV twice a day, pentamidine 380 mg IV daily, sulfadiazine 150 mg four times a day, flucytosine 2000 mg PO daily and miltefosine 150 mg PO daily treatment.[143]

Naegleria fowleri

BIOLOGY AND EPIDEMIOLOGY

The genus *Naegleria* was established by Alexeieff in 1912 for small amoebae that possess a temporary flagellate phase and the amoebae divide by promitosis during which the nuclear membrane remains intact during mitosis.[174] Currently, the genus *Naegleria* has been reported to contain 47 species[175] but only one species, *N. fowleri*, is pathogenic to humans. Two other species (*N. australiensis* and *N. italica*) are known to be pathogenic to mice after intranasal or intracerebral inoculations.

The life cycle of *Naegleria fowleri* consists of three stages: a feeding and dividing trophozoite, a transitory flagellate and a round cyst. Because of the presence of flagellates in the life cycle, *N. fowleri* is also called an ameboflagellate. The trophozoite moves rapidly by producing hemispherical bulges (lobopodia) at the anterior end and exhibits eruptive locomotion. It measures from 10–25 μm and feeds on Gram-negative bacteria and reproduces by binary fission. It has a single nucleus with a prominent, centrally placed nucleolus that stains densely with chromatic dyes. The cytoplasm contains numerous mitochondria, ribosomes, food vacuoles and a contractile vacuole. The posterior end of the trophozoite (uroid) is sticky and may have one to several trailing filaments. The trophozoite converts into a flagellate with two or more flagella, when the ionic concentration of the milieu changes. The flagellate ranges in length from 10–16 μm and usually reverts to the amoeboid form. In the laboratory, this transformation can be induced by exposing trophozoites to distilled water. Within a few minutes to an hour the trophozoites convert into flagellates with two or more flagella. The trophozoite transforms into the resistant cyst when the food supply is lacking and its environmental niche dries up. The cyst ranges in size from 6 to 12 μm, is usually spherical and double-walled with a thicker endocyst and a thinner ectocyst. The cyst wall has pores but the pores are difficult to see because they are flush with the cyst wall. Both the flagellate and cyst stages also possess a single nucleus with a prominent nucleolus.[9,174]

N. fowleri occurs worldwide and has been isolated from soil, warm fresh water, thermal effluents of power plants and hot springs, human nose and even sewage.[3,174–179] *N. fowleri* is thermophilic and can tolerate temperatures of up to 45°C. Therefore, these amoebae proliferate during summer months when the ambient temperature is high.

Since the amoebae feed on bacteria, they can be grown in the laboratory on non-nutrient agar with a lawn of bacteria, such as *Escherichia coli* or *Enterobacter aerogenes*.[28] They can also be grown in axenic medium, in a complex defined medium and on cell cultures.[28]

PRIMARY AMOEBIC MENINGOENCEPHALITIS

Clinical Features and Diagnosis

N. fowleri causes an acute and fulminating infection of the CNS called primary amoebic meningoencephalitis (PAM) primarily in children and young adults in seemingly good health, with no outward evidence of immunological deficiency. The patients usually have a history of swimming in warm freshwater lakes, streams or pools, or hot springs.[16] The portal of entry is the nasal passages because once aspirated the amoebae attach to the nasal mucosa, migrate across the cribriform plate to the brain via the olfactory nerves and proliferate in brain tissue, meninges, and CSF and cause extensive damage to the CNS.[1,3,5,6,8] This has been documented by infections via the intranasal route in the mouse model.[180] Typically, cases of PAM occur in the hot summer months when the ambient temperature increases and large numbers of people engage in recreational activities in freshwater bodies such as lakes, ponds and inadequately maintained swimming pools that may harbour these amoebae.[16]

The symptoms of PAM include sudden onset of bifrontal or bitemporal headaches, high fever, neck stiffness with positive Kernig's and Brudzinski's signs, nausea, vomiting, diplopia, photophobia, irritability and restlessness followed by neurological abnormalities including lethargy, seizures, bizarre behaviour, confusion, coma, leading to death within a week. Cranial nerve palsies (third, fourth, and sixth cranial nerves) may indicate brain oedema and herniation. Intracranial pressure is usually raised to 600 mmH_2O or higher. Cardiac rhythm abnormalities and myocardial necrosis have been found in some cases. With few exceptions, all cases of PAM reported in the literature have been fatal.[1,3,8,181–207]

No distinctive and clear-cut clinical features differentiate PAM from acute pyogenic or bacterial meningoencephalitis. CSF may vary in colour from greyish to yellowish-white and may be tinged red with few (250/mm^3) red blood cells (RBC) in the early stages of disease. As the disease progresses, RBC may increase in number to as high as 24 600/mm^3. The white blood cell count, predominantly PMN may vary from 300 cells/mm^3 to as high as 26 000 mm^3. Bacteria or fungi are not seen. The CSF pressure is usually elevated (300–600 mmH_2O). The protein concentration may range from 100 mg/100 mL to 1000 mg/100 mL, and glucose may be 10 mg/100 mL or lower.[1,3,8] Microscopic examination of CSF smear in situ will reveal the presence of actively moving trophozoites. Smears of CSF should be stained with Giemsa or Wright stains to identify the trophozoite based on its nucleus with a centrally placed large nucleolus (Figure 50.3). Gram stain is not useful. The cause of death is usually due to increased intracranial pressure with brain herniation leading to cardiopulmonary arrest and pulmonary oedema.[1,3,8] PCR and nested PCR assays for the specific identification of *N. fowleri* in CSF, cultured amoebae from patients and the environment as well as *N. fowleri* DNA in the environment have been developed.[208–211] Sequencing of the 5.8S rRNA gene and the internal transcribed spacers 1 and 2 (ITS1 and ITS2) of *N. fowleri* has been used to identify specific genotypes. As many as eight genotypes have been identified. However, only genotypes 1, 2 and 3 have been identified in the USA.[175] A real-time multiplex PCR assay developed at the CDC identifies all three genotypes present in the USA.[69] This is a quick test with short turnaround time (~4 hours), invaluable for initiating appropriate treatment.

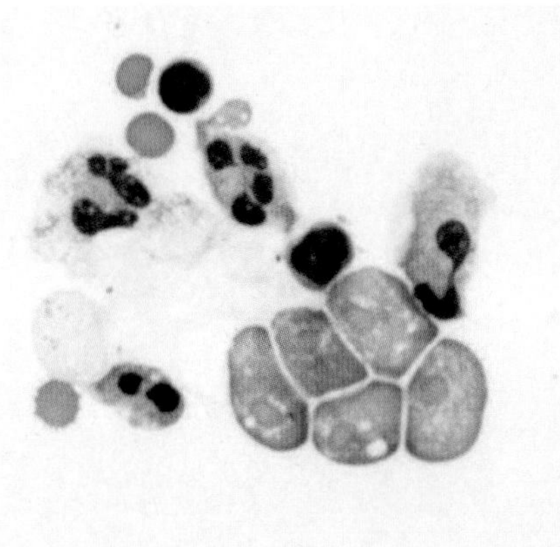

Figure 50.3 *Naegleria fowleri* trophozoites in a CSF smear interspersed with polymorphonuclear leukocytes. (Giemsa ×1500) *Courtesy of Neslihan Cetin, M.D.*

PAM can be experimentally reproduced by inoculating mice intranasally or intracerebrally with a suspension of amoebae. Mice develop the disease and usually die within a week. Continuous cultivation of clinical isolates in an axenic medium reduces the virulence of amoebae but virulence can be restored by mouse passage or via tissue culture.[3]

Pathology and Pathogenesis

PAM is characterized predominantly with acute meningeal inflammation. The cerebral hemispheres are usually soft, markedly swollen, oedematous and severely congested. The leptomeninges (arachnoid and pia mater) are severely congested, diffusely hyperaemic and opaque with limited purulent exudate within sulci, base of the brain, brainstem and cerebellum. The olfactory bulbs are characterized by haemorrhagic necrosis and are surrounded by purulent exudate. The cortex also shows numerous superficial haemorrhagic areas. Most of the lesions are found in and around the base of the orbitofrontal and temporal lobes, base of the brain, hypothalamus, midbrain, pons, medulla oblongata and upper portion of the spinal cord.[1,3,5,6,8] CT scans show obliteration of the cisternae around the midbrain and the subarachnoid space over the cerebral hemispheres. Marked diffuse enhancement in these regions may be seen after administration of intravenous contrast medium.

Microscopic examination of the CNS reveals that the cerebral hemispheres, brainstem, cerebellum, and upper portion of the spinal cord are filled with fibrino-purulent leptomeningeal exudate containing predominantly PMN, few eosinophils, few macrophages and some lymphocytes. Large numbers of trophozoites, usually in pockets without the presence of PMN, are seen within oedematous and necrotic neural tissue and in Virchow–Robin spaces usually around blood vessels with no inflammation (Figure 50.4). Amoebae ranging in size from 8–12 μm are recognizable by the presence of a large nucleus with a centrally located, deeply staining large nucleolus. Trophozoites can be identified by immunohistochemical tests by using polyclonal or

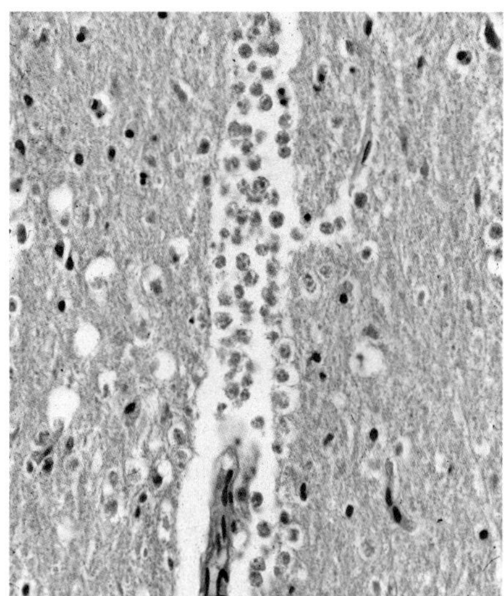

Figure 50.4 *Naegleria fowleri* trophozoites in large numbers in a CNS section. (H&E ×400)

monoclonal antibodies. *N. fowleri* does not produce cysts in the brain tissue.[1,3,5,6,8]

The portal of entry into the CNS is the olfactory neuroepithelium. It is believed that the sustentacular cells lining the olfactory neuroepithelium phagocytose the amoebae that enter the nasal passages.[180] The trophozoites pierce the cribriform plate of the ethmoid bone and penetrate into the subarachnoid space and continue on to the brain parenchyma. *N. fowleri* can be easily cultured from samples of CSF or from brain tissue obtained at postmortem by placing macerated brain tissue onto an agar plate coated with bacteria, or axenic growth medium, or inoculating the brain tissue onto tissue culture monolayers. *N. fowleri* will grow on monolayers of cell cultures and destroy them within 2–3 days.[28]

It is not clear why *N. fowleri* is so highly virulent and/or invasive, causing such extensive damage in a short period of time. Based on in vitro studies, especially using tissue cultures several possible explanations have been offered: (a) The amoebae produce sucker-like appendages or amoebostomes and 'nibble' away at the tissue culture cells and destroy the cell monolayer by causing CPE;[3] (b) produce phospholipases A and B activity or a cytolytic factor causing destruction of cell membranes; (c) neuraminidase or elastase activity facilitating destruction of tissue culture cells; (d) presence of a perforin-like, pore-forming protein that lyses target cells; and (e) the presence within amoebae of a cytopathic protein that triggers the apoptosis pathway in susceptible tissue culture cells.[3,6]

Management and Treatment

PAM is almost always fatal. Several reports of survival from PAM without adequate documentation have been published.[212–214] However, good documentation is available for three cases (one each from Australia,[195] the USA[184] and Mexico[188]) that survived. According to a recent paper a 9-year-old boy developed typical symptoms of PAM and an amoeba isolated from the CSF that was morphologically similar to *N. fowleri* was identified as *Paravahlkampfia francinae*. The patient recovered from the infection without any neurological disorders.[215] It is quite likely that some of the previously reported cases[212–214] might have been due to *P. francinae* or similar amoeba or dying leukocytes that might have been mistaken for *N. fowleri*. The 9-year-old California girl that survived was aggressively treated with intravenous and intrathecal amphotericin B, intravenous and intrathecal miconazole and oral rifampin.[184] She was followed-up for 4 years and was found to remain healthy and free of any neurological deficits. In vitro studies suggest that *N. fowleri* is highly sensitive to amphotericin B, and hence it has been the drug of choice in treating PAM cases. It is believed that this particular isolate of *N. fowleri* (ATCC 30896) is more sensitive to antimicrobials than others and this isolate is different at the molecular level from other clinical isolates.[3] Based on in vitro and in vivo testing, amphotericin B was reported to be more effective against *Naegleria* than amphotericin B methyl ester, a water-soluble form of the drug.[216] Phenothiazine compounds (chlorpromazine and trifluoperazine) inhibit growth of *N. fowleri* in vitro. Interestingly, Kim et al.[217] have shown that 75% of mice infected with *N. fowleri* survived with the administration of chlorpromazine whereas only 55% and 40% of mice survived after treatment with miltefosine and amphotericin B. Goswick and Brenner[218,219] have shown that azithromycin is not only effective in killing *N. fowleri* in vitro but also protected mice infected with *N. fowleri*. Recently, voriconazole was found to be amoeba static at ≤10 µg/mL and amoebicidal at ≥10 µg/mL.[96] A genomic study of *N. fowleri* is underway and hopefully development of molecular diagnostic tests derived from a whole genome sequence would not only allow for prompt diagnoses of PAM but also would lead to the identification of new drug targets and drug therapies leading to quicker initiation of therapies so that the patients can be saved.

Immunology

Because of the rapid onset and quick progression of PAM, most patients die within a short time (5–10 days) and there is insufficient time to mount a detectable immune response. Serologic testing as a diagnostic tool is therefore of little value, but patients that recover from PAM will develop high-titred antibody to *N. fowleri*. For example, the California patient that survived PAM developed high antibody titres (1:4096) to *N. fowleri* even at 7 days after admission to the hospital which persisted for 4 years.[184] Additionally, several individuals with a history of extensive swimming in freshwater lakes in the south-eastern USA also developed IgM antibodies.[3,5] A survey of serum samples of >80% of hospitalized patients from southeastern USA (Tennessee) revealed both IgG and IgM antibody classes to *N. fowleri* and *N. lovaniensis* and the titres ranged from 1:20 to 1:640. Additionally, IgG antibodies with titres of 1:20 to 1:80 were found in neonates indicating transplacental transmission.[3,6,220,221] Whether these antibodies have any protective activity is not clear at this time. Further, sera from some wild animals (raccoons, muskrats, squirrels, bull frogs but not toads and box turtles) have amoebicidal activity that can be destroyed upon heating, suggesting a role for complement.[3,6] Since these animals come in close contact with soil and water it is likely that they are exposed to *N. fowleri* or some other *Naegleria* sp. that is antigenically similar to *N. fowleri* and have developed antibodies. PAM does indeed occur in animals such as a South American tapir and domestic cattle.[222–224] Currently, we have no knowledge of the various factors such as the infectious dose, the virulence of the infecting isolate, the health status of the infected patient that are necessary for *N. fowleri* to cause infection. Therefore, molecular sequencing of different isolates of *N.*

fowleri reveals geographic variations but will also reveal whether the same or a different isolate infects humans as well as other animals. For example, based on an analysis of the 5.8S rRNA gene and the ITS of clinical and environmental isolates from different geographic areas of the United States it has been demonstrated that two individuals who had visited the same hot spring in California at different times were infected with the same genotype (genotype 2) of *N. fowleri*.[211] Molecular characterization of strains is also useful as an epidemiologic tool and in tracking infections to a source and recognizing potential risks for swimmers or bathers in particular locales.

Prevention

With the expected increase in global temperature due to global warming, cases of *N. fowleri* PAM may be seen even in geographic regions where it had previously not been recorded. Several recent cases of PAM infection, one in Italy[200] and the other in Minnesota,[225] a northern-most region of the USA, support this hypothesis. Since *N. fowleri* is susceptible to chlorine (one part per million (ppm)), adequate chlorination (residual chlorine level of 0.5 ppm) of swimming pools is helpful in preventing PAM. For example, 16 deaths due to PAM that occurred over a 3-year period were retrospectively traced to a swimming pool in the former Czechoslovakia with low free chlorine concentration. No deaths occurred after remedial measures were implemented.[3,6] However, it is not possible to chlorinate lakes, ponds and streams where *N. fowleri* may proliferate. The only method thought to prevent these infections would be to eliminate swimming in areas colonized by *Naegleria fowleri*; other behavioural recommendations that may reduce risk include: (1) avoiding water-related activities in warm freshwater during periods of high water temperature and low water levels; (2) holding the nose shut or using nose clips when taking part in water-related activities in bodies of warm freshwater; and (3) avoiding digging in, or stirring up, the sediment while taking part in water-related activities in shallow, warm freshwater areas. Domestic water supplies have also been implicated in contracting PAM. For example: (a) several children in South Australia with no history of swimming but 'washing out' the nose in a sun-warmed domestic bath containing tap water;[195] (b) two children in Arizona playing in a wading pool filled with untreated geothermal municipal water;[226] (c) several people in Karachi, Pakistan, using municipal water supply for irrigating the nasal passages,[192] illustrate the potential risk associated with nasal irrigation using residential tap water.

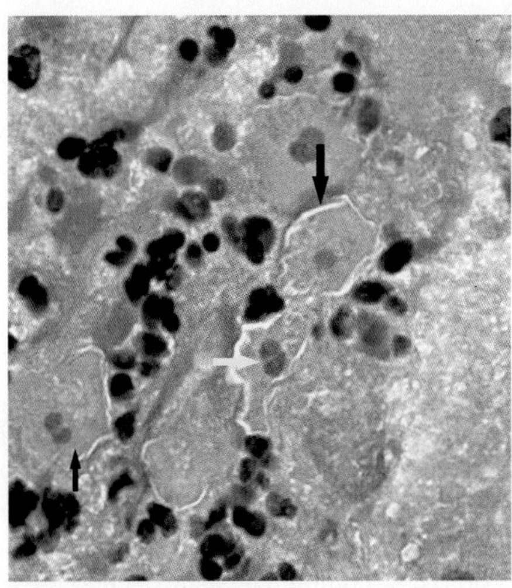

Figure 50.5 *Sappinia pedata* trophozoites (black arrows) in a CNS section. Note the abutted nuclei of the trophozoite at white arrow. (All at ×1000)

Sappinia

Sappinia is another free-living amoeba that normally lives in soil contaminated with faeces of elk, bison, and cattle. An immunocompetent male who developed headache, blurred vision, photophobia, vomiting and seizures had a single space-occupying lesion on MRI which was excised. On microscopic examination the tissue sections revealed trophozoites with the characteristic binucleate morphology but no cysts or granuloma (Figure 50.5). The patient fully recovered after treatment with azithromycin, pentamidine isethionate, itraconazole and flucytosine. The amoeba was initially identified as *S. diploidea* based on the nuclear morphology.[10] Later, it was re-identified as *S. pedata* based on sequencing of the 18S rRNA gene.[11]

Conclusions

Although encephalitis caused by the free-living amoebae is rare, it has a high mortality rate and large societal public health impact because children are often affected. Since diagnoses of most of the amoebic infections are done at autopsy it is possible that a large number of cases go undetected because autopsy is not performed routinely even in developed countries; the actual incidence of the amoebic encephalitis is not really known.[1]

REFERENCES

1. Visvesvara GS, Roy SL, Maguire JH. Pathogenic and opportunistic free-living amoebae: *Acanthamoeba* spp., *Balamuthia mandrillaris*, *Naegleria fowleri*, and *Sappinia pedata*. In: Guerrant RL, Walker DH, Weller PF, editors. Tropical Infectious Diseases Principles, Pathogens and Practice. Philadelphia: Elsevier-Saunders; 2011. p. 707–13.
3. Marciano-Cabral F, Cabral G. *Naegleria fowleri*. In: Khan ED, editor. Emerging Protozoan Pathogens. New York: Taylor & Francis; 2008. p. 119–52.
4. Schuster FL, Visvesvara GS. *Balamuthia mandrillaris*. In: Khan ED, editor. Emerging Protozoan Pathogens. New York: Taylor & Francis; 2008. p. 71–118.
14. Dart KKG, Saw VPJ, Kilvington S. *Acanthamoeba* keratitis: diagnosis and treatment update. Am J Ophthalmol 2009;148:487–99.
61. D'Auria A, Jaime L, Geiseler JP,et al. Cutaneous acanthamoebiasis post-transplantation: implication for differential diagnosis of skin lesions in immunocompromised patients. J Neuroparasitol 2012;3:1–7.
116. Schuster FL, Yagi S, Gavali S, et al. Under the radar: *Balamuthia amebic* encephalitis. Clin Infect Dis 2009;48:879–87.
117. Ghosh PS, Ghosh D, Loddenkemper T, et al. Necrotizing granulomatous meningoencephalitis due to *Balamuthia* in an immunocompetent child. Neurology 2011;77:801.

Access the complete references online at www.expertconsult.com

51 Trichomonas vaginalis

PATRICIA KISSINGER

KEY POINTS

- *T. vaginalis* is the most common treatable STI worldwide and prevalence rates vary widely.
- Risk factors include increased age, incarceration, intravenous drug use, commercial sex work and the presence of bacterial vaginosis.
- *T. vaginalis* is now gaining greater recognition as an important source of reproductive morbidity.
- *T. vaginalis* has been associated with acquisition and transmission of HIV and treatment *for T. vaginalis* may reduce *T. vaginalis*-associated transmission.
- Single dose (2 g) metronidazole therapy may not be adequate for some women including those who are HIV-positive or who have asymptomatic bacterial vaginosis.
- Scientists are focusing on better diagnostics and treatment for both index persons and their partners.
- Cost studies are needed to determine the benefit of screening for *T. vaginalis*.

Introduction

Trichomoniasis is caused by the parasite *Trichomonas vaginalis* (*T. vaginalis*). Once thought to be a nuisance sexually transmitted infection (STI), *T. vaginalis* is now being recognized as an important source of reproductive morbidity and a public health problem. In the last two centuries, scientific understanding of *T. vaginalis* has moved from discovery of the organism, recognizing it as an STI, understanding the public significance, to improved diagnostics. See Table 51.1 for a timeline of these significant developments.

Epidemiology

T. vaginalis is likely the most common non-viral sexually transmitted infection (STI) in the world. While not a reportable disease, the World Health Organization estimates that there are 174 million cases worldwide each year and nearly 90% of these infections occur among people living in resource-limited settings.[3] Compared with a global prevalence of 92 million cases of *Chlamydia trachomatis* and 62 million cases of *Neisseria gonorrhoeae*, *T. vaginalis* constitutes over 50% of the curable STIs worldwide.[4] These estimates, however, are likely underestimates, as they are based on the assumption that the sensitivity of wet mount, the diagnostic used for the estimate, ranges from 60–80% where true sensitivities may be closer to 35–60%.[5–7]

The World Health Organization estimated that in 1999, there were 76.5 million cases in South and South-east Asia; 32 million in sub-Saharan African; and 13 million in Eastern Europe and Central Asia, indicating a wide distribution of infections (Figure 51.1). These estimates are in need of updating, using more sensitive nucleic acid amplification techniques (NAAT) with prevalence rates from more population-based studies as inputs.

With no surveillance programmes in place, and the widespread use of wet mount as a diagnostic tool, the epidemiology of *T. vaginalis* is not completely known. It is known, however, to vary greatly by population and geography. Among high-risk women, rates range from 5% among female sex workers (FSW) in Pakistan,[8] to 53% among incarcerated women in the USA (Indiana).[9] Among high-risk men, rates range from 2% among jail inmates in the USA (California)[10] to 73% among male partners of women with *T. vaginalis* (South-east USA).[11] A systematic review of STIs in Papua New Guinea, found the pooled prevalence of *T. vaginalis* to be 39.3%, using various diagnostic tests.[12] Sentinel surveillance in five Central American cities found a prevalence of 11.0% among FSW.[13]

In the USA, two population-based studies that used PCR testing found rates of 2.3% among adolescents[14] to 3.1% among women 14–49 years of age.[15] Population-based studies in Africa show distinctly higher rates. In Zimbabwe, the rate was 9.5% among both genders using antibody testing.[16] Among men in Tanzania, the rate was 11% among men using NAAT.[17] Other population-based studies that used NAAT testing among reproductive aged women in other parts of the world found lower rates (e.g. 1% in Vietnam;[18] 0.37% in Flanders, Belgium;[19] 2.9% in Shandong Province in China[20]). Screening rates among women attending antenatal or family-planning clinics are often used as an indicator of the prevalence in the general population. Studies at these sites found prevalence rates from 3.2–52% in resource-limited settings and 7.6–12.6% in the USA.[4] Thus, rates of *T. vaginalis* vary greatly and are dependent on the risk factor profile of the population.

In general, Africans or persons of African descent, have higher rates of *T. vaginalis*, as evidenced by the higher rates in sub-Saharan Africa,[16,17] and among persons of African descent, such as Garifunas[21] and African-Americans in the USA.[14,15] Other risk factors for *T. vaginalis* include increased age, incarceration, intravenous drug use, commercial sex work[22] and the presence of bacteria vaginosis.[23]

Pathogenesis and Pathology

THE PARASITE

T. vaginalis is a flagellated parasitic protozoan, typically pyriform but occasionally amoeboid in shape, extracellular to genitourinary track epithelium with a primarily anaerobic lifestyle.[2]

TABLE 51.1 Scientific Developments Concerning *Trichomonas Vaginalis*[1,2]

Year	Event
1836	Alfred Donné discovered 'Animalculi' observed in purulent fluids and secretions of genital organs from men and women
1957	Culture was introduced improving the diagnosis of TV >20% compared with microscopy
1957	At a symposium on *Trichomonas* infections in Rheims, trichomoniasis deemed a venereal disease
1959	Metronidazole (Mtz) was introduced for the treatment of *T. vaginalis*
1970s	2 g Mtz recommended for treatment of *T. vaginalis*
1990s	*T. vaginalis* recognized as a co-factor for HIV transmission
1990–2000s	Nucleic acid probe, antigen detection tests, and InPouch culture introduced
2004	Tinidazole approved for use with *T. vaginalis*
2007	Draft of genome sequence
1993 and 2004	Point-of-care tests available for women
2011	First nucleic acid amplification technique (NAAT) test approved by FDA for women

The individual organism is 10–20 μm long and 2–14 μm wide. Four flagella project from the anterior portion of the cell and one flagellum extends backwards to the middle of the organism, forming an undulating membrane. An axostyle extends from the posterior aspect of the organism (Figure 51.2).[24] *T. vaginalis* has a large genome (strain G3, 176 441 227 bp) with ~60 000 protein coding genes organized into six chromosomes.[25] *T. vaginalis* is a highly predatory obligate parasite that phagocytoses bacteria, vaginal epithelial cells and erythrocytes and is itself ingested by macrophages. *T. vaginalis* uses carbohydrates as its main energy source via fermentative metabolism under aerobic and anaerobic conditions.

PATHOGENESIS

T. vaginalis primarily infects the squamous epithelium of the genital tract. Incubation time is generally between 4 and 28 days.[26] *T. vaginalis* resides in the female lower genital tract and the male urethra and prostate, where it replicates by binary fission. *T. vaginalis* is transmitted among humans, its only known host, primarily by sexual intercourse. Infection may persist for long periods, possibly months or even years in women, but it thought to persist for shorter periods in men. The parasite does not appear to have a cyst form and does not survive well in the external environment. In the absence of treatment, 54–69%[27] of men may spontaneously clear infection. While thought to be rare,[26] evidence of non-sexual transmission via fomites and possibly water has been described.[28–30] *T. vaginalis* can survive outside the human body in a wet environment for more than three hours,[31–33] though lability in laboratory environments has also been described.[1]

T. vaginalis can be infected with double-stranded RNA (dsRNA) viruses that may have important implications for trichomonal virulence and disease pathogenesis. A cross-sectional study of an STI clinic population found that 75% of the 28 isolates were infected with dsRNA and that those who were virus-positive were significantly older and more likely to be women than those who did not have the virus.[34]

T. vaginalis has been associated with mild to severe reproductive health outcomes, cancers and increased shedding of HIV and herpes simplex virus-2 (HSV-2) in the genital tract of

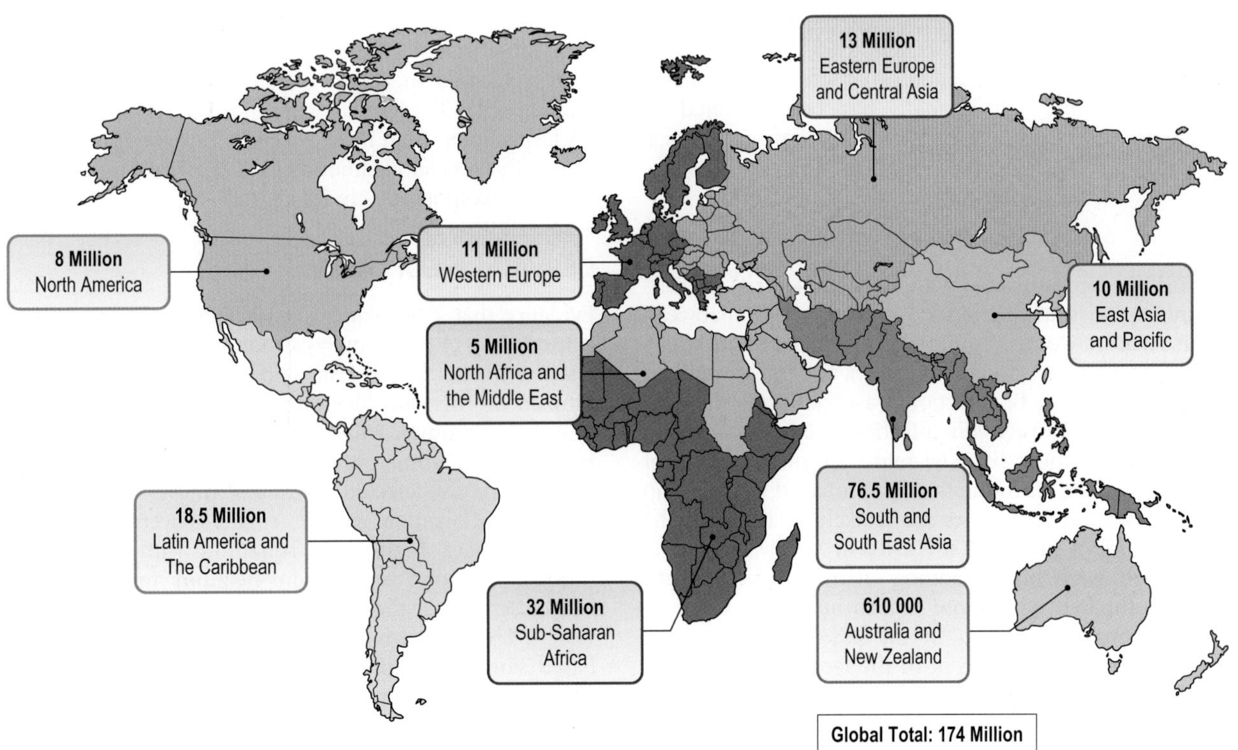

Figure 51.1 Estimated new cases of trichomoniasis among adults, 1999.

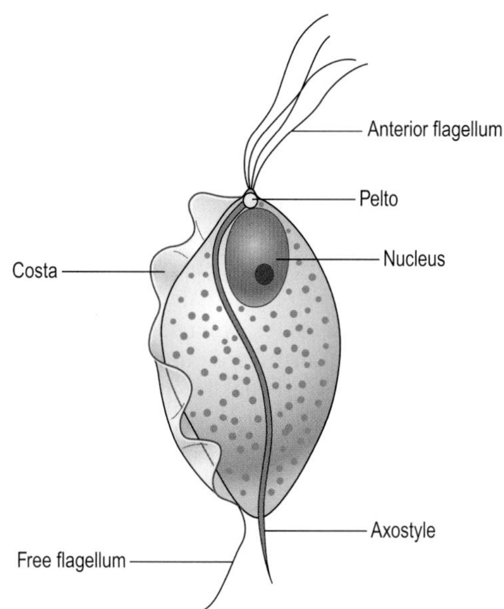

Figure 51.2 *Trichomonas vaginalis*: Trophozoite stage.

both men and women which could result in increased transmission of those STIs.

REPRODUCTIVE OUTCOMES

Among women, *T. vaginalis* has been associated with vaginitis, cervicitis, urethritis, low birth weight, premature rupture of membranes, pre-term delivery[35] and pelvic inflammatory disease.[36] Association of *T. vaginalis* with pre-term birth and low birth weight was reported throughout the 1990s. In two treatment trials, metronidazole (Mtz) cleared asymptomatic *T. vaginalis* in pregnant women but failed to prevent pre-term births.[37,38]

Among men, *T. vaginalis* is a significant cause of non-gonococcal urethritis, prostatitis and can decrease both sperm motility and viability.[39] *T. vaginalis* has been isolated in the specimens of 11–20%[40–42] of men with non-gonococcal urethritis.

HIV

T. vaginalis has been associated with an increased risk of HIV acquisition[43–45] and transmission.[46,47] A study of Zimbabwean and South African women found that *T. vaginalis* increases risk for HIV acquisition and HIV increases risk for *T. vaginalis* acquisition indicating a bi-directional association.[48] A meta-analysis found that *T. vaginalis* infection increases women's risk of HIV acquisition by 1.64-fold.[49] Another study of HIV-1 discordant couples found that HIV-infected women who had *T. vaginalis* were 2.57 times more likely to transmit the virus.[50] Among HIV+ men with urethritis in Malawi, HIV viral loads in semen were higher among men co-infected with *T. vaginalis* compared with those not co-infected.[51] Chesson and colleagues estimated that, in the USA, 747 new HIV cases a year in women are a result of the facilitative effects of *T. vaginalis* on the transmission of HIV.[52] And given that there are over 30 million cases of *T. vaginalis* in sub-Saharan African annually,[53] the impact of *T. vaginalis* on HIV transmission is considerable.

T. vaginalis infection typically elicits an aggressive local cellular immune response with inflammation of the vaginal epithelium and exocervix in women and the urethra of men.[54] The inflammatory response induces the recruitment of leukocytes, including HIV target cells such as CD4+-bearing lymphocytes and macrophages to which HIV can bind and gain access. In addition, *T. vaginalis* frequently causes punctuate mucosal haemorrhages, which potentially compromise the mechanical barrier to infection. *T. vaginalis* may also increase the risk of HIV-1 acquisition by increasing susceptibility to bacterial vaginosis or persistence of abnormal vaginal flora.[55]

Among HIV+ men with genital ulcers in South Africa, those with *T. vaginalis* diagnosed by NAAT had higher HIV viral loads in ulcers than *T. vaginalis*-negative men.[56] HIV+ women with *T. vaginalis* were more likely to have detectable HIV in cervicovaginal lavage (CVL) specimens compared to those who were *T. vaginalis* negative.[57]

Fortunately, treatment for *T. vaginalis* has demonstrated reductions in HIV genital shedding in several studies. HIV+ men with urethritis in Malawi, with *T. vaginalis* diagnosed by NAAT, experienced a decrease in seminal HIV after Mtz treatment.[27] HIV vaginal shedding was decreased after treatment in one cohort of women, diagnosed by microscopy and culture in Kenya,[47] and another, diagnosed by culture, in Louisiana, USA.[46] These data underscore the importance of screening and treatment among HIV-positive persons.

HSV-2

T. vaginalis appears to have a similar bidirectional association with herpes simplex virus II (HSV-2) as it does with HIV-1. Concomitant infection with *T. vaginalis* and previous episodes of genital herpes are associated with HSV-2 shedding. *T. vaginalis* was detected in 4.2% of women shedding HSV-2 in genital fluids versus 1.7% of women without detectable HSV-2 (p=0.001).[58] Among women attending STD clinics in the USA, in a longitudinal study, *T. vaginalis* infection was associated with a 3.7-fold increased incidence of HSV-2.[59] In Tanzania, women with *T. vaginalis* were more likely to have detectable CVL specimens than those without. *T. vaginalis* was also associated with a greater likelihood of HSV-2 shedding among women attending colposcopy clinics in Italy.[58]

CERVICAL NEOPLASIA

Evidence that *T. vaginalis* is associated with cervical neoplasia is mounting. A meta-analysis found that *T. vaginalis* was associated with a 1.9-fold risk of cervical neoplasia.[60] A study of Finnish women in cervical cancer mass screening registry found that women with *T. vaginalis* had an elevated risk for HPV.[61] Dutch women undergoing testing for cervical neoplasia had *T. vaginalis* detected in 3.2% of smears with cytology indications and women with *T. vaginalis* were two times more likely to have high-grade squamous intraepithelial lesions (HSIL).[62] Among women in Belgium undergoing cervical cancer screening, those with *T. vaginalis* diagnosed by NAAT were 1.9 times more likely to have HPV.[19] In a population-based sample of women in China (Beijing), women with *T. vaginalis* were 1.4 times more likely to have HPV and 1.7 times more likely to have cervical invasive neoplasia (CIN) I or II.[63] Yap and colleagues found an association between *T. vaginalis* and cervical cancer.[64]

Sutcliffe and co-workers found an association between *T. vaginalis* and prostate cancer in one study but not in a subsequent study.[65,66]

Clinical Features

While 73% of women infected with *T. vaginalis* are symptomatic,[67] one-third of asymptomatic women become symptomatic within 6 months.[26] Among women, common sites of infection include the vagina, urethra and endocervix. Symptoms include vaginal discharge (which is often diffuse, malodorous, yellow-green), dysuria, itching, vulvar irritation and abdominal pain. The normal vaginal pH is 4.5, but with *T. vaginalis* infection, this increases markedly, often to >5.[68] The classic presentation of *T. vaginalis* among women includes a discharge that is described as thin and frothy (Figure 51.3). *Colpitis macularis* or strawberry cervix (Figure 51.4), is seen in about 5% of women, though with colposcopy this rises to nearly 50%.[69] Other complications include infection of the adnexa, endometrium and Skene and Bartholin glands.

Whereas the majority of women are symptomatic, 77% of men are asymptomatic.[67] Among those who do have symptoms, they include urethral discharge, dysuria. In men, it can cause epididymitis, prostatitis and decreased sperm cell motility.[70] *T. vaginalis* can be isolated from men with chronic prostatitis.

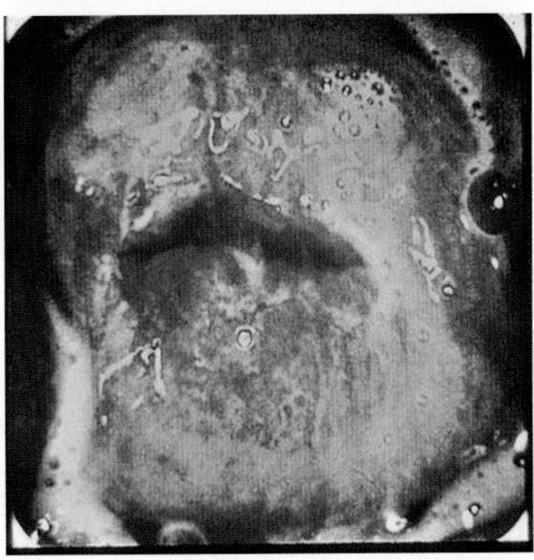

Figure 51.4 Strawberry cervix. *(Taken from: Marrazzo J, Hillier S, Sobel J. Vaginal infections. In: Morse SA, Ballard RC, Holmes KK, et al., editors. Atlas of Sexually Transmitted Diseases and AIDS. p. 76–93. © 2010, Elsevier Limited. All rights reserved.)*

BOX 51.1 CRITERIA FOR TREATMENT

FOR WOMEN

- Positive wet prep, culture, Papanicolaou smear, OSOM Rapid Test, Affirm VP III, APTIMA
- Sex partner with a diagnosis of *T. vaginalis.*

FOR MEN

- Positive wet preparation or culture from urethral, urine or semen evaluation
- Sex partner with a diagnosis of *T. vaginalis.*

Diagnosis

The criteria for treatment differ by gender, since not all Federal Drug Administration (FDA) approved tests for women have been tested with men (Box 51.1). Traditional wet mount is cheap, fast and widely available. Unfortunately, it is insensitive in both women and men. While culture has better sensitivity in women, it is more expensive, time-consuming, and demonstrates poor sensitivity in men. Two studies, one of HIV– and one of HIV+ women found that that after diagnosis by culture and treatment with 2 g Mtz, *T. vaginalis* infection was non-detectable for months and then reappeared in the absence of sexual exposure,[71,72] underscoring the need for more sensitive testing than culture.

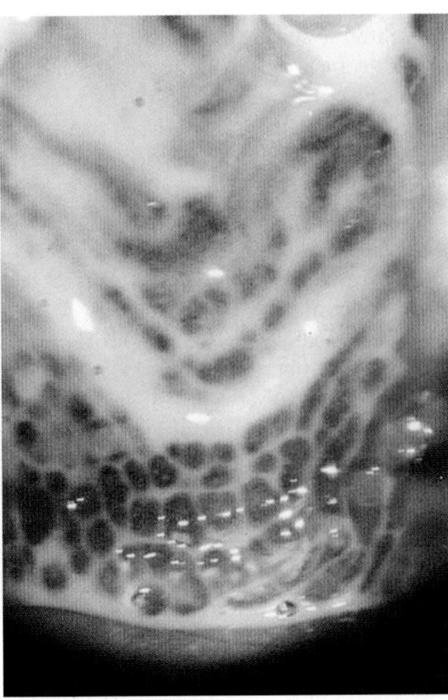

Figure 51.3 Frothy discharge. *(Taken from: Marrazzo J, Hillier S, Sobel J. Vaginal infections. In: Morse SA, Ballard RC, Holmes KK, et al., editors. Atlas of Sexually Transmitted Diseases and AIDS. p. 76–93. © 2010, Elsevier Limited. All rights reserved.)*

Nucleic acid probe techniques are moderately priced and fast, but require instrumentation. An FDA-cleared PCR assay for detection of gonorrhoea and chlamydial infection (Amplicor, Roche Diagnostic Corp.) has been modified for *T. vaginalis* detection in vaginal or endocervical swabs and in urine from women and men with sensitivity ranges from 88%–97% and specificity from 98%–99%.[7] APTIMA *T. vaginalis* Analyte Specific Reagents (ASR, Gen-Probe, Inc.) also can detect *T. vaginalis* RNA by transcription-mediated amplification using the same instrumentation platforms available for the FDA-cleared APTIMA Combo2 assay for diagnosis of gonorrhoea and chlamydial infection; published validation studies of *T. vaginalis* ASR found sensitivity ranging at 74%–98% and specificity of 87%–98%[73-75]

There are two point-of-care tests that have been approved by the US FDA for diagnosis of *T. vaginalis* among women: OSOM Trichomonas Rapid Test (Genzyme Diagnostics, Cambridge, MA), an immunochromatographic capillary flow dipstick technology[73] and Affirm VP III (Becton, Dickinson and Co., Franklin Lakes, NJ), a nucleic acid probe test that evaluates for *T. vaginalis*, *G. vaginalis* and *C. albicans.*[76] Both tests are performed on vaginal secretions and have a sensitivity of more than 83% and a specificity of more than 97%. Results of the OSOM test are available in about 10 minutes, while results of the Affirm VP III test are available within 45 minutes.

It has been generally thought that only vaginal specimens should be collected for *T. vaginalis* testing. There is, however, some evidence that endocervical specimens are suitable. Endocervical specimens have been found to be 88% sensitive and 99% specific for *T. vaginalis* by PCR, compared with 90% and 99% for vaginal swab.[7] Huppert and colleagues showed that endocervical specimens were 100% sensitive and 98% specific by TMA compared with 100% sensitivity and specificity for vaginal specimen, using latent class analysis.[73] The ability to conduct endocervical testing would simplify specimen collection should *T. vaginalis* screening become available.

Management and Treatment

CRITERIA FOR TREATMENT

T. vaginalis infection is treated with metronidazole (Mtz) as the treatment of choice.[77] Mtz belongs to the 5-nitroimidazole drug family and it and related compounds such as tinidazole (Tnz) and secnidazole are reported to have about a 95% success rate in curing *T. vaginalis*.[78] Mtz is a class B drug and several meta-analyses have found it to be safe in pregnant women in all stages of pregnancy.[79–81] Tnz has not been evaluated in pregnant women and remains a class C drug. In lactating women who are administered Mtz, withholding breast-feeding during treatment and for 12–24 hours after the last dose, will reduce the exposure of the infant to metronidazole. For women treated with Tnz, interruption of breast-feeding is recommended during treatment and for 3 days after the last dose.

TREATMENT

The Centers for Disease Control and Prevention (CDC) guidelines for treatment of *T. vaginalis* include: metronidazole (Mtz) or tinidazole 2 g single dose as the recommended regimens, and Mtz 500 mg twice a day 7-day dose as the alternative treatment regimen (Figure 51.5).[82] These recommendations, however, were based on studies conducted nearly 30 years ago and while single dose was found to be equivalent to multiple dose therapies, repeat *T. vaginalis* infection rates after single dose treatment were high (i.e. 5–20%). An RCT among HIV-infected women with *T. vaginalis* found multi-dose Mtz to be superior to single dose treatment.[83] That same group also found that the presence of bacterial vaginosis (BV) was likely a major factor in the early failure of the single dose treatment. PCR results should be negative by 2 weeks after completion of successful therapy.[6] Abstinence from alcohol use should continue for 24 hours after completion of Mtz or 72 hours after completion of Tnz.

If the patient is in contact with a sex partner with a positive diagnosis, they should be treated presumptively. Single dose therapy of Mtz was introduced in the 1960s after a series of RCTs demonstrated efficacy. There is some indication, however, that the 2 g dose may not be effective. This was found in an observational study of HIV-negative women and an RCT among HIV-positive women.[84]

If a patient fails single dose MTZ therapy, they can be given single dose Tnz or 7-day dose Mtz. If this fails, 2 g Mtz or Tnz for 5 days can be administered. If this fails and there is no history of sexual re-exposure, a consultation for medication resistance testing should be done. Consultation and *T. vaginalis* susceptibility testing are available from CDC (Tel: 404–718–4141; website: http://www.cdc.gov/std).

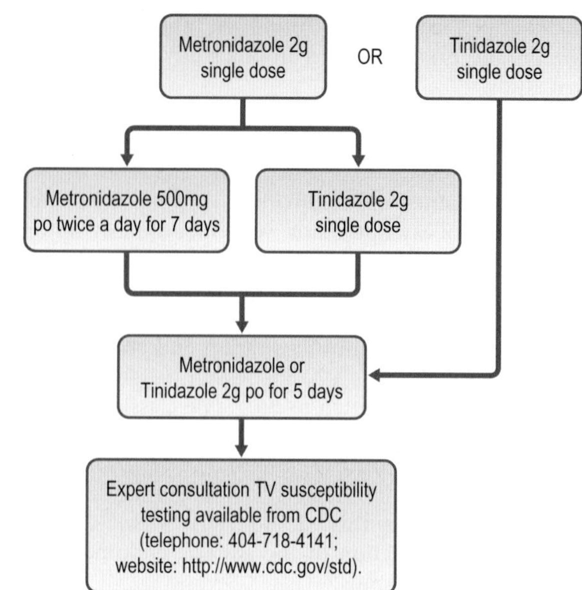

Figure 51.5 Treatment of *T. vaginalis*.

REPEATED INFECTIONS

Repeat infections are common, ranging from 5–31%,[84–94] and share similar sequelae to primary infections. Potential causes of early repeat *T. vaginalis* infections include: drug resistance, non-adherence to treatment, clinical treatment failure or reinfection from an untreated partner. Single dose therapy has removed adherence as an issue and in vitro resistance testing has consistently demonstrated low rates of insusceptibility. Resistance to Mtz is estimated to be about 5%[95] and there does appear to be in vitro evidence of cross-resistance with Mtz, Tnz and adenosine analogues.[96] The most likely sources of repeat infections, therefore, are clinical treatment failure or reinfection from an untreated partner.

T. vaginalis-infected women were given single dose Mtz and provided with medication to deliver to their sex partner(s), repeat infections rates were high (8%) and nearly all (92%) were attributed to clinical treatment failure.[84] The molecular mechanism(s) of clinical resistance are poorly understood.

Repeat *T. vaginalis* infections among HIV+ women are substantially higher with rates between 18.3% and 36.9%[84,97,98] and since these studies used culture, the true rate may be even higher. One study of HIV+ and HIV− women found that repeat infections with *T. vaginalis* among HIV-negative women was 8%, but among HIV+ women it as 18.3%. While the differences in cure rates between HIV+ and HIV− women is not completely understood, there is some indication that bacterial vaginosis may play a factor.[99] Reinfection from an untreated partner may be another source of repeat infections.

Prevention

T. vaginalis is highly prevalent and reinfections are common. Primary prevention includes promotion of condoms and other safer sex activities to reduce the chance of exposure. There is some evidence that nonoxynol-9 can be used as an anti-trichomonal agent,[100] thus condoms that contain nonoxynol-9 may also serve to prevent trichomonal infections.

Secondary prevention includes screening and prompt treatment. Periodic presumptive treatment (PPT) among female sex workers in Papua New Guinea demonstrated a twofold decrease in *T. vaginalis*.[78] Clinicians should consider diagnosis and treatment of *T. vaginalis* in men. Increased use of improved diagnostics in women is needed. Male circumcision has been associated with a reduction in *T. vaginalis* among both men and women.[101]

While infection does elicit an antibody response and produces some partial immunity, one study of HIV+ women showed no association between the prevalence of *T. vaginalis* and the use of protease inhibitors or the immune status of the woman.[97] Another study showed that HIV seropositivity does not alter the rate of infection in men.[51] Thus, while the benefits of a vaccine to prevention of *T. vaginalis* has been recognized,[78] there are presently no approved vaccines.

Since *T. vaginalis* testing for men is difficult and many *T. vaginalis*-infected men are asymptomatic,[102] partner treatment is paramount to reducing early repeat infections in women. Patient-delivered partner treatment (PDPT), or the provision of antibiotics to infected index persons to deliver to their sex partners, is a possible alternative to the standard of partner referral (PR) or telling the index woman to refer her partner for care. While PDPT has been found to be superior to standard partner referral methods for reducing repeat Chlamydia and gonorrhoea infections,[103] the efficacy of PDPT for TV is less clear. Two published RCTs of PDPT for *T. vaginalis* given to index women to deliver to their male sex partners found conflicting results[86,104] and, to-date, the CDC has not made recommendations to offer PDPT for *T. vaginalis*-infected women. However, these studies were single centred and likely underpowered, thus larger multi-centered trials are needed. Improved partner notification and partner treatment is needed.

In summary, *T. vaginalis* is now gaining greater recognition as an important source of reproductive morbidity and, possibly more urgently because of the potential for it to amplify the acquisition and transmission of HIV and possibly HSV-2. While it is not a reportable disease and screening programmes generally do not exist, scientists are focusing on better diagnostics and treatment for both index persons and their partners. Cost studies are needed to determine the benefit of screening for *T. vaginalis*.

REFERENCES

2. Harp DF, Chowdhury I. Trichomoniasis: evaluation to execution. Eur J Obstet Gynecol Reprod Biol 2011;157:3–9.
4. Johnston VJ, Mabey DC. Global epidemiology and control of *Trichomonas vaginalis*. Curr Opin Infect Dis 2008;21:56–64.
26. Petrin D, Delgaty K, Bhatt R, et al. Clinical and microbiological aspects of *Trichomonas vaginalis*. Clin Microbiol Rev 1998;11: 300–17.
54. Shafir SC, Sorvillo FJ, Smith L. Current issues and considerations regarding trichomoniasis and human immunodeficiency virus in African-Americans. Clin Microbiol Rev 2009;22:37–45.
77. Wendel KA, Workowski KA. Trichomoniasis: challenges to appropriate management. Clin Infect Dis 2007;44(Suppl 3):S123–9.

Access the complete references online at www.expertconsult.com

Schistosomiasis

AMAYA L. BUSTINDUY | CHARLES H. KING

KEY POINTS

- Schistosomiasis is a chronic inflammatory disorder that is *initiated* by infection with *Schistosoma* blood fluke parasites and which causes tissue damage and systemic pathology that often *persist* into adulthood, even after infection abates.
- Anti-schistosomal, immune-mediated pathology is the primary cause of both systemic and organ-specific morbidity.
- Presentation of disease among long-term residents of *Schistosoma*-endemic areas differs from the disease presentation seen among travellers or migrants who have had only short-term exposure to the parasite.
- Transmission of *Schistosoma* spp. parasites requires specific intermediate host snails – human prevalence is closely tied to the abundance of suitable snail host species in local freshwater habitats.
- Poverty leads to a greater risk of *Schistosoma* infection as a consequence of inadequate sanitation and limited household access to clean water.
- New dams, irrigation and urbanization can enhance local snail habitat and increase local transmission. This typically results in a dramatic increase in local prevalence of schistosomiasis.
- Diagnosis of active infection is established by detection of *Schistosoma* eggs in urine, stool or tissue biopsies. Positive antigen testing and/or serology support the diagnosis in egg-negative cases.
- Patient manifestations of schistosomiasis range from sub-clinical disease (including anaemia and growth retardation) to overt multisystem organ failure.
- Praziquantel is the drug of choice for treating all forms of established *Schistosoma* infection.
- Regular treatment with anti-schistosomal drugs decreases morbidity among endemic populations.
- Full prevention of *Schistosoma*-related disease requires interruption of transmission in order to prevent early infection and rapid recurrence of infection during childhood.

Epidemiology

Schistosomiasis refers to human disease resulting from infection by any of the parasitic blood flukes of *Schistosoma* spp. Worldwide, it is estimated that over 239 million people are acutely or chronically infected with one or more of these species, which are transmitted by specific aquatic or amphibious snails in a wide variety of freshwater habitats.[1] However, some estimates suggest that more than 400 million people worldwide may be affected. The various species of the genus *Schistosoma* are trematodes, members of the family Schistosomatidae, which are dioecious, digenean multicellular helminthic parasites whose adult habitat is the vascular system of vertebrates (Figure 52.1). Of all the mammalian blood flukes, the genus *Schistosoma* has achieved the greatest geographical distribution and diversification (Figure 52.2).[2] Of the 16 species of *Schistosoma* known to infect humans or animals, five are responsible for the vast majority of human infections. These are *Schistosoma haematobium, S. intercalatum, S. mansoni, S. japonicum* and *S. mekongi*. Very rarely, other zoophilic species or interspecies hybrid infections may be found in humans.[2]

Because the parasite is transmitted via very specific intermediate-host freshwater snails, the perpetuation of the *Schistosoma* life cycle requires suitable environmental conditions as well as water contamination by human sewage.[3] Transmission is thus linked to local ecological factors as well as to underdevelopment and lack of sanitation. Persistent exposure to reinfection is tied to a lack of safe water sources for agricultural, domestic and recreational activities,[4] a situation that is common throughout the developing world. As such, schistosomiasis is a preventable disease of poverty, with rising prevalence in rural areas and unplanned peri-urban developments.[5,6] Infection may also be common in refugee camps where transmission is often difficult to control.[7]

Prevalence estimates obtained from standard epidemiological surveys have been imprecise, because 20–30% of infections are missed by standard egg detection assays performed on stool or urine specimens.[8–10] This misclassification has resulted in a considerable underestimation of the burden of schistosomiasis and a biased view of how *Schistosoma*-related morbidity affects endemic communities.[11,12] Early childhood serosurveys, combined with the use of antigen-detection diagnostic field tests, are now providing more refined estimates of age-specific prevalence in endemic areas.[13,14] The 2011 estimated population at risk of schistosomiasis has increased to 779 million,[1] based on changing demographics in endemic countries and anthropogenic changes to the environment occurring via water project development. Based on systematic reviews, 106 million people in Africa are at high risk for schistosomiasis (both *S. haematobium* and *S. mansoni*), due to their living and working in proximity to large dam reservoirs or surface irrigation schemes.[15] In Asia, large hydroprojects such as the recently built Three Gorges Dam on the Yangtze river in central China, also have the potential to increase the prevalence of *S. japonicum* or *S. mekongi* infection by altering the river flow, local human population density, agricultural practices and their intermediate snail hosts' habitat.[16]

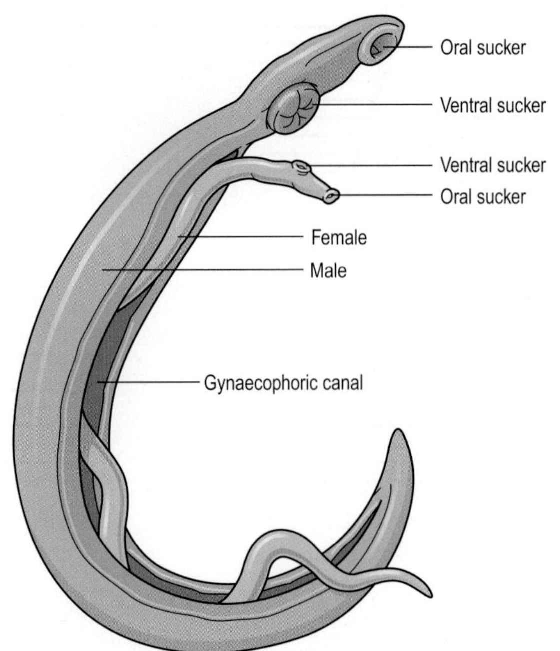

Figure 52.1 Male and female schistosomes. *(From Tropical Resources Unit: WHO.)*

Until recently, descriptions of disease and disability related to *Schistosoma* infection have focused on the late, 'pathognomonic' complications of schistosomiasis. These advanced forms of schistosomiasis involve end-organ inflammation and fibrosis of the liver and portal venous system in intestinal schistosomiasis (caused by *S. mansoni, S. japonicum, S. mekongi* or *S. intercalatum*) and bladder, ureteral and renal damage (caused by *S. haematobium*). However, based on population surveys, it is now appreciated that the occurrence of these end-organ complications is low (~10–20%) relative to more subtle, but disabling chronic morbidities of *Schistosoma* infection,[17] including anaemia, growth stunting, cognitive impairment and decreased physical fitness.[11,12]

During childhood in endemic areas, both prevalence and intensity of *Schistosoma* infection increase with age due to continuing exposure to high-risk water bodies. This increasing infectious burden is associated with a parallel increase in morbidity due to the acute inflammation induced by the ~50% of parasite eggs that remain trapped in the body.[18,19] Maximum egg excretion peaks between 12–15 years of age.[20] Intensity of infection typically decreases among older age groups, although for *S. mansoni* prevalence still tends to remain high for adults. This age-related change in infectious burden after adolescence is likely a multifactorial process,[21,22] but debate continues about whether the apparent reduction of infectious burden in adult life is related to acquired immunity, decreased exposure to contaminated water, or even decreased sensitivity of egg testing due to trapping of eggs in fibrotic tissue. The possibility of acquired anti-fecundity immunity, resulting in worms shedding fewer eggs, has also been advanced. In any event, local transmission is particularly favoured because children, who have the highest egg output in faeces or urine, are consistently more likely to be indiscriminate in terms of urination and defecation habits, thereby enhancing perpetuation of the local transmission cycle.

Schistosoma eggs (Figure 52.3) have been found in the stool or urine of children as young as 2 years old, provoking questions about the true age of onset of disease caused by *Schistosoma*

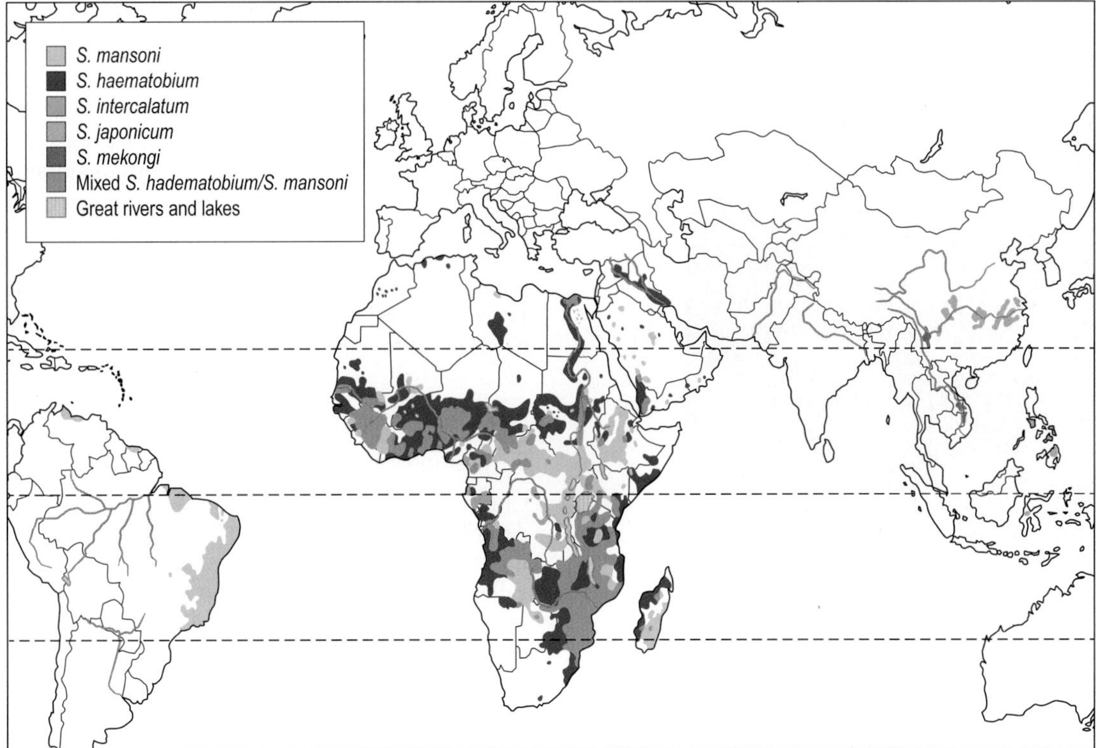

Figure 52.2 Map of worldwide distribution of schistosomiasis. *(From Gryseels B, Polman K, Clerinx J, et al. Human schistosomiasis. Lancet 2006;368(9541):1106–18.)*

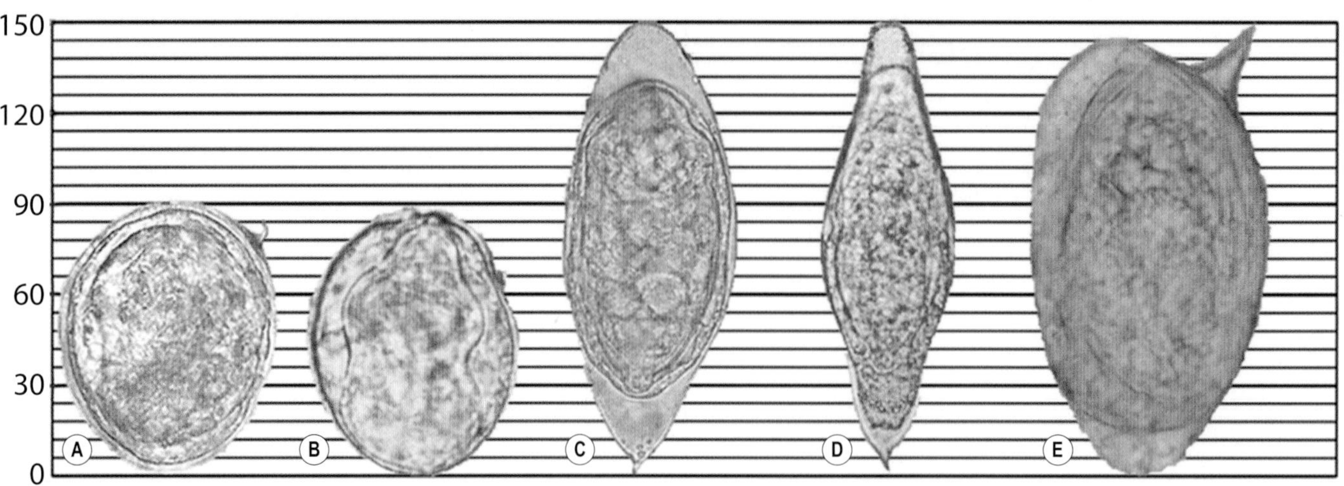

Figure 52.3 Eggs from different *Schistosoma* parasites of humans (A) *S. japonicum*, (B) *S. mekongi*, (C) *S. haematobium*, (D) *S. intercalatum*, (E) *S. mansoni*.

infection, particularly with regard to the age targets of current population-based control programmes, now focused on school-age children (5–15 years of age).[23] More extensive studies will be needed to define this issue.[14,24,25]

ANIMAL RESERVOIRS

Schistosoma japonicum is the only species having relevant animal reservoirs that contribute to environmental contamination through daily egg excretion (Figure 52.4). A total of 31 wild mammals and 13 domestic animals have been shown to carry *S. japonicum* in China,[26] and in the Philippines, cats, dogs, pigs, water buffaloes and rats were found to have a 3–31% prevalence of viable *S. japonicum* eggs in the stool.[27] In hilly environments of China, where buffalo are less common, dogs appear to be the main zoonotic reservoir, with prevalence of up to 75%.[28] In this setting, inclusion of animal infection prevention as part of schistosomiasis control campaigns has proven a more successful strategy in China.[29]

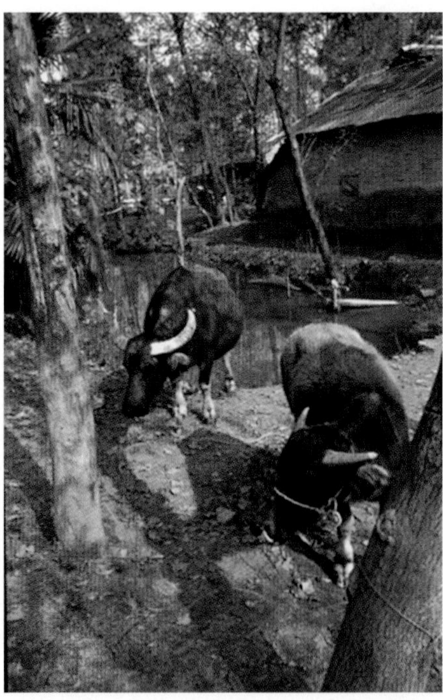

Figure 52.4 Animal reservoirs of *Schistosoma japonicum* in Hunan province, China: these buffalo used by villagers in their farm activities serve as local reservoirs for *Schistosoma japonicum* parasites, which helps to perpetuate local transmission. *(From WHO/TDR/Crump.)*

In contrast, humans are effectively the only reservoir host of *S. haematobium*. The few infections with this parasite found among non-human primates, *Arteriodactyla* or *Rodentia* can be considered as incidental and of no epidemiological importance.

S. mansoni infections have been reported in a wide range of mammals (non-human primates, *Insectivora, Arteriodactyla, Marsupilia, Rodentia, Carnivora* and *Edentata*). However, evidence implicating their role in maintenance of transmission of the parasite is, with two exceptions, lacking. In one focus in Tanzania, it is believed that baboons maintain the parasite among themselves,[30] and there is good reason to believe that the local strain of *S. mansoni* is maintained by both rats (*Rattus rattus* – a known reservoir host) and by humans in the natural habitat of Guadeloupe Island[31,32] and in some areas of Brazil. For *S. mekongi* in Cambodia, among local fauna, only dogs have been found to harbour parasite eggs in a recent survey.[33]

HISTORY

S. haematobium

Chronic haematuria and various bladder disorders were described in the earliest recorded histories, in association with the spread of agricultural civilization along the great river valleys of Egypt and Mesopotamia. Haematuria was described in the *Gynaecological Papyrus of Kahun*, written in the mid-XIIth dynasty, circa 1900 BCE. Many remedies for haematuria were recorded in the Ebers Papyrus and it can be assumed that in that era, the condition, presumably caused by *S. haematobium*, was widespread.[34] Calcified ova of the *S. haematobium* have been demonstrated in the kidneys of two Egyptian mummies of the XXth dynasty (1250–1000 BCE).[35] During

Napoleon's invasion of Egypt (1799–1801 AD), symptoms of the disease were common among French troops.[36] However, it was not until 1851, that a causal agent (a blood fluke first called *Distoma haematobium*, now *Schistosoma haematobium*), was found by Theodor Bilharz during a post-mortem examination at the Kasr-el-Aini Hospital in Cairo.[37]

S. mansoni

In 1902, Sir Patrick Manson found lateral spined eggs in the faeces of a colonial officer posted to the West Indies (then invalided to London) and postulated the existence of a second species of *Schistosoma* blood fluke parasites.[38] Subsequent controversy between A. Looss and L. W. Sambon, eminent scientists of the day, was resolved in 1915 by the work of Leiper at El Marg, a village in the present Qualyubia Governorate, just north of Cairo. Leiper established the existence of two distinct species of *Schistosoma* parasite and identified their transmission pathways via two different snail intermediate hosts belonging to two different genera and subfamilies.[39] In the New World, *Schistosoma* eggs with a lateral spine (*S. mansoni*) were identified both in Bahia State, Brazil in 1904[40] and in Venezuela in 1906.[41]

S. japonicum

In 1847, the clinical entities 'Kabure itch' and 'Katayama syndrome' were described in a village in the Hiroshima Prefecture in Japan,[42] while in 1904, Katsurada[43] recovered worms from the portal system of a cat and named the species *Schistosomum japonicum*. From 1909 to 1915, the biology of this parasite, its life cycle and the pathology it causes were elucidated and described by Japanese and other investigators.[44] The species was recognized clinically both in China[45] and in the Philippines by the early years of the twentieth century[46] and in Sulawesi (Celebes) of modern Indonesia in the 1930s.[47] *Oncomelania* intermediate host snails were identified in China in 1924[48] and in the Philippines in 1932.[49]

S. intercalatum

In 1923, suspicion arose that, because some cases of human 'intestinal' schistosomiasis in the Yakusu area near Kisangani (in present-day Democratic Republic of Congo) showed an atypical clinical picture and possessed an unusual egg morphology, a species distinct from *S. haematobium* was involved.[50] Follow-up of this work led to a description in 1934 of a new species, *S. intercalatum*, for which the snail intermediate host was a member of the *Bulinus africanus* group.[51] The recent description of a new species of human schistosome, *Schistosoma guineensis*, has led to a call for more extensive, DNA-based phylogenetic studies of the genus *Schistosoma*. This work in progress currently suggests that *S. intercalatum* and *S. guineensis* should be treated as separate taxa closely related to *S. haematobium*.[52,53]

S. mekongi *and* S. malayensis

Initially described in 1978, *S. mekongi* causes human schistosomiasis in a restricted area of Laos and Cambodia.[54] Its intermediate host, *Tricula aperta*, is aquatic and is not susceptible to infection by *S. japonicum*.[54,55] Another rare species from Malaysia, *S. malayensis*, was identified in 1987 and found to be closely related to *S. mekongi*, but genetically distinct.[56] *S. malayensis* is known to be a zoonotic disease with a vertebrate reservoir, *Rattus muelleri*.[57] The intermediate vector is *Robertsiella kaporensis*, a triculinid snail.[58] To date, little is known about the clinical significance of *S. malayensis*.

GEOGRAPHIC DISTRIBUTION OF SCHISTOSOMIASIS

According to the WHO, of the estimated 239 million people with schistosomiasis, the large majority (85%) live in sub-Saharan Africa (Figure 52.2).[1,59] Worldwide, *Schistosoma* infections are further distributed across three continents and the disease is considered to be endemic in 74 countries.[1] Some previously affected nations, such as Tunisia and Morocco have recently interrupted transmission.[60] Intestinal schistosomiasis caused by *S. mansoni* is found in 54 countries, ranging from the Arabian Peninsula, across Africa and in Madagascar. In South America, *S. mansoni* transmission still occurs at somewhat lower levels in Brazil and Venezuela and may persist in Surinam and several islands of the Caribbean (Figure 52.2).[61]

S. haematobium is now endemic in 53 countries in the Middle East, the African continent and the Indian Ocean islands Madagascar, Zanzibar and Pemba. In 40 countries, double infections with *S. mansoni* and *S. haematobium* are common.[62] *S. intercalatum* remains endemic in 10 countries in central and west Africa.[63]

S. japonicum infection is found in mainland China, Indonesia (Lindu Lake valley and the Napu valley in central Sulawesi) and in certain islands of the Philippines. There is no evidence of recent transmission in Thailand or India, where an endemic focus in Gimvi village, state of Maharashtra, was still active two decades ago. Schistosomiasis was eradicated in Japan in the 1960s.

S. mekongi is endemic on Khong Island, Lao People's Democratic Republic and in some areas of Cambodia.[64]

INFECTION BY OTHER *SCHISTOSOMA* SPECIES

Infrequently, humans are infected by schistosomes that normally infect other mammalian hosts. For example *S. bovis*, a member of the *S. haematobium* complex and a common parasite in cattle and sheep, may occasionally infect humans. Likewise *S. mattheei*, which has multiple hosts in both domestic and wild animals in southern Africa and *S. margrebowiei*, a parasite frequent in antelopes in central Africa, may possibly cause human infection.[65] Such infections in humans are seldom of pathological significance but suggestions have been advanced that they may confer a relative type of immunity (heterologous immunity) against *S. mansoni* and *S. haematobium* infections in areas where all species co-exist.[66] The cercariae of certain avian blood flukes, *Trichobilharzia, Gigantobilharzia* and *Ornithobilharzia*, may penetrate human skin producing cercarial dermatitis or 'swimmer's itch'. Outbreaks may occur in either tropical or temperate climates.[65,67]

Pathogenesis and Pathology

For a detailed description of parasite morphology, see Table 52.1.

Life Cycle

The *Schistosoma* transmission cycle is complex and highly efficient when the right environmental conditions are met (Figure

TABLE 52.1 **Comparison of Principal Features of *Schistosoma* spp. Parasites Infecting Humans**

	S. mansoni	*S. japonicum*	*S. haematobium*	*S. intercalatum*	*S. mekongi*[a]
Adult Worms					
Location of adult in host	Mesenteric veins	Mesenteric veins	Vesical plexus	Mesenteric veins	Mesenteric veins
Posterior gut caecum	Very long	Medium	Short	Short	Medium
MALE					
Length (mm)	6–13	10–20	10–15	11–14	115
Width (mm)	1.10	0.55	0.90	0.3–0.4	0.41
No. of testes	4–13 (6–9)[b]	6–7	4–5	2–7 (4–5)[b]	6–7
Tubercles	Coarse	Absent	Fine	Fine	Absent?
FEMALE					
Length (mm)	10–20	20–30	16–26	10–14	112
Width (mm)	0.16	0.30	0.25	0.15–0.18	0.23
Ovary: position in body	Front third	Middle	Rear third	Rear half	Rear half
Uterus: position in body	Front half	Front half	Front two-thirds	Front two-thirds	Front half
Length	Very short	Short	Long	Long	Short
No. of eggs	1–2	50–200	10–50	5–60	10+
Mature Egg					
Shape	Ovoid	Round	Ovoid	Ovoid	Round
Size (µm)	61×140	60×100	62×150	61×176	57×66
Spine	Lateral	Lateral (reduced)	Terminal	Terminal	Lateral (reduced)
Normally passed in	Faeces	Faeces	Urine	Faeces (and urine)	Faeces
Eggs/female per day	100–300	3500	20–300	150–400	?
Reaction of egg shell to Ziehl–Neelsen stain[c]	+ve	+ve	–ve	+ve	?

[a]From experimental animal infections.
[b]Usual range.
[c]In histological sections.
Courtesy of Sturrock RF, Department of Medical Parasitology, London School of Hygiene and Tropical Medicine. Reproduced with permission from Jordan P, Webbe G, Sturrock RF, editors. Human Schistosomiasis. Wallingford: CAB International; 1993.

52.5).[68] All species have a common pathway from sexual reproduction by adult schistosomes within the vascular system of the definitive human host, an asexual phase in the freshwater intermediate snail host and a return to the human via cercarial invasion of the skin or mucosa on a host's exposure to cercaria-infested water. Adult schistosomes are dioecious, with full separate sexes. They live as pairs within capillary blood vessels (Figure 52.6), in different anatomic locations depending on the species: *S. mansoni, S. japonicum, S. mekongi* and *S. intercalatum* in the mesenteric veins and *S. haematobium* in the vesical plexus. The slender and smooth females are held in the gynaecophoric canal of the male, where they copulate (Figure 52.1). The lifespan of the adult worm in humans is not accurately known. In the past, stress was laid on clinical evidence of longevity ranging from 18 years[69] up to 37 years, as reported in a Madagascar migrant living in France.[70] However, the average worm lifespan is estimated to be 3–5 years.[71]

The females produce non-operculated eggs daily throughout their lives, with varying numbers depending on the species. The position of the terminal spine varies among species as shown in Figure 52.3. The miracidium, or inside embryo, will develop within a period of ~16 days.

About 50% of eggs laid by the female worms are excreted into the stool or urine by ulcerating through the wall of the bowel (*S. mansoni, S. japonicum, S. mekongi, S. intercalatum*) or bladder, ureteral and genital mucosa (*S. haematobium*). The remaining 50% induce an acute and chronic inflammatory response in the host tissues that will trigger granuloma formation leading to scarring, local damage and organ dysfunction.[72] Eggs may also embolize from their initial intravascular origin to liver, lung and many other sites.[73]

When viable schistosome eggs are excreted and reach fresh water, either by direct deposition or by being washed in from a neighbouring site, in a suitable environment of warmth and light the larva within each egg becomes active and aided by osmosis the egg ruptures or 'hatches'; the larva, now termed a miracidium, emerges. Miracidia are mobile organisms swimming actively by means of ciliary movements. Miracidial behaviour is related in a general way to the ecology of the snail intermediate host and adaptive behavioural patterns have been described. On hatching from an egg in appropriate fresh water conditions, miracidia swim actively (at 2 mm/s) towards snail secretions. They remain infective to snails for 8–12 h.[74,75]

Miracidia then penetrate the soft tissues of the snail, influenced by numerous variables, including chemotaxis, the relative number of larvae and snails within a water body, length of contact time and physical characteristics of the surrounding medium, i.e. water temperature, velocity of flow, turbulence and the presence of ultraviolet light. Only a small proportion of entering miracidia develop to mature mother sporocysts.

Over the next several weeks, the sporocyst develops germinal cells that, in turn, develop into daughter sporocysts that migrate into other parts of the snail's body. After further development, each sporocyst can become a mature cercaria, which then is released from the snail. From a single miracidium, thousands

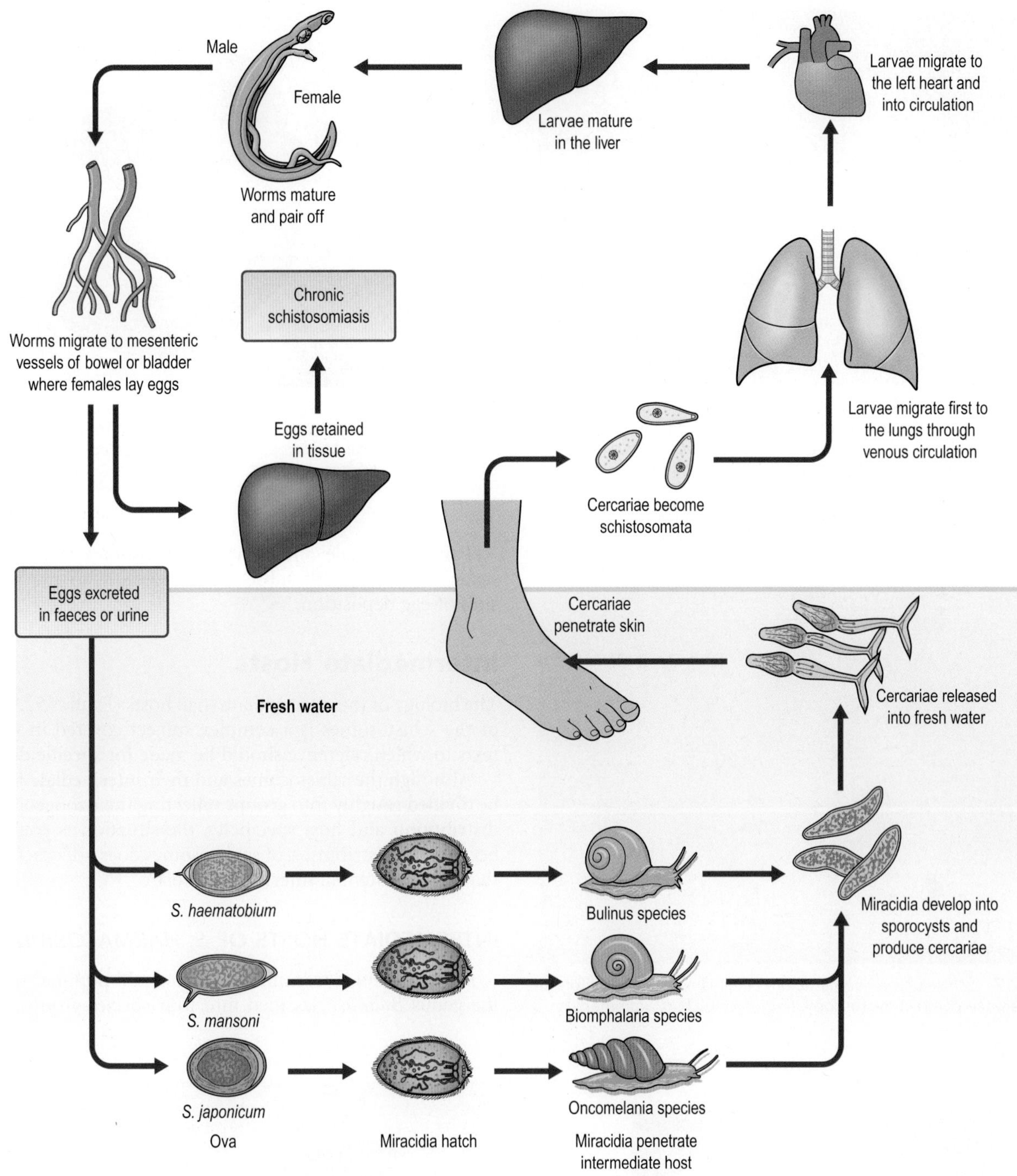

Figure 52.5 Schistosoma life cycle. *(From King CH. Toward the elimination of schistosomiasis. N Engl J Med 2009;360(2):106–9.)*

of *cercariae* are formed as a result of this asexual multiplication process.[76,77]

Free-swimming fork-tailed *cercariae*, <1 cm in length, penetrate human skin or mucosa when a person is exposed to infested water (Figure 52.7). For *S. haematobium* and *S. mansoni* the main stimulus for the release of cercariae is light, usually at temperatures between 10°C and 30°C. Cercarial lifespan is short: 36–48 h, as they are non-feeding organisms dependent on their large glycogen reserves. Throughout their long life, snails continue to produce a reasonably constant output of cercariae; many thousands can originate from a single *miracidium*.

Cercariae become schistosomules as they penetrate human skin and lose their tail (Figure 52.8). There is a remarkable transition from a 'freshwater environment' to a 'saltwater environment' as the larva moves into the human body through the tissues, lymphatics and venules making repeated circuits of the pulmonary–systemic circulation before entering a blood vessel leading to the hepatic portal system and transform into male and female adult worms.

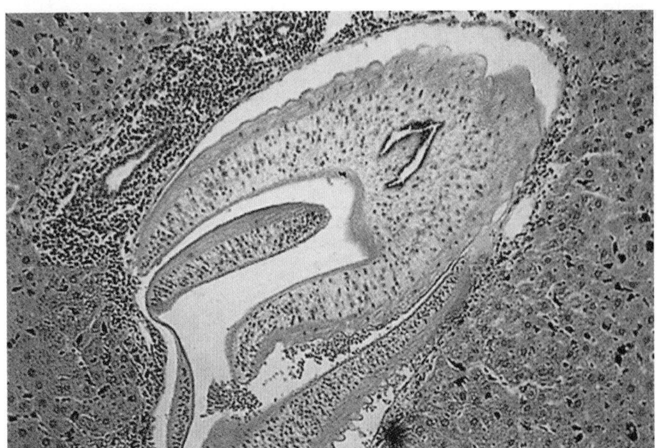

Figure 52.6 Adult *Schistosoma mansoni* in the portal circulation. The figure shows a cross-section of a male and female *S. mansoni* in a branch of the portal vein (H&E, ×44). *(From Peters W, Pasvol G. Atlas of Tropical Medicine and Parasitology, Copyright © 2006, with permission from Elsevier.)*

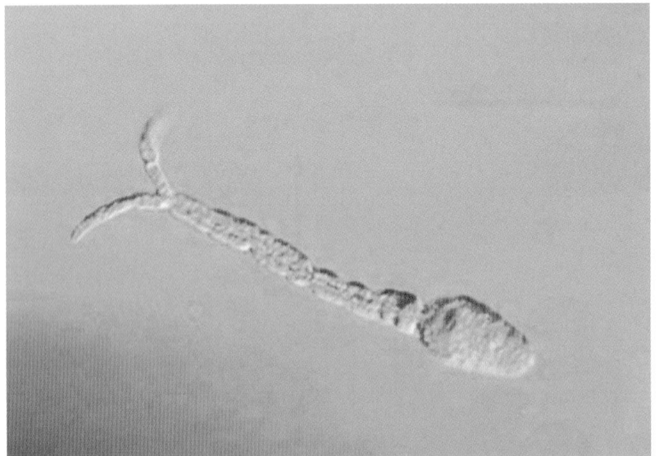

Figure 52.7 *Schistosoma haematobium* cercaria as seen on differential interference contrast microscopy. *(From WHO/TDR/Stammers.)*

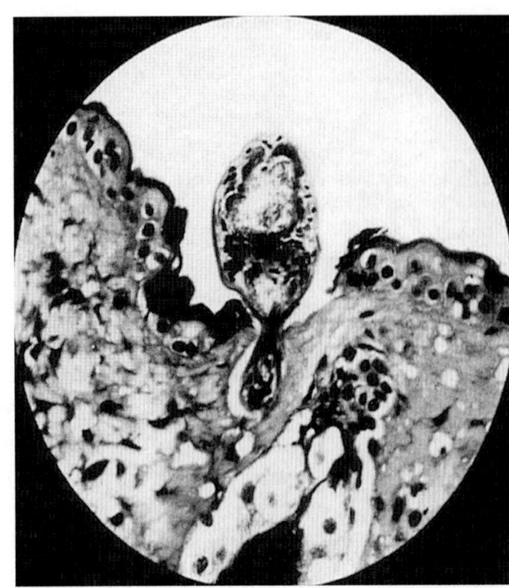

Figure 52.8 Cercarial penetration of the skin. *(From O.D. Standen.)*

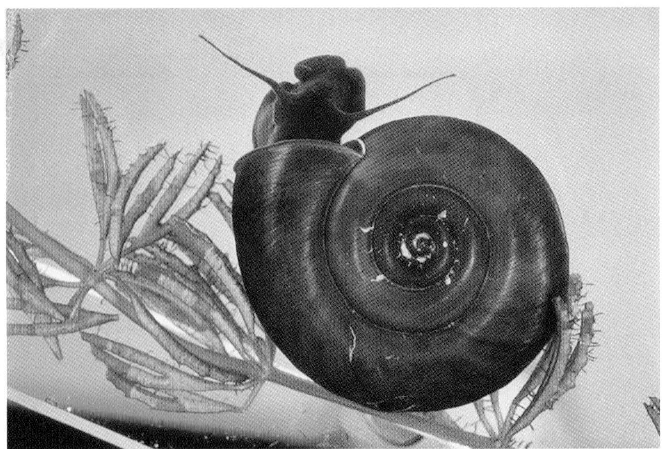

Figure 52.9 Intermediate hosts of *Schistosoma mansoni* are various species of *Biomphalaria* freshwater snails (×4). *(From Peters W, Pasvol G. Atlas of Tropical Medicine and Parasitology. Copyright © 2006, with permission from Elsevier.)*

Pairing of male and female schistosomes takes place on sexual maturity, with subsequent migration to the preferred sites of egg deposition.

Intermediate Hosts

The biology of the intermediate snail hosts (Figures 52.9–52.11) of the schistosomes is a complex subject covered in specialist texts to which reference should be made for specific details.

Although the schistosomes and their intermediate hosts can be divided roughly into groups reflecting their zoogeographical distribution and host specificity, the situation is complicated because the distribution of schistosomes does not exactly match that of the potential intermediate hosts.[78]

INTERMEDIATE HOSTS OF *S. HAEMATOBIUM*

S. haematobium is transmitted by some 30 nominal species of the genus *Bulinus*, classified into four species-groups: *Bulinus*

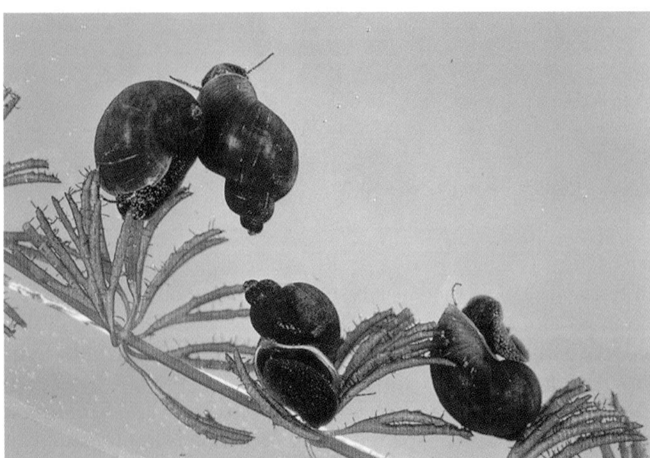

Figure 52.10 Intermediate hosts of *Schistosoma haematobium* are freshwater bulinid species within the *Bulinus africanus* complex (×3.5). *(From Peters W, Pasvol G. Atlas of Tropical Medicine and Parasitology. Copyright © 2006, with permission from Elsevier.)*

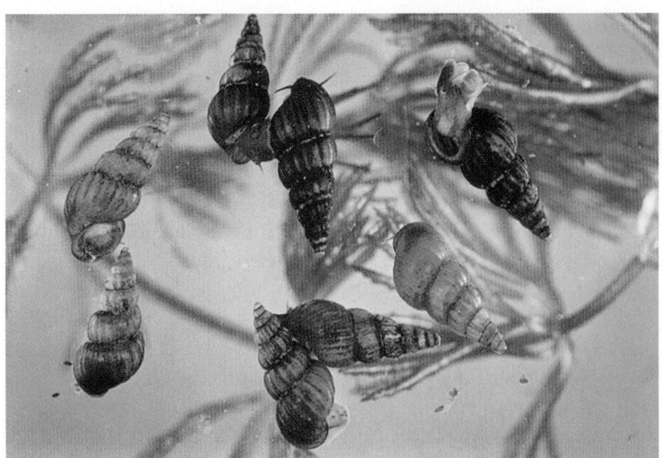

Figure 52.11 *Oncomelania*: intermediate snail host of *Schistosoma japonicum* (×3). (From Peters W, Pasvol G. Atlas of Tropical Medicine and Parasitology. Copyright © 2006, with permission from Elsevier.)

africanus, an important group medically as species within the group, namely *Bulinus nasutus* and *B. globosus* (Figure 52.10),[79,80] are intermediate hosts of *S. haematobium* in Africa south of the Sahara and, additionally, some cattle schistosomes; the *B. forskalli* group is distributed in a pan-African fashion with representatives found in Arabia and in some Indian Ocean islands; the *B. truncatus/tropicus* complex, again of pan-African distribution, extends from Malawi to east, west and north Africa and the Middle East as far as Iran; a small group, *B. reticulatus* is found patchily in Africa (e.g. in Ethiopia) and in isolated habitats in the Arabian peninsula.

INTERMEDIATE HOSTS OF *S. INTERCALATUM*

Of the two biologically distinct strains of *S. intercalatum* known to exist, one is transmitted by snails of the *Bulinus africanus* group and occurs in a restricted area of north-east Zaire; the other is transmitted by *B. forskalli* and occurs in Cameroon and Gabon. Each strain is unable to develop in a snail with which the other is compatible and, additionally, there are differences in prepatent periods and in certain enzyme patterns of the parasite.

INTERMEDIATE HOSTS OF *S. MANSONI*

S. mansoni is transmitted by snail species of the genus *Biomphalaria* (Figure 52.9), which is widely distributed throughout Africa, the Nile valley and the Arabian Peninsula, but not in Iraq or Iran. In the Americas, the genus is found in the southern USA, several Caribbean islands (notably Puerto Rico, St Lucia, Guadeloupe and the Dominican Republic) and on the South American continent in Brazil, Surinam and Venezuela.

The framework for the taxonomic status was described in 1978,[81] and four species-groups are still recognized. The *Biomphalaria pfeifferi* group has several forms and is found in all parts of Africa south of the Sahara, the Malagasy Republic, in Aden, Yemen and Saudi Arabia; the *B. choanomphala* group has only a few forms restricted to certain of the great natural African lakes; the *B. alexandrina* group has a scattered distribution in Africa and is common in the Sudan and Egypt. *B. sudanica* has both east and west African species components.

In the Americas, the genus *Biomphalaria* is represented by some 20 species but, of these, only *B. glabrata* (*Say*), *B. straminea* (*Dunker*) and *B. tenagophila* (*Orbigny*) have been found to be naturally infected with *S. mansoni*.

INTERMEDIATE HOSTS OF *S. JAPONICUM* AND *S. MEKONGI*

S. japonicum is transmitted by amphibious snails, populations of polytypic *Oncomelania hupensis* (Figure 52.11), of which there are six subspecies: *O. h. hupensis* in mainland China; *O. h. quadrasi* in the Philippines; *O. h. nosophora* in Japan; *O. h. lindoensis* in Sulawesi, Indonesia; and *O. h. formosana* and *O. h. chiui* in Taiwan, where schistosomiasis is confined to animals and does not exist in humans. A genus *Tricula aperta* from the subfamily Triculinae transmits *S. mekongi*.

The *Oncomelania* shell differs markedly in size and shape from those of the aquatic snails and *Oncomelania* snails have very different biological characteristics. In the Philippines, the average longevity is 66 days but in other endemic areas they may survive for 12 months or longer and may tolerate cold temperatures down to 0°C.[82–84]

AESTIVATION

Both aquatic and amphibious snails have the capacity to survive out of water for weeks, or in some cases, for months; this phenomenon – 'aestivation' – has important consequences on the epidemiology of the infection and its control; immature infections of both *S. mansoni* and *S. haematobium* can be carried through from one wet season to another, thus perpetuating the transmission cycle.

PARASITE–INTERMEDIATE HOST RELATIONSHIPS

If we pair a very complex parasite–intermediate host relationship with anthropogenic changes in the distribution and abundance of snails hosting schistosomes,[15,84] it becomes apparent that more detailed research in malacology must be undertaken to fully understand snail biology and the parasite–snail interaction.[85] Both environmental and genetic factors play a role in the transmission of schistosomes through particular species of snails. While snail control was a mainstay of schistosomiasis control programmes in the first part of the twentieth century, it was not particularly successful in stopping transmission in many areas. It is clear that a better understanding of snail biology and ecology is needed to provide better inputs for programmes aiming to limit transmission on the intermediate host side. The genera *Bulinus* and *Biomphalaria* are aquatic snails found in many different habitats including permanent or semi-permanent small ponds, marshes, swamps, rivers and streams and large permanent water bodies such as lakes, dams, irrigation channels and rice fields. Their biology varies with their environment and comprehensive studies are required to elucidate the details of snail survival and the factors leading to successful *Schistosoma* transmission. Cross-fertilization is usual in aquatic snails, but they are in fact hermaphrodites and capable of self-fertilization. Ova are laid in water as egg masses some

5–10 mm in diameter. Hatching of free-living snails occurs in 1–2 weeks; a steady growth ensues and maximal size and maturity is seen in 3–6 months. Like mosquitoes, snail intermediate hosts have an enormous reproductive potential because egg-laying continues throughout life and life spans have wide variations in the different species; e.g. *Bulinus globosus* infected with *S. haematobium* have lived for 400 days in captivity and *Biomphalaria pfeifferi* infected with *S. mansoni* have survived for 213 days.[78,86]

Pathogenesis and Pathology

THE ROLE OF HOST IMMUNITY

Primary Infection

In endemic areas, schistosomiasis infection occurs as early as infancy, when young children are exposed to contaminated water in bathing and playing (Figure 52.12).[24,25] Serosurveys indicate that significant exposure occurs by 3.5–4.5 years of age.[14,87] However, symptomatic acute schistosomiasis (Katayama syndrome) is seldom seen among children frequently exposed to *S. mansoni* or *S. haematobium*, possibly due to in utero imprinting of T- and B-cell responses, which has been identified among babies born to parasitized mothers.[88]

In acute schistosomiasis among short-term travellers and migrants not previously exposed to *Schistosoma* infection, patients express a considerably higher in vitro cellular response to parasite antigens than do comparable patients from endemic areas having chronic schistosomiasis. This is especially true for egg antigens. IgM and IgG against a carbohydrate epitope with the surface of larval schistosomes (KLH) is found in greater quantities in the serum of acutely exposed individuals, with a mixed Th1 and Th2 cytokine response to parasite antigens in the acute phase.[89,90] Studies in experimental animal models have long suggested that there is significant down modulation of immune responses to schistosome antigens as infection persists and exposure to egg antigens becomes chronic.[91,92] While this downregulation of immune response, with a shift towards Th2 type immune responses, may reduce the risk of morbidity caused by chronic inflammation, it is not clear if this experience-related immunity provides protection against new infections.

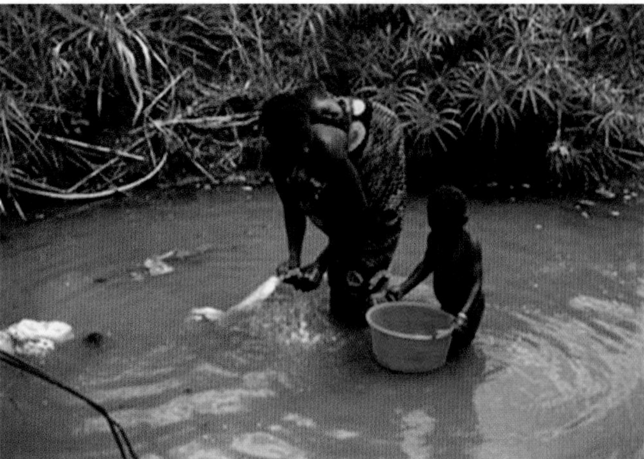

Figure 52.12 Mothers with young children do their family washing at a pond near their home. The water contains intermediate host snails for *Schistosoma haematobium* and both parent and child are significantly exposed to infection. *(From WHO/TDR/Crump.)*

Chronic Infection and Reinfection

After the primary infection in childhood, reinfection occurs regularly during subsequent years, with only limited resistance apparent at this stage of early childhood (ages 5–11). As schistosomes do not replicate within the body, it is this process of repeated exposure that results in progressive acquisition of higher worm loads, manifested by high parasite egg burdens, along with resultant pathology and morbidity. However, it is well known from community-based surveys that the prevalence and intensity of infection progressively decrease in the teenage years (>12 years) and that in successive decades of adulthood, there is a decline in egg output, suggesting a further spontaneous decline of infection intensity to much lower levels.[3,93]

There is strong evidence that disease formation is a consequence of the inflammatory immune activation that occurs during *Schistosoma* infection.[19,92] Careful studies of reinfection after successful cure have associated increased production of inflammatory cytokines IL-6, C-reactive protein and TNFα with systemic morbidities such as anaemia and growth impairment.[94–97] The pathways leading to anaemia are multifactorial, including splenic sequestration, iron loss and 'anaemia of chronic inflammation'. Chronic inflammation stimulates production of IL-6 that in turn increases the production of hepcidin, a liver hormone that regulates iron homeostasis. The downstream cascade leads to 'iron trapping' in the body storage sites, blocking its normal release and usage for haemoglobin production.[96,98]

The immune responses to chronic infection appear to vary during the course of disease progression. There are recognizable differences between those individuals without fibrosis, those with incipient fibrosis and those with recognized hepatosplenic disease. Those with early stages of fibrosis have an increased IgG (particularly IgG_4) response to soluble egg antigens (SEA), while those with established hepatosplenic disease express higher levels of immune response to soluble worm antigen preparation (SWAP).[89] In studies of cellular immune response, there is a predominantly Th2 anti-parasite response in chronic schistosomiasis that has been associated with hepatic fibrosis particularly among males[94] and production of cytokine IL-13 (as modified by IL-5) has been correlated with individual levels of fibrotic disease.[89]

An interesting observation in helminthic immunology and in particular that pertaining to *S. haematobium*, is the dramatic increase in the production of parasite-specific and non-specific IgE, which is typically associated with allergic responses (atopy) among patients in the developed world. However, in the case of parasitic infection, it has been postulated that IgE can, in fact, provide a beneficial protective effect.[99]

Concomitant immunity, in experimental terms, describes the resistance, partial or total, of an actively infected host to a subsequent challenge infection by the same type of organism. Adult worms evade the immune responses by adding a layer of host-specific antigens to their tegumental membranes. Adult worms of a primary infection are unharmed by cercarial challenge but the invading forms of the challenge infection tend to be destroyed. Concomitant immunity likely occurs to schistosome infections in many experimental hosts and in humans.[100]

Further exploratory progress was made through longitudinal field studies involving detailed quantification of egg outputs and water contact in children, allied to the technique of reinfection studies. Chemotherapy is given to remove existing infections; the levels of newly acquired infections (reinfections) are observed, quantified and related to water contact and degree of exposure. These techniques produced strong evidence that age-dependent resistance to reinfection is distinct from age-dependent exposure change in two areas, The Gambia and Kenya, for both *S. haematobium* and *S. mansoni* infection. For example, in The Gambia, changes in intensity of infection with time were compared in two communities, in one of which transmission had been interrupted by mollusciciding. In this area, the mean lifespan of the worms was 3–4 years, allowing comparison with the untreated area (control) of the numbers of eggs deposited by worms over the same 3-year period. The acquisition of new infections by adults over 25 years of age was 1000-fold less than that of 5–8-year-old children. This difference could not be attributed to a 1000-fold reduction of water contact in the adults, thus suggesting age-dependent acquisition of immunity to superinfection.[101–105] Thus, the role of immunity in limiting schistosome infections in communities in two areas endemic for *S. haematobium* and *S. mansoni* was placed on a firmer footing. However, the immunity is probably not absolute, is evident only after years of exposure to infection and some data suggest that it occurs earlier in areas of high prevalence and intensity.

The balance of the immune response in the early years of exposure to infection is directed towards production of blocking antibodies, which may be of IgM, IgG or IgG4. Protective antibodies, IgE or other immunoglobulin isotypes, are detected in both older children and adults who appear to be relatively resistant to infection.[104] Later data led to surmise that 'resistance' to acquired infection, or reinfection after successful chemotherapy, is multifactorial and compartmentalized. It may involve both humoral and cellular responses at different stages of parasitic invasion. Known influencing variables are an IgE response, high levels of interferon γ (IFNγ) and tumour necrosis factor α (TNFα) and peripheral blood mononuclear cell (PBMC) responses involving different groups of cells and various cytokines, allied to a possible genetic factor on chromosome 5q31–q33.[106,107]

Impact of Infection on Vaccine Response

Recent studies suggest a decreased response to vaccines in children born to mothers infected with schistosomiasis and other endemic helminthic parasites.[108] For children vaccinated against tuberculosis with the Bacillus Calmette-Guerin (BCG), it has been found that purified protein derivative-driven T cell IFN-γ production, evaluated 10–14 months after BCG vaccination, was significantly lower for infants who experienced prenatal sensitization to schistosomes in utero, relative to subjects who had not been sensitized.[109] These findings suggest important public health implications with respect to vaccination campaign efficacy in schistosomiasis-endemic areas.[108]

PATHOLOGY

The pathology resulting from *Schistosoma* infection is overwhelmingly due to the egg-induced inflammatory response (Figure 52.13). Adult worms are impervious to the immune system of the host and by themselves cause little or no pathology, although they excrete antigens such as the gut-associated soluble antigens found in the sera of patients with schistosomiasis and which are now used both as a marker for infection and as an indicator of therapeutic success.[110]

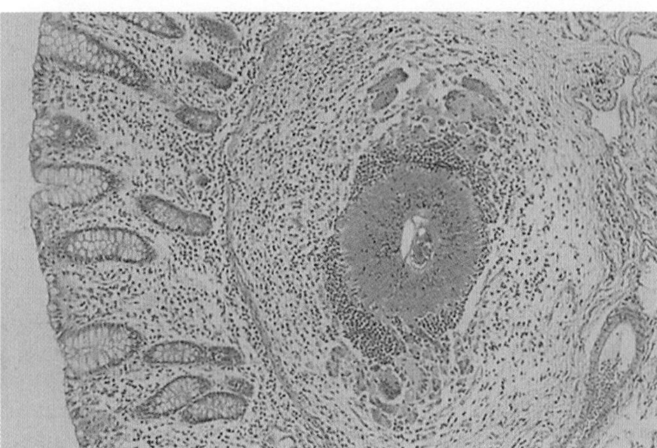

Figure 52.13 The fibrotic granuloma around this dead ovum in the colon is known as a Hoeppli reaction (H&E, ×70). *(From Peters W, Pasvol G. Atlas of Tropical Medicine and Parasitology. Copyright © 2006, with permission from Elsevier.)*

Host inflammation is essential to the reproductive success of the parasite – schistosome eggs cannot traverse capillary beds unaided because they measure up to 70 µm in width. Slightly fewer than half of the eggs laid into host venules are able to ulcerate (via host inflammatory reaction) into the lumen of the gut or urinary tract and so leave the human body. The remainder are retained in the walls of these organs or are embolized into the portal radicles or lung arterioles. Collateral vascular bypasses enable eggs to reach many other organs in the body.

At oviposition, eggs are immature, but miracidial maturation takes place within a few days. Soluble egg antigens (SEAs) originating from the secretory glands of miracidia enclosed within eggs diffuse out through submicroscopic pores in the eggshell and induce a host hypersensitivity response. The immunopathology of schistosomiasis is considered to be due to granuloma formation around tissue-deposited eggs and is a manifestation of delayed hypersensitivity through a T-cell-mediated immune response.[19] The florid granuloma is composed of the schistosome egg surrounded by cellular aggregates of eosinophils, mononuclear phagocytes, lymphocytes, neutrophils, plasma and fibroblasts (Figure 52.13). Activated macrophages cluster close to the eggshell, while lymphocytes and plasma cells are peripherally placed. Fibroblasts appear early and throughout the lengthy involution process, replace other cell types. Many granulomas are of sizes much greater than those of schistosome eggs, reducing in size as the infection shifts from acute to chronic after 3 months.

There are consistent and strong correlations of high organ and tissue egg loads and severe pathology in quantitative autopsy studies in *S. haematobium* and *S. mansoni*.[111] Other factors may operate, such as direct and indirect fibroblastic proliferation and induced abnormalities of types I and III collagen. Independent of infection intensity, individual variation in the intensity and context of host immune response may also affect the severity of tissue damage.[92]

Unlike early 'acute' granulomas, the late, obstructive and fibrous lesions of advanced chronic schistosomiasis respond poorly to antischistosomal chemotherapy.[19] Antibody and cellular immune response specific to each stage of infection are long-lived and persist after successful chemotherapy.[112] The inflammation and fibrotic injury schistosomiasis can persist long after a successful 'cure' of *Schistosoma* infection. As such, schistosomiasis should be seen as the preventable, chronic inflammatory condition caused by *present* or *previous* infection with metazoan parasitic blood flukes of *Schistosoma* species. The disease case definition then becomes: a person who has, or has previously had, infection with *Schistosoma* spp. parasites.

The pathophysiology of schistosomiasis varies within stages of the life cycle as presented below. The differences among them are clearer in non-immune affected people such as visitors, tourists, or immigrants who become infected for the first time following a defined, brief exposure in endemic areas.

Cercarial Invasion and Schistosomular Migration

Cercarial invasion of the skin or mucosal penetration on exposure to infested water, particularly when the local level of transmission is high, can occur in <15 min; the clinical consequence of cercarial dermal invasion is a cercarial dermatitis lasting for some 24–48 h.[113] The first pathophysiological response to invasion is the initiation of marked eosinophilia and an antibody-dependent cell-mediated cytotoxic response to schistosomula involving IgG.[114]

Katayama syndrome, or 'acute toxaemic schistosomiasis', is a clinical entity that appears between 14–84 days in non-immune individuals exposed to schistosome infection. It resembles serum sickness, presenting as a hypersensitivity reaction to the migrating schistosomulum and to early egg deposition by maturing female worms. In and around areas endemic for *S. japonicum*, epidemics of Katayama syndrome have been reported in communities affected by large-scale flooding (Figure 52.14).[115]

Schistosome Maturation and Egg Deposition

At variable times after infection, from some 2 months onwards, the stage of established infection occurs, with continuous egg-laying associated with the 'classical' symptoms and signs of established schistosomiasis. SEAs from miracidia in the eggs provoke a T lymphocyte-mediated host response, which, in time, results in the characteristic granuloma with eosinophils prominent in the destruction of the eggs.

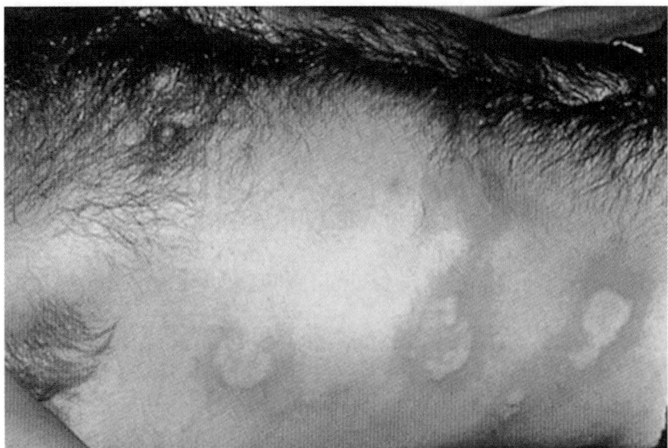

Figure 52.14 'Katayama syndrome' manifesting as massive giant urticaria soon after infection with *S. mansoni*. *(From Peters W, Pasvol G. Atlas of Tropical Medicine and Parasitology. Copyright © 2006, with permission from Elsevier.)*

Established Infection with Continuous Egg-laying

After some years, changes in clinical symptoms and physical signs appear and there is superimposition of late-stage complications such as obstructive uropathy, genital bleeding and inflammation, hydronephrosis and pyelonephritic renal failure in *S. haematobium* infection, or portal hypertension which may be 'compensated' or 'decompensated' with ascites and hepatosplenomegaly with or without gastrointestinal bleeding in *S. mansoni*, *S. japonicum* and *S. mekongi* infections. Modulation by T suppressor lymphocytes and antibody blockade diminish the host immune response over time with a more prominent Th2 response;[89] fibroblasts stimulate collagen production and fibrotic complications involving a variety of anatomical sites (e.g. periportal hepatic fibrosis and obstructive uropathy) ensue.

PATHOLOGY OF CHRONIC INFECTION

Because of differences in the *Schistosoma* species' preferred anatomic localization, many of the 'classic' manifestations of chronic schistosomiasis are species-dependent. However, all forms of schistosomiasis cause similar levels of chronic inflammation and so share common aspects of systemic morbidity that include anaemia and impaired growth and cognitive development.[12]

Schistosoma Haematobium

Urinary Bladder. The urinary bladder is the most frequently affected organ in schistosomiasis haematobia. Cystoscopy, surgery, or autopsy reveal the gross lesions, which are often multiple.[73] A hyperaemic mucosa is universal on cystoscopy.[116] 'Sandy patches' occur in one-third; these are raised greyish-yellow mucosal irregularities associated with heavy egg deposition and surrounded by dense fibrous tissue. Calcifications often occur in advanced cases. These are most commonly sighted at the trigone and near the ureteric orifices.

Other raised lesions found in the urinary and nearby genital tracts are granulomas, nodules and polyps, which may be sessile or pedunculated and are related to local heavy tissue egg loads.[18] Vesical ulcers are less common and can vary in size from a small irregular defect to an irregular deep transverse fissure. These occur mainly on the posterior wall of the bladder.

Ureters. Classic post-mortem studies have shown that though the ureters are less frequently affected than the bladder, their involvement is important for it leads to morbidity and is the forerunner of obstructive uropathy.[73] Tissue egg loads in the ureters are greater in cases with obstructive uropathy than in those without. Bilateral ureteric involvement is the rule.

The histopathological appearance of the ureteric lesions resembles that of bladder lesions and granulomatous lesions resolve and lead to ureteral fibrotic stenosis.[19] Rising back pressure leads to hydroureter, with or without hydronephrosis, causing obstructive uropathy (Figure 52.15). This may predispose to chronic or recurrent infections by enteric bacteria, including *Salmonella*.[117]

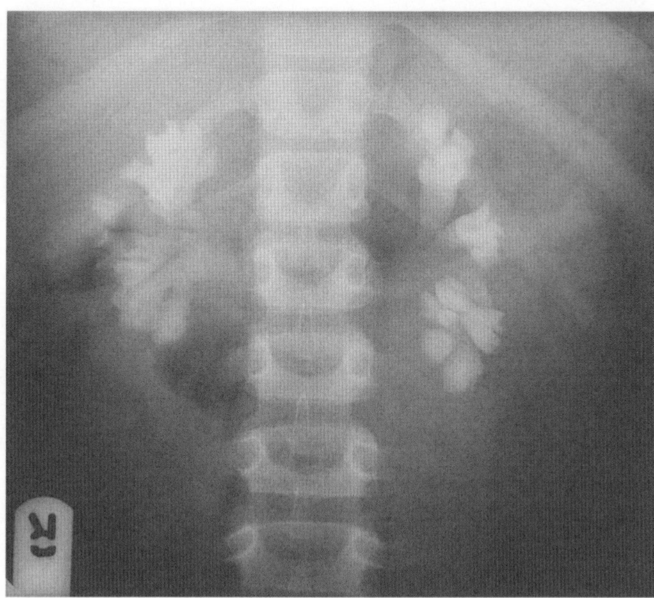

Figure 52.15 Renal contrast radiograph showing bilateral hydronephrosis in chronic urogenital schistosomiasis. *(From Peters W, Pasvol G. Atlas of Tropical Medicine and Parasitology. Copyright © 2006, with permission from Elsevier.)*

Genital Organs. Because *S. haematobium* parasitizes the vesical plexus, eggs are often found in both male and female genital organs.[73] In *males*, the mean *S. haematobium* egg count/g of seminal vesicle tissue was 20 000 in one investigation.[18] The resultant enlargement, muscular hypertrophy and fibrosis produced an increase in weight of the seminal vesicles that correlated with the presence of obstructive uropathy. Much less commonly affected were the prostate, testes, epididymis and penis. Haematospermia is often a presenting symptom of genitourinary schistosomiasis. Orchitis, prostatitis, dyspareunia and oligospermia have been associated with male genital schistosomiasis and have been shown to resolve after anti-schistosomal therapy.[118,119]

In *females*, the finding of eggs in the female genital organs is similarly frequent; eggs may be found in the vulva, vagina or cervix, where friable polypoid or nodular lesions and sandy patches may be seen (Figure 52.16).[120] Nodules in the perianal skin are not rare. The internal female genital organs – ovaries, Fallopian tubes and uterus – are much less commonly affected. However, pelvic schistosomiasis can cause reversible and irreversible female infertility.[121,122] Female genital schistosomiasis is increasingly recognized as a co-morbid condition with HIV/AIDS in sub-Saharan Africa.

Gastrointestinal Tract. *S. haematobium* eggs are found frequently in the gastrointestinal tract, their density being highest in the appendix with a decreased density in the distal tract. Polyps have been recorded in the rectosigmoid colon in an autopsy study of *S. haematobium* cases; the polyps were inflammatory and were often ulcerated.[18] *S. haematobium* eggs are often seen in rectal biopsy material, but are usually dead.

Kidney. Although schistosomal granulomas are rare in the kidney parenchyma, renal lesions occur as a sequel of obstructive uropathy and are most often manifest as pyelonephritis.

Schistosomal antigens have been observed by immunofluorescent microscopy in mesangial areas of the glomeruli in uncomplicated cases of *S. haematobium* infection. Granular deposits of IgG, IgM and C3 have also been noted, yet with a lack of basement membrane changes, an absence of clinical renal disease and with maintenance of normal renal function.[123] There remains doubt about whether *S. haematobium* causes a specific nephritis given the presence of other potential mechanisms of renal failure.[124] A reversible nephrotic syndrome in *S. haematobium* complicated by *Salmonella* infection has been described.[125]

Lung. Pulmonary arteritis and cor pulmonale are rare in pure *S. haematobium* infection, yet egg granulomas are frequently encountered in the lung at autopsy.[19]

Ectopic Lesions. Migration of *S. haematobium* within the vascular system and subsequent egg-laying may produce a variety of 'ectopic' or atypical lesions. For example, mirroring the disease caused by *S. mansoni* and *S. japonicum* (agents of intestinal schistosomiasis), low-grade liver periportal fibrosis has been detected by ultrasonography in patients with *S. haematobium* infection.[126]

The finding of eggs of *S. haematobium* in the CNS, although not as common as seen in *S. japonicum or S. mansoni* infection, seem to have few clinical sequelae; eggs appear to produce minimal or no histological reaction, in contrast to the production of inflammatory response when eggs are laid elsewhere in the body. The spinal cord is affected more often than the brain.[127]

Rare anatomic localization of parasite lesions has been described, such as multiple *S. haematobium* egg deposition in the pericardium causing a fibrous pericarditis,[128] and the demonstration of an adult *S. haematobium* worm in the choroid plexus.[129]

Bladder Cancer. The exact mechanism of bilharzial bladder carcinogenesis remains unknown. However, squamous cell

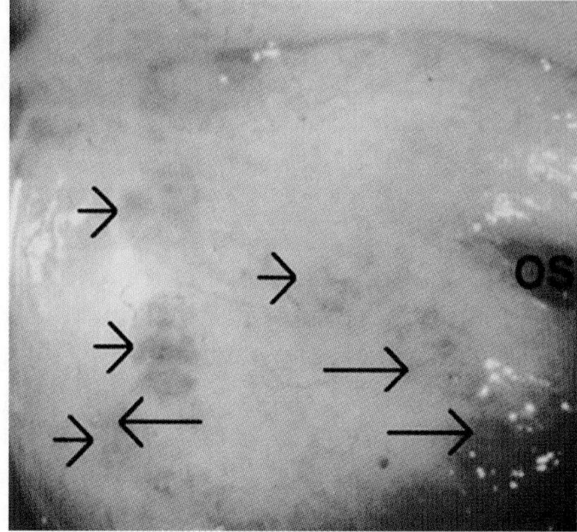

Figure 52.16 Female genital schistosomiasis: Homogenous sandy patches and abnormal blood vessels on the uterine cervix of a woman infected with *Schistosoma haematobium*. Long arrows, convoluted blood vessels; short arrows, homogenous yellow sandy patches; Os, uterine os. Some superficial sandy patches are seen next to the os. *(From Kjetland EF, Ndhlovu PD, Mduluza T, et al. Simple clinical manifestations of genital* Schistosoma haematobium *infection in rural Zimbabwean women. Am J Trop Med Hyg 2005 Mar;72(3):311–19.)*

bladder cancer associated with *S. haematobium* infection remains a major cause of morbidity in many countries. In the past, it was the most commonly diagnosed cancer of Egyptian men from parasite-endemic areas, who experienced up to 10 times the incidence of bladder cancer compared with men from non-endemic countries. The WHO International Agency for Research on Cancer has found sufficient evidence to consider *S. haematobium* a carcinogen.[130]

S. haematobium-related tumours may be differentiated from non-bilharzial tumours by their younger age of onset, a greater male-to-female ratio and by their pathology and clinical presentation. *S. haematobium*-associated tumours tend to be multifocal squamous cell cancers, as compared with the transitional cell tumours common in Europe and North America. Such bladder tumours have been successfully induced in animals (monkeys and baboons) exposed to *S. haematobium* infection.[131–133] One hypothesis postulates that the decades-long presence of chronic inflammation in the bladder facilitates DNA damage and the development of multi-centric cancers of the bladder wall. Co-factors for carcinogenesis include chronic bacterial infections and exposure to chemical carcinogens (petrochemicals, dietary nitrosamines). Raised urinary levels of β-glucuronidase related to chronic pyuria may 'retoxify' previously glucuronidated (i.e. detoxified) excreted carcinogenic chemicals, facilitating induction of bladder cancer in the presence of *S. haematobium*.[134,135]

In Iraq, coastal Kenya, Ghana, Malawi, Mozambique, Zambia and Zimbabwe, there is a consistent association between the local prevalence of *S. haematobium* infection and bladder carcinoma. However, in Nigeria, South Africa and Saudi Arabia, all countries with a moderate or high prevalence of *S. haematobium*, the association is not present. Whether this difference is due to strain differences in the parasite or to local differences in exposure to carcinogenic co-factors is not known.

Most squamous cell cancers in schistosomal bladders are fairly well-differentiated, largely indolent and localized, spreading directly through the bladder wall with late and infrequent lymphatic spread. Bloodstream metastasis is rare. This picture contrasts sharply with that of transitional cell carcinoma. Large-scale, population-based anti-schistosomal drug therapy directed at the control of morbidity would be expected to lower cancer incidence rates in the affected endemic countries and studies to this end are in place in Egypt. The critical problem will be the acquisition of accurate and acceptable population-based incidence estimates of bladder cancer.

Schistosoma mansoni

In schistosomiasis mansoni a range of chronic lesions is found, from scattered granulomas of the intestinal tract to gross hepatic periportal fibrosis (Symmer's pipe-stem fibrosis; bilharzial clay-pipe stem fibrosis) (Figure 52.17). Because of varying localization of the mature *S. mansoni* worms, focal granulomas and fibrosis may occur in any part of the intestinal tract, but these are found most frequently in the rectosigmoid colon because the preferred habitat of adult *S. mansoni* is in the tributaries of the inferior mesenteric vein. These lesions can lead to clinical symptoms of diarrhoea, haematochezia and abdominal pain. Pathology in the small bowel is not as severe as that in the large gut. In late-stage infections, particularly in Egypt and Brazil, autopsy studies suggest a shift in egg deposition from the colon to the small intestine.[136]

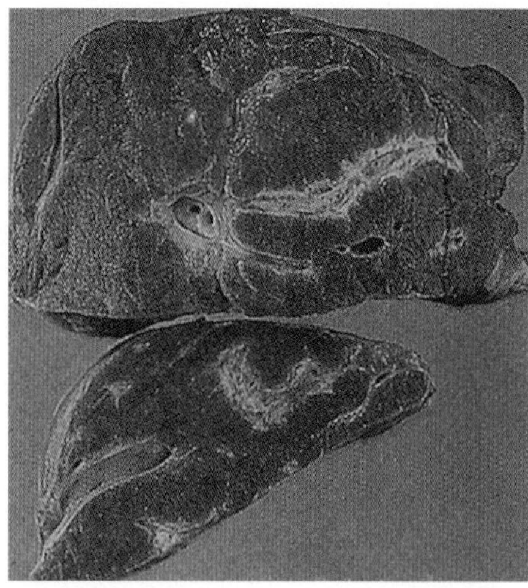

Figure 52.17 Periportal fibrosis ('pipestem fibrosis') is the classic pathological hepatic lesion of intestinal schistosomiasis. *(From Peters W, Pasvol G. Atlas of Tropical Medicine and Parasitology. Copyright © 2006, with permission from Elsevier.)*

Colonic polyposis (Figure 52.18), a syndrome often found in Egypt, occurs in younger patients and is related directly to their intensity of infection. The colon and rectum are the sites of multiple pedunculated polyps with associated mucosal swelling, hyperaemia and oedema. The concentration of eggs within the polyps is much higher than at other sites in the intestine. The clinical accompaniments are significant blood and protein losses producing anaemia, chronic diarrhoea, tenesmus and a protein-losing enteropathy.

Occasionally pseudotumours of schistosomal eggs surrounded by extensive fibrous tissue occur in *S. mansoni* infection and are termed 'bilharziomas'. Sites of predilection are the omentum, mesenteric lymph nodes, paracaecal region and infrequently the wall of the gut. Rarely, reports appear in the literature relating intestinal obstruction caused by chronic schistosomal infection.[136]

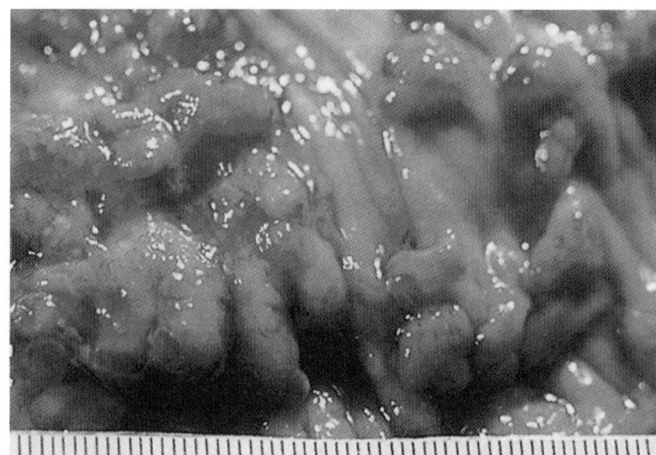

Figure 52.18 Massive *S. mansoni*-associated polyposis of the colon, with fatal intestinal haemorrhage, seen at post-mortem of an Egyptian farmer. *(From Peters W, Pasvol G. Atlas of Tropical Medicine and Parasitology. Copyright © 2006, with permission from Elsevier.)*

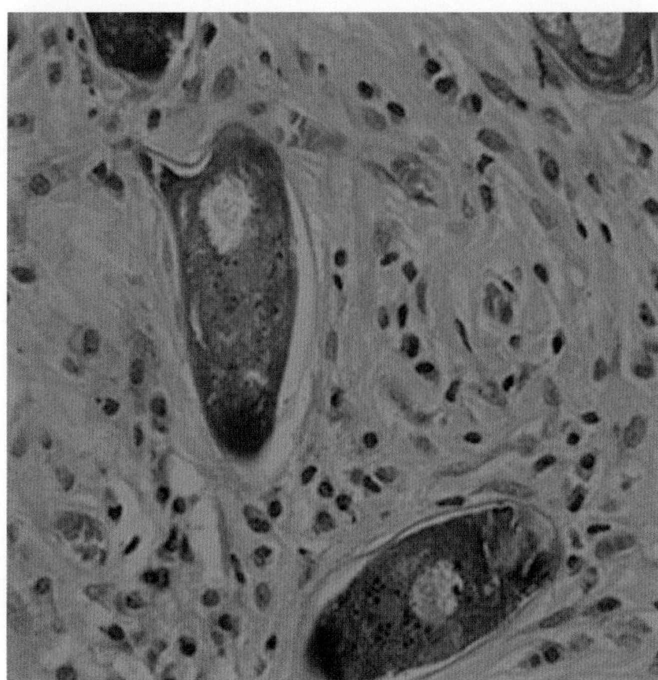

Figure 52.19 Eggs of *S. mansoni* in liver tissue, stained with H&E. *(From CDC, Images courtesy of Dr. Munaf Desai, Al Qassini Hospital, Shatjah, United Arab Emirates.)*

Hepatosplenic Schistosomiasis

The major pathognomonic complication of chronic *S. mansoni* infection is periportal hepatic fibrosis. Because the basic pathology is sited in and around the portal tracts (Figure 52.19) and the hepatic parenchyma remains normal in uncomplicated cases, the term *cirrhosis* is inappropriate for *Schistosoma*-related liver disease. A cut section of the liver, which may or may not be enlarged, shows macroscopic, wide bands of fibrosis around portal tracts, resembling the stems of a number of clay pipes (Figure 52.17). The surface of the liver may be smooth, granular or nodular. Between portal fields, the hepatic parenchyma specifically *does not* exhibit the nodularity of Laënnec's cirrhosis.

Deposited eggs produce granulomas with surrounding inflammatory infiltrates in the connective tissue that surrounds the hepatic veins, proximal to presinusoidal vessels. Affected portal tracts become blocked with granulomas and disorganized by inflammation, fibrosis and pyelophlebitis.[137] Eggs surrounded by an eosinophilic infiltrate, schistosomal pigment and/or organizing thrombi are found. The accumulation of granulomas around sites of blockage leads to further portal enlargement and simultaneously, the hepatic arteries enlarge and push out new branching capillaries. Thus the presinusoidal portal hypertension produces a compensatory arterial flow. Total intrahepatic blood flow remains within normal limits, with maintenance of hepatocellular metabolic function. The diminished portal blood flow from portal hypertension is compensated for by the increase in hepatic arterial supply and the rich capillary arterial network around the portal branches, which communicates with the portal vein.[137]

There remain unexplained discrepancies between clinical and pathological interpretations of the arterial origin of the hepatic capillary network.[138] Hepatic fibrosis results from the accumulation of collagen and may originate in the proliferation of collagen-synthesizing cells, increased synthesis by existing cells or deficiency in collagen degradation.[139,140] In experimental animals, the amount of collagen in the liver increases in parallel with egg granuloma formation. In human hepatic schistosomiasis, there is increased collagen content and marked collagen synthesis in wedge liver biopsy material when compared with control tissue. The natural course of pure periportal fibrosis is slow and is termed 'compensated' because liver cell function tests show only slight abnormalities, if any. Over time, the consequences of portal hypertension with splenomegaly and/or variceal haemorrhage, with or without ascites, appear, although hepatic decompensation does not develop until an advanced stage of the process. However, in countries where there is a high prevalence of viral hepatitis (hepatitis B, C, D or E), these may co-exist with hepatosplenic schistosomiasis and the clinical progression of decompensated hepatic fibrosis presents a much more rapid progress because hepatocellular pathology is much more severe than in the state of hepatic fibrosis due to *Schistosoma* infection alone.

Spleen. Splenomegaly is the usual accompaniment of hepatic schistosomiasis and is due to portal venous hypertension, chronic passive congestion and reticuloendothelial hyperplasia. Focal infarcts and trabecular haemorrhages may occur and the spleen is tough and fibrotic. Hypersplenism may produce pancytopenia or leucoerythroblastic anaemia. The spleen may become enormously enlarged (Egyptian splenomegaly or Banti's syndrome in the older literature), as in kala-azar (visceral leishmaniasis) or the myeloproliferative syndromes. Gamna-gandy bodies (organized foci of bleeding within the spleen caused by portal hypertension) have been found in patients with hepatosplenic schistosomiasis.[141] Lymphomas have been occasionally associated with schistosomal splenomegaly.[142]

Lungs and Heart. Pulmonary hypertension, caused by granulomatous pulmonary arteritis originating from large-scale embolization of eggs, is commonly the result of established hepatic fibrosis with extensive portocaval shunting, as occurs with chronic *S. mansoni* or *S. japonicum* infection.[136]

Granulomatous inflammation occludes distal pulmonary arterial branches and eventually produces a rise in pulmonary arterial pressure with right ventricular hypertrophy and strain; the smaller arterioles show fibrointimal sclerosis; fibrinoid necrosis and angiomatoid formation is widespread in alveolar tissue. This complication arises in long-standing cases of heavy infection and presents clinically as congestive heart failure arising in chronic cor pulmonale.

Kidney. Renal lesions, known as schistosomal nephropathy (or glomerulonephritis), occur in *S. mansoni* infection. These consist of deposition of immune complexes of host immunoglobulins with adult worm or egg antigens in the glomerular mesangium and basement membrane. A variety of glomerular lesions has been found at autopsy in hepatosplenic patients. Mild proteinuria is common in *S. mansoni* infection and in hepatosplenic cases, progressive nephropathy leading to renal failure occurs in a small proportion of patients, although the clinical course is slow and the risks are greater from the hepatic complications.[136] Amyloidosis has been demonstrated in renal biopsy material from patients with the nephrotic syndrome and schistosomiasis in Egypt.[143]

Egg deposition in the kidney is rare and is not thought to be responsible for serious renal dysfunction.

Central Nervous System. 'Cerebral' schistosomiasis has traditionally been associated with *S. japonicum* infection, but eggs of *S. mansoni* have also been found in the brain. The route of infection is thought to be via Batson's valveless intervertebral plexus or by arterial egg embolism. Eggs may be present in the CNS with little or no histological reaction and, in a randomly selected series of hepatosplenic cases of schistosomiasis coming to autopsy, one-quarter of patients had *S. mansoni* eggs in the brain;[144] these cases may be minimally symptomatic.

Myelopathy with various motor and/or sensory presentations occurs, more commonly in *S. mansoni* than in *S. haematobium* infection and cord compression or infarction with resulting paraparesis has been well described in the literature. Not infrequently, spinal cord schistosomiasis is recognized as part of the acute toxaemic syndrome that occurs in tourists and transient visitors to endemic areas.[145]

Other Ectopic Lesions. Cutaneous lesions due to *S. mansoni* are rare, although papular or nodular lesions at different sites are known. In Egypt, genital lesions are commonly found at autopsy. Placental schistosomiasis has been reported from Brazil.[146]

Cancer. According to the WHO, despite the number of case reports linking *S. mansoni* infection and different types of cancer, namely colorectal cancer, liver cancer and giant follicular lymphoma, there is inadequate evidence in humans for the carcinogenicity of infection with *Schistosoma mansoni*.[130]

Schistosoma japonicum

The intestinal and hepatic lesions of *S. japonicum* are, in general, similar to those occurring in *S. mansoni* infection, but with several specific differences. The primary lesion is a T cell-mediated granuloma formed around parasite eggs, but modulation of the granuloma size may be antibody- and T cell-mediated, whereas in *S. mansoni* infection cell mediation is the dominant mechanism.

The adult worms are located in the branches of the inferior mesenteric vein and in the superior haemorrhoidal vein.[147] An adult female deposits 1000–3500 eggs/day, with the highest density found in the large intestine and, in descending order, in the rectum, sigmoid and descending colon (Figure 52.20). The small intestine is relatively lightly affected.

Knowledge of the pathological anatomy (gross and microscopic) of *S. japonicum* lags behind that of *S. mansoni* infection because autopsy studies are fewer. Advanced schistosomiasis japonica has also been progressively declining as a cause of death for some decades.[136,148,149]

Gastrointestinal Disease. In experimental animals, gastrointestinal lesions of *S. japonicum* infection are focal and isolated and are interspersed with normal bowel. Segmental lesions occur in humans and multiple lesions are common including mucosal hyperplasia, pseudopolyposis, ulceration and thickening of the intestinal wall. Gastric schistosomiasis is seen frequently in surgical or biopsy specimens. Subclinical cases are probably common but go unrecognized owing to non-specific symptomatology and relatively insensitive diagnostic techniques for detection of *S. japonicum* infection.[8]

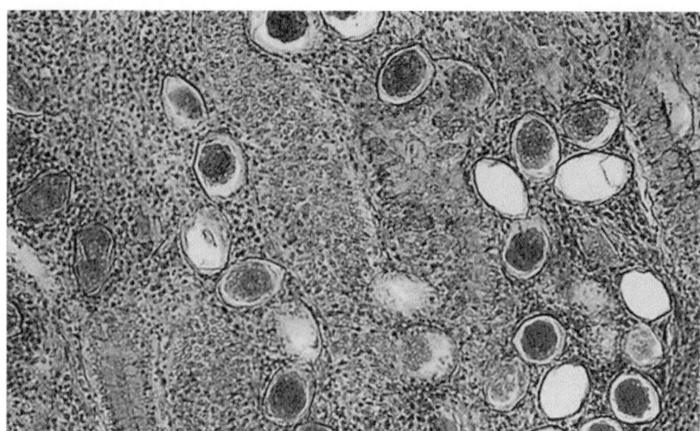

Figure 52.20 Eggs of *Schistosoma japonicum* in wall of colon (H&E, ×150). *(From Peters W, Pasvol G. Atlas of Tropical Medicine and Parasitology. Copyright © 2006, with permission from Elsevier.)*

Hepatosplenic Disease. Macroscopic hepatic changes in chronic schistosomiasis japonica parallel those in *S. mansoni* infection. The liver is frequently enlarged with an irregular surface. On cross-section, the characteristic wide bands of fibrous tissue surrounding the larger portal tracts are seen and Symmer's periportal (clay-pipe stem) fibrosis is found at autopsy (Figure 52.17). Microscopically, the picture is one of chronic pseudotubercles with chronic inflammation, cellular infiltrates around eggs, extensive fibrosis and neovascularization in the portal tracts. The accompanying manifestations of portal hypertension (i.e. splenomegaly with or without gastrointestinal varices, with or without bleeding) are common in advanced disease.

Central Nervous System. In contrast to *S. mansoni* and *S. haematobium* infections, the brain is more commonly affected in *S. japonicum* infection, although spinal cord involvement appears to be less frequent. The cerebral lesions are caused either by intracranial egg deposition or by egg embolism via a vascular route.

Lung. While cor pulmonale does occur in schistosomiasis japonica, there are fewer reports in *S. japonicum* infection than in *S. mansoni* infection, despite the similar pathogenic mechanisms.[136]

Cancer. Epidemiological studies have not demonstrated any direct relationships between gastric cancer and *S. japonicum* infection and the WHO-IARC has not found sufficient evidence to declare *S. japonicum* a human carcinogen.[130,136]

Schistosoma mekongi

Although the clinical manifestations of *S. mekongi* infection are similar to those of *S. japonicum*, the morbidity and pathology resulting from the former are compounded by the presence of *Opisthorchis viverrini* in areas endemic for *S. mekongi*. Objective descriptions of detailed pathology in humans are lacking.

Schistosoma intercalatum and S. guineensis

The distribution of *S. intercalatum* is restricted to 10 countries in central and West Africa and more information exists on experimental infection than on human infection. However, the pathology of *S. intercalatum* infection is known to be primarily due to inflammation of the sigmoid and rectum.[150] On proctoscopy of hospital inpatients, the rectal and colonic mucosa were considered abnormal in 47 out of 85 patients. Nonspecific lesions predominated: mucosal congestion, oedema, bleeding and/or ulceration. In liver biopsies, granulomatous lesions, of a size smaller than those seen in *S. mansoni* infection, were seen in the portal tracts. Tissue reaction to eggs was slight or absent in some patients. No portal hypertension was seen.[150,151]

The newly described *S. guineensis*, the only schistosome species on the island of Sao Tome, has been shown to produce 'pipestem-type' hepatic portal septal fibrosis and genital involvement. Other pathological sequelae are currently under investigation. It is suspected that hybridization with *S. intercalatum* occurs. The parasite is susceptible to treatment with praziquantel but may require increased dosage or courses of chemotherapy.[53]

Clinical Features

GENERAL PRESENTATION OF SCHISTOSOMIASIS

In the past, textbook descriptions of schistosomiasis have focused just on *Schistosoma* infection-specific pathologies and their associated symptoms. However, these 'pathognomonic' findings prove to be only a limited portion of the disease spectrum associated with schistosomiasis; we now know that such classical descriptions of schistosomiasis reflect only a minority (<10%) of patients. Not surprisingly, many *Schistosoma*-infected patients have 'nonspecific' symptoms caused by the chronic granulomatous pathology from parasite egg deposition in their tissues. There is increasing recognition of the more prevalent, but less dramatic, disabling conditions associated with chronic schistosomiasis including anaemia, growth retardation, decreased physical performance, poor school performance and sub-optimal work productivity.[11,12,152,153] Furthermore, there is now better understanding that, in terms of patient morbidity and disability, schistosomiasis is a chronic inflammatory condition that is *initiated* by infection with *Schistosoma* parasites and which causes damage that *persists* even after infection abates.[154,155]

Syndromes Common to All Schistosome Infections

For a detailed description of syndromes common to all schistosome infections, see Table 52.2.

Cercarial Dermatitis. Cercarial dermatitis occurs most commonly upon exposure to avian cercariae, with human cases reported both in schistosomiasis-endemic and non-endemic countries.[67,156,157] Itching (pruritus) of the skin is the primary symptom, arising within a few minutes of exposure and receding within 24–72 h, accompanied in some cases by erythema and/or a papular eruption.[113] The condition can occur after exposure to any of the five *Schistosoma* spp. that commonly infect humans and affects mostly non-immune visitors.

TABLE 52.2 Summary of *Schistosoma* spp. Infections of Humans, Their Impact on Health and Their Recommended Drug Treatment

Schistosoma spp.	Transmission	Geographic Distribution	Clinical Presentation	Treatment
Schistosoma mansoni	Through skin in fresh water contaminated by feces; Intermediate host: freshwater *Biomphalaria* snail	Africa; Middle East; Caribbean; Latin America	Acute: Abdominal pain, wasting, anaemia Chronic: Growth retardation, anaemia, grand mal epilepsy ascites, portal hypertension. transverse myelitis	Praziquantel 40 mg/kg/day PO for 1 day
Schistosoma haematobium	Through skin in fresh water contaminated by urine; Intermediate host: freshwater *Bulinus* snail	Africa; Middle East	Acute: Haematuria, dysuria, wasting, anaemia Chronic: Growth retardation, anaemia, decreased fitness, impaired cognition, renal failure, hydroureter/ hydronephrosis, dyspareunia, infertility, bladder carcinoma	Praziquantel 40 mg/kg/day PO for 1 day
Schistosoma japonicum	Through skin in fresh water contaminated by feces; Intermediate host: freshwater *Oncomelania* snail	China; South-east Asia; Philippines	Acute: Abdominal pain, anaemia Chronic: Growth retardation, anaemia. grand mal epilepsy, ascites, portal hypertension, transverse myelitis	Praziquantel 60 mg/kg/day divided tid PO for 1 day
Schistosoma mekongi	Through skin in fresh water contaminated by feces; Intermediate host: freshwater *Trichula* snail	South-east Asia	Acute: Abdominal pain, anaemia Chronic: Growth retardation, anaemia, grand mal epilepsy, ascites, portal hypertension.	Praziquantel 60 mg/kg/day divided tid PO for 1 day
Schistosoma intercalatum	Through skin in fresh water contaminated by feces; Intermediate host: freshwater *Bulinus* snail	Central and West Africa	Acute: Abdominal pain, wasting, anaemia Chronic: Growth retardation, anaemia, ascites, portal hypertension.	Praziquantel 40 mg/kg/day PO for 1 day

Acute Schistosomiasis. This acute illness can be found after exposure to any of the schistosomes infecting humans, but it is most marked in primary infections among non-immune individuals with *S. japonicum* infection. Also termed acute toxaemic schistosomiasis, it is also known as Katayama syndrome, or Katayama fever, after the Katayama region in Hiroshima prefecture, Japan, where it was originally described. Where *Schistosoma* transmission is coming under partial control, Katayama syndrome can also affect residents of endemic areas (Figure 52.14). In China, for example, rebound epidemics have typically been reported in endemic communities exposed to floods.[115] Acute schistosomiasis is much less commonly reported for *S. haematobium* infection and there are no data on its occurrence with *S. intercalatum* or *S. mekongi* infection.

The incubation period of acute schistosomiasis varies between 14–84 days after individuals are exposed (either to a first schistosome infection or to heavy reinfection) and symptoms are often nonspecific. This frequently poses a diagnostic challenge to the clinician. The multiple clinical manifestations are related to schistosomal migration and to early egg deposition, presenting with a constellation of systemic symptoms including nocturnal fever, non-productive cough (with diffuse pulmonary infiltrates found on radiography), myalgia, eosinophilia, headache and abdominal pain. Almost all cases have a history of water exposure.[114] Serum anti-*Schistosoma* antibodies suggest the diagnosis and schistosome egg excretion, if detected, will substantiate the presence of infection.[158] If the initial presentation includes neurological symptoms or spinal cord syndromes, this is an indication for urgent investigation and therapeutic intervention.

Systemic Effects of Established Infections

For a detailed description of systemic effects of established infections, see Table 52.2.

Anaemia. Community-based surveys in *Schistosoma*-endemic areas have frequently demonstrated associations between infection and anaemia[12,159] at both high- and low-level parasitic loads, suggesting mixed aetiologies. Iron deficiency is more commonly associated with heavy infection and is likely due to enteric blood losses in the face of poor dietary iron intake.[96] Importantly, anaemia of chronic inflammation has also been documented in schistosomiasis. The mechanism is believed to be 'iron trapping' related to persistent inflammation, the production of pro-inflammatory IL-6 and an associated release of hepcidin, a liver hormone responsible for decreased iron availability.[160] Increases in other pro-inflammatory cytokines, C-reactive protein (CRP) and TNFα, have also been associated with *Schistosoma*-induced anaemia. This has been best studied in *S. japonicum*-endemic areas.[96,98,161]

Decreased Physical Performance. Decreased aerobic capacity (an impaired ability to deliver oxygen to the tissues) has also been reported in epidemiological surveys in *Schistosoma*-endemic areas.[152] This deficit, or related reduction in physical work output, is highly correlated with anaemia and malnutrition in patients with schistosomiasis.[152,162]

GROWTH RETARDATION

There is a relationship between childhood schistosomiasis and undernutrition (growth stunting and wasting) that is becoming more clearly defined.[17] *Schistosoma* infection-related malnutrition hinders children from attaining their full growth potential if they are not treated before linear growth stops at the end of puberty.[163] Both acute and chronic malnutrition have been associated with schistosomiasis, most frequently with *S. japonicum*, but also with *S. mansoni* and *S. haematobium*.[12,98,164–166] Dramatic weight improvements have been seen in Kenya after a single therapeutic dose of praziquantel, with greatest improvements seen in children who were more severely affected at baseline.[167] Boys have frequently been found to be more affected by the nutritional complications of *Schistosoma* infection than girls.[168]

Cognitive Delays

Significant associations have been found between *S. japonicum* infection and reduced scores on tests of intellectual function among school-age children.[161] After adjustment for nutritional status, socioeconomic status (SES), haemoglobin, sex and the presence of other helminths, children with *S. japonicum* infection were specifically found to have reduced scores in tests of learning. Randomized, placebo-controlled praziquantel treatment studies for *S. japonicum* have likewise shown a treatment-related improvement in fluency, recall and visual search ability.[169] Similarly, heavy *S. haematobium* infection among Tanzanian children has been associated with poor performance in standardized tests of verbal short-term memory and reaction time,[170] and *S. mansoni* infection has been associated with poor IQ performance on Wechsler Intelligence testing in Egypt.[171]

Disability

The 1996 WHO-World Bank Global Burden of Disease Project attributed a very low disability weight to schistosomiasis (0.5%), based on that era's flawed perception that most people with current or past *Schistosoma* infection were 'asymptomatic' and only patients with advanced disease were seriously ill. As a result of this error, the Disability-Adjusted Life Year (DALY) estimates for schistosomiasis proved to be unrealistically low.[11,12,155]

Inaccurate notions about schistosomiasis were based, in part, on results of earlier case–control studies of symptoms and work productivity that compared 'infected' versus 'uninfected' persons living in *Schistosoma*-endemic communities. We have since come to appreciate the significant insensitivity of standard parasitological testing for *Schistosoma* infection,[8–10] a phenomenon that caused significant misclassification of infection status in these earlier studies, resulting in significant bias against detection of relevant infection-related symptoms.

Inaccuracies also affected many drug treatment trials: The treatment effect of anti-schistosomal therapy was most often gauged based on the outcomes of single-round treatment of overt chronic infections. The observed effects of 'causal therapy' were often minimal or temporary, leading to the false impression that treatment of the 'average' case of schistosomiasis had only minimal impact on human health.

Subsequent recognition of the long-term, 'subtle' morbidities of schistosomiasis, i.e. undernutrition, growth stunting and cognitive impairment, has led to a reassessment of the lifetime impact of chronic or recurrent infection in *Schistosoma*-endemic areas.[12] These sequelae are the cumulative result of long-term inflammatory illness and are slow to resolve. Single-treatment regimens were unlikely to reverse these pathologies immediately, nor were the benefits of therapy likely to be durable if reinfection occurred rapidly,[163,172,173] as is the norm in endemic transmission zones.[174] Finally, because disease caused by *Schistosoma* infection persists after infection abates, duration of chronic 'schistosomiasis' (i.e. the disease triggered by *Schistosoma* infection) must be viewed in terms of decades of associated morbidity. From this perspective, there is nothing 'asymptomatic' or 'benign' about the average case of schistosomiasis and its disabling impact is substantially greater than the published estimates currently in use by global health planners.[175]

LOCALIZED AND ORGAN-SPECIFIC EFFECTS

*Genitourinary Schistosomiasis (*S. haematobium*) – Common Features*

For genitourinary schistosomiasis, the cardinal complaint is recurrent haematuria. Other urinary tract symptoms may precede or be associated, for instance burning on micturition, frequency, suprapubic discomfort or pain. Bladder involvement may lead to precipitancy, dribbling or incontinence. In fact, in an endemic area, any urinary tract symptom is an indication to explore for the presence of *S. haematobium*. However, in many countries in Africa, in the young age groups and early teenagers, macroscopic haematuria may be virtually universal; in boys it provokes little comment and may be regarded as a natural sign of puberty.

In the phase of established chronic infection, it is common to recognize two stages: (1) a more active stage of disease development in children, adolescents and young adult patients, with egg deposition in many organs and egg excretion in the urine with proteinuria and haematuria, macroscopic or microscopic and (2) in older patients, where urinary egg excretion is sparse or absent but extensive pathology has developed.[176] Chronic bladder lesions may produce persistent urinary dribbling and occasionally multiple fistulas in the perineum, with the picture of the 'watering-can scrotum'; this is also seen in areas of heavy transmission in children and young teenagers where exposure is maximal, but the phenomenon is much rarer nowadays than in the past, coincidental with the more widespread use of chemotherapy.

Surveys have shown wide regional variation in co-existent bacteruria; when present, the predominant organisms are *E. coli*, *Klebsiella* spp., *Pseudomonas* spp. and *Salmonella* spp.

In Egypt, recurrent *Salmonella* bacteraemia is a well-recognized complication of *S. haematobium* infection. Patients with urinary schistosomiasis presenting with a recurrence of salmonellosis should first be treated for their *S. haematobium* infection.[125,177] In the later stages of obstructive uropathy, hydronephrosis may develop and cause renal parenchymal dysfunction which, added to urinary tract infection, leads to impaired kidney function.[178] The ominous relationship between bilateral schistosomal uropathy, bacteriuria with impairment of hydrogen ion excretion, non-functioning kidneys and death has been well described.[179]

*Genital Schistosomiasis and Infertility (*S. haematobium, S. mansoni*)*

Egg deposition in the genital tract is known to cause inflammation with easily identifiable, pathognomonic sandy patches lesions. In the female cervix, vagina and vulva sandy patches, tubercles and neovascularization can be identified by colposcopic examination (Figure 52.16). Studies in Malawi and Zimbabwe have found up to 75% of women with urinary schistosomiasis to have *Schistosoma haematobium* ova in the genitals.[120,180] Of special concern, women with female genital schistosomiasis (FGS) in rural Zimbabwean or Tanzanian communities were also found to have a three- to four-fold risk of having HIV infection.[181,182] A recent population-based study has linked FGS with female infertility and sub-fecundity in endemic communities.[122] Although rarely reported, there are cases of transitional genital schistosomiasis with *S. mansoni* in Brazil.[183] Little is known of its impact in later reproductive health.

For men, haematospermia is often a presenting symptom of genitourinary schistosomiasis. Orchitis, prostatitis, dyspareunia and oligospermia are associated with male genital schistosomiasis and have been shown to resolve after anti-schistosomal therapy.[118,119]

*Intestinal Schistosomiasis (*S. mansoni, S. japonicum, S. intercalatum *and* S. mekongi*) – Common Features*

The wider spectrum of clinical presentations in schistosomiasis has been highlighted in recent decades through the increased use of community-based surveys as a tool for investigation, in contrast with the classical descriptions of disease among hospitalized patients. The majority of persons infected with *S. mansoni* or *S. japonicum* have milder complaints and nonspecific symptoms, in agreement with the known epidemiological and biological distribution of the parasite within the human host. In general, the advanced clinical features of *Schistosoma*-related pathology are encountered in only a small proportion of patients with long-term infection.

Intestinal disease may manifest as chronic or intermittent diarrhoea with blood in the stools, by abdominal discomfort or pain, or by colicky cramps. Severe dysentery is rare but occurs. Among such patients, secondary symptoms of fever, weakness, fatigue, anorexia and weight loss are frequent.[184] In epidemiological surveys, there are significant correlations between visible or occult blood in the stools, abdominal pain and diarrhoea.[185]

S. mansoni can present with acute schistosomiasis, general 'subtle' symptoms as explained above, or with hepatomegaly (often of the left lobe) which may be combined with significant splenomegaly. In the later stages of infection, there can occur a chronic catarrhal state of the intestine, with swollen, granular mucosa and loose stools with blood and/or mucus, or an intermittent dysenteric syndrome.[186]

The anatomic complications of polyposis and hepatosplenic schistosomiasis each have their own symptomatology; polyposis produces what is, in effect, a severe, chronic dysentery with blood and protein loss (Figures 52.18, 52.21). Intussusception and/or rectal prolapse may occur. Hepatosplenic schistosomiasis presents as upper abdominal discomfort, left upper abdominal pain or a swelling of the abdomen (Figure 52.22). Physical signs include a firm enlargement of the liver, often with splenomegaly. The spleen may become greatly enlarged, sometimes extending downwards past the umbilicus into the left iliac fossa and may even at times fill most of the abdomen. Ascites may be present, but the classical signs of hepatocellular disease (cirrhosis), i.e. spider-web angiomata, gynaecomastia, palmar erythema, jaundice and alterations in hair distribution are *not* present in 'pure' schistosomal disease. They may, however, be

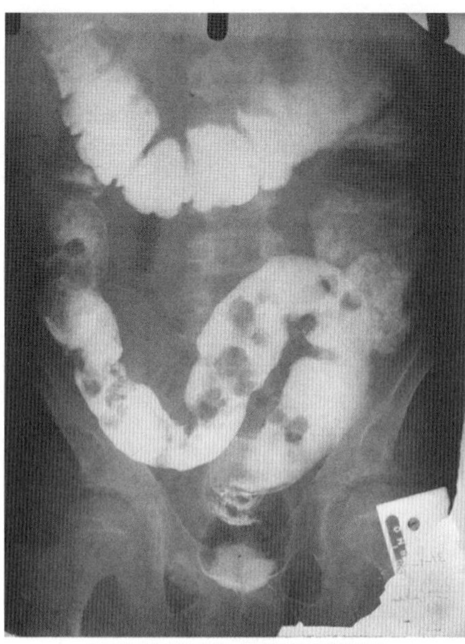

Figure 52.21 Barium contrast radiograph of colonic polyposis due to intestinal schistosomiasis. *(From Peters W, Pasvol G. Atlas of Tropical Medicine and Parasitology. Copyright © 2006, with permission from Elsevier.)*

found where hepatitis B, C, D or E co-exist with schistosomal periportal fibrosis and lead to post-hepatitic hepatocellular damage. In a recent study, co-infection with *S. mansoni* and hepatitis C (HCV) had significant worsening of fibrosis, compared with subjects with HCV infection alone.[187]

In the most advanced cases of intestinal schistosomiasis, endocrine changes can be found: growth retardation, infantilism, retarded bone age, all probably due to hypopituitarism. Amenorrhoea, early menopause, infertility and loss of libido have been attributed to a similar cause.

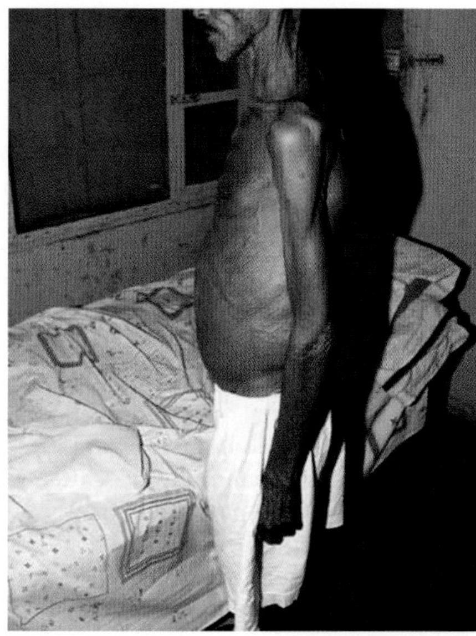

Figure 52.22 A 52-year-old man with a grossly enlarged abdomen caused by the portal hypertension of advanced chronic schistosomiasis. *(From WHO/TDR/Crump.)*

A common primary presenting sign of hepatosplenic disease in schistosomiasis is haematemesis from gastrooesophageal varices. This may occur without warning or may be preceded by a feeling of weakness or upper abdominal discomfort; patients have classical signs of acute blood loss with sweating, pallor, thirst, somnolence and a lowered blood and pulse pressure. In many cases, melaena follows and this acute episode may precipitate ascites and/or peripheral oedema. Fatalities may occur with the primary haemorrhage if treatment is not available; recurrent multiple haemorrhagic episodes are usual. Unless complicated by hepatitis B, C, D or E, liver function abnormalities and hepatic encephalopathy do not develop. Where mixed infections of *S. mansoni* or *S. japonicum* and the various hepatitis viruses co-exist, the downhill clinical course is correspondingly rapid and the typical signs of hepatocellular failure appear with, in parallel, a poor prognosis.

***S. japonicum* and *S. mekongi*.** Whereas infections with the oriental schistosomes follow a broadly similar clinical course to that of *S. mansoni*, several distinct differences are noted. In general, infection with *S. mekongi* is milder than that with *S. japonicum*. Hepatosplenomegaly is common, but cerebral and cardiopulmonary complications are not reported with *S. mekongi*.

In the past, there have been more hospital-based clinical studies of *S. japonicum* than community-based investigations. Hence, the clinical descriptions have been slanted towards advanced cases. In fact, at least half of patients infected with *S. japonicum* are not severely symptomatic. General symptoms, fatigue, weakness, nonspecific abdominal discomfort and irregular bowel movements or intermittent diarrhoea are frequent. Chronic diarrhoea is said to be a common complaint and lower abdominal pain is a frequent symptom.[115] The presence of diarrhoea is of particular importance in children, where it is a strong predictor of chronic progression to advanced disease.[188]

The later signs of hepatosplenic schistosomiasis evolve as do those of *S. mansoni* infection. Although schistosomal dwarfism was not uncommon in China in the first half of the twentieth century, it has become a rarity nowadays. Cardiopulmonary and renal complications are well known.[189]

The main difference clinically is the occurrence of cerebral schistosomiasis in *S. japonicum* infection. Spinal cord involvement appears less frequently than with *S. mansoni*, but such generalizations are difficult, if not impossible, to confirm scientifically.

In the acute phase of cerebral schistosomiasis, the presenting symptoms and signs are those of a meningoencephalitis, with pyrexia, headache, vomiting, blurred vision and disturbed consciousness. In the established or chronic phase of the infection, several distinct neurological presentations are recognized; most common is epilepsy, which may be generalized but is more frequently Jacksonian in type; signs suggestive of a space-occupying lesion or a stroke are also described. The prevalence of epilepsy in infected communities has been estimated at 1–4%, against a baseline rate of 0.3–0.5%.[189] With advances in neuroradiology, in the presence of positive serology or parasitology and with or without operational biopsy, modern imaging techniques may prove diagnostic.

***S. intercalatum*.** In comparison with *S. haematobium* or *S. mansoni* infection, clinical symptoms of disease are commonly mild in *S. intercalatum* infection and it has not been regarded as a major public health problem.[190] Active infection is most common among children and adolescents and pathology is most often detected among those with egg excretion in excess of 400 eggs/g of faeces.[151]

S. intercalatum infection can present with diarrhoea and lower abdominal pain or discomfort, but the classic presentation is that of rectal bleeding that can complicate to develop severe rectitis.[190]

Conversely, some patients may present only with haematuria. In a report from Nigeria, *S. intercalatum* eggs were found in the urine but not in faeces in 6% of the 1709 people surveyed.[151] It is believed that the natural hybridization between *S. intercalatum* and *S. haematobium* can produce an atypical clinical picture with 'ectopic' localization of worms.[191,192]

Differential Diagnosis

In an infection of such diverse clinical manifestations it is scarcely surprising that schistosomiasis in any of its forms can be confused with many other disease processes.

Acute schistosomiasis (Katayama syndrome) must be differentiated from typhoid fever, brucellosis, malaria, leptospirosis and numerous other causes of pyrexia of uncertain origin (PUO). Pyrexia and eosinophilia occur in trichinosis, tropical eosinophilia, visceral larva migrans and infections with *Opisthorchis, Paragonimus* and *Clonorchis* spp.

Urinary schistosomiasis due to *S. haematobium* must be distinguished from other causes of haemoglobinuria, including cancer of the urogenital tract, acute nephritides and other infections, including rare conditions such as renal tuberculosis with haematuria.

Abdominal symptoms commonly seen in *S. mansoni*, may suggest peptic ulcer, biliary disease or pancreatitis; in such cases, if schistosomiasis is the cause, symptoms typically abate after specific anti-schistosomal treatment. Lower abdominal conditions to be excluded are the various forms of dysentery, particularly amoebic dysentery, ulcerative colitis and non-schistosomal polyposis.

Hepatosplenomegaly can be due to multiple causes; its possible aetiology is wide and embraces all causes of hepatomegaly and splenomegaly, separately and combined. The marked splenic enlargement of portal hypertension due to periportal fibrosis must be distinguished from kala-azar (visceral leishmaniasis), certain of the chronic leukaemias or myeloproliferative syndromes, some of the haemoglobinopathies (e.g. thalassaemias) and the tropical splenomegaly syndrome.

Other Syndromes and Presentations. Schistosomiasis must always be considered as one of the causes of cor pulmonale and virtually any neurological presentation, but particularly the various forms of epilepsy and the different types of myelopathy or spinal cord compression syndromes.

A broad knowledge of local and/or regional epidemiology paired with a high index of diagnostic suspicion will contribute to the avoidance of diagnostic error.

Diagnosis

A definitive diagnosis of an active *Schistosoma* infection is made by the direct visual demonstration of parasite eggs (see Figure 52.3) in bodily excretions or secretions, usually the stool or urine or alternatively in material from rectal biopsy or biopsies from liver (see Figure 52.19) or surgically removed tissue. A sensitive direct diagnosis can also be made by hatching tests in which swimming *miracidia* originating from excreted eggs can be seen with the naked eye. This is an indication beyond doubt that the eggs are viable and have originated from living fertilized female schistosomes.

A recent addition to direct diagnostic techniques is the detection of schistosome antigens in serum or urine: circulating anodic antigen (CAA) and circulating cathodic antigen (CCA). These two glycoprotein circulating antigens associated with the gut of the adult worm are well characterized, are genus specific and their presence indicates active human infection by *S. mansoni, S. haematobium, S. japonicum,* or *S. intercalatum.* They are detected by immunoassay and have virtually 100% specificity and very high sensitivity. Patently, they offer new possibilities for epidemiological and post-chemotherapeutic monitoring. Commercial point-of-care assays for detection of CCA in the urine have been developed and are undergoing field trials for their performance characteristics in population-based control programmes.

DIRECT DIAGNOSTIC TECHNIQUES

Parasitological Diagnosis

No single diagnostic technique is optimal for all situations. Most of the currently used parasitological techniques can be interpreted qualitatively or quantitatively depending on a programme's diagnostic needs. Quantitative techniques are most often used in research studies, in experimental chemotherapy and clinical trials, in epidemiological surveys, or in the evaluation of allied intervention measures for transmission control.

In an individual clinical setting, it is customary to examine repeated specimens of excreta parasitologically (in practice, three specimens) before declaring a patient to be 'egg negative' and most likely not chronically infected by *Schistosoma* spp. Because eggs must migrate through host tissue to reach the stool or the urine, egg shedding can persist for some time after active infection is cleared. Confirmation of a diagnosis by hatching tests demonstrates that the eggs are viable and an active infection exists; the finding of only dead eggs in the excreta is not an indication for further anti-parasite treatment.

Egg Counting

The direct demonstration of eggs has an advantage over all other diagnostic measures because specificity is obviously maximal, yet an unquestioning belief in the absolute merits of quantitative diagnosis is not justified. Egg counts are indirect estimates of worm loads; they vary in time and place and between technicians and an assumed Poisson distribution of eggs in the excreta may not be valid.[193] Standard tests routinely misdiagnose as 'uninfected' those individuals who carry light infections.[194] Standard methods such as the Kato-Katz stool test for intestinal schistosomiasis are only 40–60% sensitive when performed on a single stool specimen.[8,10] This becomes relevant in adequately assessing the true burden of *Schistosoma* infection and infection-associated disease both on an individual level and within an affected community. Misclassification bias (due to this routine underdiagnosis) effectively limits our appreciation of the overall health impact of this very common human parasitic infection.[12]

Diagnosis of S. haematobium *Infection*

Ova of *S. haematobium* are most easily detected in the urine. A qualitative diagnosis can be made by the microscopic examination of a sedimented or centrifuged urine specimen of known volume. Filtration techniques, which yield a quantitative estimation of egg excretion, have mostly replaced simple sedimentation and/or centrifugation and are the norm in epidemiological studies. The preferred field test is by using the Nuclepore polycarbonate filters.[195] There are other less preferred methods using other types of polycarbonate or polyamide filters.[195–197] The principle common to all is that eggs are retained on the filter and can be counted with or without staining. Many different stains are in use and preferences are largely personal; eggs may be 'stored' in preservative or a preservative-stain mixture. As with all techniques, problems arise during field usage. False-negative epidemiological results may occur from loss of eggs during bulk transport of dried filter papers,[197] and in a small but significant proportion, eggs can be retained on polyamide filters (Nytrel) even after careful attempts to wash and reuse them. As a general rule, any filter should be used once only and then discarded.

Diagnosis of Intestinal Schistosomes

In infections with *S. mansoni, S. japonicum, S. mekongi* and *S. intercalatum*, where eggs are excreted in the faeces, simple comminution of the stool and sedimentation before microscopy is a reliable diagnostic technique. Direct saline microscopy of stool has a very low diagnostic sensitivity owing to the small amount of the faecal sample examined.

Many concentration techniques have been described.[198–201] All involve removal of fat, faecal debris and mucus and of necessity require more sophisticated laboratory facilities. They find their optimal use in the detection of 'light' infections where egg excretion is of a low intensity or is intermittent.

Presently, the cellophane thick faecal smear (the Kato technique or one of its numerous modifications) is the standard diagnostic tool[202,203] in most clinical and epidemiological studies. Essentially a semi-concentration-clearing-staining process, it is a simple microscopic method examining 20–50 mg of stool, depending on the template used and is quantitative, thus permitting the comparisons of data from site to site. It can be performed in the field and may be used at the primary healthcare level. The prepared slide takes some time to clear; this varies with ambient temperature and humidity. Slides can be stored for at least 1 week, often longer, the time again being variable, so that assessments of technicians' counts can be incorporated into a system of quality control. An advantage lies in its use in the diagnosis and counting of eggs of many intestinal nematodes or cestodes (e.g. *Ascaris lumbricoides, Trichuris trichiura, Taenia* spp. and hookworms), although to assess hookworm egg excretion, counts must be made within 15–30 min after slide preparation because hookworm eggs disappear after this period owing to breakdown and hatching within the Kato solution.

The exact details of the procedure must be calibrated for each working location, taking into account environmental variables, resources and locally available material and human resources. Disadvantages of the standard Kato-Katz technique are that watery or diarrhoeal stools cannot be processed and dietary habits may result in hard fibrous stools that are difficult to process. Additionally, there is a definite lower limit of 24–50 eggs/g of stool detectable on a single smear, with only 40–60% sensitivity for detecting active infection in a single day's stool specimen.[10] For this reason, it is common practice to examine two or three subsamples of each individual faecal specimen and to perform repeated daily exams (≥3) to more reliably detect infection. Whichever technique is used, it is vital that the amount of stool examined, whether in a single examination or by a number of subsample examinations, should be reported, so that valid comparisons can be made between areas.

A variant of the thick smear technique for *S. mansoni* infections is the glass sandwich technique[204,205] which has been used widely in the Sudan and Malawi. The technique requires no reagents and it has been suggested that it is more cost-effective than other similar quantitative methods. A small-scale experiment showed no significant differences in egg recovery or in methods, readers or slides prepared from the same stool specimens and processed by either the Kato or glass sandwich technique.[206] Further comparisons on a larger scale are needed and a major disadvantage of this technique is that it is limited to use in restricted endemic areas; hence comparison of findings with other endemic areas is, at present, invalid.

Eggs of *S. mansoni* or *S. intercalatum* are often found in the urine. In one series, 15% of patients with a sole *S. mansoni* infection had 'mansonuria', but this is an unusually high rate.[207]

Miracidial Hatching

Described originally by Fulleborn in 1921[208] and in routine use in biological and chemotherapeutic studies for decades, hatching is generally accepted as the most sensitive of all parasitological methods in all forms of schistosomiasis. The method remains essential for adequate post-treatment evaluation in clinical trials. However, its use in field studies has been less common because standardization and quantification are more difficult than for techniques where eggs can simply be counted. Diagnosis and follow-up of treated patients in the huge Chinese control programmes of the 1960s and 1970s were based on a 'nylon network running water sedimentation technique', essentially a field-adapted miracidial hatching process.[209,210]

The relative ease of isolation of eggs from urine has led to many more attempts to quantify hatching procedures in *S. haematobium* than in *S. mansoni* infections. As a rough estimate of the numbers of hatchable eggs, the miradiascope was used as a macroscopic technique routinely for surveys in southern Africa.[211] More sensitive and accurate hatching techniques have followed[212] and further refinements are appearing;[213–215] undoubtedly the use of 'wet' preparations has complicated field standardization, but hatching retains its primacy as the most sensitive diagnostic tool for *S. haematobium* infection.

In *S. mansoni* infections, many variants of hatching techniques exist, some semi-quantitative and all possessing high sensitivity.[216,217]

In *S. japonicum*-endemic areas in China, miracidial hatching is widely and routinely used for both epidemiological surveys and as an indicator of parasitological cure after chemotherapy.[136]

Rectal Biopsy

Used for decades as a simple direct diagnostic technique at the individual clinical level, rectal biopsy may be employed in addition to faecal examination and provides an effective way of visualizing eggs. Small biopsy specimens of mucosa are soaked in water and examined microscopically as a crush preparation. In the intestinal dwelling species, egg viability can often be determined by observation of flame cell or miracidial movement within the eggshell. Biopsies may be taken from rectal valves via a crocodile forceps or with a curette and proctoscope, a much simpler procedure; the mucosa is pulled over the end of the proctoscope and cut off with the curette.[218] Ova of *S. haematobium* in rectal snips are typically non-viable and will appear black.

In Brazil, the oogram technique (a quantitative rectal biopsy with division of eggs into developmental stages) is commonly used in assessment of the effects of anti-schistosomal drugs.[218]

Other Biopsy Sites

As expected, schistosome ova are frequently found in other biopsy locations, such as the liver, bladder, cervix, vagina, perineum and skin and indications for a biopsy of such sites lie at the individual clinical level.

Indirect Diagnostic Techniques

Given a high index of suspicion based on exposure history or local epidemiology, the diagnosis of active *Schistosoma* infection or persistent schistosomiasis can be based on physical or radiological signs, seroimmunological assessment, or in the case of *S. haematobium* infection, the detection of red blood cells in the urine.

Chemical Reagent Strips

Indirect diagnostic techniques are used most frequently for *S. haematobium* infections. The application of chemical reagent strips (CRSs) that are used to detect haematuria and/or proteinuria in a semi-quantitative fashion[219] is used as a diagnostic surrogate in endemic areas; a positive result is interpreted as indicating active infection. False-positive reactions occur in myoglobinuria and in the presence of bacterial peroxidases resulting from heavy bacteruria, while inhibition of the reactions may occur if urinary ascorbic acid levels exceed 10 mg/100 mL urine.

False positives for proteinuria occur in alkaline urines or when quinine or a quinine derivative is present. False negatives have occurred in strongly acid urine with Bence Jones proteinuria and in urine containing predominantly γ-globulin. In areas endemic for *S. haematobium*, there is good correlation between reagent strip reactions indicating haematuria and/or proteinuria and increasing intensity of egg output.[9,220,221]

Good predictive values resulting from high sensitivity and the relative specificity of CRSs in *S. haematobium*-endemic areas emphasize the limitations of conventional single-urine microscopic examinations at very low egg output levels and confirm the validity of CRSs in detecting those with a 'high' egg output (i.e. over 50 eggs/10 mL urine)[9] CRSs can be used in areas of both high and low transmission and typically find their optimal use in the detection of those with heavy infection.

Immunodiagnosis

Serodiagnostic techniques are used for the detection of either specific antibodies or genus-specific antigens. Antibodies to adult worm, schistosomular, cercarial or egg antigens can be detected by a number of different procedures, including the various forms of enzyme-linked immunosorbent assay (ELISA), radioimmunoassay (RIA), indirect immunofluorescence tests (IFAT), gel precipitation techniques (GPT), indirect haemagglutination (IHA), latex agglutination (LAT) and circumoval precipitin tests (COPT) which have superseded the older Cercarien-Hüllen reactions (CHR) and complement fixation tests (CFT).

In general, antibody detection techniques have been less useful to the practicing physician and epidemiologist than the techniques of direct parasitological diagnosis. Their basic disadvantage is that they all point to past exposure to mammalian or, in rare instances, avian schistosomes without indicating the duration, activity, or quantum of infection. Further disadvantages are an absence of globally agreed criteria of performance and standards; the necessity for expensive equipment, costly or labile reagents; the need for skilled technical personnel; and the slow diminution of specific antibody level after treatment, thus reducing their value as a marker of chemotherapeutic success. Each laboratory in endemic or non-endemic areas has tended to use its own particular antigen and assay procedure. The WHO has conducted several collaborative studies[222–224] in attempts to improve the technology and to standardize both antigens and procedures.

A recent field study conducted in schoolchildren in Zanzibar to evaluate the performance of the SEA-ELISA using sera from finger-prick blood was good; a sensitivity of 89% and specificity of 70%, showing promise for the SEA-ELISA as a complementary field-test.[225] Immunodiagnostics are also useful in acute schistosomiasis, where sensitivity of antibody testing for Katayama syndrome is estimated to be approximately 70–80%. A 4-year investigation of confirmed acute schistosomiasis cases among travellers reported a positive antibody diagnosis in 15 out of 23 (65%) of patients at first presentation, compared with ova detection in only five out of 23 (22%) patients.[114,158]

Advances have also been made in antigen detection tests.[13,225,226] Improvements in the production of monoclonal antibodies have led to new diagnostic tests of CAA and CCA in serum and urine. In a recent study conducted in Uganda and Zanzibar, the sensitivity and specificity of the CCA dipstick was 83% and 81% for detection of *Schistosoma mansoni*, respectively. By contrast, the antigen dipsticks failed to reliably detect *S. haematobium*-infected children, even in the presence of eggs in urine, a phenomenon perhaps related to the presence of interfering inflammatory substances in the urine. This finding limits the diagnostic use of urine-based antigen detection to *S. mansoni*-endemic areas for now.[110]

Radiology

Various imaging procedures for detecting morbidity from schistosomal infection (Figures 52.15, 52.21, 52.23) have long been in use as a form of indirect diagnosis in hospital practice. These include ultrasonography, plain abdominal radiography to detect calcification, intravenous pyelography to detect bladder and ureteral changes or obstructive uropathy, isotope renography, computed tomography for cerebral schistosomiasis, myelography for suspected cord damage and portal venography for hepatosplenic schistosomiasis with portal venous hypertensive changes. Complications, such as gastrointestinal bleeding may require the use of specialized techniques, such as splenoportography or nuclear isotopic studies of hepatic blood flow. The indications for a particular investigation lie at the individual patient level and test selection should be based on consultation between the treating physician and the radiologist.

Ultrasonography

With the introduction and expanded use of ultrasonography there have been major changes in the diagnosis of *Schistosoma*-associated morbidity, both at the individual patient level and at the community level. The technique is non-invasive, simple, portable, has no biological hazard to the patient or the operator and either complements or is an alternative diagnostic method to many older invasive techniques. With the exception of hydroureter, ureteral calculi and bladder calcification, it has, in comparison with other diagnostic procedures, high specificity and sensitivity, is superior to physical examination in measuring liver and spleen size and is the best technique for grading schistosomal periportal fibrosis, portal hypertension, hydronephrosis, urinary bladder wall lesions and renal and bladder stones.[227] WHO has published consensus guidelines for ultrasound examination in abdominal and genitourinary schistosomiasis (Figure 52.23), and an extensive review of technical and clinical experience is available.[228,229]

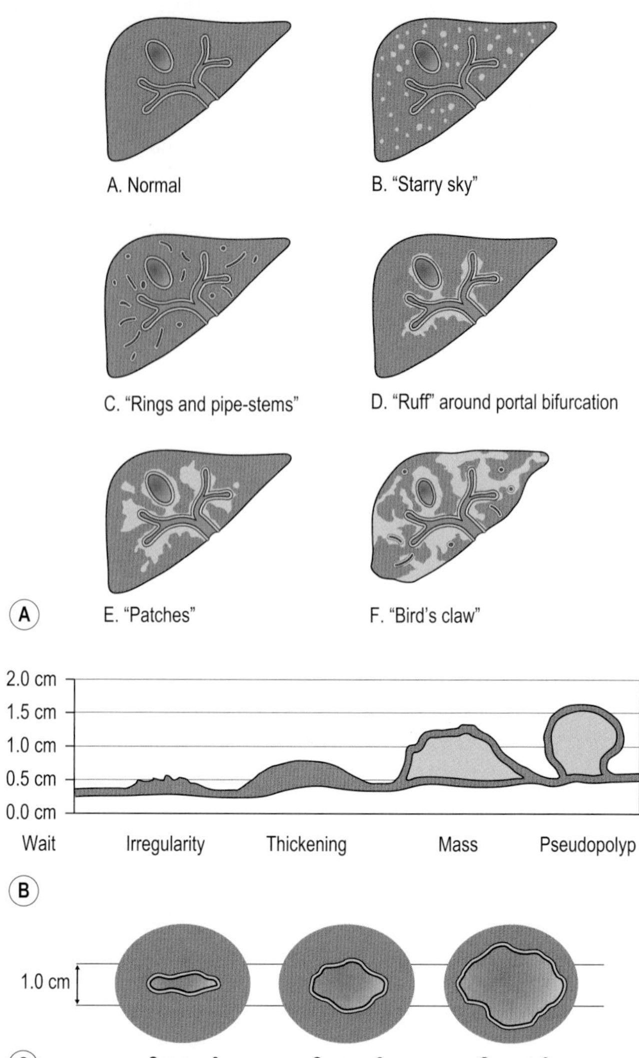

Figure 52.23 Schematic of abnormal ultrasound findings for schistosomiasis. (A) Images showing abnormal liver parenchymal patterns associated with schistosomiasis mansoni; (B) Classification of schistosomiasis haematobia-related bladder lesions. (C) Measurement of the congestive dilatation of the renal pelvis in urogenital schistosomiasis. *(From Richter J, Hatz C, Campagne G, et al. Ultrasound in schistosomiasis: A practical guide to the standardized use of ultrasonography for the assessment of schistosomiasis-related morbidity. Geneva: World Health Organization; 2000. Report No.: TDR/STR/SCH/00.1.)*

Management and Treatment

The primary objective of treatment is cure of the individual patient by eradication of the *Schistosoma* infection from which the patient suffers. Cure leads to cessation of egg deposition (the pathogenic mediator in host tissues) and this prevents additional organ damage; existing lesions will, in the vast majority of cases, improve or regress.

Since the 1960s, there have been major advances in chemotherapy for the treatment of schistosomiasis. The introduction and widespread use of the current highly effective, orally administered, well-tolerated anti-schistosomal drugs have provided physicians, epidemiologists and public health practitioners with therapeutic opportunities not available in the first half of the twentieth century. For mass drug administration programmes (now the standard in large-scale, community-based chemotherapy), the main aim is to reduce the average burden of *Schistosoma*-associated morbidity by the greatest amount possible. Individual 'cure' may or may not occur. However, in some endemic settings, the community may benefit as a whole by an important 'externality' of mass treatment – the blocking of the egg–miracidium–snail stage of the parasite life cycle, which reduces transmission by minimizing pollution of water supplies and thus diminishes cercarial exposure at human water contact sites.[68,230,231]

Praziquantel

Praziquantel is the drug of choice for schistosomiasis and is effective against all *Schistosoma* species that occur in humans. It is also effective in the other snail-borne trematode infections – clonorchiasis, paragonimiasis and opisthorchiasis – and in infections due to the adult cestodes, *Taenia solium*, *T. saginata*, *Hymenolepis nana* and *Diphyllobothrium* spp.

Although dosage is standardized in large-scale morbidity control programmes,[23] there may be variation in dose in the treatment of the individual patient.[232] In field programmes, a single oral dose of 40 mg/kg is effective in *S. haematobium*, *S. mansoni* and *S. intercalatum* infections. For *S. japonicum* infection, the dose recommended is a total of 60 mg/kg, given at 4-hourly intervals as three 20 mg/kg doses or two 30 mg/kg doses.[233] However, in some regional control programmes, current practice is to treat *S. japonicum* with a single oral dose of 40 mg/kg.

The usual total dose for *S. mekongi* is 60 mg/kg, although there is evidence that repeated treatment at this dosage may be necessary for cure of this species.[233,234]

For treatment of individual patients with heavy infections with *S. mansoni* (over 800 eggs/g of stool), a total dose of 50 or 60 mg/kg, given in two equally divided doses 4–6 h apart, may be needed; single doses are best given after food and, if possible, in the evening.

Patient tolerance is extremely good and virtually all trials have confirmed the absence of toxicity in the liver, kidney, haematopoietic system, or other body organs and functions.

However, minor side-effects do occur; those related to the gastrointestinal tract are epigastric or generalized abdominal pain or discomfort, nausea, vomiting, anorexia or loose stools. These side-effects are generally mild, transient and rarely require medication. A rare event in patients heavily infected with *S. mansoni* or *S. japonicum* is the passage of blood in the stools after praziquantel treatment. The explanation is unknown; it occurs a few hours after dosage but recovery is rapid and without clinical sequelae.

Headache and dizziness may be encountered, as may fever, pruritus or a transient skin eruption, none of which is serious or lasting. Side-effects that occur in field treatments tend to be more frequent in foci of intense transmission and should not be used as an argument for reduction of the dose.

'Cure rates' for praziquantel therapy are high; it can be expected that the rate of 'egg-positive' to 'egg-negative' conversion will be around 80% in research studies. In large-scale field operations, where supervision is less stringent and where compliance with assigned treatment may be difficult to ensure, cure rates of 50–60% are typical when a single oral dose of 40 mg/kg is scheduled to be dispensed; egg output reduction in those treated but not 'cured' should exceed 90% of pre-treatment output.[230,235]

Questions are frequently raised about the emergence of parasite resistance to praziquantel. Cure rates after praziquantel treatment in a new highly endemic focus of intense transmission of *S. mansoni* in northern Senegal in the early 1990s were alarmingly low.[236] A further increase in praziquantel dose did not improve the outcome.[237] However, a WHO consultation decided that the intensity of transmission in this focus was such as to cause the initially observed low cure rates, because praziquantel is ineffective or at least less effective against maturing worms.[238] In such a new focus, among non-immunes, experiencing a high intensity of transmission, immature worms would be present in the majority of patients. Once these 'refractory' patients were removed from any exposure to reinfection, their *Schistosoma* infections rapidly responded to standard praziquantel therapy.[239] There is good evidence from the Nile Delta that some 2–3% of patients still excrete eggs after two or three rounds of praziquantel treatment. In this setting, some 20% of field isolates transferred in to experimental mouse models of infection showed a normal susceptibility to praziquantel, but some of the remaining isolates required two to six times the normal dose to achieve a 50% reduction in worm numbers in laboratory testing. However, this reduced susceptibility was not increased upon repeated passages under drug pressure. Thus, evidence exists that certain schistosome isolates or strains of the parasite are inherently less susceptible to praziquantel. In Egypt, follow-up in areas where praziquantel has been used intensively indicates that the widespread use of the drug has not resulted in a dramatic change in its curative efficacy.[240] Although this 'resistance/tolerance' phenomenon has been reported in human *S. mansoni*, no evidence exists at present of 'resistance' in *S. japonicum* or *S. haematobium* infections. In the latter case, theoretical mathematical modelling suggests that the emergence of resistance might take some 7 years on an annual treatment coverage of 100% of an infected population. As this coverage is rarely, if ever, obtained in field practice, where a range of 25–75% compliance is more usual, emergence of resistance may take more than 20 years.[241]

Review of praziquantel treatment given in pregnancy has not shown evidence of detrimental effects to the mother or the fetus. This post-release experience, combined with available animal safety data has led to a WHO recommendation in favour of using praziquantel for treatment of *Schistosoma*-infected pregnant or lactating women after the first trimester of pregnancy.[242] A subsequent randomized, placebo-controlled trial of deworming in pregnancy has confirmed the safety of praziquantel therapy in infected pregnant women.[243]

Oxamniquine

A tetrahydroquinolone compound distantly related to hycanthone, oxamniquine is effective only against *S. mansoni*. Oxamniquine is used at all stages, from acute toxaemic to chronic and complicated *S. mansoni* infections, with good results. In animal studies, one peculiarity noted about the drug was that male worms proved more susceptible than female worms. Egg-laying by surviving females ceased in the absence of males after successful treatment, thus removing the basic pathogenic mechanism in *Schistosomiasis mansoni*.[244,245]

Oxamniquine is available as capsules of 250 mg or as a syrup containing 50 mg/mL and is marketed as Mansil® in South America and as Vansil® in Africa. It is listed in the most recent WHO Model of Essential Medicines as a 'complementary drug' for use when praziquantel treatment fails.[246] Advanced *S. mansoni* infection with hepatosplenomegaly, portal hypertension and/or ascites responds well and in schistosomal polyposis there are great improvements in both the associated anaemia and protein-losing enteropathy.[247–249] High cure rates (60–90% in different studies) are seen after oxamniquine treatment of uncomplicated *S. mansoni* infection.

From 1975 to 1979, oxamniquine was used in a major control campaign in Brazil, when some 5 million doses were given in the field programmes with high cure rates and very good tolerance.[250]

The dose of oxamniquine varies with the geographical origin of the *S. mansoni* infection, the age and hence the surface area of the patient. In South America, adults are given 15 mg/kg of body weight as a single oral dose; in children 20 mg/kg is preferred, given in two divided portions each of 10 mg/kg with an interval of 4–6 h between doses. If practicable, the drug should be given after food or just before sleep.

With the *S. mansoni* that is found on the African continent, only those with strains of West African origin are given the same doses as in South America. In Egypt, Sudan and southern Africa, a total dose of 60 mg/kg body weight is used, either as 15 mg/kg for 2 days or as 20 mg/kg once daily for 3 days. In East Africa, a total dose of 30–40 mg/kg is given in a split regimen over 1 or 2 days.

In general, oxamniquine is well tolerated. There are virtually no contraindications but classes of patients exist who require close monitoring: Patients with a history of any form of epilepsy must be supervised for 48 h after treatment because a small number of epileptiform convulsions have been reported, as have generalized seizures after the drug, fortunately without sequelae and with clinical and electroencephalographic recovery.[251,252]

Studies are lacking regarding safety of oxamniquine in pregnancy, so as a precaution, it should not be given during the first 4 months of pregnancy.

Any patient whose occupation involves care of heavy machinery or who is employed in the transport industry (e.g. pilots, truckers, dockers, crane drivers) should be placed off work for 48 h after treatment.

Side-effects are uncommon; dizziness, drowsiness and headache are most frequent but last for some 4–6 h only. Hallucinations and a state of excitement are very rare events. Although abdominal discomfort, vomiting and diarrhoea do occur, there is no constant statistical correlation and, in practice, adverse effects have had no influence on compliance in field programmes.

A harmless orange–red discolouration of the urine may occur but is transitory and a syndrome of peripheral blood eosinophilia, peaking at 7–10 days, scattered pulmonary infiltrates and increased immune complexes in serum with urinary excretion of schistosomal antigens is known in Egypt but has not been described in other locations.

In summary, oxamniquine is a highly useful drug for treatment of all forms of *S. mansoni* infection, including many advanced and complicated syndromes.

DRUG RESISTANCE

No new anti-schistosomal drugs can be expected to emerge in the international scene in the near future, as a consequence of there being little or no pharmaceutical industry profit (with slim prospects of developmental cost recovery) from anti-helmintic sales within *Schistosoma*-endemic countries. Thus, praziquantel remains the only practical treatment option for anti-schistosomal campaigns in the present day. As a result, the importance of monitoring for true praziquantel drug resistance cannot be overemphasized, although at present there are few such efforts.

Evidence for *Schistosoma mansoni* resistance to praziquantel has been sought in parasites taken from treated but uncured human patients and in laboratory isolates of *S. mansoni* subjected to successive passages under drug pressure.[253]

In community-based treatment programmes, is has been found that higher than usual doses of PZQ have been needed to effectively suppress infection levels in some areas of Egypt and Senegal[254] but the levels of drug 'tolerance' found among clinical isolates of the parasite so far are low.[253] One major problem is the precise quantitative interpretation of cure rates – without a 'gold standard' diagnostic for actual worm infection, we currently cannot make an unequivocal distinction between drug failure and the 'typical' drug performance in the presence of heavy infectious worm burden, where persistent, low-level infection is the norm after a single round of praziquantel therapy.[254]

The recent introduction of a simple new technique for assessing the effects of praziquantel on miracidia hatched from eggs may, if confirmed in different species, offer an affordable surveillance device to predict praziquantel 'resistance' or 'tolerance' in the clinical realm.[255] Undoubtedly, this in an area in need of well-designed, long-term longitudinal monitoring programmes.

Resistance to oxamniquine is known in South America but is not yet a public health problem, as such patients are treated successfully with praziquantel.[256]

FUTURE CHEMOTHERAPY

Artemisinin Derivatives (Artemether, Artesunate)

In the past decade, research in China and West Africa has focused on the potential use of artemisinin derivatives as anti-schistosomal drugs. These studies all show great promise for this group of compounds, which were initially developed as anti-malarial drugs.[257–260]

Artemisinin, first isolated in the 1970s, is the active ingredient of the herb *Artemisia annua* and is a sesquiterpene lactone containing a peroxide bridge. Several semi-synthetic derivatives including artemether and artesunate have been generated. These are among the most potent antimalarials currently available.

It has been shown that artemisinin derivatives can most effectively kill immature worms (schistosomula) during the migratory period 2–5 weeks after infection, a time when worms are relatively insensitive to praziquantel. As such, the artemesinins can have therapeutic effects against acute infection (with associated preventive effects against establishment of chronic infection) in *Schistosoma* infections. Such effects are seen both in animal models and indirectly, in human clinical trials.[261] Another randomized placebo-control trial, in an area of Cote d'Ivoire endemic for *S. mansoni*, found that oral artemether treatment resulted in lower incidence of *S. mansoni* and lower egg outputs among infected subjects, when compared with a placebo-treated group.[260]

However, because artemisinin derivatives are one of the mainstays of current antimalarial chemotherapy and because endemic malaria and endemic schistosomiasis co-exist in numerous areas, especially in Africa, wider use of these derivatives must await the clarification of their joint distribution, along with questions on the potential introduction of drug resistance among *Plasmodium* spp. through wider use of artemether drugs as 'monotherapy' for schistosomiasis without full coverage for malaria (artemisinin-combination therapy is the established norm for malaria therapy).

Assessment of Chemotherapy Outcomes

Assessment of patients treated for schistosomiasis is conducted by repeated clinical observation, evaluation of symptom improvement and diminution or disappearance of physical, radiological, particularly ultrasonographic or endoscopic signs of disease.

Direct parasitological examination of urine, stool or rectal biopsy is essential and should be performed on repeated (three) specimens of excreta at about 6–8 weeks and 4–6 months after treatment by selection of appropriate parasitological techniques detailed above.

Follow-up is simple if no reinfection risk is present; however, in endemic areas where transmission persists, the explanation of viable eggs in the excreta 4–6 months after therapy is less clear. Such post-treatment egg excretion may be due to a maturing prepatent infection that was unaffected by praziquantel chemotherapy, to a true reinfection or to a therapeutic failure. It is not always easy to decide which event, or even combination of events, is responsible. Increased use of antigen detection techniques (e.g. CAA, CCA) offers possibilities for detection of persistent low-level adult worm infection, which may provide clarification of these issues.

SPECIAL CLINICAL SYNDROMES AND MANAGEMENT

Neurological Schistosomiasis

The efficacy and safety of modern anti-schistosomal drugs has led to early treatment of encephalopathies, myelopathies or other spinal cord syndromes that are reasonably suspected (even if not proven) to be due to schistosomiasis. This improves prognosis, as risk of cord damage in myelopathy is closely related to delays in diagnosis and the time taken to provide effective therapy. Cerebral schistosomiasis has better prognosis than spinal schistosomiasis.

The presence of antibody responses to schistosomal antigens[262] or the presence of circulating parasite antigens (CCA, CAA) can be diagnostic in cases of acute schistosomiasis or light-intensity infections where eggs are not reliably excreted. These two diagnostic techniques should be used when available; unfortunately they are, as yet, restricted only to certain high-technology referral laboratories.

The use of corticosteroids in neuroschistosomiasis remains controversial but in clinical settings they are commonly used.[263] Laminectomy is an important intervention in acute paraplegia with spinal cord compression or block.

In *S. japonicum*, suspected cerebral schistosomiasis should be localized with modern imaging techniques (CT, MRI) and treated with praziquantel, which has proven safe and effective. Computed tomography demonstrates resolution of intracerebral masses, regression of cerebral oedema and the subsequent disappearance of epilepsy.[264] Appropriate neurosurgical intervention should be available in case of deterioration due to increasing intracranial pressure or hydrocephalus.

An enzyme-linked immunoassay test in cerebrospinal fluid for the diagnosis of neuroschistosomiasis has showed promising results, but needs further validation.[265]

Acute Toxaemic Schistosomiasis (Katayama Syndrome)

There is great controversy on the use of steroids, based primarily on anecdotal evidence; some case reports favour their use[266] but others do not, as clinical deterioration can follow after commencement of treatment.[267] As a general principle, Katayama syndrome patients should be treated with praziquantel, which is effective against all *Schistosoma* species.[114,158] The use of artemethers in this setting remains an area of active clinical investigation.

Associated Salmonellosis

Chronic or recurrent bacteraemia due to *Salmonella typhi* or *S. paratyphi* can be due to the presence of concurrent chronic *Schistosoma* infection. This is due to the colonization of the integument or the gut of the adult schistosome by these bacteria. Although clinical response to antibiotics is good, bacteraemia will recur unless the underlying schistosomiasis is also treated. In this setting, the therapeutic response to anti-schistosomal drugs is good.

Associated Hepatitis

Even if, in hepatosplenic schistosomiasis, there is serological or other evidence of an associated hepatitis B infection (or C, D or E) and activity of schistosomiasis is still present, it is worthwhile treating the latter with praziquantel. This is because active schistosomiasis may enhance inflammatory response to chronic hepatitis virus infections in the liver and hasten the onset of cirrhosis. Cirrhosis is not part of *Schistosoma*-related liver disease, but such co-infection may substantially hasten liver decompensation and the patient's clinical deterioration.

Portal Hypertension

Chemotherapy is but one part of patient care, as complications are mainly due to the mechanical obstructive pathology resulting from periportal fibrosis. Chemotherapy will not reverse established fibrosis and so treatment at this stage is focused on means to limit portal hypertension and prevent or control any associated variceal bleeding. Whenever *Schistosoma* eggs are still found in the excreta of such patients, treatment with praziquantel or oxamniquine is indicated and has the usual anthelmintic efficacy in reducing *Schistosoma* infectious burden.

Gastrointestinal Bleeding

Admission to a specialized centre is essential (albeit often difficult) in rural endemic areas, because that is where skills in assessment, immediate resuscitation, fibreoptic endoscopy, balloon tamponade and/or endoscopic sclerotherapy are present. The treatment of this complication is beyond the scope of the general physician and is preferably a matter for specialists in this area of intensive care. Emergency portocaval shunts have fallen into disrepute, as a high proportion of operative deaths may occur and, in the survivors, there is frequently a loss of shunt patency and/or development of an associated hepatic encephalopathy. A selective distal splenorenal shunt has been claimed to offer a lower haemorrhage recurrence rate and an improved survival rate.[268]

The clinical application of β-adrenergic blockade using non-selective β-blockers (e.g. propranolol) for the prevention of an initial gastrointestinal haemorrhage in non-schistosomal cirrhosis, has been proven beneficial.[269] However, their use for portal hypertension due to schistosomal periportal fibrosis is controversial: A randomized control trial was forced to have an early termination due to reported adverse events.[270]

'Schistosomiasis Without Eggs'

This term describes cases where no ova can be found on standard parasitological testing but there exists a high clinical suspicion of schistosomal infection, usually based upon an epidemiological history of exposure, the presence of confirmed cases among fellow members of a group, an unexplained eosinophilia after travel to an endemic area and/or a suggestive or suspicious immunodiagnostic test result.

In areas endemic for *S. haematobium*, the presence of a positive test for microhaematuria on urine examination is taken as indicative of infection.

Again, the simplicity of use of modern drugs has often clarified difficult diagnostic cases through a 'therapeutic trial' of presumptive therapy with praziquantel. Frequently, such treatment is undertaken on suspicion alone, a practice justifiable only when exhaustive efforts to reach a firm parasitological or serological diagnosis have been unsuccessful.

Prevention

RISK OF REINFECTION

Success of regional control strategies will depend, in part, on what influence local environmental and behavioural factors have on individual risk for primary infection and/or reinfection. Therefore, long-term follow-up studies post-treatment are needed to determine the true benefits of regular 'preventive chemotherapy' during a lifetime spent in *Schistosoma*-endemic areas.[230] In a 9-year follow-up study in Kenya, *S. haematobium* reinfection risks were associated with location of residence, age less than 12 years, pre-treatment haematuria and frequency of treatment, but interestingly, not cumulative duration of water exposure.[68]

Reinfection, although initially of light intensity, is not trivial. In the Philippines (in areas endemic for *S. japonicum)* follow-up studies up to 18 months post-treatment found significant associations between reinfection and increased risk for anaemia of inflammation for all infection intensities.[173] Of note, risk for reinfection appears to change over a lifetime, both as a consequence of past parasite exposures and as an effect of changing physiology related to ageing – studies in the Philippines have convincingly found endocrine-related pubertal and post-pubertal protection against infection and reinfection with *S. japonicum*.[271]

Development of fully effective prevention and control strategies for schistosomiasis will require a thorough understanding of the epidemiology and ecology of transmission, including the presence of suitable environmental factors favouring transmission in relation to patterns of human physiology, exposure behaviour and related social and economic determinants.

Control Strategies

Whereas current schistosomiasis control measures have focused on 'morbidity control' through periodic suppression of infection intensity, new interest has developed in the area of 'transmission control', with implied potential for local elimination of transmission with its attendant benefits for untreated individuals.

The basic principles for prevention and control are:

1. The reduction in the number of excreted eggs reaching waters harbouring the intermediate snail host(s); this is dependent on health education, the provision and use of adequate sanitary facilities and specific anti-schistosomal chemotherapy for infected communities and individuals
2. The reduction in the probability of miracidial/snail contact; this relies on all factors in (1) above, appropriate modification of the aquatic environment and reduction of intermediate snail host numbers by application of chemical molluscicides or the use of suitable biological control means (e.g. crayfish introduction)[272]
3. The reduction of cercarial densities, which will occur as a result of all of the preceding actions but overwhelmingly from the employment of molluscicides
4. The reduction of the probability of cercariae locating a definitive host, again due to the cumulative effects of all of the preceding factors plus the reduction of human water contact with infected water bodies by the provision of adequate, safe domestic or peri-domestic water supplies and the substitution of safe recreational water sites[273]
5. The reduction of the longevity of the adult worms in the human host, a function of chemotherapy
6. The reduction of joint water exposure with reservoir animals, such as water buffaloes, in the case of *S. japonicum*.

Multiple overlaps are obvious in these processes and, conventionally, the stress in 'prevention' initiatives is directed towards health education, behaviour modification, the provision of adequate water supplies and sanitation, as supplemented by environmental improvements. 'Control' is dominated by chemotherapy and molluscicides, yet lessons learned from China[29] and elsewhere[273] suggest that integration of these interventions is essential for success and that each endemic focus or region may require an individually tailored clinico-epidemiological, zoogeographical, sociological and environmental approach based on the common principles listed above.

Schistosomiasis and 16 other disabling conditions, including soil-transmitted helminths, lymphatic filariasis, onchocerciasis and trachoma have been placed under the broad umbrella of 'neglected tropical diseases', brought to public attention through the newly established Global Network for Neglected Tropical Diseases and by new initiatives by the WHO.[274] The ultimate aim is to integrate population-based efforts in controlling these diseases in less-developed areas. Effective and efficient integration of NTD control has been shown in state-level regional programmes in Nigeria and Zanzibar and these successes point the way towards implementation in other multi-NTD-endemic areas.[275]

Based on experience over the past decade, the rationale for the current use of 'vertical' de-worming programmes has been reinforced.[13,276,277] The Schistosomiasis Control Initiative (SCI), which started its work in 2002, has made substantial progress towards the reduction of *Schistosoma*-infection-related disease burden in seven partner nations in sub-Saharan Africa.[278] Another example of successful treatment-based control is an 8-year programme in Cambodia, where *S. mekongi* was treated with praziquantel followed with mebendazole for soil-transmitted helminths. The remarkable success of the programme was attributed to strong political commitment despite local limitations in resources.[279]

Reinfection after chemotherapy remains an ever-present risk in the context of unchanging environmental and socioeconomic conditions. This is because of practical constraints in achieving total population drug coverage and the less than complete cure rates after praziquantel therapy. This means that egg deposition continues locally and therefore transmission continues. Add this to the known hurdles in obtaining environmental modification, provision of sanitation and safe water supplies and the need for continuing health education and the 'elimination' of schistosomiasis (implying a permanent cessation of transmission) often seems a Herculean task. However, the constraining factors are political and economic, not technical.

A summary of the current rationale for control and data on its employment are provided in the latest report of the WHO Expert Committee.[59]

Mollusciciding

The use of molluscicides in the control of schistosomiasis is a highly specialized field. Synthetic chemical molluscicides are nowadays primarily restricted to one compound, niclosamide (Bayluscide; Bayer) and, although other chemicals lethal to snails exist, their practical use is minimal. Although many molluscicides of plant origin are known, isolation, characterization, toxicological screening, large-scale production and distribution of their active ingredients for use in endemic countries has not yet proven a viable alternative.

A useful specialist text on indications, technical use, application in different habitats and evaluation of molluscicides has been produced by the WHO.[280]

Molluscicides will continue in use as one of the integral specific control tools, but techniques have changed markedly from the old 'blanket application', evolving to a much more focused approach guided by the epidemiological criteria of high prevalence, high intensity and rapidity of reinfection in any particular focus or area of infection.[273]

Vaccines and Vaccination

An anti-schistosomal vaccine is far from being a reality, in that no anti-schistosomal vaccine formulation has proven capable of providing complete (100%) immunity to infection. A comprehensive review of the current status of anti-*Schistosoma* vaccines has been recently published.[281]

Whereas advances in molecular biology have led to the identification and characterization of an impressive number of anti-schistosome vaccine candidate antigens, progress in human vaccination studies has lagged far behind studies in animal models. One limiting feature is that any of the current vaccines, even those with long-term protective effects, will probably be insufficient as a sole control mechanism and will need to be given in conjunction with chemotherapy and other control methods.[282,283] The case against such vaccine development has been reviewed in detail elsewhere.[284]

Presently, the biologically relevant molecules selected as candidates for schistosomal vaccine development are: a variant of the isoenzyme glutathione S-transferase (Sm28GST); paramyosin (Sm97); an irradiation-associated vaccine antigen (IrV-5); the glycolytic enzyme triose-phosphate isomerase (TPI); the membrane antigen Sm23 and a fatty acid-binding protein (FABP) 14 (Sm14).[284] However, recent independent testing of these six antigens by two laboratories experienced in experimental schistosomiasis research showed that the modest goal of consistent induction of 40% protection or better was not reached with any of these vaccine candidate molecules tested in mice.[283] Currently, the only vaccine candidate molecule undergoing human trials is the glutathione S-transferase (Sh28GST) antigen tested for prevention of *S. haematobium* infection, although a vaccine containing the extracellular domain of the tetraspanin *Sm*-TSP-2 is about to undergo clinical testing in Brazil.[285]

There remain many unanswered questions on the immunology of schistosomiasis and on the mechanisms of protection when it exists and formidable challenges lie ahead regarding large-scale antigen production and the improvement of the modest levels of protection achieved to date in animal models. It will be some years before human vaccines evolve from the present enthusiastic hopes to realistic practical usage in the field.

REFERENCES

1. WHO. Preventive Chemotherapy Databank 2011. Online. Available: http://www.who.int/neglected_diseases/preventive_chemotherapy/databank/en/index.html.
2. Rollinson D, Southgate V. The genus Schistosoma: a taxonomic appraisal. In: Rollinson D, Simpson AJ, editors. The Biology of Schistosomes from Genes to Latrines. London: Academic Press; 1987. p. 1–3.
3. King CH. Epidemiology of schistosomiasis: Determinants of transmission of infection. In: Mahmoud AAF, editor. Schistosomiasis. London: Imperial College Press; 2001. p. 115–32.
11. King CH, Dangerfield-Cha M. The unacknowledged impact of chronic schistosomiasis. Chronic Illn 2008;4(1):65–79.
98. Friedman JF, Kanzaria HK, McGarvey ST. Human schistosomiasis and anemia: the relationship and potential mechanisms. Trends Parasitol 2005;21(8):386–92.
114. Ross AG, Vickers D, Olds GR, et al. Katayama syndrome. Lancet Infect Dis 2007;7(3):218–24.
285. Hotez PJ, Bethony JM, Diemert DJ, et al. Developing vaccines to combat hookworm infection and intestinal schistosomiasis. Nat Rev Microbiology 2010;8:814–26.

Access the complete references online at www.expertconsult.com

53 Food-borne Trematodes

PAIBOON SITHITHAWORN | BANCHOB SRIPA | SASITHORN KAEWKES | YUKIFUMI NAWA | MELISSA R. HASWELL

KEY POINTS

- Food-borne trematodes (FBTs), including liver, lung and intestinal flukes, are important 'Neglected Tropical Diseases' (NTDs).
- An estimated 85 million people worldwide are infected with FBT and more than half are in Asia.
- Humans acquire FBT infection through ingestion of viable metacercariae in second intermediate hosts in undercooked or raw food preparation.
- The diseases caused by FBTs range from asymptomatic, mild disease, to fatal bile duct cancer.
- The drugs of choice for treatment of FBTs are praziquantel and triclabendazole.

Introduction

The major human food-borne trematode infections – clonorchiasis, opisthorchiasis and fascioliasis of the liver, paragonimiasis of the lungs and intestinal fluke infections (such as *Fasciolopsis*, *Echinostoma* and *Heterophyes*) – remain Neglected Tropical Diseases (NTDs). In 1995, the WHO estimated that 40 million people harbour food-borne trematodes[1] worldwide, while more recent estimates place that figure above 85 millions.[2] Although these are commonly thought of as 'tropical' parasites, some species are not limited to hot climates. An extreme example is *Opisthorchis felineus,* which is commonly acquired through the consumption of raw frozen fish in Siberia. The availability of freshwater flora and fauna and a preference for eating them raw or incompletely cooked, are the most important factors determining their distribution in man.

These diseases most often significantly affect poverty-stricken individuals, generally in resource-limited regions, and receive very little interest from funding or government agencies. They have received less attention than other helminth infections, perhaps because of their focal distribution and lack of acute symptoms. As these diseases have complex life cycles and are rarely encountered in the West, they receive little attention in the education of physicians, which furthers their enigmatic status. However, some authors have mistakenly reported them as comparatively benign, which is certainly not the case for the liver flukes and *Paragonimus*, as reviewed here. Severity of the disease is associated with worm burden, except perhaps in the case of ectopic infections.

All food-borne trematodes belong to the subclass Digenea. Digenean trematodes have sexual reproduction in their definitive hosts (e.g. human or mammals) and asexual reproduction in their intermediate hosts (snail). Their life cycles are complex and involve one or more intermediate hosts (the first always being a snail) and several morphological stages. Eggs pass out of the definitive hosts in faeces (in some cases sputum) and those which reach freshwater can infect susceptible snails. Development in the snail results in the release of numerous cercariae which swim about until they contact a suitable plant or animal where encystment occurs to form metacercariae. The life cycle is completed and continues when viable metacercariae are ingested by susceptible definitive hosts.

Efforts to control food-borne parasites are largely dependent on chemotherapy. The drug of choice for treatment for most food-borne trematodes is praziquantel which is now inexpensive and widely available. The most effective drug for treatment of *Fasciola* is Triclabendazole. In addition to anthelmintic treatment to cure current infection, improvements in sanitation and health promotion to encourage the cooking of foods involved in transmission are important components of control to prevent reinfection. Eating habits have cultural and social significance and often are difficult to change but finding ways to reduce risk should be promoted.[3] These include the introduction of good aquaculture practices and processing in accordance with the requirements for the production of safe and quality fish particularly in the commercial sector.[4]

Liver Flukes

OPISTHORCHIASIS AND CLONORCHIASIS

Globally, 700 million people are at risk of infection with liver flukes, namely *O. viverrini*, *C. sinensis* and *O. felineus*.[5] The infections cause hepatobiliary diseases including hepatomegaly, cholangitis, fibrosis of the periportal system, cholecystitis and gallstones. They are the major aetiological agents of bile duct cancer, cholangiocarcinoma (CCA). Based on experimental and epidemiological evidence, the International Agency for Research on Cancer, World Health Organization (WHO) classified *O. viverrini* and *C. sinensis* as Group 1 biological carcinogens.[6] The highest reported incidence of the liver-fluke-associated liver cancer in the world is in Khon Kaen province, North-east Thailand.

Epidemiology

The human liver flukes, *Clonorchis sinensis, Opisthorchis viverrini and O. felineus*, remain important public health problems in many endemic areas, where they infect approximately 17 million.[1] Recent estimates suggest that about 35 million humans are infected with *C. sinensis* globally with up to 15 million in China alone.[7] Generally, prevalence and intensity of infection rise with age, with most initial infections occurring in the early teens, and may be higher in males than females.[8,9] Despite widespread availability of praziquantel and massive control efforts, these liver flukes remain common and a major public health problem in many endemic areas. Some investigators believe the number of cases of clonorchiasis in China is increasing.

In addition to their association with hepatobiliary disease, *O. viverrini* and *C. sinensis* are major aetiological agents of bile duct cancer, cholangiocarcinoma.[6] This is a leading cause of death in Khon Kaen, North-east Thailand, with the incidence (per 100 000) of intrahepatic CCA of 71.3 in males and 31.6 in females.[10,11] CCA also occurred in China (e.g. Qidong) with an incidence of 10.3 in males and 4.6 in females and in Korea the incidence in males was 5.4 and 2.5 in females.[12]

The three major liver flukes are similar in egg morphologies, life cycles and pathogenesis. Distinction between them is generally based on the adult worm morphology (Figure 53.1).[13] Genetic variations among the liver flukes, particularly *O. viverrini* and to a lesser extent *C. sinensis* in Asian countries, are associated with geographical localities.[14,15] These genetic variations are related to biological characteristics of the liver flukes, but it is unclear whether they also relate to pathogenicity.

O. felineus is prevalent in animals throughout Europe and has been reported in humans from Italy, eastern Germany, Poland, Kazakhstan, Russia and the Ukraine.[1,6] High prevalences and intensities were previously reported in Siberia, notably the Tyumen and Khanty regions.[16] Residents and immigrants to the endemic focus in Siberia enjoy eating thinly sliced frozen or lightly salted cyprinid fish.

Control efforts in northeast Thailand have achieved a drop in the prevalence of *O. viverrini* infection among the population of 20 million from approximately 35% in 1981, to 24–30% in 1992 and 18.6% in 1994 and 15.7% in 2009.[5] However, studies in northern Thailand collecting adult worms post treatment and examining metacercariae in fish have suggested that prevalence estimates for liver fluke infection may be influenced by misdiagnosis of minute intestinal fluke infections.[17] *O. viverrini* (and minute intestinal fluke) infection remains common in Laos, with an extensive distribution and a particularly high prevalence in the southern region.[18]

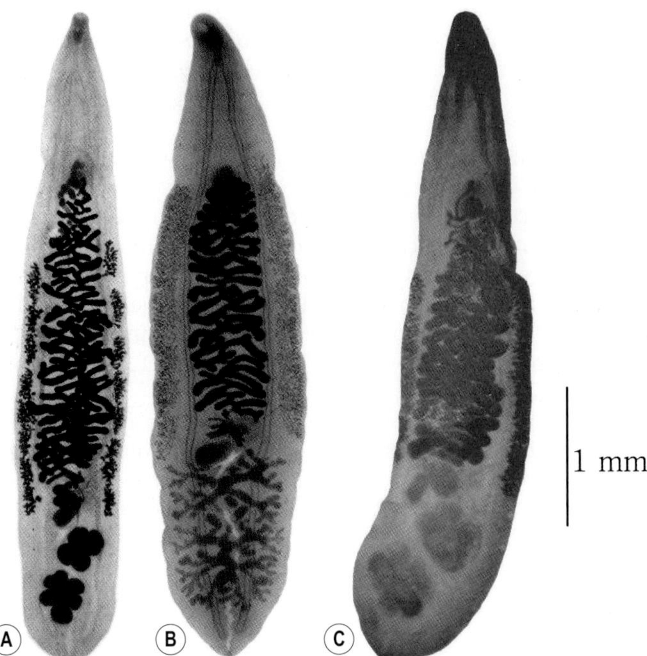

Figure 53.1 (A) *Opisthorchis viverrini.* (B) *Clonorchis sinensis.* (C) *Opisthorchis felineus.*

Raw fish dishes are a well-established dietary tradition of Laos people and the ethnic Laos in northeast Thailand. Fresh fish dishes may contain large numbers of metacercariae and are eaten occasionally. Uncooked fermented fish, which is eaten daily, may also contain metacercariae and serve as a source of infection.

Although largely eliminated from Japan and drastically reduced in Korea, *C. sinensis* remains prevalent and may be increasingly common in parts of Taiwan, Hong Kong, Vietnam, Macao and China.[19] Human infection occurs in 24 Chinese Provinces, with one major focus in the south (especially Guangdong and Guangsxi provinces) and another in the northeast (Henjian). Some Chinese people enjoy eating raw fish dipped in hot rice porridge; and children catch and eat them during play. This latter practice results in an unusual age-related pattern of infection, whereby most infections occur in children.

Life Cycle

The adult liver fluke lives in the smaller intrahepatic bile ducts of their final hosts, which include humans, cats, dogs and other wild and domestic fish-eating mammals. Eggs pass down the bile duct and into the faeces and can also be found in the gallbladder. Eggs are fully embryonated upon excretion, and hatch into miracidia after being ingested by snails. Generally fewer than 1–2% of snails are infected. The miracidia transform into sporocysts and rediae which multiply and then become free-swimming cercaria which exit the snail and attach, penetrate and encyst in susceptible species of fish. Most belong to the family Cyprinidae. Wide variation in the prevalence (up to 100%) and intensity of metacercaria is found between seasons, types of water bodies and species of fish.[20] Metacercaria are infective to humans and other mammals if consumed with uncooked fish. The metacercaria excyst, migrate up the duodenum through the ampulla of Vater and the extrahepatic biliary system to the intrahepatic bile ducts, where they mature. The pre-patent period is about 1 month and the adults may live many years.

Pathology and Pathogenesis

Liver enlargement and dilated subcapsular bile ducts with thick fibrotic walls can be seen grossly in heavily infected cases.[9] Microscopically, bile duct pathology is characterized by desquamation of epithelial cells of secondary and tertiary ducts and chronic inflammation with infiltration of lymphocytes, monocytes, eosinophils and plasma cells (Figure 53.2). Granulomatous inflammation around the eggs is occasionally observed along the bile ducts. Epithelial hyperplasia may occur at an early stage of infection. In severe cases, adenomatous hyperplasia, and goblet cell metaplasia may be seen. Periductal fibrosis is the most prominent histologic feature of chronic infection.[9,21] This corresponds to periportal echoes detected by ultrasonography. Inflammation, necrosis and atrophy of hepatic cells have also been reported.

The pathology of fluke-associated cholecystitis consists of fibrosis, infiltration of mast cells and eosinophils and mucosal hyperplasia of the gallbladder wall.[22,23] Perforation of the gallbladder wall is uncommon in liver fluke infection. Parasites and eggs have been observed in the nidus of gallbladder and intrahepatic stones (Figure 53.3).[21,24]

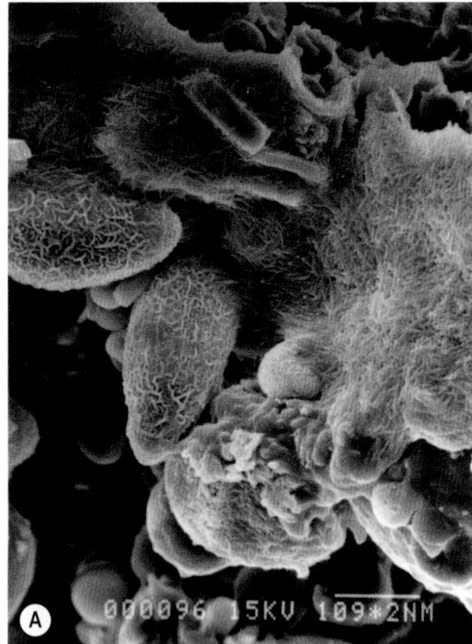

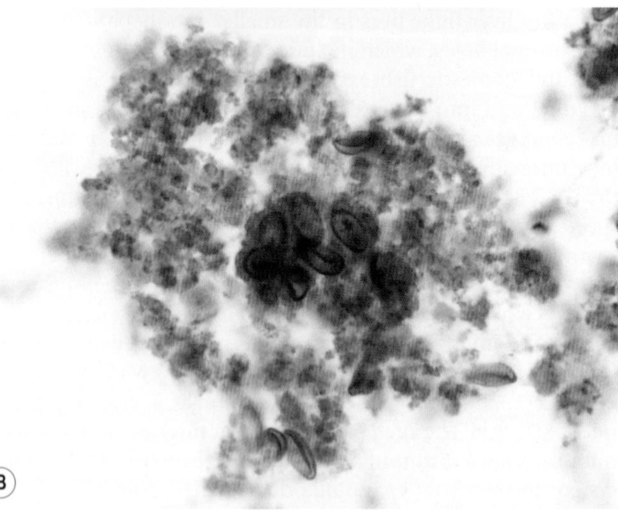

Figure 53.2 (A) Scanning electron micrograph of gallstone showing liver fluke eggs with typical mush-melon-eggshell surface in the nidus of the stone. (B) Bile sludge containing eggs of the liver fluke (*O. viverrini*).

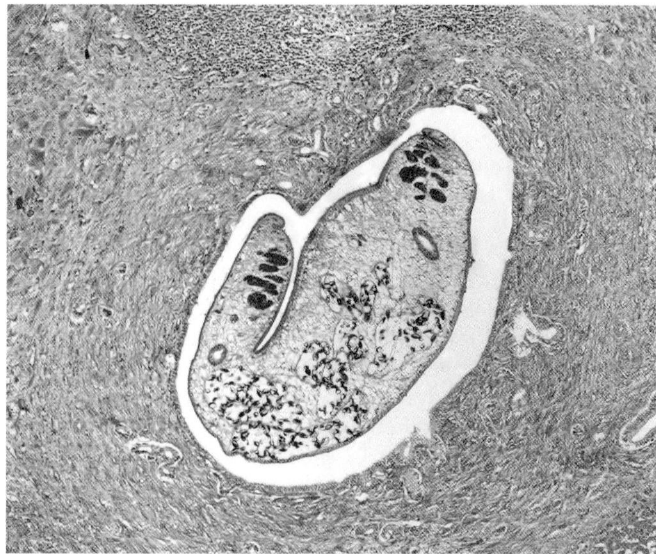

Figure 53.3 Histopathology of chronic *Opisthorchis viverrini* infection in human. An adult fluke is seen in the bile duct lumen. Adenomatous hyperplasia and inflammation with prominent periductal fibrosis are noted.

The pathogenesis of liver-fluke-mediated tissue damage may be caused directly by mechanical or chemical irritation and/or immune-mediated.[9] Mechanical injury from the activities of feeding and migrating flukes contributes to biliary ulceration through its suckers. Chemical irritation occurs as the liver fluke secretes and excretes metabolic products and wastes from the tegument and excretory openings into the bile. Some of these, such as *O. viverrini* granulin-like substance, are highly mitogenic to fibroblast, kidney or biliary cell lines cocultured *in vitro* with the flukes.[25–27] These products may cause the long-observed hyperplasia of biliary epithelial cells reported in opisthorchiasis. Moreover, the fluke excretory-secretory products are also highly immunogenic. Marked inflammatory infiltration is associated with the presence of excretory and secretory antigens in the intrahepatic and extrahepatic bile ducts in animals experimentally infected with *Opisthorchis*.[28] Nitric oxide and other reactive oxygen intermediates produced by inflammatory cells during infection might exert direct cytotoxic and mutagenic effects and increased cell proliferation.[29] Increased formation of 8-nitroguanine (8-NO_2-G) and 8-oxo-7,8-dihydro-2'-deoxyguanosine (8-oxodG) has been shown to be associated with liver fluke infection, even more enhanced in repeated infection and/or praziquantel treatment, and is considered to be mutagenic. Increased endogenous production of N-nitroso compounds and enhanced hepatic activation of carcinogens in these areas of fibrosis may create highly mutagenic conditions for the chronically proliferating bile duct epithelium.[29] In addition, a recent finding that was expression of master coregulator MTA1, an essential host component mediating inflammatory responses, was detected in stromal fibroblast in *O. viverrini*-associated CCA.[30] All of these conditions form an ideal environment for cancer development.

Clinical Features

Most chronically infected individuals have few specific signs or symptoms, except an increased frequency of palpable liver, as shown in community-based studies using physical examination.[9,31] Haematological and biochemical features are unremarkable, even in heavy infections. Ultrasonography, however, reveals a high frequency of gallbladder enlargement, sludge, gallstones and poor function in asymptomatic individuals,[31–33] which are reversed within 10 months of praziquantel treatment.[34]

Symptomatic cases of *Opisthorchis* and *Clonorchis* infection generally experience pain in the right upper quadrant, diarrhoea, loss of appetite, indigestion and fullness. Severe cases may present with weakness, lassitude, weight loss, ascites and oedema.[9,35] Complications may include cholangitis, obstructive jaundice, intra-abdominal mass, cholecystitis and gallbladder or intrahepatic stones.[24,35] Such stones are particularly frequent in clonorchiasis.

The most important clinical manifestation of liver fluke infection is an enhanced susceptibility to cholangiocarcinoma (Figure 53.4). Case–control studies in Thailand suggest a five

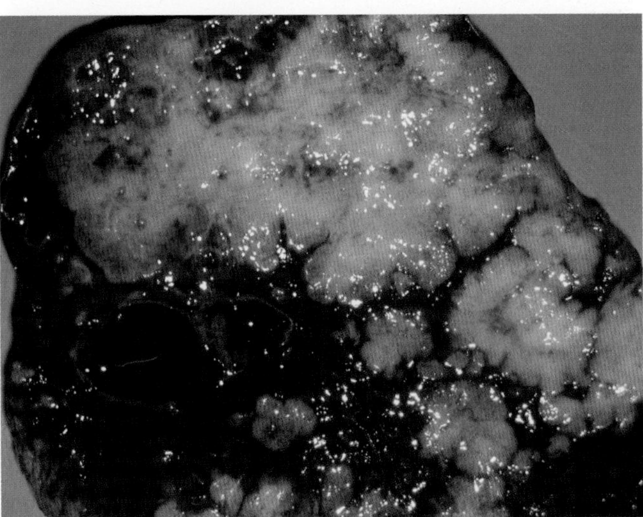

Figure 53.4 Gross morphology of intrahepatic cholangiocarcinoma in a patient from endemic areas of liver fluke (*O. viverrini*).

folds increased risk during infection of any intensity, while heavily infected people may face a 15-fold increased risk.[36] This is also reflected geographically; the population-adjusted frequency of cholangiocarcinoma was found to be six- to 10-fold higher (in females and males, respectively) in an endemic province above that of a non-endemic area in Thailand.[37,38] While such a large geographical association has not been reported for *Clonorchis* infection, there is ample evidence that this fluke is also strongly associated with cholangiocarcinoma.[6,39]

A special feature of *O. felineus* infection, not often reported for the other species, is acute opisthorchiasis associated with severe histopathology.[16] This is characterized by hepatosplenomegaly and tenderness, eosinophilia up to 40%, and chills and fever. It occurs early in infection and may be associated with primary exposure to a large dose of metacercaria.

Diagnosis

Egg counts have traditionally been used to diagnose liver fluke infection, most often using the Kato thick smear, Stoll's dilution or quantitative formalin ethyl acetate concentration technique. All three techniques effectively detect moderate and heavy infections. However, comparative studies in low-intensity areas have shown that a single reading of the concentration and dilution techniques detect about 70% of infections, while the sensitivity of Kato is considerably lower (45%). Worm burden and egg count correlate closely, with an estimated egg output of 53/g of faeces per worm (using Stoll's dilution technique).[40] Stoll's egg counts tend to be higher than those of the concentration technique.

Although egg detection is almost always used in surveys and treatment programmes, several immunodiagnostic tests have been described for *Opisthorchis* and *Clonorchis* infections. While most antigens are nonspecific and antibodies persist long after treatment, good results have been gained from new serological tests using individual antigens and detecting isotype-specific antibodies. Faecal antigen detection by enzyme-linked immunosorbent assays (ELISAs) using monoclonal antibodies against secretory antigens and molecular methods also shows promise.[41]

Management and Treatment

Treatment with praziquantel at 40 mg/kg body weight in a single dose is effective against opisthorchiasis and clonorchiasis.[42] This regimen has been used most commonly in large-scale treatment programs. Reports from China, however, indicate that higher doses (120 mg/kg over 2 days) are needed to cure heavy *Clonorchis* infections. Side-effects, such as dizziness, vomiting and abdominal pain, occur frequently but are transient and rarely severe. Most abnormalities of the gallbladder are also eliminated by elimination of the parasite. Relatively high efficacy of artesunate and artemether treatment has been reported in *C. sinensis* over *O. viverrini* in rodent models.[43] Recently, high efficacy of tribendimidine at 200 mg (age below 14 years) or 400 mg (age above 14 years) as a single dose has been reported as giving a 99% egg reduction rate equivalent to praziquantel in individuals with opisthorchiasis.[44] The drug hexachloroparaxylol (Chloxyle) has also been used extensively for the treatment of *O. felineus*, but it may be less effective than praziquantel.

Prevention

Prevention of human liver fluke infection can be facilitated by treatment (to reduce the excretion of eggs), sanitation (to prevent eggs from reaching water sources) and health education (to discourage the eating of raw fish). The application of Hazard Analysis Critical Control Point principles and procedures during fish farming can reduce metacercarial contamination of fish. Treatment of raw fish by freezing, irradiation and chemical treatment have also been suggested. Control of snail intermediate host by molluscicides is not considered feasible because of their widespread distribution and resistance to adverse conditions. To be most effective, health education should be designed and delivered in a culturally sensitive manner with the aim of effecting behaviour change as well as simply providing information. Large-scale treatment efforts in endemic areas by public health ministries have probably had a major impact on the intensity of all three infections.[5]

FASCIOLIASIS

Fascioliasis is caused by food-borne trematodes and is also considered a Neglected Tropical Disease (NTD). An estimated 17 million people are infected with the two larger human liver flukes, *Fasciola hepatica* and *Fasciola gigantica*, and 91 million people are at risk worldwide.[45] The geographical distributions cover Europe, Africa, the Americas and Oceania.[46] Infection by these liver flukes, i.e. fascioliasis, often causes serious acute and chronic morbidity.[1] These parasites commonly infect domestic ruminants and wildlife throughout the world and indirectly impact on human wellbeing through massive economic loss in the livestock industry.[47] Humans are accidental final hosts and usually become infected by eating aquatic plants grown in water that is contaminated with faeces from animals harbouring *Fasciola* (Figure 53.5).

Epidemiology

Eggs of *Fasciola* are excreted 3–4 months after ingestion of the infective metacercariae in water plants, and the entire cycle is completed in 4–6 months. High humidity, moderate temperatures and rainfall favour transmission.[48] Human infection with *Fasciola* is most common in villages and larger towns within

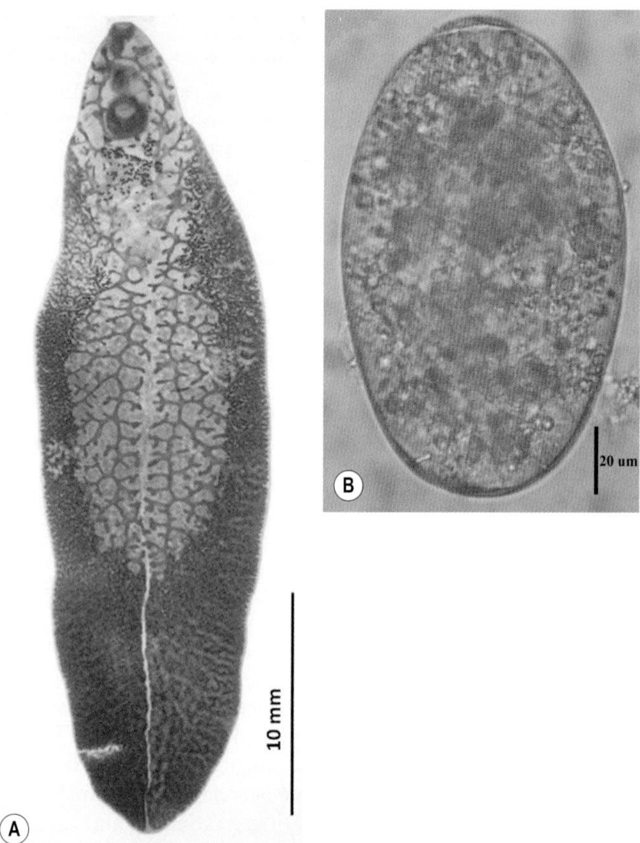

Figure 53.5 (A) *Fasciola gigantica*. (B) Egg.

rural areas, especially sheep- and cattle/buffalo grazing areas. Levels of infection depend on the frequency of humans eating plants (mainly watercress in Europe; morning glory in Asia) from water bodies contaminated with animal faeces. In most endemic areas, human infection is relatively rare, even where prevalence among domestic animals is high. Outbreaks of *F. hepatica* occur in households and communities, and are often traced to consumption of wild, rather than cultivated, watercress.[46] A high proportion of exposed people become infected but some do not have symptoms. Infection might also occur from contaminated drinking water or cooking utensils.

Fasciola infection as reported in general parasite surveys is undoubtedly underestimated, since eggs are often not detected by faecal examination. Community-based studies using improved diagnostic methods have demonstrated areas with very high prevalence and intensity of infection in Bolivia, Peru and Egypt.[49] Heavy infections found in the high altitudes of the Bolivian Altiplano region result from frequent consumption of *kjosco* (raw water-plant salad) by children tending their grazing animals.[50,51] Evidence also indicates that infection may occur by drinking water contaminated with floating metacercariae and by ingesting metacercariae attached to the surface of food or kitchen utensils washed with water contaminated with metacercariae.

Pathogenesis and Pathology

Fascioliasis is a serious medical condition due to the size of the parasite which reflects its origin as a livestock worm (adult *F. hepatica* measure 20–30 × 13 mm wide, while adult *F. gigantica* measure 25–75 × 12 mm wide). These parasites cause considerable mortality in sheep and cattle, and human morbidity which is dependent on the number of worms and stage of infection.[48] The acute phase occurs during migration of the immature flukes through the liver. Severe pathology results from parasite ingestion and destruction of parenchymal tissue, haemorrhage, parasite death and inflammatory responses largely mediated by eosinophils. Repair mechanisms can lead to extensive fibrosis, increased pressure atrophy of the liver and periportal fibrosis.

The chronic phase, during which parasites are present in the bile ducts, tends to be less severe. Progressive inflammation, including bile duct proliferation, dilatation and fibrosis, is largely caused by mechanical obstruction of the ducts, inflammatory responses and the activity of proline, which the fluke excretes in large quantities.[52] Proline may facilitate movement of the parasite through the narrow ducts. Anaemia may result from blood loss through bile duct lesions. Death is uncommon, but is usually caused by haemorrhaging in the bile duct and case reports suggest it occurs more frequently in children.[53]

Flukes that migrate out of the intestine but do not locate in the liver can form ectopic lesions in many tissues.[53,54] These nodules, granulomas or migration tracts are often misdiagnosed as malignant tumours or gastric ulcers.

Multiple yellow nodules of necrotic tissue (1–4 mm in diameter) and linear lesions through the parenchyma infiltrated with eosinophils and Charcot–Leyden crystals can be observed, probably as a result of inflammatory reaction(s) to dead parasites and migration, respectively.[54] Proliferation, dilatation, fibrosis and calcification of the bile ducts, plus sequelae of partial obstruction, may occur during the chronic phase of infection. Dead flukes are sometimes observed inside calcified areas of tissue, and granulomas and abscesses can form around eggs trapped in the parenchymal tissue. Eosinophils may infiltrate the gallbladder wall, which may be thickened and oedematous with perimuscular fibrosis. Stones are often present in the gallbladder during infection. Self-cure occurs frequently and may result from inflammation and calcification.

Clinical Features

Fascioliasis can be symptomatic or asymptomatic. More than half of cases are subclinical (asymptomatic), and human infection can be classified as acute or chronic based upon clinical manifestations and laboratory findings. Clinical manifestations include: upper abdominal pain or the right costal margin; fever; constitutional symptoms; urticaria; itching; respiratory symptoms; headache; malaise; weight loss and night sweats may begin approximately 2 months following ingestion of metacercariae and 1–2 months prior to the onset of egg excretion. The signs of acute phase of infection are hepatomegaly, splenomegaly, anaemia, weakness. Laboratory evaluations reveal eosinophilia (>500/mm^3) and leukocytosis (>10 000/mm^3) in up to 80% of egg-positive cases in faeces. In chronic infection beyond the latent phase, clinical manifestations are those of the complications of fascioliasis, namely: ascending cholangitis; cholelithiasis; cholecystitis; pancreatitis; biliary cirrhosis; and hepatic fibrosis. Unlike some other trematode infections, fascioliasis has not been associated with cancer. Typical fascioliasis results from the migration of immature worms through Glisson's capsule and the liver parenchyma en route to the bile ducts, where they mature and remain as adults. Occasionally, the juvenile worms reach ectopic destinations, resulting in a cutaneous or visceral larva migrans, similar to that observed in strongyloidiasis, taeniasis and gnathostomiasis. The clinical findings with ectopic migration depend upon the organs and tissues invaded.

Diagnosis and Investigations

Fascioliasis has been diagnosed by observation of eggs during faecal examination, by parasite-specific antibody detection in a variety of immunodiagnostic assays, by radiological methods and by laparotomy. Dietary history is helpful for differential diagnosis and in investigating outbreaks. Examination of faeces for eggs is of limited use, since eggs are not excreted during the invasive stage of infection, when many patients present with severe symptoms. Often, eggs are undetectable during the chronic phase, but it is unclear whether the techniques used are insensitive for very low egg outputs in light infections (<100 eggs/g) or if eggs are not being produced. Differentiation of eggs from *F. hepatica*, *F. gigantica*, echinostomes and *Fasciolopsis* is difficult.[55] Eggs can also be found in duodenal contents, bile and histological sections.

A further problem with faecal examination is that eggs may be passed after eating liver from infected animals. This does not indicate infection; thus positive cases should be reconfirmed if liver has been eaten recently.

Immunodiagnostic tests using every available technique have been reported in the literature, from skin tests to antibody and antigen detection assays targeting somatic and excretory/secretory antigens of adult worms. Within 2–4 weeks of becoming infected, a *Fasciola*-specific serological response ensues, allowing confirmation of infection 5–7 weeks before eggs appear in the faeces. Most claim excellent sensitivity (>90%), and problems with cross-reactivity with other trematode infections are avoided by using purified specific antigens, cystatin-treated plates or specific antibody subclasses. Positive serology can also be used to document infection in the chronic phase, when egg release may be intermittent or absent.

The advantage of immunodiagnosis over parasitological techniques is that they can detect early prepatent infections as well as chronic stages with little or no egg output. In contrast to other infections, antibody levels drop rapidly after successful treatment, so the assays tend to detect only active infection and serology should revert to negative within a year of successful treatment.

Blood cell microscopy and biochemical tests can also support diagnosis. Eosinophilia, leukocytosis, and elevated inflammatory markers are common in acute infections, while anaemia and/or elevated serum hepatic transaminases, bilirubin and alkaline phosphatase are only occasionally and transiently present during chronic infection.[56]

Clinical diagnosis is often difficult because presentations are not markedly different from hepatobiliary disease of other origin(s). Clinicians may not consider fascioliasis where human infections are uncommon. In temperate climates, outbreaks are almost invariably associated with eating wild watercress. The finding of multiple, related cases with similar diet histories and high-risk occupation (e.g. sheep farmers) may provide supporting evidence. In tropical areas where people consume water plants daily, this may be of limited use.

Laparotomy and radiological imaging by ultrasonography, endoscopic retrograde cholangiopancreatography and percutaneous cholangiography may be useful.[57] These allow visualization of the lesions of acute and chronic fascioliasis and sometimes eggs (by laparotomy) or worms in the hepatobiliary system.

Management

Triclabendazole 10 mg/kg body weight single dose is the regimen of choice against fascioliasis. The drug is active against both immature and adult parasites, with high cure rates.[42] Adverse reactions following treatment are usually temporary and mild. Praziquantel is not effective against fascioliasis even at high doses. Efficacy is often variable and difficult to assess. These problems result from differing sensitivities of the adult and migrating worms, the size and thick tegument of *Fasciola*, impaired hepatic function and varying clinical presentations.

Previously, the drug bithionol was most often used against fascioliasis at a dose of 30–50 mg/kg body weight per day in three divided doses on alternate days for a duration of 10–15 days.[58] Success against acute infection has been reported for dehydroemetine at a dose of 1 mg/kg daily for 10 days given intramuscularly or subcutaneously.[53] Moderate to severe side-effects have been observed; both drugs and multiple courses are often required. Nitazoxanide has been found to be effective in some clinical trials, with one study reporting 97% of patients free of *Fasciola* eggs in stool samples after 30 days of treatment but further studies are needed.[59]

Depending on the presentation of the patient, other drugs given before the fasciolicide may assist recovery. Prednisolone (5–10 mg/day) may alleviate toxaemia, while antibiotics are often used to treat acute cholangitis due to secondary bacterial infection. Chloroquine was previously used because it rapidly relieves symptoms of acute disease but does not kill the flukes.

Prevention

Ultimate control of *Fasciola* must focus on strategic treatment or immunization of livestock and other herbivorous animals that maintain the life cycle. Advances in the development of veterinary vaccines are very encouraging.[60] Widespread livestock immunization is being considered by some countries to reduce human infection and economic loss to the parasite. Control of the snail vectors using molluscicides is not considered practical in most situations. Health education to discourage human consumption of raw wild watercress and other edible water plants may be effective in areas where the disease is prevalent. Strict controls on commercial production of water plants, as has been instituted in some Western countries, would help to prevent the expansion of endemic areas in developing countries. Increased awareness by clinicians of the problem and its diagnostic difficulties, plus data from community-based studies assessing seroprevalence, will help quantify the extent to which fascioliasis affects human health.

Intestinal Flukes

Among the food-borne trematodes, the most diverse group comprising a total of 59 species are the intestinal flukes.[61] This review will focus on the common species of medical importance.

FASCIOLOPSIASIS

Fasciolopsiasis is caused by the infection of a giant intestinal fluke, *Fasciolopsis buski* (Figure 53.6). The geographical distribution of fasciolopsiasis is largely confined to Asian

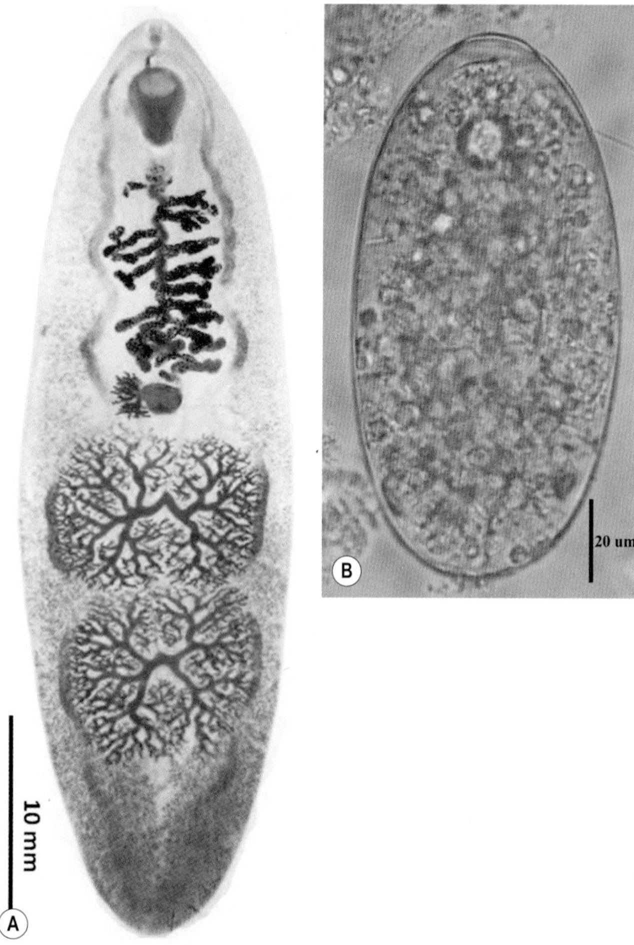

Figure 53.6 (A) *Fasciolopsis buski*. (B) Egg.

countries, namely China, India, Bangladesh, Thailand, Vietnam, Malaysia, Borneo, Sumatra and Myanmar, and may reach high prevalences within endemic focus areas. The parasite attaches to the intestinal wall of humans and pigs. Heavy infections can be severe especially in children.

Life Cycle

The final host range of *F. buski* is limited to humans and pigs.[62] They become infected through the consumption of viable metacercariae attached on the seed pods of water plants. These include the water caltrops, water hyacinth, water chestnut, water bamboo, lotus roots and wild rice shoots. Although metacercariae are not present on the edible seed of these plants, ingestion occurs during removal of pods with the teeth and lips.

F. buski metacercariae excyst in the duodenum and the escaping larvae attach to the duodenal and jejunal walls. The larvae become mature adults in 3 months and produce large numbers (an estimated 10 000–25 000 per day per worm) of large, yellow, operculated eggs. If these eggs reach water sources, further development and embryonation occurs over 3–7 weeks, then miracidia hatch and enter planorbid snail intermediate hosts in the genera *Segmentina*, *Hippeutis* or *Gyraulus* and *Indoplanorbis exustus*. After asexual reproduction as sporocysts and second generation rediae over a 3–4-week period in snails, free-swimming cercariae are released from the snail host which then attach and encyst on seed pods.[62,63]

Epidemiology

Transmission is largely confined to low-lying areas with heavy rainfall and extensive flooding, which leads to faecal contamination of the water. Use of pig or human faeces for fertilization is associated with endemicity. The highest prevalence occurs in areas with cultivation or year-round availability of water caltrops and other aquatic vegetation. Human infections occurred by the ingestion of raw or undercooked freshwater plants and their nuts, drinking unboiled water and handling or processing these raw plants. Farms where pigs are fed with raw plants and untreated water in endemic areas create the main sources of infection, and feeding fish with faeces of pigs or humans further enhances the transmission of this parasite. Fasciolopsiasis is focally endemic and prevalence peaks in school-age children.

Pathogenesis and Pathology

Eosinophils accumulate at the site of parasite attachment on the jejunal or duodenal wall, where mechanical injury and inflammation lead to ulcer formation. These ulcers sometimes bleed due to capillary damage or become abscesses. Mild infection in healthy people is associated with lower haematocrit and serum levels of vitamin B12, but no apparent change in other nutrients.[64] This may result from parasite sequestering vitamin B12 or its impaired absorption from the damaged intestinal mucosa.

Although a few parasites cause little damage, the presence of many (hundreds to thousands) is associated with severe pathology and sometimes acute intestinal obstruction. Extensive intestinal ulceration may interfere with digestion, and cause malabsorption, leading to severe malnutrition and wasting. Oedema also occurs in severe cases; it may result from toxic parasite metabolites, allergic reactions or from hypoalbuminaemia secondary to electrolyte and protein imbalance from chronic malabsorption.

Clinical Features

Symptoms are generally absent or mild, and may include diarrhoea, hunger pains, flatulence, poor appetite, mild abdominal colic, vomiting, eosinophilia and fever.[54,65] The abdominal pain may mimic that of peptic or duodenal ulcers. Late, severe cases present with ascites or oedema of the face, abdomen and legs, anaemia, anorexia, weakness and vomiting and patients may pass stools containing large amounts of undigested material. Deaths have been associated with heavy and long-standing untreated infection.

Diagnosis and Investigations

Diagnosis by faecal examination is not difficult, given the large quantity and large size of the eggs. Stoll's dilution, formalin ether concentration, direct smears and Kato techniques have been used successfully. Differentiation from *Fasciola* eggs is difficult, so that a dietary, clinical and residential history in endemic areas should also be considered.

Management

In the past, hexylresorcinol crystoids, tetrachloroethylene and dichlorophen were used for treatment of *Fasciolopsis* with varying effectiveness.[54,65,66] Praziquantel is now the drug of choice, with high efficacy at a dose of 15 mg/kg body weight. In heavily infected cases, there may be some risk of exacerbating obstruction or acute toxaemia with treatment, such that conservative treatment is advised.

Prevention and Control

The use of fermented, instead of fresh, silage for feeding pigs in endemic areas may reduce the chance of transmission since metacercariae are sensitive to both heat and salt. Drying the plants may also be effective. Treating or prohibiting the use of human and pig faeces for fertilizer and improved sanitation would help interrupt the life cycle. Refraining from using the mouth to peel vegetables, then boiling them for a few seconds, or careful washing after peeling them with hands or a knife would reduce human infection. Filtering drinking water may prevent some infections from plant-detached metacercariae in water. Health education should help people recognize the problem as well as indicate acceptable ways to avoid infection, since most infections are mild.

ECHINOSTOMIASIS

At least 20 species in eight genera (*Artyfechinostomum, Acanthoparyphium, Echinochasmus, Echinoparyphium, Echinostoma, Episthmium, Euparyphium, and Hypoderaeum*) of echinostomes have been recorded in man. The most common appear to be *E. ilocanum*, *E. revolutum*, *E. malayanum*, *E. echinatum* and *E. hortense* (Figure 53.7).[67]

Life Cycle

These parasites have a highly variable and wide host range. Humans become infected with echinostomes through the consumption of raw or incompletely cooked freshwater snails, clams, fish and tadpoles harbouring metacercaria. The parasite lives in the intestine of the definitive host, and eggs are excreted in faeces. Snails are the first intermediate host, then after a brief free-swimming stage cercariae encyst within a second intermediate host which may be mollusc, fish or amphibian larva. Aquatic birds are the most important final host of most species.

Epidemiology

Most human infections occur in Asia in areas where raw or incompletely cooked molluscs and fish are eaten. Infection is common in Korea, Indonesia, the Philippines, Malaysia, Taiwan, India, Cambodia and Thailand.[62,65] Reported prevalences in endemic communities generally range from 1% to 50%.[68,69] Infections are most prevalent in poor rural areas and may be clustered in families who prefer raw snails. Recent surveys in Cambodia found the prevalence of infections in children aged 12–14 years ranging from 7.5% to 22.4%. Adult worms were identified as *Echinostoma revolutum*.[70]

Diagnosis

The large, unembryonated, operculated eggs of echinostomes can be observed in faeces and are difficult to differentiate from those of *Fasciola* and *Fasciolopsis*. Adult worms can be recovered from faeces following treatment or retrieved through endoscopy.[71] This allows for positive differentiation based on morphology, of which the predominant feature is the circumoral disc and collar spines around the oral sucker. It should be noted that the morphology may be altered by drug treatment.

Pathogenesis, Pathology and Clinical Features

Like *F. buski*, the major pathological lesions of echinostomes are associated with parasite attachment deep between the villi of the jejunal wall. There may be inflammation and ulceration of the

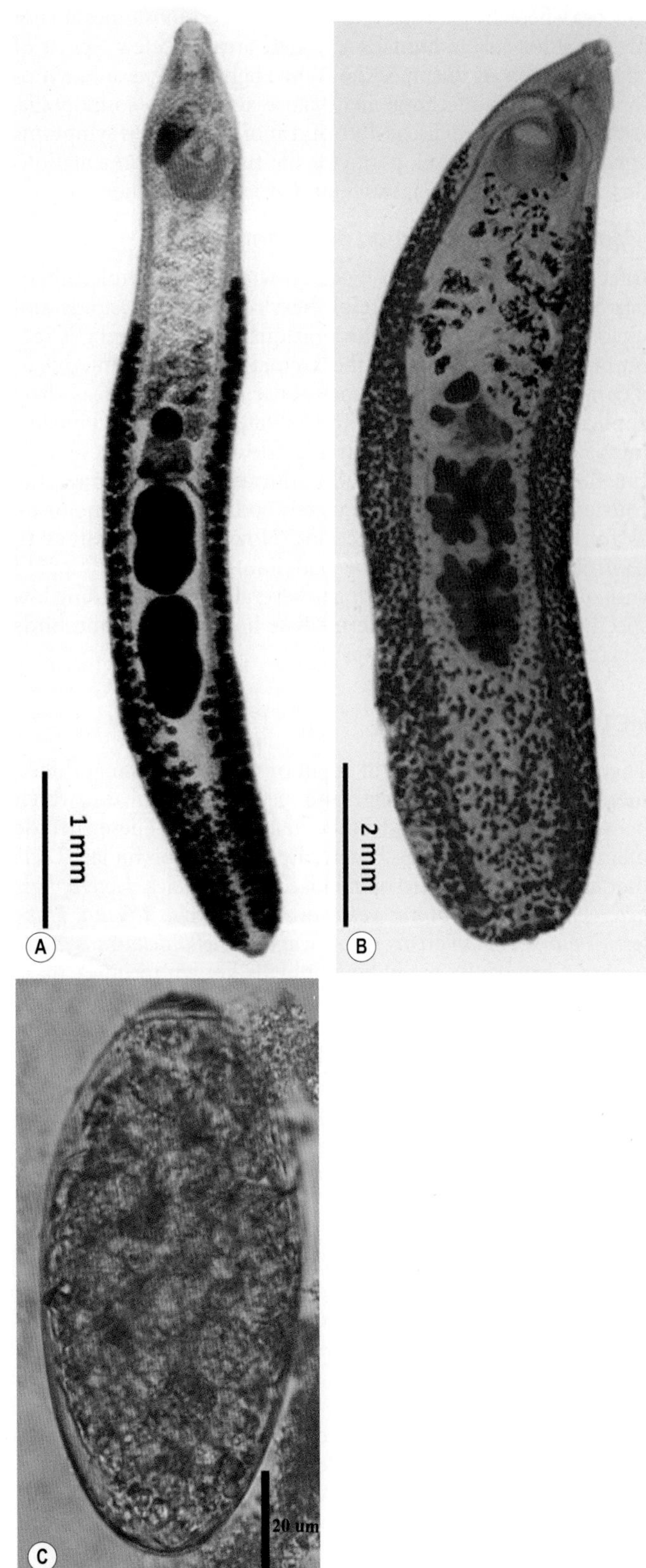

Figure 53.7 (A) *Echinostoma ilocanum*. (B) *E. malayanum*. (C) Egg of Echinostome.

mucosa where the parasites locate. However, echinostomes are not highly pathogenic to humans and there are only a few reports of clinical aspects of this infection. While light burdens are asymptomatic, heavy infections may cause diarrhoea, eosinophilia, abdominal pain and discomfort, and anorexia.[71] These symptoms apparently do not develop into the life-threatening presentations that are described (albeit rarely) in *Fasciolopsis* infection.

Management, Prevention and Control

Infections are relatively easily cured with mebendazole, albendazole, praziquantel, bithionol, hexylresorcinol crystoids and niclosamide.[72] Treatment with praziquantel at 15 mg/kg is recommended in areas where other trematodes are present, due to its broad efficacy, safety and ease of use.[65,72] In these areas, drug application may be provided to facilitate control of echinostomiasis, together with other trematode infections. Prevention can be supplemented by health education to discourage the consumption of raw or incompletely cooked fish and molluscs, as for other fish-borne infections. However, programmes to control echinostomiasis have had limited success compared with other helminthiases owing to several factors, including low specificity of the second intermediate host and common birds serving as a reservoir final host.

HETEROPHYIASIS

There are a large number of small or minute intestinal flukes, measuring <2.5 mm in length and just visible to the eye, which parasitize man, birds and other mammals.[62,73] These include members of the families Heterophyidae, Plagiorchiidae, Lecithodendriidae and Microphallidae. The species *Heterophyes heterophyes*, *Metagonimus yokogawai*, *Haplorchis taichui*, *Haplorchis pumilio*, *Haplorchis yokogawai* and *Stellantchasmus falcatus* are a few of the many heterophyids known to infect man. The first two species are thought to be the most important medically. The examination of faeces passed after treatment with praziquantel or bithionol has shown that these parasites, previously considered 'rare', may be common and very numerous in people who live in areas where raw aquatic foods and/or insect larvae are eaten.[74] Because of their similarity these parasites are covered here under the term 'heterophyids'.

Life Cycle

Adult heterophyids live deeply embedded in the intestinal mucosa of mammals and birds where they produce fully embryonated eggs which are excreted in faeces. Upon ingestion by freshwater snails (*Melanoides*, *Tarebia*, *Semisulcospira* and others), the larvae escape, undergo multiplication, then exit as cercariae. The cercariae penetrate and encyst within many species of fresh and brackish water fish or shrimps.[73] Humans become infected while eating fish or shrimps harbouring viable metacercariae, which become mature adults within 5–10 days. An average of 10 000 metacercariae of *M. yokogawai* have been found in the sweetfish (*Plecoglossus altivelis*) during the 'eating season' in Korea.[75] Metacercariae of *Haplorchis* spp. are recovered in cyprinid fish, *Stellantchasmus falcatus* in *Liza subviridis* and lecithendriids are commonly found in dragonfly larvae.[69]

Epidemiology

Heterophyids are mainly found in Asia (Japan, Korea, Laos, Thailand, Taiwan, the Philippines, China), Hawaii, Siberia, Turkey and the Balkans. The use of expulsion chemotherapy to recover adult worms has revealed the enormous number and variety of flukes that can be harboured by a person. Food habits of eating raw fish and access to rich aquatic fauna are the important determinants of human infection.

M. yokogawai and *Heterophyes nocens* infect 1.2–42% of the Korean population, respectively. High prevalences of *Haplorchis taichui* (32%) and *Haplorchis pumilio* (52%) are also reported. The prevalence of infection with fish-borne trematodes in males is frequently higher than that in females, peaked at 40–59 years in riverside localities. The relative distribution of fluke species vary by locality.[74]

Pathogenesis, Pathology and Clinical Symptoms

These are similar for the different species. Most infections are asymptomatic or accompanied by mild intestinal discomfort, which may include mucous diarrhoea, colicky pains, intermittent neurasthenia and lethargy.[54] These probably result from mild inflammation with mainly eosinophils, superficial necrosis, excessive mucus secretion and bleeding at the site of attachment. Microscopic examination of *H. taichui* infection reveals mucosal ulceration, mucosal and submucosal haemorrhages, fusion and shortening villi, chronic inflammation, and fibrosis of the submucosa.[76]

Symptoms are most frequent in heavy infections, but they subside spontaneously after one month, although the flukes remain.[75] Upon further infection, symptoms may recur, giving rise to occasional episodes of diarrhoea in endemic areas.

One special aspect of heterophyid pathogenesis is the involvement of eggs. These embed deeply in the intestinal wall, eliciting eosinophil and neutrophil infiltration. The eggs (and sometimes adult worms) may then enter nearby lymphatics or blood vessels and be transported to other sites – notably the heart, spinal cord or brain, lungs, liver and spleen.[54] Eggs become trapped and elicit granulomatous lesions and fibrosis. Signs of heterophyid myocarditis may include cardiac enlargement, cough, dyspnoea, cyanosis, fatigue, oedema and ascites, palpitation, loss of reflexes and abnormal heart sounds. Eggs or worms in the spinal cord or brain may cause neurological disease, transverse myelitis and loss of sensory and motor function.[54]

Diagnosis

Diagnosis is usually based on the recovery of eggs in faeces, however, the daily egg output per worm is low (35–45) and light infections (<100 worms) are easily missed. Extraintestinal cases of heterophyiasis may be discovered at surgery or autopsy, and then only after careful searching. Distinction between species of heterophyids and *Clonorchis* and *Opisthorchis* by egg is exceedingly difficult. The recovery of adult worms from post-treatment stools allows a definitive diagnosis, but this procedure is not routinely practical.

Management

Niclosamide, bithionol and tetrachloroethylene were previously used, but praziquantel is now the drug of choice. A single dose of 10–20 mg/kg is highly effective.[77] Recent investigation of the *in vivo* efficacy of artesunate against heterophyids in mice, using praziquantel as a therapeutic control showed 100% reduction of intestinal adult worms at a dose of 200 mg/kg per day, given for 3 successive days. The proven therapeutic efficacy of artesunate together with its reported safety, favour its use as an alternative therapy to praziquantel in human heterophyidiasis.

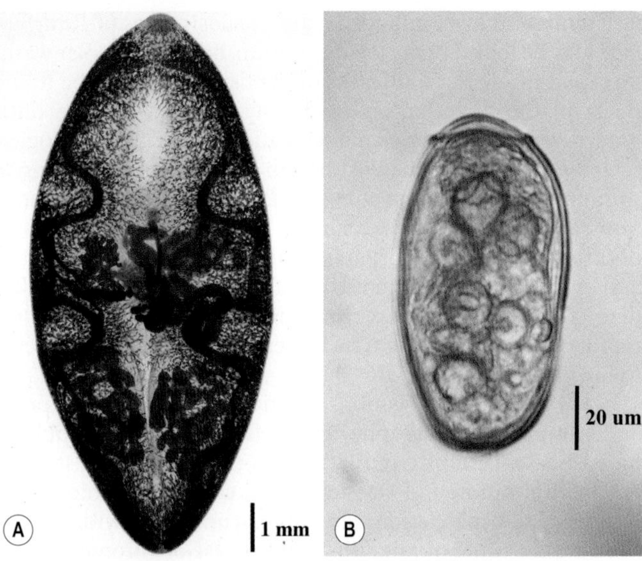

Figure 53.8 (A) *Paragonimus heterotremus*. (B) Egg.

Prevention and Control

Like other fish-borne trematodes, treatment with praziquantel, combined with health education to encourage cooking of fish and other aquatic foods, is important. More studies are required on the frequency and spectrum of clinical consequences in order to assess the amount of resources that should be allocated for control. Although these infections have been linked to fatalities, the frequency and circumstances leading to this are unclear.

Lung Flukes

PARAGONIMIASIS

Lung flukes are distributed widely, and infect an estimated 10 million people in China alone and about 20 million worldwide.[78] Infection primarily causes subacute to chronic respiratory disease, but the involvement of cutaneous, cerebral or other organs/tissues by ectopic migration of the parasites is not rare. Human infection occurs mostly by consuming raw or incompletely cooked crabs and crayfish harbouring metacercariae. Hands and utensils contaminated by metacercariae during cooking crabs or crayfish may also cause infection. Eating raw meat of wild boar, which act as the paratenic hosts harbouring juvenile worms, is an alternative route of infection and is increasingly important in Japan.[79] In addition to dietary preferences, raw crab meat and juice were thought to have medicinal properties for enhancing fertility, reducing fever and treating measles and asthma, which occasionally caused heavy infection in Korea[80] and Japan.[81]

Epidemiology

There are about 40 nominal species in the genus *Paragonimus* in Asia, and most are found in China. In addition, two species (*P. africanus* and *P. uterobilateralis*) occur in Africa; one species (*P. kelicotti*) in North America; and *P. mexicanus* and several related species in Latin America. Recent molecular phylogenetic work has revealed that *Paragonimus* species in Asia can be classified into four major species complexes: *P. westermani*, *P. skrjabini*, *P. heterotremus* and *P. ohirai* (or *P. bangkokensis*/*P. harinasutai*).[82,83] Only a few species in each complex are proven to be pathogenic to humans. In China, Japan and Korea, *P. westermani* followed by *P. skrjabini* (incl. *P. miyazakii* as a synonym or subspecies) are the most important pathogens. In South-east and South Asia, except for the Philippines where *P. westermani* is, *P. heterotremus* (Figure 53.8) is the only confirmed human pathogen, although various *Paragonimus* species are distributed in this area.[82] In addition to Thailand, recently Lao PDR,[84] Vietnam[85] and India[86,87] have been listed as the emerging endemic countries of *P. heterotremus* infection. In Africa, *P. africanus* is endemic in Cameroon,[88] and *P. uterobilateralis* is endemic in Nigeria.[89] Sporadic cases have been reported in over 10 African countries.[90] In the USA, paragonimiasis caused by *P. kelicotti* infection after eating crayfish is an emerging public health issue.[91,92] In Latin America, sporadic cases of paragonimiasis have been reported from Brazil, Columbia, Costa Rica, El Salvador, Ecuador, Guatemala, Honduras, Mexico, Nicaragua, Panama, Peru and Venezuela.[93] In this area, *P. mexicanus* and five other nominal species have been recorded, but all five are considered to be synonymous with *P. mexicanus*.[94]

Life Cycle

The life cycle of *Paragonimus* has been described in detail by Yokogawa (1969)[95] and Miyazaki (1991).[96] Adult worms live in the lungs of some mammals: mainly wild and domestic felines and canines, but some species can also infect humans. Parasite eggs are coughed up from the lungs and either expectorated in the sputum, or swallowed and excreted in the faeces. Eggs reach water and develop into miracidia, which hatch out and swim to seek snail hosts (mainly species of Thiaridae and Pleuroceridae). After penetrating the snail, asexual multiplication and development occur to produce cercariae. Cercariae merge out from snails and enter the second intermediate host, mainly potamid or other freshwater crabs and crayfish, where they become encysted metacercariae, an infective stage, in the gills, liver and muscles. When the crabs are eaten by a final mammalian host, metacercariae excyst in the small intestine, penetrate across the intestinal wall, travel from the peritoneum to the subperitoneal tissue, come back to the peritoneal cavity, pass through the liver and diaphragm, spend time in the pleural cavity, and then invade the lung parenchyma where they mature in 2 months.

Pathogenesis and Pathology

The sites of pathological change as well as clinical features of paragonimiasis depend upon the migratory route and the maturational stages of the worms.[97] During migration, pathological changes occur around juvenile worms in the extrapulmonary sites (extrapulmonary paragonimiasis). Rarely parasites become fully mature adults in extrapulmonary sites. Upon reaching the lungs, adult worms form pairs to lay eggs so that pathological changes occur around adult worms and eggs (pulmonary paragonimiasis). Basic inflammatory responses are somehow similar regardless of location and the maturation stage of the worms. In the acute and subacute stages, eosinophil-dominant inflammatory cell accumulation, often called eosinophilic abscess, is a common feature. Fibrosis progresses with time to form granulomatous lesions in the chronic stage. In the lungs, granulomatous lesions surrounding worms are destroyed by physico-chemical actions of the worms inside creating fibrotic, greyish-white capsules ('worm cyst' of 1.5–5 cm in diameter), which harbour pairs or triplets of worms, surrounded by thick, blood-streaked fluid and numerous eggs. Eggs trapped in the tissue may also provoke minute granulomas at the periphery of the nodular/cystic lesions.

Clinical Features

Chronic productive cough, with brownish purulent sputum containing streaks of blood and parasite eggs are the characteristic features of pulmonary paragonimiasis. Chest pain, fever and night sweats may occur, but are not as severe as those seen in bacterial infections. In fact, about 20% of paragonimiasis patients are asymptomatic and the infection is accidentally found in routine chest X-rays.[97] Leukocytosis is not prominent and may remain within the normal range. Eosinophilia (up to 20–25%) is characteristic in the acute to subacute phases of infection, but is reduced or disappears in the chronic stage.[79] Pleural effusion and pneumothorax with marked eosinophilia in the exudate and peripheral blood is commonly seen in the acute and subacute stages of infection when the worms move around in the pleural cavity. Although pleurisy had been considered as the unique feature of *P. miyazakii* infections in Japan[96] it commonly occurs in *P. westermani*[97–99] and *P. hetrotremus*[86,100] infections.

As an extrapulmonary paragonimiasis, cutaneous involvement is not rare and presents as painless, mobile subcutaneous swellings, most frequently on the abdomen or anterior chest. Immature worms are frequently found in surgically resected tissues. In *P. skrjabini* (including *P. miyazakii*) infections, the frequency of cutaneous involvement is relatively high and adult worms rarely mature in the lungs to cause parenchymal lesion. Cutaneous involvement is also seen in *P. westermani*[101] and *P. heterotremus*[102] infections, often associated with the lung lesions. Migration of *Paragonimus* worms into the central nervous system is rare but causes serious conditions and is occasionally fatal. During the acute phase of infection, eosinophilic meningo-encephalomyelitis can occur depending on the sites affected. In the chronic stage, the disease is characterized by convulsions of the focal Jacksonian type, often associated with hemiplegia and/or visual impairment with insidious onset.[103,104] Eosinophilic peritonitis[105] and liver abscess[106] have been reported in extremely rare cases.

Diagnosis and Investigations

The clinical signs are fairly pathognomonic, particularly when diet history and residence in an endemic area are confirmed, but misdiagnosis is common due to unfamiliarity with the disease.[97] The signs mimic pulmonary tuberculosis or lung cancer. Skin tests and sputum smear/culture are helpful in differentiation from pulmonary tuberculosis. Eggs of *Paragonimus* may be found in the faeces, sputum, bronchoalveolar washings, and rarely in plural effusion or tissue. Eggs can be found easily in the direct smear of bloody sputum, but are often missed when high-power magnification is used for cytological screening of malignancy. Although the detection of eggs in sputum/faeces is still the gold standard of diagnosis, the detection rate may be 50–70%, or lower in light infections. Immunodiagnostic tests using parasite antigens are highly sensitive and useful for surveys and in laboratory diagnosis. ELISA detects early as well as chronic infection and titres decline rapidly after cure. These tests therefore assist in assessing cure following treatment.

Radiological investigations, particularly plain radiography and computed tomography, are useful in diagnosing pulmonary disease. Lesions typically show a nodular or ring shadow, patchy infiltration and cavities.[97–99] In computed tomography, lung parenchymal lesions are often continued with pleura, showing the route of migration. In the case of chronic cerebral paragonimiasis, a 'soap bubble appearance' of dilated ventricles and multiple dense calcification and calcified cystic lesions are characteristic features.[96,107] Magnetic resonance images of the brain revealed conglomerates of multiple ring-like enhancements in the cerebral hemisphere of the brain.[107]

Management

Long regimens of bithionol, totalling 10–15 doses of 30 mg/kg body weight on alternate days, and niclofan (2 mg/kg, single dose) were used until the 1980s, but now praziquantel is a drug of choice, with a course of 3×25 mg/kg body weight/day for 3 consecutive days being nearly 100% effective against all species.[97] Side-effects are usually mild and pulmonary abnormalities decrease within 2–4 months. Urticaria may occur after praziquantel treatment for pulmonary disease. As an alternative, the efficacy of triclabendazole has been evaluated with some promising results, but was less effective in the Philippines[108] and Japan,[109] where *P. westermani* is endemic.

Prevention and Control

In addition to drug treatment, health education to discourage the consumption of raw crustaceans is recommended, particularly addressing the special danger of infection to children. Increased recognition of the problem by health workers and the population may facilitate earlier treatment and dietary change. Health promotion messages should be taken into consideration as regards beliefs in the medicinal properties of raw crabs, plus the inability of rapid dry cooking or soaking in brine, soy sauce or alcohol to kill the parasites.

REFERENCES

2. Keiser J, Utzinger J. Food-borne trematodiases. Clin Microbiol Rev 2009;22(3):466–83.
6. IARC. IARC Monographs on the Evaluation of Carcinogenic Risks to Humans. International Agency for Research on Cancer; 2011. p. 347–71.
11. Sripa B, Kaewkes S, Sithithaworn P, et al. Liver fluke induces cholangiocarcinoma. PLoS Med 2007;4(7):e201.
32. Mairiang E, Laha T, Bethony JM, et al. Ultrasonography assessment of hepatobiliary abnormalities in 3359 subjects with *Opisthorchis viverrini* infection in endemic areas of Thailand. Parasitol Int 2012;61(1):208–11.
42. Keiser J, Utzinger J. Chemotherapy for major food-borne trematodes: a review. Expert Opin Pharmacother 2004;5(8):1711–26.

Access the complete references online at www.expertconsult.com

The Filariases

PAUL E. SIMONSEN | PETER U. FISCHER | ACHIM HOERAUF | GARY J. WEIL

KEY POINTS

- Filarial worms are thread-like nematode parasites that are transmitted by insects that feed on blood. The most important filarial diseases are lymphatic filariasis and onchocerciasis, which are major causes of disability in the tropics. Although filarial diseases are uncommon in travellers, they are significant public health problems that impair the quality of life and retard economic growth in endemic communities and countries.
- Available medications can kill some species of filarial parasites, but they cannot reverse advanced clinical manifestations of filarial infections such as blindness or elephantiasis. On the other hand, simple methods have been developed for lymphoedema management that reduce the frequency of filarial fever attacks and often lead to significant improvement in patients with severe lymphoedema or elephantiasis.
- Most filarial parasite species contain intracellular bacteria called *Wolbachia* that are required for parasite development and reproduction. Antibiotic treatments that clear *Wolbachia* can sterilize and eventually kill adult filarial worms that contain *Wolbachia*.
- Large-scale programmes are using donated drugs to control and, in some cases, actually eliminate onchocerciasis and lymphatic filariasis in many disease-endemic countries. In the short term, mass drug administration programmes cure infections and prevent disease. However, the long-term goal of these programmes is global elimination of onchocerciasis and lymphatic filariasis.
- Dracunculiasis (Guinea worm) is a disabling parasitic disease caused by the nematode *Dracunculus medinensis*. People become infected when they drink water that is contaminated by small copepods that harbour larval parasites. A large public health programme has eliminated the transmission of Guinea worm infection from most countries in recent years. It is likely that dracunculiasis will be the first infectious disease to be eradicated without a vaccine or a specific medical treatment.

Introduction

The filariases result from infection with vector-borne tissue-dwelling nematodes, called filariae. The interesting history of the discovery of these parasites, their life cycles and modes of transmission has been reviewed elsewhere.[1]

Different species of adult filarial worms live in lymphatic vessels, blood vessels, skin, connective tissues or serous cavities. Adult females produce larvae (microfilariae) that live in the bloodstream or skin. All true filariae that infect humans (superfamily Filarioidea; family Onchocercidae) are transmitted by dipteran vectors. The guinea worm (superfamily Dracunculoidea) is not a true filaria, but it is included in this chapter as a related nematode with an arthropod intermediate host. A summary of the common filarial worms infecting humans and the common disease symptoms they cause is provided in Table 54.1. In addition to these, several filarial parasites of animals occasionally infect humans. The transmission of human filariae is confined to warm climates, a high temperature being necessary for parasite development in the vectors.

A general pattern of the life cycle of all filarial species is shown in Figure 54.1. Details for the species that infect humans are provided in the following sections. The infective form is the third-stage larva, which is transmitted by the vector. The rate of growth and differentiation of worms and longevity of both microfilariae and adult worms differ markedly between different species. Some adult worms may live as long as 20 years. Each filarial species requires specific arthropod and mammalian hosts for growth and maturation. Most species of filariae that infect humans contain obligatory endosymbiotic *Wolbachia* bacteria that are essential for development and reproduction of their nematode hosts.[2,3] *Wolbachia* are suspected to play a role in triggering filarial inflammatory pathology. As described later in the chapter, they also represent a promising target for development of new anti-filarial agents.

Lymphatic filariasis and onchocerciasis are the most important filarial infections in terms of public health impact, and massive international programmes have been set up to control or eliminate these diseases. These programmes hope to mirror the success of the guinea worm eradication programme, which has all but eliminated that once-dreaded parasite.

Lymphatic Filariasis

Lymphatic filariasis is a disfiguring chronic disease that is a major cause of disability in the developing world. A massive programme coordinated by the World Health Organization aims at global elimination of lymphatic filariasis by 2020.[4] Three species of lymphatic dwelling filarial worms (*Wuchereria bancrofti*, *Brugia malayi* and *B. timori*) cause lymphatic filariasis in humans. The parasites are transmitted by mosquitoes (*Anopheles*, *Culex*, *Aedes* and *Mansonia* spp.). Infection with *W. bancrofti* is also known as bancroftian filariasis, while brugian filariasis refers to infection by the other two species. *W. bancrofti* is geographically much more widespread than the *Brugia* spp.

TABLE 54.1 **Characteristics of Filarial Parasites and Guinea Worm and Common Clinical Manifestations in Humans**

Species	Distribution	Vectors	Main Location of Adult Worms	Main Location of Microfilariae	Common Disease Symptoms
Wuchereria bancrofti	Tropics	Mosquito spp.	Lymphatic vessels	Blood	Lymphangitis, elephantiasis hydrocele
Brugia malayi	South and South-east Asia	Mosquito spp.	Lymphatic vessels	Blood	Lymphangitis, elephantiasis
Brugia timori	Eastern Indonesia, Timor Leste	Mosquito spp.	Lymphatic vessels	Blood	Lymphangitis, elephantiasis
Loa loa	Central and West Africa	*Chrysops* spp.	Connective tissue	Blood	Angioedema, "eye worm"
Mansonella perstans	Africa, Central and South America	*Culicoides* spp.	Serous membranes of body cavities	Blood	Usually symptomless
Mansonella streptocerca	Central and West Africa	*Culicoides* spp.	Skin	Skin	Usually symptomless
Mansonella ozzardi	Central and South America	*Culicoides* spp. *Simulium* spp.	Serous membranes of body cavities	Blood and skin	Usually symptomless
Onchocerca volvulus	Africa, Yemen, Central and South America	*Simulium* spp.	Skin	Skin	Rash, pruritus, papules, skin atrophy, nodules, visual impairment and blindness
Dracunculus medinensis	Africa	Copepods	Connective tissue, including skin	Not applicable	Pain, ulceration, emerging worm

EPIDEMIOLOGY

Geographical Distribution

The geographical distribution of lymphatic filariasis is shown in Figure 54.2. *W. bancrofti* occurs in tropical regions of Asia, Africa, the Americas and the Pacific and is particularly prevalent in areas with hot and humid climates. *B. malayi* is found in South-east Asia and in South-western India (Kerala), whereas *B. timori* is limited to islands in eastern Indonesia.

In 1997, it was estimated that at least 128 million individuals were infected with filarial parasites (115 million with *W. bancrofti* and 13 million with the *Brugia* spp.).[5] Most of these infections were in India (48 million) and sub-Saharan Africa (51 million). These numbers were probably underestimates, because later surveys found that infection rates were much higher than expected in many areas. Population growth and mass treatment programmes have clouded the picture so that we do not have good estimates of the number of people infected or the number of people with clinically evident filariasis in the world at this time. Lymphatic filariasis disappeared with improvements in sanitation and housing in North America and Australia in the early twentieth century. More recently, Japan, Korea and China eliminated the disease with intensive control campaigns that complemented improved economic and social conditions.[6,7] Filariasis continues to be a major public health problem in Southern and Southeast Asian countries. However, prevalence rates in many of these areas are decreasing, due to rapidly escalating activities of the Global Programme to Eliminate Lymphatic Filariasis (GPELF).[4] As a counterpoint to this progress, unplanned urbanization with poor sanitary and sewerage facilities provides favourable conditions for vector breeding and transmission of urban lymphatic filariasis in many countries.

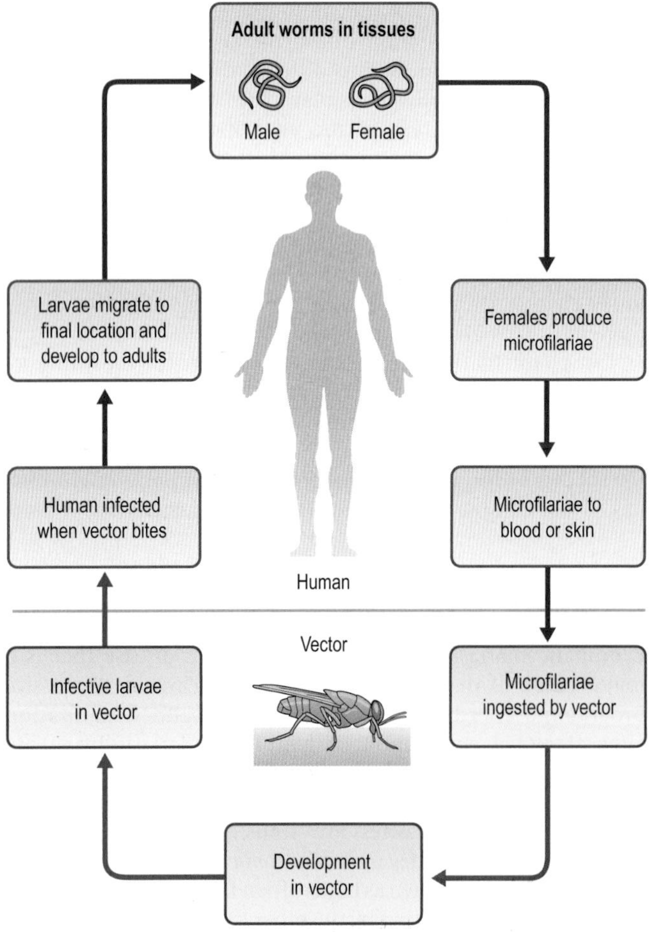

Figure 54.1 General life cycle of filariae.

Life Cycle

The adult worms reside in lymphatic vessels of the human host. Female *W. bancrofti* measure 80–100×0.25 mm and males 40×0.1 mm; adult *Brugia* spp. are about half as long. A female:male ratio of 4.5 has been reported from surgically removed adult *W. bancrofti*.[8] Microfilariae develop from eggs in the uterus of the female worm, and they are released in lymphatic vessels that drain into veins. They are sheathed and measure on average 260×8 μm (Figures 54.3–54.5). Microfilariae are ingested by female mosquito vectors during blood meals. They ex-sheath in the mosquito stomach and become first-stage larvae that penetrate the stomach wall of the

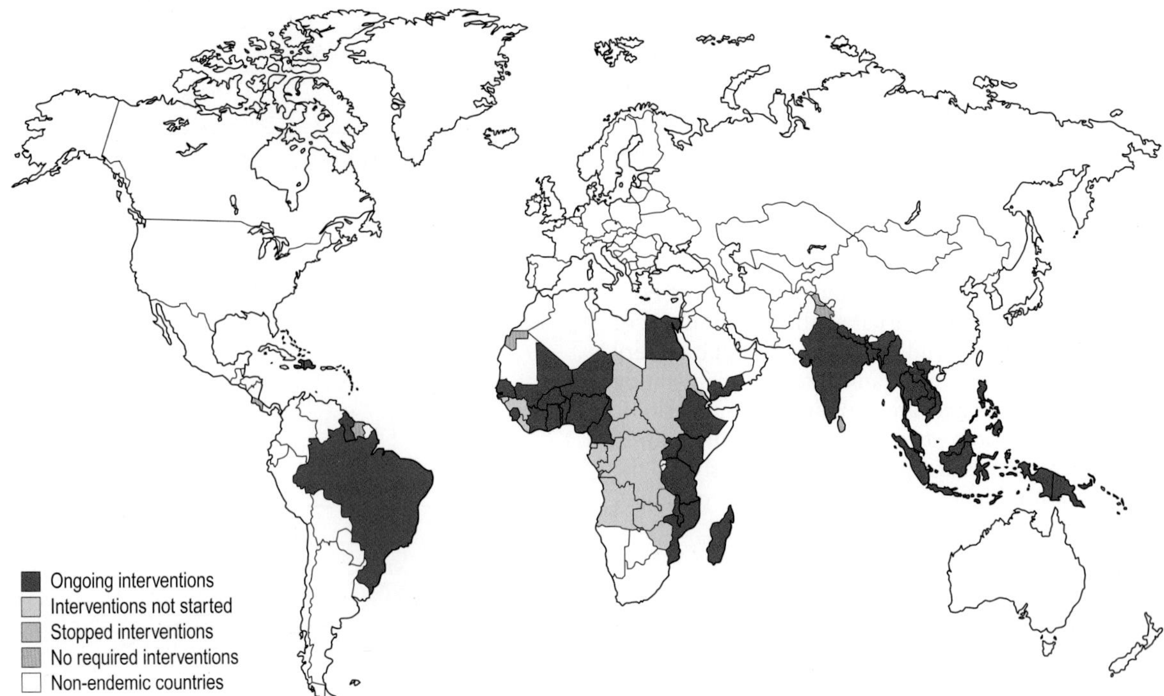

Figure 54.2 Geographical distribution of human lymphatic filariasis, and current status of national filariasis elimination programmes. *(Adapted from WHO. Lymphatic filariasis: Progress report 2000–2009 and strategic plan 2010–2020. Geneva, Switzerland: World Health Organization 2010 WHO/HTM/PCT/2010.6.)*

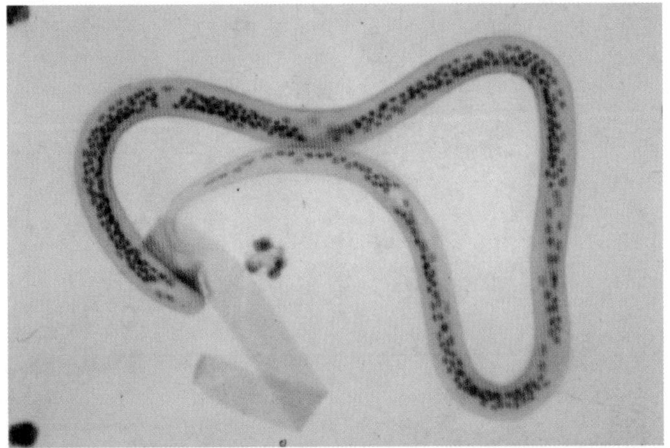

Figure 54.3 Microfilaria of *W. bancrofti* in thin blood film (haematoxylin stain).

mosquito and migrate to its thoracic muscles. There they develop through two moults to become infective third-stage larvae (1500×20 μm). The rates of development in the mosquito vary with ambient temperatures and takes a minimum of 10–12 days. Mature infective larvae migrate to the mouthparts of the mosquito from where they enter the skin of the human host, probably through the puncture wound made by the proboscis of the mosquito when it takes its blood meal. The larvae migrate to the lymphatics and develop over a period of months to become adult worms. Microfilariae appear in the blood after a minimum of 8 months in *W. bancrofti* and 3 months in *B. malayi*. The adult worms may live and produce microfilariae for more than 20 years, but their average lifespan is much shorter. Microfilariae have a lifespan of approximately 1 year. Microfilarial densities are usually between 1 and 1000/mL of blood, but they may reach 10 000/mL.

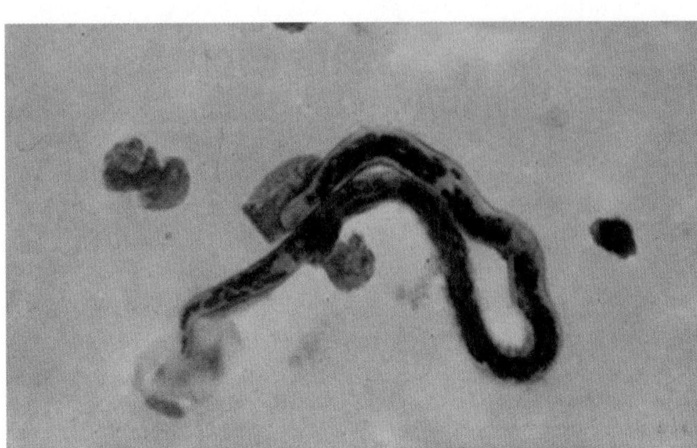

Figure 54.4 Microfilaria of *B. malayi* in thick blood film (Giemsa).

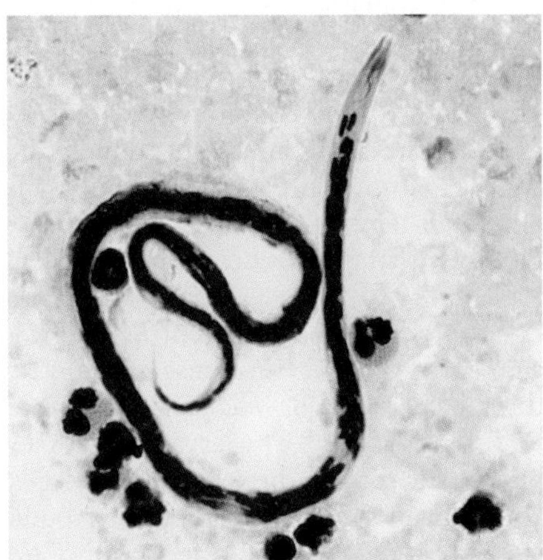

Figure 54.5 Microfilaria of *B. timori* in a thick blood film (Giemsa).

Microfilarial Periodicity

Microfilaria counts in the peripheral blood of the host vary at different times of the day and night. The periodicity patterns reflect the biting habits of the principal mosquito vector that transmits the parasites in an area. This adaptation enhances the likelihood of microfilariae being ingested and transmitted by vector mosquitoes. Periodicity is termed 'nocturnal' or 'diurnal', depending on whether the highest microfilarial density over a 24-hour period occurs during the night or the day (Figure 54.6). In most areas, the periodicity of both *W. bancrofti* and *B. malayi* is nocturnal, with peak numbers of microfilariae in the blood around midnight and none or very few at midday.[9] The parasites are transmitted by night-biting mosquitoes in these areas. There are also diurnally subperiodic and nocturnally subperiodic strains of *W. bancrofti* and *B. malayi* whose microfilariae are present continuously in the peripheral blood with higher counts during day or night, respectively (Figure 54.6).

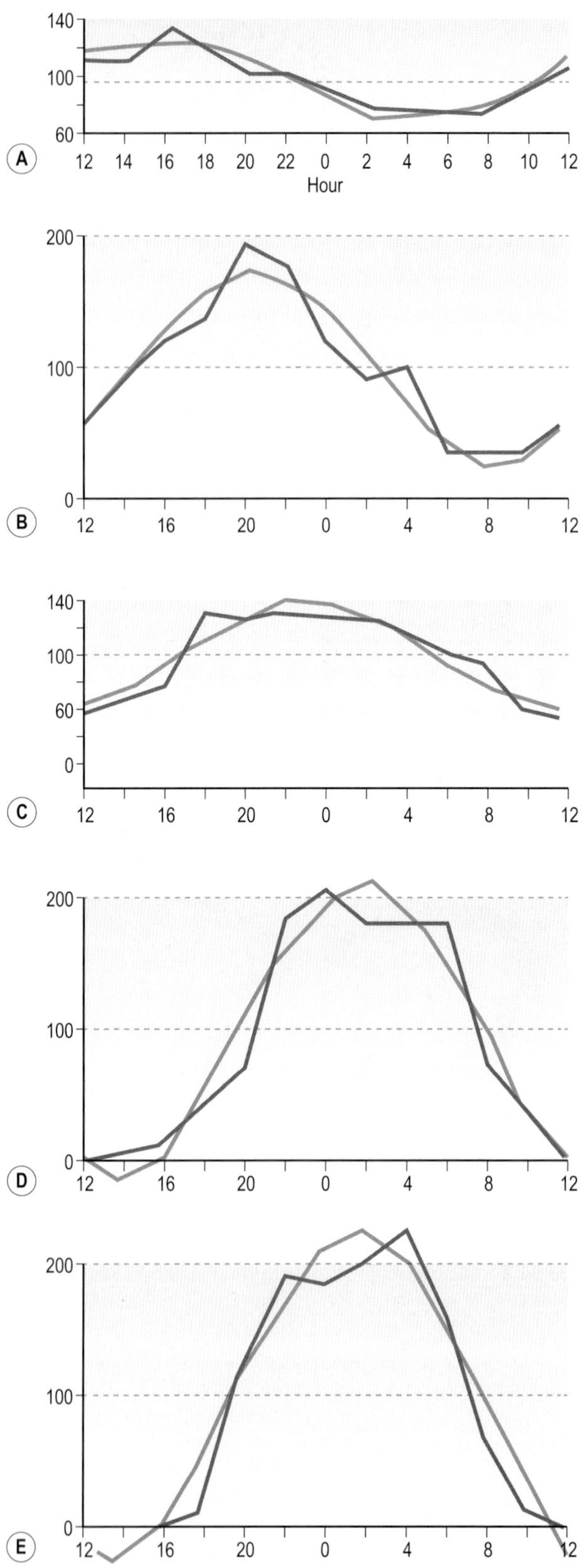

Figure 54.6 Observed (blue lines) and theoretical (green lines) periodicity of microfilariae in peripheral blood. (A) Diurnally subperiodic *W. bancrofti* in the South Pacific. (B) Nocturnally subperiodic *W. bancrofti* from west Thailand. (C) Nocturnally subperiodic *B. malayi* in the Philippines. (D) Nocturnally periodic *B. malayi* in Malaysia. (E) Nocturnally periodic *W. bancrofti* in Malaysia. *(Reproduced from Control of Lymphatic Filariasis. A Manual for Health Personnel. Geneva: WHO; ©1987.)*

Transmission

Humans are infected by mosquitoes that carry infective filarial third-stage larvae (L3). The epidemiology of filariasis varies in different geographical areas, especially with respect to infection prevalence rates and intensities, transmission patterns and clinical manifestations. Regional differences in vectorial capacity and mosquito density influence these epidemiological parameters.[10] The distribution of filariasis is often highly focal so that infection and transmission rates in a community may vary in different sectors and even from one household to the next.[11]

Geographical vector zones have been recognized for filariasis based on the predominant vector species responsible for transmission. *Culex quinquefasciatus* is the principal vector of *W. bancrofti* in urban and semiurban areas of southern and Southeast Asia, East Africa and in the Americas.[12] Increased pollution of freshwater and the introduction of pit latrines that favour breeding of this mosquito have led to increased transmission in many areas. *Cx. quinquefasciatus* mosquitoes tend to feed on humans indoors at night. *Anopheles* spp. are the main vectors for lymphatic filariasis in rural areas of Asia and Africa, with *An. funestus* and the *An. gambiae* complex being the most important vectors in Africa. These species also tend to bite indoors at night, and they breed in open, clean, water. Night-biting *Anopheles* mosquitoes are also the principal vectors for nocturnally periodic filariasis in Papua New Guinea and in parts of Indonesia.

The predominant mosquito vectors for *W. bancrofti* in islands in the South Pacific region are day-biting *Aedes* spp., especially *Ae. polynesiensis* and microfilarial periodicity is diurnally subperiodic in this region. *Aedes* mosquitoes bite outdoors and breed in small temporary water collections such as tree holes, used empty containers, coconut shells, plant axils and crab holes.

The nocturnally subperiodic form of *B. malayi* is transmitted by *Mansonia* mosquitoes in dense swampy forest areas, while nocturnally periodic *B. malayi* is transmitted by both *Mansonia* and *Anopheles* spp. The larvae and pupae of *Mansonia* spp. obtain their oxygen directly from the cells of certain species of aquatic plants present in clean water-bodies. *An. barbirostris* is the only known mosquito vector for *B. timori*, which also has nocturnal periodicity.[13]

Microfilariae of all three lymphatic dwelling filarial species can be transmitted by blood transfusions. Although transfused microfilariae do not develop further in humans, they may circulate in the recipient's blood for some weeks before they die. Congenital transmission of microfilariae has also been reported, but this is uncommon and it has no clinical significance. There is no evidence that animals are infected with *W. bancrofti* under natural conditions. The nocturnally periodic form of *B. malayi* has been reported only in humans, but the subperiodic form is found also in domestic and wild animals (monkeys, cats). There is no known animal reservoir for *B. timori*.

Infection and Disease in Endemic Communities

Characteristic patterns of microfilaraemia, adult worm infection and disease are seen in populations in filariasis-endemic areas.[10] An example from a highly endemic area in East Africa is shown in Figure 54.7. Usually, microfilaraemia starts to appear in children at about 5 years of age in areas with high transmission rates. Prevalence rates rise with increasing age and level out above age 30. Microfilaria prevalence rates rarely exceed 40% in any age group and they sometimes decrease slightly in older persons. Prevalence rates for circulating filarial antigenaemia (a molecular marker of adult worm infection) are higher than those for microfilaraemia in all age groups. Acute manifestations of filariasis typically begin to appear around the onset of puberty or in early adult life. Hydroceles also begin to develop in males at this time. Prevalence rates for clinical disease rise steadily with age, and in highly endemic areas the majority of elderly males may have hydroceles. Severe lymphoedema and elephantiasis are more common in adults, but younger persons may also be affected. The overall burden of infection and disease in endemic communities tends to be proportional to infection rates and the intensity of transmission, but this is not always the case.

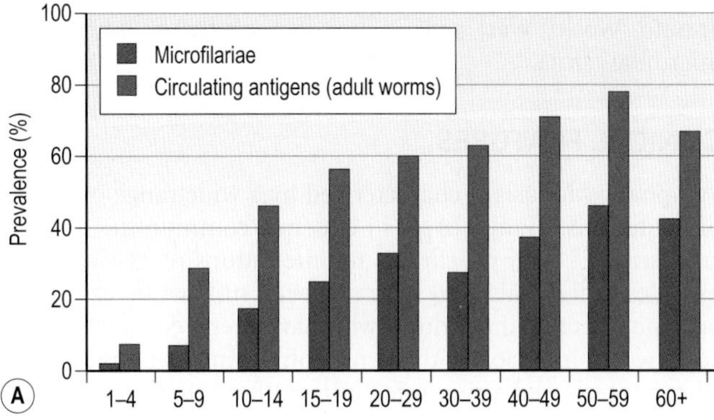

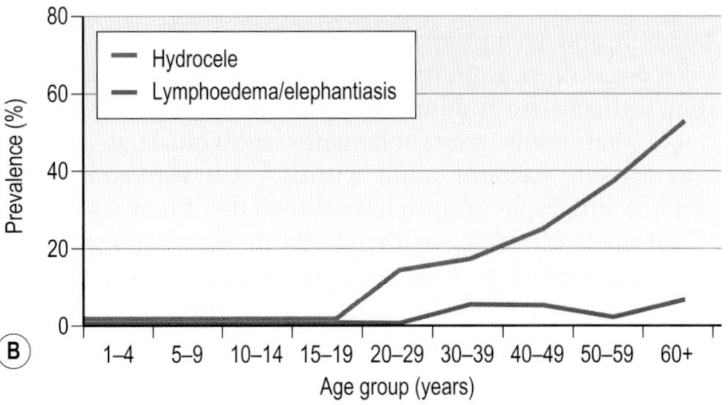

Figure 54.7 The pattern of *W. bancrofti* infection and chronic disease as seen in an endemic village on the coast of north-east Tanzania. Prevalence of (A) microfilaraemia and circulating filarial antigenaemia among all and (B) prevalence of hydrocele grade 2 and above among males and lymphoedema/elephantiasis among all. *(Based on Simonsen PE, Meyrowitsch DW, Jaoko WG, et al. Bancroftian filariasis infection, disease and specific antibody response patterns in a high and a low endemicity community in East Africa. Am J Trop Med Hyg 2002;66: 550–559.)*

Cross-sectional surveys can provide important information on the distribution of infection and disease in affected populations. However, they provide an incomplete, static view of a dynamic situation. Some people who are uninfected when a survey is performed may have been infected previously. Also, people with clinical filariasis often lack evidence of current infection with the parasite. However, a 26-year follow-up survey indicated that once infection has been acquired, the chance of ever becoming naturally free of infection is small.[14] Microfilaria prevalence rates and counts in blood tend to be higher in males than in females and this appears to be especially significant for those aged 15–40 years. It has been suggested that hormonal factors in females of reproductive age make them more resistant to infection than males of the same age group.[15] Exposure to intense transmission over long periods is necessary before a patent infection (with microfilaraemia) can be established; short-term visitors to endemic areas rarely acquire microfilaraemia. However, migrants from non-endemic areas who are first heavily exposed to filariasis as adults sometimes develop acute clinical manifestations of filariasis and accelerated disease progression. Prenatal exposure to parasite antigens (with induction of immune tolerance) may explain why children born to microfilaraemic mothers appear to have a higher chance of developing microfilaraemia in later life than children born to amicrofilaraemic mothers.[16] However, increased household exposure may also be a contributing factor. Susceptibility to infection also appears to be affected by the host's genotype.[17]

PATHOGENESIS AND PATHOLOGY

Overview

Most of the pathology in lymphatic filariasis is associated with the adult worms and their location in lymphatic vessels. A wide range of clinical manifestations is seen in endemic regions. Some people with no obvious signs of infection or disease are uninfected (so-called 'endemic normal individuals'), while others without symptoms have microfilaraemia ('asymptomatic microfilaria carriers'). Other people in endemic areas experience acute lymphadenitis and lymphangitis in response to infection. A subset of these people go on to develop chronic lymphatic pathology. People with asymptomatic infections are relatively tolerant to filarial worms and most of these will remain infected without symptoms for years. People who mount vigorous inflammatory responses to filarial worms kill the parasites with collateral damage to lymphatic vessels. This explains why most patients with chronic lymphoedema are amicrofilaraemic and have negative filarial antigen tests. Patients with tropical pulmonary eosinophilia (TPE) have exaggerated immune responses to microfilariae with immune clearance of the parasites in the lung.

The pathogenesis of lymphatic filariasis has long been a matter of debate. Many studies have tried to correlate immune responses with infection or disease phenotypes.[18–21] Persons with microfilaraemia tend to have decreased immune responses to co-infecting pathogens[22] and to some vaccines.[23] Immunologists have postulated that patients with asymptomatic microfilaraemia may experience loss of immune tolerance to filarial worms with activation of host protective immune responses that lead to death of the parasites with collateral damage to lymphatic vessels. However, several lines of evidence have challenged the idea of a central role for immunity as a driver for filarial pathogenesis. First, epidemiological data show that microfilaraemia rates tend to be similar in individuals with and without chronic clinical filariasis in most endemic communities.[10,24] Second, several studies have noted that host immune responses are more closely related to the host's infection status than to his/her disease phenotype.[25,26]

Two different pathological pathways may lead to clinically evident filariasis.[27] The first pathway emphasizes dilatation of lymphatic vessels (lymphangiectasia) as the key lesion that precedes the development of clinically evident filariasis. Lymphangiectasia is present in virtually all individuals with adult filarial worms and this is true regardless of the person's microfilaraemia status and regardless of whether or not they have clinically evident filariasis. Filarial worms appear to be capable of inducing endothelial cell proliferation and lymphatic dilatation via mechanisms that do not involve lymphatic obstruction. Dilatation may result from host proteins such as vascular endothelial growth factors, angiopoietin and matrix metalloproteinase.[28] Worm products may also play a role, since recent studies have shown that worm antigens induce proliferation of cultured lymphatic endothelial cells.[29] Proinflammatory products released from endosymbiotic *Wolbachia* bacteria (which are abundant in *W. bancrofti* and *B. malayi* adult worms), have also been suspected to play a role in the pathogenesis of clinical filariasis.[30] Lymphangiectasia caused by adult worms impairs lymphatic function and predisposes the host to microbial infections that may present as acute dermatolymphangioadenitis (ADLA). This is frequently accompanied by oedema in the affected extremity and repeated attacks of ADLA can lead to chronic lymphoedema.[27] Thus, recurrent secondary bacterial and fungal infections that are facilitated by entry lesions in the skin are believed to be important co-factors in the development of filarial lymphoedema and elephantiasis.[31,32]

The second pathway to clinically evident filariasis is driven by the death of adult filarial worms, either naturally or after drug treatment. Parasite death triggers acute inflammatory reactions in lymphatic vessels and regional lymph nodes; these episodes are called acute filarial lymphangitis (AFL). AFL episodes are typically less severe than ADLA and they rarely lead to long-term lymphoedema. AFL attacks in intrascrotal lymphatic vessels can cause acute hydroceles with temporary impairment of the lymphatic flow from the tunica vaginalis.[33] Most acute hydroceles disappear within a short time. The risk factors for progression to chronic hydrocele are still unclear, but they probably include direct effects of adult worms on lymphatic vessels, effects of increased hydrostatic pressure on the local anatomy, granuloma formation and rupture of dilated lymphatic vessels.[34]

In contrast to lymphoedema and hydrocele, there is more consensus regarding the central role of immunity in the pathogenesis of TPE. Patients with TPE have exaggerated immune responses directed against microfilariae and filarial antigens. TPE patients have very high serum levels of filaria-specific IgG and IgE antibodies and marked peripheral blood eosinophilia. Lung biopsies from TPE patients have shown inflammatory foci around degenerating microfilariae. These findings, together with the absence of circulating microfilariae, suggest that microfilariae are cleared and killed in the lungs of TPE patients. Their symptoms and pathology are caused by inflammatory responses to dying parasites and pathological effects of substances released by eosinophils and other cells in the lung.

Protective immunity is poorly understood in human filariasis. Animals develop partial immunity to new infections after repeated injections with small numbers of infective larvae or after immunization with irradiated infective larvae or certain recombinant larval antigens. Filarial infection rates in humans do not fall dramatically in older age groups, but their failure to rise to 100% suggests the possibility that some people may either be innately resistant to infection or that they develop protective immunity after repeated exposure to the parasite. One longitudinal study reported that younger people acquired new infections at a higher rate than older people.[35] The effects of human immunodeficiency virus (HIV) infection on concurrent lymphatic filariasis and vice versa are largely unknown.

Visitors to filariasis-endemic areas sometimes acquire infections with filarial worms, but they rarely develop microfilaraemia. Expatriates who are exposed to intense transmission may develop symptoms of filariasis faster than lifelong residents of the endemic area. The experience of the American military helps to illustrate these points. Thousands of cases of acute bancroftian filariasis were diagnosed in American soldiers who served in the South western Pacific region during the Second World War; only a handful of these patients had microfilaraemia.[36]

CLINICAL FEATURES

Lymphatic filariasis is characterized by a wide range of clinical presentations. Many people in endemic communities are amicrofilaraemic with no clinical manifestations of filariasis. This includes individuals who have not been sufficiently exposed to become infected, individuals who have prepatent infections or adult worm infection without microfilaraemia, and individuals who have cleared prior infections. Other people in endemic communities have circulating microfilariae but no symptoms or signs of disease. Some members of this group remain microfilaraemic and asymptomatic for many years.

Recent surveys employing diagnostic tests that detect circulating antigens from adult *W. bancrofti* worms have demonstrated that many amicrofilaraemic individuals in endemic areas actually harbour adult worms.[10] Ultrasonography and lymphoscintigraphy studies have shown that many asymptomatic infected individuals (with or without microfilaraemia) have subclinical pathology such as lymphangiectasis (dilatation of lymphatic vessels).[37,38] Clinically evident filariasis (acute and chronic) can occur in persons with or without evidence of currently active infection.

Bancroftian Filariasis

The most common clinical manifestations of bancroftian filariasis are acute adenolymphangitis, hydrocele, lymphoedema and elephantiasis. Chyluria and tropical pulmonary eosinophilia are less common. Although frequent in males, genital manifestations such as oedema of the labia majora are uncommon in females.[39]

Acute Manifestations. Acute manifestations of filariasis ('filarial fever') include ADLA and AFL (as described in the pathogenesis section, above). ADLA attacks are episodic events that start with malaise, fever and chills. Tender, enlarged lymph nodes drain the affected part (usually the lower limb), which may become warm and swollen. ADLA events usually resolve spontaneously after about a week, but they often recur several times per year. Regression of the swelling after an ADLA attack of the leg is commonly followed by superficial skin exfoliation.[40] Repeated episodes of ADLA can lead to chronic lymphoedema and elephantiasis. However, some patients with advanced disease do not report a history of prior episodes suggestive of ADLA.

In contrast to ADLA, acute filarial lymphangitis (AFL) is believed to be triggered by parasite death, which may occur spontaneously or after treatment. AFL presents as a circumscribed inflammatory nodule or cord centred around degenerating adult worms, with lymphangitis spreading in a descending (centrifugal) fashion. It usually has a mild clinical course and AFL rarely results in chronic lymphoedema.

ADLA and AFL episodes commonly involve the genitals in males and present as acute funiculitis, epididymitis and/or orchitis. These acute attacks may be unilateral or bilateral and they can occur in individuals with or without involvement of the extremities.

Hydrocele. Hydrocele is the most common chronic clinical abnormality in men with bancroftian filariasis. It results from the accumulation of clear straw-coloured fluid in the tunica vaginalis surrounding the testicles. The onset may be silent (i.e. without accompanying acute episodes), or it may be preceded by one or more attacks of funiculitis or epididymo-orchitis. The swelling around the testis may completely disappear after the first few acute episodes. However, over time the tunica vaginalis becomes thickened and there is progressive enlargement of the hydrocele (Figures 54.8 and 54.9). Most cases are unilateral, but bilateral involvement, often with different sizes on the two sides, is not uncommon. Rarely, the fluid may have a milky appearance if lymph fluid from a ruptured abdominal lymphatic vessel pours into the hydrocele to form a chylocele. Hydroceles can be graded according to their developmental stage and size.[41] Ultrasound studies have shown that many males in endemic areas with normal clinical examinations have subclinical hydroceles.[42,43] Ultrasonography is also useful for measuring and differentiating various types of filarial hydroceles.[44]

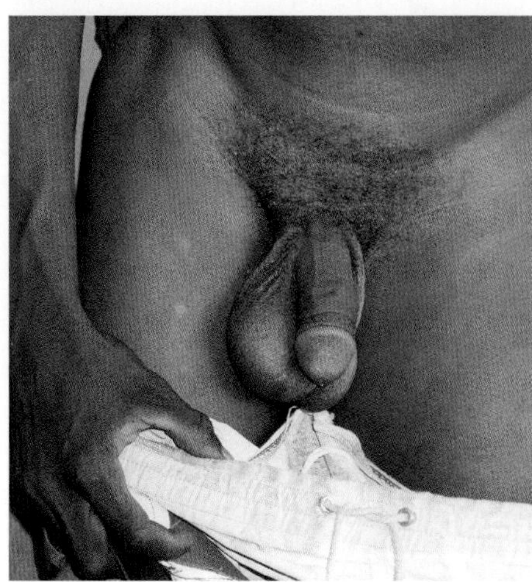

Figure 54.8 Lymphatic filariasis: early hydrocele (*W. bancrofti*).

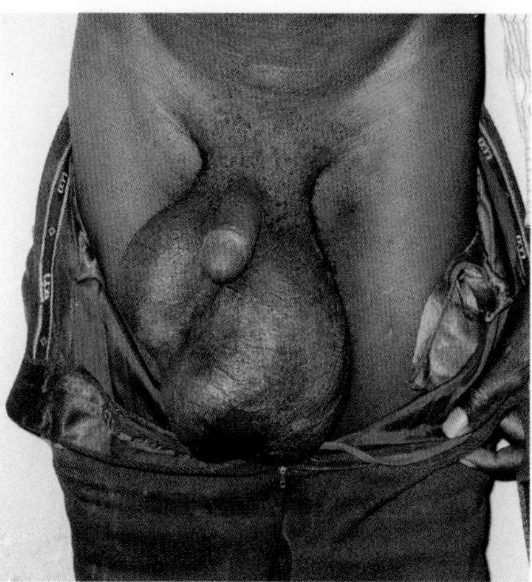

Figure 54.9 Lymphatic filariasis: advanced hydrocele (*W. bancrofti*).

Lymphoedema and Elephantiasis. Chronic lymphoedema and elephantiasis most commonly affect the lower legs (Figures 54.10 and 54.11). The arms, scrotum, penis, vulva and breasts are less commonly affected.

Lymphoedema usually starts on one side, but it often becomes bilateral. Early lymphoedema presents with loss of contour around the ankles. Limbs often return to normal after initial attacks. Over a period of years, the oedema may become non-pitting with thickening of the skin and loss of skin elasticity. Further progression leads to elephantiasis with deep skin folds, dermatosclerosis and papillomatous lesions. Secondary bacterial and fungal infections are common in lymphoedematous limbs and these probably exacerbate the progression of

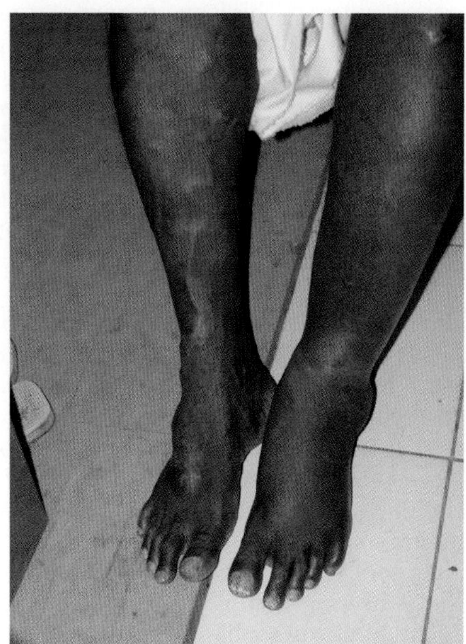

Figure 54.10 Lymphatic filariasis: early-stage lymphoedema of left leg (*W. bancrofti*).

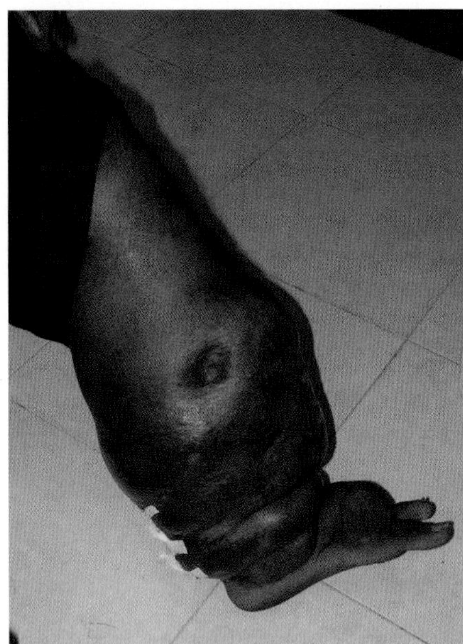

Figure 54.11 Lymphatic filariasis: advanced-stage elephantiasis of left leg (*W. bancrofti*).

elephantiasis. In severe cases pus may ooze from chronic ulcerations in the affected part and the ulcers may have a foul smell. Scarification, a common traditional treatment for body swellings in many filariasis-endemic areas, has been recognized as a risk factor for rapid progression of filarial elephantiasis.[45]

Lymphoedema of the leg is commonly classified as grade I: pitting lymphoedema, spontaneously reversible on elevation; grade II: non-pitting lymphoedema with loss of skin elasticity; grade III: obvious elephantiasis with thickening of skin and skin folds.[46] Some authorities recommend a more detailed classification with seven stages.[47]

Chyluria. Chyluria (the presence of chyle in the urine) is caused by rupture of dilated abdominal lymphatics into the urinary excretory system.[48] This is an uncommon complication of *W. bancrofti* infection. Chylous urine is milky in appearance (Figure 54.12) and blood is sometimes present. Chyluria is frequently episodic, with episodes lasting for days or weeks. The onset may be insidious or sudden. Chyle or blood clots sometimes cause urinary retention. Chyluria tends to be more pronounced in the morning or after a fatty meal. Prolonged chyluria can lead to weight loss, hypoproteinaemia, lymphopenia and anaemia.

Tropical Pulmonary Eosinophilia. Tropical pulmonary eosinophilia (TPE) is a clinical syndrome that is caused by immunological hyperresponsiveness to microfilariae in the lungs.[49,50] It occurs with low frequency in most filariasis-endemic areas. It is more common in males than in females. Microfilariae are usually absent in the blood, but they are sometimes seen in lung biopsies surrounded by inflammatory cells. Adult worms are sometimes visible in the scrotum or inguinal regions by ultrasonography. Patients present with paroxysmal coughing and wheezing that is worse at night. They have extremely high blood eosinophil counts (>3000 cells/mm^3 of blood) and very high serum levels of both total IgE and antifilarial antibodies. Chest radiographs may show focal infiltrates. Extrapulmonary manifestations such as splenomegaly, lymphadenopathy and hepatomegaly occur in some patients. Lung function is often impaired in TPE patients with reduced vital capacity, total lung capacity and residual volume. Symptoms improve in most patients after one or more courses of treatment with diethylcarbamazine. If left untreated, TPE may progress to a chronic stage with interstitial fibrosis and a permanent loss of lung function.

Other Conditions. Monoarthritis is common in filarial-endemic areas and a possible association with filariasis has long been recognized.[49,51] The knee is the most frequent joint affected and this is followed by the ankle. The joint becomes painful, warm and tender and the condition is indistinguishable from other forms of arthritis. Symptoms may improve after antifilarial treatment. Haematuria (usually microscopic) and proteinuria often accompany microfilaraemia.[49] This may be caused by immune complexes deposited on the basement membrane of the renal glomeruli. Scattered reports associate endomyocardial fibrosis, tenosynovitis, thrombophlebitis, nerve palsies and dermatoses with filariasis. These conditions sometimes co-exist with filariasis and may be atypical manifestations of other diseases conditioned by pre-existing filarial infection.

Brugian Filariasis

The main clinical difference between brugian and bancroftian filariasis is the absence of hydroceles and other genital lesions and chyluria in areas endemic for *B. malayi* and *B. timori*.[13] Lymphoedema of the legs in *Brugia* infections usually does not extend above the knee (Figure 54.13), whereas both the thigh and lower leg are often involved in bancroftian filariasis. Lymphoedema of the legs and arms seem to be both more common and less severe in brugian filariasis than in bancroftian filariasis. Acute adenitis of femoral lymph nodes is common in brugian filariasis and these may suppurate and drain pus, either spontaneously or following treatment with antifilarial medications. Scars over the femoral region from prior episodes of lymphadenitis are often seen in persons who live in areas with brugian filariasis.

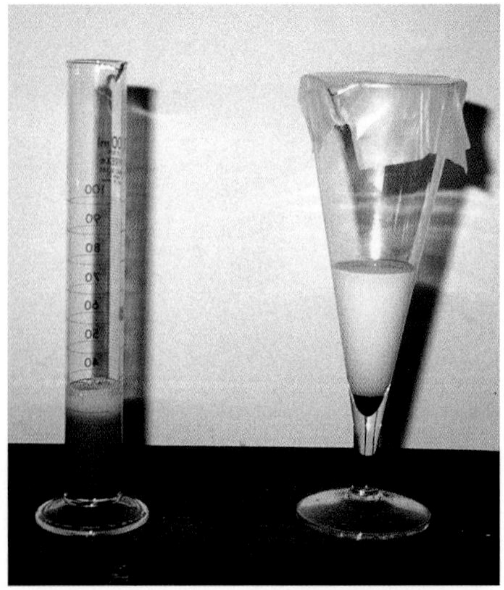

Figure 54.12 Lymphatic filariasis: chyluria – milky urine with blood. Before (left) and after (right) sedimentation.

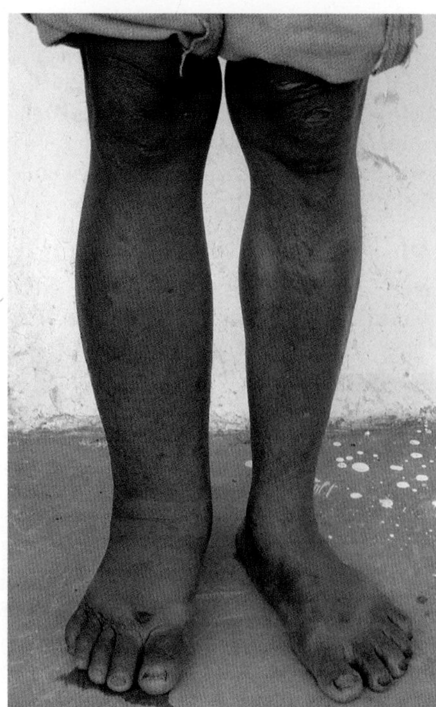

Figure 54.13 Lymphatic filariasis: lymphoedema of the right leg (*B. timori*).

Lymphatic Filariasis in Children

Although rates of clinically evident filariasis increase with age, recent studies have shown that infections with the lymphatic dwelling filariae are often acquired during childhood.[52] Children in *W. bancrofti*-endemic areas may have positive tests for circulating filarial antigenaemia without microfilaraemia. Most infected children do not have clinically evident disease, but ultrasound or lymphoscintigraphy studies sometimes show dilatation and damage of lymph vessels. These early lesions may progress to overt clinical disease over time.[53] A recent study documented improvement or complete reversal of subclinical lymphatic damage in *B. malayi*-infected children following treatment.[54]

Geographical Variation in Clinical Manifestations

Clinical manifestations of lymphatic filariasis have been reported in the past to differ considerably in different geographical areas. However, these differences have become less dramatic as examination and grading procedures have become more standardized. TPE and chyluria seem to be more common in south and South-east Asian countries; these conditions are rarely seen in Africans.[55] *W. bancrofti* microfilaria prevalence rates are very high in some areas of Papua New Guinea (60–80%). Paradoxically, clinical filariasis rates (hydrocele and lymphoedema) in these areas tend to be similar to or even lower than those seen in less highly endemic areas elsewhere in the world.[56]

Differential Diagnosis

Acute or chronic manifestations resembling those described above in individuals who live in or who have had prolonged visits to areas endemic for transmission of *W. bancrofti*, *B. malayi* or *B. timori* are strongly suggestive of lymphatic filariasis. The sudden onset of fever, accompanied by acute groin pain with swollen tender lymph glands may be difficult to distinguish from acute bacterial lymphadenitis. Filarial funiculitis and epididymitis can resemble bacterial infections in the same tissues.

Inguinal hernia is the most common scrotal swelling that needs to be distinguished from hydrocele. Unlike hydroceles, hernias can often be reduced. The diagnosis of hydrocele can often be verified by transillumination with a penlight in a dark room. Irreducible hernias and hydroceles may co-exist in the same patient. Obstructed hernias, tumours of the testis, tuberculosis and other bacterial infections of the epididymis and *Schistosoma haematobium* of the spermatic cord need to be distinguished from genital lesions caused by *W. bancrofti*.

Common conditions that need to be distinguished from filarial lymphoedema are swollen limbs due to congestive heart failure, subacute nephritis, non-filarial blockage of venous (thrombosis) or lymphatic (tuberculosis, leprosy) drainage systems and Kaposi's sarcoma. The patient's history may help to differentiate these conditions from filarial elephantiasis. The oedema of heart failure and subacute nephritis is usually painless and symmetrical (bilateral), while filariasis patients often have histories consistent with ADLA or AFL and asymmetrical swelling. Malignant lymph nodes and lymphatic obstruction due to trauma, surgery or recurrent bacterial cellulitis, may also result in elephantiasis of the limbs.

An endemic form of leg elephantiasis occurs in many parts of Africa at altitudes that preclude a filarial aetiology.[57] Silica particles from volcanic soils, absorbed through the plantar skin of bare-footed people, are believed to be the causative agents. Such non-filarial tropical elephantiasis (podoconiosis) has also been reported from South and Central America.

TPE should be differentiated from bronchial asthma and other allergic conditions, tuberculosis, paragonimiasis and eosinophilic leukaemia. TPE must also be distinguished from helminthic infections that have stages that migrate through the lungs (*Ascaris*, *Strongyloides* and *Schistosoma* spp.). A rapid improvement in symptoms after DEC therapy and a strongly positive filarial antibody test are helpful for distinguishing TPE from these other conditions.

LABORATORY DIAGNOSIS

Detection of Microfilariae

Microfilaria detection provides definitive evidence for filarial infection. In addition, microfilarial size and morphology can be used to differentiate between different filarial species. However, many patients with microfilaraemia do not have symptoms or signs of clinical filariasis and many patients with clinical filariasis are amicrofilaraemic. Also, there is no relationship between microfilaria counts in blood and disease severity. Microfilariae are often present in hydrocele fluid and they are sometimes also present in urine or other body fluids.

Blood specimens for microfilaria detection should be collected when microfilaria counts are high (e.g. between 21:00 and 03:00 hours for nocturnally periodic strains).[9] Many techniques have been described for detecting microfilariae in blood samples. The counting chamber technique is fast, quantitative and cheap.[58] An aliquot of 100 μL of finger-prick blood is added to a tube containing 0.9 mL of 3% acetic acid. Microfilariae are counted in a counting chamber using a low-power objective of a compound microscope. This technique is suitable for both routine hospital diagnosis and for field surveys in areas that are endemic for only one filarial species. This is because species identification is difficult with the counting chamber technique. Microscopic examination of stained thick blood films should be used for detecting and identifying microfilariae in areas that are endemic for multiple filarial species. Thick blood films are simple to prepare and examine, but their sensitivity may be lower than the counting chamber method, because they examine smaller volumes of blood and because microfilariae may be lost during staining. While 20 µL thick smears are often used in public health programmes, sensitivity can be increased by examination of slides with three linear 20 µL blood smears.[59] Membrane filtration and the Knott concentration method are more sensitive than routine thick blood smears for microfilaria detection, because they can be used to concentrate microfilariae from 1 mL or more of blood. However, these methods require venous blood and they are often too labour intensive (Knott) or expensive (membranes) for routine use in most endemic areas.

Microfilariae of *W. bancrofti*, *B. malayi* and *B. timori* have sheaths (Figures 54.3–54.5). Microfilariae of *W. bancrofti* measure on average 260×8 µm, whereas those of *B. malayi* are slightly shorter and can be distinguished from *W. bancrofti* by the two isolated nuclei at the tip of the tail and the absence of nuclei in the cephalic space. Microfilariae of *B. timori* are longer than those of *B. malayi* and they have an even longer nucleus-free cephalic space. Cell nuclei are more loosely spaced in microfilariae of *W. bancrofti* than in those of *Brugia*. Microscopic examination of stained blood films can also be used to differentiate microfilariae of *Loa loa*, *Mansonella perstans* and *M. ozzardi* from those of *W. bancrofti* and the *Brugia* spp.

Detection of Adult Worms by Ultrasonography

Adult *W. bancrofti* can be detected in a high percentage of infected males by ultrasonography of the scrotum.[60,61] They appear as continuously motile 'dancing worms' that are often clustered in 'worm nests' in dilated lymphatic vessels. Worm nests tend to remain in the same locations over time. Adult worms are less commonly visible in lymphatic vessels in the female breast and in the axillary and inguinal regions in males and females; *B. malayi* worms are also sometimes detectable by ultrasound in these locations.[62] Ultrasonography is also useful for assessment of hydroceles and for detecting 'subclinical hydroceles' that are not detectable by palpation.[42–44]

Detection of Filarial Parasites in Mosquitoes

Dissection with microscopy can be used to detect infection (any stage of the parasite) and infectivity (infective L3 larvae) rates in mosquitoes.[63] However, dissection is an insensitive and inefficient method for detecting filarial parasites in mosquitoes when infection rates become very low following mass drug administration.

Detection of Filarial DNA

Most assays use the polymerase chain reaction (PCR) to amplify filarial DNA sequences that are then detected by fluorometry or agarose gel electrophoresis.[64,65] Blood samples for filarial DNA detection should be collected at the same time as blood for microfilaria detection (e.g. at night in areas with nocturnally periodic filariasis). The sensitivity of DNA detection by PCR is comparable with the best microscopy methods for detecting microfilariae in blood samples. Parasite DNA detection is also superior to dissection with microscopy for detection of filarial parasites in insect vectors. Mosquito testing may be more effective for detecting human filariasis in low-endemicity settings than human blood surveys. This 'molecular xenomonitoring' has also been used to assess changes in filarial endemicity following control programmes.[66]

Detection of Circulating Filarial Antigens (CFA)

CFA tests detect antigens released by adult *W. bancrofti* worms in human blood, serum, or plasma samples. Commercially available antigen tests include a rapid format card test and an ELISA. Both of these tests are sensitive and specific for *W. bancrofti* infection and more sensitive than tests that detect microfilariae. The card test is widely used in filariasis elimination programmes for mapping endemicity and for monitoring progress.[59] Unlike tests for microfilaraemia or filarial DNA, antigen tests can be performed with blood collected during the night or day. Blood CFA levels are related to the number of adult filarial worms in the host. While filarial antigen levels decrease after treatment, CFA tests remain positive in many treated patients regardless of whether or not they have persistent microfilaraemia. There are no commercially available antigen detection tests for diagnosis of infections with the *Brugia* species.[67]

Detection of Antifilarial Antibodies

Antifilarial antibody tests that detect IgG4 subclass antibodies to recombinant filarial antigens are more specific for filariasis than earlier tests that detected IgG antibodies to native parasite antigens extracted from worms. For example, an ELISA that detects IgG4 antibodies to recombinant antigen Bm14 is sensitive for infections with *W. bancrofti* or *Brugia* infections and a rapid format cassette test for IgG4 antibodies to recombinant antigen BmR1 is sensitive for *Brugia* infections only.[59,68] These antibody tests also detect cross-reacting antibodies in sera from people with loiasis and onchocerciasis. Antibody tests have limited value for diagnosis of filariasis in individuals who live in endemic areas, because many people in such areas who do not have microfilaraemia, filarial antigenaemia, or clinical filariasis have positive antibody tests. However, some patients with clinical filariasis have burned out infections and negative antibody tests, so antibody testing cannot be used to rule out the diagnosis of clinical filariasis. Antibody testing of sentinel populations (e.g. young children) can be used to show that transmission of filariasis has been reduced or interrupted following filariasis control/elimination programmes.

Approach to Laboratory Diagnosis of Filariasis in Expatriates

Antibody or antigen testing may be the best way for non-specialists to screen for infection with lymphatic dwelling filarial parasites in expatriates with symptoms suggestive of filariasis. Many clinical laboratories do not have experience detecting microfilariae and many patients with filariasis are amicrofilaraemic.

MANAGEMENT AND TREATMENT

Drug Treatment Overview

Single-dose combination drug regimens have largely replaced traditional 12-day courses of diethylcarbamazine (DEC) for treatment of lymphatic filariasis.[69] A single dose of albendazole

(400 mg) with either DEC (6 mg/kg) or ivermectin (200 μg/kg) reduces microfilaria counts to very low levels for at least 24 months (in the absence of reinfection). Albendazole with DEC is believed to have better macrofilaricidal activity than albendazole with ivermectin. However, since DEC is contraindicated in patients with onchocerciasis, the albendazole/ivermectin regimen is preferred for treatment of lymphatic filariasis in areas that are co-endemic for onchocerciasis. Mass drug administration (MDA) programmes usually provide these medicines annually. There are no official recommendations for use of combination regimens to treat individual patients with lymphatic filariasis. However, it is reasonable to provide single-dose combination regimens at 6-month intervals until microfilaria and CFA tests are negative. There is no evidence that patients with clinically evident filariasis require more treatment than asymptomatic patients with microfilaraemia. However, for patients who live in areas with ongoing transmission, it is reasonable to repeat treatment at 6-month intervals to treat possible reinfections that might exacerbate existing lymphatic damage.

The lethal effects of antifilarial drugs on adult worms can be directly monitored in vivo by ultrasonography.[42,70] Treatment of patients with microfilaraemia (and amicrofilaraemic patients with positive CFA tests) may prevent development of lymphatic damage by killing adult worms. While some patients with early disease (pitting oedema, small hydroceles) notice clinical improvement after treatment, anti-parasite treatment may not reverse or improve advanced disease due to lymphatic damage (large hydroceles, brawny oedema or elephantiasis). The death of adult worms following treatment may trigger AFL attacks.[27] For this reason, treatment is not recommended during acute filarial fever episodes, because it may kill additional worms and further exacerbate inflammatory reactions.

Drugs Used to Treat Lymphatic Filariasis

Diethylcarbamazine citrate (DEC) has been used to treat filariasis since the 1940s. DEC kills microfilariae and it also kills a proportion of adult *W. bancrofti*, *B. malayi* and *B. timori* (Table 54.2). The mode of action of DEC is unknown. The drug does not kill microfilariae directly, but it seems to modify them so that they are cleared from the blood by the host's immune system. DEC is administered orally with food. The traditional treatment course was 6 mg/kg body weight daily for 12 days. Blood microfilaria counts decrease quickly after DEC treatment (sometimes to undetectable levels), but they tend to reappear and increase slowly a few months after treatment. CFA levels decrease after DEC treatment, but total clearance of antigenaemia is unusual after a single course of treatment. This probably indicates that some adult worms survive the treatment.[42,71]

Adverse events (AEs) are common following treatment with DEC and these may start as early as a few hours after the first dose of the drug. AEs tend to be less severe in bancroftian filariasis than in brugian filariasis.[72,73] Clinically significant AEs are not seen in uninfected individuals, so the AEs are believed to be related to systemic and local responses to dying filarial worms. Systemic AEs include fever, headache, malaise, joint and body pain, dizziness, anorexia and vomiting. The intensity of systemic AEs is correlated with microfilaria counts and the most severe reactions occur after the first treatment. Localized AEs (related to death of adult filarial worms) are less common than systemic AEs. These can include lymphadenitis (sometimes with suppuration and drainage) and transient lymphoedema. Male patients with bancroftian filariasis sometimes experience scrotal pain with funiculitis and/or epididymitis after treatment and they may develop new hydroceles that usually resolve over a period of weeks. Local AEs tend to occur later (often 1 week or more after treatment) and last longer than systemic AEs. DEC can cause severe AEs in patients with onchocerciasis and in loiasis patients with high blood microfilaria counts. DEC (6 mg/kg daily for 21 days) is effective for treating tropical pulmonary eosinophilia. Most patients respond rapidly to treatment. Symptoms recur in some patients after a period of months and these patients may benefit from retreatment.

Ivermectin (Mectizan®) is a potent microfilaricide that temporarily sterilizes adult worms of *W. bancrofti* and *B. malayi* without killing the adult worms (Table 54.2).[74] Systemic AEs after ivermectin are generally similar to those mentioned above for DEC, but localized AEs are uncommon. Ivermectin should not be used in pregnant women or in children younger than 5 years of age. The major role of ivermectin in lymphatic filariasis is for treatment and control of lymphatic filariasis in areas that are co-endemic for onchocerciasis and/or loiasis (i.e. many parts of Africa). Since it has no macrofilaricidal effect,

TABLE 54.2 Effect of Commonly Used Drugs on Microfilariae and Adult Worms of Human Filarial Parasites

Drug	Stage	*Wuchereria bancrofti* and *Brugia* spp.	*Loa loa*	*Mansonella perstans*	*Mansonella streptocerca*	*Mansonella ozzardi*	*Onchocerca volvulus*
Diethylcarbamazine	Microfilaria	++	++[a]	+	++	–	++[a]
	Adult	+	+	–	++	–	–
Ivermectin	Microfilaria	++	++[a]	–	++	++	++
	Adult	–	?	?	?	?	–?
Albendazole	Microfilaria	–	–	–	?	?	–
	Adult	+	–	–	?	?	+[b]
Doxycycline	Microfilaria	–	–	–	?	?	–
	Adult	++	–	+[c]	?	?	++

–, No effect; +, few/some are eliminated; ++, most are eliminated; ?, unknown.
[a]Severe adverse events may occur.
[b]Some effect with high doses.
[c]Assumed, because of slow reduction of microfilaraemia.

repeated annual or semi-annual treatments may be required for years to suppress microfilaraemia. Ivermectin is also effective for treating *Ascaris*, onchocerciasis, *Strongyloides* and scabies infections and it has some activity against hookworms and *Trichuris*.

Albendazole has some activity against adult filarial worms and microfilaria counts decrease slowly over a period of months by 50% or more after a single oral dose of 400 mg.[75] Treatment with high-dose albendazole (400 mg twice daily for 21 days) was effective for killing filarial worms, but this regimen caused an unacceptably high rate of local adverse events (severe scrotal pain). As noted above, albendazole is usually administered in combination with either ivermectin or DEC.[76]

Recent studies have shown that *doxycycline* is a useful option for treatment of lymphatic filariasis.[77,78] Doxycycline works by clearing *Wolbachia* bacteria from filarial species such as *W. bancrofti* and *B. malayi* that require the endosymbiont for reproduction and viability. The drug has little direct effect on microfilariae, and microfilaria counts decrease slowly over a period of months after doxycycline treatment. Long courses of doxycycline treatment are required to clear *Wolbachia* from filarial worms, but results of this treatment are impressive. For example, in one study patients were treated with 200 mg of doxycycline per day for 8 weeks and followed for 14 months.[79] This treatment cleared microfilaraemia in 87% of the study subjects. It also inactivated most adult worm nests visible by ultrasound and reduced CFA levels by 50%. Other studies have shown similar results with treatment courses as short as 4 weeks and the macrofilaricidal activity of doxycycline may be enhanced by a single dose of DEC 3 months after the course of doxycycline.[80] Although doxycycline can cause AEs such as photosensitivity, vaginal candidiasis and oesophagitis, it has not been reported to cause systemic or localized AEs related to dying filarial worms. Thus, doxycycline is an attractive option for treating individuals with lymphatic filariasis. The long treatment course required and the fact that doxycycline is contraindicated in pregnant women and children younger than 9 years of age make it unattractive for routine use in filariasis elimination programmes based on mass drug administration. Ongoing research is testing whether new drugs or drug combinations can shorten the time required to clear *Wolbachia* from filarial worms.

Lymphoedema Management

Treatment should start with antifilarial therapy that aims to kill the parasites.

Recent studies have shown that clinical manifestations of filariasis such as hydrocele and lymphoedema sometimes improve after doxycycline treatment.[28,81] This is believed to be not solely due to doxycycline activity against *Wolbachia* endosymbionts; the drug may also directly inhibit inflammation and/or angiogenesis.

Hygiene is also critically important for management of lymphoedema. Many ADLA attacks are caused by bacterial infections in limbs with compromised lymphatic drainage. Simple hygienic measures can greatly reduce the frequency of ADLA episodes. These include daily washing with soap and water with careful drying and topical treatment of fungal infections and ulcers that can serve as entry lesions for bacteria. Adjunctive measures for lymphoedema patients include massage, exercise, compressive bandages and elevation of the affected limb (especially at night). Specialized shoes or sandals should be worm to protect the foot from injury.[47,82] Patients and family members may benefit from training in basic lymphoedema management, because patients with lymphoedema may require assistance in caring for themselves. Training may be provided in primary health care centres, in specialized clinics, or during home visits. Some health systems have special clinics for filariasis patients. Others have proposed integrating management of this problem with other chronic, disabling conditions such as leprosy and diabetic foot problems.[47]

Surgical Management

Surgical procedures that aim to cure or improve lymphoedema often do more harm than good. As mentioned above, significant improvement can usually be obtained with conservative management. Small hydroceles sometimes regress after anthelmintic treatment. Large hydroceles require surgery, but this is difficult to arrange in some countries with high disease burdens. Surgery is also sometimes required for chyluria cases that do not respond to conservative measures including anthelmintic therapy and a low-fat diet.

PREVENTION AND CONTROL

As an arthropod-borne infection, lymphatic filariasis can be thought of as an environmental disease that affects the health and productivity of endemic communities.[83,84] Filariasis control programmes aim to reduce transmission and morbidity and reduce the impact of the disease as a public health problem. Mathematical models of lymphatic filariasis transmission, infection and disease within endemic communities have been developed. Such models can be used to predict the outcome of different interventions and this can provide guidance towards the most cost-effective control strategies for specific settings.[85,86]

The main methods used for filariasis control are chemotherapy, vector control and case management for patients with clinically evident disease. Successful programmes require political support and active participation by health officials at all levels. Community leaders and volunteers are often critically important for implementation of filariasis control measures. Health education emphasizing the impact of the disease, its mode of transmission and tools for control, should start at the top to secure political support. Education and social mobilization are also essential at the community level, because programmes cannot succeed without community participation.[87,88]

Chemotherapeutic Control

Traditional filariasis control programmes followed a clinical model with selective treatment of infected individuals "who were identified by mass screening programmes" plus vector control. While filariasis was controlled and even eliminated in some areas with these methods, they achieved only stalemate or lost ground in others. Problems with mass diagnosis and selective treatment were that many people are never screened, the diagnostic test (usually a 20 μL thick smear for microfilaraemia) was insensitive and infected individuals sometimes failed to return to the clinic for treatment. A paradigm shift occurred in the 1990s and most filariasis control programmes now employ selective diagnosis (limited screening to determine whether filariasis is present in a region) and mass drug administration (MDA) to entire populations in endemic areas. If high coverage rates are achieved, MDA programmes reduce the reservoir of infection in communities and this reduces transmission and prevents new infections.

Mosquito Control

Vector control can complement the effects of chemotherapy in filariasis control programmes. Effective vector control rapidly reduces transmission rates. However, since filarial parasites live for many years, vector control alone is an inefficient method for reducing filarial infection rates. The feasibility and value of vector control for filariasis programmes depend on local factors such as the vector species and density, mosquito behaviour, breeding sites, climate, etc.[12,89]

Global Programme to Eliminate Lymphatic Filariasis

Increased awareness of the public health burden of lymphatic filariasis together with technical advances (better tools for diagnosis and effective single-dose treatment regimens suitable for mass drug administration) stimulated political interest and commitment towards elimination of this disease. Other biological factors that make elimination a feasible goal for lymphatic filariasis include the absence of an animal reservoir (apart from zoonotic *Brugia* strains in limited areas in Southeast Asia), its inability to multiply in vectors and its inefficient transmission. World Health Assembly resolution 50.29 (passed in 1997) called for the elimination of lymphatic filariasis as a public health problem. While the language of the resolution left room for debate on its meaning, the filariasis community has interpreted 'elimination' to be reduction of transmission rates to levels that cannot sustain endemicity. This is because anything less would amount to temporary control rather than elimination.

The Global Programme to Eliminate Lymphatic Filariasis (GPELF) was initiated in 2000 with a target date of 2020 for completion of the programme. GPELF is a partnership of interested parties that include endemic-country health ministries, international and national development agencies, private sector donors and academic institutions, with the World Health Organization serving as the secretariat.[90] The programme helps countries to develop national filariasis elimination programmes and provides advice on financial, technical and managerial matters. The programme is supported by massive donation programmes for albendazole (from GlaxoSmithKline) and ivermectin (from the Mectizan® Donation Programme). The GPELF focuses on both transmission interruption and morbidity control. The former is accomplished with repeated, annual rounds of MDA to entire populations that live in filariasis-endemic areas (excluding very young children and pregnant women). Vector control has a secondary role in GPELF, but its use is encouraged whenever it is feasible. Filariasis-endemic zones are defined by surveys for microfilaraemia or CFA and MDA is distributed in implementation units with prevalence rates of ≥1%. Recommended MDA regimens include albendazole 400 mg plus ivermectin 200 μg/kg in African countries with co-endemic onchocerciasis and albendazole 400 mg plus DEC 6 mg/kg in other parts of the world. Annual MDA is continued until community microfilaria rates fall below 1% and until CFA rates in first grade primary school aged children fall to very low levels (below 2% with 95% certainty). WHO guidelines suggest that 4–6 rounds of MDA should be sufficient in most endemic areas. This assumes that high rates of MDA coverage and compliance (the percentage of the target population that ingests the medications) can be achieved and sustained. Health education and social mobilization are critically important for achieving high MDA compliance rates.

GPELF also supports morbidity control programmes that aim to alleviate suffering and decrease disability in filariasis patients by providing training and support for improved hygiene, treatment of secondary infections, proper limb care and increased access to hydrocelectomy. These programmes have been more difficult to implement than MDA programmes, because they require a much more sustained effort than time-limited drug distribution programmes.[91] Highly visible morbidity management programmes help to educate populations about filariasis and this can be helpful for improving compliance with MDA.

GPELF is among the most exciting global health programmes that has been implemented in this young century. According to the latest report from WHO, MDA is now being provided in 53 of 72 filariasis-endemic countries. Between 2000 and 2010, more than 3.4 billion doses of antifilarial medications were distributed to a targeted population of 897 million. Several countries have ended their MDA programmes and are now conducting surveillance to verify elimination of transmission.[92] However, other countries have not yet started their programmes and it will be difficult for GPELF to reach the goal of global elimination by 2020. But we should not lose sight of what has already been accomplished: this programme has already cured millions of filarial infections and prevented millions of new infections and clinical filariasis cases. GPELF is easily the largest infectious disease intervention attempted to date based on mass treatment. GPELF's progress has inspired the global health community and current efforts are attempting to integrate filariasis elimination with mass treatment programmes for other neglected tropical diseases to maximize benefits for affected communities.

Onchocerciasis

Onchocerciasis (river blindness) results from infection with *Onchocerca volvulus*. Humans are the only natural hosts and the vectors are species of blackflies (*Simulium* spp.). High rates of severe dermatitis, poor vision and blindness make onchocerciasis a major public health problem in endemic areas.

EPIDEMIOLOGY

Geographical Distribution

The World Health Organization estimated in 1995 that about 17.7 million individuals worldwide were infected with *O. volvulus* with 270 000 cases of blindness and 500 000 with severe visual disability (Figure 54.14).[93] More than 99% of all onchocerciasis cases are in sub-Saharan Africa. Additional mapping surveys completed in 2005 led to revised estimates for Africa with 37 million people infected and 90 million people at risk.[94]

Isolated foci of onchocerciasis exist in Latin America and in Yemen. Intensive ivermectin distribution programmes have eliminated ocular disease due to onchocerciasis in nine of the 13 known foci in the Americas. Transmission has been interrupted in Ecuador, Colombia, Mexico and in parts of Guatemala, but it is ongoing in Venezuela and an adjacent area in northern Brazil.[95]

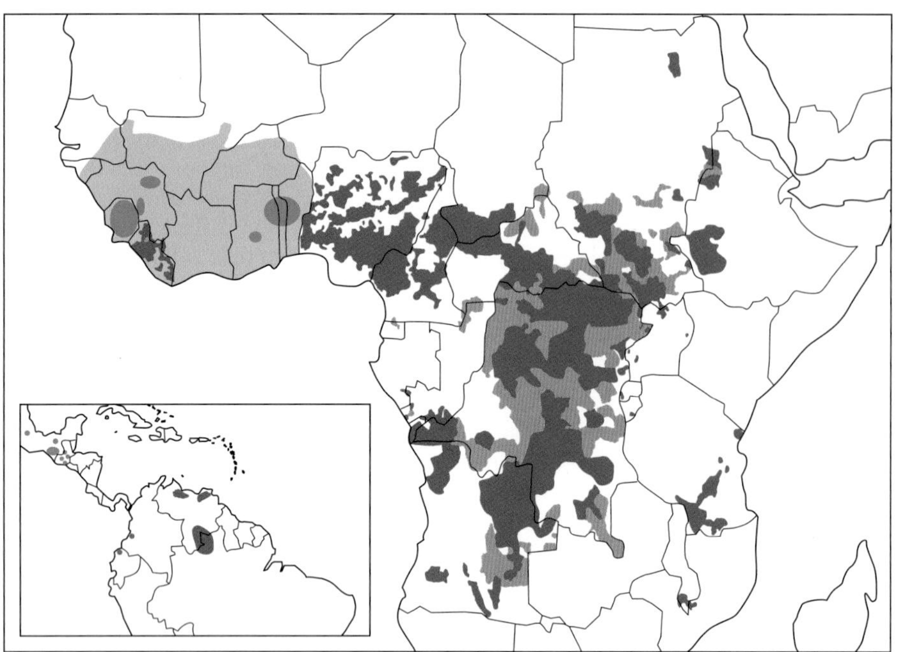

Figure 54.14 Geographical distribution of human onchocerciasis in Africa and Latin America. Red areas are under ivermectin treatment, blue areas need further mapping, orange areas are for special intervention, and ivermectin distribution has been suspended in areas shown in green. *(Modified after Basanez MG, Pion SD, Churcher TS, et al. River blindness: a success story under threat? PLoS Med 2006;3:e371 and Cupp EW, Sauerbrey M, Richards F. Elimination of human onchocerciasis: history of progress and current feasibility using ivermectin (Mectizan®) monotherapy. Acta Tropica 2011;120(Suppl 1):S100–S1008.)*

Life Cycle

The general filarial life cycle is shown in Figure 54.1. Adult *O. volvulus* worms mainly live in subcutaneous nodules (onchocercomata), but they sometimes migrate freely under the skin (especially true for male worms). The ratio of adult females to males in nodules is about 3:1. The adults are slender white worms, the male being 2–5 cm×0.2 mm and the females 35–70 cm×0.4 mm. The female produces sheathless microfilariae that are 300×8 µm with a sharply pointed tail and an expanded head that is free of nuclei (Figure 54.15).

Microfilariae are mainly found in the upper dermis (Figure 54.16) and in nodules, but they may rarely appear in blood, urine, or other body fluids, particularly in patients with heavy infections. Microfilariae are often present in the eye, with direct spread from adjacent skin as the main mode of entry. Microfilarial loads can be as high as 2000/mg of skin, but counts exceeding 100 mf/mg are now unusual because of the success of control efforts. Heavily infected individuals may have total body burdens of more than 100 million microfilariae.

Microfilariae present in the skin are ingested by *Simulium* (blackfly) vectors during feeding. Some of the ingested microfilariae migrate from the gut of the blackfly into the thoracic muscles and develop over a period of 6–12 days to become infective larvae. Transmission of infective larvae to humans occurs when the blackfly takes its next blood meal. The larvae migrate to the subcutaneous tissues, moult twice and then develop over several months to become sexually mature adult worms. They may cause the formation of new nodules or congregate with older worms in preexisting nodules. Gravid female worms release microfilariae that are first detected in the skin 10–15 months after infection. Some 500–1500 microfilariae are released per female per day in 2 or 3 reproductive periods per

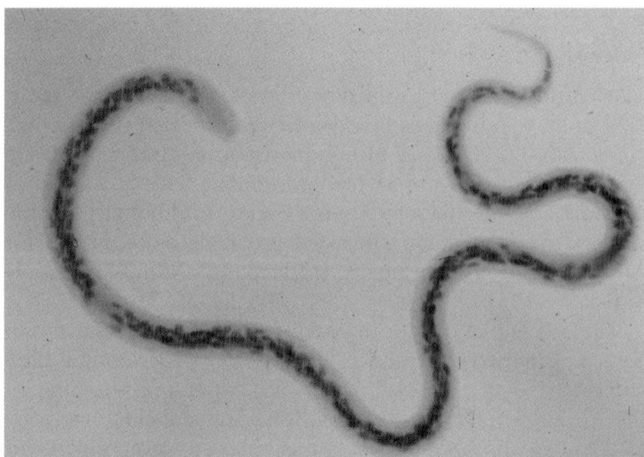

Figure 54.15 Skin microfilaria of *O. volvulus* (haematoxylin). *(Courtesy of D.W. Buttner)*

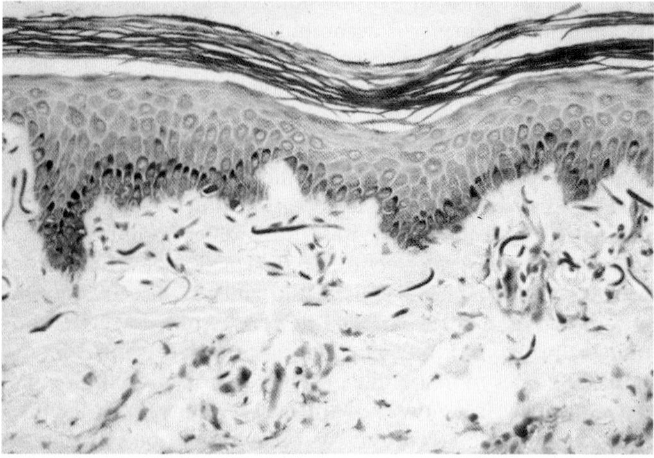

Figure 54.16 Microfilariae of *O. volvulus* in subcutaneous tissue. *(Courtesy of D.W. Buttner)*

year (each lasting 3–4 months). The reproductive life of female worms has been estimated to be 9–11 years and microfilariae have a lifespan of 1–2 years.

Despite geographical variation in pathogenicity, *O. volvulus* parasites are morphologically indistinguishable throughout their range of distribution. There are no significant animal reservoirs for onchocerciasis. Vertical transmission of *O. volvulus* microfilariae has been reported. However, these microfilariae do not undergo further development and they have no clinical significance.

African Onchocerciasis. Many species and subspecies of *Simulium* blackflies can act as vectors. Members of the *Simulium damnosum* complex are the predominant vectors in most endemic areas in Africa. Species in the *S. neavei* group also serve as vectors in areas of East and Central Africa.

S. damnosum s.l. is a complex of numerous sibling species that differ in bionomics and vectorial capacity. They are very similar morphologically, but they can be distinguished by molecular methods or by observing the banding patterns of their salivary gland chromosomes in larvae. *S. damnosum* flies breed in large rivers or small streams where there is an adequate velocity of water, adequate supply of food and suitable attachment sites (rocks, sticks, trailing vegetation). Female blackflies generally restrict their flight to within a few kilometres of breeding sites and biting rates are highest near to rivers. This explains the origin of the name 'river blindness'. Winds sometimes transport blackflies several hundred kilometres from one river basin to another. Female blackfly vectors feed mainly on humans, but they also feed on animals (bovines, horses and small ruminants) in some areas.

West Africa. A traditional hot spot for onchocerciasis, intervention programmes have reduced disease and transmission rates in many areas. Transmission remains high in parts of Liberia, Ivory Coast, Sierra Leone, Guinea, Ghana, Togo, Benin, Nigeria and Cameroon. Transmission of onchocerciasis is seasonal in dry savannah areas. This contrasts to a much longer transmission period in wet savannah and forest areas. Blinding onchocerciasis was much more common in the dry savannah than in forest areas prior to mass control programmes; genetic markers have been identified that differentiate *O. volvulus* strains in these two ecological zones.[96,97] However, in addition to parasite strain differences, it is also important to consider environmental factors – a dry atmosphere, abrasive effects of dust and sand and exposure to higher levels of ultraviolet radiation – that may damage the cornea. All of these factors are likely to be higher in the dry savannah than in rainforest zones.

East and Central Africa. *S. damnosum* complex flies are vectors in East and Central Africa, but *S. neavei* group flies are also vectors in Ethiopia, Tanzania, Malawi, Uganda and parts of the Democratic Republic of Congo. This group includes *Simulium* species with larvae and pupae that become attached to crabs of the genus *Potamonautes*. These crabs live in small rivers and streams in forests and adult *S. neavei* are restricted to densely forested areas. Several studies showed a decline of *S. neavei*-transmitted onchocerciasis due to deforestation.[98] Onchocerciasis rarely causes blindness in East Africa, but itching and dermatitis may be severe.[99,100]

Central and South America. Onchocerciasis is believed to have been introduced fairly recently in the New World, probably as a result of the slave trade.[101] The parasites are transmitted by local species of *Simulium* blackflies. In Venezuela, onchocerciasis is present in northern and eastern foci and in highland and lowland areas in the southern part of the country among some groups of Yanomami Indians.[102] There is also a focus in northern Brazil near the Venezuelan border. Onchocerciasis is no longer transmitted in Mexico, Guatemala, Ecuador or Colombia.[95]

Infection and Disease in Endemic Communities

The epidemiology of onchocerciasis varies in different regions. Different patterns of infection and disease are associated with differences in the abundance, vector competence and feeding characteristics of local blackfly populations, differences in parasite strains and differences in the human host responses to the parasites. Other human host factors that can affect the epidemiology are occupation, seasonal migration, economic or social standing, concurrent infections and genetics/racial group. Infection and disease rates in endemic areas are generally low in young children and increase gradually with age. The overall burden of infection and disease in populations is proportional to the intensity of transmission.[103] In hyperendemic communities almost all adult individuals are infected and many have clinical disease. Males and females are equally susceptible to infection and disease. Host immunity seems to limit adult worm burdens. In addition, children born from *O. volvulus*-infected mothers tend to become infected earlier in life and harbour higher loads of skin microfilariae than children of uninfected mothers.[104]

Quantitative data on transmission, infection and disease in endemic populations have been used to develop mathematical models describing the transmission dynamics of human onchocerciasis.[105,106] These models are useful for predicting the effects of control measures. Different criteria have been used to classify onchocerciasis endemicity in populations. The most common classification considers onchocerciasis to be hypoendemic, mesoendemic or hyperendemic when microfilarial prevalence rates are less than 40%, 40–59% and 60% or more, respectively. Prior to implementation of large-scale control programmes, blindness rates in hyperendemic areas sometimes exceeded 10%, with higher rates of blindness in adults. Onchocerciasis-related blindness rates in hypoendemic areas are generally below 1%.

Onchocerciasis control programmes such as the African Programme for Onchocerciasis Control (APOC) used rapid assessment methods to map endemicity so that control efforts could be focussed to areas with high endemicity and disease risk. One rapid assessment method examines a sample of 50 males per community for nodules. Nodule prevalence rates of less than 20%, 20–39% and 40% or more correspond approximately to the hypoendemic, mesoendemic and hyperendemic levels based on skin microfilarial rates. Leopard skin and blindness have also been used for rapid assessment, but these are less sensitive and specific indicators of onchocerciasis endemicity than nodule rates.

PATHOGENESIS AND PATHOLOGY

Most adult worms live in subcutaneous nodules (onchocercomata) with diameters of 0.5–3 cm (Figure 54.17). Nodules are essentially granulomatous reactions around adult worms. They often have separate chambers containing several worms. Nodules have thick fibrous walls and a variable degree of cellular infiltration with macrophages being the predominant cell

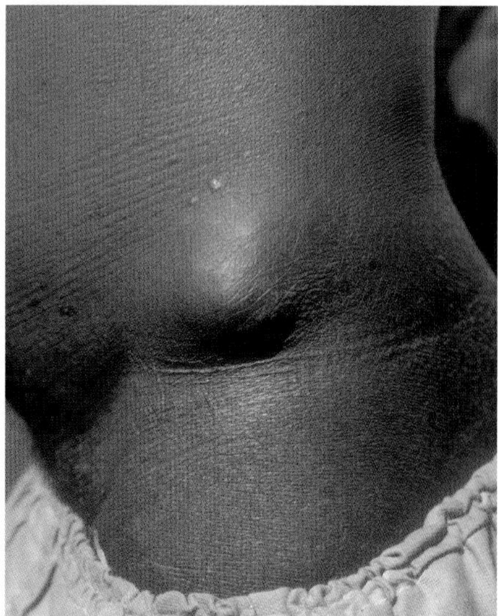

Figure 54.17 *O. volvulus* nodule on the body.

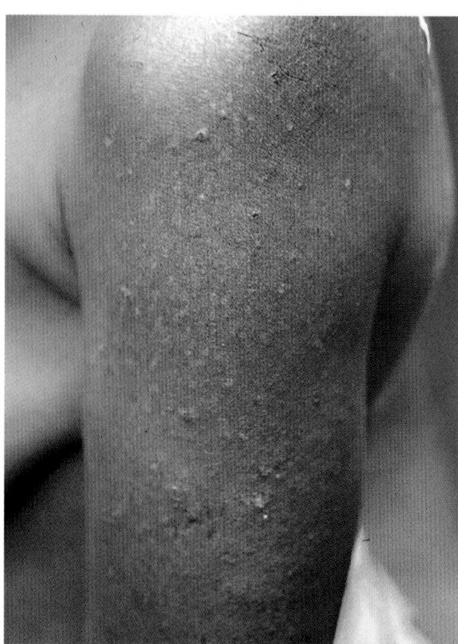

Figure 54.18 Onchocerciasis: Papular skin lesions. *(Courtesy of D.W. Buttner)*

type.[107] Nodules have their own blood supply and also induce formation of lymphatic vessels. Calcification may occur in older nodules and in dead worms.

Adult worms in onchocercal nodules contribute little to pathogenesis apart from the fact that they may be uncomfortable or cosmetically bothersome. Clinically significant onchocerciasis results from inflammatory responses to microfilariae in the skin and in the eyes. Adult worms release millions of microfilariae in the skin and some of these migrate to the cornea and intraocular tissues. In some individuals microfilariae are attacked by eosinophils, neutrophils and macrophages[107,108] that work in concert with specific antibodies and complement.[109] However, *O. volvulus* actively downregulates deleterious parasite-specific immune responses and this limits tissue damage in many individuals. Downregulation commences at the time when adult female worms become fertile and this tends to protect microfilariae. Immune downregulation associated with onchocerciasis can also reduce immune responses to BCG or tetanus vaccination and to allergens.[110–112] Patients with strongly modulated immune responses to *O. volvulus* antigens tend to have high skin microfilaria counts with little tissue reaction and little or no disease; they represent the hyporeactive end of the spectrum (so-called 'generalized onchocerciasis').[113]

Dermatitis

Skin pathology is mainly caused by reactions to dead or dying microfilariae. Microfilariae may die spontaneously or after treatment with microfilaricidal drugs such as diethylcarbamazine or ivermectin. Histopathological examination of inflammatory responses around degenerating microfilariae reveals infiltration by eosinophils, neutrophils and macrophages.[107] In early disease, the dermal tissue between the focal lesions is normal. Later, dermal fibroblasts proliferate leading to fibrosis and the normal collagen and elastic fibres of the dermis are gradually replaced by hyalinized scar tissue (Figure 54.18). There may also be loss of pigment in the skin (Figure 54.19). The histological appearance of the skin in advanced cases resembles the skin of very old subjects (i.e. presbyderma). Some of the skin damage observed in onchocerciasis patients may also be caused by the mechanical effects of scratching or by secondary infections. A minority of infected patients develop exaggerated immune responses to the parasite that may be localized or generalized. When this is unilateral, the condition is called 'sowda' (Figure 54.20). The most striking histopathological feature in biopsies from sowda patients is the presence of an extensive inflammatory cell infiltrate in the upper dermis. These immune cells kill microfilariae and microfilariae are rare or

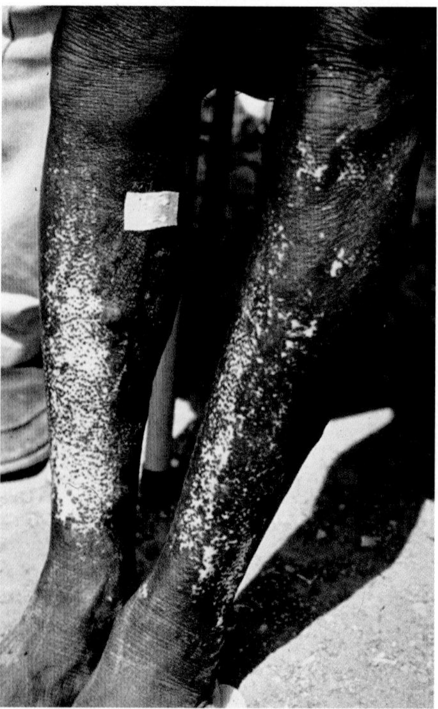

Figure 54.19 Onchocerciasis: Depigmentation and leopard skin. *(Courtesy of D.W. Buttner)*

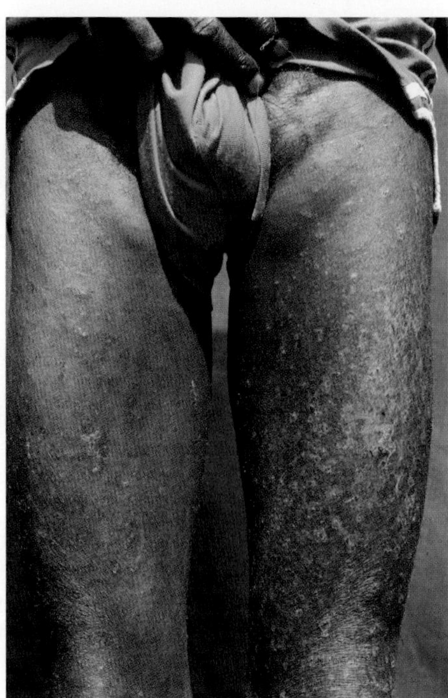

Figure 54.20 Onchocerciasis: Sowda. *(Courtesy of D.W. Buttner)*

absent in the skin of sowda patients. However, the effective antiparasitic immune response in sowda patients causes collateral damage to the skin (see below). Sowda patients do not downregulate their immune responses like those with generalized onchocerciasis. They have persistently strong Th2 responses with high IgE levels and eosinophilia but relatively little TGF-β in the peripheral blood or locally in the nodules.[114] *Onchocerca* nodules in sowda patients are surrounded by excessive numbers of inflammatory cells with ectopic lymphoid follicles.[115] Sowda tends to cluster in families and a single nucleotide polymorphism (SNP) that affects IL-13 production has been reported to be associated with this form of onchocerciasis.[116]

Ocular Disease

Live microfilariae are sometimes visible by slit lamp in the corneas of asymptomatic patients with onchocerciasis without a visible cellular response. Dead microfilariae become foci of inflammation that lead to characteristic punctate ('snowflake') keratitis, with cellular infiltrates around each microfilaria. The major pathology of the anterior segment is called sclerosing keratitis. Chronic inflammation and vascularization with scarring eventually progress to complete opacification of the cornea. This process normally starts from each side and from below and resembles an inflammatory immune response. The pathogenesis of posterior segment lesions is less clear.[117]

Antibodies mediating cellular killing of *O. volvulus* microfilariae and infective larvae in vitro are present in sera from some people who live in endemic areas and such antibodies may also be active in vivo.[109] Immunological profiles of uninfected people who have been exposed to *O. volvulus* (so-called 'endemic normals' or 'putatively immune individuals') are different from those of people with either generalized onchocerciasis or sowda. However, solid protective immunity must be uncommon in onchocerciasis, because almost all individuals are infected in hyperendemic areas.

Individuals from non-endemic areas who become infected during visits to endemic areas usually have mild disease, with dermatitis being the most common clinical presentation.[118] These patients usually have antibodies to *O. volvulus* antigens and eosinophilia, but microfilariae are often not detectable or present in low numbers and nodules or ocular lesions are unusual. HIV-infected onchocerciasis patients tend to have significantly impaired antibody responses to *O. volvulus* antigens.[119] However, HIV has not been shown to affect disease progression in onchocerciasis or to increase the risk of becoming infected with *O. volvulus*. Adverse reactions to ivermectin treatment have been reported to be less severe in HIV-positive individuals.

O. volvulus contains *Wolbachia* endosymbionts that are localized in the body walls ('hypodermal chords') of adult worms and vertically transmitted to the next generation (i.e. through oocytes) (Figure 54.21). *Wolbachia* are essential for fertility and embryo development in female worms and they are also necessary for the survival of adult worms.[120–123] Recent studies have also suggested a role for *Wolbachia* in the pathogenesis of onchocerciasis.[124] For example, direct injection of extracts from untreated *Onchocerca* adult worms induces acute keratitis in mice, but extracts prepared from worms that have been treated with antibiotics that eliminate *Wolbachia* do not induce keratitis. *Wolbachia* released from dying microfilariae may trigger the adverse events that occur after treatment with diethylcarbamazine.[125] *Wolbachia* components also attract neutrophils to microfilariae and adult worms.[126] These proinflammatory reactions are mediated by interactions between molecules present in *Wolbachia* and Toll-like receptor 2 on host cells.[127]

CLINICAL FEATURES

The main clinical manifestations of onchocerciasis are skin lesions, eye lesions and subcutaneous nodules. In general, clinical manifestations develop after a long period of exposure to infection; their severity depends on infection intensity and on host immune responses (see above). Many individuals who have microfilariae in the skin, especially those with light infections, have no symptoms or signs of onchocerciasis.

Skin Lesions

Dermatitis occurs when microfilariae die or are killed in the skin. Lesions vary from a few pruritic papules to atrophy with

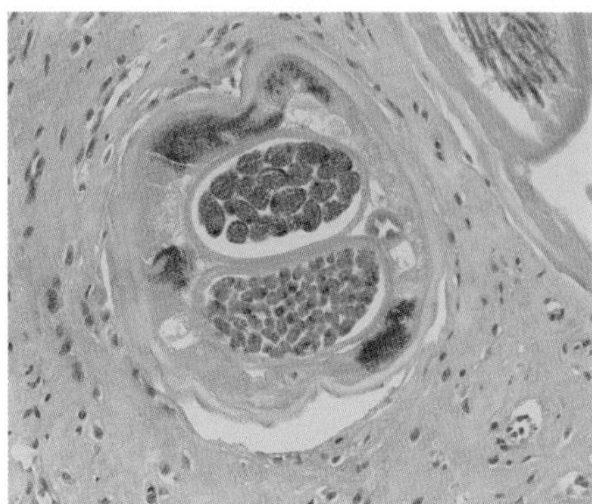

Figure 54.21 Cross-section of an adult female *O. volvulus* worm showing *Wolbachia* endobacteria stained in red.

lichenification and loss of pigment.[128] A clinical classification and grading system of cutaneous changes in onchocerciasis has been developed, with the main categories being acute papular onchodermatitis, chronic papular onchodermatitis, lichenified onchodermatitis, skin atrophy and skin depigmentation.[129] Infected individuals may have several types of skin lesions. In Africa, the skin lesions are most common over the legs, but they may cover the entire body.

Itching and rash are the most important early symptoms of onchocercal dermatitis. The rash consists of raised papules, which are localized reactions to dying or dead microfilariae. These sometimes disappear within a few days, but the rash can persist for years. The rash may be confined to one area of the skin. The resulting pruritus can be very intense (filarial itch) and the skin often becomes secondarily infected following scratching. Severe cases may have marked lichenification and thickening of the skin ('lizard skin'). Acute papular onchodermatitis can arise spontaneously or be induced by microfilaricidal treatment with ivermectin or by application of topical diethylcarbamazine (DEC; see Mazzotti reaction, below). The lesions may be papules, vesicles, or pustules. Histologically, these lesions appear as intraepidermal microabscesses and the papules often show a perivascular infiltrate of macrophages and lymphoid cells.

Chronic skin manifestations of onchocerciasis probably result from repeated acute inflammatory responses to dying microfilariae. These papules are usually larger (Figure 54.18) than those seen in early disease. In people with light-coloured skin the papules have a red appearance that was called the 'erisipela de la costa' in Guatemala. Due to chronic pruritus and scratching, the skin may become hypertrophic and lichenified (Figure 54.18); depigmentation and hyperpigmentation may be seen in the same lesions. Depigmentation with preservation of pigmentation around hair follicles is called 'leopard skin' (Figure 54.19). Leopard skin often affects the pretibial regions and this can be used as a simple epidemiological marker for mapping onchocerciasis-endemic areas. Other patients develop skin atrophy with loss of elasticity and this can cause a prematurely aged appearance (presbyderma). Loss of elastic fibres in the skin of the groin may lead to the clinical picture of 'hanging groin' (Figure 54.22) with inguinal and/or femoral glands contained in pendulous folds.

Sowda. Sowda (derived from the word for 'black' in Arabic) (Figure 54.20) is a localized form of onchodermatitis that is associated with hyperpigmentation. It is common in Yemen and some parts of Sudan, but it is also found elsewhere. However, even in those areas fewer than 3% of infected individuals have clinical Sowda. The condition is usually localized to one limb, but the legs and/or arms and the trunk may be involved. It is characterized by intense itching. The involved skin becomes oedematous, hyperpigmented and covered with scaly papules. Draining lymph glands are enlarged and microfilariae are rarely seen in biopsies. If the lesions are symmetrically distributed, the condition is called hyperreactive onchocerciasis instead of Sowda. Chronic reactive skin lesions (both Sowda and symmetrical, hyperreactive onchocerciasis) will improve following treatment that reduces microfilaria counts in skin over a long period of time[130] such as a course of doxycycline or repeated doses of ivermectin at 3-month intervals.

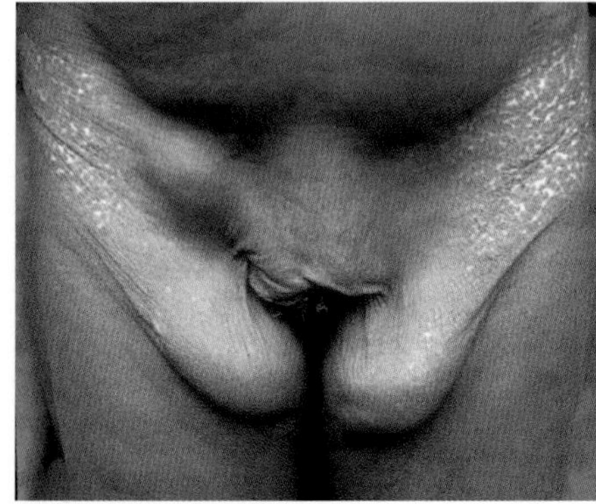

Figure 54.22 Onchocerciasis: Hanging groin. *(Courtesy of D.W. Buttner)*

Nodules

Onchocercal nodules (onchocercomata) are large granulomas that result from tissue reactions around adult worms. They are most often located in subcutaneous tissues. They are painless, round to oval in shape, firm and smooth. They can vary in diameter from a few millimetres to several centimetres. The nodules may be mobile or fixed to underlying structures and they are often matted together in clumps. As many as 25% of onchocercal nodules are in deeper tissues and not palpable. In Africa 80% of palpable nodules occur in the pelvic area. Others occur on the abdomen, chest wall, head or limbs. In Latin America, palpable nodules are commonly found on the head. It is believed that the location of the nodules reflects the biting habits of the vector flies. Nodules do not cause medical problems unless they press on vital structures such as nerves or joints. However, they may be aesthetically displeasing to patients.

Eye Lesions

Onchocerciasis can cause disease in both the anterior and posterior segments of the eye.[131]

Anterior Segment Lesions. Punctate keratitis (snowflake opacities) is sometimes visible to the naked eye, but it is best seen by slitlamp examination. These lesions are comprised of cellular infiltrates around dead or dying microfilariae and they are the corneal equivalent of the discrete papular lesions seen in the skin. Punctate keratitis is more common in younger age groups. These lesions are reversible. In sclerosing keratitis, vascular infiltrates begin at the limbus (usually at the bottom of the eye, Figure 54.23) and extend inwards. Some patients develop excessive scarring of the cornea and blindness (Figure 54.24). Microfilariae dying in the ciliary body can give rise to iridocyclitis and the formation of synechiae. Inflammation of the uveal tract also contributes to iridial pathology.

Posterior Segment Lesions. Both optic nerve atrophy and choroidoretinitis of the posterior segment may result in blindness. Choroidoretinitis includes both acute inflammatory lesions and atrophic lesions with atrophy of the retinal pigment epithelium and the choriocapillaris and hyperpigmentation of the pigment epithelial layer. Optic nerve atrophy is associated with decreased visual acuity and visual field constriction in onchocerciasis. Treatment with DEC can accelerate optic nerve damage and exacerbate other ocular lesions. For this reason, DEC is no longer recommended for treatment of

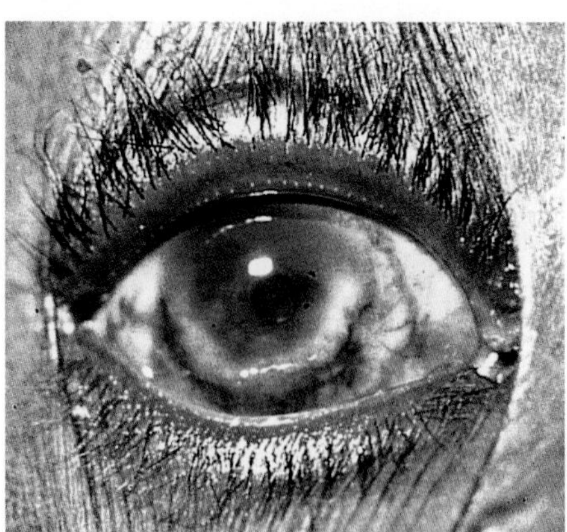

Figure 54.23 Onchoceriasis: early sclerosing keratitis. *(Courtesy of D.W. Buttner)*

onchocerciasis. Ivermectin is much less likely to exacerbate ocular disease, because it does not kill microfilariae in the eyes. Instead, they are immobilized and transported to regional lymph nodes for killing. Doxycycline treatment does not exacerbate ocular disease in onchocerciasis, because it does not acutely kill microfilariae.

Other Conditions

Onchocerciasis has been associated with weight loss and musculoskeletal pain. Several reports have indicated a higher than normal frequency of epilepsy in onchocerciasis hyperendemic areas.[132] Onchocerciasis has also been associated with a syndrome of growth arrest (dwarfism) and delayed sexual development (Nakalanga syndrome) seen in Uganda and Burundi.[133,134] However, these associations lacked statistical significance on meta-analysis.[135,136]

Geographical Variation in Clinical Disease

Clinical manifestations (skin and eye lesions) are known to differ widely in different endemic zones. Surveys in Cameroon showed that prevalence rates for sclerosing keratitis and blindness were much higher in savannah than in forest areas. This picture appears to be valid for most of West Africa, with very severe ocular disease in the dry (Sudan type) savannah, moderately severe disease in wet savannah areas and lower rates of eye disease in forest zones. The clinical picture of onchocerciasis is generally less severe in Eastern and Central Africa and severe ocular disease and blindness are uncommon in these regions.

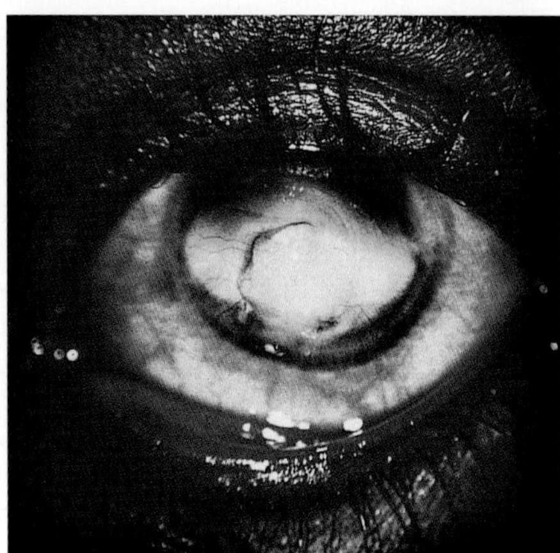

Figure 54.24 Onchoceriasis: advanced sclerosing keratitis. *(Courtesy of D.W. Buttner)*

DIAGNOSIS

Clinical Diagnosis

The presence of skin lesions, eye lesions and/or subcutaneous nodules in individuals who live in or have visited endemic areas strongly suggests the diagnosis of onchocerciasis. Pruritic onchodermatitis must be distinguished from: infection with *Mansonella streptocerca* in West and Central Africa which rarely affects the legs; scabies, where the typical burrows and mites are often present between the fingers; reactions to insect bites that are especially common in recent arrivals to the tropics; prickly heat; contact dermatitis; and herpes zoster (unilateral, segmental) in AIDS patients. Chronic onchocercal dermatitis must be differentiated from tertiary yaws, superficial mycoses, leprosy and chronic eczema. Onchocercal nodules are usually painless, firm and mobile. However, some nodules (particularly those on the head) may be fixed due to adherence to underlying tissues. Nodules must be distinguished from enlarged lymph nodes, lipomas, dermal cysts, ganglia and neurofibromas.

Ultrasonography. Although it is not often used for this purpose, ultrasonography has been used to visualize slowly-moving adult worms in onchocercal nodules.[137]

Parasitological Diagnosis. Definitive diagnosis is made by demonstrating microfilariae that have emerged from skin snips. Although most untreated persons with clinical evidence of onchocerciasis have positive skin snips, this is not always the case. The optimal site for the biopsy depends on geography; the iliac crest is the preferred site in most parts of Africa. Two to four skin snips are taken. After cleaning the skin with alcohol and allowing it to dry, a razor blade can be used to shave off the tip of a dome of skin that has been elevated with a needle. Care should be taken to avoid contamination of skin snips with blood. More uniform skin snips are obtained with a 2 mm Walser or Holth corneoscleral punch (Figure 54.25) that produces skin snips with weights of 1–2 mg. Note that punches must be carefully cleaned and autoclaved or disinfected with

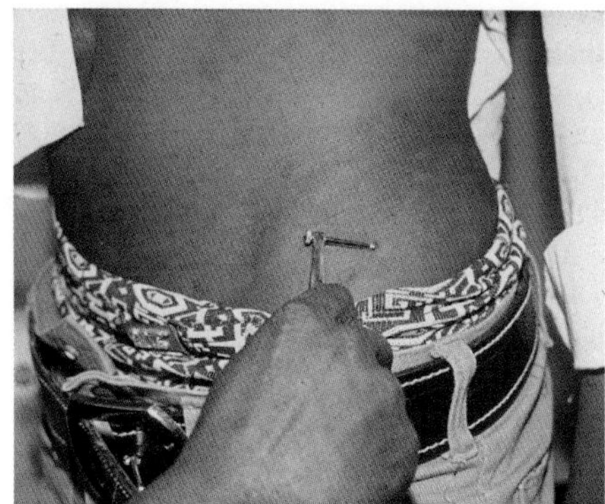

Figure 54.25 Skin snip to diagnose *O. volvulus* infection. *(Courtesy of D.W. Buttner)*

chemicals such as 1% glutaraldehyde followed by 70% ethanol and rinsed in sterile water or isotonic saline before they can be used on a different patient.

Skin snips are immersed in isotonic saline, often in wells of a 96-well microtitration plate. Microfilariae that have emerged after a period of 0.5–24 hours (preferred) are counted under the low power of a compound microscope. The sensitivity of skin snips to diagnose infection depends upon the number of skin snips taken and on the intensity of infection.

Microfilariae of *O. volvulus* are 270–320 µm long, unsheathed and they have a characteristic head and a pointed tail (Figure 54.15). They must be differentiated from the smaller skin-dwelling microfilariae of *M. streptocerca* in some areas of Africa and from *M. ozzardi* in South America. Blood microfilariae such as *W. bancrofti*, *Loa loa* and *M. perstans* are sometimes seen in skin snips that are contaminated by blood.

The Mazzotti Test. The original version of this test involved the administration of a small dose (usually 50 mg for an adult) of DEC by mouth to see whether this caused intense pruritus and skin rash 1–24 hours later. However, this test can cause serious complications and it is no longer recommended as a routine diagnostic procedure. The DEC patch test is an alternative that involves placing a gauze pad with 10% DEC lotion on the skin and covering this with a bandage. A papular rash at 48 hours is a positive test and this represents a localized Mazzotti reaction. This test detects microfilariae in the skin and it is less invasive than skin snipping.[138,139] Some experts consider this test to be more sensitive than parasitological detection of microfilariae in skin snips (especially in areas with low endemicity). However, the DEC patch test is less specific than the skin snip; false-positive reactions have been observed in uninfected persons and in individuals infected with *M. streptocerca* or other filarial species. The test is not commercially available.

Immunological and PCR-based Diagnosis

Several immunodiagnostic tests have been devised for onchocerciasis.[140] Generally, immunodiagnosis based on detection of antibodies to unfractionated native parasite antigens is of limited practical value for the diagnosis of onchocerciasis in people who live in endemic areas, because serology does not distinguish between past and present infections. In addition, cross-reactions to other nematode infections are common. However, these tests are useful for diagnosing onchocerciasis in persons who have acquired onchocerciasis after only short periods of residence in endemic areas who are unlikely to have other nematode infections.

Antibody testing may be the best way for non-specialists to screen for onchocerciasis in expatriates who have been exposed. Serum samples can be sent to specialized labs for serology testing. Skin snip examination may be unreliable when it is performed by inexperienced technicians with snips taken from lightly infected individuals. The specificity of antibody tests has been improved by the detection of IgG4 antibodies to recombinant *O. volvulus* antigens.[141] A field-applicable rapid-format card test that detected IgG4 to recombinant antigen Ov-16 in serum or whole blood specimens was shown to be sensitive and specific in laboratory and field studies.[142] Unfortunately, no recombinant antigen-based antibody test for onchocerciasis is commercially available at this time.

PCR-based tests have been developed that have high sensitivity and specificity for *O. volvulus* DNA. In addition to detecting microfilarial DNA in skin snips or skin scrapes from infected humans, this technique can also be used to distinguish between various strains of the parasite and for detecting *O. volvulus* larvae in pools of blackflies.[143,144] This is sometimes helpful, because some blackfly species serve not only as vectors of *O. volvulus* but also as vectors for morphologically similar animal filariae (e.g. *O. ochengi*). As mentioned above for antibody tests, PCR tests for onchocerciasis are not commercially available, but they are performed by several reference and research laboratories.

MANAGEMENT AND TREATMENT

Drug Treatment

Overview. DEC is no longer recommended for the treatment of onchocerciasis. It can induce severe adverse reactions, especially in heavily infected individuals and it may precipitate or aggravate ocular lesions. Ivermectin (Mectizan®) is now the drug of choice.[93] Both DEC and ivermectin are effective for killing microfilariae, but they do not kill adult worms (Table 54.2).

Suramin has activity against adult *O. volvulus*. However, it is no longer used to treat onchocerciasis, because it can cause serious adverse events including death. Conventional doses of benzimidazoles such as albendazole are not effective for onchocerciasis, but research is ongoing in this area.

Ivermectin. Ivermectin is a semisynthetic, macrocyclic lactone that was originally developed for veterinary use to treat nematode infections and ectoparasites. In the 1980s, its outstanding activity against many filarial nematode species led to its further development for human use.[145,146] A single oral dose of 150 µg/kg body weight of ivermectin causes rapid elimination of microfilariae from the skin.[147] More than 80% of skin microfilariae are eliminated in the first 48 hours. This slowly increases to 97% reduction, which lasts for a period of several months, after which there is a gradual repopulation of the skin with microfilariae. Retreatment may be necessary 6–12 months after the initial treatment. A single dose of ivermectin has no long-lasting effects on adult worms, but the drug causes temporary sterility with degeneration of intrauterine embryos. Some reports have suggested that repeated doses of ivermectin may cause long-term suppression of microfilaria production or even death of adult worms.[148,149]

Ivermectin is not approved for use in pregnant women, lactating women with infants less than 1 week old or in children shorter than 90 cm. However, an evaluation of data from women who were inadvertently treated during pregnancy suggests that ivermectin may be safe in pregnancy.[150] Ivermectin blocks glutamate-gated ion channels in nematodes. This inhibits release of uterine microfilariae by female worms and immobilizes skin and ocular microfilariae. Microfilariae are thus not destroyed in the eye, but rather transported to the regional lymph nodes where the immobilized larvae are attacked by effector cells.[151] Ivermectin is not active in vitro at concentrations that are achieved in human tissues and its activity lasts much longer in vivo than its half life in blood of 12 hours. These facts suggest that the drug may work in concert with the immune system and/or that metabolites may be important for its activity.

Adverse reactions seen with ivermectin are less common and much less severe than those associated with DEC therapy.[152]

Adverse events in descending order of frequency include itching and/or rash, muscle and/or joint pains, fever, headache, swelling of the limbs, dizziness, tender lymphadenopathy, conjunctivitis and tender nodules.[152] Adverse events are more commonly seen in heavily infected persons with more than 50 microfilariae/mg skin during the first round of treatment. They decrease in frequency and intensity after microfilarial loads have been decreased by several rounds of treatment. Adverse events can be managed with antipyretics, antihistamines or glucocorticoids. A grading scheme for these adverse events has been established.[153] There are case reports of patients who have developed severe postural hypotension and/or bronchoconstriction after ivermectin therapy.[154] These conditions were transient and they responded to symptomatic management. Patients should be instructed to stay in bed until dizziness improves. The disappearance of microfilariae from the eye is much more gradual than that in the skin. Repeated doses of ivermectin may result in improvement in early anterior segment lesions including iridocyclitis and sclerosing keratitis. Ivermectin treatment sometimes has a beneficial effect on optic nerve disease and visual field loss, but not on chorioretinitis.[155]

In infected expatriates, ivermectin treatment should be repeated at 3- to 6-month intervals and the frequency of subsequent treatments should be adjusted according to the patient's symptoms. Even in patients who are not exposed to reinfection, treatment may need to be continued for several years until the adult worms are dead or sterile. Despite reduced antibodies to *O. volvulus* in HIV-positive patients, the efficacy of ivermectin treatment is not compromised in patients with HIV.[156]

Ivermectin should be avoided in persons with heavy *Loa loa* infections (mf counts >30 000/mL) because of the risk of encephalopathy, coma and death, as discussed below. Suboptimal responses to ivermectin have recently been reported in a localized area in Northern Ghana that had received many rounds of mass treatment with ivermectin. Microfilaria counts in skin declined normally after treatment, but they repopulated the skin more rapidly than expected. This may mean that the drug has lost some of its temporary sterilizing effect on adult worms in this area.[157–159] Whether genetic changes detected in parasites from this region confer partial resistance is currently a matter of debate. However, a recent study has shown that older worms appear to be less responsive to ivermectin than younger worms.[160] More frequent treatment may be sufficient to solve this problem in Ghana, but the possible development of partial resistance to ivermectin by *O. volvulus* worms underscores the need for new treatments to control and eventually eliminate this disease.

Doxycycline. Doxycycline treatment targets a *Wolbachia* endosymbiont of *O. volvulus* that is essential for parasite reproduction and survival (see above). Six weeks of doxycycline per os at 100 mg/day (or 4 weeks of 200 mg/day) reduced *Wolbachia* by more than 99% in adult female worms.[120,161,162] This was sufficient to completely block embryogenesis and production of new microfilariae. Since doxycycline has little or no effect on microfilariae that are already in the skin or eyes, microfilaria counts decrease slowly after doxycycline treatment according to their half life. One or two doses of ivermectin separated by 3 months accelerate microfilarial clearance from the skin in patients treated with doxycycline. Since adult worms sterilized by doxycycline do not produce microfilariae, microfilariae should not reappear after these ivermectin treatments unless the patient acquires new worms by reinfection.[121]

Doxycycline treatment may be particularly beneficial for people with onchodermatitis and pruritus who would otherwise require repeated treatment with ivermectin over a period of years. In addition to its sterilizing effect, the 4-week, 200 mg/day doxycycline regimen also kills approximately 60% of adult *O. volvulus* worms. Adverse events related to doxycycline are well recognized and easily managed. Thus, doxycycline is the only available drug that can permanently clear *O. volvulus* microfilariae from the skin. This makes the drug an attractive treatment option for individual patients with onchocerciasis. Multiweek doxycycline treatment courses are too long for routine use in mass drug administration programmes for onchocerciasis control, but pilot studies have shown that they can be delivered to populations in special circumstances.[163,164]

Nodulectomy

Nodulectomy has only limited value for management of onchocerciasis, because some worms live outside of nodules and because many nodules are not palpable. Head nodules should be excised, because these nodules are associated with an increased risk of ocular disease and blindness.

PREVENTION AND CONTROL

Overview

Onchocercal skin and eye lesions can have serious social and socio-economic consequences in affected communities and this is especially true in areas with high infection rates.[165,166] Blindness reduces life expectancy by an average of 10 years in onchocerciasis-endemic areas.[167] In addition, skin microfilaria counts are significantly associated with the risk of mortality.[168] Considerable progress has been made in recent decades to establish control programmes that aim to prevent blindness and eliminate onchocerciasis as a public health problem.[169]

Vector Control

The Onchocerciasis Control Programme (OCP) was established in 1974 to control the vectors of savannah-type onchocerciasis in seven West African countries (core area with Burkina Faso, Benin, Ivory Coast, Ghana, Mali, Niger and Togo) in the Volta River Basin area. The programme expanded its operations by adding four new countries (Guinea, Guinea-Bissau, Senegal and Sierra Leone) in 1986 (Figure 54.14). The OCP used vector control to dramatically reduce *Simulium* in these areas and mass distribution of ivermectin was added in 1988.[170,171]

The OCP was an extraordinarily successful programme. By 2002 the prevalence of onchocerciasis had decreased to almost zero both in the original OCP core area and in parts of the western and southern extension zones. OCP prevented some 600 000 cases of blindness and allowed farming to resume on 25 million ha of fertile land that had been abandoned because of the risk of onchocerciasis and blindness. The total cost of the OCP (1974–2002) was estimated to have been US$560 million.[172]

Chemotherapeutic Control

Annual mass treatment with ivermectin replaced vector control as the principal strategy for onchocerciasis control after community trials in several endemic areas showed that ivermectin was acceptable for mass treatment. Ivermectin treats and prevents clinical onchocerciasis and reduces transmission of new cases in the community.[173] As noted above, ivermectin is mainly microfilaricidal and community treatment needs to continue for a period equivalent to the reproductive lifespan of the adult female worms. The manufacturer of Mectizan® (Merck & Co, Inc.) has donated ivermectin to governments and non-governmental organizations for onchocerciasis control through the Mectizan® Donation Programme.[174] There are currently two large-scale intervention programmes that cover endemic areas with clinically significant onchocerciasis.

The Onchocerciasis Elimination Programme for the Americas (OEPA) was started in 1992 and this aims to eliminate the infection in the Western hemisphere. The programme covers 13 onchocerciasis foci in six countries (Brazil, Colombia, Ecuador, Guatemala, Mexico and Venezuela), where more than 536 000 people live in endemic areas.[95] The programme used treatment with a single dose (150 μg/kg body weight) once yearly at the beginning and switched to twice-yearly treatment later. OEPA has interrupted or significantly suppressed transmission in most of the endemic foci and community-based ivermectin treatment has been or will be withdrawn in the near future from all foci outside of Venezuela and Brazil.

The African Programme for Onchocerciasis Control (APOC) was established in 1995, and this programme became the leading coordinating body of onchocerciasis control in Africa when the OCP ended in 2002. APOC focuses on hyper- (>60% infection rate) and mesoendemic (40–60% infection rate) foci with the primary goal of preventing morbidity.[175] It has used annual ivermectin treatment in most areas. In a number of countries the programme faces problems such as low coverage rates and insufficient funds to distribute the drug. Countries in Western and Central Africa where onchocerciasis is co-endemic with *L. loa* represent a special challenge for APOC. Serious adverse events including death have occurred following ivermectin treatment in a small number of people with high-intensity *L. loa* microfilaraemia.[176] Ivermectin distribution has been interrupted in some co-endemic areas and further research is currently underway to explore new treatment or distribution strategies for these areas.

Feasibility of Onchocerciasis Elimination in Africa and Integration of Onchocerciasis with Other Neglected Tropical Disease Intervention Programmes. Recent publications have presented exciting results from long-term studies of the impact of ivermectin on onchocerciasis. For example, one paper reported results from three large foci in Mali and Senegal.[177] These foci had been part of the western extension area of the OCP, but they never received vector control. Ivermectin treatment started in these areas in 1988–1989 and it was gradually phased out after periods of 10 or more years. Interestingly, no infected blackflies or infected persons were identified in sentinel villages in these foci when they were resurveyed in 2009. These results suggest that it may be feasible to eliminate onchocerciasis in Africa and some of the major donor organizations have called for changing the focus of onchocerciasis programmes from disease prevention to interruption of transmission and elimination. Some African countries such as Uganda are already working toward elimination by providing community-based ivermectin treatment in all endemic foci including hypoendemic areas.

Onchocerciasis is one of the so-called 'neglected tropical diseases' (NTD) and current efforts are focused on integrating onchocerciasis control or elimination programmes with preventive chemotherapy programmes for other NTDs. This makes sense because ivermectin has activity against *W. bancrofti*, some soil-transmitted helminths such as *Ascaris lumbricoides* and scabies mites. In addition, onchocerciasis is often co-endemic with other major NTDs including trachoma and schistosomiasis.

Other Filarial Infections

Four other filarial species commonly infect humans in addition to those that cause human lymphatic filariasis and onchocerciasis. These are *Loa loa*, *Mansonella perstans*, *M. streptocerca* and *M. ozzardi*. In addition to these, several filarial parasites of animals rarely cause infections in humans.

LOA LOA

Loa loa is commonly known as the 'African eye-worm', because adult worms occasionally move across the eyes of infected individuals.

Epidemiology and Parasitology

Humans are infected when they are bitten by infective, day-biting female tabanid or deer flies of the genus *Chrysops*, mainly *C. silacea* and *C. dimidiata*. Other *Chrysops* species are of local importance, especially in the periphery of the transmission zone. *Chrysops* flies rest in the forest canopy and are attracted mainly by movement, dark colours and wood smoke. They deposit their eggs in swamps and river banks and the larvae hatch in the mud. Fly larvae mature slowly and it may take a year or longer for them to reach the adult stage. Loiasis transmission mainly takes place during the wet season.

Infective larvae (2 mm × 25 μm) penetrate the skin of the human host when the vector takes a blood meal. They develop into adult worms over a period of months. Adult *L. loa* can live for more than 10 years and they migrate in subcutaneous and connective tissues. The females measure 50–70 × 0.5 mm and the males 30–35 × 0.4 mm. Adult female worms release microfilariae that circulate in peripheral blood. The minimum prepatent period (the interval between infection and the appearance of microfilariae in the blood) is 5–6 months, but it can be much longer. The sheathed microfilariae measure 230–300 × 6–8 μm (Figure 54.26). They exhibit diurnal periodicity that corresponds to the day-biting habits of the vectors. *Chrysops* flies ingest microfilariae when they feed on infected

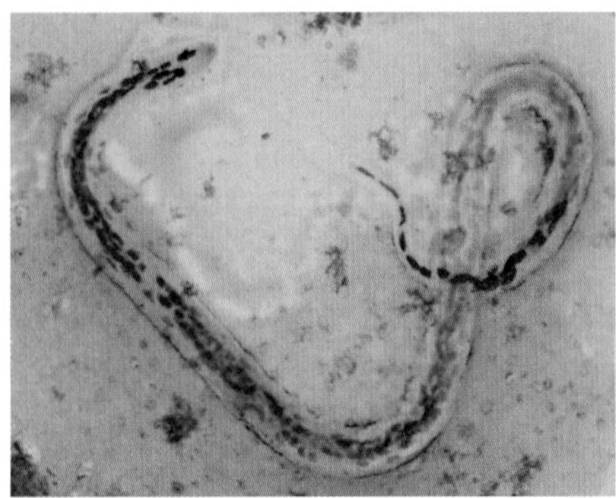

Figure 54.26 Microfilaria of *L. loa* (Giemsa).

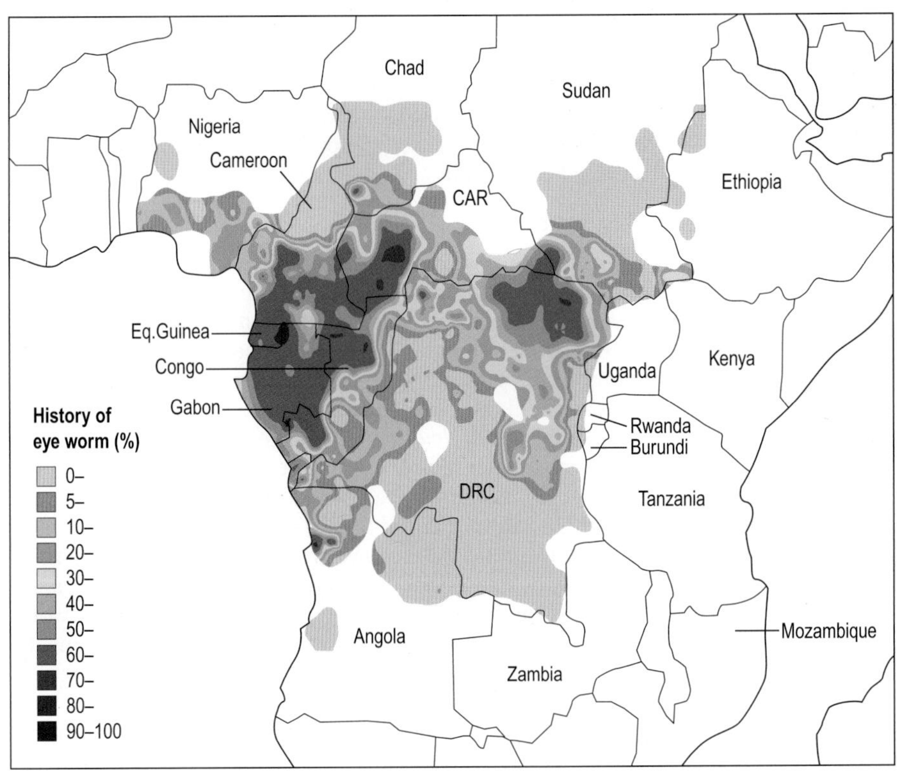

Figure 54.27 Geographical distribution of *L. loa*. *(From Zoure HG, Wanji S, Noma M, et al. The geographic distribution of Loa loa in Africa: results of large-scale implementation of the Rapid Assessment Procedure for Loiasis (RAPLOA). PLoS Negl Trop Dis. 2011;5:e1210)*

human blood. Ingested microfilariae penetrate the stomach wall of the fly vector and migrate to the fat body where they develop for 8–12 days to become infective larvae and this completes the life cycle.

Microfilaria counts in *L. loa*-infected individuals tend to be higher than in people infected with other filarial parasites. Densities of 5000/mL are not uncommon and counts may be as high as 100 000/mL. Microfilaria prevalence rates tend to be low in children; rates gradually rise with age and they tend to be higher in males than in females.[178] However, microfilaria rates in populations rarely exceed 40% even in adults.[179] Amicrofilaraemic infections are common in endemic areas and many patients with eye worms or angioedema secondary to loiasis are amicrofilaraemic.

Loiasis only occurs in Africa, where transmission is confined to rainforest and swamp forest areas of Central and Western Africa, from western Uganda to eastern Benin (Figure 54.27).[180] Recent mapping results indicate that about 90 million people live in areas that are endemic for loiasis. The parasite was previously also observed in the rainforests of Sierra Leone, Liberia, Ivory Coast and Ghana, but it has not been reported from these countries for many years.[181]

Pathogenesis and Pathology

Many cases of loiasis are asymptomatic and the pathogenesis of *L. loa* infection is poorly understood. Many infected individuals have hypereosinophilia and high antibody titres to filarial antigens.[182,183] Amicrofilaraemic infections are common. Microfilaraemic individuals have diminished cellular responsiveness to filarial antigens compared with amicrofilaraemic infected individuals.[184] Clinical signs of loiasis tend to be different in expatriates and natives of endemic areas. Infected expatriates who were first exposed to loiasis as adults often have localized angioedema (Calabar swellings) and urticaria that reflect immunological hyperresponsiveness to the parasite. In contrast, eye worms and asymptomatic microfilaraemia are more common in people who have been exposed to the parasite since childhood.[185,186]

Clinical Features

Although it is a much more geographically restricted infection than onchocerciasis or lymphatic filariasis, it is not uncommon for physicians outside of Africa to see loiasis in immigrants and travellers.[187] The first clinical signs of loiasis may occur as early as 5 months after infection.[185] The most common clinical manifestations are Calabar swellings and pruritus. Adult worms may be noticed by otherwise asymptomatic patients when the worms migrate across the eye under the bulbar conjunctiva (hence the name 'eye worm') (Figure 54.28) or under the skin (Figure

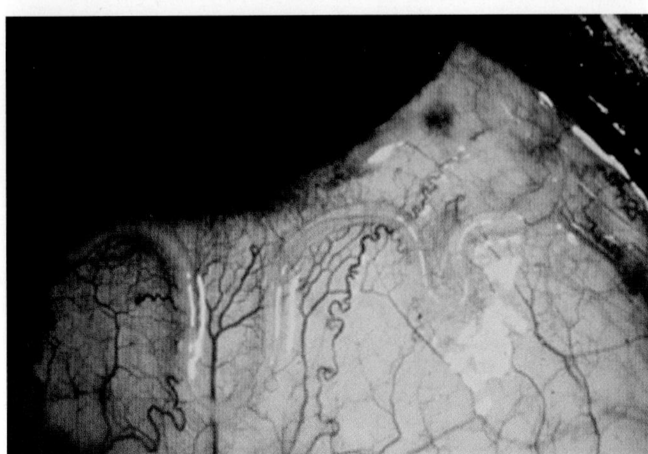

Figure 54.28 Subconjunctival migration of adult *L. loa*. *(Courtesy of J. Anderson.)*

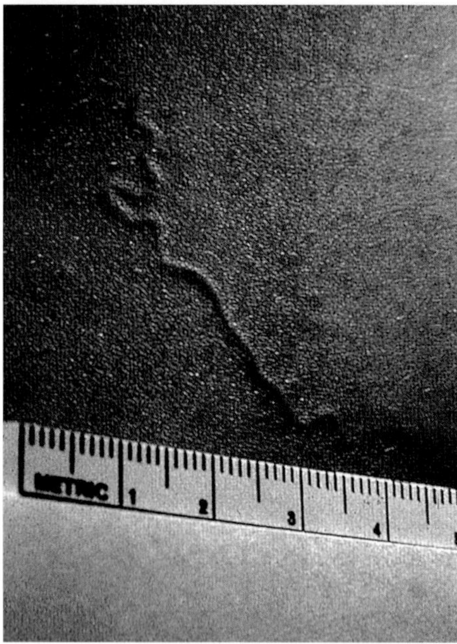

Figure 54.29 *L. loa* migrating under the skin. *(Courtesy of P.G.P. Manson-Bahr.)*

54.29).[181,188] Eye worms often leave the eye and re-enter the subcutaneous tissue less than 1 hour after they appear. Calabar swelling (Figure 54.30) most commonly occurs on the hands, wrists and forearms, but it may appear anywhere on the body. The swellings are painless, they do not pit on pressure, and they may last from a few hours to several days. They usually occur in one body location and swelling may recur at irregular intervals for years after the patient has left the endemic area. Calabar swellings occur in both microfilaraemic and amicrofilaraemic individuals. They are believed to result from host immune responses to adult worms. Loiasis can also cause generalized pruritus, fatigue and arthralgia. The death of an adult worm may occasionally cause a localized abscess. Calcified worms are sometimes seen in radiographs. An epidemiological correlation has been observed between loiasis and the occurrence of endomyocardial fibrosis. Since the latter condition can also occur in patients with extreme hypereosinophilia due to other medical conditions, it is possible that endomyocardial fibrosis associated with loiasis is also caused by toxins released into the blood by activated eosinophils.

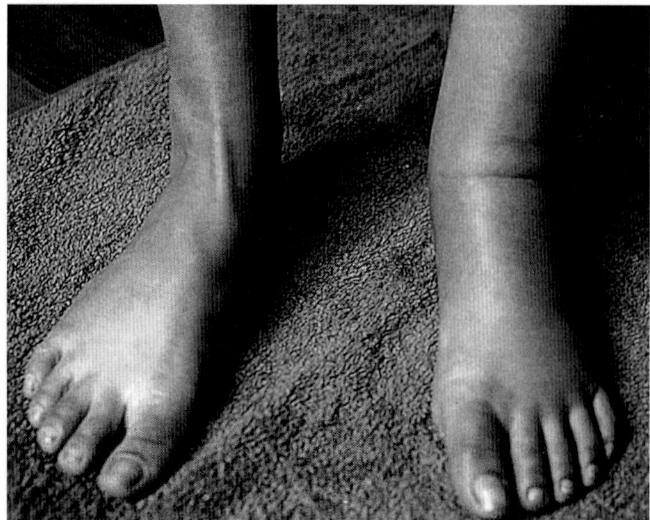

Figure 54.30 Loiasis: Calabar swelling. *(Courtesy of P.G.P. Manson-Bahr.)*

Diagnosis

The appearance of characteristic Calabar swellings in persons who have lived in endemic areas or a history of an eye worm are strongly suggestive of *L. loa* infection. Other helminths may migrate under the skin and cause cutaneous reactions. For example, *M. perstans* can cause lesions that are similar to Calabar swellings. Larva currens and cutaneous larva migrans (caused by *Strongyloides* and dog hookworm larvae, respectively) cause intense pruritus and leave tracks in the skin that may last for hours or even weeks. Guinea worms are much larger than adult *L. loa* and these parasites are now very uncommon. Subconjunctival *Loa* eye worms are easily distinguished from intraocular lesions caused by *Toxocara canis* larvae. *L. loa* infections can be parasitologically diagnosed if an adult worm is recovered from the conjunctiva or the skin. More frequently infection is diagnosed by the identification of the characteristic microfilariae in the blood (Figure 54.26). However, many persons with clinical loiasis are amicrofilaraemic (occult loiasis).[189] The optimal time for taking a blood sample for microfilaria testing is around noon, when the concentration of microfilariae in the peripheral blood is at its peak. The various techniques for concentration and examination of the blood for microfilariae mentioned under lymphatic filariasis can also be used for *L. loa*. The sheath of *L. loa* microfilariae stains with haematoxylin but not with Giemsa. The diagnosis can also be made by detecting *L. loa* DNA in blood samples by PCR.[190] A recently described antibody test is sensitive and more specific than prior tests that were based on native filarial antigens.[191] However, this test is not widely available at this time.

Management and Treatment

DEC (5–10 mg/kg daily in divided doses for 2–4 weeks) rapidly eliminates microfilariae of *L. loa* from the blood (Table 54.2). DEC also kills a proportion of adult worms and it is considered the drug of choice for loiasis when microfilaria counts are low. However, several courses of this regimen may be required for cure. Adverse events following DEC treatment often include fever, malaise, angioedema and pruritus.

Serious adverse events sometimes occur in persons with loiasis following treatment with diethylcarbamazine or ivermectin. diethylcarbamazine is no longer recommended for use in areas with onchocerciasis, but ivermectin is sometimes used for onchocerciasis control in areas with co-endemic loiasis.[176,192] Severe adverse events can include retinal haemorrhage, membranous glomerulonephritis, encephalopathy, coma and death. Brain pathology in fatal cases sometimes resembles cerebral malaria with extensive microhaemorrhages and diffuse oedema.[193] Severe adverse events are uncommon after treatment when microfilaria counts are lower than 8000/mL and neurological adverse events such as encephalopathy, coma and death are uncommon when microfilaria counts are lower than 30 000/mL. The risk of severe adverse events represents a significant barrier to control of onchocerciasis and lymphatic filariasis in areas of central Africa with co-endemic loiasis. Ongoing research is attempting to understand the pathogenesis of neurological adverse events in loiasis. They are not related to *Wolbachia*, since *L. loa* does not contain these endobacteria.[194]

Some authorities have advocated treating patients with high *L. loa* microfilaria counts with low doses of DEC plus glucocorticoids. However, this approach is not without risk. If possible, microfilaria counts should be reduced to below 8,000/mL by cytapheresis prior to treatment with DEC. If this is not possible, the benefits of therapy may not justify the potential risks of treatment.[195] Ivermectin (200 mg/kg body weight) clears *L. loa* microfilaraemia, but it does not kill adult worms and as mentioned above it can also cause severe adverse events.[181]

Albendazole was tested in patients to determine whether the drug could kill *L. loa* adult worms without causing severe adverse events. In one small study albendazole 200 mg twice daily for 21 days reduced microfilaria counts by approximately 80% at 6 months without serious adverse events.[196] No consistent benefit was observed in other studies with shorter treatment courses.

Prevention and Control

Control of *Chrysops* flies is difficult and vector control has not been implemented in large-scale programmes. *Chrysops* bites are rather painful and people usually avoid the bites wherever possible. The wearing of light-coloured clothing and frequent application of insect repellent reduces the risk of bites. Personal prophylaxis with a 300 mg dose of DEC once a week prevented loiasis in expatriates who worked in endemic areas.[197]

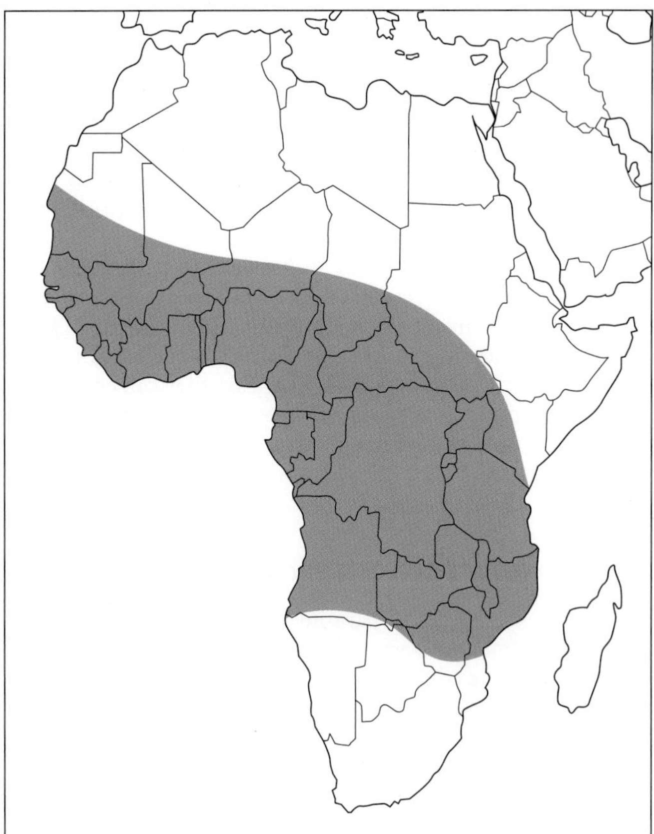

Figure 54.31 Geographical distribution of *M. perstans* in Africa.

MANSONELLA PERSTANS

Three *Mansonella* species infect humans. Microfilariae of *Mansonella* can be easily distinguished from other filariae that infect humans based on their small size and the absence of sheaths. *M. perstans* is widely distributed in sub-Saharan Africa (Figure 54.31), in parts of Central and South America and in the Caribbean. No accurate estimates are available on prevalence rates for *M. perstans* for countries or continents, but it is probably the most common filarial infection of humans in Africa.[198] *M. perstans* is transmitted by tiny biting midges of the genus *Culicoides*. Adult worms have occasionally been recovered from humans. They live in serous cavities such as the peritoneum and they usually cause no symptoms. Adult worms have been found in subcutaneous tissue in a few cases. Adult female worms measure 70–80 × 0.12 mm and male worms are 35–45 × 0.06 mm. Microfilariae (200 × 4.5 μm) are unsheathed and circulate in the blood without periodicity (Figure 54.32). The time interval between infection and the first appearance of microfilariae in the blood of humans is unknown. Only a few studies have been carried out on the epidemiology of *M. perstans* infections. Microfilaria prevalence rates are generally higher in adults than in children and males are usually more frequently infected than females.[199,200] Very high infection rates have been reported from some localities.[201]

The main vectors in Africa are *C. grahami* and *C. inornatipennis*, but other species serve as secondary vectors. The *Culicoides* species that transmit *M. perstans* in the Americas have not yet been identified. *M. perstans* is well adapted to the human host and it often causes no symptoms. However, a variety of clinical manifestations have been reported. Symptoms are more common in persons who are first exposed to the parasite as adults. Transient swellings similar to the Calabar swellings of loiasis have been reported. Other manifestations include pruritus, fever and joint pain. Some patients experience severe abdominal pain, especially in the right upper quadrant. Conjunctival nodules, oedema of the eyelids and proptosis have also been attributed to *M. perstans* infections.[198] Eosinophilia is common and cases of symptomatic hypereosinophilia have recently been reported from expatriates returning from an endemic area.[202] Diagnosis of *M. perstans* infection is usually by identification of microfilariae in the blood (Figure 54.32). Similar techniques to those used for concentration and examination of blood samples for the diagnosis of lymphatic filariasis can be used, but a smaller pore size is needed for filtration (3 μM instead of 5 μM used for lymphatic filariasis).

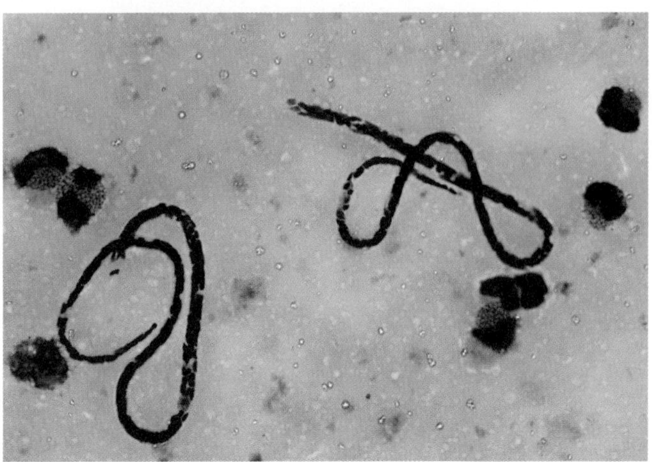

Figure 54.32 Two microfilariae of *M. perstans* (Giemsa).

Treatment

Treatments commonly used for lymphatic filariasis or onchocerciasis are not effective for *M. perstans*. Ivermectin alone or in combination with albendazole has little or no effect on microfilaria counts (Table 54.2).[203] DEC (200 mg twice daily for 21 days) and mebendazole (100 mg twice daily for 28 days) reduce microfilaria counts and combination treatment with these drugs is more effective than either drug alone.[204] Some strains of *M. perstans* contain *Wolbachia* and a study in Mali showed that doxycycline (200 mg daily for 6 weeks) was quite effective for clearing *M. perstans* microfilaraemia.[205] Since *M. perstans* microfilariae are not cleared by regimens used in MDA programmes for lymphatic filariasis, they can complicate monitoring of filarial elimination programmes that rely on microfilaria detection, although experienced microscopists can easiliy differentiate *Mansonella* microfilariae from those of *Wuchereria*.

MANSONELLA STREPTOCERCA

M. streptocerca is a filarial parasite of humans that is present in parts of Central and West Africa, although it occurs as far east as Uganda.[206] The adult worms inhabit the dermis of the upper thorax and shoulders, but they are difficult to detect in untreated patients (Figure 54.33). The adult females measure 27×0.08 mm and males are 17×0.05 mm. The microfilariae (Figure 54.34) also inhabit the dermis. They are unsheathed, measure 180–240×3–5 μm and exhibit no periodicity.

Like *M. perstans, M. streptocerca* is transmitted by *Culicoides* midges and the most common vector is probably *C. grahami*. Complete development in the vector takes 9 days. Information on the development of *M. streptocerca* in the human host is lacking and the prepatent period is unknown.

These infections are often asymptomatic. Dermatitis involving the skin over the trunk and shoulders is the most common clinical manifestation.[206] It is characterized by pruritus, hypopigmented macules and papules. Microscopic examination of skin biopsies shows dilated dermal lymphatics and it has been suggested that *M. streptocerca* may rarely cause lymphoedema and elephantiasis. The skin lesions can be similar to those seen with onchocerciasis or leprosy. Definitive diagnosis requires finding the characteristic unsheathed microfilariae in skin snips (see Onchocerciasis above, for the technique). The microfilariae have a 'shepherd's crook' tail. A sensitive and specific PCR assay for specific detection of *M. streptocerca* DNA in skin biopsies has been reported.[207]

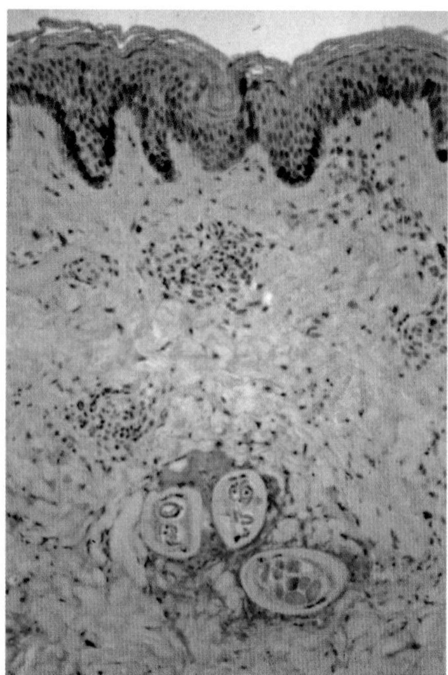

Figure 54.33 Adult worms of *M. streptocerca* in the skin.

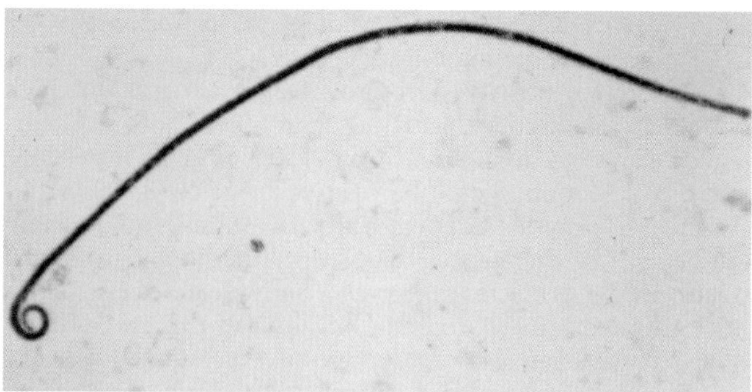

Figure 54.34 Microfilaria of *M. streptocerca* (Haematoxylin).

Treatment

Diethylcarbamazine (2–6 mg/kg body weight for 21 days) eliminates both microfilariae and adults of *M. streptocerca* (Table 54.2). DEC treatment often causes intense pruritus and patients sometimes develop cutaneous nodules around degenerating adult worms. Other adverse events similar to Mazzotti reactions associated with DEC treatment of onchocerciasis are uncommon. A single dose of ivermectin (150 mg/kg) results in sustained suppression of microfiladermia.[208] Adverse events are similar to those that are observed after DEC.[209]

MANSONELLA OZZARDI

M. ozzardi is the only human filarial parasite species that is restricted to the New World. It occurs in parts of Central America, Amazonia and the Caribbean. Adult worms have been recovered from the peritoneal cavity of humans. Females measure 50×0.15 mm and males 26×0.07 mm. The microfilariae (220×3–4 μm; see Figure 54.35) are unsheathed,

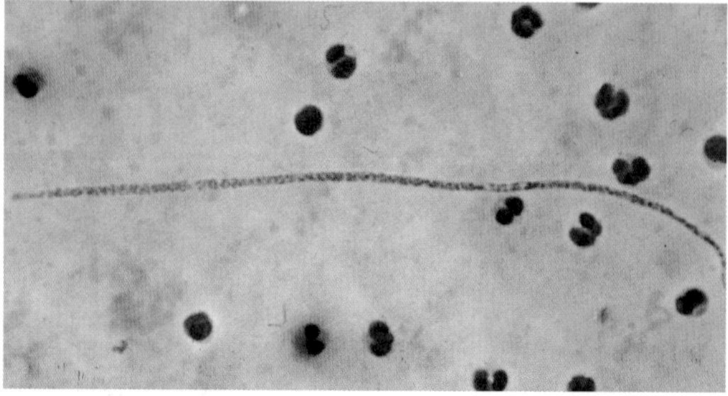

Figure 54.35 Microfilaria of *M. ozzardi* (Giemsa).

non-periodic and they can be found in the blood and in the skin. Microfilariae of *M. ozzardi* with an atypical arrangement of nuclei at the anterior end have been described from the Amazon region.[210]

Two groups of vectors have been implicated in the transmission of *M. ozzardi*. These are midges of the genus *Culicoides* in the Caribbean and blackflies of the genus *Simulium* in the Amazon basin. The prepatent period is 5–6 months in experimentally infected patas monkeys. Natural *M. ozzardi* infections have not been reported from animals. Infection rates are often very high in endemic areas and microfilaria rates increase with age.[211,212] Most people infected with *M. ozzardi* are asymptomatic. Some infected patients have experienced arthritis, headache, fever and pruritus, but causality has not been clearly established.[211,212] Eosinophilia and high titres of antibodies to filarial antigens are common.

The infection is diagnosed by identifying the microfilariae in blood or in skin biopsies.[213] The techniques described under lymphatic filariasis and onchocerciasis can be used. DEC has little or no effect on *M. ozzardi* infections (Table 54.2), but a single 6 mg dose of ivermectin provides a significant long-term reduction in microfilaria counts.[214]

Zoonotic Filarial Infections

Humans occasionally become infected with species of filariae that are normally found in animals.[215] In most cases only one or a few adult worms are found that are not reproducing. These are filarial parasites of mammals and most species belong to the genera *Dirofilaria*, *Brugia* or *Onchocerca*. These infections are not limited to tropical countries; they rarely occur in North America and Europe. Among these zoonotic infections, those due to *Dirofilaria* spp. are the most frequently reported and the most widely distributed.

DIROFILARIASIS

Dirofilaria spp. are natural parasites of various species of carnivores. Microfilariae circulate in the blood of these hosts and transmission is by mosquitoes. When humans are infected, parasite development is impaired and no microfilariae are produced.[216]

Pulmonary Dirofilariasis

D. immitis is a filarial parasite of dogs. It is transmitted in many parts of the world in tropical or temperate climates.[217] Adult *D. immitis* inhabit the pulmonary arteries and right ventricle of the heart in dogs, where they may occur in large coiled masses. *D. immitis* occasionally infects humans. Larval parasites migrate to the lung where they usually die before becoming mature adult worms. Most infections are asymptomatic, but symptoms can include cough, chest pain, eosinophilia, haemoptysis and fever. Many cases come to medical attention when a spherical nodule (a 'coin lesion') 1–3 cm in diameter is discovered in the lungs on routine radiography. These suspicious lesions are biopsied to rule out carcinoma. Typical pathological findings include a single worm (usually necrotic and sometimes calcified) in the lumen of a pulmonary arterial vessel. Serological diagnosis is not sensitive or specific enough to make biopsies unnecessary. Since the worms are usually dead, no anthelmintic therapy is required.

Subcutaneous Dirofilariasis

D. repens is a natural parasite of dogs and cats in warmer climates of the Old World. It has not been reported in the Americas. Adult worms live in the subcutaneous tissues of animal hosts. Abortive human infections typically present as subcutaneous nodules comprised of an immature worm surrounded by granulomatous tissue. Nodules or small cysts may occur in many parts of the body, especially the breasts, arms, legs, scrotum, eyelid and conjunctiva.[218] Immunodiagnosis has not proved useful and diagnosis is by biopsy. Treatment is by surgical removal of the nodule. Other *Dirofilaria* species (especially *D. tenuis* and *D. ursi*, natural parasites of racoons and bears, respectively) occasionally cause subcutaneous dirofilariasis in humans in North America.

Dracunculiasis (Guinea Worm)

Dracunculiasis or guinea worm disease in humans results from infection with *Dracunculus medinensis*, a nematode parasite closely related to filarial worms. The vectors are cyclopoid copepods (water fleas), which are tiny free-swimming crustaceans usually found in abundance in freshwater ponds. Humans acquire the infection by drinking water that contains vectors infected with guinea worm larvae. Extensive control activities over the past 20 years have reduced the incidence of guinea worm infection to nearly zero.

EPIDEMIOLOGY

Adult female *D. medinensis* (up to 60–80 cm long and 1.5–2.0 mm in thickness) inhabit human subcutaneous tissue. Most of the interior of female worms is occupied by the uterus, which contains thousands of first-stage larvae. A blister is formed on the skin of the host around the anterior end of the worm and this ruptures when it is exposed to water. The female guinea worm protrudes its anterior end from the ulcer and discharges first-stage larvae (650×20 μm) into the water. It remains protruding for the following 2–6 weeks, releasing larvae each time it is immersed in water. The worms die after they release their larvae.

The larvae are infective for copepods in freshwater for 5–6 days; they must be swallowed by a permissive species of copepod during this time if they are to survive and develop. The larvae penetrate the copepod gut wall and moult twice to become infective third-stage larvae (450×14 μm) in about 2 weeks. Vectors that contain third-stage larvae become sluggish and sink to the bottom of the water. Many species of cyclopoid copepods have been found naturally infected with *Dracunculus* species in various parts of the world.[219] Parasites resembling *D. medinensis* occur in dogs and other animals, but there is no evidence that they are a reservoir of infection for humans.[220]

Copepods ingested in drinking water are dissolved by gastric juice. *Dracunculus* infective larvae then penetrate the stomach or intestine of the human host. After a period of residence in the abdominal cavity, the larvae migrate into connective tissues, where they develop into mature worms. Mating occurs about 3 months after the initial infection and the males, which are much smaller than the females (1–4 cm×0.4 mm), die shortly thereafter. The females move about in the connective tissues and usually reach the lower extremities between 8 and 10 months after infection.

Transmission of guinea worm occurs mainly in small surface water pools used for collecting drinking water and for washing. Humans contract the infection by drinking water containing infected copepods. Humans also contribute to transmission by immersing the guinea worm ulcer in water, thereby allowing the release of first-stage larvae that infect copepods to continue the life cycle.

Transmission is frequently seasonal, with the majority of patent infections and infected copepods being present only a few months of the year. This seasonality is closely related to rainfall. In arid areas the transmission usually coincides with the rainy season, when surface water is available, whereas in wet areas transmission is most intense towards the end of the dry season, when drinking water sources are few. The transmission season often coincides with the peak period of agricultural work. In the past, guinea worm infections severely reduced agricultural output in endemic areas, because a large proportion of farmers were infected and incapacitated each year.

CLINICAL FEATURES

There are usually no symptoms in the prepatent period. The first sign appears a few days before the worm pierces the skin. The dermis becomes elevated and a blister develops (Figure 54.36). Patients experience a burning sensation and pruritus and they often place the affected part in water to relieve their discomfort. Adult worms are most frequently located in the foot or lower leg, but they may appear on arms, breasts, head, back, scrotum, or anywhere on the body surface. When worms are close to joints they may cause arthritis. Inflammatory responses or the calcification of adult worms may cause joints in the legs or feet to become stiff, thereby crippling the patient. Secondary infection of ulcers may lead to bacterial cellulitis. In addition, the ulcers can serve as entry lesions for tetanus spores.

Inflammation makes it difficult to extract adult worms from ulcers before the uterus has released its larvae. Provided there is no secondary infection, guinea worm ulcers heal spontaneously after the empty worm has been removed. If adult worms are broken, the remainder of the worm withdraws into the host tissue. This causes a severe inflammatory reaction that may result in a larger ulcer and (later) extensive fibrosis. Usually only a single worm appears in a patient per year, but several (up to ≥20) can appear at the same time in one individual. Some female worms die before they emerge through the skin. Dead or ruptured worms can lead to formation of sterile subcutaneous abscesses. Migration of worms into vital organs can cause serious problems, but such migration is rare.

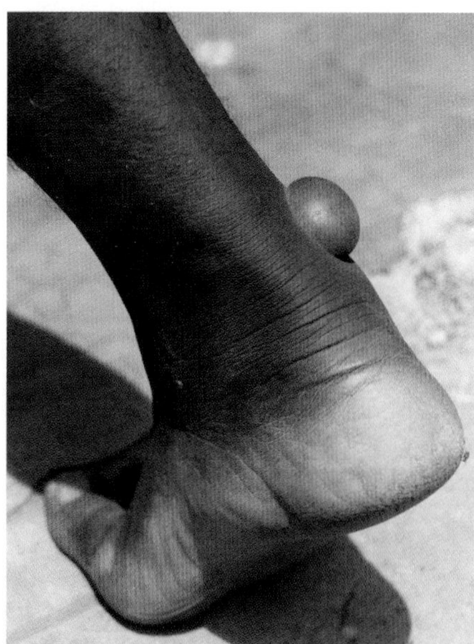

Figure 54.36 Blister on the skin related to an emerging guinea worm. *(Courtesy of P. Bloch.)*

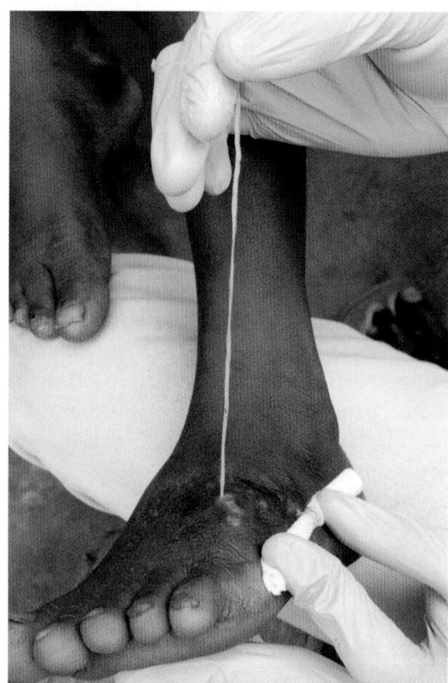

Figure 54.37 Traditional method for removing a guinea worm. *(Courtesy of The Carter Center.)*

Many people in endemic areas have antibodies to the parasite because of current or recent infections.[221,222] Infections do not confer immunity and some people in endemic areas become reinfected year after year.

DIAGNOSIS

Guinea worm infections cannot be diagnosed in the prepatent period, i.e. for the first 8–10 months of infection. Adult female worms are sometimes visible or palpable under the skin shortly before they start to emerge. A clinical diagnosis is made by examining the guinea worm ulcer and observing the female protruding from the blister (Figure 54.37). The appearance of the blister, with local itching and burning pain, makes diagnosis simple, even for the sufferer. Active larvae can be obtained by immersing the protruding adult female in a small tube or container with water. The first-stage larvae, with their characteristic pointed tails, can then be observed under the microscope. Serology is of no practical use in diagnosis. Patients with guinea worm infections often have eosinophilia. Dead calcified worms are easily seen in radiographs, but live worms are not visible.

MANAGEMENT

The traditional method of slow extraction of the emergent guinea worm is usually effective. The protruding part of the female worm is attached to a small stick which is twisted a small amount each day until the worm has been removed (Figure 54.37). Care should be taken not to break the worm.[223] Administration of antibiotics and cleaning and dressing of the ulcers are important in reducing secondary infections and tetanus vaccination is recommended.

A technique for surgical extraction of the guinea worm prior to eruption through the skin has been described.[224] Niridazole, metronidazole and mebendazole have been reported to reduce inflammation around the worm, thereby allowing easier extraction. Treatment of prepatent guinea worm infections with ivermectin had no effect.[225]

PREVENTION AND CONTROL

Provision of safe drinking water in the form of borehole wells is an expensive but effective measure for preventing infections.[226] Other measures are health education and chemical vector control.[227] Health education focuses on drinking water as the source of infection and on the importance of boiling or filtering the water before use (Figure 54.38). Special nylon material has been produced for filtering water, but effective and less expensive filters can be made from polyester cloth or even from a layer of tightly woven cotton cloth. To prevent contamination of water with guinea worm larvae, health education also emphasizes that people with guinea worm ulcers should have their wounds dressed and that they should not place infected limbs in water that is used for drinking. Vector control can be achieved in ponds and wells with the insecticide temephos (Abate™).

The guinea worm's simple life cycle and the apparent lack of an animal reservoir made elimination a feasible goal for this parasite and disease. The United Nations-supported International Drinking Water and Sanitation decade (1981–1990) raised global attention to the possibility of eradicating the infection by improving the quality of human drinking water and in 1986 the World Health Assembly adopted a resolution calling for worldwide elimination of dracunculiasis. Since then, many organizations have participated in successful control programmes that included identification and monitoring of transmission sites and provision of health education and safe water supplies.[227] Active case surveillance has been adopted in the later stages of control programmes and cash rewards have been used to identify the diminishing number of infected villages and individuals.[228] Asia was declared free of guinea worm transmission in 1997. In 2010, the global incidence had been reduced to fewer than 1800 cases (a decrease of more than 99% from 892 000 cases reported in 1989). Dracunculiasis is now confined to a few countries in Africa, with more than 90% of cases reported from South Sudan.[229]

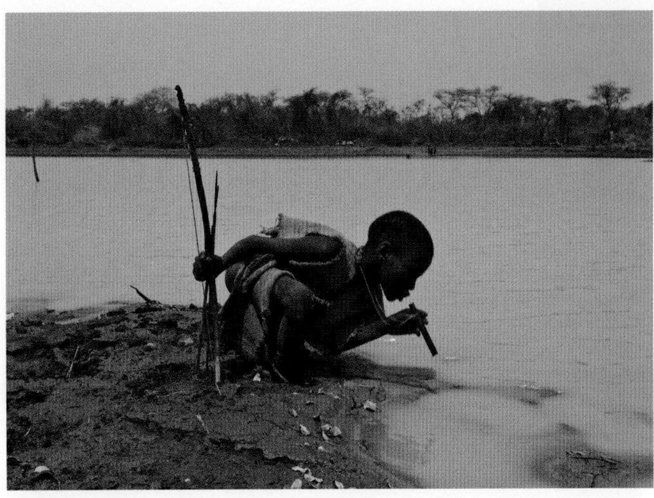

Figure 54.38 Guinea worm intervention: drinking using a handheld water filter. *(Courtesy of The Carter Center.)*

REFERENCES

4. WHO. Lymphatic filariasis: Progress report 2000–2009 and strategic plan 2010–20. Geneva: World Health Organization; 2010. WHO/HTM/PCT/2010.6.
90. Ottesen EA. Lymphatic filariasis: Treatment, control and elimination. Adv Parasitol 2006;61:395–441.
95. Cupp EW, Sauerbrey M, Richards F. Elimination of human onchocerciasis: history of progress and current feasibility using ivermectin (Mectizan®) monotherapy. Acta Tropica 2011;120(Suppl 1):S100–8.
181. Boussinesq M. Loiasis. Ann Trop Med Parasitol 2006;100:715–31.
227. Ruiz-Tiben E, Hopkins DR. Dracunculiasis (Guinea worm disease) eradication. Adv Parasitol 2006;61:275–309.

Access the complete references online at www.expertconsult.com

55

Soil-transmitted Helminths (Geohelminths)

SIMON J. BROOKER | DONALD A. P. BUNDY

KEY POINTS

- With an estimated more than 1 billion infections worldwide, soil-transmitted helminths (STH) are among the most common of all chronic infections of humans and are the most prevalent of human helminthic infections.
- Risk factors include poverty, inadequate water and sanitation and unhygienic behaviour.
- Large-scale geographical distributions are largely influenced by climatic factors, and studies using geographical information systems and remote sensing can reliably predict infection prevalence and help target national control programmes.
- The morbidity caused by STH is strongly related to the number of worms present (the intensity of infection), with most individuals harbouring only a few worms and a few people harbouring disproportionately large burdens.
- In the minority of individuals who harbour a large worm burden, chronic infection can cause anaemia, as well as impaired growth and cognition.
- In rare cases, the clinical complications of chronic infection – especially obstruction of the intestines – can result in death.
- Periodic mass anthelmintic treatment offers a cost-effective strategy to reduce the burden of STH.
- Treatment efficacy varies according to the STH species.
- Heavy infection is most common in school-aged children such that effective treatment of this age group has a disproportionately large effect on transmission, and thus this group is the natural target for school-based control efforts.

Introduction

Soil-transmitted helminths (STHs) are intestinal nematodes, part of the development of which takes place outside the body – in the soil. Infection occurs through contact with parasite eggs or larva in contaminated soil.

STHs are among the most common of all chronic human infections, occurring predominantly in areas of poverty and inadequate hygiene and sanitation in the developing world. The majority of infected individuals exhibit no or minimal signs or symptoms. This is because pathology is strongly related to the size of the number of worms present (the intensity of infection), and most individuals harbour only a few worms. In the minority of individuals who harbour a large worm burden, chronic infection can cause anaemia, impaired growth and cognition. Fortunately, however, much of this morbidity is rapidly reversible by periodic anthelmintic treatment. In rare cases, the clinical complications of chronic infection can result in death.

These nematodes are considered together since they have many similarities in biology and epidemiology and are often therefore found as multiple infections, and can be controlled using a common approach. They may be divided into three types according to their life cycle.

Type 1: Direct

Embryonated eggs are passed; they hatch and reinfect within 2–3 hours by being carried from the anal margin to the mouth and either do not reach the soil or, if they do, do not require a period of development there. This group includes *Enterobius vermicularis* (pinworm) and *Trichuris trichiura* (whipworm).

Type 2: Modified Direct

Eggs are passed out in the stool and undergo a period of development in the soil before being ingested, where they hatch, releasing larvae which penetrate the mucous membrane(s) of the stomach and enter the circulation to reach the lungs, passing up the respiratory tract to enter the oesophagus, reaching the intestine where they become adult. These include *Ascaris lumbricoides* (roundworm) and *Toxocara* spp.

Type 3: Penetration of the Skin

In this group, eggs are passed in the stools to the soil, where they hatch into larvae, which undergo further development before they are ready to penetrate the skin and reach the circulation and lungs, which they penetrate to enter the respiratory tract; they move up to enter the oesophagus and reach the small intestine, where they become adult. The hookworms, *Ancylostoma duodenale* and *Necator americanus*, and *Strongyloides stercoralis* belong to this group, but differ in that *S. stercoralis* larvae are passed in the stool and autoinfection can occur at the anal margin, or independent development takes place in the soil, where they can exist in the absence of any further cycle through humans.

Type 1: Direct (*Enterobius vermicularis, Trichuris trichiura*)

ENTEROBIASIS (PINWORM, THREADWORM, OXYURIASIS)

Enterobiasis results from infection with *Enterobius vermicularis* and is a relatively benign condition that typically affects children.

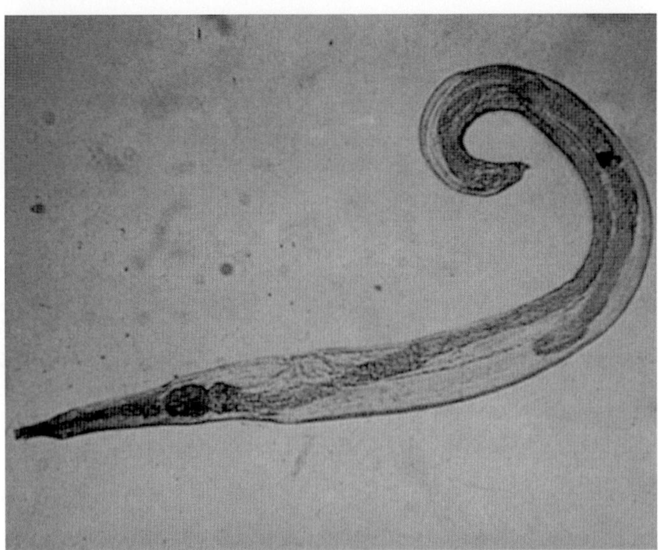

Figure 55.1 Adult *Enterobius vermicularis* (threadworm, pinworm).

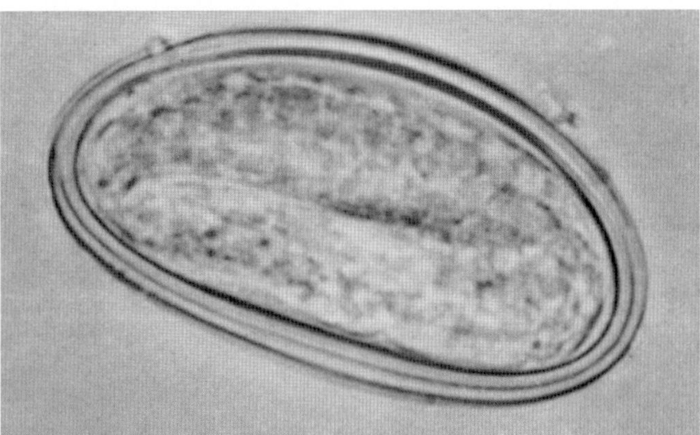

Figure 55.2 Egg of *Enterobius vermicularis*, as laid partially embryonated.

Geographical Distribution

Enterobius vermicularis has a worldwide distribution, and is one of the most common childhood helminth infections in the developed world.

Aetiology

The adult *E. vermicularis* (Figure 55.1, Chapter 10 and Appendix III) are small and white with a double bulb oesophagus and a mouth surrounded by a cuticular expansion; the skin is transversely striated. The female (9–12 mm) has a long, pointed tail and a slit-like vulva in the anterior quarter of the body. The male, which is much smaller (2.5 mm), has a posteriorly curved third and a blunt caudal extremity. The egg (Figure 55.2) measures 50–54×20–27 mm and has a characteristic shape, flattened on one side. It is almost colourless, with a bean-shaped double contour shell containing a fully formed embryo.

Life Cycle

Humans are the only hosts and there is no multiplication inside the body (see Appendix III). The mature female has a life span of 37–93 days and when the ovary is full of eggs she migrates down to the anus, from which she emerges to lay the eggs on the perianal skin and on the perineum. The eggs, which are immediately infective and are ingested in faecal material lodged under the fingernails, hatch in the stomach and larvae emerge which rapidly grow to 140–150 μm in length. They pass through the intestine to the caecum and appendix, where they invade the glandular crypts and mature. The whole cycle takes 2–4 weeks.

Transmission

There are four possible methods of transmission; the most common is by direct transmission from the anal and perianal region to the mouth by fingernail contamination and by soiled nightclothes. A second route is by exposure to viable eggs on soiled bed linen and other contaminated objects in the environment. A third way is via the mouth or nose from contaminated dust in which embryonated eggs have been detected. The fourth is by retroinfection in which eggs hatch on the anal mucosa and larvae migrate up the bowel.

Pathology

The adult worm lives in the upper part of the colon, especially the caecum and lower ileum, where minute ulcerations may develop at the site of attachment of the adult worms to the caecal and appendiceal mucosa. At times haemorrhages occur and secondary infection causes ulcers and submucosal abscesses. Symptoms are caused when gravid females migrate out of the anus on to perianal skin to deposit eggs, where they cause pruritus. *E. vermicularis* has also been implicated in nonspecific colitis in children.[1] Occasionally, ectopic infections occur in the female genital organs or urinary tract, and chronic pelvic peritonitis and ileocolitis have been described.[2] The route by which *E. vermicularis* gains access to these organs is not clear but may be via the Fallopian tubes or haematogenous spread. A case of ectopic infection in the male genital tract has been reported, with assumed entry through the urethra.[3] Aberrant infections may occur in the liver, ovary, kidney, spleen and lung as well as the appendix; however, their role in the pathogenesis of acute appendicitis remains unclear.[4] The granuloma which forms around the female and eggs consists chiefly of lymphocytes with a few eosinophils but no giant cells. Rare cases of eosinophilic granuloma of the large bowel and omentum have been ascribed to *E. vermicularis*.

Clinical Features

Natural History. In the majority of infections *E. vermicularis* lives out its normal life span in the caecum and appendix, migrates down to the anus and deposits its eggs, and the larvae re-establish themselves in the host, causing few or no symptoms.

Symptoms and Signs. Pruritus ani is the main symptom and varies from mild itching to acute pain, which occurs mainly at night. The pruritus produces scratching of the perianal region resulting in excoriation and secondary infection.

Vulvitis may be caused by worms entering the vulva, causing a mucoid discharge and pruritus vulvi.

General symptoms are insomnia and restlessness, and a considerable proportion of children show loss of appetite, loss of weight, irritability, emotional instability and enuresis. There is usually no eosinophilia or anaemia.

TABLE 55.1 Recommended Treatments for Soil-Transmitted Helminths. Note All Treatment are Administered Orally

Infection	Drugs	Dose	Duration
ENTEROBIUS			
Drugs of choice	Albendazole	400 mg	Single dose[a]
	Mebendazole	100 mg	Single dose[a]
	Pyrantel pamoate	10 mg/kg	Single dose[a]
TRICHURIS			
Drugs of choice	Albendazole	400 mg	Single dose[b]
	Mebendazole	500 mg	Single dose[b]
Alternatives	Nitazoxanide	500 mg or 200 mg for children 4–11 years or 100 mg for children 1–3 years	Daily for 3 days
ASCARIS			
Drugs of choice	Albendazole	400 mg or 200 mg for children 2–5 years	Single dose
	Mebendazole	500 mg	Single dose
	Levamisole	2.5 mg/kg	Single dose
	Pyrantel pamoate	10 mg/kg	Single dose
Alternatives	Nitazoxanide	500 mg or 200 mg for children 4–11 years or 100 mg for children 1–3 years	Daily for 3 days
TOXOCARA			
Drugs of choice	Albendazole	400 mg	Twice daily for 5 days
	Mebendazole	500 mg	Twice daily for 5 days
LAGOCHILASCARIASIS			
Drugs of choice	Albendazole	400 mg	Daily for 30 days
	Ivermectin	300 µg/kg	Weekly for 10 weeks
HOOKWORM			
Drugs of choice	Albendazole	400 mg	Single dose
	Mebendazole	500 mg	Single dose[b]
Alternatives	Pyrantel pamoate	10 mg/kg	Daily for 3 days
	Levamisole	150 mg or 2.5 mg/kg	Single dose
HOOKWORM-RELATED CUTANEOUS LARVA MIGRANS			
Drugs of choice	Albendazole	400 mg	Daily over 3–7 days to reduce recurrence
	Ivermectin	200 µg/kg	Single dose
	Thiabendazole	Topical application	Daily over 5–7 days
STRONGYLOIDES			
Drug of choice	Ivermectin	200 µg/kg	Single dose repeated after 1 week or daily for 3 days
Alternatives	Albendazole	400 mg	Daily for 3 days repeated 2 weeks later
	Mebendazole	500 mg	Single dose
TRICHOSTRONGYLIASIS			
Drug of choice	Pyrantel pamoate	10 mg/kg	Daily for 3 days
Alternatives	Albendazole	400 mg	Single dose
	Levamisole	2.5 mg/kg	Single dose

[a]Repeated every 6 weeks until environment is clear.
[b]Treatment over several days may be required for heavy infections.

Diagnosis

The diagnosis is made by finding the characteristic eggs (see Figure 55.2) in the faeces, perianal scrapings or swabs from under the fingernails, or by finding adult worms round the anus, usually at night.

Faecal examination has little practical use since eggs are present in the faeces of no more than 5–15% of infected individuals. A Sellotape swab has been devised with which it is possible to obtain eggs by scraping the perianal area, usually at night. Investigation on consecutive days increases diagnostic sensitivity. Enclosed in a container, it may be sent through the post and examined at leisure. The Sellotape is mounted in water or 0.1 mol sodium hydroxide on a slide, covered with a coverslip and examined. The Scotch tape method, in which eggs adhere to a sticky surface, is commonly used (see Appendix I).

Management

Albendazole is the treatment of choice (Table 55.1). Mebendazole, levamisole and pyrantel pamoate are as effective.

Piperazine is also effective but is less well tolerated and must be given daily for 7 days. Although it is simple to effect a temporary cure, eradication may prove difficult because of reinfection from the contaminated environment or from asymptomatic members of the same household. Repeated treatment may be necessary and other members of the family or school should also be treated.

During treatment, it is important to prevent reinfection. The child must sleep in cotton clothes and gloves and the fingernails must be kept short and scrubbed. Frequent washing of hands, bedsheets and bed clothes is essential.

Epidemiology

E. vermicularis is more common in children than adults and occurs among all socioeconomic groups. It occurs in families or institutions, such as asylums and schools, especially under crowded conditions. When one infection is found, it is likely that there are others.

TRICHURIASIS (WHIPWORM)

Trichuriasis is caused by *Trichuris trichiura*, which is one of the most prevalent human geohelminths and is commonly found in tropical areas with heavy rainfall, constant warm temperature and inadequate sanitation. Light infections give rise to few clinical symptoms, but heavy infections can cause gastrointestinal problems, rectal prolapse, anaemia, growth stunting and cognitive impairment.

Geographical Distribution

T. trichiura occurs worldwide, but is most prevalent in warm and humid tropical regions of the world.[5,6] Transmission does not typically occur in arid areas (Figure 55.3). It is estimated that 0.5 billion people were infected globally in 2010, including 35 million school-aged children harbouring high-intensity infections which cause morbidity (Pullan and Brooker, unpublished). *T. trichiura* is estimated to cause the loss of 638 000 disability adjusted life years (DALYs).[7] Owing to the generalized pathology of *T. trichiura* no reliable estimates of *T. trichiura*-associated mortality exist.

The prevalence of *T. trichiura* varies in different parts of the world and is greatest in equatorial Africa and South-east Asia. Sustained control and socioeconomic development has helped reduced prevalence levels in parts of China, East Asia and Central and South America.[8]

Aetiology

T. trichiura is a greyish-white worm, often slightly pink, which lives in the caecum and appendix. The male (30–45 mm long) has an attenuated anterior portion containing a cellular oesophagus which is half as long again as the thicker posterior portion, and a caudal extremity curved through 360° with a single spicule in the sheath which is studded with spines (Figure 55.4). The female (30–35 mm long) has the posterior half occupied by a stout uterus packed with eggs. The egg (50×22 μm) is brown with a characteristic band shape and a single cell with a plug at each end; it contains a single embryo (Figure 55.5).

Life Cycle

The worms live in the caecum, where they maintain their position by transfixing a superficial fold of mucosa and lie embedded in epithelial tunnels it creates between the intestinal villi. Eggs are laid unsegmented, and embryonation takes at least 21 days. Eggs can withstand low temperatures but not desiccation. Infection is direct from contaminated faeces. The egg hatches after being swallowed in the intestine, where the shell is digested by intestinal juices and the larva emerges in the small intestine; it penetrates the villi and develops for a week until it re-emerges and passes to the caecum and colorectum, where it attaches itself to the mucosa and becomes adult (see Appendix III).

Transmission

Transmission is direct from mature eggs to the mouth via fingers contaminated from infected soil. As well as through accidental ingestion of eggs, transmission in some settings can also occur though the practice of geophagia – eating of soil.[9]

Pathology

The pathology caused by *T. trichiura* is strongly related to the size of the worm burden: the intensity of infection. When individuals harbour only a few worms these are confined to the caecum and ascending colon, causing little damage. However, with heavy infections they spread throughout the colon to the rectum, where they cause haemorrhages, mucopurulent stools and symptoms of dysentery with rectal prolapse.[10]

The *Trichuris* dysentery syndrome (TDS) associated with heavy infections is thought to be due in part to the acute-phase immune response and a specific elevation of plasma fibronectins and plasma viscosity,[11] as well as low admission plasma levels of insulin growth factor-1 (IGF-1), low type of procollagen and high serum levels of tumour necrosis factor α (TNF-α).[11,12]

Trichuris-related mucosal damage may facilitate the invasion of other infections, including shigellosis and *Entamoeba histolytica*, causing further ulceration. Infection can exacerbate colitis caused by infection with *Campylobacter jejuni*.[13]

Immunity

Individuals living in endemic areas mount a vigorous immune response involving all antibody serotypes, including immunoglobulins (Ig) A, IgM, IgG and IgE. A negative association often exists between antibody levels and intensity of infection.[14] Cytokine response profiles are also associated with patterns of *T. trichiura* infection and reinfection.[15] However, any effects of protective immunity must be incomplete since individuals show persistent susceptibility to infection following treatment.[6]

Clinical Features

Natural History. In the vast majority of infections, which are light and asymptomatic, the worms live harmlessly in the caecum and appendix but when the infection is heavy (with worm burdens exceeding 500 worms), there can be marked and often severe symptoms and signs. In children, however, even symptomless infections may have subtle and insidious effects on nutritional status, and physical and intellectual growth.

Incubation Period. The prepatent period from ingestion of eggs to the appearance of eggs in the stool is 60–90 days.

Symptoms and Signs. The pattern and severity of symptoms and signs is positively correlated with the intensity of infection. In light infections there are no discernable symptoms, but when associated with *Ascaris lumbricoides* or hookworm mild

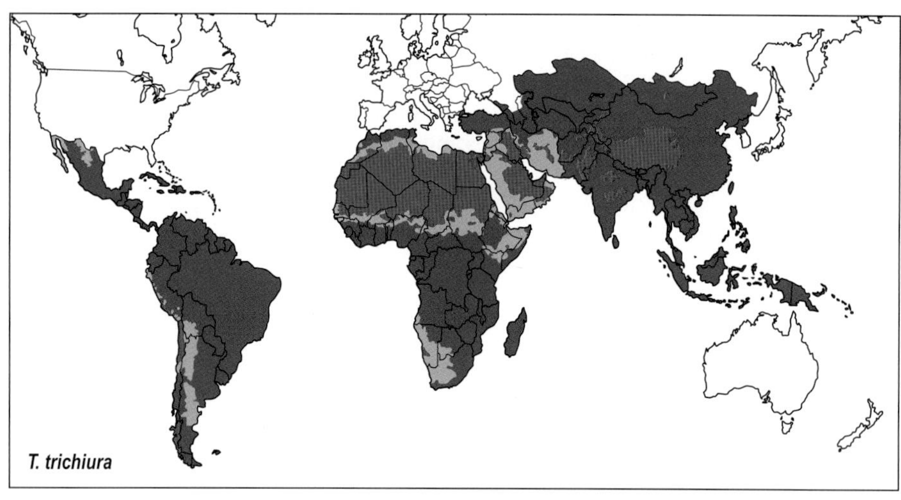

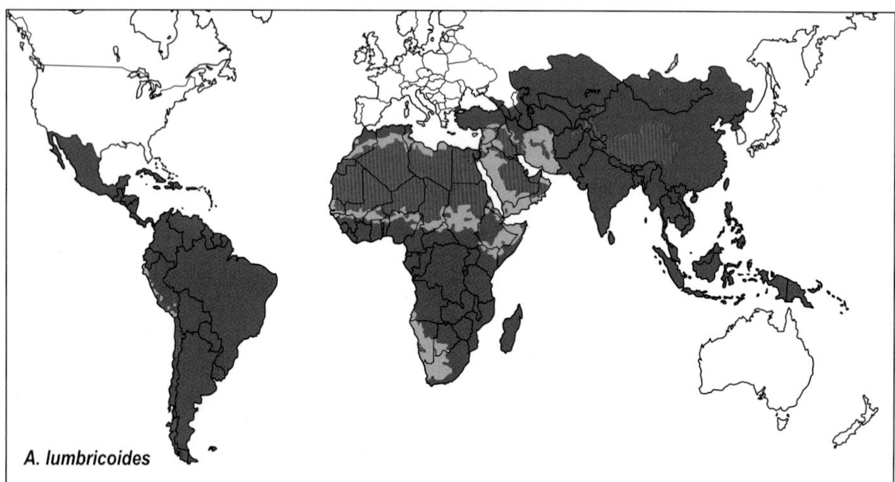

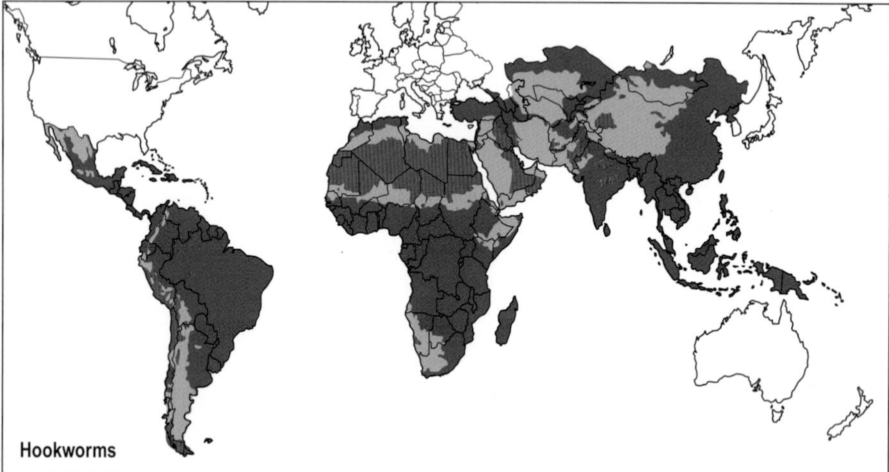

Figure 55.3 Global limits of *Trichuris trichiura, Ascaris lumbricoides* and hookworm.[5] Transmission is defined as stable (dark grey areas), unstable (hatched areas) or no risk (light grey areas), based on species-specific and continent-specific definitions. Limits are based on observed relationships between infection prevalence (from 5204 unique survey locations) and land surface temperature in the hottest quarter, rainfall in the driest season and an annual indicator of aridity. Countries defined as non-endemic on socioeconomic grounds are shown in white.

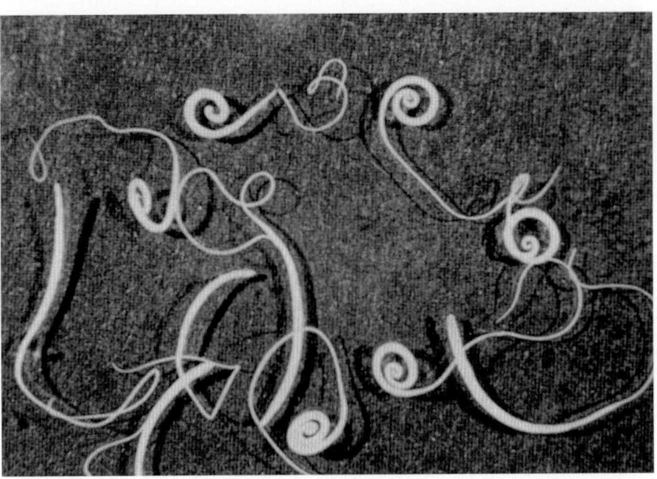

Figure 55.4 Adult *Trichuris trichiura* (whipworms), male and female. *(Courtesy H. Zaiman.)*

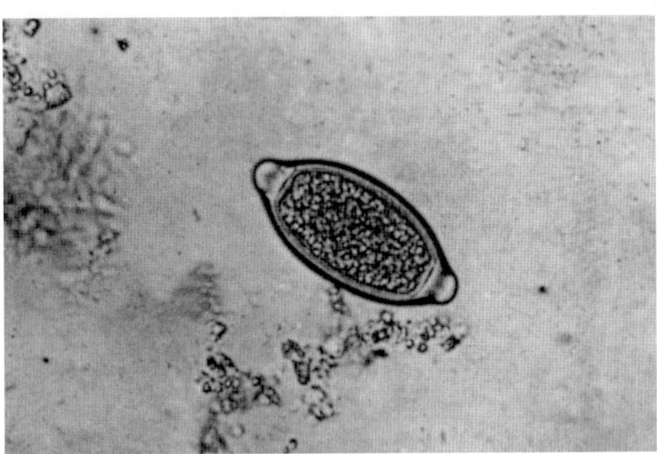

Figure 55.5 Egg of *Trichuris trichiura*. *(Courtesy of Tropical Resources Unit.)*

symptoms occur. These include epigastric pain, vomiting, distension, flatulence, anorexia and weight loss, which often may occur. Pain in the epigastrium and right iliac fossa is common. When associated with *E. histolytica*, *Balantidium coli* or shigellosis, symptoms are highly aggravated and dysenteric symptoms occur. There is usually no eosinophilia which, if pronounced, usually denotes a concurrent *Toxocara* infection, with which it is often associated.

Moderate *T. trichiura* infections can result in chronic *Trichuris* colitis, while heavy infection can cause *Trichuris* dysentery syndrome (TDS) and massive infantile trichuriasis. Typical symptoms and signs of TDS include severe dysentery with blood and mucus in the stools (Figure 55.6) and prolapse of the rectum (Figure 55.7).[16,17] In severe massive infantile trichuriasis, which typically occurs in children between 3 and 10 years, hypoproteinaemia, severe anaemia and clubbing of the fingers are common.[16,17] Both colitides can result in growth retardation and anaemia,[18] but treatment results in impressive catch-up growth.[19] Chronic heavy infection during childhood can also have a detrimental effect on cognition, educational achievement and school attendance.[20,21]

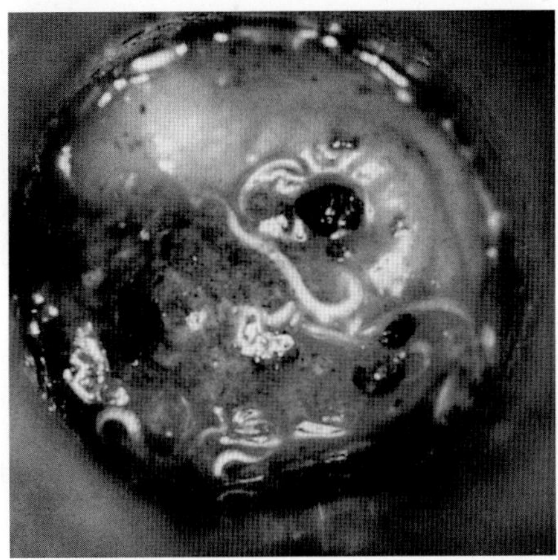

Figure 55.6 Protoscopic view of *Trichuris trichiura* worms causing dysentery.

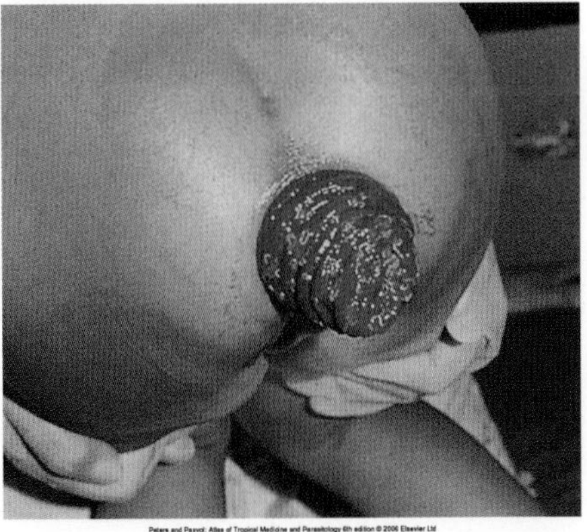

Figure 55.7 Prolapse of the rectum in *Trichuris* dysentery. *(From Peters, W., and Pasvol, G.., Atlas of Tropical Medicin and Parasitology, 6th edn, © 2006, Elsevier Ltd.)*

Diagnosis

The diagnosis is made by finding the characteristic eggs in the stool (see Figure 55.5) and the Kato-Katz method is recommended by the World Health Organization (WHO) (see Appendix I). *T. trichiura* eggs have a characteristic 'barrel' shape with two terminal polar plugs. The eggshell consists of three layers, the outermost of which is stained dark brown by host bile pigment. An egg count (see Appendix I) enables the quantification of the intensity of infection and the WHO defines a heavy infection as ≥10 000 eggs/g of faeces (Table 55.2), which is likely to be associated with morbidity.[22] Formol-ether concentration has greater sensitivity in light infections than the Kato-Katz method. FLOTAC is a new, sensitive, flotation chamber technique suitable for field settings, but is at present considerably more expensive.[23,24]

TABLE 55.2 Classification of Intensity of Infection for STH Species Based on WHO Guidelines

	Light	Moderate	Heavy
Trichuris trichiura	1–999	1 000–9 999	≥10 000
Ascaris lumbricoides	1–4 999	5 000–49 999	≥50 000
Hookworm	1–1 999	2 000–3 999	≥4 000

Proctoscopy in cases of dysentery will show numerous worms attached to the mucosa, which is reddened and ulcerated where they are responsible for the dysentery.

In some cases, a 'honeycomb' appearance of the small intestine has been seen with the appearances of Crohn's disease using radiology; deformity of the intestine is most marked in the proximal colon but also present in the ileum and appendix.

Differential Diagnosis

In severe infection, the clinical picture may resemble hookworm disease, acute appendicitis or amoebic dysentery. Many of the more subtle, indirect consequences of infection, such as undernutrition and anaemia, may be wrongly attributed to other aetiologies.

Management

Albendazole and mebendazole as single doses are recommended for the treatment of *T. trichiura* (see Table 55.1), as is a combination of albendazole 400 mg with ivermectin 200 μg/kg.[25] However, the cure rate (defined as the percentage of infected individuals who become uninfected following treatment) of single doses of benzimidazoles is not satisfactory,[26] and treatment over several days may be required, especially for heavy infections. There also seem to be regional differences in susceptibility of *T. trichiura* to benzimidazoles,[26] and it would therefore be prudent to evaluate local drug sensitivity when planning control measures.

Epidemiology and Control

T. trichiura infection is often associated with *A. lumbricoides* and *Toxocara* spp., the epidemiology of which is similar.

The development and survival of *T. trichiura* and other geohelminth free-living stages are temperature and humidity dependent. The optimum temperature is 20–30°C, with development arrested below 5°C and above 38°C.[27] Epidemiological studies demonstrate that prevalence is also associated with humidity and rainfall. Using geographical information systems (GIS) and remote sensing – which can provide spatially continuous estimates of climatic and environmental factors – it has been shown that prevalence of *T. trichiura* and of *A. lumbricoides* does not usually exceed 10% in areas where land surface temperature exceeds 38–40°C, and prevalence is thus greatest in the equatorial regions of the developing world.[27] Other important factors that determine localized transmission are poor sanitation, hygienic behaviour and socioeconomic status.[28] It is commonly assumed that both *T. trichiura* and *A. lumbricoides* are more prevalent in urban areas than in rural areas, however the evidence is equivocal, with differing urban–rural dichotomies evident in various settings.[29]

The age-dependent patterns of infection are similar for both *T. trichiura* and *A. lumbricoides*. Maximum prevalence is usually attained before 5 years of age and in low transmission settings, remains high and relatively stable throughout adulthood.[6] Mean intensity of infection is greatest in children aged 4–10 years and declines in young adults.

In common with other geohelminths, the distribution of *T. trichiura* infection within communities is highly aggregated. Thus, most individuals harbour a few parasites, while only a few harbour heavy burdens. Clustering of heavy infections within households is also common.[30] A further epidemiological observation, and one that may help explain the mechanisms of aggregation, comes from studies of reinfection which indicate that individuals tend to be predisposed to a high or low intensity of infection.[6] However, the precise reasons for observed heterogeneities in infection – genetics and/or common environmental and behavioural household factors – remain unresolved.[31,32] Control is the same as that for ascariasis: avoidance of soil pollution and periodic mass chemotherapy.

Type 2: Modified Direct (*Ascaris lumbricoides, Toxocara* spp.)

ASCARIASIS (ROUNDWORM)

Ascariasis is an infection of the small intestine caused by the roundworm *Ascaris lumbricoides*. This geohelminth is one of the most common human parasitic infections, typically found in the subtropics and tropics. Severe infection can cause a variety of clinical complications, including intestinal obstruction, and can additionally results in undernutrition and cognitive impairments.

Geographical Distribution

A. lumbricoides is one of the most common and most widespread human infections, infecting some 0.8 billion people worldwide (Pullan and Brooker, unpublished) and causing approximately 1.3 million DALYs lost annually.[7] The prevalence of *A. lumbricoides* varies in different parts of the world, and shares similar global transmission limits with that of *T. trichiura* (Figure 55.3).[5] The majority of infections occur in east and south Asia and sub-Saharan Africa.

Aetiology

A. lumbricoides (Figure 55.8) is a comparatively large worm (female 20–25 cm×3–6 mm; male 15–31 cm×2–4 mm) (the morphology is described in Appendix III).

Ascaris suum. *A. suum* is almost indistinguishable from human *A. lumbricoides* and humans are not a normal host but *Ascaris* pneumonia is common in pigs and a proportion of similar respiratory troubles in people associated with pigs may be due to *A. suum*. Although it can infect humans, man is not

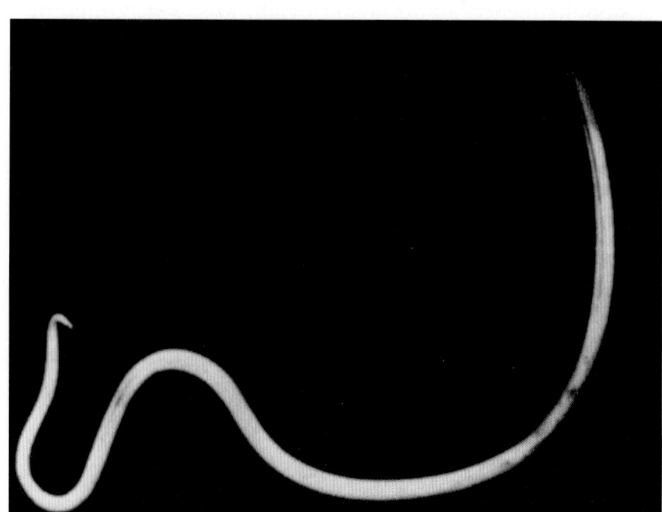

Figure 55.8 Adult *Ascaris lumbricoides* worm (roundworm). *(Courtesy of Tropical Resources Unit.)*

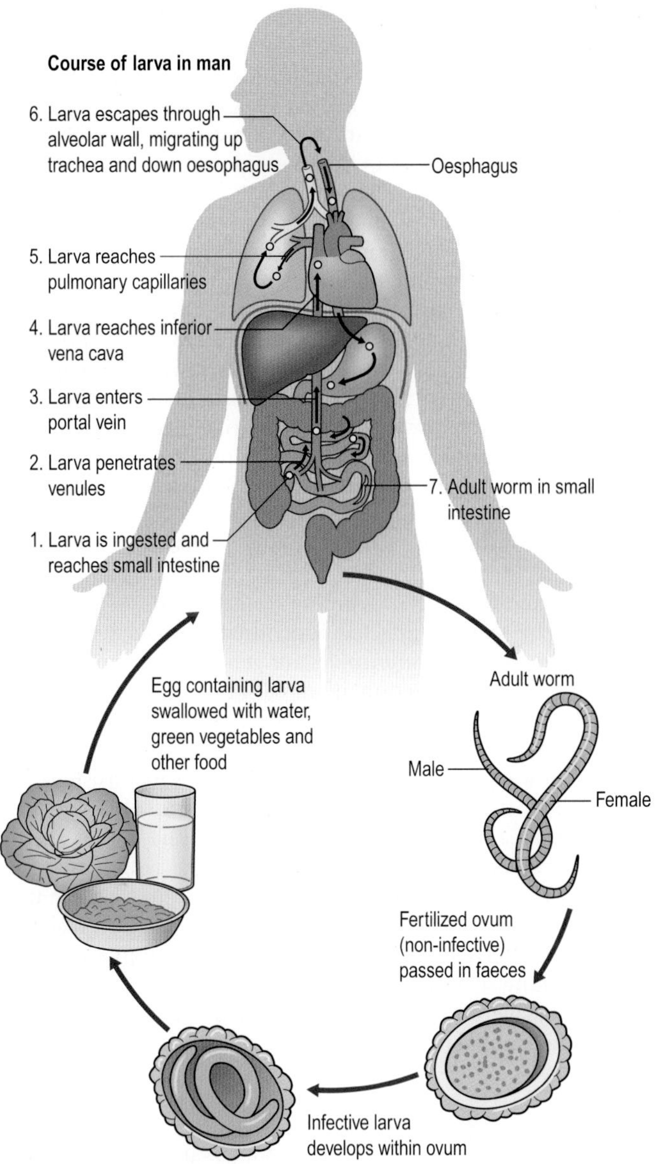

Figure 55.9 Life cycle of *Ascaris lumbricoides* (roundworm). *(Courtesy of Tropical Resources Unit.)*

its normal host; double infections may occur and eosinophilic granuloma of the bowel may be caused by *A. suum*.

Life Cycle

A. lumbricoides inhabits the small intestine and lays eggs (Figures 55.9 and 55.10) which are passed out as immature ova containing no segmented or differentiated embryo. In damp soil an embryo develops at 36–40°C in 2–4 months (at the optimum of 25°C in 3 weeks); it lies coiled up in the egg, undergoing one moult before being hatched as an infective second-stage rhabditiform larva in the small intestine when the egg is swallowed (see Appendix III). Here the rhabditiform larva penetrates the mucous membrane and enters the bloodstream, reaching the lungs via the right heart where it cannot pass through the lung capillaries, so that it burrows through the alveolar wall to enter the respiratory tract. From here it is carried up the trachea to the larynx, where it moves over the epiglottis and enters the oesophagus, and is swallowed a second

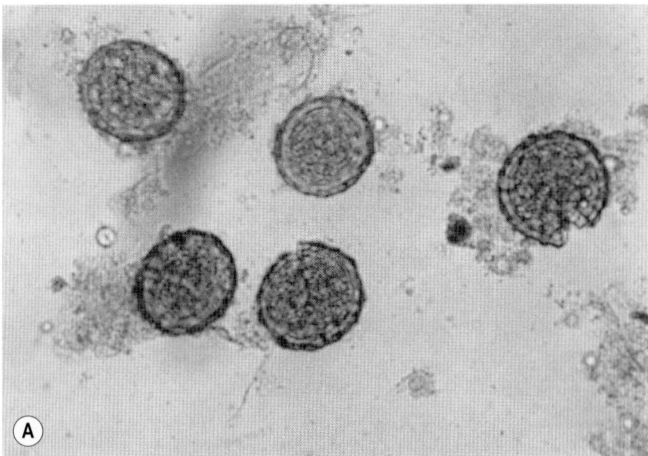

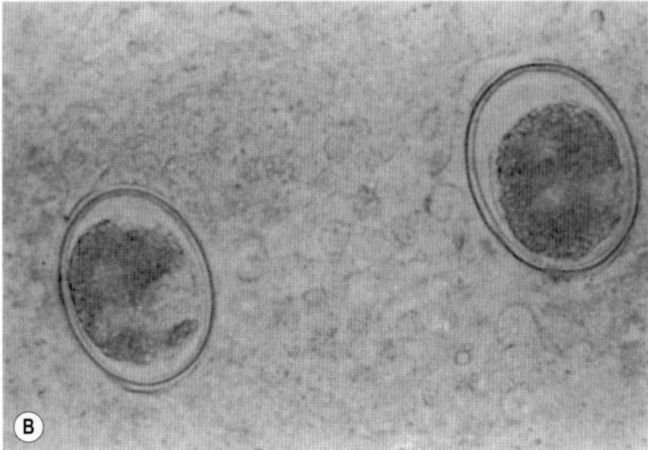

Figure 55.10 Eggs of *Ascaris lumbricoides* (roundworm). (A) Fully formed, fertile, in stool. (B) Decorticated from liver abscess. *((A) Courtesy of Tropical Resources Unit. (B) Courtesy M. L. Chu.)*

time to reach the small intestine. The whole process takes 10–14 days, during which time the larva moults twice, the fourth moult taking place between the 25th and 29th days. Larvae may reach the intestine as early as the 5th day. In humans, the period from infection to the first passage of ova in the stool is 60–70 days.

Transmission

Infection is acquired from accidental ingestion of eggs in contaminated soil, usually by children when playing around the house situated in suitable and contaminated soil. Geophagia may also contribute to the transmission.[9]

Pathology

Pathology may be caused by larvae migrating through the liver and lungs or adults residing in the intestinal tract and migrating to abnormal situations. As with other geohelminths, the severity of pathology is related to the intensity of infection.

Migrating Larvae (Larval Ascariasis). Migrating larvae cause symptoms from their actual physical presence and the eosinophilic inflammatory responses they elicit.

Damage to the lungs occurs during the migration of larvae on their way to the intestine. 'Löffler's syndrome', which can be

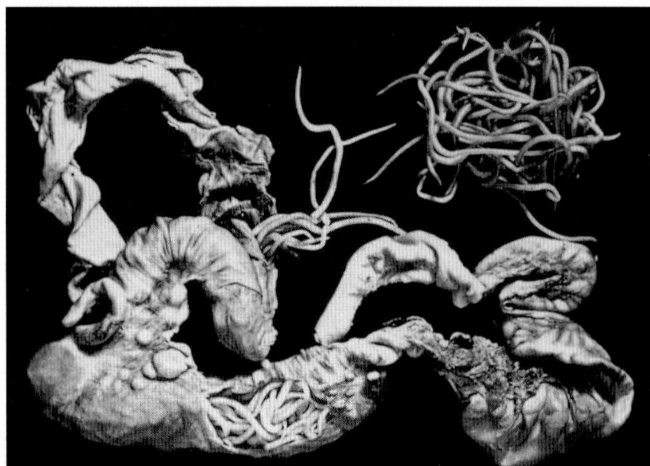

Figure 55.11 Impacted mass of adult *Ascaris* worms in the small intestine causing fatal intestinal obstruction.

potentially fatal, may be produced with fever, cough, sputum, asthma, skin rash, eosinophilia and radiological pulmonary infiltration.[33] Segments of fourth-stage larvae can be seen in the bronchioles associated with infiltration with polymorphonuclear and eosinophilic leucocytes with scattered Charcot–Leyden crystals usually associated with lysed eosinophils.

Small areas of necrosis with eosinophils may be found in the liver. Migrating larvae have been recovered from aspirated gastric juice and sputum. If the larvae reach the general circulation they may cause localized symptoms resembling those of visceral larvae migrans caused by *Toxocara* spp. Larvae may wander into the brain, eye or retina, causing granulomas simulating *Toxocara* spp. In small children, ascariasis is frequently associated with toxocariasis. Hundreds of larvae have been removed from a swelling in the neck (but see *Lagochilascaris*, below).

Adult Worms. Adult worms by themselves cause little pathology in their normal habitat (small intestine). Heavy infections can cause intestinal colic, which is the most important complaint. Aggregate masses of worms may cause volvulus, intestinal obstruction (Figure 55.11) or intussusception.

Wandering Ascarids. Adult worms tend to migrate when their environment is disturbed, for example in the presence of anaesthetics or fever. Wandering ascarids may reach abnormal situations and cause acute symptoms: ileus from mechanical obstruction, perforation of the bowel in the ileocaecal region, acute appendicitis from a worm blocking the lumen, diverticulitis, gastric or duodenal trauma, blocking of the ampulla of Vater with pancreatic necrosis, blocking of the common bile duct with obstructive jaundice, entry into the liver parenchyma and liver abscess, invasion of the genital tract and oesophageal perforation.

Liver abscesses can be caused by female *A. lumbricoides* worms migrating up the common bile duct into the liver where they die, releasing eggs. Histologically, there is a granulomatous reaction round the dead worm with release of the eggs, which can be demonstrated in the abscess as smooth, oval bodies from which the outer coat has been digested (see Figure 55.10B). In some parts of the world, *Ascaris* liver abscess is more common in young children than amoebic abscess.

Granulomatous masses may form around the eggs released from the female worms which have escaped into the peritoneum and mimic tuberculous peritonitis. An eosinophilic granuloma of the bowel may be caused by *A. suum*.

Worms entering the biliary tract can cause biliary obstruction and stasis, provoking spasm and inflammation of the biliary tree – known as biliary ascariasis.[34,35] Adult worms may be demonstrated on plain radiographs, by barium meal, by intravenous cholangiography, ultrasonography, computed tomography or magnetic resonance imaging.[36] At postmortem, cholangitis or liver abscess may be found. Adult worms, larvae and ova may all initiate stone formation and can be found in the core of many bile duct stones. Biliary ascariasis is also regarded as a possible aetiological factor for hepatolithiasis.[37] The management of biliary ascariasis is primarily medical, including analgesics and anthelminthic therapy. If medical treatment fails endoscopic extraction using biopsy forceps is successful.[38]

Immunopathological Effects. Many infected individuals manifest a sensitivity to the antigens of *A. lumbricoides*, and exhibit atopic symptoms including conjunctivitis, urticaria and asthma. The skin of infected individuals can be sensitive to minimal doses of *A. lumbricoides* antigen and gives an immediate hypersensitivity reaction, often with urticaria and erythematous lesions. Epidemiological studies point to a protective effect of *A. lumbricoides* and the development of allergy and asthma; however, the evidence for this effect is inconsistent.[39] It has been postulated that *A. lumbricoides* and other geohelminths in areas of high endemicity increase the risk of allergy but in areas of low endemicity decrease the risk. Timing of exposure in relation to maturation of the immune system may also be important. Treatment with albendazole has been shown not to be associated with an increased risk of atopy or clinical allergy among schoolchildren.[40]

The passage of adult worms in sensitive persons may give rise to intense anal pruritus, vomiting of worms and oedema of the glottis.

Nutritional and Cognitive Impairments. *A. lumbricoides* infection can cause physiological abnormalities in the small intestine,[41] resulting in malabsorption of nutrients and vitamin A and other micronutrients, nutritional deficiency and growth failure.[42] Infection may also contribute to vitamin A deficiency and children suffering from night blindness have shown rapid improvement in their eye symptoms following effective treatment. De-worming of children has been shown to increase serum retinol concentration.[43] The link between ascariasis and impaired growth and undernutrition is now well-established.[44,45] A number of studies have also implicated ascariasis in cognitive impairments,[20,21] although the mechanism by which cognitive processes are affected is uncertain. The most plausible mechanisms are indirect, operating through undernutrition.

Immunity

Humans acquire only partial immunity to reinfection, and animals can be protected using extracts of adult worms and larvae. The main immune reaction is humoral, associated with a polarized Th2-type profile,[46] and is directed against the migrating larval stage. The reaction to adult worms in unusual locations is cellular.

The antigens which elicit antibodies are released at the moulting period between the second and third larval stages when there are markedly elevated levels of IgE and a peripheral eosinophilia.[47,48] A further response is elicited in the bowel between the fourth and fifth stages, at which time there may be a marked loss of worm burden; this may be a regulatory mechanism in natural infections. It is unlikely that this humoral response confers full protection from reinfection.[14]

Adult worms in the bowel elicit no response but when they wander into tissues the reaction is cellular and results in a granuloma. Immediate hypersensitivity to adult *A. lumbricoides* antigens develops in some people.

Clinical Features

Natural History. Most *A. lumbricoides* infections are symptomless but heavy infections in childhood give rise to symptoms. These heavy infections may be controlled by immunity, or by diminished exposure, so that adults have much lighter infections, although reinfection can occur throughout life.

Incubation Period. The incubation period from infection after swallowing eggs to the first appearance of eggs in the stools is 60–70 days. In larval ascariasis pulmonary symptoms occur 4–6 days after infection.

Symptoms and Signs. Light infections do not usually cause symptoms, though a single adult worm can cause a liver abscess or block the common bile duct. Acute manifestations are roughly proportional to the number of worms harboured and serious disease may be caused when the burden amounts to 100 worms or more.

During the migratory stages the larvae cause a pneumonitis 4–16 days after infection, with fever, cough, sputum and radiological infiltration of the lungs. There is a high eosinophilia and larvae can be found in the sputum or gastric juice, especially if a quantity is collected, digested with trypsin and centrifuged. It seems that Löffler's syndrome occurs more with seasonal ascariasis, rather than with continued transmission throughout the year.[49,50] The pneumonitis is of short duration – about 3 weeks (in contrast to tropical pulmonary eosinophilia (TPE), which lasts for many months). There may be asthma, which can be so intense as to cause status asthmaticus, and the liver may be affected, becoming enlarged and tender.

On reaching the general circulation larvae may cause symptoms similar to those of *Toxocara* spp. Neurological disorders including convulsions, meningism and epilepsy, palpebral oedema, insomnia and tooth grinding during the night may occur. When the larvae wander into the brain they cause granulomas, presenting as small tumours in the eye, retina or brain.

The commonest complication of ascariasis is small bowel obstruction (Figure 55.11).[51] The incidence of *Ascaris*-induced intestinal obstruction (AI-IO) is non-linearly related to the prevalence of infection and estimated to be in the range of 0–0.25 cases per year per 1000 in endemic areas. The case fatality rate is up to 5%.[51] AI-IO is most common among children below the age of 10 years, possibly because of their narrower intestinal lumen diameter and high worm burden, and as many as 1000 worms have been removed from one patient. Gastrointestinal discomfort, colic and vomiting are quite common. Plain abdominal radiography and abdominal ultrasonography featuring the characteristic 'railway track' sign and 'bull's eye' appearance help to confirm the diagnosis.[52]

The second most common complication is biliary ascariasis, especially among adults in the Indian subcontinent. The symptoms are acute onset of right upper abdominal pain, sometimes with fever and jaundice from recurrent cholangitis.

Diagnosis

A diagnosis can be made from passage of worms in the stool or by finding eggs in faeces. Fertile eggs are oval and measure about 60×45 μm. The shell is transparent, is surrounded by an outer mamillated shell stained by bile pigments and contains an unsegmented embryo (see Figure 55.10A). Unfertile eggs are longer and narrower (90×40 μm), have a thinner shell, more irregular outer covering and are found in about two-thirds of infections, due either to a shortage or absence of males. As with *T. trichiura*, intensity of infection can be assessed by quantitative egg count methods such as the Kato-Katz, McMaster and FLOTAC methods (see Appendix I). The WHO definition of a heavy infection is ≥50 000 eggs/g of faeces (Table 55.2).

Decorticated eggs are usually found in ectopic sites where they have had the outer shell removed and present as smooth oval objects (see Figure 55.10B).

Eosinophilia. In larval ascariasis there is a high eosinophilia but in adult infections there is little or none. If a marked eosinophilia occurs in adult infections then an associated *Toxocara* spp. or *Strongyloides stercoralis* infection must be suspected.

Adult Worms. Sometimes the passage of an adult worm from the nose, mouth or anus will be reported and causes distress. The size and shape will distinguish it from other worms, especially tapeworms, which may be noticed by patients.

Radiography and Sonography. Radiographic examination 4–6 hours after an opaque meal displays the worms as cylindrical filling defects or as string-like shadows produced by the opaque substance which the worms have ingested. Ultrasound is increasingly used in the diagnosis of intestinal obstruction and biliary ascariasis.[52] On longitudinal sections, the whole worm can be seen, whilst on transverse section a single worm can be seen as a 'bull's eye', 'target mass' or 'doughnut mass'. In real-time sonography, live worms show characteristic slow, non-directional movements.

Serological Diagnosis

Since there is much cross-reactivity with other helminthic antigens, immunodiagnosis of *A. lumbricoides* infection has previously proved a challenge, but multiplex polymerase chain reaction (PCR)-based assays have recently been show to provide a promising diagnostic tool.[53,54]

Differential Diagnosis

The syndrome of pulmonary symptoms, radiological lung infiltration and hypereosinophilia is common to a number of helminthic and other infections. Larval ascariasis must be distinguished from toxocariasis, hookworm, *S. stercoralis*, schistosomiasis and tropical pulmonary eosinophilia (TPE). Essentially, larval ascariasis is a short-term illness lasting 2–3 weeks with a rapidly falling eosinophilia.

Often associated with *A. lumbricoides*, *Toxocara* spp. causes the visceral larva migrans (VLM) syndrome, which persists for many months with a persistently high eosinophilia, and lung symptoms are not prominent. Wandering *Toxocara* larvae cause almost identical lesions of the brain and eye as *A. lumbricoides* and can be diagnosed by specific serological tests (see below).

TPE may closely resemble *Ascaris* pneumonia. It occurs mainly in adults, has a much longer duration and specific filarial serological tests will be positive. It responds rapidly to diethylcarbamazine.

Pulmonary aspergillosis, drug reactions and eosinophilic leukaemia are all more chronic.

Management

Both albendazole and mebendazole are highly effective against *A. lumbricoides*[26] and the drugs of choice (Table 55.1). Levamisole and pyrantel pamoate are also effective. Treatment is best given between meals.

Clinical complications respond dramatically to prednisolone therapy. Anthelmintics should be given 2 weeks after lung involvement. Conservative treatment – antispasmodics, analgesics, gastric decompression via a nasogastric tube, administration of intravenous fluids – is usually successful. An anthelmintic, preferably in soluble form and quick-acting (levamisole, pyrantel) is given when the acute phase of the illness is over and intestinal function restored. If this fails, surgical removal is needed.[38] If surgical intervention is decreed necessary because of fever, tachycardia, visible peristalsis, severe pain or lack of remission within 48 hours of conservative treatment, this should be as conservative as possible, e.g. careful unknotting of the worm bolus and milking of the worms into the colon. Rarely is enterotomy required.

Epidemiology and Control

Biological similarities between *A. lumbricoides* and *T. trichiura* mean they share similar climatic envelopes (Figure 55.3),[27] which explains in part the close correspondence of *A. lumbricoides* and *T. trichiura* prevalence in different regions of the world.[55]

Many of the epidemiological features of *A. lumbricoides* are also similar to those for *T. trichiura*: marked age-dependency in infection patterns, highly aggregated distributions within communities,[56] household clustering of heavy infection,[29,30] and evidence of predisposition (for a review see Crompton 2001).[57]

As with *T. trichiura*, control of *A. lumbricoides* is based on a combination of personal hygiene, proper disposal of faeces, health education and periodic mass chemotherapy.

TOXOCARIASIS

Toxocariasis in humans is the result of infection with dog ascarid *Toxocara canis* or the cat ascarid *T. cati*. Infection occurs through accidental ingestion of eggs, with the larvae penetrating the intestine, and migrating through the liver, lungs and central nervous system. These geohelminths do not undergo normal development in humans, and host inflammatory responses either kill the migrating larvae or force them into a state of arrested development. Before this happens, the larvae can tissue damage the internal organs, known as visceral larva migrans (VLM) or the eye, ocular toxocariasis.[58] A third form of the infection, known as covert toxocariasis, has also been recognized.

Geographical Distribution

T. canis has a worldwide distribution; rates in humans vary from 2% to 50% in developed countries and up to 86% in developing countries, where environmental conditions favour geohelminth transmission.[59,60] The importance of *T. cati* in humans remains under-appreciated.[61]

Visceral larva migrans, which was first described in the southern USA by Beaver and colleagues in 1952,[62] has been recognized mainly in the southern and eastern USA but also in Europe, the Caribbean, Central and South America, the Philippines, Australia and Africa.

Ocular toxocariasis (granulomatous ophthalmitis), also first described in the USA,[63] has been recognized in many parts of the world.[64] Covert toxocariasis is widespread in the American south.

Aetiology

T. canis and *T. cati* are roundworm infections in dogs and cats, respectively. The morphology resembles that of *A. lumbricoides* (see above), the males being 4–6 cm long and the females 6.5–10 cm long. Eggs, which are pitted superficially, measure 85×75 μm, being larger than those of *A. lumbricoides*. They are not found in humans, only in dog and cat faeces and contaminated soil.

The ascarid *Toxascaris leonina* is commonly found in wild carnivores as well as dogs and cats that roam wild, but in rare instances can infect humans and cause VLM.

Life Cycle

In both dogs and cats, the life cycle is similar to that of *A. lumbricoides* in humans, except that transplacental infection is common and the offspring born with a patent infection shed numerous eggs from birth. In contrast, adult dogs and cats excrete few eggs. Dogs and cats are infected by ingesting the eggs from soil or through transplacental infection so that the whole cycle may be maintained in a small flat without any access to the outside.

In humans, who are not the normal host, the eggs hatch in the stomach and second-stage larvae penetrate the mucosa to enter the circulation via the mesenteric vessels, reaching the intestinal viscera and liver where they are held up in the capillaries, but may pass into the general circulation through the lungs and end up in the brain, eye and other organs. In these organs, as well as the liver, the larvae are eventually held up and destroyed by a granulomatous reaction which blocks their further migration and causes pathology. In humans, the larvae do not grow or moult but can remain alive for as long as 11 years, as has been show experimentally.

Transmission

The main source of infection is eggs passed into the environment by infected animals, mainly puppies and kittens. Infection is acquired by children playing in contaminated soil or in playgrounds and, in addition, is encouraged by the habit of earth-eating (geophagia). It has also been suggested that dogs might infect people by direct contact;[65] although this mode of transmission is not considered a major risk because embryonation of excreted *Toxocara* ova typically requires a minimum of 2 weeks.[66]

Pathology

The pathology depends on the intensity of infection. In heavy infections in childhood the syndrome of VLM is produced, whereas lighter infections can cause ocular toxocariasis, found in later life.

Visceral Larva Migrans. In heavy infections in children the second-stage larvae, which are 450 μm × 16–20 μm in diameter, are arrested mostly in the liver, where they cause few or many miliary lesions. These lesions are composed of granulomas which can be seen as white subcapsular nodules the size of millet seeds. Other sites are the lungs, kidneys, heart, striated muscle, brain and eye. Microscopically, the granulomas contain a centre of closely packed eosinophils and histiocytes surrounded by larger histiocytes with pale vesicular nuclei, sometimes arranged in a palisade-like manner. Occasionally, there is an atypical multinucleate giant cell. Living second-stage larvae may sometimes be demonstrated in recent granulomas but more usually only the remains can be seen. Less commonly they reach the lungs or brain, where similar lesions can be seen.

Ocular Toxocariasis. In the eye the granulomatous reaction forms a large subretinal mass with a superimposed patch of choroiditis, which can closely resemble a retinoblastoma.

Immunity

In dogs, immunity to reinfection develops so that adult dogs pass few or no eggs. In the abnormal host (humans) the larvae elicit both a humoral and cellular response. Antibodies are formed which cause a quantitative rise in immunoglobulins – mostly IgG but also IgM (the globulin may be so elevated that a positive formol gel test can be shown) and IgE – and there is a peripheral eosinophilia. The larvae themselves elicit a cell-mediated granulomatous response causing the granulomas so typical of the infection.

Clinical Features

Natural History. Following infection from ingested eggs, which hatch in the stomach, the larvae migrate to the liver, where they may be arrested, or continue and reach other organs. In most cases, the larvae are destroyed without causing any trouble but in some cases they can survive for many years, and on its wanderings may eventually cause a lesion. Unless the infection is heavy and the VLM syndrome is produced, most cases of infection never cause any trouble. Lesions in the eye can produce severe loss of vision and even complete loss of sight in the affected eye.

Incubation Period. An incubation period cannot be determined but in heavy infections (VLM) it is similar to that of *A. lumbricoides*. In light infections many years may pass before the ocular granuloma presents itself.

Symptoms and Signs. These depend on where in the body infection occurs. There are two main clinical presentations: VLM, where larvae spread through different organs, and ocular toxocariasis (granulomatous ophthalmitis), where larvae migrate into the eyes. Chronic exposure to migrating juvenile larvae can also result in a recognizable syndrome called covert toxocariasis.

VLM is seen most commonly in younger children. The child becomes unwell with an enlarged liver, fever and asthma. There is a marked hypereosinophilia and hypergammaglobulinemia, and there can be pulmonary signs (radiological mottling), cardiac dysfunction and nephrosis. Severe infections may cause neurological lesions (fits, epilepsy, pareses and transverse myelitis). Toxocariasis may contribute in part to the higher prevalence of epilepsy in developing countries.[67] Most cases of VLM recover naturally after 2 years but some die, and post-mortem examination will reveal extensive lesions in the liver and sometimes the brain.

Ocular toxocariasis can result in blurred or cloudy vision, sensitivity to light and a painful eye – these symptoms often affect only one eye. The retinal lesion caused by the migrating larvae presents as a solid retinal tumour often at or near the macula. In the early stages, it is raised above the level of the retina and closely mimics a retinal neoplasm. Later when the acute phase has subsided the lesion remains a clear-cut circumscribed area of retinal degeneration. If the lesion is central the visual acuity is reduced or central vision may be lost, the principal causes of which are vitritis, cystoid macular oedema or traction retinal detachment.[68] Strabismus due to macular damage is often the presenting symptom.[68] Low-grade iridocyclitis with posterior synechiae may develop and progress to general endophthalmitis and detachment of the retina. The second-stage larvae may rarely be seen with a slit-lamp microscope in the anterior chamber of the eye. Secondary glaucoma may result. Estimates of 1–7 cases of ocular toxocariasis per 100 000 have been reported.[69,70]

Symptoms and signs of covert toxocariasis include cough, sleep disturbances, headache and abdominal pain. Long-term exposure to larval migration in the lungs may also result in asthma.[71] Covert toxocariasis is also commonly associated with eosinophilia.[64]

Diagnosis

The most consistent laboratory findings in VLM are: stable persistent eosinophilia, leucocytosis, a decreased albumin: globulin ratio and an increase in IgG, IgH, anti-A or anti-B isohaemagglutinin titres. High-resolution ultrasonography reveals hypoechoic areas in the liver and, being non-invasive, is preferable to liver biopsy.[72]

Demonstration of Larvae. This is very difficult and seldom achieved. Larvae or portions of degenerate larvae may be seen at the centre of the granuloma in liver biopsy or post-mortem material. Liver biopsy may show a granuloma containing many eosinophils which can be suggestive but which must be distinguished from a *Schistosoma mansoni* granuloma. In biopsy and post-mortem material *Ancylostoma braziliense* and *Ancylostoma caninum*, which usually invade the skin, can occasionally enter the human host via the intestinal tract and form granulomas in the viscera. Autoinfection with *S. stercoralis* may cause a similar picture. Immunofluorescent staining of histological sections may be necessary to differentiate them.

Serology. Diagnosis in humans has been widely based on ELISA, using excretory-secretory (ES) antigens harvested from second-stage larvae in vitro.[73] Using larval antigens the sensitivity of ELISA at a titer of 1: 32 is >75% and specificity is >90% in VLM, provided the serum is first absorbed with *A. suum* to remove cross-reacting antibodies.[74] The sensitivity of ELISA for ocular toxocariasis is lower than for VLM.[75] In tropical areas, the difficulty with serological diagnosis has always been to obtain an antigen specific to *Toxocara* second-stage larvae which does not cross-react with other common tissue helminths. In such circumstances, serodiagnosis may be improved by ELISA based on specific IgE and IgG subclasses (IgG4)[76] and by recombinant antigen techniques.[77] Available serodiagnosis tests are generally unable to distinguish between past and present infection, and are thus not very useful for evaluating treatment success.

Ocular Toxocariasis. This is diagnosed primarily by ophthalmological examination. In addition to serum and vitreous *Toxocara* antibody determinations, fluorescein angiography, ultrasonography or computed tomography should be carried out to differentiate retinoblastoma from ocular larva migrans.

Differential Diagnosis

VLM must be distinguished from other migrating helminths, larval ascariasis (much shorter duration), strongyloidiasis (much longer duration) and TPE (pulmonary symptoms are more marked and found in adults).

Ocular toxocariasis must be distinguished from a retinal tumour (retinoblastoma) and other causes of choroiditis (toxoplasmosis). All cases of retinoblastoma in children should have a serological test to exclude toxocariasis.

Management

The drugs of choice are albendazole and mebendazole given twice daily for 5 days (Table 55.1). However, because mebendazole is not absorbed outside the gut, albendazole is generally considered the treatment of choice. Diethylcarbamazine and thiabendazole were used in the past but are no longer recommended.

In VLM, the high eosinophilia may persist for months after clinical cure, which is shown by subsidence of the fever and hepatomegaly. Once overcome, relapses do not occur and second infections are unlikely. In severe ocular toxocariasis, corticosteroids may be needed in addition. Ocular granulomas can be surgically removed or destroyed using laser photocoagulation and cryoretinopexy. Loss of vision can be arrested but lost vision is not restored.

Epidemiology and Control

Toxocara spp. is a common infection of adult dogs and cats and their offspring, who excrete eggs on to the ground which are ingested by small children. The wide range in seroprevalence in human populations is thought to reflect variation in exposure. Outdoor parks in urban and suburban areas are common sources of infection, and pet ownership and geophagia are important risk factors for infection.[60] In tropical regions toxocariasis is often associated with *A. lumbricoides* and *T. trichiura* infection, and has similar epidemiological features.[59] Seroprevalence increases throughout early childhood and equilibrium prevalence occurs around 2.5 years and the infection is patent for about 3–5 years of age. It is uncommon at a later age unless an unusual habit of dirt-eating is present, as in the mentally ill. Ocular toxocariasis is found at a later age.

Control rests upon control of infection in dogs and cats, especially puppies and kittens, which are the main agents of infection, and regular treatment of animals with anthelmintics is essential when there are children in the house. Health education about the sources of infection and means of reducing it, such as prevention of soil contamination by dog and cat faeces in areas where children play (such as sandboxes, public parks and playgrounds) and hand-washing should also be promoted.

LAGOCHILASCARIASIS

Lagochilascariasis is a rare infection of humans, who are accidental hosts.

Geographical Distribution

Cases have been described from the neotropical regions of South and Central America and the Caribbean. The majority of cases occur in the Amazon Region of South America.

Aetiology and Life Cycle

Five species of *Lagochilascaris* have been identified, but *Lagochilascaris minor* is the most common. Adult *L. minor* worms live in cavities in the submucosa of the small intestine and eggs containing infective larvae pass out in the stool, where they are ingested by mice and other small mammals. The larvae hatch in the intestine and migrate to skeletal muscle, where they mature and wait to be ingested by definitive hosts. The natural definitive hosts are unknown but opossums and wild felines, such as the cloudy leopard, have been implicated.

Transmission

Humans are thought to become infected either by ingesting eggs from the soil or eating the intermediate host. A case reported from Tobago was thought to have acquired the infection through eating the raw meat of the manakou opossum. In addition to humans, it can infect domestic animals (felines and canines) as well as silvatic or forest-dwelling carnivores. Experimental investigations suggest that wild rodents may serve as intermediate hosts.[78]

Infected humans generally live in newly deforested areas and work upon the land for subsistence and feed almost exclusively upon hunted meat.

Pathology

In humans, *L. minor* causes subcutaneous abscesses on the head and neck, and lesions in the nasopharynx. The tonsils and lymphoid tissue are replaced by granulomatous tissue containing epithelioid granulomas with larvae and eggs. Abscesses form in the neck and discharge pus. In rare cases, infection can lead to involvement of ocular globes, ears and meninges.

Clinical Features

Early symptoms are recurrent tonsillitis, a feeling of worms crawling at the back of the throat and even discharge of small white worms from the mouth. Tender tumours which swell and eventually burst discharging pus and worms form in the cervical region.

Diagnosis

Adult worms can be recognized by a longitudinal furrow along the lateral line (see Appendix III).

Management

Albendazole 400 mg/day for 30 days or ivermectin 300 μg/kg weekly for 10 weeks results in regression of the lesions with or without surgical resection.[79]

Type 3: Penetration of the Skin (*Ancylostoma, Necator, Strongyloides, Trichostrongylus*)

HOOKWORM (*ANCYLOSTOMIASIS* AND *NECATORIASIS*)

Hookworm infection is caused by two hookworm species, *Ancylostoma duodenale* and *Necator americanus*. In many cases, the nematodes, which are often present in huge numbers attached to the small intestine, ingest blood and to a lesser extent, protein, causing hookworm anaemia and hookworm disease. Globally, hookworm is estimated to infect 707 million people (Pullan and Brooker, unpublished)[8,80] and cause the loss of 3.2 million DALYs,[7] principally through its consequences for iron deficiency anaemia.

Geographical Distribution

Hookworm occurs in all tropical and subtropical countries,[5] and is particularly prevalent throughout much of sub-Saharan Africa as well as in South China, the Pacific and South-east Asia.[81]

A. duodenale is essentially a parasite of southern Europe, the north coast of Africa, northern India, northern China and Japan. It was probably introduced by migration into Latin America by a trans-Pacific route and is the predominant hookworm in coastal Peru and Chile, and in Paraguay. It has been introduced into western Australia and into areas where *N. americanus* is the predominant human hookworm, southern India, Myanmar, Malaya, the Philippines, Indonesia, Polynesia, Micronesia and parts of West Africa.

N. americanus is the predominant hookworm of sub-Saharan Africa, southern Asia, Melanesia and Polynesia. It is widely distributed in the Caribbean, Central America and northern South America, where it was introduced by slaves from Africa. It is still occasionally found in the southern USA.

Aetiology

Two species of hookworm, *A. duodenale* and *N. americanus*, infect humans. The majority of the world's cases of hookworm are caused by *N. americanus*.

Ancylostoma duodenale. *A. duodenale* is a small cylindrical white, grey or reddish-brown (from ingested blood) thread-like worm (Appendix II). Both male and female worms have a buccal capsule containing two pairs of teeth (*cf N. americanus*) for attaching to the small intestinal mucosa. The male (0.8–1.1×0.4–0.5 cm) has a copulatory bursa at the rear end consisting of an umbrella-like expansion of the cuticle (Appendix III). The female (1–1.3×0.6 cm) is slightly larger and has the body cavity occupied by the ovary and coiled uterine tubes packed with eggs. The vulva is in the posterior third of the body. The maximum egg output occurs 15–18 months after infection; the interval between infection and final disappearance of eggs from the stool with death of the worm averages 1–3 years. The female produces 25 000–35 000 eggs each day and some 18–54 million during its lifetime. (For a full morphological description, see Appendix III.) The eggs (50–60 μm×35–40 μm) are elliptical with a transparent shell and when freshly laid contain two to four segments (blastomeres) (Figure 55.12).

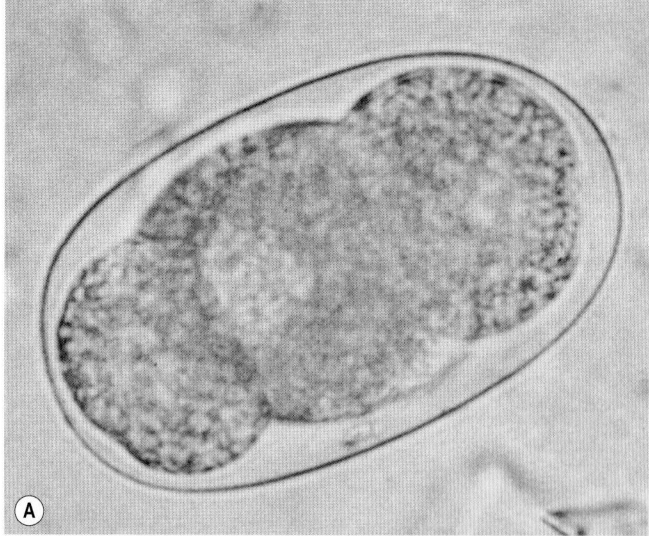

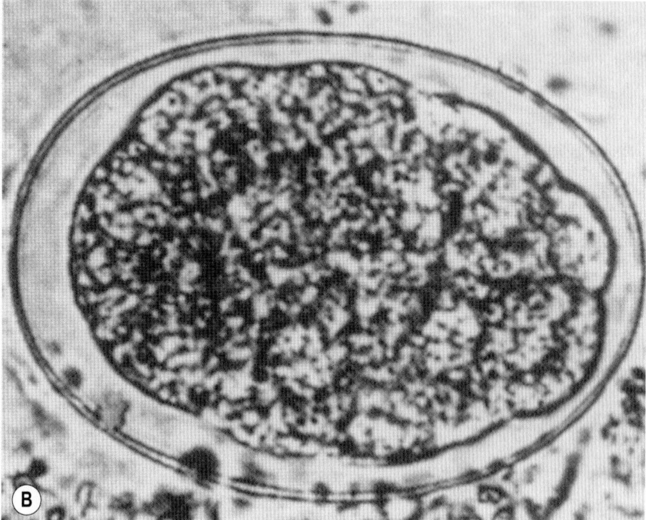

Figure 55.12 Hookworm eggs. (A) Immature egg showing developing larva. (B) Mature egg. *((A) Courtesy of J. S. Tatz. (B) Courtesy of Tropical Resources Unit.)*

Necator americanus. *N. americanus* closely resembles *A. duodenale* but it is shorter and more slender (0.9–1.1×0.4 cm) and can be distinguished from *A. duodenale* by the position of the vulva in the female, which is in the anterior third of the body (Appendix III) and the buccal capsule, which is smaller than that of *A. duodenale*, has cutting plates instead of teeth. The egg is slightly larger than that of *A. duodenale* (64–75×36–40 μm). The female lays 6000–20 000 eggs daily and has a life duration on average of 3–10 years.

Life Cycle

Adult worms live in the human intestine and each female produces eggs which are deposited into the lumen of the intestine containing two, four or eight blastomeres and exit the body in faeces which, if deposited in damp shaded soil, hatch into rhabditiform (first-stage) larvae (L1) (Figure 55.13), which are free-living and have a bulbed oesophagus. They feed avidly on organic debris and bacteria. The larva moults on the third day and the oesophagus disappears on the 5th day, the larva becoming elongated and fully developed at 20–30°C. It then moves away from the faeces into the soil and moults to form a filariform (infective) larva (L3) (Figure 55.13), which has a

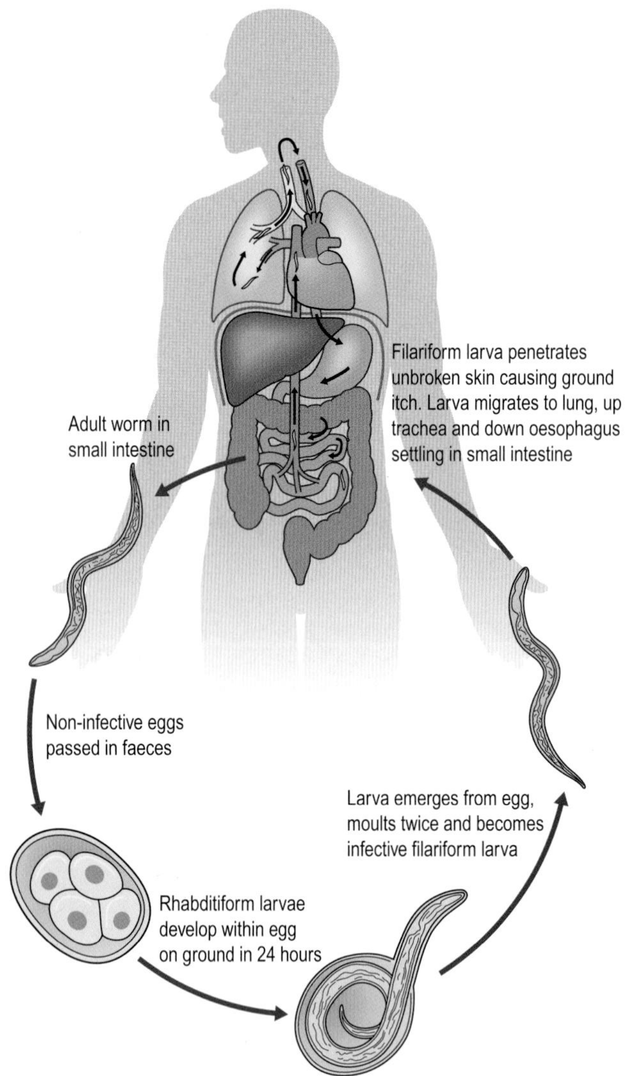

Figure 55.13 Life cycle of hookworm. *(Courtesy of Tropical Resources Unit.)*

simple muscular oesophagus and a protective sheath. The larva moves towards oxygen and cannot survive in water. The larvae are most numerous in the upper 2.5 cm of soil but can ascend from deeper layers. Protected from desiccation they can live in warm damp soil for two years. Direct sunlight, drying or salt water are fatal, although the motility of larvae means they can move downward into the soil, thereby avoiding desiccation. When the filariform larva comes into contact with the skin of the host it penetrates it and receive a signal present in mammalian serum and tissue that causes them to resume development.[82] The host-activated L3 enter the vasculature, reaching the lungs on the third day. Breaking through the alveoli it enters the bronchioles, moves up the trachea, down the oesophagus to the stomach and small intestine. During this migration the third moult takes place and the buccal capsule is formed. It arrives in the intestine on the seventh day and a fourth moult takes place, the buccal capsule assumes the adult form and the worm attaches to the mucosa of the small intestine, where it can be seen at postmortem as a small thread-like structure containing a red lining of ingested blood. In 3–5 weeks it becomes sexually mature and the female produces fertile eggs.

The life cycles of *A. duodenale* and *N. americanus* are similar, except that:

- *A. duodenale* live on average 1–3 years and *N. americanus* live 3–10 years
- *A. duodenale* can infect by ingestion as well as via the skin, whereas *N. americanus* infects only through the skin
- Migrating larvae of *N. americanus* grow and develop in the lungs, whereas those of *A. duodenale* do not
- *A. duodenale* possesses the ability to remain within the host as a larval stage for many months before finally developing to an adult, thus bridging seasons which are inappropriate for transmission.[83]

Transmission

Infection is normally acquired via the skin (percutaneous route) from filariform (infective) larvae in the soil contaminated by human faeces; or, in the case of *A. duodenale*, orally via the accidental ingestion of contaminated food or geophagia. However, other methods of transmission which are comparatively unimportant have been suggested: (1) Through eating uncooked meat containing the larvae of *A. duodenale* which have migrated into the muscles of the animal, where they can survive for 26–34 days; and (2) lactogenic transmission during breast-feeding. The migrating infective filariform larvae of *A. duodenale* are arrested in their development and migrate to the mammary gland, where they are excreted in the milk and infect the child. Third-stage infective filariform larvae of *N. americanus* have been found in the milk but none of the infected mothers was found to have infected babies.[84]

Pathology

Hookworm causes pathology at three stages of infection (the first two caused by larval hookworms usually seen only in expatriates who receive a primary infection):

1. Vesiculation and pustulation at the site of entry (ground itch). This is usually mild or absent in the tropics except in expatriates
2. Asthma and bronchitis during migration through the lungs with small haemorrhages into the alveoli and eosinophilic and leucocytic infiltration
3. Established infection, seen in the local residents of endemic areas, leading to hookworm anaemia and hookworm disease.

Hookworm Anaemia. The classical anaemia of hookworm infection is a hypochromic anaemia, the result of chronic blood loss, depletion of iron stores and deficiency of iron intake.

The attachment of hookworms' cutting organs to the intestinal mucosa and submucosa and the subsequent rupture of intestinal capillaries and arterioles causes blood loss. Hookworms have been shown to produce active suction impulses 120–200 times/min and evidence indicates that the hookworm is indeed an habitual blood-sucker and needs serum. The secretion of factor Xa and VIIa/TF inhibitors, and anti-platelet agents by the parasite helps to maintain continuous oozing of blood at the hookworm attachment site and the free flow of blood through the parasite alimentary canal.[85] The blood loss has been estimated as 0.03 mL/day per worm in *N. americanus* and 0.15 mL/day per worm in *A. duodenale* infections.[86] Where body iron stores are low, there is a significant negative relationship between the intensity of infection and blood loss[87] and haemoglobin concentration.[88] A significant negative correlation between plasma ferritin levels and hookworm burden, using the worm expulsion method, has been reported.[89] Persistent anaemia among children can result in stunted growth and impaired cognitive ability.[90] Hookworm anaemia is of the iron deficiency type and responds dramatically to iron supplementation and also to removal of the hookworm burden, but after a much longer period.

Light infections may cause anaemia where the iron intake is deficient and anaemia may also be caused in spite of the presence of an adequate iron intake, provided that the worm burden is heavy enough.[91] Light infections can have particular importance for pre-school children[92,93] and pregnant women,[94] who often have deficit iron stores. Little is known about the anaemia which develops in light primary infections, but it may be of immunological origin, similar to that which develops in dogs infected with *A. caninum*. A folate deficiency may be present, masked by the severe iron deficiency anaemia, and becomes overt only when this has been corrected. In general, children and pregnant women because of their low underlying iron reserves are considered the two populations most vulnerable to hookworm anaemia.

Hypoproteinaemia. Loss of protein is a common feature of hookworm anaemia, which is a cause of protein-losing enteropathy and in heavy infections, may result in hypoproteinaemia leading to oedema, or even anasarca. The protein loss, which is in excess of the red cell loss and is closely related to the hookworm burden, is caused by a limited capacity for albumin synthesis as well as loss caused by anaemia and other factors such as liver disease.

Immunity

Dogs are known to develop partial protective immunity towards *A. caninum* and *A ceylanicum*. Human infection with *A. duodenale* or *N. americanus* is characterized by eosinophilia and elevated serum IgE. There is also a strong IgG antibody response and detectable IgA and IgM responses. Studies in endemic populations show that infection is associated with upregulation of the T-helper 2 (Th2) cytokines controlling these antibodies, with IL-4 and IL-5 produced.[95] More recent studies reveal a more mixed cytokine response, with infected persons also producing Th-1 cytokines, interferon (IFN)-γ and IL-12.[96,97]

Whereas there is good evidence that immunity plays a role in controlling infections with *A. caninum* and *A. ceylanicum* in dogs, early observations in humans living in endemic areas were less conclusive about the existence of a vigorous, long-lasting protective immunity to human hookworm infections.[96,98] However, more recent evidence from immunoepidemiological studies indicates relationships between specific immune responses and the level of infection and reinfection,[95,99] suggestive of partial protective immunity.

Clinical Features

Natural History. After the establishment of adult worms in the intestine the females start to lay eggs. The number of eggs passed bears a direct relation to the number of female worms. The higher the worm burden the greater the blood loss. In populations with inadequate iron intake, hookworm burdens of 40–160 worms are usually sufficient to cause anaemia.[100] With worm burdens of 500–1000 significant blood loss and anaemia will result, even in the presence of an adequate iron intake.

Incubation Period. Symptoms appear 1–2 weeks after the primary infection, and in established infection eggs appear from the 42nd day onwards after infection.

Symptoms and Signs. At the site of entry of the infective larvae there is a 'ground itch', which consists of an irritating vesicular rash limited to the exposed portion(s) of the body, usually the soles of the feet or the hands. After 1–2 weeks pulmonary symptoms develop with a dry cough and asthmatic wheezing. Fever and a high degree of eosinophilia are found. Entry of larvae into the gastrointestinal tract and their development into adult hookworms frequently results in epigastric pain.[101] These symptoms generally peak at 30–45 days post-infection[102] and generally gradually disappear, and ova of hookworm can be seen on or around day 42 after infection. The whole episode is normally self-limiting, lasting not more than 2–3 months, but can persist longer due to constant stimulus by adult worms.[103] Sometimes, if many larvae enter simultaneously, symptoms are quite alarming and steroid therapy may be needed. It is not as common or as marked as larval ascariasis.

The taste may be perverted, some patients exhibiting and persistently gratifying an unnatural craving for such things as earth, mud or lime (pica or geophagy).

The essential signs of hookworm infection are connected with progressive iron-deficiency anaemia associated with gastric and intestinal dyspepsia but not wasting. The anaemia is typical of iron deficiency (see Chapter 12). The haemoglobin is reduced to a greater degree than the red cell count. The mean corpuscular volume is decreased and the mean corpuscular haemoglobin concentration may fall to as low as 22. The red cells show microcytosis and severe hypochromia. The serum iron is greatly reduced and the total iron-binding capacity of the serum greatly raised, indicating that iron stores are very low. There is no marked poikilocytosis or leucocytosis, although there may be an eosinophilia of 7–14%. The serum albumin is reduced in heavy infections.

When the iron-deficiency anaemia develops, then symptoms of anaemia occur: pallor, puffiness of the face, swelling of the feet and ankles and there may be generalized oedema caused by the hypoalbuminaemia. There is lassitude, breathlessness, palpitations, tinnitus and vertigo, and liability to syncope. The stools may contain blood, and frank melaena may occur in children. The occult blood test is always positive in the stools in cases where symptoms are caused by hookworm. There is often koilonychia. There is a high-output failure and haemic murmurs can be heard over the heart, which is seen to be enlarged on radiographic examination. Severe hookworm anaemia can, on rare occasions, result in cardiac failure and may easily be confused with rheumatic carditis. Ophthalmoscopic examination may reveal retinal haemorrhages.

The rate of progress varies in different cases. In some, a high degree of anaemia and even death may result within a few weeks or months of the appearance of the first symptoms. More frequently, the disease is chronic, ebbing and flowing or slowly progressing over a number of years.

Infantile Hookworm Disease. Most cases of hookworm in infants have been reported from China and the majority have been caused by *A. duodenale*.[84] The clinical features include diarrhoea with bloody stools, melaena, anorexia, vomiting, pallor and massive haemorrhage, which is potentially fatal if left untreated.

Diagnosis

The diagnosis is made by finding eggs in the stool (see Figure 55.12). Eggs have a characteristic thin clear shell and may appear unsegmented or show visible embryonic cleavages, usually two, four or eight cell stages. Rhabditiform larvae may be found in stale stools and may be mistaken for *Strongyloides* in which larvae only and not eggs are found in the stool (see below). The eggs may be confused with those of *Trichostrongylus* spp., which are more translucent and smaller. In light infections, concentration methods are necessary, such as zinc sulphate concentration, formol ether or the Kato-Katz direct smear (see Appendix I). Examination of Kato-Katz slides is hampered by the fact that slides must be read within 60 minutes or many of the eggs will no longer be visible. The Kato-Katz method as well as the McMaster and FLOTAC methods can provide a quantitative estimate of intensity of infection by counting the number of eggs per gram of faeces. Because of intra-specimen and day-to-day variation in egg output, diagnostic sensitivity is increased by examining multiple stool samples over consecutive days.[104] Heavy infections are defined as intensities of 4000 eggs/g of faeces or more (Table 55.1).

Adult Worms. The eggs of *A. duodenale* and *N. americanus* are morphologically almost identical. Species differentiation is achieved by morphological examination of the buccal apparatus of adult worms obtained by expulsion techniques or of larval stages cultured from eggs by the Harada-Mori method.

Serological Diagnosis

Multiplex real-time PCR-based methods are able to detect *A. duodenale* and *N. americanus* infections in faecal samples.[53,54] Such methods can distinguish infections from *Oesophagostomum bifurcum*, whose eggs are morphologically indistinguishable from hookworm.[105]

Differential Diagnosis

In countries where hookworm infection is endemic, eggs may be found in faeces in any number of conditions which are not causally related. In these conditions, an egg count is essential to determine the intensity of infection. Light infections in expatriates associated with moderate eosinophilia and mild anaemia must be differentiated from other helminth infections: *S. mansoni*, *Fasciola hepatica* and other liver flukes, and *S. stercoralis*. The epigastric pain associated with hookworm infection may suggest duodenal ulcer or pancreatitis and any patient from an endemic area with epigastric symptoms who has hookworm ova in the stool should be treated, since in many cases the symptoms will disappear without the need for any further investigation.

Severe hookworm anaemia must be distinguished from other iron-deficiency anaemias, and generalized anasarca from kwashiorkor and the nephrotic syndrome.

Management

Treatment consists of elimination of the parasites and treatment of the anaemia, if present. Treatment of the anaemia is the first priority but there is no reason why both objectives should not be proceeded with concurrently. Albendazole is highly effective against both *A. duodenale* and *N. americanus* (Table 55.1). A single dose of 400 mg will produce an 80% reduction in egg count and 200 mg daily for 3 days will give 100% cure.[26] Mebendazole is only partially effective against *A. duodenale* and *N. americanus*,[26] and treatment over several days may be required for heavy infections. Levamisole and pyrantel pamoate may also be used, although in some areas, e.g. north-western Australia, pyrantel pamoate has been found to be ineffective.[106]

The anaemia caused by hookworm is treated by the oral iron supplementation, in the form of ferrous sulphate or gluconate, 200 mg three times daily, which should be continued for 3 months after a normal haemoglobin level has been achieved. Supplementation on a weekly basis has been shown to be more practical and equally effective as daily supplementation.

After starting iron therapy, a reticulocyte response may be seen in about 1 week. In most cases, the haemoglobin will rise by 1.0 g per week. Folic acid, 5 mg daily, should be given for at least 1 month to cover the erythropoietic response. Many patients in the tropics fail to correct the haemoglobin fully and develop macrocytosis if this is not done.

Parenteral iron – iron–dextran complex or iron–poly (sorbitol gluconic acid) complex – may be used in patients who cannot tolerate oral iron, in patients where compliance is in doubt or in patients in whom regular follow-up is difficult or unlikely.

Epidemiology and Control

The main reservoir of infection is man, although *N. americanus* has been recovered on occasion from non-human primates.[107] In general, the transmission of hookworm infection depends upon an adequate source of infection in the human population, the deposition of eggs in a favourable environment for extrinsic development of the parasite, appropriate conditions of the soil (moisture and warmth) to allow larvae to develop and suitable conditions for the infective larvae to penetrate the skin.

Recent analysis employing GIS and remote sensing shows that hookworm is able to thrive better in hotter environments and has a more cosmopolitan distribution than *T. trichiura* and *A. lumbricoides* (see Figure 55.3).[27] This is suggested to be due in part to its ability to migrate downward into the soil, thereby avoiding desiccation. In addition hookworms have a longer adult life span and can find refuge from external temperatures for longer than the other geohelminth species, increasing the chances of hookworm transmission stages being deposited and developing in suitable thermal conditions. In some temperate climates local environmental conditions may allow transmission, as in the Cornish tin mines and Swiss railway tunnels in the past[108] and in the Rand in South Africa today. Cultural and agricultural practices such as the use of human faeces for fertilizer enhance opportunities for infection.[109]

Epidemiological studies show that children can be infected with hookworm as young as 6 months. Subsequently, infection prevalence typically rises monotonically with increasing age to a plateau in adulthood.[110] Increases in prevalence among the elderly have been observed in some populations.[111,112] Because of logistic and social difficulties, estimates of worm numbers by chemotherapeutic expulsion in an age-stratified host population have been very few,[110] most studies having relied on an indirect measure of intensity: quantitative egg counts. The few age-stratified estimates of hookworm burden using anthelminthic expulsion indicate that *N. americanus* worm burdens tend to increase in hosts up to age 15–25 years and remain constant thereafter.[110,113]

As with other geohelminths, the distribution of hookworms per host is highly aggregated within populations.[114] There is also evidence of household clustering and small-scale spatial variation, determined in part by local variation in socioeconomic status and environmental factors.[29,115] The basis of hookworm control is described above.

CUTANEOUS LARVA MIGRANS AND LARVA CURRENS (CREEPING ERUPTION, SANDWORM, PLUMBER'S ITCH, DUCKHUNTER'S ITCH)

Certain nematode species are incapable of growing to maturity in humans, but their larvae wander in the superficial layers of the body. Cutaneous larva migrans (CLM) is a cutaneous eruption resulting from exposure of the skin to the infective filariform larvae of the dog and cat hookworms *A. braziliense*, *A. caninum* and *Uncinaria stenocephala* – this condition is termed hookworm-related CLM.[116] A creeping eruption caused by *Strongyloides stercoralis* is called larva currens, so-called due to the fast movement of strongyloides larvae.

Geographical Distribution

Hookworm-related CLM and larva currens occur in most warm, humid, tropical and subtropical areas, being especially common in the southern USA, along the coast of the Gulf of Mexico and Florida.[117] It is also common on the coast of sub-Saharan Africa, South and South-east Asia and Latin America.

Aetiology

Creeping eruptions can be caused by animal hookworms, *Gnathostoma spinigerum*, *cutaneous myiasis* (*Hypoderma bovis* and *Hypoderma lineatum*), warble fly maggots (*Gasterophilus* spp.) cutaneous *Fasciola hepatica*, as well as *Strongyloides* (larva currens).

Ancylostoma. *A. braziliense* is the hookworm of dogs and cats. It is smaller than *A. duodenale* (female 1 cm and male 8.5 mm long), the internal pair of ventral teeth are smaller and the dorsal rays in the copulatory bursa are distinctive. The eggs are indistinguishable from those of human hookworms. The life cycle is similar to that of *A. duodenale* but man is an unsuitable host and the third-stage larva does not enter the bloodstream but wanders under the skin, causing cutaneous larva migrans.

A. caninum is the dog hookworm. Its life history is similar to that of *A. braziliense.*

Strongyloides. Filariform larvae of *S. stercoralis* can re-enter the skin as part of autoinfection around the anus and buttock, where they cause 'larva currens', a rash rather like that of cutaneous larva migrans.

S. myopotami (*Strongyloides* of the nutria) and *S. procyonis* (raccoon) produce similar lesions in the human host, in which they cannot complete their normal life cycle. The lesions are more persistent.

Transmission

Infection is acquired from damp contaminated soil through the skin of that part of the body in contact with the soil (foot, abdomen, buttock).

Pathology

The filariform larvae are unable to penetrate below the stratum germinativum of human skin, where they form a tunnel with the corium as a floor and the stratum granulosum as a roof.

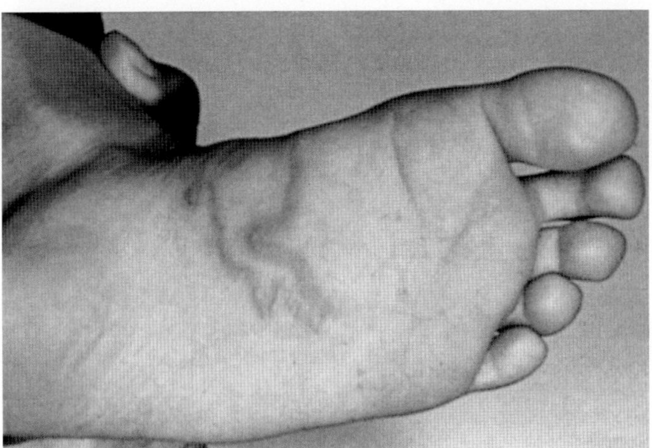

Figure 55.14 Cutaneous larva migrans (*Ancylostoma braziliense*).

Local eosinophilia and round cell infiltration occur round the tunnel and may persist for months. Rarely, the larvae reach the lungs, where they cause transitory pulmonary symptoms and eosinophilia and may be recovered from bronchial washings. They do not mature in the intestine.

Immunity

Little is known about immunity. There is no protective immunity and people can be infected more than once.

Clinical Features

Natural History. The larvae wander under the skin and can persist for months before they eventually die.

Incubation Period. Symptoms start immediately after penetration of the skin, a matter of a few hours only.

Symptoms and Signs. There is a red itchy papule at the site of entry, which becomes elevated and vesicular. The larvae move several millimetres to a few centimetres each day and leave tunnels which become dry and crusted. The track is linear and twists and turns (Figure 55.14). It causes an intense pruritus and the skin is scratched and becomes secondarily infected.[118] The lesions may be single or multiple. The most common sites are the hands and buttocks with *A. braziliense*[119] but the abdomen is often infested in plumber's itch and the lesions may be very numerous indeed (Figure 55.15). A second form of CLM associated with folliculitis has also been reported.[120]

The lesions produced by non-human hookworms are well defined, move very slowly and persist for months. There is little surrounding flare and the track is indurated. In contrast, the lesions produced by *Strongyloides* (larva currens) are less well defined, have a red flare on the outside, move much more rapidly and persist for a few hours only.

Diagnosis and Differential Diagnosis

The diagnosis is clinical, supported by travel history. Hookworm-related CLM is usually situated on the foot or toe (see Figure 55.14) and lasts for months, moving very slowly. *Strongyloides*-related larva currens is situated on the buttocks and trunk and lasts for hours only, moving comparatively quickly. Non-human *Strongyloides* is usually situated on the trunk and abdomen and

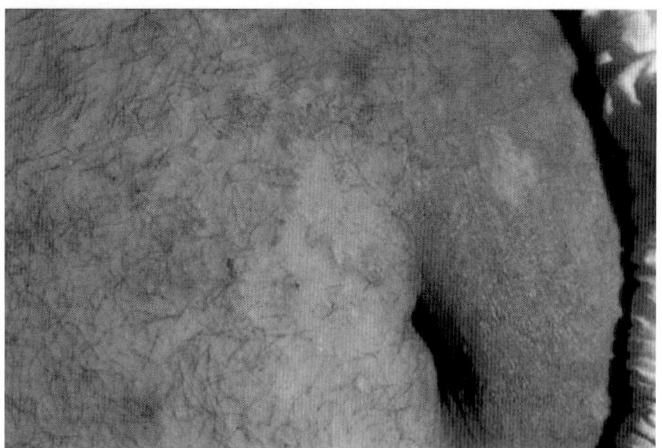

Figure 55.15 Multiple burrows of cutaneous larva migrans (creeping eruption).

can persist for many months. *Loa loa* causes no cutaneous reaction and appears and disappears in a matter of minutes. There is usually no eosinophilia but if there is then internal migration of the larvae can be suspected. It is not possible to retrieve the larva since it is invariably in advance of its track and impossible to isolate. There are no reliable serological tests at present.

Management

The drug of choice is ivermectin. A single dose (200 μg/kg body weight) provides a cure rate of 81–100%.[121] Treatment with a single dose of 400 mg oral albendazole is less effective than ivermectin, with a cure rate of 46–100%.[122] A 7-day course of 400 mg daily of oral albendazole results in fewer recurrences than single-dose treatment. Oral thiabendazole was previously recommended but is not used due to it poor tolerability, and the greater efficacy of ivermectin and albendazole. Topical thiabendazole for 5–7 days is effective and without adverse side-effects.[123] Secondary infections should be treated with a topical antibiotic.

Epidemiology and Control

The source of infection is soil contaminated with dog and cat faeces underneath beach houses on stilts, exposure taking place when people crawl underneath to repair facilities (plumber's itch) or bathe with bare feet and walk along the sand above the high water mark (sandworm) or expose themselves to mounds contaminated by nutria and racoons in the marshes (duck-hunter's itch). Hookworm-related CLM typically occurs mainly among individuals living in low-income endemic settings, but also among tourists from high-income countries visiting tropical and sub-tropical settings. In such settings exposure is most common during the rainy season. Most studies report on returning travellers. However, available population-based data indicate that in endemic areas, hookworm-related CLM is most common in children, especially those from poor households and who walk barefoot.[119,124]

Little can be done to control dogs and cats in resource-poor settings but infection can be prevented by wearing sandals above the high water mark and protective clothing when underneath houses in endemic areas. In high-income settings pets should be treated and banned from beaches and playgrounds.

STRONGYLOIDIASIS

Strongyloidiasis is a disease mostly caused by *Strongyloides stercoralis*, although in central Africa and Papua New Guinea the primate parasite *S. fulleborni kellyi* can infect humans. *S. stercoralis* is unusual among the geohelminths in that autoinfection can occur, resulting in long-lasting chronic infections. The clinical consequences of infection range from acute infection, through chronic infection, to life-threatening disseminated disease.

Geographical Distribution

Strongyloides stercoralis has a worldwide distribution, especially prevalent in parts of tropical South America, China and South-east Asia. Estimates of global prevalence are probably unreliable due to difficulties in diagnosing infection. In temperate climates it occurs at low prevalence but is not uncommon in inmates of institutions, such as mental hospitals, prisons and the mentally retarded children's homes. In recent years, it has become a serious problem in individuals who are on suppressive treatment.

Aetiology

Strongyloidiasis is caused by *S. stercoralis* (see Appendix III), a nematode worm which has two forms: one parasitic and the other free living. There are three developmental forms: adult, rhabditiform larva and filariform (infective) larva.

Life Cycle

The life cycle is complex and involves two stages in which reproduction takes place: an internal sexual cycle involving parasitic worms and the external sexual cycle involving free-living worms (Figure 55.16). Under unsuitable environmental conditions, the external sexual cycle may be omitted and autoinfection may occur.

In the internal sexual cycle, the adult female parasitic worm (2.5×0.034 mm) tapers anteriorly and ends in a conical tail. There is an oesophagus occupying a quarter of the body which has two bulbs divided by a constriction. The vulva lies in the posterior third of the body and there is a prominent uterus containing 50 eggs (50–58×30–34 μm) (Appendix III). The male exists but disappears from the bowel soon after oviposition and eggs can be produced parthenogenetically (as happens with *S. ratti*). The eggs hatch immediately in the bowel into male and female rhabditiform larvae, which pass out in the faeces to continue the external sexual cycle.

In the external sexual cycle, the free-living rhabditiform larvae develop into free-living adults which copulate in the soil and produce eggs. The free-living forms have a double-bulbed muscular oesophagus. The free-living female is smaller (1×0.05 mm) than the parasitic female, the vulva lies posteriorly and the uterus contains eggs measuring 70×40 μm (Appendix III). The male form measures 0.7×0.035 mm. The rhabditiform larvae produced by both parasitic and free-living forms are indistinguishable and develop into filariform (infective) larvae (Figure 55.17), which can remain alive in the soil for many weeks.

Autoinfection. Autoinfection can arise in one of two ways: in the first way, the filariform larvae do not pass out in the stools but reinvade the bowel or skin (external autoinfection); the other way is when the filariform larvae lodge in the bronchial

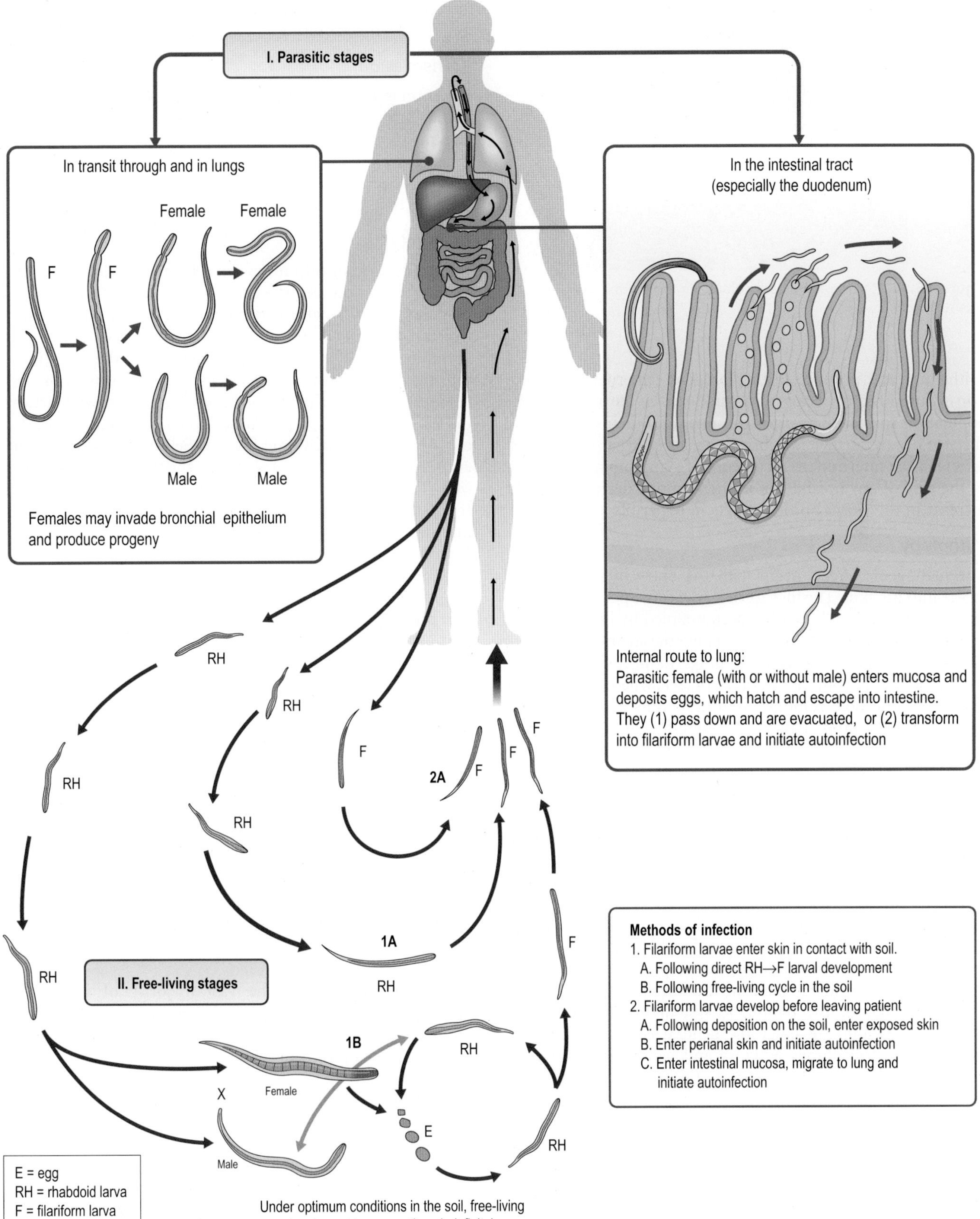

Figure 55.16 Life cycle of *Strongyloides stercoralis*.

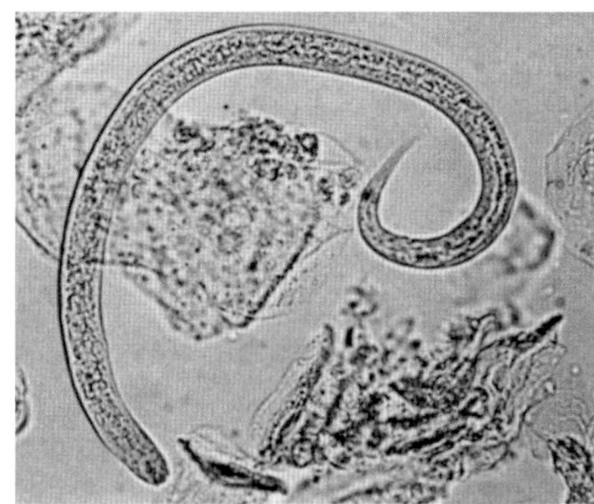

Figure 55.17 *Strongyloides stercoralis.* Rhabditiform larva in stool. *(Courtesy J. S. Tatz.)*

epithelium and produce further progeny (internal autoinfection). Autoinfection leads to a build-up in the body of the population so that the worms can maintain themselves in the absence of any further infection from an external source, and results in the intermittent recurrence of symptomatic episodes. In the case of any breakdown in the immune defences a rapid increase in the worm burden results in hyperinfection.

Pathology

The pathogenic effects begin with the entry of the infective larvae into the skin. The filariform larvae cause petechial haemorrhages at the site of invasion accompanied by intense pruritus, congestion and oedema. The larvae migrate into cutaneous blood vessels and are carried to the lungs. In the lungs they enter the alveoli and pass up the respiratory tree, where they may be delayed by the host response, become adults and invade the bronchial epithelium. Passing through the lungs the young worms may cause symptoms resembling those of bronchopneumonia with some lobular consolidation.

When they have become lodged in crypts in the intestine the females mature and invade the tissues of the bowel wall but rarely penetrate the muscularis mucosae, and move in tissue channels beneath the villi, where the eggs are deposited. The eggs hatch out and first-stage larvae work towards the lumen of the bowel and are passed out in faeces.

In heavy infections, the first-stage larvae, instead of passing out in the faeces, develop in the intestine, bore into the wall of the duodenum and jejunum and develop to the adult stage, producing ova, while encysted in the bowel. From here they spread throughout the lymphatic system to the mesenteric lymph glands and can enter the general circulation and be found in the liver, lungs, kidneys and gallbladder wall. The ileum, appendix and colon are sites of reinvasion and here the worms cause granulomas with a central necrotic area often containing a degenerate larva. The mesenteric glands may be similarly affected. The lungs may show abscesses and the liver may be enlarged with small pinpoint larval granulomas. The larvae may carry micro-organisms and an overwhelming septicaemia caused by *Escherichia coli* has been caused in this way. In light infections jejunal biopsy has shown oedema, cellular infiltration and eosinophilic infiltration of the mucosa with partial villous atrophy. At post-mortem, ulceration and atrophy of the mucosa are seen with numerous adult worms in the wall of the duodenum and jejunum. At times filariform larvae fail to break out of the alveoli, gain access to the general circulation and can invade the brain, intestine, lymph glands, liver, lungs and, rarely, myocardium.

Transmission

Infection is acquired originally from contaminated soil via free-living filariform infective larvae. Once established further infection may be acquired from the colon or anal skin from parasitic infective larvae. The transmission of *S. stercoralis* through the milk has been demonstrated in several animal species and it is possible that this occurs in humans.

Immunity

Immunity to reinfection develops in most individuals after a primary infection and the *Strongyloides* adults and larvae are confined to the small intestine and the worm burden is controlled. Immunity is both antibody- and cell-mediated. Humoral antibody-mediated immunity is elicited by the secretions of infective larvae with a Type I response, an eosinophilic tissue response, and a peripheral eosinophilia – often with urticarial rashes. Antibodies are produced which cross-react with many other helminths, including filariae. Cell-mediated immunity is elicited by adult and larval worms in the tissues, which are localized and destroyed by a cell-mediated granulomatous reaction. If cell-mediated immunity is depressed for any reason, such as immunodepressive states of drugs, then a generalized hyperinfection results, causing massive strongyloidiasis.

Among persons co-infected with human T-cell lymphotropic virus type 1 (HTLV-1) production of IFN-γ may decrease the production of antibodies that participate in the host immune response defence mechanism against infection.[125]

Clinical Features

Natural History. In the majority of cases a small population of adult worms maintains itself in the small intestine for many years (≥30) in the absence of any further infection from the outside causing recurrent symptoms when filariform larvae enter the perianal skin, and cause a recurrent rash – 'larva currens' – associated with urticaria. In a small minority of cases the defences of the body break down and a generalized severe infection ensues.

Incubation Period. The prepatent period from infection to the appearance of rhabditiform larvae in the stools is one month.

Symptoms and Signs. The vast majority of infections in endemic areas are symptomless. When for various reasons the number of *Strongyloides* present in the intestine increases then a variety of symptoms develop.

Primary Infection. This is rarely seen in endemic areas and descriptions are based on self-induced experimental infections. A pruritic erythematous eruption, which lasts about 3 weeks, occurs at the site of entry of the larvae. A dry cough or sore throat appears on the 6–9th days together with abdominal fullness, aching in the right lower quadrant of the abdomen and watery diarrhoea alternating with constipation. Larvae are first detected in the stools 27 days after infection.

Chronic Uncomplicated Strongyloidiasis. This is characterized by epigastric and right upper quadrant pain together with nausea, chronic diarrhoea and weight loss.

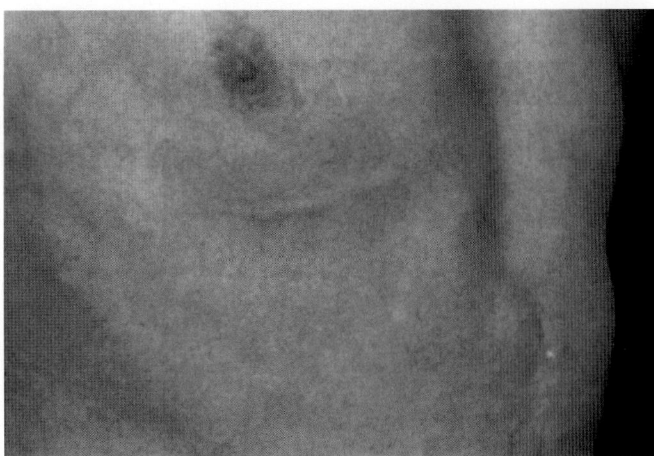

Figure 55.18 Skin rash (larva currens) of *Strongyloides stercoralis*.

Skin Rashes. There are two types of skin rashes. One, occurring around the anus and anywhere on the trunk, is a linear eruption – 'larva currens' – in which the larvae migrate under the skin causing an itching rash with a larval track which is not indurated and has a red flare at the edge which moves quite rapidly (2–10 cm/h), disappearing in a few hours (Figure 55.18), in contrast to the more indurated and persistent track of non-human hookworm (cutaneous larva migrans). The second form is urticaria caused by allergy to the larvae penetrating the skin in an individual who has already been sensitized. It occurs predominantly in the buttocks with pruritus ani and around the waist, lasts 1–2 days and recurs at regular intervals. The creeping type of eruption, which is seen mainly in infections from Indo-China and was common in prisoners of war in the Far East in the Second World War, can last for 30 years or more.[126] A strongyloides-related glomerulonephritis has been reported.[127]

Severe Complicated Strongyloidiasis. In persons debilitated by disease, malnutrition or serious illness, severe and potentially fatal complications may result from massive invasion of the tissues by *S. stercoralis* (i.e. when *S. stercoralis* disseminate). The same results can occur in immunocompromised individuals, for example, as a result of treatment with immunosuppressive drugs for lymphoma and organ transplantation and/or immunosuppression due to the effects of co-infection with HTLV-1 infection.[125] It has recently been suggested that host immunosuppression favours the direct development of infective larvae thereby promoting hyperinfection. Interestingly, it seems that in HIV-positive persons with poor immune function, indirect development – rather than direct development – of infective larvae in the gut is favoured.[128] This observation may explain the notable absence of disseminated strongyloidiasis in late-stage HIV disease.

First-stage larvae develop in the duodenum and jejunum, bore into the bowel wall, become adult and produce ova. In this way the number of *Strongyloides* is immensely increased and infective larvae invade the tissues and circulate, causing massive strongyloidiasis. Severe abdominal pain, vomiting and diarrhoea together with a sprue-like syndrome may develop: a protein-losing enteropathy, hypoalbuminaemia and generalized oedema occur. Fever, hypertension, abdominal tenderness and distension, reduced bowel sounds, paralytic ileus and a necrotizing jejunitis have been reported.

In the lungs, pulmonary symptoms resembling tropical pulmonary eosinophilia with hypereosinophilia, pneumonitis, diffuse crepitations, scattered bronchi, pleural effusion and pulmonary abscess and gross respiratory failure may occur.[129]

Neurological complications with headache, convulsions, confusion, stupor, meningitis and focal neurological signs occur. In 30% of immunocompromised patients, a Gram-negative (*E. coli*) meningitis is found. Other complications include septicaemia with enteric organisms, shock, multiple petechiae on the chest and abdomen and peri-umbilical purpura.

Laboratory Findings

Raised serum IgE levels are found. Towards the end of the early stage of infection, there is a high leucocytosis of up to 25×10^9/L; an eosinophilia of 10–12$\times 10^9$/L is characteristic. Later when the infection is chronic there is a moderate eosinophilia which may persist for years. In severe complicated strongyloidiasis the eosinophilia disappears and is an indication of poor prognosis.

Diagnosis

Only adults or rhabditiform larvae (Figure 55.17) appear in the stools, duodenal aspirate or by the Entero test capsule. They can be demonstrated, to varying degrees, by the faecal examination methods or cultured in charcoal at 26°C for a week (see Appendix III).

The Kato-Katz method, the most commonly used diagnostic method in geohelminth epidemiology, does not detect *S. stercoralis*, and this feature probably explains why the global prevalence of *S. stercoralis* is likely to be underestimated. More sensitive coprological methods include a modified agar plate[130] and the Baermann technique. However, because of low larval densities, multiple examinations are often necessary.[131] Serological methods using ELISA, which detect serum IgG against a crude extract of infective larvae,[132] are more sensitive than coprology, but are labour-intensive and prone to cross-reactions with other helminths and filariae. A gelatin particle indirect agglutination test is considered to be more practical than the ELISA for mass screening for strongyloidiasis.[133]

Differential Diagnosis

Strongyloidiasis must be differentiated from other tissue-invading helminths: *A. lumbricoides*, hookworm and liver flukes. Disseminated strongyloidiasis may closely resemble tropical pulmonary eosinophilia, especially since serology cross-reacts. 'Larva currens' resembles cutaneous larva migrans but in distinction from it in 'larva currens' the rash is situated mainly round the buttocks and on the trunk, lasts only a few hours and may occur intermittently for many years.

Management

S. stercoralis should usually be treated whether or not the infection is giving rise to symptoms. It should be looked for and treated especially in immunosuppressed patients, for example those on corticosteroid therapy, immunosuppressive drugs, HIV, or persons from endemic areas in whom transplantation is being contemplated. Ivermectin is highly efficacious and the drug of choice (Table 55.1). Albendazole, mebendazole and thiabendazole can also be used but are generally less efficacious.[134] There is often a decrease in the efficacy of treatment in persons co-infected with HTLV-1.

Epidemiology

Humans are the most important hosts of *S. stercoralis* but dogs and chimpanzees have been found infected with strains indistinguishable from those of humans. Larvae are unable to survive temperatures below 8°C or above 40°C or desiccation. Strongyloidiasis thrives in conditions of overcrowding on damp soil in tropical conditions such as in rural villages in South-east Asia and the Amazon. Due to difficulties in diagnosis, few detailed epidemiological studies exist; however, infection is normally more prevalent among males than females and increases with age.[135,136] Household clustering of infection is common.[137] It was very prevalent among prisoners of war in Burma and Indo-China in the Second World War,[126] and Vietnam veterans.

Control

Control methods are the same as for other geohelminths (see below).

Strongyloides Fülleborni. This zoonotic *Strongyloides* occurs in humans in tropical forest regions of Central and East Africa. The main source of infection is monkey faeces, although human-to-human transmission may occur. In most cases, there are no symptoms.

S. fülleborni can be distinguished from *S. stercoralis* by the prominent vulvar lips, narrowing behind the vulva and a prominent oesophagus. Eggs are passed in the stool in contrast to *S. stercoralis* and resemble those of hookworm, for which they are commonly mistaken. Treatment is as for *S. stercoralis*.

Strongyloides Fülleborni Kellyi. This is a subspecies of *S. fülleborni* confined mainly to forested areas in western Papua New Guinea, along the Fly River in the Eastern Highlands,[138] where there are no non-human primates. In low-prevalence areas, 20% of children and 5–10% of adults are infected and transmission is implicated to be percutaneous. In high-prevalence areas 100% of children aged 3–5 years are infected and 15–20% of adults. Peak intensity of infection occurs around 12 months. In these high-prevalence areas transmission is percutaneous and possibly transmammary.

Mothers carry their children in string bags lined with dried banana leaves and/or cloth which is infrequently changed and in which eggs and free-living larvae have been found. The eggs are similar to those of *S. fülleborni*.

Clinical manifestations are seen most frequently in children 2–6 months of age who present with abdominal distension, mild diarrhoea, a protein-losing enteropathy resulting in oedema and low serum protein levels – ‘swollen-belly disease’ – which can be fatal unless quickly treated. Respiratory distress may occur with a characteristic high-pitched cry. Treatment is as for *S. stercoralis* supplemented by plasma infusion, if the hypoproteinaemia is severe.

TRICHOSTRONGYLIASIS (WIREWORM)

Several species of *Trichostrongylus* infect humans, who are the accidental hosts. The majority of human infections are asymptomatic.

Geographical Distribution

Normally a parasite of sheep and goats, human infection with *Trichostrongylus* is widespread in Australia, Central Africa, Egypt and in Asia and India, Assam, Indonesia and Japan.

Aetiology and Life Cycle

At least eight species of *Trichostrongylus* have been reported to infect humans, but the main species are *Trichostrongylus colubriformis* (the species most commonly encountered in the Near and Middle East) and *T. orientalis* (the principal species in Asia) and, more rarely, *T. probulurus, T. lerouxi* and *T. axei.*

The female worm (5–8 × 0.07 mm) is slender and pink with a posterior vulva (Appendix III); the male (4–5 × 0.07 mm) has a bilobed copulatory bursa and two spicules. The mouth is unarmed. The parasites are situated in the duodenum and jejunum where they are not attached to the bowel but are a half to a third buried in mucus. The eggs, which have a transparent hyaline shell and resemble those of hookworm but are larger (85 × 115 μm), are passed in the stool in the morula stage and are remarkably resistant to desiccation and cold. The life cycle is similar to that of hookworm but they do not migrate through the lungs. Adults mature in the intestine within 25–30 days.

Transmission

Infection is either acquired through the skin or through the mouth from contaminated food or drink.

Pathology

Little is known about pathology and none has been observed, even in individuals with heavy egg counts.

Symptoms and Signs

These are few but mild abdominal discomfort and diarrhoea may result.

Diagnosis

Diagnosis is made by finding eggs in faeces and adults after treatment. However, *Trichostrongylus* eggs are most commonly mistaken for hookworm eggs, which have a similar shape. Occasionally, diagnosis can be made by finding *Trichostrongylus* larvae in duodenal aspirates. A species-specific PCR technique has recently been developed to enable species differentiation.[139]

Management

Pyrantel pamoate is the drug of choice and is given as a single oral dose of 10 mg/kg. A single dose of 2.5 mg/kg body weight of levamisole and a single dose of albendazole (400 mg) are both also effective.

Epidemiology and Control

Humans are accidental hosts and vary in their susceptibility to various *Trichostrongylus* species. *T. colubriformis* is a parasite of sheep and goats and is common where there is close contact with sheep and goats:[140] it is the species most commonly encountered in the Near and Middle East and up to 70% of the inhabitants may be infected. *T. orientalis* is common among people who look after donkeys and goats and is the principal species in Asia; the use of human excreta as fertilizer is responsible for the high level of infection.

Control is based on the sanitary disposal of human excreta and prevention of faecal contamination of the topsoil by infected animals. The treatment of infected herd animals, such as cattle or sheep, may also reduce the risk to humans. Potentially contaminated vegetables should be thoroughly cooked and water boiled before ingestion.

Community Control of Geohelminths

Effective sanitation and hygiene interrupt and prevent transmission, and control is a natural sequel to economic growth in communities. Where these conditions are absent, due to poverty, or break down, due to infrastructure failures, social shocks or emergencies, the community-level intervention of choice is chemotherapy. Infrequent, usually annual chemotherapy has been shown to be effective even in the absence of improved sanitation or hygiene education. However, improvements in hygiene have been achieved at very much lower cost than improvements in sanitation, with programmes to encourage hand-washing with soap achieving important health benefits with existing technologies and at low cost.

No practical vaccine has yet been developed, although several hookworm candidates are being investigated.[141]

ANTHELMINTICS AND DIAGNOSIS

There are now several anthelmintics active against the geohelminths (Table 55.1) which are suitable for community control. They are given orally, and are effective in a single dose if reduction in intensity of infection rather than absolute cure is the main objective. They have a broad spectrum of activity, which makes them particularly useful for community control, since polyparasitism is more common. Moreover, billions of doses have been delivered with few significant side-effects.

The clinical pharmacology of the most commonly used broad-spectrum anthelmintics is discussed above. Because of the safety profiles of these anthelmintics, screening of individuals is not required provided that the treatment can be geographically targeted. The cost of individual diagnosis is usually prohibitive except in some high-density middle-income settings (e.g. Java, Indonesia) where mass diagnosis has proven to be cost-effective.

For countries that adopt a national 'essential drugs' policy and take advantage of the joint UNICEF–WHO initiative for the procurement of 'essential drugs',[142] the cost is now low. Currently, 200 million doses of mebendazole (from Johnson & Johnson) and 400 million doses of albendazole (from Glaxo SmithKline) are available annually to low-income countries whose programmes meet quality criteria.

Geographical Targeting

In recent years, there have been significant advances in the design of chemotherapy control strategies,[143] the most important of which are the improvements in methods for identifying populations for treatment using GIS.[144] Practical, low-cost methods of using GIS for planning and targeting national programmes have now been developed and implemented at national scale.[145,146]

A global initiative has collated prevalence data against strict quality criteria, and then made the results freely available on down-loadable electronic maps.[147] These maps show the survey data in its empirical form as well as geostatistical predictions of the prevalence of STH infection based on environmental correlates (see: www.thiswormyworld.org). The maps allow policy-makers to prioritize regions for intervention and, by overlaying with national infrastructure maps, identify which specific schools should be engaged in treatment delivery. Note that in many cases the maps will need to be supplemented by actual surveys on the ground, but the maps help indicate precisely what is required, and obviate the need for very expensive national surveys.

Targeting Population Groups

WHO has identified three key groups which are given priority for treatment: (1) school-age children; (2) pre-school children and (3) pregnant women. The 2001 World Health assembly established regular treatment of 75% of school children by 2010 as the key target.[148,149]

The primary goal of chemotherapy programmes is to reduce transmission, and hence the overall worm burdens and morbidity in the community. If reduction in morbidity in individuals is the primary objective then attention may need to be paid to the age-specificity of infection with the different species: the peak intensities of *A. lumbricoides* and *T. trichiura* occur in children under 10 years of age; and at older ages for hookworm.

School-based Programmes. School-based programmes have been shown to be a cost-effective approach for controlling the intensity of intestinal helminth infection even in environments where transmission is high.[150]

The effectiveness of these programmes reflects the epidemiological observation that treatment of an intensely infected age group or subpopulation reduces transmission overall,[151] and the economic observation that this results in externalities that greatly increase the cost-effectiveness of the approach.[152–155] The increase in school participation world wide as one of the key Millennium Development Goals,[156] as well as the specific promotion of school health programmes as part of these efforts, provides an additional strong policy incentive to deliver deworming through school systems.[157,158] The sustainability of at-scale, school-based national programmes has been demonstrated in several erstwhile low-income countries that have now transitioned to middle income status or above – including Japan, Korea, Brazil and Sri Lanka.[159,160] In all of these cases the transition was from a school-based chemotherapy programme as part of a national school health system approach to management through the established health services as infection levels declined. These and other experiences show that the critical first step in developing school-based programmes is coordination between the health and education sectors. The cost advantages of the school-based approach are dependent upon the low cost of delivery through the existing education infrastructure.

School-based deworming can reduce rates of anaemia[161,162] and improve growth, particularly in weight.[161] Meta-analyses of randomized trials have given equivocal results[163] but more recent analyses demonstrate increases in growth, especially ponderal weight gain.[164] There are significant effects on school attendance,[165] but quantifying the impact on educational measures remains a challenge, with stronger evidence for impacts on cognition than on educational outcomes, probably because the latter depends on education quality.[20,21,166] Recent studies in Africa, as well as re-analysis of the extensive Rockefeller Foundation control programmes in the southern USA at the beginning of the twentieth century, have shown remarkable long-run effects on labour output, employment and wages, of treatment at school age.[167,168] An important new observation is that part of the external benefits of treating school-age children is a reduction in infection in younger children in the same community.

The demonstrated cost-effectiveness of deworming as a school-based intervention has encouraged more interest by development agencies in this intervention. The increased availability of development aid for deworming, as well as the availability of free anthelmintics through large-scale donations by the pharmaceutical industry, has resulted in a growth in community-wide programmes. These programmes are also a natural component of community-based health systems that seek to use an integrated approach to controlling the neglected tropical diseases.[169]

Programmes for Pre-school Children. These have been developed as part of micronutrient or other health campaigns, as part of health programmes delivered through pre-schools, and as an addition to 'child health days' that provide a range of health interventions to young children on a demand basis. There is evidence that all these approaches are effective in improving the growth and nutrition of pre-school children and, where they build on existing systems, are cost-effective.[161,170] Since pre-school children have relatively low rates of infection, treating them alone is unlikely to generate significant externalities or to return the level of benefits of treatment of the school-age population. An emerging recommendation is that efforts should be made to develop pre-school programmes where school-based programmes are already in place.

Maternal Care Programmes. Infection during pregnancy is widespread and affects the health of the mother, fetal development and the survival and subsequent development of the child.[171–173] Antenatal anthelmintics improve haemoglobin levels,[171] birth weight and infant survival.[173] Previous advice was that anthelmintic treatment should be avoided in pregnancy, but it is now recommended that infected pregnant mothers should be treated, ideally after the 1st trimester.[174]

RESISTANCE TO ANTHELMINTIC DRUGS

Resistance is now widespread in the gastrointestinal nematodes of ruminants, particularly sheep and goats.[175] Although resistance by human nematodes has rarely been reported, managers of control programmes should be alerted to the possibility, particularly since the current biological assays do not detect resistance until the resistance genotype is already common and fixed in the worm population. A possible genetic marker for resistance to treatment of *S. stercoralis* has been identified,[176] and the genotypic markers of resistance in veterinary nematodes have been identified in the common nematodes of humans, but not yet developed into assays appropriate for surveillance.

Mebendazole drug failure has been reported against *N. americanus* in Mali[177] and pyrantel drug failure against *A. duodenale* in Western Australia has been reported,[106] but in the absence of any definitions of resistance for these species it is difficult to interpret these findings. Careful monitoring of mass treatment programmes is therefore essential,[178] and it is very important that the available anthelmintics are used in ways that will delay or prevent drug resistance, such as ensuring the existence of refuge populations (e.g. by targeting specific age groups), by maintaining low treatment pressure through infrequent cycles of treatment, and possibly by combination therapies as is advocated for malaria. A 2007 WHO/World Bank meeting on drug resistance has developed a way forward for more structured surveillance.[179] Given the experience in the veterinary world and with malaria, this remains a major area of concern.

MONITORING AND EVALUATION

Monitoring and evaluation are essential and should be used to review or revise any control programme, demonstrate health benefits, but also to assess cost-effectiveness.[113] Since the main aim underlying geohelminth control is the prevention of disease rather than to reduce or eradicate transmission, it is important that evaluation focuses on both intensity of infection and morbidity measures where possible, and not the sole use of infection prevalence.

Clinical Pharmacology of Anthelmintic Drugs

A number of single-dose, orally administered drugs are available for the treatment and control of STH infections. There are currently five drugs on the WHO model list of essential medicines for the treatment of geohelminths: albendazole, mebendazole, pyrantel, levamisole and ivermectin. Each of these drugs is recommended by WHO for use in large-scale control programmes.[142] They are all broad-spectrum benzimidazole anthelmintics, although their efficacy against individual STH species varies (Table 55.3).[26,181,182] Because benzimidazoles are poorly

TABLE 55.3 Effectiveness[a] of Anthelminthic Drugs Given as a Single Dose

	Albendazole (400 mg Once)		Mebendazole (500 mg Once)		Pyrantel (10 mg/kg Once)		Levamisole (2.5 mg/kg Once)	
	CR[b] (%)	ERR[c] (%)	CR[b] (%)	ERR[c] (%)	CR[b] (%)	ERR[c] (%)	CR[b] (%)	ERR[c] (%)
Ascaris lumbricoides	88	87–100	95	96–100	88	88	92	92–100
Trichuris trichiura	28	0–90	36	81–93	31	52	10	42
Hookworm	72	64–100	15	0–98	31	56–75	38	68–100
Strongyloides stercoralis	40–60[d]	NA	Low effectiveness		Low effectiveness		Low effectiveness	

[a]Effectiveness measures the effect of a drug against a parasite in a field setting, whereas efficacy measures the effect of a drug in ideal settings.
[b]CR, cure rate; CR is the percentage of individuals among whom parasites are cleared, and overall CR is presented.
[c]ERR, egg reduction rate; ERR is change in mean egg count before and after treatment, and range of estimates from studies is presented (where only one estimate is available, point estimate is presented). NA, not available. Estimates based on reviews by Horton (2000)[180] and Keiser and Utzinger (2008)[181].
[d]400 mg daily for 3 days.

absorbed, they reach and kill the parasites in the intestinal tract, causing few side-effects. Since their development in the 1970s, these broad-spectrum benzimidazoles have revolutionized the community control of the geohelminths and to date, millions of individuals have been treated with minimal side-effects.[183]

ALBENDAZOLE

This is the most widely used anthelmintic for the community control of multiple STH infections. Albendazole is poorly absorbed from the gastrointestinal tract and is rapidly and extensively metabolized by the liver to sulphoxide and sulphone metabolites. The sulphoxide metabolite is an active anthelmintic and may be responsible for most of the drug effects in vivo. The drug binds to intracellular tubulin, impairing essential absorptive functions in the parasite.

It is known to be teratogenic and embryotoxic in some animals, but only after doses considerably higher than used in clinical practice. Given the fact that STH-related morbidity can develop rapidly in pregnant women and treatment confers health benefits, WHO now recommends treatment of lactating women and of pregnant women after the 1st trimester.[149] It has also recently been recommended that children as young as 12 months can be safely treated, with the recommended dose for children aged 1–2 years being 200 mg.

Adverse effects are mild and transient, and include epigastric pain, diarrhoea, headache, nausea, vomiting, dizziness, constipation, pruritus and dry mouth.

MEBENDAZOLE

Mebendazole is effective against adult worms and larval stages. It binds to nematode tubulin preventing the formation of microtubules and selectively inhibits cell division and glucose uptake in nematodes; this latter effect results in increased utilization of helminth glycogen and deprivation for the worms of their main source of energy. Oral absorption is limited by its poor solubility. The small amount absorbed is metabolized extensively by the liver to inactive compounds. As with albendazole, mebendazole is now recommended for lactating and pregnant women and young children living in endemic areas.[149]

Adverse effects are mild and transient, including gastrointestinal discomfort, headache and dizziness.

Rarely mebendazole stimulates *Ascaris* worms to emerge from the mouth and nostrils, which alarms the patients unless they are forewarned.

PYRANTEL

Pyrantel binds to acetylcholine receptors of parasites and owes its activity to its action on the neuromuscular system of the worms. It paralyses the worms, which are then expelled in the faeces. It is poorly absorbed from the gastrointestinal tract, with less than 15% excreted in the urine as unchanged drug and metabolites and 70% excreted unchanged in the faeces. Safe use in pregnancy has not been established. Pyrantel and piperazine are antagonistic and should not be administered concurrently.

Adverse effects include mild and transient gastrointestinal discomfort, headache, dizziness, drowsiness, insomnia and skin rash.

LEVAMISOLE

Levamisole has a similar mode of action to pyrantel and causes spastic paralysis followed by passive elimination of parasites. It is rapidly absorbed from the gastrointestinal tract, achieving peak plasma levels within 2 hours, and is eliminated within 3 days. Much of the absorbed drug is metabolized in the liver. There is no evidence of teratogenicity, although it should not be given in the 1st trimester.

Adverse effects include abdominal pain, nausea, vomiting, dizziness and headache.

PIPERAZINE

Piperazine is used in the treatment of *A. lumbricoides*, especially in the presence of intestinal or biliary obstruction, with reported cure rates of 60% and above.[180–181] Recommended dosage is 75 mg/kg. It is also used for the treatment of *E. vermicularis*, at a dosage of 50 mg/kg daily for 7 successive days. Safe use in pregnancy has not been established.

IVERMECTIN

Ivermectin is extensively used for the treatment and control of onchocerciasis and lymphatic filariasis and strongyloidiasis. It also has therapeutic properties against *A. lumbricoides*, but shows limited effectiveness against *T. trichiura* and hookworm.[181]

NITAZOXANIDE

Nitazoxanide is an antiparasitic drug noted for its treatment of protozoan infections[184] but has also been shown to be effective against STH infections.[185,186] Pharmaceutical compositions of nitazoxanide include both nitazoxanide and its derivative tizoxanide, as active ingredients with particle sizes of the active drug substance ranging from 5 to 200 μm. Adverse effects are mild and transient and include abdominal pain, nausea, vomiting and diarrhoea. Two daily doses (100–400 mg) are required for ≥3 days.

POTENTIAL NEW DRUGS

A number of new candidate drugs are in development for human use. The first is tribendimidine which was first synthesized in China in the 1980s and early trials in humans demonstrated that single-dose tribendimidine is effective against all STH species[187] However, before tribendimidine can be made available outside China, additional preclinical and clinical studies are required to meet the international standards. Two veterinary anthelmintics that have promising anthelmintic properties are PF1022A (and its derivative emodepside) and monepantel.[182]

Other Nematodes Orally Acquired

TRICHINOSIS (*TRICHINELLA SPIRALIS*)

Trichinosis is a disease caused by parasites of the genus *Trichinella* that can infect a diversity of mammalian and avian hosts. Humans acquire infection from eating the raw or undercooked muscle meat of domestic and wild animals. It is not a soil-transmitted helminth infection. A comprehensive review has recently been provided.[188]

Geographical Distribution

Trichinosis has been documented in 55 countries around the world, with the disease especially prevalent in the Balkans, Russia and the Baltic States, and in the Americas, especially the USA, Mexico, Argentina and Chile.[189] Large outbreaks also occur in China.[190] It was previously an important cause of disease and death in the Arctic, where polar explorers have died as a result of trichinosis; it is less important in the tropics but occurs in both east and west Africa.

Aetiology

Species and Strains of *Trichinella*. The number of species and strains of *Trichinella* has in recent years been revised, due to the advent of DNA technology. The majority of human cases are caused by *T. spiralis* and several of its subspecies. They are indistinguishable morphologically but vary in their host specificity and can be distinguished genetically and enzymatically:[191]

- *T. spiralis spiralis* of temperate regions, with domestic pigs the source of human infection
- *T. spiralis nativa* of the Arctic regions; a parasite of carrion-feeding carnivores; polar bears and walruses are the main sources of human infection
- *T. spiralis nelsoni* in Africa and southern Europe in wild carnivores, with wild pigs the source of human infection
- *T. britovi* occurs in sylvatic mammals in Europe and Asia, with wild boars, horses, foxes and jackals the sources of human infection
- *T. pseudospiralis* occurs mainly in birds and sylvatic mammals, occasionally infecting humans. It does not encapsulate in human host muscle tissue. An epidemic due to *T. pseudospiralis* was reported from Thailand, affecting 59 individuals, all of whom ate raw pork from a wild pig that was distributed to villagers by a local hunter.[192] Outbreaks have occurred in Europe.
- *Trichinella spiralis* occurs in two forms: adult and cystic. The adult *T. spiralis* (Appendix III) is a white worm just visible to the naked eye and inhabits the small intestine. The male (1.6×0.04 mm) has a cloaca situated posteriorly between two caudal papillae. The female (3–4×0.06 mm) has a vulva in the anterior fifth, an ovary in the posterior half of the body and a coiled uterine tube in the anterior portion.

Life Cycle

The female lives for 30 days and is viviparous. The eggs (20 μm) live in the upper uterus and the larvae (100×6 μm) break out, living free in the uterine cavity. One female produces more than 1500 larvae. The larvae, which emerge as early as 4–7 days after infection, continue to be produced for 4–16 weeks. They make their way via the lymphatics and blood circulation to the right heart and lungs, enter the arterial circulation and reach striated muscle, where they encyst.

Cystic Stage. The cyst is formed by the larva encapsulated by the host tissue. The capsule is an adventitious ellipsoidal sheath with blunt ends resulting from cellular reaction around the tightly coiled larva (Figure 55.19). The long axis parallels that of the muscle fibres and host amino acids nourish it so that it can remain alive for many years. In humans calcification may take place after 6 months and lead to death of the larva. When consumed by a carnivorous host the cysts are digested in the stomach and after excysting the larvae, which are resistant to gastric juice, invade the duodenal and jejunal mucosa, where they penetrate the columnar epithelium and develop into adults after 36 hours. The period between infection and the encysting stage in the muscles is 17–21 days.

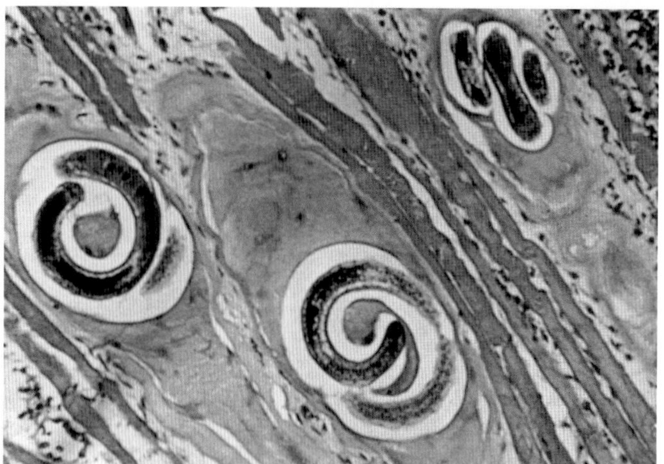

Figure 55.19 Larvae of *Trichinella spiralis* in muscle.

Transmission

Transmission is by mouth from eating raw or undercooked meat. The reservoir hosts of infection vary according to subspecies.

- *T. s. spiralis* infection is acquired from eating undercooked pork from infected pigs. The pigs are infected from eating raw garbage or perhaps from eating rats which themselves become infected from garbage.
- *T. s. nativa* infection is acquired from eating bear meat (the top predator), polar bear in the Arctic and brown bears in sub-Arctic regions of the former USSR and North America. Walrus meat can also be infective. Polar explorers have died as a result of eating polar bear meat.
- *T. s. nelsoni* infection results from eating bush pig or warthog meat which are themselves infected from carrion.
- *T. britovi* is found in sylvatic carnivores and humans can become infected from eating wild boar or horse.
- *T. pseudospiralis* is typically acquired from eating wild pig or boar meat. This species also infects birds.

Pathology

The capsule of the infective larva is digested in the intestine since it is resistant to the gastric juice and penetrates the duodenal and jejunal mucosa, where the amount of trauma and irritation depend on the number of larvae. This will cause the symptoms of the enteric phase.

After 5–7 days the worms mature and the females discharge larvae to the tissues, causing symptoms of the migratory or invasive stage. Later the larvae encyst, causing symptoms of the encystment stage. Larvae only encyst in striated muscle but travel through the brain and heart muscle, where they are unable to encyst.

Striated Muscle. Larvae, after travelling through the circulation, encyst in muscles of the diaphragm, masseters, intercostals, laryngeal, tongue and ocular muscles. At first there is a basophilic degeneration of the muscle fibres followed by formation of a hyaline capsule around the larva with an inflammatory infiltrate of lymphocytes and a few eosinophils (Figure 55.19). Foreign body giant cells may be present. The infiltrate subsides and fat is deposited at the poles and after 6 months calcification takes place, eventually leading to death of the larva.

Brain. Larvae migrate through the brain and meninges causing leptomeningitis, granulomatous nodules in the basal ganglia, medulla and cerebellum and perivascular cuffing in the cortex. They can be found in the cerebrospinal fluid with a raised cell count and increased protein.

Heart. The larvae cause considerable damage on passage through the myocardium, cellular infiltration and necrosis with subsequent fibrosis of the myocardial bundles.

Immunity

In humans, a well-marked immunity to reinfection develops after the first infection but it is necessary for the infective larvae to develop through to the adult stage before immunity is produced, which is both anti-adult and antilarval. Cell-mediated immunity is largely responsible but humoral antibodies develop. Immunized mice respond rapidly to challenge infections with an inflammatory reaction in the bowel and the elimination of adult worms. Cellular immunity can be transferred by cellular elements and diminished by corticosteroids, adrenalectomy and whole-body irradiation.

Clinical Features

Natural History. Trichinosis is a self-limiting infection lasting in light infections 2–3 weeks and in heavy ones at the most 2–3 months. Except in heavy infections mortality is low. Light infections are often asymptomatic and routine examinations of diaphragms at autopsy have shown a significant number containing calcified cysts in endemic areas.

Incubation Period. From eating infected meat the development of symptoms during the enteric phase is up to 7 days after infection and for the migratory phase from 7 to 21 days.

Symptoms and Signs. The symptomatology depends on the level of infection and can be related to the number of larvae per gram of muscle: light infections (subclinical) up to 10 larvae, moderate 50–500 larvae and severe and possibly fatal infections more than 1000. In symptomatic cases symptoms develop in three stages: enteric (invasion of the intestine) phase, migration of the larvae (invasive phase) and a period of encystation in the muscles.

Enteric Phase. Irritation and inflammation of the duodenum and jejunum where the larvae penetrate cause nausea, vomiting, colic and sweating, resembling an attack of acute food poisoning. There may be a maculopapular skin rash, and in one-third of cases symptoms of a pneumonitis occur between the 2nd and 6th days, lasting about 5 days.

Migratory (Invasion) Phase. The cardinal symptoms and signs of this phase are severe myalgia, periorbital oedema and eosinophilia. There is difficulty in mastication, breathing and swallowing due to the involvement of the muscles and there may be some muscular paralysis of the extremities. There is a high remittent fever with typhoidal symptoms, splinter haemorrhages under the nails and in the conjunctivae and blood and albumin in the urine. Characteristically, there is a hypereosinophilia from the 14th day which decreases after a week and persists at a lower level. An absence of eosinophilia denotes a poor prognosis. The lymph glands may be enlarged as well as the parotid and submental glands. Occasionally, there is splenomegaly. In severe cases, there may be subpleural, gastric and intestinal haemorrhages.

Rarely, myocardial complications can occur[193] and in 10–20% of patients neurological complications when larvae pass through the central nervous system.[194]

Encystment Phase. This is the third stage and may be severe. There may be cachexia, oedema and extreme dehydration. During the 2nd month after infection there is a decrease in muscle tenderness, fever and itching subside and congestive heart failure may appear. Damage to the brain may persist with protean neurological signs which may clear up later or persist. Gram-negative septicaemia from organisms introduced by the larvae, permanent hemiplegia and Jacksonian epilepsy 10 years after an attack of trichinosis, have been described.

Diagnosis

Diagnosis is made by demonstrating larvae, by immunological and molecular methods.[195]

Larvae have been isolated from peripheral blood in the early stages of the migration phase by mixing blood with dilute acetic acid and centrifuging. Larvae may be demonstrated in muscle by trichinoscopy. This can only be used when the encystment phase has started from 7 days after infection onwards. Samples of deltoid, biceps, gastrocnemius or pectoralis major are digested with 1% pepsin and 1% hydrochloric acid for several hours at 37°C, filtered or centrifuged and the number of larvae per gram of muscle estimated. Larvae can also be seen on muscle pressed between two slides, which is more useful in the first 3 weeks of the disease.

Xenodiagnosis can be performed by feeding diaphragmatic tissue to uninfected albino white rats and examining them 1 month later.

The following immunological and antigen detection tests have been used: indirect immunofluorescence; an enzymatic immunohistochemical technique; colorimetric sandwich ELISA; microfluorescence; enhanced chemiluminescence; dissociated enhanced lanthanide fluoroimmunoassay (DELFIA); Western blot test. DELFIA is the most sensitive for detecting antigen.[195]

Differential Diagnosis

Trichinosis resembles many conditions: typhoid, encephalitis, myositis and tetanus; due to the association with a high eosinophilia it closely resembles the tissue stages of schistosomiasis (Katayama syndrome), hookworm, *Strongyloides* and other helminthic infections. Trichinosis may also resemble collagen disorders such as periarteritis nodosa and acute rheumatoid arthritis.

Management

Treatment is directed against the larvae and the immune reaction they invoke. Ten days of oral mebendazole (200 mg twice a day) or thiabendazole 25 mg/kg twice a day for 10 days are both effective, although the former is better tolerated by patients.[196] In severe life-threatening infections the immune response must be controlled, and prednisone 20 mg three times daily is given, initially reducing and finally discontinuing over a period of 2–3 weeks. Some cases are resistant to prednisone.

Epidemiology and Control

Humans are not the normal hosts of *T. spiralis* and become infected only after eating raw or undercooked flesh. The usual type, *T. s. spiralis*, found in Europe and North America, is an infection of the black and brown rats by which it is propagated. These rats are cannibalistic and may be eaten by domestic pigs, which infect man when raw or undercooked pork is eaten. *Trichinella* infection in humans is most common in adults and is related to cultural dietary habits, with eating of raw or undercooked meat as the most important risk factor.

Clinical illness is most likely to occur when meat prepared from a single heavily infected pig is eaten by a family or community. One of the most extensive, single-source outbreaks ever recorded in China, involving more than 600 infections and over 300 clinical cases, was reported in 1997. The entire episode was attributed to the infection of undercooked pork dumplings at one restaurant.[197] Where the meat has been diluted by uninfected meat, then the disease is mild or subclinical. Garbage which contains unsterilized pig scraps and other trimmings is the most common source of infection in pigs. Another possible source is the ingestion of faeces of other infected animals, mice, rats, foxes and other pigs, at a time when mature larvae are becoming established in the intestinal wall.

T. s. nativa is found mainly in Alaska and the northern regions of the world. Here trichinosis is found in the white whale, walrus, hair seal, tree squirrel, black bear and polar bear, dog, wolf, fox and wolverine. The polar bear, which is at the top of the Arctic food pyramid, is usually heavily infected and is the usual source, along with black and brown bear, of human infections.

T. s. nelsoni is found in sub-Saharan Africa, where it has been described from East Africa and Senegal. The infection is found in bush pigs (*Potamochoerus porcus*) and in the lion, leopard, cheetah and hyena. Humans become infected by eating bush pig; domestic pigs are not infected.

T. britovi is found in Europe, Asia and parts of north and west Africa. Humans can become infected from eating wild boar and horse.

T. pseudospiralis has a cosmopolitan distribution which is found in sylvatic mammals and birds, and domestic pigs. The source of human infection is wild boar, horses and domestic pigs.

The main method of prevention is thorough cooking of all meat and regular meat inspection by means of trichinoscopy of all pork. Effective treatment of pork may be instituted by means of refrigeration. Storage of pork in deep freeze units at −18°C to −15°C is effective. The cysts are destroyed by storage at −15°C for 20 days, −20°C for 10 days, −25°C for 6 days and immediately by quick freezing at −37°C. Cooking of all rubbish will prevent the infection in pigs and dressed pork may be irradiated by cobalt-60 or caesium-137, which kill the cysts.

REFERENCES

5. Pullan RL, Brooker SJ. The global limits and population at risk of soil-transmitted helminth infections in 2010. Parasit Vectors 2012;5:81.
27. Brooker S, Clements ACA, Bundy DAP. Global epidemiology, ecology and control of soil-transmitted helminth infections. Adv Parasitol 2006;62:221–61.
53. McCarthy JS, Lustigman S, Yang GJ, et al. A research agenda for helminth diseases of humans: diagnostics for control and elimination programmes. PLoS Negl Trop Dis 2012; 6:e1601.
80. Bethony J, Brooker S, Albonico M, et al. Soil-transmitted helminth infections: ascariasis, trichuriasis, and hookworm. Lancet 2006; 367:1521–32.
164. Taylor-Robinson DC, Jones AP, Garner P. Deworming drugs for treating soil-transmitted intestinal worms in children: effects on growth and school performance. Cochrane Database Syst Rev 2007;CD000371.

Access the complete references online at www.expertconsult.com

Echinococcosis

MARIJA STOJKOVIC | BRUNO GOTTSTEIN | THOMAS JUNGHANSS

KEY POINTS

Cystic Echinococcosis (*Echinococcus granulosus*)

- Cystic echinococcosis (CE), an infection with the larval form of the dog tapeworm *Echinococcus granulosus*, causes serious disease with a worldwide geographical distribution. The liver and lungs are primarily affected, but in principle any organ can be infected.
- CE is eliminable by regular dog deworming with praziquantel, controlled slaughtering with meat inspection and appropriate disposal of infected organs in abattoirs, vaccination of the intermediate ovine host and possibly, in the future, vaccination of the definitive animal host (dogs).
- Diagnosis of CE is based on imaging, primarily ultrasound (US). Serology has largely a confirmatory role. False-negative results are frequent in early disease when the hydatid fluid is sealed off from exposure to the immune system by the intact parasite-derived cyst wall and in late disease when consolidation and calcification of the cyst again protects the parasitic material from exposure.
- CE lesions can be staged by means of US. Today, it is largely agreed to use the WHO classification of five stages: stages 1 and 2 of which are regarded as 'active'; stage 3 'transitional' and stages 4 and 5 'inactive'. MRI and CT can substitute for US if cysts are not accessible by US. CT scans, however, miss important stage-defining features, leading to misclassification.
- CE can be treated by four principal approaches: (1) surgery; (2) percutaneous sterilization techniques; (3) medical therapy (benzimidazoles, primarily albendazole) and (4) 'watch and wait', and a combination of these.
- As a rule, early, mostly small active cysts, are clinically silent. Patients do not know that they are carriers and, therefore, do not seek medical advice. CE cysts at this early stage require active screening, but they are amenable to less invasive, low-risk treatment options.
- Advanced, mostly big and multiple active cysts or cysts in anatomically critical sites often present with complications. They are difficult to treat. In low- and middle-income countries, the problem is aggravated by limited resources available to healthcare services to tackle these problems.
- As a rule, inactive CE cysts (CE4 and CE5) are clinically silent if they are not in critical sites and most likely can be left alone. However, solid evidence based on the results of formal prospective clinical studies is missing.
- There is increasing confidence in treatment decisions based on cyst stage. Slowly evolving guidelines are largely based on expert opinion. Formal trials are needed to underpin the cyst stage-based triage of patients with solid data.
- If cyst content-sterilizing techniques (as a step in surgical or percutaneous approaches) are adopted, it is necessary to take great care to exclude cysto-biliary fistulas before applying protoscolicidal (parasiticidal) agents.
- Whichever treatment approach is taken, long-term follow-up of patients is needed to detect relapses.
- CE requires interdisciplinary management. This is best done in centres specializing in CE. Formation of such centres should be encouraged. This not only contributes to significantly better care for CE patients but also promotes sharing of clinical experience and collection and analysis of data in a standardized way.

Alveolar Echinococcosis (Echinococcus multilocularis)

- Alveolar echinococcosis (AE), an infection with the larval form of *Echinococcus multilocularis*, causes serious disease in various climate zones of the northern hemisphere. The liver is primarily affected. Primary disease in other organs is extremely rare but metastases are regularly observed in advanced disease.
- Control and, more so, eradication of *E. multilocularis* is difficult to achieve due to the sylvatic parasite cycle.
- Diagnosis and staging of AE is based on imaging, primarily US, MRI and CT. Serology has largely a confirmatory role and is useful in the follow-up of patients after treatment to contribute to the verification of cure and relapse.
- As a rule, AE develops silently, and patients mostly present with advanced stages of disease.
- AE has all the features of malignancy, and patients should be cared for accordingly, i.e. with interdisciplinary management, including staging, clinical decision, therapy, long-term follow-up and psychological support. This is best done in centres specialized in AE. Formation of such centres should be encouraged. This not only contributes to significantly better care for AE patients but also promotes sharing of clinical experience and collection and analysis of data in a standardized way.

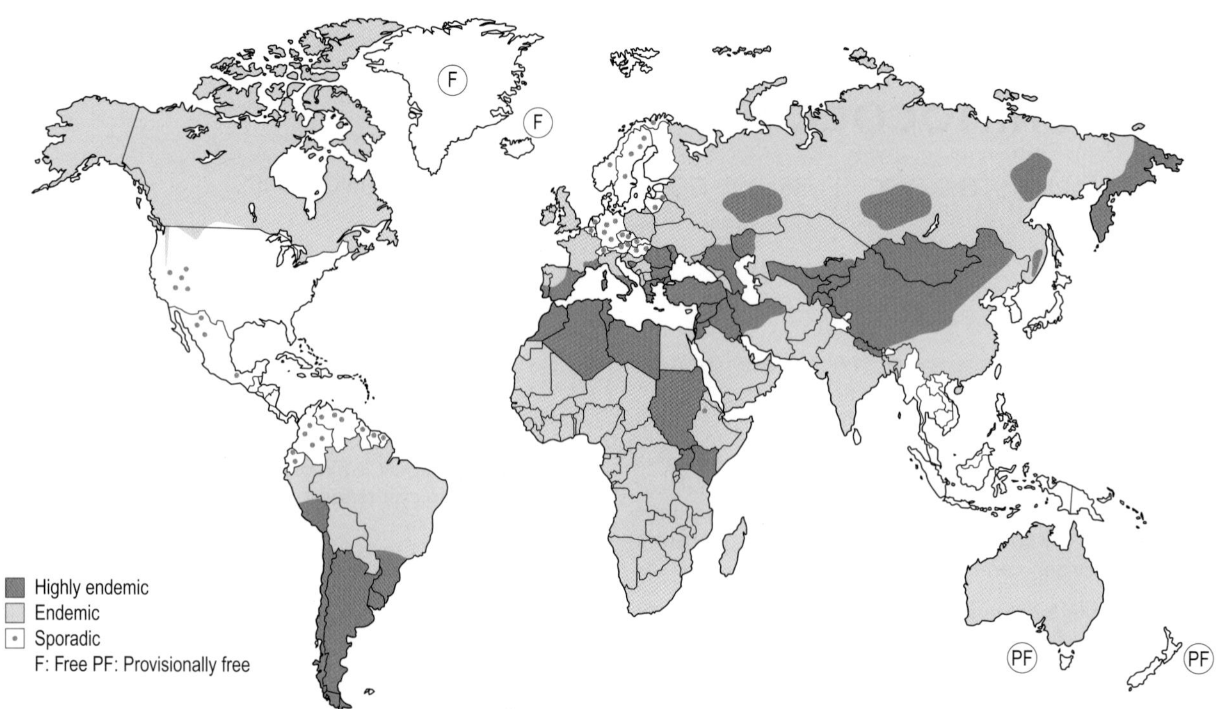

Figure 56.1 Global distribution of *Echinococcus granulosus*. (Copyright © WHO.)

Introduction

Cystic echinococcosis (CE) occurs worldwide, including tropical and subtropical regions, whereas alveolar echinococcosis (AE) is confined to the temperate northern hemisphere. The main focus of this chapter is therefore on CE.

CE (*Echinococcus granulosus*) and AE (*Echinococcus multilocularis*), although taxonomically caused by the same genus, differ profoundly in their clinical manifestations and the course of disease. CE and AE are, therefore, covered in separate sections in this chapter.

Polycystic echinococcosis (PE) is caused by *Echinococcus vogeli* and *Echinococcus oligarthus* and is confined to Latin America. The course of disease is reported to be between CE and AE. Only 100 cases of PE caused by *Echinococcus vogeli* are described in the literature, and even fewer of *Echinococcus oligarthus*. In view of this evidence base, management of PE has to be carried out on a case-by-case basis.[1–3]

Cystic Echinococcosis (*Echinococcus granulosus*)

EPIDEMIOLOGY

CE occurs on all continents except the Antarctic (Figure 56.1). By 2002, the disease had only been eradicated in a few countries, namely Iceland, New Zealand and the Australian state of Tasmania. In poorer parts of the world, the infection is highly endemic in pastoral communities, but it generally occurs in all pastoral and rangeland areas of the world.

The sheep-dog or G1 strain of *E. granulosus* accounts for 95% of human infections and has a worldwide distribution. It is transmitted between dogs and livestock, particularly sheep (Figure 56.2). High endemicity is described in the Mediterranean basin, the Near and Middle East, central Asia, western China, the Russian Federation, north and east Africa and large regions of South America.

To date, 10 genetic types of *E. granulosus* (genotypes G1–10) have been described. This may have possible implications regarding clinical manifestation, pathology and drug sensitivity.

Disease prevalence of CE is usually <2% or much lower but can be higher than 5%, as in some regions of the Tibetan

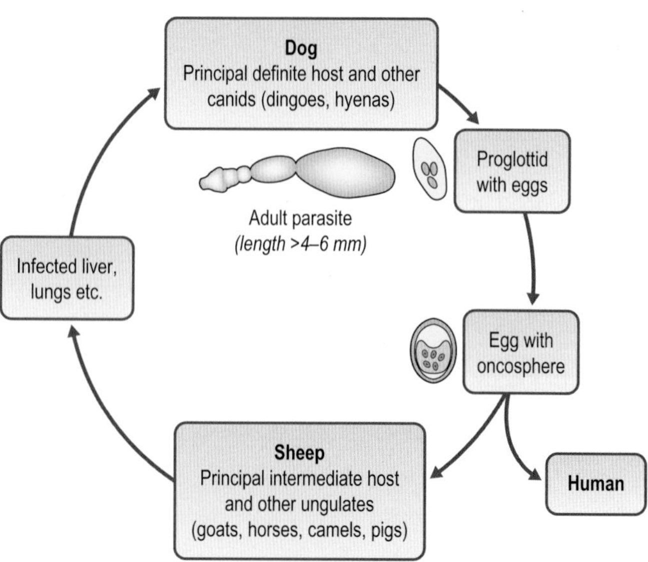

Figure 56.2 Life cycle of *Echinococcus granulosus*.

plateau. Human incidence rates can be higher than 50/100 000 person-years, e.g. in parts of Peru, Argentina, east Africa, central Asia and China.

Risk factors for acquiring human CE may vary from region to region but in general include the following: ownership of livestock (mainly sheep) or occupation (pastoralism, agriculture); dog ownership and feeding uncooked viscera to dogs (uncontrolled slaughtering); poor hygienic living conditions and poor water hygiene. In some regions, females seem to be predominantly affected possibly due to domestic activities and closer contact with dogs through feeding, herding and milking livestock.[4–9]

PATHOGENESIS AND PATHOLOGY

CE is clinically related to the presence of one or more well-delineated spherical cysts, most frequently formed in the liver and the lungs. Less usual locations of cysts include the kidneys, bones, heart, spleen, pancreas and organs of the head and neck, including the brain. Pathogenically, tissue damage and organ dysfunction result mainly from the gradual process of space-occupying compression or displacement of vital host tissue, vessels or parts of organs. Consequently, clinical manifestations are primarily determined by the site, size, number and growth rate of the turgid cysts and are therefore highly variable.

The histology of a typical CE cyst presents a thin germinal layer as the primary site of parasite development, protected by a surrounding parasite-derived thick laminated layer (Figure 56.3). The germinal layer contains the tegument and several cell types, including proliferative undifferentiated cells responsible for forming brood capsules, which develop asexually into pre-adult worms called protoscolices. Granulae and calcareous corpuscles are often observed, and occasionally free internal daughter cysts. The laminated layer is composed of mucins bearing defined galactose-rich carbohydrates and accompanied by calcium inositol hexakisphosphate deposits, as recently reviewed.[10]

The cyst induces an immune response, which basically triggers formation of a host-derived adventitious capsule. Calcifications in this peripheral compartment of the cyst correlate with degeneration of the parasite and putatively subsequent inactivation. Accidental rupture of cysts can be followed by a massive release of cyst fluid and dissemination of protoscolices, occasionally resulting in anaphylactic reactions and multiple secondary CE, as protoscolices have the potential to develop into secondary cysts within the intermediate host.

The capacity of a hydatid cyst to modulate the immune response is a prerequisite for longevity in the host; this modulation is most likely effected through parasite metabolites[11] that appear to be linked to the generation of T-suppressor populations and impairment of the accessory action of macrophages in lymphoproliferative responses. Overall, Th1 cell activation seems to be more closely related to protective immunity, whereas Th2 cell activation is more closely associated with susceptibility to infection and disease.[12]

An extensive genetic variation within this *Echinococcus (granulosus)* complex comprises a number of strains that differ in life development rate, host specificity as well as pathology (among many other factors), with important implications for the clinical outcome, diagnosis and treatment. Notably, infection with the G8 strain presents a predominantly pulmonary localization, slower and more benign growth and less frequent occurrence of clinical complications than reported for other genotypes.[13]

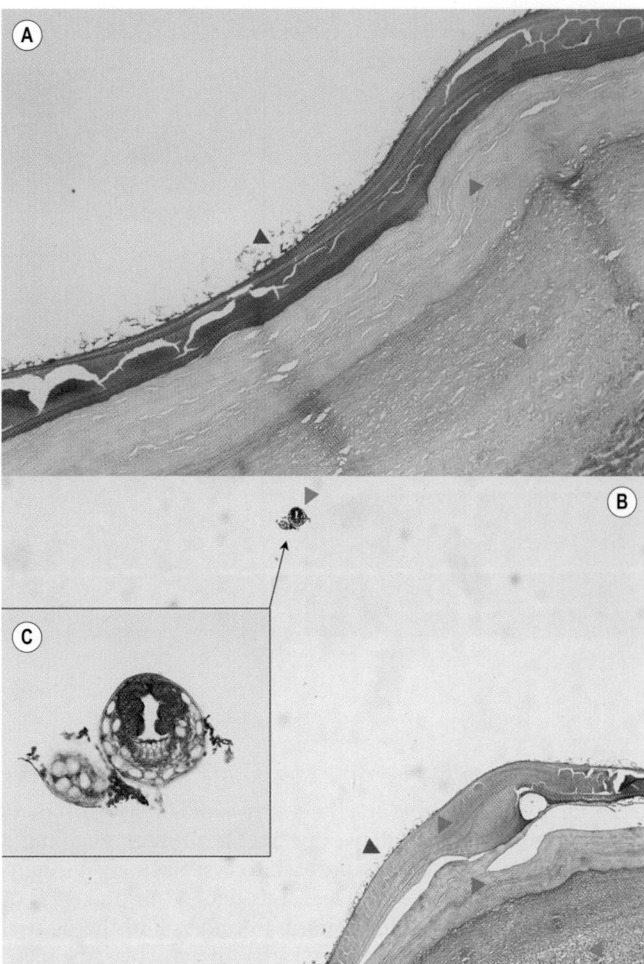

Figure 56.3 CE-histology. The fluid-filled hydatid cyst (CE-cyst) consists of an inner germinal layer (red arrowheads) supported externally by a very thick carbohydrate-rich (PAS-positive) acellular laminated layer of variable compression levels (blue arrowheads), surrounded by a very thick host-produced fibrous adventitial layer (orange arrowheads). Protoscolices (green arrowhead) are present in fertile cysts, but may not always be seen in histological specimens. PAS-stain; A,B = 40×; C = 200×. *(Copyright © B. Gottstein.)*

The Natural Evolution of CE Cysts

Imaging, and in particular ultrasound (US), opened up excellent means of observing the diversity of CE cyst features.[8,14–17] These observations led to a classification of CE cysts in five stages, with a further substratification of stage CE3 into CE3a and CE3b. Parasite 'activity' levels were then assigned to these stages, with a division into active (CE1 and CE2), transitional (CE3a and CE3b) and inactive (CE4 and CE5) (see Figures 56.4 and 56.8).[15,16] The 'activity' levels were further underpinned through viability testing with light microscopy to observe the presence, integrity (eosin staining) and motility (flame cell activity) of protoscolices,[19] the presence of intact brood capsules and the intact architecture of the cyst, in particular of the

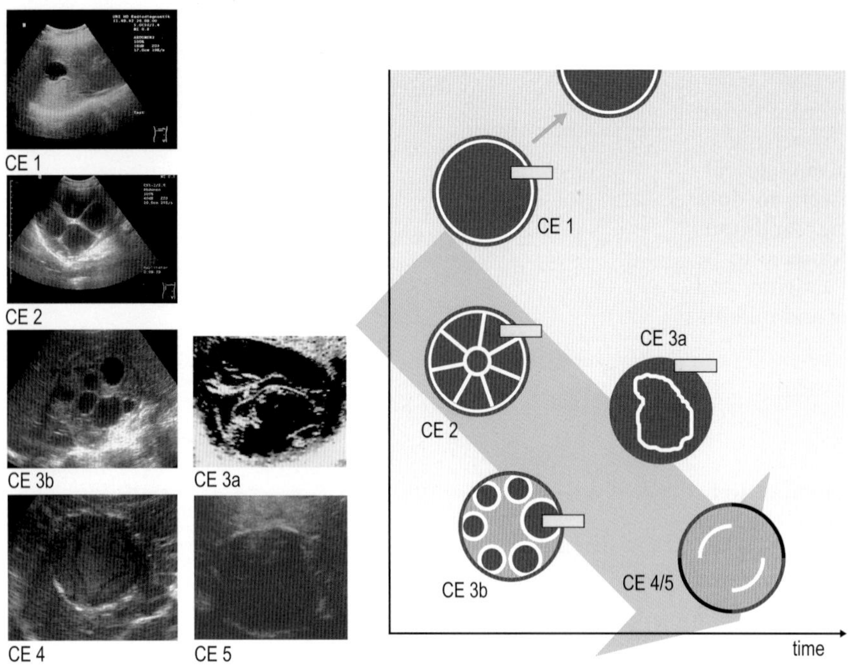

Figure 56.4 The sequence of CE cyst evolution (cyst growth) (small arrow) and involution from active to inactive, dead cysts (large arrow). The yellow bars signify cysto-biliary fistulas.

germinal layer (Figure 56.3). More recently, high-field H-MRS has been used to examine cyst fluid ex vivo and in a few instances also in vivo with quantitative metabolite profiles, enabling a multivariate metabolomics approach to cyst staging.[20–22] Aligning the individual CE cyst stages thus defined to processes of growth and decay is of importance to understand the natural evolution and involution of the CE cyst. In particular, the involutionary process has very useful applications in clinical practice for both treatment-driven involution (benzimidazoles, percutaneous sterilization techniques) as well as natural involution ('watch and wait' approach). The sequence of cyst involution from active to inactive, dead cysts is depicted in Figure 56.4.

CLINICAL FEATURES

The incubation period of CE is unclear and can range from many months to up to more than 10 years. Symptoms occur when active cysts increase in size and exert a mass effect on affected and adjacent organs. CE cysts may grow up to a diameter of 20 cm and more. Patients with CE are commonly asymptomatic, and cysts can be discovered incidentally by imaging performed for other reasons or screening of populations. These patients usually do not need immediate treatment and there is time for thorough investigations before a treatment decision is taken. A smaller proportion of patients presents with cyst-related complaints which require a timely work-up. Complications are rare, but when they precipitate they need immediate attention (Box 56.1).

Symptomatic CE has been reported from all age groups, including very young patients of less than 1 year as well as patients older than 75 years. Due to the slow-growing nature of echinococcal cysts, most patients become symptomatic above the age of 20.

Around 70% of cysts are localized in the liver, predominantly in the right liver lobe where the connective tissue reaction, forming the so-called pericyst, is most pronounced compared with other organs. Right upper quadrant pain or discomfort is the most frequent presenting symptom. Pain can be due to cyst size, but in symptomatic patients with acute onset of pain, a cysto-biliary fistula, the most common acute complication of CE liver cysts, must be considered (Figure 56.5A). Patients with cysto-biliary fistula may also present with jaundice in the case of biliary obstruction, which can be complicated by bacterial cholangitis. Raised liver enzymes (alkaline phosphatase and γ-glutamyl transferase) are a regular feature. Up to 20% of CE patients, depending on cyst size,[23] develop biliary complications ranging from mild to severe. Bacterial cyst infection and abscess formation are another, less frequent complication causing right upper quadrant pain (Figure 56.5B).[15,24,25]

The second most common CE cyst localization is in the lungs (15–30%), where cysts are predominantly located in the lower lobes (Figure 56.5H,I). Due to compression of a bronchus, cysts can cause nonspecific symptoms like retention pneumonia, atelectasis, inflammatory tissue reaction with bronchiectasis and interstitial fibrosis. In the case of a cysto-bronchial fistula, there may be abscess formation or expectoration of cyst content, which can cause asphyxia and anaphylaxis.[24,26]

BOX 56.1 CE CYST COMPLICATIONS

- Cysts with fistulas
- Biliary/bronchial obstruction (due to spillage of cyst content via cysto-biliary/cysto-bronchial fistulas)
- Bacterial infection
- Compression syndromes
  - Blood vessels (leading to thrombosis, Budd–Chiari syndrome)
  - Biliary ducts
  - Bronchi
  - Parenchyma/muscles, nerves (leading to atrophy)
- Cyst rupture
- Venous/arterial embolism

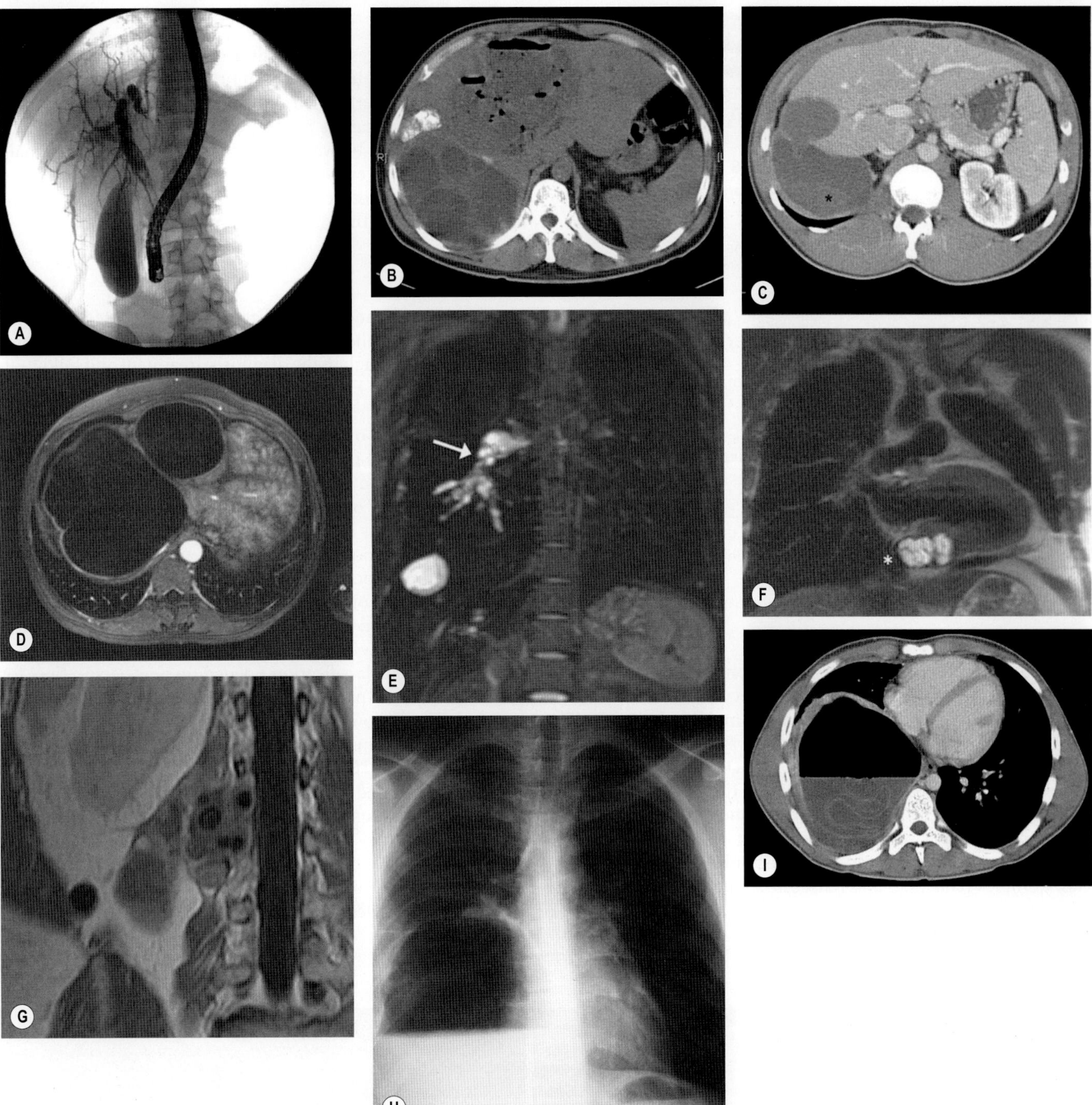

Figure 56.5 Severe and life-threatening complications of CE in different target organs. (A) Biliary obstruction/due to cysto-biliary fistula. This can be complicated by cholangitis. (B) Liver abscess formation due to secondary bacterial infection of a CE cyst. (C) Cyst rupture (*) followed by anaphylaxis and secondary CE. (D) Cyst exerting pressure on the liver veins, resulting in Budd–Chiari syndrome. (E) Embolism of the right pulmonary artery (arrow) caused by cardiac CE and vascular invasion. (F) CE infestation of the posterior wall of the left heart replacing myocardial muscle at the base of the heart. (Images from University Hospital Heidelberg; published in Brunetti, Garcia & Junghanss (2011); copyright PLoS Negl Trop Dis). (G) Spinal CE3b cyst compressing the dural sack. *(Copyright © W. Hosch, Department of Radiology, Heidelberg University Hospital.)* (H) Chest radiograph with a large CE cyst at the base of the right hemithorax. (I) CT scan showing the same pulmonary CE cyst with a free-floating membrane inside the cavity (WHO stage 3a) (Images from University Hospital Heidelberg; published in: Hosch et al (2004); copyright Chest).

Further complications of CE cysts in general are cyst rupture with anaphylaxis and/or dissemination, mostly into the peritoneal or pleural cavity (Figure 56.5C). CE cysts close to large vessels can cause impairment of blood flow and thrombotic complications (e.g. inferior caval vein, portal vein) or Budd–Chiari syndrome (Figure 56.5D).

Other locations where the parasite may establish itself and grow are the kidneys (see Figure 56.7C,D), mediastinum, skin and skeletal muscles. Involvement of the heart (Figure 56.5F), including embolization of the parasite into the pulmonary arteries (Figure 56.5E), brain and bone (Figure 56.5G) are very rare but severe manifestations.[15,27]

TABLE 56.1 Differential Diagnoses of Cystic and Solid Hepatic Space-Occupying Lesions

Cystic/Pseudocystic Space-Occupying Lesions with Liquid Content	Solid Space-Occupying Lesions
CONGENITAL SPACE-OCCUPYING LESIONS	
Simple cyst	Haemorrhagic simple cyst
VASCULAR SPACE-OCCUPYING LESIONS	
Haematoma	Haematoma Haemangioma
INFECTIOUS SPACE-OCCUPYING LESIONS	
CE [CE1, CE2, CE3a, CE3b (mixed cystic-solid)] AE with pseudocyst Abscess	CE [CE3b (mixed cystic-solid), CE4 and CE5] AE Tuberculoma
BENIGN SPACE-OCCUPYING LESIONS	
Cystadenoma	Hepatic adenoma Focal nodular hyperplasia
MALIGNANT SPACE-OCCUPYING LESIONS	
Cystadenocarcinoma Liver metastases with central necrosis	Metastatic liver tumours Hepatocellular carcinoma Cholangiocarcinoma

Differential Diagnoses of CE Cysts

The differential diagnoses of CE depend on the organ affected and the cyst stage (cystic, solid). CE liver cysts must be differentiated among others from congenital (simple) liver cysts (see Figure 56.6A), AE, in particular pseudocyst formation due to extensive necrosis (see Figure 56.20), bacterial and amoebic abscesses and benign and malignant liver tumours (see Figure 56.7A,B) (Table 56.1). Pulmonary involvement needs to be differentiated from bronchogenic cysts, post-primary cavernous tuberculosis and primary and metastatic pulmonary malignancies. Complex renal cysts and renal cell carcinoma can resemble CE cysts (see Figure 56.7).[28,29]

DIAGNOSIS

Diagnosis of CE rests primarily on imaging. Serology has a confirmatory role. In case of doubt, diagnostic puncture and aspiration can be performed. A histological diagnosis of resected parasitic material can be made. PCR can contribute to the differential diagnosis between CE and AE when doubts remain with the combined evidence of imaging, serology and histology. The viability of protoscolices, among other indicators, can be used to determine the viability of cysts.

Imaging

The development and standardization of a US-based classification[15,16] based on the Gharbi US classification of 1981 represented a breakthrough in the diagnosis, treatment and follow-up of CE patients (see Figure 56.8).[14] The classifications have been developed on CE cysts of the liver, but, in principle, they also apply for CE cysts of other organs, they may, however, not be accessible with US. In these cases, MRI fairs better than CT to identify CE-specific features (see below and Figure 56.8). An important feature of the imaging-based classification is the division of CE cysts into 'active', 'transitional' and 'inactive'. US and, if lesions are not accessible by US, other imaging modalities, with a preference for MRI (see below), are key to the diagnosis and staging of CE cysts, tailoring of treatment to cyst activity, observation of treatment response and early detection of relapse on follow-up.

The US-based classification opened up new perspectives for CE treatment, in particular for a stage-specific therapeutic approach. The following groupings are clinically very useful:

- Active and transitional cysts (CE1, CE2, C3a and CE3b) vs inactive cysts (CE4 and CE5)
- Uncomplicated vs complicated cysts, whereby small cysts are as a rule uncomplicated and patients are usually not aware that they are cyst carriers. The risk of complications increases with cyst size.[23]

The ultrasonographic features of the WHO stages CE1–CE5 are depicted and described in Figure 56.8. It is worth noting

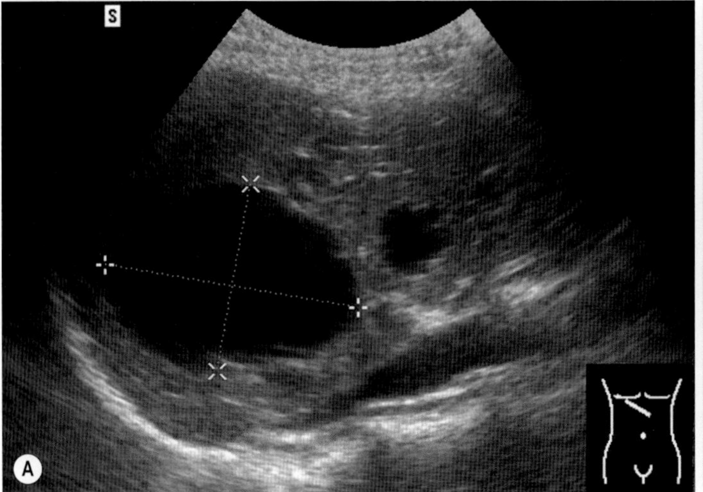

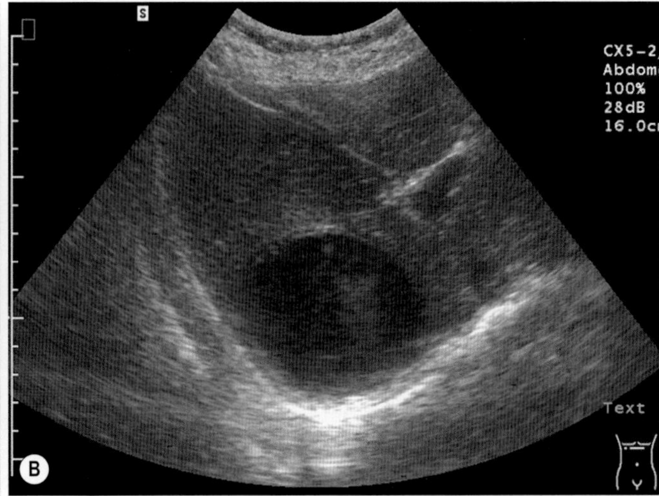

Figure 56.6 Differential diagnosis of cystic lesions: Simple cyst vs CE cyst. (A) Simple cyst: fluid filled, thin membrane at the interface to the liver tissue; often multiple. Ultrasound image. (B) CE1 cyst: fluid filled, cyst wall with double-line sign. Ultrasound image. *(Copyright © W. Hosch, Department of Radiology, Heidelberg University Hospital.)*

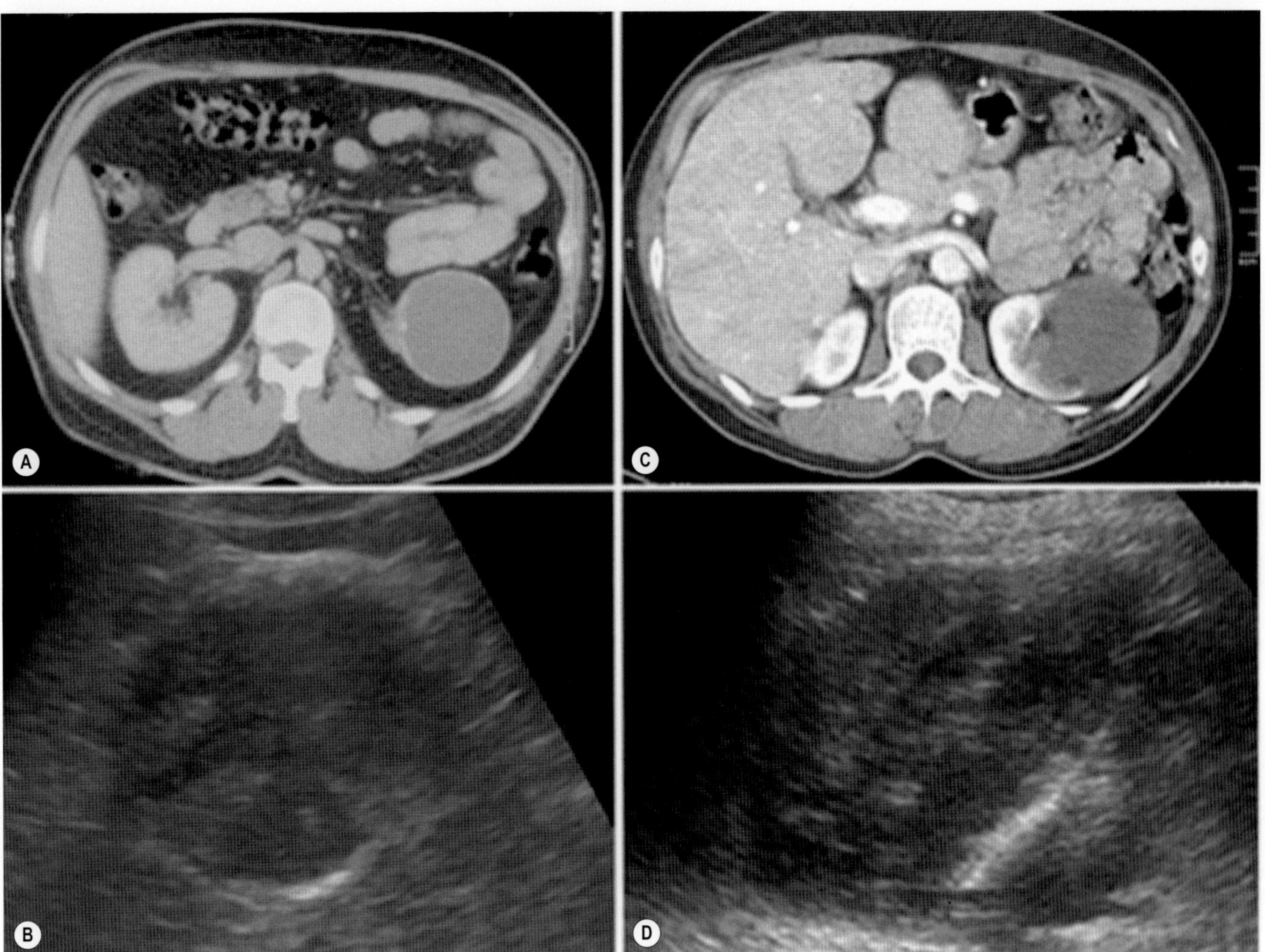

Figure 56.7 Differential diagnosis of cystic lesions. Renal cell carcinoma (A,B) vs CE (C,D). In both cases there is partial calcification of the cyst wall. Contrast-enhanced CT scans (A,C); ultrasound (B,D). *(Copyright © W. Hosch, Department of Radiology, Heidelberg University Hospital.)*

that the features of the cyst content play the major role in the assignment of a cyst to a cyst stage. The cyst wall contributes to the staging if the 'double-line sign' is visible (CE1). Care should be taken not to dismiss a CE1 cyst on the grounds that the double-line sign is not visible. Calcification of the wall is not restricted to CE5 and CE4, but may occur across all stages.[17] The cyst content regularly exhibits important cyst stage-defining features, in particular the 'water-lily sign' (CE3a), 'canalicular structures' (CE4) and 'daughter cysts in solid matrix' (CE3b). The changes in the cyst content over time often provide important clues, e.g. CE1 → CE3a with a collapse of the endocyst, CE3b → CE4 with the disappearance of daughter cysts in solid matrix and, in the reverse direction, reappearance of daughter cysts, which is regularly observed when CE4 cysts reactivate months after benzimidazole treatment (see below).

Imaging contributes also very importantly to identify cyst complications, such as cysto-biliary and cysto-bronchial fistulas and abscesses (see below).[24,30–32]

It is important to keep in mind that other 'cystic' lesions can mimic the various stages of CE cysts, in particular when the above-mentioned CE-specific features are not present.[28,29] In CE cysts of the liver the identification of a clearly visible, smooth and in advanced cysts very prominent cyst wall is of some help to differentiate CE cysts from simple cysts with a very thin lining or wall, which are very common and benign (Figure 56.6A), and from 'pseudocysts' as in AE (see below), which are basically necrotic cavities. Pseudocysts in AE show an irregular "wall" (see Figure 56.20). In most AE cases, however, there are imaging signs of an infiltrative mode of growth (see Figures 56.18, 56.19) which clearly distinguishes AE from CE lesions but not from malignancy. Malignant space-occupying lesions can also be mistaken for CE cysts. Calcification can be present in both instances (Figure 56.7). Very importantly the three imaging modalities US, MRI and CT do not reproduce the various features of the cyst wall and the cyst content equally well (see below and Figure 56.8).

If available, CT and MRI are imaging options when cysts are inaccessible by US. In these cases, MRI is preferable over CT because MRI, in particular T2-weighted series, reproduces the ultrasonographically defined features of CE cysts better than CT (Figure 56.8). The overuse of CT and MRI has to be discouraged, and the pitfalls of CTs deserve special attention.[33,34]

In case of doubt, diagnostic fine-needle puncture, which has previously been discouraged for fear of anaphylactic reactions and secondary CE, is an option in experienced hands and with the necessary precautions (see below).

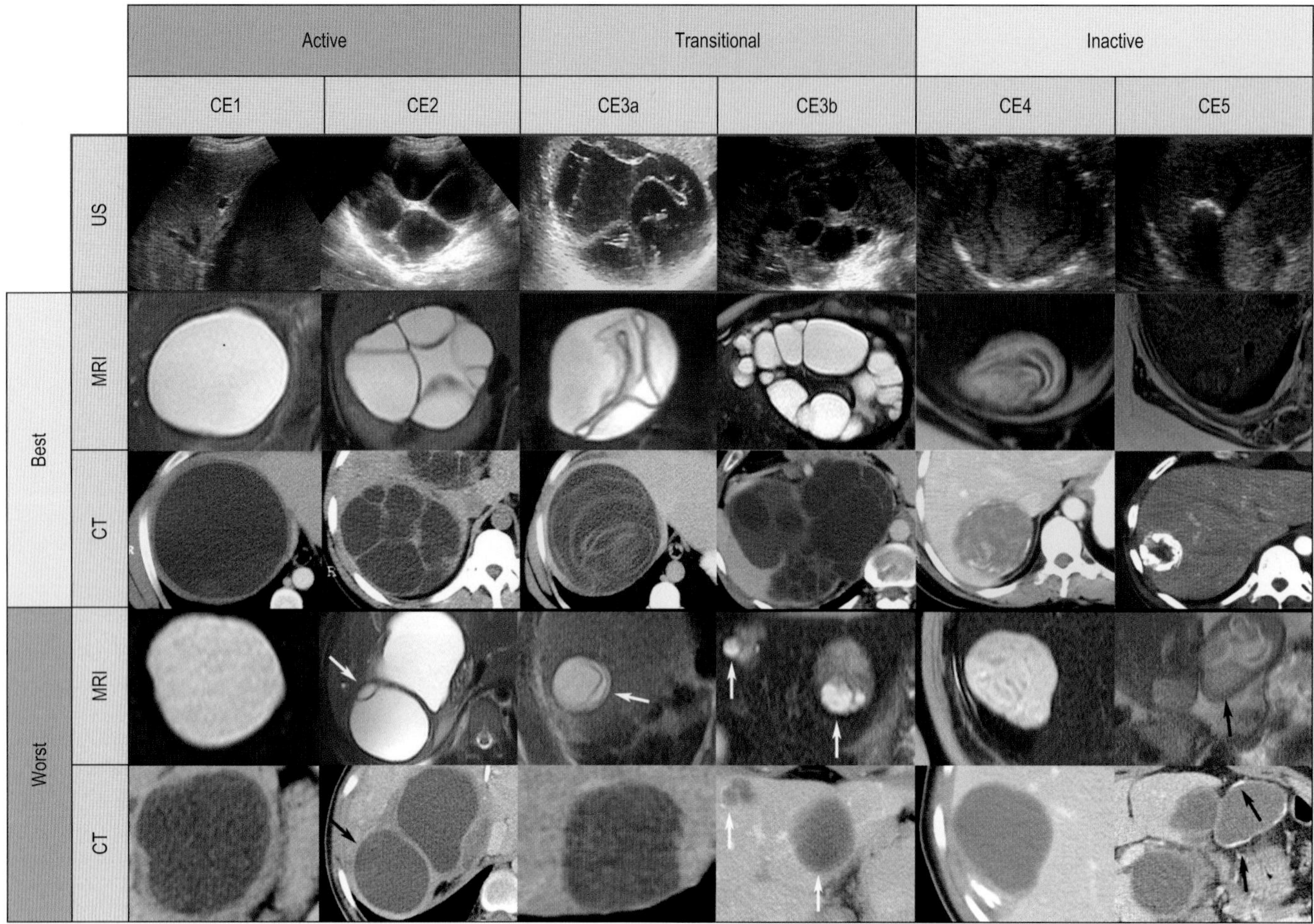

Figure 56.8 US classification of CE cysts and corresponding CT and MRI features.
US classification of CE cysts[16,18]
CE1: Unilocular unechoic cystic lesion with double-line sign
CE2: Multiseptated, 'rosette-like' 'Honeycomb' cyst
CE3a: Cyst with detached membranes (water-lily sign)
CE3b: Cyst with daughter cysts in solid matrix
CE4: Cyst with heterogeneous hypoechoic/hyperechoic contents, in particular so-called 'canalicular structures'. No daughter cysts
CE5: Solid cyst content plus always calcified wall
The WHO classification translates into the Gharbi classification as follows:
WHO-CE1 → Gharbi type I
WHO-CE2 → Gharbi type III
WHO-CE3a → Gharbi type II
WHO-CE3b → Gharbi type III
WHO-CE4 → Gharbi type IV
WHO-CE5 → Gharbi type V
'Best case' of CT/MRI.
CE1: unilocular, simple cysts with liquid content and often with the CE1-specific 'double-line sign'; CE2: multivesicular, multiseptated cysts; CE3a: cysts with liquid content and the CE3a-specific detached endocyst; CE3b: unilocular cysts with daughter cysts inside a mucinous or solid cyst matrix; CE4: heterogenous solid cysts with degenerative content, CE4-specific canalicular structure of the cyst content; CE5: cysts with degenerative content and calcified wall.
(Images from the University Hospital Heidelberg; copyright with PLoS NTD.)
'Worst case' of CT/MRI.
The 'double-line sign' typical for CE1 is often seen on US (CE1/US), but less reliably on MRI and CT. Daughter cysts and detached endocyst ('water-lily sign') are often missed by CT but clearly visible on US and MRI (CE2, CE3a, arrows). Daughter cysts inside a solid cyst matrix are often not recognized by CT (CE3b, arrows). The CE4-specific canalicular structure is often not visible on CT images. These cysts may be misinterpreted as type CE1 cysts, i.e. staged 'active' instead of 'inactive'. The identification of calcifications is the domain of CT imaging. MRI does not differentiate well between thick hyaline walls and calcifications. US picks up calcifications only when a dorsal echo shadow is produced (CE5, arrows).
MRI: HASTE sequence; CT: post-contrast-enhanced images. *(Images from the University Hospital Heidelberg; published in Stojkovic et al (2012); Copyright © PLoS Negl Trop Dis.)*

Serology

Serological diagnosis of CE is hampered by the fact that responses are highly stage-specific and depend on the location of the cyst. Early cysts, in particular CE1 and also CE2, have their antigenic components sequestered from the host's immune system by the parasite-derived multilaminated layer and thus may remain seronegative as long as it is intact. As soon as the endocyst ruptures, either during the natural involution process or induced by intervention, serology becomes positive. During the further involution process of consolidation and calcification, serology can again become negative over the course of years in a large proportion of cases (CE4 and CE5). Serological diagnosis follows a two-step approach. In the first step, diagnostically sensitive tests are employed (such as indirect haemagglutination tests and enzyme-linked immunosorbent assay using *E. granulosus* hydatid fluid antigen). However, these tests lack specificity and cross-react with other cestode infections and also gastrointestinal malignancies. In a second step, very specific tests (e.g. immunoblotting for 8 kDa/12 kDa subunits of *E. granulosus* antigen B) are used to confirm the findings of the screening tests. Regarding location, brain and lung cysts are especially problematic, with a high proportion of false-negative results. Children with CE are frequently seronegative with age as a confounder of early stages of cyst development. Serology so far cannot be used to reliably determine the post-interventional course of disease such as cure or relapse.[15,35]

Diagnostic Puncture and Aspiration of Cyst Content

In unclear cases when a diagnosis cannot be achieved by imaging and serology, fine-needle diagnostic puncture and aspiration of cyst content is a very valuable tool for differential diagnosis, in particular of malignancies. Fine-needle diagnostic punctures are regarded as safe if performed using the precautions defined for percutaneous sterilizing techniques (see PAIR, below).[36,37]

Histological Diagnosis

See Pathogenesis and Pathology, above.

Assessment of Parasite Viability

Viability of the parasite can be assessed by histopathology (intact parasite-derived cyst wall including germinal layer), by evaluation of the protoscolices (flame cell activity and morphological integrity; eosin staining) and, recently, by metabolic viability assessment using high-field H-MRS (see above) of cyst content. In specialized laboratories, viability of cyst material can be assessed by RT-PCR of several constitutively expressed genes of *E. granulosus*.

MANAGEMENT AND TREATMENT

Most CE cysts develop unnoticed until they reach a size which causes unspecific symptoms such as abdominal fullness and pain or until sudden acute complications occur such as cyst rupture or biliary obstruction due to spillage of cyst content via a cysto-biliary fistula into the biliary tree (see Clinical Features, above). This makes clinical management difficult, in particular in low-resource settings. Large cysts and complicated cysts require an interdisciplinary approach involving well-trained surgeons and anaesthetists.[15,38–41]

Early detection and treatment, in contrast, necessitate active screening, which currently would have to rely on US, with two major drawbacks. First, a substantial proportion of small early cysts do not exhibit CE-specific features. In addition, they are frequently seronegative because they have not yet elicited antibody responses due to an intact parasite-derived cyst wall (germinal layer plus multilaminated membrane), sealing off antigenic material from the host's immune system. The second problem area is the assignment of patients with small (<5–6 cm) CE cysts to the appropriate treatment option (see below).

A pragmatic approach in clinical practice is to divide CE cysts into two categories:

1. *Complicated CE cysts* which need *individualized treatment* adapted to the resources of the place where the patient needs to be treated.
2. *Uncomplicated CE cysts*, for which *standardized cyst stage-specific management* is receiving increasing support from experience and data collected in CE treatment centres.

Patients with Complicated CE Cysts

Patients with complicated cysts require individualized treatment[38,40,41] adapted to the resources of the place where the patient needs to be treated. Imaging also plays an important role in diagnosis and patient management.[24,31]

Cysts with Fistulas and Biliary/Bronchial Obstruction (Due to Spillage of Cyst Content Via Cysto-Biliary/Cysto-Bronchial Fistulas). With the liver and lungs as the two organs which carry most CE cysts, cysto-biliary and cysto-bronchial fistulas are the most common complication. Fistulas between CE cysts and the gastrointestinal tract and the gall bladder are encountered, very rarely.

Due to the significant potential of CE cysts with fistulas to cause severe complications (biliary/bronchial obstruction), these cysts should be treated early, and most experts would advise a surgical approach. The problem is, however, that it is not easy to diagnose fistulas before they become patent and active, which is mostly due to biliary obstruction or expectoration of hydatid material.

In CE cysts of the liver, a retrograde approach to the diagnosis of cysto-biliary fistulas has been proposed. The major drawback is that it carries a not negligible risk of complications, and the detection of fistulas is compromised by the fact that the intracystic pressure may be too high for the contrast media to enter. MRI with MR cholangiography (MRC) is a non-invasive imaging technique, which can detect a good number of fistulas before they cause complications.[30]

If rupture and spillage of cyst content into the biliary tree have occurred, biliary obstruction develops rapidly, which can be complicated by cholangitis. Clearance of the obstructing material and restoration of the bile flow by means of endoscopic retrograde cholangiopancreatography (ERCP) is a very elegant first step[32] (Figure 56.5A) and buys time until the fistula can be taken care of surgically in a second step. Albendazole is started as soon as possible.

With pulmonary cysts, rupture into a bronchus implicates a cysto-bronchial fistula and is accompanied by expectoration of hydatid fluid and fragments of the endocysts and asphyctic attacks. These are experienced as life-threatening by patients but are generally overcome without serious problems. Imaging studies show either an air-filled space or an air–fluid level within the cavity (Figure 56.5H,I). Again, benzimidazoles are initiated as soon as possible. The remaining cavity, which is connected to the bronchial tree via a fistula can be managed in two ways: (1) surgical removal of the remaining cyst and closure of the fistula or (2) in small cysts a conservative path may be followed. In these cases the cyst cavity must be carefully observed until it has retracted and healed. As long as the cavity remains open, it is prone to bacterial infection with consequent abscess formation. To minimize this risk, early antibiotic treatment of bacterial airway infections may help to prevent this complication until the cavity has retracted.

Bacterial Infection. In principle, all stages of CE cysts can become secondarily bacterially infected, leading to an abscess (Figure 56.5B). Bacterial infection can be blood-borne or retrograde via fistulas, e.g. cysto-bronchial, cysto-biliary, cysto-duodenal, etc.; however, this is altogether rare. Primary treatment follows the rules of abscess management with drainage and antibiotics. In a second step, specific management of the residual CE cyst/cavity follows. It appears that bacterial infection has a sterilizing effect on *E. granulosus*. To be on the safe side, benzimidazoles are administered for a few months. There are no data on the optimal length of benzimidazole therapy in these cases.

Compression Syndromes

- Blood vessels (leading to thrombosis, Budd–Chiari syndrome)
- Biliary ducts
- Bronchi
- Parenchyma/muscles, nerves (leading to atrophy).

Growing cysts exert increasing pressure on surrounding anatomic structures and tissues. This leads to critical narrowing and occlusion of blood vessels, bile ducts and bronchi. If the hepatic veins are affected, a Budd–Chiari syndrome can ensue, which requires rapid decompression to save the liver (Figure 56.5D). Narrowing of large veins such as the caval vein leads to thrombosis. Compression of bile ducts causes biliary obstruction, which may be complicated by cholangitis and compression of bronchi causes atelectases. With advanced large CE cysts of the liver and the lungs, substantial parts of these organs are lost due to pressure atrophy driven by the expanding cysts. In the liver, average growth rates of 1 cm/year are cited;[42] in the lungs, growth can be much faster.

Cyst Rupture: Allergic Reactions and Secondary CE (Figure 56.5C). Hydatid fluid is highly allergenic. If a patient is sensitized, spontaneous or trauma-induced rupture and spillage of fluid can lead to a life-threatening type 1 hypersensitivity reaction. Emergency treatment follows the standard approach to allergic reactions including anaphylactic shock. After stabilizing the patient, CE-specific treatment follows. To prevent secondary CE, e.g. of the peritoneal or pleural cavity in ruptured abdominal or lung cysts, benzimidazole treatment should be started immediately (see Benzimidazoles, below). The evidence base for the efficacy of benzimidazoles to prevent secondary CE after cyst rupture is very limited. The value of adding praziquantel based on its activity against protoscolices remains to be put on trial (see Praziquantel, below). Surgical intervention to clear CE cyst material from the site of the rupture and to remove hydatid fluid and infectious material from the peritoneal or pleural cavity should be undertaken immediately.

Venous/Arterial Embolism. When CE cyst content gains access to a vessel, either through spontaneous rupture or surgery, active CE cyst material can be widely disseminated. Rupture into the caval vein or of a right ventricular cyst of the heart leads to disseminated secondary pulmonary echinococcosis and, very rarely, to massive obstruction of the pulmonary arteries (Figure 56.5E).

Cysts in Rare Locations. CE cysts in rare locations, in particular CE cysts of the heart (Figure 56.5F), the brain and the bone (Figure 56.5G) are as a rule complicated cysts and have to be managed on an individual basis.[27,43]

Patients with Uncomplicated CE Cysts

For patients with uncomplicated cysts, a standardized cyst stage-specific approach is in sight on the basis of available data and cumulative evidence from experience collected in expert centres. Formal testing of this approach in large, well-conducted clinical trials has not yet been performed but is urgently needed, with the clinical management of CE evolving over decades without adequate evaluation of key features such as efficacy, effectiveness, rate of adverse reactions, relapse rate and cost. Currently, the 'Expert consensus for the diagnosis and treatment of cystic and alveolar echinococcosis in humans', published by the WHO-Informal Working Group on Echinococcosis[16,44–46] rests exclusively on a grading of the strength of recommendation of B and quality of evidence III.

Four treatment modalities are available:[25,39,41,46]

1. Drug treatment with benzimidazoles
2. Percutaneous sterilization techniques
3. Surgery
4. 'Watch and wait'.

The attribution of patients with uncomplicated CE cysts at the time of first presentation to the four treatment options and the risk of complications in relation to cyst stage and cyst size are depicted in Figure 56.9.

Assignment of Patients with Uncomplicated Cysts to the Four Available Treatment Options

Given the benign nature of CE, expert opinion is increasingly moving to a more careful selection of patients for surgery in the case of uncomplicated cysts (Figure 56.9).

Those centres that have stopped treating CE4 and CE5 cysts, including surgery, have reduced their surgical patient load substantially (see below).

Treatment of small active cysts with benzimidazoles (see Benzimidazoles, below) and percutaneous treatment of larger CE1 and CE3a cysts without cysto-biliary fistulas have contributed to this trend.

The decision to move in uncomplicated cysts from drug and minimal invasive treatment to surgery is not easy and continues to rest on expert opinion. More solid evidence in the absence of large and appropriately designed clinical trials is largely lacking. Patient and health facility specific factors must additionally be taken into account.

Most expert centres move to surgery in CE1 and CE3a cysts which do not respond to benzimidazole and percutaneous sterilizing procedures whereby percutaneous approaches are exploited to various degrees before this decision is taken. Some centres leave it to the classical PAIR techniques whereas others proceed to continuous catheter drainage and large-bore catheters before considering surgery. In CE2 and particularly in

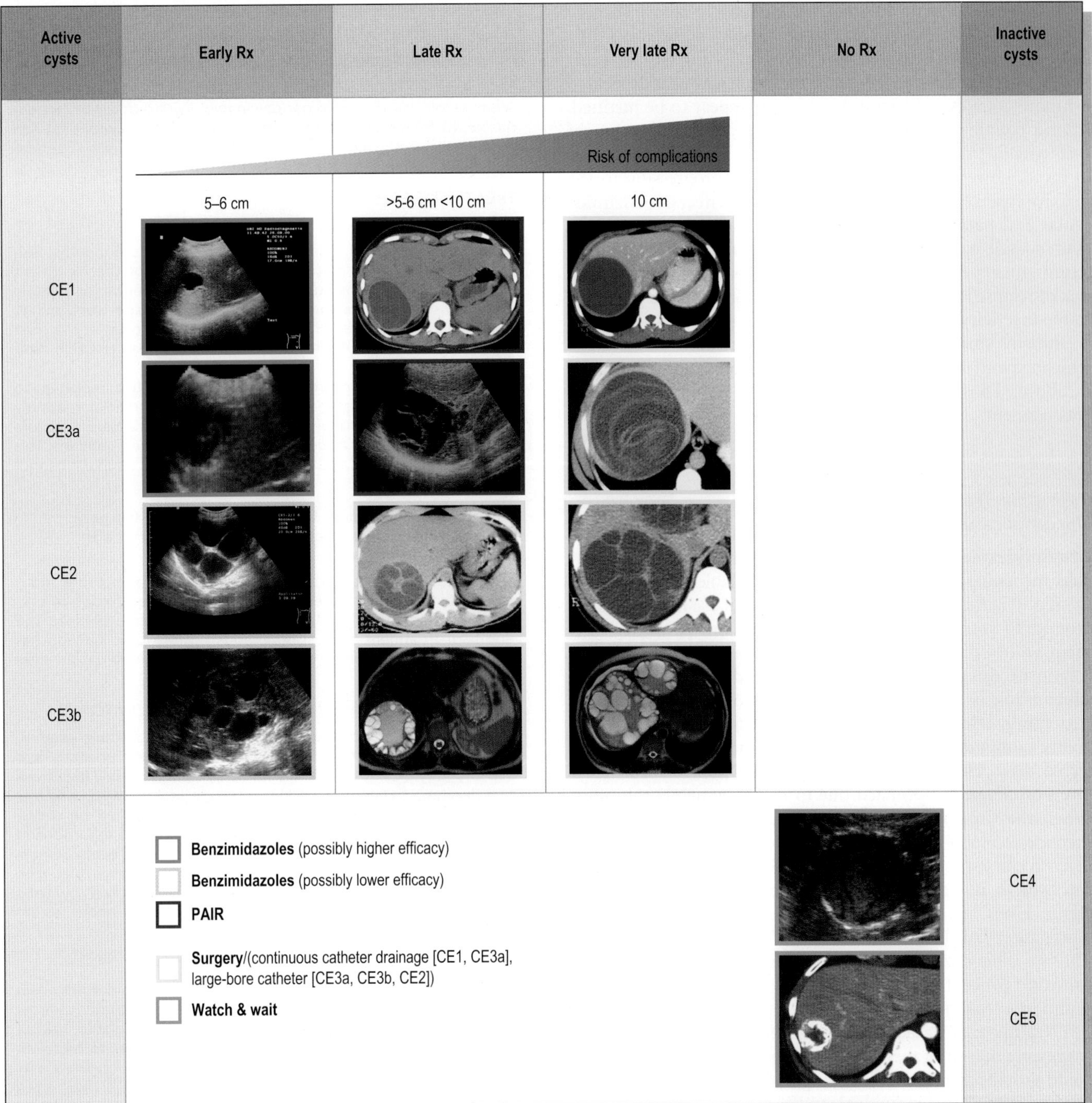

Figure 56.9 Assignment of treatment modalities to individual CE cyst stages and risk of complications in relation to cyst stage and size (for details, see text). During the involution process, CE cysts are driven from active cyst stages to inactive, dead cysts (natural involution). In the 'watch and wait' approach (CE4 and CE5), the natural involution is observed and the patient is followed-up at regular intervals to detect complications and to ensure that the patient remains relapse-free. With the use of benzimidazoles and percutaneous sterilizing techniques [mostly puncture – aspiration – injection – respiration (PAIR); in some centres continuous catheter drainage and large-bore catheters], the natural involution process is accelerated. With surgery, the parasitic material is completely removed from the patient either by removal of the parasite-derived cyst and part of the host-derived connective tissue capsule (pericyst): partial cystectomy; by removal of the parasite-derived cyst and the entire host-derived connective tissue capsule (pericyst): total cystectomy or by additional removal of the part of the organ the CE cyst is embedded in: resection *(Images copyright © W. Hosch, Department of Radiology, Heidelberg University Hospital)*. Rx = treatment.

CE3b cysts, benzimidazole treatment may be very disappointing. In these cases, the alternatives are surgery and large-bore catheter approaches.[47–51]

The further development of large-bore catheter techniques should be carefully monitored since it may become an alternative to the laparotomic approach in the future.

As long as the categories elaborated on above are not appropriately validated, a substantial degree of arbitrariness remains in the triage of patients. Of particular concern are uncomplicated small (<5 cm) CE1, CE2, CE3a and CE3b cysts in anatomically non-critical sites which cannot undergo PAIR and which do not respond to benzimidazoles.

Many experts rightly hesitate in these cases to opt for surgery straight away. If such patients can be reliably followed-up (initially by two, later by one consultation including US per year) it is justified in experienced hands to 'watch and wait'. Repeated 3-month courses of benzimidazoles also appear to be justified. After a couple of years of observation, a good proportion of cysts usually progress further to CE4 and CE5. One has to keep in mind, however, that with this approach, progression to the inactive stages (CE4 and CE5) is a combined effect of benzimidazoles and natural involution. Particular attention should be paid to CE3b cysts, which progress to CE4 under benzimidazole treatment. Experience from expert centres points to an increased risk of relapse in these cysts, even after a considerable period of stable inactivity.

Initially small (<5 cm) CE1, CE2, CE3a and CE3b cysts, which expand during the observation period should be triaged as above. Those which remain unaltered require continuing reassessment.

Individual Treatment Options for Uncomplicated Cysts

Benzimidazoles (Box 56.2). The benzimidazoles (albendazole, mebendazole) are the only drugs available for drug treatment of CE. Albendazole has been in clinical use in humans for around 30 years and is a well-established anti-parasitic treatment with a broad spectrum of activity against cestodes (i.e. echinococcosis) as well as intestinal and tissue nematodes. Albendazole is a derivative of benzimidazole carbamate and is structurally related to mebendazole. Due to its greater bioavailability compared with mebendazole, it has become the preferred drug. However, albendazole is also poorly absorbed if given on an empty stomach due to its low aqueous solubility. When the drug is taken with a fatty meal, absorption may increase 2- to 5-fold. After absorption, albendazole has an extensive first-pass effect and is almost entirely metabolized in the liver to its active metabolite albendazole sulfoxide. Peak serum levels are reached 2–5 hours after ingestion, and the elimination half-life is 8–12 hours.[52–54] Significant concentrations of albendazole are found inside CE cysts. Albendazole sulfoxide concentrations of up to 22% of serum values were found in a small patient series.[55]

Over the past decade, several studies have been published suggesting that drug therapy with mebendazole or albendazole could provide an alternative to surgery in patients with uncomplicated cysts. These individual studies were all small and inherently heterogeneous, precluding meta-analysis.[56–75]

A systematic review and pooled analysis of individual patient data collected from 6 treatment centres was recently performed to describe the long-term outcome after albendazole treatment by cyst stage and size and to derive a more robust assessment of the effectiveness of benzimidazoles in the treatment of CE.[76] The study suggests that there are substantial differences in response between cyst stages, in particular with regard to definite cure.

It appears that benzimidazoles work best in small (≤6 cm) active cysts. The more advanced CE3b cysts, in contrast, respond initially and convert into CE4 cysts, but frequently relapse after albendazole has been stopped. The overall effectiveness across all cyst stages is estimated at 40–60% in small (≤6 cm) cysts.

BOX 56.2 TREATMENT SCHEDULES AND DOSING OF BENZIMIDAZOLES

DOSING

Albendazole 10–15 mg/kg per day in two divided doses or mebendazole 40–50 mg/kg per day in three divided doses with a fat-rich meal continuously across the planned treatment interval. Albendazole is preferable because of its better bioavailability.

TREATMENT SCHEDULES

Medical treatment alone

Treatment intervals of at least 3 months and up to 6 months. Sufficient time (up to 6 months after completion of the treatment interval) should be allowed for until an effect of benzimidazoles on cysts is visible on imaging (transition of cyst stage from active/transitional to inactive). Relapses take equally long (e.g. a cyst which has reached CE4 after treatment may relapse to CE3b after many months).

Repeated courses of treatment can be given. It is important to be aware, however, that the natural decay of cysts then increasingly competes with the benzimidazole effect and that the benzimidazole therapy may be rather a suppressive than a curative treatment. This may still be an option in palliative treatment (e.g. if a patient cannot be operated on).

Prevention of secondary CE after interventions (surgery, percutaneous sterilization, diagnostic puncture) or after spontaneous rupture

Preventive treatment starting at least 4 hours before the intervention until 1 month after the intervention. The efficacy of preventive treatment is so far not based on solid evidence. The length of treatment after spontaneous rupture or if spillage has occurred during an intervention has to be decided on an individual basis.

ADVERSE REACTIONS WHICH NEED TO BE MONITORED

Liver enzymes (aminotransferases) and full blood count need to be checked initially day 5, 10, then at 2 weekly intervals and later monthly. Aminotransferase levels 2–4 times normal levels can be tolerated, depending on the intensity of follow-up, which is possible. Above this level, plasma drug levels should be determined and treatment interrupted. Treatment may be reintroduced after the aminotransferases have returned to normal levels. Switching from albendazole to mebendazole can be given a trial. The usefulness of this approach is, however, not backed by solid data. In case of myelosuppression the treatment needs to be discontinued.

CONTRAINDICATIONS

Pregnancy. Cysts which are at risk of rupture (benzimidazoles seem to soften the pericystic tissue). In patients with elevated aminotransferases and low leucocyte counts, an incalculable risk of hepatic toxicity and bone marrow suppression needs to be taken into account.

FOLLOW-UP

Follow-up after benzimidazole treatment is recommended for a minimum of 5 years after cysts have reached an inactive stage (CE4, CE5).

Albendazole treatment of early subclinical disease may allow a substantive proportion of patients to avoid complications and surgery in the future. However, this needs to be confirmed by clinical trials.

The length of treatment with albendazole has not been defined. From available data and on the basis of expert opinion it appears that a course of albendazole should be given for at least 3 months, possibly up to 6 months. It is important to know that the process of cyst involution (increasing solidification, reduction of cyst size) continues many months after termination of treatment. Enough time – up to 12 months after termination of treatment – should therefore be allowed for before the success of a course of treatment is finally assessed. Similar time spans are involved until cysts re-activate, e.g. daughter cysts reappear in the solid matrix of a cyst (reversal of CE4 into CE3b). This is one of the important rationales for long-term follow-up of CE patients (see below).

The use of albendazole for prevention of secondary CE after interventions (surgery, percutaneous sterilization, diagnostic puncture) or after spontaneous rupture is even less well established. A wide range of recommendations have been made regarding the preoperative time interval and the length of treatment after the intervention. WHO-IWGE currently recommends to start 4 hours before the intervention until 1 month after the intervention,[46] but other schedules have also been suggested.[55,77] The length of treatment after spontaneous rupture or if spillage has occurred during an intervention has to be decided on an individual basis. For combination therapy with praziquantel (see Praziquantel below).

Hepatic toxicity is the most relevant adverse reaction to albendazole in the treatment of CE. Up to 16% of patients show increased liver enzymes during albendazole treatment. In the majority of patients, the rise in liver enzymes is mild to moderate (2–4 times normal levels) and does not require interruption of treatment. Rather the opposite is true during the early phase of benzimidazole treatment of CE cyst of the liver. Benzimidazoles induce localized pericystic hepatitis with corresponding mild elevation of liver enzymes. This is a sign of good response to treatment rather than of drug hepatoxicity.[78,79] If liver enzymes go above 4 times normal levels determination of plasma drug levels and interruption of benzimidazole treatment is recommended. Liver enzyme elevation usually reverses after discontinuation of treatment within a few weeks. Reintroduction of benzimidazoles including dose adaptation and change from albendazole to mebendazole or vice versa is worth a trial. Acute liver failure of uncertain cause, as well as hepatitis have been reported. Patients with increased liver enzymes at baseline are at increased risk of hepatotoxicity.

Bone marrow suppression is an extremely rare but serious adverse reaction. Reversible leucopaenia has occurred in <1% of patients receiving the drug. Patients with underlying hepatic disease are at increased risk; furthermore, haematotoxicity is dose-dependent, as has been shown in phase I dose-finding trials for albendazole treatment in patients with advanced cancer.[80–82] Experimental studies on albendazole have indicated that it is teratogenic in rats and rabbits. Consequently its use is contraindicated during pregnancy.[83,84]

Abdominal discomfort and nausea may be a problem, in particular at the beginning of therapy. Hair loss is observed. This is, however, reversible.

Praziquantel. Praziquantel has been used in combination with albendazole in medical pre- and post-intervention therapy to prevent secondary CE based on its activity against protoscolices. Even though theoretically appealing, on the basis of currently available data, no recommendation for the use of praziquantel can be made.[85]

Percutaneous Sterilization of CE Cysts: Puncture – Aspiration – Injection – Re-Aspiration (PAIR) (Box 56.3)

US-guided percutaneous sterilization of cyst content (PAIR) is a very elegant method, which can cure patients using a minimally invasive technique.[16,45–51,86–88] Over the years, the range of cyst stages which can effectively be approached was narrowed down to CE1 and CE3a cysts of 5–6 cm to <10 cm in diameter, in which cysto-biliary fistulas are reliably excluded.[46] All protoscolicidal (parasiticidal) agents, including 95% alcohol and 20% sodium chloride, cause sclerosing cholangitis and liver failure when accidentally spilled into the biliary tree.[89] This places great responsibility on the interventionalist who performs percutaneous sterilization. A further precondition is that only cysts sufficiently covered by organ parenchyma to prevent spillage when the needle is pulled back can safely undergo percutaneous sterilization. This essentially limits the use of PAIR to liver cysts. Published clinical trials are few and are generally small. The percutaneous treatment approach is used to various degrees in hospitals in CE-endemic countries. There is still substantial reluctance to adopt it in many parts of the world, due to the fact that surgery continues to dominate the field, and also because puncturing of CE cysts is regarded as potentially dangerous, with anaphylaxis and spillage of hydatid fluid as the major threats. Additional reasons are lack of experience, training and equipment, in particular US machines. A recent systematic literature review indicates that lethal anaphylaxis related to percutaneous treatment is extremely rare.[90] However, publication bias may still obscure the picture in this context. In experienced hands, with the necessary infrastructure and equipment, including the management of major adverse events, in particular anaphylactic reactions, percutaneous cyst sterilization is minimally invasive and cost-effective and can be regarded as safe. Its use in CE1 and CE3a cysts of 5–6 cm to <10 cm in diameter in which cysto-biliary fistulas are reliably excluded can be encouraged if appropriate training in centres with the necessary infrastructure and resources can be guaranteed. Very importantly, appropriate clinical trials are overdue in view of the evidence base on which PAIR is performed. A recent systematic review found only two randomized clinical trials.[88] One compared PAIR vs surgery in 50 patients[87] and the other PAIR with or without albendazole vs albendazole in 30 patients.[86] PAIR plus albendazole was equally effective as surgery and had substantially fewer adverse events, and PAIR with or without albendazole was more effective than albendazole alone.

PAIR has also been used in large (>10 cm) CE1 and CE3a cysts with and without continuous catheter drainage.[50,91]

Percutaneous Evacuation of CE Cysts: Large-bore Catheters, Modified Catheterization Techniques (MoCat) and Percutaneous Evacuation (PEVAC)

Method: Evacuation of the entire parasite-derived cyst components (endocyst plus content). Suitable for large cysts and cysts with solid content which cannot be approached with PAIR (CE2, CE3b). So far regularly performed only in a few specialized centres. Clinical trials are urgently needed to further explore this technique because of its potential to replace surgery in the cyst stages which are not treatable with PAIR.

BOX 56.3 PAIR (PUNCTURE – ASPIRATION – INJECTION – RE-ASPIRATION)

Method: Sterilization of the germinal layer and protoscolices. Only hydatid fluid is removed; all other parasitic material remains in the cyst.

Prerequisites: Experienced interventionalist; resuscitation equipment in place to treat severe anaphylactic reactions and surgical back-up.

The Document of the WHO Informal Working Group on Echinococcosis[45] gives technical guidance on the performance of PAIR; however, it has not been updated since it was first published. Attention should be paid to the fact that indications for PAIR have meanwhile become more restrictive with regard to cyst stages, cyst size and the procedure to exclude cysto-biliary fistulas. ERCP is no longer generally recommended for excluding cysto-biliary fistulas, not least because of the danger of false-negative results due to high intracystic pressure.

PAIR is now almost exclusively used for CE1 and CE3a cysts of the liver with a diameter of 5–6 cm to <10 cm.

The major steps are (Figure 56.10):

1. Prophylaxis of secondary echinococcosis with albendazole (4 hours before until 1 month after the intervention)
2. Percutaneous puncture of the cyst under US (or CT) guidance
3. Aspiration of cyst fluid
4. Testing for bilirubin (evaluation of aspect of fluid and test strip result) and injection of contrast medium (verification of absence of cysto-biliary communications). Note that communications can only be detected when the contrast medium gains access to the fistula, which is not the case when it remains within the intact endocyst and does not enter between the endocyst and the pericyst
5. Aspiration of contrast medium
6. If fistulas are reliably ruled out: injection of protoscolicidal (parasitocidal) agent – 95% ethanol or 20% sodium chloride to remain in the cyst for 10–15 minutes
7. Re-aspiration of the fluid
8. Follow-up for a minimum of 5 years to detect relapses and secondary CE.

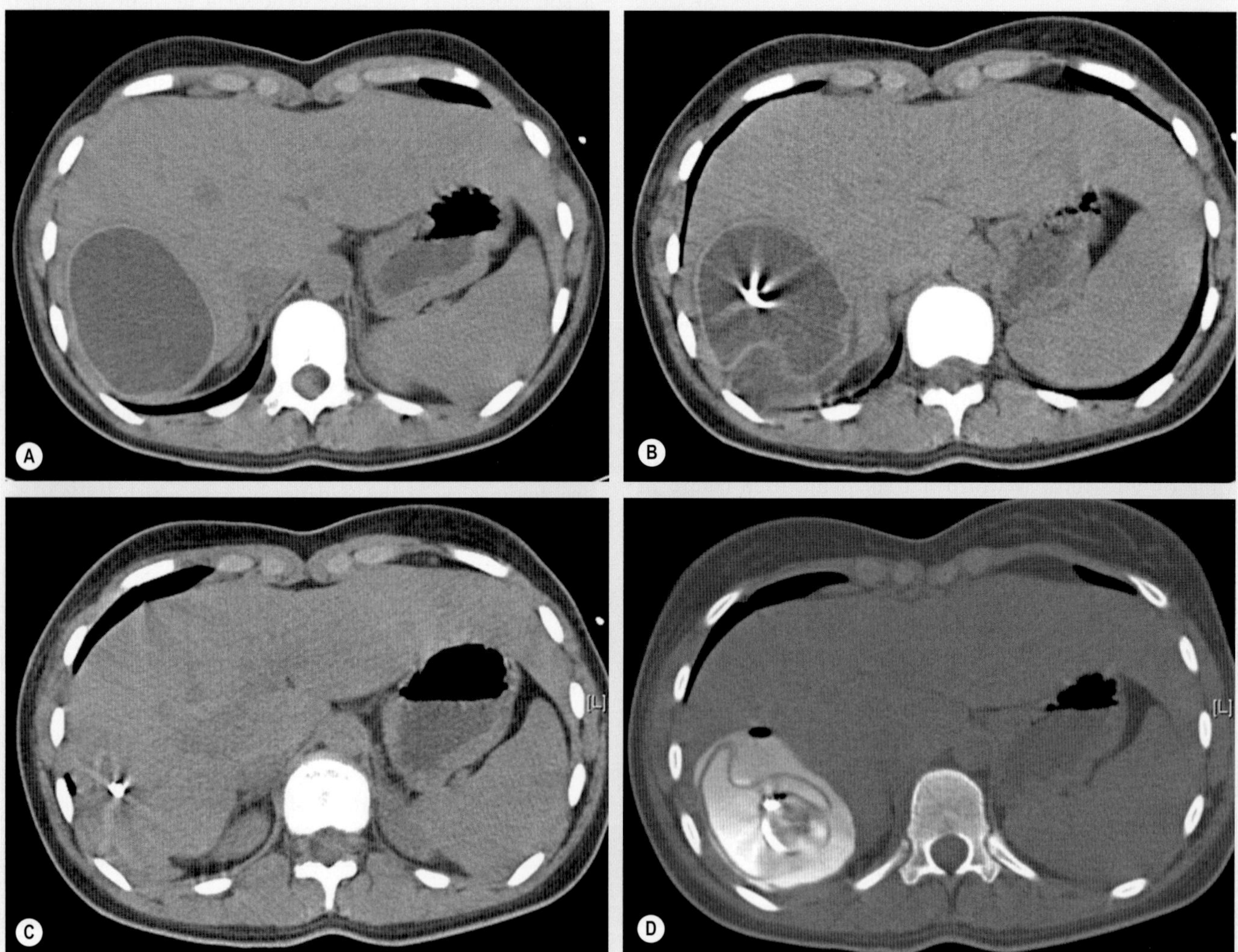

Figure 56.10 PAIR (Puncture – Aspiration – Injection – Re-aspiration). (A) CE1 cyst of the liver. (B) CT-guided puncture of the cyst. (C) Aspiration of the fluid cyst content; Testing for bilirubin (evaluation of aspect of fluid and test strip result): verification of absence of cysto-biliary communications. (D) Injection of contrast medium: verification of absence of cysto-biliary communications. Note that communications can only be detected when the contrast medium gains access to the fistula, which is not the case when it remains within the intact endocyst and does not enter between the endocyst and the pericyst.

BOX 56.3 PAIR (PUNCTURE – ASPIRATION – INJECTION – RE-ASPIRATION)—cont'd

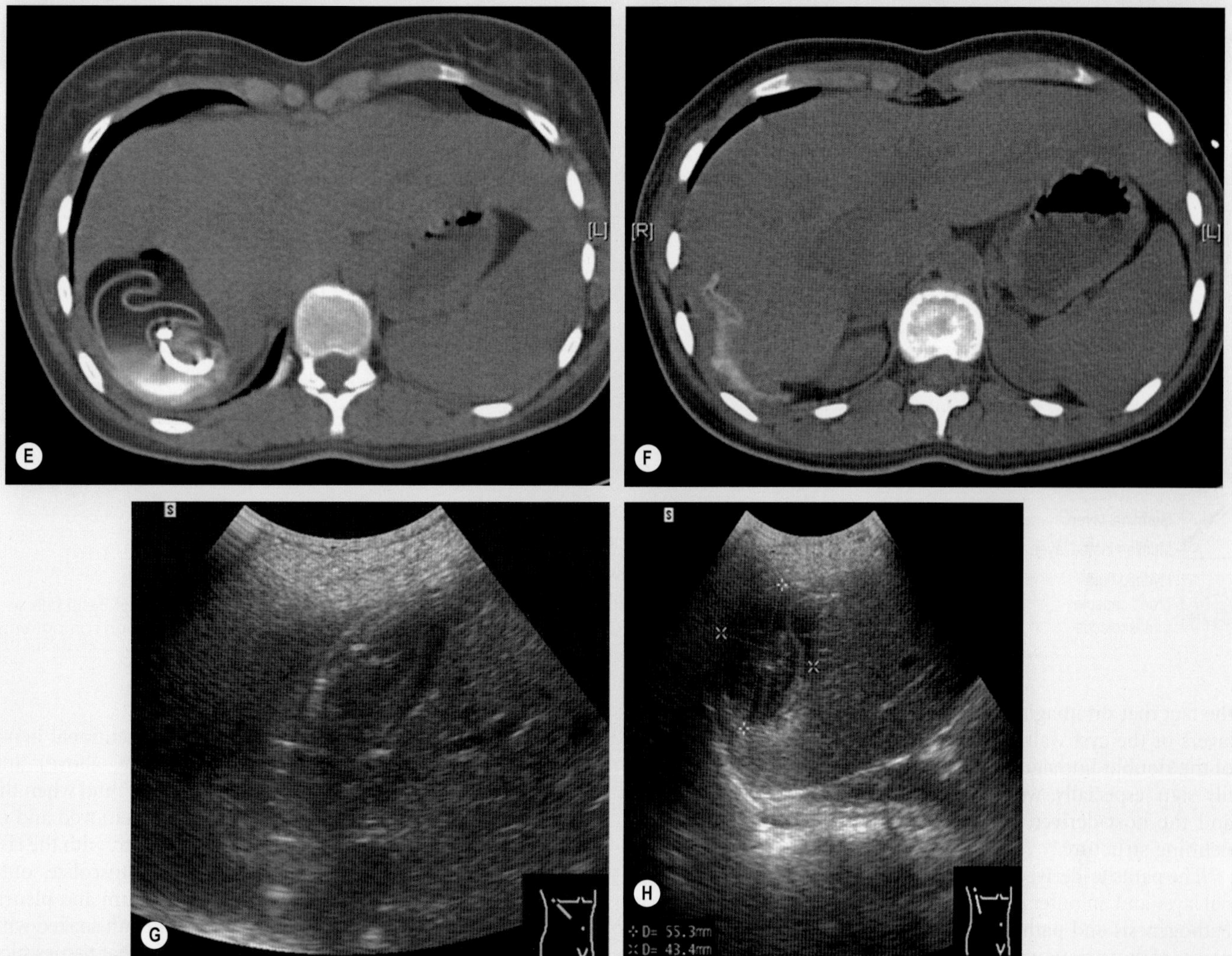

Figure 56.10, cont'd (E) After re-aspiration of contrast medium injection of 95% ethanol or 20% sodium chloride to remain in the cyst for 10–15 min. (F) Re-aspiration of 95% ethanol or 20% sodium chloride. Now only the collapsed endocyst is visible. (G,H) Ultrasonographic follow-up after the intervention which shows increasing fluid collection in the cyst cavity over a couple of weeks. This should not be mistaken for treatment failure. Further follow-up over months will show reabsorption of this tissue fluid collection (seroma) if sterilization was successful. *(Copyright © W. Hosch, Department of Radiology, Heidelberg University Hospital.)*

Prerequisites: Interventionalist experienced with this technique; resuscitation equipment in place to treat severe anaphylactic reactions and surgical back-up.[46,92–95]

Surgery (Box 56.4)

Extensive surgery, as required for CE patients, carries a certain risk depending on the available resources, infrastructure and training, is expensive and often not accessible for patients in low- and middle-income countries, where the overwhelming proportion of patients who need treatment reside.[96,97]

To understand the difference between the various surgical techniques, a thorough knowledge of the architecture of the cysts is required, which falls into two parts, parasite-derived and host-derived components (Figure 56.11).

Misconceptions about the definition of the 'CE cyst' and specifically the definition of the cyst wall may be explained by

BOX 56.4 THERE ARE TWO MAJOR SURGICAL APPROACHES

1. Partial Cystectomy: Removal of the parasite-derived cyst components (endocyst) and part of the pericyst (host-derived connective tissue capsule).
2. Total cystectomy and Resection
   a. Total cystectomy: Removal of the parasite-derived cyst components (endocyst) and the entire pericyst (host derived connective tissue capsule)
   b. Resection: additional removal of part of the organ in which the CE-cyst is embedded

FOLLOW-UP

All patients should be followed-up for a minimum of 5 years.

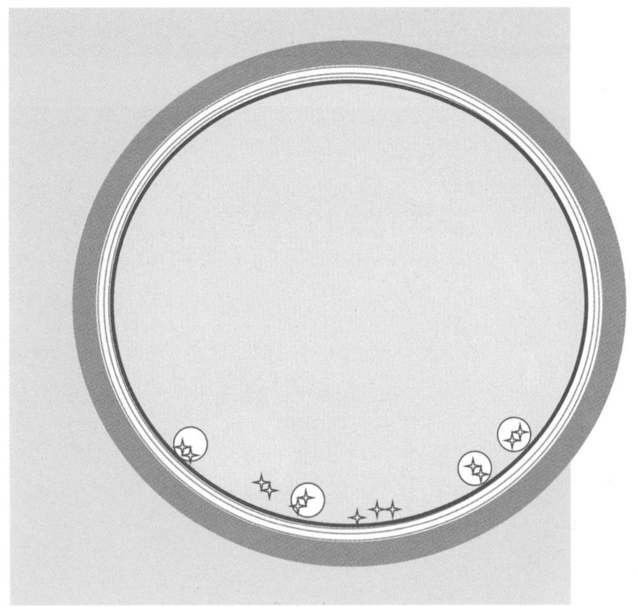

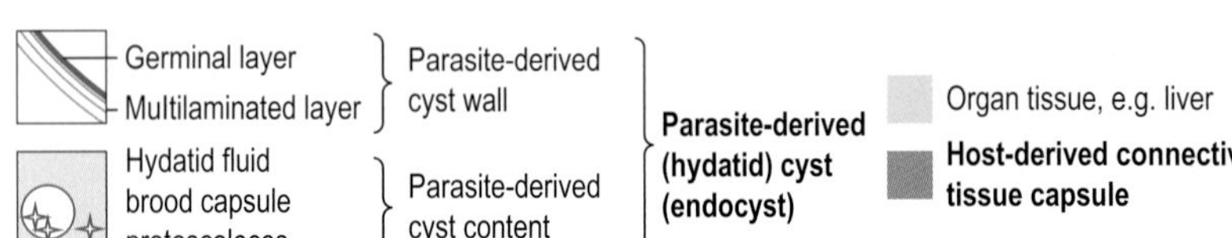

Figure 56.11 Architecture of the wall of cysts falls into two parts, parasite-derived and host-derived components.

the fact that on imaging, the parasite-derived and host-derived layers of the cyst wall cannot be separated, with the exception of the 'double-line sign' and the 'water-lily sign'. With the 'water-lily sign' especially, we see the parasite-derived cyst collapsed and the host-derived cyst wall remaining as the 'cyst' space-defining structure.

The parasite-derived cyst wall consists of an inner thin germinal layer and an outer parasite-derived thick laminated layer (see Pathogenesis and pathology and Figure 56.3). At the resolution power of the various imaging modalities, the multilaminated layer and the germinal layer cannot be separated. The endocyst is surrounded by the host-derived connective tissue layer. When operated on, the parasite-derived wall can be easily separated from the host-derived capsule in early CE cyst stages; in older cysts they may be glued together through inflammatory processes.

Depending on the cyst stage, the parasite-derived cyst content (hydatid fluid, daughter cysts, brood capsules and protoscolices or fragments thereof) is either contained within the parasite-derived cyst wall (germinal layer plus multilaminated membrane) or, as soon as this has ruptured, within the host-derived connective tissue capsule. With progressive absorption of the hydatid fluid the cyst content becomes jellylike and solid.

Fistulas are defects in the host-derived connective tissue capsule which only become active when the parasite-derived cyst wall (multilaminated and germinal layer) ruptures, giving way to the cyst content to drain via patent fistulas into the biliary tree. This can occur correspondingly in lung cysts.

The architecture of CE cysts translates as follows into the two principal surgical approaches:

Partial Cystectomy

Removal of the parasite-derived cyst components (endocyst) and part of the pericyst (host-derived connective tissue capsule) (Figure 56.12).

Main steps of partial cystectomy:

1. Prevention of secondary CE: (a) perinterventional benzimidazole prophylaxis (see Benzimidazole, above) and (b) careful prevention of spillage of hydatid fluid when the cyst is punctured and the cyst material is removed and of contamination of instruments and gloves, etc. with the risk of transferring germinal layer cells and protoscolices onto receptive tissues, in particular the peritoneum and pleura. The area around the cyst is covered with cloth soaked with 20% sodium chloride. Care has to be taken that tissues such as the peritoneum and pleura are not damaged by the protoscolicidal agent and to avoid absorption of significant amounts of sodium chloride. This is achieved by protecting these tissues with a layer of cloth soaked in normal saline.
2. Insertion of a trocar through the host-derived capsule (pericyst) into the cyst and removal of all parasite material by suction.
3. Sterilization of the cavity with 20% sodium chloride or 95% ethanol through the trocar after very careful exclusion of cysto-biliary fistulas (if in doubt, the cavity is only washed with normal saline and the sterilizing procedure is postponed until the resectable part of the host-derived capsule is removed, allowing a good view of the residual cavity for exclusion of fistulas).
4. Resection of as much of the host-derived capsule (pericyst) as possible, which allows a good view of the residual cyst cavity (Figure 56.12). Inspection of the cyst cavity to remove residual parasite-derived material and repeated or, if not yet performed, careful primary exclusion of fistulas. Additional or, if not yet conducted, primary sterilization of the residual cavity with 20% sodium chloride or 95% alcohol.
5. Closure of fistulas.
6. Filling of the residual cavity with an omentoplasty where appropriate.[98]

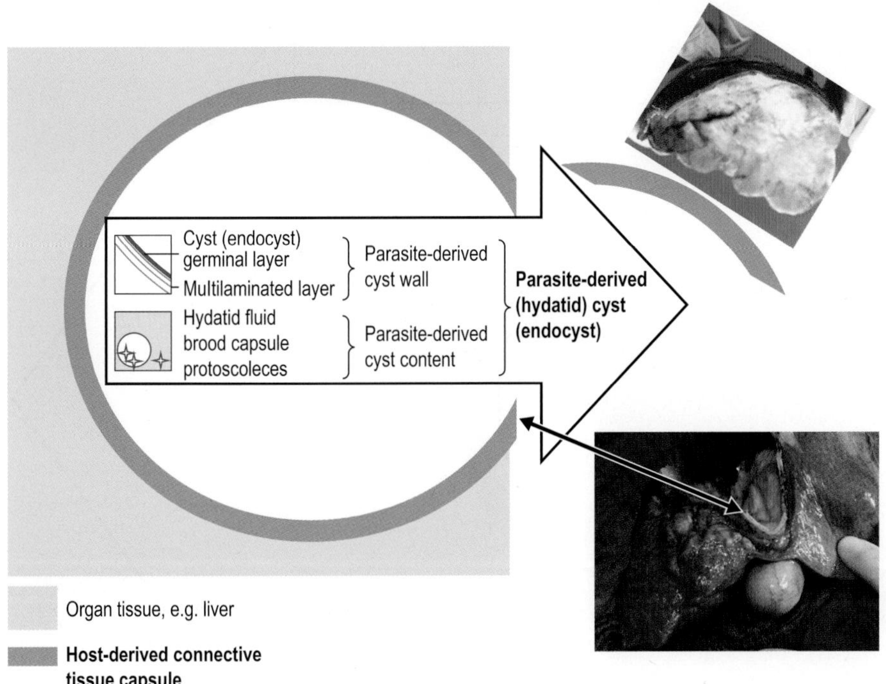

Figure 56.12 Partial cystectomy: Removal of the parasite-derived cyst components (endocyst) and part of the pericyst (host-derived connective tissue capsule). After a trocar has been inserted into the cyst and cyst content aspirated (spillage prophylaxis with cloth soaked with 20% sodium chloride to protect the peritoneum) as much of the host-derived capsule (pericyst) as possible is resected, which allows a good view of the residual cyst cavity. The layer of host-derived connective tissue which is left in place and which is firmly connected to the organ tissues – in this case the liver parenchyma – minimizes the risk of bleeding. *(Copyright © Heidelberg University Hospital.)*

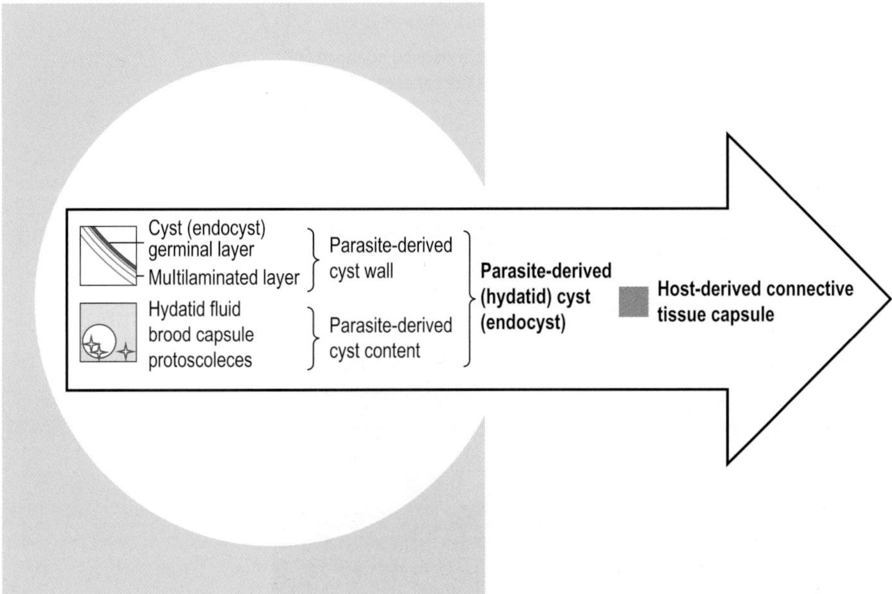

Figure 56.13 Total cystectomy (pericystectomy). The parasite-derived cyst components (endocyst) are removed together with the host-derived connective tissue capsule (pericyst), with the major advantage that the cyst remains closed and there is no exposure to infective cyst content at any time during the procedure. Risks include bleeding.

The advantages of this approach are:[96,97,99]

1. The procedure is carried out with a good view of the parasite-derived material which needs to be totally removed to ensure success and to avoid relapses.
2. The risk of bleeding is minimal due to the fact that the host-derived posterior wall of the pericyst, which is firmly connected to the organ tissues, e.g. the liver parenchyma, is left in place.
3. Parasite-derived material in anatomically critical sites can be safely removed, i.e. cysts which are intimately attached to vessels such as the portal or the caval vein, etc.

The disadvantages of the approach are:

1. Risk of secondary echinococcosis through spillage of hydatid fluid and contamination of receptive tissues through instruments and gloves contaminated with cells of the germinal layer and protoscolices.
2. Intra- and postoperative risks of extended surgery and anaesthesia, in particular in countries with limited resources.
3. Postoperative seromas and biliomas must be differentiated from recurrencies. Seromas and biliomas usually decrease in size over time. If in doubt diagnostic puncture should be considered.

Total Cystectomy and Liver Resection

Removal of the parasite-derived cyst components (endocyst) and the entire pericyst (host-derived connective tissue capsule) – total cystectomy (Figure 56.13); additionally, removal of part

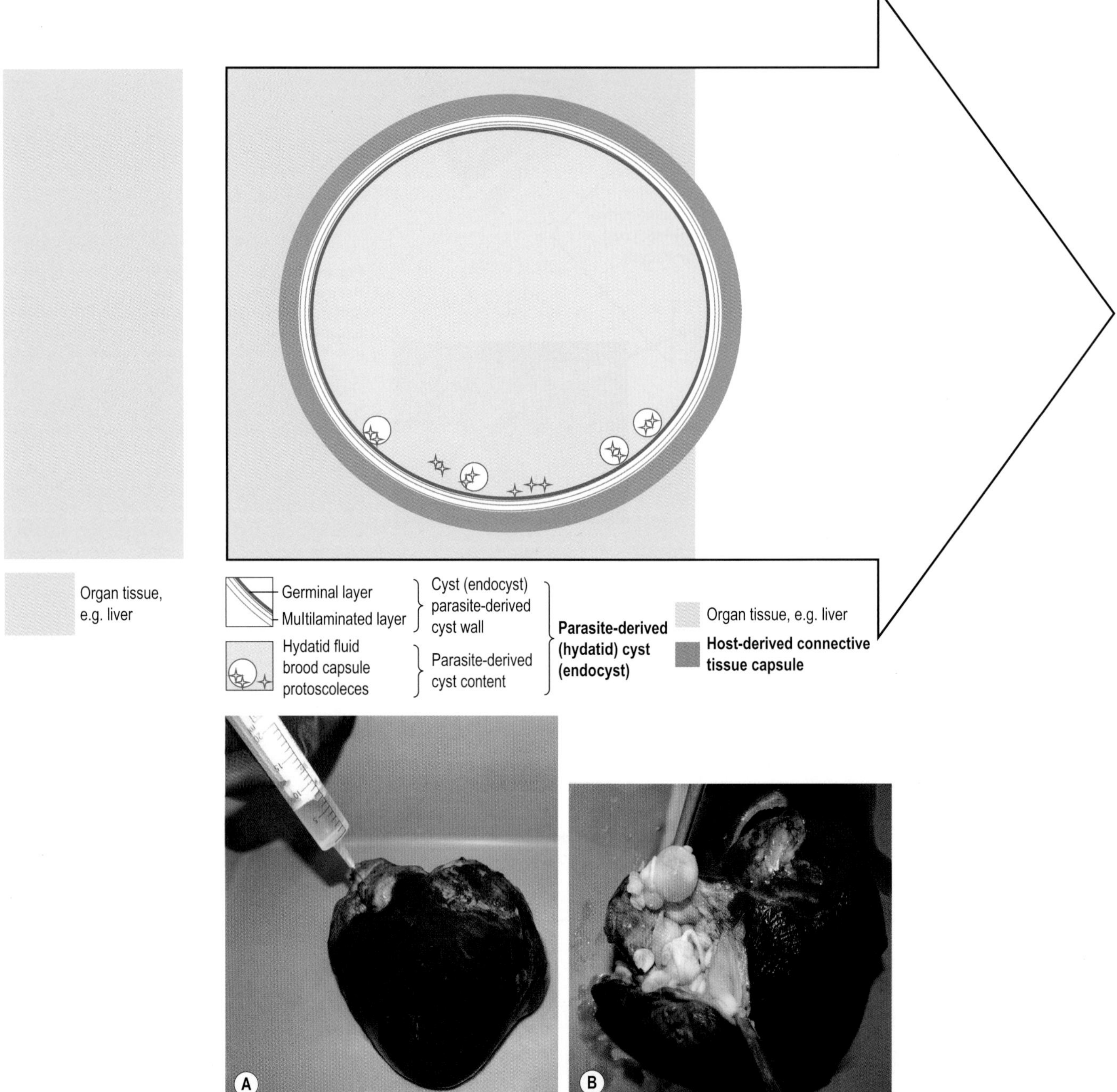

Figure 56.14 Resection: In addition to the parasite-derived cyst (endocyst) and the host-derived connective tissue capsule (pericyst) part of the organ in which the cyst is embedded is resected. Schematic and right liver lobectomy with two large CE cysts: (A) Clear hydatid fluid extracted from an active CE2 cyst; (B) Opened CE2 cyst with multiple daughter cysts. *(Copyright © Heidelberg University Hospital.)*

of the organ in which the CE cyst is embedded – resection (Figure 56.14).

In this approach, the parasite-derived cyst components (endocyst) are removed together with the host-derived capsule (pericyst), with the major advantage that the cyst remains closed and there is no exposure to infective cyst content at any time during the procedure (Figure 56.13); more specifically, this is called closed total cystectomy. Practically, this is done by resecting the cyst along the outside circumference of the host-derived connective tissue capsule (pericyst). Only when the resection plane follows the outer circumference of the pericyst is it a total cystectomy in the true sense. In practice, however, the transition to an atypical liver resection is blurred.

If, in addition to the parasite-derived cyst and the host-derived connective tissue capsule (pericyst), part of the organ in which the cyst is embedded is resected, one refers to resection. In the liver, for example, this can be a segmentectomy or lobectomy or an atypical liver resection (Figure 56.14), and correspondingly with lung cysts.

The advantages of this approach are:

1. No risk of secondary echinococcosis
2. Better control of fistulas.

The disadvantages of this approach are:

1. Higher risk of intra- and postoperative complications, in particular bleeding
2. Greater loss of the tissue in which the cyst is situated.

Partial Cystectomy versus Total Cystectomy/Resection

Since CE is, with the exception of complicated cysts (see above), a benign disease, preference should always be given to the surgical technique which holds the smallest risk for the patient.[97] Two major issues need careful consideration:

1. In hospitals of countries with limited resources, surgical and anaesthesiological infrastructure and training preference should be given to partial cystectomy
2. The amount of organ tissue which needs to be sacrificed and the risk of major complications of resections need to be carefully considered.

'Watch and Wait'

The natural evolution of an early active CE cyst (WHO stage CE1) is continuous growth, and cysts can reach an impressive size of up to 15 cm in diameter and more. At a certain point in time, involution sets in, which drives the cyst eventually to its final stage (CE5) when the parasite is dead (Figure 56.4). The stages on the way from a CE1 cyst to its final destination have various levels of activity. With the 'watch and wait' approach, one allows the cyst to progress along its natural course. Great care should be taken, however, when one decides on the 'watch and wait' approach in active and transitional cysts. There are to-date no reliable data on the success or the risks. In inactive CE4 and CE5 cysts, our centre-based experience has already generated confidence in the 'watch and wait' approach with long-term observation without relapses or complications. When opting for the 'watch and wait' approach the regional anatomical setting of the cyst has to be carefully evaluated to make sure that neighbouring organs and structures are not compromised by the space-occupying lesion. It remains important, however, to also follow-up patients with CE4 and CE5 cysts for a minimum of 5 years.

PREVENTION

The division of hydatid control into four phases is now generally accepted: (1) planning; (2) attack; (3) consolidation; and (4) maintenance of eradication. There are horizontal and vertical approaches to CE control. Horizontal approaches aim at the reduction of disease transmission through primary healthcare interventions, which include among other measures, health education, general husbandry improvements, upgrading of abattoirs and meat inspection and rely on regular deworming of dogs by their owners. This slow-track approach shows reduction in livestock and dog prevalence rates over a longer period (>25 years).

The so-called vertical or fast-track approach is so far the most successful and is targeted on the parasite. It includes mass treatment of dogs, dog registration and reduction of stray dog numbers. With this approach, ovine CE rates can be reduced significantly within 3–5 years and within 10 years human cyst rates can drop below 1 per 100 000.

Vaccination of the intermediate host is a new intervention strategy. The EG95 vaccine showed 95% effectiveness against ovine hydatidosis and needs innovative administration strategies in the future. Mathematical models have shown that a combination of vaccination and antihelmintic treatment of dogs is promising and even if antiparasitic treatment is only given 6 monthly to 60% of the dog population and 60% of sheep are vaccinated, there is a high probability of successful disease control through cumulative effects by interventions at different points in the parasite life cycle. A dog vaccine is not available at present and it is very unlikely that it will be available within the foreseeable future.[5,100–103]

Alveolar Echinococcosis (AE)

EPIDEMIOLOGY

Human infection is caused by the ingestion of tapeworm eggs originating from *E. multilocularis*-infected definitive hosts (mainly foxes and domestic dogs). Natural intermediate hosts of *E. multilocularis* include predominantly arvicolid and cricetid rodents (Figure 56.16). *E. multilocularis* is endemic in most parts of the northern hemisphere (Figure 56.15). The endemic area extends from central and eastern Europe to northern and central Eurasia and northern Japan; furthermore parts of North America (Alaska and northern Canada) are affected.[7] The geographic distribution of AE in Europe is probably wider than assumed and includes at least 12 central European countries, mainly countries bordering Switzerland, Germany and Austria. In a recent estimate of the global burden of AE, 30 of 43 European countries in all of which case reports on AE had been published, were considered endemic for AE.[7,104] In Asia, the main endemic foci of AE are in eastern Turkey, throughout the Russian Federation and adjacent countries and in northeastern, central and northwestern China as well as northern Japan.

In *E. multilocularis* there is no significant strain variability and isolates from various geographical regions show only minor genetic heterogeneity.[5]

The prevalence of AE is generally low in Europe and ranges between 0.02% and 1.4%. China is one of the major endemic regions in the world with an AE prevalence of 5% and higher. Reports on AE in several areas, such as Turkey, Lithuania and many parts of the former Soviet Union such as Kyrgyzstan and Kazakhstan are increasing. The global annual incidence of AE cases per year is estimated at 18 235; of these 91% (16 692) are considered to occur in China, 1180 in Russia and 426 in the rest of the world.[104]

The emerging number of AE cases in some regions seems to be related to environmental changes such as a decrease in ploughed fields and hedges in Europe's mid-mountain areas or overgrazing and deforestation in China. Changes in rodent and canid populations, such as increasing fox populations and fox infection rate and urbanization of foxes in Europe, and changing human behaviour may currently increase the risk of contact with parasite eggs in contaminated urban or rural areas.[105]

PATHOGENESIS AND PATHOLOGY

In infected humans the *E. multilocularis* metacestode (larva) develops primarily in the liver. In advanced stages of infection, other sites may become metastasized such as the retroperitoneum, the lungs, brain and bones, among others. The typical proliferating lesion appears macroscopically as a dispersed mass

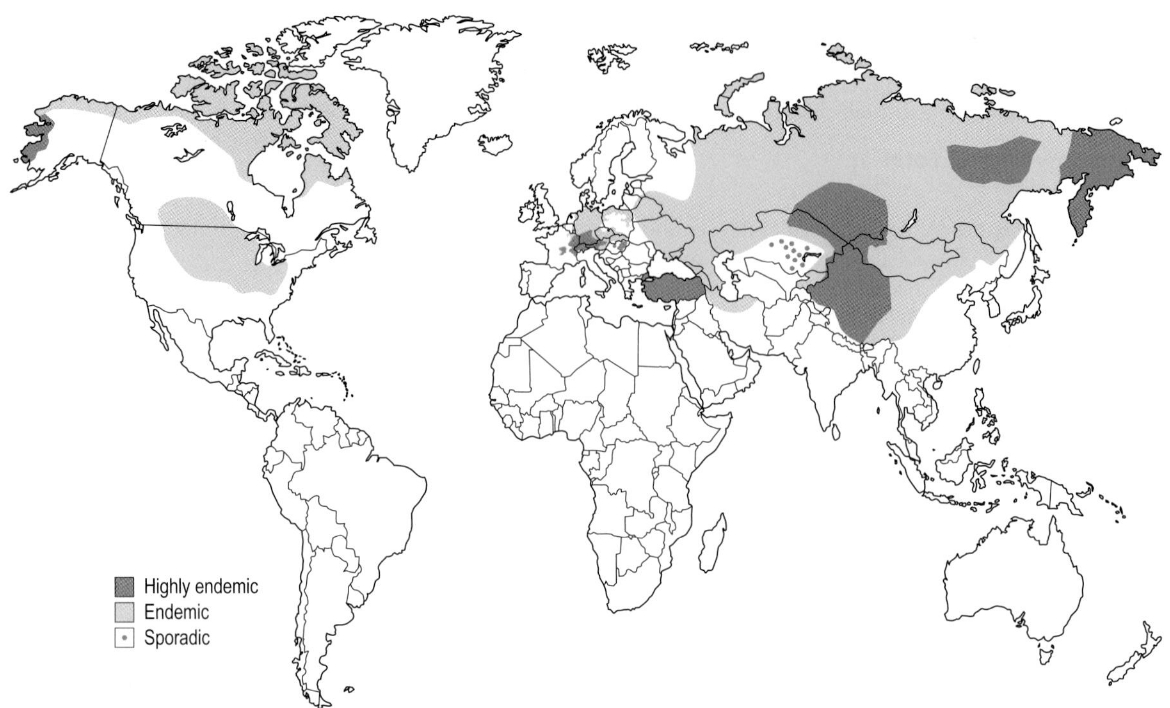

Figure 56.15 Global distribution of *Echinococcus multilocularis*. *(Torgerson et al. (2010); Copyright © PLoS Negl Trop Dis doi:10.1371/journal.pntd.0000722.g002.)*

of fibrous tissue with a conglomerate of scattered vesicles, each ranging from a few millimetres to centimetres in size. In advanced cases, central necrotic cavities can form, containing a viscous fluid which, occasionally, becomes secondarily infected by bacteria. Older lesions often contain focal zones of calcification scattered across the whole or parts of the hepatic lesion. Histologically, a conglomerate of small vesicles and cysts composed of a thin outer (PAS-positive) laminated layer and an inner germinal layer characterize the metacestode. The germinal layer represents the proliferating metacestode generating new vesicles, which leads to the tumour-like behaviour of the parasite. A granulomatous host reaction surrounds the metacestode, including a vigorous synthesis of fibrous and germinative tissue (Figure 56.17). In contrast to infections in susceptible rodent hosts, lesions from infected human patients rarely exhibit brood capsule and protoscolex formation within vesicles.

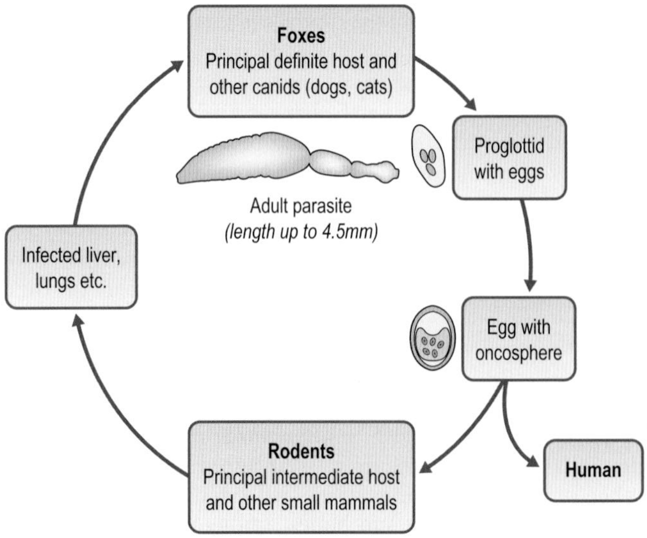

Foxes
Principal definite host and other canids (dogs, cats)
Proglottid with eggs
Adult parasite
(length up to 4.5mm)
Infected liver, lungs etc.
Egg with oncosphere
Rodents
Principal intermediate host and other small mammals
Human

Figure 56.16 Life cycle of *Echinococcus multilocularis*.

The immune response, which develops against the larval stages of *E. multilocularis*, accounts for a controlled parasite tissue development as well as for the immunopathological events. Varying innate and immunological host factors proved responsible for the occurrence of three different outcomes of infection, corresponding to three principally different clinical presentations: (1) resistance as shown by the presence of 'dying out' or 'aborted' metacestodes; (2) controlled susceptibility as shown by a slowly growing metacestode tissue – this group refers to the normal AE patients who first experience clinical signs and symptoms 5–15 years after infection; and (3) uncontrolled hyperproliferation of the metacestode due to an impaired immune response.[106] The host mechanisms modulating the course of infection include primarily T-cell interactions. Thus, the periparasitic granuloma, mainly composed of macrophages, myofibroblasts and T cells, contains a large number of CD4+ T cells in patients with abortive or died-out lesions, whereas in patients with active metacestodes the number of CD8+ T cells is increased.[107] Immunosuppressive and/or immunoregulatory processes are assumed to correlate to parasite survival and proliferation dynamics. Cytokine mRNA levels in AE show initially elevated transcription levels of pro-inflammatory cytokines, e.g. IL-1β, IL-6 and tumour necrosis factor alpha (TNFα), which are gradually re-oriented towards Th2, including elevated IL-3, IL-4 and IL-10[108] as well as TGFβ transcripts.[109] Thus, TGFβ-driven regulatory T cells are thought to play a crucial role in the parasite-modulated progressive course of AE.

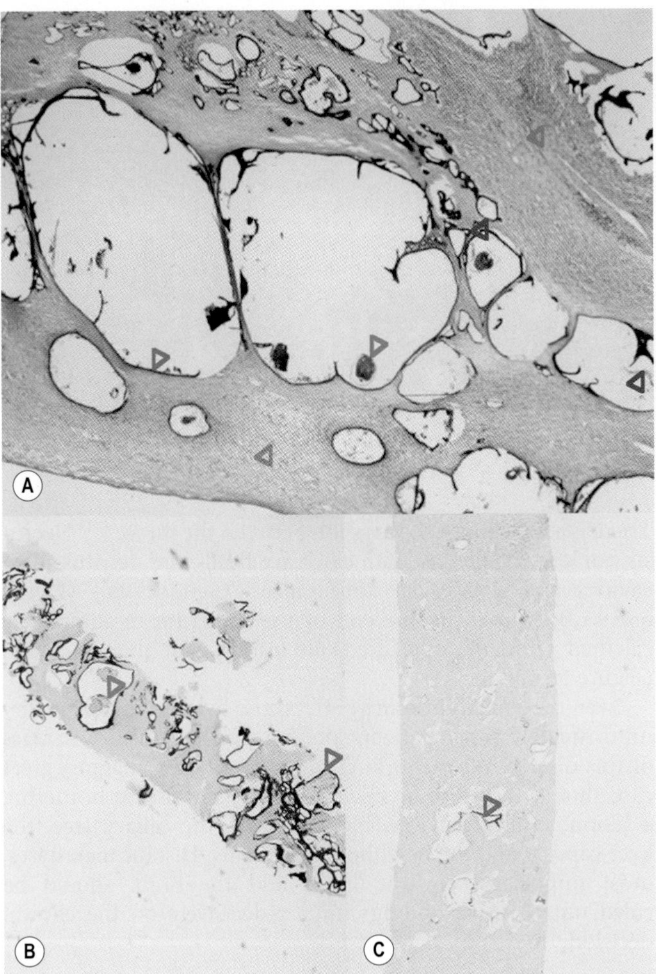

Figure 56.17 AE-histology. Multiloculated vesicles and vesiculated cystic conglomerates in the liver of an AE-affected patient. Parasitic cysts consist of an outer laminated layer (blue arrowheads), an inner germinal layer (red arrowheads) and, very rarely seen, protoscolices (green arrowheads). The acellular laminated layer presents either non-disrupted lining a cystic vesicle, or fragmented often visible as a convoluted structure. Periparasitic structures (orange arrowheads) include the presence of macrophages, neutrophilic granulocytes, lymphocytes and plasma cells, necrosis, and predominantly fibrosis. (A) Conventional histological section following surgery. (B,C) Fine-needle biopsies (FNB) from two different AE patients. While B shows a relatively heavy infection intensity of a very active AE lesion, C refers to an AE liver with a very low infection intensity, where imaging yields only vague indications for AE-specific liver lesions and where the parasite appeared to be dying out. Both FNBs were PCR-positive for *E. multilocularis*. PAS-stain; A = 40×; B,C = 100×. *(Copyright © B. Gottstein.)*

The response characteristics of AE-resistant persons could so far not be elucidated. Conversely, impairment of Th cell activity such as in advanced AIDS or other immunological disorders is associated with a rapid and unlimited growth and dissemination of the parasite in AE. CD4+ recovery in AIDS patients by means of appropriate therapy, however, reinstates control over progression of AE treated with benzimidazoles.[110]

CLINICAL FEATURES

AE patients often become symptomatic only in the 4th or 5th decade of their life after an incubation period of 5–15 years; however, there is a wide age range. In general there is no gender predominance in the distribution of AE but this may vary by region.

AE is a chronic disease affecting primarily and almost exclusively the liver. Primary infection of other organs is extremely rare. The metacestode of *E. multilocularis* shows infiltrative multivesicular growth with consecutive tissue necrosis and calcification.

In the course of disease infiltration of adjacent organs or metastases, mainly to the lung and brain, may occur. Of 559 patients reported to the European registry between 1982 and 2000, in 190 (34%) the disease had already spread by continuous growth to adjacent organs (kidneys, adrenal glands, diaphragm, pleura and lungs) or to distant organs (spleen, lungs, brain).[111,112] This indicates the importance of a complete work-up of patients who present at advanced stages of the disease.

A case series of 112 patients with AE of the liver from eastern France showed an association between the localization of the AE lesion in the liver and clinical symptoms. Jaundice was only present if the liver hilum was affected, whereas posterior localization of lesions and other hepatic localizations were not associated with jaundice. Lung metastases were most commonly seen when the hepatic veins or the vena cava were infiltrated, which was the case in 11 of 17 patients with lung involvement. In two patients, lung involvement occurred due to transdiaphragmatic growth of the AE lesion. Clinical complications, included: cholangitis, jaundice, liver abscess, ascites, pulmonary embolism, pulmonary or brain metastases, inferior vena cava thrombosis and Budd–Chiari syndrome due to hepatic vein infiltration. The main causes of death were hepatic failure, cerebral AE, gastrointestinal bleeding, septic shock or complications after liver transplantation.[113]

In summary patients with AE of the liver may present with upper abdominal pain or cholestatic jaundice, or lesions may be discovered by chance due to patient work-up for abnormal routine laboratory parameters, hepatomegaly, weight loss or fatigue. The infiltrative, tumour-like growth of AE causes a range of complications, which are mainly: (1) jaundice due to invasion of large biliary vessels at the liver hilum sometimes with (recurrent) cholangitis which may cause portal hypertension and hepatic dysfunction; (2) invasion of vascular walls with haematogenic spread of disease or vascular occlusion/thrombosis; and (3) poor vascularization of AE lesions leading to necrosis and formation of (large) necrotic cavities with irregular contours which are at risk of secondary bacterial infection and abscess formation. With regard to differential diagnoses, AE has to be distinguished from primary hepatic and metastatic malignancies as well as benign hepatic lesions, i.e. haemangiomas and cystadenomas. In the case of necrotic or pseudocystic AE lesions, the differential diagnosis includes bacterial and amoebic abscess as well as CE (Table 56.1).

A recent survival analysis from Switzerland over the last 35 years showed that recently diagnosed patients have a very good life expectancy which is only shortened by about 3 years compared with the normal Swiss population, whereas patients diagnosed in 1970 had a life expectancy of about 6–10 years only. This reflects the introduction of benzimidazole treatment and almost certainly improved disease management with increasing clinical experience in AE.[114]

Differential Diagnosis

See Table 56.1.

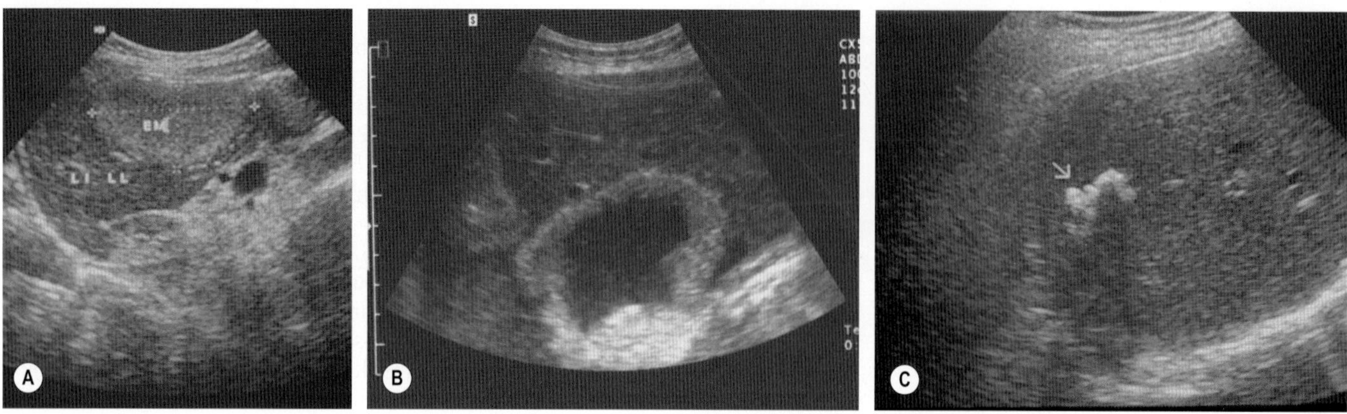

Figure 56.18 Ultrasonographic features of AE of the liver. (A) Hyperechogenic lesion. (B) Lesion with a hyperechogenic ring and hypoechogenic centre (necrosis). (C) Calcified lesion (arrow). *(Copyright © W. Hosch, Department of Radiology, Heidelberg University Hospital.)*

DIAGNOSIS

As in CE, imaging plays an important role in diagnosis. Serology has a confirmatory role and can, within limits but certainly more reliably than in CE, be used for screening. In case of doubt, diagnostic puncture and aspiration of parasitic material can be performed. A histological diagnosis can be made of resected parasitic material on the basis of characteristic structures. In histologically unclear cases, PCR is the method of choice for species-specific identification. Viability assessment can be performed with RT-PCR of biopsies and fine-needle aspirates, within the limits of the sensitivity of this method.

Imaging

US, MRI, CT. Imaging is highly sensitive and can even detect very small AE lesions. Specificity is, however, a problem with significant overlap with malignant diseases (Table 56.1). The principal features of AE space-occupying lesions are:

- Infiltrative growth at the margins of the lesions (Figures 56.18, 56.19, 56.20A, 56.21A,B)
- Necrosis in the centre of the lesion (Figures 56.18B, 56.19, 56.20A, 56.21A,B)
- Calcification (Figures 56.18C, 56.21), mostly scattered across the lesion; in contrast to CE cysts where calcifications are mostly found in the cyst wall (Figure 56.8).

There is a wide range of variation between the three.[24,115] Necrosis can lead the picture with extensive fluid- and detritus-filled cavities and a cyst-like appearance ('pseudocysts') (Figure 56.19A,B, 56.20A) at one end of the spectrum to completely calcified remnants of a died-out infection at the other end (Figure 56.18C).

Even though AE primarily affects the liver, in clinical reality unfortunately most patients present late in advanced stages of this disease. When working-up patients with imaging, great care should therefore be taken to assess the tissues bordering a lesion, infiltration into blood vessels, the biliary tree, the liver capsule and the neighbouring organs. Distant metastases, most importantly in the lungs and the brain should be ruled out. Positive findings impact decisively on the clinical decision.

PNM Classification. This resemblance to malignant diseases led to the introduction of a PNM classification for AE of the liver, as follows: P, primary mass in the liver; N, involvement of neighbouring organs including lymph nodes; M, metastases.[46,111,116]

US also has an important role in diagnostic imaging studies of AE. MRI and MRC are, however, very important assets to characterize the relationship of liver AE lesions and the very rare AE lesions in other locations with the anatomical

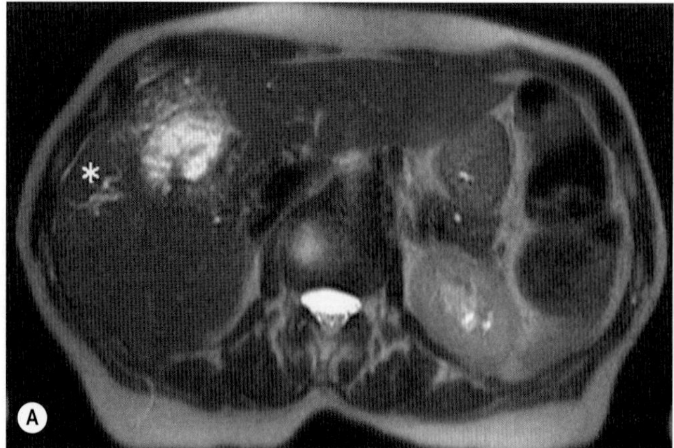

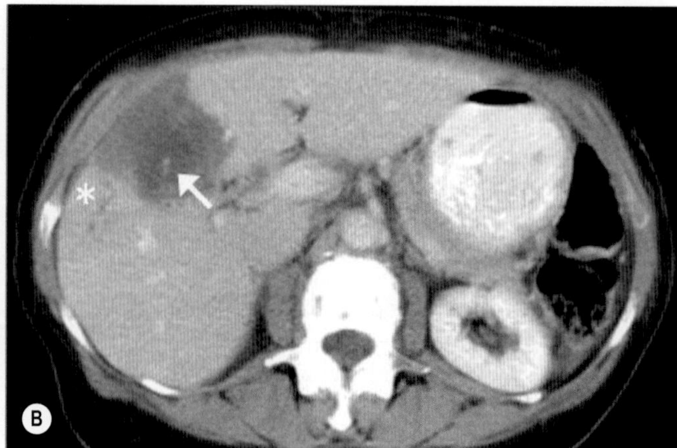

Figure 56.19 AE of the liver. MRI and CT scan of the same AE lesion. (A) T2-weighted MRI scan with dilatated biliary vessel (*). (B) Contrast-enhanced CT scan with necrotic cavity (→) and dilatated biliary vessel (*). *(Copyright © W. Hosch, Department of Radiology, Heidelberg University Hospital.)*

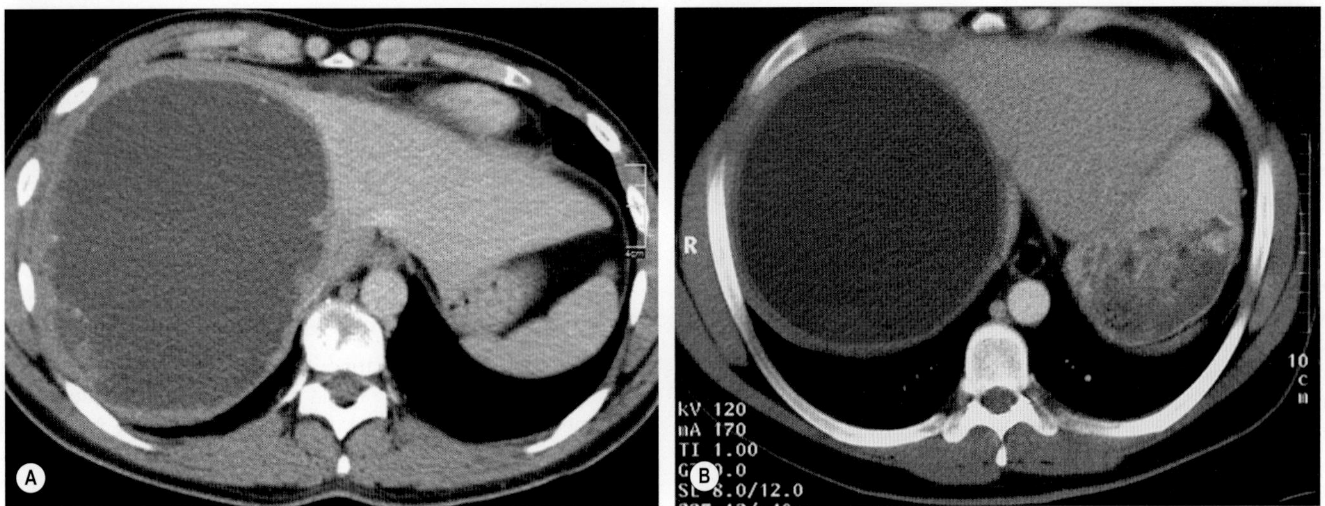

Figure 56.20 AE pseudocyst in comparison to a CE1 cyst. (A) Large AE pseudocyst: cavity with necrotic material; max. diameter 14 cm; note irregular interface between cyst content and cyst wall. (B) CE1 cyst: note smooth interface between cyst content (hydatid fluid) and cyst wall. *(Copyright © W. Hosch, Department of Radiology, Heidelberg University Hospital.)*

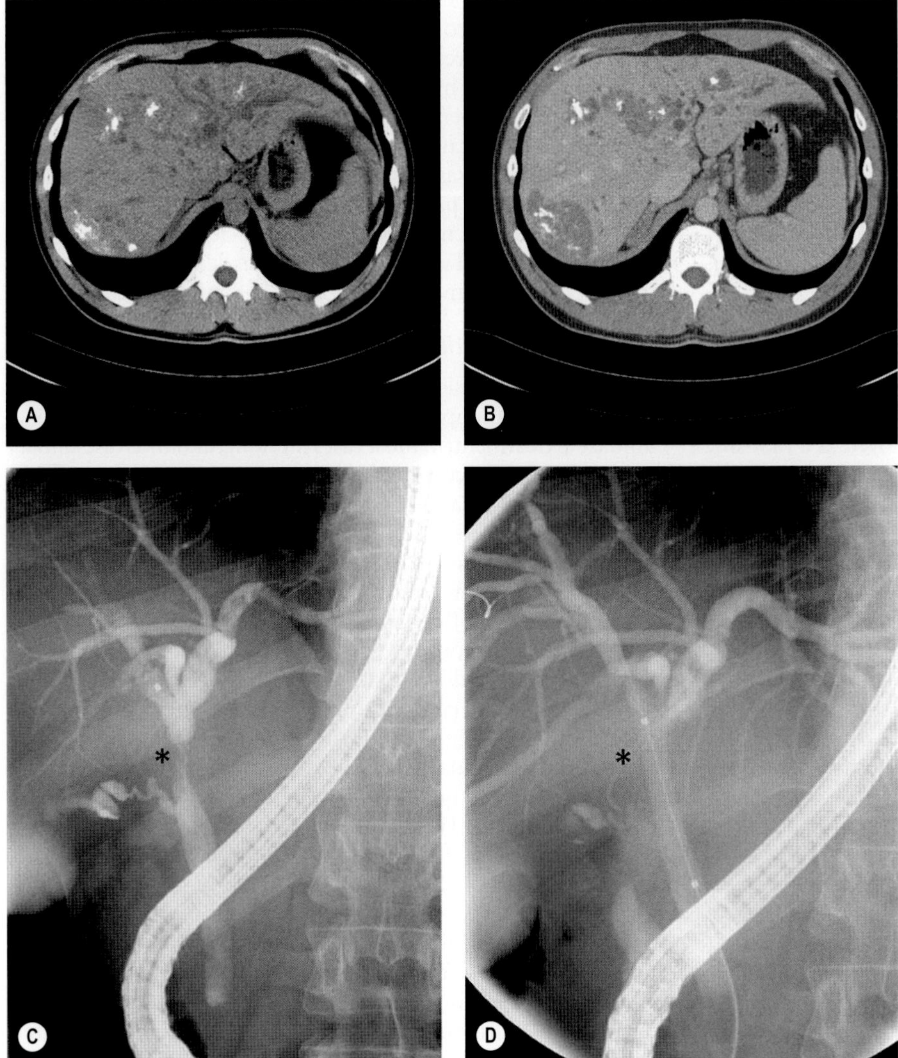

Figure 56.21 Disseminated AE of the liver. (A) CT scan without contrast enhancement. (B) Contrast-enhanced CT scan. Note the mixture of infiltrative growth, cavity formation (necrosis) and calcification. (C) Stenosis of the common hepatic duct just above the junction with the cystic duct. (D) Successful dilatation of the stenosis. *(Copyright © W. Hosch, Department of Radiology, Heidelberg University Hospital (A,B); P. Sauer, Interdisciplinary Centre for Endoscopy, Heidelberg University Hospital C,D.)*

neighbourhood, particularly in order to decide on curative resectability. T2-weighted MRI series can detect the multivesicular pattern of AE lesions which supports the diagnosis of AE (Figure 56.19A).[117] MRC can in most cases replace ERCP to clarify the involvement of bile ducts. CT detects calcifications better than MRI and also US; otherwise US and MRI (for the specific purposes listed above) are superior to CT.

PET-CT (PET-MRI). PET combined with CT or MRI picks up areas with increased glucose ([18F]fluorodeoxyglucose) turnover in inflammatory 'hotspots'. It is thus not specific for AE. In AE, focal enhancement is observed in the area immediately surrounding parasite activity. Negative findings, however, do not rule out clinically relevant infection. It only indicates absence of demonstrable periparasitic inflammation. Successful treatment with albendazole, which acts in AE mainly in a parasitostatic manner, suppresses periparasitic inflammatory activity. This feature is being used in serial PET-CT investigations where successful treatment is demonstrated by a switch from active to inactive lesions and vice versa (see Management and Treatment, below).[118–120] Apart from the fact that this technology is not available in many parts of the world, PET-CT involves a substantial radiation dose, and only a small number of patients have so far been investigated with this method.

The question is whether PET-CT could not be replaced by methods without radiation, such as contrast-enhanced ultrasound[121] or diffusion MRI. This would not only avoid radiation but would also allow more narrowly spaced serial investigations. This deserves further investigation.

Serology

Serology has a confirmatory role in lesions suspicious of AE on imaging. Furthermore, within limits but certainly more reliably than in CE, serology can also be used for screening individuals and populations at risk.

Purified and recombinant *E. multilocularis* antigens (e.g. Em2, Em2+, Em18) exhibit high diagnostic sensitivity and specificity with a high discriminatory power to differentiate between AE and CE. Immunoblotting is used in most laboratories for confirmation but can also be employed as a first-line test. In contrast to CE, some specific serologic tests are valuable to assess the efficacy of treatment in combination with imaging during follow-up of patients.[15,35,122] In this context, the Em18-ELISA showed the best correlation with PET-CT imaging and clinical findings.[123,124]

Diagnostic Puncture

In unclear cases, when imaging and serology do not lead to a diagnosis, fine-needle puncture and aspiration is a valuable tool for the differential diagnosis, in particular of malignancies, within the limits of the sensitivity of this method.

Testing of Parasite Viability

Viability assessment can be performed with RT-PCR of biopsies and fine-needle aspirates, within the limits of the sensitivity of this method.[122,125,126]

Histological Diagnosis

For a description of histopathological features, see Pathogenesis and Pathology, above.

MANAGEMENT AND TREATMENT

AE has all the features of malignancy, and patients should be cared for accordingly, i.e. with interdisciplinary management, including staging, clinical decision, therapy, long-term follow-up and psychological support. This is best done in centres specialized in AE. Formation of such centres should be encouraged. This not only contributes to significantly better care for AE patients but also promotes sharing of clinical experience and collection and analysis of data in a standardized way.

Surgical Treatment Aimed at Curing the Patient

If recognized early, curative treatment is possible with a combination therapy of radical surgery and subsequent drug treatment (benzimidazoles) for at least 2 years. Meticulous investigation of the interface between the lesion and the surrounding tissues and distant metastases is required so as to not expose the patient to major surgery without a high probability of definite cure (see Diagnosis, above).

Currently, surgery with the aim of cure is recommended if resection of the lesion including a 2 cm margin of healthy liver tissue is practicable. This is accompanied by at least 2 years of albendazole therapy.[46,127]

Follow-up after surgery is probably best life-long. Recurrences have been observed almost 20 years after surgery. After successful surgery, anti-Em18 or anti-Em2+ antibodies decline is rapid, and seroconversion to undetectable levels correlates well with curative resection.[123,128]

It remains to be investigated in appropriately designed clinical trials if further advancement can be made by cross-fertilization from cancer surgery; in particular as long as drugs with sufficient parasiticidal efficacy are not available. It was demonstrated in a patient with an AE lesion of the left lobe of the liver that macroscopically unsuspicious regional lymph nodes were infested with *E. multilocularis*, leading to the recommendation to routinely remove regional lymph nodes.[129]

Treatment of Patients Not Curable with Surgery

For patients with lesions which have advanced to a stage at which curative resection appears highly unlikely or impossible, benzimidazole treatment, in most cases life-long, and interdisciplinary management of acute problems, such as obstruction of bile ducts, abscess formation and thrombosis of major blood vessels, is recommended. Re-assessment of resectability should, however, depending on the individual case, be regularly performed.[46]

Partial debulking resection plus benzimidazole treatment does not seem to offer any advantage in addition to benzimidazole treatment alone.[130] At the level of disease control with benzimidazoles, palliative surgery should be restricted to individual cases with complications which cannot be otherwise controlled.[131]

Of the benzimidazoles (see Benzimidazoles, above), albendazole is preferred because of its better bioavailability and ease of administration. The recommended dose is 10–15 mg/kg per day in two divided doses with fat-rich meals.[113,132] Higher doses have been given.[133] Mebendazole 40–50 mg/kg per day split into three divided doses with fat-rich meals is an alternative if albendazole is not available. It can also be tried if albendazole is not tolerated and does seem to work in some cases.

Adverse reactions require regular investigation of liver enzymes and full blood count, initially at day 5, 10, 2-weekly intervals, then monthly and later every 3 months. Aminotransferase levels 5 times above normal and low leucocyte counts require discontinuation of benzimidazoles and work-up to investigate possible reasons. Benzimidazole-dose-dependent reasons can be investigated by measuring plasma drug levels (see below).

Monitoring of patients includes regular imaging with US at intervals which need to be adapted to circumstances and MRI/(CT) every 2–3 years. Albendazole sulfoxide plasma levels 4 h after the intake of the morning dose should be measured 1, 4 and 12 weeks after the start of benzimidazole therapy and 2–4 weeks after each dose adjustment. The therapeutic range is 0.65–3 μmol/L.[46]

There is emerging evidence that in a small proportion of long-term treated patients, benzimidazoles may act in a parasiticidal manner.[120,134,135] Reliable criteria for parasite death are, however, missing. What has become clear is that a negative PET-CT (see above) does not reliably indicate death of the parasite. In a series of patients benzimidazole treatment was discontinued on the basis of PET negativity alone and new PET activity or disease progression 18 months after treatment had been stopped was observed in more than half of the patients.[118] In another patient series authors recommended that patients should only be considered for discontinuation if the following combination of criteria is fulfilled: disappearance of anti-Em18 antibodies, more than 50% of the lesion calcified at initial diagnosis and a negative PET.[120] The issue needs to be further investigated.

Liver transplantation is the very last resort and should only be considered in the very late stages of the disease. Re-infestation rates are high after liver transplantation.[106] But residual or metastatic lesions are not necessarily a contraindication for liver transplantation since albendazole can control residual or recurrent AE.[124] There is controversy, however, about the success of controlling accelerated growth of AE metastases under immunosuppression with benzimidazoles.

With the advance of endoscopic techniques, biliary complications for example can, however, be managed very successfully, thus substantially delaying developments leading to liver failure (Figure 56.21).[117]

AE and Immunosuppression

There is accumulating evidence that patients with immunosuppression have an accelerated course of AE, including dissemination.[106]

PREVENTION

The main source of infection with AE is through contact with infected definitive hosts, ingestion of contaminated food, mainly raw fruit and vegetables and water. Echinococcal eggs are killed by dry heat and boiling water and are sensitive to desiccation but very resistant to freezing and are only killed by temperatures of −70 to −80°C. Individual preventive measures are based on precautionary measures when handling infected definitive hosts as well as food and water hygiene. Persons with a high risk of exposure to AE (i.e. hunters, laboratory personnel) may be serologically screened at regular intervals for early diagnosis and treatment.

Control and, more so, eradication of *E. multilocularis* is difficult to achieve due to the sylvatic parasite cycle. Anthelmintic treatment of the definitive host is so far the most effective control measure. Treatment of foxes with anthelminthic baits has been proven to be effective in reducing prevalence of infection in the definitive host in studies carried out in Germany, Japan and Switzerland. The synanthropic cycle of AE involves mainly domestic and stray dogs. In the hyperendemic setting of St Lawrence Island in Alaska mass treatment of dogs reduced environmental egg contamination dramatically. In endemic settings, the effect is less clear.[7,136,137]

REFERENCES

18. WHO/OIE. WHO/OIE Manual on Echinococcosis in Humans and Animals: a Public Health Problem of Global Concern (Eckert J, Gemmell MA, Meslin F-X & Pawlowski ZS eds.). World Organization for Animal Health (Office International des Epizooties) and World Health Organization; 2001.
41. Brunetti E, Garcia HH, Junghanss T. Cystic echinococcosis: chronic, complex, and still neglected. PLoS Negl Trop Dis 2011;5:e1146. doi:10.1371/journal.pntd.0001146.
46. Brunetti E, Kern P, Vuitton DA, writing panel for the WHO-IWGE. Expert consensus for the diagnosis and treatment of cystic and alveolar echinococcosis in humans. Acta Trop 2010; 114:1–16.
76. Stojkovic M, Zwahlen M, Teggi A, et al. Treatment response of cystic echinococcosis to benzimidazoles: a systematic review. PLoS Negl Trop Dis 2009;3:e524.
88. Nasseri-Moghaddam S, Abrishami A, Taefi A, et al. Percutaneous needle aspiration, injection, and re-aspiration with or without benzimidazole coverage for uncomplicated hepatic hydatid cysts. Cochrane Database Syst Rev 2011;(1):CD003623.

Access the complete references online at www.expertconsult.com

57 Other Cestode Infections: Intestinal Cestodes, Cysticercosis, Other Larval Cestode Infections

GUY BAILY | HECTOR H. GARCIA

KEY POINTS

- The larvae of several cestode parasites infect humans. The most frequent are *Taenia solium* (cysticercosis) and echinococcosis (see Chapter 56). More rare larval cestode infections include coenurosis, sparganosis and cysticercosis by *T. crassiceps.*
- *Taenia solium* cysticercosis is a major cause of seizures in most of the world. Diagnosis rests on neuroimaging and specific serology, and management involves symptomatic measures, antiparasitic drugs or surgery.
- Intestinal tapeworms in humans include *Taenia saginata* (beef tapeworm); *Taenia solium* (pork tapeworm); *Hymenolepis nana* (dwarf tapeworm); *Diphyllobothrium* spp. (fish tapeworm, mostly *D. latum* or *D. pacificum*) and the zoonotic tapeworms *Hymenolepis diminuta* (rat–flea cycle) and *Dipylidium caninum* (dog–flea cycle).
- *H. nana* is quite common because its life cycle can be maintained between humans without the necessity for any other host species.
- *D. latum* infections may cause macrocytic anaemia secondary to vitamin B_{12} deficit.

Introduction

Tapeworms or cestodes are an ancient class of highly specialized flatworm parasites. Their ancestors diverged from free-living flatworms to parasitize the earliest vertebrates in Cambrian times, and subsequently followed all the complexities of vertebrate evolution so that there are now innumerable species subtly adapted to the behaviour, diet and immunology of their hosts. Most cestodes require at least two host species to support the different stages of their life cycles. Adult tapeworms inhabit the gut of a vertebrate animal (the definitive host), with several species adapted specifically to humans. The tapeworm consists of a scolex equipped with suckers, grooves (bothria) or hooks which are the means of attachment to the intestinal wall. This is connected by an actively growing neck region (the strobila) to a chain of a variable number of segments or proglottids, which are progressively more mature towards the distal end of the worm. The mature proglottids, which form the bulk of the worm, are largely composed of hermaphrodite sexual organs and generate large numbers of eggs. A single *Taenia saginata* adult, for example, may produce 50 000 eggs daily for 10 years or more.

Cyclophyllidean cestodes (in humans *Taenia solium*, *Taenia saginata*, *Taenia asiatica* and *Hymenolepis nana*) typically have an exclusively terrestrial life cycle with a single intermediate host, which may be vertebrate or invertebrate. The intermediate host is infected by ingesting eggs which release invasive oncospheres in the gut. Oncospheres actively cross the intestinal mucosa and migrate into the host tissues and develop into one of the many distinctive, often cyst-like, morphologies of cestode larvae. The life cycle is completed if the intermediate host is eaten by a suitable definitive host in which the protoscolex of the larva can develop in the gut into a new adult tapeworm.

The Pseudophyllidean cestodes (in humans *Diphyllobothrium* sp.) have a more complex life cycle. The first intermediate host is typically an aquatic invertebrate which is infected by the procercoid larval stage of the parasite. When the invertebrate is ingested by a suitable second intermediate host, likely to be a fish or reptile, the parasite develops into an invasive, worm-like plerocercoid larva. This may then ascend the food chain through a series of further second intermediate hosts until finally reaching a suitable carnivorous vertebrate definitive host in which it can develop into an adult tapeworm. Tapeworms and larvae from both these cestode families can infect humans.

Because the relationship between the parasite and its host is central to the survival and propagation of the worm, but likely to be of more marginal significance to the host population, phenomena related to this ancient and highly adapted parasitism tend to have evolved predominantly according to the needs of the worm. Thus, it is in the interests of the propagation of the worm that its definitive host should be long-lived and active, disseminating eggs as widely as possible. Tapeworm infections tend therefore to be of trivial importance to the health of the host. In contrast, the worm's life cycle is only completed when the infected intermediate host is eaten, which may well occur more readily if the function of the intermediate host is disrupted. Larval cestode infections are, consequently, among the most serious helminthic diseases.

Cysticercosis

TAENIA SOLIUM

Transmission

Cysticercosis consists of infection with the small, bladder-like larvae of the pork tapeworm, *Taenia solium*. The life cycle of this parasite is maintained between man, the only definitive host able to harbour the adult tapeworm and pigs infected with cysticerci (Figure 57.1). Unfortunately, humans can also be readily infected with cysticerci and this is the cause of all the

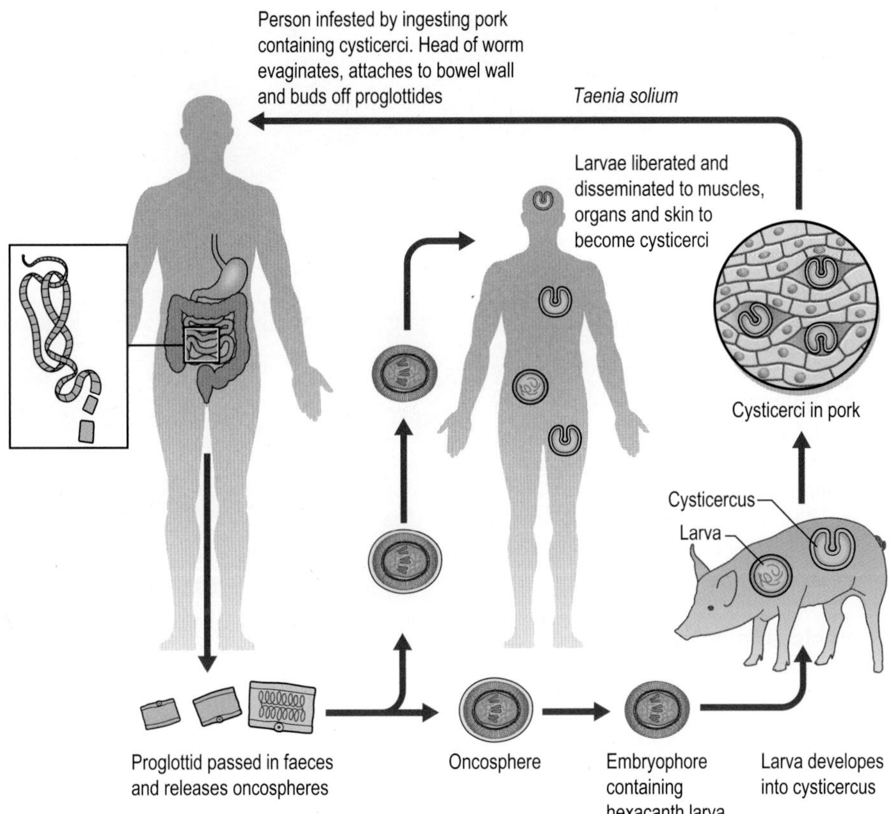

Figure 57.1 The life cycle of *T. solium*. *(Courtesy of Tropical Resources Unit, Wellcome Trust.)*

significant morbidity associated with the parasite. The tapeworms are acquired through eating undercooked pork containing cysticerci. Human cysticercosis, however, is a faecal–oral infection acquired by ingesting eggs excreted in the faeces of a human tapeworm carrier. Individuals harbouring an adult *T. solium* are at high risk of acquiring cysticercosis, probably through faecal–oral autoinfection. It has long been hypothesized that internal autoinfection might also occur as a result of reverse peristalsis, allowing taenia eggs to travel from the small bowel to the stomach and thus become activated and invasive. Little, if any, evidence has emerged to support this.

Cysticercosis was originally a ubiquitous disease occurring wherever pigs and humans existed in association and is probably of great antiquity: Aristotle gives a clear description of the condition in pigs. It was once common in central Europe, with autopsy rates of 2% in Berlin[1] in the first half of the nineteenth century, coinciding closely with the 1.9% described some years ago in Mexico City.[2] The parasite has long since been all but eradicated from the most developed countries but it remains common in Central and South America, most of sub-Saharan Africa, South Asia and China. It is rare in the Islamic countries of North Africa and South-west Asia. In the 1970s, an epidemic of cysticercosis occurred among the highland people of Irian Jaya[3] after the introduction of the parasite into a culture where pigs are of central importance and hygiene is primitive. The problem was first identified because of a dramatic increase in the incidence of severe burns related to individuals having a seizure and falling into domestic fires.

Pathology

Ingested taenia eggs, activated by gastric and duodenal environments, release invasive larvae, termed oncospheres, in the small intestine. These migrate across the intestinal wall and are probably carried by the bloodstream to the sites at which they eventually settle and mature into cysticerci, a process which takes approximately 2 months. Cysticerci may occur anywhere in the body, although they are mostly found in the central nervous system, the eye, and more rarely, in the subcutaneous tissues and muscle, probably due to improved survival in protected areas like the CNS or the eye. *Cysticerci* vary from a few millimetres to 2 cm or more across but are typically a little less than 1 cm, the largest cysts tending to be intracranial, particularly in the ventricles and the larger subarachnoid spaces. Established cysticerci that are neither actively growing nor degenerating elicit very little host immune response. The typical appearance in the brain is of the cyst surrounded by compressed, laminated host tissue with only a slight inflammatory infiltrate.[4] Dead, calcified or hyalinized cysts may be surrounded by a similar host-derived capsule. However, new, very large or degenerating cysts may all be associated with a much more extensive inflammatory response.

Clinical Features

The morbidity of cysticercosis is almost entirely due to central nervous system or ocular disease. Subcutaneous cysts are of only cosmetic significance. A heavy parasite load in muscle may give rise to some aching and altered function[5] but this is not common. Serious problems are confined to those anatomical sites where a small space-occupying lesion, with or without some inflammation, can give rise to a major disturbance in function. Such sites include the eye and, very rarely, the conducting system of the heart, but overwhelmingly, neurocysticercosis is the principal clinical problem.

Neurocysticercosis. Although autopsy rates for neurocysticercosis in areas of high prevalence may approach 2%, the majority of these cases have had no symptoms in life attributable to the infection.[2] When symptoms do occur, the most common manifestation is epilepsy. Studies from endemic areas suggest that cysticercosis is a major cause of epilepsy, accounting for one-third to a half of late-onset cases,[6–8] and it is particularly prominent as a cause of focal epilepsy in children in the Indian subcontinent. However, any neurological syndrome attributable to one or more small space-occupying lesions can occur, including focal weakness and extrapyramidal disorders. Changes in mental state, including cognitive impairment and psychiatric disease, are also very common[9,10]

The clinical expression of neurocysticercosis is mainly determined by the location of the parasites (among other factors as their number, size, evolutive stage and degree of host inflammation). Two major groups can be separated: intraparenchymal NCC, associated with seizure disorders and, generally, with a reasonably good prognosis and extraparenchymal NCC, associated with intracranial hypertension, progressive disease and significant mortality.[11]

Intraparenchymal NCC can present as any combination of viable, degenerating or calcified cysts. Initially, cysts present as non-inflamed, fluid-filled vesicles and seem to be associated with few symptoms. They can survive at this stage for years by means of a series of active immune evasion mechanisms. At some point, however, the immune system of the host detects the parasite and launches an active inflammatory response, which ends up killing the parasitic cyst. During this involutive process, the cyst contents become turbid, the vesicle shrinks and then it is gradually cleaned leaving a scar which eventually calcifies.

Single Enhancing Lesion. In the Indian subcontinent, a single small enhancing lesion on computerized tomography (CT) is commonly seen in patients presenting for the first time with epilepsy, disappearing within a few months of follow-up. Cysticercosis is the major cause of these lesions.[12]

Extraparenchymal NCC can present in the convexity of the hemispheres, Sylvian fissure, basal subarachnoid cisterns, or inside the ventricles. With the exception of cysts in the convexity, which behave as intraparenchymal cysts, cysts in other extraparenchymal locations tend to grow and infiltrate, blocking the CSF circulation and causing hydrocephalus and intracranial hypertension. This condition requires surgical management and may be lethal if untreated.

More rare presentations include chronic meningitis, with headache and global changes in cerebral function associated with markedly abnormal CSF but no fever, neck stiffness nor cranial nerve palsies,[13] or cysticercal encephalitis, when a massive cyst load is associated with a brisk and severe inflammatory response.[14] In children in particular, the inflammatory response may dominate the clinical picture, with a rapidly progressive illness over a few weeks characterized by seizures; a variety of focal neurological abnormalities; deteriorating cognitive function; and raised intracranial pressure. Also, a variety of spinal cord syndromes has been reported in association with cysts in and around the cord and the cauda equina. The most common presentation is of progressive paraplegia developing over a period of weeks.

Ocular Cysticercosis. Cysticerci are seen in the eye and annexes with some frequency.[4] The great majority of cysts are subretinal or in the vitreous humour but they could occur at any site. Clinical manifestations include altered vision and blindness. It is important to rule out intraocular cysticercosis before administering antiparasitic treatment for NCC, since the resulting inflammatory reaction can severely damage the eye.

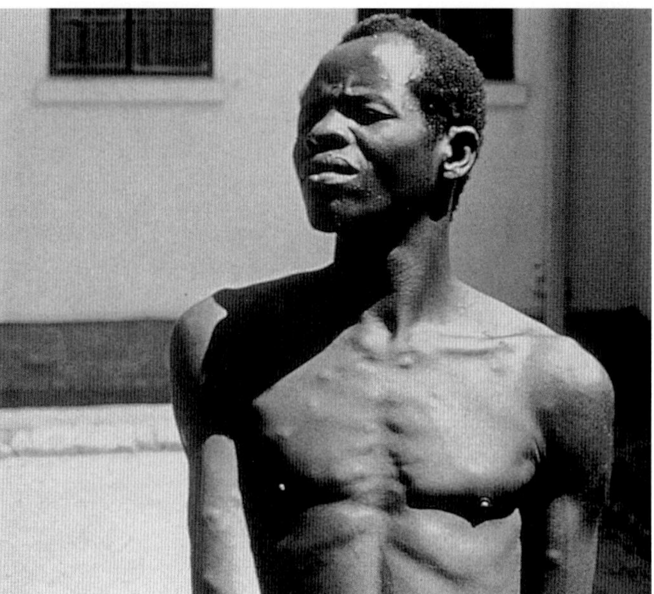

Figure 57.2 Readily visible subcutaneous cysticerci. *(Courtesy of Tropical Resources Unit, Wellcome Trust.)*

Diagnosis

The clinical diagnosis of neurocysticercosis is often difficult, as there is nothing specific about the neurological presentation. It becomes even more difficult in poor, rural endemic regions, where CT or MRI or even specific serology are not available. The presence of extracranial cysticerci, although not frequent, may provide an important clue to the diagnosis. Subcutaneous cysts (Figure 57.2) can be palpated and, if in doubt, excised for histological examination. Cysts in striated muscle are in a more stressful environment than those in the central nervous system and die and calcify more rapidly. Spindle-shaped calcifications, particularly in the large proximal muscles (Figure 57.3), may be visible on radiography. However, such clues are often absent. Spinal cysticerci may be demonstrated on myelography (Figure 57.4). Otherwise, support for the diagnosis must be obtained from brain imaging and confirmed by serology.

Imaging. Modern imaging techniques have proved very powerful in demonstrating the presence of cysticerci in the brain and have also taught us a good deal about the natural history of the disease. Either CT or MRI[15,16] can demonstrate viable or degenerating cysts, calcifications, intraventricular lesions, or cisternal cysts or membranes. Information on the number, location, size and degree of inflammation around lesions is very useful to establish the diagnosis, as well as to guide the management of the patient. MRI is particularly valuable,[16] as with other pathologies, in demonstrating posterior fossa and spinal lesions. It is also superior for imaging ventricular cysts which, having a similar radiodensity to CSF, are less easily visualized on CT. On the other hand, calcifications are poorly defined on MRI (Figure 57.5).

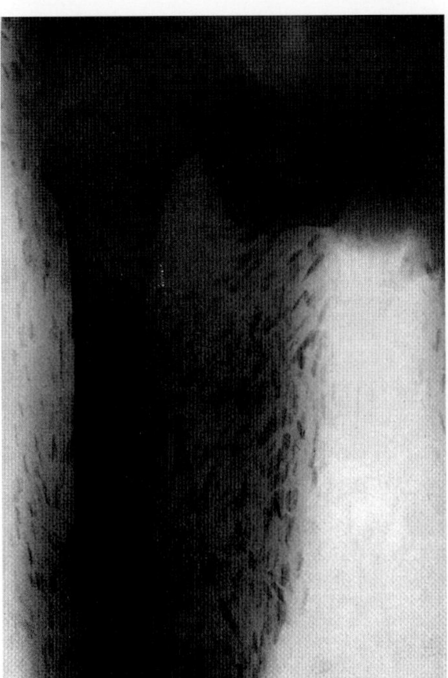

Figure 57.3 Very large numbers of calcified cysticerci in thigh muscle.

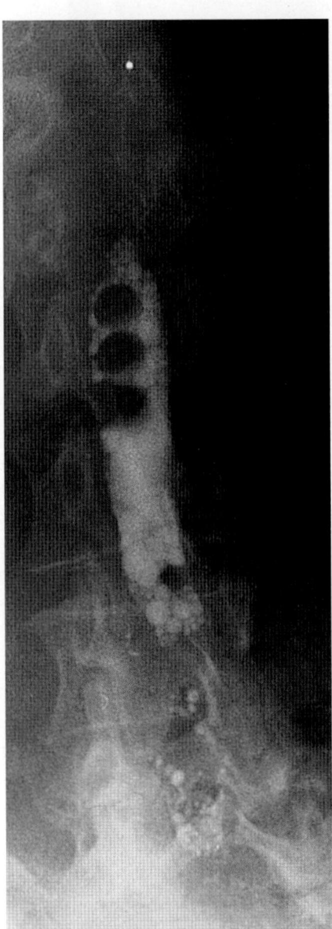

Figure 57.4 Cysticerci around the cauda equina on myelography.

Serological Diagnosis. Many serological methods have been described for cysticercosis using most of the conventional serodiagnostic techniques and a wide variety of antigens. Antigens were originally extracted from *T. solium* cysts. Glycoproteins extracted from cyst fluid have been found to be most discriminatory[17] but this is a complex process and an adequate supply of *T. solium* cysts can also be problematic. More recent developments have therefore focused on recombinant and synthetic versions of these proteins[18] or alternatively extracted homologous proteins from the animal parasite *T. crassiceps*, which are more readily obtained.[19] Cross-reactivity with other helminthic infections, particularly hydatidosis and taeniasis, remains a problem in ELISA assays but has been reduced with the use of more refined antigens. Antigen can also be detected in the blood and declining serum levels have been associated with successful treatment.[20]

Other Tests. Some abnormality of the CSF is found in approximately 50% of cases of neurocysticercosis – usually a mild pleocytosis or raised protein. A persistently high CSF protein is associated with a poor prognosis, often with progression to hydrocephalus and without surgical intervention, consequent dementia and blindness.

Management

Until the 1980s, there was no drug therapy that was known to be effective against cysticercosis. Treatment was therefore mostly symptomatic, although surgical intervention to remove cysts or to deal with their consequences, such as hydrocephalus, was sometimes appropriate. Since that time, it has been shown that anthelmintics can be effective in reducing the numbers of cysts present on CT.[21] The extent to which this leads to clinical benefit is more problematical and the exact role of anthelmintics remains the subject of debate. In parenchymal neurocysticercosis with viable cysts, there is evidence of both radiographical and clinical improvement after anthelmintic treatment.[22] In patients with only enhancing lesions, however, information is either contradictory or lacking. Patients with seizures associated with calcified cysts are unlikely to gain any benefit from anthelmintic treatment. Markedly enhancing parenchymal lesions, which constitute the most common appearance in children, have been shown to disappear spontaneously from the CT image within a year.[12] From this observation it has been suggested that such cases can generally be managed with symptomatic treatment and corticosteroids to reduce the local inflammatory response and that anthelmintics are unnecessary. This very benign view of cysticercosis reflects experience with childhood and imported disease in North America.[23] Conversely, some recent controlled studies show more rapid resolution of enhancing cysts and less frequent seizure relapses with anticysticercotics.[24] In contrast, reports from tropical countries have shown that a proportion of cases have multilesional, chronic disease and frequently relapsing symptoms, likely reflecting heavier exposure or different transmission mechanisms; some of these develop severe neurological consequences such as hydrocephalus.[25] When the inflammatory response dominates the clinical picture, as in cysticercotic encephalitis, anticysticercotics are likely to exacerbate the condition in the short term and should be avoided. Each case must be evaluated on its merits, but symptomatic treatment and close observation may sometimes be a reasonable approach.

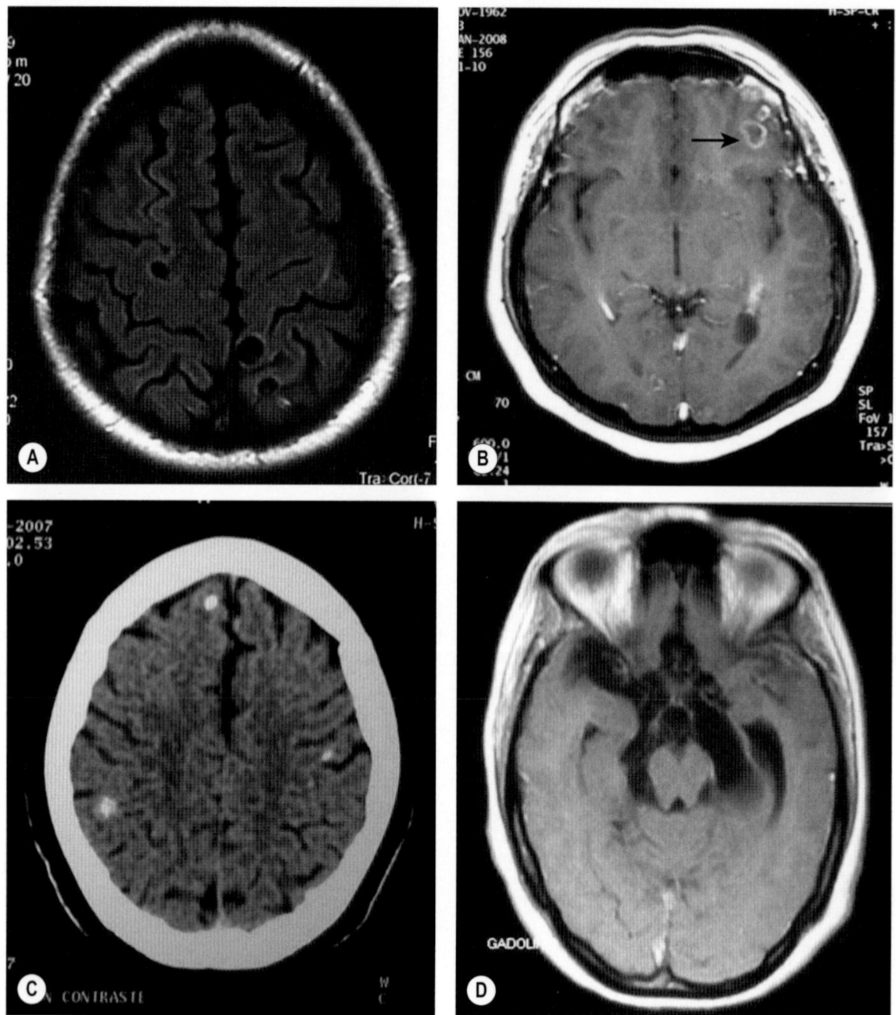

Figure 57.5 (A) Viable cysts on MRI (FLAIR protocol); (B) a degenerating cyst enhancing after contrast administration (MRI, T1 protocol); (C) multiple parenchymal brain calcifications on CT; (D) basal subarachnoid cysticercosis. Note the extensive involvement of the cisterns around the brainstem.

The first drug to be shown to be effective was praziquantel, given at 50 mg/kg daily for 15 days. Albendazole has also been studied extensively. In substantial doses (15 mg/kg daily for 30 days), it appears to have at least an equivalent effect on reducing cysts present on CT and has come to be the drug of first choice. The ideal dose of both drugs remains uncertain. Eight days of albendazole appears to be of equivalent efficacy to the original 30 days and has been widely adopted. Much shorter courses of praziquantel, e.g. 50 mg/kg daily for 8 days or even 3 doses of 25 mg/kg at 2-hourly intervals on a single day, have been shown to be effective in small numbers of cases.[26–29]

The significant adverse effects of anticysticercal therapy are similar for the two drugs. They appear to be directly related to the damage inflicted on cysticerci and the consequent acute inflammatory response. This may result in cerebral oedema and raised intracranial pressure, particularly if there are many cysts. Typically, a severe headache arises – sometimes within a few hours of commencing therapy but more often after 2–4 days. If treated symptomatically, most of these will resolve without sequelae but a minority will develop a severe acute illness with cerebral infarction and deaths have been reported. Concomitant use of corticosteroids in substantial doses is effective in suppressing this in most (though not all) cases and is almost always appropriate. The dose and type of steroid used vary considerably between centres, with dexamethasone around 0.1 mg/kg per day being the most usual regimen. Steroids have the unwanted effect of decreasing levels of praziquantel, though not albendazole.

Surgical excision is still conventionally recommended for intraventricular cysts. Neuroendoscopic removal is now the preferred technique, with multiple series reporting very good results. It may benefit from post-surgical antiparasitic treatment. Extraparenchymal disease may require protracted steroid therapy to control arachnoiditis, as well as anticysticercotics (Table 57.1).

Control. Control of the parasite has been achieved in developed countries by the interruption of its life cycle following improvements in sanitation and commercial, formal pig raising. In contrast, in developing countries, pigs often live in close association with man, rooting around for food within village compounds, with easy access to human faeces (Figure 57.6). Animals are likely to be slaughtered within the village and there may be no understanding of the health significance of 'measly' pig meat. The difficulties of introducing good sanitation and modern abattoir practices into poor communities are

TABLE 57.1 **Specific Treatment Options for Symptomatic NCC (Beyond Symptomatic Treatment)**

PARENCHYMAL NCC	
Viable cysts	Antiparasitic drugs plus steroids
Degenerating cysts	Antiparasitic drugs plus steroids/ steroids alone
Calcifications	No specific treatment
EXTRAPARENCHYMAL NCC	
Subarachnoid NCC, basal or in the convexity of the brain hemispheres	Antiparasitic drugs plus steroids, long term
Subarachnoid NCC – giant cysts or cysts clusters in the Sylvian fissure	Surgery or antiparasitic drugs with steroids
Intraventricular NCC	Neuroendoscopic exeresis when possible. If not, the decision between open surgery and antiparasitic drugs depend on the location, number and size of the cyst(s) and the risks of acute hydrocephalus and intracranial hypertension

considerable. An alternative strategy has been to reduce tapeworm carriage by mass chemotherapy and this has been shown to reduce both human taeniasis and porcine cysticercosis.[30] In Africa, there is hope that transmission could be reduced as a by-product of mass treatment campaigns using praziquantel directed against schistosomiasis. Vaccines have been developed to prevent porcine cysticercosis but it is not yet clear whether this will prove an effective control strategy.[31,32]

Other Larval Cestode Infections

COENUROSIS

Taenia multiceps is a parasite of dogs, with sheep being the principal intermediate host. The larval metacestode takes the form of a coenurus, a single cyst with multiple invaginated protoscolices in its wall, which may grow to be several centimetres in diameter. In sheep, these often develop in the hindbrain, giving rise to the condition known as 'staggers'. Other closely related *Taenia* species also give rise to a coenurus, which may be morphologically indistinguishable. Human coenurosis is a rare but often serious condition. While most cases have occurred in subcutaneous tissue, the parasite may affect the human brain and cause severe neurological disease.

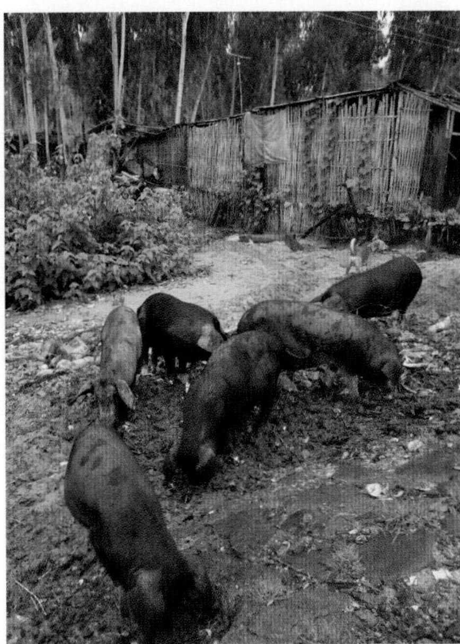

Figure 57.6 Pigs scavenging for food in an African village. *(Courtesy of Dr. Seth O'Neal.)*

Prevalence and Distribution

Cases have been reported from a wide geographical area and are rare. Most reports have been from Africa and South America but there have also been cases in Europe (notably Sardinia) and North America. Extracranial localization has been most frequent in reports from tropical Africa, while reports from South Africa and elsewhere have been almost entirely of central nervous system involvement, giving rise to the suspicion that there is some heterogeneity among the causative parasites.[33]

Clinical Features

Neurological features are those of a substantial intracranial mass lesion accompanied by varying degrees of inflammation. The cisterna magna is a particularly common site and is associated with basal arachnoiditis and hydrocephalus. Untreated, there is usually progressive neurological disease and a poor outcome. Eye involvement may result in loss of vision.

Diagnosis and Treatment

Intracranial lesions appear on computerized tomography (CT) as clear cysts 2 cm or more in diameter without a discernable internal structure. Definitive diagnosis can only be made by histology; it is distinguished from cysticercosis and hydatidosis by the presence of both multiple protoscolices and a ridged cuticle. Occasionally, the protoscolices may have degenerated, in which case the condition is difficult to distinguish from racemose cysticercosis. Surgical excision has been curative in some cases. Although praziquantel appears effective against the parasite, the clinical benefits are less clear.[34]

TAENIA CRASSICEPS CYSTICERCOSIS

Rodents are the preferred host for the *cysticerci* of this parasite but rare human infections have been reported, most recently in association with AIDS. A developing soft tissue mass is found to contain numerous cysticerci. Six months continuous praziquantel and albendazole, both in high doses, gave clinical remission in one reported case, but relapse occurred on cessation of therapy.[35]

SPARGANOSIS

Plerocercoid larvae of the *Spirometra* genus of pseudophyllidean cestodes are capable of infecting man. These organisms resemble *Diphyllobothrium* spp. in their life cycles, with canines or other terrestrial carnivores as definitive hosts, a procercoid larval stage in the water flea *Cyclops* and plerocercoids naturally infecting reptiles, amphibians and small mammals. Human sparganosis has been attributed to several species, including Spirometra *mansoni*, *S. mansonoides* and, in Africa, *S. theileri*. Human infection occurs either by the ingestion of procercoid-infected invertebrates in drinking water, by ingestion of

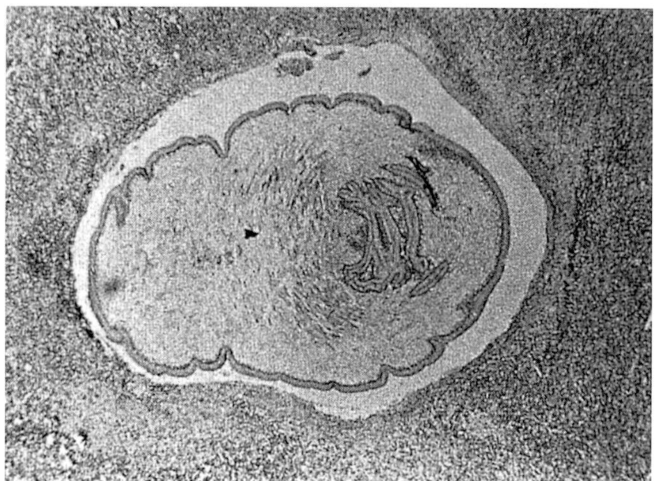

Figure 57.7 Sparganosis. Cross-section showing typical tapeworm morphology. A dense eosinophilic infiltration is present in the adjacent muscle. *(Courtesy of H. Zaiman.)*

plerocercoids through eating uncooked frogs or snakes or possibly by direct transfer of a plerocercoid from fresh frog or snake tissue applied to wounds or inflamed eyes, as is the custom in some parts of East Asia. The plerocercoid, or sparganum, is a motile worm of very variable size (1–50 cm) but is more typically a few centimetres in length and 1–2 mm in width. It excites a brisk inflammatory response as it migrates through host tissues; in some instances it is found to be contained within a cyst or abscess cavity. Multiple infections occur.

Prevalence and Distribution

A sizeable number of cases of sparganosis have been recorded very widely in the tropics and subtropics. South-east Asia and East Africa are the areas of highest prevalence. Autochthonous cases are reported from North and South America.

Clinical Features

The typical history is of inflammatory, sometimes migratory, subcutaneous swellings. These may break down to discharge the worm. Eosinophilia is common but not invariable. The most frequently described sites are the chest and legs. Involvement of the periorbital tissues may cause damage to the eye. Penetration of larvae into the brain – where they cause an intense local inflammatory lesion with invariably major neurological consequences – is uncommon but well described.[36]

Diagnosis and Treatment

The condition must be distinguished from that caused by other migratory helminths producing swellings, such as in gnathostomiasis and loiasis. Serological methods have been developed but they are not widely available. Excision and identification of the worm remains necessary for a clear diagnosis (Figure 57.7). Excision is also the only effective treatment of the parasite, wherever situated, including the brain. No drug therapy has been shown to be beneficial and the killing of the worm within the tissues may not in any case be a desirable goal, as it is likely to lead to much more intense inflammation in the short term.

Proliferative Sparganosis

A very rare variant of *sparganosis* has been described, from both Asia and the Americas, in which the parasite buds and proliferates, either as an expanding mass or as multiple small disseminated lesions. Clinically, there may be numerous small cutaneous nodules or larger painful tumours. The lesions contain worm-derived structures, some clearly resembling a typical sparganum but of very variable morphology. The condition is slowly progressive, with death resulting from deep organ involvement. There is no known treatment; praziquantel and mebendazole have failed in one case.[37]

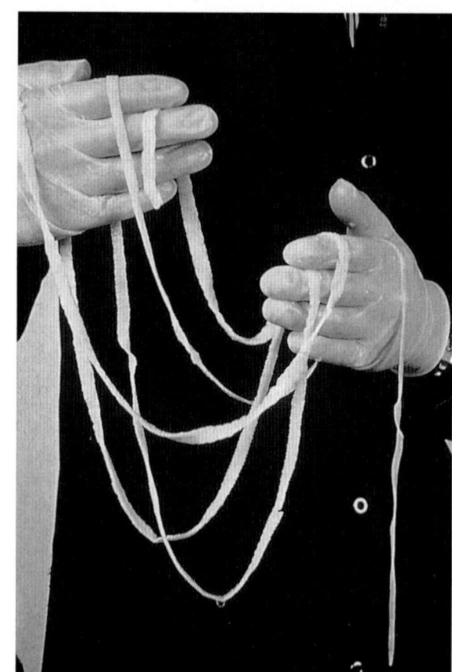

Figure 57.8 Adult beef tapeworm (*T. saginata*). *(Courtesy of G. S. Nelson.)*

Intestinal Cestodes: the Tapeworms of Humans

TAENIA SAGINATA

T. saginata is the beef tapeworm (Figure 57.8). Man is the only definitive host and cattle are the significant intermediate hosts (Figure 57.9), though a variety of ungulates have been reported as being infected. The larval stage is a translucent fluid-filled bladder or cysticercus between 5 and 10 mm in diameter but, unlike the *T. solium* cysticercus, it has never been reliably described in a human. The adult is a large, white tapeworm that can reach 10 m in length, though more typically 2–5 m, weighing around 20–30 g. The scolex is equipped with suckers but not hooks (Figures 57.10). Mature proglottids detached from the distal end of the worm are highly motile and their independent emergence from the anus is the principal cause of symptomatology. An infected individual commonly harbours more than one worm. Human infection is acquired by eating undercooked beef. Cattle are infected when their feed or grazing is contaminated by human faeces.

Prevalence and Distribution

Originally a ubiquitous parasite, transmission has been prevented in developed countries by the sanitary disposal of

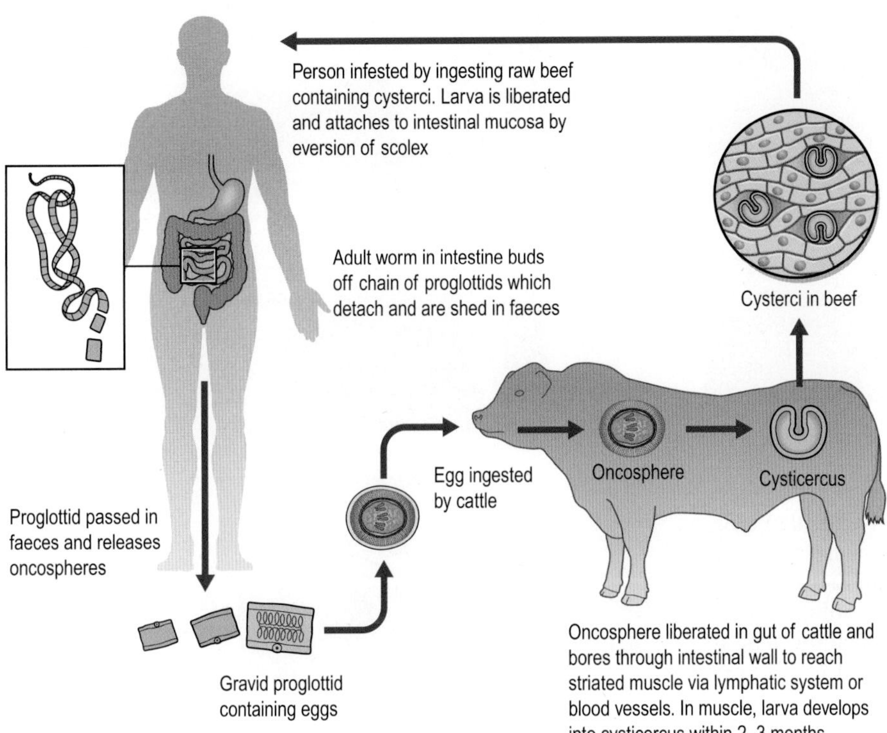

Figure 57.9 Life cycle of *T. saginata*. *(Courtesy of Tropical Resources Unit, Wellcome Trust.)*

human faeces and the detection of infected meat at abattoirs. It remains common elsewhere, especially in poorer communities where raw or undercooked beef is traditionally eaten. Highland Ethiopia is an area of intense transmission.

Clinical Features

T. saginata carriers are often aware of motile proglottids which can be felt emerging from the anus unbidden and may cause some distress. They are also conspicuous in the faeces because of their motility. Otherwise infection is largely asymptomatic. A number of 'irritable bowel-type' symptoms, particularly abdominal pain but also nausea, distension and anorexia, have been attributed to the parasite but these are so common in the general population that causality is difficult to prove. Rarely segments of worm may be vomited. Eosinophilia is not a feature of established infection.

Diagnosis and Treatment

Whenever the scolex is recovered, the absence of hooks confirms the diagnosis of species. *Taenia* eggs have a characteristic

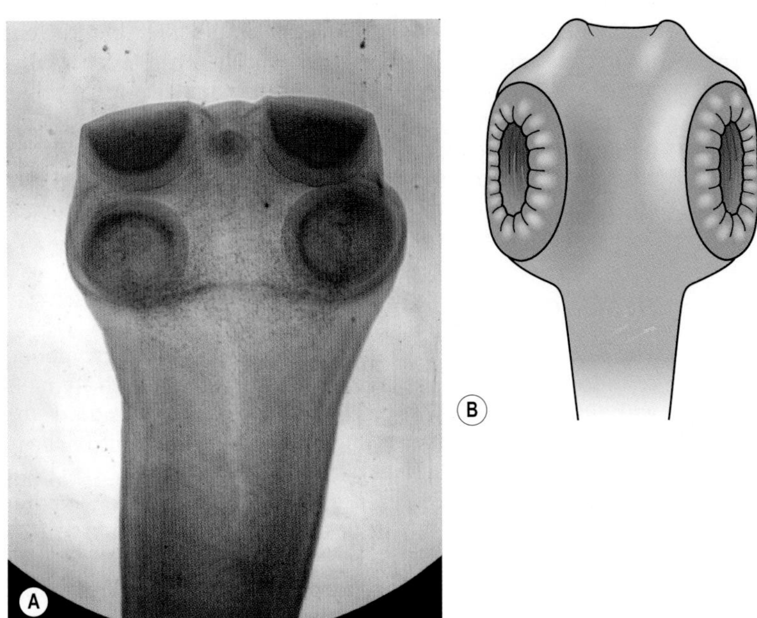

Figure 57.10 (A) *T. saginata* (unarmed tapeworm) scolex. Suckers without hooklets. (B) *Taenia saginata* head, showing suckers. *((A) Courtesy of Dr. J. Jimenez.)*

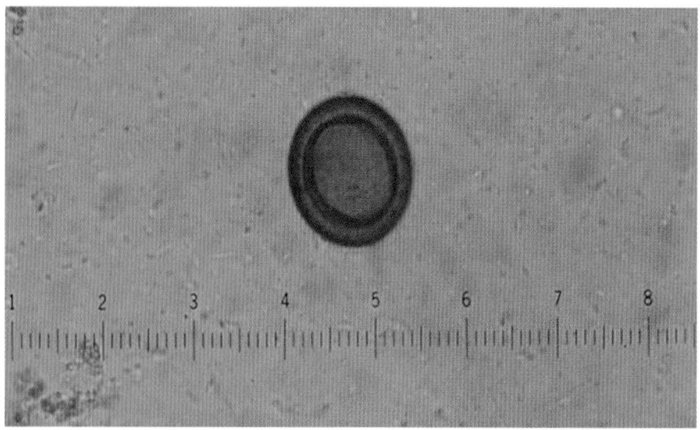

Figure 57.11 *Taenia eggs. (Courtesy of Dr. J. Jimenez.)*

appearance (Figure 57.11) and can be detected by faecal microscopy. Since all *Taenia* eggs are very similar they are not easily speciated, although they can be distinguished on Ziehl–Neelsen staining,[38] or by the use of molecular techniques. Soluble *Taenia* antigens can be detected in faeces but present methods tend to be cross-reactive between species and the value of this is principally for epidemiological surveillance.[39] Intact proglottids in reasonable condition can be speciated by the number of uterine branches. A single dose of praziquantel at 10 mg/kg is effective therapy. Niclosamide has also been used extensively.

Taenia Saginata Asiatica

An adult *Taenia* morphologically identical to *T. saginata* was discovered in indigenous highland people in Taiwan in areas where there are no cattle. The cysticerci, a little smaller than those of *T. solium* or *T. saginata*, are found in a number of mammalian species, including pigs, in which they have a strong tropism for the liver.[40] Molecular genetic studies show the parasite to be closely related to, but distinct from, *T. saginata*.[41] It has now been identified in other parts of East Asia including Korea and Indonesia. It does not appear to cause human cysticercosis.

TAENIA SOLIUM

Man is the only known definitive host for the pork tapeworm, *T. solium* – with pigs serving as the intermediate host. The adult tapeworm is somewhat smaller than *T. saginata* and the scolex is markedly different, being armed with two encircling rows of curved hooklets (Figure 57.12), which can also be identified on the protoscolex of the cysticercus. Detached proglottids are much less motile and consequently less likely to be noticed than are those of *T. saginata*. The chief significance of the parasite is that humans are readily infected by the larval cysticerci as well as the adult worm, giving rise to human cysticercosis. This is discussed above, together with the transmission, prevalence and control of the parasite.

Clinical Features

The great majority of *T. solium* carriers are unaware of their infection and it is detected only by screening. Minor abdominal symptoms may occur, as with *T. saginata*. However, carriers carry a substantial risk of acquiring cysticercosis by faecal–oral autoinfection and members of their household are also at increased risk.[42]

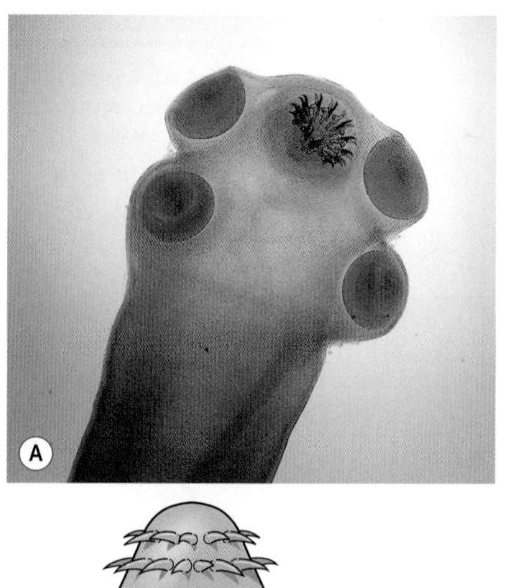

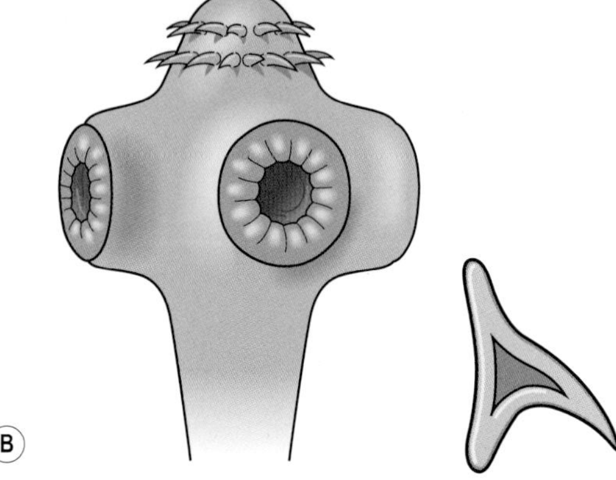

Figure 57.12 (A) *T. solium* (pig tapeworm) (armed tapeworm) scolex showing hooklets. (B) *T. solium* head, showing suckers and the arrangement of the hooklet. *((A) Courtesy of Tropical Resources Unit, Wellcome Trust. (B) Courtesy of Dr. J. Jimenez.)*

Diagnosis and Treatment

The detection and speciation of *Taenia* infections have been discussed above, under *T. saginata*. Treatment is also similar for the two infections, with niclosamide 2 g in a single dose being the drug of choice. The rationale for this is that niclosamide is not absorbed while in tapeworm carriers who also have latent viable neurocysticercosis, praziquantel could affect these silent brain cysts and cause seizures in previously asymptomatic individuals. It has previously been common practice to combine anthelmintic therapy for *T. solium* with a purgative since eggs of the dying worm were believed to constitute a risk of cysticercosis through internal autoinfection. No evidence has ever emerged to support this hypothesis and purgation is no longer regarded as necessary.

HYMENOLEPIS NANA

The dwarf tapeworm *H. nana* (Figure 57.13) is unique among cestodes in that the life cycle is maintained between humans without the necessity for any other host species; indeed, the same individual acts as intermediate and definitive host. Ingested oncospheres (Figure 57.14) are activated by the gut and invade the small intestinal mucosa where they encyst within a villus. Within 3–4 days, the protoscolex of this cercocyst evaginates to become the scolex of an adult worm. This attaches to the intestinal wall, the remainder of the worm developing to a mature length of 3–4 cm over about 1 month, after which egg

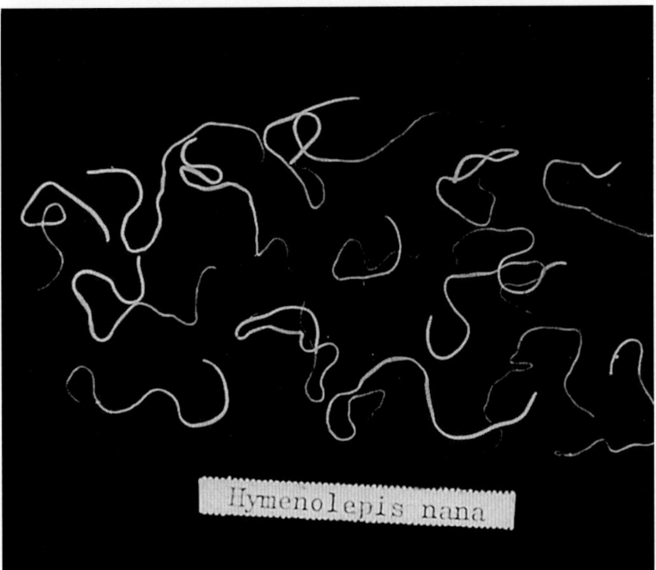

Figure 57.13 *H. nana* (dwarf tapeworm). *(Courtesy of Tropical Resources Unit, Wellcome Trust.)*

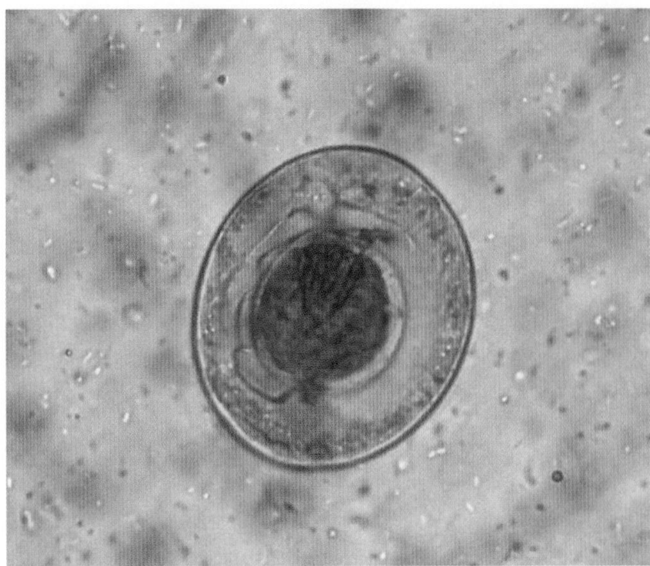

Figure 57.14 *H. nana* (dwarf tapeworm). Egg. *(Courtesy of Dr. J. Jimenez.)*

production begins. Detached proglottids degenerate during passage through the intestine, releasing their cargo of eggs and are not seen in the faeces. Infections involving several hundred worms are common. Spread is by faecal–oral transmission with autoinfection, particularly among children, amplifying the intensity of infection. Rodents may act as an alternative definitive host and insects are capable of infection with the larval stage but neither of these appears to be important in parasite transmission.

Prevalence and Distribution

H. nana is a very common parasite in warm climates where sanitation is poor, particularly in children, among whom the prevalence is often in the region of 2–3%.

Clinical Features

A variety of symptoms have been attributed to *H. nana* infection, including abdominal pain and anorexia, as well as systemic complaints such as irritability and headache. Eosinophilia is common. Several reports have associated infection with growth retardation.[43] It is difficult to be certain whether these features are truly a direct result of the parasite or whether it is acting as a marker of faecal–oral infection, insanitation and poverty,[44] but heavy infections probably do have significant clinical consequences.

Diagnosis and Treatment

Diagnosis is by detecting the characteristic egg on faecal microscopy. The cercocyst stage is in contact with the host immune system and consequently, unlike other tapeworm infections, there is a consistent humoral response for serology to be of some diagnostic value. An enzyme-linked immunosorbent assay (ELISA) has been developed with sensitivity of about 80%.[45] There is extensive cross-reaction with other cestode infections. A single dose of praziquantel is an effective therapy. At least 20 mg/kg is recommended. Niclosamide has also been widely used. Mebendazole only gives cure rates around 50%.

Control

As with other faecal–oral infections, control depends on sanitation and education.

DIPHYLLOBOTHRIUM LATUM

Man can act as definitive host for a variety of pseudophyllidean tapeworms of the genus *Diphyllobothrium* (Table 57.2). Various tiny aquatic invertebrates, especially *Cyclops* water fleas, are the first intermediate host for these parasites (Figure 57.15). The plerocercoid larvae ascend to the apex of the aquatic food chain, with species specificity in their adaptation to particular larger fish. Definitive hosts include birds and marine and terrestrial

TABLE 57.2 Species of *Diphyllobothrium* Infecting Humans

Species	Second Intermediate Host	Principal Definitive Host	Geographical Range
D. latum	Pike, perch, etc.	Man	Widespread
D. cordatum	?	Bearded seals	Greenland, Alaska
D. dalliae	Blackfish	Canines?	Alaska, Eastern Siberia
D. dendriticum	Char, salmon, trout	Gulls	Throughout sub-Arctic
D. klebanovskii	Pacific salmon	Marine mammals	Eastern Siberia
D. nihonkaiense	Pacific salmon	Marine mammals?	Japan
D. pacificum	Var. marine fish	Sea lions	Pacific South America
D. ursi	Pacific salmon	Bears	Alaska, Canada

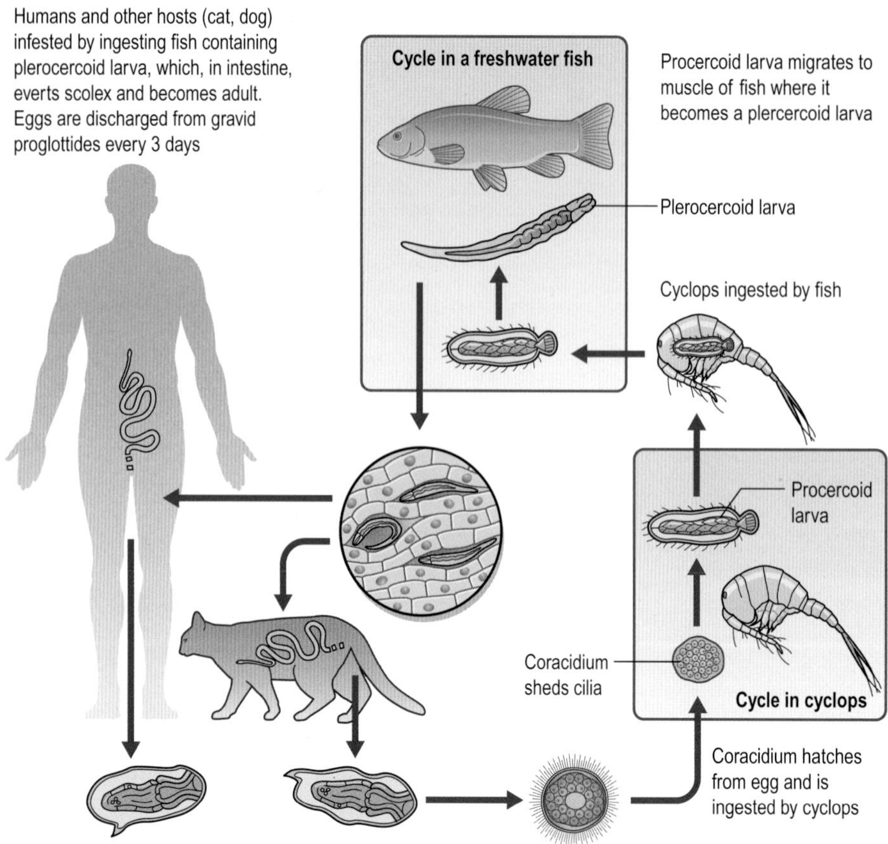

Figure 57.15 Life cycle of *D. latum*. *(Courtesy of Tropical Resources Unit, Wellcome Trust.)*

mammals. *D. latum*, the fish tapeworm, is the species most adapted to humans; bears and other terrestrial carnivores may act as paratenic hosts but man is generally the host that is significant in transmission. It is a large (up to 10 m), slightly translucent tapeworm (Figure 57.16), inhabiting the small intestine where it attaches by means of two longitudinal slit-like suckers or bothria. Infections are commonly multiple and occasionally, there may be more than 100 individual worms. The largest recorded total length of *D. latum* tapeworm(s) expelled from one patient is 330 m.[46] The preferred second intermediate hosts are temperate freshwater fish, especially pike, perch and burbot.[47,48] Human infection is acquired by eating undercooked fish. Both freezing and cooking effectively destroy the parasite.

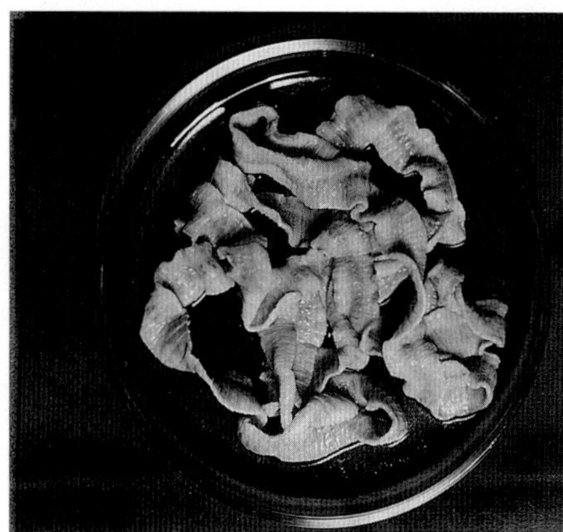

Figure 57.16 *D. latum* (fish tapeworm). Adult. *(Courtesy of Tropical Resources Unit, Wellcome Trust.)*

Prevalence and Distribution

Although the disease is reported from many parts of the world, most transmission occurs in Russia. The original heartland of *D. latum* infection extended from eastern Scandinavia across northern Russia and into western Siberia. In Finland, >20% of the entire nation was infected as recently as 1950. There have also been intense foci of transmission in the Danube delta in Romania and in the lakes of northern Italy and western Switzerland. Transmission is now uncommon in Western Europe but continues to be reported, particularly in Sweden, Finland, Switzerland and northern Italy. In Russia, there have been control programmes but also setbacks and transmission continues to be common, with some extension of the range of the parasite, due to engineering project changes in the river systems. The parasite has also been spread very widely by human migration and low-intensity transmission of *D. latum* has been recorded from many parts of the world.

A number of species of *Diphyllobothrium* other than *D. latum* have been reported as infecting humans (Table 57.1). *D. dendriticum* is the cause of human diphyllobothriasis among the indigenous people of the subarctic region, where it infects salmonid fish, especially Arctic char.[48] Gulls are the most significant definitive hosts. Prevalences of more than 30% have been recorded in Canadian Inuit communities. Several other parasites infect humans around the northern Pacific, through Pacific salmon, including *D. klebanovskii*, which is the principal

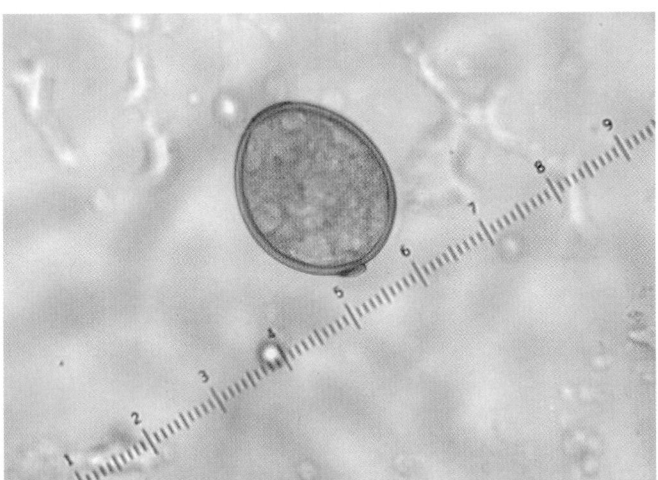

Figure 57.17 *D. latum* (fish tapeworm). Egg. *(Courtesy of Dr. J. Jimenez.)*

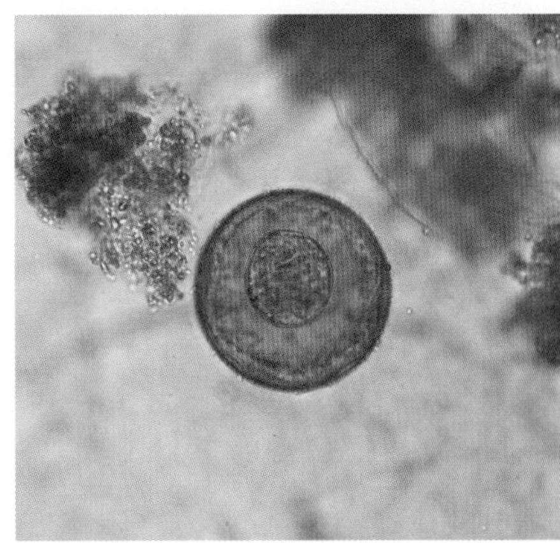

Figure 57.18 *H. diminuta* (rat tapeworm). Egg. *(Courtesy of Dr. J. Jimenez.)*

parasite in the Russian Far East, and *D. nihonkaiense* in Japan. The much smaller *D. pacificum* occurs in Chile and Peru and is acquired through the consumption of the traditional dishes of marinated raw fish known as 'ceviche'. The clinical consequences of all these infections have not been well studied but are considered to be minor.[49]

Clinical Features

As with other tapeworm infections, carriers experience few, if any, symptoms. A controlled study in Finland showed that some of the minor symptoms traditionally attributed to infection, including abdominal pain, were not significantly associated with carriage, although diarrhoea, headache and nonspecific malaise all appeared to be more common.[47] Proglottids are seldom noticed in the faeces but occasionally carriers may become aware of their infection through the spontaneous expulsion of a whole worm.

Tapeworm Anaemia. In the nineteenth century, a condition was first described, in which pernicious anaemia, at that time a fatal disease, was associated with *D. latum* infection and in some instances, improved dramatically after eradication of the worm. In the twentieth century, the condition has been described exclusively from Finland and by the time that the modern understanding of the pathogenesis of megaloblastic anaemias had become established, tapeworm anaemia was already rapidly disappearing there. Our understanding of this disease is therefore tentative and, since there has been no recognized case for many years, will probably remain so. It seems clear that tapeworm anaemia was caused by vitamin B_{12} deficiency. It was strongly associated with gastritis and achlorhydria but neither of these were necessary conditions for its development and intrinsic factor does not seem to have been deficient.[47] It is most probable that worms were simply competing with the host for vitamin B_{12}, with clinical consequences most likely to follow when absorption was already marginal. There is also some evidence of a familial predisposition.

Diagnosis and Treatment

Eggs (Figure 57.17) are detected by faecal microscopy with an estimated sensitivity of 95% for a single examination. *Diphyllobothrium* eggs are morphologically similar and cannot be speciated by microscopy. Praziquantel is the preferred therapy, a single dose of 10 mg/kg being effective. Niclosamide has been extensively used in the past.

Control

Control has been effectively achieved in many areas by the detection and treatment of human cases, improved sanitation and education with regard to dietary habits.

Zoonotic Tapeworms

HYMENOLEPIS DIMINUTA

Rats are the definitive host for this parasite, with insects, principally fleas, acting as intermediate hosts. Humans, usually children, are infected by accidentally ingesting infected fleas. Adult worms can then develop to egg-producing maturity in the human gut, reaching a length of up to 6 cm. Human infection is uncommon but probably worldwide. Known clinical consequences are limited to minor abdominal pain. Diagnosis is by stool microscopy, the eggs (Figure 57.18) differing

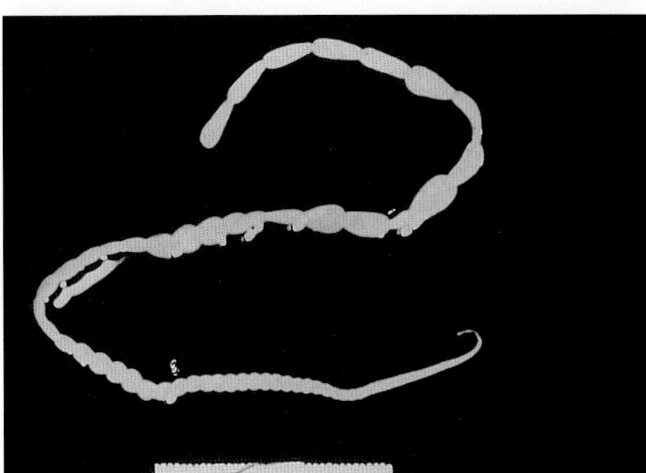

Figure 57.19 *Dipylidium caninum* (dog tapeworm). Adult. *(Courtesy of Tropical Resources Unit, Wellcome Trust.)*

slightly from those of *H. nana*. Praziquantel is said to be effective.

DIPYLIDIUM CANINUM

A ubiquitous tapeworm of dogs, with their fleas acting as the intermediate host, this parasite is very similar to *H. diminuta*, as an uncommon zoonotic infection of children who have accidently ingested dog fleas. A medium-sized tapeworm, up to 40 cm, can develop to maturity in the human gut (Figure 57.19). Motile proglottids the size of rice grains are passed intact in the stool; free eggs (Figure 57.20) are difficult to detect. Infection is most often asymptomatic and there are no known serious consequences. Treatment is with praziquantel.

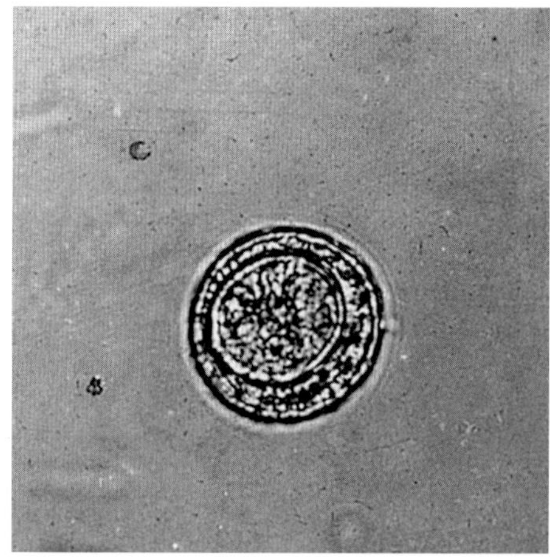

Figure 57.20 Egg of *Dipylidium caninum*.

REFERENCES

8. Ndimubanzi PC, Carabin H, Budke CM, et al. A systematic review of the frequency of neurocysticercosis with a focus on people with epilepsy. PLoS Negl Trop Dis 2010;4(11):e870.
11. Garcia HH, Gonzalez AE, Gilman RH. Cysticercosis of the central nervous system: how should it be managed? Curr Opin Infect Dis 2011;24(5):423–7.
20. Dorny P, Brandt J, Geerts S. Immunodiagnostic approaches for detecting *Taenia solium*. Trends Parasitol 2004;20(6):259–60.
22. Garcia HH, Pretell EJ, Gilman RH, et al. A trial of antiparasitic treatment to reduce the rate of seizures due to cerebral cysticercosis. N Engl J Med 2004;350(3):249–58.
48. Scholz T, Garcia HH, Kuchta R, et al. Update on the human broad tapeworm (genus diphyllobothrium), including clinical relevance. Clin Microbiol Rev 2009;22(1):146–60.

Access the complete references online at www.expertconsult.com

Scabies

BART J. CURRIE | JAMES S. MCCARTHY

KEY POINTS

- Scabies presents as an intensely pruritic rash that predominantly involves hairless and thin skin, e.g. web spaces of hands, skin creases, etc.
- A prominent cause of symptoms is sensitization to mite products. Thus, symptom onset may be delayed by weeks in the first infection.
- Secondary bacterial infection with *Staphylococcus aureus* and *Streptococcus pyogenes* frequently causes significant morbidity.
- Crusted scabies, the most severe form of scabies, presents as a hyperkeratotic rash. Lesions are loaded with mites and such patients are highly infectious.
- Direct skin-to-skin contact is the most important mode of transmission; washing of clothes and bed linen need only be done using usual methods.
- Parasitological diagnosis is difficult and therefore clinical diagnosis is usually relied upon.
- Topical permethrin cream applied to the whole body is the treatment of choice.
- Ivermectin, administered orally. is an alternative, but should be administered in two doses, one week apart.

Epidemiology

Scabies has been recognized as a contagious disease for centuries and occurs worldwide, with estimates of up to 300 million cases yearly.[1] The prevalence of scabies varies widely and fluctuates over time, but it remains endemic in many impoverished communities in less developed countries. Scabies is not restricted to tropical climates, and in industrialized countries it can be endemic in economically disadvantaged populations such as indigenous communities; institutional outbreaks continue to occur in hospitals and nursing homes.[2]

Scabies is overall most common in young children, most likely reflecting both increased exposure and, in endemic situations, a lack of immunity. In some highly endemic communities with overcrowded living conditions, the majority of children have had at least one episode of scabies in the first 2 years of life. Scabies affects both sexes similarly, although mothers of young children appear more commonly infected than other adults in some studies.

Sarcoptes scabiei affects a wide range of animal species in addition to humans. However, mite populations are generally host-species-restricted; *S. scabiei* var *canis* (dog scabies) and *S. scabiei* var *suis* (pig scabies) are rarely responsible for human cases, which result from infection with *S. scabiei* var *hominis*.

Pathogenesis and Pathology

Sarcoptes scabiei, the itch or scabies mite (*Acari*: Sarcoptidae), causes human scabies. Sarcoptid mites are obligate parasites of mammals and birds. Adult females are around 0.4 mm long and 0.3 mm wide and twice the size of males. The body is off-white opaque in colour with the legs and mouthparts brown. Adults and nymphs have eight legs and larvae have six. On the dorsal and lateral surfaces are pairs of spine like projections and some of the legs have stalked pulvilli (suckers) and/or spur-like claws.

All life cycle stages can penetrate an intact epidermis by secreting enzymes that dissolve skin, which is then ingested by the mite. Skin entry can occur in less than 30 minutes but only the fertilized female makes a permanent burrow in the epidermis. After a single mating, which results in the female being fertile for life, the male dies and the female begins to lay eggs in the skin burrow within the stratum granulosum of the epidermis. The female lays 0–3 eggs/day for up to 6 weeks before dying. Larvae hatch 2–4 days after eggs are laid, cut through to the skin surface and themselves begin to dig shallow burrows in the stratum corneum. At 3–4 days later, the larvae moult into protonymphs and 2–3 days later, these protonymphs moult into tritonymphs, from which an adult male or female emerges after a further 5–6 days. The cycle from egg to mature adult takes 10–13 days and under favourable conditions, up to 10% of eggs give rise to adult mites (Figure 58.1).

Classical studies by Mellanby showed that direct body contact person-to-person was usually necessary for transmission of scabies, with fomites such as clothing and exposure to mites shed onto surfaces such as floors or bedding unlikely to cause infection. The exception is that patients with hyperinfestation (Norwegian or crusted scabies) can shed numerous skin flakes containing hundreds of mites. Scabies mites can survive several days in humid environments at moderate ambient temperatures. Therefore, transmission by both fomites and direct skin contact may occur in nursing home outbreaks, infections in hospital staff and in crowded households if there is an undiagnosed crusted scabies patient who is the core transmitter. Intrafamilial transmission and transmission between sexual contacts account for the majority of cases worldwide.

Pathology results from sensitization of the host to the mites and their excretions, with symptom onset occurring up to 3–6 weeks after initial infection. In a normal host, the average female mite burden that develops is thought to be only 10–15, and classical burrows are often difficult to find. Both mechanical removal of mites by scratching and development of host immune responses contribute to control of the mite population, and after several months, mite numbers usually decrease rapidly. Sensitization to mite antigens can be demonstrated a month following primary infestations. In hyperinfestation (crusted scabies, see below) there is a failure of adequate cellular immune responses, but often extremely high levels of total IgE.

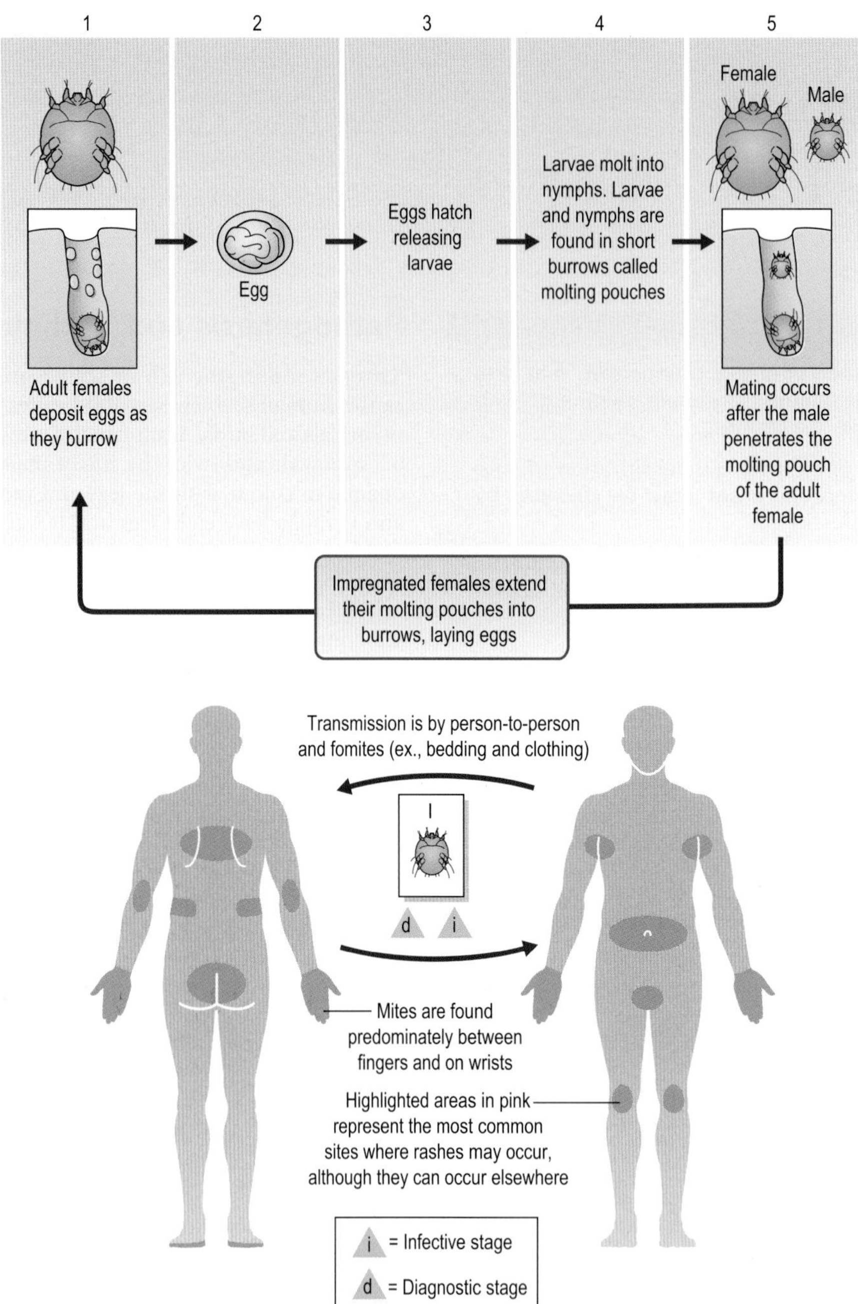

Figure 58.1 Life cycle of scabies. *(From Currie, B. and Hengge, UR., Scabies in Tyring, Tropical Dermatology, Copyright © Elsevier 2005.)*

Systemic sepsis from secondary bacterial infection and acute post-streptococcal glomerulonephritis from infection with nephritogenic *Streptococcus pyogenes* (Group A streptococcus) are the two scenarios where complications of scabies may cause death. Streptococci and staphylococci have been isolated from mite fecal pellets and from skin burrows, with mites possibly facilitating bacterial spread. The metabolic burden of scabies can contribute to malnutrition, especially in severe scabies in children and in crusted scabies.

Clinical Features

Scabies in older children and adults mostly presents as an intensely pruritic rash, with the itch classically worse at night. The symptoms develop 3–6 weeks after first infection, but can occur within 24–48 hours in those previously infected and therefore sensitized to mite antigens. The rash of scabies results from two processes: (1) papular or vesicular lesions occurring at the site of burrows made by mites (Figure 58.2) and (2) a more generalized immune-mediated pruritic and erythematous papular eruption not related to individual mites (Figure 58.3).

Mites most commonly burrow where there are few or no hair follicles and the stratum corneum is thin and soft; web spaces between the fingers and adjacent sides of the fingers; flexor surfaces of wrists; extensor surfaces of elbows; anterior axillary folds; skin around the nipples (especially in women); periumbilical region; pelvic girdle including waist and lower buttocks, upper thighs; penis (shaft and glans); extensor surfaces of knees;

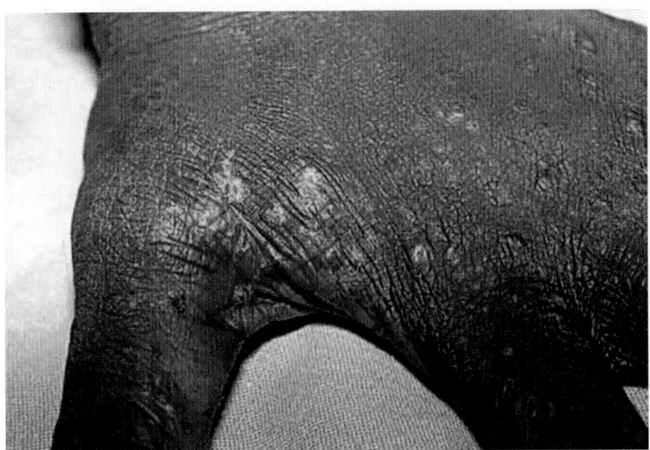

Figure 58.2 Scabies lesions of the hand. *(From Currie B. and Hengge UR. Scabies in Tyring, Tropical Dermatology, Copyright © Elsevier 2005.)*

lateral and posterior aspects of feet and toes. In infants and small children and in all ages in tropical regions, the palms, soles, face, neck, and scalp may also be involved. The more generalized immune-mediated rash is commonly seen in the axillae, chest and abdomen, buttocks and thighs.

The classical sign of scabies is the burrow made by the adult female, which can be seen by a trained unaided eye and appears as a serpiginous grey-red-brown line, up to 15 mm long, sometimes with a papule or small blood clot at the surface. Classical burrows are often absent, especially in tropical regions, in young children and in long-standing or recurrent infections, where a more intense local inflammatory response may obscure burrows and the generalized immune response-related rash may be more prominent.

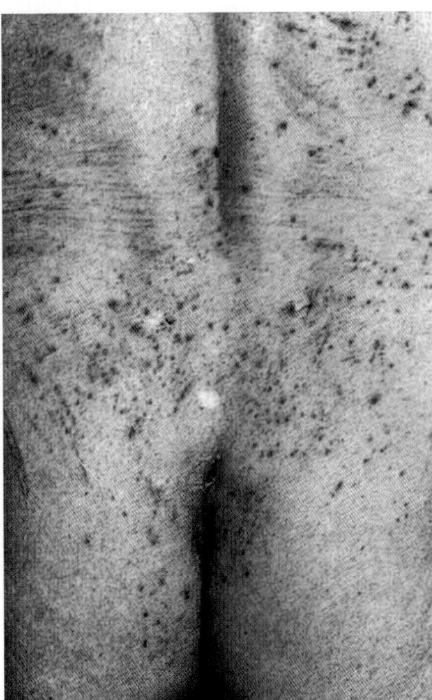

Figure 58.3 Generalized papular rash from the immunological reaction to scabies mites. *(From Currie B. and Hengge UR. Scabies in Tyring, Tropical Dermatology, Copyright © Elsevier 2005.)*

Any itchy generalized or local rash raises the possibility of scabies and young children and those with long-standing scabies can present with excoriation and eczematous rash on the limbs and trunk. In patients on topical or oral steroids, and in those with immunosuppression from disease or medication, scabies may have an atypical appearance (scabies incognito). Occasionally, a nodular reaction occurs (nodular scabies), with itchy red-brown nodules 5–8 mm in diameter, which can occur on anterior axillary folds, groin, genitalia, buttocks, or periumbilical region. The nodules may persist long after therapy has killed the scabies mites.

Secondary bacterial infection is common, and can result in pyoderma with pustular or crusted skin sores, boils and cellulitis. *Streptococcus pyogenes* and/or *Staphylococcus aureus*, including meticillin-resistant *S. aureus*, are the predominant bacteria involved and invasive bacterial infections following bacteraemic spread are a major cause of morbidity and even mortality following scabies.

CRUSTED SCABIES

Although *S. scabiei* infection and mite reproduction are usually self-limiting, hyperinfestation can develop in susceptible individuals. This potentially life-threatening condition of crusted or Norwegian scabies was first described in patients with leprosy in Norway. Crusted scabies can occur following immunosuppressive therapy in transplantation, rheumatological conditions, chemotherapy for malignancy, and in infection with HIV and HTLV-1. Crusted scabies can also occur in malnutrition, Down's syndrome and in the elderly and institutionalized, especially those with physical or cognitive disability who are unable to scratch. Patients with crusted scabies can have many thousands of mites in skin lesions and can serve as 'core transmitters' for continuing outbreaks of scabies in communities and nursing homes. Mites from crusted scabies cases are not genetically distinct, with ordinary scabies occurring in those infected from these cases.

Crusted scabies results from unfettered mite reproduction and the host reaction resulting in formation of hyperkeratotic skin crusts that may be loose and flaky or thick and adherent. Skin flakes with thousands of mites can be shed onto bed linen and floors. While hands and feet are most commonly involved, the distribution is often extensive, including neck, face and scalp as well as axillae, trunk, buttocks and limbs, especially knees and elbows. Thick deposits of debris with mites accumulate beneath the nails, which are often thickened and dystrophic. Crusting can however be limited to one or two limbs or hands or fingers. Unlike the intense itching of ordinary scabies, the presence of itch is variable in crusted scabies; it may be absent but it can also still be marked. Fissuring and secondary bacterial infection are common, and marked regional lymphadenopathy may be found (Figure 58.4). A peripheral blood eosinophilia is common but not always present, and serum IgE levels are often extremely high. There is a high mortality in crusted scabies from secondary bacterial sepsis, with polymicrobial infections sometimes occurring, including Gram-negative organisms such as *Pseudomonas aeruginosa* in addition to *S. pyogenes* and/or *S. aureus*.

The differential diagnosis of scabies includes: bites from other arthropods including mosquitoes, midges, fleas, lice, bedbugs, chiggers and other mites; tinea corporis; bacterial skin sores secondary to underlying skin damage that is not from

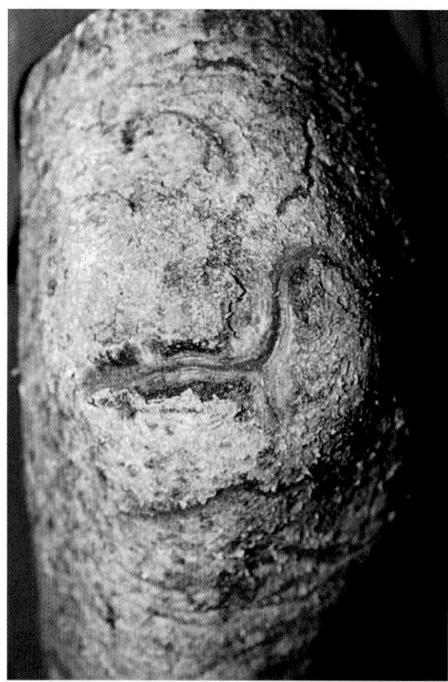

Figure 58.4 Severe crusted scabies with fissuring over the knee. *(From Currie B. and Hengge UR. Scabies in Tyring, Tropical Dermatology, Copyright © Elsevier 2005.)*

scabies, such as from trauma, tinea, eczema and insect bites; and non-infectious dermatitis, e.g. eczema, papular urticaria and other allergic skin reactions. Both disseminated herpes simplex infection (eczema herpeticum) and dermatitis herpetiformis (which is linked to celiac disease/gluten sensitivity) can mimic widespread scabies and paronychia can mimic scabies involving the fingers.

The differential diagnosis of crusted scabies includes: psoriasis, extensive tinea corporis ± nail involvement (especially with the granular variety of *Trichophyton rubrum*), skin malignancies such as the T cell lymphomas, mycosis fungoides and the Sézary syndrome, nutritional deficiencies such as pellagra, pemphigus, kava dermopathy, onchocerciasis, lepromatous leprosy and secondary syphilis.

Diagnosis

Definitive diagnosis can only be made by seeing the *S. scabiei* mite under a microscope. A drop of mineral oil is placed on a disposable scalpel blade (No. 10, 15 or 20); the suggestive skin papule, vesicle or burrow is lightly scraped to remove the superficial epidermis and the oil deposited on a microscope slide. Material from several skin lesions can be placed onto a single slide, which is then examined for mites, eggs and faecal pellets under ×40 low power, with or without 10% potassium hydroxide solution to remove skin squames. An alternative technique is to tease out a mite with a mounted needle probe or scalpel tip with the aid of a loupe, magnifying glass or dermatoscope (×10) to better view the process and suspected location within a papule or burrow. For both methods, visualization of burrows can be facilitated by placing 2–3 drops of ink over the papule for 10 seconds, then wiping clean with an alcohol swab (the burrow ink test). Lesions can also be curetted and skin biopsies performed for complex cases. In ordinary scabies few mites are present in the individual's skin and skill is required to retrieve the mite for microscopic diagnosis. In true crusted scabies however, microscopy of skin scrapings from several affected sites will almost invariably reveal scabies mites and often in large numbers.

In reality, the vast majority of diagnoses of scabies are made presumptively in scabies endemic communities and in primary care settings where microscopy is not available, with definitive diagnosis by microscopy or biopsy reserved for non-classical presentations and complex cases. Studies in scabies-endemic regions have shown that there is good sensitivity, specificity, positive predictive value and negative predictive value using the following clinical case definition:[3]

- Presence of itching involving at least two sites of the body
- Visible skin lesions involving at least two typical sites for scabies
- Presence of others in the same household with itch.

When in doubt, presumptive therapy should still be considered, as there is no definitive standard for ruling out the diagnosis of scabies.

Management and Treatment

The mainstay of scabies therapy is topical acaricides, although oral ivermectin is increasingly being used and is the therapy of choice for crusted scabies.[4]

Although not confirmed by clinical studies, two treatments 1–2 weeks apart are recommended where practicable for all cases because a second application of the topical acaricides kills residual mites that were not exposed at the time of the first treatment. Of note, the ovicidal activity of oral ivermectin may be poor. All members of the family in contact with the patient and other close personal contacts should be treated at the same time with a single therapy. Potentially exposed clothing and bed linen can be washed in the normal fashion or stored for 7 days in a bag.

Topical permethrin and oral ivermectin, where affordable, are currently considered the best treatment options (Table 58.1), although there are few high-quality studies comparing the many products available: 5% permethrin cream is probably superior to crotamiton cream, but crotamiton daily for 5 days is well tolerated and suitable therapy for infants. Permethrin is equivalent to or superior to lindane, which itself is potentially neurotoxic in young children and no longer available in many countries. Topical benzyl benzoate is more rapidly scabicidal than permethrin in vitro. There are conflicting studies comparing topical 12.5% benzyl benzoate with oral ivermectin, with the most recent study from Senegal showing superiority of benzyl benzoate. One issue with benzyl benzoate is that skin irritation is common in the first minutes after application. Although the discomfort usually rapidly decreases in severity after several minutes, the burning sensation is sometimes so severe that it requires the lotion to be washed off. This reaction appears more common with the 25% concentration. Thus, lower concentrations of 10% or more are recommended for children. To date, clinically significant resistance of *S. scabiei* to permethrin remains only anecdotal, although there are data showing prolonged in vitro knockdown times. Clinical and in vitro resistance of *S. scabiei* to ivermectin has been described in only two patients who had multiple intermittent doses of ivermectin for recurrent crusted scabies.

TABLE 58.1 Treatment of Scabies and Contacts

Syndrome	Recommended Drug	Alternative Drug	Comments
Classical scabies	Two applications of topical permethrin 5% applied in the evening and left on overnight; day 1 and between days 8–15	Oral ivermectin[a] (200 µg/kg/dose); two doses with food; day 1 and between days 8–15 *OR* Topical benzyl benzoate 10–25%; day 1 and between days 8–15	
Crusted scabies	Both topical permethrin 5% each 2–3 days initially and oral ivermectin[a] (200 µg/kg/dose), with food, for 3 (days 1,2,8), 5 (days 1,2,8,9,15) or 7 (days 1,2,8,9,15,22) doses depending on severity	Topical benzyl benzoate 12.5–25% instead of permethrin	Keratolytic creams for skin crusts Vigilance for the development of sepsis Appropriate infection control measures
Close contacts	A single application of topical permethrin 5% applied in the evening and left on overnight	Oral ivermectin[a] (200 µg/kg/dose), with food, single dose *OR* Topical benzyl benzoate 10–25%, single application	
Institutional outbreak	Treat clinical cases as above for classical and crusted scabies and ALL potentially exposed residents, staff and visitors, as above for contacts	In refractory outbreaks consider treatment of all residents with oral ivermectin[a]	Look for 'core transmitter' index cases with crusted scabies. Attention to planning and logistics of therapy. Appropriate infection control measures.
Endemic community	Multifaceted approach with education and community involvement. Treat clinical cases as above for classical and crusted scabies and all family/household members as above for contacts Consider treating all other community members as above for contacts	As above for classical and crusted scabies and contacts (community members)	Look for 'core transmitter' index cases with crusted scabies. Attention to planning and logistics of therapy. Sustainability requires addressing underlying issues of overcrowding and access to health hardware, health care and education.

[a]Not approved for this indication in some countries; insufficient safety data in pregnancy and in children under 5 years of age or under 15 kg weight.

To ensure reliable cure, topical therapy should be applied to the entire skin surface, except the eyes. This is particularly important in small children and the elderly, among whom the infestation not infrequently involves the scalp. To maximize exposure of mites to the drug, it is generally recommended that the cream be applied in the evening and left on overnight.

For crusted scabies, ivermectin administered in multiple doses is the therapy of choice. It needs to be combined with topical scabicides, alternating with keratolytic creams (such as salicylic acid or lactic acid/urea) to facilitate breakdown of the skin crusting (Table 58.1). Ivermectin is administered orally in a dose of 200–300 µg/kg. As the bioavailability of ivermectin is increased twofold with food, taking the drug with food is recommended to enhance penetration of ivermectin into the epidermis. Depending on the severity of the crusted scabies 3, 5 or 7 doses of ivermectin are recommended. At present, use of ivermectin in children under 5 years of age or weighing less than 15 kg is advised against because of theoretical concerns regarding potential passage of ivermectin across the blood–brain barrier, resulting in neurotoxicity. However, evidence for this occurring to date remains restricted to mammals other than humans. Use of ivermectin in pregnancy is also advised against. Nevertheless, reports exist documenting the inadvertent administration of the drug to pregnant women without adverse fetal outcome.

Identification and treatment with antibiotics of secondary bacterial skin infection is important, in order to prevent potential bacterial sepsis and acute post-streptococcal glomerulonephritis. This is especially important with crusted scabies, where systemic sepsis is common and can be rapidly fatal.

Prevention

Failure to diagnose scabies, lack of access to therapy or inadequately applied therapy and not treating contacts who may also be infected, all contribute to the ongoing cycles of transmission of scabies. It is critical to identify and treat cases of crusted scabies who may be core transmitters in institutional outbreaks such as in nursing homes and hospitals and in ongoing outbreaks in community settings (Table 58.1).

In small communities where scabies is endemic, whole community treatment with topical permethrin has resulted in dramatic decreases in both scabies and streptococcal pyoderma. Success and sustainability of such programmes require considerable planning, resources and follow-up.[5]

Mass drug administration programmes using oral ivermectin in those aged over 5 years, with topical permethrin for those under 5 years (or under 15 kg) have had variable success.

Failure of a community intervention reflects the known epidemiological drivers of scabies transmission from person to person, which are overcrowding, poverty, hygiene issues, sexual transmission and demographic forces such as migration, wars and displacement of populations. Ultimately, sustainability of any programme and long-term control of scabies locally, regionally and globally, requires addressing underlying fundamental issues of overcrowding and access to health hardware, health care and education.

REFERENCES

1. Chosidow O. Clinical practices. Scabies. N Engl J Med 2006;354(16):1718–27.
2. Bouvresse S, Chosidow O. Scabies in healthcare settings. Curr Opin Infect Dis 2010;23(2):111–18.
3. Mahé A, Faye O, N'Diaye HT, et al. Definition of an algorithm for the management of common skin diseases at primary health care level in sub-Saharan Africa. Trans R Soc Trop Med Hyg 2005;99(1):39–47.
4. Currie BJ, McCarthy JS. Permethrin and ivermectin for scabies. N Engl J Med 2010;362(8):717–25.
5. Taplin D, Porcelain SL, Meinking TL, et al. Community control of scabies: a model based on use of permethrin cream. Lancet 1991;337(8748):1016–18.

Access the complete bibliography online at www.expertconsult.com

59 Louse Infestation

MARIAN J. CURRIE | FRANCIS J. BOWDEN | JAMES S. McCARTHY

KEY POINTS

- Lice (*Pediculosis humanus*) have been infesting humans since antiquity.
- Infestations are most common in children (head lice), people living in crowded and unsanitary conditions (body lice) and as a result of sexual contact (pubic lice).
- Lice do not fly or jump; transmission is by human-to-human contact.
- Lice live on human blood and so cannot live for more than about 48 hours away from the human host.
- Itching is the most common symptom, but many infestations are symptomless.
- Although most infestations are merely bothersome, lice can act as a vector for diseases such as epidemic typhus, trench fever and louse-borne relapsing fever. Secondary infections with staphylococci or streptococci can enter through skin sores that result from scratching.
- Treatments can be pharmacological (topical or oral) or non-pharmacological.

Louse Infestation (Pediculosis)

Lice are ectoparasites and belong to the group called sucking lice (*Anoplura*). Three species of louse are parasitic to humans:

- *Pediculus capitis* (head louse)
- *Pediculus humanus* (body louse)
- *Pthirus pubis* (crab or pubic louse).

Biology and Description

The three species have similar life cycles comprising the egg, nymph and the adult. The fertilized female louse lays eggs which hatch in 7–9 days. The hatchlings moult their exoskeleton three times in a 7–10-day period to develop into mature adults, which survive approximately 30 days. Each female may lay 50–300 eggs in her lifetime.

Since lice have evolved with humans, their anatomy is highly specialized; each of the six legs terminates in a claw which allows the lice to move rapidly and to transfer to new hosts. Head lice are generally smaller than body lice (2–3 mm and 3–4 mm in length, respectively) and pubic lice are crab-like in shape 1.3–2 mm long and slower than the other types. All human lice are haematophagous, depending solely on human blood as a source of water and nutrition. They take a blood meal from the skin 2–5 times a day.

Transmission

For all three types, transmission is through close contact with an infested person. The role played by fomites in the transmission of head lice is unclear. Body lice are spread by contact with infested clothing. Pubic lice are usually transmitted during sexual contact, but non-sexual transmission can occur and there is some evidence that fomites play a role.

Diagnosis

The diagnosis of pediculosis is dependent on visual identification of at least one live adult louse, with detection of viable eggs on the hair shafts (for head lice) and/or clothing (for body and pubic lice). In the case of head lice, the optimal method for diagnosis is wet combing of the hair using a lubricating agent such as hair conditioner or oil (sensitivity >90%, even in children with a low infestation intensity).[1] Empty egg cases attached to hair shafts are not diagnostic of an active infection and it is important not to confuse live lice or nits with dandruff, hair casts or other debris.

PEDICULUS HUMANIS VAR *CAPITIS* (HEAD LICE)

Head lice are a dirty-white to grayish-black in colour (Figure 59.1A). They live on the scalp and attach their eggs (nits) close to the base of the hair (Figure 59.1B). They can survive for 6–24 hours away from the human host, dying of dehydration at a rate dependent on the relative ambient humidity. Eggs rarely hatch at a temperature lower than that near the scalp.

Epidemiology

Head lice infestations occur throughout the world and affect populations in every stratum of society. Systematic collection of prevalence data is not undertaken and so it is difficult to estimate the size of the problem in most countries. Prevalence rates between 0.7% and 76% have been reported in a range of settings.[2] Children aged 3–11 years are most frequently affected, with girls twice as likely to be infested, probably as a result of social behaviours (e.g. closer physical contact, sharing of hair accessories). Sociodemographic status and seasonality do not appear to affect prevalence.

Clinical Features

Pruritus is the most common symptom of infestation. Affected areas include the scalp, the back of the neck and post-auricular areas. While infestations can be asymptomatic, some people develop an allergic reaction to the saliva injected during feeding. Pruritus is more common in persistent infestations, although itch is not specific for head lice. Excoriation can accompany the pruritus and may lead to bacterial skin super-infection.

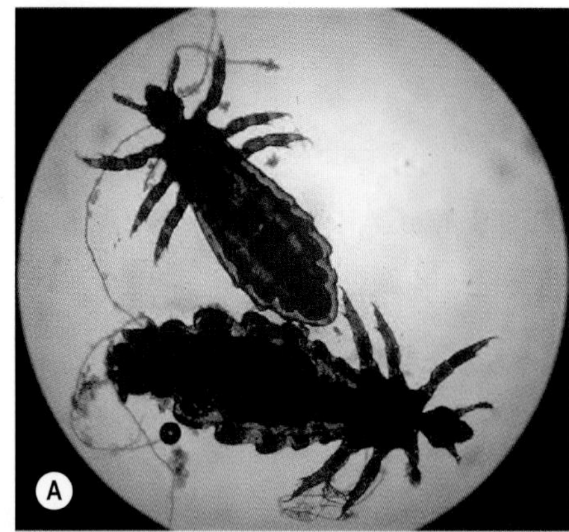

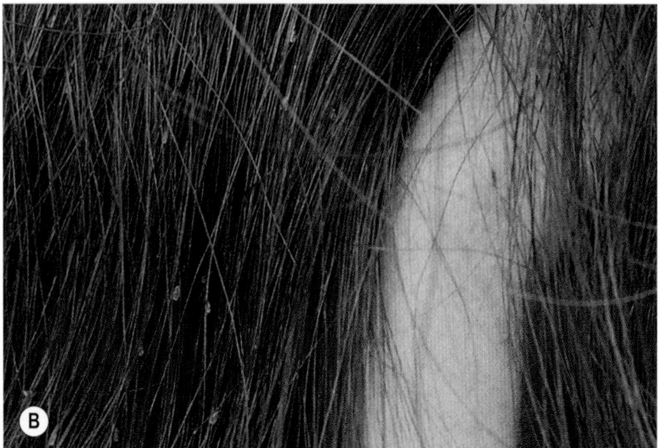

Figure 59.1 (A) Head lice. (B) Head lice eggs in hair. *(A, from Zaoutis L. Comprehensive Hospital Medicine, with permission from Elsevier. Copyright © 2007. B, from Frazier M. Essentials of Human Diseases and Conditions, with permission from Elsevier. Copyright © 2009.)*

Occasionally, cervical lymphadenopathy and conjunctivitis may occur. Rarely, glomerulonephritis may occur as a consequence of group A streptococcal super-infection of the skin.[3] Infestation can also have psychological effects and result in social stigmatisation. Persistent infestation can lead to poor performance at school secondary to sleep disturbance and difficulties in concentration.

PEDICULUS HUMANIS (BODY OR CLOTHES LICE)

The body louse almost certainly evolved from head lice with the advent of clothing and is the only parasite to evolve to fill this niche.

The adult is grayish-white, reddish or cream in colour with thinner antennae and better developed abdominal muscles than the head louse (Figure 59.2A). Females lay their nits in the seams or hems of clothes (especially underwear) that are adjacent to the surface of the skin (Figure 59.2B). They feed only when the host is resting or sleeping. Unfed body lice rarely survive longer than 10 days, while those which have fed may survive in moist clothing for 30–40 days away from a host.

Epidemiology

Body lice infestations are found worldwide, but are generally limited to persons who: live in crowded conditions; own just one set of clothes; and do not have access to hot water for regular bathing and laundering of clothes. The prevalence of body lice has declined in recent years because most people do not wear the same clothing for prolonged periods. Prevalence is greater at higher altitudes where the cold climate necessitates heavier dressing, but poverty prevents frequent changing or washing of clothes in hot water, which will kill the eggs and lice.

Clinical Features

Bites appear as minute red dots, developing into papular lesions with wheal-like inflammation. Symptoms of repeated inoculation with saliva include headache, malaise, anorexia, joint pain, fever, irritability and a Rubella-like rash. Pruritus can indicate the development of an allergy; inhalation of faeces or parts of cast skins from body lice can trigger hay fever symptoms. Secondary infections related to scratching are common. Long-lasting infestation may result in vagabond's disease (parasitic melanoderma).

Body lice are known vectors of epidemic or louse-borne typhus (*Rickettsia prowazeki*), trench fever (*Bartonella quintana*) and louse-borne relapsing fever (*Borrelia recurrentis*).

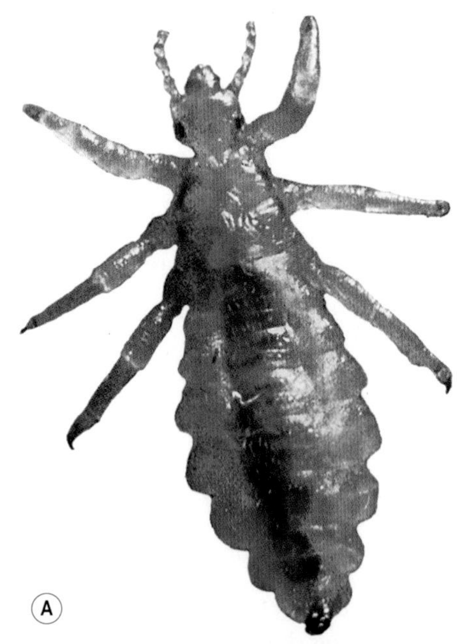

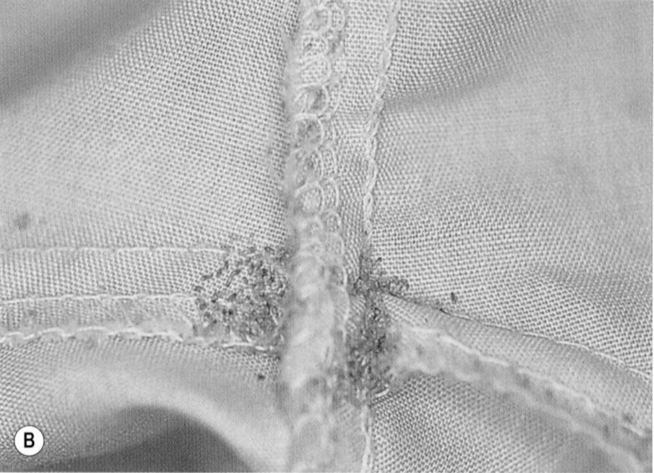

Figure 59.2 (A) Body louse. (B) Body louse eggs in seams of clothing. *(A, from Habif T. Clinical Dermatology, with permission from Elsevier. Copyright © 2010. B, from Bolognia J. Dermatology. 2nd edn., with permission from Elsevier. Copyright © 2008.)*

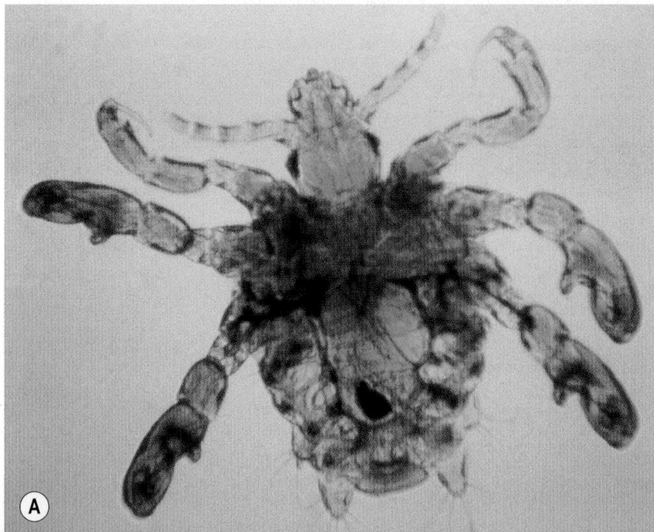

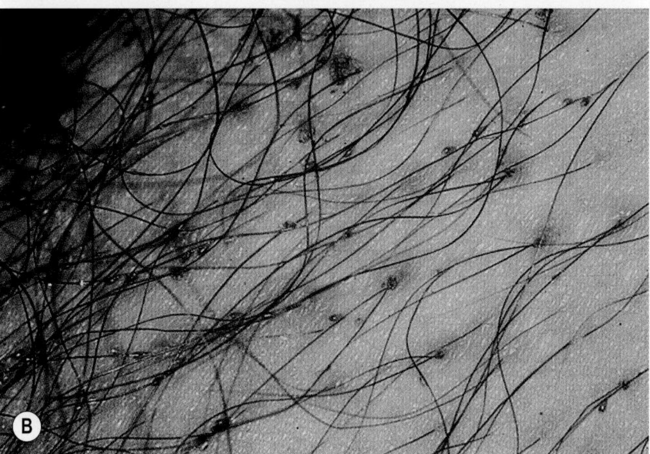

Figure 59.3 (A) Crab louse. (B) Crab lice eggs at the base of lower abdominal hairs. *(A, from Resh V. Encyclopedia of Insects. 2nd edn., with permission from Elsevier. Copyright © 2009. B from Ko CJ, Elston DM. Pediculosis. J Am Acad Dermatol 2004;50:1–12.)*

These conditions are fatal in up to 40% of patients and are most common in areas where climate, poverty, social customs, war or social upheaval prevent regular changes and laundering of clothing in hot water. Since 1995, louse-borne diseases have had a resurgence, and trench fever has been diagnosed in many developed and developing countries.[4]

PHTHIRUS PUBIS (CRAB OR PUBIC LICE)

The pubic louse is grey in colour and the nit is oval, opalescent, 0.5–0.8 mm in size and glued firmly to the hair (Figure 59.3). Pubic lice most commonly infest pubic and perianal hair, but can be found in the hair of the beard, moustache, eyelashes, armpits, chest and abdomen. The preference for these sites is due to hair spacing. The 2 mm between pubic hairs matches the space between the louse's hind legs. Pubic lice are associated with, but do not cause other sexually transmitted infections.

Epidemiology

Pubic lice are primarily found on younger sexually active adults and sex workers. Infestation rates of around 2% are usually cited. Infestation in children can be indicative of sexual abuse. Infestation is uncommon in older age.

Clinical Features

Puncture sites are red with swelling in the immediate area. Intense itching is common, but is delayed until approximately 4 weeks after the initial infestation. A characteristic grey-blue pigmentation (maculae ceruleae) appears at the feeding site. This is thought to result from altered human blood pigments or a reaction to substances excreted in louse saliva. Affected patients report rust spots (louse excrement) on clothing. Pubic lice do not transmit disease, but excoriation and secondary infection can occur in those with symptoms.

Treatment for all Types of Lice

Lice are commonly treated with over-the-counter products containing agents such as pyrethrins, permethrin, malathion, essential oils (e.g. eucalyptus oil) and products that physically suffocate the ectoparasite. The emergence of drug-resistant lice and concerns about the neurotoxic effects of malathion have created the need for new therapies. Results from trials of mechanical removal, suffocation-based pediculicide treatments, shampoos containing complex plant-based compounds, topical application of dimethicones, and home remedies (vinegar, isopropyl alcohol, olive oil, mayonnaise, melted butter and petroleum jelly) are inconsistent. Head shaving is effective but is distressing for children. Because no approved pediculicide is completely ovicidal, topical treatment failure is most commonly due to the lack of repeat treatment to ensure emerging nymphs are killed. Treatment failure can also be the result of inadequate application of the treatment product, resistance in the lice or re-infestation.[5–7] Oral and topical ivermectin have demonstrated both efficacy against head lice and acceptability in several studies,[8–11] but only the topical route of administration is currently licensed for use against lice by the United States Food and Drug Authority (FDA).

Control and Prevention

Regular surveillance, early detection and treatment may reduce the burden of lice infestation.[12] Washing of clothes, bed linen and towels used by an infested individual using a hot water laundry cycle and a high heat drying cycle is recommended for body and pubic lice infestations, but not for head lice infestation. Shaving pubic hair can be helpful and all sexual contacts should be examined and treated empirically. Household contacts should be treated only if infested. The use of fumigant sprays is not recommended because of toxicity if the agent is inhaled or absorbed percutaneously. Commonly used treatments are listed in Table 59.1. Cure rates vary between 50% and 100%.[13] Resistance to pediculicides is a growing problem.[1,14] Major types of resistance include knock-down resistance, glutathione-S-transferase-based resistance and monooxygenase-based resistance.[15]

Exclusion

Because a child with an active head lice infestation is likely to have been infested for a month or more by the time it is discovered, the child poses little additional transmission risk to classmates and so should remain in school. Parents should be discreetly notified and treatment initiated that afternoon or evening. The child may return to school the day after effective treatment has been initiated.

TABLE 59.1 Treatment for All Types of Lice

Category	Examples
Pediculicides	
Prescription	Malathion lotion 0.5%, Benzyl alcohol lotion (5%); ivermectin (topical or tablet forms)
Over-the-counter	Pyrethrins combined with piperonyl butoxide, Permethrin lotion 1%
'Natural' products	Essentials oils and other plant extracts
Occlusive agents	Petroleum jelly, hair conditioner, silicone oil (dimethicones)
Manual removal	If only a few live lice and nits are present, it may be possible to remove these with fingernails or a nit comb
Particular Interventions	
Head lice	Check family members
Body lice	More frequent changing of clothes
Pubic lice	Contact tracing and testing for other sexually transmissible infections
	Applying ophthalmic-grade petrolatum ointment (available by prescription) to the eyelid margins 2–4 times a day for 10 days is effective for infestations of the eyelashes.

No pediculicide is 100% effective in killing the eggs; resistance varies geographically.
Treatment with the organochlorine insecticide lindane is no longer recommended due to potential neurotoxic effects and low efficacy.

REFERENCES

5. Burkhart CG, Burkhart CN. Safety and efficacy of pediculicides for head lice. Expert Opin Drug Saf 2006;5(1):169–79.
6. Burgess IF. Current treatments for pediculosis capitis. Curr Opin Infect Dis 2009;22(2):131–6.
7. Heukelbach J, Speare R, Ramos AN. General considerations on treatments and treatment schemes. In: Heukelbach J, editor. Management and Control of Head Lice Infestations. Bremen: UNI-MED Verlag AG; 2010. p. 97–101.
12. Mumcuoglu KY, Meinking TA, Burkhart CN, et al. Head louse infestations: the 'no nit' policy and its consequences. Int J Dermatol 2006; 45(8):891–6.
13. Durand R, Bouvresse S, Berdjane Z, et al. Insecticide resistance in head lice: clinical, parasitological and genetic aspects. Clin Microbiol Infect 2012;18(4):338–44.

Access the complete references online at www.expertconsult.com

60

Other Ectoparasites: Leeches, Myiasis and Sand Fleas

KOSTA Y. MUMCUOGLU

KEY POINTS

- Out of 650 known leech species, few are predators, some living inland and the majority in fresh waters.
- Leeches are hermaphrodites and the majority are haematophagous.
- Myiasis is the fourth most common travel-associated skin disease, and cutaneous myiasis is the most frequently encountered clinical form.
- A higher incidence of myiasis is found in rural zones, especially in tropical and sub-tropical areas of Africa and America.
- Flies producing furuncular myiasis include *Dermatobia hominis, Cordylobia anthropophaga, Wohlfahrtia vigil* and *Cuterebra* spp.
- In humans, *Gasterophilus, Cuterebra, Cordylobia* and *Hypoderma* species can also produce creeping myiasis.
- Sand fleas, also known as jigger, chigger or chigoe fleas, are haematophagous insect parasites of humans and domestic animals.
- Sand flea infestation is considered a traveller's disease. Cases of tungiasis are also reported in tourists, missionaries and workers returning from endemic zones.

Leeches

Leeches belong to the class Hirudinea from the phylum *Annelida*. There are about 650 known species of leeches, some living inland, others in salt and fresh water. Although some are predators, most of the leeches are haematophagous. Land leeches live in the vegetation of tropical rainforests and tend to breed near springs, streams and wells frequented by cattle, horses and other vertebrates. Species from this group attacking man include *Haemadipsa zelanica, Haemadipsa sylvestris* and *Haemadipsa picta*.

Freshwater leeches, which infest humans, include *Limnatis nilotica, Limnatis maculosa, Phytobdella catenifera, Dinobdella ferox, Myxobdella africana, Hirudinea granulosa, Hirundinea viridis, Emys orbicularis, Diestecostoma mexicana* and *Haementeria ghilianii*. Leeches, which are used for the treatment of clinical symptoms in humans, are called medicinal leeches and include *Hirudo medicinalis, Hirudo verbana, Hirudo orientalis, Hirudo troctina, Hirudo michaelseni, Hirudinaria manillensi, Placobdella ornate* and *Macrobdella décora*.[1,2]

BIOLOGY AND EPIDEMIOLOGY

One of the best-studied leeches is the European medicinal leech, *H. medicinalis*, and its biology and epidemiology will be discussed below.[1,2]

The body is soft, elongated, vermiform, segmented and dorso-ventrally flattened. Their anterior and posterior suckers serve as organs of locomotion and provide firm adhesion to different objects and to the host's body at the time of feeding. They are amphibious animals, living usually in stagnant or slowly running fresh water with littoral vegetation.

Each leech is a protandrous hermaphrodite and cross-fertilizes with another leech of the same species. Eggs (10–30) are embedded in a cocoon and deposited in shady and humid places. Newborn leeches feed on plankton, young specimens on fish, frogs and toads and older leeches on the blood of warm-blooded animals. Fully mature adults can reach 20 cm in length, and are greenish-brown, with a thin red stripe on the dorsal side.

Leeches are very sensitive to vibration and when a host animal such as a human enters water, they swim towards it and attach to exposed areas of the skin. The leech attaches to the host by the apical and posterior suckers. The apical sucker surrounds the buccal cavity and is composed of three jaws, pointing in different directions. Thus, the bite of the leech leaves a mark that is an inverted Y inside a circle (Figure 60.1). Each jaw has 60–100 teeth that are connected to the salivary gland, which injects saliva into the skin during a blood meal. The posterior sucker is used for attachment only. Blood feeding lasts for about 20 minutes. Large adults can consume 5–15 mL of blood and can survive without feeding for up to 1 year and more (Figure 60.2).

PATHOGENESIS AND CLINICAL ASPECTS

Local pain is felt at the moment of leech bite, but the pain lasts for a short time only, as analgesics are injected into the skin with the saliva. Transient itching and erythema occur at the bite site, which can last for a few days. Small blood spots (ecchymoses) can develop on the bite site. When left undisturbed, the scars, which appear after the bite, disappear within 1–3 weeks. Superinfection and intensive scratching may lead to scars remaining for longer. Rare symptoms include severe itching and redness, local allergic reactions (urticaria), anaphylaxis, irritant contact dermatitis, follicular pseudolymphoma and mucosal synechiae, particularly when humans are repeatedly exposed to leeches for medicinal purposes. Bleeding of the bite site can last for several hours and longer in individuals who are being treated with anticoagulants.

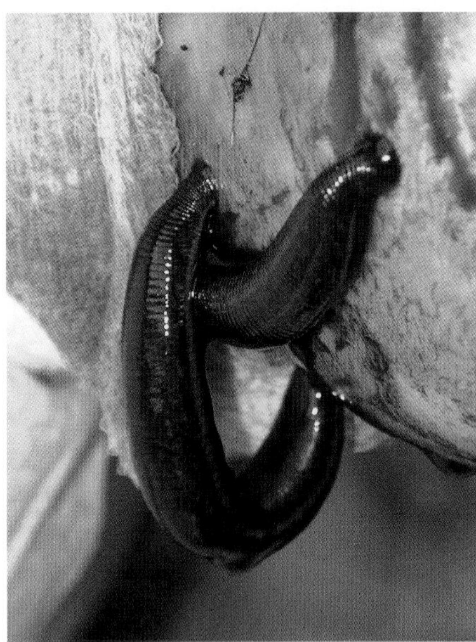

Figure 60.2 Medical leeches, *Hirudo medicinalis* taking a blood-meal from human skin.

Some species of leeches occasionally enter human orifices such as the eyes, nasopharyngeal region, urethra, vagina and rectum. In such cases, they can cause mucosal, orificial, vesical or internal hirudiniasis depending on the localization of the leech. Infestation usually occurs by drinking infested water, or bathing in stagnant streams, pools or springs. Most leech attachment is short-lived but leeches feeding on mucous membranes may stay in an orifice for days or weeks. Haematuria, haemoptysis, haematemesis, epistaxis and rectal bleeding, dysphonia, coughing, tickling sensation and dyspnoea may occur. There have been reports in Africa of severe anaemia and mortality associated with the leech *Myxobdella africana*, after it accidentally enters the human pharynx or other orifices.

PREVENTION AND TREATMENT

Application of concentrated saline, vinegar, alcohol or lidocaine or a burning cigarette on the apical part of the leech can be used for removal of the parasite. If pulled off by force during blood feeding, their jaws can remain on the skin and cause complications such as secondary infections. Internally, attached leeches may detach on exposure to gargled saline or by catheterization and normal saline infusion. Leeches in the urinary bladder can also be removed by suprapubic examination and a cystoscope.

Hirudotherapy

Access the complete Hirudotherapy section online at: http://www.expertconsult.com.

Myiasis

Myiasis is the infestation of live human and vertebrate animals with larvae (maggots) of flies from the order Diptera, which feed on the host's dead or living tissue, liquid body-substance or ingested food.[5]

A higher incidence of myiasis is found in rural zones, especially in tropical and subtropical areas of Africa and America. Animals are most commonly infested, but occasionally humans, especially those who are ill and incapacitated, can suffer from myiasis. Myiasis is the fourth most common travel-associated skin disease and cutaneous myiasis is the most frequently encountered clinical form.[6]

Myiasis may be classified in two ways: the first is according to the relationship between the host and the parasite such as obligatory, facultative or accidental; while the second pertains to the location of the affected area such as cutaneous, nasopharyngeal, ocular, intestinal or urogenital.

Some parasitic fly larvae cause obligatory myiasis, having to complete their life cycle in or on living tissue. Larvae responsible for facultative myiasis usually develop in decaying organic substrates of animal origin, but can feed on necrotic tissue from preexisting wounds or ulcers in living hosts. In accidental myiasis, eggs or larvae reach the body opportunely, via natural orifices, traumatic wounds or in the digestive tract.

Myiasis-producing flies are members of the superfamily Oestrodiae, which includes the families Oestridae, Calliphoridae and Sarcophagidae. The family Oestridae includes subfamilies such as Oestrinae, Gasterophilinae, Hypodermatinae and Cuterebrinae; all species of this family are obligatory parasites. The families of Calliphoridae and Sarcophagidae contain both obligatory and facultative agents of myiasis.

BIOLOGY AND EPIDEMIOLOGY

Female flies usually lay their eggs or larvae on the skin, inside wounds or in the opening of body cavities. The hatching larvae undergo two moults and develop to second- and third-stage larvae. The latter has to leave the host in order to pupate in a dry environment and later develop into an adult fly.

Several species are important in human disease. These include: *Wohlfahrtia magnifica* (the Spotted Flesh Fly), *Chrysomya bezziana* (the Old World Screwworm Fly), *Cochliomyia hominivorax* (the New World Screwworm Fly), *Cordylobia anthropophaga* (Tumbu Fly) and *Dermatobia hominis* (Botfly). The latter two are most common causes of human disease.

Cordylobia anthropophaga (Tumbu fly, mango fly) is common in East and Central Africa. Female tumbu flies lay their eggs in soil contaminated with faeces or urine or on damp clothing or bed linen. The larvae hatch in 2–3 days, attach to unbroken skin and penetrate the skin, producing a swelling.

Dermatobia hominis (Botfly) is commonly found in Mexico, Central and South America. The adult flies lay eggs, attaching them first to various bloodsucking insects such as mosquitoes. As the vector takes a blood meal, the botfly eggs react to the change in temperature and hatch. Cases of human *D. hominis* myiasis may only become apparent when travellers return from endemic countries.

PATHOGENESIS AND CLINICAL PICTURE

Cutaneous Myiasis (Including Dermal, Sub-dermal, Furuncular, Facial, Creeping, Wound and Traumatic Myiasis)

The flies that produce furuncular myiasis include *Dermatobia hominis*, *Cordylobia anthropophaga*, *Wohlfahrtia vigil* and *Cuterebra spec.* Flies that cause wound myiasis include screwworm flies such as *Cochliomyia hominivorax*, *Chrysomya bezziana*, *Wohlfahrtia magnifica*, *Lucilia sericata* (Figure 60.4), *Sarcophaga* spp. and many more.

In humans, the skin lesion starts as a painful red papule that gradually enlarges and develops into a furuncle (Figure 60.5). At first, the host may experience only intermittent, slight itching, but pain develops and increases in frequency and intensity as the lesions develop into a furuncle. Typically, the centre of the lesion has a regular opening, through which the larva breathes and discharges its waste products. Lesions are generally located on the backs of arms, around the waist, on the lower back or on the buttocks.

In humans, *Gasterophilus, Cuterebra, Cordylobia* and *Hypoderma* species can also produce creeping myiasis, when the path of the larvae beneath the skin can be observed. The larvae cannot develop further and produce tunnels in the epidermis, where they may wander for considerable distances.[7]

Body Cavity Myiasis

Body cavity myiasis is usually caused by *Cochliomyia hominivorax, Chrysomya bezziana* and *Wohlfahrtia magnifica.*

Oral Myiasis (Including Orofacial, Oro-maxillofacial and Orotracheal Myiasis). Oral myiasis is rare and is often associated with poor oral hygiene (e.g. advanced periodontitis) or mental disability. It is most common in rural areas in the tropical and sub-tropical zones of Africa and America.

Oral myiasis caused by *Cochliomyia hominivorax, Chrysomya bezziana, Hypoderma bovis, Oestrus ovis, Wohlfahrtia magnifica, Musca domestica, Musca nebulo, Lucilia sericata* and *Sarcophaga* spp. has been described. Orofacial myiasis caused by *C. bezziana*, oro-tracheal myiasis caused by *W. magnifica* and oro-maxillofacial myiasis caused by *C. hominivorax* have also been documented.

Ocular Myiasis (Including Ophthalmomyiasis, Orbital and Palpebral Myiasis). Ocular myiasis refers to infestations of the eye or periorbital tissue by larvae and represents less than 5% of human myiasis cases. When larvae remain outside the eye, it is termed ophthalmomyiasis externa, whereas penetration of the eye itself is termed ophthalmomyiasis interna, a severe condition that can lead to blindness. *Dermatobia hominis* very occasionally causes ophthalmomyiasis externa, with eyelid and conjunctival involvement.

Orbital myiasis in humans is commonly caused by the ovine nasal botfly, *Oestrus ovis* and the Russian botfly, *Rhinoestrus purpureus*, which are found in most sheep farming communities. Victims usually have the sensation of being struck in the eye by an insect or by a small foreign object. A few hours later, a painful inflammation develops, causing an acute catarrhal conjunctivitis. Ocular symptoms, such as foreign body sensation, irritation, redness and photophobia, have been reported. The conjunctivitis can vary from mild to severe pseudo-orbital cellulites. Features of the conjunctivitis included pale oedema, linear superficial punctate and keratopathy.

Nasal Myiasis (Including Nasopharyngeal Myiasis). Rarely, larvae of *Oestrus ovis* are deposited into the mouth and nostrils of humans, where they usually survive only a few days without further development. There are rare reports on larvae of *O. ovis*, remaining in the nasopharyngeal cavities until they reached the third larval stage. Nasal symptoms such as sneezing, nasal discharge and epistaxis may occur. Nasal myiasis by larvae of *Sarcophaga carnaria* (Figure 60.6), *Chrysomya bezziana* and *Lucilia sericata* have been reported.

Aural Myiasis (Including Otomyiasis, Myiasis of the External and Middle Ear). Aural myiasis is relatively common in warm and humid climates. In such cases, larvae feed on necrotic and living tissue until metamorphosis. Cases of otomyiasis with *Oestrus ovis, Lucilia sericata, Wohlfahrtia magnifica* and *Cochliomyia hominivorax* have been observed.

Urogenital Myiasis (Including Vaginal Myiasis, Genital Myiasis, Myiasis of the Uterine Cavity, Pelvic Organ Myiasis, Vulvo-vaginal and Vulvar Myiasis). Urogenital myiasis has been observed due to infestation by larvae of *Piophila casei, Musca domestica, Fannia canicularis, Lucilia sericata, Megaselia scalaris, Chrysomya bezziana, Cochliomyia hominivorax, Eristalis tenax, Parasarcophaga ruficornis, Psychoda albipennis* and *Scenopinus* spp.

Gastrointestinal Myiasis. Intestinal myiasis is usually an accidental phenomenon, which occurs due to the ingestion of eggs or larvae present in food. Usually, the patient is asymptomatic and the larvae are excreted harmlessly in the faeces. However, the passage of larvae may sometimes be associated with symptoms such as bleeding, diarrhoea, abdominal pain, nausea and vomiting. Larvae of species *Eristalis tenax, Muscina stabulans, Megaselia scalaris, Sarcophaga* spp. and *Lucilia* spp. may be isolated.

PREVENTION AND TREATMENT

Cutaneous myiasis is usually a self-limiting clinical condition, as the third-stage larva has to leave the skin and pupate outside the host. Spontaneous expulsion of the larvae may be precipitated by use of an asphyxiating agent, which brings larvae deposited in deeper tissue layers to the surface, thereby facilitating their surgical removal.

A cotton pellet soaked with agents such as petroleum jelly, turpentine, liquid paraffin or mineral oil should be applied in the opening and the larvae can be removed using forceps (Figure 60.7). The larva may also be expressed by gently squeezing the surrounding skin, or by enlarging the opening surgically. There are case reports of the use of ivermectin and nitrofurazone in

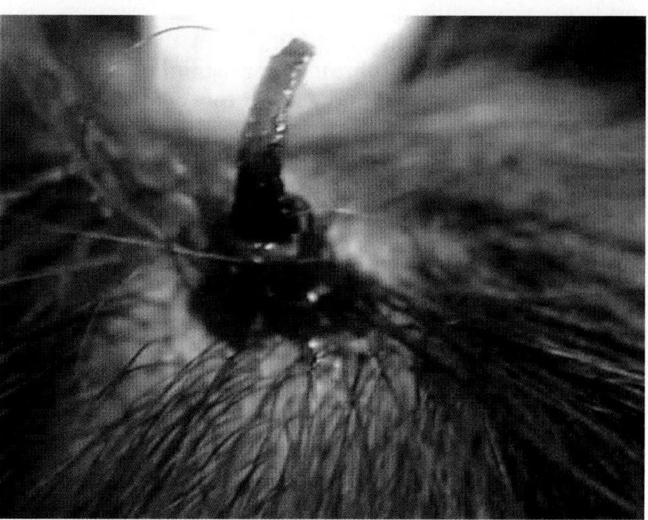

Figure 60.7 Infestation of the scalp by a larva of the botfly, *Dermatobia hominis.*

complicated cases including ocular or cavity myiasis. Patients may squash the maggots within their skin, causing foreign-body reactions, which should be treated symptomatically. Rarely, secondary infection may need systemic antibiotics. Larvae of *Oestrus ovis* in cases of ophthalmomyiasis are removed under local anaesthesia, using forceps.

Nosocomial myiasis occasionally occurs, especially in patients with impaired consciousness, infected or malodorous secretions or drainage tubes, respiratory and gastrointestinal intubations. Window screens should protect such patients from fly larva infestations.

Flypaper, electrocuting and baited traps can be used to control fly population within habitations. Keeping the area free of decaying organic matter, such as trash, decaying plants or excreta will prevent flies from being attracted to the patient's residence, and in turn, the patient. Repellents containing DEET and avoiding exposure are good preventative measures.

Access the complete Myiasis section online at: http://www.expertconsult.com.

Sand Fleas

Sand fleas, also known as jigger, chigger or chigoe fleas, are haematophagous insect parasites of humans and domestic animals. Tungiasis is a zoonotic ectoparasitosis caused by members of the Hectopsyllidae family, from the order Siphonaptera (Fleas). *Tunga penetrans* is found in resource-poor populations throughout Latin America, the Caribbean and sub-Saharan Africa, while *Tunga trimamillata* has been reported only in Ecuador and Peru. Hundreds of millions of people are at risk of infestation in more than 70 nations, mostly in developing countries.[8–10]

BIOLOGY AND EPIDEMIOLOGY

Adult sand fleas are 1 mm long and feed on human or animal blood. Males visit their hosts to take a blood meal and to copulate with females. After a blood meal, the female penetrates the skin within 40 hours. The head is embedded inside the skin, while the terminal abdominal segments with the genital and anal openings remain on the skin surface, allowing the parasite to breathe through the spiracles, to defecate, to copulate and to discharge eggs into the environment. Mating occurs after the female enters the host epidermis. Within the epidermis the body of the flea undergoes hypertrophy (neosomy) (Figure 60.8), reaching the size of up to 1 cm (Figures 60.9, 60.10).

Approximately 6 days after penetration, the female starts to oviposit. Outside the host and under optimal conditions (loose and dry soil) the larvae hatch within 6 days and feed on organic material. After two moults within 10 days, the third-stage larva starts the process of pupation. The formation of adult fleas inside the puparium lasts for 9–15 days.

Within 3 weeks, hundreds of eggs are produced. If there are no complications, the dead female is shed from the host epidermis by tissue repair mechanisms.

T. penetrans has been reported in pigs, bovines, goats, sheep, horses, donkeys, mules, llamas, dogs and cats and some wild animals. Pigs, rats, dogs and cats are the most important reservoir for human infestations. In endemic areas such as in Brazil, the prevalence of tungiasis may reach 50% in cats and 70% in dogs. Factors which influence the development of a sand flea population include sandy soil inside and around houses, the presence of organic material in the compound and presence of shade in the backyard.

PATHOGENESIS AND CLINICAL ASPECTS

In endemic areas, the preferentially affected sites in humans are the feet, especially around the nail beds of the toes, the hands, genitals, gluteus, and groin. The prevalence is highest among 5–14-year-old children. In most infested people, 5–6 adult females are found, although up to 100 fleas have been observed in heavy infestations. Lower socioeconomic status, living under poor hygienic conditions, walking barefoot or with sandals, and living in rat-infested houses with freely roaming pigs, dogs and cats predispose to infestation by sand fleas.

Cases of tungiasis imported to countries in cold or temperate climates are occasionally reported in tourists, missionaries and workers returning from endemic zones.

Early symptoms of infestation are slight and include mild local itching. As the female embedded in the skin increases in volume, the itching intensifies and slight swelling develops, accompanied by erythema and pain of variable severity. Other symptoms and signs include difficulty in walking, deformation of toenails, loss of toenails, desquamation of skin, oedema, pustule formation, ulcers, hyperkeratosis, fissures, pain and secondary infections.

The skin lesion around the embedded flea looks like a 5–10 mm blister with a blackish point (the posterior end of the flea) surrounded by a whitish halo (thinned epidermis) and by slight reddening (surrounding inflammatory zone) (Figure 60.11). Inappropriate extraction or squashing the parasite inside the skin leads to super-infection. The lesions may become septic ulcers with the formation of abscesses, lymphadenitis and thrombophlebitis. Tetanus infection has also been documented.

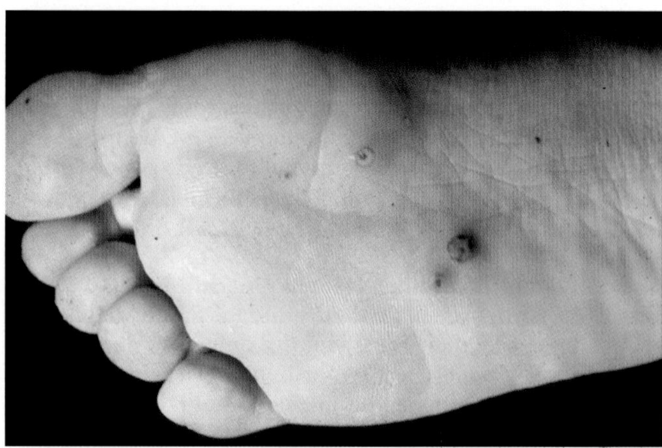

Figure 60.11 Wart-like lesions caused by the sandflea female on the sole of a patient.

The differential diagnosis includes warts, mycotic lesions, granulomas of foreign bodies, early melanoma, tick bite, ingrown toenail, fire-ant bite, dracontiasis and furuncular myiasis.

TREATMENT, PREVENTION AND CONTROL

The simplest method to treat tungiasis is to extract the flea using a sterile scalpel or needle by cutting the skin around the caudal end and pulling the entire flea out with tweezers. Antibiotics may be needed to treat bacterial infection.

Prophylaxis of human tungiasis is based on protecting the feet with closed shoes, use of a repellent such as DEET, insecticidal treatment of the soil in infested houses, control of rat populations, and the prohibition of free movement by animals inside and near houses.

Acknowledgements

I thank Jacqueline Miller for reviewing the English.

Access the following figures online at: http://www.expertconsult.com.

Figure 60.1
Leech bite, in the form of an inverted Y inside a circle, caused by the three jaws of the parasite.

Figure 60.3
The use of the medicinal leech, *Hirudo medicinalis*, to salvage a compromised free-tissue transfer.

Figure 60.4
Facultative myiasis caused by larvae of the green bottle fly, *Lucilia sericata* on the toe of a patient with a chronic wound.

Figure 60.5
Infestation of a child by larvae of Tumbu fly, *Cordylobia anthropophaga*.

Figure 60.6
Nasal myiasis caused by larvae of the flesh fly, *Sarcophaga carnaria*.

Figure 60.8
Life-cycle of *Tunga penetrans*.

Figure 60.9
A female of the sand flea, *Tunga penetrans*, with hypertrophic abdomen.

Figure 60.10
Tunga penetrans female extracted from the skin of a patient. In the middle, the anterior part of the body, which is usually embedded in the epidermis, can be seen, while in the background the swollen abdomen with the eggs is visible.

REFERENCES

1. Sawyer RT. Leech Biology and Behaviour, vol. I–III. Oxford: Clarendon Press; 1986.
2. Michalsen A, Roth M, Dobos C. Medicinal Leech Therapy. Stuttgart: G. Thieme Verlag; 2007.
5. Zumpt F. Myiasis in Man and Animals in the Old World. London: Butterworths; 1965.
6. Hall M, Wall R. Myiasis of humans and domestic animals. Adv Parasitol 1995;35:257–334.
8. Heukelbach J. Tungiasis. Rev Inst Med Trop Sao Paulo 2005;47:307–13.

Access the complete references online at www.expertconsult.com

SECTION 12 Non-communicable Diseases in the Tropics

61 Non-communicable Diseases: Equity, Action and Targets

SANDEEP P. KISHORE | K. SRINATH REDDY

KEY POINTS

- Non-communicable diseases (NCDs), including cardiovascular diseases, cancers, diabetes and lung diseases are the leading drivers of morbidity, mortality and disability globally; 80% of deaths to NCDs occur in low- and middle-income countries.
- The 'causes of the causes' of NCDs make them difficult to address; proximal causes include raised cholesterol, blood pressure and glucose; intermediate causes include tobacco, poor diet, physical inactivity and harmful use of alcohol. These risks are largely man-made and relate to how we live, age, work and play. Distal causes include urbanization, population ageing and trade. Premature death and disability due to NCDs can therefore be viewed as failures of a broader socioeconomic system.
- On the one hand, financing for NCDs with respect to overseas development assistance for health remains scarce (2.3% of all international donor assistance is focused on NCDs, US$503 million out of $22 billion). On the other, the interventions for NCDs (e.g. tobacco taxation) are highly cost-effective.
- Free trade and globalization concerns, including intellectual property and free-trade treaties surrounding access to essential medicines for the treatment of non-communicable diseases, remain a key twenty-first century priority, as observed for HIV/AIDS.
- A UN 'High Level Meeting' on NCDs in 2011, only the second such meeting on health in the UN's history, put the spotlight on NCDs as barriers to development and deserving a multidisciplinary response across all of society.

Introduction

Imagine being the Director General of the World Health Organization (WHO), a Minister of Health in a developing country or even a Head of State. In our current century of globalization and inter-dependence, where would you prioritize your attention to safeguard the health of your constituency? That is, if you have a dollar to improve your population's health, where and how would the 100 cents of that dollar be apportioned to maximize its benefit? Devastating infections such as HIV/AIDS or childhood pneumonias will compete for your attention. Both critique and applause will await your every decision. Whenever a unit of capital (whether it is financial, social, or time) is expended, it is gone. You look to population health statistics to justify and prioritize your budget – what do you find?

To respond to these critical questions, we first adopt a definition from the WHO that examines the disease burden. There are three 'buckets' or categories of disease. One bucket consists of communicable, maternal, perinatal and nutritional disorders and diseases. In developed countries, we often forget that diseases such as malaria ravished the world, including the whole southeastern seaboard of the USA, as little as 130 years ago. Strategic, focused investments in sanitation, public health and hygiene successfully diminished the burden of these disorders over the last century. This, then, helped drive an epidemiological transition towards chronic, non-communicable diseases (NCDs) such as diabetes, unipolar depression, cancers, heart disease as the second category. These are diseases that accompany globalization, are typically associated with developed countries and are driven by man-made, modifiable risk factors, which is our second bucket. Finally, the third bucket consists of physical injuries to the body. These could be traumas inflicted by war, by traffic incidents or by conscious intent (e.g. suicide).

Where is the bulk of the money going (and thus attention, time and energy currently being expended)? In the past decade, the WHO had incurred 87 cents for every dollar on 'first category' communicable diseases; 12 cents of every dollar on 'second category' non-communicable diseases; and 1 cent for every dollar on 'third category' injuries.[1] In this section, we will examine how WHO priority trend, as outlined above, has also been reflected in international development assistance budgets and Millennium Development Goals.

We next ask a very basic question: What kills us, globally? Annually, there is about a 1% turnover in the population; a global burden of 57 million human deaths.[2,3] Surprisingly, the leading driver of international mortality consists of 'second bucket' chronic, non-communicable diseases (NCDs). Cardiovascular disease, whether in the arteries of the heart (ischaemic heart disease) or brain (cerebrovascular disease), is now the leading killer worldwide. What surprises many is that nearly 80% of all global heart attacks occur in low- and middle-income countries – and this disease alone claims more than twice as many lives as HIV/AIDS, tuberculosis and malaria combined.[4] Other NCDs such as chronic obstructive pulmonary disease and lung cancer are also top-10 killers. Additionally, age-standardized mortality shows that NCDs are claiming people at increasingly younger ages in resource-poor settings, i.e. *premature mortality* (death before age 60) to NCDs, is on the rise. Death from NCDs in resource-poor settings often occurs in the backdrop of 'first category' communicable, tropical diseases, including pneumonias, HIV and tuberculosis. This constitutes the 'double' burden of disease. Finally, as a potential triple burden, traumatic traffic accidents are the ninth leading cause

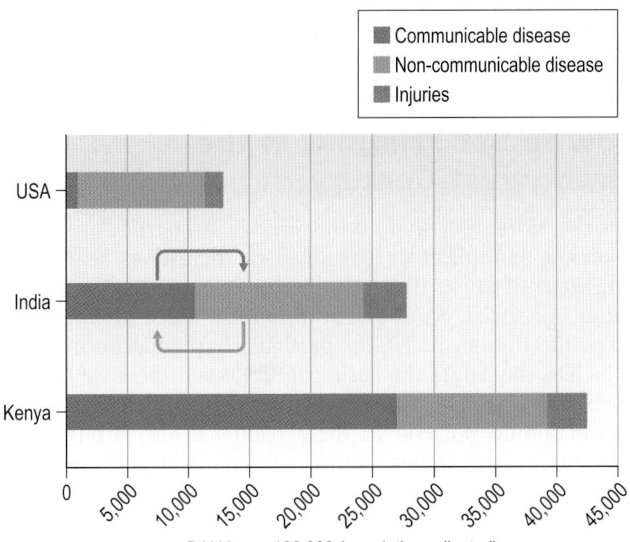

Figure 61.1 The Burden of Disease: Non-communicable Diseases. The burden of disease in terms of DALYs per 100 000. (Full explanation of figure is provided in the text.) *(Data provided by Mathers C, Fat DM, Boerma JT, World Health Organization. The Global Burden of Disease: 2004 update; Geneva, Switzerland: World Health Organization; 2008).*

of death globally, and suicides claim as many lives as malaria each year.

To quantify not just the mortality, but also morbidity of disease, we use the disability-adjusted life year (DALY) to assess the total disease burden. One DALY is equal to the number of years of life lost to disease (YLL) added to the number of years lived with disability (YLD). It is thus a more useful robust measure for chronic illnesses, in which many individuals living with their disease cannot be maximally productive during their convalescence. Figure 61.1 presents disease burden in terms of DALYs per 100 000 people in three countries with three different income settings: high-income (USA), middle-income (India) and low-income (Kenya). A higher burden of disease results in more DALYs lost. According to these data, Indians are twice as 'sick' (have twice as many DALYs lost) as the Americans; Kenyans are three times as 'sick' as the Americans (have three times as many DALYs lost).[4]

Figure 61.1 also demonstrates that for the first time in India's history, the burden of non-communicable disease has eclipsed that of communicable diseases. This same trend is playing out in other middle-income contexts including China, South Africa, Brazil, Russia and even urban environments of low-income settings. Finally, a close look at low-income settings like Kenya reveals two major points. The first point is quite unsurprising in a global health and topical medicine context: malaria, hookworm and other neglected tropical diseases continue to rage, constituting nearly three-quarters of the total burden of disease. At the same time, however, we see a second, surprising pattern: the burden of NCDs in Kenya is now equivalent to, or even slightly greater than, the burden of NCDs in the USA.

Deciding priorities on national and international health spending is critical when the health budgets of each country vary enormously. According to National Health Accounts, the USA spends close to US$8000 per person per year;[5] India spends about $43 per person per year; and Kenya spends just $19 per person per year. Based on the discussion of disease burdens above, how would you allocate your razor-thin health resources if you are the minister of health of Kenya? Would you consider prioritizing NCDs over communicable diseases?

A crucial point is that there is clear cross-talk between these categories of disease – these diseases are not isolated, but are inter-dependent and linked (as shown by the arrows in Figure 61.1) . In India, for example, type II diabetes is one of the principal risk factors for manifesting active tuberculosis.[6–8] Moreover, up to 30% of what we typically think of as chronic diseases, such as cancers, actually have an infectious origin (e.g. HPV driving cervical cancer or hepatitis B driving liver cancer). Emerging data showing the cross-links between infectious and chronic disease drivers, coined 'Endemic NCDs' provides a strong scientific, public health and clinical rationale for concerted action.[9,10] This underscores the need for a more holistic approach to address twenty-first century health – and makes it very clear that there is no need for resource 'wars' to tackle 'disparate categories' of disease burden. Resources spent on non-communicable diseases need not come out of the resources currently spent on communicable diseases. Instead, advocates of both sides should instead seek to address underlying systemic factors of all diseases together as part of a common ecology or system. To be sure, this is easier said than done!

Twenty-first Century Health: the 'Causes of the Causes'

To answer how resources could be allocated, we need to next ask what the systemic causes behind NCDs are. Globally, what is causing all the heart attacks and cancer cases? It is natural to first look towards proximal risk factors such as high blood pressure or high cholesterol levels. Indeed, when assessing the leading risk factors driving the burden of disease worldwide, blood pressure ranks at number three and high cholesterol ranks at number seven.[3] What, however, is driving the high cholesterol? What, in essence, are the causes of the causes?

Four principal risks stand above the rest: *tobacco, poor diet, inadequate physical inactivity,* and *harmful use of alcohol.* Tobacco alone accounts for 1 in 10 deaths globally, killing half of the people that use it. Moreover, its use is rising in women and youth of both genders globally.[11] Fast food and high-fat, processed diets have percolated across the globe from the West, influencing how, when and what the world consumes. Alcohol use and over-drinking have increased; in Russia in particular, it accounted for a loss of 7 years in life expectancy in the 1990s alone.[12] Tobacco use in India[13] and obesity in Egypt have been inversely correlated with education status;[14] nutritional determinants such as sugar exposure explain increased diabetes rates[15] with each 1% increase in GDP of the food service industry associated with a 1% increase in diabetes prevalence.[16] These show that the causes of the causes run deep (Figure 61.2).

It is worth noting that the impact of such changes is felt even by the world's youth. Over the past two decades, we have witnessed the slow and steady rise of childhood obesity in all income strata, regardless of country. This effectively means more children are sick early on in their lives – some even with fatty streaks in their arteries as seen in Seychelles as young as 8 years old.[17,18] Indeed, if the trajectories of earlier onset of disease patterns hold, data from the USA suggest that children born in this generation may not live as long as their parents: for the first

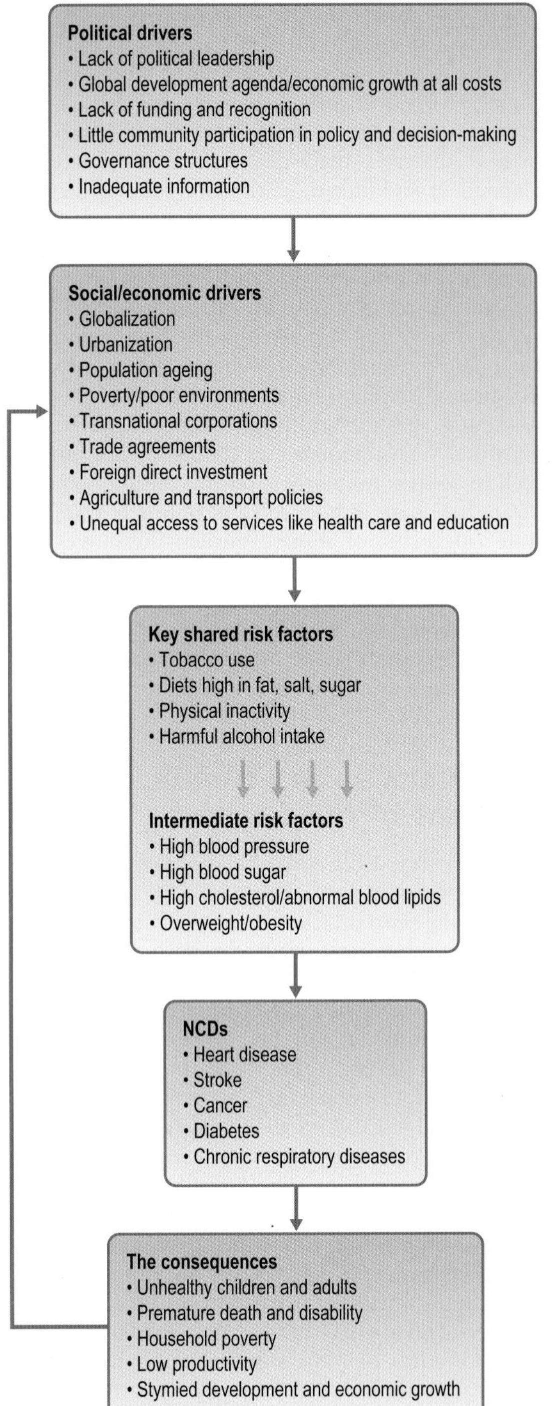

Figure 61.2 The 'Causes of the Causes'. *(Credit: Philip Baker.)*

time, life expectancy could stall or even decline.[19] This trend could be reflected in other countries in middle- and low-income settings by 2050. Furthermore, a set of compelling epidemiological data and laboratory science additionally suggests that the earliest origins of NCDs are in the womb and the first 2 years of life – demonstrating how systems biology affects predisposition to NCDs. Fetal re-programming and a 'reset' to slower metabolism in mothers without adequate nutrition and growth support causes greater rates of premature metabolic syndrome – observations that portend even greater premature mortality to NCDs for the next 2–3 decades.[20,21]

How to Set Priorities in the Twenty-first Century?

It is therefore clear that addressing NCDs, particularly in the tropics, is complicated. The diseases themselves represent a long series of causes that must be contextualized in the broader settings of social, economic and political links. Attempting to lessen the burden of NCDs, particularly premature mortality to NCDs, challenges the basic conceptions of how we live, eat, work and play. The amount of oversight private and public sectors should portend in these realms is also brought into question. We are facing a future of 'manufactured' epidemics, with global commodity producers driving increased consumption of processed foods, alcohol and tobacco. If current projections hold, the consumption of unhealthy foods in developing countries will reach that of developed countries in the next three decades.[22] What is more, proposed interventions on food policy – bans on food high in saturated fats, taxes on fizzy drinks and so on – are often shunned as the path towards a nanny state that infringes on civil liberties. How, then, do we set priorities, particularly with our limited resources?

We can begin by further understanding where money and resources currently flow. Data from Sridhar et al. (Figure 61.3) mapped the bulk of overseas donor assistance for health to the burden of disease in terms of DALYs. The mapping shows that, in the twenty-first century, major resources are locked into specific disease categories – programmes, rather than systems. Further, they are locked into *particular* diseases and programmes. The data were provocative in showing two outliers: HIV/AIDS and NCDs. The calculation, roughly, was that $1030 was spent on every HIV/AIDS death and $3 for every death to NCDs.[23] The other 'investment portfolios' of malaria, child health, clean water, tuberculosis, on the other hand, appeared to linearly correlate dollar to DALY.

Why do NCDs receive so little funding when they account for such high disease burden? A report from the Center for Global Development, entitled 'Where have all the donors gone?' demonstrated that NCDs received only 2.3% of overseas development assistance, while driving the most DALYs globally.[24] The report showed that all NCDs together were receiving only 78 cents per DALY compared with 22 dollars per DALY for HIV, tuberculosis and malaria combined.[24,25] These reports have helped animate the paucity of support for NCD control and care, particularly in development programmes. Studies from the World Economic Forum showed that, if no action is taken soon, NCDs would cost $47 trillion by 2030 in terms of lost productivity and economic toll globally.[26] Studies by the WHO showed that just $11.4 billion annually was required for effective primary and secondary prevention for NCDs.[27] Additionally, cost-effective analyses and the Disease Control Priorities Project (DCPP) highlighted that interventions for NCDs at a population level – for instance, enacting a tobacco tax of 33% – only cost $22 year[27] and were among the most cost-effective interventions a country could take.[28]

The question of whether NCDs should be perceived as a development issue by public and private donors is central to this debate. The perception is often that NCDs are diseases of the rich, diseases of the old and, critically, diseases that are

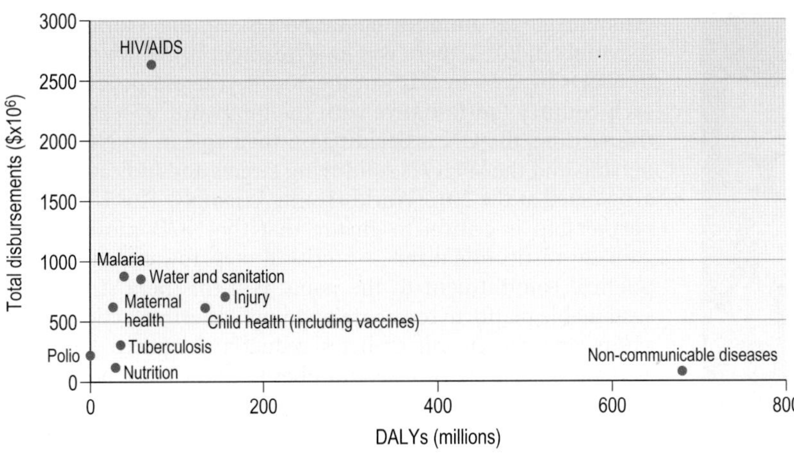

Figure 61.3 How are global health dollars spent? Distribution of the total disbursements of overseas development assistance with respect to the burden of disease (in DALYs). *(Adapted from Sridhar D, Batniji R. Misfinancing global health: a case for transparency in disbursements and decision making. Lancet 2008;372(9644):1185–1191.)*

self-indulgent. Many people assert that it is the 'fault' of the individual for living a lifestyle that resulted in an NCD. Others may simply not know that NCDs are leading causes of death in developing countries. This was shown by one study of US surveys of people's perceptions of the leading causes of death against measures of the actual disease burden from the WHO, in which little correlation between the US public's perception and the actual disease burden was found.[29]

A Social Movement Takes Root: NCDs Affirmed as a Social Justice Issue

These perceptions came to a head with the rise of a new, recently unified social movement. The vision of the movement was modelled after the HIV community's movement wherein members sought to raise the issue of HIV in the global consciousness. Further, this historical group demanded that world leaders devote attention, resources and political capital to their cause. Their effort resulted in the first-ever UN General Assembly Special Session (UNGASS) on HIV/AIDS in 2001. This meeting, the first UN meeting on any health issue, led directly to the establishment of a global fund, initially only for HIV/AIDS efforts – but which was later tapped for TB and malaria as well.

The initial NCD movement had its roots in patients' rights, with a strong constituency from the Caribbean. These patients drew the spotlight to their foot amputations, which were secondary to unchecked diabetes. By asserting that freedom from this chronic disease was a rights issue, they argued that needless suffering was resulting from global neglect of diabetes. Countries in the Caribbean, including Trinidad and Tobago, affirmed that they were spending nearly 10% of their GDP on diabetes care, with little to no improvements. This patient movement took their concerns to the ministers of a group of Caribbean countries (known as CARICOM in the UN system), to petition for greater support at the global level. The CARICOM leadership then raised the issue of diabetes and related NCDs to the UN. To the surprise of many, there was broad support from the floor, including from delegates of South-east Asia and the African Union, who cited the negative impact of NCDs on the population level. Crucially, social and economic parameters, not just health, were demonstrated to suffer with a high NCD burden. Thus, NCDs were affirmed to be a political, social and economic topic – not just a health topic. Moreover, NCDs took on a human rights angle, becoming linked to discussions of injustice and inequity.

Quickly, a proposal gained momentum to hold an UNGASS on NCDs with heads of state, a meeting analogous to the 10-year session on HIV/AIDS, was circulated and approved. The meeting, coined a 'High-Level Meeting', would position NCDs as indicators beyond just health – but social and economic processes. Further, heads of state would, for the first time, acknowledge that strategic, systems-based approaches beyond just the health sector would be required to address the global increase of NCDs. A series of consultations were held with the UN's health lead (the WHO) at six regions feeding into the first-ever WHO Global Forum in Moscow on NCDs and the first ministerial meeting on healthy lifestyles in April, 2011.[30] A series of other consultations followed, including a civil society hearing at the United Nations, and followed by the release of a zero draft on the political declaration on NCDs. This draft, initially called an 'outcomes document', was intended to provide a set of key commitments for countries to agree on so that the global attack on NCDs would be a concerted effort. Unsurprisingly, negotiation of the political declaration was mediated through a tense process with a group of 77 countries (actually representing 132), led by Suriname, accompanied by China; these countries often went head to head with developed countries for provisions on access to medicines, fighting for food/beverage policies and financing commitments. Youth, students, HIV+ patients, cancer survivors, tobacco advocates and access-to-medicine leaders converged at the UN High Level Meeting for the first-ever rally on NCDs at the UN Headquarters. Their goal was to frame NCDs as a social justice issue – they sought to petition world leaders to commit to equity promotion, action and targets (Figure 61.4). Over 300 non-governmental organizations were allowed into the UN General Assembly for this historic meeting and several representatives were allowed to make interventions from the floor. Following from the demands from people living with HIV/AIDS for access to therapies and the right to health, a newer movement has now surfaced on the rights of people living with NCDs for access to the appropriate interventions. The topic of access to medicines for NCDs, in particular, serves as a useful case study of the tensions at play that span human rights, trade policy and clinical medicine in the modern era.

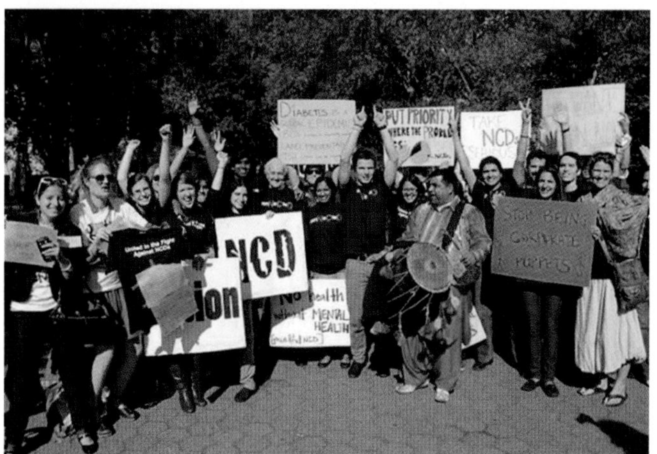

Figure 61.4 A Rally for Non-communicable Diseases: An Issue of Social Justice. A youth rally by the Young Professionals Chronic Disease Network (YP-CDN) on the date of the UN High Level Meeting on NCDs promoting Equity, Action and Targets with NCD survivors, advocates, HIV+ leaders and youth from across the globe. *(Photo Credit: Rajesh Vedanthan.)*

The Policy Tensions around NCDs: Equity, Action and Targets

Successive versions of the negotiation proceedings for the political declaration on NCDs revealed that high-income countries at one time threatened to delete any mention of access to medicines and trade-related aspects of intellectual property rights (TRIPS). This inflexibility around intellectual property restrictions prevents countries from making drugs cheaply, in generic forms, which was a major step forward for antiretrovirals in the past decade.[31,32] In fact, the previously sanctioned 2001 Doha Declaration that affirms the right of countries to except pharmaceuticals from typical trade regulations, and which allowed flexibility on intellectual property, was omitted from the draft entirely. Even the use of the word 'epidemic' to describe NCDs was viewed as a 'trigger' that would invoke the necessity of flexibility on intellectual property, construed as being relevant only to infectious diseases, and was therefore deleted.[33]

The stark contrast between the political acknowledgements of NCDs compared with communicable diseases was even more poignant to watch in the shadow of the 10-year anniversary meeting of the HIV/AIDS 2001 UNGASS session, held just months prior. Following on from the original meeting, the 2011 HIV/AIDS UNGASS included a political declaration of key commitments that Member States agreed on: while the reference to the Doha Declaration in the access to medicines section was clear, in June, 2011, for the political declaration on HIV, this same reference was conspicuously missing for the political declaration on NCDs by September, 2011. This fundamental difference in political language between HIV and NCDs reflects not just the future policy changes that must be made before appropriate resources can be allocated to tackle NCDs; it also demands that the entire global population must agree, and define, what constitutes their right to health.[33]

The final political declaration ended by calling for a set of targets to be drafted by the WHO, with a potential partnership (para. 64 of the UN declaration) proposed by the UN to help oversee a global response to NCDs.[33,34] This would lead the essential global monitoring of NCDs. At the World Health Assembly in 2012, there was an agreement to reduce mortality to NCDs by 25% by 2025 in the 30–70-year-old population of each country (an initiative with the buzzword '25×25'). As of this writing, the UN is deciding on their role in an NCD partnership and the WHO is solidifying targets and indicators to be articulated at the 2013 World Health Assembly. This UN/WHO partnership is critical to ensure that the NCD movement is globally institutionalized – a critical step towards sustaining political commitment to the issue. Will this be a strong and sustainable platform to ensure ongoing, collective, action? Indicators and targets on diabetes reduction, tobacco smoking, alcohol, dietary salt intake and obesity and cancer prevention in primary care are being considered as of this writing. The tensions on trade and health are no more salient than in the context of NCD policy.

What Happens Next?

The revision of the Millennium Development Goals (MDGs) will occur in 2015, making it an important year for the global tropical medicine community to assess development progress. At start of the last decade, NCDs were omitted from the MDGs because of the common belief that NCDs do not affect the poor at a disproportionate rate compared with tropical, communicable diseases. This decision has influenced how and why resources are spent globally today. Since then, series of meetings in Rio de Janeiro, Brazil, including the Rio+20 meeting on sustainable development, has highlighted NCDs, as a key focus. Additional support from the United Nations Development Programme has also made it clear that NCDs are a barrier to sustainable development and critical to the social determinants of health.

In the USA, data have shown that of the 30 years gained in life expectancy in the past century, only 5 of these years are directly attributable to medical care.[35] The rest followed from addressing the 'causes of the causes': the social, behavioural and economic determinants (sanitation, nutrition, hygiene) that unlocked gains in health. For addressing NCDs in the twenty-first century, medical interventions alone will not substantially decrease morbidity and mortality. Creating incentives to change how we live, how we eat and how we play are globally crucial for lifespan extension. This naturally builds upon the long legacy of public health over hundreds of years. Perhaps, particularly in light of the access to medicines, a holistic strategy of prevention (causes of the causes) and treatment will win the day. Readers of this text, whether students, teachers or field workers, must have an interdisciplinary mindset: they must seek to tackle both social and biomedical determinants of health to gain ground in global health. Re-thinking NCDs in the context of communicable diseases will require a different model of care than that used for tropical communicable diseases alone. This model will challenge the social decisions that govern our sick societies. The modern efforts observed in New York City, such as tobacco taxation, tobacco bans and soda size restrictions, may signal a new global health movement centred on regulation.

Finally, the past decade has seen the rise of social movements that are disease-orientated such as the HIV/AIDS UNGASS in 2001, the associated TB and malaria movements, the movement on neglected tropical diseases (NTDs) and the movement on maternal and child health (MCH). Now, the UN High Level

Meeting on NCDs, and the affiliated movement on global mental health, is starting to coalesce at the cusp of this new decade. We must critically ask whether these 'disease movements' are suitable for the twenty-first century – or whether such categorical campaigns result in disease 'wars' that create isolated silos for financing, political and social attention.

Importantly, does advocating for specific diseases distract from the hard work of strengthening health systems and improving social determinants that would better treat, or even prevent, a variety of diseases from all categories? For readers of this text, the challenges of transforming sick societies into healthy ones are firming up. The right to health in the tropics can, should and must be affirmed in order to address all disease categories. Indeed, to suffer is human; to suffer needlessly is not – to tackle human suffering, we must decrease morbidity across the span of human life. As we close our discussion, the final question is posed to the reader: where would you place your priorities as a Director General of the WHO or as a Head of State? How and where would you spend your 100 cents in an era of two epidemics that are equally treatable: one brought on as a by-product of modernization, the other still being waged against infectious microorganisms?

REFERENCES

2. Mathers C, Fat DM, Boerma JT, the World Health Organization. The Global Burden of Disease: 2004 update. Geneva: World Health Organization; 2008.

22. Stuckler D, McKee M, Ebrahim S, et al. Manufacturing epidemics: the role of global producers in increased consumption of unhealthy commodities including processed foods, alcohol, and tobacco. PLoS Med 2012; 9(6):e1001235.

26. Bloom DE, Cafiero ET, Jané-Llopis E, et al. The Global Economic Burden of Noncommunicable Diseases. Geneva: World Economic Forum; 2011. Online. Available: http://www.weforum.org/EconomicsofNCD (Accessed 1 Oct 2012).

27. World Health Organization and World Economic Forum From Burden to 'Best Buys'. Reducing the Economic Impact of Non-Communicable Diseases in Low- and Middle-Income Countries. Geneva: WHO; September 2011.

34. UN. Document A/66/L1 Political Declaration of the High-level Meeting of the General Assembly on the Prevention and Control of Non-communicable Diseases United Nations General Assembly, 66th session. Online. Available: http://www.un.org/en/ga/ncdmeeting2011/.

Access the complete references online at www.expertconsult.com

62

Cardiovascular and Vascular Disease in the Tropics Including Stroke, Hypertension and Ischaemic Heart Disease

NIGEL UNWIN | T. ALAFIA SAMUELS | ANGELA M. C. ROSE | ANSELM J. M. HENNIS

KEY POINTS

- Cardiovascular disease (CVD) accounts for 30% of all deaths globally, over 80% of which occur in low- and middle-income countries (LMICs).
- Rheumatic heart disease, although different in aetiology to major causes of CVD and accounting for 'only' 1% of all CVD deaths, disproportionately affects poor and young populations and remains a major cause of preventable morbidity and mortality in LMICs.
- The vast majority of CVD deaths are due to ischaemic heart disease (IHD) and stroke, and these share common behavioural risk factors that include high salt and saturated fat diet, physical inactivity, tobacco smoking and excess alcohol.
- Raised blood pressure, related to high salt diet, obesity and other factors, alone accounts for 13% of all deaths globally.
- While there is evidence for some differences between ethnic groups in salt sensitivity, the major risk factors for CVD are overwhelmingly the same in all populations.
- The management of stable hypertension and CVD is based upon an assessment of overall risk of future adverse events and utilizes both patient education and pharmacological therapy.
- Highly effective low-cost generic drugs exist for reducing CVD risk.
- The management of acute CVD events is best carried out in hospital.
- The prevention of CVD requires a dual strategy of measures to lower the risk profile of entire populations and screening to identify and treat individuals at particularly high risk.
- Successful population-wide prevention of CVD will require collaboration between different sectors of society (e.g. health, food industry, planning and transport), and governments to follow-up on commitments made at the 2011 UN High Level Meeting on non-communicable diseases.

Introduction

Cardiovascular disease (CVD) is the single largest cause of morbidity and mortality globally, and a major contributor to death and disability in all countries, whatever their level of economic development. The main focuses of this chapter are on a major risk factor and two broad categories of CVD. The major risk factor is hypertension. The two categories are ischaemic heart disease (IHD) and cerebrovascular disease, which can be further sub-divided into ischaemic stroke and intracerebral haemorrhagic stroke. In tropical countries, as elsewhere, these conditions are the major contributors to cardiovascular morbidity and mortality. While focusing on these areas, we acknowledge that other forms of CVD will be considered relevant to a textbook of tropical diseases. We have assumed that where the cardiovascular system is involved in other tropical diseases, such as in Chagas disease, this will have been covered in a relevant chapter. However, there is one condition that may not be covered elsewhere and remains a significant burden in many settings, and that is rheumatic heart disease. We have provided a description of this in Box 62.1.

It is beyond the scope of a single chapter to provide a comprehensive account of the epidemiology, pathogenesis, treatment and prevention of hypertension, IHD and stroke. What we aim to do here is to provide a comprehensive overview of these areas and to highlight aspects particularly relevant to low- and middle-income country (LMIC) settings. In the section on treatment, for example, our aim is to highlight effective interventions that are considered feasible and affordable with poor to moderate levels of resources. In aiming to keep the chapter focused in this way we have ensured that, as far as possible and appropriate, its contents are consistent with recent guidance from the World Health Organization (WHO).

Epidemiology

Diseases of the cardiovascular system are found in populations at all stages of economic development. They are a significant contributor to morbidity and mortality in populations as diverse as those of rural Africa and North America. However, the types of CVD that predominate differ with the level of economic development.[1] The epidemiological transition provides a useful framework for considering the relationships

BOX 62.1 RHEUMATIC HEART DISEASE

EPIDEMIOLOGY

Rheumatic heart disease (RHD) has almost disappeared from high-income countries (HIC), but is the most common cause of acquired heart disease, the leading cause of heart failure and CVD deaths globally in children and young adults living in poverty, and is still prevalent among some underprivileged, indigenous populations in HICs. More than 80% of the world's children (<15 years) live in endemic RHD areas. RHD accounts for 1% of CVD deaths and 4% of CVD Disability Adjusted Life Years (DALYs), yet has been mostly neglected.

The best estimates are that approximately 16 million persons have RHD and 250000 die from this disease each year, often after repeated hospitalizations, and where available, expensive heart surgery. The prevalence data are estimated from surveys of children since diagnosis is unreliable and medical records often incomplete in many high-prevalence countries. The highest prevalence rates are in young adults in sub-Saharan Africa, Pacific Islanders and Indigenous Australians of 5–10/1000 school children. In Latin America and the Caribbean, the rates are 1/1000 school children. Much of the disease is subclinical, and the recent introduction of mobile echocardiography and detection of asymptomatic disease is increasing the reported prevalence.

Although penicillin is now the primary intervention, historically, rates of acute rheumatic fever and rheumatic heart disease started declining before the advent of antibiotics, due to improvements in sanitation, overcrowding and nutrition.

PATHOLOGY

Acute Rheumatic Fever

Acute rheumatic fever occurs in children, adolescents and young adults 3 weeks after symptomatic or asymptomatic, untreated or under-treated group A streptococcal pyogenes infection of the tonsils or impetigo. Diagnosis is made by high or rising streptococcal antibody titres. It is due to an abnormal host immune response to the infection in a genetically susceptible host. Acute rheumatic fever presents with fever, painful, migratory polyarthritis affecting the large and medium-sized joints in 60–80% of cases, and carditis. Sydenham's chorea, involuntary, irregular movements, including external rotation of the hands, occurs 1–6 months later in 7–28% of cases. Carditis, including valvulitis, pericarditis and myocarditis, occur in half of patients with acute rheumatic fever, within a few weeks of the original infection. A soft, blowing, pansystolic murmur of mitral regurgitation is indicative. The pericarditis causes chest pain and a transient pericardial friction rub with small pericardial effusions. Echocardiography is able to diagnose subclinical carditis with no symptoms or signs.

Rheumatic Heart Disease

The highest prevalence is among those aged 20–50 years who present with shortness of breath, often without a history of clinical acute rheumatic fever. Women in the child-bearing years have higher prevalence, thought to be due to higher levels of exposure to group A strep from their children, health care access and genetic susceptibility.

Mitral valve incompetence is most common in the earlier phase of the disease, with mitral stenosis developing later. Aortic regurgitation may occur in tandem with mitral regurgitation, but can be an isolated and severe feature. Diagnosis is through auscultation or echocardiography, or after a presentation due to complications – infective endocarditis, atrial arrhythmias, acute heart failure or an embolic event. Mortality rates usually from severe heart failure are associated with late presentation and inadequate facilities for surgical interventions.

MANAGEMENT

Acute Rheumatic Fever

Penicillin injections should be used to clear the *Streptococcus*, which is the trigger for the sequelae. Aspirin is useful for symptomatic relief of joint pain and fever. Surgical valve repair may be necessary in cases of refractive heart failure. Education about the need for ongoing secondary prophylaxis should begin during this initial phase for better adherence.

Rheumatic Heart Disease

Antibiotic prophylaxis is the cornerstone of treatment in an effort to prevent complications, plus medical therapy for heart failure, anticoagulants for atrial fibrillation, surgery for symptomatic valvular disease. Surgery is most often indicated in areas of high prevalence of disease, which is associated with poverty and inadequately resourced health services, leading to high mortality in these settings. Monthly penicillin prophylaxis as secondary prevention, is recommended for LMIC, since primary prevention and poverty alleviation are less feasible.

PREVENTION

Rheumatic fever and rheumatic heart disease prevalence declined sharply over the last century before the advent of antibiotics in the developed world, as they made the historical transition from underdeveloped to developed status with improved housing and nutrition. Thus socioeconomic development addresses the underlying determinants, but is least feasible in the short term.

Public education and accessible health care should actively identify and promptly treat sore throats and impetigo with oral antibiotics to prevent acute rheumatic fever. However, most sore throats are viral and many bacterial causes are asymptomatic. There is no vaccine on the horizon.

Secondary prevention with monthly penicillin prophylaxis is to prevent new *Strep.* infection, with duration related to the severity of disease. Secondary prevention is best delivered based on community registries and surveillance, but compliance is often a challenge due to mobile populations, and inadequate health services. Identifying candidates for secondary prevention is also a challenge. Screening programmes have inherent limitations of differentiating RHD murmurs from functional murmurs and many cases of carditis having no murmurs. Screening is best done in communities since it is young adults who have the highest burden and school-based screening will not reach adults or children out of school. Miniature field-based echocardiography has identified 10 times as many cases as auscultation, but prevention programmes based on echo have not yet been assessed, and face the challenge of criteria for asymptomatic RHD diagnosis and guidelines on management of asymptomatic mild valvular disease.

Sources: Marijon E, Mirabel M, Celermajer DS, et al. Rheumatic heart disease. Lancet 2012;379(9819):953–64 and Mendis S, Puska P, Norrving B, editors. Global Atlas on Cardiovascular Disease Prevention and Control: Policies, Strategies and Interventions. Geneva: World Health Organization; 2011.[61]

between demography and fertility, disease patterns and social and economic development. Table 62.1 indicates the predominant forms of CVD at four different stages of the epidemiological transition,[1] and illustrates that atherosclerotic CVD predominates in the later stages of the transition, as is the case now for the vast majority of countries globally.

In 2008, CVD was estimated to account for 17 million deaths; 30% of all deaths globally. The major contributors globally to CVD death are IHD, accounting for 46% and 38% of deaths in men and women, respectively, and cerebrovascular disease or stroke, accounting for 34% and 37% of CVD deaths, respectively. Hypertensive heart disease is the next

TABLE 62.1 **Main Cardiovascular Diseases by Stages of the Epidemiological Transition**

Stage of Transition	Life Expectancy at Birth (Years)	Main CVDs
Pestilence and famine	20–40	Rheumatic fever, infectious and nutritional cardiomyopathies
Receding pandemics	30–50	As above + hypertensive heart disease and haemorrhagic stroke
Degenerative and man-made diseases	>50	All stroke, IHD at relatively young ages
Delayed degenerative diseases	>70	Ischaemic stroke and IHD at older ages

Based on Howson C, Reddy S, Ryan T, et al. Control of Cardiovascular Diseases in Developing Countries. Research, Development and Institutional Strengthening. Washington DC: National Academy Press; 1998.

largest single contributor to CVD deaths, at 6% in men and 7% in women.

Over 80% of all CVD deaths in 2008 occurred in LMICs. Not only are the vast majority of CVD deaths in LMICs, which in part reflects their larger population, but age-adjusted death rates for both IHD and cerebrovascular disease are greater than in high-income countries.[2] Although globally only responsible for 10% of the disease burden, CVDs are the main cause of death and disability considered together (as DALYs), resulting in over 150 000 million DALYs worldwide. In 2004, IHD and cerebrovascular disease accounted for 4.1% and 3.1%, respectively of all DALYs globally,[3] ranking fourth and sixth as contributors to the global burden of disease – or the single largest contributor when considered together.

In this section, we outline the epidemiology of hypertension (raised blood pressure) and its major CVD sequelae, in particular stroke and IHD. At the end of this section, we consider the common determinants, or risk factors, that underlie these conditions.

HYPERTENSION

The WHO defines hypertension as a raised systolic blood pressure (SBP) of at least 140 mmHg and/or diastolic blood pressure (DBP) of at least 90 mmHg. Using this definition, and including people with a diagnosis of hypertension who are on antihypertensive medication, the global prevalence of hypertension in adults aged 25 years and above was estimated to be around 40% in 2008.[4] Figure 62.1 shows the prevalence of hypertension by country for men and women. Note that the prevalence of hypertension tends to be higher in men than in women, with overall age-standardized prevalence being around 2–8% higher in men, depending on the setting.[4]

Blood pressure is related to the risk of both IHD and stroke, with increasing risk being evident from blood pressure >115 mmHg systolic and 75 mmHg diastolic.[5,6] In addition to IHD and stroke, raised blood pressure increases the risk of heart failure, renal disease, retinal haemorrhage and loss of vision. Compared with a range of other risk factors, including those for communicable diseases, it is estimated that raised blood pressure (based on an optimal population mean SBP of 115 mmHg) is the single biggest contributor to global mortality, accounting for around 13% (7.5 million in 2008) of all deaths. Even in low-income countries it accounts for virtually the same proportion of deaths as underweight in childhood – roughly 7.5%.[7]

The age-standardized prevalence of hypertension in LMICs is greater (a little over 40% in both sexes combined) than in high-income countries (around 35%). This pattern at a regional level also tends to be found within countries: the poorest sections of the population tend to have the highest blood pressure. This is well established in richer countries,[8] with the evidence suggesting a more mixed picture in LMICs, where risk factors for hypertension, including obesity and a high salt diet, are greater in the more affluent members of society. However, in a large study in urban Tanzania, there was some evidence for blood pressure being inversely related to socioeconomic status, a relationship that was strengthened when differences in body mass index were taken into account.[9]

An examination of global trends in SBP suggests that over the past 30 years there has been a small decline in mean blood pressure, roughly by 1 mmHg per decade.[5] However, there are marked regional differences, with evidence of greater decline in some areas, such as Western Europe and North America, and increases in others, such as in parts of Africa and Asia.[5] Globally, it is estimated that there has been an increase in those with uncontrolled hypertension over the last 30 years, from 600 million (1980) to almost 1 billion (2008).[10]

STROKE

In the 2004 update of the Global Burden of Disease Study, stroke was estimated to have caused 5.7 million deaths, or just under 10% of all deaths, second only to IHD (7.2 million deaths).[3] As well as marked geographical differences in stroke mortality (Figures 62.2) and incidence rates, there are distinct differences between high-income and LMICs. A study of trends in stroke mortality in 48 countries from 1950 to 2005, described four broad patterns.[11] In rich countries especially, including most of those of Western Europe, there was a steady decline in mortality from stroke over this period, with rates in many countries being more than halved. In some countries, including Japan, Hungary and Ireland, there was an increase followed by a decline. In others, such as in parts of central Asia and Eastern Europe, this period witnessed a rise in mortality rates. Finally, the fourth pattern represented little change over this period.

Good data on stroke incidence are relatively scarce, especially from LMICs. A recent review of available incidence studies found that, in high-income countries, stroke incidence rates have fallen dramatically over the past four decades, consistent with the trends in stroke mortality. Thus, the age-standardized incidence rate per 100 000 person years has fallen from 163 in the 1970s to 94 in the years 2000–8.[12] Over the same period, the age standardized incidence rate of stroke in LMICs rose from around 52 to 117 per 100 000 person years,[12] and therefore now exceeds rates in high-income countries.

It has only become possible to compare haemorrhagic and atherosclerotic patterns of stroke in LMICs versus high-income countries during the past decade, as pathological stroke subtype

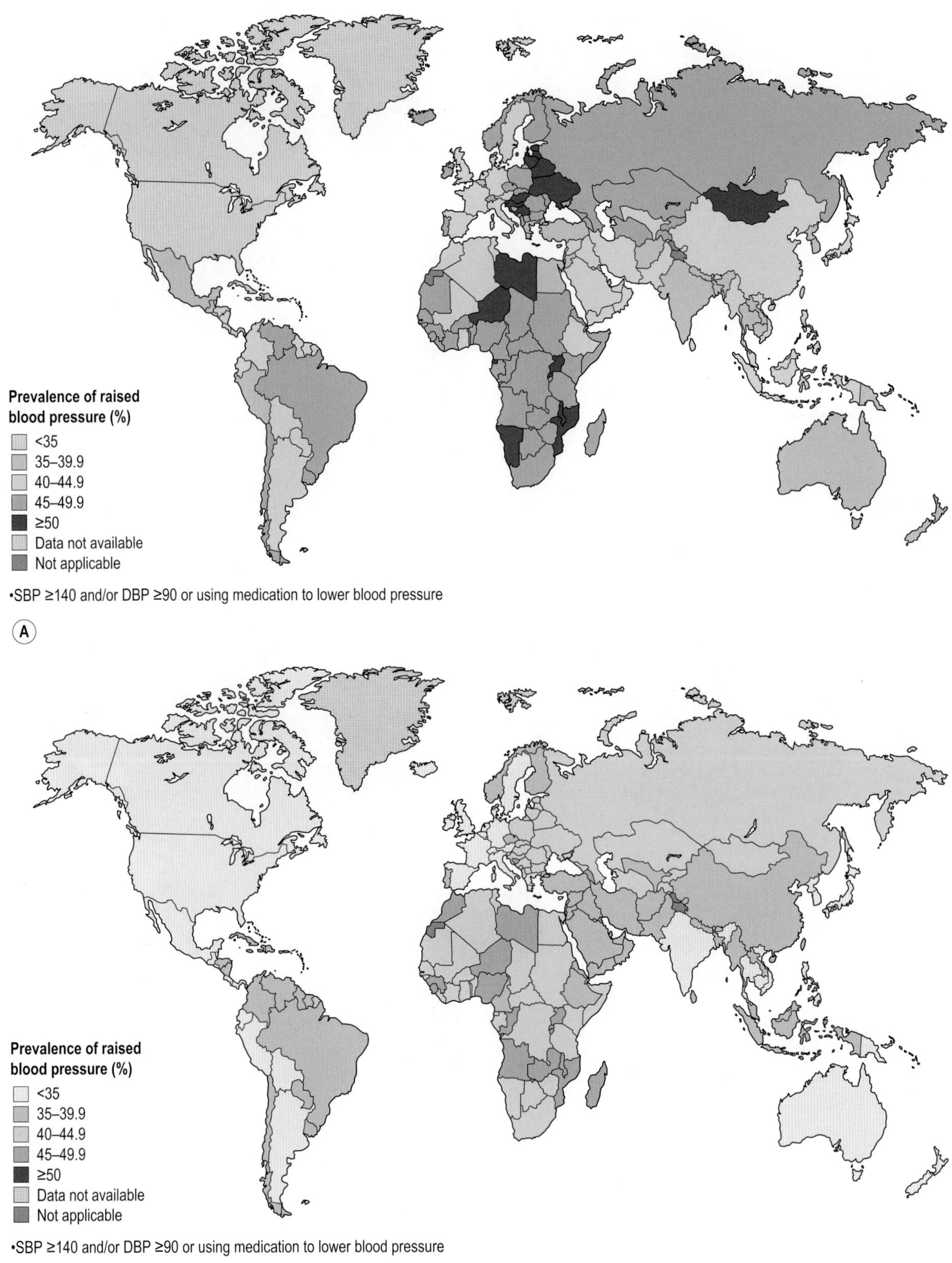

Figure 62.1 (A) Prevalence of raised blood pressure in men. (B) Prevalence of raised blood pressure in women. *(From WHO.)*

was not available in LMICs prior to the turn of this century.[12] In high-income countries in general (for whom these data were available in the published literature), between 70% and 90% of reported strokes were classified as atherosclerotic (or ischaemic), with most of the rest being classified as haemorrhagic, which includes subarachnoid haemorrhage (roughly 5–10% of all strokes). Most LMICs had a greater proportion of haemorrhagic strokes than this (e.g. Georgia and Chile reported about 35% haemorrhagic strokes).[12] Exceptions to this include Barbados, with the proportion of over 80% of strokes being ischaemic

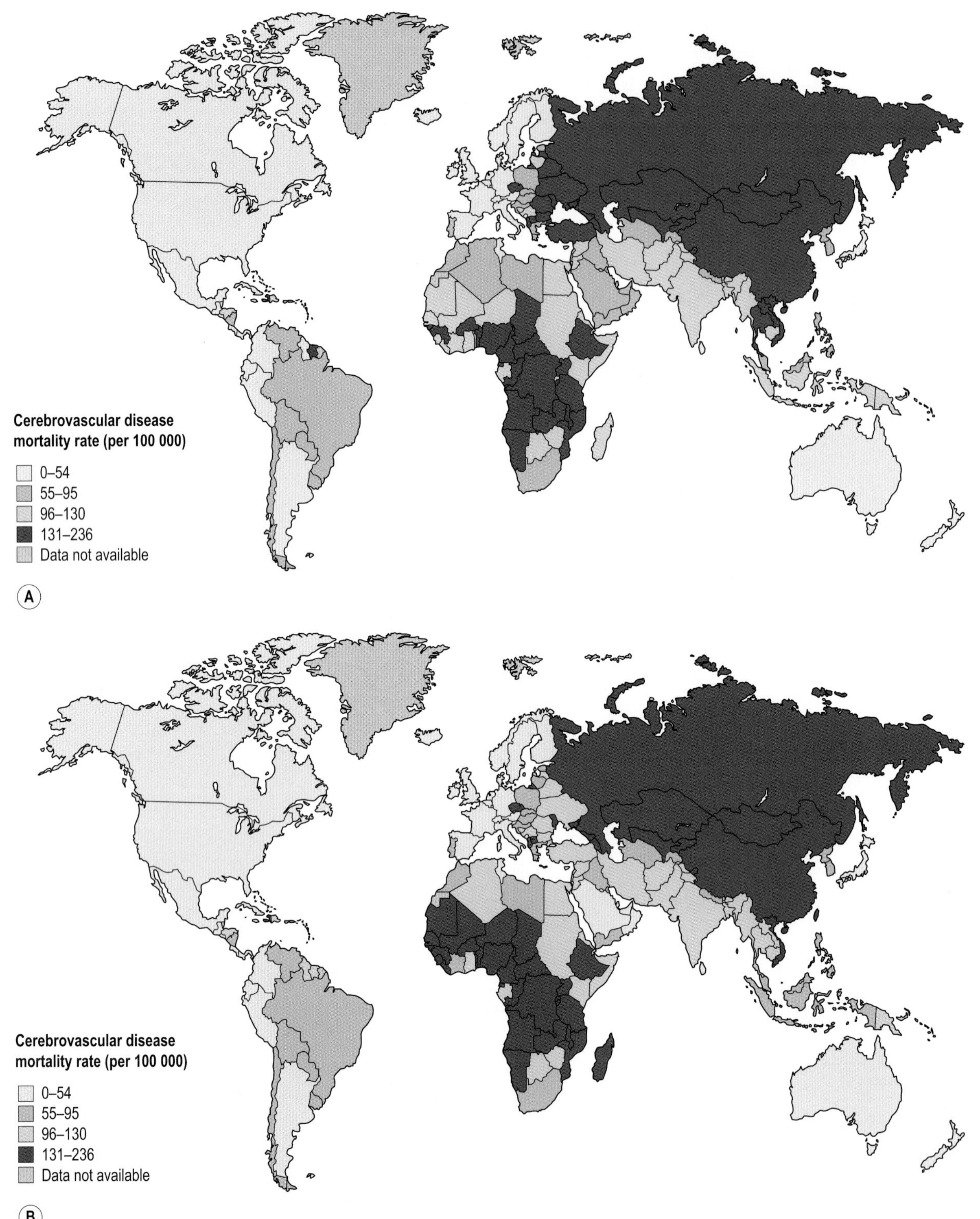

Figure 62.2 (A) Age standardized stroke mortality in men. (B) Age-standardized stroke mortality in women. *(From Mendis S, Puska P, Norrving B, editors. Global atlas on cardiovascular disease prevention and control: policies, strategies and interventions. Geneva: World Health Organization; 2011.)*

in the early part of this century.[13] In the INTERSTROKE study, a multicentre case–control study of risk factors for stroke (excluding subarachnoid haemorrhage), which suffers from potential bias of not being truly population based, the proportion with haemorrhagic stroke ranged from 9% in high-income countries to 34% in African sites.[14]

ISCHAEMIC HEART DISEASE

The beginning of the twentieth century witnessed the start of an epidemic of IHD in most industrialized countries, particularly those of northern Europe, North America, Australia and New Zealand. This epidemic was most pronounced in men, while in women, for reasons that are not fully understood, the increases in age-specific death rates were much less marked.[15,16] The evidence suggests that early in the epidemic, rates of IHD were highest in the socioeconomically more advantaged but moved across socioeconomic groups to produce the current picture, where the poorer sections of the population have the highest rates.[17] In the aforementioned Western industrialized countries, age-specific mortality rates from IHD began to fall from around 1970 and declines continue to this day, similar in magnitude to the decline in stroke mortality referred to above.

Global estimates of IHD mortality are shown in Figure 62.3, although robust data on trends in mortality from IHD in LMICs remain relatively scarce. It is a safe prediction that crude IHD rates will increase substantially over the coming years as populations age, and that age-specific IHD rates will increase as the proportion of the population living in urban rather than rural areas increases, together with the associated change in life style from urban living. For example, already in South-east Asia, modifiable risk factors in the poorer sectors of society are on the increase due to greater (unplanned) urbanization and continued consumption of unhealthy foods, compounded by low education and high stress levels.[18] Further, a study from Beijing showed a 50% increase in age-specific coronary heart disease mortality in men, and a 27% increase in women between 1984 and 1999.[19]

COMMON RISK FACTORS FOR HYPERTENSION AND CARDIOVASCULAR DISEASE

It is well known that common chronic non-communicable diseases (NCDs) share a small number of behavioural determinants or risk factors, which include physical inactivity, unhealthy diet with calories excess to needs, tobacco smoking and excessive use of alcohol.[20] Early life experience, as indicated by low birth weight and weight at age 1 year, has also been related to risk of certain chronic diseases as an adult, such as IHD and type 2 diabetes.[21] These in turn, are related to intermediate physiological risk factors, including obesity, an atherogenic lipid profile, raised blood glucose and of course, hypertension. The risk of chronic disease is also strongly determined by so-called 'unmodifiable' risk factors, with increasing age being by far the most important – the risks of myocardial infarction and stroke increase exponentially with age. Other factors include sex, family history and genetic markers. As described above, the prevalence of hypertension and risk of myocardial infarction and stroke are all higher on average in men than in women. The reasons for the sex differences are not fully understood, but are likely to reflect differences in behaviour (e.g. a higher prevalence of smoking in men in many populations) and some biological differences (e.g. the potential protective effect of female sex hormones in premenopausal women).

Figure 62.4 illustrates interrelationships between these categories of risk factors and the risk of atherosclerotic disease. Missing from this figure are the more distal determinants of behaviour, in particular the broader social and economic environments (including the influence of globalization) within which behavioural choices are shaped and made. Within any population, the socioeconomic positions of groups and individuals are strongly related to their ability to make healthy choices. There is also evidence that low self-perceived status within a social hierarchy has direct biological effects,[22] which include a tendency to central fat deposition, raised blood glucose and an atherogenic lipid profile.

Most risk factor studies have been carried out in high-income countries in White (European origin) populations, and an important question has been as to how generalizable the results from these studies are to low- and middle-income settings. Two large multinational case–control studies (INTERHEART and INTERSTROKE)[14,23] have helped to answer this question, and suggest that the major explanatory risk factors are the same in different populations throughout the world.

The INTERHEART study was a case–control study of myocardial infarction, and took place in 52 countries throughout Asia, Europe, the Middle East, Africa, Australia and the Americas. The results were similar across the world, and suggested that about 90% of first heart attacks (myocardial infarctions) can be attributed to the following risk factors: cigarette smoking; an abnormal ratio of blood lipids; high blood pressure; diabetes; abdominal obesity; stress; a lack of daily consumption of fruits and vegetables; and lack of daily exercise.

The INTERSTROKE study was conducted in 22 countries, covering a similar range of settings to the INTERHEART study. The study included ischaemic stroke and primary intracerebral haemorrhage, but excluded subarachnoid haemorrhage. Five main risk factors accounted for more than 80% of the risk of stroke (both ischaemic and haemorrhagic). These were: hypertension, current smoking, abdominal obesity, unhealthy diet (low in fresh fruit and vegetables, high in saturated fat), and physical inactivity. In the case of haemorrhagic stroke alone, hypertension, smoking, abdominal obesity, diet and alcohol intake were the key risk factors. Overall, hypertension was by far the most important risk factor for all stroke subtypes. Determinants of hypertension, including obesity, total sodium intake, the relative balance of sodium and potassium intake, and the potential influence of ethnic ancestry are discussed in the section on pathogenesis.

THE INTERACTIVE NATURE OF RISK FACTORS

As would be expected, the greater the number of risk factors an individual possesses, the higher is the probability of a CVD event, such as sudden death, myocardial infarction or stroke. The risk associated with a combination of risk factors is often greater than simply adding the risk associated with the individual risk factors together: it tends to be multiplicative. This is illustrated in Figure 62.5, which is based on a risk prediction formula from the Framingham study.[24] The figure shows how the risk of developing IHD in a 50-year-old man currently without IHD varies over sevenfold with different levels of the three main modifiable risk factors.

EXPLAINING TRENDS IN CARDIOVASCULAR DISEASE MORTALITY

As noted above, over the past few decades, high-income countries have witnessed a marked decline in age-specific mortality from CVD, both IHD and stroke. Attempting to define the reasons for this decline provides a check on the current understanding of the determinants of CVD, and can help guide future efforts aimed at prevention. Several studies have examined the reasons for the fall in mortality from IHD, including in the USA, England and Wales, Finland and New Zealand. An important finding is that the fall can be very largely explained by trends in

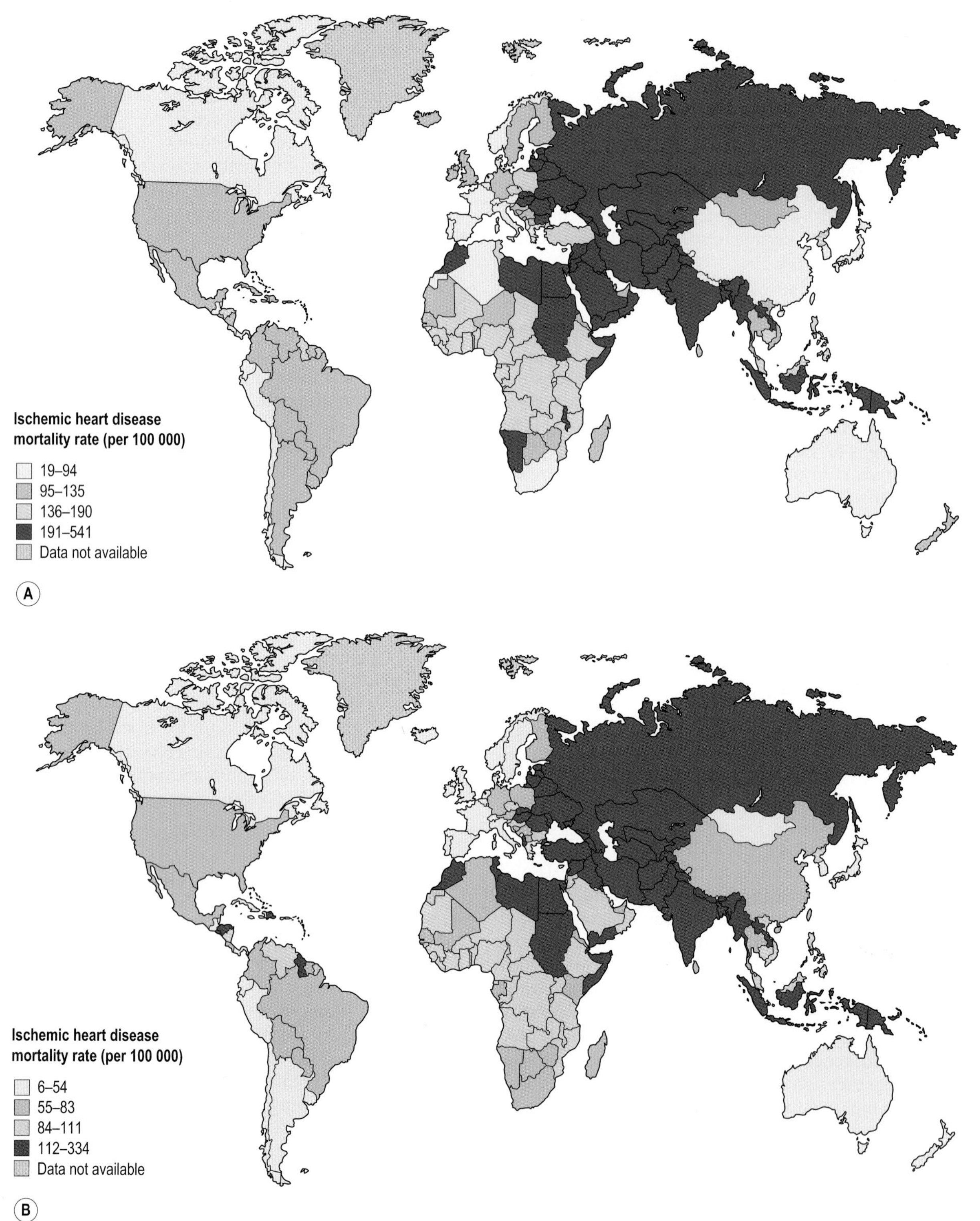

Figure 62.3 (A) Age-standardized ischaemic heart disease mortality in men. (B) Age-standardized ischaemic heart disease mortality in women. *(From Mendis S, Puska P, Norrving B, editors. Global atlas on cardiovascular disease prevention and control: policies, strategies and interventions. Geneva: World Health Organization; 2011.)*

well-established risk factors and the increased use of effective treatments. Thus, most estimates suggest that half, or a little more, of the decline can be attributed to trends in the major risk factors (smoking, dyslipidaemia and high blood pressure), and most of the rest to improvements in both the effectiveness and uptake of clinical care (particularly drug treatments for secondary prevention).[25] Data on trends from LMIC are less robust, but a study undertaken in Beijing, China, to explain the increasing rates of IHD mortality, found major explanatory factors to be considerable rises in total cholesterol levels and

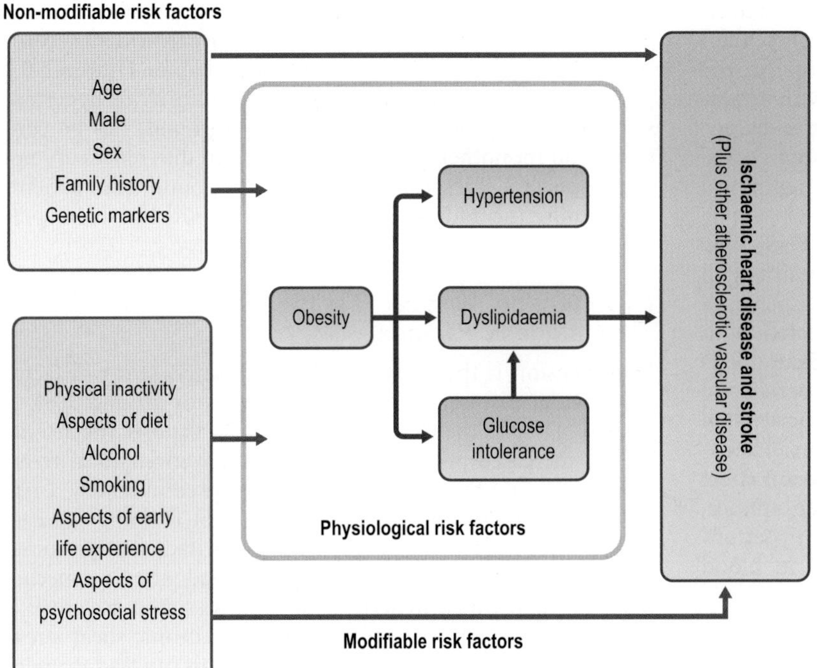

Figure 62.4 Risk factors for cardiovascular disease. *(Based on Howson C, Reddy S, Ryan T, et al. Control of Cardiovascular Diseases in Developing Countries. Research, Development and Institutional Strengthening. Washington DC: National Academy Press; 1998.)*

diabetes (reflecting substantial changes in traditional Beijing diets and lower levels of physical activity).[19]

Pathogenesis and Pathology

HYPERTENSION

Overview of Pathogenesis

Only 5–10% of hypertension is secondary hypertension, meaning that it has a specific underlying cause (e.g. renal or reno-vascular disease and tumours of the adrenal glands). Over 90% of hypertension lacks a clear underlying cause and is referred to as 'primary', 'idiopathic' or 'essential'. The use of the term 'essential' to describe hypertension reflects the now discredited notion that increasing blood pressure with ageing is essential (or compensatory) to ensure adequate perfusion of target organs.[26] In some populations, largely hunter-gatherers,

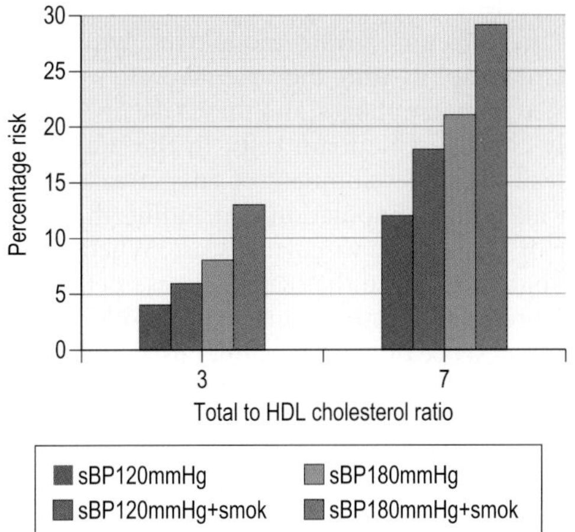

Figure 62.5 Interaction between cholesterol, blood pressure and smoking and the risk of ischaemic heart disease.

age-related increases in blood pressure are virtually absent.[27] Here, we will use the term 'primary hypertension' to refer to the increasing blood pressure associated with ageing that is found in the vast majority of modern human populations. By definition, primary hypertension lacks a specific clearly identifiable underlying cause. However, while there is much more to learn as to why one individual develops primary hypertension and another does not, epidemiological and physiological studies have identified many factors that contribute to primary hypertension.

Primary hypertension is a multifactorial disease. Epidemiological evidence suggests that an intake of sodium of >50–100 mmol/L/day (roughly 3–6 g of sodium chloride or around 1 teaspoonful/day) is necessary for the development of hypertension;[27] and that the higher the intake, the greater the increase in blood pressure. However, of itself, a high intake of sodium chloride, or sodium from other sources (e.g. in sodium monoglutamate) is necessary but not sufficient to cause hypertension. A substantial proportion of individuals in populations consuming a large amount of sodium do not develop hypertension. Part of the explanation for this will be inter-individual differences in 'salt sensitivity', defined as an increase in blood pressure in response to a higher sodium chloride intake. Differences in salt sensitivity may have a genetic basis, but evidence also suggests the importance of environmental factors. Dietary potassium intake, which comes from fruits, vegetables and other foodstuffs, has been shown to exert a powerful dose-dependent inhibitory effect on salt sensitivity. It is argued that historically, as hunter-gatherers, humans consumed 3–10 times more potassium than sodium (mmol for mmol); and that in most modern societies, the ratio is completely reversed – consuming 2–3 times more sodium than potassium.[27] High-sodium, low-potassium diets are virtually ubiquitous in modern societies. Another widespread contributor to primary hypertension is overweight and obesity, affecting well over half of all adults in many societies. Although not fully understood, several mechanisms have been implicated in the link between obesity and primary hypertension.[28] The activity of the renin-angiotensin-aldosterone system (RAAS) is greater in obese than non-obese individuals. This system has a central role in the maintenance of fluid volume and blood pressure, with activation leading to increased sodium and water retention, and vasoconstriction. Weight loss in obese individuals has been shown to lead to lower circulating levels of angiotensinogen, renin, and aldosterone.

Activation of the sympathetic nervous system (SNS) may play a role in the hypertension associated with obesity, with consequent haemodynamic and renal effects (e.g. increased sodium reabsorption). Obesity is strongly associated with insulin resistance and consequent hyperinsulinaemia, but evidence for either of these having a direct role in hypertension is at best incomplete. It is more likely that both hypertension and hyperinsulaemia/insulin resistance share common antecedents, whether environmental or genetic. A direct physical effect of obesity is the increased risk of obstructive sleep apnoea, which in turn is associated with an increased risk of hypertension, including loss of the normal nocturnal fall in blood pressure.

Ethnic/Racial Differences in the Pathogenesis of Hypertension

Within some settings, particularly with the USA and to a lesser extent with in the UK, there has been much interest in differences in the prevalence of hypertension between ethnic groups and the determinants underlying those differences. Work from the USA in particular, has tended to suggest that people of African origin are at significantly higher risk of hypertension than people of European origin.[29] In contrast, work from the UK has found much smaller differences in the prevalence of hypertension between all ethnic groups, including those of African origin. Analyses of data on both sides of the Atlantic support the suggestion that differences in environmental factors, particularly those related to socioeconomic status, explain much of the difference in blood pressure levels between ethnic groups.

However, while environmental factors appear to be of overriding importance, there is clear evidence that people of African origin tend to have lower renin activity than people of European origin[29] and, are therefore more likely to be salt-sensitive (i.e. have a greater rise in blood pressure with salt loading). The use of salt as a food preservative and flavouring is very recent in human evolutionary history, and all humans evolved in salt-scarce environments. It is plausible that those humans whose recent evolutionary history was in the tropics, with high levels of natural salt loss, became particularly efficient at salt retention, and that the pattern of low renin and high salt sensitivity in people of African origin reflects this. It is also plausible that those whose ancestors suffered and survived the transatlantic slave trade (particularly the severe deprivations of the 'middle passage') have an even greater tendency to salt retention and sensitivity. Whether other ethnic or racial groups also exhibit low renin and increased salt sensitivity is not properly known – there is a lack of comparable data. However, there is some evidence that low renin is also common in Chinese hypertensive patients,[26,29] suggesting that other ethnic/racial groups may also exhibit the pattern of low renin activity and high salt sensitivity.

A patient with low renin activity, whatever his or her ethnic background, will benefit less from antihypertensive drugs that block the renin-angiotensin-aldosterone system. This is reflected in the guidance on anti-hypertensive treatment according to ethnic group discussed later in this chapter. However, the point has also been made that as only a minority of hypertensive patients, whatever their ethnic background, can be controlled on monotherapy, such ethnic group differences are not that important. Irrespective of ethnic background, most patients will require the addition of a second- or third-line antihypertensive drug.

Hypertension, Vascular Disease and the Thrombogenic Paradox

Hypertension is the most prevalent and important risk factor for vascular disease, estimated to account for around 50% of the risk. Despite the fact that hypertension exposes the arterial tree to increased pressure, which in simple mechanical terms should increase the risk of rupture, it is predominately a risk factor for atherosclerotic/thrombotic (clot-forming) disease rather than haemorrhagic (bleeding) – a fact that is sometimes referred to as the 'thrombogenic paradox'.[26] One mechanism through which hypertension promotes atherosclerosis is through abnormalities of blood flow and chronic shear stress, particularly at the bifurcation of arteries. This can lead to endothelial damage, initiating low-grade inflammation and a procoagulant surface, which in turn promotes the atherosclerotic process as described below.

ATHEROSCLEROSIS

The Atherosclerotic Process

Atherosclerosis is a patchy, nodular type of arteriosclerosis (thickening and hardening of the arterial wall) that occurs mainly in large and medium-sized elastic and muscular arteries. At a histological level, it is characterized by lipid accumulation, hyperplasia and scarring in the arterial intima.[30] This is reflected in the derivation of the term atherosclerosis, which comes from the Greek words *athero* (meaning gruel or paste) and sclerosis (hardness). At a cellular and molecular level it is characterized by chronic inflammation, oxidation of lipids and immune cell infiltration.

Chronic inflammation of the arterial wall occurs especially at sites with disturbed laminar flow, such as branching points.[31] The activated endothelial cells secrete adhesion molecules, and smooth muscle cells secrete chemokines and chemoattractants. Together these factors attract monocytes, lymphocytes, mast cells and neutrophils into the arterial wall.[30] Monocytes are transformed in macrophages, and these take up lipids becoming the highly characteristic foam cells. In the initial stages these changes lead to the development of fatty streaks, and these are found in all human populations, including those with a low incidence of thrombotic vascular disease. Whether or not such lesions progress to those that cause disease depends upon the sustained presence of other causes of endothelial injury, and include the presence of hypertension, raised and modified LDL cholesterol levels, diabetes, the constituents of cigarette smoke and other airborne pollutants, and so on.

The American Heart Association classification of atherosclerotic lesions,[32] and the relationships between them, is shown in Figure 62.6. Lesion types I–III are always small and clinically silent, and there is evidence that all these can regress to normal. Lesion types IV–VI may or may not cause clinical consequences.

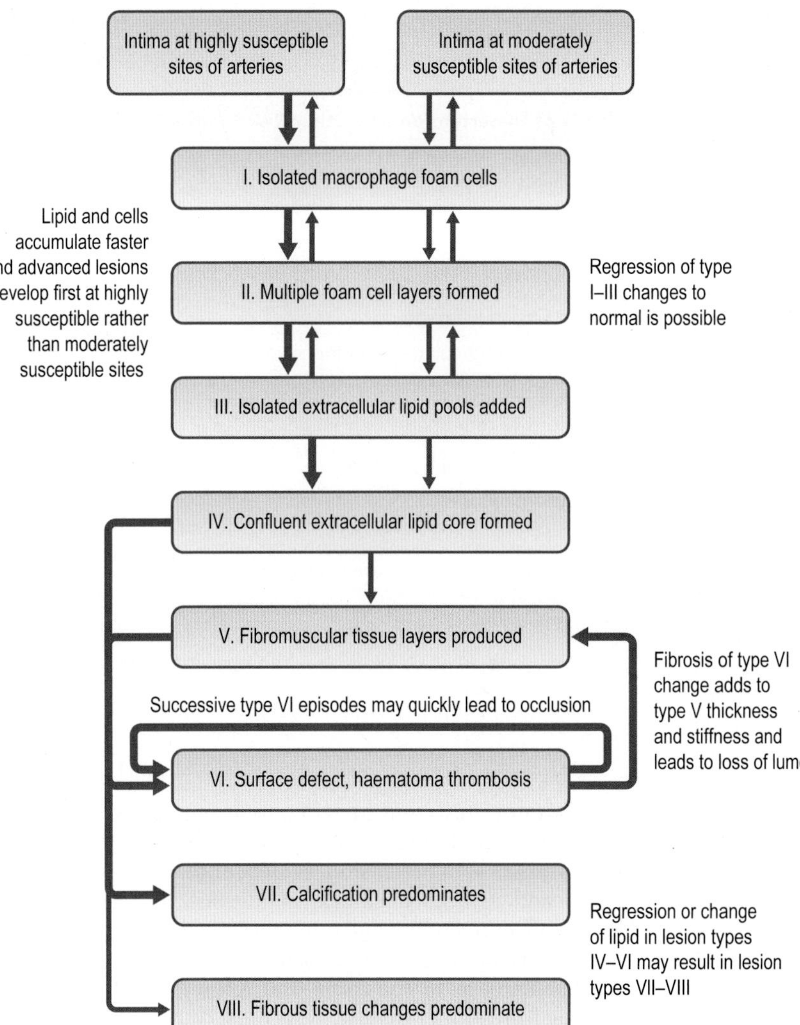

Figure 62.6 Stages of atherosclerosis. *(From Stary HC. Natural history and histological classification of atherosclerotic lesions: an update. Arterioscler Thromb Vasc Biol 2000;20(5):1177–8.)*

Some may be silent, and others may produce clinical, including fatal, events. Lesions of both types IV and V may be associated with clinical events through narrowing of the lumen. However, most clinical and fatal events involve type VI lesions. Ulceration or fissuring of the fibrous cap is the precursor of type VI lesions (also known as 'complicated lesions') in which thrombus formation occurs (Figure 62.6). Highly activated macrophages are involved in both ulceration and fissuring. Ulceration is due to endothelial denudation, exposing subendothelial connective tissue on which thrombus forms. Fissuring exposes the highly thrombogenic lipid core of the plaque. Thrombus forms initially within the plaque and may then extend into the arterial lumen.[33]

It is worth noting in the AHA classification that the key pathological step is moving from type III (always clinically silently, and capable of regression) to the potentially clinically pathological type IV lesions. As indicated in Figure 62.6, type IV may then progress in several ways, including directly to type VI, or on to more stable atherosclerotic lesions with predominant calcification or predominant formation of fibrous tissue (types VII and VIII).

Atherosclerosis and Clinical Disease

Atherosclerosis underlies the vast majority of clinical CVD. Narrowing of the arterial lumen may lead to symptoms of ischaemia, such as occurs in angina pectoris and the intermittent claudication of peripheral vascular disease. Plaque rupture and thrombus formation are a direct cause of myocardial infarction, acute coronary syndrome and ischaemic stroke.

A proportion of ischaemic strokes, roughly 20% in European-origin people,[34] result from emboli from the heart, which are associated with atrial fibrillation, left ventricular hypertrophy and previous myocardial infarction. A stroke of cardioembolic origin is also likely to have an underlying atherosclerotic origin, although there are of course also non-atherogenic causes of atrial fibrillation and left ventricular hypertrophy. So-called lacunar infarcts account for roughly 25% of all ischaemic strokes. These result from occlusion of one of the small, deep, perforating cerebral arteries.

Haemorrhagic Stroke

As described in the section on epidemiology, a significant proportion of strokes are haemorrhagic in origin, with evidence that this is between 30% and 10% in richer countries and may be more than 30% in parts of sub-Saharan Africa. Roughly three-quarters of these are classified as primary intracerebral haemorrhage, with the most common mechanism being hypertensive small vessel disease leading to small aneurysms that rupture. The other quarter of haemorrhagic strokes are subarachnoid haemorrhages, most commonly arising from saccular aneurysms in the subarachnoid space.[34]

Clinical Features, Diagnosis, Management and Treatment

The scope of this review does not permit a full description of approaches to diagnosis, management and treatment. Our goal has therefore been to indicate key principles and how approaches might differ depending on available resources, and in particular what healthcare providers can be expected to achieve in resource-constrained settings, consistent with widely accepted international guidelines, e.g. those of WHO.

HYPERTENSION

The condition is largely asymptomatic, often coming to clinical attention through manifestation of a vascular complication such as stroke or heart disease, or through screening. There are no objective criteria that delineate normal and elevated blood pressure, as cardiovascular risk occurs along a continuum. Arbitrary cut points have therefore been set to identify groups at particular risk or deemed likely to benefit from therapeutic interventions. Correct measurement of blood pressure is important to appropriate management. The patient should be comfortably seated with the arm outstretched and supported at the level of the mid-sternum with an appropriately sized arm cuff used. Standard techniques for cuff inflation and auscultation are now established.

The WHO-ISH (2003) guidelines classify hypertension[35] according to the following grades of systolic and diastolic blood pressure (SBP and DBP mmHg, respectively) in terms of increasing severity: grade I (SBP 140–159 or DBP 90–99); grade 2 (SBP 160–179 or DBP 100–109) and grade 3 (SBP≥180 or DBP≥110). There is however, recognition by the WHO-ISH and other expert bodies that blood pressure levels alone are not the sole determinants of treatment strategies, but these must be considered in terms of co-existing cardiovascular risk factors, target organ damage as well as related clinical conditions, as shown in Table 62.2.[35]

The US-based Joint National Committee 7 (JNC 7) developed criteria[36] which differ from the WHO-ISH in the recognition of a stage of pre-hypertension defined as SBP 120–139 mmHg and DBP 80–89 mmHg and also limited the hypertension staging to 2 stages: stage 1, SBP 140–159; DBP 90–99 mmHg; and stage 2, SBP≥160 and DBP≥100 mmHg. Pre-hypertension does not indicate disease, but rather identifies groups at high risk of developing hypertension. Isolated SBP is common in the elderly, and defined as a normal DBP with an elevated SBP>140 mmHg. The UK-based National Institute for Health and Clinical Excellence (NICE) guidelines also define hypertension at a cut-off point of 140/90 mmHg, but recommendations to offer ambulatory blood pressure monitoring to individuals with clinic blood pressures in excess of this value[37] are unlikely to be relevant in resource-constrained settings.[38]

When elevated blood pressure is suspected, it is important to repeat measurements on at least two further occasions. However, patients with accelerated (malignant) hypertension (BP≥180/110 mmHg with signs of papilloedema and/or retinal haemorrhage) must be referred for immediate acute care.

Comprehensive evaluation of persons with hypertension requires a complete history, thorough physical examination, and laboratory tests and imaging, to assess family history, relevant lifestyle and modifiable risk factors, identify possible secondary causes of hypertension, evidence of target organ damage (TOD) and associated clinical conditions, and other factors likely to affect treatment and outcomes (Table 62.2). It is important to carry out clinical investigations to assess the patient for diabetes, damage to the heart and kidneys, or hypertension resulting from kidney disease. Tests must be tailored to available facilities and resources, but where possible should include assessment for the presence of protein in the urine, blood tests for plasma glucose, electrolytes, and creatinine. Additional investigations should include serum lipids, and where possible an ECG. Additional tests such as chest X-rays, and more specialized tests such as echocardiography and renal imaging, can be considered in specialized settings as indicated.

TABLE 62.2 Clinical Approach to Hypertension: Evaluating CVD Risk

Grade of Hypertension and Other Risk Factors
Hypertension (grades 1–3)
Age (Males >55 years; Females >65 years)
Smoking
Dyslipidaemia
History of premature CVD in first-degree relative (age <50 years)
Obesity; Physical inactivity
Target Organ Damage
Heart – left ventricular enlargement
Microalbuminuria
Evidence of extensive atherosclerotic plaque by imaging studies
Hypertensive retinopathy (advanced; grades III or IV)
Associated Clinical Conditions
Diabetes mellitus
Cerebrovascular disease (stroke; transient ischaemic attack)
Heart disease (myocardial infarction; angina; coronary revascularization; congestive heart failure)
Renal disease
Peripheral artery disease

From Whitworth JA. 2003 World Health Organization (WHO)/International Society of Hypertension (ISH) statement on management of hypertension. J Hypertens 2003;21(11):1983–92.

Approaches to the Management of Hypertension

The approach to hypertension management in LMIC involves a risk stratification approach, based on grade of hypertension and presence of risk factors, target organ damage and/or associated clinical conditions, as shown in Table 62.3. Lowering blood pressure has been associated with reduction in incident stroke by 35–40%; reduction in myocardial infarction by 20–25% and reduction in onset of heart failure by more than 50% in clinical trials.[39] Established blood pressure control targets are set at SBP<140 mmHg and DBP<90 mmHg,[35] and management approaches are multifactorial involving lifestyle modification and therapeutic intervention.

Lifestyle Modification

Lifestyle strategies are based on reducing risk factors for blood pressure and for overall cardiovascular risk. They include, therefore, as appropriate, calorie restriction aimed at weight loss, increased physical activity, adoption of diets rich in fruits and vegetables, and reduced saturated fats, reduction of dietary

TABLE 62.3 WHO-CVD Risk Management Strategies for Low- and Medium-Resource Settings

	Blood Pressure		
Other risk Factors and Disease History	Grade 1 Hypertension	Grade 2 Hypertension	Grade 3 Hypertension
I – No other risk factors	Low risk	Medium risk	High risk
II – One or two risk factors	Medium risk	Medium risk	Very high risk
III – Three or more risk factors or TOD or diabetes	High risk	High risk	Very high risk
IV – Associated clinical conditions	Very high risk	Very high risk	Very high risk

Based on Whitworth JA. 2003 World Health Organization (WHO)/International Society of Hypertension (ISH) statement on management of hypertension. J Hypertens 2003;21(11):1983–92.

sodium intake, increased dietary potassium and moderation of alcohol intake. Smoking cessation to reduce cardiovascular risk is central.

Salt intake should be no more than 6 g/day; alcohol consumption no more than 21 units/week for men and 14 for women; and moderate to vigorous physical activity is recommended 3–5 times days per week, for at least 30–60 min/day.

Lifestyle modification is therefore a key aspect of blood pressure reduction strategies, and is recommended as first-line therapy in individuals at low to medium risk (Table 62.3), before considering pharmacological treatment (Figure 62.7). Healthcare providers monitor blood pressure responses for those at low and medium risk, with appropriate initiation of drug therapy or continued review after a suitable period of follow-up, based on clinical response. Individuals at high or very high risk commence early drug treatment.

Pharmacologic Approaches

A detailed treatment of antihypertensive drugs is beyond the scope of this chapter, although we will highlight issues we consider to be of particular importance. Based on the UK NICE guidelines, calcium channel blockers (CCB) and thiazide-type diuretics are now considered the drugs likely to confer the most benefit as first-line antihypertensive therapies.[37] UK NICE recommendations are for patients aged 55 years or older or Black people of African or Caribbean origin to be treated with CCB as first-line agents (step 1). Thiazide-type drugs are particularly indicated in settings of oedema or intolerance to CCB. Recommendations for additional treatment (step 2) in the setting of inadequate response, are the addition of angiotensin converting enzyme inhibitors (ACE inhibitors), or low-cost angiotensin II receptor blockers (ARB) to CCB treatment. UK NICE guidelines suggest ARB might be preferable for African or Caribbean individuals. Step 3 treatment is likely to result in a combination of ACE inhibitor or ARB, CCB and thiazide-like diuretic. Failure to control blood pressure with triple therapy should lead to consideration of the addition of a fourth drug such as Spironolactone (at low dose, provided plasma potassium is not elevated, and with extreme caution in persons with renal disease). Failure to control blood pressure merits referral for further care. Beta

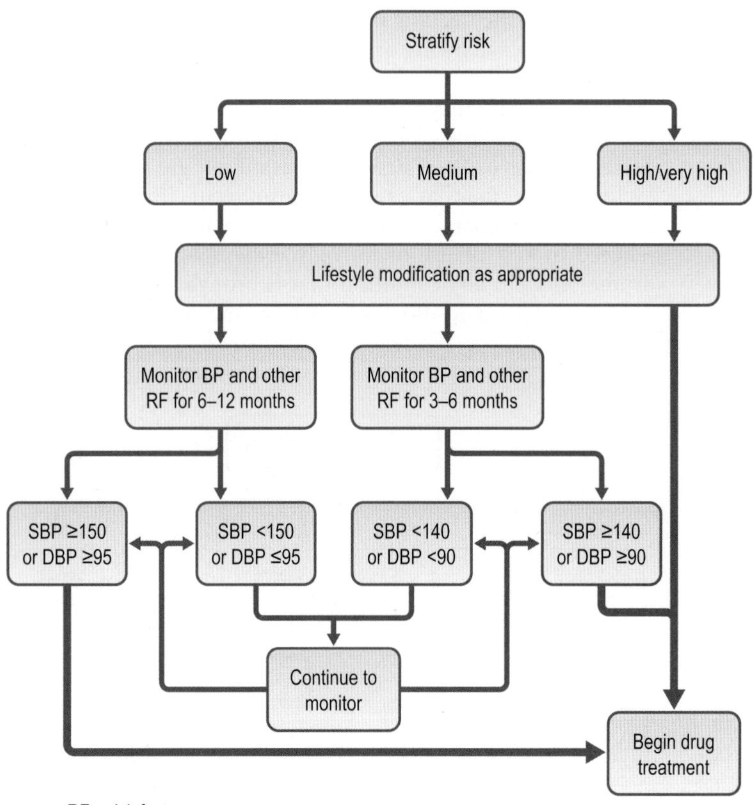

Figure 62.7 Stratified approach to CVD risk management and blood pressure treatment based on level of risk in Table 62.3.

blockers have been shown to be comparably less effective at reducing major cardiovascular events in head-to-head comparisons with other agents and are now recommended for persons intolerant of or with contraindication to ACE inhibitors or ARBs, women of child-bearing potential, and individuals with increased sympathetic drive.

This above stepwise approach must be tailored to local settings based on the availability of therapeutic options.

STROKE

The WHO definition of stroke is: 'rapidly developing clinical signs of focal (or global) disturbance of cerebral function, with symptoms lasting 24 hours or longer or leading to death, with no apparent cause other than of vascular origin'.[40] This definition excludes transient ischaemic attack (TIA), which is defined to last less than 24 hours, and patients with stroke symptoms caused by subdural haemorrhage, tumours, poisoning or trauma.

Pathology

As outlined in the section on pathogenesis above, strokes are either ischaemic or haemorrhagic in aetiology. Around 80% of all strokes are ischaemic, which results from atherosclerotic obstruction of cervical and cerebral arteries, leading to ischaemia in all or part of the vascular territory of the affected vessel. Embolic infarction results from embolization to the cerebral arteries from other sites, e.g. cardiac valve lesions or left ventricular intracavity clots formed within the heart during rhythm disturbances such as atrial fibrillation. Lacunar cerebral infarctions are tiny infarcts deep within the territory of the perforating arteries due to local vessel disease, principally related to hypertension. Other causes of infarction are much less common and can be ignored for epidemiological purposes. Following arterial occlusion, the resulting volume of structurally intact but functionally impaired tissue surrounding the ischaemic core, known as the ischaemic penumbra,[41] is a target for therapeutic interventions which may result in neurological improvement. A cascade of events takes place in the area of the penumbra beginning with energy depletion, followed by disruption of ion homeostasis, glutamate release, calcium channel dysfunction, release of free radicals, membrane disruption, inflammatory changes, with triggering of necrosis and apoptotic cell death.[42]

Haemorrhagic stroke leading to intracerebral haemorrhage is predominantly caused by hypertensive small vessel disease, which results in tiny lipohyalinotic aneurysms which rupture.[43] Approximately two-thirds of cases of primary cerebral haemorrhage are due to hypertension, whether pre-existing or newly diagnosed.[44] Intracranial vascular malformations (e.g. arteriovenous malformations), cerebral amyloid angiopathy and haemorrhage into an area of previous brain infarction might also result in intracerebral haemorrhage. Subarachnoid haemorrhages are caused by rupture of saccular aneurysms within the subarachnoid space.

Clinical Features and Management

The manifestations of a stroke are dependent on the extent of the underlying vascular injury. The most common manifestations of a stroke are sudden onset of weakness of the face, arm or leg, usually on one side of the body. There may be numbness in the affected areas, as well as confusion, difficulty speaking or understanding speech, difficulty seeing with one or both eyes, difficulty swallowing, difficulty walking, dizziness, loss of balance or coordination, severe headache without a known cause, fainting or loss of consciousness. Strokes may lead to weakness or complete paralysis of the affected limbs or side of the face, and can cause sudden death.

The diagnosis of stroke is made on clinical symptoms and signs, with neuroimaging where available by CT scan and/or MRI scan. Interventions resulting in improved blood pressure control, early mobilization, and prevention of venous thromboembolism are specific components of care for the stroke patient. Hypoxia worsens cerebral ischaemia, so patients should be positioned so as to improve ventilation, e.g. sitting up in a chair when possible. Blood glucose control is important and patients with uncontrolled hyperglycemia should be treated (with insulin if necessary) to improve control. Maintenance of fluid balance and feeding by nasogastric tube in patients unable to swallow is appropriate. Early mobilization reduces the likelihood of complications such as deep vein thrombosis, pneumonia, pulmonary embolism and pressure ulcers.

The steady decline in stroke mortality in recent decades has resulted from significant improvements in treatment and control of hypertension.[45] Other therapeutic strategies for improved outcomes in ischaemic stroke include the use of aspirin, use of statins for treatment of dyslipidaemias, and the use of warfarin for persons with cardiac arrhythmias.[46] Lifestyle modification, as for all CVDs, also remains a key element of rehabilitative care and secondary prevention.

ISCHAEMIC HEART DISEASE

Ischaemia refers to the situation where the oxygen supply to a tissue or organ is inadequate for its needs. IHD is the disturbance of cardiac function due to inadequate oxygen supply. As described in the section on pathogenesis, this is most commonly due to narrowing or complete occlusion of the coronary arteries caused by coronary atherosclerosis and associated thrombosis. IHD may manifest as stable angina pectoris, acute coronary syndrome, arrhythmias, heart failure and sudden death (Figure 62.8). These manifestations are not mutually exclusive and may co-exist and also recur (barring death). Stable angina characteristically occurs with exertion and is relieved by rest or use of nitroglycerine. Acute coronary syndrome refers to any condition that is brought on by a sudden reduction in blood flow to part of the heart. It includes

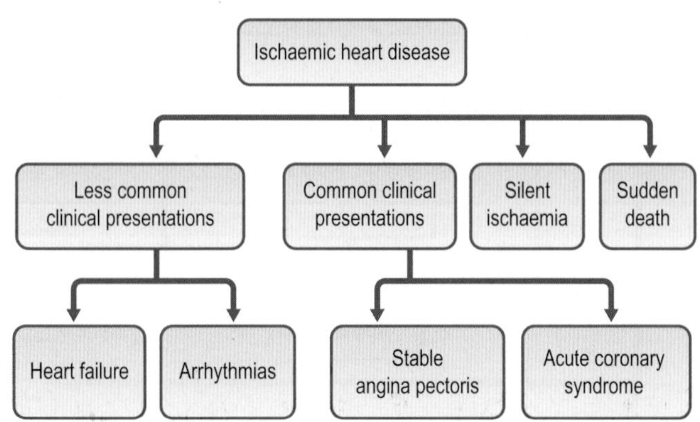

Figure 62.8 A clinical classification of ischaemic heart disease.

myocardial infarction and unstable angina. The pain of acute coronary syndrome typically occurs at rest, or with light exertion, and is poorly responsive to nitroglycerine. Symptoms of myocardial ischaemia include various combinations of chest, upper extremity, jaw or epigastric discomfort or pain as described in Table 62.4.

Myocardial infarction (MI) results from myocardial cell death due to significant and prolonged ischaemia. The diagnosis of MI has undergone significant revisions from a basis of a supporting clinical history of myocardial ischaemia, findings on the electrocardiogram (ECG), enzyme measurements in blood and postmortem findings.[47] Current universal recommendations require the detection of new biomarkers and use of imaging methods that are more specific and/or sensitive as components in the diagnosis of MI. Current best practice recommendations require a rise and/or fall in the cardiac biomarkers in a clinical setting of myocardial ischaemia. Recommended biomarkers (troponins) and imaging modalities are too expensive for widespread and sustained uptake in resource-constrained settings.[48] WHO recommendations for the diagnosis of MI are now quite comprehensive for fully resourced as well as resource-constrained environments (shown in Table 62.4),[49] with category C definitions particularly addressing the latter. Given the lack of access to new biomarkers and imaging modalities, these criteria are at best able to characterize probable rather than definite MI. The definition is based on a combination of symptoms, the new development of pathological Q waves on ECG, or incomplete biomarker data, or autopsy findings suggestive of myocardial infarction.

The pain of MI is similar in distribution to that of angina, but is typically much more severe, lasting from 30 minutes to several hours, and is relieved neither by rest nor nitroglycerine. Patients often describe it as a central crushing chest pain. Nausea, vomiting and sweating may be present, especially at the start of the pain. With large infarcts, breathlessness may be a manifestation of left ventricular failure. Although MI is usually painful, it is painless in a substantial proportion (possibly more than one-fifth) of cases, particularly in people with diabetes and in older people.[50] Manifestations may include nonspecific complaints such as transient loss of consciousness, acute confusion and complaints of weakness or nausea. Onset of an arrhythmia (such as atrial fibrillation or heart block) or an unexplained drop in blood pressure might also herald an acute MI. Arrhythmias are potentially life-threatening complications, especially ventricular fibrillation, which may lead to sudden death. By definition, this complication occurs within an hour of onset of symptoms. Early complications might include heart failure and hypotensive shock. Other potential complications in the first few days following the acute event might include myocardial rupture, rupture of the interventricular septum, mitral regurgitation following damage to the papillary muscle, and systemic and pulmonary embolism. While as many as 25% of patients admitted to hospital with acute MI die before discharge, current intensive therapy interventions can substantially reduce the mortality rate.

Overview of Management of Myocardial Infarction

Management of acute MI is best carried out in hospital. Care involves administration of aspirin, supportive care through oxygen use, intravenous access with fluids as indicated (caution in heart failure), pain relief (e.g. use of opioids), use of thrombolytics where available (within the recommended window of opportunity when myocardial salvage is still possible) and treatment of complications such as arrhythmias, heart failure, shock, etc. Specialized investigations and interventions are likely available only in specialized centres, depending on local circumstances and might include angioplasty. Optimal glycaemic control, if relevant, is important. Drugs which might have specific benefit in acute MI include beta-blockers and ACE inhibitors for heart failure, while long-term use of aspirin and statins also reduce recurrence. As for other CVDs, lifestyle changes, including tobacco cessation, are important long-term strategies.

WHERE THERE IS NO PHYSICIAN

In regions of LMICs where there is no or limited access to physicians and healthcare resources, it can still be possible to effectively manage raised blood pressure and other aspects of cardiovascular risk. This can be achieved through the training of non-physician health workers, the provision of basic equipment (most importantly equipment for measuring blood pressure), cheap generic drugs and equipment for assaying urine glucose and albumin, and ideally blood glucose and cholesterol.

The principles of management include basing decisions on an assessment of overall CVD risk, and the use of evidence-based guidelines to direct non-pharmacological and pharmacological interventions. Core to this approach, and indeed to approaches with greater resources, is patient education.

The WHO currently has two sources of guidance that are very useful for resource-poor settings, including 'where there is no physician'. One source is their pocket guidelines for the assessment and management of cardiovascular risk; and the other is their guidance on a package of essential interventions for primary health for non-communicable diseases in low-resource settings. Both can be found at: www.who.int/cardiovascular_diseases.

Prevention

In this section our focus is on the primary prevention of IHD and stroke, which means preventing new cases. Aspects of secondary prevention, which refers to limiting the progression and the prevention of further complications once the condition is present, are discussed above. It is worth noting, however, that all of the measures that support primary prevention also support secondary prevention, such as modifying environments to encourage healthier diets and increases in physical activity levels.

SOCIAL DETERMINANTS

As discussed in the epidemiology section, the main behavioural risk factors for CVD (physical inactivity, unhealthy diet, smoking, and excessive alcohol intake) arise with a broader social and economic environment. The social determinants of CVD include poverty, low health literacy, environmental degradation, poor housing and unplanned urbanization. Low socioeconomic status is associated with poorer health, lack of power and less access to resources. Social and economic structures, both between and within countries, tend to be hostile to those from the lower socioeconomic strata, and their living conditions disproportionately include risk factors for, and poor management of, CVD and other diseases. In the LMICs (as in high-income regions), it is the poorer countries, and the poorer people within countries, who have limited opportunities for healthy choices and higher age-adjusted rates of CVD.[51] The WHO's Commission on the Social Determinants of Health (CSDH) recommended strategies to improve living conditions, tackle the inequitable distribution of resources, including money and power, and to monitor health inequities. There is a need to strengthen intersectoral collaboration and to evaluate all public policies for their impact on and ability to improve health. Actions that create fairer, more inclusive societies will also create healthier societies, and that is as true for CVD as for other conditions.

TARGETING INDIVIDUALS AT HIGH RISK VERSUS POPULATION-WIDE APPROACHES

Broadly speaking, interventions that aim at the prevention of CVD can be grouped into those that target individuals at high

TABLE 62.4 World Health Organization Definition of Myocardial Infarction: 2008–2009 Revision

Category A	Category B	Category C
Definition and Diagnostic Criteria of MI for Use in Settings with No Resource Constraints	Definition and Diagnostic Criteria of MI if the Requirements for Diagnostic Tests in Category A Have Not been Met	Definition and Diagnostic Criteria of Probable MI
The term 'MI' should be used when there is evidence of myocardial necrosis in a clinical setting consistent with myocardial ischaemia (no evidence of a cause other than ischaemia). Any one of the following criteria meets the diagnosis for MI:	Whenever there is incomplete information on cardiac biomarkers (preferably troponin) and other diagnostic criteria needed to apply Category A, the term 'MI' should be used if:	In resource-constrained settings, individuals with MI may not satisfy criteria of definitions in Category A or B. This may be due to delayed access to medical services and/or unavailability of electrocardiography and/or lack of facilities for laboratory assay of specific cardiac biomarkers. The term 'probable MI' should be used when there is insufficient information to decide whether or not there was an MI based on definitions in Categories A and B above, but:
(i) Detection of rise and/or fall of cardiac biomarkers (preferably troponin) with at least one value above the 99th percentile of the upper reference limit together with evidence of myocardial ischaemia, with at least one of the following: (a) symptoms of ischaemia (include various combinations of chest, upper extremity, jaw or epigastric discomfort with exertion or at rest; the discomfort usually lasts ≤20 min, often is diffuse, not localized, not positional, not affected by movement of the region and it may be accompanied by dyspnoea, diaphoresis, nausea or syncope); (b) ECG changes indicative of new ischaemia (new ST-T changes or new left bundle branch block (LBBB)– Minnesota codes: ST-depression 4.1; 4.2; ST-elevation 9.2; LBBB 7.1); (c) development of pathological Q waves in the ECG (Minnesota codes: 1.1.1 through 1.2.5 plus 1.2.7),17 including: (1) no unequivocal pathological Q waves in the first ECG or in event set of ECG(s) followed by a record with a pathological Q wave or (2) any Q wave in leads V2–V350.02 s or QS complex in leads V2 and V3 or Q wave 50.03 s and 50.01 mV deep or QS complex in leads I, II, aVL, aVF or (3) V4–V6 in any two leads of a contiguous lead grouping (I, aVL, V6:V4–V6: II, III, aVF). (d) imaging evidence of new loss of viable myocardium or new regional wall motion abnormality. *Or*	(i) Both of the following criteria are present: (a) symptoms of ischaemia (ischaemic symptoms include various combinations of chest, upper extremity, jaw or epigastric discomfort with exertion or at rest; the discomfort usually lasts ≤20 min, often is diffuse, not localized, not positional, not affected by movement of the region, and it may be accompanied by dyspnoea, diaphoresis, nausea or syncope) and (b) development of unequivocal pathological Q waves (no pathological Q wave in the first ECG or in the event set of ECG/s followed by a record with a pathological Q wave – any Q wave in leads V2–V3 50.02 s (Minnesota code 1.2.1) or QS complex in leads V2 and V3 (Minnesota code 1.2.7). Q-wave 50.03 s and 50.1 mV deep (Minnesota codes 1.1.1; 1.2.2) or QS complex in leads I, II, aVL, aVF or V4–V6 in any two leads of a contiguous lead grouping I, aVL, V6: V4–V6: II, III, aVF (Minnesota codes 1.1.7; 1.3.6)). *Or*	(i) Either one of the following is present in a person with symptoms of ischaemia (include various combinations of chest, upper extremity, jaw or epigastric discomfort with exertion or at rest; the discomfort usually lasts ≤20 min, often is diffuse, not localized, not positional, not affected by movement of the region, and it may be accompanied by dyspnoea, diaphoresis, nausea or syncope), with no evidence of a non-coronary reason: (a) development of unequivocal pathological Q waves (no pathological Q wave in the first ECG or in the event set of ECG/s followed by a record with a pathological Q wave – Minnesota codes 4.1; 4.2; 5.1; 5.2; 9.2 – or development of new ischaemia – new ST-T changes and an equivocal change in Q waves – Minnesota code 1.2.8 or any 1.3 code – demonstrated between the ECGs associated with the event or between a previously recorded ECG and the event ECG); or (b) incomplete information on cardiac biomarkers (preferably troponin) provided that myocardial damage of other reasons and other clinical conditions that can cause a rise in cardiac biomarkers are excluded. *Or*

TABLE 62.4 World Health Organization Definition of Myocardial Infarction: 2008–2009 Revision—cont'd

Category A	Category B	Category C
Definition and Diagnostic Criteria of MI for Use in Settings with No Resource Constraints	Definition and Diagnostic Criteria of MI if the Requirements for Diagnostic Tests in Category A Have Not been Met	Definition and Diagnostic Criteria of Probable MI
(ii) Sudden unexpected cardiac death, involving cardiac arrest, often with symptoms suggestive of myocardial ischaemia (ischaemic symptoms include various combinations of chest, upper extremity, jaw or epigastric discomfort with exertion or at rest; the discomfort usually lasts <20 min, often is diffuse, not localized, not positional, not affected by movement of the region, and it may be accompanied by dyspnoea, diaphoresis, nausea or syncope) and accompanied by (a) presumably new ST elevation or new LBBB (Minnesota codes: ST-depression 4.1; 4.2; ST-elevation 9.2; LBBB 7.1) and/or (b) evidence of fresh thrombus by coronary angiography and/or at autopsy, but death occurring before blood samples could be obtained or at a time before the appearance of cardiac biomarkers in the blood, and there is no evidence of a non-coronary cause of death. (iii) Autopsy findings of an acute MI.	(ii) Death with a history of coronary heart disease and/or documented cardiac pain within 72 h before death and no evidence of non-coronary cause of death or autopsy evidence of chronic coronary heart disease, including coronary atherosclerosis and myocardial scarring.	(ii) Autopsy findings suggestive of MI but not conclusive.

From Mendis S, Thygesen K, Kuulasmaa K, et al. World Health Organization definition of myocardial infarction: 2008–09 revision. Int J Epidemiol 2011;40(1):139–46. With permission of Oxford University Press.

risk of developing CVD, and interventions that aim to lower the risk profile of the whole population. These two approaches are complementary.

Cost-effective, affordable and feasible population-wide primary prevention interventions for CVD exist for countries of all income levels, but implementation must be location-specific in collaboration with all sectors of society to address the multifactorial origin of CVD risk factors. Primary prevention depends on access to the health system, quality of the system, cost of the intervention and cultural acceptability.[4] Population-wide interventions must partner with identification and management of high-risk individuals, since the highest number of cases will come from the large population with low to moderate risk, while the highest proportion of the numerically small high-risk population will become cases.[52]

WHAT WORKS?

Population-wide interventions coupled with improved individual care have led to marked falls in CVD mortality in many high-income countries, as described in the earlier section on epidemiology. At a population level, policy measures, including fiscal and legislative interventions, have played a key role. They include measures aimed at reducing the prevalence of smoking and promoting the consumption of a healthier diet.

In LMICs, where resources are often limited, it is critical to implement feasible, cost-effective, population-based strategies based on the risk profile of the country, e.g. tackling tobacco use, excess salt in the diet and screening for and treating hypertension. As resources allow, this list would expand to include screening high-risk populations for hypercholesterolemia and diabetes, and treatment expanded to moderate-risk populations.[4]

MULTI-SECTORAL STRATEGIES

The health sector must engage with other government ministries and agencies, the private sector and civil society to tackle the range and origin of risk factors for CVD. Public health workers need new skills in multi-sectoral work, in building partnerships and networks, including with community groups, and in negotiating with the private sector around reformulation of foods to provider healthier choices, such as reducing the sodium content, workplace wellness programmes and other social supports for NCD prevention and control. However, in many low-income countries, and in some middle-income countries, the capacity of the Ministry of Health to adequately guide the implementation of 'all of society' CVD and NCD prevention is limited, and in many cases, these systems are not in place. While an inter-sectoral NCD plan is a necessary input, such a document, without the resources to implement it, has little utility.

RISK ACROSS THE LIFE-COURSE

Low birth weight is a risk factor for CVD and diabetes in adulthood, and risky behaviour acquired during childhood, e.g. tobacco and alcohol use, unhealthy diet and physical inactivity, often continues in adulthood. Childhood obesity is rising throughout the world. In addition, maternal obesity is increasing; this is recognized as causing maternal diabetes and large birth weight babies, who are also at increased risk of diabetes in adulthood. Policies that aim to improve maternal and childhood health should be part of a package of multi-sectoral action to reduce the risk of CVD in adulthood. In LMICs, CVD risk factors and CVD prevalence are higher among younger ages compared to high-income countries, thus threatening productivity and household economic security if the breadwinner suffers disability or death.

GENDER ROLES AND CVD RISK

In many LMIC settings, men have a higher prevalence of CVD risk factors than women, including smoking and excess alcohol use. Gender-sensitive interventions are therefore needed to reduce the prevalence and social acceptability of tobacco use, alcohol abuse and inadequate utilization of the health services among men. Conversely, women in many parts of the developing world are obliged by male-dominant cultures to have multiple household and social roles, which compromise their ability to address their own health needs. Some women are not permitted to wear clothing to facilitate exercise, or to leave their homes without male escorts. There are often delays in seeking preventive and curative services – including early detection and treatment – due to gender-imposed constraints, the burden of domestic and family responsibilities, unresponsive health systems and the cost of care.

TARGETING SPECIFIC BEHAVIOURS

Smoking Cessation

In addition to the well-known impact of tobacco use on cancer and CVD, there is the additional impact upon increased morbidity and mortality from tuberculosis in many low-income countries. In addition, tobacco use is associated with malnutrition, especially among women,[53] increased mortality, and mothers who smoke during pregnancy have low birth weight babies. Marketing of tobacco products to children and women in developing countries is now a major strategy of the tobacco industry, in defiance of the objectives of the Framework Convention on Tobacco Control (FCTC) which has been ratified, or acceded to, by 175 countries.[54] Despite good progress, tobacco remains the number one preventable cause of death, and more needs to be done in implementing 100% smoke-free environments, producing graphic tobacco packaging and labelling, banning advertisement, promotion and sponsorship and increasing tobacco taxes and prices (from which tax income would be a sustainable source of funding for NCD prevention and control programmes). These demand-reduction programmes can be implemented for the low cost of between 10 and 72 US cents per person per year.[55] Most of this would be for educational media campaigns, while increased tax and smoke-free environments are effective and also cheap to implement.

As Dr Margaret Chan, Director of WHO said at the United Nations High Level Meeting on NCDs in September 2011, 'Even an old dog like the tobacco industry, can still learn dirty new tricks' in referring to the latest industry tactic of litigation. The influence of the tobacco industry within and outside of government continues to cause millions of preventable deaths.

Tobacco companies are promoting the use of tobacco in many LMICs. The global youth tobacco surveys show that approximately 15% of youths (13–15 years) own products with tobacco branding, and 10% have been offered free cigarettes by a representative of the tobacco industry. As a result, the use of cigarettes or other tobacco products is >30% in Chile (Santiago), Colombia (Bogota), Cook Islands, East Timor, Latvia, and Papua New Guinea, Lebanon, Micronesia and the Northern Mariana Islands.[56]

Alcohol

Excessive use of alcohol contributes to hypertension and the risk of stroke and IHD, is widespread in many parts of the world, and is estimated to be responsible for 4% of global mortality. Decreasing the rate of harmful use of alcohol remains a major challenge, but measures that are likely to be required include limiting availability through controlling outlets, increasing the price of alcohol through taxation and controlling advertising and other means of promoting alcohol. Many economies in developing countries depend on alcohol production and revenues creating a disincentive for alcohol control. Yet the impact on alcohol abuse on violence, accidents, homicide and NCDs is undeniable.

Diet

While obesity is growing globally, including in developing countries, there are still pockets of undernutrition requiring intervention. In most middle-income countries, and among the more affluent in low-income countries, there is over-nutrition and obesity, high levels of saturated fat and trans-fatty acid consumption, approximately double the recommended salt consumption, especially from processed foods, and aggressive marketing of calorie-dense food and non-alcoholic sugar-sweetened drinks to children. Population-based action, rather than emphasis on individual choice and responsibility, will determine the chance of success in reducing the prevalence or slowing the progression of obesity. National governments need to find ways to utilize their armamentarium of regulation, taxation and legislation. Several high-income countries, for example, have taken action on controlling the advertising of fast foods to children and banning the use of trans fats. Among LMICs, Argentina and India have instituted a variety of methods for reducing the consumption of trans fat, e.g. education, product reformulation, a partial ban and required labelling for trans fat.[57]

Cost-effective and feasible dietary interventions include[4]:

- Maternity leave and flexibility at the workplace to facilitate breast-feeding
- Product labelling and education to help consumers make the right choice
- Improving the quality of food served in schools and workplaces
- Reducing salt in manufactured and prepared foods.

Consumer education on the risks associated with excess use of salt, especially for rural populations whose main source of salt is that added during cooking or at the table.

There needs to be a life-course approach that utilizes multiple cost-effective interventions. Action is needed at local and national levels, including improved communication and information strategies, improved capacity of health workers and improved family practices.

Fast food companies, who are supplying an ever-increasing proportion of meals, including in LMICs, are offering different products in developed versus developing countries. For example, some chains that offer roast chicken and/or salads in high-income countries, do not offer these options in the LMICs. Some companies claim a trans fat-free menu, yet because LMICs often lack the capacity to test for trans fats, there is no guarantee that the commitment is being honoured.

There is evidence that some transnational food corporations are moving in the right direction, with the formation in 2008 of the International Food and Beverage Alliance (IFBA). Eight CEOs of major food and beverage manufacturers committed their corporations to support the World Health Organization's 2004 Global Strategy on Diet, Physical Activity and Health. They pledged 'Five Commitments In Five Years' around: product composition and availability; nutrition information to consumers; responsible marketing and advertising to children; promotion of physical activity and healthy lifestyles and public–private partnerships. Food manufacturers in LMICs may need technical support from the IFBA in product reformulation, nutrition labelling and marketing to children.

Physical Inactivity

Physical inactivity is an independent risk factor for CVD morbidity and mortality. Populations in rural areas of low-income countries, with low levels of mechanization, remain physically active. In many middle-income countries, physical inactivity is becoming endemic in both rural and urban areas, as is the case in many high-income countries.

However, there have been great successes in increasing population physical activity in several countries in the developing world. For example, Agita Mundo in Sao Paulo has reduced inactivity in its population from 44 to 12% between 2002 and 2008.[58] Ciclovias (bicycle ways), which originated in Colombia, have been adopted across the region of the Americas and beyond. Typically, streets are closed to motorized traffic for 4–12 hours on 1 day per week, to allow space for wellness activities. Up to 1 million persons participate each Sunday in Bogota.[59] An analysis of four programmes (Bogotá and Medellín in Colombia, Guadalajara in México and San Francisco in the USA) found them to be cost-beneficial.[60]

TREATMENT OF HYPERTENSION AND DYSLIPIDAEMIA

As described in the section on epidemiology, raised blood pressure is a major contributor to mortality, being responsible for around 13% of all deaths globally, primarily through increasing the risk for IHD, stroke and heart failure. It is estimated that 18 million deaths could be averted over the next 10 years among patients already accessing the healthcare system in 23 LMICs, by use of multidrug therapy (statin, aspirin and two blood-pressure-lowering medications). Some 56% of deaths averted would be in those younger than 70 years old and the average annual per capita cost would range between US$0.43 and $2.93.[60]

The availability, access and management of essential, high-quality, low-cost generic medicines for reducing CVD risk must be coupled with programmes to improve physician adherence with evidence-based guidelines and patient compliance with medication as prescribed. In many developing countries, blood pressure screening is not routinely or easily available, despite its ranking as the number one risk factor for death globally.

Raised total cholesterol is estimated to cause one-third of all IHD and 2.6 million deaths globally. In 2008, the estimated prevalence of high total cholesterol was 40% worldwide (23% in Africa and 30% in South-east Asia). However, in most of Africa, much of South-east Asia and in some countries of Latin America and the Caribbean, routine cholesterol screening is not available. Testing capacity needs to be increased, including point of care testing, and generic statins should be made available.

PREVENTION OF DIABETES AND CVD IN PEOPLE WITH DIABETES

More than 60% of deaths in persons living with diabetes are due to CVD, related to the two- to threefold increased risk of heart disease, stroke and peripheral arterial disease in adults with diabetes. The prevention of diabetes is one of the goals of integrated NCD prevention, and is supported by a strong evidence base (see Chapter 63). The principles of preventing CVD in people with diabetes are similar to those in people without diabetes, and include the prevention of smoking, blood pressure control (to a recommended target of 130/80 mmHg), a diet low in saturated fat and sodium, and the use of statins.

Table 62.5 summarizes 'best buys' for the prevention and control of cardiovascular disease.

TABLE 62.5 'Best Buys' for CVD Prevention and Control According to the World Health Organization

Risk Factor/Disease	Interventions
Tobacco use	Raise taxes on tobacco Protect people from tobacco smoke Warn about the dangers of tobacco Enforce bans on tobacco advertising
Harmful use of alcohol	Raise taxes on alcohol Restrict access to retailed alcohol Enforce bans on alcohol advertising
Unhealthy diet and physical inactivity	Reduce salt intake in food Replace trans-fat with polyunsaturated fat Promote public awareness about diet and physical activity (via mass media)
CVD and diabetes	Provide counselling and multidrug therapy (including blood sugar control for diabetes mellitus) for people with medium–high risk of developing heart attacks and strokes (including those who have established CVD) Treat heart attacks (myocardial infarction) with aspirin

Reprinted from the Lancet. From Asaria P, Chisholm D, Mathers C, et al. Chronic disease prevention: health effects and financial costs of strategies to reduce salt intake and control tobacco use. Lancet 2007;370(9604):2044–53. © 2007. With permission from Elsevier.

International Health Priorities and Challenges for the Future

CVD PREVENTION, CONTROL AND A RE-ORIENTATION OF PRIMARY HEALTH CARE

Despite the ongoing need to address maternal and child health and communicable diseases in many LMICs, the burden from NCDs is grave, and prevention and control of CVD requires a strengthened, integrated primary health care system aligned to the needs of the country and not to donor priorities. Creating vertical silos for chosen diseases is not in the best interest of the population, whose needs span the disease spectrum. Single-purpose treatment facilities, e.g. for HIV, compromise the privacy of these patients whose diagnosis is inadvertently unmasked when they are seen entering these single-disease facilities.

Further, a balance in investment between primary and tertiary care is needed so that high-risk patients can be identified and treated as well as preventing the progress to disease among high-risk individuals. For example, Cuba is building more specialized facilities for cardiac care, whereas the demand for this facility could be reduced by increasing the price of cigarettes in order to reduce the current, very high prevalence of tobacco consumption.

Staff in primary care need to be re-trained and motivated to be proactive in screening for CVD risk factors, since these are often silent. In those low-income countries where there are insufficient physicians, other health workers need to be empowered to deliver these services. Such screening should also be done at workplaces, places of worship and in the community, with community participation and engaging with civil society, NGOs and the private sector. The chronic care model needs to be fully implemented in primary care including governance, health information systems, service delivery systems and essential medicines and technologies.

TRANSLATING EVIDENCE-BASED IMPLEMENTATION

In LMICs, as in high-income countries, there are years' long gaps between establishing evidence-based guidelines and their widespread utilization. In LMICs, there is the additional factor that there is insufficient research on how 'best buys' identified in high-income countries are applicable in LMICs, where they need to be both high-impact and affordable.

There is a need for a research agenda and impact evaluation to address these gaps.

UNITED NATIONS HIGH-LEVEL MEETING ON NCDS

Countries of the Caribbean Community led the global advocacy for the September 2011 United Nations High Level Meeting (UNHLM) on NCDs; only the second time the UN General Assembly has met on a health topic. The first time in 2001 on HIV/AIDS led to significant investment in halting that epidemic. Overseas development aid (ODA) for NCDs has always been <1% of total ODA, and by 2011, the global economic climate had become even more unfavourable. In addition, the cynic might say that because CVD in the LMICs does not threaten the health of the richer donor nations, and because many of the risk factors for CVD generate profit for multinational corporations in the developed world, there was little chance of this NCD summit achieving meaningful outcomes. There has been some movement following the UNHLM, including a process to define targets and reporting metrics. However, it seems that it will be left to the national authorities to recognize this as a priority and dedicate the resources necessary to save these lives.

REFERENCES

4. Mendis S, Puska P, Norrving B, editors. Global atlas on cardiovascular disease prevention and control: policies, strategies and interventions. Geneva: World Health Organization; 2011.
26. Messerli FH, Williams B, Ritz E. Essential hypertension. Lancet 2007;370(9587):591–603.
29. Dwivedi G, Beevers DG. Hypertension in ethnic groups: epidemiological and clinical perspectives. Expert Rev Cardiovasc Ther 2009;7(8): 955–63.
49. Mendis S, Thygesen K, Kuulasmaa K, et al. World Health Organization definition of myocardial infarction: 2008–2009 revision. Int J Epidemiol 2011;40(1):139–46.
61. Marijon E, Mirabel M, Celermajer DS, Jouven X. Rheumatic heart disease. The Lancet 2012; 379(9819):953–946.

Access the complete references online at www.expertconsult.com

63 Diabetes in the Tropics

AYESHA A. MOTALA | FRASER J. PIRIE

KEY POINTS

- The prevalence of diabetes is increasing globally, but with a greater increase in developing than in developed nations.
- Asian countries are especially affected by the increased prevalence of diabetes and by 2030, India and China will have the greatest number of persons with diabetes in the world.
- Type 2 diabetes tends to occur at an earlier age and at a lower body mass index in Asian subjects as compared to Western populations.
- Type 1 diabetes is increasingly recognized in the tropics as a disease similar to that in the Western world, especially in terms of HLA susceptibility genotypes.
- Ketosis-prone diabetes predominantly affects persons of African origin and is characterized by prolonged periods of insulin independence after initial glycaemic stabilization.
- Fibrocalculous pancreatic diabetes is an uncommon entity, most often encountered in India and is a possible consequence of tropical chronic pancreatitis.
- Data on diabetes-specific complications in the tropics are sparse, but the prevalence of complications is expected to increase as survival rates improve.

Introduction

Diabetes mellitus (diabetes) is a global disease but its prevalence varies greatly. The introduction of standardized diagnostic criteria for glucose tolerance in the 1980s by the National Diabetes Data Group (NDDG)[1] and the World Health Organization (WHO),[2,3] allowed for assessment and comparison of current and projected estimates on a global level.[4–7]

The revised classification of diabetes by the American Diabetes Association[8] and WHO[9,10] encompasses three clinical stages of glycaemia (normoglycaemia, impaired glucose regulation [impaired glucose tolerance, raised fasting glucose] and diabetes) and four aetiological types of diabetes (type 1, type 2, gestational, and other specific types).

By far, the most common forms of diabetes, globally, are type 1 and type 2, accounting for 90–95% and 5–10%, respectively.[8] Other forms of diabetes encountered in the tropics include tropical chronic pancreatitis and fibrocalculous pancreatic diabetes and ketosis-prone type 2 diabetes mellitus.[8–13]

Recent estimates of the International Diabetes Federation[14] indicate that worldwide, there were 284.6 million people with diabetes mellitus in 2010 and this is projected to increase by 54% to 438.4 million in 2030. The greatest proportional increases are estimated to occur in developing regions of the world, including Africa, South-east Asia, South and Central America, Eastern Mediterranean and Middle Eastern Crescent, in the order of 73–102%. Such increases are due in part to the projected increase in the urban and ageing populations in these regions. In sub-Saharan Africa (SSA), the burden of diabetes is projected to increase from 12.1 million in 2010, to 23.9 million in 2030; an increase of 98%. Impaired glucose tolerance in SSA is projected to increase by 75.8% over the same period, from 26.9 million to 47.3 million.[14]

Type 1 Diabetes

Type 1 diabetes, a chronic immune-mediated disease associated with selective pancreatic beta cell destruction, is regarded as a condition predominantly affecting young people in the developed world and it is clear that the highest incidence rates are found in Europe and North America. The epidemiology of type 1 diabetes in many tropical countries is unknown and in these countries, additional health issues, including HIV infection, tuberculosis and malaria, coupled with high infant mortality, frequently overshadow less common diseases, including type 1 diabetes.[15]

The WHO DIAMOND project reported the epidemiology of type 1 diabetes in children ≤14 years of age, worldwide over a 10-year period (1990–1999).[16] Although data from the developed world were extensive, there was limited information from much of the developing world, including the tropics. Except for Central America and the West Indies, the DIAMOND study showed a steady increase in incidence of type 1 diabetes. In Africa, epidemiological data on type 1 diabetes was available for a number of North African countries, but no sub-Saharan countries were represented. In North Africa, type 1 diabetes has an intermediate incidence (5–9.99/100 000/year). Incidence rates are low (1–4.99/100 000 per year) in China, Japan, Pakistan and South Korea. In Central America and the West Indies, the incidence of type 1 diabetes is highest in Puerto Rico (16.8/100 000 per year) and lowest in Barbados (2.0/100 000 per year). Annual change in incidence fell by 46.1% in Dominica – more than in any other country included in the DIAMOND study. In South America, incidence rates varied from low in Venezuela, to high (10–19.99/100 000 per year) in Argentina. This is in sharp contrast with incidence rates from Europe and North America and in particular, with those from Finland (40.9/100 000 per year), Sardinia (37.8/100 000 per year), Sweden (30.0/100 000 per year) and Canada (24.5/100 000 per year). In the majority of countries in Europe and North America, the incidence of type 1 diabetes is high to very high (≥20/100 000 per year) and annual incidence rates are increasing.[16]

Type 1 diabetes develops as a consequence of immune-mediated destruction of the pancreatic beta cells by CD4+ and CD8+ T-lymphocytes and macrophages.[17] There is considerable evidence that type 1 diabetes develops in association with genetic susceptibility, principally encoded by the human leucocyte antigen (HLA) system on located on the short arm of chromosome 6 (6p21).[18] It is estimated that approximately half of the genetic risk for type 1 diabetes resides in the highly polymorphic HLA system.[17] In high-risk populations, HLA risk is conferred by *DR4-DQ8* and *DR3-DQ2* haplotypes.[19] The evolution of new technology has led to rapid identification of additional non-HLA gene loci associated with susceptibility for type 1 diabetes and over 40 such loci have been described.[20]

Clinical expression of genetic risk requires environmental trigger factors and the steady rise in incidence of type 1 diabetes in Europe can only be explained by an increasing or an altering environmental influence, the identity of which remains unknown.[21] It has been known for many years that markers of the immune attack are specific autoantibodies. Antibodies directed at insulin, glutamic acid decarboxylase (GAD) 65 and insulinoma-associated protein 2 (IA-2) are measurable markers of the autoimmune process and also serve to identify individuals at increased risk of developing type 1 diabetes.[17]

The available data suggest that type 1 diabetes in tropical countries has a genetic and humoral immune profile broadly similar to that described in Europe and North America, but much work remains before the full characterization of type 1 diabetes in these populations is achieved.

Studies from sub-Saharan Africa have shown that type 1 diabetes HLA risk alleles and haplotypes are in general similar to those in populations in the developed world. In South African Zulu subjects, type 1 diabetes is associated with HLA *DQB*0302*, *DRB1*09*, *DRB1*0301*, *DQA*03* and *DQB*02* alleles and *DRB1*0301-DQA*0501*, *DRB1*04-DQA*03*, *DRB1*04-DQB*0302*, *DRB1*0301-DQB*0201*, *DQA*0501-DQB*0201* and *DQA*03-DQB*0302* haplotypes.[22] Similar results have been found in Zimbabwean Shona subjects.[23] In Cameroon, *DQB*0201*, *DRB1*0301* and *DQA*0301* are associated with type 1 diabetes but not *DQB*0302*.[24] In Puerto Rico, *DPB1*0301* has been shown to be associated with type 1 diabetes, with similar results found in Mexican Americans and Caucasians.[25] Very few studies have addressed the role of other genetic loci in conferring susceptibility to type 1 diabetes in populations in the tropics.

Autoantibodies have been studied in a number of populations from developing countries in tropical regions. In subjects with type 1 diabetes in South Africa, antibodies to GAD65 have been reported to occur with a prevalence of 31.8% and to IA-2 with a prevalence of 13.3%.[26] In Cameroon, GAD65 antibodies are found in 34% and antibodies to IA-2 in 6.4% of affected subjects.[27] In Northern India, 22.4% of subjects with type 1 diabetes and mean disease duration of 5.5 ± 6.0 years were positive for both GAD65 and IA-2 antibodies. Only 14.2% were positive for GAD65 alone.[28] In Brazil, GAD65 antibodies were found in 80% and IA-2 antibodies in 62.9% of subjects with short-duration type 1 diabetes.[29] It therefore appears that the prevalence of antibodies to GAD65 and IA2 in type 1 diabetes is usually, but not uniformly, lower than that reported from developed nations. It is not clear whether this represents a difference in patient selection, disease duration at the time of testing, or a real difference within different populations.

As with the developed countries, there are no clear indications as to the identity of possible environmental precipitants of type 1 diabetes in populations residing in tropical countries, although the wide disparity in living conditions between populations resident in the tropics and those in the developed world, argues against common environmental precipitants and promoters.

Type 2 Diabetes

Type 2 diabetes is the most common form encountered globally. Four major pathogenic disturbances are implicated in the development of overt (fasting) hyperglycaemia: a variety of genetic and acquired (including obesity, physical inactivity) factors influence both insulin secretion, leading to pancreatic beta cell dysfunction and insulin action, leading to insulin resistance: (a) the reduced insulin secretion decreases insulin signalling in its target tissues (liver, muscle and adipose tissue) leading to (b) increased hepatic glucose output, (c) decreased peripheral glucose uptake and (d) reduced suppression of lipolysis, with resultant hyperglycaemia and increased circulating free fatty acids characteristic of type 2 diabetes; these in turn, will feedback to worsen both the insulin secretion and resistance, i.e. *glucotoxicity*, and *lipotoxicity* and the resultant 'disharmonious quartet' involved in pathogenesis.[30,31] More recently, altered incretin responses, hyperglucagonaemia, and altered renal tubular glucose excretion, have been implicated in the pathogenesis of type 2 diabetes.[32]

Intrauterine and postnatal development can affect the future risk of diabetes and cardiovascular disease by fetal programming. Both the thrifty genotype and the thrifty phenotype hypothesis will predict that populations in some areas of the developing world would be at greater risk for diabetes. The 'thrifty phenotype' hypothesis describes the metabolic adaptations adopted as a survival strategy by a malnourished fetus; changes that may also be inappropriate to deal with the later life of affluence.

Maternal undernutrition, infant's low birth weight and rapid postnatal child growth are all associated with increased risk of diabetes in the offspring, and these factors might be especially relevant to developing countries such as India and China.

Until the 1960s, diabetes was considered to be rare in sub-Saharan Africa (SSA); however over the past few decades it has emerged as an important medical problem. Studies done in Africa prior to the 1980s suggested low diabetes prevalence, between 0 and 1%.[33–35] Using standardized 1985 WHO criteria, studies show variable prevalence, with low rates (<3%) in both urban and rural communities in West and East Africa; by contrast, moderate rates (3–10%) are reported in rural, semi-urban and urban communities in South Africa and in African-origin populations in Sudan, comparable with rates in developed countries; high prevalence (>10%) is reported in populations of mixed Egyptian ancestry in Northern Sudan.[33,35]

Using the recent ADA[8,36] and WHO[9,10] criteria, diabetes prevalence is low in rural communities in Tanzania,[37] with moderate rates in urban Tanzanians, urban and rural Ghanaians[38] and rural South Africans.[14] The WHO STEPwise chronic disease risk factor surveillance programme (STEPS) undertaken in many African countries aims to clarify the burden of diabetes in sub-Saharan Africa. Reported prevalence varies widely (Benin

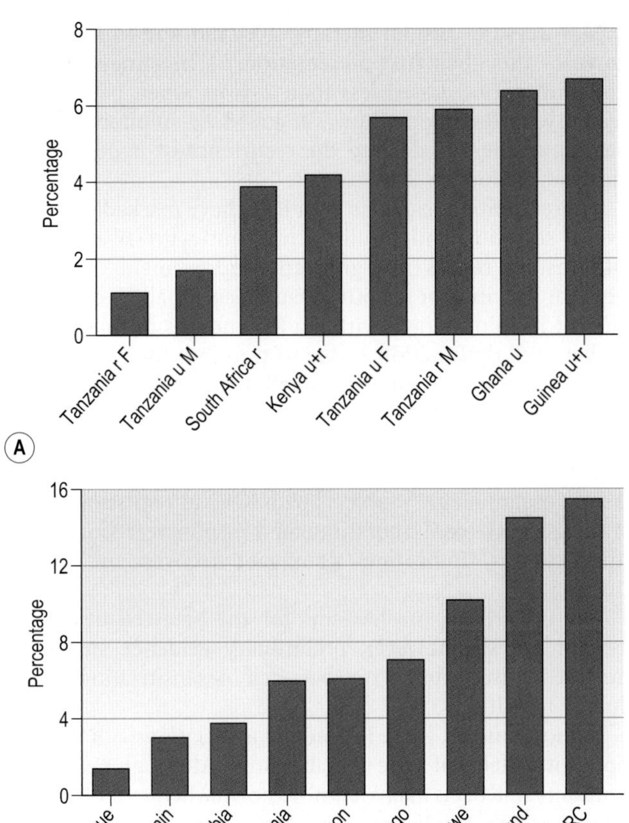

Figure 63.1 Prevalence of diabetes mellitus in sub-Saharan Africa using 1998 WHO criteria; 1B: WHO-STEPS studies. r, rural; F, female; u, urban; M, male; DRC, Democratic Republic of Congo.

3%; Mauritania 6%; Cameroon 6.1%; Congo 7.1%; Zimbabwe 10.2%; Democratic Republic of Congo 14.5%) (Figure 63.1).[35]

In most studies, diabetes prevalence is higher in urban communities and is especially striking in Tanzania, where urban rates are fivefold higher than in rural communities.[34,35,37]

Studies from Tanzania and South Africa show that diabetes prevalence is lower in the indigenous African population than in migrant Asian groups (African vs Asian, 5.3 vs 13.1% in Durban, South Africa; 1.1 vs 9.1/7.1% in Dar-es-Salaam, Tanzania) and when compared with a community of mixed ancestry (Khoi-East Indian-Europid, 8 vs 10% in the Cape Province, South Africa).[34,35,39–43]

The impact of environmental influences in populations of similar genetic origin has been confirmed in studies which showed that diabetes rates are lower in native African populations from Nigeria and Cameroon than in populations of West African origin in the Caribbean, the UK and the USA.[34,35]

Consistent with global estimates that indicate little gender difference for diabetes,[6,14] gender distribution varies widely in sub-Saharan Africa (SSA) with no discernible trend. As in other regions of the world, diabetes prevalence increases with age, both in men and women, with peak prevalence in the 45–64 year or ≥65 year age groups, and age is a significant risk factor for diabetes.[34,35]

Several African studies have examined and confirmed the association between diabetes prevalence and measures of adiposity, including body mass index (BMI) (total body obesity), waist circumference (WC) and waist:hip ratio (WHR) (upper body/abdominal obesity).[34,35] Diabetes prevalence increases with higher BMI, WHR and WC; mean BMI, WHR and WC are higher in subjects with diabetes; BMI/total body obesity and WHR/abdominal obesity are independent risk factors for diabetes.[34,35,37]

A positive family history of diabetes is a significant association in some studies.[34,35] Although physical activity was not found to be an independent risk factor for diabetes in studies in which it was examined, there is an inverse relationship between physical activity and diabetes in some populations.[34,35,37]

Using current WHO criteria, the prevalence of diabetes has risen from 2.3% in the 1980s to 4.6% in 1996 in Tanzania, with a three to seven times rise in the 35–54 years age group. In people from urban Cameroon, a four times escalation from 1.5% in the 1990s to 6.6% in 2003 was noted.[34,35,37,44]

In SSA, chronic diseases such as diabetes receive low priority due in part, to misconceptions that the adult population will be decimated by HIV/AIDS and that few will live long enough to develop chronic diseases. A recent report on the estimated impact of HIV/AIDS on projected patient load for the years 1995 and 2010, showed that the total number of people with diabetes will increase regardless of the expected impact of HIV/AIDS or the change in the prevalence of diabetes.[45]

There are no published reports of longitudinal African studies which have examined the incidence of diabetes or natural history of intermediate stages of glucose tolerance (IGT/IFG) and there is a dearth of data on the impact of dietary and genetic factors and the role of insulin from population studies.

Diabetes, already in epidemic proportions in many Asian countries, is set to further increase in the coming decades. Six of the top 10 countries are in Asia and in 2030 India and China will be the countries with the greatest number of people with diabetes (estimated at 79.4 million and 42.3 million, respectively).[46]

For India, earlier studies also reported low diabetes prevalence (1.2–3%) in both urban and rural communities.[47] Studies between 1971 and 2004, show that the prevalence in India is rising rapidly especially in urban populations, with a 10-fold increase (from 1.2–12.1%) both in national[48] and regional urban surveys.[47] In a recent national survey,[49] overall diabetes prevalence was 4.3% with higher rates in urban (5.6%) than rural (2.7%) communities. Reports from South India show that between 1989 and 2003, there has been a threefold increase (from 2.4% to 6.4%) even in rural communities;[50] important contributors include an increase in family income, educational status, motorized transport and a shift in occupational structure, i.e. socioeconomic transition.

Whereas onset is uncommon below age 40 years in the Western world, diabetes in Asian Indians appears at least 10–15 years earlier, with some reports of age of onset <50 years in up to 50%.[50]

The risk of diabetes in Asian Indians starts at lower levels of BMI than in the Western world and risk increases with small weight changes above BMI 22 kg/m^2. Despite this, the association between BMI and glucose tolerance is as strong in Asian populations, as in any other population.[51] Cut-off values for healthy BMI in Indians is <23 kg/m^2 vs <25 kg/m^2 in Europids and normal WC is <90 cm in Indian men and <80 cm in women vs 94 and 80 cm, respectively, in Europids; also, abdominal obesity is reported to occur even at lean BMI values.[51,52] In Indians, central obesity shows a stronger association with diabetes than total body obesity.[47] The excess visceral body fat and low muscle mass, even in the non-obese, may explain the high prevalence of hyperinsulinaemia and insulin resistance and high risk of type 2 diabetes in Asian Indians.[52–54]

Evidence from sub-Saharan Africa and Asia suggests that the present epidemiological transition is strongly linked with the so-called westernization of lifestyle, characterized by decreased amounts of physical activity and increased consumption of energy-dense or high-fat diets as a result of rapid urbanization. Urban populations eat more diverse diets and more micro nutrients and animal food than the rural residents but high intake of refined carbohydrates, processed foods, unsaturated and total fat and lower intake of fibre.[35,46]

Ketosis – Prone Type 2 Diabetes (KPD)

Over the past two decades, a ketosis-prone form of diabetes, which was initially observed in young African-Americans, has emerged as a new clinical entity. This syndrome of episodic diabetic ketoacidosis (DKA) without immunological markers of type 1 diabetes is characterized by insulin dependence at the time of presentation as in type 1 diabetes, but followed by absence of insulin requirements for a variable period of time. Such persons present with new diagnosis of DKA but have clinical, metabolic and immunological features of type 2 diabetes during follow-up.[13,55]

The absence of a defined pathophysiological mechanism led the ADA[8] and WHO[9] to classify this form as idiopathic type 1 or type 1B diabetes, i.e. type 1 diabetes with no known aetiologies. Because of the mixed features of type 1 and type 2 diabetes, this variant has been variously referred to as atypical diabetes, Flatbush diabetes, type 1.5 diabetes and more recently, ketosis-prone type 2 diabetes (KPD).[13,55] It is mostly observed in African-origin populations, accounting for 20–50% of African-American and 10–15% of SSA adult persons with a new diagnosis of DKA, but has also been reported in Hispanics, Native-American, Japanese and Chinese.[13,55]

Most patients with KPD are obese, middle-aged men with a strong family history of type 2 diabetes, but a lack of genetic association with HLA and a low prevalence of autoimmune markers of type 1 diabetes (antibodies to islet cell, ICA; and glutamic acid decarboxylase, GAD). From studies in migrants from SSA, mean age at diagnosis was 39.1 years; 76% were men; 75% had a family history of type 2 diabetes; mean BMI 24.9 kg/m^2 and 49.5% were overweight or obese.[13,55]

KPD typically presents with severe symptomatic hyperglycaemia (polyuria, polydipsia, weight loss) and ketosis or ketoacidosis without a precipitating cause. Insulin treatment is mandatory at onset. However, after a few days or weeks of insulin treatment, they may enter a period of near normoglycaemic remission, which may last for a few months to several years, and may be interrupted by hyperglycaemic relapses. During remission, it is possible to maintain adequate glycaemic control without insulin.[13,55] In SSA migrants, discontinuation with subsequent remission was achieved in 76% after a mean of 14.3 weeks of insulin therapy; 40% did not require insulin ten years after their first presentation.[13,55] In some studies, the remission period lasted less than 2 years when patients were treated with diet alone; however low-dose sulphonylurea and metformin therapy delayed the recurrence of hyperglycaemia and readmission for ketoacidosis.[55]

At presentation, subjects with KPD have markedly impaired insulin secretion and insulin action but aggressive treatment with insulin results in significant improvement in beta-cell function and insulin sensitivity, sufficient to allow discontinuation of insulin therapy within a few months of follow-up, i.e. the beta-cell dysfunction is due to transient functional abnormality but not irreversible beta-cell damage. In a recent study, a small number of African-American subjects with KPD in remission, subjects with type 2 diabetes and obese controls were subjected to arginine stimulation before and after 20 hours of dextrose infusion.[56] Subjects with KPD in remission demonstrated similar basal and stimulated insulin secretion to both other groups, indicating significant recovery of beta-cell function.

The underlying mechanisms for the beta-cell dysfunction are not known; however, preliminary evidence suggests an increased susceptibility to beta-cell desensitization due to glucose toxicity.[55]

In most studies, there is a lack of association with HLA susceptibility alleles of type 1 diabetes.[13,55] Although genetic susceptibility to KPD is likely, it is not known whether it is polygenic or monogenic. Studies in west Africa have shown glucose-6-phosphate-dehydrogenase (G6PD) deficiency in subjects with KPD, but no association with mutations in the *G6PD* gene or polymorphisms in the sterol regulatory element binding protein-1 (*SREBP-1*).[57]

Most studies have reported a low prevalence (0–18%) of autoimmune markers of type 1 diabetes (ICA and GAD antibodies) in KPD. In addition, there is preliminary evidence of an association between seropositivity for antibodies to *human herpesvirus 8* and subjects of African origin with KPD.[58]

Factors predictive of future near-normoglycaemic remission in adults with DKA include ethnicity (African-American, African, Hispanic), newly diagnosed diabetes, obesity, family history of diabetes, negative autoantibodies (ICA or GAD), fasting c-peptide levels (>0.33 nmol/L within 1 week after resolution of DKA or >0.5 nmol/L after 6–8 weeks of follow-up) and glucagon-stimulated c-peptide (>0.5 nmol/L at presentation and >0.75 nmol/L at follow-up).[59]

Malnutrition, Tropical Pancreatitis and Diabetes

The current WHO classification of diabetes no longer includes the clinical class of malnutrition-related diabetes mellitus (MRDM), which was previously sub-typed as fibrocalculous pancreatic diabetes (FCPD) and protein-deficient pancreatic diabetes (PDPD), also referred to as protein-deficient diabetes mellitus (PDDM). In 1995, an international workshop proposed that the term MRDM be replaced by malnutrition-modulated diabetes mellitus (MMDM) and that the previous conditions classified as PDPD (PDDM) be included in this group.[11] These conditions are distinct from FCPD, which appears in the current WHO classification under the category of other specific types.[9] FCPD is a well-characterized entity and appears to be a consequence of tropical chronic pancreatitis. MMDM, however, is less clearly defined as a distinct entity and, indeed, may encompass a heterogeneous group of specific forms of diabetes in which the clinical expression is modulated by malnutrition. Some doubt the existence of MMDM as a specific entity, whereas others have supported the need for its recognition as a unique form of diabetes.[60,61]

Tropical chronic pancreatitis (TCP) is a juvenile form of non-alcoholic pancreatitis, characterized by the presence of large intra-ductal calcium-containing calculi and a high risk of development of diabetes mellitus and pancreatic cancer.[62] Malnutrition and consumption of cassava have been implicated in the pathogenesis of this condition.[63] Much of the data on TCP are from south India, although the condition has been described in other areas of the developing world. Although the clinical disease has been well described, the epidemiology of the condition is not well understood as most descriptions are clinic-based, and few population-based studies have been reported.[62] TCP typically presents with recurrent acute abdominal pain in young persons (nearly all are <40 years of age), with subsequent development of pancreatic exocrine and endocrine insufficiency. In India, approximately half of a cohort of subjects with TCP who had normal glucose tolerance at baseline, developed diabetes after a mean follow-up of 7 years.[64] Diabetes usually requires insulin therapy but is not associated with ketoacidosis.[62] Microvascular diabetes complications, including retinopathy, nephropathy, renal failure, peripheral neuropathy and autonomic neuropathy, previously considered to be rare in FCPD, have been reported from a number of centres. Macrovascular disease, however, appears to be an uncommon complication of FCPD.[65]

A recent study conducted in a single tertiary centre in India evaluated the profile of subjects presenting with idiopathic chronic pancreatitis. Of 242 subjects seen over a 4-year period, only 5.8% of the subjects met the criteria for TCP (onset <30 years of age, BMI <18.5 kg/m^2, pancreatic calculi and dilated main pancreatic duct, presence of diabetes and absence of another cause for pancreatitis).[66] Among the group as a whole, malnutrition and cassava consumption were not risk factors for the development of chronic pancreatitis and over half of the subjects had mutations in *SPINK 1* (serine protease inhibitor Kazal type-1) and/or *CFTR* (cystic fibrosis trans-membrane conductance regulator) genes. None of the subjects in this study was shown to have mutations in *PRSS 1* (cationic trypsinogen gene).

Furthermore, in a large population-based study in Chennai, India, of 1382 subjects with known diabetes, the prevalence of FCPD was 0.36%.[67] Subjects with FCPD were younger, had an earlier age of diabetes diagnosis (36.3 ± 15.1 vs 46.0 ± 10.0 years), lower BMI and waist circumference, lower cholesterol and triglyceride levels, but higher HbA_{1c} than the other subjects with diabetes. All five subjects in whom this diagnosis had been made, were treated with insulin.

These studies suggest that even in areas where TCP and FCPD were considered common, more careful analysis indicates that they are uncommon entities that require further clarification and investigation in terms of aetiology and pathogenesis.

MMDM has been associated with polymorphisms in the MHC class 1 chain-related gene a (MIC-A) and with HLA *DR3-DQ2*.[68,69] However, more work is required to clarify whether MMDM is a form of autoimmune type 1 diabetes, with a distinctive phenotype that is influenced by nutritional deprivation.

Complications

From WHO estimates, the global excess mortality attributable to diabetes for the year 2000 was 2.9 million, equivalent to 5.2% of world all-cause mortality and similar in magnitude to those of HIV/AIDS in the same year, making diabetes the fifth leading cause of death in the world. Of the excess deaths, 1.9 million (65.5%) are from developing regions of the world where 1 in 10 excess deaths in economically productive individuals (35–65 years) can be attributed to diabetes; yet diabetes is perceived as a disease of affluent countries.[70]

The natural history and clinical course of diabetes in Africa are poorly understood due in many instances to poor follow-up.[71] From the limited evidence, mortality rates are unacceptably high and the major contributors still include preventable acute metabolic complications and infective causes. Mortality rates of 5.0–11.8% have been reported from clinic studies and of 7.6–41% from outcome studies; the major causes of death were diabetic ketoacidosis (DKA) and infection. However, reports from Ethiopia and South Africa indicate that there is a changing pattern, with renal disease accounting for 30–50% of deaths in type 1 diabetes. From earlier necropsy studies, most deaths were due to DKA (34–54%) and infection was the second leading cause. However, the limitations of these studies were that they included mixed cohorts of subjects with type 1 and type 2 diabetes and varying diabetes duration.[71] Premature mortality related to type 1 diabetes has been highlighted in rural Mozambique where life expectancy after the diagnosis is drastically reduced to only 0.6 years, whereas in urban Zambia, life expectancy is an estimated 27 years.[72]

Previous impressions that chronic complications of diabetes are rare in Africa are likely related to the decreased survival from the disease and inadequate screening.[33,71,73] Clinic-based studies on mixed cohorts of type 1 and type 2 diabetes and varying diabetes duration. have shown that where examined, the prevalence of macrovascular disease is uncommon (peripheral vascular disease, 1.7–10%; angina 0.4–10.0%), hypertension is common (19–50%) and diabetic foot disease was reported in 0.6–36.6%. Regarding microvascular complications, the prevalence of retinopathy ranges from 2.9–57.1%, of nephropathy, from 1.0–30.5%, and of neuropathy, from 5.9–69.6%.[33,71,73]

The only population-based study on the prevalence of microvascular complications in Egyptians with type 2 diabetes, showed rates among subjects with known diabetes and subjects with newly (survey) diagnosed diabetes of 41.5% and 15.7%, respectively, for retinopathy, 6.7% and 6.8% for nephropathy, 21.9% and 13.6% for neuropathy, and 0.8% for both groups for foot ulcers. Each of the microvascular complications was significantly associated with increased blood glucose.[71]

Most of the data on long-duration disease in defined patient groups are from studies in type 1 diabetes; these data have shown rates of microvascular complications ranging from 40–50% for retinopathy, 20–40% for neuropathy, and 20–30% for nephropathy.[71] In South African Indians and Africans (Blacks) with long duration (>10 year) type 2 diabetes, retinopathy was found in 64.5%, nephropathy in 25%, treatment-requiring hypertension in 68%, abnormal serum creatinine in 25%, and abnormal glomerular filtration rate in 42%. There was no significant ethnic difference for the prevalence of complications except for hypertension which was more prevalent in Africans (84.8%) than in Indians (47.4%).[74]

Therefore, the available data indicate that with improving survival rates and the emergence of larger African populations with long-duration diabetes, the prevalence of chronic complications will approach that seen in the developed world. What needs to be established however, is the apparent low frequency of macrovascular disease and the high prevalence of hypertension.

Management

As in other regions of the world, the management of diabetes in the tropics includes lifestyle modification (diet and physical activity), oral anti-diabetic agents and insulin and other injectables. Control and prevention of diabetes requires continuing access to medication, equipment (glucose-measuring strips) and trained healthcare professionals. However, in many countries in developing regions of the world, there is poor control due largely to inadequate access to care and the lack of continuous access to anti-diabetic drugs, especially insulin, at affordable cost, leading to undue and avoidable metabolic complications.[35]

REFERENCES

1. National Diabetes Data Group. Classification and diagnosis of diabetes mellitus and other categories of glucose intolerance. Diabetes 1979; 28:1039–57.
16. The DIAMOND Project Group. Incidence and trends of childhood Type 1 diabetes worldwide 1990–1999. Diabet Med 2006;23:857–66.
17. Achenbach P, Bonifacio E, Koczwara K, et al. Natural history of type 1 diabetes. Diabetes 2005;54(Suppl 2):S25–31.
32. DeFronzo RA. Overview of newer agents: where treatment is going. Am J Med 2010;123: S38–48.
33. McLarty DG, Pollitt C, Swai ABM. Diabetes in Africa. Diabetic Med 1990;7:670–84.
35. Mbanya JC, Motala AA, Sobngwi E, et al. Diabetes in sub-Saharan Africa. Lancet 2010;375 (9733):2254–66.
46. Ramachandran A, Ching Wan Ma R, Snehalatha C. Diabetes in Asia. Lancet 2010;375:408–18.
55. Umpierrez GE, Smiley D, Kitabchi AE. Narrative review: ketosis-prone type 2 diabetes mellitus. Ann Intern Med 2006;144:350–7.

Access the complete references online at www.expertconsult.com

64

Cancer in the Tropics

ROBERT NEWTON | KATIE WAKEHAM | FREDDIE BRAY

KEY POINTS

- Cancer incidence and mortality are not well measured in many parts of the developing world and so understanding of the burden of disease is based on estimates.
- Cancer incidence and mortality are increasing in the developing world.
- Infections represent the most important cause of cancer in developing countries although the impact of tobacco and other lifestyle factors, normally associated with more affluent countries, is increasing.
- Many cancers can be prevented with modification of lifestyle, screening or vaccination against oncogenic infections.
- Methods for adequate diagnosis and management of cancer are not widely available in many developing countries and palliation is widely neglected.

Introduction

This chapter aims to illustrate the key patterns and recent trends of cancer observed today, emphasizing the changing and increasing global cancer burden that is being observed as countries transit toward higher levels of social and economic development. On the basis of several metrics of the cancer burden in 2008, recorded trends in incidence from 1983–2002, and the predicted burden in 2030, we discuss the prospects for cancer prevention, and briefly examine prospects for ameliorating the disease burden via early detection and screening. We close by outlining the treatment and palliation options in low-income settings.

Routine Sources and Measures of the Global Cancer Burden

We have used a number of routine sources of information to compile, estimate and illustrate the world cancer burden in this chapter. However, it is important to note that estimation of the burden of cancer (or any other disease) in developing countries is problematic and so data should be interpreted with appropriate caution. Overall, about 4–5% of the population of developing countries is covered by routine registration of mortality statistics. Cancer registries are another important source of data on cancer occurrence, but also cover only limited geographic areas – about 3% of the population of developing countries – although they can provide information on the current cancer profile and its evolution over time. Based on these limited data, it is possible to obtain working estimates of the burden of cancer in tropical countries. The primary sources and estimation methods, for incidence, mortality, prevalence and disability-adjusted life years, are briefly described below.

INCIDENCE

Cancer incidence is defined as the frequency of occurrence of new cases of cancer in a specific population for a given period of time. It can be expressed as the absolute number of cases or as a rate per unit-time, with cancer cases as the numerator and the corresponding person-time at risk as the denominator. Comparisons of incidence rates can elucidate the underlying risk factors, aid planning and prioritization of resources for cancer control, and monitor and evaluate the impact of specific primary prevention interventions. Population-based cancer registries are the essential institutions enabling these activities. They collect and classify information on all new cases of cancer within a well-defined population and provide statistics on occurrence for the purposes of assessing and controlling the impact of cancer in the community. Registries are either national or regional in their coverage, with a high degree of completeness, accuracy and comparability of the collected data essential for making reliable inferences regarding geographical and temporal variations in the underlying rates. While incidence trends are unaffected by the impact of changes in treatment and consequently survival, changes in registration practices, definitions of malignancy and ICD classification can all impact on incidence.[1] The *Cancer Incidence in Five Continents* (CI5) series, first published in 1962 and soon to be in its 10th volume, compiles recorded cancer incidence data over a recent 5-year period from selected well-functioning population-based cancer registries around the world.[2] Inclusion in CI5 is a reliable marker of the quality of a given Registry's data as the editorial process includes numerous assessments of the comparability, completeness and accuracy of the submitted dataset. There is a substantial disparity in the availability of high-quality cancer registration data between high- and low- to middle-resource countries. While 83% of the North American population were comprehensively covered in the 9th volume of CI5, only 6%, 4% and 1% of the respective South American, Asian and African countries had registries accepted for inclusion.

MORTALITY

Mortality provides a unique measure of the outcome or impact of cancer and is expressed either as number of deaths occurring or as a mortality rate per unit-time. Mortality is a product of the incidence and the case fatality of a given cancer, and case fatality (1-survival) represents the probability that an individual with cancer will die from it. Mortality rates therefore measure the average risk to the population of dying from a specific cancer. Data are derived from vital registration systems, where usually a clinical practitioner certifies the fact and cause of death. The International Classification of Diseases (ICD) provides the uniform system for nomenclature and coding, and a suggested format for the death certificate. Mortality data are affected by both the accuracy of the recorded cause of death and the completeness of registration. Errors of death certification are well documented,[3] e.g. patients diagnosed with cancer may die of the disease without this being written on the death certificate. Mortality data remain, however, more comprehensively available than incidence. The WHO mortality databank contains national cancer mortality data on around 80 countries, available over extended periods of time for many countries. Mortality data are more readily available than incidence in South America but availability remains limited. The greater availability of mortality data in higher-resource countries might explain its common application as a surrogate for incidence in both geographic and temporal studies of cancer. Mortality can only be utilised in such a way if case fatality is constant across populations or in a specified population over time; in high-income countries where cancer treatment and management has markedly improved over time, observed incidence and mortality trends can be at considerable variance.

PREVALENCE

With breakthroughs in early detection and effective treatment, cancer has evolved into a chronic condition in higher-resource countries. Cancer prevalence helps quantify the resource needs by measuring the absolute number and the relative proportion of individuals affected by the disease that require some form of medical attention. Total prevalence is the number of persons in a defined population alive at a given time, who have had cancer diagnosed at some time in the past. This may be estimated directly in population-based cancer registries by counting the number of cases still alive at a specified point in time. As this approach requires both registration and follow-up, and the resource requirements for treating newly diagnosed patients are quite different from those for supporting long-term survivors, alternative definitions of prevalence are commonly used. Limited-duration prevalence is the number of patients diagnosed with cancer within a fixed time in the past and is likely to be pertinent in estimating the needs for cancer services relating to specific phases of cancer care from diagnosis through to palliation and death. We have estimated 5-year prevalence and partitioned it according to different phases of cancer care, e.g. initial treatment (within 1 year), clinical follow-up (2–3 years) and cure (4–5 years). The underlying methods are those used to estimate the global prevalence in 1990,[4] with the estimates built up as a product of incidence and survival at the country level. For the most recent 2008 estimates,[5] the survival dataset was updated and extended to encompass several new sets of estimates of absolute survival at the country level, including registry-specific estimates from many low- and medium-resource settings, as well as in Europe and the USA, and several country-specific estimates, including Australia and Japan.

DISABILITY-ADJUSTED LIFE YEARS (DALYS)

Information about both fatal and non-fatal cancer-related outcomes is necessary to establish priorities for cancer control. Disability-adjusted life years (DALYs) are a key measure, as they link the burden of cancer mortality in society with the degree of illness and disability among cancer patients and long-term survivors.[6] DALYs are the sum of life years lost due to premature mortality or years of life lost (YLLs) and years lived with disability (YLDs). YLLs are calculated by multiplying the number of cancer-specific deaths in a given age group with the number of years a person would be expected to live beyond the age at diagnosis. YLDs were computed by multiplying the number of incident cases at each non-fatal disease phase by the average duration of time associated with each disease phase. Disability weights were then multiplied by these life years to account for severity of each event.[6]

Measuring the Cancer Burden Worldwide – Methods of Estimation

The International Agency for Research on Cancer (IARC) is the definitive reference source for the provision of global statistics on the burden of cancer, and publishes estimates of the global cancer burden as part of the GLOBOCAN series. The most recent database contains estimates of the cancer incidence, mortality, prevalence and DALYs worldwide for all cancers combined for the year 2008, and for 26 cancer sites in 184 countries (see: http://globocan.iarc.fr).[7]

The methods used to compile the GLOBOCAN estimates have evolved with time, but the underlying principle remains one of reliance on the best available data within a country to build-up the global picture. The results are more or less accurate for different countries, depending on the extent and accuracy of locally available data. A hierarchy of methods is employed to build up the global profile, and these are dependent on the availability and the accuracy of country-specific data. The methods for estimating incidence and mortality are detailed elsewhere.[7] In brief, national sources of incidence (from cancer registries) and mortality (from the WHO databank) were used directly wherever possible to obtain information on new cases of cancer and cancer deaths, with prediction methods utilized to provide estimates for the year 2008. As cancer registries record mortality as well as incidence, a well-established method for estimating national incidence is to apply a registry-based incidence: mortality ratio to corresponding national mortality data, where available. Thus, regional data and statistical modelling were used where national incidence data were absent.

For a number of low- and medium-resource countries, no vital statistics were available, and cancer-specific mortality was estimated using the estimated incidence for 2008 and cancer survival probabilities modelled by GDP per capita; these were scaled to the WHO mortality estimates wherever possible. Adjustments were made where under-recording of mortality was suspected, and deaths recorded as uterus cancer unspecified were reallocated back to the specific sites of cervix or corpus uteri.

As well as counts and rates of cancer incidence and mortality, we also present key statistics of 5-year cancer prevalence and DALYs, partitioning the latter into its two components, YLL and YLD. The sources of data and statistical methods used to derive limited duration prevalence and DALYs at the national level are given by Bray et al.[8] and Soerjomataram et al.,[9] respectively. We present these metrics for specific cancer types by sex globally and by world region, as well as according to a country's level of the Human Development Index (HDI), a summary measure of human development. This (for the 2007 UNDP estimates) is a composite index of three basic dimensions of human development, namely a long and healthy life (based on life expectancy at birth), access to knowledge (based on a combination of adult literacy rate and primary to tertiary education enrolment rates) and a decent standard of living (based on GDP per capita adjusted for purchasing-power parity, PPP US$).

We estimated age-standardized incidence and mortality rates per 100 000 population using the world standard population[2] and estimated the lifetime cumulative risk for individuals aged 0–74 years, assuming an absence of competing causes of death.[10] We present the future burden of cancer in 2030 by sex for all cancers combined for the four levels of HDI on the basis of the rates in 2008, assuming population growth and ageing in 2030 occurs according to the UN World Population Prospects medium-fertility variant.

To examine aspects of the cancer burden according to levels of resource and extent of societal development, we used predefined categories of the distribution of HDI: *low HDI* (HDI<0.5); *medium HDI* (0.5≤HDI<0.8); *high HDI* (0.8≤HDI<0.9) and *very high HDI* (HDI≥0.9).[11] The breakdown of each country into one of these development level categories is illustrated graphically in Figure 64.1; the countries are listed in Box 64.1. We also combined high and very HDI levels, and low and medium HDI levels, to create *lower HDI* and *higher HDI* areas, as alternatives to the traditional dichotomy of 'developed' and 'developing'.

The Global Cancer Burden in 2008 by Level of Human Development

There were an estimated 12.7 million new cancer cases and 7.6 million cancer deaths worldwide in 2008 (Figure 64.2). The 5-year prevalence figure indicates there were 28.7 million persons alive with cancer at the end of 2008, who had been diagnosed within the last 5 years. Lung cancer remains the most common cancer worldwide, both in terms of incidence (1.6 million new cases, almost 13% of the total cancer incidence burden) and mortality (1.4 million deaths, 18% of the total mortality burden). Breast cancer in women is the second most frequent cancer (1.4 million new cases, 11%), although it ranks fifth in terms of mortality (458 000 deaths, 6.1%). Colorectal (1.2 million new cases, 608 000 deaths); stomach (990 000 cases, 738 000 deaths); prostate (913 000 new cases, 261 000 deaths) and liver cancer (748 000 cases and 695 000 deaths) rank third to sixth, respectively in terms of global frequency of new cases.

Within the areas defined as having higher levels of human development (high or very high HDI), lung, female breast and colorectal cancer each constituted over 800 000 new diagnoses in 2008, with prostate cancer accounting for only slightly less, about 766 000 cases (Figure 64.3A). Together, these four cancers comprise about half of the total cancer burden in these more developed countries, and the lifetime cumulative risk of

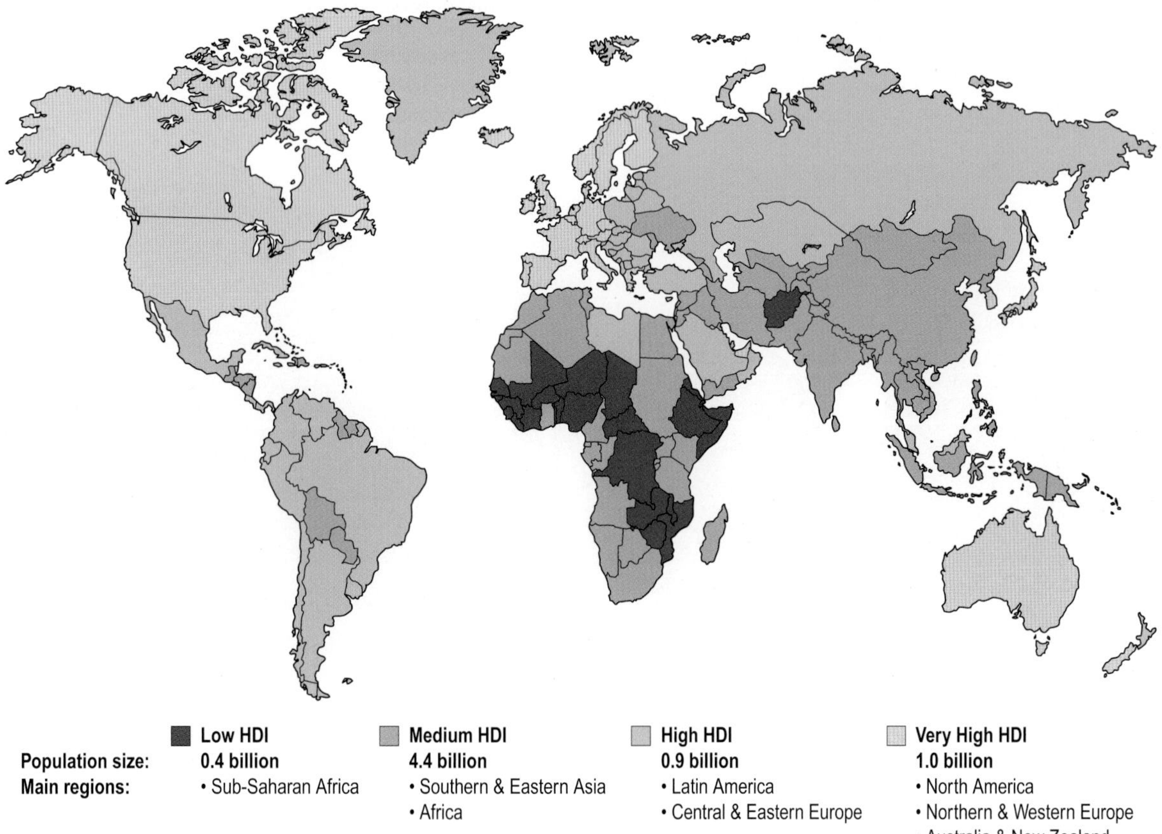

Figure 64.1 Human Development Index 2007 (4 levels).

BOX 64.1 LIST OF THE 184 COUNTRIES IN THE FOUR LEVELS OF THE HUMAN DEVELOPMENT INDEX

VERY HIGH HDI

Australia; Austria; Barbados; Belgium; Brunei Darussalam; Canada; Cyprus; Czech Republic; Denmark; Finland; France (metropolitan); France, Guadeloupe; France, La Reunion; France, Martinique; French Guyana; French Polynesia; Germany; Greece; Iceland; Ireland; Israel; Italy; Japan; Korea, Republic of Kuwait; Luxembourg; Malta; New Caledonia; New Zealand; Norway; Portugal; Qatar; Singapore; Slovenia; Spain; Sweden; Switzerland; Taiwan; the Netherlands; United Arab Emirates; United Kingdom; United States of America.

HIGH HDI

Albania; Argentina; Bahamas; Bahrain; Belarus; Bosnia Herzegovina; Brazil; Bulgaria; Chile; Colombia; Costa Rica; Croatia; Cuba; Ecuador; Estonia; Guam; Hungary; Kazakhstan; Latvia; Lebanon; Libya; Lithuania; Macedonia; Malaysia; Mauritius; Mexico; Montenegro; Oman; Panama; Peru; Poland; Puerto Rico; Romania; Russian Federation; Saudi Arabia; Serbia; Slovakia; Trinidad and Tobago; Turkey; Uruguay; Venezuela.

MEDIUM HDI

Algeria; Angola; Armenia; Azerbaijan; Bangladesh; Belize; Bhutan; Bolivia; Botswana; Cambodia; Cameroon; Cape Verde; China; Comoros; Djibouti; Dominican Republic; Egypt; El Salvador; Equatorial Guinea; Fiji; Gabon; Georgia; Ghana; Guatemala; Guyana; Haiti; Honduras; India; Indonesia; Iran, Islamic Republic of Iraq; Jamaica; Jordan; Kenya; Korea, Democratic People Republic of Kyrgyzstan; Lao People's Democratic Republic; Lesotho; Madagascar; Maldives; Mauritania; Moldova; Mongolia; Morocco; Myanmar; Namibia; Nepal; Nicaragua; Nigeria; Pakistan; Palestine; Papua New Guinea; Paraguay; Philippines; Republic of the Congo; Samoa; Solomon Islands; South Africa; Sri Lanka; Sudan; Suriname; Swaziland; Syrian Arab Republic; Tajikistan; Tanzania; Thailand; Tunisia; Turkmenistan; Uganda; Ukraine; Uzbekistan; Vanuatu; Viet Nam; Western Sahara; Yemen.

LOW HDI

Afghanistan; Benin; Burkina Faso; Burundi; Central African Republic; Chad; Cote D'Ivoire; Democratic Republic of the Congo; Eritrea; Ethiopia; Guinea; Guinea-Bissau; Liberia; Malawi; Mali; Mozambique; Niger; Rwanda; Senegal; Sierra Leone; Somalia; The Gambia; Timor-Leste; Togo; Zambia; Zimbabwe.

Source: UN 2009.

incidence of cancers of the lung, female breast, colorectum and prostate are all more than 3%, signifying that around 1 in 30 persons at risk and residing in these areas develops each of these cancer before the age of 75 (Figure 64.3B).

Lung cancer was also the most commonly diagnosed cancer (778 000 new cases) in lower (low and medium) HDI areas, although a different profile of common types of cancer is observed in these areas, including high rates of infection-related cancers of the stomach, liver and cervix (Figure 64.3A). Oesophageal cancer is also a major contributor to the cancer burden in lower HDI areas. In combination, these seven cancers account for around 62% of the total cancer burden in these lower HDI areas. The lifetime risk of lung cancer is highest at 2.3%, with the lifetime risk of cancers of the stomach, liver, female

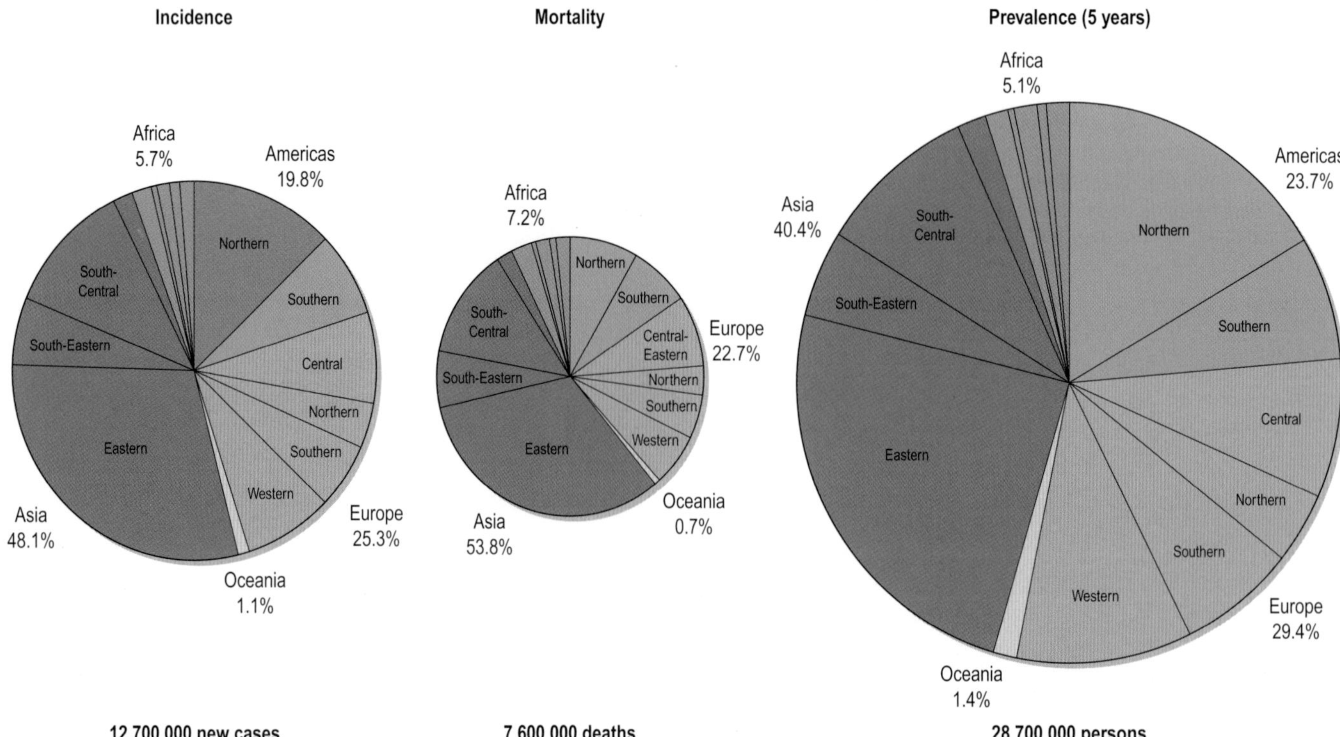

Figure 64.2 Global burden of cancer – estimated cancer incidence, mortality and 5-year prevalence by continent. (Source: *GLOBOCAN 2008*, http://globocan.iarc.fr.)

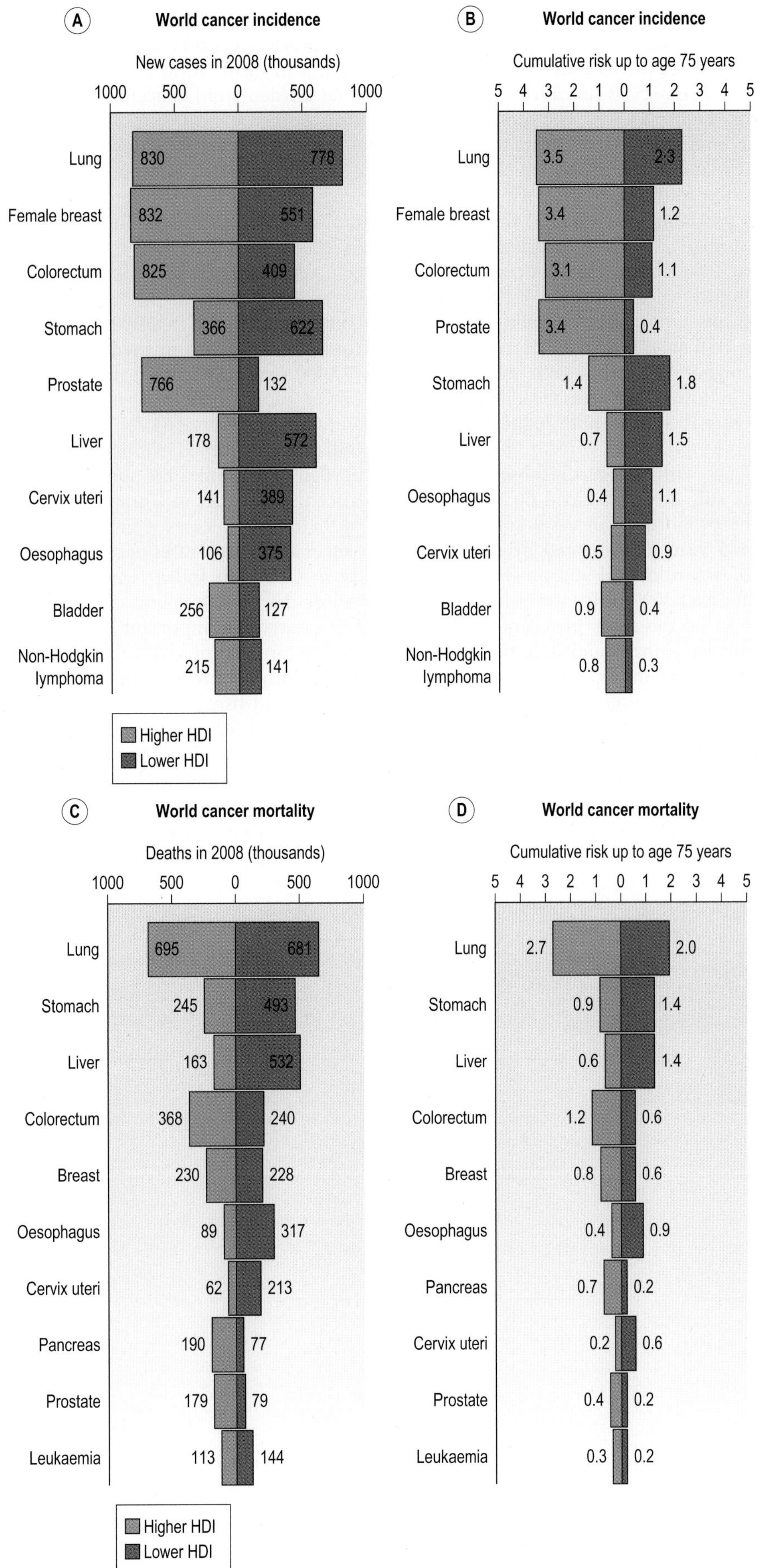

Figure 64.3 World cancer incidence: (A) new cases in 2008; (B) Cumulative risk up to age 75 years. World cancer mortality: (C) deaths in 2008; (D) cumulative risk up to age 75 years. *(Modified from Bray et al. Lancet Oncol 2012.)*

breast, colorectum, and oesophagus ranging from 1% to 2% (Figure 64.3B).

A higher relative proportion of the mortality burden is seen in low and medium HDI areas, especially for cancers of the liver, stomach, and oesophagus (Figure 64.3C). The most common causes of cancer mortality in higher HDI areas are those of the lung, colorectum, stomach and female breast, which comprise about 45% of the total cancer mortality burden. The four most common types of cancer mortality in lower HDI areas include cancers of the lung and stomach, liver and oesophageal cancer. Together, they constitute 49% of the total cancer mortality burden in these less developed regions. In terms of the cumulative risk of specific neoplasms, lung cancer mortality ranks first in both higher and lower HDI areas (Figure 64.3D). Colorectal cancer ranks second in higher HDI areas, with stomach and liver cancer equal second in lower HDI areas. The lifetime risk of stomach cancer mortality is third in both higher HDI and lower HDI areas.

The number of patients with cancer diagnosed between 2004 and 2008 who were still alive at the end of 2008 in the adult population and the proportions of cases surviving for 1 year, 2–3 years and 4–5 years is presented by cancer site in Figure 64.4. Female breast, colorectal and prostate cancers together are responsible for over 40% of the prevalence burden. Breast cancer continues to be the most prevalent cancer in the vast majority of countries globally and is responsible for 5.2 million prevalent cases; one in six cancer survivors in 2008 was diagnosed with a breast cancer within the previous 5 years. Prostate and colorectal cancers rank second and third globally, with a similar number of 5-year prevalent cases (around 3.2 million cases each). An estimated 169.3 million healthy life-years were lost because of cancer in 2008.[9] The figure indicates that an individual loses on average about 2 years of healthy life after a cancer diagnosis. Colorectal, lung, breast and prostate cancers were the main contributors to the total DALYs in most world regions, accounting for 18–50% of the total burden from cancer, with men having 6% more DALYs than women.

Examining the five most common cancers across the four categories of HDI, one notes that cancers of the colorectum, lung, female breast, prostate, and stomach are the most commonly diagnosed cancers in both very high and high HDI areas in 2008 (see Figure 64.7). With an estimated 635 000 cases, colorectal cancer is the most common cancer in very high HDI areas; and cancers of the lung, female breast, and prostate all contribute around 600 000 cases. Lung cancer is the most common neoplasm in medium HDI areas with an estimated 773 000 new cases, ahead of stomach, liver, and female breast cancer, each contributing more than half a million new cases annually (see Figure 64.7). The vast populations of China and India are contained within medium HDI, and their cancer burden and profiles are somewhat different. The incidence is three times higher in China compared with India (2.8 million vs 950 000 new cases estimated in 2008); liver and stomach cancer are major causes of cancer incidence and cancer mortality in China. In India, female cancers dominate, with cervix cancer the most frequent cancer diagnosis, and cancer of the oral cavity is an important neoplasm.

The cancer profile is rather different in low HDI areas, predominantly countries within sub-Saharan Africa. As with India, cervical and breast cancer rank as the first and second most common cancers in these low HDI areas in 2008, although a number of predominantly infection-related cancers are common including liver cancer, Kaposi sarcoma and non-Hodgkin's lymphoma. However, the incidence and mortality patterns vary markedly across countries[12] with prostate cancer

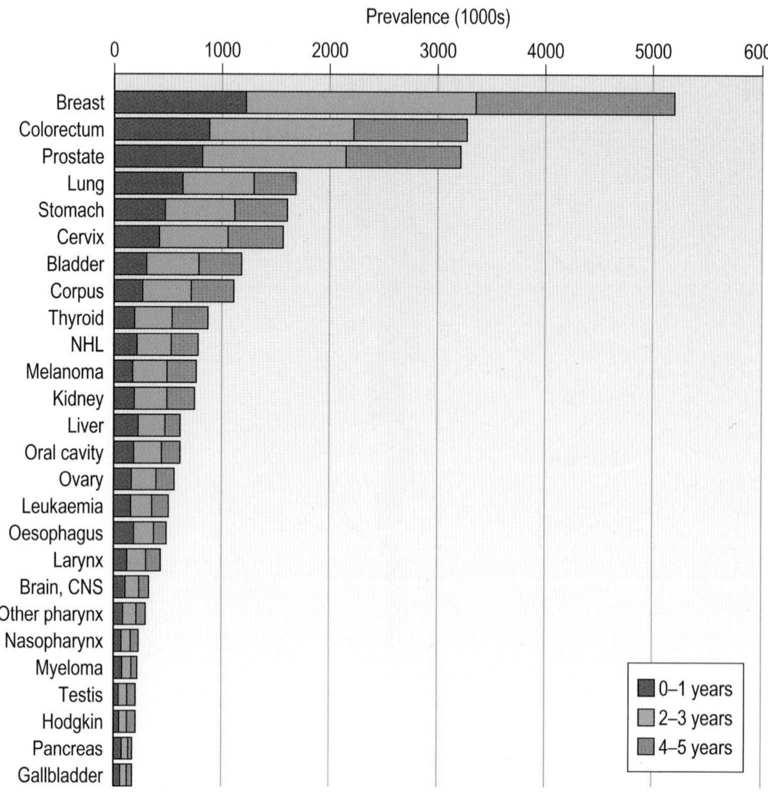

Figure 64.4 Global 5-year cancer prevalence by cancer site; stacked bars denote cancer prevalence among patients alive at end of 2008 were diagnosed in 2008, 2006–2007 and 2004–2005, respectively, both sexes and aged 15 years and older. Sorted by magnitude of prevalence.

the most common cancer in 31 of the 46 sub-Saharan countries and clusters of high incidence of male oesophageal cancer in five countries in eastern Africa and Kaposi sarcoma in nine countries (see Figure 64.7).

Indeed, in terms of age-adjusted incidence rates in men, nine different types of cancer are estimated as most often diagnosed, with prostate the most frequent cancer form in 82 countries, largely in high and very high HDI countries, but also, as stated above, in central and southern Africa (Figure 64.5). Lung cancer is the most common neoplasm in a further 47 countries, predominantly in Eastern Europe and much of Asia, including China, India and Indonesia, while liver cancer is most common in 22 countries, mainly in eastern Africa and southeast Asia. In women, either breast cancer (135 countries) or cervical cancer rank as the most frequent cancer diagnosed in almost all countries (45 countries).

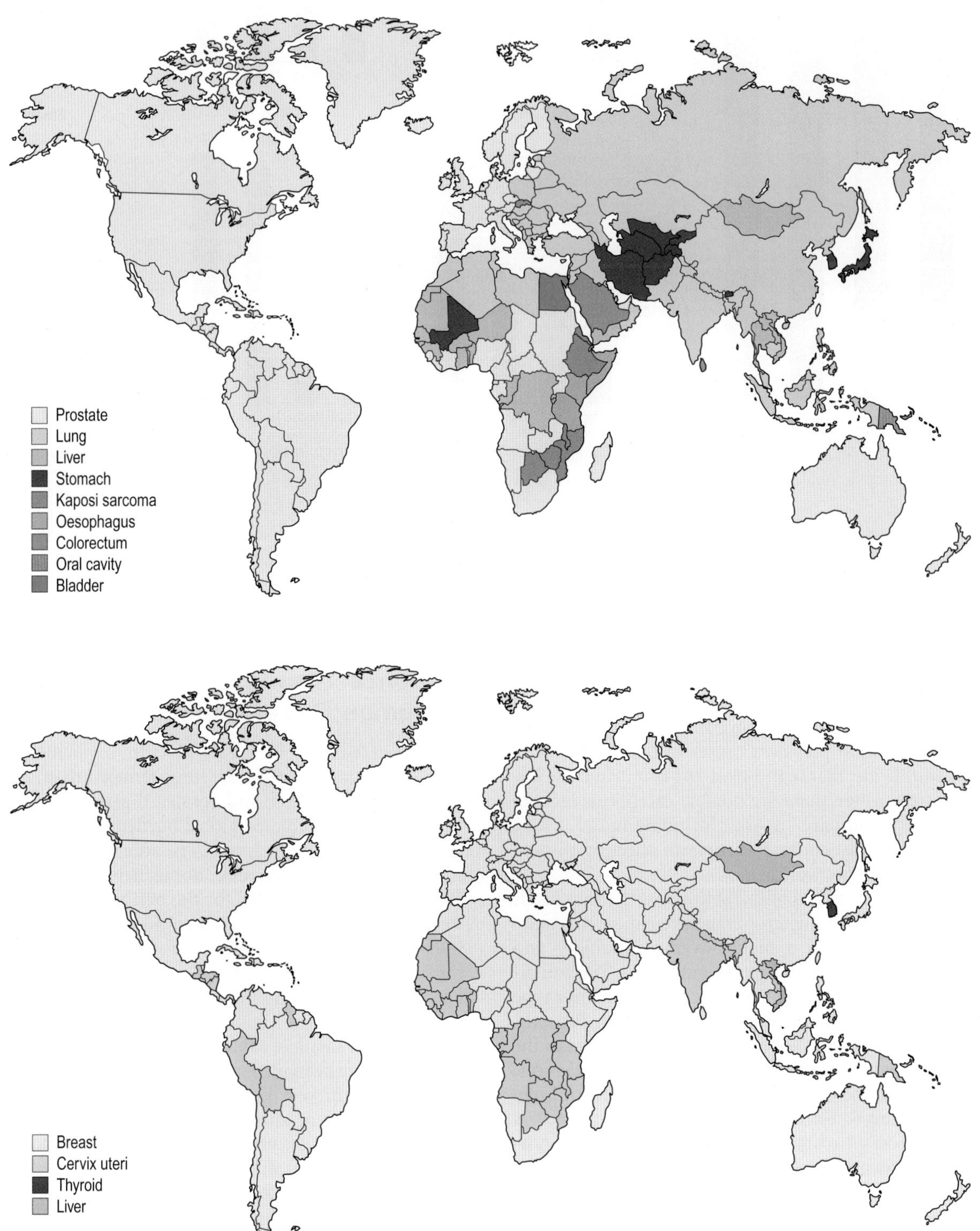

Figure 64.5 Incidence of the most common forms of cancer in 2008. *(Extracted from Bray et al. Lancet Oncol 2012.)*

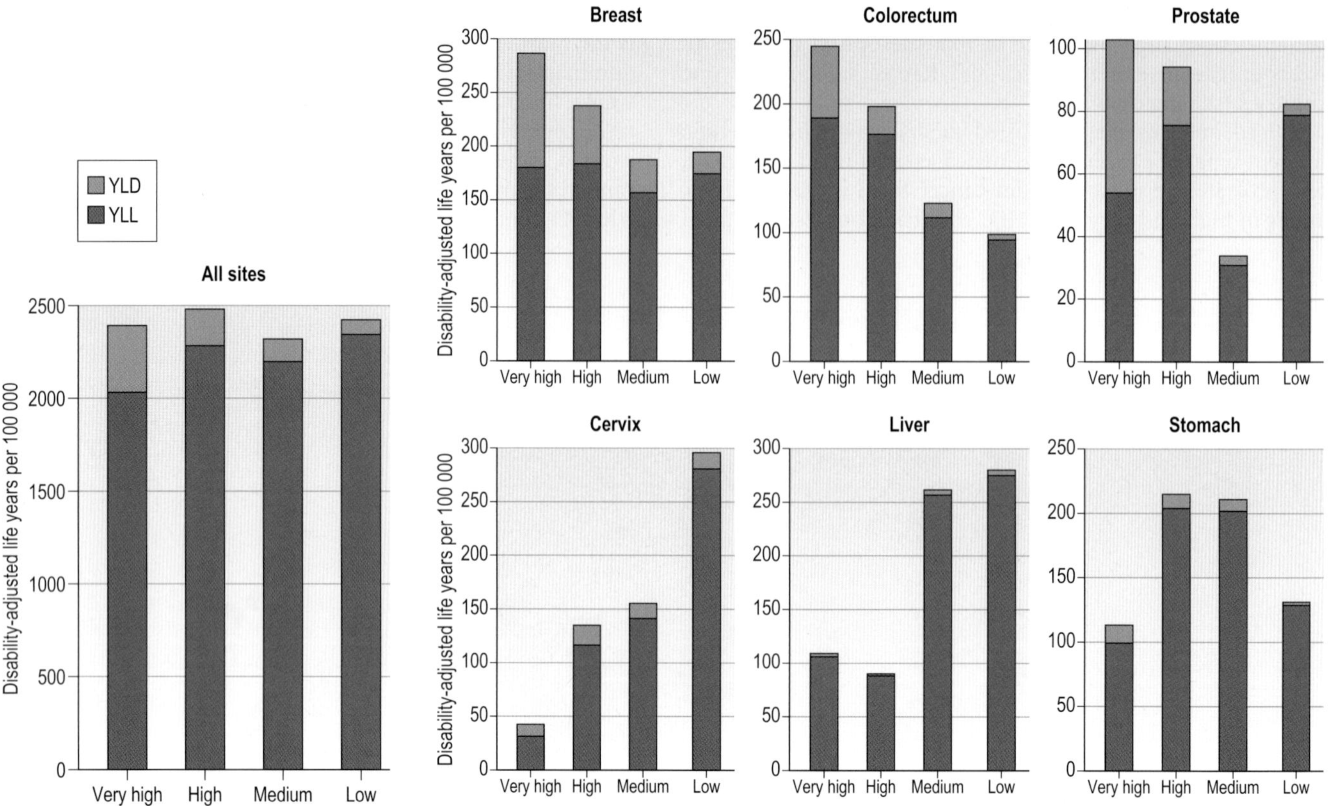

Figure 64.6 Age-adjusted DALYs per 100000 population by cancer site and level of HDI. *(Modified from Soerjomataram et al. 2012.)*

Prostate cancer is the most prevalent cancer in men in 111 of 184 countries globally, including all countries within the Americas and much of Europe.[5] Colorectal cancer ranks highest in men in 25 countries, including 13 Asian countries, stomach cancer is the most prevalent cancer in Eastern Asia including China and oral cancer is the most prevalent cancer in Indian men. Kaposi's sarcoma has the highest 5-year prevalence among males in 11 countries in sub-Saharan Africa. In women, breast cancer ranks as the most prevalent cancer in the vast majority of countries worldwide, that is, in 145 of 184 countries. The key geographical areas where there are notable exceptions include sub-Saharan Africa and parts of Asia (including India), where cervix cancer is the most common neoplasm affecting women at 5 years (in 37 countries worldwide).

Overall, DALYs tend to be comparable across the four levels of HDI, but they reflect a higher average premature mortality in low HDI countries and a higher average disability and impairment in higher HDI countries (Figure 64.6). The contribution of YLLs and YLDs to DALY totals for specific cancer type differed markedly by level of human development. Prostate, breast and colorectal cancers were the main contributors to the DALY totals in very high HDI countries, with a far greater contribution of YLDs to the total DALYs in areas of higher human development (Figure 64.6). By contrast, cancers of the cervix and liver and Kaposi's sarcoma contributed the largest proportion of disease burden in low and medium HDI countries. For these sites in these areas, the YLD contribution is rather minor; premature mortality as measured using the YLL is the major contributor to the aggregated DALYs in areas of lower human development. One also notes the major contributor of premature mortality to the total DALYs burden from prostate cancer in low HDI countries in sub-Saharan Africa.

Cancer in Transition: Recent Incidence Trends by Level of Human Development

We assessed recent incidence trends in the seven most frequently diagnosed cancers worldwide: lung, female breast, colorectum, stomach, prostate, liver and cervix. Together, these constitute over 58% of the estimated global burden. The annual percentage change of trends in annual age-adjusted incidence rates of lung, female breast, colorectal, stomach, prostate, liver, and cervical cancer were estimated for the period 1988–2002 by sex in 101 cancer registries in countries in medium, high or very high HDI were estimated. Although the absence of registries in low HDI areas, together with the few registries in medium HDI areas (six registries) and high HDI areas (11 registries) weaken the interpretation of trends, some patterns in the observed trends emerge. Incidence rates of female breast cancer and prostate cancer have been increasing in almost all countries, whether medium, high or very high HDI levels, with average increases for breast cancer of about 2%, while rises in prostate cancer varied between 3.2% and 7%. Increases in colorectal cancer were also observed in many registry populations, although the increases are more evident in registries in medium HDI areas and high HDI areas (Figure 64.7). We observed declines in the cervical and stomach cancer incidence in both sexes in almost all of the registry populations studied, with the mean annual

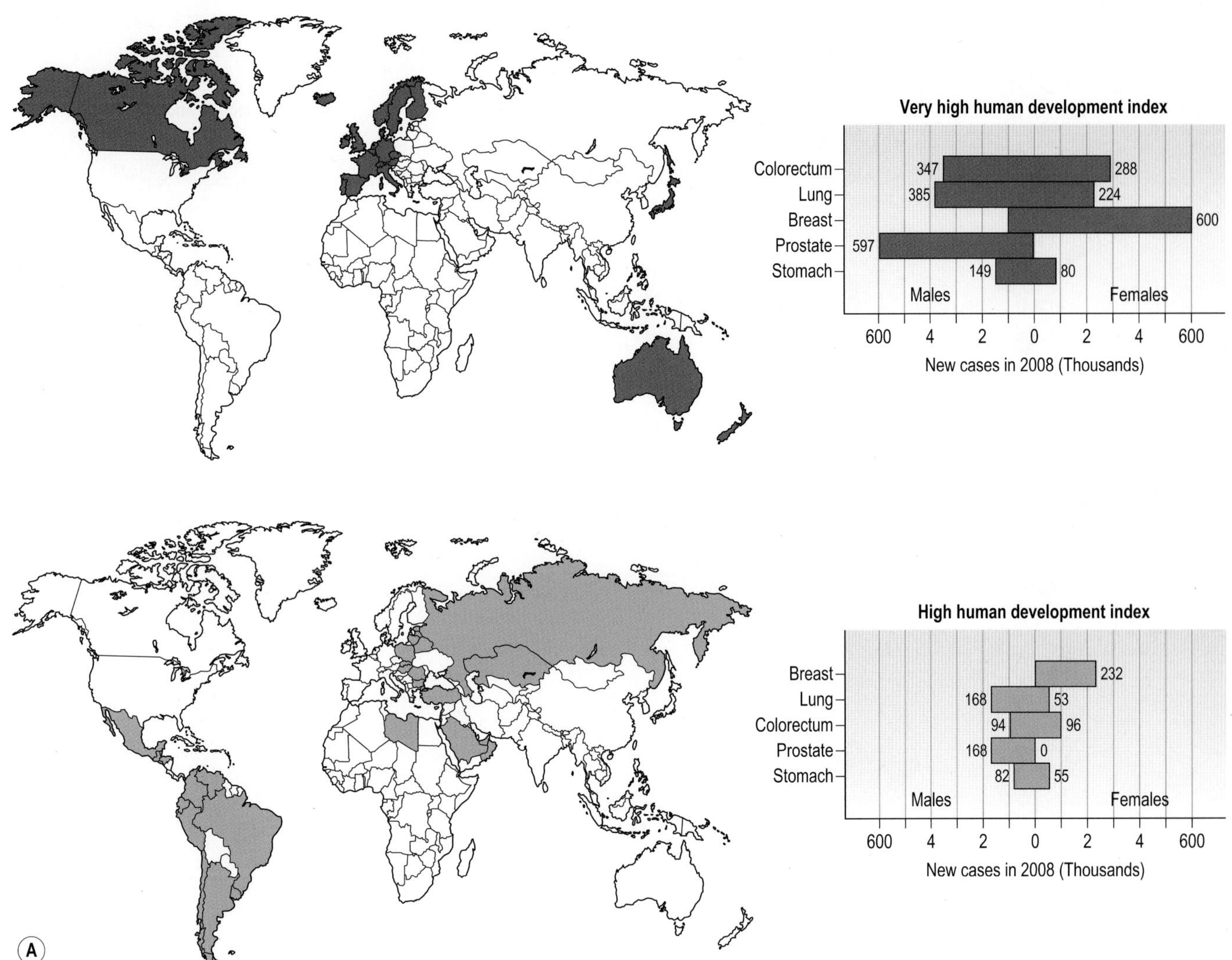

Figure 64.7 (A) Top five most common cancers in 2008 in very high and high HDI areas. Modified from Bray et al, Lancet Oncol 2012.

Continued

decreases in rates varying from around 1% to 3% in medium HDI, high HDI, and very high HDI countries. The trends for liver cancer were more heterogeneous and thus less generalizable. Lung cancer incidence rates in men tend to be decreasing in most registries, but are increasing in women – at least in populations with very high HDI levels.

The Global Cancer Incidence Burden in 2030: Demographic and Trends-based Predictions

Assuming that the overall cancer incidence remains unchanged and population growth and ageing develop to 2030 according to the United Nations *World Population Prospects* medium-fertility variant, we predict that approximately 20.3 million new cases will be diagnosed in 2030, up 61% from the 12.7 million estimated in 2008 (Table 64.1). The increases in cancer incidence are proportionally greatest in lower HDI settings, a 93% increase in both sexes. One can extend this to a trends-based scenario of the future cancer burden in 2030, on the basis of an assessment of the trends observed for several common cancers in cancer registries in medium, high, and very high HDI areas and apply the mean rate of change to the incidence in 2008.[5] Worldwide, annual average increases in the rates of colorectal (1%), female breast (2%) and prostate cancer (3%) were projected, and, in high HDI to very high HDI areas, for lung cancer in women (1%). We also projected annual decreases worldwide in stomach cancer (2.5%) and cervical cancer (2%), and, in high HDI to very high HDI areas, for lung cancer in men (1%). Assuming rates of all other cancers in 2030 remain as estimated in 2008 (including liver cancer, in view of the fact that the recorded trends are diffuse between and within HDI areas), we would see an increase in the annual incidence of 75% from 2008 to 22.2 million by 2030 (Table 64.1).

Cancer Causes and Control

TOBACCO

It is estimated that tobacco causes about five million deaths per year, corresponding to about a third of deaths in men aged 35–69 in North America and Europe and between 12–20% in the rest of the world.[13] It causes many diseases, of which the

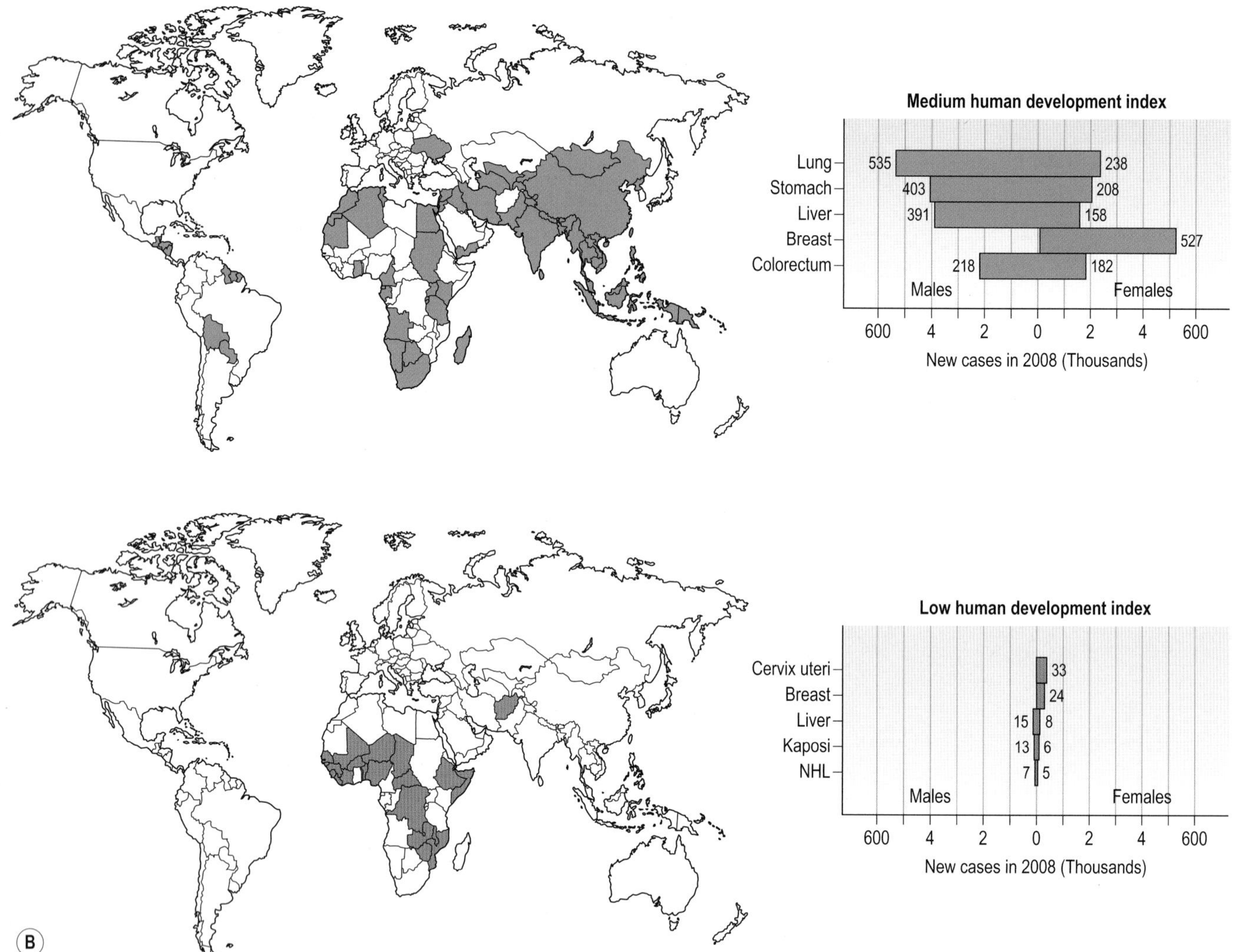

Figure 64.7, cont'd (B) Top five most common cancers in 2008 in medium and low HDI areas. Modified from Bray et al, Lancet Oncol 2012.

most important are cardiovascular disease, chronic obstructive lung disease and various cancers including a large proportion of those of the lung, pancreas, bladder, kidney, larynx, mouth, pharynx and oesophagus. It is also associated with other types of cancer, such as stomach, liver, cervix, nasal cavities, colorectum and myeloid leukaemia.[14] In parts of South-east Asia in particular, the combination of tobacco use and chewing of betel quid is an important risk factor for cancers of the mouth and pharynx.

Stopping smoking at any age has a rapid beneficial effect on cancer risk. Indeed in some developed countries, reductions in tobacco consumption have been associated with declining incidence of certain cancers, such as lung cancer. However, cigarette consumption is increasing markedly in developing countries. Because of this rising prevalence of smoking in developing countries, the incidence of many cancers and other tobacco-related diseases is rising, emphasizing the importance of tobacco control programmes. For example, in some Asian countries, lung cancer mortality rates have more than doubled in the last 30 years. Indeed, it has been estimated that if smoking rates could be halved, between 20 and 30 million premature deaths from all causes would be avoided by 2025 and about 150 million deaths by 2050. Efforts to reduce tobacco consumption are therefore central to preventing deaths from cancer and other diseases. For this reason, the WHO established the Framework Convention on Tobacco Control (see: www.who.int//fctc/FCTC-2009-1-en.pdf), to coordinate global control policies by, e.g., raising the price of tobacco products, restricting advertising, education and banning smoking in public places.

INFECTIONS

Collectively, infectious agents are the most important established cause of cancer after tobacco. Approximately 16% of cancers worldwide (about 2 million cases per year) are attributable to viral, bacterial, and helminth infections, the majority of which occur in the developing world.[13,15] In theory, if these infectious diseases were controlled, up to one in four cancers in the developing countries, and one in ten cancers in developed countries could be prevented.

More cancer cases are attributable to human papillomavirus (HPV) infection than to any other transmissible agent. It is well established that certain HPVs are the major causative agent for invasive cervical cancer. The most common HPV subtypes identified in tumours are HPV16, 18, 31, 33 and 45, although in some Asian countries the subtypes HPV52 and 58 are more

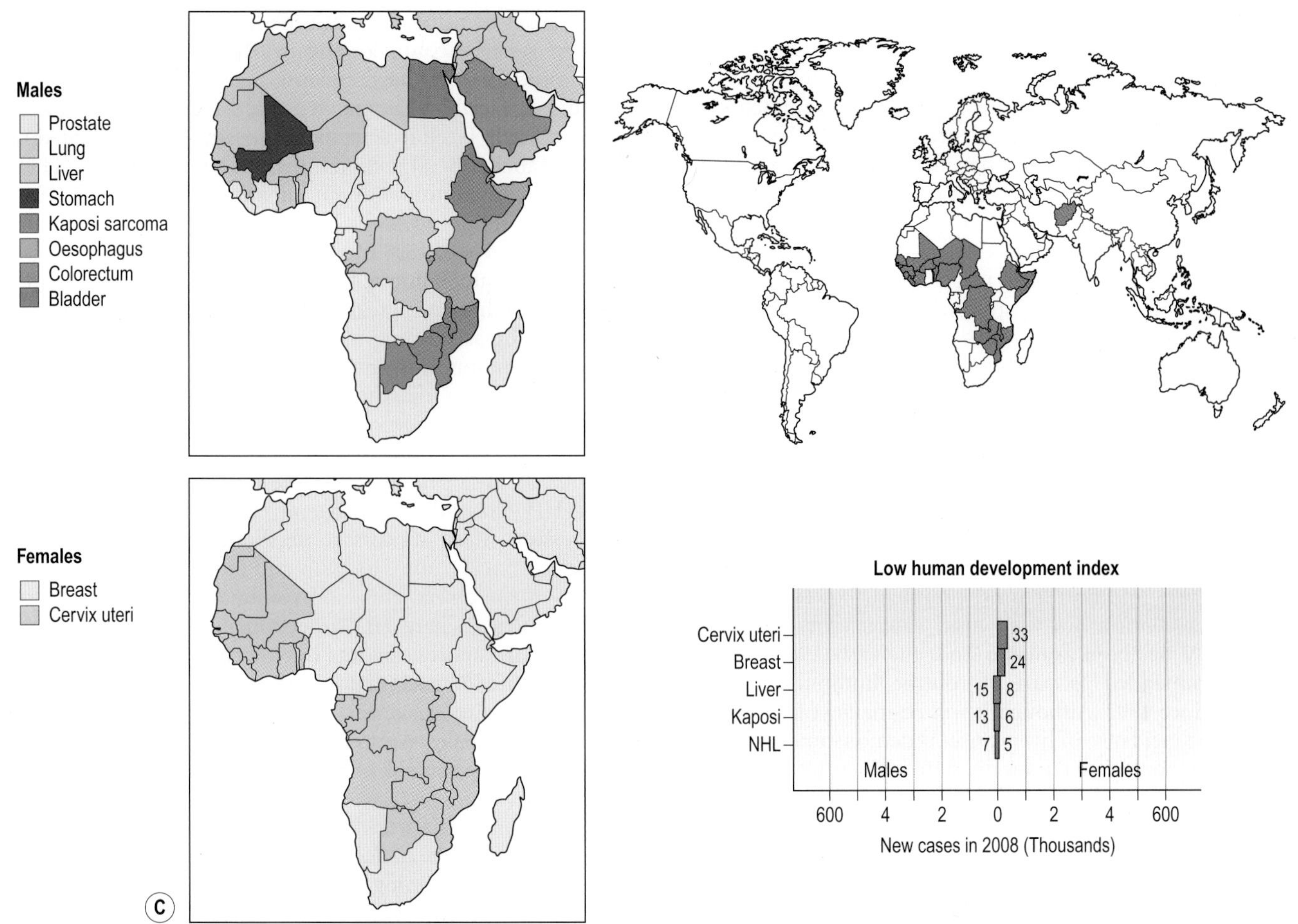

Figure 64.7, cont'd (C) Most common forms of cancer in Africa 2008. Modified from Bray et al, Lancet Oncol 2012 and Jemal et al, Cancer 2012.

common. The same subtypes also account for a significant proportion of cancers of the anus, penis, vagina and vulva. HPV infection may also cause some cancers of the head and neck (particularly cancers of the oral cavity).[16] In developed countries, cervical cancer-screening programmes, using exfoliative cervical cytology to detect treatable pre-cancerous lesions, are effective at reducing both the incidence and mortality of invasive cervical cancer. However, in many developing countries, screening procedures do not yet exist and incidence and mortality rates are still very high. Vaccination against the main HPV

TABLE 64.1 Estimated Numbers of New Cases of Cancers (All Sites Excluding Non-Melanomas) in 2008 and Predicted New Cases by 2030

	Population in 2008 (Millions [% of World Population])	Population in 2030 (Millions [% of World Population])	Incidence in 2008 (Millions [% of Total Global Burden])	Incidence in 2030[a]: Demographic (Millions [Absolute % Increase from 2008])	Incidence in 2030[b]: Demographic Plus Trend (Millions [Absolute % Change from 2008])
Low HDI	394 (5.8%)	664 (8.06%)	0.25 (2.0%)	0.48 (93%)	0.49 (100%)
Medium HDI	4442 (65.6%)	5533 (66.6%)	5.7 (45.1%)	10.1 (78%)	10.3 (81%)
High HDI	922 (13.6%)	1031 (12.4%)	1.9 (14.9%)	3.0 (60%)	3.4 (81%
Very high HDI	1010 (14.9%)	1074 (12.9%)	4.8 (38.0%)	6.7 (39%)	7.9 (65%)
Worldwide	6768	8302	12.7	20.3 (61%)	22.2 (75%)

[a]Based on demographic changes (UN) the predicted cases worldwide are derived by aggregation of the predicted cases obtained after the application of age-specific rates to the demographic forecasts within each Human Development Index (HDI) level (these numbers will not correspond exactly with those predicted from the single global figures, because the underlying rates used to derive the predictions from the two sources differ in their age structure and size).

[b]Based on demographic changes (UN) plus crude assumptions on trends in rates of six cancers on the basis of changing annual age-adjusted incidence in 101 cancer registries 1988–2002: annual decreases in stomach (2.5% [worldwide in both sexes]); cervical cancer (2% [worldwide]) and lung cancer (1% [high HDI and very high HDI areas in men only]); increases in colorectal (1% [worldwide both sexes]); lung (1% [high HDI and very high HDI areas in women only]); female breast (2% [worldwide]) and prostate cancer (3% [worldwide]). See Box 64.1 for a list of countries by HDI region.

From Bray F, Jemal A, Grey N, et al. Global cancer transitions according to the Human Development Index (2008–2030): a population-based study. Lancet Oncol 2012;13(8):790–801.

subtypes at an early age holds the most promise to substantially reduce the incidence of this cancer, although the cost remains prohibitively expensive. However, cheaper HPV DNA screening technology has emerged and this is proving to be much more cost-effective than vaccination at current costs.[17]

Chronic infection with the hepatitis B virus is responsible for causing more than 300 000 liver cancers (specifically hepatocellular carcinoma) each year, which corresponds to about 60% of all primary liver cancers across the world.[16] Approximately 10% of the population in parts of sub-Saharan Africa, China, and South-east Asia are infected with the hepatitis B virus. Transmission can occur from a mother to her child, from person to person during childhood, and via sexual or parenteral transmission during adulthood. About two-thirds of these people will develop chronic hepatitis, and a quarter of these will eventually die from primary liver cancer or cirrhosis, making liver cancer one of the most common cancers in these areas. Prospects for the prevention of hepatitis B virus associated liver cancer are good. In developed countries, screening of blood and organ donors has reduced the spread of infection among adults. In areas where infection is most prevalent, however, the best hope for prevention lies with mass vaccination – a vaccine against HBV has been available since the early 1980s and has been recommended as part of routine immunization programmes since 1992. Although it will be many years before an effect on the incidence of liver cancer is demonstrated in adults, the introduction of mass vaccination in Taiwan has already been associated with a sharp decline in the incidence of liver cancer in children and young adults.

The unrelated hepatitis C virus is also involved in the aetiology of hepatocellular carcinoma and may cause about 25% of all liver cancers, with particularly high proportions in Africa (41%), Japan (36%) and Oceania (33%). The prevalence of hepatitis C virus infection is estimated to be about 1–1.5% in Europe and North America, about 3% in Japan and Oceania (excluding Australia and New Zealand) and up to 3.6% in Africa. Transmission is commonly via the parenteral route, although sexual and perinatal transmission can also occur. However, almost half of all hepatitis C-infected individuals have no identifiable risk factors. Although a vaccine is not currently available, screening programmes have greatly reduced transmission of hepatitis C via blood transfusions in many developed countries.

Infection with the Epstein–Barr virus (EBV) is involved in the aetiology of several types of lymphoma (including Burkitt's lymphoma, Hodgkin's disease, and immunosuppression-related lymphomas) and nasopharyngeal carcinoma and may contribute up to 100 000 cancers per year worldwide.[15] Indeed, Burkitt's lymphoma (associated with both EBV and malaria) is the commonest childhood cancer in many tropical areas. EBV infects more than 90% of the world's population and is usually acquired during childhood. It is transmitted orally in saliva and establishes a latent infection with life-long persistence in the infected host. The overgrowth of virally transformed B cells is controlled by specific cytotoxic T-cell responses, the absence of which (e.g. in HIV-infected people) can result in lymphoma.

Kaposi's sarcoma associated herpesvirus (KSHV) is related to the Epstein–Barr virus and is the principal cause of Kaposi's sarcoma.[16] It also causes a rare type of lymphoma (primary effusion lymphoma) and a lymphoproliferative B cell disorder (Castleman's disease). KSHV is most prevalent in populations at highest risk of developing Kaposi's sarcoma, such as homosexual men infected with the human immunodeficiency virus in Western countries and in African populations where the tumour has long been endemic.

Human T-cell leukaemia virus type 1 (HTLV-1) is a causal agent of adult T-cell leukaemia/lymphoma. It is estimated that there are about 15–20 million individuals infected with HTLV-1 worldwide, predominantly in Japan, the Caribbean, South America, and Central Africa. Adult T-cell leukaemia/lymphoma develops in about 2–5% of HTLV-1-infected individuals and is especially frequent among those infected early in life. Perinatal transmission has been greatly reduced in Japan by avoidance of prolonged breast-feeding (i.e. more than 6 months), although this is not an option for many developing countries, where the risk of death from diarrhoeal disease rises markedly if breast-feeding is curtailed. Several countries have introduced universal screening of blood donors.

There is little evidence that the human immunodeficiency virus (HIV) has a direct oncogenic effect. Instead, its immunosuppressive effect appears to facilitate the development of Kaposi's sarcoma, non-Hodgkin and Hodgkin lymphoma and cancers of the cervix, anus and conjunctiva.[16] In areas of sub-Saharan Africa where HIV infection is highly prevalent, the incidence of Kaposi's sarcoma has increased about 20-fold with the spread of HIV, such that in Uganda and Zimbabwe it is now the most common cancer in males and among the most common in females. Antiretroviral therapy for HIV appears to reduce this increased risk of Kaposi's sarcoma and non-Hodgkin lymphoma.[18]

About half of the world's population is chronically infected with the bacterium *Helicobacter pylori*. This bacterium colonizes the stomach lining and, although many people remain asymptomatic, some go on to develop gastric or duodenal ulcers. In a very small proportion of infected individuals, gastric adenocarcinoma, and to a lesser extent, gastric non-Hodgkin lymphoma may develop.[16] The prevalence of infection is highest in developing countries and increases rapidly during the first two decades of life, such that 80–90% of the population may be infected by early adulthood; in most developed countries, the prevalence of infection is now substantially lower. Rates of infection with *H. pylori* have fallen over the last few decades, and this could explain much of the parallel decline in stomach cancer rates seen in most countries, perhaps due to improvements in living conditions. Although antibiotics are effective in eradicating *H. pylori* in about 80% of cases, this has proved to be difficult to implement on a large scale and re-infection can occur.

Infestation with the water-borne trematode, *Schistosoma haematobium*, which causes schistosomiasis (bilharzia), is associated with an increased risk of squamous cell carcinoma of the bladder, and is the predominant cause of this cancer in tropical and sub-tropical areas. Schistosomiasis affects approximately 200 million people worldwide and is endemic in Northern Africa and the Middle East. In these areas, over half of the population is at risk of infection from contaminated water supplies (lakes, rivers, swamps) that contain the larvae. There is also some evidence that *S. japonicum* and, to a lesser extent, *S. mansoni* are related to the development of cancers of the liver and colorectum in China. Although treatable, preventative measures focusing on reducing contact with contaminated water supplies are currently the best method of reducing infection. Food-borne trematodes (liver flukes), such as *Opisthorchis viverrini*, *Opisthorchis felineus* and *Clonorchis sinensis* are an established cause of cancer of the bile ducts (cholangiocarcinoma) in parts of South-east Asia, due to consumption of raw or undercooked freshwater fish that contain the infective stage of the fluke. Control of infection has been achieved in some areas by a combination of chemotherapy, health education, and improved sanitation. However, eradication programmes have had little effect on the incidence of cholangiocarcinoma in these areas and no vaccines are available.

OTHER FACTORS

Hormonal and reproductive factors play an important role in the aetiology of a number of cancers among women, in particular, breast cancer. Established risk factors include early age at menarche, older age at first birth, low parity and late age at menopause. The combination of these factors may explain much of the geographic variation in the incidence of breast cancer. Indeed, it is changes in reproductive behaviour in developing countries that are leading to substantial increases in the incidence of breast cancer. It is now known that high circulating levels of oestrogens are directly associated with breast cancer risk, at least in post-menopausal women.[19] Reproductive factors are also strongly related to ovarian cancer and, as for endometrial cancer, the most established protective factors are parity and use of hormonal contraceptives.

Several dietary factors, such as fat and meat, have been suggested to increase cancer risk, while other factors, such as fruit, vegetables and fibre, have been hypothesized to decrease risk. However, despite extensive research over the last two decades, few specific dietary determinants of cancer risk have been established, even for cancers such as colorectal cancer where dietary factors are the most obvious candidate risk factors. This is due to various reasons, the most important being the difficulty in accurately measuring dietary intake in epidemiological studies. Other problems with epidemiological studies of diet and cancer include the relatively narrow range of dietary exposures within one population, and the changes in dietary patterns over time, so that it is very difficult to determine whether dietary habits at a young age may affect cancer risk later in life. A high intake of alcoholic beverages increases the risk of cancers of the upper respiratory and digestive tracts (oral cavity, tongue, pharynx, larynx, and oesophagus). These cancers are also caused by smoking, and the increase in risk is particularly great for people who both smoke and drink heavily. Heavy and prolonged alcohol consumption is also associated with liver cancer via the development of cirrhosis and alcoholic hepatitis. Cancers of the upper gastro-intestinal tract are particularly associated with excessive alcohol consumption, although a moderate intake of 10 g of alcohol per day (approximately one drink) has been shown to increase the risk of breast cancer by around 7%.

Aflatoxins are mycotoxins produced by many species of the fungus *Aspergillus* and are among the most carcinogenic substances known. The fungi live in soil, particularly in warm and damp conditions, such as in the tropics, and are a common contaminant of cereals, oilseeds, nuts and spices. The toxin can also be found in milk from humans and livestock if the food supply is contaminated.[20] Consequences of exposure include growth retardation and hepatic necrosis leading to cirrhosis and carcinoma of the liver. Concurrent infection with hepatitis B virus increases the risk of cancer further, since it interferes with the metabolism of aflatoxins.

Overweight and obesity are usually measured in terms of an individual's body mass index (BMI) (weight in kg/height in m^2) where a BMI of >25 kg/m^2 is considered overweight and a BMI of >30 kg/m^2 is considered obese. Overweight and obesity increase the risk of colon cancer by about one-third and increase the risk of breast cancer in post-menopausal (but not pre-menopausal) women by about a half. Overweight and obesity are associated with an approximate threefold increased risk of endometrial cancer in both pre- and postmenopausal women, and may account for up to 40% of endometrial cancer worldwide. Overweight and obesity also increase the risk of cancers of the kidney and gallbladder and of adenocarcinoma (but not squamous cell carcinoma) of the oesophagus. It has been estimated that overweight and obesity account for about 5% of all cancers in Europe, most of which are cancers of the colon, endometrium and breast. Thus, up to 36 000 cases of cancer could be prevented each year if the prevalence of overweight and obesity in Europe was halved.[21] In countries such as the USA, where the prevalence of obesity is higher than in Europe, an even higher proportion of cancers may be attributable to being overweight. Furthermore, the prevalence of obesity is increasing in both developed and developing countries, and is therefore expected to lead to a greater burden of cancers in the future.

Management of Cancer

Ideally, management of cancer involves multidisciplinary services and can be both complex and expensive. Access to those services is often via screening or a primary care physician. Treatment decisions require: (1) accurate pathological diagnosis (which may involve immunohistological and genetic profiling); (2) imaging, for stage and treatment planning and monitoring; (3) biochemical markers, such as prostate specific antigen (PSA) for screening, diagnosis, prognosis, response and relapse and (4) laboratory work-up, including haematology, renal and liver function tests. In general, options for treatment include (a) surgery; (b) drugs, including hormones and chemotherapies; (c) radiotherapy; and (d) symptom control or palliative care. The outcome for the treatment of malignant disease depends, in part, on the clinical and pathological stage, metastasis, histological features and comorbidities.

Long-term survival from cancer is largely dependent on stage at diagnosis. All treatment modalities work best on small localized tumours with non-aggressive histological features. In low-income settings, presentation with cancer is often late with widespread neoplastic disease. Many factors impact access to medical care and involve patient awareness of cancer and symptoms; fear of stigmatization; preference for traditional healers; cultural barriers; health worker knowledge; healthcare infrastructure; and cost. Once accessed, the availability of diagnostic and treatment modalities is often limited, resulting in generally poor survival in these settings.[22]

Surgery is an essential part of treatment for solid neoplastic disease and the modality most likely to cure. Again, the probability of cure is increased when the cancer is small and localized, but surgery also plays a role in the management of metastasis and in palliation, for example of bowel obstruction, fistulas and gastrointestinal bleeds. There is a paucity of data from resource-poor settings on surgical oncology provision but the unmet surgical need is likely to be very high.

Cancer chemotherapies kill malignant cells by preventing cell division, disrupting DNA or RNA or nucleic acids. It is effective against systemic disease and can be used with both palliative and curative intent pre- and post-surgery and/or radiotherapy. Other forms of drug treatment include hormones (e.g. the anti-oestrogen tamoxifen for oestrogen-receptor-positive breast cancer, and LHRH antagonists for prostate cancer) and immunotherapy (for example interferon-α, used for some haematological malignancies and monoclonal antibodies, which include trastuzumab and rituximab). Drugs with different mechanisms of action are often given in combination to increase efficacy. The poor availability of cancer drugs, and drugs required to control side-effects including anti-emetics and antibiotics, is a major problem in resource-limited settings.

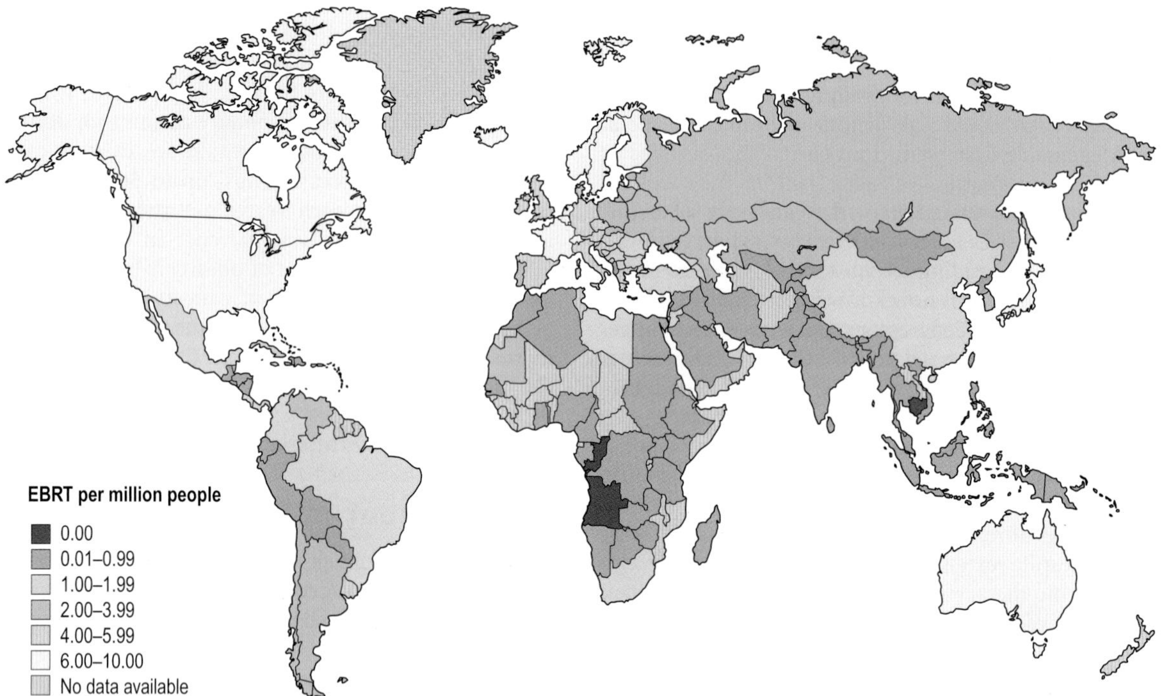

Figure 64.8 Worldwide distribution of external beam radiotherapy machines (EBRT machines).

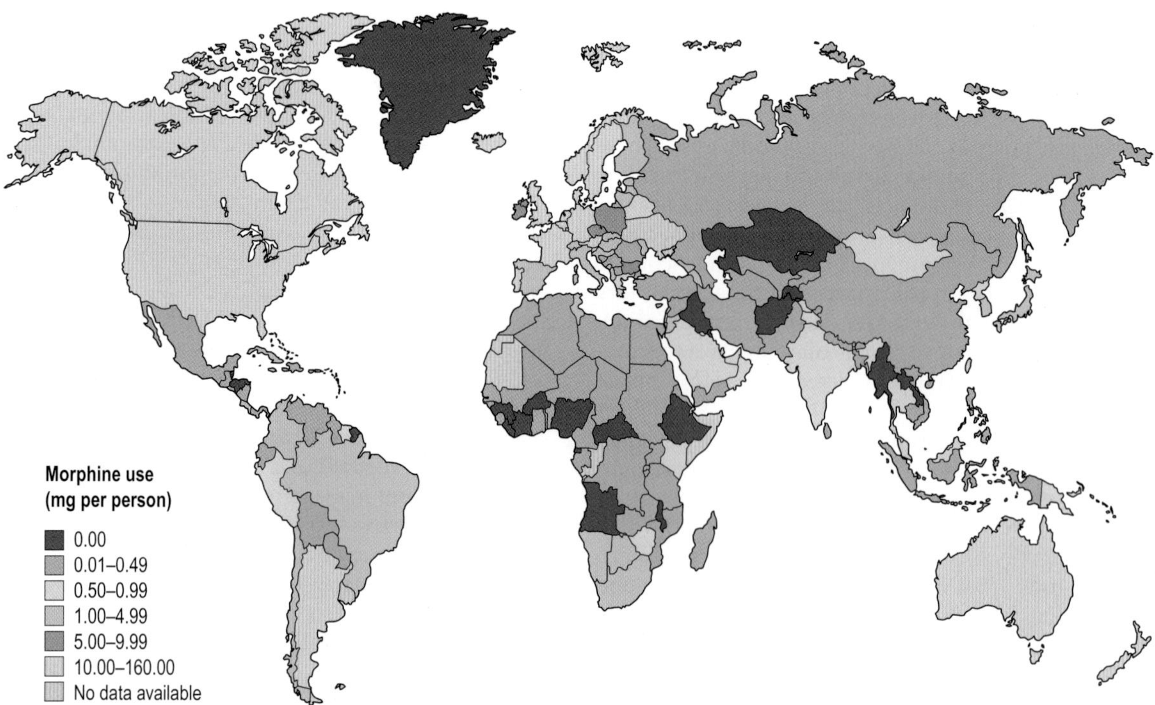

Figure 64.9 Worldwide morphine use (2010).

Radiotherapy is a common component of cancer treatment for cure or palliation and can be used alone or as an adjuvant to surgery or chemotherapy. Radiation acts by damaging cellular DNA via formation of free radicals. Cancer cells have less ability to repair DNA damage than healthy cells and lose reproductive capacity or die by apoptosis. Radiotherapy can be broadly divided into external beam or local where the radiation source is placed in the body, within or close to the cancer. Radiation can be derived from a radioactive source such as cobolt-60 or by accelerating electrons at high energy to produce photons (linear accelerator). Resource-limited settings are more likely to use a radioactive source over a linear accelerator as it is comparatively cheaper, robust, requires only limited electricity and is much easier to maintain. The Programme of Action for Cancer Therapy (PACT) is part of the International Atomic Energy Authority (IAEA). It was established in 2004 to support and monitor radiotherapy in developing countries. The IAEA advise that more than five radiotherapy machines per million people are required for adequate population coverage. Figure 64.8 shows a worldwide distribution of external beam radiotherapy machines (EBRT machines). Most low-income countries have less than one machine per million population and many have no machine at all.

The World Health Organization defines palliative care as 'an approach that improves the quality of life of patients and their families facing the problem associated with life-threatening illness, through the prevention and relief of suffering by means of early identification and impeccable assessment and treatment of pain and other problems, physical, psychosocial and spiritual' (see: http://www.who.int/cancer/palliative/definition/en). Despite the overwhelming need and the proven effectiveness of palliative care,[23] clinical models of delivery are largely absent.[24] Opioid analgesics are essential for pain relief and the keystone of palliative care. The WHO recognizes that 'inadequate management of pain due to cancer is a serious public health problem in the world'.[25] Morphine is highly effective, relatively cheap and is easy to administer, but few of those in resource-poor settings who need it, have access to it. Figure 64.9 represents countries who registered use of a strong opioid in 2007 with the international narcotics control board, where 'low levels of opioid consumption indicating inadequate medical availability'.[26]

REFERENCES

5. Bray F, Jemal A, Grey N, et al. Global cancer transitions according to the Human Development Index (2008–2030): a population-based study. Lancet Oncol 2012;13(8):790–801.
6. Soerjomataram I, Lortet-Tieulent J, Ferlay J, et al. Estimating and validating disability-adjusted life years at the global level: a methodological framework for cancer. BMC Med Res Methodol 2012;12(1):125.
9. Soerjomataram I, Lortet-Tieulent J, Parkin DM, et al. Global burden of cancer in 2008: a systematic analysis of disability-adjusted life-years in 12 world regions. Lancet 2012;380(9856):1840–50.
12. Jemal A, Bray F, Forman D, et al. Cancer burden in Africa and opportunities for prevention. Cancer 2012;118(18):4372–84.
15. de Martel C, Ferlay J, Franceschi S, et al. Global burden of cancers attributable to infections in 2008: a review and synthetic analysis. Lancet Oncol 2012;13:607–15.

Access the complete references online at www.expertconsult.com

65 Haematological Diseases in the Tropics

JECKO THACHIL | SHIRLEY OWUSU-OFORI | IMELDA BATES

KEY POINTS

- Africa and Asia have more than 85% of the world's anaemic populations and anaemia burden is highest among children and women of reproductive age.
- The accurate diagnosis of anaemia has been neglected; clinical assessment of anaemia is unreliable unless the anaemia is severe.
- In low-income countries, anaemia in an individual is often due to multiple interdependent factors. Removing or treating a single factor may not resolve the anaemia.
- Early diagnosis of sickle cell disease and rapid access to a specialist centre for emergencies such as severe pain crises, strokes and acute chest syndrome, can help to prevent permanent long-term complications.
- Beta-thalassaemia major is fatal in the first few years of life unless regular blood transfusions are given; unless they are accompanied by iron chelation, these transfusions will eventually cause death due to irreversible organ damage from iron overload.
- Malarial anaemia is a particular problem for children and pregnant women and severe anaemia can be caused by *P. falciparum* and *P. vivax*. Malarial anaemia can be reduced with chemoprophylaxis and intermittent treatment, and by anti-mosquito measures such as insecticide-treated bed nets and vector control.
- Anaemia occurs in 70% of HIV-infected patients and is an independent risk factor for death. Prompt treatment of factors associated with anaemia, such as infections and poor nutrition, and commencement of antiretroviral treatment will reduce deaths.
- Blood shortages are common in tropical countries. To increase the availability of blood, transfusions should be prescribed in accordance with guidelines and efforts made to encourage blood donors to donate regularly as repeat donors are the safest type of donor.

Introduction

Haematological disorders are common in low-income countries. They make a substantial contribution to morbidity and mortality of individuals in these regions and have a negative impact on the growth and development of under-resourced nations. Genetic red cells abnormalities are common in low-income countries because they provide protection against malaria and they often co-exist with other causes of anaemia such as malnutrition and chronic illnesses. There is a close association between haematological abnormalities and infections which are a major cause of illness and death in these populations. Morphological abnormalities of blood can often provide clues about the underlying diagnosis and blood film examination is particularly important where diagnostic facilities are limited.

Abnormal Blood Counts

Abnormal blood counts can manifest as various combinations of alterations of numbers of red cells, white cells or platelets. This section will outline some of the most common causes of abnormal blood counts likely to be encountered in clinical practice in low-income countries.

ANAEMIA

Anaemia is one of the most common causes of morbidity in the world and its impact is reflected in several of the health-related Millennium Development Goals. Although anaemia by itself is not a diagnosis, it suggests that there is an underlying disease state which needs to be recognized and treated. It is also a useful indicator of the general health of the population.

The causes of anaemia may be identified systematically by considering the life cycle of the red cells (Figure 65.1). Nutrients necessary for red cell production are absorbed from the gastrointestinal tract and carried through the portal vein to the liver and ultimately reach the bone marrow where erythropoiesis occurs. This process is regulated by erythropoietin, a hormone released from the kidneys mainly in response to hypoxia. Mature

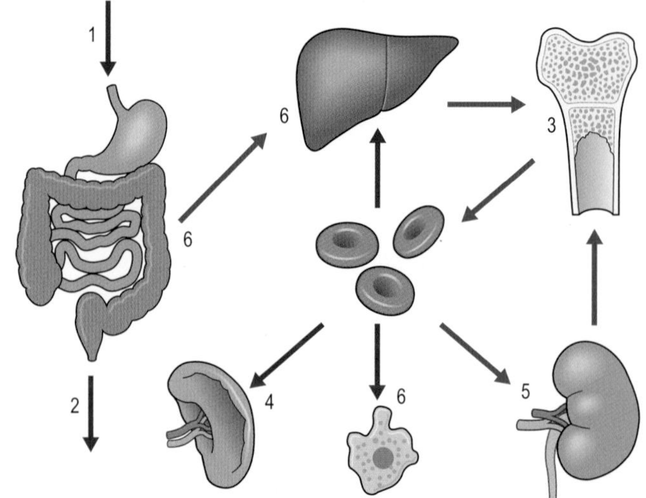

Figure 65.1 Anaemia can result from (1) inadequate nutrients; (2) blood loss; (3) inadequate or abnormal production of red cells in the bone marrow including haemoglobinopathies, myelodysplasia, or infections; (4) haemolysis in the spleen; (5) decreased erythropoietin; and (6) anaemia of chronic disease associated with inflammatory states.

red cells are released into the circulation from the bone marrow and percolate through the tissues and organs. Anaemia can result from defects in any of these stages. Inadequate production of red cells in the bone marrow can be due to lack of nutrients (e.g. iron, B_{12}, folate, vitamin A, copper or zinc), abnormal haemoglobin synthesis (i.e. haemoglobinopathies) or ineffective erythropoeisis from myelodysplasia or infections. Red cells can be lost from the body (e.g. gastrointestinal bleeding) or removed prematurely if they are abnormal or the spleen is enlarged (i.e. haemolysis). Kidney disease can result in decreased erythropoietin. Anaemia of chronic disease (or 'anaemia of inflammation') is due to an inadequate response to erythropoieitin or to increased cytokine-induced hepcidin release in inflammatory states which interferes with iron absorption or iron utilization.

Diagnostic algorithms to determine the cause of anaemia are usually based on a combination of the mean cell volume of the red cells, the reticulocyte count and blood film appearance (Figures 65.2, 65.3). This approach is based on the availability of a haematology analyser and an experienced microscopist. Several conditions which cause anaemia may co-exist in the same individual (e.g. intestinal parasites, malaria and sickle cell disease) and hence a thorough investigation is crucial to identify all potential causes of anaemia.

NEUTROPHILIA

Neutrophils released from the marrow after maturation can either enter the 'circulating pool' or they can remain in the 'marginal pool' where they are loosely attached to the blood vessel wall. Cells in the marginal pool are not sampled when blood is taken for a full blood count.[1] Neutrophilia can therefore result from increased bone marrow synthesis and also from decreased margination which increases the circulating pool. There are many causes of neutrophilia (Box 65.1) but the commonest is bacterial infection in which there is increased bone marrow production of neutrophils and release of neutrophil precursors into the peripheral blood. This 'leukaemoid reaction', characterized by circulating myelocytes and metamyelocytes, can be mistaken for leukaemia but, unlike leukaemia, there is an orderly maturation and proliferation of neutrophils. Leukaemoid reactions have also been described in patients with tuberculosis, juvenile rheumatoid arthritis and dermatitis herpetiformis.[2,3] Decreased margination of neutrophils with egress of cells into the circulation can occur with exercise, adrenaline (epinephrine) injection, emotional stress and postoperatively or in response to drugs (e.g. steroids, β-agonists). Other drugs, such as lithium and tetracycline, produce neutrophilia through increased production.

Neutrophilia is also a feature of bone marrow proliferation which occurs in myeloproliferative neoplasms, particularly chronic myeloid leukemia and myelofibrosis. Teardrop cells and nucleated red blood cells are features of myelofibrosis on the blood film; basophilia and eosinophilia are common with chronic myeloid leukaemia. Molecular testing for the JAK-2 mutation or *BCR-ABL* fusion gene can also help to differentiate between myeloproliferative neoplasms. Rebound neutrophilia can occur following treatment of megaloblastic anaemia or after recovery from neutropenia induced by drugs. Acute haemorrhage can cause neutrophilia, especially if bleeding occurs into the peritoneal cavity, pleural space, joints or adjacent to the dura. This is possibly due to the release of adrenaline and chemokines in response to local inflammation.

The presence of neutrophilia can be useful in raising suspicions about the onset of complications in infections that are not primarily associated with neutrophilia. Examples include meningitis in tuberculosis, orchitis in mumps, bowel perforation in typhoid fever and superadded bacterial infection in measles. The absence of neutrophilia can be helpful in differentiating typhoid and paratyphoid fever from pyogenic infections.

NEUTROPENIA

Neutropenia is defined as an absolute neutrophil count $<1.5 \times 10^9/L$. It is usually classified into severe ($<0.5 \times 10^9/L$), moderate

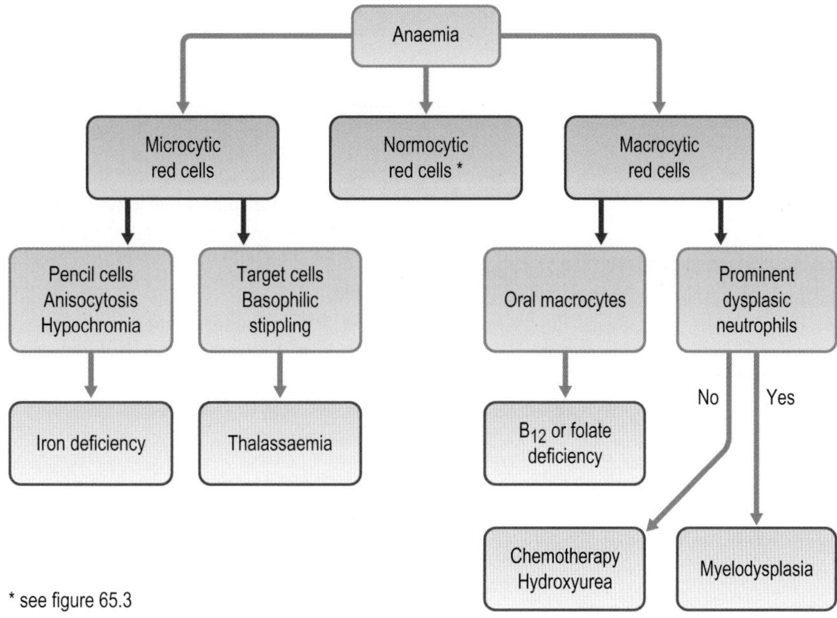

Figure 65.2 Diagnostic algorithm for investigation of anaemia.

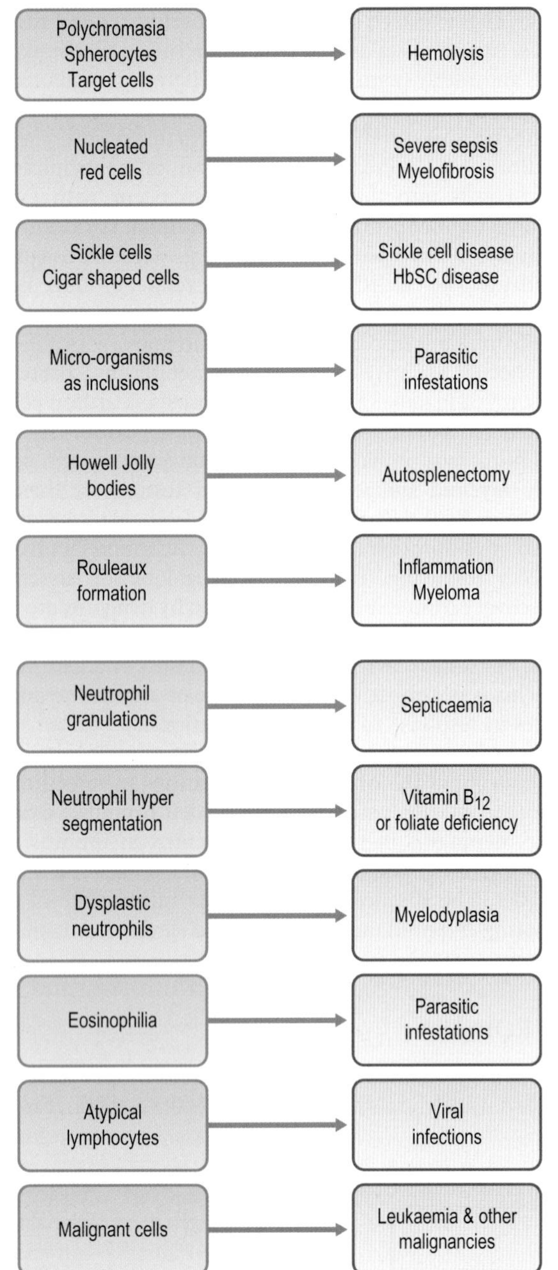

Figure 65.3 Typical appearances of blood film indicating various underlying conditions.

BOX 65.1 CAUSES OF NEUTROPHILIA

- Physical stimuli (cold, heat, exercise, fits, pain, ovulation, trauma, pregnancy, hypoxia)
- Emotional stimuli (fear, panic, depression, anger)
- Infections (all types)
- Inflammatory disorders
- Metabolic disorders (diabetic ketoacidosis)
- Haematological malignancies
- Solid tumours
- Drugs and hormones
- Smoking (commonest cause of mild neutrophilia)
- Acute haemolysis
- Poisoning
- Insect venoms.

($0.5–1.0 \times 10^9$/L) or mild ($1.0–1.5 \times 10^9$/L). The propensity to develop infections is related to the degree and duration of neutropenia, with higher risk associated with counts below 0.5×10^9/L. Africans, African Americans, Yemenite Jews, Palestinians and Saudi Arabians generally have slightly lower neutrophil counts compared with other races. This is thought to be due to an increase in the bone marrow storage pool as ethnic neutropenia is associated with good neutrophil responses to infections.

Neutropenia can be due to impaired or ineffective (intramedullary death of neutrophil precursors despite normal bone marrow production) synthesis by the bone marrow (e.g. myelodysplasia, megaloblastic anaemia, treatment with phenytoin or methotrexate); a shift from the circulating pool to marginated pool (pseudoneutropenia) and increased peripheral destruction (e.g. secondary to antibodies against the neutrophils or increased reticulo-endothelial activity in sepsis or haemophagocytic syndrome) (Box 65.2). Increased consumption of neutrophils can result from increased attachment of cells to endothelium or other leukocytes in inflammatory states. Neutropenia is often the result of a combination of several of these mechanisms.

Infants of hypertensive mothers may have moderate to severe neutropenia, which can last for several days. This is probably related to bone marrow suppression. Moderate to severe neutropenia can also occur in newborn infants as a result of the transfer of maternal IgG anti-neutrophil antibodies in a manner similar to rhesus haemolytic disease of the newborn.[4] Although neutropenia has been described with typhoid fever, minimum neutrophil count seldom falls below 0.6×10^9/L and the

BOX 65.2 CAUSES OF NEUTROPENIA

ACQUIRED

Immune

- Neonatal alloimmune neutropenia
- Autoimmune neutropenia (systemic lupus erythematosus, Felty syndrome, drugs)

Nutritional Deficiencies

- Vitamin B_{12}, folic acid, copper

Malignancies

- Myelodysplastic syndrome
- Acute leukaemia
- Myelofibrosis
- Lymphoproliferative disorders
- Bone marrow infiltration by solid cancers
- Large granular lymphocytic leukaemia

Sepsis

- Severe bacterial infections (e.g. typhoid)
- Viral: mononucleosis, HIV varicella, measles, rubella, hepatitis A&B, parvovirus and cytomegalovirus
- Rickettsial infections

Hypersplenism

CONGENITAL (examples)

- Shwachman–Diamond syndrome
- Severe congenital neutropenia
- Cyclic neutropenia
- Dyskeratosis congenital
- Chédiak–Higashi syndrome.

neutropenia may not develop until after the first week of illness. Infectious hepatitis and yellow fever can both cause neutropenia. Overwhelming infections can lead to a failure of bone marrow production of neutrophils, especially in undernourished individuals and alcoholics.

Individuals with severe neutropenia can develop life-threatening septicaemia, often from endogenous flora (e.g. oral cavity), and stringent measures should be taken to avoid situations which may predispose these individuals to infections. They may need prophylactic antimicrobials and should have rapid access to medical care. Fungal infections are less common than bacterial infections in neutropenic individuals, and viral or parasitic infections rarely occur with isolated neutropenia. Granulocyte colony stimulating factor (GCSF) injections can be helpful in raising the neutrophil count in patients with complicating infections since it stimulates the release of neutrophils from the marrow, but GCSF is only useful if there is some bone marrow reserve. Patients with some congenital or immune forms of neutropenia can tolerate persistently low counts without any increase in the incidence of infections.

MONOCYTOSIS AND MONOCYTOPENIA

Monocytosis occurs in chronic infections and inflammatory conditions. Protozoan infections such as typhus, trypanosomiasis and kala-azar may be associated with monocytosis. Chronic and juvenile myelomonocytic leukaemias are malignant disorders in which monocytosis may be severe; acute monocytic leukaemias may present with mild to moderate monocytosis. Monocytosis, and particularly a monocyte:lymphocyte ratio greater than 0.8–1.0, may indicate active progression of tuberculosis and an unfavourable prognosis. The normal ratio of 0.3 or less is restored when the healing process is complete.

A decreased absolute monocyte count occurs in bone marrow failure states such as aplastic anaemia or after chemotherapy. Low monocyte counts can occur with overwhelming sepsis and with splenomegaly. Monocytopenia is a characteristic feature of hairy cell leukaemia and is considered to be a diagnostic hallmark of this disease.

LYMPHOCYTOSIS AND LYMPHOCYTOPENIA

Peripheral blood contains only around 2% of the total body lymphocyte population since these represent the cells present in the blood during their transit into secondary lymphoid organs. Wide variations exist in lymphocyte counts between individuals especially in childhood. Lymphocyte counts exhibit a diurnal pattern; peaking at night with a nadir in the morning.

Lymphocytosis is characteristic of infectious mononucleosis and many atypical and large lymphocytes can be seen in the peripheral blood film. These atypical cells can also occur in cytomegalovirus infection and infectious hepatitis. Absolute lymphocytosis can occur with chronic infections such as brucellosis and in the recovery stages of tuberculosis. Lymphocytosis is unusual in bacterial infections except in the case of pertussis. Heavy smoking is also an often overlooked cause of lymphocytosis and is probably one of the commonest reasons for a mild to moderate increase in the lymphocyte count. Malignant bone marrow disorders, predominantly acute lymphoblastic and chronic lymphocytic leukaemia and non-Hodgkin's lymphomas, can cause lymphocytosis. These lymphocytes may have characteristic morphological changes identifiable in the blood film (e.g. smear cells with chronic lymphocytic leukaemia) and the correct diagnosis can be confirmed by immunophenotyping for specific combinations of cell markers.

Lymphopenia is due to decreased production, redistribution or increased rate of death of lymphocytes. Decreased production usually results from cytotoxic drugs and radiotherapy, while increased lymphocyte death can occur in infections such as influenza and HIV. Occasionally, an isolated low lymphocyte count in the context of an otherwise normal full blood count can be a clue to the diagnosis of HIV. This reflects the destruction of CD4+ T cells by the virus although an expansion of CD8+ T cells may raise the total lymphocyte count to normal levels. Redistribution rather than depletion of total body lymphocyte numbers occurs with steroid treatment or with endogenous secretion of corticosteroids during acute illnesses due to the retention of lymphocytes in secondary lymphoid organs.

EOSINOPHILIA

Eosinophils are involved in innate immunity and hypersensitivity. Their number in the circulation is relatively small compared to other leukocytes because they predominantly reside in tissues such as the gut, skin and lungs which are entry points for allergens and infections. The commonest causes of eosinophilia are helminthic infections, atopy and allergic diseases, and adverse drug reactions. Less common causes are classified under the umbrella term of hypereosinophilic syndromes (Table 65.1). Since parasitic infections are likely to be the commonest cause of eosinophilia in the tropics and in returning travellers, an extensive search for such infections should be undertaken in patients with persistent eosinophilia; initial investigations should be determined by the patient's history of geographical exposure (Figure 65.4).[5–7]

The absolute number of eosinophils in the peripheral blood may not correlate with their tissue distribution or with their potential to cause tissue damage from their granule release. This is because the degree of eosinophilia depends on the extent of tissue invasion and is therefore modest with tapeworms and roundworms resident in the bowel but much higher where invasion occurs, for example with, *Toxocara canis* or filaria. Schistosomiasis almost always causes eosinophilia. *Strongyloides stercoralis* has the capacity to remain in the host for decades after initial infection and causes varying degrees of eosinophilia, with or without other symptoms. Steroid treatment, which may be necessary in cases of eosinophilic tissue damage, can exacerbate clinical problems in patients with *Strongyloides* infection so this parasitic infestation should be excluded before starting steroids for hypereosinophilia.

Mild to moderate eosinophilia is common in asthma although a very high count should prompt a search for Churg–Strauss syndrome or allergic bronchopulmonary aspergillosis. Most drugs including penicillins can cause eosinophilia but the diagnosis can only be made by noting recovery when the drug is discontinued. Eosinophilia can be a feature of Hodgkin's lymphoma. It signifies a more favourable prognosis and may precede the original diagnosis of lymphoma or relapses. In immunocompromised patients, such as those with HIV infection, the finding of eosinophilia may be crucial since the success of antiretroviral treatment may depend on concomitant eradication of parasites.

TABLE 65.1 Investigations in Those with Persistent Eosinophilia Based on Travel History

Fever and respiratory symptoms	Katayama syndrome – *Schistosoma* sp. Loeffler syndrome Visceral larva migrans/acute toxocariasis Tropical pulmonary eosinophilia Pulmonary hydatid disease Paragonimiasis Coccidioidomycosis and paracoccidioidomycosis Non-parasitic causes of eosinophilia and respiratory symptoms
Gastrointestinal symptoms	Strongyloidiasis *Schistosoma mansoni* and *S. japonicum* Ascariasis Tapeworm Dwarf tapeworm Hookworm Whipworm Pin worm Trichinellosis Anisakiasis – *Anisakis* spp. and *Pseudoterranova decipiens* *Angiostrongylus costaricensis* Non-parasitic causes of eosinophilia and GI symptoms
Right upper quadrant pain/jaundice	Hydatid disease in the liver *Fasciola hepatica* and *F. giganta* *Clonorchis sinensis* and *Opisthorchis* sp. Schistosomiasis – *S. mansoni* and *S. japonicum*
Neurological symptoms	*Angiostrongylus cantonensis* Gnathostomiasis Neurocysticercosis causing meningitis Schistosomiasis/bilharzia and CNS symptoms – *Schistosoma haematobium, S. mansoni, S. japonicum* Toxocariasis Coccidioidomycosis and paracoccidioidomycosis
Skin and musculoskeletal symptoms	Onchocerca volvulus Larva currens Lymphatic filariasis Loiasis Gnathostomiasis Trichinellosis Swimmers' itch/cercarial dermatitis
Urinary symptoms	Schistosomiasis/bilharzia – *Schistosoma haematobium*

From Checkley AM, Chiodini PL, Dockrell DH, Bates I, Thwaites GE, Booth HL, Brown M, Wright SG, Grant AD, Mabey DC, Whitty CJ, Sanderson F; British Infection Society and Hospital for Tropical Diseases. Eosinophilia in returning travellers and migrants from the tropics: UK recommendations for investigation and initial management. J Infect. 2010 Jan;60(1):1-20. Copyright Elsevier 2010.

THROMBOCYTOPENIA

Thrombocytopenia is often discovered incidentally in patients during full blood count estimation. A platelet count above 20–30 × 10^9/L is usually not associated with any symptoms such as bleeding. If clinically evident haemorrhage does occur at counts above this level, other conditions such as coagulation defects, vascular problems or rarely platelet dysfunction should be suspected. Although the prime role of platelets is in haemostasis, several other important roles have been recognized in recent years including wound repair, tissue healing, antimicrobicidal properties, lymphangiogenesis, tumour metastasization and maintenance of blood vessel integrity.

Congenital platelet disorders are often part of a syndrome. Patients with Wiskott–Aldrich syndrome have small platelets in association with eczema and recurrent infections. Other congenital platelet disorders, such as MYH9-related disorders, can present with deafness or cataracts while skeletal deformities and oculocutaneous albinism are common in other syndromic presentations.

Blood film morphology can provide important clues about the causes of thrombocytopenia (Figure 65.5). Fragmented red cells (schistocytes) increase the possibility of microangiopathic haemolytic anaemia, where an altered vessel wall and fibrin formation in the blood vessels shred the erythrocytes and consume platelets. Thrombotic thrombocytopenia purpura, haemolytic uremic syndrome and disseminated intravascular coagulation can all present with thrombocytopenia. Dysplastic red or white cells should raise the suspicion of myelodysplasia which can be confirmed by bone marrow examination and cytogenetic analysis. It is important to exclude in vitro platelet agglutination as a cause for apparent thrombocytopenia. This can be an anticoagulant (EDTA)-dependent phenomenon so a repeat sample should be examined using citrate anticoagulant. Rarely, platelet satellitism where the platelets clump round the neutrophils, can cause artefactual thrombocytopenia.

Anaemia in Low-income Countries

Anaemia affects nearly two billion people globally with a much higher prevalence in developing countries compared with more wealthy nations (43% vs 9%).[8] The continents of Africa (highest prevalence) and Asia (greatest absolute burden) account for more than 85% of the anaemic population. Anaemia burden is highest among children and women of reproductive age. Anaemia contributes to more than 115 000 maternal deaths and 591 000 perinatal deaths globally per year.[9]

WHO have defined anaemia according to various haemoglobin concentrations (Table 65.2)[10] but the appropriateness of these thresholds has been questioned because there are wide variations in haemoglobin concentration among people of different races.[11] The prevalence of anaemia can be a useful indicator of public health status of a nation because:

- The prevalence of anaemia is objective and quantifiable
- Anaemia is a major complication of several infections, including malaria, HIV, tuberculosis, and the neglected tropical diseases, which are among the commonest problems in most tropical countries
- Anaemia can be measured even in the most remote areas and devices have been developed which are cheap and reliable in different climate settings

TABLE 65.2 Haemoglobin Concentration Thresholds Used to Define Anaemia in Subjects Living at Sea Level According to the World Health Organization Guidelines

Age or Gender Group	Haemoglobin Threshold (g/L)
Children (6 months to under 5 years)	110
Children (5 years to under 12 years)	115
Children (12 years to under 15 years)	120
Non-pregnant women (15 years and over)	120
Pregnant women	110
Men (15 years and over)	130

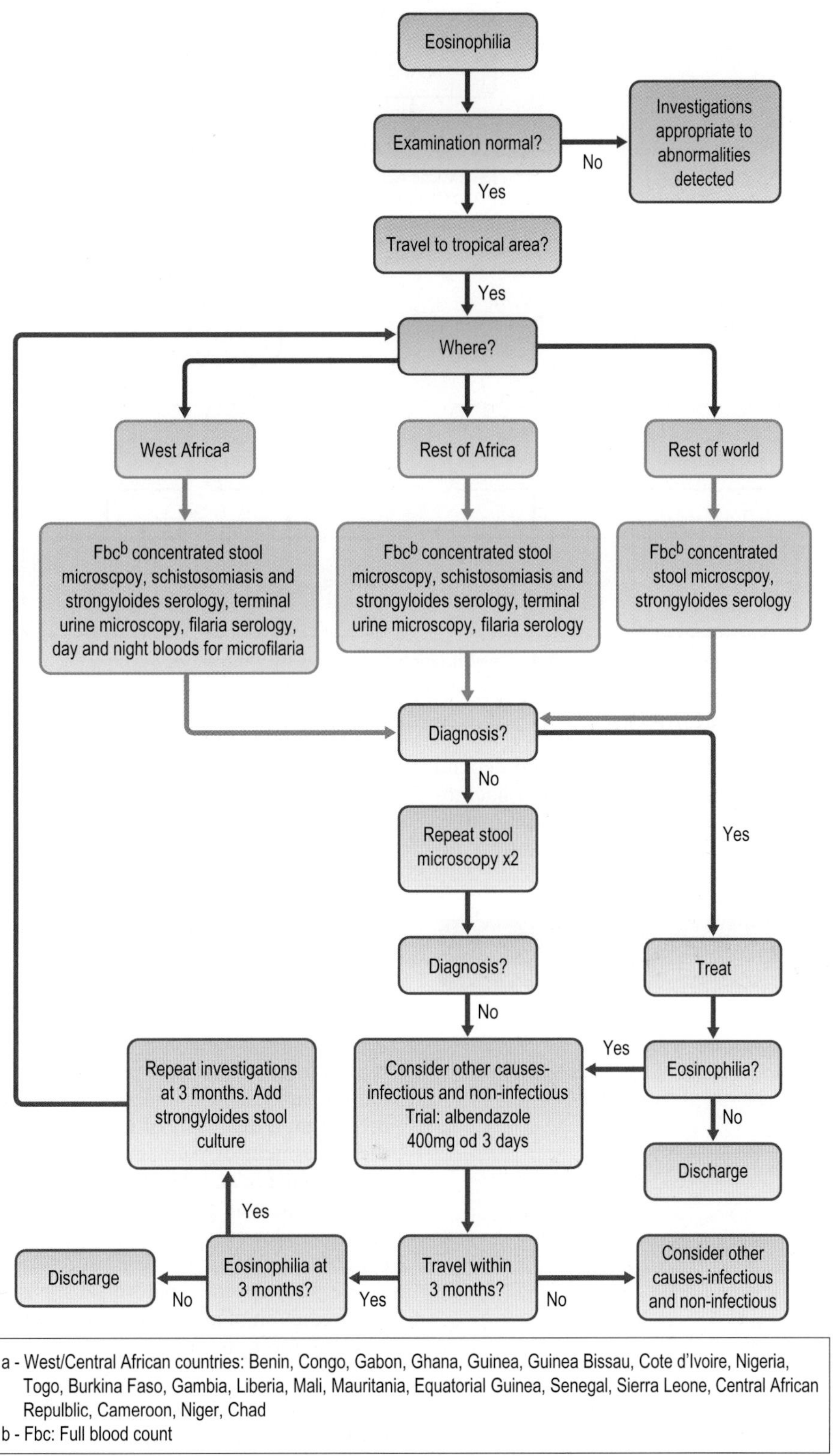

Figure 65.4 Scheme for investigation of individuals with eosinophilia. *(From Checkley AM, Chiodini PL, Dockrell DH, Bates I, Thwaites GE, Booth HL, Brown M, Wright SG, Grant AD, Mabey DC, Whitty CJ, Sanderson F; British Infection Society and Hospital for Tropical Diseases. Eosinophilia in returning travellers and migrants from the tropics: UK recommendations for investigation and initial management. J Infect. 2010 Jan;60(1):1-20. Copyright Elsevier 2010.)*

- The incidence of anaemia changes in a predictable fashion with alterations in disease burden
- The prevalence of anaemia can be used to assess whether an intervention has reached the poorest communities.

Haemoglobin concentration of <90 g/L has been recommended for disease surveillance in high-prevalence countries where changes in haemoglobin are used for monitoring the impact of interventions.[11]

Anaemia in tropical countries (Box 65.3) is often due to infections but chronic health problems, such as diabetes and chronic respiratory disease, and cancer and related complications are increasing as causes partly due to lifestyle changes.

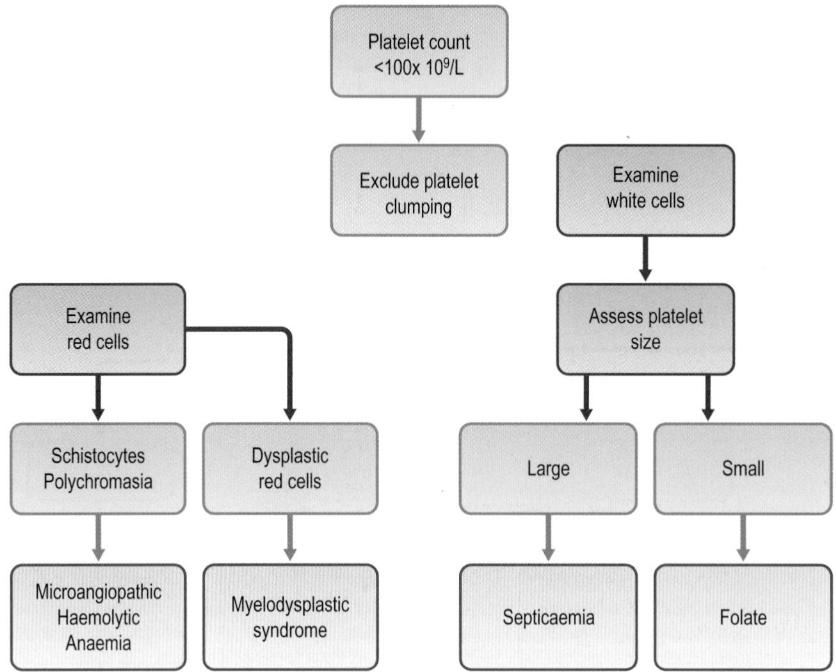

Figure 65.5 Scheme for investigation of patients with thrombocytopenia.

CLINICAL EVALUATION OF ANAEMIA

The clinical symptoms and signs of anaemia vary and depend on the cause and the speed of onset. A rapid drop in haemoglobin is much more likely to cause symptoms of anaemia than chronic anaemia. Slowly developing anaemia allows time for the body to compensate for the drop in haemoglobin content. For this reason the haemoglobin level can drop to extremely low levels before symptoms develop. Anaemia presents with symptoms such as exertional breathlessness, palpitations and in some cases, syncopal attacks. Patients with chronic anaemia may also have a multitude of nonspecific symptoms including poor concentration, decreased work performance and easy exhaustion (Table 65.3).

A thorough history and clinical examination may provide clues about the cause of anaemia but further investigations are often necessary to confirm the diagnosis and guide treatment. However, in many resource-poor settings, access to routine biochemical and haematological testing is scarce, so much reliance is placed on clinical examination. The international guidelines for the Integrated Management of Childhood Illness recommend that a diagnosis of anaemia in sick children is based on the assessment of palmar pallor. For pregnant women, symptoms of fatigue and dyspnoea, combined with signs of conjunctival and palmar pallor, and increased respiratory rate suggest anaemia. However, making a diagnosis of anaemia based on clinical assessment alone is unreliable unless the anaemia is severe.[12] No specific anatomical site is particularly accurate for the prediction of anaemia[11] though sensitivity may be increased by using multiple sites.[12]

BOX 65.3 CLASSIFICATION OF ANAEMIA IN TROPICAL COUNTRIES

NUTRITIONAL DEFICIENCIES

- Very common – Iron deficiency
- Common – Deficiencies of vitamins A, B_{12}, and folate
- Possibly common – Deficiencies of micronutrients like copper and vitamins C and E

INFECTIONS

- Malaria
- HIV
- Tuberculosis
- Hookworm infection
- Schistosomiasis
- Trichuriasis

HAEMOGLOBINOPATHIES

- Sickle cell disease
- Thalassemia
- Enzyme deficiencies (e.g. G6PD deficiency)

CHRONIC DISEASES

- Diabetes
- Chronic kidney disease due to various causes
- Chronic respiratory illnesses (e.g. chronic bronchitis, bronchiectasis)

CANCER

In many cases, there will be more than one of these conditions coexisting in the same individual. An adequate response to the treatment of anaemia requires management of ALL the contributory factors.

HAEMOGLOBIN MEASUREMENT FOR DETECTING ANAEMIA

Most central laboratories in low-income countries have automated haematology analysers and several manual methods exist for assessment of haemoglobin concentration, which are suitable for rural areas where there is no mains electricity (e.g. Haemoglobin Colour Scale; HemoCue technique).[13–15]

Haemoglobin Colour Scale[16]

Principle. The colour of a finger-prick blood sample, soaked into special chromatography paper, is compared with

TABLE 65.3 Long-Term Clinical Effects of Anaemia in Different Population Groups

Pregnant females	Increased risk of maternal morbidity Intrauterine growth retardation Increased risk of prematurity and lower birth weight Increased fetal and neonatal mortality Postpartum depression Poor maternal/infant behavioural interactions Impaired lactation
Infants and children	Cognitive defects up to two decades after iron deficiency in infancy Poor psychomotor development Decreased attentiveness, shorter attention span Poorer academic achievement in school-age children who developed iron deficiency in early childhood Breath-holding spells Increased risk of severe morbidity from malaria Increased risk of upper respiratory tract infections
All ages	Impaired physical performance Poor concentration and memory Increased irritability Poor appetite (mucositis, hypochlorhydria, oesophageal webs) worsening the nutritional status Suboptimal response to iodine in populations with endemic goitre Increased risk of chronic lead poisoning in high-lead environments Increased risk of restless legs syndrome Cardiac hypertrophy Poor fracture healing

The major cause of anaemia in most of these cases is iron deficiency. Some of the effects have been described in individuals with iron deficiency without obvious features of anaemia.

high-quality digital examples of known haemoglobin concentration. The colours are represented in 20 g/L increments from 40 g/L to 140 g/L. This method is inexpensive, does not depend on skilled scientists, is durable in dusty, hot, dry and humid conditions and is probably better than clinical diagnosis for detecting mild and moderate degrees of anaemia. The disadvantages are that it requires specific chromatography paper and good natural light and it cannot detect changes in haemoglobin less than 10 g/L.

Hemocue

This is a small battery- or mains-operated machine, which uses a drop of blood in a plastic cuvette to produce a direct read-out of haemoglobin in a few seconds. It is simple to use, produces accurate and consistent results to one decimal place and it has an in-built quality-checking mechanism. The HemoCue Hb-301 has been specifically designed for tropical conditions and operates in temperatures up to 50°C, in dusty and humid conditions. However the recurrent costs associated with disposable plastic cuvettes mean there is little opportunity for cost-saving with high-volume workloads.

PRINCIPLES OF MANAGEMENT OF ANAEMIA

(Box 65.4)

Anaemia in Infants and Children

The iron status of an infant is directly proportional to its body mass and blood volume, both of which are reflections of intrauterine growth. Thus, low birth weight and prematurity are both associated with iron depletion in the postnatal period. Several interventions have been suggested to improve infantile iron deficiency, including:[17–19]

- Delayed cord clamping at delivery; the short delay of 2–3 minutes allows a small but important amount of blood to continue to flow to the foetus from the placenta
- Improvement of infant feeding practices
- Prevention and treatment of infectious diseases
- Interventions to prevent low birth weight, such as maternal nutritional supplementation, the control of infections and chronic health problems in pregnancy.

Anaemia in young children can be due to increased nutrition requirements during periods of rapid growth; these requirements may be up to 10 times higher per kilogram of body weight than that of an adult male. In addition, infant and toddler diets often lack bio-available iron. A case–control study of preschool children in Malawi with severe anaemia (haemoglobin concentration, <50 g/L) identified bacteraemia, malaria, hookworm, HIV infections and deficiencies of vitamins A and B_{12} as the commonest causes of anaemia. Lack of folate and iron were uncommon. In low-income countries multiple interdependent causes of anaemia often operate in one individual so rectifying a single factor is unlikely to make a big impact on resolving anaemia. Interventions which are useful in preventing anaemia in younger children include micronutrient supplementation (food fortification), de-worming, prevention and treatment of infectious diseases, school nutrition programmes and community-based nutrition promotion.

Anaemia in Pregnant Women

WHO defines anaemia of pregnancy as a haemoglobin level less than 110 g/L, or haematocrit less than 33%, at any time during pregnancy. About one-fifth of maternal mortality is attributable to anaemia in pregnancy[20] and anaemia affects nearly half of all pregnant women worldwide. Maternal anaemia is associated with many factors that might also be causally associated with mortality including poverty, infections and inadequate health-seeking behaviour. Globally, the most important cause of anaemia in pregnancy is iron deficiency although hookworm, malaria, HIV infection, and deficiencies in folate and other micronutrients may contribute. Pregnancy-associated complications, including septicaemia, pre-eclampsia and other obstetric problems can precipitate anaemia.[21] It is important to note that a diagnosis of iron deficiency in pregnancy which relies on ferritin measurements may be misleading because of

BOX 65.4 PRINCIPLES OF MANAGEMENT OF ANAEMIA

- Education about the significance of anaemia and its prevention in local community, wider society and nationwide
- Manage haemoglobinopathies adequately
- Improved dietary intake (quality and quantity)
- Fortification of staple foods
- Iron and folic acid supplementation to high-risk groups[a]
- Early diagnosis and treatment of nutritional deficiencies
- Infection control
  - Treatment of infections (malaria, helminths)
  - Prevention of infections (hygiene, vaccinations)

[a]Target pre-school children, adolescent females, women of reproductive age, pregnant women, postpartum lactating women

the physiological increase in ferritin levels during the 3rd trimester.

There are three intervention strategies recommended by WHO to prevent anaemia in pregnancy:

1. Weekly iron and folic acid supplementation in women of reproductive age[22]
2. Daily iron and folic acid supplementation during pregnancy
3. Presumptive treatment of hookworm infection during pregnancy in areas where hookworm infection is known to be endemic.[23]

Several factors may interfere with the efficacy of these interventions. Under-participation in antenatal care may be common due to factors such as geographic distance, low motivation and poor interpersonal skills of health staff, poor quality of supplies and facilities, insufficient supply of iron and folic acid pills and womens' poor understanding about the daily use of supplements, especially in the face of common side effects.[23] In sub-Saharan Africa, the acute shortage and high turnover of health workers, and lack of time have also been shown to contribute to ineffective antenatal measures for reducing anaemia.[24] Interestingly, a study from Bangladesh showed that the first 20 pills (whether taken on a daily basis or less frequently) yielded most of the benefit for raising haemoglobin levels, which suggests that currently recommended doses may be higher than necessary to achieve optimal outcomes, except when anaemia is very severe.[25]

Anaemia Due to Iron Deficiency

The global burden of iron deficiency has been estimated from anaemia prevalence surveys, which include many different causes of anaemia so data may be unreliable as they are often not based on proven cases of iron deficiency. WHO estimates that globally 41% of women and 27% of pre-school children are affected by iron-deficiency anaemia, making it number 15 of selected risk factors for preventable death and disability worldwide.[20]

Iron deficiency begins in childhood, worsens during adolescence in girls and is aggravated during pregnancy. Poor iron stores at birth, low iron content of breast milk and low dietary iron intake throughout infancy and childhood result in high prevalence of anaemia in childhood. Anaemia is exacerbated by increased requirements during adolescence and iron loss from menstruation and is often compounded by the lack of adequate nutrition. The situation is worsened by pregnancy when iron requirement is approximately two times higher than in a non-pregnant state.

Iron deficiency should not be considered a diagnosis but a secondary outcome due to an underlying medical condition. Although it may be a physiological response to rapid growth or increased requirements during childhood and pregnancy, it still requires treatment due to potential deleterious consequences. Many of the chronic effects of iron deficiency may develop before the clinical and laboratory evidence of anaemia becomes apparent. The biochemical evidence for iron deficiency occurs in several steps.[26] Initially, iron stores in the bone marrow are depleted as reflected by a decreased serum ferritin. The total iron-binding capacity then starts to rise, while the serum iron saturation begins to fall before microcytosis and a drop in haemoglobin ensue. There have been attempts to identify this early iron deficiency before anaemia develops in order to improve neurological and psychomotor functions in children and work performance in adults through widespread iron supplementation. However, there are concerns that iron excess may promote infections, especially in malarious areas.

A range of laboratory investigations are usually necessary if iron deficiency is suspected (Table 65.4)[27–30] because once the diagnosis is confirmed, a search for the precise cause is necessary. A systematic approach to the investigation of iron deficiency (see below) is required based on an understanding of alterations in the iron absorption and transport cycle.

- Deficient intake (cow's milk has poor iron content and can cause gut blood loss in some infants)
- Inadequate absorption
  - *Helicobacter pylori*
  - Antacid therapy or high gastric pH (gastric acid assists in increasing solubility of inorganic iron)
  - Cereals or vegetables with high phytates (bind iron avidly)
  - Loss or dysfunction of gastrointestinal system – gastrectomy, ileal surgery, inflammatory bowel disease, coeliac disease, malabsorption syndromes
  - Cobalt or lead ingestion (share the iron absorption pathways)
- Increased demand – pregnancy, young children and adolescence, increased erythropoietic states
- Blood loss (gastrointestinal system, genitourinary system, lungs as with pulmonary haemosiderosis)
- Rare defects of haem biosynthesis and iron transport.

Iron-deficient individuals may have no symptoms. Excessive fatigue and other nonspecific signs of anaemia become more pronounced as anaemia develops. Consumption of unusual 'foods' such as ice and paint or 'pica' only occurs in a minority of individuals. Physical examination may reveal stomatitis, glossitis, koilonychia (spoon-shaped nails) and hair loss. Oesophageal webs have been described in the Plummer–Vinson syndrome but are rare and may respond to iron replacement. Since iron is important in neuromuscular development, several features of anaemia described in Table 65.3 may be related to iron deficiency.

Treatment of iron deficiency is with dietary modifications and oral or parenteral iron.[31] Blood transfusions should be reserved for those with severe symptoms especially if the anaemia developed rapidly. Haemoglobin levels alone should not be considered as a criterion for transfusion since very low levels (e.g. 10–30 g/L) may be appropriately treated with oral iron if anaemia has developed slowly. Intravenous iron should only be considered in cases of poor response or intolerance to oral iron.

Cereals, poultry and green leafy vegetables, contain non-haem iron, which is often poorly absorbed. If dietary history suggests a deficiency, diet with foods rich in haem iron, such as red meat or liver should be recommended if social and religious customs and financial status allow, ideally with a drink containing vitamin C to facilitate iron absorption. Absorption is also facilitated by taking supplements on an empty stomach although side effects of dyspepsia may not always allow this strategy. Heavy tea intake can interfere with iron absorption and should be avoided. Multivitamin or dietary supplements containing calcium, zinc or copper can also interfere with iron absorption. Absorption may be delayed by tetracyclines, milk and soft drinks. Since acid is necessary for iron absorption, antacids may account for a poor response to oral iron.

Iron is usually prescribed as a daily dose of 150–200 mg of elemental iron, commonly ferrous sulphate, 1 tablet three times

TABLE 65.4 **Tests to Confirm or Exclude Iron Deficiency**

Mean cell volume	Useful as a diagnostic clue but not confirmatory Can also be low in thalassaemia, sideroblastic anaemia and rarely lead poisoning Can be falsely normal in the presence of iron deficiency in older people or with coexistent megaloblastic anaemia Anaemia of chronic disease can occasionally cause microcytosis
Serum ferritin	The most useful laboratory measure of iron status Low value is diagnostic in the presence of anaemia Very high values (>100 μg/L) usually exclude iron deficiency' Being an acute-phase protein, it increases in inflammatory conditions, and certain malignancies, making it unreliable Also increased in tissue damage especially of the liver Levels are falsely decreased in vitamin C deficiency and hypothyroidism
Erythrocyte zinc protoporphyrin	An intermediate in haem biosynthesis and elevated concentrations indicate interrupted haem synthesis due to iron deficiency when zinc is incorporated in place of iron Can be measured on a drop of blood with a portable haematofluorometer Small sample size makes it very useful as a screening test in field surveys, particularly in children, and pregnant women where inflammatory states may not co-exist Red cells should be washed before measurement (serum bilirubin and fluorescent compounds like some drugs can give falsely high values) although not often done Lead poisoning can give falsely high values Rarely acute myeloid leukaemia and sideroblastic anaemia give slightly high values Useful in that it is not increased in thalassaemias WHO recommends normal level >70 μmol/mol haem
Iron studies	Serum iron concentration represents the iron entering and leaving the circulation. Its range varies widely with age, circadian rhythm, infections and iron ingestion Total iron binding capacity measures iron bound to transferrin. Raised levels are suggestive of iron deficiency Transferrin saturation is the ratio of serum iron and the TIBC expressed as a percentage – It is probably more useful in detecting iron overload rather than low levels.
Reticulocyte haemoglobin content	Sensitive indicator that falls within days of onset of iron-deficiency Reduced levels shown to be predictor of iron deficiency especially in the setting of renal insufficiency False normal values can occur when MCV is increased or in thalassaemia
Serum transferrin receptor	Receptors shed by iron-hungry erythropoietic cells Increased in iron deficiency It is not increased in inflammatory conditions May be upregulated by increased erythropoiesis (haemolytic diseases) giving falsely high values – serum transferrin receptor to ferritin ratio has been suggested in these cases
Bone marrow examination with special iron staining (Perl's)	Absence of stainable iron in a sample that contains particles can establish the diagnosis without other laboratory tests A simultaneous control specimen containing stainable iron should also be assessed Useful in differentiating from anaemia of chronic disorders or α-thalassaemia or milder forms of thalassaemia Can help in identifying the sideroblastic anaemias (ring sideroblasts with Perls stain), and some forms of congenital dyserythropoietic anaemia which can also cause microcytosis.

An improvement in haemoglobin and clinical symptoms with iron replacement is probably the simplest way to diagnose iron deficiency. Peripheral smear may help by demonstrating pencil cells, anisopoikilocytosis and high platelet number in cases of blood loss.

daily. The dose in children is 3–6 mg/kg per day split into divided doses. Assuming good compliance and absorption, this should result in an increase in haemoglobin within 4 weeks. Once the haemoglobin is normalized, iron should be continued for 3 months to replenish the iron stores. The major problem with oral iron is upper gastrointestinal side-effects, which can be dose-dependent. A reduction in the dose or change in the formulation to gluconate or fumarate or even liquid forms, may be successful. Liquid iron preparations may stain the teeth and should therefore be taken through a straw. Oral iron can also cause constipation or diarrhoea which is not dose-dependent. Parenteral iron is best given intravenously because intramuscular iron is painful and has been associated with development of soft tissue sarcomas.[32] High-molecular-weight iron dextran carries a low but significant risk of anaphylaxis, but the newer formulations including low-molecular-weight iron dextran, iron sucrose, ferumoxytol and iron gluconate have minimal risks.

Anaemia Due to Vitamin B_{12} Deficiency

Vitamin B_{12} or cobalamin deficiency is a well-recognized cause of macrocytic anaemia (Box 65.5). Although some microorganisms can synthesize cobalamin, humans need to obtain this essential vitamin from foods, mainly meat, poultry and dairy products. Vitamin B_{12} is an essential co-factor in DNA synthesis, serving as a co-factor in two key biochemical processes involving methylmalonic acid and homocysteine as precursors. Consequently vitamin B_{12} deficiency can interfere with DNA synthesis. Clinical manifestations include haematological (megaloblastic anaemia and pancytopenia), and neuropsychiatric disorders (paraesthesia, peripheral neuropathy, psychosis and dementia) and an increased risk of cardiovascular disease because of hyperhomocystinaemia.[32–34]

A systematic approach to the investigation of vitamin B_{12} deficiency requires an understanding of the absorption cycle.[35] Ingested vitamin B_{12} is broken down in the acidic environment of the stomach. It binds to R-binders in gastric secretions and saliva which stabilize the vitamin B_{12}. In the alkaline environment of the small intestine, vitamin B_{12} is released from R-binders to bind to intrinsic factor, synthesized in the gastric parietal cells. This vitamin B_{12}-intrinsic factor complex is absorbed from the terminal ileum. Recently, an alternative absorption system independent of intrinsic factor and the terminal ileum has been postulated which provides a rationale for

BOX 65.5 CAUSES OF VITAMIN B_{12} DEFICIENCY

REDUCED DIETARY INTAKE

- Strict vegetarians (no dairy products or eggs)
- Malnutrition
- Older individuals with poor diet (and on antacids for dyspepsia)
- Alcoholics

UNSUITABLE GASTRIC ENVIRONMENT FOR ABSORPTION

- Food-cobalamin malabsorption – probably the commonest cause; seen in older age; develops due to a decreased ability to separate cobalamin from food protein due to decreased gastric acidity
- Decreased stomach acid – atrophic gastritis, antacids (proton-pump inhibitors, H2 antagonists)
- Gastric resection

UNSUITABLE INTESTINAL ENVIRONMENT FOR ABSORPTION

- Pancreatic insufficiency (inability to transfer cobalamin from R-binders to intrinsic factor)
- Zollinger–Ellison syndrome (insufficient alkalinization in the duodenum to neutralize excess acid)
- Bacterial overgrowth due to blind-loop syndromes
- Fish tapeworm, *Diphyllobothrium latum*, competes with the host for cobalamin
- Ileal resection or bypass
- Intestinal malabsorption caused by tropical sprue, coeliac disease, Crohn's disease, or malignant infiltration of the small intestinal wall
- Medications (cholestyramine, metformin, colchicine)

DEFICIENCY OF INTRINSIC FACTOR (IF)

- Pernicious anaemia (begins after 40), increased risk of gastric carcinoma and carcinoid tumours
- Rare congenital disorders, e.g. Imerslund–Grasbeck syndrome.

increasingly popular oral replacement therapies. Once absorbed, vitamin B_{12} binds to transcobalamin II to be transported around the body.

The diagnosis of vitamin B_{12} deficiency is based on the measurement of serum vitamin levels in a patient with clinical evidence of deficiency. A note of caution is that folic acid deficiency can cause falsely low serum vitamin B_{12} levels. Diagnostic clues for vitamin B_{12} deficiency include marked macrocytosis (often >130 fl), neutrophil nuclear hypersegmentation and oval macrocytes in the peripheral blood film. Blood tests may demonstrate increased lactate dehydrogenase and low haptoglobin levels due to haemolysis within the bone marrow. The cause of the macrocytosis can be confirmed by bone marrow examination which reveals a megaloblastic picture. Although macrocytic anaemia is a typical feature of vitamin B_{12} deficiency, it can be absent in older individuals who may only have neuropsychiatric features. Measurements of methylmalonic acid and homocysteine levels, two markers which are very sensitive for detecting B_{12} deficiency, have shown that vitamin B_{12} deficiency can occur with normal haemoglobin levels and without macrocytosis.[36]

Pernicious anaemia is probably the commonest cause of vitamin B_{12} deficiency. The presence of parietal cell or intrinsic factor antibodies supports a diagnosis of pernicious anaemia.[33–36] Schilling tests are rarely performed because of the unavailability of the radio-labelled vitamin B_{12} and the difficulty in interpreting the results in the presence of renal insufficiency.

The treatment of vitamin B_{12} deficiency can be by the oral or parenteral route.[37] Increasing evidence suggests that oral supplementation may be adequate even in the presence of malabsorption or pernicious anaemia.[38,39] The recommended initial oral replacement dosage is 1–2 mg but higher doses may be needed for malabsorption or pernicious anaemia.[40] For patients with severe anaemia and/or neurological disease, daily or alternate day intramuscular injections should be initiated for the first 2–4 weeks before reverting to the maintenance three-monthly dose. Reticulocytosis is an early marker of response to treatment and is noticeable within 1–2 weeks.

Anaemia Due to Folic Acid Deficiency

Folic acid deficiency causes similar haematological manifestations to vitamin B_{12} deficiency though neuropsychiatric manifestations are less common. The ability of nerve tissue to concentrate folate to levels five times greater than those in the plasma has been suggested as a reason for the absence of neuropathy in folate deficiency. Folic acid deficiency is associated with fetal neural tube defects, and possibly with an increase in atherosclerosis and arteriovenous thrombosis, dementia and colonic cancer. Dietary folic acid is present in the form of polyglutamates, which are converted to folate monoglutamates by the enzyme folate conjugase in the intestinal brush border, prior to absorption. The monoglutamates function as a carbon transporter and are essential for DNA biosynthesis.

Folate is found in green vegetables and fruits and deficiency can result from decreased intake, impaired absorption and increased utilization, although the commonest cause is dietary insufficiency.[41] In some wealthy countries, cereals have been fortified with folic acid to successfully prevent vitamin deficiency. However folate deficiency continues to be a problem in less wealthy countries and particularly among children and pregnant women.[42,43] Exclusive feeding of goat's milk to infants can lead to folate deficiency. Other causes include alcoholism, excessive cooking of vegetables, and malabsorption (e.g. abnormalities of the small bowel). Increased demand for folic acid occurs in pregnancy because the growing foetus has a high avidity for folate. For this reason, folate supplementation has been widely recognized as an essential part of routine antenatal care to reduce the risks of neural tube defects. High folate utilization also occurs in haemolytic anaemias such as sickle cell disease due to high red cell turnover and exfoliative dermatitis. Several drugs, including sulfasalazine, trimethoprim, methotrexate, pyrimethamine and phenytoin, can also interfere with folate metabolism.

Folate-deficient individuals develop a macrocytic anaemia with peripheral blood and bone marrow findings similar to that found in vitamin B_{12} deficiency.[32] Diagnosis of folate deficiency is confirmed by the presence of low serum folate. Red cell folate levels decrease more slowly than serum levels during the 120-day turnover of the red cells. Red cell folate levels may be a better indicator of tissue folate levels than serum folate, although red cell folate can be more expensive and falsely low in vitamin B_{12} deficiency.[45,44]

Treatment of folate deficiency is with oral folate (5 mg daily) which is sufficient even in malabsorptive states. It is crucial that any co-existing vitamin B_{12} deficiency is ruled out before initiating folic acid therapy, otherwise the neurological manifestations of B_{12} deficiency may deteriorate rapidly. It is also important that the underlying cause of folate deficiency is identified and treated.

Anaemia Due to Vitamin A Deficiency

Vitamin A is important in erythropoiesis, iron metabolism (enhances iron absorption and its release from stores to the bone marrow) and for decreasing the risk of infections.[45] Vitamin A deficiency is a major public health problem in low-income countries, with an estimated 200 million preschool children affected.[47] Pregnant women and women of childbearing age also constitute high-risk groups for vitamin A deficiency.[46] Vitamin A given to Thai school children with conjunctival xerosis led to a significant increase in haemoglobin level[47] and in anaemic school children in Tanzania, vitamin A supplementation produced a marked increase in haemoglobin which was enhanced by co-administration of iron.[48] Vitamin A can also improve anaemia in pregnant women, depending on the local prevalence of deficiency[49–52] though the response may be sub-optimal in pregnant women infected with HIV.[53]

Anaemia Due to Copper Deficiency

Copper is a trace element necessary for normal haematopoiesis and myelopoiesis. Anaemia in copper deficiency is due to decreased activity of the copper-dependent enzymes, hephaestin, ceruloplasmin and cytochrome C oxidase. These are important in ferrous–ferric iron conversions and their decrease leads to abnormalities in iron absorption and its incorporation into the haemoglobin molecule. Acquired copper deficiency occurs with malnutrition and gastrointestinal malabsorption syndromes. Coeliac disease, cystic fibrosis and individuals who have had gastrectomy or surgery resulting in 'short bowel' are also at risk. Copper deficiency has also been described in persons ingesting excessive amounts of zinc-containing supplements and those who have swallowed zinc-containing coins.[54,55]

Anaemia related to copper deficiency is normocytic or macrocytic and can be associated with neutropenia; thrombocytopenia is rare. Bone marrow findings are characteristic with cytoplasmic vacuolization of both erythroid and myeloid precursor cells with ringed sideroblasts and an unusual finding of iron granules in plasma cells. These findings may be misdiagnosed as myelodysplastic neoplasm.

Measurement of serum copper levels is helpful in confirming the diagnosis although the test is fairly insensitive. Since almost complete haematological recovery can occur with copper replacement, this may be a useful diagnostic test. Oral copper supplements can be started with 8 mg of elemental copper a day slowly decreasing over the next few weeks to 2 mg until a good response is noted.

Anaemia and Zinc

Although low zinc levels do not cause anaemia they have been linked to growth retardation, heightened susceptibility to infection and male hypogonadism in relation to sickle cell disease.[56] Zinc deficiency has been described in nearly half of children and 70% of adults with sickle cell disease possibly due to increased loss of zinc in the urine and high cell turnover with decreased dietary intake.[57] In contrast zinc excess can cause anaemia through interference with copper absorption by sequestering it in the gut lumen. For this reason, zinc compounds have been used to treat Wilson's disease which is characterized by copper excess.

Anaemia Associated with Neglected Tropical Diseases

The neglected tropical diseases are a group of infections which are endemic in developing countries. Several of these neglected tropical diseases cause anaemia and many can be managed using inexpensive interventions to treat the underlying parasitic infections.[14] The mechanisms of anaemia in these conditions are predominantly blood loss from the gastrointestinal or genitourinary tracts but also poor nutrition, bone marrow suppression, inflammation, hypersplenism and haemolysis.[58]

Anaemia is a common consequence of infections with soil-transmitted helminths or schistosoma with a strong correlation between haemoglobin level and worm load or faecal egg count. Even mild infections can lead to anaemia.[59] Polyparasitism (i.e. infection with several parasites simultaneously) can be responsible for unresponsiveness of the anaemia to eradication of one organism.[60] Treatment of communities at high risk of soil-transmitted helminths improves growth and iron stores in children and reduces anaemia in pregnant women.[61]

The treatment of anaemia due to neglected tropical diseases depends on eradication of the parasite with drugs such as albendazole and praziquantel though anaemia resolution may be less successful if it is due to trichuriasis.[62–64] The addition of iron to anthelmintic treatment has met with variable success rates probably because there is associated anaemia related to inflammation. However it is still generally recommended that iron supplementation should be included with anthelmintic therapy in treatment programmes for neglected tropical diseases.[65–67]

Sickle Cell Disease

INTRODUCTION

Haemoglobin S (HbS) has a prevalence of 25–30% in many parts of Africa and also some areas in the Middle East (Figure 65.6). HbS tends to be common among ethnic groups that have traditionally had high exposure to *Plasmodium falciparum* malaria. In sub-Saharan Africa approximately 230 000 infants are born with sickle cell disease each year, mostly with HbSS. Sickle cell disease (SCD) is an autosomal recessive disorder characterized by production of an abnormal haemoglobin, sickle haemoglobin. Sickle haemoglobin (HbS) arises from a mutation in codon 6 of the β-globin gene resulting in replacement of the normal glutamic acid residue by a valine.[68] SCD is most commonly caused by the co-inheritance of two sickle cell genes (homozygous Hb SS disease) but patients who are heterozygous for HbS and for another haemoglobin mutation such as HbC (haemoglobin SC disease) or β-thalassaemia ($S\beta^0$ and $S\beta^+$) can also present with features of SCD.[69] SS disease and $S\beta^0$ disease are more severe than SC disease and $S\beta^+$ disease (Box 65.6).[70] SCD can affect multiple organs and its clinical course is punctuated by episodes of acute illness on a background of progressive organ damage, especially of the central nervous system and the lungs.[70]

HISTORY

The first description of SCD was in 1910 in an anaemic Grenadian dental student[71] and over the next 30 years it was

BOX 65.9 RISK FACTORS FOR ACUTE CHEST SYNDROME

- HbSS and HbS β^0-thalassaemia
- Lower HbF (Increase of HbF from 5–15% decreases risk by half)
- Chronic hypoxia (low nocturnal oxygen saturation)
- Bronchospasm due to asthma
- Winter months
- Smoking
- Postoperative states
- High morphine doses during pain crises
- HLA DRB1*130101haplotype
- ET-1 T8002 allele.

There is a lower risk of ACS with Arab-Indian haplotype (higher HbF levels) compared with the African haplotypes.

manifestations such as fever, cough, sputum production, tachypnoea, dyspnoea or new-onset hypoxia.[94] ACS is the most common cause of death in SCD patients and a frequent cause of hospitalization, second only to painful crisis. Mortality in patients with ACS in a wealthy country setting is 1% in children and 4.3% in adults.[95] The peak incidence for ACS is 2–4 years of age and gradually declines to 8.8 per 100 patient-years in subjects older than 20 years.[96,97]

Fever and cough are more common in children with ACS and chest pain and dyspnoea are more common in adults.[96] ACS is often preceded by febrile pulmonary infection in children and by vaso-occlusive pain crisis and lung infarction in adults. It is important to note that although tachypnoea, wheezing and features of chest infection may be identified, a third of the patients may have a normal physical examination. More than one-third of patients with ACS are hypoxaemic (oxygen saturation <90%).[98] Chest radiography is essential although infiltrates may lag behind clinical symptoms by up to 3 days. Repeat chest X-rays are recommended if there is a strong clinical suspicion of ACS. Bilateral infiltrates or involvement of multiple lobes may predict a poorer prognosis.

Risk factors for ACS (Box 65.9) include fat embolus which can be confirmed by finding stainable fat in pulmonary macrophages.[99] Chronic complications such as pulmonary hypertension occur in as many as 60% of patients and do not appear to be associated with prior episodes of ACS. High serum phospholipase A2, and the surrogate marker C-reactive protein, have been noted in patients admitted with vaso-occlusive crisis 24–48 hours before the development of ACS.[100,101]

Stroke

Neurological complications occur in at least 25% of patients with SCD and SCD is one of the most common causes of stroke in children.[102,103] In SCD, the risk of having a first stroke is 11% by the age of 20, 15% by age 30 years and 24% by age 45 years. Both thrombotic and haemorrhagic strokes occur, although the former is more common in children and those over 30 years of age, whereas the latter is more common between the ages of 20 and 30 years.[108] This age-specific pattern may be related to the higher cerebral flow rates in early childhood. Although the prevalence of clinically overt stroke is of the order of 11%, clinically silent infarction, detectable by magnetic resonance scans, affect nearly double this number by the age of 20. Silent infarcts are associated with cognitive impairment and the majority of these children require lifelong specialist care.[104] Cerebral thrombosis, which accounts for 70–80% of all strokes in SCD, results from large-vessel occlusion whereas silent infarcts are the result of microvascular occlusion or thrombosis or hypoxia secondary to large-vessel disease. In a third of SCD patients, major-vessel stenosis is accompanied by collateral vessels that appear as 'puffs of smoke' (*moyamoya*) on angiography. Risk factors for ischaemic strokes in SCD include increased cerebral blood flow velocity, previous silent infarcts, nocturnal hypoxaemia, severe anaemia, acute chest syndrome and elevated systolic blood pressure. An elevated leukocyte count is a risk factor for haemorrhagic stroke.[105–108]

DIAGNOSIS

Often the family history and clinical findings clearly point towards a diagnosis of SCD and during an acute crisis, abundant sickled red cells can be seen on a blood film. White cell counts are higher than normal in SCD disease, particularly in patients under age 10 years. The presence of sickle haemoglobin in different sickle syndromes (e.g. HbAS, HbSS, HbSC) (Table 65.5) can be confirmed by a simple sickle slide or solubility test. Haemoglobin electrophoresis will distinguish between many of these variants but high-performance liquid chromatography and iso-electric focusing are preferred for a definitive diagnosis.

TABLE 65.5 Sickle Cell Syndromes

	Hb (g/L)	MCV (fl)	Reticulocyte (%)	HbS	HbA	Others
Sickle cell disease (β^S/β^S)	80–90	70–90	6–12	>85	0	HbA2 3–3.8; HbF 2–20
Sickle cell trait (β^A/β^S)	130–150	75–90	Normal	30–40	60–70	HbA2 2.5; HbF <1
Sickle thalassemia (β^S/β^+)	80–120	65–75	4	70–90	5–30	HbA2 3.5–6; HbF 1–15
Sickle thalassemia (β^S/β^0)	70–110	60–90	4	80–95	0	HbA2 3.5–6; HbF 1–15
Sickle-HPFH	110–140	80–90	2	70–80	0	HbA2 1–3; HbF 20–30
Sickle-HbC (β^S/β^C)	80–130	75–90	4	50	0	HbA2 normal; HbF 1–7

In individuals with sickle cell trait, depending on the presence or absence of α globins, the Hb levels, MCV, and the percentages of HbS and A can vary. For example, if the genotype is –/–α, then the HB will be around 8 with MCV in the 50s and HbS and HBA demonstrating lower and higher values, respectively. Hb, haemoglobin; MCV, mean cell volume; HPFH, hereditary persistence of fetal haemoglobin

BOX 65.10 MANAGEMENT OF COMPLICATIONS OF SICKLE CELL DISEASE

RENAL IMPAIRMENT

- Inability to maximally concentrate urine (hyposthenuria) in response to water deprivation is an early finding
- Renal tubular acidosis
- Increased urinary tract infections
- Glomerular hyperfiltration, increased creatinine secretion, and a very low serum creatinine are characteristic of young patients with sickle cell anaemia, so renal dysfunction can be present even with normal serum creatinine values
- Microalbuminuria is common in childhood and up to 20% of adults develop nephrotic-range protein loss
- Gross haematuria can develop due to microthrombin in renal vessels, renal medullary carcinoma, and nocturnal enuresis
- Treatment is based on the early use of hydroxycarbamide and angiotensin-converting enzyme inhibitors in children with clinically significant albuminuria.

PULMONARY HYPERTENSION

- Noted in up to 60% of SCD cases
- No relationship to acute chest syndrome (different pathophysiology)
- Mortality risk with even mild pulmonary hypertension is high
- Regular blood transfusions and long-term anticoagulation have been tried
- Hydroxycarbamide may decrease the risk
- Prostacycline analogues (epoprostenol, and iloprost), endothelin-1 receptor antagonists (bosentan), phosphodiesterase inhibitors (including sildenafil), and calcium channel blockers are being evaluated.

PRIAPISM

- Brief but recurrent (stuttering); may occasionally last for many hours and can lead to impotence
- Usually ischaemic, or low-flow, priapism
- Patients should be educated to seek medical attention if more than 2 hours duration
- Detumescence within 12 hours is necessary to retain potency
- Intravenous hydration and analgesia initially with consideration for α-adrenergic agonists (etilefrine or phenylephrine)
- Penile aspiration and irrigation with saline and α-adrenergic agents or shunting may be required in severe cases in combination with an exchange transfusion.

Haemoglobin mass spectrometry and DNA analysis are being increasingly used.

Antenatal screening is available to women in some countries to help to identify couples who are at risk of having a baby with SCD. Community acceptance of reproductive genetic services however depends on the effectiveness of education and counselling. The use of prophylactic penicillin and the provision of comprehensive medical care during the first 5 years of life have reduced mortality related to SCD from 25% to less than 3%.[109]

MANAGEMENT (Box 65.10)

Individuals with SCD are best managed by a multidisciplinary team as they may require a variety of specialist inputs including haematology, ophthalmology, nephrology, obstetrics, orthopaedics and physiotherapy. The cornerstones of SCD therapy are disease modification and prompt and effective management of crises. Severe pain crises generally require intravenous fluids and adequate, often opiate, analgesia (Box 65.11), while disease modification is based on interventions to increase HbF levels. In steady state it is usual practice to give sickle cell patients folate supplements (1–5 mg/day) because their high rates of haemopoiesis put them at risk of deficiency. SCD is associated with functional asplenia so patients should also receive prophylactic oral penicillin (250 mg twice a day) and vaccinations against encapsulated organisms.

Hydroxycarbamide

Hydroxycarbamide is the main agent used to increase HbF (Box 65.12) and is associated with significant reductions in acute pain crises, hospitalization rate, time to first and second pain crises, episodes of acute chest syndrome, and the need for transfusions and the number of units transfused.[110] Other beneficial effects of hydroxycarbamide, which are independent of the increase in HbF, include reduced neutrophil count, increased cellular water content, decreased HbS concentration, changing expression of adhesion molecules and nitric oxide generation.[111] Hydroxycarbamide may also be an alternative to frequent blood transfusions for the prevention of recurrent stroke in children as it can lower transcranial Doppler velocities.[112,113] Under-use of this cheap, effective drug is related to concerns about leukaemogenicity but this has not been shown to be a problem when used for a non-malignant condition like SCD.

Blood Transfusions (Box 65.13)

The two main approaches to transfusion[74] in SCD are simple top-up transfusion and exchange transfusion. Target haemoglobin level in SCD therapy is 100 g/L or a haematocrit of 30%; higher target levels are associated with hyperviscosity and

BOX 65.11 MANAGEMENT OF PAIN IN PATIENTS WITH SICKLE CELL DISEASE

- Assess pain intensity
- Choose the analgesic, dosage, and route of administration
- Paracetamol and hydration should be considered in all patients
- Oral, sustained-release morphine is as good as intravenous morphine infusion in children and young adults
- Manage mild pain with rest, hydration, and weak opioids (such as codeine). Admit patients in whom pain that does not subside promptly or require opioid treatment; fever, pallor, or signs of respiratory compromise; a low likelihood of receiving appropriate care at home
- Pain management should be individualized and dosing should take into account prior pain management and use of opioids
- The pain pathway should be targeted at different points with different agents, avoiding toxicity with any one class
- Always look for a cause, e.g. infection, dehydration, etc.
- Education about avoiding exposure to precipitants
- Be empathetic, reassuring, and supportive
- Benzodiazepines may be helpful to reduce anxiety
- Re-examine the patient often to ensure adequate pain relief, to assess sedation and respiratory rate (to avoid opioid overdose). In assessing patient responses to conventional doses of analgesia, it must be remembered that those with sickle cell disease metabolize narcotics rapidly
- Re-search for evidence of any complications such as acute chest syndrome or anaemia
- Always look for a cause, e.g. infection.

BOX 65.12 HYDROXYCARBAMIDE USE IN PATIENTS WITH SICKLE CELL DISEASE

BEFORE COMMENCEMENT

- Blood counts, red cell indices, HbF level, serum chemistries, pregnancy test

PATIENT EXCLUSION CRITERIA

- Regular transfusion regimen
- Abnormal liver function tests
- Inability to attend hospital for regular follow-up

PATIENT ELIGIBILITY

Patients (HbSS or Sβ^0-thalassemia, not HbSC) with a severe clinical course as:

- Three admissions with painful crisis within 1 year *or*
- Frequent days of pain at home, leading to a lot of time off work *or*
- Recurrent acute chest syndrome.

The following predict a more severe clinical course and are additional reasons to consider offering hydroxyurea: Hb <70 g/L, WBC >15 × 10^9/L, HbF <6% and renal insufficiency due to SCD.

DOSE AND MONITORING

- Start at 10–15 mg/kg per day (to the nearest 500 mg/day)
- If no or poor response, increase dose by increments of 5 mg/kg per day every 4 weeks (max: 30 mg/kg per day). Most good responses require about 1–2 g/day in adults
- Monitor FBC, HbF%, and reticulocytes every 1 or 2 weeks initially, then every 4 weeks when on a stable dose
- Monitor biochemistry profile (hydroxyurea has renal excretion and hepatic toxicity).

GOALS OF TREATMENT

- Less pain
- Persistent increase in HbF (usually measured every 6–8 weeks) or mean cell volume
- Persistent increase in haematocrit if severely anaemic
- Decrease in LDH
- Acceptable toxicity.

Improvement in symptoms and blood parameters may take 3–4 months of therapy, but can be seen after approximately 6 weeks. If the reticulocyte count is less than expected for the degree of anaemia, erythropoietin deficiency should be considered.

worsening of complications. In exchange transfusion, the aim is to achieve an HbS% of <30%. Complications of transfusion in SCD include alloimmunization,[114] delayed haemolytic transfusion reactions and iron overload. The high rates of red cell antibody formation (30%) noted in wealthy countries are due to minor blood group incompatibilities between the recipient and the blood donor who is often of a different ethnicity. Leukocyte reduction of transfused blood, routine ABO, Rh and Kell matching for all patients and extended phenotype matching for those with alloantibodies may be useful for reducing transfusion reactions.

Management of Acute Chest Syndrome

Treatment for ACS is predominantly supportive and includes adequate pain relief, antibiotics (e.g. a macrolide with a cephalosporin), continuous pulse oximetry and delivery of supplemental oxygen to patients with hypoxaemia. Incentive spirometry can prevent atelectasis and infiltrates[115] and blood transfusion is indicated when a patient develops respiratory distress, a clinically significant fall in the haematocrit or signs of multi-organ failure.[116] Both simple transfusion and exchange transfusions have been used and neither appears to be superior. A short course of steroids may attenuate ACS but it may also increase the risk of re-hospitalization.[117] Bronchodilators may help patients with wheezing[118] but inhaled nitric oxide has not shown any clear benefits.[119] Since coagulation activation is important in the pathophysiology of acute chest syndrome, treatment with low-molecular-weight heparin may reduce clinical complications.[120]

Management of Stroke

Transcranial Doppler measurement of cerebral blood flow has been a major step forwards in identifying individuals with an increased risk of ischaemic stroke. A value more than 200 cm/second imparts a 40% risk of stroke within the next 3 years.[121] Regular blood transfusions can reduce the incidence of stroke in children.[105] Due to a high recurrence of stroke (60%) on stopping transfusions, continuation of transfusions should be guided by transcranial Doppler measurements.[122,123] Once a stroke has developed, the best therapeutic strategy is exchange transfusion which probably needs to be done monthly.[70,73] Neurosurgical re-vascularization should be considered for moyamoya-like syndromes when new strokes occur despite transfusion.

HAEMOGLOBIN SICKLE CELL DISEASE

Haemoglobin SC results from the co-inheritance of HbS and HbC and has its highest prevalence in West Africa. Clinical features and disease management are similar to those of HbSS disease but splenomegaly, splenic infarcts and splenic sequestration may occur into adulthood. Proliferative retinopathy necessitates regular ophthalmic review in those aged over 10 years. Compared with HbSS, anaemia is less marked in Hb SC (8–140 g/L) and there are fewer sickle cells and more target cells on the blood film. The diagnosis can be confirmed by haemoglobin electrophoresis, HPLC or iso-electric focussing.

BOX 65.13 BLOOD TRANSFUSIONS IN SICKLE CELL DISEASE

INDICATIONS FOR ACUTE TRANSFUSIONS

- Acute exacerbation of anaemia
- Acute chest syndrome
- Stroke or acute neurological deficit
- Multiorgan failure
- Preoperative management

INDICATIONS FOR LONG-TERM TRANSFUSIONS

- Primary and secondary stroke prevention
- Recurrent acute chest syndrome not helped by hydroxycarbamide
- Recurrent complications
- Occasionally in complicated pregnancy

SPECIAL CONSIDERATIONS

- Aim in all cases to reduce HbS level to <30%
- Exchange transfusions may be considered in cases of stroke, acute chest syndrome not responding to top-up transfusion and major surgeries
- Target haemoglobin concentration of 100 g/L may be considered in cases of organ failure and surgery.

SICKLE CELL TRAIT

Individuals with sickle cell trait (Hb AS) have 10-fold protection against severe malaria compared to individuals with normal haemoglobin (HbAA) probably due to both innate and immune-mediated mechanisms. Individuals with sickle cell trait (HbAS) are generally asymptomatic and they have a normal haemoglobin and normal life expectancy. Uncommonly, complications such as poor perfusion of the renal papillae and increased bacteruria may occur.[124] The blood film is generally normal and the diagnosis can be confirmed by haemoglobin electrophoresis, HPLC or iso-electric focusing.

Thalassaemia

HISTORY

The original descriptions of thalassaemia originated from areas round the Mediterranean and the term derives from the Greek *thalassos* (sea) and *haima* (blood).[125–127]

EPIDEMIOLOGY

Thalassaemia is one of the most common single gene disorders and approximately 5–7% of the global population are carriers. α^+-Thalassaemia occurs throughout the tropics, whereas α^0-thalassaemia, which is responsible for haemoglobin Bart's hydrops fetalis, is concentrated predominantly in South-east Asia and to a lesser extent around the Mediterranean.[128,129] β-Thalassaemia is common in the Mediterranean countries, parts of Africa, throughout the Middle East, the Indian subcontinent and South-east Asia. Haemoglobin E prevalence is highest in Cambodia, Laos and Thailand and can reach 50–60% with lower prevalence rates in Indonesia, Malaysia, Singapore and Vietnam.

MOLECULAR ABNORMALITIES

β-Thalassaemia

β-Thalassaemia is an inherited quantitative deficiency of β-globin chains which are required to make normal adult haemoglobin.[130] More than 200 mutations have been associated with the development of β-thalassaemia (a complete list is available at the Globin Gene Server website, at: http://globin.cse.psu.edu) and they affect protein synthesis[130,131] leading to reduced (designated β^+) or absent (designated β^0) production of the β-globin chains. The clinical severity of thalassaemia can be lessened by co-existing haemoglobin abnormalities such as the co-inheritance of α-thalassaemia and increased production of haemoglobin F.[132,133]

α-Thalassaemia

Normal α-globin synthesis is regulated by duplicate α-globin genes on chromosome 16. The genotype is usually represented as αα/αα and α-thalassaemia usually results from deletion of one or both α-genes. Occasionally point mutations in critical regions of the α-genes may cause non-deletional α-thalassaemia (α^T).[130] Mutations can completely abolish expression of the α-genes (i.e. α^0-thalassaemia) or partially down-regulate expression (α^+-thalassaemia).[130] Both α^0 and α^+ thalassaemias can occur in the heterozygous or homozygous state or as a compound α^0/α^+ heterozygote form (Table 65.6). Underproduction of α-globin chains due to three or four gene deletions gives rise to excess γ (fetal) or β (adult) globin chains which form tetramers, called Hb Bart's (fetal) or HbH (adult).[134] Rare forms of α-thalassaemia occur in association with other conditions such as mental retardation and myelodysplastic/leukaemia syndrome.[135,136]

TABLE 65.6 Classification of α-Thalassaemia

	Genotype	Designation
α-thalassaemia-2 trait	−α/αα	α^+/α
α-thalassaemia-1 trait	−α/−α	α^+/α^+
	αα/−	α/α^0
Hb H disease	−α/−	α^+/α^0
Hb Barts hydrops fetalis	−/−	α^0/α^0

PATHOPHYSIOLOGY

β-Thalassaemia (Figure 65.8)

Thalassaemias[131,137,138] cause an imbalance of α- and β-globin chain synthesis. In homozygous β-thalassaemia, excess α-chains precipitate in the red cell precursors and up to 75% of cells are destroyed in the bone marrow resulting in ineffective erythropoiesis and a shortened red cell survival. The red cells released from the bone marrow contain abnormal α-chains and these inclusions promote destruction of the cells by the spleen leading to clinical symptoms and signs of haemolysis. In heterozygotes, the α-chain excess and the degree of inadequate erythropoiesis is much less than in homozygous β-thalassaemia. HbF production normally tails off within a few months of birth but in β-thalassaemia HbF production can continue into adulthood. The effect of increased HbF production is to prevent precipitation of the excess globin chains and consequent ineffective erythropoiesis. However HbF has a high oxygen affinity, which can lead to increased erythropoietin production and thus, increased bone marrow expansion.

α-Thalassaemia

The pathophysiology of α-thalassaemia, and hence the clinical manifestations, is quite different from β-thalassaemia. The excess non-α-globin chains form soluble tetramers rather than precipitates so there is only minimal ineffective erythropoiesis. The only clinical abnormality in those with HbH may be splenomegaly secondary to increased work load from destruction of red cells containing inclusions. Rarely anaemia may be severe enough to require blood transfusions. The clinical manifestations of Hb Barts are the result of its very high oxygen affinity which causes severe anaemia, intrauterine hypoxia, increased capillary permeability, severe erythroblastosis with hepatosplenomegaly and cardiac failure. The grossly hydropic infant inevitably dies around the time of delivery.

CLINICAL FEATURES

β-Thalassaemia

β-Thalassaemia is categorized according to the clinical severity of the condition rather than the underlying genetic abnormality. The level of dependency on transfusions is used to

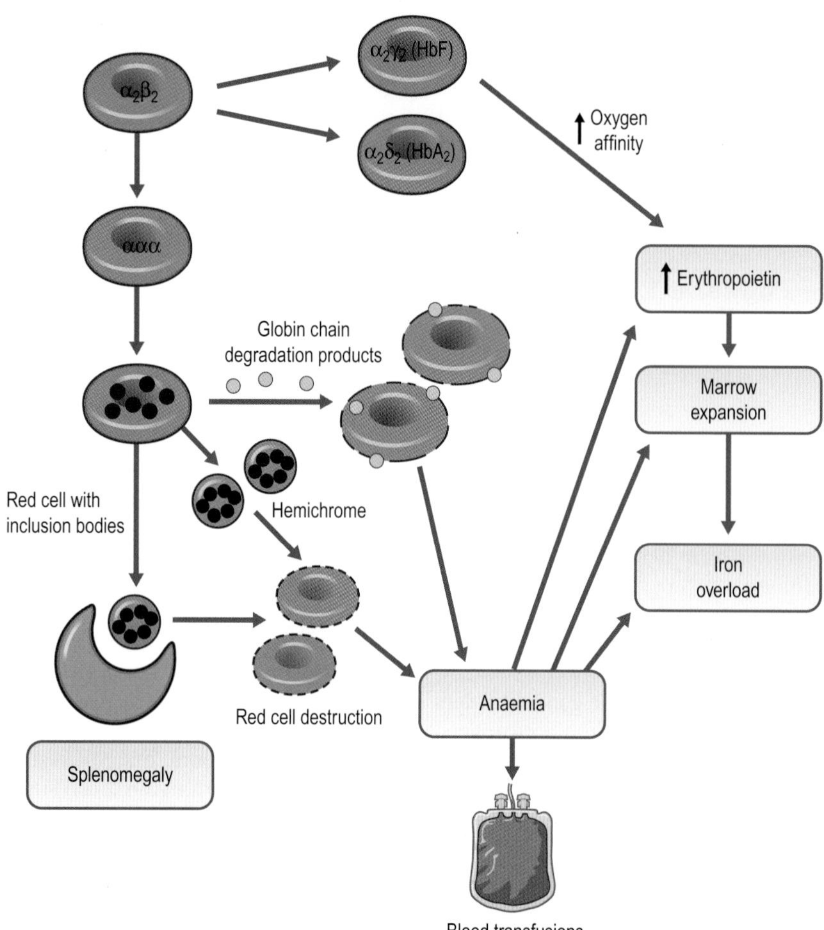

In homozygous β-thalassemia, β-globin synthesis is markedly reduced or absent. The excess α-chains cannot form a tetramer but form a precipitate in the red cell precursors leading to intra-medullary destruction of these cells. This destructive process of the red cell membrane occurs from the formation of α-chain hemichromes (shown as red cell inclusions) and degradation products of the excess α-chains. The red cells which may be released from the bone marrow are destroyed by the spleen leading to clinical symptoms and signs of haemolysis. Since only the β-chain is affected in these individuals, the synthesis of HbF and HbA_2 continues unabated. These haemoglobins have very high oxygen affinity, which can lead to increased erythropoietin production and thus, increased bone marrow expansion

Figure 65.8 Pathophysiological consequences of β-thalassaemia.

divide β-thalassaemia into thalassaemia major (transfusion-dependent), thalassaemia intermedia (able to maintain adequate haemoglobin without transfusions or requiring less than 8 units/year) and thalassaemia minor (asymptomatic).[139] Infants with β-thalassaemia are protected from severe anaemia by the presence of haemoglobin F and are usually asymptomatic. Clinical manifestations of thalassaemia major depend on whether adequate blood transfusions are available and the stringency with which iron chelation is undertaken. Untreated patients with thalassaemia major will die in late infancy or early childhood from the effects of severe anaemia. Those who receive sporadic transfusions may survive longer but suffer from the secondary effects of anaemia, bony deformities and growth retardation.

Thalassaemia Major

The clinical features of β-thalassaemia major are divided into those resulting from anaemia, bony changes and iron overload.

Anaemia from defective erythropoeisis, decreased red cell survival and increased haemolysis in thalassaemia major leads to cardiac decompensation, failure to thrive and growth retardation in children. Splenomegaly, from the increased work load of culling red cells with inclusion bodies, can cause dilutional anaemia and a further drop in haemoglobin. Compensatory extra-medullary haematopoiesis can lead to hepatomegaly and occasionally vertebral compression and neurological defects. Haemolysis from increased red cell destruction is associated with gall stones in up to 20% of individuals with β-thalassaemia.[140]

Another consequence of accelerated haemolysis is the increased incidence of thromboembolism (4% in thalassaemia major and 10% with intermedia) from the exposure of negatively charged phospholipids on the red cell membrane and the generation of red cell and platelet microparticles.[141] Splenectomy with postoperative thrombocytosis is a risk factor for thrombosis especially if combined with endothelial oxidative stress from iron overload, or procoagulant co-morbid conditions such as diabetes mellitus, hormone therapy, thrombophilic mutations and atrial fibrillation.[142] Folate deficiency, hyperuricaemia and occasionally gout have been observed in thalassaemia major due to the high turnover of red cells.

The enhanced erythropoietic drive from anaemia in thalassaemia can lead to increased marrow expansion with characteristic bossing of the skull and overgrowth of maxillary region, radiologically noted as 'hair on end' or 'sun-ray' appearance. Metatarsal and metacarpal bones are the first to expand so measurement of the metacarpal bones has been considered a good indicator for initiation of transfusion therapy.[143] Other skeletal deformities include shortening of long bones due to early epiphyseal fusion and overgrowth of the maxilla causing dental malocclusion. The marrow expansion can also lead to pathological fractures, early bone thinning and osteoporosis[144,145] while ineffective drainage of the sinuses and middle ear from skull bone overgrowth can cause chronic sinus and ear infections. Growth retardation is primarily the result of anaemia with contributions from iron overload, hypersplenism, deficiencies of thyroid and growth hormone, hypogonadism, zinc deficiency, chronic liver disease, malnutrition and psychosocial stress.[146]

Patients with β-thalassaemia have increased iron absorption mediated by reduced hepcidin and those who receive regular transfusions may also develop transfusion siderosis if they are inadequately chelated. The iron is deposited in the parenchymal tissues with a variety of clinical consequences (Box 65.14),[147–154] a process which may be modulated by variants in the haemochromatosis (HFE) gene.[155]

Thalassaemia Intermedia

Thalassaemia intermedia is characterized by haemoglobin concentrations of 70–100 g/L and children usually present at around 2–4 years of age with symptoms of anaemia, jaundice and hepatosplenomegaly.[156] There may also be skeletal changes such as expansion of the facial bones and obliteration of the maxillary sinuses.[157] Several molecular factors including: (a) coinheritance of α-thalassaemia; (b) hereditary persistence of haemoglobin F; (c) δβ-thalassaemia and (d) the specific GγXmn1 polymorphism contribute to the 'conversion' of thalassaemia from major to intermedia type.[158]

In contrast to patients with thalassaemia major, iron loading in thalassaemia intermedia occurs mainly as a result of increased intestinal iron absorption rather than transfusion therapy. Ineffective erythropoiesis with resultant chronic anaemia and hypoxia can suppress hepcidin, the regulator of iron metabolism, leading to increased iron absorption.[158] The excess iron tends to accumulate in the liver rather than the heart.[159] Other clinical complications in thalassaemia intermedia include gallstones, extramedullary haemopoiesis leg ulcers, thromboembolic events and pulmonary hypertension, which is the major cause of heart failure in these individuals.[160] Although individuals with thalassaemia intermedia do not usually need regular blood transfusions, there is some evidence that complications, particularly later in life, may be less common in regularly transfused patients.[159]

α-Thalassaemias[130,134]

Carriers of α-thalassaemia (traits, with loss of 1 or 2 α genes) are usually asymptomatic and may only be detected through a routine blood count which shows mild to moderate microcytic, hypochromic anaemia. Antenatal counselling may be indicated if the mother has αα/– as there is a possibility that the fetus may be at risk of having haemoglobin Bart's.

Haemoglobin H disease occurs mainly in Asians and occasionally in the Mediterranean population. It is the result of deletion of three α genes (α–/–) and can produce anaemia varying from 30–130 g/L. There is usually associated splenomegaly, which may be massive, and growth retardation in children. Bony changes are unusual. Other complications include infections, leg ulcers, gall stones and acute haemolysis in response to drugs and infections. The severity of the clinical features is related to the molecular basis with non-deletional types of HbH disease more severely affected.

Haemoglobin Bart's (–/–) occurs almost exclusively in Asians, especially Chinese, Cambodian and Thai populations. An infant with Hb Bart's hydrops fetalis syndrome has pallor and gross oedema with signs of cardiac failure, marked hepatosplenomegaly and skeletal and cardiovascular deformities. There is often gross hypertrophy of the placenta. Many of the clinical manifestations of this condition can be explained by the

BOX 65.14 COMPLICATIONS FROM IRON OVERLOAD IN PATIENTS WITH THALASSAEMIA

LIVER

- Earliest organ to be affected
- Liver fibrosis and cirrhosis are the commonest manifestations
- Fibrosis correlates with age, transfusion frequency, liver iron concentration (assessed by Ishak score) and transfusion-transmitted hepatitis C infection (genotype 1b)
- The prevalence of cirrhosis ranges from 10% to 20%
- 1–5% are hepatitis B surface antigen-positive (higher in Asia and South-east Asia)
- Detection techniques include transient elastography, magnetic resonance imaging and liver biopsy.

HEART

- 22% have a cardiac problem
- Heart failure and arrhythmias are the commonest manifestations
- Pulmonary hypertension may also be seen (more common in thalassaemia intermedia)
- Magnetic resonance imaging useful in the diagnosis of cardiac problems especially cardiac failure. Cardiac T2* values <10 ms associated with significantly high failure rates
- Myocardial fibrosis diagnosed by MRI more often in Italian patients who have higher prevalence of hepatitis C virus antibodies and associated myocarditis.

ENDOCRINE GLANDS

- Hypogonadism is the most frequent complication in patients with prevalence over 50% in both males and females. It is usually hypogonadotrophic suggesting iron damage to the anterior pituitary or hypothalamus. The features range from total absence of sexual development to delayed puberty. In females with normal menstrual function, fertility is normal with the ovarian function preserved in most although secondary amenorrhoea can develop. Damage of the ovaries is rare and is more likely to appear in older women (around 30) because of high vascular activity on the ovaries at this age. Secondary hypogonadism is common (50%) in older men. Serum ferritin >2000 ng/mL is a risk factor.
- Hypothyroidism is the second most common endocrine disorder (about 20%) although many of them may have the subclinical variety. Most commonly hypothyroidism is of the primary type with secondary, central hypothyroidism increasingly being diagnosed in recent years.
- The prevalence of diabetes mellitus is around 5% with the mean age of diagnosis being 18 years. Impaired glucose tolerance occurs first with microvascular damage like retinal changes being less common than the conventional form. Chronic hepatitis C infection can precipitate the onset of diabetes. Impaired glucose tolerance usually responds to oral hypoglycaemics although insulin therapy can be difficult due to difficult glycaemic control.

BOX 65.15 A STEPWISE APPROACH TO DIAGNOSIS OF THALASSAEMIAS

FAMILY HISTORY OF HAEMOLYTIC DISEASE OR THALASSAEMIA

- Ethnic background can be helpful in considering the type of thalassaemia
- Age of onset can aid in determining the severity and need for blood transfusions
- Development of the child can be useful to know the likely complications
- Late-onset complications including heart, liver and endocrine effects is also helpful.

CLINICAL EXAMINATION

- Anaemia
- Haemolysis
- Bone changes
- Splenomegaly
- Endocrine assessment.

INVESTIGATIONS

- Blood count – severe anaemia with thalassaemia major; in thalassaemia minor or trait; the mean cell volume is decreased disproportionately to the haemoglobin while the mean haemoglobin concentration is markedly reduced (20–22 pg)
- Blood film – Microcytic, hypochromic red cells; Target cells, polychromasia; Basophilic stippling; Nucleated red cells (very high levels after splenectomy); Poikilocytes in non-splenectomized patients
- Haemoglobin electrophoresis at alkaline and acidic pH – haemoglobin on a membrane is subjected to charge gradient which separates them and can be identified by special stains for haem or protein
- High-performance liquid chromatography – this procedure which separates components by their adsorption onto a negatively charged stationary phase on a chromatography column followed by elution to detect and quantify haemoglobins A, A2 and F and variants
- Isoelectric focussing – the haemoglobins are separated in a polyacrylamide or cellulose acetate gel containing molecules with different isoelectric values (when they do not have a net charge) and are identified based on comparisons with the known variants after staining.

very high affinity for oxygen for haemoglobin Bart's. The infants very often die in utero, usually after the 1st trimester due to protection from haemoglobin Portland, or shortly after birth. The morphological abnormalities of severe microcytosis and hypochromia differentiate this condition from haemolytic disease of the newborn.

DIAGNOSIS (Box 65.15)

β-Thalassaemia major, haemoglobin H disease and haemoglobin Bart's are easily diagnosed using clinical findings and basic laboratory techniques. However, the diagnosis of β-thalassaemia trait and β-thalassaemia intermedia is complex and requires considerable expertise. The haemoglobin profile varies across the spectrum of β-thalassaemia syndromes. HbF levels are increased, varying from around 10% in the more mild forms, to 100% in homozygous patients who are unable to make any HbA (ααββ). Levels of HbA2 can vary from normal to 7%. Reticulocytosis occurs but is 2–8% lower than would be expected for the extreme erythroid hyperplasia reflecting intramedullary erythroid precursor destruction. Osmotic fragility is reduced, sometimes strikingly so since in some cases the red blood cells do not haemolyse even in distilled water.[161] For this reason, if sophisticated tests are not available, osmotic fragility can be used as a screening test for thalassaemia trait. Serum zinc levels may be low and this may be related to abnormal growth.[162] Vitamin C levels may also be low due to its increased conversion to oxalic acid in the presence of iron overload.[163] Care may be needed if folic acid is commenced on a background of bone marrow failure due to folate deficiency as it may precipitate painful erythropoietic crises.[164]

MANAGEMENT

A comprehensive management plan for patients with thalassaemia may involve transfusion therapy, iron chelation, splenectomy, prevention or early treatment of complications and stem cell transplant.

Transfusion Therapy

The mainstay of treatment for the severe forms of thalassaemia is blood transfusion with the aim of reducing anaemia and erythropoietic drive. However, in many low-income settings blood supplies are inadequate and many thalassaemic patients are chronically under-transfused (Table 65.7).[165] Transfusion frequency should be guided by clinical symptoms and signs such as poor growth and facial or other bone abnormalities, and should take into account any potential disease-modifying comorbidities.[156] Although the decision to transfuse should not be based purely on haemoglobin levels, a value of <70 g/L is often used as a trigger for regular transfusions.

To prevent alloimmunization, extended red cell antigen typing for C, E and Kell in addition to ABO and Rh(D) typing should be carried out prior to the first transfusion, and before each transfusion, full cross-match and screening for new antibodies should be undertaken.[166] The risk of alloimmunization appears to be greater in patients who begin transfusion therapy after the first few years of life.[128] Development of alloantibodies and autoantibodies may result in increased transfusion requirements or haemolysis. Use of leukodepletion techniques can result in less alloimmunization and fewer febrile transfusion reactions. Since storage of red cells in anticoagulant solutions may decrease their efficacy, the use of blood that has been stored for less than 7–10 days may be beneficial for patients who require frequent transfusions. The use of 1st-degree relatives as blood donors should be discouraged, especially if the patient is a candidate for stem cell transplant.

Patients with thalassaemia major need lifelong regular blood transfusions, 15 mL/kg per month or 1–2 units of blood every 2–5 weeks, to maintain the pre-transfusion haemoglobin level above 90–105 g/L. The clinical benefits of this regular transfusion programme include normal growth, suppression of erythropoiesis and bone marrow expansion, reduced hepatosplenomegaly and an overall sense of wellbeing, which allows normal age-appropriate activities. A higher target pre-transfusion haemoglobin level of 110–120 g/L may be necessary for patients with heart disease or other medical conditions and for those patients who do not achieve adequate suppression of bone marrow activity at the lower haemoglobin level. Shorter intervals between transfusions may reduce overall blood requirements but need to be balanced against the patient's work or school schedule and other lifestyle issues.

TABLE 65.7 **Estimated Reach of Treatment for β-Thalassaemia in Each WHO Region**

	Estimated Annual Births β-Thalassaemias		Transfusion				Adequate Iron Chelation		Inadequate or No Iron Chelation	
WHO Region	Total	Transfusion-Dependent	Annual No. Starting Transfusion	% of Transfusion-Dependent Patients Transfused	Annual Deaths Because Not Transfused	**No. of Known Patients**	% with Chelation	No. with Chelation	No. of Patients	Annual Deaths Due to Iron Overload
African	1386	1278	35	2.7	1243	–	–	–	–	–
American	341	255	134	52.4	121	2750	58	1604	1146	57
Eastern Mediterranean	9914	9053	1610	17.8	7 443	39700	27	10818	28882	1444
European	1019	920	140	15.5	780	16230	91	14754	1476	74
South-east Asian	20420	9 983	962	9.6	9021	35500	19	6 621	28879	1444
Western Pacific	7 538	4 022	108	2.7	3914	3450	44	1504	1946	97
World	40618	25511	2 989	11.7	22522	97630	39	37866	59764	2988

The initiation of regular transfusion therapy for severe thalassaemia usually occurs in the first 2 years of life. Some patients with thalassaemia intermedia who only need sporadic transfusions in the first two decades of life may later need regular transfusions because of a falling haemoglobin level or the development of serious complications. Haemoglobin should be monitored to assess the rate of fall in the haemoglobin level between transfusions and this can be used to indicate the frequency of transfusions. Exchange transfusions have been tried as a way of reducing iron loading and are associated with a reduction in blood requirements by about one-third.

Iron Chelation Therapy (Table 65.8)

Since each unit of red cells can contain up to 200 mg of iron, cumulative iron burden is an inevitable consequence of a long-term transfusion programme. In addition there is increased iron absorption from the gut (0.3–0.6 mg/kg per day) as a response to severe anaemia and down-regulation of hepcidin. Iron chelation therapy[167,168] has improved survival rates for thalassaemic patients, and prevented hepatic fibrosis and iron-induced cardiac disease; most patients who are compliant with chelation therapy have normal growth and sexual development. Iron chelators (Box 65.16) are usually initiated in children over 2 years who have received 10 units of blood and/or have a steady-state serum ferritin level above 1000 ng/mL on at least two occasions. This level of iron overload typically occurs after 1–2 years of transfusions. Desferrioxamine is started at 25–30 mg/kg per day in these children initially, to avoid toxicity due to over chelation.

Splenectomy

Marked splenomegaly, often treated with splenectomy, was common in thalassaemia patients before the advent of regular transfusion programmes. Severe haemolysis in thalassaemia is related to a hyperactive spleen, which aggravates anaemia and can increase transfusion requirements. Although early

TABLE 65.8 **Features of Currently Available Iron Chelators**

	Deferoxamine	Deferiprone	Deferasirox
Chelating properties	Hexadentate binds iron in a 1-to-1 complex	Bidentate binds iron in a 3-to-1 complex	Tridentate binds iron in a 2-to-1 complex
Half-life	8–10 min	2–4 hours	12–18 hours
Excretion of iron removed	50–70% in the stool, remainder in the urine. vary with level of iron overload, dose, and erythropoietic activity	Predominantly in the urine (90%)	Predominantly (90%) faecal
Removal of iron from the liver	Very good	Good but at higher doses may be very good	Very good
Removal of iron from the heart	Mainly with 24 hour intravenous infusion	Higher than standard deferoxamine	As deferiprone
Dose	30–60 mg/kg	75–100 mg/kg	20–40 mg/kg/day
Frequency	Subcutaneous or intravenous 8–12 h, 5–7 days/week	Oral three times daily	Oral once daily
Adverse effects	1. Most common – induration at the site of infusion. 2. Aggressive chelation with lower iron levels may cause ototoxicity (bilateral high-frequency hearing loss) and visual toxicity (loss of night and colour vision, retinal atrophy, and cataract) – baseline/annual checks and adjusting the dose to ferritin level are advised 3. Growth plate deformities or cartilage dysplasia 4. Rare but serious – *Yersinia* and mucormycosis infections presenting as colitis, abdominal abscess	1. Nausea and vomiting in 33% of patients; usually resolve 2. Arthropathy with arthralgias and joint effusions in 15% 3. Agranulocytosis occurs in 1% of patients 4. Mild neutropenia in approximately 8%	1. Rare reports of fulminant hepatic failure – liver function tests every 2 weeks for 1 month after starting therapy and then monthly 2. Elevations in serum creatinine in 1/3 – kidney function monitored monthly

BOX 65.16 NEWER TREATMENTS AVAILABLE FOR THALASSAEMIA

INDUCTION OF FETAL HAEMOGLOBIN SYNTHESIS (HBF)

- Hydroxyurea – helpful in some patients with β-thalassaemia intermedia, but not as effective in thalassaemia major
- Histone deacetylase inhibitors – derivatives of butyric acid; intermittent pulses with hydroxycarbamide has been tried
- Kit ligand
- Decitabine
- Knockdown of BCL11A (regulator of γ-globin expression)
- Erythropoietin.

ANTIOXIDANTS

- Vitamins C and E
- Fermented papaya preparations.

GENE THERAPY

- Successful in β-thalassaemia animal models using a retroviral vector transferring the human β-globin gene sequence and its promoter region into mice stem cells
- β-Globin gene transfer into progenitor hematopoietic cells of humans is also being studied
- Other molecular approaches being tried include using different mutations of stop codons and aberrant splicing.

transfusion therapy can avert splenomegaly, hypersplenism still can develop, usually in children between 5 and 10 years of age. In these individuals, splenectomy can limit the complications from extramedullary hematopoiesis. Splenectomy should be considered when the annual transfusion requirement reaches 200–250 mL red blood cells/kg per year and usually results in a halving of the transfusion requirements.

Splenectomy complications include opportunistic infections with encapsulated organisms. Patients should therefore receive appropriate vaccinations preoperatively and should be advised to seek medical advice at the first sign of infection. It is advisable to delay splenectomy until patients are at least 5 years old because of the increased risk of overwhelming sepsis below this age. Thalassaemia patients can develop thromboembolic complications and pulmonary hypertension after splenectomy so partial splenectomy and splenic embolization have been attempted to minimize these complications but have not been studied in large trials.

Management of Complications

Iron overload can occur in any organ in thalassaemia patients but particularly affects the heart, liver, the endocrine system, the bone and occasionally the pancreas and lungs. Iron overload needs to be detected early and treated to prevent long-term damage. Annual assessment of the iron loading of the liver and heart can be achieved using non-invasive methods such as magnetic resonance scanning to detect early changes. Children should have regular growth and endocrine assessments and appropriate investigations should be carried out if there are any signs of developmental delay or hormonal deficiencies. Osteoporosis is increasingly being recognized and should be prevented by ensuring adequate dietary calcium intake and sun exposure. Vitamin supplementation with folic acid, zinc, vitamin E and vitamin C may be useful although the combination of vitamin C and desferrioxamine carries a risk of cardiac toxicity.

Stem Cell Transplant

Allogeneic stem cell transplant[169,170] is currently the only means of curing thalassaemia. The outcome in carefully selected patients, measured by overall event-free survival, is around 90% with a transplant-related mortality of 3%. Hepatomegaly, liver fibrosis, and inadequate iron chelation therapy predict a poor outcome. The best results from transplant have been obtained with HLA-matched siblings. Umbilical cord blood is a useful source of stem cells for young children. Other potential treatment options for thalassaemia are outlined in Box 65.16.[171–174]

Prevention of Thalassaemia

Prevention of severe thalassaemia births by prenatal diagnosis and termination of pregnancies has been successful in countries with a high prevalence of thalassaemia.[175] Early identification of couples at risk and culturally sensitive genetic counselling facilitate decision-making for termination or continuation of pregnancy. The mean corpuscular haemoglobin (MCH) is used to screen for the presence of thalassaemia using a cut-off of less than 27 pg. Rarely, silent β-thalassaemia mutation may present with an MCV over 27 pg and should be considered in those with a positive family history. At-risk couples should be referred for detailed counselling on the options for prenatal diagnosis. These include chorionic villous sampling or amniocentesis, which are used to obtain fetal DNA samples for genetic analysis. Polymerase chain reactions and precise hybridization assays to detect single point mutations using very small DNA samples have also been developed. A less invasive and less risky option is to isolate fetal DNA circulating in the maternal blood for genetic analysis. Pre-implantation genetic diagnosis is a newer technique where DNA from the blastomere is used for genetic diagnosis. Ultrasound can be used from the 2nd trimester for fetuses suspected of having α-thalassaemia to detect signs of hydrops fetalis and enlarged placenta (Figure 65.9).[175,176]

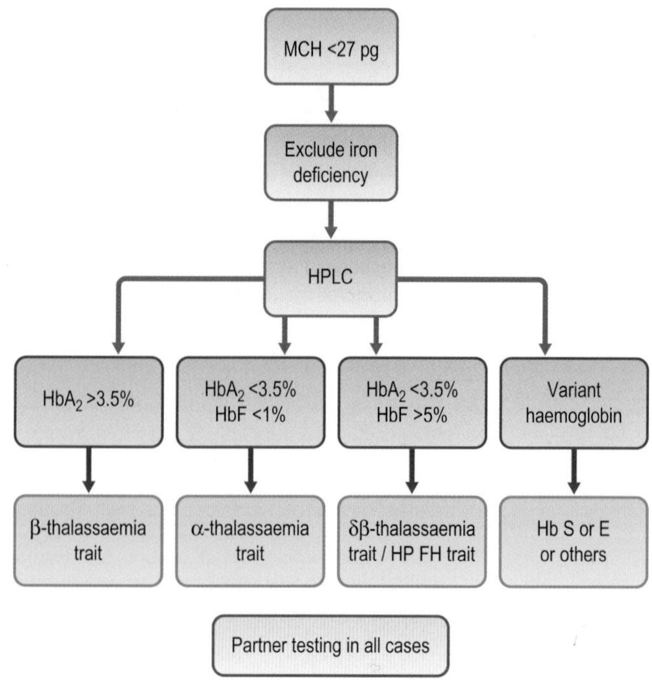

Figure 65.9 Prevention of thalassaemia births using prenatal diagnosis.

HAEMOGLOBIN E DISEASE

Hb E is caused by a substitution of glutamic acid by lysine at codon 26 of the β-globin gene.[177] This causes reduced synthesis of the β-E chain and leads to a thalassaemia phenotype. Hb E β-thalassaemia affects at least a million people worldwide and is an important health problem particularly in the Indian subcontinent and South-east Asia. In some areas, it has replaced β-thalassaemia as the most common thalassaemia disorder. The frequency of HbE reaches 60% in many regions of Thailand, Laos and Cambodia with estimates of at least 100 000 new cases of HbE β-thalassaemia expected in the next few decades in Thailand alone. The natural history of HbE thalassaemia is highly variable; some patients are asymptomatic (e.g. heterozygotes, HbE 20–30% or homozygotes HbE, 80–90%) while others (e.g. HbE with β-thalassaemia) may be transfusion-dependent.

Glucose-6-Phosphate Dehydrogenase (G6PD) Deficiency

PATHOPHYSIOLOGY

Glucose-6-phosphate dehydrogenase (G6PD) deficiency was originally recognized through its association with haemolysis related to eating fava beans ('favism') and primaquine ingestion.[178] G6PD deficiency is the most common enzyme defect in humans and is present in about 400 million people worldwide (Figure 65.10).[179,180] It is an X-linked, hereditary defect caused by mutations in the G6PD gene. G6PD is an enzyme that catalyses the first reaction in the pentose phosphate pathway, to produce NADPH, which is an important antioxidant used to preserve the reduced form of glutathione.[178,181] Reduced glutathione acts as a scavenger for oxidative metabolites thereby protecting red cells. Red cells lack any other source of NADPH and are solely dependent on the pentose phosphate pathway so G6PD deficiency leaves these cells with no defence against oxidative damage. Oxidative damage results in denatured haemoglobin aggregates which form Heinz bodies (denatured haemoglobin precipitates). These damaged cells bind to the membrane cytoskeleton resulting in decreased cellular deformability, and are also destroyed in the spleen, resulting in haemolysis. The level of enzyme activity is higher in young erythrocytes than in more mature cells so older cells are more susceptible to haemolysis.

EPIDEMIOLOGY AND CLASSIFICATION

The global distribution of G6PD deficiency mirrors that of malaria, and where malaria has historically been prevalent, and it provides a degree of protection against malaria.[181,182] The different variants of G6PD deficiency are classified according to the severity of the enzyme deficiency and resulting haemolysis.[183]

- Class I – Severely deficient with chronic non-spherocytic haemolytic anaemia as the clinical manifestation
- Class II – Severely deficient with acute haemolytic anaemia as the clinical manifestation
- Class III – Moderately deficient (10–60% enzyme activity)
- Class IV – Normal (60–150% enzyme activity)
- Class V – Increased activity (>150% enzyme activity).

G6PD enzyme variants can be distinguished by their electrophoretic mobility.[184] G6PD B, the wild-type enzyme, and G6PD A$^+$, a common variant in populations of African descent, demonstrate normal enzyme activity and are not associated with haemolysis. G6PD A$^-$ is the most common variant associated with mild to moderate haemolysis with approximately 10–25%

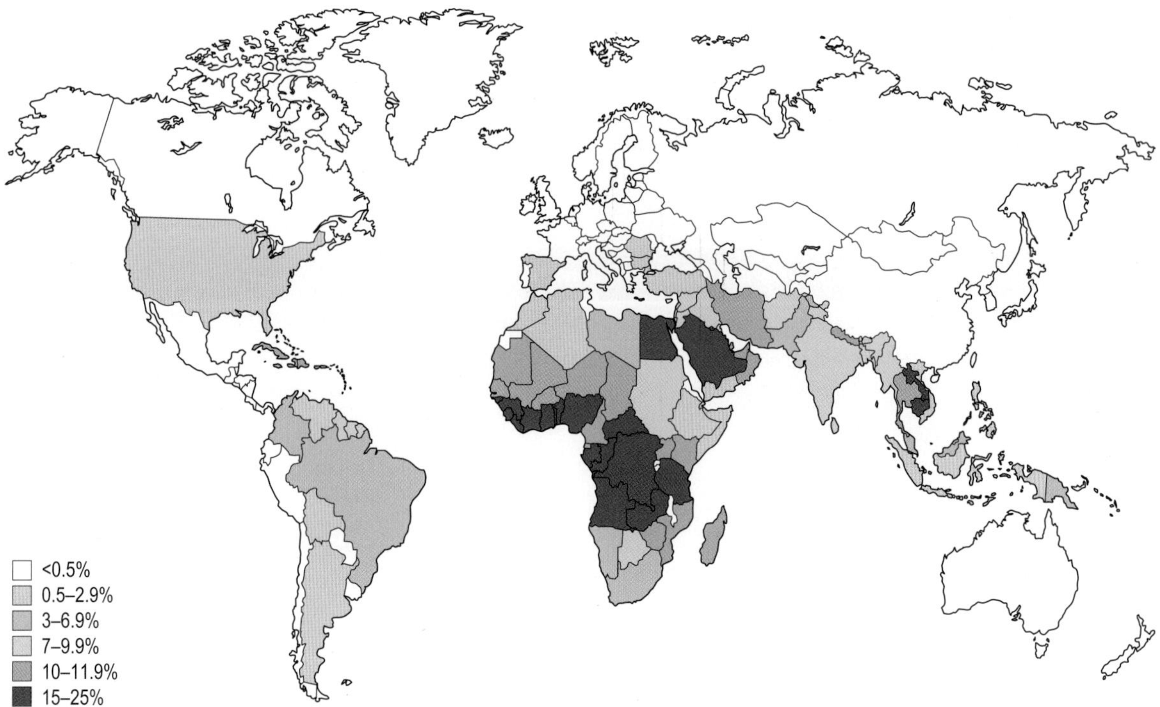

Figure 65.10 Distribution of glucose-6-phosphate dehydrogenase deficiency. *(From WHO working group. Glucose-6-phosphate dehydrogenase deficiency. Bull World Health Organ 1989; 67: 601–11.)*

of Africans carrying this variant. G6PD Mediterranean, present in all countries surrounding the Mediterranean Sea, Middle East, India and Indonesia, has the same electrophoretic mobility as G6PD B but the enzyme synthesis and catalytic activity are reduced. In several populations, G6PD A$^-$ and G6PD Mediterranean co-exist.

CLINICAL FEATURES

The clinical manifestations of G6PD deficiency can be classified into: (i) asymptomatic; (ii) acute haemolytic anaemia; (iii) favism; (iv) neonatal jaundice; and (v) chronic non-spherocytic haemolytic anaemia.

Acute Haemolytic Anaemia

Acute haemolytic anaemia in G6PD deficiency can be secondary to infection (e.g. pneumonia, hepatitis A and B, and typhoid fever) or oxidant drugs, or may be precipitated by diabetic ketoacidosis, myocardial infarction and strenuous physical exercise.[185,186] A list of the drugs which may cause haemolysis in G6PD-deficient individuals (Table 65.9)[187] can be obtained from: http://www.g6pd.org/favism/english/index.mv. A drug which is deemed to be safe for some G6PD-deficient individuals may cause haemolysis in others due to the heterogeneity of the underlying genetic variants. Haemolysis typically occurs within 1–3 days after commencing the drug and can produce intense haemoglobinuria. Fortunately, the disorder is self-limiting and most patients do not develop renal impairment or anaemia requiring transfusion. The spontaneous recovery reflects replacement of the older, enzyme-deficient red cells by younger reticulocytes which can withstand oxidative injury.[186] If the precipitating cause has been removed the haemoglobin begins to recover after 8–10 days. Acute renal failure due to acute tubular necrosis and tubular obstruction by haemoglobin casts can develop as a complication of haemolysis in G6PD deficiency. This occurs more often in adults than children and may require haemodialysis.

Favism

This occurs predominantly in boys aged 1–5 years in Mediterranean countries, but it has also been observed in the Middle East, Asia and North Africa. Both intravascular and extravascular haemolysis, occasionally severe enough to cause renal impairment, can occur after eating fresh or cooked fava beans, and favism has been reported in breastfed babies of mothers who have eaten fava beans.[179] Divicine and isouramil have been implicated as the toxic components of fava beans.[188]

Neonatal Jaundice

This occurs in one-third of male babies in areas where G6PD deficiency is common and is likely due to G6PD deficiency.[179] It presents 1–4 days after birth and can lead to kernicterus.[189,190] Maternal exposure to oxidant drugs, and even naphthalene-camphor mothballs, can precipitate haemolysis in affected babies. Breast-feeding mothers should therefore be warned to avoid offending drugs, umbilical potions containing fava, triple dye or menthol, and should not apply henna to the skin or use clothes that have been stored in naphthalene.[190] Premature infants and babies who have co-inherited the mutation for Gilbert's syndrome are at particular risk. Phototherapy and exchange transfusion therapy may be required to reduce the level of unconjugated bilirubin. The diagnosis may be easily missed so assessment of G6PD status should be undertaken for any jaundiced infant whose family history or ethnic or geographic origin suggest the likelihood of G6PD deficiency, and in infants who respond poorly to phototherapy.[191]

Congenital Non-spherocytic Haemolytic Anaemia

This is an unusual manifestation of G6PD deficiency and usually presents in childhood.[179,184] There may be a history of severe neonatal jaundice, episodic or worsening anaemia which requires blood transfusions, and complications from gallstones. Although these individuals usually have a well-compensated anaemia, and require transfusions only for exacerbations, rarely some may become transfusion-dependent. Antioxidants such as vitamin E and selenium may be of benefit in some cases. The haemolysis does not resolve following splenectomy. Folic acid supplementation is necessary to support the increased compensatory erythropoiesis.

DIAGNOSIS

The diagnosis of G6PD deficiency is usually suspected when neonatal jaundice occurs in an area where G6PD deficiency is

TABLE 65.9 Drugs Which May Cause Haemolysis in G6PD-Deficient Individuals

	Definite Haemolysis	Possible Haemolysis	Doubtful Haemolysis
Antimalarials	Primaquine Pamaquine	Chloroquine	Mepacrine Quinine
Sulfonamides	Sulfanilamide Sulfacetamide Sulfapyridine Sulfamethoxazole	Sulfadimidine Sulfasalazine Glibenclamide	Aldesulfone Sulfadiazine Sulfisoxazole
Sulfones	Dapsone		
Nitrofurantoin	Nitrofurantoin		
Antipyretic or analgesic	Acetanilide	Aspirin	Paracetamol Phenacetin
Other drugs	Nalidixic acid Niridazole Methylthionium Phenazopyridine Co-trimoxazole	Ciprofloxacin Chloramphenicol Vitamin K analogues Ascorbic acid Mesalazine	Aminosalicylic acid Doxorubicin Probenecid Dimercaprol
Other chemicals	Naphthalene 2,4,6-trinitrotoluene	Acalypha indica extract	

common or when an episode of non-immune haemolytic anaemia occurs in association with an infection or drug. The appearance of the red cells on the blood film is characteristic because denatured haemoglobin concentrates in one area within the cell creating 'helmet' or 'bite' cells.[192] Denatured haemoglobin precipitates in peripheral red blood cells as Heinz bodies which can be detected by staining with methyl violet. Definitive diagnosis of G6PD deficiency is by quantitative spectrophotometric analysis of the rate of NADPH production. Point of care tests for G6PD deficiency are being developed but have not yet been validated for routine use. Measuring enzyme activity during an episode of acute haemolysis is not helpful since reticulocytosis, which is a feature of acute haemolysis, produces a false-negative result because of the high enzyme levels in younger erythrocytes.[179,186]

MANAGEMENT

The most effective management strategy for G6PD deficiency is to prevent haemolysis by avoiding triggering agents like infections, drugs and fava beans. For the milder variants (e.g. Class III and IV), drugs known to trigger haemolysis may be given to individuals with G6PD deficiency if the benefits outweigh the risks and the blood count is closely monitored (e.g. use of low-dose primaquine for individuals with G6PD A-variant). Screening programmes have been established in some Mediterranean and other populations where G6PD deficiency is prevalent.[193]

Haematological Complications of Malaria (see Chapter 43)

MALARIAL ANAEMIA

Pathophysiology

The pathophysiology of anaemia in malaria is multi-factorial and influenced by the age of the individual and their anti-malarial immune status. Anaemia mechanisms in malaria involve:

- Haemolysis with increased red cell destruction of both infected and bystander erythrocytes
- Dyserythropoiesis
- Hypersplenism
- Haemolysis
- Co-existent conditions which can cause anaemia.

Haemolysis is more common in non-immune individuals with acute malaria, whereas dyserythropoiesis is the predominant mechanism for anaemia in recurrent falciparum malaria.[207,194] Haemolysis is the result of red cell phagocytosis by the reticuloendothelial system and is triggered by damage to the red cell membranes and exposure of abnormal surface antigens on their surface.[195–198] Ten uninfected red cells are removed from the circulation for each infected red cell destroyed,[199] possibly related to loss of red cell complement regulatory proteins and increased levels of circulating immune complexes.[200] This may partly explain the persistent or worsening anaemia following parasite clearance and the poor correlation between parasitaemia and the severity of anaemia noted in some studies.[207] An increased incidence of anaemia has been noted in malaria vaccine trials possibly due to enhanced clearance of uninfected red blood cells.[201]

Decreased erythropoeisis with abnormalities in red cell precursors and reticulocytopenia is found consistently on examination of bone marrow from malaria-infected patients.[202] The decreased erythropoiesis is due to many factors including low levels of TNF-α, high levels of interleukin-10, abnormalities of erythropoietin, a decrease in burst colony forming units, cytokine-induced suppression of red cell production and the inhibitory effect of the malarial pigment haemozoin.[203–206]

Epidemiology

Malaria-related anaemia is most commonly seen in children and pregnant women. The prevalence of malarial anaemia in sub-Saharan Africa in children is 30–90% and in pregnant women it is 60–80%.[207] The highest prevalence is in infants and children less than 3 years of age. Infants may acquire malaria through the placenta.[208,209]

Individuals living in malarious areas may have multiple reasons for anaemia such as bacteraemia, hookworm infections and vitamin A deficiency[208] making it difficult to assign anaemia solely to malaria. However, animal studies and the fact that anaemia improves with anti-malarial treatment suggest a direct relationship between malaria infection and anaemia.[210,211] For example, in Tanzanian children about 60% of anaemic episodes were thought to be caused by malaria.[212]

WHO defines severe anaemia attributable to malaria as: (i) haemoglobin concentration <50 g/L or haematocrit <15%; (ii) parasitaemia with >10 000 parasites/μL of blood and (iii) normocytic blood film (to exclude other common causes of anaemia).[213] However, aspects of this definition have been criticized because blood films are not examined routinely and parasite density varies with endemicity and age.[207] Although traditionally it is *P. falciparum* that has been associated with the most severe malaria-related anaemia, *P. vivax* is also a major risk factor for severe anaemia especially in young children or those with chronic and recurrent infections. *P. vivax* anaemia is associated with recurrent bouts of haemolysis of predominantly uninfected erythrocytes with increased fragility.[214]

Clinical Features

Symptoms of malarial anaemia can vary from negligible to profound depending on the degree of anaemia and the rapidity of onset. Splenomegaly is a common feature of malarial anaemia because of the role of the spleen in the removal of both infected and uninfected red cells.[215] Blackwater fever, characterized by intense intravascular haemolysis with haemoglobinuria and occasionally renal failure in a patient with malaria, may be related to underlying glucose-6-phosphate deficiency.[216,217] Factors such as poor nutrition, deficiencies of vitamins and micronutrients, bacteraemia, and hookworm or HIV infection may co-exist with malaria and contribute to anaemia[209] so non-malarial causes of anaemia should be considered in patients whose anaemia does not respond to malaria treatment.

Management and Prevention

The management of severe malarial anaemia involves supportive care and treatment of the malaria and any other underlying conditions. Recovery from malaria-associated anaemia can be slow, taking 6 weeks or even longer if there are episodes of re-infection.[212] In children, blood transfusion is usually reserved for those with haemoglobin levels of less than 40 g/L (<50 g/L if there are complications such as respiratory distress[207]). There have been some concerns about a possible increased risk of infection associated with iron supplementation for children in malarious areas[218,219] but current recommendations advocate that where iron deficiency and malaria are common, iron supplements should not be withheld and appropriate anti-malarial treatment or prevention should also be offered.[220]

The best way to prevent malarial anaemia is to prevent malaria infection by avoiding mosquito bites (e.g. through the use of bed nets) or through chemoprophylaxis. Malaria chemoprophylaxis during infancy can reduce both malaria and anaemia.[221] Children who have been hospitalized with severe malarial anaemia may benefit from intermittent preventive malarial therapy after discharge to prevent recurrence of anaemia.[222] Daily co-trimoxazole prophylaxis which is used for HIV-infected individuals has been shown to reduce malaria parasitaemia and anaemia.[223]

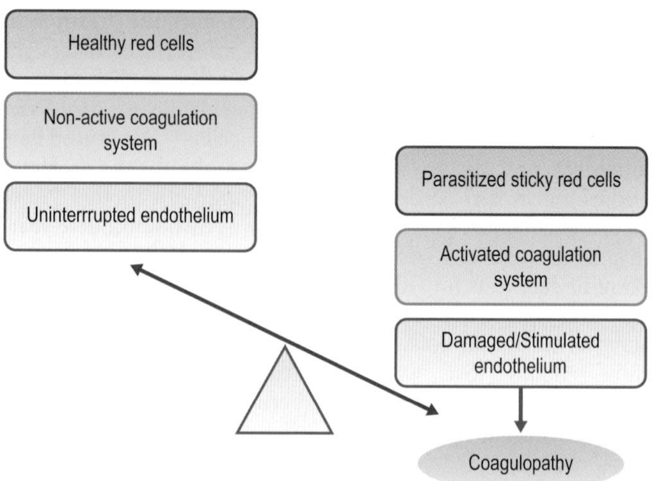

Figure 65.12 Coagulopathy induced by malaria infection.

THROMBOCYTOPENIA IN MALARIA

The normal platelet life span of 7–10 days is reduced to less than 4 days in malaria infection.[224] Several factors are responsible for thrombocytopenia in malaria infection, the most common being increased platelet activation and aggregation (Figure 65.11).[225] Platelet activation is by parasitized red cells which express surface tissue factor and initiate coagulation and platelet aggregation. The resultant activated endothelium binds platelets and sequesters them in vascular beds including in the cerebral vasculature.[226,234] These platelets facilitate the adhesion of parasitized red cells[227] and the release of von Willebrand factor multimers which cause widespread platelet aggregation leading to thrombocytopenia[228,84,231] Platelet synthesis by the bone marrow is relatively well maintained during infection[231,229] but antiplatelet antibodies, immune complexes and splenomegaly all contribute to thrombocytopenia.[230]

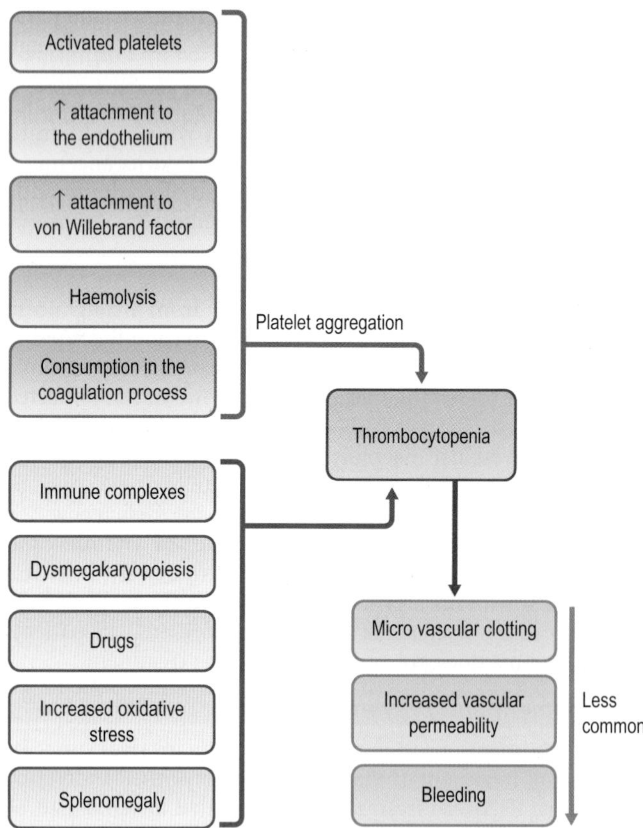

Figure 65.11 Factors associated with thrombocytopenia in malaria infection. The more significant mechanisms are given in bold. The mechanisms described in the top half cause thrombocytopenia by platelet aggregation, which is the major consequence on platelets.

Thrombocytopenia occurs in 60–90% of individuals infected with malaria irrespective of the species of plasmodium.[214,231] Thrombocytopenia in febrile patients in an endemic area increases the probability of malaria by a factor of 5[232] and in individuals returning from tropical countries with a fever, thrombocytopenia is highly specific for malaria infection.[233] Profound thrombocytopenia is unusual and malaria-associated thrombocytopenia is rarely associated with haemorrhagic manifestations.[234]

The clinical consequences of platelet aggregation and endothelial binding are primarily microvascular ischaemia. This may manifest as renal impairment, cerebral ischaemia, and occlusion of retinal vasculature or even in some cases, skin necrosis. Bleeding is unlikely, although in severe thrombocytopenia, petechiae or purpura may develop which denotes extravasation of red cells into the subcutaneous tissue.[235] Continued platelet activation and consumption can exacerbate bleeding and decreased circulating platelets are associated with increased vascular leakage and the development of oedema.[236] Platelet transfusions are rarely required because the platelet count generally rises rapidly on treating the underlying malaria.

COAGULOPATHY IN MALARIA

Coagulopathy is a disturbance of the whole coagulation system involving not just coagulation factors but platelets, anticoagulant factors, fibrinolytic system and, in the case of malaria, the parasitized red cells and the vascular endothelium. Parasitized red cells induce expression of tissue factor on endothelial cells and monocytes, release of microparticles, cytokine release and platelet clumping, all of which initiate blood coagulation and tilt the balance towards the pro-coagulant state (Figure 65.12).[234,237–242] Anticoagulant factors are severely depleted in malaria. Protein C and antithrombin levels are inversely correlated with severity of falciparum malaria and return to normal with treatment of the malaria.[245]

Coagulopathy in malaria infection is unusual, occurring in less than 5% of cases. It appears to be most common in adults with cerebral malaria who may present with gastrointestinal bleeding[243] or with microvascular ischaemia in the brain, kidneys, retina and occasionally, the dermal vasculature.[244] Prolongation of prothrombin time and activated partial thromboplastin time only occur in 4–8% of patients with *P. falciparum* infection and coagulopathy does not appear to be a feature of *P. vivax* infection.[245] Since coagulation factors need to be depleted to less than 20% of normal to prolong the clotting times, these tests can be normal despite active coagulopathy.

Management of coagulopathy aims to restore the balance between pro- and anticoagulant processes. This is complex and requires input from a coagulation specialist and ideally, access to plasma, heparin and factor concentrates and a well-equipped coagulation laboratory.

Haematological Complications of HIV Infection (see Chapter 10)

ANAEMIA

Anaemia is very common in HIV-infected individuals occurring in up to 20% at initial presentation and about 70% at some stage during their disease.[246] Thirty-seven percent of patients with clinical AIDS have a 1-year incidence of anaemia (haemoglobin <100 g/L)[246] and high rates of anaemia persist despite combination anti retroviral treatment (ART).[247] Anaemia is directly related to mortality in HIV infection and is independent of other risk factors including CD4 count.[248]

There are multiple reasons for anaemia in HIV-infected patients (Box 65.17), which often co-exist in individual patients. Bone marrow infection by mycobacteria species, *Histoplasma*, *Cryptococcus* and *Penicillium marneffei* can all decrease red cell production[249] and can be detected by bone marrow examination and cultures. Parvovirus has a predilection for the erythroid progenitor cells and can cause severe anaemia in HIV-infected patients. Serological tests for parvovirus are unhelpful in HIV-infected patients and viral polymerase chain reaction is needed to confirm the diagnosis.[250] The likelihood of parvovirus-induced anaemia increases with the severity of anaemia and has been found in 31% of individuals with HIV and haemoglobin less than 70 g/L.[251] Haemophagocytosis occurs in HIV infections and may be secondary to co-infection with mycobacteria, cytomegalovirus, Epstein–Barr or other herpesviruses.

Poor nutrition due to socioeconomic reasons, HIV-related anorexia, malabsorption from conditions affecting the gastrointestinal tract, and achlorhydria may contribute to anaemia. Haemolytic anaemia occurs secondary to drugs or concomitant glucose-6 phosphate dehydrogenase deficiency and because reticulocytopenia is common in those with HIV infection, reticulocyte counts cannot be used to exclude haemolysis. Although the direct Coombs test may be positive in patients with HIV infection, autoimmune haemolysis is not a common cause of anaemia. A reduction in red cell precursors has also been noted in children in Africa with severe anaemia.[252]

Treatment of HIV-related anaemia should focus on starting ART and eliminating any other factors, such as infections or vitamin deficiencies, which may contribute to the anaemia. In wealthy countries ART has been shown to reduce anaemia prevalence from 65% to 53% within 6 months of starting treatment, and to 46% after a year.[253,247] Although transfusions may be required in severe life-threatening cases of anaemia, aggressive transfusion therapy has been associated with fatal pulmonary emboli due to accelerated haemolysis and disseminated intravascular coagulation.[254]

In those who do not respond to ART, erythropoietin may be considered since reduced responsiveness to this hormone and antierythropoietin antibodies have been noted in HIV patients. Erythropoietin is particularly useful in individuals whose erythropoietin levels are less than 500 IU/L[255] because in addition to increasing the haemoglobin it can also improve the quality of life.[256] Erythropoietin may take several weeks to achieve full effect and patients should be replete in haematinics. Erythropoietin can very rarely be associated with thrombosis or pure red cell aplasia.

BOX 65.17 CAUSES OF ANAEMIA IN HIV INFECTION

INFECTIONS
- Mycobacteria (tuberculosis or atypical forms)
- Parvovirus
- Opportunistic viruses – cytomegalovirus
- Histoplasma capsulatum
- Malaria
- HIV itself

MALIGNANT INFILTRATION OF THE BONE MARROW
- Lymphoma
- Other malignancies

HAEMOLYSIS
- Drug-induced
- Autoimmune haemolysis
- Microangiopathic haemolysis

INSUFFICIENT NUTRIENTS
- Iron
- Vitamin deficiencies (folate, B_{12}, A)

GASTROINTESTINAL BLEEDING
- Gastritis (e.g. *Candida*)
- Gastric and duodenal ulcers
- Intestinal Kaposi's sarcoma or lymphoma
- Viral infections such as cytomegalovirus

DRUGS
- Bone marrow suppression (e.g. ganciclovir)
- Glucose-6-phosphate dehydrogenase deficiency haemolysis (e.g. Dapsone)

HAEMOPHAGOCYTOSIS
- Infection related

HYPERSPLENISM

ANAEMIA OF CHRONIC DISEASE

CO-EXISTENT HAEMOGLOBINOPATHIES

HYPOGONADISM.

THROMBOCYTOPENIA

Thrombocytopenia is a common finding in HIV-infected patients and it may be the initial manifestation of HIV infection in as many as 10% of patients. Data from wealthy countries demonstrate platelet counts less than 150 × 10^9/L in 11% of patients, and less than 50 × 10^9/L in 1.5%. Overall the 1-year incidence of moderate thrombocytopenia ($<50 \times 10^9$/L) is 3.7%, though this is higher in those with clinical AIDS (8.7%).[257,258] Thrombocytopenia is more common in those who abuse drugs, have opportunistic infections and malignant disorders of the bone marrow (e.g. lymphoma), and it may also be a side-effect of therapeutic drugs.[259]

The most common cause of thrombocytopenia in HIV infection is immune thrombocytopenia which may be associated with hepatitis C co-infection, and produces decreased platelet survival, particularly at CD4 counts below 200/μL. The anti-platelet antibodies, immune complexes and cross-reacting antibodies to HIV envelope proteins and platelets, which occur in HIV-associated thrombocytopenia[259,260] may also contribute to generation of reactive oxygen species.[261] Platelet production can also be affected in HIV infection and may explain the high levels of thrombopoietin that have been documented in HIV-related thrombocytopenia.[262]

Some cases of HIV-related thrombocytopenia may undergo spontaneous remission so treatment of thrombocytopenia is usually only initiated if it is associated with bleeding, which is unusual.[259] The first line of treatment involves antiretroviral therapy with the aim of achieving undetectable plasma HIV viraemia.[263,264] Any drugs that may be associated with causing thrombocytopenia should be withdrawn and opportunistic infections or secondary malignancies treated. The treatment of immune thrombocytopenia is the same as in non-HIV cases and options include a short course of steroids, intravenous immunoglobulin (short-lived response), anti-D, interferon-α or splenectomy.

THROMBOTIC THROMBOCYTOPENIC PURPURA

Although there are multiple causes of thrombocytopenia in HIV-positive individuals, one of the most devastating is the thrombotic microangiopathy of thrombotic thrombocytopenic purpura (TTP). This is because the combination of haemolytic anaemia and microthrombi has a very poor prognosis. Symptoms are nonspecific and may include fever, headache, bleeding and changes in consciousness. If TTP is suspected, an urgent blood film should be requested and the combination of thrombocytopenia with red cell fragmentation is highly suggestive of TTP. TTP associated with HIV infection was more frequent before the introduction of ART and is more common if adherence to treatment is poor or resistance to therapy has developed.[265] TTP is thought to be due to endothelial damage, but unlike the situation in non-HIV-infected individuals, low levels of ADAMTS-13 are not a useful predictor of outcome.[266]

Treatment of TTP involves plasma exchange, and although refractoriness may occur, this can be corrected by ART in some cases.[266] If ART is administered in these cases it is important to maintain adherence throughout the period of plasma exchange. If apheresis facilities are limited, plasma infusions alone (30 mL/kg per day) may also produce a response.[267] ART should also be administered immediately after plasma exchange to minimize drug removal. Patients with a viral load of less than 500 000 copies/mL generally require fewer plasma exchanges for remission than those with a higher load.[265] Survival of patients with HIV-associated TTP in the pre-ART era was rarely longer than 2 years, even with plasma exchange and steroid treatment, but for patients who are compliant with ART the mortality is around 4%.[268,269]

HIV-RELATED LYMPHOMA

Non-Hodgkin's lymphoma (NHL) was noted to be associated with HIV infection early in the epidemic and is an AIDS-defining illness.[270] The incidence of NHL is up to 200 times greater in HIV-infected adults than in those who are not infected, and it is responsible for nearly one-sixth of the deaths attributable to AIDS. Since the introduction of HAART, the incidence of all types of NHL has decreased by approximately 30–50%[271,272] and the outcome of HIV-infected patients with lymphoma has improved. In the setting of clinical trials, the 60% 1-year survival rate is comparable to those without HIV infection.[273] The incidence of Hodgkin's lymphoma has increased in the post-HAART era, possibly due to immune reconstitution and increased CD4 cells.[274,275] Evidence of Epstein-Barr virus (EBV) infection can be found in virtually all cases of Hodgkin's disease.[276]

HIV-related lymphomas (Box 65.18)[277] (see also Lymphomas, below), are broadly divided into systemic lymphomas (80%) and primary central nervous system lymphomas.[278] The incidence of highly aggressive lymphomas, either Burkitt's lymphoma (approx. 25%) or diffuse large B-cell lymphoma (approx. 75%), is much higher in HIV-infected patients than in those without infection.[279] Although T-cell lymphomas are uncommon in HIV disease (1%), there has been an increase in recent years. The incidence of primary central nervous system lymphoma in HIV-affected individuals is 2–6% and it is 1000 times more common than in the general population.[280]

The pathogenesis of NHL in HIV infection is related to the inadequate host immune responses to viruses with oncogenic potential, predominantly EBV and human herpesvirus 8 (HHV8)/Kaposi's sarcoma-associated herpesvirus. This allows unregulated lymphoid growth and an accumulation of genetic abnormalities in B cells.[272] Markers of B-cell activation such as serum immunoglobulins and free light chains, and CD4 cell count have been suggested as predictive markers for the development of NHL in HIV infection.[281,282]

Extranodal and leptomeningeal involvement, and B-symptoms occur in the majority of HIV-infected patients with NHL and the bone marrow is commonly involved. The most common extranodal site to be involved is the

BOX 65.18 LYMPHOMAS ASSOCIATED WITH HIV INFECTION

LYMPHOMAS ALSO OCCURRING IN IMMUNOCOMPETENT PATIENTS

- Diffuse large B-cell lymphoma
- Burkitt's lymphoma
- Extranodal marginal zone B-cell lymphoma of mucosa associated
- Mucosa-associated lymphoid-tissue (MALT) lymphoma
- Peripheral T-cell lymphoma

LYMPHOMAS OCCURRING MORE SPECIFICALLY IN HIV+ PATIENTS

- Primary effusion lymphoma
- Plasmablastic lymphoma of the oral cavity type

LYMPHOMAS ALSO OCCURRING IN OTHER IMMUNODEFICIENCY STATES

- Polymorphic B-cell lymphoma
- 'Post-transplant lymphoproliferative disorder (PTLD)-like'.

gastrointestinal tract, often the stomach or the perianal region.[283] Hepatic involvement, seen in a quarter of cases, is associated with a particularly poor prognosis. CNS disease may be asymptomatic so diagnostic lumbar puncture may be required.[284] HIV-related lymphomas frequently present with poor prognostic features such as elevated serum lactate dehydrogenase levels.[285,286] Older age, lowest nadir CD4 cell counts prior to NHL diagnosis, developing NHL while on ART, and cumulative HIV viraemia are also poor prognostic features.[282] A formal prognostic scoring system has been developed which takes into account the CD4 count (<100 cells/μL).[287]

Some types of HIV-related lymphoma are associated with characteristic clinical and laboratory features. Primary effusion lymphoma is an aggressive lymphoma characterized by effusions in serosal cavities in the absence of any other tumour masses.[288,289] It is strongly associated with HHV8 infection and the virus can be identified in the nuclei of the malignant cells. Plasmablastic lymphoma mainly affects the oral cavity and the mucosa of the jaw and is typically associated with Epstein–Barr virus.[290]

Histological examination of biopsied tissue is necessary to confirm the diagnosis and type of lymphoma. Diagnostic difficulties may arise because HIV-related hyperplasia in lymph node biopsies may be confused with lymphoma, the histological appearance of HIV-related lymphomas may be different from those of non-infected individuals[291] and many opportunistic pathogens may mimic the appearances of NHL, or co-exist with it, and will need to be identified or excluded before making a diagnosis of lymphoma.

Prior to the widespread use of ART, conventional lymphoma chemotherapy resulted in considerable toxicity, increased opportunistic infections and high mortality. ART has facilitated the use of conventional doses of chemotherapy in conjunction with haematopoietic growth factor support. This has markedly improved the outcome of patients with HIV-related lymphomas who now have overall response rates of 60%.[292] The concomitant use of ART and chemotherapy is therefore recommended, especially in those with CD4 counts of less than 100/μL. Anti-CD20 antibody is now included in treatment regimens for NHL, and studies that include patients with HIV-related lymphomas all report favourable outcomes.[293,294] Some antiretroviral agents such as zidovudine are best avoided in combination with chemotherapy, because it adds to the myelosuppression of chemotherapy. Didanosine may worsen the peripheral neuropathy caused by taxanes and vinca alkaloids. HIV-infected patients undergoing chemotherapy should receive adequate anti-infective prophylaxis due to the high risk of opportunistic infections such as pneumocystis, herpes simplex and zoster and candida. Consolidation chemotherapy and stem cell transplant have been used successfully in relapsed HIV-related lymphomas.

Abnormalities of Coagulation

PATHOPHYSIOLOGY

Haemostasis is maintained by interactions between vessel walls, platelets and a balance between pro- and anticoagulant factors. Although the process of haemostasis is usually considered to occur in a stepwise fashion, in vivo the steps happen virtually simultaneously. Activation of the lining of the endothelium by trauma, cancer cells or cytokines triggers vasoconstriction, which immediately limits the amount of blood loss. Exposure of the subendothelial space releases factors such as von Willebrand factor multimers which bind to platelets and initiate platelet adhesion to the endothelium. The adherent platelets release their granules and attract more platelets, which in combination with fibrinogen, form an aggregate. The activated platelets also attract coagulation factors thereby promoting the clotting process. The critical parts of clot formation are the conversion of prothrombin to thrombin and the thrombin-facilitated conversion of fibrinogen to fibrin (Figure 65.13). Haemostatic control mechanisms operate throughout the clotting process to prevent excessive clot formation and involve proteins C and S, and anti-thrombin and antifibrinolytic systems. Any alteration in these regulatory pathways can lead to either bleeding or thrombotic complications.

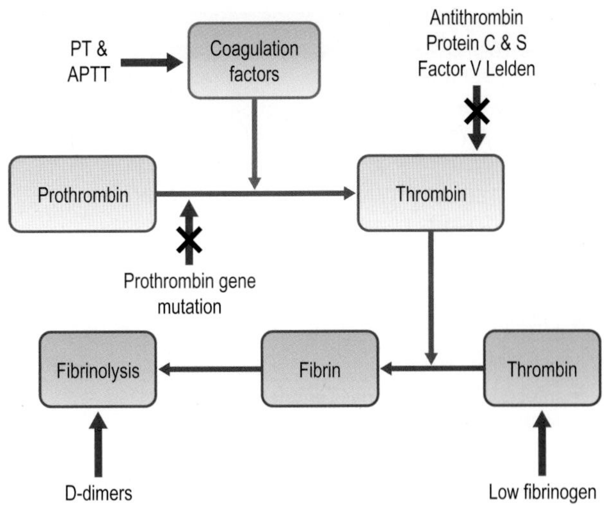

Figure 65.13 Critical processes in clot formation.

Bleeding can result from:

- Inadequate vasoconstriction, due to vascular problems which can be acquired (e.g. viral haemorrhagic fevers or immune vasculitis) or congenital (e.g. collagen vascular disorders)
- Qualitative or quantitative abnormality of von Willebrand factor causing von Willebrand's disease
- Decreased number or function of platelets which can be either acquired (e.g. aspirin, NSAIDs) or congenital (e.g. platelet function defects)
- Qualitative (e.g. caused by inhibitors to coagulation factors, commonly factor VIII) or quantitative (e.g. haemophilia) abnormality of coagulation factors
- Increased fibrinolysis (e.g. viral haemorrhagic fevers, snake bites).

ACQUIRED BLEEDING DISORDERS

Acquired bleeding disorders are commonly caused by vitamin K deficiency, disseminated intravascular coagulation (DIC) or platelet disorders (Box 65.19) but may sometimes be due to acquired inhibitors of coagulation factors. The initial laboratory tests in a patient with excessive bleeding should therefore include a platelet count, clotting screen (prothrombin time (PT) and activated partial thromboplastin time (aPTT)), and

BOX 65.19 ACQUIRED BLEEDING DISORDERS

VITAMIN K DEFICIENCY

- Dietary deficiency or malabsorption
- Systemic illness (e.g. liver disease)
- Haemorrhagic disease of newborn

DISSEMINATED INTRAVASCULAR COAGULATION

- Viral and bacterial infections
- Obstetric disorders (e.g. septic abortion, placental abruption)
- Shock (e.g. trauma, surgical, burns)
- Envenomation

PLATELET DISORDERS

- Infections (e.g. malaria, dengue)
- Hypersplenism
- Immune (e.g. ITP, drugs, HIV)
- Others (e.g. cyclical, congenital, cytotoxic or non-steroidal drugs).

fibrinogen levels, which may be helpful in cases of excessive fibrinolysis (Table 65.10). A difficult venepuncture can cause in vitro activation of the clotting system resulting in a shortened PT or aPTT. Similar findings may occur in chronic DIC due to in vivo activation. The PT and aPTT are not necessarily good predictors of the bleeding risk because some clotting disorders associated with thrombosis (e.g. anti-phospholipid antibodies) can prolong the aPTT. A shortened aPTT can be associated with marked elevation of factor VIII levels (e.g. pregnancy) and may be a predictor of deep vein thrombosis. A prolonged thrombin time is caused by quantitative or qualitative fibrinogen deficiency, heparin and fibrin degradation products. Reptilase time is helpful to distinguish between fibrinogen abnormalities (prolonged reptilase time) and heparin therapy (normal reptilase time).

Vitamin K Deficiency

Deficiency of vitamin K can be due to poor diet, small bowel disease or bile flow obstruction. Clotting factors (II, VII, IX and X) are dependent on vitamin K which is a fat-soluble vitamin. Vitamin K deficiency therefore causes prolongation of the PT and APTT. In newborn infants, vitamin-K-dependent clotting factors can drop precipitously within a couple of days of birth. This causes haemorrhagic disease of the newborn which particularly affects infants that are premature, exclusively breast fed or have been exposed to drugs for tuberculosis, convulsions or anticoagulation in utero. These babies develop bleeding into the skin and gut, or bleeding from the umbilical stump or circumcision.

Vitamin K deficiency will respond to intravenous vitamin K (10 mg/day for 3 days orally or by intravenous injection) and in severe bleeding the clotting abnormality can be treated with fresh frozen plasma. Haemorrhagic disease of the newborn can be prevented with 1 mg of intramuscular vitamin K given at delivery.

Disseminated Intravascular Coagulation

Disseminated intravascular coagulation (DIC) is characterized by activation of haemostasis with widespread fibrin formation, activation of fibrinolysis and consumption of platelets and clotting factors. It may be precipitated by tissue injury, obstetric complications, malignancies and infections and is a serious condition with a high mortality. Patients present with spontaneous bruising or excessive bleeding from minor wounds such as venepuncture sites, and they may also have signs of complications such as renal failure, acute respiratory distress syndrome and microangiopathic haemolytic anaemia. DIC is associated with a combination of depleted clotting factors (i.e. prolonged PT and APTT), a falling platelet count, red cell fragments on the blood film, raised D-dimers or fibrin degradation products, and reduced fibrinogen levels. Management of disseminated intravascular coagulation includes treating or removing the underlying cause, and correcting the haemostatic abnormalities with combinations of platelets, cryoprecipitate and fresh frozen plasma.

Acquired Platelet Disorders

Although bleeding due to thrombocytopenia is unusual unless the platelet counts falls below 10–20 × 10^9/L, bleeding may occur with a normal platelet count and normal clotting screening tests (i.e. PT and aPTT) if platelet functions are impaired (e.g. myelodysplastic syndromes). Platelet transfusions are generally not required unless there is active bleeding or prior to surgery.

Idiopathic Thrombocytopenic Purpura. Idiopathic thrombocytopenic purpura is due to immune destruction of platelets. It is usually primary but can be associated with conditions such as lymphomas and infections including HIV. It may present incidentally or with petechiae, bruising or bleeding from the nose or gums, especially if the platelet count is less than 20 ×

TABLE 65.10 Interpretation of Clotting Tests

PT	aPTT	Plt	Condition
N	N	N	Common – Normal haemostasis, vascular abnormalities[a] Rare – Platelet dysfunction, dysfibrinogenaemia, mild coagulation factor defect[b] Extremely rare – Factor XIII deficiency, alpha 2 antiplasmin deficiency
Long	N	N	Common – Early oral anticoagulation, early vitamin K deficiency Rare – Factor VII deficiency
N	Long	N	Common – Antiphospholipid antibody, Heparin, Factors VIII, IX, XI, XII, deficiency, vonWillebrand's disease Rare – inhibitors to the above factors
Long	Long	N	Common – Vitamin K deficiency[c], oral anticoagulants[c] Rare – Factors V, VII, X and II deficiency
Long	Long	N	Heparin[d], liver disease, fibrinogen deficiency, hyperfibrinolysis
Long	Long	Low	DIC, acute liver disease

Plt, Platelet count; N, normal; DIC, disseminated intravascular coagulation.

[a]Vascular abnormalities include scurvy, Cushing's disease and Ehlers Danlos.

[b]A mild coagulation defect below the detection of the routine tests or which has been masked by the administration of blood products (e.g. mild factor VIII deficiency; some cases of von Willebrand's disease).

[c]PT is relatively more prolonged than aPTT.

[d]TT is extremely sensitive to heparin and a normal reptilase time is useful to confirm the presence of heparin.

10^9/L. Spontaneous recovery occurs less commonly in adults than in children. It is important to exclude other causes of thrombocytopenia such as drugs, DIC or sepsis. The diagnosis can be suspected from a bone marrow examination which shows increased numbers of platelet precursors. Treatment with prednisolone (0.25–0.5 mg/kg) is usually only necessary if there is bleeding or excessive bruising and the dose should be reduced slowly once the platelet count improves. Second-line treatments include immunosuppressive agents and danazol. Splenectomy may also be beneficial but carries an increased risk of infection. Platelet transfusions or intravenous gammaglobulin can temporarily increase the platelet count in an emergency or prior to surgical procedures.

INHERITED BLEEDING DISORDERS

Inherited bleeding disorders can be classified broadly into coagulation factor deficiencies (e.g. factor VIII and factor IX deficiencies), von Willebrand's disease and platelet disorders. The frequency of genes for inherited bleeding disorders is the same throughout the world. Haemophilia A has a prevalence of about 10/10 000, von Willebrand's disease of >10/10 000 and haemophilia B of <0.1/10 000. These conditions occur more frequently among populations where consanguineous marriage is common and where prenatal diagnostic facilities are unavailable.

In general, individuals with inherited coagulation factor deficiencies present with soft tissue bleeds such as haemarthroses or intramuscular bleeds. Those with platelet disorders or von Willebrand's disease tend to present with mucosal bleeds, however severe (type III) von Willebrand's disease can present with severe soft tissue bleeds. Many of these conditions are diagnosed following excessive and uncontrolled bleeding after trauma or surgical procedures. Menorrhagia and delayed severe postpartum haemorrhage may be presenting features of bleeding disorders, particularly von Willebrand's disease or hypothyroidism, which can cause decreased synthesis of von Willebrand factor. Some inherited platelet function disorders are associated with characteristic syndromes (e.g. oculocutaneous albinism or skeletal defects) which may provide a clue to the diagnosis.

Early recognition of symptoms by clinicians, teachers and the public is important so that early treatment can be established. Patients with inherited bleeding disorders are usually managed with blood products (Box 65.20) or chemotherapy designed to reduce bleeding and associated complications.[295,296,298,299] Clotting factor concentrates may be imported or produced locally by fractionation of plasma and are included in the WHO list of essential medicines.[297,298] One international unit (IU) of FVIII clotting factor concentrate per capita is recommended as the minimum requirement for countries wishing to achieve optimal survival for their haemophilia population but only about 25% of the estimated 400 000 people in the world with haemophilia receive adequate treatment. Management of patients with bleeding disorders relies on a well-equipped and quality assessed laboratory for accurate diagnosis and monitoring of treatment and access to plasma and components for replacement therapy. Appropriate support services such as physiotherapy, orthopaedics and counselling should also be available. In many countries inherited bleeding disorders are associated with stigma, which is particularly directed against the mothers of affected children,[297] so educational interventions are an important intervention.

BOX 65.20 PRINCIPLES OF MANAGEMENT OF HAEMOPHILIA AND RELATED CONDITIONS IN LOW-INCOME SETTINGS

EDUCATION

- For the individual
- For the family
- For the healthcare providers

DIAGNOSIS

- Local laboratories
- Central laboratories to ensure quality control and provide training

ANCILLARY TREATMENTS

- Soft tissue bleeds – PRICE: Protection, Rest, Ice packs, Compression and Elevation (avoid compression in children who may not be able to report adverse symptoms like paresthesiae)
- Mucosal bleed – tranexamic acid mouthwashes (better than tablets)
- Regular physiotherapy

DEFINITIVE TREATMENT

Early factor replacement for soft tissue bleeds may limit prolonged product requirement and long-term damage

- Musculoskeletal bleeds – 5–15 U/kg daily until resolution of symptoms
- Serious bleeds (e.g. intracranial haemorrhage) – 30–40 U/kg for at least 3–5 days
- Major surgery – target level of 100% maintained for 3 days followed by decrease by 20–30% every 3 days
- Minor surgery – target level of 40–60% levels with further decrease over the next few days

DRUG THERAPY

- Desmopressin (DDAVP)
- Danazol
- Oestrogens in von Willebrand's disease.

Desmopressin (DDAVP) is a relatively inexpensive drug that increases FVIII levels and vWF activity within 30 minutes of administration. It is useful in mild haemophilia and mild von Willebrand's disease.[299] The major side effects are headaches and hyponatraemia so fluid intake should be restricted to 1.5 L/day. Tranexamic acid mouthwashes may be helpful for oral mucosal bleeding. Danazol can increase both factor VIII and IX levels within 5–7 days[300] and has therefore been recommended for patients with recurrent haemarthrosis or with central nervous system bleeding which both carry a high risk of recurrence.

THROMBOEMBOLISM

Most thromboembolic episodes are single events and may be associated with precipitating events or underlying risk factors. Thrombophilia is the clinical state of hypercoagulability and should be suspected in patients who have a strong family history of thrombosis, or who have recurrent or unusual thromboses.

Increasing affluence and consequent lifestyle changes mean that the prevalence of thromboembolism is rising in some low- and middle-income countries. Risk factors such as sedentary work, obesity, excessive alcohol intake, smoking and additional cardiovascular risk factors are compounded by other conditions that are associated with thrombosis such as HIV infection, and chronic infections including tuberculosis[301,302] and helminth-induced eosinophilic myocarditis.[303] African Americans are more likely to be diagnosed with pulmonary embolism rather than deep-vein thrombosis compared to other racial groups[304] and African patients with thrombosis tend to be younger than those reported in literature[305] with higher mortality rates (around 28%) possibly due to late presentation and poor access to health facilities. Asian populations[306–308] seem to have a lower prevalence of symptomatic venous thrombosis compared to African Americans.[304]

Very little is known about the prevalence of prothrombotic factors such as mutations of the prothrombin gene or deficiencies of antithrombin, protein C and protein S in tropical countries, although high rates of factor V Leiden, a risk factor for venous thrombosis, have been described in Tunisia.[309,310] Lupus anticoagulant and anti-phospholipid syndrome, which are associated with increased thrombosis risk, are increased in Afro-Caribbean populations, especially in the presence of HIV, and have also been described in Nigerian women with pre-eclampsia.[311,312]

The management of venous thrombosis is initially with heparin and then with warfarin for 3–6 months. Compliance may be difficult in low-resource settings because of the requirement for regular monitoring of warfarin. It is therefore important to try to prevent thromboses by removing any underlying risk factors and by treating individuals at risk of thrombosis with a short course of prophylactic heparin to cover procedures known to be associated with thrombosis risk.

Thrombophilia

This can present as venous or arterial thromboembolism and it may be inherited (e.g. deficiencies of thrombin, protein S or protein C) or acquired (e.g. antiphospholipids). The patient's personal and family history, and the results of clinical and imaging examinations to confirm thrombosis, may suggest the diagnosis. The laboratory tests needed to determine the cause and classify the type of thrombophilia, and their interpretation, are complex, so patients with recurrent or unusual thromboses should be referred to a specialist centre.

Haematological Malignancies in the Tropics

Haematological malignancies are predominantly leukaemias, lymphomas and myelomas. Some of the general approaches for managing these conditions in low-income countries are outlined in Box 65.21[313] but definitive treatment should be undertaken by a specialist haematology unit.

LEUKAEMIAS

Clinical Features

Leukaemias can be broadly classified as acute or chronic, and lymphoid or myeloid. The presenting symptoms and signs are related to the disturbed blood cell production from the bone marrow due to the effects of the malignant cell clone (Box 65.22). Acute leukaemias are characterized by rapid progression and poor prognosis if left untreated whereas chronic leukaemias generally follow a much slower course.

BOX 65.21 MEASURES WHICH MAY BE ADOPTED TO IMPROVE CARE OF PATIENTS WITH HAEMATOLOGICAL MALIGNANCIES IN AN UNDER-RESOURCED SETTINGS

- Mobilization of the community (especially parents and families) to raise awareness among local councils and government bodies about the treatability of the cancers and benefits from curing them
- Find an external partner unit locally, nationally or internationally which is already well-established and willing to help but will not dictate terms
- Improvement of supportive care facilities, especially protection from those with infectious diseases
- Development of a safe and reliable blood transfusion service
- Provision of subsidized travel, and satellite clinics to lessen the burden
- Development of appropriate protocols for each disease entity which is locally practicable with minimum cost and maximum efficacy
- Development of medical, nursing and paramedical expertise in the diseases to be treated – initially by offering visiting fellowships and in the long term for the trained individuals to arrange regional and local teaching programmes
- Formation of a cooperative group bringing together all the professionals involved in the speciality within a country or region to share expertise and develop training programmes.

Diagnosis

Acute and chronic leukaemias are usually associated with a high white cell count but acute leukaemias can present with normal or even sub-normal white cell counts. Morphology of peripheral blood and bone marrow specimens is crucial to confirm the diagnosis. This is particularly important in the case of acute leukaemia in children which may be mistaken for an acute viral infection. Staining methods including Sudan black B, myeloperoxidase and nonspecific esterase are important to distinguish between the different subtypes of acute myeloid and lymphoid leukaemias and therefore to guide treatment.

Management

Acute Myeloid Leukaemia (AML). Prevalence of this increases with age and the success rate with chemotherapy protocols is not high even in the most sophisticated centres. Neutropenia and myelosuppression requiring intensive blood component support occur during chemotherapy[314] and bone marrow transplantation offers the best option for cure for patients who relapse. Management of AML is therefore complex and expensive. Hydroxycarbamide or subcutaneous cytarabine may be used as a palliative treatment.

Acute Promyelocytic Leukaemia (AML Subtype M3). This must be distinguished from other types of acute myeloid leukaemia because it has a high cure rate with early treatment. It predominantly affects young adults and it has a high incidence in certain ethnic groups especially those of Latin American descent.[315] A treatment protocol which includes all-transretinoic acid with combination chemotherapy has been developed which is feasible in low-income countries.[315,315] Another regimen based on intravenous arsenic trioxide has been developed in India,[316,317] which has an 86% response rate with good disease-free and overall survival.

BOX 65.22 CLINICAL FEATURES OF LEUKAEMIAS

ACUTE LEUKAEMIAS

- Fatigue and cardiac symptoms from anaemia
- Bleeding from thrombocytopenia
- Increased risk of infections despite a higher number but dysfunctional white cells
- Lymphadenopathy and hepatosplenomegaly occur with ALL although lymphadenopathy may be observed in the monocytic variety of AML
- Blindness due to hyperviscosity from hyperleukocytosis
- Tumour lysis syndrome due to spontaneous cell lysis presents as renal failure
- Pustules or pyogenic infections of the skin from minor wounds
- Bleeding gums are a characteristic feature of acute monocytic leukaemia
- Disseminated intravascular coagulation can occur with acute promyelocytic leukaemia
- Gout can arise from breakdown of the excess white cells and release of uric acid
- Oral aphthous ulceration is seen with severe neutropenia in both AML and ALL
- Granulocytic sarcoma or chloroma represent extramedullary deposits of leukaemic cells in any organ but mainly the skin. This may occur in the absence of peripheral blood involvement and is more common with chromosomal translocation (8; 21) of AML
- Central nervous system manifestations due to sludging of the cerebral circulation by the malignant cells or increased intracranial pressure due to ventricular blockade can occur. Monocytic myeloid leukaemia can also involve the meninges
- Intracranial haemorrhage can occur in ALL with very high white cell counts (>400 × 10^9/L)
- Bone pain and arthralgia can be a presenting feature of ALL in children in more than a quarter. These children may present with a limp or unwillingness to walk due to marrow infiltration by leukaemic cells. Rarely, they may have normal blood counts delaying the diagnosis of ALL
- Anterior mediastinal mass (thymus enlargement) can also occur in children and young adults with ALL which may present as superior venocaval obstruction
- Painless enlargement of scrotum is a sign of testicular leukaemia or hydrocele from lymphatic obstruction. Priapism can result from hyperleukocytosis rarely.

CHRONIC LEUKAEMIAS

- Most often asymptomatic and usually suspected on blood counts
- The chronicity of CML or CLL tends to cause gradual-onset symptoms since the patients get adjusted to the slowly developing anaemia
- Abdominal discomfort and early satiety are a feature of CML due to excessive splenomegaly compressing the stomach and reducing the luminal volume
- Sternal tenderness may be noted in CML
- Hyperleukocytosis in CML can occur more often than with AML or ALL due to the gradual increase in white cells. This can cause symptoms like hyperuricaemia and gout, tinnitus, priapism or central nervous system disturbances
- Left shoulder tip pain can arise from splenic infarction from the massive splenomegaly in CML
- CML can rarely present with features of thyrotoxicosis (heat intolerance, weight loss and excessive sweating) due to hyper-metabolism
- CLL is often associated with lymphadenopathy and rarely with mild to moderate splenomegaly.

ALL, acute lymphoid leukaemia; AML, acute myeloid leukaemia; CLL, chronic lymphocytic leukaemia; CML, chronic myeloid leukaemia.

Acute Lymphoblastic Leukaemia (ALL). This is the most common type of leukaemia in children. It has a good prognosis when treated with modern chemotherapy protocols with cure rates in the best centres exceeding 80%.[318] In low-income countries, cure rates are much lower at around 35%[319] primarily because of failure to complete therapy and deaths caused by treatment. Considerable improvements in ALL outcomes have been achieved by twinning institutions in developing countries with specialist centres elsewhere in the country or internationally.[313] Measures that may improve outcomes focus on preventing abandonment of therapy (e.g. providing funding for transport, satellite clinics and support groups) and prompt treatment of infection.[320] Treatment in a dedicated paediatric oncology unit using a comprehensive multidisciplinary team approach and protocol-based therapy, is also associated with improved outcomes in resource-poor settings.[321]

Chronic Myeloid Leukaemia (CML). Management has been revolutionized by tyrosine kinase inhibitors (e.g. imatinib) which can produce complete remission in over 80% of cases. Once the diagnosis of CML is established, hydroxycarbamide can be used to reduce the white cell count, followed by treatment with a tyrosine kinase inhibitor. Manufacturers will provide the drug free of charge to patients in low-income countries with confirmed CML and generic forms of tyrosine kinase inhibitors are now becoming available.

Chronic Lymphocytic Leukaemia (CLL). This occurs predominantly in older people and usually presents with lymphadenopathy and recurrent infections. Treatment is with chlorambucil and prednisolone although aggressive forms require combination therapy with rituximab, fludarabine and cyclophosphamide. Treatment is generally not curative but the disease may be indolent and drugs may only be required if the patient has symptoms or if there is a risk of hyperviscosity from a very high lymphocyte count.

LYMPHOMAS

Epidemiology and Clinical Features

Approximately 30 000 cases of non-Hodgkin lymphoma (NHL) occur in the equatorial belt of Africa each year (Table 65.11).[322] There are marked geographical variations in prevalence but up to 50% are thought to be related to HIV infection.[322] Burkitt's lymphoma, a B-cell NHL, was originally described in children from Africa and has an estimated incidence of 30–70 per million. Lymphomas are broadly classified into Hodgkin's lymphoma and NHL; NHL are divided into B-cell, T-cell and NK-cell, and immunodeficiency-associated types.

The clinical presentation of lymphomas is characterized by enlargement of the lymphoid organs and subsequent compression of the adjacent structures, infiltration of organs by the malignant lymphoid cells and a dysfunctional immunological system which can manifest as immunosuppression or excessive but dysregulated immune activation associated with, for example, autoimmune conditions.

Diagnosis

The diagnosis and management of the various types of lymphomas are complicated and should be undertaken in a specialist

TABLE 65.11 **Types of Lymphomas Identified from Selected Countries in Sub-Saharan Africa**

	Paediatric And Adolescent Cases	Adult Patients
Type of non-Hodgkin's Lymphoma		
Precursor lymphoid neoplasms	3%	4.7%
Mature B-cell neoplasms	92.5%	91.3%
Burkitt	82%	9%
Diffuse large B-cell	7.5%	55%
Mature T-cell and NK cell neoplasms	2.2%	3%
Type of Hodgkin's Lymphoma		
Nodular lymphocyte predominant	5%	9.4%
Nodular sclerosing classical	37%	53%
Mixed cellularity classical	37%	31.2%
Lymphocyte-depleted classical	21%	3%
Lymphocyte-rich classical	0%	3%

centre. Diagnosis depends on clinical history and examination, radiological investigations to document the extent of disease, and morphology, immunohistochemistry and molecular studies on tissue samples to confirm the lymphoma subtype. Guidance on the diagnosis and treatment of lymphoma in settings where resources are limited includes recommendations about panels of immunostains and chemotherapy regimens that minimize the need for supportive care.[322] Tele-pathology, which involves transmitting histological images via the internet to experts overseas, may be helpful in certain circumstances though it is dependent on the quality of the histology preparations and the images of appropriate diagnostic regions in the sample.

Management

Treatment regimens for lymphomas differ according to the subtype but may involve chemotherapy and radiotherapy. High remission rates can be achieved in Burkitt's lymphoma with a combination of cyclophosphamide, vincristine and methotrexate and progressive disease can be managed with ifosfamide, mesna and cytosine arabinoside.[322,323]

ADULT T-CELL LEUKAEMIA-LYMPHOMA (ATLL)

Adult T-cell leukaemia-lymphoma (ATLL) is an uncommon lymphoid malignancy which occurs in patients infected with human T-lymphotropic virus type I (HTLV-I).[324] HTLV-1 is endemic in the Caribbean, western Africa, Peru and southern Japan. Less than 5% of those infected with HTLV-I develop ATLL and up to 30 years can elapse between the primary infection and the development of ATLL suggesting additional factors are needed for malignant transformation.[325]

ATLL presents acutely in approximately 60% of cases, although chronic forms have also been described.[326] The clinical presentation is with generalized lymphadenopathy in most cases and hepatosplenomegaly in over half.[324] ATLL is associated with a high risk of hypercalcaemia which occurs in more than two-thirds of patients during the course of their disease and may be associated with central nervous system disturbances and renal impairment. Lytic bone lesions occur as a para-neoplastic phenomenon due to production of parathormone-like peptides. As with other T-cell disorders, ATLL can involve the skin, producing, e.g. erythrodermic plaques.

The diagnosis of ATLL can be suspected from a high peripheral blood white blood cell count in combination with hypercalcaemia and characteristic lymphocytes with convoluted and hyperlobulated nuclei.[324] The diagnosis is confirmed by histological examination of a tissue (lymph node or bone marrow), immunophenotyping for specific cell markers and proof of HTLV infection, usually by serological methods.

Management of ATLL is primarily with combination chemotherapy with intrathecal prophylaxis.[327,328] A combination of zidovudine and interferon, as agents against HTLV, has also been tried with some success.[329] Hypercalcaemia and opportunistic infections should be sought and treated early in these patients. The high white cell count is associated with a significant risk of tumour lysis syndrome and should be prevented by adequate hydration and the judicious use of allopurinol and other urate-reducing agents.

MULTIPLE MYELOMA

Myeloma is a monoclonal proliferation of plasma cells and it particularly affects older people. Myeloma appears to be less common in Asian countries than elsewhere, although during the last 25 years, an almost four-fold increase in incidence of myeloma has occurred in Taiwan.[330] In the United States, the incidence of multiple myeloma in the black population is twice that of the white population.

Pathophysiology and Clinical Features

The abundant plasma cells infiltrate the bone marrow and interfere with normal haematopoiesis. This leads to anaemia, which is a presenting feature in 70% of individuals. Bony infiltration by the malignant plasma cells can produce osteoporosis, lytic lesions and pathological fractures in 60% of patients with myeloma. Involvement of the bones can lead to hypercalcaemia, which may be a presenting feature, and vertebral fracture leading to spinal cord compression. The malignant plasma cells produce a paraprotein which can cause renal impairment in 20–50% and hyperviscosity may ensue in 10% of patients if the paraprotein production is not controlled.

Management

Patients with myeloma may need a variety of supportive interventions including management of anaemia, renal failure, hypercalcaemia, hyperviscosity, infections and bone pains. Specific anti-myeloma treatment should be managed within a specialist unit and has undergone a radical change in the last decade with the use of thalidomide and its newer formulations, and the more expensive, proteasome inhibitors (e.g. bortzomib). Thalidomide is relatively safe and effective although somnolence and constipation can sometimes be troublesome. There is a risk of thrombosis with thalidomide especially at the initiation of therapy, and prophylaxis with heparin, warfarin or antiplatelet agents, depending on an assessment of the risk, may be warranted. Melphalan may also be useful, particularly if resources are limited and there is no specialist centre. However it is myelosuppressive, so regular monitoring of the blood count is essential.

Blood Transfusion

Maintaining an adequate blood supply is a major challenge for low-income countries. Only 39% of the global blood supply is donated in the poorest countries where 82% of the world's population lives.[331] Blood transfusion is a vital component of every country's health service. It can be a life-saving intervention for illnesses such as severe acute anaemia, but mistakes in the transfusion process can be life-threatening, either immediately or years later through transmission of infectious agents. Clinicians need to understand how blood is acquired and its risks and benefits, and to use it appropriately. Governments and transfusion services need to put measures in place to ensure that blood is safe for transfusion and that it reaches those who need it in a timely manner.

BLOOD TRANSFUSION AT THE NATIONAL LEVEL

Only 16% of member states meet all the World Health Organization's (WHO) recommendations for a national quality blood transfusion system.[331] At the national level the transfusion service should have a director, an advisory committee and clear transfusion policies and strategies (Table 65.12).[331] WHO recommend standardization of blood collection, testing and distribution. Although centralization of these services may offer the best guarantee of quality, it is often not practical in countries with poorly developed communications and transport infrastructure.

Two systems, centralized and hospital-based, exist in low-income countries for managing blood supply. In the centralized system, voluntary blood donors are recruited, screened and bled by regional centres and the blood collected is distributed to peripheral hospitals. Hospital-based systems are the predominant source of blood across sub-Saharan Africa. Hospital-based systems obtain blood predominantly from relatives of patients, and blood is screened and used within the local vicinity.[332]

TABLE 65.12 Components of National Strategies for Blood Safety

Essential Element	Supporting Strategy
Well-organized, nationally coordinated blood transfusion service	Government commitment; specific, adequate budget; implementation of national blood policy and plan; legislative and regulatory framework
Quality systems covering all aspects of activities	Organizational management; quality standards; documentation systems; staff training; quality assessments
Blood collection only from voluntary, non-remunerated donors	Effective donor recruitment programmes; stringent donor selection criteria; donor care programme
Quality assured testing of all donated blood	Testing for transfusion-transmissible infections; accurate blood group serology and compatibility testing procedures
Reduction in unnecessary use of blood	Use of appropriate component therapy; safe administration of blood and blood products

Blood from the centralized system costs at least three times as much per unit as that from a hospital-based system.[333] Although centralized systems can save costs through batching and bulk purchasing, the quality assurance processes and donor recruitment components are expensive and difficult to maintain without dependence on external funds. In hospital-based transfusion services, testing quality is variable and the families of patients bear the cost of finding blood donors.

SEPARATION OF WHOLE BLOOD INTO COMPONENTS

The vast majority of blood in low-income countries is transfused as whole blood. In high-income countries it is standard practice to optimize the use of each donation of blood by separating it into individual components but whether this approach is cost-effective in low-income countries, where indications for transfusion are different, is not known. These components, which may include plasma, platelets and cryoprecipitate, are prepared by centrifugation using a closed, sterile system and each component has different storage requirements. Plasma and cryoprecipitate are kept frozen, red cells are stored at 1–5°C, and platelets at 18–22°C with constant agitation. Recent evidence suggests that warm, fresh, whole blood may be better than component therapy for resuscitation of acidotic, hypothermic and coagulopathic trauma patients[334] and for patients needing massive transfusions.[335]

ENSURING SAFETY OF BLOOD FOR TRANSFUSION

Many infections can be transmitted through blood transfusions and transfusion of infected blood causes morbidity and mortality in the recipients, and has an economic and emotional impact on their families and communities. Those who become infected through blood transfusion are infectious to others and contribute to the spread of disease thereby increasing the burden on health services and reducing productive labour.

Selecting Low-risk Blood Donors

Strategies for recruiting blood donors have to provide blood for all who need it in a timely manner while ensuring that the blood is as safe as possible. The safest type of blood donor is one who donates regularly (i.e. repeat donors). WHO states that the safest source of blood is altruistic, voluntary, unpaid donors. Only 32% of WHO member states report having at least 90% of their blood supply from voluntary donors, and low-income countries have not been able to increase the recruitment of voluntary donors for several years.[331] Recent evidence from sub-Saharan Africa indicates that the focus on voluntary donors may be misplaced since first-time voluntary donors have a similar prevalence of transfusion-transmitted infections as family replacement donors.[336] In order to limit blood shortage and maintain constant blood supply in poorer countries, both voluntary and replacement donors should be accepted and encouraged to donate regularly. Mechanisms to convert family replacement donors into repeating voluntary donors have the potential to significantly increase blood donations in Africa. Political will and open-mindedness about ways to improve the supply and safety of blood are essential to promote more evidence-based approaches to blood transfusion practice in poorer countries.[337]

High-risk donors, such as commercial sex workers and their contacts, intravenous drug abusers, or those with an itinerant lifestyle such as traders, drivers and military personnel, should be deterred from donating.[338] Even in areas where HIV infection rates in the general population are high, donor deferral can be effective in excluding HIV-infected donors.[339] The whole donation process, including tests for HIV and other infections, should be explained to the donor before blood is collected and donors should have the option of knowing the results and receiving counselling. It is imperative that complete confidentiality is maintained throughout all procedures.

Screening for Transfusion-transmitted Infections

Infections with organisms such as HIV, hepatitis viruses, cytomegalovirus, syphilis, lyme borreliosis, malaria, babesiosis, American trypanosomiasis (Chagas disease) and toxoplasmosis can all be acquired through blood transfusions. Some 5–10% of HIV infections worldwide are thought to have been transmitted through the transfusion of infected blood and blood products. There have also been reports of transmission of variant Creutzfeldt–Jakob disease through blood transfusion and there is a theoretical risk of transmission of severe acute respiratory syndrome (SARS).[340,341] WHO recommends that all donated blood should be screened for HIV, hepatitis B and syphilis and, where feasible and appropriate, for hepatitis C, malaria and Chagas disease.

Malaria can be transmitted by blood transfusion and, depending on the local infection prevalence, 2–55% of blood donors in Africa screen positive for malaria.[342] However, there is very little evidence to suggest that these donors transmit malaria to transfusion recipients. Although WHO recommends screening donors in endemic areas for malaria, none of the screening methods that would be practical for transfusion services are sufficiently sensitive. Furthermore, in some countries with high malaria transmission, exclusion of parasitaemic donors could result in deferral rates exceeding 50% which would have a major impact on blood supply.[343] There is no evidence to support the widespread practice of routine treatment of transfusion recipients for malaria.

Fresh blood is potentially infectious for syphilis, but storage at 4°C for more than 5 days can inactivate *Treponema pallidum*. The high demand for blood in low-income countries means that blood is generally not stored for long enough to inactivate *T. pallidum* and syphilis seroconversion associated with transfusion has been reported from Africa.[344]

Globally, the prevalence of hepatitis C, HTLV-1 and -2 and Chagas disease is variable and the decision to introduce donor screening for these infections should be based on local assessments of the risks, benefits, feasibility and costs. Blood should not be separated into components if the residual risk of infection is high, as this will increase the number of potentially infected recipients. A unit of blood is usually stored until screening tests for infections have been completed. This means that potentially infected blood may be mixed up with units that have already been screened, and costly blood collection bags are wasted. Screening potential donors before venesecting a unit of blood may therefore be a more cost-effective way of ensuring safe blood.[345]

Tests for screening blood donors need to be highly sensitive, and infected blood should be rejected. Before informing the donor of the outcome, all positive results should be confirmed using a test with a high degree of specificity. Where blood donation is organized locally, the confirmatory test is often performed at a central laboratory, so there may be a delay in informing the donor of the result. There is evidence that nucleic acid amplification techniques (NAT) may be cost-effective in low-income countries where infection prevalence is high.[346]

CLINICAL USE OF BLOOD

Reasons for Transfusion in Low-income Countries

In wealthy countries, the majority of transfusions are carried out electively. By contrast, in poorer countries, and particularly those where the malaria transmission rate is high, most transfusions are given for life-threatening emergencies. In low-income countries, 50–80% of transfusions are administered to children, predominantly for malaria-related anaemia, and pregnant women. Transfusion can significantly reduce the mortality of children with severe anaemia within the first 2 days of hospital admission[347] and successful malaria control can reduce paediatric transfusion requirements.[348] In sub-Saharan Africa, 26% of in-hospital maternal deaths from severe bleeding were due to lack of blood for transfusion.[349] Other specialities which are significant users of blood are surgery, trauma, emergency medicine and general medicine.

Avoiding Unnecessary Transfusions

In low-income countries the most effective way to avoid transfusions is to reduce the prevalence of anaemia. More studies on the efficacy and cost of combinations of interventions including insecticide-treated bed nets, nutritional supplements and anthelmintic drugs to prevent anaemia are needed. When resources are very limited, governments may need to make some difficult decisions in order to achieve an equitable balance between investing in a transfusion service and public health measures to reduce anaemia.

Whether a patient needs a blood transfusion or not is ultimately a clinical decision. Emergency transfusions can be lifesaving for patients in whom anaemia has developed too quickly to allow physiological compensation, as in severe malaria-related anaemia in children, and sudden, severe obstetric bleeding. In contrast, if the anaemia has developed slowly, for example due to hookworm infestation or nutritional deficiency, patients can generally be managed conservatively by treating the cause of the anaemia and prescribing haematinic replacements. Iron supplements should be continued for at least 3 months after the haemoglobin has returned to normal, so that body stores can be replenished.

Clinical Guidelines. It is possible to avoid unnecessary transfusions by adhering to clinical transfusion guidelines. Most institutions have developed guidelines to help clinicians make rational decisions about the use of blood transfusions (Box 65.23)[344,350] and strict enforcement of transfusion protocols can significantly reduce avoidable transfusions.[351] The principles underlying most transfusion guidelines are similar and combine a clinical assessment of oxygenation, with haemoglobin measurement being used as a surrogate measure for intracellular oxygen concentration. Increasingly, transfusion guidelines are making use of evidence which shows that adequate oxygen delivery to the tissues can be achieved at haemoglobin levels that are significantly lower than the normal range.[352]

Implementation of transfusion guidelines is particularly difficult if clinicians do not have access to reliable haemoglobin

BOX 65.23 PRESCRIBING BLOOD: A CHECKLIST FOR CLINICIANS

Always ask yourself the following questions before prescribing blood or blood products for a patient:

1. What improvement in the patient's clinical condition am I aiming to achieve?
2. Can I minimize blood loss to reduce this patient's need for transfusion?
3. Are there any other treatments I should give before making the decision to transfuse, such as intravenous replacement fluids or oxygen?
4. What are the specific clinical or laboratory indications for transfusion in this patient?
5. What are the risks of transmitting HIV, hepatitis, syphilis or other infectious agents through the blood products that are available for this patient?
6. Do the benefits of transfusion outweigh the risks for this particular patient?
7. What other options are there if no blood is available in time?
8. Will a trained person monitor this patient and respond immediately if any acute transfusion reactions occur?
9. Have I recorded my decision and reasons for transfusion on the patient's chart and the blood request form?

Finally, if in doubt, ask yourself the following question:

If this blood were for me or my child, would I accept the transfusion under these circumstances?

measurements. When they doubt the haemoglobin result, clinicians rely entirely on clinical judgement to guide transfusion practice which can lead to significant numbers of inappropriate transfusions.[353] A lack of investment in the quality of a critical test, such as haemoglobin measurement, can waste significant resources downstream in the transfusion process, and unnecessarily expose recipients to the risk of transfusion-related infections.

Minimizing Surgical Blood Loss. Where blood is in short supply, it is particularly important to ensure that the best anaesthetic and surgical techniques are used, to minimize blood loss during surgery. Drugs which improve haemostasis or reduce fibrinolysis, such as aprotinin and cyklokapron, and fibrin sealants, can be effective in reducing perioperative blood loss. These drugs can therefore reduce the need for blood transfusion but they may be too expensive for use in low-income countries. A cost-effectiveness study of surgical bleeding in four sub-Saharan countries indicates that the antifibrinolytic, tranexamic acid, could save lives in countries with blood shortages, reduce healthcare costs and prevent transmission of infections.[354]

Preoperative Autologous Blood Deposit. Patients undergoing planned surgery who are likely to require a blood transfusion can have units of their own blood removed and stored in case they have significant intraoperative blood loss and need a transfusion. This process, known as preoperative autologous donation, can reduce the need for allogeneic transfusions by 46–74%[355] but it requires careful organization: the surgeon needs to predict how much blood will be required, the patient has to be fit enough to withstand removal of one or more units of blood over the weeks preceding the surgery and the surgery must take place within the shelf-life of the blood. As the blood has to be stored in the blood bank there is still a risk that the patient may receive blood which is not their own or that the blood may become infected with bacteria during the process.

Intraoperative Blood Salvage. This involves collecting blood lost during the operation and reinfusing it into the patient either during or after surgery. Although this technique is practical and safe, and reduces the need for donor blood by 27–53%,[355] it requires specialized equipment and training, and may be more expensive than routinely donated blood.[356]

Other Measures. Normal saline or intravenous replacement fluids can be used judiciously in acute blood loss, and in certain circumstances may be as effective as whole blood, red cells or plasma. Erythropoietin, which stimulates endogenous red cell production is well-established for use in chronic anaemias such as those due to renal failure, cancer and HIV infection but its delayed action makes it unsuitable for use in acute anaemias. Synthetic oxygen carriers, such as perfluorocarbons, are not yet routinely available.[357]

Haemoglobin Thresholds for Transfusion

In low-income countries, the recommended haemoglobin threshold for transfusions is often well below that which would be accepted in more wealthy countries. Randomized controlled studies in wealthy countries indicate that for most adults and children undergoing critical care, a haemoglobin threshold of 70 g/L for transfusion is safe[358] whereas paediatric blood transfusion protocols in sub-Saharan Africa often recommend transfusions for stable children only when the haemoglobin level is less than 40 g/L.[351] Complications such as cardiac failure or infection may necessitate transfusion at a higher haemoglobin level. Transfusion should be combined with adequate haematinic replacements and underlying conditions should be treated.[359] Early evidence suggests that intermittent preventive treatment with anti-malarials may reduce the high hospital readmission rates experienced by children post-transfusion.[360]

COMPLICATIONS OF BLOOD TRANSFUSION

Complications can occur immediately during transfusion, within a few hours of its completion, or be delayed for many years, as in the case of viral infections (Box 65.24).

BOX 65.24 COMPLICATIONS OF BLOOD TRANSFUSION

- Febrile non-haemolytic transfusion reactions. Haemolytic reactions include chills, headache, backache, dyspnoea, cyanosis, chest pain, tachycardia and hypotension
- Risk of severe bacterial infection and sepsis
- Transmission of viral infection (hepatitis B, HIV or hepatitis C)
- Transmission of blood-borne trypanosomes, filaria, malaria, etc.
- Cardiac failure
- Air embolism
- Transfusion-associated acute lung injury (TRALI) – a syndrome of acute respiratory distress, often associated with fever, non-cardiogenic pulmonary oedema, and hypotension, which may occur as often as 1 in 2000 transfusions
- Other risks: volume overload, iron overload (with multiple red blood cell transfusions), transfusion-associated graft-versus-host disease, anaphylactic reactions (in people with IgA deficiency), and acute haemolytic reactions (most commonly due to the administration of mismatched blood types).

Acute and Delayed Haemolysis Due to Red Cell Incompatibility

Transfusion of blood into a recipient who possesses antibodies to the donor's red cells can cause an acute, and occasionally fatal, intravascular haemolysis. This could occur, e.g. if group A cells are transfused into a group O recipient who has naturally occurring antibodies to group A cells. The profound haemolysis induces renal vasoconstriction and acute tubular necrosis. Treatment involves stopping the transfusion, cardiorespiratory support and inducing a brisk diuresis. In addition to abnormalities indicating renal failure, laboratory findings include haemoglobinuria and haemoglobinaemia. Proof of the diagnosis involves rechecking the whole transfusion process including all documentation stages, regrouping the donor and the recipient, and screening for antibodies on red cells with a direct antiglobulin test. These tests are usually available in any hospital laboratory capable of providing a transfusion service. Delayed haemolysis has a similar physiological basis to acute intravascular haemolysis but it tends to be less severe, it occurs 7–10 days after the transfusion and it is less likely to present as a clinical emergency.

Bacterial Contamination

Limited data from sub-Saharan Africa show rates of bacterial contamination in donated blood of around 9%[361,362] but the clinical consequences for transfusion recipients are unknown. Bacteria can enter the blood bag during venesection or if the bag is breached, e.g. when reducing the volume for a paediatric recipient or during component preparation. Gram-negative bacteria, including *Pseudomonas* and *Yersinia*, grow optimally at 4°C and infected blood may not necessarily appear abnormal to the naked eye. Reactions following infusion of infected blood are often due to endotoxins and may occur several hours after the transfusion has finished. Although these reactions are rare, they can be severe and fatal. If bacterial contamination is suspected, the transfusion should be stopped and samples from the patient and the blood bag sent to the laboratory for culture. Cardiorespiratory support may be needed and broad-spectrum antibiotics should be started immediately and continued until culture results are available.

Non-haemolytic Febrile Reactions

Non-haemolytic febrile reactions are episodes of fever and chills associated with transfusion and for which no other cause can be found. They are due to the recipient's antibodies reacting against antigens present on the donor's white cells or platelets. These reactions are most common in patients who have had transfusions in the past and have therefore been exposed to allo-antigens. Mild febrile reactions usually respond to simple antipyretics such as paracetamol. More severe reactions may be the first indication of a haemolytic transfusion reaction or bacterial contamination and should be investigated and managed accordingly.

Allergic Reactions

Allergic reactions are due to infusion of plasma proteins and manifestations include erythema, rash, pruritus, bronchospasm and anaphylaxis. The transfusion should be stopped and the patient treated with antihistamines. If the reaction is mild and the symptoms and signs completely disappear, the transfusion can be restarted. If this type of mild reaction occurs repeatedly with more than one unit of blood, the red cells can be washed before transfusion. This should only be done if absolutely necessary, as it carries the risk of introducing potentially fatal bacterial infection. Severe allergic reactions with evidence of systemic toxicity should be managed as acute anaphylaxis.

Circulatory Overload

Blood should always be transfused slowly to avoid overloading the circulation, unless the patient has active and severe bleeding. Fluid overload may be a particular problem when paediatric blood bags are not available, as children may be over-transfused due to miscalculation of the required volume, lack of accurate infusion devices or inadvertent administration of an adult-sized unit of blood.

Haemosiderosis

Four units of blood contain the equivalent amount of iron stored in bone marrow (approx. 1 g). Repeated transfusions for chronic haemolytic anaemia, as in thalassaemia major and sickle cell disease, lead to iron deposition in parenchymal cells. Eventually failure of the heart, liver and other organs supersedes. Adequate doses of iron chelators, such as injectable desferrioxamine or oral deferiprone, are able to maintain acceptable iron balance in patients with chronic anaemia who need regular transfusions.

Hypothermia

It is not usually necessary to warm blood unless large quantities are transfused rapidly. This may lower the temperature of the sino-atrial node to below 30°C at which point ventricular fibrillation can occur. If blood needs to be warmed, an electric blood warmer specifically designed for the purpose should be used. This keeps the temperature below 38°C and avoids the haemolysis associated with overheating blood.

Graft-Versus-Host Disease

Graft-versus-host disease occurs when donor lymphocytes engraft in an immune-suppressed recipient. The lymphocytes recognize the recipient's bone marrow as foreign and induce aplasia. Graft-versus-host disease is almost universally fatal and can be prevented by irradiating the donor blood, which inactivates the donor lymphocytes.

REFERENCES

11. Balarajan Y, Ramakrishnan U, Ozaltin E, et al. Anaemia in low-income and middle-income countries. Lancet 2011;378(9809):2123–35.
70. Rees DC, Williams TN, Gladwin MT. Sickle cell disease. Lancet 2010;376:2018–31.
129. Weatherall DJ. The inherited diseases of hemoglobin are an emerging global health burden. Blood 2010;115:4331–6.
156. Rachmilewitz EA, Giardina PJ. How I treat thalassaemia. Blood 2011;118(13):3479–88.
346. Van Hulst M, Hubben GAA, Sagoe KWC, et al. Blood donors and blood collecton: Web interface–supported transmission risk assessment and cost-effectiveness analysis of postdonation screening: a global model applied to Ghana, Thailand, and the Netherlands. Transfusion 2009;49(12):2729–42.

Access the complete references online at www.expertconsult.com

66

Renal Disease in the Tropics

RAJ THURAISINGHAM | DWOMOA ADU

KEY POINTS

- Infections remain an important cause of kidney disease in the tropics.
- Kidney disease is best assessed by using an estimated GFR (the MDRD equation) and urine tests for proteinuria (urine protein to creatinine or urine albumin to creatinine ratio).
- Most glomerulonephritides in the tropics are idiopathic, although there is more infection-related glomerulonephritis in these areas.
- Strong associations have been found between polymorphisms in the non-muscle myosin heavy chain 9 gene (MYH9) and apolipoprotein L1 (APOL1) gene and HIV-associated nephropathy (HIVAN), focal segmental glomerulosclerosis (FSGS) and chronic kidney disease in African Americans.
- The main cause of acute kidney injury (AKI) in the tropics is acute tubular necrosis, often as a result of infection, with glomerulonephritis presenting less commonly.
- Infections, haemolysis and nephrotoxins are important causes of AKI in tropical countries.
- Hypertension, diabetes and glomerulonephritis are important causes of chronic kidney disease in the tropics.
- There is now compelling evidence that good blood pressure control, especially with angiotensin blockade, reduces proteinuria and slows the progression of chronic kidney disease.

Introduction

There are variations in the causes of renal diseases in different parts of the world and this is most marked between temperate and tropical regions. Even within tropical regions, differences are seen in the pattern of renal diseases. The main factor that differentiates renal disease in the tropics from that in temperate regions of the world is the much higher frequency of an infectious aetiology. Much renal disease in the tropics is, however, idiopathic and similar to renal disease found elsewhere in the world.

ASSESSMENT OF KIDNEY DISEASE

Abnormalities in the kidneys are assessed by estimating glomerular filtration rate (GFR) using serum creatinine levels and determining the presence of blood or protein in urine. This is complemented by imaging techniques and in particular, ultrasound. The normal GFR is approximately 130 mL/min per 1.73 m^2 in young males and 120 mL/min per 1.73 m^2 in young females and these values decline with age at a rate of approximately 0.9 mL/min per year from the age of 40.

SERUM CREATININE CONCENTRATION

Serum or plasma creatinine determination is widely used, however there is a non-linear relation between the concentration of creatinine in the blood and GFR. This means that GFR must decline to approximately half the normal level before the serum creatinine concentration rises above the upper limit of normal. Correspondingly, many patients with chronic kidney disease (CKD) maintain serum creatinine levels in the normal range, despite having significantly impaired renal function. Serum creatinine levels are dependent on dietary protein intake, total muscle mass and the use of medications such as cimetidine and trimethoprim, which interfere with renal creatinine handling. Additionally, several substances can interfere with the laboratory measurement of creatinine. Glucose, uric acid, ketones, plasma proteins and cephalosporins may lead to falsely high creatinine values when the Jaffe reaction method is used. The effect of non-creatinine chromogens in serum is markedly reduced in the kinetic rate Jaffe reaction, which is used in many autoanalysers.

GFR ESTIMATION USING PREDICTION EQUATIONS

In an attempt to overcome the drawbacks using serum creatinine alone, several equations have been developed to estimate GFR.[1] The most widely used equations for estimating GFR are the Cockcroft and Gault (CG) equation and the Modification of Diet in Renal Disease (MDRD) equation. The MDRD equation has been widely validated in several groups including African Americans with hypertension (Box 66.1).[2]

The equation is not valid in children and has not been validated in the setting of acute kidney injury (AKI). The original MDRD equation was derived from a population of patients with impaired renal function. It is less accurate with estimating the GFR when applied to serum creatinines in the normal range. Recognizing this, the Chronic Kidney Disease Epidemiology Collaboration derived a new equation (CKD-EPI)[3] and this equation may well supercede the MDRD equation in future (Box 66.1).

PROTEINURIA

Proteinuria[4] is a marker of renal damage. Physiologically, the glomerular basement membrane provides both a mechanical and a charge barrier to the passage of plasma proteins into the glomerular filtrate. Nevertheless, some plasma proteins cross this barrier in concentrations that are related to the protein's

BOX 66.1 GFR EQUATIONS

MDRD EQUATION FOR GFR

$$GFR = 186 \times (Creatinine/88.4)^{-1.154} \times age^{-0.203}$$

- Creatinine: µmol/L
- Women: Multiply by 0.742
- Black: Multiply by 1.210

Calculator on: http://www.renal.org/eGFRcalc/GFR.pl

CKD EPI EQUATION FOR GFR

$$GFR = 141 \times \min(Scr/1) \times \max(Scr/1)^{-1.209} \times 0.993^{age}$$

- Scr, Serum creatinine: µmol/L
- Women: Multiply by 1.018
- Black: Multiply by 1.159

Calculator on: http://mdrd.com

size, charge, deformability and concentration in the plasma. Under normal circumstances, the mechanical barrier to filtration excludes large molecules like globulins from entering the glomerular filtrate, only low-molecular-weight proteins, such as peptide hormones, insulin and derivatives of immunoproteins cross the glomerular basement membrane. Normal persons usually excrete very small amounts of protein in the urine. Increased excretion of protein is therefore a sensitive marker for glomerular disease. Proteinuria is not only a marker of kidney damage but also a strong predictor of clinical progression of kidney disease[5] and can be of considerable value in assessing the effectiveness of therapy and the progression of the disease.[6]

The assessment of proteinuria in clinical practice is generally carried out using dipstick methods and/or quantification of proteinuria. The quantitative methods widely used are the untimed (spot) urine and the timed (overnight or 24 h) urine specimen. The standard commercial dipsticks measure total protein or albumin, they are simple to use and provide high specificity. This is advantageous for clinicians because only few false-positive results are identified. The standard urine dipstick is insensitive for low concentrations of albumin (microalbuminuria) and to positively charged serum proteins, such as immunoglobulin light chains. Quantification of proteinuria based on the timed urine collection over 24 h is a definitive measure of protein or albumin excretion. However, the 24 h urine collection is time-consuming, subject to collection error and requires good compliance. In recent years, the ratio of protein or albumin to creatinine in an untimed ('spot') urine specimen has replaced protein excretion in a 24-hour collection, as the preferred method for measuring proteinuria.[6] These ratios correct for variations in urinary concentration due to hydration and provide a more convenient method of assessing protein and albumin excretion. Many studies have found that values for urine protein/creatinine ratios measured in random urine samples correlate well with measurements of protein excretion in 24-hour urine collections from the same patients.[7,8] Most guidelines recommend the use of first morning urine sample but when not available, a random urine sample to estimate protein creatinine ratio is acceptable.

Glomerulonephritis

Glomerulonephritis is more common in the tropics than in temperate countries. It has been calculated that the incidence of nephrotic syndrome is 60–100 times higher in some tropical countries than in the USA and UK.[9] In tropical areas, infections are a major cause of both acute and chronic glomerulonephritis. Only a minority of individuals with a given infection develop a glomerulonephritis, demonstrating the importance of host factors in pathogenesis. Often with a single infecting organism, a variety of glomerulonephritides is seen in different individuals (Table 66.1). In most instances infection-induced acute glomerulonephritis resolves when the infection is cured, although glomerulonephritis resulting from chronic infection (e.g. quartan malaria and schistosomiasis) is not reversed following measures that eradicate the infection.

TABLE 66.1 Infection-Associated Glomerulonephritis

Glomerulonephritis	Infection
Membranous nephropathy	Hepatitis B *Schistosoma mansoni* Leprosy Loa loa Syphilis
Mesangiocapillary glomerulonephritis	*Schistosoma mansoni* Leprosy Loa loa Onchocerciasis Tuberculosis Candidiasis
Focal segmental glomerulosclerosis	HIV *Schistosoma mansoni*
Proliferative glomerulonephritis	*Streptococcus* spp. *Staphylococcus* spp. *Schistosoma mansoni* Leprosy *Wuchereria bancrofti* Onchocerciasis Syphilis
Amyloid	Leprosy *Schistosoma mansoni*

CLASSIFICATION

The most helpful classification is one based on aetiology and histology. The histological changes may be of unknown aetiology (idiopathic), or secondary to well-defined aetiological factors. The types and clinical features of idiopathic glomerulonephritis have been reviewed elsewhere.[10–12]

CLINICAL PRESENTATION

The ways in which glomerulonephritis may present are fairly limited and are summarized in Box 66.2.

BOX 66.2 CLINICAL PRESENTATION OF GLOMERULONEPHRITIS

- Persistent microscopic haematuria
- Persistent proteinuria
- Nephrotic syndrome
- Acute nephritic syndrome
- Acute renal failure
- Chronic renal failure.

DIAGNOSIS

Definitive diagnosis of most forms of glomerulonephritis is dependent on a renal biopsy with careful interpretation of the renal histology in the light of clinical, biochemical and immunological features of the disorder.

OVERVIEW OF MANAGEMENT OF GLOMERULONEPHRITIS

Conservative management of the nephrotic syndrome is with salt restriction, careful use of diuretics and of angiotensin-converting enzyme inhibitors (ACEI) or angiotensin receptor blockers. There is now good evidence that a reduction in blood pressure and in urine protein retards the rate at which renal function deteriorates. ACE inhibition is more effective than other antihypertensive drugs in reducing proteinuria and the rate of decline in renal function in patients with a glomerulonephritis and proteinuria.[13–15] The treatment of glomerulonephritis is often with steroids and immunosuppressants and these drugs have major toxicities, which need to be offset against any benefit. The aims of treatment of glomerulonephritis are the induction of remission, the maintenance of remission and the prevention of progression of glomerular injury.

PATTERN OF GLOMERULAR DISEASE IN THE TROPICS

This has been reviewed by Jha and Chugh.[16] In most tropical countries, primary glomerular diseases are more common than secondary glomerular disease. In Jamaica, however, 54% of patients with a nephrotic syndrome have secondary glomerular disease, usually lupus nephritis.[17] The aetiopathogenesis of glomerulonephritis in tropical countries does seem to be changing. Over the last two decades there have been only infrequent reports of quartan malarial nephropathy,[18] which had been a common cause of the nephrotic syndrome in children in Nigeria and Uganda.[9,19] In Ghana, Kenya, the Indian subcontinent and South-east Asia, however, 70–90% of adults and children with a nephrotic syndrome have a primary glomerular disease.[16,20–23] Indeed, there is now increasing evidence that idiopathic glomerulonephritis is common in tropical countries, making the diagnosis and treatment of these disorders important. Children aged between 1 and 8 years with a nephrotic syndrome are no longer subjected to renal biopsy and instead treated with a trial of steroids. In the tropics, it is important to exclude infections with hepatitis B, hepatitis C and HIV prior to starting steroids.

IDIOPATHIC GLOMERULONEPHRITIS

Minimal-change Nephropathy

In this condition, the glomeruli are normal on light microscopy and there are no glomerular deposits of immunoglobulin and complement. The incidence varies in tropical Africa, where it is found in 4–46% of cases.[21,22,24–26] In India and Pakistan, over 30% of children with a nephrotic syndrome have minimal-change nephropathy.[27–29]

Recent reports show that 50–80% of children with a nephrotic syndrome in tropical Africa are steroid-responsive.[22,30,31]

Management: Children

Steroids.[32] Meta-analysis showed that treatment with prednisolone for 3 months or more during the first episode of a nephrotic syndrome in children significantly reduced the risk of relapse at 12–24 months as compared with treatment for 2 months (RR 0.70, 95% CI 0.58–0.84). It is therefore recommended that children receive at least 6 weeks of treatment with daily oral prednisolone 60 mg/m^2 BSA/day followed by 6 weeks of alternate day prednisolone 40 mg/m^2 BSA/day.

Treatment of Frequent Relapsers.[33] Approximately 30–50% of children with steroid-sensitive nephrotic syndrome have frequent relapses. An 8-week course of cyclophosphamide (2–3 mg/kg per day) or chlorambucil (0.2 mg/kg per day) significantly reduced the risk of further relapse, as compared with prednisolone alone, RR 0.44, 95% CI 0.26–0.73 and RR 0.15, 95% CI 0.02–0.95, respectively. Approximately 50% of treated children are in remission at 2 years and 40% at 5 years. Cyclophosphamide has been carefully evaluated in these children and is the drug of choice. Ciclosporin (6 mg/kg per day) was as effective as cyclophosphamide or chlorambucil but the effect was maintained only during treatment. We prefer a lower dose of ciclosporin (5 mg/kg per day) as the drug is nephrotoxic. Levamisole, which is also anthelminthic, has also been used and is more effective in reducing relapses than prednisolone alone (RR 0.15, 95% CI 0.02–0.95) but again the effect was only restricted to the period of treatment. Levamisole can cause a reversible neutropenia.

Steroid-Resistant Nephrotic Syndrome in Children.[34] In children presenting with a first episode of nephrotic syndrome, about 90% go into remission with steroid treatment. Steroid-resistant children will, if biopsied, have minimal-change nephrotic syndrome, mesangioproliferative glomerulonephritis or focal segmental glomerulosclerosis. In these patients, ciclosporin is more effective in inducing complete remission than placebo or no treatment (RR 7.66, 95% CI 1.06–55.34).

Management: Adults

Minimal-change Nephropathy in Adults. About 20% of adults with a nephrotic syndrome have minimal-change nephropathy. The mean age of onset is 40 years but the condition can occur at any age. The histology is identical to that found in children, with the exception of a higher incidence of globally sclerosed glomeruli that are a feature of ageing. As in children, the clinical presentation is with a nephrotic syndrome, although this is not generally as severe.

Diagnosis. A renal biopsy is essential to make the diagnosis in adults with a nephrotic syndrome.

Treatment of Minimal-change Nephropathy in Adults. Treatment is with prednisolone at an initial dose of 60 mg/day: response occurs slightly less often than in children and also more slowly. Response to steroid treatment takes longer and is also less complete in adults at 75% at 6 months. Up to 60% of patients who go into a remission have a relapse and 39% have frequent relapses. In frequent relapsers treatment with cyclophosphamide induces a sustained remission of 60% over a five-year period. Ciclosporin is also of benefit in frequent relapsers but most patients relapse when this is discontinued.

New Treatments. Mycophenolate mofetil and also tacrolimus have been reported in uncontrolled trials to be effective in inducing and maintaining remission in patients with steroid-resistant or relapsing minimal-change disease and in focal segmental glomerulosclerosis (FSGS).

FOCAL SEGMENTAL GLOMERULOSCLEROSIS

This is particularly common in Ghana, Senegal, Zaire and South Africa.[20,22,35,36]

As with other glomerulonephritides it can be idiopathic or secondary to a variety of conditions.

Secondary FSGS. Segmental scarring of glomeruli is the end-product of a variety of pathological processes. These include sickle cell anaemia, reduced renal mass, HIV infection, inherited mutations of podocyte-related genes and immune complex nephritis. Some of these causes lead to well-defined glomerular lesions, e.g. collapsing glomerulopathy in HIV-associated nephropathy and prominent hilar segmental lesions in reduced renal mass. Mutations in genes encoding slit diaphragm proteins are found in up to 20–30% of children with steroid-resistant nephrotic syndrome but not in patients with steroid-sensitive nephrotic syndrome and are uncommon in adults.[37] Importantly, patients with a genetic cause for their nephrotic syndrome show no response to steroids or immunosuppressants and these should not be used.

Pathology (Figure 66.1)

The histological lesions of FSGS comprise segmental areas of glomerular sclerosis with hyalinization of glomerular capillaries, the segmental areas usually being adherent to Bowman's capsule.[38] In childhood with FSGS, these lesions predominantly affect juxtamedullary glomeruli. One suggested classification is the Columbia FSGS classification.[39] Several variants have been described based on the site of the segmental sclerosing lesion (perihilar variant and glomerular tip lesion), the presence of glomerular collapse (collapsing variant) and endocapillary cellularity with visceral epithelial cell hyperplasia (cellular variant). Having excluded these variants, this leaves FSGS (not otherwise specified). Typically, the areas of segmental sclerosis are randomly distributed within the glomerular tuft with a predilection for the hilar regions. Focal areas of tubular atrophy and interstitial nephritis are prominent. On immunofluorescent microscopy, deposits of IgM and C3 may be seen in the sclerotic areas.

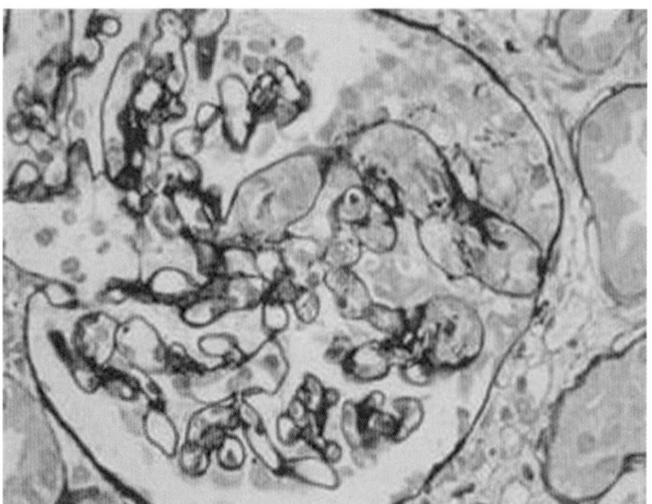

Figure 66.1 Early focal segmental sclerosing glomerular disease. *(Courtesy of Professor A.J. Howie.)*

Management

Steroids. Cohort studies report that 40–60% of patients treated with a 6-month course of prednisolone go into complete or partial remission.[40] Complete as well as partial remissions are associated with a significant reduction in the risk of developing end-stage renal failure from 94% to 53% as compared with no remission. Relapses are common and found in 40–56% of patients. All patients with idiopathic FSGS and a nephrotic syndrome should be treated with prednisolone for 6 months. Children are treated with prednisolone at an initial dose of 60 mg/m^2 BSA/day and adults with a dose of 60 mg/day with tapering of the steroid dose.

Ciclosporin. Patients whose nephrotic syndrome is resistant to 6 months' treatment with prednisolone should receive ciclosporin for 26–52 weeks.[41] A meta-analysis of three studies in patients with FSGS who were resistant to an 8-week course of prednisolone indicates that ciclosporin was more effective than prednisolone or placebo in inducing complete or partial remission[42] but there is a risk of nephrotoxicity from this drug.

Other Immunosuppressants. There is no evidence that cyclophosphamide or chlorambucil are of benefit in the treatment of FSGS.

ACE Inhibition/ARB

Children. Angiotensin-converting enzyme inhibitors have been shown to be of benefit in reducing proteinuria in patients with a steroid-resistant nephrotic syndrome.[43]

Prognosis. There is no difference in prognosis between adults and children. Adverse prognostic factors include tubulointerstitial fibrosis, renal impairment and a failure of remission with treatment.

MEMBRANOUS NEPHROPATHY

This is common in children in Zimbabwe,[44] Namibia[45] and South Africa,[26,46] and also in adults in Mali,[47] Thailand,[48] India,[49] Sudan[24] and Pakistan.[50] In both Africa and Asia, it is frequently a complication of hepatitis B infection. The glomerular basement membranes are uniformly thickened in membranous nephropathy with regular spikes on the epithelial side when stained with periodic acid–methenamine silver. Immunohistology shows uniform granular deposition of IgG and complement on the epithelial side of glomerular basement membranes.

Aetiology

In about 20–25% of adults and 35% of children with membranous nephropathy, there is an identifiable associated condition. These include systemic lupus erythematosus, malignancy (particularly in patients aged over 65) and hepatitis B infection.[12] A recent study showed that 70% of patients with an apparently idiopathic membranous nephropathy had autoantibodies to the M-type phospholipase A2 receptor (anti-PLA2R), which is found in podocytes.[51] These antibodies were not present in secondary forms of membranous nephropathy due to lupus and hepatitis B. These observations may allow monitoring of treatment and also explain the effect of immunosuppressants and B-lymphocyte depletion in membranous nephropathy.

Renal Vein Thrombosis in Membranous Nephropathy. Patients with membranous nephropathy are at particular risk of developing renal vein thrombosis, although this risk is not as high as originally suggested.[52] Most such patients are asymptomatic, but they may present with pulmonary emboli. Detection is by Doppler ultrasound of the renal veins or computed tomography (CT).

Management

About 70% of patients with membranous nephropathy and a nephrotic syndrome survive free of end-stage renal failure at 10 years.[53] Therefore, any therapy that benefits the 30% of patients who develop renal failure exposes the other 70% to unnecessary toxicity. The twin aims of treating membranous nephropathy are first to induce a remission of the nephrotic syndrome and second to prevent the development of end-stage renal failure. Despite several careful studies using steroids and immunosuppressants, there is still no agreement that these aims can be achieved.

Meta-analysis of the Treatment of Membranous Nephropathy. There have been several meta-analyses on the treatment of idiopathic membranous nephropathy.[54] These show that steroids alone are of no benefit in inducing remission or preventing end-stage renal failure. Treatment with cyclophosphamide or chlorambucil, together with prednisolone, leads to more complete remissions (RR 2.37; 95% CI 1.32–4.25) and more partial remissions (RR 1.22; 95% CI 0.63–2.35) than prednisolone alone. No beneficial effect was seen on end-stage renal failure (RR 0.56; 95% CI 0.18–1.68). In this meta-analysis, ciclosporin as compared with prednisolone or no treatment, did not appear to be associated with any important clinical benefit. Between 40% and 60% of patients with a membranous nephropathy and a nephrotic syndrome go into spontaneous remission. Our current strategy is to wait for 12 months and then only treat those patients who are still nephrotic or who have deteriorating renal function, with prednisolone and cyclophosphamide.

MESANGIOCAPILLARY (MEMBRANOPROLIFERATIVE) GLOMERULONEPHRITIS

This has been described in Indonesia,[55] Pakistan,[50] India,[56] Ghana,[57] Nigeria[58] and South Africa,[59] and may be idiopathic but is also commonly seen in post-infectious glomerulonephritis.[60] Most cases of mesangiocapillary glomerulonephritis (MCGN) in the tropics are of the Type I (subendothelial) variety. Immunohistology reveals subendothelial deposits of IgG and less frequently IgM and IgA and C3. In Type II MCGN (dense-deposit disease), basement membrane and mesangial deposits of C3 are found.

Management

Randomized controlled trials of steroids in MCGN showed no benefit. At present, treatment with angiotensin blockade and diuretics is recommended.

IGA NEPHROPATHY

This is common in Singapore, Malaysia, Hong Kong and Taiwan; in Singapore 75% of patients with more than 1 g of proteinuria per 24 hours have IgA nephropathy.[61] IgA nephropathy is, however, uncommon in Blacks in Africa,[59] although it has been recently reported in patients with HIV infection. Renal histology is characterized by the presence of mesangial proliferation and diffuse mesangial deposits of IgA and C3.

Management

Between 20% and 30% of patients with IgA nephropathy will develop end-stage renal failure in 20 years. Adverse prognostic features for renal function include proteinuria in excess of 1.0 g/24 hours, renal impairment at the time of diagnosis and possibly hypertension. The options for treatment of patients with IgA nephropathy, and proteinuria >1.0 g/24 hours and serum creatinine <250 µmol/L are: (a) supportive treatment only with ACE inhibitors; (b) prednisolone (methylprednisolone 1 g intravenously daily for 3 days at 0, 2 and 4 months and oral prednisolone 0.5 mg/kg on alternate days for 6 months or (c) fish-oil (MaxEPA) 6 g twice daily for 2 years. Further randomized clinical trials are necessary to establish the effectiveness of these treatments.

MESANGIAL IgM PROLIFERATIVE GLOMERULONEPHRITIS

Mesangial IgM proliferative glomerulonephritis is a major cause of the nephrotic syndrome in Thailand and other parts of South-east Asia and in parts of Africa. This type of glomerulonephritis can also present with asymptomatic proteinuria and haematuria.

SECONDARY GLOMERULONEPHRITIS

Systemic Lupus Erythematosus

Lupus nephritis is common in Malaysia and Singapore and other parts of South-east Asia, and in these areas is found mostly in people of Chinese origin.[62] Lupus nephritis is also common in Jamaica[17] and also in black Americans.[63] More recently, lupus has been found to be common in Blacks in Africa.[64–66] Clinically apparent nephritis develops in about 40–75% of patients with systemic lupus erythematosus. The renal manifestations of lupus nephritis are heterogeneous both in clinical presentation and in histology. Patients with minimal changes or mesangial glomerulonephritis usually have an inherently low rate of progressive renal failure. Patients with membranous nephropathy have an intermediate prognosis for renal function. In contrast, patients with focal or diffuse proliferative glomerulonephritis have a high risk of progressive renal failure.

Management

Lupus Mesangial Proliferative Glomerulonephritis. In the absence of controlled trials to guide treatment, it is reasonable to treat such patients with corticosteroids in the hope that this will prevent progression to a more severe glomerulonephritis, although that is not certain.

Lupus Membranous Nephropathy. A recent pooled analysis of patients with lupus membranous nephropathy from two randomized controlled studies showed that prednisolone and mycophenolate mofetil were as effective as prednisolone and intravenous cyclophosphamide in terms of remission induction and stabilization of renal function and survival.[67]

Focal and Diffuse Lupus Proliferative Glomerulonephritis: Cyclophosphamide for Remission Induction. The careful randomized controlled studies from the NIH made intravenous cyclophosphamide and oral prednisolone the accepted method for the management of severe lupus nephritis (WHO Classes III and IV).[68] A recent study[69] showed that a shorter 12-week course of intravenous cyclophosphamide every 2 weeks at a dose of 500 mg followed by azathioprine, was as effective as an abbreviated NIH regimen (six monthly pulses of 0.5 G/m^2) followed by two quarterly pulses. In a recent meta-analysis of randomized controlled studies,[70] when compared with prednisolone, cyclophosphamide and prednisolone reduced the risk of doubling of the serum creatinine (RR 0.59; 95%CI 0.4–0.88), while azathioprine did not (RR 0.98; 95% CI 0.36–2.68). However, azathioprine reduced the risk of death (RR 0.60; 95% CI 0.36–0.99), while cyclophosphamide did not (RR 0.95; 95%CI 0.53–1.82). Lupus affects predominantly women of child-bearing age and the documented gonadotoxicity of cyclophosphamide (RR 2.18 95%CI: 1.10–4.34) makes it an inherently unattractive agent for therapy and one that could only be justified by its effectiveness in reducing the risk of reducing renal failure.

Mycophenolate mofetil (MMF) is a powerful immunosuppressant that is licensed for renal transplantation. Pilot studies suggested that it might be effective together with steroids in the induction treatment of lupus nephritis and this has now been tested by randomized controlled trials.[71,72] The Aspreva Lupus Management Study (ALMS) randomized 370 patients with either class III, IV or V nephritis to treatment with mycophenolate 3 g/day or intravenous cyclophosphamide 0.5–1 g/month for 6 months.[73] The results showed no difference in renal response between groups (56.2% with mycophenolate and 53% with cyclophosphamide), serious adverse events (28% mycophenolate and 23% cyclophosphamide) or infections (69% mycophenolate and 62% cyclophosphamide).

Remission Maintenance. Two recent studies compared the effectiveness of azathioprine and mycophenolate mofetil maintenance of remission in patients with proliferative lupus nephritis with discrepant results. The MAINTAIN study showed no benefit of MMF over azathioprine,[74] while the ALMS study showed that MMF was significantly better than azathioprine.[75] Where resources are constrained it seems reasonable to use azathioprine in the remission phase of this disease.

Crescentic Glomerulonephritis

Most renal biopsy series from the tropics report that between 4% and 7% of patients have a crescentic glomerulonephritis with extracapillary proliferation.[59] This is seen in a wide variety of disorders, including post-streptococcal glomerulonephritis, hepatitis B- and C-associated glomerulonephritis, microscopic polyarteritis (polyangiitis), Wegener's granulomatosis and lupus nephritis. The importance of a crescentic glomerulonephritis is that it is usually associated with a rapid decline in renal function. Treatment is usually with prednisolone and cyclophosphamide.

INFECTION-ASSOCIATED GLOMERULONEPHRITIS

Acute Endocapillary Proliferative Glomerulonephritis

The most common cause of acute proliferative glomerulonephritis (APGN) is an infection with group A streptococci. This is common in Africa,[25] the Caribbean countries[76] and in India.[77] A similar type of glomerulonephritis has been reported with other bacterial infections in patients with infective endocarditis, shunt nephritis and visceral abscesses. APGN commonly develops 1–2 weeks after a streptococcal pharyngitis and 3–6 weeks after a skin infection (impetigo). With both sites of infection the risk of an ensuing glomerulonephritis is higher in children aged between 2 and 12 years. APGN has become quite rare in Western countries but epidemic outbreaks following skin infections with streptococci still occur in tropical countries.[78]

Pathogenesis.[79] Only certain M types (cell wall protein antigens) of Lancefield group A streptococcal infections are followed by the development of glomerulonephritis. This is an immune-mediated nephritis and would by convention be termed an immune complex nephritis.

Pathology. This is the classical endocapillary proliferative glomerulonephritis. There is increased hypercellularity of glomeruli from mesangial proliferation and an influx of polymorphonuclear leucocytes, monocytes and T lymphocytes (Figure 66.2). Subepithelial humps on electron microscopy are characteristic of this disorder. Extracapillary proliferation (crescents) is infrequent. Renal biopsies show deposits of C3, IgG and sometimes IgM in the glomerular mesangium and also large subepithelial deposits (humps) on immunofluorescence and electron microscopy.

Serology. Antibodies to various streptococcal antigens form the basis of diagnosis in culture-negative cases: after pharyngitis 95% of children will have an antibody response to streptolysin O, deoxyribonuclease, deoxyribonuclease B, hyaluronidase and streptokinase. After pyoderma antibody responses to

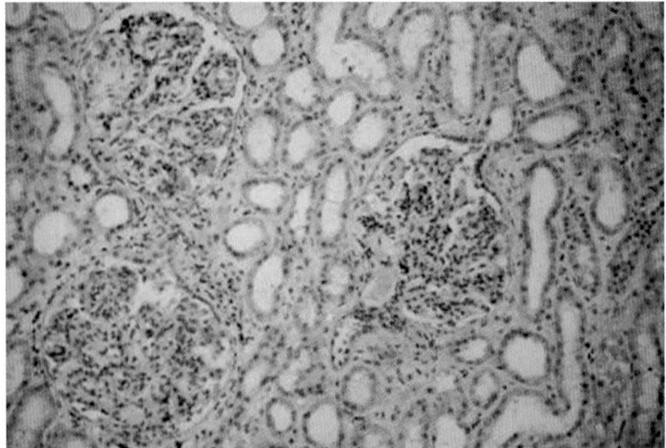

Figure 66.2 Acute post-infective glomerulonephritis. Solid-looking glomeruli filled with neutrophil polymorphs. *(Courtesy of Professor A.J. Howie.)*

deoxyribonuclease B are found, while responses to streptolysin O are infrequent.

Clinical. The clinical presentation ranges from asymptomatic haematuria and proteinuria, through to an acute nephritic syndrome, at times accompanied by a nephrotic syndrome, and rarely a rapidly progressive glomerulonephritis. The patient with an acute nephritic syndrome presents with oliguria, reddish-brown urine due to haematuria, proteinuria, a puffy face and ankle oedema and this is often accompanied by hypertension. Hypertension and cardiac failure are usually due to salt and water overload. Headache, vomiting and fits may complicate the rise in blood pressure. A full-blown nephrotic syndrome is infrequent and acute renal failure from extracapillary glomerulonephritis is rare, being found in less than 2% of affected children.

Management. All patients should be given a 10-day course of penicillin or erythromycin to eradicate the organism and prevent secondary spread, although this treatment has no effect on the outcome of the renal illness. The management of the acute nephritic illness is based on conventional treatment, with meticulous attention to fluid balance, together with diuretics and antihypertensive drug therapy as necessary. Rarely, there may be the development of a crescentic glomerulonephritis and if renal failure is severe, then treatment with prednisolone and cyclophosphamide should be considered.

Outcome. The long-term prognosis of post-streptococcal glomerulonephritis is good and there are few reports of end-stage chronic renal failure as a long-term sequel. Long-term prospective studies of epidemic post-streptococcal glomerulonephritis following skin infection showed little evidence of progressive chronic renal failure or hypertension. Other studies of sporadic post-pharyngitic glomerulonephritis, however, showed that up to 50% of patients have some evidence of chronic renal damage.

EOSINOPHILIC PROLIFERATIVE GLOMERULONEPHRITIS IN UGANDA

An eosinophilic diffuse proliferative glomerulonephritis was reported by Walker et al.[80] from Uganda in children with proteinuria. Immunostaining showed granular deposits of C3 and IgG and electron microscopy revealed subepithelial and intramembranous dense deposits. The eosinophilia raised the possibility of a parasitic contribution to the cause of the glomerulonephritis. There was no clear association with streptococcal infection or evidence of malaria or HIV infection in the whole series.

HEPATITIS B INFECTION AND RENAL DISEASE

The renal complications of hepatitis B infection[81] are found mainly in individuals who are chronically infected. The major renal lesions of hepatitis B infection are membranous nephropathy, which is more common in children, and less commonly a mesangiocapillary glomerulonephritis, IgA nephropathy (more common in adults) and polyarteritis.

HEPATITIS-B-ASSOCIATED MEMBRANOUS NEPHROPATHY

This is seen particularly in children who are chronic carriers of hepatitis B virus. The frequency of hepatitis B as a cause of membranous nephropathy parallels the general carrier rate of this virus in the population. Between 60% and 100% of children with membranous nephropathy in Jamaica, Japan, Hong Kong, South Africa and Zimbabwe have HBsAg.[17,46,60,82,83] By contrast this is infrequent in the USA and the UK. In children, the age of onset is between 2 and 12 years, and over 80% of affected children are male. The clinical presentation is usually with a nephrotic syndrome. Most affected children have no clinical evidence of liver disease; this is more common in adults.

Serology

Sera from almost all patients with hepatitis-B-associated membranous nephropathy show evidence of infection in the form of HBsAg, HBc antibodies, HBeAg and HBe antibodies.

Pathology

The histological lesion of hepatitis-B-associated membranous nephropathy differs from the idiopathic variety, in that in addition to subepithelial immune deposits there are often subendothelial and mesangial deposits (Figure 66.3). Glomerular capillary deposits of the hepatitis B antigens HBsAg, HBcAg and HBeAg have been demonstrated in renal biopsies.

Management and Outcome

There is no evidence that corticosteroids are of benefit and indeed, their use and withdrawal may lead to rebound hepatitis. In a recent study, Tang et al.[84] treated 10 patients with hepatitis-B-associated membranous nephropathy with lamivudine. As compared with historical controls, lamivudine increased the proportion of patients going into complete remission from 25% to 60% and reduced renal failure from 60% to nil. There was a need for long-term treatment, as cessation of this at 2 years leads to a relapse of the nephrotic syndrome. The prognosis in children is good, with reported spontaneous remissions of the nephrotic syndrome in up to two-thirds of cases. Approximately 5% of children progress to end-stage renal failure, while adults fare worse with 10% developing renal failure. Vaccination of all neonates has been shown to reduce the rate of hepatitis B carriage and hepatitis-B-associated glomerulonephritis.[85]

HEPATITIS-B-ASSOCIATED POLYARTERITIS NODOSA

HBsAg[86] has been reported in 10–40% of patients in the USA, 18–50% of patients in France and 4–8% of patients in the UK who have classical polyarteritis. This association is uncommon in tropical countries.

HEPATITIS-C-ASSOCIATED NEPHROPATHY

Hepatitis C virus infection[87] is found in less than 0.6% of the population of North America and Northern Europe but is more common in southern Europe and Africa and has a high prevalence in haemophiliacs and intravenous drug abusers. Hepatitis C infection may lead to chronic active hepatitis and cirrhosis. Hepatitis C infection is the main cause of mixed essential

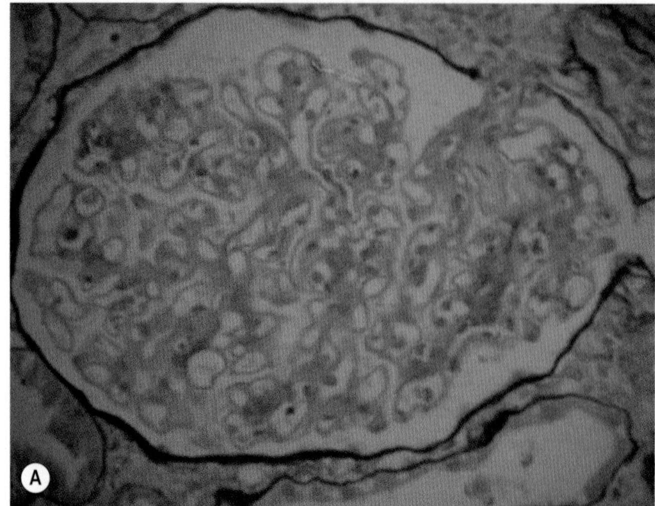

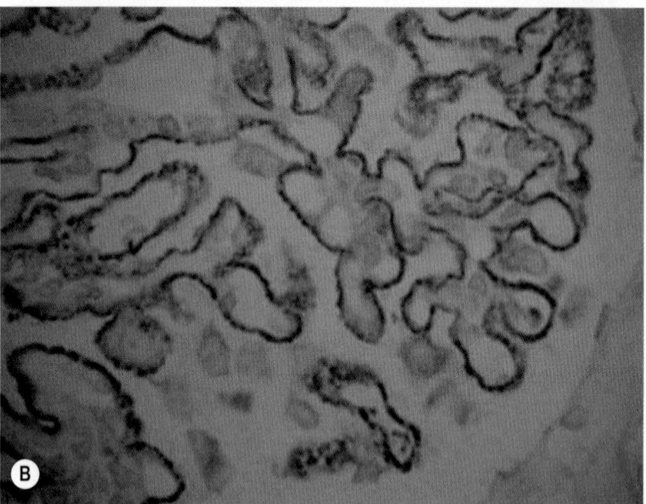

Figure 66.3 (A) Glomerulus showing thickening of the basement membrane in hepatitis-B-associated membranous nephropathy. (B) Immunoperoxidase staining showing sub-epithelial deposits of IgG in hepatitis-B-associated membranous nephropathy. *(Courtesy of Professor A.J. Howie.)*

cryoglobulinaemia. The clinical presentation is with a fever, purpuric rash particularly over the shins, arthralgia and peripheral neuropathy. The renal presentation is with proteinuria or a nephrotic syndrome often accompanied by mild to moderate renal impairment.[87–90]

Pathology

The renal lesion in cryoglobulinaemic glomerulonephritis is a type of membranoproliferative glomerulonephritis characterized by intraluminal and subendothelial deposits but other types of glomerulonephritis, e.g. mesangioproliferative glomerulonephritis, have been reported and rarely, there is a renal arteritis. Immunofluorescent microscopy shows subendothelial as well as mesangial and capillary wall deposits of IgM, IgG and C3. On electron microscopy these deposits may show the characteristics of cryoglobulins.

Management

Treatment of HCV infection is pegylated interferon α-2a/2b in combination with ribavirin.[87] Treatment of acute cryoglobulinaemic glomerulonephritis and vasculitis has usually been with prednisolone and cyclophosphamide and more recently with rituximab. Interpretation of these studies of treatment is complicated by the lack of controlled studies. Plasma exchange reduces cryoglobulin and immune complex levels and has been reported to lead to an improvement of renal function. However, the effects are usually temporary, since depletion of cryoglobulins leads to rapid rebound immunoglobulin synthesis.

HUMAN IMMUNODEFICIENCY VIRUS (HIV)-ASSOCIATED GLOMERULONEPHRITIS

The major renal syndromes associated with HIV infection are HIV-associated nephropathy (HIVAN), HIV-associated immune complex disease (HIVICK), thrombotic microangiopathy (TMA) and drug-induced nephrotoxicity.[91] In addition, acute deterioration of renal function may develop as a result of volume depletion from renal salt wasting or from diarrhoea and vomiting. There may also be renal disease from co-existent hepatitis B or C infection, post-infectious glomerulonephritis or an IgA nephropathy. A major clinical problem in these patients is the development of proteinuria, a nephrotic syndrome and renal impairment.[92–94] In Africa, in addition to HIVAN, other lesions are commonly found.[93] In a recent study from South Africa, HIVAN was found in only 27% of cases.[94] An HIV immune complex deposition disease (HIVICK) was found in 21% of cases and other glomerular lesions such as membranous nephropathy and IgA nephropathy were also frequently seen.[94]

Clinical Presentation

The clinical presentation of HIVAN and HIVICK is usually with a nephrotic syndrome and renal impairment. Hypertension is uncommon and ultrasound examination shows large echogenic kidneys. Without antiretrovirals, these lesions carry a poor prognosis with at least a 50% mortality within 2 years and it is now clear that antiretroviral treatment markedly improves the prognosis.

Pathology

Collapsing glomerulopathy was initially described in patients with HIV-associated nephropathy (HIVAN), where it was associated with a severe nephrotic syndrome and rapid progression to end-stage renal failure. There are two characteristic glomerular histological lesions in HIV. The first, HIVAN, is a type of focal segmental sclerosing glomerulonephritis, characterized by segmental or global collapse of glomerular capillaries with basement membrane wrinkling and podocyte proliferation (Figure 66.4).[95–97] There is often a marked interstitial infiltrate of lymphocytes and plasma cells with microcysts. In addition, there are endothelial tubuloreticular inclusions. On immunofluorescent microscopy, mesangial and capillary wall deposits of IgM and C3 are seen. Collapsing glomerulopathy may also be seen in patients without HIV infection and may be idiopathic or associated with parvovirus B19 infection. The second lesion, HIVICK, results in mesangial proliferation and immune complex deposition. Large subepithelial deposits are present often with a mesangial reaction giving a characteristic 'ball in cup' appearance. IgA, IgM and IgG may be present along with C3 and, in some cases, the immunohistochemical appearances may be similar to those seen in lupus nephritis.[94]

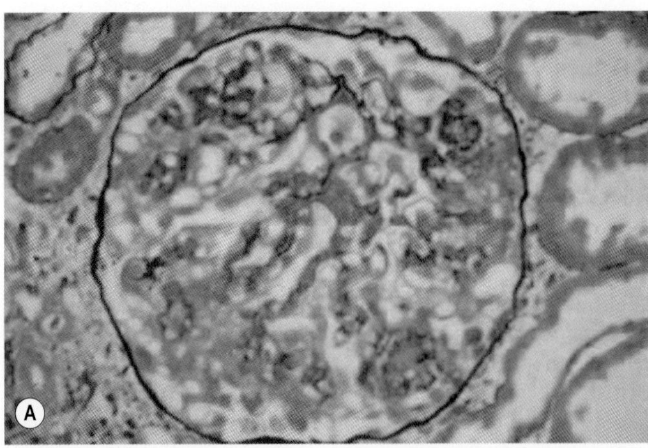

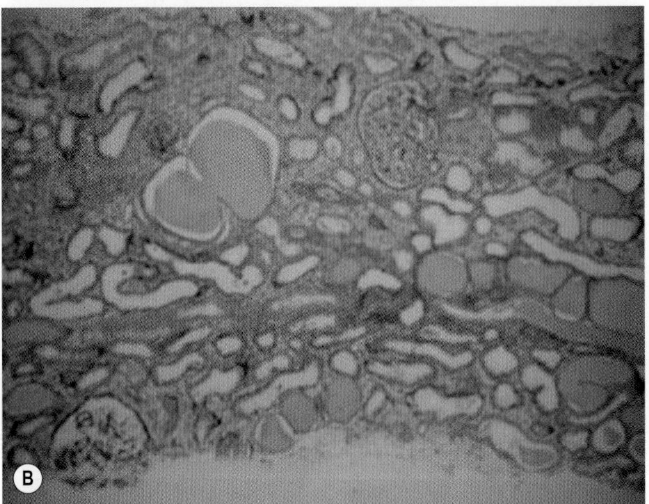

Figure 66.4 (A) HIV-associated nephropathy: Glomeruli have changes of collapsing glomerulopathy. (B) Renal cortex in HIV nephropathy. Tubules are dilated and contain casts. *(Courtesy of Professor A.J. Howie.)*

Genetics

Recent genetic studies provide some insight into the observation that most individuals with HIVAN are African Americans or Africans. Strong associations have been found between some polymorphisms in the non-muscle myosin heavy chain 9 gene (MYH9) and apolipoprotein 1 (APOL1) gene and HIVAN and also FSGS. These polymorphisms are common in African Americans but not in Caucasian Americans. In particular, variants of the APOL1 gene are strongly associated with FSGS and HIVAN.[98–100]

Management

There is increasing evidence to suggest that treatment with highly active antiretroviral drugs improves both the renal and overall prognosis of affected patients.[92,101] As with other proteinuric renal diseases, there is evidence that treatment with ACEI may be of long-term benefit. Haemodialysis is safe in patients with HIV-associated renal failure and in those patients with undetectable viral loads and preserved CD4 counts transplantation can also be considered if the patient is stable on anti-retroviral treatment.

Some of the antiretroviral drugs used in the treatment of HIV are nephrotoxic[102,103] and these effects are summarized in Table 66.2.

SCHISTOSOMIASIS

Schistosomiasis (see also Chapter 52) is widespread in the tropics. *Schistosoma haematobium* affects the urinary tract, and *S. mansoni* and *S. japonicum* the intestine(s) and liver. Significant glomerular disease has been reported only in patients with *S. mansoni* infection and hepatosplenic disease.[104–106] Overall, just fewer than 5% of patients with *S. mansoni* infection have hepatosplenic disease, and of these about 10–15% develop glomerular lesions over a period of up to 10 years. The clinical presentation is with proteinuria or nephrotic syndrome. In Egypt, there is evidence that schistosomal glomerulonephritis is more common in individuals with concomitant chronic *Salmonella* infections.[107,108]

Pathology

A mesangial proliferative glomerulonephritis is seen in mild or early cases and the most common histological change in advanced cases is a mesangiocapillary glomerulonephritis, seen in about 50% of patients. The next most frequently seen histological lesion is a focal segmental glomerulosclerosis. There are also infrequent reports of a membranous nephropathy and a proliferative glomerulonephritis. Immunofluorescent microscopy of renal biopsies shows granular deposits, predominantly of IgM but also of IgG, IgA, IgE and C3 in the mesangium and the subepithelial and subendothelial sites. Renal amyloidosis has been described in patients with *S. mansoni* infection in Sudan and in Egypt.[109,110]

TABLE 66.2 Nephrotoxicity of Highly Active Antiretroviral Drugs

Antiretroviral Class	Name	Renal Abnormalities	Histology
Protease inhibitors	Indinavir	Renal calculi, crystalluria, ARF, CRF	Tubulointerstitial nephritis with crystals
	Nelfinavir	Renal colic	
	Ritonavir	ARF	
Nucleoside reverse transcriptase inhibitors	Abacavir	ARF	Interstitial nephritis
	Didanosine	Proximal tubular dysfunction	
	Lamivudine	Proximal tubular dysfunction	
	Stavudine	Proximal tubular dysfunction	
Nucleotide reverse transcriptase inhibitors	Tenofovir	Proximal tubular dysfunction, ARF nephrogenic diabetes insipidus, nephritic syndrome	
HIV-1 fusion inhibitor	Enfuvirtide	Glomerulonephritis	Membranoproliferative nephritis

Management

Treatment of schistosomal glomerulonephritis with antischistosomal drugs, prednisolone and cyclophosphamide has been of no benefit and progression to renal failure is usual.

LEPROSY

The major renal lesions found in leprosy (see also Chapter 41) are amyloidosis and glomerulonephritis, although chronic interstitial nephritis has also been described.

Amyloidosis

Renal amyloid is a complication of long-standing leprosy and has been most often described in patients with lepromatous leprosy and rarely in patients with tuberculoid leprosy.[111,112] In earlier autopsy studies, renal amyloid was described in up to 30% of cases in North and South America, but is relatively uncommon (<10% of cases in India, Papua New Guinea and Africa). The amyloid fibrils in leprosy are of the AA variety, which is derived from the acute-phase reactant serum amyloid A (SAA). Serum levels of SAA rise in patients with erythema nodosum leprosum (ENL) reactions and there are suggestions that amyloidosis is more common in patients with recurrent ENL.[111] The clinical presentation is with proteinuria, microscopic haematuria and the nephrotic syndrome, and progression to renal failure is common.

Leprosy and Glomerulonephritis

Glomerulonephritis is found in up to 10% of patients with leprosy at autopsy. It tends to be more common in patients with lepromatous than with tuberculoid leprosy, and the onset of glomerulonephritis may coincide with an episode of ENL. The most common glomerular lesions are a mesangial proliferative glomerulonephritis and a focal or diffuse proliferative glomerulonephritis. Rarely a membranous nephropathy or mesangiocapillary glomerulonephritis is seen. Immunofluorescent microscopy shows granular glomerular deposits of IgG, IgM and C3 in the mesangium or on capillary walls.[112,113] The renal disease progresses to renal failure and it is unclear whether treatment for leprosy influences progression.

FILARIASIS

There are several reports of an association between filariasis and glomerulonephritis from India and Cameroon.[114,115] The clinical presentation is usually with nephrotic syndrome and rarely with an acute nephritic syndrome. Patients with *Wuchereria bancrofti* infection may develop a mesangial proliferative or a diffuse proliferative glomerulonephritis.[115] In patients with Loa loa infections, a membranous and a mesangiocapillary glomerulonephritis have been reported. Onchocerciasis have been reported to be associated with a nephrotic syndrome due to minimal-change nephropathy, mesangial proliferative glomerulonephritis and a mesangiocapillary glomerulonephritis.[115]

Pathology

On immunofluorescent microscopy, glomerular deposits of IgG, IgM and C3 are seen in the mesangium and capillary walls, and in one study onchocercal antigens were identified on glomerular capillaries.

Management

Treatment with diethylcarbamazine probably hastens recovery in those patients with an acute nephritic presentation but has no effect in patients presenting with nephrotic syndrome.

MALARIA

Malaria (see also Chapter 43) is widespread in the tropics and is a major cause of death. In the 1930s in British Guyana, Giglioli established the long-suspected association between *Plasmodium malariae* infection and a nephrotic syndrome. Proteinuria, nephritis and deaths from nephritis were common in British Guyana. Patients with nephrotic syndrome in this area had a higher incidence of *P. malariae* parasitaemia than unaffected individuals, who more often had *P. vivax* and *P. falciparum* infection. In 1962, Giglioli[116,117] summarized his observations that following eradication of malaria from British Guiana, there was a reduction in the incidence of proteinuria and nephritis and deaths from malaria.

QUARTAN MALARIAL NEPHROPATHY

The association between *P. malariae* infection and glomerulonephritis was confirmed by clinicopathological studies from Nigeria and Uganda in children with nephrotic syndrome. These children mostly had an incidence of *P. malariae* parasitaemia (up to 88% of children) that was significantly higher than in healthy controls (20%).[9,118,119] Most recent studies from tropical Africa do not report quartan malarial nephropathy.[18,22]

SICKLE CELL DISEASE

Patients with sickle cell disease[120,121] often have an impaired ability to concentrate and acidify urine and to excrete a potassium load but these changes are minor and usually of no clinical significance. Glomerular filtration rate (GFR) and effective renal plasma flow are increased in children with sickle disease and it is suggested that the increased GFR may lead to glomerular damage in later life.

Haematuria

Microscopic haematuria is common in patients with both sickle cell disease and trait, and less commonly macroscopic haematuria, that may be persistent, is seen.[122] The management is with conservative measures only. It is worthwhile screening for other causes of haematuria in these patients, e.g. schistosomiasis.

Renal Papillary Necrosis

Renal papillary necrosis[123] is found in both sickle cell disease and sickle cell trait. The clinical presentation is with haematuria that on occasion may be complicated by clot colic. Diagnosis is confirmed by intravenous pyelography, showing changes ranging from clubbing of calyces to a ring sign in which an often-calcified, partly attached papilla is surrounded by a ring of contrast.

Medullary Renal Cell Carcinoma

This has been rarely reported in individuals with sickle cell trait and carries a poor prognosis.

Glomerulonephritis

Focal Segmental Glomerulosclerosis.[124] This is the most frequently described lesion. It is found in older patients, usually aged over 30 years. The incidence of this lesion is unclear. Histologically, the glomeruli are larger than normal and show segmental areas of glomerular sclerosis. Because the GFR is raised in early life in patients with sickle cell disease, it has been suggested that the segmental sclerosis is a consequence of hyperfiltration and intraglomerular hypertension. The clinical presentation is with proteinuria and the clinical course is with progressive renal impairment. The proteinuria reduces with treatment with angiotensin-converting inhibitors and it is possible that these agents, by reducing intraglomerular pressures, might reduce the rate at which renal function declines.

Mesangiocapillary Glomerulonephritis.[125] The second most commonly described lesion in patients with sickle cell anaemia and proteinuria is mesangiocapillary glomerulonephritis. The pathogenesis of this is unclear and suggestions that it is caused by the glomerular deposition of renal tubular epithelial cell antibodies and antigen await confirmation.

Acute Proliferative Glomerulonephritis.[126] An increased predisposition to post-streptococcal glomerulonephritis from infected leg ulcers has also been reported in older patients with sickle cell anaemia.

End-Stage Renal Failure in Sickle Cell Anaemia.[121] Both continuous ambulatory peritoneal dialysis and haemodialysis have been successfully used in these patients. Anaemia is a major problem and does not respond well to erythropoietin. It is necessary to perform exchange transfusion with AA blood prior to renal transplantation to prevent sickling of the renal graft.

Acute Kidney Injury (AKI)

Acute renal failure is being increasingly referred to as acute kidney injury (AKI).[127–131] It is a process that complicates a wide variety of diseases. The incidence varies in published series from different countries; ranging from 4.1/year per million population in a Kuwaiti series[132] to 6.4/1000 admissions in an Indian series.[133] The abrupt cessation of renal function leads to uraemia, with abnormalities of fluid and electrolyte balance. Patients with AKI do not necessarily present in neat diagnostic categories but more often as unexplained acute uraemic emergencies. The priorities in this early phase are to manage acute uraemia and electrolyte abnormalities, in particular hyperkalaemia, to establish the reversibility of the renal failure and to define its cause.

The main differences in the epidemiology of AKI in the tropics compared with temperate countries are the cause of AKI (discussed below) and the age of onset, as patients generally present in their mid-30s compared with their 70s in temperate countries.[134,135]

CAUSES OF ACUTE URAEMIA

The main cause of AKI in the tropics is acute tubular necrosis, often as a result of infection, with glomerulonephritis presenting much less commonly. Of all cases of AKI in the tropics, 60% have a medical cause, 25% a surgical cause and 15% an obstetric cause.[128,134,136] In the more developed areas, the pattern is akin to that found in the West, where medical and surgical causes predominate and obstetric cases are rare. The differences in aetiology are largely dependent on socioeconomic factors and the availability of therapeutic pregnancy termination services. The classification of the causes of AKI into pre-renal, intrinsic and post-renal categories remains clinically useful in that it allows a structured approach to diagnosis and management. In an Egyptian series, 38% had pre-renal, 24% post-renal and the rest intrinsic renal disease, as a cause of their AKI.[137] The major causes of AKI are summarized in Box 66.3. This list is not exhaustive and is meant to emphasize the importance of seeking an aetiology in a patient with unexplained AKI.

BOX 66.3 CAUSES OF ACUTE RENAL FAILURE

PRE-RENAL

- Renal hypoperfusion (leading to acute tubular necrosis)
- Hypovolaemia
- Septicaemia
- Obstetric accidents
- Massive intravascular haemolysis
- Rhabdomyolysis

RENAL

- Acute tubular necrosis
- Acute interstitial nephritis
- Diffuse extracapillary glomerulonephritis
- Acute pyelonephritis
- Nephrotoxins
- Haemolytic–uraemic syndrome

POST-RENAL

- Obstructive uropathy
- Renal tubule blockage
- Myeloma (light chains)
- Uric acid, sulfadiazine
- Bilateral urinary tract blockage
- Calculi
- *Schistosoma haematobium*
- Urethral stricture
- Prostatic hypertrophy
- Pelvic malignancy
- Posterior urethral valves.

CLINICAL SYNDROMES

Acute Tubular Necrosis

A variety of infections and hypovolaemia may lead to renal ischaemia with renal vasoconstriction and tubular cell damage with a reduction in GFR. In addition there may be tubular obstruction and back-leakage of filtrate. A similar outcome may be the result of nephrotoxic drugs, such as aminoglycosides, and also traditional herbal remedies. There has been considerable research into the mediators involved in this injurious process. Nitric oxide, oxygen radicals, endothelin and free iron have all been implicated. To-date, there have been little convincing data to suggest that manipulation of these systems improves outcome. Although some early studies included in a meta-analysis in 2003 suggest beneficial outcomes with N-acetylcysteine in preventing acute tubular necrosis (ATN) secondary to radio contrast-induced AKI[138] more recent trials suggest that adequate hydration and careful attention to fluid management provides similar results.[139]

The clinical consequence of ATN is uraemia, which is usually associated with oliguria, although some patients may be non-oliguric, producing urine volumes of ≥1–2 L. In the vast majority of cases, acute tubular necrosis is self-limiting and with spontaneous recovery occurring between 10 days and 6 weeks, provided the initial insult is treated. When the initial insult is very severe, cortical necrosis may occur, leading to irreversible renal failure, although this is rare in infection-associated ATN.

Renal Parenchymal Causes

Acute glomerulonephritis, especially when accompanied by extracapillary proliferation (crescent formation), may lead to AKI. Acute interstitial nephritis is seen in leptospirosis and may also be a complication of drugs such as the penicillins, sulfonamides, thiazide diuretics and frusemide as well as non-steroidal anti-inflammatory drugs.

Obstructive Uropathy

Obstruction to the urinary tract is a common and potentially reversible cause of AKI. The most common site of obstruction is at the bladder outlet due to prostatic hypertrophy or cancer and urethral stricture. Urethral stricture is more common in tropical Africa than in developed countries.[140] Pelvic tumours in women (cervical and disseminated ovarian tumours), and in both sexes bladder cancer and less commonly retroperitoneal fibrosis or malignancy, may also obstruct the urinary tract. Obstruction at the level of the ureters or higher must be bilateral, unless there is a solitary functioning kidney, to cause AKI. This is usually due to renal calculi or schistosomal-induced ureteric stenosis.[141,142] Renal tubules may become blocked by uric acid crystals, particularly in patients with hyperuricaemia following chemotherapy for lymphoma, leukaemia or myeloma. Prophylactic treatment with allopurinol, hydration and alkalinization of urine in these patients now make this an infrequent cause of AKI. Rasburicase, a urate oxidase, has been shown to be effective in reducing renal injury in tumour lysis syndrome.[143] Other causes of renal tubular obstruction include sulfadiazine therapy, antiretrovirals (outlined above) and high-dose methotrexate treatment.

CAUSES OF AKI IN THE TROPICS

AKI in Pregnancy

AKI from obstetric causes is common in the tropics. In the West, 3% of all causes of AKI have an obstetric aetiology, whereas this figure is much higher in the tropics: 25% in Ghana[136] and 9–15% in India.[134,144] A recent study looking at obstetric admission to ITU comparing a centre in India and one in the USA demonstrates the differences between the tropics and the West.[145] The actual cause varies according to the different stages of pregnancy. In the 1st trimester, septic abortions account for the vast majority of cases. This is commoner than it is in the West because of the lack of legal abortion services in some tropical countries. In the 3rd trimester, causes include pre-eclampsia and eclampsia, HELLP syndrome, puerperal sepsis, haemorrhage and abruptio placentae. The most common histological lesion found is acute tubular necrosis, although cortical necrosis is found more frequently in the tropics. The striking decline in the incidence of AKI during pregnancy in some developing countries can be attributed to improved obstetric care and also to liberalization of abortion laws.[146]

Massive Intravascular Haemolysis.

Glucose-6-phosphate Dehydrogenase Deficiency. Glucose-6-phosphate dehydrogenase (G6PD) deficiency is an inherited sex-linked red cell abnormality affecting more than 400 million people across the tropics. There are over 180 different variants mainly resulting from mutations in the G6PD gene and conferring varying levels of deficiency. The product of the G6PD reaction is NADPH, which is essential for the function of enzymes that protect against oxidants (catalase and glutathione peroxidase). Hence in G6PD deficiency, erythrocytes are susceptible to oxidant stress. The major clinical consequence of this is haemolysis due to infections and drugs. AKI has been reported in G6PD-deficient individuals following massive haemolysis (so-called blackwater fever) due to drugs[147,148] and infections such as typhoid fever, malaria and hepatitis.[149,150]

Malaria.[151,152] AKI is a well-recognized complication of severe *P. falciparum* infections in adults.[153–157] The pathogenesis of AKI is unclear but reduction in microcirculatory flow leading to ATN is thought to be the main factor variably compounded by dehydration and sometimes massive haemolysis (blackwater fever).[158–160] The latter may be a consequence of severe infection alone but may also be triggered by drugs such as quinine, or caused by G6PD deficiency. AKI usually occurs together with other manifestations of severe malaria and can be either of the oliguric or non-oliguric type. Most patients are hypercatabolic. Jaundice, acidosis, oliguria, hypotension and multi-organ failure signify a poor prognosis.[152]

P. falciparum infection results in the expression of red cell surface proteins that increase red cell adherence. Erythrocytes containing *P. falciparum* become adherent to adjacent uninfected red cells,[161] capillary endothelium[162] and platelets[163] and are sequestered in organs such as the kidney, causing alterations in the microcirculation. The infected red cells also display reduced deformability, which results in predominantly extravascular haemolysis. The combination of these two phenomena causes renal vasoconstriction, renal tubular toxicity and activation of intravascular coagulation.[164] Activation of cytokines may also contribute to the increased adhesion and alteration of the renal microcirculation.

The histological changes are those of acute tubular necrosis, more marked in the distal tubule, and there may be casts of haemoglobin and malaria pigment. Artesunate has now replaced quinine as the treatment of choice for severe malaria.[165–167] The renal failure should be treated along standard lines with early renal replacement. Haemofiltration is superior to peritoneal dialysis and is associated with a lower mortality.[168] In established renal failure, renal function usually returns to normal within 3 weeks. There is no residual renal damage.

Diarrhoeal Diseases. Diarrhoea is the second commonest cause of death in children under the age of 5 in the world; according to the WHO, the vast majority come for tropical countries. Many sufferers die because of malnutrition and AKI. The AKI that occurs with diarrhoeal disease is usually due to volume depletion.

Typhoid Fever. Renal complications are unusual in uncomplicated typhoid fever.

AKI. AKI may be caused by massive intravascular haemolysis and this is particularly common in patients with G6PD deficiency.[149,150] There have been reports of haemolytic–uraemic syndrome[169] and rhabdomyolysis[170] in association with *Salmonella* species infections and also of a transient mesangial proliferative glomerulonephritis.

***Shigella* Species.** *Shigella* dysentery can lead to childhood AKI[171,172] with severe *Shigella* species infection resulting in volume depletion and toxaemia. AKI may also occur from a haemolytic–uraemic syndrome during the diarrhoeal phase of the illness. Mortality from this condition is high at 70%, with 14% of the survivors going on to develop chronic renal impairment as a result of chronic interstitial nephritis and cortical necrosis.[173]

Cholera.[174] The WHO received reports of over 310 000 cases of cholera worldwide in 2010, of which there were over 7500 deaths. The rise was highest in the Americas, largely due to the cholera outbreak following the earthquake in Haiti. The vast majority of deaths are due to AKI secondary to volume depletion as a result of the profuse diarrhoea. Given the degree of diarrhoea in cholera, hypokalaemia is frequently present, and in addition to acute tubular necrosis, there may also be evidence of vacuolation of the proximal tubular epithelium. These complications can usually be prevented by adequate fluid replacement in most cases, using oral rehydrations solutions.

Leptospirosis.[175–177] Leptospirosis is contracted following exposure to contaminated water, either in rivers or sewage. The clinical presentation is with myalgia, pyrexia, conjunctival congestion and haemorrhages, headache and jaundice. There may be a bleeding diathesis with gastrointestinal and pulmonary haemorrhage. AKI occurred in nearly 15% of patients in a recent well-characterized outbreak of leptospirosis in Sri Lanka.[178] AKI occurs during the acute leptospiraemia stage and is usually accompanied by jaundice (Weil's syndrome). The renal lesion appears to progress from tubular cell swelling to acute tubular necrosis to severe interstitial nephritis.[179] Minor glomerular mesangial proliferation may be seen. The AKI is usually hypercatabolic complicated by hyperuricaemia and hyperkalaemia and a rise in blood urea disproportionate to the serum creatinine. Dark-field microscopy of urine may reveal leptospires and they may also be grown from blood culture specimens in the early phase of the disease if antibiotics have not been given. The diagnosis may also be established by serological tests (the MAT; rapid tests have been developed but are insufficiently reliable). Treatment of leptospirosis when there is renal failure, is with penicillin, doxycycline or cefotaxime.[180] Treatment may sometimes be complicated by a Jarisch–Herxheimer reaction and may not prevent the need for dialysis.[181] Patients with severe renal failure require dialysis and there is some evidence to suggest blood purification techniques provide patients with a better outlook compared with peritoneal dialysis.[182]

Post-streptococcal Glomerulonephritis

Beta-haemolytic streptococcal infections of the throat or skin can be complicated by an endocapillary proliferative glomerulonephritis. In Ethiopia, 5% of children with these infections developed renal complications.[183] There is evidence that the incidence is decreasing in some tropical countries; however, it still accounts for up to 13% of all paediatric AKI cases.[184] This disease is discussed in more detail above.

Heatstroke

Heatstroke[185,186] occurs in hot climates, usually in association with exertion and poor fluid input, and can lead to AKI. The mechanism of the renal failure is rhabdomyolysis and disseminated intravascular coagulation. Fulminant hepatic failure may also occur, contributing to the coagulopathy and renal failure. Investigations reveal evidence of haemoconcentration with a raised creatinine kinase, hyperuricaemia, myoglobinuria, hyperkalaemia, hypocalcaemia, proteinuria and often microscopic haematuria. Renal failure is treated along standard lines.

Melioidosis

This infection is caused by *Burkholderia pseudomallei*, an organism found in soil and water, and the infection is endemic in South-east Asia, and Northern Australia with sporadic cases reported elsewhere.[187] Patients with diabetes mellitus, chronic renal disease, cirrhosis and immune suppression have an increased susceptibility to this infection. There is a marked seasonal variation in this disease, with the majority of cases occurring in the rainy season. In Northern Thailand the incidence ranges from 4.9 to 14.9 per 100 000 population with a corresponding mortality of around 36%.[188] AKI is more common in patients with septicaemia (60%) than in those with the localized form of the infection (35%). In the septicaemic form the presentation is usually one with a short history of a high temperature which may be accompanied by, shock and a metabolic acidosis. There is usually radiological evidence of pneumonia, although there may be no symptoms or signs to support this. Microabscesses are sometimes seen in the skin. In patients with AKI the mortality is high. In most patients melioidosis occurs in patients with pre-existing renal disease (in SE Asia chronic nephrolithiasis secondary to renal tubular acidosis is a common predisposing factor). Occasionally, ATN or renal microabscesses may occur. Initial treatment is with high-dose ceftazidime or meropenem.[189] Imipenem can also be used. The organism is resistant to gentamicin and penicillin.

Snake Bite

Snake bites (see also Chapter 75) are a relatively common event in the tropics. In Papua New Guinea snake bite victims account for 60% of all ventilator bed-days in intensive care units.[190] AKI is a well-recognized complication of snake bite. In a series from Chandrigah in India, out of 1862 patients with snake bites 3% developed AKI.[191] AKI has been reported in patients bitten by snakes of the viper, colubrid and sea snake classes. Russell's viper envenomation results in AKI in 3% and 30% of patients, with a recent study indicating a figure of 7%;[192] the figure following rattlesnake envenomation is around 15%. The risk of developing AKI depends on the venom dose and the time between the bite and the administration of antivenom. Gastrointestinal bleeding and also bleeding into the muscle, viscera and subarachnoid space may develop. AKI develops within hours to 3 days after envenomation. The mechanism for the AKI differs among the various snake families. Vipers cause intravascular haemolysis and disseminated intravascular coagulation but there is also evidence for direct nephrotoxicity.[193] The mechanism whereby sea snake bites cause AKI is rhabdomyolysis and myoglobinuria. The most common renal histological change seen is acute tubular necrosis, but cortical necrosis may be seen in up to 3% of cases.[193] Other renal lesions reported include proliferative glomerulonephritis (occasionally with crescents), arteritis and renal infarcts. The main aim of treatment is adequate volume replacement and the administration of a specific antivenom as soon as possible. Treatment of renal failure is along standard lines.

Nephrotoxins

A wide variety of plants used as herbal remedies in the tropics have been reported to be nephrotoxic (see also Chapter 76).[194,195] Renal failure has also been reported following multiple bee and wasp stings, spider bite and scorpion sting. In addition to direct nephrotoxicity the causes of AKI include haemolysis and disseminated intravascular coagulation. Other causes of nephrotoxic AKI include paraquat and copper sulphate poisoning. More recently, ingestion of the hair dye paraphenylene diamine has been reported to cause AKI in North Africa and in India.[196] This is associated with neck and upper respiratory oedema, rhabdomyolysis and respiratory failure.

Haemolytic–Uraemic Syndrome

This is a syndrome of thrombocytopenia, microangiopathic haemolytic anaemia with fragmented red blood cells and AKI. The main cause of epidemic diarrhoea-associated haemolytic–uraemic syndrome (HUS) is Shiga toxin-producing *Escherichia coli* (STEC) in the West and in countries in South America but in South Asia and Africa it is more often associated with *Shigella dysenteriae*.[197] Mortality from this condition can be as high as 40% in some countries. Sporadic cases of HUS also occur and this is more common in adults. Rare infective causes of HUS include neuraminidase-producing pneumococci and also *Salmonella typhi* infection.[169] Most cases of endemic HUS occur in infants and young children. The clinical syndromes of STEC infections include mild diarrhoea, haemorrhagic colitis and in 7–24% of patients, HUS. Hypertension is common and focal neurological abnormalities such as fits and strokes may develop.

Once ingested, the Shiga toxin is transported to the kidney where the A subunits are internalized causing cell death, activation of platelets and the coagulation casade[198,199] leading to the characteristic microangiopathic haemolytic anaemia. Histological abnormalities on renal biopsy include glomerular changes such as endothelial swelling, proliferation and capillary loop thrombosis. Afferent glomerular arterioles may show fibrin deposition and may be thrombosed. Whether antibiotics prevent or worsen HUS is controversial, with some studies showing benefit and others a detrimental effect.[200]

INVESTIGATIONS IN AKI

These are aimed at establishing the presence and severity of AKI and its aetiology, together with the history and physical examination; it is then possible to plan rational management for these patients.

Urine

Microscopic haematuria with red cell casts in the presence of proteinuria points strongly to a glomerulonephritis, while eosinophiluria suggests a drug-induced acute interstitial nephritis. The presence of urinary myoglobin is diagnostic of rhabdomyolysis.

Haematology

In AKI, an elevated neutrophil count usually suggests underlying sepsis while in STEC or *Shigella*-associated HUS it correlates with disease severity. Anaemia with thrombocytopenia and fragmented red cells in the presence of normal clotting indices is also indicative of HUS, whereas the presence of a coagulopathy and raised serum levels of fibrinogen degradation products suggests disseminated intravascular coagulation. In severe drug-induced interstitial nephritis there may be an increase in the peripheral blood eosinophil count. Blood should also be examined for the presence of malaria parasites.

Chemistry

An elevation of blood urea and creatinine will be found in AKI. An inappropriately elevated urea compared to creatinine suggests volume depletion and a prerenal aetiology or gastrointestinal haemorrhage. If rhabdomyolysis is suspected the blood creatinine phosphokinase concentrations should also be measured as these will be grossly elevated.

Radiological Investigations

A chest radiograph should be performed in all patients with AKI and a plain abdominal radiograph may reveal renal or ureteric calculi. An ultrasound examination of the kidneys helps to exclude obstruction and determine renal size. In patients with an obstructive uropathy, percutaneous antegrade pyelography allows visualization of the pelvis and ureter, defines the site of obstruction and allows both drainage and decompression, allowing recovery of renal function. If access to the renal pelvis is not achieved the site of the obstruction may be determined using retrograde pyelography. Computed tomography is another useful tool for defining the nature and the level of obstruction in obstructive nephropathy. Radionuclide scanning with DTPA or DMSA demonstrates renal perfusion.

Renal Biopsy

Renal histology is useful in all patients with unexplained AKI and normal-sized unobstructed kidneys, especially if they have features suggestive of glomerulonephritis or other systemic diseases.

MANAGEMENT

Prevention of Acute Tubular Necrosis

Many patients develop acute tubular necrosis after a severe infection. It is likely that many of these cases can be prevented by paying careful attention to fluid balance and avoiding nephrotoxic drugs. In this early phase AKI may be potentially reversible. Oliguria, with a low urinary Na+ (<10 mmol/L), a low fractional excretion of Na+ and urine that is more concentrated than plasma, is indicative of incipient or pre-renal AKI. The ability of these urinary indices to differentiate reversible from established renal failure is imprecise and is invalidated by loop diuretics so their use is limited. In patients with oliguria the first step is to correct hypovolaemia and a low cardiac output. Low-dose dopamine improves renal blood flow but not renal oxygen extraction and does not improve the outcome of patients with AKI.[201] Frusemide may make fluid overload easier to manage and avoid the need for dialysis but some studies suggest a poorer outcome for patients treated in this way.

Fluid Balance

A daily weight chart is valuable in assessing the fluid balance of patients with AKI. Volume depletion is usually present if the jugular venous pressure is not visible, there is a resting tachycardia and a postural drop in blood pressure. Skin turgor is more difficult to interpret as it depends on other factors such as age. The amount of fluids given to a patient in AKI is based on: (1) measured fluid losses; (2) insensible losses, which can be considerable in febrile patients in tropical climates minus metabolically produced water (about 600 mL/day in an adult); (3) fluid removed by dialysis. Crystalloids such as normal saline and isotonic sodium bicarbonate or more physiologically balanced solutions such as Hartmann's should be used unless there has been blood loss, in which case blood transfusions are required.

Hyperkalaemia and Acidosis

Serum potassium can rise rapidly in patients who are hypercatabolic or acidotic or who have rhabdomyolysis. Hyperkalaemia is cardiotoxic and the electrocardiographic features include tall peaked T waves, prolongation of the PR interval, broadening of the QRS complex, which merges into the T wave, and ventricular arrhythmias with cardiac arrest. The plasma or serum potassium must be measured daily in patients with AKI and more frequently in patients who are hypercatabolic. With milder degrees of hyperkalaemia (K+ less than 6.0 mmol/L) cation exchange resins may be used to increase faecal potassium excretion, although these can lead to severe constipation and should be administered with laxatives. Plasma potassium levels higher than 6.0 mmol/L are an indication for urgent haemofiltration or dialysis. Intravenous glucose and soluble insulin are helpful in reducing serum potassium pending dialysis. If available, electrocardiographic monitoring should be performed. Most patients with AKI have a metabolic acidosis and this can be severe in patients who are hypercatabolic. Intravenous isotonic sodium bicarbonate is useful in that it can be administered peripherally, corrects the acidosis and by doing so also lowers serum potassium. It should only be used in patients who are volume-depleted and should not be used in the presence of hypocalcaemia as it will lower ionized calcium and provoke tetany and convulsions.

Dialysis

There are now a variety of techniques for treating uraemia and removing fluid from patients with AKI. These include haemodialysis, peritoneal dialysis, haemofiltration, continuous arteriovenous haemofiltration, and continuous veno-venous haemodialysis (CVVHD).

Peritoneal Dialysis. This has the advantage of being widely available, easy to set up and easy to run. The advent of percutaneous peritoneal dialysis catheter insertion techniques has made this procedure safer. It is effective in patients with milder degrees of renal failure who are not hypercatabolic. It has the advantage of not needing specialized equipment, avoids anticoagulation and is carried out at the bedside. Because it is a continuous process, it is suitable for patients who are cardiovascularly unstable. The main complication of peritoneal dialysis is peritonitis.

Haemofiltration and Haemodialysis. Haemofiltration or haemodialysis are now the mainstay of treatment for AKI in the non-ITU setting. Haemofiltration is superior to peritoneal dialysis being more rapidly effective and thus life-saving.[168] Access to the circulation is achieved by central venous catheters. Tunnelled semi-permanent venous catheters should be employed if prolonged dialysis is likely to be required.

Patients are usually dialysed for between 3 and 4 hours, either daily or every other day. This is an extremely efficient form of treatment, as it has the ability to clear large quantities of catabolic products and fluid over a relatively short period of time. Its intermittent nature also means that patients do not require the continuous anticoagulation needed for the other forms of dialysis (discussed below). The disadvantages of intermittent haemodialysis are that patients who are hypotensive or cardiovascularly unstable may not tolerate the procedure.

In the unstable patient, continuous forms of dialysis are better tolerated. Peritoneal dialysis has been discussed above. Continuous forms of dialysis are also available but require intensive care. The standard mode of continuous haemodialysis is continuous veno-veno haemodiafiltration with fluid replacement. It requires continuous anticoagulation. Fluid removal takes place constantly, making this suitable treatment for unstable patients.

Nutrition

Patients with AKI should be given adequate nutrition in an attempt to minimize muscle catabolism and reduce malnutrition, with the added risks of delayed wound healing and impaired resistance to infection.

Sepsis

Sepsis is important both as a cause and as a complication: most studies show that sepsis is still a major cause of death in patients with AKI. The major sites of sepsis are intra-abdominal and pulmonary, and septicaemia is a frequent complication. Antibiotic doses may need to be adjusted, as many are cleared by the kidney. More importantly, if drugs such as gentamicin and vancomycin are required, strict monitoring of trough levels is required almost on a daily basis.

Drugs

Many drugs used in patients with AKI are excreted by the kidneys and, unless their dose is modified, will accumulate with potentially toxic effects. It is therefore essential to know the precise pharmacokinetics of any drug before it is given to a patient with AKI. Detailed guidelines of drug treatment in these patients are available.

Chronic Kidney Disease

DEFINITION

Chronic renal failure is now referred to as chronic kidney disease (CKD). CKD results from the progressive and irreversible loss of kidney function. When the GFR is <10 mL/min, then uraemic symptoms develop and dialysis and/or transplantation

TABLE 66.3 **KDOQI Stages of Chronic Kidney Disease**

Stage	Description	GFR (mL/min per 1.73 m²)
1	Kidney damage with normal or increased GFR	>90
2	Kidney damage with mild decrease in GFR	60–89
3	Moderate decrease in GFR	30–59
4	Severe decrease in GFR	15–29
5	Kidney failure (ESRD)	<15 or dialysis

The stages of chronic kidney disease are set out above. Stage 1 and 2 refers to patients with known proteinuria or haematuria or structural abnormalities, e.g. polycystic kidneys.

is required for survival. The estimated MDRD GFR was used by the KDOQI (Kidney Disease Outcomes Quality Initiative) committee to define the stages of CKD as shown in Table 66.3.[202] In studies from the USA, Europe, Asia and Australia, CKD affects between 5% and 15% of the adult population,[203–206] making this a major public health problem.[207] The more severe stages of CKD (3–5) are a major risk factor for cardiovascular disease, as well as for more severe renal failure (CKD stages 4 and 5).[208] There are few data on the prevalence of CKD from the tropics. Reported prevalence from the tropics are 4.2% in India;[209] 8.6% in Indonesia;[210] 9.6% in Brazil;[211] 10.4% in Nigeria[212] and 14% in the Democratic Republic of the Congo.[213] In hypertensive patients in Ghana, the prevalence of CKD was 46.9%.[214] In the tropics, economic factors determine the availability of dialysis, and in low-income societies most patients with end-stage renal failure die as dialysis is unavailable or unaffordable.

AETIOLOGY

In tropical countries, glomerulonephritis, hypertension and diabetic nephropathy are major causes of CKD, as are nephrolithiasis and obstructive uropathy.[215–218]

Diabetic Nephropathy

Diabetic nephropathy has been reported in tropical Africa, the Caribbean, the Indian subcontinent and South-east Asia. In most areas, the prevalence of diabetic nephropathy in patients with diabetes mellitus varies between 10% and 20%. The prevalence of diabetic nephropathy as a cause of CKD in most countries in the tropics is around 20% or higher.[219–221] In one report from Malaysia, 57% of patients with end-stage renal failure had diabetic nephropathy.[222]

Hypertension

Hypertension is a major cause of CKD and an important determinant of progression, regardless of the cause of renal disease. Worldwide, hypertension is common[223] and this is a major cause of CKD in tropical countries.[214,215,221,224,225]

PATHOPHYSIOLOGY

When a critical proportion of functioning nephrons is lost, glomerular hypertrophy is accompanied by glomerular hyperperfusion, hyperfiltration and hypertension and these in turn lead to progressive glomerular sclerosis, tubulointerstitial atrophy and scarring.[226] In rats, reduction of intraglomerular pressures, either by a low protein diet or by an angiotensin-converting enzyme inhibitor (ACEI) (which reduces intraglomerular pressures by efferent arteriolar vasodilatation), slowed down the rate at which renal failure progressed. A common consequence of hyperfiltration injury is proteinuria, which is associated with the development of tubulointerstitial injury. Patients with proteinuria are more likely to progress to end-stage renal failure, independent of the initial diagnosis.[227]

EARLY DETECTION AND MANAGEMENT

Recent guidelines and public health campaigns have focused on early detection and treatment of CKD as treatments that are initiated early in the disease course, will slow the progression of kidney disease and delay the onset of kidney failure.

TREATMENT OF CHRONIC KIDNEY DISEASE

The management of CKD focuses on identifying CKD-related risk factors and stages of kidney disease, and intervening appropriately. Specific treatment for CKD should depend on the cause of kidney disease and a thorough search for reversible causes, e.g. obstruction to the renal tract and nephrotoxic drugs should be carried out in each patient. There is now compelling evidence that inhibiting the effects of angiotensin using angiotensin-converting enzyme inhibitors (ACEi) or angiotensin-2-receptor blockers is important in slowing the progression of diabetic as well as non-diabetic kidney disease.[2,13,14,228–231] The blood pressure target aimed for is 130/80 mmHg or lower in patients with proteinuria (Box 66.4), as this reduces the rate of progression of renal disease. A low salt intake reduces blood pressure and probably slows progression of renal failure. Good glycaemic control has been shown to slow down the progression of CKD in patients with type 1 diabetes.[232]

BOX 66.4 MANAGEMENT OF CHRONIC KIDNEY DISEASE

1. Maintain blood pressure <130/80 mmHg and 125/75 for patients with significant proteinuria.
2. ACE inhibitors (ACEi) and angiotensin II receptor blockers (ARBS) are effective in slowing progression of renal failure and should be used when there is proteinuria.
3. Check creatinine and potassium 2 weeks after starting an ACEi or ARB and after any increase in dose. There is usually a slight decline in GFR. Discontinue drugs only if GFR drops by more than 20 mL/min and exclude renal artery stenosis.
4. In patients with impairment of renal function who are on ACEi or ARBS, do not use potassium sparing diuretics (spironolactone/amiloride) or NSAIDs because of the risk of hyperkalaemia.
5. Treat hyperkalaemia (K^+ 5.5–6.0) with frusemide and re-check in 2 weeks. Discontinue angiotensin blockade if K^+ still ≥6.0 mmol/L.
6. Discontinue non-steroidal anti-inflammatory drugs in patients with renal impairment.
7. Annual mortality from cardiovascular disease is 10–100 times higher with kidney failure, so monitor and treat risk factors.
8. Patients with type 1 or 2 diabetes mellitus and microalbuminuria or proteinuria should be managed with an ACEi or ARB.
9. Arrange urgent ultrasound kidneys and bladder in patients with urological symptoms.

CONSEQUENCES OF CKD

Hyperkalaemia and Acidosis

These are not marked until the GFR falls below 20 mL/min. Exceptions to this are patients with tubulointerstitial disorders.

Bone

Increased blood levels of parathormone are found in very early renal failure when GFR falls below 50–60 mL/min. This is probably due to inappropriately low levels of 1,25-dihydroxycholecalciferol and not to hyperphosphataemia with consequent hypocalcaemia, as previously thought. With advanced renal failure there is impaired renal synthesis of 1,25-cholecalciferol from its precursor 25-cholecalciferol. A reduction in intestinal absorption of calcium and also hyperphosphataemia increase the tendency to hypocalcaemia. This stimulates the parathyroid glands to hyperplasia and in severe cases to adenoma formation. The consequences of this are renal osteodystrophy. Vitamin D deficiency leads to osteomalacia, and hyperparathyroidism to the development of bone erosions and osteitis fibrosa.[233,234]

Anaemia

Haemoglobin concentrations tend to be maintained until the GFR falls below 30 mL/min. There are several reasons for the anaemia of CKD. Perhaps the most important is the failing kidney's inability to produce sufficient quantities of erythropoietin, the hormone that drives the bone marrow to produce red blood cells. Other factors such as reduced red cell survival are also important. Recombinant human erythropoietin is now readily available but at considerable cost and there is evidence that it improves the quality of life. However, using erythropoietin to target higher levels of haemoglobin has now been shown to increase the risks of hypertension, stroke, vascular access thrombosis and probably the risk of death and progression to renal failure.[235] In patients with CKD stages 3 and 4, normalization of haemoglobin did not reduce the risk of cardiovascular events.[236] In the CHOIR study, patients randomized to a target haemoglobin of 13.5 g/dL had a significantly higher risk of cardiovascular events than patients randomized to a target haemoglobin of 11.3 g/dL with no improvement in the quality of life.[237] Finally, the TREAT trial of darbepoetin alfa in patients with diabetes mellitus and CKD reported that as compared with placebo darbepoetin alfa did not reduce the risk of either of the two composite end-points of either death or a cardiovascular event or death or a renal event but was associated with an increased risk of stroke.[238] Erythropoietin should be considered in patients with chronic kidney disease who are symptomatic or who have haemoglobin of <9 g/dL. Other causes of anaemia such as blood loss, iron folate and B12 deficiency should be sought for and treated. The European Best Practice Guidelines now suggest a target haemoglobin of 10–12 g/dL in patients with CKD.[239] Adequate utilizable iron is required to minimize erythropoietin dosage and many centres in the West now administer regular intravenous iron to dialysis patients.

MANAGEMENT

The causes of CKD are varied and its clinical presentation differs between patients. Management must therefore be guided by the assessment of individual patients.

Conservative Management

This is effective in individuals with a GFR of ≥10 mL/min. The first objective is to identify and correct potentially reversible causes of progressive renal failure. Examples of this include obstructive uropathy and the use of potentially nephrotoxic drugs such as non-steroidal anti-inflammatory drugs.

There is now good evidence that control of blood pressure will slow down the progression to end-stage renal failure of both diabetic and non-diabetic renal disease.[240] In African Americans, intensive blood pressure control slowed the rate of decline in renal function in patients with significant proteinuria and had no effect in patients without proteinuria.[241] In diabetes, large studies in both type 1 (DCCT)[232] and type 2 (UKPDS)[242] have shown that good glycaemic control will slow the rate of progression of CKD. The UKPDS further emphasizes the importance of blood pressure control in retarding progression of CKD in type 2 diabetes.[243]

Most nephrologists now advocate the use of ACEIs in the treatment of hypertension in CKD. Caution, however, needs to be exercised in patients with both large- and small-vessel renal disease, as in this setting, these drugs may cause an acute but usually reversible deterioration in renal function. Because of this, high-risk patients require close monitoring of renal function after the initiation of therapy. In a recent study of patients with CKD who mostly had an eGFR of <20 mL/min per 1.73 m^2, there was often a sustained increase in eGFR when ACE is or angiotensin receptor blockers were discontinued.[244,245] In areas where dialysis is unavailable or unaffordable this approach is reasonable.

A low-protein diet reduces the progression of renal damage in rats but there is no evidence that it does so in humans. We, however, advise against excessive protein intake in patients with renal impairment.

The maintenance of GFR in advanced renal failure is critically dependent on salt and water balance. Salt and water overload leads to heart failure, a reduction in cardiac output and worsening of renal function. Salt and water depletion leads to volume depletion, a reduction in cardiac output and a reduction in GFR. Each patient must have careful regular assessments of their fluid status and salt and water intake and this is then optimized, if necessary, using diuretics. Once the GFR falls below 20 mL/min plasma potassium tends to rise, justifying a reduction in dietary potassium intake. Expert dietetic help adjusted to the local foods is invaluable in the management of these patients.

Renal osteodystrophy was relatively uncommon in most parts of the tropics but is becoming more of a problem, as more patients are now receiving maintenance dialysis. Key principles in management include control of hyperphosphataemia with phosphate binders, which binds ingested phosphate and the use of 1α-hydroxycholecalciferol or 1,25-dihydroxycholecalciferol in patients who are: (1) hypocalcaemic; (2) have a raised alkaline phosphatase; and/or (3) have a raised parathormone.[233,234] The dose of calcium carbonate must be adjusted to avoid hypercalcaemia.

Dialysis and Transplantation

Once the GFR falls below 10 mL/min, renal replacement with either dialysis or a renal transplant is necessary if life is to be maintained. The costs of dialysis – both continuous ambulatory dialysis and haemodialysis – are substantial but increasingly, tropical countries are providing chronic dialysis facilities. In the more developed tropical countries, the level of dialysis provision approaches that of the West. Renal transplantation once set up is less costly in the long term.

Haemodialysis. This is the most popular method for the delivering of long-term dialysis worldwide. In the USA, nearly 90% of all patients on dialysis receive haemodialysis. In the UK, the proportion receiving haemodialysis is somewhat lower at 60%. In tropical countries, the majority with chronic dialysis programmes have more patients on haemodialysis.

Peritoneal Dialysis. Several techniques are now on offer: continuous ambulatory peritoneal dialysis (CAPD), automated peritoneal dialysis (APD) and intermittent peritoneal dialysis (IPD). Both CAPD and APD are domiciliary treatments and hence, are less dependent on staff or space. Patients living far from dialysis centres may benefit from these modalities, although provision and delivery of dialysate may prove difficult. Unfortunately, most commercially produced dialysates are expensive and hence render this treatment no cheaper than haemodialysis.

Transplantation.[246] This form of renal replacement therapy provides patients with the best long-term outlook, with living donation providing the best graft survival. Many tropical countries have established live donor programmes but cadaveric programmes are also being established in some. The previous practice of 'organ trade' is now illegal in countries such as India following the passage of Act 42: The Transplantation of Human Organs Act. Transplantation provides patients with a near-normal lifestyle, most of the complications occurring as a result of side-effects of the immunosuppressive therapy. The mainstay of immunosuppression is steroids, azathioprine or mycophenolate mofetil and calcineurin inhibition, with drugs such as cyclosporin and tacrolimus. The patent on calcineurin inhibitors has recently expired, resulting in numerous cheaper generic forms. This will hopefully afford greater access to this drug. This is especially important when graft failure secondary to poor compliance, for economic reasons, is common.

Obstructive Uropathy

RENAL TUBERCULOSIS

Tuberculosis can affect the urinary tract in many ways.[247] Most commonly, there is parenchymal renal involvement with ureteric and bladder involvement. Parenchymal renal involvement often leads to cavitation, seen on intravenous urography as papillary ulceration or cavities in the parenchyma and these may communicate with the pelvicaliceal system. Advanced parenchymal lesions lead to a non-functioning kidney – so-called autonephrectomy. On plain abdominal radiographs, renal calcification is often a clue to the diagnosis of tuberculosis. Bladder involvement leads to ulceration and there may be inflammation of the ureters. In advanced disease, the bladder becomes obstructed and fibrosed and this, together with ureteric stricture or incompetence of the vesico-ureteric junction, can lead to an obstructive uropathy. Extrarenal tuberculosis may lead to the late development of glomerular amyloid. The clinical presentation is that of renal amyloid from any other cause. Rarely tuberculosis has been associated with the development of an interstitial nephritis.[248]

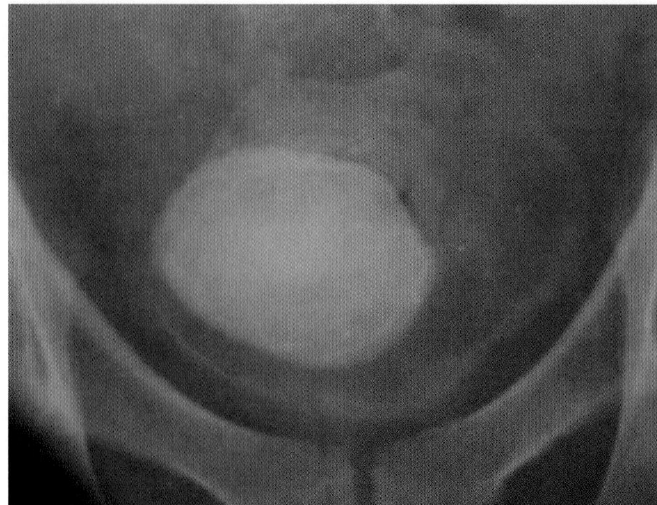

Figure 66.5 Bladder wall calcification and a bladder stone in schistosomiasis.

RENAL CALCULI

Renal and ureteric calculi tend to be uncommon in Blacks in tropical Africa but are common in the Middle East, the Indian subcontinent and the rest of Asia. The overall probability of forming stones ranges from 1–5% in Asia to 20% in Saudi Arabia, compared with 5–9% in Europe and 13% in North America.[249]

A high prevalence of renal calculi is commonly seen in countries such as Egypt, Pakistan, India, Myanmar, Thailand, Indonesia and Philippines. It is suggested that a high temperature, inadequate fluid intake and low urine volume predispose to stone formation in some areas. Bladder stones are common in Central Africa and parts of South-east Asia.

SCHISTOSOMA HAEMATOBIUM

S. haematobium infections are widespread in the tropics.[105] Schistosoma-mediated inflammation of the bladder and ureters can lead to fibrosis and to obstructive uropathy. The bladder and the juxtavesical ureter are initially involved by granuloma formation. Ureteric involvement leads to ureteric dilatation, stricture and vesico-ureteric reflux. Functionally, these abnormalities may lead to renal failure. Diagnosis is by examining the urine for *S. haematobium* ova. A calcified bladder or ureters may be seen on abdominal radiographs (Figure 66.5). Schistosomiasis predisposes to bladder calculi. Intravenous urography shows a variety of changes, including segmental dilatation of the ureter, ureteric stenosis and dilatation of the upper tracts. More recently, the ultrasonographic features have been described and this technique is gaining popularity. Treatment with praziquantel results in high cure rates and when used community-wide in endemic areas, has been shown to reduce the prevalence of urinary tract abnormalities. There is good evidence of an association between *S. haematobium* infection and the subsequent development of bladder cancer. The majority of these tumours are squamous cell carcinomas.

REFERENCES

1. Stevens LA, Coresh J, Greene T, et al. Assessing kidney function – measured and estimated glomerular filtration rate. N Engl J Med 2006;354(23):2473–83.
16. Jha V, Chugh KS. Glomerular disease in the tropics. In: Davison AM, Cameron JS, Grunfeld J, editors. Oxford Textbook of Clinical Nephrology. New York: Oxford University Press; 2005. p. 639–55.
133. Cerda J, Lameire N, Eggers P, et al. A. Epidemiology of acute kidney injury. Clin J Am Soc Nephrol 2008;3(3):881–6.
224. Barsoum RS. Chronic kidney disease in the developing world. N Engl J Med 2006;354(10):997–9.
226. Remuzzi G, Benigni A, Remuzzi A. Mechanisms of progression and regression of renal lesions of chronic nephropathies and diabetes. J Clin Invest 2006;116(2):288–96.

Access the complete references online at www.expertconsult.com

67

Ophthalmology in the Tropics and Sub-tropics

NICHOLAS A. V. BEARE | ANDREW BASTAWROUS

KEY POINTS

- Resource-poor countries bear a disproportionate burden of eye disease and blindness.
- 80% of blindness is preventable, curable or treatable.
- Blindness due to age-related disease, e.g. cataract and glaucoma and non-communicable disease, e.g. diabetes, is increasing.
- Blindness due to infectious disease, mainly trachoma and onchocerciasis, is decreasing.
- Systematic examination of the eyes can yield a great deal of information on eye and neurological disease, without specialist equipment.
- Fundoscopy through dilated pupils can provide valuable insights into systemic diseases such as AIDS, diabetes, cerebral malaria and tuberculosis.
- Two mass population measures to prevent eye disease: vitamin A supplementation and oral azithromycin have each been shown independently to reduce infant mortality of all causes by one-third and one-half, respectively.

World Blindness

The World Health Organization (WHO) Programme for the Prevention of Blindness estimates that there are 285 million visually impaired people worldwide, 39 million of whom are blind and 246 million of whom have low vision (moderate and severe visual impairment).[1] About 90% of blind people live in developing countries and around 80% of all visual impairment could be avoided or cured.[2]

Worldwide, visual impairment has decreased in the past 20 years despite an overall ageing population. This is due to reduction in blindness due to infectious disease (primarily onchocerciasis and trachoma), improved cataract surgical coverage, particularly in Asia, and improved prevention such as preventing vitamin A deficiency.

WHO CATEGORIES OF VISUAL IMPAIRMENT

Blindness is defined as a binocular visual acuity of <3/60 (less than counting fingers at 3 metres); or a visual field of less than 10° around fixation in the better eye (Table 67.1).

In the past, the WHO has used *best-corrected* visual acuity to define 'blind' and 'visually impaired'. However, most people with poor vision do not have access to the best spectacle correction and many people are visually impaired or blind for want of spectacles. Therefore, the 'presenting' visual acuity is now used – the visual acuity with the glasses normally worn.

COMMON CAUSES OF WORLDWIDE BLINDNESS

The majority of blindness is preventable, curable or treatable. Most blindness is due to exclusively ocular conditions: cataract, refractive error, glaucoma and age-related macular degeneration (AMD) (Table 67.2). Blindness due to infectious disease, mainly trachoma and onchocerciasis is reducing. Diabetic retinopathy is increasing due to changing lifestyles and previous estimates probably underestimate this as a problem. Apart from vitamin A deficiency, blindness due to other systemic disease is low in global numbers.

PATTERNS OF BLINDNESS

The prevalence of blindness is substantially higher in tropical zones than in temperate countries because of factors predominantly related to poor resources. These allow ophthalmic infectious diseases to flourish and mean that interventions that cure blindness, such as cataract surgery, are inadequately provided.

Age

Life expectancy is increasing in many developing countries and with the increase in elderly numbers, there is a corresponding increase of those who are blind. The WHO estimates that two-thirds of the visually impaired and 82% of blind people are over the age of 50.[2] Increased longevity has resulted in more older people with chronic blinding diseases, e.g. cataract, glaucoma and macular degeneration and diabetic retinopathy. Many elderly have multiple ocular pathologies.

Gender

Women suffer from more blinding eye diseases throughout the world than men. Women account for nearly two-thirds of all blindness and in some locations, the imbalance is even greater.[3] For chronic, slowly debilitating disease such as cataracts, a large part of the variation is due to differing access to eye services, attitudes to women's health and decision-making.[4] However, some diseases have differing preponderances for the sexes. Trachoma trichiasis is four to five times more common among women compared with men, due to the recurrent cycle of reinfection affecting children and mothers. Onchocerciasis is more often blinding in men, who are more exposed to the bites of the black fly (genus *Simulium*).

Ethnic Origin

Glaucoma shows considerable ethnic variation around the world.[5] Angle closure glaucoma is more common among the

TABLE 67.1 Definitions of Visual Impairment

Category	Presenting Distance Visual Acuity	
	Worse than:	Equal to or Better than:
Mild or no visual impairment	–	6/18
	–	20/70
	–	0.3
Moderate visual impairment	6/18	6/60
	20/70	20/200
	0.3	0.1
Severe visual impairment	6/60	3/60 (finger counting at 3 m)
	20/200	20/400
	0.1	0.05
Blindness[a]	3/60 (finger counting at 3 m)	No light perception
	20/400	–
	0.05	–

The first line gives the notation in the Snellen 6-metre scale; the second line gives the equivalent notation in the 20-foot scale; the third gives the decimal notation.

[a]Blindness is sub-divided into three categories by the International Classification of Diseases: 3/60 to 1/60, 1/60 to light perception and light perception to no light perception.

Mongols and Chinese, but open angle glaucoma is more common in Africans, including Afro-Americans and Afro-Caribbeans, and presents at a younger age. Age-related macular degeneration is more common in Caucasians. These variations are due to differences in genes encoding ocular structures and other systems such as the immune system.

Environmental Factors

Environmental factors overlap with socioeconomic ones, but often relate to how infectious eye diseases are transmitted. They are usually amenable to preventative intervention, e.g. trachoma is found in communities with poor sanitation and inadequate water supplies.

Socioeconomic Factors

The prevalence of blindness in developing countries is higher than in industrialized countries and the proportion of blindness caused by different diseases differs. Infectious causes such as trachoma and onchocerciasis are more common in developing countries, although disease-specific interventions have reduced these significantly. Corneal scarring from vitamin A deficiency, trauma and corneal ulcers are also more common in resource-poor settings. Cataract remains the commonest cause of blindness, although surgical coverage has improved, particularly in India and China where the disadvantaged are most affected.

In middle-income countries, better perinatal care allows premature neonates to survive, but at a risk of retinopathy of prematurity because of poor oxygen control and ophthalmic screening. In countries where obstetric and neonatal care is less advanced, premature babies do not survive.

Low literacy rates and poverty are linked to a greater risk of blindness, and being visually impaired or blind increases the risk of being in poverty.[6]

TABLE 67.2 Major Causes of Blindness Worldwide[1]

Cause of Visual Impairment	% of 39 Million Blind	% of 246 Million with Low Vision
Cataract	51	33
Glaucoma	8	2
Age-related macular degeneration	5	1
Corneal opacity	4	1
Childhood blindness	4	1
Refractive error	3	42
Trachoma	3	1
Diabetic retinopathy	1–4.6[a]	1
Undetermined	21	18

[a]4.6% is WHO estimate of 1.8 million blind from diabetic retinopathy.

EYE CARE SERVICES

There is a huge disparity in the provision of eye care services between the developed and the developing world. In Europe and North America, there is one ophthalmologist per 20 000–100 000 of the population. In sub-Saharan Africa, on average, there is one ophthalmologist for 1 million people and these are disproportionately represented in urban centres. There is also gross under-provision of eye care services in rural areas of Asia.

There is a clear need to increase the capacity of eye care in developing countries, particularly in Africa and to increase access to eye care for those most in need. This involves increasing the number of ophthalmologists who are trained and retained within the continent and who will lead the eye care teams of the future; as well as increasing the number of ophthalmic clinical officers (medical assistants), ophthalmic nurses and primary eye healthcare workers who can widely deliver eye care.

In order to meet the needs of the huge numbers of cataract blind patients in Africa, surgeons who are not medically qualified, are being trained in eye care. These surgeons need on-going training and support in order to be effective; but, as this is often not available, it is estimated that 30–50% do not therefore practice as cataract surgeons. Three-quarters of those that do practice, do so in a hospital with an ophthalmologist and on average, they perform 250 surgeries a year.[7] Despite enthusiasm in some quarters it is not yet clear that training non-medical cataract surgeons is the most effective way to increase cataract surgery rates.

It is clear that ophthalmic clinical officers and other cadres are required to deliver eye care to the vast majority of the population and to recognize cases that require referral or surgery. They also need support, continual training and professional development in order to remain up-to-date, enthusiastic and engaged. There is certainly potential for increasing cataract surgery rates per surgeon in Africa by allowing more operating time and enhancing efficiency. This has already been achieved in many units in India, pioneered by Aravind Eye Hospitals.

Eye Camps

Ophthalmology lends itself to the provision of eye services by mobile units, co-called eye camps. These ophthalmic outreach programmes may be described in two broad categories:

- Screening/diagnostic eye camps with transport to a base hospital primarily for surgery
- Surgical eye camps, with operating in a temporary theatre on-site.

Although eye camps can deliver services to populations who would otherwise have no access to eye services, the results of surgery are worse in eye camps than in static units.[8] The provision of free surgery may undermine local attempts to achieve sustainable cost-recovery and short visits of external ophthalmologists can undermine efforts to build local capacity. It is now recommended that eye camps should be used primarily for screening/diagnosis rather than surgery.

VISION 2020: THE RIGHT TO SIGHT

Vision 2020: The Right to Sight is the joint WHO/International Agency for the Prevention of Blindness (IAPB) initiative to eliminate avoidable blindness by 2020. This global partnership involves governments and leading international non-governmental development organizations in eliminating the main causes of blindness. This is through integrated and sustainable national plans for equitable and excellent eye care.

Vision 2020 focuses on three areas requiring action:

- Disease control
- Human resource development
- Infrastructure development and appropriate technology.

Disease Control

The priorities are conditions which are treatable or preventable and are major causes of blindness and visual impairment. They include:

- Cataract
- Refractive error
- Trachoma
- Childhood blindness
- Low vision
- Onchocerciasis
- Glaucoma
- Diabetic retinopathy
- Age-related macular degeneration (AMD).

Human Resource Development

Vision 2020 promotes the training of more ophthalmologists, ophthalmic clinical officers and nurses. Other specialist personnel requiring training include refractionists, managers and equipment technicians. Basic eye care should be taught in medical schools worldwide by 2020.

Infrastructure and Appropriate Technology

Vision 2020 promotes the development of infrastructure and appropriate equipment to deliver its objectives. It provides a procurement platform for the eye care sector. It has standard lists of equipment and consumable materials that are affordable and effective. Local production of instruments and consumables for eye examination, ophthalmic surgery and spectacles has been encouraged. Mass production in developing countries has reduced the price of a standard rigid intraocular lens from approximately US$200 in 1990 to about US$2 in 2012.

Achievements

While it is clear that Vision 2020 will not meet its ambitious aim by 2020, it is through its ambition and endeavour that it has had an impact. There are 15 million fewer blind people than projections made when the initiative was launched in 1999 and 91 countries now have national eye care plans. Most of the gains have come from scaling up of cataract surgery and reductions in infectious causes of blindness. However, its emphasis on integration with local healthcare provision and sustainable improvements will reap benefits for many with eye disease in the future.

Examination of the Eyes

One of the advantages of ophthalmology is the opportunity to directly visualize eye abnormalities and disease. With a torch, the cornea, iris and anterior chamber (anterior segment) can be examined; and with slit lamp magnification, the anterior eye can be seen in more detail. With an ophthalmoscope, the vitreous, optic nerve, retina and blood vessels (posterior segment) can be seen.

BASIC EQUIPMENT AND DIAGNOSTIC MATERIALS

For effective examination of the eyes, only a few basic items are required:

- Test chart, e.g. Snellen's E chart
- Pin-hole disc to overcome refractive errors
- Pen torch, an LED torch with long battery life is ideal
- Magnifying lens or loupe (uniocular or binocular)
- Direct ophthalmoscope
- Tonometer, e.g. Schiotz tonometer, to measure intraocular pressure
- Eye drops: local anaesthetic drops, e.g. proxymetacaine, benoxinate; short-acting mydriatics (to dilate the pupil), e.g. tropicamide, cyclopentolate, fluorescein dye or paper strips
- Sterile hypodermic needles
- Cotton-wool 'buds'.

CLINICAL EXAMINATION OF THE EYES

This chapter cannot describe the methods of examination in detail, some of which are best taught by demonstration. However, a systematic approach to examination will provide a framework for clarity and completeness.

Measurement of Visual Acuity

Assessing visual acuity is critical to quantify function. Distance visual acuity should be measured for each eye individually with a Snellen chart (or similar) at a distance of 6 m (Figure 67.1). If distance spectacles are worn, visual acuity should be tested with these on. If visual acuity is reduced, it should be repeated using a pin-hole. Pin-holes act as universal glasses and an improvement in vision in one or both eyes using them indicates a likely refractive error – spectacles should improve vision. If the patient cannot see the largest letter then re-test at 3 m and 1 m; test ability to see fingers (count fingers, CF), hand movements (HM), a torch light (perception of light, PL) or no light perception (NPL).

Examine the Periorbital Region of Each Eye

Identification of orbital disease should lead to specific examination of eye movements, optic nerve function (vision, visual fields, colour vision and pupil reactions) and ophthalmoscopy of the optic nerve head. Pyrexia should also be sought in acute swelling (orbital cellulitis). Palpable orbital masses should be measured and their relation to anatomy noted, such as the lacrimal gland. Is there evidence of proptosis or displacement of either eye (Figure 67.2)? Are the eyelids

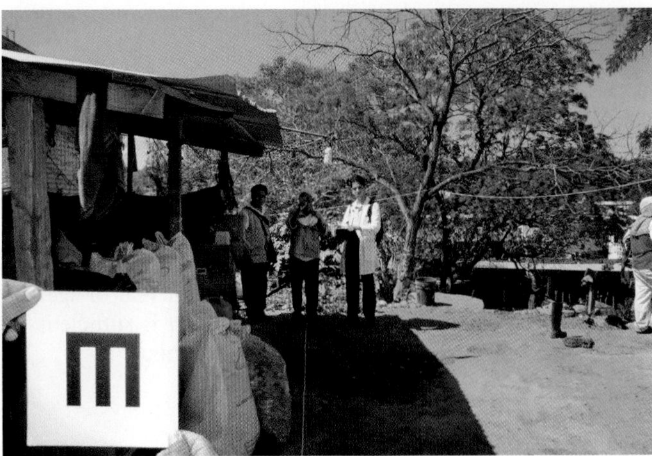

Figure 67.1 Measuring visual acuity with Snellen 'tumbling Es' in Mexico. Patient points in direction of 'legs' of the E without necessarily having to be able to read letters. Note cord to measure 6 metres. *(Courtesy of Pedro Gómez Bastar.)*

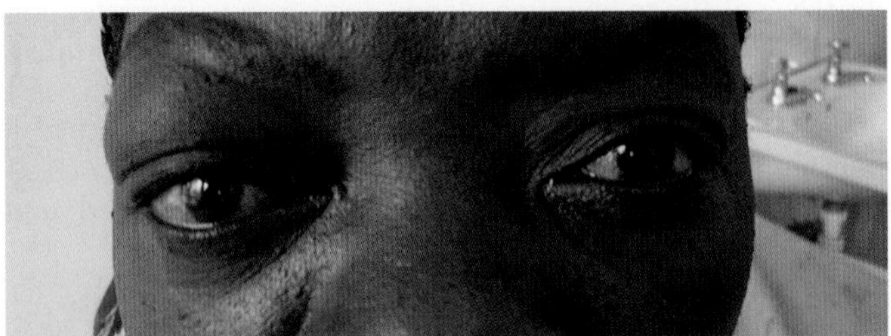

Figure 67.2 Patient with right superior orbital mass displacing the eye inferiorly. *(Courtesy of Nicholas A. V. Beare.)*

in the normal position, or are they everted (ectropion) or inverted (entropion)?

Examine Eye Movements

This has three purposes. In orbital disease or blow-out fracture it elicits any involvement of extra-ocular muscles. In neurological disease, it will reveal III, IV or VI cranial nerve palsies (Figure 67.3). A patient presenting with diplopia may of course have either problem. In long-standing squint there is no diplopia and the angle of squint is usually constant in all positions of gaze (concomitant strabismus).

Examine the Anterior Segment

Use a torch and a magnifier if available, to examine the anterior segment – the conjunctiva (bulbar and inferior tarsal by pulling the lower lid down), cornea, anterior chamber, iris and pupil. Evert the upper lid to examine the tarsal conjunctiva.

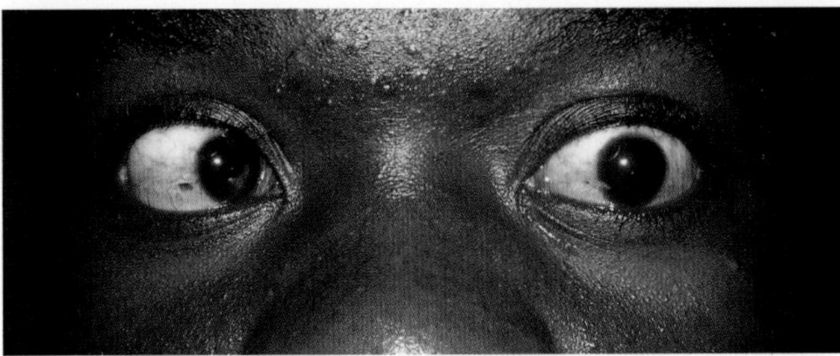

Figure 67.3 Patient with left VIth cranial nerve (lateral rectus) palsy looking to left (pupils have been pharmacologically dilated). *(Courtesy of Nicholas A. V. Beare.)*

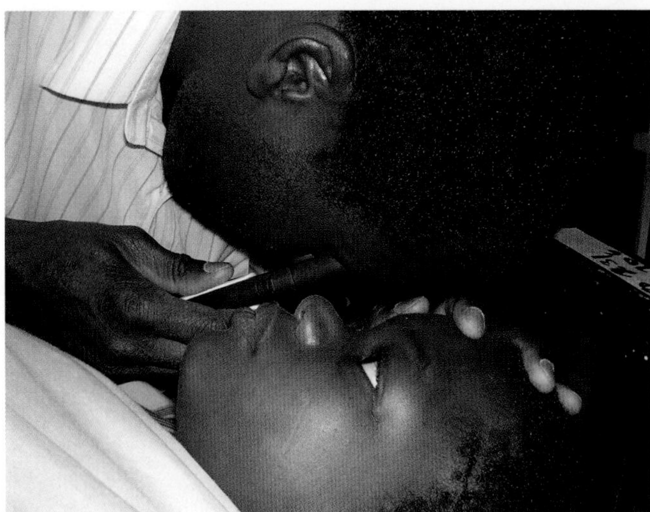

Figure 67.4 Funduscopy with a low-cost direct ophthalmoscope. Note the proximity required to obtain a reasonable field of view. *(Courtesy of Ajib Phiri and Nicholas A. V. Beare.)*

Examine the Posterior Segment

Using the ophthalmoscope, examine the clarity of the lens against the red reflex, then the retina, optic nerve and retinal blood vessels (Figure 67.4). It is essential to dilate the pupils with tropicamide 1% and, if possible, phenylephrine 2.5% to obtain a reasonable view of the fundus. This is only one part of an ocular examination, but one that non-specialists often rush to and then struggle with because the pupils are not dilated, or they are not close enough to the patient's eye.

Examine the Intraocular Pressure

A very crude estimate of the intraocular pressure can be obtained by gently palpating the eyeball through the upper eyelid, using the two index fingers, with alternating compression. This will indicate only a very hard eye with increased intraocular pressure, or a very soft eye. Much more accurate readings may be obtained using a tonometer. Extreme care should be observed in manipulation should there be an eye injury, particularly if perforation is a possibility.

Acute Ophthalmology

It is important to distinguish between serious causes of an acute red eye from minor, self-limiting conditions. Serious causes can cause permanent damage to vision and include acute glaucoma, uveitis, corneal ulcers and orbital cellulitis. Infective and allergic conjunctivitis are common but rarely cause blindness. All these conditions can usually be diagnosed confidently without specialist equipment.

WARNING SIGNS

- **The vision is affected**. The vision remains reduced after using a pin-hole to overcome refractive error and any copious discharge is removed.
- **Severe eye pain** as opposed to discomfort or foreign body sensation. Photophobia is a feature of uveitis and keratitis,

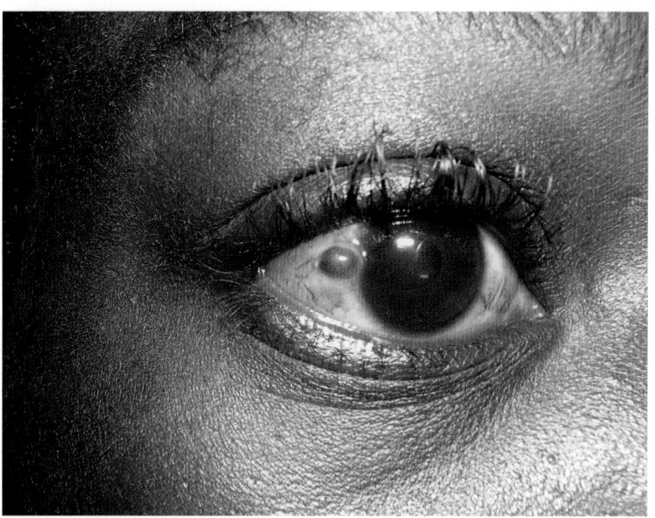

Figure 67.5 Pupil is ovoid and distorted because the iris has plugged a penetrating injury. This has been epithelized by conjunctiva. *(Courtesy of Nicholas A. V. Beare.)*

but not exclusive to them. Debilitating pain and nausea are cardinal features of an attack of acute glaucoma.

- **A pattern of redness around the cornea** usually indicates corneal or intraocular inflammation. In infective or allergic conjunctivitis the redness is most intense on the tarsal conjunctiva.
- **The cornea is not clear**. When examined by a torch the cornea appears dull or hazy, or details of the iris are not clearly visible.
- **The pupil is not round and reactive**. The pupil may be fixed mid-dilated in acute glaucoma and may be adherent to the lens (posterior synechiae) in an irregular pattern in uveitis. In corneal injury with perforation the iris may be incarcerated in the wound, distorting the pupil (Figure 67.5).

DISORDERS OF THE ORBITS AND EYELIDS

Orbital Cellulitis

Infection within the orbital cavity leads to tense swelling of the eyelids and proptosis. Eye movements are reduced. The patient usually has a fever and is unwell. Eyelid swelling without these other signs may be infection anterior to the orbital septum (pre-septal cellulitis) which can be treated with oral antibiotics.

Orbital cellulitis requires high-dose intravenous antibiotics. The most common pathogens are staphylococci and streptococci species, so antibiotics covering Gram-positive cocci with β-lactam resistance are preferred (e.g. co-amoxiclav) or a 3rd generation cephalosporin. If MRSA is prevalent, add vancomycin. If response is poor to first-line antibiotics, the infection may be caused by anaerobic organisms and suitable antibiotics such as metronidazole should be added. If the lids cannot be opened, or there is a relative afferent papillary defect, the patient's optic nerve is at risk from compression. Complications include intra-orbital abscess (usually subperiosteal), cerebral abscess, meningitis, cavernous sinus thrombosis and optic nerve compression leading to optic atrophy.

Dacryocystitis

Tears drain through the canaliculi, lacrimal sac and naso-lacrimal duct into the nose. Blockage of the naso-lacrimal duct prevents drainage of the lacrimal sac, which may lead to infection, causing a painful swelling at the side of the nose below the medial canthus. This may present as a chronically watery, discharging eye, or as an acutely inflamed abscess. This should be treated with oral broad-spectrum antibiotics. The problem may recur unless drainage into the nose is re-established. In children a congenital blockage is very likely to clear by 1 year of age and thereafter a probing of the naso-lacrimal duct is sufficient. In adults a dacryocystorhinostomy can achieve this.

Stye (Hordeolum)

A localized staphylococcal abscess may form at the base of an eyelash. Epilation of the eyelash may speed resolution of the infection.

Chalazion (Meibomian Cyst)

Blockage of the meibomian glands ducts results in a retention cyst with ensuing inflammatory reaction and sometimes infection (acute phase). This is treated with twice daily hot compresses to encourage discharge of the gland. Once settled a non-tender granuloma forms in the lid (chronic phase). If present for more than 3 months, it can be incised and curetted.

Ectropion and Entropion

Abnormal positions of the eyelids, such as an eyelid which turns out (ectropion) or turns in (entropion), may cause discomfort, inflammation and even corneal scarring.

Ectropion usually involves the lower eyelid and can follow facial nerve paralysis. Eyelid scarring can cause a cicatricial ectropion.

Entropion can affect both upper and lower eyelids. The scarring of trachoma leads to upper eyelid entropion. In older age, eyelid laxity can lead to ectropion or entropion. Lid surgery is required for definitive treatment.

Other Eyelid Inflammations

Inflammation and scarring of the eyelids may be caused by conditions such as anthrax, actinomycosis, Leishmaniasis and yaws.

DISEASES OF THE CONJUNCTIVA

Infectious Conjunctivitis

Both bacteria and viruses may cause suppurative conjunctivitis, characterized by foreign body sensation, conjunctival injection and a purulent discharge.

Most bacterial conjunctivitis is self-limiting and does not affect vision. Gonococcal conjunctivitis may affect adults, particularly young men who may transfer genital gonorrhoea to their conjunctiva. This causes a very severe conjunctivitis, with a profuse purulent discharge and may lead to corneal ulcers and perforation.

Viral conjunctivitis is highly infectious and can be unilateral. Occasionally viral conjunctivitis may be associated with transient corneal opacities, which can affect the vision.

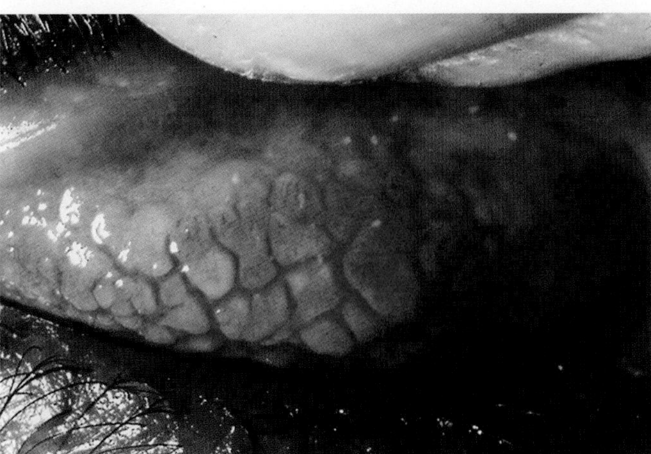

Figure 67.6 Upper tarsal conjunctiva in vernal conjunctivitis. Large papillae or cobblestones are evident. *(Courtesy of John Anderson.)*

Allergic Conjunctivitis

Allergic conjunctivitis is characterized by a slightly red eye, itching and a watery or mucous discharge. Treatment is with cold compresses and sodium cromoglycate 2% eye drops.

Vernal Keratoconjunctivitis

This disorder, which mostly affects children and teenagers, is common in the more temperate parts of the tropics (e.g. highlands of East Africa). The aetiology remains obscure but IgE and cell-mediated immune mechanisms play an important role. The upper tarsal conjunctiva and the limbus (corneoscleral junction) are inflamed. The eyes are itchy, red, irritable and discharge mucus. Conjunctival papillae may be large and often have an appearance like 'cobblestones' (Figure 67.6).

Treatments for vernal conjunctivitis include topical or systemic antihistamines. Topical mast cell stabilizers, such as sodium cromoglycate or nedocromil 2%, may alleviate symptoms if used continuously over several weeks. Symptomatic relief may be obtained with cold compresses and artificial tears to irrigate the conjunctiva.

Topical corticosteroids are an effective treatment of vernal keratoconjunctivitis; however, these should only be used under ophthalmic supervision. Topical corticosteroids can induce glaucoma and exacerbate infection, particularly herpes simplex corneal ulcer with catastrophic results. Although the symptoms of vernal catarrh are troublesome and irritating, they are self-limiting, as the condition goes into remission in adulthood and very rarely affects the sight.

Pinguecula

Yellow-white fatty deposits at the nasal or temporal conjunctival limbus are a common finding in middle or older age. Occasionally, the pinguecula may become inflamed, when a topical anti-inflammatory agent may be used. No treatment is the best treatment, but they need to be distinguished from squamous cell carcinoma of the conjunctiva.

Pterygium

A pterygium is a projection of fibrovascular conjunctival tissue which grows across the cornea from the temporal or nasal side. Although poorly understood, it is associated with exposure to sunlight and dust. Most pterygia cause few problems and do not encroach on the visual axis. If they are simply excised, they are likely to recur. If surgery is required because they are encroaching on the visual axis, a conjunctival autograft reduces the risk of recurrence.

Phlyctenulosis

A phlyctena appears as a raised, pale nodule with vascularization at the limbus or on the cornea. It is a lymphocytic infiltrate; evidence of a hypersensitivity reaction to staphylococci or other bacterial allergens including tuberculosis. It responds quickly to a short course of topical corticosteroids.

Keratoconjunctivitis Sicca (Dry Eye)

Keratoconjunctivitis sicca (KCS) is a common condition where dryness of the eyes causes symptoms of irritation, with grittiness and burning. It is more common in patients over 50 years. It can be associated with dry mouth (Sjögren syndrome) and rheumatoid arthritis. Dry eyes can follow trachoma, in which the lacrimal gland ducts and conjunctival goblet cells, are damaged.

Poor tear film and drying of the cornea is revealed by a drop of fluorescein and blue light. Corneal desiccation leads to punctate staining.

Treatment is with artificial tears, such as hypromellose eye drops, as required. In severe cases, temporary occlusion of the lacrimal canaliculi (using plugs) or permanent occlusion (using cautery) can be effective.

DISEASES OF THE CORNEA

Suppurative Corneal Ulceration

Suppurative corneal ulceration (keratitis), due to either bacteria or fungi, is a common problem, which frequently leads to unilateral loss of vision (Figure 67.7). Epithelial ulceration, without stromal involvement, can heal without scarring. However, ulceration involving the stroma will leave a corneal scar on healing. If the infection penetrates the eye, it can result in endophthalmitis and phthisis bulbi. In tropical countries, corneal trauma is a common precedent to suppurative keratitis.

Many organisms cause suppurative keratitis. Bacterial causes are more common and the most frequent causes are *Staphylococcus* spp, *Streptococcus pneumoniae* and *Pseudomonas*. The frequency of cultured organisms varies widely in different locations, even within countries. The most common fungi are *Aspergillus*, *Fusarium* and *Candida albicans*. Fungal keratitis is more frequent in resource-poor settings and not in relation to climate or humidity.[9] Agricultural accidents and injuries with vegetable matter predispose to fungal infection.

Clinical Appearance

The eye will be red, painful and photophobic, with profuse lacrimation. A whitish corneal opacity with overlying ulcer which stains with fluorescein is the characteristic feature of suppurative keratitis. A hypopyon, which appears as a white or yellow fluid level in the anterior chamber, may be present.

It is not easy to determine whether a corneal ulcer is due to bacterial or fungal infection on clinical grounds alone. However, serrated margins, a raised slough and coloured infiltrate suggest infection due to a fungus.

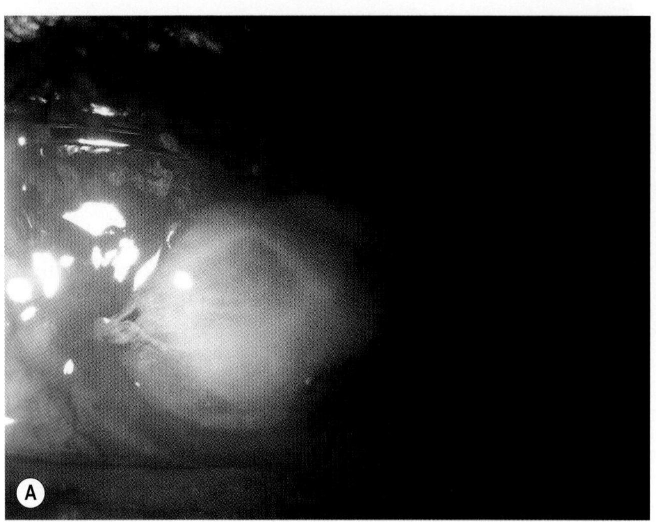
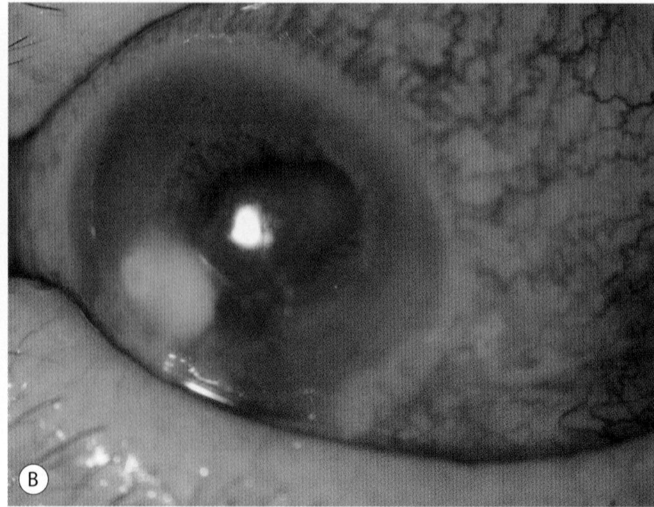

Figure 67.7 (A) Suppurative keratitis with corneal abscess and semi-opaque peripheral cornea. (B) Less advanced corneal ulcer with dense corneal inflammatory infiltrate and distorted pupil from posterior synechiae. *(A, Courtesy of Nicholas A. V. Beare; B, Courtesy of Manon Owen and William Hooley.)*

Laboratory Diagnosis

Urgent Gram staining and microscope examination are required by corneal sampling. The procedure for obtaining and examining material from a corneal scrape is shown in Table 67.3. This may demonstrate the presence of bacteria or fungi, but additional examinations may be required (such as potassium hydroxide wet mount) for fungal identification. The interpretation of corneal scrapes requires skill and experience and it may be impossible to detect any organism.

Management

The treatment of suppurative keratitis is urgent with frequent (½ to 1-hourly) antibiotic eye drops. Treatment is often presumptive but should be guided by knowledge of the locally common causes of infectious keratitis and Gram stain results, if available. For example, fungal keratitis is common in South India, so an antifungal should be given when the organism is unknown. Treatment can be modified if culture and sensitivity results become available later. Different regimens of treatment are given in Table 67.4.

Fluoroquinolones, such as ciprofloxacin or ofloxacin, have good activity against all Gram-negative organisms, including *Pseudomonas*. They are also effective against many Gram-positive species and are recommended as monotherapy.

Natamycin or an imidazole, such as econazole, are the antifungals of choice. Natamycin has limited corneal penetration, but has been shown to be effective in randomized clinical trials.

A cycloplegic, such as atropine, should be given once daily.

A bacterial ulcer should be sterilized within 48 hours of intensive treatment, but healing may take much longer. Bacterial ulcers should be healed in 10–14 days and fungal ulcers within 21–28 days. If the ulcer does not heal, a temporary tarsorrhaphy should be performed. If perforation is imminent, a conjunctival flap can save the eye.

TABLE 67.3 Materials and Procedure for a Corneal Scrape

Materials

- Topical anaesthetic (ideally preservative-free if culture is to be performed)
- Sterile gloves
- Scalpel blades (or sterile needles as alternative)
- Alcohol or gas burner for sterilization
- Clean glass microscope slides (labelled)
- Wax or diamond marker
- Culture media (labelled)

Procedure

- Explain the procedure to the patient (children require sedation)
- Instill topical anaesthetic and don sterile gloves
- Use sterile, cooled blade to sample central ulcer by wiping blade gently over ulcer at the slitlamp. One hand holds the blade and one hand controls the slitlamp; an assistant is helpful to ensure the head is still and hold the eye lids. Alternatively loupes can be used
- Avoid touching lids and lashes
- Use each scrape to prepare one smear or culture
- Spread material thinly on to microscope slides (one for Gram stain and one for fungi)
- Use new scalpel blade, or re-sterilize and cool between scrapes
- Fix slides for Gram stain with gentle heat (or alcohol)
- Place blade into transport medium for microbiology examination, or directly inoculate culture plates
- Label slides and cultures with name and date

TABLE 67.4 Topical Treatment of Suppurative Keratitis According to Results of Gram Stain

	Eyedrops in Ideal Circumstances	Practical Alternatives
Gram-positive cocci	Cefuroxime 50 mg/mL or fluoroquinolone[a]	Chloramphenicol
Gram-negative rods	Fluoroquinolone[a] or gentamicin[b] 8 mg/mL	
Fungi	Econazole 1% or natamycin 5%	Chlorhexidine gluconate 0.2%
Unknown organism	Fluoroquinolone[a] + antifungal if indicated	Gentamicin 8 mg/mL

All antibiotics should be given hourly for 48 hours and then reduced to every 6 hours. Frequent eyedrops are preferred to ointment as the diffusion of antibiotic out of ointment can be unpredictable.

[a]E.g. ciprofloxacin or ofloxacin.

[b]Can be given as a subconjunctival injection.

Herpes Simplex Keratitis

The herpes simplex virus (HSV) is distributed worldwide and can have severe effects on the eye. HSV is a cause of recurrent keratitis and unlike 'cold sores' on the face, heal with scarring, which can have a detrimental effect on vision. Unilateral, recurrent keratitis with initially mild, but progressive scarring with recurrences, strongly suggests HSV.

The inappropriate use of topical corticosteroids (which are contraindicated in this infection unless used by an eye specialist) can lead to a disastrous exacerbation. Most HSV keratitis is caused by HSVI infection, although occasionally HSVII infections occur, particularly in the newborn – when infection occurs in the mother's birth canal (see below).

The virus remains latent in the ganglion of the 5th cranial nerve between bouts of keratitis. HSV infection is more severe in immunocompromised individuals and may complicate the picture of measles keratitis and malnutrition. It is a common cause of keratitis in malnourished children. The primary infection is more severe in malnourished or immunosuppressed children affecting the lids, nose and lips, but keratitis usually comes later (Figure 67.8).

Clinical Appearance

Symptoms of HSV keratitis include pain, photosensitivity and lacrimation with circumcorneal injection. HSV keratitis classically causes a branching dendritic ulcer, obvious with fluorescein staining (Figure 67.9); however the infection often has an atypical appearance with late presentation or immunosuppression. When healing occurs, a scar results in loss of corneal transparency. Later recurrences may not have a dendritic ulcer, but localized infiltrates and nonspecific ulceration. Blood vessels often invade the cornea, causing vascularization. A valuable sign is diminished corneal sensation in the affected eye. Atypical features include a large geographic ulcer and destruction of the stroma.

Complications

Corneal hypoaesthesia may cause a chronic neurotrophic ulcer. HSV can cause uveitis and secondarily raised intraocular pressure. Recurrence may be stimulated by a number of factors including fever, exposure to ultraviolet light, minor trauma, measles and psychological factors.

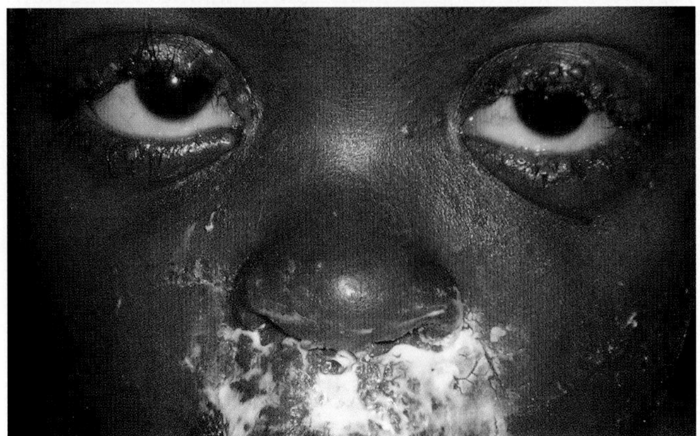

Figure 67.8 Primary HSV infection in child with lid vesicles, nasal crusting and lip lesions. *(Courtesy of Nicholas A. V. Beare.)*

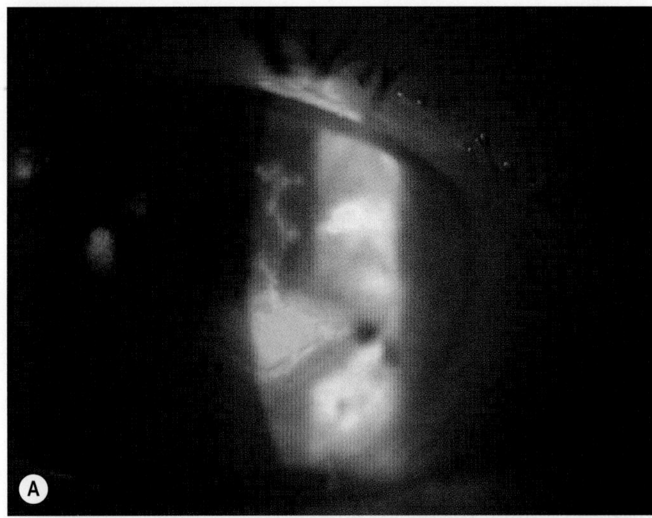

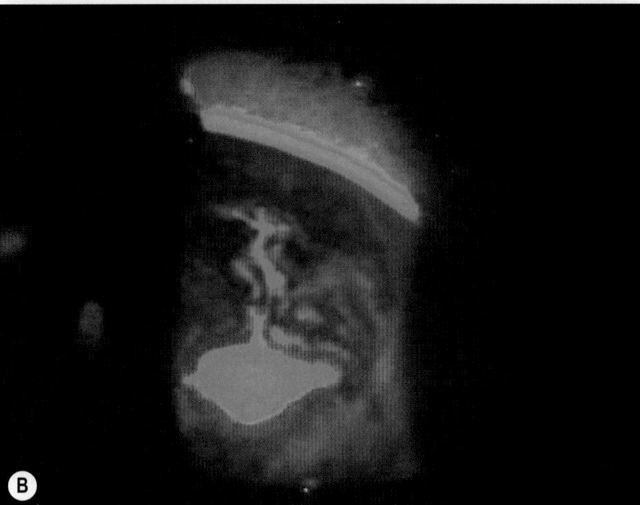

Figure 67.9 Herpes simplex keratitis with dendritic ulcer outlined by fluorescein on the right. *(Courtesy of Micheal Briggs.)*

Management

Previously, superficial HSV keratitis affecting only the corneal epithelium was treated with debridement of the infected epithelial cells. Other treatments are now more commonly used, including aciclovir 3% ointment, or trifluorothymidine 1% drops, five times daily. Cycloplegic eye drops should be given while the eye is painful.

Topical corticosteroids may be required when there is an immune response resulting in a deep stromal keratitis. The weakest effective dose of steroid should be used and must be given with an antiviral agent under supervision of an eye specialist.

Eye health workers should refer any patient with geographic or stromal HSV keratitis to an ophthalmologist, after beginning treatment with a topical antiviral agent, if this is available. An unhealed HSV ulcer may require a conjunctival flap or a tarsorrhaphy to effect healing.

INFLAMMATION OF THE EYEBALL

Endophthalmitis

Endophthalmitis is the term for suppurative infection inside the eye and can occur when a corneal ulcer perforates, following a penetrating injury, from haematological spread or intraocular surgery. This causes a severe intraocular inflammatory reaction which may destroy the eye. The eye is red and painful with reduced vision. There is fibrin in the anterior chamber, a hypopyon (a fluid level in the inferior anterior chamber formed by white cells) may be visible and the red reflex is reduced. Urgent treatment is required with antibiotics given systemically and by intravitreal injection as soon as possible. Intravitreal ciprofloxacin and vancomycin from intravenous preparations are suitable.

Scleritis

Inflammation of the sclera causes severe pain and redness. The redness is deep to the conjunctiva and described as violet-tinged. The eyeball is tender and there may be secondary inflammation of the lids and orbit. Occasionally, scleritis may lead to scleral necrosis and perforation. It is associated with rheumatoid arthritis and systemic vasculitis. Infective conditions associated with scleritis are leprosy, tuberculosis and ophthalmic herpes zoster.

Scleritis requires systemic treatment, either with non-steroidal anti-inflammatory agents or oral prednisolone. Other immunosuppressive agents may be required. Subconjunctival injections of corticosteroids are contraindicated as they may cause focal scleral necrosis. When the scleral inflammation has settled, the area of sclera may be thinned.

Inflammation of the Anterior Uvea (Anterior Uveitis, Iritis)

Inflammation of the anterior uveal tissue, the iris and ciliary body, may be described as anterior uveitis, iritis or iridocyclitis.

Clinical Appearance

Iritis presents typically with tender pain, redness and photophobia. The condition may be unilateral or bilateral. Torch examination will reveal redness around the cornea (circumciliary injection) and sometimes blurred iris details. Examination with magnification will reveal hazy aqueous fluid in the anterior chamber due to circulating proteins and visible inflammatory cells. Deposits of cells may be found on the inferior endothelium of the cornea (keratic precipitates, KP). If there is very severe inflammation, a hypopyon can occur particularly in Behçet's disease.

Inflammation of the iris may result in adhesion of the pupil to the anterior lens surface (posterior synechiae, PS) resulting in poor or irregular pupil dilation. Synechiae may also occur at the base of the iris to the cornea (peripheral anterior synechiae, PAS). Synechiae can lead to secondary glaucoma.

Causes and Associations

Most cases of anterior uveitis are idiopathic and further investigation is not required. The granulomatous type of anterior uveitis with large keratic precipitates can occasionally be due to systemic diseases including sarcoidosis and tuberculosis (Figure 67.10). HLA-B27 antigen is associated with uveitis, ankylosing spondylitis and Reiter syndrome (nonspecific urethritis, polyarthritis and anterior uveitis). Syphilis can cause uveitis and as

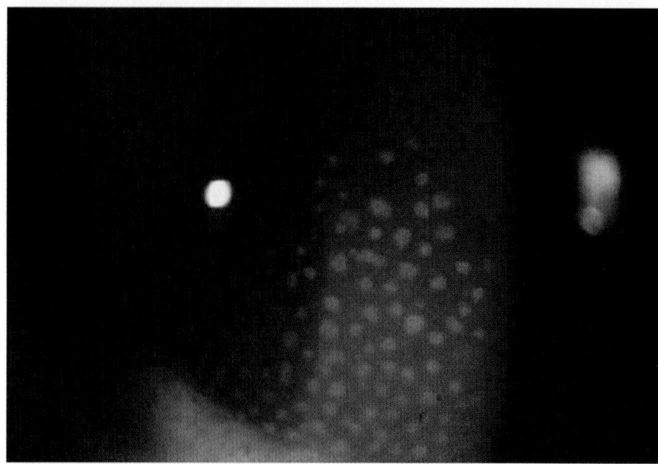

Figure 67.10 'Mutton-fat' granulomatous keratic precipitates (KP) in anterior uveitis *(Courtesy of Micheal Briggs.)*

a curable cause should be included in any investigations in areas where the disease is common. Injury to an eye can rarely result in a 'sympathetic' inflammation of the undamaged eye. This may occur weeks, months or even years after the original injury. Behçet's disease, sarcoidosis, tuberculosis and syphilis can all cause posterior uveitis threatening vision, requiring systemic treatment.

Management

Anterior uveitis is treated with corticosteroid and cycloplegic eye drops. The intraocular pressure should be measured and treated if very high. Dilated funduscopy should be performed to look for signs of posterior uveitis including a hazy vitreous. If severe, subconjunctival injections of corticosteroid and mydriatics may be required. Once the inflammation is reducing the frequency of steroid eye drops can be tapered slowly.

EYE INJURIES

Trauma is a common cause of uniocular red eye and sometimes blindness. Injuries to the eye are classified as 'closed globe' and 'open globe', which includes globe ruptures, penetrating injuries and intraocular foreign body (Table 67.5). It is important to identify occult open globe injuries such as posterior globe rupture. Eye injuries, particularly corneal injuries can be complicated by secondary infection.

Corneal Abrasion

This is a superficial injury involving the corneal epithelium, causing pain, lacrimation and photophobia. The corneal stroma is clear and intact, but the abrasion stains with fluorescein drops.

Management. Instill topical antibiotics for 5 days and stat dose of cycloplegic, e.g. cyclopentolate 1%. Padding is not generally recommended.

Superficial Retained Foreign Body

These are often metallic but may also be stone or wood. The foreign body may lie on the upper tarsal conjunctiva, where it will be revealed by everting the eyelid.

TABLE 67.5 Emergency Assessment and Treatment of Major Eye Injuries

	Assessment	Treatment
Chemical injury	Patient should be triaged to immediate irrigation with copious water over at least 15 minutes before assessment	Topical antibiotic and examine for conjunctival ischaemia and corneal haze; also give prednisolone drops if present and review the next day to release any conjunctival adhesions
Blunt injury	Signs of blow-out facial fracture: diplopia on up gaze, maxillary hypothesia, enophthalmos (sunken eye)	Advise patient not to blow nose and give prophylactic antibiotics. If enophthalmic or diplopia persists for a week refer for facial surgery if available
	Signs of ocular injury: reduced vision, hyphaema, iris root dislocation, lens dislocation, vitreous haemorrhage.	Give the patient prednisolone drops, cycloplegia and monitor intraocular pressure
	Globe rupture indicated by soft eye, extensive subconjunctival haemorrhage without posterior edge, hyphaema, vitreous haemorrhage. Perforation may occur at scleral/corneal junction or posterior globe	Give stat antibiotic eye drop, cover eye with shield and refer for surgical repair
Sharp, low-velocity injury	Penetrating injury indicated by corneal or scleral laceration; incarceration of iris in cornea with pupil distortion, extrusion of brown pigmented iris/uveal tissue, soft eye, shallow or flat anterior chamber, hyphaema, traumatic cataract or vitreous haemorrhage	Give stat antibiotic eye drop, systemic antibiotics (e.g. ciprofloxacin), cover eye with shield and refer for surgical repair
Sharp, high-velocity injury, e.g. from hammering or drilling metal	Globe penetration indicated by sealed corneal laceration (staining with fluorescein), iris damage, traumatic cataract. Small intraocular foreign bodies may leave no obvious sign of entry. Ocular X-rays with the patient looking up and down for metal FB	Unless specialist vitreous surgical techniques are available attempted removal of a vitreous FB may do more harm than good. Ferrous FBs may cause a progressive retinal toxicity. Specialist magnets may be used to remove them

Management. Instill local anaesthetic drops. Remove the foreign body with a cotton-wool bud or a sterile hypodermic needle. If the foreign body is ferrous, there may be some surrounding rust. Do not attempt to remove this without a microscope, as the cornea is only about 0.5 mm thick. Give topical antibiotics for 5 days and a single dose of a cycloplegic.

Penetrating Injuries

A penetrating injury may be due to any sharp object such as a thorn, which penetrates the eye. Signs include extruded brown uveal tissue, distorted pupil, hyphaema and a soft eye, however the evidence of injury may not always be obvious. A retained foreign body, which is radio-opaque, may be seen on X-ray.

Management. As soon as a penetrating injury is recognized, the patient should be given antibiotic cover, both topically and systemically and referred immediately to the eye specialist for surgical repair. Further examination is unnecessary and may even harm the eye. The damaged eye should be protected with a shield.

Blunt Injury

A blunt injury caused by objects such as a stone or a fist can result in an open or closed globe injury.

Following a blunt injury, examine the eye systematically from the front to the back, beginning with the periorbital region. Fractures of the bony floor of the orbit (a blow-out fracture), can lead to entrapment of the inferior rectus muscle and diplopia and pain on upgaze. Bruising affecting the eyelids can make it difficult to open the eye. There may be bleeding into the anterior chamber of the eye (hyphaema); a hyphaema of more than 50% of the anterior chamber, carries a risk of secondary glaucoma. Intraocular tissues such as the root of the iris may be torn (iridodialysis). The lens may be dislocated. Bleeding in the posterior segment of the eye may result in vitreous haemorrhage. Retinal oedema and haemorrhages may be apparent on ophthalmoscopy.

Management. A patient with a blow-out fracture should be advised not to blow their nose (surgical emphysema of the orbit can result) and be given prophylactic antibiotics. In most closed globe injuries the correct treatment is observation, until the condition resolves. A hyphaema with a high intraocular pressure forces blood into the corneal stroma, leading to corneal staining; so for a large hyphaema, the intraocular pressure must be monitored carefully. Treat with a topical antibiotic, steroid and cycloplegic eye drops. Raised pressure should be treated with topical agents and oral acetazolamide. If medical treatment is insufficient the patient should be referred urgently for surgical removal of the hyphaema.

Chemical Burns of the Eye

Chemical injury may be caused by acid or alkali. Alkali burns, e.g. cement, are generally more serious.

Management. When a chemical injury has occurred, immediately irrigate the eye with copious water (any water, not necessarily sterile). Keep washing for 15–20 min, until all traces of the chemical have been washed out. Remember to irrigate under the eyelids as well. Any fragments of cement or solid material may be picked off with forceps. Antibiotic and steroid drops should be applied hourly for 2 days and then reduced in frequency. Eyelids should be kept mobile with deliberate movement of the lids a number of times each day. Corneal haze, conjunctival fluorescein staining or ischaemia suggests a severe alkali burn and should be urgently referred to the eye specialist.

Snake Venom Conjunctivitis

Spitting cobra venom can cause a painful conjunctivitis. Management is the same as any chemical injury. Severe damage is rare and is more likely to be caused by frantic attempts to remove the venom than by the toxin itself.

Tarantula and Caterpillar Hair Conjunctivitis (Ophthalmia Nodosum)

Caterpillar hairs in the conjunctiva provoke a foreign body reaction known as ophthalmia nodosum. A granuloma forms around each caterpillar hair. Treatment requires removal of the hair, or deeper invasion may occur. Tarantula hairs can penetrate through the cornea and progress into deeper ocular tissues causing inflammation.

Non-infectious Ophthalmic Disease

CATARACT

Cataract is any opacification of the lens in the eye and will have varying degrees of impact on vision from blinding (Figure 67.11), to an incidental finding with no visual consequence. Cataract is the most common cause of blindness, responsible for half of blindness globally (Table 67.2). About 18 million people are blind due to cataract and many millions more have visual impairment. Most blind people requiring surgery are in Asia and Africa.

The number of cataract blind people is increasing worldwide because of population growth and increasing longevity. The number of people over 60 in developing countries will rise from 8% in 2006 to 20% in 2050.

The treatment for cataract is surgical removal of the lens, usually with insertion of an intraocular lens implant. This has been shown to be one of the most cost-effective healthcare interventions.

Aetiology

The main risk factor for cataract is age, which is obviously non-modifiable. Associations with the following factors have been described: diabetes, smoking, severe dehydration, nutrition, ultraviolet light, genetics and medications.

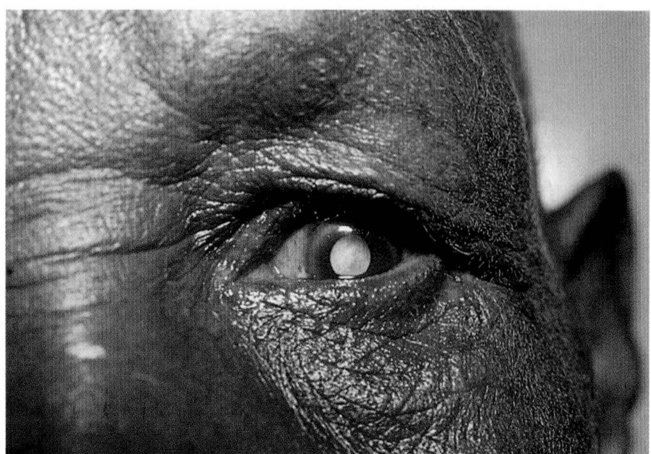

Figure 67.11 Mature white cataract. *(Courtesy of Murray McGavin.)*

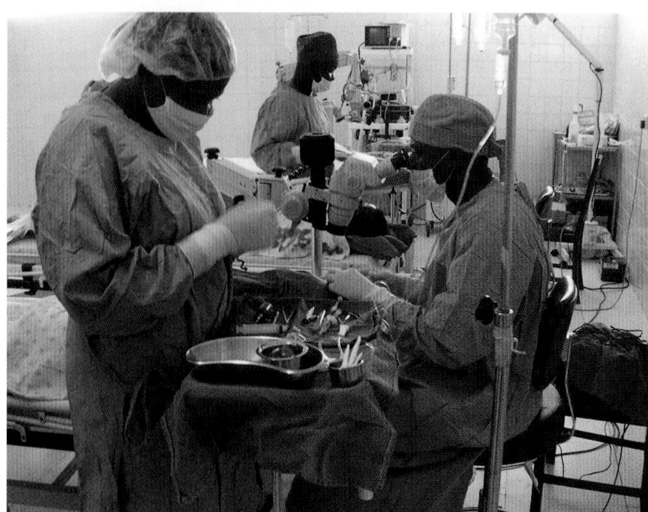

Figure 67.12 Performing small incision cataract surgery in an ophthalmic theatre in Malawi. Note the next patient is prepared in the background to minimize time between operations and maximize efficiency. *(Courtesy of Gerald Msukwe and Nicholas A. V. Beare.)*

CATARACT SURGERY

There are three surgical techniques for removing a cataract: intracapsular cataract extraction (ICCE), extracapsular cataract extraction (ECCE) (Figure 67.12) and phacoemulsification. In ICCE, the lens is removed whole and the patient is left without a lens, aphakic. This can be performed without an operating microscope, but the results are poor and the patient is reliant on thick glasses with distortion of peripheral vision. In extracapsular cataract extraction (ECCE), the lens capsule is opened and the nucleus and the cortex of the lens are removed, leaving the posterior capsule in place. This can be done through a standard 120° incision closed by sutures, or a small incision which does not usually require sutures (Small Incision Cataract Surgery or SICS) (Figure 67.13). The lens is replaced with a prosthetic lens, generally placed in the lens capsule restoring normal vision. Better optical correction leads to better surgical outcomes, allowing earlier intervention and eliminates the use of thick spectacles. Nevertheless, reading spectacles are often necessary to compensate for the lack of accommodation (presbyopia).

In phacoemulsification (phaco), an ultrasound probe is used to fragment the lens, which is aspirated through a small incision. Phacoemulsification is not available widely in developing countries due to the high cost of equipment and consumables. It may be available in high-fee private clinics or to wealthier patients as part of a cost-recovery programme.

The disadvantages of ECCE and IOL include the need for an operating microscope, additional skills of microscopic surgery and the retention of the posterior capsule, which may opacify, causing loss of vision years after the cataract surgery. However the limited data on posterior capsular opacification (PCO) in Africa and Asia suggests that it is not frequent, possibly due to the advanced nature of the cataract at the time of surgery. In those with PCO it is rarely blinding.

ECCE with a small-incision (SICS) involves a self-sealing tunnel incision through the sclera. No sutures are required and the procedure causes less astigmatism than a standard

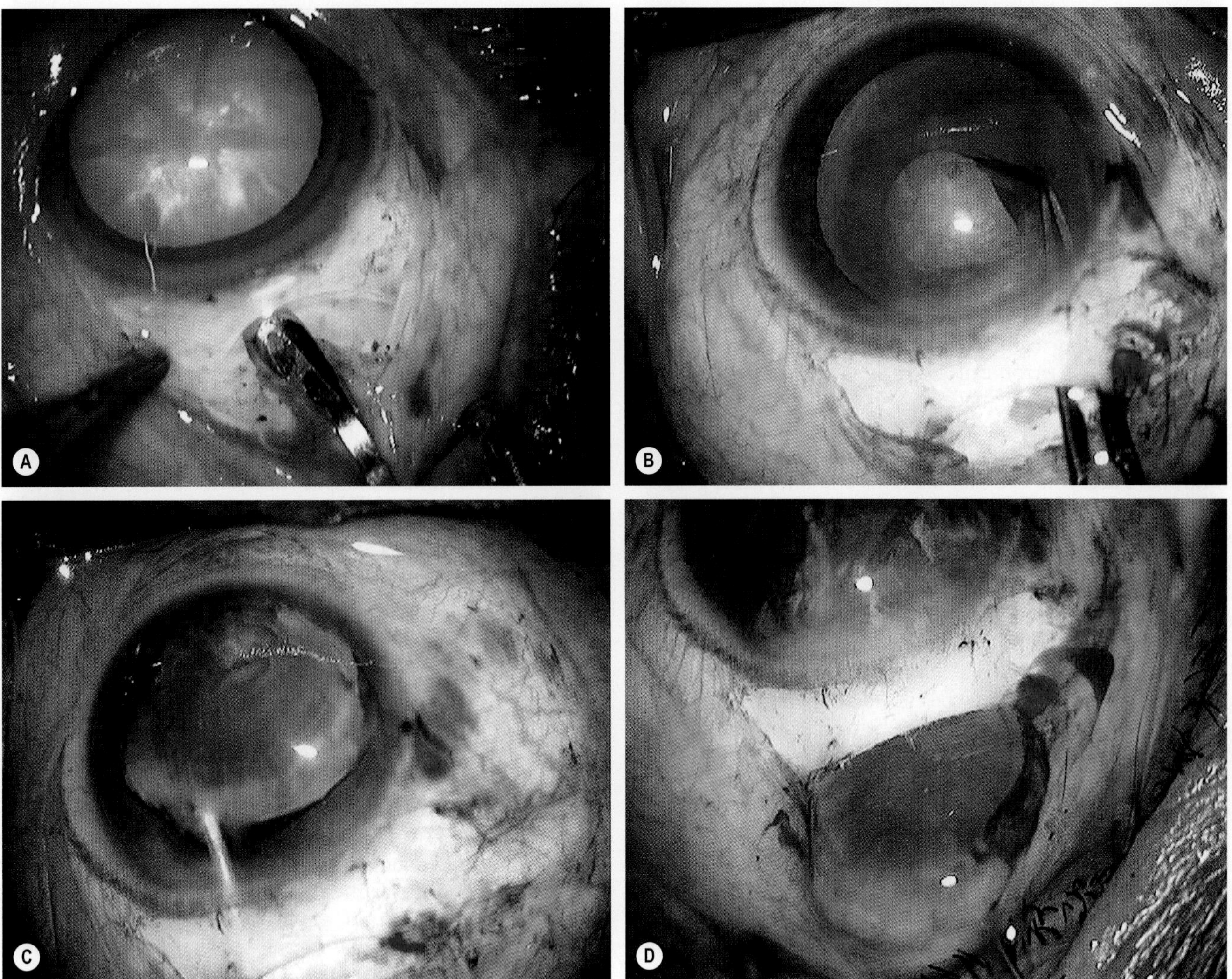

Figure 67.13 Stages of small incision cataract surgery (SICS). (A) Creating a tunnelled incision through the sclera into the eye. (B) Performing a capsulotomy in the lens capsule to remove the cataractous lens material. The capsule has been stained blue with a vital dye to aid the surgery. (C) Mobilization of the lens nucleus out of the lens capsule. (D) Expressing the cataractous lens nucleus through the scleral tunnel. The remaining lens cortex is aspirated and an intraocular lens is inserted into the lens capsule. The tunnelled incision is self-sealing without sutures. *(Courtesy of K. Hennig.)*

ECCE and IOL. The surgery is very cost-effective and has been widely adopted. Recent results are comparable with phacoemulsification in terms of visual outcome and corneal endothelial cell loss.

A further intervention for cataract is 'couching', a traditional method whereby the cataractous lens is dislocated in to the back of the eye. The outcome of this procedure is very poor, however in a national survey in Nigeria, it was found to be the most common procedure for cataract (see below).

Improving Outcomes

Community-based studies show that visual outcomes from cataract surgery can be disappointing.[8] In order to implant the correct power of IOL an individual eye's parameters have to be accurately measured, a process termed biometry. Biometry requires additional time from trained personnel and equipment.

Unsurprisingly, outcomes may be improved by monitoring results of surgery.[10] Postoperative refraction and provision of glasses will reduce poor outcomes due to uncorrected refractive error.

Cataract Surgical Rate and Coverage

In order to eliminate cataract blindness, it is necessary to at least operate on the number of people who become blind every year. The cataract surgical rate (CSR) is the number of operations performed per year, per million population. In industrialized countries, the CSR is between 4000 and 6000. India has significantly increased its CSR in recent years, from less than 1500 to over 4000. However, in most of Africa, the CSR remains below 1000.

Cataract surgical coverage (CSC) is the number of individuals (or eyes) who had cataract surgery divided by the number who needed it, as a percentage. This indicator is used to assess how well cataract services meet the need and provides information on the impact of cataract intervention programmes. In population-based surveys data are usually obtained using standardized methodology known as Rapid Assessment of Cataract

Surgical Services (RACCS)[11] or Rapid Assessments of Avoidable Blindness (RAAB).[12]

REFRACTIVE ERRORS

Uncorrected refractive error is the commonest cause of visual impairment worldwide, but is less commonly severe enough to render the person blind (Table 67.2). This position reflects the woeful under-provision of spectacles in developing countries.

An eye with no refractive error is 'emmetropic' and can focus parallel light from distant objects (taken as 6 metres for spectacle purposes) on to the retina, an eye with refractive error cannot. Refractive error can be myopia (short-sightedness), hypermetropia (long-sightedness) and astigmatism (non-spherical error).

It is estimated that 500 million people with refractive errors do not have access to eye examinations and affordable glasses. Of those, 153 million are significantly visually impaired and 8 million are blind as a result. Patients who are aphakic after cataract surgery are effectively blind again if they do not have appropriate glasses. Refractive error can also affect the performance of children in school.

Patients with a high degree of myopia are predisposed to degeneration of the macula which affects corrected vision, sometimes severely. This may be chorioretinal atrophy, or choroidal neovascularization, which can be treated in a similar way to neovascular AMD.

THE GLAUCOMAS

Glaucoma is a progressive optic neuropathy usually associated with raised intraocular pressure (IOP). There are several mechanisms of raised IOP and therefore the group of conditions is best described as 'the glaucomas'. The pathophysiology of the characteristic optic nerve atrophy (Figure 67.14) and corresponding visual field defects is not fully understood.

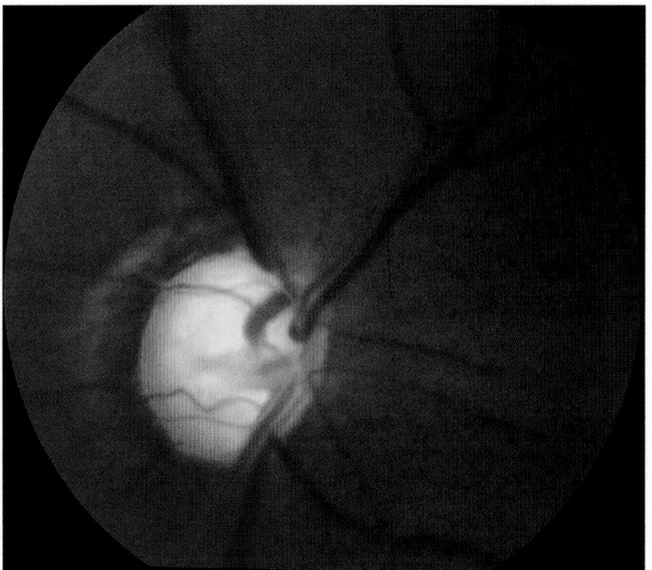

Figure 67.14 Cupped optic disc due to glaucoma. *(Courtesy of Nicholas A. V. Beare.)*

There are two fundamental types of glaucoma which may be primary or secondary:

- Open angle glaucoma
- Angle closure glaucoma.

Epidemiology of the Primary Glaucomas

Glaucoma is a blinding disease largely because it presents late or is not treated adequately. The 4.5 million blind with glaucoma include those with open angle glaucoma who are not symptomatic until almost all the vision is lost and those with angle closure whose acute attacks are not treated promptly.

Open angle glaucoma has a higher prevalence among people of African origin, in whom it occurs at a younger age. The prevalence of open angle glaucoma among African-Americans is 8–10 times higher than white Americans. Current estimates of glaucoma prevalence in sub-Saharan Africa are 6.5 million with a projected increase to 8.4 million by 2020. It is likely these figures underestimate the true numbers.

Very late presentation of open angle glaucoma is the norm in most resource-poor countries. Typically, patients are already completely blind in one eye (i.e. light perception or none) and reduced to counting fingers in the other. Once vision is lost no treatment can restore it.

Angle closure glaucoma is most prevalent in central Asia, e.g. China and Mongolia. It can be prevented with a single laser treatment (iridotomy) but patients in remote communities again often present after the vision is lost.

Anatomy and Physiology of Aqueous Fluid Circulation

Aqueous fluid is produced by the ciliary body. It circulates around the lens and through the pupil. Most of the fluid drains through the trabecular meshwork at the angle of the anterior chamber. Any obstruction, whether at the pupil, root of the iris, or due to blood, inflammatory cells or pigment, can reduce the drainage of aqueous from the eye, leading to raised IOP.

Open Angle Glaucoma

In open angle glaucoma, raised IOP leads to progressive visual field loss and enlargement of the optic disc cup, as nerve fibres are lost. Raised IOP without apparent optic neuropathy is termed ocular hypertension (OHT). Occasionally, the optic neuropathy can progress with normal IOP – normal or low tension glaucoma (LTG). Primary open angle glaucoma (POAG) is typically a bilateral condition. As peripheral vision is lost first, central vision and visual acuity are only affected very late.

In open angle glaucoma, the anterior chamber is deep and the angles are open. The anterior chamber depth can be assessed with a torch beam shone from the temporal side. The ocular angle can only be assessed by a slit-lamp and gonioscopic lens.

Ophthalmoscopy of the optic nerve head is required to diagnose open angle glaucoma. The cup within the optic nerve head is enlarged with loss of the neuroretinal rim (Figure 67.15). Visual field defects correspond to the loss of optic nerve cells. Detailed examination of visual fields for glaucoma requires field testing equipment, which is usually automated. However, in resource-poor settings, there is often complete loss or only tunnel vision remaining.

Management. The treatment of open angle glaucoma is to lower the intraocular pressure, either by medication or by surgery. No treatment can restore vision, just minimize

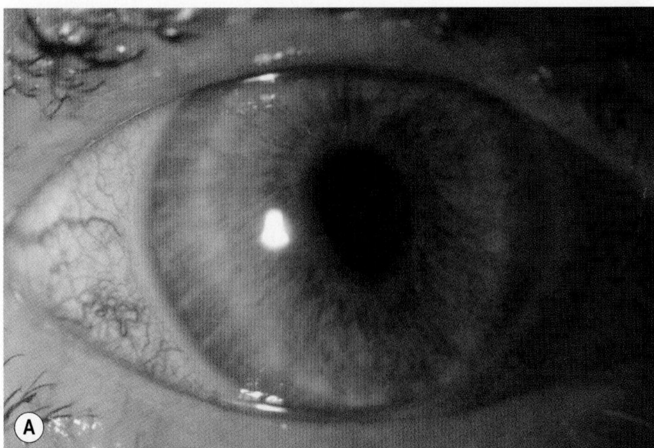

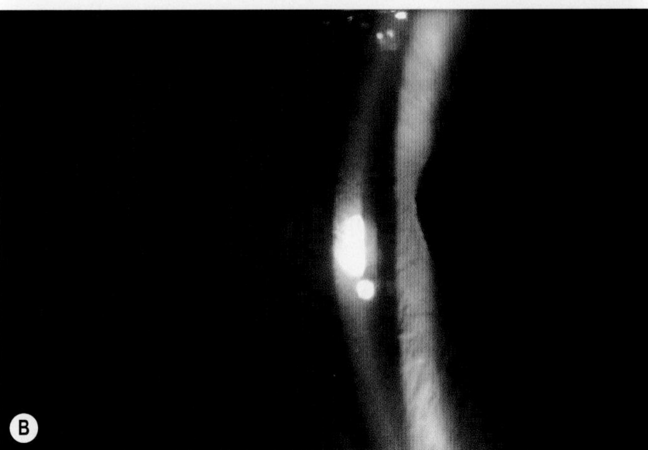

Figure 67.15 (A) Angle closure glaucoma. Note distorted ovoid pupil and shadowing of nasal iris due to anterior position of iris and temporal illumination. (B) Slit image shows very shallow anterior chamber. *(Courtesy of Ade Garrick and Martin Hodson.)*

progression. The problem with topical treatments is that they have to be continued and monitored indefinitely to prevent deterioration. They offer no improvement in vision, are costly and some require refrigeration. Regular and indefinite monitoring of IOP, optic disc and visual field tests are often not practical in resource-poor settings.

The following topical medications are available:

- Beta-blocker, e.g. timolol, levobunolol, carteolol or metipranolol
- Prostaglandin analogue, e.g. latanoprost, travoprost or bimatoprost
- Carbonic anhydrase inhibitor, e.g. dorzolamide or brinzolamide
- Alpha-agonist, e.g. brimonidine.

Previously pilocarpine or epinephrine were used, but have more side-effects.

Surgery for open angle glaucoma involves increasing aqueous outflow in order to lower IOP. Trabeculectomy is the most established operation for this and allows the aqueous fluid to drain into the subconjunctival space. African patients may have an unwanted postoperative healing response with fibrosis and blockage of the filtering site. This can be dealt with by using antimetabolites (e.g. mitomycin C or 5-fluorouracil) at the time of surgery, but these increase the risk of complications. Beta-irradiation application during surgery is inexpensive and improves the effectiveness of trabeculectomy in African eyes, but increases the risk of cataract. Glaucoma surgery which does not fully penetrate the eye (termed deep sclerectomy or canalostomy) has fewer complications and may be more appropriate in resource-poor settings with poor patient retention.

Angle Closure Glaucoma

In angle closure glaucoma, occlusion of the angle by the iris root in eyes with a narrow anterior chamber obstructs aqueous outflow. It may be acute or chronic. Acute angle closure glaucoma is an emergency – delay will result in permanent loss of vision. Furthermore, without treatment, the second eye has a >50% chance of developing angle closure glaucoma within 5 years.

Clinical Presentation. In acute glaucoma, the patient is distressed with severe pain and nausea. The eye is red with a hazy cornea and reduced vision. The anterior chamber is very shallow or flat, with the iris apposed to the peripheral cornea (Figure 67.15). The pupil is semi-dilated and unreactive. The intraocular pressure is very high (over 40 mmHg). Episodes of acute angle closure may be intermittent, delaying diagnosis.

Chronic angle closure is usually asymptomatic and painless. Visual acuity is lost only after the optic nerve has been severely damaged. Chronic angle closure is the most common presentation in Asia.

Angle closure glaucoma usually occurs in eyes which are anatomically predisposed by 'crowding' of the ocular angle. This most often occurs in hypermetropia and is exacerbated by lens growth with increasing age.

Management. In acute angle closure, treatment should be immediate. Give acetazolamide 500 mg stat and 250 mg four times daily, orally or by intravenous infusion initially. Topical IOP-lowering treatment is also required with timolol, apraclonidine and other IOP-lowering agents as necessary. Pilocarpine should be given to overcome the angle closure when the intraocular pressure has started to come down.

The definitive treatment for angle closure is iridotomy, which can be performed with a laser or surgically. This procedure creates another opening through which aqueous fluid can pass and deepens the anterior chamber of the eye by equalizing the pressure anterior and posterior to the iris. The second eye should have prophylactic surgery, as it is at high risk of developing angle closure.

Chronic angle closure glaucoma is usually treated similarly to open angle glaucoma, by trabeculectomy or topical medication. In eyes predisposed to angle closure, iridotomy will reduce the risk of developing chronic or acute angle closure. As the lens pushes the iris forward cataract surgery is sometimes used to treat angle closure and will certainly prevent it.

Secondary Glaucomas

There are a number of secondary forms of glaucoma, most commonly:

- Uveitic, with inflammatory products obstructing aqueous outflow
- Traumatic, acutely due to blood obstructing outflow and chronically due to damage to the angle
- Phacolytic, where lens proteins from a hypermature cataract clog aqueous outflow

- Neovascular, due to new vessel growth in the angle secondary to diabetes or retinal vasculopathy
- Steroid-induced from chronic steroid use, more usually topically.

Congenital Glaucoma (Buphthalmos)

Glaucoma in childhood is rare and may be present at birth or develop during the first few years. The trabecular meshwork does not develop normally, leading to a reduction in aqueous fluid outflow and raised IOP. As the sclera is still elastic, the eyeball enlarges (buphthalmos). Other features, which may be more obvious than the enlarged eye(s) in a small child, include excess lacrimation, photosensitivity and hazy cornea. On examination the cornea is enlarged (>11 mm diameter) and may be oedematous.

Management is mainly surgical. Children should be treated by a specialist paediatric ophthalmologist.

DIABETES MELLITUS

The prevalence of diabetes worldwide is increasingly dramatically, with the fastest increase in developing countries. The number of adults with diabetes is projected to rise from 336 million in 2011 to 522 million in 2030. Most of this increase will occur in resource-poor settings, which are least equipped to deal with this chronic disease with multiple microvascular and macrovascular complications, especially diabetic eye disease.

The prevalence of diabetes in some Middle Eastern and Pacific Island countries is already 20% of adults. Africa currently is the region with the lowest prevalence of diabetes, estimated to affect 14.6 million people, but with the highest projected growth to 2030.[13,14]

A 2010 WHO community-based study of non-communicable diseases in Malawi found raised fasting blood sugar in 5.6% in a nationally representative sample of 3056 adults.[15] This is comparable with the prevalence of diabetes in the UK (6.8%) but with a much higher proportion undiagnosed. There was no difference in the prevalence between rural and urban areas. A separate study found the prevalence of sight-threatening retinopathy in a tertiary diabetic clinic in Malawi to be high (19%).[16]

WHO estimates that about 1.8 million people are blind due to diabetic retinopathy and it is still the leading cause of blindness in people under 65 in wealthy countries. As the risk of blindness from diabetes rises steeply after 15 years duration, the epidemic of sight-loss in developing countries from DR will follow the rise in diabetes, unless improvements in care are made.

Diabetic Retinopathy

Diabetes damages retinal capillaries through prolonged exposure to hyperglycaemia. This leads to leakage from capillaries resulting in retinal oedema; and to capillary closure and ischaemia. Widespread retinal ischaemia results in new vessel growth (proliferative diabetic retinopathy, PDR).

Visual loss results from:

- Oedema or ischaemia affecting the macula (diabetic maculopathy)
- Vitreous haemorrhage from new vessels, or traction retinal detachment from fibrovascular proliferation and contracture – complications of PDR
- Rubeotic glaucoma from neovascularization of the angle.

The detailed classification of diabetic retinopathy using standard photographs is beyond the scope of this chapter. However, an outline of a classification including the clinical features is given below:

Pre-proliferative Retinopathy

1. Background diabetic retinopathy: at least one microaneurysm
2. Mild pre-proliferative retinopathy: microaneurysms and dot, blot or flame-shaped haemorrhages in all four fundus quadrants
3. Moderate pre-proliferative retinopathy: dense microaneurysms and haemorrhages in one to three quadrants. Cotton-wool spots and venous calibre changes, including venous beading and small intraretinal microvascular abnormalities (IRMA) may be seen
4. Severe pre-proliferative retinopathy (Figure 67.18), at least one of the following:
   - Dense haemorrhages and microaneurysms in all four quadrants
   - Clear venous beading in at least two quadrants
   - Prominent IRMA in at least one quadrant.

American terminology is slightly different referring to non-proliferative diabetic retinopathy, which can be mild (background) to severe.

Proliferative Diabetic Retinopathy

New vessels grow from the retina along the scaffold provided by the posterior vitreous surface. Fans of new vessels progress to fibrovascular bands and sheets (Figure 67.17). These may bleed, causing vitreous haemorrhage (sudden onset of floaters and loss of vision), or contract, leading to traction retinal detachment (progressive visual loss). Treatment for proliferative retinopathy should therefore commence within 2 weeks.

Diabetic Maculopathy

This is the most common cause of visual loss in diabetes mellitus. If retinal oedema or ischaemia involves the fovea (centre of the macula) it will no longer function effectively and vision will be blurred. Macular ischaemia is not treatable, but if retinal oedema or exudates threaten (Figure 67.18), or involve the fovea (Figure 67.16), macular laser treatment is indicated. Macular oedema which meets the threshold for laser is termed clinically significant macular oedema (CSMO).

Macular ischaemia is harder to recognize clinically. There may be dense blot haemorrhages and small IRMAs on the macula and the visual acuity is reduced with foveal involvement. It often co-exists with macular oedema and moderate to severe pre-proliferative or proliferative retinopathy (Figures 67.16 and 67.18).

Treatment of Diabetic Retinopathy

Good control of blood sugar (in type I and type II diabetes) and tight control of blood pressure (in type II diabetes) delay the onset of retinopathy and slow the progression of the disease. There is also evidence that long-term treatment with statins and another lipid-lowering agent, fenofibrate, reduces the progression of DR and need for laser.

Laser photocoagulation is the mainstay of treatment for diabetic retinopathy reducing the risk of vision loss (Table 67.6).

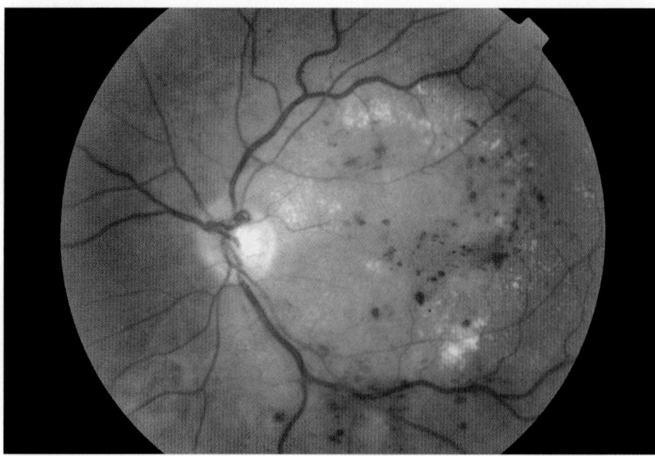

Figure 67.16 Diabetic maculopathy with macular oedema, exudates and multiple blot haemorrhages. *(Courtesy of Nicholas A. V. Beare and William Hooley.)*

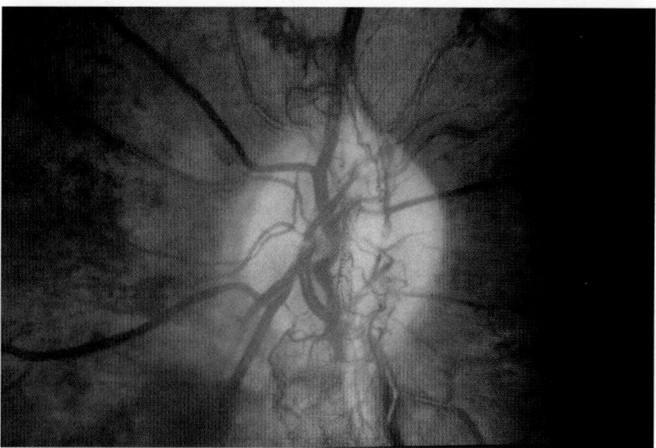

Figure 67.17 Proliferative diabetic retinopathy. New vessels over the optic disc. *(Courtesy of Clare Gilbert.)*

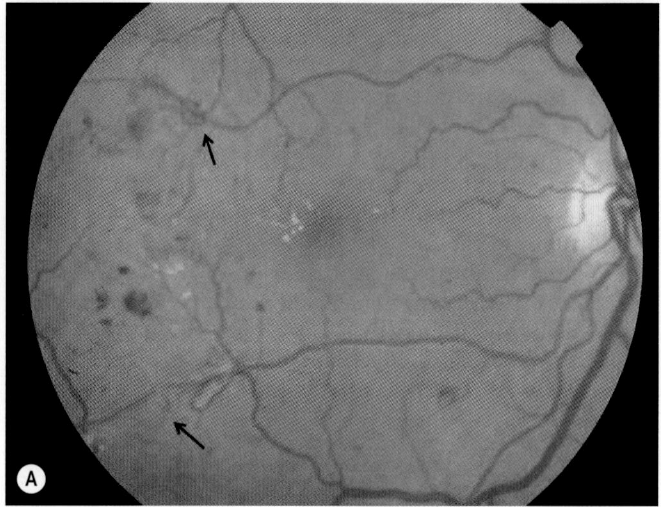

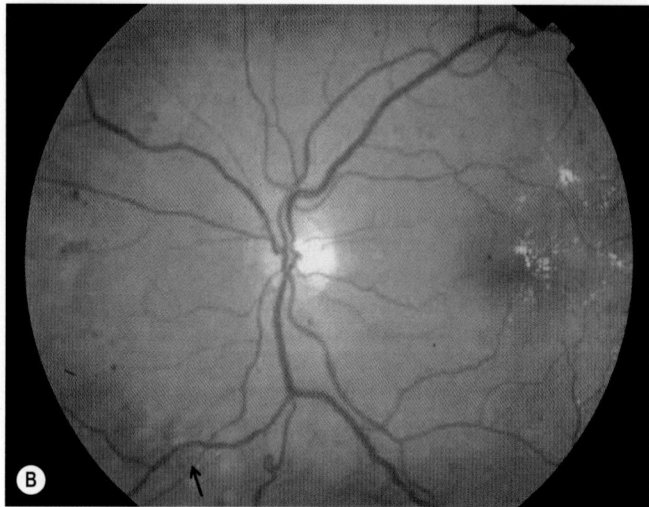

Figure 67.18 Severe preproliferative and proliferative diabetic retinopathy with maculopathy. This patient's vision is good, but they are at high risk of visual loss without treatment. (A) Right eye with severe pre-proliferative retinopathy and maculopathy. As well as exudates on the macula there are signs of ischaemia with multiple IRMAs (examples arrowed) on the temporal macula, venous loop and multiple deep blot haemorrhages. (B) New vessels elsewhere (arrow) with nearby venous beading, venous loop and IRMA; dilated arcade retinal veins and exudates on temporal macula. *(Courtesy of Nicholas A. V. Beare and Martin Hodson.)*

Laser Treatment. Peripheral retinal (pan-retinal) photocoagulation (PRP) involves multiple, small burns (200–400 μm) to the peripheral retina. PRP is the treatment for severe pre-proliferative and proliferative DR (Figure 67.19). It coagulates a proportion of the peripheral retina, reduces the cytokine produced by hypoxic cells which stimulates new vessel formation (VEGF). Non-response indicates too small proportion of the peripheral retina has been treated and further PRP is required. Side-effects of reduced night vision and peripheral vision become more likely after 3000 burns. Macular oedema

TABLE 67.6 Laser Treatment for Diabetic Retinopathy and Maculopathy

	Indications for Laser	Type of Laser	Method of Application	Risks and Side Effects of Laser
Diabetic retinopathy (DR)	Severe pre-proliferative DR; or proliferative DR	Peripheral retinal laser (PRP)	1500–5000 burns in the peripheral fundus	Reduced night/peripheral vision. Worsening of macular oedema
Diabetic maculopathy	Oedema involving the fovea; or CSMO[a]	Macular laser (focal or grid)	150–300 burns directly to MAs or in grid to oedematous area	Foveal burn Poor response

CSMO, Clinically significant macular oedema.

[a]CSMO defined as retinal oedema, or exudates with oedema, within 500 μm of the foveal centre; or oedema larger than 1 disc area within 1 disc diameter of the foveal centre. 500 μm is approximately one-third of a disc diameter.

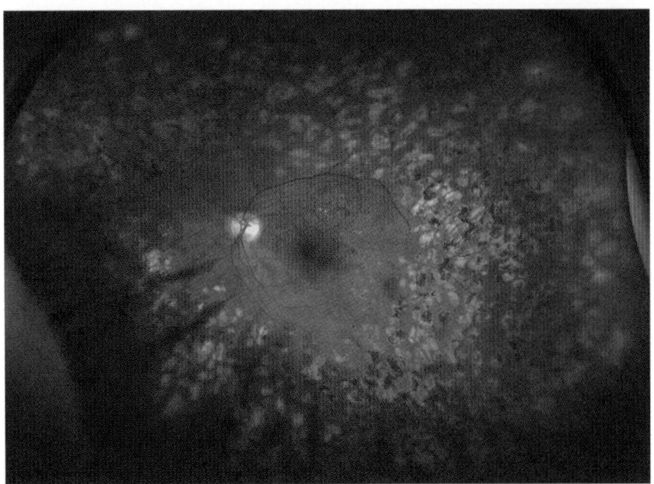

Figure 67.19 Wide-field colour fundus photograph of diabetic who has been treated with peripheral retinal laser (PRP) and macular laser (within the vascular arcades). There is lash artefact inferiorly. *(Courtesy of Nicholas A. V. Beare and Jerry Sharpe.)*

can be worsened by PRP and so should be treated first or concurrently with the PRP fractionated in several sittings.

Laser treatment of macular oedema involves direct photocoagulation of leaking microaneurysms and/or a grid of light burns to oedematous areas, or all around the fovea (Figure 67.19). Its effect is less reliable, but still halves the risk of moderate visual loss. The mode of action is unknown but may involve stimulation of the RPE. Once a macular grid is complete, further macular laser is unlikely to be effective and may damage remaining macular function.

Both forms of photocoagulation are most effective if delivered early, before there is a decrease in visual acuity.

Intravitreal Treatments. Anti-VEGF drugs (ranibizumab and bevacizumab) injected into the vitreous are effective in diabetic macular oedema but have to be repeated monthly for an uncertain period.

Pars Plana Vitrectomy. Vitrectomy is indicated for vitreous haemorrhage, or if the macula is detached or threatened by tractional retinal detachment. The timing of surgery for vitreous haemorrhage depends on the risk of active proliferative disease behind the haemorrhage. Relatively few eye clinics in developing countries have the expertise and equipment to perform this complex surgery.

Screening for Diabetic Retinopathy

Diabetic retinopathy is suitable for a systematic screening programme, because laser treatment is most effective before vision is affected. Retinal photography is the most consistent method of screening, but otherwise clinicians caring for diabetics should perform ophthalmoscopy through dilated pupils for diabetic retinopathy at least annually.

SICKLE CELL DISEASE

Sickle cell disease can cause a proliferative retinopathy which is most severe in heterozygotes with haemoglobin C (SC), rather than homozygous patients with haemoglobin SS. Other ocular manifestations include conjunctival vascular abnormalities (truncated, comma-shaped vessels), focal iris ischaemia and retinal vascular tortuosity.

Vascular occlusion in the peripheral retina causes ischaemia which can lead to arteriolar-venous anastomoses and new vessel formation. Neovascularization is in a 'sea-fan' pattern, which extends circumferentially. This can cause vitreous haemorrhage and occasionally retinal detachment, but regression can also occur from infarction of hypoxic retina.[17]

Laser photocoagulation should be used to treat proliferative disease. Treatment of peripheral ischaemic retina can either be local to new vessels, or 360° if reliable follow-up is not possible.

AGE-RELATED MACULAR DEGENERATION

Age-related macular degeneration (AMD) is the most common cause of blindness in the industrialized world, where it accounts for about 50% of blindness. It occurs in people over 60 years old and its prevalence increases with age. As people live longer, AMD prevalence is increasing. It is a bilateral degenerative disease of the central retina (macula) with atrophy and neovascularization accounting for most of the visual loss.

The features of AMD are predominantly on the macula:

- Drusen: yellowish deposits of accumulated debris (lipofuscin) beneath the retinal pigment epithelium (RPE), the layer beneath the retina
- Pigment deposits within the RPE
- Atrophy of the RPE
- Subretinal fibrosis suggests previous neovascularization
- Signs of active neovascularization such as elevation, retinal oedema and haemorrhage.

The first two have little effect on vision; the latter three reduce vision if they involve the central macula or fovea.

Aetiology

As the name suggests, longevity is the greatest risk factor for developing AMD. There appears to be an inflammatory component and there is a strong association between a nucleotide polymorphism coding for complement factor H and AMD. Relative hypoxia in the retina also plays a role and smoking is another important risk factor and the only modifiable one.

Clinical Appearance

Age-related changes on the macula are initially asymptomatic. As changes accumulate in the central macula there may be some loss of acuity. This may lead to slowly progressive atrophy of the RPE and photoreceptors. This is termed dry AMD, which causes slow deterioration in vision, with severe visual loss only if atrophy involves the fovea (Figure 67.20). Wet (neovascular) AMD is heralded by symptoms of distortion and rapid loss of central vision. Choroidal or retinal neovascularization occurs causing subretinal haemorrhage, RPE detachment, macula oedema and scarring (Figure 67.21).

There is a haemorrhagic variant of AMD termed polypoidal choriovasculopathy (PCV) which is more common in Asia. There is a paucity of data from Africa on AMD, but AMD is much less common in African Americans and Afro-Caribbeans. Its prevalence by age group appears to be similar in Indians and Caucasians.[18] AMD is likely to become a more prevalent cause of visual impairment in developing countries, particularly as cataract coverage increases.

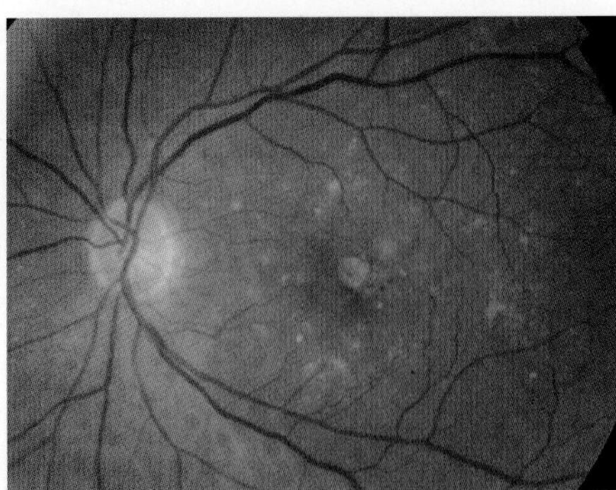

Figure 67.20 Dry age-related macular degeneration (AMD). A small area of atrophy of the retina and underlying retinal pigment epithelium (RPE) at the fovea (central macula) has reduced vision to 6/48. Multiple drusen (lipofuscin deposits beneath the RPE) are another feature of dry AMD but tend not to affect vision. *(Courtesy of Nicholas A. V. Beare and Stephen Pearson.)*

Management

There is no treatment for dry AMD. Patients who smoke should be encouraged to give up as a preventative measure.

Active neovascular AMD can be treated with repeated intraocular injections of anti-VEGF drugs such as bevacizumab or ranibizumab. These are effective at inhibiting new blood vessel growth, reducing macular oedema and causing regression of early neovascularization. They do not reverse fibroatrophic changes. However, they need to be given every month and are very expensive, making them inaccessible to most living outside the industrialized countries. Without treatment fibrosis and atrophy usually progress until central vision is lost. However, peripheral navigational vision remains intact.

TOXINS AND THE OPTIC NERVE

The optic nerve is susceptible to toxic damage, particularly in patients with nutritional deficiency of the vitamin B complex. Thus, optic neuropathy can result from heavy tobacco smoking, excess alcohol consumption and other toxins combined with poor nutrition. One such toxin is methanol and poisoning can lead to blindness.

Inadequately prepared cassava can cause optic neuropathy and peripheral nerve abnormalities due to cyanide toxicity. Cyanide is found particularly in the skin of the tubers. Water used for soaking cassava must be discarded, together with any fermenting cassava.

Drugs which may cause a toxic optic neuropathy include ethambutol, quinine and isoniazid.

Epidemics of bilateral optic neuropathy have occurred in West and East Africa without known cause. There tends to be acute onset, with impairment of colour vision and temporal pallor of the optic discs. There may be associated peripheral neuropathy and sensorineural hearing loss.

TRADITIONAL EYE MEDICINES

Many patients will go to the local traditional healer before attending a health centre or eye clinic. It should be recognized that traditional healing can provide benefit to patients. However, some applications to the eyes used by these local healers can cause severe adverse reactions.

The clinical features of the original condition may be confused by the application of harmful eye medicines into a diseased eye. The patient, or the parent, may be very reluctant to admit that traditional eye medicine has been used.

A variety of harmful substances, organic and chemical, may be used: the liquor of plant leaves, lime juice, kerosene, toothpaste and animal or human urine. A chemical or caustic keratoconjunctivitis may occur (Figure 67.22), or infection, such as with *N. gonorrhoea* from urine. Infectious keratitis is common after the use of traditional eye medicines. Topical therapy with an antibiotic every 2–6 hours and a cycloplegic such as atropine sulphate once daily, should be used. Steroid eye drops may be added once any infection is treated. The underlying eye disease should be treated as usual.

Programmes to develop a constructive approach of dialogue and cooperation with traditional healers have been developed in Zimbabwe, Malawi and Nepal, where it has been demonstrated that traditional healers can have a role in the prevention of blindness.

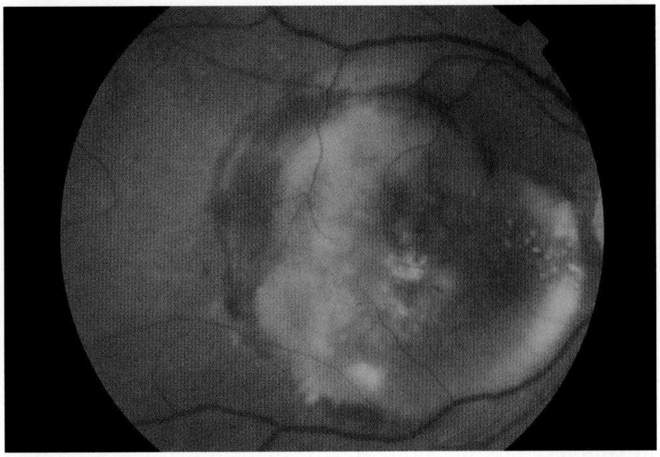

Figure 67.21 Wet (neovascular) age-related macular degeneration (AMD). New vessels proliferate under the retina and retinal pigment epithelium (RPE) causing RPE detachment, retinal oedema and haemorrhage which progresses to fibrosis. *(Courtesy of Nicholas A. V. Beare and Gill Lewis.)*

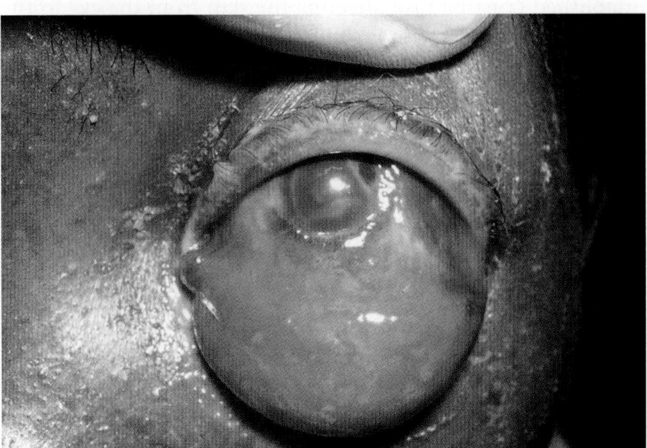

Figure 67.22 Severe keratoconjunctivitis with conjunctival prolapse from harmful traditional eye treatment. *(Courtesy of Nicholas A. V. Beare.)*

Couching

Couching is a traditional procedure for the treatment of cataract in which the opaque lens is displaced from the visual axis. The procedure often leads to blinding complications.

Two methods of couching are reported:

1. The 'Sharp' method: the eye is perforated and the lens is pushed backwards by a sharp instrument, e.g. a long thorn.
2. The 'Blunt' method: the lens is pushed into the vitreous by vigorous massage or by blunt injury.

Infectious Ophthalmic Disease

VIRAL OPHTHALMIC DISEASE

HIV/AIDS AND THE EYE

The HIV epidemic in resource-poor countries, particularly in sub-Saharan Africa, has affected the pattern of eye disease commonly dealt with in these areas. The commonest manifestations of HIV presenting to eye departments in Africa are squamous cell carcinoma of the conjunctiva, herpes zoster ophthalmicus, Kaposi's sarcoma of the eyelids, viral retinitis and uveitis.

Preventing Transmission in the Eye Clinic. HIV has been found in the tears, conjunctiva, cornea, aqueous humour and retinal vessels. Tears are a theoretical mode of transmission, although there is no report of transmission occurring through tears. However, decontamination of instruments which come into contact with the eye such as tonometers is essential. Immersion in sodium hypochlorite (2%) or dichloroisocyanurate (1000 ppm) between patients is adequate.

The transmission of HIV by corneal transplantation is possible and standard donor transplant precautions should be in place.

HIV and Herpes Zoster Ophthalmicus

Herpes zoster ophthalmicus (HZO) is a marker for HIV infection in Africa and should prompt an HIV test if HIV status is not already known.[19] The course of this disease is more severe in HIV-positive patients, with more neuropathic pain, keratouveitis and corneal damage. It also occurs in a younger age group. In resource-poor areas, HZO often presents with an established crusting rash affecting the skin from the eye to the vertex of the skull without crossing the midline, but this is preceded by dermal hyperaemia and vesicles. There may be conjunctivitis, episcleritis, scleritis, keratitis and loss of corneal sensation, anterior uveitis, secondary glaucoma, extraocular nerve and muscle involvement and optic neuritis.

Treatment is aimed at limiting the damage from lid and corneal involvement, uveitis and secondary glaucoma. Lubricating eye ointment (chloramphenicol ointment is most readily available) should be given at least four times a day if the lids are involved. Anterior uveitis is more common if the rash is present on the nose indicating nasociliary nerve involvement (Hutchinson's sign). It should be treated with topical aciclovir, minimal steroid eye drops and a mydriatic such as cyclopentolate 1%. For superficial keratitis topical aciclovir alone is sufficient. However, neuropathic corneal ulcers can develop and can perforate. Treatment of corneal ulcers involves adding topical antibiotics, lubricating ointment and temporary lid closure with taping or a tarsorrhaphy. HZO can also cause scleral and orbital inflammation, cranial nerve palsies and optic disc swelling.

Oral antiviral drugs, such as aciclovir, valaciclovir or famciclovir if available, reduce the severity of the rash and complications if started within 3 days of the onset of the rash. Intravenous aciclovir (or oral valaciclovir) may be required in HIV and other immunosuppressed patients.

Herpes zoster virus, in-keeping with other herpes viruses, can cause viral retinitis. This usually occurs as painless loss of vision in AIDS patients unrelated to HZO (see below).

HIV Retinal Microangiopathy

The most common fundus manifestation of HIV-infected patients is microangiopathy, or abnormalities of the small vessels of the retina. Microangiopathy consists of cotton-wool spots and small intraretinal haemorrhages and is asymptomatic. Microangiopathy can be found in around one-third of AIDS patients and has been associated with a high viral load. HIV retinopathy does not cause visual loss.

AIDS and Cytomegalovirus (CMV) Retinitis

Cytomegalovirus is a *Herpes* virus whose latent infection is very prevalent in the adult population. In HIV patients with severe immunosuppression (CD4 count <50/mm^3), reactivation of latent CMV infection may cause gastrointestinal disease, pneumonitis, encephalitis and retinitis. CMV retinitis affected up to 30% of AIDS patients in the industrialized world prior to highly active antiretroviral therapy (HAART), while in sub-Saharan Africa the prevalence seems to be lower.[20] This is unlikely to be just because AIDS patients in Africa die from other opportunistic infections before they develop CMV retinitis. It may be that lack of specialist infrastructure has resulted in many cases going unrecognized or undiagnosed. The prevalence of CMV retinitis is higher in Asia.[21]

The classical appearance of CMV retinitis is that of a haemorrhagic retinal necrosis – sometimes described as tomato ketchup on cottage cheese or pizza fundus, with extension of the lesions along the vascular arcades (Figure 67.23). There is little vitritis or inflammation, as the patient is unable to mount an immune response. The disease is bilateral in about 50% of patients. It is slowly progressive and, if no treatment is provided, the whole retina and vision may be destroyed within 6 months.

The optimum treatment of CMV retinitis is daily intravenous ganciclovir or foscarnet. Ganciclovir suppresses the bone marrow, while foscarnet is nephrotoxic. An alternative drug is cidofovir, which does have the advantage of once-weekly treatment, but can cause severe uveitis. Oral valganciclovir is an alternative to intravenous ganciclovir for initial treatment and preferred for maintenance therapy. Ganciclovir intraocular implants can be used to maintain suppression of CMV for 6–9 months. These drugs are very expensive, toxic and inconvenient. An option is to use weekly intravitreal injections of 2 mg of ganciclovir until active inflammation resolves.[22] This is relatively inexpensive and stabilizes the disease, maintaining the vision, provided central vision has not already been affected, until antiretroviral treatment takes effect.[23] CMV retinitis will regress once a patient's immune system reconstitutes and is able to suppress the infection. Treated or regressed CMV retinitis leaves a necrotic retina with a speckled or salt-and-pepper appearance. The retina frequently detaches at this stage, even with regression of the infection and this requires specialist surgery to salvage any vision.

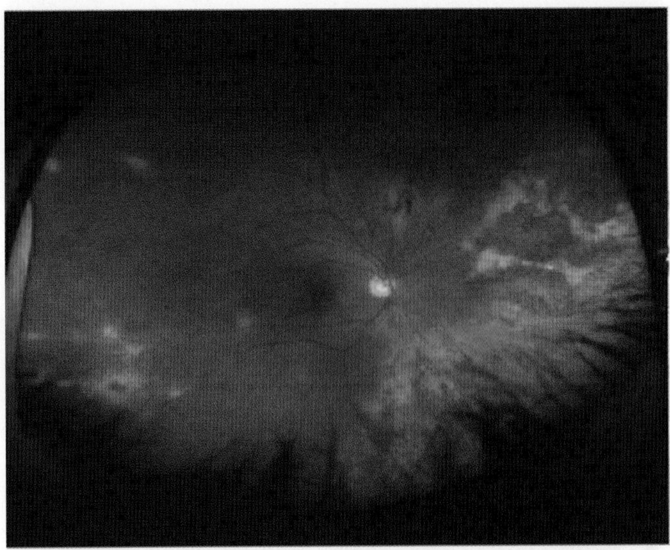
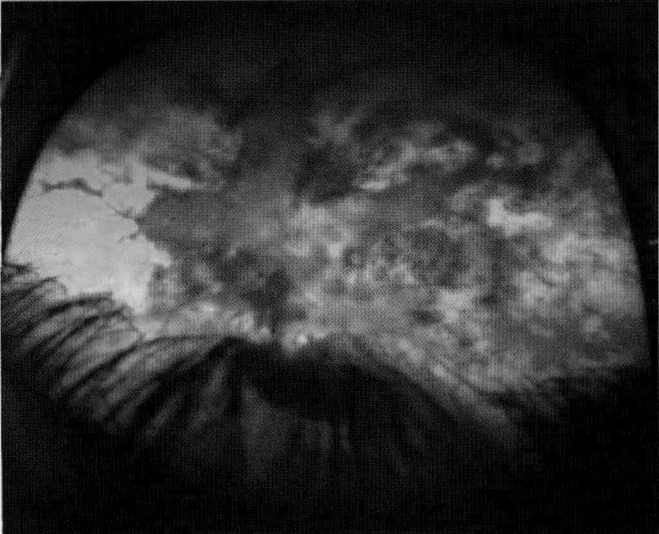

Figure 67.23 Wide-field fundus image of CMV retinitis in patient with HIV. Left eye has no perception of light with extensive retinal necrosis and haemorrhage (pizza fundus). Note vitreous is clear despite severe retinitis. Right eye had good vision with only peripheral retinal involvement, but subsequently developed a retinal detachment. Eyelash artefacts are present inferiorly. *(Courtesy of Nicholas A. V. Beare and Stephen Pearson.)*

Paradoxically, improvement in the patient's immune system with HAART can lead to a worsening of vision as part of the immune reconstitution inflammatory syndrome (IRIS). This is because the inactivated cytomegalovirus provokes an immune response that may cause uveitis and macular oedema, so-called immune-recovery uveitis. If severe, this can be treated with steroid treatment as with macular oedema from endogenous uveitis.

HIV and Other Herpes Viruses

Herpes simplex virus (HSV) and varicella zoster virus (VZV) can also cause retinitis in immunocompromised patients, which can be difficult to distinguish clinically from CMV retinitis. Varicella zoster retinitis tends to be unilateral, less haemorrhagic and spreads in a circumferential pattern around the retinal periphery. This appearance is termed 'progressive outer retinal necrosis', while retinitis due to HSV is termed 'acute retinal necrosis' and is not exclusive to immunocompromised patients. Both cause an occlusive vasculitis with occluded vessels, perivascular haemorrhage and areas of opacification due to retinal necrosis. The only certain way to distinguish HSV, VZV and CMV retinitis is for an eye specialist to take a sample of aqueous fluid which is analysed for the presence of viral DNA by PCR.

HSV and VZV are sensitive to aciclovir (whereas CMV is not) and ganciclovir. Aciclovir should be given IV initially and continued orally (as aciclovir, or preferably as the pro-drug valaciclovir) for 3–6 months. As in CMV retinitis, retinal detachment is a frequent complication once the initial infection has been treated.

HIV and Syphilis

Syphilis has a high prevalence in resource-poor, particularly urban, settings. It is frequently a co-infection with HIV, so all patients should be tested for HIV. Ocular manifestations of syphilis are uncommon but include anterior uveitis, posterior uveitis, retinitis, retinal vasculitis (Figure 67.24) and optic nerve disease.

The recommended treatment for ocular syphilis in HIV-seropositive patients is 12–24 million units of aqueous crystalline penicillin G intravenously per day for 10–14 days. Clinicians should have a low threshold for testing for syphilis, testing all patients with posterior uveitis, retinitis or retinal vasculitis.

HIV and Tuberculosis

The alarming rise in the prevalence of tuberculosis parallels the spread of the HIV pandemic. In developing countries, 30–50% of adults have latent tuberculosis that may be reactivated in the presence of HIV infection. Because of the profound depression of cell-mediated immunity in HIV/AIDS patients, there may be rapid dissemination of the infection to multiple organs (miliary disease). In patients with profound immunosuppression, the presentation may be atypical, with extrapulmonary involvement and a negative tuberculin test. In patients with AIDS, massive choroidal invasion may lead to secondary retinal necrosis and blindness; these patients die within a few months. More common are single or multiple small, pale, elevated choroidal lesions representing choroidal granulomas, which are associated with mycobacteraemia.[20]

The treatment of tuberculosis is the same as in patients who are not HIV-infected.

HIV and Pneumocystosis

Pneumocystis is an opportunistic pathogen which causes pneumonia (PCP) in immunosuppressed individuals, particularly in HIV/AIDS.

Pneumocystis jirovecii can rarely cause choroiditis characterized by yellow-white subretinal plaques in the posterior pole that enlarge and coalesce into irregular multilobular lesions. Exudative retinal detachments may develop. It is important to recognize *Pneumocystis choroiditis* as it indicates disseminated disease. Treatment is with high-dose co-trimoxazole or atovaquone.

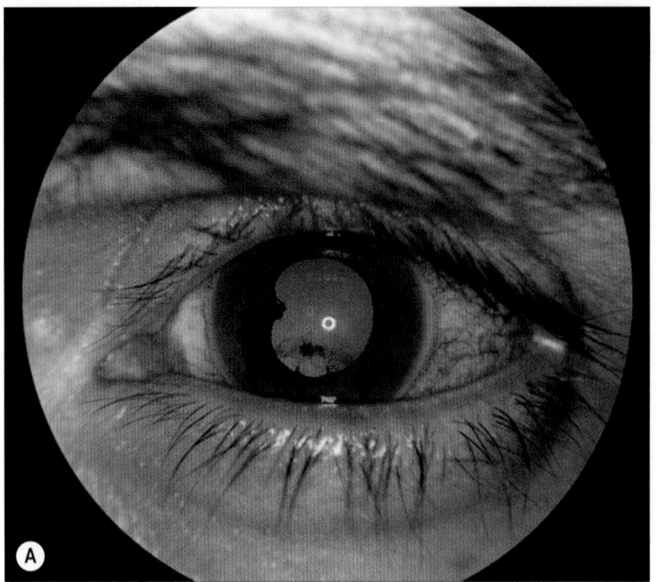

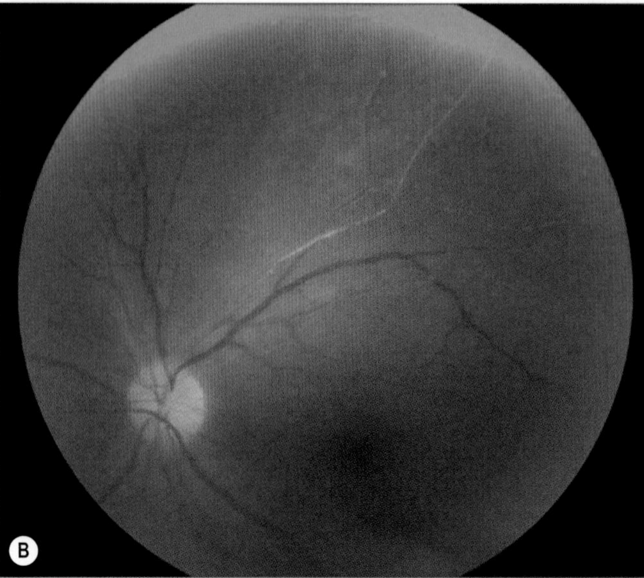

Figure 67.24 Uveitis due to syphilis in patient with HIV. (A) Circumciliary injection, posterior synechiae and fibrinous inflammatory reaction in the anterior chamber due to anterior uveitis. (B) Retinal vasculitis prominently affecting an arteriole (frosted branch angiitis), but also venules. *(Courtesy of Albert Anderson and Chris Berstrom, Lancet Infectious Diseases, Volume 9, Issue 7, Page 453, July 2009.)*

HIV and Cryptococcal Meningitis

The yeast *Cryptococcus neoformans* is a common cause of meningitis in patients with AIDS. Papilloedema due to raised intracranial pressure is common and can cause visual loss if it is prolonged (Figure 67.25). *Cryptococcus* infection can itself damage the optic nerve causing optic atrophy and loss of vision. Diplopia can occur because of oculomotor nerve palsies. *C. neoformans* var. *gattii* infections are more likely to cause invasive disease in immunocompetent individuals.

HIV and Squamous Cell Carcinomas of the Conjunctiva

Squamous cell carcinoma of the conjunctiva (SCCC) has been reported with greater frequency in HIV-infected individuals. An increased incidence of 5–10-fold, in parallel with the HIV epidemic, has created a substantial burden on the surgical capacity of eye units in sub-Saharan Africa. Cutaneous human papilloma viruses (HPV), in combination with HIV, have been implicated in the aetiology of SCCC, however HPVs are only detected in less than half of cases.[24] It is likely that the aetiology is multifactorial, including HPV, HIV and ultraviolet light exposure.

Typical clinical appearance of SCCC is of a greyish-white elevated mass surrounded by a blood supply of engorged conjunctival vessels, sometimes with pigmentation (Figure 67.26). SCCC arises in the palpebral conjunctiva, often at the conjunctival-corneal junction (the limbus). The tumour spreads to involve the whole conjunctiva, lids, local tissue and lymph nodes. Treatment is prompt and complete surgical excision,

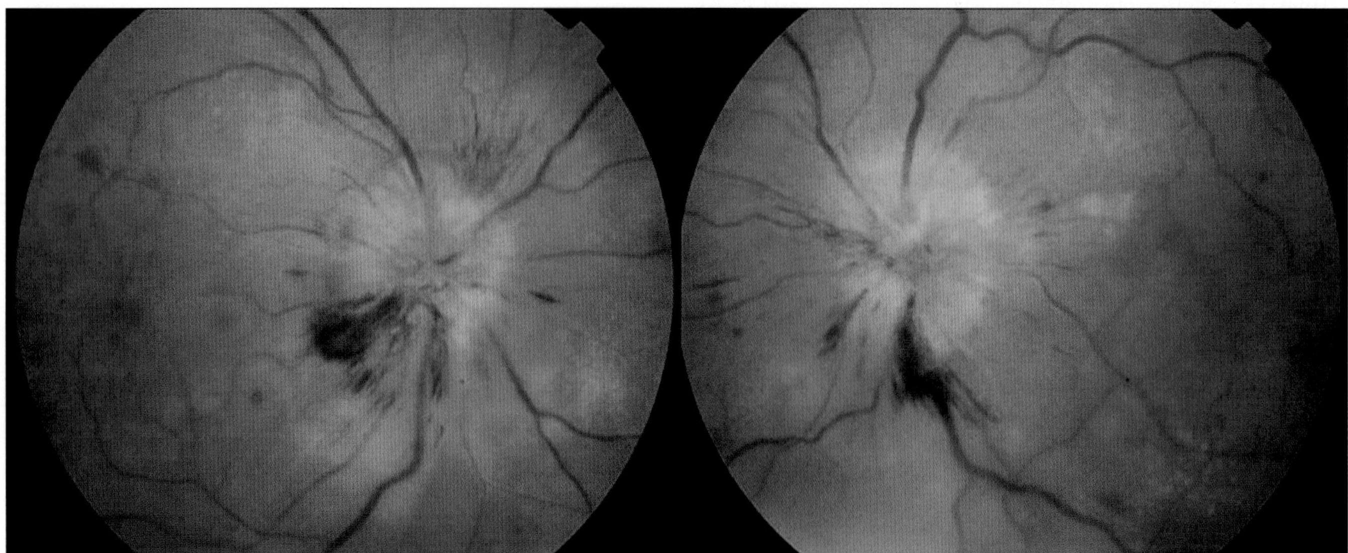

Figure 67.25 Severe papilloedema. Bilateral disc swelling due to raised intracranial pressure with blurring of disc margins, elevation, loss of cup and superficial haemorrhages. *(Courtesy of Nicholas A. V. Beare and Jerry Sharp.)*

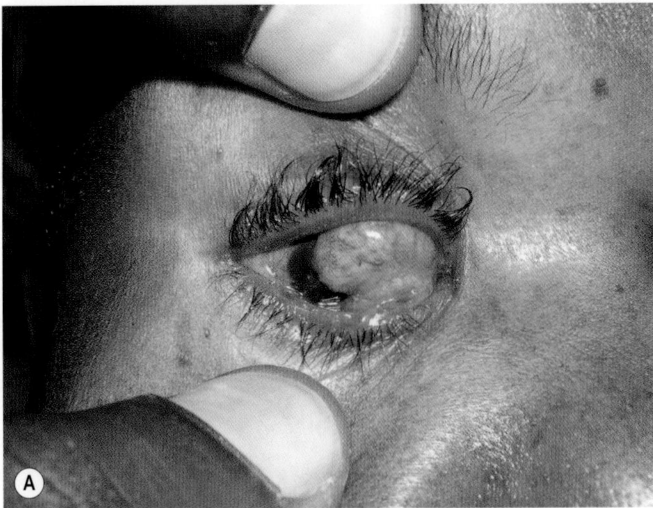

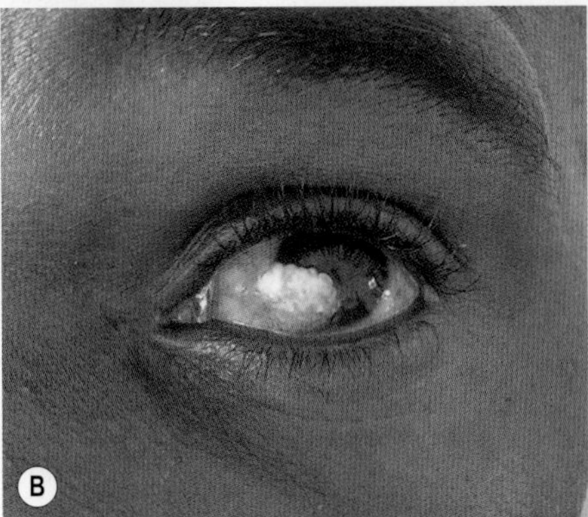

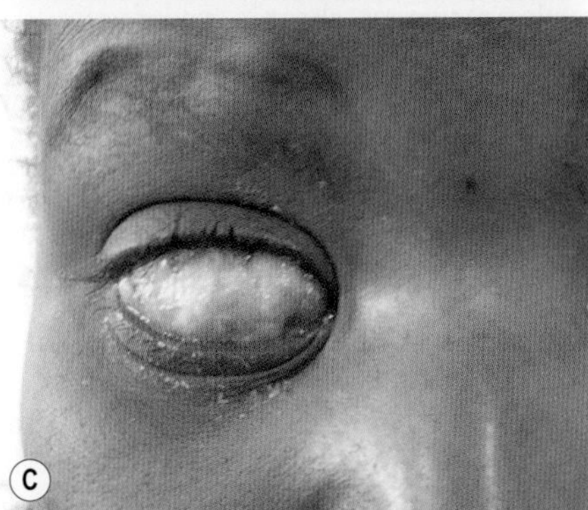

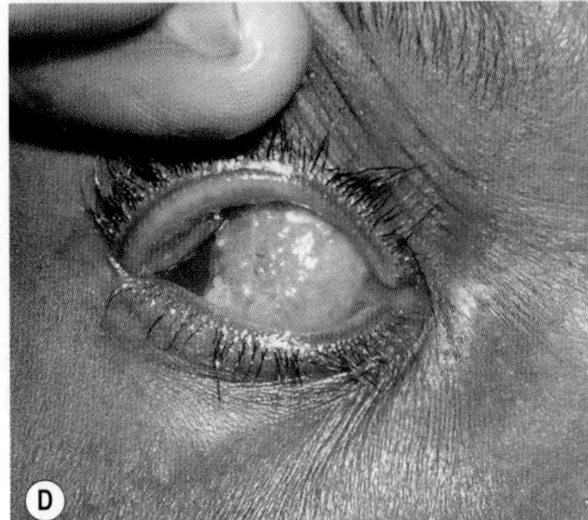

Figure 67.26 (A–D) Examples of squamous cell carcinomas of the conjunctiva. *(Courtesy of Nicholas A. V. Beare and Nkume Batumba.)*

preferably at an early stage. As more conjunctiva is involved surgical excision becomes more difficult and may involve enucleation of the eye or exenteration of the orbit.

Simple excision is associated with high recurrence rates of 30–40%, which have been reported to be reduced by adjuvant treatments. These include topical chemotherapy with antimetabolites (mitomycin C or 5-fluorouracil), cryotherapy[25] and intraoperative β-irradiation.[22] None have been subject to a randomized trial.[26] All have logistical difficulties in developing countries, but a β-radiation source, once obtained, is long-lasting and stored relatively easily.

HIV and Kaposi's Sarcoma

Kaposi's sarcoma is a malignant vascular tumour which occurs in 15–24% of patients with AIDS in the developing world. This tumour can present on the skin or mucous membranes. It may develop on the eyelid skin, eyelid margins, conjunctiva and rarely, within the orbit. The clinical presentation of the tumour appears as a deep purple-red nodule (Figure 67.27). Typically, multifocal skin lesions appear, which later ulcerate. They are usually slow-growing and rarely invasive. The tumours can be excised or given focal radiation therapy.

Herpes Simplex Keratitis

For details of herpes simplex keratitis, see above.

Measles

For details of measles and the eye, see later.

Rubella

Rubella is frequently subclinical or presents with an erythematous maculopapular rash on the face, trunk and extremities, often in epidemics. Maternal infection during the 1st trimester has an 80% chance of affecting the unborn child. Cataract may occur in around half of all children affected by rubella in utero. The virus may remain in the lens for some years after birth and surgical removal of the cataract causes uveitis. Other eye defects include congenital glaucoma, retinopathy with a 'salt and pepper' appearance, optic atrophy, squint, nystagmus and microphthalmos. Congenital cataract due to rubella has a poor prognosis.

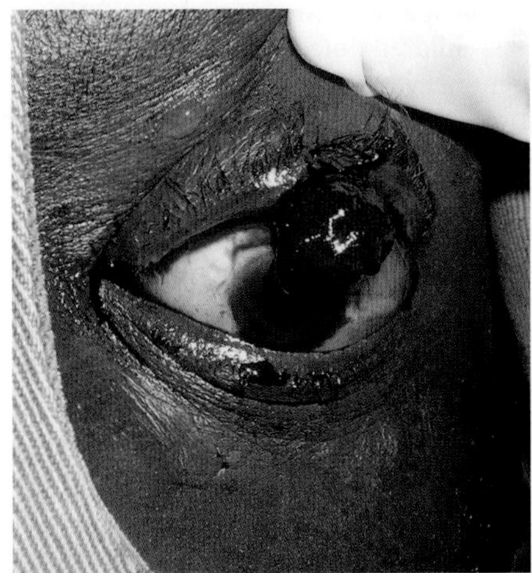

Figure 67.27 Kaposi's sarcoma of the eyelid. *(Courtesy of Nicholas A. V. Beare and Nkume Batumba.)*

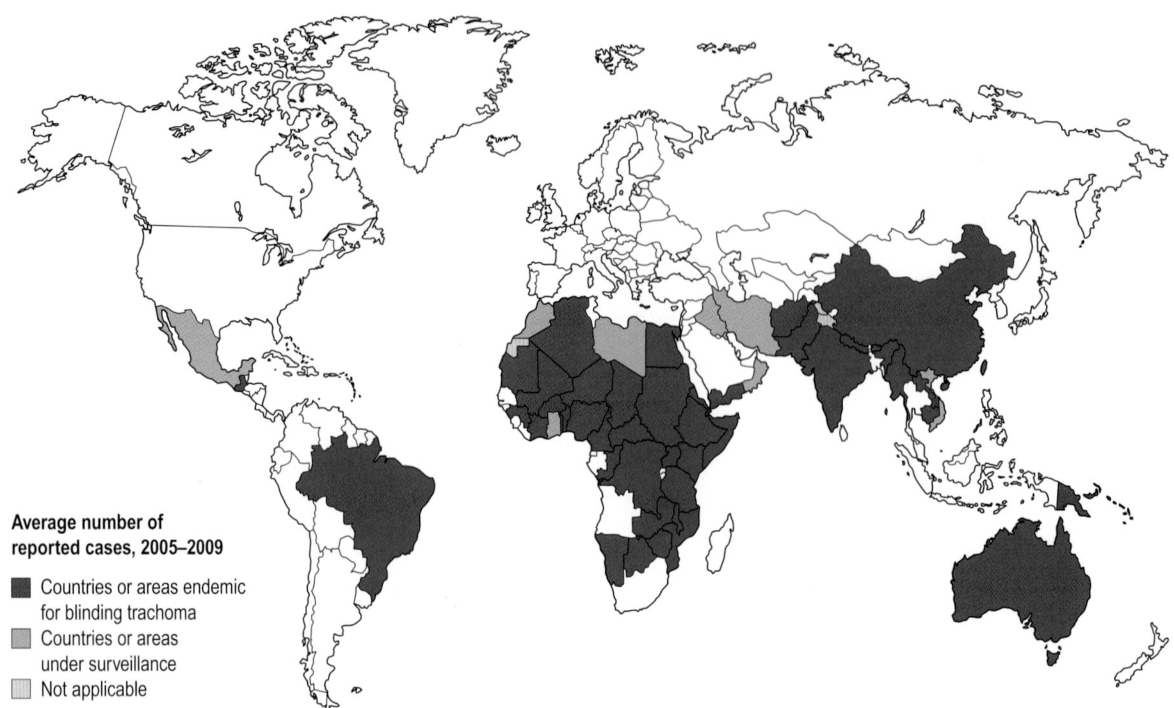

Figure 67.28 Worldwide distribution of trachoma. *(Courtesy of WHO:* http://gamapserver.who.int/mapLibrary/Files/Maps/Global_trachoma_2010.png.*)*

Rubella can be prevented by immunization of females achieving at least 80% coverage of the population.

Mumps

An acute fever with parotitis is the typical presentation, sometimes involving other organs, causing orchitis, oophoritis and pancreatitis. Following infection, the patient has long-term immunity.

Eye complications are uncommon but include lacrimal gland swelling (dacryoadenitis), conjunctivitis, keratitis, iritis, scleritis, retinitis and optic neuritis. Treatment is supportive with analgesics and appropriate treatment of any eye complications.

Molluscum Contagiosum

Molluscum contagiosum is caused by a DNA virus which usually infects children. Infection in adults, especially in Africa, may be a sentinel lesion for HIV infection. A small papule with a central umbilicus is typical. The lesion may be isolated or in clusters. Lesions on the eyelid may cause a follicular conjunctivitis or sometimes a keratitis. Curetting of the lesions with the application of iodine or carbolic acid is usually successful.

BACTERIAL OPHTHALMIC DISEASE

Chlamydia and Trachoma

Trachoma is one of the major blinding diseases of the world. It is the most common infectious cause of blindness. Active trachoma is believed to affect 40.6 million people and 8.2 million have trichiasis putting them at risk of blindness as a consequence of trachoma.[27] This eye disease is a serious public health problem in many parts of Africa, the Middle East and Asia (Figure 67.28). However, the prevalence is declining and the year 2020 has been earmarked as the target for Global Elimination of Trachoma.

Trachoma is a recurrent, chronic eye infection. The infecting organism is *Chlamydia trachomatis*, an obligate intracellular bacterium. Serotypes A, B, Ba and C cause the eye infection. Serotypes D–K mainly cause urogenital infection, but can also involve the eyes.

Eye infection begins in early childhood in endemic areas, which are typically dry with inadequate water supply and sanitation. This begins a cycle of recurrent episodes of inflammation, secondary bacterial infection and eventually scarring of the tarsal conjunctiva. With conjunctival fibrosis the upper eyelid turns inwards (entropion) and distortion of the eyelashes occurs (trichiasis). These cause severe irritation by rubbing on the eyeball. The trichiasis repeatedly degrades the corneal surface leading directly to corneal scarring or through secondary infection. After a long painful process, blindness results.

Risk Factors. Communities with a high prevalence of trachoma typically have a dry and dusty environment, a poor water supply, inadequate sanitation, overcrowding in the homes and a large fly population.

Flies carry the organism from child to child (Figure 67.29). They are attracted by discharging eyes and noses. Dirty, unwashed faces create an environment which predisposes to trachoma.

Exposed faeces attract the flies. Well-designed pit latrines, properly used, will reduce the prevalence of trachoma within a community. An inadequate water supply is another risk factor. There is a correlation between the distance travelled to collect water and the prevalence of trachoma. Poor education, especially of mothers, is another risk factor.

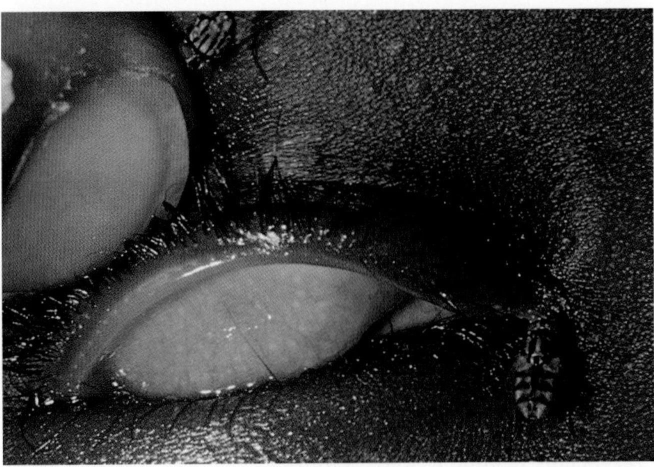

Figure 67.29 Everted upper eyelid of a Gambian child with follicular trachoma and a feeding female bazaar fly (*Musca sorbens*). *(Courtesy of Paul Emerson and Robin Bailey.)*

Health education emphasizing facial cleanliness reduces the transmission.

Clinical Examination

1. Look for evidence of any discharge and to see if any eyelashes are touching the cornea.
2. It should be noted if any eyelashes have been removed (epilation).
3. The cornea is examined for evidence of inflammation and corneal opacity.
4. Evert the upper lid by asking the patient to look down, keeping the eyes open. The eyelashes are gently grasped between finger and thumb, while the other hand places a glass rod or similar object on the superior eyelid skin, above the skin crease. The eyelid is rotated against the slim rod and everts, revealing the upper tarsal conjunctiva.
5. The tarsal conjunctiva is examined for evidence of follicles, intense inflammation or conjunctival scarring.

Grading System. A simplified grading classification for trachoma looks for five selected signs (Figure 67.30):

- **Trachomatous inflammation – follicular (TF)**: five or more follicles at least 0.5 mm in diameter in the upper tarsal conjunctiva. Follicles are accumulations of lymphoid cells, like small yellowish or white lumps (like grains of rice) within the conjunctiva.
- **Trachomatous inflammation – intense (TI)**: pronounced inflammatory thickening of the upper tarsal conjunctiva obscuring more than half of the deep tarsal vessels. In severe inflammation, the tarsal conjunctiva appears red, rough and thickened. There is diffuse inflammatory infiltration, oedema and vascular papillary hypertrophy. This is the most infective stage.

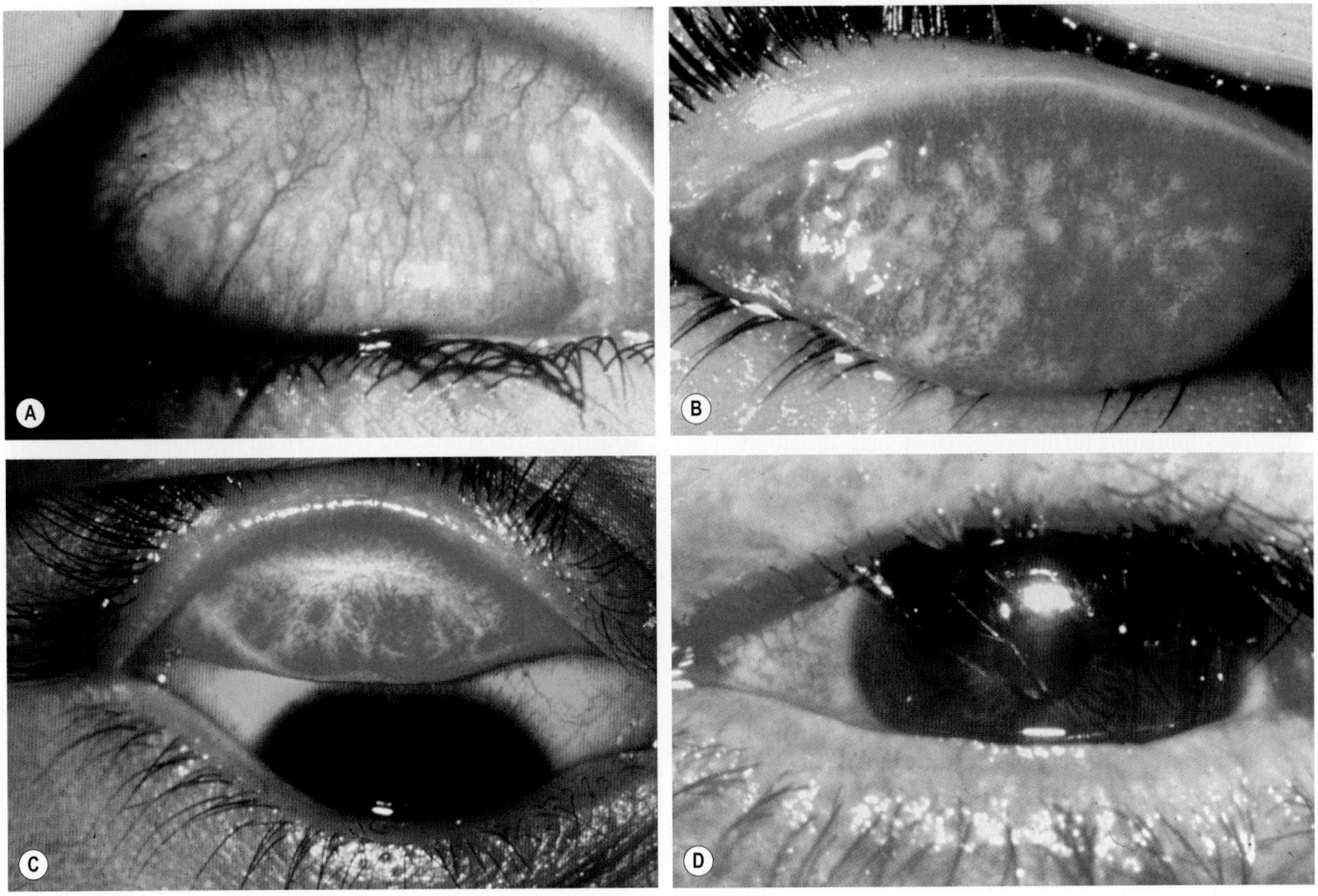

Figure 67.30 Stages in the development of trachoma. Clockwise from top left: (A) Follicles of trachoma (TF). (B) Intense inflammation of trachoma (TI). (C) Trichiasis of trachoma (TT). (D) Conjunctival scarring of trachoma (TS). *(Courtesy of International Centre for Eye Health, London.)*

- **Trachomatous scarring (TS)**: scarring in the tarsal conjunctiva. White lines in the tarsal conjunctiva show early signs of the scarring stage of trachoma. The scarring may also appear as bands or sheets.
- **Trachomatous trichiasis (TT)**: at least one eyelash rubbing on the eyeball. Evidence of removal of eyelashes (epilation) is included in this category.
- **Corneal opacity (CO)**: corneal opacity obscuring at least part of the pupil. This leads to visual impairment.

Trachoma Control and the SAFE Strategy. The SAFE strategy provides an appropriate and focused approach to control measures albeit in reverse order of healthcare stratification. S stands for surgery required to prevent corneal scarring in those with trichiasis/entropion; A is for antibiotic treatment as secondary prevention (tetracycline eye ointment or azithromycin orally); F is for facial hygiene; E is for environmental change (primary prevention). Of these interventions repeated mass distribution of single-dose oral azithromycin is the most effective in delivering trachoma control. The WHO recommends 3 years of azithromycin distribution as part of a trachoma control programme where active trachoma is present in 10% or more of children. Trachoma surveillance programmes are required after 3 years of population treatment because trachoma prevalence can recur to levels above 10% of children within 3 years.[28]

Management

Medical Treatment. Both tetracyclines and macrolides are effective against trachoma in its acute stages (TF and TI), e.g. tetracycline eye ointment twice daily for 6 weeks. In practice, compliance with this regimen is poor. A single dose of oral azithromycin (adults, 1 g; children 20 mg/kg) is as effective as treatment with topical tetracycline and more convenient. Mass treatment of endemic communities may interrupt the transmission of infection, but at present, it is not known how frequently treatment must be repeated, nor which populations require mass treatment.

As azithromycin has activity against causative organisms of respiratory disease, diarrhoea and malaria, mass distribution of azithromycin reaching 80% of the population on a 6-monthly or yearly basis has been found to reduce child mortality by half in trachoma-endemic areas.[29] This supports the need to continue trachoma control programmes with the goal of elimination, while stimulating further research on mass distribution of antibiotics and its effect on community disease burden and mortality.

Trichiasis and Epilation. When an eyelash touches the cornea, causing extreme irritation, many patients remove it using forceps. Unfortunately, eyelashes will grow again in 4–6 weeks; however, epilation does provide temporary symptomatic relief.

Surgery for Trachomatous Entropion. Surgery to evert the lid margin and rotate the lashes away from the cornea may provide a permanent cure for trichiasis and reduce the risk of visual loss. Several procedures have been described, but there is a significant risk of recurrence following any operation. Uptake of trichiasis surgery is poor and most patients never have an operation. Access to surgery may be improved by using ophthalmic nurses or clinical assistants to perform the surgery in the patient's own village.

Corneal Graft Surgery after Corneal Opacity. The outcome of corneal transplantation in advanced trachoma is usually poor, as there is a poor conjunctival surface and ocular surface, with an unstable tear film and possible corneal epithelial stem cell deficiency.

Prevention. Treatment of an entire community with azithromycin reduces transmission of trachoma; however reinfection is likely. Without additional preventive measures, antibiotic treatment will not have a permanent effect.

Communities need to be educated in the prevention of trachoma and government or NGO agencies enlisted to enable community-wide prevention measures. Community development eliminates the factors in which trachoma flourishes. Communities need to:

- Secure a suitable water supply
- Keep children's faces clean
- Build and use well-designed ventilated pit latrines
- Rubbish should not be left lying in the open
- Animals, especially cattle, should be housed some distance from the family home.

In many countries of the world, trachoma prevalence is falling even in the absence of a control programme, due to improved environmental and socioeconomic conditions.[30] However, foci of severe disease remain, particularly in the most marginalized and disadvantaged groups in severely resource-poor settings. Trachoma will only be eradicated when we improve the quality of life of these communities.

Lymphogranuloma Venereum

Lymphogranuloma venereum is caused by the L1, L2 or L3 serotypes of *Chlamydia trachomatis* and is transmitted by sexual contact. The organism is widespread geographically.

The initial lesion, the primary sore, is usually in the genital region and within days, there follows a regional lymphadenitis, with fever, headache and malaise.

Eye Complications. Lymphogranuloma venereum is one cause of Parinaud's oculoglandular syndrome: follicular conjunctivitis with pre-auricular lymphadenopathy. A keratitis can occur with corneal infiltration and new vessel formation. Anterior uveitis, panuveitis and scleritis have been described.

Management. The treatment of lymphogranuloma venereum is with a tetracycline and is described in Chapter 23.

RICKETTSIA

Typhus

Typhus fever is caused by *Rickettsia* or *Orientia*, which are obligate intracellular bacteria, transmitted by lice, ticks, mites or fleas.

Eye Complications. Eye complications associated with typhus fever include conjunctivitis, anterior uveitis, retinal haemorrhages and optic nerve oedema, which may lead to optic atrophy.

Management. See Chapter 24.

Boutonneuse Fever (Mediterranean Spotted Fever)

Boutonneuse fever is caused by *Rickettsia conorii* and is transmitted by a tick infesting dogs and rodents. It has a widespread distribution including Africa and India but is endemic to the countries around the Mediterranean Sea. After an incubation of 7–10 days, the patient has fever, headache, malaise and myalgia with a maculopapular rash and a black crust developing at the site of the tick bite.

Eye Complications. Posterior uveitis complicates around a third of cases with vitritis, retinal haemorrhages including white-centred haemorrhages, retinal vasculitis, serous retinal detachment, macular oedema and a macular star of exudates.

Management. Treatment is with tetracyclines, usually doxycycline.

Cat-scratch Disease

This is caused by intracellular bacteria of the genus *Bartonella*. Patients develop a lymphadenopathy in the region of the scratch.

Eye Complications. *Bartonella* is a rare cause of uveitis and neuroretinitis. It causes the characteristic combination of optic disc swelling and deposition of exudates in a star-shaped pattern on the macular which is oedematous. A history of a scratch from a cat is required to consider the diagnosis.

Bartonella is sensitive to tetracyclines and to macrolides such as erythromycin and azithromycin.

MYCOBACTERIA

Tuberculosis

There has been an epidemic of tuberculosis (TB) in combination with HIV in Africa, however elsewhere the incidence is decreasing. The WHO estimates that there are 8.8 million new cases each year, with nearly 1.4 million deaths (WHO, 2010). A quarter of deaths from TB are in HIV-positive patients, accounting for a quarter of HIV-related deaths.[31]

Eye Complications. The disease may affect all systems of the body, including the eyes. Infection of the skin (lupus vulgaris) can result in eyelid scarring and secondary corneal involvement due to exposure. Phlyctenular keratoconjunctivitis is due to a hypersensitivity reaction to the tuberculoprotein, presenting as small yellow/pink nodules, often on the corneoscleral margin. A phlyctena nodule generally responds quickly to topical corticosteroid therapy.

TB can cause scleritis which may be associated with marked thickening of the sclera due to granuloma formation.

A granulomatous anterior uveitis with large keratic precipitates (described as ‘mutton fat’) may occur but is not specific to TB (Figure 67.10). Examination with magnification may reveal small white inflammatory nodules at the pupil margin (Koeppe nodules). Posterior uveitis can take the form of choroidal tubercles, pale elevated fundus lesions which indicate disseminated disease (Figure 67.31). Both optic neuritis and optic atrophy are described.

Tuberculosis is an important infectious cause of retinal vasculitis and should be included in the differential diagnosis with non-infectious causes, e.g. sarcoidosis, Behçet’s disease, Wegner’s granulomatosis and multiple sclerosis. The vasculopathy may be non-occlusive with vascular sheathing, perivascular exudates or haemorrhage; or occlusive with retinal ischaemia leading to new vessel formation, traction retinal detachment and vitreous haemorrhage.

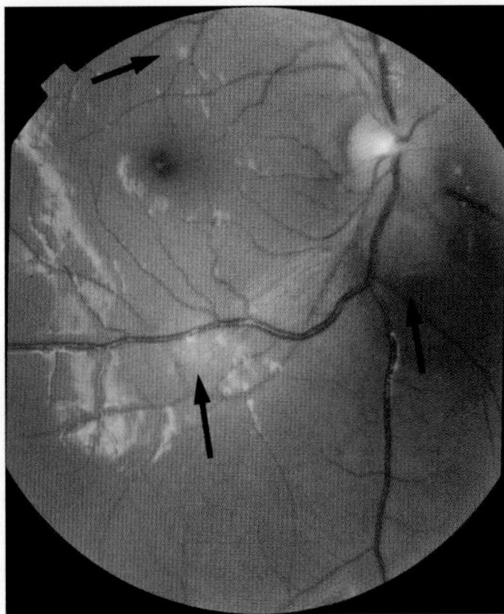

Figure 67.31 Tubercular choroidal granulomas in child with TB meningitis (arrowed). *(Courtesy of Nicholas A. V. Beare.)*

Management. The systemic treatment of tuberculosis is described in Chapter 40. A TB-associated anterior uveitis should be treated with topical steroids and pupil dilation (cyclopentolate 1% or atropine 1% eye drops) alongside systemic treatment for TB. Choroidal granulomas do not require specific treatment in addition to systemic anti-tuberculous therapy. Retinal vasculitis may require additional systemic corticosteroids if affecting the macula and threatening vision. However, steroids should be used with caution and in liaison with the treating clinician. Substantial areas of ischaemia (best delineated with fluorescein angiography if available) require treatment with scatter laser photocoagulation to reduce neovascularization. If occluded, vessels are present clinically and fluorescein angiography or laser are not available, it is satisfactory to observe for early neovascularization before referral.

Eales’ Disease

Eales’ disease is a form of occlusive retinal vasculitis in the peripheral retina of otherwise healthy young adults, predominantly men. It is particularly common in South Asia and has been associated with TB infection or exposure. It is postulated that the disease is due to an immune response to tuberculin protein, but human leucocyte antigens (HLA type) are also implicated and the aetiology is likely to be multifactorial. There is no diagnostic test, so other causes of retinal vasculitis should be excluded.

In the early inflammatory stage, periphlebitis is the predominant feature, but in later stages retinal ischaemia and its consequences predominate. Treatment is with oral corticosteroids in the acute inflammatory stage, coupled with a search for TB infection and appropriate treatment. In the ischaemic phase, retinal laser photocoagulation to ischaemic zones is beneficial in preventing neovascularization and vitreous haemorrhage.[32] Intravitreal injection of vascular endothelial growth factor inhibitors (anti-VEGF agents, e.g. ranibizumab, bevacizumab) will regress new vessels but also cause tractional retinal detachment so should be used with caution and close monitoring.

They do not eliminate the need to photocoagulate ischaemic retina.

Leprosy

Epidemiology. It is estimated that around 100 000 leprosy patients are blind due to the disease and thousands more are blind due to other eye disease but have poor access to eye services.

Clinical Presentation. Leprosy (see Chapter 41) is caused by *Mycobacterium leprae*, an acid-fast bacillus of low-grade infectivity. It has a preference for cooler temperatures, thus the anterior eye and eyelids are more affected.

The clinical picture of leprosy depends on the immune response; a strong cellular immune response will result in paucibacillary (PB) leprosy with a low bacterial count. A weak immunity allows multibacillary (MB) leprosy to develop with a high bacterial count. MB patients are contagious. Two mechanisms are responsible for nerve damage and disabilities in leprosy, type I and type II reactions.

Type I Reaction (Reversal Reaction). If cellular immunity increases in MB patients acute inflammation in skin lesions and peripheral nerves causes motor and sensory deficits. Cranial nerve involvement leads to corneal hypoaesthesia (5th nerve) and lagophthalmos (7th nerve paresis). Lagophthalmos, inability to close the eyes, is a common complication (Figure 67.32). The combination of inadequate lid closure and corneal insensitivity poses a grave risk to the eye through exposure keratopathy and corneal trauma. Permanent tarsorrhaphy may be required to protect the cornea.

Type II Reaction (Erythema Nodosum Leprosum: ENL). In MB patients immune complex deposition leads to subcutaneous nodules, nerves swelling and fever. A type II reaction can cause anterior uveitis, episcleritis and scleritis. Infiltration with *M. leprae* can cause tissues atrophy, leading to madarosis (loss of eyebrows), collapse of the nose and thin earlobes.

Eye Signs and Complications.

- Acute anterior uveitis (AAU): Treatment of anterior uveitis is the same as idiopathic AAU, pupil dilation and corticosteroid eye drops.

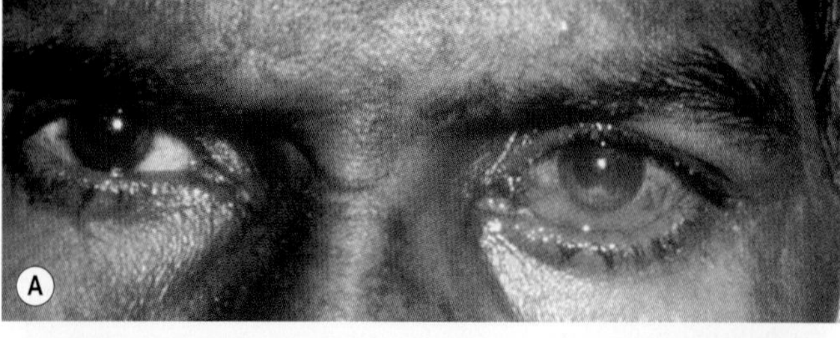

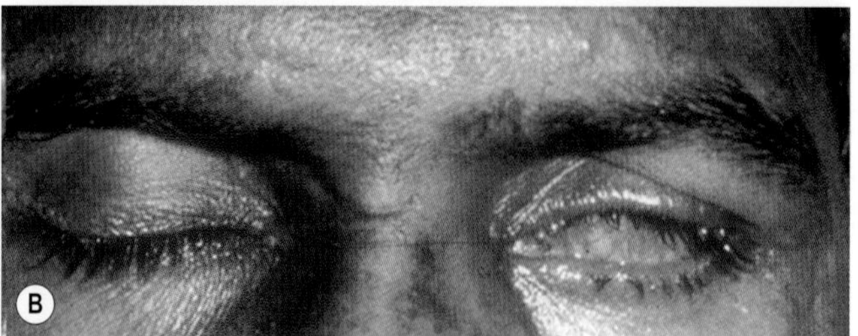

Figure 67.32 Left lagophthalmos due to leprosy. *(Courtesy of Margreet Hogeweg.)*

- Episcleritis and scleritis: Episcleritis responds quickly to corticosteroid drops. The deeper inflammation of scleritis, particularly severe bilateral scleritis, is a complication of type II reactions. Treatment is with short courses of systemic corticosteroids, together with clofazimine and topical frequent (1 or 2 hourly) corticosteroids drops. There is a risk of staphyloma (bulging of the thinned sclera with adherent choroid) or scleral perforation associated with scleral thinning. A very thin sclera or staphyloma can also allow bacterial infection into the globe causing a blinding endophthalmitis.
- Chronic anterior uveitis: Posterior synechiae are uncommon, but keratic precipitates may be found. When treating chronic anterior uveitis, keep the pupil as dilated and active as possible, using phenylephrine 2.5–5% eye drops.
- Limbal leproma: A painless pink or yellowish nodule at the corneoscleral margin (limbus). This resolves slowly with systemic treatment.
- Leprous keratitis: Chalky deposits in the upper temporal quadrant of the cornea due to invasion by *M. leprae*, which usually do not affect vision.
- Iris atrophy: In MB leprosy, the iris stroma and pupil dilator muscle become atrophic, leading to a fixed small (miotic) pupil. Irregular atrophy of the iris may result in pupil distortion.
- Iris pearls: Small white nodules on the surface of the iris which are calcified foci of dead leprosy bacilli and pathognomonic for leprosy.

Age-related Cataract in Leprosy Patients. Management of cataract in leprosy patients can be complicated by intraocular inflammation and small rigid pupils. Surgery should be delayed until after 6 months of systemic treatment, without reaction. Intraocular lenses may be used provided there is no active inflammation.

Intraocular Pressure in Leprosy Patients. Intraocular pressure (IOP) may be raised in association with anterior uveitis, or low owing to atrophy of the ciliary body. Raised IOP may lead to secondary glaucoma and chronically very low IOP can lead to phthisis and loss of vision.

Approach to the Eyes in Leprosy. Take particular note of the following:

- Visual acuity
- Eye lid closure and corneal sensation. Test the corneal sensation with a tip of 'rolled' cotton wool from the side
- Corneal scarring
- Red eye – predominantly circumlimbal in AAU, localized in episcleritis, extensive and deep in scleritis. Examine with magnification for evidence of anterior uveitis
- Cataract and pupil dilation in response to mydriatic.

Eye health education and referral:

- Refer patients to an eye specialist for visual acuity of 6/18 or worse, or acute red eye.
- Ask the patient to close the eyes gently and forcibly. If there is a lid-gap >5 mm the patient should be referred.
- Patients with lagophthalmos should be encouraged to 'think-blink' or close lid manually, frequently.

The success of leprosy control has resulted in the closure of some specialized leprosy programmes. Collaboration or integration between former leprosy control and prevention of blindness programmes will be required to prevent blindness in leprosy.

BACILLI AND COCCI

Brucellosis (Undulant Fever; Mediterranean Fever)

Brucellosis is caused by infection with the Gram-negative bacilli: *Brucella abortus*, *B. melitensis* or *B. suis*. The disease is widely distributed throughout the world but is particularly common in the Middle East where infections usually occur in people handling hoofed livestock or drinking unpasteurized milk. It presents as an acute febrile illness with a chronic period of often vague symptoms. Diagnosis is by blood culture or serology.

Eye Complications. These include a chronic uveitis which may be anterior or involve the posterior segment. It is a cause of granulomatous uveitis with choroidal granulomas appearing as multifocal, well-circumscribed elevations with haemorrhage. Epithelial opacities may occur in the cornea. An optic neuritis is rare but papilloedema indicates neurological involvement. Extraocular muscle abnormalities can appear, as a result of either local inflammation or 6th cranial nerve paralysis due to a basal meningoencephalitis.

Management. A Brucellosis-associated anterior uveitis should be treated with topical steroids and pupil dilation (cyclopentolate 1% or atropine 1% eye drops) alongside systemic treatment for Brucellosis. Posterior uveitis requires systemic treatment with antibiotics as described in Chapter 28.

Tularaemia

Tularaemia is caused by a small Gram-negative bacillus, *Francisella tularensis* (*Pasteurella tularensis*). The disease is transmitted from intermediate hosts, mainly rabbits, but also other rodents, foxes and cats and possibly via tick bites. Definitive diagnosis relies on rising titres of antibodies, or isolation of the bacteria in special medium.

Eye Complications. Ocular infection with tularaemia causes a severe conjunctivitis, after an incubation of up to 2 weeks. The conjunctiva is red, oedematous and discharging, with granulomas and regional lymph nodes become enlarged (Parinaud's oculoglandular syndrome).

Treatment. Treatment is with streptomycin or the tetracycline class of antibiotics which reduce the associated mortality.

Bacterial Meningitis

Epidemics of meningococcal meningitis caused by *N. meningitidis* occur in tropical countries, although the disease is found worldwide. Other organisms (*S. pneumoniae*, *N. meningitidis*, *H. influenzae*, *S. suis*) can cause meningitis with similar ocular manifestations.

Ocular Manifestations. Cranial nerve palsies can occur resulting in incomitant strabismus. A 6th nerve palsy results in horizontal diplopia most pronounced when looking to the side of the lesion and is often an indicator of raised intracranial pressure. In 3rd nerve paralysis, the eye looks down and out resulting in vertical diplopia diminishing on downgaze; there may be ptosis and pupil enlargement. In the comatose patient pupil dilation and lack of reaction to light, initially in one eye then bilaterally, indicates critically raised intracranial pressure, brain stem coning and imminent death. Gaze palsies may result in persistent gaze in one direction. These indicate involvement of the eye movement fields in the frontal lobe and are not prognostic.

The optic nerve may be involved resulting in vision loss from optic atrophy on recovery from meningitis. Vision loss can also occur from occipital cerebral lobe infarcts involving the visual cortex.[33]

Management. The treatment of meningitis is described in Chapter 27. As with any comatose patient eye care is important to avoid exposure keratopathy. Carers should be asked to frequently close the eye lids manually. If the cornea is persistently dry apply chloramphenicol ointment four to six times per day.

Diphtheria

Diphtheria is caused by toxin produced by infection with a Gram-positive bacillus, *Corynebacterium diphtheriae*. The disease is virtually unknown in many countries because of immunization. Where immunization is lacking, e.g. in Somalia and areas of Indonesia, outbreaks can occur.

Eye Complications. Infection of the conjunctiva causes a membranous conjunctivitis with eyelid oedema, discharge and local lymph node enlargement. The classical sign of ocular diphtheria is a grey membrane on the mucous membrane of the conjunctiva as well as the throat. On removal of the membrane, the uncovered surface is raw with petechial haemorrhages. Corneal ulceration with stromal infiltrate can occur. Membranous conjunctivitis may be caused by other infections, such as *Streptococcus*, *Pneumococcus* or adenovirus.

The diphtheria toxin damages the heart, kidneys and central nervous system causing cranial nerve paralysis, particularly the 6th cranial nerve.

Management. Refer to Chapter 35.

Anthrax

Cutaneous anthrax caused by *Bacillus anthracis* can involve the eyelids and periorbital regions. Infection is by direct contact with contaminated skins and other animal products, most often among those who work with live or dead animals. The organism may also be transmitted by insects. A red papule forms at the site of inoculation with the organism, *Bacillus anthracis*. The area becomes black (eschar) and gangrenous – often with development of a vesicle (the malignant pustule).

Eye Complications. Eschar formation affecting the eyelids can progress to severe scarring, resulting in dramatic cicatricial ectropion – the eyelid can turn inside out. Exposure keratitis may cause corneal scarring and blindness. Where there is eye involvement early referral to an eye specialist is advised.

Management. See Chapter 31. Correction of the ectropion requires division of the scar tissue and a full-thickness skin graft.

SPIROCHAETES

Syphilis

Syphilis is caused by the spirochaete *Treponema pallidum*. It is transmitted by sexual contact or across the placenta to the unborn child. The prevalence is high in resource-poor countries. In sub-Saharan Africa, a prevalence between 2% and 12% has been reported in antenatal women, and co-infection with HIV is common.

Ocular Manifestations of Syphilis. Ocular disease is primarily associated with secondary syphilis. Manifestations include anterior uveitis, vitritis, neuroretinitis, multi-focal chorioretinitis, retinal vasculitis (Figure 67.24) and papillitis, but there are no specific diagnostic features. In anterior uveitis inflammation of the iris (iritis) may be obviously hyperaemic (roseolae). In neuroretinitis the retina becomes opacified with a ground-glass appearance.

In primary syphilis, a conjunctival chancre can occur. Tertiary syphilis may ensue after a variable period of time and can have similar ocular features to secondary syphilis. Rarely the Argyll–Robertson pupil may occur, with small irregular pupils which do not react to either direct or consensual light stimulation but will constrict on accommodation. Optic atrophy may be found as a sequelae to papillitis.

Given that syphilis is a curable and potentially debilitating or fatal cause of uveitis clinicians should have a low threshold for serological testing for syphilis and include it in any patient in whom investigations for uveitis are instigated. Venereal Disease Research Laboratory (VDRL) and rapid plasma reagent (RPR) antibody tests can give false-positive results in the presence of connective tissue disease, Lyme disease, pregnancy, leprosy and mononucleosis.

Congenital Syphilis. In congenital syphilis, anterior uveitis may be present from birth to 6 months and after 6 months chorioretinitis with pigment clumps (classical salt and pepper fundus) or multi-focal choroiditis can occur. Other ocular manifestations of congenital syphilis include inflamed eyelids, dacryocystitis, conjunctivitis, extraocular muscle paresis, interstitial keratitis, pupil abnormalities, papillitis and optic atrophy. Typically, congenital syphilis becomes latent and then reactivates, often during the teenage years and may reappear as an interstitial keratitis. The patient complains of discomfort with photosensitivity and a red eye. New blood vessels grow into the deep corneal stroma differentiating interstitial keratitis from the superficial neovascularization of other chronic keratitides. The affected, inflamed area of oedematous cornea may appear pink, which has been described as a 'salmon patch'. The keratitis can lead to corneal scarring with empty blood vessels or 'ghost vessels'.

Management. Treatment of anterior uveitis eye is with pupil dilation with atropine or cyclopentolate eye drops and topical corticosteroids. As ocular disease in syphilis implies neurological involvement a treatment regimen for neurosyphilis is advised.

Leptospirosis

Leptospirosis is caused by spirochaetes of the genus *Leptospira*, which are widespread. Domestic and wild animals (typically rodents) with chronic renal infections act as reservoirs. Man can be infected by contact with urine or contaminated water and soil. After an incubation of 8–12 days, the patient develops fever and chills with general malaise. Jaundice and meningitis can develop. Diagnosis requires rising serum titres of *Leptospira* antibodies or culture from blood or urine.

Eye Complications. Leptospirosis is a rare cause of uveitis. Anterior uveitis, vitritis, retinal and papillary haemorrhages have all been reported (see Chapter 37).

Relapsing Fever

Louse-borne relapsing fever is caused by the spirochaete *Borrelia recurrentis* and occurs in resource-poor tropical countries where living conditions are poor. Tick-borne relapsing fever caused by *Borrelia duttonii* occurs in East Africa. Relapsing fever causes a high fever with generalized muscle aches and malaise which may recur after defervescence for several days.

Eye Complications. Relapsing fever can cause acute or chronic, anterior uveitis. Retina haemorrhages and exudates have been described. Meningitis may result in papilloedema and cranial nerve palsies.

Management. See Chapter 37.

FUNGAL OPHTHALMIC DISEASE

Filamentous fungi, yeasts and dimorphic organisms have all been associated with eye infections, predominantly keratitis. Difficulties in the diagnosis of oculomycosis and inadequate availability of antifungal agents make the management of ocular fungal infections problematic.

Fungi can cause a suppurative keratitis which is indistinguishable from bacterial keratitis on clinical grounds alone. Feathery margins to corneal infiltrates seen with magnification suggest fungal keratitis. Gram staining can distinguish bacterial and fungal infections and fungal organisms can be seen with hematoxylin and eosin staining used in histopathology.

Fungi causing eye infections are most commonly filamentous fungi and yeasts. Filamentous fungi are multicellular organisms with projections known as hyphae. Hyphae may have divisions or be non-septate. The most common causes of fungal eye infections are septate filamentous fungi: *Fusarium* and *Aspergillus*. Non-septate filamentous fungi, e.g. *Rhizopus* and *Phycomycetes*, less commonly involve the eye.

Candida albicans and *Cryptococcus neoformans* are unicellular yeasts that reproduce by budding and may be involved in eye infections. Dimorphic fungi such as *Blastomyces dermatitidis* may be responsible for ocular and orbital disease following blood and lymphatic spread.

Oculomycoses are found worldwide but particularly in hot and humid climates. In some parts of the tropics, between a third and a half of adult corneal ulcers are caused by fungi.

Fungal Keratitis

The most significant anatomical site of fungal eye infections is the cornea, where suppurative keratitis, ulceration, hypopyon and possible corneal perforation mean that early diagnosis and prompt treatment are vital. Fungi causing keratitis include *Aspergilli* and *Fusaria*. As with any suppurative keratitis, corneal scarring is likely when the area of infection and inflammation heals. Later, corneal grafting may be indicated for scarring affecting vision particularly if the better eye has been affected.

A fungal corneal ulcer is suggested by feathery margins with a raised slough and a coloured infiltrate, particularly if the ulcer fails to respond to antibiotic treatment. However, these signs are not consistently present.

Fungi are associated with eye injuries with vegetable matter. So secondary infections following corneal abrasions with twigs, stalks and husks must raise suspicion of possible fungal infection.

Fungal Vitritis or Endophthalmitis

Fungi can also infect the eye through haematological spread and cause a vitritis or endophthalmitis. This usually results from intravenous drug abuse and associated poor hygiene such as the use of lemon juice to acidify and dissolve heroin. Fungal vitritis can also occur from indwelling intravenous catheters or abdominal surgery in a debilitated patient.

Fluffy white balls form in the vitreous with vitreous haze resulting in a relatively indolent onset of blurred vision. *Candida* and *Aspergilli* are the commonest causative organisms. Other fungi infections can lead to endogenous endophthalmitis, including *Blastomyces dermatitidis* and *Coccidioides immitis.*

Fungal Orbital Cellulitis

The nose and paranasal sinuses may harbour *Aspergillus*, which can lead to orbital infection with extraocular muscle palsies, particularly if the orbital walls are breached such as by a fracture.

Blastomycosis and Coccidioidomycosis

Blastomyces dermatitidis and *Coccidioides immitis* are usually contracted through inhalation of organisms. Blastomycosis occurs in the Americas and Africa, whereas coccidioidomycosis is restricted to the Americas. Coccidioidomycosis in particular seems to be associated with dust inhalation making agricultural and construction workers more prone.

Infection of the skin by *Blastomyces dermatitidis* is characterized by suppurative granulomas, which may be found in the mouth, nose and the eyelids. Keratitis occurs presumably from local infection. Both saprophytes can spread to the eye haematologically and cause choroiditis and endogenous endophthalmitis.

Immunocompetent patients can be affected, but disseminated disease is more likely in immunocompromised patients such as those with AIDS. Diagnosis is through specialized culture or direct identification of the organisms by histopathology.

Histoplasmosis

Histoplasma capsulatum is endemic in the Americas and the Caribbean. The fungus is present in soil, particularly nitrogen-rich soil from bird or bat droppings. Infection occurs from inhalation of the spores. *Histoplasma capsulatum* can cause a disseminated disease in which the eye is involved through haematological spread; or more commonly, a distinctive chorioretinitis in otherwise well patients described as 'presumed ocular histoplasmosis syndrome' (POHS). 'Presumed' based on serological evidence of infection, but no organism has been isolated from the eye. However, similar fundus findings can occur in patients who have never travelled to endemic areas. Disseminated histoplasmosis and endophthalmitis are more common in immunosuppressed patients.

POHS is characterized by multiple well-demarcated lesions of chorioretinal atrophy with pigment in the posterior pole. These are frequently accompanied by a ring of pigment and atrophy around the disc (Figure 67.33). There is no anterior uveitis or vitritis. Chorioretinal lesions close to the fovea are prone to developing choroidal neovascularization with macular oedema and haemorrhage. Patients present with visual distortion and central scotoma, which often leads to loss of central vision from subretinal scarring. The neovascularization is best treated with intravitreal injections of anti-VEGF agents, or photodynamic therapy with verteporfin, or even surgical removal.

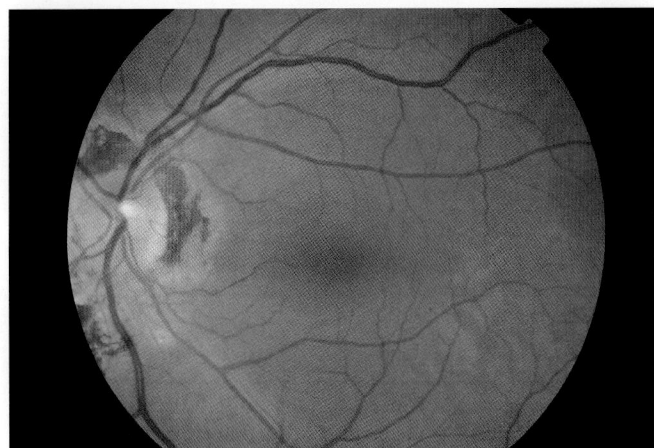

Figure 67.33 Presumed ocular histoplasmosis syndrome (POHS) with characteristic pigment round the optic disc with surrounding halo. *(Courtesy of Nicholas A. V. Beare and Lisa Cairns.)*

Diagnosis and Treatment of Fungal Infections

If fungal keratitis is suspected initially, or when there has been no response to antibiotics after 48 hours, examination of a corneal scrape should be done if possible to try to identify the organism. Internal elements of hyphae stain variably with Gram stain and yeasts stain Gram positive. Giemsa stain can be helpful to identify fungal hyphae and yeasts but has to be freshly prepared and the slide immersed for 1 hour. Potassium hydroxide 10% wet mount is straightforward, cheap and sensitive in detecting fungi.[34] However, antifungal treatment often has to be empirical.

Natamycin eye drops are most effective against filamentous fungi, including *Aspergillus* and *Fusarium*. Dosage is one drop half-hourly, then six to eight times per day after 3–4 days. It is expensive and supply is erratic. Amphotericin B is most effective against yeasts, particularly *Candida* and *Cryptococcus*, but also has activity against filamentous fungi. It is used intravenously or intravitreally (10 μg) for endophthalmitis, or may be diluted to 1–2.5 mg/mL solution for use topically in keratitis.

The azoles have a broad spectrum of antifungal activity and can be used topically or orally. Econazole and clotrimazole (Aurolab, Madurai, India) are available as ophthalmic preparations; econazole appears to be more effective. Fluconazole is preferred as an oral agent (400–800 mg daily), as it has excellent absorption and penetration into the eye with few side-effects. It can also be used topically. If available, both agents can be used orally as adjunctive treatment in fungal keratitis or as the primary treatment of fungal endophthalmitis. However, fluconazole has poor activity against *Aspergillus* species. Voriconazole is a triazole with a broad spectrum of activity which has become the treatment of choice for invasive *Aspergillus*. There is evidence of its effectiveness in fungal keratitis. It is available for topical use as a 1% solution or as a 0.1% solution for intravitreal injection (Aurolab, Madurai, India).

Flucytosine is an oral agent that has also been given topically. It is synergistic with amphotericin B and azoles against yeasts, including *Candida* and *Cryptococcus*. However, resistance is common or develops readily, so it must therefore be given in combination.

Reports of topical caspofungin (0.5%; prepared from intravenous preparation), an echinocandin, suggest it is effective in fungal keratitis. However, its ocular penetration is poor when given systemically.

Where anti-fungal agents are not available antiseptics have been used for fungal keratitis. Despite in vitro activity povidone iodine does not seem to be effective, but chlorhexidine gluconate 0.2% has been shown to be at least as effective as natamycin.[35] Chlorhexidine can be diluted to the appropriate concentration with sterile water.

Any improvement in fungal keratitis is slow so antifungal treatment has to be continued for at least 3 weeks and about one-third of fungal ulcers will not heal within 1 month. Bacterial ulcers respond more rapidly. Topical corticosteroids exacerbate fungal keratitis so should be avoided for 2 weeks after commencing antifungal treatment.

PROTOZOAL OPHTHALMIC DISEASE

Toxoplasmosis

Toxoplasmosis is caused by *Toxoplasma gondii*. It is an extremely common infection worldwide with seroprevalences of over 50% commonly reported in healthy populations. Prevalence of toxoplasmosis varies depending on consumption of undercooked, cured or raw meat; and the presence of cats, which are the definitive hosts. It is particularly common in South and Central America and southern Europe. In Asia prevalences of 30–60% of healthy individuals are reported with evidence that infection has increased from the 1960s.[36] What little data exist for sub-Saharan Africa suggest no less endemicity than in other regions,[37] although clinical toxoplasmosis or fundus evidence of toxoplasmosis is uncommon.

Toxoplasmosis is an opportunistic infection which can occur or recrudesce in patients with reduced immunity such as AIDS. As well as a severe chorioretinitis, immunocompromised patients can be afflicted by toxoplasma encephalitis.

Ocular Toxoplasmosis. Toxoplasma causes an intense, localized chorioretinitis with variable associated vitritis, which is usually unilateral (Figure 67.34). This leaves a pigmented chorioretinal scar (Figure 67.35). If this is in the peripheral retina the acute episode may go unnoticed leaving an incidental scar as clinical evidence of infection. If the chorioretinitis involves the macula, the patient may complain of distortion or reduced vision. Vitritis may cause hazy vision or marked floaters. If chorioretinal scarring involves the macula vision may be permanently affected.

An acute episode is characterized by focal, necrotizing retinitis, often arising at the border of a previously healed scar, a so-called satellite lesion. The foci of inflammation are 'fluffy' white with hazy margins. Local retinal haemorrhage may be present and occlusive vasculitis of nearby retinal vessels occurs. The vitreous is hazy due to vitritis and there is an anterior uveitis. Vitritis may partially obscure the focus of retinitis, the so-called 'headlight in the fog' appearance. Cystoid macular oedema can develop.

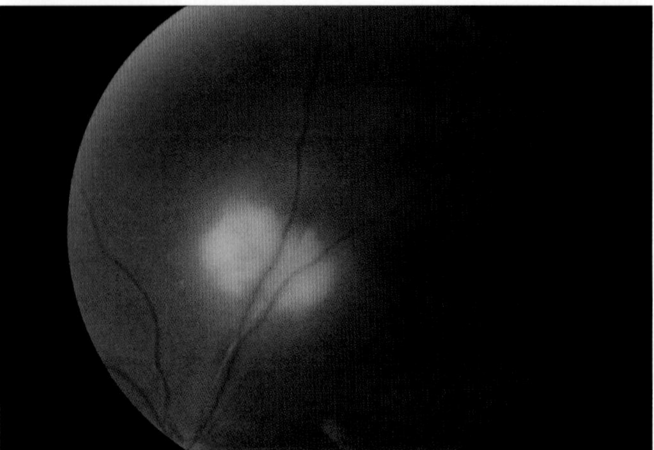

Figure 67.34 Primary toxoplasmosis chorioretinitis acquired in Brazil and preceded by a prodromal illness. Note retinal arteriolar vasculitis remote from chorioretinitis. *(Courtesy of Nicholas A. V. Beare and Lisa Cairns.)*

In patients with HIV/AIDS, the disease may be bilateral, multifocal with lesions at different stages of evolution. The chorioretinitis may progress relentlessly whereas an intact immune system will contain toxoplasmosis to a localized, short-lived insult. In HIV/AIDS patients, toxoplasma can cause encephalitis and other systemic manifestations.

Treatment. Treatment of toxoplasma chorioretinitis is controversial. Focal chorioretinitis in the peripheral retina without complications does not require treatment. Treatment is required when vision is threatened by chorioretinitis on, or close to the macula, symptomatic dense vitritis, or macula oedema.

Established antiprotozoan therapy for toxoplasmosis is with a combination of pyrimethamine (two 50 mg loading doses, then 25 mg twice daily) and sulfadiazine (1 g 4 times a day). High dose pyrimethamine is toxic to bone marrow which should be reduced by folinic acid (calcium folinate 10–15 mg daily). Folic acid is a competitive antagonist so should be avoided. Sulfadiazin crystallizes in the renal tubules and can cause crystal nephropathy or renal colic, so fluid intake should

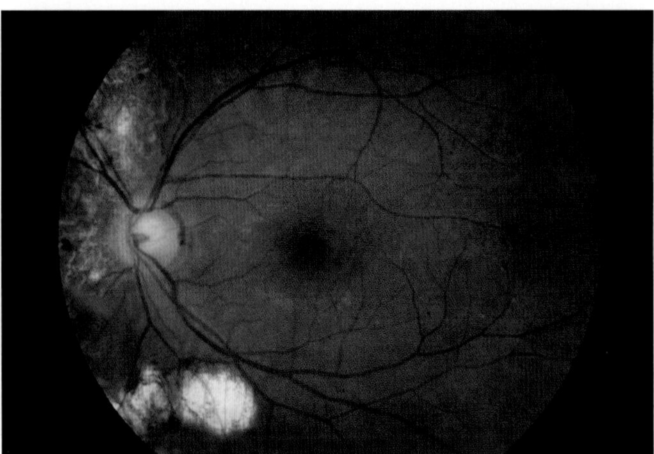

Figure 67.35 Inactive toxoplasmosis scar inferior and nasal to the optic disc. *(Courtesy of Nicholas A. V. Beare and William Hooley.)*

be increased. It can also rarely cause Stevens–Johnson syndrome.

Clindamycin (300 mg 4 times a day) is effective and more straightforward to take than the above regime. Clindamycin should be discontinued if diarrhoea develops because it is associated with pseudomembranous colitis. Azithromycin (500 mg stat, followed by 250 mg daily) is regarded as an effective alternative treatment. The combination of trimethoprim and sulfamethoxazole has been used as acute and preventative treatment (Bactrim DS 60 mg/160 mg every 3 days). Atovaquone (750 mg four times a day) is also advocated as an alternative treatment. Antibiotic therapy should be continued for 4–6 weeks. In immunocompromised patients preventative antiprotozoan therapy should be continued until immune function has improved, but the optimal regimen is yet to be determined.

Corticosteroids are often used concomitantly with antibiotics for toxoplasmosis to limit the damage from chorioretinitis and reduce vitritis. They should not be used without antibiotics, but prednisolone (0.5 mg/kg) commenced after 48 hours of antiprotozoan therapy then tapered to nil to coincide with cessation of antibiotic therapy is a suitable regimen.

Leishmaniasis

Leishmaniasis is a protozoan disease caused by parasites of the genus *Leishmania* transmitted by the sandfly. It occurs in many tropical and sub-tropical countries, with up to 2.5 million cases of 'visceral' disease and 9.5 million of the cutaneous form estimated.

Eye Complications (Visceral Leishmaniasis). The visceral form of leishmaniasis is known as kala-azar. Retinal haemorrhages have been described, typically multiple and bilateral. These are likely to be due to the anaemia and thrombocytopenia secondary to hypersplenism.

Eye Complications (Cutaneous Leishmaniasis). Cutaneous leishmaniasis causes skin disease with varied manifestations including nodules, ulcers, lepromatous lesions and subsequent scarring. Unusually, the eyelids may be affected with associated conjunctivitis and keratitis.[38]

Treatment. Ocular treatment should aim at minimizing corneal damage from cicatricial scarring and secondary infection. Chloramphenicol ointment is suitable for this initially, along with removal of aberrant lashes impinging on the cornea and surgery for lid malposition (see Chapter 47).

African Trypanosomiasis

African trypanosomiasis (sleeping sickness) is caused by *Trypanosoma brucei gambiense* and *T. b. rhodesiense*, transmitted by the tsetse fly.

Eye Complications. Neuro-ophthalmic signs occur in the severe form of the disease with meningoencephalopathy. These include ptosis, cranial nerve palsies, optic neuritis and papilloedema. Interstitial keratitis has been reported.

Management. See Chapter 45.

American Trypanosomiasis

American trypanosomiasis (Chagas' disease) is caused by *T. cruzi* in Central and South America.

Eye Complications. Characteristic evidence of Chagas' disease is unilateral oedema of the eyelids (Romana's sign), which typically occurs when the inoculation site is close to the eye. The lacrimal gland can be involved in the inflammation.

Management. See Chapter 46.

Malaria

Malaria is common throughout the tropics and remains an important fatal disease particularly in Africa where WHO estimates 90% of the 850 000 malaria deaths occur, with 85% in children (2008 data). It is caused by infection with one of the five *Plasmodium* spp. (*P. falciparum*, *P. vivax*, *P. ovale*, *P. knowlesi*, *P. malariae*). *P. falciparum* causes most complicated infections and deaths from malaria. Severe malaria causes a distinct retinopathy termed malarial retinopathy.[39] Malarial retinopathy is seen in two-thirds of children with cerebral malaria and is also seen to a lesser extent in children with less severe forms and in adults.[40]

Eye Complications. The fundus signs in cerebral malaria reflect the pathology in the cerebral circulation, where infected erythrocytes sequester by cytoadherence to microvascular endothelium. The retinal signs of malarial retinopathy are retinal haemorrhages, retinal whitening due to ischaemia, retinal vessel discolouration (Figure 67.36) and cotton-wool spots. Papilloedema also occurs and is a particularly poor prognostic sign.[41]

Retinal haemorrhages are mostly white-centred, but blot and flame intraretinal haemorrhages also occur. In severe cases haemorrhages can be numerous and confluent. Retinal whitening is often seen around the fovea and temporal macula and is caused by ischaemia due to capillary non-perfusion in the retina.[42] Retinal vessels can be discoloured to orange or white and this tends to be in the retinal periphery. White vessels are occluded and discolouration is thought to be due to the sequestered erythrocytes in which the haemoglobin (the red pigment in blood) has been consumed by the parasite.

These retinal signs are diagnostic of severe malaria. This is of importance in endemic areas where malaria infection is common and may not be the cause of coma in an unconscious patient with parasitaemia. Also the severity of malarial retinopathy is prognostic for death in children with cerebral malaria. Patients with cerebral malaria without retinopathy have better survival rates and shorter coma duration than those with retinopathy. In adults the severity of retinopathy is related to severity of malaria, but white retinal vessels have not been reported.

Fluorescein angiograms of the retinal circulation in cerebral malaria show multiple small areas of capillary closure corresponding to retinal whitening. In some patients there are larger areas of ischaemic retina (Figure 67.36). As the retina is part of the central nervous system with a similar microvasculature it can be inferred that similar pathological processes are occurring in the brain.

After an episode of cerebral malaria there may be cranial nerve palsies or cortical blindness as a result of cerebral damage.

Management. Malarial retinopathy does not require treatment in addition to management of severe malaria. It does not appear to cause any visual deficit after recovery unless a haemorrhage

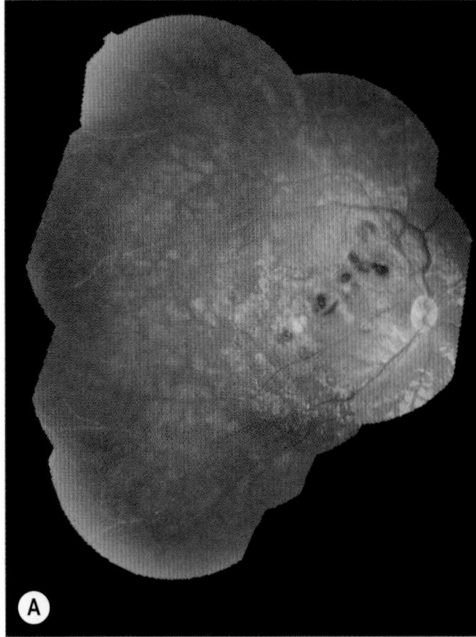

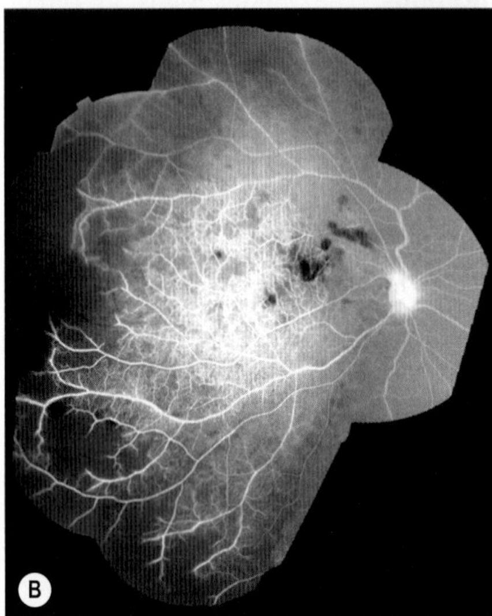

Figure 67.36 Malarial retinopathy in Malawian child with cerebral malaria. (A) Composite retinal photograph showing severe malarial retinopathy with white-centred haemorrhages, macular and peripheral retinal whitening and white discolouration of retinal vessels, including capillaries. (B) Fluorescein angiogram shows multiple small areas of non-perfusion in the central retina corresponding to macular whitening and extensive non-perfusion in parts of the peripheral retina. *(Courtesy of Simon Glover and Nicholas A. V. Beare. Lancet Infect Dis 2010; 10(6):440.)*

affects the fovea. Bilateral visual failure after cerebral malaria is due to cortical impairment and often accompanied by other neurological deficits. The treatment of malaria is described in Chapter 43.

NEMATODAL OPHTHALMIC DISEASE

Onchocerciasis

Onchocerciasis, or river blindness, is caused by the filarial worm *Onchocerca volvulus*. The worm is transmitted by the *Simulium* blackfly, which breeds in fast-flowing rivers. Both the skin and eyes are affected. The eye problems are insidious but progressive, with chronic inflammation that leads to scarring in both the anterior and posterior segments. Visual field is gradually lost in each eye from optic nerve involvement, eventually leading to blindness.

Epidemiology. The WHO estimates that 18 million people are infected by *O. volvulus*, of whom 270 000 are blind. The vast majority of these are in Central and West Africa (Figure 67.37) but there are foci of infection in Central and South America and Yemen. After successes in control of onchocerciasis in West Africa, the Vision 2020 initiative has the goal of elimination of blindness due to onchocerciasis by 2020.

In endemic areas, the social and economic consequences of this disease are huge. A large proportion of people of productive age are often affected after repeated infection with the larvae of *O. volvulus* from *Simulium* fly bites. Once blind, infected individuals have a reduced life-expectancy with most dying within 10 years. In untreated populations, the prevalence of blindness near fast-flowing rivers may reach 50% and in the past, this led to migration away from fertile river valleys.

The WHO Onchocerciasis Control Programme had success in eliminating onchocerciasis as a public health problem in 10 West African countries. This led to renewed efforts by the African Programme for Onchocerciasis Control in the other 26 endemic African countries and by the Onchocerciasis Elimination Programme for the Americas. Mass treatment of populations over 15 or more years with ivermectin has achieved complete elimination of onchocerciasis in endemic foci in Africa,[43] demonstrating eradication is possible.

In the Americas, endemic foci are much more limited and the coverage of ivermectin treatment is over 85%. Thus four of the six affected countries have halted transmission. In the

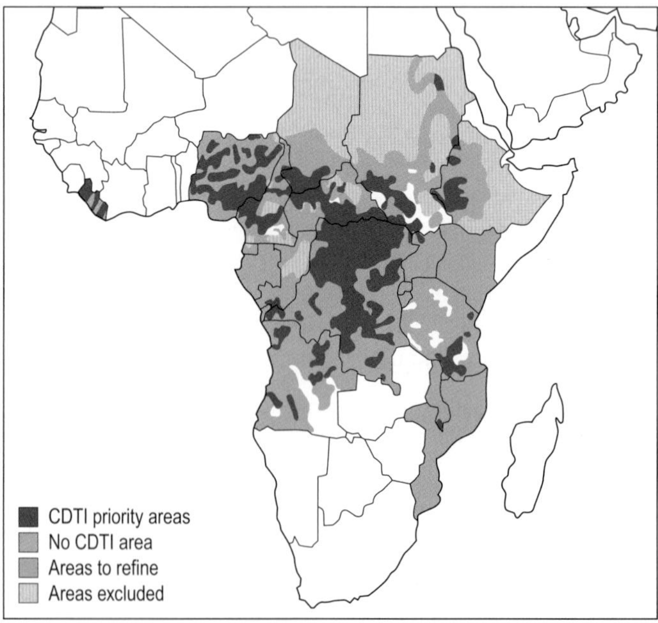

Figure 67.37 Rapid epidemiological mapping of onchocerciasis in countries covered by the African Programme for Onchocerciasis Control (APOC). Of the West African states covered by the Onchocerciasis Control Programme in West Africa (OCP), only in Sierra Leone is onchocerciasis still a public health problem. CDTI indicates community-directed treatment with ivermectin. *(Courtesy of WHO: http://www.who.int/apoc/onchocerciasis/status/en/index.html.)*

remaining two, efforts are focusing on the Yanomami population who migrate through the rainforest of Brazil and Venezuela.

The Vector: the* Simulium *Fly. The disease is spread from person to person by the *Simulium* blackfly. The female *Simulium* lays eggs on rocks and vegetation, where rivers are fast flowing with whitewater, because the eggs and larvae need highly oxygenated water for their development.

The female fly tends to stay 5–10 km from a river, although she can fly up to 80 km in 1 day. During the rainy season, flies may travel to new breeding sites, but in the dry season they are restricted to permanent rivers. The female fly requires a blood meal to develop her eggs, preferring human blood at dawn or dusk.

***Life Cycle of* O. Volvulus.** When a *Simulium* fly bites an infected person, the small embryo worms (microfilariae) present in the skin enter the gut of the fly. They pass through the gut wall and enter the thoracic muscles. After about 7 days, the larvae move to the head of the fly, ready to be transmitted to the next human host when the fly takes another blood meal.

They will take 1–3 years to develop into adult worms and before symptoms develop. Female worms can produce 0.5–1 million microfilariae per year. Microfilariae densely infest the skin infecting the next biting *Simulium* fly and the cycle of transmission continues.

Pathogenesis. Large numbers of microfilariae migrate into the skin and into the eye. Microfilariae live for 6–24 months eliciting very little immune response. They enter the cornea from the conjunctiva and the uvea probably by direct penetration and blood-borne spread. When microfilariae die, they provoke an immune response which leads to inflammation and scarring.

Wolbachia species are bacterial symbionts of *O. volvulus*, which appear to require the intracellular infection for normal development of larvae and embryos. The release of *Wolbachia* antigens from dead microfilariae has been recognized as a major factor in the host inflammatory response. *Wolbachia* surface antigens activate Toll-like receptors (TLR 2 and 4) on leucocytes triggering inflammatory cascades and are now recognized as major drivers of the disease pathology.[44]

Clinical Presentation.

Skin Manifestations. Itching is one of the first symptoms of onchocerciasis and this can be severe, disturbing sleep. There is a papular rash on any part of the body but often affecting the buttocks. Obvious scratch marks may indicate the severity of the pruritus. Repeated episodes of dermatitis lead to depigmentation, described as 'leopard skin'. There is subcutaneous fibrosis, skin atrophy and pigmentary changes. The skin may look and feel like the skin of an old person or a 'lizard skin'.

Lymphoedema results in chronic thickened skin. Lymph node enlargement in the inguinal areas can lead to folds of skin known as the 'hanging groin' of onchocerciasis.

Subcutaneous nodules containing adult worms are often found over bony prominences. They are firm, discrete and painless. There is a fibrous reaction around the coiled adult worms which evade an immune response. Surgical removal of nodules (nodulectomy) may be considered, particularly where nodules are situated in the region of the head or shoulders.

Eye Manifestations. As with the skin changes, it is the dead microfilariae which cause most inflammatory reaction within the eye. Live microfilariae are widely distributed through ocular tissues and may be seen in the anterior chamber with a slit lamp microscope.

Blinding disease is mainly through inflammation and scarring of the cornea and inflammation leading to atrophy of the chorioretina and optic nerve.

- Punctate or 'snowflake' keratitis: Fluffy white-grey spots, about 0.5 mm in diameter, may be seen in the superficial cornea, indicating an inflammatory reaction to dead microfilariae. The eye may be red and photophobic. Topical corticosteroids may be used, with ophthalmic supervision. The lesions can completely regress.
- Sclerosing keratitis: Sclerosing keratitis is a progressive opacification of the cornea which typically begins in an inferior arc from nasal to temporal aspects and extends to include all the lower cornea. Advanced sclerosing keratitis can result in complete corneal opacification and blindness (Figure 67.38).
- Anterior uveitis: The degree of anterior uveitis is very variable and may be granulomatous or non-granulomatous. The pupil may be dragged inferiorly, like an inverted tear drop, due to inflammation caused by accumulated dead microfilariae. In chronic anterior uveitis there may be loss of iris architecture, pupil synechiae, cataract and secondary glaucoma. Anterior uveitis should be treated with atropine 1% and steroid eye drops.
- Posterior uveitis or chorioretinitis: Posterior uveitis manifests initially as granular atrophy of the retinal pigment epithelium with intraretinal pigment. In more advanced disease lobular coalescing zones of retinal pigment and choroidal atrophy are commonly seen. Occasionally, pale elevated swellings of the choroid, believed to be granulomas, can be seen; or active retinitis or vasculitis. However, atrophic changes mostly predominate.
- Optic neuritis and atrophy: Optic nerve involvement is presumed to be due to death of microfilariae in the optic nerve, but extensive retinal atrophy will also result in optic atrophy. Visual field defects progress to complete loss of vision with severe optic atrophy apparent as a white optic disc. Once established there is no treatment for chorioretinal or optic atrophy, which are leading causes of blindness in onchocerciasis.

Diagnosis. The clinical signs are often sufficient to make a diagnosis: onchodermatitis, signs of scratching, depigmentation of the skin, 'lizard' skin and subcutaneous nodules. Characteristic eye changes and microfilariae in the anterior chamber confirm the diagnosis.

The Skin Snip. A small piece of skin is removed from the iliac crest or shoulder, using a sterile needle and blade, or specific skin punch. The skin fragment is placed on a microscope slide and a drop of saline added. After at least 30 minutes, the slide is examined using ×40 magnification. Mobile microfilariae can be seen in the saline. Skin snips are used less frequently today, as treatment is largely based on community prevalence.

Treatment and Control

Ivermectin (Mectizan®). Ivermectin is a broad-spectrum antihelminthic agent which has proved an extraordinarily successful treatment for this disease. It binds to glutamate-gated chloride channels causing hyperpolarization of invertebrate

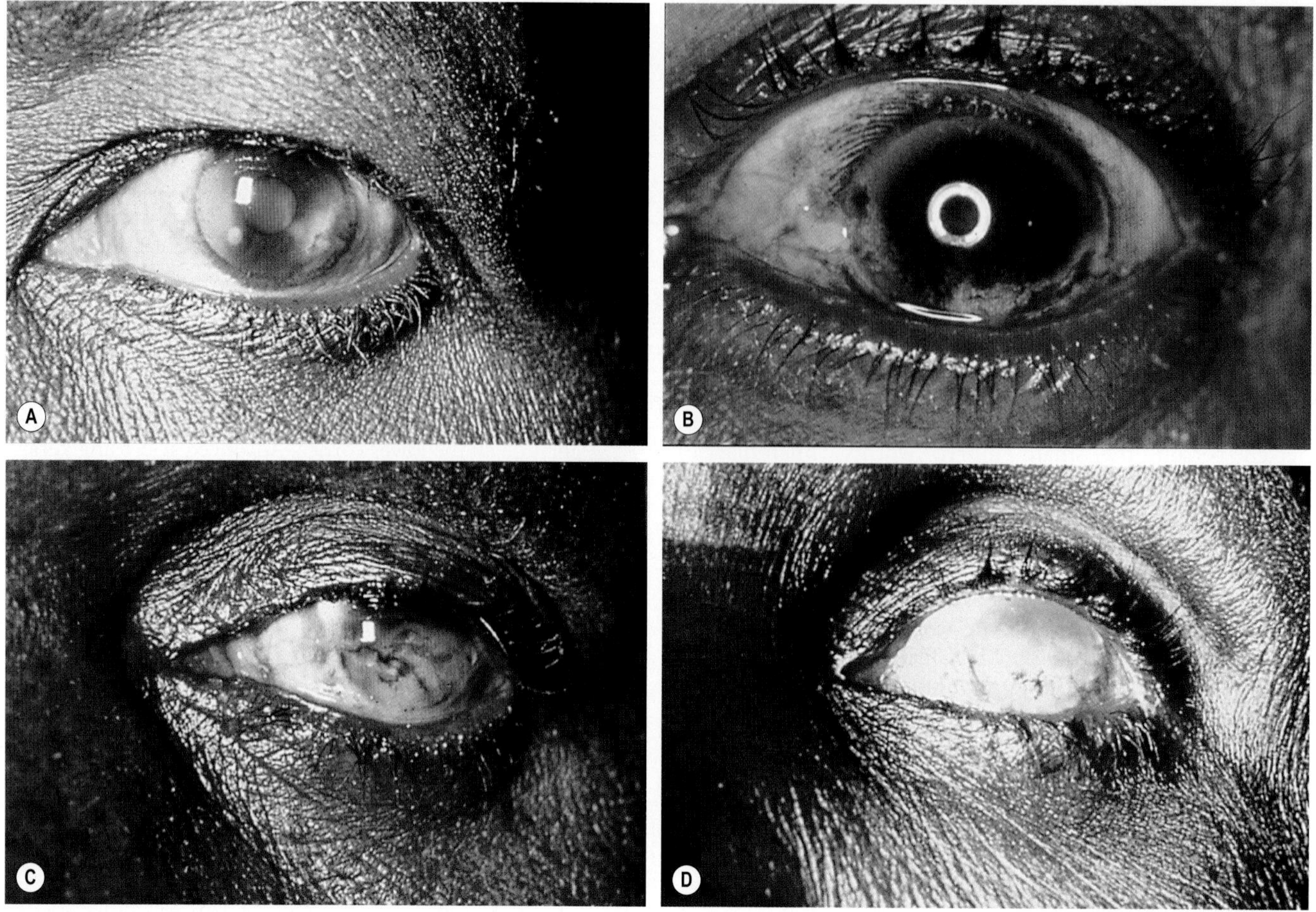

Figure 67.38 (A–D) Sclerosing keratitis in onchocerciasis with increasing severity from top left, clockwise. *(Courtesy of Ian Murdoch and Allen Foster.)*

nerve and muscle cells and death of the parasite. It has a direct effect on the microfilariae causing paralysis and death but does not kill the adult worm. It does however, halt production of microfilariae by female worms for many months. Thus, it only needs to be given as a single dose once every 6–12 months.

Ivermectin dose not cause the severe inflammatory reactions incited by older treatments which could cause further ocular damage. This may be because its primary effect is to paralyse the microfilariae without their sudden mass death.

Because ivermectin is safe and effective, treatment can be aimed at the whole community, in order to reduce the prevalence of the infection, rather than targeting symptomatic individuals. Rapid epidemiological mapping techniques identify the communities at greatest risk. The usual strategy is community-directed treatment with ivermectin (CDTI). This involves the affected communities in the planning, implementation and monitoring of treatment activities. Local people are trained to distribute the ivermectin and to monitor its use.

Since 1987, ivermectin has been donated free of charge by the manufacturer (Merck) for everyone who needs it for as long as it is needed. Merck has worked with WHO and other agencies to supply hundreds of millions of doses which are distributed by the onchocerciasis control programmes to remote areas through CDTI.

The dose of ivermectin is 150 mg/kg, every 6–12 months by mouth. A simplified dosage schedule uses patient height as a proxy for weight. It should not be given to:

- Children under 5 years old, or weighing less than 15 kg, or less than 90 cm in height
- Pregnant women
- Women breast-feeding a child under 1 week old.

Paracetamol or an antihistamine may be given for minor side-effects, such as pruritus or fever. More severe reactions are rare. Although ivermectin is safe, there have been rare cases of encephalopathy in patients who have heavy infection with *Loa loa* (>30 000 mf/mL). Ivermectin should be used with caution where loiasis is endemic.

Vector Control. Vector control uses larvicides to kill the *Simulium* larvae. The Onchocerciasis Control Project (OCP) in West Africa has carried this out effectively, but unfortunately, vector control is very expensive. Selective larvicides must be delivered to all breeding sites, including the most remote and inaccessible.

Obsolete Treatments. Diethylcarbamazine (DEC) was the mainstay of treatment for many years. However, the resulting sudden death of millions of microfilariae often caused a severe systemic reaction with intense itching, a skin rash, fever, headache and joint pains. This is known as the Mazzotti reaction and it causes further ocular inflammation and loss of sight.

The macrofilaricide, suramin was used by weekly intravenous injections, but it is toxic and can cause serious systemic and ocular reactions. It is no longer used.

Toxocariasis

Toxocariasis is the ocular manifestation of *Toxocara canis* larval infection, which also causes visceral larva migrans, but rarely together. Infection results from ingesting soil or faeces containing eggs of the canine roundworm. Toxocariasis is found in both developing and industrialized countries and a history of eating soil or contact with a puppy that is not house-trained arouses suspicion. It is not only important as a cause of unilateral visual loss, but also because it can mimic retinoblastoma.

Eye Complications. Ocular toxocariasis typically occurs in children between 6 and 11 years. It may present as a squint or a white pupil (leucocoria). It may manifest as a chromic endophthalmitis with dense vitreous cellular reaction; or as a choroidal granuloma which is usually solitary in the posterior pole or fundal periphery. Chronic endophthalmitis may be accompanied by pre-retinal exudate, vitreous membranes, retinal detachment or cataract. This is the form that may be confused with an exophytic retinoblastoma.

Retinoblastoma tends to occur in younger children (around 2 years old), can have a family history, is more often bilateral and frequently has calcification within the tumour. Ultrasound or a CT scan can detect calcification. Toxocariasis is excluded by a negative serum ELISA and supported by a positive test, but false positives in exposed individuals are common.

Management. Most choroidal granulomas are quiescent and no therapy is indicated. Chronic endophthalmitis or severe uveitis is treated with systemic or periocular corticosteroids. Anthelminthics are not required as the larvae are dead and the disease is caused by a severe inflammatory reaction. Vitreous membrane formation and traction retinal detachment can be addressed by specialist surgery involving vitrectomy, division of membranes and retinal detachment surgery.

Loiasis

Loiasis is found in West and Central Africa and is caused by the filarial helminth *Loa loa*. It is primarily a cutaneous pathogen, but is known as the eye worm because of the ability of the adult worm to live in the ocular adnexa and subconjunctivally. The vector is the fly of the genus *Chrysops*. The microfilariae are blood-borne and can cause a generalized myalgia, low-grade fever and paraesthesia.

Eye Complications. A subconjunctival *Loa loa* worm causes irritation and redness and may be visible, or only as a granuloma. Alternatively, there may be considerable eyelid swelling due to oedema (Calabar swelling), caused by the subcutaneous worm. Usually this swelling will settle in a few days. Microfilariae may invade the uveal tract causing uveitis. Diagnosis is by demonstration of microfilariae on a blood film.

Loiasis complicates the treatment of onchocerciasis, as treatment of mixed infections with ivermectin can be associated with severe neurological adverse effects.

Management. The removal of a subconjunctival worm requires topical or subconjunctival anaesthesia which may help to immobilize the worm. A suture is passed under the worm and tied tightly and the worm is dissected out. Alternatively, cryotherapy may help immobilize the worm or be used for removal. The worms can move with surprising agility!

Thelaziasis

The eye worm, *Thelazia callipaeda*, has principally been reported from countries in the Far East and *Thelazia californiensis* in western USA. It is a zoonosis transmitted from the eye secretions of animals directly to human hosts by flies that are intermediate hosts.

Eye Complications. Typically, the patient complains of irritation and watering with a congested eye. The thread-like white worms may be seen within the conjunctival sac.

Management. Worms can be removed from the conjunctival sac with forceps after the application of a local anaesthetic.

Bancroftian and Brugian Filariasis

Lymphatic filariasis caused by *Wuchereria bancrofti* has a widespread distribution in Africa, Asia and Latin America, with 119 million infected (WHO), whereas *Brugia malayi* occurs principally in South-east Asia and *Brugia timori* in Indonesia. Transmission is by mosquitoes.

Eye Complications. Adult worms have been isolated in the conjunctiva, with associated pain and redness. Larvae can infiltrate the anterior chamber, iris, lens capsule, retina and choroid. A subretinal adult worm has been reported. Worms have been found in the eyelid and also the lacrimal gland.

Management. An adult worm may be removed from beneath the conjunctiva after the application of topical anaesthetic. Treatment is described in Chapter 54.

Trichinosis

Trichinosis is a myositis caused by the larvae of *Trichinella spiralis* commonly affecting the extraocular muscles. Infection is commonly the result of eating uncooked meat, most often pork or game meats. The disease is found worldwide, except Australia. After an acute illness, myositis ensues affecting active muscles including extra-ocular muscles, diaphragm, intercostals, tongue and gastrocnemius. Central and peripheral nervous system disease may develop.

Eye Complications. The ophthalmic manifestations are primarily bilateral periorbital oedema, conjunctival chemosis, subconjunctival haemorrhages, proptosis and pain on eye movement related to invasion of the extraocular muscles by the organism. Optic nerve compression may cause disc swelling and later atrophy.

Management. Treatment of the eyes is predominantly symptomatic with cycloplegic drops, such as atropine sulphate 1% and topical corticosteroids. Systemic treatment of trichinosis is with thiabendazole. Optic nerve compression may require concurrent oral steroids.

Gnathostomiasis

Gnathostomiasis is due to infection with *Gnathostoma spinigerum* usually from eating uncooked freshwater fish. Infection results in initial nonspecific symptoms followed by cutaneous and/or visceral larva migrans. Central nervous system involvement carries a high morbidity and mortality. Gnathostomiasis has foci of endemicity in South-east Asia, central and south America and is now reported in southern Africa and northern Australia.

Eye Complications. Cutaneous gnathostomiasis is the most common manifestation and may involve the eyelids with nodular migratory swellings and pathognomonic subcuticular haemorrhages. The commonest intraocular manifestation is anterior uveitis with larvae visible in the anterior chamber with magnification, but posterior uveitis with larvae in the posterior chamber, intraocular haemorrhage and secondary glaucoma are described. A subretinal worm may cause inflammatory changes along the track made by the moving worm.

Management. Treatment is with albendazole 400 mg twice a day for 21 days; or ivermectin 0.2 mg/kg as either a stat dose or on two consecutive days.[45] Effective drug treatments should negate the need to surgically remove the worm.

Dirofilariasis

Dirofilariasis is a zoonotic disease transmitted from raccoons, dogs and cats by mosquitoes. It is caused by filarial worms of the genus *Dirofilaria* with cases reported from the Americas, Asia, Europe and North Africa. The worms can grow up to 15 cm long and are usually found as encapsulated non-viable subcutaneous nodules.

Eye Complications. *Dirofilaria conjunctivae* has a tendency to locate in peri-ocular tissues, but all species can affect the orbit, peri-ocular tissues, conjunctiva, anterior chamber, vitreous and sclera. Patients present with inflammation, pain and/or a mass effect such as proptosis or diplopia. Treatment is by surgical excision and diagnosis may be in retrospect on histopathology of an excised mass.

Diffuse Unilateral Subacute Neuroretinitis

Diffuse unilateral subacute neuroretinitis (DUSN) is caused by a subretinal motile roundworm of various species, a subretinal visceral lava migrans. It is usually unilateral and presents with loss of vision. There can be successive crops of retinitis with grey-white, deep retinal or subretinal lesions, progressive retinal pigment epithelium depigmentation, vasculitis and disc oedema which may be accompanied by vitritis. The diagnostic clues are tracks of retinal or retinal pigment epithelium lesions, or even a visible subretinal worm. Later there is optic atrophy and diffuse subretinal pigmentary changes, with attenuation of the retinal vessels and severe visual loss.

Attempts have been made to remove the worm surgically, but the preferred treatment is to kill it with laser photocoagulation. High-dose oral albendazole (400 mg od) for 30 days has been reported to be effective.[46]

CESTOIDAL OPHTHALMIC DISEASE

Cysticercosis

Cysticercosis is the encysted form of the tapeworm larvae *Taenia solium* and occasionally *T. saginata*. Infection is by the faecal contamination of food and water or consumption of raw pork or beef. Cysticerci have been found in many tissues, with predilection for subcutaneous tissues, the central nervous system and eyes. It is widespread but more common in South and Central America.

Eye Complications. Ophthalmic cysticercosis can occur in the orbit, lids, subconjunctival space and intraocularly, most commonly subretinally. It can mimic an orbital tumour or occur as a translucent cyst subretinally, or free floating within the vitreous or anterior chamber. The typical form of the intraocular cyst may show amoeboid movements and the protoscolex may move 'in or out' of the cyst. Symptoms depend on site of the cysticerci, but patients may have flashes of light and visual loss from subretinal lesions. There is little inflammation while the larva is alive, but death of the larva induces a granulomatous inflammatory reaction.

Management. Treatment of the intraocular cyst is by surgical removal if possible, before systemic treatment. The systemic treatment of cysticercosis is with praziquantel, albendazole or metrifonate, with corticosteroids in neurocysticercosis to reduce the inflammatory response (see Ch. 58). Praziquantel has been reported to be ineffective in intraocular cysticercosis, possibly because of poor penetration into the eye.

Echinococcosis

Also termed hydatid disease, this infection is most often due to the larvae of the tapeworm *Echinococcus granulosus*. The disease is widespread and other species are found in particular geographical locations. Most cysts are found in the liver and lungs.

Eye Complications. Echinococcosis can cause a space-occupying lesion within the bony orbit with proptosis and conjunctival chemosis. Cysts may also be found within the eye.

Management. Treatment of the orbital cyst is by surgical removal. The systemic treatment is described in Chapter 56.

Sparganosis

Sparganosis is due to infection with larvae of the *Spirometra* tapeworms and is mostly found in East Asia. Infection can occur through drinking contaminated water or eating infected snakes, birds or animals. Infection by direct contact can occur through the practice of using the flesh of an infected frog or snake to poultice open wounds. This practice occurs in the Far East and eye problems are usually caused by direct contact. For example in China, raw flesh may be applied to the eyes of patients who have fever.

Eye Complications. Direct infection with the parasite causes eyelid oedema, watering and pain. There may be periocular nodules and extreme irritation. A worm may be found subconjunctivally and retrobulbar invasion can occur. The larva has been identified in the anterior chamber of the eye.

Management. The worm or nodule should be removed surgically.

TREMATODAL OPHTHALMIC DISEASE

Paragonimiasis

This infection is caused by a number of lung flukes of the genus *Paragonimus*, mainly in the Far East in relation to raw fish consumption.

Eye Complications. Orbital and intraocular involvement is rare but visual sequelae from cerebral infection occur. Invasion of the worm into periocular or intraocular tissue typically causes severe inflammation and pain which is intermittent. The uveitis is brisk and may cause hypopyon formation with vitreous and retinal haemorrhages.

Management. In ocular paragonimiasis, the worm should be removed surgically if possible. The systemic disease is described in Chapter 67.

Schistosomiasis

Schistosomiasis (bilharzia) is caused by *Schistosoma* spp. (Chapter 52). Infection occurs by contact with infected freshwater containing the snail which is the intermediate host.

Eye Complications. Eye involvement is extremely rare considering the many millions infected. Schistosome egg granulomas occur in the conjunctiva and are reported in the choroid and lacrimal gland.

OCULAR DISEASE CAUSED BY ARTHROPODS

Myiasis

The larvae of *Diptera* flies (maggots) may cause ocular myiasis. These infestations are widely distributed in association with poor hygiene or neglect.

Eye Complications. *Diptera* flies lay their eggs directly on the lid margins, or the patient's hand or secondary vectors may deposit them there. The hatched larvae burrow under the conjunctiva causing irritating subconjunctival nodules and discharge. This may progress to affect the orbits and ocular adnexa. Less commonly larvae may penetrate the sclera resulting in internal ocular myiasis and uveitis, which can be severe. A subretinal larva can cause retinal tracks similar to diffuse unilateral subacute neuroretinitis (DUSN).

Management. Treatment is by surgical debridement and removal of larvae. It may be possible to carefully remove larvae from the lid margins after applying local anaesthetic eye drops. Subconjunctival larvae will require surgical removal. The extent of surgery becomes more drastic with increasing penetration of the larvae. Systemic antibiotics are required to deal with secondary bacterial infection.

Internal ocular myiasis requires treatment of any inflammation with corticosteroids. Occasionally it may be necessary to remove the larvae surgically.

Paederus Dermatitis and Conjunctivitis

The rove beetle – a red and black beetle of the genus *Paederus* – causes a severe vesicular dermatitis 24–48 hours after being squashed on the skin because of a toxin in its haemolymph. Indirect contact with the eye causes an intense periorbital dermatitis and keratoconjunctivitis.

In different parts of the world, different species of rove beetle cause *Paederus* dermatitis. In East Africa it is known as 'Nairobi eye', but it also occurs in West Africa, South America and India and in outbreaks elsewhere.

The dermatitis tends to be more severe than the conjunctivitis and can be treated with topical steroid and oral antihistamine. Oral antibiotics such as ciprofloxacin may speed healing because of symbiotic Gram-negative bacteria which contaminate the dermatitis.[47] Severe keratitis has been reported in patients hit in the eye by rove beetles while motorcycling.

Paediatric Ophthalmic Disease

It is estimated that the number of blind children is approximately 1.4 million and 75% live in Africa and Asia. Children have a much lower prevalence of blindness than adults and there are few surveys large enough to estimate the prevalence of childhood blindness with any precision.

Although childhood blindness accounts for less than 4% of global blindness, blind children have a longer life expectancy than blind adults who are generally elderly. The 1.4 million blind children accounts for 70 million blind years (blind-years is the number of years lived with blindness) compared with 120 million blind years from adult cataract globally. Childhood blindness is the second leading cause of blindness in terms of blind-years. Blind children have a higher mortality than their sighted counterparts and the economic costs are significant.

Major Causes and Strategies for Prevention

The realization of childhood blindness as a major source of blind-years has led to increased efforts in recent years to prevent, treat and mitigate it. Childhood blindness is commonly caused by vitamin A deficiency, measles, congenital cataract, conjunctivitis in the newborn and retinopathy of prematurity (ROP). The relative prevalence of these causes varies in different resource settings (Table 67.7).[48]

VITAMIN A DEFICIENCY DISORDERS (VADD) AND THE EYE

Severe vitamin A deficiency kills and blinds hundreds of thousands of children every year, but every tragedy is preventable. Subclinical vitamin A deficiency can impact on immune status, growth, haemopoiesis, morbidity and mortality of young children. Malnourished children in the poorest countries are affected. When the eye is affected, it is known as xerophthalmia ('dry eye'). Countries with a history of widespread VADD have shown improvement in vitamin A status in recent years, particularly India, Indonesia and Bangladesh.

Vitamin A (Retinol)

Stores of vitamin A are found in the liver, where 90% of the body's vitamin A is retained. Vitamin A deficiency is typically associated with other nutritional deficits, which make the child

TABLE 67.7 **Prevalence and Causes of Childhood Blindness by Income Category**

	Low-Income Countries	Middle-Income Countries	High-Income Countries
Prevalence of blindness/1000 children	1.2	0.6	0.3
Number blind children/million total population	600	180	60
Primary causes	Corneal scar Congenital cataract (including rubella) Ophthalmia neonatorum	Retinopathy of prematurity Inherited retinal disease Congenital cataract	Cognitive visual impairment Retinopathy of prematurity Congenital anomalies and genetic diseases

vulnerable to disease. Deficiency results in an impaired immune response and epithelial metaplasia, with decreased resistance to infection.

Measles infection is important in vitamin A deficiency. The measles virus affects all epithelial surfaces. Following an acute infection with measles, the body stores of vitamin A are quickly exhausted and corneal necrosis (keratomalacia) may occur.

In older children and adults, chronic vitamin A deficiency may result in night blindness. Vitamin A is required for the photosensitive pigment of the retinal rods, rhodopsin.

Eye Changes in Vitamin A Deficiency (Xerophthalmia)

The symptoms and signs of xerophthalmia are listed in Table 67.8. Blindness results from bilateral severe corneal disease. In corneal xerosis (X2) the cornea appears dry and dull and may ulcerate due to epithelium break down (X3A). The cornea may melt dramatically (keratomalacia, X3B), with an acute onset, sometimes over a few hours. Children aged 1–3 years are particularly at risk. Keratomalacia usually leads to irreversible blindness from corneal scarring (XS) (Figure 67.39).

Apart from vision loss, many children with severe VADD will die because they are susceptible to infections, such as respiratory infections and diarrhoea. If a child has vitamin A deficiency, others in the same family and community are also at risk.

Treatment of Xerophthalmia

The treatment of xerophthalmia is given in Table 67.9. If there is vomiting, an intramuscular injection of 100 000 IU of water-soluble vitamin A (not an oil-based preparation) may be used instead of the first oral dose.

Once vitamin A treatment is started for xerophthalmia, a topical antibiotic prevents secondary infection and patients with corneal involvement should be referred to an eye specialist.

Prevention of Vitamin A Deficiency

A schedule for prevention of vitamin A deficiency is given in Table 67.9. High doses of vitamin A are contraindicated in pregnancy, because of concerns about the effects on the unborn child. Breast milk provides an adequate supply of vitamin A.

TABLE 67.8 **Eye Changes and Vitamin A Status**

Eye Lesion	Vitamin A Status	Comments	Proportion of Children 6 Months to 6 Years Affected to Constitute a Public Health Problem[a]
Night blindness (XN)	Mild–moderate decrease	Sensitive sign of low body vitamin A stores associated with increased illness and mortality Vitamin A is part of rhodopsin so deficiency affects rod function Prevalence increases into early school years.	Over 1 per 100
Conjunctival xerosis (X1A)	Mild–moderate decrease	Dryness of conjunctiva due to decrease in goblet cells and epithelial change Difficult to diagnose reliably by clinical examination	Not used
Bitot's spots (X1B)	Mild–moderate decrease	White 'foamy' or 'cheese-like' lesions on the conjunctiva: usually temporal Caused by change in squamous epithelium with underlying xerosis May persist after vitamin A treatment	Over 5 per 1000
Active corneal changes (X2 – xerosis/X3 – ulceration)	Severe decrease	Danger signs of permanent loss of sight Cornea may 'melt' (keratomalacia) in a few hours Most common at age 2–4 years	Over 1 per 10 000
Corneal scars (XS)	Persist regardless of Vitamin A status	End-stage of malnutrition eye damage Scarring (leukoma) often allows some residual vision Blinded eyes may be protuberant (anterior staphyloma) or shrunken (phthisis)	Over 5 per 10 000

[a]*Source:* WHO Programme for Prevention of Blindness.

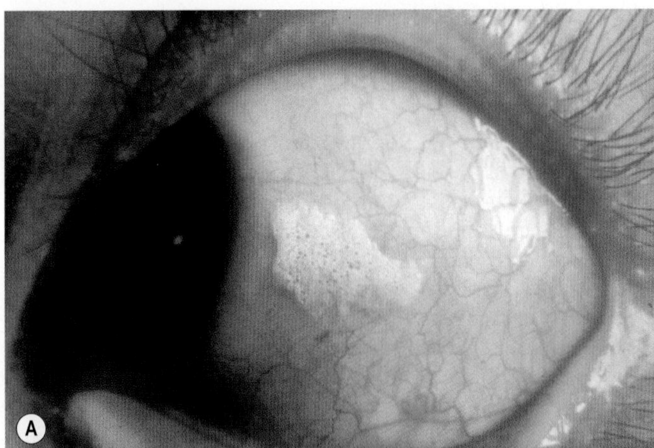
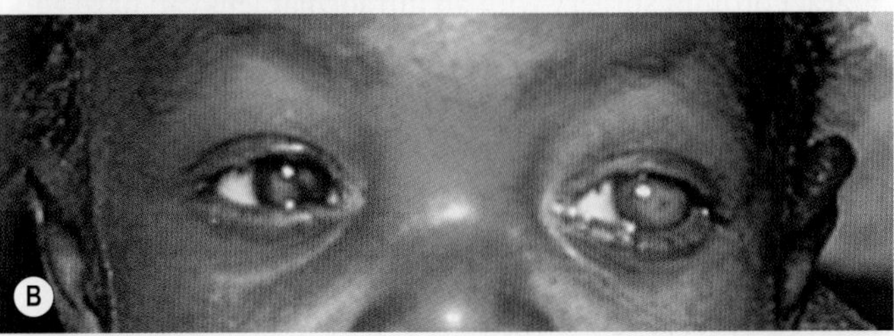
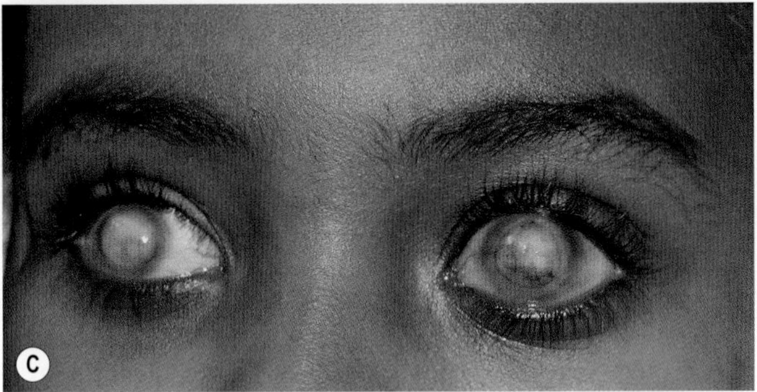

Figure 67.39 Vitamin A deficiency and xerophthalmia. (A) Bitot's spot indicating vitamin A deficiency. (B) keratomalacia (X3B). (C) 12-year-old Ethiopian girl who is blind from vitamin A deficiency (XS). She has had a corneal graft in her left eye; this has unfortunately failed. *(A, Courtesy of ICEH; B, Courtesy of John Anderson; C, Courtesy of Lance Bellers.)*

Communities which have endemic vitamin A deficiency should receive additional nutritional education. Vitamin A-rich foods may be available, but for cultural or other reasons are not consumed by children. Mango, papaya, dark-green leafy vegetables, sweet potatoes and red palm oil are all rich in vitamin A. Vitamin A supplementation can be combined with immunization.

MEASLES AND THE EYE

In 2008, there were 164 000 global deaths from measles. A safe and cost-effective vaccination is available and in 2010, 85% of children globally had been immunized (72% in 2000). Measles infection may trigger the onset of eye problems in children with vitamin A deficiency.

Clinical Presentation

Measles virus causes high fever, cough and conjunctivitis, causing photosensitive, watery, red eyes. There may be evidence of a punctate keratitis. However, measles conjunctivitis is self-limiting and it is the complications of measles which can cause blindness.

In a child with low reserves of vitamin A, measles infection can result in corneal ulceration and keratomalacia. A depressed immune response may lead to severe herpes simplex keratitis.

Treatment of Measles and its Eye Complications

Treatment with vitamin A can prevent blindness and has been shown to reduce the number of deaths from measles by half. A topical antibiotic should be given to each eye at least four times each day. Supportive treatment should be given as appropriate for gastroenteritis or respiratory infection.

Prevention

Routine measles immunization is associated with a reduction in severe vitamin A deficiency. The fourth Millennium Development Goal aims to cut the infant mortality rate by two-thirds and measles vaccination is an indicator of progress towards this goal.

NEWBORN CONJUNCTIVITIS (OPHTHALMIA NEONATORUM)

In newborn conjunctivitis, infection occurs during the birth of the child and presents within 28 days as a severe conjunctivitis with purulent discharge. There is a danger of corneal ulcer and perforation. The common causative organisms are *Neisseria gonorrhoea* and *Chlamydia trachomatis*.

Between 25% and 50% of infants exposed to *N. gonorrhoea* or *C. trachomatis* during birth develop conjunctivitis, if no eye prophylaxis is given. The prevalence of gonorrhoea among antenatal attenders in African countries is high: between 4%

TABLE 67.9 Vitamin A Prevention and Treatment Schedule for Xerophthalmia

Timing and Age	Treatment Dosage[b]	Preventative Dosing[b]
Immediately on diagnosis:		
<6 months of age	50 000 IU	50 000 IU orally
6–12 months of age	100 000 IU	100 000 IU orally every 4–6 months
>12 months of age	200 000 IU	200 000 IU orally every 4–6 months
Women[a] with XN, X1A, X1B	25 000 IU	
Women with X2 or X3	200 000 IU	
Mothers		200 000 IU orally within 8 weeks of delivery
Next day	Same age-specific dose[c]	
At least 2 weeks later	Same age-specific dose[d]	

[a]Of reproductive age.
[b]For oral administration, preferably in an oil-based preparation.
[c]The mother or carer can administer the next-day dose at home.
[d]To be administered at a subsequent health service contact with the individual.

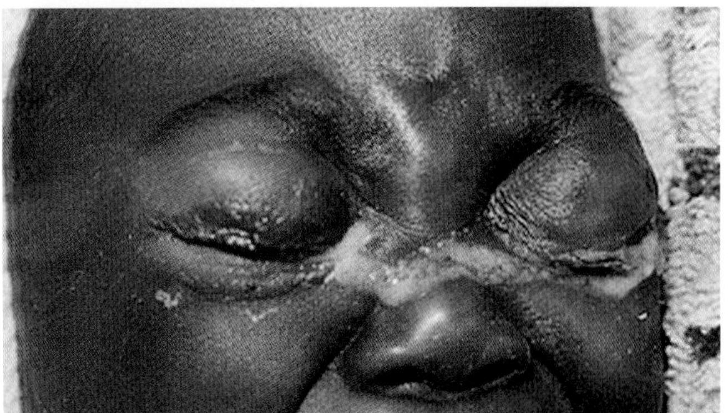

Figure 67.40 Gonococcal conjunctivitis in a 14-month-old child. *(Courtesy of Harjinder Chana.)*

and 15%. Ideally, pregnant mothers and their partners should be treated at this stage, which avoids infection of the newborn.

Newborn conjunctivitis due to *N. gonorrhoea* has a rapid onset with profuse discharge of pus and tense, swollen eyelids (Figure 67.40). Neonatal conjunctivitis usually presents after 5 days in *N. gonorrhoea* and from 3 days to 2 weeks with *C. trachomatis* infection.

Neonatal conjunctivitis is an emergency and treatment must be started immediately with hourly topical antibiotic drops (e.g. ofloxacin or gentamicin), repeated cleaning of the eyes and systemic anti-gonococcal treatment (parenteral penicillin). *C. trachomatis* has similar clinical features, but does not lead to corneal ulceration. As the causative organism is not known immediately, treatment should be started for both. Treatment for *C. trachomatis* is a systemic macrolide (erythromycin or azithromycin). Systemic treatment must also be given to both parents, who may have other sexually transmitted diseases.

Other pathogens, which may cause newborn conjunctivitis include *Haemophilus*, *Streptococcus pneumoniae*, *Staphylococcus aureus*, *Pseudomonas* and herpes simplex virus (HSVII).

To prevent newborn conjunctivitis, prophylactic treatment should be instilled. Povidone iodine, 2.5% solution, given once as eye drops at birth, is effective and cheap. Silver nitrate drops, or tetracycline or erythromycin ointment are alternatives. Povidone iodine may be safely used by traditional birth attendants as well as hospital midwives.

CONGENITAL CATARACT

The treatment of congenital cataract in children is much more problematic than cataract in adults. In children under the age of 8, cataract leads to failure of visual development, or amblyopia (lazy eye). If surgery is delayed, the amblyopia may be irreversible and the vision will not recover, despite successful surgery.

Causes of Congenital Cataract

- Maternal infection: rubella most commonly, chickenpox, cytomegalovirus and toxoplasmosis.
- Genetic: as an isolated defect or part of a syndrome including Down syndrome.
- Metabolic disorders, e.g. galactosaemia.
- Idiopathic: in most cases, no cause is found and exhaustive investigations are unnecessary.

Management

A child with bilateral cataract should be referred as soon as possible for surgery, ideally to a paediatric ophthalmologist in a specialist unit.

Most infants in developing countries are left aphakic after surgery and will require aphakic spectacles (or contact lenses). Intensive follow-up is required with refraction at least every 6 months as the child's eye is growing. An intraocular lens may be implanted at a later date or in older children. Despite surgery and adequate refractive correction, the child often has residual visual impairment and will require additional support for schooling. Low-vision services are an integral part of the management of childhood cataract.

Unilateral congenital cataract causes profound amblyopia and surgery is not justified. Whereas in childhood traumatic cataract prompt surgery with an intraocular lens can have good results.

CONGENITAL GLAUCOMA (BUPHTHALMOS)

See above.

RETINOPATHY OF PREMATURITY

Retinopathy of prematurity (ROP) is a leading cause of childhood blindness in middle-income countries. Better neonatal care has increased the survival of premature babies who are at risk of this condition. In industrialized countries, premature neonates are screened for ROP and careful oxygen management means that blinding ROP is rare in babies with a birth weight over 1000 g, or gestational age of greater than 28 weeks. However, in the middle-income countries of Asia and Latin America, heavier, more mature babies are at risk.[49]

ROP is a proliferative retinopathy of retinal blood vessels which have not yet matured. The vessels fail to develop to the periphery of the retina, dilate with new vessel formation. This can progress to vitreous haemorrhage and retinal detachment.

Early detection, by screening neonates at risk, followed by photocoagulation or cryotherapy of ischaemic retina, has been shown to reduce the risk of blindness. Premature babies at risk of ROP should be examined by an ophthalmologist with indirect ophthalmoscopy. Local guidelines should be developed to identify babies at risk. In middle-income countries, examining all neonates under 1750 g may be a reasonable strategy.

RETINOBLASTOMA

This is a malignant tumour of retinal precursor cells, which arises in children because of mutations in the tumour-suppressing gene *RB1*, on the long arm of chromosome 13. Two-thirds of children with retinoblastoma have random mutations which arise in their retina (somatic). These children present with a single tumour, typically at a relatively older age (peak 2–3 years), than multifocal disease. If they survive, these children do not pass on a genetic defect to their offspring.

The remaining third of children with retinoblastoma have a mutation in the *RB1* gene in every cell in the body. Either the defect is inherited or the mutation occurs in an early germline. This mutation requires a sporadic mutation to occur at the same gene locus to disable the second *RB1* gene, which often

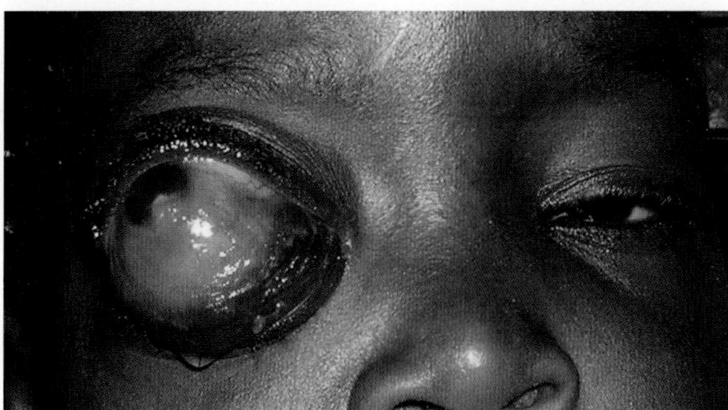

Figure 67.41 Retinoblastoma. *(Courtesy of Nicholas A. V. Beare.)*

occurs in multiple retinal cells. This causes bilateral, multiple tumours occurring at a younger age (peak 6 months). These children are also at risk of other tumours.

Retinoblastoma may present with a white pupil (leucocoria), but many children in resource-poor settings present late, with an advanced tumour. The eye is grossly enlarged and commonly extraocular or extraorbital spread has occurred (Figure 67.41). The tumour extends along the optic nerve to the brain and metastasizes to other parts of the body. Retinoblastoma may present with squint, glaucoma, visual loss, a painful red eye and proptosis. The tumour may present at any time during the first 5 years of life.

Adults who have survived multiple retinoblastomas, should be advised of a 50% risk of their children being affected. Parents of a child with retinoblastoma have a 1–2% risk of retinoblastoma in subsequent children and there is a 1% chance in the offspring of an adult who survived unilateral disease.

The differential diagnosis of intraocular retinoblastoma includes toxocariasis, toxoplasmosis, ROP, Coat's disease, congenital cataract and other conditions. Investigations should include ultrasonography or computed tomography (if available), because a mass with calcification in a child under 3 is virtually diagnostic of retinoblastoma. In Africa, the differential of severe unilateral proptosis in a child is Burkitt's lymphoma.

Management

Following the discovery of a single tumour, both eyes must be examined carefully. Examinations should continue regularly, every 3–6 months, until at least the age of 5 years.

Treatment of advanced tumours is with enucleation, with removal of as long a length of optic nerve as possible. Cryotherapy and laser have been used for small tumours. Some specialist centres will be able to provide chemotherapy, which is very effective.

TABLE 67.10 Essential Eye Drugs[a]

Topical antimicrobial agents	Antibiotic[b]	0.5% Chloramphenicol drops 1% Tetracycline ointment 0.3% Gentamicin drops
	Antiherpetic	0.1% Idoxuridine drops or 3% aciclovir ointment
	Antiseptic[b]	5% Povidone-iodine or 0.2% chlorhexidine gluconate
Local anaesthetic	Topical[b]	0.5% Amethocaine hydrochloride or 0.4% Oxybuprocaine hydrochloride drops
Mydriatic	Diagnostic and short-acting[b]	1% Tropicamide or 1% Cyclopentolate hydrochloride drops
	Therapeutic and long-acting[b]	1% Atropine sulphate drops
Topical steroids	Weak[b]	0.1% Prednisolone drops
	Normal[b]	0.5% Prednisolone drops
	Strong[b]	1.0% Prednisolone drops
Corneal stain	Diagnostic	Fluorescein paper strips or 1% drops
Subconjunctival drugs	Antibiotic	Gentamicin 40 mg/mL
	Steroid	Hydrocortisone succinate 100 mg ampoule Methylprednisolone 40 mg/mL (Depo-prep)
	Mydriatics	Atropine sulphate 1 mg/mL Adrenaline hydrochloride 1/1000
Oral agents		Tab. Acetazolamide 250 mg Tab. Prednisolone 5 mg Tab./Amp. Vitamin A 200 000 IU Tab. Ivermectin (in areas where onchocerciasis occurs)

[a]Many of these can be locally made and are already in use by some National Prevention of Blindness programmes.
[b]These drops can be locally prepared from raw materials.

Essential Eye Drugs

Table 67.10 gives details of medications routinely used in ophthalmic practice. Many of these drugs can be locally manufactured from ready-prepared materials.[50]

Acknowledgements

We would like to acknowledge David Yorston and Murray McGavin as the authors of this chapter in the previous, 22nd edition of Manson's Tropical Diseases, on which this revision is based.

REFERENCES

9. Shah A, Sachdev A, Coggon D, et al. Geographic variations in microbial keratitis: an analysis of the peer-reviewed literature. Br J Ophthalmol 2011;95(6):762–7.
16. Glover SJ, Burgess PI, Cohen DB, et al. Prevalence of diabetic retinopathy, cataract and visual impairment in patients with diabetes in sub-Saharan Africa. Br J Ophthalmol 2012;96(2):156–61.
29. Porco TC, Gebre T, Ayele B, et al. Effect of mass distribution of azithromycin for trachoma control on overall mortality in Ethiopian children: a randomized trial. JAMA 2009;302(9):962–8.
39. Beare NA, Taylor TE, Harding SP, et al. Malarial retinopathy: a newly established diagnostic sign in severe malaria. Am J Trop Med Hyg 2006;75(5):790–7.
44. Tamarozzi F, Halliday A, Gentil K, et al. Onchocerciasis: the role of *Wolbachia* bacterial endosymbionts in parasite biology, disease pathogenesis and treatment. Clin Microbiol Rev 2011;24(3):459–68.

FURTHER READING

Sandford-Smith J. Eye Disease in Hot Climates. Oxford: Butterworth-Heinemann; 1997.

An excellent short textbook of ophthalmology that is particularly relevant to the developing world.

The Journal of Community Eye Health. Online. Available: www.cehjournal.org

A freely accessible online Journal which contains a wealth of useful articles. The paper edition is sent free of charge to health workers in developing countries.

Access the complete references online at www.expertconsult.com

68 Dermatological Problems

FRANCISCO VEGA-LOPEZ | SARA RITCHIE

KEY POINTS

- Skin disease may represent a primary condition or be a secondary manifestation of systemic illness and the history and examination should be directed towards both.
- Both infective and non-infective inflammatory conditions need to be considered when formulating a differential diagnosis for skin problems in the tropics.
- Skin malignancies should always be considered in the differential diagnosis.
- Superimposed pyogenic infection can complicate many other tropical skin infections.
- Syphilis occurs worldwide and should be considered in the differential diagnosis of tropical skin presentations.
- Leprosy should always be considered in individuals who have lived for several years in endemic areas.
- Infection with tuberculous mycobacteria or atypical mycobacteria should be considered with either a history of travel to areas of endemicity or a history of high-risk activities.
- Fungal infection, either superficial or deep, should be considered in the differential, particularly in the immunocompromised.
- Cutaneous leishmaniasis can have protean manifestations and should be considered with a history of travel to any endemic region.
- Detailed knowledge of geographical endemicity patterns is vital in formulating the correct differential diagnoses of skin conditions presenting in or from the tropics.

Introduction

Poverty and disability characterize a number of skin diseases in the tropics. A number of studies support the aetiological role of poverty in skin conditions such as fungal diseases, leprosy, scabies and impetigo. A vicious circle can arise as chronic or recurrent skin disease results in further disability and loss of economic activity. Clear examples of this complex problem are overtly manifest in those individuals suffering from mycobacterial infections, cutaneous leishmaniasis, leprosy and deep fungal infection.

Skin infections and tropical diseases may present as a primary condition or as a secondary manifestation of systemic illness. Cutaneous larva migrans and localized cutaneous leishmaniasis are examples of the former, whereas the latter can be exemplified by systemic conditions such as disseminated leishmaniasis secondary to kala-azar and coccidioidomycosis. The clinical approach to a patient with tropical skin disease involves a thorough history-taking that leads to establishing a morphological and topographical diagnosis. Table 68.1 shows examples of lesions and symptoms that suggest or establish a particular diagnosis in clinical practice.

The history must include detailed information on previous skin disease, travel history, activities while travelling, occupation, drugs, wild or domestic animal contacts, precipitating factors, duration of signs and symptoms, evolution of clinical signs, symptoms in relatives or household contacts and an assessment of the patient's immune status. The examination must include extracutaneous signs such as fever, enlarged lymph nodes, hepatosplenomegaly and general malaise, which may indicate systemic illness. In-depth epidemiological knowledge of global geographical pathology is also required in the practice of tropical dermatology.

Skin Diseases Caused by Bacteria

PYOGENIC INFECTIONS

Aetiology and Pathogenesis

Staphylococcus and *Streptococcus* spp. are ubiquitous in both urban and rural environments worldwide. Healthy and immunocompromised hosts may develop pyogenic infections of the skin following direct inoculation of bacteria. Less commonly, haematogenous dissemination or even bacteraemia may develop as a result of a minor skin injury. The portal of entry for these pathogenic organisms is often unnoticed by both the patient and doctor, but minor injuries, insect bites, friction blisters or superficial fungal infection are the commonest found in clinical practice.

Pyogenic bacteria cause damage by the pathogenic action of proteases, haemolysins, lipoteichoic acid and coagulases. Erythrogenic toxins are responsible for the erythema commonly observed in infections by *Streptococcus* spp.

Clinical Findings and Diagnosis

The clinical spectrum of skin pyogenic infections includes folliculitis and furunculosis on hair-bearing skin, plaques of impetigo (Figure 68.1), with thickened dermis commonly affecting the lower limbs (Figure 68.2) and abscess formation, cellulitis and necrotic ulceration at the more severe end of the spectrum.

The perimalleolar regions are commonly affected as they are exposed to mechanical trauma, however pyogenic infections may present on the upper limbs, face (Figure 68.3) and trunk. Common clinical signs of pyogenic infection include erythema, inflammation, pus discharge, abscess formation, ulceration,

TABLE 68.1 Skin Lesions and Symptoms Suggesting a Variety of Diagnoses

Clinical Features	Working Diagnosis
Itchy papules in clusters	Arthropod bites
Asymptomatic palmoplantar papules	Syphilis
Single ulcerated nodule on exposed skin	Cutaneous leishmaniasis
Asymptomatic chronic verrucous plaque	Tuberculosis or chromoblastomycosis
Dysautonomic changes and ulceration	Leprosy
Hyper/hypopigmented patch/plaques with atrophy and ulceration	Leprosy
Erythematous or hypopigmented plaques or nodules with peripheral neuropathy	Leprosy
Excoriated papules and burrows	Scabies
Ulcerated nodule and lymphangitis	Sporotrichosis or cutaneous leishmaniasis
Chronic scarring and sinus tracts	Mycetoma
Itchy serpiginous track	Cutaneous larva migrans
Haemorrhagic eschar, rash and fever	Tick typhus, Lyme disease
Pruritic lichenification, nodules and dyschromic changes	Onchocerciasis
Recurrent swellings	*Loa loa* or gnathostomiasis
Patchy alopecia and boggy inflammation	Scalp ringworm
Acute urticaria, fever and abdominal pain	Acute schistosomiasis (Katayama fever)
Painful, pruritic, plantar blisters	Acute tinea pedis or acute eczema
Furunculoid painful lesions	Myasis
Erythema or urticaria or exfoliative skin lesions with/without mucosal involvement	Drug reactions

blistering, necrotizing lesions and gangrene. Severe scarring may result from pyogenic ulcers (Figure 68.4). Most pyogenic skin infections are painful and the diagnosis is often clinical. Bacteriological investigations and antibiotic sensitivity profile should be requested if available.

Management

Mild infections are successfully treated with bathing or soaking the affected skin in potassium permanganate solution (1 : 10 000 dilution in water) for 20 minutes daily. Necrotizing soft tissue infections can have a high mortality and pose one of the few dermatological emergencies, with early diagnosis being crucial. The optimum treatment is surgical debridement combined with antimicrobial therapy; additional therapies that may be

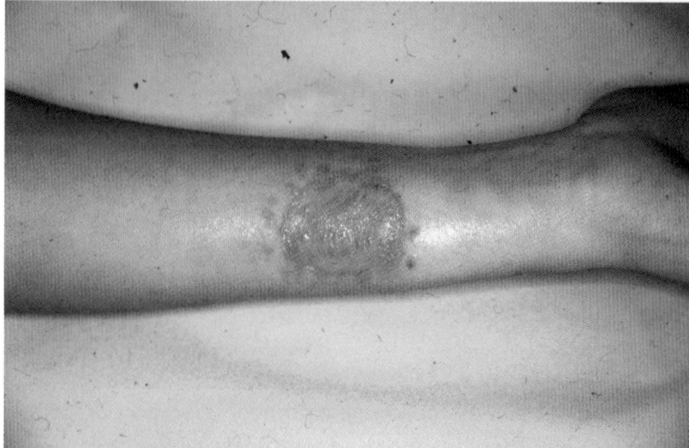

Figure 68.1 Erythematous plaque of superficial impetigo with satellite lesions.

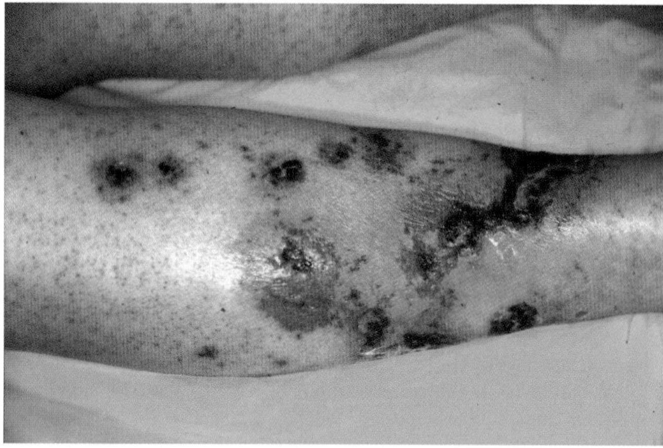

Figure 68.2 Pyogenic superficial lesions with purpuric plaques of cellulitis and proximal dissemination.

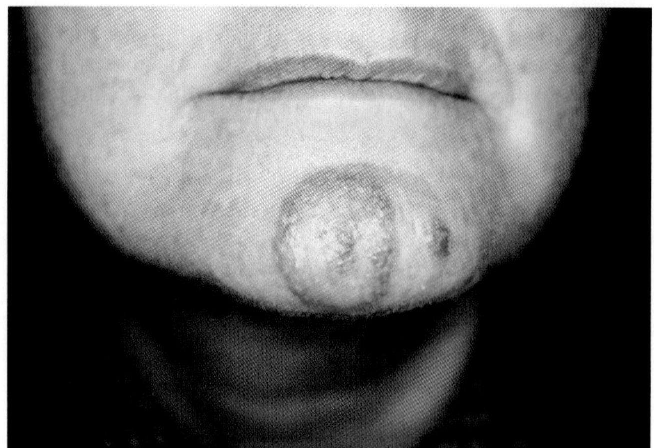

Figure 68.3 Circular plaque of staphylococcal pustular impetigo on the chin, with satellite lesions.

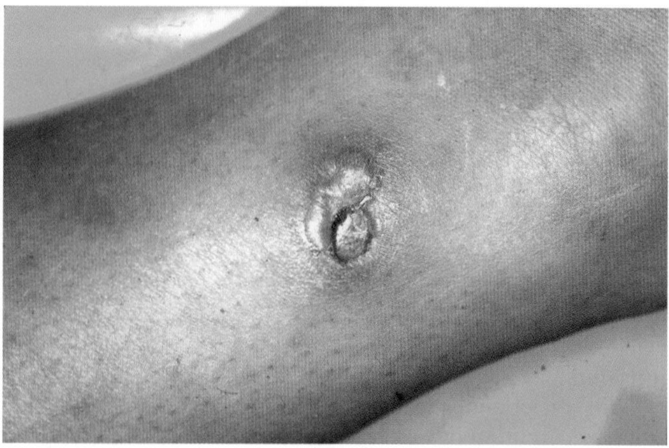

Figure 68.4 Localized ecthyma with surrounding cellulitis on the lower limb.

considered include hyperbaric oxygen and intravenous immunoglobulin.

Treatment

Mild superficial infections such as isolated plaques of impetigo or impetiginized eczema respond well to antiseptic creams and ointments containing cetrimide, chlorhexidine, fucidic acid or mupirocin. Acute or chronic eczema requires treatment with potent topical steroids in order to eliminate risk factors for infection. Infections with multiple lesions or those involving larger areas of the skin require a complete course of systemic beta-lactam or macrolide antibiotics. Recurrent infections may require an antimicrobial soap substitute and screening and eradication of colonizing MSSA or MRSA.

Prevention

Prevention of pyogenic infections in the tropics requires careful attention to cleaning and hygiene of even minor wounds, as the tropical environment can predispose to the early spread of bacterial infection.

TREPONEMAL INFECTIONS

These spirochaetal infections consist of venereal syphilis, non-venereal endemic syphilis, yaws and pinta. The non-venereal *Treponema* species may be transmitted among children living in tropical and subtropical climates, primarily by direct contact.[1]

Syphilis (see Chapter 23)

Primary syphilis is typically characterized by the appearance of a painless chancre at the point of infection, usually the genital or oral mucosa.

If the primary form is untreated, secondary syphilis may develop from 20 to 60 days after infection, resulting in an erythematous maculopapular rash with common palmoplantar involvement. The differential diagnosis of this rash may include HIV seroconversion or other viral infections. There may be a scarring alopecia, ulceration of mucous membranes and characteristic condylomata lata in the flexures. Condylomata lata are whitish grey and, due to their presence in flexures, tend to be moist. Systemic symptoms include fever, lethargy, myalgia and arthralgia.

Tertiary syphilis may develop from 3–5 years after infection. Tuberous syphilids with grouped red-brown papules occur on the skin. Such lesions may develop central regression and atrophy. Gummata may be localized on the forehead, scalp, lips, tongue, genitals (Figure 68.5) or any part of the body. Morphologically, the gummata are various shades of red and may ulcerate and heal with extensive scarring.

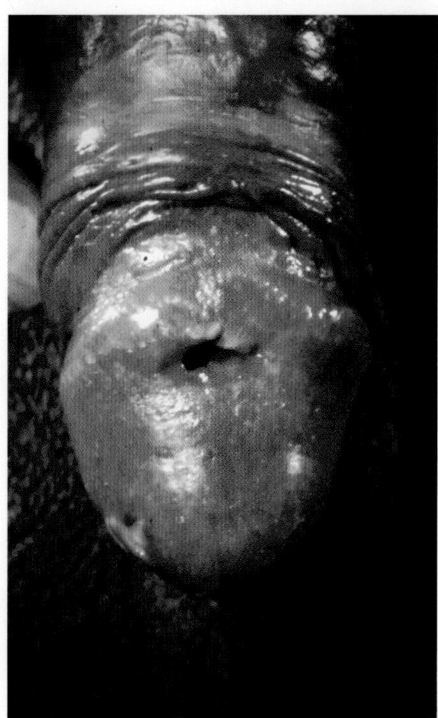

Figure 68.5 Asymptomatic exudative gummata of the penis in syphilis.

Treatment. The treatment of choice is penicillin and allergic individuals respond to tetracyclines or erythromycin.

Yaws

Yaws tends to begin in childhood and is associated with overcrowding, as the main form of transmission is skin-to-skin contact. Propagation of the causative organism *Treponema pertenue* is dependent on a hot humid climate and is seen throughout the tropics. The clinical presentation is divided into four stages: primary, secondary, latent and tertiary. The primary stage is characterized by a single papule, which enlarges to become a papilloma at the site of inoculation. The average incubation period is 20 days. Deceptively, this papilloma resolves spontaneously, only for the same papilloma to appear 6 months later in a disseminated distribution in the secondary phase. These secondary-stage papillomata tend to heal spontaneously, leading to an asymptomatic latent phase with sporadic appearance of papillomatous skin lesions which also spontaneously heal. Both secondary and latent phases may be associated with characteristic palmoplantar hyperkeratosis, which makes it painful for the patient to walk and, hence, the associated 'crab gait'. The tertiary stage may occur in up to 10% of patients, with scarring of the skin manifesting in:

- juxta-articular nodules, which are hard nodules around joints, mainly on the extensor side of elbows and wrists and also on hips, ankles and sacrum
- the appearance of gummata on the nose, palate and upper lip, causing soft tissue destruction that results in scarred areas called gangosa.

There can also be inflammation of the bones of the nose and upper jaw, leading to destruction of bone and cartilage that results in scarred mutilated areas called goundou.

Treatment. The prognosis of primary and secondary yaws is excellent, with a single dose of penicillin causing healing of cutaneous lesions within weeks. Alternative antibiotics are tetracyclines and erythromycin. Unfortunately, once the scarring lesions of tertiary yaws have been established these remain permanent.

Pinta

This is endemic in parts of Latin America and caused by *Treponema carateum*. It is characterized by chronic skin lesions only, with no systemic involvement and occurs mainly in young adults. There are four stages: primary, secondary, latent and tertiary. Three weeks after inoculation, a papule or verrucous

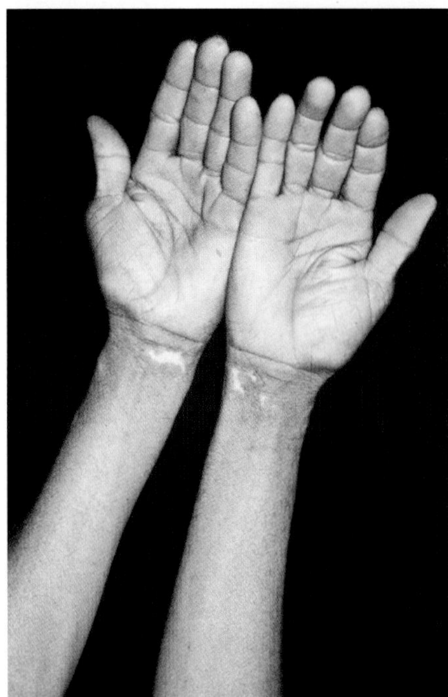

Figure 68.6 Circumscribed patches of hypopigmented skin on the wrists in 'mal del pinto'.

plaque appears on the periphery of the limbs, which enlarges and becomes gradually hyperkeratotic. Secondary pinta is said to occur 9 months later, when there is dissemination of such lesions throughout the skin. Years later, the tertiary form may develop, with hypo- and hyperpigmented scarred areas throughout the skin (Figure 68.6).

In both yaws and pinta, treponemal organisms can be found by dark-field microscopy from early skin lesions. Both give identical cross-reactive positive serology to syphilis.

Treatment. Benzylpenicillin is the treatment of choice for all of these treponemal infections, with tetracyclines and erythromycin being alternatives in penicillin allergy (see Chapter 36).

MYCOBACTERIAL INFECTIONS

The main disease-causing mycobacteria are *M. tuberculosis* and *M. leprae*. Atypical mycobacteria can also cause skin disease, including *M. marinum, M. ulcerans, M. chelonae* and *M. abscessus*.

Clinical Findings and Diagnosis

M. marinum. Fish tank granuloma commonly affects the fingers or dorsum of the hand, but has also been described on the foot and other anatomical sites. *M. marinum* frequently infects freshwater fish and, hence individuals handling fish tanks represent the main population at risk. The dorsal aspects of the hand, foot and the malleolar regions are exposed to trauma and direct inoculation. The disease manifests as a localized progressive swelling with variable pain and the appearance, within a few weeks, of nodular or ulcerated skin lesions measuring a few millimetres up to 2 or 3 cm on the affected area (Figure 68.7). These lesions may resolve spontaneously after a few months or disseminate proximally by haematogenous or lymphatic spread. Once the condition is suspected, skin biopsies for microbiological and histopathological investigations are the most sensitive tests to confirm the diagnosis. Combination therapy with at least two antibiotics for several months is recommended and should be continued for 4–6 weeks after clinical resolution.

M. ulcerans. (See Chapter 42) This causes the Buruli ulcer, which mainly affects young individuals in rural Africa, in particular West Africa. More than two-thirds of all cases present in children below the age of 15. The initial lesions present as papules or nodules that increase in size to cause painless ulceration of the skin. The ulcer characteristically presents with undermined edges and can progress via a toxin-mediated process to involve a large area of the affected limb or trunk. Oedematous forms may progress rapidly and cause a panniculitis with destruction of underlying tissues such as fascia and bone. Significant contractures of the affected limb result from scarring and some patients will require amputation of the deformed limb. Dual therapy with rifampicin and streptomycin for 8 weeks is the current standard chemotherapeutic regimen in addition to surgery.[2]

***M. chelonae* and *M. abscessus*.** These can cause local infection after trauma. Iatrogenic infections due to *M. chelonae* are well documented, with the source of contamination commonly tap-water or contaminated medical instruments. Lesions can be varied, with ulcers, subcutaneous nodules and fistula formation. Disseminated infections usually only occur if the patient is immunocompromised.

Tuberculosis of the Skin

Aetiology. Tuberculosis of the skin is caused by *M. tuberculosis*. Those infected usually come into contact with the bacteria during childhood and have usually been in direct contact with people who are bacteriologically positive.

Primary Tuberculosis. This form of the disease manifests 3–4 weeks after infection, appearing as a papule which becomes a plaque (Figure 68.8) or in a nodular inflammatory form which

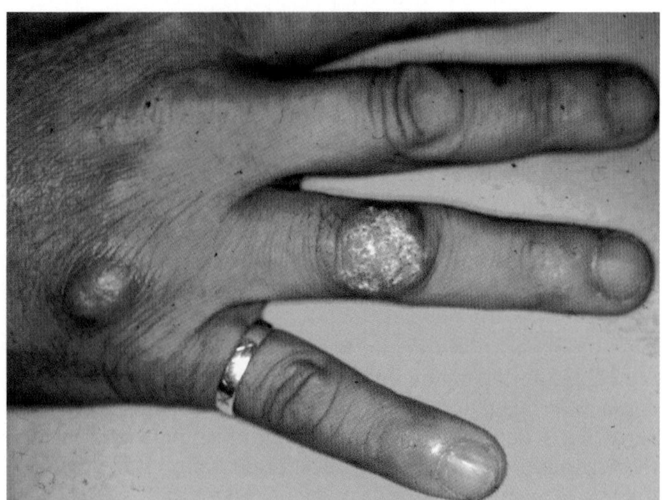

Figure 68.7 Nodular verrucous violaceous lesions with proximal dissemination caused by *Mycobacterium marinum*.

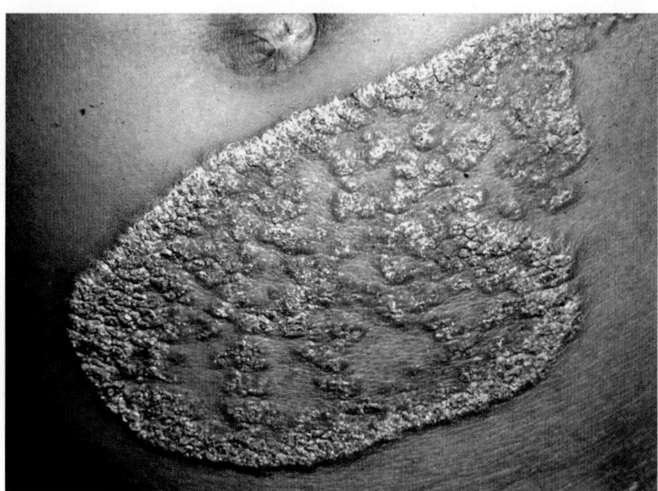

Figure 68.8 Circumscribed large verrucous plaque with erythematous islets in chronic tuberculosis verrucosa cutis. *(Courtesy of Professor Amado Saúl, Mexico.)*

evolves into an ulcer. The tuberculin test is usually negative initially but becomes positive as the disease progresses.

Secondary Tuberculosis. This form of tuberculosis occurs in patients previously infected. The patient will have some level of immunity and will have a positive result to a tuberculin test.

Types of Skin Tuberculosis

Lupus Vulgaris. Indolent, erythematous nodules form plaques that may be scaly, ulcerated or crusted. These are most commonly found on the face, nose and ears, but may occur at any site. The tuberculin test is strongly positive. An SCC may develop on the surface of a chronic lesion.

Scrofuloderma. This is the most common form of multibacillary skin tuberculosis. Skin infection occurs due to an underlying focus of TB, usually from lymph nodes or bone, with sinuses draining onto the surface of the skin.

Acute Haematogenous Miliary Tuberculosis. This form of tuberculosis is very rare. It normally occurs in children, but is also seen in immunocompromised adults, presenting as multiple papules, plaques or nodules (Figure 68.9). The presence of these severe symptoms helps in making this diagnosis.

Orificial Tuberculosis. This is a rare form of tuberculosis of the mucous membranes and periorificial skin as a result of auto-infection in patients with advanced progressive visceral tuberculosis. Patients with tuberculosis of the lungs will develop lesions in their mouth and on their lips. Patients with intestinal tuberculosis will develop lesions in the anus and patients with urogenital tuberculosis will have lesions in the genital area. It is easier to diagnose this form of the disease if the doctor is aware that the patient has visceral tuberculosis.

The clinical appearance of cutaneous tuberculosis is also dependent on the immunity of the patient. A hypersensitivity state may occur in patients with good immunity, causing tuberculids, which are a cutaneous hypersensitivity reaction to TB infection. Papulonecrotic tuberculid, Bazion's erythema induratum and lichen scrofulosorum are the skin manifestations of this. A diagnosis of a tuberculid should prompt further investigation to identify the underlying focus of TB infection.

Papulonecrotic Tuberculid. This hypersensitivity reaction presents as crops of papules with central pustules which develop necrotic centres and finally atrophic scars. Lesions are found characteristically in acral areas such as the elbows, knees and ears.

Bazin's Erythema Induratum. This form may resemble erythema nodosum, but in contrast tends to be seen on the calves rather than the shins. The lesions are tender red nodules that break down and ulcerate, discharging onto the surface of the skin and healing with atrophic scars. It is more common in females.

Lichen Scrofulosorum. This is a rare form, occurring in children and teenagers with primary tuberculosis or tuberculosis after vaccination. This form normally appears in the lateral part of the chest in the form of erythematous plaques, which sometimes can be followed by peeling.

Diagnosis. A tuberculin test is likely to be positive unless the patient is immunocompromised, although this is not diagnostic. Culture is the gold standard investigation, but can take a number of weeks to become positive. Culture has a low sensitivity in paucibacillary cases. PCR may be more sensitive, however PCR, microscopy and culture can each be negative.[3] If there is strong clinical suspicion, a trial of antituberculous therapy should be considered. Tuberculids can be diagnosed by positive tuberculin test and skin biopsy for histopathology.

Treatment Summary. All forms of skin tuberculosis respond to standard WHO antituberculosis regimens with 4 drugs for 2 months, followed by dual therapy for 4 months (see Chapter 40). Atypical mycobacteria must be treated with at least two antituberculous drugs, such as with rifampicin and streptomycin for 8 weeks for *M. ulcerans*. The main drugs with antimycobacterial activity are rifampicin, ethambutol, pyrazinamide,

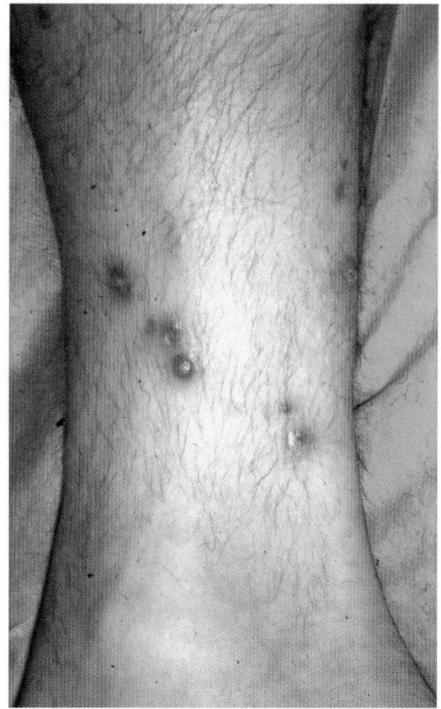

Figure 68.9 Erythematous papules, nodules and scarring caused by MAI complex infection in a patient with HIV.

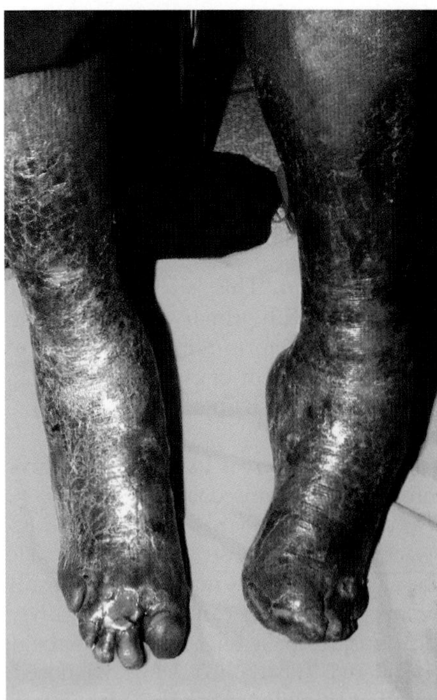

Figure 68.10 Pigmentary atrophic changes of the skin and mutilation in severe bilateral leprosy neuropathy.

clofazimine, sulfone, isoniazid, macrolide antibiotics, tetracyclines and quinolones.

Leprosy

Leprosy is a chronic disease caused by *M. leprae* which affects the skin and peripheral nerves (see Chapter 41). Untreated, it can cause severe deformity (Figure 68.10) and stigmatization.

Aetiology. *M. leprae* is a Gram-positive, alcohol–acid-resistant bacillus. Analysis using the Ziehl–Neelsen staining method will show that the bacilli are arranged in a unique pattern called globi in polar lepromatous cases.

Transmission and Evolution. Transmission is by close person-to-person contact, via nasopharyngeal secretions or via contact with an area of damaged skin. *M. leprae* is infectious but has low pathogenicity. Only a small number of those infected will develop signs of disease. The average incubation period varies from 2 to 5 years. The majority of the population in geographical areas where the disease is prevalent is immune to infection by *M. leprae*. Immunity can be tested for classification purposes using an intradermal injection of dead bacilli in the Mitsuda test.

Classification. The World Health Organization (WHO) classification divides leprosy into two groups for purposes of treatment:

- Paucibacillary cases – negative bacilloscopy. This group includes tuberculoid and indeterminate leprosy.
- Multibacillary cases – positive bacilloscopy. This group includes lepromatous and borderline leprosy.

There are WHO protocols for administering multi-drug therapy and countries in which the disease is endemic are strongly advised to adopt those policies, available on the WHO website.

Clinical Manifestations

Nerve Damage. The peripheral nervous system is compromised in all forms of the disease,[4] and leprosy is often initially diagnosed as a result of the patient experiencing sensitivity disorders. The patient will first lose the ability to detect heat, cold or a change in temperature. This will be followed by loss of the ability to feel pain and finally the patient will lose the ability to experience touch.

Cutaneous nerves can be palpably thickened, including the great auricular nerve in the neck, the superficial branch of the radial nerve at the wrist, the ulnar nerve at the elbow, the lateral popliteal nerve at the knee and the sural nerve on the lower leg. Both the sensory and motor function of each nerve should be tested. 'Tinel's sign' is paraesthesia reproduced by percussion over the nerve. Nerve damage may occur before signs of skin disease, leading to late diagnosis.

Skin Damage. The following skin manifestations are determined by the host immune response.

Indeterminate Leprosy. Indeterminate leprosy may consist of a single early poorly demarcated macule with minor sensory or vasomotor change, which may be difficult to diagnose. The macules may be erythematous or hypopigmented and there are no bacilli on smear testing.

Tuberculoid Leprosy. Tuberculoid leprosy is paucibacillary and is characterized by up to four macules or plaques with raised borders. Generally the disease in this form will appear as one or more single anaesthetic lesions asymmetrically distributed over the body. Negative bacilloscopy will be seen, but there will be an extremely positive result to a Mitsuda test.

Borderline Leprosy. This may consist of numerous erythematous plaques with moderate sensory loss.

Lepromatous Leprosy. Lepromatous leprosy is multibacillary and characterized by polymorphic lesions; the skin and the nervous system are both severely affected by multiple lesions which are symmetrically distributed. Nerve damage occurs late but the patient may suffer from a total loss of sensitivity.

The patient may develop leonine facies, hair loss from the eyebrows and eyelashes, a misshapen nose, thickened deformed earlobes, ichthyosis of the calves, glove and stocking anaesthesia with skin ulcers and deformity of fingers and toes. Males suffer from testicular damage and sexual dysfunction.

Reactions in Leprosy. There are two distinct types of reaction that can occur after becoming infected with *M. leprae*. These are classified as type 1 and type 2 reactions. Type 1 or reversal reactions appear in patients who have some level of cellular immunity such as in tuberculoid and borderline leprosy. The skin lesions all become both more erythematous and oedematous and new lesions may appear. This reaction may appear before, during or after treatment. Reversal reactions may cause acute inflammation causing rapid loss of nerve function and require prompt initiation of treatment with oral steroids.

Type 2 is known as erythema nodosum leprosum (ENL) and most commonly occurs during the course of treatment, although it can appear after the course of treatment has been completed.

ENL is a systemic illness due to immune complex deposition and symptoms can include fever, nausea, neck pain, erythema nodosum, arthralgia, epididymo-orchitis, lymphadenopathy and painful hepatosplenomegaly. ENL requires treatment with thalidomide and variable doses of oral prednisolone.

In HIV co-infection, relapse rates of leprosy appear unchanged, however leprosy may become apparent as part of immune reconstitution and these patients appear to be at increased risk of reactions.[5]

Diagnosis. Leprosy is a clinical diagnosis, supported by epidemiological data, microscopy, histology and molecular techniques. The investigation of choice is a slit skin smear to look for acid-fast bacilli. Biopsy may show granulomata or foamy cells. PCR is very sensitive and can detect *M. leprae* in skin before any visible signs.

Treatment Summary. WHO recommends the following multi-drug antilepromatous therapy regimens for adults:

- Paucibacillary leprosy: a 2-drug regimen of rifampicin 600 mg once a month (supervised) and dapsone 100 mg daily. At least 6 months of treatment must be taken within a period of 9 months.
- Multibacillary leprosy: a 3-drug regimen of rifampicin 600 mg once a month (supervised), clofazimine 300 mg once a month (supervised) and 50 mg daily and dapsone 100 mg daily. At least 12 months of treatment must be taken within a period of 18 months.

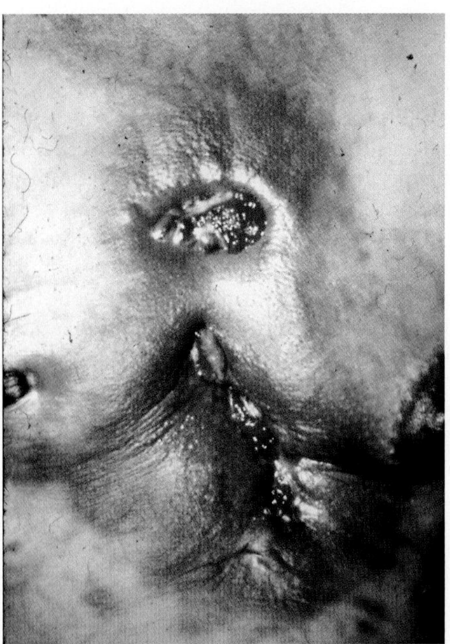

Figure 68.11 Sinus tract formation and severe scarring in chest actinomycetoma. *(Courtesy of Dr Ruben López, Mexico.)*

Management and Prevention of Mycobacterial Infections

Most mycobacterial diseases represent public health priorities not only for the endemic countries where they occur, but also at an international level. Combination antimycobacterial therapy for each disease should be administered according to international and local guidelines. The management of all mycobacterial diseases must consider not only the medical treatment but also a full range of educational initiatives aimed at the patient, the community and health personnel.

BACTERIAL MYCETOMA

Aetiology and Pathogenesis (see Chapter 38)

'Madura foot' encompasses both fungal eumycetoma and bacterial actinomycetoma. *Nocardia, Actinomadura* and *Streptomyces* spp. are the common aetiological agents of actinomycetoma. Actinomycetoma occurs in tropical countries within the 'mycetoma belt' from 15° south to 30° north of the equator. The infection is acquired by direct inoculation via the skin. Mycetomas are a disease of poverty and young male individuals living in endemic regions engaged in agricultural activities have the highest incidence of actinomycetoma. Mycetoma does not seem to represent a risk for travellers. Bacteria causing actinomycetoma are thick-walled, with compounds such as lipoarabinomannan and mycolic acids in the cytoplasmic membrane having been identified as virulence factors. They are considered to have low pathogenic potential however and most of them live as saprophytes in the soil.

Clinical Findings and Diagnosis

Actinomycetoma runs a chronic course, with nodular or verrucous lesions, inflammation, formation of sinus tracts discharging pale, red or yellow 'grains' and progressive deformity of the affected foot. Healing of discharging sinus tracts over years causes scarring, with atrophy and secondary pigmentary changes. It can be asymptomatic, however pain often results from superimposed pyogenic infection, acute inflammation or the development of osteomyelitis. Actinomycetoma may result in severe disability (Figure 68.11). The clinical picture on one foot is highly suggestive of the diagnosis.

The main differential diagnosis includes mycetoma caused by fungi (see Eumycetoma, below), histoplasmosis, chromoblastomycosis, cutaneous tuberculosis and sarcoidosis. Correct species identification greatly aids management. Direct KOH microscopy of the grains, via fine-needle aspiration or deep-tissue biopsy, can determine fungal or bacterial cause. Cultures may identify the causative species, but prolonged culture is necessary and culture is frequently negative. Serological tests such as ELISA are also used by some centres to support diagnosis and assess treatment response. X-ray, USS, CT or MRI may detect bone involvement.

Treatment

Actinomycetomas respond more favourably to drug therapy than eumycetomas, but cure rates still vary widely from 60–90%. Combined therapy is advocated to reduce drug resistance. The mainstay of treatment for nocardial infections has been with sulphonamide combinations, such as co-trimoxazole, for 6 months to several years. The addition of aminoglycosides such as amikacin to co-trimoxazole gives higher efficacy and shorter treatment duration. This is particularly advocated for severe unresponsive cases and for cases where there is a danger of dissemination to adjacent organs. A long period of follow-up is recommended to detect relapse. Actinomycetomas are not usually managed surgically.[6–8]

OTHER BACTERIAL INFECTIONS

Tropical sea-borne infections by *Vibrio vulnificus* can produce localized or systemic disease manifested by painful erythema, purpura, oedema and necrosis, particularly of the lower limbs. Cases of returning travellers presenting in inland metropolitan areas can be very difficult to diagnose and these patients carry a high mortality risk. Septicaemia manifests with coalescing purpuric patches on one or both lower limbs that subsequently spread to the periumbilical region. The infection is acquired by direct traumatic inoculation in estuaries and seawater or by ingestion of raw seafood, particularly oysters. Severe cases require immediate referral to a specialist hospital for intravenous antibiotics and early surgical debridement.[9]

Exfoliation of the face, truncal and palmoplantar skin is part of the complex and severe picture of staphylococcal scalded skin syndrome (SSSS), whereas necrotic ulceration on a limb can result from tropical cutaneous diphtheria caused by *Corynebacterium diphtheriae*. Cutaneous diphtheria commonly manifests as a non-healing single ulcerated lesion on the toe or toe cleft lasting between 4 and 12 weeks.[10]

Skin Diseases Caused by Parasites

CUTANEOUS LARVA MIGRANS

Aetiology and Pathogenesis

This dermatosis results from the accidental penetration of the human skin by hookworm larvae. Various animals pass these helminth ova with the stools and larval stages develop in soil or beach sand. Close contact with human skin allows the infective larvae to burrow into the epidermis. The main aetiological agents are *Ancylostoma braziliense*, *A. caninum*, *A. ceylanicum* and *Uncinaria stenocephala* but other species can also cause human disease. Following penetration into the skin, the larvae are incapable of crossing the human epidermodermal barrier and migrate slowly in the epidermis at a rate of 1–2 cm/day, until they die a few days or weeks later. Multiple infections can, however, last for several months. Cases of systemic invasion with a Loeffler syndrome have been exceptionally described.

Clinical Findings and Diagnosis

The feet are the main anatomical site affected (Figure 68.12), but any part of the body in contact with infested soil or sand can be involved. The disease is a common problem for tourists on beach holidays where they walk on bare feet or lie on infested sand. The initial lesion is a pruritic papule at the site of penetration that appears within a day following the infestation. An erythematous, raised larval track measuring 1–3 mm in width starts progressing in a curved or serpiginous fashion. Commonly, the larval track measures between a few millimetres up to several centimetres in the region adjacent to the penetration site. Localized infections on the toes may present with only papular lesions, but other presentations include eczematous plaques, blisters and urticarial wheals. Secondary complications include eczematization, impetigo and even deeper pyogenic infections. Intense pruritus and burning sensation are the main symptoms. The diagnosis is clinical based on history and examination.[11]

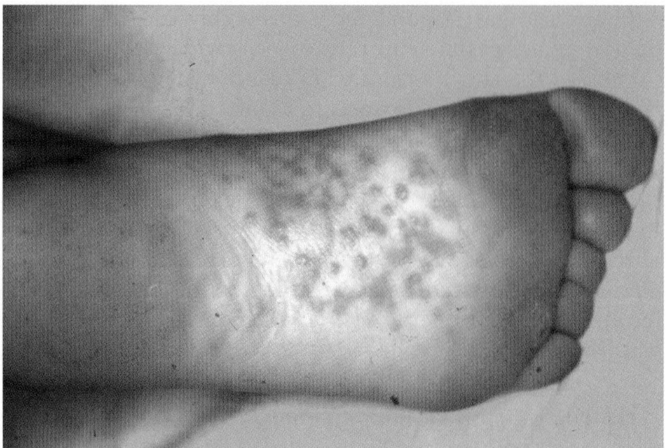

Figure 68.12 Erythematous larval track and papulovesicular eruption in unilateral cutaneous larva migrans of the plantar region.

Treatment Summary

Treatment is with albendazole 400–800 mg (according to body weight) daily for 3 days or ivermectin 200 μg/kg stat dose. Topical tiabendazole (1 g tiabendazole in 10 g yellow soft paraffin applied under an occlusive dressing for up to 10 days) may be used for early localized lesions or single tracks or in children. These drugs should be avoided in pregnancy. Liquid nitrogen cryotherapy can also be used, applied near the head of the track.

Prevention

Prevention is by avoiding walking barefoot on soil or sand in the tropics.

LEISHMANIASIS

Introduction

See Chapter 47.

Aetiology and Pathogenesis

Leishmania spp. are protozoal parasites transmitted to humans by the bite of female sandflies of the genera Phlebotomus or Lutzomya. Most *Leishmania* spp. can cause skin or mucocutaneous disease and a few can also cause visceral disease. It is estimated that 12–14 million individuals are infected by *Leishmania*, which is endemic in 88 countries. The main endemic foci are found in South Asia, the Middle East, the Mediterranean basin, North and Central Africa and Central and Latin America. A hot and humid environment such as that found in rainforest jungles provides adequate habitat for the animal reservoirs and vectors in Latin America. In contrast, desert conditions favour breeding sites for the vectors in the Middle East and North Africa.

Leishmania spp. causing skin disease in humans have been classified in geographical terms as Old World or New World cutaneous leishmaniasis. Old and New World lesions are often not distinguishable morphologically, however most of the New World species can cause potentially severe mucosal disease. *Leishmania* parasites can resist phagocytosis and damage by complement proteins from the host by the action of lipophosphoglycan and glycoprotein antigens. Following phagocytosis, the intracellular forms of *Leishmania* parasites induce a granulomatous reaction which adds to the tissue damage. This may be due to exaggerated production of IFN-γ and TNF-α which can be harmful to the tissue; the same cytokines involved in killing the parasite may be associated with the pathogenesis of cutaneous leishmaniasis and mucocutaneous leishmaniasis. Lesions may heal spontaneously or develop localized or disseminated disease, dependent on a number of factors including the species, inoculum load and host immunity.

Clinical Findings and Diagnosis

The bite of a sandfly may induce an inflammatory papule or nodular lesion that slowly progresses for several weeks. The incubation period can be as short as 15 days (or as long 20 years due to immunosuppression causing reactivation), but commonly is estimated at around 4–8 weeks. Only one area of exposed skin may be affected or multiple infective bites or disseminated forms may present with lesions on several anatomical regions. Common inoculation sites include bony prominences on the face, external aspects of the wrists and malleolar regions. On average 6–8 weeks after the sandfly bite the nodule starts to ulcerate. The ulcer is partially or completely covered by a thick crust that following curettage reveals a haemorrhagic and vegetating bed. Cutaneous leishmaniasis can be clinically manifest as nodules covered with crust, ulceration with a raised inflamed solid border, tissue necrosis and lymphangitic forms. The differential diagnosis of lymphangitic forms may include atypical mycobacterial infection or subcutaneous fungal infection. Advanced late forms present with scarring and skin atrophy. A particular localized form caused by *L. mexicana* or *L. braziliensis* is called 'chiclero ulcer' (Figure 68.13) and affects the helix of one ear, although *L. braziliensis* more commonly manifests as a single destructive ulceration of the skin (Figure 68.14).

The clinical form called post-kala-azar dermal leishmaniasis (PKDL) can present in the early stages with hypopigmented macules or papules as a delayed immune response to latent dermal parasites after an episode of visceral leishmaniasis by *L. donovani* in cases originating from India and Africa. Other common and characteristic clinical pictures include a dry, single oriental sore by *L. tropica* (Figure 68.15), a wet destructive single ulcer by *L. major*, a diffuse presentation by *L. aethiopica* and cases of mucocutaneous leishmaniasis by *L. braziliensis*. In HIV co-infection leishmaniasis can present atypically, be more severe and may present as immune reconstitution.[12]

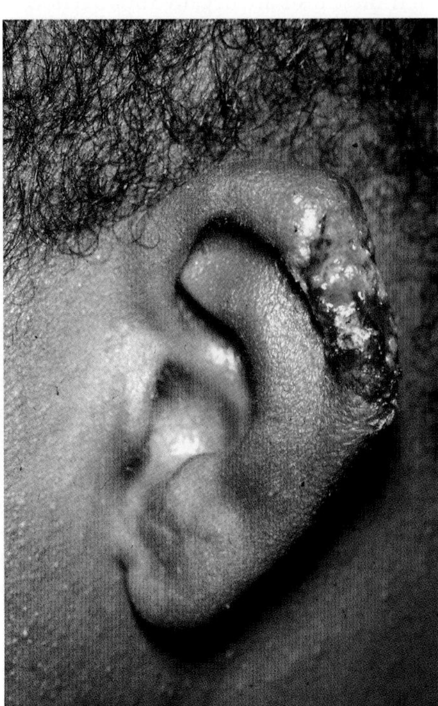

Figure 68.13 Chiclero ulcer in American cutaneous leishmaniasis caused by *Leishmania braziliensis*.

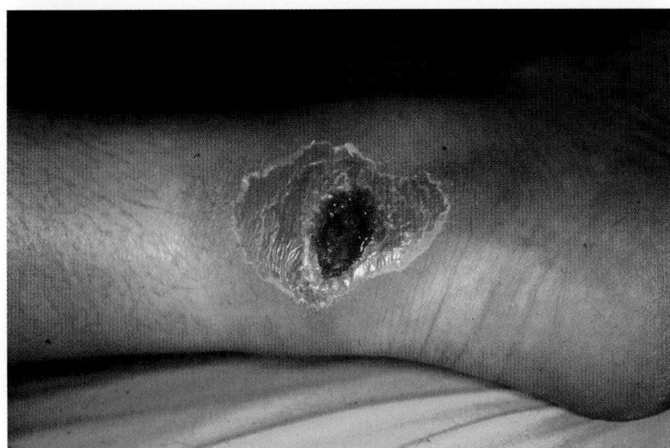

Figure 68.14 Erythemato-violaceous nodular ulceration with surrounding cellulitis caused by *Leishmania braziliensis*.

The clinical picture and history of exposure in an endemic area suggest the diagnosis. Investigation includes skin biopsies showing granulomata on HE histology, direct microscopy with Giemsa stain to reveal amastigotes and culture in NNN medium to allow for the growth of promastigotes. Determination of the infecting species by PCR has a major role helping to determine optimum treatment and the establishment of prognosis.

Management

Not all cutaneous lesions need treatment – many Old World species may heal spontaneously and single or improving lesions may simply be observed. New World species of the *L. viannia* sub-genus or New World lesions that cannot be speciated require systemic therapy because of the risk of subsequent development of mucosal disease. Physical treatments including cryotherapy and thermotherapy have been used with occasional success for simple lesions. Intralesional stibogluconate can also be used for Old World or non-*Viannia* New World lesions.

Antimonials, particularly intravenous sodium stibogluconate, are the most commonly used systemic therapy. The usual

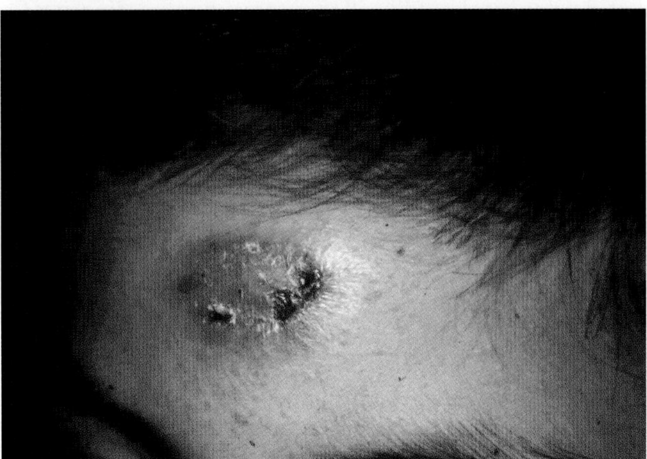

Figure 68.15 Single scarring erythematous sore with crusting in Old World leishmaniasis caused by *Leishmania tropica*.

regimen is 20 mg/kg intravenously daily for 20 days although 10 days therapy may be sufficient for Old World disease. Adverse effects are common and include hepatotoxicity and cardiotoxicity. Pentamidine is an alternative second-line agent which may possibly have fewer adverse effects than antimonials, but may have similar efficacy for *L. aethiopica* and some New World species. Oral agents that may be considered include azoles such as fluconazole or itraconazole, which have shown efficacy of 55–79% to treat Old World species. The efficacy of miltefosine has been inconsistent and may vary according to the species. Other approaches include allopurinol in combination with low-dose (e.g. intra-lesional) antimonials which has achieved similar results for mucocutaneous leishmaniasis to those obtained using full-dose antimonials, newer agents such as topical imiquimod as an adjunct to systemic antimonials and enhanced topical paromomycin formulations.[13,14]

Treatment Summary

Species identification is important for the correct management of cutaneous leishmaniasis. Localized infections with Old World species may respond to intralesional antimonials, but many New World species require parenteral therapy because of the potential to develop mucocutaneous disease. Parenteral antimonials are generally used as first-line systemic therapy.

Prevention

Individual prevention of cutaneous leishmaniasis relies on bite avoidance, with application of DEET and use of bed nets when the risk of the vector sandfly bites is highest from dusk till dawn. Public health control programmes may also be aimed at control of the local animal reservoir.

ONCHOCERCIASIS

Aetiology and Pathogenesis

This filarial disease affecting the skin and eyes is acquired through the inoculation into the skin of *Onchocerca volvulus* microfilariae by black flies of the genus *Simulium* (See also Chapter 54). It is found only in humans. Also named 'river blindness', it is primarily found in a wide band across equatorial Africa (between latitudes 15°N and 15°S), although it also affects tropical countries in Central and South America and the Yemen. It extends from Savannah regions to rainforest, with fast-flowing brooks and small rivers providing breeding sites for the black fly vectors. The female blackflies bite principally those pursuing outdoor activities throughout the day. Travellers are at risk, but it is the local population that suffers the highest toll from both clinical disease and subsequent disability.

Following an incubation period of approximately 1 year, the adult worms live freely in the skin or within fibrotic nodules or cysts named onchocercomata. The female adult worm releases microfilariae into the dermis, which are disseminated by the lymphatic system. Adult worms may live and reproduce for up to 15 years in the human host.

Clinical Findings and Diagnosis

The skin manifestations include pruritus, with lichenified papules or plaques or nodular prurigo, atrophic changes and pigmentary abnormalities. Early symptoms include fever, arthralgia and transient urticaria affecting the face and trunk. The trunk, lower limbs and buttocks are commonly involved

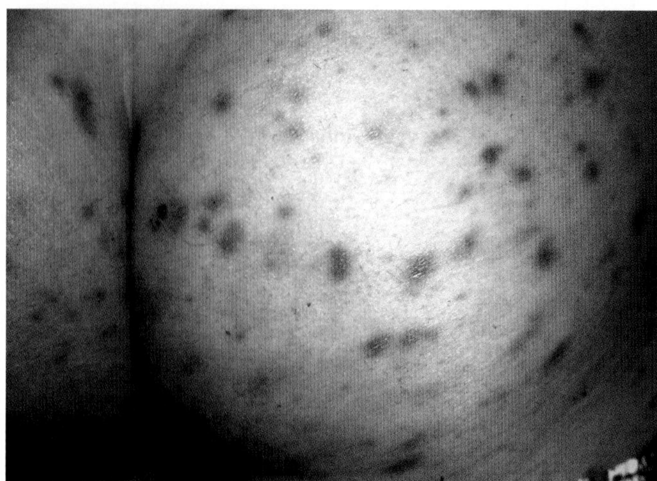

Figure 68.16 Pruritic papules and nodules on the buttocks in a patient with eosinophilia caused by onchocerciasis.

(Figure 68.16) and oedematous plaques are characteristic in Latin American cases, locally named 'mal morado'. Late skin lesions show atrophy with hyper- and hypopigmented patches giving the appearance of 'leopard skin' described in African cases. The differential diagnosis includes leprosy, syphilis, pinta and yaws. The earliest symptoms of eye involvement are redness and irritation, with late ocular lesions leading to photophobia, corneal lesions, optic atrophy and blindness.[15]

Diagnosis by microscopy for microfilariae from skin snips taken from the back, hips and thighs is less useful for early infections and has lower sensitivity than newer biochemical methods such as skin-snip PCR, serology and antigen dipstick tests. Antigen dipstick tests have a reported 100% sensitivity and 100% specificity in urine. Most patients develop peripheral eosinophilia. If these tests are negative but onchocerciasis is still strongly suspected the 'Mazzotti patch test' can be considered, by applying topical DEC (oral DEC must only be given after ophthalmological examination, as it can risk loss of visual acuity). Resolution of pruritic papular eruption may be a better indicator of cure than resolution of eosinophilia.[16]

Treatment

A single dose of 150 µg/kg oral ivermectin arrests late-stage microfilarial production, but does not fully kill the adult worms. Further research has shown that doxycycline kills *Wolbachia* endosymbiotic bacteria which sterilize adult female worms. Doxycycline has a dose-dependent macrofilaricidal effect, which is strongest at a dose of 200 mg/day for 6 weeks. A single dose of ivermectin 6 months later then appears to eradicate remaining microfilariae initially too immature to be sensitive. Doxycycline can be used for macrofilaricidal effect outside transmission areas, but is not routinely considered appropriate in areas of endemicity due to the long duration of administration and because new infections would require repeated rounds of doxycycline. The surgical excision of nodules is indicated and all patients require a comprehensive ophthalmological assessment.[17,18]

Prevention

In areas of endemicity a single annual dose of 150 µg/kg oral ivermectin is given to prevent disease progression. As it significantly reduces the microfilarial load, this reduces transmission and the prevalence of onchodermatitis and blindness. Other control strategies in endemic regions include the rotational spraying of breeding sites with insecticides.

GNATHOSTOMIASIS

Aetiology and Pathogenesis

Humans can acquire this nematode worm as accidental hosts by eating contaminated uncooked fish, shellfish, frogs, chicken, cats or dogs. The larval stages do not reach maturation in the human body, however they can cause disease in several internal organs as well as in the skin. The disease is prevalent in South-east Asia, China, Japan, Indonesia, Central and South America and in Mexico.

Clinical Findings and Diagnosis

Episodes of migrating subcutaneous oedema with pruritus can be protracted over years. The trunk and proximal limbs are commonly affected. The episodes of oedema can be inflammatory and painful. If the migratory lesions are on the face, there is a serious risk of CNS or ocular invasion. Cough, pleuritic chest pain or pleural effusion can indicate pulmonary infestation. The onset of symptoms may be delayed for months or even years. The differential diagnosis includes erythema nodosum, leprosy or the Calabar swellings of *Loa loa* infection; the travel history may help to differentiate these. Peripheral eosinophilia is common although it may subside in the chronic stages. Positive serology supports the clinical diagnosis. MRI and lumbar puncture may be necessary in suspected CNS disease.

Treatment

Albendazole has been proven to be efficacious for gnathostomiasis, with cure rates of over 90% at a dose of 400 mg bd for 21 days. Small studies of ivermectin 200 µg/kg either as a stat dose or on two consecutive days seem to show similar efficacy to albendazole. Initial treatment is not always successful and second courses of treatment have been needed in some cases. Either albendazole or ivermectin may be used sequentially in such patients. Further trials are needed to determine whether relapse rates are lower with combination drugs than with monotherapy. Follow-up should be for at least 1 year.[19,20]

LOA LOA

Aetiology, Clinical Findings and Diagnosis

Loa loa is a filarial helminth infection transmitted in the Central African rainforests by bites from the *Chrysops* fly, which can affect the skin and eyes (see also Chapter 54). As the larvae mature they migrate away from the bite site around the body in the subcutaneous tissues or deep fascial layers, at intervals producing transient, itchy oedematous lumps called calabar swellings. These can last from between a few hours to a few days. Some patients may present with recurrent migratory angio-oedema. Adult worms may be clearly visible migrating beneath the conjunctiva. Diagnosis is clinical, parasitological or serological. Microfilaria may be found on a blood smear collected around midday. Eosinophil count may be normal initially but is often raised. Symptoms may not appear until several years after the patient has left an area of endemicity.

Treatment

The surgical removal of adult worms may be possible. Microfilariae can be treated with diethylcarbamazine or ivermectin at standard doses of 150 µg/kg, however there is a risk of severe neurological reactions such as meningoencephalitis or encephalopathy due to dying microfilaria in patients with a high microfilaraemia load. These patients should therefore have their microfilaraemia load reduced with albendazole initially.[21]

TRYPANOSOMIASIS

African Trypanosomiasis

African trypanosomiasis is a protozoal parasitic infection occurring in tropical Africa transmitted by the bite of the tse tse fly. It causes a neurological disease also known as sleeping sickness, but the initial bite can produce a pruritic or painful inflammatory reaction at the site of inoculation called a chancre. This is characteristically an indurated red or violaceous nodule 2–5 cm in diameter that usually appears 48 hours after the bite and is accompanied by regional lymphadenopathy. A central necrotic eschar may form before the chancre desquamates within 2–3 weeks, leaving no trace. Many patients think of it as an isolated 'boil'. Chancres are rare in *Trypanosoma gambiense*, but occur in 70–80% of people infected with *Trypanosoma rhodesiense*. Erythematous, urticarial or macular rashes on the trunk called trypanids, which may have a haemorrhagic component, may occur in up to 50% of light-skinned individuals 6–8 weeks after the onset of illness. Diagnosis requires the identification of the parasite in blood, lymph nodes or CSF.

South American Trypanosomiasis

South American trypanosomiasis, also known as Chagas disease, occurs in Central and South America due to transmission of *Trypanosoma cruzi* from the bite of triatomine bugs in poor, rural areas. The domestic cycle is the result of human invasion in wild areas, where the vector bugs invade mud huts or shacks with crude wooden walls or palm leaf roofs in search of a blood meal. They are also known as 'kissing bugs' due to their habit of biting human faces and the parasite penetrates the skin wound or conjunctiva, leaving a local inflammatory lesion. When *T. cruzi* penetrates through the conjunctiva the local periorbital swelling with conjunctivitis and local lymphadenopathy is referred to as Romana's sign. When entry occurs through the skin wound, the erythematous or violaceous furuncle-like area of induration is called a chagoma. This may last for several weeks and be accompanied by regional lymphadenopathy. Other signs include fever, malaise, headache, myalgia, hepatosplenomegaly and transient skin rashes. The main organs affected in Chagas disease are the heart, oesophagus and intestine, although the CNS can also be invaded. Acute myocarditis may lead to cardiac insufficiency and the chronic stages can cause cardiomegaly and severe heart failure. Diagnosis requires a history of exposure to *T. cruzi* and in the early stages microscopy for identification of the parasite. In the later stages culture, serology, PCR or xenodiagnosis are required.

Treatment

Treatment (see also Chapters 45 and 46) depends upon the species and stage of disease. For *T.b. gambiense*, pentamidine or suramin is used in early-stage disease and melarsoprol or eflornithine for CNS disease. For *T.b. rhodesiense*, suramin and melarsoprol are recommended for early and CNS disease, respectively.[22]

Treatment of South American trypanosomiasis is difficult, but in the early stages nifurtimox and benznidazole may be used for a period of 30–90 days.[23]

Prevention

Measures to prevent African trypanosomiasis include vector control with insecticides, repellents and protective clothing. Prevention of South American trypanosomiasis involves residual insecticides directed at domiciliary vectors to interrupt transmission.

TUNGIASIS

Aetiology and Pathogenesis

Tungiasis is a localized skin disease commonly affecting one foot and caused by the burrowing flea *Tunga penetrans* (see also Chapter 60). This is also known as sandflea, jiggers or chigoe infestation. It has been found in Central and South America, the West Indies, Africa, Madagascar, India and Pakistan. It is the smallest known flea, measuring approximately only 1 mm in length and lives in soil near pigsties and cattle sheds. The females require blood and penetrate to the superficial dermis. After nourishment through several days, eggs are laid to the exterior and the flea dies.

Clinical Findings and Diagnosis

These fleas usually penetrate the soft skin on the toe-web spaces, but the toes and plantar aspects on the foot can be affected. The initial burrow and the flea body can be evident in early lesions, but within 3–4 weeks a crateriform single nodule develops with a central haemorrhagic punctum (Figure 68.17). Superimposed bacterial infection may cause impetigo, ecthyma and cellulitis.[24]

The differential diagnosis of a haemorrhagic nodule by *Tunga penetrans* may include an inflamed wart or a melanoma, but the short duration and history of exposure suggest tungiasis.

The diagnosis is clinical, but skin specimens for direct microscopy and histopathology with H&E stain reveal structures of the flea and eggs.

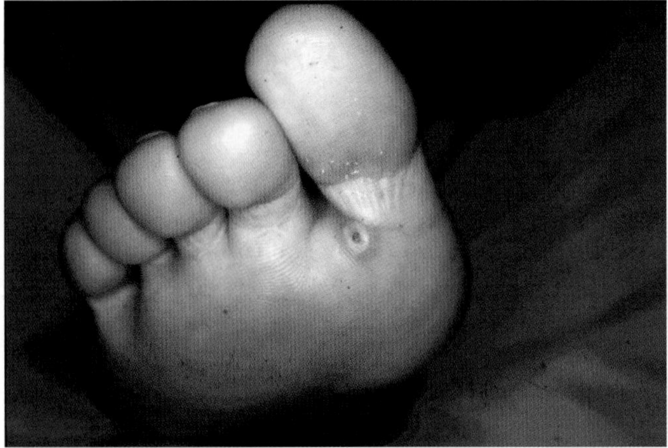

Figure 68.17 Single nodular lesion with central haemorrhage caused by *Tunga penetrans* acquired in Tanzania.

Treatment

Curettage, cryotherapy, surgical excision or application of Vaseline® and then careful removal of the flea and eggs with a sterile needle are curative. Medical management in the form of drugs such as ivermectin has not proved successful.[25] Avoidance of secondary infection is vital, particularly in individuals with diabetes, leprosy or other debilitating conditions of the feet.

MYIASIS

Aetiology and Pathogenesis

Several worldwide dipteran species in larval stages (maggots) are capable of colonizing the human skin (see also Chapter 60). This involves direct deposition of eggs, contamination by soil or dirty clothes, other insects acting as vectors or penetration of larvae into the skin. Drying clothes on a line can enable eggs to become attached and subsequently reach contact with human skin (*Cordylobia*). Species of *Dermatobia* and *Cordylobia* are the commonest found in the tropics, in the Americas and Africa, respectively.

Clinical Findings and Diagnosis

Elderly and debilitated individuals with exposed chronic wounds or ulcers are at higher risk, however most affected hosts are in good general health. In children, the scalp is a commonly affected site. Larvae feed on tissue debris and may not cause discomfort, however they can result in secondary local or systemic pyogenic infections. The diagnosis is usually clinical.

Treatment

The treatment of choice for myiasis is the mechanical removal or surgical excision of the larvae. Single furunculoid lesions can be covered by thick Vaseline or paste to suffocate the larvae, which, following death, can subsequently be extracted via a cruciform incision. Superficial infestations respond to repeated topical soaks or baths in potassium permanganate at a 1:10 000 dilution in water carried out for a few days. Cases with secondary pyogenic infection require a full course of β-lactam or macrolide antibiotics. Research has shown that it is possible to perform chemotherapy of myiasis with a single dose of ivermectin 150–200 µg/kg, however this is off-label and the larva may still need extraction.[26–28]

Prevention

Cases are observed throughout the year in tropical regions where the standards of hygiene, nutrition and general health are poor. Sleeping under mosquito nets helps prevent flies from reaching the skin. Drying clothes in bright sunlight and ironing clothes can destroy eggs laid in clothing. Other precautions include covering wounds and wearing long-sleeved clothing.

SCABIES (Chapter 58)

Aetiology and Pathogenesis

Scabies is a cosmopolitan problem but individuals in poor tropical countries with low standards of hygiene and overcrowding can suffer from cyclical outbreaks of severe and chronic forms. Direct skin contact is required for transmission. The mite burrows into the superficial epidermis, where eggs are laid. Females live up to 6 weeks and lay up to 50 eggs. A new generation of fecundated females penetrate the skin in adjacent

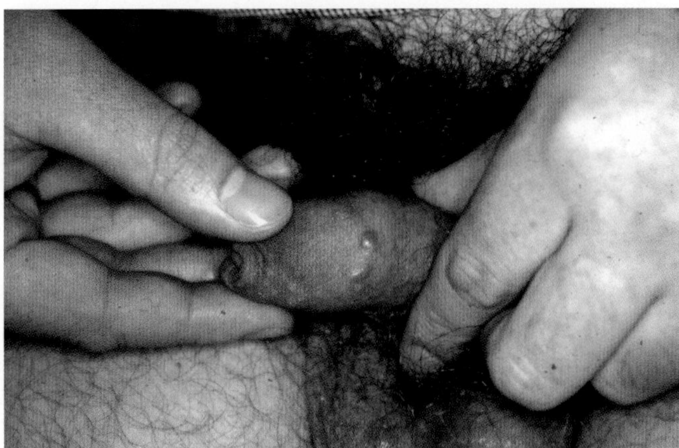

Figure 68.18 Pruritic erythematous papules of scabies on the prepuce and scrotum.

regions to the nesting burrow and the mite infestation can also be perpetuated by clothes or by reinfestation from another household host.

Clinical Findings and Diagnosis

Papules and S-shaped burrows are the classical lesions of scabies. In infants and young children both feet are commonly affected. In contrast, adults rarely manifest scabies on the lower limbs below the knees (Hebra lines), but exceptional cases of crusted scabies may present with lesions on both feet. Lesions are usually on the fingers, finger web spaces, anterior wrists, upper limbs, anterior axillary lines, areolae, periumbilical region, external genitalia, inner thighs and buttocks. A high proportion of males suffer involvement on prepuce and scrotum (Figure 68.18). Chronic crusted scabies may present with eczematization, impetiginized plaques and hyperkeratosis masking the typical clinical signs of this infestation. Large crusts (Figure 68.19) covering inflammatory papular lesions contain a high number of parasites and a careful examination is required to prevent health personnel from acquiring the infestation.

The clinical findings and intense pruritus support the diagnosis. Confirmation may be obtained by direct microscopy of skin scrapings from a burrow on a glass slide under low power although it has a low sensitivity (potassium hydroxide should not be used since it can dissolve mite pellets). Dermoscopic mite identification with a handheld dermascope can also be a useful diagnostic tool, with high sensitivity.[29]

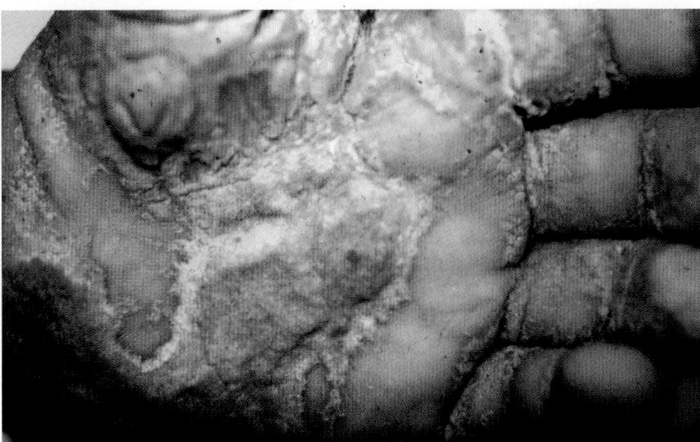

Figure 68.19 Disseminated crusted scabies in an immunodeficient child. *(Courtesy of Dr Edmundo Velázquez, Mexico.)*

Treatment

Treatment of scabies is with topical permethrin, benzyl benzoate, malathion or oral ivermectin. The patient should apply 5% permethrin cream to the whole body, including the scalp, all folds, groin, navel, external genitalia and skin under the nails, washing it off after 12 hours. In adults with classical scabies, treatment of the face is controversial, but in babies the skin of the face should also be treated. A second application 7 days after the original treatment must be prescribed and all the affected members of a household require treatment at the same time to prevent cyclical reinfestations. Oral ivermectin is being increasingly used as a first-line treatment. Severe outbreaks require a second dose of ivermectin at a 2-week interval (200 μg/kg body weight). Treatment of secondary bacterial infection and antihistamines may be required. Washing clothes and linen at 60° will kill all the young fecundated female mites (an alternative is to keep these in a plastic bag for 48–72 hours, as mites separated from the human host die within this time). It is important to explain that pruritus commonly lasts for several weeks after cure, which may be partially alleviated by non-sedating or sedating antihistamines.[30]

Skin Diseases Caused by Ectoparasites and Bites

TICKS

Ticks are cosmopolitan ectoparasites capable of transmitting severe viral, rickettsial, bacterial and protozoal diseases. The transmission of infectious agents takes place at the time of taking a blood meal from a human host that becomes infested accidentally. Infections and diseases transmitted by ticks include arboviruses, spirochaetes, spotted fever, tick typhus, relapsing fever, anaplasmosis, tularaemia, ehrlichiosis, babesiosis, tick paralysis and encephalitis. Rickettsia may also be transmitted by fleas, lice and mites. Ticks may carry more than one pathogen. Co-infection may increase disease severity and duration.

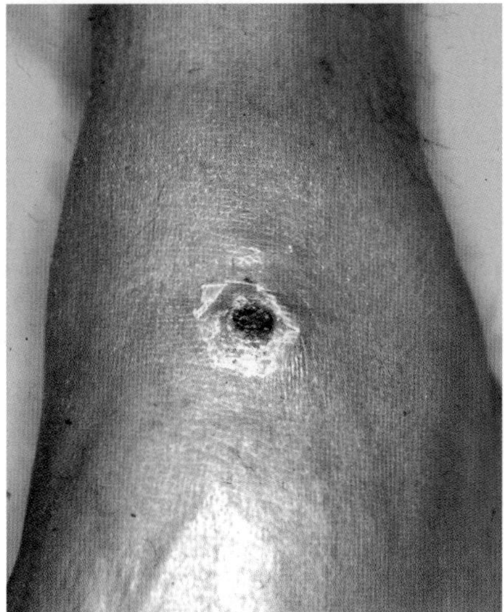

Figure 68.20 Small erythematous patch surrounding a haemorrhagic ulceration characteristic of an eschar produced by tick bite.

The bite characteristically produces an eschar (Figure 68.20). An area of circular scaling of the skin surrounding the original haemorrhagic bite can be seen after 7–10 days, although extensive subcutaneous haemorrhages can be caused by the anticoagulant inoculated with the saliva. Bites may result in necrotic ulceration, vesiculobullous lesions or oedema of the extremity. Tick bites may also be associated with local secondary bacterial infection, foreign body granuloma due to retained mouthparts, local contact dermatitis and rarely even anaphylaxis at the time of the bite.

The tick should be removed carefully with very fine forceps held as close to the skin as possible and pulled firmly out from the skin. The bite site should be thoroughly disinfected with a skin antiseptic. Squeezing of the tick during removal should be avoided as this may inject infectious material into the skin. Use of chloroform, petroleum or other organic solvents to suffocate ticks should be avoided as this can cause delay in removal with increased risk of transmission.[31]

Careful follow-up and self-surveillance are indicated, as systemic illness may start a few days or weeks following the tick bite. Symptoms such as a fever, skin rash, lymphadenopathy and fatigue indicate systemic disease. Initial investigations include serology and PCR of tissue and thick and thin films if the protozoa *Babesia* is suspected.

Treatment

Empirical antibiotic therapy should be started early before awaiting confirmation of diagnosis if rickettsial infection is suspected. The drugs of choice for treatment of rickettsial infection are doxycycline (100 mg twice a day) or tetracycline (500 mg four times a day). The duration of antibiotic therapy is related to clinical response and should be continued for at least 3 days after the patient becomes afebrile to prevent recrudescence. If infected individuals are not improving with initial treatment, co-infection should be considered.[32]

MITES

Mites can transmit *Orientia tsutsugamushi*, the causative agent of scrub typhus, which is endemic in South-east Asia, northern Australia and the western Pacific, in a geographical area known as the scrub typhus triangle. This is bounded to the north by northern Japan and southeastern Siberia, to the south by Queensland in Australia and to the west by Pakistan. The mites inhabit rural areas such as scrub forests, tall grasslands and plantations. An eschar may occur at the site of infection, with flu-like symptoms, a maculopapular rash, lymphadenopathy and a lymphocytosis. This is a potentially severe infection which can cause pneumonia, myocarditis and meningoencephalitis, with a potentially high mortality rate in untreated patients. Empirical treatment should be started if the diagnosis is suspected, pending serological results, with doxycycline 200 mg daily for 14 days.

FLEAS

The human flea *Pulex irritans* is cosmopolitan, but a number of other species show preference for tropical climates, such as the tropical rat flea *Xenopsylla cheopis*. Fleas bite humans in order to obtain a blood meal. The history may reveal an individual or family members recently moving house or acquiring second-hand wooden furniture where fleas can live for months without taking blood meals. Fleas may travel from one location to another in an individual's belongings. Fleas may be the vectors of plague or typhus and some may also transmit *Bartonella*.

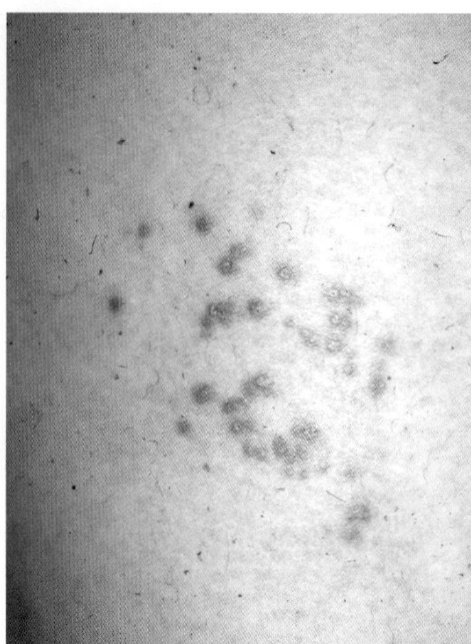

Figure 68.21 Cluster of pruritic erythematous papules on a thigh caused by *Pulex irritans*.

Pruritic papules, vesicles or small nodules of prurigo on the feet and lower legs are characteristic and the lesions are often found in clusters (Figure 68.21). The papules may reveal a central haemorrhagic punctum. Modification of the initial pruriginous lesions may result from intense scratching and superimposed secondary bacterial infection.

Management

Fumigation to eradicate fleas can be successfully achieved by using common insecticide products approved for domestic use. Severe reactions of prurigo require a topical steroid cream and impetiginized cases topical or systemic antibiotics. Antihistamine lotion or tablets may provide symptomatic relief. Severe cases are treated with a single dose or short course of systemic corticosteroids.[33]

BEDBUGS

The common bedbug *Cimex* hides during the day in cracks and crevices of walls or thatched roofs and feeds at night. Three or more bites are often inflicted in a cluster or linear fashion ('breakfast, lunch, dinner') and vary from urticated wheals to haemorrhagic blisters. There is no evidence for disease transmission by bedbugs.[34]

BEETLE DERMATITIS

Epidemics of bullous disease due to a contact dermatitis from flying beetles in hospital wards have been described in tropical climates worldwide, where windows are left open at night. 'Nairobi eye' or 'night burn' is due to a blister beetle found in Northern Kenya. Blister beetle dermatosis comprises extensive erythema, vesicles, pustules and sometimes bullae. Treatment with topical steroids may be required.

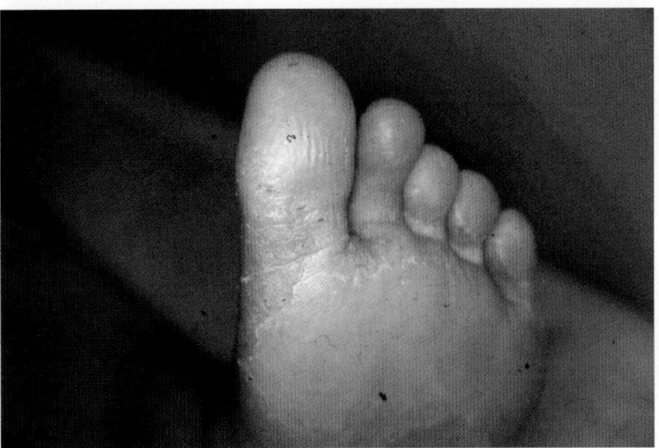

Figure 68.22 Scaling and diffuse erythema in tinea pedis.

SWIMMER'S ITCH, SEABATHER'S ERUPTION, JELLYFISH AND CORAL INJURIES

Cercarial dermatitis (swimmer's itch) is caused by penetration of the skin by the free-living larval stages of the helminth schistosomiasis in freshwater lakes. It occurs in sub-Saharan Africa, South-east Asia and parts of Brazil and Venezuela. It is a clinical diagnosis, presenting with an itchy, papular rash and a history of swimming in infected freshwater. Treatment with praziquantel should be offered. At this stage, serology may be negative and in addition urine and stool may also be negative in the first 8 weeks after infection.

Seabather's eruption is a relatively common dermatitis which occurs after swimming in sea water. Larvae of particular sea anemones become trapped in the bathing suit or wet-suit and pressure results in toxin release. Pruritic, monomorphic, erythematous papules or vesicles develop within hours on areas which were covered by the bathing suit and new lesions may continue to occur for days after the initial exposure. The rash may persist for 2 weeks or longer. Treatment is symptomatic, with topical steroids.

Jellyfish stings can cause a persistent contact dermatitis with eruptions that may recur for several months after the initial sting. Injuries to the skin from swimming in contact with coral can cause a contact dermatitis or mycobacterial infection. Seaweed can also cause a contact dermatitis.

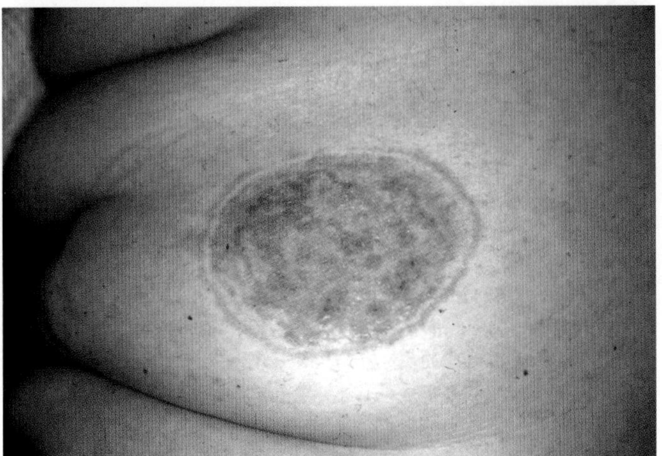

Figure 68.23 Pruritic erythematous and inflammatory localized plaque of tinea corporis.

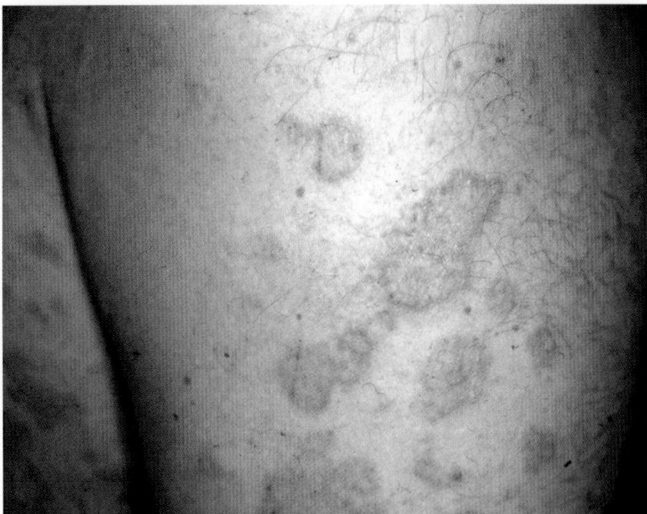

Figure 68.24 Coalescing small erythematous plaques with a microvesicular border in tinea corporis.

Skin Diseases Caused by Fungi (Chapter 38)

DERMATOPHYTES AND MALASSEZIOSIS

Aetiology and Pathogenesis

Superficial fungal infections by dermatophytes are cosmopolitan and affect any anatomical site, including scalp and nails, however they commonly occur on one or both feet. These fungi are transmitted to humans by direct skin contact from soil, vegetation, animals or other individuals. Local conditions prevalent in the tropics such as a moist and hot environment are predisposing factors. The main genera involved in human infections are *Trichophyton*, *Epidermophyton* and *Microsporum*, although there are more than 25 pathogenic species. Dermatophytes are keratinophilic, but only involve keratin and do not penetrate living tissue. They exert their pathogenesis through attachment to the skin, nails or hair by the action of acid proteinases, keratinase, elastase and lipolytical enzymes.

Clinical Findings and Diagnosis

The main clinical pictures of dermatophytes are those of localized tinea pedis (Figure 68.22), intertrigo, tinea capitis and onychomycosis. Common names for these conditions include ringworm and athlete's foot. Dermatophyte infections can manifest as localized single (Figure 68.23) or multiple coalescing circinate plaques with erythema and variable degrees of scaling such as in tinea corporis (Figure 68.24). Patients with a history of atopy are predisposed to superficial dermatophyte infections and in these cases fungal lesions may co-exist with patches of eczema. A particular form of toenail infection by *T. rubrum* manifests clinically as a subungual white onychomycosis. Scalp infections in children can manifest with the kerion clinical form with patches of non-scarring alopecia and boggy inflammation of the skin (Figure 68.25). Less commonly, adults manifest granulomatous inflammation or pustular eruptions caused by species of *Trichophyton* (Figure 68.26).

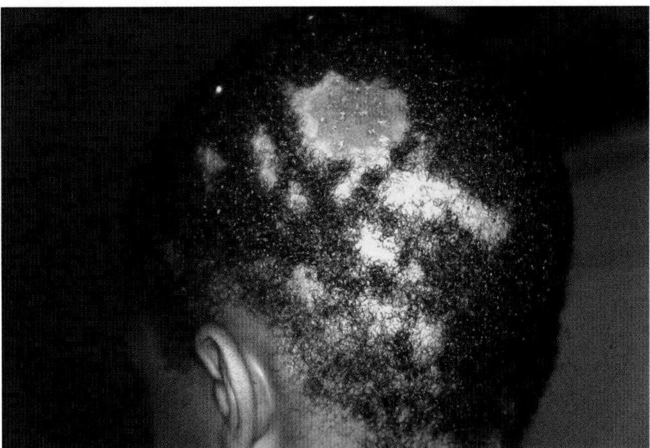

Figure 68.25 Non-scarring patchy alopecia and boggy inflammation in Celsus' kerion.

Granuloma annulare or discoid eczema should be considered in the differential diagnosis of localized ringworm and fungal infection can co-exist with plaques of psoriasis. The commensal yeast *Malassezia furfur* can cause a superficial infection called pityriasis versicolor (Figure 68.27) which is characterized by small coalescing patches or plaques on upper truncal skin and shoulders showing hyper- or hypopigmentation and furfuraceous scaling.

The diagnosis of dermatophyte infection on the skin is usually made on clinical grounds. Additional diagnostic investigations include direct microscopy of skin scrapings in 10–12% KOH solution and the identification by culture in Sabouraud's medium of the causative organism. A similar strategy is recommended for the laboratory diagnosis of pityriasis versicolor (malasseziosis) that requires special oily additives for a successful isolation in culture.

Treatment

Therapy includes the use of topical and/or systemic antifungals. Dermatophytes respond to terbinafine or griseofulvin. Malasseziosis responds to topical selenium sulphur shampoo and azole antifungals such as ketoconazole shampoo oral fluconazole or itraconazole. Localized infections require topical therapy for 3–4 weeks but cases with intertriginous athlete's foot may require up to 6–8 weeks. Oral antifungals are indicated in severe or disseminated skin infections, tinea capitis and onychomycosis. Tinea capitis (scalp ringworm) in children requires oral terbinafine (or griseofulvin) 15–20 mg/kg for 6–8 weeks. Superficial lesions and broken skin on the lower limbs can be the port of entry for pyogenic or other bacteria and superimposed bacterial infection should also be treated. This is particularly important in patients with diabetes and leprosy.

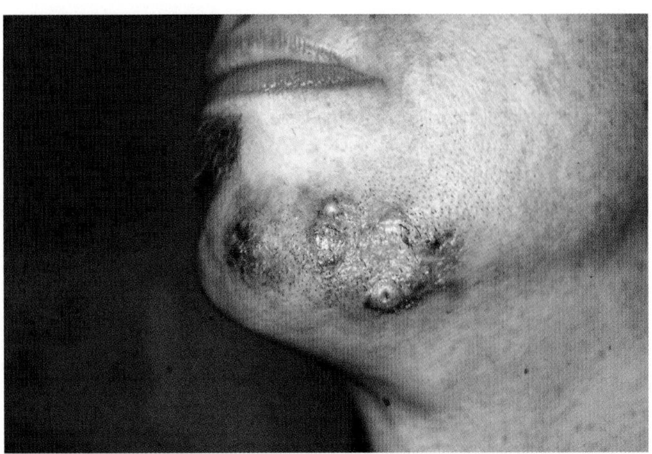

Figure 68.26 Erythematous plaque with nodules and pustules in tinea barbae caused by *Trichophyton mentagrophytes*.

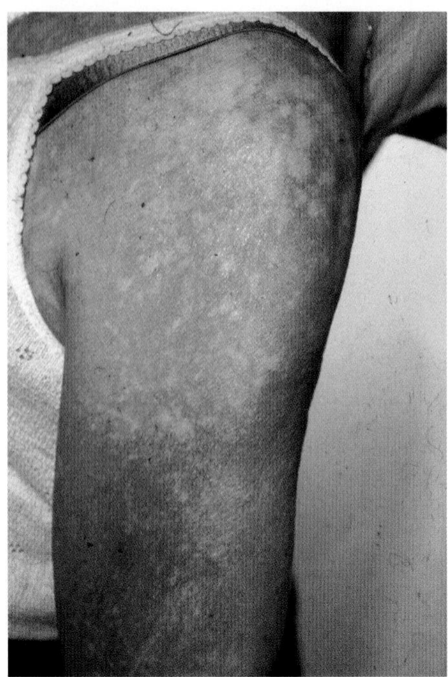

Figure 68.27 Hypo- and hyperpigmented small coalescing patches of pityriasis versicolor.

Prevention

General hygiene and appropriate footwear can be useful to treat and prevent infections, however reinfection, particularly onychomycosis and athlete's foot, is a common problem in the tropics.

SPOROTRICHOSIS

Aetiology and Pathogenesis

Sporotrichosis is a subcutaneous or deep fungal infection acquired by either direct inoculation or inhalation of *Sporothrix schenckii* as a result of outdoor contact involving thorns, splinters, straw or wood shavings. This dimorphic fungus is ubiquitous at both tropical and temperate latitudes and lives in soil, tree bark, shrubs and plant detritus. It therefore poses a risk for travellers. *S. schenckii* has low pathogenic potential but virulence factors include extracellular enzymes, polysaccharides and thermotolerance. The infective structures display strong acid phosphatase activity and mannan compounds are capable of inhibiting phagocytosis by macrophages.

Clinical Findings and Diagnosis

Sporotrichosis may manifest as a systemic pulmonary illness, but in most cases is limited to the skin, subcutaneous and lymphatic tissues. The upper and lower limbs are the usual sites of inoculation. The inoculation chancre develops into a suppurative and granulomatous infection that can disseminate proximally via the lymphatic system. Satellite lesions may develop along the path of the lymphatic vessels (sporotrichoid spread). Definitive diagnosis of sporotrichosis is based on isolation and identification in culture. However, direct microscopy, histopathology and serological tests, in the context of clinical correlation, may enable an earlier presumptive diagnosis.

Treatment

Oral itraconazole at 200–400 mg daily for 3–6 months is the drug of choice for treatment of localized cases of sporotrichosis. Intravenous amphotericin B is the drug of choice for disseminated sporotrichosis or CNS involvement. Pulmonary disease can be treated with either agent.[35,36]

Prevention

Protective footwear, clothing and gloves to avoid skin contact with splinters, rough bark, plant detritus and soil when gardening, handling hay or planting seeds or trees are the most efficient methods to prevent sporotrichosis.

EUMYCETOMA

Aetiology and Pathogenesis

Madurella mycetomatis, *Pseudallescheria boydii* and *Leptosphaeria senagalensis* are the main aetiological agents of fungal mycetoma, also known as eumycetoma. Eumycetoma occurs in Sudan, Senegal and Saudi Arabia, particularly in arid or semi-arid regions. Cases also occur in India, Central and South America and in the south of the USA. Transmission is by direct traumatic inoculation.

Clinical Findings and Diagnosis

Eumycetoma affects predominantly young males between 20 and 50 years of age. The classic clinical triad is the presence of a subcutaneous mass, sinus tract formation and granular discharge affecting particularly one foot (Figure 68.28) or other parts of the body. The perimalleolar region and the foot dorsum are the most commonly affected sites. Mycetomas should be considered as part of the differential diagnosis of all subcutaneous swellings in endemic regions. Pigmentary changes of the skin and scarring result from chronic inflammation over months or years. Periosteal involvement can progress to bone resorption, osteolysis and irreversible osteomyelitis.

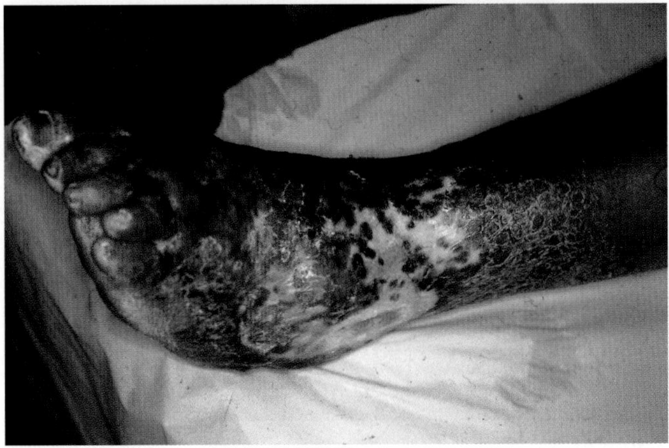

Figure 68.28 Deformity, atrophy, sinus tract formation, scarring and pigment disorder in fungal mycetoma.

Diagnosis is by direct microscopy and histological sections of deep skin specimens revealing pale or black grains between 0.5 and 1 mm in size containing fungal structures. This material grows in agar containing glucose and peptone. Fungal culture can be particularly difficult. Serology is not always sensitive and can be prone to cross-reactivity. A species-specific PCR has now been developed for identifying *M. mycetomatis*, the commonest black grain causing eumycetoma. Radiological investigation identifies periosteal involvement, cortical resorption and osteolysis.

Treatment

Eumycetoma usually responds less well than actinomycetoma to medical management and is therefore combined with aggressive surgery. Surgical excision of lesions or debulking together with medical therapy started before surgery and continued afterwards is the preferred therapeutic strategy. Typically, drug therapy is long-term lasting 18–24 months or longer. A poor response is not uncommon however despite high-dose antifungals and long therapy duration. Small lesions that can be easily excised have a more favourable prognosis, whereas osteomyelitis often requires amputation. Itraconazole (300–400 mg daily) and ketoconazole (400–800 mg daily) are the mainstays of therapy for eumycetoma. There is some evidence that the newer azoles, voriconazole (up to 600 mg daily) and posaconazole (at 800 mg daily in divided doses) may be more efficacious, although expensive long-term therapy is still required.[37]

Prevention

Education and use of protective footwear are important strategies for prevention.

CHROMOBLASTOMYCOSIS

Aetiology and Pathogenesis

This is a chronic infection caused by pigmented fungi of *Fonsecaea*, *Cladosporium* and *Phialophora* spp. The disease is widely distributed in the tropics and affects predominantly agricultural workers, who acquire the infection through direct inoculation into the skin. Numerous cases have been reported mainly from Costa Rica, Cuba, Brazil, Mexico, Indonesia and Madagascar.

Clinical Findings and Diagnosis

The initial lesion starts as a papule or nodule that subsequently develops a warty appearance. This is characteristically slow to develop and becomes a large verrucous asymptomatic plaque. The commonest sites affected are the foot dorsum or perimalleolar region. The plaque may become very thick over several years, causing gross deformity of the affected foot. Varying degrees of disability and recurrent secondary infections and/or infestations are a common problem for the foot with chromoblastomycosis. Less characteristic clinical forms include psoriasiform, rupioid and sporotrichoid localized pictures.

The diagnosis is confirmed by direct microscopy of a scraping taken from the characteristic black dots visible on the surface of skin lesions. This will show thick-walled, multiseptate brown sclerotic cells known as 'copper pennies', 'Medlar bodies' or 'muriform cells', which are pathognomonic of chromoblastomycosis, irrespective of the causative species. The histopathology of skin specimens is characteristic, showing acanthosis with a granuloma formation and the presence of typical fungal structures known as fumagoid or muriform cells. Culture in glucose–peptone agar may be inconclusive. ELISA has proved to be a valuable tool for the diagnosis and follow-up of patients with chromomycosis (due to *C. carrionii*). PCR assays have been developed for the identification of Fonsecaea species and *C. carrionii.*

Treatment

Localized early cases respond successfully to complete surgical excision. In extensive disease a more realistic goal may be disease reduction and control, as even years of continuous drug therapy may fail to clear the lesions. First-line medical agents are itraconazole (200–400 mg daily) or terbinafine (500–1000 mg daily) given for a minimum of 6–12 months, preferably at the higher dose if tolerated. These drugs in combination may be synergistic. A single small study has demonstrated effectiveness with long-term posaconazole in refractory cases and voriconazole has also shown promise. Drug therapy can be combined with surgery or physical destructive treatments such as cryotherapy or thermotherapy. Ideally antifungal chemotherapy should be started before surgery and continued afterwards. Drug therapy should be continued for several months after cure in order to prevent relapse.[38–40]

SYSTEMIC MYCOSIS MANIFESTING ON THE SKIN

Infections by *Coccidioides immitis, Histoplasma capsulatum* and *Paracoccidioides brasiliensis* commonly manifest with pulmonary disease, but haematogenous dissemination results in the appearance of skin lesions.

Coccidioidomycosis

Coccidioidomycosis is acquired through inhalation of infective spores in subtropical desert regions of the world, most commonly in urban areas in the Americas. South and western states in the USA and north-western regions of Mexico are well-recognized endemic regions. This systemic mycosis presents a risk particularly for the immunocompromised traveller. The skin becomes involved in a small proportion of cases and lesions manifest as erythematous, verrucous, scarring or scaling nodules on the face, trunk (Figure 68.29), upper or lower limbs. A history of exposure in endemic regions followed by an episode of erythema nodosum supports the diagnostic possibility. Microscopy, serology, chest X-ray and culture may confirm the diagnosis. Culture of agents causing systemic mycoses should only be carried out in specialized laboratories as they represent a serious biological hazard.

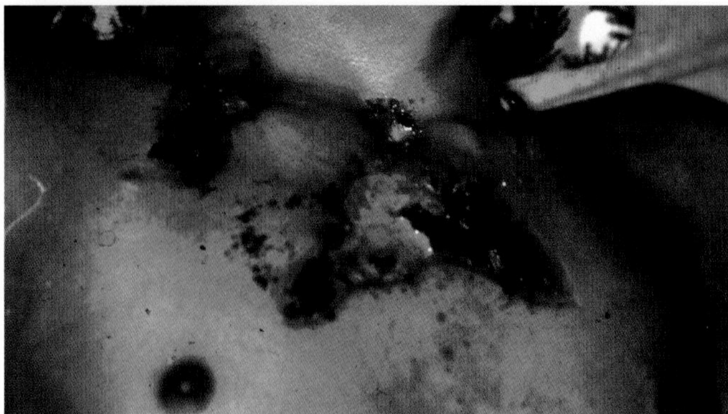

Figure 68.29 Ulcerated plaques and scarring of the trunk in coccidioidomycosis. *(Courtesy of Dr Sergio González, Monterrey, Mexico.)*

Treatment. Systemic therapeutic options for coccidioidomycosis include triazole compounds such as fluconazole (400–800 mg daily) or itraconazole (200 mg bd) or amphotericin B in severe cases, with surgical intervention sometimes being required as an adjunctive measure.[41]

Histoplasmosis

Histoplasmosis is a worldwide mycosis found in birds' and bats' excreta (guano) and is highly prevalent in caves and abandoned mines. This infection is caused by the dimorphic fungus *Histoplasma capsulatum* var. *capsulatum* (American) or var. *duboisii* (African), acquired by inhalation. Acute or chronic pulmonary forms may be asymptomatic or severe, with high mortality rates. The main differential diagnosis is pulmonary tuberculosis. A low proportion of chronic forms may result in haematogenous dissemination to the skin and mucosal regions, presenting as ulcerations or erythematous exudative nodules (Figure 68.30). Diagnosis is made by history of exposure, clinical picture, chest X-ray, direct microscopy and culture in Sabouraud's medium. Immunocompromised individuals are at higher risk.

Treatment. Preferred systemic therapeutic agents for histoplasmosis include itraconazole and amphotericin B.[42]

Paracoccidioidomycosis

Paracoccidioidomycosis occurs only in the American continent, particularly in Mexico and Central and South America. It

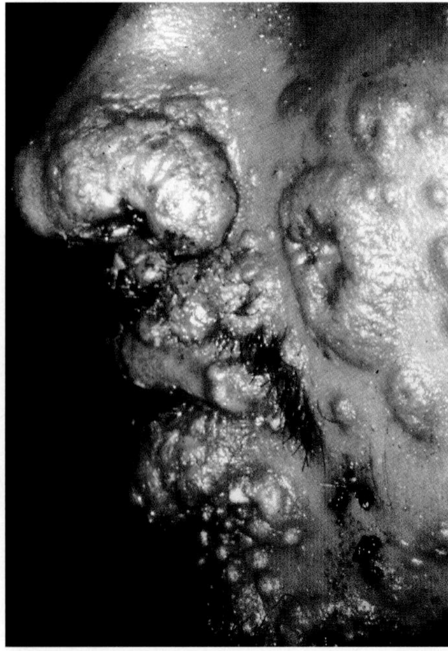

Figure 68.30 Nodular lesions and plaques with exudate on the face in a case with histoplasmosis. *(Courtesy of Dr Alexandro Bonifaz, Mexico.)*

predominantly affects male agricultural workers, but can occur in urban environments. Infection is via inhalation or direct inoculation into the skin. It may present many years after an individual has left an endemic region, with an average latency period of 15 years, but up to 60 years has been reported. Following a chronic picture of lung involvement, weight loss and fatigue, the skin of the face, particularly periorificial or else of other anatomical location on lower limbs, becomes affected. Painful nodular, haemorrhagic, ulcerated and verrucous lesions can be observed covered by a thick crust (Figure 68.31) and advanced forms of the disease can result in severe disability. The adrenal glands may be involved causing Addison's disease. A chest radiograph and lumbar puncture are necessary in all cases. Direct microscopy from skin lesions or bronchoalveolar lavage is more sensitive than H&E preparations for histology, which reveal the presence of the typical large budding yeast cells. These may also be identified in culture. PCR is a sensitive and specific method for rapid diagnosis and may also be useful for monitoring response to treatment.[43]

Treatment. Treatment of paracoccidioidomycosis is with oral itraconazole 200–300 mg daily for 6–12 months, depending on clinical response or intravenous amphotericin B for severe or resistant cases.[44]

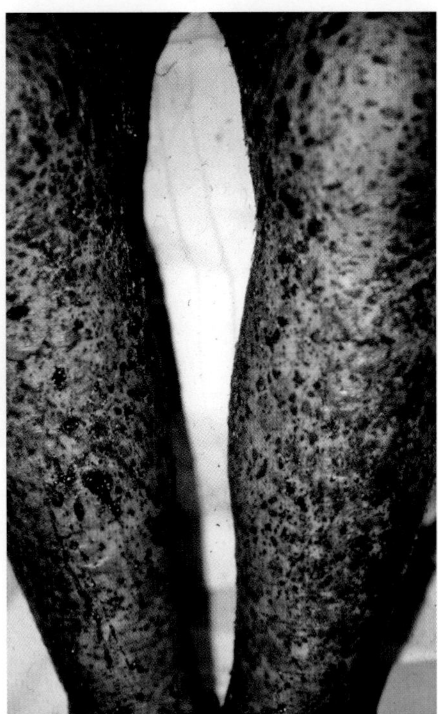

Figure 68.32 Disseminated blistering and crusting in a case of varicella infection.

Diseases Caused by Viruses

Most common viral skin diseases are cosmopolitan, but the onset may coincide with a trip to the tropics and pose problems in the differential diagnosis of the returning traveller. Viral infections that are prevalent in the tropics include molluscum contagiosum in children, plantar warts in adults, Kaposi's sarcoma in patients with HIV infection and severe blistering forms of varicella (Figure 68.32). Severe cases require a full diagnostic protocol with specimens for culture, electron microscopy, serology and histopathology, followed by specialized treatment in tertiary referral centres.

Patients with HIV infection commonly suffer from one or more skin conditions, including pruritus, xerosis, eczema, seborrheic dermatitis, recalcitrant viral warts (Figure 68.33) or worsening of psoriasis. The frequency and number of infectious skin disorders increase with progressing HIV infection and include cytomegalovirus, severe dermatophyte infections, cutaneous cryptococcosis (Figure 68.34) and Kaposi's sarcoma (Figure 68.35). With antiretroviral therapy, inflammatory skin disorders predominate in HIV infection and the incidence of cutaneous non-AIDS-defining cancers may be increased, particularly in Caucasian individuals (Figures 68.36, 68.37).

Non-infectious Skin Problems in the Tropics

The clinical expression of tropical skin disease may vary with ethnicity and socioeconomic and environmental factors, leading to differing presentations and different approaches to treatment.

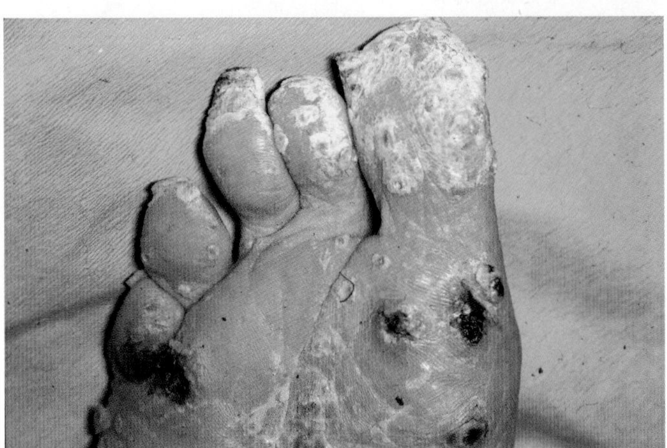

Figure 68.31 Hyperkeratotic, verrucous, ulcerated and crusted lesions on the feet in a patient with paracoccidioidomycosis.

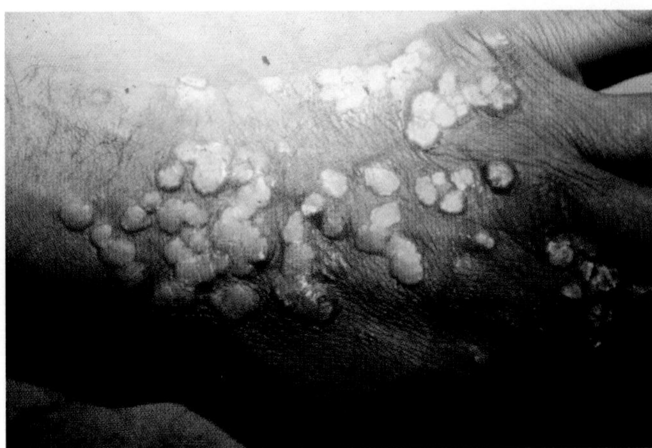

Figure 68.33 Chronic warty plaques on the dorsum of the hand caused by human papillomavirus in a patient with HIV.

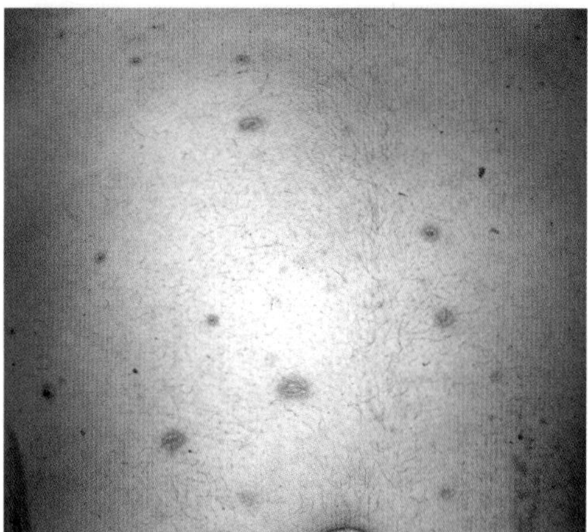

Figure 68.34 Erythematous lesions with central ulceration in cutaneous cryptococcosis.

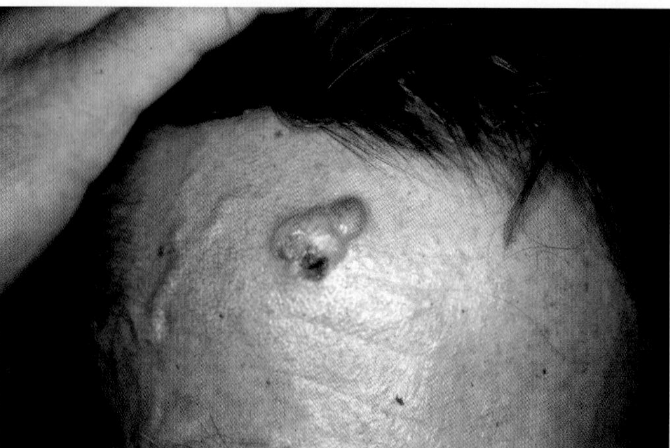

Figure 68.36 Large nodular basal cell carcinoma in a Caucasian patient with HIV infection.

ACNE VULGARIS

Acne is a disorder of the pilosebaceous unit involving four interrelated pathophysiological factors: excess sebum production, blockage of the pilosebaceous duct, proliferation of the commensal bacterium *Propionibacterium acnes* and resulting inflammation. The underlying aetiology is hormonally mediated via androgens. Clinically, the excess sebum production and blockage results in either a comedone or an inflammatory lesion. This is an ideal environment for the proliferation of *Propionibacterium acnes*, which results in the release of pro-inflammatory mediators. The comedones present as blackheads and whiteheads and the inflammatory lesions present as inflamed papules, pustules and cystic nodules. A patient may have a mixture of all lesions or a predominance of either comedones or inflamed lesions. A tropical environment causes increased sebum production and patients may find either an exacerbation or the first initial presentation of acne when they travel from a temperate zone to a tropical zone. There is considerable ethnic variation in the incidence of acne, with South-east Asians having less sebaceous gland activity and decreased incidence of acne as well as it being less severe. Black-skinned patients are more likely to form comedones and white-skinned patients more likely to have inflammatory acne. Patients with black skin may respond to inflammatory acne by forming keloid scars which can result in gross disfigurement. The distribution of acne occurs where the density of sebaceous glands is greatest, namely the forehead, cheeks, chin (Figure 68.38), upper chest and upper back.

Management of Acne Vulgaris in the Tropics

Early treatment of acne is essential to prevent cosmetic disfigurement associated with scarring.

Comedonal Acne. Topical tretinoin or adapalene used once daily at night is now first-line. Topical retinoids are used at night as they can photosensitize the skin and are washed off in the morning. If topical retinoids are not available, salicylic acid up to 2% in numerous formulations may be used as a comedolytic and mild anti-inflammatory agent. Topical azelaic acid can also be effective. A specific form of comedomal acne that is

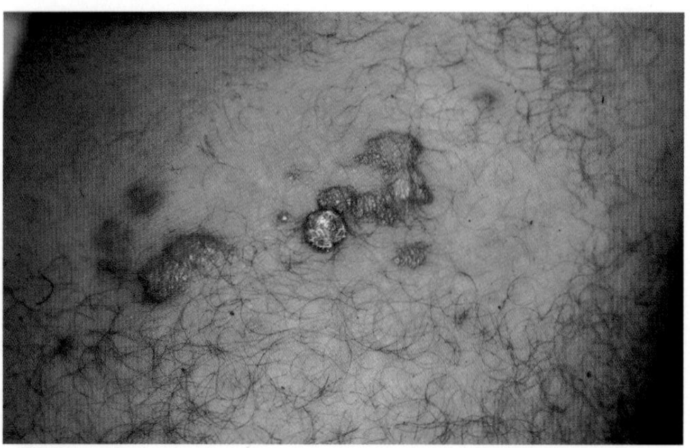

Figure 68.35 Violaceous plaques and nodules of Kaposi's sarcoma in a patient with HIV infection.

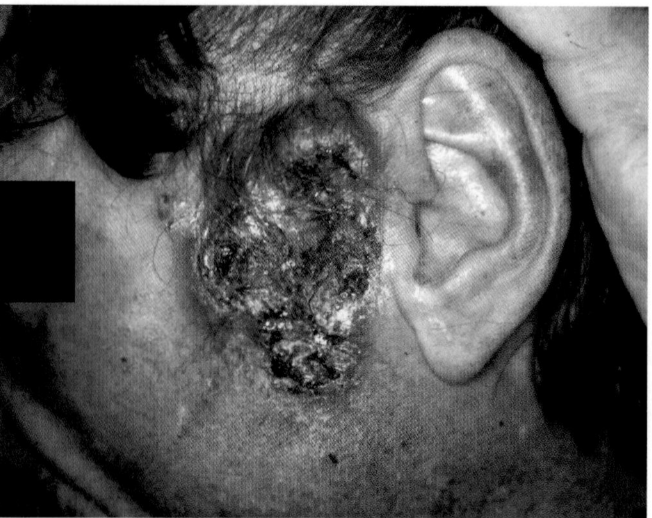

Figure 68.37 Ulcerated and exophytic large squamous cell carcinoma in a Caucasian patient with HIV infection.

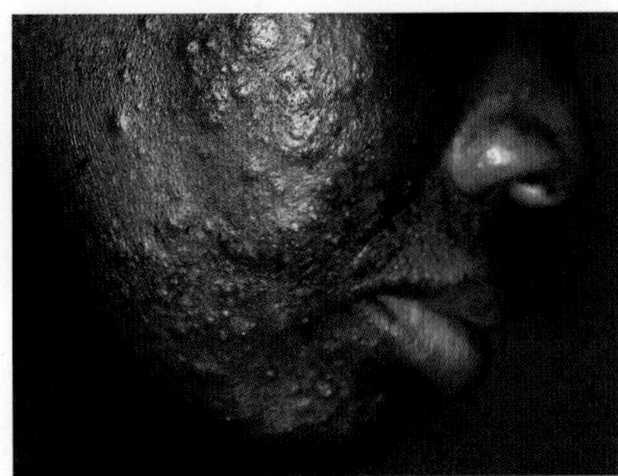

Figure 68.38 Papular, nodular and cystic facial late-onset acne.

very common in black patients is pomade acne, due to the application of waxes, greases and oils to the hair, resulting in pilosebaceous duct blockage and therefore comedogenesis. Ideally, the patient should cease using such materials on the hair.

Inflammatory Acne. Mild inflammatory acne may be treated by either 5–10% benzoyl peroxide on its own or benzoyl peroxide combined with erythromycin or topical clindamycin twice daily. More severe inflammatory acne will require systemic antibiotics such as tetracyclines or erythromycin or trimethoprim if tetracyclines are contraindicated. Systemic retinoids in the form of roaccutane are the treatment of choice for severe cases. A 4–6-month course of 0.5–1.0 mg/kg per day causes complete remission in most cases. Hormonal therapy with cyproterone combined with an oestrogen can be very effective in female patients, even when serum androgens are normal.

ECZEMA/DERMATITIS

Eczema is not a single disease, but rather a family of conditions, the hallmark of which is epidermal oedema (spongiosis), trans-epidermal water loss and pruritus. Both endogenous and exogenous factors may interact in the pathogenesis. The main exogenous eczema is contact dermatitis, either irritant or allergic. Endogenous forms of eczema include atopic dermatitis, seborrhoeic dermatitis, pompholyx, varicose eczema, xerotic eczema and discoid eczema.

Pruritus leads to chronic scratching and the epidermis becomes hyperkeratotic and lichenified. The epidermal oedema of acute eczema manifests clinically as vesicles; if these rupture the extracellular fluid accumulates and evaporation of water leaves protein behind, leading to crusting.

ATOPIC DERMATITIS

Atopic dermatitis itself is increasingly being recognized as a collection of disorders, with differing genetic predisposition. The clinical expression of atopy is dependent on the interaction of genetic and environmental factors. Bacterial colonization with *Staphylococcus aureus* can occur in exacerbations of atopic dermatitis. A small section of the atopic population may have reactions to *Malassezia furfur*. Indeed, in some atopics, exacerbations may be controlled with topical ketoconazole or oral itraconazole. *Trichophyton rubrum* infection has been similarly implicated. Since fungal infections are extremely common in the tropics, fungal infection is an important factor in the exacerbation of atopic dermatitis.

Presentation

Presentation may be classic or can be very varied. The earliest manifestations of atopic dermatitis are dryness and transient redness of the skin, however most clinical manifestations of atopic dermatitis are a result of the secondary skin lesion caused by the patient continually scratching. The distribution is symmetrical and varies with age at presentation. Infants have involvement of areas where they can reach to scratch, such as the extensor extremities, the scalp, neck and face. Once the child is over 4 years old, facial involvement is less common and lesions present in the antecubital and popliteal fossae, the neck, wrists and the ankles. Adult involvement tends to be flexural. In darker-skinned patients, scratching may produce follicular papules instead of lichenification and it is important to note that the reaction may be entirely follicular, often found para-umbilically and on the extensor surface of the elbows. Darker-skinned patients may also undergo postinflammatory hyperpigmentation, which may take several years to resolve.

Complications

Abnormal cell-mediated immunity may lead to ocular herpes simplex virus infection and corneal damage. Generalized infection with herpes simplex virus can occur and can be rapidly fatal if not treated. Such an infection is called eczema herpeticum; the patient is unwell with a fever and has the appearance of multiple monomorphic punched-out erosions on the skin. Atopics are also more susceptible to infection with molluscum contagiosum virus, as well as the human papillomavirus.

Management

Avoidance of precipitating factors for pruritus such as heat and perspiration is especially relevant in the tropics. Some 90% of patients are intolerant to wool and this should be avoided, with cotton being the clothing material of choice.

Topical Therapy

Regular emollients and intermittent topical steroids are the mainstays of therapy for atopic dermatitis. Topical steroids are classified into weak, moderate and potent strengths. The patient is instructed to apply the required strength of topical steroid sparingly twice a day until the symptoms have subsided. Topical steroids are then slowly tapered to reduce the potency. In general, weaker steroids should be used on the face and flexures, with stronger steroids being used on the more lichenified areas. In adults, where flexures are more likely to be colonized by fungi, it may be wise to use a preparation that contains an antifungal, such as Daktacort® or Trimovate®.

Unfortunately, steroids are associated with folliculitis, telangiectasia, striae, cataracts and glaucoma (when used around the eyes). Tachyphylaxis and systemic absorption can also occur.

The phosphatase calcineurin enzyme inhibitors tacrolimus and pimecrolimus prevent the dephosphorylation activity crucial for the transcription of numerous cytokines involved in inflammation and are now used topically as steroid-sparing agents in moderate to severe atopic eczema, particularly on the face and neck in children.

Systemic Therapies

PUVA or UVB phototherapy is very effective in atopic dermatitis but requires the use of specialized facilities often not available in the tropics. However, one of the advantages of the tropics is that such radiation is freely available and, if cultural factors permit, the patient should be instructed to expose the body to sunlight, beginning with small periods of time such as 10–15 minutes and building up over weeks to 1 or 2 hours.

Azathioprine is used in the treatment of severe atopic dermatitis. The risk of myelosuppression is increased in those with low levels of the enzyme TPMT which metabolizes azathioprine and TPMT should be measured before commencing therapy.

Ciclosporin has been shown to be highly effective in both childhood and adult atopic dermatitis in clinically controlled trials. It is started at a dose of 2.5–5 mg/kg and the dose adjusted according to clinical efficacy and safety. Ciclosporin may be nephrotoxic and requires regular monitoring of renal function.

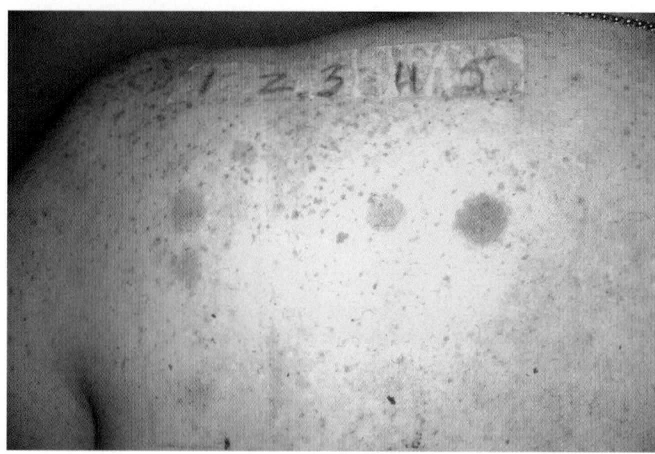

Figure 68.40 Erythema and induration of positive patch testing read at 96 hours.

CONTACT DERMATITIS

This is divided into irritant and allergic contact dermatitis. The vast majority of cases of contact dermatitis are of the irritant type. Irritant contact dermatitis occurs due to the application of a normally irritant substance to the skin and is most often occupationally related, involving contact with detergents or chemicals. Individuals vary in their susceptibility to such irritation, however all irritants when applied in sufficient concentration in frequent-enough applications will cause an irritant dermatitis.

About one-quarter of all contact dermatitis is due to allergy to a specific substance, which is a type IV delayed hypersensitivity reaction. In such cases, patch-testing has to be performed to identify the causative antigen. A DTH reaction may occur in response to metal such as nickel (Figure 68.39) and fragrances.

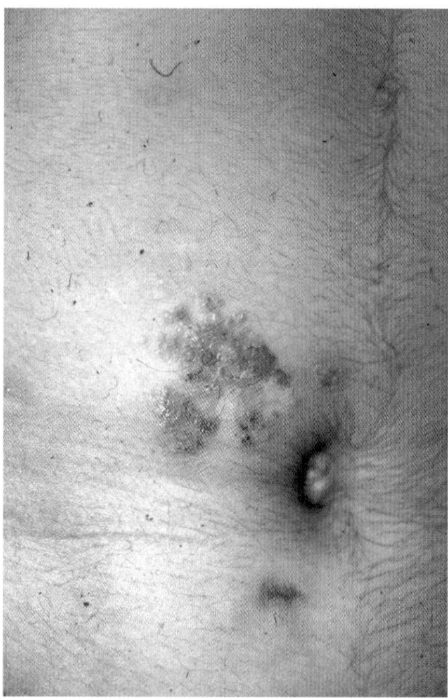
Figure 68.39 Acute allergic contact dermatitis to nickel from the metal button and buckle of blue jeans.

In Europe, there is a standard battery of the commonest allergens in the form of a patch-test. Patch-tests are applied on a suitable anatomical location which is usually the back, for a period of 48 hours and then removed and patches are then reviewed again a further 48 hours later in order to identify a positive reaction. Any area of redness under each patch is graded as a positive result (Figure 68.40). Treatment requires avoidance of irritant or allergen as well as using emollients instead of soap and topical steroids.

POMPHOLYX

This is very common in the tropics, being associated with sweating of the hands and feet. The initial pathophysiological process of epidermal oedema causes superficial vesicles and since the keratin layer of the palmoplantar skin is especially thick they do not burst or form crusts. The condition usually begins on the sides of the fingers and is intensely itchy. It may be associated with other forms of endogenous eczema and with tinea pedis. Treatment is to avoid sweating of the hands, use of emollients instead of soap and potent topical corticosteroids. Calcineurin inhibitors have been shown to be effective as well. Secondary fungal infection can be a complication.

DISCOID ECZEMA

This consists of symmetrical coin-shaped patches which are atypical of most eczemas in that they are well defined and up to 2 cm in diameter. When they first present as solitary lesions they may be mistaken for cutaneous fungal infection. They are commonly found on the arms and legs and vary in the degree of pruritus. Treatment should be followed as for atopic dermatitis.

Treatment Summary

Emollients should be used as a soap substitute and to moisturize the skin several times daily. Topical steroids are the mainstay of therapy for relapses. Topical calcineurin inhibitors can be considered as maintenance treatment to reduce long-term use of topical steroids. Secondary infections require therapy with antibiotics and/or antifungals. Sedating antihistamines are commonly required. Treatment of contact dermatitis requires avoidance of the irritant or allergen. Oral immunosuppressant medication may be required for severe eczema.

KELOID

Keloid scars result from an abnormal wound-healing process in which the normal regulatory pathways of tissue regeneration and scar remodeling are disrupted, although the pathogenesis continues to be investigated. Incidence is increased in darker skin types. Keloids may occur after surgical procedures and are defined by their extension beyond the area first traumatized. Clinically, keloids are raised, dense and hard, with a shiny erythematous or hyperpigmented surface, with borders which are usually smooth and may have claw-like extensions. The commonest sites are the earlobes, mid chest, upper back and shoulders. They can be painful or itchy.

Acne keloidalis nuchae is a chronic progressive keloidal scarring process on the nape of the neck that affects mainly black men who have their hair cut short. Follicular inflammation elicits a foreign body inflammatory reaction in the dermis, where scarring leads to keloidal formation. Clinically, a follicular pustular eruption is found on the nape of the neck and this may cause a scarring alopecia.

Treatment

Treatment of keloids may be medical and/or surgical. Keloid scars may be excised as long as there is not too much tension on the postoperative wound. They may be shaved down to follicular level and then injected with a single dose of potent intralesional steroids postoperatively, followed-up by monthly injections until control of the scar is attained. Intralesional steroids may be used on their own in order to induce atrophy of smaller scars. Active inflammatory pustules in acne keloidalis nuchae may be controlled with oral tetracyclines combined with a potent topical steroid twice daily. Residual keloid lesions of acne keloidalis nuchae may be injected with intralesional steroid.

PSORIASIS

Epidemiology and Aetiology

Psoriasis is a chronic autoimmune disease which is now known to include systemic features. Activated T cells play a major role in the pathogenesis. Psoriasis predominantly affects the skin and joints, but can also be associated with an increased risk of cardiovascular disease, particularly in severe psoriasis and an increased risk of metabolic syndrome and lymphoma. The incidence is around 1%, with a global distribution. It has a genetic basis, but environmental factors are heavily implicated in first presentation and exacerbations. Aetiological environmental factors can include smoking, alcohol, medications such as chloroquine, HIV disease, psychological stress and sunlight. It tends to arise in two different age groups: between 20 and 30 years and between 50 and 60 years.

Clinical Features

Psoriasis can present with a number of morphological forms and can affect a distribution of a few areas to total skin surface involvement. The diagnosis is clinical, from the morphology and distribution of skin lesions. In some patients it may go into complete remission, whereas in others it may continue to remit and relapse in a chronic form. The classic psoriasis lesion is a well-defined, erythematous, raised plaque with a thick white silvery scale on its surface.

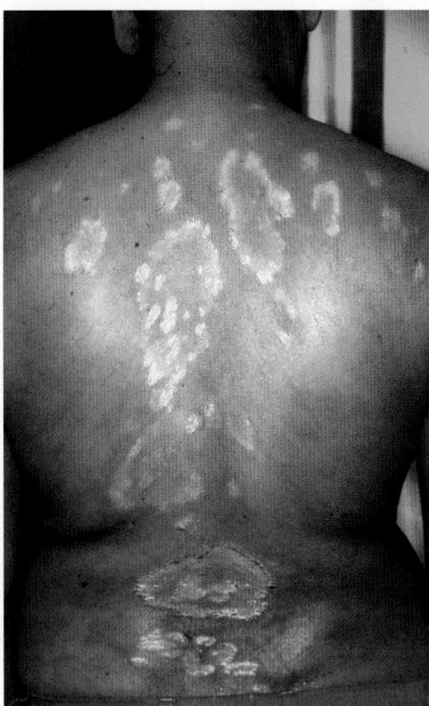

Figure 68.41 Circumscribed plaques of erythema, thickening and scale in plaque psoriasis.

Clinically, psoriasis may be divided into the following general forms:

- Plaque psoriasis (psoriasis vulgaris). This is the commonest form, with involvement of the scalp, trunk (Figure 68.41), elbows and knees, the sacrum and the nails.
- Flexural psoriasis. This occurs in the skin folds and genital area and typically presents with much less scale.
- Guttate psoriasis. This is characterized by the sudden onset of scaly pink macules or flat papules (Figure 68.42). It is strongly associated with recent or active β-haemolytic streptococcal infection.
- Pustular psoriasis. This may be a localized form on the palms and soles or it may be generalized. The palmoplantar form is relatively common, with the appearance of sterile yellow pustules on an erythematous background on the palms and soles (Figure 68.43). The generalized form may be precipitated by sudden withdrawal of oral or potent topical steroids and may be fatal. In the generalized form there are extensive sheets of painful sterile yellow pustules and the patient may have systemic symptoms such as a fever and tachycardia.
- Erythrodermic psoriasis. The skin is red and has a fine scale over at least 80% of the skin surface. This form commonly arises in a patient with pre-existent plaque psoriasis, but may occur as a first presentation. It may also occur as a result of medication with corticosteroids, β-blockers, non-steroidal antiinflammatory drugs, lithium and antimalarials. The condition can be fatal and the patient

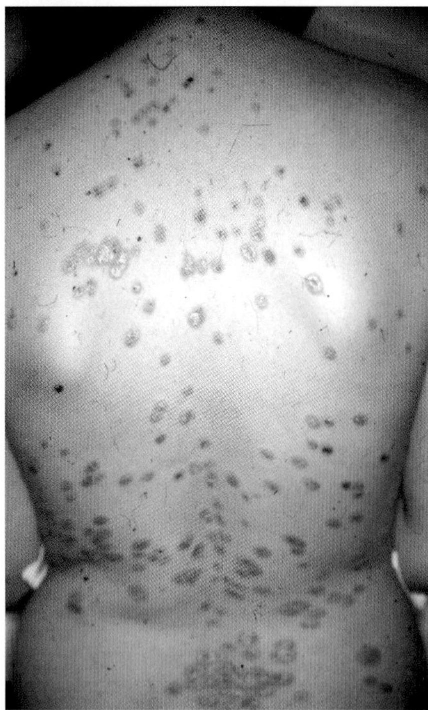

Figure 68.42 Guttate erythemato-scaling small plaques of guttate psoriasis.

should be hospitalized and kept warm, with particular attention paid to fluid and electrolyte imbalance, as well as the risk of infection and septicaemia. Etanercept has been demonstrated to be an effective treatment.

Psoriatic Arthropathy

There are five clinical patterns of joint involvement:

1. An arthritis similar in distribution to osteoarthritis, with distal interphalangeal joint involvement and the clinical manifestations of Heberden's nodes
2. Rheumatoid arthritis distribution with involvement of the metacarpal and metatarsal joints
3. Mono- or oligo-arthropathy with one joint being involved, most commonly the knee or ankle
4. Sacroiliitis
5. Arthritis mutilans. This is a particularly severe form of psoriatic arthritis where the phalanges are eroded leading to telescoping of the skin of the fingers and a destructive arthropathy.

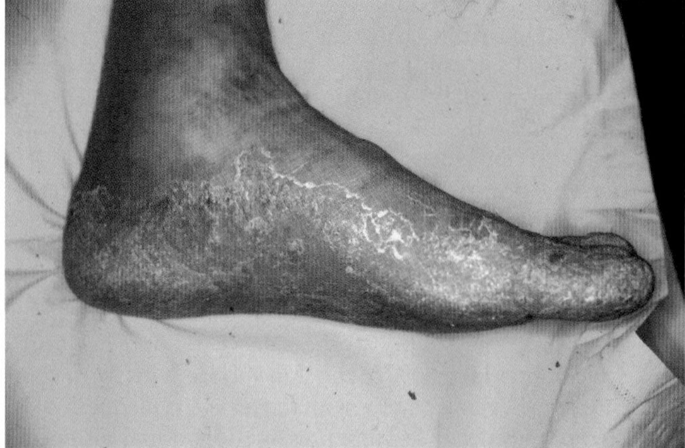

Figure 68.43 Erythema, scaling, hyperkeratosis and pustules in pustular plantar psoriasis.

Management

There is no cure for psoriasis and treatment is aimed at control. Treatments are tailored to the extent of the disease. A soap substitute and regular application of emollients are important.

Potent topical steroids should only be used for very small periods of time in psoriasis as rapid withdrawal can lead to a rebound effect with a more severe psoriasis. They can be useful on the scalp and palmoplantar skin and moderate-strength topical steroids can be used on the face and flexures. The vitamin D analogue, calcipotriol, can be used alone or synergistically in combination with topical steroids (such as Dovobet®) for flare-ups or as intermittent weekly maintenance treatment alternately with calcipotriol used alone.

Tar has been used for several decades in a solution of 5%, 10% or 20% in some form of vehicle such as Lassar's paste or paraffin. This is applied once or twice daily but has the disadvantage of being extremely smelly and also tends to stain clothing. It can be especially effective in combination with ultraviolet therapy or simple sun exposure. It may be combined with a topical steroid for added potency.

Dithranol is derived from the bark of the araroba tree. It has been used in psoriasis for several decades and is often made up in Lassar's paste in different concentrations varying from 0.1% to 1%, with higher concentrations being used for in-patients. The dithranol treatment may be applied for 24 hours and then washed off with arachis oil the next day. Short-contact dithranol protocols require contact for 30 minutes and then the dithranol is washed off. Dithranol has several disadvantages and causes erythema and burning, it stains clothing and the patient's skin tends to have a characteristic staining which lasts for up to 2 weeks. It cannot be used in flexures or on pustular psoriasis.

Phototherapy with PUVA or UVB is effective in psoriasis, although it may not be available in the tropics. Graduated sun exposure may be beneficial for psoriasis, although it can rarely cause an exacerbation. If psoralens are available locally, a methoxypsoralen may be considered and the patient instructed to expose their skin to sunlight for 30–60 minutes, three times weekly.

Systemic therapy for psoriasis involves the use of agents such as methotrexate, ciclosporin, hydroxyurea or mycophenolate. Methotrexate is given weekly, ranging from 2.5 mg to up to 25 mg per week. Baseline liver function tests and levels of procollagen peptide should be performed and monitored throughout therapy. A full blood count has to be performed regularly as methotrexate can cause bone marrow aplasia. Ciclosporin has been shown to be highly effective in psoriasis but it is very expensive, nephrotoxic and often not available in the tropics. Systemic retinoids have been used successfully in the form of acitretin at a daily dose of 30–40 mg daily, however these are expensive drugs that require close monitoring for renal and liver toxicity and teratogenesis is a significant concern.

The biological agents are an effective major advance in treatment in terms of less widespread immunosuppression, but currently are only indicated for severe disease owing to cost and lack of data on long-term safety profile and there is also a significant risk of reactivation of latent TB.[45]

Treatment Summary

Therapy for psoriasis should be aimed at balancing treatment efficacy with potential toxicity. In general, the more efficacious the treatment for psoriasis, the greater the potential for harmful side-effects. Interventions comprise topical therapy, phototherapy, systemic agents and the newer biological agents. Type of psoriasis, extent of involvement and previous treatment must be taken into consideration. Topical treatments may be sufficient to control many cases of psoriasis. When there is more than 10% body surface area involvement however it may be preferable to combine topical treatments with a systemic treatment, which requires specialist initiation.

PHOTOSENSITIVITY DISORDERS

These dermatoses are characterized by the development of a cutaneous eruption after exposure to UVB, UVA and/or visible light. Photodermatoses can be classified into four main groups: idiopathic; dermatoses that are made worse by sunlight; those due to exogenous agents, such as phototoxicity and photoallergy; and those secondary to endogenous conditions, such as the porphyrias. The classic photoreactive eruption occurs on exposed sites such as the forehead, nose, cheeks, the V of the neck (Figure 68.44), the forearms and the dorsa of the hands.

Clinical Evaluation in Photosensitivity

It is important to ask if a rash is photoexacerbated and whether the eruption occurs seasonally. It is also important to assess how much sun exposure is required to produce the eruption, how long after exposure the eruption occurs and how long it lasts. An occupational and social history should be taken to exclude any topical photosensitizers that have been applied. A family history is sought of autoimmune disorder, porphyrias or any genetic disorders. Morphology is a very good clue as to aetiology, with urticarial plaques being common in erythropoietic porphyria, papules occurring in solar urticaria and vesicles and plaques being common in polymorphic light eruption. Vesicles, scarring and pigment disorder are commonly found in porphyria cutanea tarda.

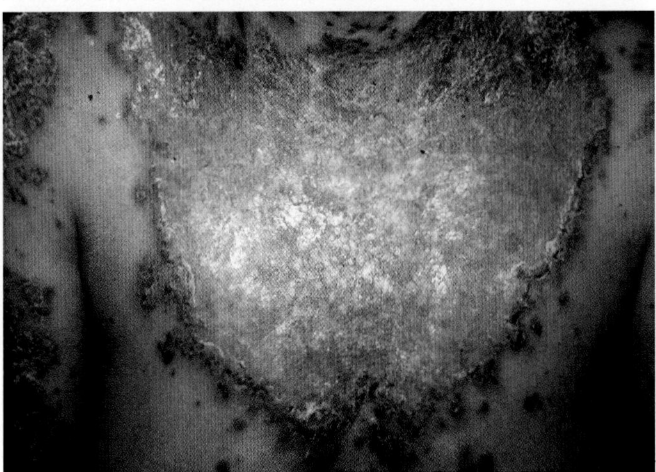

Figure 68.44 Severe erythema and inflammation on the neck 'V' following sun exposure in a case of photosensitive dermatosis.

Polymorphic Light Eruption

This is the most common idiopathic photodermatosis, appears to be a delayed type IV hypersensitivity reaction and occurs when a patient is exposed to the first seasonal sunshine of the year. Its onset is commonly from childhood to late adult life and is more common in women than men. It is common in all races and skin types. It presents clinically with polymorphic lesions, including erythematous papules, vesicles, nodules, plaques, purpura and target-like lesions. Only one type of lesion tends to predominate in any one patient. Unfortunately, it tends to recur each year on sudden exposure to sunlight. It is crucial that serology be performed to exclude systemic lupus erythematosus.

Treatment

Treatment includes photoprotection as topical steroids are only partially effective, although systemic corticosteroids may be used for severe flares. UVB phototherapy may be used prophylactically. Prednisolone, 20 mg od, may suppress the eruption for the duration of a short two-week holiday or hydroxychloroquine, 200 mg bd, may provide partial protection for 1 week prior to and during travel. Azathioprine has been used for severe cases.

Porphyria Cutanea Tarda

This is the most common type of porphyria and is due to defective hepatic uroporphyrinogen decarboxylase activity. Most cases are sporadic, with a small number being autosomal dominantly inherited. Precipitating factors may include alcohol, exogenous oestrogens, subclinical haemochromatosis, iron and chlorinated hydrocarbons. It may also be associated with hepatitis C and HIV infection. Clinically, it presents with skin fragility, vesicles, milia on sun-exposed areas, periorbital hypertrichosis, mottled hyperpigmentation, hypopigmentation and sclerodermatous changes of the hands. Investigations reveal an elevated neuroporphyrin in the urine and elevated isocoproporphyrin in the stool.

Treatment

Treatment is with avoidance of precipitating factors or drugs, venesection, low-dose hydroxychloroquine, cholestyramine or erythropoietin.

Drugs that Cause Photosensitivity

There is a large group of drugs that may cause photosensitivity; the commonest are the tetracyclines, antimalarials, retinoids, thiazide diuretics, antipsychotics and sulfamide compounds.

Skin Malignancies

Cutaneous cancer is rare in very dark-skinned patients, however a major hazard of light-skinned people travelling to the tropics, even for short periods, is skin carcinogenesis. Skin cancer is divided into non-melanoma skin cancer and melanoma skin cancer, as prognosis differs greatly between these.

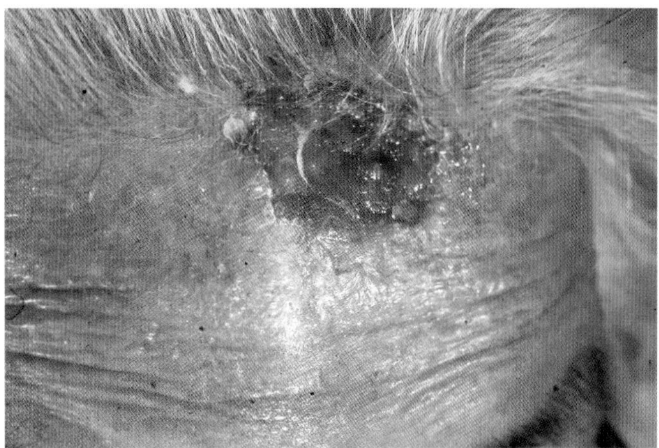

Figure 68.45 Erythema, superficial ulceration and scaling in actinic keratosis.

NON-MELANOMA SKIN CANCER

This includes actinic keratoses, basal cell carcinomas and squamous cell carcinomas.

Actinic Keratoses

These are pre-cancerous, poorly circumscribed scaly erythematous macules and flat plaques variable in diameter from several millimetres to a few centimetres (Figure 68.45). Lesions arising from the ears, dorsum of hands and forearms tend to be thicker and more hyperkeratotic than those on the face. Actinic keratoses can be tender or hyperpigmented. Actinic keratoses arising on the lip present as confluent scaliness with focal erosion and fissures and loss of definition of the vermilion border. The natural history of actinic keratosis is controversial, but studies indicate that progression to squamous cell carcinoma may be approximately 1 in 1000.

Treatment. Isolated lesions may be treated using cryotherapy, with two freeze/thaw cycles required. If the lesions are widespread, topical 5-fluorouracil (Efudix®) may be used once daily to the rough areas for 4 weeks. The patient should be warned there may be an intense inflammatory response and that this is a normal part of the treatment. If the inflammation causes these areas to become painful, a moderate topical steroid may be used in the mornings, with Efudix applied at night. A more expensive alternative is imiquimod 5% cream, which up-regulates cytokines to invoke both a nonspecific immune response and a specific immune response. It is applied three nights a week for 6 weeks. Photodynamic therapy can also be used if there is field change.

Squamous Cell Carcinoma (SCC)

Incidence of SCC is dependent on cumulative sun exposure. The classic SCC is a hyperkeratotic, skin-coloured or erythematous exophytic, warty nodule arising on sun-damaged skin.

Aetiology. SCCs arise from epithelial keratinocytes whose cells usually show some degree of maturation toward keratin formation. Most actinic keratoses and SCCs contain mutations of the *p53* tumour suppressor gene. *p53* is a negative cancer regulator and normally prevents keratinocytes from uncontrolled proliferation. Ultraviolet radiation may cause mutations in the *p53* gene.

Metastases and Natural History. The actinic keratosis is the initial lesion in a disease continuum that progresses to in situ SCC (Bowen's disease) and invasive SCC. Invasive SCC may metastasize to the regional lymph nodes. Local recurrence and regional metastasis are dependent on treatment modality, previous treatment, location, size, depth, histological differentiation, histological evidence of perineural involvement, precipitating factors other than ultraviolet light and host immunosuppression. Lesions found on the ears and lip are known to be at higher risk of local recurrence and metastasis. SCCs presenting on the lip have an especially high recurrence and metastatic rate.

Treatment. The surgical treatment of SCC requires a 4 mm margin. Certain tumour characteristics are associated with a greater risk of subclinical tumour extension and include large size, aggressive histology – especially invasion of the subcutaneous tissue and perineural spread – and location in high-risk areas, in which case at least a 6 mm margin is recommended. Carcinomas with a diameter of more than 2 cm involve a much higher risk of recurrence, due to local micrometastases, and may require more generous local excision with a safety margin of approximately 10 mm and should be treated by specialists in the management of skin cancer.

Basal Cell Carcinoma (BCC)

BCCs are the most common human cancer worldwide. BCCs derive from the keratinocytes and stroma of the pilosebaceous follicle.

Aetiology. The vast majority present on the head and neck, with the inner canthus and eyelids also frequently involved. Inactivation of the tumour suppressor gene *PTCH* by UV radiation exposure is thought to be important in the pathogenesis.

Metastasis, Progress and Clinical Features. The course of BCCs is slow but steady at approximately 1 mm every 3 months and progression results in local destruction of structures if left untreated. In immunosuppressed patients, tumours may be more aggressive. Metastases are extremely rare, with an estimated risk as low as 0.1%. There are six main clinical types of BCC:

1. Nodular BCC (Figure 68.46) begins as a small papule that becomes nodular with central ulceration. The margins of the tumour are well defined, slightly raised with a rolled border and with a pearly, shiny appearance. Blood vessels traversing over the margin give it a telangiectatic appearance.
2. Pigmented BCC is clinically similar but the margins of the tumour are pigmented. Such pigmented BCCs may be mistaken clinically for malignant melanoma.
3. Cystic BCC is a well-defined papule which attains a pearly coloured lobulated appearance with a telangiectatic surface, with subsequent ulceration of the central part of the tumour.
4. Morphoeic (sclerosing) BCC may have the clinical appearance of a scar, although the pearly colour may be

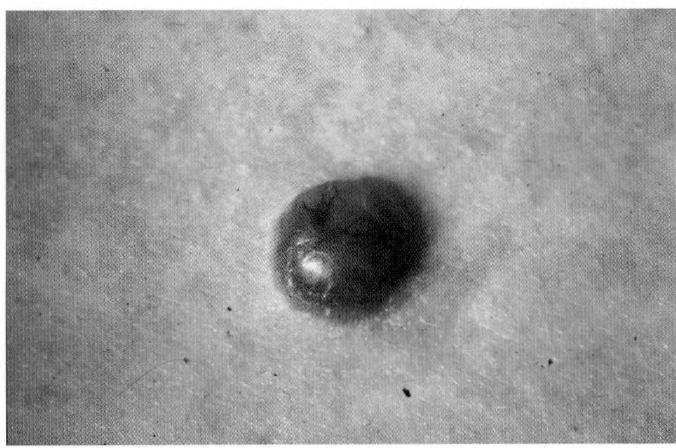

Figure 68.46 Nodular basal cell carcinoma on the chest.

maintained in certain areas of the tumour and telangiectasia is often present.

5. Superficial BCC often occurs on the trunk or limbs. It is a well-defined, slightly raised red plaque with an adherent scaly surface. Most lesions are solitary and may be pigmented.
6. Linear BCC is an uncommon variant, which is a linear, pearly and telangiectatic lesion located most often on the head and neck and may be a more aggressive subtype.

Diagnosis. The diagnosis of BCC is usually clinical or dermoscopic, however if doubt exists a preoperative biopsy is advised.

Treatment. Treatment is with surgical excision, Mohs surgery (pathological examination of tissue during surgery), 5-FU, imiquimod or sometimes by curettage and cautery, depending on the histological type, number of BCCs present and patient age and comorbidities. Tumours in certain sites have a higher risk of recurrence, including the nasal alae, nasolabial fold, tragus and retro-auricular area.

Follow-up. The aims of follow-up are detection of recurrence and early detection of new lesions. Some 36% of patients who have a previous BCC will develop a further BCC. Most BCCs that will recur do so within 3 years. Frequency and duration of follow-up surveillance depend on resources available. Patients with multiple BCCs should be followed up at least 6-monthly for life.

MALIGNANT MELANOMA

The incidence of malignant melanoma is increasing in developed countries. Although pale-skinned patients are most at risk, rare forms such as the acral lentiginous malignant melanoma are equally distributed throughout all skin types. Other risk factors include sun-damaged skin, family history, previous melanoma, the existence of numerous dysplastic naevi, higher than average number of benign naevi, the existence of a congenital naevus and immunosuppression. Mutations have been found in susceptibility genes such as the *CDKN2A* gene or in genes implicated in control of the cell cycle or maintenance of cell integrity. The molecular basis of each type of malignant melanoma continues to be elucidated.

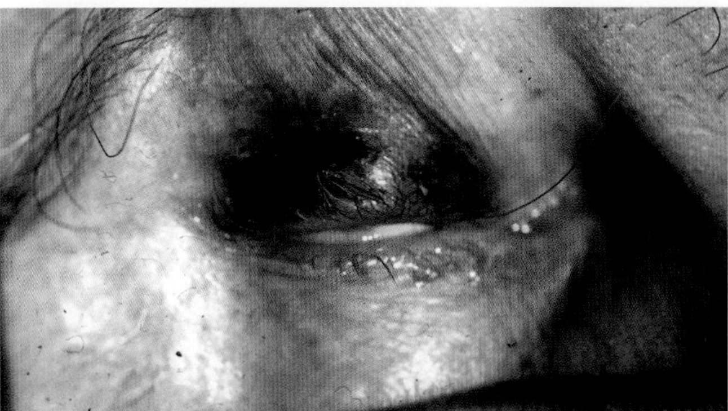

Figure 68.47 Chronic lentigo maligna melanoma on the upper eyelid of an elderly patient.

Metastasis and Natural History of Malignant Melanoma

There is an inverse relationship between tumour thickness and survival. The thickness of the tumour is defined by the Breslow scale, which is measured in millimetres from the granular cell layer of the epidermis to the deepest tumour cells. Those tumours that have a Breslow thickness of ≤1.5 mm have a 93% 5-year survival rate, whereas those with a Breslow thickness of >3.5 mm have a 5-year survival rate of 37%. Metastasis is first to regional lymph nodes and then to lung, liver, brain, bone and peritoneum.

Clinical Presentation

Most malignant melanomas appear de novo, rather than from pre-existent naevi. Asymmetry, an irregular border, a variegated or dark colour, enlarging diameter and rapid elevation may suggest malignant melanoma. The four major types of malignant melanoma are superficial spreading melanoma, lentigo maligna melanoma, acral lentiginous melanoma and nodular melanoma. Lentigo maligna appears as an irregularly bordered tan-coloured patch which enlarges slowly over many years and is found mainly on sun-damaged skin of the head and neck (Figure 68.47). Superficial spreading melanoma often has a diameter more than 1 cm and is usually palpable. There may be great variability in the colour of melanoma, from pink, red and brown to black (Figure 68.48). Nodular melanoma appears as a rapidly growing papule or a nodule, commonly on the trunk in men and on the leg in women. Acral lentiginous melanoma is found on the palms, soles and nail-beds. Although this is a rare tumour, it is of equal incidence in all races and therefore may be seen in the tropics. This form of malignant melanoma has the poorest prognosis and it is vital that it is recognized early.

Treatment

The definitive treatment for melanoma is excision. Diagnosis must be made early if this is to be curative. The margins for excision are dependent on the Breslow thickness. Once the melanoma has metastasized there are currently no known therapies at present which affect long-term prognosis. The management of melanoma should be left to experts and multidisciplinary teams.

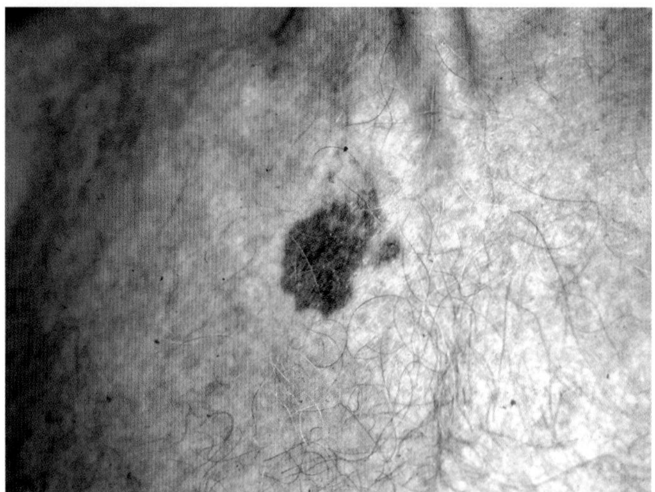

Figure 68.48 Superficially spreading malignant melanoma of the chest.

Urticaria

Urticaria is a common family of conditions characterized by raised itchy wheals. The wheals themselves are transient, vary considerably in shape and size and can occur at any site (Figure 68.49). In the Caucasian patient, they may be pink or red in colour, but this erythema may not be apparent in the darker-skinned patient. By definition, an urticarial attack will last <24 hours. Clinically, urticaria can be divided into acute and chronic forms.

ACUTE URTICARIA

This is defined as urticaria occurring for less than 6 weeks. The commonest causes are drugs, including aspirin, non-steroidal anti-inflammatory drugs, opiates and ACE inhibitors. A minority of patients may have a food allergy and the commonest precipitants are nuts, fish, shellfish, eggs and milk. When a patient's urticaria appears during spring and summer, the role of inhaled allergens such as pollens and spores should be considered as a cause. Certain infectious agents such as viral infections and streptococcal pharyngitis in children may also cause a transient urticaria over weeks. The commonest acute contact urticarial reaction is to latex.

Treatment

Always discontinue any causative medication. A non-sedating antihistamine is usually sufficient to treat an acute urticaria. If the patient is non-responsive, treat as for chronic urticaria.

CHRONIC URTICARIA

This is defined as urticaria lasting more than 6 weeks. Chronic urticarias may be divided into the physical urticarias, chronic idiopathic urticaria, angio-oedema and urticarial vasculitis.

Physical Urticaria

This may be caused by pressure, sweating, heat, cold, sunlight or water. In most cases, the type of physical urticaria can be elucidated by the history, with pressure urticaria (Figure 68.50), occurring under tight clothing and cholinergic urticaria occurring at times of emotion and sweating. Patients with cold urticaria may complain of lesions as soon as they exit a hot bath. Cold urticaria may be tested for by placing an ice cube on the skin for 10 minutes and then observing a wheal appearing 5–10 minutes later. In aquagenic urticaria the wheals occur in response to contact with water. Solar urticaria is very rare and occurs in response to sunlight.

Chronic Idiopathic Urticaria

This is the largest group within the chronic urticarias, however it is a diagnosis of exclusion. In the tropics, common causes of chronic urticaria may be hookworm, tapeworms and roundworms and stool microscopy: serology for filariasis and strongyloides is therefore important. Some patients labelled as having chronic idiopathic urticaria have been found to have histamine-releasing autoantibodies to mast cell receptors.

Angio-oedema

This is a deeper dermal form of urticaria and results in swollen lips, eyelids, tongue, hands and feet, with involvement of the upper airways causing respiratory arrest and fatal respiratory failure. Less than 1% of cases of angio-oedema may be hereditary, in an autosomal dominant fashion, in which case complement C4 should be measured. If this is low, more detailed investigations of C1 esterase activity are required.

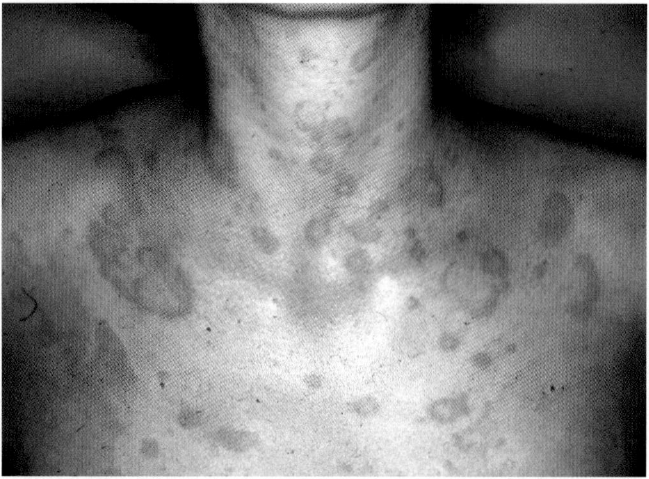

Figure 68.49 Pruritic urticarial wheals on the trunk.

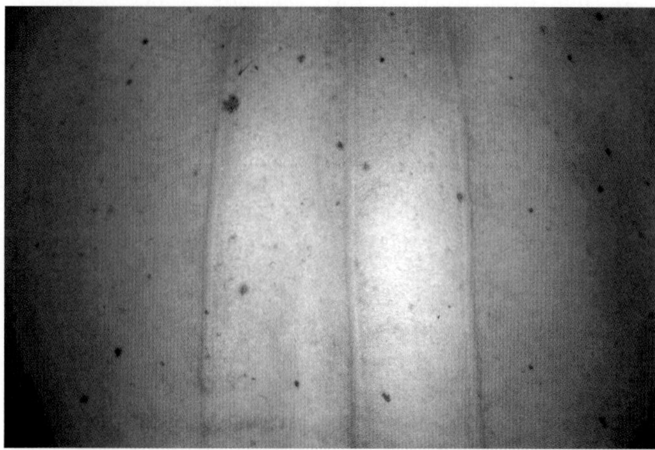

Figure 68.50 Pressure urticaria or dermographism.

Urticarial Vasculitis

This is defined as urticarial lesions lasting longer than 24 hours. Histological investigation is required and the biopsy should include both lesional and non-lesional skin. The biopsy will show a vasculitis or a leukocytoclastic vasculitis. A leukocytoclastic vasculitis is more likely to be associated with systemic diseases such as the autoimmune connective tissue diseases or drugs.

Management of Chronic Idiopathic Urticaria

Any identifiable causes should be removed and the patient should avoid drugs that may cause histamine release, such as aspirin, non-steroidal antiinflammatory drugs and opioids. The patient should be started on a non-sedating antihistamine; if there is a poor response the dose can be doubled or a sedating antihistamine can be added at night. If the patient still has not responded, an H_2 antagonist may be added. Resistant forms of urticaria may need short courses of systemic steroids and patients with hereditary angio-oedema or severe angio-oedema may need adrenaline (epinephrine) pens for emergency situations. Refractory cases may require immunosuppression with ciclosporin, intravenous immunoglobulin and even, in extreme cases, plasmapheresis.

DELUSIONAL INFESTATION

Delusional infestation manifests an intense and often incapacitating pruritus, in which the patient has a fixed delusion that they are infested with insects, parasites or fibrous material. A variety of names have previously been attributed to this syndrome including delusory parasitosis, Ekbom syndrome, parasitophobia and the lay term, Morgellons disease. The belief that they have an infestation leads to these patients suffering from dermatitis artefacta. They scratch the affected parts until the skin breaks down and further skin damage may be caused by the overuse of disinfectants or insecticides. Such cases may follow an actual infestation by fleas or other arthropods or secondarily as a result of psychiatric disorders or drug or alcohol abuse. Treatment is difficult, but every effort should be made to establish that there are in fact no minute biting insects or allergen-producing mites or insects, particularly of the type bearing or shedding urticating hairs and samples brought by the patient should always be sent for analysis. A full examination of the skin should be undertaken, including the nails and scalp. It is extremely important to engage with the patient, but avoid collusion with their delusion. There is little merit in trying to challenge the nature of the delusion and instead, it can be more successful to explain that even though you may not have found any parasites, you will keep looking for these but nonetheless would like to offer the patient treatment for their skin.

Treatment

Risperidone 1 mg daily has shown success in some studies for 6 months to 2 years duration, although it must be explained to the patient at the outset that this is an antipsychotic medication, but is being used in much lower doses than normal. Amisulpride may have the same effect with a better side-effect profile. Coexistent affective disease can occur, so if the patient will not engage with an antipsychotic, an SSRI can be tried instead. An occasional feature of these cases is that the problems in the sufferer can result in other members of the household presenting with similar symptoms and in these circumstances the family members should be treated with emollients.

Other Non-infective Dermatoses Mainly Limited to the Tropics

ARSENISM

The commonest form of arsenism is now due to water contamination and cases have been reported in Chile, Taiwan, Mexico, Argentina, Thailand and the Ganges delta in India. Arsenic is normally detoxified in the liver and excreted in the urine. This detoxification process may be subject to genetic polymorphisms, which can cause carcinogenicity in a proportion of the human population. Cutaneous changes begin with hyperpigmentation in the groin and areolae. These areas may develop hypopigmented areas within them, giving rise to a characteristic raindrop appearance. As many as 30% of patients may have pigmentation in the oral cavity. Hyperkeratotic papules on the palms and soles occur in up to 70% of patients, however patients may have an associated cutaneous malignancy such as Bowen's disease, BCC, SCC or keratoacanthomas. These tumours mainly occur on sun-exposed sites and suspicion of arsenism should be aroused as such tumours are rare in dark-skinned patients.

Treatment

Long-term monitoring for the development of cutaneous neoplasms and also associated internal malignancy is required. The palmoplantar hyperkeratotic areas may be treated by a 10% salicylate ointment twice daily. Systemic retinoids may prevent the onset of cutaneous malignancy.

BRAZILIAN PEMPHIGUS FOLIACEUS

This is an autoimmune bullous dermatosis, known locally as fogo selvagem (wildfire). It is characterized by antibodies to the epidermal desmosomes, specifically desmoglein 1 (Dsg1). It is clinically identical to the non-endemic global form of pemphigus foliaceus. Pemphigus foliaceus itself is a variant of pemphigus vulgaris. Fogo selvagem is endemic to certain regions of Brazil and some areas of Colombia, Bolivia, Paraguay and Argentina. The incidence decreases with increasing urbanization and the vast majority of patients are found living near rivers within flying range of black flies (*Simulium pruinosum*). Clinically, the lesions are superficial vesicles which can be mistaken for impetigo. The blisters rupture easily, leaving superficial erosions. Unlike in pemphigus vulgaris, oral or mucosal lesions are uncommon in pemphigus foliaceus. Fogo selvagem may present in a localized form on the seborrhoeic areas of the face which may be distinguished from discoid lupus erythematosus by skin biopsy. The localized form may stay localized or gradually become generalized. Patients with generalized fogo selvagem may present in one of three ways. An acute aggressive form has a predominance of blisters which may be associated with fever, arthralgias and malaise and increased susceptibility to life-threatening HSV infections. An exfoliative erythrodermic form has superficial erosions and crusting. The third more slowly aggressive form clinically consists of keratotic plaques and nodular lesions in the seborrhoeic and acral areas. There is a rarer, hyperpigmented, form of fogo selvagem, which often occurs when the patient is recovering after treatment.

It is important that this condition is diagnosed early in childhood as delay can lead to dwarfism and azoospermia as an adult. It is thought that fogo selvagem may also have psychiatric effects. The gold test for diagnosis is indirect and direct immunofluorescence for Dsg1. If such investigations are not available, a Tzank smear or skin biopsy may show acantholytic cells.

Treatment

Untreated pemphigus foliaceous has a high mortality rate of 40% within 2 years. High-dose systemic steroid is the treatment of choice and is slowly tapered in dosage according to response. Steroid-sparing agents such as azathioprine are useful and cyclophosphamide has been used with good results. Useful adjunctive therapies include antimalarials and dapsone. Both tuberculosis and strongyloidiasis must be excluded before starting systemic steroids in these patients.[46]

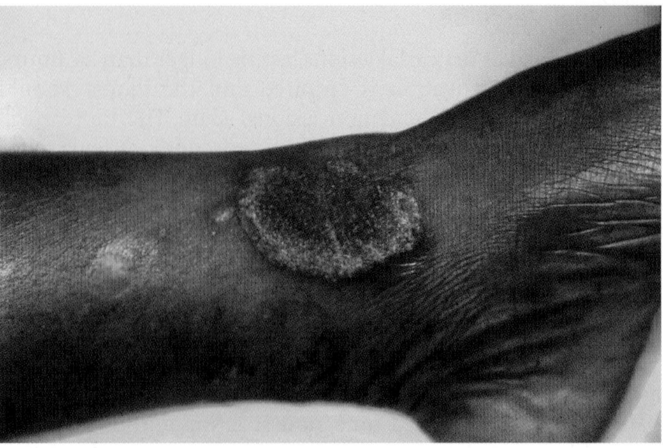

Figure 68.52 Isolated papules and large plaque of lichen planus with Wickham's striae.

LICHEN PLANUS AND LICHENOID ERUPTIONS

Lichen planus is an inflammatory T-cell-mediated mucocutaneous disease of unknown cause. It can affect the skin, mucosa and nails. The prevalence is estimated at approximately 1%. Cutaneous lesions present with flat-topped, polygonal, pruritic shiny papules with a violaceous hue. In darker skin, purple, brown or black are more typical colours than violet (Figure 68.52). Post-inflammatory hyperpigmentation is prominent and persistent in darker-skinned patients. It is thought that lichen planus is more common in darker-skinned patients. Lichen planus classically presents on the wrists and ankles. Involvement of the oral cavity may present with white Wickham's striae or as erosive painful lesions (Figure 68.53). The two types of lichen planus, which are most relevant to the tropical physician, are hypertrophic lichen planus and actinic lichen planus.

Hypertrophic Lichen Planus

This presents with red, brown or violaceous lichenified verrucous plaques which are extremely itchy. The lesions primarily occur on the lower legs and ankles (Figure 68.51). It is especially common in inhabitants of southern India and Sri Lanka.

Actinic Lichen Planus

This occurs in a photodistribution and is induced by sun exposure. In countries such as India, actinic lichen planus forms as little as 5% of all cases of lichen planus, whereas in the Middle East it can be as high as 30–40% of cases. Children and young adults are primarily affected. There are three clinical presentations: annular, dyschromic and pigmented. The commonest form is the annular type. This presents as brownish plaques with an annular configuration, most commonly affecting the lateral aspects of the forehead, dorsum of the hands, forearms, lower lip, cheeks and the V-shaped area of the neck. With time, the annular lesion can develop central hypopigmentation and some subtle atrophy. This form of lichen planus typically affects women more than men and occurs at a younger age than classic lichen planus.

Treatment. Spontaneous remissions of cutaneous lichen planus may occur in up to 70% of cases after 1 year. Mucous membrane lichen planus tends not to resolve spontaneously however and may be recurrent and resistant to treatment. Scratching should be avoided and a broad-spectrum, high-factor sunscreen used. Topical steroids, topical steroids with

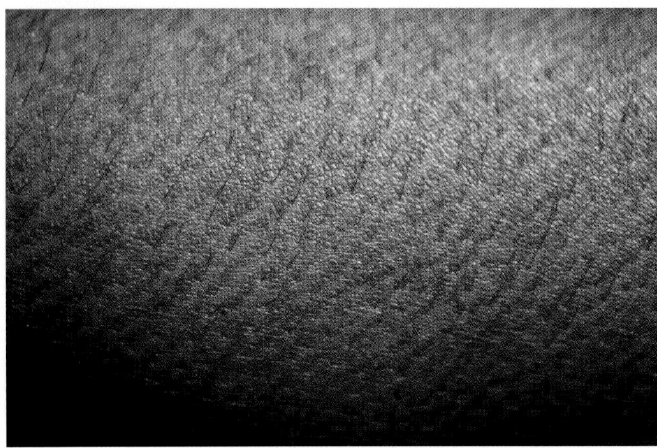

Figure 68.51 Pruritic plaque of lichen amyloid on the shin.

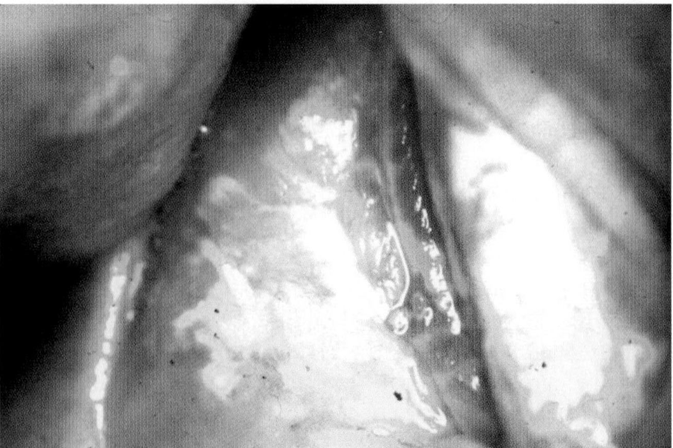

Figure 68.53 Erosive oral lichen planus.

occlusion and intralesional steroids are all used. Systemic steroids may be used when lichen planus is severe, rapidly progressive or for erosive oral lichen planus. Acitretin has been used successfully in widespread lichen planus, as have ciclosporin, dapsone and antimalarials.

Actinic lichen planus has been reported to respond particularly well to systemic antimalarials. Hypertrophic lichen planus can be treated with intralesional steroids and topical steroids under occlusion. The authors find that a potent steroid combined with 5% or 10% salicylate is particularly effective applied twice a day for a period of at least 4–6 weeks. Phototherapy can be used to treat most cutaneous forms of lichen planus, with the exception of actinic lichen planus.

Treatment Summary. Potent topical steroids, if necessary under occlusion, can be used to treat localized lichen planus. Cases with extensive disease or erosive mucosal lichen planus will require systemic therapies, such as oral steroids, acitretin, ciclosporin, dapsone or antimalarials.

DISORDERS OF PIGMENTATION

The majority of the world's population is brown-skinned and therefore postinflammatory hyper- or hypopigmentation is of major concern to dermatologists worldwide and to tropical physicians. The unfortunate and widespread use of depigmenting creams in Africa and parts of Asia in order to lighten the complexion has in some cases led to permanent disfigurement.

Vitiligo

This is an autoimmune condition characterized by the complete loss of pigment within skin. Males and females are equally affected. Depigmentation starts suddenly, with the commonest sites being the hands, feet, genitalia and periocular and perioral areas of the face. The pigmentation may form a generalized symmetrical pattern or a segmental pattern which follows a dermatome (Figure 68.54). The focal form may be an isolated lesion which progresses slowly. Diagnosis is clinical although it can be confused with pityriasis versicolor, postinflammatory hypopigmentation, scleroderma and lichen sclerosus et atrophicus.

Treatment. Treatment success in vitiligo is very variable and may not be permanent. Very potent topical steroids used for 1 month's duration only may cause repigmentation in between 15% and 55% of patients. Narrow-band UVB has been found to be up to 60% successful in vitiligo, however due to the slow mobility of melanocytes, treatment may need to be prolonged for more than 1 year. Melanocytes migrate from the margins and also from hair follicles and therefore when repigmentation occurs, it is around hair follicles and the periphery of the lesion.[47] Sun protection is important for the depigmented areas to reduce risk of skin neoplasia.

Melasma

Of the affected patient, 90% are women, although men can be affected in the same way. This condition is most common in Hispanic and Asian people. Black-skinned patients may be affected but melasma may not be easily noticed. Up to 70% of

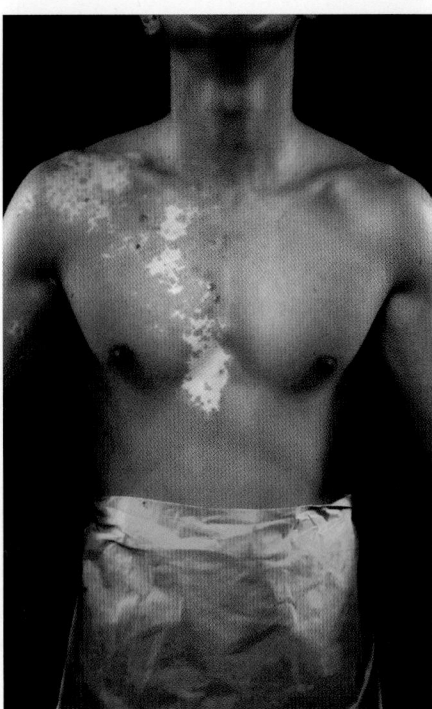

Figure 68.54 Segmental hypopigmentation of trunkal vitiligo.

patients can have a family history, with UV exposure, oestrogen contraceptives, hormone replacement therapy, pregnancy and, rarely, thyroid dysfunction being other aetiological factors. Clinically, the lesions are symmetrical, well-demarcated, tan-coloured macules and patches on the face. Rarely, melasma can be more widespread, affecting the chest, upper back and the sun-exposed side of the arms.

Melasma may be predominantly epidermal or dermal or mixed, with the epidermal type being much more amenable to therapy. Clinically, the epidermal type of melasma is accentuated by Wood's light examination of the skin. African women are more likely to have melasma of the dermal-type pathology.

Treatment. Hydroquinone may be helpful in epidermal-type melasma. Concentrations vary from 2% to 10% and hydroquinone may be used twice daily for 12 weeks. Hydroquinone may cause local skin irritation, however, and thereby leading to post-inflammatory hyperpigmentation, making the skin pigmentation worse. The patient should also be warned that if the hydroquinone happens to go onto surrounding normal skin, this may lighten as well and may give the patient leopard-skin appearance. Monobenzyl ether of hydroquinone, which is a permanent depigmentating agent, should never be used to treat melasma, as it causes irreversible loss of pigment. Exogenous ochronosis is also thought to be a rare side-effect of hydroquinone therapy.

Hydroquinone may be combined with topical tretinoin and 1% hydrocortisone in an ointment known as Kligman's solution, which may be applied once a day at night for a minimum of 4–6 months. There may be an irritant dermatitis about which the patient should be warned.

Azelaic acid may be used twice daily for 6 months and is tolerated very well, with very few side-effects.

More recent therapy for melasma has included glycolic acid peels, tretinoin peels and laser treatment.[48]

Treatment Summary. Melasma is difficult to treat in darker skin types as treatments have very variable effects and may make the appearance worse. The most important treatment for melasma is to avoid any exacerbating medication such as oestrogen contraceptives and sun protection is also vital to prevent deterioration of the pigmentation.

Post-inflammatory Hyperpigmentation

This is an acquired excess of pigment in skin that can develop after any cause of inflammation (Figure 68.55), reactions to medications, phototoxic eruptions and physical agents. It is much worse in conditions that disrupt the basement membrane layer, such as discoid lupus erythematosus and lichen planus. It is difficult to treat and patients should be reassured that it will slowly fade with time.

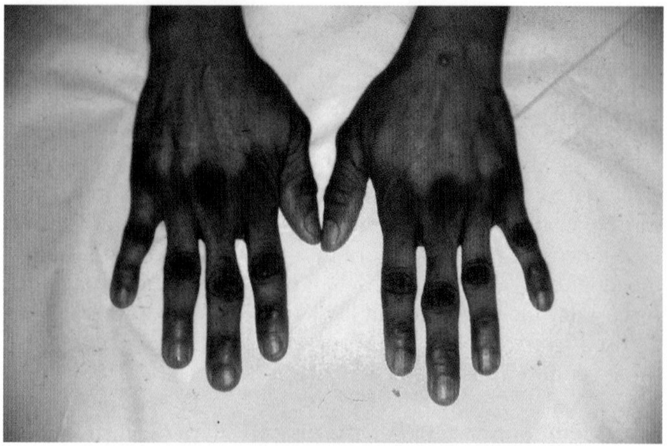

Figure 68.55 Postinflammatory hyperpigmentation of the hands in a patient with atopic eczema.

PHRYNODERMA

This is a distinctive form of follicular hyperkeratosis, usually appearing on extensor surfaces. It was initially described in association with vitamin A deficiency, however there is no good evidence that adults with vitamin A deficiency respond to replacement therapy. Children with phrynoderma however seem to show signs of deficiency of both vitamins A and B and a study from Thailand has shown that children with vitamin deficiency may respond well to vitamin A therapy. Those that do not have a vitamin A deficiency can be treated with a 5–10% salicylate ointment twice a day, a potent topical steroid on its own or in a combination with salicylate and 10–20% urea has also been used effectively. Most of the lesions tend to disappear by the age of 18 without treatment.

REFERENCES

3. Abdalla CMZ, Prado de Oliveira ZN, Sotto MN, et al. Polymerase chain reaction compared to other laboratory findings and to clinical evaluation in the diagnosis of cutaneous tuberculosis and atypical mycobacteria skin infection. Int J Dermatol 2009;48:27–35.
6. Ameen M, Arenas R. Emerging therapeutic regimes for the management of mycetomas. Expert Opin Pharmacother 2008;9(12):2077–85.
13. Goto H, Lindoso JAL. Current diagnosis and treatment of cutaneous and mucocutaneous leishmaniasis. Expert Rev. Anti Infect Ther 2010;8(4):419–33.
17. Udall DN. Recent updates on onchocerciasis: diagnosis and treatment. Clin Infect Dis 2007; 44:53–60.
32. Parola P, Paddock CD, Raoult D. Tick-borne rickettsioses around the world: emerging diseases challenging old concepts. Clin Microbiol Rev 2005;18(4):719–56.

Access the complete references online at www.expertconsult.com

69 Musculoskeletal Disorders

INOSHI ATUKORALA | THASHI CHANG

KEY POINTS

- Musculoskeletal diseases afflicting low-income populations in the tropics have previously been of little relevance to doctors practicing medicine in non-tropical regions. However, with increased international travel and globalization, the gap between the spectrum of diseases seen in tropical and temperate regions has narrowed, increasing the need to universally recognize these conditions previously confined to, or most prevalent in, the tropics.
- Musculoskeletal disorders encountered in the tropics are not very different to the disorders encountered in temperate regions, albeit differences in frequency of some diseases. Unsurprisingly, diseases associated with infections prevalent in the tropics are more common. However, non-infectious musculoskeletal disorders related to 'Western' lifestyles are now emerging as significant socioeconomic problems in the tropics.
- In addition, musculoskeletal diseases associated with reactivated infections and atypical infections in patients with impaired immunity due to malnutrition, diabetes mellitus, HIV infection and immunosuppressive drugs present both diagnostic and therapeutic challenges in the often resource-poor settings of the tropics.[1]
- This chapter will highlight the musculoskeletal disorders commonly encountered in the tropics with special emphasis on diseases of the joints, muscle, bone and soft tissue related to infections, and discuss some of the dilemmas that arise in diagnosis and management of inflammatory musculoskeletal diseases in the tropics.

Infectious Diseases

BACTERIAL INFECTIONS

Among infective aetiologies, bacteria account for most of the tropical musculoskeletal diseases associated with articular manifestations. In addition to direct infection, articular disease may arise as an immunological manifestation of bacterial infection. Bones, joints and muscle can be infected by a multitude of organisms including *Staphylococcus aureus,* resulting in clinical syndromes such as osteomyelitis, septic arthritis and pyomyositis. Tuberculosis, leprosy and brucellosis manifest typical articular syndromes.

Tuberculosis

Epidemiology. Tuberculosis (TB) continues to be a global health problem, and a particular problem in the tropics. Although the highest incidence of tuberculosis is in sub-Saharan Africa, the absolute burden of tuberculosis is condensed to the densely populated areas in China and South Asia, with India and China notifying approximately 40% of incident cases.[2] Osteoarticular tuberculosis affecting the spine and joints accounts for only 1–3% of all cases of tuberculosis and 10–11% of extra-pulmonary tuberculosis.[3] However, given the high prevalence of TB in the tropics, osteoarticular tuberculosis adds significantly to the burden of musculoskeletal disease in the region.[4]

BOX 69.1 CLINICAL SYNDROMES OF MUSCULOSKELETAL TUBERCULOSIS

- Tuberculous spondylitis (Pott disease)
- Peripheral arthritis
- Tenosynovitis, dactylitis and bursitis
- Osteomyelitis
- Poncet disease.

Clinical Features. Osteoarticular tuberculosis (OTB) has an insidious onset with often little or no systemic symptoms.[5] It occurs frequently without evidence of pulmonary or other primary organ involvement.[6,7] The clinical syndromes of OTB are legion (Box 69.1). However, the condition continues to be a chameleon mimicking other common tropical infections and tumours.

Tuberculous spondylitis or Pott disease is the commonest presentation of musculoskeletal tuberculosis, accounting for 50% of cases. The commonest region involved is the dorsal spine. However, lumbar spinal involvement is not uncommon, particularly in HIV-infected patients. The typical description is of severe spinal pain or stiffness accompanied by night sweats, profound constitutional symptoms and tenderness of affected vertebrae.[8] However, in high-prevalence countries, patients may present with minimal constitutional symptoms. Nonetheless, the backache is usually relentlessly progressive and severe enough for the patient to seek medical attention. In patients with poor access to healthcare, late presentations are seen with angular kyphosis (gibbus deformity) and spastic or flaccid paraplegia.

The differential diagnosis of spinal TB includes malignancy and spondylitis due to other infections. Staphylococcal and other pyogenic infections have an acute onset with prominent systemic manifestations unlike spinal TB. Malignancy including multiple myeloma, metastases from prostate, breast and the gastrointestinal tract need to be excluded if the clinical and radiological findings are not typical of TB (see below).

Tuberculosis of the joints presents as a chronic monoarthritis affecting weight-bearing joints such as the hips, knees and ankles. The joints of the feet including the ankle, talocalcaneal and mid-tarsal joints may also be involved. However, signs of inflammation are minimal in most with profound joint swelling with effusion, abscess, chronic sinus formation and systemic symptoms of fever, weight loss and night sweats being infrequently documented.[9] Dactylitis, the swelling of an entire digit or tenosynovitis may occur with or without joint involvement.[10] The differential diagnoses for TB of joints include monoarticular presentation of inflammatory arthritides such as rheumatoid arthritis, spondyloarthropathy or crystal arthritides.

Tenosynovitis and bursitis arising from TB are rare, particularly after the advent of anti-tuberculous treatment. Tenosynovitis tends to affect the hands and wrists, especially on the dominant side.[11] Bursitis is commoner in sites of repetitive trauma, i.e. olecranon, trochanteric and prepatellar bursae.[12]

Poncet disease has been defined as a 'non-destructive, parainfective, symmetric polyarthritis occurring in patients with active visceral or disseminated TB'.[13,14] In this condition, there is no evidence of joint infection by tuberculosis or any other cause of joint inflammation. Poncet disease may be accompanied by episcleritis and/or erythema nodosum on the shins, thighs or upper limbs. The condition resolves completely with anti-TB therapy.[15]

Pathogenesis and Pathology. The pathogenesis of tuberculosis has been discussed elsewhere. Tuberculous infection of bones and joints occurs after haematogenous, lymphatic or contiguous spread of bacilli from a primary focus of infection. Typically, there is a long latent period between primary tuberculosis and joint involvement, usually spanning several years. The primary focus is usually the lung, kidney or a lymph node.[9] However, only 30% of patients with OTB have radiographic evidence of current or previous pulmonary TB. In 50% of patients, the primary focus cannot be identified.[16]

Tuberculous disease of the spine and dactylitis starts in the subchondral bone and spreads to the disc space, adjacent vertebral bodies, ligaments and tissues. This disease process is accelerated in the presence of a co-existent bacterial infection with rapid joint destruction. Vertebral bodies become progressively destroyed with disc space narrowing.[8] The granulomatous inflammation and necrotic debris can result in a paraspinal mass or a draining sinus (Figure 69.1).

In articular and periarticular tuberculosis, the synovium is the focus of original infection.[19] The articular disease starts as low-grade granulomatous synovitis. This invades the articular cartilage, separating it from the bone. Fibrin in the synovial fluid and articular cartilage may precipitate, forming 'rice-bodies'.[3]

In contrast, Poncet disease is a non-destructive, parainfectious arthritis occurring as a consequence of hypersensitivity to tuberculous infection in another part of the body. There is no bacteriological or radiological evidence of infection of the joint *per se* and the condition subsides completely without recurrence after anti-tuberculous therapy.[15]

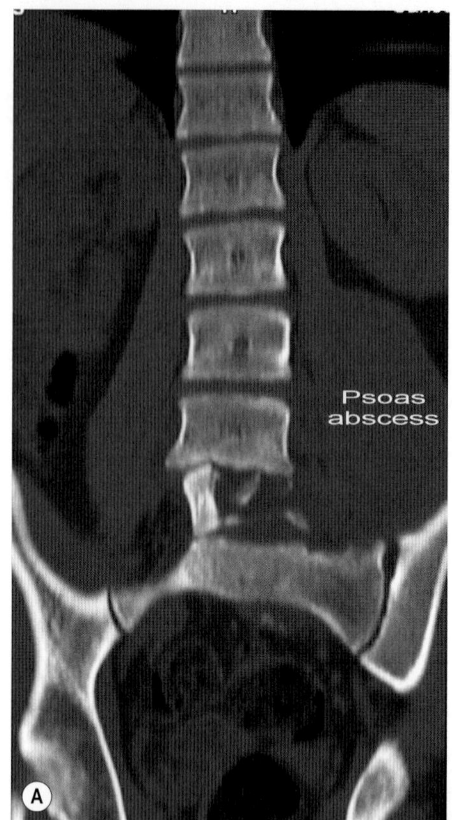

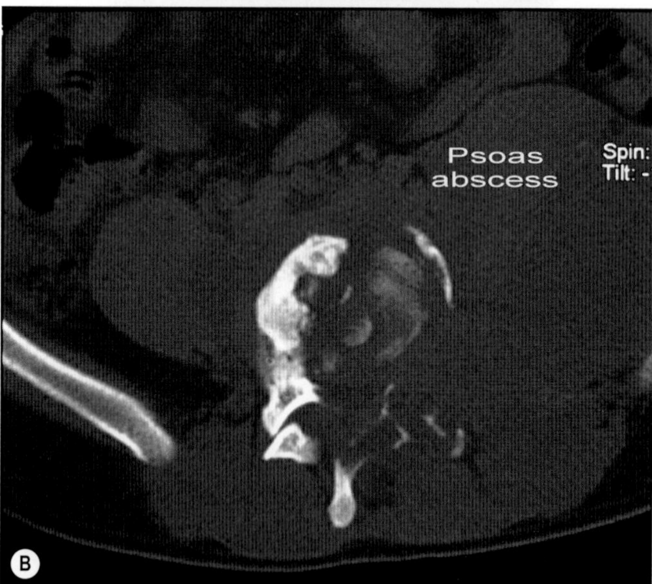

Figure 69.1 (A,B) CT images showing vertebral destruction and formation of paraspinal (psoas) abscess in a patient with tuberculous spondylitis in the lumbar spine. *(Courtesy of Dr Priyangee Arambepola.)*

Diagnosis. Early diagnosis of OTB is essential to preserve articular cartilage and joint integrity. However, the diagnosis of TB in resource-poor settings is difficult, but the delay in diagnosis is partly due to varied clinical presentations and even more challenging in immunocompromised individuals.

Radiographic changes are minimal in the early stages. Therefore, if OTB is suspected, radiography must be repeated after a time lapse. In spinal tuberculosis, the earliest radiographic changes are erosions particularly in the antero-superior or antero-inferior parts of the vertebral body, followed by erosions of the endplate culminating in disc narrowing, contiguous spread and collapse of adjacent vertebral bodies. Paraspinal abscess formation occurs in about 65% of patients (Figure 69.1), commonly in the cervical and dorsal spines. However, as initial radiographs can be normal or equivocal, magnetic resonance imaging (MRI) and computerized tomography (CT) are useful for early diagnosis in such cases. MRI is of particular value in assessing abscess formation, soft tissue involvement and cord compression and instructive for guided aspiration of abscess and planning surgical intervention.[17] It is noteworthy that the radiological findings of spinal TB contrast with those of its differential diagnoses: pyogenic infections involve a single vertebral body with disc space involvement and frequent presence of bone sclerosis, while malignancy involves non-contiguous vertebral bodies affecting the vertebral body pedicles.[18]

Soft tissue swelling and periarticular osteopaenia are the initial findings in TB arthritis. In contrast to other inflammatory joint diseases, joint space narrowing is a late feature. The classical triad of juxta-articular osteoporosis, peripheral osseous erosion and intra-articular joint space narrowing occurs only with articular TB that remains untreated for months.[19,20] In contrast to pyogenic arthritis where reactive sclerosis occurs early, in TB, sclerosis occurs later, usually with treatment.

Routine blood tests, including blood counts are unhelpful in diagnosis. The sedimentation rate and C-reactive protein are elevated in most patients, but are nonspecific. However, if elevated, inflammatory markers are useful in monitoring response to treatment. Although Mantoux skin testing for TB is positive in 90% of patients with OTB, this test is of limited value in countries with a high prevalence of TB.[21] In countries with routine BCG immunization, a higher cut-off is required for a positive Mantoux. Furthermore, the Mantoux is likely to be negative in patients with general debility, HIV infection and immunosuppressive therapy. The synovial fluid in articular TB demonstrates an inflammatory pattern with high white cell counts over 10 000/mm^3 (predominantly neutrophils), protein levels higher than 3.5 g/dL and blood : synovial fluid glucose gradients >40 mg/dl. However, synovial fluid cultures are positive in only 20–40% of patients.[22] The more expensive polymerase chain reaction (PCR) is both sensitive and specific in detecting TB from tissues and synovial fluid.[23] However, histological confirmation remains the gold standard in diagnosis with synovial biopsies demonstrating caseating granulomata in 80% of patients.

Pitfalls in diagnosis are common in patients with a background of inflammatory arthropathy especially if these patients are using disease-modifying anti-rheumatic drugs or biologics.[22] In tropical countries, articular tuberculosis must be suspected if a patient with well-controlled arthritis develops an isolated monoarthritis. In such situations, it is imperative to conduct synovial fluid aspiration and biopsy to investigate for joint TB. Similarly, a diagnosis of tuberculosis must be excluded in patients with unilateral sacroiliitis before a diagnosis of spondyloarthropathy is reached.

Treatment. Anti-tuberculous drug therapy (ATT) will cure most patients with joint and non-paralytic spinal tuberculosis. Treatment commences as an initial intensive phase with essential first-line anti-tuberculosis drugs: isoniazid, rifampicin, ethambutol and pyrazinamide with or without streptomycin. This is followed by a continuation phase with two or three drugs (including isoniazid and rifampicin depending on national protocols) for 9–10 months. The treatment is continued until clinical improvement with normalization of acute-phase reactants and radiological signs of bony fusion. However, effectiveness of treatment depends on patient compliance for long-term treatment. This is particularly problematic in situations where regular patient follow-up is difficult due to lack of communication facilities. Directly observed therapy (DOTS) and a single poly-pill are mechanisms utilized to improve patient adherence. Since side effects of ATT are relatively common, vigilance for them are essential, but is difficult in countries lacking well-structured health care delivery systems.

Early detection of spinal (before extensive neurological involvement) and joint disease (before joint surfaces are severely destroyed) is associated with a better prognosis. Although a variety of surgical interventions are used in late-stage OTB their outcome is variable.[24] In spinal tuberculosis, anterior spinal decompression and fusion is useful in selected patients.[25] However, in established paraplegia, surgical outcome is generally poor.

In joint tuberculosis, operative intervention by synovectomy and debridement are required if the patient is not responding to over 5 months of ATT. In addition, 'palliative' surgical procedures such as excisional arthroplasties of hip and elbow joints or joint fusion in the shoulder or ankle are useful in improving joint function and reducing pain in end-stage joint damage.[24] However, in advanced joint failure, joint replacement remains the only option.[24] Unfortunately, such major surgical procedures are not widely available in countries with a high prevalence of tuberculosis. The prognosis is worse in HIV-infected patients, particularly those with AIDS. In such situations, the response to chemotherapy is usually poor, and the outcome of surgery is variable.

Leprosy

Epidemiology. Leprosy is a chronic granulomatous disorder caused by *Mycobacterium leprae* that typically manifests cutaneous and neurological disease. However, musculoskeletal disease occurs in approximately 75% of cases (Box 69.2) and is occasionally the only presenting manifestation.[26] With the advent of multidrug therapy (MDT), leprosy has been eradicated from many countries, but continues to be a problem in Asia, Africa and South America.[27]

Epidemiological data on the prevalence of arthritis in leprosy vary depending on the reporting centre ranging from 1–78%.[28–30] The disease expression can be minimal in the tuberculoid form of leprosy where the T cell response is predominant. Alternatively, the disease can cause severe skin, nerve, joint and bone damage in the lepromatous form of leprosy that occurs in impaired immune states. The disease can be polarized to one of these extreme clinical states or remain in intermediate states. Musculoskeletal disease can occur with disease flares that occur spontaneously or with MDT (reactional states). Lepra reactions triggered by vaccines, pregnancy, surgery, physical and mental stresses have been documented.[31]

Pathogenesis and Pathology. The pathogenic process underlying articular disease in leprosy (see Chapter 41) is yet to be ascertained. However, multiple mechanisms including

BOX 69.2 TYPES OF RHEUMATOLOGICAL INVOLVEMENT IN LEPROSY

- Acute polyarthritis of lepra reaction
- Bacterial septic arthritis
- Chronic/subacute polyarthritis
- Charcot arthropathy (neuropathic arthropathy)
- 'Swollen hand' syndrome.

reactional states (Type I and II lepra reactions),[32,33] direct infiltration of synovium and neurological deficits leading to joint destruction have been implicated.

Clinical Features. The clinical features of leprosy depend on the intensity of the T cell response. A vigorous T cell response causes tuberculoid leprosy to be limited to single or few well-defined, skin lesions which are hypopigmented and anaesthetic. Here, nerve involvement is restricted to isolated thickened cutaneous nerves or to mononeuritis multiplex. Musculoskeletal involvement in tuberculoid leprosy is limited to muscle wasting from nerve damage or to tenosynovitis adjacent to skin lesions.

At the other end of the spectrum, lepromatous leprosy is characterized by many, widespread, skin lesions, and extensive infiltrative nerve, cartilage and joint damage. *M. leprae* septic arthritis results from bone invasion extending to joints, and occurs in classical forms of leprosy, without superadded lepra reactions. Approximately 10% of leprosy patients with long-standing peripheral neuropathy develop Charcot arthropathy,[32] or neuropathic joint damage, which is characterized by joint dislocations, bone resorption, digital loss, fractures and gross deformities of the weight-bearing joints. Despite its decline in recent times, leprosy remains a leading cause of neuropathic joints in the tropics. However, other causes of Charcot joints such as diabetes mellitus, tabes dorsalis and syringomyelia must be considered in the differential diagnosis.

Chronic tenosynovitis has also been described in lepromatous and borderline leprosy. The majority of patients have thickened nerves in addition to skin lesions.[33,34] In addition, a chronic symmetrical polyarthritis has been described. This pattern of arthritis can occur in the absence of lepra reactions.[35] Most patients with the symmetrical polyarthritis are patients with long-term joint symptoms and chronic leprosy for decades without current active disease.[36]

The majority of articular manifestations in leprosy are associated with lepra reactions. Fever, worsening skin lesions, numbness and joint pains dominate the clinical picture in both types of lepra reactions. An acute-onset, 'rheumatoid-like', symmetrical swelling of small joints of the hands and feet, wrists and knees is the commonest manifestation. The arthritis typically settles within a few weeks. In addition, acute onset of oedema with nodules on the dorsum of hands and feet has been described in lepra reactions. The nodules present in this 'swollen hand syndrome' when biopsied contained bacilli and granulomatous inflammation.

Diagnosis. Diagnosis of articular forms of leprosy requires a high index of clinical suspicion. It must be noted that the rheumatoid factor and anti-nuclear antibodies (ANA) can be falsely elevated in leprosy. The typical 'rheumatoid-like' arthritis, nodules and positive rheumatoid factor may lead to a misdiagnosis of rheumatoid arthritis. Further complicating diagnosis is the similarity of erosions in leprosy to those in rheumatoid arthritis. Anti-cyclic citrullinated (Anti-CCP) antibodies which are highly specific for rheumatoid arthritis may not be widely available in resource-poor settings to aid differentiation. Similarly, the presence of photosensitive skin lesions, a positive ANA and a symmetrical arthritis may prompt an incorrect diagnosis of systemic lupus erythematosus (SLE). Therefore, the presence of a symmetrical arthritis with or without tenosynovitis in the tropics should prompt the search for thickened nerves and anaesthetic skin lesions suggestive of leprosy. Suspicious skin lesions should be biopsied if nerve thickening is contentious. The diagnosis is more challenging when rheumatological manifestations occur in purely neuritic leprosy in which skin lesions are minimal. In such situations nerve biopsy may be required to ascertain diagnosis.[35]

Demonstrating the presence of *Mycobacterium leprae* in the synovium or joint tissues remains the gold standard in diagnosis of musculoskeletal leprosy. However, *M. leprae* bacilli are difficult to isolate in routine practice. It is envisaged that a recently developed serological test to identify antibodies for phosphoglycolipid-1 specific to *M. leprae*[37] or PCR to detect genes or DNA sequences unique to the bacilli[38] would assist in diagnosis. However, these investigations are not widely available in the tropics, where the diagnosis is still reliant on clinical acumen.

Treatment. All musculoskeletal manifestations of leprosy, apart for Charcot joints, respond well to WHO multi-drug therapies (MDT) for leprosy.[39] Early diagnosis is essential as prompt treatment is associated with good prognosis.

For lepra-reaction-associated arthritis the mainstay of therapy is corticosteroids. Prednisolone is usually commenced at 1 mg/kg per day, followed by a gradual taper. The total duration of corticosteroids varies from 4–6 months. Erythema nodosum leprosum may additionally require clofazimine or thalidomide. The potential for anti-TNF therapy is now being evaluated.[37]

Rickettsiosis

Rickettsial infections (see Chapter 22) are bacterial infections transmitted to the human host by ticks, fleas, mites and other arthropods. The clinical syndrome is characterized by fever, headache, maculopapular exanthema, arthralgia and an eschar at the inoculation site of tick-borne rickettsioses. Frank arthritis is unusual. In recent times, an array of rickettsial pathogens has been described in the tropics causing myalgia and articular manifestations in the local populations and travellers. Personal protective measures that prevent insect bites are effective in preventing rickettsioses.[40–43]

Brucellosis

For detailed information on Brucellosis, see Chapter 28.

Rheumatic Fever

Rheumatic fever (RF) is a post-infectious immunological complication of group A streptococcal infection. It is characterized by an acute febrile illness, arthritis and carditis giving rise to late sequelae of rheumatic valvular heart disease and chorea. RF usually afflicts children and young adults manifesting as arthritis in 80% and arthralgia in 10%. The articular involvement of RF is generally a polyarticular flitting arthritis involving one to two joints at a time with a single joint involved for less than one day. Residual joint sequelae are rare. The incidence of RF in the tropics has declined due to the widespread use of penicillin antibiotics for sore throat and improved socioeconomic conditions.[44,45]

Osteomyelitis and Septic Arthritis

Osteomyelitis and septic arthritis continue to be significant problems in the tropics. The infection reaches the bone by haematogenous spread or by direct inoculation with the former being the more common route. The commonest causative organism is *Staphylococcus aureus*, followed by *Escherichia coli* and *Klebsiella*. However, certain organisms have been implicated in specific patient populations. For example, *Pseudomonas* species are common in intravenous street drugs users (IVDU) and in patients with sharp penetrating injuries. Persons with sickle cell disease have a propensity for non-typhoid *Salmonella* infections. The increasing incidence of HIV infection in the tropics has led to an unprecedented increase in bone, muscle and joint infections, particularly that of infections by uncommon organisms.[46,47] In addition, reactivation of previous osteomyelitis has been documented in adults with AIDS. Furthermore, gonococcal arthritis has re-emerged and is considered to be virtually pathognomonic of HIV infection in high prevalence countries.

Bone infection in children is particularly common in long tubular bones, while in adults, osteomyelitis affects flat bones, preferentially targeting the pelvis, clavicle or spine, particularly in IVDU. Osteomyelitis or bone infection typically presents with bone pain, local swelling, warmth and fever. A fluctuant subfascial abscess may be detected in some patients.[46]

Joint infection or septic arthritis presents as a monoarthritis. This diagnosis is easily evident in the presence of a hot, swollen joint in a febrile patient. The differential diagnosis of septic arthritis includes crystal arthritis and inflammatory arthritis. Discrimination between these conditions is based on analysis of synovial fluid. Elevated inflammatory markers and high white cell counts are commonly present in both osteomyelitis and septic arthritis. It is noteworthy that HIV infection-associated osteomyelitis and septic arthritis have a less abrupt onset and less florid physical signs.[48,49]

Blood cultures are usually positive in both osteomyelitis and septic arthritis. Radiography demonstrates variable degrees of osteoporosis, periosteal reaction and bone destruction in the latter stages. However, in the early stages, radiography is usually normal. MRI scanning and three-phase bone scanning (with or without gallium or indium) are useful in early diagnosis, but are not widely available in the tropics.[50]

The clinician is guided by antibiotic sensitivity reporting and minimum inhibitory drug concentrations when treating. In resource-poor settings in the tropics, empirical antibiotic treatment is common. Cloxacillin, flucloxacillin and ciprofloxacin are the usual empiric choices. Treatment of osteomyelitis and septic arthritis requires protracted courses of antibiotics with or without drainage of accumulated pus. Since facilities for outpatient-based intravenous antibiotic therapy are scarce in the resource-poor tropics, patients are often treated as in-hospital patients with substantial economic consequences for both the patient and healthcare service. In HIV-infection-associated osteomyelitis and septic arthritis, the response to treatment is usually poor. Drainage of pus and intravenous antibiotics produce only a temporary response in HIV-infected patients who end up often necessitating limb amputation to control infection and to save life.[47]

Myositis

Primary diseases of skeletal muscles (myopathies) are uncommon. More commonly, myopathies occur in association with other disease processes of which infections are a relatively common cause in the tropics. Muscle has a limited range of responses to a wide range of disease and most commonly presents with either muscle weakness or muscle pain, or both. However, it must be noted that diseases of the motor nerves (motor neurone disease) and neuromuscular junction (snake bite envenomation[51] and organophosphate poisoning,[52] which are common in the tropics) can clinically mimic a myopathy.

Infectious myositis occurs due to a wide variety of pathogens, including bacteria, fungi, parasites and viruses. The commonest causative bacteria are staphylococcal and streptococcal species.[53] Although the definitive diagnosis of the causative agent requires cultures or tests to detect microbial antigens or nucleic acid, the clinical presentation can suggest the general category of the aetiological agent. For example, bacterial myositis usually presents as a focal muscle infection while viruses and parasites are often more diffuse and present as generalized myalgias or multifocal myositis.

Pyomyositis

Pyomyositis is an intramuscular suppurative infection that arises from haematogenous spread, which was classically seen in the tropics but is now increasingly recognized in temperate climates.[54,55] Tropical pyomyositis mostly occurs in otherwise healthy children (ages 2–5) and adults (ages 20–45), while the majority of temperate pyomyositis cases occur in immunocompromised adults.[56] *Staphylococcus aureus* is the causative organism in up to 90% of cases in tropical areas and 75% of cases in temperate countries followed by group A streptococci and less commonly, non-group A streptococci, pneumococci and Gram-negative enteric bacilli.[57]

Pyomyositis presents with fever and pain localized to a single muscle group. The disease commonly affects large muscles of the lower extremity (thigh, calf and glutei), but any muscle group can be involved. Multifocal infection involving more than one muscle group has been observed in up to one-fifth of cases.[56] The disease then evolves to the stage of intramuscular abscess formation characterized by high spiky fever, exquisite muscle tenderness and oedema. However, the classical signs of abscess may not be clinically apparent due to the overlying tense muscle. If untreated, pyomyositis evolves to a stage of septicaemia and systemic toxicity.

MRI and CT are the modalities of choice for early diagnosis in pyomyositis while ultrasonography is useful to diagnose intramuscular abscesses and to guide percutaneous needle drainage.[58] Lack of availability of these imaging modalities may delay the diagnosis in tropics. Blood cultures have a low positivity,[59] but are essential in all cases. Laboratory tests show neutrophil leucocytosis and raised inflammatory markers. Muscle enzymes (CPK, LDH) are only slightly raised despite muscle destruction. HIV and other immunodeficient states must be investigated.

Treatment involves drainage of abscess and parenteral antibiotics directed against staphylococci and streptococci in immunocompetent patients with additional antibiotic coverage directed against Gram-negative and anaerobic organisms in immunocompromised patients.

VIRAL INFECTIONS

Viral arthritides seen in the tropics are caused by agents similar to those causing disease in temperate regions. However, arthritogenic arboviruses, in particular alphaviruses, and HIV infection, cause most of the clinically distinct virus-associated musculoskeletal disorders in the tropics.

Alphaviruses

Epidemiology. Mosquitoes are not just a nuisance in the tropics; they transmit several viruses which cause disabling musculoskeletal disease in humans. Foremost among them are arboviruses, which share the common feature of transmission by arthropod vectors. Of these viruses belonging to the genus *alpha*, family Togaviridae are of special interest by virtue of their potential to cause significant joint involvement. These viruses are unique in causing vast outbreaks followed by a complete disappearance for years or decades. Most of these viruses have a typical geographical distribution, but international travel has obscured these boundaries. A typical example of this globalization is an Italian outbreak of chikungunya triggered by a man travelling from India carrying an African strain of the virus, disseminated by an Italian vector mosquito.[60]

Clinical Features. Alphavirus infections are characterized by the triad of fever, arthralgia and rash. These clinical features occur abruptly after an incubation period of 2–10 days. In the early phase, fever, muscle pains, malaise and headache dominate the clinical picture. This can be followed by grave manifestations such as petechiae, purpura, haematemesis, melaena and bleeding of the gums in a minority with severe infections of Chikungunya, O'nyong-Nyong, and Mayaro virus infections.[61]

The joint symptoms of these diseases are severe and debilitating, as reflected in the graphical descriptions of these diseases in colloquial language (Tables 69.1). The joints affected commonly are the ankles, wrists and phalanges. The symptoms are similar to other inflammatory joint diseases and it is difficult to differentiate clinically without further investigation. In the 2006 chikungunya outbreak, virtually all the patients had joint involvement.[62] Previous reports have indicated that the arthritis can persist for 4 months in 33%;[63] 20 months in 15%;[64] and 3–5 years in 10%.[65] In our experience, a small percentage of patients from the 2006 outbreak of chikungunya continue to have an inflammatory arthropathy more than 5 years later, amenable to conventional disease-modifying drugs. Data from the COPCORD study (see below) have indicated a doubling in the percentage of rheumatic musculoskeletal disease in certain communities in the aftermath of the chikungunya outbreak.[66,67]

The differential diagnosis of chikungunya includes dengue fever, transmitted by *Aedes* mosquitoes with a similar epidemiological distribution in Asia. The clinical features of both infections are similar, but profound arthritis has been a discriminatory feature of chikungunya.[68] Leucopaenia was common to both infections though severe thrombocytopaenia was limited to dengue infection.

TABLE 69.1 Arthritic Alphaviruses and Their Typical Geographical Distribution

Chikungunya (Makonde: 'He who walks doubled up')	Africa, India, Indian Ocean islands (2005/2006 outbreak in Mauritius, Sri Lanka, etc.), South-east Asia
O'nyong-Nyong (Acholi tribe Uganda: 'weakening of the joints')	Africa
Mayaro fever	Rural South America
Igbo-Ora ('the disease that breaks your wings')	Africa (Ivory Coast)

Real-time polymerase chain reaction (RT-PCR) is valuable in the early confirmation of arbovirus infections, particularly chikungunya. However, the value of RT-PCR is limited to diagnosis in the viraemic phase, with later infection requiring serology. Direct immunofluorescence assay to detect chikungunya IgM has a high sensitivity and specificity and is used in the latter stages.[69] However, the use of these tests in the tropics may be limited by financial constraints.

A normal erythrocyte sedimentation rate and a negative rheumatoid factor are useful to differentiate chikungunya arthritis from rheumatoid arthritis. Extensive, symmetrical joint involvement, particularly of the metacarpophalangeal and proximal joints, the presence of rheumatoid nodules or anti-cyclic citrullinated peptide (anti-CCP) antibodies favours rheumatoid arthritis over chikungunya with chronic arthropathy. The presence of lower limb asymmetrical joint involvement with axial skeletal affliction favours the diagnosis of spondyloarthropathy over chikungunya.

Pathogenesis and Pathology. For detailed information on the pathogenesis and pathology of Arbovirus infections, see Chapter 14.

Treatment. Treatment is symptomatic. Non-steroidal anti-inflammatory drugs can be used if dengue is excluded. The anecdotal reports of treating acute/subacute infection with hydroxychloroquine are now disputed.[70] Protection from mosquito bites and controlling vector breeding remain the most effective strategies in preventing disease.

Human Immunodeficiency Virus (HIV) Infection

At the end of 2010, an estimated 24 million people were living with HIV infection, of whom more than 80% were residing in tropical and sub-tropical regions. Although rheumatic disorders associated with HIV infection are rare, increased numbers of HIV patients make this disease burden a significant socio-economic problem in the tropics.[71] In some parts of sub-Saharan Africa and India, HIV infection continues uncurtailed from the initial viraemic stage to florid AIDS due to the unavailability of highly active anti-retroviral treatment (HAART). Patients with early stages of HIV infection present with bone, muscle and joint infection as a consequence of trauma. In later stages, patients present with spontaneous musculoskeletal infections or with reactivation of previous infections (see below).

Rheumatic Syndromes Associated with HIV Infection. A wide range of articular manifestations with HIV infection has been reported.[72] These conditions include arthralgias, arthritis and HIV-associated inflammatory articular syndromes (Box 69.3).

Of inflammatory articular syndromes associated with HIV, the most common are spondyloarthropathies (SpA), which have features distinct from the classical SpA not associated with HIV. The classical SpA not associated with HIV are a cluster of inflammatory joint disorders associated with HLA-B27 gene positivity, with predilection for axial skeletal inflammation, sacroiliitis and enthesitis. The spondyloarthropathy family includes reactive arthritis (an immunological consequence of infection elsewhere), psoriatic arthritis (with its hallmark psoriatic skin and nail lesions) and enteropathic arthritis. The articular involvement of these conditions is typically an asymmetrical oligoarthritis of lower limbs.

BOX 69.3 TYPES OF RHEUMATOLOGICAL INVOLVEMENT IN HIV INFECTION

- Expected increase in bone, joint and muscle infection
- Unexpected increase in rheumatic disorders
- Arthralgia (5–45%)
- Painful articular syndrome
- HIV-associated arthritis (10–12%)
- Spondyloarthropathies
- Reactive arthritis (0.4–10%)
- Psoriatic arthritis (1.5–2%)
- Undifferentiated spondyloarthritis
- Hyperuricaemia and gout
- Osteonecrosis
- Immune reconstitution inflammatory syndromes.

It is noteworthy that classical SpA was uncommon in the tropics prior to the HIV epidemic: a phenomenon attributed to low prevalence of HLA B27 in indigenous populations and SpA disease suppression by parasitic diseases, particularly malaria.[73] However, HIV-associated SpA (HIV SpA) occurs in these populations despite the absence of the HLA B27 gene. The commonest forms of HIV SpA are reactive arthritis and psoriatic arthritis (see below). The explanation for the increase in this particular form of inflammatory joint disease in HIV remains elusive, although its association with HLA-B57, a gene associated with slow progression of HIV, is a matter of considerable research interest.[74] Advanced clinical and radiological features of spinal inflammation are rare, presumably due to the shortened life span of these patients.

Another feature of HIV SpA is the increase in florid skin manifestations. Reactive arthritis with prominent mucocutaneous features of circinate balanitis and keratoderma blenorrhagicum is particularly common in HIV infection. Similarly psoriatic arthritis associated with HIV is associated with florid psoriatic skin lesions of a guttate-psoriatic plaque mixture.[72]

The mainstay of treatment of HIV-associated SpA is non-steroidal anti-inflammatory drugs (NSAIDs). Intra-articular/entheseal steroids, sulfasalazine[75] and hydroxychloroquine[76,77] have proved beneficial and safe in these immunocompromised populations. However, more potent agents such as methotrexate are best avoided or used with extreme caution.[78,79] HAART is very effective in treating SpA and increasing the availability of HAART in the tropics will reduce the disease burden of HIV-associated SpA.[72]

The prevalence of arthralgia in HIV is 5% in retrospective studies and 45% in prospective studies.[80,81] Arthralgia affects particularly the knees, shoulders and elbows. The arthralgia of HIV infection settles with NSAIDs. An intermittent painful articular syndrome lasting a few hours, but severe enough to warrant opioid analgesics has been reported.[82] This syndrome has become less common with the increasing use of HAART.

HIV-associated arthritis is an inflammatory arthropathy that occurs in HIV infection. These patients do not fulfil the diagnostic criteria for SpA or rheumatoid arthritis and are HLAB27, ANA, rheumatoid factor and anti-CCP antibody negative. In contrast to European studies where HIV-associated arthritis is a predominantly lower limb oligoarthritis, the African variety tends to be polyarticular, symmetrical and 'rheumatoid'-like.[83] HIV-associated arthritis has a good prognosis, settling within 2–5 weeks of NSAIDs in the majority.

PARASITIC INFECTIONS

Parasitic diseases are common in the tropics. However, associated rheumatological syndromes are rare. This phenomenon may be attributed to early detection of parasitic infections combined with improved accessibility to appropriate treatment. Musculoskeletal diseases associated with parasitic infections occur mostly due to nematode infections (Table 69.2). Infections due to other parasites are rare.[84]

FUNGAL INFECTIONS

Musculoskeletal diseases caused by fungi are rare. Some subcutaneous and deep tissue mycoses are commoner in the tropics and cause arthritis, which occurs from direct joint infection or spread from an adjacent bone focus. Arthritis may also occur as a result of an immunological response to fungal infection.

TABLE 69.2 Parasitic Diseases Causing Musculoskeletal Involvement

Parasite	Clinical Syndromes
LYMPHATIC FILARIASIS	
Bancroftian filariasis (*Wuchereria bancrofti*, *Brugia malayi* and *Brugia timori*) In tropical regions of Asia and Africa	Sterile monoarthritis of knee Associated features: inguinal lymphadenopathy Chylus effusion is an early feature Acute lymphatic inflammation Chronic stage: lymphatic obstruction with elephantiasis of limb, chyluria or hydrocele
TISSUE FILARIASIS	
Loiasis (*Loa loa*)	Microfilarial septic arthritis, arthritis or periarthritis of the large joints of lower limbs (eosinophilic synovial fluid) Associated features: microfilaria containing subcutaneous nodules (Calabar swelling), conjunctivitis
ONCHOCERCIASIS	
Onchocerca volvulus Africa, South and Central America	Microfilaria monoarthritis of hips, knees and elbows Associated features: nodules adjacent to affected joint, dermatitis, keratitis and chorioretinitis ('river blindness') Rheumatoid arthritis-like polyarthritis Associated features: precipitated or worsened by treatment with diethylcarbamazine
DRACUNCULIASIS (GUINEA WORM INFECTION)	
West and Central Africa, India South East Asia	Acute microfilarial eosinophilic monoarthritis (usually of knee) Can progress to a destructive arthropathy ('Ibadan knee') Sterile arthritis or periarthritis (reaction to adjacent filarial worm)
STRONGYLOIDIASIS	
Strongyloides stercoralis	Reactive arthritis, asymmetric oligoarthritis with or without sacroiliitis (with or without eosinophilia) Treatment of rheumatological conditions may be associated with disseminated strongyloidosis

Fungal bone and soft tissue infection is less common, but causes substantial disability and morbidity. Among this group of disorders are mycetoma, a chronic infection of bones, joints and soft tissue, often of the foot.[85]

Fungal musculoskeletal disorders have an insidious course. Treatment involves the use of an appropriate antifungal agent in combination with surgical debridement.

Metabolic Bone Diseases

Metabolic bone diseases pertaining to the tropics include fluorotoxic bone disease and vitamin D deficiency. In addition, increased life expectancy and sedentary lifestyles consequent to rapid urbanization have increased the magnitude of problems associated with osteoporosis in tropical countries.

FLUOROTOXIC METABOLIC BONE DISEASE

Fluorosis is endemic in over 20 countries worldwide, but is focused in particular tropical regions, with India and China among the worst affected. Chronic fluoride toxicity occurs mainly through consumption of ground water with a fluoride concentration in excess of 1.5 mg/L.

Fluorosis primarily affects skeletal tissue with a majority of patients presenting with bone deformities, bone pain and proximal muscle weakness. A third of patients develop fluorotic dental mottling. Radiologically, fluorosis is characterized by osteosclerosis and ligamentous calcification (Figure 69.2). Renal tubular damage leading to secondary nephronal loss and chronic kidney disease has been attributed to excess fluoride ingestion, particularly in hot dry climates of the tropics where greater dehydration and acidification of urine occurs.[86]

The skeletal and dental effects of chronic fluorosis are irreversible. Prevention is the key and is directed towards keeping fluoride intake within safe limits. This goal is achieved by defluoridation of water or by using an alternative source of water. Improving the nutritional status of children in affected regions and dietary supplementation of calcium and vitamin C is useful in minimizing the effects of fluorosis.

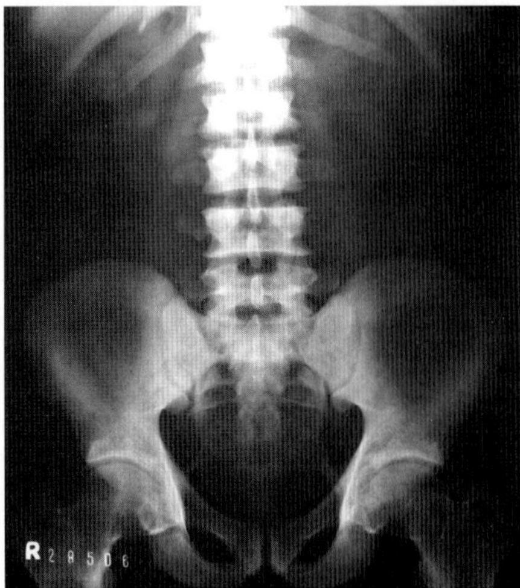

Figure 69.2 Radiograph showing osteosclerosis of vertebral and pelvic bones, and calcification of sacroiliac ligaments in a patient with fluorosis. *(Courtesy of Dr Priyangee Arambepola.)*

RICKETS AND OSTEOMALACIA

Rickets in children and osteomalacia in adults are metabolic bone diseases, resulting from vitamin D deficiency. Poor dietary intake of vitamin D, highly pigmented skin with reduced sun exposure in certain communities wearing a garment called a 'Abhaya' are contributory factors for vitamin D deficiency in the tropics where sunshine is plentiful. However, increasingly, secondary causes such as renal tubular acidosis are recognized as causes of rickets/osteomalacia. Maternal vitamin D deficiency causing rickets in babies has been reported. Vitamin D deficiency typically presents with bony deformities (rickets) or with nonspecific musculoskeletal pains or weakness in adults. The treatment of this condition is with high-dose calciferol for 8–12 weeks followed by vitamin D supplementation in the long term.[87]

Haemoglobinopathy-associated Bone Disease

SICKLE CELL DISEASE

Sickle cell disease is caused by a point mutation in the β-globin chain of haemoglobin (Hb). This results in formation of Hb polymers with de-oxygenation and sickling of red blood cells Homozygotes for the disease have severe haemolytic anaemia and joint pains from bone infarcts. The characteristic musculoskeletal involvement of sickle cell disease is shown in Box 69.4. Management of the conditions includes symptomatic treatment, including hydration and opioids in sickle cell crises. Transfusion reduces the amount of abnormal Hb. Antibiotic prophylaxis and vaccination are useful in minimizing infection. Bone marrow transplant or stem cell transplant is useful when facilities are available.[88]

Soft Tissue Rheumatism and Osteoarthritis in the Tropics

Diseases of the musculoskeletal soft tissues (ligaments, tendons and peri-articular structures) are equally common in tropical and temperate regions. However, it is generally believed that patients living in the tropics do not seek medical attention as often as their Western-world counterparts, as demonstrated in some studies.[89] This may be due to poor accessibility to

BOX 69.4 BONE AND JOINT INVOLVEMENT IN SICKLE CELL DISEASE

ACUTE BONE PROBLEMS

- Painful vaso-occlusive crises
- Osteomyelitis
- Septic arthritis
- Bone marrow necrosis, stress fractures
- Dental infections.

CHRONIC PROBLEMS

- Avascular necrosis
- Osteopaenia and osteoporosis
- Growth retardation.

healthcare services and sickness absence-related financial repercussions. The consequences of daily wage loss are particularly marked in communities where the bread winners are employed as manual labourers.

Knowledge on the magnitude of soft tissue rheumatism in the tropics was previously limited. However, initiatives such as the Community Oriented Program for the Control of Rheumatic Disorders (COPCORD) have provided epidemiological data on musculoskeletal disorders from several tropical regions including Asia, Asia-Pacific, South America and Africa. The overall prevalence of musculoskeletal pain in these studies averaged at 25%.[1,90] Knee osteoarthritis, mechanical back pain, soft tissue rheumatism and low back pain were the dominant causes of musculoskeletal pain.[90] Common soft tissue problems in the tropics include repetitive strain injuries, osteoarthritis, pain from generalized hypermobility and chronic widespread pain syndromes.

Repetitive strain injuries (RSI) in the tropics occur from contrasting circumstances to those in the West. The association of RSI with agricultural practices dependent on manual labour, religious practices such as repetitive kneeling and domestic practices such as scraping and extracting coconut milk, etc., indicate the need to appreciate the sociocultural circumstances of the individual when treating their complaints.

Another disease entity common in the tropics is hypermobility resulting from joint laxity. Generalized benign hypermobility syndromes are characterized by the presence of musculoskeletal complaints in subjects who have generalized hypermobility of joints without demonstrable systemic rheumatological disease. These conditions are commoner in populations from the Indian and African subcontinents than Caucasian populations,[91] with the highest prevalence reported among Oriental Asians.[92] Joint hypermobility is most marked in children and reduces in severity with increasing age. The majority of patients are asymptomatic (Figure 69.3). Symptomatic individuals present with widespread or localized pain without arthritis. It has been noted that these patients have repetitive strain injuries with normal levels of activity and recurrent joint dislocations. Treatment is by reassurance, counselling towards joint protection, and exercise therapy to improve muscle tone, joint stability and proprioception.[92]

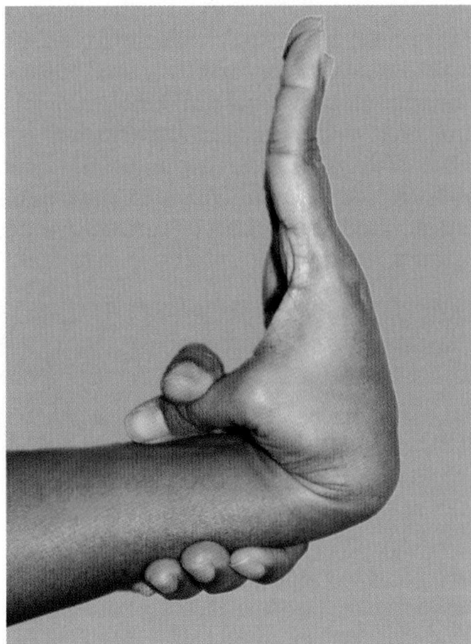

Figure 69.3 Joint hypermobility in an asymptomatic young Asian female.

Another common problem is chronic widespread pain, which is defined as pain arising from muscles and periarticular soft tissues that lasts for more than 3 months. This group includes syndromes such as fibromyalgia (FM) and is characterized by the presence of normal investigations, poor treatment response and chronic ill-health and disability. The COPCORD study revealed varied prevalence rates of FM in different communities with higher prevalence rates in rural populations.[92–95] It is important to note that these studies are limited by difficulties in assessing pain and disability in cultural and social circumstances very different from the original Western applications. These limitations are further compounded by problems of poor literacy.[94] This may account for a plethora of aches and pains of undetermined aetiology reported in an Indian COPCORD study;[96] a possible result of varied cultural and social experiences in different communities.

Osteoarthritis (OA) of the knees, neck and back are common in all communities, with the tropics being no exception. Moreover, the COPCORD studies revealed comparable epidemiology to studies done in temperate regions.[97–99] However it is noteworthy that curious forms of premature OA have been described in certain tropical populations in China (Kashin-Beck disease),[100] India (Malnad disease)[101] and Zululand, South Africa (Mseleni disease).[102] The role of genetic and environmental factors for these premature OA syndromes is under investigation, the results of which may shed new light on the pathogenesis of OA.

The prevalence rates of OA from the COPCORD studies varied from country to country.[96] Knee OA was the commonest form of OA while hip and hand OA were less common in most communities. In addition to risk factors described in temperate countries, residing in multi-storied building (possibly without elevators), squatting (for toilet use or working), rickshaw pulling, earth digging[97] and occupations with a high physical workload on the knees were associated with OA in the tropical setting.[96]

The determinants of neck pain in tropical countries are yet to be determined. Casual passers-by in the tropics will note inhabitants carrying heavy loads on heads and necks, seemingly without complaint (Figure 69.4). Studies have shown increased neck pain[103] and radiological cervical spondylosis[96] in these groups. A similar phenomenon has been observed with other musculoskeletal complaints. Low back pain was previously perceived as being rare in tropical countries. However, recent studies in the tropics show that the prevalence of low back pain is comparable to that of developed nations. This was particularly notable in agricultural communities in Africa.[103] However, the causal relationship between occupational load-carrying and back pain needs to be further explored.[104]

Traditional and complementary medicine continues to be popular in the tropics. The COPCORD studies observed that traditional healthcare practices are used by nearly 80–90% of persons in both rural and urban settings. Moreover, self-medication was as high as 58.8% in certain studies.[105] These practices may contribute to the underestimation of the burden of musculoskeletal diseases in the tropics. Furthermore, the clinical features may alter with herbal medications, further hampering the diagnostic process.

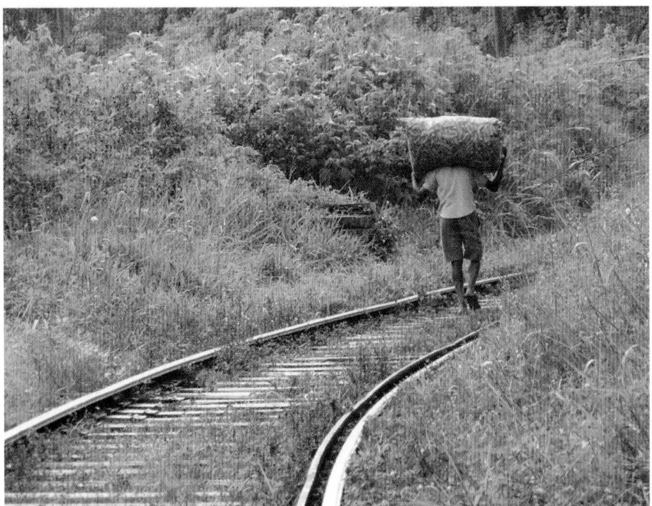

Figure 69.4 A villager carrying a heavy load in rural Sri Lanka. *(Courtesy of Mr Priyanjan De Silva.)*

The COPCORD studies have highlighted the global nature of soft tissue rheumatic disorders. However, the contributory and causative factors varied widely from country to country and region to region within individual tropical countries. This phenomenon is attributed to the socio-cultural variations in each region. Thus, an in-depth knowledge of the personal circumstances of each patient is required to understand and treat their musculoskeletal problem meaningfully.

Challenges in Managing Inflammatory Musculoskeletal Diseases in the Tropics

The management of rheumatic diseases in the tropics is difficult. In addition to infections and infection-related articular disorders, there is varied expression of more universal rheumatological syndromes such as rheumatoid arthritis (RA), systemic lupus erythematosus (SLE), gout and spondyloarthropathies (SpA). The prevalence of these conditions appears to be more in urban tropical settings.[106–108] However, this observation may be confounded by adverse socio-economic conditions in rural areas which limit health service accessibility and general longevity. Furthermore, the premise that genes protective against multiple parasitic infections, including malaria, are selected over genes associated with autoimmune disease, may account for the rarity of these rheumatological diseases in rural communities in malarial-endemic areas.

In general, the clinical features and activity of inflammatory diseases are comparable with those of non-tropical developed countries. However, diagnosis is frequently delayed. Diagnostic antibody assays and investigations for assessment of target organ damage are not widely available. Cheaper drugs such as methotrexate and hydroxychloroquine are preferred. Cytokine and other targeted therapies are not regularly available due to financial constraints. Moreover, delayed diagnosis, poor health-seeking behaviour, inadequate drug compliance and erratic follow-up increase disease-related complications in the tropics.[106] In addition, an estimated 5% of persons aged 15–49 years in sub-Saharan Africa are HIV-positive,[71] with similar trends being observed in other HIV-prevalent regions in the tropics. This is the same age group in which most classical inflammatory joint diseases occur. Therefore differentiating HIV-associated rheumatic disorders from the classic disorders of RA, SLE, SpA, assessing disease activity and using immune suppression is a challenge for clinicians.

Rheumatoid arthritis (RA) is a chronic inflammatory arthropathy characterized by severe joint destruction and propensity to affect the small joints of the hands and feet. While, the developed world is focusing on diagnosing and treating early arthritis, the situation is strikingly different in the tropics. Viral infections such as chikungunya, hepatitis B and C and HIV have similar joint symptoms, making the diagnosis of early rheumatoid arthritis difficult, especially when immunological and serological investigations are unavailable. Furthermore, management of established arthritis in resource-poor tropical countries is often suboptimal in comparison to more affluent developed countries. In an era when tight disease control is achieved in developed countries, late and advanced presentations of RA are occurring in developing countries. Long-term patient compliance is hindered due to the limited availability of anti-rheumatic drugs in the tropics. Inadequate monitoring for side-effects of multiple drug therapies occurs due to lack of infrastructure to ensure regular patient follow-up.

The increased prevalence of HIV in the tropics has compounded difficulties in management of RA. The conundrum of using disease-modifying drugs in HIV has been discussed earlier. However, it is important to be aware that HIV may cause a remission in RA or mimic its clinical manifestations. Disease-modifying anti-rheumatic drugs (DMARDS), particularly methotrexate, increase the risk of opportunistic infections in HIV. Therefore, HIV testing before DMARDS and at regular intervals in patients on potent immunosuppressive agents is necessary. However, anti-TNF agents are believed to be safe and effective in patients with CD4 counts >200/mm^3.[71]

Systemic lupus erythematosus (SLE) is a multisystem autoimmune disease commoner in young females. However, fever, constitutional symptoms with a falsely positive ANA can be seen in a multitude of other viral and mycobacterial infections common in the tropics (Table 69.3). Furthermore, in countries with increased prevalence of HIV infection, there is a potential for diagnostic confusion as arthritis, oral ulcers, serositis, lymphadenopathy, alopecia and similar patterns of neurological, haematological and renal involvement are seen in both SLE and HIV. This diagnostic conundrum is compounded by falsely positive ANA, extractable nuclear antigens, antiphospholipid antibody tests in HIV and falsely positive HIV

TABLE 69.3 Autoantibodies Associated with Malaria and Tuberculosis

Autoantibody	Malaria (prevalence, %)	Tuberculosis (prevalence, %)
Rheumatoid factor	22	20
Antinuclear	30	40
Single stranded DNA	10	30
Anti-phospholipid antibodies	35	43
ANCA	<5	<5

Source: Adebajo AO, Charles P, Maini RN, et al. Autoantibodies in malaria, tuberculosis and hepatitis B in a west African population. Clin Exp Immunol 1993;92(1):73–6.

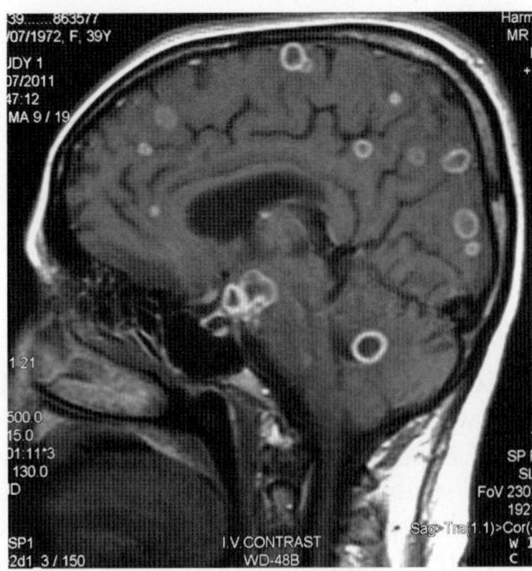

Figure 69.5 Contrast-enhanced brain MRI showing multiple tuberculomas in a patient taking immunosuppressive drugs for SLE.

ELISA in SLE. The only unique test for SLE in this setting is C3/C4 hypocomplementaemia.

Idiopathic inflammatory myopathies (IIM) such as dermatomyositis, polymyositis and inclusion-body myositis occur as uncommonly and present with typical clinical features as seen in non-tropical regions. Diagnosis is based on the clinical presentation of muscle weakness with myalgia and muscle tenderness, typical rash of dermatomyositis, elevated muscle enzymes, myopathic changes on electromyography, specific autoantibodies and characteristic histopathology on muscle biopsy. Glucocorticoids and other immunosuppressants remain the mainstay of treatment. This presents an added challenge in the tropics because of opportunistic and reactivated infections (Figure 69.5). Moreover, the association of tuberculosis with IIM is relatively commoner than with other autoimmune rheumatic diseases.[109,110] This not only presents a diagnostic dilemma in a patient with IIM who presents with pyrexia of unknown origin, but one of therapeutic challenge in treating the infection while preventing relapse of the IIM. The dose of corticosteroids may require increase to counteract the effect of hepatic enzyme induction by rifampicin used in the treatment of tuberculosis.

Gout is an inflammatory arthropathy triggered off by synovial monosodium urate crystal deposition. In certain Indonesian, Polynesian and Micronesian communities, gout is a significant problem due to a genetic predisposition.[111] However, the prevalence of gout is increasing in most urban tropical settings associated with excess alcohol consumption and unhealthy dietary habits.

The problems in management of inflammatory joint disorders are further compounded by increased self-medication practices. Self-medication with potent corticosteroids and non-steroidal anti-inflammatory drugs without prescription and the incorporation of these agents to widely accepted herbal remedies is a cause for concern and a contributory factor to drug-related complications.

Conclusion

Tropical rheumatology continues to be of interest to doctors practicing in the tropics and elsewhere. Insight to different disease presentations in the tropics has led to new insights into the pathogenesis of several diseases. Furthermore, the changing epidemiology of non-communicable diseases, the decline of some infections and the problems with new and re-emerging infections, have made this topic to be a subject-in-evolution. For doctors practicing in the tropics, limited laboratory facilities, infectious mimics of disease and the predisposition to typical and atypical infections with immune suppression places a premium on honed clinical acumen and sound clinical judgement.

REFERENCES

1. Adebajo A, McGill P, Tikly M. Tropical rheumatology – a global issue. Rheumatology (Oxford) 2009;48:599–601.
3. Halder S, Gosht P, Ghosh A. Tuberculous arthritis – the challenges and opportunities: observations from a tertiary center. Indian J Rheumatol 2011;1:62–8.
26. Chauhan S, Wakhlu A, Agarwal V. Arthritis in leprosy. Rheumatology (Oxford) 2010;49:2237–42.
72. Walker UA, Tyndall A, Daikeler T. Rheumatic conditions in human immunodeficiency virus infection. Rheumatology (Oxford) 2008;47:952–9.
93. Rahman A, Haq SA. Chronic widespread pain: North and South: Are the factors similar in both developed and developing countries? Rheumatology (Oxford) 2010;49:404–5.

Access the complete references online at www.expertconsult.com

70 Respiratory Problems in the Tropics

STEPHEN B. GORDON | KEVIN J. MORTIMER | REFILOE MASEKELA

KEY POINTS

- In an average tropical hospital, 20–50% of outpatients attend with respiratory complaints, and 20–30% of hospital medical admissions are for disorders predominantly affecting the lungs.
- The incidence is highest in infants and young children, especially for those living in urban areas and causes 20% of deaths in all children. It is estimated that acute respiratory infection (ARI) is responsible for one-third of deaths of children under 5 years of age globally and the majority of these deaths occur in children from tropical countries.
- The major burden of adult disease has traditionally been due to pneumonia and tuberculosis (see Chapter 40) but the incidence of chronic obstructive pulmonary disease is rising globally, due to the increasing use of tobacco and continuing use of biomass fuel.
- Occupational lung disease and asthma are problems of polluted and urban environments and the pulmonary complications of HIV infection include empyema, bronchiectasis and pulmonary hypertension as well as opportunistic infections.

Clinical Assessment in Children

HISTORY

Most of the morbidity and mortality due to ARI in children occurs in infants and young children. This influences the clinical approach as there is less detail of symptoms than for older children and adults, and abnormalities of auscultation or percussion may be absent or hard to define in small chests. The child usually presents with cough and/or difficulty breathing. Factors that increase the incidence and severity of childhood pneumonia include young age, low birth weight, malnutrition, exposure to indoor smoke and underlying disease such as HIV infection, cardiac abnormalities or cerebral palsy. Poor immunization coverage for measles and whooping cough may be a factor in some regions.

EXAMINATION

A raised respiratory rate is consistently the most reliable clinical sign for lower respiratory tract infection. There is some clinical overlap with the presentation of other common childhood illnesses such as malaria or septicaemia. More severe pneumonia is indicated by chest indrawing, difficulty with feeding in infants or cyanosis. School-aged children often present with acute lobar pneumonia and initially cough may not be a prominent symptom. They may complain of pleuritic chest pain and sometimes present with acute abdominal pain or with headache and neck pain, depending on the site of lobar involvement. The presence of stridor suggests large airway obstruction (e.g. croup), whilst wheeze indicates small airway obstruction (e.g. bronchiolitis in the infant or asthma in the toddler or older child). The presence of hyperinflation with loss of cardiac dullness, inferior displacement of the liver and the presence of a Hoover's sign are all indicative of small airways disease.

In children with persistent cough or wheeze not responding to standard treatment consider pulmonary TB (PTB), foreign body, HIV-related lung disease or cardiac failure. A review of the growth chart is often helpful. Mild asthma or recurrent viral respiratory infection causing persistent symptoms usually occurs in thriving well-nourished children while TB is marked by significant failure to thrive or weight loss. A history of TB contact (or of household contacts with chronic cough), particularly close contact with sputum smear-positive PTB, is important. In HIV-endemic regions, consider *Pneumocystis jerovicii* pneumonia (PcP) in an infant with severe pneumonia not responding to standard antibiotic treatment. PcP can be the first presentation of HIV-related disease. In young infants under 6 months the presence of a severe pneumonia, hypoxaemia and a clear chest on auscultation are suggestive of PcP. Lymphocytic interstitial pneumonitis (LIP) is an HIV-related lung disease that usually presents in older children and is often misdiagnosed as PTB. Look for features suggestive of HIV infection such as generalized lymphadenopathy, extensive oral candidiasis, parotid swelling, digital clubbing or typical skin rashes. A history of a choking episode in a child with persistent wheeze suggests foreign body aspiration. Children with congenital or acquired heart disease often present with recurrent or persistent respiratory symptoms.

Clinical Assessment in Adults

HISTORY

The most common respiratory symptoms are cough and dyspnoea. Carefully determine the duration of cough and degree of dyspnoea. In a patient with cough, ask for associated symptoms such as fever, chest pain, haemoptysis, night sweats and weight loss. Ask about previous anti-TB therapy, the basis for the diagnosis of PTB and successful completion of treatment. In a patient with dyspnoea, determine the speed of onset and a careful smoking and occupational history. In a patient with a short history of dyspnoea, consider pneumothorax or an inhaled foreign body; in all patients with cough, fever and dyspnoea, consider the possibility of HIV infection. HIV infection is suggested by chronic ill health of either the patient or their partner, and is particularly common in migrant workers and truck drivers.

In your differential diagnosis, remember that cardiac disease can present with dyspnoea. Mitral valve disease and pericardial tamponade (often due to TB) are much more common in developing than in industrial countries and cardiomyopathy is not uncommon.

EXAMINATION

Always start by assessing a patient with respiratory symptoms from the end of the bed in order to observe the severity of respiratory distress, as well as the symmetry of chest movement. Many patients have advanced disease by the time they reach medical attention, and have florid signs rarely seen in developed countries. Abnormalities of chest movement or shape and mediastinal (tracheal) shift may indicate contraction from chronic fibrosis within the chest. Hydropneumothorax or pyopneumothorax can be identified clinically by the succussion splash and shifting dullness (percussion over the 5th intercostal space anteriorly is dull with the patient erect, and hollow when supine). Amphoric breathing and post-tussive crackles may be heard over a large pulmonary cavity. Look for features suggestive of chronic lung disease such as a barrel-shaped chest or finger clubbing. Marked wasting, generalized lymphadenopathy and enlarged non-tender parotid glands are consistent with HIV infection but may also occur with disseminated TB or malignancy. Severe fungal infections such as histoplasmosis, cryptococcosis or paracoccidioidomycosis can also present as pneumonia in an emaciated patient and occur more commonly, but not exclusively, in HIV-infected individuals (see Chapter 19). Palpable lymph nodes may provide a source of diagnostic material and should be sought routinely.

Finally, look carefully for evidence of cardiac or abdominal abnormalities. Pericardial constriction or effusion may mimic or complicate pulmonary diseases such as TB. Right ventricular hypertrophy with cor pulmonale may develop secondary to chronic pulmonary disease, e.g. pulmonary schistosomiasis or chronic pulmonary histoplasmosis.

Pulmonary Investigations in Children and Adults

The diagnosis of bacterial pneumonia is clinical. Blood culture is often not available, has a low sensitivity (<30%) and a decision to treat with antibiotics must be made before the result is available. Transthoracic needle aspiration of consolidated lung has a higher yield and has been an important research technique for studies of aetiology, particularly in children, that guide standard management policy, but is not practical or recommended for routine clinical management.

Sputum smear microscopy for acid-fast bacilli is the initial investigation of choice for PTB diagnosis. Appropriate patient selection, proper sputum collection and optimal specimen processing are all important.[1] HIV-infected patients have increased susceptibility to TB (both reactivation and new infections) but PTB is more likely to be sputum-negative in HIV-infected patients than in other people due to the decreased immune response and hence decreased cavitation seen in the HIV-infected group. Children under eight years of age are usually unable to expectorate sputum and so the diagnosis of PTB can be particularly difficult. Improved samples can be obtained in adults by initiating a deep cough using physiotherapy or nebulized hypertonic saline to induce sputum production. In children, the use of two induced sputum samples provides a yield that is equivalent to three early morning nasogastric aspirate samples.[2]

Good sputum samples may yield other information, depending on available microbiology services. Bacterial culture is of very limited value because of the plentiful commensal flora in the pharynx but culture for tubercle bacilli yields a delayed diagnosis in some smear-negative subjects. Nocardiosis is difficult to distinguish clinically and radiologically from PTB but *Nocardia asteroides* is identifiable by Gram stain or culture of the sputum. Other organisms that are identifiable from sputum include *Burkholderia pseudomallei* (causing melioidosis), *Pneumocystis jerovicii*, *Histoplasma capsulatum*, *Cryptococcus* spp. and *Paracoccidioides brasiliensis*. Sputum microscopy may occasionally reveal larval helminths, *Strongyloides*, *Paragonimus ova*, hydatid scolices or fungal hyphae (aspergilloma).

Bedside lung function testing is not available in many parts of the tropics and under-used elsewhere. A peak flow meter provides an index of airways obstruction, both for diagnosis and for observing changes and response to treatment. Duration and force of blowing a full breath out can yield similar information (duration more than 4 s indicating severe obstruction). Pulse oximetry is a useful method for determining severity of hypoxia and response to oxygen therapy.

Chest radiographs are important but expensive. They should be used with discretion and not simply to prove what is clearly deducible from clinical features, such as in lobar pneumonia, massive pleural effusion or sputum smear-positive PTB. It is better to reserve radiography for circumstances such as the management of pneumothorax or the investigation of unresolving pneumonia. HIV infection has affected the specificity and sensitivity of chest X-ray abnormalities for patients with PTB. The appearance may be atypical, e.g. lower zone infiltrates, or even normal, especially in the severely immunocompromised patient (see Chapters 19 and 56).

Lymph node aspiration and biopsy can provide useful diagnostic information, particularly if TB or disseminated malignancy is suspected. If a large effusion is present, a pleural tap is often helpful to differentiate causes such as TB (straw-coloured fluid, by far the most common cause of effusion in TB-endemic areas), empyema (thick purulent fluid) or pulmonary Kaposi's sarcoma (bloody tap in the presence of palatal KS). Pleural biopsy, using an Abrams' needle and taking two or three specimens in different directions at the same site, may assist with histological diagnosis. HIV testing is widely available and should be considered in all patients: caution must be used in order not to miss multiple diagnoses in HIV-infected patients.

If available, fibreoptic bronchoscopy may provide useful additional diagnostic information, by identifying causes of local bronchial obstruction (e.g. foreign bodies, tumours) or obtaining secretions and specimens by bronchoalveolar lavage and transbronchial biopsy. As for sputum sampling, the value of fibreoptic bronchoscopy is limited by the quality of laboratory facilities that can be applied to fluid or tissues obtained. It is rarely indicated in young children except for foreign body removal.

ACUTE RESPIRATORY INFECTION IN CHILDREN

The urban child suffers an average of five to eight episodes of ARI per year and the rural child three to four episodes per year, whether in the tropics or non-tropics. The majority are mild upper respiratory tract infections due to viruses. In HIV-infected children the shedding of respiratory syncytial virus (RSV) is prolonged and presentation of bronchiolitis may be outside the RSV season. The important difference in epidemiology between the regions is that acute lower respiratory tract infection (pneumonia) is more common, more frequently due to bacteria, more severe and much more likely to be lethal in the tropics. Although respiratory diseases are seasonal, especially in temperate regions, the contrast in severity is a reflection of socioeconomic differences rather than differences in climate.

Simple clinical criteria, such as respiratory rate and the presence of subcostal indrawing are very useful in determining severity of ARI. In children the presence of integrated management of childhood illness (IMCI) danger signs, i.e. difficulty in drinking/breastfeeding, lethargy, convulsions and vomiting everything necessitate admission to hospital. Bacteria are responsible for up to 60% of severe pneumonia cases and for the majority of pneumonia-related deaths. The most common bacteria in children over 2 months of age are *Streptococcus pneumoniae* and *Haemophilus influenzae*. These facts provided the foundation for the case management approach that aimed to reduce pneumonia deaths by identification and appropriate antibiotic (and supportive, i.e. oxygen/feeding) management of children with severe pneumonia and to reduce unnecessary use of antibiotics in children with mild ARI.[1]

There is increasing resistance of pneumococcus and *Haemophilus* to co-trimoxazole, penicillin and chloramphenicol, common first-line antibiotics for children with suspected acute bacterial pneumonia in low-income countries. As the bacteria are rarely isolated in cases of pneumonia, useful information of the pattern of resistance in the community can be obtained from nasopharyngeal sampling of healthy young children or by reviewing the pattern of resistance among isolates from children with bacterial meningitis. However, unlike for meningitis, in vitro resistance may not necessarily affect treatment response for pneumococcal pneumonia.

Pneumonia is due to a wider range of bacteria in neonates, malnourished children and HIV-infected children, and they are at greater risk of death. *Staphylococcus aureus* and Gram-negatives, such as *Klebsiella*, *Escherichia coli* or *Salmonella* are also important in these children. Staphylococcal pneumonia with pneumatoceles seems to be less common than previously and this may in part be due to less frequent and less severe measles in many countries. Non-typhoidal *Salmonella* is a common isolate from young children presenting with pneumonia in tropical Africa.[3]

WHO recommendations for first-line treatment for acute childhood pneumonia in tropical countries are aimed at reducing deaths due to bacterial pneumonia and are currently under review. A recent meta-analysis concluded that amoxicillin is superior to co-trimoxazole for the outpatient treatment of non-severe pneumonia and that penicillin and gentamicin is superior to chloramphenicol alone for hospitalized children with severe pneumonia.[4] The use of shorter courses of antibiotics of 3–5 days with high-dose amoxicillin is adequate in treating children with community-acquired pneumonia. The WHO/UNICEF guideline on the Integrated Management of Childhood Illness (IMCI) recommends the use of ceftriaxone for children with very severe pneumonia who fail first-line therapy with amoxicillin, particularly in those who require hospitalization. There is a lack of good-quality data comparing ceftriaxone versus penicillin and gentamicin.[5]

Of the responsible viruses causing pneumonia, RSV, the influenza and parainfluenza viruses, human metapneumovirus and measles are numerically most important. Bronchiolitis and croup occur but are less seasonal and less common than in cooler climates. Again, nutritional state affects presentation and outcome. RSV is the commonest viral cause of childhood pneumonia in tropical countries. The typical clinical picture of RSV bronchiolitis in infants is recognized, but in malnourished and HIV-infected children wheeze is unusual and secondary bacterial infection more common. Common and often fatal complications of measles were severe laryngotracheitis and/or pneumonia. However, measles is now less common owing to effective immunization and vitamin A supplementation and treatment has further reduced the frequency of such complications in children with measles.

Mycoplasma pneumoniae and *Chlamydia pneumoniae* cause atypical pneumonia, particularly in school-aged children, usually not severe, and characterized by a protracted course over a few weeks and fine crackles on auscultation. Their relative importance in the tropics is not clear. Treatment of choice is erythromycin. *Chlamydia trachomatis* causes pneumonia in up to 20% of infants born to infected women and presents between 1 and 3 months of age. There is often a history of neonatal conjunctivitis. Finally, remember that TB can present as acute pneumonia, particularly in infants and HIV-infected children. The contact will usually be the mother.

Immunization against measles and pertussis, breast-feeding and improved socioeconomic circumstances can reduce the incidence and mortality of childhood ARI. The successful development of effective conjugate vaccines against invasive pneumococcus and *Haemophilus influenzae* type b (Hib) means that there is great potential for prevention of severe bacterial pneumonia in the tropics. Following efficacy studies, the Hib vaccine has already been added to routine immunization in a number of low-resource countries with great effect in reducing the burden of Hib meningitis and pneumonia.[5] More recent field trials of a 9-valent pneumococcal conjugate vaccine in South Africa and The Gambia showed similar efficacy against invasive pneumococcal disease due to vaccine serotypes resulting in significant improvements in child survival and making a very strong case for routine implementation of bacterial conjugate vaccines in developing countries.[6] The use of the pneumococcal vaccines in African children has also been found to reduce viral pneumonia in children.

ACUTE RESPIRATORY INFECTION IN ADULTS

Acute pneumonia is common in adults in tropical countries and as in developed countries, the most common cause is *Streptococcus pneumoniae*. The higher incidence of pneumonia in tropical countries is primarily due to immunocompromise due to HIV infection but is also due to increased carriage of pneumococci by children and adults, large family size, crowding in small houses, exposure to domestic and tobacco smoke and the impaired immunity due to poor diet and parasitic diseases. Individuals with increased susceptibility to pneumonia include those with reduced splenic function (sickle cell disease, post-splenectomy), pregnant women, patients with diabetes mellitus and those with excess alcohol intake. Bacterial pneumonia may be preceded by a viral infection such as influenza that damages mucosal defence mechanisms.

The symptoms and signs of lobar pneumonia may be confusing. In early pneumonia, the diagnosis may have to be made in a patient with symptoms, fever and shallow tachypnoea in the absence of any auscultatory signs. The patient will often point to the place where pain occurs when asked to cough. When pleurisy is diaphragmatic, the patient may present with suspected abdominal disease. In some populations a considerable proportion of patients with lobar pneumonia develop jaundice.

The aetiological cause of pneumonia cannot usually be determined at the bedside but a clinical assessment of severity is more important as it can be used to guide management. In particular, young patients with uncomplicated lobar pneumonia can be managed at home with oral therapy. Patients with indicators of severity (age, co-existing disease, multi-lobar disease, shock, hypoxia) should be managed in hospital with broad-spectrum antibiotic cover to include likely (*Streptococcus pneumoniae, Haemophilus influenzae*) and atypical organisms.

Mycoplasma pneumoniae, Chlamydia pneumoniae and *Legionella pneumophila* also cause pneumonia in adults but are rare in Africa. In South-east Asia and northern Australia, melioidosis should be considered as a possible cause of both acute and unresolving pneumonia, especially in the debilitated or immunocompromised. Appropriate media are needed to culture the organism *Burkholderia pseudomallei*. Paracoccidioidomycosis is common in Latin America and may present with pulmonary disease. Histoplasmosis and blastomycosis are also endemic in the Americas. It is important to remember that PTB may present with a clinical syndrome indistinguishable from acute bacterial pneumonia. William Osler recognized this when working in Boston in 1900, and PTB was the second most common cause of pneumonia described in Kenyan adults in 2000.[7]

Pulmonary Tuberculosis in Children and Adults

Mycobacterium tuberculosis is now the second leading cause of death due to infectious disease in the world after HIV infection. The epidemiology and clinical management of TB in children and adults are covered in detail in Chapter 40. The differential diagnoses of PTB include a range of fungal diseases, parasitic diseases and non-infectious granulomatous disorders (Table 70.1).

HIV Infection and Pulmonary Presentations in Children and Adults

HIV infection is common in many regions of the tropics, particularly in sub-Saharan Africa. (This subject is dealt with in detail in Chapter 10.) The peak prevalence is among young adults, and mother-to-child transmission is common. Respiratory disease, acute or chronic, is the commonest cause of morbidity and mortality in HIV-infected adults and children. Pulmonary symptoms are often the first clinical manifestation of the disease, but clinical evidence of underlying immunosuppression should be sought.

There are important differences in the pattern of HIV-related pneumonia between adults and children within the tropics, and in comparison to non-tropical regions (Table 70.2).[8,9] The incidence of bacterial pneumonia is greatly increased in both HIV-infected children and adults, but is highest in children.[10] The range of causative organisms is similar to that which occurs in HIV-uninfected children of similar nutritional status. Although HIV-infected children are more susceptible to PTB, the actual incidence of PTB is low. A common cause of chronic lung disease in HIV-infected children, which is often misdiagnosed as PTB or miliary TB, is LIP.[9] LIP is an HIV-related disease that usually occurs in children. Common clinical markers include marked generalized lymphadenopathy, finger clubbing, enlarged parotid glands and massive hepatomegaly. The typical radiographic abnormalities are diffuse reticulonodular infiltration with bilateral hilar lymphadenopathy, which contrasts with the focal and often unilateral abnormalities of PTB. Bronchiectasis presents with a chronic cough productive of copious purulent and sometimes blood-stained sputum, finger clubbing and halitosis. Bronchiectasis may complicate LIP or PTB. Any person who presents with persistent infiltrates for more than six months on chest X-ray that do not resolve with appropriate treatment should be suspected of having bronchiectasis.

TABLE 70.1 Differential Diagnoses of Pulmonary Tuberculosis

Fungal disease	PCP Cryptococcosis Aspergillosis Histoplasmosis Candidiasis Paracoccidioidomycosis[a] Coccidioidomycosis[a] Penicilliosis[b]
Bacterial disease	Nocardiosis Melioidosis[b] Lung abscess Brucellosis Actinomycosis
Parasitic disease	Paragonimiasis Amoebiasis Echinococcosis Strongyloidiasis
Non-infectious disease	Sarcoidosis Emphysema Cardiac disease Neoplasm

[a]In Central and South America.
[b]In South-east Asia.

TABLE 70.2 Causes of HIV-Related Lung Disease in Low-Income Tropical Regions

Age Group	Most Common	Less Common
Infants	Bacterial pneumonia PCP	Viral pneumonia (e.g. CMV) Tuberculosis
Children	Bacterial pneumonia LIP Tuberculosis	Viral pneumonia (e.g. measles) Pulmonary Kaposi's sarcoma Nocardiosis Candidiasis
Adults	Bacterial pneumonia Tuberculosis	PCP Cryptococcosis Nocardiosis Pulmonary Kaposi's sarcoma[a] Penicilliosis[a] Melioidosis[a] Paracoccidioidomycosis[b] Histoplasmosis[b]

[a]In South-east Asia.
[b]In Central and South America.

With the availability of highly active antiretroviral therapy (HAART), more young children are presenting with complications of immune-reconstitution. BCG disease is becoming more common and may present as either regional lymphadenitis or disseminated BCG infection with multi-organ involvement. This condition is difficult to diagnose and requires mycobacterial culture species identification which may not be available.

PTB and bacterial pneumonia are the major causes of respiratory morbidity in HIV-infected adults living in the poorer regions of the tropics. The clinical features of bacterial pneumonia are similar to those in HIV-seronegative patients, although bacteraemia is more common.[7] The HIV pandemic has had a profound effect on the epidemiology, clinical presentations, diagnosis, drug treatment and treatment response in TB. In many HIV-infected adults, the clinical presentation is atypical (e.g. diffuse, miliary or basal in its distribution) due to the impaired Th1 type immunity in HIV-infected adults that prevents formation of the usual granulomatous inflammation followed by cavitation. Drug reactions are more common among patients with HIV-related disease and there is a high mortality in early treatment. The introduction of appropriate antiretroviral therapy during TB treatment makes management of HIV/TB more difficult than TB alone with difficulties with drug interactions and maintaining follow-up. Cure rates are lower in HIV-infected patients than in individuals without HIV.

Less common diseases in HIV-infected adults living in tropical Africa include cryptococcosis, pulmonary Kaposi's sarcoma and PcP.[8] The clinical presentation of pneumonitis caused by *Pneumocystis jerovicii* is described in Chapter 39. This is a common cause of severe pneumonia in HIV-infected African infants but is rare beyond 6 months of age.[9] In comparison to bacterial pneumonia, PcP is characterized by a low-grade or absent fever, a clear chest with good air entry or diffuse rather than focal abnormalities, severe and persistent hypoxia, and a poor clinical response to usual broad-spectrum antibiotics (e.g. chloramphenicol) and to oxygen. Hyperinflation and diffuse interstitial infiltration are the usual radiographic abnormalities. PcP is often fatal even when treated with high-dose co-trimoxazole, prednisolone and oxygen. Co-trimoxazole prophylaxis is very effective in preventing PcP in HIV-infected infants and is recommended by WHO for all HIV-exposed infants until HIV infection can be excluded. Co-trimoxazole prophylaxis is also effective in improving survival for HIV-infected adults and children and in some studies improved outcome has been due to reduction in non-PcP pneumonia.[11]

HIV-related infections in other tropical regions include paracoccidioidomycosis in tropical America and penicilliosis due to *Penicillium marneffei* in South-east Asia.[12,13] Although a variety of parasites causes lung problems in the tropics (see below), these infections do not appear to be increased in frequency or altered in their clinical manifestations by concomitant HIV infection or AIDS.

Asthma and Allergy in Children and Adults

Asthma is less common in the tropics than in some temperate regions and there are differences in the patterns of presentation.[14] The prevalence of asthma in tropical countries however is increasing, particularly in urban communities. Many asthmatics first develop symptoms in adult life and are less likely to have a history of other atopic conditions. The low but increasing incidence of atopic disease and asthma in tropical countries is an area of current research, with the hope that it may provide important information as to why such diseases have become so common in more affluent countries. Nutrition is likely to be one factor: asthma is rare in malnourished children. The relationship to infections more prevalent in the tropics such as the higher burden of parasitic disease may also be important.

Patients with asthma should be assessed for possible precipitating factors, including seasonal allergy, nocturnal and exertional exacerbation, dust including house-dust, farm and industrial dusts, fumes including perfumes, drugs (e.g. salicylates and beta blockers), cigarette smoking and animals. A history to reveal other atopic manifestations like eczema and allergic rhinitis should be obtained. Growth parameters in children are usually normal; this aids in differentiating asthma from other conditions, e.g. TB nodal airway obstruction. Clinical examination may reveal evidence of air trapping with hyperinflation. Many patients may present late with a chest deformity (Harrison's sulcus). Wheezing may be present on auscultation. A thorough inspection for other atopic manifestations should be done, namely for allergic shiners, nasal obstruction, mouth breathing and eczema. Measurements of peak expiratory flow rate and a sleep diary can help to monitor health status and response to treatment.

In children, the diagnosis of asthma may be limited by inability to perform peak flow measurements. A bronchodilator response test should be done in a symptomatic child by counting the respiratory rate and auscultation for wheezing. A bronchodilator is administered via a spacer device and clinical measurements repeated 10–15 minutes following the bronchodilator to assess for improvement. In the child with suspected asthma who is asymptomatic at presentation, the use of a trial of oral steroid for 7–14 days may aid in clinching the diagnosis.

Treatment should be appropriate to the frequency and severity of symptoms but often the range of therapeutic options available is limited. Oral salbutamol or aminophylline are perhaps the most widely available but have limited efficacy and often cause systemic side effects. Inhaled β2-agonists such as salbutamol or terbutaline are very useful in symptom relief, particularly if patients are taught to use the inhaler effectively either by direct delivery or via a spacer. Low-cost spacer devices can be fashioned where none are available, as these are critical in medication delivery, particularly in young children and the elderly. The mainstay of asthma management is inhaled corticosteroid therapy, which is stepped up and down in response to symptom control and peak expiratory flow rate. Combination therapy with long-acting inhaled β2-agonists and steroid preparations is highly effective. Cromoglycate may be assessed for prophylactic efficacy over a period of weeks for those suffering frequent attacks of exercise-induced asthma – it is particularly useful in children. The availability of effective asthma therapy in developing countries is still poor and is being addressed by global initiatives including the Global Initiative for Asthma (GINA) (see: www.ginasthma.org) and The International Union Against Tuberculosis and Lung Disease (IUATLD). Severe episodes of asthma can be treated with oxygen, nebulized β2-agonists and short courses of oral corticosteroids. Subcutaneous adrenaline (epinephrine) can be very useful for the life-threatening episode especially as it is usually available. User-friendly guidelines for the management of asthma in low- and middle-income countries are available from the IUATLD website (see: www.theunion.org).

Chronic Obstructive Pulmonary Disease (COPD)

WHO estimates that in 2004, 64 million people were living with, and 3 million died of, COPD, worldwide. By 2030, COPD is expected to become the third leading cause of death globally. Around 90% of this burden of disease will be seen in low- and middle-income countries. Currently, many cases of COPD are not diagnosed because patients do not present to healthcare facilities, spirometry is not available or the debilitation is dismissed as an effect of ageing.

COPD varies in prevalence and severity according to the distribution of risk factors. Tobacco smoke is the most significant of these. Household air pollution from biomass fuel combustion and occupational exposures are increasingly recognized as major causes of COPD. Other risk factors include in utero exposures, childhood lower respiratory tract infections, tuberculosis, asthma and outdoor air pollution.

The pathogenesis of COPD is that inhalation of noxious gases and fumes induces chronic inflammation in the airways and distal alveolar destruction. Neutrophils, macrophages and lymphocytes predominate and tissue damage occurs owing to high oxidative stress, protease release and impaired defence against infections. Physiological consequences include hypersecretion of mucus, airflow obstruction, air trapping and impairment of gas exchange.

The clinical features of COPD tend to be seen in people over the age of 35 with sufficient cumulative exposure to inhalational exposures. Gender and racial group are not major determinants. People with COPD commonly experience exertional breathlessness, chronic cough, sputum production and wheeze. Clinical examination may be normal particularly in mild disease but as the disease progresses, chest hyper-inflation, a prolonged expiratory phase, pursed-lip breathing, use of accessory muscles of respiration, elevated respiratory rate, central cyanosis and lower limb oedema can be seen. The clinical features are similar wherever the disease is seen in the world. Differences between tobacco smoke-induced and non-smoking-related COPD are poorly characterized.

The clinical course of COPD is often gradually progressive and punctuated by exacerbations that are usually triggered by viral or bacterial lower respiratory tract infections. As the disease progresses, respiratory failure and cor pulmonale can develop. COPD is also associated with systemic features including cachexia, muscle wasting, heart disease, osteoporosis, anxiety and depression that can be prominent in severe disease.

The diagnosis of COPD is made using post bronchodilator spirometry. Attention to quality control and assurance is important. Unfortunately access to spirometry is poor in many areas making the task of confirming a diagnosis of COPD difficult. The Global Initiative for Chronic Obstructive Lung Disease (GOLD) (see: http://www.goldcopd.org/) defines airflow obstruction as the presence of an FEV1/FVC ratio <0.70. The FEV1 as a percentage of the predicted value (accounting for age, height, gender and race) is useful for grading severity of impairment (mild ≥80 %; moderate 50 to <80%; severe 30 to <50%; very severe <30%). Asthma is the main differential diagnosis. Chronic unproductive cough, variable symptoms and nocturnal awakening due to breathlessness, coughing or wheezing are more in-keeping with asthma than COPD. Bronchiectasis is less common than asthma or COPD but does have some overlapping clinical features. TB should also be considered.

COPD is a highly preventable condition and treatment is only partially effective in established disease. Avoiding or minimizing exposure to the major inhalation risk factors of tobacco smoke and household air pollution from biomass fuel combustion, is of key importance. For relief of symptoms, bronchodilators (β2-agonists, anticholinergics and methylxanthines), are taken as required or regularly. Inhaled corticosteroids have little effect compared with their prominent place in asthma management and are used mainly for patients with severe disease and repeated exacerbations. Regular oral corticosteroids should be avoided. Non-pharmacological interventions such as exercise programmes can be very helpful and inexpensive. Long-term oxygen therapy where available can help improve survival when respiratory failure has occurred.

Exacerbations of COPD are characterized by acute changes in breathlessness, cough and sputum that are beyond the patient's usual day-to-day variations. Inhaled bronchodilators, together with a short course of oral corticosteroid and controlled oxygen therapy when needed, are the mainstays of treatment. Antibiotics should also be given when there are pointers to bacterial infection.

Bronchopulmonary Dysplasia

There are high maternal infection and pre-eclampsia rates in the tropics. This increases the numbers of premature infants born, who are often also low weight for age. With increasing availability of technologies and improved survival of premature infants, survivors of prematurity may present with chronic lung disease of infancy (CLDI). CLDI (previously referred to as bronchopulmonary dysplasia) survivors may present with persistent tachypnoea, hyperinflation, poor weight gain and pulmonary hypertension. These children may be oxygen-dependent and difficult to treat. Careful attention should be paid to increasing caloric intake as somatic growth generally improves the pulmonary status. Diuretics may be used where available and a short course 5–7-day trial of steroids may be attempted to wean the child from respiratory support.

Lung Cancer and Mesothelioma

The geographic distribution of lung cancer and mesothelioma varies markedly according to the distribution of risk factors, particularly tobacco, biomass, coal smoke and asbestos exposure. Occupational exposure to asbestos can be considerable in mining, engineering, ship-building and demolition. Both lung cancer and mesothelioma are largely preventable through risk factor avoidance. Common presenting symptoms are cough, haemoptysis, breathlessness, chest pain and weight loss. Clinical examination findings vary from no abnormalities to features due to the local tumour (e.g. lobar collapse, pleural effusion) to consequences of metastatic disease (e.g. lymphadenopathy, hepatomegaly, cachexia). Tuberculosis and Kaposi's sarcoma are important differential diagnoses in the tropics particularly in areas with a high HIV prevalence. The diagnosis and staging requires pathological assessment of a biopsy specimen and investigations, particularly chest X-ray and CT thorax. Unfortunately access to these investigations and treatments such as surgical resection, chemotherapy and radiotherapy is often limited. A clinical diagnosis based on exclusion of treatable alternative diagnoses, clinical assessment, disease course and simple imaging may be all that can be carried out diagnostically. Establishing a definite diagnosis of mesothelioma can be important if industrial compensation is payable. Careful attention to communication with the patient and relatives and control of symptoms is essential.

Biomass Fuel Use and Respiratory Health

Biomass fuel (burned organic products such as wood, charcoal or animal dung) is used by 2 billion people daily for cooking, heating and lighting. This form of energy produces particulate smoke that is often poorly vented resulting in very high exposures to smoke, particularly among women and young children. Biomass fuel smoke increases susceptibility to acute and chronic pulmonary infection in children and is associated with chronic obstructive pulmonary disease (COPD) and lung cancer in adults.[15] The impact of indoor smoke on the incidence of respiratory disease in developing countries is likely to be enormous but has been poorly documented.[16]

Although effective strategies for reducing smoke exposure have existed for decades (e.g. ventilation, improved stoves, cleaner fuels, behaviour modification), they have been out of reach for the majority of biomass fuel users due to a wide range of largely poverty-related factors. Many new forms of environmentally sensitive cooking stoves have been designed in the last 50 years (see: http://stoves.bioenergylists.org/), primarily with the aim of reducing deforestation and consumption of fossil fuel. It is likely that stoves which substantially reduce smoke exposure will also have a beneficial health effect but health impact assessments have only been described in a few studies to date.[17,18] The Global Alliance for Clean Cookstoves (see: http://cleancookstoves.org) is a new international public–private initiative that will hopefully lead to improvements in health and save lives by making improved and acceptable cooking solutions more widely available and affordable.

Tobacco and Health

Many developing countries have a tobacco industry that was created hoping to create revenue, employment and trade but it is now realized that the economic cost of this industry exceeds its benefit. In particular, poor agricultural practice leads to loss of soil fertility, pesticide toxicity and green tobacco leaf-related illnesses are a major problem in the workforce and curing the leaf requires large amounts of firewood, making this process a major cause of deforestation. Furthermore, the processed end-product is expensive and tobacco companies curtailed by strict advertising regulations and costly litigation in rich countries are now targeting middle- and low-income countries as their future market. Particularly alarming, are figures from secondary schools: 30–40% of pupils in some areas have been found to be regular smokers.[19]

Smoking-related diseases have increased in tandem. Emphysema and lung cancers are becoming more common in China, Nigeria, India and Malaysia. Because of the delayed effects of smoking, a great increase of these and other smoking-related diseases can be expected within the coming decade in tropical countries. COPD is still primarily related to the use of biomass fuel in many developing countries but tobacco smoking-related COPD will increase dramatically as tobacco consumption increases.

Occupational Lung Diseases

Respiratory disease often relates to occupation. In particular, mining dusts may cause pulmonary fibrosis, a wide variety of aerosolized compounds cause asthma and rare infections are common in exposed professional groups.

Work in mines, even in the distant past, may have been responsible for fibrotic lung disease (e.g. silicosis, asbestosis or berylliosis) or anthracosis and is associated with an increased risk of lung cancer. Retired miners are often debilitated if they have worked in poorly regulated conditions and the pulmonary damage sustained is increased by concomitant cigarette smoking. Exposure to asbestos and industrial air pollutants (e.g. diesel fumes, acid fumes such as SO_2 and NO_2) is associated with mining and other heavy industry.

Several hundred causes of occupational asthma have now been described including both high-molecular-weight compounds (flour, seafood proteins, starch) and low-molecular-weight compounds (glutaraldehyde, isocyanates). It is important to enquire about both current and past places and conditions of work, with particular emphasis on the relation of symptoms to the time of work. The 'healthy worker effect' where affected workers leave the workplace, can result in poor association between current exposure and symptoms in exposed workforces.

Infectious occupational lung disease is common. Most cases of melioidosis in South-east Asia occur in rice farmers. A patient who works with animals or birds may be exposed to zoonotic diseases that sometimes have a pulmonary component: histoplasmosis, brucellosis, tularaemia, Q-fever, leptospirosis or psittacosis. In areas where paragonimiasis and gnathostomiasis occur, enquire about eating raw or undercooked fish; where schistosomiasis is prevalent, consider the likelihood of environmental contact (e.g. fishermen and bus-washers in Lake Victoria).

Pulmonary Problems in Parasitic Diseases and Tropical Pulmonary Eosinophilia

Parasitic infection often involves the lung. In paragonimiasis, the lung is the predominant organ involved. Paragonimiasis may present with cough, haemoptysis and cavitating lung disease. It is often mistaken for PTB and must be considered in areas where raw fish is eaten.

More usually, however, parasitic disease is systemic, with lung symptoms presenting with other features. Hydatid cysts (see Chapter **56**) may produce a variety of lung problems as a result of mechanical compression of intrathoracic structures. In schistosomiasis, especially where portal hypertension has led to venous shunts bypassing the liver, eggs may be deposited in pulmonary capillaries and arterioles, eliciting a granulomatous reaction resulting either in pulmonary hypertension or the accumulation of large masses of granulation tissue (see Chapter **52**). In a number of helminth infections (hookworm, ascaris, strongyloides, schistosomiasis) a larval stage of the parasite migrates through the lungs, when it may cause cough, fever, dyspnoea and sometimes wheeze or haemoptysis (see

Chapter 55). The severity of the illness probably depends on how many larvae are migrating at one time; the classical self-experiment of Koino illustrated this. He swallowed 2000 viable Ascaris eggs, and within a week, suffered a severe illness with high fever, dyspnoea, cyanosis, severe cough and frothy, blood-stained sputum lasting for 7 days. There was eosinophilia, and many Ascaris larvae were recovered from his sputum. It would be unusual for such a large number of eggs to be ingested simultaneously in natural circumstances.

Malaria may be complicated by pulmonary problems; cough is not uncommonly a symptom, even in moderately severe malaria, and in severe *Plasmodium falciparum* malaria pulmonary problems have been reported in 5–15% of cases. Although pulmonary oedema due to therapeutic fluid overload, or bronchopneumonia complicating deep coma, may occur, a more specific malarial lesion indistinguishable from adult respiratory distress syndrome has been recognized in which there is septal oedema, endothelial cell swelling and hyaline membrane formation within the alveoli. In children in endemic areas, anaemia and acidosis with resultant tachypnoea are common in severe malaria, but respiratory distress syndrome is rare.

TROPICAL PULMONARY EOSINOPHILIA

In areas where *Wuchereria bancrofti* and *Brugia malayi* are common, patients with cough or wheeze may have tropical pulmonary eosinophilia, in which marked eosinophilia (eosinophil count often >3000/mm^3) and lung shadows on radiography are supported by a positive filarial antibody test. The condition improves rapidly with antifilarial treatment (see Chapter 54).[20,21] Filariasis is most common in southern and eastern Asia, the Pacific and Brazil. The condition is uncommon in Africa, but a similar combination of cough, wheeze and eosinophilia may occur due to the migrating larval stages of *Ascaris*, hookworm, schistosomiasis or *Strongyloides* infection.[22]

Pleural Diseases – Pneumothorax, Effusion and Empyema

PNEUMOTHORAX

Primary pneumothorax (air in the pleural space) occurs in the absence of any previous lung pathology and has a good prognosis; secondary pneumothorax occurs on a background of damaged lung (e.g. chronic obstructive pulmonary disease; PcP) and the prognosis is often poor. The immediate management of pneumothorax depends on the size and complications of the pneumothorax. Small primary pneumothoraces can be managed conservatively or with simple aspiration. Large or tension pneumothoraces require urgent aspiration and if this is unsuccessful, a drain must be used. Secondary pneumothoraces are often very slow to respond and may require prolonged drainage for up to several weeks. Prolonged drainage carries a high risk of secondary infection.

EFFUSION

Pleural effusion (fluid in the pleural space) is most commonly caused by TB in endemic areas. Parapneumonic effusion and malignant effusion (often blood-stained) are the important differentials. The cause of the effusion must be diagnosed and treatment designed to relieve symptoms while treating the underlying cause. Asymptomatic effusion due to tuberculosis need not be drained.

EMPYEMA

Empyema (infection in the pleural space) is a common complication of pleural effusion and can occur as a primary presentation of TB. Empyema must always be removed either by repeated aspiration, drainage or surgery. Full recovery requires prolonged (≥6 weeks), appropriate antibiotic therapy. Intercostal drainage of empyema can result in super-infection; mixed pleural infections in AIDS patients are difficult to cure and sometimes long-term drainage or fistula is the best that can be achieved.

Vascular Diseases – Pulmonary Embolism and Pulmonary Arterial Hypertension

THROMBOEMBOLIC PULMONARY EMBOLISM

Thromboembolic pulmonary embolism is a potentially life-threatening complication of immobilization and dehydration that can be prevented by anticoagulant prophylaxis. Large thrombi form in deep veins, typically of the pelvis and legs, and embolize to the pulmonary circulation. Large pulmonary emboli present with sudden cardiac collapse and death, and smaller emboli may present with dyspnoea and chest pain. Patients have few signs or present with tachycardia, prominent pulmonary heart sounds or abnormal ECG features. Due to resource constraints, many immobilized in-patients in tropical hospitals do not receive prophylactic heparin or low-molecular-weight heparin and so thromboembolism is common. This is a particular problem in obstetrics, orthopaedics and among medical patients recovering from dehydrating conditions such as diabetic ketoacidosis.

PULMONARY ARTERIAL HYPERTENSION

Pulmonary arterial hypertension can be primary or secondary. The most common causes of secondary pulmonary arterial hypertension in tropical hospitals are as a complication of pulmonary thromboemboli and HIV infection. Sickle cell disease should be ruled out particularly in subjects of African origin where no other cause for pulmonary hypertension is found. Patients present with shortness of breath and signs of right heart failure but definitive diagnosis and treatment are difficult. Treatment with high-dose calcium channel blockers (e.g. diltiazem) or sildenafil may be of benefit.

Interstitial Lung Disease in Adults and Children

In the tropics the approach to both adults and children with interstitial lung disease (ILD) should include a history of duration of symptoms, effort tolerance, haemoptysis and potential exposures including occupational exposures particularly mining. It is vital to exclude HIV infection as a potential cause as this has implications in terms of investigations for a potential cause.

The presentation of ILD is similar in both adults and children with the presence of chronic dry cough, tachypnoea, progressive dyspnoea, recurrent pulmonary infections and progressing to respiratory failure if untreated. On clinical examination finger clubbing, hypoxaemia, fine basal crepitations, wheezing and failure to thrive in children may be present.

In HIV-infected children and adults, infectious causes including fungal infection, chronic PcP and tuberculosis should be ruled out. Kaposi's sarcoma may also present with pulmonary infiltrates. In the HIV-negative patient causes of ILD are similar to those of patients in non-tropics.

In many tropical countries, sarcoidosis has never been identified. However, in temperate countries, Africans, West Indians and Asians have a much higher incidence of sarcoidosis than do Caucasians living in the same vicinity. Caucasians are also found to have less severe disease, with fewer systemic manifestations, than the other ethnic groups. There is now evidence that sarcoidosis has been under-reported from tropical countries and is often misdiagnosed as TB.[23] The possibility of sarcoidosis should be considered in patients 20–50 years of age with unresolving lung disease, especially if there are accompanying extrathoracic features such as iridocyclitis, lymphadenopathy, central nervous system complications or hypercalcaemia. In young children sarcoidosis usually presents with extrapulmonary manifestations with rash, uveitis and arthritis being more common.[24]

Diagnosis of ILD depends on the presence of typical interstitial infiltrates on chest X-ray or a ground-glass appearance, increased inter-lobar septae and fibrotic changes on CT scanning. A lung biopsy is necessary to make a definitive diagnosis. Specialized sputum and immunological tests are often not available. The management involves avoidance of environmental triggers especially in extrinsic allergic alveolitis and occupational diseases, use of steroids in some cases, and supportive measures. Immunomodulatory drugs, which have some efficacy for specific disease entities, are generally expensive and often unavailable.

REFERENCES

4. Kabra SK, Lodha R, Pandey RM. Antibiotics for community acquired pneumonia in children. Cochrane Database Syst Rev 2006;(3):CD004874.
5. WHO. Recommendations on the management of diarrhoea and pneumonia in HIV-infected infants and children: integrated management of childhood illness (IMCI) 2010. Online. Available: http://whqlibdoc.who.int/publications/2010/9789241548083_eng.pdf.
7. Levine OS, O'Brien KL, Knoll M, et al. Pneumococcal vaccination in developing countries. Lancet 2006;367:1880–2.
18. Romieu I, Riojas-Rodriguez H, Marron-Mares AT, et al. Improved biomass stove intervention in rural Mexico impact on the respiratory health of women. Am J Respir Crit Care Med 2009; 180:649–56.
19. Smith KR, McCracken JP, Weber MW, et al. Effect of reduction in household air pollution on childhood pneumonia in Guatemala (RESPIRE): a randomised controlled trial. Lancet 2011;378:1717–26.

Access the complete references online at www.expertconsult.com

71

Tropical Neurology

JEANNINE M. HECKMANN | AHMED I. BHIGJEE

KEY POINTS

- Acute encephalitis can be infectious, post-infectious or antibody-mediated.
- Mortality from tuberculous meningitis remains high.
- Tuberculomas may present as focal brain lesions with a wide range of appearances on brain imaging.
- Complex interactions between tuberculosis and HIV in co-infected subjects present diagnostic and therapeutic challenges.
- Paradoxical clinical worsening or new symptoms consistent with an inflammatory process after antiretroviral treatment initiation in HIV-infected patients, suggests an immune reconstitution syndrome.
- HIV-associated neurological complications may simultaneously affect the nervous system at multiple anatomical levels and involve more than one pathogenic process.
- Cerebral malaria is best treated with artesunate.

Introduction

Tropical neurology traditionally includes 'exotic' diseases prevailing between the tropics of Cancer and Capricorn, and neurological diseases arising from socioeconomic circumstances such as poverty, malnutrition, high population growth and overcrowding, which are so prevalent in these regions. The spread of the human immunodeficiency virus (HIV) epidemic has resulted in diverse neurological manifestations of the HIV infection and fuelled other epidemics associated with deprivation, such as tuberculosis.

Diagnosis in tropical neurology requires a detailed history as well as a sound knowledge of neuroanatomy. With this in mind, we have used neuroanatomical compartmentalization (Table 71.1) to present an overview of clinical conditions that may form part of the differential diagnosis of tropical infections of the nervous system. We conclude the chapter by discussing a more traditional, focussed approach to specific pathogens that affect the nervous system.

MENINGITIS

Neck stiffness is the clinical hallmark of acute meningeal inflammation although this sign may rarely disappear in a deeply comatose patient with meningitis. Headache and fever in an acute illness developing over hours should alert one to the possibility of bacterial meningitis caused by *Streptococcus*, *Meningococcus* (accompanying skin purpura) or *Haemophilus*. *Listeria monocytogenes* should be considered in older, pregnant or immune-compromised subjects. Neonatal meningitis may be associated with almost any organism but Gram-negative bacteria such as *Escherichia coli* and other enteric bacilli are the most frequent cause. Confirmatory cerebrospinal fluid (CSF) examination should not delay treatment as early treatment is critical. In the search for an appropriate antibiotic in a high-incidence part of Africa, an Angolan study showed children with pneumococcal meningitis treated with early cefotaxime infusions had a better outcome compared with bolus doses.[1] As pneumococcal resistance is increasing to more than 5% in certain tropical areas, a third generation cephalosporin with vancomycin is recommended until antibiotic sensitivity is available.

Symptoms in tuberculous meningitis (TBM) may have a subacute onset (1–3 weeks),[2] whereas in cryptococcal meningitis it may be chronic and indolent. CSF in TBM typically shows a mild to moderate lymphocytosis, raised protein and a low serum/CSF glucose ratio (<0.5) (Table 71.2).[2] In HIV-infected subjects there are a number of conditions that can closely mimic TBM: cryptococcal meningitis, CMV encephalitis, toxoplasmosis and primary CNS lymphoma.[2]

Cryptococcal meningitis should be considered in those with persistent low-grade headaches persisting over months, especially in those who are immunocompromised due to immunosuppressants for autoimmune disease, underlying malignancy or HIV infection. It is important to bear in mind that even immunocompetent subjects are at risk if, for instance, there is close contact with pigeon droppings.

ENCEPHALITIS

Patients with acute encephalitis have fever, altered consciousness with or without seizures, and CSF pleocytosis. Acute encephalitis can be infectious, post-infectious or antibody-mediated. In many cases, the illness is short-lived and no cause is found.

Arboviruses have caused outbreaks of Japanese encephalitis and West Nile virus-related encephalitis.[3] Other viruses that have caused epidemics in Asia include enterovirus 71 (resulting in hand, foot and mouth disease and associated with aseptic meningitis, encephalitis or myelitis), and Nipah virus.[4] Among immunocompromised hosts, cytomegalovirus (CMV), human herpes virus type 6 and *Toxoplasma gondii* are the most common causes of encephalitis,[3] whereas in the developed world, herpes simplex viruses (HSV)-1 and -2 and varicella zoster virus (VZV) are viruses usually implicated. Rabies encephalitis (which is invariably fatal) remains endemic in many countries whilst measles virus and *Mycoplasma pneumonia* are the commonest causes of post-infectious encephalitis.[3]

HSV-1 is a treatable cause of viral encephalitis. The temporal lobe(s) is predominantly involved and the patient often experiences a prodrome of headache and fever for 5 days followed by

TABLE 71.1 A Neuroanatomical Compartmentalized Approach to Acute or Subacute Neurological Disorders

		Symptoms and Signs	Aetiological Examples
Encephalopathy		Confusion/behavioural changes Delirium Dementia	Infective encephalitis/meningitis, metabolic/deficiencies, autoimmune/antibody-mediated
Grey matter	Cortical	Seizures Myoclonus Eloquent cortical function	Cysticercosis, toxoplasmosis, herpes simplex, prions, measles, syphilis
	Deep (basal ganglia)	Hyperkinesia Hypokinesia	Toxoplasmosis
White matter	Multifocal	Spasticity ± psychomotor slowing	Autoimmune (ADEM), HIV, metabolic, PML
Focal brain lesions		Hemiparesis, seizure, aphasia	Space-occupying lesions
Cerebellar		Anterior Pancerebellar	Alcohol, nutritional, PML in HIV, metabolic-Leigh's disease
Brainstem encephalitis		Spasticity/cranial Ns ± cerebellar	Post-infectious, listeria
Myelopathy		Spasticity ± incontinence	Post-infectious, HTLV1, syphilis
Myeloradiculopathy	Conus medullaris and cauda equina	Sphincters + leg paraparesis (UMN/LMN signs)	TB, schistosomiasis, CMV in HIV
Radiculopathy		Proximal/distal weakness/areflexia	Schistosomiasis, post-infectious autoimmune
Neuropathy		Small fibre – pain Large fibre – areflexia/weakness	HIV, nutritional and drugs Vitamin B12 deficiency, diabetes
Neuromuscular junction		Fatiguable proximal weakness ± ocular	Myasthenia gravis, botulism
Myopathy		Girdle weakness	Myositis, drugs

behavioural changes, seizures, motor deficits, amnestic symptoms and altered consciousness. Brain imaging shows increased signal in the cortical and subcortical regions of one, rarely both, temporal lobes on MRI T2 and FLAIR sequences. Electroencephalography (EEG) may show lateralized slowing. As the mortality of HSV encephalitis is high, acyclovir is often initiated empirically before the diagnosis can be excluded with a negative CSF HSV PCR. Early (<48 hours of symptoms) CSF HSV PCR may be falsely negative and acyclovir should be continued until a confirmatory negative PCR is performed at least 72 hours after symptom onset.[3] HSV encephalitis should be treated with acyclovir for 14–21 days.

The recently identified immune-mediated limbic encephalitides, which are important to recognize, as they generally respond well to steroids and immunosuppression, also occur in the tropics and frequently has a flu-like prodrome. Antibody targets in children and young adults may differ from older individuals.[5]

Syphilitic vasculitis rarely presents with a syndrome resembling limbic encephalitis with focal motor or complex partial status epilepticus, memory disturbance, periodic lateralized epileptiform EEG discharges and hyperintense MRI signals in the temporal lobes.[6,7]

Immunocompromised patients presenting with focal motor status epilepticus with or without generalized seizures and evidence of focal MRI T2 signal changes in the cortical ribbon should raise suspicion for subacute measles encephalitis (see later; Figure 71.1).[8] In contrast, post-infectious acute disseminated encephalomyelitis (ADEM) usually presents as a syndrome with symptoms and signs involving predominantly white matter (Table 71.1). An opsoclonus-myoclonus syndrome has also been described in HIV-infected individuals and presents subacutely, much like the childhood paraneoplastic form, with chaotic eye movements together with myoclonus, ataxia and behavioural disturbance.[9] The clinical course is monophasic with virtually complete recovery occurring over months.[9]

Seizures are generally an important indicator of cortical involvement (Table 71.3). Neurocysticercosis is the most common cause of adult-onset epilepsy in the developing world,[10] while other infections known to result in seizures are listed in Table 71.3. One should be alerted to the possibility of parasitic infections in recent travellers who present with features of acute meningoencephalitis and seizures, altered consciousness, focal neurological deficits and blood eosinophilia >10% or a CSF eosinophil count of ≥10 cells/μL, although not all parasites present in this fashion in the first instance.[11]

TABLE 71.2 Differences in the Cerebrospinal Fluid Parameters Between Subjects Who are HIV-Uninfected with Tuberculous Meningitis (TBM) and Those Who are HIV-Infected with TBM

CSF Parameter	TBM : HIV –ve	TBM: HIV +ve
Mean cell count	223	230
>50% neutrophils	27%	42%
Acellular	6%	11%
Mean protein (g/L)	2.2	1.2
Normal protein	6%	43%
Low glucose	72%	69%
+ve smear	25%	12%
+ve culture	61%	23%

Adapted from Garcia-Monco JC. Central nervous system tuberculosis. Neurol Clin 1999;17:737–59 and Katrak SM, Shembalkar PK, Bijwe SR, et al. The clinical, radiological and pathological profile of tuberculous meningitis in patients with and without human immunodeficiency virus infection. J Neurol Sci 2000;181:118–26.

FOCAL BRAIN LESIONS

Focal signs of brain dysfunction such as hemiparesis, hemianaesthesia, language disturbance and seizures suggest one or more focal brain lesion(s) (Table 71.3). Brain abscess or subdural empyema can present with such focal signs, often associated

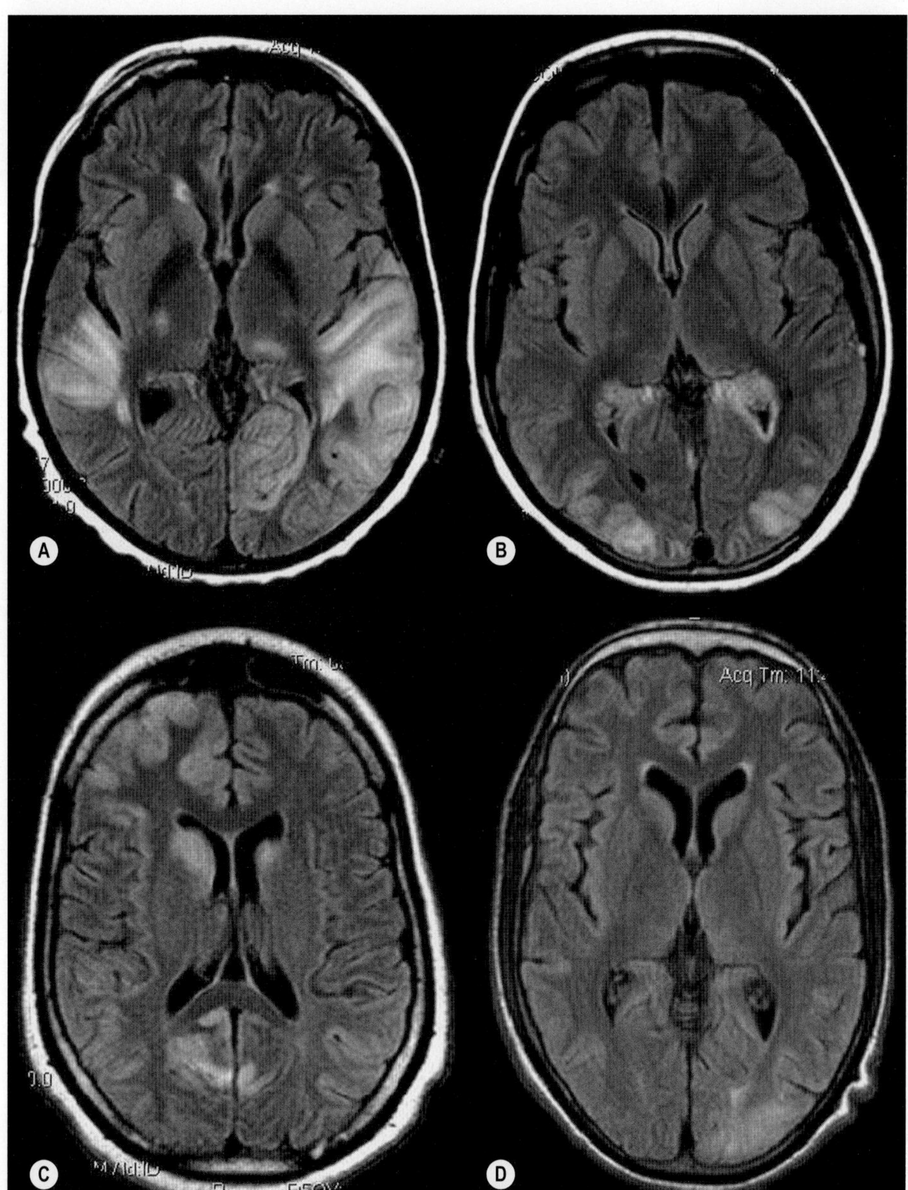

Figure 71.1 Axial T2 FLAIR images demonstrating the characteristic polioencephalopathy (grey matter) in subacute measles encephalitis. (A) Bilateral temporal-parietal cortical hyperintensities; (B) parieto-occipital cortical hyperintensities; (C) superficial cortical (left frontal and bilateral occipital) and deep grey matter (bilateral head of caudate) hyperintense signal abnormalities and (D) hyperintense signal changes in the right occipital cortex. *(From Albertyn C, van der Plas H, Hardie D, et al. Silent casualties from the measles outbreak in South Africa. S Afr Med J 2011;101:313–4, 6–7.*[8]*)*

TABLE 71.3 **Causes of Seizures/Epilepsy**

Infections	Bacterial meningitis Cerebral malaria TB meningitis Cryptococcal meningitis Neurocysticercosis Schistosomiasis Cerebral hydatid disease Paragonimiasis Cerebral toxoplasmosis Cerebral amoebiasis Neuroangiostrongyliasis Gnathostomiasis Baylisascariasis Tetanus (pseudoepilepsy)
Focal brain lesions	Tumours, cysts, granulomas, tuberculoma
Toxins/drugs/metabolic	Alcohol, opiates, altered glucose levels
Metabolic	Hypoglycaemia
Stroke	Haemorrhage, intracerebral/ subarachnoid

with headaches and spiking temperatures. Organisms such as *Staphylococcus aureus*, streptococci (e.g. *S. pyogenes*, *S. pneumoniae*, *S. milleri*) and anaerobes such as *Bacteroides fragilis*, can be seeded into the CNS through penetrating traumatic injuries and neurosurgery, as well as through haematogenous (e.g. endocarditis) or contiguous spread (e.g. mastoiditis, paranasal sinusitis).[3]

In developing countries, tuberculomas constitute a significant proportion of focal brain lesions. Brain imaging shows either solid or ring-enhancing lesions with variable surrounding oedema. Most immunocompetent patients with tuberculomas do not have evidence of meningitis or pulmonary tuberculosis.[12] Anti-tuberculous treatment tends to reduce surrounding oedema rather than affect lesion size during the first 2 months, whereas a definite reduction in tuberculoma size is expected after 6 months of treatment and complete resolution after 12 months.[12] Some tuberculomas transiently increase in size after treatment initiation, often with accompanying meningeal reaction.[12]

In the era before antiretroviral therapy (ART), toxoplasmosis was the commonest cause of a focal brain lesion in HIV-infected individuals.[13] Other causes include tuberculoma, primary CNS lymphoma (PCNSL) and cryptococcoma. With the advent of ART, the frequency of cerebral toxoplasmosis has declined remarkably.[14] On brain imaging, toxoplasmosis shows multiple nodular or ring-enhancing lesions, commonly involving the basal ganglia, with surrounding oedema. Imaging findings of meningeal involvement suggest PCNSL.[15]

MYELITIS

Acute or subacute myelitis is often non-infectious inflammatory, tends to affect the mid-thoracic cord and may include post-infectious and post-vaccination myelitis. Infectious myelitis may be the result of HSV or VZV, *Mycoplasma pneumonia* and *Borrelia burgdorferi* (Lyme disease),[3] whereas Japanese encephalitis, West Nile and Coxsackie viruses are causes of an acute flaccid paralysis.[3]

Spinal epidural abscess due to pus between the dura and vertebral periosteum causes localized back pain and tenderness followed by radicular symptoms, and myelopathy. In most cases the organism is *S. aureus*.[3] This condition requires urgent neurosurgical attention.

Multiple sclerosis is rare in the tropics, but neuromyelitis optica (NMO) (or Devic's syndrome) is relatively common in Africa, Asia and the Pacific region. This inflammatory disorder results in optic neuritis and a longitudinal myelitis which are temporally closely related.[16] It is important to distinguish between the two because NMO responds to immunosuppression (prednisone, azathioprine), but poorly to immunomodulatory treatment. NMO can be monophasic or recurrent.[16] There are several reports of monophasic NMO occurring as a para-infectious syndrome associated either with viral infections or tuberculosis.

MYELORADICULOPATHY

Lower limb pareses/paralysis presenting with mixed upper motor neurone (myelopathy) and lower motor neurone (root/cauda equina) involvement together with sphincter dysfunction indicates a lumbar-sacral radiculomyelopathy. This may be due to schistosomiasis, tuberculosis, fungal infections or carcinomatous meningeal involvement.

The CSF findings in TB radiculomyelitis and meningitis are similar with low glucose. In TB radiculomyelitis symptoms usually develop over weeks, but may occur over days. Pathologically, the tuberculous inflammatory infiltrate may invade the underlying cord parenchyma and the pial vessels may thrombose causing cord and root infarction. The longer intradural/meningeal course of the lumbosacral nerve roots increases their vulnerability to damage. Chronic inflammation (arachnoiditis) may provoke a constrictive fibrosis of structures which may only become symptomatic after anti-tuberculous treatment.[17]

Parasitic infections such as schistosomiasis, neurognathostomiasis and *Angiostrongylus cantonensis* can all cause a myeloradiculopathy.

PERIPHERAL RADICULOPATHY/NEUROPATHY

Involvement at this neuroanatomical level presents with combinations of proximal (ventral root) and distal (nerve) weakness with or without dermatomal and/or peripheral sensory nerve disturbance.

Shingles causes an eruption of a vesicular rash in one or more dermatomes, often in the thoracic area, typically preceded by tingling or dysaesthetic pain in the affected dermatome before the eruption. The ophthalmic division of cranial nerve V is also frequently affected. This condition often occurs when cell-mediated immunity is compromised through ageing, drugs, malignancy or HIV infection, resulting in the reactivation of latent VZV in the sensory and autonomic nerve ganglia.[3] Rarely, there may be associated paralysis of the myotome corresponding to the dermatomal rash resulting in neuropathies, radiculopathies and even myelitis.[3] VZV vasculopathy can result in stroke months after the rash or even without a preceding rash. A histopathological study supports the notion that VZV can spread transaxonally from the ganglia to the arterial adventitia, and from there, transmurally to damage the vessel media and intima.[18] Prompt treatment with oral aciclovir or valaciclovir reduces the incidence of post-herpetic neuralgia although in immune-suppressed patients and in those with ophthalmic zoster, intravenous therapy may be necessary. Steroids are ineffective in preventing the development of post-herpetic neuralgia.[3]

An acute lumbosacral polyradiculopathy has been seen in HIV-infected subjects. This syndrome has a predilection for the legs and can be confused with variations of Guillain–Barré syndrome. Patients present over a few days with progressive flaccid paraplegia accompanied by areflexia, sphincter dysfunction and saddle-distribution anaesthesia. In a small series of HIV-infected patients with low CD4+ counts, the aetiology was shown to be CMV invasion of the lumbar-sacral roots (>50 cells/L in CSF, predominantly neutrophils), lymphoma (mild/moderate CSF lymphocytosis) or presumed immune-mediated with spontaneous recovery.[19] CMV lumbosacral polyradiculopathy can be painful and aggressive, even fatal if not treated with empiric ganciclovir.[19] A motor variant has been described in which HIV-infected patients with relatively preserved CD4+ counts develop paraparesis without sensory deficits or sphincter abnormalities. Spontaneous recovery has been shown to occur.[20,20a]

NEUROMUSCULAR JUNCTION

Botulism causes symmetrical cranial nerve palsies with ophthalmoparesis and ptosis followed by descending flaccid paralysis which may result in respiratory muscle compromise and death. The toxin released from *Clostridium botulinum* arises from wounds infected with the bacteria or from the consumption of contaminated foods. The toxin interferes with the presynaptic release of acetylcholine causing neuromuscular failure, but unlike myasthenia gravis, the autonomic nervous system is also involved, resulting in altered pupillary responses, dry mouth and postural hypotension.[21] Treatment includes intensive care support and early antitoxin administration to mop up unbound toxin.

Myasthenia gravis occurs world-wide and generalized disease is potentially fatal if unrecognized. The characteristic feature is fatigability which in the extraocular muscles and eyelids show characteristic flutter-like dysconjugate eye movements and weakness in proximal muscles after brief periods of exercise with full recovery within seconds. Drugs frequently used in the tropics such as quinine and certain antibiotics (fluoroquinolones, tetracyclines, aminoglycosides) can impair neuromuscular transmission.

MYOPATHIES

Bacterial myositis is usually the result of penetrating injury or haematogenous spread due to *Staph. aureus*. Parasitic infections such as trichinosis or cysticercosis are accompanied by eosinophilia. Muscle cysts may cause myalgia, weakness and rarely pseudo-hypertrophy. Viruses may cause benign diffuse myalgia such as with influenza or dengue, although fulminant cases have been described.[22,23]

Polymyositis is the commonest myopathy in HIV-infected subjects and resembles that in non-HIV-infected subjects. However, HIV-infected patients may be younger and have a greater likelihood of normal serum creatine kinase levels which does not reflect burnt-out disease.[24] Treatment includes steroid therapy and antiretrovirals.[24]

STROKE

In the tropics, infectious causes should be considered in ischaemic or haemorrhagic stroke presentations.[25] Viral infections associated with stroke include HIV (infarcts, vasculitis, aneurysmal vasculopathy),[26] Dengue shock syndrome,[27] West-Nile virus, Japanese encephalitis and VZV.[25] Bacterial infections such as TBM, syphilis, and infective endocarditis can involve large and small cerebral vessels whereas in leptospirosis, a large intracranial arteriopathy has been described. Parasitic infections associated with stroke include malaria, Chagas' disease and gnathostomiasis. Sickle-cell disease can result in parenchymal and subarachnoid haemorrhages in Africa and Central/South America.[25]

Specific Bacterial Diseases

TUBERCULOSIS

The HIV epidemic has had a major impact on the incidence of tuberculosis (TB), particularly in the developing world. In sub-Saharan Africa and South-east Asia where TB is endemic and HIV prevalence is high, TB has become the major opportunistic infection among HIV-infected subjects.[2]

Tuberculosis involving the CNS may result in spinal cord compression secondary to osteitis, TB meningitis (TBM) and intracranial tuberculomas. Patients with TBM frequently have evidence of pulmonary tuberculosis on chest radiography (see Chapter 40).[2] Although most studies have shown similar CSF findings between HIV-infected and uninfected patients, a few have shown differences (Table 71.2): lower cell counts among HIV-infected subjects not on antiretrovirals, lower protein levels and neutrophil predominance when TBM occurs in HIV-infected subjects.[2] Culture confirmation of TBM can be elusive although increasing the CSF volume sent for culture, especially in HIV-uninfected subjects, will increase the yield of a confirmatory result; 1.5 mL in HIV-infected subjects yielded positive results compared with 4 mL from HIV-uninfected subjects.[2] The mortality in HIV-infected subjects is almost double that in uninfected subjects and those with severe hyponatraemia are particularly at risk.[2] The current treatment recommendation is rifampicin and isoniazid for 9–12 months, in addition to pyrazinamide plus ethambutol or streptomycin or ethionamide during the first two months.[2] Unlike isoniazid, rifampicin poorly penetrates the blood–brain barrier.[2] If it is suspected that tuberculomas show poor apparent responses to standard tuberculous therapy, inadequate CSF rifampicin levels should be considered.

Corticosteroids improve the prognosis in subjects with TBM who are HIV-uninfected; dexamethasone 0.4 mg/kg per day gradually weaned over 8 weeks, improves survival.[3] Presently, there is no evidence of benefit amongst HIV-infected patients. Common complications of TBM are hydrocephalus, stroke and expanding tuberculoma (even in HIV-negative individuals). Obstructive hydrocephalus may develop at any stage, sometimes acutely, as a sudden neurological deterioration. It should be treated promptly by surgical drainage.

The optimal timing of ART initiation in a patient with HIV/TB co-infection is complex and influenced by the degree of immunosuppression.[28] Simultaneous institution of treatment for TB and HIV has the potential of overlapping drug toxicities, drug–drug interactions and paradoxical TB immune reconstitution syndrome (IRIS). Recent evidence suggests that in patients with advanced immunosuppression a lower mortality can be achieved by starting ART within 2–4 weeks of anti-tuberculous treatment.[28] However, severely immunocompromised subjects with TBM did not benefit from starting ART early (≤7 days) compared with an 8-week delay.[28]

HIV/TB co-infected patients may develop new or worsening meningitis, tuberculoma, tuberculous brain abscess or radiculomyelitis as part of a paradoxical reaction to TB treatment (paradoxical TB-IRIS). TB-IRIS is more likely to occur in a patient with a low CD4+ count; the median time of symptom presentation is 14 days (up to 3 months) after starting ART.[29] TB-IRIS has significant morbidity and mortality; prednisone (1.5 mg/kg daily for 2 weeks, then 0.75 mg/kg daily for 2 weeks) has shown benefit.[30] Importantly, TB drug resistance must be excluded before administering corticosteroids.

Tuberculous osteitis may occur at any spinal level and rarely involve the calvarium.[31] Vertebral compression is usually anteriorly, although posterior cord compression due to tuberculous osteitis in the laminae and pedicles can occur. Epidural tuberculomas can be confused with tumours.

LEPROSY

For details on leprosy, see Chapter 41.

BRUCELLOSIS

Brucellosis mainly involves bones/joints, but the nervous system may be rarely affected. It can cause an acute meningoencephalitis with papilloedema, seizures and coma. Spinal presentation is with spastic or flaccid paraparesis due to cord compression or myeloradiculopathy secondary to osteitis of the spine or epidural abscess. Diagnosis depends on blood or CSF culture of brucella, or more commonly on an enzyme-linked immunosorbent assay of the blood and CSF. Treatments with rifampicin, tetracycline and streptomycin should be for 3 months (see Chapter 28).

Protozoal Diseases

CEREBRAL MALARIA

Plasmodium falciparum, the predominant species in tropical countries, can result in the major life-threatening complication of cerebral malaria. The diagnosis is based on the presence of parasitaemia on a blood smear and altered consciousness or coma often with seizures and motor signs. Meningism is not a feature and the CSF is normal; plasmodium is never seen in CSF. Malaria should be excluded in any patient with fever and a history of travel to a malaria-endemic region within the past 6 months, even if they took antimalarial prophylaxis which is only 80–90% effective.[3] Children, pregnant women and non-immune adults are more susceptible to cerebral malaria. Although humans in endemic areas become immune to malaria this natural immunity is relatively inefficient.

Cerebral malaria-associated neurological sequelae and systemic complications such as hypoglycaemia, hypovolaemia, hyperpyrexia, renal failure, bleeding disorders, anaemia, lactic acidosis and respiratory distress, may contribute to the pathogenesis of coma. The mechanisms underlying the fatal cerebral complications of *P. falciparum* are still not fully understood. Even with treatment the mortality in children approaches 20%.[32]

A Cochrane review concluded that severe malaria is best treated with artesunate (2.4 mg/kg at 0, 12 and 24 hours), rather than intravenous quinine.[33] Quinine can cause hypoglycaemia and neurotoxicity.[3,32] A study comparing intravenous mannitol with placebo for the treatment of cerebral oedema, found no difference in the mortality and neurological sequelae at 6 months.[34]

TOXOPLASMOSIS

Cerebral toxoplasmosis is thought to be due to the reactivation of latent brain infection in immunocompromised hosts (CD4+ <100 cells/μL). These patients present as a subacute encephalopathy with altered consciousness and focal signs such as hemiparesis or seizures. Severely immune-suppressed patients may present with rapidly fatal diffuse necrotizing encephalitis.

On brain imaging it can be difficult to distinguish toxoplasmosis from the lesions of PCNSL. About 20% of AIDS-related toxoplasmosis patients can have negative toxoplasmosis serological tests. However, the response to anti-toxoplasmosis treatment is relatively rapid with >90% of patients responding significantly by 14 days (median 5 days) (Figure 71.2).[15] A combination of pyrimethamine and sulfadiazine is the therapy of choice. An effective alternative is high-dose cotrimoxazole.[35] As the drugs do not eradicate tissue cysts, 50–80% of those not maintained on therapy will relapse within 1 year. In patients on ART, prophylactic therapy can be stopped once the CD4+ count is maintained at >200 cells/μL for 3 months.

TRYPANOSOMIASIS

Two major diseases have been identified: human African trypanosomiasis (HAT) or sleeping sickness and American

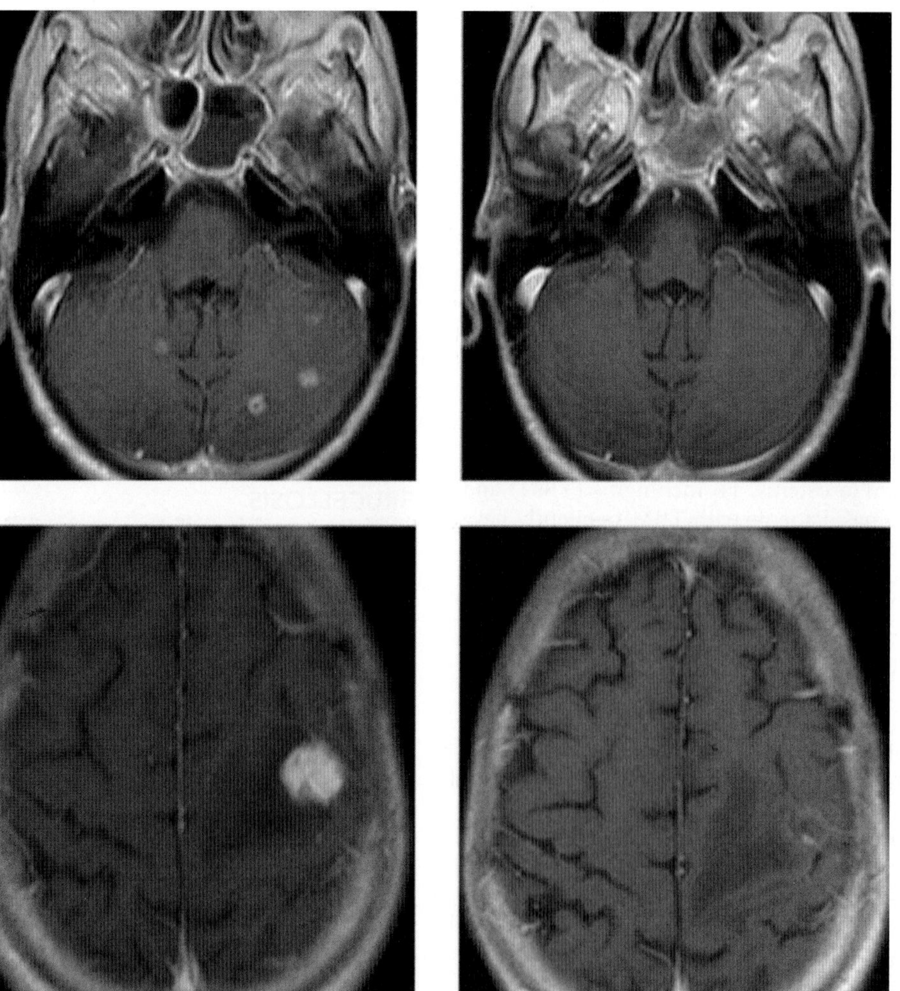

Figure 71.2 Cerebral toxoplasmosis. MR images on the left show several discrete contrast-enhancing lesions in the cerebellum and a focal frontal-parietal region mass lesion with surrounding oedema. The images on the right show resolution after 11 days of treatment.

trypanosomiasis or Chagas' disease (see Chapters 45 and 46). HAT produces progressive CNS damage which is fatal if untreated. HAT is spread by the bite of an infected tsetse fly and the symptoms occur within weeks in the case of *Trypanosoma brucei* (*T.b.*) *rhodesiense*, but usually takes much longer with *T.b. gambiense*, i.e. months to years. Intermittent bouts of fevers follow the incubation period and then the insidious classical symptoms of sleeping sickness: somnolence, persistent headaches, psychiatric symptoms and behavioural changes, and a chronic lymphocytic meningoencephalitis.[36] The diagnosis is based on identifying the trypanosomes in blood smears, lymph node aspirates or CSF. The CSF white cell count is normal in the early stages, but later rises to >5 cells/µL.[36] The treatment for early-stage *T.b. rhodesiense* is suramin and in the late stage when the trypanosomes reside in the CSF treatment is dependent exclusively on melarsoprol. Early-stage *T.b. gambiense* is treated with pentamidine and late-stage with either eflornithine or melarsoprol.[36] Six-monthly LPs are required for 2 years to monitor for the recurrence of trypanosomes in the CSF necessitating further treatment. Melarsoprol is effective but 5–10% of patients develop a post-treatment encephalopathy which can be fatal and thought to be due to reactive immune-mediated CNS vasculitis induced by dying trypanosomes. Eflornithine kills the trypanosomes slower and therefore is better tolerated, but requires 6-hourly intravenous administration for 2 weeks.[36]

Chagas' disease (CD) (Chapter 46) has an acute phase lasting 6–8 weeks which can involve the CNS. CD is a major cause of cardiomyopathy 10–20 years after infection. CD can reactivate in patients with HIV/AIDS and present as a focal brain lesion or acute meningoencephalitis.

Spirochaetal Diseases

SYPHILIS

Sexually acquired syphilis, caused by *Treponema pallidum*, presents as primary, secondary, latent and tertiary or neurosyphilis. The neuropathological consequences can be broadly divided into: (a) meningovascular complications such as subacute meningitis with strokes in the brain or spinal cord or (b) parenchymal disease manifesting as dementia (syphilitic encephalitis or general paralysis of the insane) or tabes dorsalis. However, pathologically many cases show meningeal, vascular, and parenchymal involvement.[37]

A large retrospective series showed half the cases presented with delirium, dementia and other neuropsychiatric conditions and less frequently stroke, myelopathy and seizures.[37] The average age at presentation ranged from 36–43 years. Although worldwide there appears to be resurgence in neurosyphilis, tabes dorsalis has become rare.

Serological tests identify specific IgG and IgM to *T. pallidum* haemagglutination assay (TPHA) and *T. pallidum* particle agglutination assay (TPPA), whereas the indirect serological tests indicate disease activity; Venereal Disease Reference Laboratory (VDRL) test or Rapid Plasma Reagin (RPR) test.[3] A CSF examination is mandatory; a positive CSF VDRL or RPR confirms neurosyphilis, but a negative result does not exclude it (CSF VDRL/RPR is negative in 10–27%).[3,37] However, a negative CSF TPHA or TPPA excludes neurosyphilis. Neurosyphilis should be treated with 17 days of either intramuscular procaine penicillin with probenecid or IV benzylpenicillin.[3] Adjuvant prednisone (40–60 mg/day for 3 days) started 24 hours prior to antibiotics is recommended to prevent the Jarisch–Herxheimer reaction.[3]

OTHER SPIROCHAETES

Other spirochaetal infections affecting the nervous system include borreliosis or relapsing fever (*Borrelia recurrentis*, louse-borne, *B. duttonii*, tick-borne), usually presenting as a febrile meningoencephalitis. Leptospirosis may affect any part of the nervous system. Lyme disease (*B. burgdorferi*) is spread to man by infected ticks. The neurological manifestations span from meningitis, encephalitis, focal cranial neuropathies, polyradiculitis, and post-borreliosis syndromes.

Viruses

The acute exanthemas of childhood – measles, mumps and chickenpox – are still major killers, especially during epidemics in the presence of severe malnutrition.

GEOGRAPHICALLY RESTRICTED VIRAL ENCEPHALITIS

Viral encephalitis should be suspected if a patient with a flu-like prodrome develops high fever, severe headache, nausea and vomiting, altered consciousness or behaviour and seizures. Many of these viruses are restricted to geographic areas, thus a history of travel is critical.[4]

Dengue, especially the haemorrhagic variety, still causes considerable morbidity and fatality in South-east Asia, and *yellow fever* similarly in Africa and South America. Dengue virus is transmitted by mosquito bites. The neurological complications include meningitis, encephalitis, ADEM, transverse myelitis, and Guillain–Barré syndrome.[23]

Eastern equine encephalitis – mainly on the Atlantic and Gulf Coasts of America – tends to occur in summer and autumn and the mortality may be as high as 70%. *Western equine encephalitis*, which despite its name occurs throughout the USA and eastern South America, tends to be less severe.

Japanese encephalitis is a mosquito-borne infection which still claims many lives in South-east Asia. This arbovirus is antigenically related to the flaviviruses of St Louis encephalitis and Murray Valley encephalitis and to the *West Nile virus*. The illness is usually severe, fatal in 25% of cases and with neuropsychiatric sequelae in 30%. Involuntary movements due to basal ganglia involvement may occur.[4] West Nile virus affects the young, but early immunization may be shifting it to the elderly. CT and MRI show thalamic involvement (Figure 71.3).

The clinical features of *Rift Valley fever* include fever, nausea, vomiting, abdominal pain, diarrhoea, jaundice, encephalitis, haemorrhagic manifestations, retinitis and uveitis. Haemorrhagic fever, encephalitis and jaundice were independently associated with high mortality.

HUMAN IMMUNE DEFICIENCY VIRUS (HIV)

More than 30 million people worldwide live with HIV infection, of whom 68% are in sub-Saharan Africa. HIV-1 and HIV-2 infection affects both the central and peripheral nervous system with very similar presentations.[38] HIV enters the CNS compartment early in primary infection, setting the stage for a low-grade chronic inflammation. However, acute meningitis,

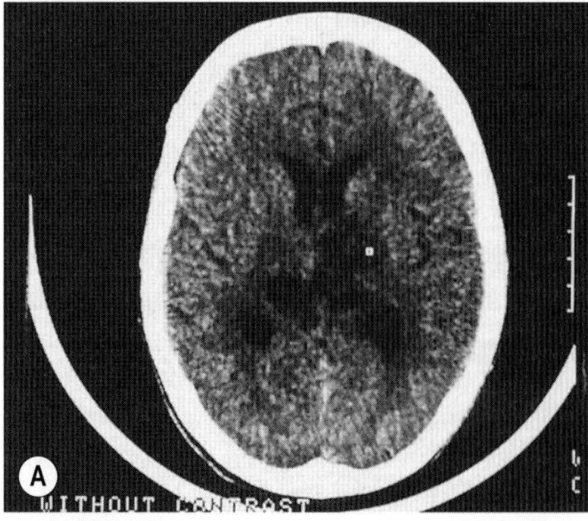

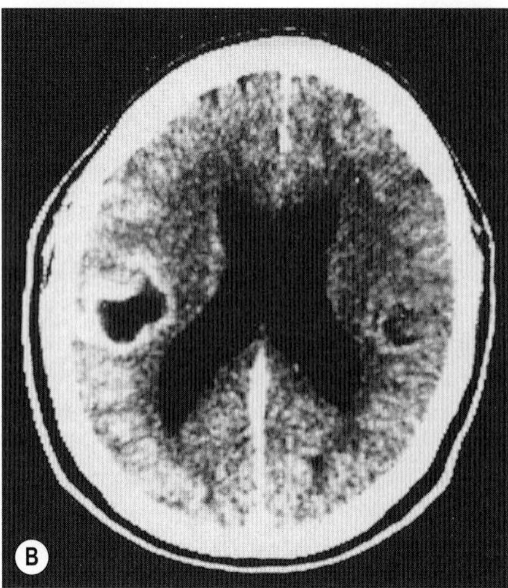

Figure 71.3 Japanese encephalitis. CT brain scan showing: (A) uncontrasted thalamic lesions and (B) ring-enhancing lesions.

encephalitis, Bell's facial palsy (often bilateral) and Guillain–Barré syndrome can occur at seroconversion. Before the era of combination ART (cART), frequent neurological complications of chronic HIV infection were HIV-associated dementia (HAD) and distal sensory polyneuropathy (DSP).

HAD is a progressive subcortical encephalopathy with slowing of both mental and motor function, apathy and memory loss.[39] The examination may show increased tone and hyperreflexia that is more prominent in the legs than arms, suggesting a degree of myelopathy. As the disease progresses the patient develops varying combinations of myelopathy, incoordination and parkinsonian-like bradykinesia and eventually becomes mute with ataxia giving way to paraparesis with incontinent sphincters.[39] The latter may reflect an accompanying HIV-related vacuolar myelopathy. Brain imaging shows atrophy and T2 and FLAIR MRI show diffuse periventricular hyperintensity. CSF examination may show non-specific lymphocytosis with increased protein and antibody production. However, excluding opportunistic infections such as cryptococcal and tuberculous meningitis is the most useful aspect of analysing CSF.[39]

The spectrum of HIV-associated neurocognitive/psychiatric disorders (HAND) may range from mild, asymptomatic cognitive changes (increasing in the post-ART era) to severe HAD described above. There is a concern that the burden of HAND will increase as a result of the following: an ageing HIV-infected population; the brain may serve as a long-term reservoir for HIV with associated ongoing inflammation despite cART; and the variability of drug penetration efficacy into the CNS.[40]

DSP is a common peripheral neuropathy in HIV-infected subjects. Almost all patients dying from AIDS show some histological peripheral nerve pathology.[41] The clinical relevance of DSP is that neuropathic pain is present in 10–37% of HIV-infected subjects prior to ART, and incident neuropathy occurs in 4–25% within a few months of starting cART.[41,42] The symptoms are those of symmetrical dysaesthesia in the soles of the feet, hot, burning and occasionally numb pain, as well as hyperalgesia. The symptoms gradually creep up the legs accompanied by neuropathic signs of areflexia, length-dependent stocking and glove loss of pin-prick sensibility and vibration sense. Proprioceptive dysfunction and weakness rarely occurs. The incidence of DSP is thought to be reduced with the early introduction of cART. Where the onset is temporally related to cART initiation, it is generally attributed to drug toxicity. The drugs most often associated with neuropathy are the nucleoside reverse transcriptase inhibitors (or 'd-drugs': stavudine, didanosine, zalcitabine) and possibly some protease inhibitors (indinavir, saquinavir, ritonavir). Discontinuing the neurotoxic drug is reported to result in symptom improvement in many cases.[41] Nutritional deficiencies and co-morbid anti-tuberculous treatment such as isoniazid, appear to increase the risk of developing DSP.[43] Adequate attention to nutrition and micronutrient supplementation may reduce the incidence of painful neuropathy, particularly where there is a high incidence of HIV/TB co-infection.[44]

Inflammatory demyelinating neuropathy, either acute (AIDP) or chronic (CIDP) occur with increased frequency among HIV-infected people. These immune-mediated neuropathies more commonly manifest in the earlier stages of HIV infection when the immune system is dysregulated rather than depleted.[41] The clinical and electrophysiological features, as well as treatment responses are similar to non-HIV-infected subjects. Although the CSF shows a protein : cell dissociation characteristic of demyelination, HIV-infected subjects often have lymphocytosis (<50 cells).[45] Less common neuropathies such as mononeuritis or mononeuritis multiplex occur either as a manifestation of vasculitis or, in advanced disease, as opportunistic CMV and VZV infections.[41] Progressive cauda equina syndrome in immune-compromised patients can be due to CMV and VZV infection, neurosyphilis or leptomeningeal lymphoma.[41] Subacute painful asymmetrical sensorimotor neuropathy associated with enlarged salivary glands due to CD8+-lymphocytic infiltration and sicca symptoms also known as diffuse infiltrative lymphocytosis syndrome (DILS), responds well to prednisone treatment and/or ART.[20a]

The introduction of cART has had a significant positive impact on the epidemiology and neurological manifestations of HIV infection. However, it poses new challenges in neurological management and treatment such as the development of IRIS and drug–drug interactions, for example between antiepileptic drugs and cART. First-generation anti-epileptic drugs such as phenytoin, carbamazepine and phenobarbital are enzyme inducers and should be avoided in combination with ART as they will reduce drug levels. Valproate, not an enzyme inducer, is useful in combination with cART. Gabapentin, lamotrigine and topiramate are alternatives although lamotrigine doses must be increased when in combination with lopinavir/ritonavir.

IRIS is a potential complication in patients with low CD4+ counts starting cART and usually occurs within weeks of initiating cART.[30] It should be suspected where there is a paradoxical worsening of a patient's condition in the setting of a rapid restoration of immune function and control of HIV plasma viral load. Neurological manifestations of HIV-IRIS can be due to mycobacteria, cryptococci, herpesvirus, cytomegalovirus and JC virus (JCV). Treating TB-IRIS with prednisone has been shown to be beneficial. However, glucocorticoids should be avoided in patients with Kaposi's sarcoma and a diagnosis of TB-IRIS being considered, the possibility of drug resistance should first be excluded.[30]

Up to 5% of AIDS patients will develop progressive multifocal leukoencephalopathy (PML) caused by JCV reactivation in an immunocompromised host. JCV infects oligodendrocytes and astrocytes, resulting in progressive, non-inflammatory demyelination, necrosis, and cell death. CSF analysis is often normal. Clinical and radiological involvement of the cerebellum and brainstem is common in HIV-infected subjects. Reconstituting immune function with cART has a relatively good prognosis. However, PML may develop or worsen with cART causing an IRIS, which often demonstrates MRI contrast-enhancement of the white matter lesions.[46] It is uncertain whether or not additional prednisone cover in the context of PML-IRIS is beneficial. Where features suggest a significant inflammatory component in PML-IRIS, such as CSF lymphocytosis or mass effect with gadolinium enhancement on MRI, this may sway towards empiric prednisone cover.[47]

HUMAN T-CELL LYMPHOTROPIC VIRUS-1 (HTLV-1)

The aetiology of tropical spastic paraparesis (TSP) remained elusive until the serendipitous discovery of an association between TSP and HTLV-1 and the Japanese description of HTLV-1-associated myelopathy (HAM). This condition is now commonly known as HAM/TSP. HTVL-1 is endemic in Latin America, the Caribbean Basin, sub-Saharan Africa and Japan.[48] Transmission may occur by sexual contact, blood transfusion or vertically from mother to child. It is estimated that 10 million people are infected worldwide but only about 5% develop myelopathy implying that viral- and host-related variables are important. While the virus is detected in the spinal cord, much of the damage is thought to be immune-mediated.[49]

HAM/TSP appears more often among females between 30 and 60 years as a subacute, progressive paraparesis with variable sensory disturbance and bladder dysfunction. Spasticity is present in all and weakness (96%), bladder dysfunction (80%), backache (60%), numbness or paraesthesiae (66%) and bowel dysfunction (47%) occur in descending frequency. HTLV-1 is also associated with adult T-cell leukaemia/lymphoma, polymyositis, peripheral neuropathy, uveitis, pneumonitis and dermatitis.

In the appropriate setting, the finding of HTVL-I-specific antibodies in the serum and CSF using Western blot supports the diagnosis.[50] Nonspecific laboratory features include anaemia, raised ESR, and a CSF lymphocytic pleocytosis, raised IgG index and oligoclonal bands. In HAM/TSP the radiological findings are of cord atrophy or arachnoiditis although imaging is of most value in excluding other causes of myelopathy.

There is no specific treatment for HAM/TSP. Steroids, intravenous immunoglobulins and zidovudine have been tried. Some patients appear to transiently respond but relapse soon after therapy is stopped. Few patients stabilize, but the majority have a slow progressive course. Preventative measures include blood donation screening and avoidance of breast-feeding by infected mothers.

LASSA FEVER

The Lassa virus, spread by the urine and droppings of the rodent *Mastomys natalensis*, is endemic in West Africa. It causes an acute haemorrhagic fever with myalgia, sore throat, oral ulcers (sometimes bleeding gums), nausea, vomiting, chest and abdominal pain.[51] Blood vessels bear the brunt of the disease with increased capillary permeability, peripheral vasoconstriction, disseminated intravascular coagulation and a haemorrhagic syndrome affecting various organs including the brain.[51] Although less than one-third present with bleeding, this is a grave prognostic sign. Neurological features may include encephalitis, meningitis, hearing loss and seizures. Neurological symptoms such as deafness may also occur during convalescence.[51]

A combined ELISA Ag/IgM assay is found to be highly sensitive and specific for the diagnosis of Lassa fever. Treatment with a 10-day course of intravenous ribavirin is effective; treatment within the first week of fever onset had a case-fatality rate of 5% compared with >20% if started later. Lassa fever is highly contagious. Human transmission must be avoided by strict barrier nursing and infection control measures.

MEASLES

The measles virus is highly contagious and outbreaks are fuelled by overcrowding and poor vaccine coverage. Measles may infect the CNS as an acute encephalitis or cause post-infectious ADEM 2–4 weeks later. Two rare forms resulting from latent measles infection of the CNS are recognized; subacute sclerosing panencephalitis (SSPE) is seen after years of viral persistence in an immunocompetent host, and subacute measles encephalitis (SME) in an immunocompromised host.[8]

With a large population of people living with HIV, South Africa experienced a measles outbreak in late 2009 tailing off 18 months after a mass vaccination campaign.[8] The aftermath was a clustering of cases with SME in immunocompromised HIV-infected subjects, almost all with a fatal outcome 4–8 weeks later. These patients presented 1–7 months after acute measles with seizures, and not infrequently with acute blindness and deafness. SME is an elusive diagnosis: the preceding measles rash may be absent in an immunocompromised host; CSF analysis may be normal and specific measles testing using antibodies and more sensitive PCR may be negative. Absence of measles virus DNA in the CSF is likely due to the intraneuronal location of the virus and unlike non-neuronal cells, viral budding and shedding does not occur in the CNS. Measles viral transmission occurs via trans-synaptic neuronal spread in the CNS. MRI of the brain shows focal or multi-focal hyperintensity of the cortical ribbon.[8]

SSPE, due to a chronic infection with a defective measles virus, is usually acquired before the age of 2 years. Years later, the disease manifests with insidious behavioural and schooling difficulties, which progress relentlessly over months to a fatal myoclonic-dementia.[52] The EEG shows periodic complexes and the CSF contains high levels of measles-specific antibodies.

POLIOMYELITIS

In 2010, the WHO reported that, as a consequence of the Global Polio Eradication Initiative, only four countries in the world remain polio-endemic: Afghanistan, India, Nigeria and Pakistan. Polio mainly affects children under 5, with 1/200 infections leading to irreversible paralysis, usually affecting the legs. Prevention strategies include high-coverage infant immunization with four doses of oral poliovirus vaccine (OPV) in the first year of life; supplementary OPV doses to all children under 5 when other vaccinations are administered; surveillance for wild poliovirus through reporting and laboratory testing in all cases of acute flaccid paralysis affecting children under 15 years.

RABIES

This rapidly progressive, fatal viral encephalitis is transmitted by infected saliva from animal bites, especially of dogs, foxes, bats and raccoons. It remains a significant public-health threat, especially in Africa and Asia where infected domestic dogs are endemic. The encephalitis presents in 80% with hydrophobia or a paralytic syndrome in 20%. Rabies can be prevented with prompt post-exposure prophylaxis if the skin integrity has been breached by the bite (even without bleeding) of an infected animal. The wound should be cleaned and post-exposure vaccination (PEV), as well as rabies immunoglobulin, should be urgently administered. PEV derived from cell cultures are now much safer than vaccines derived from nerve-tissue. The WHO recommends either intramuscular PEV (4- or 5-day regimen) or intradermal (4-day dosing).[53]

RICKETTSIA

This group of illnesses are transmitted to man via the bites of ticks or mites. Mediterranean spotted fever (*Rickettsia conorii*) in Africa, Asia and the Mediterranean, scrub typhus (*R. tsutsugamushi*) in Asia and the Pacific, typhus (*R. prowazekii*) and Q fever (*Coxiella burnetii*) are all ubiquitous diseases. Whereas the incubation period and clinical features vary between organisms, all manifest with high fever, rash and headache. Meningoencephalitis develops during the 2nd week of the illness, which may be associated with meningism, photophobia, confusion, altered consciousness and seizures. The distinctive eschar at the site of the bite may suggest the diagnosis. CSF examination is rarely helpful and treatment with tetracycline or chloramphenicol should be started on clinical suspicion.

Fungal Infections

CRYPTOCOCCUS

Cryptococcal meningitis (CM) can occur in immune-competent persons, but in HIV-infected persons, it is an important AIDS-defining illness and major cause of death.[54,55] CM occurs when there is advanced HIV infection (CD4+ counts <100 cells/μL) and 20% of these cases present shortly after ART initiation.[56] The mortality of CM is ~33% in the first 10 weeks.[56] In HIV-infected patients CM can relapse which tends to occur at a higher CD4+ cell count and is less severe.

Patients with CM may present with headaches, fever, meningism, features of raised intracranial pressure, seizures and focal neurological signs. The LP opening pressure is almost invariably elevated. CSF is generally colourless with lymphocytic pleocytosis. Between 70–90% will have a raised CSF protein and low glucose while India ink preparations show the organism in 50–70% of cases. The most sensitive and specific test is the cryptococcal latex agglutination test (CLAT) which detects antigen and is positive in over 90% of cases. Importantly, in advanced HIV disease the CSF may show no abnormality apart from a positive CLAT. Similarly, brain imaging can be normal.

Treatment for HIV-infected patients with CM is amphotericin B (1.0 mg/kg per day IV) plus flucytosine (100 mg/kg per day in 4 doses) for ≥2 weeks followed by fluconazole (400 mg/day) for 8 weeks.[57] An alternative is fluconazole >1200 mg/day for 10–12 weeks.[57] Maintenance therapy is fluconazole (200 mg/day) which can be stopped after 12 months if the CD4+ count is >100/μL and plasma HIV has been undetectable for >3 months. Daily LPs may be required to reduce symptomatic raised intracranial pressure. IRIS should be treated with antifungal agents and corticosteroids. Antiretroviral therapy may be initiated as soon as the patient shows improvement or 4 weeks after initiation of antifungal therapy to reduce the risk of IRIS.

Helminthic Infections

With increasing international travel and the natural desire to sample exotic cuisine, which is often improperly processed, parasitic infections are being detected in returning tourists. The more important or common ones affecting the nervous system are summarized in Table 71.4 and only a few will be discussed. The life cycles of these parasites are considered elsewhere.

NEUROCYSTICERCOSIS

Cysticercosis develops when humans accidentally ingest ova of *Taenia solium*; the commonest source apparently being contact with faeces from a household member with an asymptomatic tapeworm.[10] Ova show a predilection for brain, muscle and eye where they mature in ±3 months. Viable cysts avoid destruction by actively modulating the host's immune system. Symptoms are produced when a dying cyst 'leaks' antigens thereby provoking an inflammatory response. In neurocysticercosis it is important to differentiate parenchymal cysts lodged within the brain from those extraparenchymal to brain tissue. The parenchymal forms have several stages: vesicular (hypodense on CT); colloidal (degenerating cyst; ring enhancing on imaging); granular (advanced degeneration) and the calcified stage. Extraparenchymal cysts in the ventricles, fissures or basal cisterns can result in abnormal growth of the parasitic membranes with degeneration of the parasite's scolex forming a racemose cyst(s) (Figure 71.4).

The commonest clinical presentation is seizures, but may include headache, focal deficits, movement disorders and cognitive impairment. Rarely, an encephalitic picture results from multiple cerebral cysts causing a severe host response. Racemose cysts often result in arachnoiditis, ependymitis, mass effect and hydrocephalus. Infrequently the cysts localize to the spine presenting as myelitis or compressive myelopathy.

Where there are ≥2 vesicular or enhancing lesions the serological assay of choice is the serum or CSF enzyme-linked immune-electrotransfer blot (EITB) with a sensitivity of 98% and 100% specificity.[10] EITB is not useful for solitary lesions. An alternative is the CSF ELISA with a sensitivity of 87% and 95% specificity.

TABLE 71.4 Helminths that May Infect the Central Nervous System

Organism	Main Areas of Distribution	Presentation	Management
CESTODES			
Neurocysticercosis	Latin America, sub-Saharan Africa, India	Seizures, mass lesion, hydrocephalus	Albendazole 15 mg/kg/day in 2 divided doses for 8 days. Cover with corticosteroids (see text)
E granulosus (Hydatid disease)	Worldwide	Mass lesion, seizures	Surgical resection. Pretreat: albendazole 15 mg/kg/day in 2 divided doses (40 days) to shrink cyst. If unresectable: albendazole 10–15 mg/kg/day in two divided doses twice a day ≥3 months
Taenia multiceps (coenurosis)	Worldwide	Hydrocephalus	Surgical removal
Spirometra sp. (Sparganosis)	Far East and S-e Asia, East Africa	Seizures, infarcts	Surgical removal
NEMATODES			
Angiostrongylus cantonensis	S-e Asia, Caribbean, Southern USA	Meningoencephalitis	Repeated LPs to reduce ICP. Corticosteroids + Albendazole 10–15 mg/kg/day in two divided doses – 2 weeks
Gnathostoma spinigerum	S-e Asia, Mexico, Ecuador, Japan	Meningoencephalitis, seizures, myeloradiculopathy	Albendazole 10–15 mg/kg/day in 2 divided doses – 21 days + corticosteroids. Surgical removal if accessible
Onchocerca volvulus	West Africa, Yemen, Latin America	Chorioretinitis, keratitis, seizures	Ivermectin single oral doses of 0.15 mg/kg single oral dose
Baylisascaris procyonis	Worldwide	Meningoencephalitis	Corticosteroids, albendazole 10–15 mg/kg/day in 2 divided doses
Trichinella sp.	Worldwide	Myopathy, strokes, meningoencephalitis	Corticosteroids, repeated LPs
TREMATODES			
Schistosomiasis	Africa, Asia, Brazil	cauda equina/conus syndrome/ cerebral granuloma	*S. mansoni*, *S. haematobium* and *S. intercalatum* - Praziquantel 40 mg/kg/day – 3 days, corticosteroids (see text) *S. japonicum* and *S. mekongi* – Praziquantel 60 mg/kg/ day – 3 days, corticosteroids (see text)
Paragonimus sp.	Latin America, Asia, West Africa	Encephalitis, mass lesion, infarcts, seizures, myelopathy	Praziquantel 25 mg/kg three times a day – 3 days, corticosteroid
Fasciola hepatica	Worldwide	Meningitis, mass lesion, infarct	Triclabendazole 10 mg/kg single dose or 20 mg/kg in two divided doses

S-e, South-east; LP, lumbar puncture; ICP, intracranial pressure; meningoencephalitis in this table refers to an eosinophilic meningoencephalitis.

There has been controversy as to whether or not all patients require anti-cysticercal therapy (ACT). Generally, calcific lesions do not require ACT, while those with an isolated lesion can probably get by without ACT. ACT should be avoided in cysticercal encephalitis where corticosteroids are administered to decrease intracranial pressure. Most patients may be treated with albendazole (superior to praziquantel) with/without steroids. The albendazole dose is 15 mg/kg per day for a week.[10] Higher dosages (≤30 mg/kg per day in divided doses) for a month may be required for extraparenchymal disease. Surgical

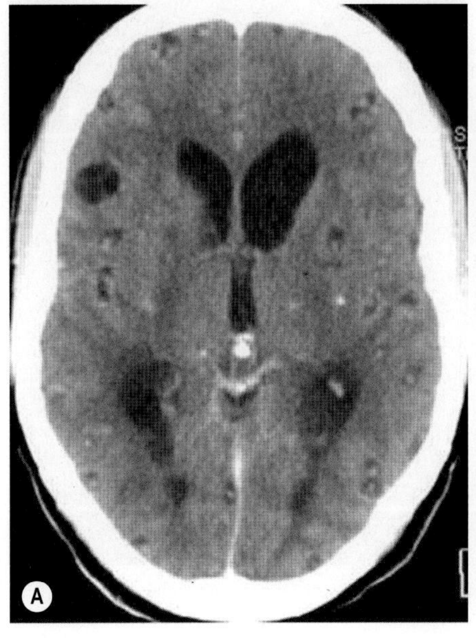

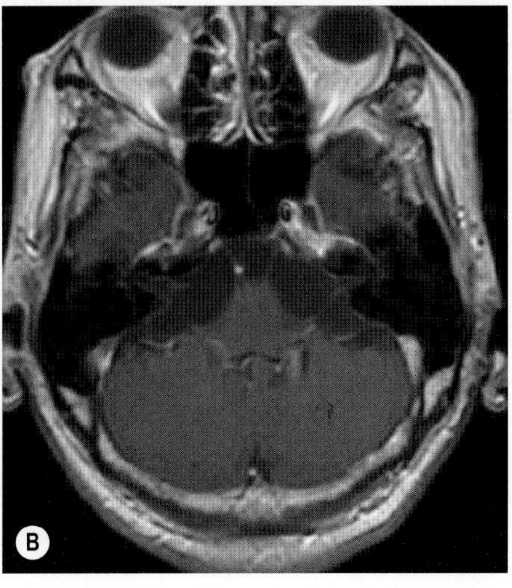

Figure 71.4 (A) Neurocysticercosis. Cysts in different stages of maturation. Some cysts contain central scolices. Note asymmetry of the anterior horns of the lateral ventricles suggesting intraventricular cysts causing a degree of obstruction. (B) Neurocysticercosis. Racemose cysts in the prepontine cistern.

management may be indicated for hydrocephalus and in selected cases, endoscopic removal of ventricular and accessible arachnoid cysts.

GNATHOSTOMIASIS

The disease is common in Asia, especially Thailand, southern China and Bangladesh. Humans become infected by consuming raw, under-cooked or marinated amphibians, crustaceans and fish infected with encysted larvae. After ingestion, there is a prodromal gastrointestinal illness lasting 2–3 weeks followed by a variable incubation period (weeks to years), during which there is cutaneous and neural migration. CNS invasion may manifest as an eosinophilic meningoencephalitis, subarachnoid haemorrhage, cranial neuritis or focal signs. A classical presentation is with painful radiculomyelitis due to invasion of the spinal cord via the spinal nerves.

Peripheral eosinophilia is common. Imaging may show the larval tracks within the brain and cord parenchyma (Figure 71.5A) and antibody testing is highly specific.[58] The usual treatment is albendazole 400 mg twice a day for 21 days under prednisone cover (1 mg/kg per day for 7 days). An alternative drug is ivermectin 200 mg/kg orally as a single dose. The larva may be removed if located in a surgically accessible site (Figure 71.5B).

SCHISTOSOMIASIS

This disease is endemic in Africa, the Middle and Far East, South America and the Caribbean. Neuroschistosomiasis is caused by ectopic ova. Eggs released in the porto-caval system reach the spinal veins via Batson's venous plexus, explaining why the lower spinal cord is a favoured site, whereas those reaching the brain probably arise via porto-pulmonary venous shunts.[59] *S. haematobium* almost exclusively affects the spinal cord, while *S. japonicum* localizes to the brain. *S. mansoni* may produce lesions in both brain and spinal cord.

Myelopathy most frequently results from an intramedullary granulomatous mass (ova surrounded by cellular infiltrates) usually between T12 and L1 with surface nodules ± a meningeal reaction (Figure 71.6). The clinical presentation is a conus/cauda equina syndrome characterized by subacute progressive paraparesis ± sphincter disturbance. Less commonly, an acute lumbar transverse myelitis results from a combination of inflammation, vasculitis and ischaemia. Symptoms develop over 24–48 hours.[60,61] *S. japonicum* causes an encephalitis with delirium, coma, visual disturbance, hemiparesis and seizures whereas more chronic symptoms may be due to the mass effect of granulomas.

Peripheral blood eosinophilia is frequently seen. Serological tests in endemic areas are of limited value. The key investigation is neuro-imaging; CT myelography and MRI may show an expanded cord with enhancement of the lesion (Figure 71.6B) or clumping of the roots indicating arachnoiditis. Findings of ova in the urine, faeces or rectal snip will provide further support for neuroschistosomiasis obviating the need for a cord biopsy. The CSF shows a lymphocytic response, elevated protein and a normal or slightly reduced glucose. Ova are not seen. The differential diagnosis includes other granulomatous diseases such as tuberculosis and syphilis, and neoplasms. A presumptive diagnosis may be made and treatment started without a biopsy if there is the characteristic clinical and radiological presentation and evidence of extra-neurological

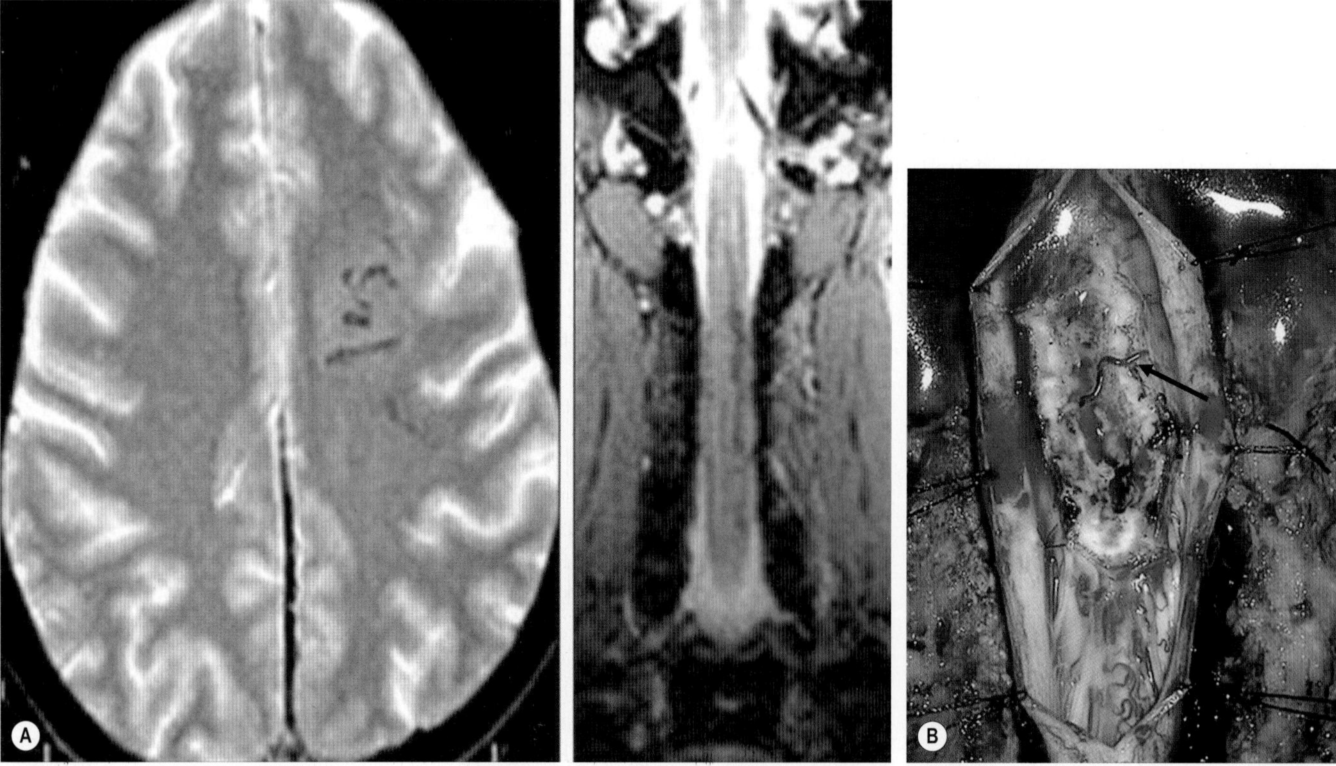

Figure 71.5 (A) Gnathostomiasis; larval tracks evident on brain and spinal cord MRI. (B) Gnathostomiasis; larvae can be surgically removed if in an accessible site (see arrow). *(Courtesy of R Shakir & N Poungvarin.)*

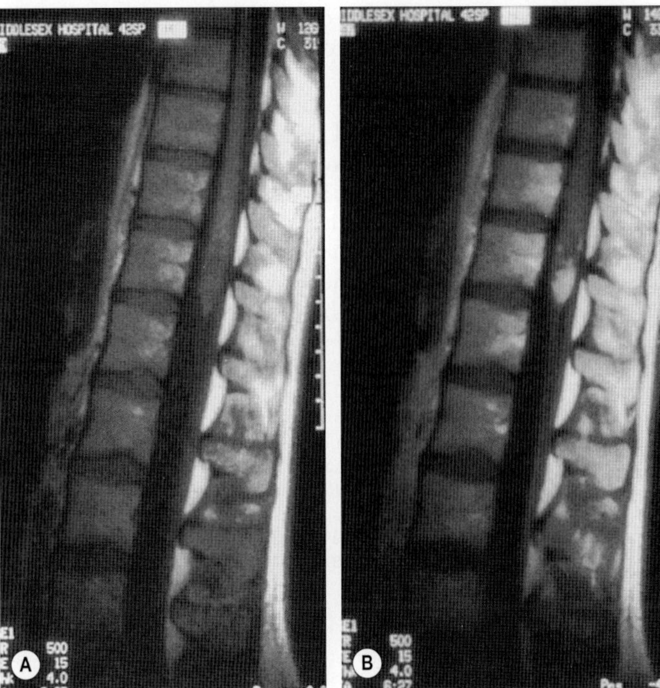

Figure 71.6 Schistosomiasis of the lower spinal cord and conus. (A) Before contrast and (B) irregular contrast-enhancing lesion with surrounding oedema.

schistosomiasis.[60] Some advocate treating with concomitant steroids, initially intravenously followed by oral prednisone (1 mg/kg daily).[61]

Nutritional and Toxic Factors

Malnutrition and micronutrient deficiencies are also still common in many parts of the world, especially in chronically ill populations such as those suffering from HIV and tuberculosis.

The vitamin B complex is particularly important in the development and functioning of the nervous system. Deficiencies may result in weakness and paresthesiae or burning pain in the feet, ataxia, nerve deafness, disturbances of vision and absent or exaggerated reflexes. Beriberi due to thiamine (vitamin B1) deficiency, which is often attributed to discarding of the thiamine-rich germinal layer when polishing rice, presents clinically in wet (cardiac) or dry (neuropathic) forms: the salient neurological features are painful polyneuropathy with tender calves and sensitive soles. Wernicke's encephalopathy (B1 deficiency) may be acute or insidious and chronic with confusion, ophthalmoplegia and ataxia, whereas Korsakoff's syndrome presents more dramatically with amnesia and confabulation. Alcoholism is the most frequent predisposing factor for Wernicke's encephalopathy. Severe thiamine deficiency may be encountered with malabsorption syndromes such as occur with severe AIDS or persistent vomiting such as in hyperemesis gravidarum which can also result in neuropathic beriberi. The latter condition requires urgent administration of high doses of intravenous thiamine (>100 mg daily).

Pellagra, due to niacin deficiency in those eating white maize as staple food, presents clinically with diarrhoea, erythematous rash in sun-exposed areas, atrophic glossitis, diplopia, dysarthria, myelopathy, neuropathy and dementia. Strachan's syndrome manifesting with visual failure, neuropathic feet and oral, peri-anal and scrotal dermatitis and ulceration, is another consequence of multiple nutritional deficiencies including riboflavin (B2), thiamine, niacin and pyridoxine (B6).

There are many drug-associated peripheral neuropathies, but here brief mention will be made only of a few widely used agents. A painful neuropathy, particularly in those genetically disposed to slow acetylation of isoniazid, is well known, as is optic neuritis related to ethambutol. Both drugs are used in the treatment of tuberculosis. There is some evidence to suggest that HIV-infected subjects, who are at increased risk of developing or re-activating tuberculosis, may be at increased risk of developing a painful neuropathy shortly after starting tuberculous treatment.[43] Multivitamin supplementation including 25 mg daily pyridoxine has been associated with a reduced incidence of painful neuropathy in both TB, and HIV/TB co-infected subjects.[62] Clioquinol, previously widely used in the treatment of diarrhoea and intestinal amoebiasis, is now known to cause subacute myelo-optic neuropathy whereas aromatic diamidines, used in the treatment of leishmaniasis and trypanosomiasis, have been associated with trigeminal neuropathy.

Heavy metals such as arsenic, lead and thallium are often used in traditional folklore medications. Arsenical toxicity presents with acute symptoms such as vomiting, diarrhoea, burning eyes, tearing and photophobia, congestion and facial swelling, followed by a predominantly sensory polyneuropathy. Mees' lines (transverse white bands across fingernails), pigmentation of the extremities with patchy depigmentation, hyperkeratosis and desquamation of palms and soles may occur. Demonstrating high concentrations of arsenic in scalp hairs or nail clippings confirms the diagnosis. Illicit liquor, crude abortifacients and deliberate contamination of well-water and opium have been reported as sources of arsenic. Certain ocean fish and marine crustaceans, such as the pomfret, plaice, halua and hilsa, may also contain relatively high concentrations of arsenic. Dimercaprol and/or penicillamine must be given early as the response is poor after delay.

Lead may cause an encephalopathy in children and a peripheral neuropathy in adults. This is predominantly motor, more evident in the arm extensors and associated with abdominal colic. The characteristic anaemia with punctuate basophilia suggests the diagnosis. Potential sources include reconditioning of car batteries, burning lead-containing batteries for cooking, illicit liquor distillation by means of lead pipes or radiators, and contaminated water. Thallium may induce both neuropathy and encephalopathy. The acute painful neuropathy may be associated with nonspecific gastrointestinal symptoms and the occurrence of alopecia within 3 weeks should suggest the diagnosis. Oral potassium ferrocyanide is the treatment of choice.

Cassava sustains millions of people in Africa and the toxic effects are well documented. Flour made from cassava roots may contain a high concentration of linamarin, a cyanogenic glycoside, which results in chronic cyanide intoxication presenting as a progressive 'tropical ataxic neuropathy'. In addition to painful neuropathy and ataxia the patient may develop blurred vision and impaired hearing; occasionally spasticity also develops. Konzo, caused by long-term intake of cassava, is a distinct syndrome with a relatively abrupt onset of non-progressive spastic paraparesis. It has been reported that linamarin is enzymatically converted to cyanide by intestinal bacteria. The absorbed cyanide then damages neural cells.

Lathyrism, endemic in parts of India, Bangladesh and Ethiopia, is caused by excessive consumption of chickpeas of the lathyrus family. It presents as a slowly progressive spastic paraparesis. The neurotoxin, β-N-oxalyl amino-L-alanine, an excitatory amino acid, acts as an AMPA receptor agonist and ultimately causes toxic inhibition of mitochondrial complex I. This, in turn, mediates neuronal damage in the motor cortex and lumbar spinal cord. In a similar manner, excessive consumption of the seed of the false-sago palm – either as food or medicinal component – may induce excitatory neurotoxicity. This is thought to be one of the factors responsible for the occurrence of amyotrophic lateral sclerosis and Parkinsonism–dementia complex in the Pacific Mariana Islands.

Rarer plant toxins include that associated with *Gloriosa superba* (glory lily): accidental ingestion may cause alopecia, aplastic anaemia and polyneuropathy due to colchicine, which impairs exoplasmic transport in peripheral nerves and also damages skeletal muscle. Another poisonous shrub belonging to the buckthorn family (*Karwinskia humboldtiana*), grows freely in Mexico and Texas, and may cause a polyneuropathy progressing to respiratory and bulbar paralysis.

REFERENCES

2. Marais S, Pepper DJ, Marais BJ, et al. HIV-associated tuberculous meningitis – diagnostic and therapeutic challenges. Tuberculosis (Edinb) 2010;90:367–74.
3. Davies N, Thwaites G. Infections of the nervous system. Pract Neurol 2011;11:121–31.
4. Solomon T, Hart IJ, Beeching NJ. Viral encephalitis: a clinician's guide. Pract Neurol 2007;7:288–305.
28. Torok ME, Farrar JJ. When to start antiretroviral therapy in HIV-associated tuberculosis. N Engl J Med 2011;365:1538–40.
40. Vivithanaporn P, Gill MJ, Power C. Impact of current antiretroviral therapies on neuroAIDS. Expert Rev Anti Infect Ther 2011;9:371–4.

Access the complete references online at www.expertconsult.com

72 Psychiatry

CHARLOTTE HANLON | ABEBAW FEKADU

KEY POINTS

- Mental disorders are common across the world and associated with high levels of suffering and disability.
- Physical and mental health are intertwined; comorbid mental disorders contribute to poorer prognosis, quality of life and survival in physical health conditions.
- Mental disorders increase mortality through suicide, accidents and poorer physical health.
- Stigma and discrimination mean that persons with mental disorders get worse health care.
- Effective and affordable treatments for mental disorders are available for all countries of the world but awareness and implementation is low.
- General health professionals can safely and effectively deliver care to persons suffering from mental disorders using evidence-based guidelines.
- The World Health Organization (WHO) has identified priority mental disorders for focused action and many LAMICs are scaling up mental health care.

Introduction

Mental disorders affect people in every country of the world. Despite this, psychiatry is often a marginalized and neglected specialty within low- and middle-income countries (LAMICs). There are, however, compelling reasons why action should be taken to provide better care for those with mental disorders. Mental disorders are common: 10–30% of people worldwide are estimated to be affected by a mental disorder over any 12-month period.[1] Mental disorders cause immense suffering to the person, their family and the wider community. Often this suffering is compounded by the effects of stigma, discrimination and human rights abuses, all of which are exacerbated by a lack of access to known effective treatments. This situation has been described as a 'global emergency on a par with the worst human rights scandals in the history of global health'[2] and a 'failure of humanity'.[3] The public health argument recognizes that mortality alone is not an adequate measure of the adverse consequences of disease and illness. When disability is also taken into account, neuropsychiatric disorders top the list of the most disabling disorders worldwide.[4] Even these figures ignore the substantial contribution of mental disorders to death by suicide (800 000 deaths/year, worldwide)[5] and accidental death, and to poorer health outcomes when mental disorders are comorbid with a range of physical health conditions. There is, indeed, 'no health without mental health'.[5] Mental disorders also have important economic consequences for the person and their family: effective treatment of mental disorders is one way to alleviate poverty.[6]

Effective, culturally appropriate and affordable interventions exist that could help to treat distressing symptoms, and to rehabilitate and reintegrate persons with mental disorders into society. The problem is largely one of coverage: in many LAMICs, over 75% of persons with severe mental disorders never receive effective treatment during their lifetime.[7] Given the dearth of specialist mental health professionals in LAMICs,[8] task sharing with general healthcare professionals is one workable way to reduce this scandalous treatment gap. The WHO advocates that the care for priority mental disorders should be integrated into the primary and general healthcare system, with support from specialist mental health services.[1] New evidence-based guidelines (the WHO mental health Gap Action Programme Implementation Guide; mhGAP-IG) exist to support this process and will form the basis of guidance given within this chapter.[9]

Diagnosis and Epidemiology of 'Priority' Mental Disorders

Mental disorders are diagnosed according to international, standardized criteria. The two most widely used diagnostic systems are the WHO's International Classification of Disease, currently in its 10th revision (ICD-10)[10] and the Diagnostic and Statistical Manual of Mental Disorders, version V (DSM-V).[11] Both systems operationalize diagnosis by specifying constellations of symptoms and signs that appear to define a specific mental disorder and discriminate that disorder from other disorders. Review of the DSM has just been completed and review of the ICD is currently underway with the expectation that diagnostic criteria will become more closely aligned, although current differences are not substantial. The WHO recommends that general health workers focus their attention on selected 'priority disorders',[1] namely the common mental disorders (CMDs), which include depression, anxiety and medically unexplained somatic symptoms, the severe mental disorders (SMD), which comprise the psychoses and bipolar disorder, as well as developmental and behavioural disorders in children and adolescents, dementia, and alcohol and drug use disorders. In addition, the cross-cutting issue of suicide and self-harm is prioritized for action.

The estimated global prevalence of the WHO priority conditions is as follows:[12] depression 1.9% in men, 3.2% in women; psychosis 0.4%; bipolar disorder 0.4%; child development disorders 1.0–3.0%;[13] child behavioural disorders 10.0–20.0%; dementia 0.6% in the total population, ranging from 1.6% (sub-Saharan Africa) to 6.4% (USA) in those over 60 years;[14] alcohol use disorders 2.8% in men, 0.5% in women; drug use disorders 0.4–4.0%.

It should be noted that the combined estimates of prevalence of SMD is conservative and likely to be closer to 2%.[15,16] Cross-country studies show a comparable prevalence of priority mental disorders in general population samples in LAMICs and high-income countries,[17,18] although individual countries show some variation. In primary and general healthcare settings, the prevalence of depression is substantially higher than that found in the general population, with most countries in a WHO cross-country study finding around 20–40% prevalence.[19]

Culture, Mental Health and Disorder

Most diagnostic categorizations of mental disorder are based upon Western conceptualizations of mental health and illness. In the absence of gold standard tests for mental disorders, there is concern that mental pathology in non-Western cultures may be diagnosed where none truly exists; Kleinman's so-called 'category fallacy'.[20] For example, it has been hypothesized that postnatal depression is a culture-bound disorder of the West, arising because of certain societal changes, including the dominance of biomedical management of childbirth and the alienation of women from important cultural rites of passage.[21] Although plausible, the evidence accumulating from well-conducted, culturally sensitive studies in LAMICs rather supports the opposite: women in LAMICs appear to be at higher risk of postnatal depression, which is recognized within the culture and has public health relevance due to adverse effects on both mother and child.[22]

Some mental disorder categories are more controversial than others and the risk of category fallacy might vary across categories of mental disorder; higher for CMDs and lower for the SMD and dementia, whose manifestations appear less variable across cultures. Despite variation in presenting symptoms, however, the core syndromes of the WHO's priority mental disorders appear to be present across cultures.

Nonetheless, culture remains highly relevant to mental health and disorder in a number of ways. Cultural factors may affect vulnerability to mental disorder, the way that symptoms are expressed, detection by health professionals, the illness attribution of the person and their family, as well as the favoured help-seeking behaviour. For example, in South Asia, the societal pressure to deliver a boy baby has been shown to lead to increased levels of postnatal depression in women who give birth to girl babies.[23]

Mental Health and Physical Health

Mind and body are inextricably linked. Mental disorders can be risk factors for physical disorders or may arise as a consequence of physical ill-health. In some cases, a common predisposition may underlie the occurrence of both conditions. All too often, mental disorders remain undetected, and therefore untreated, in general and primary healthcare settings. Findings from a recent comprehensive global review of the complex inter-relationships between physical and mental ill-health will now be summarized in relation to physical conditions that command a high public health priority in LAMICs.[5]

CHRONIC COMMUNICABLE DISEASES

The prevalence of HIV/AIDS is increased in persons with SMD in high-income countries, with mental disorder thought to increase the risk of HIV infection. Findings from LAMICs are less clear. However, alcohol and drug use are associated with risky sexual behaviours,[24] as well as direct risk of HIV transmission for injecting drug users, worldwide. There is strong evidence that the risk of CMDs is increased in persons with HIV/AIDS, both in high-income countries[25] and LAMICs.[5] CMDs co-morbid with HIV have been associated with decreased help-seeking and uptake of treatment services for HIV/AIDS, poorer treatment adherence, more rapid disease progression, increased disability, poorer quality of life and increased mortality. Cognitive deficits and alcohol and drug use also adversely affect the outcome of HIV/AIDS.

Similar consequences of undetected CMDs are also found in tuberculosis (TB), particularly in those suffering from multi-drug resistant TB (MDR-TB).

CHRONIC NON-COMMUNICABLE DISORDERS (NCDs)

As reviewed by Prince and co-workers,[5] CMDs increase the risk of a person developing hypertension, ischaemic heart disease and stroke, and may increase the risk of diabetes. The risk of diabetes is also raised substantially in persons with psychosis, related in part to lifestyle and the side-effects of medication. NCDs also increase the risk of developing CMDs, so that overall comorbidity between NCDs and mental disorders is high. CMDs comorbid with NCDs are associated with poorer prognosis, including higher risk of complications (e.g. diabetic retinopathy) and death. CMDs appear to worsen self-care, responsiveness to advice about lifestyle change and adherence to medication regimens that need to be sustained over a long period of time. CMDs have a large negative impact on overall health status and functioning, consistently greater in magnitude than that arising from the chronic and disabling diseases of diabetes, arthritis, angina and asthma.[26]

REPRODUCTIVE AND CHILD HEALTH

In LAMICs, pregnant women appear to have an elevated risk of CMDs.[27] Untreated CMD has been associated with poorer antenatal care attendance, increased use of alcohol and cigarettes, poorer weight gain during pregnancy and increased risk of preterm birth and low birth weight in high-income countries.[28] To date in LAMICs, antenatal CMDs have been associated with prolonged labour, delayed initiation of breast-feeding[29] and low birth weight.[30,31] Although not appearing to be more prevalent than at other times in the life course, postnatal CMDs have been found to be associated with early cessation of breast-feeding; infant undernutrition;[22] ill-health and decreased vaccine uptake;[32] poorer cognitive development;[33] and increased child mortality[33] in LAMICs.

Aetiology

Known aetiological mechanisms for specific priority mental disorders will be considered later. In this section, we introduce a widely used aetiological framework for conceptualizing possible reasons for the presence of a particular mental disorder in a particular person at a given moment in time; the so-called biopsychosocial formulation.[34] The biopsychosocial approach recognizes that mental disorders often arise due to a

TABLE 72.1 Example of Possible Biopsychosocial Framework for Psychosis

	Predisposing	Precipitating	Perpetuating
Biological	Genetics/family history	Cannabis use	Non-adherence with antipsychotic medication
Psychological	Developmental delay	Conflict in the family	High expressed emotion within the family
Social	Migration	Social isolation	Stigma and discrimination

combination of biological, psychological and social factors, some leading to a vulnerability or resilience to mental disorders, others triggering the onset of the disorder, and perhaps others contributing to the maintenance of a mental disorder once started. Elucidating the contribution of these factors can be important in guiding appropriate management of mental disorders. See Table 72.1 for a possible biopsychosocial formulation of psychosis in an individual.

In this case, the predisposing factors may give us important prognostic information, whereas the precipitating and perpetuating factors will be essential to address to maximize the person's clinical and functional recovery from psychosis.

Attributions for the causes of mental disorders vary widely across cultures and need to be understood by the healthcare workers. Even within cultures, marked individual variation in illness attribution is apparent, meaning that healthcare workers should take care not to make assumptions about an individual person's illness model. Spiritual and supernatural explanations of mental disorder, e.g. due to the evil eye of an envious neighbour; bewitchment; spirit possession; influence from ancestral spirits; divine punishment for wrong-doing – are more commonly found in LAMICs, particular for SMD. Such illness models may guide help-seeking, affect the acceptability of interventions and contribute to non-adherence with biomedical treatments.

General Principles of Assessment

Psychiatric assessment follows the same structure as any medical assessment, with systematic exploration of signs and symptoms of disorder. Unlike other fields of medicine, assessment of mental disorder relies more heavily upon the person's report of their experiences, collateral history from those in a good position to observe the development of disorder in the person, and the observations of the health worker during the interview. The health worker's observations are collected systematically in a 'mental state examination', which looks at abnormalities of general appearance and behaviour, speech, mood, thoughts, perceptions, cognition and the patient's level of awareness about their condition (insight). The health worker's communication and observational skills are, therefore, of paramount importance in order to make a correct diagnosis.

ACUTE BEHAVIOURAL DISTURBANCE

If a person has acutely disturbed behaviour, they need to be seen straight away. A basic guideline for assessment is given in Figure 72.1.

On occasion, the person may be too disturbed for an adequate physical examination to be carried out. Emergency tranquilization may then be required (Figure 72.2) but should not diminish the urgency of investigation of the underlying cause of disturbance.

SCREENING AND DETECTION

When a person presents to a general healthcare setting suffering from a CMD, the symptoms rarely fit neatly into the distinct diagnostic categories for a psychiatric disorder.[35] With all patients, be attentive to emotional clues and non-verbal communication of distress. For example, does the person look sad or miserable, unduly worried, or preoccupied beyond what would be expected given their complaint? The presenting complaint may give some clue to psychosocial problems: a woman with multiple injuries may be a victim of intimate partner violence and at high risk of a CMD; a man who keeps getting injured in fights may have an alcohol problem. Other clues to underlying CMDs include nonspecific, vague or multiple complaints which do not easily map onto known illness. Forgetfulness is most often secondary to the difficulty in concentrating that comes with CMD, but in an older person it should raise the possibility of dementia. Psychotic illness is often indicated by behaviour or beliefs that are outside the norms of the society.

COMMUNICATION AND PRIVACY

The patient's willingness to disclose emotional concerns will depend partly on the ability of the healthcare professional to

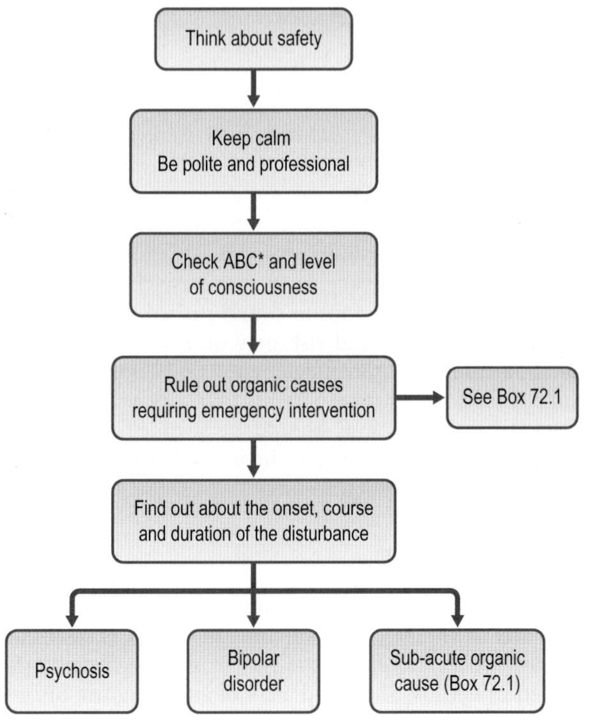

Figure 72.1 Flowchart for assessment of acute behavioural disturbance.

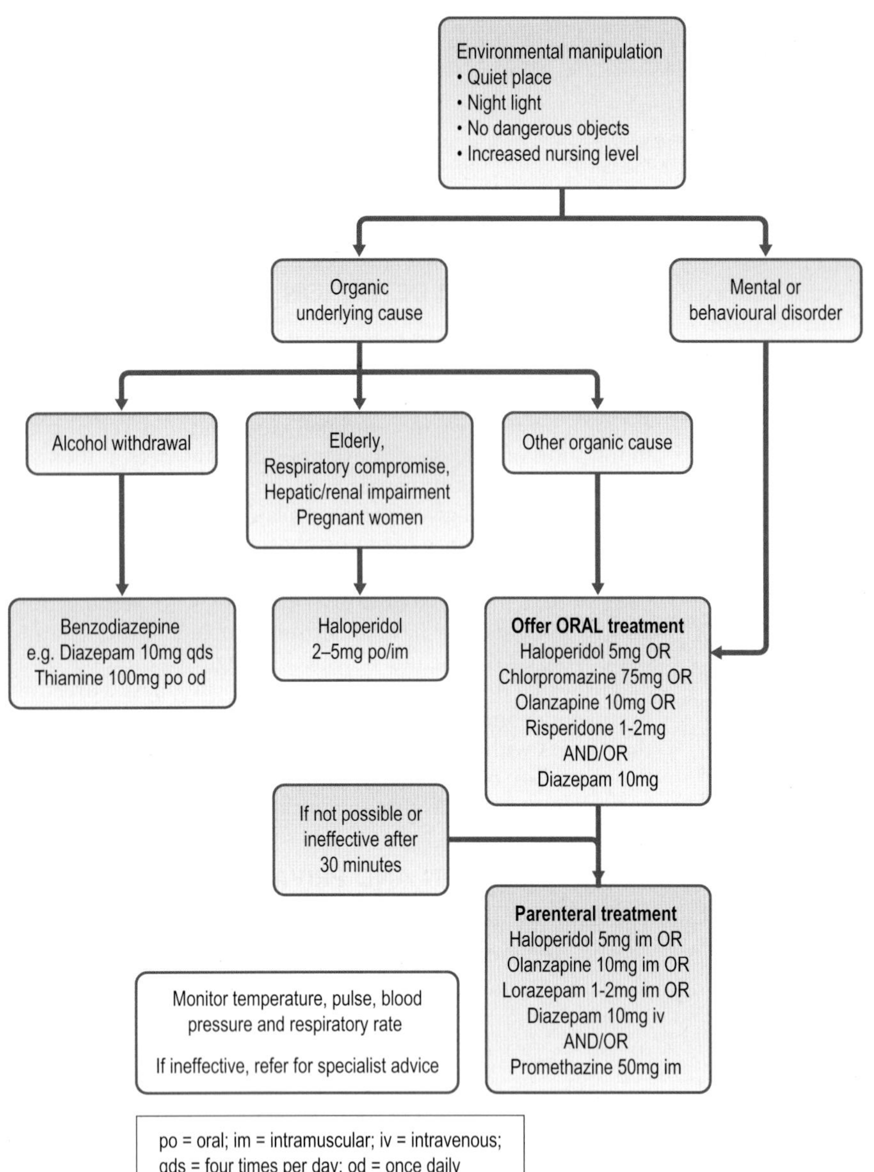

Figure 72.2 Management of acute behavioural disturbance. *(Based on Taylor D, Paton C, Kapur S, editors. The Maudsley Prescribing Guidelines in Psychiatry, 11th ed. Chichester: Wiley-Blackwell; 2012.)*

make them feel comfortable to do so. This includes ensuring that the patient has privacy. Even in a busy clinic, it is crucial for health workers to try not to sound rushed. Important indicators of severe illness and risk may otherwise be missed, e.g. suicidal ideation. A non-judgemental and non-stigmatizing attitude will also encourage patients to be open about their difficulties. Closed questions should be avoided. For example, 'You're not feeling sad, are you?' invites a 'No' response, even if the patient does have such feelings.

RISK ASSESSMENT

In any patient presenting with signs of mental disorder, and particularly in the case of a suicide attempt, it is essential for the health worker to assess the risk of suicide. Suicide risk is increased in CMDs, SMD and alcohol and drug use disorders. Asking about suicidal thoughts does not increase the risk of a person attempting suicide and for many, it will be a relief to share their distress. Be sensitive in your questioning, starting with more neutral questions, e.g. 'Have you ever thought that life was not worth living?', and proceeding to 'Have you ever thought of harming yourself in some way or trying to end your life?'. Past suicide attempts and current suicide plans or intent indicate high risk of suicide. Other important risk factors for completion of suicide include: chronic pain or a debilitating medical condition; presence of a priority mental disorder; social isolation; male sex; and unemployment.

IDENTIFYING ORGANIC CAUSES OF MENTAL DISTURBANCE

A number of general medical conditions can give rise to symptoms of mental disorder due to direct physiological consequences of the medical condition (Box 72.1). The underlying condition must be identified and treated.

General Principles of Management

Just the process of being listened to by a health worker can be therapeutic and help to relieve some patients of their mental

BOX 72.1 SOME OF THE ORGANIC CAUSES OF MENTAL DISTURBANCE

- *Non-infectious, CNS*: Sub-dural haematoma, tumour, aneurysm, epilepsy (status epilepticus, post-ictal), severe hypertension, normal pressure hydrocephalus, head injury, multiple sclerosis, Parkinson's disease
- *Metabolic/Endocrine*: Hyper-/hypoglycaemia, hyper-/hypothyroidism, Addison's disease, Cushing syndrome, hyper-/hypoparathyroidism, renal or hepatic disorders, Wilson's disease, electrolyte derangement, vitamin deficiency (thiamine, vitamin B12, folate), porphyria
- *Infectious*: Viral, e.g. HIV, HSV, Japanese encephalitis, rabies; bacterial, e.g. meningococcal meningitis, syphilis, typhoid fever, sepsis; mycobacterial, TB; parasitic, e.g. malaria, human African trypanosomiasis; mycotic, e.g. cryptococcosis
- *Cardiopulmonary*: hypoxia, myocardial infarction, congestive cardiac failure
- *Systemic*: systemic lupus erythematosus, vasculitis, anaemia
- *Exogenous Substances*:
  - Alcohol or drug misuse
  - Prescribed medications: e.g. beta-blockers, methyldopa, reserpine, oral contraceptive pill, steroids, histamine-2 blockers, opiate analgesia, benzodiazepines, barbiturates, antimalarial drugs (especially mefloquine), antiretroviral therapies (e.g. efavirenz)
  - Poisoning: e.g. heavy metals (lead, mercury, organophosphates, manganese, arsenic).

Adapted from Williams E, Shepherd S. Medical clearance of psychiatric patients. Emerg Med Clin North Am. May 2000; 18:2;193

distress. The principles of management of mental disorders follow from the biopsychosocial assessment. In this section, we outline some common principles of interventions for priority mental disorders, divided into biological and psychosocial interventions. A summary of the WHO evidence-based guidelines is presented in Table 72.2.

BIOLOGICAL INTERVENTIONS

Physical Health and Nutritional Status

Attending to the person's physical as well as mental health needs is a necessary component of intervention. Self-neglect may have led to undernutrition and poorer general health status, which in turn may be contributing to worse mental health status. Prior to commencing psychotropic medications, a physical examination, measurement of blood pressure and pulse, and some basic laboratory investigations are usually required. For details, see Taylor and colleagues,[36] but in summary: for antipsychotic medication, baseline full blood count, renal and hepatic function tests, prolactin level, plasma lipids, fasting blood glucose and, ideally, an ECG (mandatory for haloperidol) are recommended; with lithium, renal function and thyroid function tests are essential baseline investigations; and other mood-stabilizers require baseline hepatic function and full blood count.

TABLE 72.2 Summary of Evidence-Based Treatment Approaches for Priority Mental Disorders Treated in General Healthcare Settings

COMMON APPROACH FOR ALL PRIORITY DISORDERS	
BIO	Monitoring of physical health and medication side-effects
PSYSOC	Psychoeducation
	Risk management
	Family/carer support
	Regular follow-up
DEPRESSION AND ANXIETY	
BIO	Antidepressants
	Tricyclic (e.g. amitriptyline)
	Selective serotonin reuptake inhibitor (e.g. fluoxetine)
	Short-term anxiolytic medication
	Diazepam
PSYSOC	Addressing current psychosocial stressors
	Reactivate social networks
	Structured physical activity
	If available, can also consider: behavioural activation, cognitive behavioural therapy, interpersonal therapy, problem-solving therapy, relaxation training
PSYCHOSIS	
BIO	Antipsychotics
	High-potency first-generation antipsychotics (FGAs) (e.g. haloperidol, trifluoperazine)
	Low-potency FGAs (e.g. chlorpromazine)
	Second-generation antipsychotics (SGAs) (e.g. risperidone, olanzapine)
	Second-line only antipsychotic medication (clozapine)
	Depot medication (e.g. fluphenazine)
	Anticholinergic medication
	Biperiden, benzhexol
PSYSOC	Community-based rehabilitation

Continued on following page

TABLE 72.2 Summary of Evidence-Based Treatment Approaches for Priority Mental Disorders Treated in General Healthcare Settings—cont'd

BIPOLAR DISORDER	
BIO	Acute mania Antipsychotics (FGA or SGA) and/or mood-stabilizer (lithium, valproate or carbamazepine) Consider short-term benzodiazepine (diazepam) Depressive relapse Mood-stabilizer alone or in combination with antidepressant Prevention of relapse Mood-stabilizers (lithium, valproate or second-line carbamazepine)
PSYSOC	Reactivate social networks Rehabilitation
DEMENTIA	
BIO	Reduce cardiovascular risk factors, where relevant Treat associated physical conditions For behavioural and psychological symptoms associated with imminent risk and not responding to psychosocial approach, consider low-dose haloperidol/atypical antipsychotic If specialist supervision and support is available and specific diagnosis of Alzheimer's disease, anticholinesterases may be appropriate
PSYSOC	Sensitive communication of assessment findings Psychosocial interventions for cognitive symptoms and functioning Promote independence, functioning and mobility Manage behavioural and psychological symptoms
CHILD DEVELOPMENTAL DISORDERS	
BIO	Manage nutrition problems and medical conditions, e.g. epilepsy
PSYSOC	Advice to teachers Community-based rehabilitation Promoting and protecting human rights If available, consider parent skills training
CHILD BEHAVIOURAL PROBLEMS	
BIO	If specialist supervision and support is available and specific diagnosis of hyperkinetic disorder present, consider methylphenidate
PSYSOC	Advice to teachers If available, consider parent skills training, cognitive behavioural therapy, social skills training and problem-solving for family issues
ALCOHOL USE DISORDERS	
BIO	Alcohol intoxication Supportive treatment and observation Exclude methanol poisoning Alcohol withdrawal if dependent Diazepam Thiamine Hydration Haloperidol for psychotic symptoms Alcohol dependence Planned withdrawal as above Relapse prevention If specialist supervision and support is available, acamprosate, naltrexone or disulfiram may be considered
PSYSOC	Brief intervention Self-help groups Attend to social problems, e.g. housing and employment If available, consider family therapy, cognitive behavioural therapy, problem-solving therapy, motivational enhancement therapy, contingency management therapy
DRUG USE DISORDERS	
BIO	Sedative overdose Naloxone if opioid Stimulant overdose Diazepam Short-term antipsychotics Manage physical complications of intravenous drug use Opioid withdrawal Supportive treatment, e.g. antiemetic With specialist support, reducing dose of methadone, buprenorphine, clonidine or lofexidine
PSYSOC	Brief intervention Self-help groups Attend to social problems Harm-reduction strategies

From World Health Organization. Mental Health Gap Action Programme Intervention Guide (mhGAP-IG) for mental, neurological and substance use disorders in non-specialized health settings. Geneva: WHO; 2010.

Psychotropic Medications

Medication is recommended in the treatment of several priority conditions, although the effectiveness often depends on accompanying psychosocial support. Where the patient lacks insight into their condition, they may be ambivalent about taking medication. Psychoeducation (below), including honest information about side-effects, and a flexible, but supportive approach can help. Patients will often need encouragement to continue medication, even when they feel well. Response to medication needs to be reviewed. Health workers should not be tempted to prescribe placebo medication or ineffective treatments. Evidence-based treatments do exist.

PSYCHOSOCIAL

Psychoeducation

Explaining to patients and family/care givers about the nature of the mental disorder and the availability of interventions can help to instil hope and reduce the stigma associated with the condition. Providing information can empower families and patients to maximize self-help strategies to bring about symptom relief and rehabilitation.

Risk Management

If a risk to the patient, or to others, is identified, then appropriate steps need to be taken to minimize the risk of harm. Management strategies may include referral for in-patient psychiatric care, continuous monitoring by family members and appropriate treatment for the underlying condition.

Family/Care Giver Support

The psychological impact of caring for a person with a mental disorder puts care givers at increased risk of developing mental disorders, particularly CMDs or alcohol or drug use disorders. Provide support through listening, giving information and screening for mental disorders where indicated.

Regular Follow-Up

Scheduling regular appointments allows monitoring of the patient's mental state, response to medication and problems with side-effects. In addition, regular follow-up fulfils an important supportive function, helping to motivate and engage the patient and give encouragement to the care givers.

Common Mental Disorders

PATHOGENESIS

A modest contribution of genetic factors to the aetiology of depression is supported by twin and adoption studies.[37,38] The best evidence to date is of a gene–environment interaction between a polymorphism in the promoter region of the serotonin transporter gene and child maltreatment.[39] Other factors have also been implicated in the aetiology of CMDs, including: poverty; stressful experiences (e.g. death of a loved one, unemployment, marriage/divorce); female gender; increasing age; physical ill-health, especially if associated with chronic pain and disability; and alcohol or drug use.[35] Disability associated with poor physical health appears to explain most of the prevalence of depression in later life.[5]

CLINICAL FEATURES AND DIAGNOSIS

Medically unexplained somatic symptoms are the commonest way that people express mental distress worldwide and are often culture-specific. For example, in many sub-Saharan African settings, somatic complaints may take the form of burning or crawling sensations on the head or body. Somatic symptoms are a manifestation of underlying depression or anxiety in about two-thirds of cases.[40] However, on direct enquiry, the classic features of depression and anxiety (see below) are usually straightforward to elicit. Somatic symptoms may also communicate subconsciously understood distress, e.g. the woman who presents with medically unexplained genital pain following sexual assault.

The cardinal features of depression in Western settings are sad mood and loss of interest or enjoyment of life's usual pleasures. In the young and the old, irritability may predominate over sadness. Other features are also present, including: somatic symptoms (loss of appetite, weight loss, sleep disturbance, loss of libido) and cognitive symptoms (hopelessness, worthlessness, poor self-esteem, suicidal ideation, unjustified guilt, impaired concentration and memory). General aches and pains, headache and constipation are also frequently seen. In situations of precarious survival, moderate levels of poor energy and motivation may be overcome due to necessity and not manifest as impaired functioning. Where communal religious beliefs prevail, there are often strong societal sanctions against admitting feelings of worthlessness or suicidal ideation. Sensitivity is required. In such settings, irritability, somatic symptoms and feelings that one is being punished for perceived wrong-doing can be pointers to an underlying depression.

Anxiety is characterized by persistent worry or fear, out of proportion to the level of threat or difficulties faced, and associated with impairment. In anxiety, physiological effects of noradrenaline and adrenaline lead to somatic symptoms such as palpitations, shortness of breath, light-headedness, tremor and chest tightness. Other physical consequences of anxiety include muscle aches and headache secondary to tension, diarrhoea, nausea and stomach discomfort.

Isolated CMD symptoms are experienced by most people within the general population. To be considered an illness, symptoms should be present most of the time, enduring (present for more than 2 weeks) and should not occur in the immediate aftermath of bereavement or be directly attributable to a general medical condition or medication side-effect (see Box 72.1). Furthermore, impairment should be present, in terms of relationships, work and/or daily functioning. Life difficulties may make CMDs understandable, but not all people with psychosocial problems develop CMDs – the key is to look for symptoms that the person or their associates consider to be excessive or out of keeping with their usual reactions.

MANAGEMENT AND TREATMENT

Somatic Symptoms

Where the presentation is predominantly somatic, it is important to carry out a proper medical investigation. If screens for comorbid anxiety, depression, alcohol or drug use are negative, the main principles of management for somatic symptoms are as follows: (1) gain the patient's trust; (2) facilitate a shift in the patient's understanding of the causes of their symptoms from medical to psychosocial; (3) minimize disability and restore functioning; and (4) minimize the adverse effects of multiple visits to healthcare providers in terms of cost and receiving ineffective/potentially harmful investigations and treatments.

Gaining the patient's trust requires listening sympathetically to all of their symptoms and investigating them appropriately, but not excessively. Shifting the patient's model of illness is a greater challenge. Avoid confrontation and statements such as, 'it is all in your head', or 'there is nothing really wrong with you'. Ask about psychosocial stressors and discuss with the patient how these may link to their symptoms. Give examples of how the close links between mind and body could give rise to symptoms: 'when you worry a lot, your muscles become tense and that can lead to headache'. In longstanding cases, a pragmatic approach may be required, admitting that there is no medical intervention for the person's symptoms, but that the person will feel better if they can distract themselves by doing some activities. Regular follow-up appointments and a trusting health worker–patient relationship help to reduce 'doctor-shopping' and the associated harms. Low-dose tricyclic antidepressant (e.g. amitriptyline 25 mg at night) can help with chronic pain.

Depression and Anxiety

Where depression and/or anxiety disorders are present, evidence-based treatment protocols (Table 72.2) should be followed. If an antidepressant is prescribed, psychoeducation involves explaining that the medication takes 3–6 weeks before having a noticeable effect. Side-effects are usually transient and tolerable.

Address psychosocial stressors by asking the patient about difficulties in their life and listening with compassion. People with CMD may feel overwhelmed by even relatively small difficulties. Reactivating social networks, by asking the person about the people who have supported them in the past and encouraging them to resume contact, can be one way to bolster coping with psychosocial stressors. Behavioural activation may be helpful, e.g. encouraging the person to structure their day, spend some time outside the house and try to do things that previously held meaning for them.

PREVENTION

There is preliminary evidence that targeted and universal depression primary prevention programmes are effective in reducing the incidence of depression in children and adolescents.[41] A population-based approach to primary prevention of CMDs across the age span, e.g. by reducing social risk factors such as poverty, has been advocated, but little explored, to-date.[42] Psychological but not antidepressant therapy may prevent depression post-stroke.[43]

Psychotic Disorders

In its simplest form, psychosis is a symptom rather than a disorder, but even in isolation, psychosis symptoms indicate a potentially severe problem. Psychosis may occur de novo (primary psychotic disorder) or as a secondary manifestation of other disorders (e.g. secondary to mood disorders, general medical conditions or alcohol or drug use). Schizophrenia is the prototypical example of primary psychosis. In this section, schizophrenia will be discussed in detail with reference to other psychotic disorders where relevant.

EPIDEMIOLOGY

Almost all psychotic disorders affect both men and women equally. These disorders start early in life, most between 15 and 45 years of age, and tend to follow a chronic course, meaning that psychoses make a disproportionate contribution to population disease burden. Historically, the prognosis of schizophrenia was thought to be better in LAMICs[44] but recent studies have challenged this finding.[45–47]

PATHOGENESIS

Imaging studies of untreated persons with schizophrenia have identified characteristic structural brain changes. The 'neurodevelopmental' model of schizophrenia, whereby developmental genes and early neurological insults (e.g. secondary to obstetric complications) are hypothesized to interact and bring about psychosis, has been expanded to incorporate the role of later environmental insults (e.g. chronic social adversity and drug use).[48] This multifactorial model of schizophrenia is hypothesized to bring about dopamine dysfunction within the brain as a final common pathway.[49] Other neurotransmitter abnormalities, e.g. serotonin and glutamate, have also been implicated.[50]

CLINICAL FEATURES

There are three main symptom dimensions of schizophrenia: positive, negative and general symptoms.[51] Positive and general symptoms occur predominantly during an acute episode of schizophrenia. Positive symptoms include delusions, hallucinations, psychomotor disturbance, such as agitated behaviour and formal thought disorder. Delusions are defined as fixed, false beliefs that are not shared by people of the same educational and cultural background. Delusional beliefs are most commonly persecutory but referential delusions and grandiose delusions are also common. Hallucinations, referring to perceptions without external stimuli in any of the sensory modalities, are most often auditory. Impairment in reality testing is probably the key psychopathological feature of psychosis, in which the affected person has lost a fundamental ability to distinguish between reality and fantasy.

The negative symptoms of schizophrenia relate to loss of functions necessary for relating with the external world. The person tends to be withdrawn and in their own world, with reduced affective expression or blunted affect, and markedly reduced verbal output, which is considered to be an expression of a reduced ability to think (alogia).

ICD-10 requires the occurrence of characteristic symptoms for at least 1 month for a diagnosis of schizophrenia.[52] The main differential diagnoses of schizophrenia are other psychotic disorders: schizoaffective disorder, delusional disorder and acute and transient psychotic disorders. In schizoaffective disorder, psychotic episodes are associated with clear mood episodes that may be depressive or manic in nature. In delusional disorder, there are systematized delusions in the absence of persistent hallucinations or other psychotic symptoms. In acute and transient psychotic disorders, 'delusions, hallucinations, incomprehensible or incoherent speech, or any combination of these' develop over a maximum of 2 weeks.[52]

TREATMENT AND MANAGEMENT

The WHO's evidence-based guidelines (Table 72.2) mean that treatment for psychosis can begin in primary or general health-care settings, with appropriate review by specialist mental health workers if the person does not respond to first-line interventions. Whenever possible, persons with psychosis should be managed in the community.

The WHO guidelines assume that only first-generation antipsychotics will be available in most LAMICs. The typical effective dose of haloperidol is 3–20 mg, although doses above 10 mg rarely bring extra benefit but carry a high risk of serious extrapyramidal side effects (EPSE), including Parkinsonian symptoms, dystonia, dyskinesia and akathisia. Second-generation antipsychotic medications have an equal efficacy to the older medications and may be better tolerated, although they can also have troublesome side effects.

PREVENTION

There are no established primary prevention strategies. There is an accepted link between duration of untreated psychosis (DUP) and poor outcome. Therefore, secondary prevention strategies to reduce DUP are important. Community rehabilitation and recovery strategies, as well as prevention of relapse through maintenance treatment, are also important strategies to reduce the impact of the disorder on functioning.

Bipolar Disorder

Bipolar disorder (BD) is a recurrent condition characterized by episodes of severe fluctuation in mood.

EPIDEMIOLOGY

The mean age of onset of BD is 21 years and the disorder affects both men and women equally. In primary care settings, up to 10% of patients may have a bipolar spectrum condition.[53] Comorbidity with substance abuse and anxiety disorders is in the order of 50–60%.[15]

PATHOGENESIS

Genetic factors are important in BD: the risk of BD in monozygotic twins is 40–70%, while in dizygotic twins and all other 1st degree relatives it is 5–10%.[38] However, the mode of inheritance is complex, mediated by multiple genes of small effect. Neuroimaging studies show an increase in size and reduction in glucose utilization in the amygdala and basal ganglia.[54] Grey matter volume appears to be reduced in the subgenual prefrontal cortex. Neuropsychological tests have shown impairment in memory and concentration during illness episodes that also persist after recovery.

CLINICAL FEATURES

The central feature of mania is severely elated or irritable mood lasting for at least a week. Associated behavioural and cognitive symptoms include increased energy and hyperactivity, ranging from semi-purposeful activity to disruptive and restless behaviour. Disinhibition, with increased sexual energy, excessive socializing and over-talkativeness, indiscrete and inappropriate behaviour, overspending and reckless decision-making are additional behavioural symptoms. Optimism and self-confidence generally gives way to grandiosity and grandiose delusions. The depressive phase of the illness shares similar symptoms to that of a depressive disorder. Reversal of biological symptoms (increased appetite and weight, hypersomnia and mood reactivity) and excessive tiredness, so-called leaden paralysis, are said to be more characteristic of a bipolar depression.

TREATMENT AND MANAGEMENT

The treatment of BD may be viewed in three phases: acute, continuation and maintenance. See Table 72.2 for evidence-based guidelines. Treatment invariably requires medication but psychosocial interventions will also be required. Medication options for an acute episode of mania include mood stabilizers or antipsychotic medications. All these drugs require careful monitoring, but lithium requires the most intensive monitoring because of its narrow therapeutic margin and potential renal toxicity and neurotoxicity. Continuation treatment is the treatment phase that follows the achievement of remission and lasts about 6 months. Almost 90% of persons with a first episode of mania will experience relapse. Therefore, maintenance treatment is required. Often longer-term management of BD requires specialist input or the input of a practitioner with a special interest in mental health. In particular, management of the depressive phase of the illness can be complicated. It is important that the affected person and care givers are educated about the illness. The person needs to be advised to modify their lifestyle and maintain routine, e.g. in terms of dietary and sleep habits.

PREVENTION

Prevention should be considered in terms of prevention of relapse and recurrence as described above. This should extend to addressing issues of substance abuse, careful physical health monitoring and monitoring for risk of suicide, which can affect up to 15% of patients.

Dementia

EPIDEMIOLOGY

After the age of 65 years, the prevalence of dementia doubles every 5 years.[55] Diagnosis of dementia remains a challenge in non-Western settings with low levels of educational attainment, leading to probable underestimation of prevalence.[56] Almost 60% of persons with dementia are found in LAMICs, projected to increase to 71% by 2040.[14] Dementia is highly burdensome, for the affected person as well as for care givers.[57] Early diagnosis and evidence-based interventions can help to alleviate this burden, even in LAMICs.[57]

Alzheimer's disease (AD) accounts for the majority of confirmed diagnoses of dementia at postmortem (over 50%), followed by vascular dementia (25%), dementia with Lewy bodies (15%) and other dementias including frontotemporal dementias (5%).[58]

PATHOGENESIS

Most is known about the pathogenesis of AD.[55,59] Around 70% of the risk of AD is attributable to genetic factors, with dominant transmission of genetic mutations explaining about 5% of cases (mostly early-onset AD), and multiple, interacting genes of small effect increasing the risk of late-onset AD.[59] Of the latter, polymorphisms of the gene encoding apolipoprotein E are associated with the biggest increased risk.[59] The core pathological findings in AD are amyloid plaques and neurofibrillary tangles, which are associated with neurotoxicity and neuronal death. There is substantial overlap in the pathological changes seen in AD and vascular dementia.[55,59]

In HIV-associated dementia (HAD), neurotoxicity due to direct effects of HIV infection, coupled with indirect effects due to neurotoxins from infected or immune-activated microglia or macrophages are implicated in the pathogenesis.[60] Even following the introduction of highly active antiretroviral therapy, HAD remains an important feature of AIDS.[60,61]

CLINICAL FEATURES

Dementia is characterized by global, chronic and progressive cognitive decline (affecting memory, orientation, speech and language), which is associated with impaired functioning; e.g. in the activities of daily living such as washing, dressing, eating and personal hygiene. The presenting complaint for dementia, particularly AD, is often forgetfulness, but can also be depressed mood or deteriorating social behaviour, emotional control and motivation or symptoms of psychosis.[9,58] The affected person may not appreciate the symptoms of the disease and so a detailed history from a reliable informant is also necessary.

Other forms of dementia have some distinguishing features, although there is much overlap in the clinical picture. In vascular dementia, the classical presentation is with executive dysfunction rather than forgetfulness, and the disease follows a stepwise progression, which may even be associated with periods of improvement or stabilization of symptoms.[58] In Lewy body dementia, motor symptoms and visual hallucinations may be prominent, associated with sensitivity to antipsychotic medication.[58] In frontotemporal dementias, personality and behavioural changes are often the first manifestations of disorder, with onset usually before 60 years of age. In HIV-associated dementia, a sub-cortical picture of deficits is often seen, characterized by mental and motor slowing, poor attention and memory, apathy, reduced emotional responsivity and social withdrawal.[61]

TREATMENT AND MANAGEMENT

The first priority is to exclude delirium and screen for potentially reversible causes of cognitive decline, including severe depression (see Box 72.1). Clinical features favouring delirium rather than dementia include an abrupt and recent onset, worsening at night-time and disorientation to time and place. Three simple cognitive screening tests for dementia are: testing memory by asking the person to repeat three common words immediately and after 5 minutes (memory), assessing orientation to time and place, and asking the person to point to parts of the body and explain their function (language skills).[9] Principles of intervention are outlined in Table 72.2.[9] Supporting care givers also brings benefits to the patient, including delaying institutionalization.[62] Although rare, challenging behaviours in the affected person may provoke abusive practices from others.

PREVENTION

A recent expert consensus panel using data from systematic reviews of the best available evidence concluded that there were insufficient data to guide preventive interventions for dementia at the current time.[63] However, tackling probable lifestyle risk factors for dementia, e.g. by increasing physical activity, improving diet and stopping smoking, would in any case bring other health benefits.[59] Increasing cognitive reserve through cognitive activities is a promising disorder-specific intervention to reduce the risk of dementia.[59]

Alcohol and Drug ('Substance') Use Disorders

EPIDEMIOLOGY

Alcohol consumption alone is associated with an estimated 3.8% of all global deaths and 4.6% of global disability-adjusted life-years (DALYs).[64] Worldwide, around 15.3 million persons are estimated to suffer from drug use disorders.[65] Many more use illicit substances: in 2008, an estimated 155–250 million persons worldwide used drugs, mostly cannabis, followed by amphetamine-type stimulants, cocaine and opioids.[65] As well as adverse health effects, the social costs of illicit drugs are high, estimated to be around 2% of GDP in countries, where this has been measured.[66] Patterns of alcohol and drug use vary across countries and over time, but new fashions can quickly spread due to global interconnectedness. Drug use is expanding particularly fast in LAMICs, e.g. heroin use in East Africa.[65]

CLINICAL FEATURES

Alcohol and drug use disorders include the syndromes of dependence and harmful use[10] or abuse.[11] Dependence is less common but more severe and is characterized by a strong desire or compulsion to take the substance, difficulty controlling the substance misuse, physiological or psychological withdrawal, escalating intake due to tolerance to the effects, continuing to use the substance despite obvious harm, dominance of the substance use over all aspects of life, and fast reinstatement of the substance use to previous levels following a period of abstinence.[52] Harmful use occurs when a person's substance use is associated with clear physical, interpersonal, social or legal harm.

In general healthcare settings, alcohol and substance use disorders commonly present with trauma, secondary to accidents or violence, or physical consequences of the substance use (e.g. acute pancreatitis in binge-drinkers, hepatic impairment in persons with alcohol dependence, blood-borne disorders such as HIV and abscesses in injecting drug users). Healthcare workers therefore have an opportunity to identify a group of persons who are at high risk of complications from substance use.

TREATMENT AND MANAGEMENT

Emergency interventions may be required for acute intoxication or withdrawal (Table 72.2). In the majority of cases, safe withdrawal from alcohol and/or benzodiazepines requires active medical management in order to minimize the risk of seizures, delirium and death. Although not life-threatening, opiate withdrawal is unpleasant and symptomatic treatment of symptoms is helpful. For all substances, the process of withdrawal is the easy part; the true challenge lies in remaining abstinent. To achieve this goal, psychosocial support and rehabilitation are the mainstays of intervention. Self-help groups, e.g. alcoholics anonymous or narcotics anonymous, where available, can also be highly beneficial for some individuals.

PREVENTION

For legally available substances such as alcohol, successful primary prevention strategies involve reducing access, e.g. through price regulation or reducing opening hours of retail outlets selling alcohol.[67] Alcohol-related harm is directly related to the per-capita consumption in a country.[64] Secondary prevention measures include legislation to stop drink-driving and individual-based brief psychological interventions for persons identified to be 'at-risk'. In persons with harmful use of alcohol, this simple intervention has been shown to reduce alcohol intake.[68] Providing injecting drug users with sterile needles and swapping injectors onto long-term use of oral opiate substitutes, e.g. methadone, can reduce injecting behaviour and the harms associated with injecting, particularly transmission of blood-borne diseases.[69]

Child Mental Health Problems

The WHO's mhGAP-IG provides specific guidelines for the detection and management of: (a) developmental disorders and (b) behavioural disorders in children.[9] CMDs and substance use disorders are also problems for children and adolescents, but covered in the general sections with specific advice for when these conditions occur in young people.

EPIDEMIOLOGY

Mental health and developmental problems are a leading cause of disability in the child and adolescent age group.[70] Timing of risk factor exposure can be usefully divided into preconceptional, perinatal, infancy or early childhood, school age and adolescence, superimposed upon lifelong risk factors such as genetic predisposition, physical health problems, mental health problems within care givers, problems in the care-giving environment, exposure to harmful substances or toxins, and exposure to violence, abuse or neglect.[71]

CLINICAL FEATURES AND DIAGNOSIS

Developmental disorders encompass the categories of intellectual disability (formerly known as mental retardation) and pervasive developmental disorders, including autism. Intellectual disability (ID) is characterized by delays in broad domains of development, including cognitive, social, language and motor development, which are associated with impaired functioning in activities of daily living. Care needs to be taken when applying intelligence quotient tests from other cultures in order to make a diagnosis of ID; comparison to other children and evaluation of adaptive functioning are usually better indicators of developmental delay. Pervasive developmental disorders (PDD) are indicated by more specific deficits in social behaviour, communication and language, together with a narrowed range of activities or interests that are often carried out repetitively. ID is also present in about two-thirds. Investigations need to exclude visual or auditory impairment, impoverished psychosocial stimulation within the home and maternal depression, all of which can lead to apparent developmental delay in the child. Epilepsy and co-morbid priority mental disorders, especially depression and psychosis, are more common in children with developmental disorders and can lead to episodic behavioural disturbance or deterioration in functioning. The presentation of these comorbid conditions will often be atypical, requiring a high index of suspicion in clinicians and greater reliance upon observable symptoms, e.g. appetite and weight loss in depression.

Behavioural disorders in children include attention deficit hyperactivity disorder (ADHD) and conduct disorder. The main features of ADHD are: (a) difficulty maintaining attention, e.g. getting distracted in the middle of activities and leaving things undone, and (b) an increased level of activity, shown as excessive restlessness, fidgeting, noisiness and talkativeness. For ADHD to be present, these symptoms must have started before the age of 6 years, have persisted for more than 6 months and be causing difficulties in more than one setting, e.g. at school and in the home. Conduct disorder manifests as severe temper tantrums, persistent disobedience and antisocial acts that go far beyond normal naughtiness or rebellious behaviour, e.g. bullying others, stealing, setting fires, cruelty to animals; destruction of property; lying; and running away from home. To be considered a disorder, these behavioural problems should have been present for at least 6 months and lead to difficulties in several domains of life.

TREATMENT AND MANAGEMENT

See the WHO's mhGAP guidance for treatment of developmental and behavioural conditions,[9] summarized in Table 72.2. Simple tips for general health workers to provide support and psychoeducation to care givers of children with developmental disorders are provided in freely downloadable training materials being piloted in Ethiopia, see: http://labspace.open.ac.uk/mod/oucontent/view.php?id=451962&direct=1.

Brief psychosocial interventions can be highly effective in improving behavioural disorders in children, but care givers and teachers will need clear guidance and support to enable them to implement changes. Consistently rewarding good behaviour yields better results than punishing bad behaviour. Withdrawal of treats or attention, e.g. using a strategy of 'time-out', can also be effective.

PREVENTION

A public health approach to the primary prevention of ID is required, including: improving nutrition; reducing infections (including rubella, HIV and toxoplasmosis) and alcohol consumption in pregnant women; improving obstetric care; and reducing the risk of central nervous system infections (including malaria, epidemic meningitis, HIV, and measles); head injury; malnutrition (stunting, iodine- and iron-deficiency); and exposure to environmental pollutants (e.g. arsenic and lead) in infants and young children.[72] Maternal depression, particularly in the postnatal period, is an important and remediable risk factor for onset and maintenance of poorer development and both emotional and behavioural disorders in children.[73]

Post-humanitarian Crises

Increasingly, mental health interventions are being included in the standard responses to humanitarian crises.[74] Although this is largely a welcome development and provides opportunities for improving mental health care in previously underserved communities (e.g. see: http://internationalmedicalcorps.org/page.aspx?pid=313), there is also the potential for inappropriate targeting of scarce resources to culturally insensitive, ineffective or even harmful interventions.[74] To avoid such outcomes, sound guidance has been issued by an inter-agency taskforce of experts in the field.[75] There are two main mental health issues post-humanitarian crisis: (1) (re-)establishing protection and treatment for those with known SMD and (2) responding to any trauma-related mental health problems. In both cases, it is critical not to neglect the basic needs of food, shelter and safety. Much mental distress will be alleviated by attending to these necessities. For mental distress arising due to the crisis, the need for cultural sensitivity is paramount. Giving time and allowing society to heal its wounds collectively may be most helpful in the longer term. Indeed, immediate 'debriefing' of traumatized persons has been found to increase, not decrease, subsequent development of mental disorders.[76] However, severe or persistent reactions may need immediate intervention, following the WHO's mhGAP[9] or IASC guidelines.[75]

REFERENCES

5. Prince M, Patel V, Saxena S, et al. Global mental health 1: no health without mental health. Lancet 2007;370:859–77.
9. WHO. Mental Health Gap Action Programme Implementation Guide (mhGAP-IG) for mental, neurological and substance use disorders in non-specialized health settings. Geneva: World Health Organization; 2010.
12. WHO. The world health report 2001. Mental health: new understanding, new hope. Geneva: WHO; 2001.
71. Kieling C, Baker-Henningham H, Belfer M, et al. Child and adolescent mental health worldwide: evidence for action. Lancet 2011;378(9801):1515–25.
75. Inter-Agency Standing Committee (IASC). IASC Guidelines on Mental Health and Psychosocial Support in Emergency Settings. Geneva: IASC; 2007.

Access the complete references online at www.expertconsult.com

73 Tropical Oral Health

RAMAN BEDI | CRISPIAN SCULLY

KEY POINTS

- Oral health poses a major health burden for many countries, and some forms of oral disease are specific to tropical countries.
- Oral diseases are the most common non-communicable diseases and share risk factors with many other non-communicable diseases.
- Some 90% of the world's population is affected by tooth decay.
- A high proportion suffer from periodontal disease.
- Oral cancer rates are high among smokers and tobacco users.

Introduction

The importance of oral health as part of general health is now well established and this is true not only in industrialized countries but also tropical and subtropical climates. Global Oral Health as a specific discipline is beginning to take shape, with support from the World Health Organization (WHO) and World Dental Federation. The focus for the early part of the twenty-first century, for international oral health, will be dental caries, and the commitment to eradicate dental cavitation (or at least confine to <10%) in the child cohort born in 2026.[1]

It is also important to recognize that tropical dentistry is not just dentistry (oral health) in the tropics, but with migration and global travel, oral diseases traditionally restricted in some developing countries have manifested themselves within all areas of the global community. This chapter will cover oral conditions common in all parts of the world, as well as tropical region-specific conditions and risk factors.

Dental Caries

Together with the common cold, dental caries is perhaps the most prevalent disease of modern man, but unlike the cold, its effects leave behind defects that are permanent.[1] The general consensus of international epidemiological studies is that non-milk extrinsic sugars are the most important dietary factor in the aetiology of dental caries. The role of nutrition during tooth development is considered to be minimal in industrialized countries.[2,3] However, in tropical and subtropical areas where malnutrition is evident, delayed tooth eruption is observed, especially in the primary dentition,[4] but there is inconclusive evidence that malnutrition during tooth development can influence subsequent levels of dental caries.[5]

In the last few decades, there has been enormous progress in development, with decreased infant mortality and increased life expectancy, literacy and sanitation in developing countries. Such development is all too often coupled with increasing access to sugars, commonly in the form of confectionery or carbonated drinks. The WHO's global databank on oral health established in 1969, and continuing to monitor dental caries levels across different countries, demonstrates two clear trends: first the ongoing decline in dental caries for the industrialized world and, second, the increasing prevalence of caries in the developing world.[6]

The treatment of dental caries has not essentially changed over the past few decades, although tooth cavity design and filling materials have changed the practical approach to dental restorative treatment. The Atraumatic Restorative Technique (ART) has produced promising results in developing countries, especially those with a shortage of suitably qualified manpower.[7]

There have been a number of studies that have demonstrated significant caries reduction as a result of fluoride toothpaste. The major barrier to the implementation of fluoride toothpaste to the developing world has been cost; however, the new WHO programmes to introduce locally produced affordable fluoridated toothpaste to many developing countries are producing encouraging results.[8]

The evidence base for addressing dental caries in children has been documented and the predictive models and policy options to managing this clarified.[1] It is clear that each health economy needs to document its fluoride policy and preferably adopt either a water fluoridation or improving the child oral health.[1] Cultural habits such as the use of smokeless tobacco are known to have an effect on dental caries.[9] A significantly higher number of cariogenic bacteria are found at the site of smokeless tobacco placement, attributed to the sugar content in these products which enhance the growth of bacteria such as *Streptococcus mutans*.[10] Although there is some evidence of an association between smokeless tobacco and dental caries, a cause and effect relationship cannot be conclusively established.

Periodontal Disease

There is no evidence that inflammatory periodontal disease in developed and developing countries is in principle different in character.[11] There are indeed more similarities in periodontal conditions globally than differences. Evidence shows however, that periodontal diseases are more prevalent in developing countries in terms of poorer oral hygiene and greater calculus retention but not in terms of periodontal destruction in adults.[11]

The WHO has published guidelines on prevention.[12] Limited resources, in many developing countries, often inhibit the purchase of toothbrushes, and traditional cleaning materials such as the miswak chewing stick which is still widely used and has been shown to be an effective tooth-cleaning agent, comparable in effectiveness with some agents used in Western societies.[13] In addition, tobacco products (powder and paste), charcoal and ash have been used as cleaning agents in parts of southern Asia and Africa. They are used by applying tobacco to the teeth and gums, usually with the index finger. Other specific tobacco products used as dentifrices are Gul, Mishri, Bajjar, Gudakhu and tobacco water (used as a mouthwash).[14]

Oral Cancer

Most oral cancer is squamous cell carcinoma (SCC), and it is customary to include cancers of the lip (ICD 140), tongue (ICD 141), gum (ICD 143), floor of the mouth (ICD 144) and unspecified parts of the mouth (ICD 145).[15] There is clear inter-country variation in both the incidence and mortality from oral cancer and also ethnic differences, which are attributed mainly to specific risk factors such as alcohol and tobacco (smoking and smokeless), betel use, and, in the case of lip cancer also sunlight exposure, but dietary factors as well as the existence of genetic predisposition may play a part. Variations in availability and access to care services are also evident.[16]

The incidence of oral cancer varies widely between countries and geographical areas of the world and is generally most common in developing countries, particularly in Asia, though Eastern Europe and France have some of the highest recorded rates globally. Mouth cancer worldwide is the 12th most common cancer but it is the 8th most common in males.[17] Annually, there are 197 000 deaths worldwide from cancer of the mouth and pharynx, with the highest mortality from mouth cancer in Melanesia and South-Central Asia. The gender ratio is 2:0 (M:F). Mouth cancer in men is most common in Eastern Europe, South Asia, Melanesia, southern Africa and Australia/NZ. In females, it is most common in South-Central Asia, Melanesia and Australia/NZ. Lip cancer is particularly common in white Caucasians in the tropics and subtropics.[17]

The aetiology of oral cancer has been attributed to specific risk factors: tobacco[18] and/or alcohol in southern Africa, and betel quid in people of South-Central Asian and Melanesian cultures.[19] Smokeless (chewing) tobacco use is an important factor for South Asian populations. The areca (betel) nut habit is important in the development of oral submucous fibrosis and of mouth cancer. Some chew the nut only and others prefer 'paan', which includes tobacco, and sometimes lime and catechu. Studies from India have confirmed the association between 'paan' tobacco chewing and oral cancer, particularly cancer of the buccal and labial mucosa. There is growing evidence associating increased alcohol consumption with risk of oral cancer. The role of alcohol drinking is observed in a negative social class gradient and for many countries, follows a similar pattern to tobacco use. Finally, there is an increasing predisposition of younger (<45 years) people to oral and pharyngeal cancer in many countries, and in this respect, human papillomaviruses (HPV) are increasingly linked.[20]

The molecular changes found in oral carcinomas from Western countries (UK, USA, Australia), particularly p53 mutations, are infrequent in the East (India, South-east Asia), where the involvement of ras oncogenes, including mutation, loss of heterozygosity (H-ras) and amplification (K- and N-ras) are common, suggesting genetic differences. It is also evident that there can be genetic differences in the metabolism of

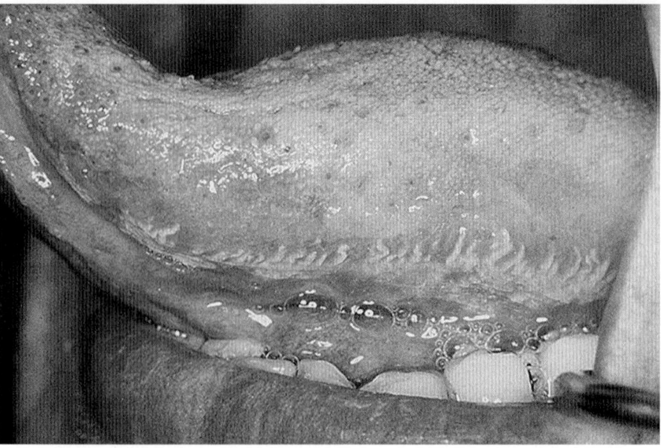

Figure 73.1 Hairy leukoplakia associated with HIV.

pro-carcinogens and carcinogens by xenometabolizing enzymes or ability to repair the DNA damage in different ethnic groups.

Carcinomas present anywhere in the oral cavity, commonly on the posterolateral margin of the tongue and floor of the mouth – the 'coffin' or 'graveyard' area – and in the buccal mucosa in betel users. It is crucial, therefore, not only to examine visually and manually the whole oral cavity, but also to take particular care to inspect and palpate the posterolateral margins of the tongue and the floor of the mouth (Figure 73.1). There is usually solitary chronic:

- Ulceration
- Red lesion
- White lesion
- Indurated lump
- Fissure
- Cervical lymph node enlargement.

Anterior cervical lymph node enlargement may be detectable by palpation. Of presenting patients, 30% present with palpably enlarged nodes containing metastases and, of those who do not, a further 25% will go on to develop nodal metastases within 2 years.

Lip carcinoma presents with thickening, crusting or ulceration, usually of the lower lip. Potentially malignant lesions or conditions may include actinic cheilitis, erythroplasias, dysplastic leukoplakias (about 50% of oral carcinomas have associated leukoplakia), lichen planus, oral submucous fibrosis and chronic immunosuppression.

Too many patients with oral SCC present or are detected late, with advanced disease and lymph node metastases. With early detection and treatment, the cosmetic and functional results and survival are better. There should be a high index of suspicion, especially of a solitary lesion present for over 3 weeks, particularly if it is indurated, there is cervical lymphadenopathy and the patient is in a high-risk group.

It is essential to confirm the diagnosis, and determine whether cervical lymph nodes are involved or there are other primary tumours, or metastases (Figure 73.2). Therefore, almost invariably indicated are:

- Lesional biopsy: an incisional biopsy is usually indicated but an oral brush biopsy is now available mainly for cases where there are widespread potentially malignant lesions, and for revealing malignancy in lesions of more benign appearance

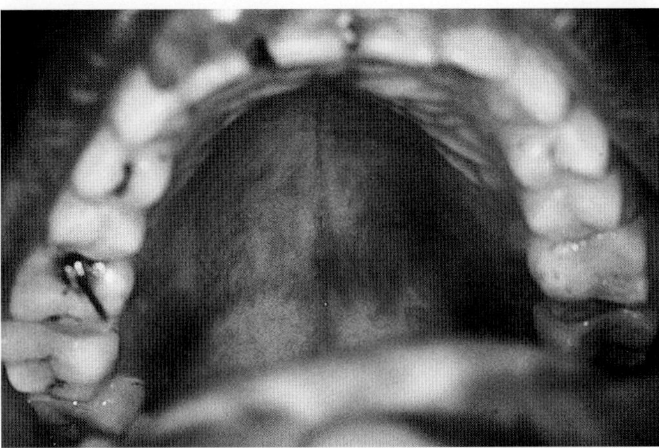

Figure 73.2 Kaposi's sarcoma associated with HIV.

- Jaw radiography
- Chest radiography and endoscopy of the upper aerodigestive tract to exclude second primary tumours
- Fine needle aspiration biopsy of palpable cervical lymph nodes; full blood count and liver function tests, in some indications.

Oral cancer is still treated largely by surgery and/or irradiation, though chemotherapy is an emerging modality, especially using inhibitors of epidermal growth factor receptor.[21] There have been few unequivocal controlled trials of the conventional treatment modalities. Multidisciplinary clinics, with surgeons, oncologists and support staff, usually have an agreed treatment policy and offer the best outcomes. However, mortality rates for oral cancer have substantially increased in many countries. Although the efficacy of screening for oral cancer to increase survival and reduce mortality remains unproven, it is believed that Cuba's ongoing oral cancer screening programme has resulted in a higher proportion of cancers being localized at diagnosis and a comparatively high survival rate.[22] The WHO has published guidelines on prevention,[23] and studies have shown reduction or reversal in pre-cancerous lesions by primary prevention or abstinence from tobacco. There is a considerable body of evidence indicating a protective effect on oral cancer and pre-cancer, of diets rich in fresh fruits and vegetables and of vitamin A in particular. The prognosis is very site-dependent. For intra-oral carcinoma, 5-year survival may be as low as 30% for posterior lesions presenting late, as they often do, while for lip carcinoma, there is often more than a 70% 5-year survival.

Erythroplasia (Erythroplakia)

Erythroplasia is a rare, isolated, red, velvety lesion which affects patients mainly in the 6th and 7th decades. Erythroplasia usually involves the floor of the mouth, the ventrum of the tongue or the soft palate. This is one of the most important oral lesions because 75–90% of lesions prove to be carcinoma or carcinoma in situ, or are severely dysplastic. The incidence of malignant change is 17 times higher in erythroplasia than in leukoplakia. Erythroplasia should be excised and sent for histological examination. Prevention is by avoidance of lifestyle habits of tobacco, betel and alcohol use.[24]

Leukoplakia

All oral white lesions were formerly called leukoplakia and believed often to be potentially malignant. The term leukoplakia is now restricted to white lesions of unknown cause. Most white lesions are innocuous keratoses caused by cheek biting, friction or tobacco, but can be:

- Infections (e.g. candidosis, syphilis, and hairy leukoplakia)
- Dermatoses (usually lichen planus)
- Neoplastic disorders (e.g. leukoplakias and carcinomas).

Other conditions must be excluded, usually by biopsy.

Keratoses are most commonly uniformly white plaques (homogeneous leukoplakia), prevalent in the buccal (cheek) mucosae, and usually of low malignant potential. More serious are nodular and, especially, speckled leukoplakias, which consist of white patches or nodules in a red, often eroded, area of mucosa. The presence of severe epithelial dysplasia indicates a considerable risk of malignant development. The overall prevalence of malignant change is 3–33% over 10 years, but a percentage (about 15%) regress clinically.

It can be difficult to be certain of the precise diagnosis of a white patch, as even carcinoma can present as a white lesion. Incisional biopsy is indicated, sampling indurated, red, erosive or ulcerated areas rather than the more obvious whiter hyperkeratinized areas; staining with toluidine blue may help highlight the most appropriate area.

Management can be difficult, especially in extensive lesions of leukoplakia, and those with areas of erythroplasia. Obvious predisposing factors need to be reduced or eliminated. Prevention is by avoidance of lifestyle habits of tobacco and alcohol use.[25] Dysplastic lesions should certainly be excised and the patient should then be followed-up regularly at intervals of 3–6 months. Unfortunately, more than one-third recur.

Oral Submucous Fibrosis

Oral submucous fibrosis (OSMF), though not regarded as a connective tissue disease, has pathological changes closely similar to those of scleroderma. Unlike the latter, which has severe effects on the skin but minimal effects on the oral mucosa, OSMF causes severe and often disabling fibrosis of the oral tissues alone.

OSMF affects virtually only those from the Indian subcontinent.[26] There is some evidence it is premalignant. The condition appears to be related to the chewing of areca nut and the 5A genotype of matrix metalloproteinase 3 (MMP3) promoter is associated with the risk of OSMF.[27] Iron-deficiency anaemia may be present but this is not uncommon in Asians in the absence of submucous fibrosis.[28]

Clinically, OSMF causes symmetrical fibrosis of such sites as the cheeks, soft palate or inner aspects of the lips. The fibrosis is often so severe that the affected area is almost white and so hard that it literally cannot be indented with the finger. Frequently the buccal fibrosis causes such severe restriction of opening that dental treatment becomes increasingly difficult and finally impossible. Ultimately, tube feeding may become necessary.

Intralesional corticosteroids and regular stretching of the oral soft tissues with an interdental screw or 'therabite' may delay fixation in the closed position. Medical therapies range from topical medication (e.g. with COX-2 inhibitors); to intralesionally injected medicaments such as corticosteroids, collagenase, or hyaluronidase; to systemic medication with lycopene or pentoxifylline. Surgical therapies range from laser release to excision of the bands and split skin, radial forearm or other flap repair.

Tobacco and Areca Nut Use

SMOKELESS TOBACCO

Tobacco (both smoking and smokeless) had been a part of the Native American culture even before Columbus discovered America, after which this habit has spread worldwide. In the Middle Ages, tobacco was used as medication in ointments, mouth rinses and poultices. Some communities continue to believe in its perceived medicinal value.

Smokeless tobacco use is on the increase among young individuals, particularly, after the smoking ban, and the general misconception that it is less harmful than smoking tobacco. There is an ever-increasing market of smokeless tobacco products, which have diverse and varied patterns of use,[29] e.g. insufflation (of snuff) or mastication and sucking (of gutka). Smokeless products are currently used in many parts of the world, including America and Sweden, however, the most harmful products are available from southern Asia, particularly, the Indian subcontinent. The habit is most prevalent in the south Asian communities and, despite substance control via point of sale legislation, is culturally acceptable among all ages, with the habit commencing from as young as 5 years.[30,31]

Data on the prevalence of this habit in the UK are limited. The Health Survey of England 2004 observed that smokeless tobacco was most widespread among the Bangladeshi community, with a prevalence of 9% in men and 16% in women, followed by Indians (mainly Punjabi and Gujarati; 1–4% in men and 1% in women) and Pakistanis (1–2% in men and 1% in women).[32]

This habit is associated with an increase in cardiovascular risk factors including hypertension, increased heart rate, brain damage from stroke and cancers of the pancreas, stomach, bladder and lungs, decrease in sperm quality, increased risk of stillbirth, decreased gestational age at birth and decreased birth weight independent of gestational age in pregnancy.[33] Different smokeless products have a range of health risks, depending on the ingredients used, varying widely from minor reddish-orange discolouration/staining of teeth to more serious effects including oral birth defects like cleft palate and cancer of the oral cavity. These products contain variable quantities of proven carcinogens such as tobacco-specific nitrosamines, benzo(a) pyrene and toxic metals. Although some users associate it with oral cancers, knowledge of precancerous lesions, such as leukoplakia and oral submucous fibrosis, are relatively low.[34] The risk of pre-cancerous lesions and mouth cancers are known to increase when used as a 'night quid', i.e. placed in the cheek pouch overnight, combination with other habits such as alcohol and cigarette smoking has a synergic effect, further increasing these risks.[35]

Typical lesions, i.e. 'the Indian Oral Cancer' refer to cancer in the buccal mucosal, gingival and retromolar trigonal region, caused by placement of smokeless products in this area. As the name suggests, these patterns are particularly prevalent in southern Asia. Poor oral health is another trait often seen among users, characterized by increased periodontal pocket depth, gingival inflammation and bleeding.[36] While insoluble particulate matter in smokeless products leads to attrition and abrasion of dental hard tissues, there is also some indication of association between smokeless tobacco and dental caries, although, a cause and effect relationship cannot be conclusively established.

Recent smoking bans have highlighted an increased incidence of smokeless use, as an alternative to smoking. Although, interventions proven to be effective for smoking cessation, such as nicotine replacement and bupropion SR are ineffective among smokeless users, behavioural interventions have had a positive impact.[37,38]

ARECA NUT

Areca nut, the fourth most common addiction globally following tobacco, alcohol and caffeine, is estimated to be used by 600 million people, particularly among South, East and South-east Asian communities. It is considered to be a 'fruit of divine origin' in Hindu religious ceremonies, as it is a vital ingredient of idol worship. In southern Asia, it is perceived to have medicinal values, including as an aphrodisiac, breath-freshener and with digestive properties. It is common practice to offer these products to guests in important social gatherings, weddings and other religious events.[39] This habit is widely accepted among all strata of society, including vulnerable populations such as women and children, making this habit a significant part of the cultural and ethnic identity.

Although there are regional variations, the habit is generally practiced by chewing or holding areca nut typically with slaked lime (calcium hydroxide), spices and other flavouring agents wrapped in a betel pepper leaf between the gum and cheek. The saliva produced can be either swallowed or spat out. While habitual users add tobacco to the quid in parts of the Indian subcontinent, this is not the norm in other countries such as Taiwan and Papua New Guinea.[40] In the last few decades, an estimated 20–40% of the Indian, Nepali and Pakistani populations were reported to be habitual users. While trends appear to be changing, with a decrease in the habit in Thailand, this habit is shockingly high in other countries, such as Palauans, where 70–80% of the population use areca nut. Areca nut is not only common throughout Asia but is becoming increasingly widespread in the Western society where these communities have settled. There has been a reported increase in the prevalence of areca nut among the minority immigrant population in the USA and UK.[41]

Areca nut with/without tobacco is carcinogenic to humans. It contains about 11–26% tannins and 0.15–0.67% alkaloids, known to be both cytotoxic and genotoxic. It is associated with the development of potentially malignant disorders with high potential for malignant transformation, including oral lichen planus, oral leukoplakia and oral submucous fibrosis. The risk of malignancy further increases with the addition of smokeless tobacco.[42]

Lime used in the quid has high concentrations of arsenic, a toxic metal also known to be carcinogenic.[43] Other additional ingredients used are known to cause lichenoid lesions, the premalignant potential of which is not fully understood. While areca nut consumption is associated with oral, pharyngeal and oesophagus cancers (due to p53 gene mutation), and to some extent liver cancers, it is also linked to metabolic syndrome, obesity, cardiovascular disease, diabetes, chronic kidney disease, liver cirrhosis and low-birth-weight infants.[44–48]

Areca nut users have poor oral hygiene, halitosis, poor periodontal health with an increase in gingival lesions, recession, periodontal pockets and bleeding of gums. Mild to severe attrition is another common finding among users, in severe cases it can be accompanied by periapical periodontitis and alveolar bone resorption. The severity of attrition is directly proportional to length and frequency of the habit. Although there appears to be little evidence on effective interventions, cessation advice along with behavioural support and counselling may be effective for abstinence from areca nut use.[49]

NASWAR

Naswar (Nass, niswar, kap) is a form of smokeless tobacco containing powdered tobacco, slaked lime, indigo, cardamom and menthol. It is practised primarily among Central Asian, Afghani, Pakistani, Iranian and also in some Swedish and South African communities. Typically, it is used by sniffing through the nose, but is also used orally by placing a pinch under the tongue or in the buccal vestibule.

Naswar is chiefly manufactured in Pakistan and is available as green, grey and black variants. Like most smokeless products, it contains unionized nicotine (13.2 mg/g), carcinogenic tobacco-specific N-nitrosamines (TSNAs), a relatively high pH of 9.0, potential to induce cell mutations due to the presence of cyclic aromatic compound as well as toxic metals including cadmium, arsenic and lead which contributes to the adverse effects on both oral and general health.[50] While it is used as herbal medicines, especially in children, naswar is associated with peptic ulcers, potentially malignant disorders such as oral submucous fibrosis and cancers of the mouth and oesophagus.[51] Although users associate this habit to poor oral health (toothache, dental caries as well as bleeding gums), many fail to link its use to more serious life-threatening conditions such as oral cancers.

There are limited data on effective interventions and hence, culturally acceptable education materials, to increase the awareness of the adverse health effects associated with this habit, as well as behavioural interventions, to support the long-term abstinence, should be used for cessation interventions among these communities.

HOOKAH

Hookah, a type of smoking tobacco, is increasing in prevalence among young individuals and is considered to be a global epidemic. Although the use of hookah is culturally associated with eastern Mediterranean and western Asia, it is increasingly becoming popular worldwide, including developed countries such as the UK and the USA. Depending on the region of the world, this habit is also known as shisha, waterpipe, nirghile, arghile, hubble-bubble and galyan. Each hookah smoking session last about 20–80 minutes and releases the same quantity of smoke as an individual smoking 100 cigarettes, exposing hookah users to an eightfold increase in carbon monoxide, increasing the adverse effects of this habit.

This habit is perceived to be a less harmful alternative to smoking; however, its use has both oral and general health implications. Users are at a significantly increased risk of lung cancer, heart disease, respiratory illness, periodontal disease and adverse effects during pregnancy such as low birth weight. Although there is some evidence of its association with hepatitis C and tuberculosis, particularly because it is a shared habit, this evidence is inconclusive. While there is a dearth in the current evidence-base for prevention and treatment of the long-term abstinence of this habit, evidence suggests that hookah users should be made aware of its addictive and harmful effects in order to influence behaviour change.[52]

Coca Chewing

Despite legal restriction, coca, a plant native to South America, is a significant part of the Andean culture and religious identity, as it is believed to be a protector of health. The coca plant is popularly known as the plant responsible for the production of cocaine, globally. The habit of chewing coca leaves has been prevalent since before the Middle Ages and the plant is grown in Peru, Bolivia, Colombia, Argentina, Ecuador and Chile.[53] While these leaves have religious connotations and are used as offerings among indigenous communities in the Andean regions, coca leaves are also infused in water and imbibed as tea. Coca users adapt to cold, fatigue, hunger and are able to perform prolonged periods of strenuous physical activity, making the habit more prevalent among manual workers, including farmers and mine workers as well as at high altitudes.[53]

Traditionally, the coca leaves are used as a stimulant, as well as for various ailments including gastrointestinal problems, altitude sickness, depression, toothache (for its anaesthetic effects) and obesity. Some of the associated oral ill-effects of coca use are an increased risk of dental attrition, cervical root caries and periapical abscess.[54,55]

Although coca is one of the drugs on the UN's list of prohibited drugs, South American countries such as Bolivia are keen on protecting the indigenous cultural practices among the Andean communities. The use of coca by the indigenous people is comparable with caffeine consumption in Western culture and despite the increased dental health risks, and international disapproval, prohibition of coca is currently under dispute to protect the cultural identity and heritage of these communities.

Dental Mutilation

Dental mutilation, including chipping and filing of teeth as well as intentional extraction of teeth, is a common traditional practice in many African countries, including Tanzania, Uganda, Sudan, Ethiopia and Kenya. Adult dental mutilations, primarily involving the maxillary incisors and canines, have been observed among many African tribes. Evidence from Cameroon suggests six patterns of adult dental mutilation – loss of incisors; inverted V-shaped central incisors; V-shaped central incisors; T-shaped anteriors; rectangular and hourglass-shape of at least one of the anteriors.[56] The tribe-specific adult dental mutilation is a cultural form of beautification and is associated with puberty ceremonies in both sexes, where the inverted V-shaped pattern is particularly observed. Clinical implications of these traditional practices are pulpal exposure, radicular cysts and extensive bone loss of the labial cortical plate.[56]

Infant dental mutilations differ from adult dental mutilations, as they are performed for their perceived medicinal benefits, however, they can have devastating health implications leading to death due to sepsis. Two patterns of infant dental mutilations have been observed – extraction of mandibular primary canines; and rarely extraction of permanent mandibular incisors. The strong cultural belief that during infancy, the

TABLE 73.1 Odontogenic Infections

Condition	In Non-Allergic Individuals, Antimicrobial for >3 Days or until Symptoms Resolve	Comments
Acute necrotizing gingivitis	Metronidazole or amoxicillin	Only if systemic involvement
Bites	Co-amoxiclav	
Cellulitis	Benzyl penicillin plus flucloxacillin	
Periapical abscess	Amoxicillin or metronidazole for 5 days	Only if systemic involvement or cellulitis
Pericoronitis	Metronidazole or amoxicillin	Only if systemic involvement or trismus
Periodontal abscess	Amoxicillin or metronidazole for 5 days	Only if systemic involvement or cellulitis
Periodontitis	Metronidazole or doxycycline	Only for severe disease
Sinusitis	Amoxicillin, or doxycycline or erythromycin for 7 days	Only for symptoms >7 days

swelling in the area associated with unerupted primary canines is the cause of persistent fever, vomiting, loss of appetite, diarrhoea and gastroenteritis, make this procedure acceptable. Children as young as 1 month undergo extractions of primary teeth by traditional healers, without topical anaesthetics. Tools used for these traditional customs are not sterilized and include knives, metal blades, bicycle spokes as well as sharp fingernails. A salt or herbal pack is sometimes placed over the operated area.

The traditional healers extract the primary teeth after which a hot knife is inserted into the socket to destroy the permanent tooth. The procedure is successful if the 'toothworm' (dental follicle of the permanent tooth) is removed along with the primary teeth. The consequences of infant oral mutilation are mainly due to the damage of the permanent teeth during this procedure; these range from enamel defects, loss of teeth, decreased mandibular arch size, hypoplasia of adjacent primary and permanent teeth, retention of primary teeth, malpositioned, displaced or impacted permanent successors, odontomas, to serious infection and death from sepsis.[57,58]

Although there have been efforts made to reduce the prevalence and associated adverse health consequences of infant dental mutilations, it is still practised in many African countries due to the strong cultural beliefs associated to it.[59]

Infections

Infections are suspected and/or antimicrobial therapy is indicated in immunocompetent patients with fascial space infections in the neck, necrotizing fasciitis (surgical osteomyelitis, removal of affected tissue is mandatory) or other serious, or life-threatening infections. In ill or immunocompromised persons, antimicrobial therapy should be considered in acute sinusitis, acute ulcerative gingivitis, dental abscess, dry socket, pericoronitis and to cover oral surgery.

ODONTOGENIC INFECTIONS

Odontogenic infections are mainly a consequence of pulpitis, leading initially to periapical infection and a dental abscess. Most odontogenic (and many orofacial) infections arise from the commensal oral mixed flora, with a substantial proportion of anaerobes. Most odontogenic and orofacial infections respond to drainage, either by endodontic treatment, incision, or tooth extraction. Analgesics also may be required. Antimicrobials may be indicated in a number of circumstances.

Most odontogenic infections respond well to penicillin or metronidazole, but increasing rates of resistance due to production of β-lactamase enzymes, which degrade penicillins, have lowered the usefulness of penicillins (Table 73.1). Co-amoxiclav and clindamycin, because of broad spectrum of activity and resistance to beta-lactamase, are increasingly first-line antimicrobials. Other bacterial infections are shown in Table 73.2.

Acute Necrotizing Ulcerative Gingivitis

Acute necrotizing ulcerative gingivitis (ANUG) is characterized by painful ulceration of the gum between the teeth (interdental papillae) (Figure 73.3), a pronounced tendency to gingival bleeding and halitosis. Anaerobic fusiform bacteria and spirochaetes are implicated, predisposing factors including poor oral hygiene, smoking, malnutrition and immune defects including HIV and other viral infections and leukaemias. ANUG not infrequently follows a respiratory tract infection presumably being predisposed by the transient immune defect consequent upon some such infections, particularly viral. ANUG is increasingly seen in viral infections such as HIV disease; in some other persons with ANUG only more subtle immune defects, such as reduced salivary immunoglobulin A and neutrophil dysfunction, have been described. However, there are patients who suffer from ANUG in the absence of any clear immune defect, malnutrition or other systemic factor and, in these, poor oral hygiene and tobacco-smoking may be factors. It is seen primarily in early childhood, young adults and HIV disease.[60]

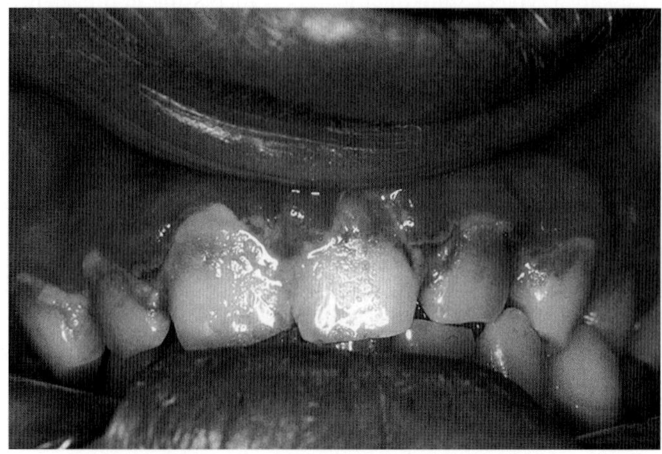

Figure 73.3 Acute necrotizing ulcerative gingivitis.

TABLE 73.2 Bacterial Infections which May Have Implications on Oral Health

Infecting Organism	Main Features	Orofacial Lesions
Treponema pallidum	Bejel	Mucous patches/sores in the mouth, destruction of palate in late stages
Treponema pallidum carateum	Pinta	Flattened, red, itchy patches on the face
Treponema pallidum	Yaws	Soft nodules on the face, which may ulcerate, destructive, disfiguring growths (gangosa), especially around the nose, mouth, and palate
Klebsiella granulomatis	Granuloma inguinale	Secondary to genital lesions, chronic, granulomatous ulceration in the oral cavity
Chlamydia trachomatis	Lymphogranuloma venereum	
Bacillus anthracis	Anthrax	Painful or ulcerated swellings mainly on palate
Brucella, melitensis, suis and abortus	Brucellosis	Rare infections or cranial nerve palsies
Clostridium botulinum	Botulism	Xerostomia, parotitis, muscle weakness
Clostridium perfringens (Cl. welchii), Cl. sporogenes, Cl. oedematiens, Cl. septicum	Gas gangrene	Gas gangrene
Escherichia coli	Enteric infections mainly Also urinary tract, wound, and other infection	Found in some oral infections, especially in denture-wearers and immunocompromised
Francisella tularensis	Tularaemia	Pharyngitis Stomatitis (often ulcerative) Faucial membrane Cervical lymphadenopathy
Mycobacterium leprae	Leprosy	In lepromatous leprosy, yellow-red, soft to hard, sessile lesions that ulcerate and heal to form fibrous scars, seen on gingiva, palate and tongue
Mycoplasma hominis and pneumoniae	Pneumonia	Rare infections or cranial nerve palsies? Reiter's syndrome
Neisseria meningitidis	Meningitis Septicaemia	Petechiae Occasionally: herpes labialis Facial palsy
Nocardia asteroides, brasiliensis and caviae	Nocardiosis	Ulceration Cheek or gingivae
Proteus vulgaris		Occasional infections
Pseudomonas mallei	Glanders (acute pneumonia)	Ulceration from nasal glanders Ulcers
Pseudomonas pseudomallei	Melioidosis (lung or other localized infections or septicaemia)	Oral abscesses, or other infections Parotitis
Rickettsia ricketssiae	Rocky mountain spotted fever	Faucial gangrene
Rickettsia akari	Rickettsialpox	Vesicles
Salmonellae typhi, paratyphi, choleraesuis and enteritidis	Typhoid and paratyphoid fever	Occasional infections

ANUG is typically seen where plaque control is poor. A mixed flora dominated by fusobacteria and spirochaetes such as *Treponema* species, *Bacteroides* (*Porphyromonas*) *melaninogenicus* species intermedius, *Fusobacterium* species, *Selenomonas* species and *Borrelia vincentii* is invariably present and the condition improves dramatically when treated with penicillin or metronidazole, suggesting a significant role for these bacteria. Viruses may play a role,[61] possibly also by inducing immune suppression.

Management includes oral debridement and hygiene instruction, peroxide or perborate mouthwashes and metronidazole 200 mg three times a day for 3–5 days.

Gangrenous Stomatitis (Cancrum Oris; *Noma*)

Noma is derived from the Greek *nomein*, which means to 'devour'; essentially it is a gangrenous stomatitis, which starts in the mouth as a benign oral lesion and rapidly destroys both the soft and hard tissues of the mouth and face (Figure 73.4). Most noma sufferers are under 6 years of age and it has been estimated that the case-fatality rate is probably between 70% and 90%. It is estimated that 100 000 African children under the

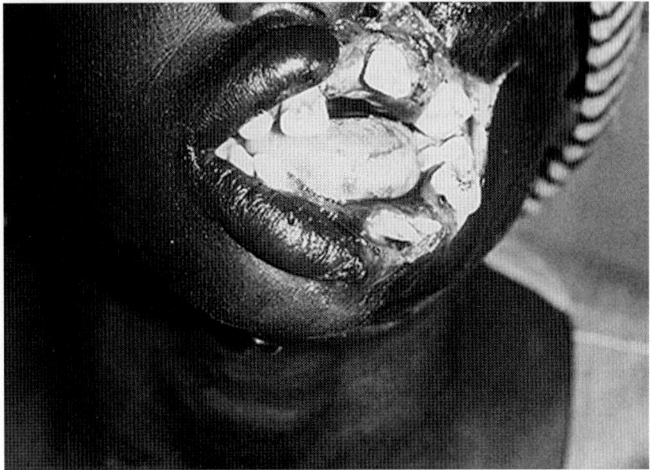

Figure 73.4 Noma.

age of 6 years contract noma every year.[62] Factors which predispose to the development of gangrenous stomatitis include protein–energy malnutrition and deficiencies of vitamins A, B, C, iron or magnesium. Therefore, poor living environment, exposure to debilitating childhood diseases, poor oral hygiene and malnutrition all appear to put children at risk for noma. In the developed world, gangrenous stomatitis is rare, and typically seen in immunocompromised persons such as those with HIV infection, leukaemia and diabetes.[63] The condition is seen especially in sub-Saharan Africa. Nigeria probably has the highest incidence, although The Gambia, Algeria, Uganda, Senegal, Madagascar, South Africa, Sudan and Egypt are also areas of high prevalence, as are Afghanistan, India, the Philippines, China, Vietnam, Papua New Guinea and South America.

Anaerobes, particularly *Bacteroides* (*Porphyromonas*) species, *Fusobacterium necrophorum* (an animal pathogen), *Prevotella intermedia*, Actinomyces and alpha haemolytic streptococci, have been implicated. In cases following ANUG, *Streptococcus anginosus* and *Abiotrophia* spp. are predominant species. In early noma, predominant species include *Ochrobactrum anthropi*, *Stenotrophomonas maltophilia*, an uncharacterized species of *Dialister*, and an uncultivated phylotype of *Leptotrichia*. A range of species or phylotypes are found in advanced noma, including *Propionibacterium acnes*, *Staphylococcus* spp., *Stenotrophomonas maltophilia*, *Ochrobactrum anthropi*, *Achromobacter* spp., *Afipia* spp., *Brevundimonas diminuta*, *Capnocytophaga* spp., *Cardiobacterium* spp., *Eikenella corrodens*, *Fusobacterium* spp., *Gemella haemolysans*, and *Neisseria* spp. Phylotypes unique to noma infections include those in the genera *Eubacterium*, *Flavobacterium*, *Kocuria*, *Microbacterium*, and *Porphyromonas*, and the related *Streptococcus salivarius* and genera *Sphingomonas* and *Treponema*. Spreading necrosis penetrates the buccal mucosa, leading to gangrene and an orocutaneous fistula and scarring.

The presenting feature may be a painful red or purplish-red spot (an indurated papule), usually on the gingiva in the premolar–molar region, which enlarges and ulcerates rapidly and spreading to the labiogingival or mucobuccal fold, and exposing the underlying bone. There is pain and often fetor. A blue-black area of discoloration appears on the skin and leads to a perforating wound. Sequestration of the exposed bone and loss of teeth are rapid and then the wound heals slowly by secondary intention, often leaving a defect. In former times, noma was often a lethal condition.

Gangrenous stomatitis does not respond readily to treatment unless the underlying disease is controlled, especially nutritional rehabilitation. The wound should be cleaned regularly with chlorhexidine and/or saline and/or hydrogen peroxide. A soft cotton gauze or tulle gras dressing may be used but changed frequently. Any loose slough, loose teeth and bony fragments should be removed. Parenteral fluids should be given to correct any dehydration and electrolyte imbalance. Management includes improving nutrition, systemic antibiotics (clindamycin, penicillin, tetracyclines or metronidazole) and plastic surgery. Folic acid, iron, ascorbic acid and vitamin B complex may be required.

Syphilis (Venereal Treponematosis)

In 1995, it was estimated that there were approximately 12 million new cases of syphilis among adults worldwide, with the greatest number of cases occurring in South and South-east Asia, followed by sub-Saharan Africa.

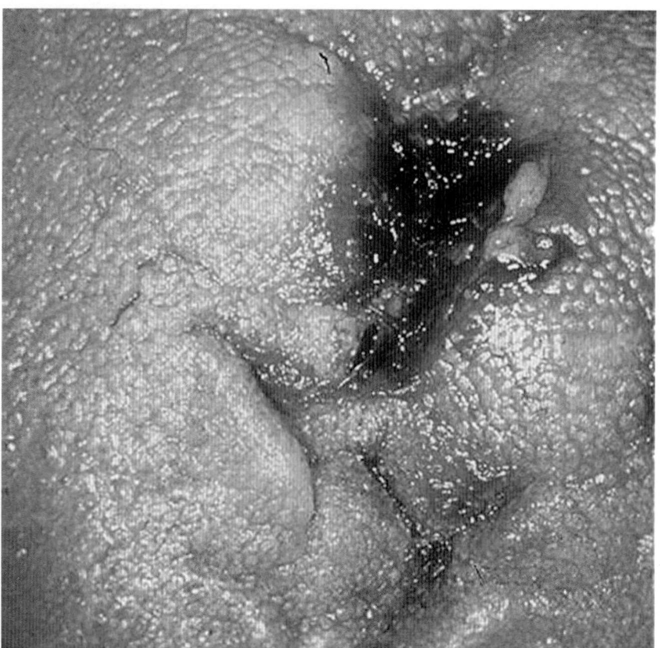

Figure 73.5 Oral lesion associated with syphilis.

The lip is the most common extragenital site of primary infection with *Treponema pallidum*. It causes a chancre (primary, hard or Hunterian chancre) which begins as a small, firm, pink macule, changes to a papule and then ulcerates to form a painless round ulcer with a raised margin and indurated base (Figure 73.5). About 60% of oral cases affect the lip or may present at the angles of the mouth.[64] Other oral sites affected may include the tongue and to a lesser extent the gingivae and fauces. Lymph nodes in the submaxillary, submental and cervical regions are usually enlarged. Chancres heal spontaneously within 3–8 weeks. Secondary syphilis follows the primary stage after 6–8 weeks but a healing chancre may still be present. As in the primary stage, the mucosal lesions are highly infectious. The typical signs and symptoms are fever, headache, malaise, a rash (characteristically symmetrically distributed coppery maculopapules or lesions on the palms) and generalized painless lymph node enlargement. It is this stage that classically causes oral lesions. Painless oral ulcers (mucous patches and snail-track ulcers) are the typical lesions and are slightly raised, greyish white, glistening patches seen on the fauces, soft palate, tongue, buccal mucosa and, rarely, gingivae. Cervical nodes are enlarged and ‘rubbery’ in consistency. Latent syphilis follows secondary syphilis and persists until late syphilis (tertiary syphilis) develops. The characteristic lesion of tertiary syphilis is a localized midline granuloma (‘gumma’) varying in size from millimetres to several centimetres, which breaks down to form a deep punched-out painless ulcer. The most common oral site for a gumma is the hard palate although the soft palate, lips or tongue are commonly involved. The gumma starts as a small, pale, raised area which ulcerates and rapidly progresses to a large zone of necrosis with denudation of bone and, in the case of a palatal gumma, may eventually perforate into the nasal cavity.[65]

The presence of clinical manifestations together with a history of contact may suggest the diagnosis but serodiagnostic tests, and sometimes dark-field microscopy is required for confirmation. There is no specific oral management except general palliative care if there is soreness of oral soft lesions, but the general management is straightforward: procaine penicillin intramuscularly for 10 days (erythromycin for 14 days) should be given.

Gonorrhoea

Oral, pharyngeal and tonsil involvement is being reported with increasing frequency particularly among homosexuals and heterosexuals practising oral sex. Infection of these sites is acquired primarily by fellatio and infrequently by cunnilingus.[66] The tonsils become red and swollen with a greyish exudate and there is cervical lymphadenitis. Lesions in other parts of the mouth are described as showing fiery erythema and sometimes oedematous, perhaps with painful superficial ulceration of the tongue, gingiva, buccal mucosa, hard or soft palate. The inflamed mucosa may also be covered with a yellowish or greyish exudate, which when detached may leave a bleeding surface.

A throat swab should be taken for Gram staining to show polymorphs containing Gram-negative diplococci. Confirmation is by culture and sugar fermentation to aid differentiation of species. Rapid identification of gonococci by fluorescent antibody techniques is possible.

Penicillin is the drug of choice, given as 2 g ampicillin plus 1 g probenecid as a single oral dose. Patients hypersensitive to penicillin can be treated with co-trimoxazole. Many strains are resistant to penicillin in parts of Africa and the Far East. Tetracycline or cefazolin–probenecid and streptomycin or spectinomycin may be used.

Actinomycosis

A breach in the continuity of mucosa caused either by trauma or surgery is the prerequisite for the majority of actinomycotic infections. Cervicofacial actinomycosis occurs predominantly in adult males following trauma either accidentally or rarely from dental treatment such as exodontia or endodontics.[67] Rarely, a periodontal pocket with suitable anaerobic conditions predisposes to the disease. The perimandibular area appears to be the commonest site. A relatively painless reddish-purple indurated mass appears at the angle of the jaw or in the vicinity of the parotid gland. It may drain through sinuses, the material containing the so-called sulphur granules. Actinomycosis may rarely involve the oral cavity, tongue, mandible, maxilla, paranasal sinuses, eye, ear, face, neck or salivary glands.

Sulphur granules may be seen by direct vision or after staining with Gram stain. Actinomycosis should be confirmed by the isolation of *A. israelii* in anaerobic culture. Penicillin is the first-choice antimicrobial. Alternatives include cephalosporin, clindamycin and lincomycin.

Tuberculosis

It is estimated that over 1.5 million tuberculosis cases per year occur in sub-Saharan Africa. HIV and tuberculosis speed each other's progress, with the latter contributing about 15% of AIDS death worldwide.

Oral lesions are seen mainly in pulmonary tuberculosis although systemic symptoms suggestive of lung disease are by no means always present.[68] Apart from pain, typically the main symptom of tuberculosis is chronic ulcers or granular masses. These are usually on the dorsum/base of the tongue, gingivae or occasionally in the buccal mucosa, floor of the mouth, lips and the hard and soft palates.

Primary oral lesions develop when bacilli are directly inoculated into the oral tissues of a person who has not acquired immunity. Primary tuberculosis of the mouth is more common in children and adolescents than adults. It usually presents as a single painless indolent ulcer commonly on the gingiva with enlarged cervical lymph nodes, or the gingivae, tooth extraction sockets and the buccal folds. Occasional cases of primary jaw tuberculosis have been reported, usually resulting from extension of a gingival lesion, from an infected post-extraction socket, from an extension from a tuberculous granuloma at the apex of the tooth or haematogenous spread. Tuberculous osteomyelitis may involve the maxilla particularly, or the mandible. The same general pattern as seen in other affected bones is common, with a slow rarefying osteitis resulting in sequestration of bone. Pain is not a prominent early feature but is seen later. Secondary infection may lead to difficulty in making a diagnosis. Tuberculous involvement of the mandible causes symptoms of pain, swelling, difficulty in eating, trismus, paraesthesia of the lower lip and enlargement of the regional lymph nodes. The infection may spread throughout the jaw, producing multiple sinuses, which drain intra- or extra-orally. The posterior mandible and ascending ramus are typically affected, and radiographical appearances include irregular linear calcifications along the lower border and irregular radiolucencies within the jawbone. In the maxilla the infra-orbital region, particularly in the young, is the usual site affected. Typically, a cold abscess develops and may eventually drain through fistulae but occasionally a firm intra-bony lesion may be present. TB in AIDS may affect the salivary glands.[69–71]

The diagnosis of pulmonary tuberculosis, suggested by a chronic cough, haemoptysis, loss of weight, night sweats and fever, is confirmed by physical examination, chest radiography, sputum smears and culture, and tuberculin testing (Mantoux or Heaf test). A lesional biopsy should be examined histologically, and with acid-fast stains and culture of the organism is the absolute proof of the disease.

Conventional chemotherapy of tuberculosis consists of administering two or more active drugs for 18 months to 2 years. Isoniazid in combination with ethambutol, thiacetazone or para-aminosalicylic acid and, depending on the severity of the disease, streptomycin intramuscularly for a period of the first 2–3 months, may be necessary. Other available drugs include rifampin, pyrazinamide and ethionamide. In tropical countries, directly observed treatment strategies may be adopted which use multiple drugs for shorter durations.

NON-TUBERCULOUS MYCOBACTERIAL INFECTIONS

Non-tuberculous (atypical) mycobacteria (NTM) include *Mycobacterium avium* and *M. intracellulare* (*M. avium-intracellulare* complex: MAC), *M. scrofulaceum* and *M. haemophilum*. Infections with NTM are being increasingly reported, especially in immunocompromised individuals. Cervical lymphadenopathy is occasionally caused by NTM but oral lesions are rare.

Atypical mycobacteria may be resistant to conventional antituberculous chemotherapy, although in children with cervical lymphadenitis caused by NTM conventional drug therapy alone or cycloserine for very resistant cases may be effective, and only occasionally is surgical excision necessary.[72,73]

VIRAL INFECTIONS

Viral infections affecting the oral region are briefly reviewed in Table 73.3.

TABLE 73.3 Viral Infections with Orofacial Manifestations

Virus	Orofacial Lesions
Cytomegalovirus	Oral ulcers with necrotic borders
Epstein–Barr virus	Oral hairy leukoplakia
Hepatitis B	Lichenoid lesions
Hepatitis C	Lichen planus
Herpes simplex	Primary infections, gingivitis, oral ulcers
	Recurrent oral
	Recurrent peri-oral, herpes labialis
HIV	Opportunistic fungal and viral infections, bacterial periodontitis, neoplasms (Kaposi's sarcoma, lymphoma), salivary gland disease and xerostomia
Influenza	Vesicles, erosive lesions, particularly in children
Papillomaviruses	Leukoplakia, oral cancers
Severe acute respiratory syndrome	Lesions not common, site of early replication
Varicella zoster	Chickenpox
	Zoster
	Zoster in immunocompromised

FUNGAL INFECTIONS

Superficial Mycoses

Candidosis. Candidosis (candidiasis) is the most common oral superficial mycosis. Caused mainly by *Candida albicans*, the condition typically reflects an underlying change in oral flora, depressed salivation, or immune defect. Increasingly, infections with variants of *C. albicans*, with other and sometimes new *Candida* species and of organisms resistant to antifungal agents, are now seen especially in immunocompromised persons.[74]

Pseudomembranous candidosis or thrush may be seen in neonates and among terminally ill patients, particularly in association with immunocompromising conditions (Figure 73.6).[75] Thrush is characterized by white patches on the surface of the oral mucosa, tongue, gingivae and elsewhere. The lesions form confluent plaques that resemble milk curds and can be wiped off the mucosa with gauze. Oral candidosis in the form of thrush is classically an acute infection, but it may recur for many months or even years in patients using corticosteroids topically or by aerosol, in HIV-infected individuals and in other immunocompromised patients. The term chronic pseudomembranous candidosis has been used for chronic recurrence. Erythematous or atrophic candidosis is an uncommon and poorly understood condition. It may arise as a consequence of persistent acute pseudomembranous candidosis, when the pseudomembranes are shed, or in HIV infection may precede pseudomembranous candidosis. Erythematous areas are seen mainly on the dorsum of the tongue, palate, gingivae or buccal mucosa. Lesions on the dorsum of the tongue present as depapillated areas. Midline or median rhomboid glossitis, or glossal central papillary atrophy, is characterized by an area of papillary atrophy that is rhomboid in shape, symmetrically placed centrally at the midline of the tongue, anterior to the circumvallate papillae. Red areas are often seen in the palate in HIV disease. Hyperplastic candidosis (*Candida* leukoplakia) is typified by chronic, discrete raised lesions that are typically found at the commissures, rarely on the gingivae. Angular stomatitis (perlèche, angular cheilitis) is a clinical diagnosis of lesions that affect, and are restricted to, the angles of the mouth, characterized by soreness, erythema and fissuring, and is commonly associated with denture-induced stomatitis. Both yeasts and bacteria are involved, as interacting, predisposing factors. It is occasionally an isolated initial sign of anaemia or vitamin deficiency, and resolves when the underlying disease has been treated. Angular stomatitis may also be seen in HIV disease and Crohn's disease.

Chronic multifocal oral candidosis is a term given when there are several lesions in the absence of predisposing drugs (except tobacco smoking) or medical conditions, typically angular stomatitis that is unilateral or bilateral, retrocommissural leukoplakia, which is the most constant component of the tetrad, median rhomboid glossitis, and palatal lesions where the lesions are of more than 1 month duration.

Clinical diagnosis can be supported by culture from saliva or an oral rinse. Antifungal therapy is initially with topical agents, especially the polyenes (nystatin, amphotericin), except in immunocompromised persons in whom the azoles, especially fluconazole, may be required systemically.[76]

Systemic (Deep) Mycoses. The systemic mycoses are potentially serious, sometimes lethal fungal infections seen mainly in the developing world, or in those who have visited endemic areas. Cases have been recorded as long as 34 years after visits to endemic areas.[77] Infections are increasingly seen in immunocompromised persons, especially in HIV infection.[78–80] In otherwise healthy persons, infection with these fungi is typically subclinical although some have pulmonary infection. The increase in mycoses in immunocompromised persons is accompanied by significant morbidity and mortality and 'new' opportunists are appearing.

Orofacial lesions are mainly chronic ulcers or maxillary sinus infection, which are typically associated with respiratory lesions. Most of the mycoses may mimic carcinoma or tuberculosis, and are diagnosed on the basis of a history of travel to endemic areas, or an immunocompromising state, confirmed by taking a smear, biopsy or culture of the affected tissues. Serodiagnosis, physical examination and chest radiographs may be indicated. Most systemic mycoses can be treated with systemic amphotericin or azoles.

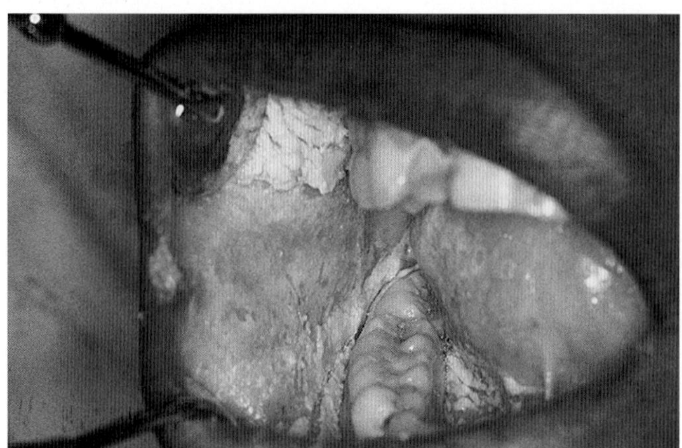

Figure 73.6 Thrush associated with HIV.

PARASITIC INFECTIONS

Malaria is the most important parasitic disease of man, and like many parasitic infestations has few oral complications. However, the lack of reporting of oral lesions in parasitic infestations may simply be a reflection of their under-diagnosis.

Myiasis

Myiasis is caused when fly maggots invade living tissue or when they are harboured in the intestine or bladder. In oral lesions they are seen mainly in the anterior maxillary or mandibular gingivae.[81,82] An opening burrow is usually patent, with induration of the marginal tissues and is raised, forming a dome-shaped 'warble', or an extraction wound may be effected. Often several larvae are present and there is a severe inflammatory reaction in the surrounding tissues.

Larvae can be seen with the naked eye. A few drops of turpentine oil or chloroform in light vegetable oil should be instilled in the lesion and the larvae removed with blunt tweezers. It may be prudent to give an antibiotic, as there is often a superimposed secondary infection. Ivermectin may be effective in some cases.[83]

Ciguatera Poisoning

Ciguatera, the most common form of fish poisoning, occurring in most tropical and subtropical seas, may result in oral or perioral paraesthesiae or dysaesthesiae.[84,85]

REFERENCES

20. Kumaraswamy KL, Vidhya M. Human papilloma virus and oral infections: An update. J Cancer Res Ther 2011;7:120–7.
24. Villa A, Villa C, Abati S. Oral cancer and oral erythroplakia: an update and implication for clinicians. Aust Dent J 2011;56:253–6.
38. Ebbert J, Montori VM, Erwin PJ, et al. Interventions for smokeless tobacco use cessation. Cochrane Database Syst Rev 2011;(2): CD004306.
43. Al-Rmalli SW, Jenkins RO, Haris PI. Betel quid chewing elevates human exposure to arsenic, cadmium and lead. J Hazard Mater 2011;190 (1–3):69–74.
50. Stanfill SB, Connolly GN, Zhang L, et al. Global surveillance of oral tobacco products: total nicotine, unionised nicotine and tobacco-specific N-nitrosamines. Tob Control 2011;20 (3):e2.

Access the complete references online at www.expertconsult.com

74 Environmental Stress

BUDDHA BASNYAT | JENNIFER O'HEA | KEN ZAFREN

KEY POINTS

Heat Illness

- Heat illness is a spectrum of disorders that range in severity from mild cardiovascular and central nervous system disturbances to severe cell damage in multiple organs. This spectrum includes heat cramps, heat syncope, heat exhaustion, prickly heat rash and heat stroke.
- Risk factors include poverty, extremes of age, isolation, chronic disease, athletes, military recruits and multiple recreational and prescription medications.
- The imbalance of heat gain and heat loss (through the methods of evaporation, convection, conduction and radiation) can lead to hyperthermia.
- Heat stroke is defined by both a core body temperature >40°C and neurological dysfunction.
- Heat exhaustion and heat stroke are medical emergencies. Rapid cooling should begin in the pre-hospital setting.
- Evaporative cooling is the most effective, well-tolerated method for treating heat stroke.
- Prevention of heat illness involves simple measures of shade, hydration and breaks from exertion. Acclimatization can be accomplished prior to entering a hot environment.

Accidental Hypothermia and Local Cold Injuries

- Hypothermia is defined as a core temperature <35°C. It can occur in countries with temperate and tropical climates, where it is often underdiagnosed. Hypothermia is a special risk during disasters and in ill or immobile patients, even when temperatures are mild or warm.
- Hypothermia is neuroprotective. Some hypothermic patients without cardiac activity can be resuscitated with normal neurological outcome. Dependent lividity, apparent rigor mortis and fixed dilated pupils are not contraindications to advanced life support (ALS) with cardiopulmonary resuscitation (CPR) in hypothermic patients.
- In moderate or severe hypothermia, core temperature is best measured by oesophageal probe. Epitympanic temperature measurement may also be used. Tympanic, rectal, oral and bladder temperatures are not reliable.
- Hypothermic patients should be handled gently to avoid provoking ventricular fibrillation (VF). They should be removed from a cold environment and covered to decrease further heat loss. Cardiac and core temperature monitoring should be initiated as soon as possible to help guide resuscitation.
- Moderately and severely hypothermic patients (core temperature <32°C) cannot re-warm themselves. They require active re-warming. Cardiopulmonary resuscitation and extracorporeal re-warming may be required for hypothermic patients who are apnoeic and pulseless.
- Hypothermia can mask signs and symptoms of underlying diseases. If neurological findings or vital signs are not consistent with the degree of hypothermia, underlying conditions should be sought.
- In spite of the common saying that 'No one is dead until they are warm and dead', some people are cold and dead.

Drowning and Tsunamis

- Drowning refers to respiratory impairment after submersion in liquid (usually water). Drowning kills about 500 000 people annually.
- Death by drowning is due to hypoxia. Survivors are at risk of hypoxic brain damage and lung injury.
- Immediate water rescue and rapid resuscitation are critical to ensure the best possible outcome for drowning victims.
- Patients who are alert or arousable on arrival at a medical facility usually survive without neurological sequelae. Almost half of comatose patients will also survive with good neurological outcome.
- Lung injury may be delayed. The initial chest X-ray may be normal, even in patients with lung injury.
- A tsunami is a series of waves caused by displacement of a large volume of water, most commonly by an earthquake or volcanic eruption. Drowning is the most common cause of death due to tsunamis. The 2004 tsunami in the Indian Ocean killed about 230 000 people.
- Many drowning deaths and deaths in tsunamis may be preventable with water-safety measures and tsunami warning systems.
- People in coastal areas who observe a 'drawback' or feel an earthquake should run for higher ground if possible.

Altitude Illness in Pilgrims

- Altitude illness comprises of the benign acute mountain sickness (mainly, headache and nausea) and the life-threatening high altitude cerebral and pulmonary edemas.
- Although altitude illness is well described among trekkers, mountaineers and the porters who accompany them, there is a dearth of literature on local pilgrims to high altitude.
- Unlike most tourists sojourning to high altitude, pilgrims are often elderly people with comorbidities and hence may require more care.
- There may be genetic polymorphism involved in better acclimatization/adaptation to high altitude, but a specific gene has yet to be found.

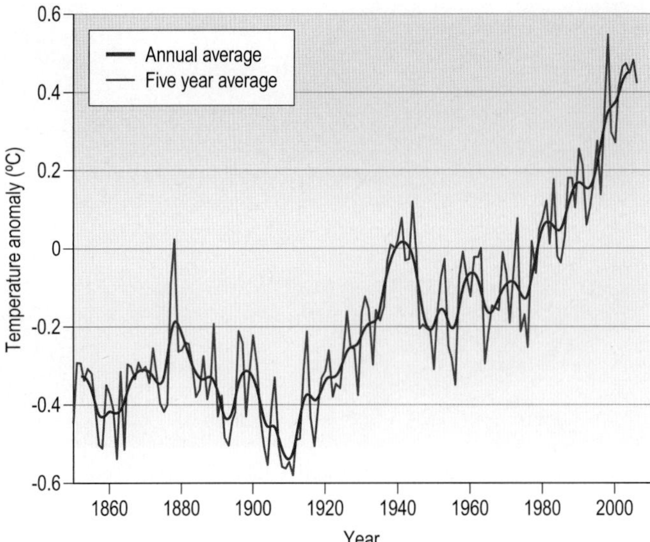

Figure 74.1 Global temperature change.

Heat Illness

EPIDEMIOLOGY

Despite humans' physiological adaptation to heat attained from our origins in tropical Africa, heat illness (and heat stroke at its extreme) continues to be a medical burden in most countries. With the rise of global temperatures in the last 100 years, knowledge of heat illness by medical providers will become increasingly more important (Figure 74.1).

Environmental heat stress includes the effects of temperature, humidity and solar radiation. Most national weather service websites publish a heat index chart, allowing for a daily measure of temperature and humidity in order to assess the risks of outdoor exposure.

Heat illness is a spectrum of disorders that range in severity from mild cardiovascular and central nervous system disturbances to severe cell damage, including brain, kidney and liver.[1] This spectrum includes heat cramps, heat syncope, heat exhaustion, prickly heat rash and heat stroke.

Many risk factors need to be considered with heat illness. Globally, indigenous people in the tropics with limited access to clean water and adequate shelter are at high risk. In Saudi Arabia for *Hajj*, millions of pilgrims journey annually to Mecca. When this gathering occurs in the summer, temperatures can reach over 45°C.[2] There, heat illness is common with extended hours standing outside, crowded accommodations and lack of acclimatization. Other groups at risk worldwide include the poor, elderly and socially isolated, infants, military recruits and athletes.

Prescription and recreational drugs often contribute to heat illness. Anticholinergics impair sweating, diuretics and alcohol predispose to dehydration, and beta-blockers can blunt the increase in cardiac output needed to adapt. Methamphetamine and cocaine not only lead to illogical choices of heat exposure, but they impair the body's ability to vasodilate and transfer heat to the environment.

Finally, chronic diseases predispose to heat illness. These include heart disease, diabetes, Alzheimer's disease, psychiatric disease, renal failure, obesity, chronic lung disease, infections and skin diseases such as scleroderma.

PATHOGENESIS AND PATHOLOGY

Heat Regulation

Heat production under resting conditions is about 1 kcal/kg per hour (1500–1700 kcal/day in an average person). Exercise can increase this to as high as 6000 kcal/day. Without heat loss, body temperature at rest would rise by 1°C/hour. The body maintains normothermia by balancing heat production with heat dissipation. The anterior hypothalamus detects elevations in core body temperature; in response it stimulates the autonomic nervous system to produce *cutaneous vasodilatation* and *sweating*.[3]

As core temperature rises, peripheral blood vessels dilate and skin blood flow increases (up to 8 L/min).[4] This leads to increased heat delivery to the ambient air for convective exchange. The cardiovascular system must increase heart rate and stroke volume (up to a cardiac output of 20 L/min in extreme cases), in order to compensate for the peripheral blood pooling. Those with cardiovascular disease or on certain medications that prohibit this compensation, will do poorly.

Principles of Cooling

Four mechanisms for heat transfer are responsible for cooling the body.[5]

Evaporation

As ambient temperature rises, evaporation becomes the dominant mechanism for heat dissipation (about 70%). The rate of thermal sweating can be as high as 1–2 L/h. As 1 L of sweat evaporates from the skin, it leads to a loss of 580 kcal of heat from the body. If sweat drips off the body or is wiped away, no heat loss occurs. Evaporative heat loss becomes less effective in humid environments.

Convection

Heat can be lost from the body surface to a gas or fluid, such as moving air and water molecules in direct contact with the skin. This is a minimal source of heat loss (and possibly heat gain) as ambient temperature rises. Wind velocity allows for more rapid convective heat loss.

Conduction

Here, heat is lost between two surfaces in direct contact, such as sitting on a cool surface. This is another minimal source of heat loss normally, except in the case of heat stroke treatment.

Radiation

Heat is exchanged between the body and its surroundings by electromagnetic waves. This is an important mode of heat loss in cooler weather, but a source of heat gain in warmer weather. Up to 300 kcal can be gained from direct exposure to summer sun.

Hyperthermia

Hyperthermia is defined as an elevation in core body temperature above normal range (36–37.5°C) due to a failure of thermoregulation (too much heat gain or too little heat loss). This must be differentiated from fever, which is an alteration of the hypothalamic thermal set point triggered by cytokines in response to illness. The effects of hyperthermia begin at a molecular level. Tissue damage appears to be a function of temperature and length of exposure time. Cellular damage and death occur at a 'critical thermal maximum', which is

41.6°C–42°C for 45 minutes to 8 hours.[4] This results from denatured enzymes, liquefied membrane lipids, damaged mitochondria, impaired coding of proteins, and uncoupling of oxidative phosphorylation. Hepatocytes, neural tissue, and vascular endothelium appear to be the most sensitive. Meanwhile, acute phase and heat shock proteins combine to protect against heat-induced tissue injury and promote repair.

The combined failure of these processes – heat regulation and altered expression of heat shock and acute phase proteins – lead to a progression to heat stroke. As the peripheries vasodilate, splanchnic vasoconstriction leads to intestinal ischaemia and hyperpermeability. Endotoxins enter the circulation and increase production of inflammatory cytokines, procoagulants, and endothelial vasoactive factors such as nitric oxide. This precipitates hypotension and hyperthermia. Cooling the body to a normal temperature does not result in an immediate cessation of this process. The time to intervention in this process and the host's risk factors dictate the severity of the disease.[6]

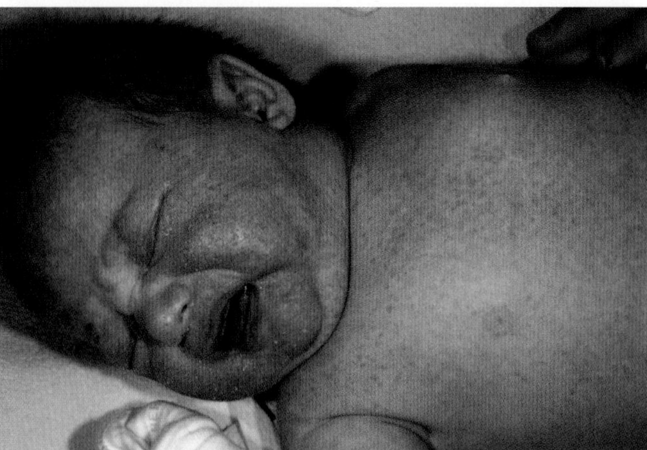

Figure 74.2 Heat rash. *(From Habif T. Skin Disease, Diagnosis and Treatment, 3rd edn. Copyright © Elsevier 2011.)*

CLINICAL FEATURES

In the spectrum of heat illness, the various forms range in severity from the mild, common heat cramps and heat rash to potentially fatal heat stroke.[5]

Heat cramps are caused by low salt levels in muscles in persons who have been sweating excessively and drinking hypotonic fluid. Large muscle groups in the abdomen, arms and legs are most affected, and this occurs after exertion when at rest. The incidence is highest in the first few days of work or exercise in a hot environment. Construction workers and miners are at high risk. Lab abnormalities include hyponatraemia, hypochloraemia, and low urinary Na and Cl.

Heat tetany can be confused with heat cramps. Hyperventilation in a hot environment leads to respiratory alkalosis, which then causes a relative hypocalcaemia. Carpopedal spasm, perioral and distal paresthesias, and myalgias may occur as a result.

Heat syncope occurs with prolonged standing or upon standing. Peripheral blood pooling causes reduced cardiac output and cerebral blood flow. Dehydration, poor acclimatization, and certain cardiovascular medication pose an increased risk.

Heat rash (prickly heat, lichen tropicus, miliaria rubra) is a skin inflammation caused by excessive sweating, especially in hot, humid weather leading to blockage of sweat glands by stratum corneum. It begins as a red cluster of pruritic pimples or small blisters as obstructed sweat glands dilate and rupture (Figure 74.2). Most common areas include the neck, upper chest, groin, elbow creases and under the breasts. Keratin plugs can form leading to a secondary deeper obstruction in dermis that lasts for weeks as white papules. A secondary staphylococcal infection may also occur. Heat rash is more commonly seen in children.

Heat exhaustion is the body's response to excessive loss of water and salt through sweating. Symptoms include heavy sweating, extreme weakness, dizziness, nausea, pale or flushed complexion, muscle cramps, hyperventilation and a slightly increased body temperature. No alteration in mental status is an important distinguishing factor between heat exhaustion and heat stroke. However, there are often blurred boundaries between the two. If the diagnosis is unclear, it is safest to treat a patient as having heat stroke.

Heat stroke requires both a core body temperature greater than 40°C *and* central nervous system dysfunction that results in delirium, convulsions or coma. This is the final result of impaired heat load dissipation. Most patients have tachycardia and hyperventilation. Other symptoms include hot dry skin or profuse sweating, hallucinations, headache, slurred speech and confusion. Cessation of sweating is a late finding. As the cascade of heat stroke progresses, symptoms in almost every organ system are evident, such as haemorrhage, pulmonary oedema and compartment syndrome from rhabdomyolysis.

DIAGNOSIS

Mild manifestations of heat illness can be diagnosed clinically, and no further testing is required. Heat stroke can be divided into two main types: classic (non-exertional) and exertional heat stroke (Table 74.1), each with distinguishing characteristics of epidemiology and laboratory abnormalities.[3,7] Identifying the type can aid in determining the most appropriate treatment regimen.

A typical patient with classic (non-exertional) heat stroke may be the poor, elderly patient with multiple medications and comorbidities who was without air conditioning for days before being found unresponsive. As another example, the homeless, schizophrenic patient abusing cocaine found confused outside in the heat could also be a victim of classic heat stroke. A victim of exertional heat stroke, in contrast, would be the young military recruit exercised to the point of collapse on a hot summer day. Certainly, some crossover can occur, and the laboratory abnormalities on presentation may help to differentiate.

MANAGEMENT AND TREATMENT

Heat cramps can be managed with the administration of salt solutions (commercial electrolyte solutions/sports drinks or a 0.1–0.2% salt solution). If the patient is intolerant to oral fluids, IV normal saline is an option.

Heat syncope is self-limited. Rest the patient in a recumbent position with the legs up.

Heat rash can be prevented by keeping the area dry and clean, and wearing loose-fitting clothing. Avoid lotions and talc. To treat, use chlorhexidine lotion with 1% salicylic acid TID.[5] A course of antibiotics may be necessary if a superinfection is suspected.

TABLE 74.1 Comparison of Classic and Exertional Heat Stroke

	Classic	Exertional
Age group	Elderly	Men (15–45 years old)
Health status	Chronically ill	Healthy
Activity	Sedentary	Strenuous exercise
Drug use	Anticholinergics, diuretics, antipsychotics, antihypertensives, antidepressants	Usually none
Sweating	Usually absent	Often present
Lactic acidosis	Usually absent	Common, may be marked
Rhabdomyolysis	Unusual	Frequently severe
Hyperuricaemia	Modest	Severe
Acute renal failure	<5% of patients	25–30% of patients
Hypocalcaemia	Uncommon	Common
DIC	Mild	Marked
CPK/aldolase	Mildly elevated	Markedly elevated
Hypoglycaemia	Uncommon	Common
Mechanism	Poor dissipation of environmental heat	Excessive endogenous heat production

From Khosla R, Guntupalli KK. Heat-related illnesses. *Crit Care Clin* 1999;15(2):251–63.

Heat exhaustion and heat stroke should be considered a medical emergency. The basic tenets of circulation, airway and breathing should be followed. Mortality correlates with the degree of temperature elevation, time to initiation of cooling and number of organ systems affected. Since delay in treatment can increase morbidity, heat exhaustion should be treated as heat stroke, until better clarified. Rapid cooling and management of distributive shock should be instituted according to Table 74.2.

Evaporative methods are the primary method of heat dissipation, but no evidence exists to support the superiority of any one cooling technique in classic heat stroke.[7] Although slow in cooling (up to 5 h), evaporation is the most well-tolerated, especially for the elderly. Spraying the body with cool or tepid water and warm air (45°C) fans is effective and minimizes shivering. This is the concept behind the Makkah cooling unit, a bed widely used in the Middle East to treat heat stroke pilgrims in Mecca.[8]

Conductive methods such as ice packs can be used, but as an adjunctive tool with evaporation. Convection via Cool (not ice) water immersion is more effective with faster (<60 min) cooling times, but should only be employed in exertional heat stroke such as a military recruit, where it is better tolerated. As every patient should be evaluated for the need for intubation for airway protection, a patient must have a patent airway for safe cool water immersion. Gastric, bladder and peritoneal lavage are less effective, time-consuming and sometimes dangerous. Alcohol sponge baths should be avoided, as the alcohol can be

TABLE 74.2 Management of Heat Stroke

Condition	Intervention	Goal
OUT OF HOSPITAL		
	Measure core temperature with a rectal probe, assess for neurological symptoms	Diagnose heat stroke
	If core temperature >40°C: Move the patient to a shaded, cooler place. Remove clothing, raise legs. Initiate external cooling: – continuous fanning – cover with a thin wet sheet – tepid water 25–30°C spray mist – cold packs on the neck/axillae/groin – open ambulance windows	Lower core temperature to <39.4°C Promote cooling by evaporation and conduction
	Airway – position unconscious patient on side, clear airway	Minimize risk of aspiration
	Administer oxygen at 4 L/min	Increase arterial oxygen saturation to >90%
	IV normal saline	Provide volume expansion
	Rapidly transfer the patient to an emergency department	
IN HOSPITAL		
Cooling period	Confirm diagnosis with thermometer calibrated to record high temperatures (40–47°C)	
Hyperthermia	Monitor rectal and skin temperatures, continue cooling	Keep rectal temperature <39.4°C and skin temperature 30–33°C
Seizures/shivering	Give benzodiazepines	Control seizures, minimize heat generation
Respiratory failure	Consider elective intubation	Protect airway and augment oxygenation (arterial oxygen saturation >90%)
Hypotension	Administer fluids, consider vasopressors, central venous pressure monitoring	Volume expansion, increase mean arterial pressure to >60 mmHg and restore organ perfusion
Rhabdomyolysis	IV normal saline, sodium bicarbonate	Prevent myoglobin-induced renal injury, promote renal blood flow, alkalinization of urine
Hyperkalemia, hypocalcaemia	Monitor serum potassium and calcium levels, treat abnormalities	Prevent life-threatening cardiac arrhythmia
Multiorgan dysfunction	Supportive therapy	Recovery of organ function

Adapted from Bouchama A, Knochel JP. Heat stroke. *N Engl J Med* 2002;346:1978–88.

absorbed through the skin. Vigorous skin massage can be employed to increase blood flow to the skin. Shivering should be treated with benzodiazepines; dantrolene has not been shown to effectively treat shivering and should not be used. If possible, avoid pressors (especially alpha agonists) during cooling which will increase vasoconstriction. The blood pressure may rise spontaneously as the patient cools. Consider isoproterenol if the cardiac output is not compensating to a hyperdynamic state as predicted. If renal failure or rhabdomyolysis is severe, dialysis will need to be employed. Compartment pressures should be measured in limbs that have sustained prolonged pressure, feel tense or lack pulses. There is no indication for routine antibiotics or corticosteroids. Antipyretics are not effective, since pyrogens only play a role in fever, not hyperthermia.[4] The endpoint of cooling is not well-defined, but a rectal temperature of 39°C is generally accepted.

PREVENTION

All forms of heat illness should be considered preventable, often with simple measures. Shade, hydration, salt and frequent breaks are the mainstay in hot, humid environments. One should maximize voluntary fluid intake and gastric emptying, so that fluid can rapidly enter the small intestine to be absorbed. Gastric emptying is hastened by large, cool fluid volumes (500–600 mL at 10–15°C) of low osmolality (<200 mOsm/L).[5]

Education of coaches, foremen and military instructors has become more common. Heat wave warnings via the print and audiovisual media are now methods of communication between villages in rural areas. However, more rural outreach is needed. Showing some promise is vulnerability mapping, which provides a template for determining local and regional heat vulnerability. After validation using health outcome data, interventions can be targeted at the most vulnerable populations.[9]

Acclimatization is a tool of prevention that can be used by a traveller planning to visit an area with a high heat index such as the tropics. It is possible to quickly develop physiological adaptations to warmer environments after repeated exposures to heat stress. Daily exposure to work and heat for 100 min/day results in near-maximal acclimatization in 7–14 days.[5] Increased sweat and plasma volume and earlier aldosterone release all contribute. The acclimatized person exhibits a lower rise in rectal temperature and oxygen utilization, and an increased maximal oxygen consumption during exercise. Heat exposure needs to continue intermittently at 4-day intervals to maintain acclimatization.

Physical fitness also predicts easier acclimatization. In general, the higher the maximal oxygen uptake (indicating aerobic fitness) of an individual, the lower the heat strain observed in a warm humid climate. Caffeine and alcohol have both been shown to increase susceptibility to heat illness.[10]

SUMMARY

The spectrum of heat-related illnesses is common, yet highly preventable. Healthcare providers in areas of high heat and humidity must be able to diagnose the disorders in the heat illness spectrum, especially heat stroke. Rapid treatment can reduce morbidity and mortality, especially when a high-risk patient is identified. More global outreach is needed to identify isolated communities who lack resources to adapt to increasing global temperatures.

Accidental Hypothermia and Local Cold Injuries

EPIDEMIOLOGY

Accidental hypothermia refers to unintentional core temperature <35°C. Therapeutic hypothermia refers to deliberately cooling comatose patients with return of spontaneous circulation after cardiac arrest, to improve neurological outcome. There are few statistics in developed countries regarding deaths due to hypothermia and virtually no data from less developed countries. Details on local cold injuries, such as frostbite and non-freezing cold injuries (trench foot or immersion foot) are unfortunately beyond the scope of this chapter.

Primary hypothermia results from inability to maintain core temperature above 35°C, usually in cold or wet conditions. These conditions can occur even in tropical climates, especially at high altitudes and during rainy seasons. Famine and malnutrition limit metabolic rate and can contribute to hypothermia, even in moderate environmental conditions. Immersion in water can cause hypothermia. Primary hypothermia is a disease of wars.[11] It is also associated with homelessness and the use of alcohol and other drugs. In the aftermath of natural disasters, hypothermia can be a major killer. The 2005 earthquake in Pakistan killed about 80 000 people outright and left 3.5 million people homeless. The death toll due to hypothermia was significant, but is unknown.

Secondary hypothermia has many causes, including sepsis and trauma. Diseases that decrease metabolic rate and conditions such as tumor and stroke that decrease hypothalamic function can cause hypothermia. Elderly and ill patients can become hypothermic indoors in well-heated houses.[12]

Iatrogenic hypothermia is a common problem in neonates and during surgery. Hypothermia can result from resuscitation with room temperature fluids or refrigerated blood products.

PATHOGENESIS AND PATHOLOGY

Normal core temperature: about 37–37.5°C, is the result of a balance between heat production and heat loss. Heat production increases with increasing metabolic rate. Hypothermia increases metabolic rate by stimulating the thyroid and adrenal glands. Shivering, mediated by the hypothalamus in response to skin temperature, is the most effective way to increase heat production, but causes increased metabolic demands.[12,13]

Heat is lost by radiation, conduction, convection and evaporation. Radiation is the exchange of radiant energy with the surrounding environment. Conduction is the exchange of heat by direct contact with a warmer or cooler object. Convection is the transfer of heat to a moving liquid or gas. Evaporation removes heat from the body by conversion of liquid to gas. Insensible heat loss due to breathing and evaporation of sweat are the two main forms of evaporative heat loss. Cutaneous vasoconstriction can limit heat loss from skin. The main mechanisms by which humans avoid becoming hypothermic are behavioural responses, putting on clothing and seeking shelter.[12]

CLINICAL FEATURES

Decreased core temperature initially leads to increased catecholamine secretion, peripheral vasoconstriction and shivering.

TABLE 74.3 Hypothermia Staging and Clinical Findings

Core Temp.	Thermoregulatory Capacity	Signs and Symptoms		Classifications
37°C	Control and responses fully active	May feel cold and be shivering		Normal
35–32°C	Control and responses fully active	Vital signs decrease linearly.	Physical (gross and fine motor) and mental impairment	Mild
32–28°C	Responses attenuated or extinguished	Vital signs reduced Below 30°C: Shivering stops. Loss of consciousness		Moderate
Below 28°C	Responses absent	Rigidity Vital signs markedly reduced or absent Risk of VF (rough handling)		Severe
Below 25°C	Responses absent	Spontaneous ventricular fibrillation cardiac arrest		

Adapted with permission from Alaska Cold Injuries Guidelines (revised 2005).

Shivering is maximal at 35–31 °C, increasing with cooling until it rapidly ceases at about 30°C.

Heart rate, blood pressure and cardiac output increase initially. Below 35°C, these parameters decrease nearly linearly. Below 28°C, the myocardium becomes irritable, decreasing the threshold for ventricular fibrillation. Death in accidental hypothermia usually results from decreased cardiac output, especially due to ventricular tachycardia (VT) or ventricular fibrillation (VF).[14,15]

Hypothermia decreases cerebral blood flow, but also decreases cerebral metabolism, protecting the brain from ischaemic injury. Initially, patients are clumsy and have decreased fine motor coordination. They may be anxious and irritable. Further decreases in core temperature cause confusion, dysarthria, problems with judgement and memory and eventually stupor and coma. Most patients are unresponsive at 30°C, but some may be alert.[12,15]

The respiratory system responds to mild hypothermia with tachypnoea followed by decreased minute ventilation and lowered oxygen consumption as core temperature decreases. Bronchospasm and bronchorrhoea caused by decreased ciliary function predispose to aspiration and pneumonia.

The renal system responds to mild hypothermia with cold-induced diuresis, decreasing intravascular volume. Further cooling causes lowered sensitivity to antidiuretic hormone, limiting water reabsorption. Glomerular filtration rate decreases. In severe hypothermia, decreased tubular hydrogen secretion predisposes to metabolic acidosis.

Afterdrop is the continuing decrease in core temperature after the patient is removed from the cold environment, mainly due to loss of heat from the warm core to the cool peripheral tissues. Afterdrop can be as much as 0.5°C, even with optimal re-warming.

DIAGNOSIS

Diagnosis of hypothermia is made by core temperature measurement.[12,16] Investigations are done to guide treatment and to diagnose underlying conditions. Underlying conditions associated with hypothermia include acute spinal cord transection, toxic exposures, including medications, central nervous system conditions, endocrine dysfunction, iatrogenic causes, infection, decreased cardiac output, abdominal catastrophes and skin conditions that allow abnormal heat loss.

Hypothermia is generally classified into mild (35–32°C), moderate (32–28°C) and severe (<28°C).[12,16] In the field, core temperature can be estimated by observing level of consciousness and the presence of shivering (Table 74.3).[11,16] Alert, shivering patients have mild hypothermia. Confused patients may or may not be shivering and have moderate hypothermia. Unconscious patients have severe hypothermia. Profoundly hypothermic patients may have clinically undetectable vital signs and lack all reflexes, including corneal reflexes. In some respects, the field staging system is more useful than the actual core temperature measurements, because symptoms at a given core temperature vary markedly among individuals.

Core temperature is best measured by an oesophageal probe in the lower third of the oesophagus.[14] In conscious patients, epitympanic probe (thermistor) temperature correlates well with core temperature, but may be falsely lowered by a number of factors. Tympanic (infrared), rectal, oral and urinary bladder temperatures are unreliable. During re-warming, oesophageal temperature tracks changes in core temperature, while other sites lag considerably behind. This may mislead the clinician into thinking that core temperature is still decreasing, when it is actually rising. If other methods are not available, rectal temperature can be measured using a low-reading thermometer. Most standard thermometers do not read below 34°C.[16]

Neurological findings or vital signs that are not consistent with the degree of hypothermia should prompt consideration of underlying causes such as head injury, hypoglycaemia, hypovolaemia, infection (especially CNS infection) or overdose. Tachypnoea suggests metabolic acidosis. Fingerstick glucose should be determined as soon as possible. Continuous pulse oximetry is helpful. Probes often work better on an ear lobe than on vasoconstricted fingers or toes.

Electrocardiographic monitoring is critical. Hypothermia causes prolonged PR, QRS and QT intervals. Muscle tremors may cause artifacts that complicate ECG interpretation. Osborne (J) waves are a common finding, but have no prognostic significance. Sinus tachycardia is usual in mild hypothermia. In moderate to severe hypothermia, dysrhythmias include: sinus bradycardia; atrial fibrillation or flutter; AV blocks; nodal rhythms; premature ventricular contractions; VT; VF or asystole. Atrial dysrhythmias seldom require treatment and resolve with re-warming.

Arterial blood gases are only needed in mechanically ventilated patients. Blood gas values that are 'corrected' for temperature are misleading and should not be used. Only 'uncorrected' blood gas values should be used to guide treatment.[12]

Haematology. For every 1°C decrease in temperature, haematocrit decreases about 2%. A severely hypothermic patient with a 'normal' haematocrit is probably anaemic. White blood cell and platelet counts decrease due to sequestration. Hypothermia produces a coagulopathic state, but coagulation testing is unreliable.

Blood chemistries. Potassium levels are not affected by temperature, but hyperkalaemia is more dangerous in hypothermia. Blood glucose is increased due to inactivity of insulin below 30–32°C. Creatine kinase should be checked to rule out rhabdomyolysis.

Radiological studies are based on clinical presentation. Hypothermia can cause abdominal findings that mimic acute abdomen.

MANAGEMENT AND TREATMENT

Patients with mild hypothermia retain the ability to re-warm themselves with supportive treatment. Shivering is an effective means of increasing heat production. Patients who are shivering should be allowed to eat or drink, if they can do so safely, in order to replace calories used by shivering. Medications that decrease shivering, such as pethidine (USA – meperidine) and phenothiazines, should not be used. In the field, mildly hypothermic patients may be allowed to walk after wet clothing is replaced with dry clothing and they have consumed adequate calories to support exercise.[16]

Treatment of patients with moderate and severe hypothermia begins with the ABCs: Airway, Breathing and Circulation. Handle patients gently to limit the risk of ventricular fibrillation. Keep the patient horizontal to avoid fluid shifts away from the core. Cut off wet clothing rather than pulling it off. Insulate the patient, including covering the head and neck to prevent further heat loss. Begin forced air re-warming if available.[17] Resuscitation rooms should be heated to 28°C.

The American Heart Association (AHA) and the European Resuscitation Council (ERC) have each published guidelines for advanced life support (ALS) with special considerations for hypothermia. Dependent lividity, apparent rigor mortis and fixed dilated pupils are not contraindications to ALS with cardiopulmonary resuscitation (CPR) in hypothermic patients. However, the axiom that 'No one is dead until they are warm and dead' is a myth. Some people are cold and dead. Contraindications to CPR include core temperature <10°C, obvious fatal injuries or obstructed airway. In patients who have been asphyxiated, including avalanche victims, serum potassium >12 mEq/L correlates with generalized cell lysis and is a contraindication to CPR.

In the field, if there is no pulse, begin CPR. Once cardiac monitoring is available, if the heart rhythm is VF or VT, one attempt should be made to defibrillate the patient. Further attempts to defibrillate can be made once the patient is re-warmed to 30°C. Patients have survived neurologically intact even after several hours of CPR.

If necessary, secure the airway with an endotracheal tube or extraglottic airway. Monitor the temperature using an oesophageal probe inserted to 15 cm. Intravenous access can be difficult. Intraosseous access or a femoral central line are usually the best means of vascular access. Central lines reaching the heart or pulmonary arteries are contraindicated.

Most hypothermic patients are volume-depleted. Initial volume replacement should use normal saline with 5% dextrose (D5NS). Lactated Ringer's solution is contraindicated because the hypothermic liver cannot metabolize lactate. All IV and IO fluids should be heated to 40–42°C to prevent further heat loss. Although many texts state that the heat content of warmed parenteral fluids is too low to be effective in re-warming, the circulating blood volume in moderate hypothermia may be only one-third normal. Giving 1–2 L can cause significant increase in core temperature.

Medications should be given intravenously or by the intraosseous route. Medications are ineffective at low temperatures due to decreased activity and increased protein binding. Medications accumulate in the bloodstream during hypothermia and may reach toxic levels during the warming process. Defer administration of medications until the core temperature is above 30°C, except for thiamine and glucose given empirically.

When environmental exposure alone cannot account for hypothermia, underlying and contributing causes should be sought. Work-up and treatment for sepsis are indicated if infection is suspected.

After initial resuscitation, re-warming[12,15,16] should begin (Table 74.4). Passive re-warming methods use heat generated by the patient. Active re-warming methods involved adding heat to the patient. Mildly hypothermic patients can be treated by passive re-warming, utilizing their own metabolism with adequate caloric intake to support shivering. They also should receive active external re-warming using warm blankets or heated forced air. Other external re-warming methods include plumbed blankets, tub bath and arteriovenous anastomosis

TABLE 74.4 Summary of Treatment Approaches. (Recommended Methods in Italics)

Active External Re-Warming	Active Core Re-Warming
Warmed blankets	*Warm IV or IO fluids* (40–42°C)
Forced air warming	*Thoracic or peritoneal lavage* 40–42°C (Thoracic lavage preferred)
Plumbed (water-filled) blankets	*Arteriovenous (AV) or Venovenous (VV)*
Tub bath (37°C)	*Extracorporeal Circulation (ECC) (Cardiopulmonary Bypass, ECMO)*
Arteriovenous Anastomosis (AVA) re-warming[a] (42–45°C)	*Open cardiac massage*. Other methods include: thoracic lavage, stomach or bladder irrigation.
Other external devices, such as the Norwegian heater	Experimental: endovascular catheter[b]
	Heated, humidified oxygen (40–42°C) (adjunctive method only)

[a]AVA Re-warming method: The lower arms and hands (distal to the elbow) and the lower legs and feet (distal to the knees) are immersed in water between 42–45°C. This opens the arteriovenous anastomosis (AVA). This method is only for use in mildly hypothermic patients.

[b]The endovascular catheter, was developed to produce therapeutic hypothermia, but shows promise for re-warming as well.

Adapted with permission from Alaska Cold Injuries Guidelines (revised 2005).

re-warming. A device, known as the Norwegian heater is useful for field re-warming. Patients with core temperatures below 32°C require active core re-warming, especially if they exhibit cardiovascular instability or have comorbid conditions.

The choice of method for active core re-warming[12,16,18] will depend on the cardiovascular status of the patient and institutional resources. Thoracic lavage and blood re-warming techniques are the most effective methods. Warm saline irrigation of the stomach and urinary bladder are ineffective.

Blood re-warming techniques include arteriovenous (AV) or venovenous (VV) re-warming, haemodialysis, extracorporeal circulation (ECC). AV or VV re-warming can be done in low-resource centres. The patient must have a systolic blood pressure ≥60 mmHg, which can be achieved using chest compressions. Patients without spontaneous circulation are likely to benefit from ECC[19] (cardiopulmonary bypass or ECMO) or open chest cardiac massage with warm saline irrigation. Fluid and electrolyte fluxes require active management during re-warming.

During re-warming, atrial arrhythmias are common and should not be treated. Coagulopathy responds to re-warming and generally does not require specific treatment. There is little potential harm in giving an empiric dose of dexamethasone 10 mg IV in patients who are not responding to re-warming. In patients who may be hypothyroid, levothyroxine 250 μg IV can be given after blood has been obtained for thyroid function tests.

PREVENTION

Shelter for homeless people, provision of warm clothing and avoidance of intoxication with alcohol or other drugs are the most helpful preventive measures. Persons who are active in outdoor environments should take measures to avoid wet clothing, including avoidance of sweating. They may want to seek shelter during wet and windy conditions, even when temperatures are moderate. Changing into dry clothes may be necessary if clothing gets wet. In temperate and tropical climates, it is important to recognize that hypothermia is possible in order to take steps to prevent it.

Drowning and Tsunamis

EPIDEMIOLOGY

The World Congress on Drowning in 2002 defined drowning as 'the process of experiencing respiratory impairment from submersion/immersion in liquid'. The term near-drowning is no longer used. Drowning may be non-fatal or cause immediate or delayed death.

Drowning kills about 500 000 people annually. About 97% of deaths occur in developing countries. Almost half of the victims are under 20 years old. This estimate does not include drowning deaths from catastrophic events such as tsunamis, transportation incidents, assaults and suicides. Accurate statistics are not available. For each drowning death, there are multiple injuries warranting hospital admission.

A tsunami is a series of waves caused by displacement of a large volume of water, typically by an earthquake or underwater volcanic eruption. Underwater landslides and explosions can also generate tsunamis. As a tsunami wave nears the shoreline, it slows down and increases in height to as high as 30 metres. Rarely, in confined areas, a tsunami wave may be as high as 500 metres (a megatsunami).

The 2004 tsunami in the Indian Ocean was generated by a magnitude 9.0 undersea earthquake. It killed at least 230 000 people in 15 countries, mostly by drowning.

PATHOGENESIS AND PATHOLOGY

Some drowning victims die rapidly due to 'immersion syndrome', which is thought to be due to a fatal dysrhythmia after exposure to cold water (<10°C). Others die as a result of 'cold shock', involuntary gasping in response to sudden immersion in cold water, causing aspiration. Long QT syndrome can cause cardiac arrest that may be precipitated by swimming. Seizure disorders or alcohol may cause altered levels of consciousness resulting in drowning.

Drowning causes death by hypoxia. In drowning victims who are rescued alive, aspiration of water causes lung injury, causing non-cardiogenic pulmonary oedema. Lung injury is augmented by contaminants in water, such as bacteria, particulate or organic matter, chemicals and vomitus.

A victim of a tsunami may drown due to sudden submersion. Injuries may cause loss of consciousness or inability to swim, resulting in drowning. Alternatively, death may be due to injury without drowning.

Survivors of tsunamis are at risk of infection from organisms in the water. After the 2004 Indian Ocean tsunami, many survivors developed 'tsunami lung', necrotizing pneumonia due to *Burkholderia pseudomallei* (melioidosis), as well as pneumonia or abscesses due to a variety of other microorganisms. Many infections were polymicrobial.[20] Skin infections, including cutaneous melioidosis, were also reported. Many infections were subacute or chronic.

CLINICAL FEATURES

The drowning victim may appear well or ill. Tachypnoea, respiratory distress or abnormal lung sounds predict lung injury, but a clear chest does not rule out aspiration. Victims should be carefully examined for trauma, including marine envenomations. Shock is uncommon in drowning and suggests illness or injury. Drowning victims may be hypothermic.

Patients who are alert or arousable on arrival at a medical facility usually survive neurologically intact. Almost half of comatose patients survive without neurological damage. The remainder survive with neurological sequelae or die from hypoxic-ischaemic brain injury or pulmonary complications. Drowning in cold water (<20°C) is associated with greater survival than drowning in warm water.[21]

Although most drownings are obvious, drowning should be suspected in any victim found near water. Differential diagnosis includes all medical and traumatic causes of altered mental status.

DIAGNOSIS

Asymptomatic drowning patients do not need any investigations, except possibly an ECG. An ECG should be obtained in all drowning victims with a sudden loss of consciousness or symptoms suggesting cardiovascular disease. Pulse oximetry and chest X-ray should be obtained in all symptomatic drowning patients. Initial chest X-ray may be normal, even in patients who later develop lung injury. Other imaging and laboratory investigations should be guided by clinical presentation and associated conditions.

MANAGEMENT AND TREATMENT

Prolonged hypoxia is the primary insult in drowning. Immediate resuscitation at the scene is critical for survival and protection against neurological injury. The European Resuscitation Council 2010 guidelines describe four phases of treatment: aquatic rescue, basic life support, advanced life support and post-resuscitation care.[22] In the aquatic rescue phase, the safety of the rescuers is the first consideration. Rapid removal of drowning victims from the water with rapid resuscitation is the next priority. Basic life support with rescue breathing can begin in the water, but chest compressions must be done with the victim on a firm surface. Victims should be removed from the water in a horizontal position to prevent circulatory collapse. Automated external fibrillation, if available, should be used once CPR is underway. Vomiting is common during resuscitation. Advanced life support follows standard guidelines.

Post-resuscitation care is largely supportive.[23,24] Therapeutic hypothermia may be helpful in comatose patients after cardiac arrest.[25] Prophylactic antibiotics are indicated only after submersion in highly contaminated water.

If there is a history of sudden loss of consciousness or an uncertain history, genetic analysis may reveal a cause of cardiac rhythm disturbances that can be used to prevent future problems in survivors or family members.[26]

Patients with symptoms prior to arrival or on arrival to a medical facility should be observed for at least 4 hours. If the chest X-ray and oxygen saturation remain normal, they may be safely discharged. Asymptomatic patients with normal oxygen saturation on arrival may be discharged safely.

PREVENTION

Many drowning incidents could be prevented by measures such as the use of personal flotation devices, swimming and water-safety awareness and training, swimming and boating regulations, avoidance of alcohol and use of lifeguards.

Tsunami warning systems with signs showing evacuation routes can decrease deaths and injuries due to tsunamis. Receding water observed at a shoreline signifies that the trough of a tsunami wave has reached land. This is referred to as a 'drawback' and may be the only warning that a tsunami is imminent. If an earthquake is near a coastal area, even the best warning system may be ineffective. If a drawback is observed or an earthquake is felt, people in coastal areas should immediately run to higher ground if possible. Upper stories of sturdy buildings may offer protection if higher ground is not available, but buildings can be swept away.

Altitude Illness in Pilgrims

BUDDHA BASNYAT

EPIDEMIOLOGY

Altitude sickness, which generally occurs >2500 metres comprises of AMS (acute mountain sickness), the benign form of the disease and the two life-threatening forms: high-altitude cerebral oedema (HACE) and high-altitude pulmonary oedema (HAPE).[27,28] The subject of altitude illness is relevant to tropical medicine because about 38 million people live permanently at altitudes >2400 metres and about 100 million travel to high altitude locations annually. Many of these high-altitude regions are in the 'tropics'. For example, all of the 8000 metre peaks (14 in total) are in South Asia.

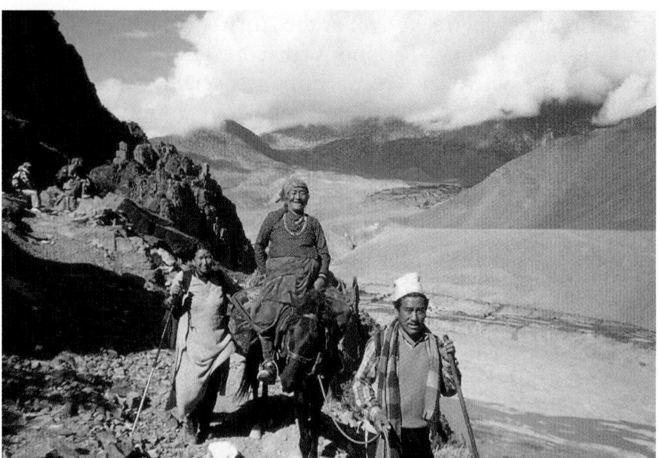

Figure 74.3 Pilgrims on their way to Mukti Nath (3710 m) in Nepal.

For many local people, these mountains at high altitude (>2500 m) are sacred sites; the abode of the gods.[29] In the Himalayan region, some of these places where pilgrims travel by foot, horseback, motor vehicle or aircraft are Damodar Kunda in the Mustang region at 4890 m; Mukti Nath (3900 m) (Figure 74.3); Kedar Nath (3584 m); Lake Tilicho (4900 m) in Manang; and Lhasa (3650 m) in Tibet. Probably the most sacred and popular high altitude site in the Himalayan region is Mount Kailash (6714 m), with the adjoining Lake Mansarovar located in Tibet.

At about 4300 metres, almost 50% of people will suffer from AMS and some (about 1–5%) who do not listen to their body and continue to ascend may suffer from the life-threatening forms, HACE and HAPE.[27,28]

Although there is an important body of literature about altitude sickness in trekkers, mountaineers and porters,[30,31] there is mostly anecdotal documentation about altitude sickness in pilgrims to high altitude. Since time immemorial, pilgrims have been travelling to high-altitude sacred sites with comorbidities like heart, lung and metabolic diseases. Many wish to seek a cure for these diseases by praying at these sacred sites. Every year, there are many 'narrow escapes' and deaths, predominantly due to altitude sickness, reported by travel agents in these pilgrim cohorts, especially among the tens of thousands that annually ascend to the region of Kailash and Mansarovar (about 5000 m) in Tibet. Pre-existing medical problems are common, as many pilgrims are elderly with diabetes, hypertension and coronary artery disease. These diseases may not per se predispose pilgrims to altitude illness, but these diseases could be worsened by the hypoxia and exertion.

Although altitude sickness is common in all sojourners at high altitude, this section will focus on pilgrims, so that attention can be drawn to the plight of this vulnerable group.

Treatment and rescue of pilgrims is more challenging because many pilgrims are fatalistic and may think that the sacred site is a good place to die. Hence, preventive measures in this group may be even more important.

The most important risk factor for altitude sickness is the rate of ascent. Many sojourners, especially pilgrims rapidly ascend to high altitude in motor vehicles, helicopters or airplanes and become predisposed to this illness. A prior history of altitude illness is also a risk factor. Exertion is a risk factor, but lack of physical fitness is not. Everyone, children and adults, men and women, are equally vulnerable to AMS. A protective factor may be sleeping at high altitude in the preceding 2 months. Being well hydrated (not overhydrated) may also be helpful at high altitude.

PATHOGENESIS

Acclimatization is the term used to describe the process by which a sojourner adapts to high altitude. With the decrease in barometric pressure with increasing altitude, hyperventilation mediated chiefly through the carotid bodies is the cornerstone of acclimatization. Hyperventilation causes respiratory alkalosis and may actually inhibit respiration, but in 2–3 days time at altitude, the kidneys excrete more bicarbonate and tend to bring the PH back to normal. However, with normal acclimatization, maximum exercise tolerance decreases at high altitude. When people climb up too high too fast without giving the body a chance to properly acclimatize, altitude sickness sets in. Other physiological changes during normal acclimatization are increased erythropoietin leading to increased haemoglobin levels and red blood cell mass, increased tissue capillary density and mitochondrial numbers and higher levels of 2-3-bisphosphoglycerate, enhancing oxygen utilization.[27,28]

Acute Mountain Sickness and High-Altitude Cerebral Oedema

Headache, nausea, fatigue, dizziness and insomnia are the nonspecific symptoms that characterize AMS. Some have described these symptoms being akin to a hangover. The differential diagnosis, especially in the pilgrim population is dehydration, as pilgrims may ascend to high altitude in a fasting state, sometimes avoiding liquids as well. Exhaustion, hypothermia, hyponatraemia are other considerations in the differential diagnosis of AMS. HACE may be a continuum of AMS with predominantly neurological features. Ataxia and altered consciousness with diffuse cerebral involvement without focal neurological signs are features of HACE, which are absent in AMS. Retinal haemorrhages are also commonly seen in sojourners at >5000 metres regardless of the presence of AMS. Features of AMS may gradually progress to HACE, but they may be rapid if ascent is continued.

The exact mechanism causing AMS or HACE is not known,[27,28] but at high altitude, there may be some vasogenic cerebral oedema, even in those without AMS and HACE. Hypoxia is the most important trigger for impaired cerebral autoregulation with altered permeability of the blood–brain barrier and increased sympathetic activity, which may play important roles in causing AMS and HACE. The most common prominent symptom of AMS is headache, which may be brought about by chemicals and mechanical factors which influence the trigeminovascular system of the brain.

High-Altitude Pulmonary Oedema

HAPE is primarily a pulmonary problem, unlike AMS and HACE, which are more neurological. HAPE usually does not develop on the first night at altitude, and that may be why in some high-altitude pilgrimage sites, we rarely encounter HAPE, as pilgrims do not spend more than a night at the site and rapidly descend the next day. HAPE develops within 2–4 days after arrival at high altitude. Excessive shortness of breath even after rest may be a sign of HAPE, which is not always accompanied by headache and nausea. Fatigue on minimal exertion is another clue for HAPE. Cough may be present but the causes of cough at high altitude are multifactorial. Hypoxaemia, which can be easily detected by a handheld pulse oximetry, is a helpful objective finding for corroboration. In the past, many pilgrims who may have died of HAPE were thought to have succumbed to pneumonia due to the cold at high altitude. The chest X-ray features of HAPE and pneumonia can be very similar.

HAPE is a non-cardiogenic oedema similar to acute respiratory distress syndrome (ARDS). Hypoxia is a powerful trigger for pulmonary hypertension, which is mandatory for the processes of HAPE to begin. At the cellular level endothelial dysfunction due to the hypoxaemia may impair the release of nitric oxide, an endothelium-derived vasodilator.[32,33] It has been shown that at high altitude, HAPE-prone persons have decreased levels of exhaled nitric oxide. The role of nitric oxide in HAPE is supported by the effectiveness of phosphodiesterase-5 inhibitors in decreasing high-altitude pulmonary hypertension.[32]

Besides hypoxia, exercise and cold temperatures-triggered increase in sympathetic drive, may also lead to pulmonary vasoconstriction and extravasation of fluid into the alveoli from the pulmonary capillaries.

Inflammation is also thought to play an important role in HAPE because of fever and peripheral leucocytes which often accompany HAPE. But numerous studies have now shown that inflammation may not be a primary problem in HAPE, except when respiratory tract infections predispose patients to HAPE.[33] Finally, impaired transepithelial clearance of sodium and water from the alveoli has also been proposed to cause HAPE. In a double-blind, randomized, placebo-controlled trial of HAPE, susceptible mountaineers, prophylactic inhalation of adrenergic agonist salmeterol (which upregulates the clearance of alveolar fluids) reduced the incidence of HAPE by 50%.[34]

PREVENTION AND TREATMENT

In general, for the prevention of altitude sickness, it is best to ascend gradually with adequate time for acclimatization (see Table 74.5). Although there is no concrete proof, it is said that above 3000 metres, a graded ascent of not more than 300–500 metres from the previous day's sleeping altitude is recommended and using every 3rd day of gain in sleeping altitude as a day of rest, is useful. However in our experience, the pilgrim population may not listen to this advice, partly for logistic reasons. Clearly an itinerary with extra days for acclimatization will help. People should be discouraged from ascending further with symptoms of altitude sickness. HAPE or HACE mandate descent.

AMS and HACE

Pharmacological prophylaxis is warranted for people with a history of AMS or when people do not ascend gradually for logistic reasons, e.g. journey by plane to a high-altitude region

TABLE 74.5 Summary of Prevention and Treatment Approaches.

Problem	Prevention	Treatment
Acute mountain sickness (AMS), mild (Mild or moderate forms are dependent on the severity of headache, nausea, fatigue, dizziness and insomnia)	Gradual ascent (see text) Adequate hydration (2–3 L/day) Acetazolamide (125–250 mg every 12 hours) In people allergic to acetazolamide, dexamethasone 4 mg every 12 hours	Discontinuation of ascent Treatment with acetazolamide (250 mg every 12 hours) Descent (No fixed altitude. Even 300–500 m descent may improve symptoms)
AMS, moderate (Mild or moderate forms are dependent on the severity of headache, nausea, fatigue, dizziness and insomnia)	As for mild AMS (see above)	Immediate descent for worsening symptoms Use of low-flow oxygen if available Treatment with acetazolamide (250 mg every 12 hours) and/or dexamethasone (4 mg every 6 hours) Hyperbaric therapy (see text)
High-altitude cerebral oedema (HACE)	As for mild AMS (see above)	Immediate descent or evacuation Administration of oxygen (2–4 L/min) Treatment with dexamethasone (8 mg PO/IM/IV; then 4 mg every 6 hours) Hyperbaric therapy (see text) if descent is not possible
High-altitude pulmonary oedema (HAPE)	Gradual ascent (see text). Adequate hydration (2–3 L/day) All of these drugs are known to work individually (see text) Nifedipine (30 mg extended release every 12 hours) Salmeterol (125 μg inhaled twice daily) Tadalafil (10 mg twice daily) Dexamethasone (8 mg twice daily)	Immediate descent or evacuation Minimization of exertion while patient is kept warm Administration of oxygen (4–6 L/min) to bring O_2 saturation to >90% Adjunctive therapy with nifedipine (30 mg, extended-release, every 12 hours) Hyperbaric therapy (see text) if descent is not possible

like Lahsa (3650 m), Tibet or La Paz (4061 m), Bolivia. For people who are not allergic to sulphas, acetazolamide (125–250 mg twice a day is adequate) is administered and continued for 3 days. Paraesthesias are well-known side-effects of acetazolamide. Dexamethasone (4 mg bd) is also effective. Gingko biloba is ineffective in the prevention of AMS.[30]

For the treatment of mild AMS, rest may be sufficient. In the face of increasing symptoms, even a descent of about 500 metres may be sufficient to relieve symptoms.

For HACE, use of dexamethasone (8 mg orally or parenterally) and prompt descent are very helpful. In a pilgrimage setting such as Kailash, where for logistical reasons immediate descent may not be possible, a simulation of descent in a portable hyperbaric chamber (Figure 74.4) is very effective. Carrying a hyperbaric chamber which weighs about 5 kg may be an important precaution for pilgrims going to remote pilgrimage sites where electricity may not be available. The use of the hyperbaric chamber and dexamethasone has been life-saving in high-altitude locales. Like nifedipine (see below), phosphodiesterase-5 inhibitors have no role in the treatment of AMS or HACE.

HAPE

Gradual ascent is the best way to prevent HAPE. Sustained-release nifedipine (30 mg) given once or twice daily prevents HAPE in people susceptible to HAPE or those who have to ascend rapidly. Dexamethasone has recently been shown to prevent HAPE,[32] but its side-effects have to be kept in mind, especially in a remote setting. Acetazolamide has been shown to blunt hypoxic pulmonary vasoconstriction,[35] and this observation warrants further study in HAPE prevention; but one study[36] failed to show a decrease in pulmonary vasoconstriction in partially acclimatized individuals who were given acetazolamide.

Almost 50% of the time HAPE is not preceded by AMS symptoms of headache and nausea, hence early recognition in detecting HAPE is important. Fatigue and dyspnoea may be the only symptoms to start with. Hyperbaric therapy as for HACE is very effective as a temporizing measure if descent and oxygen are not available. Physical exertion should be minimal and the patient needs to be kept warm. Oral sustained-release nifedipine (30 mg once or twice daily) can be used as adjunctive therapy. Inhaled beta agonists may also be useful. Although used in the prevention of HAPE, no studies have investigated phosphodiesterase inhibitors in the treatment of HAPE. Although dexamethasone may prevent HAPE, it is ineffective in treatment.

GENETICS

To date, we do not know of an altitude illness gene, but we know that there are both altitude-tolerant and altitude-sensitive

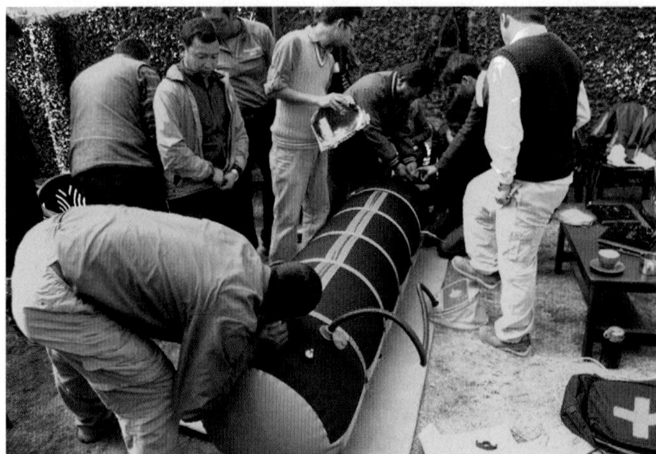

Figure 74.4 Demonstrating the easy usage of an inflated Gamow bag (a brand of hyperbaric bag), which simulates lower altitude pressure. A simple foot pedal helps to inflate the bag.

BOX 74.1 ADVICE FOR PILGRIMS TRAVELLING TO HIGH ALTITUDE

1. Pre-existing medical problems (heart and lung disease, diabetes, history of seizures, strokes, etc.) need to be carefully addressed by a physician experienced in high-altitude medicine prior to departure.
2. Useful travel vaccinations including influenza vaccine should be administered prior to departure.
3. Sojourners should be advised to drink adequate amount of fluids at high altitude (2–3 L/day).
4. Awareness of the clinical symptoms and signs of altitude illness including the importance of descent needs to be emphasized.
5. The usage of acetazolamide and its side-effects need to be explained.
6. If a health professional is travelling with the group, a medical kit which includes acetazolamide, dexamethasone, nifedipine should be included in addition to a hyperbaric chamber.
7. If travellers have health problems, a concise, legible summary of their illness including the generic names of all the drugs needs to be on their person.

individuals, and traditional physiological explanations appear inadequate to explain this difference, hence this is one of the reasons for the ongoing interest in altitude illness genes. Gene polymorphism has been implicated in HAPE, but the data are unclear at present. Although angiotensin-converting enzyme gene polymorphism appears to confer a performance advantage at high altitude, an association with susceptibility to HAPE is lacking.

While studying high-altitude natives, one of the most striking recent findings[37] has been the difference in the frequency of the gene EPAS1, which codes for HIF-2a, a transcriptional regulator that plays a role in the host of responses to hypoxia including erythropoiesis, angiogenesis, carotid body function, anaerobic metabolism and energy metabolism. In one study, the frequency of one variant of the EPAS1 gene differed between Tibetans and Han Chinese by 78%. It is well known that Tibetans have adapted well to altitude compared with the Han Chinese. Another important gene (EGLN1) described by Indian scientists[38] may play an important role in high-altitude hypoxic adaptation in accordance with Ayurvedic concepts. Finally, suggestions for pilgrims ascending to high altitude are summarized in Box 74.1.

REFERENCES

3. Khosla R, Guntupalli KK. Heat-related illnesses. Crit Care Clin 1999;15(2):251–63.
4. Bouchama A, Knochel JP. Heat stroke. N Engl J Med 2002;346:1978–88.
5. Platt M, Vicario S. Heat illness. In: Marx J, Hockberger R, Walls R, editors. Rosen's Emergency Medicine. 7th ed. Philadelphia: Mosby; 2009. p. 1882–92.
13. Danzl DF, Pozos RS. Accidental hypothermia. N Engl J Med 1994;331(26):1756–60.
16. Copass M, Nemiroff MJ, Bowman WD, et al. State of Alaska Cold Injuries Guidelines. Juneau: Section of Community Health and EMS; 2005.
37. Beall CM, Cavalleri GL, Elston RC, et al. Natural selection of EPAS1 (HIF2alpha) associated with low hemoglobin concentration in Tibetan highlanders. Proc Natl Acad Sci 2010;107(25): 11459–64.

Access the complete references online at www.expertconsult.com

75 Venomous and Poisonous Animals

DAVID A. WARRELL

KEY POINTS

- Envenomings and poisonings with animal toxins are unusual medical emergencies in most Western temperate countries but, especially in rural areas of tropical developing countries, they may be a common occupational and environmental hazard.
- Snakebites kill over 100 000 people each year, many of them children. In India, a well-designed national survey discovered 46 000 deaths in 1 year. Survivors of snakebites may be left with permanent physical handicap, mainly as a result of necrosis of the bitten part.
- Scorpion stings and anaphylactic deaths in people hypersensitized to Hymenoptera (bees, wasps and ants) venoms account for several thousand deaths each year. In some countries, they cause more deaths than snakebites.
- Antidotes to envenoming are antivenoms, refined plasma from horses or sheep that have been hyperimmunized with selected venoms. They are effective in reversing snake venom-induced anti-haemostatis, shock and post-synaptic neurotoxicity and, if given early, may prevent local necrosis, pre-synaptic neurotoxicity and rhabdomyolysis. They cause many early anaphylactic and pyrogenic and late serum sickness-type reactions, are expensive, in short supply and have a limited shelf-life.
- Marine poisoning from fish and shellfish is prevalent and endemic among populations of many oceanic islands but occurs sporadically even in Western temperate countries. Ciguatera fish poisoning may cause persisting morbidity but has a low case fatality.

Introduction

Venoms are complex mixtures of proteins, polypeptides and other molecules that exert toxic, irritant or allergic properties when injected into prey or squirted at enemies. Some poisonous and venomous animals are distinctively (aposematically) coloured, conferring protection both on their own species and on other harmless species that mimic their appearance or behaviour (Batesian or Müllerian mimicry). Venoms or poisons secreted on to the skin of some amphibians protect their moist respiratory integument against infection and are distasteful, poisonous and therefore a deterrent to predators. Animals have evolved various methods of injecting venom. Mammals (e.g. monotremes, Insectivora and vampire bats), snakes, lizards, spiders, ticks, leeches and octopuses inject their venoms by biting with teeth, fangs, venom jaws, beaks or other hardened mouth parts; centipedes sting with a pair of modified claws (forcipules) on the post-cephalic segment; male duck-billed platypuses are armed with venom-injecting spurs; fish, cnidarians (coelenterates), echinoderms, cone shells, insects and scorpions have different kinds of stinging apparatus. Some snakes, toads, scorpions and other arthropods can squirt their venom at enemies. Poisoning results from the ingestion of toxins from the skin of amphibians or the flesh and viscera of aquatic animals. Allergic reactions to injected venoms (e.g. of Hymenoptera: bee, wasp and ant venoms – and cnidarians) are in some cases far more frequent and life-threatening than their direct toxic effects and recurrent ciguatera fish poisoning may be associated with hypersensitivity.[1,2]

VENOMOUS MAMMALS

Bisonalveus browni, an extinct Palaeocene mammal, possessed grooved canines suggesting that it might have been venomous, although some non-venomous animals have similar teeth.[3] Several extant mammals are venomous.[4] Male duck-billed platypuses (*Ornithorhynchus anatinus*), aquatic egg-laying mammals (Family Ornithorhynchidae, Order Monotrema) of eastern Australia, can sting one another when fighting. They have venomous spurs on their hind limbs fed by venom glands on the thighs.[5] The venom contains C-type natriuretic peptides, defensin-like peptides, nerve growth factor, an L-to-D-peptide isomerase, hyaluronidase and proteases. The venom gland transcriptome contains 83 novel putative platypus venom genes from 13 toxin families homologous to known toxins from fish, reptiles, insectivores, spiders, sea anemones and starfish.[6] Only 17 stings have been recorded in the last 100 years. They cause agonizing local pain, persistent local swelling and inflammation with regional lymphadenopathy but are neither necrotic nor life-threatening. Persistent local weakness, stiffness and muscle wasting have been reported. In experimental animals, the venom causes haemolysis, coagulopathy, local haemorrhage, oedema and fatal hypotension.[5]

Haitian (*Solenodon paradoxus*) and Cuban (*S.* [*Atopogale*] *cubanus*) solenodons, the European water shrew (*Neomys fodiens*), Mediterranean shrew (*N. anomalous*) and short-tailed shrews of the eastern USA and Canada (*Blarina brevicauda*, *B. hylophaga*, *B. carolinensis*, Order Insectivora) secrete venomous saliva from enlarged, granular submaxillary salivary glands that discharge at the base of the grooved lower incisors. Their venom immobilizes invertebrate, amphibian or rodent prey and may be used, lethally, in internecine fights. *Blarina brevicauda* venom is lethal to rodents, lagomorphs and cats but in humans, bites cause only local burning pain, swelling and inflammation.

While vampire bats (Order Chiroptera, Desmodontinae) are taking their blood meal, salivary toxins promote blood flow by inhibiting platelet aggregation and activated factors X and IX and by activating plasminogen of the animal on which they are feeding.

Brachial glands of slow lorises (*Nycticebus coucang*) (Family Lorisidae, Order Primates) secrete a toxin that resembles Fel d 1 cat allergen. They lick it up and inject it when they bite, causing pain, swelling, tissue damage, infection and anaphylaxis.

VENOMOUS SNAKES

Taxonomy, Identification and Distribution

Of the 3346 species of snakes, 667 belong to the three families of venomous snakes: Lamprophiidae subfamily Atractaspidinae (burrowing asps); Elapidae (cobras, kraits, mambas, coral snakes, sea snakes, etc.) and Viperidae (old world and pit vipers).[7] Only about 200 species have caused death or permanent disability by biting humans.[8] The largest family, Colubridae, includes 1748 species of which 100 are capable of producing mild envenoming in humans, but only a few have caused fatalities.[9]

The giant constrictors (family Boidae) are potentially dangerous to man. There are reliable reports of fatal attacks by South-east Asian (especially Indonesian) reticulated pythons (*Python reticulatus*), African rock pythons (*Python sebae*), South American anacondas (*Eunectes murinus*) and an Australian scrub python (*Morelia amethistina*). Some of the victims were swallowed.

Snake Taxonomy. Snakes are classified according to morphological characteristics (numbers and arrangement of their scales – lepidosis, dentition, osteology, myology, sensory organs, the form of the hemipenes) and, increasingly, by sequence analysis of DNA encoding important mitochondrial and other enzymes.[10–12]

Snake-like Animals. Legless lizards, such as slow worms, glass lizards (family Anguidae), worm-like geckos (family Pygopodidae) and legless skinks, may be distinguished from snakes by their external ears, eyelids (in some cases), fleshy tongues, long friable tails and by the lack of enlarged ventral scales. Some lizards have vestigial limbs. Amphisbaenid lizards have worm-like annular grooves along the length of their bodies and caecilians (legless amphibians) lack obvious eyes and scales. Eels (order Anguilliformes), especially snake eels (family Ophichthidae), and pipe-shaped fish must be distinguished from snakes by their gills and in most cases their fins.

Medically Important Snakes. Medically important snakes possess enlarged grooved or cannulated teeth (fangs) in their upper jaws through which venom is injected into prey or human victims. About 400 species of *Colubridae* have short, immobile opisthoglyphous (posteriorly placed) fangs or enlarged solid aglyphous (lacking groove or canal) teeth at the posterior end of the maxilla (Figure 75.1). The African and Middle Eastern burrowing asps or stiletto snakes (genus *Atractaspis*, subfamily *Atractaspidinae*), also known as burrowing or mole vipers or adders, false vipers, side-stabbing or stiletto snakes, have very long solenoglyphous (hinged erectile) front fangs on which they impale their victims by a side-swiping motion, the fang protruding from the corner of the partially closed mouth (Figure 75.2). The *Elapidae* (cobras – *Naja*; kraits – *Bungarus*; mambas – *Dendroaspis*; shield-nosed snakes – *Aspidelaps*; Asian and American coral snakes – *Calliophis, Maticora, Sinomicrurus, Micrurus*; African garter snakes – *Elapsoidea*; terrestrial venomous Australasian snakes and sea snakes) have relatively short, fixed proteroglyphous (fixed erect) front fangs (Figure 75.3). The *Viperidae* (vipers, adders, rattlesnakes, moccasins, lance-headed vipers and pit vipers) have long, curved, hinged, solenoglyphous (hinged erectile) front fangs containing a closed venom channel (Figure 75.4). The subfamily *Crotalinae* (pit vipers) includes rattlesnakes (genera *Crotalus* and *Sistrurus*), moccasins (*Agkistrodon*) and lance-headed vipers (genera *Bothrops, Bothriechis, Porthidium, Lachesis*, etc.) of the Americas and the Asian pit vipers (genera *Gloydius/Agkistrodon, Deinagkistrodon, Calloselasma, Hypnale, Trimeresurus* – now divided into several different genera including *Cryptelytrops, Himalayophis, Parias, Peltopelor, Popeia, Protobothrops, Viridovipera*).[12]

The pit of crotaline snakes is an infrared/heat-sensitive organ, situated between the eye and nostril, which detects

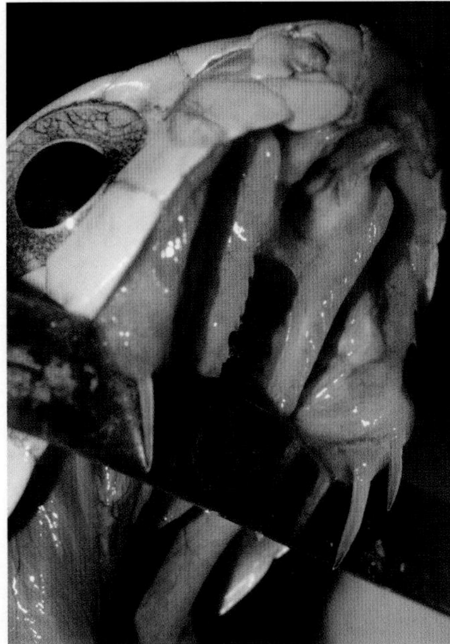

Figure 75.1 Rear fangs of the boomslang (*Dispholidus typus*: family Colubridae). Specimen at Bio-Ken, Watamu, Kenya. *(Copyright D. A. Warrell.)*

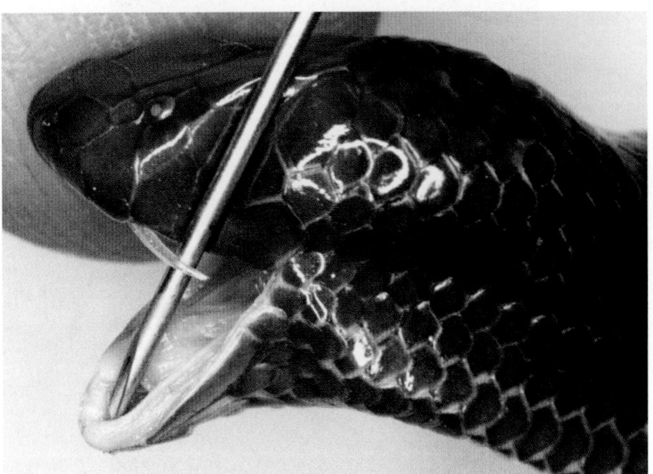

Figure 75.2 Very long front fang of a West African burrowing asp (*Atractaspis aterrima*: subfamily Atractaspidinae). Specimen from Zaria, Nigeria *(Copyright D. A. Warrell.)*

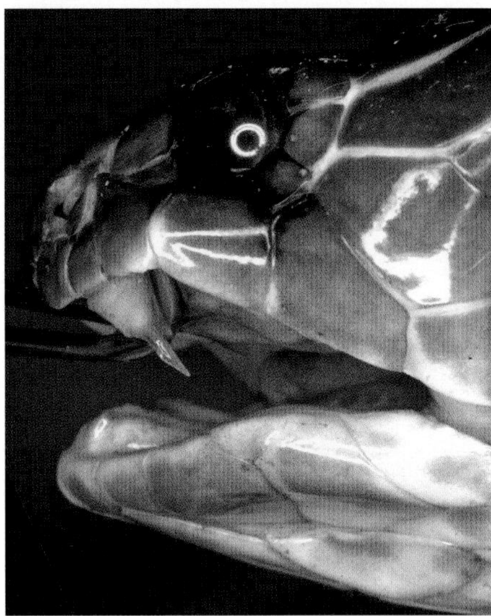

Figure 75.3 Short front fangs of the Indian spectacled cobra (*Naja naja*: family Elapidae). Specimen from Anuradhapura, Sri Lanka *(Copyright D. A. Warrell.)*

warm-blooded prey (Figure 75.5A).[13] Snakes of the subfamily Viperinae, the Old World vipers and adders, lack this pit organ (Figure 75.5B). The words viper (strictly a snake producing live young – ovoviviparous) and adder (laying eggs) are not used rigorously.

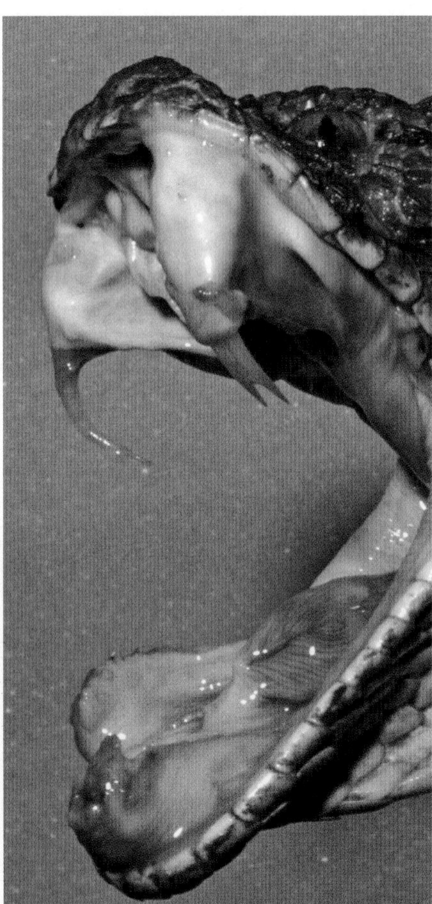

Figure 75.4 Long hinged front fangs of the puff adder (*Bitis arietans*: family Viperidae; subfamily Viperinae). Specimen from Garki, Nigeria *(Copyright D. A. Warrell.)*

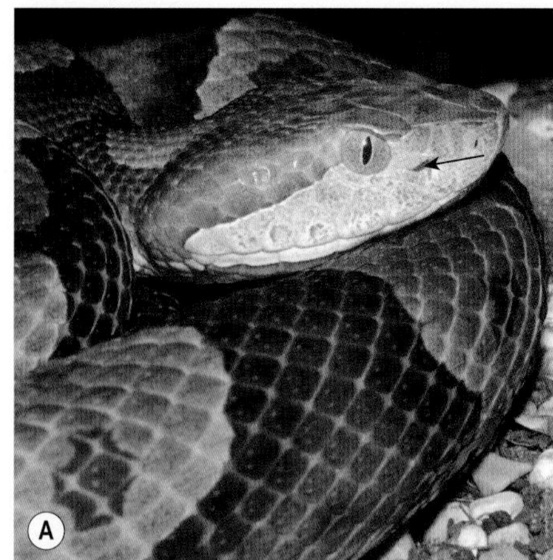

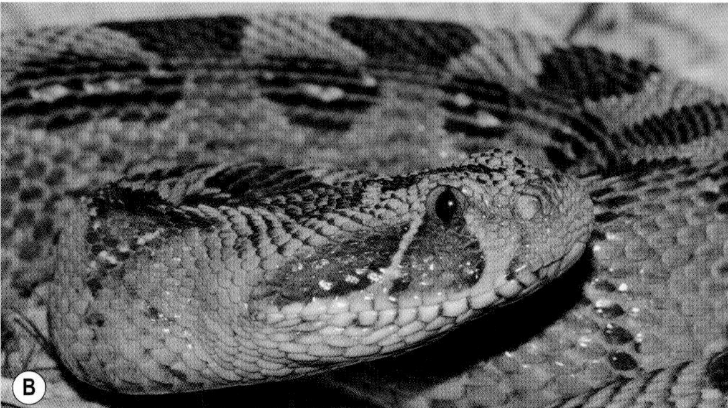

Figure 75.5 (A) North American copper head (*Agkistrodon contortrix*: family Viperidae; subfamily Crotalinae), a typical pit-viper showing heat-sensitive pit (arrow). (B) Ethiopian mountain viper (*Bitis parviocula*; family Viperidae; subfamily Viperinae), a typical Old World viper *(A,B, Copyright D. A. Warrell.)*

Snake Identification. There is no simple and entirely reliable method for distinguishing venomous from non-venomous snakes. The shaft of a needle passed forward along the maxilla from the angle of the jaw may engage upon and reveal the fangs but these may be very small in elapids and folded back inside a sheath in vipers. The characteristic hood of cobras and some other elapids is erected only when the snake is rearing up in a defensive attitude (Figure 75.6). Vipers may be identifiable by a colourful and sometimes distinctive dorsal pattern (Figure 75.7). Russell's vipers (*Daboia russelii* and *D. siamensis*) and puff adders (*Bitis arietans*) make a loud hissing sound by expelling air through their large nostrils; the saw-scaled or carpet vipers (genus *Echis*), lowland viper (*Proatheris superciliaris*) and desert horned vipers (*Cerastes*) produce a characteristic rasping sound by rubbing their coils together (Figure 75.8); rattlesnakes produce an unmistakable sound like castanets. Some harmless snakes are easily mistaken for the venomous species that they mimic, e.g. *Telescopus* (cat snakes) and *Dasypeltis* (egg-eating snakes) resemble *Echis* (saw-scaled vipers) in Africa; *Boiga multomaculata* resembles *Daboia siamensis* in Thailand; *Dryocalamus*, *Dinodon* and *Lycodon* species resemble kraits in South Asia; *Xenodon* species resemble *Bothrops* species in the Amazon region and the colourful venomous coral snakes (*Micruroides*, *Micrurus*) of the Western Hemisphere have many non-venomous mimics. The adage 'red on yellow kills a fellow, red on black venom lack' distinguishes corals from their mimics only in North America (Figure 75.9). Table 75.1 lists the species

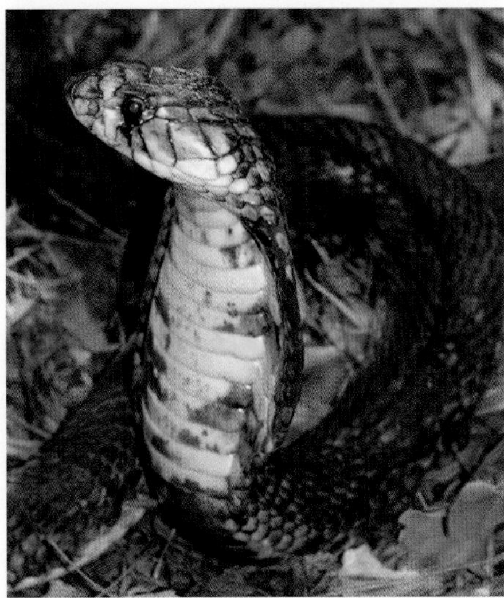

Figure 75.6 Egyptian cobra (*Naja haje*: family Elapidae), showing spread hood in threatening/defensive attitude. Specimen at Bio-Ken, Watamu, Kenya. *(Copyright D. A. Warrell.)*

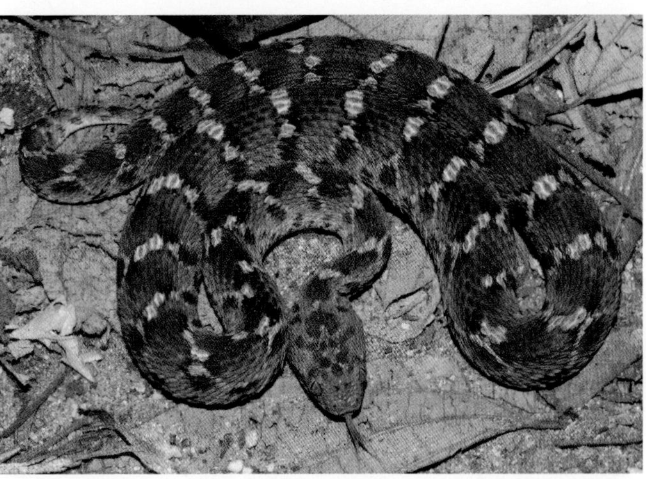

Figure 75.8 East African saw-scaled viper (*Echis pyramidum*) coiling to produce a rasping sound. Specimen from Baringo at Bio-Ken, Watamu, Kenya. *(Copyright D. A. Warrell.)*

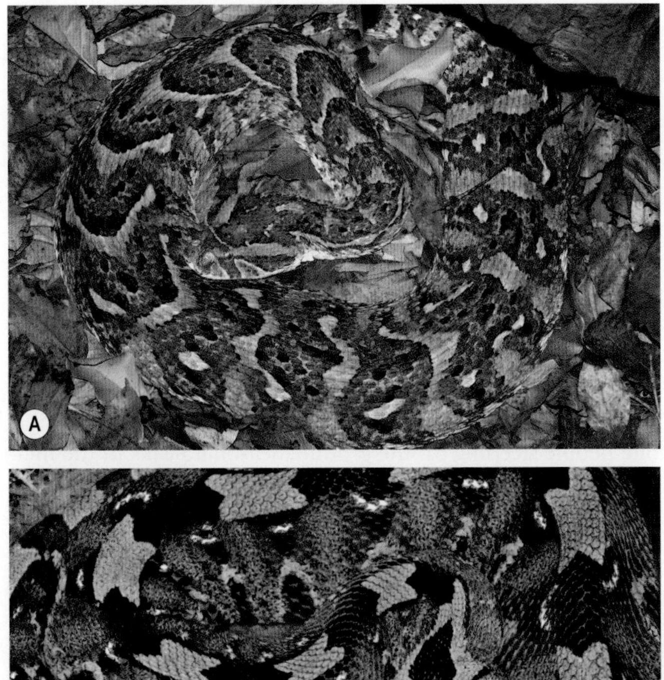

Figure 75.7 (A) Puff adder of the African savanna (*Bitis arietans*), showing distinctive repeated 'V' or 'U' dorsal pattern. Specimen at Bio-Ken, Watamu, Kenya. (B) Rhinoceros or nose-horned viper of the African rain forest (*Bitis nasicornis*) showing distinctive repeated dorsal pattern. *(A,B, Copyright D.A. Warrell)*

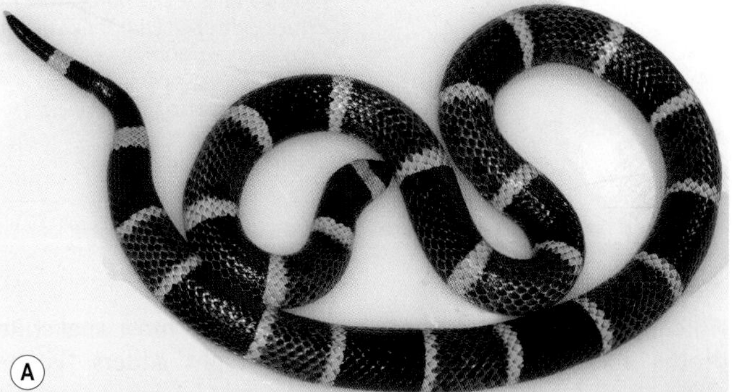

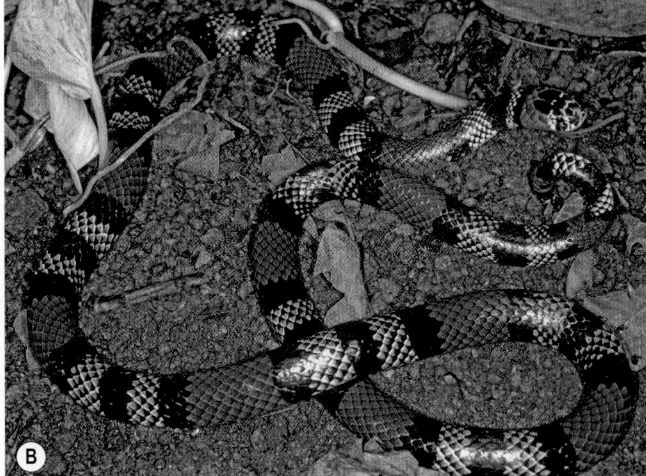

Figure 75.9 (A) Texas coral snake (*Micrurus tener*). Specimen from Kingsville. (B) South American coral snake (*Micrurus frontalis*: family Elapidae). Specimen from Brazil. *(A,B, Copyright D. A.Warrell.)*

TABLE 75.1 Species of Snake Responsible for Most Human Snakebite Deaths and Morbidity

Area	Scientific Name	Common Name
North America	*Crotalus adamanteus*	Eastern diamondback rattlesnake
	Crotalus atrox	Western diamondback rattlesnake
	Crotalus oreganus and *Crotalus helleri*	Western rattlesnakes
Central America	*Crotalus simus* subsp.	Central American rattlesnakes
	Bothrops asper	Terciopelo
South America	*Bothrops atrox, B. asper*	Fer-de-lance, barba amarilla
	Bothrops jararaca	Jararaca
	Crotalus durissus subsp.	South American rattlesnakes, cascabel
Europe	*Vipera berus, V. aspis*	Vipers, adders
	Vipera ammodytes	Long-nosed or nose-horned viper
Africa	*Echis ocellatus, E. leucogaster, E. pyramidum, E. jogeri*	Saw-scaled or carpet vipers
	Bitis arietans	Puff adders
	Naja nigricollis, N. mossambica, etc.	African spitting cobras
	Naja haje	Egyptian cobra
Asia, Middle East	*Echis* spp.	Saw-scaled or carpet vipers
	Macrovipera lebetina	Levantine viper
	Daboia palaestinae	Palestine viper
	Naja oxiana	Oxus cobra
Indian subcontinent and South-east Asia	*Naja naja, N. kaouthia, N. siamensis*, etc.	Asian cobras
	Bungarus spp.	Kraits
	Daboia russelii, D. siamensis	Russell's vipers
	Calloselasma rhodostoma	Malayan pit viper
	Echis carinatus	Saw-scaled or carpet viper
Far East	*Naja atra* etc.	Asian cobras
	Bungarus multicinctus	Chinese krait
	Protobothrops (Trimeresurus) flavoviridis	Japanese habu
	Protobothrops (Trimeresurus) mucrosquamatus	Chinese habu
	Gloydius blomhoffii, G. brevicaudus	Mamushis
Australasia, New Guinea	*Acanthophis* spp.	Death adders
	Pseudonaja spp.	Brown snakes
	Notechis spp.	Tiger snakes
	Oxyuranus scutellatus	Taipan

which, in each continent, are responsible for most snakebite deaths and severe morbidity. African night adders (genus *Causus*) and burrowing asps (Atractaspis), Asian green pit vipers (genus *Trimeresurus* sensu lato), North American copperheads (*Agkistrodon contortrix*) and Latin American hog-nosed vipers (e.g. *Porthidium* species) bite many people but rarely cause severe envenoming. Electronic images of snakes responsible for bites may be sent, for example by mobile phone, to expert herpetologists for identification.

Distribution of Venomous Snakes. Venomous snakes are widely distributed (Figure 75.10) from sea level to altitudes of 4000 m (*Gloydius himalayanus*). European adders (*Vipera berus*) are found inside the Arctic Circle but no other venomous species occurs in cold regions such as the Arctic, Antarctic and north of about latitude 51°N in North America (Newfoundland, Nova Scotia). There are no venomous snakes in the islands of Crete, Ireland and Iceland, in the western Mediterranean, Atlantic and Caribbean (except for Martinique, Santa Lucia, Margarita, Trinidad and Aruba), New Caledonia, New Zealand, Hawaii and elsewhere in the Pacific. Madagascar and Chile have only mildly venomous colubrid snakes. Sea snakes, sometimes in vast numbers, occur in the Indian and Pacific Oceans between latitudes 30°N and 30°S, as far north as Siberia (*Pelamis platura*) and as far south as Easter Island and the North Island of New Zealand and in estuaries, rivers and some freshwater lakes (e.g. *Hydrophis semperi* in Lake Taal, Philippines; *Enhydrina schistosa* in Ton Ley Sap, Cambodia).

Epidemiology of Snakebite (Table 75.2)

Most snakebites are inflicted on the lower limbs of agricultural workers and their children in rural areas of tropical developing countries. Asian kraits (*Bungarus* spp.) and African spitting cobras (*N. nigricollis*) enter human dwellings at night and may bite people sleeping on the ground. Seasonal peaks in the incidence of snakebite are associated with rainfall and increased agricultural activities. Floods have caused epidemics of

TABLE 75.2 Determinants of Snakebite Incidence and Severity of Envenoming

Incidence of Bites	Severity of Envenoming
1. Frequency of contact between snakes and humans, depends on: (a) Population densities (b) Diurnal and seasonal variations in activity (c) Types of behaviour (e.g. human agricultural activities) 2. Snakes' 'irritability' – readiness to strike when alarmed or provoked – varies with species	1. Dose of venom injected – depends on mechanical efficiency of bite and species and size of snake 2. Composition and hence potency of venom – depends on species and, within a species, the geographical location, season and age of the snake 3. Health, age, size and (?) specific immunity of human victim 4. Nature and timings of first aid and medical treatment

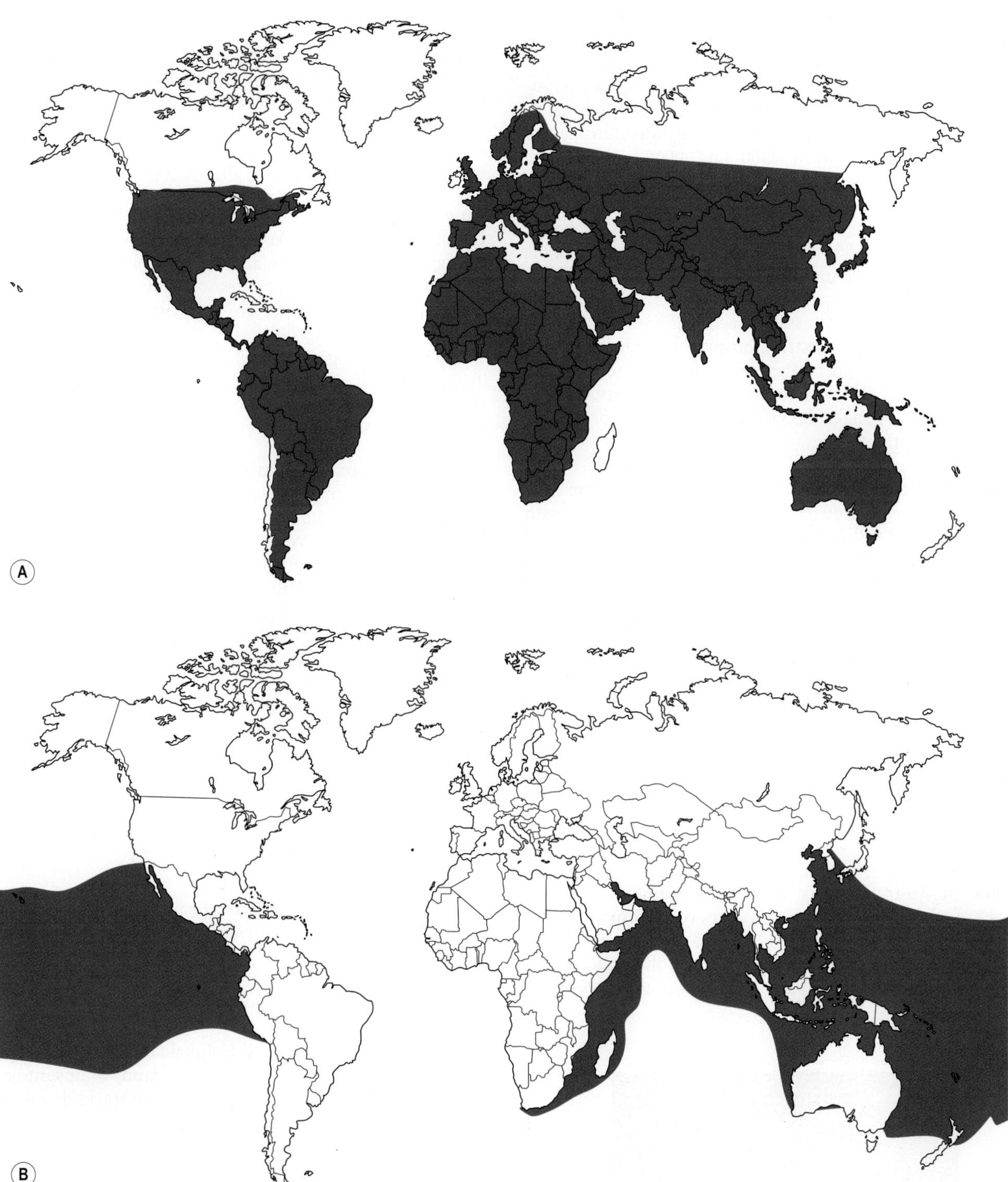

Figure 75.10 (A) Distribution of venomous terrestrial snakes. (B) Distribution of venomous sea snakes. *(A,B Copyright D. A. Warrell.)*

snakebite in Bangladesh, Nepal, Burma, Vietnam, Pakistan, India and Colombia. In tropical developing countries, most snakebite victims seek traditional treatment and so evade hospital records, the main source of snakebite reporting. Properly designed community surveys, assessing randomly selected households, give the most accurate picture of the incidence of snakebite in the area surveyed. However, the results cannot be extrapolated to provide national incidences because of wide heterogeneity within countries.

Asia. In India, 46 000 people (99% CI 41 000–51 000) die from snakebite each year, a figure based on verbal autopsy of all deaths in 6671 randomly chosen sample areas (average population ~1000 each) throughout the whole country.[14] Snakebite was responsible for 0.5% of all deaths, 3% in the age group 5–14 years; 97% of the victims died in rural areas, only 23% in a health facility.[14] A cross-sectional study in Bangladesh estimated 590 000 bites with 6000 deaths in one year.[15] The highest recorded focal incidence in Asia is 162 deaths per 100 000 population per year in the Eastern Terai of Nepal, where only 20% of the deaths occurred in hospitals. Being bitten inside the house while resting between 2400 and 0060 h carried an increased risk of fatality, suggesting bites by kraits.[16] Other risk factors were an initial visit to a traditional healer and delayed transport to hospital. In Burma, mortality from snakebite exceeds 1000 (3.3 per 100 000) per year. Russell's viper (*Daboia siamensis*) bite was once the fifth most important single cause of all deaths. In Sri Lanka, there are about 37 000 snakebite admissions to government hospitals each year with 80 fatalities. However, in Monaragala District, hospital records underestimated by 63% the number of snakebite fatalities reported by death certification.[17] This discrepancy was partly explained by the fact that 36% of snakebite victims did not seek or achieve hospital treatment.

Africa. In the Benue Valley of north-eastern Nigeria, the incidence of snakebites was 497/100 000 population per year, with a mortality of 12.2%.[18] Most bites and deaths were attributed to saw-scaled vipers (*Echis ocellatus*). In Bandafassi, south-east Senegal, in a population of 10 509, snakebite mortality was 14 per 100 000 per year. Saw-scaled vipers (*E. ocellatus*), puff adders (*Bitis arietans*) and spitting cobras (*Naja katiensis*) were implicated.[19]A community survey of snakebites by the black-necked spitting cobra (*N. nigricollis*) in Malumfashi, northern Nigeria, found that in a population of 43 500 there were 15–20 bites/100 000 per year. Only 8.5% of the victims had visited a hospital. The case fatality was 5%, and 19% of survivors had persistent physical disability from the locally necrotic effects of the venom.[20] A community-based study in the coast in Kilifi district, Kenya, discovered 15 adult snakebite fatalities per 100 000 population per year.[21]

Oceania. In Australia, there are 1000–2000 bites, with an average of three to four deaths, per year. Brown snakes (*Pseudonaja* species; Figure 75.11) are the most important. In the Central Province of Papua New Guinea, the incidence of bites, mainly by Papuan Taipans (*Oxyuranus scutellatus*) was 215, and of deaths 7.9/100 000 population per year, while in Kairuku subprovince there were 526 bites per 100 000 per year.[22]

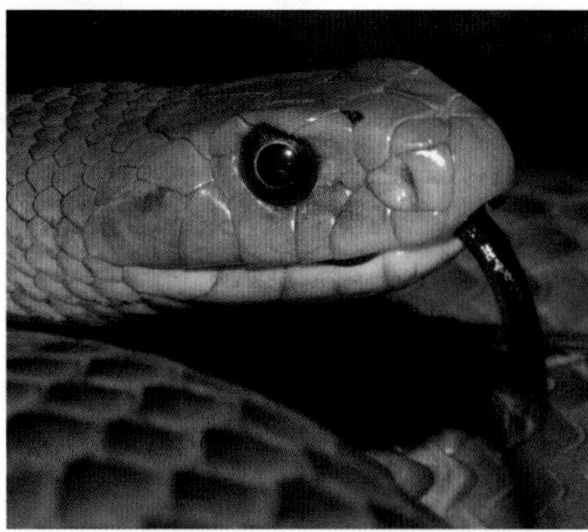

Figure 75.11 Australian Eastern brown snake (*Pseudonaja textilis*: family Elapidae). Specimen from Ballarat, Victoria. (*Copyright D. A. Warrell.*)

Europe. In Britain, there are an estimated 100 hospital admissions for adder (*Vipera berus*) bites each year, but there have been only 14 deaths during the last hundred years, the last in 1975.[23] There were 44 deaths caused by this species in Sweden between 1911 and 1978; and, in Finland, 21 deaths in 25 years, with an annual incidence of almost 200 bites.

Americas. Snakebite is common in Latin America.[24] In Brazil, the case fatality of snakebites in the pre-antivenom era was thought to be about 25%, and the total number of bites 19 200 each year. By 2005, 28 711 bites were reported with 114 deaths (0.4 %). In the USA there are 7000 bites by venomous snakes each year, with 12–15 deaths.

Some hunter–gatherer tribes are at high risk of snakebite. Two per cent of adult deaths among the Yanomamo of Venezuela, 5% among the Waorani of Ecuador and 24% among adult Kaxinawa of Acre, Brazil, were attributed to snakebites.[25]

Snakebite as an Occupational Disease. Farmers, especially rice farmers, plantation workers, herders and hunters are at high risk of snakebite in many tropical developing countries.[26] In the savannah of West Africa, farmers are bitten by *Echis* species as they dig the fields at the start of the rainy season.[18] Rubber-tappers in South-east Asia are bitten by Malayan pit vipers (*Calloselasma rhodostoma*) as they make their early morning rounds of the rubber trees in the dark. In the jungles of western Brazil, collectors of natural rubber ('seringueiros') are bitten by *Bothrops atrox*.[25]

When hand nets were widely used throughout South-east Asia,[27,28] sea snakebites were an occupational hazard of fishermen but are now uncommon because snakes caught in drift or trawl fishing nets are drowned before they are landed.

Bites by Exotic Pet Snakes. In Western countries, venomous snakes are increasingly popular as exotic or 'macho' pets. Many are kept illegally.[29]

Bites Inflicted on Sleepers. Kraits, in India,[30] Sri Lanka,[31] Nepal,[16] Thailand and Malaysia,[32] and African spitting cobras,[33] enter human dwellings at night in pursuit of their prey (rodents, lizards, toads) and may strike at people who move in their sleep.

Venom Apparatus[34]

Colubridae. In back-fanged Colubridae, the posterior part of the superior labial gland (Duvernoy's gland) drains into a peri-odontal fold of buccal mucosa. The venom tracks down grooves in the anterior surfaces of the several enlarged posteriorly situated fangs (Figure 75.1).[9] Human envenoming is uncommon, as the snake must seize and chew the finger of its victim, often a herpetologist, in order to inject enough venom to cause symptoms.

Atractaspidinae. The long fangs of *Atractaspis* species are protruded out of the corner of the mouth to allow a side-swiping strike at their prey encountered underground in a burrow (Figure 75.2).

Elapidae (Including Sea Snakes) and Viperidae. The venom glands are surrounded by muscles in Elapidae (*adductor superficialis*) and Viperidae (*compressor glandulae*) allowing venom to be squeezed through the venom duct to the base of the fang.

Venom is transmitted to the tip of the fang through a partially or completely closed canal. In African spitting cobras and the ringhals or rinkhals (*Hemachatus haemachatus*) and Asian spitting cobras, the fang is modified to allow the snake to eject a spray of venom forwards for a metre or more, into the eyes of an aggressor.[35–37]

Venomous Snakebite without Envenoming ('Dry Bites'). Between about 10% (in the case of *Echis ocellatus*)[38] and 80% (Australian eastern brown snake, *Pseudonaja textilis*)[39] of people bitten by venomous snakes, with puncture marks confirming that the fangs penetrated the skin, develop no signs of envenoming.

Venom Composition[40,41]

Snakes have evolved the most complex of all venoms, each containing more than 100 different components.[42,43] The variation in venom composition between species and within a single species throughout its geographical distribution, at different seasons of the year and as a result of ageing, contributes to the clinical diversity and unpredictability of snakebite. More than 90% of the dry weight is protein, comprising a variety of enzymes, non-enzymatic polypeptide toxins and non-toxic proteins such as nerve growth factor and cobra venom factor. Non-protein ingredients include carbohydrates and metals (often part of glycoprotein metalloprotein enzymes), lipids, free amino acids, nucleosides and biogenic amines such as serotonin (5-hydroxytryptamine) and acetylcholine.

Enzymes. Approximately 89–95% of viperid and 25–70% of elapid venoms consist of enzymes (molecular weight 13–15 kDa), including digestive hydrolases, hyaluronidase, and activators or inactivators of the prey's physiological mechanisms. Most venoms contain L-amino acid oxidase, phosphomono- and di-esterases, 5′-nucleotidase, DNA-ase, NAD-nucleosidase, phospholipase A_2 and peptidases. Elapid venoms, in addition, contain acetylcholine esterase, phospholipase B and glycerophosphatase, while viperid venoms have endopeptidase, arginine ester hydrolase kininogenase which releases bradykinin from bradykininogen, oligopeptide ACE-inhibitors/bradykinin-potentiating peptides, thrombin-like serine proteases, and factor X- and prothrombin-activating enzymes. Phospholipases A_2 are the most widespread venom enzymes. They damage mitochondria, red blood cells, leukocytes, platelets, peripheral nerve endings, skeletal muscle, vascular endothelium and other membranes, produce presynaptic neurotoxic activity, opiate-like sedative effects and the autopharmacological release of histamine. Hyaluronidase promotes the spread of venom through tissues. Proteolytic enzymes (endopeptidases or hydrolases) are responsible for local changes in vascular permeability leading to oedema, blistering and bruising, and to necrosis. Metalloproteinases cause local and systemic haemorrhage and local myonecrosis, blistering and oedema through their actions on vascular endothelium, platelets,[44,45] muscle and other tissues.

Neurotoxins. Polypeptide toxins are low-molecular-weight, non-enzymatic proteins found almost exclusively in elapid venoms. Post-synaptic (curaremimetic) neurotoxins, or α-neurotoxins, such as α-bungarotoxin and cobrotoxin bind to nicotinic acetylcholine receptors at the motor end-plates of skeletal muscles, causing generalized flaccid paralysis and death from bulbar and respiratory muscle weakness. They have a distinctive 'three-finger' structure, complementary in shape to their receptor, and have also been found in some colubrid venoms.[46] Presynaptic phospholipases A_2, or β-neurotoxins, such as β-bungarotoxin, crotoxin and taipoxin, contain a phospholipase A subunit. These damage nerve endings at neuromuscular junctions, targeting voltage-gated potassium channels and causing sequential suppression, enhancement and finally complete failure of acetylcholine release. Clinical effects are similar to those caused by postsynaptic toxins except that the latter may be ameliorated rapidly by specific antivenoms and anticholinesterase drugs. Some of the neurotoxic phospholipases A_2 and other phospholipases have myotoxic activity. Mamba (*Dendroaspis*) venoms contain unusual neurotoxins.[40,41] Dendrotoxins bind to voltage-gated potassium channels at nerve endings, causing acetylcholine release, and calcicludine blocks calcium channels. Two 'three-finger' neurotoxins are unique to mamba venoms. Fasciculins inhibit some acetylcholinesterases, causing persistent muscle fasciculations, while calciseptine binds to calcium channels. Krait venom toxins are important tools for experimental neuropharmacologists: presynaptic phospholipases A_2, β-bungarotoxins; and postsynaptic α-bungarotoxins; and κ-bungarotoxins, which bind to some specific nicotinic acetylcholine receptors in the brain and various ganglia.

Cardiovascular Toxins. Snake venom toxins can lower blood pressure by various mechanisms. Permeability factors cause extravasation and hypovolaemia. An oligopeptide from the venom of the Brazilian jararaca (*Bothrops jararaca*) that activates bradykinin, potentiates its action and inhibits the conversion of angiotensin I to angiotensin II was the basis for synthetic angiotensin-converting enzyme (ACE) inhibitors. Sarafotoxins in the venom of the Israeli burrowing asp (*Atractaspis engaddensis*: Atractaspidinae) have 60% sequence homology with endogenous mammalian endothelins.[47] They cause coronary artery vasoconstriction and delay atrioventricular conduction. Natriuretic peptides in snake venoms are also being used as blue-prints or 'scaffolds' for drug design.

Clinical Features of Envenoming

Symptoms and signs in victims of snakebite are caused by anxiety and effects of first-aid and other treatments as well as direct action of venom toxins.[8,24,48,49]

Local Swelling. In the bitten limb, increased vascular permeability and extravasation of plasma or blood causes swelling and bruising. Venom metalloproteinase haemorrhagins, membrane-damaging polypeptide toxins, phospholipases, and endogenous autacoids such as histamine, serotonin and kinins are responsible. Tissue necrosis is caused by myotoxins and cytotoxins, and secondary effects of first-aid methods such as tight tourniquets. Most myotoxins are phospholipases A_2, either enzymatically active (aspartate-49) or enzymatically inactive (lysine-49). Cobra 'cardiotoxins' are cytotoxic low-molecular-weight polypeptides.

Hypotension and Shock. Extravasation of plasma or blood into the bitten limb and elsewhere or massive gastrointestinal or uterine haemorrhage may cause hypovolaemia after viper bites. Vasodilatation, especially of splanchnic vessels, and a direct effect on the myocardium may contribute to hypotension after viper and rattlesnake bites. Acute profound hypotension with or without other features of anaphylaxis is part of the autopharmacological syndrome which may occur within minutes of bites by *Vipera berus*, *Daboia* species, *Bothrops* species, *Lachesis* species, *Actractaspis engaddensis* and *A. microlepidota* and some Australasian elapids. It may be caused by release of endogenous vasoactive compounds such as nitric oxide, kinins, histamine, serotonin and endothelins (see Cardiovascular toxins, above). Snake handlers who have become sensitized to snake venoms may develop life-threatening anaphylactic reactions within minutes of being bitten.

Bleeding and Clotting Disturbances.[50,51] Incoagulable blood, resulting from consumptive coagulopathy or venom anticoagulants, thrombocytopenia with platelet dysfunction, and vessel wall damage by haemorrhagins combine to cause life-threatening haemorrhage after snakebite. These anti-haemostatic effects are a feature of envenoming by vipers, pit-vipers, Australasian elapids and colubrids.

Procoagulant enzymes activate intravascular coagulation which, combined with activation of endogenous fibrinolysis by plasmin, results in consumptive coagulopathy and incoagulable blood. Prothrombin activators are present in venoms of Colubridae, *Echis* species and Australasian elapids; factor X activators occur in *Daboia*, *Echis*, *Bothrops* and other viperid venoms; thrombin-like enzymes are common in pit-viper venoms.

Haemorrhagins are zinc metallo-endopeptidases (reprolysins) which damage vascular endothelium causing spontaneous systemic bleeding. Some have disintegrin-like, cysteine-rich and lectin domains.

Venom anticoagulants found in Australian elapid and other venoms are phospholipases.

Platelet Activators/Inhibitors. Snake venom toxins activate or inhibit platelets through GPVI, GPIb, GPIbα, GPIa-IIa and other platelet receptors. Thrombocytopenia is a common accompaniment of systemic envenoming. In patients bitten by Malayan pit vipers and green pit vipers (*Cryptelytrops albolabris*) there was initially inhibition of platelet agglutination followed by activation and the appearance of circulating clumps of platelets.[52]

Intravascular Haemolysis. Most snake venoms are haemolytic in vitro, but its clinical significance is uncertain. In victims of envenoming by Sahara horned-vipers (*Cerastes cerastes*),[53] Australian brown snakes (*Pseudonaja*),[54] taipans (*Oxyuranus*), *Bothrops* and some other species, fragmented erythrocytes (schistocytes/helmet cells) are observed in the blood film, indicating microangiopathic haemolysis. This is associated with acute kidney injury, a clinical picture similar to haemolytic uraemic syndrome or thrombotic thrombocytopenic purpura.

Complement Activation and Inhibition.[55] Elapid and some colubrid venoms activate complement via the alternative pathway ('cobra venom factor' is cobra C3b),[33] whereas some viperid venoms activate the classical pathway. Complement activation may also affect platelets, the blood coagulation system and other humoral mediators.[44,45]

Acute Kidney Injury (AKI).[56] Acute kidney injury is a common consequence, causing many deaths following bites by Russell's vipers,[26] tropical rattlesnakes (*Crotalus durissus* subspecies)[24] and sea snakes.[28] Mechanisms of acute tubular necrosis include prolonged hypotension and hypovolaemia, disseminated intravascular coagulation, microangiopathic haemolysis, a direct toxic effect of the venom on the renal tubule, haemoglobinuria, myoglobinuria and hyperkalaemia. Russell's viper venom produces hypotension, disseminated intravascular coagulation, direct nephrotoxicity[57] and, in Sri Lanka[58] and India, intravascular haemolysis, sometimes with evidence of microangiopathy. In Burmese patients envenomed by Russell's vipers (*D. siamensis*), high urinary concentrations of β_2-microglobulin, retinal binding protein and N-acetyl glucosaminidase suggested failure of proximal tubular reabsorption and tubular damage. High plasma concentrations of active renin suggested that renal ischaemia with activation of the renin–angiotensin system was involved in the development of AKI. A massive transient capillary and glomerular leak of albumin was an early sign of oliguric renal failure. The mechanism of renal failure in victims of *Crotalus durissus* is most likely to be generalized rhabdomyolysis, combined with hypotension in some cases.[59] A variety of renal histopathological changes have been described after snakebite, including proliferative glomerulonephritis, toxic mesangiolysis with platelet agglutination, fibrin deposition, ischaemic changes, acute tubular necrosis, distal tubular damage ('lower nephron nephrosis') suggesting direct venom nephrotoxicity, and bilateral renal cortical necrosis with subsequent calcification.[56,]

Neurotoxicity. The neurotoxic polypeptides and phospholipases of snake venoms cause paralysis by blocking transmission at peripheral neuromuscular junctions. Paralytic symptoms are characteristic of envenoming by most elapids, such as kraits, coral snakes, mambas and cobras, but not of the African spitting cobras which, unusually among elapids, cause local tissue destruction without detectable neurotoxicity.[33] Venoms of terrestrial Australasian snakes, sea snakes and a few species of Viperidae, notably *Crotalus durissus terrificus*, mamushi (*Gloydius blomhoffii*, *G. brevicaudus* etc.) in Japan, China, Korea and Russia, *Daboia russelii* in Sri Lanka and South Indian, the southern African berg adder (*Bitis atropos*), some other small *Bitis* species of southern Africa (*B. peringueyi*, *B. xeropaga*), and European *Vipera ammodytes* and *V. aspis* from southern France, Hungary, Bulgaria and Rumania and the European Montpellier snake (*Malpolon monspessulanus*) are neurotoxic in humans. Patients with paralysis of the bulbar muscles may die of upper airway obstruction or aspiration, but the most common mode of death after neurotoxic envenoming is respiratory paralysis. Anticholinesterase drugs, by prolonging the activity of acetylcholine at neuromuscular junctions, may improve paralytic symptoms in patients bitten by snakes whose neurotoxins are predominantly postsynaptic in their action (e.g. Asian cobras,[60] Australasian death adders genus *Acanthophis*, and Latin American coral snakes *Micrurus frontalis*). Some patients bitten by elapids or vipers become pathologically drowsy in the absence of respiratory or circulatory failure. This may be caused by endogenous opiates released by a venom component. Intracerebral injection of β-RTX (receptor-active protein) or 'vipoxin' from *Daboia russelii* venom produced sedation in rats.[61]

Rhabdomyolysis. Generalized rhabdomyolysis with release into the bloodstream of myoglobin, muscle enzymes, uric acid, potassium and other muscle constituents, is an effect in man of phospholipase A_2 presynaptic neurotoxins of most species of sea snakes;[28] many of the terrestrial Australasian elapids such as tiger snake (*Notechis scutatus* and *N. ater*), king brown or mulga snake (*Pseudechis australis*), taipan (*Oxyuranus scutellatus*), rough-scaled snake (*Tropidechis carinatus*) and small-eyed snake (*Cryptophis nigrescens*); at least three species of krait (*Bungarus niger*, *B. fasciatus* and *B. candidus*); at least three species of coral snake (*Micrurus fulvius*, *M. laticollaris* and *M. lemniscatus*) and several species of Viperidae; tropical rattlesnake (*Crotalus durissus terrificus*),[56] canebrake rattlesnake (*Crotalus horridus atricaudatus*), Mohave rattlesnake (*Crotalus scutulatus*)[62] and Sri Lankan Russell's viper (*Daboia russelii*).[58] Patients may die of bulbar and respiratory muscle weakness, from acute hyperkalaemia or later AKI.

Venom Ophthalmia. Venoms of the spitting cobras and rinkhals are intensely irritant and even destructive on contact with mucous membranes such as the conjunctivae and nasal cavity. Corneal erosions, anterior uveitis and secondary infections may result.[37,63]

Envenoming by Different Families of Venomous Snakes

Colubridae (Back-Fanged Snakes).[8,9,24] Mild local envenoming has been described after bites by many colubrid species but only a few species have caused severe or fatal envenoming: in Africa, boomslang (*Dispholidus typus*) and vine, twig, tree or bird snake (*Thelotornis* species; Figure 75.12); in Japan – yamakagashi (*Rhabdophis tigrinus*); and in South-east Asia – red-necked keelback (*R. subminiatus*). Symptoms may be delayed for many hours or even days after the bite. There is nausea, vomiting, colicky abdominal pain and headache. Bleeding develops from old and recent wounds such as venepunctures, and there is spontaneous gingival bleeding, epistaxis, haematemesis, melaena, subarachnoid or intracerebral haemorrhage, haematuria and extensive ecchymoses. Intravascular haemolysis and microangiopathic haemolysis have been described. Most of the fatal cases died of AKI many days after the bite. Local effects of the venom are usually trivial, but several patients showed some local swelling and one bitten by *Dispholidus typus* had massive swelling with blood-filled bullae. Investigations reveal incoagulable blood, defibrination, elevated fibrin(ogen) degradation products (FDPs), severe thrombocytopenia, anaemia, and complement activation by the alternative pathway.[64] Venoms contain prothrombin activators.

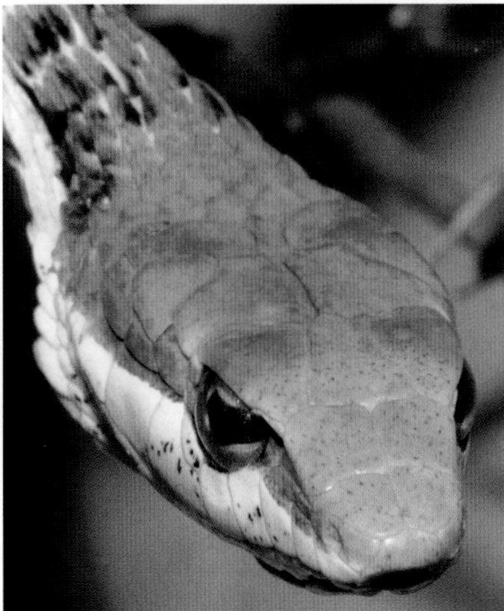

Figure 75.12 Twig, vine, tree or bird snake (*Thelotornis mossambicanus*: family Colubridae) Specimen at Bio-Ken, Watamu, Kenya. (*Copyright D. A. Warrell.*)

Atractaspidinae (Burrowing Asps or Stiletto Snakes and Natal Black Snake). A total of 17 species of the genus *Atractaspis* and one species of *Macrelaps* have been described in Africa and the Middle East. All are venomous, but fatal envenoming has been described by only three species: *A. microlepidota*, *A. irregularis* and *A. engaddensis*. Local effects include pain, swelling, blistering, necrosis, tender enlargement of local lymph nodes, local numbness or paraesthesiae. The most common systemic symptom is fever. Most of the fatal cases died within 45 minutes of the bite, after vomiting, producing profuse saliva and lapsing into coma.[65] Severe envenoming by *A. engaddensis* may produce violent autonomic symptoms (nausea, vomiting, abdominal pain, diarrhoea, sweating and profuse salivation) within minutes of the bite. One patient developed severe dyspnoea with acute respiratory failure; one had weakness, impaired consciousness and transient hypertension; and in three there were electrocardiographic changes (ST–T changes and prolonged PR interval).[66] Mild abnormalities of blood coagulation and liver function have also been described. *Atractaspis* venom has very high lethal toxicity.

Elapidae (Cobras, Kraits, Mambas, Coral Snakes, Sea Kraits and True Sea Snakes)

Local Envenoming. In the case of kraits, mambas, coral snakes, most of the Australasian elapids (see below), some of the cobras (e.g. Philippine cobra, *Naja philippinensis*; Cape cobra, *N. nivea*) and sea snakes, local effects are usually mild although exceptions do occur. However, patients bitten by African spitting cobras commonly develop tender local swelling, blistering surrounding a demarcated pale or blackened anaesthetic area of necrotic skin and regional lymphadenopathy. The lesion smells putrid and eventually breaks down with extensive loss of skin and subcutaneous tissue. Skip lesions, separated by areas of apparently normal skin, may extend proximally up the limb. Prolonged morbidity may result and some patients may lose a digit or the affected limb if there is secondary infection. Severe envenoming by the king cobra (*Ophiophagus hannah*) results in swelling of the whole limb and formation of bullae at the site of the bite, but local necrosis is minimal or absent.[67]

Neurotoxic Effects. Descending flaccid paralysis is seen in patients envenomed by Asian cobras (it is the main feature in victims of *N. philippinensis*), king cobras and most other elapids, but not in victims of African spitting cobras. The earliest symptom of systemic envenoming is repeated vomiting. Use of emetic herbal medicines may confuse the interpretation of this symptom. Other early pre-paralytic symptoms include contraction of the frontalis (before there is demonstrable ptosis), blurred vision, paraesthesiae especially around the mouth, hyperacusis, loss of sense of smell and taste, headache, dizziness, vertigo, and signs of autonomic nervous stimulation such as hypersalivation, congested conjunctivae and 'goose-flesh'. Paralysis is first detectable as ptosis and external ophthalmoplegia (Figure 75.13). These signs may appear as early as 15 minutes after the bite (cobras or mambas), but may be delayed for 10 hours or more following krait bites. Later, the facial muscles, palate, jaws, tongue, vocal cords, neck muscles and muscles of deglutition may become paralysed. The pupils are dilated. Many

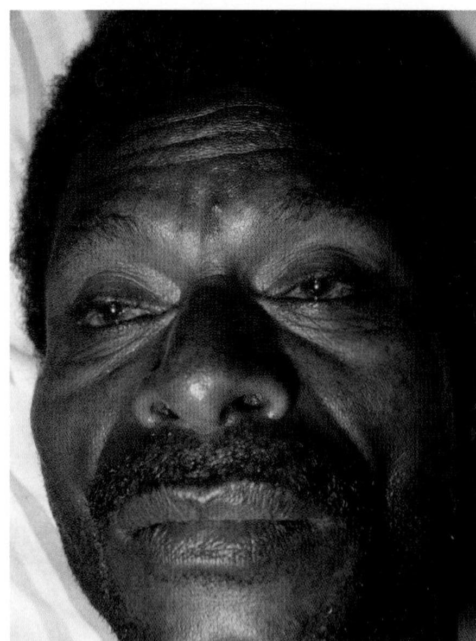

Figure 75.13 Early bilateral ptosis in a patient bitten by a Papuan taipan (*Oxyuranus scutellatus*) in Papua New Guinea. *(Copyright D. A. Warrell.)*

patients are unable to open their mouths, but this can be overcome by force. In a minority, the jaw is said to hang open. Respiratory arrest may be precipitated by obstruction of the upper airway by the paralysed tongue or inhaled vomitus. Intercostal muscles are affected before the limbs, diaphragm and superficial muscles, and, even in patients with generalized flaccid paralysis, slight movements of the digits may be possible, allowing the patients to signal. Loss of consciousness and generalized convulsions are usually explained by hypoxaemia in patients who have respiratory paralysis. Drooping eyelids from tiredness may be misconstrued as ptosis, unless the extent of lid retraction with upward gaze is formally assessed. Patients with systemic envenoming suffer from headache, malaise and generalized myalgia. Intractable hypotension can occur in patients envenomed by Asian cobras, despite adequate respiratory support. Neurotoxic effects are completely reversible, either acutely in response to antivenom or (e.g. in Asian cobra, South American coral snake and Australasian death adder bites) to anticholinesterases,[6] or they may slowly wear off spontaneously. In the absence of specific antivenom, patients supported by mechanical ventilators recover sufficient diaphragmatic movement to breathe adequately in 1–4 days. Ocular muscles recover in 2–4 days and there is usually full recovery of motor function in 3–7 days.

Bites by Australasian Elapids.[5,68,69] Venoms of these snakes result in four main groups of symptoms: neurotoxicity similar to that seen with other elapid bites (Figure 75.13),[68–70] generalized rhabdomyolysis, haemostatic disturbances and AKI associated with microangiopathic haemolysis.[54] Local signs are usually mild, but extensive local swelling and bruising with necrosis has been reported, especially after bites by the king brown or mulga snake (*Pseudechis australis*). Painful and tender local lymph nodes are a common feature in patients developing systemic envenoming. Early symptoms include vomiting, headache and syncope. Electrocardiographic changes were common in patients envenomed by taipans (*Oxyuranus scutellatus*) in Papua New Guinea, and some had raised cardiac troponin-T levels suggesting myocardial damage.

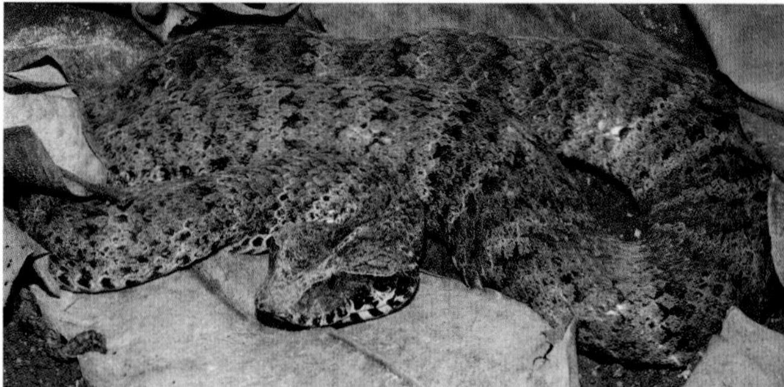

Figure 75.14 Death adder (*Acanthophis* species). Specimen from Gomore, Papua New Guinea. *(Copyright D. A. Warrell.)*

Persistent bleeding from wounds and spontaneous systemic bleeding from gums and gastrointestinal tract is found in association with incoagulable blood following bites by many Australasian species. Haemostatic abnormalities are particularly frequent and serious in patients bitten by tiger snakes (*Notechis* species), taipans (*Oxyuranus* species) and brown snakes (*Pseudonaja* species), uncommonly with bites by black snakes (*Pseudechis* species) and rare with bites by death adders (*Acanthophis* species; Figure 75.14).

Snake Venom Ophthalmia.[37,63] When venom is spat into the eye, there is intense local pain, blepharospasm, palpebral oedema and leukorrhoea (Figure 75.15). Slit-lamp or fluorescein examination reveals corneal erosions in more than half the patients spat at by *Naja nigricollis*.[37,63] Secondary infection of the corneal lesions may result in permanent opacities causing blindness or panophthalmitis with destruction of the eye. Rarely, venom is absorbed into the anterior chamber, causing hypopyon and anterior uveitis. Seventh (facial) cranial nerve paralysis is a rare complication.

Bites by Sea Snakes.[5,27,28,71] The bite is usually painless and may not be noticed by the wader or swimmer. Teeth may be left in the wound. There is minimal or no local swelling, and involvement of local lymph nodes is unusual. Generalized

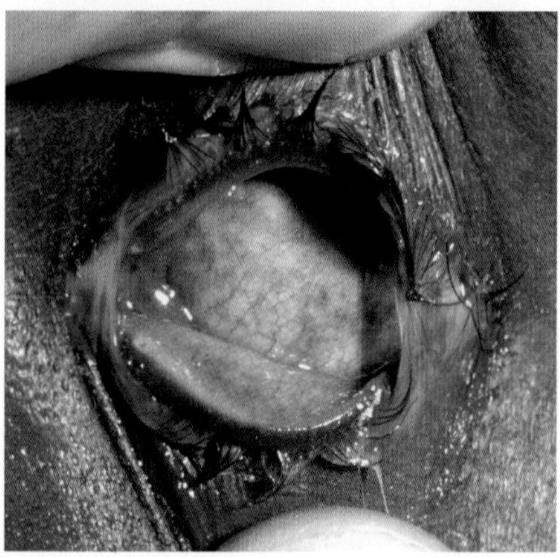

Figure 75.15 Intense conjunctivitis with leukorrhoea in a patient 'spat' at 3 hours previously by an African black-necked or spitting cobra (*Naja nigricollis*). *(Copyright D. A. Warrell.)*

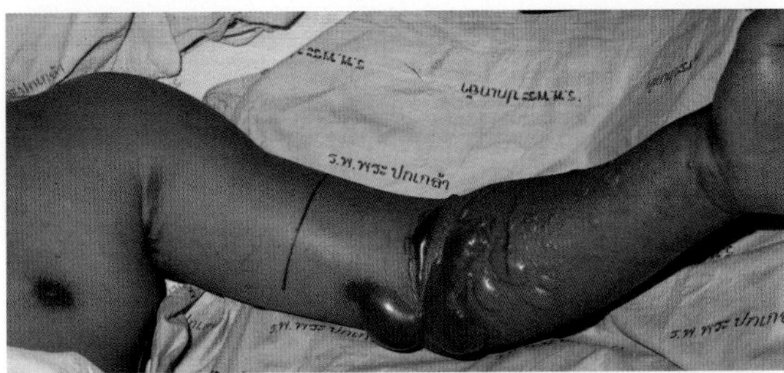

Figure 75.16 Extensive swelling and bulla formation in a Thai patient 13 hours after being bitten by a Malayan pit viper (*Calloselasma rhodostoma*). (*Copyright D. A. Warrell.*)

rhabdomyolysis is the dominant effect of envenoming by these snakes. Early symptoms include headache, a thick feeling of the tongue, thirst, sweating and vomiting. Generalized aching, stiffness and tenderness of the muscles becomes noticeable between 30 minutes and 3.5 hours after the bite. Trismus is common. Passive stretching of the muscles is painful. Later, there is progressive flaccid paralysis starting with ptosis, as in elapid envenoming. The patient remains conscious until the respiratory muscles are sufficiently affected to cause respiratory failure. Myoglobinaemia and myoglobinuria develop 3–8 hours after the bite. These are suspected when the serum/plasma appears brownish and the urine dark reddish brown ('Coca-Cola-coloured'). 'Stix' tests will appear positive for haemoglobin/blood in urine containing myoglobin. Myoglobin and potassium released from damaged skeletal muscles may cause renal failure, while hyperkalaemia developing within 6–12 hours of the bite may precipitate cardiac arrest.

Viperidae (Old World Vipers and Adders, New World Pit Vipers, Rattlesnakes, Moccasins and Lance-Headed Vipers, Asian Pit Vipers)

Local Envenoming. Venoms of vipers and pit vipers often produce severe local effect. Swelling may appear within 15 minutes, but rarely is delayed for several hours. It spreads rapidly, sometimes to involve the whole limb and adjacent trunk. There is associated pain, tenderness and enlargement of regional lymph nodes. Bruising, especially along the path of superficial lymphatics and over regional lymph nodes, is common (Figure 75.16). There may be persistent bleeding from the fang marks. Swollen limbs can accommodate many litres of extravasated blood, leading to hypovolaemic shock. Blistering may appear at the bite site as early as 12 hours after the bite (Figures 75.16, 75.17). Blisters contain clear or bloodstained fluid. Necrosis of skin, subcutaneous tissue and muscle (Figure 75.17) develops in up to 10% of hospitalized cases, especially following bites by North American rattlesnakes, South American lance-headed vipers (genus *Bothrops*), bushmasters (genus *Lachesis*), Asian pit vipers (e.g. *Calloselasma rhodostoma, Deinagkistrodon acutus* and *Protobothrops flavoviridis*), African vipers (genus *Bitis*), saw-scaled vipers (genus *Echis*) and Palestine viper (*Daboia palaestinae*). Bites on the digits and in areas draining into the tight fascial compartments, such as the anterior tibial compartment, are particularly likely to result in necrosis. High intracompartmental pressure may cause ischaemia which contributes, together with direct effects of the venom, to muscle necrosis.[72]

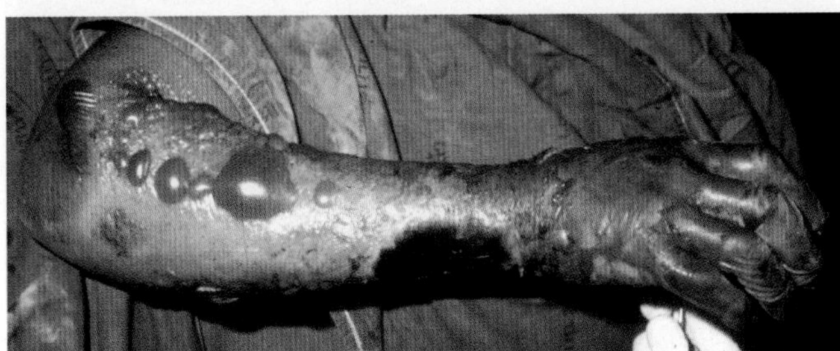

Figure 75.17 Swelling, blistering and necrosis in a woman 4 days after being bitten by a Malayan pit viper (*Calloselasma rhodostoma*) in Thailand. Amputation was unavoidable. (*Copyright D. A. Warrell.*)

The absence of detectable local swelling 2 hours after a viper bite usually means that no venom has been injected. However, there are important exceptions to this rule: fatal systemic envenoming by the tropical rattlesnake (*Crotalus durissus terrificus*), Mohave rattlesnake (*Crotalus scutulatus*) and Burmese Russell's viper (*Daboia siamensis*) may occur in the absence of local signs. Victims of *C. d. terrificus* and other South American *Crotalus* species may develop local erythema, but rarely more than mild swelling.[24]

Haemostatic Abnormalities. These are characteristic of envenoming by Viperidae, but are usually absent in patients bitten by the smaller European vipers (*V. berus, V. aspis, V. ammodytes*, etc.) and some species of rattlesnakes. Persistent bleeding (>10 minutes) from the fang puncture wounds and from new injuries such as venepuncture sites and old partially healed wounds is the first clinical evidence of consumption coagulopathy. Spontaneous systemic haemorrhage is most often detected in the gingival sulci (Figure 75.18). Bloodstaining of saliva and sputum usually reflects bleeding gums or epistaxis. True haemoptysis is rare. Haematuria may be detected a few hours after the bite. Other types of spontaneous bleeding are ecchymoses, intracranial and subconjunctival haemorrhages, bleeding into the floor of the mouth, tympanic membrane, and gastrointestinal and genitourinary tracts, petechiae and larger discoid (Figure 75.19) and follicular haemorrhages. Bleeding into the anterior pituitary (resembling Sheehan's syndrome) may complicate envenoming by Russell's vipers in Burma, India and Sri Lanka, and one case has been reported following a bite

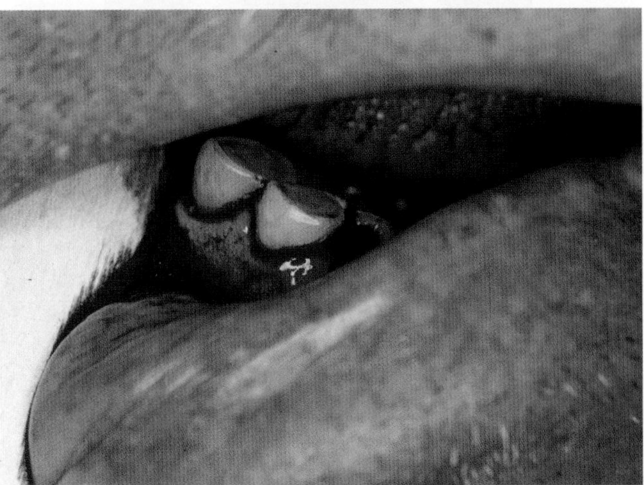

Figure 75.18 Bleeding from gingival sulci in a patient bitten by a jararaca (*Bothrops jararaca*) in Brazil. (*Copyright D. A. Warrell.*)

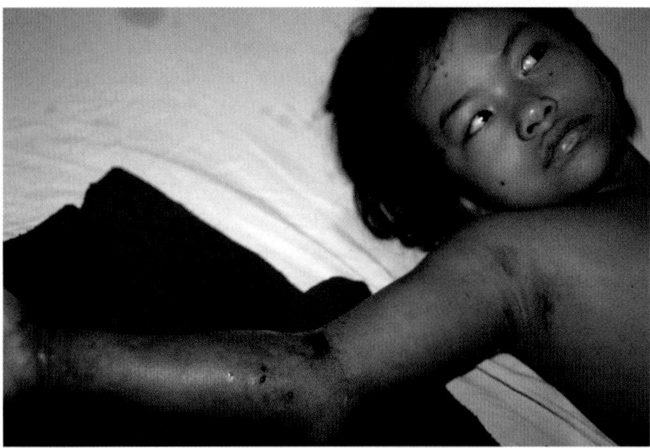

Figure 75.19 Extensive swelling, bruising and facial discoid haemorrhages in a 9-year-old Vietnamese girl 12 hours after being bitten on the elbow by a Malayan pit viper (*Calloselasma rhodostoma*). (*Copyright D. A. Warrell.*)

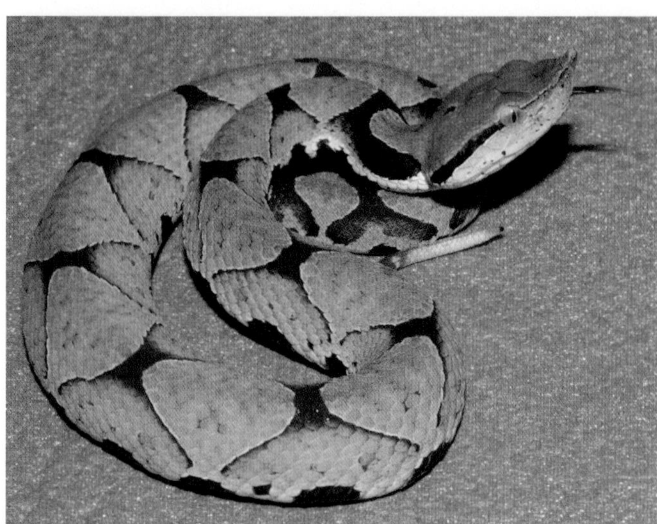

Figure 75.21 Juvenile 'hundred pacer' (*Deinagkistrodon acutus*). (*Copyright D. A. Warrell.*)

by a *Bothrops* species in Southern Brazil. Menorrhagia and antepartum and postpartum haemorrhage have been described after envenoming by vipers. Severe headache and meningism suggest subarachnoid haemorrhage; evidence of a developing central nervous system lesion (e.g. anisocoria, hemiplegia), irritability, loss of consciousness and convulsions suggest intracranial haemorrhage (Figure 75.20) or cerebral thrombosis. Abdominal distension, tenderness and peritonism with signs of haemorrhagic shock but no external blood loss (haematemesis or melaena) suggest retroperitoneal or intraperitoneal haemorrhage. Incoagulable blood resulting from defibrination or disseminated intravascular coagulation is a common and important finding in patients systemically envenomed by members of many genera: *Atheris*, *Daboia*, *Vipera*, *Echis*, *Lachesis*, *Agkistrodon*, *Gloydius*, *Ovophis*, *Bothrops*, *Calloselasma*, *Crotalus*, *Deinagkistrodon* (Figure 75.21) and *Trimeresurus* sensu lato. In situ thrombosis of major arteries (cerebral, pulmonary, coronary, etc.) is an important feature of envenoming by the 'fer-de-lance' (*B. lanceolatus*) of Martinique and *B. caribbaeus* in adjacent St Lucia (Figure 75.22)[24] and has been described in envenoming by other *Bothrops* species, *Daboia siamensis* (Taiwan), *D. russelii* (India and Sri Lanka), *Bitis arietans*, *Crotalus helleri* and some other *Crotalus* species.[73]

Intravascular Haemolysis. This presents as haemoglobinaemia (pink plasma) and black or greyish urine (haemoglobinuria or methaemoglobinuria). The presence of fragmented erythrocytes (schistocytes, helmet cells) in the blood film may indicate microangiopathic haemolysis, associated with progressive severe anaemia and acute kidney injury (see above).[53,54]

Circulatory Shock (Hypotensive) Syndromes. A fall in blood pressure is a common and serious event in patients bitten by vipers, especially in the case of some of the North American rattlesnakes, South American pit-vipers (e.g. *Lachesis muta* and *Bothrops* species – Figure 75.23) and Old World Viperinae (e.g.

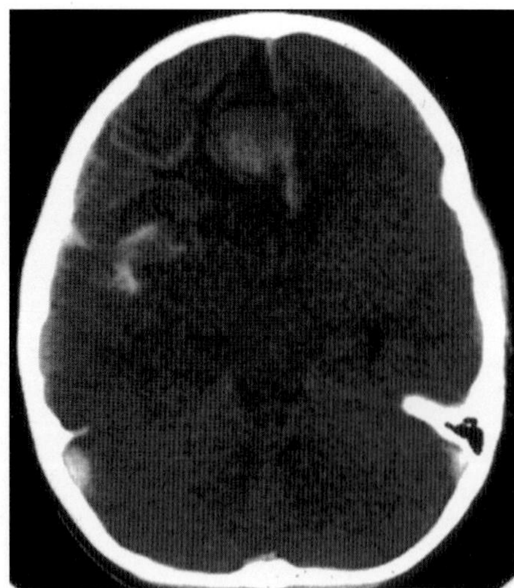

Figure 75.20 Cerebral CT scan of a 7-year-old Ecuadorian girl who had developed sudden headache followed by loss of consciousness 25 hours after being bitten by a common lancehead (*Bothrops atrox*). (*Copyright D. A. Warrell.*)

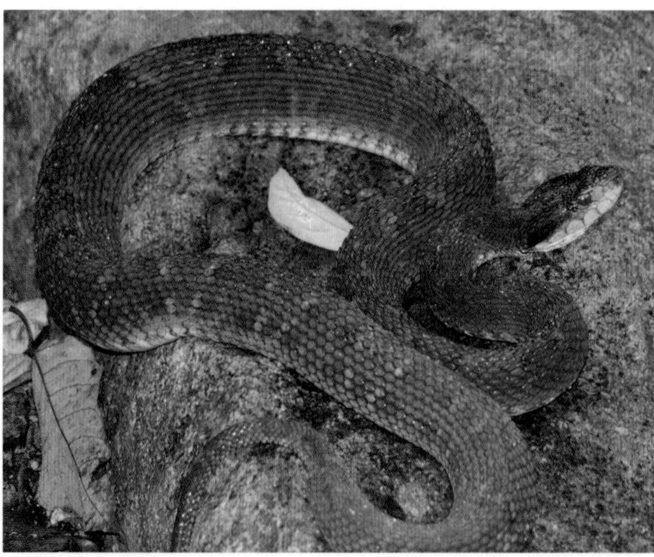

Figure 75.22 St Lucian 'fer-de-lance' (*Bothrops caribbaeus*). (*Copyright D. A. Warrell.*)

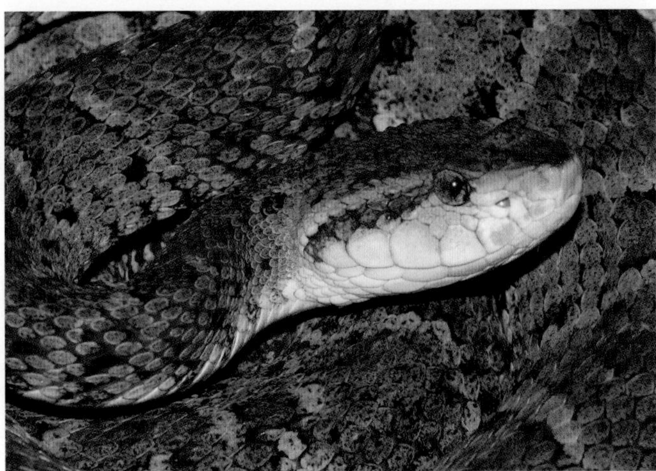

Figure 75.23 Colombian lancehead pit-viper (*Bothrops colombiensis*). *(Copyright D. A. Warrell.)*

Daboia russelii, D. palaestinae, Vipera berus, Bitis arietans, B. gabonica and *B. rhinoceros*). Sinus tachycardia suggests hypovolaemia resulting from extravasation into the tissues of the bitten limb, external haemorrhage, or generalized increase in capillary permeability. Patients envenomed by Burmese Russell's viper (*Daboia siamensis*) may develop conjunctival oedema (Figure 75.24), serous effusions, pulmonary oedema, haemoconcentration and a fall in serum albumin concentration, evidence of increased vascular permeability.[26] The pulse rate may be slow or irregular if the venom is affecting the heart directly or reflexly and vasovagal syncope may be precipitated by fear and pain. Early, repeated and usually transient syncopal attacks with features of anaphylaxis develop in patients bitten by some Viperidae, notably *Daboia palaestinae* and European *Vipera*. Hypotension is an important feature of anaphylactic reactions to antivenom (see below) and in cases of venom hypersensitivity.

Acute Kidney Injury. This is most common in victims of Russell's viper, tropical rattlesnake (*Crotalus durissus*

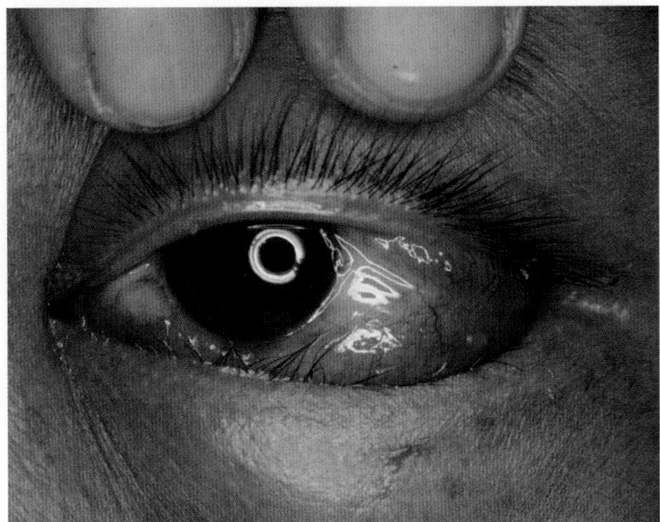

Figure 75.24 Conjunctival oedema (chemosis) in a Burmese man bitten 36 hours previously by an Eastern Russell's viper (*Daboia siamensis*). *(Copyright D. A. Warrell)*

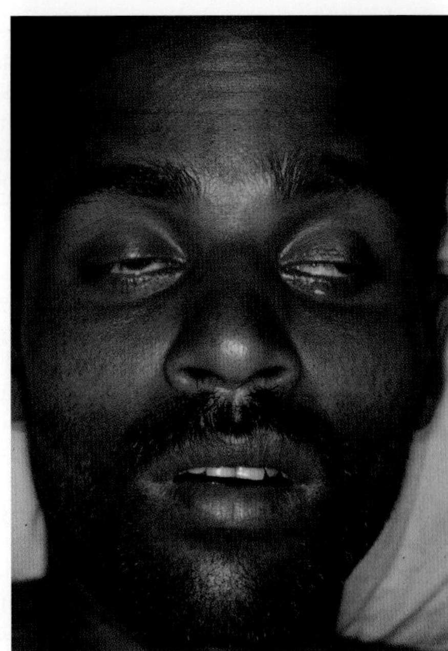

Figure 75.25 Sri Lankan man with neurotoxic envenoming by a Western Russell's viper (*Daboia russelii*). There is ptosis, ophthalmoplegia, facial paralysis and inability to open the mouth and protrude the tongue. *(Copyright D. A. Warrell.)*

subspecies) and some species of *Bothrops*. Patients bitten by Russell's vipers may become oliguric within a few hours of the bite. Loin pain and tenderness may be experienced within the first 24 hours and, in 3 or 4 days, the patient may become irritable and hypertensive and may convulse and become comatose with evidence of metabolic acidosis.

Neurotoxicity. Viperid neurotoxicity is usually attributable to venom phospholipases A_2. It is a feature of envenoming by *Crotalus durissus terrificus, Gloydius blomhoffii, G. brevicaudus, Vipera aspis* and other European *Vipera, Bitis atropos* and other small South African *Bitis* species, and Indian and Sri Lankan Russell's vipers (*Daboia russelii*) (Figure 75.25). Paralysis descends as with elapid envenoming and may progress to involve bulbar and respiratory muscles. Associated generalized myalgia and muscle tenderness suggest rhabdomyolysis. Mydriasis, causing visual disturbance from loss of accommodation, is a feature of severe envenoming by tropical rattlesnakes and small *Bitis* species (e.g. *B. peringueyi*) and may be a permanent neurological sequela. In North America, severe envenoming by some populations of Mohave rattlesnakes (*Crotalus scutulatus scutulatus*), Southern Pacific rattlesnakes (*C. helleri*), timber rattlesnakes (*Crotalus horridus horridus*) and Western diamondback rattlesnakes (*C. atrox*) causes weakness and facial or generalized fasciculations (myokymia). In the case of *C. helleri* envenoming in south-west California and Baja California, neurotoxic clinical effects may be dramatic. There is a metallic taste in the mouth, generalized weakness, ptosis, diplopia, dysphagia, dysphonia, respiratory distress progressing to respiratory paralysis and persisting muscle fasciculations of the face, tongue, and upper extremities, as well as local swelling, shock, coagulopathy and rhabdomyolysis.[74,75]

Clinical Course and Prognosis

Local swelling is usually evident within 2–4 hours of bites by vipers and cytotoxic cobras, and may evolve very rapidly after rattlesnake bites. Swelling is maximal and most extensive on the 2nd or 3rd day after the bite. Resolution of swelling and restoration of normal function in the bitten limb may be delayed for months, especially in older people. The earliest systemic symptoms such as vomiting and syncope may develop within minutes of the bite, but even in the case of rapidly absorbed elapid venoms, patients rarely die within 1 hour of the bite. Defibrinogenation may be complete within 1–2 hours of the bite.[76] Neurotoxic signs may progress to generalized flaccid paralysis and respiratory arrest within a few hours. If the venom is not neutralized by antivenom, these effects may be prolonged. Defibrinogenation can persist for weeks in untreated patients. Patients with neurotoxic envenoming have recovered after being artificially ventilated for as long as 10 weeks. Tissue necrosis becomes obvious within a day of the bite. Sloughing of necrotic tissue and secondary infections including osteomyelitis develop during subsequent weeks or months. Fatal neurotoxic envenoming results from airway obstruction or respiratory paralysis, whereas later deaths may result from technical complications of mechanical ventilation, aspiration pneumonia or intractable hypotension. Late deaths, more than 5 days after the bite, are usually the result of acute kidney injury.

Risk of Death from Envenoming

Even when the fangs of a venomous snake have pierced the skin, envenoming is not inevitable (see above 'Dry bites'). The case fatality of *Crotalus durissus terrificus* bites is said to have been 74% before and 12% after introduction of antivenom.[24] Mortality of *Echis ocellatus* bites was reduced from about 20% to 3% with antivenom.[38]

Interval between Bite and Death

Death after snakebite may occur as rapidly as 'a few minutes' (reputedly after a bite by the king cobra *Ophiophagus hannah*) or as long as 41 days after a bite by the saw-scaled or carpet viper (*Echis carinatus*). The speed of killing has been exaggerated. Most elapid deaths occur within hours of the bite, most sea snakebite deaths between 12 and 24 hours, and viper bite deaths within days.[8,18,71]

Laboratory Investigations

Systemic envenoming is usually associated with an inflammatory neutrophil leukocytosis: counts above 20×10^9/L indicate severe envenoming. Initially, haematocrit may be high from haemoconcentration resulting from a generalized increase in capillary permeability. Later, haematocrit falls because of bleeding into the bitten limb and elsewhere, and from intravascular haemolysis or microangiopathic haemolysis in patients with disseminated intravascular coagulation. Thrombocytopenia is common in viper, colubrid and Australasian elapid envenoming.

The 20-minute Whole Blood Clotting Test (20WBCT).[38,76] Incoagulable blood is a cardinal sign of systemic envenoming by most of the Viperidae and many of the Australasian elapids and medically important Colubridae. For clinical purposes, a simple, bed-side, all-or-nothing test of blood coagulability is adequate. A few millilitres of blood taken by venepuncture is placed immediately in a new, clean, dry, glass vessel; left undisturbed at room temperature for 20 minutes; and then tipped once to see if there is clotting or not. The vessel must be glass in order to activate Hageman factor (FXII).

Depending on the availability and speed of laboratory services, more sensitive tests may be appropriate, such as whole blood or plasma prothrombin times (INR) and detection of elevated concentrations of fibrin degradation products (FDP) by agglutination of sensitized latex particles or of D-dimer.

Serum concentrations of creatine kinase, aspartate amino transferase and blood urea are commonly raised in patients with severe envenoming, because of local muscle damage at the site of the bite. Generalized rhabdomyolysis causes a steep rise in serum creatine kinase and other muscle-derived enzymes, myoglobin and sometimes potassium concentrations. Plasma is stained brownish by myoglobin and pink by haemoglobin. Heparinized blood should be allowed to sediment spontaneously (without centrifugation) to reveal these pigments which cannot be satisfactorily distinguished by eye or by simple tests. Blood urea or serum creatinine and potassium concentrations should be measured in patients who become oliguric, especially in patients bitten by species whose venoms cause acute kidney injury (Russell's vipers, *Crotalus durissus terrificus*, *Bothrops* species, terrestrial Australasian snakes, sea snakes and Colubridae). Severely sick, hypotensive and shocked patients develop lactic acidosis (suggested by an increased anion gap). Those with renal failure will also develop a metabolic acidosis (decreased plasma pH and bicarbonate concentration, reduced arterial PCO_2), and patients with respiratory paralysis will develop respiratory acidosis (low pH, high arterial PCO_2, decreased PO_2) or respiratory alkalosis if they are mechanically overventilated. Arterial puncture is contraindicated in patients with incoagulable blood but oximetry is usually adequate to assess oxygenation.

Patients should be encouraged to empty their bladders on admission to allow examination for blood/haemoglobin/myoglobin (all positive for 'blood') and protein (by 'stix' test) and for microscopic haematuria and casts.

Other Investigations

Electrocardiographic abnormalities include sinus bradycardia, ST–T changes, various degrees of atrioventricular block, evidence of hyperkalaemia and myocardial ischaemia or infarction secondary to shock.

Chest radiographs will help to detect pulmonary oedema, pulmonary haemorrhages and infarcts, pleural effusions and secondary bronchopneumonias. CT and MRI imaging are increasingly available for assessment of haemorrhages and infarcts in the brain and elsewhere.

Ultrasound will detect pericardial effusion and myocardial dysfunction and bleeding into the pleural and peritoneal cavities.

Immunodiagnosis

Detection and quantitation of venom antigens in body fluids of snakebite victims using enzyme immunoassays (EIA) has proved a valuable research tool for confirming the species responsible for envenoming (immunodiagnosis), as a prognostic index of the severity of envenoming and to assess the effectiveness of antivenom teatment.[77–80] Commercial venom detection kits for rapid clinical diagnosis are available in Australia. They are highly sensitive but their specificity may be inadequate to distinguish between envenoming by different species in the same genus or in closely related genera. Relatively high venom antigen concentrations (e.g. from wound swabs or wound aspirates) can be detected within 15–30 minutes. For retrospective diagnosis, including forensic cases, tissue around the fang punctures, wound and blister aspirate, serum and urine should be stored for EIA. PCR detection of venom gland mitochondrial DNA in wound swabs is being developed as a highly specific method for determining the identity of the biting species.

Management of Snakebite[8,24,48,49]

First Aid. First aid must be carried out by bite victims themselves or bystanders, using skills and materials that are immediately available.

1. Reassure the victim, who may be terrified.
2. Do not tamper with the bite wound in any way. Remove tight rings and bracelets from the bitten limb. Immobilize the whole patient, especially their bitten limb, using a splint or sling. Application of pressure-immobilization or a pressure-pad may be possible to delay the systemic absorption of venom (see below). Transport the patient as quickly and as passively as possible to the nearest health clinic, dispensary or hospital where medical treatment can be given. Movement (muscular contraction) will promote spread of venom and so it must be reduced to a minimum. Ideally, the patient should be transported by motor vehicle or boat or carried on a stretcher (ideally in the recovery position, in case they vomit), or by motor bike or bicycle (as a passenger).
3. Avoid harmful and time-wasting treatments.
4. If the snake has already been captured or killed, it should be taken with the patient as potentially valuable evidence. However, if the snake is still at large, neither risk further bites nor waste time searching for it. Snakes, even those apparently dead, should not be touched with the bare hands. Some species (e.g. the rinkhals *Hemachatus haemachatus*) sham death, and even a severed head can inject venom!

Pressure-immobilization (PI). Classic experiments by Struan Sutherland in Australia proved this technique effective in limiting the absorption of Australian elapid toxins in restrained monkeys.[81] Unfortunately, the method was never subjected to formal clinical trials, but it has proved successful, judging by anecdotal reports of delayed systemic envenoming and rapid deterioration after release of the bandage, in some cases supported by measurements of venom antigenaemia. There have been practical difficulties in implementing this discovery. Even in Australia, only a minority of the bandages in place when patients arrived in the hospital had been correctly applied. Some experienced physicians remain skeptical of the benefit of PI and it is impracticable in rural areas of tropical countries such as India, where snakebite is common.[82,83] The aim is to exert a pressure of about 55 mmHg, that of a venous tourniquet, which is sufficient to occlude both veins and lymphatic vessels through which larger-molecular-weight toxins spread from the bite site and veins. Elasticated bandages are more effective than the crepe bandages originally recommended.[83] In practice, it is difficult to judge how tightly to apply the bandage. Most are applied too loosely. It may be impossible for the victim to apply it unaided. External compression will increase intracompartmental pressure, potentiating intracompartmental ischaemia and, by localizing the injected venom, PI might accentuate the necrotic effects of some snake venoms. However, these concerns have not been confirmed clinically or experimentally.[84,85]

The broad (10 cm) elasticated bandage should be applied firmly, but not so tightly as to cause ischaemic pain, cyanosis of the extremity or obliteration of peripheral arterial pulses. Lymphoscintigraphy studies showed that excessive pressure (>70 mmHg) and movement of the other limbs increased lymphatic flow.[86]

Pressure-pad Method. A foam rubber or folded fabric pad approximately 5 × 5 × 3 cm, bound firmly over the bite wound, slowed lymphatic flow and delayed spread of a 'mock venom' in human subjects.[87] In victims of Russell's viper bite in Burma, systemic envenoming was delayed, as assessed by measurements of venom antigenaemia.[88] The method appeared safe and effective in a preliminary field trial in Burma and deserves further attention.[89]

Victims of neurotoxic elapid envenoming may develop respiratory paralysis before reaching medical care. PI or pressure-pad should therefore be applied immediately in all cases of snakebite in which a bite by an elapid snake cannot be confidently excluded.

Inhibition of the Lymphatic Pump. In rats, application of glyceryl trinitrate ointment to the bitten limb reduced lymphatic clearance of venom and prolonged life. In human subjects this treatment slowed lymphatic flow.[90]

Rejected First-Aid Methods. Cauterization, incision or excision, amputation of the bitten digit, suction by mouth, vacuum pumps[91] or 'venom-ex' apparatus, instillation of chemical compounds such as potassium permanganate, application of ice packs (cryotherapy), 'snake stones' or electric shocks are absolutely contraindicated as they are harmful and have no proven benefit.[92] Incisions provoke uncontrolled bleeding when the blood is incoagulable and may damage nerves, blood vessels or tendons and introduce infection. Suction, chemicals and cryotherapy can cause tissue necrosis. Tight (arterial) tourniquets have been responsible for terrible morbidity and even mortality in snakebite victims and should never be recommended or used.

Treatment of Early Symptoms. Distressing and dangerous effects of envenoming may appear before the patient reaches hospital.

Local pain may be intense. Oral paracetamol, codeine phosphate or stronger opiates are preferable to aspirin or non-steroidal antiinflammatory agents, which carry the risk of gastric bleeding in patients with incoagulable blood. *Vomiting* is a common early symptom of systemic envenoming. Patients should be placed in the recovery position (prone on their left side) with their head down to avoid aspiration. The airway should be protected (see below). Persistent vomiting can be treated with intravenous or rectal chlorpromazine (25–50 mg in adults, 1 mg/kg in children).*

Postural hypotension should be prevented by keeping the patient in the prone position.

Syncopal Attacks and Anaphylactic Shock. Patients who collapse within minutes of the bite may suffer transient profound hypotension. Some show features of either a vasovagal attack with profound bradycardia or of anaphylaxis with tachycardia, hypotension, angio-oedema, urticaria, asthma, abdominal colic and diarrhoea. These patients must be laid down supine or prone. Anaphylaxis should be treated with adrenaline (epinephrine) 0.1% (1 in 1000) (0.5 mL in adults,

*In patients with incoagulable blood, injections will cause haematomas. Pressure dressings should be applied to all injection sites to prevent oozing.

0.01 mL/kg in children) by intramuscular* injection. The value of histamine H_1-blockers such as chlorphenamine maleate (10 mg in adults, 0.2 mg/kg in children) by intravenous or intramuscular* injection and hydrocortisone is unproven.

Respiratory Distress. This may result from upper airway obstruction if the jaw, tongue and bulbar muscles are paralysed or from paralysis of the respiratory muscles. Patients should be placed in the recovery position, the airway cleared, if possible using a suction pump, an oral airway inserted and the jaw elevated. If the patient is cyanosed, in respiratory distress, or respiratory movements are very weak, oxygen should be given by any available means. If clearing the airway does not produce immediate relief, artificial ventilation must be initiated. In the absence of any equipment, mouth-to-mouth or mouth-to-nose ventilation can be life-saving. Non-invasive manual ventilation by Ambu bag and anaesthetic mask is rarely effective. Ideally, a cuffed endotracheal tube should be introduced, using a laryngoscope, or a cuffed tracheostomy tube inserted. Laryngeal mask airways and i-gel supraglottic airways have proved effective in some situations. The patient can then be ventilated by Ambu bag. If no femoral or carotid pulse can be felt, external cardiac massage must be started.

Treatment at Health Clinic, Dispensary or Hospital by Medically Trained Staff

Clinical Assessment. Snakebite is a medical emergency. The history, symptoms and signs must be elicited rapidly so that urgent and appropriate treatment can be given. Four important preliminary questions are:

- Show me in which part of your body you were bitten? (Quickly observe any local signs – fang marks, swelling, bruising, persistent bleeding)
- When were you bitten? (If the bite was very recent, there may not have been time for signs of envenoming to develop)
- Where is the snake that bit you or what did it look like? (If it was killed and left at home, ask someone to fetch it)
- How are you feeling now? (Have any symptoms of envenoming developed).

Patients should be asked whether they have taken any herbal or other treatment, whether they have vomited, fainted or have noticed any bleeding, weakness, visual disturbance or other ill-effects of the bite and whether they have passed urine since being bitten. Before removing any compression bandage or tourniquet, put up an intravenous line and be prepared to resuscitate the patient, as they may deteriorate dramatically. Paired puncture marks suggest a bite by a venomous snake but fang marks are sometimes invisible and may be confused with bites by other animal. Local swelling, tenderness and lymph node involvement are early signs of envenoming. The gingival sulci are an early site of detectable spontaneous bleeding. Persistent bleeding from venepuncture sites, recent wounds and skin lesions suggests incoagulable blood. If the patient is shocked (collapsed, sweating, cold, cyanosed extremities, low blood pressure, tachycardia), the foot of the bed should be raised immediately, and intravenous fluid should be infused. The jugular or central venous pressure should be observed. The earliest symptom of neurotoxicity after elapid bites is often blurred vision, a feeling of heaviness in the eyelids and drowsiness. The earliest sign is contraction of the frontalis muscle (raised eyebrows and puckered forehead) and tilting back the head, even before true ptosis can be demonstrated. Signs of respiratory muscle paralysis (dyspnoea, 'paradoxical' abdominal respiration, use of accessory muscles and cyanosis) are ominous. Patients with generalized rhabdomyolysis may have trismus and muscles that are stiff, tender and resistant to passive stretching. Urine output may dwindle or cease very early after Russell's viper bites. Black urine suggests myoglobinuria or haemoglobinuria.

If the responsible snake was brought and can be identified confidently as non-venomous, the patient can be discharged after a booster dose of tetanus toxoid. All other patients giving a history of snakebite should be admitted for 24 hours observation, even if there is no evidence of envenoming when they first arrive. Symptoms, level of consciousness, ptosis, pulse rate and rhythm, blood pressure, respiratory rate, extent of local swelling and other new signs should be recorded every hour. If there is any evidence of neurotoxicity, the ventilatory capacity or expiratory pressure should also be recorded every hour. Useful investigations include the 20-minute whole blood clotting test (or other tests of coagulation), peripheral leukocyte count, haematocrit, urine microscopy and 'stix' testing, and electrocardiography.

Antivenom (also known as Antivenin, Antivenene, Anti-Snakebite Serum, Anti-Snake Venom – ASV). Antivenom is the immunoglobulin of animals, usually horses or sheep, which have been immunized with one or more venoms. It is the only specific antidote available and has proved effective against many of the lethal and damaging effects of venoms. In the management of snakebite, the most important clinical decision is whether or not to give antivenom. Only a minority of snake-bitten patients require antivenom, which may cause severe reactions, is expensive and is often in short supply.

Indications for Antivenom

Systemic Envenoming:

1. Haemostatic abnormalities: spontaneous systemic bleeding (including evidence of internal haemorrhage – antepartum, intracranial, gastrointestinal etc.), incoagulable blood (20WBCT) or prolonged clotting time, elevated FDP or D-dimer, thrombocytopenia.
2. Cardiovascular abnormalities: hypotension, shock, cardiac arrhythmia, reduced ejection fraction (echocardiogram).
3. Neurotoxicity (paralysis, fasciculations).
4. Black urine indicating generalized rhabdomyolysis or intravascular haemolysis.
5. In patients with definite signs of local envenoming, the following confirm systemic envenoming: neutrophil leukocytosis, elevated serum enzymes such as creatine kinase and aminotransferases, haemoconcentration, uraemia, hypercreatininaemia, oliguria, hypoxaemia and acidosis.

Severe Local Envenoming. In the absence of 1–5 above, the development at any stage of local swelling involving more than half the bitten limb or extensive blistering or bruising, especially in patients showing the abnormalities listed above under (5) and in patients bitten by species known to cause local necrosis (e.g. Viperidae, Asian cobras, African spitting cobras). Bites on the digits by these species carry a high risk of necrosis.

Wealthy countries can afford a wider range of indications for the use of antivenom. The following *additional* indications have been suggested.

*In patients with incoagulable blood, injections will cause haematomas. Pressure dressings should be applied to all injection sites to prevent oozing.

USA and Canada. Following bites by the most dangerous rattlesnakes (*Crotalus atrox*, *C. adamanteus*, *C. viridis*, *C. helleri*, *C. horridus* and *C. scutulatus*), antivenom is recommended if there is rapid spread of local swelling, even without evidence of systemic envenoming, and after bites by coral snakes (*Micruroides euryxanthus*, *Micrurus fulvius*, *M. tener*) if there is immediate pain or any other symptom or sign of envenoming.

Australia. Antivenom is recommended in any proved or suspected case of snakebite if there is any evidence of systemic spread of venom, including tender regional lymph nodes, and if there has been an effective bite by any identified highly venomous species.[5]

Europe. To improve the rate of recovery of local swelling after bites by *Vipera berus*, antivenom has been recommended in adults with swelling extending up the forearm or leg within 2 hours of the bite.[23,93]

Contraindications. There is no absolute contraindication to antivenom treatment in severely envenomed patients. However, atopic patients and those who have had reactions to equine antiserum on previous occasions have an increased risk of developing severe antivenom reactions. In such cases, antivenom should not be given unless there are definite signs of severe (potentially life-threatening) systemic envenoming. Pretreatment with adrenaline (epinephrine) 0.25 ml of 0.01% solution subcutaneously (see below) followed by empirical histamine H_1-blocker and corticosteroid by intravenous injection is recommended. The patient should be closely observed for 3 hours after antivenom has been given. Rapid desensitization is not recommended.

Prediction of Antivenom Reactions. Hypersensitivity testing by intradermal or subcutaneous injection or intraconjunctival instillation of diluted antivenom has been widely practised in the past. However, these tests delay the start of antivenom treatment, are not without risk of sensitizing the patient, and have no predictive value. Most early (anaphylactic and pyrogenic) antivenom reactions are the result of direct complement activation by aggregates, other physicochemical properties of the antivenom or endotoxin contamination and are not manifestations of IgE-mediated (reaginic) type I hypersensitivity.[94,95]

Prevention of Antivenom Reactions. In a large, well-designed randomized, double-blind trial, subcutaneous adrenaline (epinephrine) (0.1%; adult dose, 0.25 mg), given just before antivenom administration, reduced the rate of severe adverse reactions over the first hour by 43% and over the first 48 hours by 38%.[96] Intravenous promethazine and hydrocortisone, compared alone and in all possible combinations, were ineffective.

Monovalent and Polyvalent Antivenoms. The range of venoms neutralized by an antivenom is usually stated in the package insert and is to be found in compendia of antivenoms.[97] If the biting species is known or strongly suspected, an appropriate monospecific (monovalent) antivenom can be used. However, in most parts of the world, polyspecific (polyvalent) antivenoms are used to cover the venoms of the most important species in the region. Polyvalent antivenoms are no less specific than monovalent ones and may have a wider range of paraspecific activity extending to the venoms of closely related species.

Expiry Dates. Useful neutralizing activity of antivenoms may be retained for years after the manufacturers' stated expiry dates. Liquid lyophilized antivenoms stored at below 8°C usually retain most of their activity for 5 years or more.[98,99] Solutions that are opaque or contain visible particles should not be given, as precipitation of protein indicates loss of activity and an increased risk of reactions.

Timing of Antivenom Administration. Antivenom should be given as soon as it is indicated, but it is almost never too late to give it as long as signs of systemic envenoming persist (e.g. up to 2 days after a sea snakebite and many days or even weeks for prolonged defibrinogenation following bites by Viperidae). In contrast, local effects of venoms are probably not reversible or preventable by antivenom delayed more than a few hours after the bite.

Intravenous Administration. The intravenous route is the most effective. An infusion over 30–60 minutes of antivenom diluted in isotonic fluid may be easier to control than a slow intravenous 'push' injection of reconstituted but undiluted antivenom given over 10–20 minutes. There is no difference in the incidence or severity of antivenom reactions in patients treated by these two methods.[94] In the rural tropics, the intravenous push method has the advantage that it involves less expensive equipment, is quicker to initiate, and compels someone to remain with the patient at least while the injection is being given.

Intramuscular Administration. Bioavailability of antivenom, even Fab fragments, given intramuscularly is very slow and incomplete. However, in case of emergency and in the absence of anyone capable of giving an intravenous injection, antivenom might be given by this route. Deep intramuscular injection (e.g. at several sites into the anterolateral aspect of the thighs but not into the gluteal region) could be followed by massage to promote absorption and application of pressure dressings over the injection sites to restrict bleeding. However, the volumes of antivenom normally required would make this route impracticable, especially in children, as would the risk of haematoma formation in patients with incoagulable blood. Local injection of antivenom, for example into the fang marks, seems rational by analogy with local infiltration of rabies immune globulin but it is difficult, painful, hazardous (especially when the bite is on a digit or other tight compartment) and has not proved effective in animal studies.

Initial Dose. The average initial dose of antivenom required for envenoming by different species should be based on results of clinical studies, but few data are available. Most manufacturers base their recommendations on the mouse assay, which may not correlate with clinical findings.[100] Initial doses of some important antivenoms are given in Table 75.3. The apparent serum half-lives of antivenoms in envenomed patients range from 26 to 95 hours, depending on which IgG fragment they contain.[100,101] Children must be given the same dose of antivenom as adults since the same amount of venom has been injected.

Recurrent Envenoming. Recurrence of clinical and laboratory features of systemic envenoming, including recurrent venom antigenaemia several days after an initially good response to antivenom, was clearly documented in patients envenomed by Malayan pit vipers (*Calloselasma rhodostoma*) in Thailand in the 1980s and the phenomenon was rediscovered after the introduction of CroFab in the USA.[102] Recurrent envenoming is probably the result of continuing absorption of venom from the injection site after antivenom has been largely cleared from the circulation or perhaps by redistribution of venom from tissue in response to antivenom.[103] Venom absorption may increase after a hypotensive, shocked patient has been

TABLE 75.3 **Guide to Initial Dosage of Some Important Antivenoms**

Species		Antivenom	
Latin Name	English Name	Manufacturer, Antivenom (Abbreviations Explained at Foot of Table)	Approximate Initial Dose
Acanthophis spp.	Death adders	CSL, death adder or polyvalent	6000–18 000 units (1–3 vials)
Bitis arietans	African puff adders	SAVP, polyvalent	80 mL
		Sanofi-Pasteur ('Fav Afrique' and 'FaviRept'), polyvalent	80 mL
Bothrops asper	Terciopelo	ICP polyvalent	5–20 vials
		LBS Antivipmyn Trivalent	
Bothrops atrox	Common lancehead	Brazilian manufacturers, *Bothrops* polyvalent	2–12 vials
Bothrops bilineatus	Papagaio	Butantan polyvalent	2–4 vials
Bothrops jararaca	Jararaca	Brazilian manufacturers, *Bothrops* polyvalent	2–12 vials
Bungarus caeruleus	Common krait	Indian manufacturers, polyvalent	100 mL
Bungarus candidus	Malayan krait	TRC Malayan krait antivenin monovalent or 'neuro-polyvalent'	50 mL
Bungarus fasciatus	Banded krait	TRC Banded krait antivenin or 'neuro-polyvalent'	50 mL
Calloselasma (Agkistrodon) rhodostoma	Malayan pit viper	TRC monovalent or 'haemato-polyvalent'	100 mL
Cerastes species	Desert (horned) vipers	NAVPC polyvalent	30–50 mL
		Vacsera AntiViper or polyvalent	30–50 mL
Crotalus adamanteus	Eastern diamondback rattlesnakes	Protherics ('CroFab')	7–15 vials
Crotalus atrox	Western diamondback rattlesnakes		
Crotalus viridis, C. oreganus, C. helleri	Western rattlesnakes		
Crotalus durissus	Tropical (South American) rattlesnakes	Brazilian manufacturers *Crotalus* or *Bothrops-Crotalus*	5–20 vials
Crotalus simus	Central American rattlesnakes	ICP polyvalent	5–15 vials
		LBS polyvalent	5–15 vials
Cryptelytrops (Trimeresurus) albolabris and *C. macrops*	White-lipped green pit viper and dark green pit viper	TRC Green pit viper antivenin or 'haemato-polyvalent'	50–100 mL
Daboia (Vipera) palaestinae	Palestine viper	Rogoff Medical Research Institute, Tel Aviv, Palestine viper monovalent	50–80 mL
Daboia (Vipera) russelii	Western Russell's viper	Indian manufacturers, polyspecific	100 mL
Daboia (Vipera) siamensis	Eastern Russell's viper (Thailand)	TRC Russell's viper antivenin 'haemato-polyvalent'	50 mL
Daboia (Vipera) siamensis	Eastern Russell's viper (Burma)	Myanmar Pharmaceutical Factory monovalent	80 mL
Dendroaspis species	Mambas	SAVP Dendroaspis or polyvalent	50–100 mL
Dispholidus typus	Boomslang	SAVP boomslang monovalent	1–2 vials
Echis carinatus Asia	Asian saw-scaled viper	Indian manufacturers polyvalent	50 mL
Echis species Africa	African saw-scaled or carpet vipers	MicroPharm EchiTAb-G	10 mL
		ICP EchiTAb-Plus	30 mL
		SAVP Echis monospecific	20 mL
		Sanofi-Pasteur ('Fav Afrique')	100 mL
Echis species Middle East	Middle Eastern saw-scaled vipers	NAVPC polyvalent	50 mL
		Vacsera polyvalent or antiViper	50 mL
Hydrophiinae	Sea snakes	CSL, sea snake	1000 units
Lachesis species	Bushmasters	ICP polyvalent	10–20 vials
		FED Bothrops Lachesis	10–20 vials
		Butantan polyvalent	10–20 vials
Micrurus species Central America	Central American coral snakes	ICP coral snake antivenom	1–5 vials
Micrurus species South America	South American coral snakes	Butantan anti Elapid antivenom	1–5 vials
Naja kaouthia and *N. siamensis* etc.	Monocellate Thai cobra and SE Asian spitting cobras	TRC cobra antivenin or 'neuro-polyvalent'	100 mL
Naja haje, N. nigricollis and other African cobras	Egyptian cobra, black-necked spitting cobra, Cape cobra etc.	SAVP polyvalent	100 mL
		Sanofi-Pasteur FaviRept and Fav Afrique	100 mL
Naja arabica and *N. haje* (Egypt and Middle East)	Arabian and Egyptian cobras	Vacsera polyvalent	100 mL
		NAVPC bivalent Naja/Walterinnesia or polyvalent	100 mL
Naja naja, N. oxiana	Indian cobras	Indian manufacturers, polyspecific	100 mL
Notechis scutatus	Tiger snake	CSL tiger snake or polyvalent	3000–6000 units 1–2 vials
Oxyuranus scutellatus	Taipan	CSL taipan or polyvalent	12 000 units
Pseudechis species	Australian black snakes and king brown snake	CSL black snake antivenom or polyvalent	18 000–54 000 units 1–3 vials

TABLE 75.3 Guide to Initial Dosage of Some Important Antivenoms—cont'd

Species		Antivenom	
Pseudonaja species	Australian brown snakes	CSL brown snake or polyvalent	1000 units
Rhabdophis tigrinus and *R. subminiatus*	Japanese yamakagashi and red-necked keelback	Japanese Snake Institute Nitta-gun Yamakagashi antivenom	1–2 vials
Vipera berus	European adder	Immunoloski Zavod-Zagreb, Vipera polyvalent	10–20 mL
		Therapeutic Antibodies Inc. ('ViperaTAb'), Fab monospecific	100–200 mg
Walterinnesia species	Black desert cobras	NAVPC bivalent Naja/Walterinnesia or polyvalent	50 mL

Brazilian Manufacturers – Instituto Butantan, São Paulo and Fundação Ezequel Dias (FED), Belo Horizonte; CSL, Commonwealth Serum Laboratories, Australia; ICP, Instituto Clodomiro Picado, San José, Costa Rica; Indian Manufacturers – Bharat Serums and Vaccines, Mumbai – Premium Serums and Vaccines and Biological Evans, Hyderabad – Vins Bioproducts, Hyderabad; LBS, Laboratorios Bioclon/Silanes, Mexico City; NAVPC, National Antivenom and Vaccine production Center, National Guard Health Affairs, Riyadh, KSA; SAVP, South African Vaccine Producers (formerly SAIMR); TRC, Thai Red Cross Society, Bangkok.

resuscitated and the bite site becomes better perfused. Recurrent envenoming is more likely when a rapidly eliminated small IgG fragment antivenom is used, such as Fab, or an antivenom of low potency. In this case, an initial dose of antivenom, however large, may not prevent late or recurrent envenoming.

Repeated Dosing. The response to antivenom will determine whether further doses are required. Where post-synaptic neurotoxins are involved, as in the case of envenoming by cobras and Australasian death adders, signs may improve as early as within 30–60 minutes of antivenom treatment. Hypotension, sinus bradycardia and spontaneous systemic bleeding may respond within 10–20 minutes and blood coagulability is usually restored within 6 hours, provided sufficient specific antivenom has been given. A second dose of antivenom should be given if severe cardiorespiratory symptoms persist for more than about 30–60 minutes, and incoagulable blood persists for more than 6 hours, after the start of the first dose.

The '6-Hour Rule'. Studies of envenoming by several species of snakes whose venoms cause coagulopathy have demonstrated that, once an adequate neutralizing dose of antivenom has been given, blood coagulability (assessed by 20WBCT, see above)[38,76] will be restored within a median of 6 hours.[104] This reflects the ability of the liver, highly activated by circulating fibrin(ogen) breakdown products and inflammatory mediators, to restore coagulable levels of clotting factors in patients with consumption coagulopathy. This important observation is the basis for a simple method of titrating antivenom dosage in individual patients whose blood is initially incoagulable. The 20WBCT is performed at 6-hourly intervals and the initial dose of antivenom is repeated every 6 hours until blood coagulability is restored. After that, the 20WBCT is checked at 12-hourly intervals for at least 48 hours to detect recurrent envenoming (see above).

Antivenom Reactions. Early (anaphylactic), pyrogenic, or late (serum sickness-type) reactions may occur.

Early antivenom reactions are not predicted by hypersensitivity tests (see above) because they are not type I IgE-mediated hypersensitivity reactions to equine serum protein.[94] Itching, urticaria, fever, tachycardia, palpitations, cough, nausea and vomiting develop within 10 to 180 minutes of starting antivenom. Incidence, which varies from 3% to 84%, increases with dose and decreases when highly refined antivenom is used and intramuscular rather than intravenous injection is used. Unless patients are watched carefully for 3 hours after treatment, mild reactions may be missed. Up to 40% of patients with early reactions show features of severe systemic anaphylaxis – bronchospasm, hypotension or angio-oedema – but deaths are rare, although they might be misattributed to the envenoming itself. Adrenaline (epinephrine) in an initial dose of 0.5 mL of 0.1% (1:1000, 1 mg/mL) for adults (children, 0.01 mL/kg) should be given at the first sign of a reaction, followed by histamine H_1-blockers such as chlorphenamine maleate (adult dose, 10 mg; children, 0.2 mg/kg) by intravenous injection.

Pyrogenic reactions are caused by contamination during antivenom manufacture. High fever and rigors develop 1–2 hours after treatment, followed by vasodilatation and a fall in blood pressure. Febrile convulsions may be precipitated in children. Patients should be cooled using physical methods and given antipyretic drugs such as paracetamol.

Late (serum sickness-type) reactions develop 5–24 (mean, 7) days after treatment. Their incidence and speed of development increase with the dose of antivenom. They are underreported because patients have usually left hospital by the time they occur. Symptoms include fever, itching, urticaria, arthralgia, which may involve the temporomandibular joint, lymphadenopathy, periarticular swellings, mononeuritis multiplex, albuminuria and, rarely, encephalopathy. Treatment is a histamine H_1-blocker such as chlorphenamine (adults, 2 mg four times a day; children, 0.25 mg/kg per day in divided doses), or, in more severe cases, prednisolone (5 mg four times a day for 5 days in adults; 0.7 mg/kg per day in divided doses for 5 days for children).

Supportive Treatment (in Addition to Antivenom). Artificial ventilation was first suggested for neurotoxic envenoming more than 120 years ago but patients continue to die for lack of respiratory support. Antivenom alone cannot be relied upon to reverse established bulbar and respiratory paralysis. However, neurotoxic effects are fully reversible with time: a patient bitten by *Bungarus multicinctus* in Canton recovered completely after being ventilated manually for 30 days, and a patient probably envenomed by a rough-scaled snake *Tropidechis carinatus* recovered after 10 weeks of mechanical ventilation in Queensland, Australia.

Anticholinesterase drugs may produce a rapid, useful improvement in neuromuscular transmission in patients envenomed by some species of Asian and African cobras, death adders

(*Acanthophis* species), coral snakes (*Micrurus* species) and kraits.[60] It is worth trying the 'Tensilon test' in all cases of severe neurotoxic envenoming, as with suspected myasthenia gravis. Atropine sulphate (adults, 0.6 mg; children, 50 µg/kg) is given first by intravenous injection to block unpleasant muscarinic effects of acetylcholine such as increased secretions and abdominal colic. Edrophonium chloride (Tensilon®) is then given by slow intravenous injection in an adult dose of 10 mg, or 0.25 mg/kg for children, or neostigmine bromide or methylsulphate (Prostigmin®) by intramuscular injection, 0.02 mg/kg for adults, 0.04 mg/kg for children. A simple alternative might be the 'ice test' in which an ice-filled plastic glove is applied to the closed lid of one eye for 2 minutes. If this improves the ptosis on that side compared to the other, effectiveness of anticholinesterase may be inferred.[105] Patients who respond convincingly can be maintained on neostigmine methylsulphate, 0.5–2.5 mg every 1–3 hours up to 10 mg/24 hours maximum for adults or 0.01–0.04 mg/kg every 2–4 hours for children, by intramuscular, intravenous or subcutaneous injection.

Hypotension and Shock. Hypovolaemia is the commonest cause in patients with extensive local swelling. It is confirmed by detecting a postural drop in blood pressure (from supine to 45° or sitting) and treated with intravenous isotonic saline. Central venous pressure monitoring or observation of jugular venous pressure can be used to control volume replacement. Dopamine, initial dose 2.5 µm/kg per minute by intravenous infusion, restored blood pressure in patients envenomed by Burmese Russell's vipers.[26]

Acute Kidney Injury (AKI).[48,56] If urine output drops below 400 mL/24 hours, urethral and central venous catheters should be inserted. If urine flow fails to increase after cautious rehydration, diuretics should be tried, e.g. furosemide (frusemide) by slow intravenous injection, 100 mg followed by 200 mg if urine output fails to increase, and then mannitol, but these are of no proven benefit. If these measures fail to restore urine flow, the patient should be placed on strict fluid balance. Renal replacement therapy (peritoneal dialysis, haemodialysis or haemoperfusion) will be required in most patients with AKI.

Local Infection. A booster dose of tetanus toxoid should be given. A variety of bacteria have been isolated from snakebite wounds.[106,107] Local wound abscesses are common after bites by some species such as South American pit vipers (*Bothrops*)[24] and Malayan pit vipers (*Calloselasma rhodostoma*).[107] Prophylactic antibiotics are not justified unless the wound has been incised or there is evidence of necrosis.[108] Penicillin, erythromycin or chloramphenicol are appropriate, or an antibiotic effective against the bacterial flora of the buccal cavity and venoms of local snakes.[106] An aminoglycoside such as gentamicin should be added for 48 hours.

Intracompartmental Syndrome and Fasciotomy. In a snake-bitten limb, swelling of muscles within tight fascial compartments, such as the anterior tibial compartment, may raise the tissue pressure to such an extent that perfusion is impaired. Ischaemic damage (as in Volkmann's contracture of the forearm) is added to direct effects of the venom. Excessive elevation of the bitten limb reduces arterial perfusion pressure in the compartment decreasing muscle PO_2 and nerve conduction velocity.[72] The classic signs of intracompartmental syndrome include excessive pain, weakness of the compartmental muscle, pain on passive movement, hypoaesthesia of skin supplied by nerves running through the compartment and obvious tenseness of the compartment. These features have been characterized as 'the 7 Ps': Pain at rest, Pain on passive movement, Paralysis, Pallor, Paraesthesiae, Poikilothermia and Pulselessness. However, local envenoming can cause these features in the absence of greatly increased compartment pressure. Inexperienced surgeons may proceed to fasciotomy, at which the discovery of black-looking muscle fasciculi may reassure them that the operation was necessary. However, envenomed but viable muscle often looks black because of haemorrhage and may regenerate. Dangers of fasciotomy include severe persistent bleeding if the venom-induced haemostatic abnormalities have not been corrected by adequate doses of antivenom, delayed recovery of function, prolonged hospital admission and persistent morbidity from damage to sensory nerves and contractures from keloid formation or hypertrophic scarring especially in African patients. Detection of peripheral pulses by palpation or Doppler ultrasound does not exclude intracompartmental ischaemia. However, direct measurement of intracompartmental pressure is reasonably simple, using a perfusion pump and saline manometer system or a commercial transducer such as the Stryker apparatus. An intracompartmental pressure of more than 45 mmHg in an adult or 30 mmHg in a child is associated with a high risk of ischaemic necrosis. In these circumstances, fasciotomy might be justified to relieve the pressure in the compartment. However, decompression did not prove effective in saving envenomed muscle in animal experiments.[109] Necrosis occurs most frequently after digital bites. Fasciotomy must never be embarked upon until blood coagulability has been restored by adequate doses of specific antivenom, followed by the transfusion of fresh whole blood, clotting factors or platelets to hasten restoration of haemostasis.

Unproven Treatments. Corticosteroids, heparin, antifibrinolytic agents such as aprotinin (Trasylol®) and ε-aminocaproic acid, antihistamines, trypsin and a variety of traditional herbal remedies have been used and advocated for snakebite. Most are potentially harmful and none has been proved to be effective.

Snake Venom Ophthalmia.[37] Urgent decontamination is achieved by irrigating the affected eye or mucous membrane as soon as possible using large volumes of water or other bland fluids (saline, milk or even urine, in an emergency). Pain is relieved by instilling adrenaline (epinephrine) eyedrops (0.1%) or cautious temporary use of local anaesthetic drops such as tetracaine. Corneal abrasions must be excluded by fluorescein staining or slit lamp examination or prevented by application of prophylactic topical antibiotics such as tetracycline, chloramphenicol, framycetin ('Soframycin'), ciprofloxacin, penicillin-streptomycin ointment, polymixin B sulphate, gatifloxacin or moxifloxacin. Posterior synechiae formation and ciliary spasm are prevented with topical cycloplegics. In cases of allergic kerato-conjunctivitis in snake keepers, systemic antihistamines are indicated. Topical or intravenous antivenom and topical corticosteroids are contraindicated.

Prevention. Greater efforts should be made through community education to reduce the risk of snakebites. Safer walking could be encouraged by wearing solid footwear such as the light-weight boot tested in rice farmers in Burma[110] and using a light when moving about after dark. Sleeping could be made safer by sleeping on a raised bed, or, where this is impracticable, by sleeping under a well tucked-in mosquito bed net.[111] High-risk habitats, times of day and seasons of the year should be identified, together with the increased danger following floods. Unfortunately, many obvious preventive strategies are impracticable for those, such as farmers in tropical countries, who have to do hard physical work in hot snake-infested areas. Snakes should never be disturbed, attacked or handled unnecessarily even if they are thought to be harmless species or appear to be dead. Venomous species should never be kept as pets or as performing animals. Particular care should be taken while collecting firewood, moving logs, boulders, boxes or debris likely to conceal a snake, and climbing rocks and trees covered with dense foliage or swimming in overgrown lakes and rivers.

Domestic animals such as chickens and rodent pests attract snakes into human dwellings. Snakes can be discouraged by rodent-proofing, by removing unnecessary junk and litter, and by using solid building materials. Various toxic chemicals such as naphthalene, sulphur, insecticides (e.g. DDT, dieldrin and pyrethrins) and fumigants (e.g. methyl bromide, formaldehyde, tetrachloroethane) are lethal to snakes and some plants, such as 'Indian snake root' (*Rauvolfia serpentina*), are said to repel them.

VENOMOUS LIZARDS

Two species of venomous lizard[112] (genus *Heloderma*) have proved capable of envenoming humans. Venom from glands in the mandible is conducted along grooves in the lower teeth. The Gila monster (*H. suspectum*), which occurs in the south-western USA and the adjacent areas of Mexico, grows up to 60 cm in length and is striped (Figure 75.26). The Mexican beaded lizard or escorpión of western Mexico and Central America as far south to Guatemala (*H. horridum*) reaches 80 cm in length and is spotted. *Heloderma* venoms contain lethal glycoprotein toxins, phospholipase A_2 and five interesting bioactive peptides: vasoactive intestinal peptide (VIP) analogues – helospectins I and II and helodermin and glucagon-like peptide-1 (GLP-1) analogues – exendins-3 and -4 which have been developed for the treatment of type 2 diabetes mellitus.[113] Bites are rare and almost always provoked by attempts to handle or molest the animals. These lizards have a powerful grip making the bite difficult to disengage. Radiolucent teeth may be left in the wound. There is immediate severe local pain with tender swelling and regional lymphadenopathy. Both species cause similar symptoms. Pain starts immediately and radiates up the bitten limb to the shoulder, chest and epigastrium. It is often excruciating in intensity and may persist for 24 hours or more. Swelling may extend to involve the whole limb. Red lymphangitic lines extend up the limb and regional lymph glands may become tender and enlarged. Local paraesthesia, hyperaesthesia and paralysis have been described. Systemic symptoms start within 5 minutes of the bite. They include dizziness, weakness, nausea, vomiting, profuse generalized sweating and breathlessness. Hypotension and tachycardia are common. Less commonly, there is angioedema (swelling of lips, tongue, throat and upper airway), increased secretions, chills, fever and tinnitus. Leukocytosis, coagulopathy, electrocardiographic changes, myocardial infarction and acute kidney injury are reported but there have been no confirmed fatalities. Antivenom is not available. A powerful analgesic may be required. Hypotension should be treated with plasma expanders and adrenaline (epinephrine) or a pressor agent such as dopamine.

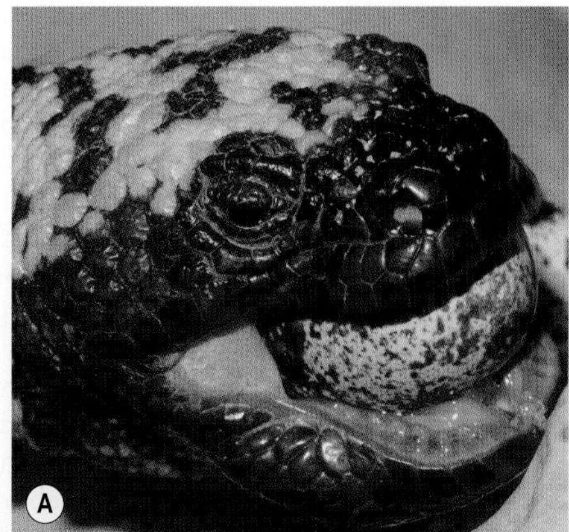

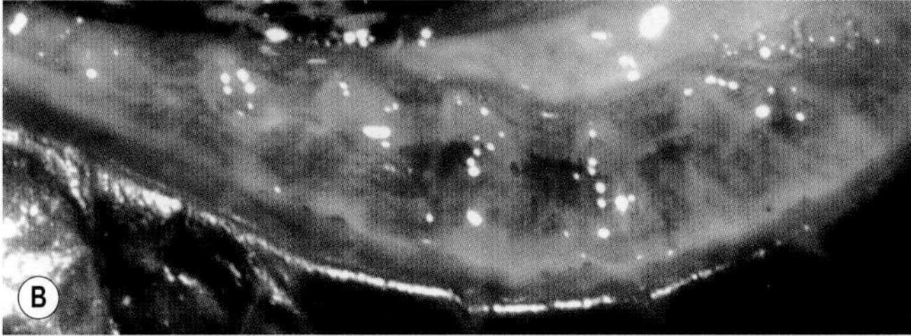

Figure 75.26 (A) Gila monster (*Heloderma suspectum*: family Helodermatidae) eating a bird's egg. (B) Detail – showing venom-conducting lower incisor teeth. *(B, Copyright D. A. Warrell.)*

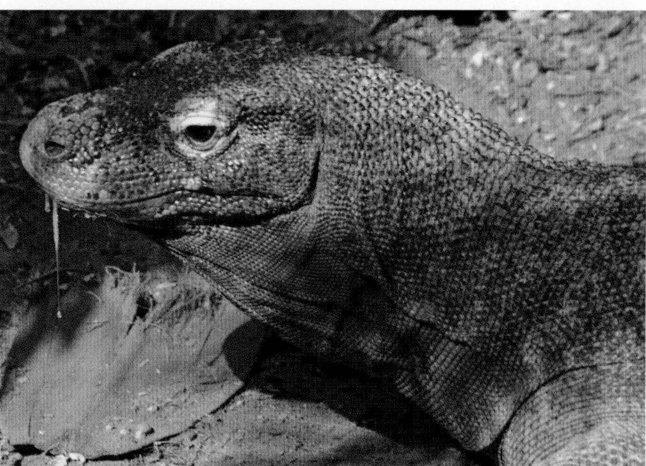

Figure 75.27 Komodo dragon (*Varanus komodoensis*) dribbling venom-containing saliva. *(Copyright D. A. Warrell.)*

Salivary venom secretion has been discovered in two other groups of lizards, iguanas (Iguanidae) and monitors (Varanidae), notably the Komodo dragon (*Varanus komodoensis*, Figure 75.27).[114]

VENOMOUS FISH

Taxonomy

About 200 species of fish,[5,115,116] inhabiting temperate and tropical seas, possess a defensive venom-injecting apparatus that can inflict dangerous stings, but more than 1200 species are now thought to be venomous.[117] Fatal stings have been reported from cartilaginous fish (class Chondrichthyes) such as sharks and dogfish (order Squaliformes) and stingrays and mantas (order Rajiformes); and bony fish (superclass Osteichthyes), such as ray-finned fish (class Actinopterygii) of the orders Siluriformes (catfish), Perciformes (families Trachinidae, weever fish; Uranoscopidae, stargazers or stone-lifters; and others) and Scorpaeniformes (scorpion fish, stonefish).

Venom Apparatus

Venom is secreted around spines or barbs in front of the dorsal, anal or pectoral fins and tail and opercular spines in the gill covers.[115,116] The venom gland in stingrays lies in a groove beneath a membrane covering the barbed precaudal spine up to 30 cm long. The most advanced venom apparatus is found in the genus *Synanceia* (stonefish, family Synanceiidae): bulky venom glands drain through paired ducts to the tips of the short, thick spines.

Venom Composition

Fish venoms are unstable at normal ambient temperatures and so have been difficult to study. Proteinaceous toxins with potent haemolytic and lethal activities have been purified from stonefish (*Synanceia*): trachynilysin releases catecholamine from chromaffin cells and acetylcholine from atrial cholinergic and motor nerve terminals; stonustoxin and verrucotoxin and neoverrucotoxin are proteins of unknown function. Venom of the toad fish (*Thalassophryne nattereri* order Batrachoidiformes), a marine stinging fish of the Brazilian coast, contains a kininogen-like protein. Venoms of the North American round stingray (*Urolophus halleri*) and weever fish (*Trachinus*) contain peptides, protein, enzymes and a variety of vasoactive compounds (kinins, serotonin, histamine, adrenaline and noradrenaline).[118] Toxic effects include local necrosis, direct actions on cardiac, skeletal and smooth muscle, causing electrocardiographic changes, hypotension and paralysis, and central nervous system depression.[115,116]

Epidemiology of Fish Stings

There are hundreds of weever fish stings around the British coast each year, especially in Cornwall. The peak incidence is in August and September. Some 58 cases were seen at a hospital in Pula on the Adriatic over 13 years. In the USA, 1500 stings by rays and 300 stings by scorpion fish are thought to occur each year. A total of 81 cases of stonefish sting were seen over a 4-year period at a hospital in Pulau Bukom, an island near Singapore. Stings by venomous freshwater rays (*Potamotrygon* species) are common in the Amazon region and equatorial Africa.[119] Ornate but highly venomous and aggressive members of the genera *Pterois* and *Dendrochirus* (zebra, lion, tiger, turkey or red fire fish or coral or fire cod, family Scorpaenidae) are popular aquarium pets. Fatal fish stings are very rarely reported. Stings occur when people wading near the shore tread on fish which are lying in the sand or shallow water. Most victims are stung on the sole of the foot, but stingrays lash their tails upwards and impale the ankle. Fishermen, scuba divers and aquarium enthusiasts are stung on the fingers while handling or attempting to fondle the fish.

Symptoms of Envenoming

Immediate, sharp, agonizing pain is the dominant symptom. Bleeding may be seen from single or multiple puncture sites. Hot, erythematous swelling extends rapidly up the stung limb.

Stingrays. These fish are widely distributed in oceans and rivers. The large barbed spine can cause fatal lacerating injuries, usually to the lower part of the legs but occasionally penetrating the body cavities, heart and viscera when the swimmer falls on, or swims over, the ray (as in the case of Steve Irwin, the Australian wildlife presenter). Systemic effects include hypotension, cardiac arrhythmias, muscle spasms, generalized convulsions, vomiting, diarrhoea, sweating and hypersalivation.[115,120]

The venom produces local swelling and sometimes necrosis, with a high risk of secondary infection with unusual marine bacteria capable of causing fatal septicaemias, such as *Photobacterium*, *Vibrio vulnificus* and other *Vibrio* species, *Shewanella putrefaciens*, *Staphylococcus* and *Micrococcus* species and *Halomonas venusta*.

Weevers. Stings by Trachinidae produce intense local pain with slight swelling. Systemic symptoms are rare but some patients develop severe chest pain simulating myocardial ischaemia, cardiac arrhythmias and hypotension.[121]

Scorpion Fish and Stonefish. The family Scorpaenidae comprises more than 350 species which are widely distributed in some temperate and all tropical seas and are especially abundant around the coral reefs of the Indo-Pacific region. Stonefish (genus *Synanceia*) are the most dangerous venomous fish. They occur from East Africa, across the Indian Ocean, to the Pacific. Stings are excruciatingly painful and symptoms may persist for 2 days or more. There is local swelling, discolouration, sweating and paraesthesia and sometimes local lymphadenopathy and necrosis.[122] Systemic symptoms include nausea, vomiting, hypotension, cardiac arrhythmias, respiratory distress, neurological signs, convulsions and evidence of autonomic nervous system stimulation.[122] Fatalities are very rare.

Treatment

The most effective treatment for pain is to immerse the stung limb in water that is uncomfortably hot but not scalding (i.e. just under 45°C). Temperature can be assessed with the unstung limb. Injection of local anaesthetic such as 1% lidocaine, for example as a ring block in the case of stung digits, is less effective. The spine, membrane and other foreign material must be removed from the wound. Prophylactic antibiotics and tetanus toxoid should be given to patients stung by rays or scorpion fish. In the rare cases of severe systemic envenoming, an adequate airway should be established and cardiorespiratory resuscitation instituted when necessary. Severe hypotension can be treated with adrenaline (epinephrine) and bradycardia with atropine. The only antivenom now available commercially is manufactured by the Commonwealth Serum Laboratories in Australia. It neutralizes the venoms of *Synanceia trachynis*, *S. verrucosa* and *S. horrida* and has paraspecific activity against venoms of the North American scorpion fish (*Scorpaena guttata*) and other members of the Scorpaenidae family. One 2 mL ampoule (2000 units) is given intravenously for each two puncture marks found at the site of the sting. The dose is increased in patients with severe symptoms.

Prevention

Bathers and waders should adopt a shuffling gait to reduce the risk of stepping on a venomous fish skulking in sand or mud. Footwear protects against most species except stingrays.

VENOMOUS MARINE INVERTEBRATES

Cnidarians (Coelenterates): Hydroids, Stinging Corals, Medusae, Portuguese Men-O'-War or Bluebottles, Jellyfish, Blubbers, Box-Jellies, Stinging Algae, Sea Anemones and Sea Pansies

Cnidarian stinging capsules or nematocysts are triggered by physical contact or chemicals. They evert at enormous speed, acceleration and force, plunging a thread-like tubule with a sharpened tip into the skin as far as the dermo-epidermal junction and injecting toxin. The tentacles of cnidarians are armed with millions of these nematocysts which produce lines of painful irritant wheals on the skin of swimmers unlucky enough to be embraced by them. Cnidarian venoms contain peptides together with vasoactive compounds such as serotonin, histamine, prostaglandins and kinins which cause immediate severe pain, inflammation, urticaria and sometimes cardiovascular or peripheral vascular problems.[5,115,116]

Epidemiology. Cnidarian stings are common in most parts of the world. The most dangerous, the Australian box-jellyfish (*Chironex fleckeri*), occurs along the north coast of Australia from Broome to Port Curtis. It has caused more than 70 deaths since 1883. Most stings occur in December and January. Other lethal chirodropid cnidarians such as *Chiropsalmus quadrigatus* occur in the Indo-Pacific Ocean.

During a 3.5-year period, 116 cases of marine stings were seen in Cairns, north Queensland.[123] Some 40% of the patients had clinical features of 'Irukandji sting' caused by *Carukia barnesi*. Fatal stings by *Stomolophus nomurai* have been reported from China. Prodigious swarms of the scyphomedusa *Pelagia noctiluca* appeared along the northern Adriatic coast during the summers of 1977–1979. In 1978, it was estimated that 250 000 swimmers had been stung. The North American sea nettle (*Chrysaora quinquecirrha*) (Figure 75.28) is widely distributed throughout the Atlantic and Indo-Pacific oceans and is especially abundant in Chesapeake Bay on the Maryland coast. There are millions of stings each year but no fatalities.

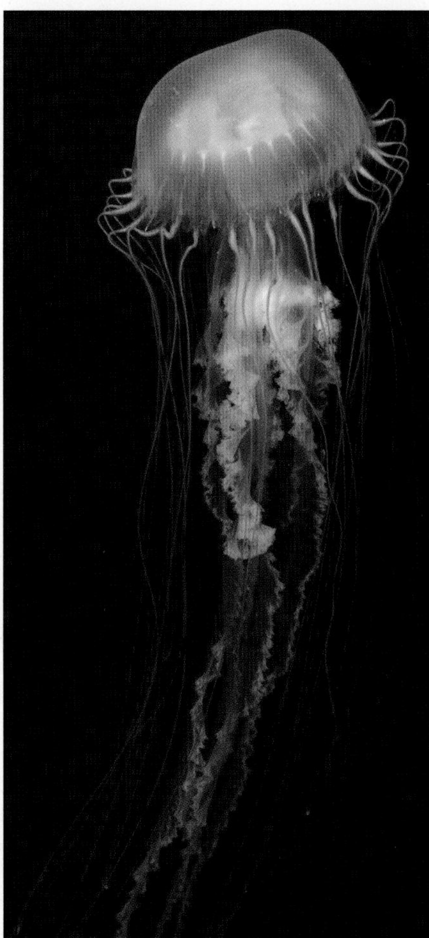

Figure 75.28 East Coast sea nettle (*Chryasaora quiquecirrha*) an abundant jellyfish in Chesapeake Bay, USA. *(Copyright D. A. Warrell.)*

Clinical Features. The imprint of nematocyst stings on the skin may have a diagnostic pattern. *Chironex fleckeri* produces immediate brownish or purplish wheals 8–10 mm wide with cross-striations. More extensive swelling, erythema and vesiculation develop, with areas of necrosis and eventual healing with scar formation. *Carukia barnesi* produces an oval erythematous area about 7 cm in diameter and then transient papules with surrounding hyperhidrosis. Portuguese man-o'-war (*Physalia*) stings produce chains of oval wheals surrounded by erythema. These lesions persist for only about 24 hours. Histological sections of the skin lesions may reveal identifiable nematocysts, allowing differentiation between stings by different genera.

Severe pain is the dominant symptom. Systemic symptoms are most severe following stings by cubomedusae (box-jellyfish), genera *Chironex* and *Chiropsalmus*. The victim, usually a child swimming in shallow water, suddenly screams with pain and within minutes becomes cyanosed, suffers generalized convulsions and is found to be pulseless. The whole jellyfish or a length of tentacles may still be adherent to the patient's skin. Autopsies reveal pulmonary oedema suggesting a cardiac death. *Carukia barnesi* stings cause severe systemic effects minutes to hours after the sting, attributed to catecholamine-induced hypertension, but with little or no local effect. Systemic effects of cnidarian stings include cough, nausea, vomiting, abdominal colic, diarrhoea, rigors, severe musculoskeletal pains, syncope and signs of autonomic nervous system stimulation such as profuse sweating. The Portuguese man-o'-war (*Physalia*) stings may cause local vasospasm leading to gangrene and occasionally cause systemic symptoms, intravascular haemolysis, haemoglobinuria, AKI and rare fatalities. The sea anemone *Anemonia sulcata* produces painful local papules, erythema, oedema and vesiculation and occasional systemic symptoms such as sleepiness, dizziness, nausea, vomiting, myalgia and periorbital oedema.[124]

Treatment. Appropriate first aid is urgent as patients may die within minutes of the sting by box-jellyfish. The victim is taken out of the water, adherent tentacles are washed off with sea water or removed by shaving the skin and hot water is applied to relieve pain (see above, as for fish stings).[125]

Undischarged nematocysts in adherent tentacles should be inhibited. For *Chironex* and other cubozoans, including Irukandji, commercial vinegar or 3–10% aqueous acetic acid inhibits further nematocysts discharge but is not recommended for stings by *Physalia* or *Stomolophus*. For *Chrysaora stings*, baking soda and water (50% w/v) is used. In vitro, several popular remedies, such as alcohol (in sun lotion), ammonia, acetic acid and meat tenderizer, caused massive discharge of *Chrysaora quinquecirrha* and *Physalia physalis* tentacles. However, 5–15% lignocaine hydrochloride prevented discharge and relieved the pain of *Chiropsalmus quadrumanus* and *Chrysaora quinquecirrha* stings, in proportion to the concentration applied.[126]

Pressure immobilization with a crepe bandage may increase the amount of venom injected and is not recommended.[127]

CPR on the beach has proved life-saving in several patients who collapsed, cyanosed and pulseless. Verapamil is not recommended.

A specific 'sea wasp' antivenom is manufactured by the Commonwealth Serum Laboratories in Australia for *Chironex fleckeri* stings. Its effectiveness is uncertain.

Prevention. People, and especially children, should keep out of the sea at times of the year when dangerous cnidarians are most prevalent and especially when they have been sighted and warning notices are being displayed on beaches. Wet suits and other clothing, including fine mesh nylon stockings, are protective.

Echinoderms (Starfish and Sea Urchins)

Echinoderms[5,115,116,128] have hard protective exoskeletons. Starfish (Asteroidea) sprout numerous sharp spines which can penetrate human skin, releasing a violet-coloured liquid that stains the wound. The crown of thorns starfish (*Acanthaster planci*) of the Red Sea and Indian and Pacific Oceans is up to 60 cm in diameter and possesses venomous spines 6 cm long. The venom causes severe local pain, redness and swelling, severe vomiting that may be persistent and, in cases of severe systemic envenoming, hepatic dysfunction, muscle weakness, hyper/hypoaesthesia, facial oedema, cardiac arrhythmias, and paralysis. There is a risk of secondary infection of the wound.[5,116,129]

Sea urchins (Echinoidea), especially of the tropical families Diadematidae and Echinothuridae, have brittle, articulated spines (30 cm long in the black or long-spined sea urchin *Diadema setosum,* Figure 75.29) and grapples (globiferous pedicellariae). Both contain venom which is released when they are embedded in the skin. Impalement and stings by *D. setosum* and the flower sea urchin (*Toxopneustes pileolus*) cause severe local pain and swelling and, if there is severe systemic envenoming, nausea, syncope, numbness, generalized paralysis, aphonia, and respiratory distress. Fatalities have occurred among indigenous peoples.[5,116] The fragments of spines embedded in the skin may cause secondary infection, and granuloma formation several months later. Penetration of bones and joints may be destructive.

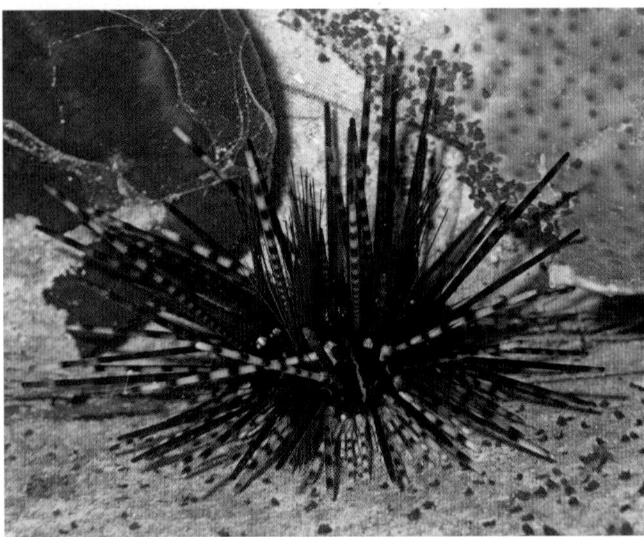

Figure 75.29 Long-spined sea urchin (*Diadema setosum*) Madang, Papua New Guinea. *(Copyright D. A. Warrell.)*

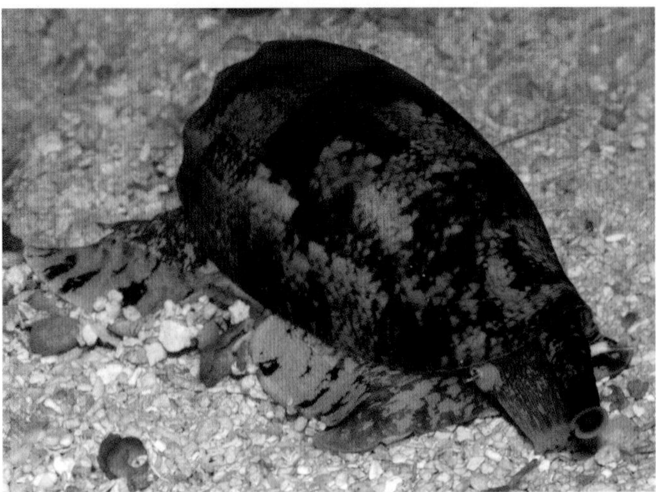

Figure 75.30 Geography cone (*Conus geographus*). *(Copyright D. A. Warrell.)*

Treatment. Spines and pedicellariae must be removed as soon as possible as they may continue to inject venom and give rise to later complications. The sites of penetration are usually on the soles of the feet. The superficial layer of thickened epidermis should be pared down and 2% salicylic acid ointment applied for 24–48 hours to soften the skin. Most spines can then be extruded, but deeply embedded ones may require surgical removal under local anaesthetic.

Molluscs (Cone Shells and Octopuses)

Cone shells (family Conidae) (Figure 75.30) of the Pacific and Indian Oceans and blue-ringed octopuses of Australia and New Guinea (genus *Hapalochlaena*) (Figure 75.31) are rare causes of marine envenoming but there have been a few fatalities. No antivenoms are available.[5,115,116,130]

ARTHROPOD BITES AND STINGS (PHYLUM ARTHROPODA)

Insect Stings (Class Insecta) – Hymenoptera Stings (Bees, Wasps, Yellow Jackets, Hornets, Ants) (Order Hymenoptera)

Fatal sting anaphylaxis in those who have become hypersensitized to the venoms is reported from most parts of the world and is a leading cause of anaphylactic deaths in Western countries. Hymenoptera venoms also have direct toxic effects but these are not seen in man unless there have been many, usually hundreds of, stings, as in the case of mass attacks by Africanized honey-bees (*Apis mellifera scutellata*) in the Americas.[132,133] Apidae (e.g. honey-bees *Apis mellifera*), Vespidae (e.g. wasps, yellow jackets and hornets), fire ants (*Solenopsis*) in the

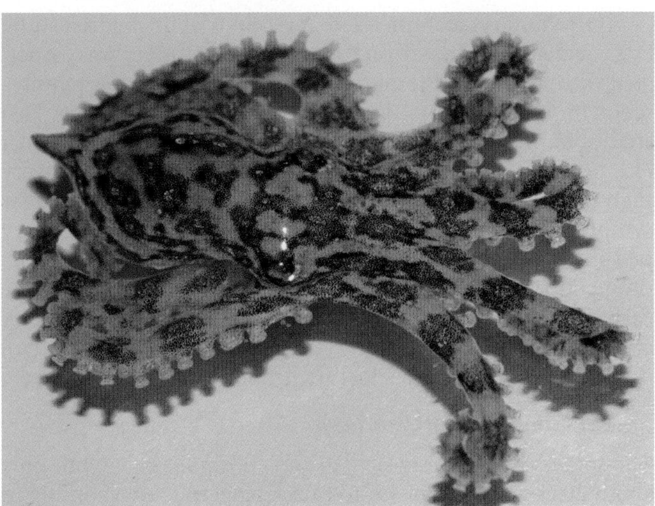

Figure 75.31 Southern blue-ringed octopus (*Hapalochlaena maculosa*) Point York, South Australia. *(Copyright D. A. Warrell.)*

Americas and jumper ants (*Myrmecia*)[131,135] in Australia are important causes of sting anaphylaxis.[5,134]

Venom Apparatus and Composition.[131,135] Venoms are injected through a barbed sting. Bees leave the stings embedded in the skin, but wasps and hornets can sting repeatedly. The venoms contain biogenic amines (histamine, serotonin and acetylcholine), enzymes such as phospholipase A and hyaluronidase, and toxic peptides; kinins in the case of Vespidae; apamin, melittin and antiinflammatory compounds such as mast-cell degranulating peptide in Apidae.

Clinical Features

Direct Toxic Effects in Non-allergic Subjects. Single stings produce only local effects attributable to venom biogenic amines. Pain, and an area of heat, redness, swelling and wealing develop rapidly but rarely exceed 2–3 cm in diameter or last more than a few hours. These effects are dangerous only if the airway is obstructed, e.g. following stings on the tongue.

Fatal systemic toxicity can result from as few as 30 stings in children, while adults have survived more than 2000 stings by *Apis mellifera*. Clinical effects of massive envenoming may resemble histamine overdose: vasodilatation, hypotension, vomiting, diarrhoea, throbbing headache and coma. Mass attacks by Africanized bees in Latin America can cause intravascular haemolysis, generalized rhabdomyolysis, hypertension, pulmonary oedema, myocardial damage, bleeding, hepatic dysfunction and AKI.[133] Hepatic dysfunction and rhabdomyolysis followed by myoglobinuria and AKI can occur after multiple hornet stings (*Vespa affinis*). Intravascular haemolysis with haemoglobinuria (*Vespa orientalis*), thrombocytopenic purpura, myasthenia gravis (*Polistes* species) and various renal lesions, including nephrotic syndrome, have also been described.

Allergic Effects.[136] Between 3% and 4% of the population may be hypersensitive to *Hymenoptera* venoms. Clinical suspicion of venom hypersensitivity arises when systemic symptoms follow a sting. Most patients allergic to bee venom are bee-keepers or their relatives. Systemic symptoms include tingling scalp, flushing, dizziness, visual disturbances, syncope, wheezing, abdominal colic, diarrhoea and tachycardia developing within a few minutes of the sting, progressing to urticaria, angio-oedema, oedema of the glottis, bronchospasm, profound hypotension and coma may develop. Patients may die within minutes of the sting. Raised serum concentrations of mast-cell tryptase, which may persist for up to 6 hours, confirm the diagnosis of anaphylaxis. Serum sickness may develop a week or more after the sting. Atopy does not predispose to sting allergy but asthmatics who are allergic to venom are likely to suffer severe reactions. Reactions are enhanced by β-blockers. The diagnosis of venom hypersensitivity can be confirmed by intradermal prick skin testing with dialysed venoms, or by detecting specific IgE antibodies in serum by the radioallergosorbent test (RAST). A postmortem diagnosis of insect sting anaphylaxis is supported by detecting specific IgE in the victim's serum. Pathological findings in cases of fatal systemic anaphylaxis include acute pulmonary hyperinflation, laryngeal oedema, pulmonary oedema and intra-alveolar haemorrhage.

Treatment. The embedded bee sting must be extracted as quickly as possible.

Toxic Effects of Mass Attacks. Adrenaline, bronchodilators, histamine H_1-blockers and corticosteroids may be needed. No antivenoms are commercially available. AKI is prevented by correcting hypovolaemia and giving mannitol and bicarbonate or treated with renal replacement therapy.

Allergic Effects. Adrenaline (epinephrine) (initial adult dose 0.5 ml of 0.1% solution, children 0.01 mL/kg) is given by intramuscular injection. Those known to be hypersensitive should wear an identifying tag (e.g. 'Medic-Alert') as they may be discovered unconscious after a sting. They should be trained to self-administer adrenaline (e.g. 'EpiPen' delivering 0.3 mg adult, or 0.15 mg child, doses of 0.1% adrenaline). Injection of a histamine H_1-blocker (e.g. chlorphenamine maleate, 10 mg intravenously or intramuscularly) will alleviate the mild urticarial symptoms, and combat the effects of massive histamine release during the reaction. Corticosteroid may prevent recurrence of anaphylaxis, which is said to occur after about 6 hours in up to 10% of cases. Severe reactions may require cardiorespiratory resuscitation, fluid volume replacement and vasopressor drugs. β2 agonists such as salbutamol are needed if there is marked bronchospasm. Respiratory tract obstruction is the main cause of death.

Prevention of Hymenoptera Sting Anaphylaxis. Patients with histories of systemic anaphylaxis and demonstrable venom-specific IgE can be desesensitized.[137]

Scorpion Stings (Order Scorpiones)[131]

Scorpions capable of inflicting fatal stings in humans belong to the families Buthidae (thick-tailed scorpions) and Hemiscorpiidae (rock, creeping or tree scorpions). The most important species include:

- Family Buthidae – *Androctonus, Buthus* and *Leiurus* species in North Africa and the Middle East; *Parabuthus* species in East and South Africa; *Centruroides* species in Arizona and Mexico (Figure 75.32); *Tityus* species in Latin America and *Hottentota* (*Mesobuthus*) *tamulus* in India and Nepal.
- Family Hemiscorpiidae – *Hemiscorpius lepturus* (Middle East).

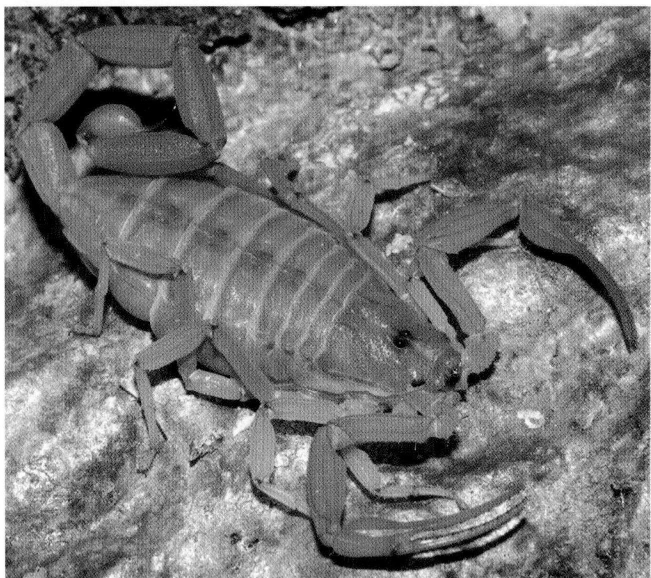

Figure 75.32 Arizona bark scorpion (*Centruroides sculpturatus*) Tucson, Arizona. *(Copyright D. A. Warrell.)*

Epidemiology. Painful scorpion stings are a common event throughout the tropics but fatal envenoming is frequent only in parts of Latin America, North Africa, the Middle East and India. In Mexico, about 250 000 stings are reported each year throughout the country with 70 fatalities. In Brazil, among 36 558 reported stings there were 50 deaths.

Clinical Features. Rapidly developing, excruciating local pain is the most common symptom. Local blistering and necrosis occur only after stings by *Hemiscorpius lepturus*. Systemic symptoms may develop within minutes, but may be delayed for as much as 24 hours. Features of autonomic nervous system excitation are initially cholinergic and later adrenergic. There is hypersalivation, profuse sweating, lacrimation, hyperthermia, vomiting, diarrhoea, abdominal distension, loss of sphincter control, and priapism. Massive release of catecholamines, as in phaeochromocytoma, produces piloerection ('gooseflesh'), tachycardia, hyperglycaemia, hypertension and toxic myocarditis with arrhythmias (most commonly sinus tachycardia), electrocardiographic S–T segment changes, cardiac failure and pulmonary oedema. These cardiovascular effects are particularly prominent following stings by *Leiurus quinquestriatus*, *Tityus* species[138]and *H. tamulus*.[139]

Fasciculation, muscle spasms that can be misinterpreted as tonic-clonic convulsive movements, and respiratory distress are a particular feature of stings by *Centruroides* species. *Parabuthus transvaalicus* envenoming is more likely to cause ptosis and dysphagia. Strokes are described after stings by *Nebo hierichonticus* and *H. tamulus*. Hypercatecholaminaemia could explain hyperglycaemia and glycosuria but, in the case of stings by Trinidadian black scorpions (*T. trinitatis*), there is acute pancreatitis.

Treatment. Pain is most effectively treated by local infiltration of 1% lidocaine or xylocaine, using digital block for stings on digits. Parenteral opiate analgesics such as pethidine and morphine may be required.

Antivenom is recommended. A recent trial in children stung by *C. sculpturatus* in Arizona, antivenom treatment was associated with more rapid resolution of symptoms and less requirement for midazolam sedation than placebo.[140] In India, two studies found that addition of a new antivenom raised against *H. tamulus concanensis* venom produced more rapid recovery than prazosin alone.[141,142] For patients with cardiovascular symptoms (hypertension, bradycardia and early pulmonary oedema) vasodilators such as the α_1-blocker prazosin are recommended. Patients who develop left ventricular failure despite early prazosin therapy benefit from dobutamine.[143] The use of atropine (except in cases of life-threatening sinus bradycardia), cardiac glycosides and β-blockers is not recommended.[138]

Spider Bites (Order Aranea)

The spiders (Order Aranea)[144] are an enormous group but only about 20 species are known to cause dangerous envenoming in humans. Many others have been wrongly accused of inflicting harmful bites.[145] Spiders bite with a pair of fangs, the chelicerae, to which the venom glands are connected.[131] A central venom duct opens near the tip of the fang. In Brazil, in 2005, 19 634 spider bites were reported, with nine deaths (0.05%).

Clinical Features. Spider bites can cause two main clinical syndromes, 'necrotic loxoscelism' and 'neurotoxic araneism'.

Necrotic Loxoscelism. Skin lesions, varying in severity from mild localized erythema and blistering to extensive tissue necrosis, have been falsely attributed to species of familiar peri-domestic species, such as the Australian white-tailed spider (*Lampona cylindrata*), North American hobo spider (*Tegenaria agrestis*), European and South American wolf spiders (*Lycosa*, including the Italian 'tarantula' *L. terentula*) and cosmopolitan sac spiders (*Cheiracanthium*).[145] Only members of the genus *Loxosceles* (American recluse spiders) have proved capable of causing 'necrotic arachnidism/araneism'. *Loxosceles* species are extending their geographical ranges in Central and South America, the USA and in the Mediterranean region, North Africa, Israel and elsewhere.

Some 80% of patients are bitten indoors, usually in their bedrooms while asleep or dressing. The bite may be painless initially but a burning pain develops at the site over the next 12–36 hours with local oedema. An ischaemic lesion ('red-white-and-blue' sign), coloured red (vasodilatation), white (vasoconstriction) and blue (pre-necrotic cyanosis) appears (Figure 75.33) and, over the course of a few days, becomes a black eschar (Figure 75.34), which sloughs in a few weeks, sometimes leaving a necrotic ulcer. Rarely, the necrotic area may cover an entire limb. In 12% of cases there are systemic effects including fever, methaemoglobinaemia, haemoglobinuria and jaundice resulting from haemolytic anaemia, scarlatiniform rash, respiratory distress, collapse and AKI. The case fatality is less than 5%.[146]

Neurotoxic Araneism. Widow, hour-glass, button or red-back spiders (genus *Latrodectus*) are the most widespread and numerous of all venomous animals dangerous to man. *L. mactans* (black widow spider) occurs in the Americas. *Latrodectus tredecimguttatus*, widely but incorrectly known as a 'tarantula', lives in fields in the Mediterranean countries, where it has been responsible for epidemics of bites. The Australian red-back spider or New Zealand katipo (*L. hasselti*) causes up to 340 reported bites each year in Australia, where 20 deaths are known to have occurred.[5,39] This adaptable species has settled in Japan,

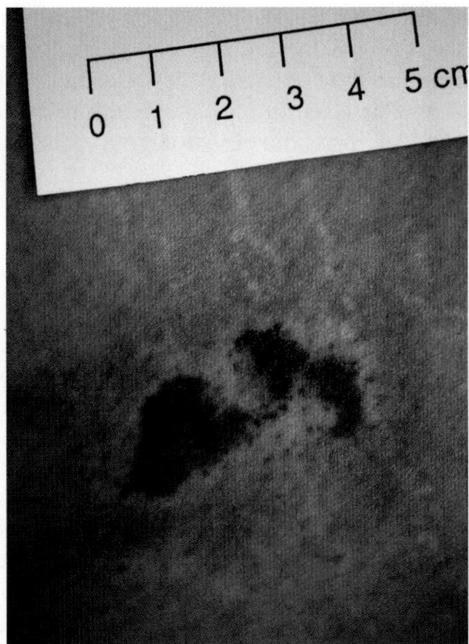

Figure 75.33 Early lesion at the site of the bite of a Brazilian recluse spider (*Loxosceles gaucho*), showing the 'red-white-and-blue' sign. *(Copyright D. A. Warrell.)*

the Middle East, New Caledonia and elsewhere. *Latrodectus mactans* and the brown widow (*L. geometricus*), cause bites in South and eastern Africa. *Latrodectus hasselti* bites produce local heat, swelling and redness, which is rarely extensive. Intense local pain develops in about 5 minutes; after 30 minutes, there is pain in local lymph nodes, and after about an hour, headache, nausea, vomiting and sweating occur. Tachycardia and hypertension may follow but muscle tremors and spasms are uncommon.[5,39] *Latrodectus mactans* bites produce minimal local changes. Local dull aching or numbness may develop after 30–40 minutes. Painful muscle spasms and lymphadenopathy spread and increase in intensity during the next few hours until the trunk, abdomen and limbs are involved and respiration may be embarrassed. An acute abdomen may be simulated by the painful spasms and rigidity. Other features include profuse generalized sweating, tachycardia, hypertension, irritability, psychosis, vomiting and priapism.[144] Similar effects are produced by the Brazilian 'banana', 'armed' or 'wandering' spider (*Phoneutria nigriventer*) and related species, which cause bites and deaths in South American countries. These spiders may be exported in bunches of bananas to temperate countries, where they have been responsible for bites and a few deaths.

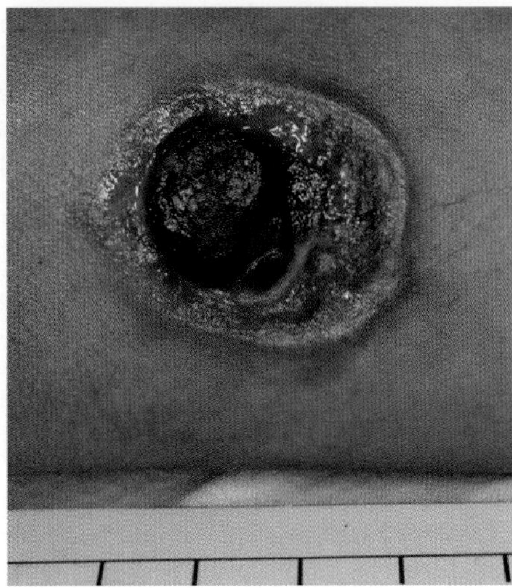

Figure 75.34 Necrotic eschar at the site of a bite by a Brazilian recluse spider (*Loxosceles gaucho*). (Scale in cm.) *(Copyright D. A. Warrell.)*

Funnel web spiders, genera *Atrax* and *Hadronyche*, are confined to south-eastern Australia, the Adelaide area and eastern Tasmania.[5] *Atrax robustus*, the Sydney funnel-web spider, occurs within a 160 km radius of Sydney. Unusually among spiders, the aggressive male is more dangerous to man than the larger female. The powerful chelicerae of this large spider produce a painful bite but there is minimal local envenoming. Numbness around the mouth and spasm of the tongue may develop within 10 minutes, followed by nausea and vomiting, abdominal colic, profuse sweating, salivation and lacrimation, dyspnoea and coma. There are local or generalized muscle fasciculations and spasms, hypertension, and, in some of the fatal cases, pulmonary oedema, thought to be neurogenic in origin. Thirteen deaths, occurring between 15 minutes and 6 days after the bite, were reported between 1927 and 1980.[5]

Treatment

First-Aid Treatment. Pressure-immobilization (see Snakebite above) is recommended for bites by Australian funnel web spiders.[5]

Specific Treatment. Neurotoxic araneism seems more responsive to antivenom than does necrotic loxoscelism.[147] *Atrax robustus* antivenom is effective against the venom of other *Atrax* and *Hadronyche* species.

Supportive Treatment. The use of dapsone for necrotic loxoscelism and intravenous calcium gluconate for *Latrodectus* bite muscle spasms is not evidence based. Antihistamines, corticosteroids, β-blockers and atropine have also been advocated. Surgical debridement for necrotic lesions caused by *Loxosceles* species is not recommended, and corticosteroids, antihistamines and hyperbaric oxygen have not proved helpful.

Tick Bite Paralysis (Order Acari or Acarina, Superfamily Ixodoidea)[148,149]

Taxonomy and Epidemiology. Adult females of about 30 species of hard tick (family Ixodidae) and immature specimens of six species of soft tick (family Argasidae) have been implicated in human tick paralysis. The tick's saliva contains a neurotoxin which causes presynaptic neuromuscular block and decreased nerve conduction velocity.[148,149] The tick embeds itself in the skin with its barbed hypostome, introducing the salivary toxin while it engorges with blood.

Although tick paralysis has been reported from all continents, including Europe, most cases occur in western North America (*Dermacentor andersoni*), eastern USA (*D. variabilis*) and eastern Australia from north Queensland to Victoria (*Ixodes holocyclus*, known as the bush, scrub, paralysis or dog tick). In British Columbia, there were 305 cases with 10% mortality between 1900 and 1968. About 120 cases have been reported in the USA, and in New South Wales there were at least 20 deaths between 1900 and 1945.

Clinical Features.[150] Ticks are picked up in the countryside or in the home from domestic animals, particularly dogs. Most victims are children. After the tick has been attached for about

5 or 6 days, a progressive ascending, lower motor neurone paralysis develops with paraesthesiae. Often, a child, who may have been irritable for the previous 24 hours, falls on getting out of bed first thing in the morning, and is found to be weak or ataxic. Paralysis increases over the next few days: death results from bulbar and respiratory paralysis and aspiration of stomach contents. Vomiting is a feature of the more acute course of *Ixodes holocyclus* envenoming. In the past, this clinical picture was misinterpreted as poliomyelitis. Other neurological conditions, including Guillain–Barré syndrome, paralytic rabies, Eaton–Lambert syndrome, myasthenia gravis or botulism, may also be suspected. Diagnosis depends on finding the tick, which is likely to be concealed in a crevice, orifice, or hairy area of the body such as the scalp or external auditory meatus.

Treatment. The tick must be detached without being squeezed. It can be painted with ether, chloroform, paraffin, petrol or turpentine, or prised out between the partially separated tips of a pair of small curved forceps. Following removal of the tick, there is usually rapid and complete recovery. Ventilatory support may be needed. No antivenom is currently available.

Centipede Stings and Millipede Envenoming (Subphylum Myriapoda)[131]

Centipedes (Class Chilopoda). Many species of centipede (Chilopoda) can inflict painful stings through venomous claws (forcipules) arising from the first thoracic segment just behind the mouth parts. Local pain, swelling, inflammation and lymphangitis may develop. Systemic effects such as vomiting, headache, cardiac arrhythmias and convulsions are extremely rare and the risk of mortality was greatly exaggerated in the older literature. The most important genus is *Scolopendra*, which is distributed throughout tropical countries. Local treatment is the same as for scorpion stings. No antivenom is available.

Millipede Envenoming (Class Diplopoda).[151] Venom glands in each of the body segments secrete or squirt out irritant liquids for defensive purposes. These contain hydrogen cyanide and various aldehydes, esters, phenols and quinonoids. Members of at least eight genera of millipedes have proved injurious to man. Children are particularly at risk when they handle or try to eat these large arthropods. When venom is squirted into the eye, intense conjunctivitis, corneal ulceration and blindness may result. Skin lesions are initially stained brown or purple, blister after a few days, and then peel. First aid is generous irrigation with water. Eye injuries should be treated as for snake venom ophthalmia.

Poisoning by Ingestion of Marine Animals

A variety of illnesses, usually categorized as 'food poisoning', are caused by eating seafood.[115,116,152,153] The best known are attributable to bacterial or viral infections, including *Vibrio parahaemolyticus*, *V. cholerae*, non-O1 *V. cholerae*, *V. vulnificus*, *Aeromonas hydrophila*, *Plesiomonas shigelloides*, *Salmonella typhi*, *Campylobacter jejuni*, *Shigella* species, hepatitis A virus, Norwalk virus and astro- and caliciviruses. Botulism has been reported in people eating uneviscerated, smoked and canned fish.

Various clinical syndromes are associated with ingestion of flesh or viscera of marine animals containing toxins derived from marine microalgae or bacteria (e.g. ciguatera, tetrodotoxic or paralytic shellfish poisoning) or resulting from bacterial decomposition of fish during storage (scombrotoxic fish poisoning).[154,155]

GASTROINTESTINAL AND NEUROTOXIC SYNDROMES

Nausea, vomiting, abdominal colic, tenesmus and watery diarrhoea may precede the development of neurotoxic symptoms.[152,153] Paraesthesiae of the lips, buccal cavity and extremities are early symptoms. Other neurotoxic manifestations include a peculiar distortion of temperature perception so that cold objects feel hot (like dry ice) and vice versa, dizziness, myalgia, weakness starting with muscles of phonation and deglutition and progressing to respiratory paralysis and flaccid quadriplegia in some cases, ataxia, involuntary movements, convulsions, visual disturbances, hallucinations and psychoses, cranial nerve lesions and pupillary abnormalities. Cardiovascular abnormalities include hypotension and bradycardia and some patients develop florid cutaneous rashes.

Ciguatera Fish Poisoning

Ciguatera fish poisoning[156] results from ingestion of any of more than 400 species of warm-water, shore or reef fish between latitudes 35°N and 34°S, especially in the South Pacific and Caribbean (including Florida). These fish are now widely available in fish markets in temperate northern countries to meet the demands of immigrant populations. Overall, there must be more than 50 000 cases in the world each year, with an incidence of up to 2% of the population each year and a case fatality of about 0.1%. The fish most often associated with ciguatera are ray-finned fish (order Perciformes) of the families Serranidae (sea basses and groupers); Lutjanidae (snappers); Scaridae (parrot fish); Scombridae (mackerels, tunas, skipjacks and binitos); Sphyraenidae (barracudas) and Carangidae (jacks, pompanos, jack mackerels, scads) and eels (order Anguilliformes), notably Muraenidae (moray eels).

Causative polyether ciguatoxins, maitotoxins and scaritoxins originate from benthic dinoflagellates such as *Gambierdiscus toxicus* that are ingested by herbivorous fish and in turn become the prey of the carnivorous fish eaten by humans. They excite Na^+ channels and voltage-independent Ca^{2+} channels. Ciguatoxins are concentrated in the fishes' intestine, gonads and viscera. The risk of poisoning is greater with some species, e.g. moray eels and parrot fish (*Scarus sordidus*) and increases as the fish gets older and larger.

Clinical Features. Symptoms first appear minutes to 30 (mean 1–6) hours after eating the poisoned fish. In many cases, especially with milder poisoning, the earliest symptoms are gastrointestinal: sudden abdominal colic, nausea, vomiting and watery diarrhoea. The earliest neurotoxic symptom is numbness or tingling of the lips, tongue, throat and extremities, a metallic taste, and a dry mouth or hypersalivation. Reversed perception of heat and cold is a distinctive symptom. Myalgia, ataxia, vertigo, visual disturbances and pruritic skin eruptions develop later. In severely neurotoxic cases, flaccid paralysis and respiratory arrest may develop. Gastrointestinal symptoms resolve

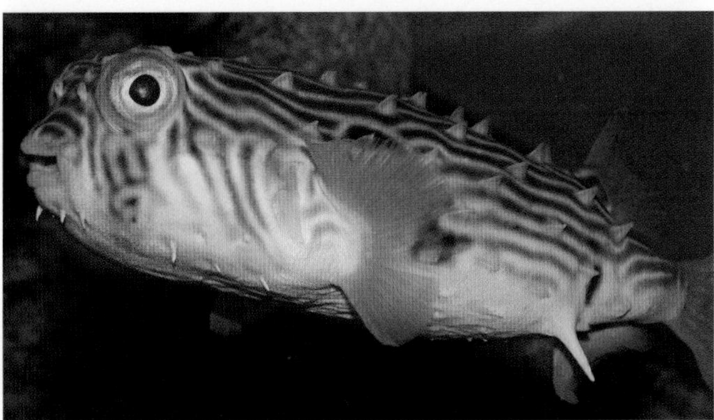

Figure 75.35 Striped burrfish or spiney box-fish (*Chilomycterus schoepfi*: family Diodontinae). *(Copyright D. A. Warrell.)*

within a few hours but paraesthesiae and myalgias may persist for a week, months or even years.

Chelonitoxication from ingestion of marine turtles (Chelonia) resembles ciguatera poisoning. Most outbreaks have been in the Indo-Pacific area. The species usually implicated are green hawksbill and leathery turtles. The case fatality among reported cases is 28%.[115, 116, 156]

Tetrodotoxic (Puffer Fish) Poisoning

More than 50 species of tropical scaleless fish (Order Tetraodonitiformes) have proved poisonous. They include porcupine fish (*Chilomycterus*; Figure 75.35), molas or sunfish (*Mola*), and puffer fish or toadfish (Tetraodontidae – genera *Arothron*, *Fugu*, *Lagocephalus*, etc.). The flesh of the puffer fish (Japanese fugu) is a delicacy in Japan, where, despite stringent regulations and skilful fugu cooks, tetrodotoxin poisoning continues to occur, causing around four deaths each year. Cases have been reported in Thailand and many other Indo-Pacific countries. Tetrodotoxin, an aminoperhydroquinazoline, is one of the most potent non-protein toxins known. It is concentrated in the fishes' ovaries, viscera and skin. There is a definite seasonal variation in toxin concentration, reaching a peak during the spawning season (May–June in Japan). Tetrodotoxin impairs nervous conduction by blocking the sodium ion flux without affecting movement of potassium, producing neurotoxic and cardiotoxic effects. It may be synthesized by *Pseudomonas* bacteria and acquired through the food chain. An identical toxin has been found in the skin of newts (genus *Taricha*), frogs (genus *Atelopus*) and salamanders, the saliva of octopuses (genus *Hapalochlaena*), in the digestive glands of several species of gastropod mollusc and in xanthid and horseshoe crabs, starfish, flat worms (*Planorbis*) and nemertine worms in Japan. Paralytic fresh-water puffer fish poisoning attributable to saxitoxin has been reported in Thailand.

Clinical Features. Paraesthesiae, dizziness and ataxia become noticeable within 10–45 minutes of eating the fish. Generalized numbness, hypersalivation, sweating and hypotension may develop. Some patients remain aware of their surroundings despite appearing comatose while others may appear brain dead. Gastrointestinal symptoms may be completely absent. Death from respiratory paralysis usually occurs within the first 6 hours and is unusual more than 12 hours after eating the fish. Erythema, petechiae, blistering and desquamation may appear.

Paralytic Shellfish Poisoning[114,115,152–154]

Bivalve molluscs such as mussels, clams (*Saxidomus*), oysters, cockles and scallops may acquire neurotoxins such as saxitoxins from the dinoflagellates *Alexandrium* species (formerly *Gymnodinium catenatum*) and *Pyrodinium bahamense* which occur between latitudes 30°N and 30°S. These dinoflagellates may be sufficiently abundant during the warmer months of May–October to produce a 'red tide'. The dangerous season is announced by the discovery of unusual numbers of dead fish and sea birds. Symptoms develop within 30 minutes of ingestion. They include perioral paraesthesia, gastrointestinal symptoms, ataxia, visual disturbances and pareses, progressing to respiratory paralysis within 12 hours in 8% of cases. Milder gastrointestinal and neurotoxic symptoms without paralysis have been associated with ingestion of molluscs contaminated by neurotoxic brevetoxins from *Gymnodinium breve*, which act on sodium channels. These microalgae also produce a 'red tide'.

Histamine Syndrome (Scombrotoxic Poisoning)

The dark red flesh of scombroid fish such as tuna, mackerel, bonito and skipjack, and of canned non-scombroid fish such as sardines and pilchards, may be decomposed by the action of bacteria such as *Proteus morgani*, decarboxylating muscle histidine into histamine, saurine, cadaverine and other toxins. Toxic fish may produce a warning tingling or smarting sensation in the mouth when eaten. Between minutes and up to 24 hours after ingestion, flushing, burning, urticaria and pruritus of the skin, headache, abdominal colic, nausea, vomiting, diarrhoea, hypotensive shock and bronchial asthma may develop. Exogenous histamine may be detected in patients' plasma and urine and in the fish.[155] Identical symptoms have been described in Sri Lankan patients who ate fish while taking the antituberculosis drug isoniazid, which inhibits the enzyme normally responsible for inactivating histamine.[157]

Poisoning by Ingestion of Carp's Gallbladder[158]

In parts of the Far East, the raw bile and gallbladder of various species of freshwater carp are believed to have medicinal properties. Patients develop acute abdominal pain, vomiting and watery diarrhoea 2–18 hours after drinking the raw bile or eating the raw gallbladder of these fish. Hepatic and renal damage may develop, progressing to hepatic failure and oliguric or non-oliguric AKI. The hepatonephrotoxin has not been identified, but is heat-stable and may be derived from the carp's diet.

TREATMENT OF MARINE POISONING

The differential diagnosis includes bacterial and viral food poisoning and allergic reactions. No specific treatments or antidotes are available. If ingestion was recent, gastrointestinal contents should be gently eliminated by emetics and purges. Activated charcoal absorbs saxitoxin and other shellfish toxins. Atropine is said to improve gastrointestinal symptoms and sinus bradycardia in patients with gastrointestinal and neurotoxic poisoning. Oximes, such as pralidoxime and 2-pyridine aldoxime, have been claimed to benefit the anticholinesterase features of ciguatera poisoning, but the evidence is not convincing. Calcium gluconate may relieve mild neuromuscular symptoms. In scombroid poisoning, adrenaline (epinephrine), histamine H_1-blocker, corticosteroids and bronchodilators

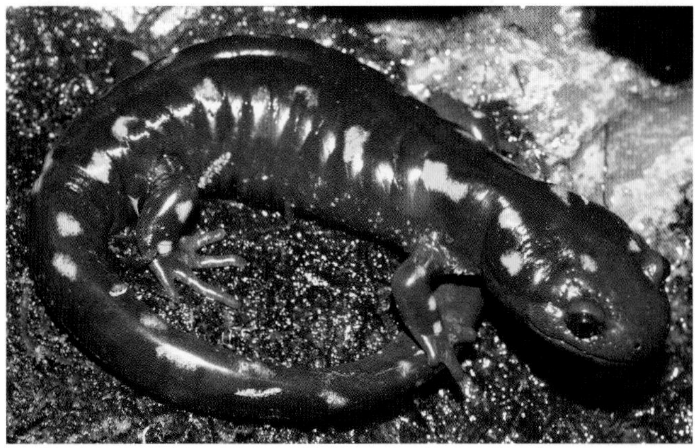

Figure 75.36 Spotted salamander (*Ambystoma maculatum*: family Ambystomatidae). *(Copyright D. A. Warrell.)*

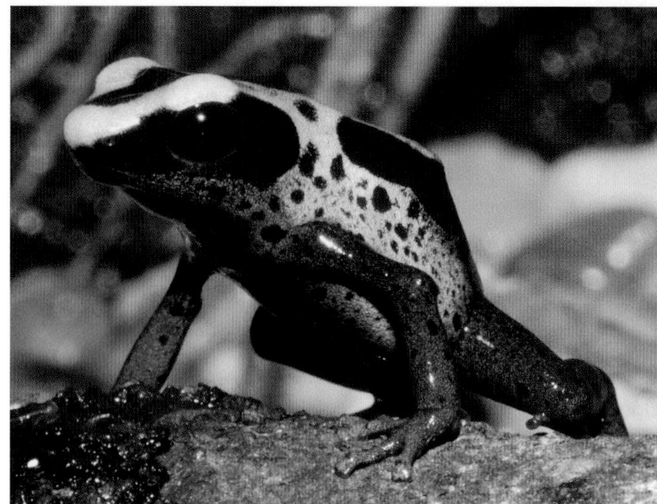

Figure 75.37 Dyeing dart frog (*Dendrobates tinctorius*: family Dendrobatidae). *(Copyright D. A. Warrell.)*

should be used, depending on severity. In cases of paralytic poisoning, endotracheal intubation and mechanical ventilation and cardiac resuscitation have proved life-saving. In Malaysia, a patient with tetrodotoxin poisoning developed fixed dilated pupils and brain stem areflexia, so appearing brain dead, but made a complete recovery after being mechanically ventilated.[159] The use of mannitol intravenously in acute ciguatera poisoning is not supported by convincing evidence.[160,161]

Gabapentin has been suggested as a treatment for chronic persisting paraesthesiae after ciguatera poisoning.[162]

PREVENTION OF MARINE POISONING

Ciguatera, tetrodotoxin and histamine are heat-stable, so cooking does not prevent poisoning. In tropical areas, the flesh of fish should be separated, as soon as possible, from the head, skin, intestines, gonads and other viscera, which may have high concentrations of toxin. All scaleless fish should be regarded as potentially tetrodotoxic, while very large fish carry an increased risk of being ciguateratoxic. Tetraodontiform fish, Moray eels and parrot fish should never be eaten. Some toxins are fairly water-soluble and may be leeched out, so water in which fish are cooked should be thrown away. Scombroid poisoning can be prevented by prompt freezing or by eating the fish fresh. Shellfish should not be eaten during the dangerous season and when there are red tides.

POISONOUS AMPHIBIANS[163]

The moist skin of amphibians such as frogs (Figure 75.37), toads, newts, and salamanders (Figure 75.36) is an accessory respiratory organ that is protected from micro-organisms by highly toxic secretions containing amines, peptides, proteins, steroids, and alkaloids. Ingesting these animals can be fatal. Some toads can squirt from their parotid glands venom containing bufadienolides which affect membrane Na^+/K^+-ATPase. When licked or put in the mouth by dogs or children or when ingested as Chinese traditional medicines, the poisons can cause fatal digoxin-like poisoning. Symptoms include hypersalivation, cyanosis, cardiac arrhythmias, and generalized convulsions. Antidigoxin antibodies ('Digibind', 'DigiTAb') have some therapeutic effect.

REFERENCES

5. Sutherland SK, Tibballs J. Australian Animal Toxins. The Creatures, their Toxins and Care of the Poisoned Patient. 2nd ed. Melbourne: Oxford University Press; 2001.
8. Meier J, White J, editors. Handbook of Clinical Toxicology of Animal Venoms and Poisons. Boca Raton: CRC Press; 1995.
24. Warrell DA. Epidemiology, clinical features and management of snakebites in Central and South America. In: Campbell J, Lamar WW, editors. Venomous Reptiles of the Western Hemisphere. Ithaca: Cornell University Press; 2004. p. 709–61.
81. Sutherland SK, Coulter AR, Harris RD. Rationalization of first-aid measures for elapid snakebite. Lancet 1979;i:183–6.
115. Halstead BW. Poisonous and Venomous Marine Animals of the World. 2nd ed. New Jersey: Darwin Press; 1988.

USEFUL WEBSITES

Envenoming

General: http://vapaguide.info

General, especially in Australasia: http://www.toxinology.com/

WHO Snakebite in Africa: http://www.afro.who.int/en/clusters-a-programmes/hss/essential-medicines/highlights/2731-guidelines-for-the-prevention-and-clinical-management-of-snakebite-in-africa.html

WHO Snakebite in South and South-east Asia: http://www.searo.who.int/entity/emergencies/documents/9789290223774/en/index.html

Antivenoms General

Global crisis: http://globalcrisis.info/latestantivenom.htm

Munich AntiVenomINdex (MAVIN): http://toxinfo.org/antivenoms/

WHO Venomous snakes distribution: http://apps.who.int/bloodproducts/snakeantivenoms/database/

WHO Guidelines for the Production, Control and Regulation of Snake Antivenom Immunoglobulins: http://www.who.int/bloodproducts/snake_antivenoms/snakeantivenomguide/en/

European Antivenoms

Zagreb Immunology Institute in Croatia: http://www.imz.hr/english/products/Description-European-Viper-Venom-Antiserum.pdf

Australian Antivenoms

CSL antivenom handbook: http://www.toxinology.com/generic_static_files/cslavh_antivenom.html

South African Antivenoms

South African Vaccine Producers: http://www.savp.co.za/

Venomous Snake Taxonomy Updates

School Of Biological Sciences: http://pages.bangor.ac.uk/~bss166/update.htm

Scorpions

Norwegian University of Science and Technology: http://www.ub.ntnu.no/scorpion-files/index.php

Access the complete references online at www.expertconsult.com

76 Plant Poisons and Traditional Medicines

JEFFREY K. ARONSON

KEY POINTS

- The recreational use of plants for their stimulant, aphrodisiac, or hallucinogenic effects is ancient, and throughout the ages plants have been used as poisons.
- Many plants that are regarded as poisonous have been used for their supposed therapeutic properties, but while many can still be found in herbals, not all have found their way into modern formularies. In contrast, many tropical plants are used herbally, although evidence of efficacy is often poor or lacking.
- Traditional medicines exist in many forms and lack standardization; very few have been rigorously tested for toxicity, especially for their long-term effects.
- Traditional medicines are often prescribed as complex mixtures with uncertain pharmacology, or are prepared and taken by patients themselves. Poisoning occurs because the herb is itself toxic, has been mistaken for another plant, mislabelled, mixed accidentally or deliberately with other, poisonous, plants and medicines, contaminated with insecticides or herbicides, or, as in the Asian kushtays, mixed with appreciable amounts of heavy metals. Herbal medicines are also used in combination with allopathic drugs, and the often unpredictable effects of such combinations add to the hazards.
- Plant poisoning can occur as a result of accidental, unknowing, or deliberate poisoning from contaminated foodstuffs or from toxic seeds and fruits; from the misuse of traditional or herbal medicines; or from the deliberate use of plants for their psychotropic or supposedly aphrodisiac properties.

Introduction

Since ancient times, people have used plants as sources of chemicals, for therapeutic and recreational purposes and for poisoning.[1] Curare (from *Chondodendron tomentosum* Figure 76.1), a toxin used by South American Indians as an arrow poison (the word *toxin* comes from a Greek word meaning 'a bow'), is a good example of a poison that has been harnessed therapeutically.[2] Its pharmacological action on skeletal muscle was demonstrated by Claude Bernard in 1856,[3] and curare was introduced into anaesthetic practice in 1942.[4]

Many plants that are regarded as poisonous have been used for their supposed therapeutic properties, but while many can still be found in herbals, not all have found their way into modern formularies. Some therapeutically useful chemicals found in plants are listed in Table 76.1. However, the list is relatively short and although ethnopharmacology aims to remedy that, there are difficulties.[5] There have been few successes. When the US National Cancer Institute, in collaboration with the US Department of Agriculture initiated a plant screening programme for anticancer drugs from 1960 to 1981, over 114 000 plant extracts from an estimated 15 000 species were screened, representing about 6% of the world's plant species; only about 4% of the extracts had any activity and of those, only taxol eventually got beyond phase II studies.[6] In contrast, many tropical plants are used herbally, although evidence of efficacy is often poor or lacking. Recent harnessing of ancient remedies has also been singularly unimpressive, a rare exception being the development of artemisinin derivatives from qinghao (*Artemisia annua*; Figure 76.2).[7]

The recreational use of plants for stimulant, aphrodisiac, or hallucinogenic effects is also ancient.[1,8,9] In contrast to most of the therapeutic plants listed in Table 76.1, many of these plants are native to the tropics. Examples include absinthe (*Artemisia absinthium*);[10] ayahuasca (a combination of *Banisteriopsis* spp. and a plant such as *Psychotria viridis* or *Diplopterys cabrerana*, as a source of dimethyltryptamine, a 5-HT_{2A}, 5-HT_{2C} and 5-HT_{1A} receptor agonist;[11] betel leaves (*Piper betle*) taken with areca (betel) nuts (*Areca catechu*); cannabis; cocaine; Jimson weed (*Datura stramonium*); kava (*Piper methysticum*); khat (*Catha edulis*); mescalin or peyotl (*Lophophora williamsii*); morning glory (*Ipomoea tricolori*); nicotine (from many plants, including *Nicotiana tabacum*); nutmeg (*Myristica fragrans*; Figure 76.3); ololiuqui (*Rivea corymbosa*); opioids; and pituri (*Duboisia hopwoodii*). The ascomycete *Ophiocordyceps sinensis* (or *Cordyceps sinensis*),[12] also called Chinese caterpillar fungus and more recently Himalayan Viagra, is a parasitic fungus that grows in symbiosis with the ghost moth genus *Thitarodes* in the mountains of Tibet and Nepal, where it is called 'yarchagumba'; it is a prized Chinese traditional medicine and a Tibetan folk remedy and has been used as an aphrodisiac.

Plants are also sometimes used for culinary purposes; examples include *Papaver rhoeas*, whose seeds are used to decorate bread and as a filling in the delicious Jewish pastry called Hamantaschen (literally Haman's ears), eaten in remembrance of the events in Persia that are recounted in the book of Esther; tansy (*Tanacetum vulgare*) used to make tansy cakes, for consumption at Easter time; cannabis in hashish fudge (a recipe for which can be found in *The Alice B Toklas Cook Book*[13]), space cakes or hash brownies (which featured in the 1968 movie *I Love You, Alice B Toklas*); and a wealth of vegetables (such as cassava and yams) and culinary herbs and spices, too numerous to be listed.

TABLE 76.1 Some Commonly Used Therapeutic Agents that Originally Derived from Plants (see also Tables 76.2 and 76.3)

Drug	Example of Medical Use	Plant of Origin
Artemisinin derivatives	Malaria	*Artemisia annua* (qinghao)
Atropine	Anticholinergic	*Atropa belladonna* (deadly nightshade)
Cannabinoids	Palliative care	*Cannabis sativa* (cannabis)
Capsaicin	Painful neuropathies	*Capsicum* spp. (peppers)
Cephaeline	[Emetogenic]	*Cephaelis ipecacuanha* (ipecacuanha)
Cocaine	Local anaesthetic	*Erythroxylon coca* (coca)
Colchicine	Gout, Familial Mediterranean Fever	*Colchicum autumnale* (autumn crocus)
Curare	Anaesthesia	*Chondodendron tomentosum* (pareira)
Digoxin/digitoxin	Atrial fibrillation and heart failure	*Digitalis lanata/purpurea* (foxgloves)
Ephedrine	Sympathomimetic	*Ephedra sinica* (sea-grapes)
Gamolenic acid	Mastodynia	*Oenothera biennis* (evening primrose)
Hyoscine (scopolamine)	Anticholinergic	*Datura stramonium* (thorn apple)
Ispaghula	Laxative	*Plantago ovata* (ispaghula)
Opioid alkaloids	Analgesia	*Papaver somniferum* (poppies)
Physostigmine	Myasthenia gravis	*Physostigma venenosum* (Calabar bean)
Pilocarpine	Glaucoma	*Pilocarpus jaborandi* (jaborandi)
Quinine	Malaria	*Cinchona pubescens* (cinchona)
Salicylates	Analgesics	*Spiraea ulmaria* (meadowsweet) *Salix alba* (willow) *Gaultheria procumbens* (wintergreen)
Sennosides	Purgative	*Cassia acutifolia* (senna)
Taxanes	Cytotoxic	*Taxus* spp. (yew trees)
Theophylline	Asthma	*Camellia sinensis* (tea plant)
Topoisomerase inhibitors	Cancers	*Camptotheca acuminata (cancer tree)*
Vinca alkaloids	Cytotoxic	*Catharanthus rosea* (Madagascar periwinkle)

And, of course, throughout the ages plants have been used as poisons. Socrates, for example, executed himself at the behest of the state, supposedly using hemlock (*Conium maculatum*), although the exact poison that was used is disputed.[14] We do not know what the hebenon was that Hamlet's uncle poured in the elder Hamlet's ear, but it may have been from henbane (*Hyoscyamus niger*; Figure 76.4) or some form of yew (*Taxus*; German Eibenbaum). And aconite (from *Aconitum napellus*; Figure 76.5) is a toxin that has been used as an arrow poison and was a favourite of professional poisoners in the Roman empire; it is still to be found in some Chinese herbs[15] and has been used as a homicidal poison in modern times.[16] Poisons were so commonly used as weapons of assassination that Mithridates, King of Pontus (120–63 BC), tried to prepare a universal antidote for poisoning (hence called a 'mithridate') by combining many substances in a single formulation, which he then took in increasing doses, in an attempt to achieve immunity to their toxic effects.[17]

Traditional medicines exist in many forms and lack standardization; very few have been rigorously tested for toxicity, especially for their long-term effects. They are often prescribed as complex mixtures with uncertain pharmacology or are

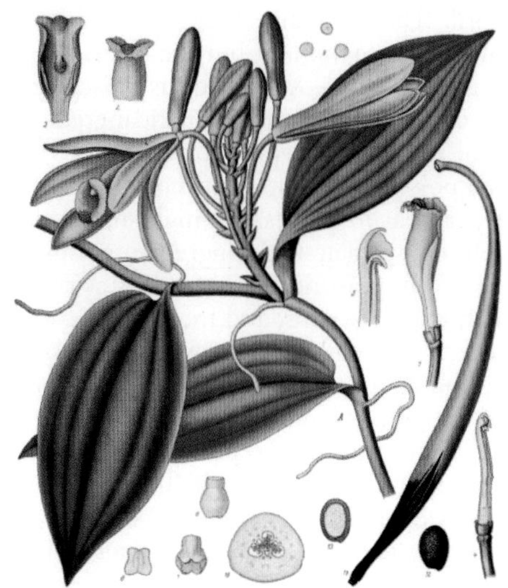
Figure 76.1 *Chondodendron tomentosum* (curare).

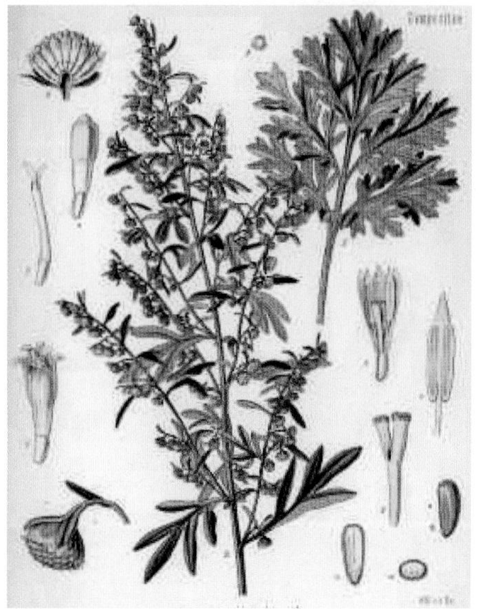
Figure 76.2 *Artemisia absinthium* (wormwood).

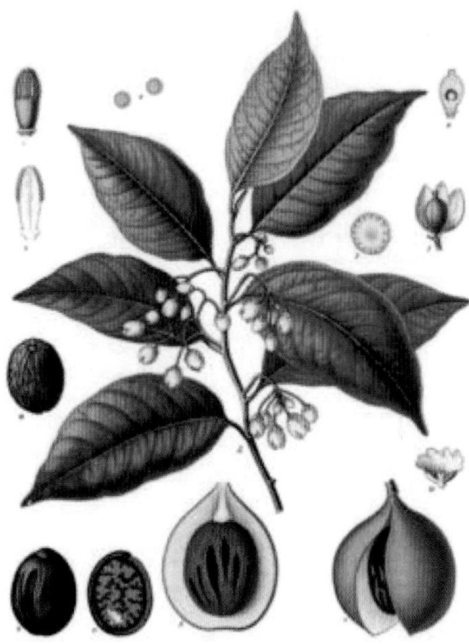

Figure 76.3 *Myristica fragrans* (nutmeg).

prepared and taken by patients themselves. Poisoning occurs because the herb is itself toxic, has been mistaken for another plant, mislabelled, mixed accidentally or deliberately with other, poisonous, plants and medicines, contaminated with insecticides or herbicides, or, as in the Asian kushtays, mixed with appreciable amounts of heavy metals.[18] Herbal medicines are also used in combination with allopathic drugs, and the often unpredictable effects of such combinations add to the hazards.[19]

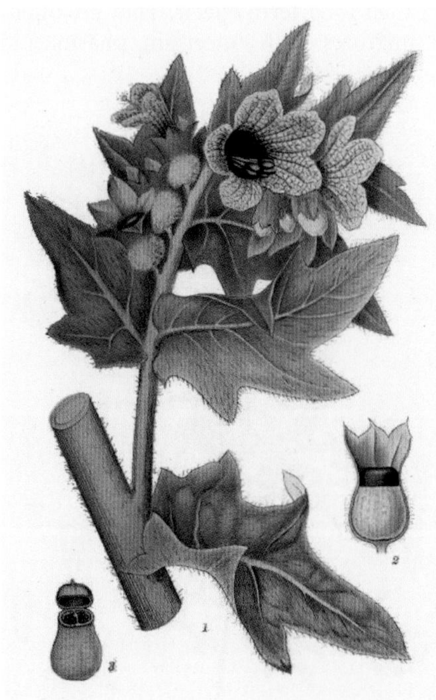

Figure 76.4 *Hyoscyamus niger* (henbane).

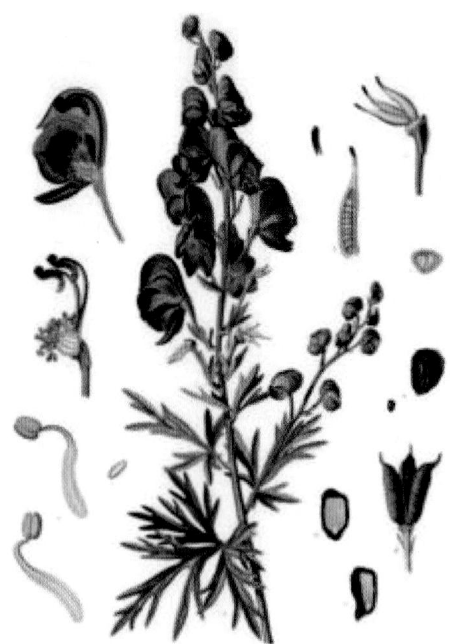

Figure 76.5 *Aconitum napellus* (monkshood).

Plant poisoning can occur as a result of accidental, unknowing, or deliberate poisoning from contaminated foodstuffs or from toxic seeds and fruits; from the misuse of traditional or herbal medicines; or from the deliberate use of plants for their psychotropic or supposedly aphrodisiac properties. Contact dermatitis can occur from contact with irritant plants.[20] A report from the Uppsala Monitoring Centre of the WHO has summarized all suspected adverse reactions to herbal medicaments reported from 55 countries worldwide over 20 years.[21] A total of 8985 case reports were on record. Most originated from Germany (20%), followed by France (17%), the USA (17%), and the UK (12%). Allergic reactions were the most frequent serious adverse events and there were 21 deaths. The relative lack of reports from tropical countries may have been because of poor reporting.

Not all parts or constituents of a poisonous plant are poisonous. The stalks of rhubarb can be eaten, but the leaves contain toxic oxalates; all parts of the yew are poisonous except the fleshy red aril. The purgative castor oil is expressed from the beans of *Ricinus communis*, but the beans also contain the highly toxic alkaloid ricin. Ackee fruit is poisonous only when unripe. Furthermore, the amount of toxic ingredient in a single part of a plant varies from season to season.

Nor are all poisonous plants poisonous to all species. Goats, for example, can eat foxgloves and nightshade with impunity, since they eliminate their toxic ingredients rapidly; bees can harvest pollen from poisonous plants, such as rhododendrons, which contain grayanotoxins, and the honey so produced may be poisonous to humans (see below).[22] One should not be misled by seeing an animal feed on a plant, into thinking that it is safe for human consumption.

The frequency of exposure to poisonous plants is difficult to assess. Many reports are anecdotal. In one series of 912 534 plant exposures in the USA, *Philodendron* spp. were the most commonly implicated, followed by *Dieffenbachia*, *Euphorbia*, *Capsicum*, and *Ilex*.[23] In a series of 135 cases of severe plant poisonings (23 children, 112 adults) in Switzerland, including five deaths, 12 plants were the most commonly involved: *Atropa belladonna* ($n = 42$); *Heracleum mantegazzianum* (18); *Datura stramonium* (17); *Dieffenbachia* (11); *Colchicum autumnale* (10); *Veratrum album* (8); *Aconitum napellus* (4); *Aesculus hippocastanum* (3); *Hyoscyamus niger* (3); *Ricinus communis* (3); *Oenanthe crocata* (2); and *Taxus baccata* (2).[24] Of 277 cases of acute poisoning in South Africa during 12 months, 18% were due to ingestion of traditional medicines; 26% were fatal.[25] In 1306 cases of acute poisoning during 5 years, 16% were due to traditional medicines; 15% of these were fatal and poisoning with traditional medicines resulted in the highest mortality, accounting for 52% of all deaths due to acute poisoning.[26]

In a review of the American Association of Poison Control Centers (AAPCC) 1983–2009, there were 668 111 reported exposures to plants during 2000–2009, of which 621 109 were exposures to single substances.[27] In all, 8.9% of all exposures involved plants in 1983, 6.0% in 1990, 4.9% in 2000, and 2.4% in 2009. Male subjects accounted for 52% of ingestions and over 60% of the moderate and major outcomes; children aged 5 years or under accounted for 81% of plant exposures. Only 45 deaths were recorded between 1983 and 2009; *Datura* and *Cicuta* species were responsible for 36%.

There is no simple way of classifying poisonous plants, other than by the scientific names of their genera and species and even those change from time to time. Furthermore, many disparate plants contain compounds with similar effects. This chapter contains a mixture of headings, using either the names of the plants or their chief constituents; or terms that describe their chemical or pharmacological characteristics or their clinical effects. The following discussion will not be restricted to plants that are found only in tropical areas.

Alcohol

The history of alcohol is as ancient as human history, and plants play a central part in its production. Rum (65–72% alcohol) is distilled from fermented molasses in the West Indies and South America; arrack or sake (50–60%) is manufactured from fermented rice in India, China, Java, and Japan. Toddy, made from the sweet sap of various palms, such as coconut, is drunk in India, Sri Lanka, and West Africa. A potent drink, pulque, is made in South America from the juice of agaves.

The main medical and psychiatric problems caused by alcohol are:

- acute alcohol intoxication;
- chronic alcoholism associated with chronic organ damage (e.g. cirrhosis, cardiomyopathy);
- alcohol withdrawal reactions (delirium tremens).

In the brain, alcohol acts as a dose-dependent depressant, producing the well-known features of intoxication. At plasma concentrations of around 40 mg/dL (400 mg/L or 8.7 mmol/L) learned skills are impaired, including the ability to maintain self-restraint. Other early effects include loss of attentiveness, loss of concentration, and impaired memory, and there may be lethargy. At progressively higher concentrations, there are further changes in mood, behaviour, and a variety of sensory and motor functions. The effects on mood depend on the individual's personality, mental state, and social environment. Commonly, there is euphoria, but any kind of mood change can occur. Libido is often enhanced, but sexual performance is impaired. Alcohol generally increases confidence, often resulting in aggressive or silly behaviour; loss of self-restraint leads to increased loquacity with immoderate speech content, such as swearing or the use of lewd language. Unsteadiness of gait, slurred speech, and difficulty in carrying out even simple tasks, with impaired coordination, become obvious at plasma concentrations of about 80 mg/dL (the concentration above which driving is illegal in many countries). Driving skills are therefore impaired and are affected even at concentrations below 80 mg/dL. Recovery from dazzle is delayed, which can impair night-time driving. Visual acuity, peripheral vision, colour vision, and visual tracking are impaired. Hearing and taste may also be impaired. The pain threshold is increased. At high concentrations, there may be vertigo and nystagmus. Alcohol causes acute drowsiness and deep sleep; in high concentrations it causes coma and respiratory depression. In some individuals, sleep may later be impaired. On waking, there is the characteristic 'hangover', which usually consists of irritability, headache, thirst, abdominal cramps, and bowel disturbance. The cause of hangover is not known.

Delirium tremens is an acute withdrawal reaction that can be fatal. The symptoms come on within a few hours after the last drink and mount over the next 2–3 days. At first, there is anxiety, agitation, tremulousness, and tachycardia. These are later accompanied by confusion, severe agitation, and hallucinations (often visual). The patient is tremulous, sweating, and tachypnoeic and may be pyrexial, dehydrated, hypoglycaemic, and vitamin-deficient. The blood pressure may be high, low or normal. Nausea and vomiting are common. Seizures can occur and can be prolonged and potentially life-threatening.

The medical management of alcohol withdrawal (including delirium tremens) involves the maintenance of fluid and electrolyte balance, the administration of vitamins (particularly thiamine to prevent Wernicke's encephalopathy), a high-carbohydrate and high-calorie diet, and the use of sedating drugs to suppress symptoms and prevent seizures. Treatment is with a benzodiazepine (such as chlordiazepoxide) or clomethiazole.

For many years, disulfiram (Antabuse®) and calcium carbamide have been prescribed in an attempt to prevent relapse in abstinent alcoholics. They act by inhibiting the enzyme aldehyde dehydrogenase, which results in a rapid build-up of blood acetaldehyde if the subject drinks. This produces severe vomiting and diarrhoea, along with potentially dangerous alterations in blood pressure. However, adherence to therapy is usually poor and the evidence of effectiveness probably does not justify the unpleasant adverse reactions that these drugs can cause.

Two newer drugs show some promise. Naltrexone is a μ-opioid (MOR or OP_3) receptor antagonist, whose use was suggested by demonstrated links between alcohol and opioid receptors. Small uncontrolled and placebo-controlled trials have suggested that it significantly reduces the likelihood and severity of relapse in comparison with placebo.[28,29] Acamprosate is derived from the amino acid taurine and has structural similarities to GABA. In the brain it reduces the effects of excitatory amino acids, such as glutamate, and alters GABA neurotransmission. Clinical trials have suggested that it is significantly better than placebo in preventing or delaying relapse, with a very low incidence of adverse reactions.[30] It can cause diarrhoea, nausea, vomiting, or abdominal pain; occasionally it causes pruritus or a maculopapular rash. However, behavioural interventions may be at least as good as either naltrexone or acamprosate[31] or even better.[32]

Allergic Reactions to Plants

Some people are allergic to certain fruits (avocado, banana, chestnut, fig, kiwi, lychee, mango, melon, olives, papaya, passion fruit, peach, pineapple, and tomato),[33,34] nuts (such as chestnuts[35]), vegetables (such as celeriac, carrots, turnips,[36] zucchini,[36] or cassava[37]), or even spices.[38] This is one expression of the so-called pollen–food allergy syndrome. Allergy can be acquired by either direct sensitization via the gastrointestinal tract or by primary sensitization to plant pollen or latex.[39] There are at least 13 latex allergens found in the rubber tree *Hevea brasiliensis* and recognized by the International Union of Immunological Societies; they are known as Hev b 1, 2, 3, etc.[40,41] Latex-fruit allergy may be associated with the enzyme β-1,3-glucanase (Hev b 2),[42] since the glucanase in some fruits and vegetables has allergenic properties mediated by well-conserved IgE-binding epitopes on the surface of the enzyme, which might account for the IgE-binding cross-reactivity that is often reported in people with the latex–fruit syndrome.[43] Other enzymes that have been implicated include UDP glucose pyrophosphorylase,[44] fructose-bisphosphate aldolase and glyceraldehyde-3-phosphate dehydrogenase.[45] Hevein (Hev b 6.02)[46] and a latex profilin (Hev b 8)[47] have also been implicated. Some fruit and vegetable allergies have been related to allergens in other forms of pollen, such as birch (*Betula* spp.),[48,49] grass,[50] mugwort,[51–53] and ragweed.[54,55] The clinical manifestations of latex-fruit allergy range from urticaria to angio-oedema, rhinoconjunctivitis, bronchial asthma, and anaphylactic shock.[56–59] The prevalence depends on the method used to identify it; in 182 children 16 of 26 latex-sensitized children cross-reacted to fruits.[60]

Many tropical plants cause contact dermatitis, with erythema, vesiculation, or urticaria. Contact with the leaves of *Toxicodendron* (formerly *Rhus*) spp. (poison ivy, poison oak, or poison sumach) causes intense irritation and inflammation.[61,62] In Japan severe dermatitis can follow contact with lacquer made from *Toxicodendron verniciffluum*.[63] Treatment consists of thorough washing of the skin with soap and water and removal of the poison from the clothes by soaking in 1% hypochlorite solution.

Dermatitis can be caused by pyrethrum in *Chrysanthemum* spp.[64] Exposure to the leaves and flowers causes itching, usually beginning at the corners of the eyes, and lachrymation, followed by an irritating vesicular rash, peeling of the skin, and the formation of painful fissures. Sweating and exposure to sunlight exacerbate the lesions. Urticaria and photosensitivity have also been reported.

Many plants and flowers, such as the Euphorbias (which contain phorbol esters), orchids, primulas, lilies, and mangos, can cause allergic dermatitis in sensitive people. The juice of some of the umbelliferae contains photosensitizing furanocoumarin derivatives that on contact with the skin cause erythema and vesication after exposure to light.

The manchineel, *Hippomane mancinella* (Figure 76.6), like many other members of the Euphorbiaceae, produces a highly irritant latex.[65] This small tree is common along the coastlines of South and Central America, the West Indies, and India. Both varieties, one with leaves like holly and the other like laurel, are poisonous. The attractive fruit resembles a crab-apple and sensitive people who touch it develop erythema, bullae, and vesiculation. The wood and even the sawdust are irritant and can cause dermatitis, frequently of the genitalia and anus, with a vesiculopustular eruption, sometimes confined to the glans penis. In the eye the latex causes keratoconjunctivitis, with pain, photophobia, and blepharospasm. If the fruit is eaten it causes vesiculation of the buccal mucosa, with superinfection, bloody diarrhoea, and sometimes death. Latex on the skin should be washed off at once; blisters should be protected against infection and, if extensive, treated like second-degree burns.

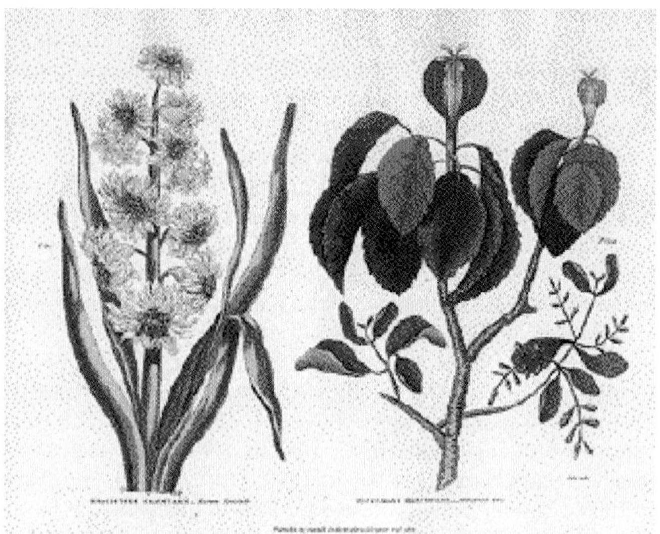

Figure 76.6 *Hippomane mancinella* (manchineel).

Seaweed dermatitis has been reported from Hawaii, probably as a result of contact with an alga, *Microcoleus lyngbyaceus*, which produces a rash in persons bathing in the sea off windward beaches.[66]

The dust from certain trees, such as iroko (African teak), pine, mahogany, satinwood, and obeche, can cause skin irritation, facial oedema, blepharospasm, acute coryza, and pharyngitis.[67] Asthma and rhinitis have also been reported.

In 361 of 76 697 patients with rosacea, there were positive reactions to the resin of *Myroxylon pereirae* (balsam of Peru) in 5.9%.[68]

The crushed leaves of henna (*Lawsonia inermis*) are used as a cosmetic agent world-wide, particularly in the Middle East. It causes a red-brown coloration of the skin. The name is also used for other dyes, such as black henna or neutral henna, which do not derive from the plant. Traditionally, henna is used as a pure dye prepared from the stems and the leaves of the plant, with the addition of coffee or tea to enhance the colour. Contact allergy and immediate hypersensitivity reactions are rare and when contact dermatitis after the use of henna tattoos has been reported it has often been attributed to the sensitizer para-phenylenediamine, which is used as an anti-oxidant and favours a long-lasting effect of the henna.[69] The use of para-phenylenediamine in henna is responsible for early sensitization to it in children and in some cases local hypopigmentation occurs in the tattoo.[70]

ARGEMONE MEXICANA AND EPIDEMIC DROPSY

Epidemic dropsy is caused by sanguinarine, an alkaloid constituent of several plants, including the Mexican poppy, *Argemone mexicana* (Figure 76.7). The small, black, oily seeds of

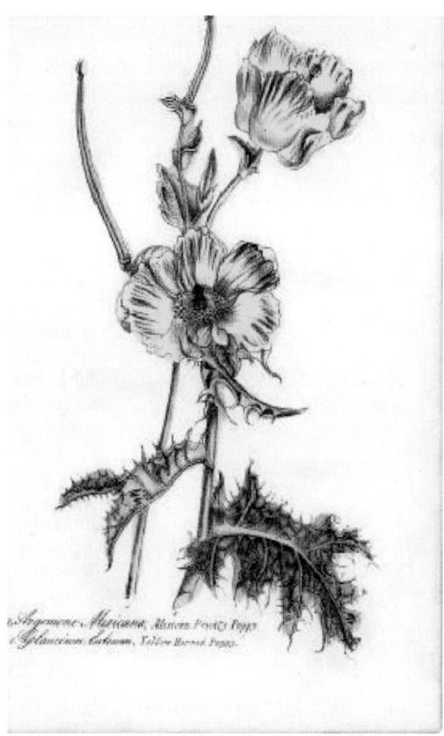

Figure 76.7 *Argemone mexicana* (Mexican poppy).

Argemone resemble those of mustard and can become mixed with them accidentally or by deliberate adulteration. Village boys in India can collect up to 8 kg of *Argemone* seeds a day in summer and may sell them to unscrupulous dealers. As a contaminant of a widely used cooking oil derived from mustard seed, *Argemone* has led to outbreaks of so-called 'epidemic dropsy' in many tropical countries. Sanguinarine is absorbed from the gut and through the skin if oil containing it is used for massage.[71] It causes capillary dilatation and increased permeability.

Epidemic dropsy is seen mostly in India,[72] but has also been reported in Mauritius, Fiji, South Africa, and Nepal.[73] It presents with gastrointestinal symptoms a week or so before the onset of pitting oedema of the legs, fever, and darkening of the skin, often with local erythema and tenderness. Perianal itching is common and severe myocarditis and congestive cardiac failure can occur. Other features include hepatomegaly, pneumonia, ascites, alopecia, and sarcoid-like skin changes. Glaucoma can occur, as can visual field disturbances independent of any rise in intraocular pressure.[74] Haemolytic anaemia occurs when oxidative stress causes methaemoglobin formation by altering pyridine nucleotides and glutathione redox potential; treatment with antioxidants has been suggested to be effective.[75]

A decoction of *Argemone mexicana*, used as a traditional medicine, has also been used in the treatment of malaria.[76]

CARDIOTOXIC GLYCOSIDES IN PLANTS

The number of plants worldwide that contain cardiac glycosides (cardenolides or bufadienolides) is legion – one incomplete list[77] runs to nearly 400 compounds and spans genera such as the Apocynaceae, Asclepiadaceae, Cruciferae, Liliaceae, Moraceae, Ranunculaceae, and Schrophulariaceae. Some examples are given in Table 76.2 and Figure 76.8.

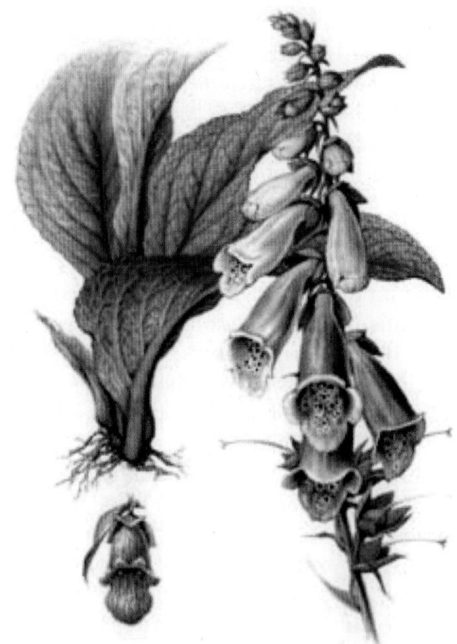

Figure 76.8 *Digitalis purpurea* (purple foxglove).

Some cardenolides (such as digoxin and digitoxin, obtained from foxgloves; Figure 76.8) are used therapeutically, but even then adverse reactions are common, because these drugs have a low therapeutic index.[78] Poisoning with plants containing cardenolides is not uncommon. One example is the current

TABLE 76.2 Some Plants that Contain Cardiac Glycosides (Cardenolides or Bufadienolides)

Scientific Name	Common Name(s)
Acokanthera ouabaio/schimperi	Olmorijoi/ Murichu
Adenium multiflorum	Impala lily
Adonis vernalis	False hellebore, yellow pheasant's eye
Antiaris toxicaria	Upas tree
Apocynum cannabinum	Black Indian hemp
Asclepias curassavica	Redheaded cotton-bush
Asclepias fruiticosa	Balloon cotton
Asclepias syriaca	Milkweed
Bowiea kilimandscharica	Climbing potato
Calotropis procera	King's crown
Carissa acokanthera	Bushman's poison
Carissa spectabilis	Wintersweet
Cerbera manghas	Sea-mango
Cerbera odollum	Pong pong
Convallaria majalis	Lily of the valley
Cotyledon orbiculata	Pig's ears
Cryptostegia grandiflora	Rubber vine
Digitalis lanata	Woolly foxglove
Digitalis purpurea	Purple foxglove
Euonymus europaeus	Spindle tree
Gloriosa superba	Glory lily
Helleborus niger	Christmas rose
Homeria pallida	Homeria
Nerium oleander	Oleander
Periploca sepium	Silkvine
Plumeria rubra	Frangipani
Scilla maritima	Squill
Strophanthus spp.	Various
Tanghinia venenifera	Ordeal tree
Thevetia peruviana	Yellow oleander
Urechites suberecta	Savannah flower
Urginea maritima	Squill

epidemic of self-poisoning with the seeds of oleander trees in South India and Sri Lanka. In one series of 300 cases of self-poisoning with *Thevetia peruviana* (yellow oleander) (mostly women aged 11–20, of whom 97% took crushed seeds), the main symptoms were vomiting, palpitation, epigastric pain, a burning sensation in the abdomen, shortness of breath, and diarrhoea; sinus bradycardia, sinus arrest, sinoatrial block and heart block were common.[79]

In Madagascar, the ordeal tree (*Tanghinia venenifera*) was used to test the innocence or guilt of an accused person; death on eating it signified guilt. The odollam tree, *Cerbera manghas*,[80] another ordeal tree of former times, which contains the cardenolide cerberin, is responsible for about 50% of cases of plant poisoning and 10% of total poisoning cases in Kerala, India, and has been used both for suicide and homicide;[81] cases have also been reported in Sri Lanka.[82] Poisoning can also occur by eating crabs that have eaten *Cerbera manghas* fruits.[83]

In one series of 4556 cases of self-poisoning in Sri Lanka, 2.5% were caused by plants and mushrooms; the glory lily *Gloriosa superba*[84] was responsible in 44% of those (i.e. 50 cases);[85] the toxic effects of *Gloriosa* are due to both cardenolides and colchicine alkaloids. Plants containing cardenolides that have been used as arrow poisons include *Acokanthera schimperi* in Africa[86] and the upas tree (*Antiaris toxicaria*; Figure 76.9) in Malaysia and China.[87,88] *Boophone distichia* (candelabra flower), used as an arrow poison in southern Africa, may have antidepressant properties.[89]

Treatment of cardenolide poisoning is largely supportive, but special attention should be paid to potassium balance, since cardenolides inhibit Na/K-ATPase (the Na/K pump), inhibiting the influx of potassium into cells; the severity of toxicity and therefore the prognosis, is related to the degree of hyperkalaemia that results. Fab fragments of antidigoxin antibody are effective not only in poisoning with digoxin but also with many other cardiac glycosides;[90] they have been used in oleander poisoning, but without evidence of an effect on mortality.[91] In contrast, repeated doses of activated charcoal (50 g 4-hourly) reduced mortality in a large randomized study from 8.0% to 2.5%, probably by encouraging the intestinal secretion of the toxic cardenolides that oleander seeds contain.[92] In another study of patients with less severe poisoning and an overall lower mortality, this treatment did not reduce mortality,[93] and it is probably most effective in those with severe poisoning.

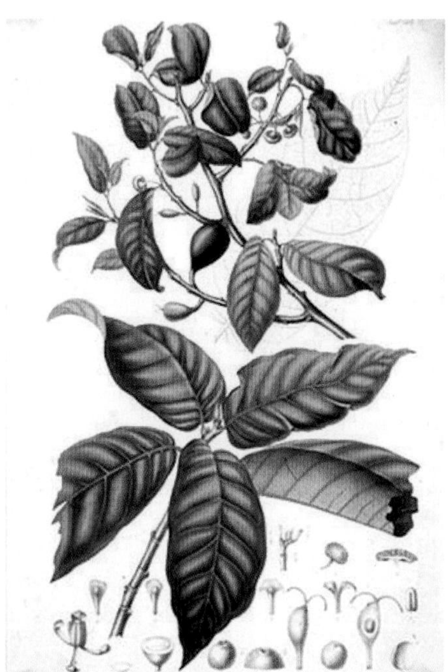

Figure 76.9 *Antiaris toxicaria* (upas tree).

TABLE 76.3 Some Species that Contain Cyanogenic Glycosides

Species	Glycoside
Acacia	Acaciapetalin
Deidamia	Deidaclin
Gynocardia	Gynocardin
Linum	Linamarin
Loyus	Lotaustralin
Lucuma	Lucumin
Macadamia	Proteacin
Manihot	Lotaustralin
Nandina	Proteacin
Pangium	Gynocardin
Prunus	Amygdalin, prunasin
Sambucus	Sambunigrin
Sorghum	Dhurrin
Taxus	Taxiphyllin
Tetrapathaea	Tetraphyllins
Trifolium	Linamarin
Triglochin	Triglochinin
Vicia	Vicianin
Zieria	Zierin

CYANOGENIC GLYCOSIDES IN PLANTS

Cyanogenic glycosides are found in several plants,[94,95] and in certain butterflies,[96] protecting them against predators. Some of their sources are listed in Table 76.3.

Cassava (*Manihot esculenta*; Figure 76.10) is a native of South America and sub-Saharan Africa, which is widely grown in the tropics for the production of flour and tapioca. The grated roots must be thoroughly washed to remove the toxic material. Badly prepared cassava causes signs of hydrocyanic acid poisoning: nausea, vomiting, abdominal distension and respiratory difficulty. Chronic cassava ingestion can cause an ataxic neuropathy, with bilateral primary optic atrophy, bilateral perceptive deafness, myelopathy and peripheral neuropathy.[97] Previous reports of goitre and pancreatitis as chronic effects have not been confirmed.

Konzo ('tired legs'), a symmetrical, non-progressive, non-remitting spastic paraparesis, which occurs in epidemic and endemic forms in several African countries,[98] and is invariably associated with consumption of inadequately processed bitter cassava roots and minimal protein; it may be associated with thiamine deficiency.[99] It has also been proposed that konzo, tropical ataxic neuropathy (also associated with cassava consumption), and lathyrism (associated with consumption of the grass pea, see below) are all caused by the fact that they contain cyano groups with direct neurotoxic actions not mediated by systemic cyanide release.[100]

The Bio Cassava Plus programme in sub-Saharan Africa aims to develop and deliver genetically engineered cassava containing increased amounts of nutrients, such as zinc, iron, protein, and vitamin A, to increase shelf-life, reduce the cyanogenic glycoside content, and improve resistance to viruses.[101]

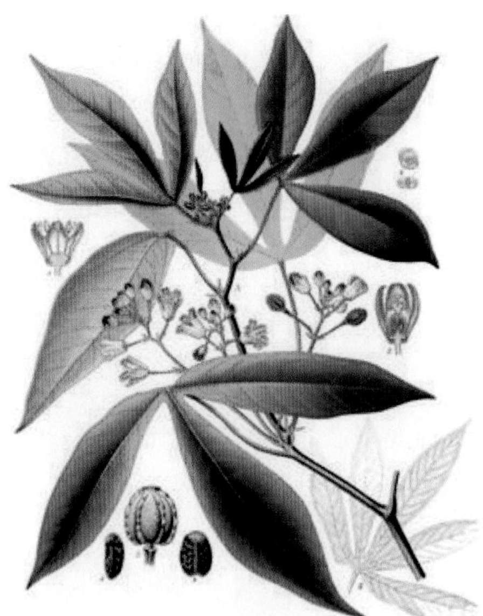

Figure 76.10 *Manihot esculenta* (cassava).

The broken kernels of certain fruits also contain cyanogenic glycosides, particularly *Prunus* spp. (plums, peaches, cherries, apricots, almonds) and loquats (*Eriobotrya japonica*; Figure 76.11). The active principle, amygdalin (laetrile), has been used in patients with cancer; however, it is ineffective and adverse reactions have been not uncommon.[102]

Yams are the tubers of *Dioscorea* of many varieties, including bitter toxic species, such as *D. dumetorum* and *D. hirsuta*, which contain cyanogenic glycosides, such as diosgenin. They can be steeped and washed in water and eaten sliced, but if badly prepared they are toxic. Bitter yams are sometimes interplanted with edible varieties in order to deter theft by strangers. Deaths have occurred from the consumption of bitter yams.[103]

Treatment of acute cyanide poisoning includes gastric lavage with 5% sodium thiosulfate within 1 hour if possible; 300 mL of 25% sodium thiosulfate should be left in the stomach. Dicobalt edetate (dicobalt EDTA, 600 mg in 40 mL over 1 min) should be given intravenously as soon as possible in all cases of poisoning. If recovery does not occur within 1–2 min, another 300 mg of dicobalt edetate should be given. Oxygen (100%) should also be given and acidosis should be corrected with sodium bicarbonate. If dicobalt edetate is not available, give 10 mL of 3% sodium nitrite over 3 min intravenously, followed by 25 mL of 50% sodium thiosulfate over 10 min intravenously.

ERGOT

Ergot (*Claviceps purpurea*) is a fungus whose sclerotia contain ergotoxine and related alkaloids that stimulate smooth muscle. It is harvested with the ears of rye and other grasses. Chronic consumption of small amounts causes uterine and vascular contraction, resulting in abortion, arterial occlusion, and painful gangrene.[104] In the Middle Ages, this was called St Anthony's fire, because it was relieved by a pilgrimage to the shrine of St Anthony, in an area that was not affected by the fungus. Acute consumption of large amounts can cause headache, vertigo, hallucinations, and convulsions; the Salem witches may have been victims of this. Ergot poisoning, although easy to prevent, still occurs from careless harvesting in times of food shortage; it can also occur with deliberate hallucinogenic or abortifacient use. Vasodilators, such as sodium nitroprusside, ease ischaemic pain and help to prevent gangrene.[105] Derivatives of ergot are used therapeutically (e.g. bromocriptine in Parkinson's disease) and as hallucinogens (e.g. LSD).

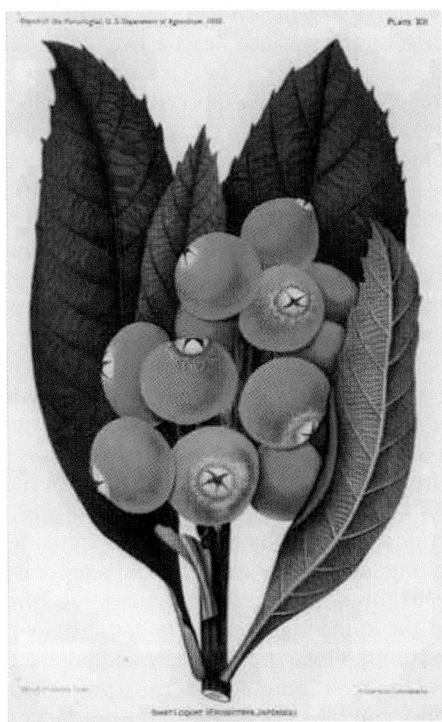

Figure 76.11 *Eriobotrya japonica* (loquat).

Gastroenteritis due to Compounds in Plants

Jequirity beans (*Abrus precatorius*; Figure 76.12) and castor oil beans (*Ricinus communis*; Figure 76.13)) are bright and attractive and are sometimes made into necklaces. *Ricinus* is the source of the purgative castor oil and *Abrus* has been used to treat schistosomiasis. However, these beans contain poisons that, after a delay of 1–48 hours, can cause fatal gastroenteritis; their toxic principles, abrin and ricin, are among the most poisonous substances known;[106] one bean can kill a child. Acute poisoning is treated by gastric lavage, demulcents and adjustment of fluid and electrolyte balance. Abdominal pain may require analgesics. In serious cases ventilation or haemodialysis may be needed. Modeccin, a lectin found in *Adenia digitata*, the wild granadilla,[107] may have similar properties to those of abrin and ricin.[108]

Abrin and ricin both consist of two components, an α chain and a β chain; the former is toxic and is carried into cells by the latter, from which it then dissociates.[109] This action has been put to use therapeutically, by conjugating the β chain of ricin to monoclonal antibodies for use, for example, in the treatment of leukaemias.[110] The dose is limited by the risk of a vascular leak syndrome.

Because ricin is so easily prepared from castor oil beans, there has been some concern in recent years that it might be

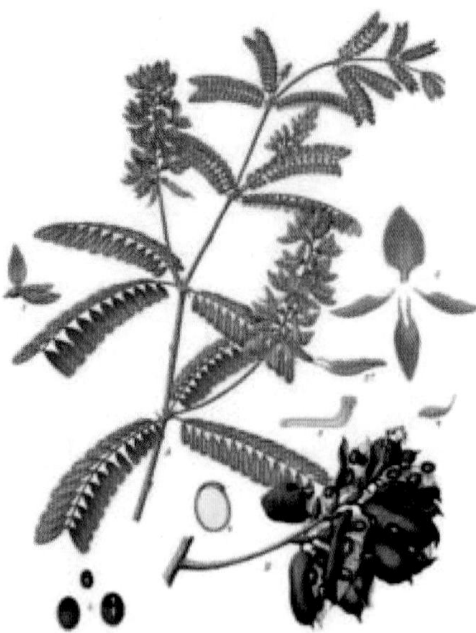

Figure 76.12 *Abrus precatorius* (jequirity).

used as a weapon of mass terror, particularly because it was supposed to have been the agent that was used to kill the Bulgarian dissident Georgi Markov, who was thought to have had it injected into his leg in a metal pellet via the medium of an umbrella tip.[111] However, this fear is largely unfounded.[112] Although ricin is highly toxic, oral administration results only in effects on the gut and impracticably large amounts would be needed (e.g. to contaminate water supplies); mass parenteral or inhalational delivery is unrealistic. On 15 October 2003, a metal canister was found in a package in a Post Office in Greenville, South Carolina, with a note threatening to poison water supplies if certain demands were not met; there was ricin in the canister, but the threat came to nothing.[113]

Many other plants can cause gastrointestinal disturbances, such as nausea, vomiting, and diarrhoea. These include the

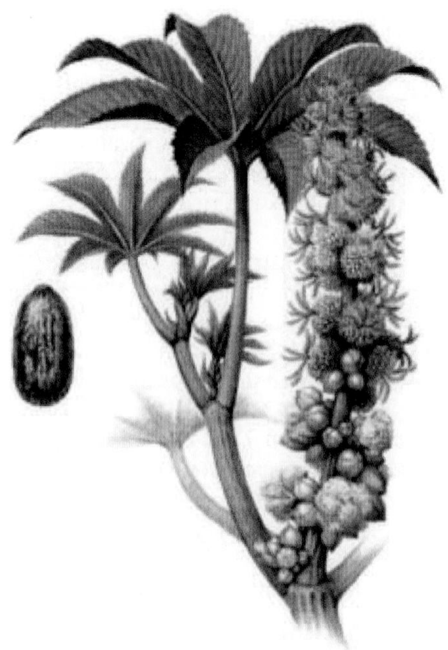

Figure 76.13 *Ricinus communis* (castor bean).

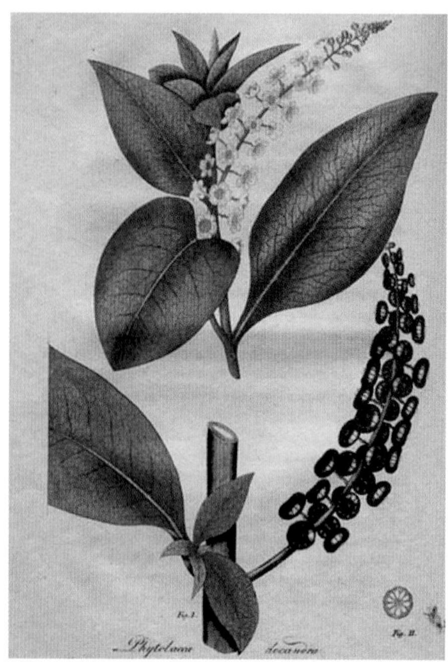

Figure 76.14 *Phytolacca americana* (pokeweed).

Euphorbia spp., *Phytolacca americana* (Figure 76.14), and all plants that contain cardiac glycosides (Table 76.2) or cucurbitacins (such as *Bacopa monnieri*, *Begonia heracleifolia*, *Bolbostemma paniculatum*, *Bryonia aspera*, *Cayaponia racemosa*, *Citrullus colocynthis*, *Coutarea hexandra*, *Cucurbita pepo*, *Ecballium elaterium*, *Elaeocarpus hainanensis*, *Gratiola officinalis*, *Hemsleya endecaphylla*, *Kageneckia oblonga*, *Leucopaxillus gentianeus*, *Luffa operculata*, *Momordica balsamina*, *Morierina montana*, *Neopicrorhiza scrophulariiflora*, *Physocarpus capitatus*, *Picrorrhiza scrophulariaeflora*, *Picria fel-terrae*, *Trichosanthes tricuspidata*, and *Wilbrandia ebracteata*). Severe gastrointestinal toxicity can sometimes cause heart block, secondary to vagal stimulation.[114]

The leaves of *Dieffenbachia* spp. cause damage to the mucosa of the gastrointestinal tract if chewed or swallowed; this has been attributed to their oxalate content.[115] The sap can also cause corneal damage.

The attractive red berries of *Arum maculatum* (cuckoo-pint or lords and ladies) can cause burning of the mouth, tongue, and oesophagus, followed by nausea, haematemesis, and intestinal and other smooth muscle spasm.[116] However, poisoning is rarely serious.

Lectins are phytohaemagglutinins that are resistant to digestion in the gut but are removed from food by proper cooking. They affect the integrity of the intestinal epithelium and the absorption of dietary antigens and cause release of allergic mediators from mast cells in vitro. Many plants, such as *Jatropha macrorhiza* (Figure 76.15)[117] and *Euonymus europaeus*, contain lectins,[118] which, if not destroyed by cooking, can cause severe vomiting and bloody diarrhoea, in some cases followed by damage to the central nervous system, the cardiovascular system, and the kidneys. Coral plants, *Jatropha curcas*, *J. glandulifera*, and *J. multifida*, grow rapidly and are used as hedges in Africa and the West Indies. Their fruits, physic nuts, taste like sweet almonds but have been reported to cause colic, cramps, thirst, and hypothermia. Another species, *J. gossypifolia*, is

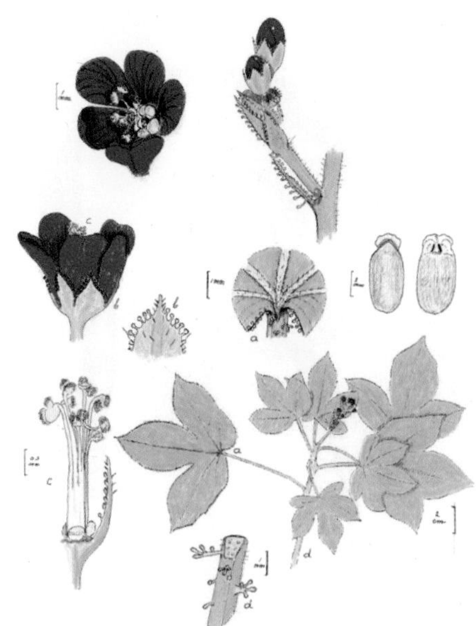

Figure 76.15 *Jatropha gossypifolia* (bellyache bush).

known in the West Indies as the bellyache bush. The potential uses of lectins, such as those found in *Viscum album* (mistletoe), *Phaseolus vulgaris* (common beans), *Robinia pseudoacacia* (black locust), and *Agaricus bisporus* (button mushrooms), in the treatment of cancers have been investigated.[119]

Croton spp., which are widespread in the tropics cause violent purgation. They contain phorbol esters, which activate protein kinase C,[120] are carcinogenic, and can cause contact dermatitis.[121]

The ackee, *Blighia sapida* Figure 76.16; (named after Captain Bligh of the Bounty) is a native of West Africa but is common in the West Indies and South America. The fruit has a large fleshy aril and is eaten when ripe; however, the unripe fruit is poisonous and has caused 'vomiting sickness' in Jamaica and other islands.[122] Unripe ackee fruits contain toxic hypoglycins, hypoglycin A (L-α-aminomethylenecyclopropylpropionic acid) and its γ-glutamyl conjugate, the less toxic hypoglycin B.[123] Hypoglycin A is metabolized to methylenecyclopropylacetic acid, which reduces several cofactors that are essential for β-oxidation of long-chain fatty acids and inhibits the transport of long-chain fatty acids into mitochondria. Accumulation of short-chain fatty acids in the serum results from suppression of short-chain acyl-CoA dehydrogenases and β-oxidation, leading to omega-oxidation of long-chain fatty acids in the liver. Reduced fatty acid metabolism causes increased use of glucose and hypoglycaemia.[124,125] Anaphylaxis and cholestatic jaundice have also been reported. Typically, poisoning presents with abdominal discomfort and vomiting, usually within 6–48 hours of ingestion, and a few hours later convulsions and coma. Extreme hypoglycaemia occurs and unless glucose is given promptly, death usually occurs within 12 hours of the initial vomiting. The liver shows fatty changes, with almost complete absence of glycogen.

GRAYANOTOXINS IN PLANTS

Certain species of rhododendron contain grayanotoxins (andromedotoxins), which open sodium channels. In the heart, this effect can trigger the Bezold–Jarisch reflex and cause bradycardia, heart block, asystole, and hypotension.[126] There have been many anecdotal reports of these complications in people who have eaten honey prepared by bees from *Rhododendron luteum*, *Rhododendron mucronulatum*, *Rhododendron ponticum*, or *Castanea sativa*;[127–142] myocardial infarction has also been reported.[143] In one case, poisoning from *Rhododendron simsii* occurred when a baby's grandmother prepared a decoction of the plant in milk.[144] Poisoning with *Agauria salicifolia* has also been reported in a series of cases from Reunion Island[145] and a case from the Mascarene Islands.[146]

In the eastern Black Sea region of Turkey, where most cases have been reported, such honey is called 'bitter honey' or 'mad honey'. It is often used as a household remedy for various conditions, including stomach pains, bowel disorders, hypertension, and erectile dysfunction.[147] Because of variations in the plant content of grayanotoxins, poisoning with honey made in the spring is more severe.[147] However, honey poisoning is rarely fatal and the effects generally last for no more than 24 hours.

Common adverse reactions that have been reported in case series include nausea, vomiting, salivation, sweating, dizziness, and weakness several hours after ingestion and in some cases hypotension, sinus bradycardia, or complete atrioventricular block.[148–152] Blurring of vision and diplopia have also been reported.[153] Deliberate self-poisoning has been used as a means of enhancing sexual performance.[154]

Muscarinic M_2 receptors in the vagus are involved in the cardiotoxicity of grayanotoxins,[155,156] and bradycardia and heart block in these cases respond to atropine, as in toxicity with Veratrum alkaloids. However, temporary pacing may sometimes be required.[157]

Haemotoxicity due to Compounds in Plants

HAEMOLYSIS IN GLUCOSE-6-PHOSPHATE DEHYDROGENASE DEFICIENCY

Deficiency of the enzyme glucose-6-phosphate dehydrogenase (G6PD) in erythrocytes results in reduced production of NADPH. Consequently, oxidized glutathione (and to a lesser and insignificant extent methaemoglobin) accumulates. If the erythrocytes are then exposed to oxidizing agents, haemolysis occurs, probably because of unopposed oxidation of sulphydryl

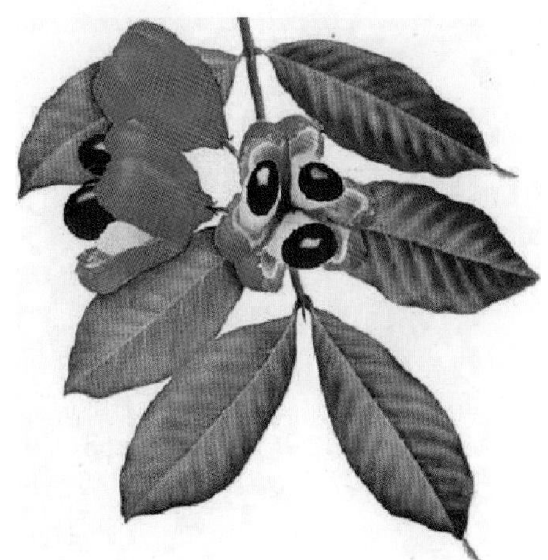

Figure 76.16 *Blighia sapida* (ackee).

groups in the cell membrane, which are normally kept in reduced form by the continuous availability of reduced glutathione. The prevalence of this defect varies with race. It is rare among Caucasians and occurs most frequently among Sephardic Jews of Asiatic origin, of whom 50% or more are affected. It also occurs in about 10–20% of Blacks. Inheritance of the defect is sex-linked but complex, the genetic basis for the abnormal enzyme being heterogeneous; most of the variations produce an unstable enzyme. In the variety that affects Blacks (but is not confined to them) G6PD production is probably normal, but its degradation is accelerated, so that only erythrocytes older than about 55 days are affected; acute haemolysis occurs on first administration of the drug and lasts for only a few days, after which continued administration causes chronic mild haemolysis. In the Mediterranean variety the enzyme is abnormal and both young and old erythrocytes are affected; in this form severe haemolysis occurs on first administration and is maintained with continued administration. Occasionally methaemoglobinaemia can also occur.[158] The reaction is sometimes called favism, because it can result from eating broad beans (*Vicia faba*; Figure 76.17), which contain oxidant substances such as divicine and isouramil.[159] In a high proportion of patients with the Mediterranean form there is a mutation in the G6PD gene, G6PD(C563T).[160] The condition is rare in Thailand, probably because the G6PD mutants that occur there are different.[161]

IMPAIRED PLATELET AGGREGATION

Some plants contain compounds that inhibit platelet aggregation,[162] e.g. *Ginkgo biloba*, the maidenhair tree, extracts from the leaves of which are marketed in some countries for the treatment of cerebral dysfunction and of intermittent claudication, garlic (*Allium sativum*; Figure 76.18) and saw palmetto (*Serenoa repens*; Figure 76.19). As a result, bleeding complications can occur, including strokes.

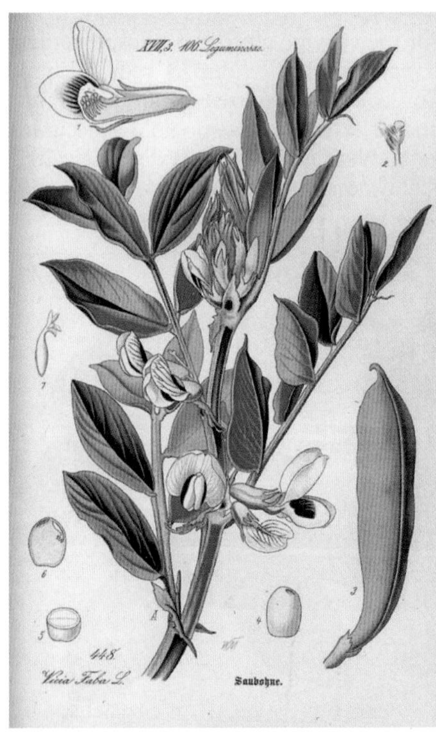

Figure 76.17 *Vicia faba* (broad bean).

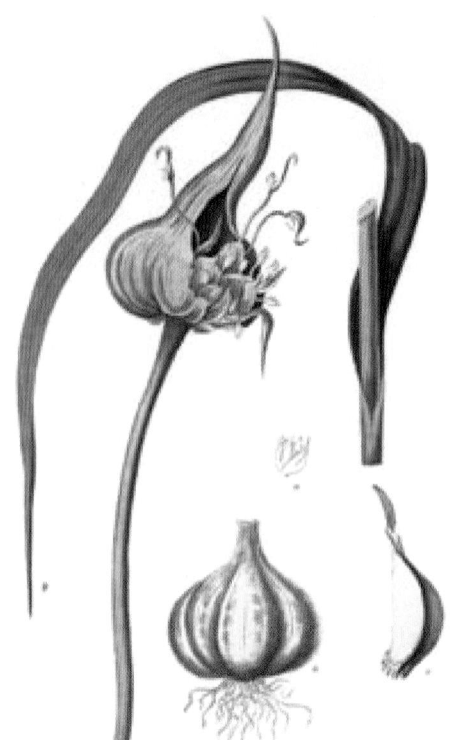

Figure 76.18 *Allium sativum* (garlic).

Hepatotoxicity due to Compounds in Plants

HEPATITIS

The number of plants that have reportedly caused acute liver damage is legion.[163] The pattern is a rise in serum activities of the so-called liver enzymes (aspartate and alanine aminotransferases), which is usually rapidly reversible; occasionally death

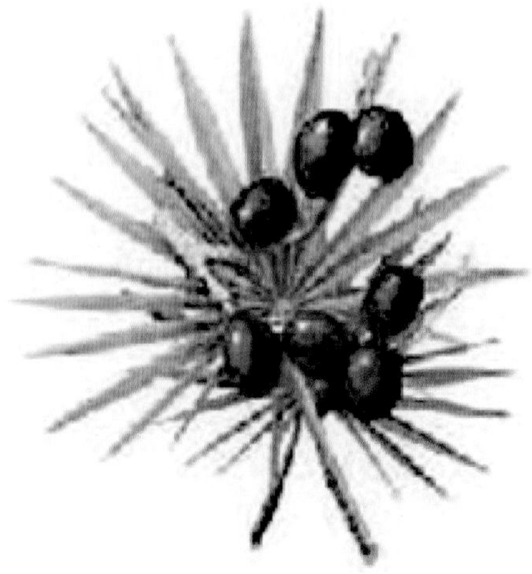

Figure 76.19 *Serenoa repens* (saw palmetto).

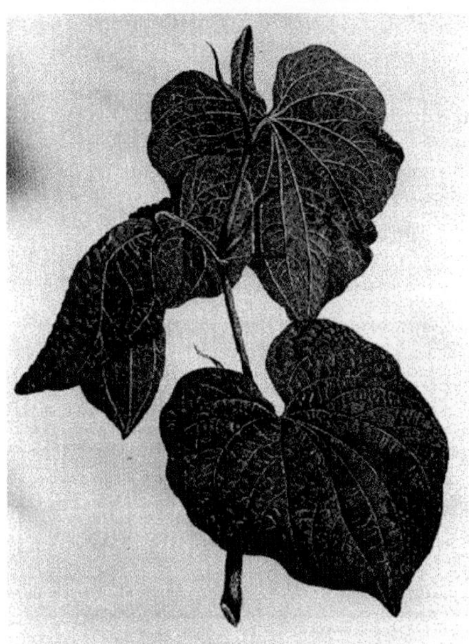

Figure 76.20 *Piper methysticum* (kava).

can occur. Plants that have been reported to cause acute liver damage include *Breynia officinalis*,[164] *Callilepis laureola* (ox-eye daisy),[165] *Camellia sinensis* (green tea),[166] *Chelidonium majus* (celandine),[167] *Cimicifuga racemosa* (black cohosh; Figure 76.21),[168,169] *Larrea tridentata* (chaparral),[170] *Piper methysticum* (kava; Figure 76.20; see below under Psychotropic drugs), *Polygonum multiflorum*,[171] *Symphytum officinale* (comfrey; see below under Sinusoidal obstruction syndrome)[172,173] and *Teucrium* spp.[174,175] Of these, black cohosh, chaparral, comfrey, and kava are the most common culprits.

Hepatic Carcinoma

Aspergillus flavus and *A. parasiticus* produce aflatoxins that are toxic to the liver and are carcinogenic;[176] e.g. the consumption of contaminated groundnuts has been linked with hepatic carcinoma in Africa and Asia.[177]

Sinusoidal Obstruction Syndrome (Veno-Occlusive Disease) and Pyrrolizidine Alkaloids

Pyrrolizidine alkaloids occur in a large number of plants, notably the genera *Crotalaria* (Figure 76.22), *Cynoglossum*, *Eupatorium*, *Heliotropium*, *Petasites*, *Senecio* (Figure 76.23), and *Symphytum* (Table 76.4).[178] They can contaminate foodstuffs;[179] examples include *Senecio jacobaea* in Europe and *Ageratum conyzoides* in Ethiopia.[180] They may contaminate pollen and hence honey.[181,182] They may also be found in certain plants that are used in some forms of traditional medicine.[183]

Certain representatives of this class and the plants in which they occur, are hepatotoxic as well as mutagenic and carcinogenic. They can cause the sinusoidal obstruction syndrome (veno-occlusive disease of the liver),[184] with clinical features that

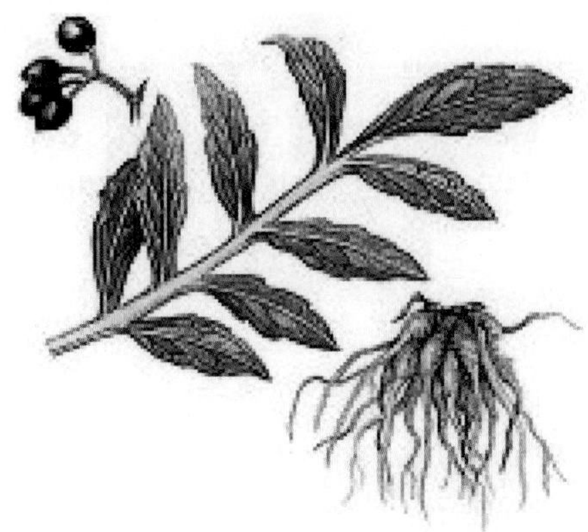

Figure 76.21 *Cimicifuga racemosa* (black cohosh).

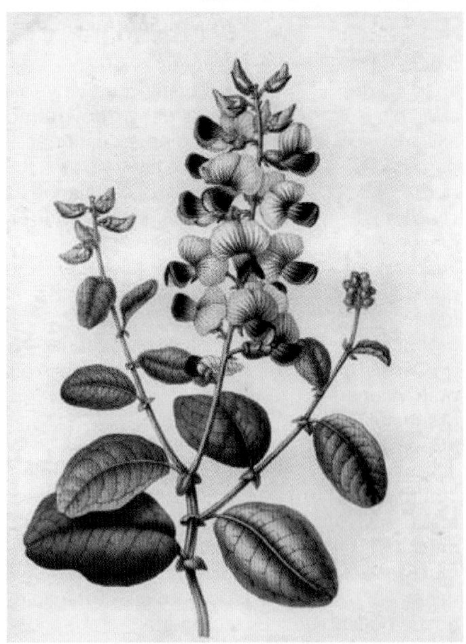

Figure 76.22 *Crotalaria verrucosa* (blue rattlesnake).

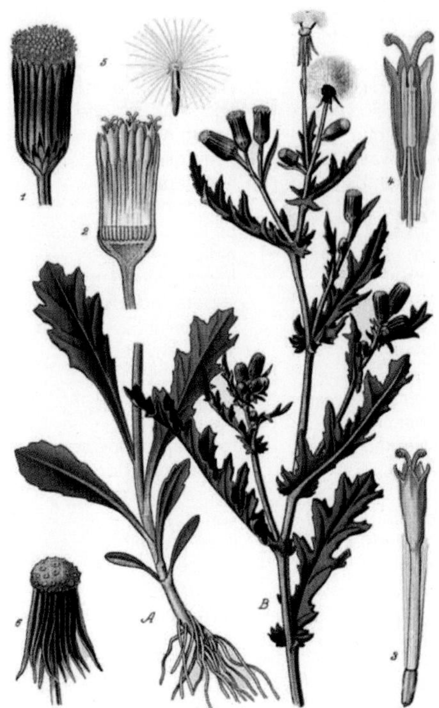

Figure 76.23 *Senecio vulgaris* (groundsel).

TABLE 76.4 **Plants that Contain Pyrrolizidine Alkaloids**

Genus	Pyrrolizidine Alkaloids
Crotalaria albida	croalbidine
Crotalaria anagyroides	anacrotine, methylpyrrolizidine
Crotalaria aridicola	various dehydropyrrolizidines
Crotalaria axillaris	axillaridine, axillarine
Crotalaria barbata	crobarbatine
Crotalaria burha	croburhine, crotalarine
Crotalaria candicans	crocandine, cropodine
Crotalaria crassipes	retusamine
Crotalaria crispata	crispatine, fulvine
Crotalaria dura	crotaline
Crotalaria fulva	fulvine
Crotalaria globifer	crotaline, globiferine
Crotalaria goreensis	hydroxymethylenepyrrolizidine
Crotalaria grahamiana	grahamine
Crotalaria grantiana	grantianine
Crotalaria incana	anacrotine
Crotalaria intermedia	integerrimine, usaramine
Crotalaria laburnifolia	crotalaburnine, hydroxysenkirkine
Crotalaria madurensis	crotafoline, madurensine
Crotalaria mitchelii	retusamine
Crotalaria mucronata	mucronitine, mucronitinine
Crotalaria nana	crotaburnine, crotananine
Crotalaria novae-hollandiae	retusamine
Crotalaria retusa	retusamine
Crotalaria semperflorus	crosemperine
Crotalaria spectabilis	retronecanol
Crotalaria stricta	crotastrictine
Crotalaria trifoliastrum	various alkylpyrrolizidines
Crotalaria usaramoensis	usaramine, usaramoensine
Crotalaria virgulata	grantaline, grantianine
Crotalaria walkeri	acetylcrotaverrine, crotaverrine
Cynoglossum amabile	amabiline, echinatine
Cynoglossum glochidiatum	amabiline
Cynoglossum lanceolatum	cynaustine, cynaustraline
Cynoglossum latifolium	latifoline
Cynoglossum officinale	heliosupine
Cynoglossum pictum	echinatine, heliosupine
Cynoglossum viridiflorum	heliosupine, viridiflorine
Eupatorium cannabinum	echinatine, supinine
Eupatorium maculatum	echinatine, trachelantimidine
Heliotropium acutiflorum	heliotrine
Heliotropium arguzoides	trichodesmine
Heliotropium curassavicum	angelylheliotridine
Heliotropium dasycarpum	heliotrine
Heliotropium eichwaldii	angelylheliotrine
Heliotropium europeum	acetyl-lasiocarpine, helioitrine
Heliotropium indicum	acetylindicine, indicine, indicinine
Heliotropium lasiocarpum	heliotrine, lasiocarpine
Heliotropium olgae	heliotrine, incanine, lasiocarpine
Heliotropium ovalifolium	heliofoline
Heliotropium ramosissimum	heliotrine
Heliotropium strigosum	strigosine
Heliotropium supinum	heliosupine, supinine
Heliotropium transoxanum	heliotrine
Petasites japonicus	fukinotoxin, petasinine, petasinoside
Senecio adnatus	platyphylline
Senecio alpinus	seneciphylline
Senecio amphibolus	macrophylline
Senecio angulatus	angulatine
Senecio aquaticus	aquaticine
Senecio argentino	retrorsine, senecionine
Senecio aureus	floridanine, florosenine, otosenine
Senecio auricula	neosenkirkine
Senecio borysthenicus	seneciphylline
Senecio brasiliensis	brasilinecine
Senecio campestris	campestrine
Senecio cannabifolius	senecicannabine
Senecio carthamoides	carthamoidine
Senecio cineraria	jacobine, seneciphylline
Senecio cissampelinum	senampelines
Senecio crucifolia	jacobine
Senecio doronicum	doronine
Senecio erraticus	erucifoline, floridanine
Senecio filaginoides	retrorsine,ionine
Senecio franchetti	franchetine, sarracine
Senecio fuchsii	fuchsisenecionine
Senecio gillesiano	retrorsine, senecionine
Senecio glabellum	integerrimine, senecionine
Senecio glandulosus	retrorsine, senecionine
Senecio glastifolius	graminifoline
Senecio hygrophylus	hygrophylline, platyphylline
Senecio ilicifolius	pterophine, senecionine
Senecio illinitus	acetylsenkirkine, senecionine
Senecio incanus	seneciphylline
Senecio integerrimus	integerrimine, senecionine
Senecio isatideus	isatidine, retrorsine
Senecio jacobaea	jacobine, jacoline, jaconine, jacozine, otosenine, renardine
Senecio kirkii	acetylsenkirkine, senkirkine
Senecio kubensis	seneciphylline
Senecio latifolius	senecifolidine, senecifoline
Senecio leucostachys	retrorsine, senecionine
Senecio longibolus	integerrimine, longiboline, retronecanol, retrorsine, riddelline, senecionine, seneciphylline
Senecio macrophyllus	macrophylline
Senecio mikanoides	mikanoidine
Senecio nemorensis	nemorensine, oxynemorensine
Senecio othonnae	floridnine, onetine, otosenine
Senecio othonniformis	bisline, isoline
Senecio palmatus	seneciphylline
Senecio paucicalyculatus	paucicaline
Senecio petasis	bisline
Senecio phillipicus	retrorsine, seneciphylline
Senecio platyphylloides	neoplatyphylline, platyphylline, sarracine, seneciphylline,
Senecio platyphyllus	platyphylline, seneciphylline
Senecio pojarkovae	sarracine, seneciphylline
Senecio procerus	procerine
Senecio propinquus	seneciphylline
Senecio pseudoarnica	senecionine
Senecio pterophorus	pterophine
Senecio ragonesi	retrorsine, senecionine, uspallatine
Senecio renardi	renardine, seneciphylline, senkirkine
Senecio retrorsus	isatidine, retrorsine
Senecio rhombifolius	neoplatyphylline, platyphylline, sarracine, seneciphylline
Senecio Riddellii	riddelline
Senecio rivularis	angeloyloxyheliotrine
Senecio rosmarinifolius	rosmarinine
Senecio ruwenzoriensis	ruwenine, ruzorine
Senecio sarracenicus	sarracine
Senecio scleratus	isatidine, scleratine
Senecio seratophiloides	senecivernine
Senecio spartioides	seneciphylline, spartoidine
Senecio squalidus	senecionine, squalidine
Senecio stenocephalus	seneciphylline
Senecio subalpinus	seneciphylline
Senecio subulatus	retrorsine, senecionine
Senecio swaziensis	swazine
Senecio triangularis	triangularine
Senecio uspallatensis	senecionine, uspallatine
Senecio vernalis	senecivernine
Senecio vira-vira	anacrotine, neoplatyphylline
Senecio viscosus	senecionine
Senecio vulgaris	senecionine
Symphytum asperum	asperumine, echinatine, heliosupine
Symphytum caucasicum	echinatine, heliosupine, lasiocarpine, symphytine, viridiflorine
Symphytum officinalis	echinatine, heliosupine, lasiocarpine, symphytine, viridflorine
Symphytum orientale	anadoline
Symphytum tuberosum	heneicisane, tricosane
Symphytum uplandicum	acetylintermedine, acetyl-lycopsamine, uplandicine

include abdominal pain, ascites, hepatomegaly and splenomegaly, anorexia, nausea, vomiting, and diarrhoea. Sometimes there is also damage to the lungs. The primary pathological change of hepatic sinusoidal obstruction syndrome is subendothelial oedema, followed by intimal overgrowth of connective tissue, with narrowing and occlusion of the central and sublobular hepatic veins. Atrophy or necrosis of liver cells, with consequent fibrosis, leads to gross changes similar to those seen in cardiac cirrhosis; portal hypertension results.[163]

In the West Indies[185] sinusoidal obstruction syndrome is related to the consumption of bush tea made from plants such as *Crotalaria* and *Senecio*.[186] Hepatotoxic compounds in *Crotalaria*, *Senecio*, and *Heliotropium*, and other composite plants can also enter the diet through contamination of cereals with weed seeds. For example, 28 of 67 patients died with sinusoidal obstruction syndrome in central India after consuming a local cereal, gondii, contaminated with the seeds of *Crotalaria*.[187] *Heliotropium popovii* has been implicated in outbreaks in villages in north-western Afghanistan, with high mortality.[188]

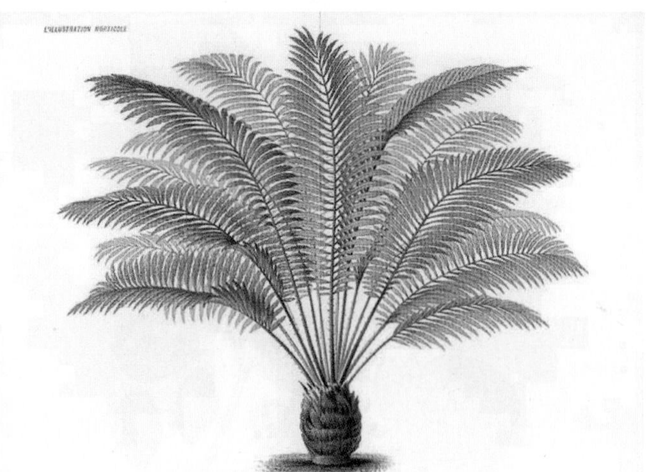

Figure 76.24 *Cycas circinalis* (cycad).

Nephrotoxicity due to Compounds in Plants

Djenkol beans (*Pithecolobium*) cause poisoning in Malaysia, Java, and Thailand. Blood and casts appear in the urine and the renal tract may be blocked, causing acute kidney damage;[189] crystals of djenkolic acid can form urinary calculi.[190] Treatment is by alkalinizing the urine (pH 8) by giving sodium bicarbonate by intravenous infusion (250 mL of a 3.5% solution four times in a single day for a 70-kg adult).

Aristolochia fangchi (Chinese snakeroot), and perhaps other constituents of Chinese herbal slimming remedies, can cause a nephropathy[191] through progressive interstitial fibrosis. It may also cause urothelial carcinoma.[192] Nephrotoxicity has been incorrectly attributed to *Stephania tetrandra* (Chinese: *fang-ji*) through confusion with *Aristolochia* (Chinese: *quang-fang-ji*). Other species of *Aristolochia* are used medicinally elsewhere.[193] The active ingredient, aristolochic acid, has also been implicated in Balkan endemic nephropathy, a chronic tubulointerstitial disease associated with urothelial cancer, which affects people living in the alluvial plains along the tributaries of the River Danube.[194]

Oxalate-rich foods (spinach, rhubarb, beets, nuts, chocolate, tea, wheat bran, and strawberries) increase urinary oxalate excretion, predisposing to renal calculi.[195] Rarely acute oxalate toxicity can occur, e.g. due to ingestion of raw rhubarb stalks or leaves.[196]

Neurotoxicity due to Compounds in Plants

In some countries, the root stocks of cycads (*Cycas* and *Zamia*) are used as foodstuffs. The seeds of *Cycas circinalis* (Figure 76.24), eaten by the Chamorro people of Guam and neighbouring islands[197] contain a neurotoxic amino acid, β-*N*-methylamino-l-alanine, which is thought to cause amyotrophic lateral sclerosis, Parkinsonism, and dementia.[198]

A related condition, lathyrism, is caused by *Lathyrus sativus* (Figure 76.25), the grass pea, which contains the neurotoxin β-*N*-oxalylamino-l-alanine.[199] It causes a symmetrical motor spastic paraparesis, with a pyramidal pattern and greatly increased tone in the leg muscles, causing sufferers to walk on the balls of their feet with a lurching gait. The arms can also be affected. Sensory signs are absent. Grass pea is a profitable cash crop that is used as a cheap adulterant in flour from other pulses; lathyrism is likely to occur in places remote from grass pea cultivation and follows food shortages in India and Africa. Strains with low toxin content have been developed.[200]

The poison-nut (*Strychnos nux-vomica*; Figure 76.26) is the source of poisonous alkaloids (strychnine, vomicine, icajine, brucine). Strychnine is an antagonist of the actions of the inhibitory neurotransmitter glycine in the spinal cord and causes painful convulsions.[201]

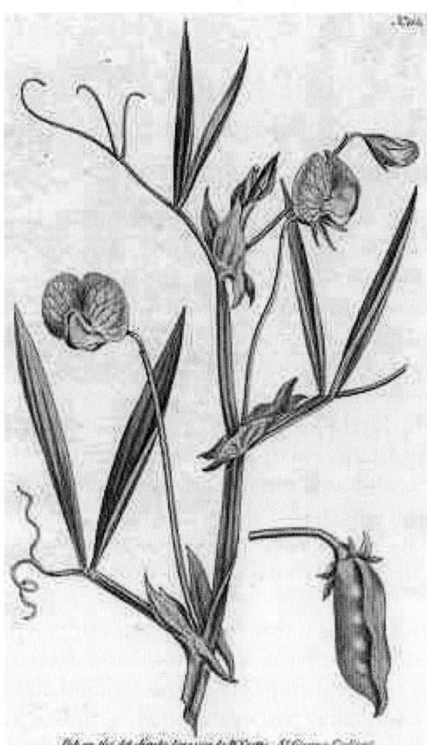

Figure 76.25 *Lathyrus sativus* (grass pea).

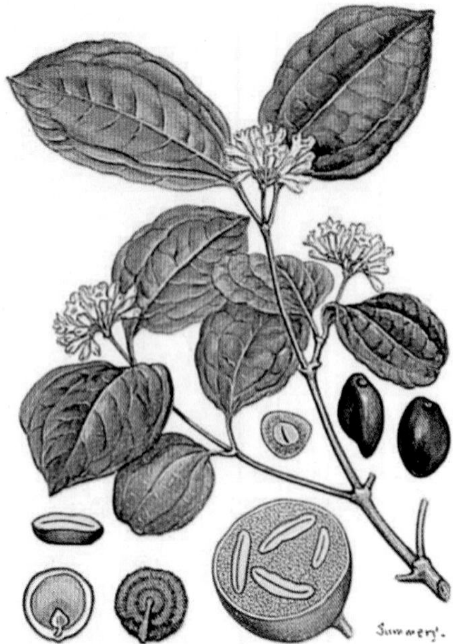

Figure 76.26 *Strychnos nux-vomica* (poison-nut).

The fruit of *Diospyros mollis* (maklua) contains a derivative of hydroxynaphthalene and is used in Thailand for treating intestinal worms. It is oculotoxic[202] and has been reported to cause optic neuritis in children.

Water hemlock is the common name that is given to two genera of plants, *Cicuta* and *Oenanthe*, which contain the conjugated polyacetylenes cicutoxin and oenanthotoxin, which are non-competitive gamma-aminobutyric acid (GABA) antagonists and can cause seizures, which can be fatal.[203] Other features include nausea, vomiting, diarrhoea, tachycardia, mydriasis, rhabdomyolysis, renal failure, coma, respiratory impairment, and cardiac dysrhythmias.

Parasympathetic Nervous System Actions due to Compounds in Plants

ANTICHOLINERGIC COMPOUNDS

Anticholinergic compounds, such as atropine, hyoscine (scopolamine), and semisynthetic derivatives, are widely used therapeutically (for example, in Parkinson's disease and as adjuncts to anaesthesia). Poisoning causes tachycardia, a dry mouth and hot dry skin, dilated pupils (mydriasis), blurred vision and loss of accommodation, difficulty in micturition, confusion, an acute psychosis with hallucinations, and convulsions; glaucoma can occur in elderly people, as can acute urinary retention in men with prostatic enlargement. Treatment of poisoning is symptomatic; although physostigmine has been used to reverse anticholinergic effects,[204,205] it has a short duration of action, tolerance to its beneficial effects occurs, and it can cause adverse reactions – it should not be used except in life-threatening poisoning.[206]

The thorn apple or Jimson weed, *Datura stramonium* (Figure 76.27), grows in most parts of the world and is a frequent cause of poisoning in cereal crops. The seeds contain alkaloids of the tropane series, notably hyoscyamine. One outbreak of poisoning in Tanzania involved the consumption of porridge made from millet distributed by a local branch of the National Milling Corporation.[207] Jimson weed has also been used as a drug of abuse, because of its hallucinogenic properties.[208,209]

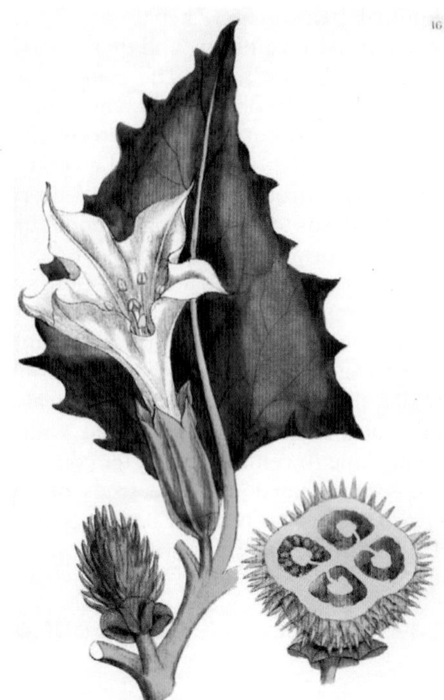

Figure 76.27 *Datura stramonium* (Jimson weed).

Other plants that can cause anticholinergic poisoning include angel's trumpet (*Brugmansia* spp., now called *Datura*),[210] found in Central and South America and prepared as a tea for its hallucinogenic effects and jessamine (*Gelsemium sempervirens*; Figure 76.28),[211] which is native to North and Central America.

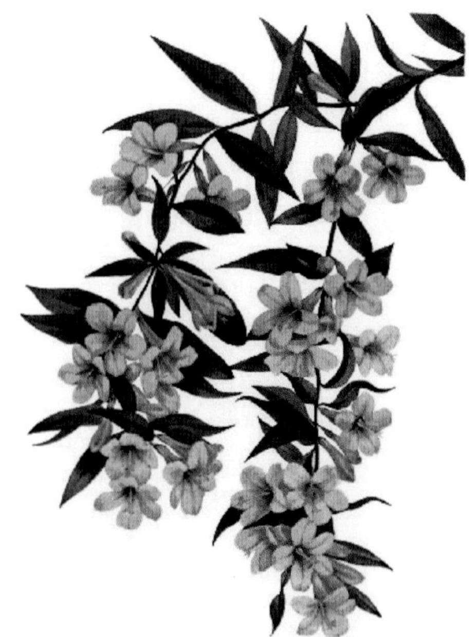

Figure 76.28 *Gelsemium sempervirens* (jessamine).

The seeds of various species of *Datura* have been used in cases of criminal poisoning in tropical countries. *D. fastuosa* was a favourite poison of practitioners of thagi in India, *D. sanguinea* is used in Colombia and Peru, *D. ferox* and *D. arborea* in Brazil, and the leaves of *Hyoscyamus fahezlez* by the Tuareg in the Sahara. The seeds of *D. stramonium* with *D. metel* have been used in East Africa for criminal purposes, as an inebriant to facilitate robbery or to elicit confessions of witchcraft.

CHOLINERGIC COMPOUNDS

Drugs can cause cholinergic effects either by stimulating acetylcholine receptors or by inhibiting acetylcholinesterase.

Drugs that stimulate acetylcholine receptors, of which nicotine and muscarine are the prototypes, are used therapeutically (e.g. pilocarpine in glaucoma) and are found in a wide variety of plants. The effects of poisoning are constricted pupils (miosis); hypersalivation and sweating; nausea, vomiting, and diarrhoea; bradycardia; and headache, vertigo, confusion, delirium, hallucinations, coma, and convulsions. Bronchorrhoea, bronchospasm, and pulmonary oedema produce respiratory failure, the usual cause of death. Most cases of cholinergic poisoning with flowering plants have been reported with laburnum in temperate zones; other cases have been reported with hemlock (*Conium maculatum*; Figure 76.29).[212]

Many fungi contain cholinergic compounds, and muscarinic poisoning can occur with, for example, jack o'lantern (*Omphalotus olearius*), *Clitocybe* spp., and *Inocybe* spp. In severe cases of poisoning with *Amanita* spp. there may be cholinergic symptoms, but the main effects are due to the GABAergic compound muscimol.[213]

Anticholinesterases potentiate the actions of acetylcholine by inhibiting its breakdown. Solanine is one such compound, found in plants of the *Solanum* spp., including the unripe berries of the bittersweet nightshade (*S. dulcamara*) and greened tubers of potatoes (*S. tuberosum*). However, *S. dulcamara* poisoning can also present with anticholinergic effects.[214] Accidental or suicidal poisoning can occur with anticholinesterase organophosphorus insecticides;[215] treatment is with atropine[216] and cholinesterase reactivators, such as pralidoxime and obidoxime.[217]

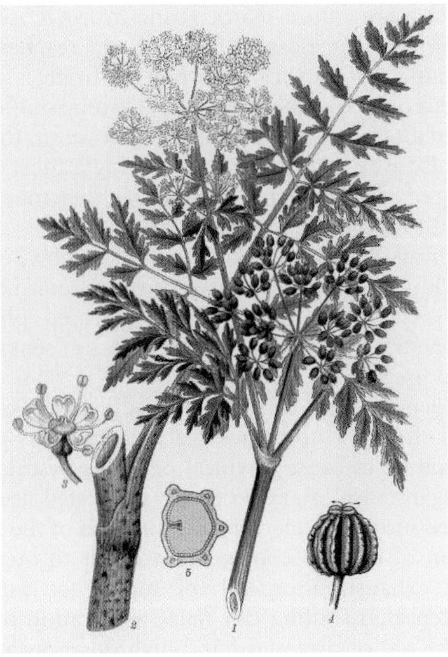

Figure 76.29 *Conium maculatum* (hemlock).

Psychotropic Drugs in Plants

AYAHUASCA

Ayahuasca[218] (*Quichua aya* = spirit, *huasca* = vine) is a hallucinogenic beverage that is prepared by boiling the bark of the liana *Banisteriopsis caapi*, which contains the beta-carbolines harmine, harmaline, and tetrahydroharmine, with the leaves of various plants, such as *Psychotria viridis* (chacruna or jagé), *Psychotria carthagenensis*, or *Diplopterys cabrerana* (chagropanga), which contain N,N-dimethyltryptamine, a potent hallucinogen. Dimethyltryptamine is inactive orally, because it is metabolized by gut monoamine oxidase. However, the β-carbolines are highly active reversible inhibitors of monoamine oxidase; they inhibit the deamination of dimethyltryptamine, making it orally active. In vitro, ayahuasca inhibits monoamine oxidase in proportion to the concentrations of β-carbolines.[219]

Ayahuasca induces a psychedelic, visionary state of mind and is used for medical and religious purposes. Shamans may use it to inspire diagnoses. At South American shamanic ceremonies people gather to take ayahuasca and sing themselves into a collective trance. After oral administration, its dose-related hallucinogenic effects first occur after 30–60 minutes, peak at 60–120 minutes and resolve by 240 minutes.[220] The experience is generally regarded as pleasant, although nausea is not uncommon and diarrhoea can occur; there are occasional dysphoric reactions, with transient disorientation and anxiety.

Drug interactions are to be expected between ayahuasca and drugs that would be expected to interact with monoamine oxidase inhibitors, such as selective serotonin reuptake inhibitors (SSRIs).[221]

BETEL

Chewing betel, the leaves of *Piper betle* [sic] (Figure 76.30), together with lime and areca (betel) nuts (*Areca catechu*) is a common practice in India, Sri Lanka, and other Eastern countries. It may act by inhibiting GABA uptake. The mouth, lips, and cheeks are stained bright red and the face is flushed; there is euphoria, heightened alertness, sweating, salivation, a hot sensation in the body, and an increased capacity to work; there are increases in heart rate, blood pressure, sweating, and body temperature.[222] Betel chewers can also develop manganese toxicity through contamination of the plant.[223] The presence of the codon 326 polymorphism in the hOGG1 gene may confer a greater risk of oral cancer in betel chewers.[224]

CANNABIS

Cannabis sativa (Figure 76.31), the hemp plant, yields marijuana and hashish. A cannabis smoker inhales at least 60 mind-altering chemicals, but the main psychoactive ingredient is delta-9-tetrahydrocannabinol (delta-9-THC), an antiemetic, antispasticity agent, appetite stimulant, analgesic, anxiolytic,

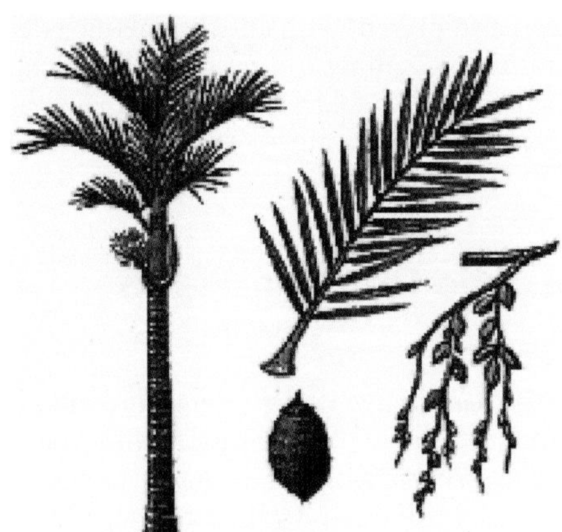

Figure 76.30 *Piper betle* (betel).

hypnotic, and antipyretic, which also lowers intraocular pressure. However, its beneficial effects in terminal disease are disappointing.

Marijuana ('grass', 'weed', 'bush', 'herb') is the dried mixture of crushed leaves and stalks of the plant. The flowering tops of the plant secrete a resin that can be compressed to form hashish ('hash', 'blow', 'puff', 'draw', 'ganja', 'dope', 'pot') or dissolved into an oil or tincture. Marijuana is usually rolled in home-made cigarettes ('spliffs', 'joints' or, if enormous, 'blunts'), with or without tobacco. Hashish is heated and crumbled on to tobacco in spliffs or smoked in a wide variety of pipes. In many parts of the world cannabis is an ingredient of a range of culinary preparations.

Cannabis has physical and mental effects that begin within minutes.[225] The physical effects include an increase in heart rate, peripheral vasodilatation, conjunctival suffusion, bronchodilatation, dryness of the mouth and, in large doses, tremor, ataxia, nystagmus, nausea, and vomiting. The mental effects vary from person to person, depending on such variables as personality, mood, surroundings, expectations, and previous cannabis experience. Generally, there is a feeling of wellbeing, accompanied by feelings of enhanced sensory perception. There may be drowsiness or hyperactivity. Ideas flow rapidly and may be disconnected. Time seems to pass slowly. Motor performance may be altered, as it may be by any sedative drug, and driving skills may be impaired.[226]

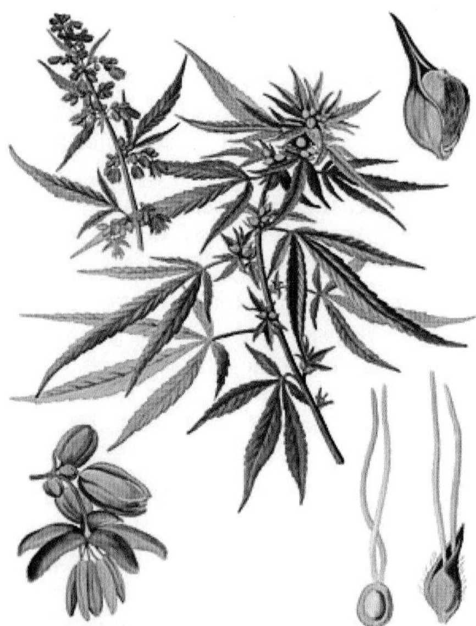

Figure 76.31 *Cannabis sativa* (hemp).

There may be mild tolerance and a mild withdrawal syndrome, rather like a mild benzodiazepine withdrawal syndrome. Physical dependence does not seem to be a big problem, but psychological dependence does occur.

Heavy use of marijuana is associated with social apathy, but this often precedes drug use and may not be an adverse effect. Adverse psychological reactions include anxiety, acute panic reactions, and paranoid ideas. Large doses can cause an acute toxic psychosis with confusion and hallucinations. There is controversy as to whether marijuana can produce a prolonged psychosis, but it can certainly aggravate pre-existing mental disease. Cannabis smoke contains more insoluble particulates and carcinogens than tobacco smoke, so lung and airways damage can be anticipated in heavy regular consumers. Birth defects occasionally follow use in pregnancy.

Although cannabis causes little acute toxicity, long-term use is associated with cognitive impairment and can lead to dependence in a proportion of regular users.[227] Smoking cannabis involves the additional risks of chronic lung damage and possibly cancer.

COCA

Erythroxylon coca (Figure 76.32) is widely grown in South America and India. The leaves are dried in the sun and are chewed with lime or, in India, with betel. Cocaine powder can be sniffed, prepared as a solution for intravenous injection, or separated from its hydrochloride and smoked as the free base or as 'crack' (so-called because of the popping and clicking of exploding impurities when it is burnt). Crack vaporizes at a much lower temperature than cocaine hydrochloride, so that the active ingredient escapes pyrolysis and reaches the lungs intact. Because the transfer from lung to brain is so fast, the impact of smoked cocaine gives a 'rush' comparable with that experienced after intravenous injection. However, the euphoriant effect also wears off quickly, producing a most unpleasant downswing of mood in many users, which they may attempt to fend off with repeatedly larger and larger doses.

The clinical effects of cocaine ('coke', 'snow', 'charlie', or 'crack') include euphoria, increased drive, increased confidence, increased sociability, loquacity, and increased physical and mental capacities. After chewing there is loss of sensation in the tongue and lips.

The tendency to take cocaine repeatedly to fend off rebound effects and the rapid tolerance that occurs to its euphoriant effects, combine to cause a typical pattern of escalating doses terminating in 'crash', characterized by exhausted sleep followed by depressed mood, which fuels the initiation of the next binge. Termination of a binge comes about either through physical or mental exhaustion or lack of money or further drug supplies. Repeated sniffing can cause perforation of the nasal septum. The use of prolonged and high dosages can lead to a cocaine-induced psychosis, not dissimilar from acute paranoid schizophrenia. There are no major physiological withdrawal

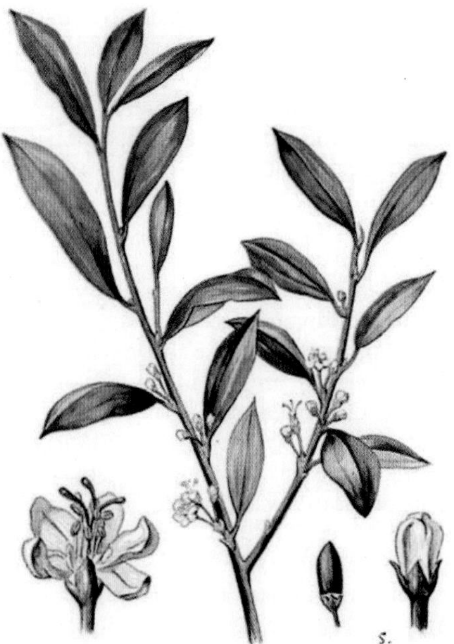

Figure 76.32 *Erythroxylon coca* (coca).

reactions, but troublesome dysphoria and craving can persist for months or even years. When it is taken during pregnancy, cocaine can cause constriction of the uterine and placental blood vessels and damage the fetus by depriving it of oxygen and other nutrients.[228] Besides its adverse neuropsychiatric effects,[229,230] long-term cocaine abuse also has adverse effects on other organs, including the heart and skin.[231,232]

IBOGAINE

Ibogaine is the main active ingredient of *Tabernanthe iboga*, a West African shrub that grows in the Congo and Angola,[233] and is isolated from the root bark. It has been used traditionally as a hallucinogen, to suppress hunger and fatigue, and as an aphrodisiac. In high doses it can cause convulsions and paralysis, and deaths have been reported. It is an indole that is an antagonist at serotonin and NMDA receptors. Another constituent, tabernanthine, is an antagonist at $GABA_A$ receptors. *Tabernanthe iboga* has been used in Gabon to induce a near-death experience for spiritual and psychological purposes.[234] It has been used for anti-addictive purposes,[235] leading to the development of a congener, 18-methoxycoronaridine.[236]

KAVA

The powdered root of *Piper methysticum*, prepared as a beverage, is drunk on festive occasions throughout Polynesia.[237] Formerly, the root was prepared by mastication by selected girls, a practice that caused the spread of tuberculosis. The actions of some of its constituents include altered activity at $GABA_A$ receptors and inhibition of voltage-dependent sodium channels. Over-indulgence in kava causes a state of hyperexcitement, with loss of power in the legs. Chronic intoxication leads to weight loss, raised liver enzymes, nausea, loss of appetite and a reversible ichthyosiform eruption (kava dermopathy).[238] In the west hepatotoxicity has often been reported;[239] this may be partly related to the fact that western formulations are prepared by lipid rather than aqueous extraction,[240] although the evidence is not conclusive,[241] and it has been suggested that it may be due to contamination of kava formulations with hepatotoxic moulds.[242]

KHAT

Khat or qat (cafta, miraa, muiragi) is a stimulant commonly used in East Africa, Yemen, and southern Saudi Arabia and is derived from a small tree, *Catha edulis*.[243] The leaves and twigs are chewed while fresh, but can also be smoked, infused in tea, or sprinkled on food. The khat alkaloids are absorbed first from the oral cavity and then from the gut, justifying slow chewing.[244] It produces euphoria and loquaciousness, with a misleading sensation of sharpened mental processes, because it contains cathinone (S[−]alpha-aminopropiophenone) and cathine (norpseudoephedrine), phenylalkylamines that are related to ephedrine and have amphetamine-like properties.[245] Cathinone increases dopamine release and reduces dopamine re-uptake.[246]

Khat is often used in social gatherings called 'sessions', which can last 3–4 hours. They are generally attended by men, although khat use among women is growing. Men are also more likely to be daily users. Users pick the leaves, chew them on one side of the mouth, swallow only the juice and add fresh leaves periodically. About 100–300 g of khat may be chewed during each session and 100 g of khat typically contains 36 mg of cathinone.

It is estimated that 10 million people chew khat worldwide and it is used by up to 80% of adults in Somalia and Yemen. It is also used by immigrant African communities in the UK and USA. It is banned in Saudi Arabia, Egypt, Morocco, Sudan, Kuwait, the USA, and European countries. However, in Australia its importation is controlled by a licence issued by the Therapeutic Goods Administration, which allows up to 5 kg of khat per month per individual for personal use.

Khat has many adverse effects.[247] It increases blood pressure and heart rate and may increase the risk of acute myocardial infarction. It can cause headaches. Psychosis has been reported with heavy use. Constipation is common, and anorexia, stomatitis, gastritis, and oesophagitis can also occur. Khat use can lead to dependence, and khat users may devote significant amounts of time to acquiring and using it, to the detriment of work and social responsibilities. The physical effects of early khat withdrawal are generally mild. Chronic users may experience craving, lethargy, and a feeling of warmth during early khat abstinence. Chronic consumption may be genotoxic.

NICOTINE

The leaves and flowers of *Nicotiana* spp. (Figure 76.33) have been universally smoked, snuffed, or chewed for their stimulant effects. Preparations of the leaves applied to the chest to relieve respiratory complaints have sometimes given rise to toxic effects by percutaneous absorption of nicotine. However, nicotine is much more widespread in plants and occurs in such diverse species as *Acacia* spp., *Aesculus hippocastanum*, *Asclepias* spp., *Duboisia* spp. *Echeviria* spp., *Erythroxylon coca*, *Juglans regia*, *Mucuna pruriens*, *Prunus* spp., *Sempervivum arachnoideum*, and *Urtica dioica*. During the nineteenth and early part of the twentieth century, Australian Aborigines used pituri, a

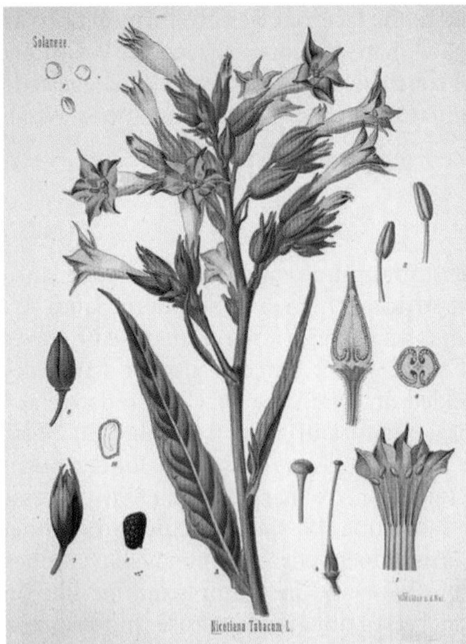

Figure 76.33 *Nicotiana tabacum* (tobacco).

nicotine-containing preparation from the cured leaves of *Duboisia hopwoodii*.[248]

Green tobacco sickness is an occupational illness reported by tobacco workers worldwide.[249] It causes nausea, vomiting, headache, weakness, and dizziness.[250,251] Among farm workers in shade tobacco fields in Connecticut 15% had diagnoses that could be attributed to possible green tobacco sickness (ICD-9);[252] using a stricter case definition, the frequency fell to 4%. Non-smokers were significantly more likely than smokers to report symptoms, particularly isolated symptoms of headache and dizziness.

An unusual nostrum made by the Yoruba people of Nigeria is 'cow's urine mixture', which consists of green tobacco leaves, rock salt, citron (*Citrus medica*), the leaves of the bush basil, *Ocimum viride*, and cow's urine.[253] The remedy is swallowed or rubbed into the skin for prevention and treatment of epileptic or eclamptic fits; the toxic effects are those of nicotine – central nervous excitation, with vomiting, diarrhoea, dehydration, and hypoglycaemia, followed by depression and coma, sometimes with permanent neurological damage or death. Convulsions must be controlled and glucose given intravenously. The poison is removed by gastric lavage or cleansing of the skin; blood glucose, electrolytes, and fluid balance should be monitored.

OPIUM ALKALOIDS AND THEIR DERIVATIVES

Opioid dependence is a worldwide public health menace associated with a great deal of criminal activity. Heroin ('smack,' 'junk', 'gear', 'brown') is the opiate chosen by 75% and heroin-related referrals are increasing by at least 15% per year. On initial use there may be nausea, vomiting, and anxiety, but these symptoms disappear with subsequent use and euphoria becomes predominant. As tolerance develops and the cost of the habit increases, the addict may switch to the intravenous route to maximize value for money. In an attempt to retain the euphoria (the 'rush') that results from rapidly increased concentrations of the drug in the brain, larger and larger doses will be used. Tolerance to constipation and pupillary constriction does not occur to any great extent. Eventually the addict becomes most concerned with combating withdrawal symptoms and needs a regular supply of the drug to avoid them.

Withdrawal symptoms begin at about 8 hours after the last dose and reach a peak at about 36–72 hours. Symptoms occur in the following order:

- Psychological symptoms: anxiety, depression, restlessness, irritability, drug craving
- Lachrymation, rhinorrhoea, mydriasis, yawning, sweating, tachycardia, and hypertension
- Restless sleep, after which the above symptoms are accompanied by sneezing, anorexia, nausea, vomiting, abdominal cramps, diarrhoea, bone pain, muscle pain, tremor, weakness, chills and goose-flesh ('cold turkey'), twitching and jerking of the legs ('kicking the habit'), and insomnia. Hypotension, cardiovascular collapse, and convulsions occur rarely.

These symptoms gradually fade over about 5–10 days, during which time, general malaise, and abdominal cramps persist. This withdrawal syndrome is not as bad as has been widely depicted in literature and is not fatal.[254]

With methadone, the onset of withdrawal symptoms is delayed for 24–48 hours and peaks at 3–4 days; because of this slower effect, methadone is often used to help an addict withdraw, by substituting it for morphine or heroin.

PSILOCYBIN

Psilocybin was isolated in 1957 from the *Psilocybe mexicana* mushroom and it has since been identified as a component of over 75 distinct mushroom species.[255] Psilocybin-containing mushrooms, also called 'magic mushrooms', are used recreationally.[256] Psilocybin and psilocin are listed as Schedule I drugs under the United Nations 1971 Convention on Psychotropic Substances.

Psilocybin content varies based on such factors as species and preparation. The most commonly used mushroom is *Psilocybe cubensis*, which contains 10–12 mg of psilocybin per gram of dried mushrooms; effective oral doses range from 6 to 20 mg and about 40 μg/kg is considered the threshold level for intoxication.[257]

Psilocin is a high-affinity agonist at serotonin 5-HT_{2A} receptors, which are especially prominent in the prefrontal cortex. It increases cortical activity secondary to down-stream post-synaptic glutamate effects. It is also active at 5-HT_{1A}, 5-HT_{1D}, and 5-HT_{2C} receptors, although these are thought to play a lesser role in its effects. In the presence of the 5-HT_{2A} antagonist ketanserin, the changes in mental state that psilocybin typically causes do not occur.[258] Although psilocybin has no affinity for dopamine D_2 receptors, a PET study using the D_2 receptor ligand raclopride showed that psilocybin increases dopamine transmission in the striatum, probably through secondary increases in dopamine.[259,260] Some psilocybin-containing mushrooms contain phenylethylamine, which may contribute to sympathomimetic effects.

Psilocybin alters mood, perception and cognition. In healthy volunteers, changes in emotion, consciousness, perception, and thought begin within 20–30 min, peak at 30–50 min, persist for 2 hours, and resolve within 6 hours. Lower doses may produce shorter-lasting effects of 1–2 hours. Moderate oral doses (12–30 mg) alter consciousness, increase introspection, and induce derealization, dream-like states, illusions, complex hallucinations, synaesthesia, and altered perceptions of time and space. Muscle relaxation also occurs during intoxication. Altered attention causes difficulty in disengaging from prior stimuli and impairment in monitoring several simultaneous visual stimuli.[261] Euphoria, grandiosity, and other amplifications of affective experience are common. Most psilocybin users experience a pleasant alteration in mood, but some panic or become dysphoric. A user's expectations and environment very strongly influence the hallucinogenic effects. Settings with more interpersonal support reduce panic and paranoia and increase positive experiences.[262]

Adverse reactions to psilocybin include hypertension, exacerbation of pre-existing psychosis, and hallucinogen persisting perceptual disorder.[263] Trauma can occur if people believe that they have superhuman powers.[264]

Treatment of Poisoning

This is not the place for a thorough description of the treatment of poisoning,[265] but a few simple principles are summarized in Table 76.5.

Drug Interactions with Compounds in Plants

Drug interactions can occur between plant medicaments and allopathic medicines.[266–268] Some of these are summarized in Table 76.6. Many of these interactions are poorly attested, being anecdotal. However, interactions with grapefruit and St John's wort are well described and are dealt with below.

PHARMACODYNAMIC INTERACTIONS

If a herbal medicine shares a pharmacological action with an allopathic remedy, it may potentiate its therapeutic or adverse effects; the following are examples:

- Digitalis and plant remedies containing cardioactive glycosides (*Strophanthus*, *Convallaria*, *Cytisus*, *Scilla*); furthermore, some herbal medicines can interfere with serum digoxin radioimmunoassays[269–271]
- Antihypertensive drugs and hypotensive herbs (*Rauwolfia*, *Crataegus*, *Viscum*)
- Oral hypoglycaemic drugs and karela, the fruit of *Momordica charantia*; karela, which has a hypoglycaemic action,[272] is used in curries and is a traditional Indian remedy for diabetes
- Oral hypoglycaemic drugs and plants that contain alpha-glucosidase inhibitory activity, such as chancapiedra (*Phyllanthus niruri*), zarzaparrilla (*Smilax officinalis*), yerba mate (*Ilex paraguayensis*), and huacatay (*Tagetes minuta*)[273]
- Antiasthma drugs and betel nut, which is thought to have a bronchoconstricting effect, attributed to arecoline[274]
- ACE inhibitors and *Capsicum* spp. ACE inhibitors increase the amount of bradykinin in the lung and enhance the cough response to capsaicin, which acts by depleting substance P from nerve endings.

TABLE 76.5 A Summary of the Management of Acute Self-Poisoning

Target		Therapeutic Action
1.	Respiratory function	Check gag reflex Remove dentures Clear out oropharyngeal obstructions, debris, secretions Lay on the left side with head down Insert oral airway or, if cough reflex lost, an endotracheal tube Give oxygen if hypoxic Assist respiration if required
2.	Circulatory function	Check heart rate and blood pressure If systolic blood pressure below 80 mmHg (young patients) or 90 mmHg (old patients): Raise end of bed If ineffective, give volume expanders If fluid overload and oliguria: Give dopamine and/or dobutamine
3.	Renal function	Monitor urine output
4.	Consciousness	Assess level of consciousness (Glasgow Coma Scale)
5.	Temperature	Take temperature rectally; if below 36°C reheat slowly Warm all inspired air and intravenous fluids
6.	Convulsions	Treat with diazepam, clomethiazole, phenytoin, or anaesthesia with assisted ventilation
7.	Cardiac arrhythmias	Treat as required
8.	Gastric lavage	Not now recommended
9.	Activated charcoal	A single dose or repeated doses for some poisons
10.	Fluid and electrolyte balance	Dehydration: oral fluids usually enough Unconscious patients: use intravenous fluids and insert a central venous line Treat hypokalaemia
11.	Emergency measures	Specific to the poison
12.	Chest radiography	In drowsy or comatose patients who vomit After endotracheal intubation
13.	Collection of specimens	Gastric aspirate (drugs) Urine (drugs, renal function) Blood (drugs, arterial gases, electrolytes)

TABLE 76.6 Some Reported Interactions of Medicinal Compounds with Plants and Herbal Products; Many of These Associations Have been Reported Anecdotally and Some Have not been Confirmed in Small Formal Studies

Plant(s)	Drug(s)	Outcome
Areca catechu (areca nut)	Neuroleptic drugs	Exacerbation of extrapyramidal effects
Berberis aristata (berberine)	Tetracycline	Prolonged diarrhoea in cholera
Citrus paradisi (grapefruit juice)	Amiodarone	Risk of amiodarone toxicity (e.g. cardiac arrhythmias)
	Antihistamines (astemizole, terfenadine)	Prolongation of QT interval; risk of ventricular tachycardia
	Ciclosporin	Risk of ciclosporin toxicity (immunosuppression)
	Benzodiazepines (alprazolam, diazepam, midazolam, triazolam)	Increased drowsiness; altered psychometric tests
	Calcium channel blockers (felodipine, nifedipine, nisoldipine)	Reduced blood pressure, increased heart rate, headaches, flushing, light-headedness
	Lovastatin	Risk of lovastatin toxicity (including rhabdomyolysis and renal insufficiency)
	Quinidine	Prolongation of QT interval; risk of ventricular tachycardia
	Saquinavir	Risk of saquinavir toxicity
	Sertraline	Risk of sertraline toxicity (serotonin syndrome)
Cyanopsis tetragonolobus (guar gum)	Digoxin, glibenclamide, metformin, phenoxymethylpenicillin	Reduced absorption
Eleutherococcus senticosus (Siberian ginseng)	Digoxin	Increased plasma digoxin concentration
Gingko biloba (maidenhair)	Thiazide diuretics	Hypertension
Glycyrrhiza glabra (liquorice)	Corticosteroids	Increased risk of hypokalaemia
	Spironolactone	Reduced potassium-sparing effect
Hypericum perforatum (St John's wort)	Amitriptyline, ciclosporin, digoxin, finasteride, HIV protease inhibitors, irinotecan, oral contraceptives, phenprocoumon, theophylline	Induction of metabolism by CYP3A4, causing reduced effects (e.g. increased risk of transplant rejection with ciclosporin, reduced anticoagulation with warfarin); induction of P glycoprotein, increasing intestinal and renal secretion of drugs
	Digoxin, indinavir	Induction of P glycoprotein, increasing clearance and reducing effects
	Serotonin reuptake inhibitors	Serotonin syndrome
Panax ginseng (ginseng)	Antidepressants	Risk of mania
	Cocaine	Tolerance inhibited
	Digoxin	Increased plasma digoxin concentration
	Metamphetamine	Tolerance inhibited
	Opioids	Reduced pharmacological effects of opioids
	Phenelzine	Headache, tremulousness, hyperactivity
Pausinystalia yohimbe (yohimbine)	Tricyclic antidepressants	Increased risk of hypertension
Plantago ovale (bran, ispaghula husk)	Digoxin, iron, lithium, lovastatin, tricyclic antidepressants	Reduced absorption
Tamarindus indica (tamarind)	Aspirin	Increased systemic availability
Shankhapushpi (an Ayurvedic mixture of herbs)	Phenytoin	Decreased concentrations of phenytoin, leading to seizures
Xaio chai hu tang (sho-salko-to)	Prednisolone	Reduced effect of prednisolone

Anticoagulants

Many alternative medicines interact with oral anticoagulants (principally warfarin) and interactions with plants are listed separately in Table 76.7. Drug interactions of warfarin with herbal preparations have been reviewed.[275,276]

In a retrospective analysis of the pharmaceutical care plans of 631 patients, 170 (27%) were taking some form of complementary or alternative medicine and 99 were using a medicine that could interact with warfarin, the commonest being cod-liver oil and garlic.[277] The risk of bleeding associated with the use of alternative medicines has been evaluated in 171 patients taking warfarin in a prospective study in an acute-care academic research hospital in Canada.[278] The patients completed a 16-week diary by recording bleeding events; 87 (51%) reported at least one bleeding event and 73 (43%) indicated that they had used at least one alternative medicine previously reported to interact with warfarin. The therapies associated with an increased risk of self-reported bleeding included cayenne, ginger, willow bark, St John's wort, and ubidecarenone (co-enzyme Q10). Use of more than one alternative medicine while taking warfarin was also a significant susceptibility factor.

In a systematic review, warfarin was the most common cardiovascular drug involved in interactions with herbal medicines.[279] In a meta-analysis of interactions of warfarin with other drugs, herbal medicines, Chinese herbal drugs, and foods, 642 citations were retrieved, of which 181 eligible articles contained original reports on 120 drugs or foods.[280] Of all the reports, 72% described potentiation of the effect of warfarin, and the authors considered that 84% were of poor quality, 86% of which were single case reports. The 31 incidents of clinically significant bleeding were all single case reports. Relatively few anecdotal reports of adverse event–drug associations are

TABLE 76.7 **Some Reported Interactions of Warfarin and Other Coumarin Anticoagulants with Plants and Herbal Products**[a]

Plant	Effect on Anticoagulation
Allium sativum (garlic)	Reduced (altered platelet aggregation)
Angelica sinensis (dong quai)	Potentiated
Camellia sinensis (green tea)	Reduced (contains vitamin K)
Carica papaya (papaya)	Potentiated
Citrus paradisi (grapefruit juice)	Potentiated (inhibition of warfarin metabolism)
Cucurbita pepo	Potentiated (contains vitamin E)
Ginkgo biloba (maidenhair)	Potentiated
Harpagophytum procumbens (devil's claw)	Potentiated
Hypericum perforatum (St John's wort)	Reduced (induction of warfarin metabolism)
Lycium barbarum (Chinese wolfberry)	Potentiated
Mangifera indica (mango)	Potentiated
Matricaria chamomilla (chamomile)	Potentiated
Panax ginseng (ginseng)	Reduced platelet aggregation
Panax quinquefolium (American ginseng)	Reduced anticoagulation
Peumus boldus (boldo)	Potentiated
Punica granatum (pomegranate juice)	Potentiated
Salvia miltiorrhiza (danshen)	Potentiated (?altered pharmacokinetics)
Trigonella foenum graecum (fenugreek)	Potentiated
Vaccinium macrocarpon (cranberry juice)	Potentiated
Zingiber officinale (ginger)	Potentiated

[a]Many of these associations have been reported anecdotally and some have not been confirmed in small formal studies.

followed-up with formal studies,[281] and reports of interactions of warfarin with herbal medicines are no exception – most are based on anecdotal reports.

Medicines that resulted in increased anticoagulation include *Allium sativum* (garlic[282–284]), *Angelica sinensis* (dong quai[285]), *Carica papaya* (papaya), curbicin[286] (from *Cucurbita pepo* seed and *Serenoa repens* fruit), *Ginkgo biloba* (maidenhair[287–290]), *Harpagophytum procumbens* (devil's claw), *Lycium barbarum* (Chinese wolfberry[291,292]), *Mangifera indica* (mango),[293] *Matricaria chamomilla* (chamomile[294]), *Salvia miltiorrhiza* (danshen[295–297]), *Trigonella foenum graecum* (fenugreek[298]), *Vaccinium macrocarpon* (cranberry[299–301]), and *Zingiber officinale* (ginger[302,303]). Medicines that result in reduced anticoagulation include *Camellia sinensis* (green tea[304]), *Hypericum perforatum* (St. John's wort[305–308]), *Panax ginseng* (ginseng[309–312]), and *Panax quinquefolium* (American ginseng[310]).

Other plants and herbal products that have been reported to increase or reduce the actions of warfarin[313] include angelica root, anise, arnica flower, asafetida, bogbean, borage seed oil, bromelain, capsicum, celery, clove, feverfew, green tea, horse chestnut, liquorice root, lovage root, meadowsweet, melilot, onion, parsley, passion-flower, poplar, quassia, red clover, rue, sweet clover (in which coumarin anticoagulants were originally discovered), sweet woodruff, tonka beans, turmeric, vitamin E, and willow bark.

The mechanisms vary: for example, garlic reduces platelet aggregation; some plants (e.g. dong quai) contain anticoagulant coumarins; and some (e.g. tonka beans) contain vitamin K, a natural antagonist of the actions of coumarin anticoagulants.

Warfarin has also been reported to interact with Chinese medicines, which often contain mixtures of herbs; in such cases it is difficult or impossible to identify the precipitant plant or the mechanism. For example, Quilinggao, a mixture that contains numerous herbal ingredients (including *Fritillaria cirrhosa* and other *Fritillaria* species, *Paeoniae rubra*, *Lonicera japonica*, and *Poncirus trifoliata*, in many different brands), has been reported to enhance the actions of warfarin.[314]

Citrus Fruits

Various isoforms of the enzyme cytochrome P450 are responsible for the oxidative metabolism of many drugs.[315] One of these isoforms, CYP3A4, is responsible for the metabolism of several drugs in the gut wall while they are being absorbed after oral administration. Inhibition of the enzyme by something in grapefruits (*Citrus paradisi*) and Seville oranges (*Citrus bigaradia*) causes more of the drug to escape presystemic metabolism and enter the circulation unchanged, potentially leading to drug toxicity. The compounds in grapefruit juice and Seville oranges responsible for these interactions may be, at least in part, bergamottin and dihydroxybergamottin, which are furocoumarins.[316] Lime juice, which contains bergamottin but not dihydroxybergamottin, has a smaller effect.[317] In some countries, a drug label has been introduced, alerting patients to potential drug interactions with grapefruit.[318] In the UK in 1997, the antihistamine terfenadine was withdrawn from over-the-counter sales because of cardiac arrhythmias,[319] and a year later another antihistamine, astemizole, was withdrawn for similar reasons.[320] Drugs whose effects can be increased by grapefruit juice, causing toxicity[321] are listed in Table 76.6.

Grapefruit juice probably also inhibits the P glycoprotein and organic anion transporting polypeptides that are responsible for the intestinal secretion and active absorption of many drugs,[322] and therefore other drug interactions are to be expected. This effect is at least partly due to furocoumarins[323] and partly to naringin.[324]

Ginseng

Reported drug interactions with ginseng (*Panax ginseng*) are listed in Table 76.6. The root has been used in China, Korea, and Japan for centuries in the belief that it counters fatigue and stress and confers health, virility, and longevity; it is supposed to enhance immunity and to combat the effects of oxidative free radicals that cause chronic diseases and ageing.[325] The pharmacological basis for its reputation is slender, but ginseng is in fashion worldwide. It is often adulterated with *Eleutherococcus senticosus* (Siberian ginseng, Table 76.6), *Mandragora*, *Rauwolfia*, and other roots of similar appearance. Ginseng contains a complex mixture of steroids and saponins; it can cause insomnia, tremor, headache, diarrhoea, hypertension, and oestrogen-like effects.[326] It may also increase the risk of gastric cancer.[327]

St John's wort

As an antidepressant, St John's wort[328] may enhance the effects of other antidepressants; since it is an inhibitor of 5-HT reuptake, combination with serotonin reuptake inhibitors can cause

TABLE 76.8 Some Adulterants and Contaminants that Have Been Found in Herbal Products

Type of Adulterant/Contaminant	Examples
Allopathic drugs	Albendazole, analgesic and anti-inflammatory agents (for example aminophenazone, cocaine, diclofenac, diethylpropion, indometacin, paracetamol, phenylbutazone), benzodiazepines, chlorphenamine, ephedrine, glucocorticoids, ketoconazole, sildenafil, sulfonylureas, tadalafil, thiazide diuretics, thyroid hormones
Botanicals	*Aristolochia* spp., *Atropa belladonna, Digitalis* spp. (see Table 76.2), *Colchicum, Rauwolfia serpentina*, pyrrolizidine-containing plants (see Table 76.4)
Fumigation agents	Ethylene oxide, methyl bromide, phosphine
Heavy metals	Arsenic, cadmium, lead, mercury
Microorganisms	*Escherichia coli, Pseudomonas aeruginosa, Salmonella* spp., *Shigella* spp., *Staphylococcus aureus*
Microbial toxins	Aflatoxins, bacterial endotoxins
Pesticides	Carbamate insecticides and herbicides, chlorinated pesticides (for example aldrin, dieldrin, heptachlor, DDT, DDE, HCB, HCH isomers), dithiocarbamate fungicides, organic phosphates, triazine herbicides
Radionuclides	^{134}Cs, ^{137}Cs, ^{131}I, ^{103}Ru, ^{90}Sr

the serotonin syndrome. Hyperforin, an ingredient of St John's wort (*Hypericum perforatum*), is an enzyme inducer and increases the metabolism of certain drugs, principally through CYP3A4, reducing their effects; St John's wort also induces intestinal P glycoprotein, leading to increased clearance of some drugs by intestinal and renal secretion.[305] Examples of these pharmacokinetic interactions are listed in Table 76.6.

Adulteration of Herbal Products

There have been many reports that Chinese herbal remedies have been adulterated or contaminated with conventional drugs, heavy metals, and even other herbal substances not announced on the label.[329] Some examples are listed in Table 76.8.

BIBLIOGRAPHY

Aronson JK, editor. Meyler's Side Effects of Herbal Drugs. Amsterdam: Elsevier; 2009. Online. Available: http://www.elsevier.com/wps/find/books_browse.cws_home.

Burkill HM. The useful plants of West tropical Africa. 2nd edition. Volumes 1-6. London: Crown Agents for Oversea Governments and Administrations; 1985, 1994, 1995, 1997, 2000, 2004.

Caius JF. The Medicinal and Poisonous Plants of India. Jodhpur: Scientific Publishers; 2003.

Everist SL. Poisonous Plants of Australia. 2nd ed. Sydney: Angus & Robertson; 1981.

Nelson LS, Shih RD, Balick MJ. Handbook of Poisonous and Injurious Plants. 2nd ed. New York: The New York Botanical Garden/Springer; 2007.

Schmidt RJ. Botanical Dermatology Database. Online. Available: http://www.botanical-dermatology-database.info.

Watt JM, Breyer-Brandwijk MG. The Medicinal and Poisonous Plants of Southern and Eastern Africa. 2nd ed. Edinburgh: E & S Livingstone; 1962.

Wink M, van Wyk B-E. Mind-Altering & Poisonous Plants of the World. Portland Oregon: Timber Press; 2008.

Access the complete references online at www.expertconsult.com

Nutrition-associated Disease

STEPHEN ABRAMS | BERNARD J. BRABIN | JOHN B. S. COULTER

KEY POINTS

- About one-third of children <5 years old in developing countries are stunted. Stunting is usually well established by 2 years of age.
- Mortality of children hospitalized for severe acute malnutrition is also markedly increased in HIV-positive children and is likely due to a higher rate of medical complications.
- Two-thirds of deaths from acute severe malnutrition occur within the first week of admission. To reduce the mortality rate, special care has to be given during this period.
- The prevalence of micronutrient deficiencies in children may be decreased with micronutrient supplementation using powders or ready-to-use therapeutic foods.
- Nutritional rickets is still a major problem in many developing countries and is common in North Africa and the Middle East.

Introduction

The interrelationship between nutrition and disease has long been recognized as fundamental. Diets in low-resource areas often have inadequate micronutrients as well as being deficient in macronutrients and there may be the added burden of bacterial and parasitic infections, especially hookworm and other nematodes. These infections can cause loss of appetite and malabsorption, which result in growth retardation, weight loss and micronutrient deficiencies. Seasonal and climatic variations have an enormous influence on disease transmission, agricultural potential and food security, which all affect nutritional status. This concurrence may also result in the 'hungry season', which describes the time between the exhaustion of the previous year's food stores and the new harvest which generates a state of nutritional stress in many developing countries. Traditional practices and cultural and religious food customs may lead to further dietary limitations or deficiencies in key nutrients such as iron or vitamin D.

Malnutrition in Children

Malnutrition is common in children in most resource-limited countries. Over 50% of deaths in children less than 5 years of age are associated with malnutrition. The prevalence of severe acute malnutrition is approximately 1–2% depending on the level of poverty and limitations in food supply. The interactions between infection and nutrition are key factors in determining this rate.[1–4]

PREVALENCE

The prevalence of malnutrition may be measured according to rates of stunting, underweight and wasting. Table 77.1 outlines the geographical distribution in developing countries. Approximately 34% of children less than 5 years old in developing countries are stunted. Stunting is usually well established by 2 years of age and improvements after that in final achieved height percentile may be incomplete. Causes are multifactorial and reflect socioeconomic, educational and health status of society. Prenatal factors and low birth weight are also important causes. Approximately 22% of children less than 5 years of age in developing countries are underweight. Wasting (low weight-for-age or weight-for-height ratios) affects approximately 12% of children and usually occurs between 6 months and 2 years of age. Rates increase during famine, war, forced migration and economic depression. Socioeconomic causes of malnutrition vary geographically and are outlined in Table 77.2. Nutritional causes are difficult to assess. Wasting may be due more to deficient quantity and stunting to deficient quality of food.[2,5]

SEVERE ACUTE MALNUTRITION

Severe acute malnutrition is manifest by wasting and/or oedema. Major factors are nutritional deficiency and recurrent infections, both of which have underlying socioeconomic causes, particularly poverty and lack of hygiene and education. Infant-feeding practices of concern including improper complementary (weaning) foods are compounded by infections associated with anorexia and increased metabolic demand. Many children with severe organic diseases, e.g. cardiac and renal disorders and mental and physical handicap, have variable degrees of malnutrition and are frequently stunted and underweight.

MEASUREMENT AND CLASSIFICATION

There are various methods of classifying malnutrition which depend on the type of information required and the prevalence of oedema; also the level of training of health workers undertaking measurements. Methods for assessment of underweight (WAZ), wasting (WHZ), stunting (HAZ), thinness (MUAC) and microcephali (head circumference) using Z-scores are available. WHO child growth standards have replaced the National Centre for Health Statistics (NCHS)/WHO reference values. This shift from NCHS to WHO growth standards will identify more children at high risk for mortality.[2,3]

Weight for Age

Weight for age as a percentage of the median standard is useful for assessment at child health clinics. Disadvantages include inaccuracy of age of the child for some uneducated mothers and

TABLE 77.1 Percentage of Underweight, Stunting and Wasting for Children Less Than 5 Years Old 2003–2009 According to WHO Child Growth Standards[2,3]

	Underweight	Wasting	Stunting
Sub-Saharan Africa	22	9	40
Middle East and North Africa	14	10	31
Asia	27	17	35
South Asia	42	19	48
East Asia and Pacific	11	–	22
Latin American and Caribbean	4	2	14
CEE/CIS	4	4	16
Developing countries	22	12	34

CEE/CIS, Central and Eastern Europe/Commonwealth of Independent States.
Underweight is defined as weight-for-length <5th percentile based on the CDC gender-specific weight-for-length reference for children less than 2 years of age and Body Mass Index (BMI) for age – <5th percentile for children 2–20 years of age. Wasting is defined as weight for height Z-score less than –2.0 and stunting is defined as height for age Z-score less than –2.0.

it also does not take into account lightness in weight due to stunting. Inaccuracy of scales used to measure weight in many settings is also a problem.

Mid Upper Arm Circumference (MUAC)

This measurement is useful for screening children between 6 months and 5 years of age and only requires a measuring tape. Severe malnutrition is usually defined as <115 mm[3]. Standard deviations of MUAC in relation to age and standards for MUAC related to height (QUAC stick) are available.[3]

Weight for Height

This is used in criteria for admission of children with acute malnutrition. It may be described as percentage of standard, standard deviations or standard deviation (or Z) scores.

WHO Classification

This uses weight for height, MUAC and presence of bilateral oedema (see Table 77.3). A weight for height below –3 SD and a MUAC <115 mm for children 6–60 months should both be used as independent criteria for admission to therapeutic feeding programmes.[2,3]

TABLE 77.2 Socioeconomic Causes of Malnutrition

General	Food	Infection
Lack of education Poverty Frequent pregnancies Low birth weight Intrafamilial • divorce, separation • working mothers • unemployment • sending a child away for care by a relative Inadequate medical and nutritional support	Food insecurity • general • seasonal Cultural practices and taboos Maldistribution within the family	Poor hygiene and sanitation HIV infection Failed measles immunization Tuberculosis

TABLE 77.3 Recommended Diagnostic Criteria for Severe Acute Malnutrition in Children 6–60 Months of Age[2,3]

Indicator	Measure	Cut-off
Severe wasting[b]	Weight-for-height[a]	<–3 SD
Severe wasting[b]	MUAC	<115 mm
Bilateral oedema[c]	Clinical sign	

[a]Based on WHO child growth standards.
[b,c]Independent indicators of severe acute malnutrition that require urgent action.

AETIOLOGY OF MALNUTRITION

Nutrient Deficiency

Breast-feeding. In many traditional societies, prolonged breastfeeding for up to 2 years or longer is common. However, rarely is it exclusive; additional foods/fluids may be introduced as early as the 1st month of life. In resource-limited societies, absence of breastfeeding or cessation before 6 months of age is associated with early onset of malnutrition, especially wasting and high mortality rates. Breast-feeding provides important sources of energy and protein and anti-infective factors, but if not supplemented by age-appropriate complementary feeds after about 6 months of age, the child's weight becomes static or falls. In the latter situation, severe malnutrition may follow quickly upon stopping of breastfeeding, commonly associated with recurrent infections, e.g. diarrhoea or measles (Figure 77.1).[6,7]

Infant Diets. Diets often consist of single staples, e.g. millet, sorghum, maize or rice, which are usually bulky with high water content, low energy density and high phytate levels (especially maize). High phytate concentrations reduce the

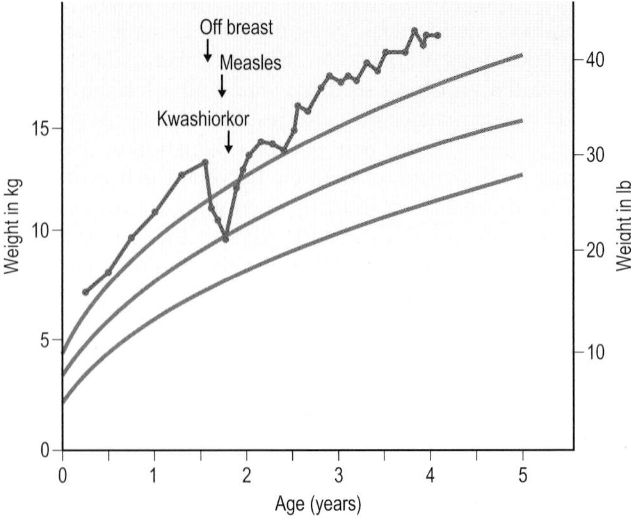

Figure 77.1 Effect of measles on weight gain. *(From Morley D. Prevention of protein-calorie deficiency syndromes. Trans R Soc Trop Med Hyg 1968; 62:200–8.)*

bioavailability of nutrients such as zinc, iron and calcium. Contamination by pathogenic microorganisms is common. Where the major component of diet is root crops, e.g. cassava, yams, potatoes or bananas, there is a low protein : energy ratio. Single-cereal diets may be deficient in a specific essential amino acid, e.g. tryptophan (maize) or lysine (cereals in general) and require to be balanced by a complementary plant protein source like legumes, e.g. beans, lentils, chickpeas and groundnuts or even better, animal protein which has a high biological value, e.g. milk (human or animal), meat and eggs. Sick children require frequent meals during and for 2 weeks or more after the infection to assist catch-up growth.

Infection. Infection may cause severe weight loss through anorexia, catabolic loss and tissue depletion. There are few prospective studies on the immunological effects of infection on growing children. Most studies are preformed on hospitalized children with severe malnutrition. Of the latter, children with oedematous malnutrition tend to have more immune suppression than those with wasting only. Cell-mediated immunity is often severely depressed. Their B lymphocytes and immunoglobulins are usually normal or raised due to recurrent infections (polyclonal stimulation), but the immune response to infections may be suboptimal. Complement is reduced. Activity of neutrophils in 'killing' ingested bacteria may also be depressed. An important factor in depression of the immune system associated with recurrent infections is failure of the system to recover because of nutrient deficiency, e.g. defective protein metabolism and micronutrient deficiency, especially zinc. Zinc is also important in promoting growth during rehabilitation and in the prevention and management of persistent diarrhoea.[8–10]

Most children have gut and/or respiratory infections and bacteraemia is common, often due to Gram-negative bacteria, including *Salmonellae*. Septicaemia and shock are important causes of death. Urinary tract infection is not infrequent. Tuberculosis and HIV may be underlying factors. Infections may be difficult to diagnose clinically as the temperature may be normal (or subnormal), the pulse not increased nor the neutrophil count raised and acute phase protein response is impaired. Hydration may be difficult to assess and clinical signs of pneumonia may be minimal despite radiological changes.[11]

Malnutrition itself is a risk factor for recurrent infections. Newborns and small children with severe protein malnutrition have atrophied thymi and poorly developed peripheral lymphoid organs. T cell counts may be low, with an increased undifferentiated lymphocyte count and decreased serum complement activity.[12] This malnutrition-induced immunodeficiency promotes infections that, as mentioned earlier, exacerbate malnourishment.

HIV Infection. HIV infection has a direct effect in worsening children's nutrition status. Malnutrition occurs, despite apparently appropriate breast-milk intake. In communities where chronic childhood undernutrition is common, stunting and decreased weight-for-age are more common in HIV-positive than HIV-negative children.[13] Mortality of children hospitalized for severe acute malnutrition is also markedly increased in HIV-positive children and is likely due to a higher rate of medical complications.[14] Common infections include pneumonia, tuberculosis, extensive skin infections, oral thrush and persistent diarrhoea.[15]

Treatment of severe acute malnutrition in the setting of HIV is more difficult. Whereas appetite can be used to assess recovery in HIV-negative malnourished children, it may not be useful in HIV-positive children in whom persistent anorexia is common.[15] HIV infection not only appears to lengthen hospital stay for re-nutrition but also may promote malnutrition relapse, increasing the number of hospitalizations.[16] Mortality remains higher in HIV-positive children when compared with HIV-negative children despite adequate nutrition treatment. Further research to determine more effective treatment of severe acute malnutrition in HIV-positive children is warranted.[14–16]

In areas of high HIV prevalence, the nutritional status of HIV-negative children can also be affected. Their mothers or caretakers may be infected; they may be symptomatic, depressed and have difficulty in coping. The children who become orphans are less able to feed themselves.[15] Nutritional status often worsens as children mature because more attention is given to younger siblings. They often take on family responsibilities like caring for siblings and fetching water, which expends more energy in a setting of decreased meal frequency.[13]

EPIDEMIOLOGY

The onset of frank malnutrition frequently dates from the time that breast-feeding stopped and/or of a severe infection. If the infant is bottle-fed, onset is usually in the first 6 months of life, usually with wasting. Artificial milk including whole cow's milk is often over-diluted and infected. Otherwise, in breast-fed children, malnutrition usually presents in the 2nd and 3rd years. However, malnutrition may occur in the first 6–12 months of age associated with tuberculosis and HIV infection despite apparent adequate breast milk intake.

Geographical Distribution

Kwashiorkor is associated with areas where staples have a low protein : energy ratio, e.g. root crops and bananas or a maize diet (poor bioavailability of protein). These foods may also be deficient in micronutrients. Kwashiorkor is not common in fish-eating or cattle-herding communities if diets are supplemented by animal protein. Comparison between village children in Keneba, The Gambia and the Baganda area of southern Uganda showed distinct differences in nutrition, growth and endocrine response.[17] In The Gambia, where the predominant type of malnutrition is marasmus, the main staple is a low-energy millet gruel. In the Baganda area of Uganda, kwashiorkor is the predominant type of malnutrition, the major staple is bananas and their diet has a lower protein : energy ratio than that in The Gambia. However, the energy intake was inadequate in both communities.

There are reports of kwashiorkor in middle-class American infants without significant infection. The majority of cases are caused by severely restricted diets after parents' concern for adverse reaction to certain foods like milk.[18]

Season

In many parts of the world, there is an increased rate of malnutrition in the wet (or hungry) season. There is deficiency of food as the previous year's crop has been consumed and families may have to survive on a limited diet of fruits or vegetables, while awaiting the harvest. Admissions for malnutrition often increase following an epidemic of measles. During the rains there is an increase in some infections, e.g. diarrhoea and malaria. The roads are often inaccessible and this limits travel for medical care. Women are often busy working on the land and leave the younger children at home to be looked after and fed by siblings or relatives. They may only breastfeed at night or not at all.

AETIOLOGY OF KWASHIORKOR

The aetiology of hypoalbuminaemia and oedema in kwashiorkor has been debated since the 1930s when the theory of dietary protein deficiency was proposed by Cecily Williams who coined the name kwashiorkor. Kwashiorkor is the name given by the Ga people in Ghana for 'the disease of the child displaced from the breast'. Recent associations include excess free radical generation,[18a] deranged amino acid metabolism[19] and aflatoxin toxicity.[20,21,32,33] Essentially, in malnutrition there is adaptation to an inadequate diet by a reduction in metabolic activity, 'reductive adaption'. This adaptation is stressed and compromised by infection.

The cause of hypoalbuminaemia is multifactorial and includes: catabolism of albumin due to infection and stress, transient loss from capillary leak and in some cases from a damaged gut. Malnourished children appear to maintain their ability to synthetize albumin. In nutritionally vulnerable children, a fall in serum albumin and lipoprotein levels commonly occurs in response to infections. Tumour necrosis factor-α, interleukin (IL)-1 and IL-6 released from macrophages may depress albumin synthesis and divert amino acids to production of acute-phase reactants. Capillary leak is associated with increased levels of leukotrienes.[22]

Oedema occurs essentially due to retention of sodium and water. Capillary leak may also be a factor during the initial stages associated with inflammation and release of cytokines. However, the cause of sodium and water retention in hypoalbuminaemic states, e.g. oedematous malnutrition and the nephrotic syndrome, is still debated.[23–25]

In kwashiorkor, oedema may resolve during the initial stages of management on a low-protein diet (0.6 g/kg) before serum albumin levels rise. However, serum albumin may not reflect total vascular albumin mass or oncotic pressure. Factors involved in clearance of established oedema may include restoration of homeostasis with stabilization of intracellular metabolism and cellular membranes of the kidney and other cells and provision of energy and potassium.

Free Radicals and Amino Acid Deficiency

It is proposed that many of the features of kwashiorkor are caused by an imbalance between the production of free radicals (FR) and their safe disposal.[18a] Children with oedematous malnutrition tend to have lower levels of trace elements, e.g. zinc, copper or manganese required for formation of a major antioxidant, superoxide dismutase and selenium for glutathione peroxidase; also lower levels of other antioxidants including the vitamins β-carotene, E, C and riboflavin. Whether this is due to deficient intake (suggesting differential diets between kwashiorkor and marasmus), reduced binding capacity of serum proteins, maldistribution because of the metabolic disorder or increased loss, is not certain. Free iron can catalyse FR reactions and high levels of stored or free iron are detected in severe malnutrition.[26–28] Reduced glutathione (γ-glutamylcysteine glycine or GSH) and glutathione peroxidase are important intracellular compounds in protection against FR damage and low levels are considered to be a marker of FR activity. Lower erythrocyte levels of reduced GSH have been detected in kwashiorkor than marasmus and levels of thiobarbituric acid-reactive substances, a marker of lipid peroxidation, are raised in kwashiorkor. These findings suggest there is more FR activity in children with kwashiorkor than marasmus. However, some studies have shown an overlap in reduced glutathione and glutathione peroxidase levels between kwashiorkor and marasmus. In addition, there is a very slow restoration of reduced glutathione to normal levels despite a clinical response. Conversely, low glutathione levels could be partly due to dietary deficiency of sulphur-containing amino acids, e.g. methionine, which are low in kwashiorkor. Methionine is important for synthesis of cysteine. GSH is synthesized de novo from glycine, cysteine and glutamate. Methionine is also essential for functions of the Na^+/K^+/ATPase pump (sodium pump). Impaired sodium pump activity results in a large excess of intracellular sodium and a huge deficit in intracellular potassium. However, these intracellular electrolyte changes also occur in marasmus.[29,30]

Decreased rates of synthesis of GSH have been demonstrated in children with oedematous malnutrition compared with non-oedematous patients. Supplementation of oedematous children with N-acetylcysteine restored the synthesis rate of erythrocyte GSH and increased erythrocyte cysteine concentration.[30] This suggests that the low GSH levels in kwashiorkor may be, at least in part, due to limited availability of dietary essential amino acids and/or suppression of protein breakdown. However, a randomized placebo controlled trial of supplementation of 1–4-year-olds in Malawi over a 5-month period with antioxidant powder containing riboflavin, vitamin E, selenium and N-acetylcysteine (three times the recommended dietary requirement of each micronutrient), failed to prevent development of oedematous malnutrition.[30] Although excess FR activity may have a role in the demise of sick children with severe malnutrition, these studies suggest that there are other explanations for low GSH levels in kwashiorkor.

The difference in metabolism between children who develop oedematous and non-oedematous malnutrition (demonstrated in the recovered state) might support an interindividual genetic variation in susceptibility[31] but this would not explain the different geographical distribution of kwashiorkor and marasmus.

Aflatoxins

Aflatoxins are common contaminants of foods in tropical countries where the fungus *Aflatoxin flavus* thrives in the warm humid climate. Aflatoxins are commonly detected in urine of healthy adults and children in tropical countries and they have also been detected in cord blood and breast milk. Large doses administered to animals may be lethal and result in liver damage, profound metabolic disorders including hypoalbuminaemia and immunosuppression.

Studies in malnourished children in some (but not all) areas have demonstrated higher frequency and concentration of aflatoxins in blood of kwashiorkor than marasmus patients and aflatoxicol, a reversible derivative of aflatoxin B_1, has been detected in blood of kwashiorkor patients only. Studies of livers from children have demonstrated that aflatoxin detection is virtually confined to oedematous children. The above findings suggest there is a clear difference in liver metabolism of aflatoxins between kwashiorkor and marasmus. This is most likely due to liver dysfunction in kwashiorkor. However, in sick kwashiorkor children aflatoxin toxicity may be an additional aetiological factor in the metabolic disturbance.[32,33]

Growth Difference between Kwashiorkor and Marasmus Patients

Kwashiorkor patients tend to be taller, heavier (more fat) and have a larger head circumference and fewer delayed milestones than marasmic children. This may be due to the chronicity of disease, poorer socioeconomic background and, in some cases, low birth weight in marasmus (and some marasmic kwashiorkor). However, the better growth of children predisposed to develop kwashiorkor may be a factor in aetiology by increasing the demand for energy, protein and micronutrients, thus making them more vulnerable when infection and acute deficits of nutrients occur. Genetic factors may also be operative where the demand for nutrients may be higher in some children than others.

CLINICAL FEATURES

In marasmus the main findings are growth failure with severe wasting of muscle and fat (Figure 77.2). There may be hair changes in longstanding cases. In kwashiorkor there is oedema, hair changes, skin changes (not always) and often an enlarged liver. Kwashiorkor tends to have an acute onset (Figure 77.3). Marasmic kwashiorkor has similar features to kwashiorkor, but there is more wasting and they are also more stunted and often have a higher mortality rate. The main biochemical difference between marasmus and kwashiorkor is hypoalbuminaemia (present in kwashiorkor). The following signs should be looked for.[11,34,35]

Sepsis and Shock. Invasive bacteraemia and electrolyte imbalance are important causes of peripheral circulatory failure and death. Lethargy and impaired consciousness are common features. Though cardiac function is impaired there may be few clinical signs.

Anaemia. Anaemia is common but is not usually severe, e.g. mean Hb 8 g/dL. It is due to a mixed deficiency of micronutrients, e.g. iron, folic acid and riboflavin and general depression of metabolism. An acute fall in haemoglobin may follow malaria or other disease including those associated with worm infections, such as hookworm. It may also be due to inhibitors of iron absorption such as phytic acid in foods and use of elemental iron with poor bioavailability in many foods.

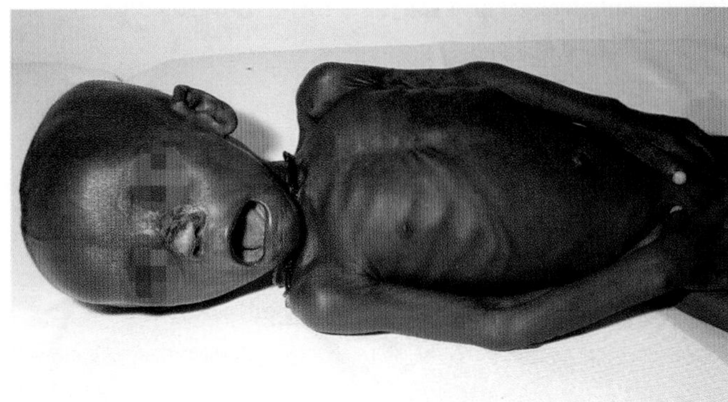

Figure 77.2 Child with marasmus (marked wasting, prominent ribs, increased axillary skin folds, 'old man' face). *(From Walton E and Allen S. Malnutrition in developing countries. Practice points. Paediatrics and Child Health, 2011–09–01, Volume 21, Issue 9, Pages 418–424. With permission from Elsevier. Copyright © 2011.)*

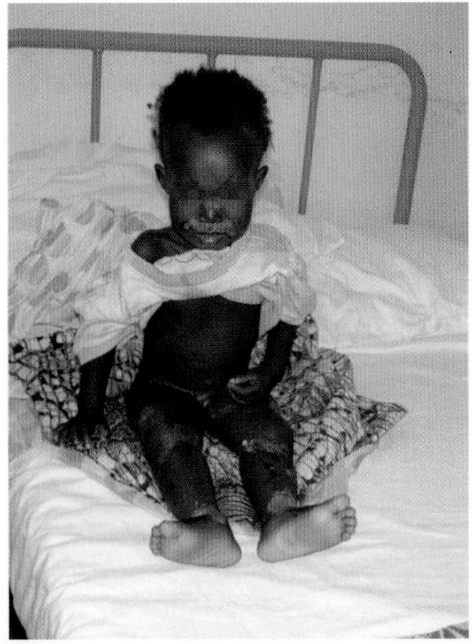

Figure 77.3 Child with kwashiorkor (lower limb oedema, sparse depigmented hair, dermatitis with areas of hypo- and hyperpigmentation, angular stomatitis). *(From Walton E. and Allen S. Malnutrition in developing countries Practice points. Paediatrics and Child Health, 2011–09–01, Volume 21, Issue 9, Pages 418–424. With permission from Elsevier. Copyright © 2011.)*

Oedema. Oedema may vary from slight in the feet and legs with some swelling of the cheeks (moon facies) to marked and generalized. It can be exacerbated by giving excess oral rehydration fluid. Ascites is rare. Severe ileus may give an impression of ascites.

Hair Changes. Hair changes, especially in colour, may antedate the florid appearance of malnutrition by some months. There may be dyspigmentation (change of colour to red or fair), sparseness (loss of hair), dry and thin hair fibres, loss of curls and easy-pluckability. The flag sign, alternating depigmented and normal hair, may be seen in children with long hair (not curly). Hair changes are common in longstanding malnutrition.

Eyes. The eyes may show pathological changes including conjunctivitis due to measles, herpes simplex, trachoma or bacterial infection. Xerophthalmia should be treated immediately.

Skin Changes. Skin changes may vary from slight dryness and cracking or mild 'speckled' hyperpigmentation to marked hyperpigmentation with generalized peeling, e.g. flaky paint dermatosis. Ulcers may develop in flexures and around the perineum. Purpura may occur. Peeling is usually only seen in those with oedema or with a history of oedema. There may be generalized loss of skin pigment or in areas where peeling has occurred, localized hypopigmentation. Consider HIV infection if there is severe ulceration and multiple infected areas.

Mucosal Changes. Mucosal changes include angular stomatitis, cheilosis and glossitis (smooth red tongue). Angular stomatitis is an important cause of anorexia. Oral thrush is common.

Liver. Liver size may vary from impalpable to grossly enlarged. It is more likely to be enlarged in those with oedema. In kwashiorkor, the liver is usually fatty (whether enlarged or not). Fatty change is considered to be due to reduced lipoprotein production and thus inability to transport lipids (triglycerides) from the liver. Fat clears spontaneously with rehabilitation and there is no residual liver damage. Serum bilirubin and transaminases are usually normal except in severe or lethal cases.

Lymphadenopathy. Lymphadenopathy is uncommon except in cases of local infection, e.g. tuberculosis or HIV infection. Other lymphoid tissues, e.g. tonsils, are also small.

Gut. There may be a chronic enteropathy, with variable degrees of villous atrophy due to infection, nutrient deficiency and possibly bacterial overgrowth. Protein loosing enteropathy may complicate measles and probably also other gut infections.

Brain. Mental changes vary from just irritability and lethargy to profound apathy (especially in kwashiorkor) or semi-consciousness. Reversible shrinkage of cerebral tissue has been demonstrated on brain imaging in kwashiorkor and less frequently in marasmus. Long-term effects are related to age of onset, longevity of malnutrition, poverty and lack of education and intellectual stimulation in the child's home environment.

TABLE 77.4 Criteria for in-Patient or Community-Based Therapeutic Care in Severe Acute Malnutrition

In-Patient Care for Complicated Cases	Out-Patient Care for Uncomplicated Cases
Generalized oedema *or* MUAC <115 mm + mild oedema *or* MUAC <115 mm or mild oedema *and one of the following*: Anorexia Temperature >38.5°C Severe dehydration Pneumonia Severe anaemia Drowsy, lethargic or clinically unwell	MUAC <115 mm *or* MUAC ≥115 mm + mild oedema *and* Alert Appetite present Clinically well

Adapted from Collins S, Dent N, Binns P, et al. Management of severe acute malnutrition in children. Lancet 2006;368:1992–2000.

MANAGEMENT OF ACUTE SEVERE MALNUTRITION

Community-based Therapeutic Care

An initial decision needs to be made regarding whether the child requires in-patient treatment or is suitable for community-based therapeutic care (CTC). CTC has recently been developed in a number of countries using ready-to-use therapeutic foods (RUTF).[1,31,36,37] Advantages of CTC include wide coverage, earlier presentation, reduced cost compared with in-patient care and a satisfactory outcome for most. Criteria for admission to in-patient care or an outpatient CTC programme depends on severity of oedema and/or presence of complications (Table 77.4). Recommendations for the management of severe acute malnutrition can be found in Table 77.5.[2,3]

RUTFs are based on F-100 catch up feeds with the addition of peanut butter (Table 77.6 and typical ingredients in RUTF, Table 77.7). They have a greater energy and nutrient density than F-75 initial formula feeds for malnutrition. RUTF are lipid-based pastes with a very low water activity and thus are resistant to bacterial contamination. They can be kept in silver foil packaging for several months unrefrigerated and can be consumed directly from the package without additional preparation.

Children attend out-patients weekly or fortnightly and in addition to RUTF (200 kcal/kg per day) receive a broad-spectrum oral antibiotic, vitamin A, folic acid, anthelmintics and if required antimalarials. Patients are discharged after a minimum of 2 months when clinically well, free of oedema, with sustained weight gain and MUAC >110 mm. RUTF are also appropriate for HIV-infected children either after discharge from in-patient care or primarily for care in the community. Weight gain is demonstrated in over 50% of HIV-infected patients.[37] RUTF are also useful for supplemental feeds for children with moderate malnutrition and appear to be more effective than corn-soya flour diets.[31]

Although RUTF are produced in low-resource countries their cost and distribution are important factors in the sustainability of CTC programmes. The role of RUTF in malnutrition prevention is controversial and warrants further investigation.[38]

In-patient Care

Two-thirds of deaths from acute severe malnutrition occur within the first week of admission. To reduce the mortality rate,

TABLE 77.5 Recommended Severe Acute Malnutrition Management[2,3]

Independent Additional Criteria	No Appetite	Appetite
	Medical Complications ↓	No Medical Complications ↓
Type of therapeutic feeding	Facility-based	Community-based
Intervention	F75 ® F100/RUTF and 24 hour medical care	RUTF, basic medical care
Discharge criteria (Transition criteria from facility to community-based care) ⟵	Reduced oedema Good appetite (with intake of at least 75% of calculated RUTF ration for the day)	15–20% weight gain

TABLE 77.6 F-100 Feed (in Bold) and Alternatives[a]

	Milk (g)	Sugar (g)	Vegetable Oil (g)	Electrolyte/Mineral mix (mL)	Water (mL)
Dried skimmed milk[b]	80	50	60	20	to 1000
Fresh cow's milk	880 (mL)	75	20	20	to 1000
Whole dried milk	110	50	30	20	to 1000

[a]If milk is unavailable a precooked corn-soya or wheat-soya blend (150 g) may be used with sugar (25 g), oil (40 g), electrolyte/mineral mix (20 mL) made up to 1000 mL water.
[b]Contains 2.9 g protein and 100 kcal/100 mL.

TABLE 77.7 Typical Recipe for RUTF[37]

Ingredient	% Weight
Full-fat milk	30
Sugar	28
Vegetable oil	15
Peanut butter	25
Mineral-vitamin mix	1.6

TABLE 77.8 Modified WHO Oral Rehydration Solution (ORS): (Low Sodium)

Water	2 L
WHO–ORS	1 packet
Sugar	50 g
Electrolyte/mineral solution[a]	40 mL

[a]If electrolyte/mineral solution is not available give additional potassium, 40 mmol/L.

special care has to be given during this period. The basic principle is, after initial resuscitation, to give high energy feeds with increased protein so that the child regains weight as rapidly as possible compatible with safety. Measles vaccination should be given to children >6 months of age who are not immunized or if the child is >9 months and has been immunized before 9 months. Delaying immunization should be done if the patient is in shock. Resuscitation of children with kwashiorkor is often more difficult than those with marasmus, but the principles described below are important regardless of etiology with exceptions as noted related to oedema.

Resuscitation (First 1–7 Days)

Intravenous therapy should be avoided unless there is evidence of severe dehydration or shock. Give modified WHO oral rehydration solution (ORS) (Table 77.8) over 4–10 h, 5 mL/kg every 30 min for 2 h, then 5–10 mL/kg hourly for 4–10 h. It has lower sodium than standard ORS and additional potassium and minerals. Great care must be taken to prevent overhydration. When hydrated (usually 4–6 h), commence Phase I with F-75 formula (Table 77.9), 130 mL/kg per day (100 mL/kg per day for oedematous children) as per the feeding regimen. If IV therapy is required, give Ringer lactate with 5% dextrose 15–20 mL/kg over 1 h, then 10 mL/kg per hour over the next 5 h or so. Whole blood may be required for septic shock not responding to above.

Also:

- *Diarrhoea* usually settles over 3–5 days. Lactose intolerance may be treated with yoghurt and/or a cereal/oil/sugar mix. In the rare situation where milk protein sensitivity is considered, alternative sources of protein include chicken, fish or soy protein. Give metronidazole if *Giardia lamblia* is detected or if treatment of anaerobic bacterial colonization of bowel is considered.
- *Hypothermia* (rectal temp <35.5°C): Use a low reading thermometer. Clothe child, including the head and keep in a warm room. Check for hypoglycaemia. Commence feeding as soon as possible.
- *Hypoglycaemia* (blood glucose <3 mmol/L): Use glucose test strip. If able to drink, give 50 mL of 10% glucose solution or sugared water (1 teaspoon sugar to 3½ tablespoons of water) followed by the first feed of F-75. If blood glucose remains low repeat glucose or sugar solution. If unconscious/convulsing, give 5 mL/kg 10% dextrose IV or if unable to have IV access, give 50 mL of 10% glucose by nasogastric tube.
- *Infection*: For mildly sick children showing no signs of infection, amoxicillin may be given for 5 days. For ill children, give ampicillin (50 mg/kg parenterally 6-hourly for at least 2–3 days), then oral amoxicillin (15 mg/kg 8-hourly for 5 days) + once daily gentamicin (7.5 mg/kg) for 7 days. If there is still a poor response by 48 h, add

TABLE 77.9 F-75 Feed (in Bold) and Alternatives[a]

	Milk (g)	Sugar[b] (g)	Vegetable Oil (g)	Electrolyte/Mineral mix (mL)	Water (mL)
Dried skimmed milk[c]	25	100	30	20	to 1000
Fresh cow's milk	300 (mL)	100	20	20	to 1000
Whole dried milk	35	100	20	20	to 1000

[a]If milk is unavailable a precooked corn-soya or wheat-soya blend (50 g) may be used with sugar (85 g), oil (25 g), electrolyte/mineral mix (20 mL) made up to 1000 mL water.
[b]A low osmolar feed can be prepared by replacing 30 g sugar with 35 g cereal/flour solution which is cooked for 4 min. It is useful for osmotic diarrhoea.
[c]Contains 0.9 g protein and 75 kcal/100 mL.

chloramphenicol or cefotaxime or a fluoroquinoline. Consider tuberculosis or HIV infection in children who fail to respond to nutritional rehabilitation.

- *Blood transfusion*: 10 mL/kg whole blood should be given over 3 h plus furosemide 1 mg/kg at commencement of transfusion, to anaemic children, i.e. Hb <4 g/dL or 4–6 g/dL in those who are very sick or have respiratory distress. If heart failure is suspected, give 10 mL/kg of packed cells.
- *Electrolytes and minerals*: Potassium 6–8 mmol/kg per day should be given for 1–2 weeks or so. When high-protein and -energy formula is given only 1–2 mmol potassium supplements are then required. An electrolyte/mineral solution containing potassium, magnesium, zinc and copper (Nutriset, France) should be added to modified ORS, F-75 and F100. If this solution is unavailable, give zinc 2 mg/kg per day and one intramuscular (IM) injection of 50% magnesium sulphate 0.3 mL/kg (max. 2 mL).
- *Vitamin A*: If vitamin A has not been given in the last month, give as capsules as per the doses listed in Table 77.10.[39] If unable to take orally, give 100 000 units (55 mg) IM (water miscible). Additional doses are required for measles and xerophthalmia.
- *Anti-malarials*: Administer in endemic areas as clinically indicated.
- *Intestinal parasites*: Mebendazole (500 mg, single dose or 100 mg twice a day for 3 days) may be indicated in children older than 12 months in areas where parasites such as hookworm and *Ascaris lumbricoides* are prevalent.

Rehabilitation

This is the phase of gradual increase in energy and protein intake until values such as 150–220 kcal/kg per day (normal requirement 100–110 kcal) and protein 4–6 g/kg per day (normal 1.5–2 g/kg per day) are reached. To supply this amount of energy and protein without increasing the volume of fluid to excessive amounts, energy-rich foods, such as vegetable oil and sugar are added to the energy/protein source, which is preferably milk-based (Tables 77.6 and 77.9).

Feeding Regimen (Phase I and II)

In Phase I, F-75 formula is given 2-hourly, including during the night. Unless the child is able to take all the milk by cup, it should be given wholly or partly by nasogastric tube. Frequency of feeds is increased to 3–4-hourly over the next week or so. Mothers should be taught to give milk by spoon/syringe. A gradual switch from Phase I to Phase II with F-100 should take approximately 3–4 days commencing after about 1 week. The volume of feed is gradually increased from 100 mL in Phase I, up to a maximum of around 200 mL/kg body weight in Phase II.

TABLE 77.10 Suggested Vitamin A Supplementation Scheme for Infants and Children 6–59 Months[39]

Age	Dose	Frequency
Infants 6–11 months	100 000 IU (30 mg RE)	Once
Children 12–59 months	200 000 IU (60 mg RE)	Every 4–6 months

As soon as the child wants food, they are offered a normal diet in addition to their full requirement of F-100. Mothers should continue breast-feeding preferably after the formula feed. For infants under 6 months, if breast milk is insufficient it can be supplemented by commercial infant formula or F-100 diluted with 1.5 L of water.

The mother should receive advice on infant feeding and health education and should be encouraged to participate as much as possible in the feeding of her child.

Additional Treatment

Folic acid 5 mg is started on day 1 and 1 mg daily is provided for 2–3 months. Iron-ferrous sulphate or gluconate 3 mg/kg per day are given for 3 months. Typical guidance is to start iron 2 weeks after admission when the child has regained an appetite and starts to gain weight. Multivitamin solution should also be administered. Extra vitamin K should be given if purpura or bleeding tendency is present.

Discharge

When the child has regained an appetite and ideally is over 90% weight for height, it is safe to discharge. However, this usually takes ≥4–6 weeks. In practice, when the appetite returns, there is weight gain (15–20% weight gain recommended), infection is controlled, oedema is resolving and guardians are able to cope, the child can be discharged to community-based care (see above). Emotional (as well as medical) support for the child is essential during rehabilitation, especially in children of socially disrupted families. Encourage the family to stimulate and play with their child.

PROGNOSIS

Case fatality rates may range from 5% to 50%, with a median of 20–30%. The highest mortality rates occur in oedematous malnutrition, especially marasmic kwashiorkor and also in HIV-infected children. The aim should be around 5–10% mortality. High mortality rates reflect both the severity of malnutrition on admission and the management and prevalence of HIV infection.

Mortality rates after discharge may be 10% or more. This depends on a number of factors, including the condition of the child on discharge, the level of education of the mother, her ability to afford the necessary additional foods and nutrients for catch-up growth and facilities for and compliance with follow-up.

The prevalence of micronutrient deficiencies in children may be decreased with micronutrient powders (MNP). A powdered form of iron and other micronutrients are packaged into single-dose sachets and can be sprinkled onto foods prepared in the home. In one formula of MNP, iron is encapsulated within a lipid layer to prevent changes to taste, colour or texture to the food when it is added.[40] MNP are an effective intervention for anaemia and iron deficiency in children and infants older than 6 months of age, but their effects on other micronutrient deficiencies have not been demonstrated yet.[41] In some situations there may be safety concerns about iron containing MNP. An association with malaria risk has been shown with iron supplements alone, and an association with bloody diarrhoea has been reported from Pakistan.[41a,b] Other than iron, the vitamins and minerals within MNP can vary. Micronutrient supplementation may reduce morbidity of certain diseases. A study in China studied the effects of three different combinations of micronutrient seasoning powder on infectious morbidity in preschool children. When compared to children receiving vitamin A alone and children receiving vitamin A plus iron, the children receiving vitamin A plus iron, thiamine, riboflavin, folic acid, niacinamide, zinc and calcium had decreased rates of diarrhoea and respiratory infectious disease.[42]

Malnutrition in Adults

The aetiology of malnutrition in adults is similar to children, although clinical manifestations may differ, e.g. effusions into serous cavities and ascites may be seen in adults.[6] The stresses that cause malnutrition may also differ, e.g. the necessity to continue manual work despite dietary inadequacy and/or infections; prison and concentration camps; famine, where adults may have to continue to use energy in obtaining food and caring for the young; psychiatric disorders and in postsurgical or secondary malnutrition. In areas where kwashiorkor in children is common and adults are subject to extreme dietary, physical and mental stress as in war, typical cases of kwashiorkor including skin changes are seen in adolescents and adults.

A considerable amount of research has been undertaken on famine oedema in adults occurring during the First and Second World Wars in Europe and in Japanese prisoner camps and famines in Asia and Africa. The main controversy concerned the importance of hypoalbuminaemia.[18a] When serum albumin levels are borderline, a dilute, salted vegetable diet may precipitate oedema, as may excess ORS in children with marasmus. Hypoalbuminaemia was less common in studies of oedematous subjects after the Second World War in Europe than in famine oedema in Asia and Africa. This may have been due to more prolonged dietary protein and micronutrient deficiency in the latter. Other causes of oedema in adults include dropsy caused by consumption of contaminated cottonseed or mustard oil and beriberi.

IODINE DEFICIENCY DISORDERS

The term iodine deficiency disorders (IDD) replaces the terms 'endemic goitre' and 'cretinism' and emphasizes the wider spectrum of disorders which occurs as a result of iodine deficiency or the effect of goitrogens. The disorders include, apart from cretinism and varying degrees of brain damage, goitre and hypothyroidism in neonates, children and adults.

Epidemiology

Low iodine intake is related to lack of iodine in the environment. Areas of iodine deficiency are usually those far away from the sea, where iodine originally present in soil was leached by high rainfall and snow. The amount of iodine returned to the soil by rainwater is small and, as a result, many areas have insufficient iodine in the environment. It is estimated that globally 2.2 billion people live in areas with iodine deficiency and that this is the single most common cause of preventable mental retardation and brain damage in the world.[43] In the tropics it is found in Africa, Central and South America and in Asia and Papua New Guinea. Those exhibiting goitre are estimated at between 200 and 300 million. Goitre becomes endemic when the total goitre rate is ≥10% or the visible goitre rate is ≥1%.

Goitre is a problem in the Atlas Mountains, Nile Valley, highland areas of Kenya, Tanzania, Rwanda, Burundi, Cameroon and The Gambia. Central Africa contains some of the most severely affected populations in the world. Goitrogens in the diet, which interfere with thyroid metabolism, can be an important contributory cause, in particular thiocyanates which are found in the widely used tuber cassava (maniac). In Central and South America, IDD occurs widely. Ecuador, Peru and Bolivia are particularly affected. The most affected populations in Asia are China, India, Indonesia, Nepal, Myanmar and Bangladesh.

Aetiology

Inadequate intake of iodine leads to reduced production of thyroid hormone and stimulation of thyroid-stimulating hormone (TSH) production. TSH increases thyroid hormone production resulting in the thyroid gland becoming hyperplastic and goitrous. The cause of endemic goitre is a failure of the thyroid gland to obtain adequate iodine to maintain its natural structure and function. Apart from iodine deficiency, other factors also influence iodine balance. Thiocyanate, a metabolic product of several factors, competitively inhibits active transport and is goitrogenic. Dietary goitrogens are found in cassava, lime beans, sweet potatoes, cabbage and broccoli and certain types of millets. Cassava has been implicated as an important contributing factor in Zaire. Goitrogenic factors seem to be superimposed on primary iodine deficiency.

Pathology

In the later chronic stages when iodine stores are exhausted, the thyroid gland becomes soft and enlarged (goitre) with a large number of colloid follicles. Nodular formation takes place and haemorrhage and calcification may occur. The gland does not become 'toxic' and malignancy does not occur.

The term 'endemic cretinism' refers to a combination of mental deficiency, deaf mutism and motor rigidity or, less commonly, to severe hypothyroidism. The two forms are often referred to as neurological cretinism and hypothyroid cretinism and can occur separately or together. They should be distinguished from 'sporadic cretinism' which results from congenital hypothyroidism and occurs worldwide. Endemic cretinism is associated with iodine deficiency that is sufficiently severe to cause goitre in 3% or more of the population, reaching 5–10% in areas with severe iodine deficiency. It appears that severe deficiency may be responsible for the impaired neurological development of the fetus from early in pregnancy.[44]

Clinical Features

Goitre. Large goitres are easily recognized. Sizes are classified as shown below.[45] Tracheal pressure may interfere with the recurrent laryngeal nerve and produce hoarseness. Choking may occur with monstrous goitres. The patient is almost always euthyroid.

Classification of goitre:
0 – No goitre
IA – Goitre detectable only by palpation
IB – Goitre palpable and visible when neck fully extended. Includes nodular glands if not goitrous
II – Goitre visible with neck in normal position
III – Very large goitre recognizable from a distance.

Endemic Cretinism. This includes severe mental deficiency and there is a characteristic facies. Neurological cretinism includes defects of hearing, speech, squint and spastic dysplasia of varying degrees. Myxoedematous cretinism includes the predominant feature of profound hypothyroidism and short stature. Neuromotor deficits are less profound than in the neurological cretin and hearing is preserved.

Reproductive Failure. There is higher risk of abortions, miscarriages, stillbirths, low birth weight and increased perinatal and infant mortality.

Diagnosis. Measurement of iodine in the urine is the most precise index of dietary iodine intake. Mild IDD occurs with iodine excretion ranging from 50–100 mg daily and in severe IDD the excretion is below 20 mg daily. In endemic goitre, serum T_4 levels are often low with a normal or slightly elevated serum T_3 and an increased TSH. In some countries newborns are screened for blood thyroxine and if low levels are identified immediate thyroxine replacement therapy is required.

Treatment. Cretinism with its associated mental deficiency cannot be reversed through treatment. For the myxoedematous type thyroxine and iodine supplementation reduce the effects of hypothyroidism. Goitres in older children and adults may disappear completely following iodine administration. Beneficial results will be observed in 4–6 weeks. Advanced goitres must be treated surgically if causing symptoms.

Prevention. Fortification of salt for human and animal consumption is the method of choice for the prevention of IDD. In Africa, virtually all edible salt is iodized in several countries. The level of iodine in salt must be enough to meet the minimum daily iodine requirement of 150 mg per person. Iodination of irrigation water has also been used in China.[46] Iodinized oil (lipiodol) is the major alternative and is the best option for severely afflicted areas. It is administrated by intramuscular injection or the oral route. The recommended dose is 480 mg iodine (1 mL) for subjects 1 year or older and 240 mg iodine in infants. This is effective for at least 1–2 years.[47] Priority should be given to improving the iodine status of adolescent girls and young women before they begin pregnancy.

Scurvy. The disease is due to lack of vitamin C, which is essential for collagen formation.

Epidemiology. Scurvy does not commonly affect any population as it did in the past and therefore may be overlooked. Frank scurvy is uncommon and is most likely to occur in tropical areas where fresh fruit and vegetables are sparse. Babies are especially vulnerable when they are fed on dried cereals and boiled milk. Soldiers, prisoners and refugees in camps in dry desert areas are particularly vulnerable[48] and it can occur in epidemics in non-refugee populations. The possibility of widespread subclinical deficiency in these areas cannot be ruled out. A form of scurvy has been extensively studied in South Africa among Bantu male labourers who developed haemochromatosis attributed to drinking large quantities of beer. It was thought that vitamin C in the body was irreversibly oxidized by large deposits of ferric iron in tissues.[49]

Pathology. Vitamin C is required for the formation of fibrous collagen in connective tissue and bone. This leads to extravasation of blood, loosening of teeth and easily fractured bones with subperiosteal haemorrhage. Autopsy shows extensive haemorrhage in internal organs.

Clinical Features

Infantile Scurvy. The majority of cases present in the second half of the first year, especially in premature and artificially fed infants. The three main features are: irritability, leg tenderness and pseudoparalysis. The baby lies in a characteristic position with legs partially flexed at the knees and hips and internally rotated due to pain from subperiosteal haemorrhages. This may be mistaken for rheumatic fever, polio or osteomyelitis because of pain. These extravasations may be palpable at the proximal end of the tibia and distal end of the femur. Costochondral beading (scorbutic rosary) is also usually palpable. The arms are rarely involved. There may be bleeding around erupting teeth and gingival lesions. Bleeding into the skin is rarely a presenting sign. Hypochromic microcytic anaemia is commonly present. The anaemia may be megaloblastic due to accompanying folate deficiency resulting from lack of folate coenzymes associated with vitamin C. *Pyrexia* is frequent with associated infections, especially tuberculosis. The combination of gingival lesions, pseudoparalysis and irritability strongly suggests a diagnosis of scurvy.

Adult Scurvy. There is an insidious onset with weight loss, progressive weakness and aching in bones, joints and muscles especially at night and characteristic stiffness in the leg muscles or other muscles in extensive use. Haematomas form in calf and thigh muscles. Perifollicular haemorrhages occur with subcutaneous petechiae on the limbs and trunk producing scorbutic purpura. Haemorrhage into the myocardium may be life-threatening. Splinter haemorrhages may form a crescent on the fingernails. In extreme deficiency the gums become affected with swelling and sponginess of the alveolar margin, which is friable and bleeds readily. Secondary infection, gangrene and loose teeth supervene. Wounds fail to heal and scars break down.

Diagnosis. The main differential diagnosis is from rickets which may coexist as 'scurvy rickets'. Radiography reveals a characteristic ground-glass appearance due to generalized osteoporosis and atrophy of the trabeculae. Epiphyseal ends are sharply outlined. Widening of the zone of provisional calcification causes a dense shadow at the end of the shaft (the white line of Frankel) and this is also seen at the periphery of ossification centres ('halo epiphysis' or pencilled effect). With treatment, even the grossest deformities resolve. The capillary permeability test of Hess using a sphygmomanometer to occlude venous return to the arm results in petechiae appearing. Laboratory tests on plasma or leucocyte levels of ascorbic acid are sensitive, although plasma levels are influenced by recent dietary intake.

Treatment. In infant scurvy ascorbic acid (50 mg four times daily) should be given for 1 week, followed by 50 mg twice daily for 1 month. In the adult, the usual dose is 100 mg administered three to five times daily until 4 g has been administered. If the patient is critically ill, 1 g can be given daily by intravenous infusion. Vitamin C may also be given as fresh daily orange juice. Severe weakness and bleeding rapidly resolve (48 h) and haematomas heal within 2 weeks. Radiological evidence may persist for years.

Prevention. Foods steamed and cooked rapidly retain much of their vitamin C which is destroyed by prolonged cooking. Artificially fed infants require supplements (e.g. fresh orange juice).

RICKETS AND OSTEOMALACIA

Nutritional rickets is still a major problem in many developing countries and is common in North Africa and the Middle East. The terms 'rickets' and 'osteomalacia' refer to the histological and radiological abnormalities seen in a variety of under-mineralization conditions although they are not identical to osteoporosis. Rickets is only present in children and adolescents whereas osteomalacia is generally seen in adults.

Aetiology

Vitamin D deficiency results from inadequate dietary intake and/or cutaneous biosynthesis of vitamin D. Rickets describes the disordered growth and mineralization of the growth plate of the long bones. Osteomalacia describes abnormalities resulting from delayed and reduced mineralization of mature bone. Calcium deficiency has been implicated as a cause of rickets in African children who often have adequate vitamin D status. After weaning, the staple food of many young African children is maize porridge, which has low calcium and high fibre content. The fibre content, as well as the phytate content of many of the foods used as weaning foods may inhibit calcium absorption, although this has not been clearly demonstrated. It is much more likely that the overall low calcium intake, combined with genetic factors and low vitamin D status leads to an inadequate absorption of calcium in most African children.

Epidemiology

In the tropics, rickets may occur where sunlight is reduced by urban high-rise buildings and in crowded areas of cities where there are few play areas. It is sometimes described in higher socioeconomic groups because these mothers tend to keep their babies indoors and may be likely to continue to breast-feed without vitamin D supplementation into the second year of life. Other factors are weaning diets with inadequate vitamin D supplementation, high phytate diets and low birth weight. Mothers with low sunshine exposure, vegetarians, dark-skinned mothers, cultural habits which limit the amount of skin exposed to sunshine.[50]

Of note is that usually human milk is a very limited source of vitamin D, providing <20% of the daily requirement of about 400 IU/day (10 μg/day). Human milk may have higher vitamin D levels when maternal supplementation is done with >6000 IU/day of vitamin D, but there is little evidence specific to this approach in developing countries.[51]

Pathology

Defective calcification of developing long bones results in slowing of calcium and phosphorus precipitation in the newly formed matrix. A mass of uncalcified osteoid tissue causes enlargement of the growing ends of bone and a softening of all bones in both rickets and osteomalacia.

Clinical Features

Rickets. The onset during the first 2 years of life is later than that in scurvy. The child becomes ill, pale, flabby and irritable and prone to tetany and laryngeal stridor. There is general physical and mental retardation and deformity of ribs ('rachitic rosary'), spine, pelvis and limbs (widening of wrists and ankles) and short stature (Figure 77.4). Craniotabes occurs due to thinning of the outer table of the skull. The muscles are poorly developed and lack tone. In calcium-deficient rickets neither muscle hypotonia nor bone pain are features and cases tend to be older (4–16 years of age). As the child grows, the skeletal changes heal, but marked deformities remain, such as pigeon chest, spinal curvature, knock-knees and bow legs (Figure 77.5). Clinical rickets is less common in malnourished children, probably because they have less demand for calcium and phosphorus due to slow growth.

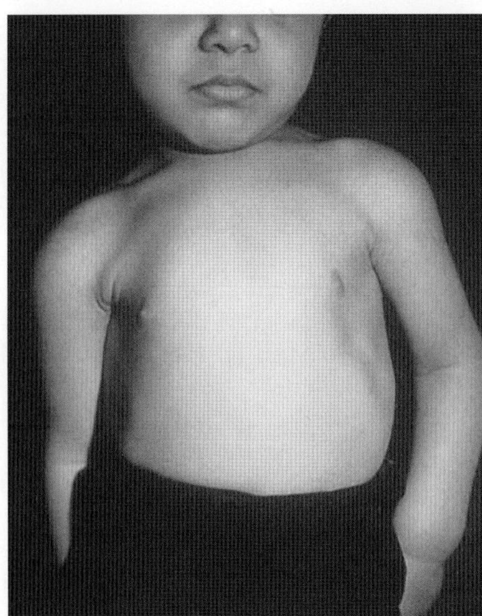

Figure 77.4 Rachitic rosary and chest deformity in a 2-year-old child.

Osteomalacia. This occurs in women of child-bearing age, usually in their first pregnancy. The bones of the pelvic girdle, ribs and femora become soft, painful and deformed. The gait is

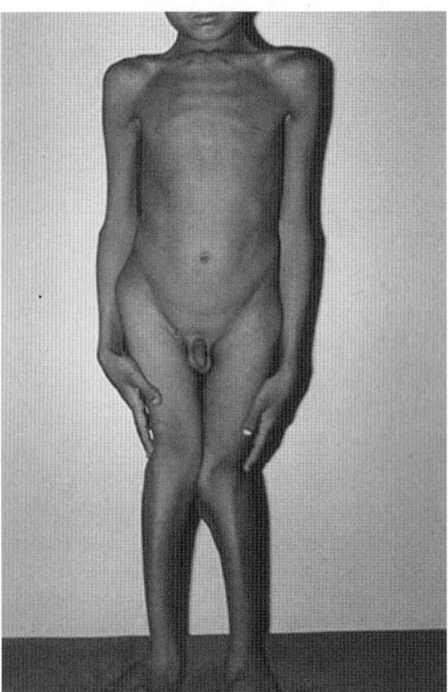

Figure 77.5 Stunting and limb deformity in a boy with rickets from northern Pakistan.

characteristic. Tetany is common, anaemia is present and spontaneous fracture(s) occur. Fetal bones do not generally show signs of rickets as calcium is transported across the placenta independent of vitamin D.

Complications

Rickets may have severe consequences. It is strongly associated with pneumonia in young children in developing countries.[52] The relative risk of death for the children with rickets compared with those without is one in seven. Bony deformity of the pelvis in women leads to obstructed labour and increased perinatal morbidity and mortality rates.

Diagnosis

The distinction from infantile scurvy may be difficult, but rickets usually occurs in infants over 6 months of age and there are no subperiosteal haemorrhages; other possibilities are congenital syphilis, achondroplasia and osteogenesis imperfecta. Radiographs show characteristic epiphyseal changes (cupping, fraying and decreased density; Figure 77.6). Early in vitamin D deficiency, the following values are typically seen: a normal fasting serum calcium; low-normal to low phosphorus; low 25(OH)D; elevated levels of alkaline phosphatase.

A challenging clinical issue is the level of 25(OH)D that may be associated with rickets. An evidence-based review as well as other clinical studies have not been able to clearly identify such a level and it remains controversial. In general, it is likely that the risk of rickets is increased with 25(OH)D levels <25 nmol/L, but many infants below this level do not develop rickets if calcium intake is adequate and many cases of rickets, especially in children with low calcium intake are associated with much higher levels of 25(OH)D.[51,52]

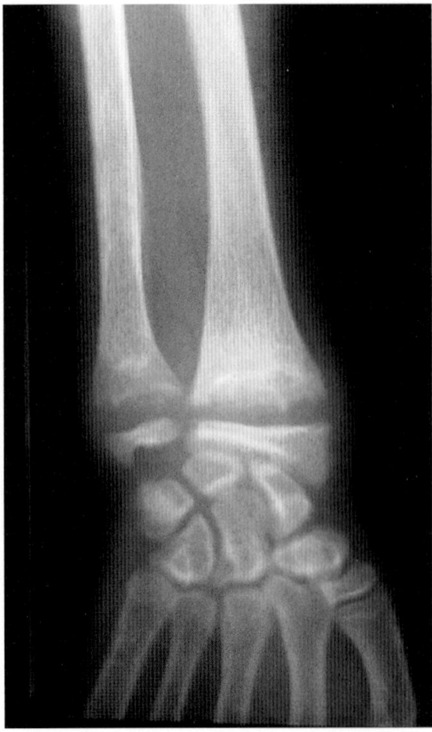

Figure 77.6 Radiological changes of rickets showing fraying, cupping and decreased density.

Treatment

Guidelines for the evaluation and therapy of nutritional rickets have been published.[53] Therapy is primarily based on providing an adequate calcium and vitamin D intake. The guidelines suggest providing 20 μg (800 IU) per day for 3–4 months. Many will choose to use higher doses of 1000–10 000 IU/day for 8–12 weeks depending on the age of the child. In teenagers and adults, 50 000 IU/weekly of vitamin D can also be provided. Calcium is often given at 30–75 mg/kg elemental calcium split over several doses each day.

Whether vitamin D2 or vitamin D3 should be the preferred form of vitamin D that is used, as well as whether so-called 'stoss therapy' in which over 100 000 IU of vitamin D are given at one time or similar extremely high doses are given, is controversial. In general, it is recommended for most situations to try to provide vitamin D3 when available, and not to use stoss therapy if daily or weekly moderate dose therapy as described above is likely to have high compliance. If compliance may be poor, then stoss therapy may be considered.

VITAMIN B1 DEFICIENCY (BERIBERI)

Epidemiology

Until recently, beriberi was common in many tropical and subtropical areas and was endemic in countries of Asia and the Far East, where highly milled rice was the staple cereal. It was the scourge of plantations in Malaysia, China and Indonesia and caused enormous mortality and morbidity rates. Outbreaks have occurred in ships' crews, mining communities, institutions, such as mental homes and among prisoners of war in the Far East. Endemic beriberi can show a seasonal pattern with increasing incidence in the pre-harvest farming months, possibly related to physical exertion at this time. Incidence has decreased with improved eating habits, but the reappearance of thiamin deficiency has been reported in Japan, The Gambia and South Africa. It remains endemic in Thailand, China, Myanmar, Laos and Vietnam.[54] Cases of infantile beriberi have been frequently seen in refugee camps in Thailand. Antihistamine factors in the diet of breast-feeding mothers (e.g. freshwater fish) can increase the risk of infantile beriberi.

Aetiology

Thiamin is present in the tissues in the phosphorylated form and a continuous supply is required to satisfy the body's relatively high turnover rate as little is stored. It acts as a co-enzyme for carbohydrate metabolism in the Krebs citric acid cycle and exerts a role in the oxidative breakdown of pyruvic acid. Since the brain nervous tissue and heart muscle use large amounts of glucose, it is in these tissues that carbohydrate metabolism is especially deranged in thiamin deficiency. Thiamin is also involved in acetylcholine synthesis and in neurotransmission. Lactic acid accumulates with breakdown of the Krebs cycle, producing a metabolic acidosis.

The germ and bran portions of cereal grains contain the most thiamin. Highly milled rice is particularly low in thiamin (60 mg/100 g), although parboiling, prior to milling, retains much of the thiamin. The discovery that milling of rice was an aetiological factor was of great value in the prevention of beriberi. However, any factor leading to an increased thiamin demand may be aetiological. For example, young men are often affected possibly because they work hardest. Onset may be associated with fever, infections including dysentery and HIV infection; other factors such as pregnancy, lactation and rapid growth may exacerbate sub-clinical deficiency. Thiamin levels in the milk secreted by thiamin-depleted mothers will be inadequate to prevent beriberi in the suckling infant. Anti-thiamin factors (thiaminases) occurring in foods can alter thiamin structure and reduce biological activity. Thiaminases are found in raw freshwater fish and shellfish, in several microorganisms and in some vegetables, plants and tea.

True alcoholic beriberi is a form of oedematous cardiac disease with high output failure in severe alcoholics. It has been described as 'palm-wine tappers heart' in Gambia, as palm tappers work strenuously climbing trees and consume substantial quantities of fermenting sap. Drug-induced beriberi has been reported from the use of nitrofurazone (which interferes with pyruvate metabolism) in the treatment of trypanosomiasis.

Pathology

The pathological anatomy of beriberi involves changes in the nervous system, the heart and muscle fibres. Microscopically, the nerve trunks show changes ranging from slight medullary degeneration to complete neural destruction (Wallerian degeneration). In Wernicke's encephalopathy, foci of congestion and haemorrhage are scattered symmetrically in the grey matter of the brain stem, mamillary bodies and hypothalamic regions. There are also numerous perivascular haemorrhages and widespread degenerative brain changes.

In the heart, there is fatty degeneration of varying severity and loss of contractility due to water retention. The essential features of 'beriberi heart' are: a hyperkinetic circulation, peripheral vasodilation, right side enlargement and high output failure. The cause of the hyperkinetic circulation deficiency is low peripheral arterial resistance from vasodilation due to loss of muscular arteriolar tone. Post-mortem appearances are those of severe right heart failure.

Clinical Features

Beriberi assumes various clinical forms but can be grouped into five major types:[55]

1. Subacute cardiac (wet beriberi)
2. Acute fulminant
3. Neurological (dry beriberi)
4. Infantile
5. Wernicke's encephalopathy.

The two main forms, dry and wet beriberi, constitute the same disease and a mixture of the two forms is usual. The onset is insidious, but may be acute with death within hours without nervous system symptoms occurring.

Subacute Cardiac Beriberi. Symptoms include anorexia, fatigue, irritability, depression and abdominal discomfort. These may be associated with fever. Cardiovascular features are prominent with warm extremities, tachycardia, palpitations and breathlessness. Oedema may occur at the end of a working day and calf muscles have a sensation of fullness.

Acute Fulminant Beriberi. When heart failure appears, the hands may be cold. Blood pressure is low with a high pulse pressure producing a 'pistol shot' sound over larger arteries. There is cardiomegaly with right- and left-sided enlargement and a loud pansystolic murmur is audible over the pericardium

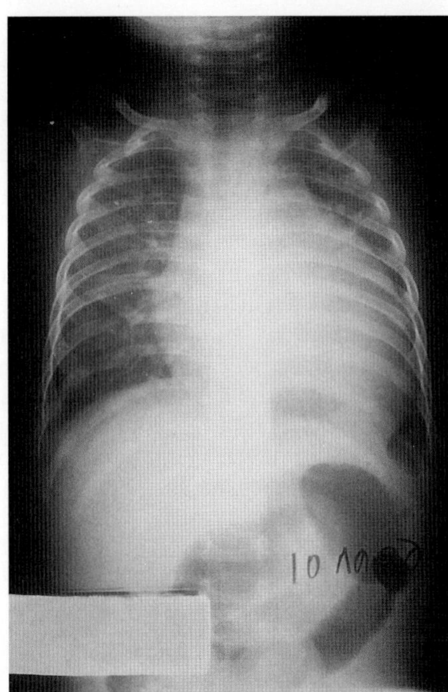

Figure 77.7 Chest radiograph showing cardiomegaly in an infant from Thailand.

(Figure 77.7). Atrial enlargement may cause paralysis of the recurrent laryngeal nerve. The liver is enlarged and tender. Pericardial effusion is unusual unless it is late-stage disease. Hydrothorax and ascites are frequent. The ECG shows inversion of T waves, a decreased P-R and increased Q-T interval, which rapidly revert to normal with treatment. Sudden cardiac failure is common. Death occurs from right heart failure and the patient usually dies fully conscious.

Neurological Beriberi. The clinical features are those of a peripheral neuropathy of mixed motor and sensory type. There is peripheral neuritis with tingling, burning and paraesthesias of the feet. Glove and stocking anaesthesia may spread from the feet to the thighs or from the tips of the fingers. There is loss of vibration sense and tenderness and cramping of the leg muscles. The gait becomes ataxic due to loss of postural sensation. The cranial nerves are not involved, although ptosis of the eyelids may occur. Motor signs include: flaccid weakness and wasting with foot, toe and wrist drop, difficulty in standing from the squatting position and loss of tendon reflexes and deep sensation. Paralytic symptoms are more common in adults than children.

Infantile Beriberi. This occurs in breast-fed infants of thiamin-deficient mothers, especially in those babies receiving a high-carbohydrate diet. Nearly all cases have infections before developing the symptoms of thiamin deficiency. These include pneumonia, diarrhoea, upper respiratory infections and cellulitis. The cases can be classified into three groups as: the cardiac form, the aphonic form and the pseudomeningitic form. It is not unusual to find features of two or three forms together. Characteristically, the cardiac form has its onset during the second or third month of life. The symptoms are dyspnoea, fever, cyanosis, vomiting and irritability with convulsions. The cardiorespiratory phase is most dramatic with rapid onset and physical examination reveals tachycardia, hepatomegaly and peripheral circulatory failure (Figure 77.7). Cardiac arrest may occur in a significant number of cases and infants may expire on the way to hospital. The overall mortality rate is between 5% and 20%. Blood chemistry shows metabolic acidosis. Survivors respond to parenteral thiamin within 24–48 h. The aphonic form occurs in slightly older infants (4–6 months). There is anorexia, weight loss and constipation. Left recurrent laryngeal nerve involvement from left atrial pressure gives rise to a characteristic cry (crying but no sound is heard). This may last a few days before restlessness, oedema and dyspnoea develop. The pseudomeningeal form occurs in older infants (6–12 months). There is vomiting and irritability. The infant develops nystagmus, a bulging fontanelle, twitching of muscles and convulsions followed by unconsciousness. The illness resembles meningitis or encephalitis but the CSF is normal.

WERNICKE'S ENCEPHALOPATHY

This is characterized by cerebellar degeneration, peripheral and optic neuropathy and is caused primarily by thiamin deficiency in alcoholics by causing reduced absorption of the vitamin from the gastrointestinal tract. Outbreaks of this disease, unrelated to alcohol, occurred in the Far East during the Second World War. Diagnosis was established at autopsy by demonstration of mamillary body haemorrhages. Recent surveys suggest that the disease may have a prevalence of about 3% in all chronic alcoholics. Predisposing factors include diarrhoeal infections, sepsis and malaria. Clinical features of this syndrome include paralysis of one or more eye muscles, horizontal nystagmus, a wide gait, clouding of consciousness, insomnia, disorientation and semi-coma. Brain stem damage is associated with haemorrhage and necrosis and myelosis. Retinal haemorrhages occur. Wernicke's encephalopathy may be reversed with injection of thiamin, but the accompanying psychosis (Korsakoff's) is irreversible.

Laboratory Diagnosis

The erythrocytes are among the first tissues affected in thiamin deficiency. The erythrocyte transketolase can be stimulated by TPP (thiamin pyrophosphate) and values >20% are found in deficient subjects. Urinary excretion of thiamin is low in subjects with thiamin deficiency but is not highly sensitive. The pyruvic acid concentration in blood is raised in acute beriberi and falls after thiamin administration.

Differential Diagnosis

Wet beriberi must be distinguished from other causes of right heart failure with high output, e.g. severe anaemia and hookworm disease. Dry beriberi must be distinguished from other causes of flaccid paralysis and neuropathy: alcoholic, tabes dorsalis, chronic arsenic and lead poisoning, lathyrism, triorthocresyl phosphate paralysis in which there is a pure motor flaccid paralysis and nutritional neuropathies, e.g. vitamin B_{12} deficiency.

Treatment

In acute beriberi, patients may die without treatment. There is usually a dramatic improvement within hours of receiving parenteral thiamin (50 mg). In adult beriberi oral treatment with 50 mg thiamin given three times daily should continue for some days followed by oral supplements of 10 mg/day for several weeks. In infants, 25 mg of thiamin should be given intravenously and a further 25 mg intramuscularly once or twice daily until symptoms have improved when oral supplements (10 mg) can be given daily. Breast-feeding mothers should also be treated with 50 mg daily for several days.

Prevention

Health education and improved milling methods in which the germ is retained have reduced incidence in some Middle Eastern countries. Hand pounding of rice would improve thiamin content, but this traditional practice is unpopular and many rice eaters have strong preferences for particular types of milled rice. A maternal diet containing adequate thiamin prevents deficiency in breast-fed infants. Thiamin requirements increase with a high carbohydrate diet. General dietary improvement may increase intake, but this is not easy to achieve in poor developing countries. Mixed diets with other sources of thiamin are important, e.g. with pulses, groundnuts, whole wheat, vegetables and fruits.

PELLAGRA

Pellagra is a nutritional disease caused by the combined deficiency of the vitamin niacin and the essential amino acid tryptophan.

Epidemiology

While pellagra has vanished from most parts of the world where it was formerly present, it continues to be a problem in southern and central Africa. Recent reports of outbreaks in refugee camps and following civil strife[56] highlight that its presence often follows social disturbances with the establishment of large camps.

Aetiology

The spread of pellagra largely followed the introduction of maize as a dietary staple. The reason maize predisposes to pellagra is that the proteins of maize are poor in tryptophan required for nicotinic acid (niacin) synthesis. Pellagra has never been a problem in Central America, the original home of maize, because in preparation, rather than milling, maize is soaked in lime water which hydrolyses nicotinoylesters releasing nicotinic acid. It is likely that other factors play a role: marginal intakes of other vitamins (B_2 and B_6) required for endogenous synthesis of nicotinamide from tryptophan; prolonged exposure to mycotoxins which can deplete the body of nicotinamide; dietary excess of leucine causing an amino acid intolerance; and the impairment of tryptophan metabolism by oestrogens and progesterone which may be sufficient to precipitate pellagra more commonly in women than men. Pellagra may occur due to malabsorption, inborn errors of metabolism, following prolonged isoniazid treatment for tuberculosis (due to inhibition of kynureninase) and with faddist diets. It may follow intestinal surgery and be associated with gastrointestinal pathology, e.g. oesophageal stricture, carcinoma of the colon or stomach, Crohn's disease, chronic amoebiasis and tropical sprue. Alcoholic pellagra may complicate gastritis.[56]

Pathology

The epidermis becomes hyperkeratotic and later becomes atrophic and these changes are also present in the tongue, vagina and mucous membranes. The colonic mucous membrane is inflamed and pseudomembranes form; later, the mucosa atrophies. The viscera show fatty degeneration and a characteristic deep pigmentation. Haemorrhages may occur in the renal medulla. Nervous system changes occur late. Demyelination in the spinal cord may involve the posterior and lateral columns. Myelin degeneration in the peripheral nerves is common. Increased intracellular pigment is present in frontal lobes and basal ganglia.[57]

Clinical Features

The main features comprise the triad: 'diarrhoea, dermatitis and dementia'. Since it is also fatal, a fourth 'D' is death. The classic symptoms are usually less well developed in infants and children.

Pre-Pellagrin State. The early symptoms are vague: anorexia, lassitude, joint pains, dizziness and burning sensations which recur periodically for years. The complexion is 'muddy' with bluish leaden-coloured sclerae. The personality changes with irritability and character changes. There may be associated vitamin deficiencies and many people in endemic areas suffer from chronic poor health. In children with parasites or chronic disorders manifestations may be severe.

Dermatitis. The cause of the photosensitive dermatitis in pellagra is unknown, but it may relate to low histidine levels in skin. This amino acid may absorb ultraviolet light and minimize skin damage from sunlight. Dermatological lesions appear on sites exposed to sun and/or pressure. An erythema initially occurs which may develop suddenly or insidiously; it is symmetric and can resemble sunburn. Mild cases may escape recognition. The lesions are usually sharply demarcated and are often on the neck (Casal's necklace), backs of the hands and feet (pellagrin glove or boot) (Figure 77.8) and sometimes on the scrotum, female genitalia or anus. The affected area is swollen, pruritic with burning sensations which become acute on exposure to the sun. Petechia, bullae and vesicles (wet type) may develop. The skin then becomes dry, rough, thickened, cracked with scaling, a shiny surface and brown pigmentation. Erythema becomes blackish (or purplish) on black skin and is sepia in olive-skinned races. Hyperkeratosis may affect the malar or supraorbital regions and can involve the whole body. The cutaneous lesions are sometimes preceded by stomatitis, glossitis, vomiting or diarrhoea. Swelling of the tongue may be followed by intense redness, ulceration, fissuring with atrophy of lingual papillae.

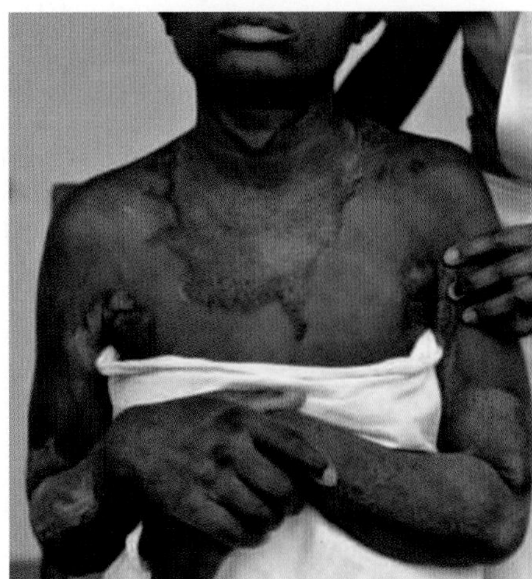

Figure 77.8 Characteristic skin lesions of pellagra on hands and lesions on the neck (Casal necklace). *(Courtesy of Dr. J.D. MacLean, McGill Centre for Tropical Diseases, Montreal, Canada, From Kleigman R., et al., Nelson Textbook of Pediatrics , Nineteenth Edition, Chapter 46, 191–198.e1. With permission from Elsevier. Copyright © 2011.)*

Diarrhoea. Diarrhoea is common in pellagrins, but is not a constant feature and in some cases there may be constipation. The cause is probably related to atrophy of intestinal mucosa. A characteristic symptom is pyrosis – a burning sensation in the oesophagus causing dysphagia. The stools are often pale, resembling those of tropical sprue.

Dementia. The psychiatric disturbances range from mild hallucinations with psychomotor retardation, insomnia, through confusion, to severe dementia, anxiety psychosis, intermittent stupor and possibly epileptiform convulsions and catatonia. Confusion and acute mania may herald death. The cause of the psychiatric disturbance is likely to be deficiency of tryptophan which is a precursor of the neurotransmitter serotonin. It has been estimated that 4–10% of patients with pellagra become permanently insane and pellagrins were formerly numerous in lunatic asylums.

The time of appearance of mental symptoms varies widely; they may be present from the start or occur during convalescence. In the later stages peripheral neuropathy or ataxic or spastic paraplegia may develop. Tremors and rigidity (extra pyramidal) may occur. The cranial nerves may be involved (8th nerve deafness, retrobulbar neuritis, central scotomas). Some features of these late manifestations may be caused by vitamin B deficiencies. Corneal dystrophy and lens opacities may occur.

Acute encephalopathy is described to consist of cogwheel rigidity, clouding of consciousness, uncontrollable gasping and sucking. Stupor, delirium and acute psychotic symptoms may be present and a mild pellagrin rash. These patients may respond dramatically to intravenous nicotinic acid.

Course. Symptoms may abate after 2–3 months although the skin remains dark and rough. It re-occurs the following year if the diet is similar. The eruption darkens and mental symptoms develop with melancholia, maniacal interludes and a suicidal tendency. The gait deteriorates and is of the paraplegic type. Body pains increase and may be acute with cramps, twitches and tremors. Symptoms may persist or deteriorate further unless treatment is given or the diet improved.

Diagnosis

This depends essentially on the history and physical examination. A rapid clinical response to niacin is an important confirming test. N-methylnicotinamide, a metabolite of niacin, is almost undetectable in urine in niacin deficiency (<0.5 mg/g creatinine).

Treatment

An adequate balanced diet is essentially supplemented with nicotinic acid at 50–150 mg daily for 2 weeks. In a severe case or in cases of poor intestinal absorption, the dose can be doubled and 100 mg may be given intravenously. Administering large doses is usually followed within half an hour by sensations of local heat, flushing and burning of skin. Overdosage may cause numbness of the tongue and lower jaw. Intravenous nicotinic acid at high dose (1000 mg daily in divided doses) may produce rapid recovery in acute mania. Chronic psychotic and spinal symptoms respond poorly to nicotinic acid.

The diet should be supplemented with other vitamins, especially riboflavin (1–3 mg daily). The diet of the cured pellagrin should be continuously supervised to prevent recurrence. Isoleucine (5 g daily) can counteract the metabolic effect of leucine on the metabolism of tryptophan and nicotinic acid. Leucine is present in large quantities in maize and sorghum. Sun exposure should be avoided during the active phase and skin lesions covered with soothing applications.

Prevention

Pellagra may be prevented through improved socioeconomic conditions among populations dependent on subsistence agriculture. In institutions, the diet should not be confined to maize meal but must include fresh fruit and vegetables, milk and eggs. Hard physical labour should be avoided.

ARIBOFLAVINOSIS

Epidemiology

Riboflavin deficiency without deficiencies of other vitamin B complex vitamins is rare. Deficiency is present in many developing countries and it was common in prisoner-of-war camps.

Aetiology

Riboflavin is not synthesized by higher animals and is therefore an absolute dietary requirement. The co-enzymes of flavin mono- and dinucleotide are synthesized from riboflavin, forming the prosthetic groups of several enzymes important in electron transport. Riboflavin is destroyed on exposure to light and signs of deficiency occur if daily intake is less than 0.2–0.3 mg, although 2 mg is considered ideal for an adult. Riboflavin-poor staple diets, such as polished rice, are common in developing countries. Large amounts of riboflavin occur in liver, kidney, milk, cheese and eggs.

Clinical Features

Cheilosis (sore red lips), vertical fissuring of lips (perlèche) and corners of the mouth (angular stomatitis) and a purplish raw, smooth tongue with loss of papillary structure are well-described features. Other features are scrotal dermatitis, keratitis, conjunctivitis, photophobia, corneal vasculation and seborrheic dermatitis. The skin has a roughened appearance due to hyperkeratosis (toad's skin or phrynoderma). Cheilosis epidemics occur in families and institutions on inadequate diets. A normocytic normochromic anaemia is common. Ariboflavinosis often complicates pellagra and PEM.

Diagnosis

Biochemical status estimates are based upon urinary excretion or measurements of erythrocyte glutathione reductase.

Treatment

Treatment consists of the oral administration of 3–10 mg of riboflavin daily. If no response occurs within a few days, intramuscular injections of 2 mg of riboflavin in saline may be used. Meat and fish are good sources of riboflavin and certain fruit and dark green vegetables.

VITAMIN A DEFICIENCY

Vitamin A deficiency is a major problem in developing countries and deficiency is usually diagnosed with a serum retinol <0.70 μmol/L, which often occurs well before clinical signs of deficiency such as night blindness or xerophthalmia.

Aetiology and Epidemiology

Vitamin A deficiency typically results from inadequate dietary intake of vitamin A. Deficiency in childhood is caused by low levels of vitamin A in breast milk due to maternal vitamin A deficiency, insufficient intake of vitamin A during and after weaning and frequent bouts of infections that worsen vitamin A status. Pre-school children and pregnant women are at higher risk of vitamin A deficiency, likely due to their increased demand for vitamin A. Globally, about 33% of pre-school children and 15% of pregnant women are vitamin A deficient, with the highest burdens of both groups in Africa and South-east Asia.[39]

Vitamin A is necessary for normal vision, maintenance of cell function for growth, epithelial integrity, erythrocyte production, properly functioning immune system and reproduction.[39] Night blindness is a typical indicator of the vitamin A status of a population. It affects 5.2 million pre-school children and 9.8 million pregnant women worldwide.[39] Night blindness is reversible with increased vitamin A intake. Xerophthalmia indicates more severe vitamin A deficiency and can range from reversible Bitot's spots to irreversible blindness. Xerophthalmia is the leading cause of preventable childhood blindness in the world. Vitamin A deficiency also may decrease immunity by delaying normal regeneration of damaged mucosal barriers, decreasing function of leukocytes.

Prevention

Vitamin A supplementation (VAS) in children ≥6 months of age is a widely accepted, cost-effective intervention that reduces mortality in children 6–59 months old.[48] Controversy exists over supplementation in infants <6 months. VAS in infants younger than 6 months may reduce early child mortality and studies on VAS effect on mortality when given in the neonatal period have conflicting results.[48a] Furthermore, it is uncertain if VAS, when administered concomitantly with vaccines in early infancy, alters vaccine response, further research is warranted. VAS in HIV-positive patients may also be associated with increased mortality and transmission of HIV. Table 77.10 lists the recommendations for VAS in children.

Special Groups

PREGNANT WOMEN

In addition to the usual requirements, pregnancy incurs extra energy costs. It is, however, difficult to prescribe precise energy intakes for individual women, as their metabolic and behavioural responses (activity and food intake) cannot be predicted. Inadequate pregnancy weight gains have been associated with lower birth weights in undernourished women. It has long been recognized that pregnant and lactating women are especially vulnerable for mild xerophthalmia.

Low vitamin A content of breast milk will also contribute to the increased susceptibility of the infant. A high proportion of pregnant women in developing countries are at risk of inadequate intakes of zinc, iron, vitamin B_{12}, folic acid and other micronutrients. Improving the diets of pregnant women and adolescent girls before their first pregnancy is therefore important for primary prevention of nutritional disorders. Practical methods include modifying the diets to improve bioavailability and provision of appropriate micronutrient supplements during pregnancy which may yield substantial benefits. Maternal arm circumference can be used as an indicator of risk in non-pregnant and pregnant women because of its high correlation with maternal weight for height.

VEGETARIANS

In poor populations of tropical countries, the meat intake in the diet may be very low or absent. Despite this the macronutrient composition is unremarkable. Vegetarians are prone to iron deficiency due to low iron bioavailability. Combined deficiencies of vitamin B_{12} and folate can lead to megaloblastic anaemias. Consumption of unleavened breads such as chapattis and brown rice may predispose to rickets and osteomalacia, particularly in Asian vegetarians. Leavening of bread with yeast destroys phytic acid which binds to calcium and this ameliorates this effect. Intake of high dietary fibre and phytates may modify zinc absorption. In general, vegetarians have lower rates of some cancers (mouth, prostate and possibly colon), but there is little evidence relating this to the absence of meat in the diet. The beneficial effects of a vegetarian diet may relate to cancer-preventive substances such as antioxidants and phytochemicals.

REFUGEES

Nutrition deficiencies in refugees and other uprooted people are well documented. Scurvy, xerophthalmia, anaemia, pellagra and beriberi are described in people dependent on refugee rations. Refugees are prone to anaemia because their food rations are often low in vitamin C which enhances iron absorption. Control of deficiency diseases among refugees has largely depended on the distribution of supplementary tablets and additional food, e.g. fruits, dried fish, meat. Nutrient fortification of bulk food to improve the quality of rations has been successfully exploited, e.g. micronutrients in cereals, vitamin A in oil and iron in sugar.[58]

Acknowledgements

The authors would like to acknowledge Lynda Aririguzo for her assistance.

REFERENCES

1. Prudhon C, Prinzo ZW, Briend A, et al. Proceedings of the WHO, UNICEF and SCN informal consultation on community-based management of severe malnutrition in children. Food Nutr Bull 2006;27(Suppl. 3):S99–S104.
4. Svedberg P. How many people are malnourished? Annu Rev Nutr 2011;31:263–83.
8. WHO. Management of Severe Malnutrition: a Manual for Physicians and Other Senior Health Workers. Geneva: World Health Organization; 1999.
35. Collins S, Dent N, Binns P, et al. Management of severe acute malnutrition in children. Lancet 2006;368:1992–2000.
41. De-Regil LM, Suchdev PS, Vist GE, et al. Home fortification of foods with multiple micronutrient powders for health and nutrition in children under two years of age. Cochrane Database Syst Rev 2011;(9)CD008959.

Access the complete references online at www.expertconsult.com

78 Obesity in the Tropics

SOPHIE HAWKESWORTH | ANDREW M. PRENTICE

KEY POINTS

- Obesity is the excess accumulation of body fat and is commonly assessed at the population level by the body mass index (BMI). A BMI ≥30 kg/m^2 indicates obesity but other measures of adiposity may be used.
- The highest rates of obesity in the world are currently experienced in Oceania, although the prevalence is rising throughout the tropics.
- Obesity occurs when energy intake exceeds energy expenditure over a number of years. Although sedentary lifestyles contribute to obesity, most of the imbalance occurs through over-consumption of energy.
- Populations are increasingly living in 'obesogenic' environments driven in part by the nutrition transition occurring across the tropics, particularly in urban areas.
- Obesity is a strong predictor for a wide range of comorbid conditions, including type 2 diabetes mellitus. Healthcare costs associated with the treatment of obesity and its comorbidities place a strain on health services across the tropical region.
- Effective treatment strategies for obesity must focus on weight loss and even modest loss is associated with important reductions in risk. Successful weight loss programmes involve the setting of individual, realistic and achievable goals and require a high level of patient motivation.
- It is increasingly recognized that a whole system approach to obesity prevention encompassing both the individual and population level will need to be adopted to account for the complex, interacting and multi-level causes that underpin the current epidemic.

Epidemiology

Obesity is a condition characterized by the excess accumulation of body fat (adiposity) and represents an important risk factor for death and disability, currently ranking as the fifth leading cause of death in the world. Traditionally viewed as a disease of affluence, obesity is now recognized as a global issue and rates are increasing across the tropics in both low- and middle-income countries. Within this region however, there is marked heterogeneity with some of the South Pacific islands reporting rates of overweight and obesity in excess of 90% (the highest in the world) while countries in sub-Saharan Africa, such as Zambia, are currently experiencing much lower rates of around 8% for men and 23% for women (Figure 78.1).[1] In 1980, the global age-standardized prevalence of obesity was 4.8% for men and 7.9% for women, by 2008 this had risen to 9.8% and 13.8%, respectively; the range of increase varies greatly across the globe with the greatest increases in Oceania.[1] While the rapid increases in obesity rates observed in higher-income countries in recent decades are slowing down, the burden will increasingly fall on low- and middle-income countries (LMICs), which may be ill-equipped to deal with the associated health burden.

Although obesity is increasingly recognized as an important risk factor for ill health, routine statistics are not commonly collected, which makes international comparisons challenging. While heights and weights are often measured in health surveillance studies and occasionally during national surveys, these are not conducted regularly, resulting in an extremely patchy evidence base. For example, a recent attempt was made to summarize worldwide trends in BMI, by the Chronic Diseases Collaborating Group but they were unable to identify any usable data for 30 countries, many of which were in the Caribbean. High-quality health statistics are essential for planning and implementing health policy in all settings and accurate obesity statistics at a country-level will enable us to understand the epidemic and to evaluate prevention strategies. Inter-country comparisons allow insights into the epidemiology of the disease and can be used to highlight the growing burden. The WHO Global Infobase (see: https://apps.who.int/infobase) is an important resource in this field, with easily accessible national data.

Obesity rates are not uniform within populations and in all settings, women exhibit a higher body mass index (BMI, see definition below) than men. Obesity rates increase with age but childhood obesity is a strong predictor of obesity in adulthood. Globally, over 179 million children are classified as overweight and obese;[2] the prevalence of obesity in pre-school children is predicted to experience the greatest rise in Africa from current levels of around 8.5–12.7% by 2020, representing an increase of 49%.[3]

In many countries in the tropics, obesity co-exists with a high prevalence of under-nutrition. Countries that have experienced rapid rates of epidemiological and nutrition transitions witness the emergence of obesity as a public health problem on top of a background of intergenerational cycles of under-nutrition, leading to a so-called 'double-burden' of disease (Figure 78.2). This double burden may even occur within the same household and poses a considerable challenge to policy-makers and healthcare practitioners. In Indonesia, it has been estimated that around 10% of households experience simultaneous obesity and undernutrition among family members[4] and a separate study in Benin revealed 16% of families suffered from this double burden.[5] The links between malnutrition and obesity are themselves complex because stunted children may be at increased risk of developing overweight/obesity as adults.

Although nationally representative statistics are often used to provide a picture of obesity rates at a macro-level, they mask

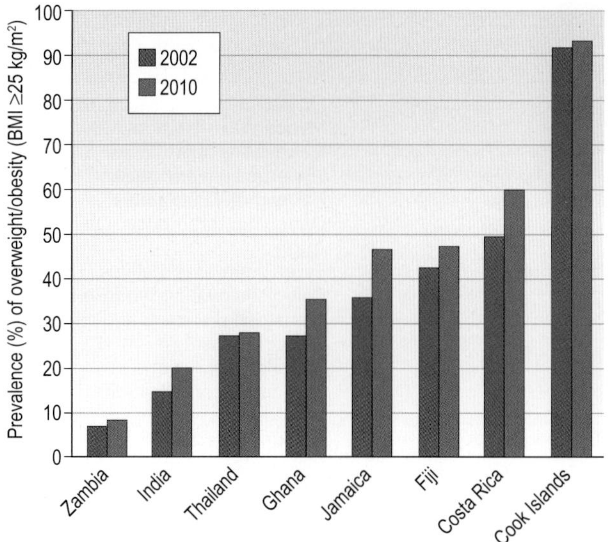

Figure 78.1 The rising prevalence of overweight and obesity across the Tropics. *(Data derived from: WHO Global Infobase (https://apps.who.int/infobase), which contains health statistics provided by WHO Member States. Prevalence displayed for overweight and obesity combined and defined by BMI cut-off of ≥25 kg/m²)*

important differences that occur within populations. Obesity rates often show a distinct socioeconomic gradient although the direction of this relationship depends upon the stage of economic development for a given area; for higher-income countries obesity rates are higher among individuals from the lower socioeconomic classes, whereas the opposite relationship can be observed for countries at earlier stages of their economic transition. In addition, there are often rural–urban differences with higher rates observed in the urban areas than in rural settings where more traditional ways of life prevail.

Pathogenesis and Pathology

Obesity occurs when energy intake exceeds energy expenditure over a number of years (i.e. individuals are not in energy balance). Under normal circumstances, energy balance is maintained within very fine limits. For instance many people maintain a constant body weight to within ±1–2 kg over years or decades, which require maintaining energy balance to within a fraction of a percent of the total energy consumed during this time. This regulation is orchestrated by a complex system of orexigenic (appetite stimulating) and anorexigenic (appetite suppressing) neural and hormonal systems. Regulatory signals arising primarily in the gut, liver and adipose tissue, are integrated in the hypothalamus.[6] Primary among these signals is the adipokine hormone leptin, which provides the hypothalamus with signals regarding the size of adipose tissue stores and the state of energy flux within them.

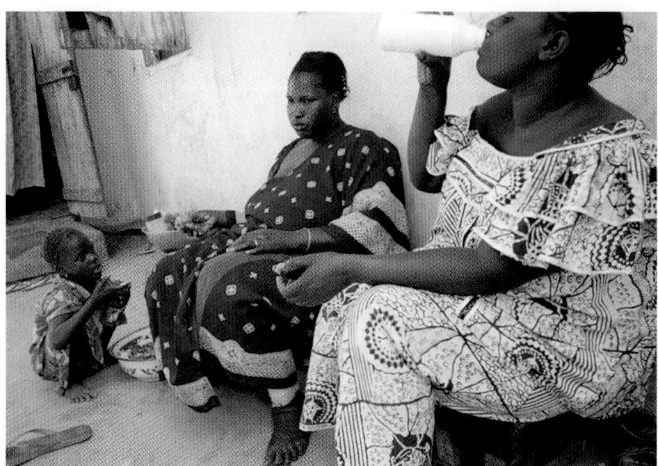

Figure 78.2 The double burden of malnutrition and obesity facing families in the Tropics. Urban obesity in The Gambia. *(Reproduced by permission of Felicia Webb.)*

Imbalances on either side of the energy balance equation (energy consumed or energy expended) or both, can lead to obesity. Some decades ago, it was believed that obese people do not overeat and that the defect must involve a super-efficient metabolism. This has now been disproved and it is clear that, although sedentary lifestyles contribute to obesity (see below), most of the imbalance occurs through over-consumption of energy. Interestingly, all of the genetic defects known to contribute to obesity cause errors in the regulation of food intake rather than expenditure.

Survival depends upon a regular supply of energy and nutrients and hence, the pathways regulating hunger and appetite have evolved to be very efficient and there are multiple redundancies in the control mechanisms in case one should fail. This is not true for satiety mechanisms, since over-feeding would have been an advantage rather than a peril during evolutionary times when food was generally scarce.[7] Consequently, there is an asymmetry in appetite regulation, which means that weight gain is more likely than weight loss. Experiments have shown that humans are ill-equipped to recognize changes in the energy density of foods.[8] This leads to 'passive overconsumption' when people are exposed to high-fat, high-energy diets. Such over-consumption leading to fat gain is not intentional and is usually unrecognized; it arises as an accidental outcome of poor physiological regulation combined with major dietary changes.

Many nations in the tropics are experiencing rapid economic development, which results in a 'demographic transition' that is usually associated with profound changes in diet (both quantitative and qualitative) and a move towards sedentariness.[9] As people emerge from conditions of poor and irregular food supply combined with high levels of physical labour it is not surprising that they seek out rich and prestigious foods and value items associated with a more sedentary lifestyle. This so-called nutrition transition results in profound changes in diet composition and underlies the rapid increases in obesity experienced across lower- and middle-income countries today. In general terms, a pattern of infrequent high-volume, low-fat, high-complex-carbohydrate meals is replaced by frequent meals that are high in fat and energy-dense, rich in refined carbohydrates and animal protein and deficient in complex carbohydrates. These changes are themselves driven by upstream complex and interacting determinants including urbanization, globalization and profound changes to the agriculture and food systems.[10]

The very rapid increase in obesity in populations in which there has been a minimal infusion of new genes through immigration and inter-marriage provides unequivocal proof of the importance of these environmental factors. This, however, does not diminish the importance of understanding genetic susceptibility to obesity. Not all individuals exposed to the current obesogenic environment will develop obesity and understanding the underlying genetic susceptibility to disease may help to elucidate important and as yet poorly understood mechanisms. It has long been clear that overweight and obesity cluster in families; obesity is 2–8 times higher in the families of obese individuals than in the population at large and estimates of heritability of BMI ranges between 64% and 84%.[11] In rare cases, it is possible to determine single-gene (monogenetic) causes of obesity such as Prader–Willi and Bardet–Biedl syndromes, but progress on the identification of common genetic polymorphisms that underlie susceptibility to obesity in the general population has been much slower.[12] Recent advances in genetics have allowed rapid increases in the identification of genotypes associated with BMI through genome-wide association studies. This approach has so-far identified 15 new loci influencing BMI, with the strongest association observed for variants within the FTO (the fat-mass and obesity-related) gene.[13] However, the public-health impact of these genotypes is small and depends on the prevalence of risk alleles within a population. Within a large UK cohort, eight of the common obesity loci explained only 0.84% of the difference in BMI between individuals.[14] It is likely that an increased understanding of gene–environment interactions, which may help to identify individuals at high risk and to inform prevention strategies, will be the more useful application of genetic research from a public health standpoint.

Clinical Features

Obesity is a strong predictor for a very wide range of other comorbid conditions (see Table 78.1) and hence, is associated with a lowering of life expectancy. BMI in the range 30–35 kg/m^2 is associated with a reduction in median survival of 2–4 years and a BMI of 40–45 kg/m^2 with a reduction of 8–10 years.[15] Life expectancy is reduced most in those with early-onset obesity. The association with mortality has a reversed-J shape with somewhat higher mortality and lower survival for BMI <20 kg/m^2. This arises from the strong relationship between thinness, lung cancer and severe respiratory diseases.

Obesity is one of the defining criteria for the 'metabolic syndrome'; a commonly observed confluence of excess weight (especially central body fat), hypertension, dyslipidaemia and insulin resistance. The metabolic syndrome is defined by the presence of central obesity (defined by waist circumference, see below) and at least two of the other risk markers.[16] An individual with the metabolic syndrome is at increased risk of cardiovascular disease and assessment of the metabolic syndrome is often included in algorithms for determining which patients qualify for antihypertensive and cholesterol-lowering medications.

Although obesity represents a significant risk factor for many life-threatening conditions its strongest association is with type 2 diabetes mellitus (T2DM). This association is so strong that it is often described as 'diabesity'. Numerous studies have confirmed that obesity is a very strong predictor of incident T2DM. Studies in the USA showed that severe obesity increases the risk of T2DM by over 40-fold in men and over 90-fold in women (Figure 78.3).[17,18] Remarkably, a BMI in the range 28–30 kg/m^2 (i.e. not even classified as clinically obese) increases the risk by

TABLE 78.1 Medical Conditions Significantly Increased in Obesity

Cardiac and vascular	Ischaemic heart disease (IHD) Myocardial infarction (MI) Congestive heart failure Hypertension and stroke Hypercholesterolaemia Deep vein thrombosis (DVT) Angina
Endocrine	Type 2 diabetes mellitus (T2DM) Polycystic ovarian syndrome (PCOS) Menstrual disorders and infertility Hypogonadism Erectile dysfunction Pregnancy complications Birth defects
Neurological	Stroke sequelae Migraines Dementia
Orthopaedic	Osteoarthritis Reduced mobility Gout Back pain
Cancers	Almost all cancers
Respiratory	Obstructive sleep apnoea Asthma Anaesthetic complications
Gastrointestinal	Reflux disease Fatty liver Gallstones
Dermatological	Acanthosis nigricans Lymphoedema Cellulitis Hirsutism
Urological	Chronic renal failure Incontinence
Psychiatric and social	Depression Social stigma and isolation
Economic	Reduced earnings

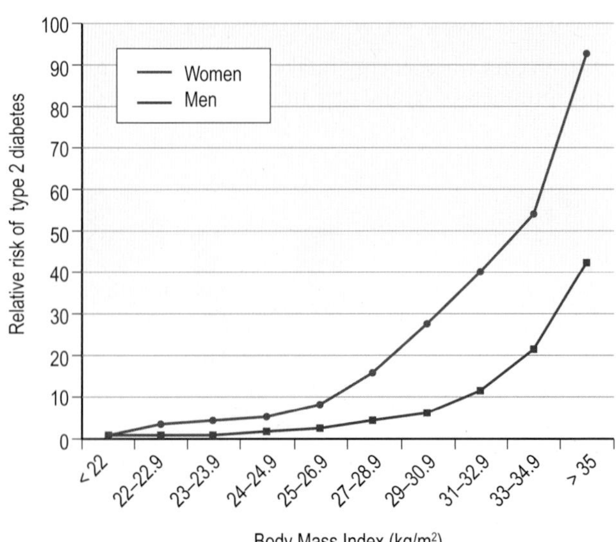

Figure 78.3 Obesity and risk of incident type 2 diabetes mellitus. Association between body mass index and risk of type 2 diabetes displayed for men and women separately. *(Modified from: Chan JM et al. Obesity, fat distribution and weight gain as risk factors for clinical diabetes in men. Diabetes Care 1994;17:196–9 and Colditz GA et al. Weight gain as a risk factor for clinical diabetes mellitus in women. Ann Intern Med 1995;122:481–6.)*

around 20-fold in women and even a few extra BMI points significantly increases the odds of developing T2DM.

RESOLUTION OF OBESITY-RELATED COMORBIDITY

In most cases, it is clear that there is a direct causal pathway between excess body fat and disease with weight loss and related health interventions being very effective in ameliorating the condition, especially if the obesity has not been of very long duration. For instance trials of diet and lifestyle intervention in people with impaired glucose tolerance (the first step towards T2DM) have shown that, despite relatively modest weight loss of only a few kilograms, the risk of progressing to T2DM can be reduced by 40–60%.[19] Some other conditions can show even more impressive resolution; for instance, weight loss resolves obesity-related infertility in most cases. However, it is important to recognize that obesity is a progressive disease and for many comorbid illnesses the condition reaches a point of no return if not treated soon enough. For example, knee joint damage caused by the wear-and-tear of supporting excess weight, will not self-resolve with weight loss, even though pain may be reduced.

The transition towards T2DM is shown in Figure 78.4. Initially, the insulin resistance caused by excess adipose tissue is well compensated by post-meal hyperinsulinaemia and patients appear normoglycaemic. As the condition progresses, even high levels of insulin production fail to compensate and patients become hyperglycaemic. Over a number of further years, the requirement for greatly increased insulin production causes beta-cell exhaustion and progression towards insulin-dependent diabetes. In the early stages of development, hyperinsulinaemia is fully reversible by weight loss, but only islet transplants or possible future stem cell treatments can be effective once islet exhaustion has occurred.

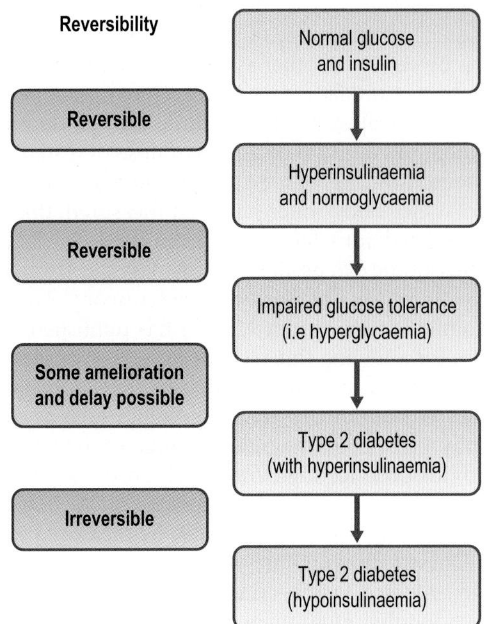

Figure 78.4 Progressive stages in the development of type 2 diabetes mellitus.

TABLE 78.2 The International Classification of Adult Underweight, Overweight and Obesity According to BMI

Classification	BMI (kg/m²) Principal Cut-Off Points	Additional Cut-Off Points
Normal range	18.50–24.99	18.50–22.99
Overweight	25.00–29.99	25.00–27.49
Obese	≥30.00	
Obese class I	30.00–34.99	30.00–32.49
Obese class II	35.00–39.99	35.00–37.49
Obese class III	≥40.00	

BMI, body mass index.

Modified from: WHO Expert Consultation. Appropriate body-mass index for Asian populations and its implications for policy and intervention strategies. Lancet 2004;363:157–63.

In certain conditions, and especially in patients with severe monogenic causes for their obesity, the excess adipose tissue may be more coincident with, than causal of, their comorbidities. In such circumstances, weight loss may improve quality of life in some respects (e.g. improved mobility and exercise tolerance) but cannot be expected to improve all conditions.

Diagnosis

As it is not possible to directly measure an individual's body fat in vivo, proxy measurements must be adopted. The most widespread and simple method of assessing obesity is by calculating body weight adjusted for height. This is known as the body mass index (BMI) and is calculated as weight(kg)/height(m)^2. A BMI ≥30 kg/m^2 is considered obese, while 25–29.9 kg/m^2 is considered overweight (Table 78.2). These classifications are themselves based on increased mortality and morbidity at higher BMI and, at a population level, BMI strongly predicts all-cause and disease-specific mortality. However, BMI may not correspond to the same degree of fatness in different populations due, in part, to different body proportions. There is evidence that individuals of Asian origin experience increased risk of mortality at lower BMI values than Caucasian populations and there have been several international consultations to determine if a separate classification system is warranted. The most recent WHO Consultation in 2002, reviewed the evidence and concluded that the international classification should be retained for all populations but with additional cut-off points that can be applied if relevant. It was, therefore, recommended that countries should use all categories (i.e. 18.5, 23, 25, 27.5, 30, 32.5 kg/m^2, and in many populations, 35, 37.5 and 40 kg/m^2) for reporting purposes, with a view to facilitating international comparisons.[20]

The definition of overweight and obesity in children is more challenging than for adults, when height remains fairly stable. In contrast to adults, BMI in childhood changes substantially with age making the adult cut-off definitions inapplicable. Various methods of assessing obesity have been suggested often utilizing defined weight-for-height percentiles in an analogous method to the assessment of undernutrition. However, these centiles are not based on disease risk per se and it is now recommended to utilize age- and sex-specific cut-offs developed by the International Association for the Study of Obesity, which

TABLE 78.3 International Cut-Off Points for Body Mass Index (BMI) for Overweight and Obesity in Children and Adolescents

	BMI 25 kg/m^2		BMI 30 kg/m^2	
Age (years)	Males	Females	Males	Females
2	18.41	18.02	20.09	19.81
2.5	18.13	17.76	19.80	19.55
3	17.89	17.56	19.57	19.36
3.5	17.69	17.40	19.39	19.23
4	17.55	17.28	19.29	19.15
4.5	17.47	17.19	19.26	19.12
5	17.42	17.15	19.30	19.17
5.5	17.45	17.20	19.47	19.34
6	17.55	17.34	19.79	19.65
6.5	17.71	17.53	20.23	20.08
7	17.92	17.75	20.63	20.51
7.5	18.16	18.03	21.09	21.01
8	18.44	18.35	21.60	21.57
8.5	18.76	18.69	22.17	22.18
9	19.10	19.07	22.77	22.81
9.5	19.46	19.45	23.39	23.46
10	19.84	19.86	24.00	24.11
10.5	20.20	20.29	24.57	24.77
11	20.55	20.74	25.10	25.42
11.5	20.89	21.20	25.58	26.05
12	21.22	21.68	26.02	26.67
12.5	21.56	22.14	26.43	27.24
13	21.91	22.58	26.84	27.76
13.5	22.27	22.98	27.25	28.20
14	22.62	23.34	27.63	28.57
14.5	22.96	23.66	27.98	27.87
15	23.29	23.94	28.30	29.11
15.5	23.60	24.17	28.60	29.29
16	23.90	24.37	28.88	29.43
16.5	24.19	24.54	29.14	29.56
17	24.46	24.70	29.14	29.69
17.5	24.73	24.85	29.70	29.84
18	25	25	30	30

Cut-off values provided by sex, between 2 and 18 years and defined to pass through BMI of 25 and 30 kg/m^2 at age 18. Obtained by averaging data from Brazil, Great Britain, Hong Kong, Netherlands, Singapore and the USA.

Modified from: Cole TJ, Bellizzi MC, Flegal KM, et al. Establishing a standard definition for child overweight and obesity worldwide: international survey. BMJ 2000;320:1240–3.

link childhood BMI to the adult cut-off points for overweight and obesity (Table 78.3).[21]

Despite its usefulness at predicting health risks at a population level, there are challenges to the interpretation of BMI for individuals.[22] BMI provides information on excess weight only and this weight may be attributable to a variable combination of fat and lean mass. Thus, individuals with a large amount of muscle mass (such as athletes) may have a relatively high BMI, but in this particular case, their BMI does not confer increased risk of disease. For individuals, other assessments of adiposity, each with their own set of limitations, may be used[23] and are outlined below.

Of the various alternatives to BMI in a clinical setting, perhaps the simplest is the measurement of waist circumference and this is becoming increasingly popular as a public health tool. WHO guidelines specify that the circumference should be measured at the midpoint between the lower margin of the last rib and the top of the hip bone: cut-offs associated with high risk of disease are still under development but values of ≥90 cm for men and ≥80 cm for women have been suggested, based on Caucasian populations.[24] An individual's waist circumference provides information on the distribution of fat in the body, a feature that has been shown to be an important risk factor for disease. A large waist circumference is now recognized as an important contributor to the metabolic syndrome, partly because the measurement correlates with visceral fat area, the metabolically dangerous fat store. Waist circumference is also associated with type 2 diabetes.

Other anthropometric prediction techniques can also be used to estimate body fatness. Traditionally skinfold thickness measurements are a popular technique, particularly in lower-income country settings, where resources are scarce. Skinfolds are measured using calipers at defined sites on the body which often include the triceps, biceps, subscapular and suprailiac sites. The appropriate site must be identified carefully by trained personnel, taking care to only measure the adipose skinfold in order to minimize measurement error. While skinfolds can be measured on individuals of all ages, they are often harder to accurately measure in obese individuals. Once the raw data have been obtained, these can be converted into estimates of body density and thence body fatness but as the applied equations are highly population-specific, the raw data may represent a more useful resource with which to assess individual or population-level adiposity.

The final field-friendly prediction technique utilizes the technology of bioelectrical impedance and is becoming an increasingly popular technique in both the clinical and research setting. The measurement is based on the relative impedance of tissues to a small electric current that is passed through the body. Machines encompassing a variety of shapes and sizes have now been developed but all utilize the same principles; they provide contact points for the electric current, measuring the tissue impedance and converting this into an estimate of fat mass. The impedance values are converted it into an estimate of total body water using prediction equations that are population- and manufacturer-specific. Estimates of body water are then converted into fat-free mass and finally fat mass is calculated by the difference from body weight. Precision and accuracy are usually in the range of ±1–2 kg for body fat.

There are a variety of other assessment methods that are able to indirectly measure fat mass and therefore do not need to rely on prediction equations. These include isotope dilution techniques, where the dilution of a known dose of a stable isotope (usually deuterium, ^{2}H) can be used to measure the total body water pool. Once body water has been measured, this estimate can be converted into fat-free mass and thence fat mass as before. The isotope can be analysed by mass spectrometry or by the less costly process of infra-red spectroscopy. The International Atomic Energy Agency (IAEA) has published standardized guides for applying this technique (see: www.iaea.org).

Techniques are also available that use other sophisticated but very expensive state-of-the-art technologies such as computed tomography (CT) and magnetic resonance imaging (MRI). Both methods produce high-resolution cross-sectional images allowing total fat volume and percentage fat to be estimated. The area of visceral fat depots can also be measured with good accuracy. These techniques are very expensive, require patients to travel to a medical facility and may be problematic for people with claustrophobia. Dual-energy X-ray absorptiometry (DXA) is a widely used imaging technique that utilizes the principal that transmitted X-rays at two energy levels are differentially attenuated by bone mass and soft tissue. It is possible to obtain abdominal fat estimates with DXA, although these cannot be separated into subcutaneous and visceral components.

Management and Treatment

As stated previously, the disease of obesity is caused at the individual level by a fundamental imbalance between energy intake and energy expenditure. Therefore any effective treatment strategy must focus on weight loss and even modest reductions in weight have been shown to have important health benefits. However, helping people to manage their weight is difficult and can be discouraging and time-consuming both for the health professional and for the patient involved. Motivation for weight loss in obese individuals is a key component of effective treatment but is often lacking partly because it depends on the acceptance and recognition that obesity is a medical disorder. Motivation for change may also be reduced if the obese individual is yet to develop comorbidities and does not yet conceive their health is compromised. Proper identification and classification of obesity through body composition assessment (see above) are important steps to initiate before beginning weight-loss treatment. Dietary management, physical activity, surgery, pharmacotherapy and psychosocial and familial support must be considered as part of obesity assessment. Before beginning a weight-loss programme, a detailed case-history should be collected (Box 78.1) and patients should be evaluated for the number and severity of cardiovascular risk factors and conditions that may require treatment, in addition to weight-loss strategies.

One of the most important aspects of a successful weight-loss programme is to help the patient set individual, realistic and achievable goals such as 5–10% loss over 3–6 months. After weight loss has been achieved, weight maintenance strategies are also vital and patients require ongoing support in this phase to prevent rebound weight gain. In many countries, obesity is associated with stigma and a non-judgemental and supportive environment will be required to underpin a successful weight loss strategy. After initial assessment and goal setting, group-based support has been found to be successful. The scale of the obesity epidemic has turned weight loss programmes into a multi-billion pound business with a constant stream of fad diets in the press. It is therefore important for the physician to be able to provide professional advice on what constitutes effective lifestyle changes. A recent review of dietary weight-loss interventions found that reduced-calorie diets were equally effective weight-loss strategies, regardless of the macronutrients they targeted.[25] Thus, the patient can be allowed to choose whether a low-fat or low-carbohydrate diet is most effective for them, provided they are continually monitored for any adverse effects and/or the likelihood of rebound weight gain.

While data on effective treatment strategies in certain settings cannot be assumed to be applicable elsewhere, due to the paucity of information from many LMICs, it can be argued that while we wait for context-specific information, it is still necessary to act on what we do already know. Due to the global nature of the obesity epidemic and the long-term health consequences associated with the disease, effective prevention and/or treatment strategies have become an important and well-funded focus of research at least in higher-income countries. Where a lot of studies exist, health practitioners and policy-makers can become overwhelmed by information and systematic reviews of the evidence base can be especially important in identifying effective treatment strategies. Recent reviews have highlighted the effectiveness of a range of lifestyle, pharmaceutical and surgical interventions for treating overweight and obesity. Exercise has been shown to be effective at inducing modest weight reduction, particularly when combined with dietary advice, and also demonstrates important reductions in cardiovascular risk factors such as blood pressure and fasting glucose. Exercise and regular self-monitoring of weight have been shown to be important predictors of successful long-term maintenance of weight loss.

Despite massive investment, very few anti-obesity drugs have been licensed for the management of the disease and only orlistat remains on the market following the withdrawal of sibutramine and rimonabant following post-marketing observations of adverse events. A recent meta-analysis demonstrated modest weight-loss for patients on long-term (>1 year) treatment with orlistat[26] but the use of obesity drugs should only be prescribed following the assessment of risks and benefits and with regular monitoring. Effective management of obesity must be life-long and focussed on weight loss maintenance. Studies that have compared the relative effectiveness of lifestyle and pharmaceutical interventions have found additional benefit from combined strategies. In one study, an intensive lifestyle intervention was found to be as effective as sibutramine treatment but the combined effect of both the lifestyle and drug treatment was doubly effective for an individual's weight loss.[27]

Recently, particularly in higher-income countries, surgery has been increasingly used as a treatment of obesity when other treatments have failed. Weight loss surgery, known as bariatric surgery, can encompass a variety of different procedures, including gastric banding, gastric bypass and vertical banded gastroplasty. Bariatric surgery has been shown to result in greater weight loss than conventional treatment and improvement in obesity-associated comorbidities such as type 2 diabetes but it is not without complications and the evidence base is too limited to effectively compare the different types of surgery. Furthermore, the clinical treatments such as pharmacotherapy and bariatric surgery may not currently be available in some tropical countries due to limited resources and cost-effectiveness

BOX 78.1 IMPORTANT PATIENT HISTORY FACTORS TO ASSESS IN THE MANAGEMENT OF OBESITY

- Is the weight problem recent or longstanding (e.g. since childhood)?
- Consider the patient's successful and unsuccessful attempts at losing weight and establish what s/he thinks about them.
- What is the patient's attitude to smoking? Do they feel that stopping smoking will cause them to gain weight?
- How does the patient feel about illness and medication and how they relate to weight gain?
- Is there a family history of weight problems? Does the patient's partner have weight problems?
- Does the patient believe that their medical, social or psychological problems are related to their obesity?
- What is the patient's motivation for weight loss or stability?

Modified from: Lean M, Finer N. Obesity management: part II – drugs. BMJ 2006; 333:794–7.

TABLE 78.4 **Strength of the Evidence for Factors that Might Promote or Protect Against Weight Gain and Obesity Derived from Expert Committee Reviews**

Evidence[a]		Decreased Risk	Increased Risk
Convincing	WHO	Regular physical activity High dietary intake of non-starch polysaccharides (fibre)	Sedentary lifestyles High intake of energy-dense micronutrient-poor foods
	WCRF	Physical activity	Sedentary living
Probable	WHO	Home and school environments that support healthy food choices for children Breastfeeding	Heavy marketing of energy-dense foods and fast-food outlets High intake of sugars-sweetened soft drinks and fruit juices Adverse socioeconomic conditions (in developed countries, especially for women)
	WCRF	Low energy-dense foods Breast-feeding	Energy-dense foods Fast foods Sugary drinks Television viewing

[a]Evidence level ranked by expert scientific committee review.
Modified from: WHO/FAO 2003 Diet, nutrition and the prevention of chronic diseases: report of a joint WHO/FAO Expert Consultation. WHO Technical Report Series: 916. Geneva: World Health Organization and World Cancer Research Fund/American Institute for Cancer Research 2007 Food, Nutrition, Physical Activity and the Prevention of Cancer: a Global Perspective. Washington DC: WCRF/AICR.

studies are required to assess what can be implemented in these settings.

Treatment for childhood obesity is particularly important, as childhood obesity affects both the physical and psychosocial health of children in addition to putting them at risk of ill health in adulthood. Evidence on effective treatment strategies for children and adolescents is currently limited and more information is required, particularly in low- and middle-income country settings. A recent Cochrane review concluded from the current evidence base that combined behavioural lifestyle interventions can produce a clinically meaningful reduction in weight for this age group but that more information is required.[28]

Prevention

Countries across the tropics are experiencing the obesity epidemic at different stages but all are also faced with a large burden of the more traditional 'tropical' infectious diseases. In settings where resources are scarce, access to healthcare is limited and where communicable diseases are still rife, population-based prevention strategies will be particularly important. However, the current evidence base is limited by a lack of good-quality data, particularly when looking at the community rather than the individual level; there is currently no consensus on effective population strategies. This is particularly true for low- and middle-income countries, which often lack information on population-specific individual-level risk factors (diet and physical activity) or routine statistics on BMI that are needed to provide achievable targets for effective interventions. It is arguable that even while further good-quality evidence on effective interventions is being gathered a 'do nothing' scenario is not acceptable due to the rising costs of obesity and its comorbidities. In wealthy nations, obesity causes a very significant drain on health services. Studies in both the USA and UK have concluded that, at current levels of obesity, the condition accounts for 9% of the total health expenditure. Obesity is also a major contributor to lost productivity and is the leading reason for disability pensions in the UK. Such burdens will soon start to mount up in emerging nations. A recent analysis suggests the cumulative economic losses to low- and middle-income countries from non-communicable diseases will surpass 7 trillion US dollars between 2011 and 2025.[29] In contrast, population-based measures for reducing unhealthy diets and physical inactivity will be relatively inexpensive.

Effective prevention strategies must target the root causes of rising obesity rates and there is current consensus on the major causes of weight gain. Two comprehensive expert reviews of the evidence base within the past decade have highlighted the role of sedentary lifestyle and a high intake of energy-dense foods, including sugar-sweetened beverages and fast foods, as being strongly related to weight gain (Table 78.4).[30,31] It is increasingly recognized that individual behaviour change against a background environment that promotes these lifestyles is particularly challenging and ineffective. Thus, the 'obesogenic' environments themselves must be tackled. An analysis by the International Obesity Taskforce in 2010 revealed that the UK and Brazil are leading the way in obesity prevention (www.iaso.org). In Brazil, this has taken the form of policies that target the regulation of food marketing, the provision of healthy school meals, the monitoring of obesity trends and the promotion of breast-feeding.

Interventions against the rise of obesity will be most effective if they are targeted at early life cycle stages. The earlier that excess weight is present, the greater the long-term risk to health and the magnitude of weight loss required in childhood is likely to be more achievable than that in later life. In addition, behaviour patterns tend to track throughout life so that the earlier healthy choices can be adopted the greater the likely impact. Schools have been a popular target for prevention strategies because they are more easily regulated than other environments and they are guaranteed to reach most of the target population. Strategies have focussed on the provision of healthy school meals, removal of vending machines selling sugar-sweetened beverages and walk-to-school programmes, among others. Evaluation is often poor however, hampering conclusions on what works, and effective strategies are also likely to be very context-specific which again highlights the urgent need for good-quality evaluation studies.

Screening for high-risk individuals has been proposed as a way of targeting prevention strategies but is not without controversy. Singapore adopted a national childhood screening programme in 1993, making it a legal requirement for all children to undertake BMI screening. Children in the upper range of the distribution were then required to undergo specific healthy lifestyle education sessions and were provided with targeted diets. The initiative was associated with a reduction in national obesity levels but has now been stopped due to parental pressure from individuals who felt their children were being stigmatized. Advertisement of foods and beverages has been shown to be an important determinant of increasing obesity rates and strategies aimed at the prevention of marketing to schoolchildren have been adopted as preventative measures in a number of countries. There is now a consensus on the advertising of unhealthy foods to children led by the WHO but enforcement in different settings can be challenging.

Tackling the current burden of obesity will require prevention strategies to be directed across the ages in a life-course approach. The complexity of the multilayered causes of obesity and the variety of approaches that are required to stem the epidemic can be quite overwhelming for policy-makers. Cost-effective evaluations help to focus resources and may be particularly important in LMICs, where resources are stretched. A recent Australian study identified taxation on unhealthy foods and beverages as the most cost-effective policy of the current options in terms of cost per disability-adjusted life years saved (Table 78.5).[32,33]

TABLE 78.5 Cost-Effectiveness of Selected Interventions Evaluated in Australia

Intervention	Target Population	DALYs Saved	Gross Costs (A$ million)
Unhealthy food and beverage tax (10%)	Adults	559 000	18.00
Front-of-pack traffic light nutrition labelling	Adults	45 100	81.00
Reduction of advertising of junk food and beverages to children	Children (0–14 years)	37 000	0.13
School-based education programme to reduce television viewing	Primary schoolchildren (8–10 years)	8600	27.70
Multi-faceted school-based programme including nutrition and physical activity	Primary schoolchildren (6 years)	8000	40.00

DALY, Disability adjusted life years; Gross costs, intervention costs; A$, Australian dollars.
Modified from: Gortmaker SL, Swinburn BA, Levy D, et al. Changing the future of obesity: science, policy and action. Lancet 2011;378:838–47.

BOX 78.2 CORE ACTIONS FOR GOVERNMENTS TO ADOPT FOR THE PREVENTION OF OBESITY

LEADERSHIP AND GOVERNANCE

- Show high-level leadership by supporting actions to reduce obesity
- Introduce cross-sectoral structures to ensure support
- Establish mechanisms that limit the influence of commercial interests in policy-making.

HEALTHY PUBLIC POLICIES

- Protect and promote health and sustainable food security as over-riding priorities in food policy development
- Ensure trade agreements and agricultural and food fiscal policies (e.g. subsidies, taxes, import tariffs and quotas) protect and promote health
- Prioritize public transport, walking and cycling environments, and safe recreation spaces in transport and urban planning policies and budget allocations
- Ensure taxation and social policies support the reduction of socioeconomic inequalities that contribute to health inequalities.

RESOURCES

- Commit funding for preventive health including targeted effective direct and structural actions
- Include health promotion activities within other existing budgets (e.g. treatment services, education and local government)
- Establish health promotion foundations and fund through taxes on tobacco, alcohol or unhealthy food and beverages.

INTELLIGENCE SYSTEMS

- Create monitoring systems to track obesity trends in children and adults and key aspects of the food and physical activity environments (e.g. nutrient composition of foods, and exposure of children to marketing)
- Identify and support centres with expertise in obesity prevention research and assessment within academic institutions
- Establish knowledge-exchange mechanisms to share evidence and experiences.

SUPPORT SYSTEMS FOR POLICY IMPLEMENTATION

- Adopt nutrient profiling systems to underpin food and nutrition policies (e.g. front-of-pack traffic light labelling, and regulations on marketing to children)
- Support healthy food-service policies implemented by public and private sector organizations and support physical activity
- Set standards and guidelines for local authorities to create environments for active transport and recreation.

WORKFORCE CAPACITY AND DEVELOPMENT

- Employ sufficient, skilled staff within the prevention workforce
- Include nutrition, physical activity and the prevention of obesity within curricula for health and related professionals (e.g. planners, teachers, child care workers)
- Expand quality postgraduate courses, including PhD opportunities, within LMICs.

PARTNERSHIPS, ORGANIZATIONAL RELATIONSHIPS AND NETWORKS FOR COORDINATION

- Instigate cross-sectoral structures at the national and state level to coordinate activities across governments, non-governmental organizations, private sectors and at the local level.

COMMUNICATIONS

- Communicate and update national guidelines for individuals on healthy eating and physical activity
- Establish and communicate national targets for the food industry on food composition, marketing to children and food claims
- Provide consistent messages through effective social marketing communications that motivate individuals to adopt healthy lifestyles and create healthy environments for others, especially children.

Modified from: Gortmaker SL, Swinburn BA, Levy D, et al. Changing the future of obesity: science, policy and action. Lancet 2011;378:838–47.

BOX 78.3 KEY ACTIONS FOR INTERNATIONAL AGENCIES, THE PRIVATE SECTOR, CIVIL SOCIETY, HEALTH PROFESSIONALS AND INDIVIDUALS FOR THE PREVENTION OF OBESITY

INTERNATIONAL AGENCIES

- The UN, its Member States and agencies, should provide global leadership through commitments for increased funding and policy support for prevention of obesity and non-communicable diseases
- The protection and maintenance of public health should be considered in relevant trade, economic, agriculture, environment, food and health agreements and policies
- The UN should implement and coordinate policies and funding to prevent obesity and non-communicable diseases across its agencies
- WHO should develop global standards, particularly for food and beverage marketing to children and for nutrient profiling.

PRIVATE SECTOR

- Processed food and beverage industries should reformulate existing products and develop new ones with healthier nutrient compositions, particularly through feasible reductions in sugar, salt, and unhealthy fat
- Food and beverage, and communications industries should apply voluntary restrictions on all forms of marketing promotions of foods high in sugar, salt and unhealthy fat to children and adolescents
- Food and beverage industries, and food retailers should ensure food labelling, packaging and health claims meet high standards in all countries
- The private sector needs to use all available strategies to support public health efforts to create healthier food systems
- Relevant industries need to support efforts to monitor progress towards healthier food systems by the sharing of relevant data, which helps governments to assess progress towards targets while protecting commercially sensitive information.

CIVIL SOCIETY

- Alliances and networks could be formed to share information, build the constituency for change, and advocate for the policies and programmes to reduce obesity
- Policies and practices of the other parties should be monitored. Civil society should hold these parties to account for their actions, inactions, or counteractions in relation to promotion of healthier environments and reduction of obesity and chronic disease.

HEALTH PROFESSIONALS

- Health professionals need to monitor the weight of patients and offer suitable evidence-informed advice about maintaining a healthy body weight
- Physicians should provide continuing support (or refer for support) to those patients ready to undertake a weight-loss programme.

INDIVIDUALS

- Parents and caretakers should act as role models for health-promoting behaviours for children and adolescents
- Individuals need to make healthy food and activity choices, and help to create healthy food and physical activity environments in homes and other settings, such as schools, workplaces, sports clubs, churches and community organizations.

Adapted from The Lancet. Gortmaker SL, Swinburn BA, Levy D, et al. Changing the future of obesity: science, policy and action. Lancet 2011;378:838–47. Copyright 2011, with permission from Elsevier.

Comprehensive prevention strategy analyses, such as the UK Foresight project,[34] now recognize the need for a whole system approach to obesity prevention encompassing both the individual and population levels. The challenge of tackling obesity has been likened to that of tackling climate change, recognizing the enormous challenge facing societies in stemming the rise of disease involving such multifaceted causes. Both require whole societal change with cross-governmental commitment and action by industry, communities, families and society as a whole. A recent summary of a systems approach to obesity prevention identified important core actions for governments and wider society to adopt if prevention strategies are to be successful (Boxes 78.2, 78.3).[35] As identified by this review, country-level policies are not on their own sufficient to stem the rising tide of obesity in a world where the food system is increasingly globalized and dominated by powerful multinational companies. Again, in common with climate change, global strategies and consensus will be required for the root causes of the epidemic to be addressed and for changes to be maintained in the long term.

REFERENCES

1. Finucane MM, Stevens GA, Cowan MJ, et al. National, regional, and global trends in body-mass index since 1980: systematic analysis of health examination surveys and epidemiological studies with 960 country-years and 9.1 million participants. Lancet 2011;377:557–67.
10. Popkin BM, Adair LS, Ng SW. Global nutrition transition and the pandemic of obesity in developing countries. Nutr Rev 2012;70:3–21.
15. Whitlock G, Lewington S, Sherliker P, et al. Body-mass index and cause-specific mortality in 900 000 adults: collaborative analyses of 57 prospective studies. Lancet 2009;373:1083–96.
23. Wells JCK, Fewtrell MS. Measuring body composition. Arch Dis Child 2006;91:612–17.
35. Gortmaker SL, Swinburn BA, Levy D, et al. Changing the future of obesity: science, policy, and action. Lancet 2011;378:838–47.

Access the complete references online at www.expertconsult.com

Obstetrics in the Tropics

ROSE MCGREADY | GLEN D. LIDDELL MOLA | MARCUS A. J. RIJKEN | FRANÇOIS H. NOSTEN | THEONEST MUTABINGWA

KEY POINTS

- Based on data from 2005, the average lifetime risk of dying from complications related to pregnancy or childbirth increases 300-fold and the lifetime risk of women dying due to pregnancy-related issues increases up to 1000-fold in the least developed countries.[1] Maternal deaths could be mostly preventable with the well-known prevention or management solutions, which can be implemented when there is an accessible, equitable and basically functional health system.
- In the rural tropics, pregnant women are just as susceptible to the common infections observed in pregnancy in developed countries, e.g. pyelonephritis. However, in the tropics, there are many more challenging infections, e.g. malaria, TB, syphilis, HIV, etc. that need to be diagnosed and treated with effective medicines.
- In tropical countries, cultural and socioeconomic issues commonly have more impact on women in pregnancy. In developing countries, many women do not have access to services or the capacity to control their fertility, which can lead to unplanned and inappropriately timed pregnancies which can sometimes be life-threatening. High-resource settings support planned caesarean section for breech presentation and post-term induction but caesarean section may be less safe in low-resource settings. Caesarean section increases the risks for pathological placental conditions and the risk of uterine rupture or dehiscence in the next pregnancy. Hence, a different risk–benefit assessment due to restricted access and finance in low-resource settings is required.
- Tropical infections in pregnant women require prompt treatment. In severe disease, the aim of treatment is to save the life of the mother and prevent functional disability. Life-saving presumptive treatments should not be withheld because of an inability to obtain rapid results to diagnostic tests or for fear of fetal compromise.
- Constructive and well-timed antenatal visits provide a window of opportunity to identify high-risk pregnancies, optimize the woman's health and to assist in delivery planning and postpartum family planning, before the woman goes into labour.
- Access to safe delivery and planning for expected and unexpected events is associated with reduced maternal and neonatal death. Waiting rooms can be ideal for rural or difficult-to-access areas; however, the resources required to provide food and care during this period are usually the main constraints on their effective use.
- Staff who train and practice emergency obstetric care in clean facilities with simple but working equipment, will provide better maternal and neonatal outcomes than home-birthed women, even when there is a health worker in attendance, because of the difficulties in transferring women to referral facilities if complications arise.
- Neonatal survival is closely linked with antenatal, peripartum and postnatal care. Correct resuscitation and appropriate use of antibiotics will greatly increase neonatal survival. The prospect of improved neonatal survival is one of the most important advocacy tools for encouraging women to come to facilities for a supervised birth.
- Maternal health care starts before pregnancy begins and strengthening pre-pregnancy counselling (in developing countries this should take place in the community and in part, a component in the primary school curricula), post-abortion care and family planning, will impact significantly on maternal and neonatal mortality and morbidity.
- Promising 'low-tech' interventions for pregnant women in developing countries include use of the partograph, with continuous support in labour, symphysiotomy, therapeutic manoeuvres for shoulder dystocia, improved management of intra-amniotic infections and vacuum extraction to assist vaginal delivery comes.[2]

Introduction

This chapter cannot attempt to provide all the obstetric or perinatal knowledge that is needed to work in the tropics. The Millennium Development Goals have led to a wealth of freely available online materials addressing maternal and infant mortality and health, many of which are referred to at: http://www.who.int/topics/maternal_health/en/ (Table 79.1).[3]

This chapter highlights the common pitfalls related to obstetrics in the tropics and provides readers with the core approaches to providing effective maternity care at each level to reduce maternal and perinatal mortality and morbidity.

Geographic Distribution of Obstetrics Indicators in the Tropics

It is generally accepted that high maternal mortality is the dominant problem in reproductive health in most places in developing countries. The solutions to problems relating to

TABLE 79.1 Reference Resource List of Reading Materials on Maternal and Newborn Care

WEB ACCESS SITE AND TYPE OF DOCUMENT AVAILABLE (ALL ACCESSED 4 AUG 2013)
HTTP://PORTAL.PMNCH.ORG/EFFECTIVE-INTERVENTIONS.
The Partnership for Maternal, Newborn & Child Health. 2011. A Global Review of the Key Interventions Related to Reproductive, Maternal, Newborn and Child Health (RMMCH).[3] Joint document led by the World Health Organization, Switzerland and the Aga Khan University, Pakistan. Experts in maternal, newborn and child health participated in meetings in Geneva in April 2010 and September 2011 and provided inputs to the development and finalization of this document.
HTTP://RIGHTTOMATERNALHEALTH.ORG/
The International Initiative on Maternal Mortality and Human Rights site with documents on maternal mortality, field projects and resources.
HTTP://WWW.PIH.ORG/PRIORITY-PROGRAMS/WOMENS-HEALTH
Partners in Health site with documents on maternal health, projects and resources.
HTTP://WWW.FPAINDIA.ORG
Family Planning India site with documents on Maternal and Child Health, Family Planning, Adolescent Reproductive and Sexual Health, Management of RTI/STI.
HTTP://WWW.POPCOUNCIL.ORG/TOPICS/MNH.ASP
The Population Council site with documents on a wide range of Maternal and Newborn Health Issues.
HTTP://WWW.RCOG.ORG.UK/GUIDELINES?UTM_SOURCE=QL&UTM_MEDIUM=QL&UTM_CAMPAIGN=GTG
Guidelines developed by the Royal College of Obstetrics and Gynaecology (RCOG) are an educational aid to good clinical practice. They present recognized methods and techniques of clinical practice, based on published evidence, for consideration by obstetricians/ gynaecologists and other relevant health professionals. While the standard of clinical investigations and treatment are for resource-rich settings a surprising proportion of the guidelines can be used directly in resource-poor settings.
HTTP://WWW.GFMER.CH/000_HOMEPAGE_EN.HTM
The Geneva Foundation for Medical Education and Research (GFMER) is a non-profit organisation established in 2002 with the objective of furnishing health education and research programmes that can be applied by developing countries, and countries in economic transition, and to establish collaboration between entities from the public and private sectors.

maternal mortality are not technically difficult. They tend to be brought about by insufficient political leadership, commitment and will to implement integrated maternal health programmes.[4,5]

Maternal mortality is highest in developing countries, especially in sub-Saharan Africa and South-east Asia (Figure 79.1), where an estimated 1000 women die every day from complications relating to childbirth.[6] Predominantly, economic disparity with inequities in access to health services such as antenatal (Figure 79.2), delivery and postpartum care (including family planning), increase the risk of maternal death in low-income people living in rural and urban areas, even within the same country.[7] In many areas, adolescents face a higher complication and death rate than other pregnant women.[8] The definition of maternal death extends from conception to 42 days after the end of pregnancy regardless of the duration and site of the pregnancy, from any cause related to or aggravated by the pregnancy or its management but not from accidental or incidental causes.[6] The risk of death is highest close to birth, with 60% of deaths occurring in the immediate postpartum period and in deliveries attended by unskilled birth attendants with the highest maternal mortality ratio (Figure 79.3).

According to WHO, severe bleeding, infections, high blood pressure during pregnancy (pre-eclampsia and eclampsia), obstructed labour and unsafe abortion, are the major complications responsible for 80% of all maternal deaths.[9] HIV has aggravated maternal mortality in some countries.[10] In the WHO systematic review of maternal deaths,[9] only 37 of 126 datasets in the analysis for individual causes were able to confirm the cause of death. While a lack of data on the cause of pregnancy-related death in rural and resource-poor settings probably results in under-estimation of the contribution from tropical and infectious diseases, as there are difficulties obtaining robust data.

Organization of Maternity Care in Developing Countries

Pregnancy-related death is complex, difficult to count comprehensively and large regional differences exist. For developing countries, international agencies have given more credence to estimates based upon mathematical modelling rather than local empirical data. Local deaths need to be counted and documented accurately in order for change to occur.[11]

A study in Mozambique noted that violence was the fourth highest cause of maternal death.[12] Sadly, most women remain silent about violence by an intimate partner and do not seek help.[8]

In order to obtain improvements in maternal and perinatal health, health systems, health workers and health promotion are crucial components to provide a continuum of care and universal coverage with skilled care at every birth. Too often, these components are not well integrated in low-income countries resulting in drainage of meagre resources from those who can least afford it. The 56 components of essential interventions to reduce maternal and neonatal mortality are summarized in Table 79.2.

Family planning is another crucial part of effective maternity care to minimize maternal and perinatal mortality and morbidity.[11] Family planning decision-making counselling and availability of contraceptives should be available at every point of care in the health system.

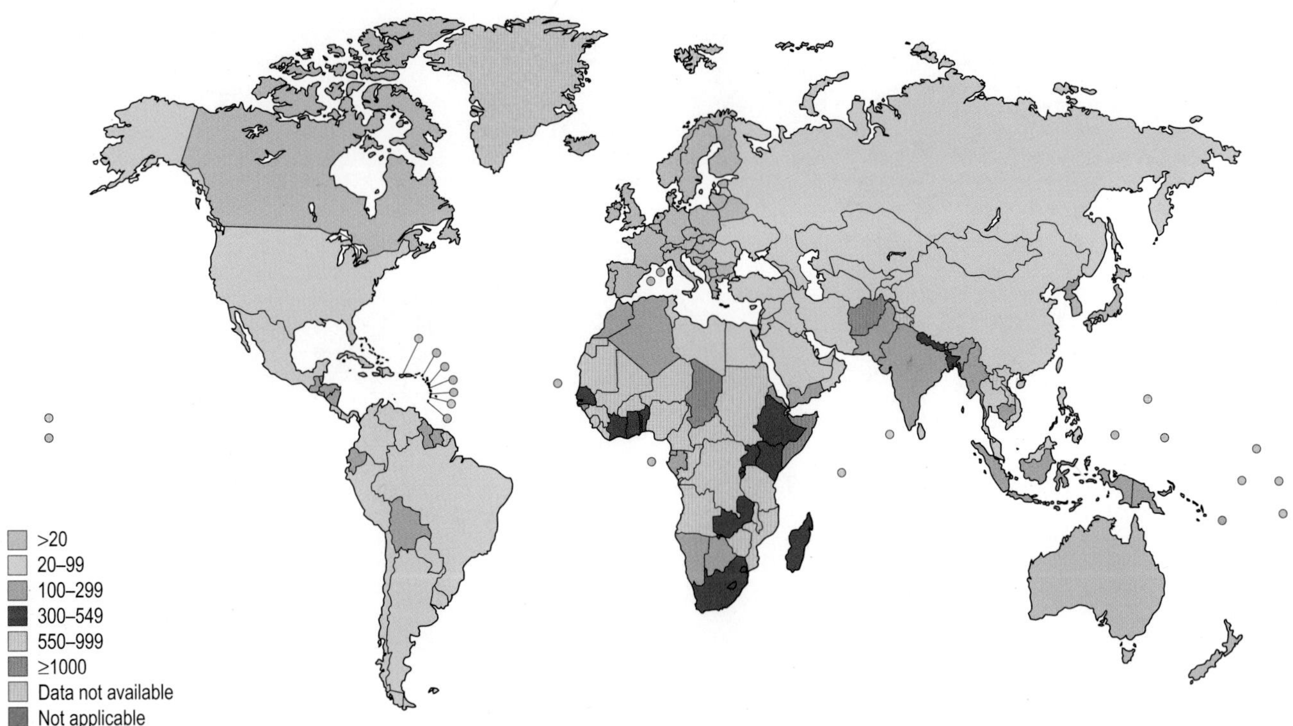

Figure 79.1 Maternal mortality ratio (per 100 000 live births), 2008. *(Reproduced with permission from World Health Organization, http://gamapserver.who.int/mapLibrary/Files/Maps/Global_MDG5_2011_MaternalMortality.png.)*

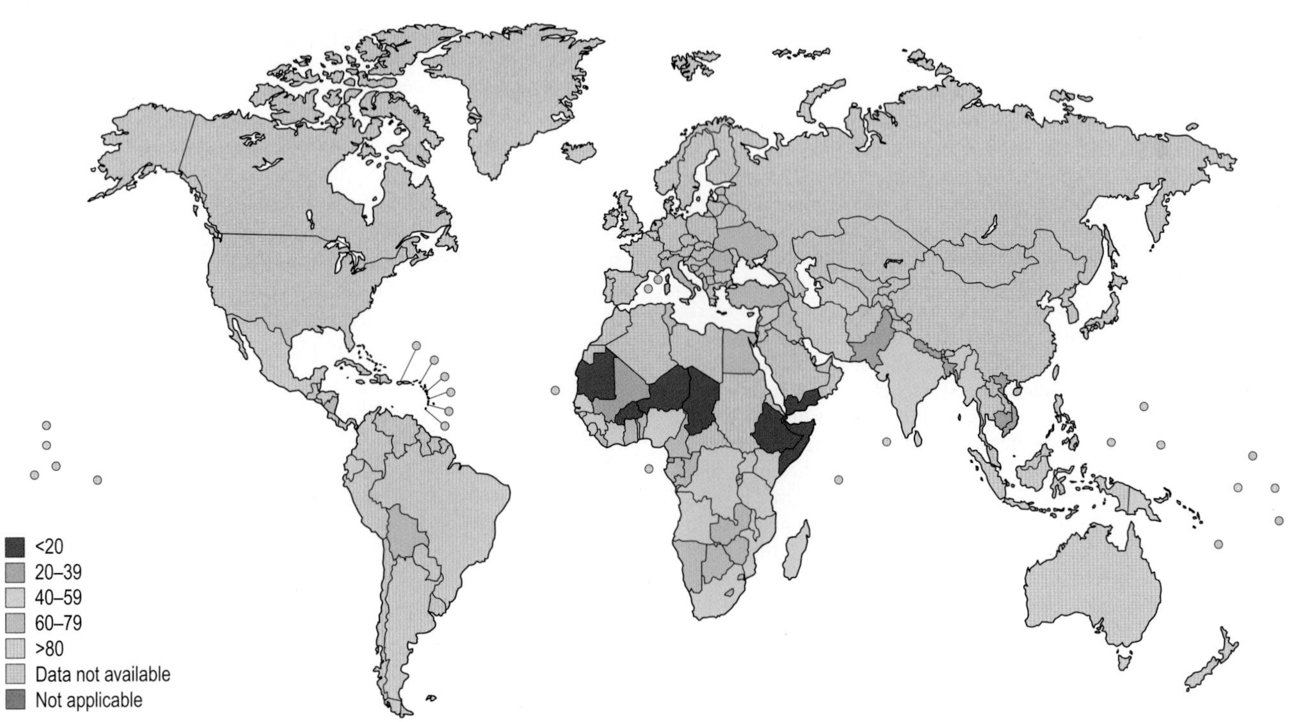

Figure 79.2 Antenatal coverage (% of women reporting 4+ visits), 2000–2010. *(Reproduced with permission from World Health Organization, Figure:* http://gamapserver.who.int/mapLibrary/Files/Maps/Global_MDG5_2011_Antenatal.png.*)*

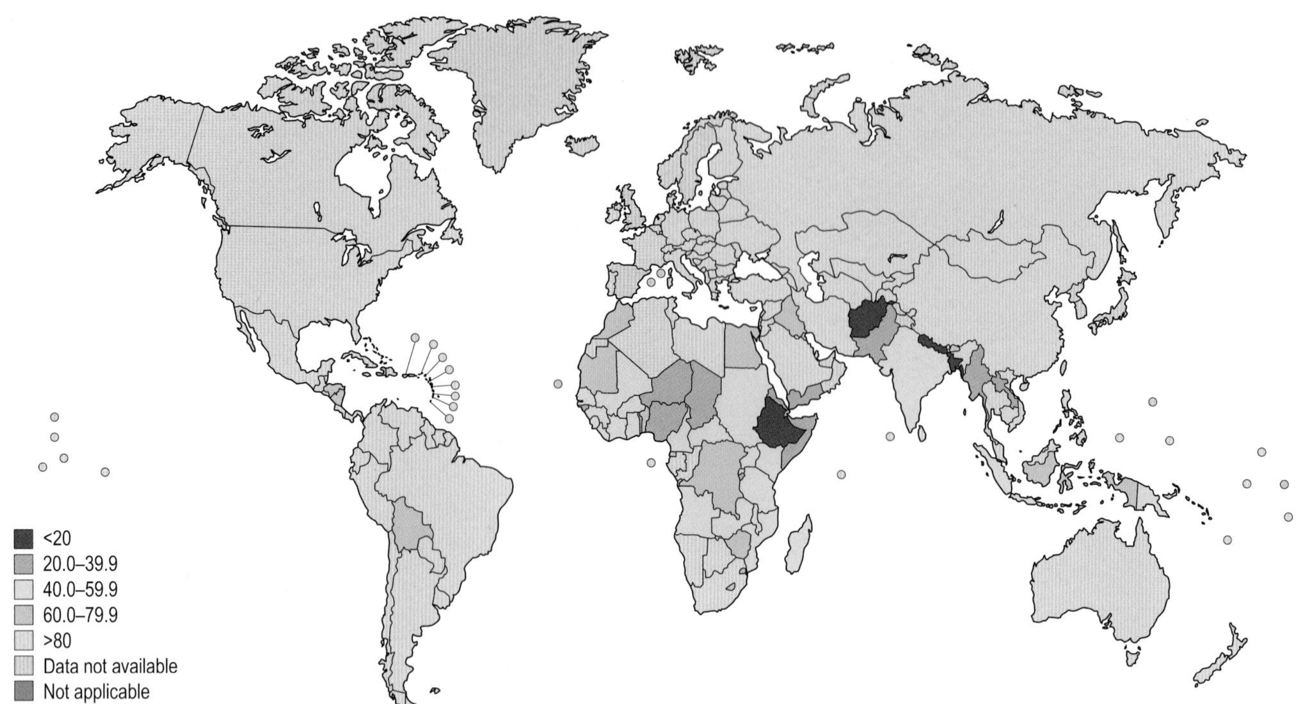

Figure 79.3 Proportion of births attended by skilled health personnel (%), 1993–2010. *(Reproduced with permission from World Health Organization, http://gamapserver.who.int/mapLibrary/Files/Maps/Global_MDG5_ProportionBirth_1993_2010.png.)*

CASE STUDY

A mother of two in Myanmar goes to the antenatal clinic on Monday. It takes 1.5 hours to get there and costs half a daily wage for transport costs but the baby is due in the next month. On Tuesday, she feels unwell and goes to have her malaria smear checked at the nearest out-patient department. Her malaria smear is negative so she returns home still feverish. On Wednesday, she returns to the antenatal clinic where they find she has pyelonephritis and admit her for treatment. It is difficult to look after her youngest child while unwell as her husband is doing farm work and cannot help and they do not have relatives in the village. Unfortunately, she has HIV and has to request discharge against medical advice to get her monthly ARVs, supplied by a different hospital. Missing the scheduled appointment makes her fearful of being seen as unreliable and she wants to keep taking the medication. Luckily, the hospital staff understand her predicament and ask her to continue oral treatment for the pyelonephritis. It costs twice the daily wage to reach the HIV clinic but she only has to go once per month. On Friday, her youngest child has a high fever and a cough and again half a daily wage goes towards the cost of reaching the clinic. The blood smear of the child is positive for malaria and is treated free of charge. She feels the trip was worth it because he already looks a bit better. On Friday night, her husband becomes angry that she used so much money this week; he beats his wife up. Thereafter, she develops abdominal pain and collapses. There is not enough money left to pay for a taxi to take her to the clinic. She dies. Nobody follows-up when she does not turn up at antenatal care because they think she had a home birth and the PMTCT team think she has defaulted by moving from the catchment area, like many others before her. Her death is never registered.

ADOLESCENT AND PRE-PREGNANCY CARE

The role of adolescent and pre-pregnancy care is to provide friendly, accessible services for the provision of family planning and pre-pregnancy supplements in preparation for a healthy pregnancy. The ability of the service to diagnose and treat STI and HIV (or referral to appropriate centres) is important in this group of potential pregnant women who are at high risk in some parts of the world.[8] In many sub-Saharan African countries more than 70% of young women have sexual encounters in their teenage years and more than 20% of adolescents have their first child by the age of 18.[13] Glasier et al. reported that in the developing world, girls aged under 15 years are more likely to have premature labour and are four times more likely to die from pregnancy-related causes than women aged 20 years and above.[8] In the developed world, where contraceptive use is high, governments are concerned about teenage pregnancy, as this often leads to single motherhood, disrupted education, social isolation and repeat cycles of unintended pregnancy. While the uptake of contraception in developed countries is not a major problem, there is widespread failure to use a method consistently and correctly.[14]

ANTENATAL CARE

The role of antenatal care in determining pregnancy outcome depends on the location.[4] In much of the rural tropics, living standards are poor, much of the population is malnourished, literacy and education rates low and health is undermined by many prevalent endemic diseases. Antenatal care provides an

TABLE 79.2 Essential, Evidence-based Interventions to Reduce Reproductive, Maternal Newborn and Child Mortality, and Promote Reproductive Health

ontinuum of Care	Adolescence and Pre-Pregnancy	Pregnancy (Antenatal)	Childbirth	Postnatal (Mother)	Postnatal (Newborn)	Infancy and Childhood
ALL LEVELS COMMUNITY PRIMARY REFERRAL	• Family planning (advice, hormonal and barrier) • Prevent and manage sexually transmitted infections, HIV • Folic acid fortification/ supplementation to prevent neural tube defects	• Iron and folic acid supplementation • Tetanus vaccination • Prevention and management of malaria with insecticide treated nets and antimalarial medicines • Prevention and management of sexually transmitted infections and HIV, including with antiretroviral medicines • Calcium supplementation to prevent hypertension (high blood pressure) • Interventions for cessation of smoking	• Prophylactic uterotonics to prevent postpartum haemorrhage (excessive bleeding after birth) • Manage postpartum haemorrhage using uterine massage and uterotonics • Social support during childbirth	• Family planning advice and contraceptives • Nutrition counseling	• Immediate thermal care (to keep the baby warm) • Initiation of early breast feeding (within the first hour) • Hygienic cord and skin care	• Exclusive breast feeding for 6 months • Continued breastfeeding and complementary breastfeeding from 6 months • Prevention and case management of childhood malaria • Vitamin A supplementation from 6 months • Routine immunization plus *H.influenzae*, meningococcal, pneumococcal and rotavirus vaccines • Management of severe acute malnutrition • Case management of childhood pneumonia • Case management of diarrhoea
PRIMARY AND REFERRAL	• Family planning (hormonal, barrier and selected surgical methods)	• Screening for and treatment of syphilis • Low dose aspirin to prevent pre-eclampsia • Antihypertensive drugs (to treat high blood pressure) • Magnesium sulphate for eclampsia • Antibiotics for preterm prelabour rupture of membranes • Corticosteroids to prevent respiratory distress syndrome in preterm babies • Safe abortion • Post abortion care	Active management of 3rd stage of labour (to deliver the placenta) to prevent postpartum haemorrhage (as above) Management of postpartum haemorrhage (as above	• Screen for and initiate or continue antiretroviral therapy for HIV • Treat maternal anaemia	• Neonatal resuscitation with bag and mask (by professional health workers for babies who do not breathe at birth) • Kangaroo mother care for preterm (premature) and for less than 2000g • Extra support for feeding small and preterm babies • Management of newborns with Jaundice ("yellow" newborns) • Initiate prophylactic antiretroviral therapy for babies exposed to HIV	• Comprehensive care of children infected with, or exposed to , HIV
REFERRAL*	• Family planning (surgical methods)	• Reduce malpresentation at term with External Cephalic Version • Induction of labour to manage prelabour rupture of membranes at term (initiate labour)	• Caesarean section for maternal/fetal indication (to save the life of the mother/ baby) • Prophylactic antibiotic for caesarean section	• Detect and manage postpartum sepsis (serious infections after birth)	• Presumptive antibiotic therapy for newborns at risk of bacterial infection • Use of surfactant (respiratory medication) to prevent respiratory distress syndrome in preterm babies • Continuous positive airway pressure (CPAP) to manage babies with respiratory distress syndrome • Case management of neonatal sepsis, meningitis and pneumonia	• Case Management of meningitis
COMMUNITY STRATEGIES	• Home visits for women and children across the continuum of care • Women's groups			*Family planning interventions at Referral level include those provided at the Primary level		

Detailed online http://www.who.int/pmnch/knowledge/publications/201112_essential_interventions/en/index1.html

TABLE 79.3 **Antenatal Interventions Known to be Effective**[16]

Condition/Stage	Test/Treatment	Effect
Reduced number of antenatal care visits	Reductions to 4–5 antenatal visits, including proven effective interventions	Similar maternal results
Delivering antenatal care visits	Midwife/general practitioner-managed care compared with obstetrician/gynaecologist-led shared care	Similar clinical effectiveness
Prevention of anaemia	Routine supplementation with iron and folate during pregnancy	Reduces or prevents fall in haemoglobin. Reduces percentage of anaemic women
	Malaria chemoprophylaxis	Reduces percentage of women who become anaemic
Detection and investigation of anaemia	Copper sulphate densitometry test	Detects haemoglobin level below chose cut-off point
	Colorimetric tests	Estimates haemoglobin concentration
	Coulter counter	Diagnosis of type of anaemia
	Blood film microscopy	Diagnosis of type of anaemia and of malaria
Treatment of iron-deficiency anaemia	Oral iron and folate	Can raise Hb by 0.4–0.7 g/dL per week
	Intramuscular and intravenous iron	Can raise Hb at same rate as oral. Avoids problems of compliance but need IM or IV equipment and trained staff. Danger of anaphylaxis
	Packed cell transfusion	Raises Hb immediately. Hazards of blood transfusion-infection (HIV-hepatitis) and fluid overload. Need for equipment and trained staff
Detection and investigation of HDP	Measurement of blood pressure with sphygmomanometer using fifth Korotkoff sound	Detects hypertension
	Urinalysis of clean catch urine	Detects proteinuria. Indicative of pre-eclampsia in presence of hypertension
Treatment of severe pre-eclampsia	Transfer to first referral level for expert care	Control of disease. Reduces case fatality
Treatment of eclampsia	Supportive first aid maintaining airway and preventing injury during fit	Reduces case fatality
	Magnesium sulphate (IM or IV)	Reduces recurrent convulsions and maternal mortality
	Recognition and speedy transfer to fully equipped facility	Reduces case fatality
	Expedited delivery	Only definite treatment
Prevention of obstructed labour	External cephalic version at term	Reduces caesarean section
Screening for infection	Serological screening and treatment for syphilis	Detects asymptomatic disease. Coupled with effective treatment, contact tracing and follow-up, reduces fetal loss and maternal and infant morbidity
	Microbiological screening for gonorrhoea	Detects asymptomatic disease. Coupled with effective treatment, contact tracing and follow-up, reduces fetal loss and maternal and infant morbidity
	Screening for bacteriuria with quantitative culture of urine	Detects asymptomatic disease. Coupled with effective treatment prevents pyelonephritis and preterm delivery/low birth weight
Prevention of infection	Tetanus immunization in pregnancy and/or women of child-bearing age	Prevents maternal and neonatal tetanus
	Induction of labour in uncomplicated pre-labour rupture of membranes	Prevents maternal infection

important opportunity to improve the health of pregnant women and provide prophylaxis and treatment for common but dangerous conditions in pregnancy such as malaria and anaemia. Gestational assessment is also critical to assist women in making effective plans for safe labour and delivery and to gain their trust and confidence, so that when pregnancy complications requiring interventions develop, such procedures take place at the right time, right place and under optimal conditions. The number of antenatal visits that provide this in developing country settings is still contentious,[15] however, it is clear that for antenatal care to be effective, it must be focused and goal-orientated.

Antenatal care has three main components:

Screening for Risk Factors and Care Referral

Risks include both pregnancy complications and associated diseases and socioeconomic and demographic factors that cause pregnancy complications to occur more commonly.

Accurate gestational assessment is absolutely critical to effective pregnancy care; the best opportunity for accurate gestational assessment is as early in the pregnancy as possible. This is one of the reasons that women should be encouraged to book at the antenatal clinic as soon as they think they might be pregnant (Table 79.3).[16]

The history taken at the booking visit is the most important source of information on obstetric risk and is crucial in planning prenatal, labour and delivery and postpartum care, including appropriate advice for family planning decision-making.[17] Structured methods of taking the antenatal history used during the first antenatal visit generates more and better information and leads to improved clinical responses. This may be the first examination a female in a tropical country has received since childhood at which some congenital abnormalities, e.g. congenital heart disease, or childhood acquired diseases, e.g. rheumatic heart disease, may be detected. Other serious medical conditions may be diagnosed, e.g. tuberculosis, or become more overt due to pregnancy-related physiological changes, e.g. hyperthyroidism.

Monitoring of BP and proteinuria for the detection of pre-eclampsia, weight gain or loss for nutritional assessment or as a measure of poor or deteriorating placental function[11] or other disease, e.g. tuberculosis, haematocrit or haemoglobin for anaemia, measurement of symphysis-fundal height for fetal growth, abdominal palpation for malpresentation and multiple pregnancy, screening for malaria at every antenatal visit by microscopy of malaria smear or rapid detection test, all constitute routine care. Screening for syphilis and HIV can be life-saving for the fetus. Screening for STIs, diabetes and ABO blood group system and early (1st trimester) ultrasound examination for accurate estimation of gestational age, placental location, multiple pregnancy and viability would also occur subject to availablility.[17,18]

The concept of four antenatal visits in low-risk women has been recommended without considering malaria.[15]

Identification of risk factors to assist with appropriate counselling about the appropriate facility for supervision of the labour and delivery:

1. First pregnancy
2. Age younger than 19 or older than 40 years
3. Five or more previous births
4. Short or small stature
5. History of caesarean section (or other uterine surgery, e.g. myomectomy)
6. Previous history of major obstetric complications, subfertility, complicated deliveries, vesicovaginal fistula repair, blood transfusion, fetal, neonatal death or child loss.
7. Pre-existing medical conditions, e.g. diabetes

Disease Prevention, Detection and Treatment

Specific measures against anaemia, malaria, tetanus, syphilis, HIV, helminthic infestations (e.g. schistosomiasis, hookworm) and STI are efficacious out-patient-based interventions which are cost-effective.[17,18] In sub-Saharan Africa, health education on the prevention of these diseases is normally delivered to all attendants of reproductive child health (RCH) as the first activity of the clinic before dispersion to individual units, e.g. antenatal, family planning, immunization, etc. Advice to cease or at least reduce smoking, alcohol, recreational drugs and/or betel nut use is recommended but has limited success.[17,18]

Health Education and Health Promotion

Packages should include:

- Basic hygiene
- Nutrition
- Routine haematinics
- Traditional cultural practices in relation to reproductive health
- Encouraging appropriate and safe delivery place
- Breast-feeding
- Newborn care
- Child vaccination
- Decision-making on postpartum family planning
- Instructions on danger signs in pregnancy such as vaginal bleeding
- Preterm premature rupture of membranes
- Sudden generalized oedema
- The use of support persons in labour
- Caesarean risks
- Compliance with treatment and prophylaxis.

All these issues are more effectively handled when partners (men) are involved in the discussions and decision-making. For this reason, it is important that men are specifically invited to attend antenatal clinics and be present (also as support persons where appropriate) for their wives.[19]

MEDICAL EMERGENCIES IN PREGNANT WOMEN

After stabilization of the patient the obstetric team needs to be consulted for all admitted pregnant women with severe medical problems such as cerebral malaria, pyelonephritis or undifferentiated febrile illness, to monitor the condition of the fetus, advise on optimal timing of delivery or provide management for expected pre-term labour. A multidisciplinary team approach can be beneficial in big hospitals and when carried out in a coordinated manner, can reduce maternal and neonatal mortality and long-term disabilities. In some district hospital settings, it is often more efficient to care for pregnant women with medical problems in the antenatal ward where the nursing staff are more knowledgeable and experienced in pregnancy and labour issues.

UNBOOKED EMERGENCIES

These are the women who fail to receive antenatal care and arrive at the healthcare facility for the first time when labour is already complicated or worsened with coincidental disease. For example, obstructed labour can be complicated by haemorrhage, septic shock and a ruptured uterus. Neglected medical problems such as moderate anaemia and untreated malaria become very significant complications when the woman is brought to hospital with a retained placenta. Unbooked emergencies have high anaesthetic and operative risks. In areas where resources are limited, a disproportionate share of resources can be spent on unbooked emergencies compromising the care of booked healthy women in labour, with adverse effects on their labour outcomes.

Each obstetric team needs to have a protocol for rapid work-up of these patients. More peripheral facilities need standard management and referral protocols for effective triage, emergency resuscitation and stabilization prior to urgent transfer.

PREGNANT MOTHER HOUSE OR MATERNITY VILLAGES

Accommodation located near to or inside the hospital can provide a safe place where women with complicated pregnancies or those who live in remote areas can wait for delivery; their presence on site for extended periods can be an opportunity to give detailed health education and promotion. Local cultural and economic needs may not always permit this arrangement to occur. These houses need security, supervision and clean water, adequate food, cooking, washing and toilet facilities.

DELIVERY CARE

The ability to reduce maternal and neonatal mortality is heavily dependent on having trained personnel to attend to women in labour. While intrapartum care aims to avert intrapartum-related hypoxic injury, rigorous evidence is lacking, especially in the settings where most deaths occur.[3]

Every woman who commences care in the labour room must have her antenatal card scrutinized for relevant information and for the special care required in labour. Personal and family data, demographic status, results of laboratory tests, past obstetric history and progress during the current antenatal period, should be reviewed. Progress in labour charted on a partograph is an action-oriented tool that can lead to early effective management for prolonged labour and appropriate referral to the next level of care in cases that require augmentation of poor contractions, assisted vaginal delivery, or caesarean section. Clean birthing (the woman, the attendants and the place of birth) and attention to asepsis during birthing care and quick recourse to antibiotics, including parenteral ampicillin, gentamicin and metronidazole treatment when there is evidence of endometritis or puerperal sepsis, can have a major impact on reducing the risk of serious morbidity and mortality from postpartum sepsis. In a supervised birth with trained attendants, it is possible to provide active management of the third stage with syntocinon and resuscitation, as well as added measures to staunch blood loss and referral if needed, which can be life-saving for woman suffering postpartum haemorrhage. Delayed cord clamping may be more useful in the tropics than in developed countries where it is now being promoted to reduce infant anaemia. Early detection of pre-eclampsia, control of dangerously high BP with methyldopa, nifedipine or hydralazine, prevention of fits with magnesium sulphate and proper management of the rest of the pregnancy and birth, can prevent many deaths from severe pre-eclampsia and eclampsia. Correct identification and repair of perineal injuries should be incorporated to routine delivery room care.

All staff need constant reminding of the importance of completing the details of the birth register and hospital records. For auditing purposes, a weekly summary of perinatal events is useful feedback to staff. This should include details of low-birth-weight infants, perinatal deaths, multiple births, operative deliveries, vaginal breech delivery and intrapartum complications and their treatment. The formal presentation of these perinatal events should take place at regular perinatal audit session that should be compulsory for medical, midwifery and nursing staff.

NEONATAL CARE

The principles of neonatal resuscitation, umbilical cord care to avoid haemorrhage and infection, the provision of warmth, establishment of breast-feeding and early transfer to the special care baby unit if the need arises, are core components of neonatal care and must be taught to all health workers supervising labour and delivery care.

The first 30–60 seconds of a baby's life are critical. Many neonates will be saved if standard evidence-based care for the neonate is practiced by birth attendants. This will include fairly vigorous drying of the baby's skin to dry it and stimulate respiration. If there is thick meconium present and the baby has not yet taken a breath, the upper airway, nose and pharynx can be gently sucked out before bag and mask resuscitation is commenced. During the first 30–60 seconds of the baby's life and while the attendant is drying the baby, assessment is also being made as to its condition. If there is any doubt whether the baby is breathing normally at the end of 60 seconds, active resuscitation with bag and mask should begin with five slow inflation breaths.

Other routine neonatal care that should be carried out routinely immediately after birth includes:

- Hepatitis B vaccination
- Tetracycline (or chloramphenicol) ophthalmic ointment to prevent gonococcal ophthalmitis (when this is a problem in the community)
- Vitamin K injection to prevent haemorrhagic disease of the newborn
- Weighing, recording and completion of maternal and neonatal vital registration.

POSTNATAL CARE

In the absence of antenatal, delivery and postpartum problems and complications, early discharge can be encouraged. Primigravidae should stay at least 48 hours (or until breast-feeding is established), but multiparas (with a history of successful postnatal care) can be discharged after 24 hours. The baby should be breast-fed early, preferably in the first hour.

Instructions on postpartum care should be given to the woman and her family and a routine postnatal check on day 3–5 postpartum is useful to screen for babies with feeding problems, to encourage continuation of exclusive breast-feeding and to screen for neonatal sepsis. The woman should be told when to report back to the healthcare facility/hospital if she has excessive vaginal bleeding, fever, breast-feeding problems or the baby becomes jaundiced, drowsy or is not feeding well, or if they have any other problems.

Women with complicated deliveries are required to stay longer on the wards to ensure full recovery. At the end of the immediate postpartum period, health education should continue. The woman should be encouraged to return to the postnatal clinic for a postnatal check at 5–7 weeks to check again on exclusive breast-feeding, commence family planning, immunization for the baby and follow-up any problems that were found antenatally. It makes sense to time the post-natal visit with the neonatal vaccination at 6–8 weeks.

ACCESS TO LIFE-SAVING SKILLS, EMERGENCY OBSTETRIC AND NEONATAL CARE (EMONC)

Access to people trained in life-saving skills is highly relevant in reducing pregnancy mortality and morbidity.[5] Poor transportation and communication; poverty and lack of client-focused care that deter women from using available healthcare facilities; inadequately trained staff; failure to deliver prompt effective care and shortage of essential drugs and equipment, all contribute to a failure to access life-saving skills. To address transportation barriers, operational research is being contemplated in some African countries to assess the impact of providing subsidized transport vouchers to pregnant women near-term to enable them to attend the healthcare facility when labour starts.

Attempts to improve the lack of adequately trained and competent staff has been met with an array of materials and courses.[20] These include: *Advanced Life Support in Obstetrics* (ALSO) (see: http://www.also.net.au/ALSO-in-Developing-Nations), devised by the American Academy of Family Physicians and *Basic Life Support in Obstetrics* course (BLSO) for more junior staff. Theoretical and practical components are included: bleeding during pregnancy, pre-term labour, fetal monitoring, post-partum haemorrhage, forceps & vacuum delivery, shoulder dystocia, malpresentations, neonatal resuscitation, maternal resuscitation and all levels of maternity care providers are encouraged to participate, recognizing the multidisciplinary work of maternity care. In the UK, *Managing Obstetric Emergency and Trauma* (MOET) (see: http://www.alsg.org/uk/node/6) is more designed for tertiary facilities where there are specialists in every field and high-tech back-up is available in areas such as blood bank, intensive care and anaesthesia and the *Practical Obstetric Multi-Professional Training* course (PROMPT) (see: http://www.prompt-course.org) emphasizes teamwork. Some of these programmes have been assessed in developing countries, including a package of *Life Saving Skills – Essential Obstetric and Newborn Care Training* (LSS-EOC and NC) (see: http://www.rcog.org.uk/international/projects/life-saving-skills) designed specifically around the basic signal functions (maternal hypovolaemia and neonatal resuscitation, manual removal of the placenta, assisted vaginal delivery, parenteral antibiotics and magnesium sulphate administration and the extra two functions essential for the first referral level: blood transfusion and caesarean section) including seven countries in sub-Saharan Africa.[21] The *Pacific Emergency Obstetric and Newborn Care* programme (PEmOC) (see: http://www.psrh.org.nz/), which has recently been piloted in a number of remote Pacific island countries, has been designed so that it can be modified for roll out to various levels of health care workers from community health workers to doctors.

Developing countries should adapt international emergency obstetric and newborn training packages to suit their own circumstances and needs. These can be used in both pre-service and in-service training scenarios to improve the quality of emergency and neonatal care in facilities. Criteria-based clinical audit and regular perinatal audit can also be used to measure and improve quality of obstetric care for five life-threatening obstetric complications and should be encouraged.[22,23]

Obstetric Problems

There are many obstetric problems which are more common in the tropics than in developed countries and are often associated with worse outcomes:

ANAEMIA IN PREGNANCY

Anaemia is by far the most common complication of pregnancy worldwide and contributes significantly to maternal mortality.[3] Pregnancy is a period of high iron requirement. It is critical to address this as early as possible in pregnancy and preferably prenatally. However, there is still a problem with the definition of anaemia in pregnancy. The proposed WHO definition of anaemia in pregnancy is a haemoglobin of <110 g/L, or haematocrit of <33%, but haemoglobin levels vary with gestation and there is also doubt as to whether First World levels of haemoglobin have the same clinical significance in developing countries. Some studies suggest that optimal levels of haemoglobin in areas where malaria and chronic anaemia are common may be lower.[24] In tropical countries, accurate gestation and anaemia data are scarce. The prevalence of anaemia in the 3rd trimester when anaemia is more likely to affect the risk of mortality, is unknown in most areas.[25]

In women of reproductive age, as for other anaemic populations, iron deficiency is the main cause of anaemia due to a low intake of iron, poor absorption of iron from diets high in phytate or phenolic compounds, heavy hookworm burdens and frequent and closely spaced pregnancies. Acute and chronic infections, including malaria, tuberculosis, schistosomiasis and HIV, can also lower blood Hb concentrations. The presence of other micronutrient deficiencies, such as vitamins A and B12, folate, riboflavin, zinc and copper can increase the risk of anaemia.[25] Furthermore, the impact of haemoglobinopathies on anaemia prevalence needs to be considered within some populations. Since iron-deficiency anaemia develops slowly, dangerously low haemoglobin levels may be reached before women become symptomatic. Pregnancy complications can suddenly tip the balance from coping to catastrophic consequences.

IRON SUPPLEMENTATION

The dosage for iron supplementation in pregnancy is 60 mg elemental iron/day. Health promotion for pregnant women to comply with the supplements is useful. As the efficiency of absorption of iron increases as iron-deficiency anaemia becomes more severe, this dose should provide adequate supplemental iron to women who do not have clinically severe anaemia if it is given for an adequate duration. However, if the duration of supplementation during pregnancy is short, a higher dose (120 mg/day) is recommended. The ideal duration of iron therapy in pregnancy is long (6 months) and if this cannot be achieved in pregnancy supplementation into the postpartum period should be continued.

Iron overload in thalassaemia needs to be considered (see Haemoglobinopathies, below). In women unable to tolerate oral iron or with malabsorption, parenteral iron can be given while adhering to the necessary precautions in case of an allergic response. Iron levels with parenteral iron do not build up more quickly than with oral iron. Either way, a response in haemoglobin levels should be evident within 4 weeks. Death from cardiac failure may occur with haemoglobin levels below 4 g/dL if the onset of the anaemia is acute; however, it is not uncommon to see women with levels below this figure who are oligosymptomatic when the anaemia has been very slow in onset and the compensatory right shift in the oxygen dissociation curve occurred. When blood transfusion needs to be administered to a very anaemic woman with complications (such as heart failure or evidence of anoxia) fluid balance must be carefully monitored and intravenous furosemide administered with each bag, preferably of packed cells, to ensure at least twice as much urine is passed as the volume of transfusion given, otherwise the patient may be tipped over into heart failure with fatal consequences.

Women whose haemoglobin level is between 4 and 7 g/dL are also at greater risk of dying from malaria infection or from the effects of perinatal haemorrhage. Blood losses of 500 mL that may be easily tolerated by a woman with a normal haemoglobin level may be fatal in the presence of severe anaemia. Other effects of severe anaemia in pregnancy include stillbirth, fetal growth restriction, fetal distress in labour and premature labour.[26] When a woman with moderate to severe anaemia comes into labour, venous access should be established and blood cross-matched in case she suffers a postpartum haemorrhage. Transfusion in resource-poor settings should be reserved for life-saving events because of the high incidence and prevalence of HIV, hepatitis B and C, syphilis and malaria. The mainstay of anaemia treatment should be to treat the cause and provide family planning to give time to rebuild iron stores and revert to normal haemoglobin concentrations.

Other local causes of anaemia, e.g. high hookworm loads or thalassaemia, should be considered in anaemic pregnant women. Dietary deficiencies may necessitate extra folate and B12 supplementation. The blood film is a useful tool for anaemia diagnosis. The microscope is also a valuable tool for identifying soil-transmitted helminths and assessing worm loads. A useful clinical approach is to give standard treatment for women with mild and moderate anaemia (which should include iron, folic acid, albendazole for women likely to have hookworm infestation and provide malaria treatment or prophylaxis as appropriate) and to investigate women who have severe anaemia (Hb <6 g/dL) or who fail to respond to 4 weeks of iron supplements and other standard treatment for anaemia in the local setting.

HAEMOGLOBINOPATHIES

Sickle cell anaemia and the thalassaemias are the most important inherited abnormalities of haemoglobin synthesis.[4]

Sickle Cell Disease

Sickle cell disease complications during pregnancy include sickle cell crisis affecting the bones and joints which can occur at any time during pregnancy, labour and the puerperium. Crises during the last 4 weeks of pregnancy and the first 4 days after delivery are more severe, necessitating immediate partial exchange blood transfusion and rapid delivery, by induction of labour or caesarean section as necessary, according to the clinical scenario: delay may cause fatality in a sickle cell crisis situation. The most serious clinical scenario is bone marrow embolism, which has been called pseudotoxaemia. It is characterized by systolic hypertension and proteinuria, without oedema and it is important not to mistake pseudotoxaemia for pre-eclampsia, as inappropriate treatment such as heavy sedation may be given, which can be fatal. Sickle cell crisis can also affect the lungs and brain causing headaches or in the kidneys causing low backache.

Sickle cell disease is associated with anaemia and coupled with malaria and further haemolysis significantly increases the demand for folic acid; 5 mg should be given daily in all pregnant women with sickle-cell disease.

Aplastic crisis is typically a paediatric problem but can be seen in adolescent pregnant girls with sickle-cell disease. A high level of alert for bacterial infection, particularly in the puerperium is required for these patients. Obstetric complications such as haemorrhage, fetal malpresentation, pre-eclampsia and multiple pregnancy in these complicated patients require impeccable obstetric care.[4]

Thalassaemia

As a group, the thalassaemias are not nearly as catastrophic for the mother as sickle-cell disease. Supplementation with folate (5 mg) throughout the pregnancy is usually sufficient to control maternal anaemia, but thalassaemic women may be either iron overloaded or iron-deficient. This is impossible to determine without sophisticated testing such as measurement of serum ferritin. Obstetric complications such as labour dystocia may occur in women with β^0-thalassaemia because of pelvic deformity due to poor bone growth. In most less developed tropical countries, advances made in developed countries in relation to genetic counselling and investigations of 'at-risk couples' are not yet available. However, in the absence of any routine testing, thalassemia major may be diagnosed in women with microcytic anaemia unresponsive to routine iron therapy, or later at term because of polyhydramnios or fetal hydrops.

PRE-ECLAMPSIA AND ECLAMPSIA

A 2005 WHO analysis of maternal deaths showed that hypertensive disease was responsible for about 10% of all maternal deaths but in Latin America and the Caribbean, hypertensive disorders were responsible for the highest proportion of deaths (25.7%, 7.9–52.4).[9] Timely provision of effective care to women presenting with pre-eclampsia and eclampsia could avoid many of these deaths. A WHO Technical Consultation on the Prevention and Treatment of Pre-eclampsia and Eclampsia (in April 2011) made 23 recommendations to optimize management and minimize maternal death and morbidity.[27] The summary list of these recommendations can be accessed at: http://whqlibdoc.who.int/hq/2011/WHO_RHR_11.30_eng.pdf. It is timely here to remind tropical health workers that 25% of eclamptic cases occur in the postpartum period and these tend to be particularly severe. Autopsies of deaths from eclampsia incriminate intravascular cerebral haemorrhage as the main cause of death, emphasizing the importance of aggressive antihypertensive therapy when the blood pressure reaches dangerous levels (>160/110 mmHg) and protection of women from convulsions with magnesium sulphate ($MgSO_4$) therapy.[4]

A safe simple regimen for eclampsia is 4 g of intravenous (IV) $MgSO_4$ administered slowly (over 20 min), followed directly by 10 g intramuscular injection (IM) (5 g in each thigh) and then maintenance doses of 5 g every 6 hours. The next dose of $MgSO_4$ is withheld if the urine output is less than 30 mL/hour, the respiratory rate less than 14/min or the reflexes are absent.

When resources permit, a loading dose of 4 g IV of $MgSO_4$ administered over 20 min (diluted with normal saline) is followed by 1 g IV dose $MgSO_4$ per hour for 24 hours. Fitting after the loading dose can be treated with 2 g IV dose of $MgSO_4$ administered over 10 min. $MgSO_4$ therapy should be continued for at least 24 hours postpartum.

The BP can be controlled by hydralazine 5–10 mg IV every 4–6 hours. More effective management of severe pre-eclampsia and eclampsia can be facilitated by having an 'Eclampsia Kit' in the labour ward; this kit can just be a box which contains everything necessary to manage a case.

If the woman is at term (or pre-term and there is evidence of maternal organ dysfunction – kidneys, brain, lungs, placenta, liver or dropping platelet count), the pregnancy should be terminated by induction of labour. If the cervix is unripe, oral Misoprostol is a safe and effective way to ripen the cervix and induce labour: one 200 µg tablet can be dissolved in 200 mL of water and aliquots of 25 mL (25 µg) given 2-hourly until the cervix is ripe or labour commences (occasionally this small dose has no effect after 4 aliquots and needs to be increased to 50 µg or 100 µg). Intrauterine Foley catheter with intravenous oxytocin is an alternative method of induction when the cervix is unfavourable. When the cervix is favourable for induction, artificial rupture of membranes and IV syntocinon can be used.

OBSTETRIC HAEMORRHAGE

Haemorrhage is the leading cause of maternal mortality worldwide, accounting for 34% of maternal deaths in Africa; 31% in Asia; 21% in Latin America and 13% in developed countries.[28] Primigravidae and grandmultiparae are at higher risk, as are women who have had retained placenta or postpartum haemorrhage in the past or suffer prolonged labour (particularly prolonged 2nd stage) in the current labour. Women with severe pre-eclampsia and anaemia are more at risk because they tolerate blood loss less well.

From a social perspective, lack of access to adequate obstetric care; the existence of strong social pressures (e.g. cultural and religious reasons to marry too early or to have large families) which can interfere with the proper use of healthcare services where these exist; poor transportation and gross infrastructural inadequacies can all mean that many women will succumb to both antepartum and postpartum haemorrhage. With regard to delay in effective treatment within the healthcare system, lack of access to adequate supplies of safe blood is an important factor (Figure 79.4).[29] Lack of blood transfusion directly affects maternal mortality. Countries in sub-Saharan Africa with the highest maternal mortality rates have the lower blood donation rates (<5 units/1000 population vs >30/1000 in many developing countries).[29]

Correct management of obstetric haemorrhage will not be repeated here as this can be found on a number of websites (Table 79.1). Active management of the 3rd stage of labour should be practiced in every delivery room for every delivering woman. Practical ways to assess blood loss by weighing are important, as it is very common for birth attendants to underestimate blood loss. Indeed 'under-resuscitation' because of under-estimation of blood loss is an important contributory factor in maternal death and morbidity associated with facility births.

Having a PPH kit (containing everything necessary to handle a major obstetrical haemorrhage including oxytocin, ergometrine and misoprostol), and practising drills for postpartum haemorrhage and assigning team members who come on shift duty to a particular role in the event of PPH, audits of haemorrhage-related maternal death and near-miss events, can improve clinical competence and confidence and reduce the need for blood transfusion and prevent maternal mortality.

Certain infectious diseases, such as malaria and dengue are associated with reduced platelet count in pregnancy, as are abruption and severe pre-eclampsia cases. While the fall in platelet count is probably at its lowest at the peak of parasitaemia in malaria and so is likely to improve once treatment starts, the most critical phase in dengue infection is the defervescent phase when the fever subsides but the patient develops life-threatening thrombocytopenia due to complement activation by viral antigens binding to platelets. A ready supply of cross-matched blood for any woman with a recent history of fever and for cases who might be at increased risk of PPH is a useful clinical strategy. The timing of induction of labour requires careful planning in these cases.

DIFFICULT AND OBSTRUCTED LABOUR

Maternal mortality and serious maternal morbidity including ruptured uterus,[30] vesico-vaginal fistula[31] and PPH are the major serious maternal outcomes of prolonged labour. These outcomes are rare in high-income countries and most of these events are preventable. Again, delay in seeking appropriate care

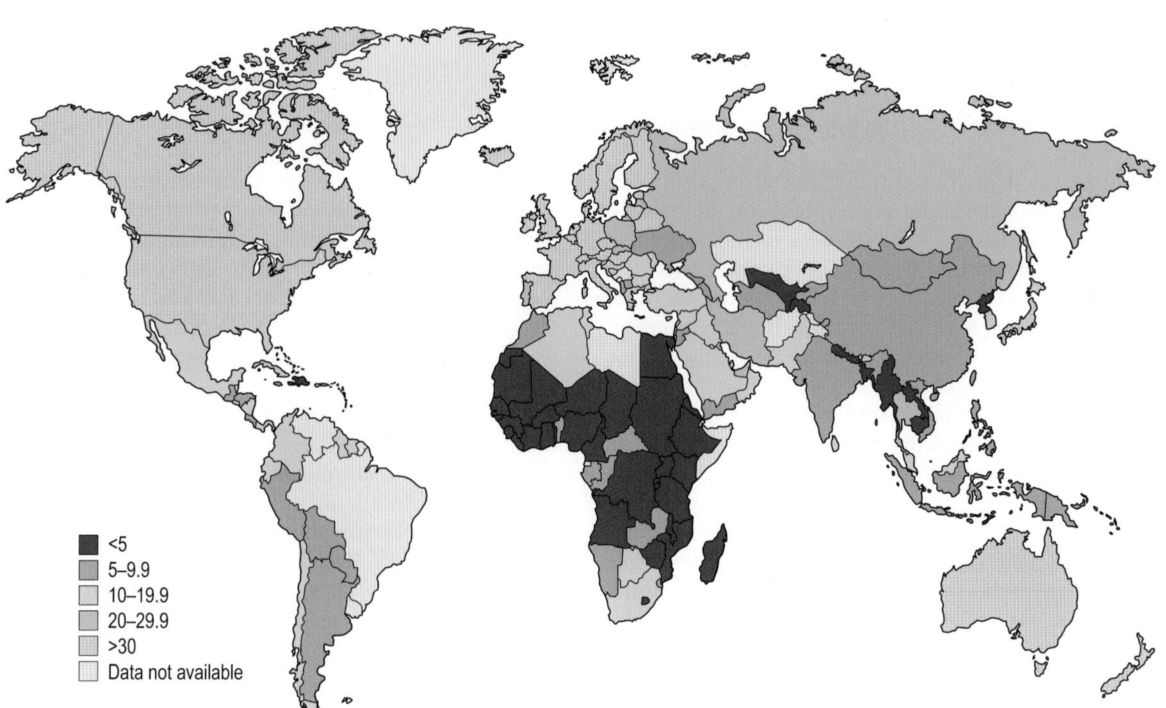

Figure 79.4 Blood donations per 1000 population (2007). *(Reproduced with permission from World Health Organization, http://www.who.int/mediacentre/factsheets/donations_per1000_population_20091110.pdf.)*

at the onset of labour, cephalopelvic disproportion, illiteracy, poverty, young maternal age and low status of women, a poor or non-existent referral system, non-attendance for antenatal care, delayed interventions due to a combination of factors such as lack of skilled human resources and medical supplies contribute to these poor outcomes. Midwives and nurses at primary health centres are encouraged to use partographs to monitor the progress of labour to help them identify poor progress and when to refer such cases for further management. Oxytocin to improve uterine contractions is indicated if there are no contraindications such as suspected fetal compromise, a malpresentation (importance of antenatal care), a previous caesarean delivery and obstructed labour. When, despite adequate contractions for 4–6 hours with oxytocin augmentation, labour fails to progress, intervention by caesarean section or vacuum extraction (± symphysiotomy) if the woman is in the second stage of labour, is required.[32]

From a public health point of view, vesico-vaginal fistula prevention requires social change, particularly avoidance of child marriage and unplanned early teenage pregnancy and the widespread development of timely referral infrastructure within developing countries.[33] Treatment and subsequent reintegration of fistula patients requires a team of specialists, including surgeons, nurses, midwives and social workers, which is largely unavailable in developing countries. However, there is increasing support for training of fistula surgeons through standardized programmes as well as establishment of rehabilitation centres in many nations. The eradication of fistula is dependent upon building programmes that target both prevention and treatment.[31]

One of the components of emergency obstetric care is instrumental birth (also called assisted vaginal delivery with a vacuum extraction device (ventouse) or with forceps), which applies traction to the fetal head in cases of obstructed or prolonged second stage of labour to accelerate birth.[2] Safety relies on the skill of the operator for both devices. Based on its association with lower maternal morbidity, fewer caesarean deliveries and its superiority for managing certain fetal malpositions (e.g. deflexed occipital posterior), vacuum extractor may be preferable[2] but there is a lack of evidence on its use from low-resource settings.

Symphysiotomy is strongly recommended where caesarean section is not available, culturally unacceptable or the balance of risks outweighs the adverse consequences of not providing symphysiotomy.[34] In some clinical scenarios, e.g. when there has been a failed trial of assisted delivery, or in the presence of intrauterine sepsis, a symphysiotomy is a much safer operation than caesarean section for both mother and baby. In the review of more than 5000 symphysiotomy cases, Bjorklund[35] reported that it: (1) compares favourably with caesarean delivery in terms of risk for the mother's life and is equal to caesarean delivery in terms of risk to the newborn's life (PMR in four studies from 1973 to 1995 was 37 out of 307 symphysiotomy (12.1%) vs 66 out of 571 (11.6%) caesarean); (2) confers a permanent enlargement of the mother's pelvic outlet while avoiding a caesarean scar and risk of subsequent uterine rupture; and (3) is rarely associated with severe long-term complications. Partial symphysiotomy (Zarate procedure, developed in the early 20th century) has very low risk of maternal morbidity and mortality. To perform symphysiotomy, instructions can be found at: http://helid.digicollection.org/en/d/Js3015e/9.11.html#Js3015e.9.11.[36,37]

AVOIDING DEVELOPED COUNTRY TRENDS FOR RISING CAESAREAN SECTION RATES

The risks and benefits to both mother and baby of caesarean delivery compared with vaginal delivery should be carefully considered in low-resource settings, particularly where caesarean delivery facilities and capabilities are suboptimal or where women may not have ready access to safe repeat caesarean delivery during subsequent pregnancies, placing them at risk for uterine rupture and maternal death.[2] A review of caesarean delivery in the developing world found diverging trends: in the least developed countries, access to the procedure remains limited at levels much less than 5% of all births. This limited access is linked with increases in maternal and neonatal mortality, but safety concerns are equally valid when more than half of women in certain socioeconomic strata are having surgical delivery, as in the more advanced developing economies of Latin America and China.[38] In developing countries, rising rates portend more danger for future pregnancies. As clearly stated by Ibekwe 'there should be a clear and unquestionable indication for caesarean section in every case'.[39] Quality clinical obstetric practice, which aims to maintain a caesarean section rate of about 5% in booked cases (i.e. non-referred problem cases) cannot be found in any modern textbook written for developed country practice; one of the few texts which describes a balanced view appropriate for district hospitals in developing countries can be found in the Marie Stopes International Guide to Safe Motherhood.[40]

To propose and implement effective measures to reduce or increase caesarean section rates where necessary, an appropriate classification is required but there is a dearth of information on the indication for caesarean section in developing countries.[2] A systematic review of systems to classify the indication for caesarean section recommended women-based classifications – Robson's classification,[41] which is suitable for both local and international comparisons.[41–43]

NON-PUERPERAL AND PUERPERAL SEPSIS

An unknown number of women in resource-poor settings die of infection due to non-puerperal sepsis.[44] The details of these infections are rarely known due to lack of access to microbiological facilities in most resource-limited settings. In addition, therapy is usually empirical and local antimicrobial resistance is rarely examined. Innovations in microbiology diagnostics that permit access at a low cost are a high priority for resource-poor settings.[45,46] Recent guidelines on antibiotic use in bacterial sepsis in and following pregnancy[47,48] are provided (Table 79.4).

Deaths due to postpartum sepsis were higher in Africa (odds ratio 2.71), Asia (1.91) and Latin America and the Caribbean (2.06), than in developed countries.[9] Even in developed countries, substandard care has been identified as a contributing factor to maternal deaths, and studies in the non-pregnant population have found that the survival rates following sepsis are related to early recognition and initiation of treatment.[47,48] Bacterial sepsis in pregnancy is a medical emergency which requires administration of intravenous broad-spectrum antibiotics (ampicillin plus gentamicin plus metronidazole or gentamicin plus clindamycin plus ciprofloxacin plus metronidazole if penicillin allergic) within 1 hour of suspicion of severe sepsis in the woman, with or without septic shock. This should be

TABLE 79.4 **Antimicrobials Spectra for Bacterial Sepsis in Pregnancy**[47,48]

		Anaerobes		Gram-Positive		Gram-Negative	
Antimicrobial	**Limitations of Antimicrobial**	*Clostridia/ Bacteroides/ Peptostreptococci*	**MRSA**	*Staph. aureus* (fluclox. sensitive)	Group A Strep/ Group B Strep	Coliform	Pseudomonas
Ampicillin	–	<50%	No	<30%	Yes	<30%	No
Cefuroxime/ Cefotaxime	–	No	No	Yes	Yes	Yes	No
Clindamycin	Covers most streptococci and staphylococci, including many MRSA and switches off exotoxin production with significantly decreased mortality. Not renally excreted or nephrotoxic.	Yes	<50%	Yes	Yes	No	No
Co-amoxiclav	Does not cover MRSA or *Pseudomonas* and there is concern about an increase in the risk of necrotizing enterocolitis in neonates exposed to co-amoxiclav in utero	Yes	No	Yes	Yes	Yes	No
Erythromycin	–	Yes	No	Yes	Yes	No	No
Gentamicin	Gentamicin (as a single dose poses no problem in normal renal function but if doses are to be given regularly serum levels must be of 3–5 mg/kg) monitored	No	Yes	Yes	No	Yes	Yes
Metronidazole	Only covers anaerobes	Yes	No	No	No	No	No
Imipenem/ Meropenem and Tazocin	Covers most organisms except MRSA. Tazocin (Piperacillin–tazobactam) covers all except MRSA and are renal sparing (in contrast to aminoglycosides)	Yes	No	Yes	Yes	Yes	Yes
Trimethoprim	–	No	<30%	>50%	>50%	>50%	No
Vancomycin/ Teicoplanin/ Linezolid/ Daptomycin	–	Yes	Yes	Yes	Yes	No	No

No, no cover; Yes, close to 100% cover; when expressed as %, only that proportion of organisms would be expected to be covered by the antibiotic.

administered along with a sepsis resuscitation bundle, including: treating the source, e.g. with uterine evacuation or drainage of abscess; aggressive fluid replacement in the case of hypotension and oliguria; and blood replacement if severe anaemia due to haemorrhage is also a problem.[47,48]

The presence of a large denuded area of the uterus post-delivery predisposes to the development of endometritis and subsequent puerperal sepsis.[4] Sepsis may also occur secondary to laceration of the genital tract, which is more likely when there is poor personal perineal hygiene and in the presence of retained products of conception. The presence of untreated sexually transmitted diseases during pregnancy, poor hygiene on the part of the birth attendant and inadequate sterilization of instruments inserted into the genital tract during delivery or abortion pose a particular risk.[4] The presence of a puerperal genital tract infection is suspected by the presence of fever, lower abdominal pain in the presence of foul-smelling lochia or discharge. Less specific symptoms include vomiting, headache and loss of appetite. Examination reveals pyrexia and a tender bulky uterus. In more advanced stages of the disease, tender masses in the adnexa or in the posterior fornix may be found, suggesting the presence of tubo-ovarian or pouch of Douglas abscesses. Septicaemia may also occur. Treatment in the early stages is by the use of broad-spectrum intravenous antibiotics (ampicillin, gentamicin and metronidazole or ceftriaxone and metronidazole) followed by evacuation of the uterus after approximately 24 hours if retained products of conception are suspected because of continuing vaginal bleeding.[49,50]

PYELONEPHRITIS

Screening for urinary tract infection with urine culture and dipstick for leucocyte esterase and nitrite and subsequent treatment of positive cases will reduce the risk of pyelonephritis and appears to be cost-effective.[18] *Escherichia coli* infection can be transmitted to the fetus and increase the risk of late fetal death, while untreated haematogenous spread can cause septic shock and maternal death. Stock out of urine dipsticks and limited ability to culture urine often means that screening and laboratory assisted management are not feasible in resource-poor rural settings and antimicrobial drug resistance (if known) can complicate treatment in pregnant women.[51] Treatment can be initiated with ceftriaxone if oral antibiotics are not tolerated or preferably oral ciprofloxacin 500 mg twice daily 10–14 days when tolerated.

TROPHOBLASTIC DISEASE

Gestational trophoblastic disease (GTD) comprises a spectrum of chorionic tumours from the benign hydatidiform mole to the highly malignant choriocarcinoma. GTD is more likely to develop in women of Asian origin, teenagers and women over 40 years with a variable incidence of 0.2–2 per 1000 pregnancies.[4] Survival has changed drastically in developed countries since the 1970s, due to early detection and effective evacuation, as previously the mortality rate for invasive mole approached 15%, most often because of haemorrhage, sepsis, embolic phenomena or complications from surgery.[52] Untreated choriocarcinoma has a mortality rate of almost 100% when metastases were present and approximately 60% even when hysterectomy was done for apparent non-metastatic disease. Gestational trophoblastic neoplasms are now one of the most curable of all solid tumors, with cure rates >90% even in the presence of widespread metastatic disease. Nevertheless, the lack of early detection in resource-poor tropical countries makes it a significant contributor to pregnancy-related death.

Women with hydatidiform mole typically present with vaginal bleeding and crampy lower abdominal pain (like an incomplete abortion) and sometimes with a history or passing vesicles; large-for-dates uterine size, anaemia, pre-eclampsia (complicates about 10% or cases), hyperemesis due to very high serum β-hCG levels and rarely clinical hyperthyroidism. The passage of typical vesicles is diagnostic, but in threatened abortion cases, ultrasound is very helpful, as it provides a diagnostic, classic, 'snowstorm appearance'. Prognosis and monitoring of treatment are aided by measurement of quantitative serum β-hCG measured by radioimmunoassay, but where this is not available, pregnancy tests have to suffice. Treatment is by suction curettage, usually with an oxytocic drip running to limit haemorrhage from uterine atony.[53] When suction curettage is performed on a uterus greater than 14 weeks in size, it is wise to schedule a visit 1 week later for the woman, so a repeat ultrasound can rule out incomplete removal of trophoblastic tissue. When ultrasound is unavailable, sharp curettage of the uterus is recommended.

Hydatidiform mole evacuation can be complicated by severe haemorrhage; perforation of the uterus; acute right ventricular failure with alarming collapse during or post-evacuation due to massive pulmonary embolization of trophoblastic tissue. In such cases, supportive therapy with positive pressure ventilation may save the patient. The development of choriocarcinoma post-uterine evacuation occurs in about 1–2% of cases. Patients have previously been monitored with serial serum β-hCG (or urinary pregnancy tests) measured monthly up to 12 months. Later onset of malignancy has been reported in a small number of cases and reliable family planning, e.g. Depo medroxyprogesterone acetate or a tubal ligation if the woman does not wish to have a further pregnancy, has usually been advised for at least 12 months. Contraception does not affect the risk of choriocarcinoma developing: the reason why contraception is advised, is that β-hCG levels due to normal pregnancy could not be distinguished from those due to recurrent mole or the development of choriocarcinoma. Now normal pregnancy can be documented as early as 2 weeks after conception by radio receptor assay for β-hCG, combined with serial ultrasound.[54]

Cases of choriocarcinoma diagnosed by rising or recrudescent β-hCG levels or return of a positive pregnancy test can usually be cured by high-dose parenteral methotrexate therapy with folinic acid rescue; however, high-risk cases with metastases require multiple drug chemotherapy to effect a cure. A recent review on molar pregnancy provides a simple schedule for the use of methotrexate with folinic acid rescue.[55]

ECTOPIC PREGNANCY

Ectopic pregnancy may be responsible for nearly 5% of maternal deaths in developing countries compared with <1% in developed countries.[9] As in industrialized countries, pelvic inflammatory disease (PID) associated with sexually transmitted diseases (STDs) is the most important risk factor for ectopic pregnancy in developing countries. Late diagnosis, leading in almost all cases to complications requiring emergency surgical intervention account for high fatality rates in women suffering from ectopic pregnancy in Africa.[56] Clinicians should be suspicious of ectopic pregnancy in any woman of reproductive age presenting with acute abdominal or pelvic symptoms. The diagnosis of ectopic pregnancy can be difficult and protracted, but may be aided by ultrasound and serum β-hCG. A positive pregnancy test and no visible gestational sac in the uterus on ultrasound should always make for a presumptive diagnosis of ectopic pregnancy and if the diagnosis is not immediately obvious should trigger further investigations and follow-up until the final outcome of the pregnancy is known.[57] A culdocentesis that produces any amount of dark blood is virtually diagnostic of a ruptured or leaking ectopic pregnancy; this test is very simple and can be performed as part of the original gynaecological examination of the patient in the outpatient's department. The treatment of ectopic pregnancy is primarily surgical removal of the ectopic pregnancy, but medical management with methotrexate is successful for small, stable ectopic pregnancies with serum β-hCG concentrations <3000 IU/L.

UNWANTED PREGNANCY

Maternal mortality from abortion is highest in Latin America and the Caribbean (as high as 30% of all deaths in some countries in this region) but are also common in sub-Saharan Africa, especially in countries where legal abortion is difficult to obtain.[9] In addition, a far larger number of women experience short- and long-term health consequences such as gynaecological infections and chronic pelvic pain.[58] Some 40% of the world's women are living in countries with restrictive abortion laws, consequently, women resort to clandestine interventions to terminate unwanted pregnancy.[58] To address the harmful health consequences of unsafe abortion, a post-abortion care model has been developed and implemented with success in many countries where women do not have legal access to abortion.[58] This involves treatment of incomplete abortion and provision of post-abortion contraceptive services. To enhance women's access to post-abortion care, focus is increasingly being placed on upgrading mid-level providers to provide emergency treatment, as well as implementing misoprostol as a treatment strategy for complications after unsafe abortion[1] and early bacterial sepsis treatment.[47,48]

FETAL GROWTH RESTRICTION (FGR)

The concept of developmental origins of health and disease, the Barker hypothesis,[59] and the epidemic of non-communicable diseases in low- and middle-income countries has increased the focus on fetal growth restriction (FGR). Worldwide epidemiological and experimental animal studies demonstrate that adversity in fetal life, resulting in FGR, programmes the offspring for a greater susceptibility to ischaemic heart disease, diabetes and hypertensive disease in adulthood.[60] FGR and preterm labour can be distinguished only if the gestational age is known with some accuracy and this can be difficult in resource-poor settings.[61] The estimate of a substantially higher number of LBW pre-term babies has important policy implications in view of special health care needs of these infants but there is a relative lack of population-based studies.[62]

Small for gestational age (SGA) refers to a fetus that has failed to achieve a specific biometric or estimated weight threshold by a specific gestational age. The threshold of the 10th centile for abdominal circumference and estimated birth weight is commonly used. SGA fetuses are a heterogeneous group comprising fetuses that have failed to achieve their growth potential (fetal growth restriction, FGR) and fetuses that are constitutionally small (50–70% of fetuses with a birth weight below the 10th centile for gestational age) and the vast majority of term SGA infants have no appreciable morbidity or mortality. Expert opinion suggests that detection and management of FGR with the help of maternal BMI, symphysial-fundal height measurement (3 cm below gestationally expected height) and targeted ultrasound could be effective in reducing FGR related stillbirths by 20% in a review of related studies (all bar one from developed countries).[63] This is one of the reasons why early booking at the ANC and even in later booking gestation, careful attention to gestational assessment (including the documentation and correlation of menstrual history, quickening and uterine size at the first visit) is so important. Some effort to produce local thresholds to identify pregnant women at risk at booking have been introduced, e.g. in India (wt <40 kg, BMI <19.8 mg/kg^2, haemoglobin <7 g/dL)[64] and in South Africa (short stature (<145 cm), low body weight (<45 kg) and/or MUAC <22 cm).[65] Well-constructed fundal height growth charts, or population-specific fetal biometry growth charts could also contribute to identification of these infants.[66] The problem for resource-poor settings is acting upon the findings. With the caveat 'when the gestation is known', pregnancy with significant FGR and particularly if there is evidence of poor placental function (like static or falling weight in the 3rd trimester[67] or oligohydramnios (AFI<5 cm) on ultrasound measurement of the amniotic fluid index) should be induced in consultation with the paediatric team.

After poor placental function and calorie/energy malnutrition, maternal anaemia is probably the next contributor to impaired fetal growth. Infections such as falciparum malaria and HIV, maternal medical conditions of pre-eclampsia and hypertension, multiple pregnancy, smoking and indoor air pollution also contribute. Antenatal care, including ferrous and folic supplements and deworming and prevention of common contributors such as malaria[68] and smoking cessation as early as possible in the pregnancy may help to alleviate some of these problems. When a fetus is approaching term (37–38 weeks) or earlier if there is evidence of fetal compromise (i.e. 34–38 weeks), induction of labour may save the baby.

PREMATURE LABOUR

In the tropics, fever and the underlying disease are the main preventable risk factors for premature labour. Treatment should be with antipyretics and specific therapy. Oral nifedipine to reduce contractions may be started in women with premature labour before 34 gestational weeks to maximize the effect of corticosteroid therapy given to reduce the risk of respiratory distress syndrome, intraventricular haemorrhage and necrotizing enterocolitis in the premature neonate. Concerns that corticosteroids may increase the risk of chorioamnionitis, postpartum endometritis, or neonatal sepsis are not supported by evidence.

PRE-LABOUR RUPTURE OF MEMBRANES (PROM)

The diagnosis of PROM is usually made on the basis of maternal history and confirmed by speculum examination and simple tests, e.g. fern test or inspection of a clean perineal pad is often sufficient to make the diagnosis. Once PROM is confirmed, both the mother and the fetus are at increased risk of ascending infections, such as group B *Streptococcus*. When there are signs of chorioamnionitis (maternal fever, fetal tachycardia, uterine tenderness, foul-smelling or purulent vaginal discharge, maternal leucocytosis or raised C-reactive protein (CRP)), treatment should be with broad-spectrum intravenous antibiotics, e.g. ceftriaxone and metronidazole and induction of labour. If there are no signs of infection, antibiotic therapy with a 7-day course of ampicillin, amoxicillin or erythromycin, is indicated for premature PROM. At 34 weeks' gestation, labour may be induced. If the membranes rupture at less than 28 weeks and ultrasound shows that there is no liquor in the uterus, obstetricians in developing countries would consider termination of the pregnancy due to the danger of infection and the extreme unlikelihood of getting to a viable gestation.

Obstetrics and Tropical Diseases

While each of the following infections are referenced to the relevant chapter, these tropical infections are associated with an increased susceptibility and/or severity in pregnancy and in some, treatment in pregnancy is controversial (Table 79.5). Obstetric management issues are discussed. Fever is dangerous in pregnancy; it has been associated with miscarriage, congenital abnormality and premature labour.[69,70] Each febrile episode in pregnancy should be recognized and treated with paracetamol 1 g 4–6-hourly or as needed, with immediate clinical examination and investigations so the diagnosis is made to treat the underlying disease promptly and effectively.

MALARIA IN PREGNANCY

The burden of malaria in pregnancy in sub-Saharan Africa, the Asia Pacific Region and South America is significant.[71,72] In a recent review on malaria in pregnancy in the Asia-Pacific region,

TABLE 79.5 **Drugs for Common Tropical Parasites with Recommendations for Pregnancy**

Disease	Drug Contraindications or Recommendations
Flukes and tapeworms (including *Diphyllobothrium, Dipylidium, Clonorchis, Fasciolopsis, Hymenolepis, Paragonimus, Opisthorchis*)	Praziquantel and niclosamide – benefits likely to outweigh the risk and no well controlled trials in pregnancy
Loa loa, gnathostomiasis	Diethylcarbamazine (DEC): avoid in pregnancy. Albendazole must be avoided in the 1st trimester. If more than a single adult worm, the required 21 days of therapy and risk benefit are likely to be in favour of using drug therapy after delivery.
Malaria	Doxycycline or tetracycline, Halofantrine and Primaquine or Tafenoquine are contraindicated in ALL trimesters. All antimalarials except quinine, chloroquine and clindamycin are contraindicated in the 1st trimester in *uncomplicated malaria*. Artesunate (IV) is the drug of choice for *severe malaria* and should NOT be withheld for fear of harming the fetus, as the mortality is lower than with quinine (IV).
Schistosomiasis	Despite a lack of safety data on praziquantel in pregnant women, the WHO recommends that pregnant women are treated based on experience in mass treatment campaigns and review of the veterinary and human evidence.
Soil-transmitted helminths	Mebendazole, Albendazole, Pyrantel pamoate and Ivermectin are contraindicated in the 1st trimester mostly due to a lack of safety data.
Strongyloidiasis	Albendazole – avoid in the 1st trimester in uncomplicated infection. In hyperinfection syndrome and disseminated strongyloidiasis, albendazole therapy can be life-saving.
Toxoplasmosis	The pyrimethamine component of pyrimethamine-sulfadiazine (1st line therapy) is contraindicated in the 1st trimester. Women who develop toxoplasmosis during the 1st trimester of pregnancy should be treated with spiramycin (3–4 g/day). If there is no documented transmission to the fetus, spiramycin can be continued until term. If transmission has occurred in utero, therapy with pyrimethamine and sulfadiazine should be started.
Visceral leishmaniasis	Due to the high mortality treatment with Amphotericin B or antimonial sodium stibogluconate should be instituted according to local availability and efficacy. Observational data suggests Amphotericin B is associated with lower rates of pregnancy loss.

it was pointed out that detailed malaria-attributable maternal mortality rates are rarely reported, but 39% of pregnant women with severe malaria died. In three districts in India, 22 (23%) of 95 maternal deaths were attributed to malaria between 2004 and 2006, which is a total mortality rate of 722 per 100 000 live births and on the Thai–Burmese border, before the introduction of malaria-control programmes for pregnant women, five (1%) of 500 pregnant women died of malaria in 1 year; an estimated maternal mortality rate of 1000 per 100 000.[72] A review of the burden of malaria in pregnancy reported rates of maternal death in Africa as: 0.5–23% in hospital-based studies, 2.9–17.6% in community-based reports and in low-endemicity areas 0.6–12.5% in hospital-based studies; and in Papua New Guinea, an estimated 9 per 100 000 live births.[71] Furthermore, successful prevention of maternal malaria is thought to reduce the risk of severe maternal anaemia by 38%, low birth weight by 43% and perinatal mortality in paucigravidae by 27%.[71] Recent longitudinal cohort studies in Africa indicate that malaria in pregnancy impacts negatively on child survival and malaria-related morbidity.[73,74]

The WHO recommendation for prevention of malaria with chemoprophylaxis or intermittent preventive treatment (IPTp) is problematic. There are very few areas where chloroquine chemoprophylaxis is effective and no suitable replacement for sulphadoxine-pyrimethamine for IPTp, to which there are now significant rates of resistance in many areas, has been identified.[75] In a systematic review of published trials in 1998–2009 of parasitological failure rates following antimalarial treatment in pregnancy, there were 23 treatment studies where 17 different antimalarial drugs were delivered in 53 study arms; 43.4% (23/53) reported a failure rate of <5%; 83.3% of sulphadoxine-pyrimethamine (SP) arms and 9% of artemisinin combination therapy (ACT) arms had failure rates ≥10%. Placenta-positive rates (mostly reported in the context of IPT in pregnancy) were >10% in 68% (23/34) of SP trial arms and >15% in all seven chloroquine arms. When ACT was used for treatment (not intermittent preventive treatment), this provided lower parasitological failure and gametocyte carriage rates.[76] ACTs are safe in the 2nd and 3rd trimesters and more likely to be complied with than quinine (preferably with clindamycin) due to significantly fewer side-effects and shorter duration of therapy, making them more efficacious and safe.[76] ACT for confirmed malaria is also likely to be relatively safe in the 1st trimester, however, there are insufficient data to recommend them categorically at this stage.[77]

Recent data highlight the considerably increased risk of early pregnancy loss from asymptomatic (three-fold higher) and symptomatic malaria (four-fold higher) than in women without malaria and no increased risk with antimalarials including artesunate treatment.[75] Frequent screening of pregnant women offers the chance of early detection and treatment. A policy of opportunistic screening of pregnant women, e.g. while waiting for delivery and treatment with an effective regimen, decreases vertical transmission.[78] Screening tools in pregnancy are limited as microscopy and rapid tests fail to detect low-level parasitaemia seen in pregnancy. Operational effectiveness of the policy assumes high utility of antenatal services and availability of RDTs, which may not be the case in some poor-resource countries.

Chloroquine-resistant *P. vivax* is a problem in pregnancy in some areas and these women should be treated with the ACT locally available and followed-up closely.[79,80] Malaria-related anaemia needs timely and appropriate treatment to prevent deleterious effects to both the mother and the fetus.

The clinical picture of cerebral malaria can be confused with eclampsia and where there is any doubt, the diagnosis should be verified by making a malaria smear. It is important to give the correct treatment, as the consequences can be fatal. Rarely, the two can occur together. Pregnant women with severe malaria are at higher risk of hypoglycaemia that may be exacerbated by IV quinine treatment, pulmonary oedema, severe anaemia and secondary bacterial infections, e.g. pneumonia and urinary tract infection.

Malaria in pregnancy is associated with decreased platelet counts for both *P. falciparum* and *P. vivax* and greater decreases are observed with increasing parasitaemia. Platelet counts need to be verified before epidural anaesthesia and caesarean section: there is conflicting evidence on the risk of PPH with malaria. Preventive obstetrics should be practiced in any case with active management of the third stage. Acute malaria at the time of labour is associated with more adverse maternal and neonatal outcomes and staff should prepare for delivery of a small-for-dates infant with meconium-stained liquor and low Apgar scores.[81] Stillbirth, pre-term fetal distress, premature labour and maternal mortality, especially in severe malaria, have also been reported.

Common sense obstetrics needs to be practiced in severe malaria with the aim of treatment focused on preserving the life of the mother.[82] The first course of action is to stabilize the patient's condition (which may be very difficult) with IV artesunate (or IV quinine if artesunate is unavailable), fluid resuscitation, blood for severe anaemia, glucose for hypoglycaemia and antipyretics for hyperpyrexia. Labour often starts spontaneously. It has been suggested that removing the fetus, even if not viable, helps the mother's condition but much of this evidence is anecdotal. Major haemodynamic changes occur with delivery and as the uterus receives 20–30% of cardiac output at term, considerable benefit to maternal cardiorespiratory function may be gained by delivery if uncomplicated by severe haemorrhage. If the pregnancy is at or near term and the patient is stabilized, induction (with blood on stand-by) seems a reasonable option as placental function is likely to be compromised.

Congenital malaria should be treated aggressively because it can develop rapidly into severe disease. As the absorption of orally administered antimalarials in very young infants is unknown and may be variable, it is better to give the first dose parenterally and a full treatment course should be completed. There is a paucity of data on ACT treatment in children <5 kg. Congenital *P. vivax* or *P. ovale* does not need treatment with primaquine, but only with the standard antimalarials used in the area.

VIRAL HEPATITIS

Acute viral hepatitis is sporadic and can be due to Hepatitis E, B or A virus. In pregnancy, the disease can progress rapidly to fulminant hepatitis carrying a high maternal mortality, particularly in the 3rd trimester.[83] Hepatitis E virus occurs in areas which lack safe sewerage disposal. High attack rates and increased severity in pregnancy have been reported. Uncomplicated cases can be managed with supportive therapy but in fulminant hepatitis, treatment aims to sustain life. Once hepatic failure develops, premature labour is to be expected. It may be recognized late in women with coma. Since infected mothers become carriers transmitting the infection to their infants, hepatitis B vaccination (within 12 hours of birth) of the child is indicated as routine. The carrier state causes a high risk of chronic hepatitis, cirrhosis and hepatocellular carcinoma. Most resource-poor settings do not have hepatitis B immunoglobulin for the newborn when the mother is core antigen positive.

DIARRHOEAL DISEASES

Uncomplicated watery diarrhoea usually causes mild constitutional disturbance and oral treatment that prevents dehydration and electrolyte disturbance will usually suffice. If there is little response in 48 hours or miscarriage threatens, hospitalization is indicated. Antibiotics are not needed for viral gastroenteritis, e.g. rotavirus.

COMPLICATED ACUTE WATERY DIARRHOEA

Complicated watery diarrhoea worsens the effects of coincident infections such as anaemia, obstetric haemorrhage and puerperal sepsis. Low circulating blood volume can impair placental circulation and cause fetal death. In these cases, rapid rehydration with intravenous fluids is required and specific antimicrobial treatment depends on the causative agent (Table 79.4). Blood cultures are the key investigation, although treatment is usually empirical as laboratory testing can be difficult. Toxic shock syndrome caused by staphylococcal or streptococcal exotoxins can produce confusing symptoms, including nausea, vomiting and diarrhoea (Table 79.4).

BLOODY DYSENTERY

Stools with mucous and blood should be examined microscopically for cysts of *Entamoeba histolytica*. Amoebiasis can be fatal in pregnancy due to delayed diagnosis. Metronidazole should be instituted rapidly irrespective of the duration of pregnancy. If intestinal perforation occurs, the prognosis is poor. If amoebic dysentery has been covered or excluded, the cause of the illness can be bacterial such as *Shigella*, *Escherichia coli*, or *Campylobacter*, in which case, locally available effective antimicrobials are needed. While short-course ciprofloxacin has been the drug of choice fluoroquinolone resistance is highly problematic.

CHOLERA

The attack rate and severity of cholera are increased in pregnancy and an increased rate of pregnancy loss (stillbirth and late miscarriage) is well documented, even when prompt adequate treatment is given.[84,85] Fluid loss from vomiting and diarrhoea can be profound and lead to severe dehydration and peripheral circulatory collapse. Other serious complications are acute renal failure, acute pulmonary oedema from inappropriate fluid therapy that do not contain alkalis and hypokalaemia. Short-course oral antibiotics to limit the spread to contacts are appropriate usually with ciprofloxacin but fluoroquinolone resistance is reported.

SCHISTOSOMIASIS

Schistosomes infect approximately 40 million women of childbearing age, yet little is known about schistosome-associated morbidity in pregnant women and their offspring.[86] In 1994 and 2002, respectively, the World Health Organization proposed that treatment for hookworm and schistosomiasis could be provided during the 2nd and 3rd trimesters of pregnancy. It was hoped that this might have benefits on maternal anaemia, fetal growth and perinatal mortality; a beneficial effect on the infant response to immunization was also hypothesized. Of three trials recently reviewed and conducted in areas of high prevalence but low intensity of helminth infection: two examined the effects of benzimidazoles; one (the Entebbe Mother and Baby Study) the effects of albendazole and praziquantel. Under adequate provision of haematinics the benefit of routine anthelminthics during pregnancy for maternal anaemia may be small and none of the other expected benefits were demonstrated.[87]

SOIL-TRANSMITTED HELMINTHS

Over 50% of pregnant women in low- and middle-income countries suffer from iron-deficiency anaemia. Intestinal helminths are associated with blood loss and decreased supply of nutrients for erythropoiesis. High hookworm loads are a major contributor to iron deficiency in women of reproductive age in endemic areas. Anthelmintics (mebendazole or albendazole) remain efficacious in treating helminths although reinfection after treatment can be expected in endemic areas.

Malaria and soil-transmitted helminths have complex interactions. A recent Cochrane review suggested more well-designed, large-scale randomized controlled trials are needed to establish the benefit of anthelmintic treatment during pregnancy.[88] In practice, anaemia that fails to respond to haematinics should be treated with anthelmintics ideally after a direct stool examination. Albendazole is the anthelmintic that has been used most widely and is effective against hookworm and other helminths: it is safe in pregnancy.

SCRUB AND MURINE TYPHUS

There are very little published data on scrub and murine typhus in pregnancy. On the Thai–Burmese border, rickettsial infections (murine and scrub typhus) were one of the leading causes of fever in pregnancy. Previously reported associations with stillbirth and low birth weight were confirmed.[89] The problem is the nonspecific symptoms and signs of this illness compared with other febrile illness in the rural tropics and a lack of diagnostic tools. A thorough search for an eschar (diagnostic of scrub typhus), high index of suspicion and a low threshold to treat with azithromycin in febrile pregnant women from endemic areas may reduce the adverse effects of the disease.

LEPTOSPIROSIS

The impact of leptospirosis on pregnancy is not well understood as the literature comprises case studies or small series reports, in which there is always a potential for bias. In these reports, poor pregnancy outcomes were common and included abortion, fetal death and vertical transmission through blood and breast milk (one case), while other series report no problem when the infection was treated.[90] Again, no single clinical feature is pathognomonic of leptospirosis and a therapy should be initiated on the basis of clinical judgement, as laboratory confirmation is difficult and may be delayed. Early treatment is essential to reduce mortality.

DENGUE

A systematic review of 30 published studies (19 case reports, 9 case series and 2 comparative studies) assessed the impact of dengue infection during pregnancy on birth outcomes. Case reports report high rates of caesarean deliveries (44.0%) and pre-eclampsia (12.0%), while the case series showed elevated rates of pre-term birth (16.1%) and again caesarean deliveries (20.4%), among women with dengue infection during pregnancy. One comparative study found an increase in low birth weight among infants born to women with dengue infections during pregnancy, compared with infants born to non-infected women. Vertical transmission was described in 64.0% and 12.6% of women in case reports and case series respectively, as well as in one comparative study. The authors concluded that there was a risk of vertical transmission, but whether maternal dengue infection is a significant risk factor for adverse pregnancy outcomes remain inconclusive and more comparative studies are needed.[91]

BRUCELLOSIS

Brucellosis is a worldwide zoonosis and a common cause of economic loss and ill health among animal and human populations; it is a major problem in the Middle East, including Egypt. The identification of acute disease is challenging due to the diverse clinical presentations and the need for a specialized laboratory for confirming the diagnosis. In a longitudinal cohort study conducted in Egypt, higher rates of abortion and IUFD were observed than in women who were serologically negative.[92] The recommended treatment in pregnancy is rifampicin or alternatively rifampicin with cotrimoxazole.[93]

INFLUENZA

Pregnant women and infants suffer disproportionately from severe influenza and WHO recommends that pregnant women should be vaccinated to reduce complications of influenza disease during pregnancy.[94] Two recent prospective, controlled trials of maternal influenza vaccination in Bangladesh and US Native American reservations demonstrated that inactivated influenza vaccine given to pregnant women can decrease laboratory-confirmed influenza virus infection in their newborn children. These studies support consideration of the feasibility of targeted influenza vaccine programmes in resource-constrained countries. Vaccination seems a somewhat more feasible possibility than recent recommendations for the management of influenza A-H1N1 in 2009 to treat pregnant women systematically with oseltamivir or zanamivir. The early symptoms of influenza are nonspecific: sore throat, cough or dyspnoea, with fever, myalgias and exhaustion.[95]

TUBERCULOSIS

There were an estimated 8.8 million new tuberculosis cases with 1.4 million deaths in 2010,[96] which explains why TB is a significant contributor to maternal mortality and among the three leading causes of death among women aged 15–45 years in high-endemicity areas.[97] Diagnosis of tuberculosis in pregnancy may be challenging, as the symptoms may initially be ascribed to the pregnancy and the normal weight gain in pregnancy may temporarily mask the associated weight loss associated with early disease. Obstetric complications of TB include spontaneous abortion, pre-term labour, low birth weight (IUGR) and increased neonatal mortality. Congenital TB, though rare, is associated with high perinatal mortality. The prognosis for the pregnancy is directly related to the duration of treatment that can be attained before term, so diagnosis as early as possible in pregnancy is vital.[98] Rifampicin, isoniazid and ethambutol are the first-line drugs while pyrazinamide use in pregnancy is becoming more common.

Isoniazid preventive therapy is a WHO innovation aimed at reducing the infection in HIV-positive pregnant women. Babies born to an HIV-positive mother should be started on isoniazid prophylaxis for 6 months, after which the baby can be vaccinated with BCG if they test negative to HIV. Successful control of TB demands improved living conditions, public awarness, primary prevention of HIV/AIDS and BCG vaccination.[97]

HIV

Whereas mother-to-child transmission (MTCT) has been virtually eliminated in North America and Western Europe, 390 000 (210 000–570 000) children are infected each year in sub-Saharan Africa, with 90% as a result of MTCT.[99] Without interventions, over one-third of infants will be infected with HIV by 2 years of age, half of them as a result of breast-feeding. Research has shown clearly that breast-feeding transmission rates are significantly increased if there is mixed feeding and less if breast-feeding is exclusive.[100] Significant changes have occurred recently to WHO guidelines,[101,102] with infant and postpartum maternal prophylaxis now recommended to support and minimize the risk of breast-feeding, as well as starting antenatal antiretroviral therapy (ART) at an earlier stage of gestation and irrespective of the CD4 count. There are many excellent online references[101,102,103] on diagnosis, prevention, treatment with HAART and counselling for HIV and PMTCT.[3]

Repeat HIV testing towards term is important to detect HIV infection acquired during pregnancy, as new infections acquired in pregnancy are much more likely to lead to transmission to the fetus and the breast-feeding baby.

HIV interacts with other diseases, e.g. malaria where HIV infection seems to compromise malarial immunity such that HIV-infected multigravidae have at least as high a risk of placental infection as non-HIV-infected primigravidae. Thus, HIV essentially eliminates the typical gravidity-specific pattern of malaria risk in stable malaria transmission areas by shifting the burden from paucigravidae to all pregnant women.[71]

Some antiretroviral drugs (ARVs) used in HIV interact with drugs used for other disease conditions and having a common metabolic pathway. For example, artemether-lumefantrine and nevirapine are metabolized by cytochrome P450 3A4 enzyme system, which nevirapine induces, with a potential drug interaction. Consideration of possible drug interactions should be part of the management package for HIV-positive pregnant women who are being treated for other disease conditions.[104]

SEXUALLY TRANSMITTED INFECTIONS (STI)

Sexually transmitted infections require detection and prompt treatment in pregnancy, as vertical transmission can occur. Some STIs are associated with pregnancy complications such as ectopic pregnancy, chorioamnionitis, premature rupture of membranes, pre-term labour, stillbirth, congenital abnormality, puerperal sepsis and infertility resulting from chronic pelvic inflammatory disease. For example, untreated early syphilis in pregnancy will result in a stillbirth rate of 25% and be responsible for 14% of neonatal deaths – an overall perinatal mortality of about 40%.[105] Syphilis prevalence in pregnant women in Africa ranges from 4% to 15%.[105] In the absence of prophylaxis, 30–50% of infants born to mothers with untreated gonorrhoea and up to 30% of infants born to mothers with untreated chlamydial infection will develop ophthalmia neonatorum, which can lead to blindness. An estimated 1000–4000 newborn babies worldwide are blinded every year because of this condition.[105] For this reason, it is advisable that an appropriate antibiotic ointment (usually chloramphenicol or tetracycline) is put in the eyes of all newborns in areas of significant *Chlamydia* and/or gonorrhoea prevalence and the local antibiotic resistance pattern is known.

Bacterial vaginosis, although not actually an STI, but a result of alterations in the normal vaginal flora, is a very common reproductive tract infection: it is the most prevalent cause of vaginal discharge in many developing countries. Up to 50% of pregnant women have bacterial vaginosis in sub-Saharan Africa.[105] Bacterial vaginosis has been implicated as a cause of pre-term birth, low birth weight, pre-term pre-rupture of membranes, postpartum sepsis and spontaneous miscarriage. Bacterial vaginosis has also been implicated in the transmission of HIV infection.[105] Trichomonas vaginalis is also an extremely common vaginal infection and is sexually transmitted; however, its significance as a threat to perinatal health is not known; however, like bacterial vaginosis, it can cause inflammation of the genital tract and increase the risk of HIV transmission and should be promptly treated.

IMPROVING THE USE OF AND ACCESS TO USEFUL TOOLS IN OBSTETRICS IN THE TROPICS

The tools necessary to reduce maternal death are available. Many of these fail to be implemented however, which compounds the problems of access, poverty and inequity. Evidence-based guidelines and clinical practice guidelines;[3] the partogram;[106] population validated fundal height curve as a tool to identify growth restricted and macrosomic infants[66] and ultrasound;[107] and use of clinical practice guidelines, can all be taught to local health workers to improve maternal and fetal outcomes.

Experience in many developing countries has shown that use of locally produced evidence-based standard management protocols (or clinical practice guidelines as they are more commonly called in developed countries) can assist health workers deliver quality care. Papua New Guinea has been a pioneer in the development of standard treatment manuals, and in obstetrics and gynaecology and child health, these have been updated every 5 years since the early 1970s.[108]

TRAINING SKILLED BIRTH ATTENDANTS

WHO advocates for 'skilled care at every birth' because among the more than 130 million births that take place each year, approximately 358 000 women die while pregnant or giving birth; 3.1 million newborns die in the neonatal period and 1 million intrapartum-related stillbirths occur.[109] The highest incidence of maternal and perinatal mortality occurs around the time of birth, mostly occurring within the first 24 hours after birth.[109] WHO, ICM and FIGO advocate for 'An accredited health professional – such as a midwife, doctor or nurse – who has been educated and trained to proficiency in the skills needed to manage normal (uncomplicated) pregnancies, childbirth and the immediate postnatal period and in the identification, management and referral of complications in women and newborns' to be present at every birth.[109] Such health professionals should be motivated and located in the right place at the right time and need to be supported by appropriate policies, essential supplies including medicines and should operate under appropriate regulatory frameworks.[109]

The training and deploying of skilled birth attendants and the upgrading of emergency obstetric care facilities do not address the immediate safe-delivery needs of the estimated 45 million women who are likely to deliver at home, without a skilled birth attendant.[110] More than half of all births in 28 countries from four major global regions are attended by unskilled birth attendants and together contribute to 69% of maternal deaths, despite the fact that these countries only constitute 34% of the total population in these regions.[110] There is no indication for imminent change judging from the proportion of births with skilled attendants in these 28 countries over the last 15–20 years. Solutions to rapidly reduce maternal mortality in regions where delivery at home without skilled birth attendants are common, requires initiative and willingness of governments and community-based organizations to implement a cost-effective, complementary strategy involving the health workers who are likely to be present when births in the home take place. Unfortunately, the training of community-based birth attendants has not been shown to be effective in preventing maternal death. Recently however, there have been some studies to show that certain technologies aimed at specific interventions that are known to prevent maternal deaths, e.g. misoprostol to reduce maternal blood loss in cases of PPH, family planning to assist women defer births or limit the total numbers of births and postpartum care focused on identifying women developing endometritis and administering antibiotics in the home, will increase the chance that women in the lowest economic groups benefit from global safe motherhood efforts.[110]

Conclusion

Many obstetric clinical conditions common in Africa, Asia and tropical South America receive little attention in regular textbooks and many texts on tropical infections refer to pregnancy in a short paragraph only.[4] This gap can be partly explained by a failure of integration of not only the healthcare system but the network of health professionals involved in the care of pregnant women. Excellent other sources specifically written to assist health workers provide care in developing countries using appropriate technologies[4,32] and online resources[1] are available. While high technologies have invaded developed country obstetrics, these are generally unavailable in the resource-poor rural tropics, although there are some changes. Nevertheless, many of the serious clinical conditions that are seen in the rural tropics are preventable using simple tools, e.g. comprehensive antenatal care and safe delivery. Prompt action is also needed and treatment can go from being simple to extremely complicated in a short space of time, e.g. uncomplicated and severe malaria in pregnancy, unruptured and ruptured ectopic, normal labour and ruptured uterus, hence the WHO emphasis on skilled birth attendants.

REFERENCES

1. United Nations Children's Fund. The state of the world's children 2009. New York: United Nations Children's Fund; 2009.
2. Hofmeyr GJ, Haws RA, Bergstrom S, et al. Obstetric care in low-resource settings: what, who and how to overcome challenges to scale up? Int J Gynaecol Obstet 2009;107(Suppl 1):S5, S21–44.
3. The Partnership for Maternal, Newborn & Child Health. A Global Review of the Key Interventions Related to Reproductive, Maternal, Newborn and Child Health (RMNCH). Geneva: RMNCH; 2011.
4. Lawson JB, Harrison KA, Bergstrom S. Maternity Care in Developing Countries. London: RCOG; 2001.
6. WHO. Trends in maternal mortality: 1990 to 2008. Estimates developed by the World Health Organization, UNICEF, UNFPA and The World Bank. Geneva: World Health Organization; 2010 NLM Classification: WQ 16.

Access the complete references online at www.expertconsult.com

Paediatrics in the Tropics

ZULFIQAR A. BHUTTA

KEY POINTS

- About 7.6 million children died globally in 2010 before reaching their 5th birthday; an improvement from 9.6 million in the year 2000.
- Newborn deaths are an increasing proportion of the under-5 deaths: 43% in 2011 up from 37% in 1990.
- The major causes of neonatal deaths are complications of prematurity, intrapartum-related deaths ('birth asphyxia') and severe neonatal infections (pneumonia, sepsis or meningitis).
- Most deaths in post-neonatal, under-5 children are due to infectious causes with the three major killers being diarrhoea, pneumonia and malaria.
- Effective interventions exist to address all of the main causes of child deaths, but the infrastructure required to make these available on a timely basis is not present.
- A holistic approach to provide a continuum of care from conception to adulthood is needed to ensure that the progress is made towards the millennium development goals.
- Ending preventable child deaths requires global commitments to ambitious and achievable targets through evidence-based country plans, expanding country/stakeholder engagement, creating transparency and accountability and devising new approaches when needed.

Introduction

Unlike more industrialized countries, developing countries continue to carry a large childhood mortality burden due to preventable causes. The highest risk of death is at the youngest ages, with neonatal deaths accounting for a greater proportion of deaths in all regions of the world, reflecting an urgent need to focus resources not only on the young child, but also on the pregnancy and peripartum period. To address the goals of health, equity and development, 189 heads of state signed the Millennium Declaration consisting of eight Millennium Development Goals (MDGs) in 2000.[1] The goals defined included specific targets eradicating extreme poverty and hunger; achieving universal primary education; promoting gender equality and empowering women; reducing child mortality rates; improving maternal health; combating HIV/AIDS, malaria and other diseases; ensuring environmental sustainability; and developing a global partnership for development, all by the target date of 2015. These MDGs form a blueprint agreed to by all the world's countries and leading development institutions. They have galvanized unprecedented efforts to meet the needs of the world's poorest people. The MDGs break down into 21 targets that are measured by 60 indicators. Working together, governments, the UN and partners, the private sector and civil society have succeeded in saving many lives and improving conditions for many more, but with the deadline approaching rapidly, it is essential to monitor both achievements and progress towards the MDGs in order to map which indicators need additional efforts.

Since specific diseases are covered in other chapters, the aim here is to focus on child health in tropical countries by reviewing two of the MDGs in some detail.

- MDG 4: Reduce by two-thirds, between 1990 and 2015, the under-5 mortality rate
- MDG 5: Reduce by three-quarters, between 1990 and 2015, the maternal mortality ratio.

Summarizing the progress in over 130 countries is difficult because a good assessment of progress towards MDGs must go beyond averages and aggregates, to consider strategies, implementation and pace of change in indicators. A discussion of child survival also requires consideration of two other MDGs, because of their impact on child health.

- MDG 1: Reduce by half the proportion of people living in extreme poverty and people who suffer from hunger, by 2015.
- MDG 7: Reduce by half the proportion of people without sustainable access to safe drinking water and basic sanitation and achieve a significant improvement in the lives of at least 100 million slum dwellers by 2015.

The MDG 7 of environmental sustainability has far-reaching consequences towards climate change, agricultural productivity and food security, the latter being important in preventing hunger and malnutrition and thus safe-guarding two other vital goals, i.e. MDG 4 and MDG 5, effectively reducing both child and maternal mortality. In essence, the scope of one goal reaches beyond its own effect and provides solutions, which impact other goals. By investing in national programmes that provide dignified access to facilities for the poor and the marginalized, a link between MDG 1 and MDGs 4 and 5 can be established wherein the fulfilment of the former goal can effectively serve to deliver the latter two goals. Essentially, simple interventions at the policy level can serve more complex tasks at the level of implementation.

Global Burden and Trends

Aspirational goals were set at the Millennium Summit for reducing child and maternal mortality. Numerous policies have been influenced to meet these goals by directing the focus to neglected global health challenges. However, even with major accelerated efforts, most countries are unlikely to achieve the targets for MDGs 4 and 5. This might be seen as a failure, but it is worthwhile to view the pace of progress. Most countries are progressing on reducing maternal and child mortality but will take many years past 2015 to achieve the targets of MDGs 4 and 5. Immediate determined action is needed for a large number of countries to achieve MDG 4 and MDG 5 by 2015 or as shortly as possible thereafter.[2]

The data from 74 *Countdown* countries shows that 23 are on track to achieve MDG 4. Bangladesh, Brazil, Egypt and Peru reduced the under-5 mortality rate 66% or more and China, Lao People's Democratic Republic, Madagascar, Mexico and Nepal reduced it 60–65%, 13 countries made no progress and 38 made insufficient progress. Therefore, much remains to be done.

Since 2000, there has been an increased focus on neonatal deaths.[3] Rapid policy changes have been driven after recent assessments demonstrating that an increasing proportion of under-5 deaths were neonatal, coupled with evidence that effective measures were possible even in low-resource settings. From 1990–2011, the early neonatal, late neonatal, post-neonatal and childhood (ages 1–4 years) death rates declined annually by 1.7%, 2.7%, 2.5% and 2.4%, respectively. Globally, 43% of under-5 deaths happen in the first 28 days of life. The pace of reduction for neonatal mortality is a third slower than for older children, limiting progress to MDG 4. Newborn deaths comprise an increasing proportion of under-5 deaths – 43% in 2011 up from 37% in 1990.[4,5] The trends show that of the 3.07 million deaths annually in the newborn period, 1.08 million of these are attributable to pre-term birth complications and 0.72 million to intrapartum complications. The chief preventable causes of post-neonatal deaths among children are pneumonia (1.07 million deaths annually), diarrhoea (0.75 million deaths) and malaria (0.56 million deaths).[6]

Maternal deaths, which significantly impact morbidity in children, declined at 1.9% per year on average, from 1990 to 2011, dropping from 409 000 in 1990 to 274 000 in 2011. The subset due to direct and indirect obstetric causes seemed to decline steadily at an annual pace of 2.8% from 1990 to 2011; from 393 000 to 218 000. Over the same timeframe, the number of HIV-related deaths during pregnancy rose to a peak of 81 000 in 2003 and has since declined to 56 000 in 2011, because of the scale-up of antiretroviral drugs and the epidemic curve for HIV. From 2005 to 2011, 28.6% (21 000 of 74 000) of the decrease in maternal deaths was in India, whereas Ethiopia, Pakistan, Nigeria, Indonesia, China and Afghanistan accounted for a further 32.1% (24 000 of 74 000) (Figure 80.1). To achieve MDG-5, the annual rate of decrease in maternal mortality must be 5.5%, much greater than the rate of 1.9% since 1990. Furthermore, one in eight births in low-income settings is in girls aged 15–19 years old, who account for a large proportion of unsafe abortions and therefore, high mortality rates. Overall, only three countries (Equatorial Guinea, Nepal and Vietnam) reduced the maternal mortality ratio 75% or more from 1990 to 2010, though Cambodia, Bangladesh, Egypt, Eritrea and Lao People's Democratic Republic came close, reducing it 70–74%.

NEONATAL MORTALITY

Estimates from 2010 show 3.1 million newborn deaths compared with the nearly 4 million neonatal deaths in 2000 (17% reduction). Over half of under-5 deaths are newborns in all regions except sub-Saharan Africa and Oceania. More than three-quarters of the world's newborn deaths occur in South Asia and sub-Saharan Africa. Ten countries alone make up for 65% of the total 2 955 000 annual newborn deaths in 2011. In

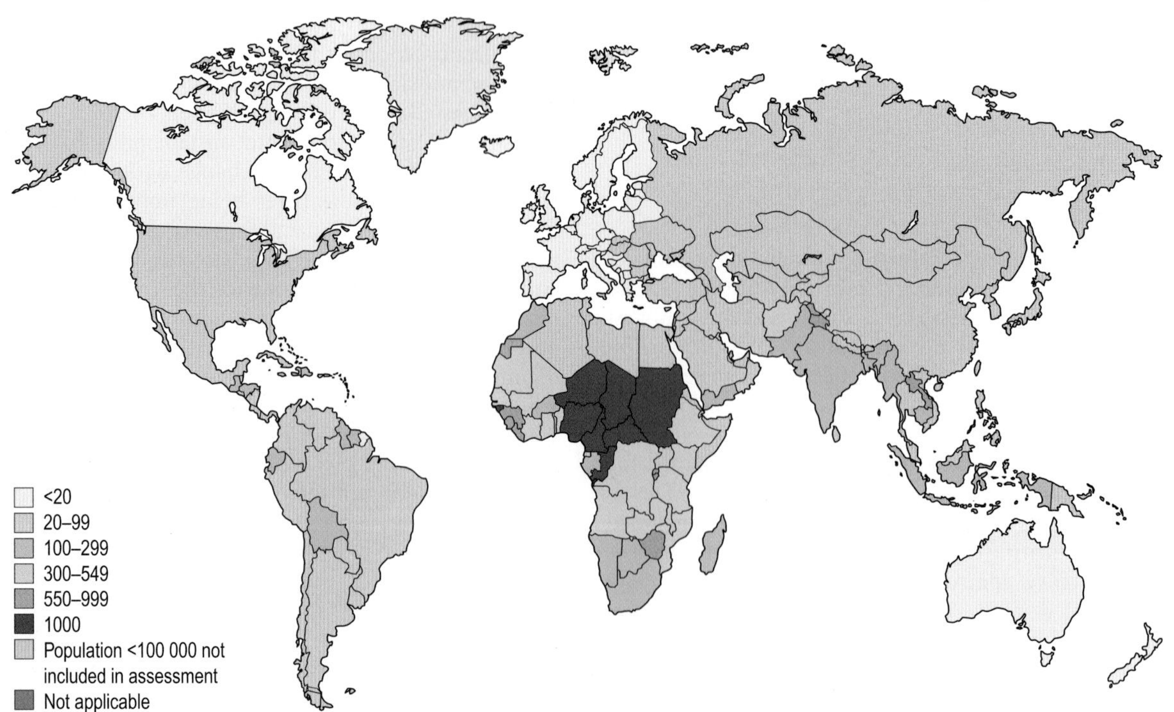

Figure 80.1 Global map for Maternal Mortality Ratio (MMR, deaths per 100 000 live births), 2010. (Source: *Adapted from WHO, UNICEF, UNFPA and the World Bank, Trends in Maternal Mortality: 1990 to 2010. Geneva: WHO; 2012.*)

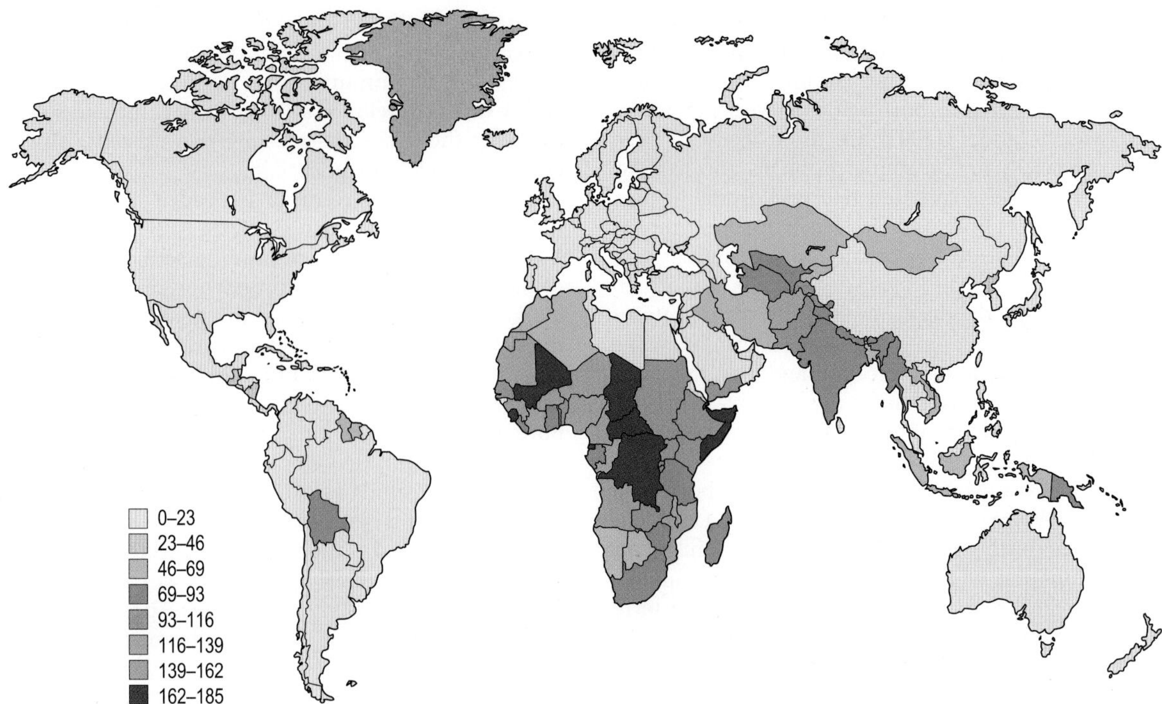

Figure 80.2 Global map for Under-5 Mortality Rate (probability of dying under age 5 per 1000 live births) 2011. (Source: *Adapted from UNICEF, Levels and Trends in Child Mortality Report 2012.*)

sub-Saharan Africa alone, an estimated 1 122 000 babies die before they reach 1 month of age.[7] Some countries have achieved notable progress in reducing neonatal mortality. Five countries have been able to more than halve their neonatal mortality rates between 2000 and 2010 (Turkey, Oman, Greece, Belarus and Estonia). Sub-Saharan Africa was the region with the least progress, which has had, on average, no significant change in neonatal mortality rate during the last decade.

UNDER-5 MORTALITY

About 7.6 million children died globally in 2010, before reaching their 5th birthday, an improvement from 9.6 million in the year 2000 (Figure 80.2). The majority of the 7.6 million unacceptable child deaths that occur each year could be prevented using effective and affordable interventions.[8] South Asia accounted for one-third of worldwide deaths of children younger than 5 years, with the proportion of deaths in sub-Saharan Africa increasing from 33% (3.9 million of 11.6 million) in 1990 to 49% (3.5 million of 7.2 million) in 2011, while the number of deaths in North Africa and the Middle East declined from 5.7% (0.66 million of 11.6 million) to 3.7% (0.27 million of 7.2 million).

Causes of Child Death

NEONATAL DEATHS

The distribution of direct causes of death shows the major causes of neonatal deaths are complications of: prematurity – 1 078 000; intrapartum-related deaths ('birth asphyxia') – 717 000; and severe neonatal infections (pneumonia, sepsis or meningitis) – 717 000 (Figure 80.3).

Prematurity

Pre-term birth is a syndrome with a variety of causes which can be classified into two broad subtypes: (1) *spontaneous* pre-term birth (spontaneous onset of labour or following pre-labour premature rupture of membranes) and (2) *provider-initiated* pre-term birth (defined as induction of labour or elective caesarean birth before 37 completed weeks' gestation for maternal or fetal indications (both 'urgent' or 'discretionary')) or other non-medical reasons.[9]

Approximately 29% of neonatal deaths globally are attributable to pre-term birth complications. Most pre-term infants are

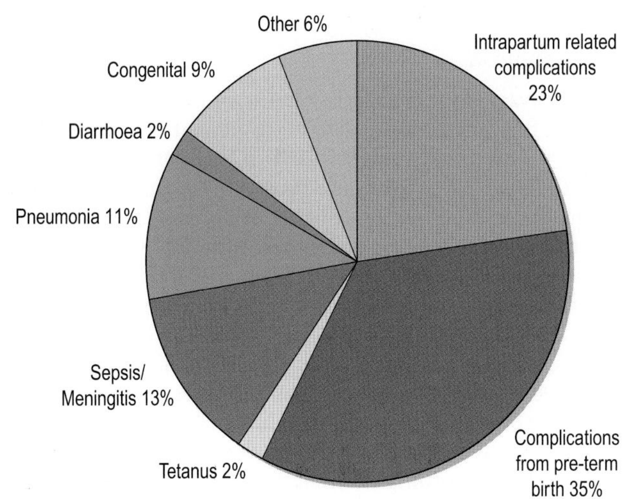

Figure 80.3 Estimated distribution of direct causes of newborn deaths. (Source: *Liu L, Johnson H, Cousens S, et al. Global, regional and national causes of child mortality: an updated systematic analysis. Lancet 2012;379(9832):2151–61.*)

born between 33 and 37 weeks' gestation. With careful attention to feeding, warmth and early treatment of problems, including breathing problems, infections and jaundice, these babies should be able to survive. Babies born before 33 weeks' gestation or with birth weight under 1500 g are more likely to need advanced care, especially for breathing problems and feeding. These babies should receive care in a referral hospital, if possible. Pre-term birth acts both as a risk factor for mortality as well as a direct cause of death.[10] According to the International Classification of Disease, the direct cause of death is only attributed to pre-term birth if the death results from complications specific to pre-term birth or is in a severely pre-term baby. If a moderately pre-term baby has an infection and dies, the death is most appropriately attributed to infection and pre-term birth acts as a risk factor. Thus, many infants recorded as dying from infection are also pre-term.

An average of 14% of babies born worldwide are born with low birth weight (LBW), a weight at birth of <2500 g. LBW may be due to pre-term birth or growth restriction of full-term babies or a combination of the two causes. Pre-term infants are at 13 times greater risk of neonatal death than full-term infants. Furthermore, at least one-half of neonatal deaths are in pre-term babies. Babies who are both pre-term and growth-restricted have an even higher risk of death.

LBW infants in Africa are at greater risk of being born pre-term; around 12%. This is almost double the frequency of pre-term birth in European countries and probably related to infections, particularly sexually transmitted infections, malaria and HIV/AIDS. The situation in South Asia is markedly different. The LBW rate there is almost twice that in Africa but most LBW babies are term infants who are small for gestational age.

In any setting, co-infection during pregnancy with HIV and malaria is of major concern. These two infections act synergistically resulting in serious consequences for maternal and newborn health, especially increasing the LBW rate. To date, strategies to prevent LBW and pre-term birth have not resulted in significant progress and remain a critical discovery research gap for both high- and low-income countries. Identifying small infants and providing extra support for feeding, warmth and care, particularly kangaroo mother care, has great potential to reduce neonatal deaths in the short term.

Birth Asphyxia

Birth asphyxia is the fifth largest cause of under-5 child deaths (8.5%), after pneumonia, diarrhoea, neonatal infections and complications of pre-term birth. It is estimated that around 23% of all newborn deaths are caused by birth asphyxia, with a large proportion of these being stillbirths. The incidence of birth asphyxia has reduced significantly following improvements in primary and obstetric care in most industrialized countries and accounts for less than 0.1% of newborn infant deaths. In developing countries, rates of birth asphyxia are much higher, ranging from 4.6/1000 in Cape Town to 7–26/1000 in Nigeria and case fatality rates may be 40% or higher. Exact epidemiological data are lacking and the precise burden of severe neurological disability in developing countries is unknown. According to the World Health Organization (WHO), between 4 and 9 million newborns develop birth asphyxia each year. Of those, an estimated 1.2 million die and at least the same number develop severe consequences, such as epilepsy, cerebral palsy and developmental delay. The numbers of disability-adjusted life years (DALYs) for birth asphyxia estimated by WHO exceed those due to all childhood conditions preventable by immunization. Community-based data on disability in less developed settings are lacking and studies reliably assessing the cause are virtually non-existent. This makes the estimates essentially uncertain.

Epidemiological research is needed to accurately estimate the contribution of birth asphyxia to perinatal morbidity and mortality, especially in community settings where the burden of disease, due to the high proportion of unattended deliveries, is likely to be larger than in the hospital setting. One of the major difficulties in collecting accurate epidemiological data on birth asphyxia is the lack of a standard definition of the condition. This has added to the difficulties in assessing the true burden of the condition, especially at the community level. Historically, asphyxia was categorized into two grades of severity; asphyxia pallida and livida, signifying varying degrees of affliction. Infants with asphyxia pallida or pale asphyxia were generally regarded as more severely affected, requiring immediate resuscitation. This definition was, however, replaced by more objective measures such as the Apgar score, proposed in 1952.[11] The Apgar score is universally accepted on the basis that a low score, especially at 5 min, can predict survival. The Apgar score has come under criticism for its inability to correctly diagnose perinatal asphyxia and predict long-term neurodevelopmental disabilities.[12,13] The seemingly weak relationship between low Apgar scores and several indicators of perinatal asphyxia is not surprising, since the Apgar score was not intended to be a measure of perinatal asphyxia. Just as the Apgar score alone is a poor predictor of outcome, metabolic acidosis in isolation has also proved to be a poor predictor of significant perinatal brain injury. Similarly, a combination of low Apgar score and acidosis at birth was found to have poor predictive value for neonatal neurological morbidity.[14] According to the American College of Obstetricians and Gynecologists and the American Academy of Pediatrics, a neonate is labelled to be asphyxiated if the following conditions are satisfied: (1) Umbilical cord arterial pH <7; (2) Apgar score of 0–3 for longer than 5 min; (3) Neonatal neurological manifestations (e.g. seizures, coma or hypotonia); and (4) Multisystem organ dysfunction, e.g. cardiovascular, gastrointestinal, haematological, pulmonary or renal system. Thus, hypoxia or asphyxia should be labelled as a cause of disability and handicap only when the neonate demonstrates the four perinatal findings listed above and in whom other possible causes of neurological damage have been excluded. In the absence of such evidence, subsequent neurological deficiencies cannot be ascribed to perinatal asphyxia or hypoxia.

Birth asphyxia can be caused by events in the antepartum, the intrapartum or the postpartum periods or combinations of all three.[15] A recent review suggests that asphyxia is probably primarily antepartum in 50% of cases, intrapartum in 40% and postpartum in the remaining 10% of cases. In developed countries where intrapartum complications are rare events, cases of perinatal asphyxia are more commonly related to antepartum causes or to the superimposition of intrapartum insults over an already at-risk situation. Given the higher incidence of serious complications in labour and reduced availability of skilled care during delivery, intrapartum causes account for a larger proportion of cases in developing countries. The consequences of asphyxia range from no ill effects to multi-organ complications and death. This huge variation in the outcome diverges with the severity and duration of asphyxia. Despite identification of many possible predictors of outcome, little is known of the long-term developmental outcome of asphyxiated term neonates.[16] Furthermore, the evaluation of long-term outcome is stalled by the lack of a consensus on standard case definitions of birth asphyxia, difficulties in assessing asphyxia in non-hospital births and in measuring disabilities, especially among young children and the difficulty of attributing aetiology in the wake of malnutrition and disease.[17]

Although neonatal encephalopathy is the most commonly accepted marker of birth asphyxia, studies show that over 75% of the cases of neonatal encephalopathy have no clinical signs of intrapartum hypoxia. Assessing the proportion of neonatal encephalopathy that is due to birth asphyxia is difficult because of problems in defining both asphyxia and neonatal encephalopathy and in recognizing the cause of neonatal neurological illness.[18,19] It was previously believed that birth asphyxia is a primary cause for one to two cases of cerebral palsy per 1000 live births. Cerebral palsy is a chronic nonprogressive neuromuscular condition that results in muscular spasticity or paralysis and may have associated mental retardation. Earlier studies concluded that up to 50% of cerebral palsy was attributable to birth asphyxia. Further studies reduced this figure to under 10% of cases. Clinical epidemiological studies also show that in most cases, the events leading to cerebral palsy occur in the fetus before the onset of labour or in the newborn after delivery.[20] With the importance ascribed in the past to hypoxia in asphyxia and the role of oxygen in resuscitation, the relationship of asphyxia to cerebral palsy may also be related to aggressive and inappropriate treatment strategies.

Neonatal Infections

Infections, including sepsis, pneumonia, tetanus and diarrhoea, are estimated to be the most common causes of neonatal mortality.[21] The early neonatal period, which includes the period from birth to the 7th day of life, is the most dangerous period for a neonate, with increased risk of morbidity and mortality from perinatal causes, including birth asphyxia, prematurity and infection. Three-quarters of neonatal deaths occur during this period; early-onset neonatal sepsis (EONS) is typically defined as sepsis occurring within the first 3 or 7 days after birth. Seven days is typically used for Group B streptococcal (GBS) sepsis; 3 days is more commonly used in epidemiological studies.[22]

Determining the true burden of EONS in the developing world is not an easy task. Most births and deaths in developing countries take place at home and are unrecorded. Limited community-based surveillance and inadequate laboratory resources to identify EONS hinder assessment of the burden of disease.[23] Most of the available information comes from Demographic and Health Surveys, which are believed to underreport early neonatal deaths. Precise diagnosis of EONS and EONS-related deaths is further complicated by the uncertainties involved in distinguishing the clinical syndrome of sepsis from those of birth asphyxia and prematurity in the early neonatal period. Because hospitals in developing countries with high neonatal mortality capture only a small proportion of all cases of neonatal sepsis, the data do not reflect population-based incidence estimates. Other factors responsible for uncertainty in the data, include the lack of standardization of case ascertainment, limited laboratory facilities for blood culture, problems with sensitivity of blood cultures in detecting true bacteraemia in neonates and inherent limitations of verbal autopsy tools, which make the cause of death unclear for most neonatal deaths in developing countries. Three studies reported incidence of culture-confirmed EONS, which ranged from 2.2 to 9.8 per 1000 live births. The fourth study reported the incidence of clinical EONS of 20.7 per 1000 live births.[24–27] A more recent study from Bangladesh reported the incidence of EONS observed during a home-based newborn surveillance programme. The rate of clinical EONS was 50 per 1000 live births and blood culture-confirmed EONS was 2.9 per 1000 live births. All of these studies were from the South Asian region. Two of the studies also reported case fatality rates for EONS in the range of 18–19%.

Reviews have shown that the bacteriological profiles of organisms responsible for EONS have evolved over time, highlighting the need for constant surveillance to identify predominant organisms. Knowledge of pathogens that are likely to cause sepsis guides empiric therapy while awaiting culture and antimicrobial susceptibility results.[28,29]

The longest running database on neonatal sepsis in the developed world has been maintained by the Yale-New Haven Hospital. Published findings for a 75-year period, from 1928 to 2003 showed that *Streptococcus pneumoniae* and group A streptococci account for almost half the cases from 1933 to 1943.[30] The incidences of infections due to *S. pneumoniae* or group A streptococci have shown a steady decrease and have been replaced by GBS and *Escherichia coli.* The recommendation of intrapartum use of antibiotics, since the 1990s, to reduce vertical transmission of GBS, has significantly contributed to a decline in the percentage of EONS secondary to GBS in recent years.[31]

Aetiological information on causes of EONS in developing countries is again limited. A recent review shows 44 studies that reported the causes of EONS in developing countries. Only four focused on community-acquired infections, the rest were facility-based studies not representative of home environments with high neonatal mortality rates. The limited data available in the review showed that 25% of all episodes of EONS were caused by *Klebsiella*; 15% were caused by *E. coli*; 18% were caused by *Staphylococcus aureus*; 7% were caused by GBS; and 12% were caused collectively by *Acinetobacter* and *Pseudomonas* (Table 80.1).

In the global dataset, the overall ratio of Gram-negative organisms to Gram-positive organisms was 2:1. In African countries, the ratio of Gram-positive organisms to Gram-negative organisms was equal, due to a larger proportion of infections caused by *Staphylococcus aureus* and GBS, as compared with other regions of the world. *Pseudomonas* and *Acinetobacter* were more common in East Asia, Pacific and South Asian countries and *S. aureus* was uncommon in East Asia and Latin America, as compared with other regions. Although GBS is one of the predominant organisms causing EONS in developed countries, it was uncommon in developing countries. In developing countries, South Asia had the lowest rates of GBS. The reason for this difference in distribution of GBS between developed and developing countries is not clearly understood. Stoll and Schuchat[31] reviewed 34 studies published between 1980 and 1996 that evaluated GBS colonization rates in women in developing countries. Studies using adequate culture methods found differences in the prevalence of colonization in different

TABLE 80.1 **Causes of Sepsis in Neonates up to 7 Days of Age in Developing Countries**

Organisms Isolated	≤3 Days of Life (%)	≤7 Days of Life (%)
Total	100	100
S. aureus	17.3	17.5
S. pyogenes	0.4	1
GBS	13.1	6.5
Group D streptococci	5.3	2.5
Group G streptococci		0.03
Viridans streptococci	0.04	0.2
S. pneumoniae	1.1	1.5
Other *Streptococcus* species	2.3	1.1
ALL GRAM POSITIVES	40.2	32.4
Klebsiella species	26.4	25.3
E. coli	12.6	15.3
Pseudomonas species	5.9	7.0
Enterobacter species	3.6	4.4
Serratia species	0.5	0.3
Proteus species	0.6	0.8
Salmonella species	0.7	1.2
Citrobacter species	0.4	1.3

Source: Zaidi AK, Thaver D, Ali SA, et al. Pathogens associated with sepsis in newborns and young infants in developing countries. Pediatr Infect Dis J 2009;28(Suppl 1):S10–18.

regions (Middle East/North Africa, 22%; Asia/Pacific, 19%; sub-Saharan Africa, 19%; Americas, 14%; and India/Pakistan, 12%). Other factors contributing to observed differences in GBS rates in different populations include strain virulence, maternally derived antibody levels or cultural practices. Another reason for lack of information could be that in developing countries GBS is a very early-onset illness causing death within a few hours of birth, it is possible that data miss the vast majority of GBS cases.

A number of factors contribute to the high incidence of infections and mortality. These include: immediate causes such as lack of antenatal care; unsupervised or poorly supervised home deliveries; unhygienic and unsafe delivery practices and cord care; prematurity; low birth weight; lack of exclusive breast-feeding and delays in recognition of danger signs in both mother and baby.[32] Furthermore, underlying factors such as health system inefficiencies, infrastructural, logistic or economic constraints also contribute to high rates of infection and infection-associated mortality. In addition, wide inequities exist in health service provision, such that the lowest coverage rates of known effective maternal and child interventions are in the poorest income groups.

In developing countries, blood cultures and adjunct laboratory tests are often not possible, so the diagnosis of neonatal sepsis is often based solely on clinical signs. The signs of sepsis in the neonate are often nonspecific and include lethargy or irritability, poor feeding, vomiting, jaundice, respiratory distress, apnoea, fever or hypothermia. These symptoms overlap with those of perinatal asphyxia and with normal findings in pre-term infants, further complicating the diagnosis. Neonatal pneumonia and meningitis may be included within the term, neonatal sepsis, particularly in the developing world where microbiology laboratories are not available. In addition, the clinical syndromes overlap and pneumonia and meningitis are variably accompanied by bacteremia.

There are a number of factors that put newborns in developing countries at an even greater risk for developing sepsis compared with the newborns in industrialized countries. These can be categorized into intrinsic and extrinsic factors in the antenatal, intrapartum and the early neonatal period. Intrinsic factors in the developing world include higher rates of prematurity, intrauterine growth restriction, birth asphyxia, premature and prolonged rupture of membranes and maternal peripartum infections. The most important extrinsic factors contributing to the high risk of sepsis are the lack of antenatal care and unhygienic birth practices. According to WHO estimates, only 35% of births in least developed countries are attended by a skilled health professional.

THE UNDER-5 CHILD

Diarrhoea and pneumonia are responsible for 29% of under-5 deaths globally. This is greater than the mortality caused by measles (1%), meningitis (2%), malaria (7%) and AIDS (2%) combined (Figure 80.4). Successful vaccination programmes have reduced the worldwide total for deaths caused by measles and tetanus, but each of these diseases was still responsible for about 1% of deaths worldwide in 2008. Other causes of death such as vector-borne diseases (e.g. malaria, dengue and Japanese B encephalitis), meningitis and HIV/AIDS are relatively small. AIDS, however, remains a substantial threat since so many HIV-infected people remain undiagnosed. It is remarkably striking that all-cause child deaths and deaths due to some specific causes, such as diarrhoea, pneumonia, malaria and AIDS are heavily concentrated in some countries. This is partly related to the large populations of children younger than 5 years in these countries, but also due to the concentration of diseases in these settings because of epidemiological and social conditions. Success in disease control efforts in these countries is essential if MDG 4 goals are to be achieved.

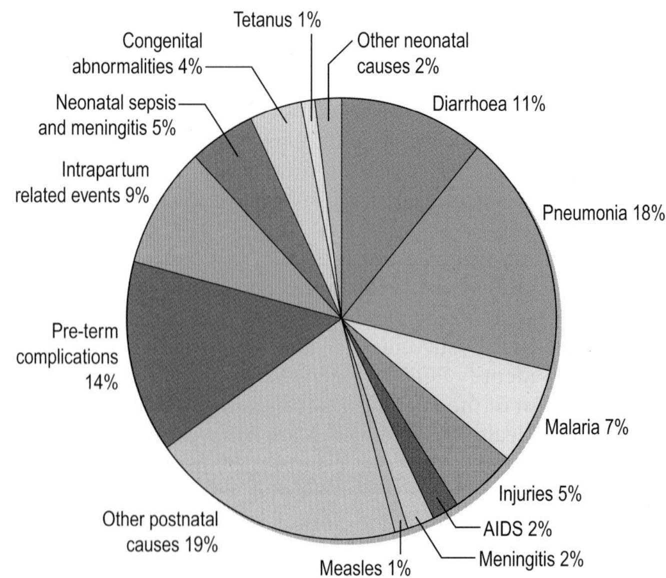

Figure 80.4 Causes of under-5 mortality worldwide. (*Source: Liu, et al. Child Health Epidemiology Reference Group of WHO and UNICEF. Global, regional and national causes of child mortality: an updated systematic analysis for 2010 with time trends since 2000. Lancet 2012;379(9832):2151–61.*)

TABLE 80.2 The 15 Countries with the Highest Estimated Number of Deaths due to Clinical Pneumonia and Diarrhoea

Country	Predicted No. of Deaths (Thousands)	Total No. of Annual Deaths due to Diarrhoea
India	408	386 600
Nigeria	204	151 700
Democratic Republic of the Congo	126	89 900
Ethiopia	112	73 700
Pakistan	91	53 300
Afghanistan	87	82 100
China	74	40 000
Bangladesh	50	50 800
Angola	47	19 700
Niger	46	151 700
Uganda	38	29 300
United Republic of Tanzania	36	23 900
Mali	32	20 900
Kenya	30	27 400
Burkina Faso	25	24 300

Source: World Health Organization, Global Burden of Disease estimates. (The totals were calculated by applying the WHO cause of death estimates to the most recent estimates for the total number of under-5 deaths, 2007 and Liu et al. 2012.)

A total of 95% of disease deaths preventable by the Expanded Programme on Immunization (EPI) vaccines are caused by measles (67%) and tetanus (28%); protection is higher for diphtheria and pertussis, as deaths from these diseases are rare. The low rate overall of deaths from vaccine-preventable diseases relates to the high rates of EPI coverage, measuring 80–95% in most countries. However, EPI coverage continues to be a problem in some countries, particularly those with poor public health infrastructure and in settings with difficult-to-reach populations such as indigenous groups.

Malnutrition is a major contributor to child deaths, in 61% of diarrhoea, 57% of malaria, 53% of pneumonia and 45% of measles deaths. Overall, 53% of all deaths may not have occurred in the under-5 age group if the child was well nourished.[33]

To summarize, pneumonia and diarrhoea are the leading killers of children and each year more than 2 million children die due to these illnesses. This toll is highly concentrated in low-income countries (Table 80.2). The persistent importance of these infections as immediate causes of death relates to predisposing factors: a lack of access to basic health facilities, unsafe and unhealthy environments. Unsafe water for drinking and food preparation, inadequate availability of water for hygiene and lack of access to sanitation contributes to around 88% of deaths from diarrhoea. Indoor air pollution is implicated in over 50% of deaths of children 0–4 years old, largely related to pneumonia and bronchitis.

Pneumonia

Pneumonia kills more children under the age of 5 than any other illness, yet it is a forgotten pandemic. Around 18% of deaths in children under the age of 5 are caused by pneumonia, 20% in low-income countries and only about 4% in high-income countries. Among these, 14% occur in the postnatal period, whereas 4% occur in the neonatal period. The relative importance of the causes differ among different regions, however, pneumonia remains a major killer of children under the age of 5 worldwide. Two-thirds of these deaths are concentrated in just 15 countries.

About 156 million new cases of pneumonia occur worldwide every year, with 74% of these new cases in just 15 countries and more than half in just six countries: India, China, Pakistan, Bangladesh, Indonesia and Nigeria. This can be attributed to high rates of malnutrition, poverty and inadequate access to health care.

Region-specific data indicate that about 50% of worldwide deaths from pneumonia in children under the age of 5 occur within the African region; less than 2% occur in the European region; and less than 3% in the region of the Americas. Figure 80.5 represents the trends in global mortality from pneumonia in children under 5 years of age over the last 2 decades. Although there has been some reduction in mortality rates, the global burden of pneumonia has remained unchanged since these composite figures hide the significant differences that exist in pneumonia mortality rates between various socioeconomic groups and countries.

Many low-income countries have introduced new vaccines against the common agents of pneumonia in children. These include the *Haemophilus influenzae* b vaccine and pneumococcal conjugate vaccine. By 2011, nearly all GAVI-eligible countries had introduced Hib vaccines with GAVI support, immunizing a cumulative 124 million children and preventing an estimated 697 000 future deaths.

Once children develop pneumonia, prompt and effective treatment saves lives. Data from a subset of countries with comparable data for around 2000 and 2010, indicate that progress in appropriate care seeking for suspected childhood pneumonia has been limited, with appropriate care seeking rising from 54% to 61%. Sub-Saharan Africa showed the most progress, although it still has the lowest level of appropriate care seeking.

It is therefore important that developing countries look at a combination of strategies for reducing the burden and mortality from pneumonia. These include the important role of preventive strategies such as control of environmental factors (e.g. indoor air pollution) dealing with prevalent micronutrient deficiencies such as zinc and vitamin A deficiencies and promotion of household behaviors such as exclusive breast-feeding and hand washing. Many of these preventive strategies have health

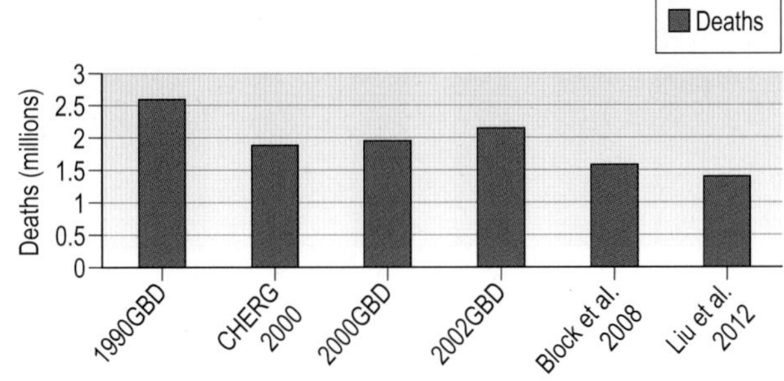

Figure 80.5 Trends in mortality from pneumonia. (Source: *Bhutta et al. 2007; Black et al. 2008; Liu et al. 2012; GBD, Global Burden of Disease; CHERG, Childhood Epidemiology Reference Group.)*

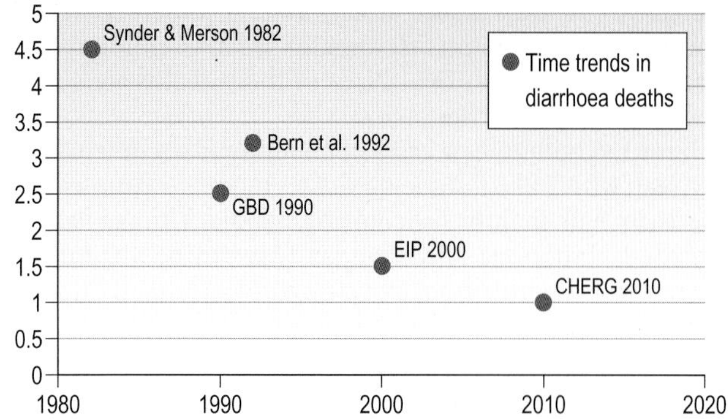

Figure 80.6 Time trends in diarrhoea deaths. (Source: *Snyder and Merson 1982 4 3; Bern et al, 1992; GBD 1990 2; EIP 2000 1; CHERG 2010 0 1975 1980 1985 1990 1995 2000 2005 2010.* Source: *Boschi-Pinto C, Tomaskovic L. For CHERG (2006) and Fischer-Walker et al. (2013).*

benefits that far exceed mere reduction in respiratory infections, such as reduction in diarrhoea burden and improvement in nutrition indices.[34]

More than 1 million lives could be saved if both prevention and treatment interventions for pneumonia were implemented universally. Around 600 000 children's lives could be saved each year through universal treatment with antibiotics alone, costing around $600 million.

Diarrhoea

About 2.5 billion episodes of diarrhoea occur per year across the world in children under 5 years of age. Every year, nearly 1 in 5 child deaths – about 1.5 million child deaths each year – are due to diarrhoea. Although mortality from diarrhoea has declined over the past three decades (Figure 80.6), it still remains the second most common cause of death among children under the age of 5, globally.

Diarrhoea incidence rates have not changed substantially over the years. Incidence rates in sub-Saharan Africa and Latin America are greater than in Asia or the Western Pacific (Figure 80.7). Walker et al. in 2012, estimated that diarrhoea incidence

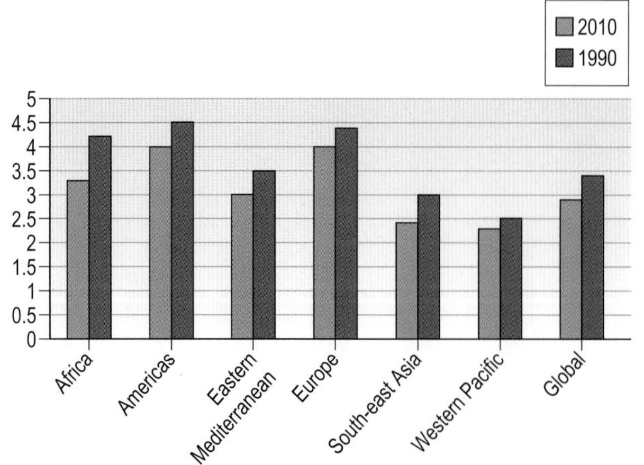

Figure 80.7 Trends in diarrhoea incidence rates in under-5 children by WHO region in low- and middle-income countries (1990–2010). (Source: *Walker et al. 2012.*)

in children under 5 years of age has declined from 3.4 episodes/child year in 1990, to 2.9 episodes/child year in 2010, with the highest incidence rate of 4.5 episodes/child year in the age group 6–11 months.[35]

Diarrhoea is more prevalent in the developing world due, in large part, to the lack of safe drinking water, sanitation and hygiene, as well as poorer overall health and nutritional status. A total of 783 million people still do not use an improved drinking water source and 2.5 billion do not use an improved sanitation facility, mostly in the poorest households and rural areas; 90% of people who practice open defecation live in rural areas. Another important cause is the reduced rates of optimal breastfeeding. Only about 40% of children under 6 months of age are exclusively breast-fed. Malnutrition has a bidirectional relationship with diarrhoea. It reduces the immunity and makes children susceptible to infections, including diarrhoea and can also be caused as a result of persistent or severe diarrhoea.[36] Childhood malnutrition is prevalent in low- and middle-income countries. According to an estimate, 20% of children <5 years of age in these countries are underweight (weight for age Z score <–2). The prevalence of both underweight is highest in Africa and South-Central Asia. Most children with diarrhoea are not managed appropriately, with only around one-third of them given oral rehydration solution (ORS). Moreover, despite the evidence of benefit, widespread introduction of zinc for diarrhoea treatment has been limited. UNICEF's zinc procurement began in 2006 and has increased substantially. Despite this progress, global zinc supply is dismally low compared with global need.

Rotavirus, responsible for at least one-third of severe and potentially fatal episodes of diarrhoea, is potentially preventable through rotavirus vaccine. In developing countries, around 440 000 deaths occur every year due to vaccine-preventable rotavirus infection.[37] Thus, cost-effectiveness and increase in access to the vaccine can potentially lead to remarkable reduction in diarrhoea mortality in developing countries.

Social Determinants of Health

Social conditions and circumstances are major determinants of health. Social factors affect health and risk behaviours, environmental exposures and access to resources that protect good health. It is generally seen that there is an inverse relationship between social position and health status of people. Developing a better understanding of the social determinants of health is essential to reduce health disparities and to design policies to address social and economic factors associated with poor health.[38] Statisticians use the term socioeconomic position (SEP) to describe the social and fiscal resources available to individuals. There is clear evidence to suggest that health indicators are inferior in lower SEP groups as compared with higher SEP groups, and this classification could be used to target resources.

EDUCATION

Education is a lifelong process starting at birth and increase in formal educational attainment is an important social goal. A causal link has been established between education and a range of health outcomes. One of the most consistent and powerful findings in public health is the strong association between mothers' education and child mortality. Results of studies show that a 1-year increment in the mother's education is associated with a 7–9% reduction in mortality in children younger than 5 years and that child mortality rates among mothers with at least 7 years of schooling were 58% lower than among those without any education. Increases in educational attainment have also been linked to reductions in fertility, which in turn contributes to reduced child and maternal mortality rates.

Considerable progress has been made in education in the past 40 years, especially in developing countries, where the mean number of years of education has increased in men and women aged 15 years and older between 1970 and 2009. For women of reproductive age (15–44 years) in developing countries, the increase is much greater. This rapid advancement in educational attainment in women has resulted in significant reductions in the gender gap in education. The impact on child health has been enormous, with an increase in women's education estimated to avert 4.2 million deaths. The expansion of women's education will have serious implications for global health in the next few decades. Increases in educational attainment will probably lead to more rapid reductions in the total fertility rate, even in sub-Saharan Africa. Research shows that education is associated with a reduction in the demand for children and thus increased demand for family planning services.

Early childhood offers huge opportunities to reduce health inequities within a generation. The importance of early child development and education for health across the lifespan provides a strong imperative to start action at the grass-roots level.[39] Inaction will have detrimental effects that can last more than a lifetime. A new approach is needed that embraces a more comprehensive understanding of early child development and includes not just physical survival but also social, emotional and cognitive development.

INEQUITY

Inequities in intervention coverage are generally unfair, yet avoidable. Within-country inequities in the health of mothers and children in low-income and middle-income countries are generally indiscernible from the global medical literature. The assumption has been that all mothers and children in low-income and middle-income countries were equally poor and that there was no need to account for subnational inequalities when strategies were designed for the scaling-up of health interventions. Practical difficulties in the stratification of health status by socioeconomic position contributed to this lack of visibility. The most inequitable indicators are skilled birth attendant, followed by four or more antenatal care visits, whereas the most equitable was early initiation of breast-feeding. These analyses confirm previous findings that, unlike in high-income countries, in many low-income countries, breast-feeding is more prevalent in poor than in rich individuals.

Interventions that are usually delivered in fixed health facilities, particularly those that need constant access to secondary-level or tertiary-level care, tend to be the most inequitably distributed in the population (e.g. skilled birth attendant and four or more antenatal care visits). Interventions that are often delivered at community level (e.g. vaccinations or vitamin A supplementation) tend to be much more equitable than are those delivered in health facilities (Figure 80.8). Cost might also be a factor. Some interventions are usually provided free of charge, such as vaccinations and vitamin A, but others might need out-of-pocket spending by families, either for services or because families need to travel to a health facility. For example, in Uzbekistan, Kyrgyzstan and Brazil, where maternity hospitals are accessible and free of charge, coverage for skilled birth attendant is almost universal.[40] Cultural perceptions might affect care-seeking patterns and the choice of whether to adopt specific interventions, such as contraceptives or breast-feeding, despite counselling or information campaigns.

SOCIAL SECURITY

Lack of basic and social security is an important determinant of health. Extending social protection to all people will eventually pave the way towards securing health equity. This is not just a matter of social justice; it is also the key to social protection

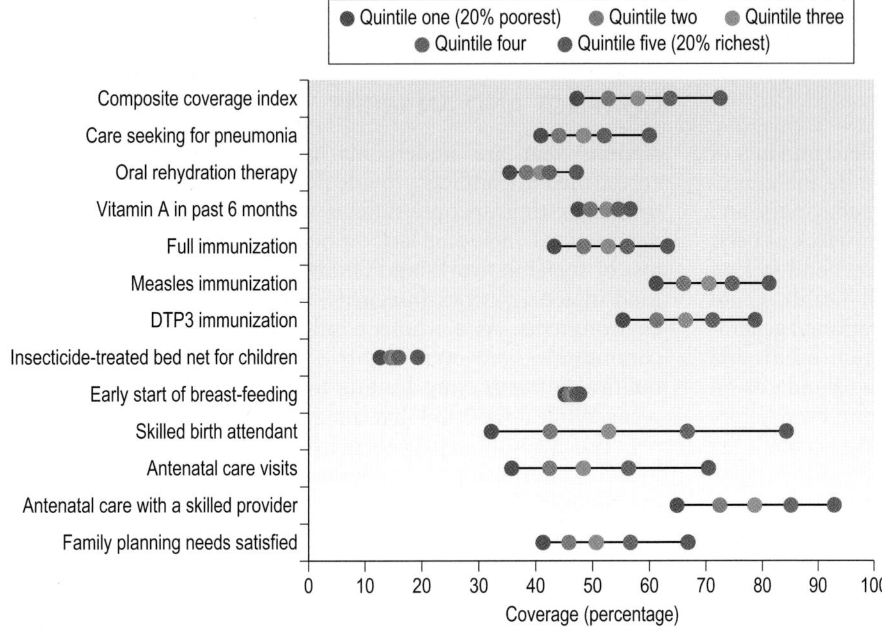

Figure 80.8 Mean coverage in respective wealth quintile for studied interventions in the 54 Countdown countries. Coloured dots show the average coverage in each of the respective wealth quintile. Q1 is the 20% poorest quintile; Q5 is the 20% richest quintile. The distance between quintiles 1 and 5 represents absolute inequality. (*Source: Adapted from Barros et al, Lancet 2012.*)

and can be instrumental in realizing developmental goals. Social protection can cover a broad range of services and benefits, including: basic income security; entitlements to non-income-based benefits such as food and other basic needs; services such as health care and education; and labour protection and benefits such as maternity leave, paid leave, childcare and health insurance. Countries with more generous social protection systems tend to have better population health outcomes. Data on the association between the magnitude of health inequities within countries and social protection policies remain scarce, however, and more investment in comparable data sources and methods is needed. The existing data from high-income countries show that while relative mortality inequities are not smaller in states with more generous, universal, social protection systems, absolute mortality levels among disadvantaged groups are lower.

Universal social protection systems should safeguard the health and rights of all people across their lifespan – as children, in working life and in old age. Women and children are among the most vulnerable in terms of the population, especially when it comes to health and diseases. Women do most of the household work, have a reproductive role as well and more often than not, assist their male counterparts in work outside the home, especially those from lower-incomes groups. Their work is not subject to maternity leave or benefits. A national strategy to eradicate child poverty needs to be enacted upon, which should ideally encompass as least financial security, employment support and security, housing security and opportunities to avail public amenities.

Addressing health equity through a social determinants framework is a long-term investment. Low- and middle-income countries cannot be expected to implement a fully comprehensive suite of universal social protection policies overnight. It is, however, feasible gradually to develop these systems by developing and implementing pilot projects. Many low- and middle-income countries are starting to experiment with social protection programmes. These include social pension schemes and cash transfer programmes. Administrative and institutional capacity remains a critical barrier in many poor countries. Nevertheless, poor countries can progressively expand such systems by starting pilot projects and by gradually increasing the system's generosity, where necessary, with help from donors.

POVERTY

Poverty and low living standards are powerful determinants of ill-health and health inequity. They have significant consequences towards determining health-related behaviours and poor health outcomes. Crowded living conditions, lack of basic amenities, unsafe neighbourhoods, parental stress and lack of food security are all contributors towards ill health. Child poverty and transmission of poverty from generation to generation are major obstacles to improving population health and reducing health inequity. The influence of living standards on healthcare behaviour is a process that begins from even before a child is conceived and continues until he or she becomes the cause of another birth.

LACK OF EMPOWERMENT

Any serious effort to reduce health inequities will involve political empowerment, as in changing the distribution of power within society from the leaders and community stakeholders to people themselves. Health equity depends vitally on the empowerment of individuals and groups to represent their needs and interests and also to challenge and change the inequitable and skewed distribution of social resources and material resources. It is important to have the freedom to participate in economic, social, political and cultural opportunities. Restriction in participation can result in deprivation of fundamental human capacities, setting the grounds for unequal distribution of employment, education and health care.

A special mention should be made of the indigenous population, the lives of whom continue to be governed by specific and particular laws, regulations and conditions that apply to no other members of civil states. They continue to live on bounded or segregated lands and are often at the heart of jurisdictional divides between levels of governments, particularly in areas concerning access to financial allocations, programmes and services. The enactment of legal changes to recognize and support community empowerment initiatives will ensure the comprehensive inclusion of disadvantaged groups in action at global, national and local levels concerned with improving health and health equity.

DEFICIENT AUTONOMY

The global growth in precarious employment and child and bonded labour both reflects and reinforces a disempowerment of workers and their industrial and political representatives. Such a system jeopardizes the autonomy of people to exercise control and their free will in decisions regarding health, education and living conditions.

Autonomy of women for decision-making and resource utilization needs to be recognized. The support of women's efforts to coordinate through resourcing via private donors and government is very important for ensuring gender equity. For instance, building their own organizations has been one of the ways that women have chosen to promote solidarity, offer support and collectively work for change. These organizations are of various sizes, from small village-based or neighbourhood groups to large movements. It is imperative to support and encourage such organizations and movements in a way that preserves and protects their autonomy and promotes their long-term sustainability, and self-reliance.

CONFLICT AND ANARCHY

Nations that are undergoing rapid power shifts and are entrenched in conflicts provide poor security to individuals. In conflict settings, people suffer a variety of physical and social deprivations, including lack of social security, displacement and loss of social networks and family structure, loss of livelihood, food insecurity, work insecurity, and poor physical and social environments. As a whole, conflict disempowers individuals, communities and even countries and cripples the social and political infrastructure leading to a multitude of health concerns. While it is critical that community members share control over processes that affect their lives, without political commitment and leadership and allocation of resources such initiatives can be short-lived.

Evidence-based Solutions

Priorities across the continuum of care need to be emphasized to move the agenda of the MDGs forward. Current recommendations target reproductive health (contraceptive information and services, sexual health and safe abortion services); maternal health (skilled birth attendants; facility-based delivery, emergency obstetric care and postpartum care); stillbirths (addressing the complications of childbirth, maternal infections and diseases and maternal undernutrition); newborn health (addressing the complications of pre-term birth), child health (targeting pneumonia, diarrhoea and malaria); and adolescent health (sexuality education and universal access to reproductive health services).

Across the world, many children from the most deprived and impoverished groups are still dying of easily preventable diseases due to poor access to quality health services. Effective interventions exist to address all of the main causes of child deaths, yet the infrastructure required to make these available on a timely basis is not present.[41] Enhancing access to and use of life-saving commodities is essential, as is investing in neonatal and maternal health and nutrition. At the moment, it is an essential need to focus on those simple and cost-effective intervention issues that will bring about the greatest morbidity and mortality benefit, particularly those due to pneumonia, diarrhoea and malaria. Urgent efforts are needed in health system capacity to take care of newborns, particularly in the field of human resources, such as training nurses and midwives for newborn and premature baby care and ensuring reliable supplies of commodities and equipment.

INTERVENTIONS IN THE NEWBORN

About 60 million of the world's 130 million births occur at home. Many more take place in facilities without adequate resources to prevent stillbirth. Figure 80.9 shows the estimates of the global number of babies undergoing resuscitation at birth. Thus, we need to focus on ways to improve healthcare systems to increase coverage of key, life-saving perinatal interventions. The components of such systems include facilities, equipment and supplies, but also involve various healthcare

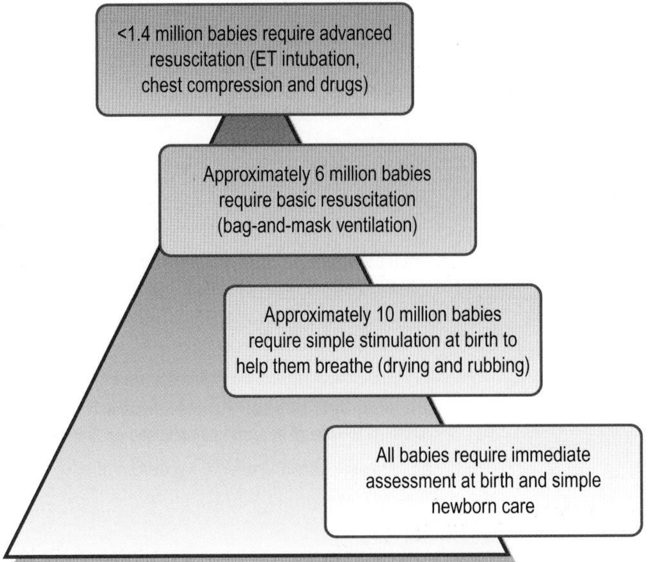

Figure 80.9 Estimates of global number of babies undergoing resuscitation at birth. (Source: *Wall SN, et al. Int J Gynecol Obstet 2009;107(S47–64)*.

providers. Studies show that the linking of community birth attendants to referral systems and facility-based clinical care is beneficial.[42] Evidence also indicates that the mobilization and empowerment of communities to increase demand for and implement improvements in pregnancy-related care can facilitate reductions in the large stillbirth burden in low-income and middle-income countries.

At the level of the international community, several steps can be taken to reduce stillbirths.[43] To enumerate, stillbirth reduction should be included in all relevant maternal and neonatal health initiatives and international health reports. Reporting of accurate stillbirth rates and cause-of-death data should be established. Furthermore, a universal classification system and implementation of an effective business model to reduce stillbirths is necessary. Key actions at the level of individual countries should include: empowerment for women and families; setting-up pregnancy improvement committees; providing birth plans and transportation; reducing the stigma associated with stillbirths; and provision of bereavement support.

Strengthening family-community and outreach services, including health education to improve homecare practices and preventive services such as tetanus immunization, can be done relatively quickly and can reduce neonatal deaths by 20–40%. High coverage of clinical care, which includes skilled maternal and immediate newborn care, emergency obstetric care and emergency newborn care, is needed to achieve the larger reductions in child mortality required to meet MDG 4. Postnatal care and intrapartum care both have the potential to save 20–40% of newborn lives, but postnatal care costs about half the amount of skilled care during childbirth. Postnatal care for mothers and newborns has not received much emphasis in public health programmes. Care at birth and in the first days of life can not only save the lives of mothers and newborns, but also reduces serious long-term complications.[44] Progress is slow, especially in reaching poor families. Currently, only about half of women worldwide deliver with a skilled attendant. The variation between countries is extreme, ranging from 5% to 99%. Skilled attendance and institutional delivery rates are lowest in countries with the highest neonatal mortality rates.

Simple immediate newborn care should be provided to newborns in all settings as part of essential newborn care. These include warming, drying, stimulation, hygiene and thermal care. These are the first and immediate steps in neonatal resuscitation and can even be performed by family members. Training in essential newborn care, either before or concurrent with training in basic and advanced neonatal resuscitation should be ensured at all levels.[45] Basic neonatal resuscitation training can be performed by a wide range of health providers (from traditional birth attendants (TBAs), community health workers (CHWs), nurses and midwives to physicians), resulting in reductions in intrapartum-related mortality in both the facility and home settings (Table 80.3).

There is evidence from India and Indonesia that community-based neonatal resuscitation may be both feasible and effective in reducing intrapartum-related mortality in settings with high rates of home birth and delivery attendance by community cadres, ranging from TBAs and CHWs to midwives.[46] Training for community-level neonatal resuscitation should not occur in isolation. It should be paralleled with efforts to strengthen health systems and the quality of, and linkages to, facility-based skilled emergency obstetric care.

Several key considerations are required for an effective and sustainable programme, including:

TABLE 80.3 Interventions to Save Newborn Lives

	Interventions
Immediate essential newborn care – at the time of birth	Promotion and provision of thermal care for all newborns to prevent hypothermia (immediate drying, warming, skin to skin, delayed bathing) Promotion and support for early initiation and exclusive breast-feeding (within the first hour) Promotion and provision of hygienic cord and skin care Neonatal resuscitation with bag and mask for babies who do not breathe at birth Newborn immunization
Neonatal infection management	Presumptive antibiotic therapy for the newborns at risk of bacterial infection Case management of neonatal sepsis, meningitis and pneumonia Initiation of ART in babies born to HIV-infected mother
Small and ill babies	Kangaroo mother care for pre-term and for <2000 g babies Extra support for feeding the small and pre-term baby Prophylactic and therapeutic use of surfactant to prevent respiratory distress syndrome in pre-term babies Continuous positive airway pressure (CPAP) to manage pre-term babies with respiratory distress syndrome Management of newborns with jaundice

Source: The Partnership for Maternal, Newborn & Child Health. A Global Review of the Key Interventions Related to Reproductive, Maternal, Newborn and Child Health (RMNCH). Geneva: PMNCH; 2011.

1. A trained attendant must be present at birth, to recognize and assist a baby who does not breathe and attend an adequate number of cases to maintain skills
2. Training should focus on essential newborn care first
3. Adequate systems should be in place for equipment procurement, cleaning/maintenance, resupply
4. Systems are required for supervision, refresher training and monitoring of skills retention
5. Functional referral systems should exist for post-resuscitation care and to follow-up resuscitated newborns.

A range of preventive strategies can reduce the burden of neonatal infections in community settings and must be implemented at scale. Preventive strategies can be implemented in all cases and in at-risk populations (Figure 80.10). However, the key to treating neonatal infections successfully in community settings is the appropriate rapid diagnosis and triage to therapy. The onset of illness and course of progression is much more rapid in newborns, thus both clinical diagnosis, as well as empirical therapy are the mainstay for management of neonatal sepsis.[47] Appropriate strategies are needed for prevention of infections, as well as interventions for the domiciliary care and referral of newborn infants who develop bacterial infections. In several resource-poor situations, where prompt referral to a facility is not possible, health workers may have no alternative but to provide domiciliary care, which entails visiting households to provide care for the treatment of serious neonatal bacterial infections (Table 80.4). To prevent EONS in low-resource settings, cost-effective interventions must be introduced at the community level, with prevention strategies applied during the antenatal, intrapartum and early neonatal period. It is estimated that implementation of these interventions with coverage of 99% can prevent 41–72% of neonatal deaths globally. The knowledge and implementation of these interventions, however, is lacking in the poorest countries, where they are most needed.

The benefits of breast milk in preventing neonatal infections and infection-related neonatal mortality are well established. Early and exclusive breast-feeding should be encouraged in developing country settings, since it is perhaps the most important postnatal intervention to prevent EONS.[48] Hygienic newborn care also needs to be encouraged to prevent infections in the early neonatal period. This includes sanitary disposal of waste, provision of clean water in homes and hand washing by care providers. Appropriate cord and skin care is also essential with recent trials showing the benefit of cord and skin cleansing with chlorhexidine. Similarly, massage of newborns with topical sunflower oil, a traditional practice in some communities, has been shown to produce substantial reductions in hospital-acquired neonatal infections among pre-term infants in randomized controlled trials in developing countries. Kangaroo care by mothers is another intervention that can decrease EONS. Kangaroo care involves skin-to-skin contact between mother and infant in a strict vertical position between a

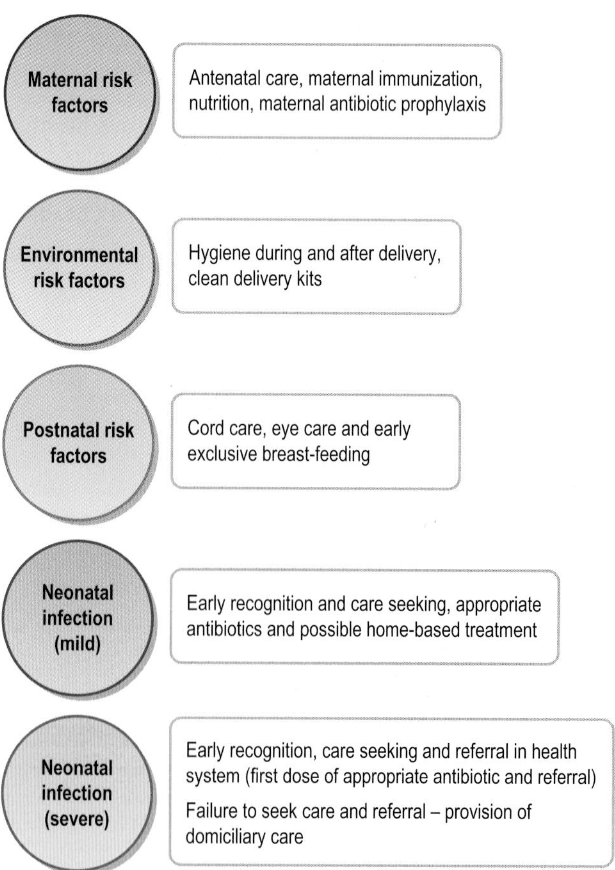

Figure 80.10 Risk factors and intervention strategies for serious neonatal infections. *(Source: Bhutta ZA, et al. Pediatr Infect Dis J 2009;28:S22–30.)*

TABLE 80.4 Factors Determining Approaches to Community Management of Neonatal Sepsis

Overarching Considerations	Health System Preparedness	Availability of Community Healthcare Providers	Family and Household Factors	Information Determining Antibiotic Choice and Route of Therapy
Development of an overall strategic plan for managing serious neonatal infections Epidemiological data suggestive of high burden of neonatal sepsis in domiciliary settings Patterns of care seeking and access suggestive of the need for community-based care	Outreach services capable of supporting community health workers Linkages with various tiers of the health services for referral and effective care Health information systems capable of supporting community care strategies	Community health workers available for household visits and case detection Community health workers trained to detect serious neonatal infections Community health workers trained in recognition of serious infections in newborns and young infants Community health workers authorized to treat with oral or injectable antibiotics	Care-seeking practices for newborns and gender-related behaviours Access to health services and emergency transport Willingness to sustain regular access and supervised treatment in community clinics/health centres Acceptance of home care	Local microbiology and antimicrobial resistance patterns Availability of common antibiotics effective for above pathogens Availability of antibiotics for daily delivery, preferably once-daily dosages in suitable form (e.g. Uniject)

Source: Bhutta ZA, et al., Pediatr Infect Dis J 2009;28:S22–S30.

mother's breasts and frequent and exclusive breast-feeding. Kangaroo care provides the benefits of increasing body temperature and weight of the child and reducing the stress level of the infant. These factors, combined with the increased rate of exclusive breast-feeding, might be responsible for the lower rates of infections in neonates receiving kangaroo care.

In developed countries, the standard of care for management of EONS is in-patient administration of parenteral antibiotics and supportive care, often in an intensive care unit setting. Hospitalization provides supportive care, such as intravenous fluids; oxygen therapy, when needed; and a controlled thermal environment. The WHO recommends the same standard of care for newborns in developing countries. Unfortunately, most newborns with severe illness in developing countries never reach a healthcare facility. Treatment strategies, therefore, in developing countries, need to be tailored to deliver care at the community level (home or primary care facility), with close interaction between the community health workers, mothers and other family members and linkages with the formal health system. WHO and United Nations Children's Fund (UNICEF) have developed the Integrated Management of Neonatal and Childhood Illnesses (IMNCI) programme, which trains community health workers to identify severely ill infants and provide treatment and referral.[49]

A recent review on the management of neonatal sepsis in primary care settings shows that there is a deficiency of data on community-based management options. However, the use of parenteral antibiotics integrated into home- or community-based packages is an effective option. There is a lack of aetiological data for EONS from community settings, which makes it difficult to design empiric antibiotic regimens. Among the various parenteral antibiotic options, penicillins, cephalosporins and aminoglycosides are most commonly used in health-facility settings of developed and developing countries. For many families in the developing world, living in remote communities, even injectable antibiotic therapy is not easily accessible. Administration of oral antibiotics is preferred in such situations as an alternative in affected neonates and is superior to no therapy. Furthermore, added information on antimicrobial resistance patterns of pathogens causing EONS in the community in different regions of the world is needed to devise appropriate empiric treatment regimens.

INTERVENTIONS IN THE UNDER-5 CHILD

Effective interventions to reduce pneumonia and diarrhoea and the morbidity and mortality associated with them includes primary prevention by reduction of environmental risk factors, as well as immunization and secondary prevention by effective case management once the infection has been acquired. These strategies could save the lives of innumerable children that die of preventable causes of pneumonia and diarrhoea each year.[50] There is an overlap between many of the prevention and treatment strategies of diarrhoea and pneumonia (Figure 80.11).

Pneumonia

Adopting strategies to achieve targets for effective immunization against measles and pertussis via national immunization programmes is central to prevention of preventable causes of pneumonia. Vaccinations against other pathogens such as *Streptococcus pneumoniae* and *Haemophilus influenzae* type b have only recently been introduced. The latter has been integrated into the national immunization programme of many countries but the integration of the former is still just a recommendation in most countries. Progress in this area is expected, especially in the least developed countries.[51] However, introducing a vaccine does not necessarily translate into high and equitable coverage within countries and inequities in uptake greatly reduce the impact of vaccines.

Simple measures for primary prevention basically include exclusive breast-feeding and zinc supplementation.[52] These strategies reduce rates of low birth weight and undernutrition, which helps prevent pneumonia. Indoor air pollution is a well-known risk factor for pneumonia in children under 5 because of special susceptibility factors that place children at particular risk – their lungs and immune systems are not fully mature,

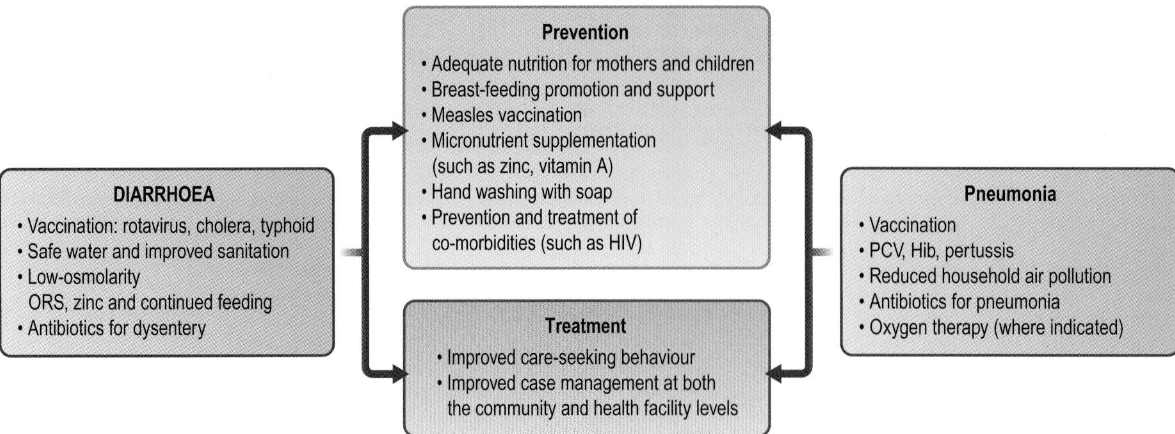

Figure 80.11 Prevention and treatment strategies for diarrhoea and pneumonia are identical. (Source: *Gupta GR. Tackling pneumonia and diarrhoea: the deadliest diseases for the world's poorest children. Lancet 2012;379(9832):2123–4.)*

they breathe more in proportion to their body size and they spend most of their time inside the home. Indoor air pollution in developing countries is due largely to the use of solid fuels for cooking or heating purposes in poorly ventilated and closed home units. Material used most often for fuels to light fires and stoves in most rural and many urban areas include wood, crop waste, animal dung and coal. Statistics show that around 3 billion people worldwide use solid fuels as their main cooking fuel and more recent studies show that the use of this solid fuel contributes to as many as 2 million premature and preventable deaths, with as many as half of them attributable to childhood pneumonia alone. The use of these solid fuels is disproportionally higher in rural areas as compared with urban households. Now, with increased spending in research, newer technologies have become available that can reduce indoor air pollution that may help prevent pneumonia. In addition to this, allocation of funds for additional research is needed to demonstrate the health benefits of these interventions.

Overcrowding in homes is also associated with increased risk of childhood pneumonia because disease-causing pathogens can spread to more people faster in the small vicinity of a house. Houses in rural areas and urban slums are typically devoid of shutters and windows. This leads to entrapment of indoor pollutants and bacteria that in turn make the inhabitants of the house more susceptible to both upper and lower respiratory tract infections.

Once infection has been acquired, case management following the appropriate guidelines is imperative. Countries with a high under-5 mortality rate should strive to implement strategies to ensure adequate pneumonia case-management at hospitals, healthcare facilities and community levels, to achieve sufficient coverage within a predetermined timeframe. In low-income settings, elaborate laboratory investigations such as chest radiographs, blood sampling and sputum analysis and culture are not easily available to confirm diagnosis, identify the underlying pathogen and determine the severity of illness or direct treatment guidelines.[53] Even without these tools, pneumonia can be easily classified and treated based on symptoms and physical examinations according to IMNCI guidelines. Based on these guidelines, pneumonia can be classified by a fast respiratory rate counted by a trained healthcare worker. Children diagnosed with pneumonia should receive a full course of effective antibiotics because most severe cases have a bacterial cause. WHO recommends amoxicillin given twice daily for 3–5 days. In cases of severe pneumonia and if infrastructure for a healthcare setup more advanced than the very basic is available, then pulse oximetry to improve the diagnostic specificity for pneumonia, oxygen systems for providing as needed oxygen as an emergency measure, injectable antibiotics and other supportive measures for continued care may help children with severe acute respiratory syndromes.

Diarrhoea

Primary preventive strategies are both simple and effective for the prevention of diarrhoea. A clean home and surrounding environment are indispensible to reduce disease. Access to safe and clean drinking water and adequate sanitation are necessary to prevent diarrhoea. Improving home and personal hygiene helps prevent diarrhoea. Nearly 90% of deaths due to diarrhoea worldwide have been attributed to unsafe water, inadequate sanitation and poor hygiene. Water, sanitation and hygiene programs include several interventions including promoting safe disposal of human faeces, encouraging hand washing with soap, improving water quality and advancing household water treatment and safe storage.[54] Supply of potable water is again an equity-based issue and requires an equity-based solution in that poor households and marginalized areas require more attention.

Hand washing with water and soap is the most cost-effective health intervention for reducing the incidence of not only diarrhoea in children under age 5 but also other diseases like pneumonia. There is consistent and dependable evidence to suggest that hand washing with soap at necessary times such as before eating a meal, before preparing food and feeding a child and after using the lavatory can effectively reduce the risk of diarrhoea. Monitoring of correct hand washing techniques by supervised healthcare personnel in the community can help in the assessment of community behaviour with respect to hand washing, and thus serve as an effective preventive strategy in the defence against diarrhoeal pathogens.[55]

Maternal and child malnutrition is also a contributing factor to the morbidity and mortality associated with diarrhoea. While all undernourished children are at higher risk of death, severely under-weight, wasted and stunted children are at greatest risk. Undernutrition generally weakens the immune system, that itself requires adequate protein for antibody and interferon formation in addition to energy, vitamins and minerals for proper functioning. For diarrhoea, undernutrition places children at higher risk of more severe frequent and prolonged illness. Undernutrition is also a consequence of repeated bouts of illness such as diarrhoea itself and in effect malnutrition and diarrhoea are linked to one another by a vicious cycle that further worsens a child's crippling nutritional status at a time when they have higher caloric requirement. Beliefs associated with diarrhoea, that if feeding is stopped then it might actually improve the diarrhoea, need to be dispelled.

Repeated diarrhoeal episodes in young children lead to stunting and hence adequate and effective control of diarrhoea in the first few months of life reduces the prevalence of stunting among children. Undernutrition and infection interact to create a potentially lethal cycle of worsening illness and deteriorating nutritional status. Critical nutrition interventions to break this cycle include encouraging optimum breast-feeding practices such as early initiation, exclusive breast-feeding for the first 6 months of life and continued breast-feeding to age ≥2, encouraging micronutrient supplementation and also reducing the incidence of low-birth-weight newborns through interventions to improve maternal health and nutrition. Infants who are cared for in this manner develop fewer infections and suffer less severe illness. Underlying the inculcation of this health-conscious behaviour are other interventions such as improving maternal education, provision of healthcare workers and improving empowerment through policy-making and implementation.

In addition, micronutrient supplementation such as zinc and vitamin A are critical for normal growth and development in young children. However, the coverage remains low. Zinc deficiency places children at greater risk of illness and death due to pneumonia and diarrhoea, particularly in low-income countries. There is evidence that zinc is beneficial in managing acute or persistent diarrhoea in children under 5, especially with respect to reduction in duration of illness.[56] In addition, vitamin A supplementation reduces all-cause and diarrhoea-related mortality among children less than 5 years. Vitamin A therapy during an episode of measles has also been demonstrated to reduce the child's risk of post-measles diarrhoea and other measles-associated complications. Coverage for these two supplements, although not ideal at the moment does show a promising trend towards increasing coverage in developing countries.

Rotavirus results in higher diarrhoea-related death in children less than 5 years of age, than any other single agent. This is especially true of low- and middle-income countries. Although the vaccine is available, it is not yet part of the National Immunization Programme in many countries. The number of countries planning to introduce vaccination, however, is increasing.

Once diarrhoea has occurred, prompt recognition and treatment are essential. The UNICEF/WHO joint recommendation for the treatment of diarrhoea under the IMNCI strategy includes encouraging universal access and provision of the oral rehydration solution, continued feeding, recommended home-made fluids and zinc treatment for children with acute diarrhoea. A recent change has been the modification of the original high-osmolarity ORS to the new low-osmolarity solution, which reduces stool output and the overall duration of diarrhoea. Zinc treatment for 10–14 days, in addition to low-osmolarity ORS, is an adjunct therapy that reduces the duration and severity of a diarrhoea episode and the likelihood of subsequent infections in the 2–3 months following treatment. At the policy level, many strategies have been implemented, yet at the implementation level, many gaps still need to be filled.

The role of probiotics needs emphasis. Daily intake of a probiotic drink can play a role in prevention of acute diarrhoea in young children, as shown in community-based trials.[57]

Delivery Strategies

The comprehensive goal of child health interventions is to improve child survival and reduce the overall burden of childhood diseases. Policies that govern the improvement of child survival need periodic renewal and assessment, since changing geo-political situations put the continuity of implementation strategies at risk.

In this chapter, we aim to present the tasks or the core solutions required for the improvement of child survival and the implementation strategies that are required to channel a task on paper into a task in action. Beginning from the care of the expecting mother all the way to the adolescent child, solutions need to be focused around interventions and scaling-up those interventions to reach all sections of society equitably.

REDUCING POVERTY-ASSOCIATED BARRIERS

The structure of national health systems in many countries continues to direct most resources away from their poorest citizens. Unless the bottlenecks faced by poor and marginalized people in access to and use of health interventions and services are explicitly addressed, inequities will probably worsen, as more expensive and elaborate interventions are introduced. Expansion of coverage by empowering women, removing financial and social barriers to accessing basic services, developing innovations that make the supply of critical services more available to the poor and increasing local accountability of health systems are policy interventions that would allow health systems to improve equity and reduce mortality.[58]

Reduction or elimination of user fees increases the use of curative services and facility-based deliveries, although the effect sizes vary depending on study site and outcome examined. Equity also seems to improve, with the greatest increases in access noted in households from the poorest quintiles. Legislation mandating universal access to maternal healthcare services and eliminating user fees in low- and middle-income countries also have been shown to be an important prerequisite to ensuring all women receive antenatal care. However, quality of care can be negatively affected by difficulties in meeting increased demand and in provision of drugs to more patients, poor staff morale, decreasing health service revenues and the creation of unofficial fees to replace user fees.

A programme that provides monetary transfers to households on the condition that they comply with a set of behavioural requirements can serve to bring equity-based health care to target disadvantaged groups. As low-income individuals usually face the greatest barriers to access, such conditional cash transfer mechanisms can also help redistribute resources to reduce health inequities. They can potentially increase the use of health services by low-income individuals, by providing funds to help overcome some financial barriers to access, including costs related to seeking health care or sending children to school. Such programmes have been used effectively in Latin America to provide tangible benefits to marginalized groups. For instance, an incentive such as free provision of food supplements on the condition that children would be brought for preventive health examinations where they would have the opportunity to receive vaccinations, deworming agents, vitamins and supplements, is an excellent means to bring about a health-related behavioural change in a local community.[59] Other reasonable incentives can be cash transfers contingent on enrolment and regular attendance at primary school. This approach has the capacity to scale-up existing resources for measurable outcomes. However, success depends upon a working and effective infrastructure that can provide services.

COMMUNITY APPROACHES AND TASK SHIFTING

Robust evidence shows that delivery of several key interventions can be safely and effectively transferred from clinical services (i.e. provided by qualified health professionals) to community health workers. For example, training of TBAs and other CHWs to dispense simple immediate preventive and curative actions for neonatal care, including neonatal resuscitation and injectable antibiotics, is likely to reduce stillbirths and perinatal mortality in various settings. Additional evidence suggests that CHWs can effectively provide treatments and care to reduce morbidity and mortality prenatally and in children under 5. More recent evidence for the effect of community-based malaria treatment on child health outcomes suggests a reduction in malaria prevalence and a fall in under-5 mortality when combined with delivery of insecticide-treated nets and antimalarial chemoprophylaxis.

Subcontracting of services, such as obstetric care, maintenance of health services and administration, to private sector providers is another strategy that could reduce bottlenecks associated with geographical access, particularly for isolated districts.[60] More intensive and extensive use of outreach services is another strategy to change how interventions are delivered. Studies show that increasing the number of locations such as local health set-ups and schools offering immunization services can lead to moderate-to-high gains in coverage. Additionally, provision of specialist outreach services can substantially improve access without compromising the quality of care and might improve the skills and morale of the health workers in remote settings.

Transference of interventions that necessitate little optional action – such as immunization, vitamin A supplementation, insecticide-treated nets and deworming medicines – from clinical services to large-scale campaigns, is also an effective way to boost coverage. These campaigns are regularly used by low-income and middle-income countries to deliver key child survival interventions more efficiently, overcome coverage bottlenecks such as distance to health clinics, and improve equity of coverage by targeting groups most at risk of missing out on these services.

Evidence suggests that mass media campaigns can directly and indirectly produce positive changes or prevent negative changes in health-related behaviours across large populations and thereby substitute for individual care and attention. Social marketing has positive effects on promotion of awareness and use of insecticide-treated nets and adoption of recommended practices for dengue prevention.[61]

The establishment and enhancement of partnerships with councils, health organizations and non-governmental organizations as well as the private sector offers an opportunity to develop more effective tools to reach out to the indigenous population. Public support on regulatory issues can be enhanced through partnerships by increasing the understanding of the partner organizations and the regulatory process associated with the development and implementation of various policies.

MONITORING AND ACCOUNTABILITY

To maximize the impact of multiple initiatives in women and children's health and to ensure coordination and coherence in their implementation, a more formal global governance framework for women and children's health needs to be established. At present, there is a governance gap that must be filled by a mechanism that includes partner countries, multilateral agencies, donors, non-governmental organizations, health professionals, researchers, foundations and the private sector.

Scarcity of data is still a major obstacle for identifying where the real burden of disease rests. Medically certified vital registration data need to be made available for future health initiatives to progress. Where mortality rates and the need for data are the highest, resources and data are least available. Global, regional and national childhood cause-of-death estimates should enable the setting of priorities for scaling up child survival interventions and guide national and international resource allocation.[62] The attainment of the MDGs is possible only if life-saving maternal, newborn and child health interventions are rapidly scaled-up in high-burden regions. Continued efforts to gather high-quality data are essential and require strengthening of national health information systems to enable better accountability. The potential for digital technology to accelerate improvements in women and children's health is great – notably, in supporting country civil registration and vital statistics systems.

POLICY AND EDUCATION

Workplace policies are important to promote healthy pregnancies and reduce the risk of pre-term birth, including regulations to protect pregnant women from physically demanding work. Studies have shown that carrying heavy workloads and working more than 5 days a week is associated with pre-term birth. Environmental policies to reduce exposure to potentially harmful pollutants, such as from traditional cook stoves and second-hand smoke are also necessary. Examples include time off for antenatal care visits, paid pregnancy leave and exemption from nightshifts and tasks requiring heavy lifting or standing for long periods of time.[63] Measures that can improve general working conditions are especially important for pregnant women in low- and middle-income countries, where they are more likely to be engaged in agricultural labour and other physically demanding tasks.

Human rights-based approaches have a crucial, but neglected part to play in the delivery of global strategy.[64] In 2011, the Committee on the Elimination of Discrimination against Women became the first UN human rights body to state that countries have an obligation to guarantee and take responsibility for women's timely and non-discriminatory access to maternal health services. Individual or group education or knowledge-transfer interventions (e.g. counselling, training and education) applied to specific services or practices, such as breast-feeding and complementary feeding, can greatly improve coverage.

ALLOCATION OF FUNDS

Identification of a budget that would ensure the sustainability of existing and upcoming projects is critical. Allocation of funding in the right direction is an imperative through which implementation of policies can be accomplished.

Cash transfers are an effective way to increase use of health and nutrition services and have moderate effect sizes depending on the indicator. Cash transfers have clear effects on health outcomes, particularly morbidity and on some longer-term outcomes, such as stunting and anaemia. Despite the quality of some studies, reviewers noted that disentanglement of the effects of different programme components (especially non-cash components) was difficult. Some evidence suggests that vouchers, which are distributed free or at low cost, provide an entitlement to a good or service and then reimburse the facilities or providers, can substantially improve use and quality of services and reduce care-seeking delays.

IMCI, IMNCI (INTEGRATED STRATEGIES)

Globally, a limited number of childhood illnesses, such as pneumonia, diarrhoea, measles, malaria and malnutrition are the cause of children dying under the age of 5 years. Focusing specifically on these illnesses and training personnel in their specific management can help save innumerable lives. The WHO and UNICEF therefore came up with the idea of an integrated management of childhood illness (IMCI) strategy, which relied upon using simple clinical signs for case detection without the use of sophisticated laboratory investigations. As soon as a case is labelled, empirical treatment is started. Further, the 'integrated' approach entails the combination of major childhood illnesses with involvement of parents in provision of home-based care, prevention of disease through immunization, improved nutrition and breast-feeding.[65]

Initially, the programme focused just on childhood illness, but now it has also integrated a neonatal component (IMNCI). This includes care of the newborn child in the first week of life. The implementation of this programme requires home visits to all newborns in the first week of life by the CHWs, for the promotion of optimal care practices and identification of severe illness and referral. Health workers assess the newborns, ensure breast-feeding, counsel on warmth and danger-signs, treat local infections and refer to appropriate facilities for possible serious bacterial infections.[66] In addition, the workers are expected to assess sick children, manage children with minor illness and refer severely ill children.

In addition, the programme has shifted focus from a facility-based healthcare service to a community-based workers' programme. The sustainability of this programme depends upon allocating reasonable funds and providing a framework for accountability to ensure transparent dealings and quality of care. As part of the programme, the community health workers receive training and are provided with basic drugs and supplies required for treating identified children. Their work is supervised and they are to be provided feedback.

A general observation has been that children presenting with one illness often suffer from more than that one condition and the secondary disease is frequently the underlying cause of the illness that caused the child to present to the community health centre. As an example, a child presenting with diarrhoea may also be malnourished and may not have received immunization as per schedule. Thus, assessment of nutritional, as well as vaccination status of all children reporting to a community health facility, is indispensable. Any contact of the sick child with the health system is an incredible opportunity to complete unfinished tasks.

Conclusions

With only a short time left to achieve the MDG targets, extensive and evidence-based strategies are imperative to improve child survival. Unless addressed urgently, not only will the MDGs for women and children not be met, but also the gains that have been made so far will not be protected and secured for the future. The grounds for moving fast to implement recommendations are strong. Evidence is gradually growing to show that investing in adolescent, women's and children's health has important economic as well as health returns. This emerging evidence should give confidence to Ministries of Finance to invest in adolescents, women and children for long-term economic prosperity. The past few years have seen many new and welcome initiatives launched to accelerate progress towards improving women's and children's health, e.g. on child survival, family planning and life-saving commodities.

Since most of the MDGs are interlinked and dependent on one another, a holistic approach is necessary. For example, strategies targeting improvement in water and sanitation can potentially reduce the incidence of diarrhoea, thereby reducing child mortality. A child's full potential for survival, normal growth and development is predetermined by conditions in intrauterine life, beginning at conception and indirectly, it is also dependent on preconception care. Therefore, the approach that emphasizes pre-pregnancy and pregnancy care of women can potentially reduce many perinatal and newborn deaths. Other interventions that can reduce newborn deaths include antibiotics to combat neonatal sepsis, resuscitation with room air for a newborn who is not breathing and other measures to protect the newborn, including promotion of home-based neonatal care.

Most developing countries have high fertility rates, which indirectly has an adverse impact on maternal and child health. No programme will make sustainable progress without urging women to have later and fewer pregnancies with a birth interval of 3 years. This will mean contraceptives as public health interventions directed at young women and men.

Presently, the coverage of IMCI is lowest in poor countries and among poor and difficult-to-reach populations. In some countries, there are currently no specific programmes that tackle pneumonia and diarrhoea, since older programmes were integrated as part of the IMCI or discontinued. An approach that targets these two leading killers of children under the age of 5 should be implemented until the rate of IMCI training and coverage expands.

The lack of equity is a growing issue, particularly in those countries where a transition is occurring from planned to free-market economies.[67] Improved quality of care, starting with women- and child-friendly services; improved financial access to high-quality public services through social security mechanisms; free education and subsidized water – all must be viewed by governments as public goods, where the benefit to one individual cannot be separated from the benefit of the whole society. The strategic focus must be on prevention more than cure, particularly for those populations that live outside areas with easy access to healthcare facilities. Because prevention demands fewer medical skills than cure, the focus will bring in new partners, many of them outside of the health system and Ministries of Health, in civil society, the NGO community, women's and youth groups, religious groups, etc. Hence, community-based programmes for outreach, monitoring, education and communication will need to be emphasized.[68] Health workers must extend outreach immunization activities to remote areas. These outreach programmes can use combined interventions to cover immunizations, vitamin A dosages as well as provide other micronutrients, family planning interventions, promotion of breast-feeding, water purification or test kits, general health examinations, counselling of pre-pregnant women and so on. They should always include communication materials in local language with illustrations, preferably those derived from community inputs.

In addition to the preventive approaches mentioned above, curative approaches are equally important for child survival. For diarrhoeal diseases this means use of oral rehydration therapy using a hypo-osmolar solution along with zinc. For respiratory infections, it means early diagnosis of respiratory difficulties and treatment with appropriate antibiotics. Where logistical as well as financial access to new vaccines exists, they can be used to reduce the mortality from diarrhoea (rotavirus vaccine) and respiratory infections (conjugate pneumococcal and Hib vaccines). Governments should implement water, sanitation and hygiene (WASH) strategies where the burden of diarrhoea is high. The effectiveness of a 'Diarrhoea Pack' (comprising low-osmolarity ORS, zinc, water purification tablets and pictorial instruction sheet in a single pack) has been tested in a trial and was acceptable in the community for the treatment of diarrhoea.

Revision of curriculum of community workers, laying emphasis on the recognition of signs, appropriate management and counselling of caregivers for diarrhoea and pneumonia is required. Awareness regarding the recent guidelines for diarrhoea and pneumonia should also be increased and updated by refresher courses. Special emphasis should also be made to recognize the need to complete the duration of treatment.

A key element of any implementation strategy is the provision of an adequate supply of essential commodities for the community and for primary health facilities; for health care, nutrition (including essential vitamins and minerals), water and sanitation. Often the availability of these within the public sector can reduce out-of-pocket expenses to the family, reduce health-seeking behaviour that leads families to the unregulated private sector and improve utilization of public facilities. Distribution and supply, quality checks on medicines and equipment, referral systems and transport are all critical to ensure accessible equitable health care.

Thus, ending preventable child deaths requires global commitments to ambitious and achievable targets through evidence-based country plans, expanding country/stakeholder engagement, creating transparency and accountability and devising new approaches for countries that are lagging.

REFERENCES

4. Lozano R, Wang H, Foreman KJ, et al. Progress towards Millennium Development Goals 4 and 5 on maternal and child mortality: an updated systematic analysis. Lancet 2011;378 (9797):1139–65.
6. Liu L, Johnson HL, Cousens S, et al; Child Health Epidemiology Reference Group of WHO and UNICEF. Global, regional and national causes of child mortality: an updated systematic analysis for 2010 with time trends since 2000. Lancet 2012;379(9832):2151–61.
33. Black RE, Allen LH, Bhutta ZA, et al. Maternal and child undernutrition: global and regional exposures and health consequences. Lancet 2008;371(9608):243–60.
47. Darmstadt GL, Bhutta ZA, Cousens S, et al. Evidence-based, cost-effective interventions: how many newborn babies can we save? Lancet 2005;365:977–88.
50. Gupta GR. Tackling pneumonia and diarrhoea: the deadliest diseases for the world's poorest children. Lancet 2012;379(9832):2123–4.

Access the complete references online at www.expertconsult.com

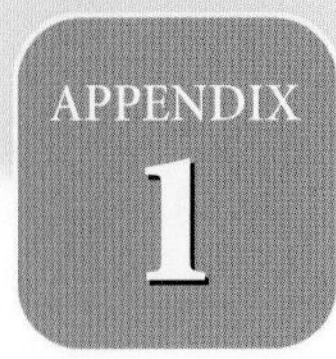

Clinical Laboratory Diagnosis

JANET ROBINSON

Health and Safety

GOOD LABORATORY PRACTICE: GENERAL RULES

Overall safety in the laboratory remains the responsibility of all laboratory staff but the head of department and the laboratory supervisor must ensure that the safety guidelines are implemented. The prevention of exposure to hazardous substances must be the main aim. This can be achieved by engineering controls and documented processes such as use of protective equipment, personal protective clothing, adequate training and good laboratory practice (GLP). A health and safety statement, and procedures to implement it, are required to ensure a safe environment in the laboratory for staff, patients and visitors.

Safety Matters

All staff should be aware of their responsibilities relating to health and safety. This can be necessitated by the use of appropriate Personal Protective Equipment (PPE). The choice of PPE to be used must be evaluated to give maximum protection. In the case of facemasks for instance, the choice would consider the size of the face of those who will be using them and for what they will be used. Staff will be required to train on how to don and doff gloves in order to avoid contaminating the rest of the body.

Health and Safety Procedure(s) that should be in Place

The laboratory must have systems and actions in the event of fire; a major spillage of dangerous chemicals or clinical material; inoculation accident; and reporting and monitoring of accidents and incidents. These must be followed by proper documented reports indicating corrective and preventive action.

Other essential procedures for documentation are: Control of Substances Hazardous to Health (COSH)/risk assessments; disinfection processes; decontamination of equipment; chemical handling; storage and disposal of waste. (Examples of these can be located at: http://www.hse.gov.uk/coshh/ and also at the World Health Organization's Laboratory Biosafety Manual: http://www.who.int/csr/resources/publications/biosafety/WHO_CDS_CSR_LYO_2004_11/en/).

Close attention to laboratory discard procedures for: biological material; paper; contaminated or uncontaminated glassware; broken glassware; disposable pipettes or plastic ware; solvents; toxic chemicals; sharps; and radioactive material should be made. Liquid wastes that are drained down the sink must be well decontaminated and comply with local regulations for decontamination, dilution and release before disposal in the sink or into the sanitary sewer.

Some General Points for Good Clinical Laboratory Practice (GCLP)

METHOD VALIDATION AND VERIFICATION

A laboratory applying a specific method should have documented evidence that the method has been appropriately validated. This holds for methods developed in-house, as well as for standard methods. Method validation is the process used to confirm that the analytical procedure employed for a specific test is suitable for its intended use. Results from method validation can be used to judge the quality, reliability and consistency of analytical results, which is an integral part of any good analytical practice. Analytical methods need to be validated or revalidated before their introduction into routine use, or whenever the conditions change for which the method has been validated (e.g. an instrument with different characteristics or samples with a different matrix); and whenever the method is changed and the change is outside the original scope of the method. The following eight steps must be considered for validation success. These are:

- Accuracy
- Precision
- Specificity
- Limit of detection
- Limit of quantitation
- Linearity and range
- Ruggedness
- Robustness.

This involves defining the scope of the user's method, validation parameters and limits, performing validation and suitability testing.

Tools to assist with method validation are available through the Clinical Laboratory Standards Institute (http://www.clsi.org/) and the College of American Pathologists (http://www.cap.org/apps/cap.portal).

LABORATORY TRAINING

Technical staff should be well trained for the tasks they are to perform and supervised before being allowed to handle clinical samples. Training should include knowledge of potential hazards that various clinical samples present, including the risk of aerosols and droplet formation. Microbiological samples should be processed away from other laboratory areas, particularly samples that carry a risk of viral or bacterial transmission.

All staff should possess a personal authenticated log of procedural competence.

STANDARD OPERATING PROCEDURES (SOPs)

Each method used in the laboratory should be written into an SOP with additional information on interpretation of the results obtained and any special precautions necessary for handling the reagents or chemicals made available.

Written instructions on how to deal with breakage or spillage involving specimens should be clearly available and a suitable laboratory disinfection procedure followed.

Apparatus used in the laboratory should have clear written instructions for proper use and maintenance.

Instructions for disinfection and disposal of clinical specimens by incineration should be available.

A procedure for disposing of needles and other 'sharps' into a suitable impervious pot, with appropriate provision for incineration, should be in place.

QUALITY CONTROL AND EXTERNAL QUALITY ASSURANCE

Quality is vital to ensure reliable, accurate and timely diagnosis of disease. For the laboratory diagnosis of disease both internal quality control (IQC) and external quality assurance (EQA) are requirements expected by all international standards.

IQC is the method of verifying in real time that the tests have been performed correctly and that the correct results are obtained. Typically, samples of known value, such as positive and negative controls, are included with each batch of testing or on each day that tests are performed. If the control samples provide the expected results, then the patient results can be reported with confidence. If the control samples do not provide the expected results, then the cause of the problem should be investigated and corrected and the controls and patient samples re-tested until the correct results are obtained. Patient results should never be released if the control samples fail.

In the case of the laboratory diagnosis of tropical diseases, IQC is important when new batches of stains or culture media are prepared to check that they stain or grow the organisms of interest. IQC is also important when using reagent test kits, ELISA and any other qualitative or quantitative test. Always refer to the manufacturer's kit insert to learn what IQC tests must be performed and how frequently.

EQA is the method of evaluating the trends in quality performance over time. It cannot tell you on a day-to-day basis whether the results are correct but by charting data over time, you can detect trends in performance and from there, identify emerging issues. EQA allows for a retrospective review of quality.

One way to perform EQA is to participate in an External Quality Assurance Scheme (EQAS). These schemes send out blinded (unknown) samples to laboratories for testing. After testing, the laboratory sends their results back and then learns how they performed individually and compared with laboratories performing the same method. EQAS schemes are widely available and cover most of the specimen types and diseases expected. Examples of EQAS providers are the UK National External Quality Assessment Service (http://www.ukneqas.org.uk/content/Pageserver.asp) and the College of American Pathologists (www.cap.org) but many others are available globally. If a laboratory cannot participate in an EQAS for any reason, then sharing samples of known value or identity with a partner laboratory that tests them blind is another way to evaluate performance. This alternative method is called an inter-laboratory comparison.

Using the Laboratory

The laboratory is an essential tool for the diagnosis of infectious diseases in most countries and much of the work is still performed manually, requiring good observation skills. Bacteria, blood cells and parasitic organisms are recognized by their size, colour and morphological appearance, often with the assistance of stains and in the case of scanty infections, after concentration.

Diagnosis may be made more appropriately by serological means, particularly for viral infections and chronic bacteriological or parasitological infections. In a few cases, the diagnosis may be made by only histological examination. Molecular techniques, notably using the polymerase chain reaction (PCR), are becoming important tools for diagnosis of viral (human immunodeficiency virus; HIV), microbiological (*Mycobacterium tuberculosis*) infections and some parasitic infections such as malaria and leishmaniasis as well as many viruses that can cause human disease. The introduction of rapid diagnostic tests using labelled monoclonal antibody tests based on immunochromatography has improved the ability to screen for several important infections at clinic or small laboratory level.

CLINICAL PARASITOLOGY DIAGNOSIS

Essential Equipment

For routine diagnosis of intestinal and blood parasites, a microscope, preferably equipped with a binocular head and ×10 eyepiece is required. A good quality sub-stage Abbe condenser with a diaphragm to control the entry of light and objectives with ×10, ×40 and ×100 magnification are most suitable. Sub-stage illumination using electric lighting is the better option, although several microscopes are available with a sub-stage plano-convex mirror that gives the alternative option of using reflected sunlight. A calibrated graticule should be available for one of the eyepieces. The graticule can be left in situ or inserted as required. It should be calibrated for each objective using a slide micrometer.

LABORATORY INVESTIGATION OF DIARRHOEA

Diarrhoea may be defined as a change in bowel habits different to that normally experienced. Faecal appearance can be categorized as solid, unformed or liquid, depending on its consistency. Causes of diarrhoea may be bacterial, parasitic, viral or dietary, and specific procedures may be needed to determine the cause, including microscopic examination, enzyme-linked immunosorbent assay (ELISA) and molecular methods.

Investigation of the causes of diarrhoea (Figure A1.1). Steps of diarrhoea investigation in the laboratory.

DIRECT MICROSCOPIC EXAMINATION OF FAECES

Direct examination of a suspension of fresh faeces in warm saline enables the presence of motile trophozoites of protozoa to be seen (*Entamoeba histolytica, Giardia lamblia, Chilomastix mesnili, Trichomonas hominis*). It will also show protozoan cysts and helminth larvae and ova when present in sufficient numbers.

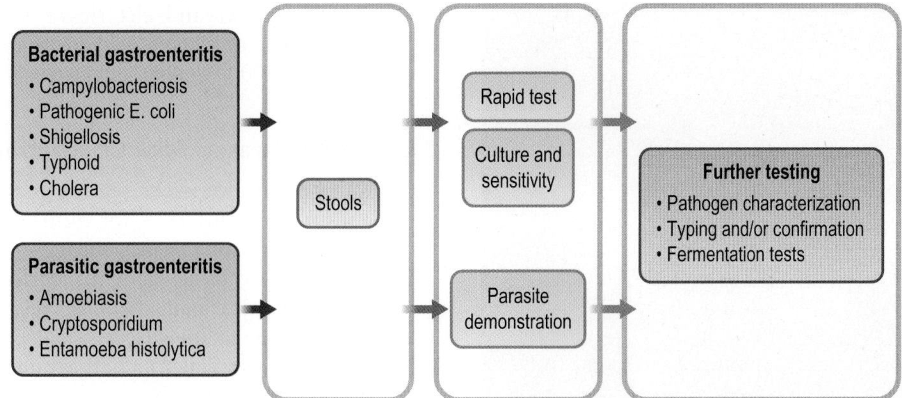

Figure A1.1 Steps of diarrhoea investigation in the laboratory (Cholera *dysenteriae*).

The presence of cellular exudate, white blood cells, red blood cells and macrophages may help to confirm a diagnosis of amoebic or bacillary dysentery. Excess fat globules may be apparent in cases of malabsorption seen in parasitic or viral infections of the small bowel (*G. lamblia*, *Cyclospora cayetanensis*, *Isospora belli*, *Cryptosporidium parvum*, Rotavirus, etc.). Faecal smears may be prepared and stained to show the characteristic morphological features of trophozoites or spores of *Microsporidia* spp. and to describe the exudate content (Figures A1.2–A1.5).

Preparation of Direct Faecal Smear

Materials

- Physiological saline (0.9% sodium chloride)
- Lugol's iodine.

Method

1. Take a microscope slide and label one end with the patient's name.
2. Place a drop of warm saline (37°C) at each end of the slide.
3. Using an applicator stick, select a small piece of faecal material and emulsify the faeces into the two drops of saline on the slide. If the faeces contains any blood or

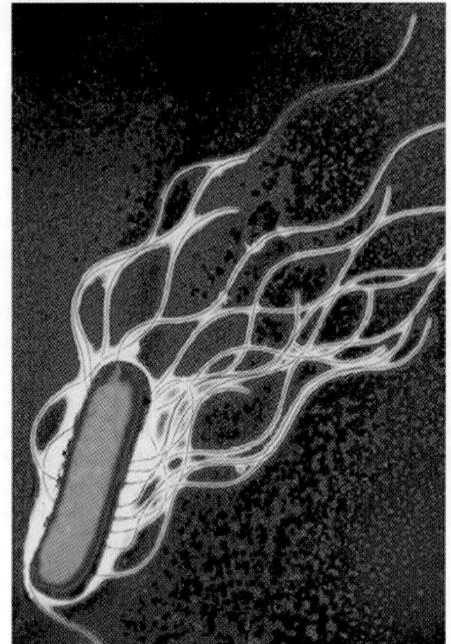

Figure A1.3 *Cyclospora cayetanensis.*

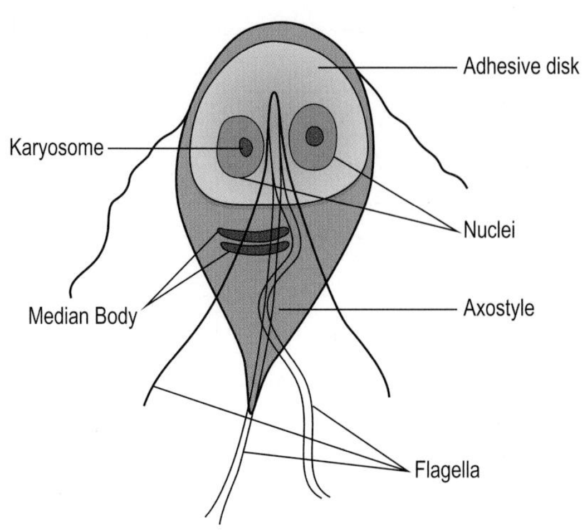

Figure A1.2 *G. lamblia.* k, MB, Fg, AD, Nu, Ax

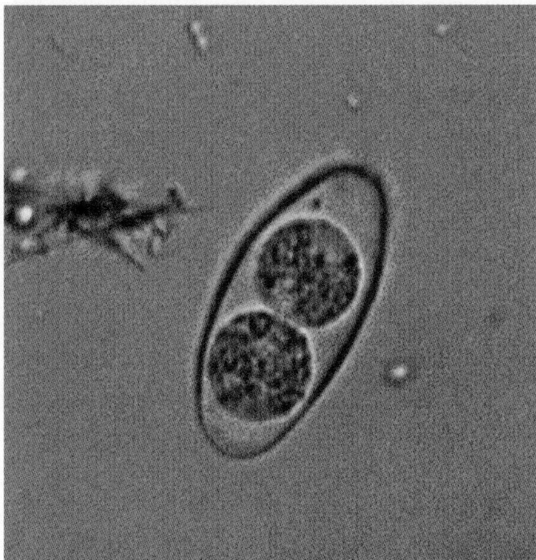

Figure A1.4 *Isospora belli. (From: Diagnosing Medical Parasites Through Coprological Techniques, Vol 2, M. Arcari, A. Baxendine and C.E. Bennett, The Ciliates, Coccidia and Microsporidia, Copyright© 2000, with permission from University of Southampton.)*

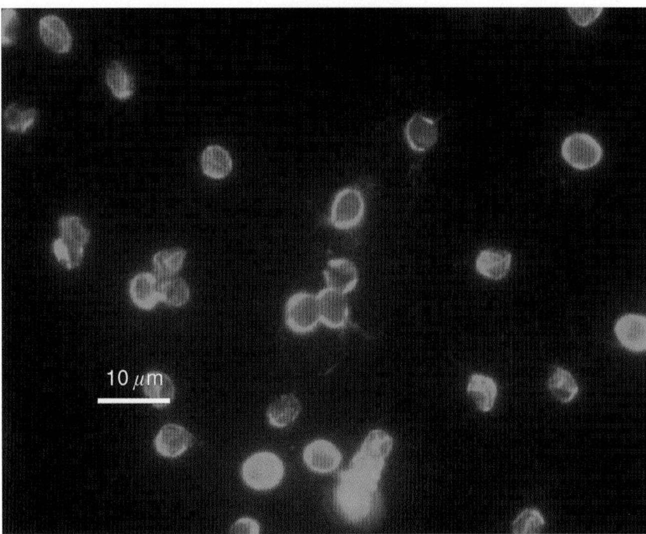

Figure A1.5 *Cryptosporidium parvum.*

mucus, prepare a separate slide for this. Add one drop of Lugol's iodine solution to the right-hand suspension. Correct thickness allows printed material to be seen through the preparation.

4. Place a 22 mm^2 coverslip on to each preparation and scan the coverslip areas using the ×10 and ×40 objectives.

Motile organisms seen in the saline preparation will be identified by characteristic movement and morphology. Confirmation can be made with one of the staining methods described. Larger helminthic stages may be seen at lower power. Staining with Lugol's iodine solution enhances the internal structure of protozoan cysts but will kill active trophozoites. Cells present can be stained and identified by running a little 1% methylene blue stain beneath the saline suspension coverslip.

FAECAL CONCENTRATION METHODS

Concentration methods are necessary when cysts or ova are present in low numbers; these methods will not show motile trophozoites, as the use of 10% formalin to suspend and fix the faeces will kill vegetative forms (Figure A1.6).

Standard Protocols

1. Direct impression
2. Flotation methods
3. Sedimentation. This technique is currently the method of choice and can be illustrated with the formol-ethyl acetate method.

Formal-ether/Ethyl Acetate Concentration for Ova and Cysts

Materials

- *Parasep* midi or mini faecal concentrators (other commercial varieties are available) are filters that provide an enclosed system, adding safety to the use of flammable solvents
- 10% v/v formalin (100 mL formaldehyde + 900 mL distilled water) or SAF fixative
- Diethyl ether or ethyl acetate
- A vortex mixer and electric or battery-powered centrifuge capable of receiving 15 cm centrifuge tubes and operating at 1000 g also required (2000 rpm for bench centrifuge).

Method for Parasep *Midi Concentrator*

1. Using applicator sticks, select a quantity of faeces (approx. 1 g for midi and 1/2 g for mini) to include external and internal portions of the faeces.
2. Emulsify the faeces in 7 mL of formalin or SAF in the bottom conical half of the device, add 3 mL of ether or ethyl acetate to the suspension.
3. Screw the conical top half containing the filter tightly onto the bottom half.
4. Vortex the tube vigorously for 15 seconds or by hand for 1 min.
5. Invert the tube and centrifuge at 2000 rpm for 1 min.
6. Separate the two halves, discard the top part containing the filter and pour the supernatant away by quickly inverting the tube. It is necessary to dispose of ether/ethyl-acetate safely, as these are flammable substances.
7. Allow the fluid on the side of the tube to drain on to the deposit; mix well, and transfer a drop to a slide for examination under a coverslip.
8. Use the ×10 and ×40 objectives to examine the whole of the deposit for ova and cysts.

Parasep SF (Diasys Europe), a modified version of the device that has a secondary filter and does not require a solvent extraction step is available.

Small bowel parasites, such as *Giardia* or *Strongyloides* can be specifically recovered using a procedure known as the 'Entero-Test' capsule (the string test) (Figures A1.7, A1.8).

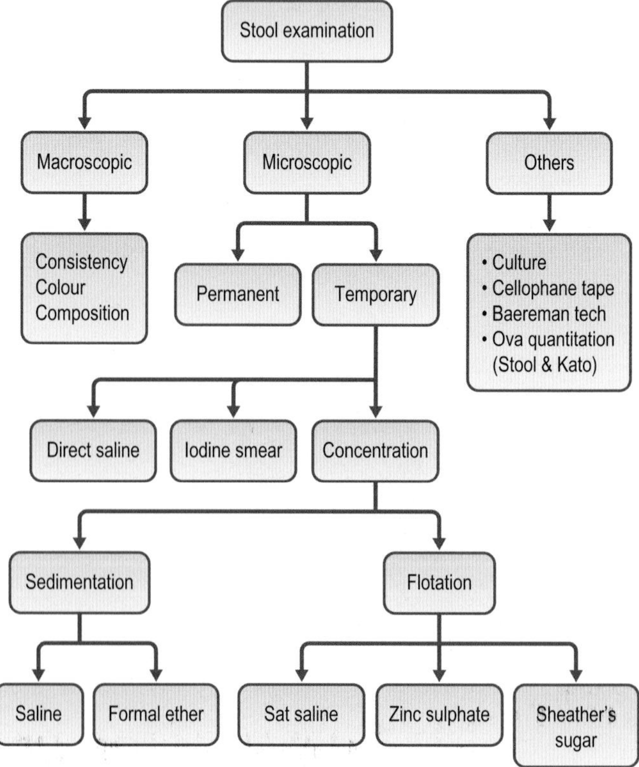

Figure A1.6 Flowchart showing concentration method.

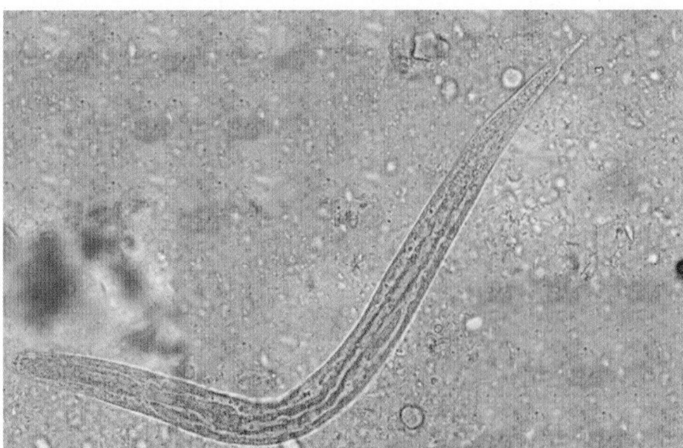

Figure A1.7 *Strongyloides stercoralis. (From: Oregon State Public Health Laboratories, public.health.oregon.gov)*

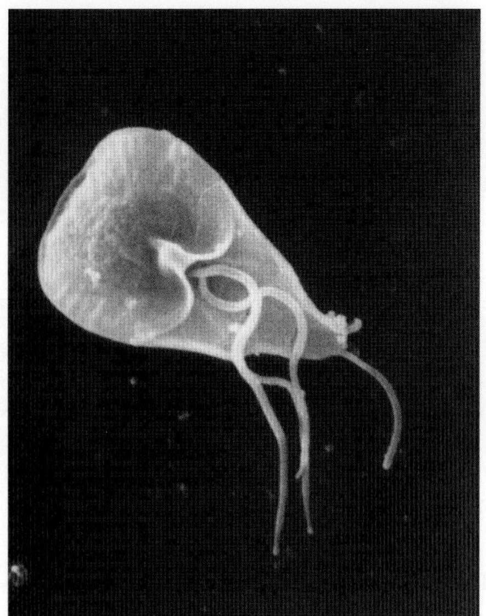

Figure A1.8 *Giardia lamblia.*

This procedure utilizes a length of thread in a weighted gelatin capsule. The end of the string is taped to the patient's face and the capsule is swallowed. The patient lies on the right side so that the capsule will travel to the duodenum. After 4 hours, the string is pulled up (the weight is passed out in the faeces). The string will be stained yellow with bile and mucus where it has been in the duodenum. If no part of the string is yellow, the test should be repeated.

1. The string is placed in a pot and covered with 5 mL of saline.
2. Agitate the string and saline, preferably using a vortex mixer, to remove mucus from the string.
3. Wind the string around an applicator stick, pressing it against the side of the container to remove mucus and excess saline, and then discard it.
4. Centrifuge the saline at 2000 rpm for 2 min.
5. Discard the supernatant and transfer the deposit to a microscope slide and examine using the ×10 and ×40 objectives for trophozoites of *G. lamblia* and active larvae of *Strongyloides* spp. Ova from flukes in the biliary tract may also be found.

Staining Methods for Intestinal Protozoa

Table A1.1 lists the identifying features of common protozoan cysts. Particular stains can be used to identify these features; the stains may be applied to the wet suspension or to an air-dried, fixed faecal smear.

TRICHOMONAS SPP. DIAGNOSIS PROCEDURE

The following procedure will be used to diagnose *Trichomonas* sp. and *Trypanosome* sp.

1. Detect antibodies serologically. Several techniques (immunofluorescence etc.) have been developed
2. A direct agglutination reaction of trypanosomes is a cheap and practical method. A direct agglutination reaction of trypanosomes on a plastic card, with macroscopic read-off (Card Agglutination Test for Trypanosomiasis, CATT)
3. A drop of blood (finger prick) and a drop of reagent that contains blue-coloured parasites of a known serotype are mixed on a white plastic card
4. The card is mechanically shaken for 5 min and then immediately read. When the test is positive (presence of antibodies) the trypanosomes agglutinate and form a blue clot. CATT must not be confused with the CIATT (Card Indirect Agglutination Test for Trypanosomiasis)
5. Another method is to take a blood drop on very small filter papers (confetti) and examine this later in a laboratory

TABLE A1.1 **Identification of Cysts of Common Protozoa**

Protozoan Cyst	Size	Nuclear Pattern	Inclusions
Entamoeba histolytica/dispar	1–4 nuclei, 9–14 μm	Fine chromatin, central karyosome	Diffuse glycogen, chromidial body
Entamoeba hartmanni	1–4 nuclei, 7–9 μm	Fine chromatin, central karyosome	Diffuse glycogen, chromidial body
Entamoeba coli	1–8 nuclei, 14–30 μm	Fine chromatin, eccentric karyosome	Diffuse glycogen, chromidial body rare
Iodamoeba bütschlii	1 nucleus, 9–15 μm	Coarse chromatin, no karyosome	Compact glycogen vacuole
Endolimax nana	3–4 nuclei, 6–9 μm	3–4 granules forming refractile nuclei	Nil
Giardia lamblia	Oval, 4 nuclei, 8–12 μm (not obvious unless stained)	No diagnostic significance	Refractile axoneme and flagellar remnants
Chilomastix mesnili	Lemon-shaped, 1 nucleus, 5–6 μm	Fine chromatin	Refractile axoneme

6. The patient should be called back later if the result is positive. Antigen-detection methods (ELISA) have also been developed, but are not yet in routine use
7. A problem arises in persons who have a positive serology, but who are asymptomatic and in whom no parasites are
8. After successful treatment the antibodies remain for years. Antibody detection therefore cannot be used for detecting relapse or reinfection
9. Circulating antigens can be detected either directly by ELISA or by PCR or variants of these.

It is at best 60% sensitive, however, and is best used as a screening tool. Wet mount is the most conventional procedure for detecting *Trichomonas* spp. A microscope slide is prepared by suspending a specimen in saline solution. The slides are then visually examined for trichomonads.

POTASSIUM HYDROXIDE (KOH) 'WHIFF TEST'

The 'whiff' test is a rudimentary technique that may be used as part of a clinical diagnosis. The test is conducted by mixing a swab of vaginal fluid with a 10% potassium hydroxide solution, then smelling it. A strong amine (fishy) smell could be an indication of trichomoniasis or bacterial vaginosis.

PAPANICOLAOU TEST (PAP SMEAR)

The Papanicolaou test is a microscopic examination of a stained specimen. It is mainly used as a diagnostic test for the screening of various cervical abnormalities and genital infections. While it may occasionally detect trichomonads, it has a high diagnostic error rate and is not suitable for screening unless used in conjunction with a more sensitive test.

TEMPORARY STAINS

These stains are applied to wet preparations from concentrations or direct faecal suspensions; their purpose is to enhance diagnostic features within the cysts such as glycogen or refractile components.

Lugol's Iodine Solution (Double Strength)

Reagent 1

- Potassium iodide 20 g
- Iodine 10 g
- Distilled water 100 mL.

Add potassium iodide to the distilled water; when dissolved, add the iodine crystals.

Reagent 2

- 25% glacial acetic acid.

For use, mix equal parts of reagents 1 and 2. Store in a brown bottle. Remains stable for many weeks.

Iodine stains glycogen brown and the nuclear chromatin of amoebic cysts brown/black.

Burrows' Stain for Chromatoid Inclusion of Entamoeba *Cysts*

- Thionin 20 mg
- Acetic acid 3 mL
- Ethanol 3 mL
- Distilled water 94 mL.

Add an equal volume of the stain to the faecal concentrate and allow to stand for 12–18 hours. After this period, examine one drop of the stained deposit under the microscope.

Chromidial bars within the cysts of *Entamoeba* spp. stain deep blue.

PERMANENT STAINS

Trichrome Stain

The trichrome method for staining protozoa is especially recommended for identifying features of amoebic cysts and trophozoites.

Formula: Trichrome Stain (Modified)

- Chromotrope 2R 1 g
- Aniline blue 0.5 g
- Phosphotungstic acid 0.7 g.

Mix the components together with 3 mL glacial acetic acid in a flask and allow to stand for 30 min.

Add 100 mL distilled water and mix well.

Acid/Alcohol Decolourizer

- 4.5 mL glacial acetic acid in 995.5 mL 95% industrial methylated spirit.

Fixation. Most smears from faeces or pus can be fixed by placing immediately into methanol for 5 min.

Staining

1. Methanol 5 min
2. Wheatley's formula trichrome stain 30 min
3. Rinse in tap water
4. Acid alcohol decolourizer 2–3 seconds
5. 95% Ethanol dip twice
6. 95% Ethanol 5 min
7. 95% Ethanol 5 min
8. 100% Ethanol 3 min
9. Xylene or substitute 5 min
10. Mount with DPX mountant – do not allow xylene to dry on the slide.

Nuclei, chromidial bars, chromatin, red cells and bacteria stain red. Cytoplasm stains blue-green. Background and yeasts stain green.

Modified Trichrome Formulation for Spores of Microsporidia

- Chromotrope 2R 6 g
- Aniline blue 0.5 g
- Phosphotungstic acid 0.7 g.

Mix the components together with 3 mL glacial acetic acid in a flask and allow to stand for 30 min.

Add 100 mL distilled water and mix well. (A pink/red granular aggregate may be found; this is not important.)

Method

1. Suspend approximately 1 mg of faecal material in a drop of 10% formalin at a ratio of 1:3.
2. Using an applicator stick in a rolling motion, spread a drop of the faecal suspension very thinly over two-thirds of the slide surface.
3. Dry the smear and fix in methanol for 5 min.
4. Stain with modified trichrome stain for 90 min at room temperature, or for 30 min at 50°C in a waterbath.
5. Rinse in acid alcohol decolourizer for 3–5 seconds.

TABLE A1.2 Types and Classes of Helminths

Cestode	Trematodes	Nematodes
Taenia solium, Taenia saginata, Hymenolepis nana, Hymenolepis diminuta, Diphyllobothrium latum, echinococcus granulosus	Schistosoma species (blood flukes), *Clonorchis sinensis, Fasciola hepatica, Fasciolopsis buski, Heterophyes heterophyes, Metagonimus yokogawai, Paragonimus westermani*	*Enterobius vermicularis, Trichuris trichiura, Ascaris lumbricoides, Strongyloides stercoralis, Trichinella spiralis, Brugia malayi, Loa loa*

6. Rinse in 95% ethanol until excess stain has washed off the slide.
7. Dehydrate in two changes of 99% ethanol.
8. Clear in xylene or substitute for 10 min and mount in DPX mountant.
9. Examine with the oil immersion objective.

Spores of *Microsporidia* species appear pinkish red and are 0.5–1.0 µm, and oval in appearance. They frequently exhibit a central band-like structure flanked on either side by non-staining areas (polar vacuoles).

Modified Field's Stain

This is a useful rapid stain for identifying protozoa in faecal smears.

- Field's stain A
- Field's stain B (diluted 1:4 with distilled water).

Method

1. Prepare thin faecal smears and air dry.
2. Fix with methanol for several minutes.
3. Remove the methanol and flood the slide with 1 mL of diluted Field's stain B.
4. Immediately add 1 mL of undiluted Field's stain A and mix the two stains.
5. Stain for 1–2 min before rinsing in water and allowing to drain dry.

Nuclei and flagella stain red, cytoplasm stains blue.

Morphological features of inflammatory cells can be seen by means of this method (Table A1.2).

TABLE A1.3 *Shigella* spp. *Serogroups* Designation and Serotypes

Species	Serogroup	Serotypes
S. dysenteriae	Serogroup A	1–13
S. flexneri	Serogroup B	1–6
S. boydii	Serogroup C	1–18
S. sonnei	Serogroup D	1

TABLE A1.4 Reaction of *Shigella* in Screening Biochemical Tests

Screening Medium	*Shigella* Reaction
KIA	K/A
TSI	K/A
H2S (on KIA or TSI)	Negative
Motility	Negative
Urea	Negative
Indole	Positive or negative
LIA	K/A (Purple slant/yellow butt)

Bacterial Culture of Intestinal Pathogens

The common intestinal pathogens that are infectious to humans are *E. coli* 0157: H7, *Salmonella* sp., *Cholera* sp. and *Campylobacter* sp. The genus *Shigella* is divided into four species: *dysenteriae*, *S. flexneri*, *S. boydii* and *S. sonnei*. Each of the species, with the exception of *S. sonnei* has several serotypes. *Shigella* sp. has several serogroups designation and serotypes (see below) (Table A1.3).

Isolation of Suspected *Shigella*

Colonies of *Shigella* on MacConkey appear as convex, colourless colonies about 2–3 mm in diameter. *Shigella* colonies on xylose lysine desoxycholate agar are transparent pink or red smooth colonies 1–2 mm in diameter. Screening media such as Kligler iron agar (KIA) or triple sugar iron agar (TSI) are commonly used on suspected colonies (Tables A1.4, A1.5).

There are several typing systems and serogroups and they are epidemic associated as shown in Table A1.6.

Vibrio cholera grows on commonly used agar media. Isolation from faecal specimens is more easily accomplished with specialized media. Alkaline peptone water (APW) is recommended as an enrichment broth and thiosulphate citrate bile salts sucrose agar (TCBS) is a selective medium of choice (see Tables A1.7, A1.8 and Figure A1.9).

TABLE A1.5 The Appearance of *Shigella* Colonies on Selective Plating Media

Selective Agar Medium	Colour Colonies	Size of Colonies
MAC	Colourless	2–3 mm
XLD	Red or colourless	1–2 mm
DCA	Colourless	2–3 mm
HE	Green	2–3 mm

Vibrio cholera serogroups O1 are classified into two biotypes namely, El, Tor and classical on the basis of several phenotypic characteristics.

TABLE A1.6 Typing Systems and Serogroups, Epidemic Associated

Typing Systems	Serogroups: OI, O139	Serogroup: Non-O1 (>150 exist)
Biotypes for serogroup O1	Classical and El Tor	Biotypes are not applicable to non-OI strains)
Serotypes for serogroup O1	Inaba, Ogawa and Hikojima	These 3 serotypes are not applicable to non-OI strains
Toxin production	Produces cholera toxin	Usually do not produce cholera toxin; produce other toxins

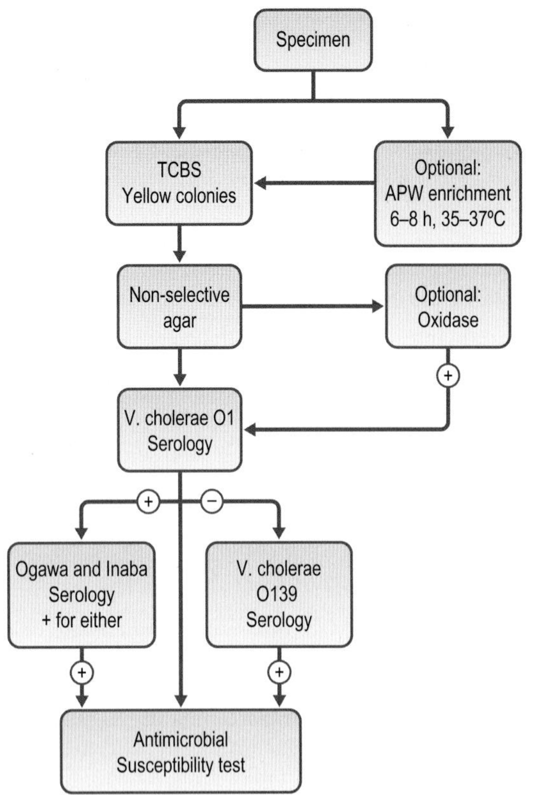

Figure A1.9 Isolation and identification of *Vibrio cholera* serogroups O1 and O139.

Salmonella

Salmonella is a Gram-negative facultative rod-shaped bacterium in the same proteobacterial family as *Escherichia coli*, the family Enterobacteriaceae, trivially known as 'enteric' bacteria. *Salmonella* is nearly as well-studied as *E. coli* from a structural, biochemical and molecular point of view, and as poorly understood as *E. coli* from an ecological point of view. *Salmonellae* live in the intestinal tracts of warm and cold blooded animals. Some species are ubiquitous. Other species are specifically adapted to a particular host. In humans, *Salmonella* are the cause of two diseases: salmonellosis – enteric fever (typhoid), resulting from bacterial invasion of the bloodstream; and acute gastroenteritis – resulting from a food-borne infection/intoxication. They are chemo-organotrophs, obtaining their energy from oxidation and reduction reactions using organic sources, and are facultative anaerobes. Most species produce hydrogen sulfide, which can readily be detected by growing them on media containing ferrous sulfate, such as TSI.

SALMONELLA sp.

Many different diseases are caused by more than 1400 serotypes of this bacteria genus (Box A1.1).

Laboratory Investigation for Blood and Tissue Parasites

The blood or tissue parasites are transmitted during vector insect blood feeds and usually continue their life cycle in the human host. The common blood or tissue parasites found belong to the genus of *Plasmodium* (Table A1.9), *Trypanosoma* (African and South American trypanosomes), *Babesia* and the *Leishmania* complex and a few blood spirochaetes (Table A1.10 and Figure A1.10).

Blood parasites can be identified from peripheral blood, bone marrow aspirate, splenic aspirate and gland aspirate or from tissue biopsy material (Table A1.11).

Routine procedures for identification include:

- Direct staining of blood or impression smears
- Concentration methods
- Culture of appropriate sample

TABLE A1.7 Reactions of *V. Cholerae* in Screening Tests

Screening Test	*Vibrio Cholerae* Reactions
Oxidase test	Positive
String test	Positive
KIA	K/A, no gas produced (red slant/yellow butt)
TSI	A/A, no gas produced (yellow slant/yellow butt)
LIA	K/K, no gas produced (purple slant/purple butt)
Gram stain	Small, Gram-negative curved rods
Wet mount	Small, curved rods with darting motility

K, alkaline; A, acid.

BOX A1.1 COMMON SALMONELLA SEROTYPES

Species	*S. enterica*
Salmonella	*Typhimurium, Enteritidis* *Salmonella enterica serovar Typhi.* (Also called *Salmonella Typhi* or abbreviated to *S. Typhi*) *Salmonella enterica serovar Typhimurium.* (Also called *Salmonella Typhimurium* or *S. Typhimurium*) *Salmonella enteric serovar Enteritidis.* (Also called *Salmonella Enteritidis* or *S. Enteritidis*)

TABLE A1.8 Identification of *Campylobacter*

	Campylobacter Jejuni	*Campylobacter Lari*	*Campylobacter Coli*
Gram staining	Gram-negative curved rod	Gram-negative curved rod	Gram-negative curved rod
Test for catalase	+	+	+
Test for oxidase	+	+	+
Hippurate hydrolysis	+	–	–
Hydrolysis of indoxyl acetate	+	–	–

This organism can be isolated in stool cultures using media containing selective growth supplements (e.g. various anti-infective agents). The cultures are incubated at 48 hours at 42°C in a microaerophilic atmosphere. Identification is based on growth requirements as well as detection of catalase and oxidase.

TABLE A1.9 Identification of Malaria Parasites

	Plasmodium Falciparum	*Plasmodium Vivax*	*Plasmodium Ovale*	*Plasmodium Malariae*
Red blood cell	Normal size and shape	Enlarged	Enlarged, fimbriate, oval	Small, older
Inclusions	Maurer's clefts in mature trophozoite	Schüffner dots, fine stippling	James' dots, coarse stippling	Ziemann dots, not seen unless overstained
Trophozoite	Delicate fine rings, accolé forms	Larger, thicker rings	Thick compact rings	Small compact rings
Developing trophozoites	Compact ring, cytoplasm vacuolated	Large amoeboid parasite with central vacuole	Slightly amoeboid but smaller than *P. vivax*	Sometimes seen as a band across red cell
Schizont	2–24 merozoites; single, large, brown pigment clump	12–24 merozoites almost filling red blood cell	8–12 merozoites fill three-quarters of red blood cell	6–12 merozoites around central pigment mass
Gametocyte	Crescent-shaped aggregated chromatin and pigment in centre	Large, round, almost fills red blood cell	Smaller, round, fills half red blood cell	Round, may fill between one-half and two-thirds of red blood cell
Pigment	Single clump in schizont	Several fine clumps from late trophozoites	Coarse granules from late trophozoites	Dark fine granules at all stages

TABLE A1.10 Blood and Tissue Parasites

	Species	Infective to Humans
Trypanosome	*Trypanosoma brucei gambiense*	Yes
	Trypanosoma brucei rhodesiense	Yes
Babesia	*Babesia* spp	Yes
Leishmania	*L. donovani*	Yes
Spirochaetes	*Treponema pallidum*	Yes

- Detection of parasite DNA using PCR
- Immunochromatographic rapid tests for the detection of parasite antigen.

STAINING OF BLOOD FILMS

Giemsa Stain

Giemsa stain is a Romanowsky stain and stains chromatin material red and cytoplasm blue. Inclusion bodies within the cell stain red or blue according to their origin.

Materials

- Giemsa stain: a good quality stain is necessary (e.g. Gurr's R66 formulation, E. Merck/BDH, Poole, UK)

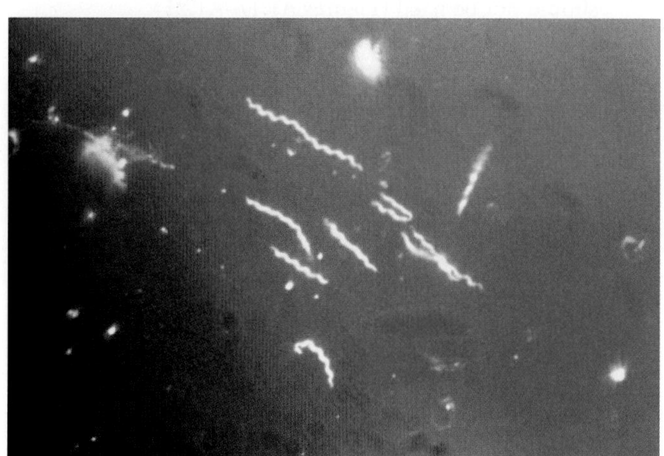

Figure A1.10 Photographs of spirochaetes that infect humans (*Borrelia* spp.).

TABLE A1.11 Human Samples Used for Disease Detection

Sample Type	Parasites Detected
Cerebral spinal fluid	Bacteria (*N. meningitis*)
Whole blood	Protozoan spp (*P. falciparum*)
Plasma	Viruses
Sputum	Bacteria (*Mycobacterium tuberculosis*)
Skin snips	Fungus
Stool	Intestinal parasites
Urine	Flukes (*S. hematobium* and *S. mansoni*)

- Solvent methanol
- Buffered water pH 6.8 and pH 7.2; tablets are available for the preparation of 1-L volumes.

Method. Allow thin smears prepared from blood, aspirates or cerebrospinal fluid (CSF) deposits to dry thoroughly before staining.

1. Flood the dry smear with solvent methanol and allow fixing for 1 min.
2. Tip off the alcohol.
3. Prepare a 1:10 dilution of Giemsa stain (5 drops of stain and 45 drops of appropriately buffered water). Use buffered water pH 7.2 for staining for malaria and pH 6.8 for the other blood parasites.
4. Flood the fixed slide with diluted stain and allow to stain for 30 min.
5. At the end of this time, rinse the stain from the slide with buffered water and allow the slide to drain dry.
6. Slides are examined using the oil immersion objective of the microscope.

Parasite nuclear chromatin stains red, cytoplasm stains blue and cellular inclusions stain red. Red cell nuclear remnants (Howell–Jolly bodies) stain deep blue, the nucleus of white blood cells stains purple and the granules stain red.

CONCENTRATION OF PARASITES FROM BLOOD

- Parasites that are scanty can be concentrated before staining by several methods
- Thick blood film, suitable for concentrating malaria parasites, trypomastigotes and spirochaetes

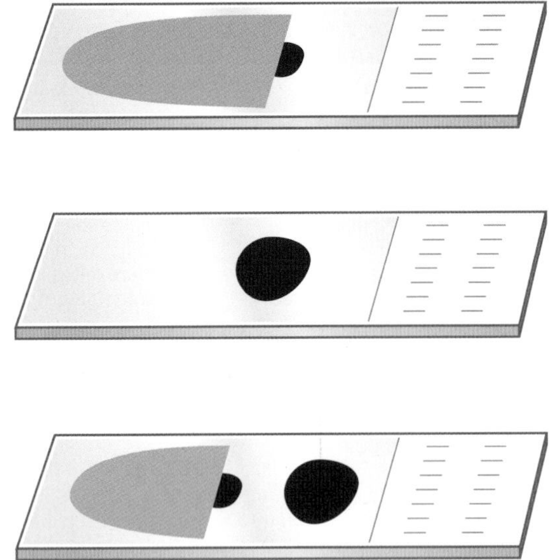

Figure A1.11 Preparation of thin and thick film on a slide.

- 'Buffy coat', suitable for concentrating malaria parasites, trypomastigotes and spirochaetes
- Mini anion exchange column, suitable for concentrating trypomastigotes.

Thick Blood Films

Preparation. Using an applicator stick to remove blood from an anticoagulated tube or directly from a finger prick, place two or three drops of blood on to one end of a slide. Using the applicator stick or the edge of a glass slide, spread the blood over an area of 1 cm^2 and allow to dry thoroughly. Appropriate thickness is judged by seeing printed material through the slide.

Do not fix the slide with methanol.

Field's Stain for Thick Blood Films. Field's stain consists of the two components of the Romanowsky stains in separate solutions. These are called Field's stain A and Field's stain B. Used to stain unfixed thick blood films, the procedure will stain white blood cells, platelets and parasites but will haemolyse the red blood cells. It is a useful method for the concentration of malaria parasites, *Trypanosoma* spp. and *Borrelia* spp.

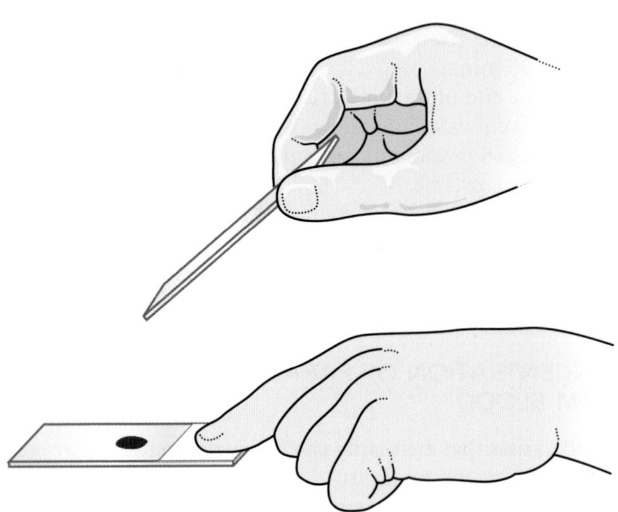

Figure A1.12 Method of making a blood slide.

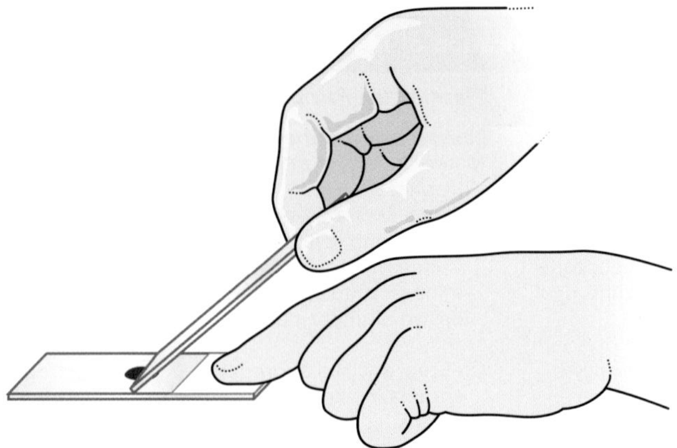

Figure A1.13 Method of spreading blood on slide.

Figure A1.11 shows how to prepare good thick and thin films for malaria and gives photographs of the different species and life stages.

Procedure

1. Whenever possible, use separate slides for thick and thin smears.
2. Thin film (a): Bring a clean spreader slide, held at a 45° angle, toward the drop of blood on the specimen slide (Figure A1.12).
3. Thin film (b): Wait until the blood spreads along the entire width of the spreader slide (Figure A1.13).
4. Thin film (c): While holding the spreader slide at the same angle, push it forward rapidly and smoothly (Figure A1.14).
5. Thick film: Using the corner of a clean slide, spread the drop of blood in a circle the size of a 5p coin (diameter 1–2 cm). Do not make the smear too thick or it will fall off the slide (you should be able to read newsprint through it) (Figure A1.15).
6. Wait until the thin and thick films are completely dry before staining. Fix the thin film with methanol (100% or absolute) and let it dry completely before staining. The thick film should not be fixed (Figure A1.16).
7. If both thin and thick films need to be made on the same slide, fix only the thin film with methanol. The thick film should not be fixed (Figures A1.17–A1.21).

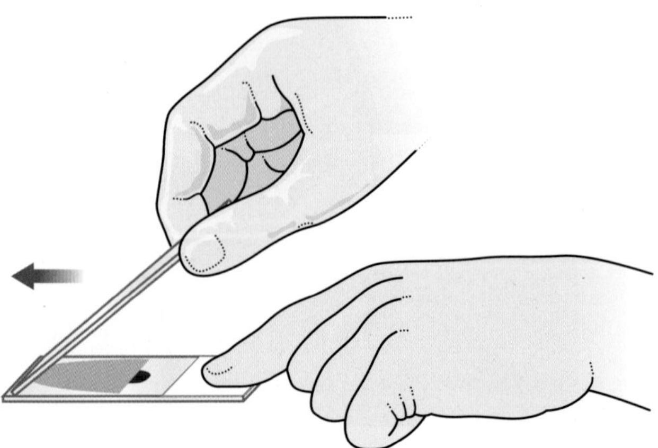

Figure A1.14 Typical thin blood film.

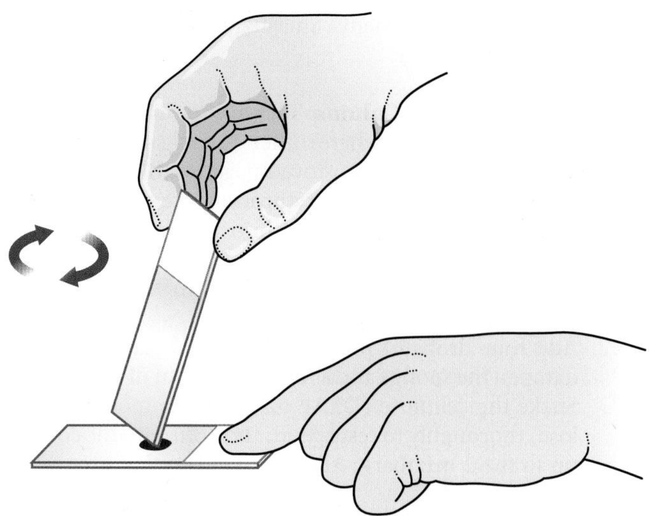

Figure A1.15 Preparation of thick blood film.

- Materials Field's stain A solution (purchased as prepared stain or prepared as 2.5 g% (25 g/L) in distilled or filtered water, from the powder form)
- Field's stain B solution (prepared as for Field's stain A).

Method

1. Dip the dried, unfixed, thick blood film in Field's stain A for 3–5 seconds.
2. Carefully rinse the slide in a beaker of tap or buffered water for 3 seconds.
3. Dip the slide in Field's stain B for 3 seconds.
4. Rinse the slide in water again and then stand vertically to thoroughly dry.

Erythrocytes will be haemolysed, parasite chromatin stains red and cytoplasm blue; inclusion dots (Schüffner or James), if seen, stain red.

Buffy Coat Examination. Parasites are concentrated near to the band of WBC/platelets (buffy coat).

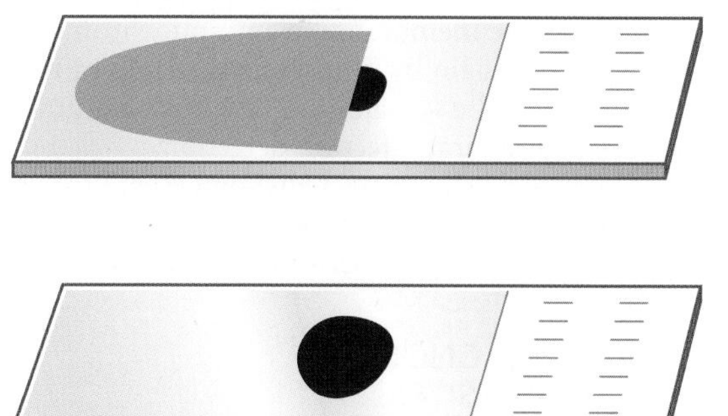

Figure A1.16 Preparation of both thick and thin films on different slides.

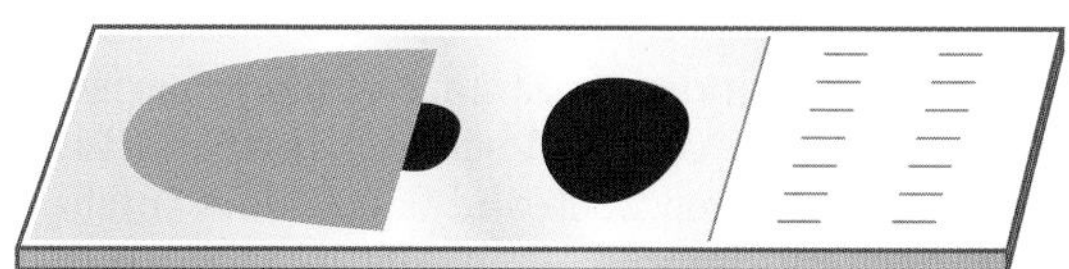

Figure A1.17 Preparation of thick and thin film on one slide.

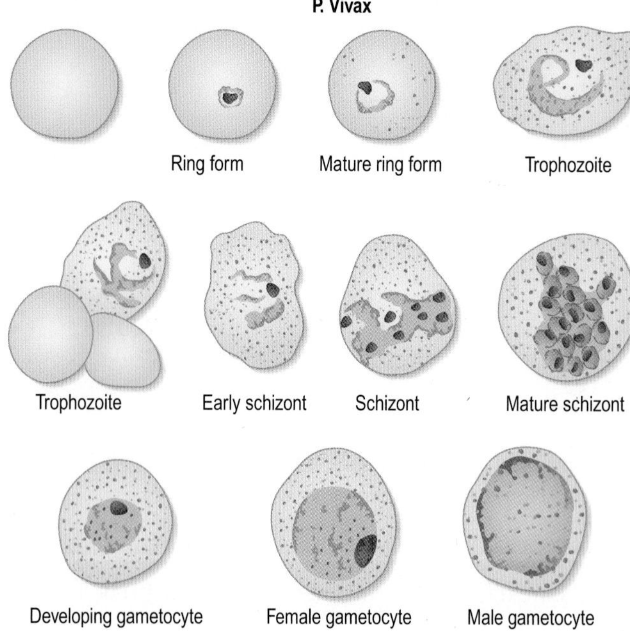

Figure A1.18 *P. vivax* with salient features.

Method

1. Collect peripheral blood into capillary tubes containing ethylenediamine tetra-acetic acid (EDTA) anticoagulant, filling the tube three-quarters full with blood and rotating to mix the anticoagulant. Seal the end with plasticine and place the tube into a microhaematocrit centrifuge with a corresponding balance tube opposite.

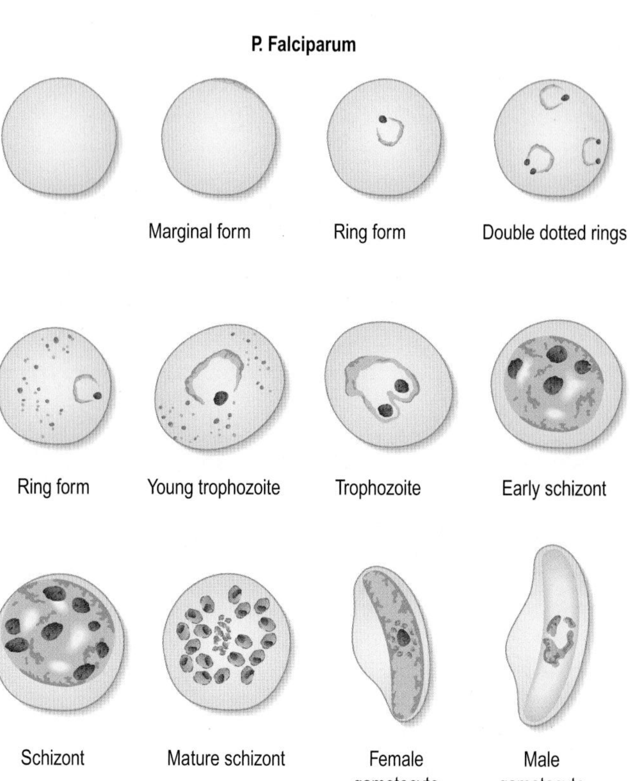

Figure A1.19 *P. falciparum* with salient features.

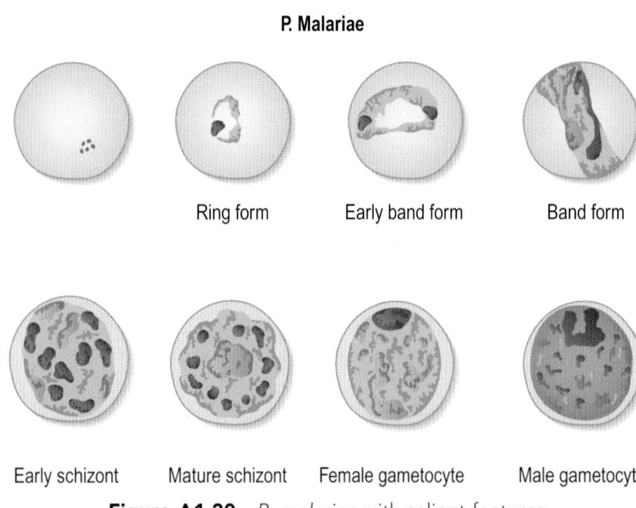

Figure A1.20 *P. malariae* with salient features.

2. Secure the lid and centrifuge the blood at 10 000 rpm for 5 min.
3. Remove the tube and, using an ampoule blade or a diamond marker, score the tube just below the layer of white cells and platelets (buffy coat) at the junction of the plasma layer. Break the tube at this point and expel the buffy coat by tapping on to the end of several slides.
4. Prepare a thin slide from the buffy coat.
5. When dry, fix the slide in methanol for 5 min and stain with Giemsa stain, as described previously.

Malaria parasites, spirochaetes and trypanosomes may be concentrated at the buffy coat and may demonstrate parasites when none can be seen in the thick or thin film. It may also concentrate abnormal white blood cells which are too few to see in the peripheral blood. When applied to the peripheral blood of immunocompromised patients, amastigotes of *Leishmania* spp. can sometimes be found.

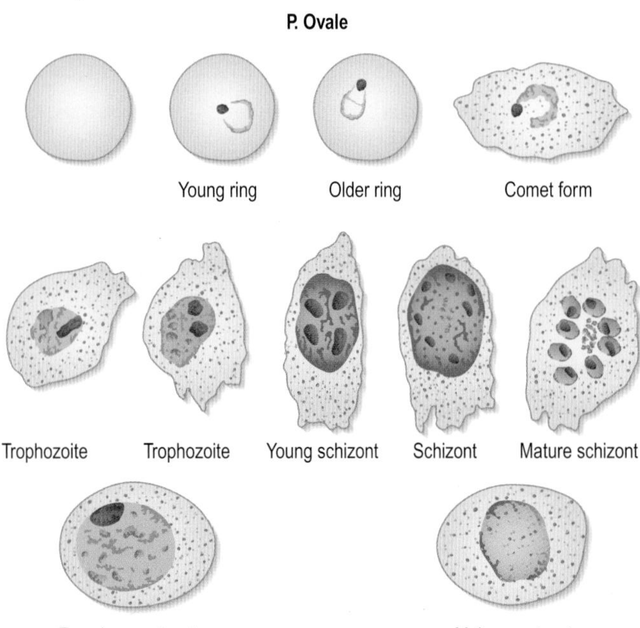

Figure A1.21 *P. ovale* with salient features.

Mini Anion Exchange Column Technique. This is a useful concentration technique where other investigations for trypanosomes in the blood have proved negative. Blood is passed through a column of cellulose; erythrocytes are retained in the column and trypanosomes pass out into a collecting tube.

Method

1. Place a piece of dry sponge into a 2 mL syringe barrel. (This is now termed the column.)
2. Add four drops of phosphate-buffered saline (PBS) to dampen the sponge and allow to drain out of the column.
3. Shake the cellulose (DEAE 52-diethylaminoethyl cellulose) thoroughly to resuspend, and pour into the column up to the 2 mL mark. Allow to stand so that excess PBS will drain out.
4. Add a few millilitres of PBS plus glucose (PBSG) to the top of the column and allow it to drain through.
5. Take 150–200 μL of blood (from a finger prick) and drop on to the top of the column. Allow the blood to soak into the column. Attach a collecting pipette to the base of the column.
6. Pipette a few drops of PBSG on top of the blood and immediately attach the reservoir and fill with PBSG (approx. 1.5 mL). This will drip slowly on to the column.
7. Leave until all the PBSG has washed through the column. (This should take approx. 4 min.)
8. The collecting pipette will now be full of PBSG plus any trypanosomes that were present in the blood.
9. Centrifuge the collecting pipette (in its plastic cover) at 2000 rpm for 10 min.
10. Place the pipette on a slide or viewing chamber and, using the ×20 objective, examine its tip within 20 min for motile trypanosomes.

RAPID DIAGNOSTIC TESTS (RDT) FOR PARASITE ANTIGEN DETECTION

Rapid diagnostic tests utilize gold-labelled monoclonal antibodies to capture parasite antigen from blood, transport it along cellulose nitrate membranes by immunochromatography where it is captured again by immobilized stripes of monoclonal antibody and can be visualized. These tests are now widely used for malaria and viral infection detection.

Devices are available that detect Histidine Rich Protein (HRP 2) from *P. falciparum* or parasite specific lactate dehydrogenase (pLDH) or aldolase from all four malaria species.

LABORATORY DIAGNOSIS OF THE *FILARIA* PARASITES

Filariasis is diagnosed either serologically or by finding the L3 microfilariae in peripheral blood, urine, hydrocele fluid or skin snips. Occasionally, adult worms can be removed as they cross the eye (*Loa loa*) or from a subcutaneous nodule (*Onchocerca volvulus*).

Because of the periodic appearance of microfilariae, peripheral blood samples are collected between 1000 and 1400 hours (day blood) and between 2200 and 0200 hours (night blood). An early morning sample of urine is most suitable for

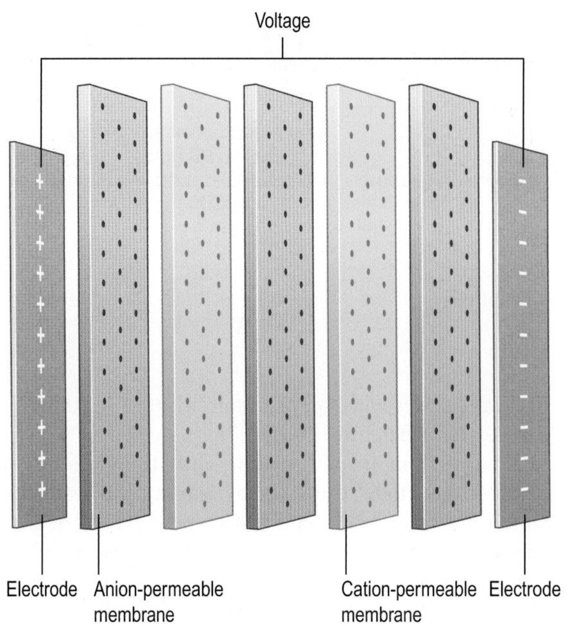

Figure A1.22 Polycarbonate membrane. *(Lawrence Livermore National Laboratory – Science and Technology Review, www.llnl.gov)*

examination. Urine may show a milky appearance, called chyluria, if filariasis is present.

Examination of Blood for Microfilariae

Membrane Filtration Method

1. Collect 20 mL blood into sodium citrate anticoagulant at the appropriate time.
2. Draw the blood up into a syringe and connect it to a Swinnex® holder containing a 5 µm pore size Nuclepore® polycarbonate membrane (Figure A1.22).
3. Gently push the blood through the membrane, collecting the filtrate into a container of disinfectant.
4. Draw up 10 mL normal saline into the syringe and push this through the membrane in a similar manner.
5. Draw several millilitres of air into the syringe and push this through to clear the membrane.
6. Carefully dismantle the holder and, using forceps, remove the membrane and place it on to a slide.
7. Add a drop of normal saline to the membrane and cover with a coverslip.
8. Scan the whole area of the coverslip using the ×10 objective to search for the motile microfilariae.
9. Closer inspection using the ×40 objective and by allowing a drop of 1% methylene blue dye to run under the coverslip will help to show whether the microfilariae possess a sheath.

Modification of Knott's Method for Examining Blood for Microfilariae

1. Collect 20 mL blood into sodium citrate anticoagulant, as described above.
2. Add the blood to an equal volume of 1% saponin in saline (or 2% formalin if saponin is not available).
3. Mix well and allow to stand for 15 min before transferring to centrifuge tubes and centrifuging for 20 min at 2000 rpm.

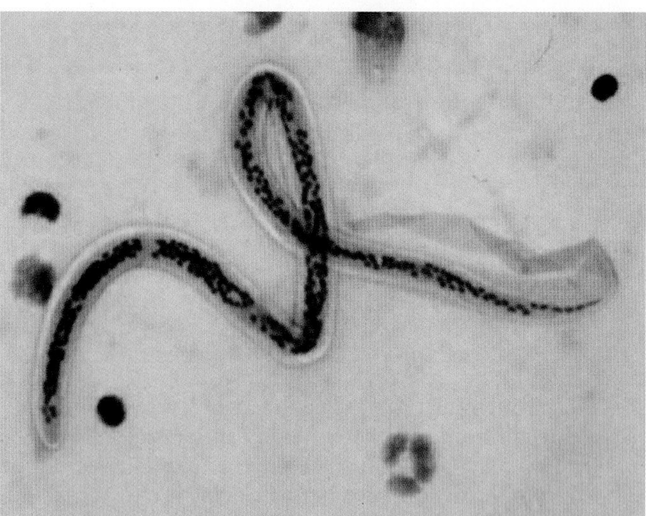

Figure A1.23 *W. bancrofti.*

4. Pour off the supernatant into a container of disinfectant and mix the deposit well before transferring a drop to a slide, covering with a coverslip, and scanning for microfilariae. The saponin preparation will show actively moving larvae; those in the formalin preparation will not be moving (Figures A1.23–A1.25).

Examination of Urine and Hydrocele Fluid. Urine and hydrocele fluid can be filtered in a similar manner to blood to show any microfilariae present. Alternatively, they can be put into a clean centrifuge tube and centrifuged at 2000 rpm for 5 min, the supernatant discarded and a drop of the deposit transferred to a slide. Cover with a coverslip and examine in the same way as for blood above.

Identification of Microfilariae

Staining of Microfilariae

Reagents

- Giemsa stain
- Delafield's haematoxylin.

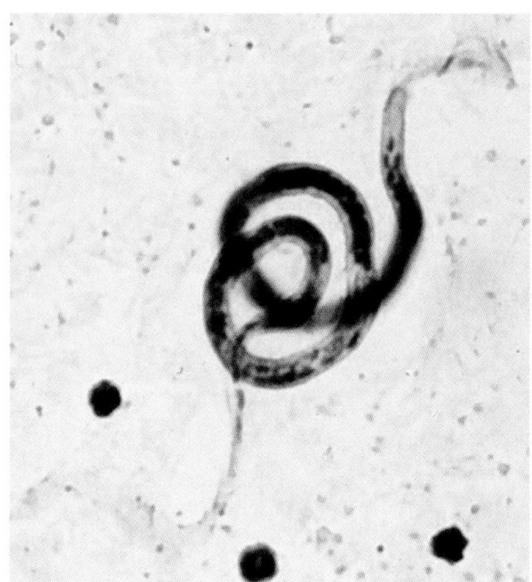

Figure A1.24 *B. malayi.*

TABLE A1.12 Identification of Microfilariae

Microfilariae	Sheath	Tail	Other Features
Loa loa	Yes, stains pale blue	Blunt, large nuclei to tip	Found in peripheral blood 1000–1200 hours
Wuchereria bancrofti	Yes, stains pink, lies in gentle curves	Pointed, nuclei small, discrete; stop short of tail	Nocturnal, found in peripheral blood 2200–0200 hours
Brugia malayi	Yes, stains deep pink, lies in sharp angles	Blunt, with two large discrete nuclei in tail	Nocturnal
Mansonella perstans	No	Blunt, one large nucleus in tail	
Mansonella ozzardi	No	Pointed, nuclei stop short of tail	

If sufficient microfilariae (Table A1.12) are present, films prepared directly from peripheral blood can be used. If not, the blood can be prepared as a thick film or microfilariae can be washed from the membrane filter by placing it into a small pot of saline and agitating. The saline can then be centrifuged at 2000 rpm for 5 min and the deposit pipetted on to a slide and dried (Figures A1.26, A1.27).

Method. Fix the thin blood film or the film prepared from the deposit with methanol for 5 min. If a thick blood film is used, it is necessary first to haemolyse the dried slide by placing it vertically in water for 5 min. Dry the slide well before fixing in methanol for 5 min.

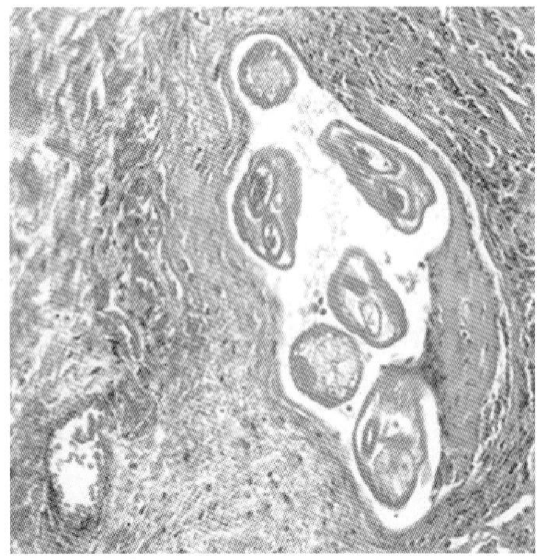

Figure A1.25 *Brugia* spp.

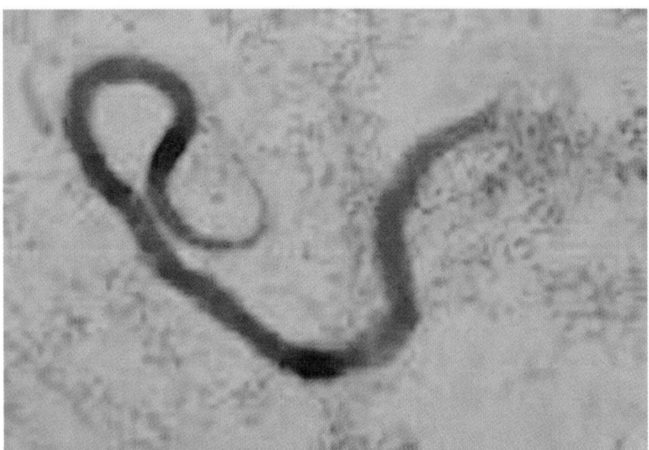

Figure A1.26 *Microfilaria* spp.

1. Stain the slides with Giemsa stain diluted 1 : 10 with buffered water pH 6.8 for 20 min.
2. Wash the stain from the slide with the buffered water, then 'differentiate' the stain by leaving the water on the slide for 5 min. At the end of this period look at the slide to see whether the nuclei of the microfilariae are clear and discrete. If not, repeat the process, reducing the time of 'differentiation' until nuclei are clearly seen.
3. Tip the buffer from the slide and flood the slide with undiluted Delafield's haematoxylin for 15 min.
4. Wash the stain from the slide using buffered water and allow the slide to remain in the water for 5 min to reach the maximum intensity of staining (called 'blueing' the slide).

Giemsa stain will stain the nuclei of the microfilariae purple and the haematoxylin will stain the sheath grey (Figures A1.28, A1.29).

Examination of Skin Snips for Microfilariae of Onchocerca Volvulus. *Onchocerca volvulus* is a filaria worm found in subcutaneous tissue nodules. The discharge of microfilariae into the surrounding tissue occurs. Laboratory diagnosis is made by examining small pieces of skin tissue taken from various parts of the body which contain the migrating larvae.

Method

1. Using a corneal punch, collect small pieces of skin and subcutaneous tissue to a depth of 1 mm. Alternatively, use

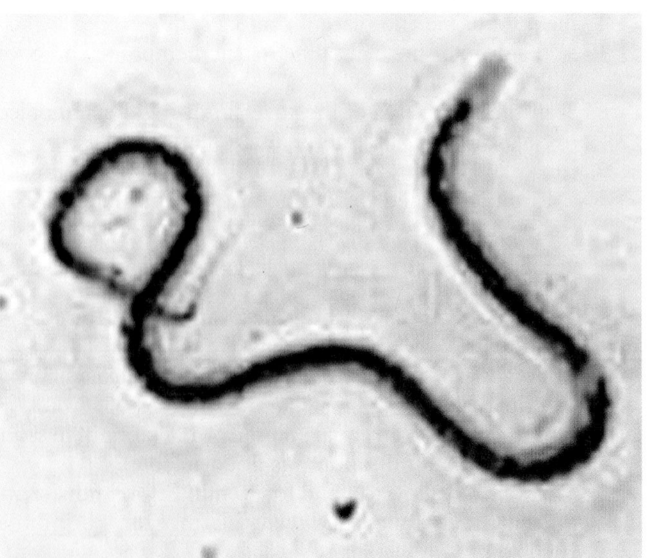

Figure A1.27 *Microfilaria* spp. stained with Giemsa.

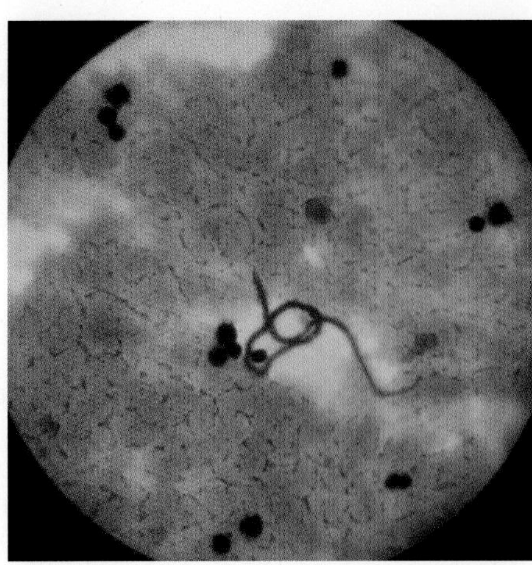

Figure A1.28 Giemsa stain of sheathed Brugia malayi microfilaria in blood smear; 180 to 230 μm long × 5 to 6 μm wide. From Murray P.R., Medical Microbiology 7th edition, Copyright © 2013 by Saunders, an imprint of Elsevier Inc.

a needle point to lift the skin and cut it using a sharp scalpel blade.

2. Place the skin snips into a microtitre tray containing a few drops of saline. Alternatively, place them individually on to a slide with a drop of saline and cover with a coverslip.

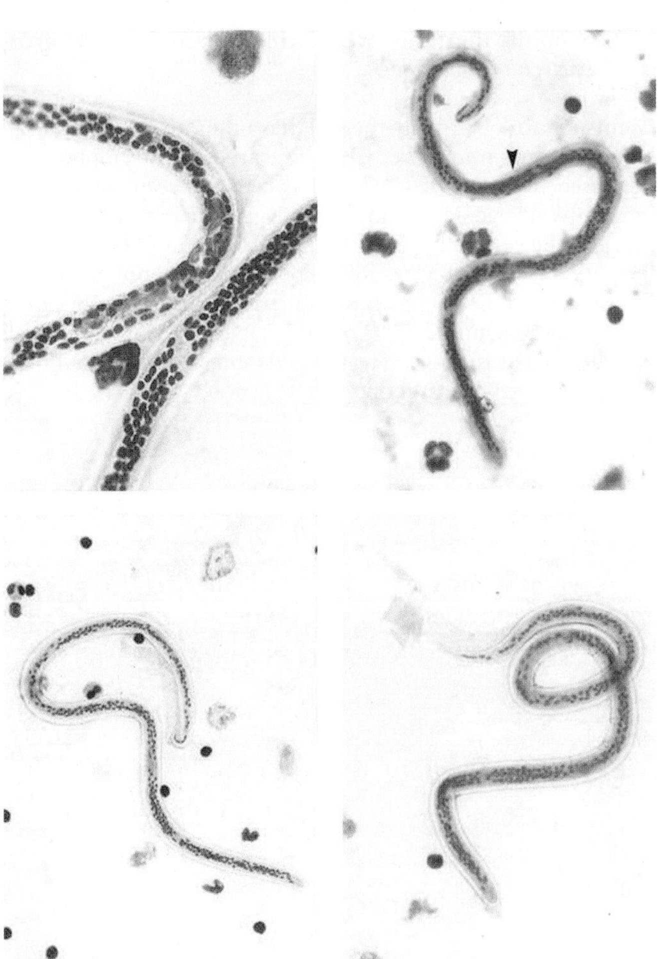

Figure A1.29 Giemsa stain of sheathed Wuchereria bancrofti microfilaria in blood smear; 245 to 295 μm long × 7 to 10 μm wide. From Murray P.R., Medical Microbiology 7th edition, Copyright © 2013 by Saunders, an imprint of Elsevier Inc.

3. Leave the snips in the saline for at least 4 hours and examine under the microscope using the low-power (×10) objective or by using an inversion or dissecting microscope, looking for microfilariae that swim out from the snips.
4. Areas of the body that can be 'snipped' are usually the back, buttocks and calves of the legs, but any area exhibiting urticaria or itching should be included.

LABORATORY DIAGNOSIS OF LEISHMANIASIS

The *Leishmania* genus comprises intracellular organisms that include a wide range of species responsible for a variety of clinical responses from self-healing ulcers to deep cutaneous or mucocutaneous invasion and visceral infection. Laboratory diagnosis is made by identifying the organism in tissue or from cells of the reticuloendothelial system. *Leishmania* is categorized into complex groups of organisms. *L. donovani* complex and *L. braziliensis* complex are the biggest groups. Other groups include *L. tropica*, *L. major* and *L. aethiopica*, and *L. mexicana* in South America. An important subgroup of organisms called the *Viannia* subgroup are found in South America and are primarily responsible for mucocutaneous leishmaniasis.

Confirmation of the diagnosis is made in the laboratory by demonstrating the amastigote stage using direct smear examination from material obtained from bone marrow or spleen, or from a cutaneous ulcer or by culture or molecular identification of specific DNA using the PCR.

Serology is applicable only to the widely disseminated visceral infection as insufficient antibodies are produced by the localized ulcers. Specific antibodies when high titres of antibody are present can be detected using the direct agglutination test (DAT) or an RDT using recombinant rK39.

Culture is an important diagnostic aid; culture media are varied but NNN media, a rabbit blood-agar base using a salt-based (e.g. Locke's solution) or water overlay and a liquid tissue culture medium (e.g. *Schneider's Drosophila* medium) with added fetal calf serum, are useful. Cultures are incubated at 23°C for up to 28 days with weekly subculture. On examination, they will show a conversion from amastigote stage to motile promastigote stage.

Methods of Identification

Cutaneous Leishmaniasis

- Slit-skin smears from an ulcer edge: the edge of the ulcer is compressed to provide a blood-free area, then, using a fine point (no. 15) scalpel blade, a slit is made into the subcutaneous tissue and the base is gently scraped. The tissue juice and cells are transferred to a slide and smeared over an area of 1 cm^2. The preparation is allowed to dry before being fixed in methanol and stained with Giemsa stain (see above). Cultures can also be made from the slit-skin smear material.
- Biopsies of the ulcer edge may provide a more satisfactory sample: impression smears are made by dabbing the tissue several times on to a slide to deposit the cells. These are then dried and fixed in methanol before staining with Giemsa stain. Other portions of the biopsy can be used for diagnosis by histological or molecular examination.

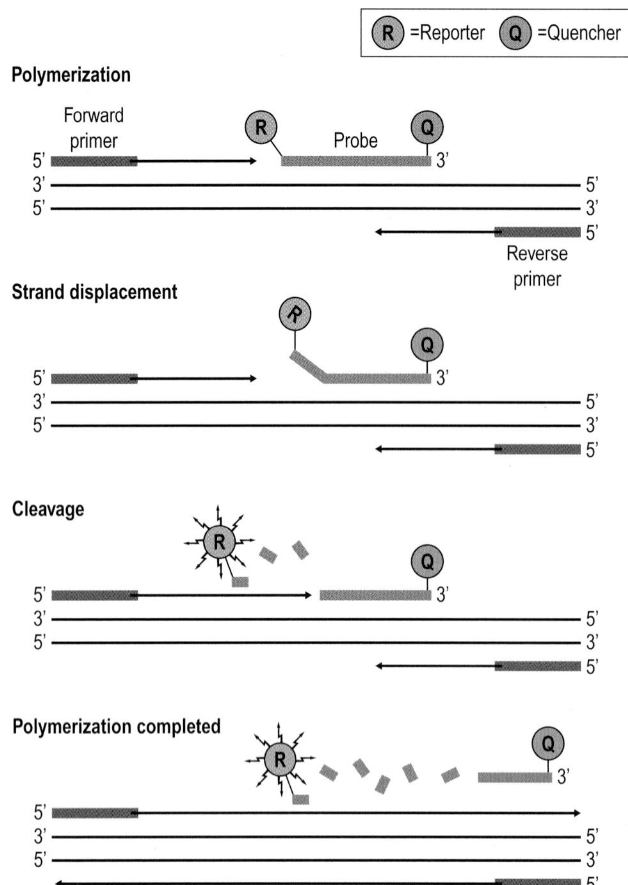

Figure A1.30 Taqman probe-based assay chemistry. *(Asuragen.com)*

Visceral Leishmaniasis

- Smears are made from bone marrow, splenic aspirate or lymph node aspirations and fixed in methanol before being stained with Giemsa stain.
- Cultures are prepared by inoculation of material into NNN medium and incubated at 24°C for up to 21 days.

Identifying the Species of Leishmania

Identification of specific species of *Leishmania* can be made using two principal techniques:

1. Zymodeme: using the isoenzyme pattern
2. Polymerase chain reaction (PCR) using complex specific primer sets for the organism's minicircle DNA (Figure A1.30).

CSF collected by lumbar puncture can be used to search for parasites or bacteria causing meningitis. The procedures attempt to identify the causative organisms of cerebral malaria or trypanosomiasis, or to demonstrate bacteria causing meningitis. CSF is collected into two clean sterile containers; one sample is sent for bacteriological culture, the second sample is used for (a) cell count, (b) examination of stained deposit after centrifugation and (c) biochemical tests on the supernatant, if possible.

Method

1. Examine the CSF visually and report one of the following appearances:
   a. Clear
   b. Opalescent or cloudy – this specimen is likely to have a raised cell count
   c. Blood-stained-red blood cells that have disintegrated as a result of age may give a yellow tinge to the fluid, known as xanthochromia.
2. Note any fibrin clot that may form on standing.
3. Remove the clot carefully using a small wire loop and spread it over a small area of a slide. Allow to dry and, after fixation, stain the slide by the Ziehl–Neelsen method for *Mycobacterium*.
4. Transfer the CSF to a centrifuge tube and centrifuge at 2000 rpm for 5 min.
5. Carefully tip off the supernatant into a second tube for biochemical analysis (glucose, protein).
6. Mix the deposit well by tapping the tube and use a clean Pasteur pipette to transfer a drop to each of three slides. (At this point, larval stages of helminths (*Strongyloides*) or motile amoeba should be looked for by direct microscopy if suspected, or for preparations to look for opportunistic infections with *Cryptococcus neoformans*.)
7. Spread the drops over a small area and allow the slides to dry well before staining (Figure A1.31).

Staining Procedures

1. Stain one slide with Giemsa stain in order to differentiate any blood cells or haemoflagellated parasites present.
2. Stain the second slide with Gram stain to detect any microorganisms present.
3. Stain the third slide with Ziehl–Neelsen stain for *Mycobacterium tuberculosis*.

Giemsa Stain. Normally the CSF has no more than five white blood cells per microlitre (μL); these are usually lymphocytes. Increased numbers of white blood cells are seen in bacterial infections. Pyogenic meningitis will give an increase in polymorphonuclear cells, and tubercular meningitis gives an increase in lymphocytes. Red blood cells are not a normal finding and indicate an accidental traumatic tap or bleeding into the subarachnoid space.

Malaria parasites or *Trypanosoma* may also be found in Giemsa-stained preparation.

Gram Stain

Materials

- Gram stain – 1 g gentian or crystal violet dissolved in 100 mL distilled water

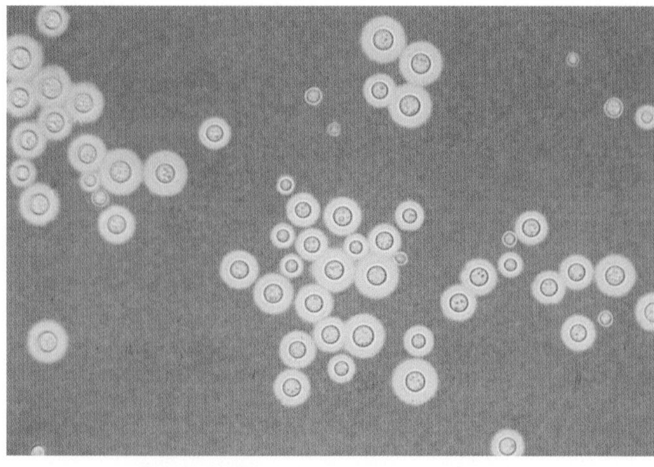

Figure A1.31 *Cryptococcus neoformans.*

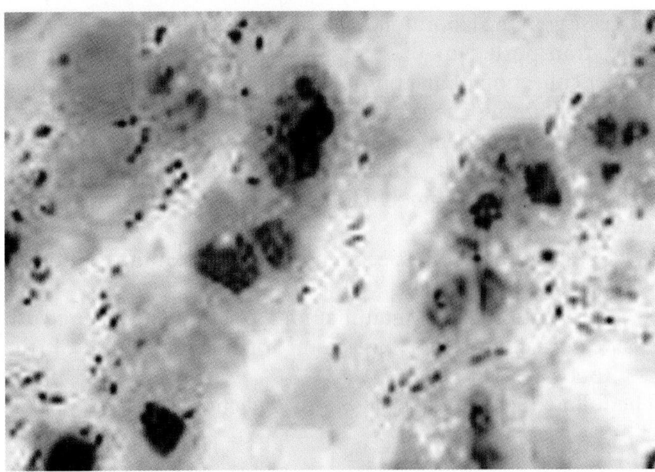

Figure A1.32 *Pneumococci.*

- Lugol's iodine (see above)
- Acetone or methylated spirit
- Neutral red – 0.5 g neutral red dissolved in 100 mL distilled water.

Method

1. Fix the slide by passing it quickly through the flame of a spirit lamp.
2. Place the slide on a rack and flood with Gram stain for 1 min.
3. Wash the stain from the slide.
4. Flood the slide with Lugol's iodine for 1 min.
5. Tilt the slide and pour on acetone or alcohol to decolourize; allow the decolourizing agent to stay on the slide for a short time only (3–5 s) before washing off with tap water.
6. Flood the slide with the neutral red counterstain for 30 seconds.
7. Wash the stain carefully from the slide with water and stand the slide vertically to dry.

Although almost any group of bacteria can be responsible for meningitis, some are seen more commonly:

- Pneumococci – Gram-positive cocci in pairs (diplococci) (Figures A1.32, A1.33)
- *Haemophilus influenzae* – small, slender, Gram-negative bacilli

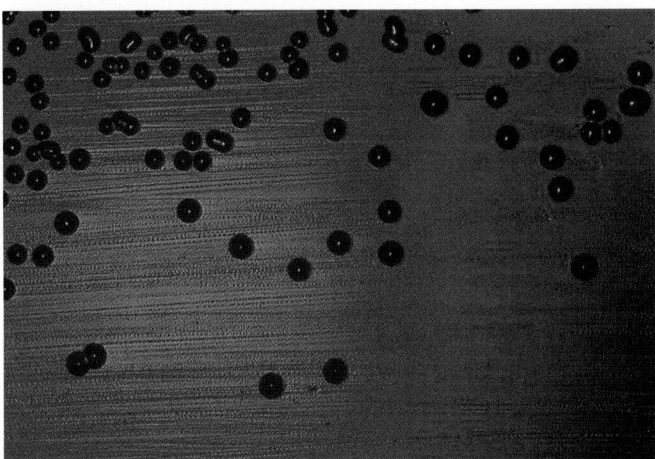

Figure A1.33 *Haemophilus influenza.*

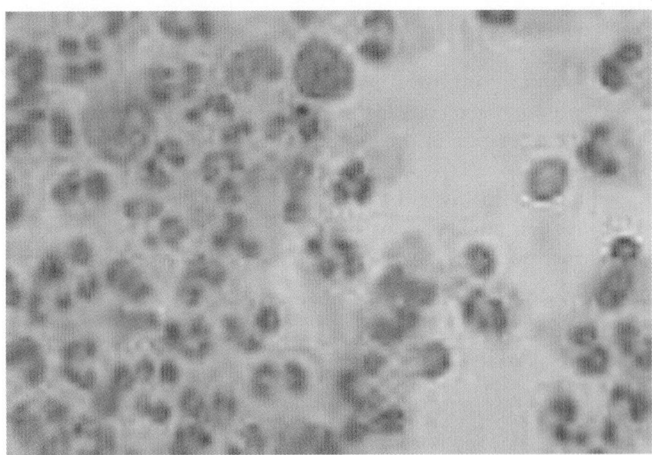

Figure A1.34 *Meningococci* in an infected cell.

- *Meningococci* – Gram-negative intracellular diplococci seen inside the polymorphonuclear cells (Figure A1.34).

Other bacteria will vary in morphological shape and Gram-stained appearance. *Cryptococcus neoformans*, a capsulated yeast organism seen frequently as an opportunistic organism in the immunocompromised patient, may also be seen.

Ziehl–Neelsen Stain for Mycobacteria

Materials

- Strong carbol fuchsin stain
- 1% acid alcohol (1 mL concentrated hydrochloric acid in 99 mL methylated spirit)
- 0.5% malachite green (0.5 g malachite green dissolved in 100 mL distilled water).

Method

1. Fix the smear by passing it through the flame of a spirit lamp.
2. Flood the slide with carbol fuchsin and, using the spirit lamp, gently warm the slide until the surface begins to steam.
3. Stain for 15 min.
4. Wash the slide with water.
5. Flood the slide with 1% acid alcohol and gently rock until no more colour will come out.
6. Wash the slide with water.
7. Flood the slide with malachite green counterstain for 1 min.
8. Wash the slide with water and drain dry.

Mycobacteria are acid-fast bacilli and stain as red bacilli against a green background. (This stain can also be used to demonstrate *Cryptosporidia* oocysts in faecal smears.)

How to Perform Auramine Stain. The auramine-rhodamine stain (AR), also known as the *Truant auramine-rhodamine stain*, is a histological technique used to visualize acid-fast bacilli using fluorescence microscopy, notably species in the *Mycobacterium* genus. Acid-fast organisms display a reddish-yellow fluorescence. Although the auramine-rhodamine stain is not as specific for acid-fast organisms (i.e. *Mycobacterium tuberculosis* or *Nocardia*) as the Ziehl–Neelsen stain, it is more affordable and more sensitive, therefore it is often utilized as a screening tool. AR stain is a mixture of Auramine O and Rhodamine B.

Examination of Sputum

Sputum is commonly examined for parasites of the respiratory tract and for bacteria causing pulmonary infections such as tuberculosis or pneumonia. Sputum is usually described by its appearance as:

- Salivary: frothy, white and watery
- Purulent: thicker consistency, often with a greenish colour
- Mucopurulent: thick, sticky consistency, containing pus; may be blood stained.

EXAMINATION FOR PARASITES

Paragonimus westermani and other *Paragonimus* species discharge ova with the sputum and usually cause 'rusty' blood-stained sputum.

Ova can be recovered after dissolving mucus in the sputum by mixing a portion with an equal portion of 10% potassium hydroxide or other mucus-dissolving reagent, and, after mixing thoroughly, standing for 15 min before centrifuging at 2500 rpm for 5 min. The deposit is examined for ova under the microscope using the ×10 objective.

The sputum can also be concentrated after dissolving the mucus, using the formol-ether method, as described.

Pneumocystis carinii: although now reclassified as a fungal organism, demonstration of this parasitic organism of the immunocompromised host requires specialized laboratory techniques. Grocott's silver stain or PAP stains are commonly used, but a fluorescent method using specific labelled monoclonal antibodies is available.

Strongyloides stercoralis larvae (seen in wet preparation) and oocysts of *Cryptosporidium parvum* (seen by Ziehl–Neelsen stain) may be found in sputum in patients with severe immunosuppression.

EXAMINATION FOR BACTERIA

Many alternative techniques are now entering the diagnostic field and these may be reviewed for further information. Microscopic examination remains a primary diagnostic method for many areas.

Two thin smears of sputum are made using a wire loop that can be sterilized in a flame afterwards, or an applicator stick that can be burned. The smears can then be fixed when dry by passing the back of the slide through a flame twice.

One smear is stained for acid-fast bacilli using the Ziehl–Neelsen method (see above). The second is stained for other bacteria using the Gram stain (see above).

Concentration of sputum using a mucus solvent such as KOH or dilute sodium hypochlorite solution and centrifugation is often helpful for concentrating tubercle bacilli. Smears are made from the neutralized deposit and stained in a similar way.

Sputum should be sent for routine culture if available, and for culture for *Mycobacterium tuberculosis* if required.

Microbiological Examination of Other Specimens for Presence of Bacteria

The laboratory diagnosis of an infectious disease begins with the collection of a clinical specimen for examination or processing in the laboratory (the right one, collected at the right time, transported in the right way to the right laboratory). Proper collection of an appropriate clinical specimen is the first step in obtaining an accurate laboratory diagnosis of an infectious disease. Guidelines for the collection and transportation of specimens should be made available to clinicians in a lucidly written format. The guidelines must emphasize two important aspects:

- Collection of the specimen before the administration of antimicrobial agents
- Prevention of contamination of the specimen with externally present organisms or normal flora of the body.

The following samples are used for detection:

BLOOD

Whole blood is required for bacteriological examination. Serum separated from blood is used for serological techniques. Skin antisepsis is extremely important at the time of collection of the sample. Tincture of iodine (1–2%), povidone iodine (10%) and chlorhexidine (0.5% in 70% alcohol) are ideal agents. However, some individuals may be hypersensitive to iodine present in some of these. While collecting blood for culture, the following points must be remembered:

- Collect blood during the early stages of disease since the number of bacteria in blood is higher in the acute and early stages of disease
- Collect blood during paroxysm of fever since the number of bacteria is higher at high temperatures in patients with fever
- In the absence of antibiotic administration, 99% culture positivity can be seen with three blood cultures.

CEREBROSPINAL FLUID (CSF)

Examination of CSF is an essential step in the diagnosis of any patient with evidence of meningeal irritation or affected cerebrum. Almost 3–10 mL of CSF is collected and part of it is used for biochemical, immunological and microscopic examination and remaining for bacteriological or fungal examination. The following important precautions need to be taken for CSF collection and transportation:

- Collect CSF before antimicrobial therapy is started, if possible.
- The volume of CSF taken is crucial, diagnostic yields increase with greater volumes.
- Collect CSF in a screw-capped sterile container and not in an injection vial with cotton plug.
- Do not delay transport and laboratory investigations.
- Transport in a transport medium if delay in processing is unavoidable.
- CSF is a precious specimen, handle it carefully and economically. Coordinate between laboratories to ensure the most efficient use of the sample to gain the most information. It may not be possible to get a repeat specimen.
- Perform physical inspection of the CSF immediately after collection and indicate findings (particularly colour) on laboratory requisition form.
- Store at 37°C, if delay in processing is inevitable.

SPUTUM

Sputum is processed in the laboratory for aetiological investigation of bacterial and fungal infections of the lower respiratory tract. It is of utmost importance in the diagnosis of pulmonary tuberculosis.

- Select a good wide-mouthed sputum container, which is preferably disposable, made of clear thin plastic, unbreakable and leak-proof material.
- Give the patient a sputum container with the laboratory serial number written on it. Show the patient how to open and close the container and explain the importance of not rubbing off the number written on the side of the container.
- Instruct the patient to inhale deeply 2–3 times, cough up deeply from the chest and spit in the sputum container by bringing it closer to the mouth.
- Make sure the sputum sample is of good quality. A good sputum sample is thick, purulent and sufficient in amount (2–3 mL).

Give the patient an additional container with laboratory serial number written on it for an early morning specimen. Explain to the patient to rinse his/her mouth with plain water before bringing up the sputum.

URINE

Under normal circumstances, urine is sterile. The lower part of the urethra and the genitalia are normally colonized by bacteria, many of which may also cause urinary tract infection. Since urine is a good growth medium for all sorts of bacteria, proper and aseptic collection assumes greater importance for this specimen.

For microbiological examination, urine must be collected as a 'clean catch-mid-stream' specimen.

Urine specimens should be transported to the laboratory within 1 hour for bacteriological examination, because of the continuous growth of bacteria in vitro, thus altering the actual concentration of organisms.

STOOL

Faecal specimens for the aetiological diagnosis of acute infectious diarrhoeas should be collected in the early stage of illness and prior to treatment with antimicrobials. A stool specimen rather than a rectal swab is preferred.

- The faeces specimen should not be contaminated with urine.
- Do not collect the specimen from bed pan.
- Collect the specimen during the early phase of the disease and as far as possible before the administration of antimicrobial agents.
- 1–2 g quantity is sufficient.
- If possible, submit more than one specimen on different days.
- The fresh stool specimen must be received within 1–2 hours of passage.
- Store at 2–8°C.
- Modified Cary and Blair medium (see Chapter 5) is recommended as a good transport medium. It is a very stable medium and can be stored for use in screw – capped containers. It is a semi-solid transport medium. At least two swabs should be inoculated. Most pathogens will survive for up to 48 hours at room temperature. Specimens are unacceptable if the medium is held for more than 1 week or if there is detectable drying of the specimen.

THROAT SWAB

- Depress the tongue with a tongue blade.
- Swab the inflamed area of the throat, pharynx or tonsils with a sterile swab, taking care to collect the pus or piece of membrane.
- Transport in sterile transport tube.

The following lists some of the less commonly encountered bacterial pathogens which require special isolation or detection conditions.

Pneumococcus

- Sample – throat swab, sputum, blood, CSF
- Media – blood agar, solid or liquid infusion agar
- Special atmospheric requirements – 5% CO_2
- Incubation time – 2–3 days
- Temperature: 37°C
- Alternative ways to diagnose – serotyping (Quellung reaction)
- Appear on Gram stain as lancet-shaped diplococci.

Leprosy

- Sample – skin scrapings, slit skin smear
- Media – liquid media, chemically defined media
- Special atmospheric requirements – N/A
- Incubation time – N/A
- Temperature: room temp.
- Alternative ways to diagnose – definitive diagnosis of leprosy by doing a test called a skin biopsy or slit skin smear
- Appear dark-blue color when stained with Gram stain.

Listeria

- Sample – blood, urine, CSF
- Media – cultured aerobically in blood agar
- Special atmospheric requirements: 5–10% CO_2
- Incubation time – 18 hours
- Temperature: 20–37°C
- Alternative ways to diagnose – Serological tests.

Neisseria

- Sample – urethral and cervical swabs, joint fluid, eye swabs, CSF
- Media – selective enriched medium (modified Thayer–Martin)
- Special atmospheric requirements – in 5% CO_2 overnight
- Incubation time – 2 days
- Temperature: 35–37°C
- Alternative ways to diagnose – nucleic acid amplification test
- Appear as Gram-negative diplococci.

Anthrax

- Sample – skin lesions, blood, CSF, stool
- Media – standard media or 5% Sheep blood agar
- Special atmospheric requirements – 5% CO_2

- Incubation time – 2 days
- Temperature: 35°C
- Gram-positive bacilli, non-motile and non-hemolytic on blood agar
- Alternative ways to diagnose – hanging drop method, ZN, induction of capsule formation, gamma bacteriophage test
- Appear as bamboo sticks at swollen ends.

Procedure for Isolation and Identification of *B. Anthracis* and Confirmation of Diagnosis (Figure A1.35)

Tetanus

- Sample – wound swab, pus, blood, CSF
- Media – toxin peptone free media
- Special atmospheric requirements – anaerobic
- Incubation time – 2–5 days
- Temperature: 35°C
- Alternative ways to diagnose – spatula test is done to diagnose tetanus
- Gram-positive beaded (appearance) rods with blunt and tapered ends.

Brucella

- Sample – blood, urine, sputum, breast milk, lymph node biopsy, bone marrow aspirate
- Media – Blood agar enriched with animal serum and glucose
- Special atmospheric requirements – 5–10°C CO_2
- Incubation time – 3–5 days
- Temperature: 20–30°C
- Alternative ways to diagnose – biopsies in cultures, slide agglutination reaction (Gruber–Widal), complement binding reaction and direct Coombs test
- On Gram stain they appear as dense clumps of Gram-negative coccobacilli.

Mycoplasma

- Sample – throat swab, sputum
- Media – isotonic nutrient mediums
- Special atmospheric requirements – 5% CO_2
- Incubation time 2–8 days
- Temperature: 37°C
- Alternative ways to diagnose – CFT, IgM-Specific EIAs
- Appear as bacteria (within capsule): when stained with safranin appear as red capsule (outer layer of bacteria): clear background of organism: stained dark with nigrosin.

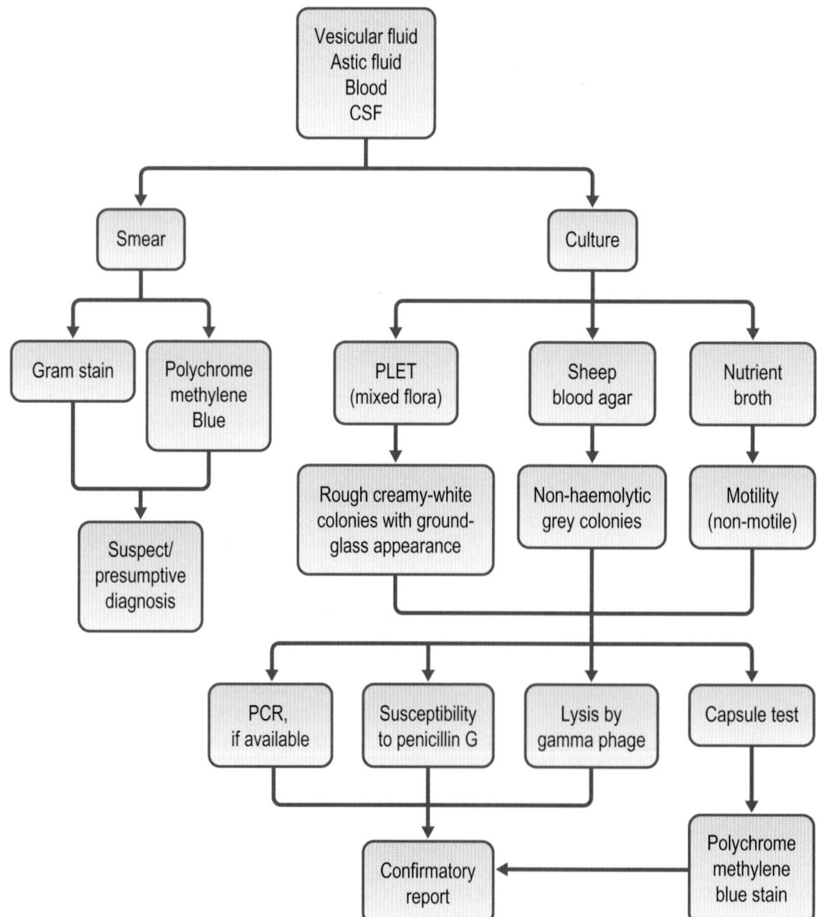

Figure A1.35 Procedure for isolation and identification of *B. anthracis* and confirmation of diagnosis.

Yersinia

- Sample – stool, blood
- Media – cultured on standard nutrient medium
- Special atmospheric requirements – require standard medium
- Incubation time – 2–3 days
- Temperature: 20–30°C
- Alternative ways to diagnose – ELISA and immunoblot can be used to detect the antibodies
- Gram-negative rods, colonies may have deep red centres.

Nocardia

- Sample – bronchial washings/lavages, sputum, pus, wound drains, tissue biopsy and CSF
- Media – standard blood culture media, nonselective media
- Special atmospheric requirements – 8% CO_2
- Incubation time – 2 weeks
- Alternative ways to diagnose include staining samples and cultures with modified acid fast stains
- Nocardia colonies may be smooth and moist, or have a 'mold-like' verrucous grey-white waxy or powdery appearance from aerial hyphae.

Rickettsia

- Sample – blood, CSF
- Media – embryo yolk sacs in suitable experimental animals or cell cultures
- Special atmospheric requirements – 5% CO_2
- Incubation time – 3–15 days
- Temperature: 37°C
- Alternative ways to diagnose – PCR, immunofluorescence test, Weil Felix agglutination test.

BARTONELLOSIS

- Sample – blood, CSF, tissue biopsy
- Media – Columbia blood agar
- Special atmospheric requirements – 5% CO_2
- Incubation time – 7–100 days
- Temperature: optimum 35–37°C
- Alternative ways to diagnose – antibody assay with IF or EIA, indirect immunofluorescence techniques, PCR.

LEPTOSPIRA

- Sample – blood, CSF, peritoneal dialysate, urine
- Media – special culture medium under aerobic conditions
- Special atmospheric requirements – 5% CO_2
- Incubation time – 4 weeks
- Temperature: 27–37°C
- Alternative ways to diagnose – dark field microscopy, lysis agglutination reaction with specific set sera, antibody assay.

Diphtheria

- Nasopharyngeal aspirate/swab
- Media – blood agar
- Special atmospheric requirements – 5% CO_2
- Incubation time – 2–5 days
- Temperature: 36–37°C
- Alternative ways to diagnose – Passive haemagglutination test in serum or PCR
- The 'barred' appearance is due to the presence of polyphosphate inclusions called metachromatic granules.

Spirochaetes

- Sample – fluid exudates, genital specimens and ulcer fluids, CSF
- Media – in vitro culturing not yet achieved
- Special atmospheric requirements – N/A
- Incubation time – N/A
- Temperature: N/A
- Alternative ways to diagnose – antibody assays (TPPA, TPHA, VDRL)
- Dark field and immunofluorescent stains.

*Fungal infections (*Candida *and* Pneumocystis*)*

- Sample – swab, skin scrapings, CSF, fluid exudates
- Media – blood culture media, biphasic media incorporating both agar and broth phases, glucose, Peptone (Sabouraud's agar) or malt agar, brain heart infusion agar
- Special atmospheric requirements – 5–10% CO_2
- Incubation time – up to 28 days
- Temperature: 25–30°C
- Alternative ways to diagnose – serological tests to detect fungal antigens, ELISA, complement fixation tests, immunodiffusion, PCR
- Appear red and blue when stained using H&E stain.

Examination of Blood for Haematological Assessment

Haematological values are necessary in the diagnosis of infection or anaemia. The most useful criteria include:

- Total white cell count, differential white blood cell count, haemoglobin
- Haematocrit, mean corpuscular haemoglobin concentration (MCHC) and mean corpuscular volume (MCV)
- Platelet count
- Examination of the blood film picture can give much useful information even when other parameters are not available.

METHOD

1. Fix thin blood films in methanol and stain with Giemsa stain.
2. Examine the slide under the microscope using the oil immersion objective (×100).

OBSERVATIONS

Red Blood Cells

1. Note the size: a normal erythrocyte measures 7 μm in diameter. The cell may be enlarged (macrocyte) or appear smaller (microcyte).
2. Note the colour; in a normal erythrocyte the haemoglobin is stained pink with a small area of pallor in the centre. An enlarged area of central pallor (hypochromia) indicates an iron deficiency.

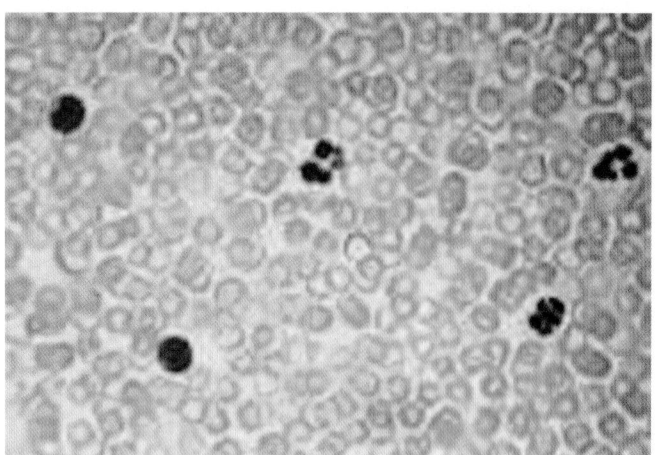

Figure A1.36 Thin film showing red blood cells and blood cellular components.

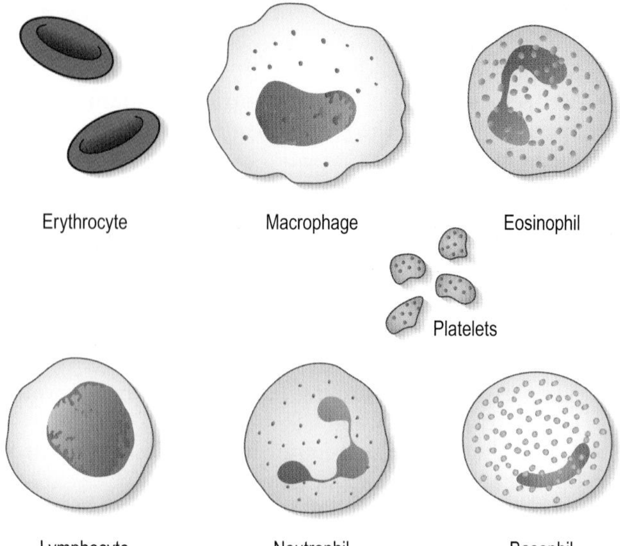

Figure A1.37 The elements of blood. *(Fotosearch.com)*

3. Note the presence of any abnormal erythrocytes; target cells or sickle cells may indicate an abnormal haemoglobin type.
4. Note any inclusions of the erythrocytes; basophilic stippling and nucleated cells or spherocytes may indicate a haemolytic process.
5. Note any intracellular or extracellular parasites which may be present: malaria, *Trypanosoma*, *Babesia*, *Borrelia*, microfilariae.

White Blood Cells

An impression of the number of white cells present can be gained from the thin blood film; an average of 1–2 cells in each field is normally seen. A differential count will indicate the types of cells present.

Note the morphological appearance of the cells. Neutrophils may show a shift to the left or to the right. Mononuclear cells may be 'atypical', and any primitive cells must be recorded. Increases in the number of eosinophils should be recorded as this can be linked to a number of different infectious, non-infectious and autoimmune conditions (Figures A1.36–A1.38).

Platelets

These are normally seen in every field, either singly or in small clumps. A decrease in platelets (thrombocytopenia) is noted when platelets are scanty and only seen in every 3–5 fields.

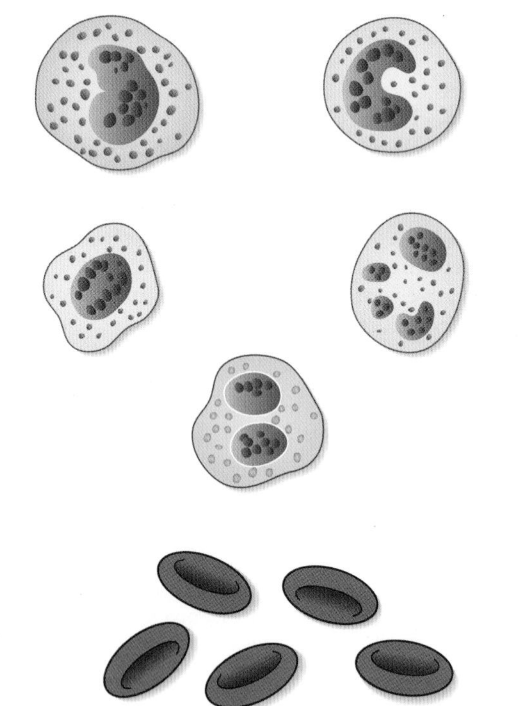

Figure A1.38 *P. ovale* and red blood cells. *(Fotosearch.com)*

BIBLIOGRAPHY

1. Health and Safety Commission's Health Service Advisory Committee. Safety in Health Service Laboratories: Safe Working and the Prevention of Infections in Clinical Laboratories. London: Health and Safety Executive; 1991.
2. Muhumuza J, Asiimwe BB, Kayes S, et al. Introduction of an in-house PCR for the routine identification of *M. tuberculosis* in a low-income country. Int J Tuberc lung Dis 2006;10(11):1262–7.
3. Helmy MM, Rashed LA, Abdel-Fattah HS. Co-infection with *Cryptosporidium parvum* and *Cyclospora cayetanensis* in immunocompromised patients. J Egypt Soc Parasitol 2006;36(2):613–27.
4. Haque R, Mollah NU, Ali IK, et al. Diagnosis of amoebic liver abscess and intestinal infection with the TechLab *E. histolytica* II antigen detection and antibody tests. J Clin Microbiol 2000;38(9):3235–9.
5. Haque R, Ali IK, Akther S, et al. Comparison of PCR, isoenzyme analysis, and antigen detection for diagnosis of *E. histolytica* infection. J Clin Microbiol 1998;36(2):449–52.
6. Clarke SC, McIntyre M. Acid-fast bodies in faecal smears stained by the modified Ziehl–Neelsen technique. Br J Biomed Sci 2001;58(1):7–10.
7. Muller A, Bialek R, Kamper A, et al. Detection of microsporidia in travellers with diarrhoea. J Clin Microbiol 2001;39(4):1630–2.
8. Srinivasan S, Moody AH, Chiodini PL. Comparison of blood-film microscopy, the OptiMAL dipstick, Rhodamine 123 staining and PCR, for monitoring antimalarial treatment. Ann Trop Med Parasitol 2000;94(3):227–32.
9. Moody A. Rapid diagnostic tests for malaria parasites. Clin Microbiol Rev 2002;15(1):66–78.

10. Chilton D, Malik AN, Armstrong M, et al. Use of rapid diagnostic tests for diagnosis of malaria in the UK. J Clin Path 2006;59(8):862–6.
11. Iqbal J, Hira PR, Sher A, et al. Diagnosis of imported malaria by *Plasmodium* lactate dehydrogenase (pLDH) and histidine-rich protein 2 (PfHRP-2)-based immunocapture assays. Am J Trop Med Hyg 2001;64(1–2):20–3.
12. Schuetz A, Addiss DG, Eberhard ML, et al. Evaluation of the whole blood filariasis ICT test for short-term monitoring of treatment. Am J Trop Med Hyg 2000;62(4):502–3.
13. Sanchez-Tejeda G, Rodriguez N, Parra CI, et al. Cutaneous leishmaniasis caused by members of *Leishmania braziliensis* complex in Nayarit, State of Mexico. Mem Inst Oswaldo Cruz 2001;96(1):15–19.
14. Venazzi EA, Roberto AC, Barbosa-Tessmann IP, et al. Detection of Leishmania (Viannia) DNA in blood from patients with American cutaneous leishmaniasis. Exp Parasitol 2007;115(4):399–402.
15. Alborzi A, Rasouli M, Nademi Z, et al. Evaluation of the rK39 strip test for the diagnosis of visceral leishmaniasis in infants. East Mediterr Health J 2006;12(3–4):294–9.
16. Zijlstra EE, Nur Y, Desjeux P, et al. Diagnosing visceral leishmaniasis with the recombinant rK39 strip test: experience from the Sudan. Trop Med Int Health 2001;6(2):108–13.
17. Perkins MD, Roscigno G, Zumla A. Progress towards improved tuberculosis diagnostics for developing countries. Lancet 2006;367:942–3.
18. Richardson MD, Warnock DW. Fungal Infection Diagnosis and Management. 3rd ed. Chichester: John Wiley & Sons; 2003.
19. Chiodini PL, Moody AH, Manser DW. Atlas of Medical Helminthology and Protozoology. Edinburgh: Elsevier Science Health Science Division; 2001.
20. Kayser FH, Bienz KA, Eckert J, et al. Medical Microbiology 1st ed. New York: Thieme; 2004.

APPENDIX 2

Parasitic Protozoa

HONORINE WARD | SITARA S. R. AJJAMPUR

Introduction and Classification

Protozoa or protists refer to unicellular eukaryotic microbes with animal-like nutrition (holozoic) patterns. Although more than 50 000 species have been described, most are free living with a few that are parasitic for humans and animals and can cause a range of mild to life-threatening infections. Most parasitic protozoa in humans are <50 μm in size with the largest being up to 150 μm (*Balantidium coli*). Some have locomotory organs like pseudopodia, cilia and flagella and a cytostome or cell 'mouth' for ingesting fluids or solid particles. Several developmental stages of a protozoan parasite may participate in the life cycle, and more than one host (definitive, intermediate, vector or reservoir hosts) may be required. The trophozoite stage is a general term for the active, multiplying stage of many protozoa and is usually the infective form. Some protozoa also produce environmentally resistant, dormant cyst forms. Reproduction is asexual in most cases while sexual reproduction occurs in some protozoa (e.g. Apicomplexa).

The previous classification of Kingdom Protozoa into six phyla, mostly based on morphology, has been revised, based on genomic and phylogenetic evidence with inclusion of most human parasites into four of six eukaryotic supergroups.[1] Although supportive data for these groups is variable, a working classification is provided (Table A2.1).[2] In this chapter, an overview of parasites causing blood and tissue infections followed by enteric protozoa is provided.[3,4]

APICOMPLEXAN PARASITES

Apicomplexa are a diverse group of protists that have an apical complex, a cluster of organelles including rhoptries, micronemes and dense granules specialized for host cell invasion. Apicomplexans also display a unique substrate-dependent 'gliding' motility which propels them across the surface and aids in active host cell invasion. This phylum includes a wide range of human parasites such as enteric parasites *Cryptosporidium*, *Isospora* and *Cyclospora*, the tissue cyst forming parasite *Toxoplasma gondii* and parasites such as *Plasmodium* spp. and *Babesia* spp. specialized in infecting red blood cells (RBC).

Malarial Parasites

The four species of genus *Plasmodium* associated with malaria in humans include *P. vivax*, *P. falciparum*, *P. malariae* and *P. ovale*; *P. vivax* has the broadest geographical range due to its ability to replicate in more temperate climates. More recently, *P. knowlesi*, morphologically similar to *P. malariae* and originally described in macaques, has emerged as a human parasite in Malaysia. Malarial parasites are transmitted by ~60 different species of the female *Anopheles* mosquito with different biting patterns and efficiency of transmission contributing to varying epidemiological patterns. *Anopheles gambiense* is one of the most efficient, anthropophilic vectors and is found mainly in Africa.

Infection is initiated by the bite of an infected mosquito which injects sporozoites along with saliva into the bloodstream. Within 30–60 minutes, the sporozoites invade hepatocytes and then over the next 1–2 weeks (duration varies with species, see Table A2.2), each parasite commences nuclear division (exoerythrocytic schizogony) to produce several thousand meronts followed by cytoplasmic division to form merozoites. *P. vivax* and *P. ovale* also produce dormant forms called hypnozoites that cause relapses following a primary attack. Merozoites freed by the rupture of the infected hepatocytes enter the circulation, where they invade erythrocytes and reside within a parasitophorous vacuole. Early trophozoites are disc-shaped with a central vacuole and one nucleus which when viewed through a microscope in optical section resembles a signet ring and are termed 'ring forms' (Figure A2.1). As the trophozoite grows, the central vacuole disappears and the characteristic black or brown hemozoin pigment appears. In this erythrocytic stage repetitive rounds of invasion, growth and division (producing schizonts and merozoites) occur resulting in an exponential increase in parasite numbers and appearance of symptoms. Acute febrile episodes and rigors that occur within a 48–72 hour periodicity (24 hours in *P. knowlesi*) coincide with the synchronized lysis of infected cells releasing merozoites, parasite debris and malarial pigment.

Some merozoites develop into gametocytes (Figure A2.2) whose continued development depends on their being ingested by a feeding female *Anopheles* mosquito. In the mosquito gut, male and female gametes emerge from the infected RBC. The male gametocyte produces eight long motile gametes (microgametes), by a rapid process known as 'exflagellation', which break free and swim through the blood meal in search of a female gamete. The gametes fertilize in the gut, give rise to motile, diploid ookinetes that burrow into the gut wall and develop into oocysts where they produce several thousand haploid sporozoites. These travel to the salivary gland of the mosquito to continue the life cycle. The mosquito becomes infectious to its next blood meal donor in ~2 weeks.

Most bites from infected *Anopheles* result in no infection, asymptomatic infections or uncomplicated malaria presenting with fever and nonspecific symptoms, such as vomiting and/or diarrhoea. Severe malaria develops only in a few cases and may present as cerebral malaria, severe anemia or acidosis-driven respiratory distress. Susceptibility to and outcome of infection is determined by a wide range of factors including the mosquito inoculation rate, sporozoite dose, immunity acquired from previous exposure, stable or unstable transmission patterns,

TABLE A2.1 Classification of Protozoan Parasites into Supergroups

Supergroup	Group	Subgroup		Human Pathogens
Amoebozoa	Archamoebae	Entamoebae		*Entamoeba histolytica*
	Amoebae	Acanthamoebae		*Acanthamoebae* spp.
				Balamuthia mandrillaris
		Thecamoebae		*Sappinia diploidea*
SAR clade/Harosa	Alveolates	Apicomplexa	Haemosporidia	*Plasmodium* spp.
(Chromoalveolata)			Piroplasmida	*Babesia* spp.
			Coccidiasina	*Cryptosporidium* spp.
				Toxoplasma gondii
				Cyclospora cayetanensis
				Isospora belli
				Sarcocystis spp.
		Ciliophora	Litostomatea	*Balantidium coli*
	Stramenopiles	Opalinata		*Blastocystis hominis*
Opisthokonts	Fungi	Microsporidia		*Nosema* spp.
				Encephalitozoon spp.
				Enterocytozoon spp.
Excavates	Metamonads	Diplomonads		*Giardia lamblia*
		Parabasalia		*Trichomonas vaginalis*
	Discoba	Heterolobosea	Vahlkampfiidae	*Naegleria fowleri*
		Euglenozoa	Kinetoplastids	*Trypanosoma brucei*
				Trypanosoma cruzi
				Leishmania spp.

SAR clade: Stramenopila, Alveolata and Rhizaria.
Based on Walker G, Dorrell RG, Schlacht A, et al. Eukaryotic systematics: a user's guide for cell biologists and parasitologists. Parasitology 2011;138(13):1638–63.

parasite virulence, host genetic polymorphisms and nutritional status, housing conditions and accessibility to prompt diagnosis with effective treatment.

In *P. falciparum*, rosetting of RBC and cytoadherence results in sequestration in tissues, capillary blockage and rupture, with haemorrhage into the surrounding tissue. Other consequences of sequestration include avoidance of splenic removal and disappearance of mature forms from peripheral blood such that only ring-form trophozoites and gametocytes are seen. Increased levels of proinflammatory cytokines contribute to manifestations of severe malaria. Anaemia in malaria arises due to increased destruction and removal of parasitized RBCs, dyserythropoiesis and occasionally, acute hemolysis. In pregnant women, malaria causes fetal growth restriction, preterm delivery, or fetal loss due to infection of the placenta.

Diagnosis. Clinical diagnosis of malaria is based on fever and splenomegaly. Microscopy remains the gold standard and involves the examination of thick and thin blood films. A thick

Figure A2.1 *Plasmodium falciparum* ring forms in peripheral blood thin film (Giemsa stain): small rings with 1 or 2 chromatin dots, appliqué or accole forms at the edge of the RBC; multiple rings, heavy parasitaemia seen.

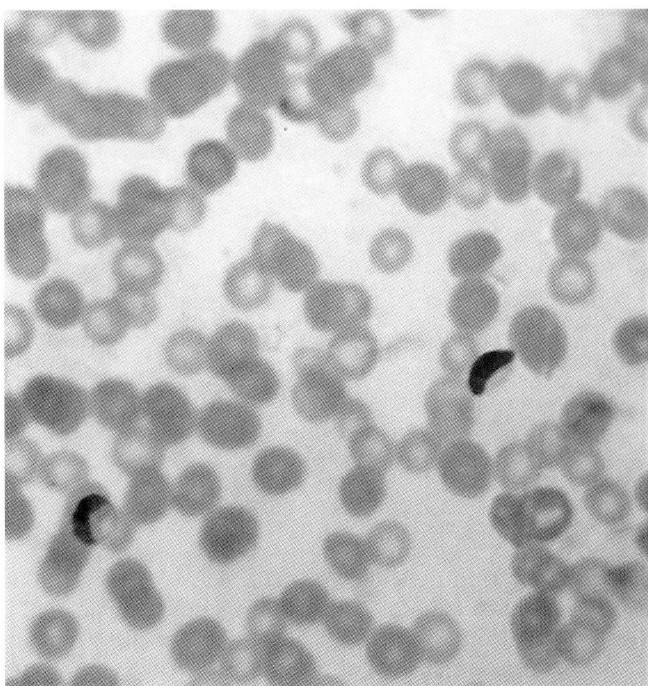

Figure A2.2 *Plasmodium falciparum* gametocytes in peripheral blood thin film (Giemsa stain): Crescentic or banana shaped with outline of RBC seen, also called Laveran's bib.

TABLE A2.2 **Comparison of Human *Plasmodium* Species**

Species	*P. vivax*	*P. ovale*	*P. malariae*	*P. falciparum*
Geographic distribution	Worldwide tropical and sub-tropical areas, Asia, South America	West Africa, South Asia	Scattered, pockets in Africa, South Asia and South East Asia	Tropical and sub-tropical areas Africa and Asia
CLINICAL CHARACTERISTICS				
Incubation period (days)	8–17	18–40	10–17	8–11
Initial fever	Irregular	Irregular	Regular	Continuous
Periodicity (hours)	48	48	72	36–48
Illness	Benign tertian malaria	Ovale tertian malaria	Quartan malaria	Malignant tertian malaria
Severity of paroxysms	Mild to moderate	Mild	Mild to moderate	Severe
Duration of primary attack (weeks)	3–8	2–3	3–24	2–3
Duration of infection (years)	5–7	1	20+	0.5–1
Anaemia	Mild to moderate	Mild	Mild to moderate	Severe
CNS disease	Rare	Rare	Rare	Common
Nephrotic syndrome	Rare	Rare	Common	Rare
Relapse (persistent exoerythrocytic cycle)	Yes (hypnozoites) e.g.: *P. vivax subspecies hiberans*	Rare (hypnozoites)	No, recrudescence seen	No
PERIPHERAL BLOOD FILMS				
Stages seen	All (often in same blood film)	All	All, more mature forms	Early ring, gametocyte only – other stages appear only in heavy infections
'Ring' form	Delicate, signet ring, ~2.5 µm	Smaller, delicate ring	Thick ring, ~2.5 µm	Small, ~1.5 µm, multiple rings, 2 chromatin dots, accole/applique forms
Trophozoite	Amoeboid	Compact, non-amoeboid	Compact, rounded often band-like	Compact, rarely seen in peripheral blood
Merozoites/RBC	12–24	8–12	6–12	Rarely seen in peripheral blood
Hemozoin pigment	Fine, light brown	Coarse, dark brown	Coarse, dark brown, abundant	
Schizont	Merozoites in clusters fill entire RBC	Merozoites in clusters	Merozoites in cluster around central pigment	
Gametocyte appearance	3 days (early)	4–18 days	Several weeks	7–10 days
Macrogametocyte	Rounded or oval, darker than microgametocyte, compact chromatin, pigment present	Similar to *P. vivax* but smaller and fewer in number	Similar to *P. vivax* but smaller and fewer in number. Pigment more conspicuous	Crescentic, with central chromatin, darker cytoplasm, dark brown pigment
Microgametocyte	Light blue cytoplasm with diffuse chromatin and pigment			Crescentic, diffuse chromatin, lighter staining, scattered pigment
PARASITIZED RBC				
Parasitaemia	1–2%	1%	<1%	>5%
Limitations of RBC	Young RBC	young RBC	old RBC	All RBC
Size	Enlarged (1.5 times)	Enlarged, easily deformed and some have fimbriated edges	Normal	Normal
Cell surface	Schüffner's dots	Schüffner's dots (larger and darker than *P. vivax*, appear earlier)	Fine stippling (Ziemann's dots)	Maurer's clefts (larger, rarely seen)

film is highly sensitive and detects as few as 50 parasites/µl of blood in field conditions. The accompanying thin film allows for better description of morphology and provides clinically useful information on level of parasitaemia. While microscopy remains an important tool for diagnosis, it is labour intensive, provides delayed results and requires a skilled microscopist and quality control. Laboratory diagnosis in clinics without microscopy has now become possible through the development of rapid diagnostic tests, based on detection of parasite antigens (lactate dehydrogenase, histidine rich protein and aldolase). These tests can differentiate *P. falciparum* (HRP) and *P. vivax* (pLDH) and detect as few as 100–200 parasites/µl of blood. Although sensitivity is variable and not as high as microscopy, higher negative predictive values than clinical diagnosis in remote, endemic regions allows for better use of limited therapeutic options.

Babesia

Babesia are tick-borne intraerythrocytic Apicomplexan parasites. This emerging infection has over the last few decades become endemic in the northeastern and midwestern regions of the USA and is caused by *Babesia microti*. Sporadic reports of other species include *B. duncani* (USA), *B. divergens* and *B. venatorum* (Europe). Clinical features range from asymptomatic infection or mild viral-like illness to severe disease in people with underlying immunosuppressive conditions, including splenectomy, malignancies and HIV.

Diagnosis. In Giemsa-stained thin blood films, *Babesia* appear as round or oval parasites of 1–2 μm with blue cytoplasm and red chromatin and often appear as paired forms. The tetrad form referred to as a Maltese cross is pathognomic for *B. microti* and *B. duncani*. PCR and Immunofluorescence assays (IFA) are also available for diagnosis.

Toxoplasma gondii

Toxoplasma gondii is an Apicomplexan parasite with members of the cat family as the definitive host. This widespread infection can be acquired by ingestion of oocysts shed in cat faeces in contaminated soil or water, ingestion of tissue cysts containing bradyzoites of intermediate hosts present in undercooked meat, solid organ transplant with infected donor organs and congenital infection with tachyzoites from a mother who became infected during or just prior to delivery. During an infection, rapidly dividing tachyzoites (2–4 μm wide and 4–8 μm long) multiply in host cells (macrophages referred to as pseudocysts) and use these as a 'Trojan horse' to spread and infect cells in other tissues such as the CNS, eye, skeletal, muscle and placenta) Following the acute phase, the infection becomes chronic with the development of spherical tissue cysts of up to 60 μm in size that contain several thousand slowly dividing bradyzoites. In immunocompetent adults, the acute phase results in asymptomatic or mild to moderate febrile illness with lymphadenopathy followed by a lifelong symptomless chronic phase. In immunocompromised persons especially those with AIDS, reactivation of chronic infection most often results in encephalitis but can also cause ocular and disseminated multi-organ disease. Congenital toxoplasmosis with severe neurological and ocular disease is rare and usually associated with transmission during the first trimester.

Diagnosis. Diagnosis in pregnancy and neonates is carried out with EIA tests detecting IgG, IgM, IgA and avidity of IgG using prescribed algorithms,[3] as no single test can be interpreted as evidence of recent infection. In immunocompromised hosts, direct detection with PCR and microscopic examination of brain tissue, CSF, vitreous and aqueous fluid, bronchoalveolar lavage (BAL) fluid or blood is preferred due to low antibody levels.

Sarcocystis spp.

Sarcocystis hominis and *S. suihominis* are related to *Toxoplasma*, and employ humans as definitive hosts to cause asymptomatic infections or mild to moderate, self-limiting diarrhoea. Oocysts may be found in human faeces and measure 15–20 μm long by 15–20 μm wide. Humans may also become dead-end hosts for non-human *Sarcocystis* spp. after the accidental ingestion of oocysts resulting in tissue cysts in muscle that are usually symptomless, but can cause myalgia, muscle weakness and transitory oedema.

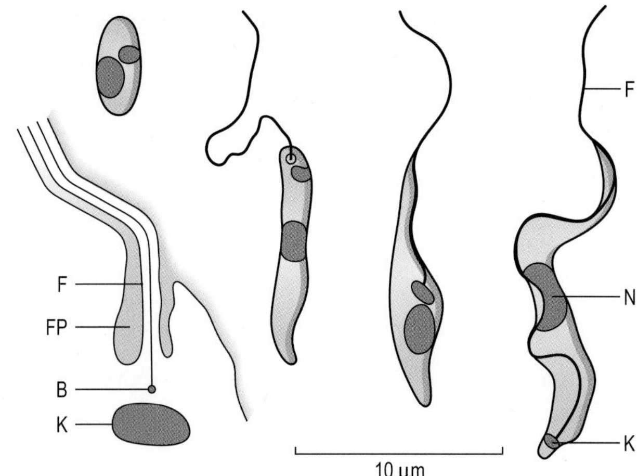

Figure A2.3 Morphological stages of Kinetoplastidae. (A) Trypomastigotes – elongate, motile and extracellular with flagellum originating near the posterior end of the cell which pulls out the surface membrane of the cell into a thin membrane-like structure called the undulating membrane. (B) Epimastigotes – flagellar origin is close to the nucleus near the centre of the elongated cell and extends forward to form an undulating membrane. (C) Promastigotes – flagellar origin is anterior to the nucleus with no undulating membrane, and (D) Amastigote – non-motile, intracellular, more or less spherical cell with a very short, rudimentary flagellum. B, basal body; F, flagellum; FP, flagellar pocket; K, kinetoplast; N, nucleus.

KINETOPLASTID PARASITES

Trypanosoma and *Leishmania*, motile kinetoplastid protozoans, contain kinetoplastid DNA in a single large mitochondrion close to the base of a flagellum, undergo morphological changes during their life cycle and are transmitted by insect vectors. The morphological stages that may develop during the life cycle are differentiated based on the presence or absence of a flagellum and the location of the kinetoplast in relation the nucleus (Figure A2.3). Although highly similar at the genomic level, these parasites cause distinct human diseases.

Trypanosomes

Two species of trypanosomes are associated with disease in humans and include *Trypanosoma brucei,* which causes human African trypanosomiasis (HAT) or sleeping sickness and *Trypanosoma cruzi* which causes American trypanosomiasis or Chagas disease (Table A2.3).

Trypanosoma brucei

Trypanosoma brucei is transmitted by the tsetse fly (*Glossina* spp.) and three subspecies are described: *Trypanosoma brucei gambiense* (*T. b gambiense*), *Trypanosoma brucei rhodesiense* (*T. b rhodesiense*) and *Trypanosoma brucei brucei* (*T. b. brucei*), among which only the first two affect humans while *T. b. brucei* affects cattle. *T. b. brucei* are susceptible to trypanolytic activity of apolipoprotein L-I (APOL1) in human sera, while *T. b*

TABLE A2.3 Comparison of African and American Trypanosomiasis

	Trypanosoma brucei (HAT)		*Trypanosoma cruzi* (Chagas Disease)
Species	*T. b. gambiense*	*T. b. rhodesiense*	*T. cruzi*
Stages in human host	Trypomastigotes	Trypomastigotes and amastigotes	
Geographic distribution	Western and Central Africa	Eastern and Southern Africa	South and Central America
Habitat	Forested rivers and shores	Savannah	Usually peridomestic in roofs and palm trees
Vector	*Glossina palpalis* group	*Glossina morsitans* group	*Triatoma infestans* (sub Amazonian regions) *Rhodnius prolixus* and *Triatoma dimidiate* (northern south America and Central America)
Transmission	Salivarial – infected fly bite, congenital transmission and blood transfusion		Stercorarial – defaecation of infected bug, congenital transmission, blood transfusion and organ transplant and rarely ingestion
Reservoir	Mostly human	Cattle, wild ungulates	Domestic and wild animals including dogs, cats, rodents, marsupials and armadillos
Disease	Chronic, anthroponotic, endemic	Acute, zoonotic, epidemic	Acute self limiting illness followed by chronic disease in 15–30%
Host cells/tissue	Blood, CSF, cervical lymph nodes		Blood, muscle, ganglion cells, adipose tissue
Site of infection	Chancre – more often in *T. b. rhodesiense*		Chagoma, Romana's sign (swollen eyelid)
Stages of disease	Haemolymphatic stage – acute febrile illness with lymphadenopathy, Winterbottom's sign (cervical lymph node) Meningoencephalitic stage – sleep disorders (sleeping sickness), neurological symptoms with progressive dementia		Acute stage – self-limiting febrile illness or asymptomatic Poor demarcation between stages Chronic stage Cardiac – arrhythmias, cardiac failure, thromboembolism, sudden death Digestive – megaoesophagus and megacolon
Progression of disease	Several months to years	Progression within weeks to months	2–3 decades

rhodesiense (mediated by the serum resistance associated gene, SRA) and *T. b gambiense* are resistant. This parasite is restricted to ~300 micro-foci in sub-Saharan Africa with suitable habitats for the vector along with contact with susceptible hosts. Despite near elimination of HAT in the 1960s, resurgence in the disease occurred in the 1990s due to dismantling of surveillance and control efforts.

The *T. brucei* subspecies are morphologically similar and in the vertebrate host (humans and other mammals) only extracellular trypomastigotes are seen in the blood, CSF and other body fluids. Trypomastigotes range in length from 14 to 33 μm, appear long and slender with a considerable length of free anterior flagellum and an undulating membrane. Non-replicating trypomastigotes present in the peripheral blood are ingested by the male or female tsetse fly during a blood meal and over a course of 4 weeks undergo morphological and physiological changes as epimastigotes in the alimentary tract and salivary gland of the fly to become infective metacyclic trypomastigotes. Only ~0.1% flies sustain a mature salivary gland infection. All three *T. brucei* subspecies have numerous (~1000) variant surface glycoprotein (VSG) genes with periodic recombination and switching of expression sites allows antigenic variation and immune escape of the parasite with resultant waves of parasitemia, polyclonal B cell activation and elevated IgM (both trypanosome specific and nonspecific) levels in the mammalian host. The disease has two distinct stages. The first stage is the haemolymphatic stage with a chancre at the site of the bite, followed by spread of trypanosomes throughout the blood and lymph systems. In the second stage, the meningoencephalitic stage, the parasites penetrate the CNS and multiply in the capillaries, tissue fluid and CSF, leading to severe neurological and sleep disorders and death if untreated.

Diagnosis. Diagnosis of HAT is based on screening, parasitological confirmation and staging of disease. Screening for *T. b. gambiense* in the field is carried out with the Card Agglutination Test for Trypanosomes (CATT), based on the major VSG antigen. Screening for *T. b. rhodesiense* is based on nonspecific clinical symptoms (fever, cervical lymph node) and a history of exposure to tsetse fly bites. More recently, PCR oligochromatography dipstick tests based on the SRA protein have been developed for *T. b. rhodesiense*. Confirmation of infection prior to initiating treatment is necessary due to low positive predictive value of CATT test and high drug toxicity and is by microscopic examination of chancre smear, lymph node fluid, blood or CSF. Due to the low density of parasites in *T. b. gambiense* infections, concentration techniques are recommended for blood and CSF samples. These include the microhaematocrit centrifugation technique and the micro-anion exchange centrifugation technique, which have been adapted for the field. Motile trypanosomes can be seen in fresh or stained preparations of blood, lymph or CSF. Staging by CSF examination in patients with HAT is essential as treatment of first and second stage disease is significantly different. Second stage HAT is defined by the presence of trypanosomes and/or >5 WBC/μL of CSF along with high CSF IgM levels. Foamy plasma cells or Mott's morular cells may also be seen in CSF.

Trypanosoma cruzi

T. cruzi is transmitted by the reduviid bug and is found mostly in South and Central America. Chagas disease is associated with poor-quality housing and bug infestation. Successful vector control programmes have led to a decline in transmission in recent years. Six phylogenetic lineages of *T. cruzi* have been reported based on multi-locus typing. Types I and II are the most common and associated with different geographical distribution, transmission cycles and varying disease symptoms. Another species, *T. rangeli* also occurs in South America, is considered non-pathogenic but may be incorrectly diagnosed as *T. cruzi*, either in human or insect hosts.

In the mammalian host, non-replicative trypomastigotes in the bloodstream (see Figure A2.5) and replicative intracellular amastigotes in macrophages and tissues are seen (see Figure A2.5). *T. cruzi* trypomastigotes in peripheral blood films often adopt a curved C shape and are about 20 μm long with a sharply pointed posterior end with an intensely staining kinetoplast and an anterior extension of the flagellum beyond the end of the cell (undulating membrane). Trypomastigotes ingested by a feeding reduviid bug develop into epimastigotes in the midgut, undergo division and migrate to the hindgut where they transform into small metacyclic trypomastigotes. Infective trypomastigotes are released onto the skin of the mammalian host in faeces of the bug and enter through the wound made by the bug's proboscis while feeding or through permissive mucosal surfaces or the conjunctiva. Early in the infection, *T. cruzi* trypomastigotes differentiate into replicative amastigotes within macrophages before differentiating back to bloodstream-form trypomastigotes that leave one cell type and invade others. The trypomastigotes invade adjacent tissues and spread via blood and lymphatics to other tissues, affecting mainly muscle and ganglion cells in the heart and gut, smooth muscle and adipose tissue.

Clinical manifestations begin with inflammation at the site of infection, leading to an oedematous swelling known as a 'chagoma'. The acute phase of infection lasts for 4–8 weeks and can be asymptomatic or self-limiting, though rarely, fatal febrile illness, usually in young children, can occur. The chronic phase of illness occurs decades later due to persistence of parasites in tissues. In the indeterminate form, patients have antibodies to *T. cruzi* (≥2 *T. cruzi* specific serological tests are positive) but are asymptomatic. The determinate form occurs in 15–30% of cases 10–25 years after initial infection resulting in cardiac and/or digestive symptoms. Cardiac symptoms arise due to destruction of myocardial cells, fibrosis and scarring of the conduction system. Gastrointestinal disease occurs due to destruction of intramural autonomic ganglia in the oesophagus and colon.

Diagnosis. Direct detection of parasites in the acute phase of disease can be carried out by examination of blood films, both fresh preparations and stained slides. Examination of concentrated cord blood and peripheral blood by the microhematocrit centrifugation technique is recommended in suspected congenital infections. Parasite culture, xenodiagnosis with uninfected reduviid bugs, and PCR have also been used. In the chronic phase, in addition to symptomatic diagnosis, serological tests including indirect haemagglutination, indirect immunofluorescence, and ELISA techniques are available.

Leishmania spp.

Leishmania are obligate intramacrophage kinetoplastids with more than 20 species belonging to two sub-genera *Leishmania* and *Viannia* differentiated based on location in the sandfly gut, which are associated with a wide clinical spectrum of disease (Table A2.4). They are transmitted by the bites of sandfly vectors belonging to two genera: *Phlebotomus* spp. of the 'Old World' and *Lutzomyia* spp. of the 'New World'. During its life cycle, procyclic promastigotes (15–20 μm, elongate, flagellate forms) differentiate in sandflies into infective, non-dividing metacyclic promastigotes, which are located in the foregut. During blood feeding by female flies, the sandfly regurgitates metacyclic promastigotes which are phagocytosed by dendritic cells, monocytes or macrophages and early in infection, even by neutrophils in the dermis. Once phagocytosed, metacyclic promastigotes transform into flagellate amastigotes, which undergo replication within the phagolysosome of the host cells that rupture when too many amastigotes are present (Figure A2.4) allowing re-infection of local phagocytes. The transmission cycle is complete when infected phagocytes are taken up by another sandfly with the blood meal.

Leishmania spp. display preferential tissue tropisms, including viscerotropism, dermotropism and mucocutaneous tropism (Table A2.4). Cutaneous leishmaniases (CL) are relatively benign with chronic, slow-to-heal ulcers and may develop into serious clinical disease such as diffuse (DCL) or mucocutaneous leishmaniasis (MCL). Visceral leishmaniasis (VL), also known as kala-azar, is the most severe form and is nearly always fatal if left untreated. VL is characterized by undulating fever, loss of weight, splenomegaly, hepatomegaly and/or lymphadenopathies and anaemia. In India, 5–15% of patients develop a chronic cutaneous form called post-kala-azar dermal leishmaniasis (PKDL) within 2 years of complete cure. In HIV co-infection, in addition to recurrence and increased susceptibility

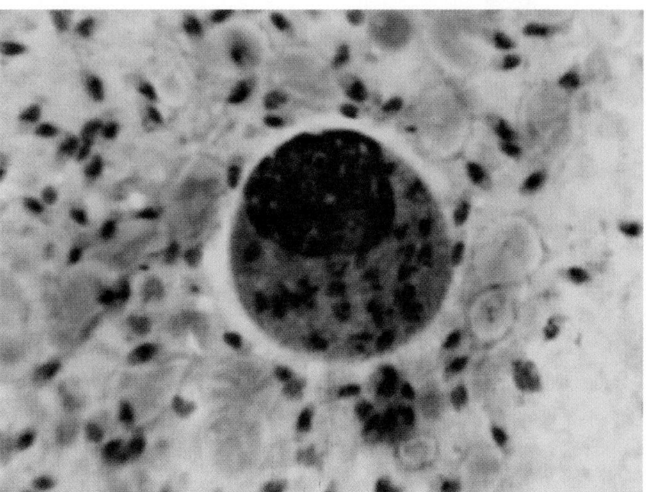

Figure A2.4 *Leishmania donovani* amastigotes in spleen (Giemsa stain): ovoid, 2.5–5 μm diameter, intracellular amastigotes with no flagellum, prominent kinetoplast and nuclei seen.

TABLE A2.4 *Leishmania* spp. Associated with Human Disease

	Clinical Disease	Specific Lesions	Vectors	Transmission	Reservoir	Geographic Distribution	HIV
OLD WORLD LEISHMANIASIS							
L. (Leishmania) donovani	VL, CL, PKDL	Kala-azar	*P. argentipes, P. orientalis, P. martini*	Anthroponotic in India	Dogs and rodents in Africa, Humans with PKDL	South and central Asia and Africa	MCL Gastrointestinal symptoms
L. (Leishmania) infantum/Chagasi	VL, CL, PKDL		*P. (Larroussius) ariasi/ Lutzomyia (Lutzomyia) longipalpis*	Zoonotic (peridomestic)	Dogs	Europe, north Africa (*L. chagasi* in South America)	MCL
L. (Leishmania) tropica	LCL	Oriental sore	*P. (Paraphlebotomus) sergenti, P. papatasi* and *P. chaudaudi*	Anthroponotic	Dogs	South and central Asia, north Africa, Middle East, Mediterranean	
L. (Leishmania) major	LCL	Oriental sore	*P. papatasi, P. duboscqi* and *P. salehi*	Zoonotic	Rodent, gerbil	Central Asia, north and east Africa	MCL
L. (Leishmania) aethiopica	LCL, DCL		*P. longipes, P. pedifer*	Zoonotic	Rock hyraxes	Ethiopia, Kenya	
L. (Leishmania) killicki	LCL		*? P. sergenti*	Zoonotic		North Africa	
NEW WORLD LEISHMANIASIS							
L . (Leishmania) amazonensis	LCL, DCL	Recidivans	*L. flaviscutellata*	Zoonotic	Rodents, marsupials, foxes	South and Central America, Mexico	MCL, VL
L. (Leishmania) mexicana	LCL, DCL	Chiclero ulcer	*L. olmeca, L. anthophora*	Zoonotic	Forest rodents	Central America, Mexico, United States	VL
L. (Leishmania) pifanoi	DCL, LCL			Zoonotic		South America	
L. (Leishmania) venezuelensis	LCL		*L. olmeca*	Zoonotic	Not known	Northern South America	
L. (Leishmania) garnhami	LCL		*L. youngii*	Zoonotic	Marsupials	South America	
L. (Viannia) braziliensis	LCL, MCL	Espundia/ tapir nose (naso-pharynx and palate)	*L. (Psychodopygus) carrerai, L. wellcomei, L. intermedius, L. pessoai*	Zoonotic	Rodents, sloths, porcupines, ant-eaters	South and Central America, Mexico	VL
L. (Viannia) panamanensis	LCL, MCL		*L. trapidoi, L. ylephiletor, L. gomezi*	Zoonotic	Sloths	South and Central America	
L. (Viannia) peruviana	LCL	Uta (dry sore)	*L. peruensis, L. verrucarum*	Zoonotic	Dogs	Peru, high altitudes	
L. (Viannia) guyanensis	LCL	Pian-bois, recidivans	*L. umbratilis*	Zoonotic	Sloth, ant-eater, rodents, opossums	South America	MCL
L. (Viannia) lainsoni	LCL		*L. ubiquitalis*	Zoonotic	Rodents	South America	
L. (Viannia) columbiensis	LCL		*L. hartmanii, L. gomezi, Psychodopygus panamensis*	? Zoonotic		Northern South America	
L. (Viannia) shawi	LCL		*L. whitmani*	Zoonotic	Monkey, sloth, coatimundi	South America	
L. (Viannia) naifii	LCL		*Psychodopygus ayrozai*	Zoonotic	9-banded armadillo	South America	

LCL, localized cutaneous leishmaniasis; DCL, diffuse cutaneous leishmaniasis; MCL, mucocutaneous leishmaniasis; PKDL, post-kala-azar leishmaniasis; VL, visceral leishmaniasis.

(geographic opportunistic infection), unusual forms of leishmaniasis have been reported. (Table A2.4).

Diagnosis. Confirmatory diagnosis is based on parasite detection by microscopic examination of Giemsa-stained smears, culture of biopsy material on diphasic culture media with a 4-week follow-up, where parasites grow as promastigotes, or PCR on blood or biopsy material. In VL, appropriate specimens are splenic puncture or lower risk bone marrow biopsy, and in CL or MCL, material obtained by puncture of the margin of a suspect lesion with a hypodermic needle attached to a syringe containing a small amount of physiological saline. More recent tests for VL are a latex agglutination test for detection of antigen in urine, serological tests including the rK39 immunochromatographic dipstick test, which is recommended for point-of-care testing in south Asia, and the direct agglutination test (DAT) and IFNγ assays for T-cell responses (Quantiferon).

FREE-LIVING AMOEBAE

Among the several free-living (amphizoic) amoebae, three genera have been associated with human disease and include *Acanthamoeba* spp (Figure A2.5), *Balamuthia mandrillaris* and *Naegleria fowleri* (Table A2.5). Although encephalitis caused by these amoebae is rare, disease is severe and usually fatal. Recently, another genus, *Sappinia diploidea* has been linked with encephalitis in a single case.

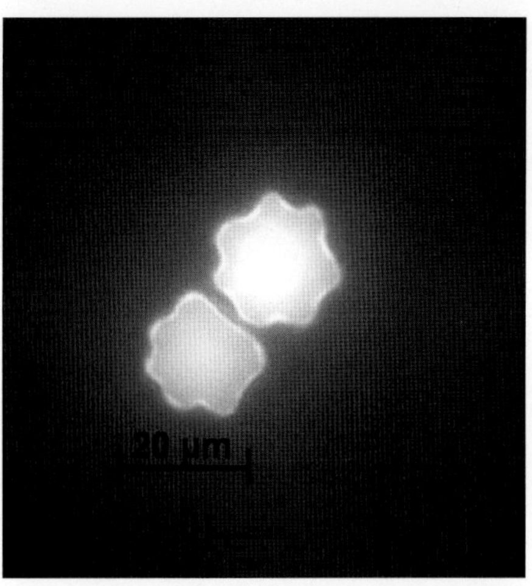

Figure A2.5 *Acanthamoeba* cyst in culture (Calcofluor stain under UV).

INTESTINAL PROTOZOA (TABLE A2.6)

Entamoeba histolytica

E. histolytica primarily inhabits the colon but can also disseminate via the bloodstream to extra-intestinal sites. Luminal infection is usually asymptomatic or associated with mild diarrhoea and abdominal pain. Invasive disease results in amoebic dysentery or colitis and extra-intestinal infection

TABLE A2.5 Comparison of Free-Living Amoebae Associated with Disease in Humans

	Naegleria spp.	*Acanthamoeba* spp.	*Balamuthia* spp.
Species associated with disease	*Naegleria fowleri*	*A. castellanii, A. culbertsoni, A. polyphaga, A. astronyxis, A. healyi*	*Balamuthia mandrillaris*
Taxonomic classification	*Excavata; Heterolobosia; Vahlkampfiidae*	*Amoebozoa: Acanthamoebidae*	*Amoebozoa: Acanthamoebidae*
Stages			
Trophozoite	Rapidly moving with lobopodia, 10–25 µm, uninucleate with centrally placed nucleolus	Fine tapering thorn like acanthopodia, 15–50 µm, uninucleate with granular cytoplasm	Pleiomorphic, 12–60 µm, usually uninucleate
Flagellate	Temporary, pear shaped, 2 flagella, 10–16 µm – seen in water	–	–
Cyst	Spherical, single walled, 7–15 µm – not seen in human tissue	Double walled, 10–25 µm, uninucleate with wrinkled outer ectocyst wall. Inner endocyst may be polygonal, stellate, spherical or oval	Spherical, 12–30 µm, appear double walled in light microscopy with wavy outer wall
Stages in human tissue	Trophozoite	Trophozoite and cyst	Trophozoite and cyst
Habitat	Fresh water	Ubiquitous, soil, water	Soil
Route of entry	Enter through olfactory epithelium while swimming	Enter through abrasions; possible hematogenous spread	Enter through abrasions
Risk	Children and young adults	Immunocompromised individuals, corneal trauma or contact lens (for keratitis)	Immunocompromised and immunocompetent children and elderly
CNS disease	Primary amoebic meningoencephalitis- acute, fulminant	Granulomatous amoebic encephalitis – chronic, insidious; cutaneous, sinus and lung infections also reported	
Ocular	–	Keratitis with non-healing corneal ulcers	–
Diagnosis	Wet mount examination of CSF for motile trophozoites, stained smears	Imaging (CT and MRI scan), microscopic examination of brain biopsy or corneal scrapings for trophozoites or cysts, IFA and culture on non-nutrient agar with bacterial lawn; Confocal microscopy for amoebic keratitis	Imaging (CT and MRI scan), microscopic examination of brain biopsy, IFA and culture on mammalian cell lines

TABLE A2.6 **Intestinal Protozoa**

Species	Developmental Stages	Transmission	Clinical Features	Diagnosis
E. histolytica	Cyst Trophozoite	Faecal–oral Water-borne Food-borne Anthroponotic	Asymptomatic (cyst carrier), Diarrhoea, abdominal pain dysentery Extraintestinal liver abscess, rarely lung or brain abscess	Stool microscopy for cysts or trophozoites
G. lamblia	Cyst Trophozoite	Faecal–oral Water-borne Food-borne Anthroponotic	Asymptomatic Diarrhoea, nausea, flatulence Malaise, weight loss May become chronic and associated with malabsorption	Stool microscopy for cysts or trophozoites Duodenal aspirate for trophozoites ELISA IFA
D. fragilis	Trophozoite	Unclear	Asymptomatic	Stool microscopy for trophozoites
C. hominis *C. parvum*	Oocyst Sporozoite Trophozoite Merozoite Gametocyte	Faecal–oral Water-borne Food-borne Anthroponotic Zoonotic	Immunocompetent: Asymptomatic Self-limiting watery diarrhoea Immunocompromised: Severe chronic diarrhoea and wasting	Microscopy of modified acid fast stained stools for oocysts ELISA IFA PCR
C. cayetanensis	Oocyst Sporozoite Trophozoite Merozoite Gametocyte	Faecal–oral Water-borne Food-borne	Immunocompetent: Asymptomatic Self-limiting diarrhoea Immunocompromised: Severe diarrhoea and wasting	Microscopy of modified acid fast stained stools for unsporulated oocysts
I. belli	Oocyst Sporozoite Trophozoite Merozoite Gametocyte	Faecal–oral Water-borne Food-borne	Immunocompetent: Asymptomatic Self-limiting diarrhoea Immunocompromised: Severe diarrhoea and wasting	Microscopy of modified acid fast stained stools for unsporulated oocysts
B. coli	Cyst Trophozoite	Faecal–oral Water-borne Food-borne Anthroponotic ? Zoonotic	Asymptomatic Mild gastrointestinal symptoms Dysentery	Stool microscopy for cysts or trophozoites
B. hominis	Pleomorphic, polymorphic forms	? Faecal–oral	Asymptomatic ? Mild gastrointestinal symptoms ? pathogen ? commensal	Stool microscopy

leads to liver (and rarely lung or brain) abscesses. *E. histolytica* is transmitted via the faecal–oral route through ingestion of contaminated water or food or by direct person-to-person contact.

The cyst is the environmentally resistant, infective stage, which is round to oval in shape, contains up to four nuclei and is characterized by the presence of 'chromatoid' bodies, which are aggregated ribosomes, and a refractile cyst wall. Following ingestion, cysts excyst in the lower small intestine to release trophozoites which are amorphous or 'ameboid' in shape, and move by extruding pseudopodia, exhibiting 'amoeboid' movement. Trophozoites reproduce by binary fission and may invade the colonic mucosa or differentiate into cysts, which are passed via the faeces into the environment where they can survive in moist, warm conditions and are immediately infectious when ingested by a new host.

Diagnosis. Diagnosis is made by microscopic demonstration of cysts or trophozoites (Figure A2.6) in faecal samples. Cysts are generally found in formed stools, whereas trophozoites are identified in freshly passed diarrhoeal or dysenteric stools and

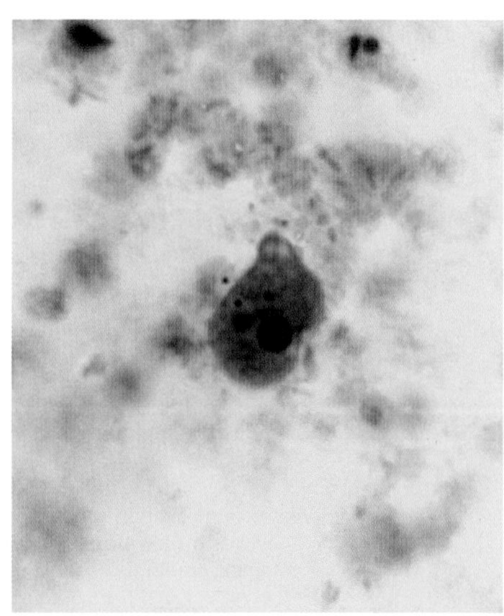

Figure A2.6 *Entamoeba histolytica* trophozoite stage in human faecal smear (Trichrome stain).

may contain ingested erythrocytes, demonstrating 'erythrophagocytosis'. PCR-based tests, though not widely used clinically, are more sensitive and can distinguish the morphologically similar but non-pathogenic *E. dispar* from *E. histolytica*. Serological tests do not distinguish current from previous infections but may be useful in the diagnosis of liver abscesses. Other tests for liver abscesses include imaging techniques and abscess aspiration.

Giardia lamblia

Giardia lamblia (also called *G. intestinalis* or *G. duodenalis*) colonizes the upper small intestine, where it adheres to epithelial cells or intestinal mucus. It is one of the commonest intestinal protozoans infecting humans and is prevalent worldwide. Infection is generally asymptomatic but may result in acute or chronic diarrhoea and possibly malabsorption. Transmission occurs most commonly via the faecal–oral route. Zoonotic transmission has also been suggested but not confirmed experimentally. Recent molecular studies have identified several genetic groups or 'assemblages', two of which, A and B, infect humans.

The infectious cyst stage is oval in shape, quadrinucleate and characterized by 'axonemes', 'median bodies' and a well-defined cyst wall. Infection is initiated by ingestion of cysts in contaminated water or food. Exposure to gastric acid in the stomach stimulates excystation which leads to release of trophozoites, the motile replicative stage. Trophozoites have a characteristic pear or teardrop-shaped appearance with two nuclei, 'axonemes' (which are the proximal regions of the flagella) 'median bodies' and four pairs of flagella, which aid in motility (Figure A2.7). The ventral surface of the trophozoite contains an adhesive or suction disk, which is believed to aid in adhesion to host cells. Median bodies are thought to be involved in formation of the disk. Trophozoites adhere to intestinal epithelial cells but do not invade them and replicate by binary fission. Upon exposure to bile in the small intestine, trophozoites differentiate into cysts, which are then excreted via the faeces into the external environment.

Diagnosis. Diagnosis is made by detection of cysts or trophozoites upon microscopic examination of stool samples. Since excretion of cysts is variable from day to day, examination of more than one sample on different days is recommended. Trophozoites may also be seen in duodenal aspirates or in duodenal biopsies. ELISA or IFA are also currently used for detection of antigen in stool samples.

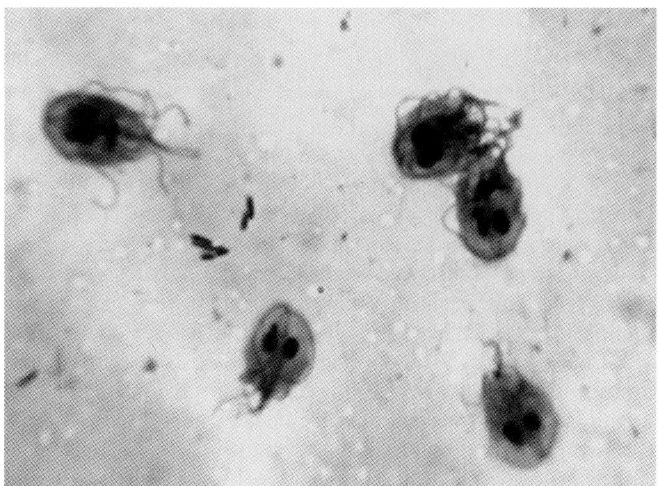

Figure A2.7 *Giardia duodenalis* trophozoites in human faecal smear (Fields' stain).

Cryptosporidium spp.

Cryptosporidium spp. are Apicomplexan parasites which colonize the small intestine. Several species with differing host specificities have been identified but those most commonly found in humans include *C. parvum* which infects humans as well as animals, and *C. hominis* which almost exclusively infects humans. In immunocompetent hosts, infection is generally asymptomatic or associated with self-limiting diarrhoeal symptoms. However, in immunocompromised hosts such as AIDS patients, infection can result in severe, chronic diarrhoea and wasting which can ultimately be fatal. Another vulnerable group in resource-limited areas are malnourished children in whom cryptosporidiosis is associated with delayed growth and cognitive development. Transmission is faecal–oral via ingestion of contaminated water or food, or by direct person to person contact. Zoonotic transmission from infected farm animals or pets can occur with *C. parvum*. *Cryptosporidium* spp. have been responsible for several outbreaks of water-borne diarrhoeal disease worldwide.

The life cycle of *Cryptosporidium* involves asexual as well as sexual cycles, which occur within a single host. The infectious oocyst stage is round, 4–6 μm and surrounded by a thick cyst wall. Infection is initiated by ingestion of sporulated oocysts which excyst in the small intestine to release sporozoites, the invasive stage of the parasite. Sporozoites attach to and invade the microvillus brush border of intestinal epithelial cells where they develop into trophozoites within a parasitophorous vacuole in a unique intracellular but extracytoplasmic niche. Trophozoites undergo asexual replication to form Type I merozoites which can re-infect adjacent cells or undergo additional rounds of merogony to form Type II merozoites which initiate sexual replication (gametogony). The resultant gametocytes form gametes, which fuse to form zygotes that differentiate into oocysts which then undergo sporulation. Oocysts are released into the intestinal lumen where they can excyst and initiate an auto-infection cycle or be excreted via the faeces into the environment.

Diagnosis. Diagnosis is made by microscopic identification of oocysts in faecal samples stained by modified acid fast staining (Figure A2.8). Intracellular stages can also be identified in H&E-stained intestinal biopsies. Currently, ELISA and IFAs are widely used for diagnosis. PCR-based assays are the most sensitive but are not yet widely used in clinical practice.

Isospora belli

Isospora belli is an opportunistic Apicomplexan parasite that inhabits the small intestine, is prevalent worldwide and is transmitted via the faecal–oral route. Humans are the only known hosts of *Isospora belli*. Infection in immunocompetent hosts is asymptomatic or associated with a self-limiting gastrointestinal illness, but in AIDS patients can cause severe diarrhoea and weight loss. Unlike *Cryptosporidium* oocysts which are small, round and undergo sporulation in the host, *Isospora belli* oocysts are larger, oval in shape and undergo sporogony

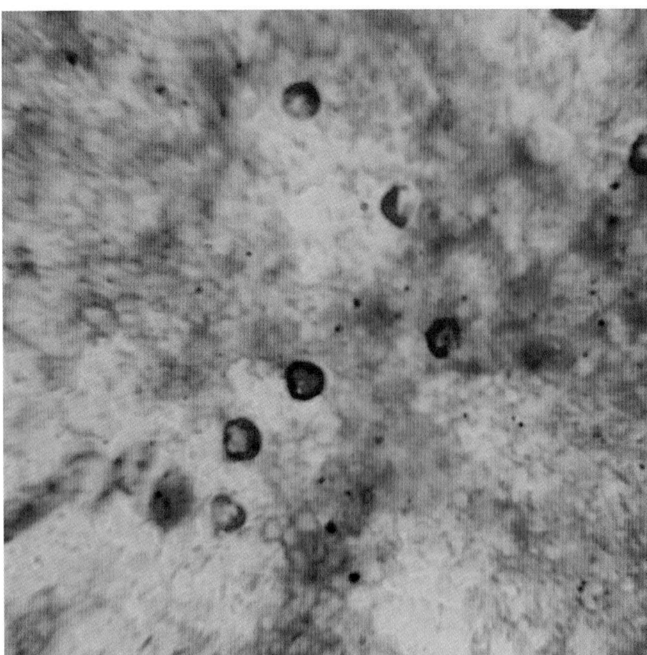

Figure A2.8 *Cryptosporidium* spp. oocysts in human faecal concentrate (Modified acid fast stain).

within 2–3 days in the soil. Ingestion of sporulated oocysts, which are the infectious stage, by a human host is followed by excystation to release sporozoites, which invade epithelial cells and undergo further intracellular development in a parasitophorous vacuole, which is situated within the cytoplasm of the host cell. *Isospora* replicates asexually via merogony and sexually via gametogony.

Diagnosis. Unsporulated *Isospora belli* oocysts are easily detected by microscopic examination of modified acid fast stained-stool samples (Figure A2.9).

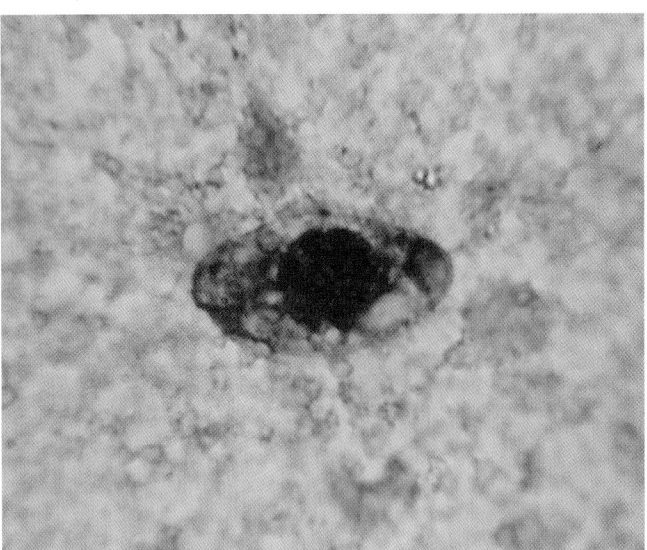

Figure A2.9 *Isospora belli* oocysts in human faecal concentrate (Modified acid fast stain).

Cyclospora cayetanensis

Cyclospora cayetanensis is an Apicomplexan parasite that inhabits the small intestine, is prevalent worldwide and is transmitted via the faecal–oral route. Humans are the only known host for *Cyclospora cayetanensis*. In the USA, outbreaks of cyclosporiasis have been associated with ingestion of contaminated fruit (particularly raspberries) and vegetables. Cyclosporiasis is asymptomatic or self-limiting in immunocompetent hosts but can result in prolonged or severe diarrhoeal illness in the immunocompromised.

The life cycle of *Cyclospora cayetanensis* is similar to that of *Isospora belli,* with infection being initiated by ingestion of sporulated oocysts. Replication occurs within the parasitophorous vacuole, which is located in the cytoplasm by asexual (merogony) and sexual (gametogony) cycles. Sporulation of oocysts (sporogony) occurs in the soil and takes 7–15 days, longer than that of *Isospora belli.*

Diagnosis. Diagnosis is made by microscopic identification of unsporulated oocysts in modified acid fast stained-stool samples. The oocysts (8–10 μm) are smaller than those of *Isospora belli* but larger than those of *Cryptosporidium* spp.

Balantidium coli

Balantidium coli is a ciliated protozoan, which inhabits the colon. It is prevalent worldwide, though more common in resource-poor tropical areas. In addition to humans, *B. coli* infects a variety of mammals, particularly swine. Transmission occurs by the faecal–oral route through ingestion of contaminated water or food or by person-to person contact but may also be zoonotic through contact with infected animals. Infection is usually asymptomatic or associated with mild gastrointestinal symptoms but invasive disease resulting in dysentery may occur.

Trophozoites are oval in shape and display the characteristic features of ciliates such as cilia, nuclear dimorphism (a large macronucleus and adjacent micronucleus), a cystosome and contractile vacuole. Cysts are smaller, rounder and surrounded by a cyst wall. *B. coli* replicates asexually via binary fission and sexually via conjugation.

Diagnosis. *B. coli* can easily be identified by its characteristic morphology in fecal samples in a wet preparation.

Microsporidia

Although included in this section, Microsporidia are not protozoa but are currently classified as fungi. This phylum contains over 1200 species which infect all animals, with over 15 species infecting humans. Four species predominantly infect humans: *Enterocytozoon bieneusi, Encephalitozoon cuniculi, Encephalitozoon intestinalis* and *Encephalitozoon hellum. Microsporidia* are single-celled intracellular organisms which are opportunistic pathogens associated with a wide range of clinical syndromes in humans. Microsporidial infections are mostly asymptomatic in immunocompetent hosts but can cause self-limiting disease in children or in travelers to endemic regions. In the immunocompromised, mainly in AIDS patients with low CD4 cell counts, Microsporidia like other opportunistic pathogens, can cause severe and chronic disease. *E. bieneusi* or *E. intestinalis* primarily infect the small intestine but can disseminate to the hepatobiliary tract (*E. bieneusi*) or widely to almost every organ system (*E. intestinalis*).

The infectious forms of Microsporidia are the spores which are small and surrounded by an outer glycoprotein layer and an inner chitinous layer. A structure unique to the Microsporidia is the coiled polar tube which facilitates infection of host cells by injecting its sporoplasm into the host cell cytoplasm. The sporoplasm undergoes replication by merogony or schizogony within a parasitophorous vacuole (*E. intestinalis*) or in direct contact with the host cytoplasm (*E. bieneusi*). Sporogony occurs within the host cell to form environmentally resistant spores which are released into the environment when the cell ruptures.

Diagnosis. Microsporidiosis[5] can be diagnosed microscopically in stool samples or fluids such as urine in cases of dissemination, with trichrome staining used alone or in combination with the Gram stain, and the Warthin–Starry silver stain or more accurately with fluorescent stains such as Calcofluor White or Uvitex 2B, which bind to the chitinous layer in the spore wall. PCR-based methods are more sensitive but are not yet widely used in clinical practice.

Trichomonas vaginalis

T. vaginalis is the only urogenital protozoan parasite in humans. It is sexually transmitted and inhabits the vagina and urethra. The trophozoites are oval, 14–17×5–15 μm and have a single nucleus, a prominent axostyle, four anterior flagella and a single lateral flagellum, which runs back along the surface of the cell and forms an undulating membrane. Multiplication is by binary fission and no cyst is formed. In women, vaginitis with purulent discharge accompanied by vulvar and cervical lesions, abdominal pain, dysuria and dyspareunia is seen, while men may be asymptomatic or have mild urethritis or prostatitis. *Trichomonas* pathology may also result in increased efficiency of HIV transmission and therefore requires prompt diagnosis and treatment of both partners.

Diagnosis. Clinical diagnosis may be confirmed by demonstration of the trophozoites in Giemsa-stained smears made from swabs of vaginal or urethral discharge or culture with the Tv InPouch diagnostic system. Point-of-care tests include the nonspecific pH and KOH amine tests and more recent dipstick and nucleic acid probe tests.

REFERENCES

1. Adl SM, Simpson AG, Farmer MA, et al. The new higher level classification of eukaryotes with emphasis on the taxonomy of protists. J Eukaryot Microbiol 2005;52(5):399–451.
2. Walker G, Dorrell RG, Schlacht A, et al. Eukaryotic systematics: a user's guide for cell biologists and parasitologists. Parasitology 2011; 138(13): 1638–63.
3. NCCLS. Clinical Use and Interpretation of Serologic Tests for *Toxoplasma gondii*; Approved Guideline. NCCLS document M36-A. Wayne: NCCLS; 2004.
4. Wiser MW. Protozoa and Human Disease. London: Garland Science; 2010.
5. Didier ES, Weiss LM. Microsporidiosis: current status. Curr Opin Infect Dis 2006;19:485–92.

APPENDIX 3

Medical Helminthology

MALCOLM K. JONES | JAMES S. McCARTHY | VAUGHAN R. SOUTHGATE | RODNEY A. BRAY

Introduction

Helminths contribute substantially to human morbidity. Some hundreds of helminth species have been recorded as parasites of humans. This section of the book provides inclusive lists of the parasites that are known to occur, or have been recorded historically, in humans. Detailed information on the most significant helminths parasites of humans are found in the chapters in Section 10 of this volume. In this appendix, we provide a brief record in tabular form of the broad range of helminths parasites infesting humans, their primary recognition features and their life cycles. Eggs or early larval stages of these parasites in faeces, other excreta or some tissues are the stages most frequently observed in a diagnostic setting. The stage of development of these transmissive stages and sites where they are encountered in the human host are listed in the tables.

For the first time, this appendix covering medical helminthology will be presented in two forms – as a brief synopsis for inclusion in the printed book, and a longer detailed treatise of species and their biology that will be published online. In this printed version, the primary characteristics of the major taxonomic groups of helminths will be presented, along with species lists, sites of infestation in the human host, and sites of passage from the host. We will not list the specific intermediate hosts or vectors of these helminths, but will indicate the higher level taxa to which the intermediate hosts belong. Geographical distribution for each parasite is presented broadly as continent or major geographical region. It is recognized that the distribution of individual species of parasites within their geographic range can be quite focal. The general distribution data presented in the Tables below will, as with other detailed information on helminth species, be provided in the more extensive online version of this appendix (see: http://www.expertconsult.com).

Phylum Platyhelminthes

This phylum contains the 'flat worms', a group of soft-bodied worms that inhabit a range of environments, both free-living and parasitic. Three of the four classes of platyhelminths are strictly parasitic. Of these, two, the Class Trematoda and Class Cestoda contain species that infect humans. Platyhelminths are acoelomate worms and have a generally simple body plan. The species are usually fecund and much of their bodies in adults are given over to organs involved in egg synthesis. Platyhelminthes are almost invariably hermaphroditic and are quite often protandrous.

Major taxa of the Phylum are recognized primarily by their mode of attachment to the host. The flukes (Class *Trematoda*, Subclass *Digenea*) are flatworms that possess in most species two attachment suckers, termed the oral and ventral suckers. The tapeworms (Class *Cestoda*) have an anterior holdfast, the scolex, that attaches to the intestinal musca. The scolex is equipped with suckers and accessory holdfast structures.

Class *Trematoda*

SUBCLASS *DIGENEA*.

The subclass Digenea of the Class Trematoda (see also Chapters 52 and 53) is a large and diverse clade of organisms, commonly referred to as the flukes or trematodes. Digeneans have complex multi-host life cycles involving at least two hosts. In the first intermediate host, the parasite follows a multigenerational form of reproduction involving usually two generations that reproduce by asexual proliferation. Almost exclusively, digeneans use gastropod molluscs as first intermediate host. The sexual adults are found in the vertebrate, definitive host. Sexual reproduction results in the generation of intra-ovular embryos that pass from the hosts in faeces, urine or sputum.

Some 6000 species of digeneans have been described. Some 80 species are known from humans, many of which are recorded here (Tables A3.1, A3.2). The majority of the anthropophilic digeneans are found in the intestine of humans. Some, among them the more pathogenic species, occur in body tissues of humans. Digeneans infect humans either by direct invasion (percutaneous penetration) or as cystic forms within food of humans (food-borne). The species of digeneans infesting humans are listed in Table A3.1. Diagrammatic representation of a representative adult trematode is shown in Figure A3.1. See Figure A3.3 for illustrations of eggs from faeces of some trematodes and other helminths. Characteristics of the different superfamilies of trematodes are taken from a recent series edited by David Gibson, Arlene Jones and Rodney Bray.[1–3]

SCHISTOSOMATIDS RESPONSIBLE FOR CERCARIAL DERMATITIS IN HUMANS

In addition to the parasites listed above, members of the family Schistosomatidae and related families can cause a condition in humans termed cercarial dermatitis or swimmer's itch. Humans are infected by these schistosomatids by exposure of skin to bodies of water containing cercariae, the infective larvae. Cercariae penetrate the skin of humans by percutaneous penetration. All species use a snail, predominantly of the Order *Pulmonata*, as first intermediate host.

A wide range of schistosomatid species has been implicated as agents of cercarial dermatitis.[4] List of such genera their geographic range, types of waterbodies in which the parasites are

TABLE A3.1 List of Digeneans Infecting Humans, Showing Their Broad Geographic Range, Site of Patent Infection in the Human Host, Mode of Human Infection, the Intermediate Hosts and Sites of Transmission of Eggs or Larvae from the Human Host

Species	Geographic Range	Site in Human	Mode of Human Infection	Intermediate Host	Site of Parasite Transmission
Superfamily Echinostomatoidea. This group contains some of the most well-known flukes of humans and domestic animals. Defining features of the family are based on the structure of the excretory system, features that will not be discussed here. Digeneans of the Echinostomatoidea are parasites in a wide range of hosts. Humans become infected by ingesting encysted metacercariae with food.					
Fasciola hepatica	AFR, EUR, NA, OCE, SA	Liver, Bile ducts	FB	1^0 Mollusca-Gast; 2^0 Plants	Eggs, F
F. gigantica	AFR, IND, SEA	Liver, Bile ducts	FB	1^0 Mollusca-Gast; 2^0 Plants	Eggs, F
Fasciolopsis buski	AS, IND	SI	FB	1^0 Mollusca-Gast	Eggs, F
Echinostoma lindoensis	SEA	SI	FB	1^0Mollusca-Gast; 2^0 Mollusca-Gast; Bivalvia	Eggs, F
Echinostoma revolutum	AS, SEA	SI	FB	1^0 Mollusca-Gast; 2^0 Mollusca-Gast; Bivalvia; FW fish	Eggs, F
Echinostoma hortense	AS	SI		1^0 Mollusca-Gast; 2^0 Amphibians; fish	Eggs, F
Echinostoma malayanum	SEA	SI	FB	1^0 Mollusca-Gast; 2^0 Mollusca-Gast; Bivalvia; FW fish	Eggs, F
Euparyphium ilocanum	SEA	SI	FB	1^0 Mollusca-Gast; 2^0 Mollusca-Gast; Bivalvia	Eggs, F
Euparyphium jassyense	EUR	SI	FB	1^0 Mollusca-Gast; 2^0 Amphibian; fish	Eggs, F
Other echinostomatoids: *Echinostoma cinetorchis* (AS), *E. macrorchis* (AS), *Echinochasmus perfoliatus* (AS), *E. japonicas* (AS), *E. jiufoensis* (AS), *Himasthla muehlensis* (SA), *Episthmium caninum* (SEA), *Euparyphium melis* (AS, EUR), *Hypoderaeum conoideum* (AS).					
Superfamily Opisthorchioidea. These are often lanceolate flukes. Cercariae of this group almost always penetrate fish as second intermediate host. The egg, which passes from the definitive host with faeces, must be ingested by the first intermediate host, a gastropod, for the life cycle to proceed.					
Clonorchis sinensis	AS, SEA	Liver, Bile ducts	FB	1^0 Mollusca-Gast; 2^0 Numerous species of fish	Eggs, F
Opisthorchis felineus	AS	Liver, Bile ducts	FB	1^0 Mollusca-Gast; 2^0 Numerous species of fish	Eggs, F
Opisthorchis viverrini	SEA	Liver, Bile ducts	FB	1^0 Mollusca-Gast; 2^0 Numerous species of fish	Eggs, F
Heterophyes heterophyes	AFR, AS, EUR, SEA	SI	FB	1^0 Mollusca-Gast; 2^0 Numerous species of brackish water fish	Eggs, F
Additional species infecting humans: *Heterophyes continua, Haplorchis pumilio, H. vanissimus* and *Procerovum calderon*					
Metagonimus yokogawai	AS, SEA	SI	FB	1^0 Mollusca-Gast; 2^0 Numerous species of freshwater fish	Eggs, F
Superfamily Gorgoderoidea. This is a morphologically diverse group of trematodes, with constituent members linked by molecular evidence. Two families, the Paragonimidae and Dicrocoeliidae have species that infect humans.					
Genus: *Paragonimus*					
Many species of *Paragonimus* occur and can be divided into four groups on the nature of the cuticular spines and the ovary					
1. Westermani: *P. westermani, P. pulmonalis*					
2. Compactus: *P. compactus, P. siamensis*					
3. Kellicotti-miyazaki: *P. kellicotti, P. miyazakii, P. heterotremus, P. caliensis, P. amazonicus, P. mexicanus* (*peruvianus*).					
4. Ohirai-ilokstuenensis: *P. ohirai, P. ilokstuenensis.*					
Other species include: *P. tuanshenensis, P. szechuanensis, P. hueitungensis, P. bangkokensis, P. philippinensis, P. sadoensis, P. skrjabini* and the African species *P. africanus* and *P. uterobilateralis.*					
Paragonimus	AFR, AS, IND, OCE, SA, SEA	Lungs, additional sites	FB	1^0 Mollusca-Gast; 2^0 Numerous species of decapod crustaceans	Eggs, SP, F
Dicrocoelium dendriticum	AS, EUR, IND, NA, SA, SEA	SI	FB	1^0 Mollusca-Gast; 2^0 Insecta-Formicidae	Eggs, F
Dicrocoelium hospes	AFR	SI	FB	1^0 Mollusca-Gast; 2^0 Insecta-Formicidae	Eggs, F
Superfamily Schistosomatoidea. This group contains the blood flukes. In humans, blood flukes are elongate worms, with separate sexes. The males carry females within a canal on their ventral surface. The male forms this gynaecophoric canal by wrapping the lateral margins of its body around the female. Eggs of schistosomes are distinctive, possessing a spine but lacking an operculum.					
Schistosoma haematobium	AFR, ME	Veins of systemic circulation	AP		Eggs, U (rarely F)
Schistosoma mansoni	AFR,ME, SA	Mesenteric veins	AP	1^0 Mollusca-Gast	Eggs, F (rarely U)
Schistosoma japonicum	AS, SEA	Mesenteric veins	AP	1^0 Mollusca-Gast	Eggs, F
Schistosoma intercalatum	AFR	Mesenteric veins	AP	1^0 Mollusca-Gast	Eggs, F
Schistosoma mekongi	SEA	Mesenteric veins	AP	1^0 Mollusca-Gast	Eggs, F

Continued on following page

TABLE A3.1 List of Digeneans Infecting Humans, Showing Their Broad Geographic Range, Site of Patent Infection in the Human Host, Mode of Human Infection, the Intermediate Hosts and Sites of Transmission of Eggs or Larvae from the Human Host—cont'd

Species	Geographic Range	Site in Human	Mode of Human Infection	Intermediate Host	Site of Parasite Transmission
Schistosoma guineensis	AFR	Mesenteric veins	AP	1^0 Mollusca-Gast	Eggs, F
Schistosoma mattheei	AFR	Mesenteric veins	AP	1^0 Mollusca-Gast	Eggs, F
Schistosoma bovis	AFR	Mesenteric veins	AP	1^0 Mollusca-Gast	Eggs, F
Schistosoma curassoni	AFR	Mesenteric veins	AP	1^0 Mollusca-Gast	Eggs, F
Schistosoma malayensis	SEA	Mesenteric veins	AP	1^0 Mollusca-Gast	Eggs, F
Superfamily Paramphistomoidea. This superfamily are characterized by the absence of an oral sucker and by positioning of a ventral sucker at the posterior extremity of the body. Infection of the definitive host is through ingestion of metacercariae on vegetation.					
Gastrodiscoides hominis	AFR, AS, IND, SEA	CAE, LI	FB	1^0 Mollusca-Gast; 2^0 Plants	Eggs, F
Watsonius watsoni	AFR	CAE, LI	FB	1^0 Mollusca-Gast; 2^0 Plants	Eggs, F
Superfamily: Brachylaimoidea. These parasites are mostly parasites of birds and mammals. The parasites have a very short oesophagus, or lack one altogether. The cercarial tail of brachylamoids is either absent or very short.					
Brachylaima cribbi	OCE (Australia)	SI	FB	1^0 Mollusca-Gast; 2^0 Mollusca-Gast	Eggs, F

Abbreviations – Geographic range: AFR, Africa; AS, Asia; EUR, Europe; IND, Indian subcontinent; ME, Middle East; NA, North America; OCE, Oceania including Australia; SA, South America; SEA, South-east Asia. Site in human: CAE, caecum; LI, large intestine; SI, small intestine. Mode of human infection: AP, active penetration by percutaneous penetration; FB, food-borne. Intermediate host: Gast, gastropod snail; 1^0, first intermediate host; 2^0, second intermediate host. Site of parasite transmission: F, faeces; SP, sputum; U, urine.

TABLE A3.2 Genera Containing Species Responsible for Cercarial Dermatitis (CD) in Humans, Their Distribution and Waterbodies in Which Cercariae Occur[4]

Genera	Geographic Range	Waterbodies	Class of Definitive Host
Austrobilharzia	C	BR, SW	B
Bivitellobilharzia?	AFR, IND	FW	M
Gigantobilharzia	C	BR, SW	B
Heterobilharzia?	NA	FW	M
Macrobilharzia	C	FW	B
Orientobilharzia	A	FW	M
Ornithobilharzia?	NH	BR, SW	B
Schistosoma	AFR, AS, IND, ME, SA, SEA	FW	M
Schistosomatium?	NA	FW	M
Bilharziella	AFR, EUR, IND, NA	FW	B
Trichobilharzia	C	FW	B
Jilinobilharzia?	AS	FW	B
Dendritobilharzia?	C	FW	B

Genera marked with a question mark contain species suspected, but not confirmed, as agents of CD.
Abbreviations – Geographic range: AFR, Africa; C, cosmopolitan; IND, Indian subcontinent; EUR, Europe; AS, Asia; SEA, South-east Asia; NA, North America; SA, South America. Waterbodies: BR, Brackish water; SW, saltwater; FW, freshwater. Class of definitive host: B, birds; M, Mammals.

usually found and class of normal definitive hosts, are shown in Table A3.2. It is noted that the vast majority of human infections do not reach patency (that is, production of parasite eggs by adult schistosomatids and their excretion from the host). These infections, which are typified by intense pruritic irritations on the skin of humans, represent the response of host to dead or dying cercariae of the parasites. While these parasites do not develop in humans, there is always potential that they may cause breakthrough infections, where the parasites develop to sexual maturity in the host. Species of *Schistosoma* that are

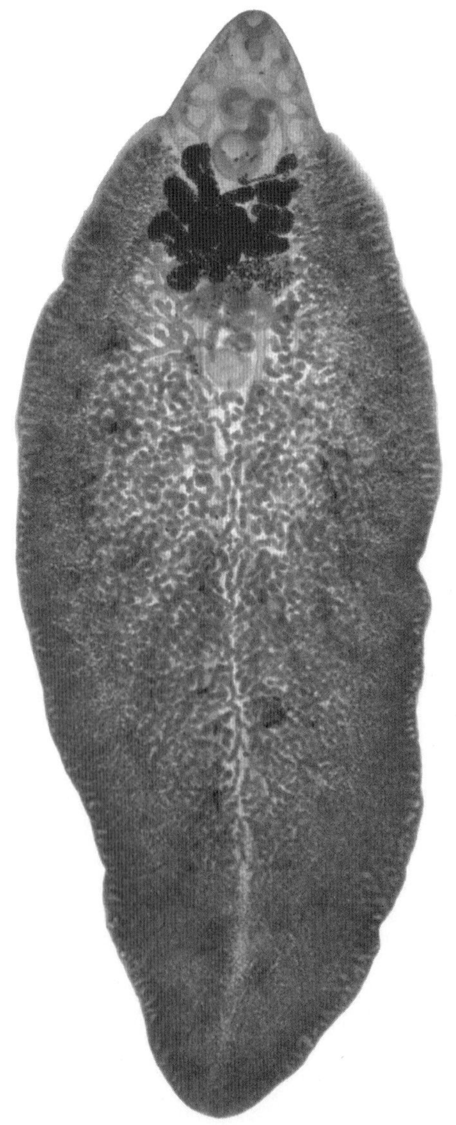

Figure A3.1 Representative digenean – *Fasciola hepatica*.

normally parasites of humans (Table A3.2) can also cause cercarial dermatitis.

Class *Cestoda*

The name cestode is derived from *kestos* (Greek meaning 'a girdle') (see also Chapters 56 and 57). The anterior attachment organ is known as the scolex, and the 'tape', also known as the 'strobila', is usually divided into serially-repeated reproductive units, the proglottids. The worms can live for several years and absorb nutriment through the body wall. Cestodes are hermaphroditic, with a single set of male and female gonads in each proglottis. Male organs often develop before the female. Cestodes infecting humans have been recorded from two orders.

1. Order Pseudophyllidea: with slit-like bothria, oval scolex (two long grooves with muscular walls); no hooks on scolex. Genital pores open in the mid-line of the proglottis (flat surface). A uterine pore may be present.
2. Order Cyclophyllidea: Two cup-like or round suckers on the scolex; accessory holdfast (rostellum) with hooks or adhesive glands present. Genital pore is marginal on proglottis (opens laterally). No uterine pore is present.

The cestodes parasiting humans are shown in Table A3.3. Representative illustrations of cestodes from the orders *Pseudophyllidea* and *Cyclophyllidea* are shown (Figure A3.2). See

TABLE A3.3 List of Cestodes Infecting Humans, Showing Their Broad Geographic Range, Site and Stage of Infection in Humans and Means of Human Infection

Species	Geographic Distribution	Stage and Site of Infection	Mode of Infection
Order: Pseudophyllidea. These tapeworms are characterized by an anterior holdfast in adults that consists of a pair of simple muscular slits or bothria. The life cycle traces through three hosts. The first intermediate host is a crustacean and the second usually occurs in fish. Pseudophyllideans are predominantly found as adults in fish, but some species are found in other hosts.			
Diphyllobothrium latum, Diphyllobothrium nihonkaiense, D. yonagoense, D. pacificum, D. dendriticum (minus), D. alascense	AFR, AS, EUR, SA	AD, SI	Ingestion of fish
Spirometra erinaceieuropaei (S. erinacei, S. mansonoides), S. theileri or S. pretoriensis in Africa	AS, EUR, NA, OC, SEA,	MC, subcutaneous, intramuscular, walls of the alimentary canal, mesentery, kidney, lung, heart and brain	Ingestion of second intermediate or paratenic hosts; direct tissue transfer.
Order Cyclophyllidea. The most abundant order of tapeworms, the Cyclophyllidea contains species that have a scolex with four cup-shaped suckers and reduced vitelline glands in the female reproductive system. The life cycle involves typically two hosts. The intermediate host is usually an invertebrate species, although in the family Taeniidae, the intermediate host is a mammal. Cyclophyllideans usually parasitize mammals or birds as definitive hosts.			
Family Taeniidae. Generally large tapeworms (except for *Echinococcus*). These worms have a scolex with four suckers and in most species a hooked rostellum. The metacestode of taeniids are always found in mammals. Hence, humans can serve as intermediate or definitive host for one taeniid.			
Taenia asiatica	AS	AD, SI MC?	AD, ingestion of pork
Taenia solium	AFR, AS, EUR, IND, SA, SEA	AD, SI MC, skeletal muscles, subcutaneous, CNS	AD, ingestion of pork MC, ingestion of eggs
Taenia saginata	AFR, AS, EUR, OC, SA	AD, SI	Ingestion of bovine meat
Rare infections in humans: *Taenia multiceps, T. serialis brauni* and *T. serialis serialis*			
Echinococcus granulosus	C (eliminated in some countries, island states)	MC, liver, many other sites	Ingestion of eggs
Echinococcus multilocularis	AS, EUR, NA	MC, liver	Ingestion of eggs
Family Hymenolepididae. This family has many species infecting a wide range of warm-blooded hosts. They are generally small worms with an armed or unarmed rostellum. Their metacestodes are found in arthropods, usually insects.			
Rodentolepis nana	AFR, AS, EUR, IND, SA, SEA	AD, SI MC in mucosa	AD, ingestion of insects; autoinfection
Hymenolepis diminuta	C	AD, SI	Ingestion of infected insects
Family Davaineidae. This family contains species found often in birds. The scolex is characterized by possessing rostellar hooks with a distinctive morphology.			
Raillietina asiatica *R. celebensis* *R. demerariensis*	AFR, EUR, IND	AD, SI	Ingestion of arthropods
Family Anoplocephalidae. The scolex of anoplocephalids has presence of 4 suckers and the absence of a rostellum or apical organ.			
Bertiella studeri, B. mucronata	SA	AD, SI	Ingestion of mites
Inermicapsifer madagascariensis (Im), I. cubensis (Ic)	AFR (*Im*) SA (*Ic*)	AD, SI	Ingestion of mites
Family Dilepididae. The scolex of dilepidids has four suckers and a rostellum that is saccate.			
Dipylidium caninum	C	AD, SI	Ingestion of insects (fleas)

Eggs will only be observed in human faeces if the human is infected with an adult parasite. For many cyclophyllidean parasites, gravid proglottids may be shed by the adult parasite and may emerge intact on the periphery of faeces.

Abbreviations – Geographic range: AFR, Africa; AS, Asia; EUR, Europe; IND, Indian subcontinent; ME, Middle East; NA, North America; OCE, Oceania including Australia; SA, South America; SEA, South-east Asia. Stage and site of infection: AD, adult; SI, small intestine; MC, metacestode (larval); CNS, central nervous system.

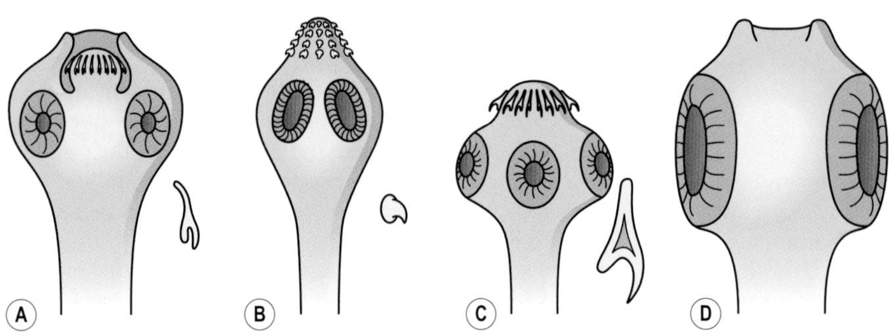

Figure A3.2 Representative *scoleces* of some human tapeworms showing suckers and when present, the arrangement of rostellar hooks. (A) *Hymenolepis nana.* (B) *Dipylidium caninum.* (C) *Taenia solium.* (D) *T. saginata.*

TABLE A3.4 List of Nematodes Parasitizing Humans, Showing Their Broad Geographic Range, Site of Patent Infection in the Human Host, the Mode of Human Infection Including, Where Relevant, the Intermediate Hosts and the Sites of Transmission of Eggs or Larvae from the Human Host

Species	Geographic Range	Site in Human	Mode of Human Infection	Site of Parasite Transmission
Superfamily Ascaridoidea. Ascaridoids are large nematodes that occur in the small intestine of their definitive hosts. The mouth of ascarids has 3 lips.				
Ascaris lumbricoides	C	SI	Ingestion of eggs	Eggs, F
Ascaris suum	C	SI	Ingestion of eggs	Eggs, F
Toxocara canis	C	Lungs, liver and other viscera, and eyes	Ingestion of eggs	?
Toxocara cati	C	Lungs, liver and other viscera, and eyes	Ingestion of eggs	?
Lagochilascaris minor	SA	Head and neck	Ingestion of mammals	–
Anisakis simplex	C	Larvae in intestine	Ingestion of infected fish	–
Other anisakids infecting humans: *A. pegreffii, A. simplex* s.s., *A. simplex* C, *A. typica, A. ziphidarum, Anisakis* sp., *A. physeteris, A. brevispiculata, A. paggiae, Pseudoterranova decipiens*				
Superfamily: Gnathostomatoidea				
Gnathostoma spinigerum	AS, SEA, EUR, NA	Subcutaneous tissues, viscera	Ingestion of vertebrate host	–
Physaloptera caucasica (Pc), P. transfuga (Pt)	AFR, ME, SA (*Pc*) EUR (*Pt*)	Anterior digestive tract	?Ingestion of insect	Eggs, F
Gongylonema pulchrum	NA, EUR, SEA, AS, OCE	Anterior digestive tract	Ingestion of insect	No eggs in human faeces
Superfamily Ancylostomatoidea. Commonly called the hookworms, members of this superfamily of strongylid nematodes have a large capsular buccal capsule possessing teeth or cutting plates. The buccal capsule is reflexed, giving the adult parasites a characteristic hook-like appearance.				
Ancylostoma duodenale, A. ceylanicum, A. caninum	AFR, SEA, AS, SA (*Ad*), IND, SEA (*Ace*), C (*Aca*)	Digestive tract. Larvae can arrest in tissue	Percutaneous penetration	Eggs, F
A. braziliense	SA, NA	Cutaneous agent of larva migrans	Percutaneous penetration	–
Necator americanus	SA, NA, AFR, IND, SEA, OCE	Digestive tract.		
Other rare human infections: A. malayanum, A. japonica, Necator suillus and *N. argentinus*				
Superfamily Strongyloidea. Strongyloids possess a buccal capsule that is not reflexed, as in hookworms, and bears anteriorly a ring of spines emerging from the border of the labial region, the corona radiate. Strongyloids usually occupy posterior regions in the gastrointestinal tract.				
Oesophagostomum apiostomum	AFR,	SI, CAE	Ingestion of larval parasites	Eggs, F
Oesophagostomum stephanostomum	AFR, SA	SI, CAE	Ingestion of larval parasites	Eggs, F
Ternidens diminutus	AFR	SI, CAE	Ingestion of larval parasites	Eggs, F
Superfamily Metastrongyloidae. These strongylids are commonly called lungworms, although not all species live in the lungs. The Metastrongyloidea includes parasites affecting a wide range of mammal hosts. Species infecting humans are vascular parasites.				
Angiostrongylus cantonensis (Parastrongylus cantonensis)	AS, IND, NA, OCE, SA, SEA,	CNS	Ingestion of molluscs, paratenic hosts	–
Angiostrongylus costaricensis (Parastrongylus costaricensis)	SA	Abdominal organs	Ingestion of molluscs, paratenic hosts	–?

TABLE A3.4 List of Nematodes Parasitizing Humans, Showing Their Broad Geographic Range, Site of Patent Infection in the Human Host, the Mode of Human Infection Including, Where Relevant, the Intermediate Hosts and the Sites of Transmission of Eggs or Larvae from the Human Host—cont'd

Species	Geographic Range	Site in Human	Mode of Human Infection	Site of Parasite Transmission
Superfamily Trichostrongylidae. Members of this superfamily of strongylids occur in anterior regions of the gastrointestinal tracts of a variety of animals. These parasites have a direct life cycle. The buccal capsules of species in this group are vestigial.				
Trichostrongylus colubriformis	AFR, AS, EUR, OCE	SI	Ingestion of larvae	Eggs, F
T. orientalis (Jimbo 1914), *T. capricola* (Ransom 1907), *T. probolurus* (Railliet 1896) and *T. skrjabini* (Kalantarian 1928) are said to be common in humans in parts of the world.				
Superfamily Rhabditoidea. Rhabditoids contain many free-living species. Features of the group include a bulbous pharynx. Members of *Strongyloides* have a free-living cycle where adults are found in faeces or soil.				
Strongyloides stercoralis	AFR, AS, IND, NA, OCE, SA, SEA	SI	Percutaneous penetration by larvae, invasion of buccal capsule, autoinfection	Larvae, F
Strongyloides fülleborni	AFR, OCE	SI	Percutaneous penetration by larvae, invasion of buccal capsule, autoinfection	Eggs, F
Superfamily Oxyuroidea. These nematodes of the order Oxyurida are parasites of the digestive tracts. The adults possess an oesophagus with a distinct bulb. Eggs, which are elongate and flattened on one side, are ingested directly by the host.				
Enterobius vermicularis	C	CAE, LI	Ingestion of eggs	Adult females lay eggs on perianal regions
Superfamily Trichinelloidea. These nematodes are characterized by a peculiar oesophagus consisting of an elongate glandular region consisting of distinct cells forming the oesophagus and a set of three large glandular cells that open by pores into the lumen of the oesophagus.				
Trichuris trichiura	AFR, AS, OCE, SA, SEA	CAE, LI	Ingestion of eggs	Eggs, F
Calodium hepaticum (*Capillaria hepatica*)	C (in rodents)	Liver	Ingestion of eggs from soil or infected animals	Eggs, Liver
Paracapillaria (*Crossicapillaria*) *philippinensis*	AFR, AS, IND, SA, SEA,	SI	Ingestion of infected fish, autoinfection	Eggs, F
Trichinella spiralis (Ts)	AFR, AS, IND, NA, SA, SEA	SI (adults), skeletal muscles (larvae)	Ingestion of skeletal muscle of infected host	First stage larvae in skeletal muscle
T. nelsoni	AFR	As for *Ts*	As for *Ts*	As for *Ts*
T. nativa	AS, EUR, NA	As for *Ts*	As for *Ts*	As for *Ts*
T. pseudospiralis	AFR, AS, IND, NA, SA, SEA	As for *Ts*	As for *Ts*	As for *Ts*
T. britovi	AS, EUR, NA	As for *Ts*	As for *Ts*	As for *Ts*
T. papuae	OCE	As for *Ts*	As for *Ts*	As for *Ts*
T. murrelli	AS, EUR, NA	As for *Ts*	As for *Ts*	As for *Ts*
Superfamily Filarioidea. Filarioids are tissue parasites of tetrapods, transmitted in their life cycle by blood-feeding arthropods. The worms are generally elongate and have much reduced buccal cavities.				
Wuchereria bancrofti	AFR	Lymphatics	Bite from infected mosquito	Microfilariae, Blood
Wuchereria bancrofti var. pacifica	OCE	Lymphatics	Bite from infected mosquito	Microfilariae, Blood
Brugia malayi	AS, SEA	Lymphatics	Bite from infected mosquito	Microfilariae, Blood
Onchocerca volvulus	AFR, SA	Subcutaneous tissues	Bite from infected simuliid fly	Microfilariae, Skin
Other species: *Onchocerca gutturosa* – rare parasite of humans				
Mansonella ozzardi	SA	Mesenteries, body cavity	Bite from infected simuliid or *Ceratopogonid* fly	Microfilariae, Blood
Mansonella (*Esslingeria*) *perstans*	AFR, SA	Mesenteries, body cavity	Bite from infected *Ceratopogonid* fly	Microfilariae, Blood
Mansonella (*Esslingeria*) *streptocerca*	AFR	Mesenteries, body cavity	Bite from infected *Ceratopogonid* fly	Microfilariae, Skin
Meningonema peruzzii	AFR	Subarachnoid space		
Loa loa	AFR	Subcutaneous connective tissues	Bite from tabanid flies	Microfilariae, Skin
Zoonotic filariae: *Dirofilaria*, *Brugia*, *Dipetalonema*, *Loaina*				
Superfamily Dracunculoidea. These nematodes live as adults within tissues of their hosts. The female worms liberate larvae that are infectious to copepods.				
Dracunculus medinensis	AFR (ME, IND – now eradicated)	Subcutaneous tissues	Ingestion of infected freshwater copepods	Larvae expelled from sores on skin
Superfamily Thelazioidea. These spiruroid nematodes have generally rounded mouths, as opposed to compressed or ornamented mouth regions of other groups. Species of *Thelazia* are parasites of the orbits of humans and animals.				
Thelazia callipaeda	AS, EUR, IND, SEA	Eyes	Dipteran flies	Larvae in lachrymal secretions
Thelazia californiensis	NA, SA	Eyes	Dipteran flies	Larvae in lachrymal secretions
Superfamily Gnathostomatoidea. This group of spirurid nematodes include species that have massive complex false lips in the mouth (pseudolabia) and often inflated spinous inflations of the head regions.				

Continued on following page

TABLE A3.4 List of Nematodes Parasitizing Humans, Showing Their Broad Geographic Range, Site of Patent Infection in the Human Host, the Mode of Human Infection Including, Where Relevant, the Intermediate Hosts and the Sites of Transmission of Eggs or Larvae from the Human Host—cont'd

Species	Geographic Range	Site in Human	Mode of Human Infection	Site of Parasite Transmission
Gnathostoma spinigerum	AS, EUR, NA, SEA	Subcutaneous tissues, viscera	Ingestion of vertebrate host	–
Physaloptera caucasica, P. transfuga (Pt)	AFR, ME, SA (*Pc*) EUR (*Pt*)	Anterior digestive tract	?Ingestion of insect	Eggs, F
Gongylonema pulchrum	AS, EUR, NA, OCE, SEA	Anterior digestive tract	Ingestion of insect	No eggs in human faeces
Superfamily Muspiceioidea. This superfamily contains a group of highly specialized species that are found in the tissues of a range of hosts. Very little is known of transmission and life cycles of these parasites.				
Haycocknema perplexum	OCE	Skeletal muscles	?	?

Abbreviations – Geographic range: AFR, Africa; AS, Asia; EUR, Europe; IND, Indian subcontinent; ME, Middle East; NA, North America; OCE, Oceania including Australia; SA, South America; SEA, South-east Asia. Site in infection in humans: CAE, caecum; SI, small intestine. Site of parasite transmission: F, faeces. A question mark indicates that information is not available.

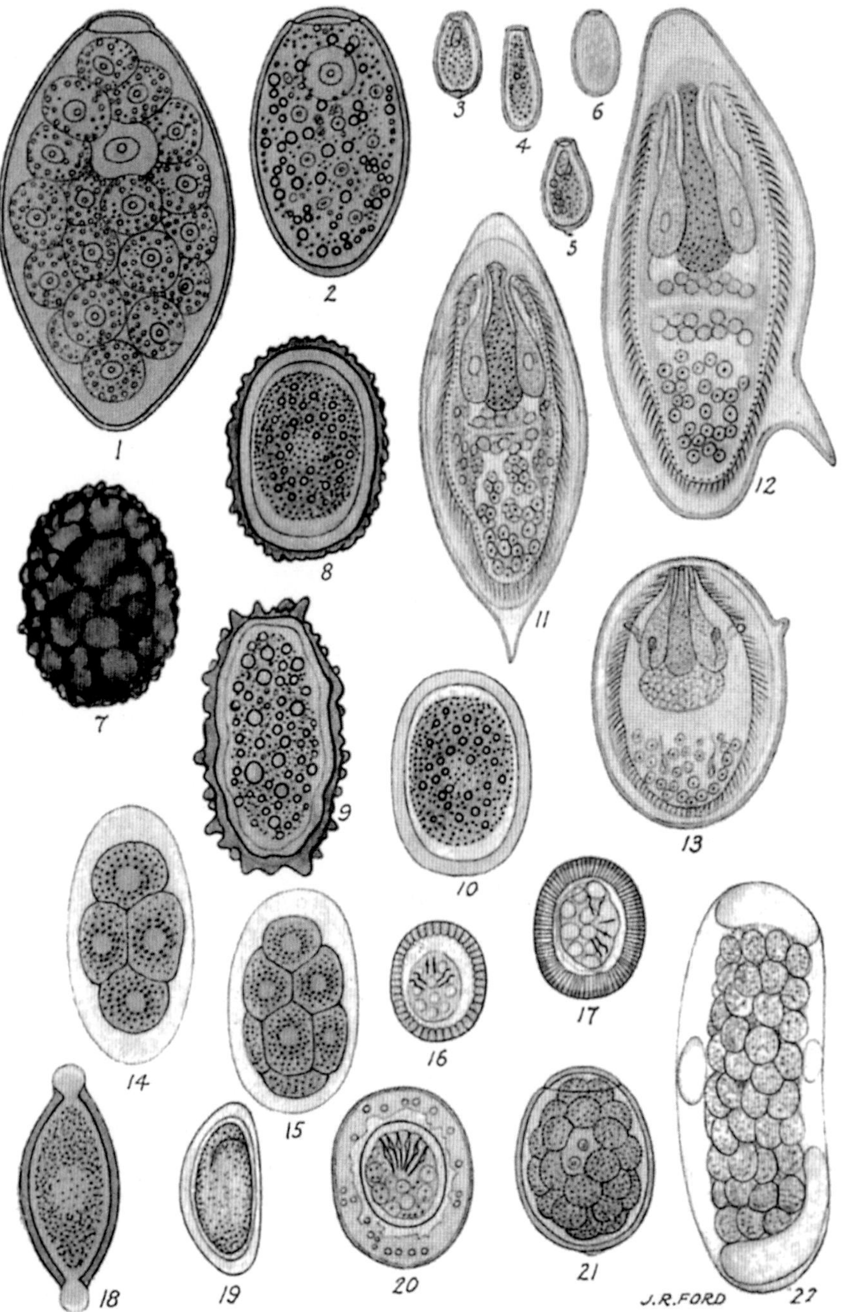

Figure A3.3 Eggs of representative helminths. 1, *Fasciolopsis buski*. 2, *Paragonimus westermani*. 3, *Heterophyes heterophyes*. 4, *Opisthorchis felineus*. 5, *Clonorchis sinensis*. 6, *Metagonimus yokogawai*. 7, 8, *Ascaris lumbricoides*, external aspect. 9, *Ascaris lumbricoides*, unfertilized egg. 10, *Ascaris lumbricoides*, decorticated egg. 11, *Schistosoma haematobium*. 12, *Schistosoma mansoni*. 13, *Schistosoma japonicum*. 14, *Ancylostoma duodenale*. 15, *Trichostrongylus colubriformis*. 16, *Taenia solium*. 17, *Taenia saginata*. 18, *Trichuris trichiura*. 19, *Enterobius vermicularis*. 20, *Vampirolepis nana*. 21, *Diphyllobothrium latum*. 22, *Heterodera radicicola*, non-parasitic, ingested with vegetables. *(Courtesy of Tropical Resources Unit.)*

Figure A3.3 for illustrations of eggs from faeces of some trematodes and other helminths. Cestodes infect humans either as adult worms or as developing larvae. Adult forms have the true tapeworm appearance and are found in the small intestine. The larval form, termed a metacestode, is found in a variety of tissues, and its distribution in a host is often specific to that species. In humans, metacestodes will possess a scolex that is withdrawn or invaginated into the body of the larval form. Metacestodes do not possess the strobila found in adults.

In Table A3.3, the species name, taxonomic group, stage and site of infection and geographic distribution of the parasite are shown. All cestodes infecting humans, with the exception of the sparganum worm *Spirometra*, are transmitted to humans with food, or through ingestion of eggs from the environment. For each cestode species, we identify mode of infection of humans – whether by ingestion of eggs or of the intermediate host (Table A3.3).

Phylum *Nematoda*

This phylum contains the roundworms, which are pseudocoelomate, non-segmented worms. Nematodes are limited externally by an extracellular cuticle. Nematodes are cylindrical, tapering at both ends and they are white or yellow, sometimes semitransparent. The sexes of these worms are separate. Progeny are passed from the host as characteristic eggs or as first stage larvae. These progeny are encountered diagnostically in faeces or in human tissues; their location is characteristic and governed by the sites in the hosts occupied by the adult parasite. Thus, eggs of gastrointestinal roundworms usually pass from the host with faeces. Agents of lymphatic filariasis inhabit the lymphatic system and their larvae are found in peripheral blood where they are taken up by mosquitoes during feeding.

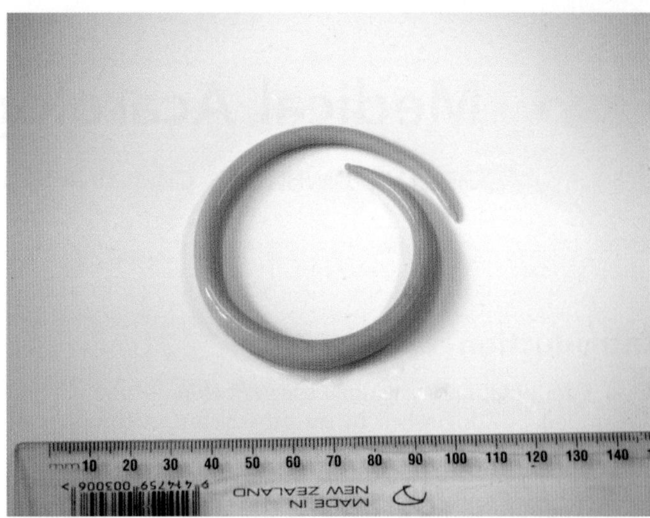

Figure A3.4 Representative nematode – *Ascaris* species. *(Photo courtesy of Ms Lyn Knott, University of Queensland.)*

Nematodes grow by moulting and there are five stages in the life cycles. The third-stage larva is most often the stage that infects the definitive host. Humans can be infected with nematodes in a variety of ways, by ingestion of eggs or larvae from the environment, by direct invasion of human skin, through ingestion of infected intermediate hosts or by transfer by a vector that feeds on blood. Nematodes infecting humans are listed in Table A3.4. Representative forms of adults are shown in Figure A3.4, while illustrations of eggs commonly seen in human faeces are presented in Figure A3.3. Characteristics of the different superfamilies of trematodes are taken from Anderson[5] and Anderson and colleagues.[6]

REFERENCES

1. Gibson DI, Jones A, Bray RA. Keys to the Trematoda, Vol. 1. New York: CABI and The Natural History Museum; 2002.
2. Jones A, Bray RA, Gibson DI. Keys to the Trematoda, Vol. 2. New York: CABI and The Natural History Museum; 2005.
3. Bray RA, Gibson DI, Jones A. Keys to the Trematoda, Vol. 3. New York: CABI and The Natural History Museum; 2008.
4. Kolářová L. Schistosomes causing cercarial dermatitis: a mini-review of current trends in systematics and of host specificity and pathogenicity. Folia Parasitologica 2007;54:81–7.
5. Anderson RC. Nematode parasites of vertebrates: their development and transmission. 2nd ed. Wallingford: CABI; 2000.
6. Anderson RC, Chabaud AG, Willmott S. Keys to the Nematode Parasites of Vertebrates: Archival Volume. Wallingford: CABI; 2009.

APPENDIX 4

Medical Acarology and Entomology

GRAHAM B. WHITE | CHRISTINA FAUST

Introduction

Over 90% of all known animal species belong to the phylum Arthropoda, distinguished by an exoskeleton. Arthropods of medical interest belong to three classes: Arachnida (ticks, mites, etc.), Crustacea (copepods, etc.) and Insecta (insects). This review will provide an overview of the life cycle, distribution and human diseases caused by a diversity of arthropods. Arthropods can either cause direct pathology or serve as vectors for viral, bacterial, filarial or protozoan pathogens. Vectors can pass infections to host through bites or other methods, but can maintain infections within species by trans-stadial (stage to stage, i.e. from larva to nymph to adult) and transovarial (through eggs to larvae of the next generation) transmissions. Control of arthropods is often the most effective method of controlling a disease (Table A4.1), but understanding their biology is essential.[57] This review only attempts to give a glimpse at the diversity of important arthropods and an introduction to their role in human health (see 1, 2, 6, 29, 46 for more detail). A large literature is devoted to specific taxa and we urge readers to consult these (some cited throughout the appendix, others found online) for specific keys and clearer ecological insights.

Class: *Arachnida*

SUBCLASS *ACARINA*

Arachnids have unsegmented bodies without antennae or wings. They undergo incomplete metamorphosis: eggs hatch into six-legged larvae, which develop through eight-legged nymphal stage(s) to eight-legged adults (no pupal stage). Ticks and mites are grouped within subclass Acarina, which has 30 000 species in 2000 genera. Some of these acarines are of medical importance and are outlined below.

Order Sarcoptiformes

Family Sarcoptidae. *Sarcoptes scabei* is the most important species of Sarcoptidae (Figure A4.1). It is the causative agent of scabies (Chapter 58). Adult females make permanent burrows in horny layers of skin and excrete large eggs and faeces within the tunnels (Figure A4.2). Eggs hatch and live within the follicles, molting into larvae and then two nymph stages. The life cycle from egg to egg takes about 10–14 days, with high mortality (90%), but adults can live for several weeks to months in skin, and females lay eggs daily. *Sarcoptes scabei* is one causative agent of mange in humans and a variety of wild and domestic animals.

Family Acaridae. Forage mites (family Acaridae) are pests of stored food products, such as cheese, vanilla pods and flour. Handling infested products results in bites or a simple contact allergy, sometimes referred to such as grocer's itch, copra itch and baker's itch . Forage mites may also be swallowed or inhaled and can cause gastric disturbances or respiratory symptoms.

Order Trombidiformes

Family Demodicidae. Follicle mites (*Demodex* species) are extremely small (0.1–0.4 mm; Figure A4.3) and, as the name would suggest, undergo their entire life cycle within follicles. *Demodex* spp. infect a variety of mammalian hosts, but are usually very host specific. Humans can be infected by multiple species that specialize on different tissues: *D. folliculorum* (hair follicles) and *D. brevis* (sebaceous glands). Human infestations are usually benign and occur in eyelids, nose and facial areas. Blepharitis or granulomatous acne may occur because of infestations.

Family Trombiculidae. Larvae of trombiculid mites, known commonly as chiggers, is the only stage that is parasitic on vertebrates. Eggs are laid in damp, well-drained soil and upon hatching, larvae crawl upwards to the tips of grass stems and await in clusters for carbon dioxide from passing hosts (Figure A4.4). Larvae attach and feed by partially digesting host tissue with saliva and sucking it up. After feeding a minimum of 3 days, larvae drop from hosts and enter a quiescent stage before molting into nymphs and then to adults. The length of the life cycle varies from 40 days in tropical regions, to an entire year temperate regions.

Of 1200 described species, only 50 are known to utilize humans or livestock as hosts. Larvae usually parasitize rodents and birds, but will feed on humans given the opportunity and can cause dermatitis. Trombiculid species are widespread; regionally important species include *Neotrombicula autumnalis* (Europe, 'harvest mite'), *Eutrombicula alfreddugesi* (America) and *Eutrombicula batatas* (Central America).

Trombiculid mites within the genus *Leptotrombidium* also act as vectors for scrub typhus (*Orientsia tsutsugamushi*) (Chapter 22). Transmission is maintained through trans-stadial and transovarial transmissions. *L. deliense* is the main vector over most of the distribution of the disease and is typically associated with ecologically disturbed vegetation (Figure A4.5). Other important human vectors species include: *L. akamushi* (Japan, Figure A4.6), *L. fletcher* (Malaysia, Borneo, New Guinea and Philippines); *L. arenicola* (Malaysia); *L. pallidum* (Japan, Korea and the Primorye region of Russia); *L. pavlovskyi* (Siberia and the Primorye region of Russia); and *L. scutellare* (Mt. Fiji, Japan).

Order Acariformes

Family Pyroglyphidae. House-dust mites in the family Pyroglyphidae (i.e. *Dermatophagoides pteronyssinus*, Figure A4.7) are commonly found in dust in tropical and temperate regions, where they feed mainly on shed human skin. Inhalation of

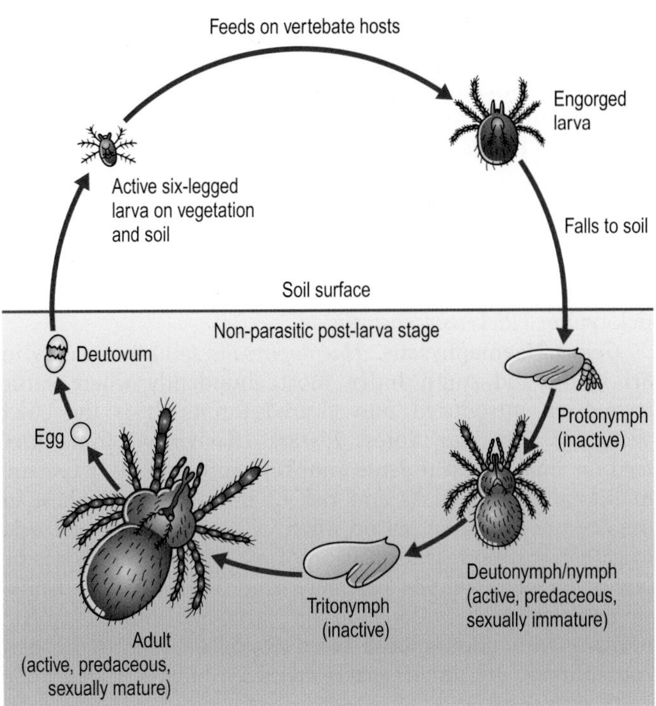

Figure A4.4 Summarized life cycle of trombiculid mites.

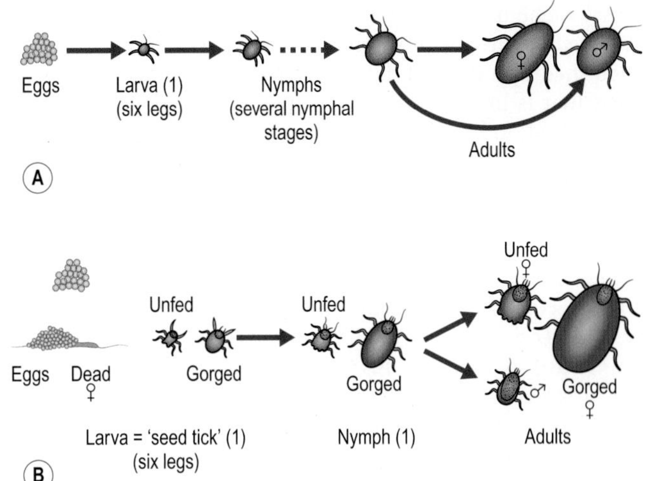

Figure A4.10 Tick life cycles: (A) Argasidae. (B) Ixodidae.

allergens associated with these mites (live and dead mites and their faeces) can cause asthma and extensive dermatitis in sensitized individuals.

Order Mesostigmata

Families Dermanyssidae and Macronyssidae. Species in the families Dermanyssidae and Macronyssidae are blood-sucking mites. In the absence of their natural hosts, they will parasitize humans and can cause dermatitis. Rat mites (i.e. *Ornithonyssus bacoti*) are associated with groceries and warehouses. Bird mites (i.e. *Dermanyssus gallinae*) are often found in the eaves of houses and in air-conditioning ducts.

Order Ixodida

All species of ticks are obligate ectoparasites of vertebrates. They are large (3–20 mm) and lack prominent hairs found on mites. Ticks have a gnathosoma which is well development for firm attachment to hosts, preventing easy dislodgement during grooming (Figure A4.8, A4.9). Both families of ticks undergo three stages of development (larval, nymphal and adult) but hard (Ixodidae) and soft (Argasidae) ticks differ in their life cycles and blood meal source (Figure A4.10, Table A4.2). Most ixodids also have a high reproductive potential, laying several thousands of eggs to offset considerable mortality during the life cycle.

Ticks parasitize a wide range of wild and domestic hosts and many appear to have a preferred host, although this apparent preference may be due to availability rather than choice. Both male and female adult ticks ingest large quantities of blood: a fully engorged female ixodid may reach a length of over 20 mm and weigh 2.0 g or more. Large infestations can cause physical damage in addition to considerable blood loss. Ticks can also act as vectors for viruses and bacteria (Table A4.3). Lastly, ticks can also cause paralysis, although removal of the tick will result in immediate recovery.

Family Argasidae. Soft ticks, family Argasidae, are tough, leathery ticks that lack a dorsal plate or scutum (Figure A4.9), hence their common name. Argasids are nocturnal rapid feeders, usually taking only 2–3 minutes to engorge. The coxal gland, located between the first and second pairs of legs, is essential for rapid feeding; it concentrates the blood meal by filtering out fluid and excreting it from the glands. Soft ticks live in habitats close to their hosts to allow easy access for feeding and can utilize the same host their entire life. There are three to six nymphal stages: each stage feeds once and molts to the next stage. Adult males and females feed repeatedly and mate on the hosts; the female lays a batch of 100–200 eggs after each blood meal. Some argasids can live for many years with prolonged periods of starvation.

TABLE A4.2 Differences Between *Argasid* Ticks and *Ixodid* Ticks

Morphology	Argasidae	Ixodidae
Scutum	Absent	Present; anterior in larva, nymph and female, covering dorsal side in male
Capitulum	Ventral, not visible from above	Anterior, visible from above
Palps	Long, movable	Short, rigid
Life cycle	Several nymphal stages	One nymphal stage
	Multiple batches of eggs: 100–200 per blood meal	One batch of eggs (several–1000)
Habits	Rapid feeders, usually nocturnal; male and female feed repeatedly	Slow feeders, day and night, several days; only females feed once
	Restricted habitat, burrows or nests of hosts	Diffuse habitat, pasture, etc. where hosts forage

Argasidae has about 150 species in three genera. *Argas* and *Ornithodoros* are the most medically important and can be distinguished by a distinct flattened lateral margin of the body in *Argas* that is present even when fully engorged. *Argas* species usually feed on birds or bats, but can attack humans and cause painful bites. The coxal glands of soft ticks have an important role in disease transmission: coxal fluid often contains pathogens, which can enter the bite wound (Figure A4.11, A4.12). Species of *Ornithodoros* can transmit *Borrelia* species spirochetes through salivary secretion or contamination of the bite through coxal fluid. *Borrelia* cause relapsing fevers in humans by *B. parkeri* (*O. parkeri*), *B. turicatae* (*O. turicata*), *B. hermsi* (*O. hermsi*), *B. venezuelensis* (*O. rudis*) and *B. persica* (*O. tholozani*) (Table A4.2). High rates of trans-stadial and transovarial *Borrelia* transmission, long vector life spans and the ability of the vector to starve for long periods lead to the perpetuation of natural foci in the absence of vertebrate hosts. Ticks are the main reservoirs of infection, while other animals, such as rodents, probably serve only as amplifiers of infection.

Family Ixodidae. Hard ticks are easily distinguished from soft ticks by the presence of a capitulum in all stages (Figure A4.13). They are also characterized by slow feeding, attaching to their host for several days, anchored by their chelicerae, hypostome and 'cement' from their salivary glands. Each stage (except the eggs) feed on a vertebrate host for 4–12 days: three mobile stages of larva, one nymphal stage and adults. Much smaller adult males live on host for weeks or months and mate with several females. Fertilized and engorged females drop off hosts to lay a mass of several thousand eggs on the ground before dying. The whole life cycle takes 2–4 months in the tropics and up to 3–5 years in cold or temperate climates.

Coxal glands are absent in ixodid ticks and the ingested blood is concentrated during the slow feeding by passage of fluid from the stomach into the body cavity, from where it is processed through the salivary glands back into the host. A few ticks are host-specific, but the majority use a wide range of hosts. Immature stages usually feed on smaller mammals (rodents, etc.), whereas adult ticks feed on large mammals. Most ixodid ticks parasitize a different animal of the same or different species at each stage. Ixodidae has about 800 species in 13 genera, of which *Ixodes*, *Amblyomma*, *Hyalomma*, *Haemaphysalis*, *Dermacentor* and *Rhipicephalus* transmit diseases to humans.

***Genus* Ixodes.** *Ixodes scapularis* (*I. dammini*) (American deer tick) is widely distributed in the USA and adjacent Canada; the range appears to be extending, probably due to proliferation of deer, hosts of the adult ticks. Larvae and nymphs parasitize rodents (particularly the white-footed mouse) as well as humans. The adult ticks feed mostly on white-tailed deer, or occasionally on humans. *I. scapularis* is the vector of human babesiosis (*Babesia microti*; Chapter 44) and Lyme disease (*Borrelia burgdorferi*) in eastern USA. *I. ricinus* (European sheep tick or castor bean tick) is distributed widely in rough pasture and woodland across Europe to the Caspian Sea and northern Iran. *I. ricinus* is the vector of three human flaviviruses: louping ill (primarily of sheep and cattle but affecting humans also) in the British Isles, tick-borne viral encephalitis (TBE) in central Europe and Lyme disease (*Borrelia burgdorferi*) which is becoming increasingly widespread in areas with deer populations as hosts for adult *I. ricinus*. Immature ticks are found on rodents and birds; adults attack deer, sheep, cattle and also humans. The life cycle takes 2–4 years to complete. *I. persulcatus* (the *taiga* tick) is widespread from the Baltic to Japan, its distribution overlapping with that of *I. ricinus*. It is more cold-hardy than *I. ricinus*. In Russia, *I. persulcatus* is associated with the taiga forest. The life cycle extends over 2–4 years. It is the chief vector of Russian spring-summer encephalitis (flavivirus). Transovarial transmission occurs, but the rate is variable. *I. holocyclus* occurs in the humid densely vegetated coastal areas of Queensland and New South Wales in Australia where it infests a variety of mammalian hosts. Its bites may cause tick paralysis in dogs and humans. It is the vector of Queensland tick typhus (*Rickettsia australis*).

***Genus* Haemaphysalis.** *Haemaphysalis spinigera* occurs in Sri Lanka and south India, most abundantly where cattle have been introduced into cleared forests. It is the chief vector of Kyasanur Forest disease (flavivirus). Immatures feed on small forest rodents, monkeys and humans. Exposure of humans to the ticks and risk of infection are highest in the dry pre-monsoon period when villagers go into the forest to gather firewood. Transmission of infection to humans is by bite by infected nymphs and there is no transovarial transmission. *H. leachi* is widespread on carnivores but can infect humans with boutonneuse fever (*Rickettsia conori*) through contamination of skin or eyes from infected ticks crushed while de-ticking dogs.

***Genus* Rhipicephalus.** *Rhipicephalus appendiculatus* parasitizes cattle and wild game animals in wooded and shrubby grassland from southern Sudan to South Africa, but is absent from West Africa. In East Africa, it is the vector of the protozoan disease East Coast fever (*babesiosis*) in cattle, but in the South African veld it is the chief vector of African tick typhus (*Rickettsia*) and an avid human-biter. *R. sanguineus* is the chief vector of boutonneuse fever to humans in the Mediterranean basin.

***Genus* Dermacentor.** Species of *Dermacentor* can transmit several rickettsias via bite and trans-stadial and transovarial transmission occur (Chapter 22). *Dermacentor andersoni* (Rocky Mountain wood tick) and *D. variabilis* (American dog tick) are the primary vectors for Rocky Mountain spotted fever (*Rickettsia rickettsi*) in central and eastern USA, respectively. It may take hours or a day before the attached tick can transmit the rickettsiae, therefore risk of infection is considerably reduced if tick is removed hours after attachment. *D. andersoni* also transmits Colorado tick fever virus to humans. *D. marginatus*, *D. silvarum* and *D. nuttalli* are the chief vectors of Siberian tick typhus (*Rickettsia sibirica*) from central Europe to central Asia. *R. sibirica* can survive for long periods in the ticks.

***Genus* Amblyomma.** *Amblyomma* species have especially long mouthparts, increasing the difficulty of removal from hosts. *Amblyomma hebraeum* (the South African bont tick) is the vector of boutonneuse fever (*Rickettsia conori*) in Southern Africa. *A. americanum*, the lone-star tick and *A. cajennense*, the Cayenne tick, can transmit Rocky Mountain spotted fever in the USA and Latin America, respectively. *A. variegatum* is the vector of *R. africae* in the Caribbean and Africa (Figure 4.13).

***Genus* Hyalomma.** *Hyalomma marginatum* is a hardy tick adapted to living under arid or semi-arid conditions in Eurasia. Birds are important hosts of the immature stages and the ticks have been carried to many parts of Europe and Africa by migrating birds. It is the vector of the arbovirus responsible for Crimean-Congo hemorrhagic fever arbovirus (Chapter 14).

Class *Maxillopoda* (Subphylum *Crustacea*)

SUBCLASS *PENTASTOMIDA*

Pentastomids, also called linguatulids or 'tongue worms', have arthropod-like characteristics and current taxonomy classifies them as endoparasitic crustaceans.[3] Four species, belonging to two families, can affect humans as dead-end infections.

Family Linguatulidae. The body of adult *Linguatula* (Figure A4.14) is club-shaped, flattened ventrally, convex dorsally and transversely striated into about 90 superficial annulations. Two pairs of simple retractile hooks aid in attachment to host tissue. *Linguatula serrata* is found worldwide, adults infect the nasal passages of canids (dogs, foxes, wolves).[4] Transmission occurs through nasal discharge of eggs or passage through the intestine. Both eggs and infective stages of larvae can establish in humans and domestic animals through consumption or accidental inhalation. The larvae may attempt to migrate to the nasal passages, but humans are a dead-end host and cannot transmit fertilized eggs. They usually do not cause symptoms in humans and are found incidentally during autopsy.

Family Armilliferidae. The life history of *Armillifer* (Figure A4.15) is broadly similar to that of *Linguatula*. Eggs remain viable on soil for at least 3 months and, when ingested, hatch in the intestine; the larvae immediately bore through the intestinal wall to lodge in any tissue. At least six moults occur over a period of 6 months to 1 year, to form infective nymphs. Adult parasites inhabit the lungs of pythons and large African vipers, but larval forms encyst in the tissues of many mammal species, including monkeys and humans. Humans can act only as a dead-end intermediate host and acquire the infection by eating poorly cooked snake meat, or by drinking water contaminated by snake faeces. Nymphs commonly encyst in or on the liver, intestinal tract and lungs in humans. *Armillifer armillatus* infects humans in tropical Africa. In Oriental regions, *A. moniliformis* is the usual cause of human infection and has been recorded in Malaysia, Manila, Java, Sumatra and China.

Class *Insecta*

All insects have an exoskeleton of chitin, three body segments (head, thorax, abdomen), three pairs of legs and a pair of antennae. It is the most diverse group of animals on the planet, with over 1 million described species but many more species undiscovered or not yet described. Insects can be very beneficial to humans, but in this section we will discuss species that cause nuisance or disease in humans.

Order Diptera

The Order *Diptera* includes over 120 000 species true flies, characterized by a pair of wings and a pair of halteres (knobbed structures modified from hind wings). In addition to causing myiasis Chapter 60), true flies can vector or serve as intermediate hosts for many pathogens and is one of the most medically important orders.[47]

Family Psychodidae. Phlebotomine sandflies are small (1.5–3.5 mm), delicate, hairy flies with long, filamentous antennae (Figure A4.16).[8] Up to 70 eggs are laid at a breeding site with high moisture and organic detritus; eggs hatch after 1–2 weeks. Larvae go through four instar stages, with the possibility of diapausing in the four instar stage in cooler climates. Length of larval instars varies greatly, within and between species and is largely determined by temperature. Pupae are inactive and emerge within 5–10 days during the night, often before dawn. Relatively little is known about the immature stages of sandflies because breeding sites and larvae are difficult to find. Adults are easy to distinguish from other small fly species because they hold their wings above their body, like a vertical 'V' (Figure A4.17). Adults of both sexes feed on nectar and other plant sugars, but females can also be haematophagous on vertebrates to obtain nutrition for egg production. Eggs are laid 5–10 days after a blood meal. Usually one blood meal is taken for each batch of eggs, but autogeny (ability to lay eggs without a blood meal) has been recorded in some human-biting species.

Phlebotomine sandflies are found mainly in the tropics and subtropics, with a few species penetrating into temperate regions in both the northern (to 50°N) and southern (to about 40°S) hemispheres.

They only fly at night. Little is known about their long range movements but they can fly over 2 km in a few days in open habitats. Biting, then, is also crepuscular, with different feeding times associated with particular species. Few species are endophilic and these are mostly peridomestic species. Resting places are cool, relatively humid dark niches. Vertical stratification within the canopy has been noted.

Phlebotomine sandflies can transmit viruses, bacteria and protozoa, but not helminths, to vertebrates. They are vectors of visceral leishmaniasis (kala-azar; see Chapter 47), various forms of cutaneous leishmaniasis (oriental sore, espundia, etc.), bartonellosis (Oroya fever, Carrión's disease, Chapter 30) and sandfly fever (papataci or papatasi fever).[30,47]

Leishmania transmission is usually highly focal, probably related to the ecological constraints of the vectors (Figure A4.18). Transmission of pathogens takes place during blood feeding. Human involvement in *Leishmania* transmission can be very variable: there can be occasional zoonotic spillover to completely anthroponotic cycles (only humans and sandflies).[7] Not all infected sandflies can transmit to humans: i.e. in southern Eurasia *L. major* infections are maintained among rodents by *P. mongolensis*, *P. caucasicus* and *P. andrejevi*, but only *P. papatasi* transmits the parasite to humans. Vector-parasite specificity of sandflies and the *Leishmania* spp. they transmit is affected by several factors, including behaviour (e.g. propensity of a vector to bite a particular species of reservoir host), ecological factors and biochemical factors (e.g. enzyme activity) operating in the sandfly gut (Table A4.4). Natural infection rates in wild flies are usually very low (below 1%), but may be exceptionally high in some foci (e.g. up to 20% in the Jordan Valley).

Genus* Phlebotomus *(Old World). Vectors of visceral leishmaniasis in the Old World are distributed through several subgenera: *Larroussius* (Mediterranean basin and Sahel); *Synphlebotomus* (East Africa); *Euphlebotomus* (India); and *Adlerius* (Near East, northern China). Species of *Phlebotomus* (*sensu stricto*) are associated with *L. major* transmission in arid environments of East Africa, the Middle East and the former USSR. The subgenus *Paraphlebotomus* contains many species living in rodent burrows in central Asia and transmitting *L. major* between rodents and occasionally to humans. One species, the peridomestic *P. sergenti*, is a vector of *L. tropica* in western Asia and the Middle East. Vectors of visceral leishmaniasis in the Old World are distributed through several subgenera: *Larroussius* (Mediterranean basin and Sahel); *Synphlebotomus* (East Africa); *Euphlebotomus* (India); and *Adlerius* (Near East, northern China). Species that bite humans and are vectors of disease are confined to the subtropics in the Old World; very few anthrophilic phlebotomine sandflies exist in tropical Africa. However, the range of *Phlebotomus* extends from very low elevations (i.e. Dead Sea) to altitudes of 2800 m in Ethiopia. Different species have unique ecological requirements, but the group exists in a diversity of habitats from deserts to savannahs to tropical rainforests. Foci of cutaneous leishmaniasis are in dry, semi-arid areas.

Phlebotomus perniciosus transmits *Toscana* virus in the northern Mediterranean and other viruses have been isolated. Sandfly fever (papataci or papatasi fever) is common during the summer months throughout the Mediterranean basin, the Middle East, Pakistan and parts of India (Chapter 14). *Phlebotomus papatasi* was incriminated as the vector in Egypt and is generally thought to transmit sandfly fever throughout the Old World range of the disease. Natural infection rates are between 0.015 and 0.5% in sandflies. No natural vertebrate reservoir is known.

Genus* Lutzomyia *(New World). The genus *Lutzomyia* is much more diverse than its Old World counterpart; some subgenera contain several vector species (e.g. *Nyssomyia* and *Psychodopygus*), whereas many other subgenera and species groups contain only one or two species that are involved in the transmission of *Leishmania* spp. In contrast to Old World, transmission of cutaneous leishmaniasis occurs mainly within forests (Figure A4.18). Land clearance has reduced the incidence of cutaneous leishmaniasis, but has increased opportunities for transmission of visceral leishmaniasis.

In valleys of the central Andean Cordilleras of Peru, Colombia and Ecuador *Lutzomia* species also transmit *Bartonella bacilliformis* (Oroya fever, verruga peruana). Not all vector species are known, but some species involved may be *Lutzomyia verrucarum* (Peru) and *L. colombiana* (Colombia). The disease is thought to circulate only in humans and sandflies, without any other hosts or reservoirs. Viruses are also spread by sandflies in the New World: *Lutzomyia trapidoi* and *L. ylephiletor* transmit *Chagres*' and *Punta Toro* viruses.

Family Culicidae. Mosquitoes are sometimes considered the most dangerous animals on earth because of their abundance, distribution and role as vectors for many potent diseases. All mosquitoes breed in water: whether it is moist soil, in containers or in pools of water. Most eggs hatch within a few days of being laid, but members of *Aedini* can go into diapause and withstand drying out or overwintering. In the tropics, larvae develop in a week, whereas temperate larvae usually overwinter in that stage. Most larvae are filter feeders, but some species are predatory (i.e. *Toxorhynchites*, *Aedes* subgenus *Mucidus*, *Culex* subgenus *Lutzia*) (Figure A4.19). Four instar larval stages are followed by a pupal stage (Figure A4.20). Pupae emerge as adults after a few days and the adults flies to rest under shelter for several hours (Figure A4.21). Males are not able to copulate for about a day, until their external genitalia have turned upside down (Figure A4.22). Mating occurs within or near swarms of males that have distinct characteristics and form at particular times of the day. Once females engage in copulation, the sperm is sufficient for fertilizing all the eggs she may produce in her lifetime.

Adult mosquitoes of both sexes feed on nectar and other plant fluids. Adult anopheline and culicine females also suck blood from mammals, birds, amphibians and other vertebrates and usually show a host preference towards a particular species (Figures A4.23–A4.25). Anophelines show the most regular cycles of blood-feeding and egg-laying; most species require a blood meal before egg-laying (Figures A4.26–A4.28). Toxorhynchites and some culicines produce eggs autogenously (i.e. without having fed on blood). Male and female mosquitoes may well live for several weeks, feeding repeatedly, under natural conditions.

The majority of mosquitoes hunt and feed at night, although many aedine, mansoniine and sabethine species do so by day. Females hunt for hosts by flying upwind and following scent cues. Each blood meal generally provides enough nutrition for the female mosquito to produce a batch of 30–150 eggs. Each species has a well-defined activity cycle: some attack at dusk, others around midnight or at other hours. Species showing strong attraction to humans are said to be anthropophilic, or more strictly anthropophagic when the human is bitten, as opposed to zoophilic or zoophagic species which attack other creatures. Endophilic mosquitoes are those that favour houses or animal sheds for resting indoors, whereas exophilic species prefer to remain outdoors. Outdoor biting behaviour is termed exophagy, as opposed to the endophagy of mosquitoes that enter dwellings to bite people or animals.

Approximately 3300 species of *Culicoides* in three subfamilies and 35 genera have been described.[13,15,16,18,19,21,28,33–35,37–43,45] Anopheline and culicine subfamilies encapsulate all species of medical concern (Figures A4. 29, A4.30). Their range extends from tropical regions to the Arctic Circle.

Mosquitoes are important vectors of many human diseases. Vectors of malaria all belong within *Anopheles* (Table A4.5). Various anophelines and especially culicines transmit arboviruses and filariasis of humans (Tables A4.6–A4.8). Mosquitoes also serve as the vectors of enzootic infections (i.e. restricted to animals or birds) and some zoonotic diseases due to pathogens transmitted from animals to humans (e.g. yellow fever and subperiodic *Brugian filariasis*).

In order to quantify amounts of human–mosquito contact for epidemiological purposes, it is necessary to estimate: (1) the number of bites/person per 24 h, (2) the percentage of mosquito blood meals obtained from human compared with other animals and (3) the feeding interval, expressed as the mean number of days between times when successive blood meals are taken by a given species of mosquito. These data can be combined with the probability of mosquito daily survival, estimated from the proportion of parous females, in order to calculate an index of vectorial capacity.[30,31,48]

Identifying mosquitoes to genera is straightforward (Table A4.7), whereas correct species identification is a challenge. Some species of mosquito are morphologically identical, or nearly so, and so it may be necessary to look at chromosomes, DNA, proteins or behaviour in order to distinguish between species (Figure A4.30). Eggs and larval stages can also be essential in differentiating species (Figure A4. 31). Groups of such closely related species are known as sibling species complexes. Genetic evidence shows that these biologically distinct species do not normally interbreed in nature. The significance of

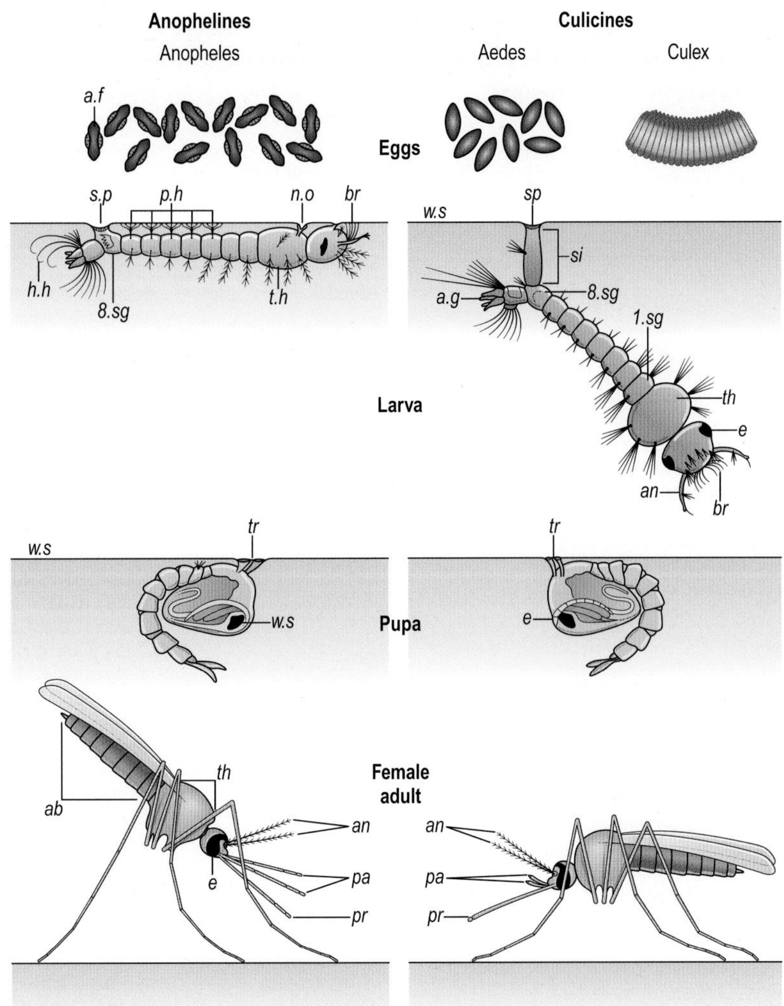

Figure A4.29 Chief distinguishing features of anophelines and culicines. *a.f*, air floats; *a.g*, anal gills; *ab*, abdomen; *an*, antenna; *br*, mouth brushes; *e*, eye; *h.h.*, hooked hairs or caudal setae; *n.o*, notched organ; *pa*, palps (maxillary palpi); *p.h*, palmate hairs or float hairs; *pr*, proboscis; *1.sg*, first abdominal segment; *8.sg*, eighth abdominal segment; *si*, siphon; *sp*, spiracles; *th*, thorax; *tr*, respiratory trumpets; w.s, water surface.

species complexes is that some of the species are pests and vectors of disease, whereas others are not.

Subfamily Anophelinae. The wings of most anophelines have a characteristic pattern of pale and dark spots of scales (Figure A4.32). Palps are as long, or nearly as long, as the proboscis (Figure A4. 33). The most important genus in the subfamily is *Anopheles* – vectors of human malaria (Table A4.5). Medically important anthropophilic species belong to the subgenera *Anopheles* (mostly Northern Hemisphere); *Cellia* (Old World Tropics); *Kerteszia* (New World Tropics); and *Nyssorhynchus* (New World Tropics) of the genus *Anopheles.* Neither of the other two anopheline genera, *Bironella* and *Chagasia*, nor the *Anopheles* subgenera *Lophopodomyia* and *Stethomyia* are of any applied interest. The capability of any particular species of *Anopheles* to transmit malaria is regulated by a number of factors, such as the numbers present, the degree of anthropophily (human blood index), the probability of survival to a potentially infective age and whether the parasites of malaria can complete their development in the mosquito.[9,10,11,12,17,44]

In addition to malaria, *Anopheles* spp. transmit *Wuchereria bancrofti*, many of the malaria-carrying species are also implicated in transmission (Table A4.6).[26,27] Timor filariasis, caused by *Brugia timori*, is transmitted by *A. barbirostris* on Flores.[14] *Anopheles* also transmit several arboviruses, such as eastern equine encephalitis, western equine encephalitis, Venezuelan equine encephalitis, *o'nyong-nyong*, *tataguine* and others (Table A4.7).

Subfamily Culicinae. This subfamily has over 2500 species in 40 genera divided into 11 tribes. Culicines have flat scales covering their entire abdomens and usually rest with proboscis and abdomen more or less parallel with the supporting surface (Figure A4.34).

Tribe Aedinii. Although many genera are within Aedinii, the most important is *Aedes*, with over 100 species distributed globally. *Aedes* eggs are capable of withstanding dessication and can survive in artificial containers. Medically important *Aedes* are active during the day: they spread arboviruses, *Brugia malayi* and *Wuchereria bancrofti. Aedes aegypti* originated in Africa, but now is found in tropical and subtropical regions globally.[23,24,32] *A. aegypti* can transmit yellow fever virus, Chikungunya and dengue (Figure A4.35, Tables A4.6, A4.7). Species of *Haemagogus* can be vectors of sylvatic yellow fever (Figure A4.36).[20]

Text continued on p. 1268

TABLE A4.7 Important Mosquitoes and the Arboviruses They Transmit

Arbovirus And Endemic Area	Natural Vector (*Indicates Principal Species)
Togaviridae	
ALPHAVIRUS (GROUP A)	
Barmah Forest Virus (BFV)	
Australia	*Aedes (Ochlerotatus) vigilax Culex (Culex) annulirostris* Aedes (Diceromyia) furcifer
Chikungunya (CHIK)	
Africa	**Aedes (Stegomyia) aegypti* *Aedes (Stegomyia) africanus* *Coquillettidia (Coquillettidia) fuscopennata* *Culex (Culex) quinquefasciatus* *Mansonia (Mansonioides) africana* *Mansonia (Mansonioides) uniformis*
South-east Asia	**Aedes (Stegomyia) aegypti* *Aedes (Stegomyia) albopictus?* *Culex (Culex) gelidus* *Culex (Culex) quinquefasciatus* *Culex (Culex) tritaeniorhynchus*
Eastern equine encephalitis (EEE)	
North America	*Aedes (Aedimorphus) vexans* *Aedes (Ochlerotatus) atlanticus* *Aedes (Ochlerotatus) fulvius* *Aedes (Ochlerotatus) mitchellae* **Aedes (Ochlerotatus) sollicitans* *Aedes (Ochlerotatus) sticticus* **Aedes (Ochlerotatus) taeniorhynchus* *Anopheles (Anopheles) crucians* *Coquillettidia (Coquillettidia) perturbans* *Culex (Culex) nigripalpus* *Culex (Culex) quinquefasciatus* *Culex (Culex) restuans* *Culex (Culex) salinarius* **Culiseta (Climacura) melanura* **Culiseta (Culicella) morsitans*
South America	**Aedes (Ochlerotatus) taeniorhynchus* *Culex (Culex) nigripalpus* *Culex (Melanoconion) caudelli* *Culex (Melanoconion) spissipes* *Culex (Melanoconion) taeniopus*
Europe	*Culex (Culex) pipiens*
Everglades (EVE)	
Florida	*Aedes (Ocherotatus) taeniorhynchus* *Aedes (Ocherotatus) crucians* *Culex (Culex) nigripalpus* *Culex (Melanoconion) spp.*
Mayaro (MAY)	
South and Central America	*Culex spp.* **Haemagogus spp.* *Coquillettidia (Rhynchotaemia) venezuelensis* *Psorophora (Janthinosoma) ferox* *Sabethini spp.*
Mucambo (MUC)	
South America	*Aedes spp.* *Aedes (Ochlerotatus) serratus* *Culex spp.* **Culex (Melanoconion) portesi* *Haemagogus spp.* *Sabethini spp.* *Wyeomyia spp.*
O'nong-nyong (ONN)	
Africa	*Anopheles (Cellia) funestus* *Anopheles (Cellia) gambiae (sensu lato)*
Ross River (RR)	
Australasia	*Aedes (Ocherotatus) vigilax* *Culex (Culex) annulirostris*
Semliki Forest (SF)	
Africa	*Aedes (Aedimorphus) abnormalis group* *Aedes (Aedimorphus) argenteopunctatus* *Aedes (Aedimorphus) denatus* *Aedes (Neomelaniconion) palpalis* *Anopheles (Cellia) funestus* *Eretmapodites grahamii*
Sindbis (SIN)	
Africa	*Aedes (Aedimorphus) cumminsi* *Aedes (Neomelaniconion) circumluteolus* *Anopheles (Celia) pharoensis* *Coquillettidia (Coquillettidia) fuscopennata* **Culex (Culex) antennatus* **Culex (Culex) perexiguus* *Culex (Culex) pipiens (sensu lato)* **Culex (Culex) univittatus* *Mansonia (Mansonioides) africana*
Australasia	*Aedes (Ochlerotatus) normanensis* *Aedes (Ochlerotatus) vigilax* **Culex (Culex) annulirostris* *Mansonia (Mansonioides) septempunctata*
Orient	**Culex (Culex) bitaeniorhynchus* *Culex (Culex) pseudovishnui* **Culex (Culex) tritaeniorhynchus*
Venezuelan Equine Encephalitis (VEE)	
Tropical Americas about 40 species implicated, including:	*Aedes (Ochlerotatus) angustivittatus* *Aedes (Ochlerotatus) scapularis* **Aedes (Ochlerotatus) serratus* *Aedes (Ochlerotatus) sollicitans* **Aedes (Ochlerotatus) taeniorhynchus* *Aedes (Ochlerotatus) thelcter.* *Aedes (Stegomyia) aegypti* *Anopheles (Anopheles) aquasalis* *Anopheles (Anopheles) crucians* *Anopheles (Anopheles) neomaculipalpus* *Anopheles (Anopheles) pseudopunctipennis* *Anopheles (Anopheles) punctimacula* *Culex (Culex) corniger* *Culex (Culex) coronator* *Culex (Culex) nigripalpus* *Culex (Culex) tarsalis* **Culex (Melanoconion) spp.* *Culex (Melanoconion) iolambdis* *Culex (Melanoconion) acossa/panocossa* *Culex (Melanoconion) portesi* *Culex (Melanoconion) taeniopus* *Culex (Melanoconion) vomerifer* *Deinocerites pseudes* *Haemagogus spp.* *Limatus flavisetosus* *Mansonia (Mansonia) indubitans* *Mansonia (Mansonia) titillans* **Psorophora (Grabhamia) confinnis* *Psorophora (Grabhamia) discolor* *Psorophora (Janthinosoma) albipes* *Psorophora (Janthinosoma) cyanescens* **Psorophora (Psorophora) ciliate* *Psorophora (Psorophora) cilipes* *Sabethes spp. Wyeomyia spp.*

TABLE A4.7 **Important Mosquitoes and the Arboviruses They Transmit—cont'd**

Arbovirus And Endemic Area	Natural Vector (*Indicates Principal Species)
Western Equine Encephalitis (WEE)	
North and South America	Mainly Culex (Culex) tarsalis in western USA; Culiseta (Climacura) melanura in eastern USA; occasionally Aedes, Anopheles, Culex, Culiseta and Psorophora spp.
FLAVIVIRUS (GROUP B)	
Banzi (BAN)	
Africa	Culex (Culex) nakuruensis *Culex (Eumelanomyia) rubinotus Mansonia (Mansonioides) africana
Bussuquara (BSQ)	
South and Central America	Coquillettidia (Rhynchotaenia) venezuelensis *Culex (Melanoconion) spp. Culex (Melanoconion) epanatasis (crybda) Culex (Melanoconion) taeniopus Culex (Melanoconion) vomerifer Mansonia (Mansonia) titillans Trichoprosopon sp.
Dengue (DEN) Types 1–4	
between 40°N and 40°S	Aedes (Finlaya) niveus group Aedes (Stegomyia) spp. *Aedes (Stegomyia) albopictus Aedes (Stegomyia) polynesiensis Aedes (Stegomyia) scutellaris
Ilheus (ILH)	
South and Central America	Aedes (Ochlerotatus) angustivittatus Aedes (Ochlerotatus) Aedes (Ochlerotatus) scapularis fulvus Aedes (Ochlerotatus) serratus Aedes (Stegomyia) aegypti Coquillettidia spp. Culex (Culex) nigripalpus Culex (Culex) quinquefasciatus Culex (Melanoconion) spp. Culex (Melanoconion) caudelli Culex (Melanoconion) spissipes Culex (Melanoconion) taeniopus Haemagogus (Conopostegus) leucocelaenus Hemagogus (Haemagogus) janthinomys (falco) Psorophora (Janthinosoma) albipes *Psorophora (Janthinosoma) ferox Psorophora (Janthinosoma) lutzii Sabethes (Sabethoides) chloropterus Trichoprosopon sp. Wyeomyia sp.
Japanese Encephalitis (JE)	
South-east Asia to India and Japan and former USSR	Aedes (Aedimorphus) vexans Aedes (Cancraedes) curtipes Aedes (Finlaya) koreicus Aedes (Finlaya) togoi Anopheles (Anopheles) barbirostris group Culex (Culex) bitaeniorhynchus group Culex (Culex) epidesmus Culex (Culex) gelidus Culex (Culex) pipiens group Culex (Culex) pseudovishnui *Culex (Culex) tritaeniorhynchus Culex (Culex) vishnui (annulus) Culex (Culex) whitmorei
Kunjin (KUN)	
Borneo, Australia	*Culex (Culex) annulirostris Culex (Culex) pseudovishnui Culex (Culex) squamosus
Murray Valley Encephalitis (MVE)	
Australasia	Aedes (Ochlerotatus) normanensis *Culex (Culex) annulirostris Culex (Culex) bitaeniorhynchus
Septik (SEP)	
Australasia	Armigeres sp. Mansonia (Mansonioides) septempunctata Mimomyia (Mimomyia) flavens
Spondweni (SPO)	
Africa	Aedes (Aedimorphus) cumminsi Aedes (Aedimorphus) fowleri? *Aedes (Neomelaniconion) circumluteolus Aedes (Ochlerotatus) fryeri? Culex (Culex) univittatus Eretmapodites spp. Eretmapodites silvestris Mansonia (Mansonioides) africana Mansonia (Mansonioides) uniformis
St Louis Encephalitis (SLE)	
North America	Aedes (Ochlerotatus) dorsalis/melanimon Aedes (Ochlerotatus) scapularis Aedes (Ochlerotatus) serratus Anopheles (Anopheles) crucians *Culex (Culex) nigripalpus Culex (Culex) peus *Culex (Culex) pipiens *Culex (Culex) quinquefasciatus Culex (Culex) restuans Culex (Culex) salinarius Culex (Culex) tarsalis *Culex (Culex) pipiens *Culex (Culex) quinquefasciatus Culex (Culex) restuans Culex (Culex) salinarius Culex (Culex) tarsalis
South America	*Culex (Culex) coronator Culex (Culex) declarator (as virgultus) Culex (Culex) nigripalpus Culex (Melanoconion) candelli Culex (Melanoconion) spissipes Culex (Melanoconion) taeniopus Psorophora (Janthinosoma) ferox Sabethes (Sabethes) belisarioi Sabethes (Sabethoides) chloropterus Trichoprosopon sp. Wyeomyia sp.
Wesselsbron (WSL)	
Africa	Aedes (Aedimorphus) hisutus Aedes (Aedimorphus) minutus Aedes (Aedimorphus) tarsalis group Aedes (Neomelaniconion) spp. Aedes (Neomelaniconion) circumluteolus Aedes (Neomelaniconion) lineatopennis Aedes (Ochlerotatus) caballus Anopheles (Cellia) gambiae (sensu lato) Anopheles (Cellia) pharoensis Culex (Culex) telesilla Culex (Culex) univittatus Mansonia (Mansonioides) uniformis

Continued on following page

TABLE A4.7 Important Mosquitoes and the Arboviruses They Transmit—cont'd

Arbovirus And Endemic Area	Natural Vector (*Indicates Principal Species)
Thailand	*Aedes (Aedimorphus) mediolineatus* *Aedes (Neomelaniconion) lineatopennis*
West Nile (WN)	
Africa	*Coquillettidia (Coquillettidia) metallica* *Culex (Culex) theileri* **Culex (Culex) univittatus* *Culex (Culex) weschei*
Europe	*Culex (Barraudius) modestus*
Middle East	*Anopheles (Anopheles) coustani* *Culex (Culex) antennatus* *Culex (Culex) perexiguus (as univittatus)* *Culex (Culex) pipiens group*
Asia	*Anopheles (Cellia) subpictus* *Culex (Culex) quinquefasciatus* *Culex (Culex) tritaeniorhynchus* *Culex (Culex) vishnui group*
Yellow Fever (YF)	
Africa	*Aedes (Aedimorphus) vittatus* *Aedes (Diceromyia) taylori* **Aedes (Stegomyia) aegypti* **Aedes (Stegomyia) africanus* *Aedes (Stegomyia) luteocephalus* *Aedes (Stegomyia) metallicus* **Aedes (Stegomyia) simpsoni*
South and Central America	**Aedes (Stegomyia) aegypti* *Haemagogus (Conopostegus) leucocelaenus* *Haemagogus (Haemagogus) janthinomys (falco)* **Haemagogus (Haemagogus) spegazzinni* *Sabethes (Sabethoides) chloropterus*
Zika (ZIKA)	
Africa	*Aedes (Stegomyia) luteocephalus* *Aedes (Stegomyia) aegypti*
Malaysia	**Aedes (Stegomyia) africanus*
Bunyaviridae (Bunyavirus)	
BUNYAMWERA GROUP	
Bunyamwera (BUN)	
Africa	**Aedes (Neomelaniconion) circumluteolus* *Aedes (Skusea) pembaensis* *Culex* spp. *Mansonia (Mansonioides) africana* *Mansonia (Mansonioides) uniformis*
Calovo (CVO)	
Europe	*Anopheles (Anopheles) maculipennis (sensu lato)* *Coquillettidia (Coquillettidia) richiardii*
Germiston (GER)	
Africa	*Aedes (Neomelaniconion) circumluteolus* *Anopheles (Cellia) arabiensis* *Anopheles (Cellia) funestus* *Culex (Culex) theileri?* **Culex (Eumelanomyia) rubinotus*
Guaroa (GRO)	
South America	*Anopheles (Kerteszia) neivai*
Ilesha (ILE)	
Africa	*Anopheles (Cellia) gambiae (sensu lato)* *Mansonia (Mansonioides) uniformis*
Tensaw (TEN)	
South-east USA	*Aedes (Ochlerotatus) atlanticus* *Aedes (Ochelerotatus) infirmatus* *Aedes (Ochelerotatus) mitchellae* **Anopheles (Anopheles) crucians* *Anopheles (Anopheles) punctipennis* *(Anopheles) quadrimaculatus* *Coquillettidia (Coquillettidia) perturbans* *Culex (Culex) nigripalpus* *Culex (Culex) salinarius*
Wyeomyia (WYO)	
South and Central America	*Aedes (Howardina) septemstriatus* *Aedes (Howardina) sexlineatus* *Aedes (Ochlerotatus) fulvus* *Aedes (Ochlerotatus) scapularis* *Aedes (Ochlerotatus) serratus* *Aedes (Protomacleaya) argyrothorax* *Anopheles* spp. *Anopheles (Stethomyia) nimbus* *Coquillettidia (Rhynchotaemia) arribalzagae* *Culex (Aedinus) amazonensis* *Culex (Culex) nigripalpus* *Haemagogous (Conopostegus) leucocelaenus* *Limatus durhamii* *Limatus flavisetosus* *Psorophora (Grabhamia) cingulata* *Psorophora (Janthinosoma) albipes* *Psorophora (Janthinosoma) ferox* *Trichoprosopon (Runchomyia) leucopus* *Trichoprosopon (Runchomyia) longipes* *Trichoprosopon (Trichoprosopon) digitatum* *Wyeomyia (Dendromyia) aporonoma* *Wyeomyia (Dendromyia) complosa* *Wyeomyia (Dendromyia) melanocephala*
BWAMBA GROUP	
Bwamba (BWA)	
Africa	*Anopheles (Cellia) funestus* *Anopheles (Cellia) gambiae (sensu lato)*
C GROUP	
Apeu (APEU)	
Brazil	*Aedes (Howardina) arborealis* *Aedes (Howardina) septemstriatus* *Aedes (Ochlerotatus) serratus* *Culex (Melanoconion) acossa/panocossa (aikenii)*
Caraparu (CAR)	
South America	*Culex (Melanoconion)*spp. *Culex (Melanoconion) caudelli* **Culex (Melanoconion) portesi* *Culex (Melanoconion) spissipes* *Culex (Melanoconion) vomerifer* *Limatus durhamii* *Wyeomyia* sp.
Itaqui (ITQ)	
Brazil	*Culex (Melanoconion)* spp. *Culex (Melanoconion) portesi* *Culex (Melanoconion) vomerifer*
Madrid (MAD)	
Panama	*Culex (Melanoconion) vomerifer*
Marituba (MTB)	
Brazil	*Culex (Melanoconion) ocossa/panocossa (aikenii)* *Culex (Melanoconion) portesi*

TABLE A4.7 Important Mosquitoes and the Arboviruses They Transmit—cont'd

Arbovirus And Endemic Area	Natural Vector (*Indicates Principal Species)
Murutucu (MUR)	
South America	Coquillettidia (Rhychotaenia) venezuelensis Culex (Melanoconion) ocossa/panocossa (aikenii) Culex (Melanoconion) portesi other Culex spp. and Sabethini
Oriboca (ORI)	
South America	Aedes spp. Aedes (Ochlerotatus) taeniorhynchus Culex spp. Culex (Melanoconion) portesi Mansonia spp. Psorophora (Janthinosoma) ferox Sabethini
Ossa (OSSA)	
Panama	Culex (Melanoconion) taeniopus Culex (Melanoconion) vomerifer Restam (RES)
South America	Culex (Melanoconion) portesi
CALIFORNIA GROUP	
California Encephalitis (CE)	
South-western USA	Aedes (Aedimorphus) vexans *Aedes (Ochlerotatus) dorsalis *Aedes (Ochlerotatus) melanimon Aedes (Ochlerotatus) nigromaculis Anopheles (Anopheles) pseudopunctipennis Culex (Culex) tarsalis Culiseta (Culex) inornata Psorophora (Grabhamia) signipennis
Inkoo (INK)	
Finland	Aedes (Ochlerotatus) communis/punctor
La Crosse (LAC)	
USA	Aedes (Ochlerotatus) canadensis Aedes (Ochlerotatus) communis Aedes (Promacleaya) triseriatus Culex (Culex) pipiens
Melao (MEL)	
South America	Aedes (Ochlerotatus) scapularis Aedes (Ochlerotatus) serratus Psorophora (Janthinosoma) ferox
Tahyna (TAH)	
Africa Europe	Aedes (Skusea) pembaensis *Aedes (Aedimorphus) vexans Aedes (Ochlerotatus) cantans Aedes (Ochlerotatus) caspius Aedes (Ochlerotatus) cinereus Anopheles (Anopheles) hyrcanus (sensu lato) Anopheles (Anopheles) maculipennis (sensu lato) Culex (Barraudius) modestus Culex (Culex) pipiens (sensu lato) Caliseta (Culiseta) annulata
GUAMA GROUP	
Catu (CATU)	
South America	Anopheles (Stethomyia) nimbus Coquillettidia (Rhynchotaemia) venezuelensis Culex (Aedinus) majuensis Culex (Culex) declarator (virgultus) *Culex (Melanoconion) portesi Culex (Melanoconion) vomerifer
Guama (GAM)	
South and Central America	Aedes (Howardina) sexlineatus Coquillettidia (Rhynchotaenia) venezuelensis Culex (Aedinus) mojuensis Culex (Melanoconion) spp. Culex (Melanoconion) epanatasis (crybda) *Culex (Melanoconion) portesi Culex (Melanoconion) spissipes Culex (Melanoconion) taeniopus Culex (melanoconion) vomerifer Culex (Tinolestes) spp. Limatus durhamii Wyeomyia sp.
NYANDO GROUP	
Nyando (NDO)	
Africa	Anopheles (Cellia) funestus
SIMBUGROUP	
Oropouche (ORO)	
South America	Mainly Ceratopogonidae Aedes (Ochlerotatus) serratus Coquillettidia (Rhynchotaenia) venezuelensis Culex (Culex) quinquefasciatus
Shuni (SHU)	
South Africa	Culex (Culex) theileri
PHLEBOTOMUS FEVER GROUP	
Chagres (CHG)	
Panama	Sabethes (Sabethoides) chloropterus and phlebotomine sandflies
Rift Valley Fever (RVT)	
Africa	Aedes (Aedimorphus) dentatus Aedes (Aedimorphus) tarsalis Aedes (Aedimorphus) triseriatus Aedes (Neomelaniconion) circumluteolus Aedes (Neomelaniconion) lineatopennis *Aedes (Ochlerotatus) caballus Aedes (Ochlerotatus) juppi Aedes (Stegomyia) deboeri Aedes (Stegomyia) aegypti Aedes (Stegomyia) africanus Aedes (Stegomyia) dendrophilus Anopheles (Anopheles) coustani Coquillettidia (Coquillettidia) fuscopennata Coquillettidia (Coquillettidia) microbannulata Coquillettidia (Coquillettidia) versicolor Culex (Culex) neavei *Culex (Culex) pipiens (sensu lato) *Culex (Culex) theileri Culex (Culex) univattatus Culex (Culex) zombaensis Eretmapodites chrysogaster group Mansonia (Mansonioides) africana Mansonia (Mansonioides) uniformis?
GANJAM GROUP	
Gamjam (GAN)	
India	Culex (Culex) vishnui group and ticks (Ixodidae)

Continued on following page

TABLE A4.7 Important Mosquitoes and the Arboviruses They Transmit—cont'd

Arbovirus And Endemic Area	Natural Vector (*Indicates Principal Species)	Arbovirus And Endemic Area	Natural Vector (*Indicates Principal Species)
***ANOPHELES* A GROUP**		**Poxviridae**	
Tataguine (TAT)		Cotia (COT)	
Africa	*Anopheles (Cellia) funestus* *Anopheles (Cellia) gambiae (sensu lato)*	South America	*Aedes (Ochlerotatus) serratus* *Coquillettidia (Rhynchotaenia) venezuelensis* *Culex (Melanoconion) portesi* *Limatus pseudomethysticus* *Psorophora (Janthinosoma) ferox*
UNGROUPED			
Zinga (ZGA)			
Africa	*Aedes (Neomelaniconion) palpalis* group *Mansonia (Mansonioides)africana*		

Tribe Culicini. The genus *Culex* contains 800 species within 21 subgenera, which are mainly night-biting. Many species acting as vectors of enzootic arboviruses, protozoa and filariae (Figure A4.37).[25] Japanese encephalitis virus is transmitted mainly by *Culex* spp. in the Oriental region. *C. theileri* in southern Africa and members of the *C. pipiens* complex in Egypt are important vectors of Rift Valley fever virus from livestock to humans and bancroftian filariases transmission. Eastern and western equine and St Louis encephalitis viruses in America are transmitted by *C. nigripalpus*, *C. pipiens*, *C. restuans* and other mosquitoes that occasionally pass infection to humans as dead-end hosts. *C. pipiens* serves the same function for Eastern equine encephalitis virus in Europe (Figure A4.38).

Tribe Culisetini. The genus *Culiseta* has 35 species, most of which are harmless. However, in North America, both eastern and western equine encephalitis circulate among birds through *Culiseta inornata*, *C. melanura* and *C. morsitans*. The latter may also be involved as a vector in Old World situations.

Tribe Mansoniini. The genus *Coquillettidi*, with 55 species, occurs on all continents. *C. perturbans* in North America and *C. venezuelensis* in South America are some of the most important pests and the latter has been implicated as a vector of several arboviruses (see Table A4.7, Figure A4.21). *Mansonia* is also in the tribe (Figures A4.39–A4.41); *M. titillans* is an important vector of Venezuelan equine encephalitis and may contribute to transmission of *W. bancrofti*. Other species of *Mansonia* are important vectors of *brugian filariasis* (Table A4.6).

Tribe Sabethini. Mosquitoes in the genus *Sabethes* live in forested areas and transmit yellow fever and other arboviruses in South America (a common vector is *S. chloropterus*).

Tribe Toxorynchitini. The 60 species of *Toxorhynchites* are the largest mosquitoes, but they do not suck blood. They are container breeders and their larvae are important predators on dangerous culicinae (namely *Aedes aegypti*), therefore they can be considered beneficial to human health.

Family Ceratopogonidae. Biting midges, belonging to the family Ceratopogonidae, are very small (1–4 mm), compact flies. Larvae live in wet or moist habitats: ranging from decomposing vegetation, bovine faeces, to fresh or brackish water or mud. Females suck blood and can attack in huge numbers- they can elicit a prolonged reaction in sensitive individuals. Males only feed on plant sugars.

Biting midges are found worldwide in a variety of habitats. There are over 6000 species in 60 genera: but only three contain species of medical importance. Species of *Leptoconops* and *Forcipomyia* are biting pests. *Culicoides* species can spread nematodes and virus of veterinary importance and are vectors of *Mansonella* spp. in humans (Figure A4.42). *Culicoides* transmit *M. perstans* (Africa) and *M. ozzardi* (Caribbean and Central America). Viruses (i.e. *Oropouche* virus, Japanese B encephalitis, Dugbe viruses and others) have been isolated from ceratopogonoids, but it is not thought that these midges transmit these viruses.

Family Simuliidae. The Simuliidae, usually known as blackflies, are small robust flies (1–5 mm long) (Figure A4.43).[49] Females lay their eggs in running (oxygenated) water, in masses of 300–500. The eggs hatch in 1–2 days and emerge larvae attach to substrate in the water column- species often have specific niches on stones, leaves, etc. There are six to eight larval instars, ending in 1–2 weeks or more. Before pupation, the larva spins a tent-like, silken cocoon. The pupal period is 2–10 days.

Although they are abundant in tropical areas, blackflies occur in especially large numbers in late spring and early summer in northern countries and are abundant in the north temperate and subarctic zones. Female adults suck blood during the daytime, but do not enter houses. Because of the shear population size, they can be a severe biting nuisance but they also are intermediate hosts for filariae and blood-borne protozoa of birds and mammals.

Onchocerciasis, caused by *O. volvulus*, is transmitted to humans in Africa, Central America and South America by members of Simuliidae. The *Simulium damnosum* and *S. neavei* complexes are African groups with sibling species that have been separated into a number of different species by biological and chromosome studies.[1] More importantly, these species differ in their ecology (breeding, adult habitat choice) and feeding preferences, affecting transmission of onchocerciasis. The *S. damnosum* complex (jinja fly) contains at least 40 sibling species found in habitats ranging from savannah to forest. Species vector only *O. volvus* strains endemic to their ecozones. Despite larvicide control efforts, onchocerciasis control has been made very difficult by the long flight capabilities of females (200–400 km). The *S. neavei* complex is confined to small streams in hilly forest and have a much smaller flight range. Eradication of *S. neavei* has been much more successful. In the Americas, the main vectors are as follows: *S. ochraceum* complex (Mexico and Guatemala), *S. metallicum* (Venezuela), *S. exiguum* (Colombian Andes) and *S. guyanense*, *S. limbatum* and *S.*

oyapockense (Brazilian and Venezuelan Amazonia). Minor vectors include *S. metallicum* and *S. callidum* in Central America.

Family Tabanidae. Tabanidae contains the largest species of hematophagous flies, with wingspans greater than 60 mm (Figure A4.44). Only females bite and, because of their large size, they take a large blood meal, from 20 to 200 mg. The mouthparts are short and stout; they project downwards below the head and inflict a painful bite. There are about 3000 species of Tabanidae, in numerous genera, but medically important species occur only in the genera *Tabanus*, *Haematopota* (subfamily Tabaninae) and *Chrysops* (subfamily Chrysopsinae) (Figures A4.45, A4.46). Aside from a significant biting nuisance, Tabanidae species can transmit tularemia, loaiasis, anthrax, viruses and more pathogens to humans (Table A4.9, Figure A4.47). They are also important vectors for many animal diseases (Table A4.10) and can be such a nuisance to drive migration.

Family Glossinidae. The genus *Glossina* contains about 30 species and subspecies of tsetse flies (Figures A4.48–A4.51). Like higher insects, *Glossina* undergo viviparous reproduction: a single larva is produced at a time and nourished within the female for 8–12 days. Females usually mate only once and store sufficient viable sperm throughout its 2–3 month life span, producing up to 20 larvae. The mother extrudes larvae when they are a third instar and larvae burrow into shady, moist soil to pupate. After emerging, unfed flies (known as teneral flies) enter a quiescent period and then seek their first blood meal. Both sexes feed on vertebrate blood at intervals of 3–4 days, sometimes less and hunt their hosts by sight and scent. Species that feed on humans actively feed during daylight, with activity decreasing during overcast weather. Resting places are in woody elements of vegetation with a good field of view. Males have a much shorter lifespan than females (Figures A4.52, A4.53).[54] The scissor-like folding of the wings over the back of the resting fly is a very characteristic feature of *Glossina* (Figure A4.54).

The range of tsetse flies is restricted to the African continent between 15°N and 30°S (Figure A4. 55). Modern taxonomists usually divide the genus into three species groups (sometimes given subgeneric status) as follows: the *fusca* group (subgenus *Austenina*), the *palpalis* group (subgenus *Nemorhina*) and the *morsitans* group (subgenus *Glossina*) (Table A4.11).[52,53] This taxonomic separation is reflected in the ecological requirements and distribution of the species included in each group. Flies of the fusca group are associated with dense humid tropical forest or forest edges. Members of the palpalis group are dependent on more or less dense riverine or lacustrine vegetation but their distribution extends into savannah zones well away from forested, or formerly forested, areas. Species of the morsitans group are the least hydrophilic and occupy vast areas of bushland and thicket vegetation often far from lakes and rivers.

Glossina species are intermediate hosts for African trypanosomes (Chapter 45). Infective metacyclic trypanosomes of the *Trypanosoma brucei* subgroup are found in the salivary glands of the tsetse fly.[51,55,56] To reach their final station in the glands, trypanosomes undergo a complex migration in the fly that takes nearly 3 weeks to complete; hence only flies >3 weeks old can be infected with trypanosomes infective to humans (Table A4.12). Even among older flies, infection rates with the *T. brucei*

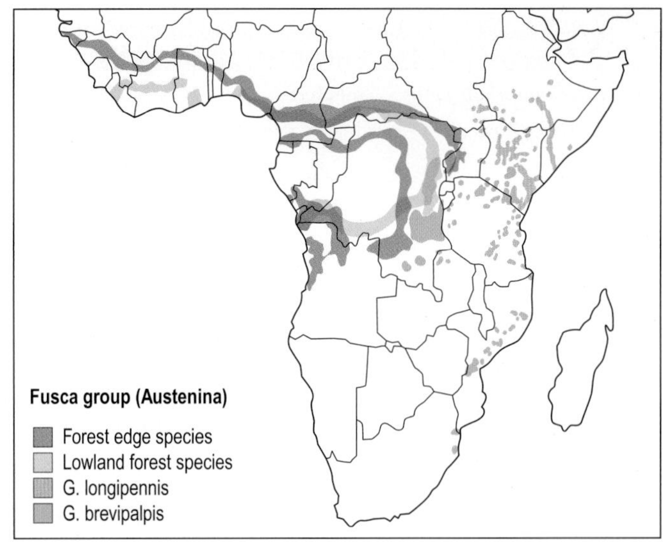

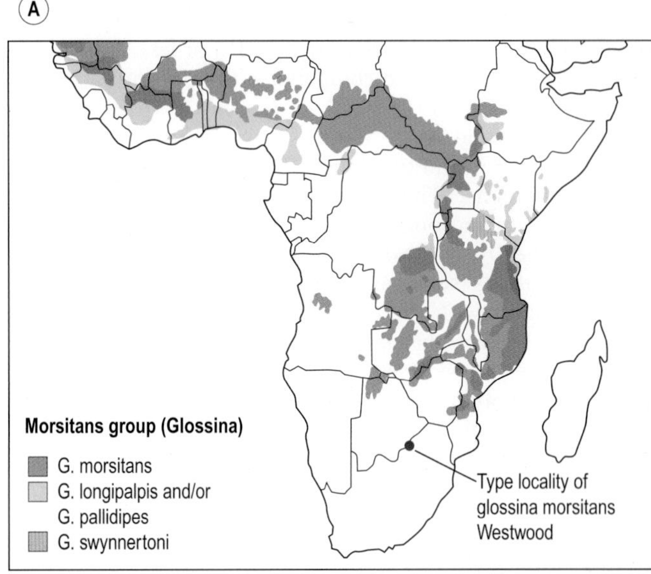

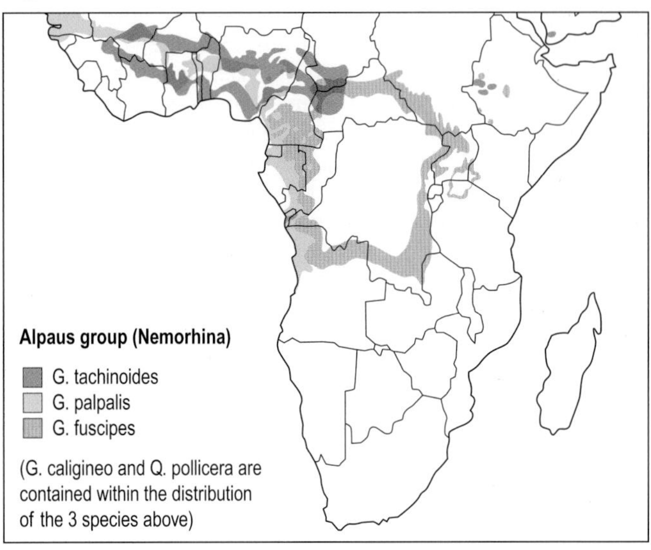

Figure A4.55 Distribution of the important species of *Glossina*. (A) *fusca* group; (B) *palpalis* group; (C) *moristans* group (see also Chapter 45).

TABLE A4.11 Biotype, Distribution and Medical Importance of *Glossina*

Species Group/Subgenus	Habitat Type	Distribution	Species of Medical Importance
Fusca group (*Austenina*)	Mainly rainforest areas	Chiefly forest areas of West and Central Africa; Relict species in dry areas of East Africa	None. But several vectors of livestock trypanosomiasis
Palpalis group (*Nemorhina*)	Mainly linear: shores of lakes and rivers in forested or formerly forested areas	15°N to 12°S, approx.; 17°W to 40°E, approx. 10°N to 12°S, approx.; 10°E to 40°E, approx. 12°N to 4°N, approx.; 12°W to 40°E, approx.	*G. palpalis*, vector of *T. brucei gambiense* in West Africa *G. fuscipes* (and subspecies), vectors of *T. brucei gambiense* (West Africa, Central Africa) and *T. brucei rhodesiense* (East Africa) *G. tachinoides*, vector of *T. b. gambiense* in West Africa and of *T. b. rhodesiense* in South-west Ethiopia
Morsitans group (*Glossina*)	'Game' tsetse of the savannah zones; open woodland ('miombo'), bushland and thicket	15°N to 20°S, approx.; 17°W to 45°E, approx. 8°N to 20°S, approx.; 25°E to 48°E approx. Limited area south-east of Lake Victoria; mainly in Tanzania	*G. morsitans* (and subspecies), vectors of *T. b. rhodesiense* in East and South-east Africa *G. pallidipes*, vector of *T. b. rhodesiense* in East Africa *G. swynnertoni*, vector of *T. b. rhodesiense*

subgroup are always low (commonly 0.1% or less, rarely more than 1%), especially when compared with infection rates with the *T. vivax* (*Duttonella*) and *T. congolense* (*Nannomonas*) groups in the same flies.

Tsetse flies transmit trypanosomiasis to a variety of animals, including humans.[50] Flies of the fusca group include important vectors of trypanosomes pathogenic to livestock, especially species of the *Trypanosoma vivax* (subgenus *Duttonella*) and *T. congolense* groups (subgenus *Nannomonas*), but they have never been associated with the transmission of trypanosomiasis to humans. *T. brucei gambiense* and *T. b. rhodienese* cause chronic and acute sleeping sickness, respectively. Several species within the moritans and palpalis group are responsible for the transmission of these pathogens (Table A4.10). Exposure to *T. b. rhodesiense* strains is largely occupational: hunters, honey-gatherers, pole-cutters and charcoal-burners are among groups likely to enter fly-infested bush.

Order Hemiptera

Family Cimicidae. Bed-bugs have a worldwide distribution with over 70 species. All are wingless and dorsoventrally flattened. They are large, about 1 mm in diameter, yellowish-white and easily visible to the naked eye. The females deposit eggs in daily batches from 10 to 50, totaling 200–500 over their lifetime. The five successive nymphal stages resemble adults, but have no hemielytra; they mature in about 6 weeks if fed at each stage, but can resist starvation for up to 2 months. Under less favourable conditions, development may be protracted for 6 months or more. Adults may live for many months. Bed-bugs are sensitive to high temperatures: even 37.8°C with a fairly high humidity will kill many. The mouthparts consist externally of a segmented rostrum (proboscis) and are normally folded back under the head. The maxillae are serrated at the tip. On the thorax of the adults are short pad-like hemielytra, which are vestigial forewings. Both sexes of *Cimex* feed only on blood and can resist starvation well. Bed-bugs are nocturnal in their feeding habits, hiding in crevices during the daytime.

The species parasitic on humans are: *Cimex lectularius*, the cosmopolitan bed-bug and *C. hemipterus* (*rotundatus*), the common bed-bug of the tropics, which is distinguished by its elongated narrow abdomen and the shape and proportion of the thorax (Figure A4.56). In West Africa, a species of another genus, *Leptocimex boueti*, attacks humans. Although bed-bugs can cause a great deal of irritation by their bites, it has not actually been proved that they disseminate disease, with the possible exception of viral hepatitis (see Chapter 13).

Family Reduviidae. The family includes insect predators, but all the haematophagous species of medical importance are within the subfamily Triatominae (Table A4.13, Figure A4. 57). Female *triatomines* commence egg laying 10–30 days after copulation; eggs are laid singly or in small groups, either unattached or cemented to the substrate, depending on species. The number of eggs laid in life by a female depends upon species and external factors, but about 500 is normal and 1000 not uncommon. Eggs hatch after 10–30 days; the emerging first-stage nymph is initially pink and soft-bodied but hardens sufficiently to take its first blood meal within 48–72 h of leaving the egg. At least one full blood meal is required by each nymphal stage, sometimes more, before the molt to the next stage can be initiated. Their blood meals are very large relative to their own body weight: first stage nymphs can take up 10 times their own body weight. All stages of triatomines, in particular the larger nymphal stages, have a remarkable ability to endure long periods of starvation (up to several months). The adults are in general poor fliers and probably take flight only when their nutritional status is poor and their weight lowest, to disperse at random to seek new habitats with new hosts on which to feed. All triatomines have a long life cycle, even in hot climates; the average is about 300 days from egg to adult, although some species may take up to 2 years.

The bulk of the Triatominae (four of the five tribes) occur exclusively in the neotropical region: the Rhodniini (the important genus *Rhodnius* and the genus *Psammolestes*) are found from Central America to Argentina.

All triatomines are dependent on the blood of vertebrates (principally mammals and birds, occasionally reptiles) for survival, development and reproduction.[58] The primary habitat of triatomines is thus in or near the shelters, roosts, burrows and nests of a variety of wild animals, prominent amongst which are marsupials (e.g. *Didelphis* (Figure A4.58), *Marmosa*), edentates (e.g. *Dasypus*), rodents (*Rattus*, *Neotoma*), carnivores, bats and birds. Many of the animals and birds find their main shelter in palm fronds or in arboreal epiphytic bromeliads under fallen logs or in hollow trees (Figures A4.59, A4.60). Triatomines do not seem to have host preferences and are more governed by proximity to suitable hosts. Some species have the ability to colonize human settlements. Species such as *Rhodnius prolixus* or *Triatoma infestans* thrive in areas of poverty, where they live in houses made from local materials- hiding during the day in dark moist places and emerging at night to feed on humans (Figures A4.61, A4.62).

Triatomines are important in the epizootiology and epidemiology of an important neglected tropical disease, Chagas' disease, caused by *Trypanosoma cruzi* (Chapter 46). Although all triatomines can probably support the development of *Trypanosoma cruzi* (well over half the species have been found infected in the wild), only a few species have the capacity to colonize human dwellings and have overriding medical importance as the domiciliary vectors of Chagas' disease to humans. *T. cruzi* is transmitted through the faeces of a triatomine; it is an inefficient transmission method because high levels of trypanosomes are necessary and the faeces must contaminate the bite wound (Figure A4.63). By virtue of their wide geographical distribution and large domiciliary populations, together with the large human population in the areas they occupy, the three species *Rhodnius prolixus*, *Triatoma infestans* and *Panstrongylus megistus* are of prime importance (Figures A4.64–A4.66). Other species of the same three genera (particularly *Triatoma* spp. and especially *T. dimidiata*) are of considerable importance on a smaller geographical scale (e.g. *T. dimidiata*, *T. barberi*, *T. brasiliensis*, *T. pallidipennis*, *T. phyllosoma*, *R. pallescens* and *R. ecuadorensis*).

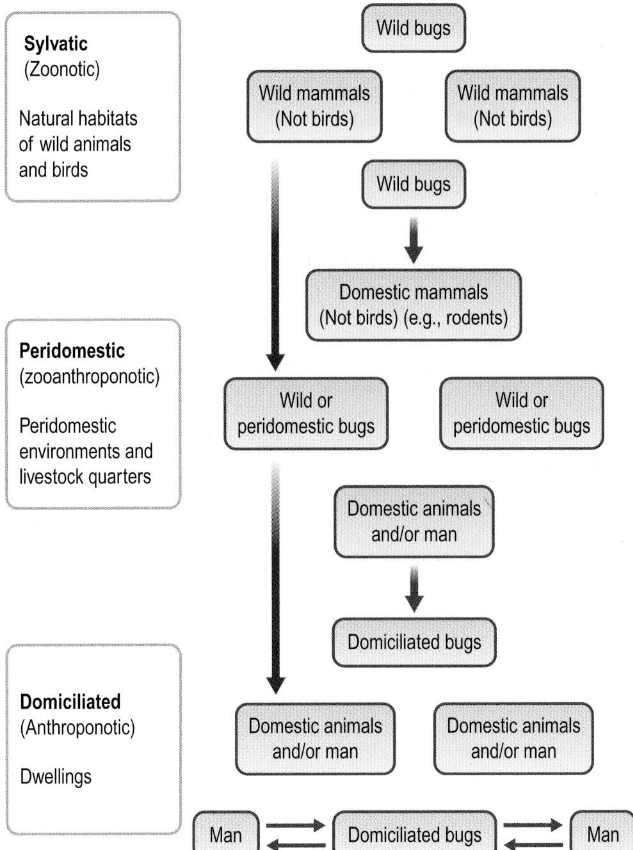

Figure A4.63 Transmission cycles of bug-mediated *Trypanosoma cruzi* infection.

Order Siphonaptera

Fleas are small (1–4 mm) and wingless, with laterally compressed bodies composed of a blunt head, compact thorax and a relatively large rounded abdomen (Figure A4.67).[59,60] All three pairs of legs are strongly developed, allowing fleas jump to several meters in height to reach hosts or evade capture. The period of development from egg to pupa is 2 weeks or more, depending on temperature (Figure A4.68). The active white larvae have sparse hairs and develop in nests of hosts or indoors among fabrics or between floorboards. There are two larval instars before the pupal stage. Hatching of the adult may be delayed for months until the proximity of a host (vibration, warmth) stimulates emergence. Adult fleas can survive actively and away from the host for many weeks, provided that the climate is not too harsh. In general fleas thrive at temperatures of 20–30°C and humidity of 60–90%.

Adult fleas of all species are obligate, temporary ectoparasites of birds (6%) or of mammals (94% of flea species). More than 2000 species of flea have been described and are classified into some 200 genera. They are moderately host-specific, meaning that each kind of flea tends to infest only one or a few kinds of host. Humans are frequently attacked by fleas from domestic or wild animals, as well as by the human flea *Pulex irritans*.

People suffer localized dermal reactions to flea bites and generalized allergic sensitization is not uncommon. Both sexes feed regularly on blood and so become liable to transmit pathogens from host to host. Various flea species may be involved in the transmission cycles of tularaemia, brucellosis, lymphocytic choriomeningitis and possibly other diseases. Murine typhus, the causative agent *Rickettsia typhi*, depends on fleas as vectors. Some fleas also serve as the intermediate hosts for tapeworms found in animals: *Dipylidium caninum* of dogs and cats; *Hymenolepis diminuta* of rodents; *H. nana* strains endemic in rodents. These occasionally cause diarrhoea in humans, especially children who may have eaten infected fleas.

More than 50 genera and numerous species of fleas have been implicated as vectors of enzootic plague in various parts of the world, meaning that they maintain the transmission of *Yersinia pestis* bacilli among rodents. Plague vectors, such as *Xenopsylla* spp., have large proventricular spines on which plague bacilli accumulate and multiply, tending to promote thrombus formation and blocking of the proventriculus. Bacilli may then be regurgitated when the flea next tries to feed, so that transmission to another host occurs. Humans are seldom infected primarily through the bites of zoophilic fleas, except when infected *Xenopsylla* move on to a human after plague-stricken rats have died (Chapter 33). Rarely are conditions conducive for person-to-person transmission by *Pulex* or *Ctenocephalides* to reach epidemic proportions.

Family Pulicidae. The members of this family, being fleas without ctenidia (combs), include several species of medical importance both as pests and as disease vectors. *Pulex irritans*, the human flea, is a ubiquitous pest of humans, prevailing in many temperate and tropical situations. Occasionally suspected of bubonic plague transmission from human to human,

P. irritans is definitely the vector responsible for vesicular and tonsillar plague outbreaks in Ecuador. Five other *Pulex* spp. are known, of which *P. simulans* also sometimes attacks humans in North and South America.

Xenopsylla cheopis, the oriental or black rat flea, normally infests *Rattus rattus* in urban situations throughout the world, but is scarce in parts of the northern temperature zone (Figure A4.69). It frequently attacks people in rat-infested buildings and is the classical vector of epidemic plague (*Yersinia pestis*) and of murine typhus (*Rickettsia mooseri*) from rat to rat and from rat to human. Other *Xenopsylla* species fulfill similar roles regionally, notably *X. brasiliensis* (India and South America) and *X. astia* (India).

Echidnophaga gallinacea, the sticktight flea of poultry, sometimes also infests dogs, cats, rabbits and other animals and can be a nuisance to people. Ctenocephalides is a small genus of nine species found mainly on carnivores in Africa and Eurasia, with two species that have become generally distributed: *C. canis* and *C. felis*, the dog and cat flea, respectively (Figure A4.70). Each of these species actually infests both cats and dogs interchangeably and *C. felis* tends to be found more often on both kinds of host. In modern centrally heated homes in temperate countries, *C. canis* and *C. felis* often thrive, sometimes in the temporary absence of cats and dogs and can transmit tapeworm.

Family Leptopsyllidae. *Leptopsylla segnis*, the European mouse flea, is frequently found indoors in various parts of the world. It also infests rats and sometimes transmits enzootic plague, but seldom bites humans.

Family Ceratophyllidae. *Ceratophyllus gallinae*, the European chicken flea, has spread to many parts of the world, has a wide range of bird hosts and occasionally invades houses and attacks people. It is a particularly large flea with a painful bite. *Nosopsyllus fasciatus*, the brown rat flea, has also become widespread with its main host *Rattus norvegicus*. Like *Ctenocephalides*, *N. fasciatus* serves as an intermediate host of the dog tapeworm, *D. caninum*.

Family Hectopsyllidae. *Tunga penetrans*, the sand flea or jigger (chigoe, chique), has females adapted for intracutaneous permanent attachment on the host (Chapter 60). *T. penetrans* regularly infects humans, pigs, poultry and other creatures in Central America, West and East Africa and parts of the Indian subcontinent.

BIBLIOGRAPHY

1. Eldridge BF, Edman JD, editors. Medical Entomology: A Textbook on Public Health and Veterinary Problems. Dordrecht: Kluwer Academic; 2003.
9. Sinka ME, Rubio-Palis Y, Manguin S, et al. The dominant Anopheles vectors of human malaria in the Americas: occurrence data, distribution maps and bionomic précis. Parasit Vectors 2010;3:72.
10. Sinka ME, Bangs MJ, Manguin S, et al. The dominant Anopheles vectors of human malaria in Africa, Europe and the Middle East: occurrence data, distribution maps and bionomic précis. Parasit Vectors 2010;3:117.
11. Sinka ME, Bangs MJ, Manguin S, et al. The dominant Anopheles vectors of human malaria in the Asia-Pacific region: occurrence data, distribution maps and bionomic précis. Parasit Vectors 2011;4:89.
13. Knight LL, Stone A. A Catalog of the Mosquitoes of the World. The Thomas Say Foundation. Vol. VI. College Park: Entomological Society of America; 1977(Suppl 1978).
49. Crosskey RW. The Natural History of Black Flies. John Wiley, Chichester: NY; 1990.
52. Potts WH. Systematics and identification of Glossina. In: Mulligan HW, editor. The African Trypanosomiases. London: Allen & Unwin; 1970.
55. Molyneux DH, Ashford RW. The Biology of Trypanosoma and Leishmania, Parasites of Man and Domestic Animals. London: Taylor and Francis; 1983.
58. Schofield CJ. Triatominae – Biology & Control. Bognor Regis: Eurocommunica; 1994.

Access the complete references online at www.expertconsult.com

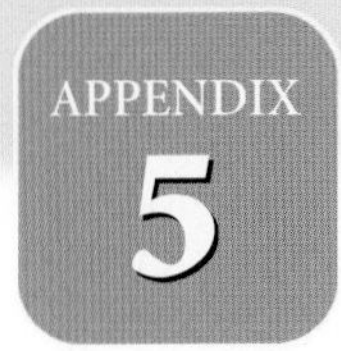

Sources of Information in Tropical Medicine

TRUDIE LANG | LAURA MERSON

Summary

Information is a vital driving force behind health sciences and the use and source of information in *Tropical Medicine* have important distinctions and special circumstances.

Recent advances in technology, medicine and funding have rapidly increased the quantity and access to information with direct health benefits. But challenges remain in understanding the varied sources of information, in ascertaining quality among them and in ensuring access to those limited by resources and geography.

Here, we provide comprehensive guidance on what sources of information are available, how to seek the most relevant information and how to judge quality and credibility. We will also discuss how information can be most effectively used and shared.

Media has evolved far from the papyrus and hieroglyphics of historical medical practitioners and scholars. Different types of media lend themselves to varied purposes, such as patient education, health worker training, dissemination of research findings and influencing government and international bodies to change and improve healthcare policies. We examine who needs access to information within the field of tropical medicine, what type of information they need and for what roles and purposes and describe different types of information used in this field and their relative merits and limitations. We describe the most reliable mediums available in tropical medicine and give advice on how to determine quality between them. A large proportion of this section will focus on using digital technology and how it might be harnessed to enhance progress in tropical medicine. Finally, recommended sources of information are included, with more online.

Introduction: Why Information is Important

The generation and distribution of information and the sharing and implementation of knowledge has always been of significant consequence in health sciences. This is especially true throughout the history of tropical medicine due to geography and the limitations that are brought about by different people interested in the same disease or health issue being located thousands of kilometers apart.

Early Egyptian, Greek and Roman scholars developed rudimentary papyri records of apparent emergent new diseases documenting the characteristics of disease and suggested remedies. Later in the 1800s the founders of what we know as 'tropical medicine' were concerned with understanding illnesses that were not encountered in the northern hemisphere. In these times, transferring information between researchers in far regions of the globe in order to understand, manage and treat illness was slow and cumbersome. Characterization and peer consensus building on identification and then later treatment and prevention of specific disease or health issues, such as snakebites, took literally decades. Theoretically now, in the twenty-first century, we can do all this in real-time, in vast groups – at the click of a button.

It might seem as though we do not need to concern ourselves too much with information in our field of tropical medicine. Surely it is all straightforward these days with access to scientific papers and educational materials being universal and easy? Furthermore, we are over a century out of the times when we did not understand malaria, leprosy, dengue and other common foes, or know how to treat and manage them. But this is true only to a limited extent. There are important gaps in the understanding of each of these diseases and continued research including vaccinology, diagnosis, treatment, and genetics will fill some gaps and identify new ones. For some diseases, especially neglected tropical diseases, the gaps far outweigh the knowledge. Moreover, we are in an era of larger and higher-density populations with increased mobility and access to global travel, therefore more rapid spread of disease and increased risk of epidemics and pandemics. Any new or emergent disease 100 years ago might have remained contained by geography. This however, is no longer the case. Today, our ability to combat the challenges that modern tropical medicine faces will depend in no small way on our willingness and capacity to rapidly share and exchange information and use novel mechanisms and technology to achieve this. We will also benefit from a change of attitudes and behaviour in the way we store, share, capture and use information.

What Information is Needed and What are the Challenges to Access?

The large diversity in scientific disciplines, diseases, pathogens and geography within the field of tropical medicine calls for complex and wide-ranging information needs from varied stakeholders. Patients, healthcare workers, researchers, educators, governments, non-government and inter-government organizations, private sector and media all require rapid access to reliable and relevant resources.

The availability of information has seen a sharp increase over the past couple of decades as a result of globalization, economic development and advances in technology. However, both the supply and the understanding of the potential of rapid access and information sharing, still lag the needs of players in the health arena. The following takes a look at the scope of information needs and some of the challenges of meeting those needs.

INFORMATION ACCESS FOR INDIVIDUALS

Populations within the tropical zone, for whom information on risks, prevention, diagnosis and management of tropical disease is vital, are among the fastest growing populations in the world; but diseases within the 'tropical' classification are no longer confined by latitudes. Effects of international travel, climate change, migration, drug resistance and changes in land use have dissolved geographic and cultural barriers to this multidisciplinary and diverse field. The information needs at the level of the individual are increasingly challenging to deliver as the number, diversity and geography of these users continues to increase. But providing access to information and access to informed health providers is a necessary foundation for improving health.

Delivering information to communities through effective health education programmes is essential to promote prevention and appropriate health seeking behaviour. Motivating the adoption of interventions such as bed nets, sanitation and condoms relies on effective transmission of information about the risks of the diseases the interventions prevent. Communities also require education on the identification of signs, symptoms and severity of disease in order to inform decisions on self-treatment and when to seek a health professional. Key areas of high mortality, such as maternal and early infant death require focused community education programmes in order to encourage mothers to seek trained birth attendants or deliver their babies in government clinics. Giving communities access to this information is an effective approach to reducing morbidity and mortality because individuals become engaged and empowered to make educated decisions about their health. To make efficient use of community health education resources, the message must be culturally appropriate and targeted to the correct user. It must also reflect the economic context of the community as the availability of resources will determine the individual's ability to use the information. The onus of delivering this information is on governments and in some cases, is supported by non-government and/or inter-government organizations. Investing in overcoming the geographic, cultural and language obstacles to effective delivery of health information to the communities that need it will provide returns of a healthier and more productive society.

For much of the world's population, the primary source of reliable health information is a healthcare provider. Implicit in access to an informed health provider is the assurance that recent and reliable information is available to that provider. Up-to-date research publications, health policies, diagnostic tools and treatment guidelines are necessary for doctors, nurses, clinical officers, midwives and pharmacists to make informed decisions and give good advice. Outbreak reports and current incidence data must reach emergency rooms, laboratories, pharmacies and care facilities rapidly to inform the response of the health workers who will encounter them and allow for resource planning. Existing real-time information dissemination networks must overcome technology and language barriers to deliver urgent information to a larger community. Training and continuing education should be made accessible to multidisciplinary health fields so that individuals can update their knowledge with current resources. The potential for digital technology to be harnessed effectively in the area is tremendous and as yet, largely untapped. Concerted efforts to address this could bring more significant healthcare changes in developing countries than have been seen in recent history.

The largest supplier of medical information to healthcare providers and the lay public is industry. There are ubiquitous sources of sensationalized, unreliable and profit-driven information available from media and marketers including pandemic panic campaigns, pharmaceutical marketing and advertisements for products including infant formula and cigarettes. These messages may complement or contradict health promotion and should be synergized or challenged by public health campaigns and education. Tipping the supply of new information towards reliable evidence-based knowledge is the charge of educational institutions and the academic community.

INFORMATION FOR EDUCATIONAL, PROFESSIONAL AND ACADEMIC INSTITUTIONS

Academic, health and professional institutions are responsible for generating and disseminating much of the world's new scientific information. They are additionally the organizations that deliver primary and continuing health education to healthcare professionals. Digested information is distributed in many formats ready for implementation, including lectures and training courses, reports, guidelines, websites and presentations. But the most extensive supply of reliable undigested information is research results published in scientific journals. Access to these publications is essential for healthcare providers, but also essential between institutions to feed the cascade of scientific discovery. Lack of information can lead to duplication of studies and poorly planned or executed research, and therefore inadequate research conclusions. A strong global foundation of scientific literature requires contribution from researchers in developing and developed countries, robust peer review systems and access for all. The recent open-access trend in health research publication has increased the availability of quality information to many individuals and institutions that require it. But there is progress still to be made as the number of journals that are open access remain limited and the ability to access them is strongly divided by the limitations of internet access in general. The gap in ability to exchange information that exists between resource-rich and resource-limited settings is further widened by this unequal access. The information supply from resource-limited settings may be restricted by the requirement for authors, their institutions or funding bodies to cover the cost of publication. However, some journals waive publication fees for developing countries and reliable internet access continues to expand through technology and investment. As these improvements increase the availability of information, there is hope that the open access movement will expand further to include protocols, data collection tools and datasets on which the publications are based.

INFORMATION FOR GOVERNMENTS, NON-GOVERNMENT AND INTER-GOVERNMENT ORGANIZATIONS

The planning and delivery of health care, health policy and health governance is the responsibility of governments.

Non-government and inter-government organizations often support these efforts in degrees inversely correlated to the level of national development. In order to know what to deliver, these groups require access to high quality health statistics, which address the unique epidemiology and health-systems of the nation. In order to expedite the response to outbreaks and epidemics, governments require real-time data on disease incidence, diagnostic capacity and trends in drug sales. Availability of health economic data is necessary to develop treatment guidelines, plan budgets and funding, focus advocacy and allow rationalization of services. Collection of core epidemiological data and health indicators is key to strategic planning of logistics, provision and utilization management of healthcare services and to create the public information campaigns discussed above. And finally, evaluation of healthcare outcomes and the impact of health policy are imperative to improve the systems in place and provide better quality care with greater access.

The challenges to health system improvements are many, and include the difficulties in collecting and analysing reliable information to inform decisions. The collection of reliable data is limited by political instability and availability of resources such as diagnostics, communication infrastructure and skilled healthcare workers. Data comparison is compromised by differences in collection methods, terminology and classifications, statistical methods and population coverage. There is an urgent need to address the reporting gaps, so that reliable health indicators can be analysed to determine effective health interventions.

The global relevance of tropical medicine is increasing and unprecedented volumes of information are now available to meet the needs of individuals, institutions and governments. But large gaps remain in the effort to improve the quality and maximize the health benefits derived from that information. Addressing the barriers to transmission and uptake of information will empower individuals to make informed decisions about health. Removing geographic, technology and resource barriers will cause a cycle of positive feedback within the research community and fuel the generation of further research. Harmonizing international data collection through standardization and a systematic approach to coordination will allow for the design of health policy with the greatest possible benefit. Making this information readily available will promote the evaluation and development of those policies. Information is fundamental to decisions that improve health.

Types of Information Relevant and Important to Tropical Medicine

The scale of relevant information ranges from a single case report to global trends in pharmaceutical trade. This information is increasingly abundant and rapidly distributed in diverse and vociferous forms of variable quality. It is important for individuals at all levels of health engagement to have access to, and be able to identify reliable and relevant resources.

In tropical medicine, information takes many forms and can be obtained from varied sources between the main mediums of print and digital form. This section describes the main forms of information that are of most benefit to tropical medicine practitioners and researchers and considers the benefits and limitations of each in the context of tropical medicine.

PEER-REVIEWED BIOMEDICAL PAPERS PUBLISHED IN JOURNALS

There are specialized yet cross-cutting journals dedicated to tropical medicine, such as the *Transactions of The Royal Society of Tropical Medicine and Hygiene* and the *American Journal of Tropical Medicine and Hygiene*. Other journals have specific titles that focus more on diseases of poverty, neglected disease or one specific tropical disease such as malaria. Others have a focus that is very relevant to tropical medicine, such as parasitology or infectious disease. The broad interest high impact medical journals such as *The Lancet*, *BMJ* and *Nature* also publish papers within the tropical medicine field as all have a strong interest in global health and neglected diseases. The most widely used search resource for medical journal papers and books is PubMed (see: www.ncbi.nlm.nih.gov/pubmed/), which accesses MEDLINE, the vast bibliographic database of the US National Library of Medicine.

Implicit hierarchy exists among journals, often based on perceived quality of peer review (including rejection rates) and coverage by popular databases, which enhances international visibility. Impact factor, an indicator of the annual number of citations a journal receives per article has become *de facto* status symbol for scientific journals despite popular dispute. Impact factor is assigned to all journals listed on the Institute for Scientific Information Web of Knowledge citation databases (Thompson Reuters, see: apps.webofknowledge.com), but neglects valuable regional journals covered by PubMed.

Advances in journal publishing have emulated the electronic communication revolution. Advantages of online publishing include decreased length restrictions, the possibility of multimedia inclusion, reduced publishing time and the ability to link directly to references and related editorials. Electronic publishing has also made open access publishing possible due to the elimination of manufacturing and shipping costs of paper journals. Such access is free and unrestricted to all internet users. Some journals, such as the *Public Library of Science* group (PloS) and *Bio Medicine Central* are entirely open access. Other journals have certain papers designated as open access or allow the authors to pay a fee to make access open to all. Open access publishing shifts the cost of publication to the authors and in spite of reduced fees for low and middle income countries, it may limit publication access in these media.

To improve access to subscription-based journals, the World Health Organization has set up Hinari (see: www.who.int/hinari), a program supported by many publishers to enable no or low-cost access to medical literature in developing countries. Institutions in more than 100 countries and territories can register to access more than 7500 journals and 8000 electronic books. Other organizations provide document delivery services in low income settings.

BOOKS

The rapidly increasing amount of information available free on the internet endangers the popularity of printed books, but the value and reliance placed on formal textbooks still forms a major part of the search for information. This source was once reliant on the resources available to the individual, institution and/or library, which are often limited in areas where tropical medicine is especially relevant. Two valuable initiatives working to address this deficit are worthy of mention here.

First, the World Health Organization distributes a standard collection of 150 essential health sciences books named 'Blue Trunk Library' in developing countries (see: www.who.int/ghl/mobile_libraries/bluetrunk). Second, the shift to digital format for libraries allows subscription access to online editions of texts, often at a discount to the printed version or supported by mechanisms such as Hinari for institutions in developing countries. Online textbooks are a recent and welcome development, which overcomes the inherent challenge of information quickly becoming outdated in large volume printed texts whose subsequent editions may be published years apart. Some electronic versions of textbooks, e.g. the Oxford Textbook of Medicine, 5th edn., and the text you are currently reading, undergo systematic updates and addition of key developments by authors after publication.

GREY LITERATURE

Beyond the bibliographic databases and publisher's lists lie additional sources of information critical to tropical medicine. Grey literature is a broad classification for works released outside of commercial publication, which covers vital resources including treatment guidelines, diagnostic tools, reports, technical and working papers, patents, conference proceedings and curriculum. The broad range of sources and topics included in this classification means that the materials cover a wide spectrum of find-ability and validity. An informed approach to these issues can yield some of the best resources on health statistics, healthcare delivery and policy development.

Access to grey literature has been transformed by the internet. It has simultaneously reduced the relevance of find-ability and increased the importance of deciphering the validity of this material. What was previously buried within government, library and institutional repositories can now be found in abundance with a comprehensive internet search using a popular engine. Appropriate search strings can overcome the limitations imposed by the absence of standard bibliographic identifiers and irregular (or absent) publication schedules. But there is opportunity for libraries to contribute further to the accessibility and persistence of quality grey literature by identifying the most relevant works of academic quality from reliable sources and cataloguing them, or details of where to find them, within their collections.

All major health players regularly publish and update collections of grey literature. Governments, inter-government organizations and recognized academic institutions and non-government organizations are good starting points for recent and locally relevant publications. When searching on popular topics, established experts can be prioritized, but when the focus is more obscure, it may be necessary to consider lesser-known sources. In this case, the vital step is in the discernment of reliability of the material.

How to Determine if Publications are Reliable

With an abundance of available publications, it is important to be able to determine the quality of information presented. This is often done by reputation alone, but that limits perceived credibility to well-known publishers, journals and authors. There is an abundance of reliable new or lesser-known resources, which are necessary to provide the full scope of tropical medicine literature. Easy targets for books are university libraries where dedicated staff select and review materials stock material determined to be a credible source. Basic markers of journal quality are robust peer review processes, impact factor of the journal and a listing on MEDLINE.

This does not mean that every book in the library or article in a top paper is reliable. Publications do have errors, misinterpretations, omissions and bias. The best policy is to read all available information critically and compare it with other sources in a full literature review. This is ideal, but may not be realistic to pursue. When evaluating the quality of a publication you may consider if the publisher is reputable and when it was published. Has the information has been independently reviewed and are the authors known experts? What else have they published, who is the work is funded by and have authors declared any conflicts of interest? If it is a trial publication, methodological considerations need to be taken into account: was the trial registered on an international registry before recruitment began and does the reporting match the registered methods and analysis? Does the reporting format fit international standards such as STROBE (Statement for cohort, case–control and cross-sectional studies, available at: www.strobe-statement.org) or CONSORT (Statement for reporting clinical trials, available at: www.consort-statement.org)? When reading through, consider if there is a good background with relevant and reliable references. Also, do the authors discuss assumptions or statistical modelling used to generate results? Are the authors open about the limitations of their work? Is the information presented enough to allow you to determine if you agree with the authors' conclusions – and do you?

Literature on tropical medicine is spread through general and specialized sources, so it is necessary to look at both when searching. When searching for literature you may wish to avoid starting with one source, and spreading the scope of the search based on the references in that source, then further from the references in those sources. This can lead to a biased selection of results, as authors may not include references to all work that does not support their own. Instead, look for literature reviews published by recognized and respected authors and groups who have conducted systematic reviews of all available literature. The leading example of such a resource is the Cochrane Collaboration (see: cochrane.org) who has more than 4600 reviews available at no or low cost to many countries through funded provisions.

The Use and Potential of Digital Technology

The internet has rapidly accelerated the ease and speed of information dissemination in a variety of formats, as detailed above. In the field of tropical medicine, the effect of such access is revolutionary due to the conquering of geographical barriers. But there remain limitations to access and a need to discern quality and other sources of information, which have yet to be exploited online.

Accessing information digitally is going to be (and for many already is) the primary source for obtaining information. In medicine and medical research, the ability to access information via the internet has transformed the ability to gain knowledge by the immediateness and sheer quantity of information available. From the perspective of tropical medicine, access to a fast internet connection is the key factor, because in many regions of the world, fast and reliable connectivity is still not yet a reality or still relatively new. In these areas, information is limited primarily to books and printed journals and is dependent on the quality or wealth of the library and the speed and expense of the postal service. However, this is changing rapidly and internet access is increasing in Africa, Asia and South America. People are increasingly using mobile phone networks to access the internet and ongoing infrastructure advances continue to rapidly improve access. One such example is the internet cable programme in Africa that was completed in South Africa in 2011. This huge length of cable now connects West Africa with Southern Africa, Eastern Africa and Europe.

In many developed regions, the internet has been easily accessible for decades and it is now second nature to use facilities such as PubMed to access research papers and texts. Most universities and medical institutions in these regions have subscriptions that allow immediate access for staff and students, to a requested paper. This has made a dramatic impact on how medical personnel and researchers can access and apply current data and reports to their working practices. As developing countries improve access and speed of the internet, it is increasingly important that journals and/or funding agencies provide open access to journals, as the greatest barrier to access shifts from infrastructure to subscription costs.

Formal information released on the websites of organizations such as the World Health Organization, The World Bank, Ministries of Health, funding bodies, Medical Research Councils and regulatory bodies (such as the US Food and Drug Administration or European Medicines Agency) are very important and these institutions use the internet as their primary source of releasing information. The great advantage of digital release of such information is that it can be kept current. Previously, the release of guidelines or recommendations via printed form, or even via CD-ROMS became outdated very quickly, and the danger was that these old versions remained on shelves and were referred to well beyond the time they remained relevant.

Other very useful materials are those put up by organizations working in a specific field. This might be disease-specific or cross-cutting. These websites may be operated by University departments, medical research organizations or funders. The best of these provide resources and learning materials as well as links to other websites that they recommend. While the large volume of different websites might be overwhelming, there are some simple considerations that can help distinguish quality material from that which is less useful. Below, we provide some examples of the diverse and high quality resources that are available.

In terms of establishing whether or not the material is of high quality, the following points are helpful to consider:

- Who has set up the website? This may be obvious (e.g. the World Health Organization website) or you might need to look for an 'about' page. The latter is more typical if the website has been set up by a network or collaboration. Then, consider whether this is a respected group or organization. If the material comes from a network or collaboration it is often reassuring to see several partners and at least one or two from a reputable organization. If the website has been set up by an individual or a group of people, this may be less reliable. Authors should be listed on the materials they write, either by name or by organization.
- Is the website of high quality? Does the website look credible and have those involved ensured that required statements on privacy and data are present as well as a terms and conditions policy? These statements are important and also give reassurance that the site is being responsibly managed and maintained.
- Is the material moderated or reviewed? Consider the nature of the material; is it a discussion forum or a paper or similar written piece? Good websites will have a statement about how the material has been reviewed and or moderated. Discussion forums and blogs often allow users to post straight on the website, which is good practice provided those operating the website have a process for quality management and moderation. Also check for references. Information published as fact should be substantiated and the source of the information made available.
- Is the material free and open access? Is feedback and contribution invited and encouraged? These elements are not necessarily a mark of quality and accuracy but as we will go on to explain, open access and interactive-type sites can be beneficial, as other users might have rated the material and this will help establish whether it will be of use and relevant to you.
- Can you see how up-to-date the material and the overall site is? If articles are dated or if there are members or discussions, you can see how often material is updated and when others have recently contributed. This is a good way to see whether the site is current, up-to-date and being used by others.

In many areas of modern life, the latest advances in digital technology are being applied. Most people are well aware of successful use of these types of website and good global examples are Facebook, LinkedIn and Amazon. These companies have successfully exploited the interactive elements to build communities and to determine what information the user is trying to find. The online social and professional networking sites work because they use digital technology to find people who know each other or share common interests, connect them together and allow people to share various types of media and communications in an instant. Commercial platforms like Amazon work by learning from users' searching and browsing history. The Amazon website learns about its customers each time they visit and over time, builds up a comprehensive picture of the user's interests.

The fields of tropical medicine and global health should also exploit this digital technology and there is a vast potential gain to be had by doing so. Those working in tropical medicine are typically located in diverse areas and people working in the same field can be separated by thousands of miles. Resources are also limited for training and meetings because many tropical diseases are neglected or are rare diseases that attract limited commercial funding. In this environment, linking researchers together on the internet, rather that face-to-face would be valuable. People can meet and connect far more often than the limited opportunities they may or may not get to attend meetings or go on training courses. There are active initiatives on the use these highly interactive applications on websites to create professional communities throughout the world, in the field of tropical medicine. The aims of these platforms are to share knowledge and methods and to support better practice and research via the open access to peers and knowledge.

One example is The Global Health Network (see: www.theglobalhealthnetwork.org), which could be described as an online science park and it is striving to use the latest digital technology to support research in tropical medicine. It is a collection of websites located together on a digital 'e-hub' and those using any of the member websites can move between them to seek reliable information, methods and tools for research and practice.

Websites such as The Global Health Network have taken cutting edge digital technology to create platforms that can link researchers and research groups with the shared aim of supporting research or improving practice. Within The Global Health Network, the many constituent websites each focus on their own topic but are located together on a shared hub, all built from the same digital template, to provide a familiar format for the user. The Global Health Network and its constituent websites have the shared ethos of supporting research, and aims to achieve this by increasing the opportunity and access for individual scientists and research groups to collaborate and by open sharing of knowledge, training and research methods. Each research community focuses on a specific therapeutic area (e.g. respiratory disease, reproductive health or oncology); type of research (e.g. diagnostics or microbiology); or are cross-cutting research support communities (e.g. clinical trials and research ethics). These types of communities are successful because they are built and led by researchers from these fields, who have built these sites because of their realization that there is a need for a space online where scientists can access each other to share knowledge, methods and tools, as well as to build collaborations and work on joint activities.

These types of websites, including general sites such as Facebook and Amazon, as well as those specifically for working in tropical medicine and international health (see below for examples) are utilizing the second generation website technology. This is known as Web 2.0. Across the industrialized world, Web 2.0 communities are growing and leading change. The philosophy of Web 2.0 is about communities of practice and tacit knowledge sharing.

Communities of practice are where people with a similar interest or need come together, and in the context of this discussion, these groups would come together online, to improve 'practice' in whatever area they share a common interest. Communities of practice explain to each other how to do something, often by sharing their experiences or solutions. In tropical medicine, the ethos of 'community of practice' has always been present however, the greatest limitation has been the cost of travel. The result has been that most efforts to share skills, resources and methods have been limited to better funded diseases, health issues, locations. Now a much greater impact may be made if there is greater sharing of knowledge between therapy areas and across varied regions. The combination of the Web 2.0 technology and the philosophy of community of practice make this possible. Community of practice is not about companies or organizations telling customers what they want, or large institutions setting guidelines and delivering downward cascades of dictated instruction. Using Web 2.0 technology to apply the philosophy of community of practice concerns those involved in an activity telling others how they did it and sharing their methods. This has only been harnessed as yet to a limited extent in tropical medicine but doing so fully could bring about and speed up major advances in both treatment practices and research in resource-limited settings.

This new way of learning and accessing knowledge and information may appear too informal and fraught with risks of unreliability and of being undisciplined. However, rigour and quality are achievable and these are largely obtained democratically and by the way in which people use these online platforms. Wikipedia was developed as an online encyclopaedia and the term 'wiki' is now in general use. A wiki is defined (on Wikipedia) as a website whose users can add, modify, or delete its content via the internet. A powerful wiki feature that could bring significant advances to tropical medicine if applied and taken up correctly, is that a wiki enables communities to write documents collaboratively. This could be used for developing new treatment guidelines perhaps, or for collaborative protocol writing.

The concerns over the use of wiki's in science and medicine are about quality and validity. Normally there is no prior review or modification before an entry to a wiki is posted live, and this could result in low quality submissions. Having users register and create a user account can mitigate this problem. Users who post using their real name and affiliation will be motivated to submit high quality entries as people's reputations are involved. If others disagree with a post then they are able to comment and suggest corrections and modifications. Experience has shown that users do write high quality and valid comments on these types of professional sites because they are open and can be read by peers. Therefore, the concern that information found on these platforms is inferior due to the lack of traditional peer review is unfounded and conversely it could be claimed that if these sites are well-read then the quality of the review could be higher, as it is entirely open and democratic.

Digital access to information then offers the tropical medicine practitioner, student or researcher an exciting, varied and expanding wealth of information. How this information is sought and used needs to be considered in terms of the quality of the website from which it was accessed. Determining whether material can be trusted is achievable by considering some straightforward points.

The future for accessing knowledge and information will be increasingly dependent on the internet and so providing equitable access across the globe is becoming more important. It is not just a matter of countries having access to fast internet cables or satellite technology but the end-user, clinician, student or researcher having access to some form of screen that will determine true ability to use this powerful resource.

Where to Find Information

This section aims to list and summarize varying types of information that is available and relevant in varying forms and how to find it. This is a generic summary and gives links and short summaries where possible about the nature and scope of the source.

ONLINE SEARCH ENGINES, DATABASES AND PUBLIC ACCESS CATALOGUES

There are several catalogues of literature available on the internet that are particularly relevant to tropical medicine practitioners and researchers. In order to use these, an understanding of the structure and indexing of databases, while not critical, would be beneficial, alongside an understanding of various search strategies. Tutorials in how to use these databases are available. For example, see: www.nlm.nih.gov/bsd/disted/pubmed.html

Online public access catalogues (OPACs) are among the most common and highly accessed databases of information on tropical medicine. Most OPACs are for single libraries or institutions, such as those at universities. Some, however, are catalogues for *national libraries*, which often have large holdings. An index of national libraries, such as the British Library and the Library of Congress, is available via Wikipedia. Some OPACs are *union catalogues* covering more than one library, for example all of the libraries in a multi-university system or a consortium. Some excellent examples include: (a more extensive list is available in the electronic version of this text)

ClinicalTrials.gov US National Institutes of Health. This online resource describes over 145 000 clinical studies in over 185 countries. This is useful for recruiting trials and complements Cochrane Library's bibliography of (published) clinical trials – www.clinicaltrials.gov

The Cochrane Library A major online resource (updated quarterly) for evidence-based medicine. Included is a database of over 7800 full-text systematic reviews, with an increasing number on infectious and tropical diseases; a database of abstracts of reviews of effectiveness; a comprehensive bibliography of clinical trials as well as a handbook on critical appraisal and the science of reviewing research – www.thecochranelibrary.com This is free to many developing countries via HINARI. For further details of the Cochrane Collaboration and its specialist groups (particularly the Infectious Diseases Group) – www.cochrane.org

Global Health Network A network of health-related websites connected together on a shared digital hub, all aiming to support research – www.theglobalhealthnetwork.org

Google Scholar Based on the popular Google search engine, Google Scholar indexes a substantial part of the scientific literature. It contains an internal mechanism for linking citations and is free. – www.scholar.google.com

ITM Institute of Tropical Medicine, Antwerp, Belgium. One of the world's leading institutes for training, research and services delivery in tropical medicine and health care in developing countries. It has a highly specialized library facility – www.itg.be

PubMed National Library of Medicine, Bethesda MD, USA. A free database accessing the MEDLINE database of references and abstracts on life sciences and biomedical topics – www.pubmed.gov

WHOLIS World Health Organization Library Information System An index of all WHO publications – http://dosei.who.int

Wiley An academic and professional publisher with an extensive multidisciplinary collection of online resources covering life, health, social and physical sciences and humanities – www.wiley.com

OPEN ACCESS MEDICAL LITERATURE

A fundamental factor which affects information access is whether the material is freely available or has a cost. The following links provide access to medical literature that is free. Alternatively, several donor agencies finance access to medical journals and books. (a more extensive list is available in the electronic version of this text)

BMC BioMed Central Publisher of over 250 open access journals – www.biomedcentral.com

Google Books Excellent database of available texts, many with sections or full content available for preview or download – www.books.google.com

HINARI Health Inter Network Access to Research Initiative Allowing free or low cost access for developing countries to major journals in biomedical and related social sciences – www.who.int/hinari/en

INASP/PERI International Network for the Availability of Scientific Publications Program for the Enhancement of Research Information. Access to full text journals (incl. extensive bibliographic database information and document delivery) for not-for-profit institutes in developing countries – www.inasp.info/peri/

National Academies Press Created by the United States National Academy of Sciences, has over 4,000 books on science, engineering and medicine available free for download – www.nap.edu

Open J-Gate Informatics (India) Ltd Promoting free and unrestricted access to scholarly and research journals – www.openj-gate.org

PLOS Public Library of Science journals A collection of access journals, including 'PLOS Neglected Tropical Diseases' – www.plos.org

PMC PubMed Central (US National Library of Medicine – National Institutes of Health) A free full text archive of biomedical and life sciences journal literature. Many long established high impact journals (as well as new journals, including the BMC series of online journals) offer their back-sets free – several stretching back many decades to their very first volume – but there is generally an embargo for the most recent issues – www.ncbi.nlm.nih.gov/pmc/

SciVerse ScienceDirect A leading full-text scientific database offering journal articles and book chapters from more than 2,500 peer-reviewed journals and more than 11,000 books – www.sciencedirect.com

ONLINE ACCESS TO TREATMENT AND PRACTICE GUIDELINES

Communities rely on their healthcare providers to have up-to-date access to the current best practice and the latest guidelines, recommendations and treatment protocols. Here are some examples of guidelines that are available online and other sources of information where the latest recommendations or practices are made available. Several of these general tropical medicine-related websites (e.g. WHO) contain excellent information on individual diseases. Country specific treatment guidelines are often available on the websites of the country's Ministry of Health or National Institute of Health. (additional links are available in the electronic version of this text)

Agency for Healthcare Research and Quality, National Guideline Clearinghouse – www.ahrq.gov

IDSA Infectious Disease Society of America – www.idsociety.org/IDSA_Practice_Guidelines

WHO World Health Organization Guidelines– www.who.int/rpc/guidelines

WHO World Health Organization Health Topics – http://www.who.int/topics

WHO TDR Special Programme for Research and Training in Tropical Diseases – www.who.int/tdr

ONLINE LEARNING, E-SEMINARS AND INTERACTIVE MECHANISMS FOR GAINING KNOWLEDGE AND INFORMATION

In addition to resources such as journals, books, guidelines and reports, there is also an increasing amount of interactive teaching, learning and knowledge resources. Many are free and are very useful mechanisms for increasing knowledge and skills – especially in regions or situations where access to training and learning is limited by geography or access to funding. (a more extensive list is available in the electronic version of this text)

Medicus Mundi A list of postgraduate training programs in international health – www.healthtraining.org

Institute of Tropical Medicine (ITM), Antwerp, Belgium Illustrated Lecture Notes on Tropical Medicine. The English edition is freely available from this website; English and Spanish editions can be obtained on CD-ROM at a low price. Mail to: info@itg.be – www.itg.be/ILNtropmed/

KABISA Interactive Training Software A computer-based training tool for diagnostic skills in tropical and subtropical medicine. Available in eight languages and three levels of competency. Free download or CD-ROM available – www.kabisa.be

TALC Teaching Aids at Low Cost Slide sets and books for sale at low cost, as well as a series of free CD-ROMs containing teaching materials, articles and other full-text information. PO Box 49, St Albans, Herts AL1 5TX, UK – www.talcuk.org

Wellcome Trust Topics in International Health, London (now distributed by **TALC**, see above). A CD-ROM series each containing interactive tutorials, hundreds of photographic images and a glossary of terms: Acute Respiratory Infection; Dengue; Diarrhoeal Diseases; HIV/AIDS; Human African Trypanosomiasis; Leishmaniasis; Leprosy; Malaria; Nutrition; Schistosomiasis; Sexually Transmitted Infections; Sickle Cell Disease; Trachoma; Tuberculosis. Prices discounted for individuals and users from developing countries – www.wellcome.ac.uk

DISEASE OUTBREAK AND EPIDEMIOLOGY INFORMATION

Up-to-date information on disease outbreaks, epidemics and general disease epidemiology data is of great importance to tropical medicine. The following is a list of organizations or sources where information in this area can be accessed: (additional links are available in the electronic version of this text)

GAR Global Alert and Response (WHO) An integrated global alert and response system for epidemics and other public health emergencies based on strong national public health systems and capacity and an effective international system for coordinated response – www.who.int/csr

ProMed Program for Monitoring Emerging Diseases An internet-based reporting system dedicated to rapid global dissemination of information on outbreaks of infectious diseases and acute exposures to toxins – www.promedmail.org

WHO Weekly Epidemiological Record – www.who.int/wer/

WHO The Global Health Atlas Giving statistics on infectious diseases – http://apps.who.int/globalatlas Also see DengueNet and FluNet via links on this site

ONLINE RESEARCH AND PUBLIC HEALTH COMMUNITIES

There are an increasing number of online platforms being set up to enable researchers and health practitioners in tropical medicine to establish professional networks and online communities. The aim of these digital communities is broadly to facilitate collaboration and the sharing of knowledge. The following are some examples of established online scientific communities in the field of tropical medicine:

Afro-NETS African Networks for Health Research and Development – www.afronets.org

E-DRUG An electronic discussion group on essential drugs – www.essentialdrugs.org

The Global Health Network This network operates like an online science park and is a collection of varied collaborations and projects – each aiming to support and enhance research in Global Health via the sharing of knowledge and methods – www.theglobalhealthnetwork.org

HIFA Health Information for All by 2015 Established to progressively meet the information needs of all healthcare providers, HIFA hosts five online discussion networks linking health professionals, publishers, policy-makers, researchers, librarians, information professionals and citizen representatives. Focus on health students, nurses and midwives, mothers and care givers, community health workers – www.hifa2015.org

HRWEb A web-based, interactive platform aimed at improving health, equity and development through research. Particularly aimed at research focusing on improving health in low- and middle-income countries and populations, but it will be useful to high income countries as well – www.healthresearchweb.org

ORGANIZATIONS AND INSTITUTIONS WORKING IN TROPICAL MEDICINE

Various organizations are highly influential in the field of tropical medicine through their roles as funders, regulators, educators or in research. These organizations can be valuable sources of information. This could be in the form of their own reports and guidance materials, or as publications or recommendations. A sample of organizations is listed below. (a more extensive list is available in the electronic version of this text)

Global Fund to Fight AIDS Tuberculosis and Malaria – www.theglobalfund.org

MSF Médecins sans Frontières – www.msf.org

TDR UNDP/UNICEF/World Bank/WHO Special Programme for Research and Training in Tropical Diseases – www.who.int/tdr

UNAIDS Joint United Nations Program on HIV/AIDS – www.unaids.org

WHO World Health Organization – www.who.int

WHO Regional and Other Offices – www.who.int/regions

Organizations providing funding opportunities in tropical medicine:

Bill and Melinda Gates Foundation – www.gatesfoundation.org
Foundation Center – www.fdncenter.org/funders
GrantsNet – www.grantsnet.org
Wellcome Trust – www.wellcome.ac.uk
WHO TDR Grants – www.who.int/tdr/grants

KEEPING UP-TO-DATE: USING INFORMATION FEEDS

Many organizations that provide information operate digital information feed services. These can be very helpful in ensuring access and awareness of the latest relevant information. Setting up alerts that are sent to you via e-mail, or that you can read as personalized alerts on websites, is a sophisticated and intelligent way to sort through the immense and seemingly endless amount of information, to ensure you are aware of important developments in your field. A common example is 'really simple syndication' (RSS) feeds. RSS feeds are software programs that regularly aggregate the latest information on set topics (usually identified by tags) and make it available for access via web pages. Another example is eTOCs. These are simply an electronic table of contents that can be e-mailed to subscribers and can be set up to include or exclude specific areas or topics. Simple e-mail alerts can also be a useful mechanism for being made aware of new information and being able to sort and screen the nature of these notifications. In this era of ever increasing digital information, the use of information feeds is recommended and is likely to become more sophisticated. Feeds are available from many of the sources listed above.

Conclusion

Sources of information in tropical medicine are highly dynamic within a rapidly changing scientific environment. Much of the information suggested here are digital and therefore able and likely to change often compared with printed material. The links given are current at the point of publication but may change and, while every effort has been made to give a broad and representative list of information sources, it certainly will have omissions.

With the rapid uptake and lowering access costs, internet access to information should become faster and easier. A major factor in tropical medicine for seeking information will be the availability of fast internet connection and access to a computer, smart phone, tablet – or future hardware. If costs continue to fall, relative to the cost of living, then this will make specialist and high quality tropical medicine information more widely accessible to healthcare workers and research staff, which will be of great benefit to public health.

A significant change in access and availability of information in tropical medicine would come if more data, methods and knowledge were to be made free and open access to all online. If protocols, operating procedures, data and methods were more widely shared then research and standards would be raised and practitioners would have better access to evidence and guidelines. Information is a vital driving force behind health sciences. It is important to ensure access to information in the settings where it is most critical.

INDEX

Page numbers followed by 'f' indicate figures, 't' indicate tables, and 'b' indicate boxes.

Notes
vs. indicates a differential diagnosis or comparison.

A

B

D

F

G

I

N

O

P

Q

R

S

W

X

Y

Z